AF700756

Roberts and Hedges'
Clinical Procedures in Emergency Medicine and Acute Care

ASSOCIATE EDITORS

Arjun Chanmugam, MD, MBA
Vice Chair
Department of Emergency Medicine
The Johns Hopkins School of Medicine
Baltimore, Maryland

Carl R. Chudnofsky, MD, FACEP
Professor and Chair
Department of Emergency Medicine
Keck School of Medicine of USC
Los Angeles, California

Christopher Colwell Sr, MD, FACEP, FAEMS
Professor and Vice Chair
Department of Emergency Medicine
University of California at San Francisco
Chief
Department of Emergency Medicine
Zuckerberg San Francisco General Hospital and Trauma Center
San Francisco; California

Peter M.C. DeBlieux, MD, FACEP
Professor of Clinical Medicine
Assistant Dean of Advanced Learning and Simulation
Louisiana State University Health Sciences Center
Professor of Clinical Surgery
Tulane University School of Medicine
New Orleans; Louisiana

Kevin Hanley, MD
Associate Physician
Department of Emergency Medicine
University of California San Francisco
San Francisco, California

Michael Hayoun, MD, MPhil, MRO, FACEP, FAAEM
Associate Site Medical Director
Department of Emergency Medicine
Tristar Hendersonville Medical Center
Hendersonville, Tennessee;
Assistant Clinical Professor
Integrated Clinical Education
Thomas F. Frist, Jr. College of Medicine at Belmont University
Core Faculty, Emergency Medicine
Tristar Skyline Medical Center
Nashville, Tennessee

Siamak Moayedi, MD, FAAEM
Professor
Department of Emergency Medicine
University of Maryland School of Medicine
Baltimore, Maryland

Maria C. Raven, MD, MPH, FACEP
Professor and Vice Chair
Chief of Emergency Medicine
University of California San Francisco School of Medicine
San Francisco, California

Alfred Sacchetti, MD, FACEP
Director
Clinical Services Emergency Medicine
Virtua Our Lady of Lourdes Hospital
Camden, New Jersey;
Assistant Clinical Professor
Department of Emergency Medicine
Thomas Jefferson University
Philadelphia, Pennsylvania

Amanda Smith, DMSc, MMS, PA-C, CAQ-EM
Emergency Medicine Physician Assistant
Johns Hopkins Bayview Medical Center
Baltimore, Maryland

Jeffrey Tabas, MD, FACEP
Professor
Department of Emergency Medicine
University of California San Francisco School of Medicine
San Francisco, California

VIDEO EDITORS

Martha A. Roberts, ACNP, PNP, BCEN, CPEN
Associate Professor of Nursing
Clinical Instructor, Chamberlain University
Lead Faculty, The Center for Medical Education
Adult and Pediatric Critical Care and Primary Care Nurse Practitioner
Department of Public Health
Department of Emergency Medicine
Zuckerberg San Francisco General Hospital and Trauma Center
San Francisco, California

Jessica Mason, MD, FACEP
Associate Professor of Clinical Emergency Medicine
Department of Emergency Medicine
Texas Christian University
Fort Worth, Texas

Christine Butts, MD
Clinical Instructor of Emergency Medicine
Director of Division of Emergency Ultrasound
Department of Emergency Medicine
Louisiana State University Health Sciences Center
New Orleans, Louisiana

PHARMD EDITOR

Zlatan Coralic, PharmD
Emergency Medicine Clinical Pharmacist
Clinical Professor of Pharmacy and Emergency Medicine
University of California San Francisco
San Francisco, California

Elsevier
1600 John F. Kennedy Blvd.
Ste 1600
Philadelphia, PA 19103-2899

ROBERTS AND HEDGES' CLINICAL PROCEDURES IN
EMERGENCY MEDICINE AND ACUTE CARE, EIGHTH EDITION ISBN: 978-0-323-77922-7
Copyright © 2026 by Elsevier Inc. All rights are reserved, including those for text and data mining, AI training, and similar technologies.

Chapter 32 is modified with permission from Roberts JR. Intravenous regional anesthesia. *JACEP*. 1977;6:261-265.

For accessibility purposes, images in electronic versions of this book are accompanied by alt-text descriptions provided by Elsevier. For more information, see https://www.elsevier.com/about/accessibility.

Books and Journals published by Elsevier comply with applicable product safety requirements.
For any product safety concerns or queries, please contact our authorized representative, Elsevier B.V., at productsafety@elsevier.com.

Publisher's note: Elsevier takes a neutral position with respect to territorial disputes or jurisdictional claims in its published content, including in maps and institutional affiliations.

No part of this publication may be reproduced or transmitted in any form or by any means, electronic or mechanical, including photocopying, recording, or any information storage and retrieval system, without permission in writing from the publisher. Details on how to seek permission, further information about the Publisher's permissions policies and our arrangements with organizations such as the Copyright Clearance Center and the Copyright Licensing Agency, can be found at our website: www.elsevier.com/permissions.

This book and the individual contributions contained in it are protected under copyright by the Publisher (other than as may be noted herein).

Notice

Practitioners and researchers must always rely on their own experience and knowledge in evaluating and using any information, methods, compounds or experiments described herein. Because of rapid advances in the medical sciences, in particular, independent verification of diagnoses and drug dosages should be made. To the fullest extent of the law, no responsibility is assumed by Elsevier, authors, editors or contributors for any injury and/or damage to persons or property as a matter of products liability, negligence or otherwise, or from any use or operation of any methods, products, instructions, ideas contained in the material herein.

Previous editions copyrighted 2019, 2014, 2010, 2004, 1998, 1991, and 1985 by Elsevier, Inc.

Senior Content Strategist: Lauren Boyle
Senior Content Development Manager: Joanie Milnes
Publishing Services Manager: Catherine Jackson
Senior Project Managers: Carrie Stetz, Rachel McMillan
Design Direction: Ryan Cook

Printed in Canada

Last digit is the print number: 9 8 7 6 5 4 3 2 1

ELSEVIER Book Aid International Working together to grow libraries in developing countries
www.elsevier.com • www.bookaid.org

Roberts and Hedges'

Clinical Procedures in Emergency Medicine and Acute Care

EIGHTH EDITION

EDITOR-IN-CHIEF

Diane M. Birnbaumer, MD, FACEP

Emeritus Professor
Department of Emergency Medicine
David Geffen School of Medicine at UCLA
Emeritus Faculty
Department of Emergency Medicine
Harbor-UCLA Medical Center
Torrance, California

ELSEVIER

IN MEMORIAM

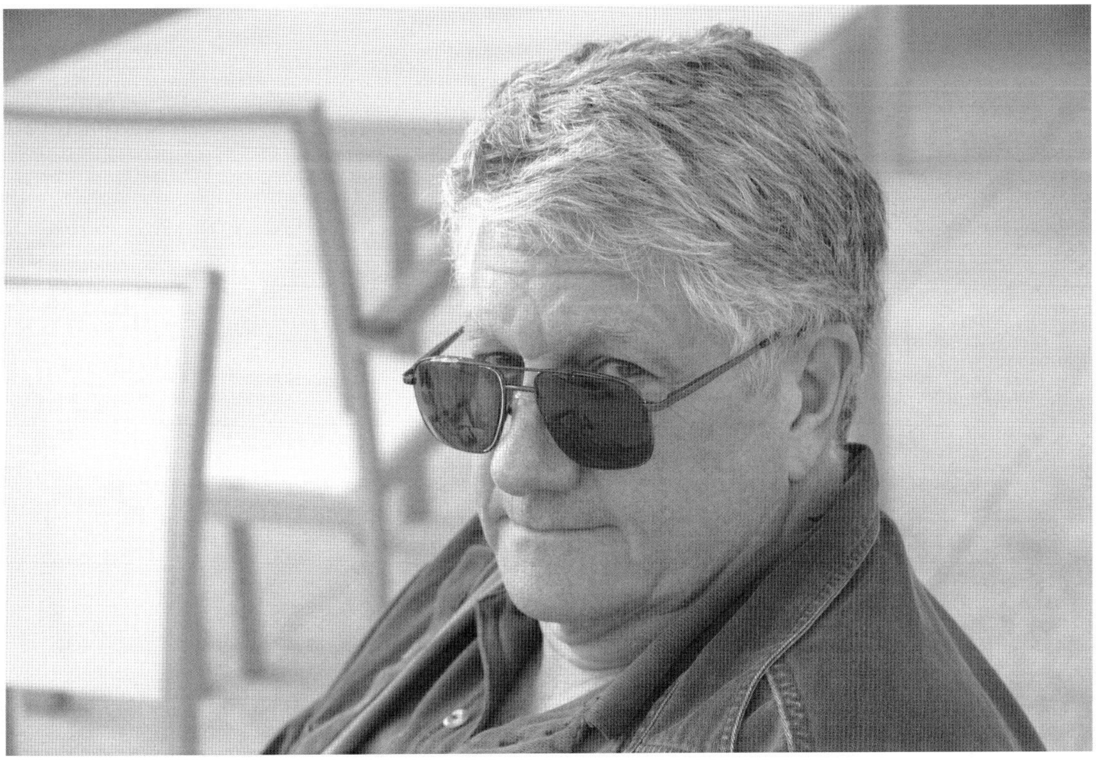

James R. Roberts, MD, FACMT, FACEP, FAAEM, CMRO
February 9, 1946 to July 22, 2022

"I've learned that people will forget what you said, people will forget what you did, but people will never forget how you made them feel."
Maya Angelou

To J.D.T., for the selfless patience and support he gave me while I worked on this book, and to all the extraordinary people providing medical care for people in their moments of greatest need.

Diane M. Birnbaumer

With sincere thanks to my beloved wife, Karen, who has been a remarkable partner throughout our life journey, as well as to our children, Sydney, Nathan, William, and Travia. Thank you to Amanda Smith for her steadfast efforts in helping produce this work and to the students and teachers everywhere who help continue the mission of lifelong learning.

Arjun Chanmugam

As I pondered my dedication for this edition, I realized that it will likely be my last. As such, I would like to dedicate this book to the things that I hold most dear: my wife, Marcy, the nicest, most caring, and generous person I have ever known and who I have loved forever. To my children, Adam, Arielle, and Allison, the kind of children every parent dreams about having; they make me proud every day. And to my grandchildren, Ayla, Amira, Austin, Andrew, and "Shelly"; their unconditional love has changed me in ways I could not have imagined. I would also like to dedicate this edition to Jim Roberts. To me Jim was first a mentor, then a friend and colleague. He was a truly amazing physician and very special human being who transformed the practice of emergency medicine.

Carl R. Chudnofsky

To my wife, Jane, my children, Christopher, Peter, and Ana, and my parents, Carolyn and Cliff Colwell, who have supported me in both my medical career and my life more than I deserve or could ever adequately thank them for. You are the reason I am where I am today, and you have my eternal love and gratitude.

Christopher Colwell Sr

In appreciation to my wife, Karen, and my sons, Joshua and Zachary, for their patience, support, and love. To my healthcare colleagues, students, residents, patients, and their families, who remind me daily what an amazing opportunity we have to reduce suffering. You inspire me to educate and serve others with compulsion and compassion. What an amazing team-oriented mission we practice each day. Great love and gratitude.

Peter M.C. DeBlieux

Thank you to my wonderful wife, Nicole, for being my best friend and my source of strength and humor in all of life's endeavors. And thank you to Jeff Tabas, for being a kind and supportive mentor throughout this process.

Kevin Hanley

To our patients, who grant us the privilege of practicing our craft; to our students, residents, and colleagues, from whom we learn; and to our families past and present, without whose support this would not have been possible.

Michael Hayoun

For our students, who in turn will be teachers and care for us in the near future. For our patients, for whom we strive mastery of procedures. My gratitude to Amal Mattu, who mentors so many of us. And for Mercedes, my partner in everything.

Siamak Moayedi

Thank you to my amazingly supportive husband, Bobby, and to my kids, Max and Sophie, who teach me things every day. Thank you to the truly wonderful faculty at Parnassus who keep me excited about coming to work every day and motivated to advocate for emergency medicine. And thanks to our patients, who are the reason I went into this field.

Maria C. Raven

To my wife, Lisa, for her continuous encouragement and support. To my children, and especially my grandchildren, for always making me feel like their hero. And to my father, who taught me there was no problem we could not solve. Thank you J.R.R. for inviting a young emergency physician to be a part of this amazing project from the beginning.

Alfred Sacchetti

To my beloved family: my daughters, Kira and Quinn, who are the greatest joys of my life; my husband, Paul, for his unrelenting love and support of my many pursuits; my parents, William and Denise, for their steadfast guidance and belief that I could accomplish anything; my grandmother, Nancy, for being the best cheerleader; and my siblings, Adam, Amber, and Austin, who are my oldest and most treasured friends.

Amanda Smith

To my wife, Michiko, and children, Kenzo, Kai, and Maya. Your love has kept me inspired and sane. To the people we care for—I truly hope that the learning from this resource helps us to take better care of you. And to all our physicians and trainees—hopefully this inspires and assists you in your care.

Jeffrey Tabas

This edition is dedicated to my father, Dr. James R. Roberts (1946–2022). Jim was an incredible man and the brick and mortar of this text from the beginning. He was also my hero, best friend, and mentor. Jim's dedication to the specialty and teaching of emergency medicine impacted students, colleagues, and patients for over 40 years. His legacy and teachings will continue to live on through this text and from the memories of his kind and generous soul. Dad, I miss you more with every passing day and with every ED shift. For my brother, Matthew J. Roberts, and mother, Lydia Forte Roberts. You make my life worthwhile. Thank you. To Dr. W. Richard Bukata: without you in my life, I am truly not sure where I would be now. Thank you for your incredible support, love, and guidance. To Dr. Diane Birnbaumer, thank you for all your work on this edition. You have taught me more than you will ever know. For my dearest husband, Jason Weaver. My light, love, and laughter. And to Eleanor, my darling daughter and the inspiration for all things truly important in this life. I love you. Finally, to the future of emergency medicine and to Jeanne Forte, of course.

Martha Roberts

To my colleagues: the physicians, residents, and students that I have had the pleasure of working alongside in the service of our patients. I hope I have taught you a fraction of what you have taught me. A special thank you to Jim Roberts, who saw the need for including more ultrasound content in the text years ago and entrusted me to create it. A giant in our field and an inspiration. Finally, to the love of my life, my son Danny.

Christine Butts

To my husband, Dave, for his relentless support of this piece of work.

Jessica Mason

To our patients, who grant us the privilege of learning from their care. To our students, residents, nurses, and faculty, for the continuous infusion of thoughtful questions that renew my passion for clinical practice. And to my wife and son, Kora and Zak, who provide an unlimited supply of love and support.

Zlatan Coralic

Contributors

Benjamin S. Abella, MD, MPhil
Mount Sinai Professor and System Chair
Department of Emergency Medicine
Icahn School of Medicine at Mount Sinai
New York, New York

Michael K. Abraham, MD, MS
Associate Professor
Department of Emergency Medicine
University of Maryland School of Medicine
Baltimore, Maryland

Pablo Aguilera, MD, MBA
Associate Professor
Department of Emergency Medicine
Director
Continuing Medical Education and Global Outreach
Pontificia Universidad Católica de Chile;
Director
Department of Emergency Medicine
Christus Health
Santiago, Chile

Robert Allen, MD
Clinical Assistant Professor
Department of Emergency Medicine
Los Angeles General Medical Center
Los Angeles, California;
Clinical Assistant Professor
Keck School of Medicine of USC
Studio City, California

Kathlene T. Babalola, MD
ED Ultrasound Director
Department of Emergency Medicine
University of Maryland Shore Regional Health
Easton, Maryland

Kimberly Bambach, MD
Assistant Professor
Department of Emergency Medicine
Wexner Medical Center at The Ohio State University
Columbus, Ohio

Kenny Vinh Banh, MD
Assistant Dean
Undergraduate Medical Education
Professor
Department of Emergency Medicine
University of California San Francisco
Fresno, California

David K. Barnes, MD, FACEP
Health Sciences Clinical Professor
Department of Emergency Medicine
UC Davis Health
University of California Davis
Sacramento, California

Marc T. Bartman, MD
Associate Professor
Department of Emergency Medicine
Medical University of South Carolina
Charleston, South Carolina

Ryan Bateman, MD
Attending Physician
Department of Emergency Medicine
Virtua Our Lady of Lourdes Hospital
Camden, New Jersey

Lance B. Becker, MD, FAHA
Hofstra/Northwell School of Medicine Chair
Department of Emergency Medicine
North Shore University Hospital & Long Island Jewish Medical Center
Manhasset, New York

Solomon Behar, MD
Director
Pediatric Emergency Medicine Resident Education
Long Beach Memorial/Miller Children's Hospital
Voluntary Faculty
Department of Pediatrics
UC Irvine and David Geffen UCLA School of Medicine
Long Beach, California

Diane M. Birnbaumer, MD
Emeritus Professor
Department of Emergency Medicine
David Geffen School of Medicine at UCLA
Rancho Palos Verdes, California;
Emeritus Faculty
Department of Emergency Medicine
Harbor-UCLA Medical Center
Torrance, California

Chad Bleske, MD
Resident
Emergency Department
Henry Ford Health
Detroit, Michigan

Barbara K. Blok, MD
Associate Professor
Department of Emergency Medicine
University of Colorado School of Medicine
Aurora, Colorado;
Executive Associate Program Director
Denver Health Residency in Emergency Medicine
Denver Health
Denver, Colorado

Michael Joseph Bono, MD
Professor of Emergency Medicine
Vice Chair
Department of Emergency Medicine
Macon & Joan Brock Virginia Health Sciences at Old Dominion University
Norfolk, Virginia

Heather A. Borek, MD
Associate Professor (Retired)
Department of Emergency Medicine
University of Virginia School of Medicine
Charlottesville, Virginia

William J. Brady, MD
Professor of Emergency Medicine and Medicine (Cardiovascular)
Vice Chair and Medical Director
David A. Harrison Distinguished Educator
Department of Emergency Medicine
University of Virginia Health System
Charlottesville, Virginia

Meghan Breed, MD
Assistant Professor
Department of Emergency Medicine
Georgetown University School of Medicine
Attending Physician
Surgical Critical Care
MedStar Washington Hospital Center
Washington, DC

W. Rick Bukata, MD
Medical Director
Center for Medical Education
Adjunct Professor of Clinical Emergency Medicine
Keck School of Medicine of USC
Los Angeles, California

Caroline W. Burmon, MD
Associate Quality Improvement Director
Emergency Department
Mount Sinai Beth Israel
New York, New York

Christine Butts, MD
Clinical Instructor of Emergency Medicine
Director of Division of Emergency Ultrasound
Department of Emergency Medicine
Louisiana State University Health Sciences Center
New Orleans, Louisiana

Michele Callahan, MD
Assistant Professor
Department of Emergency Medicine
University of Maryland School of Medicine
Baltimore, Maryland

Merle Carter, MD, FACEP
Executive Vice Chair
Department of Emergency Medicine
Albert Einstein Healthcare Network
Philadelphia, Pennsylvania

Stephanie A. Caterson, MD
Section Chief, Plastic Surgery
Department of Surgery
Christiana Care Health
Newark, Deleware

Theodore C. Chan, MD
Professor and Chair of Emergency Medicine
Department of Emergency Medicine
University of California San Diego
San Diego, California

Wan-Tsu W. Chang, MD
Associate Professor
Departments of Emergency Medicine, Neurology, and Program in Trauma
University of Maryland School of Medicine
Baltimore, Maryland;
Chair
Department of Critical Care
University of Maryland Capital Region Health
Largo, Maryland

Jason Chu, MD
Associate Professor of Emergency Medicine
Columbia University Vagelos College of Physicians & Surgeons
Department of Emergency Medicine
Columbia University Irving Medical Center
New York, New York

Carl R. Chudnofsky, MD
Professor and Chair
Department of Emergency Medicine
Interim Chair
Department of Radiology
Keck School of Medicine of USC
Los Angeles, California

Ilene Claudius, MD
Professor
Department of Emergency Medicine
David Geffen School of Medicine at UCLA
Los Angeles, California;
Physician Specialist
Department of Emergency Medicine
Harbor-UCLA Medical Center
Torrance, California

Wendy C. Coates, MD
Emeritus Professor
Department of Emergency Medicine
David Geffen School of Medicine at University of California Los Angeles
Los Angeles, California

Jonathan S. Cohen, MMSc, MBA, PA
Physician Associate
Department of Emergency Medicine
Johns Hopkins Bayview Medical Center
Baltimore, Maryland

Alessandra Conforto, MD
Physician
Department of Emergency Medicine
University of Southern California
Long Beach, California

Jonathan Davis, MD
Professor
Department of Emergency Medicine
Senior Associate Dean & DIO
Graduate Medical Education
Georgetown University & MedStar Health
Washington, DC

Nida F. Degesys, MD
Assistant Professor
Department of Emergency Medicine
University of California San Francisco
San Francisco, California

Ken Deitch, DO
VA Salt Lake City Health System
Attending Physician, Emergency Medicine
George E. Whalen Emergency Department
Mountain West Medical Center
Tooele, Utah;
St. Mark's Hospital
West Valley Emergency Center
West Valley City, Utah;
Adjunct Assistant Professor
Spencer Fox Eccles School of Medicine
University of Utah
Salt Lake City, Utah

Brian E. Driver, MD
Faculty Emergency Physician
Department of Emergency Medicine
Hennepin County Medical Center
Associate Professor
Department of Emergency Medicine
University of Minnesota
Minneapolis, Minnesota

Joshua Easter, MD, MBA, MHA, MSc
Associate Professor of Emergency Medicine
University of Virginia Health System
Charlottesville, Virginia

Erick Eiting, MD, MPH, MMM
Professor of Emergency Medicine and Medical Education
Icahn School of Medicine at Mount Sinai
New York, New York

Brian Euerle, MD
Professor
Department of Emergency Medicine
University of Maryland School of Medicine
Baltimore, Maryland

Alison N.A. Fedigan, MD
Resident Physician
Department of Emergency Medicine
Los Angeles General Medical Center
University of Southern California
Los Angeles, California

Michael T. Fitch, MD, PhD
Professor and Vice Chair for Academic Affairs
Department of Emergency Medicine
Wake Forest University School of Medicine
Winston-Salem, North Carolina

Kerry A. Forrestal, MD, MBA, FACEP
Attending Physician
Department of Emergency Medicine
TidalHealth
Salisbury, Maryland

Timothy S. Forsythe, DO, FACEP
Associate Program Director
Department of Emergency Medicine
Riverside Regional Medical Center
Newport News, Virginia

Mark T. Foster, MD, MS, FACEP
Associate Clinical Professor
Department of Emergency Medicine
UT Health San Antonio
San Antonio, Texas

Robert T. Gerhardt, MD, MPH
Director
Trauma and Clinical Care Research
Science and Technology Division
JBSA-Lackland
Lackland, Texas;
Adjunct Faculty
Department of Emergency Medicine
Brooke Army Medical Center
JBSA-Fort Sam Houston
Sam Houston, Texas

John C. Greenwood, MD
Assistant Professor
Department of Emergency Medicine
Assistant Professor
Department of Anesthesiology & Critical Care
Perelman School of Medicine at the University of Pennsylvania
Philadelphia, Pennsylvania

Kerry E. Gregory, DPA, PA-C
Physician Associate
Plastic and Reconstructive Surgery
Christiana Care Health System
Newark, Delaware

Neeraj Gupta, MD, FACEP, FAAEM, FPD-AEMUS
Attending Physician
Emergency Department
Jefferson Einstein Philadelphia Hospital
Philadelphia, Pennsylvania

Emily Haley, MHS, PA-C, CAQ-EM
Lead Physician Assistant
Department of Emergency Medicine
Medstar Franklin Square Medical Center
Rosedale, Maryland

Aaryn Hammond, MD
Assistant Professor
Department of Emergency Medicine
Wake Forest University School of Medicine
Winston-Salem, North Carolina

Michael Hayoun, MD, MPhil, MRO, FACEP, FAAEM
Clinical Assistant Professor
Thomas F. Frist, Jr. College of Medicine at Belmont University
Nashville, Tennessee

Randy B. Hebert, MD
Clinical Assistant Professor
Emergency Medicine
University of Illinois at Chicago
Attending Physician
Department of Emergency Medicine
Advocate Illinois Masonic Medical Center
Chicago, Illinois

Christopher Peter Holstege, MD
Professor
Departments of Emergency Medicine and Pediatrics
Chief
Division of Medical Toxicology
University of Virginia School of Medicine
Director
Blue Ridge Poison Center
University of Virginia Health
Charlottesville, Virginia

Kaitlen Howell, MD
Associate Physician
Volunteer Clinical Instructor
Department of Emergency Medicine
University of California San Francisco
San Francisco, California;
Director
Resident Ultrasound Education
Department of Emergency Medicine
Highland Hospital/Alameda Health System
Oakland, California

Ayo Igun, MD
Department of Emergency Medicine
University of Maryland Capital Region Health
Largo, Maryland

Paul Jhun, MD
Assistant Clinical Professor
Department of Emergency Medicine
University of California San Francisco
San Francisco, California

Russell F. Jones, MD
Professor
Department of Emergency Medicine
University of California Davis
Sacramento, California

Colin G. Kaide, MD, FACEP, FAAEM
Clinical Associate Professor
Department of Emergency Medicine
Wexner Medical Center at The Ohio State University
Columbus, Ohio

Caroline Kaigh, MD
Assistant Professor of Clinical Emergency Medicine
Lewis Katz School of Medicine at Temple University
Philadelphia, Pennsylvania

Bonnie Kaplan, MD
Associate Professor
Department of Emergency Medicine
University of Colorado
Aurora, Colorado

Danya Khoujah, MBBS, MEHP
Attending Physician
Department of Emergency Medicine
Tampa AdventHealth
Tampa, Florida;
Volunteer Adjunct Assistant Professor
Deparment of Emergency Medicine
University of Maryland School of Medicine
Baltimore, Maryland

John Kiel, DO, MPO, FACEP, CAQSM
Associate Professor
Department of Emergency Medicine
University of South Florida Morsani College of Medicine
Tampa General Hospital
Tampa, Florida

Thomas D. Kirsch, MD, MPH, FACEP
Adjunct Professor
Department of Emergency Medicine
George Washington University School of Medicine
Washington DC

Samantha S. Klein, MD
Attending Physician
Department of Emergency Medicine
Division of Medical Toxicology
Hackensack University Medical Center
Hackensack, New Jersey

Kevin J. Knoop, MD
Emeritus Program Director
Department of Emergency Medicine
Riverside Regional Medical Center
Newport News, Virginia;
Clinical Professor
Military and Emergency Medicine
Uniformed Services University of the Health Sciences
Bethesda, Maryland

Pavitra Kotini-Shah, MD
Associate Professor
Department of Emergency Medicine
University of Illinois Chicago
Chicago, Illinois

J. Michael Kowalski, DO, FACEP
Medical Toxicologist
Department of Emergency Medicine
Medical Director
Vice-Chair, Quality and Safety
Associate Professor
Department of Emergency Medicine
Jefferson Einstein Hospital
Philadelphia, Pennsylvania

Alex Koyfman, MD
Attending Physician/Core Faculty
Department of Emergency Medicine
UT Southwestern Medical Center
Parkland Health and Hospital System
Dallas, Texas

Thomas W. Kramer, MD
Assistant Professor
Department of Emergency Medicine
University of Pennsylvania Perelman School of Medicine
Philadelphia, Pennsylvania

Diann M. Krywko, MD
Professor and Chair
Department of Emergency Medicine
Medical University of South Carolina
Charleston, South Carolina

Jeremy Lacocque, DO, FACEP, FAEMS
Assistant Professor
Department of Emergency Medicine
University of California San Francisco
Medical Director
San Francisco Fire Department
San Francisco, California

Steven Lai, MD
Associate Clinical Professor
Department of Emergency Medicine
Ronald Reagan UCLA Medical Center
Olive View-UCLA Medical Center
Los Angeles, California

Richard L. Lammers, MD
Emeritus Professor
Department of Emergency Medicine
Western Michigan University Homer Stryker MD School of Medicine
Kalamazoo, Michigan

Bárbara Lara, MD, MPH
Assistant Professor
Department of Emergency Medicine
Pontificia Universidad Católica de Chile
Santiago, Chile

Danielle Levine, MD, MEd
Clinical Assistant Professor
Department of Emergency Medicine
Christiana Hospital
Newark, Delaware

Shan W. Liu, MD, SD
Associate Professor
Department of Emergency Medicine
Harvard Medical School
Geriatric Emergency Medicine Fellowship Director
Massachusetts General Hospital
Boston, Massachusetts

Brit Long, MD
Professor of Emergency Medicine
University of Virginia Medical Center
Charlottesville, Virginia

Angelica Loza-Gomez, MD
Adjunct Clinical Associate Professor of Emergency Medicine
Keck School of Medicine of USC
Los Angeles General Medical Center
Los Angeles, California

Wendy L. Macias-Konstantopoulos, MD, MPH, MBA
Director, Center for Social Justice and Health Equity
Department of Emergency Medicine
Massachusetts General Hospital
Associate Professor
Department of Emergency Medicine
Havard Medical School
Boston, Massachusetts

Thomas Mailhot, MD, FPD (AEMUS)
Director of Emergency Ultrasound
Department of Emergency Medicine
Los Angeles General Medical Center
Volunteer Clinical Associate Professor of Emergency Medicine
Keck School of Medicine of USC
Los Angeles, California

David Manthey, MD
Professor
Department of Emergency medicine
Wake Forest University School of Medicine
Winston-Salem, North Carolina

Asa Matthew Margolis, DO, MPH
Associate Professor
Department of Emergency Medicine
Johns Hopkins University School of Medicine
Baltimore, Maryland

Anthony Santo Mazzeo, MD, FACEP, FAAEM, FACHE
Professor of Clinical Emergency Medicine
Vice-Chair of Clinical Operations
Department of Emergency Medicine
Perelman School of Medicine at the University of Pennsylvania
Philadelphia, Pennsylvania

Sean McCann, MD
Assistant Professor
Department of Emergency Medicine
University of Illinois
Chicago, Illinois

Daniel McCollum, MD, FACEP
Director of Teaching and Learning and Professor
Department of Emergency Medicine
Louis Katz School of Medicine at Temple University
Philadelphia, Pennsylvania

Douglas L. McGee, DO, FACEP
Vice Dean of Graduate Medical Education
Sidney Kimmel Medical College
Vice Provost
Clinical Affiliates
Thomas Jefferson University
Philadelphia, Pennsylvania

Jillian McGrath, MD
Associate Professor
Department of Emergency Medicine
Wexner Medical Center at The Ohio State University
Columbus, Ohio

Rita McKeever, MD
Assistant Professor of Clinical Emergency medicine
Emergency Medicine
Louis Katz School of Medicine at Temple University
Philadelphia, Pennsylvania

Rohit Menon, MD
Clinical Instructor
Department of Emergency Medicine
University of Maryland Medical System
Baltimore, Maryland

Mary Mercer, MD, MPH
Clinical Professor
Department of Emergency Medicine
University of California San Francisco
San Francisco, California

Andrew F. Miller, MD
Assistant Professor of Pediatrics
Harvard Medical School
Assistant Medical Director
Division of Emergency Medicine
Boston Children's Hospital
Boston, Massachusetts

Robin Naples, MD
Professor
Department of Emergency Medicine
Sidney Kimmel Medical College at Thomas Jefferson University
Philadelphia, Pennsylvania

Mark J. Neavyn, MD
Department of Emergency Medicine
MaineHealth Maine Medical Center
Portland, Maine;
Associate Professor
Department of Emergency Medicine
Tufts University School of Medicine
Boston, Massachusetts

Emily Neill, MD
Associate Physician
Department of Emergency Medicine
University of California San Francisco
San Francisco General Hospital
San Francisco, California;
Physician
Department of Emergency Medicine
Marin Health Medical Center
Greenbrae, California

Jeanne Noble, MD
Associate Professor
Department of Emergency Medicine
University of California San Francisco
San Francisco, California

Jeanhyong Park, MD, FACEP
Assistant Professor
Department of Emergency Medicine
Medical University of South Carolina
Charleston, South Carolina

Brian Parker, MD
Associate Professor
Department of Emergency Medicine
UT Health San Antonio
San Antonio, Texas

Arielle C. Paul, MD
Assistant Professor of Clinical Emergency Medicine
Assistant Medical Director
Evaluation and Treatment Clinic
Department of Emergency Medicine
Keck School of Medicine of USC
Los Angeles, California

Christopher Peabody, MD, MPH
Associate Clinical Professor
Department of Emergency Medicine
University of California, San Francisco
San Francisco, California

Margarita E. Pena, MD, FACEP
Associate Residency Director
Department of Emergency Medicine
Henry Ford St. John Hospital
Wayne State University School of Medicine
Detroit, Michigan

Rebecca C.R. Plante, MHS, PA-C, CAQ-EM
Advanced Practice Manager
Department of Emergency Medicine
Johns Hopkins Bayview Medical Center
Baltimore, Maryland

Michael Podell, DVM, MSc, Diplomate ACVIM (Neurology)
Distinguished Fellow, National Academies of Practice
Board of Directors, MedVet
Columbus, Ohio

Amelia Y. Pousson, MD, MPH, CTropMed
Assistant Professor of Emergency Medicine
The Johns Hopkins University School of Medicine
Baltimore, Maryland

Heather M. Prendergast, MD, MPH, MHA, FACEP
Professor
Department of Emergency Medicine
University of Illinois
Chicago, Illinois

Robert F. Reardon, MD
Faculty Emergency Physician
Department of Emergency Medicine
Hennepin County Medical Center
Professor
Department of Emergency Medicine
University of Minnesota
Minneapolis, Minnesota

Kathryn E. Redinger, MD
Associate Professor
Departments of Emergency Medicine and Medical Education
Western Michigan University Homer Stryker M.D. School of Medicine
Kalamazoo, Michigan

Salvador Rios, MD
EMS Fellow
Department of Emergency Medicine
University of Southern California
Los Angeles, California

Emanuel P. Rivers, MD, MPH
Clinical Professor
Department of Emergency Medicine and Surgery
Wayne State University/Michigan State
Vice Chairman and Research Director
Department of Emergency Medicine
Senior Staff Attending Physician
Emergency Medicine and Surgical Critical Care
Henry Ford Hospital
Detroit, Michigan

Ralph J. Riviello, MD
Professor and Chair
Department of Emergency Medicine
UT Health San Antonio
San Antonio, Texas

Aaron E. Robinson, MD, MPH
Faculty Emergency Physician
Department of Emergency Medicine
Hennepin County Medical Center
Physician, Hennepin EMS
Assistant Professor
Departments of Emergency Medicine and Medical Education
Western Mich Univ Homer Stryker MD School of Medicine
Minneapolis, Minnesota

Emily Rose, MD
Associate Professor of Clinical Emergency Medicine (Educational Scholar)
Department of Emergency Medicine
LA County and USC Medical Center
Director for Pre-Health Undergraduate Studies
Department of Medical Education
Keck School of Medicine of the University of Southern California
Los Angeles, California

Lea Rowson, DO
Attending Physician
Department of Emergency Medicine
Virtua Our Lady of Lourdes Hospital
Camden, New Jersey;
Affiliate Faculty
Department of Medicine
Rowan Virtua School of Osteopathic Medicine
Stratford, New Jersey

Alexis Salerno, MD
Assistant Professor
Department of Emergency Medicine
University of Maryland School of Medicine
Baltimore, Maryland

Bryan Salvato, MD
Resident Physician
Department of Emergency Medicine
University of Florida
Jacksonville, Florida

Leonard E. Samuels, MD
Clinical Associate Professor
Department of Emergency Medicine
Sidney Kimmel Medical College at Thomas Jefferson University
Philadelphia, Pennsylvania

Christopher E. San Miguel, MD, Med, FAAEM, FACEP
Clinical Associate Professor
Department of Emergency Medicine
Wexner Medical Center at The Ohio State University
Columbus, Ohio

Stephen Sanko, MD
EMS Fellowship Director
Adjunct Associate Professor
Department of Emergency Medicine
Keck School of Medicine of the University of Southern California
Former Chief Physician and EMS Bureau Commander
Los Angeles Fire Department
Los Angeles, California

Jairo Santanilla, MD
Specialist
Department of Emergency Medicine
University of New Orleans
New Orleans, Louisiana

Genevieve Santillanes, MD
Physician Specialist
Los Angeles General Medical Center
Adjunct Associate Professor of Clinical Emergency Medicine
Keck School of Medicine of USC
Los Angeles, California

Steven G. Schauer, DO
Physician
Department of Emergency Medicine
Brooke Army Medical Center
JBSA Fort Sam Houston
Fort Sam Houston, Texas

Richard B. Schwartz, MD, FACEP
Chairman and Professor
Department of Emergency Medicine
Medical College of Georgia at Augusta University
Augusta, Georgia

David Scordino, MD, MPH, FACEP, FAWM, FAAEM
Department of Emergency Medicine
Alaska Regional Hospital
Anchorage, Alaska

Lovita Scrimshaw, DO
Emergency Physician
Department of Emergency Medicine
CHI St. Alexiums Health
Dickinson, North Dakota

Michael J. Shallcross, MD
Chief Resident
Department of Emergency Medicine
Riverside Regional Medical Center
Newport News, Virginia

Kristen Hart Shanahan, MD, MPH
Attending Physician in Pediatric Emergency Medicine
Department of Emergency Medicine
Massachusetts General Hospital
Assistant Professor of Emergency Medicine and Pediatrics
Harvard Medical School
Boston, Massachusetts

Ross Allen Simcoe, MD
Clinical Director
Department of Emergency Medicine
Virtua Our Lady of Lourdes Hospital
Camden, New Jersey

Daniel Simpson, DO, FACEP, FAAEM
Attending Physician
Department of Emergency Medicine
Virtua Our Lady of Lourdes Hospital
Camden, New Jersey

Peter E. Sokolove, MD
Professor and Chair
Department of Emergency Medicine
University of California San Francisco School of Medicine
San Francisco, California

Ricaurte Solis, DO, AAS
Associate Professor
Department of Emergency Medicine
Medical College of Georgia at Augusta University
Augusta, Georgia

Ryan Spangler, MD
Assistant Professor
Department of Emergency Medicine
University of Maryland School of Medicine
Baltimore, Maryland

Morgan Sweere, MD, MPH
Resident Physician
Department of Emergency Medicine
University of Florida Jacksonville
Jacksonville, Florida

Rebecca J. Teague, MD, FACEP
Assistant Professor
Department of Emergency Medicine
Emory University School of Medicine
Atlanta, Georgia

Semhar Z. Tewelde, MD
Associate Professor
Department of Emergency Medicine
University of Maryland School of Medicine
Baltimore, Maryland

Daniel Thomas, MD
Senior Physician
Department of Emergency Medicine
Duke Regional Hospital
Durham, North Carolina

Eric Tizzard, MD
Emergency Medicine Specialist
Department of Emergency Medicine
University of Florida Jacksonville
Jacksonville, Florida

Craig Torres-Ness, MD, MPH, MST
Associate Professor
Department of Emergency Medicine
University of Southern California
Los Angeles, California

Scott R. Votey, MD
Emeritus Professor of Emergency Medicine
David Geffen School of Medicine at UCLA
Los Angeles, California

Jonathan G. Wagner, MD
Associate Professor
Department of Emergency Medicine
Keck School of Medicine of USC
Attending Physician
Department of Emergency Medicine
Los Angeles General Medical Center
Los Angeles, California

Kara E. Ward, MD
Critical Care Physician
Department of Pulmonary & Critical Care
St. Tammany Hospital System
Covington, Louisiana

Jonathan Watson, MD
Assistant Professor
Department of Emergency Medicine
Georgetown University School of Medicine
Washington, DC

Susan R. Wilcox, MD
Vice Chair for Academic Affairs
Department of Medicine
Medical Director of 5c ICU
Pulmonary and Critical Care
Lahey Hospital
Professor of Medicine
UMass Chan-Lahey Medical School
Burlington, Massachusetts;
Associate Chief Medical Officer
Boston MedFlight
Bedford, Massachusetts

George Willis, MD
Vice Chair of Faculty Affairs
Emergency Medicine
UT Health Science Center at San Antonio
San Antonio, Texas

Mike Winters, MD, MBA, FACEP, FAAEM
Professor of Emergency Medicine
Vice Chair for Clinical and Administrative Affairs
Department of Emergency Medicine
University of Maryland School of Medicine
Baltimore, Maryland

Preface

This eighth edition of *Roberts and Hedges' Clinical Procedures in Emergency Medicine and Acute Care* reflects both the tried-and-true and the cutting edge in its content as well as its editorial board and authors.

Dr. James Roberts, a visionary who created this eponymous core textbook that has educated decades of clinicians around the world, passed away early in the development of this edition. Before his passing he updated the table of contents. He gave his thanks to the long-time associate editors who stepped down and he oversaw the expansion of the Editorial Board to include new associate editors and many new authors. He also brought me on as a co-Editor-in-Chief. Since his death it has been my goal to assure the quality of this text continues to meet Dr. Roberts' exacting standards.

This edition continues the book's ongoing dedication to providing complete, highly detailed, and up-to-date descriptions of both common and uncommon procedures encountered during emergency and acute care practice. Highly complicated or invasive procedures such as open thoracotomy, troubleshooting implantable cardiac devices, and dealing with complicated obstetrical deliveries are discussed in detail, including when to intervene—and when *not* to intervene. As some of the procedures in the text are frequently performed in urgent care clinics and clinician's offices, this book is also useful to those who practice in those settings. To that end, detailed discussions of procedures such as of wound closure and burn care, treatment of soft tissue injuries, and drainage of cutaneous abscesses are just a few of the more minor procedures applicable to the outpatient setting that are covered in this book.

This edition is heavily illustrated. The figures have been expanded and updated to reflect the patient population served and to add clarity to the text. This edition also continues the use of procedure boxes that can be viewed as a "mini-atlas" that allows the clinician to see the entire procedure at a glance.

While one could haul this massive physical text to the bedside to use to illustrate procedures while teaching, it may be preferable to use the online version of the book, which can be called up on a computer, laptop, tablet, Kindle, or smartphone. For ease of use, the online version is fully searchable.

The video library for this edition has been vastly enlarged thanks to the tireless efforts of Martha Roberts, NP, and Jessica Mason, MD. A special thanks goes to the enormous contributions from Larry Mellick, MD, whose generosity in sharing his expansive library of procedure videos enhances this edition significantly.

This edition also includes information on the continuously expanding use of ultrasound in medical procedures, and many of the chapters include an ultrasound section. These sections, presented in easily found and readily deciphered boxes within the chapters, are the result of the efforts of ultrasound editor Christine Butts, MD.

To the editors and authors of this edition, my heartfelt thanks. Transitioning from a singularly visionary editor like Dr. James Roberts to a new Editor-in-Chief is never easy, and it was particularly difficult as we all dealt with not only the loss of one of the true icons of emergency medicine, but, for many of us, the death of a long-term friend. I thank them for their patience as I took over the reins mid-update and for their incredibly hard work in maintaining the extraordinarily high standards of this text.

I would like to thank the Associate Editors individually. Many are names you may recognize, as they are highly accomplished physicians, educators and leaders. I am also honored to call many of them friends. The all embody the pinnacle of emergency medicine and acute care excellence. The erudite and capable editors of this edition are Arjun Chanmugam, MD, MBA; Carl R. Chudnofsky, MD, FACEP; Christopher Colwell Sr, MD, FACEP, FAEMS; Peter M.C. Deblieux, MD, FACEP; Kevin Hanley, MD; Michael A. Hayoun, MD, MPhil, MRO, FACEP, FAAEM; Siamak Moayedi, MD, FAAEM; Maria C. Raven, MD, MPH, FACEP; Alfred Sacchetti, MD, FACEP; Amanda Smith, DMSc, MMS, PA-C, CAQ-EM; Jeffrey Tabas, MD, FACEP; and Zlatan Coralic, PharmD, the pharmacology editor. I can never repay the time they spent on this book but can only offer them my deepest thanks.

The content of this edition is the layered work of hundreds of authors and editors over multiple editions. They contributed their expertise, experience, time, and energy filtering through the massive medical literature to ensure the content is as current and accurate as possible, often building on the work of the authors and editors who came before.

There are, of course, many ways to approach any individual patient or procedure, so this text is not a dictum and is not truly authoritative. This book does not attempt to define the standard of care. The clinician should remember these caveats if involved in a medicolegal scenario. This book contains practical hints and successful tactics gleaned from the literature and years of practice, adeptly described by skilled clinicians. As with previous versions, this edition incorporated the personal opinions and experience of the authors and editors.

This text should be viewed as a clinical guide, not a legal document. Do not reference this book if you testify in court for either the defense or the plaintiff.

If any of the editing changed, altered, or misinterpreted the original thoughts of the contributors (an unavoidable consequence of multiple layers of review), my apologies. Hard decisions had to be made to ensure clear recommendations to the users of this book.

This book attempts to help readers learn not just what to do, but how and when to do it, but it cannot always fit into every clinical situation. It is at the bedside and in the care of any given patient that the combination of medical knowledge and clinical experience is best put to use.

Diane Birnbaumer, MD, FACEP

Foreword

It is a great honor to be asked to write the foreword to *Roberts and Hedges' Clinical Procedures in Emergency Medicine and Acute Care*. Dr. Jim Roberts, the principal author and a dear friend for over 40 years, had been well on his way to editing the eighth edition when he passed away unexpectedly. Leaving huge shoes to fill, Dr. Diane Birnbaumer and Jim's daughter, Martha Roberts, NP, both colleagues and great friends of mine, took up the challenge of finishing the book with a focus on maintaining the quality and thoroughness that Jim would have expected. Even a casual review will indicate that the work of all three of these individuals has resulted in an extraordinary text—one that is required to be on every emergency clinician's bookshelf and referred to regularly.

The legacy of this book mirrors the essence of the emergency department itself—a place where precision, adaptability, and swift decision-making converge to save lives. It is within this dynamic realm that countless procedures are performed every day, often under extraordinary pressure. Whether it's securing an airway in the chaos of a trauma bay, reducing a dislocated joint in the middle of the night, or providing meticulous wound care for a frightened child, mastery of procedural skills is the cornerstone of emergency medicine and acute care.

For decades, *Roberts and Hedges' Clinical Procedures in Emergency Medicine and Acute Care* has served as the definitive guide for emergency medicine practitioners. Now in its eighth edition, this textbook remains unparalleled in its scope, depth, and utility. With over 1,500 meticulously curated pages and contributions from decades of leading experts, it continues to set the gold standard for procedural education. The inclusion of linked references and hundreds of procedural videos in its online version only enhances its value, making it an indispensable resource for learners and seasoned clinicians alike.

The importance of this book cannot be overstated. It is more than just a collection of techniques; it is a comprehensive repository of knowledge that blends evidence-based medicine with the art and science of procedural practice. Each chapter provides not only step-by-step instructions but also critical insights into the indications, contraindications, and potential complications of every procedure. From the foundational skills of wound management and splinting to the nuanced complexities of procedural sedation and regional anesthesia, this book covers it all with remarkable clarity and thoroughness.

Emergency medicine demands a relentless pursuit of excellence, and this text embodies that ethos. It empowers clinicians to approach every procedure—whether routine or high-stakes—with confidence and competence. By integrating the latest advancements and evidence into this edition, the authors and editors have ensured that it remains at the forefront of medical education and practice. The addition of hundreds of procedural videos further bridges the gap between theory and application, offering an invaluable visual guide to complement the written material.

To those new to emergency medicine, this book will be your trusted companion as you develop and refine your procedural skills. To the experienced practitioner, it serves as a reliable reference and a source of continual learning. And to the educators, it provides an unparalleled tool to inspire and train the next generation of emergency care clinicians.

Roberts and Hedges' Clinical Procedures in Emergency Medicine and Acute Care is not just a textbook; it is the bible of emergency department procedures. It is a testament to the dedication, expertise, and passion of the well over 100 authors who have poured their collective wisdom into its pages. This edition, fully updated and revised, solidifies its place as the ultimate resource for procedural mastery in emergency and acute care settings.

For those of us who strive daily to make a difference in the lives of our patients, this book is a beacon—a guide that illuminates the path to excellence in procedural care. It is an honor to introduce this essential work, and I am confident it will continue to inspire and elevate our practice for years to come.

Rick Bukata, MD
Chief Medical Officer
The Center for Medical Education
Adjunct Clinical Professor of Emergency Medicine
Department of Emergency Medicine
Keck School of Medicine at USC
Los Angeles, California

Acknowledgements

Although it seems intuitive that putting together and publishing a nearly 2000-page book full of graphics and videos is a massive undertaking, the reality of the endeavor eclipses any preconceptions. These factual masterpieces that grace your bookshelf or office countertop—or, more and more commonly, live out in cyberspace and visit the interior of your device—come together as the result of the gargantuan efforts of literally hundreds of people.

Each chapter got a thorough review and update by the current set of nearly 100 authors. Most are updates from chapters in previous editions, many written by previous authors. The cumulative effort of years of expertise and hundreds of brilliant minds shines from these pages. They all deserve the deepest thanks for their hard work invested in this text.

While a more robust thanks is offered to these individuals in the Preface, I would also like to take this opportunity to acknowledge the mind-boggling amount of work put in by the Editorial Board of this edition and give them my heartfelt thanks: Video Editors Martha Roberts and Jessica Mason; Ultrasound Editor Christine Butts; Associate Editors Arjun Chanmugam, Carl R. Chudnofsky, Chris Colwell, Peter M.C. Deblieux, Kevin Hanley, Michael Hayoun, Siamak Moayedi, Alfred Sacchetti, Maria C. Raven, Amanda Smith, and Jeffrey Tabas; and PharmD Editor Zlatan Coralic. A special thanks goes to Dr. Larry Mellick, who selflessly shared countless videos from the expansive library he has accumulated during his career. To this illustrious group of remarkable individuals, I can never repay the time they spent on this book but can only offer them my deepest thanks.

This book would never be published without the extensive planning and tireless efforts at Elsevier. When Dr. Roberts started working on this edition and before he brought me on board, he worked with Senior Content Strategist Kayla Wolfe to determine content and make a game plan for the updated version. She helped Dr. Roberts bring me on board as Co-Editor-in-Chief. When she received a promotion to Executive Content Strategist, Kayla passed the reins into the capable hands of Senior Content Strategist Lauren Boyle, with whom I have worked through the rest of the development of this edition since Dr. Roberts' passing. The lion's share of the credit for the high editorial content of this book goes to Joanie Milnes, Senior Content Development Specialist. I could not have done what I needed to do for this text without her expert guidance.

Throughout the process of creating this edition, every effort was made to maintain the high standard set by Dr. Roberts. Through this work we honor his memory.

Diane Birnbaumer, MD, FACEP

Contents

Video Contents

Video 44.1
Paracentesis: Fluid Wave Demonstration. (Courtesy Martha Roberts, NP, and Dr. Fishman.)

Video 44.2
Paracentesis: Using Ultrasound to Identify Fluid. (Courtesy Martha Roberts, NP, and Dr. Fishman.)

Video 44.3
Paracentesis Simulation. (Courtesy Jared Novack, MD, and Ernest Wang, MD.)

Video 44.4
Paracentesis Without Ultrasound Guidance. (Courtesy Alfred Sacchetti, MD.)

Video 44.5
Paracentesis Demonstration on a Patient With Ascites. (Courtesy Martha Roberts, NP, and Dr. Fishman.)

Video 45.1
Hernia Reduction. (Courtesy Jessica Mason, MD. Mackenzie Brown, MD, Nicole Bigot, MD, and Martha Roberts, NP.)

Video 46.1
Equipment Review of Anoscope and Rectal Exams. (Courtesy Martha Roberts, NP, and James Roberts, MD.)

Video 46.2
Thrombosed Hemorrhoids Treatment. (Courtesy Martha Roberts, NP, and James Roberts, MD.)

Video 47.1
Cervical Collar Application.

Video 47.2
Spinal Immobilization Backboard Use.

Video 47.3
Traction Splint Field Application.

Video 47.4
Hare Traction Splint Placement.

Video 48.1
Emergency Management of Amputated Toes. (Courtesy Larry B. Mellick, MD.)

Video 48.2
Fingertip Amputation Treated With Cyanoacrylate Tissue Adhesive. (Courtesy Larry B. Mellick, MD.)

Video 48.3
Field Amputation: Upper Extremity. (Courtesy Steven Zils, MD, Panna Codner, MD, and Ronald Pirallo, MD.)

Video 48.4
Field Amputation: Lower Extremity. (Courtesy Steven Zils, MD, Panna Codner, MD, and Ronald Pirallo, MD.)

Video 48.5
Field Amputation: Introduction and Clinical Pearls. (Courtesy Steven Zils, MD, Panna Codner, MD, and Ronald Pirallo, MD.)

Video 50.1
Fun and Interesting Joint Reductions. (Courtesy Center for Medical Education and W. Richard Bukata, MD.)

Video 50.2
Anterior Shoulder Dislocation: Lidocaine Intraarticular Traction and Countertraction. (Courtesy Martha Roberts, NP, and James Roberts, MD.)

Video 50.3
Intraarticular Lidocaine for Anterior Shoulder Dislocation Reduction. (Courtesy Larry B. Mellick, MD.)

Video 50.4
Shoulder Dislocation Reduction: Using Ultrasound to Guide Intraarticular Injection. (Courtesy Michael Stone, MD.)

Video 50.5
Difficult Dislocation: Using Sedation for Spasm. (Courtesy Neil Cunningham, MD, and Gerard Fennessy, MD.)

Video 50.6
Can't Adduct: Troubleshooting Positioning. (Courtesy Neil Cunningham and Gerard Fennessy.)

Video 50.7
Stimson Technique With Scapular Manipulation. (Courtesy Jessica Mason, MD.)

Video 50.8
Scapular Manipulation. (Courtesy Neil Cunningham and Gerard Fennessy.)

Video 50.9
Anterior Shoulder Dislocation Reduction: External Rotation Technique. (Courtesy Daneil Gromis, MD.)

Video 50.10
Shoulder Dislocation and External Rotation Maneuver. (Courtesy Larry B. Mellick, MD.)

Video 50.11
Anterior Shoulder Dislocation Reduction: Spaso Technique. (Courtesy George Douros, MD.)

Video 50.12
Fares Method for Anterior Shoulder Dislocation. (Courtesy Larry B. Mellick, MD.)

Video 50.13
Davos Method for Shoulder Dislocation. (Courtesy Larry B. Mellick, MD.)

SECTION I

Vital Signs and Patient Monitoring Techniques

CHAPTER 1

Vital Signs Measurement

Jillian L. McGrath and Kimberly Bambach

Measuring the temperature, pulse, respiratory rate (RR), blood pressure, and pulse oximetry is generally recommended for all emergency department (ED) patients, in addition to assessment of pain in the appropriate patient population. For very minor problems or for some fast-track patients (e.g., suture removal), a full set of vital signs may not be required, and this is best decided on a case-by-case basis rather than by strict protocol. Vital signs may indicate the severity of illness and dictate the urgency of intervention. Although a single set of abnormal values suggests pathology, findings on triage or the initial vital signs may be spurious and related to stress, anxiety, pain, or fear. It is prudent to repeat vital signs when initial triage vital signs are abnormal, as it would not reflect standard of care to attribute abnormal vitals to a specific pathology based on a single measurement. It is incorrect to retrospectively assume that diagnostic or treatment interventions should have been initiated based solely on these readings.[1] An abnormal vital sign may constitute the patient's entire complaint, as in a febrile infant, or it may be the only indication of the potential for serious illness, as in a patient with resting tachycardia.[2]

Emergency medical service (EMS) personnel begin assessment of the patient's status and vital signs in the prehospital setting. Surges of epinephrine and norepinephrine commonly occur during transport by the EMS, and these catecholamines are known to alter vital signs and lead to increases greater than 10% in the heart rate (HR).[3] Vagus nerve stimulation may also influence EMS-derived vital signs. Prehospital vital signs should always be interpreted with the entire clinical scenario in perspective. The greatest utility of vital signs is in their continued observation and trends over time. Deteriorating vital signs are an important indicator of a compromised physiologic condition, and improving values provide reassurance that the patient may be responding to therapy. When a patient undergoes treatment over an extended period, it is essential that the vital signs be repeated as appropriate to the clinical scenario, particularly those that were previously abnormal. In some clinical circumstances, it is advisable to monitor the vital signs continuously. Vital signs should be measured and recorded at intervals as dictated by clinical judgment, the patient's clinical state, or after any significant change in these parameters.

The implementation of medical emergency teams or rapid response systems has invigorated investigation into the clinical significance and predictive value of abnormal vital signs in an inpatient setting.[4] Two metaanalyses demonstrated significant reductions in nonintensive care unit (non-ICU) in-hospital cardiac arrests in children and adults (>33% reduction) and of mortality in children (>20% reduction) related to rapid response systems that rely heavily on vital sign abnormalities.[5,6]

Abnormal vital signs during the ED encounter may increase the likelihood of adverse events including in-hospital mortality, unexpected ICU admission, and return visits or readmission.[7–9] One analysis identified vital sign cutoffs that were associated with twice the odds of admission within 7 days after discharge: systolic blood pressure (SBP) <97 mm Hg, HR >101 beats/min, body temperature >37.3°C, and pulse oximetry <92 SpO_2; concluding that ED providers should recognize and remeasure abnormal vital signs and consider arranging for closer outpatient follow-up for such patients.[9]

Blood pressure and pulse are frequently evaluated together as a measure of blood volume. Capillary refill is discussed as an assessment of overall perfusion, circulatory volume, and blood pressure. Although body temperature is usually the last vital sign measured during resuscitation, it has special importance for patients suffering from thermal regulatory failure. With these considerations in mind, this chapter is organized according to the priorities of patient resuscitation and evaluation. Assessment of pain as a vital sign is a controversial and relevant construct that is discussed briefly at the end of this chapter.

BACKGROUND
CAN BE FOUND AT ELSEVIER EBOOKS+

NORMAL VALUES

The range of normal resting vital signs for specific age groups must be appreciated by the clinician to enable identification of abnormal values and their clinical significance. The normal ranges for vital signs are also influenced by gender, race, pregnancy, and residence in an industrialized nation. These ranges have not been validated in ED patients, who have many reasons for abnormalities in vital signs, including anxiety, pain, and altered physiology as a result of their disease states. Ranges of normal vital signs, commonly quoted as normal or abnormal in other settings, serve only as a guide and not an

TABLE 1.1 Pediatric Heart Rate Limits Based on Age Group and Percentile

AGE GROUP	5TH PERCENTILE	50TH PERCENTILE	95TH PERCENTILE
0–3 months	113	140	171
3–6 months	108	135	167
6–9 months	104	131	163
9–12 months	101	128	160
12–18 months	97	124	157
18–24 months	92	120	154
2–3 years	87	115	150
3–4 years	82	111	146
4–6 years	77	106	142
6–8 years	71	100	137
8–12 years	66	94	129
12–15 years	61	87	121
15–18 years	57	82	115

Adapted from Bonafide CP, Brady PW, Keren R, et al. Development of heart and respiratory rate percentile curves for hospitalized children. *Pediatrics*. 2013;131(4):e1150-e1157, Table 3.

TABLE 1.2 Pediatric Respiratory Rate Limits Based on Age Group and Percentile

AGE GROUP	5TH PERCENTILE	50TH PERCENTILE	95TH PERCENTILE
0–3 months	27	41	62
3–6 months	25	38	58
6–9 months	23	35	54
9–12 months	22	33	51
12–18 months	21	31	48
18–24 months	20	29	45
2–3 years	18	27	42
3–4 years	18	25	40
4–6 years	17	24	37
6–8 years	16	23	35
8–12 years	15	21	31
12–15 years	13	19	28
15–18 years	13	18	26

Adapted from Bonafide CP, Brady PW, Keren R, et al. Development of heart and respiratory rate percentile curves for hospitalized children. *Pediatrics*. 2013;131(4):e1150-e1157, Table 4.

absolute criterion for diagnosis, treatment, further observation, or intervention in the ED.

Published vital sign norms for children are not as well accepted as those for adult patients. Tables 1.1 and 1.2 report HR and RRs by age grouping and percentile for children from birth to 18 years of age. These data represent a large cross-sectional study using 6 months of nurse-documented HRs and RRs from the electronic records of 14,014 children on general medical and surgical wards at two tertiary-care children's hospitals. Up to 54% of HR observations and up to 40% of RR observations in this sample were outside textbook reference ranges.[14] During the newborn period, normal arterial blood pressure rises rapidly. Values for pulse and respiration in children older than 3 years reflect an average of male and female values for 0 to 1-, 3-, 9-, and 16-year-old populations. The values for blood pressure reflect an average of male and female values for the 1- to 6-month-old and the 3-, 9-, and 16-year-old populations.[15] Other studies have assessed the reference values for RR in children demonstrating the same variability of pediatric "normal" vital sign ranges.[16–18]

For the adult population, normal blood pressure values have been better established. Although SBP increases with age, *normotensive* or *normal SBP* is defined as 90–140 mm Hg, and normotensive or *normal diastolic blood pressure* is defined as 60–90 mm Hg. The recent literature suggests defining an "optimal" blood pressure as 115/75 mm Hg because values at or below this level have been associated with minimal vascular mortality.[19,20] Hypertension is further integrated into a global cardiovascular risk assessment.[21–23] Although most patients have similar blood pressure in both arms, Pesola and colleagues found that 18% of their hypertensive population[24] and 15% of their normotensive population had a difference of greater than 10 mm Hg in SBP between arms.[25] Within the adult population, optimal definitions for normal SBP probably vary with age, and particular differentiation should be made in regard to geriatric patients in the emergency setting. The recent literature suggests redefining values representative of hypotension in the elderly, especially in the setting of trauma. SBP readings ranging from approximately 90 to 120 mm Hg have been associated with occult hypoperfusion and increased mortality in geriatric trauma patients.[26–28]

In 1928 the New York Heart Association, by consensus, established the normal limits for the resting HR as 60 and 100 beats/min. Later data indicate that 45 and 95 beats/min may better define the HR limits of normal sinus rhythm in adults. Spodick and colleagues recommended that the operational definition for the limits of the resting HR in adults should be 50 and 90 beats/min.[29,30] This view is widely supported among cardiologists,[31,32] but these ranges have not been validated in the ED setting. A compilation of baseline ECGs of 79,743 individuals offered a reference range for HR of 48–98 beats/min with differences based on age and gender (using 2nd and 98th percentiles).[33] There is currently no consensus on what constitutes a normal adult RR; however, an RR range of 12–24 breaths/min is generally accepted in the existing literature as the norm for adults.[34–36]

Pregnancy results in alterations in the normal adult values of pulse and blood pressure. Pregnancy is characterized

TABLE 1.3 Vital Signs During Pregnancy in the Lateral Decubitus Position (Means ± SD)

	Trimester		
PARAMETER	1ST	2ND	3RD
Pulse rate (beats/min)	77 ± 2	85 ± 2	88 ± 2
Systolic BP (mm Hg)	98 ± 2	91 ± 2	95 ± 2
Diastolic BP (mm Hg)	53 ± 2	49 ± 2	50 ± 2

BP, Blood pressure; *SD*, standard deviation.
Adapted from Katz R, Karliner JS, Resnik R. Effects of a natural volume overload state (pregnancy) on left ventricular performance in normal human subjects. *Circulation*. 1978:58:434. By permission of the American Heart Association.

by significant increases in minute ventilation and is thought to be due to the combined facilitatory effects of progesterone and estrogen on central and peripheral chemoreflex drives to breathe.[37] The resting pulse rate increases throughout pregnancy from 10% to 15% over baseline values. The norms for SBP and diastolic blood pressure are dependent on patient positioning. When a pregnant patient is sitting or standing, systolic pressure is essentially unchanged. Diastolic pressure declines until approximately 28 weeks' gestation, then it begins to rise to nonpregnant levels. When a pregnant patient is in the lateral decubitus position, both SBP and diastolic pressure decline until the 28th week and then rise to nonpregnant levels (Table 1.3).[38]

RESPIRATION

Breathing is initiated and primarily controlled in the medullary respiratory center of the brainstem. The respiratory center is modulated by the pneumotaxic center, which limits the length of the inspiratory signal and greatly influences the RR and apneustic center in the pons.[39] Respiratory frequency reveals only a glimpse of the entire clinical picture. The pattern, effort, and volume of respiration may be more indicative of altered respiratory physiology. An abnormality in respiration may be a primary complaint or a manifestation of other systemic diseases. Increased RRs may be seen in patients with a variety of pulmonary or cardiac diseases, and acidosis, anemia, temperature, stress, and drugs (such as stimulants and salicylates) can significantly alter the RR in the absence of cardiopulmonary dysfunction.

Indications and Contraindications

The only contraindications to careful measurement of RR are the scenarios of respiratory distress, apnea, and upper airway obstruction, which require immediate therapeutic intervention. RR and respiratory effort should be assessed as soon as patient care demands allow. The respiratory status of both adults and children plays a crucial role in determining the overall assessment of illness. Although it is a sensitive yet nonspecific indicator of respiratory dysfunction, the RR can also predict nonpulmonary morbidity. Several prehospital and hospital-based illness or injury severity scores feature the RR as a cardinal value. A prehospital RR of less than 10 breaths/min or greater than 29 breaths/min is associated with major injury in 73% of children.[40] Using tachypnea alone as a predictor of pulmonary pathology, infants with an RR higher than 60 breaths/min are found to be hypoxic 80% of the time.[41] Pediatric studies have linked abnormal RRs to in-hospital mortality and the level of care required in the ED.[42,43] In a retrospective study exploring predictors of critical care admission for adult ED patients who were initially triaged as having low to moderate acuity, an abnormal RR at the first nursing assessment increased the odds of critical care admission by a factor of 1.66.[44] An RR higher than 25 breaths/min in prehospital trauma patients was associated with increased mortality.[45] Prearrest respiratory insufficiency (RR >36 breaths/min or pulse oximetry <90%) was an independent predictor of mortality (odds ratio [OR], 4.2) in patients with EMS-witnessed cardiac arrest.[46] Although some studies have associated abnormal RRs in adult ED patients with increased mortality,[47,48] a 2011 large prospective cohort study of adult patients found that an initial abnormal RR on triage in the ED was not an independent predictor of hospital mortality.[49] More recently, Barfod showed abnormal vital signs were associated with in-hospital mortality in the acutely ill patients admitted through the ED, especially RR and SpO_2.

Procedure

To measure RR (inspirations per minute), count the respirations when the patient is unaware that their breathing is being observed. Count for a full minute to most accurately determine the RR. The frequency of breathing is less regular than the pulse, and inaccurate measurement is more likely to occur if the count is taken for a shorter interval. It is common to measure respirations over 15 seconds and multiply by 4, and this can significantly alter the true RR per minute. An infant's RR can easily be determined by observing or palpating the excursion of the chest or the abdominal wall.[50] Infants should be observed for grunting respirations that are produced by expiring against a partly closed glottis (an attempt to maintain positive airway pressure).

Interpretation

Respiratory Rate

The reproducibility of RR measurements may be limited by significant interobserver variability.[1,51] Clinicians should recognize this inherent variability and interpret the RR with caution. Rates obtained by nurses versus medical students varied significantly, as did those obtained by medical students versus residents and attending clinicians. Interobserver variability may account for a difference of up to 6 breaths/min, and variability in the same observer may account for up to 5 breaths/min.[52] A study comparing RRs obtained by triage nurses with an electronic monitor found that neither provided an accurate measurement of the RR in the ED, suggesting that new clinical strategies for obtaining this vital sign may be necessary.[53] RR is an independent risk marker for in-hospital mortality in community-acquired pneumonia and should be measured when patients are admitted to the hospital with pneumonia and other acute conditions.[54]

Current texts vary considerably in their definition of a normal RR and cite published values that range from 8 to 24 breaths/min. In a study that specifically investigated normal RRs in an ED (afebrile ambulatory patients without respiratory complaints), females had a mean RR of 20.9 breaths/min and males had a mean RR of 19.4 breaths/min. The researchers concluded that a normal RR in the adult patient population was 16 to 24 breaths/min.[52] Other studies have provided additional information on normal resting and sleeping RRs in children younger than 7 years.[8–12 B-R] RRs obtained with a stethoscope were higher than those obtained by observation (mean difference, 2.6 breaths/min in awake and 1.8 breaths/min in asleep children). Smoothed percentile curves demonstrated a larger dispersion at birth (5th percentile, 34 breaths/min; 95th percentile, 68 breaths/min), whereas dispersion was less at 36 months of age (5th percentile, 18 breaths/min; 95th percentile, 30 breaths/min).

The RR will generally increase in the presence of fever. It is often difficult to determine whether tachypnea is a primary finding or is simply associated with hyperpyrexia. A study of children younger than 2 years in whom pneumonia was subsequently diagnosed found that age-appropriate limits for resting tachypnea in the presence of fever could be defined. A sensitivity of 74% and specificity of 77% for pneumonia were found when children 6 months of age had an RR higher than 59 breaths/min, when those aged 6–11 months had an RR higher than 52 breaths/min, and when those 1–2 years old had an RR higher than 42 breaths/min.[55] Even in the face of physiologic compensation for fever, interpretation of the RR alone can help predict the presence of pulmonary disease.

Respiratory Pattern and Amplitude

Hyperventilation and hypoventilation can result from an extensive variety of disorders and may be related to pulmonary or extrapulmonary pathology. Abnormal respiratory patterns can be characteristic of metabolic or central nervous system pathologic conditions (Fig. 1.1) and may aid in the differential diagnosis. Kussmaul respirations, deep inspiratory, and expiratory efforts describe the hyperventilation pattern seen in diabetic patients with ketoacidosis. Decreased RR is commonly seen with opiate toxicity. Hyperpnea, or a normal RR with

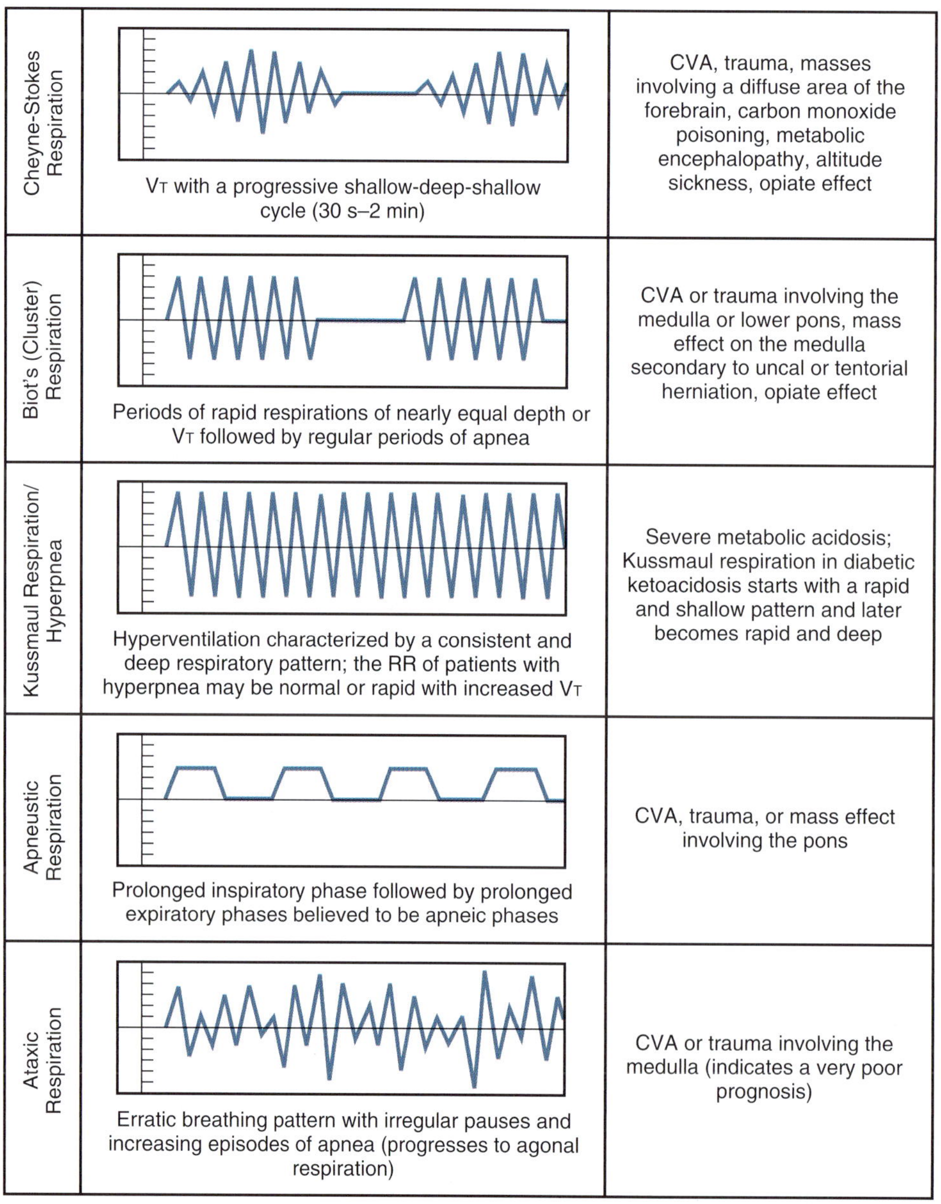

Fig. 1.1 Abnormal respiratory patterns. *CVA*, Cerebrovascular accident; *RR*, respiratory rate; *VT*, tidal volume. (Modified from D'Urbano J. Breathing Patterns, Breath Sounds 2011. http://www.BreathSounds.org.)

clinically significant hyperventilation secondary to increased tidal volume, may be seen with salicylate poisoning.[56]

Recognition of subtle tachypnea can be difficult in the emergency setting, although it can be the solitary indicator of disease. Another instance of pathology that can confuse routine measurement of the RR is diaphragmatic breathing or retractions. The variability in counting respiratory effort versus effective respirations is not generally appreciated in a single recorded value.

Observe the respiratory patterns carefully in children. In infants, it is essential to distinguish normal *periodic breathing* from *apnea*. By definition, periodic breathing consists of three or more respiratory pauses longer than 3 seconds in duration with less than 20 seconds between pauses. There is no associated bradycardia or cyanosis. This contrasts with apnea and is a particular problem in preterm infants. Apnea is defined as a respiratory pause longer than 20 seconds. It may be associated with bradycardia and hypoxia.[50] Periodic breathing and apnea are believed to be disorders on a continuum, both stemming from abnormal physiologic control of respiration. Periodic breathing is considered a benign disorder. Infants with symptomatic apneic episodes that result in apparent life-threatening events were previously considered at increased risk for sudden infant death syndrome.[57] This is more recently defined as a brief resolved unexplained event. These observed events occur in an infant younger than 1 year of age where the observer reports a sudden, brief, yet resolved episode of one or more of the following: cyanosis or pallor, absent, decreased, or irregular breathing, marked change in tone (hyper- or hypotonia) or altered level of responsiveness.[58]

For BRUE (Brief Resolved Unexplained Event) patients who have been evaluated in the ED and determined to be at lower risk, a metaanalysis showed that their risk is about the same as the baseline for death during the first year of life.[59]

PULSE

Examine the pulse to establish the cardiac rate, regularity of the rhythm, and strength of the pulsations. Though rarely diagnostic, peripheral pulses may yield clues about cardiac disease, such as aortic insufficiency, dysrhythmia, and information about the integrity of the peripheral vascular supply. Doppler ultrasound has utility in locating a pulse, assessing fetal heart tones beyond the first trimester of pregnancy, evaluating peripheral lower extremity vascular insufficiency with an ankle-brachial index, and assessing blood pressure in infants or in patients with low-flow states.

Physiology

Blood flowing into the aorta with each cardiac cycle initiates a pressure wave. Blood flows through the vasculature at approximately 0.5 m/sec, and pressure waves in the aorta move at 3–5 m/sec. Therefore palpated peripheral pulses represent pressure waves, not blood flow.

Indications and Contraindications

Assessment of blood flow by palpation of the pulse can be used to gauge the presence of cardiac contractility and not just the electrical rhythm. Caution should be taken to not overgeneralize the presence or strength of a pulse when predicting blood pressure. The necessity for repeated pulse evaluations is dictated by the clinical complaint and the status of the patient. Continuous monitoring is not routine and may be helpful when the clinical situation predicts significant variability in HR, as in the setting of sepsis.[60–62] An association between absence of a radial pulse or absence of both radial and femoral pulses and hypotension has been demonstrated in hypovolemic trauma patients. The variability in individual response prohibits the use of this parameter as an absolute gauge of blood pressure.[63]

No contraindications exist to assessment of the pulse rate. Keep in mind a few cautionary notes about examination of the carotid pulse. Avoid concurrent bilateral carotid artery palpation because this maneuver could theoretically endanger cerebral blood flow. Massage of the carotid sinus, found at the bifurcation of the external and internal carotid arteries at the level of the mandibular angle, may result in reflex slowing of the HR. To avoid inadvertent carotid sinus massage and carotid hypersensitivity syndrome, palpate the carotid pulse at or below the level of the thyroid cartilage. In adults with atherosclerotic disease, there is a rare risk of precipitating a cerebrovascular event by vigorous palpation of the carotid artery. Minimize this risk by prior auscultation of the carotid artery. If a bruit is present, gently palpate the carotid pulse while avoiding vigorous palpation or use a Doppler ultrasound probe to assess carotid flow.

Procedure

Depending on the clinical scenario, pulses are palpable at numerous sites, although for convenience the radial pulse at the wrist is routinely used. Pulses are easily palpated at the carotid, brachial, femoral, posterior tibial, and dorsalis pedis arteries as well. Use the tips of the first and second fingers to palpate the pulse. The two advantages of this technique are that (1) the fingertips are quite sensitive, thereby enabling the pulse to be located easily and counted and (2) the examiner's own pulse may be erroneously counted if the thumb is used.[64] Determine the pulse rate by counting for 1 minute, particularly if any abnormality is present. In the acute care setting, it is conventional to count a regular pulse for 10 or 15 seconds and multiply the resulting number by 6 or 4 to determine the beats per minute.

Palpation of the carotid pulse is recommended for a child. For an infant, check the brachial pulse with two fingers on the inside of the upper arm.[65] In neonates, direct heart auscultation and umbilical cord palpation are standard methods for determining the HR.[66] In unstable children, palpate the central arteries, particularly the femoral and brachial pulses, instead of the more peripheral arteries. In a comparison of four methods of determining the HR in infants, listening at the apex of the heart was found to be more accurate than palpation of the brachial, carotid, or femoral pulses.[67] Of the sites for palpation of the HR, the femoral artery has proved most valuable, especially in hypotensive infants.[68]

Interpretation

Pulse Rate

Consider the individual's physiology when interpreting the pulse. In infants and children, interpret the pulse rate with reference to age (see Table 1.1). Pulse varies with respiration: it increases with inspiration and slows with expiration. This is known as sinus dysrhythmia and is physiologic. Although *bradycardia* is most commonly defined as a HR lower than 60 beats/min in adults, a well-conditioned athlete may have a normal resting HR of 30–40 beats/min.[69,70] As discussed earlier, a redefinition of bradycardia to less than 45 beats/min and tachycardia to greater than 95 beats/min has been proposed based on a normal healthy population.[30,71] Such definitions include 95% of the population and do not address any given individual's normal baseline rate.

Consider whether a patient's abnormal pulse rate is a primary or secondary condition. Examine the entire set of vital signs when attempting to discern the cause of the abnormal rate. For example, hyperthermia causes sinus tachycardia. Drug fever, typhoid fever, and central neurogenic fever are considerations when no corresponding tachycardia is found in a patient with elevated body temperature. Hypothermia, with its reduced metabolic demands, may be associated with bradycardia. Some disease states are defined by their effect on HR, such as thyrotoxicosis with tachycardia or myxedema coma with bradycardia.

Consider the medications that the patient may be taking or the presence of a mechanical pacemaker. Digitalis compounds, β-blockers, and antiarrhythmic medications may alter the normal HR and the ability of this vital sign to respond to a new physiologic stress. The effect of such medications may cause the abnormality in the patient's HR. Nonprescription drugs can be equally significant in their effect on HR. Sympathomimetic drugs such as cocaine and methamphetamine increase HR, as do anticholinergic drugs.

Heart Rhythm

In addition to determining the pulse rate, obtain information about the regularity of the pulse by palpation. An irregularly irregular pulse suggests atrial fibrillation or flutter with variable block, and accurate assessment of the pulse should be carried out by auscultation of the apical cardiac sounds. The apical pulse is frequently greater than the peripheral pulse because of inadequate filling time and stroke volume, with resultant nontransmitted beats. A greater pulse deficit generally reflects more severe disease.[72]

Pulse Amplitude and Contour

Accurate examination and description of pulse amplitude and contour can provide additional clinical information and aid in decision-making. Superimposition of one pathophysiologic state on another may modify the pulse. For example, sepsis may result in variable pulse amplitudes, depending on the stage in the development of the disease. Early in sepsis, cardiac output increases and vascular resistance decreases, causing bounding pulses. In advanced sepsis or septic shock, falling cardiac output and increased vascular resistance are seen, diminishing pulses.[73] Definable age-related changes in pulse amplitude and contour can be identified. Such changes are due to an increase in arterial stiffness, resulting in increased pulse wave velocity and progressively earlier wave reflection. This leads to increased pulse amplitude in the elderly at all commonly measured sites (carotid, femoral, and radial).[74] In addition to these age-related changes, pulse wave analysis may be useful in determining arterial stiffness and the likelihood of atherosclerotic disease.[75] If present globally, weak pulses can be a significant finding in hypotensive patients, or an indication of limb ischemia if isolated to one extremity. Bounding pulses can be seen with a widened pulse pressure and are discussed later in the section on blood pressure. Routine measurement of pulse amplitude is not reproducible by simple palpation and requires instrumentation unavailable in EDs.

Pulses During Cardiopulmonary Resuscitation

Palpated femoral pulses during chest compression may represent either forward arterial blood flow or "to-and-fro" movement of blood from the right side of the heart to the venous system. A carotid pulse is preferred when assessing the adequacy of chest compressions during cardiopulmonary resuscitation (see Chapter 17).

ARTERIAL BLOOD PRESSURE

SBP changes with each heartbeat. Changes in arterial blood pressure over time may indicate success of treatment or worsening of the patient's overall condition. An abrupt reduction in a patient's arterial blood pressure usually indicates the need for immediate reassessment and intervention. The current section discusses indirect blood pressure monitoring; intraarterial techniques are considered elsewhere. Discussion of the specific use of the Doppler device for measurement of pulse and blood pressure and for measurement of orthostatic blood pressure and changes in pulse follow this section. Despite an association between the absence of hypotension and the presence of a radial pulse, or between hypotension and the absence of both radial and femoral pulses in the setting of trauma, the variability in individual responses prohibits the use of this parameter as an absolute gauge of blood pressure.[63]

Physiology

Arterial blood pressure indicates the overall state of hemodynamic interaction between cardiac output and peripheral vascular resistance. Arterial blood pressure is the lateral pressure or force exerted by blood on the vessel wall. It indirectly measures perfusion, and blood flow equals the change in pressure divided by resistance. Because peripheral vascular resistance varies, a normal blood pressure does not confirm adequate perfusion.[76] Mean arterial blood pressure (MAP) can be estimated by adding one-third of the pulse pressure (i.e., the difference between SBP and diastolic blood pressure) to diastolic pressure or by using the following measure[77]:

$$\text{MAP} = \frac{\text{Diastolic pressure} \times 2 + \text{Systolic pressure}}{3}$$

MAP is determined by cardiac output, systemic vascular resistance, and a critical closing pressure at the level of the arterioles.[78] Many modern bedside telemetry monitors automatically incorporate MAP measurements into the blood pressure systolic and diastolic pressure readings.

Indications and Contraindications

Patients with minor ambulatory complaints unrelated to the cardiovascular system may not necessarily need their blood pressure measured in the ED, and those with hemodynamic instability need frequent monitoring of blood pressure. In children, there is a significant amount of variability regarding standard situations that require measurement of blood pressure. In general, the younger the patient, the less likely blood pressure will be measured.[79,80] In newborns, infants, and even toddlers, capillary refill is sometimes substituted for standard blood pressure measurement, although viewing these tests as equivalent can lead to significant errors.

In low-flow states, Doppler measurement of blood pressure may be obtained rapidly. Repeated measurements will provide an evaluation of the adequacy of resuscitation in patients whose blood pressure cannot be auscultated by standard techniques and in those in whom intraarterial blood pressure measurements are either contraindicated or technically unobtainable.[81,82] Placing a catheter for direct intraarterial measurement of blood pressure may be performed safely in the ED and is not standard of care in most clinical scenarios, associated with a higher risk of complications.

Direct measurement of arterial pressure during pulseless electrical rhythms may help discriminate between a severe shock state and otherwise nonresuscitatable status.[83,84] Alternative noninvasive devices for continuous blood pressure measurement (CBPM) have been clinically introduced, with varying success. One common method of CBPM uses finger cuffs equipped with infrared (IR) photoplethysmography and sophisticated technology for quantification of finger blood pressure levels. Finapres (Ohmeda, Madison, WI) was the first commercial product utilizing this technique, and several newer products are on the market today. A number of commercial systems use an alternative method of arterial applanation tonometry to measure CBPM. Further study is needed for the validation of devices using these techniques.[85,86] Rapid technological advances have led to the development of optical, electrical, pressure, and ultrasonic sensors in searching for the standard noninvasive blood pressure (NIBP) replacement that can capture data continuously in real time and can be accessed remotely.[87]

Relative contraindications to specific extremity blood pressure measurement include an arteriovenous fistula, ipsilateral mastectomy, axillary lymphadenopathy, lymphedema, and circumferential burns over the intended site of cuff application.

Equipment

Two types of blood pressure monitoring equipment are currently available and used in EDs: cuff type and noninvasive waveform analysis.

Cuff Type

The equipment required for indirect blood pressure measurement includes a sphygmomanometer (cuff with an inflatable bladder, inflating bulb, controlled exhaust for deflation, and manometer) and a stethoscope, Doppler device (for auscultation), or oscillometric device.[88–90] A common practice in the prehospital and interhospital transport setting is to forego auscultatory blood pressure measurements with a stethoscope and instead obtain systolic values only by palpation of the first Korotkoff sound. This practice, though sometimes the only feasible method of obtaining any value in a noisy environment, poses a significant potential for error.

According to the American Heart Association guidelines, the sphygmomanometer cuff should be an appropriate size for the patient to ensure an accurate reading. The width of the bladder should be at least 40% of the distance of the limb's midpoint (i.e., from the acromion process to the lateral epicondyle). This published figure of the ideal width, when studied in a validation review, may be higher, up to approximately 50%.[91] The length of the bladder should be 80% of the midarm circumference or twice the recommended width.[81] Discrepancies in matching upper arm size with cuff size have been demonstrated to produce significant errors in critically ill populations when compared with invasive intraarterial blood pressure measurements.[91] The availability of appropriately sized cuffs appears to be a pervasive problem, especially as approximately 80% of patients do not fit the standard 12-cm large cuffs.[92] In one study, 90% of aneroid devices had only one size of cuff available.[93]

The manometers in common use are either aneroid, digital, or mercury gravity column, though the mercury type is much less common in modern use. All three types of manometers are convenient for bedside use, although the mercury gravity column must be placed vertically to ensure accurate measurements. An aneroid manometer uses a metal bellows that elongates with the application of pressure. This elongation is mechanically amplified and transmits the motion to the indicator needle.

Manometers require annual servicing. Mercury columns may require the addition of mercury to bring the edge of the meniscus to the zero mark. The air vent or filter at the top of the mercury column should also be checked for clogging. An aneroid manometer should be calibrated against a mercury column at least yearly. If the aneroid indicator is not at zero at rest, the device should not be used.[94] Digital manometers may not be validated for all patient groups and could give inaccurate readings.

Automatic sphygmomanometers may improve physiologic monitoring with their alarm and self-cycling capabilities. They offer indirect arterial blood pressure measurement with little pain and without the risks associated with invasive arterial lines.[95] Accuracy of measurements does not suffer during rapid cycling, and the potential for vascular injury from nearly continuous arterial compression dictates that most automated blood pressure units will revert back to less frequent (i.e., every 15–20 minutes) cycling as a safety precaution. Oscillometric blood pressure monitors detect motion of the blood pressure cuff transmitted from the underlying artery. A sudden increase in the amplitude of arterial oscillations occurs with systolic pressure and MAP, and an abrupt decrease occurs with diastolic pressure.[96]

There appears to be less variability with the oscillometric blood pressure method than with the auscultatory method in children. These results are not generalizable to the neonatal population, and errors are commonly encountered even when exhaustive measures are taken to control the environment.

In adult patients, numerous studies have focused on the reliability of auscultatory versus automated blood pressure measurements. Mercury column versus Dinamap readings showed increased disparity when SBP was greater than 140 mm Hg, the range at which accuracy should be most rigorously sought to correctly identify hypertension. In general, automated blood pressure devices yield higher SBP and lower diastolic blood pressure.[97] The range of error in automated devices was, on average, 4.0–8.6 mm Hg.[98,99] Unfortunately these studies represent populations without critical illness and do not reflect the accuracy of readings at the extremes of hypertension and hypotension, making generalization to an ED population difficult.[99,100] Like most durable medical equipment, sphygmomanometers are subject to deterioration with use. Automatic sphygmomanometer validation is a form of calibration and offers quality control and traceability to ensure accurate results.[100]

Procedure

Obtain indirect blood pressure measurements at the patient's bedside by palpation, auscultation, Doppler, or oscillometric methods. The technique is straightforward and accurate when the equipment is well maintained, calibrated, and used by clinicians who follow accepted standards. The patient may be lying or sitting, as long as the site of measurement is at the level of the right atrium and the arm is supported.[81,90] Unless the arm is kept perpendicular to the body with the elbow resting on a desk, measurements will be 9–14 mm Hg higher, regardless of body position.[91,99] Allowing the arm to be parallel to the body when supine and supporting the arm perpendicular to the body when measuring blood pressure may create a pseudo-drop in blood pressure.[100] These changes are thought to be dependent on the mechanical properties of the arteries themselves and not associated with hydrostatic pressure alone.[101]

To palpate arterial blood pressure, inflate the cuff to 30 mm Hg above the level that the palpable pulse disappears. Once properly inflated, palpate directly over the artery and deflate the cuff at a rate of 2–3 mm Hg/sec. Report the initial appearance of arterial pulsations as the palpable blood pressure. This practice, known as the Riva-Rocci palpatory technique, has shown mixed results in yielding accurate estimations of blood pressure. One study determined that the average underestimation of SBP was 6 mm Hg.[102] Another operative study looking at the combination of palpated SBP and observed visual return of continuous pulse oximetry reported an underestimation of 10–20 mm Hg.[99] The same technique is used with the Doppler device, and the palpated pulse is replaced with the Doppler auditory signal. Measurement of arterial pressure by palpation and Doppler yields only estimates of SBP. The Doppler method is preferred when determining blood pressure in infants.[100]

When auscultating blood pressure at the brachial artery, apply the blood pressure cuff approximately 2.5 cm above the antecubital fossa with the center of the bladder over the artery.[76] Apply the bell of the stethoscope directly over the brachial artery with as little pressure as possible.[103,104] *Systolic arterial blood pressure* is defined as the first appearance of faint, clear, tapping sounds that gradually increase in intensity (Korotkoff phase I). *Diastolic blood pressure* is defined as the point at which the sounds disappear (Korotkoff phase V).[105] In children, phase IV defines diastolic blood pressure (Fig. 1.2).[64] Phase IV is marked by a distinct, abrupt muffling of sound when a soft, blowing quality is heard.

It is best to auscultate over the brachial artery because of accepted standardization of the measured values. Alternative sites include the radial, popliteal, posterior tibial, or dorsalis pedis arteries, although any fully compressible extremity artery may be used. Studies evaluating direct and indirect blood pressure measurements have demonstrated good correlation between these methods.[106,107]

Occasionally it may not be feasible to obtain proximal upper extremity blood pressure measurements because of patient access issues, particularly those encountered in the prehospital setting. Forearm measurements may be obtained more easily, though correlation to standard proximal upper extremity values has been controversial. An earlier study showed fair correlation to a brachial cuff measurement (within 20 mm Hg in 86% of systolic measurements and 94% of diastolic measurements).[108] A subsequent study demonstrated that forearm measurements cannot routinely replace upper arm measurements to determine blood pressure (the potential variance from an upper arm measurement is ±19 mm Hg for systolic pressure).[109] Alternatively, noninvasive finger blood pressure measurements have shown promise when compared with standard upper extremity readings. The overall discrepancy in an ED study was 0.1 mm Hg with a standard deviation of ±5.02 mm Hg when comparing finger blood pressure and invasive MAP via radial artery cannulation.[84]

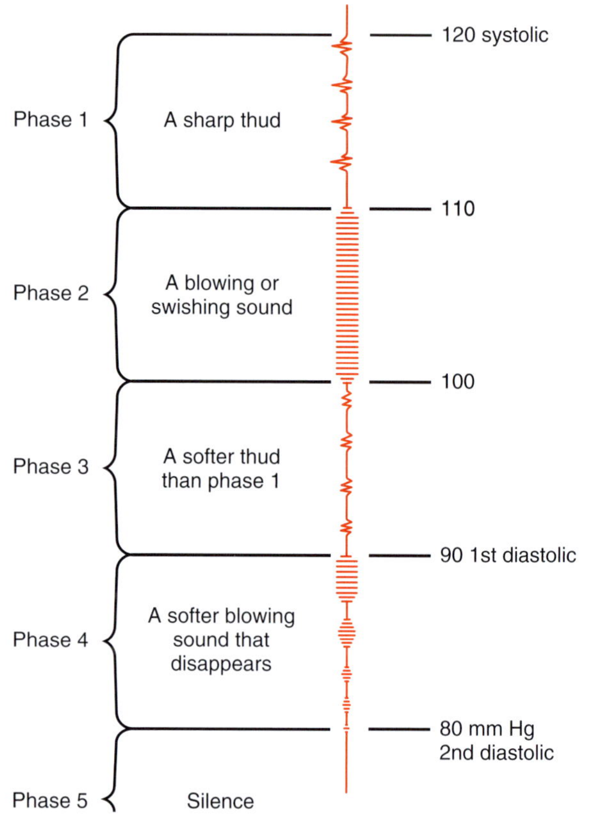

Fig. 1.2 Korotkoff sounds. The first audible sound occurs in systole, and the sound disappears in diastole. (From Burnside JW, McGlynn TJ. *Physical Diagnosis*. 17th ed. Baltimore: Williams & Wilkins; 1986.)

Novel noninvasive continuous finger cuff technology offers the benefit of uninterrupted monitoring and has the advantage over invasive techniques of being safer and immediately available. Noninvasive finger cuff measurements have shown reasonable correlation, even in critically ill populations in the ED.[85] Wrist blood pressure has been shown to have good average accuracy in the surgical environment when compared with oscillometric devices. Patient comfort is reported to be greater with these devices. The typically stated contraindications to the acquisition of upper arm blood pressure (limitation after mastectomy, etc.) may not apply.[110]

The accuracy of the palpatory, Doppler, and oscillometric methods has also been investigated.[111–113] When phase I and V Korotkoff sounds are used, indirect methods typically underestimate SBP and diastolic pressure by several millimeters of mercury.[111–114] During shock, the palpatory and auscultatory methods underestimate simultaneous direct arterial pressure measurements.[115] The flush method, in which the return of color after deflation of the cuff is used to estimate blood pressure in infants, may underestimate SBP by up to 40 mm Hg.[116] This method is unreliable and not recommended.

Complications

Complications of indirect blood pressure measurements are minimal when the proper procedure is followed. Inadvertent prolonged application of an inflated blood pressure cuff may result in falsely elevated diastolic pressure and ischemia distal to the site of application.[91] Invasive blood pressure monitoring is associated with a number of potential problems (see Chapter 20).

Interpretation

Normal blood pressure increases with decreasing distance from the heart and aorta. Blood pressure tends to increase with age and is generally higher in males. Individual factors that influence blood pressure include body posture, emotional or painful stimuli, environmental influences, vasoactive foods or medications, and the state of muscular and cerebral activity. Exercise and sustained isometric muscular contraction increase blood pressure in proportion to the strength of the contraction. A normal diurnal pattern of blood pressure consists of an increase throughout the day with a significant, rapid decline during early, deep sleep.[117]

Normal lower limits of SBP in infants and children can be estimated by adding 2 times the age (in years) to 70 mm Hg. The 50th percentile for a child's systolic arterial blood pressure from 1 to 10 years of age can be estimated by adding 2 times the age (in years) to 90 mm Hg. Children older than 2 years are considered hypotensive when SBP is less than 80 mm Hg.[118] Children are able to maintain MAP until very late during shock.[119] The finding of a normal blood pressure in a child with signs of poor perfusion should not dissuade the clinician from appropriate treatment. Most adults are considered hypotensive if SBP is lower than 90 mm Hg, and some individuals normally exhibit a systolic pressure in that range. In the elderly, the presence of normotension within defined or published limits may not be reassuring. When considering SBP cutoffs for trauma patients, 85 mm Hg for patients aged 18–35 years, 96 mm Hg for patients aged 36–64 years, and 117 mm Hg for those older than 65 years have been proposed as new standards for hypotension.[26] When accompanied by signs of shock, immediate treatment is indicated. In patients with shock, blood flow cannot be reliably inferred from HR and blood pressure values.[120,121]

Hypertension

Adults are hypertensive if either systolic or diastolic pressure consistently exceeds 140 or 90 mm Hg, respectively.[122,123] A metaanalysis showed strong correlation of blood pressure to vascular (and overall) mortality down to at least 115/75 mm Hg.[124] Some authors have suggested altering the blood pressure definitions to include an "optimal" blood pressure of 115/75 mm Hg.[19] Other authors have suggested incorporating blood pressure into a global cardiovascular risk assessment that includes other associated risk factors.[21,22] The applicability of population norms for hypertension in a stressful emergency situation is controversial. One should not make diagnostic or therapeutic decisions based solely on an abnormal initial measurement. Patients with hypertension require repeated measurements to assess whether therapy is required in the ED. Because sustained hypertension may be seen in more than one-third of initially hypertensive ED patients, careful evaluation and follow-up are required.[125] Unfortunately, elevated blood pressure readings are almost uniformly ignored or unrecognized in the emergency setting, particularly in children.[126] The phenomenon of *white coat hypertension* (WCH) is defined as a persistent elevation in blood pressure in the clinical setting only. The prevalence of WCH is between 20% and 94%, depending on the frequency of reassessment in the clinical setting.[127] It is unclear whether patients who have isolated hypertension in the clinical setting (WCH) are at increased risk for the development of hypertension and subsequent end-organ damage.[128]

Measurement Errors

Erroneous blood pressure measurements may result from several factors.[129] Falsely low blood pressure may be caused by using an overly wide cuff, by placing excessive pressure on the head of the stethoscope, or by rapid cuff deflation.[130,131] Falsely high blood pressure may be caused by the use of an overly narrow cuff, anxiety, pain, tobacco use, exertion, an unsupported arm, or slow inflation of the cuff.[132] There appears to be a statistically significant difference in the error rate associated with patients weighing more than 95 kg, whether from obesity or as a result of muscular upper arms from body building.[133,134]

Of note, 41% of adults observed at the University of Pittsburgh required nonstandardized cuffs, and the use of small cuffs was associated with a mean error of 8.5 and 4.6 mm Hg in SBP and diastolic pressure, respectively.[131] Other studies have confirmed relatively high rates of inappropriately diagnosed hypertension in obese patients based on erroneous cuff size.[133] Other specific study populations in this area have been critically ill patients, in whom disparate cuff size can lead to significant inaccuracies based on arm circumference.[91]

Hypotensive patients have unreliable Korotkoff sounds, and Doppler measurements are well correlated with direct arterial systolic pressure measurements in these patients.[135] An auscultatory gap can be appreciated in hypertensive patients and may mislead the clinician. It is heard during the latter part of phase I and should not be confused with diastolic readings. Auscultation until the manometer reading approaches zero should prevent misinterpretation. In patients with aortic insufficiency or hyperthyroidism, in those who have just finished exercising, and in children younger than 5 years, measurement of diastolic blood pressure should occur at Korotkoff phase IV. Extremes of blood pressure, both hypotension and hypertension, have been found to be factors contributing to measurement errors in critically ill pediatric patients. Predictably, falsely high readings for noninvasive versus invasive measurements have been obtained in hypotensive patients and falsely low values in hypertensive states.[136]

Irregular HRs may also interfere with accurate determination of blood pressure. Take a second or third reading, with 2 minutes of deflation between recordings, and obtain an average when premature contractions or atrial fibrillation are present.

Hemiplegic patients may exhibit different blood pressures in the affected and unaffected arms.[137] A flaccid extremity tends to yield lower systolic and diastolic pressure, whereas a spastic extremity tends to yield higher values than the extremity with normal motor tone. Although these differences are generally small, it is preferable to monitor blood pressure in the unaffected limb.

Numerous errors may occur in the accurate measurement of blood pressure. The only way to combat these errors is to first be cognizant of practices contributing to them. Unfortunately, few nurses can identify the causes of potentially erroneous readings. In a study examining nurses' ability to obtain accurate readings, proper technique in determining SBP could be identified 61% of the time; diastolic blood pressure, 71% of the time; and an auscultatory gap, 54% of the time. Nurses were able to correctly identify faulty equipment 58% of the time, assess cuff size 57% of the time, determine appropriate inflation pressure 29% of the time, note the appropriate deflation rate 62% of the time, and determine correct arm positioning 14% of the time.[138]

An increasing number of patients with heart failure are receiving bridging measures to transplantation or treated with long-term circulatory augmentation devices in the form of left ventricular assist devices (LVADs); therefore it is useful to understand the difficulty in interpreting blood pressure measurements in these patients. All types of VADs fit into two categories: (1) pulsatile and (2) nonpulsatile. Pulse and blood pressure readings in patients with pulsatile VADs (Thoratec, HeartMate XVE, Novacor, C-Pulse) are comparable to values in the general non-VAD population. Nonpulsatile VADs (HeartAssist 5, Incor and Excor, Jarvik 2000, VentriAssist, MTIHeart LVAD, HVAD/MVAD, DuraHeart, DeBakey LVAD, HeartMateII/III) function by either centrifugal or axial blood flow, and this has a significant impact on the ability to detect pulses.[139] Typically these patients appear to be well-perfused with adequate skin warmth and capillary refill even though pulses may be absent. Blood pressure readings can be obtained with these nonpulsatile flow devices, and diastolic blood pressure, pulse-pressure values, and MAP vary significantly depending on the speed of the pump.[140]

Pulse Pressure

The difference between SBP and diastolic pressure is termed pulse pressure. For example, if the blood pressure is 120/80 mm Hg, the pulse pressure is 40 mm Hg. Increased pulse pressure (i.e., ≥60 mm Hg) is commonly observed with anemia, exercise, hyperthyroidism, arteriovenous fistula, aortic regurgitation, increased intracranial pressure, and patent ductus arteriosus. A narrowed pulse pressure (≤20 mm Hg) may be a manifestation of hypovolemia, increased peripheral vascular resistance (as seen in early septic shock), or decreased stroke volume. A narrowed pulse pressure is classically noted in aortic stenosis and pericardial tamponade. Traditional vital sign measurements, such as SBP and oxygen saturation, often fail to predict mortality or indicate the need for life-saving interventions or reductions in central blood volume until after the onset of cardiovascular collapse. There is evidence that an early indicator of reduced central blood volume in the presence of stable vital signs is the reduction in pulse pressure.[141]

Differential Brachial Artery Pressure

The presence of a SBP difference of 10–20 mm Hg between the arms suggests a normal condition. If greater, it may indicate advanced focal atherosclerosis, coarctation of the aorta proximal to the left subclavian artery, type A aortic dissection, aortic arch syndromes, or other vascular processes preferentially affecting one extremity. The utility of upper extremity bilateral blood pressure measurements has recently come into question. One study found a 10-mm Hg systolic or diastolic difference in 53% of patients in the emergency setting and a 20-mm Hg or higher difference in 19% of patients.[142] Although these numbers have not generally been found to be of this magnitude in metaanalyses,[143] the unique setting of the study in the ED makes correlation particularly salient for the emergency physician. The reliability of peripheral pulse deficits in diagnosing or excluding type A aortic dissection is a frequently cited reason for evaluating blood pressure in both arms. In a metaanalysis, Teece and Hogg noted that the successful use of the absence of a clinical pulse deficit to exclude thoracic dissection in patients with chest pain was just 31%, and the authors concluded that peripheral pulse deficits are far too insensitive to warrant their use as a means of excluding thoracic aortic dissection in patients with chest pain.[144] Given that many in the general population have significant differences in blood pressure in each arm, the diagnostic value of this frequently cited indication for obtaining bilateral brachial blood pressure is unproven. Essentially most patients with a type A aortic dissection will not have a measurable blood pressure discrepancy between the arms, and most of those who do have such a finding will not have dissection.

Brachial pressure differences did not appear to be linked to age, gender, race, MAP, cardiovascular risk, or final discharge diagnosis. Smaller interarm differences have been reported in the ED setting (18% in hypertensive patients and 15% in normotensive patients when a cutoff greater than 10 mm Hg was used).[24,25] Though not tested, a method proposed to minimize these differences in the ED is to take simultaneous blood pressure readings from both the left and right extremities with two calibrated automated blood pressure units.[145]

Pulse Pressure Variation

Fluid resuscitation is an integral piece of the management of patients with circulatory failure, though administration of the proper amount and rate of parenteral fluids can be challenging. Fluid responsiveness, or the ability of the left ventricle to increase stroke volume in response to fluid administration, is an emerging concept that helps to address this challenge.[146] This concept is based on the physiology of the Frank-Starling curve and the knowledge that pulse-pressure (systolic pressure minus diastolic pressure) is directly proportional to stroke volume. The variation in pulse pressure seen with the respiratory cycle, or *pulse-pressure variation*, reflects the magnitude of respiratory change on stroke volume. This is best demonstrated by the influence of mechanical ventilation on right ventricular preload. Studies have shown that a pulse-pressure variation of greater than 13% is highly predictive of fluid responsiveness in mechanically ventilated patients.[147]

Though many methods exist to assess fluid responsiveness, the standard method is done with passive leg raising (PLR). This "self-volume challenge" increases preload through translocation of venous blood from the lower extremities to the thorax. A patient who exhibits a rise of more than 10% in their aortic blood flow (measured with esophageal Doppler) or cardiac index (measured with thermodilution) is considered a "fluid responder," indicating the need for further fluid administration.[146] This concept is becoming increasingly useful in optimizing the fluid management of critically ill patients.

Pulsus Paradoxus

Normal respiration briefly decreases SBP by approximately 10 mm Hg during inspiration. Pulsus paradoxus occurs when there is a greater than 12-mm Hg decrease in SBP during inspiration. Pulsus paradoxus may occur in patients with

A
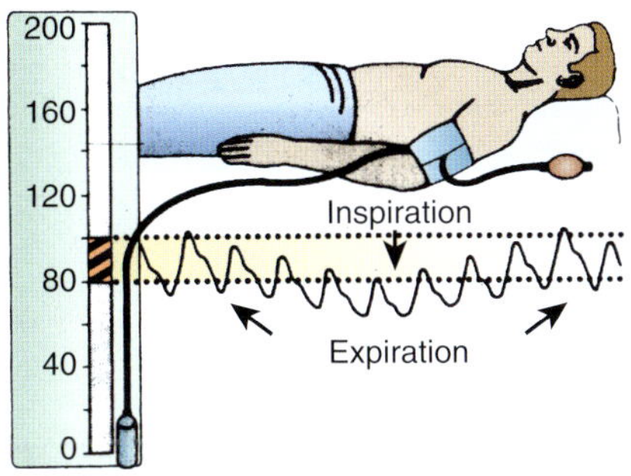

B

PROCEDURE FOR THE MEASUREMENT OF PULSUS PARADOXUS

The patient should be reclining at a 30° to 45° angle and instructed to breathe normally.

1. Inflate a standard blood pressure cuff until Korotkoff sounds over the brachial artery disappear.
2. Lower pressure in the cuff a few millimeters of mercury per second until the first Korotkoff sounds appear during expiration.
3. Maintain pressure at this level and observe the disappearance of sounds during inspiration. Record this cuff pressure.
4. Very slowly lower cuff pressure until Korotkoff sounds are heard throughout the respiratory cycle. Record this cuff pressure.
5. The difference between pressures recorded in the two previous steps is then recorded as the measurement (in millimeters of mercury [mm Hg]) of pulsus paradoxus. A pulsus paradoxus >12 mm Hg is abnormal but nonspecific (see text).

Fig. 1.3 (A) Measurement of pulsus paradoxus. Note that systolic pressure varies during the respiratory cycle. Inspiration normally decreases systolic blood pressure slightly (termed paradoxical pulse), but if the difference between inspiratory and expiratory systolic pressure is greater than 12 mm Hg, the paradoxical pulse is abnormally wide. (B) Technique for measurement of pulsus paradoxus. (A, Reproduced with permission from Stein L, Shubin H, Weil M. Recognition and management of pericardial tamponade. *JAMA*. 1973;225:504. Copyright 1973, American Medical Association.)

chronic obstructive pulmonary disease, pneumothorax, severe asthma, or pericardial tamponade.[115]

To measure a paradoxical pulse, have the patient lie comfortably in the supine position at a 30- to 45-degree angle and breathe normally in an unlabored fashion (typically unusual conditions in a patient suspected of having cardiac tamponade, severe asthma, chronic obstructive pulmonary disease, or pneumothorax).[148] Inflate the blood pressure cuff well above systolic pressure and slowly deflate it until the systolic sounds that are synchronous with expiration are first heard (Fig. 1.3). Initially, the arterial pulse will be heard only during expiration and will disappear during inspiration. Deflate the cuff further until arterial sounds are heard throughout the respiratory cycle. Palpation at the radial or femoral arteries may yield complete disappearance during inspiration. When present, this technique is a quick bedside confirmation of the possibility of severe tamponade or pulmonary dynamic hyperinflation.

An alternative method for determination of pulsus paradoxus is by visually observing the loss of the pulse oximetry waveform and then its reappearance.[149] The plethysmographic method has been validated in ICU settings.

If the difference between inspiratory and expiratory pressure is greater than 12 mm Hg, the paradoxical pulse is abnormally wide.[148,149] Most patients with proven tamponade have a difference of 20–30 mm Hg or greater during the respiratory cycle.[148–150] This may not be true of patients with very narrow pulse pressures (typical of advanced tamponade), who have a "deceptively small" paradoxical pulse of 5–15 mm Hg.[150–152] Point-of-care ultrasound can also be used to measure mitral valve inflow variation, a surrogate marker for pulsus paradoxus.[153]

Pulsus paradoxus has been correlated with the level of impairment of cardiac output by tamponade. In an uninjured patient with pericardial effusion, a pulsus paradoxus greater than 25 mm Hg (in the absence of relative hypotension) is both sensitive and specific for moderate or severe versus mild tamponade.[133,154] An echocardiographic study found that an abnormal pulsus paradoxus had a sensitivity of 79%, a specificity of 40%, a positive predictive value of 81%, and a negative predictive value of 40% for right ventricular diastolic collapse.[154–156] The absence of a paradoxical pulse does not rule out tamponade.

In the pediatric population, pulsus paradoxus has been studied to determine the severity of obstructive and restrictive pulmonary disease,[155] most commonly asthma. A value of 15 mm Hg or greater correlates well with the clinical score, peak expiratory value, flow rate, oxygen saturation, and subsequent need for admission.[156]

Despite the disease entities that a widened pulsus paradoxus may suggest, it is a difficult test to perform adequately with only a sphygmomanometer. Because it is a useful clinical tool, new aids should be developed and used to reliably predict this important vital sign.[157]

Shock Index

The ratio of pulse rate to SBP has been suggested as a measure of clinical shock. The shock index (SI) has a normal range of 0.5–0.7. Although calculating the SI is not standard of care in the ED, a number of clinical scenarios have been studied in which the SI can be used as a predictor of severe illness or injury. An SI above 0.85–0.90 suggests acute illness in medical patients and a marked increase in the potential for gross hemodynamic instability in trauma patients.[158–161] The SI has been studied for use in a variety of clinical scenarios from severe pneumonia to first-trimester risk for ectopic pregnancy to sepsis. It has been found to be a valid gauge of the severity of illness.[162,163] Some studies have found that the initial pulse rate alone had nearly the same predictive power as the SI for the severity of illness. Although the SI appears to correlate with the left ventricular stroke work index, it has little correlation with systemic oxygen transport in patients with hemorrhagic and septic shock.

DOPPLER ULTRASOUND FOR EVALUATION OF PULSE AND BLOOD PRESSURE

Principles of Doppler Ultrasound

Doppler ultrasound is based on the Doppler phenomenon. The frequency of sound waves varies depending on the speed of the sound transmitter in relation to the sound receiver. Doppler devices transmit a sound wave that is reflected by flowing erythrocytes, and the shift in frequency is detected. Frequency shift can be detected only for blood flow greater than 6 cm/sec.

Indications and Contraindications

Doppler ultrasound is commonly used in the ED for the measurement of blood pressure in low-flow states, evaluation of lower extremity peripheral perfusion, and assessment of fetal heart sounds after the first trimester of pregnancy. Doppler's sensitivity allows detection of SBP down to 30 mm Hg in the evaluation of a patient in shock. In a patient with peripheral vascular disease in whom there is concern about the adequacy of peripheral perfusion, the ankle-brachial index provides a rapid, reproducible, and standardized assessment.[164] Fetal heart sounds provide a baseline assessment of any pregnant patient with 12 weeks' gestation or longer in the setting of abdominal trauma or fetal distress as a result of a complication of pregnancy. The use of Doppler ultrasound for the evaluation of deep venous thrombosis is a valuable tool, and specific training and experience are required to attain proficiency. Discussion of this topic is beyond the scope of this chapter.

Equipment

A nondirectional Doppler device has a probe that houses two piezoelectric crystals. One crystal transmits the signal and the other receives it. Reflected signals are converted to an electrical signal and fed to an output that transforms them to an audible sound.

Probes with a frequency of 2–5 MHz are best for detecting fetal heart sounds. Frequencies of 5–10 MHz are appropriate for limb arteries and veins. The probes should be monitored periodically for electrical damage and integrity of the crystals. The sphygmomanometers used in conjunction with the Doppler device should be calibrated periodically, as described in the section on "Doppler Ultrasound for Evaluation of Pulse and Blood Pressure."

Procedure

Place the Doppler probe against the skin with acoustic gel used as an interface. The gel ensures optimal transmission and reception of the ultrasound signal and protects the crystals. In an emergency, water-soluble lubricant (e.g., Surgilube or K-Y Jelly) may be substituted for commercial acoustic gel. Angle the probe at 45 degrees along the length of the vessel to optimize frequency shifts and signal amplitude.

To evaluate peripheral perfusion, place a sphygmomanometer cuff proximal to where the arterial pulse is being evaluated and inflate it. Place the probe over the arterial pulse and slowly deflate the cuff. The pressure at which flow is first heard is the systolic pressure under the cuff, and not the pressure at the level of the Doppler probe.

In the evaluation of peripheral vascular disease, one may determine the ankle-brachial index. It is standard for this procedure to be performed in a formal vascular laboratory, and an approximation of pressures can be determined in the ED (Fig. 1.4 and Video 1.1). Usually, only the ankle-brachial index is considered for ED purposes. Examine both brachial arteries at the medial aspect of the antecubital fossa. Angle the probe until the most satisfactory signal is obtained. Inflate the cuff and slowly deflate it until the systolic pulse is heard. Repeat the procedure for the posterior tibial and dorsalis pedis arteries of both lower extremities. This procedure may be done with oscillometric devices and lacks sensitivity in identifying disease.[165]

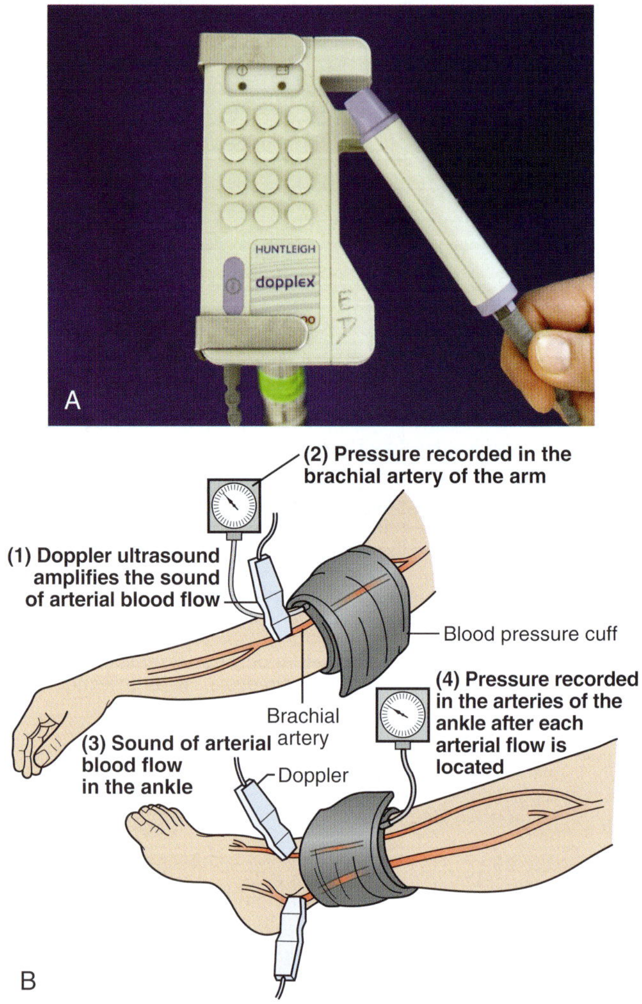

Fig. 1.4 (A) Handheld Doppler device with a speaker. Devices with an attached stethoscope are also used. (B) Peripheral vascular testing is performed in a vascular laboratory, but an approximation of the integrity of the peripheral arterial circulation can be gleaned in the emergency department by using Doppler to determine systolic blood pressure in the foot and arm and calculate the ankle-brachial index.

In evaluating fetal heart tones, because of variable positioning of the fetus, an examination of several locations and angles over the uterus must be performed in search for the optimal signal. It is best to begin in the mid-suprapubic area and then explore the uterus via angulation of the probe. Once tones are located, move the probe along the abdomen to reach a position closer to the origin of the sound. Distinguish fetal heart tones from placental flow by differentiating the quality of the fetal heart tones that will not match the maternal pulse. The placental flow and maternal pulse should be identical.

Interpretation

As noted earlier, in low-flow states, Doppler ultrasound can detect blood pressure as low as 30 mm Hg. Calculate the ankle-brachial index (Video 1.1) of each limb by dividing the higher systolic pressure of the posterior tibial or the dorsalis pedis artery of the limb by the higher systolic pressures in the brachial arteries. In normal individuals, the index should be greater than 1.0 (Fig. 1.5). Patients with mild to moderate claudication have values between 0.4 and 0.9. Values

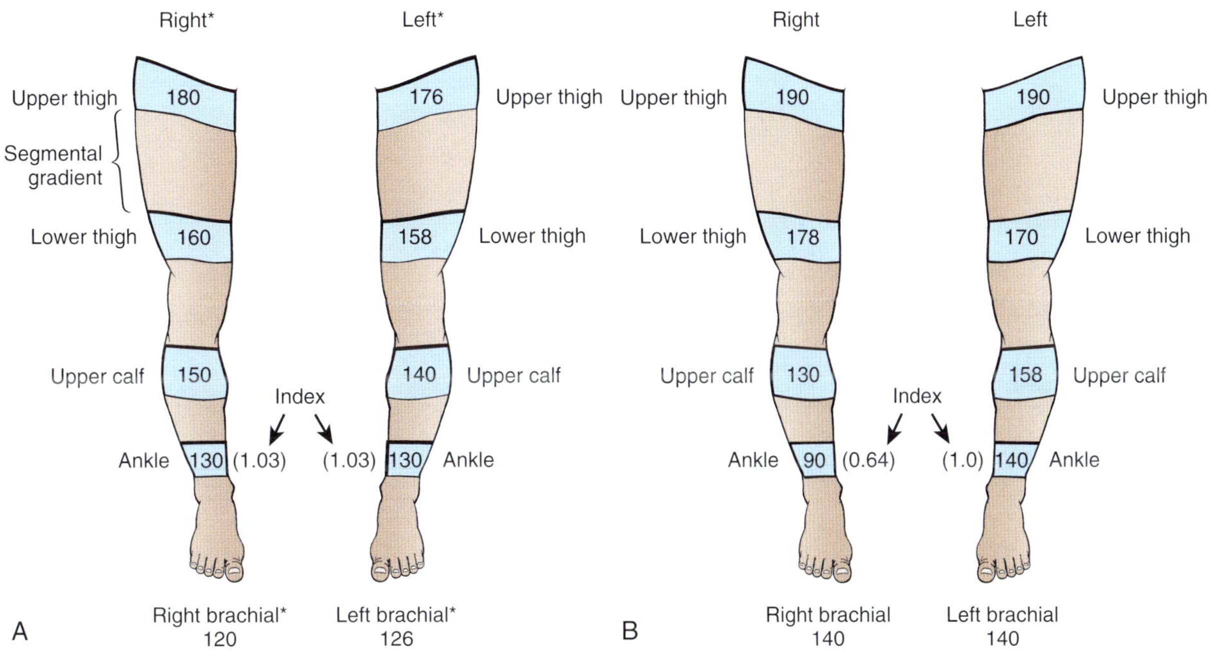

Fig. 1.5 (A) Typical pressures in a normal individual. Findings, based on resting pressure, show no evidence of occlusive disease of the large- or medium-sized arteries. Normal findings are as follows: (1) ankle-to-brachial pressure index of 1.0 or higher; (2) all segmental pressure gradients lower than 30 mm Hg; and (3) upper thigh pressure at least 40 mm Hg above brachial pressure. *Systolic pressure in mm Hg. (B) Typical pressures in a patient with obstruction of the right popliteal or tibial arteries. Significant findings are as follows: (1) ankle-to-brachial pressure index less than 0.9 in the right leg; (2) abnormally high gradient from the ankle to below the knee and again from below to above the knee in the right leg; and (3) upper thigh pressure 50 mm Hg higher than brachial pressure, consistent with normal flow at the aorta-iliac level. Findings are suggestive of right popliteal occlusion or right anterior and posterior tibial occlusion, or both. (Reproduced with permission from Barnes RW, Wilson MR. *Doppler Ultrasonic Evaluation of Peripheral Arterial Disease: A Programmed Audiovisual Instruction*. Iowa City: University of Iowa; 1976.)

lower than 0.4 indicate severe impairment and are consistent with critical limb ischemia.[166] When the lower extremity has been amputated or injured, brachial-brachial indices can be used (i.e., comparison of SBP in the injured or diseased upper extremity with the other extremity). Patients with ankle-brachial index values of 0.9 or lower have increased cardiovascular morbidity and mortality.[167] One study of 323 penetrating extremity wounds found that an ankle-brachial index (or brachial-brachial index) lower than 0.9 was 72.5% sensitive and 100% specific for vascular injuries.[168] Segmental lower extremity pressure measurements may help identify the level of the obstruction (Table 1.4).[169] Obese patients, diabetic patients, or those with calcified vessels that are not compressible may have abnormally high systolic pressure (e.g., 250–300 mm Hg) and indices that do not accurately reflect flow. Normal fetal heart tones should be between 120 and 140 beats/min. Fetal heart tones may be heard as early as the 12th week of gestation.

VITAL SIGN DETERMINATION OF VOLUME STATUS

Many techniques have been advocated to assess volume status. Unfortunately, most procedures lack a database to judge their reliability. Recommended methods include evaluation of skin color; skin turgor; skin temperature; supine, serial, and orthostatic vital signs; neck vein status; transcutaneous oximetry; and hemodynamic monitoring (e.g., monitoring of central venous pressure). Serial vital sign measurements have been used for assessing blood loss, but they do not reliably detect small degrees of blood loss.[166,170,171] Up to 15% of the total blood volume can be lost with minimal hemodynamic changes or any alteration in supine vital signs.[170,171] A decrease in pulse pressure occurs with acute blood loss,[172] and the patient's baseline blood pressure values are often unknown. Clinical examination of neck veins adds useful information and is less precise than measurement of central venous pressure. Most clinicians use skin color, temperature, and moisture as a reflection of skin perfusion and sympathetic tone. This is not an accurate guide to circulatory volume because the vasomotor tone of the skin is affected by numerous diseases, as well as by emotional and environmental factors. Capillary refill has been advocated as a noninvasive test for hypovolemia, and it has been found to be inaccurate in adults (see the following discussion regarding its use in children).[172] The ideal test for determining volume status would rapidly and accurately detect 5% or greater depletion of volume with a noninvasive technique. At present, no such test exists.

ORTHOSTATIC VITAL SIGNS MEASUREMENT

Orthostatic vital signs have historically been used to evaluate patients with fluid loss, hemorrhage, syncope, or autonomic dysfunction. They are also used to assess the patient's response to therapy. The clinician is often concerned with accurate detection of acute blood loss or volume depletion. When the clinical syndrome of shock exists, assessment of a deficit in blood volume poses little difficulty. It is preferable that loss of

TABLE 1.4 Use of Segmental Lower Extremity Pressure to Identify the Level of Obstruction

	UPPER THIGH	LOWER THIGH	UPPER CALF	ANKLE
Normal[a]				
Right	180	160	150	130
Left	176	158	140	130
Arm	124	124	124	124
ABI	1.45	1.29	1.21	1.05
Obstruction at the Right Popliteal Artery[b]				
Right	190	178	130	90
Left	190	176	158	140
Arm	140	140	140	140
ABI	1.36	1.27	R 0.92 L 1.12	R 0.64 L 1.0
Obstruction at the Abdominal Aorta or Bilateral Iliac Obstruction[c]				
Right	140	126	112	94
Left	130	120	110	100
Arm	135	135	135	135
ABI	1.03	0.91	0.82	0.71

[a]Typical pressures in a normal individual. The findings, based on resting pressures, show no evidence of occlusive disease of the large- or medium-sized arteries. Normal findings are as follows: (1) ABI of 1.0 or higher; (2) all segmental pressure gradients lower than 30 mm Hg; and (3) upper thigh pressure at least 40 mm Hg above brachial pressure.
[b]Typical pressures in a patient with obstruction of the right popliteal or tibial arteries. Significant findings are as follows: (1) ABI less than 0.9 in the right leg; (2) abnormally high gradient from the ankle to below the knee and again from below to above the knee in the right leg; and (3) upper thigh pressure 50 mm Hg higher than brachial pressure, consistent with normal flow at the aorta-iliac level. The findings are suggestive of right popliteal occlusion or right anterior and posterior tibial occlusion, or both.
[c]Typical pressures in a patient with obstruction of the abdominal aorta or bilateral iliac obstruction. Significant findings are as follows: (1) ABI of less than 0.9 in both legs; (2) all segmental gradients lower than 30 mm Hg; and (3) both upper thigh pressures relatively low with respect to brachial pressure. The findings are suggestive of severe aortoiliac occlusive disease.
ABI, Ankle-brachial index.

volume be detected before loss of physiologic compensation and clinical shock occur.

Although orthostatic testing is commonly cited as a method to detect hypovolemia, it is frequently misleading and has less clinical value than often touted. The medical literature is inconsistent regarding values representative of a positive or negative orthostatic test, and its value for estimating volume status is probably overstated. In patients with an acute loss of less than 20% of total blood volume, orthostatic vital signs have been shown to lack both sensitivity and specificity.[171]

Physiologic Response to Hypovolemia

Acute blood loss or severe hypovolemia related to dehydration decreases venous return.[173] This can be seen with acute blood loss (usually greater than 20% of blood volume), severe burns, or prolonged vomiting or diarrhea that depletes body fluids. As a result, cardiac output falls and clinical manifestations of shock ensue. Several compensatory mechanisms are initiated by acute hypovolemia (Box 1.1). The dominant compensatory mechanism in shock is a reduction in carotid sinus baroreceptor inhibition of sympathetic outflow to the cardiovascular system. This increased sympathetic outflow results in several effects: (1) arteriolar vasoconstriction, which greatly increases peripheral vascular resistance; (2) constriction of venous capacitance vessels, which increases venous return to the heart; and (3) an increase in the HR and force of contraction, helping maintain cardiac output despite significant loss of volume.[170]

BOX 1.1 Homeostatic Mechanisms in Hemorrhagic Shock

- Sympathetic reflex compensation
  - Arteriolar vasoconstriction
  - Venous capacitance vasoconstriction
  - Increased inotropic and chronotropic cardiac activity
  - Central nervous system ischemic response
- Selective increase in cerebral and coronary perfusion by means of local autoregulation
- Increased oxygen unloading in tissues
- Restoration of blood volume
  - Renin-angiotensin-aldosterone axis activation
  - Antidiuretic hormone secretion
  - Transcapillary refill
  - Increased thirst resulting in increased fluid intake
  - Increased erythropoiesis

The value of sympathetic reflex compensation is illustrated by the fact that 30%–40% of blood volume can be lost before death occurs. When sympathetic reflexes are absent, a loss of only 15%–20% of blood volume may cause death.[170] Increased sympathetic nerve activity results in the commonly recognized physical signs of shock, including pallor, cool clammy skin, rapid HR, muscle weakness, and venous constriction. An inadequate immediate compensatory response will result in dizziness, altered mental status, or loss of consciousness.[174] The central nervous system response to ischemia further stimulates the sympathetic nervous system after arterial pressure falls below 50 mm Hg.[170] Subsequent compensatory mechanisms that work to restore blood volume to a normal level include the release of angiotensin and antidiuretic hormone (vasopressin). This causes arteriolar vasoconstriction, conservation of salt and water by the kidneys, and a shift in fluid from the interstitium to the intravascular space.[174]

Several investigators have examined the changes in blood pressure and pulse that occur in supine patients with blood loss.[158,159,171,175] Collectively, these studies have shown variable individual hemodynamic responses to acute blood loss of up to 1 L. The frequent inability to detect significant loss of volume with supine vital signs, and the observation that syncope frequently develops in patients with acute volume loss on rising, led to the investigation of the use of orthostatic vital signs to detect occult hypovolemia.

Physiologic Response to Changes in Posture

When an individual assumes the upright posture, complex homeostatic mechanisms compensate for the effects of gravity on the circulation to maintain cerebral perfusion with minimal change in vital signs. These responses include (1) baroreceptor-mediated arteriolar vasoconstriction; (2) venous constriction and increased muscle tone in the legs and the abdomen to augment venous return; (3) sympathetic-mediated inotropic and chronotropic effects on the heart; and (4) activation of the renin-angiotensin-aldosterone system.[176] These compensatory mechanisms preserve cerebral perfusion in the upright position with minimal changes in vital signs. When a normal individual stands, the pulse increases by an average of 13 beats/min, SBP falls slightly or does not change, and diastolic pressure rises slightly or does not change.[177] In patients with vasodepressor syncope, the normal compensatory reflexes that preserve cerebral perfusion with changes in posture are altered. The normally increased sympathetic tone on standing is paradoxically inhibited, and an exaggerated enhancement of parasympathetic activity (bradycardia) occurs and can lead to syncope.[178]

Few data exist regarding the true effect of acute blood loss on postural vital signs, and this parameter varies greatly among individuals experiencing hypovolemia. One study of 23 young adult volunteers from whom 500 to 1200 mL of blood was withdrawn found no reliable change in postural blood pressure, and a consistent postural increase in pulse of 35%–40% was noted after 500-mL blood loss.[169] Of the six individuals from whom approximately 1000 mL of blood was withdrawn, only two were able to tolerate standing, and each had a postural increase in pulse of greater than 30 beats/min. The other four individuals experienced severe symptoms on standing, followed by marked bradycardia and syncope if they were not allowed to lie down.

Following phlebotomy of 450–1000 mL of blood from healthy volunteers, the criterion of an increase in pulse of 30 beats/min or the presence of severe symptoms (syncope or near-syncope) during a supine-to-standing test accurately distinguished between 1000-mL blood loss and no blood loss. The sensitivity and specificity of using the aforementioned criteria for detecting 1000-mL blood loss (Box 1.2) were both 98%, for an accuracy of 96% (2% false-negative results and 2% false-positive results). The investigators were unable to consistently detect blood loss of 500 mL with these criteria.[171] In a similar study, the change in HR with postural changes after 500-mL phlebotomy was more discriminatory for blood loss than were changes in blood pressure or a change in the bioimpedance-based stroke index. Of note, these authors found that a change in HR of 30 beats/min or greater was 13.2% sensitive and 99.5% specific for 500-mL blood loss and that a change in HR of 20 beats/min or greater was 44.7% sensitive and 95.4% specific. The finding of a significant rise in pulse, though insensitive for 500-mL blood loss, was relatively specific in these healthy adult blood donors.[179] In a metaanalysis evaluating orthostatic vital signs, the authors concluded that a large postural pulse change (>30 beats/min) or severe postural dizziness precluding the completion of vital sign measurements is required to clinically diagnose hypovolemia secondary to acute blood loss. The analysis demonstrated that orthostatic vital signs are often absent after moderate amounts of blood loss, thus significantly limiting the test's sensitivity (22%) in this scenario.[180] A consensus statement defined orthostatic hypotension as a reduction in SBP of at least 20 mm Hg or a reduction in diastolic blood pressure of at least 10 mm Hg within 3 minutes of standing and reinforces the theory that this is a physical finding rather than a disease process.[174]

BOX 1.2 Summary of Orthostatic Tilt Testing[a]

TEST PROCEDURE

1. Blood pressure and pulse are recorded after the patient has been supine for 2–3 minutes.
2. Blood pressure, pulse, and symptoms are recorded after the patient has been standing for 1 minute; the patient should be permitted to resume a supine position immediately if syncope or near-syncope develop.

POSITIVE TEST

1. Increase in pulse of 30 beats/min or more in adults or
2. Presence of symptoms of cerebral hypoperfusion (e.g., dizziness, syncope)

[a]*The predictive ability of orthostatic vital signs to assess volume status is often overestimated in clinical practice. This suggested guide is based on the ability of the change in pulse and patient symptoms to distinguish between no acute blood loss and 1000-mL acute blood loss in healthy, previously normovolemic volunteers (sensitivity of 98% for detecting 1000-mL acute blood loss).[159] This guide may not be applicable to elderly patients, sick children, medicated patients, and those with autonomic dysfunction.*

Variables Affecting Orthostatic Vital Signs

Many conditions affect the compensatory mechanisms that allow patients to assume the upright posture. Most of the conditions that affect postural blood pressure regulation involve a pathologic condition that affects the sympathetic nervous system or the use of medications that alter normal cardiovascular compensatory functions. Orthostatic hypotension caused by autonomic insufficiency is not usually accompanied by tachycardia, and the orthostatic hypotension produced by acute volume depletion is commonly accompanied by a pronounced reflex tachycardia. Even in normal individuals, passive tilting generates a high incidence of orthostatic syncope.[181]

Because of decreased vasomotor tone, limited chronotropic response, and other factors, the elderly have a higher incidence of orthostatic hypotension leading to syncope and fall-related injuries.[182] Carotid sinus hypersensitivity may play a greater role than orthostasis in geriatric syncope.[183] Note that drugs that antagonize the normal autonomic compensatory mechanisms can also produce orthostatic changes. These changes can be severe enough to produce frank syncope, especially in the elderly. A study of patients with syncope seen in an ED found that orthostatic hypotension was considered to be the cause of the syncope in 24%, and that the largest proportion of these cases were drug related. Patients with orthostatic hypotension as the cause of syncope were older, had more comorbid conditions, and were found to be more frequently taking antihypertensive medications.[184] Advanced patient age is an independent risk factor for orthostatic blood pressure changes and does not appear to have a direct correlation to the presence of chronic cardiovascular disease, disability, or body mass index.[185] A study assessing vital sign changes prior to cardiac arrest found significant differences between elderly and nonelderly patients in the predictive value of the Modified Early Warning Score, noting more accurate detection of cardiac arrest by vital sign changes in nonelderly patients.[186]

Patients with hypertension may also have abnormal vasomotor responses to tilt testing and demonstrate more instability.[187] Chronic anemia patients, who exhibit compensated blood volume, seem to have the same postural response as normal individuals.[188] Ethanol ingestion exaggerates postural pulse changes and mimics the hemodynamic changes seen with acute blood loss.[189]

The utility of orthostatic vital signs in children has been questioned. Healthy adolescents had changes in HR of 21.5 ± 21.2 beats/min and variable changes in SBP (+19 to −17 mm Hg) after 2 minutes of standing.[190] A study comparing mildly dehydrated children with normal children found a significant difference in the orthostatic rise in pulse, and no difference in orthostatic blood pressure. The investigators concluded that an orthostatic increase in pulse of greater than 25 beats/min constitutes a positive tilt test and less than 20 beats/min constitutes a negative test (sensitivity of 75%, specificity of 95%, and predictive value of 92% when using near-syncope or an increase in HR greater than 25 beats/min).[191]

Another complicating factor in interpreting orthostatic vital signs is the development of paradoxical bradycardia in the presence of blood loss. Bradycardia in the face of hemorrhage has generally been considered a preterminal finding of irreversible shock, and bradycardia has been documented in hypovolemic, conscious trauma patients as well. It has been reported that when orthostatic syncope occurs, it is accompanied by hypotension and often bradycardia.[168,171] Many central nervous system factors can contribute to vagally mediated syncope in ED patients with acute traumatic blood loss, including pain, the sight of blood, anxiety, and nausea. This paradoxical bradycardia may be more frequently associated with rapid and massive bleeding. Patients with more gradual blood loss tend to have a more typical tachycardic response. When the patient's clinical findings are consistent with loss of volume or shock, the clinician should not allow the absence of tachycardia to change the assessment.

Indications and Contraindications

When the volume status of a patient is assessed with the use of orthostatic vital signs, several points should be remembered. Many factors influence orthostatic blood pressure, including age, preexisting medical conditions, medications, and autonomic dysfunction. It must be emphasized that data relating the effect of blood loss to orthostatic vital signs are limited to phlebotomized healthy volunteers. Great care must be used when extrapolating these data to patients with anemia, comorbid conditions, dehydration, or painful trauma. The clinician must consider the patient's clinical condition when interpreting orthostatic vital signs in the evaluation of a patient with potential volume depletion.

Orthostatic vital signs can be considered an adjunct for the evaluation of any patient with known or suspected loss of blood volume or a history of syncope. Contraindications to orthostatic measures include supine hypotension, the clinical syndrome of shock, severely altered mental status, the setting of possible spinal injuries, and lower extremity or pelvic fractures.

The use of medications that block the normal vasomotor and chronotropic response to orthostatic tests is also a contraindication to using this test for the assessment of volume status. When the patient's volume status is believed to be adequate and the clinician seeks to determine whether specific medications may have affected the patient's ability to respond to postural changes, the test may be useful. In these situations, the primary finding may be the sensation of near-syncope with little or no change in vital signs.

Orthostatic vital signs are often used to assess a patient's response to therapy. In patients receiving intravenous rehydration therapy, serial orthostatic vital signs are widely used to judge the end point of therapy before release. In one study, individual orthostatic vital sign response to saline infusion in women with hyperemesis gravidarum was associated with other measures of rehydration, including weight gain and decreased urine specific gravity.[192] Although the individual improvement in orthostatic vital signs in response to rehydration was of clinical value, the initial orthostatic vital signs were considered insufficient as the sole indicator of clinical dehydration in this population.

Technique

To obtain orthostatic vital signs, record the blood pressure and pulse after the patient has been in the supine position for 2–3 minutes (see Box 1.2). Allow the patient to rest quietly and do not perform any painful or invasive procedures during the test.

Next, ask the patient to stand and be prepared to assist if severe symptoms or syncope develop. A supine-to-standing test is more accurate than a supine-to-sitting one. If severe symptoms develop on standing, defined as syncope or extreme dizziness requiring the patient to lie down, the test is considered positive and should be terminated. If not symptomatic, allow the patient to stand for 1 minute and then record the blood pressure and pulse. A 1-minute interval resulted in the greatest difference between control and 1000-mL phlebotomy groups in one study.[171]

A number of studies have been conducted on normotensive, normovolemic patients to assess end points for orthostatic vital sign parameters. Such studies have included sitting-to-standing methods and varying rates of postural changes,[193] including supine times of 5–10 minutes and standing times of 0–2 minutes.[194] Arm position may affect postural changes in blood pressure and should be held constant to accurately assess orthostatic change.[88] Complications include syncope with resulting falls and injuries.

Interpretation

The most sensitive criteria for orthostasis are tachycardia or symptoms of cerebral hypoperfusion (e.g., near-syncope). Although changes in blood pressure may be seen, they are too variable to be an indicator of blood loss. Specific population-based thresholds for changes in pulse rate and blood pressure have some value in identifying patients at high risk for significant blood loss, and great individual variability limits the use of this technique as a screening test. A loss of 500 mL, and occasionally more, may be associated with a negative orthostatic vital sign assessment.[183,195] The use of serial measurements to ascertain the response to therapy in patients considered to be at risk for loss of volume appears to have clinical utility.[196]

In the setting of suspected blood loss, if the patient has a rise in pulse of 30 beats/min or manifests severe symptoms, and if other complicating factors have been excluded, blood loss is highly likely (2% false-positive rate). The presence of a negative test indicates only that acute blood loss of 1000 mL is unlikely (2% false-negative rate) and that blood loss of 500 mL cannot be excluded (43%–87% false-negative rate).[171,183,195,197] Orthostatic changes in the SI were no more sensitive than established tilt test criteria in discriminating normal individuals from those with moderate acute blood loss (450 mL).[196]

Criteria for significant orthostatic changes in blood pressure cannot be definitively set for the following reasons: (1) large variability in postural blood pressure has been found in the adult ED population[197,198]; (2) the results of studies using passive tilt tables cannot be extrapolated to the bedside use of orthostatic vital signs; (3) studies using healthy patients with acute blood loss may not reflect the orthostatic changes seen in the elderly, those with chronic bleeding, dehydration, other medical problems, or in association with certain medications; and (4) many studies of orthostatic changes did not use a criterion standard in their determinations.

In summary, orthostatic vital sign testing is common in the ED and has limited proven clinical value. The clinical interpretation of orthostatic changes in blood pressure and pulse varies widely. Although this intervention may occasionally yield information not obtained through other means, the authors do not consider orthostatic blood pressure testing a standard of care in the evaluation of ED patients.

CAPILLARY REFILL

The capillary refill test is a measurement of the interval of time from the release of pressure on the nail bed or soft tissue sufficient to blanch the nail bed or superficial soft tissue, until the return to normal coloration. Delayed capillary refill is an indication of reduced skin turgor, often as a result of volume depletion or limited perfusion. Measurement of capillary refill time (CRT) appears to be somewhat accurate in children, and its accuracy in assessing dehydration and reduced perfusion in adults is highly suspect.[172,199] Skin elasticity is the characteristic that allows skin to spring back to its original shape after it has been deformed, and the speed of refilling the capillary bed after compression is responsible for the return of color to the skin.

Indications and Contraindications

CRT should not be determined from a dependent extremity, from a recently burned or injured extremity, or at the site of an infection or acute injury. Because CRT can be used without additional equipment and takes only a few seconds to perform, it can be a useful bedside assessment of perfusion and dehydration when used in conjunction with other objective signs of the adequacy of perfusion. It should not be considered accurate as a stand-alone tool. Capillary refill is not an appropriate alternative to measuring blood pressure in pediatric patients.

Procedure

The preferred sites for determining CRT are the nail bed, the thenar surface of the palm, and the heel. Alternative sites may have different CRTs, and the current standards are best developed for capillary refill determined at the nail bed.[200] Regardless of the site chosen, position the extremity at approximately the level of the right atrium. The minimum pressure necessary to produce blanching yields the most reproducible values. Release the nail bed and begin timing with a stopwatch or simply by counting out "one-thousand-one, one-thousand-two" for an approximation of the interval. Stop the clock when the nail bed becomes pink again. Interobserver reliability has been shown to be moderate, with kappa values of less than 0.5 in the evaluation of both adults and children.[201,202]

Interpretation

The normal CRT increases with age and is slightly longer in female patients. It is further increased by degrees of dehydration or hypoperfusion. Hypothermia, hyponatremia, congestive heart failure, malnutrition, and edema all increase CRT. Environmental conditions such as ambient air temperature can falsely alter capillary refill.[203] Fever alone did not appear to prolong or shorten CRT in children,[204] and a study of healthy adults found a 5% decrease in CRT for each degree Celsius rise in patient temperature.[203]

The main difficulty in interpreting CRT is that normal values in healthy patients fall into a wide range. In 30 normal infants 2–24 months of age, mean CRT was 0.8 ± 0.3 seconds. Measurements obtained from the nail bed were more reproducible than those from the heel.[201] Combined results from four studies evaluating capillary refill revealed a pooled sensitivity of 0.60 (95% confidence interval [CI], 0.29–0.91) and a specificity of 0.85 (95% CI, 0.72–0.98) for detecting 5% dehydration in children.[205] The presence of a 2-second or longer delay in CRT when combined with any two or more of the findings of absent tears, dry mucous membranes, or ill general appearance predicted clinical dehydration (>5% deficit in body weight) in children (1 month to 5 years of age) with 87% sensitivity and 82% specificity.[204] A 2015 systematic review including 21 studies suggests applying a cutoff of 3 seconds or more to define abnormal CRT in infants and children over 7 days of age.[206]

Frequent monitoring of capillary refill may be useful in assessing responses to rapid fluid resuscitation in children. A normal CRT of 2 seconds or less has been shown to correlate with superior vena cava oxygen saturation of 70% or higher in critically ill children.[200] The role of serial CRT measurements for assessing the response to rehydration in adults is unknown, and it does not appear to be useful for assessing acute loss of blood volume. Lima and colleagues studied the prognostic value of the subjective assessment of peripheral perfusion in critically ill patients following initial resuscitation.[207] When an abnormal CRT was defined as greater than 4.5 seconds, coupled with extremity coolness, these parameters identified patients who had been hemodynamically stabilized and continued to have more severe organ dysfunction and higher lactate levels. In adults, CRT was found to be less sensitive and less specific than orthostatic vital signs in detecting 450-mL blood loss during blood donation.[170] However, a 2014 study showed CRT, measured as a continuous variable in a cohort of admitted medical patients, was associated with an increased 1- and 7-day all-cause mortality.[208]

In summary, assessment of CRT is a common technique used in the ED. This procedure has limited proven value, with a clinical interpretation that is very subjective. Although this intervention may occasionally yield information not obtained through other means, predominantly in children, the authors do not consider such testing an absolute standard of care in the evaluation of ED patients.

TEMPERATURE

Detection of abnormal body temperature may facilitate proper diagnosis and evaluation of patients' complaints in the ED. An inability to maintain normal body temperature is indicative of a vast number of potentially serious disorders, including infections, neoplasms, shock, toxic reactions, and environmental exposures.[209–213] Fever in neutropenic, immunocompromised, or intravenous drug-using patients may be more reliable than laboratory tests or clinician assessment in diagnosing serious illness.[209,214] Infants are particularly sensitive to thermal stress and may demonstrate lower body temperatures during critical illness.[211,215] In one study, although higher rates of serious bacterial infection were found in neonates who had documented fever (OR, 3.23) on admission, only 8.4% of neonates with historical fever were later diagnosed with serious bacterial infection.[213] Pretriage or home assessment of body temperature is fraught with difficulty and unreliability. Whether taken by the oral, rectal, or tympanic routes, reports of fever at home are very difficult to interpret in the clinical setting.[210,213] Some studies report rates as low as 13% in frequency when measuring temperature in the critically ill or injured,[216] and temperature and Glasgow Coma Scale were the least frequently documented physiologic observations (less frequent than RR, oxygen saturation, HR, and SBP) across ED, critical care, and medical/surgical unit settings despite temperature representing a key sign of systemic inflammatory response syndrome.[217]

Physiology

Under normal conditions, the temperature of deep central body tissues (i.e., core temperature) remains at 37 ± 0.6°C (98.6 ± 1.08°F).[218] Core body temperature can be maintained within a narrow range, whereas environmental temperature varies from as much as 13 to 60°C (55 to 140°F),[218] and surface temperature rises and falls with environmental and other influences. Mean oral temperature is 36.8 ± 0.4°C (98.2 ± 0.7°F).[219] Maintenance of normal body temperature requires a balance of heat production and heat loss. Heat loss occurs by radiation, conduction, and evaporation by approximately 60%, 18%, and 22%, respectively. Heat loss is increased by wind, water, and lack of insulation (e.g., clothing). Sweating, vasodilation, and decreased heat production serve to decrease temperature. Piloerection, vasoconstriction, and increased heat production serve to increase body temperature. Heat production is increased by shivering, fat catabolism, and increased thyroid hormone production.

Temperature is controlled by feedback mechanisms operating through the hypothalamus. Heat-sensitive neurons in this area increase their rate of firing during experimental heating. Receptors in the skin, spinal cord, abdominal viscera, and central veins primarily detect cold and provide feedback to the hypothalamus that signals an increase in heat production. Stimuli that change core body temperature result in reflex changes in mechanisms that increase either heat loss or heat production.[218,219]

Indications and Contraindications

Clinicians generally measure body temperature to determine whether it is outside the normal range and as an indication of pathologic conditions that can affect core body temperature. Measurement of actual core body temperature requires the placement of invasive monitors, such as a bladder, esophageal, or pulmonary artery (PA) probe. Clinicians commonly use estimates of core body temperatures to conveniently and safely assess abnormalities in core temperature. All noncore body sites and methods have inherent limitations in accuracy, and clinicians have come to accept these shortcomings in assessing most patients.

Measurement of oral temperature requires a cooperative adult or child. Patients who are uncooperative, hemodynamically unstable, septic, or in respiratory distress (with an RR >20 breaths/min) require a method of measuring temperature other than the traditional oral route.[220] This group includes children younger than 5 years and patients who are intubated. Ingestion of hot or cold beverages has shown that they can alter oral temperature readings for 5–30 minutes and can falsely elevate a normal temperature or mask a fever.[221]

Special techniques of measuring core body temperature may be indicated in certain patients (e.g., those with profound hypothermia, frostbite, or hyperthermia). Measurement of core body temperature is indicated in these individuals because it accurately measures the effects of treatment. This is the group of patients who will benefit the most from continuous temperature measurements.[222]

Measurement Sites

Core Body Temperature

The following sites accurately reflect core body temperature and changes in it: the distal third of the esophagus, the tympanic membrane (TM) (with a direct thermistor in contact with the anterior inferior quadrant of the TM),[223,224] and the PA.[225,226] Other sites may represent core body temperature under certain conditions; for example, (1) the rectum when the temperature is obtained at least 8 cm from the anus with an indwelling thermistor and the body temperature is relatively constant, and (2) the bladder when measured with an indwelling thermistor.[227]

Rectal temperature is often considered the criterion standard for body temperature in ambulatory patients, and it is often used routinely in children younger than 3 years.[228] Advantages include accuracy, sensitivity, and availability. One ICU study found that rectal probe temperatures demonstrated limited variability or bias when compared with PA temperatures.[229] Disadvantages include longer intervals for measurement, safety concerns, and inconvenience. Neutropenia and recent rectal surgery represent relative contraindications to measurement of rectal temperature. Thermistor probes (i.e., small thermocouples with instantaneous readouts) for esophageal and vascular temperature measurement provide continuous temperature readouts when attached to a potentiometer. Thermistor probes are available for measurement of esophageal, bladder, and rectal temperature with appropriate monitors.

Peripheral Body Sites Approximating Core Temperature

A body temperature measurement by IR radiation can be detected from the ear, including the auditory canal and TM; it is easy to use, hygienic, convenient, and quick. It can be used as a general screening technique, particularly in cases when temperature is not of great importance, such as in minor trauma. Though clearly superior to axillary temperature readings,[230] controversy remains regarding the sensitivity and specificity of IR TM readings in the ED. In a cohort of ICU patients, agreement of tympanic with PA temperature was inferior to that of urinary temperature. Compared with PA temperatures, Δ (limits of agreement) were 0.36°C (–0.56 to 1.28°C), –0.05°C (–0.69 to 0.59°C), and 0.30°C (–0.42 to 1.01°C) for tympanic, urinary, and axillary temperatures, respectively.[231] It is possible that alterations of regional blood flow accompanying critical illness (TMs may behave as an extension of the skin or the mucous membrane in the critically ill) and the peripheral vasoconstriction that occurs with inotropes and some forms of shock may occur in the TM, making such measurements less accurate in this population.

More work is being done in the pediatric population, with an overall sensitivity of between 50% and 80% and a specificity of 85%. The lower sensitivities are found in newborns and infants younger than 3 years.[232–234] Systematic reviews of pediatric studies have pooled data suggesting 65% sensitivity, which is unacceptable in the clinical setting.[235] One study found that neither TM nor skin thermometers could reliably predict rectal temperature, and it concurred that these methods could not replace rectal temperature measurement as the "gold standard" for detecting fever in the pediatric population.[236] Adult studies, though generally more favorable in recommending TM temperatures, have shown gaps in reliability.[237] Alternatively, a systematic review suggested that TM and oral thermometry provides an accurate measure of core temperature in critically ill adults with fever.[238] Temporal artery scanning to detect fever is increasingly being examined. In general, these devices show better sensitivity in detecting fever in infants than TM thermistors do (66% versus 49% sensitivity) and may be useful in excluding fever,[239] defined as a rectal temperature higher than 38.3°C if the temporal artery readings are lower than 37.7°C.[240] The point can be argued that a sensitivity of 60% in any population lacks the required sensitivity to be useful clinically. A theoretical disadvantage of TM temperatures might be a falsely elevated estimate of the core temperature in the presence of otitis media. In one study, TM thermometers accurately reflected oral temperatures in children with otitis media.[241]

In a group of pediatric patients receiving anesthesia, measurements taken at the temporal artery were similar to nasopharyngeal thermometer recordings, and the axillary temperature was lower than the temporal artery and nasopharyngeal temperatures.[242]

Prehospital providers who might wish to measure IR TM temperature at low ambient temperatures should be aware that below 24.6°C, the TM readings will greatly underestimate core temperatures.[243] EMS personnel should also be aware that in a cohort of exhausted marathon runners, rectal and IR TM temperatures have only moderate correlation.[244] External thermometry may be unreliable in the setting of heat-related illness or hypothermia; if these diagnoses are clinically suspected and the IR TM temperature does not confirm an abnormal temperature, a measurement by rectal or esophageal probes should be obtained for diagnosis and during treatment.[245]

Axillary and tactile temperature assessments have been demonstrated to be unreliable and insensitive. They should not be used as screening methods for core temperature abnormalities in the ED.[246–248] Single-use Tempa-DOT thermometers show progressive temperature dot darkening with increasing temperature, and these thermometers have been adopted by many EDs. These temperature devices have been shown to have 100% sensitivity and approximately 80% specificity for identification of fever when temperature was obtained orally in both adults and children.[249] The most rudimentary method for temperature measurement, parental assessment by tactile touch, is associated with a measured fever approximately 75% of the time.[250] Clinician estimation of fever is almost identical (70%).[251]

Procedure

Begin the temperature measurement by selecting the body site. Consider the accuracy of using a certain site to reflect core temperature, the sensitivity of the site to changes in temperature, the convenience, the time required, the safety, and the availability of the site.[252] Insert the temperature probe and allow the probe to equilibrate with the temperature of the local body tissues.

Proper placement of the temperature probes significantly influences the results of oral, rectal, esophageal, and vascular temperatures.[253–256] Obtain sublingual oral temperatures in either the right or the left posterior sublingual pocket with the mouth closed.[253] Though anxiety-producing for parents, biting and breaking a mercury thermometer is generally inconsequential with regard to ingestion of either glass or mercury. Obtain a rectal temperature with the patient in the left or right lateral decubitus position and advance the probe gently to a depth of 3–5 cm to ensure accurate, atraumatic results.[257] Complications associated with rectal temperature measurements are extremely rare and include rectal perforation, pneumoperitoneum, bacteremia, dysrhythmias, and syncope.[253] Falsely low supranormal rectal temperature measurements may be seen during shock.[258] Rectal temperature may also lag behind changes in core temperature. An esophageal catheter or PA probe can be placed for measurement of core body temperature, and these techniques are not typically used in the ED.

Though not commonly used, measurement of the temperature of a freshly voided urine specimen can validate measurement of temperature at other body sites.[259] Urinary bladder temperature measurement has been demonstrated to be similar to PA catheter temperature.[260]

Digital electronic probes are commonly used for the measurement of oral temperature in ambulatory patients.[261] Electronic methods of temperature measurement are based on the thermocouple principle. Modern electronic thermometers signal when extrapolation of the temperature–time curve has occurred. Current in vitro standards call for an accuracy of ±0.1°C (±0.18°F) over the range of 37–39°C (98.6–102.2°F). Disadvantages include factors that affect clinical accuracy and sensitivity. Disposable single-use oral thermometers are now available and are as reliable as mercury or TM thermometers.[262] In the pediatric population, pacifier thermometers record supralingual readings in infants. The average time needed to record a reading with a pacifier thermometer is 3 minutes and 23 seconds, thus making its application in emergency medicine limited, although its sensitivity (72%) and specificity (98%) rival that of alternative methods.[263] Various IR ear thermometers are available commercially with varying operating temperature ranges, features, and reported accuracy.[264] Complications associated with axillary, oral, ear IR, and liquid crystal thermometers are rare or unreported. TM perforation and pain have been reported as complications of placement of the thermistor probe in the auditory canal.

Interpretation

Normal values for body temperature are affected by the following variables: (1) site and methods used for measurement; (2) perfusion; (3) environmental exposure; (4) pregnancy; (5) activity level; and (6) time of day. Clinicians must interpret body temperature with knowledge of the range of normal values at the intended site of measurement. Although core body temperature remains nearly constant (37.0 ± 0.6°C or 98.6 ± 0.18°F), surface temperature rises and falls with changes in ambient temperature, exercise, and time of day. The definition of fever varies by the site of measurement and is defined by a temperature greater than 2 standard deviations above the mean. Fever has been defined as an oral temperature of 37.8°C or higher (100.0°F),[257] a rectal temperature of 38.0°C or higher (100.4°F),[265] or an IR ear temperature of 37.6°C or higher (99.6°F).[257] Based on measurement of temperatures in normal, healthy infants, it is recommended that fever be defined as a rectal temperature of 38°C or higher in infants younger than 30 days, 38.1°C or higher in infants 30–60 days (1–2 months), and 38.2°C or higher in infants 60–90 days old (2–3 months).[266] Hypothermia has been defined as a core body temperature lower than 35°C (<95°F), and hyperthermia has been defined as a core body temperature higher than 41°C (>105.8°F) with accompanying symptoms and signs.[267] A useful nomogram and formulas for conversion of centigrade to Fahrenheit are provided in Fig. 1.6.

Temperature probes that depend on transfer of heat energy from local tissues to the probe require a period of equilibration and reliable tissue contact at the intended body site. Acceptable equilibration times for mercury-in-glass thermometers in oral, rectal, and axillary sites are 7, 3, and 10 minutes, respectively. Used in a predictive mode, electronic digital thermometers generally require 30 seconds for oral or rectal temperature equilibration. The predictive mode uses temperature changes versus time to predict an equilibration temperature.

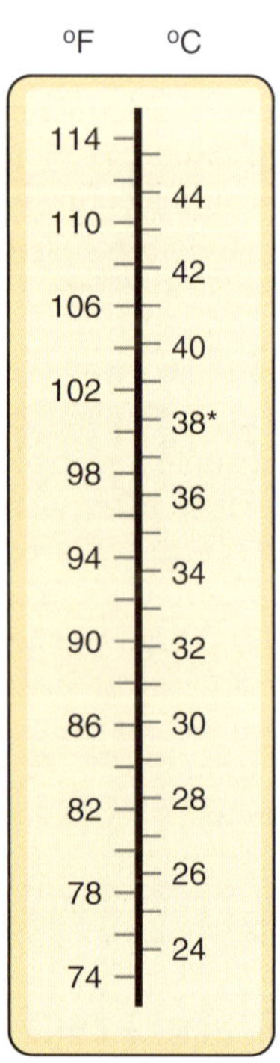

Fig. 1.6 Temperature conversion scale. To change Celsius (centigrade) to Fahrenheit, multiply the Celsius temperature by 9/5 and add 32. To change Fahrenheit to Celsius, subtract 32 from the Fahrenheit number and multiply by 5/9.

Normal ranges and suggested febrile thresholds for common body sites and methods should be considered in the interpretation of temperature values (Table 1.5). Interpretation of temperature measurements during clinical assessment must consider the use of antipyretics, level of activity, pregnancy, environmental exposure, and patient age. Body temperature is increased during sustained exercise, pregnancy, and the luteal phase of the menstrual cycle. Temperature also increases in the late afternoon because of diurnal variation. Body temperature is generally reduced with advanced age, and age may have an impact on the magnitude of fever. Axillary temperatures have a low sensitivity and a high specificity for fever. Axillary temperatures should not be used to screen for fever.

Oral temperature measurements are affected by the ingestion of hot or cold liquids,[238] tachypnea,[268] and cold ambient air.[269] Before taking an oral temperature the examiner should inquire about these features and possibly delay taking the temperature. A 2.7°C (4.9°F) reduction in oral temperature measurement was found when the probe was placed under the tip of the tongue instead of under the posterior sublingual pocket.[253] Given the extrapolation that occurs with rapidly reading thermocouple devices and IR detectors, it is not surprising that the sensitivity of these devices for detection of fever is only 86%–88%.[270] Many clinicians have adopted the adage that when an elevated temperature is suspected or crucial in decision-making and not evident with an oral thermocouple probe or IR TM thermometer, measurement with a mercury-in-glass thermometer is indicated.

When rapid changes in body temperature occur, oral and TM temperature measurements appear to be more reliable than rectal temperature. In 20 adults examined during open-heart surgery, oral temperatures showed a better correlation with blood temperature during rapid cooling and rewarming.[254] Additionally, esophageal temperature measurements showed a faster response rate compared to the temperature

TABLE 1.5 Normal Ranges and Suggested Febrile Thresholds for Human Body Temperature (in Healthy Resting Patients)

BODY SITE	TYPE OF THERMOMETER	NORMAL RANGE (°C)	FEVER (°C)
Core[a]	Electronic	36.4–37.9	38.0
Oral	Mercury in glass, electronic	35.5–37.7	37.8
Rectal	Mercury in glass, electronic	36.6–37.9	38.0
Ear	Infrared emission	35.7–37.5	37.6[b]

[a]Temperature obtained with a properly positioned pulmonary artery, esophageal, or tympanic membrane thermistor.

[b]For unadjusted ear temperature using the Thermoscan Pro-1 (Thermoscan, Inc., San Diego, CA).

measured in the bladder when cold saline infusion was used to induce mild hypothermia in cardiac arrest patients.[255]

Infrequently, ED patients require constant monitoring of temperature (e.g., in cases of profound hypothermia or hyperthermia). This can usually be performed by using a bladder or esophageal probe attached to a potentiometer. Patients with indwelling central venous or PA catheters may have electronic thermistors inserted into the central circulation to measure core body temperature. As noted earlier, rectal temperature measurements are less desirable for monitoring patients undergoing rapid changes in core temperature. Periodic IR TM temperature monitoring may represent one useful option in a hypothermic patient.[271]

Interpretation of ear IR temperatures requires knowledge of the mode of thermometer operation and ambient temperature. Occlusion of the ear canal by cerumen may produce a falsely low reading.[272] Most IR ear thermometers have different modes that allow users to predict the equivalent temperature at other body sites. IR ear thermometers appear to be moderately sensitive for fever.[273] If these devices are used, the clinician must be aware of the potential for a falsely low temperature. When in doubt the measurement should be repeated with a more standard method.

Patients, parents, and caregivers often misinterpret the significance of a fever, and the term "fever phobia" has been coined to describe the ubiquitous and unsubstantiated fear that fever, by itself, is harmful or has diagnostic or prognostic significance.[211] Some of the highest fevers are the result of benign viral infections. Fever has been demonstrated to increase the body's immune response, making aggressive fever reduction counterproductive. Most individuals, especially children, feel better when a high fever is lowered. Uninitiated medical personnel may contribute to the incidence of fever phobia. Routine administration of antipyretics in the ED for any fever, regardless of the degree of discomfort, has fueled unwarranted concern and may result in potentially harmful interventions, unnecessary testing and treatments, avoidable side effects of medications, and additional patient anxiety. Mandatory medical evaluation for any fever, the use of alcohol sponge baths, waking a sleeping child to administer antipyretics, alternating ibuprofen with acetaminophen, around-the-clock use of antipyretics, and misconceptions about fever causing brain damage are some of the myths that still exist in some EDs and throughout the general population. An ED protocol stating that any child should be afebrile, demonstrate a significant decrease in hyperpyrexia, or even have a temperature reading repeated before discharge has no scientific validity.

PAIN AS A VITAL SIGN

Background

One of the goals of modern medicine has been to understand, accurately assess, and adequately treat pain. A paradigm shift has occurred in which pain is viewed as a mechanism to provide a mechanical warning of actual or potential damage to cells and tissues in a specific area. An individual's pain should be addressed as early as possible in the ED encounter, and reflex interventions aimed at immediately or completely relieving a patient's pain are inappropriate and potentially counterproductive. Importantly the concept of using pain as "the fifth vital sign" can be problematic, and this concept has not met with universal agreement.[274] Literal interpretation of this concept can be fraught with problems, and because of the subjective nature of pain, measurement and interpretation are imprecise. An overemphasis on rigorously quantifying pain and aggressively treating a specific number on the pain scale has the potential to expose patients to unneeded opioids, result in unrealistic expectations by patients, and lead to opioid dependence or addiction.

Pain can cause sympathetically mediated changes in vital signs, and standard vital signs (pulse, respiration, blood pressure) do not meaningfully correlate with the level of perceived pain. It is a common error to relate changes in vital signs, or lack thereof, as an indication of a patient's true level of pain. A retrospective study of patients with confirmed painful diagnoses showed no clinically significant associations between self-reported triage pain scores and HR, blood pressure, or RR.[275] Contentions that the judicious use of analgesics will obscure a clinical condition or otherwise adversely affect clinical care are antiquated and unscientific. Adequate pain control may facilitate the overall ED encounter for both the patient and clinician.

Initiatives mandating documentation of pain as the fifth vital sign have not been associated with improvement in pain management.[274] A prospective, multicenter study evaluating the current state of ED pain management practices concluded that there is high pain intensity, as demonstrated by intense pain on arrival (median rating, 8 of 10), and suboptimal pain management practices. It also showed assessment of pain occurring in 83% of patients, 40% of patients receiving no analgesics, lengthy delays in analgesic administration, and a large proportion of patients reporting moderate to severe pain at discharge (74%).[276] Assuming weight-based dosing for acute pain management, analgesic regimens did not conform to the recommended regimens in a study of ED patients.[277] Mandating the recording of a triage pain score has been shown to improve time to initial analgesic treatment.[276] Acute or chronic pain is the most common chief complaint of more than 50% of ED patients, with the figure approaching 75% in some studies.[278] Reliably quantifying pain should be the goal of ED clinicians and is an appropriate step in the triage process.

Procedure/Interpretation

The Joint Commission goals mandate that all hospitals develop comprehensive programs for the measurement, treatment, and documentation of pain. There is no perfect measurement tool suitable for the wide variety of patients and clinical scenarios experienced in EDs.[278,279] Pain is a complex, subjective, multifaceted, personal experience that is difficult to easily quantify in all individuals. The perfect pain assessment tool for the ED setting would be simple and rapid to administer while providing a precise, reliable, and valid measure of pain regardless of a patient's age, cultural background, and cognitive or physical impairments. Currently no tool meets all the criteria necessary to satisfy this definition. The primary focus should be to allow patients to report and rate their pain from a personal viewpoint, as it is widely accepted that health professionals cannot rate pain intensity as accurately as patients themselves.[280,281] A patient's self-report of the pain is considered the gold standard for the initial assessment of pain and tracking of a response to interventions, although such reporting does not mandate specific interventions.[282]

Multiple unidimensional acute pain measurement instruments have been published and many have been independently validated. Common instruments include the verbal rating scale, numerical rating scale, visual analog scale (VAS), and graphic rating scales. The most used pain scale in the ED is the 1–10 VAS. The VAS uses a 10-cm line bounded on each end by perpendicular stops and descriptors. Zero equates to no pain, and 10 equates to the worst pain ever experienced. The initial score is not as important as change during treatment. Generally a change in VAS scores has been shown to be valid and reliable if self-completion is appropriate.[283] There is wide variability in this technique, and at least a 13- to 30-mm (1.3–3 cm) change on the scale is required to validate clinically relevant worsening or relief.[282] Low completion rates may be seen in patients with visual or cognitive impairment.[284] Graphic rating scales are useful for patients with limited cognitive and expressive ability, especially children. They may also be helpful to overcome language or cultural differences. A systematic review recently evaluated a variety of graphic scales in pediatric patients and supported use of the Faces Pain Scale (FPS), the Faces Pain Scale-Revised (FPS-R), the Oucher Pain Scale, and the Wong-Baker Faces Pain Rating Scale (WBFPRS).[285] In an ED survey, the WBFPRS was the most common (81.7% of responding facilities) pain measurement tool used for pediatric pain assessment.[284] Scale ratings may overestimate or underestimate pain in certain patients and do not mandate a specific pain reduction approach.[286] This is better driven by clinician evaluation and consideration of the entire scenario. Such ratings rarely correlate with the seriousness of a patient's medical condition. It is not uncommon for patients to rate their pain higher than 10 on a scale of 1–10 in an attempt to emphasize their personal experience, anxiety, or fear of receiving inadequate analgesia. It may be a patient's perception that a higher rating will expedite treatment, prompt higher doses of medications, or otherwise engender more compassionate care. A common erroneous tactic or subterfuge of litigation proceedings is to incriminate a clinician's diagnosis, treatment, or disposition based on the patient's rendition of the pain scale.

Overall Goal of Pain Relief

The goal of pain management in the ED is to adequately relieve or control pain without compromising diagnosis, treatment plans, or the safety of the patient and population. Although the theoretically ideal objective is to totally relieve pain, this goal is difficult to consistently achieve in the complex ED milieu and should not be the standard of care. Pain relief is best accomplished by combining clinician experience, real-time clinical judgment, repeated evaluation, and discussion with the patient and family. Concerns about safety and the potential for abuse of addictive pharmaceuticals often weigh into the decision-making process for emergency physicians, and universal prescriptive reporting services can be used to assist in patient care and safe prescribing practices.[287–289] Strict adherence to protocols, patient self-reporting on any pain scale, or reliance on a dogmatic approach to relief of a patient's pain can be fraught with peril. A recent ACEP policy statement emphasized that optimal acute pain management is patient-specific and pain syndrome-targeted when feasible, using a multimodal approach that includes pharmacological and nonpharmacological interventions. They recommend the assessment of pain and need for therapy be based on an overall accounting of patient status, including functional assessment, rather than solely on patient-reported pain scores.[290]

In summary, although the routine use of patient-reported pain scales may facilitate the administration of analgesics and be somewhat useful in trending response to analgesia, experienced clinicians and the authors recognize their limitations in an ED clinical setting. Specific pain scales do not have diagnostic or prognostic value. Pain scales are best used to assist in recognition of pain and prompt the most prudent management in the ED.

REFERENCES ARE AVAILABLE AT ELSEVIER EBOOKS+

CHAPTER 2

Devices for Assessing Oxygenation and Ventilation

Kristen Hart Shanahan and Andrew F. Miller

SPIROMETRY

For patients with acute exacerbations of asthma and chronic obstructive pulmonary disease (COPD), accurately estimating the severity of airflow obstruction is a critical component of their care. Although a focused history plus physical examination is the cornerstone of this assessment in the practice of emergency medicine, wide variation exists in the ability to accurately diagnose airway obstruction, and a significant proportion of patients with marked airflow obstruction present without dyspnea. This blunted perception of disease severity may be a contributor to fatal and near-fatal asthma attacks.[1,2] Similarly, patients presenting with acute exacerbations of asthma may experience subjective resolution of their symptoms after therapy, even when severe airflow obstruction is still present. Given these difficulties in recognizing airflow obstruction, objective measurement provides valuable information.

Spirometry is the measurement of the volume of air exhaled during forced expiration. It can be interpreted as a function of time to determine the flow rate. Spirometry gives the most complete picture of lung mechanics and is the centerpiece of pulmonary function testing. Some of the most useful parameters derived from a spirogram including forced vital capacity (FVC), which is the total volume exhaled during a forced expiratory maneuver, and forced expiratory volume in 1 second (FEV_1), which is the average flow rate during the first second of the forced expiratory maneuver (Fig. 2.1).

The advent of small handheld devices allows convenient spirometric evaluation in the emergency department (ED). The most common objective measurement of respiratory mechanics used in the ED is peak expiratory flow rate (PEFR). PEFR is the maximum flow of gas achieved during a forced expiratory maneuver. It correlates well with standard spirometry and has been studied extensively in the ED and outpatient setting.[3–5]

Indications

Evaluation of Acute Asthma Attacks

Currently, no standards exist for the measurement of pulmonary function parameters in ED patients, and practices vary widely. Most patients with asthma exacerbations can be evaluated, treated, and given a disposition with no further pulmonary function testing other than PEFR if quantitative assessment is deemed prudent. The 2019 American College of Emergency Physicians (ACEP) policy statement suggests that the decision to measure PEFR in patients with acute asthma should be individualized. There is no evidence that demonstrates improved outcomes with PEFR use in the emergency setting.[6] It is reasonable that asthma exacerbations be evaluated and treated according to clinical judgment. If any pulmonary function parameters are to be utilized, their use should be optimized, including measurements at arrival, after initial treatment, and periodically thereafter.[7–9]

Evaluation of Exacerbations of COPD

PEFR and spirometry testing can yield objective data on airflow obstruction during the ED evaluation of COPD exacerbations. Though used by some ED practitioners, consensus guidelines do not recommend routine use of these tests in the acute setting.[10]

Differentiating Causes of Dyspnea

PEFR has been studied for its ability to differentiate between COPD and congestive heart failure (CHF).[11,12] Insufficient data exist to recommend its routine use for this purpose in the ED.

Evaluation of Neuromuscular and Chest Wall Disease

Diseases of the chest wall and neuromuscular system can cause respiratory compromise. Though not commonly done in the ED, pulmonary function testing and assessment of negative inspiratory force can quantify the degree of impairment and help determine the level of ventilatory support required.

Contraindications

Need for Immediate Intervention

Patients with severe respiratory compromise should receive aggressive therapy without delaying care for pulmonary function testing. Although portable pulmonary function testing may guide management, providing immediate intervention for those in distress should be the priority. Formal pulmonary function testing has limited value for acute exacerbations, and such assessments are most predictive when patients are at their baseline functional status.

Conditions That May Be Worsened by Increased Intrathoracic Pressure

Significant elevations in intrathoracic pressure will develop in patients performing a forced expiratory maneuver. Pneumothorax and pneumomediastinum may be exacerbated by the forced expiratory maneuver and aneurysms of the aorta or the cerebral vasculature could theoretically be affected with increased pressures. The presence of these conditions should be considered a relative contraindication to pulmonary function testing.

Equipment

Spirometers can be divided into two categories. Volume spirometers measure the amount of gas exhaled as a function of time. These devices tend to be cumbersome and are not ideally suited to the ED. Flow spirometers measure the flow of gas past a certain point and use that information to extrapolate volume and time data. These machines are smaller, simpler to use, and more portable. Flow spirometers determine gas flow by measuring the difference in pressure between two points in a tube (pneumotachograph), cooling of a heated wire (hot wire anemometer), or revolutions of a rotating vane. Most handheld spirometers also measure PEFR.

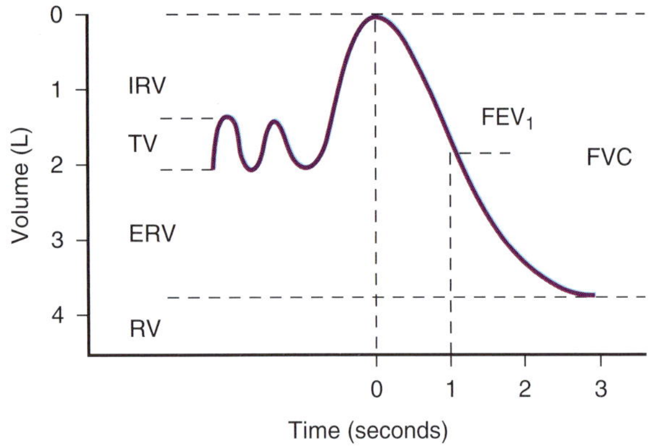

Fig. 2.1 Diagrammatic representation of spirometry values. *ERV,* Expiratory reserve volume; *FEV₁* forced expiratory volume in 1 second; *FVC,* forced vital capacity; *IRV,* inspiratory reserve volume; *RV,* residual volume; *TV,* tidal volume.

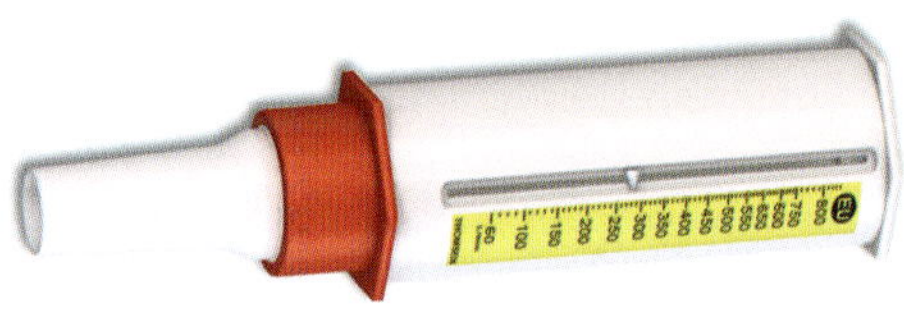

Fig. 2.2 "Mini-Wright" peak flow meter.

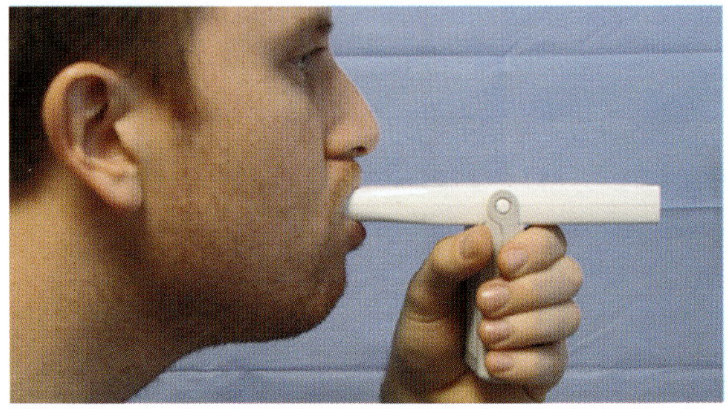

Fig. 2.3 Measurement of the peak expiratory flow rate (PEFR) with a portable disposable peak flow meter. Ask the patient to take a maximal inspiration with the lips sealed around the mouthpiece and then initiate a rapid, forceful expiration immediately afterward. Three separate measurements should be obtained. Be sure to zero the device before each test. PEFR is the easiest and most common pulmonary function test used to evaluate asthma in the emergency department. Trends are more important than actual values because individual baselines vary widely. PEFR alone cannot be used to make accurate clinical decisions on admission or discharge.

The most commonly used device to measure PEFR is the "mini-Wright" peak-flow flow meter (Fig. 2.2). These meters provide accurate and reproducible measurements of PEFR.[13] Variation exists between types and brands of peak-flow flow meters, so comparative measurements should be recorded with the same brand of peak-flow flow meter when possible.

Procedure

See Video 2.1. Calibrate the spirometer in accordance with the manufacturer's directions and examine the peak-flow meter to ensure that the measurement bar is resting at the zero line before beginning the procedure. For multipatient devices, attach a disposable mouthpiece to the input orifice.

Before starting the test, explain the procedure and allow unfamiliar patients to practice a few times. Ideally, the patient should be in the standing position or, if not feasible, be seated upright in bed. Ask the patient to elevate the chin and hold the neck in a slightly extended position. A nose clip is not required for PEFR measurements, but may be useful when performing formal spirometry testing.

After a period of normal breathing, ask the patient to take a maximal inspiration with the lips sealed around the mouthpiece while taking care to keep the tongue from partially obstructing the mouthpiece. Because airflow is greatest when the lung volumes are highest and the airways are larger, the test is accurate only if performed after maximal inspiration. Request the patient to initiate a rapid, forceful expiration as soon as possible after reaching maximal inspiration (Fig. 2.3). Coach the patient throughout the procedure and remind the patient to continue to make a forceful and complete exhalation. The PEFR usually occurs during the first 100 ms of expiration. In contrast, when performing spirometry, it is essential that the patient exhale fully. With both tests it is important to have a rapid, forceful exhalation rather than a slow, sustained effort. Obtain three separate measurements for both spirometry and PEFR.

PEFR measurements are very sensitive to technique and patient effort. Even a small decrease in effort can lead to considerable degradation of results.[8] In addition, any deviation from technique can lead to inaccurate results and a faulty estimation of the degree of airway obstruction. Therefore emergency physicians should directly observe and guide their patients when performing this testing.[14]

Interpretation

Obstructive diseases are characterized by a disproportionate decrease in airflow (FEV_1) in relation to the volume of gas exhaled (FVC).[10] A decreased FEV_1/FVC ratio with preservation of FVC indicates the presence of airflow obstruction. Restrictive diseases decrease total lung capacity and therefore decrease FVC to a greater degree than FEV_1. Decreased FVC with a normal or increased FEV_1/FVC ratio is indicative of restriction. It is useful to consider the FEV_1/FVC ratio when attempting to determine whether a patient has airflow obstruction. In patients with an established diagnosis of obstructive disease, FEV_1 is the test that best reflects changes in lung function. Typical values are shown in Table 2.1. These values are dependent on age, sex, and height and can be predicted from mathematical equations.[15–17] These reference ranges are based on equations with race/ethnicity as a variable. Recent evidence suggests that race-neutral equations should be used to create new reference ranges for predicted PEFR values.[18,19]

Isolated measurements of PEFR are not reliable in making the diagnosis of asthma because of significant variation between individuals. It is appropriate to use PEFR to monitor the degree of airflow obstruction in patients with known asthma.

Although measures of airflow obstruction are not standalone tests, they can provide additional objective information when considered along with other clinical factors. The highest of three PEFR or FEV_1 measurements should be

TABLE 2.1 Approximate Values

	FEV_1 (L)	FVC (L)	FEV_1/FVC RATIO (%)
Male	3.0–5.0	3.5–6.0	75–85
Female	2–3.5	2.5–4.0	75–85

FEV_1, Forced expiratory volume in 1 second; *FVC*, forced vital capacity.
Modified from Hankinson JL, Odencrantz JR, Fedan KB. Spirometric reference values from a sample of the general US population. *Am J Respir Crit Care Med.* 1999;159:179.

TABLE 2.2 Severity of Asthma Exacerbations According to Objective Measures of Airflow Obstruction

% OF PERSONAL BEST OR PREDICTED (FEV_1 OR PEFR)	SEVERITY OF EXACERBATION
≤30	Life-threatening
31–50	Severe
51–80	Moderate
>80	Mild

FEV_1, Forced expiratory volume in 1 second; *PEFR*, peak expiratory flow rate.

used and, whenever possible, compared with the patient's personal best.[7,8] In circumstances where previous best values are unknown or thought to be inaccurate, comparison with predicted values is appropriate. References are available for predicted PEFR values for adults.[15,18–20] These references are also based on equations with race/ethnicity as a variable, and new reference ranges are called for.[18,19] The National Asthma Education and Prevention Program has used the results of FEV_1 and PEFR testing to classify the severity of asthma exacerbations (Table 2.2).[9]

Multiple guidelines and articles have advocated specific cutoff values for PEFR and FEV_1 to guide decisions on disposition; however, there is variation within these guidelines and spirometry has not been shown to alter outcomes in the ED.[6–9] Spirometric values including PEFR and FEV_1 should be viewed as additional data points to be considered, along with other clinical variables such as response to inhaled bronchodilators in determining the disposition of patients with asthma seen in the ED. Poor response to treatment or failure to recover PEFR or FEV_1 to greater than 70% of personal best are examples of factors that might favor admission rather than outpatient management of acute asthma exacerbations.

NONINVASIVE OXYGENATION MONITORING: PULSE OXIMETRY

Pulse oximetry, or noninvasive measurement of the percentage of hemoglobin bound to O_2, provides real-time estimates of arterial saturation in the range of 80% to 100% and gives early warning of diminished capillary perfusion while avoiding the discomfort and risks associated with arterial puncture. Pulse oximetry is the standard of care in well-resourced clinical settings.

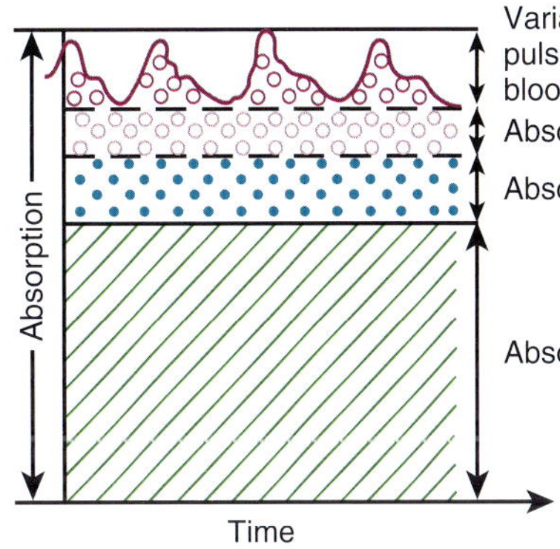

Fig. 2.4 Factors influencing light absorption through a pulsatile vascular bed. (From McGough EK, Boysen PG. Benefits and limitations of pulse oximetry in the ICU. *J Crit Illness*. 1989;4:23.)

Technology

Oximetry is based on the Beer-Lambert law, which states the concentration of an unknown solute dissolved in a solvent can be determined by light absorption. Pulse oximetry combines the principles of optical plethysmography and spectrophotometry. The probe, set into a reusable clip or a disposable patch, is made up of two photodiodes, which produce red light at 660 nm and infrared (IR) light at 900 nm to 940 nm, and a photodetector, which is placed across a pulsatile vascular bed. Pulse oximeter sensors are typically placed on the finger, with the light centered over the nailbed, not the fat pad. Other locations such as the toes and earlobes are used in some settings, including pediatrics. These particular wavelengths are used because the absorption characteristics of oxyhemoglobin and reduced hemoglobin are quite different at the two wavelengths. The majority of the light is absorbed by connective tissue, skin, bones, and venous blood. The amount of light absorbed by these substances is constant with time and does not vary during the cardiac cycle. A small increase in arterial blood occurs with each heartbeat, thereby resulting in an increase in light absorption (Fig. 2.4). By comparing the ratio of pulsatile and baseline absorption at these two wavelengths, the ratio of oxyhemoglobin to reduced hemoglobin is calculated.

Because the pulse oximeter uses only two wavelengths of light, it can distinguish only two substances. Pulse oximeters measure "functional saturation": the concentration of oxyhemoglobin divided by the concentrations of oxyhemoglobin plus reduced hemoglobin. The disadvantage of functional saturation is that the denominator *does not include other hemoglobin species that may be present, such as carboxyhemoglobin and methemoglobin*. The advantage of using only two wavelengths in the oximeter is that the cost, size, and weight of the device are reduced. Alternative devices, such as the CO-oximeter, use four or more wavelengths to measure "fractional saturation" and quantify additional hemoglobin species.

Physiology

Arterial O_2 saturation (Sao_2) measures the large reservoir of O_2 carried by hemoglobin, 20 mL of O_2/100 mL of blood, and arterial O_2 partial pressure (Pao_2) measures only the relatively small amount of O_2 dissolved in plasma, approximately 0.3 mL of O_2/100 mL of blood. Sao_2 correlates well with Pao_2, but the relationship is nonlinear and is described by the

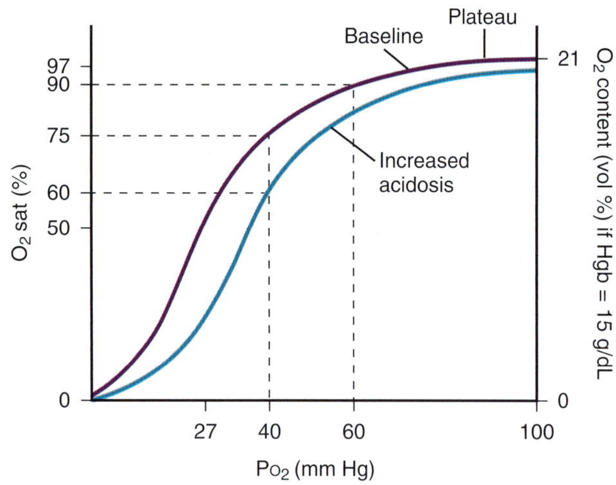

Fig. 2.5 Oxyhemoglobin dissociation curve. Measurements of Sao_2 are relatively insensitive in detecting significant changes in Pao_2 at high levels of oxygenation because these Sao_2 values fall on the plateau portion of the curve (labeled). Hence, O_2 saturation is an insensitive way of detecting early compensation in patients with asthma.

BOX 2.1 Clinical Applications of Pulse Oximetry

Assessing the adequacy of preoxygenation before endotracheal intubation
Monitoring oxygenation during emergency airway management
Monitoring the ventilator and changes in Fio_2
Providing an early indicator of ventilator dysfunction
Assisting in routine weaning from O_2 therapy
Monitoring patients in acute respiratory distress
Monitoring during procedural sedation and analgesia
Monitoring during interhospital and intrahospital transport

Fio_2, *Fractional concentration of inspired O_2.*

oxyhemoglobin dissociation curve (Fig. 2.5). In hypoxemic patients, small changes in Sao_2 represent large changes in Pao_2 because these Sao_2 values fall on the steep portion of the curve. Conversely, measurements of Sao_2 are relatively insensitive in detecting significant changes in Pao_2 at high levels of oxygenation because these Sao_2 values fall on the plateau portion of the curve.

Currently available pulse oximeters are accurate and precise when saturation ranges from 70% to 100% in patients with low melanin content in the skin and are more likely to overestimate blood oxygenation in patients who have higher melanin content (see section on "Racial Bias in Pulse Oximetry").[20] The range of 70% to 100% is considered satisfactory because for most patients an O_2 saturation of 80% or less requires urgent intervention.

Racial Bias in Pulse Oximetry Measurement

Racial and ethnic disparities in the overestimation of blood oxygenation by pulse oximetry lead to inequitable delivery of care in the management of hypoxia. The sources of this bias likely include inadequate enrollment of subjects with high melanin concentrations in the skin during testing and calibration and failure to adjust for melanin interference in measurement during device development.[21] The biased blood oxygen overestimation leads to more occult hypoxia in Black and Hispanic patients monitored with pulse oximetry. Occult hypoxia impacts clinical decision-making and leads to lack of intervention and treatment delays in Black and Hispanic patients. Because occult hypoxia affects treatment eligibility, racial bias in the accuracy of pulse oximetry is an important form of systemic racism in medicine, leading to inequitable delivery of care and racial and ethnic inequities in health.[22–24]

Clinical Utility

Pulse oximetry peripheral oxygen saturation (Spo_2) offers an advantage in assessing the adequacy of oxygenation over arterial blood gas analysis by providing continuous measurements. Direct measurement of Sao_2 requires blood gas values coupled with knowledge of the actual hemoglobin levels in a patient's blood. Sao_2 measurement is estimated with pulse oximetry. In this chapter, we equate Sao_2 and Spo_2.

There are limited data on the clinical efficacy of pulse oximetry monitoring in the ED.[25–27] Anesthesia studies have demonstrated that continuous monitoring of saturation can improve detection of hypoxemia and related events, though this practice has not been shown to impact major clinical outcomes such as mortality or transfer to the intensive care unit (ICU).[28] There may be benefit to use in emergency medicine, particularly in those with primary cardiopulmonary disease or critically ill patients. Rapid recognition of adverse physiologic events should allow prompt initiation of therapeutic interventions.

Indications

Recommended uses for pulse oximetry fall into two broad categories: (1) as a real-time indicator of hypoxemia, continuous oximetry monitoring can be used as a warning system because many adverse patient events are associated with arterial desaturation, and (2) as an end point for titration of therapeutic interventions to avoid hypoxia (Box 2.1).

Pulse oximetry can also be used to assess peripheral perfusion and evaluate for possible ischemia in the extremities. Although clinical experience validates its use, minimal data are available for such utilization in the ED. Vascular surgeons will use a pulse oximetry probe on a finger or toe to assess the results of vascular surgery on the arm or leg. Peripheral artery occlusion from peripheral artery disease may be suggested by comparison of pulse oximetry readings in the extremities. Decreased peripheral oxygenation may be detected in patients with compartment syndrome, traumatic arterial injury, and external compression of the proximal circulation, such as inflated blood pressure cuffs (Fig. 2.6; Video 2.2).

Procedure

The location for the probe is determined by the clinical situation and the types of probes available (Fig. 2.7). A reusable clip-on probe works well on digits that are easily accessible. Other sites include the earlobe, the nasal bridge, the septum, the forehead/temporal artery, and the foot or palm of an infant. More central locations may provide better readings in cold ambient temperature or during movement. Tape and splints can be used to secure oximetry probes and minimize motion.

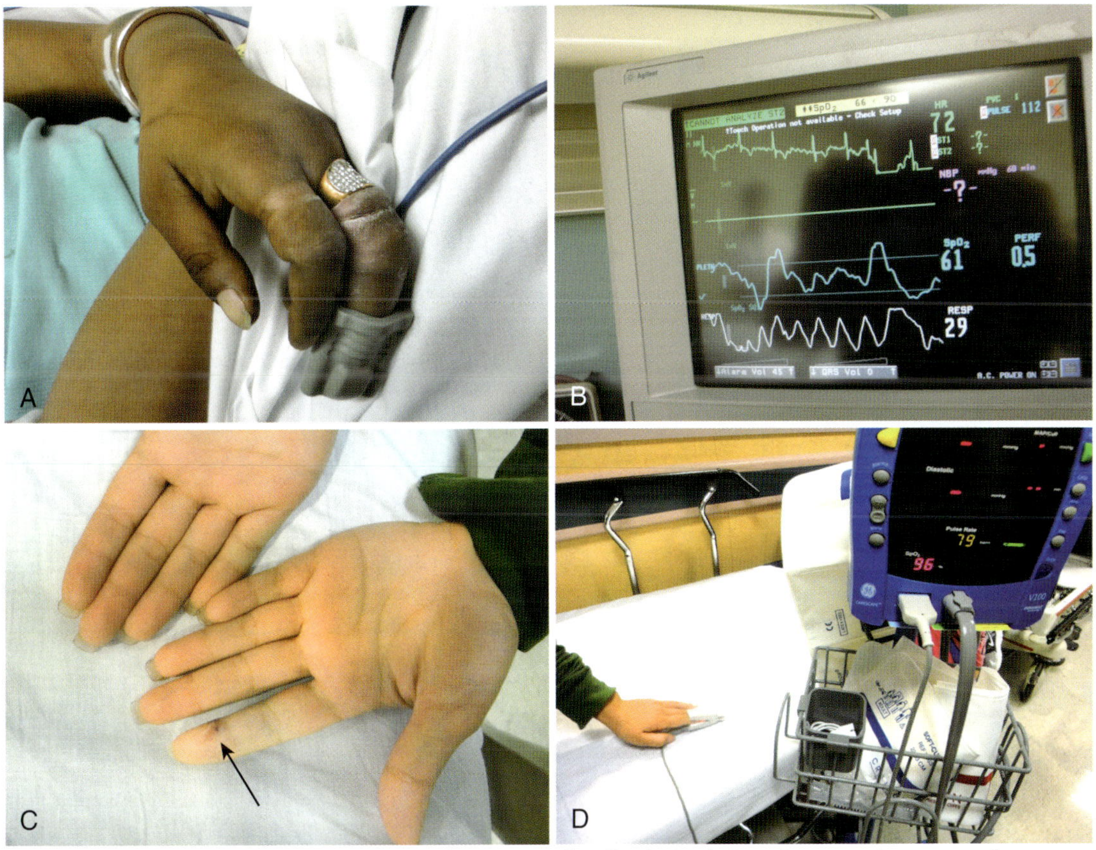

Fig. 2.6 Pulse oximetry can be used to assess the distal circulation after vascular surgery for trauma and to initially evaluate other causes of decreased peripheral perfusion. (A) This patient had a markedly swollen and ischemic finger from a tight ring. (B) Although the need for immediate removal of the ring is clinically obvious, a pulse oximetry probe confirmed ischemia with an O_2 saturation of 61%. The uninvolved fingers registered 99%. Following ring removal the saturation returned to normal, thus suggesting that fasciotomy need not be performed. (C) When a discharged EpiPen caused a pale finger, injection of phentolamine was considered. (D) When pulse oximetry demonstrated a saturation of 96% (97% to 98% in the other fingers), injection was not performed and the circulation spontaneously normalized over a period of 30 minutes.

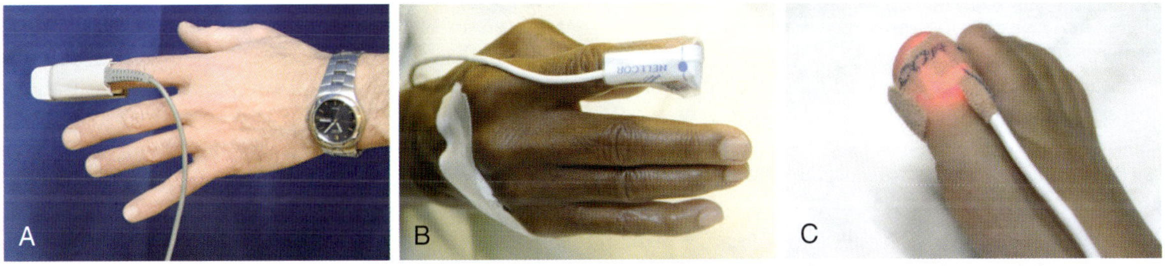

Fig. 2.7 Pulse oximeter sensors. (A) Reusable adult sensor, attached to finger. (B) Single-use adult sensor, attached to finger. (C) Single-use pediatric sensor, attached to toe. Note that the light source is centered over the nail, not the fat pad. See text for various parameters that affect pulse oximetry readings.

The computer analyzes the incoming data to identify the arteriolar pulsation and displays this parameter as beats per minute. Newer devices also display a pulse plethysmograph (Fig. 2.8). Simultaneously, O_2 saturation is displayed on a beat-to-beat basis. Machines differ in their display when a pulsatile flow is not detected. Either the reading will not display at all, or the SaO_2 value will be given along with a poor-signal quality warning. It is important to evaluate serial measurements and to verify that the measurements correlate with other clinical markers.

Interpretation

Patients with normal physiologic gas exchange have an O_2 saturation between 97% and 100%. When SaO_2 falls below 95%, hypoxemia may be present, which may be baseline for some patients with cardiac or lung disease. O_2 saturation below 90% represents hypoxemia. As with spirometry, an isolated, low early measurement of SaO_2 does not mandate admission because of the potential for rapid response to therapy. Low

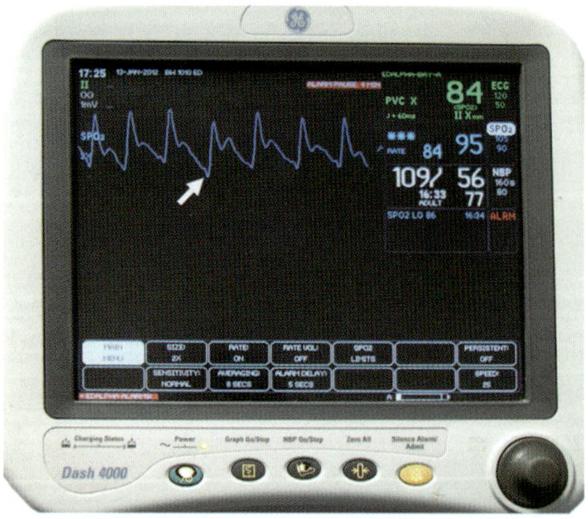

Fig. 2.8 Patient monitor displaying a pulse plethysmograph *(arrow)*. The patient's heart rate (84) and O_2 saturation (95) are also displayed *(blue numbers)*.

BOX 2.2 Factors Affecting Pulse Oximetry Readings

Racial bias: Underestimates hypoxia due to melanin in skin
Severe anemia: Satisfactory readings obtained down to a hemoglobin level of 5 mg/dL
Motion artifact: See text regarding probe sites
Dyes: Transient effect unless resulting in methemoglobinemia
Light artifact: Minimize by covering the probe with opaque material
Hypoperfusion: An inadequate pulse signal will be displayed
Electrocautery: Minimize by increasing the distance of the sensor from the surgical site
Dark nail polish: Remove with acetone or place a sensor sideways on the digit
Dyshemoglobinemias (e.g., carboxyhemoglobin and methemoglobin): Falsely elevate true oxygen saturation readings
Elevated bilirubin: Accurate up to a bilirubin level of 20 mg/dL in adults; no problem reported in jaundiced children
High saturation: Pulse oximetry not useful for monitoring hyperoxemia in neonates
Fetal hemoglobin: No effect on pulse oximetry; falsely reduced CO-oximetry readings
Venous pulsations: Artificially lower O_2 saturation; choose a probe site above the heart
Dialysis graft (arteriovenous fistula): No difference from the contralateral extremity unless the fistula is producing distal ischemia.

Sao_2 readings should be heeded as important clinical warning signs. Pulse oximetry may be affected by numerous extrinsic factors, and a decline in O_2 saturation with serial measurements should always prompt an evaluation of respiratory status and adequacy of circulation.

Although pulse oximetry represents a significant advance in noninvasive monitoring of oxygenation, clinicians must recognize and understand its limitations.[20,29] Pulse oximetry overestimates oxygenation in people with high concentrations of skin melanin and introduces racial bias in the evaluation and management of hypoxia in this group (see section on "Racial Bias in Pulse Oximetry").[22,23] In addition, pulse oximetry measures only O_2 saturation. In contrast to arterial blood gas determination, pulse oximetry provides no direct information on pH or the arterial partial pressure of CO_2 ($Paco_2$). Nonetheless, a room-air Sao_2 value of 97% or higher strongly rules against hypoxemia and moderate to severe hypercapnia. A room-air Sao_2 value of 96% or less has been demonstrated to be 100% sensitive and 54% specific for detecting hypoxemia (Pao_2 <70 mm Hg), and 100% sensitive and 31% specific for detecting hypercapnia ($Paco_2$ >50 mm Hg). Using a cutoff value of 92% or less for room-air Sao_2 is more accurate in identifying hypoxemia in patients with COPD.

Pulse oximetry is not a substitute for monitoring ventilation because of the variable lag time between the onset of hypoventilation or apnea and a change in O_2 saturation. During procedural sedation, monitoring of ventilation is a more desirable goal for prevention of hypoxemia and hypercapnia than simple pulse oximetry (see section on "Procedural Sedation and Analgesia" under "Carbon Dioxide Monitoring" later in this chapter). Hypoventilation and the resultant hypercapnia may precede a decrease in hemoglobin O_2 saturation by many minutes. Supplemental O_2 may mask hypoventilation by delaying the eventual O_2 desaturation that pulse oximetry is designed to monitor and recognize. Other limitations of pulse oximetry are summarized in Box 2.2.

Sources of Interference

Melanin

The accuracy of pulse oximeters is affected by melanin in the skin, leading to an overestimation of blood oxygenation in patients with more melanin (see section on "Racial Bias in Pulse Oximetry"). This effect may be due to a shift in the light-emitting diode's output spectrum as the light output is increased. By overestimating blood oxygenation in patients who are Black or Hispanic and misinforming clinical decisions by healthcare providers, this phenomenon may lead to treatment delays and lack of interventions, contributing to racial inequities in the delivery of healthcare.[22,23]

Effects of Dyshemoglobinemias

In patients with methemoglobinemia or elevated carboxyhemoglobin levels, pulse oximetry does not accurately depict quantitative changes in hemoglobin O_2 saturation.[20] Carboxyhemoglobin results in falsely elevated Sao_2 estimates of hemoglobin O_2 saturation. Low quantities of methemoglobin will reduce pulse oximetry readings by approximately half the actual methemoglobin percentage. Large quantities of methemoglobin (>10%) can result in a stable pulse oximetry reading of 85% regardless of the actual Sao_2. Because pulse oximetry will variably underestimate the percentage of abnormal hemoglobin, a CO-oximeter or blood gas sample for quantitative analysis is required for confirmation of these conditions.

Fetal Hemoglobin

Full-term newborns can have up to 75% of total hemoglobin in the form of fetal hemoglobin and up to 5% in the form of carboxyhemoglobin. Although fetal hemoglobin interferes with the spectrophotometric method, pulse oximetry will remain accurate. A CO-oximeter may erroneously interpret the carboxyhemoglobin level as elevated and the oxyhemoglobin level as artificially reduced. When fetal hemoglobin levels are high, CO-oximetry readings should not be used to confirm pulse oximetry readings.

Low Perfusion

To function properly, pulse oximeters require a pulsating vascular bed. Vasoconstriction related to hypotension, hypothermia, or the administration of vasoconstricting drugs may reduce the pulsatile component to less than 0.2% of the total signal. At this level, the true signal cannot be distinguished from background noise. Modern pulse oximeters have signal strength detectors and will display a message indicating an inadequate pulse signal when perfusion is compromised. Changing the location of the sensor to an area with higher perfusion, such as an earlobe or the forehead, may improve the pulse signal.

Intravenous Dyes

A number of dyes and pigments interfere with the accuracy of pulse oximetry.[30] Methylene blue, the treatment for methemoglobinemia, absorbs light at 660 nm, which is similar to the absorption of reduced hemoglobin, and can significantly decrease pulse oximeter saturation readings to as low as 1%. Low readings can also be seen with other intravenous dyes such as indigo carmine, indocyanine green, and fluorescein, although the rapid clearance of these agents minimizes this phenomenon.

Bilirubin

Hyperbilirubinemia does not affect the accuracy of pulse oximetry, but it may have an effect on absorption at the lower wavelengths used by CO-oximeters and result in a discrepancy between pulse oximeter and CO-oximeter readings.

Nail Polish and Synthetic Nails

Data suggest that some nail polishes may affect the accuracy of pulse oximetry.[31–33] Turning the probe sideways on the finger may improve accuracy, although removing any nail polish with acetone is the favored solution. The accuracy of Sao_2 readings in the setting of synthetic nails is unknown. If a poor signal is obtained through a synthetic nail, either the nail should be removed or an alternative site should be used for placement.

High Saturation

Because the O_2 dissociation curve plateaus at saturation levels greater than 90%, a large increase in Pao_2 results in only a small increase in saturation. An error of a few percentage points could represent a large error in Pao_2. Although inconsequential for most adults, this is of extreme importance for neonates, who are at risk for retinopathy and other pathologies caused by hyperoxemia.

Venous Pulsations

The increased venous pulsations resulting from right heart failure and tricuspid regurgitation can interfere with accurate readings and lead to artificially lower O_2 saturation because the pulse oximeter interprets any pulsatile measurement as arterial. Placing the probe on a site above the heart may improve accuracy. Some pulse oximeters have the capability of synchronizing pulsations at the probe site to electrocardiographic (ECG) signals, thus enhancing the signal-to-noise ratio.

Anemia

Because pulse oximetry depends on light absorption by hemoglobin, it becomes less accurate and less reliable in conditions of severe anemia.

Ambient Light

Because the pulse oximeter's photodetector is nonspecific, high-intensity ambient light can produce interference. Surgical, fluorescent, and heating lamps are common sources of light interference. This problem can be corrected by wrapping the probe with a light barrier, such as a dark cloth or other opaque material.

Motion

Motion of the probe can produce considerable artifact and inaccurate readings. Correlating a pulse oximetry signal with an ECG waveform or using alternative probe sites, such as the ear or toe, may reduce motion artifact. Newer-generation pulse oximetry signal processing technology has greatly reduced the effect of motion artifact.[34]

Probe Site

The finger is the most common probe site used for adult pulse oximetry. If the finger is inaccessible or unsuitable, other probe sites, such as the earlobe, nose, and forehead (using reflectance instead of transmittance), may be used. It should be noted, though, that forehead and nasal bridge probes may be less accurate than finger and ear probes. In infants and small children, an adhesive sensor unit is preferred and frequently placed on the fingers and toes. Probes can also be secured in place over the palm, heel, or lateral aspect of the foot with a gauze or wrap.

Electrocautery

Electrical interference from devices such as electrocautery can impair the accuracy of pulse oximetry. Such interference can be reduced by increasing the distance between the surgical site and the probe.

Conclusions

Pulse oximetry is a widely available technology that provides an easy and noninvasive method of monitoring oxygenation. Pulse oximetry leads to racial inequities in the evaluation and management of hypoxia due to the effects of increased concentrations of skin melanin causing in the overestimation of blood oxygenation on treatment initiation in Black and Hispanic patients. Because measurements are continuous, pulse oximetry allows earlier detection of hypoxic episodes than intermittent arterial blood gas analysis. Frequent measurements can lead to earlier corrective interventions and prevention of adverse consequences.

Future Directions

New technologies including polarization-based oximetry are being studied to noninvasively monitor oxygen saturations regardless of race or skin pigmentation to eliminate racial bias introduced by current methods.[35] Devices that focus on regional detection of O_2 saturation, specifically cerebral oximetry, are being studied for various clinical applications relevant to emergency medicine. This technology uses near-IR spectroscopy to obtain tissue-level O_2 saturations. Data are emerging to support cerebral oximetry monitoring to assess quality of cardiopulmonary resuscitation (CPR) and to predict return of spontaneous circulation for these patients.[36–44] Early studies have also suggested a role for cerebral oximetry in monitoring patients with altered mental status, including pharmacologically induced sedation.[45–48] Currently, there are no clear guidelines on when this technology should be used in an ED setting, and its growing experience may direct future applications in end-organ perfusion monitoring.[49]

CARBON DIOXIDE MONITORING

Capnography is a noninvasive measurement of the partial pressure of CO_2 in an exhaled breath. Measurement of CO_2 at the airway can be displayed as a function of time (CO_2 concentration over time) or as an exhaled tidal volume (CO_2 concentration over volume). This chapter focuses on the use of time-based capnography because it can be adapted for use in both patients with and without and endotracheal (ET) tube and is the only form of CO_2 monitoring used by the emergency medical service (EMS) and the predominant form used in the ED.

The relationship of CO_2 concentration to time is graphically represented by the CO_2 waveform or capnogram (Fig. 2.9). The maximum CO_2 concentration at the end of each tidal breath is the end-tidal CO_2 pressure (P_{ETCO_2}). Changes in the shape of the capnogram are diagnostic of disease conditions, and changes in P_{ETCO_2} can be used to assess disease severity and response to treatment.

Oxygenation and ventilation are distinct physiologic functions that are assessed in both patients who are intubated and spontaneously breathing. Pulse oximetry provides real-time feedback about oxygenation, and capnography provides breath-to-breath information about all of the following: ventilation (how effectively CO_2 is being eliminated by the pulmonary system); perfusion (how effectively CO_2 is being transported through the vascular system); and metabolism (how effectively CO_2 is being produced by cellular metabolism).

Terminology

The ancient Greeks believed that there was a combustion engine inside the body that gave off smoke (*capnos* in Greek) in the form of a breath. A capnometer is a CO_2 monitor that displays a number (i.e., P_{ETCO_2}). A capnograph is a CO_2 monitor that displays a number and a waveform (i.e., the capnogram).

Technology

Capnography became a routine part of anesthesia practice in Europe in the 1970s and in the United States in the 1980s. Capnography was incorporated into the American Heart Association (AHA) guidelines in 2000 and the ACEP guidelines in 2001 and has become the standard of care for verification of ET tube placement.

Most capnography technology is built on IR radiation techniques. These techniques are based on CO_2 molecules that absorb IR radiation at a very specific wavelength (4.26 μm), with the amount of radiation absorbed having a close to exponential relationship to the CO_2 concentration present in the breath sample. Detecting these changes in IR radiation levels by using appropriate photodetectors sensitive in this spectral region allows the CO_2 concentration in the gas sample to be calculated.

CO_2 monitors measure gas concentration or partial pressure by using one of two configurations, depending on the location of the sensor: mainstream or sidestream (Fig. 2.10). Mainstream devices measure CO_2 directly from the airway, with the sensor located at the proximal end of the ET tube. Sidestream devices measure CO_2 by aspirating a small sample from the exhaled breath through tubing and a sensor located inside the monitor. Mainstream systems are configured only for intubated patients because the sensor is located on the ET tube. Sidestream systems do not require an ET tube because the sensor is located inside the monitor and may therefore be used in either intubated or nonintubated patients. The airway interface for intubated patients is an airway adapter placed on the hub of the ET tube. For spontaneously breathing patients, a nasal-oral cannula is used. This allows concomitant CO_2 sampling and delivery of low-flow O_2 to the patient.

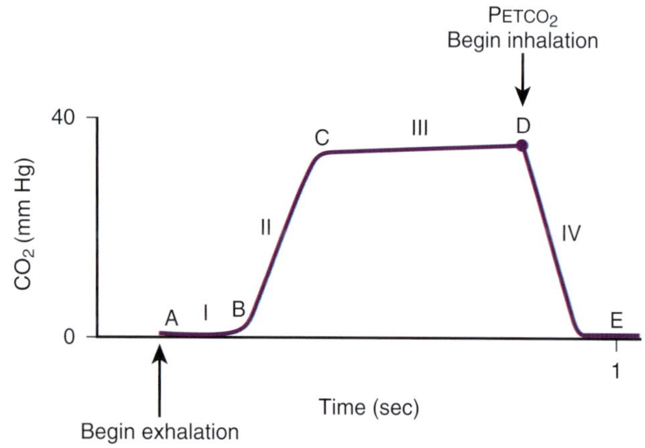

Fig. 2.9 Normal capnogram. The maximum CO_2 concentration at the end of exhalation of each tidal breath and at the beginning of inhalation is the end-tidal CO_2 pressure (P_{ETCO_2}), depicted by *D* on this graph. CO_2 pressure at *D* will be displayed numerically on the screen. See text for further explanation of the physiology of this graph. (From Krauss B, Hess DR. Capnography for procedural sedation and analgesia in the emergency department. *Ann Emerg Med.* 2007;50:172.)

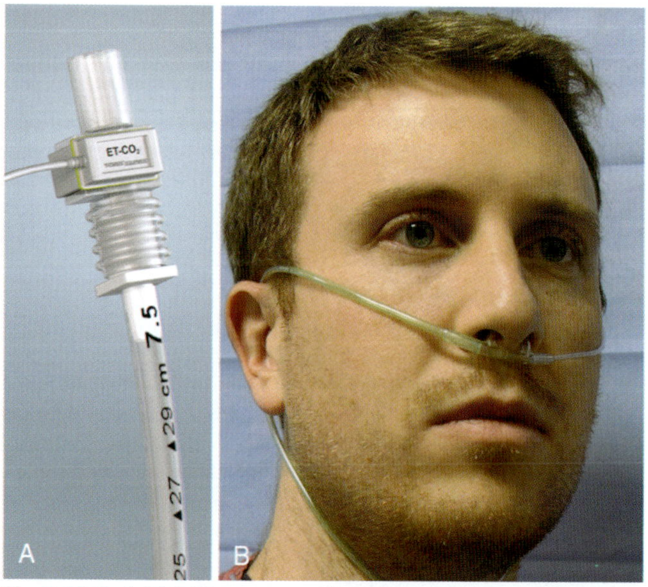

Fig. 2.10 End-tidal CO_2 sensors. (A) Mainstream sensor. This device measures CO_2 directly from the proximal end of an endotracheal tube. (B) Sidestream sensor. This cannula-type device allows concomitant CO_2 sampling and low-flow O_2 delivery to the patient.

Sidestream systems can be high-flow (requiring 150 mL/min of CO_2 in the breath sample to obtain an accurate reading) or low-flow (requiring 50 mL/min of CO_2). Low-flow sidestream systems have a lower occlusion rate (from moisture or patient secretions) and are more accurate in patients with low tidal volumes (neonates, infants, and patients with hypoventilation and low–tidal volume breathing).[50]

CO_2 monitors can be either quantitative or qualitative (Fig. 2.11). Quantitative devices measure the precise P_{ETCO_2} as either a number (capnometry) or a number and a waveform (capnography). Qualitative devices measure the range in which P_{ETCO_2} falls (e.g., 0 to 10 mm Hg, >35 mm Hg) as opposed to a precise value (e.g., 38 mm Hg). The most commonly used qualitative device is the colorimetric P_{ETCO_2} detector, consisting of a piece of specially treated litmus paper that turns color when exposed to CO_2. Its primary use is for verification of ET tube position. If the tube is in the trachea, the resultant exhalation of CO_2 will change the color of the litmus paper; if the tube is in the esophagus with no CO_2 in the breath, no change in color will take place.

Physiology

The capnogram, which corresponds to a single tidal breath, consists of four phases (ascending phase, alveolar plateau, inspiratory limb, and dead space ventilation; see Fig. 2.9). Each phase has conventionally been approximated as a straight line.[51,52] Phase I (dead space ventilation, A to B) represents the beginning of exhalation in which dead space is cleared from the upper airway. Phase II (ascending phase, B to C) represents the rapid rise in CO_2 concentration in the breath stream as CO_2 from the alveoli reaches the upper airway. Phase III (alveolar plateau, C to D) represents the CO_2 concentration reaching a uniform level in the entire breath stream (from alveolus to nose) and concludes with a point of maximum CO_2 pressure (P_{ETCO_2}). *This is the number that appears on the monitor display.* Phase IV (D to E) represents the inspiratory cycle in which the CO_2 concentration drops to zero as atmospheric air enters the airway.

A normal capnogram, for patients of all ages, is characterized by a specific set of elements: it includes the four distinct phases just described, the CO_2 concentration starts at zero and returns to zero (i.e., there is no rebreathing of CO_2), a maximum CO_2 concentration is reached with each breath (i.e., P_{ETCO_2}), the amplitude is dependent on P_{ETCO_2}, the width is dependent on the expiratory time, and there is a characteristic shape for all subjects with normal lung function.

Patients with normal lung function, irrespective of age, will have a characteristic rectangular- or trapezoidal-shaped capnogram and a narrow P_{ETCO_2}-P_{CO_2} gradient (0 to 5 mm Hg), with P_{ETCO_2} accurately reflecting Pa_{CO_2}. Patients with obstructive lung disease will have a more rounded ascending phase and an upward slope in the alveolar plateau (Fig. 2.12).[53] In patients with abnormal lung function from ventilation/perfusion ($\dot{V}/\dot{Q}$) mismatch, the gradient will widen depending on the severity of the lung disease, and P_{ETCO_2} will be useful only for trending ventilatory status over time and not as a spot check because it may not correlate with Pa_{CO_2}.

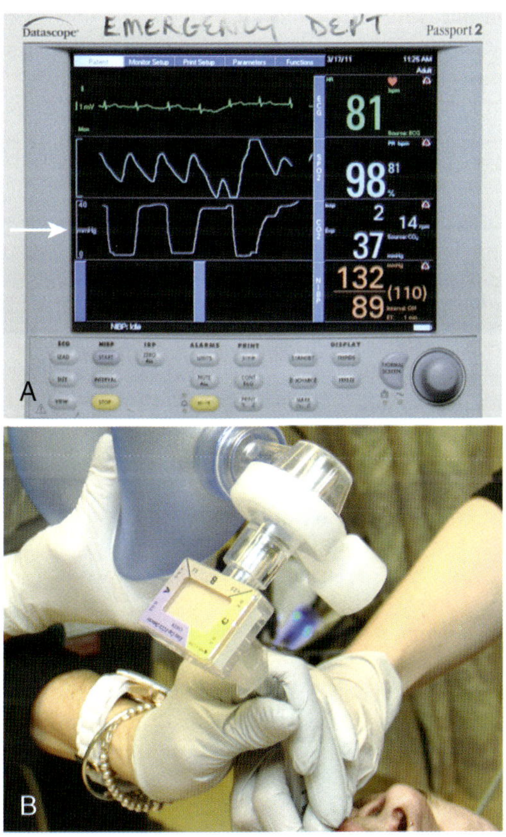

Fig. 2.11 CO_2 monitors. (A) Quantitative monitor. A capnography waveform *(arrow)* is displayed, as is a capnometry numerical reading (37). (B) Qualitative device. This simple colorimetric detector is used to verify endotracheal tube position and changes color when exposed to CO_2.

Indications for Intubated Patients

- Verification of ET tube placement
- Continuous monitoring of tube location during transport
- Gauging the effectiveness of resuscitation and prognosis during cardiac arrest
- Titrating P_{ETCO_2} levels in patients with suspected increases in intracranial pressure
- Determining prognosis in patients after trauma
- Determining the adequacy of ventilation

Verification of Endotracheal Tube Placement

Unrecognized misplaced intubation (UMI) is placement of an ET tube in a location other than the trachea that is not

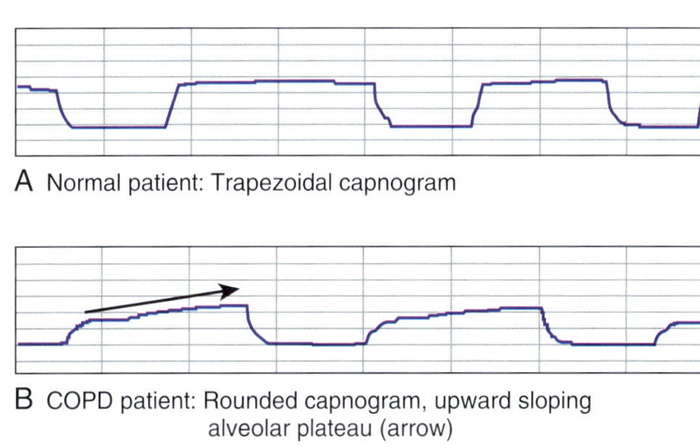

Fig. 2.12 Capnogram shape in (A) normal subjects and (B) patients with chronic obstructive pulmonary disease *(COPD)*. (From Krauss B, Deykin A, Lam A, et al. Capnogram shape in obstructive lung disease. *Anesth Analg.* 2005;100:884.)

recognized by the clinician. This life-threatening condition has been extensively documented in the EMS literature, with reported UMI rates most commonly between 7% and 10%.[54]

After intubation, the presence of a waveform with all four phases indicates that the ET tube is through the vocal cords. A flatline waveform following intubation indicates esophageal placement except in selected conditions, including obstruction of the ET tube, complete airway obstruction distal to the tube, tracheal placement with inadequate pulmonary blood flow as a result of poor chest compressions, or prolonged cardiac arrest with no circulating CO_2 because of cessation of cellular metabolism.

The accuracy of P_{ETCO_2} in confirming the tracheal location of an ET tube varies according to the type of CO_2 technology used. In adult patients who are not in cardiac arrest, qualitative colorimetric P_{ETCO_2} and quantitative capnography studies have demonstrated 100% sensitivity and specificity for tracheal placement.[55] In delivery room settings with preterm infants, the colorimetric verification may fail to perform accurately.[56] The use of clinical signs for ET tube verification has been shown to be unreliable. Fogging or condensation of the tube, chest wall movement, and auscultation for breath sounds have all been demonstrated to incorrectly identify tube location in some cases, including esophageal intubations.

Although the accuracy of P_{ETCO_2} in verifying ET tube placement is 100% in adult patients with spontaneous circulation or low-perfusion states, sensitivity for tracheal placement in cardiac arrest patients ranges from 57% to 100%, depending on the type of CO_2 monitoring used and the duration of the arrest.[55,57] Data are limited regarding specificity of capnography to detect esophageal intubations in cardiac arrest. When a waveform is present in an intubated patient in cardiac arrest, the ET tube can be assumed to be in the trachea. Absence of a waveform may result from esophageal intubation or a correctly placed ET tube in a patient with insufficient pulmonary blood flow.

Colorimetric studies have shown variable sensitivity because the exhaled CO_2 concentration can fall below the detection threshold. It is particularly important when evaluating P_{ETCO_2} studies to distinguish those involving qualitative colorimetric detection from those using capnography.

Monitoring Tube Position During Transport

UMI (as a result of either initial misplacement of the ET tube or subsequent dislodgment during transport) can have catastrophic consequences and is largely preventable. Capnography has been demonstrated to help prehospital providers recognize ET tube dislodgement leading to more rapid correction of tube position.[58] Continuous monitoring of tube position during transport (prehospital to hospital, interhospital, or intrahospital) is essential for patient safety. P_{ETCO_2} confirmation of initial ET tube placement with continuous monitoring of tube position is an accepted standard of care by the American Society of Anesthesiologists and is recommended by other national organizations.[59]

Gauging the Effectiveness of Cardiopulmonary Resuscitation

Studies using animal models in the 1980s demonstrated that P_{ETCO_2} levels reflect cardiac output during CPR and can be used as a noninvasive measure of cardiac output. A landmark study in 1988 demonstrated this principle in humans (Fig. 2.13).[60] During cardiac arrest, when alveolar ventilation and metabolism are essentially constant, P_{ETCO_2} reflects the

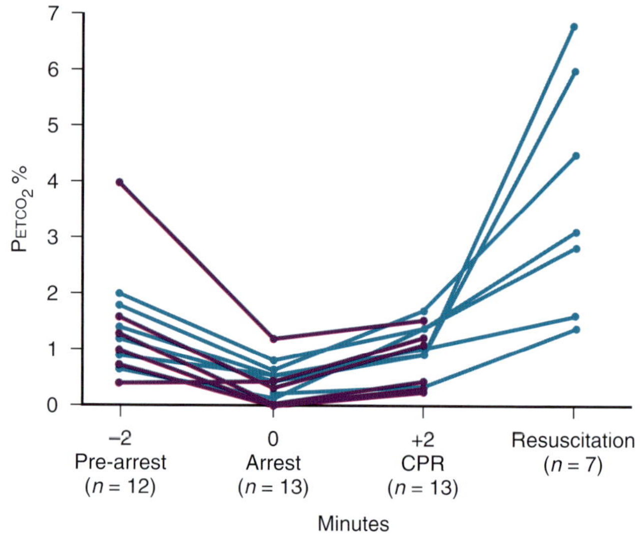

Fig. 2.13 End-tidal carbon dioxide concentration *(P_{ETCO_2})* pattern during cardiac arrest. *CPR*, Cardiopulmonary resuscitation. (Modified from Falk JL, Rackow ED, Weil MH. End-tidal carbon dioxide concentration during cardiopulmonary resuscitation. *N Engl J Med* 1988;318:607.)

degree of pulmonary blood flow. Therefore P_{ETCO_2} can be used as a gauge of the effectiveness of cardiac compressions. Effective cardiac compression leads to higher cardiac output, and the resultant increase in perfusion corresponds to a rise in P_{ETCO_2} from baseline.[61] The 2020 AHA Guidelines recommends monitoring end-tidal CO_2 ($ETCO_2$) during CPR to improve chest compression performance if $ETCO_2$ is <10 mm Hg, and titrating to a goal $ETCO_2$ of >20 mm Hg.[61,62] While this goal $ETCO_2$ has clearly been shown in adult populations to be beneficial, there has not been clear data to suggest this in pediatrics, yet this is still the recommendation by the AHA.[63]

Indicator of Return of Spontaneous Circulation

A peak in P_{ETCO_2} is the earliest sign of return of spontaneous circulation (ROSC) and may occur before palpable or measurable hemodynamic signs (pulse or blood pressure).[60] When the heart resumes contractions, the dramatic increase in cardiac output and the resulting increase in perfusion lead to a rapid increase in P_{ETCO_2} from baseline as the CO_2 that has built up in the blood during cardiac arrest is effectively transported to the lungs and exhaled.

The AHA guidelines emphasize the importance of continuing chest compressions without interruption until a perfusing rhythm is reestablished. Experimental evidence indicates that interruptions in chest compressions are followed by sustained periods during which flow gradually returns to preinterruption levels. Capnography provides a means of monitoring the patient's physiological response to ongoing resuscitative efforts with minimal interruption to compressions for the purpose of checking for pulses. Reestablishment of a perfusing rhythm will be immediately accompanied by a dramatic increase in P_{ETCO_2}, albeit in young infants the increase in $ETCO_2$ may not be as dramatic as in adults or older children.[64]

Assessing Prognosis After Initiation of Cardiac Arrest Resuscitation

Multiple factors can affect the recorded $ETCO_2$ values during cardiac arrest resuscitations.[65] P_{ETCO_2} can be used as a prognostic indicator of ROSC and survival in adult cardiac arrest patients. In multiple studies, P_{ETCO_2} levels of 10 mm Hg or lower measured 20 minutes after the initiation of advanced cardiac life support accurately predicted death in patients with cardiac arrest.[61] Newer studies suggest that a P_{ETCO_2} level of 20 mm Hg or higher at intubation during cardiac arrest coupled with a positive trend of the P_{ETCO_2} at 10 minutes of CPR is a predictor of survival to hospital discharge with good neurologic outcome.[66]

Identifying the Cause of Cardiac Arrest

Though not generally used clinically, differences in P_{ETCO_2} may be seen depending on the cause of the cardiac arrest. Animal studies reported higher P_{ETCO_2} values at the onset of cardiac arrest caused by primary asphyxia than after arrest caused by ventricular fibrillation. Prehospital cardiac arrest studies have demonstrated higher P_{ETCO_2} results in patients with cardiac arrest secondary to respiratory or asphyxia causes than for those with primary cardiac etiologies.[65,67]

Titrating $ETCO_2$ in Patients With Suspected Increased Intracranial Pressure

P_{ETCO_2} monitoring has been shown to play a role in controlled ventilation in patients with head injury and suspected increased intracranial pressure. CO_2 levels affect blood flow to the brain, with high CO_2 levels resulting in cerebral vasodilation and low CO_2 levels resulting in cerebral vasoconstriction. Sustained hypoventilation (P_{ETCO_2} ≥50 mm Hg) is detrimental to patients with increased intracranial pressure because it results in increased cerebral blood flow and potential worsening of intracranial pressure.

Sustained hyperventilation is also detrimental and associated with worse neurologic outcome in severely brain-injured patients. Unless a patient is actively herniating, ventilation with CO_2 monitoring to achieve normocapnia is recommended. The benefit of continuous P_{ETCO_2} monitoring for this indication has been demonstrated in many prehospital-based studies. Severe head-injury patients monitored with continuous P_{ETCO_2} have better-controlled ventilation, linked to improved outcomes.[68]

P_{ETCO_2} monitoring has also demonstrated prognostic value in determining outcome in trauma patients requiring prehospital ET intubation. Specifically, lower P_{ETCO_2} levels 20 minutes after intubation are associated with poor survival and may predict the need for massive transfusion.[69,70]

Indications for Capnography in Spontaneously Breathing Patients

In patients who are spontaneously breathing and nonintubated, capnography can be used in a variety of clinical indications, including:

- Rapid assessment of critically ill, injured, or seizing patients through assessment of the airway, breathing, and circulation (ABCs)
- Assessment and triage of victims of chemical terrorism and mass casualty
- Gauging the severity and response to treatment in patients with acute respiratory distress
- Determining the adequacy of ventilation in patients with altered mental status
- Detecting metabolic acidosis (including diabetic ketoacidosis and gastroenteritis)

Assessment of Critically Ill, Injured, or Seizing Patients

The ABCs of critically ill or injured patients can be assessed rapidly by using the capnogram and P_{ETCO_2}. The presence of a normal waveform denotes a patent airway and spontaneous breathing. Normal P_{ETCO_2} (35 to 45 mm Hg) signifies adequate perfusion.

Capnography can be used to assess and triage critically ill or injured patients and actively seizing patients. When used to triage undifferentiated patients, capnography outperforms other vital signs when predicting intensive care admission.[71] Unlike pulse oximetry, capnography is not affected by motion artifact and provides reliable readings in low-perfusion states.

Capnography is a reliable, accurate monitoring modality for actively seizing patients. Capnographic data (respiratory rate [RR], P_{ETCO_2}, and capnogram) can be used to distinguish among:

- Seizing patients with apnea (flatline waveform, no P_{ETCO_2} readings, and no chest wall movement)
- Seizing patients with ineffective ventilation (small waveforms, low P_{ETCO_2})
- Seizing patients with effective ventilation (normal waveform, normal P_{ETCO_2})

Assessment and Triage of Victims of Chemical Terrorism and Mass Casualty

EDs and EMS systems have focused on training to identify and effectively manage mass casualty and chemical terrorism events. Capnography can serve as a noninvasive assessment tool to quickly identify the common life-threatening complications of chemical terrorism.[72] It can rapidly detect the common airway, respiratory, and central nervous system adverse events associated with nerve agents, including apnea, upper airway obstruction, laryngospasm, bronchospasm, respiratory failure, seizures, and coma (eTable 2.3).

eTABLE 2.3 CAPNOGRAPHIC IDENTIFICATION OF LIFE-THREATENING COMPLICATIONS OF NERVE AGENTS
AVAILABLE AT ELSEVIER EBOOKS+

Gauging Severity and Response to Treatment of Patients in Acute Respiratory Distress

Capnography provides dynamic monitoring of ventilatory status in patients with acute respiratory distress from any cause, including asthma, bronchiolitis, CHF, COPD, croup, and cystic fibrosis. By measuring P_{ETCO_2} and RR with each breath, capnography provides immediate information on the clinical status of the patient. RR is measured directly from the airway (nose and mouth) with an oral-nasal cannula and provides a more reliable reading than does impedance respiratory monitoring. In upper airway obstruction and laryngospasm, impedance monitoring detects chest wall movement, interprets this as valid breathing, and displays a RR even though the patient is not ventilating. In contrast, capnography will detect absence of air movement and therefore shows a flatline waveform.

P_{ETCO_2} trends can be assessed rapidly, especially in tachypneic patients. For example, a patient with an RR of 30 breaths/min will generate 150 P_{ETCO_2} readings in 5 minutes. This provides sufficient information to determine whether the patient's ventilation is worsening despite treatment (increasing P_{ETCO_2}), stabilizing (stable P_{ETCO_2}), or improving (decreasing P_{ETCO_2}) (Fig. 2.14).

Procedural Sedation and Analgesia

Pulse oximetry is the standard technique for monitoring procedural sedation in the ED, and capnography is more likely to detect the common adverse airway and respiratory events associated with procedural sedation and analgesia.[73–76] In 2014, ACEP gave capnography during procedural sedation a Level B recommendation: "Capnography may be used as an adjunct to pulse oximetry and clinical assessment to detect hypoventilation and apnea earlier than pulse oximetry and/or clinical assessment alone in patients undergoing procedural sedation and analgesia in the ED."[76]

Capnography is the earliest indicator of airway or respiratory compromise and will show an abnormally high or low P_{ETCO_2} well before pulse oximetry detects a falling oxyhemoglobin saturation, especially in patients receiving supplemental oxygen (Fig. 2.15).[76,77] Capnography provides a non–impedance-based RR directly from the airway, that is more accurate than impedance-based respiratory monitoring, especially in patients with obstructive apnea or laryngospasm.

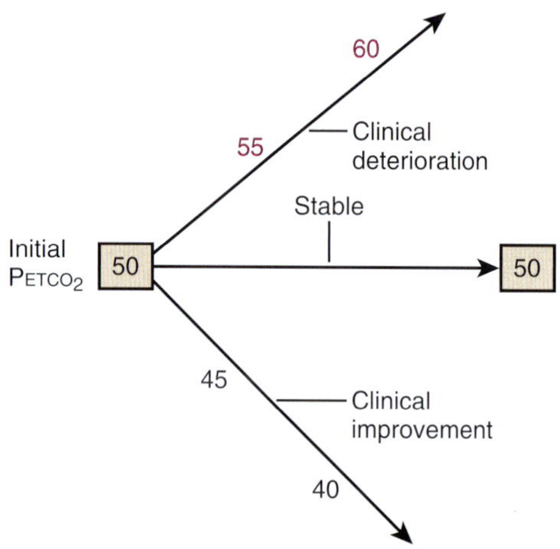

Fig. 2.14 End-tidal carbon dioxide concentration *(P_{ETCO_2})* trending in patients with acute respiratory distress. The dynamic ventilatory information provided by P_{ETCO_2} trends can be used to gauge response to treatment in patients with acute respiratory distress. Trends show worsening despite treatment (increasing P_{ETCO_2}), stabilized (stable P_{ETCO_2}) ventilatory status, or improving (decreasing P_{ETCO_2}) ventilatory status.

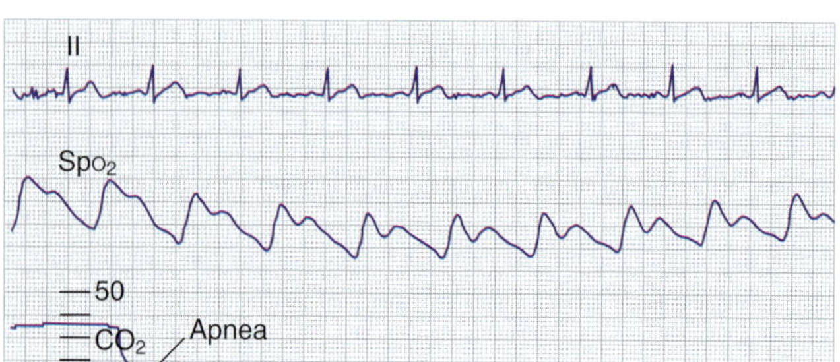

Fig. 2.15 Capnographic detection of apnea. The CO_2 flatline indicates complete absence of air movement. Note that the ECG and pulse oximetry initially appear normal in this patient with a respiratory arrest.

Both central and obstructive apnea can be detected almost instantaneously by capnography (Table 2.4). Loss of the capnogram, in conjunction with no chest wall movement and no breath sounds on auscultation, confirms the diagnosis of central apnea. Obstructive apnea is characterized by loss of the capnogram with continued chest wall movement and absent breath sounds. The response of the capnogram to airway alignment maneuvers can further distinguish upper airway obstruction from laryngospasm.

Capnography is more sensitive than clinical assessment of ventilation in detecting apnea along with other respiratory complications. This leads to more awareness of respiratory complications associated with procedural sedation, which is followed by appropriate and timely interventions.[74–77]

Because the amplitude of the capnogram is determined by P_{ETCO_2} and the width is determined by the expiratory time, changes in either of these parameters affect the shape of the capnogram. Hyperventilation (increased RR, decreased P_{ETCO_2}) results in a low-amplitude and narrow capnogram. Classic hypoventilation (decreased RR, increased P_{ETCO_2}) results in a high-amplitude and wide capnogram (see Table 2.4.). Acute bronchospasm results in a capnogram with a curved ascending phase and an upsloping alveolar plateau (Fig. 2.12). A P_{ETCO_2} reading higher than 70 mm Hg in patients without chronic ventilation problems indicates respiratory failure.

Two types of drug-induced hypoventilation occur during procedural sedation and analgesia (see Table 2.4).[78] Bradypneic hypoventilation (type 1), commonly seen with opioids, is characterized by increased P_{ETCO_2} and increased Pa_{CO_2}. RR is depressed proportionally greater than tidal volume, resulting in bradypnea, an increase in expiratory time, and a rise in P_{ETCO_2}, graphically represented by a high-amplitude, wide capnogram (see Table 2.4).

Bradypneic hypoventilation follows a predictable course, with P_{ETCO_2} increasing progressively until respiratory failure and apnea occur. Although there is no absolute threshold at which apnea occurs, patients with acute increases in P_{ETCO_2} to above 80 mm Hg are at significant risk.

Hypopneic hypoventilation (type 2), commonly seen with sedative-hypnotic drugs, is characterized by normal or decreased P_{ETCO_2} and increased Pa_{CO_2} because airway dead space remains constant (e.g., 150 mL in the normal adult lung) and tidal volume decreases. Tidal volume is depressed proportionally greater than RR, thereby resulting in low tidal volume breathing and leading to an increase in the fraction of airway dead space (dead space volume/tidal volume). As tidal volume decreases, the airway dead space fraction increases, resulting in an increase in the Pa_{CO_2}-P_{ETCO_2} gradient. Even though Pa_{CO_2} is increasing, P_{ETCO_2} may remain normal or decrease, graphically represented by a low-amplitude capnogram.

Hypopneic hypoventilation follows a variable course. Three possibilities exist: (1) ventilation may remain stable with the low tidal volume breathing resolving over time as drug levels in the central nervous system decrease following redistribution, (2) hypoventilation may progress to periodic breathing with intermittent apneic pauses (that may resolve spontaneously or progress to central apnea), or (3) hypoventilation may progress directly to central apnea.

The low tidal volume breathing that characterizes hypopneic hypoventilation increases dead space ventilation as a result of inhibition of the normal compensatory mechanisms by drug effects. Minute ventilation, which normally increases to compensate for an increase in dead space, does not change

TABLE 2.4 Capnographic Airway Assessment for Procedural Sedation and Analgesia

DIAGNOSIS	WAVEFORM	FEATURES		MANAGEMENT
Normal	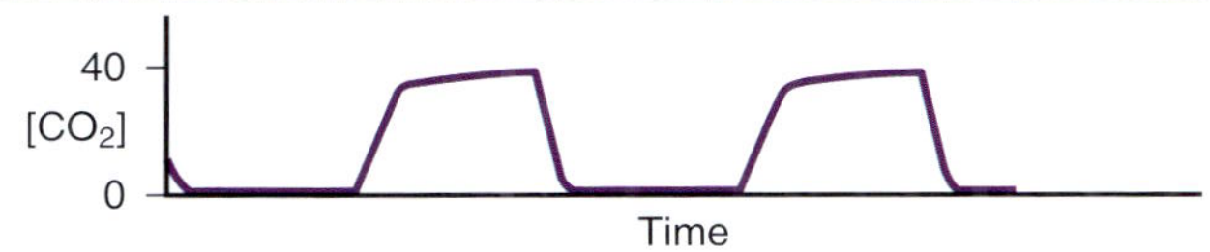	Spo_2 P_{ETCO_2} Waveform RR	Normal Normal Normal Normal	• No intervention required • Continue sedation
Hyperventilation	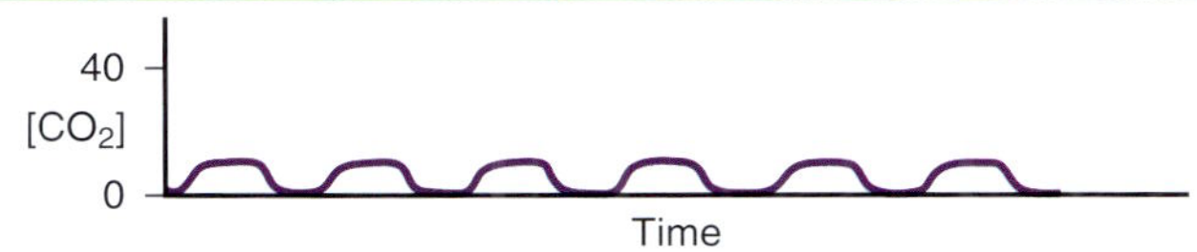	Spo_2 P_{ETCO_2} Waveform RR	Normal ↓ Decreased amplitude and width ↑	
Bradypneic hypoventilation (type 1)	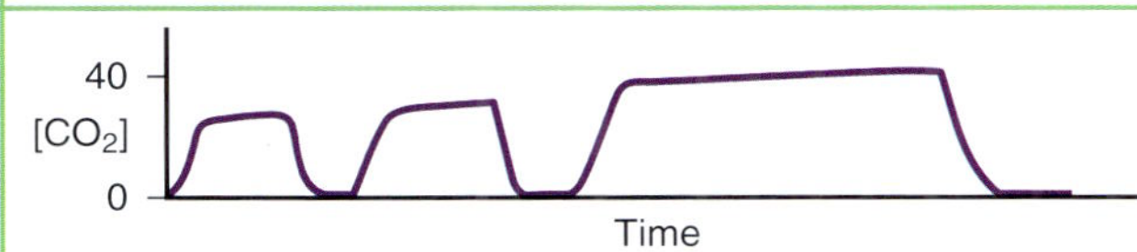	Spo_2 P_{ETCO_2} Waveform RR	Normal ↑ Increased amplitude and width ↓↓↓	• Reassess patient • Continue sedation
		Spo_2 P_{ETCO_2} Waveform RR	↓ ↑ Increased amplitude and width ↓↓↓	• Reassess patient • Assess for airway obstruction • Supplemental oxygen • Cease drug administration or reduce dosing
Hypopneic hypoventilation (type 2)	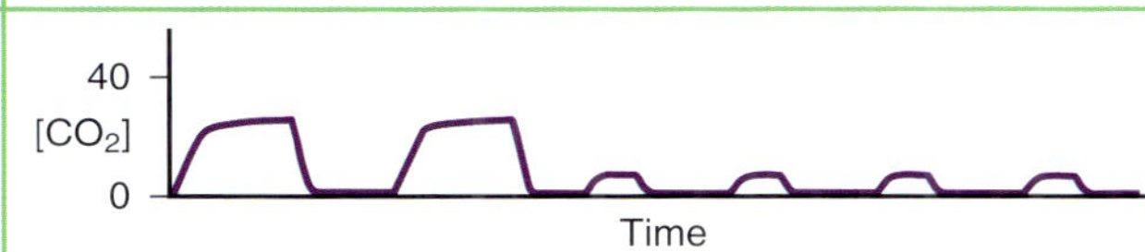	Spo_2 P_{ETCO_2} Waveform RR	Normal ↓ Decreased amplitude ↓	• Reassess patient • Continue sedation
		Spo_2 P_{ETCO_2} Waveform RR	↓ ↓ Decreased amplitude ↓	• Reassess patient • Assess for airway obstruction • Supplemental oxygen • Cease drug administration or reduce dosing
Hypopneic hypoventilation with periodic breathing	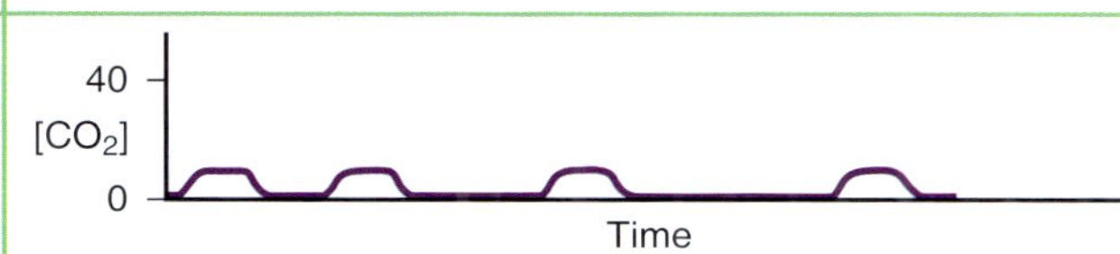	Spo_2 P_{ETCO_2} Waveform RR Other	Normal or ↓ ↓ Decreased amplitude ↓ Apneic pauses	

Continued

TABLE 2.4 Capnographic Airway Assessment for Procedural Sedation and Analgesia—cont'd

DIAGNOSIS	WAVEFORM	FEATURES		MANAGEMENT
Physiologic variability	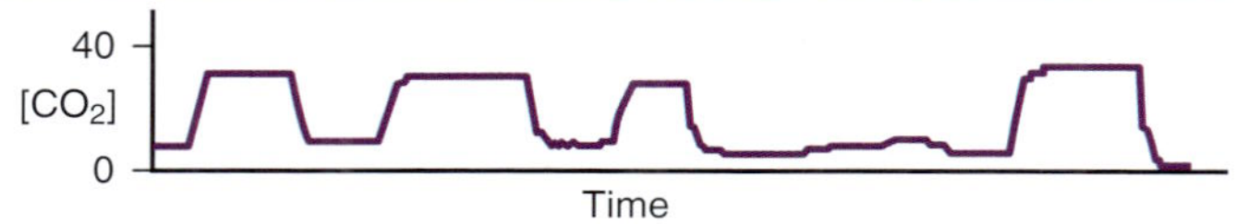	Spo_2 P_{ETCO_2} Waveform RR	Normal Normal Varying[a] Normal	• No intervention required • Continue sedation
Bronchospasm	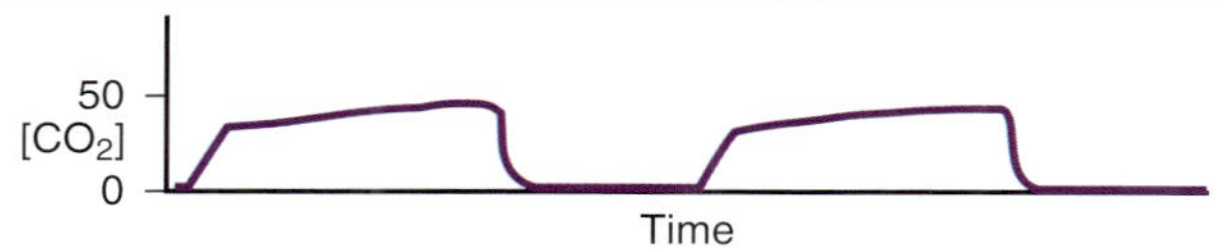	Spo_2 P_{ETCO_2} Waveform RR Other	Normal or ↓ Normal, ↑, or ↓[b] Curved Normal, ↑, or ↓[b] Wheezing	• Reassess patient • Bronchodilator therapy • Cease drug administration
Partial airway obstruction Partial laryngospasm	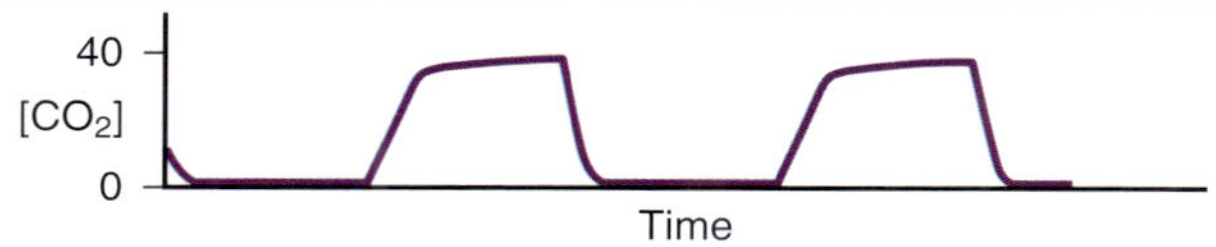	Spo_2 P_{ETCO_2} Waveform RR Other	Normal or ↓ Normal Normal Variable Noisy breathing and/ or inspiratory stridor	• Reassess patient • Establish IV access • Supplemental O_2 (as needed) • Cease drug administration • Full airway patency restored with airway alignment • Noisy breathing and stridor resolve • Airway not fully patent with airway alignment • Noisy breathing and stridor persist
Apnea	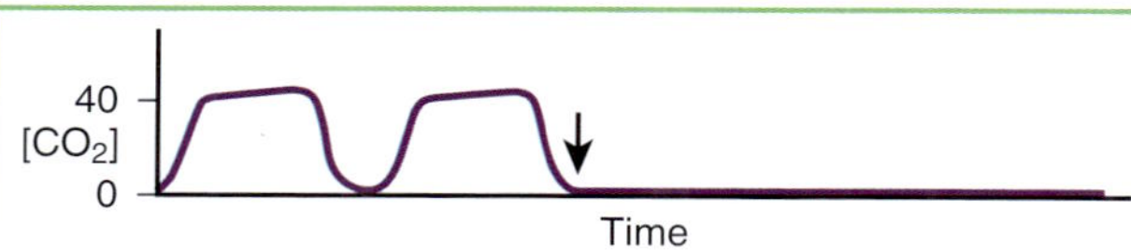	Spo_2 P_{ETCO_2} Waveform RR Other	Normal or ↓[c] Zero Absent Zero No chest wall movement or breath sounds	• Reassess patient • Stimulation • Bag-mask ventilation • Reversal agents (as appropriate) • Cease drug administration
Complete airway obstruction		$Spo_2 P_{ETCO_2}$ Waveform	Normal or ↓[c] Zero Absent	• Airway patency restored with airway alignment • Waveform present
Complete laryngospasm		RR Other	Zero • Chest wall movement and breath sounds present	• Positive pressure ventilation • Airway not patent with airway alignment • No waveform

[a]Varying waveform amplitude and width.
[b]Depending on the duration and severity of bronchospasm.
[c]Depending on the duration of the episode.
P_{ETCO_2}, End-tidal carbon dioxide pressure; *RR*, respiratory rate; *Spo_2*, oxygen saturation as measured by pulse oximetry.

or may decrease. As minute ventilation decreases, arterial oxygenation decreases. P_{ETCO_2} may initially be high (bradypneic hypoventilation) or low (hypopneic hypoventilation) without significant changes in oxygenation, particularly if supplemental O_2 is given. Therefore a drug-induced increase or decrease in P_{ETCO_2} does not necessarily lead to O_2 desaturation and may not require intervention.

Determining the Adequacy of Ventilation in Patients With Altered Mental Status

Patients with altered mental status, including those with alcohol intoxication, intentional, or unintentional drug overdose, patients requiring chemical restraint, and postictal patients (especially those treated with benzodiazepines) may have impaired ventilatory function. Capnography can differentiate between patients with effective ventilation and those with ineffective ventilation, as well as provide continuous monitoring of ventilatory trends over time to identify patients at risk for worsening respiratory depression.[79]

Detection of Metabolic Acidosis

In addition to its established uses for assessment of ventilation and perfusion, capnography is a valuable tool for assessing metabolic status by providing information on how effectively CO_2 is being produced by cellular metabolism.

Studies have shown that P_{ETCO_2} and serum bicarbonate (HCO_3) are well correlated in patients with diabetes, gastroenteritis, as well as undifferentiated patients in a triage setting. P_{ETCO_2} can be used as an indicator of metabolic acidosis in these patients (Fig. 2.16).[71,80–83] As the patient becomes acidotic (i.e., HCO_3 decreases), a compensatory respiratory alkalosis develops with an increase in minute ventilation and a resultant decrease in P_{ETCO_2}. By increasing minute ventilation, these patients are able to lower arterial CO_2 tension to help correct the underlying acidemia. The more acidotic, the lower the HCO_3, the higher the RR, and the lower the P_{ETCO_2}.

P_{ETCO_2} can be used to distinguish diabetics in ketoacidosis (metabolic acidosis, compensatory tachypnea, low P_{ETCO_2}) from those who are not (nonacidotic, normal RR, normal P_{ETCO_2}).[80,82] Capnography should be considered as a potential triage tool to determine the need for intravenous access and rapid assessment by a physician versus delayed physician assessment and may be a predictor of need for intensive care hospitalization as well as mortality.[71]

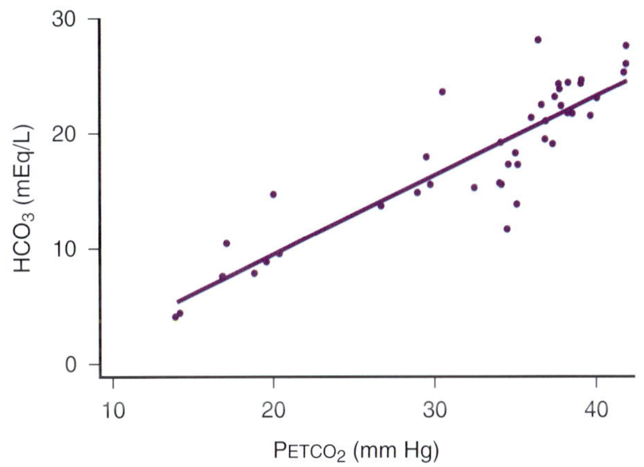

Fig. 2.16 End-tidal carbon dioxide concentration *(P_{ETCO_2})*-HCO_3 correlation in patients with diabetes. (From Fearon DM, Steele DW. End-tidal carbon dioxide predicts the presence and severity of acidosis in children with diabetes. *Acad Emerg Med.* 2002;9:1373.)

Limitations

Significant technical problems have historically restricted the effective clinical use of capnography. Such problems include interference with the sensor by condensed water and patient secretions in both mainstream and high-flow sidestream devices, cross-sensitivity with anesthetic gases in conventional CO_2 sensors, lack of ruggedness for intrahospital and interhospital transport, and power consumption issues related to portable battery operation time. These issues have largely been resolved in the newer-generation capnography monitors.

Problems with accuracy continue to affect high-flow sidestream systems. When the tidal volume of the patient drops below the flow rate of the system (e.g., neonates, infants, hypoventilating patients with low tidal volume breathing), the monitor will entrain room air, thereby falsely diluting P_{ETCO_2} and slurring the ascending phase of the waveform.[84]

Early capnography airway interfaces (i.e., nasal cannula) had difficulty providing consistent measurements in mouth-breathing patients and those who alternated between mouth and nose breathing; however, oral-nasal interfaces have addressed these problems.

Capnography is most effective when assessing a pure ventilation, perfusion, or metabolism problem. Capnographic findings in patients with mixed ventilation, perfusion, or metabolism problems are difficult to interpret. For example, in patients with complex pathophysiology, a ventilation problem may elevate P_{ETCO_2}, and a perfusion problem may simultaneously lower P_{ETCO_2}. Absolute values and even trends over time may be difficult to interpret in these situations.

Although capnography in patients in cardiac arrest is 100% specific for tracheal placement of the ET tube, its sensitivity for esophageal placement is uncertain.

CONCLUSION

Capnography is a versatile noninvasive diagnostic modality for monitoring ventilation, perfusion, and metabolic status in both intubated and nonintubated patients. Clinical applications include verification and continuous monitoring of ET tube placement; determination of the efficacy of CPR in cardiac arrest; ventilatory monitoring of head-injured patients; assessment of vital signs in patients who are critically ill, injured, seizing, or undergoing procedural sedation or have altered mental status; evaluation of patients in acute respiratory distress; and detection of metabolic acidosis.

REFERENCES AVAILABLE AT Elsevier eBooks+ .

SECTION II

Respiratory Procedures

CHAPTER 3

Basic Airway Management and Decision-Making

Aaron E. Robinson, Brian E. Driver, and Robert F. Reardon

Basic airway procedures, though often overlooked in favor of more exciting intubation devices and techniques, are critically important and generally more lifesaving than advanced techniques. Establishing a patent airway, administering oxygen, and performing bag-mask ventilation (BMV) are the cornerstones of good emergency airway management.[1,2] These techniques can be used quickly in any setting. They allow practitioners to keep apneic patients alive indefinitely until a definitive airway can be established.[2]

Extraglottic devices (EGDs), such as laryngeal mask airways (LMAs) and the King laryngeal tube (LT), are also important for the initial resuscitation of apneic patients and for rescue ventilation when intubation fails.[3–5]

This chapter describes basic airway skills, including opening the airway, oxygen (O_2) therapy, BMV, and EGDs. These are foundational skills that clinicians can use at any time—they can also be relied upon when other airway techniques are difficult or impossible. Mastery of these basic skills will help clinicians manage difficult, anxiety-provoking emergency airways.

CHALLENGE OF EMERGENCY AIRWAY MANAGEMENT

Most emergency airways are managed by emergency clinicians rather than by other specialists.[6] Airway management in the emergency department (ED) is different from airway management in the controlled setting of an operating room. Major challenges include hypoxia, shock, a full stomach, and the presence of emesis, blood, or excessive secretions in the airway. Many patients are uncooperative and combative, making it impossible to thoroughly examine the airway before choosing an intubation technique. Medical history, allergies, and even the current diagnosis are often unknown before emergency airway management begins. Time constraints, lack of patient cooperation, and risk for emesis and aspiration limit the use of some techniques, such as awake intubation. In trauma patients, the risk for cervical spine injury limits optimal head and neck positioning for BMV and laryngoscopy. All these factors increase the risk for complications from emergency airway management,[6,7] and approximately 0.5% to 1% of all emergency airways require a surgical approach.[6,8]

STANDARDIZING THE APPROACH TO AIRWAY MANAGEMENT

This may be the most important element affecting the safety of critically ill patients undergoing emergency airway management. Emergency airway management is often a stressful event and involves multiple team members—a consistent approach leads to better teamwork, less stress, and fewer mistakes. Individual practitioners *and* departments should adopt a standard approach to emergency airway management that standardizes basic airway management, preparation, medications, techniques, and devices for nearly all patients who require intubation. This standard approach should use the best available techniques and equipment, ensuring that the standard approach will be successful for difficult cases. Using new, unfamiliar, or rarely used techniques or devices for difficult or unusual airways will often translate to unanticipated challenges or intubation failure.

All clinicians in a department should have uniform practice in opening the airway, applying oxygen, performing BMV (using a two-hand technique), and all should be comfortable placing EGDs. A departmental clinician should act as the *airway lead* and be responsible for keeping up with advances in the literature, maintaining up-to-date airway equipment, organizing airway training, and overseeing airway management to ensure best practices are followed. High-performing centers that use this framework have demonstrated high intubation success and safety.

BASIC AIRWAY MANAGEMENT TECHNIQUES

Opening the Airway

The upper airway must be patent for oxygenation and ventilation to occur (Video 3.1). Upper airway obstruction commonly occurs when patients are unconscious or sedated. It can also be caused by injury to the mandible or muscles that support the hypopharynx. In these scenarios, the tongue and related structures fall posteriorly, or the hypopharynx relaxes circumferentially, and the passage of air is obstructed. Upper airway obstruction caused by the tongue and hypopharynx can be relieved by positioning maneuvers of the head, neck, and jaw; the use of nasopharyngeal or oropharyngeal airways; or the application of noninvasive ventilation (NIV).

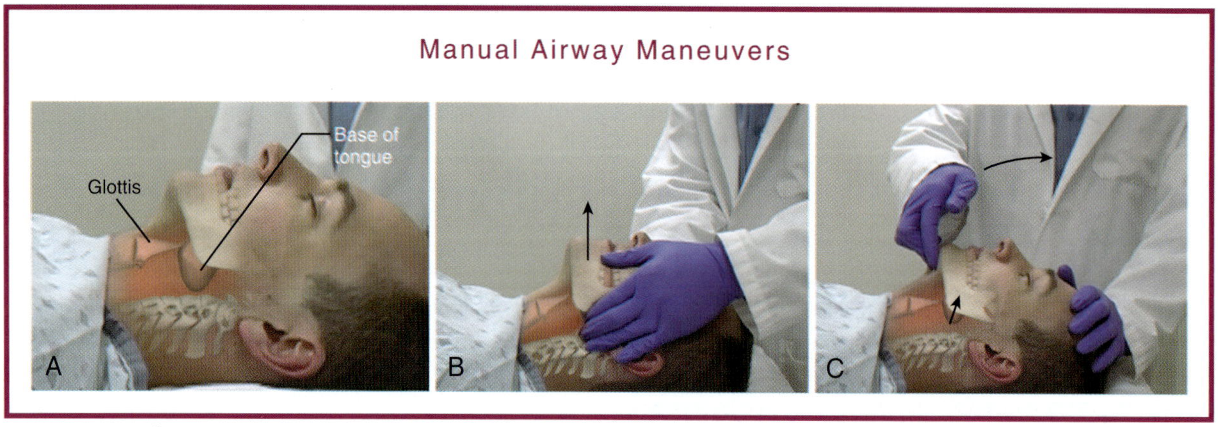

Fig. 3.1 Manual airway maneuvers. (A) The most common cause of airway obstruction in an unconscious patient is the tongue. Initial maneuvers for opening the airway include (B) jaw thrust and (C) head-tilt/chin lift. The jaw-thrust maneuver is the most important technique.

Manual Airway Maneuvers

Airway obstruction in unconscious patients is often due to posterior displacement of the tongue (Fig. 3.1A). Upper airway obstruction often causes obvious snoring or stridor, and when obstruction is complete there are no abnormal sounds and no air movement, despite the patient's effort to breathe. All unconscious patients are at high risk for upper airway obstruction.

More than 40 years ago, Guildner[9] compared different techniques for opening obstructed upper airways and found that the jaw-thrust and head-tilt/chin-lift techniques were both effective (Fig. 3.1B–C). The jaw-thrust maneuver (anterior mandibular translation to bring the lower incisors anterior to the upper incisors) is the most important technique for opening the upper airway because it can be performed on any patient.[2,10]

It is widely accepted that the jaw-thrust-only (without head-tilt or chin-lift) maneuver should be performed in patients with suspected cervical spine injury.[11] There is no evidence that it is safer than the head-tilt/chin-lift maneuver.[12] The American Heart Association (AHA) concluded that airway maneuvers are safe during manual inline stabilization of the cervical spine and highlighted evidence that all airway maneuvers cause some spinal movement. Both the chin-lift and the jaw-thrust maneuvers have been shown to cause similar substantial movement of the cervical vertebrae.[13–17] There is no evidence that this movement worsens existing spinal cord injury or causes new spinal cord injury in patients with cervical spine fractures. Most experts believe that airway interventions performed for patients with cervical spine injury are safe.[18–20] The AHA recommends that "if healthcare providers suspect a cervical spine injury, they should open the airway using a jaw thrust without head extension. Because maintaining a patent airway and providing adequate ventilation are priorities in cardiopulmonary resuscitation (CPR), use the head-tilt/chin-lift maneuver if the jaw thrust does not adequately open the airway."[4,21]

Jaw-Thrust Maneuver

The jaw-thrust maneuver is the most important technique used to open the upper airway. To perform the jaw-thrust maneuver, place the tips of the middle or index fingers behind the angle of the mandible (see Fig. 3.18). Lift the mandible toward the ceiling until the lower incisors are anterior to the upper incisors. This maneuver can be performed in combination with the head-tilt/chin-lift maneuver or with the neck in the neutral position during inline stabilization.

Head-Tilt/Chin-Lift Maneuver

To perform the head-tilt/chin-lift maneuver, place the tips of the index and middle fingers beneath the patient's chin (see Fig. 3.1C). Lift the chin cephalad and toward the ceiling. The upper part of the neck will naturally extend when the head tilts backward during this maneuver. Apply digital pressure on only the bony prominence of the chin and not on the soft tissues of the submandibular region. The final step in this maneuver is to use the thumb to open the patient's mouth while the head is tilted and the neck is extended.

Triple Airway Maneuver

The "triple airway maneuver" is described by some authors as a valuable method for maintaining a patent upper airway.[2,11] The most common description of this maneuver is head tilt, jaw thrust, and mouth opening.[2,11] Evidence demonstrates that the upper airway is more patent when the mouth is closed.[22–24] Although the triple maneuver is commonly mentioned in the anesthesia literature as a valuable technique, no studies exist to support the assertion that this technique is more effective than the head-tilt/chin-lift or jaw-thrust maneuvers.

Patient Positioning

The best way to position a patient's head and neck for opening the upper airway is to mimic how patients position themselves when they are short of breath, with the neck flexed relative to the torso and with atlanto-occipital extension.[2] This is known as the *sniffing position* and was described by Magill almost 100 years ago.[25] In normal-sized supine adults, this is accomplished by elevating the head approximately 10 cm while tilting the head back, so that the plane of the patient's face tilts slightly toward the clinician at the head of the bed (see Chapter 4, Fig. 4.10).[2,26–28] Patients with a markedly elevated body mass index (BMI) require much more head elevation to achieve the proper sniffing position. This can be accomplished by building a ramp of towels and pillows under the upper torso, head, and neck or by using a Troop Elevation Pillow (Mercury Medical) or similar device (Fig. 3.2).[29–32] The head of the bed can be raised to about 15 to 20 degrees to minimize the number of towels and pillows needed. Rather than elevating the head by a standard height, the goal of head elevation is to achieve horizontal alignment of the external auditory meatus with the sternum. This is the best position for opening the upper airway in patients with markedly elevated BMI (Fig 3.2).[31–34]

The sniffing position is contraindicated in patients with cervical spine injuries. The best technique for opening the airway in this situation is a simple jaw-thrust maneuver with anterior mandibular translation to bring the lower incisors anterior to the upper incisors (see Fig. 3.18).[2,10] In patients with elevated BMI, fat deposition on the upper back results in neck extension when the patient's head is resting on the bed.

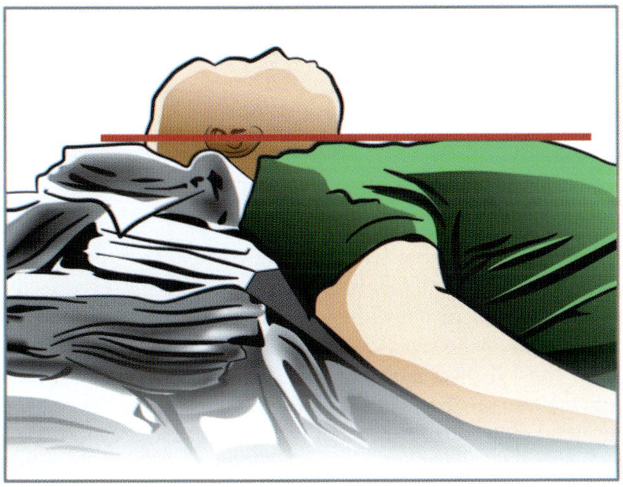

Fig. 3.2 The best position for opening the upper airway in patients with a markedly elevated body mass index is elevation of the head, neck, and shoulders so that the external auditory meatus is aligned with the sternum. This can be accomplished with purpose-built pillows; however, similar results may be achieved with other devices or a ramp of towels and pillows.

In these patients, it is acceptable to carefully elevate the head with a towel or pillow to move the head and neck into a more neutral position even in the setting of cervical spine trauma.

In young children, the sniffing position is often achieved without lifting the head and can be achieved with the head and body in the same horizontal plane (Fig. 3.3). In infants, the torso needs to be elevated in relation to the head to achieve the sniffing position because their large occiput creates flexion of the lower cervical spine when they are lying supine on a flat surface (Fig. 3.4).

Airway management is usually easiest when patients are in the supine position, and the left lateral position may be best for patients who are actively vomiting and those with excessive upper airway bleeding or secretions. Some evidence suggests that rotating patients to the lateral position may not prevent aspiration.[35] Patients with suspected cervical spine injury should have their head immobilized with manual inline stabilization if they need to be rolled to the lateral position. Airway management maneuvers will be more difficult when patients are in the lateral position.

Foreign Body Airway Obstruction

Awake patients with partial airway obstruction can usually clear a foreign body on their own. Intervention is required when the patient is not moving air or has altered mental status. Some patients with upper airway obstruction can be ventilated and oxygenated with aggressive high-pressure BMV, so always try this if standard BMV fails. Massive aspiration of vomitus is often a fatal event because of inability of the patient and clinician to adequately clear the airway.

Abdominal Thrusts (Heimlich Maneuver), Chest Thrusts, and Back Blows (Slaps)

AHA guidelines[36] recommend first administering back slaps for awake adults with an ineffective cough, then moving to abdominal thrusts if those are not effective. Manual removal of the foreign body with a finger or hand sweep can be effective

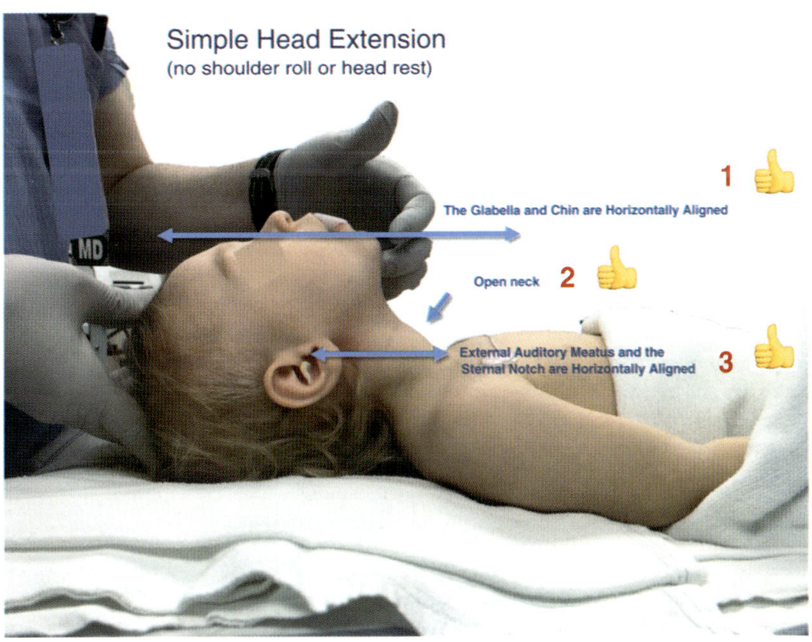

Fig. 3.3 Sniffing position in a young child without the need for elevation.

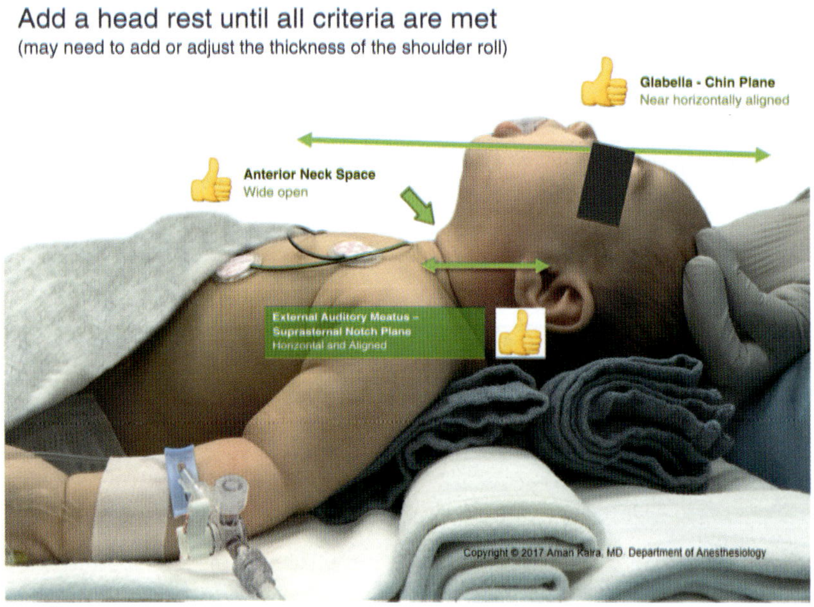

Fig. 3.4 Torso elevation in relation to the head in an infant due to large occiput.

if the foreign body is large enough and not deeply lodged. When someone is unconscious, chest thrusts should be attempted, and a clinician should attempt to remove the foreign body with Magill forceps or any tool capable of grasping.

The technique of subdiaphragmatic abdominal thrusts to relieve a completely obstructed airway was popularized by Dr. Henry Heimlich and is commonly referred to as the *Heimlich maneuver*.[37] The technique is most effective when a solid food bolus is obstructing the larynx. In a conscious patient, stand behind the upright patient. Circle the arms around the patient's midsection with the radial side of a clenched fist placed on the abdomen, midway between the umbilicus and xiphoid. Then grasp the fist with the opposite hand and deliver an inward and upward thrust to the abdomen (Fig. 3.5A). A successful maneuver will cause the obstructing agent to be expelled from the patient's airway by the force of air exiting the lungs. Abdominal thrusts are relatively contraindicated in pregnant patients and those with protuberant abdomens. Potential risks associated with abdominal thrusts include stomach rupture, esophageal perforation, and mesenteric laceration, compelling the rescuer to weigh the risks and benefits of this maneuver.[38–43] Use a sternal hand position for pregnant patients (Fig. 3.5B).

If a choking patient loses consciousness, use chest compressions in an attempt to expel the obstructing agent (Fig. 3.5C).[4] The theory is the same as the Heimlich maneuver, with high intrathoracic pressure created to push the obstruction out of the airway. Some data suggest that chest compressions may generate higher peak airway pressure than the Heimlich maneuver.[44] After 30 seconds of chest compressions, remove the obstructing object if seen, attempt two breaths, and then continue CPR at 30 compressions to two breaths. Every time you open the airway to give breaths, look for the object and remove it if possible, then continue CPR if necessary.

Back blows are recommended for infants and small children with a foreign body obstructing the airway. Some authors have argued that back blows may be dangerous and may drive foreign bodies deeper into the airway, however, there is no convincing evidence of this phenomenon.[45,46] Anecdotal evidence suggests that back blows are effective.[47–49] No convincing data indicate that back blows are more or less effective than abdominal or chest thrusts. The AHA guidelines suggest back blows in the head-down position (Fig. 3.5D) and head-down chest thrusts in infants and small children with foreign body airway obstruction (Fig. 3.5E).[4] The AHA does not recommend abdominal thrusts in infants because they may be at higher risk for iatrogenic injury. From a practical standpoint, back blows should be delivered with the patient in a head-down position, which is more easily accomplished in infants than in larger children. It is recommended that suction be performed on newborns rather than giving them back blows or abdominal thrusts.[50]

Any patient with a complete airway obstruction may benefit from chest compressions, abdominal thrusts, or back blows. It is important to realize that more than one technique is often required to clear obstruction of the airway by a foreign body, so multiple techniques should be applied in a rapid sequence until the obstruction is relieved. A finger sweep might help remove an obstructing object, even if it is not visible. It is even better to look with a laryngoscope and use a grasping tool to remove foreign material.

Perform CPR on all unconscious patients with airway obstruction. Aggressive high-pressure BMV should be attempted, as this may distend the trachea enough to allow air to bypass the obstruction. In cases in which obstructive foreign bodies cannot be removed under direct visualization and aggressive positive pressure ventilation has failed, practitioners with advanced airway skills and proper equipment can perform cricothyrotomy or try to push a subglottic foreign body beyond the carina, usually into the right main stem bronchus.

Suctioning

Patient positioning and airway-opening maneuvers are often inadequate to achieve complete airway patency. Ongoing hemorrhage, vomitus, and particulate debris frequently require suctioning. Several types of suctioning tips are available. A

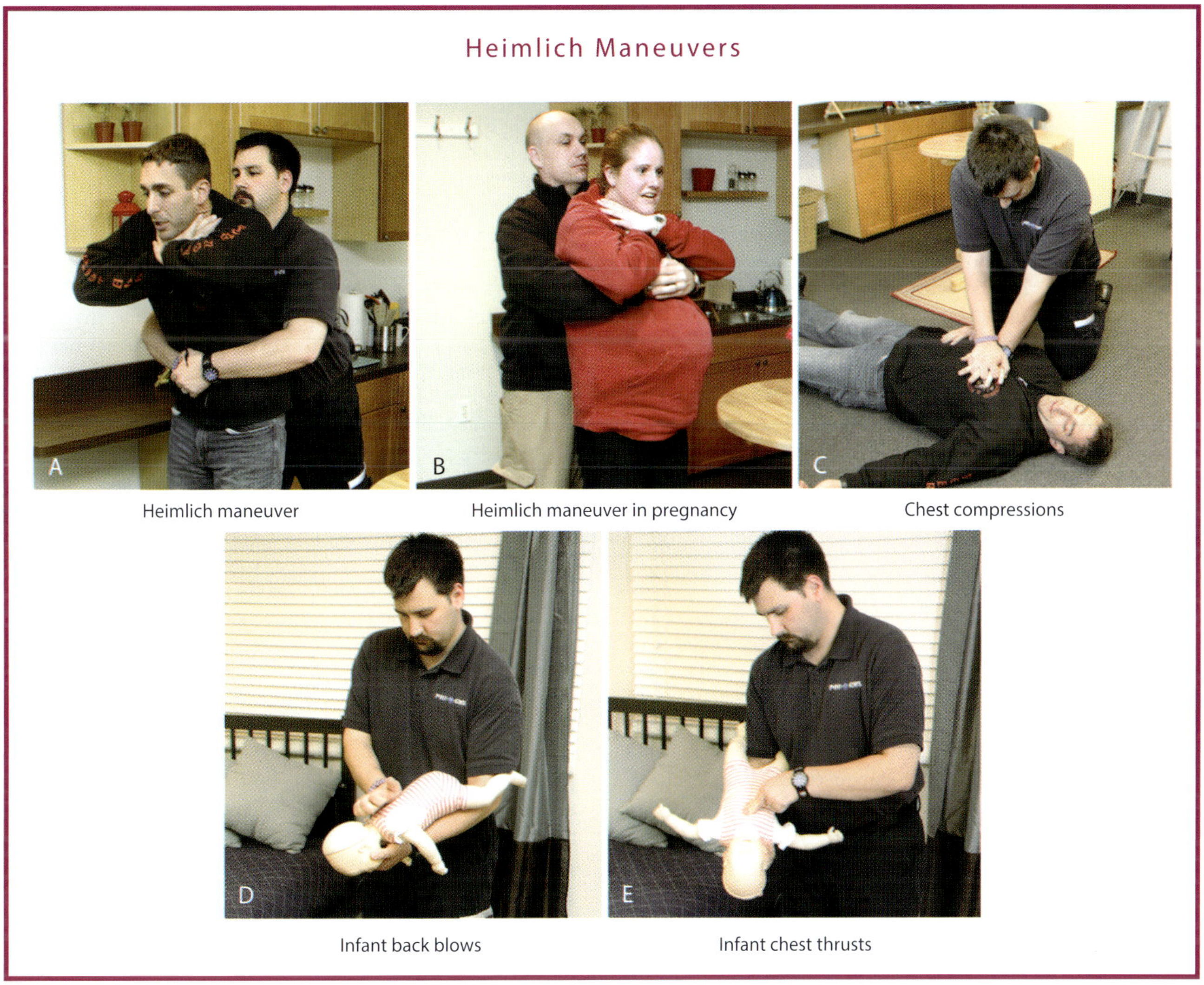

Fig. 3.5 (A–E) Heimlich maneuvers (see text).

large-bore dental-type suction tip is the most effective in clearing vomitus from the upper airway because it is less likely to become obstructed by particulate matter. The tonsil tip (Yankauer) suction device can be used to clear thin secretions. Its rounded tip is less traumatic to soft tissues, and the tonsil tip device is not large enough to effectively suction anything apart from thin liquids.

A large-bore open tip device, such as the HI-D Big Stick (SSCOR Inc.) suction tip, should be readily available at the bedside during all emergency airway management (Fig. 3.6). The large-bore tip allows rapid clearing of vomitus, clots, blood, and secretions.

A limiting feature of many suction catheters is the diameter of the tubing. Vomitus may obstruct the standard ¼-inch-diameter catheter.[51] A ⅝- or ¾-inch-diameter suction tube (Kuriyama Tubing, 5⁄16-inch inner diameter, 0.44-inch outer diameter, clear) has been shown to significantly decrease suction time for viscous and particulate material (see Fig. 3.6).[52]

Keep suctioning equipment connected and ready to operate. Everyone participating in emergency airway management should know how to use it. Interposition of a suction trap close to the suction device prevents clogging of the tubing with particulate debris.

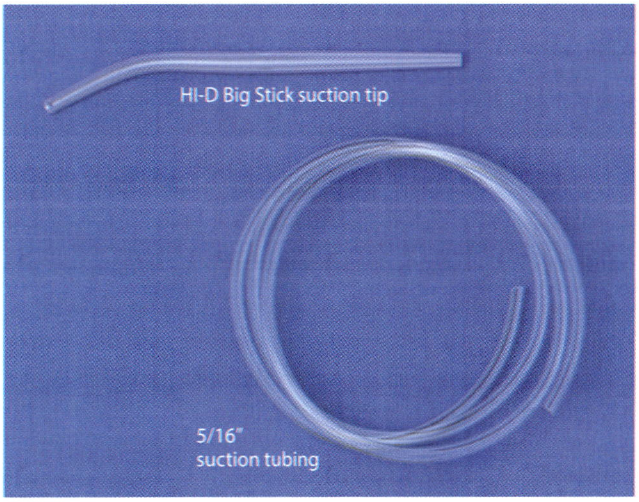

Fig. 3.6 HI-D Big Stick suction tip (SSCOR, Inc.) and 5⁄16-inch tubing.

No specific contraindications to airway suctioning exist. Complications of suctioning may be avoided by anticipating problems and providing appropriate care before and during suctioning maneuvers. Nasal suction is seldom required, except in infants, because most adult airway obstruction occurs in the mouth and oropharynx.

Avoid prolonged suctioning because it may lead to significant hypoxia, especially in children. Do not exceed 15 seconds for suctioning intervals and administer supplemental O_2 before and after suctioning. Naigow and Powaser[53] found that suctioning consistently induced hypoxia in dogs and that it was best avoided by hyperventilation with high-concentration O_2 before and after suctioning. Hypoxia was also prevented in children by preoxygenation prior to attempting tracheal intubation with suctioning attempts.[54]

When feasible, perform suctioning under direct vision or with the aid of the laryngoscope. Forcing a suction tip blindly into the posterior pharynx can injure tissue or push foreign material into the airway, converting a partial obstruction to a complete obstruction.

Oropharyngeal and Nasopharyngeal Artificial Airways

Indications and Contraindications

Once the airway has been opened with manual maneuvers and suctioning, artificial airways, such as nasopharyngeal and oropharyngeal airways, can facilitate both spontaneous breathing and BMV (Review Box 3.1 and Video 3.2). In semiconscious patients who require a head-tilt/chin-lift or jaw-thrust maneuver to open their airways, hypoxia may develop because of recurrent obstruction if these maneuvers are discontinued. Oxygen supplementation and a nasopharyngeal airway may be all the support that is necessary to maintain a functional airway.

Patients who are unresponsive or apneic are usually easier to ventilate with a bag-mask device when an oropharyngeal airway is in place. In the ED, patients who tolerate an oropharyngeal airway should generally be intubated.

Artificial Airway Placement

The simplest and most widely available artificial airways are the oropharyngeal and nasopharyngeal airways (Fig. 3.7). Both are intended to prevent the tongue from obstructing the airway by creating a passage for air between the base of the tongue and the posterior pharyngeal wall. The oral airway may also prevent teeth clenching. In cases of severe upper airway edema, such as angioedema, these devices may not function properly or be able to bypass the obstruction. The oropharyngeal airway may be inserted by either of two procedures. One approach is to insert the airway in an inverted position along the patient's hard palate (Fig. 3.7, *step 2*). When it is well into the patient's mouth, rotate the airway 180 degrees and advance it to its final position along the patient's tongue, with the distal end of the artificial airway lying in the hypopharynx (Fig. 3.7, *step 3*). A second approach is to open the mouth widely and then either use a tongue blade to displace the tongue or simply grasp and lift the jaw and tongue with the left hand. Then advance the artificial airway into the oropharynx (Fig. 3.7, *step 4*). No rotation is necessary when the airway is placed in this manner.

The nasopharyngeal airway is easy to place. It may be easiest to place it on the patient's right naris so that the bevel is facing the septum on insertion. Be sure to lubricate the device before insertion (Fig. 3.7, *step 6*). Simply advance it into the nostril and direct it along the floor of the nasal passage in the direction of the occiput, *not* cephalad (Fig. 3.7, *step 7*). Advance it fully until the flared external tip of the airway is located at the nasal orifice (Fig. 3.7, *step 8*).

Both oropharyngeal and nasopharyngeal airways are available in multiple sizes. To find the correct size of either device, estimate its size by measuring along the side of the patient's face before insertion. An oropharyngeal airway of the correct size will extend from the corner of the mouth to the tip of the earlobe (see Fig. 3.7, *step 1*); a nasopharyngeal airway of the correct size will extend from the tip of the nose to the tip of the earlobe (see Fig. 3.7, *step 5*).

Oropharyngeal and Nasopharyngeal Airways

Indications

Facilitation of spontaneous breathing and bag-valve-mask ventilation in patients requiring head-tilt/chin-lift or jaw-thrust maneuvers

Contraindications

Nasopharyngeal

Significant facial and basilar skull fractures

Complications

Oropharyngeal

Vomiting (in patients with an intact gag reflex)

Airway obstruction (if the tongue is pushed against the posterior pharyngeal wall during insertion)

Nasopharyngeal

Epistaxis

Deterioration requiring intubation (semiconscious patient)

Equipment

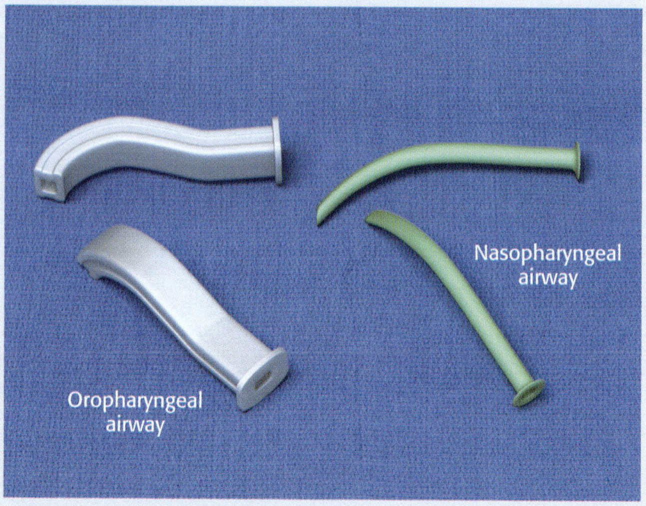

Review Box 3.1 Oropharyngeal and nasopharyngeal airways.

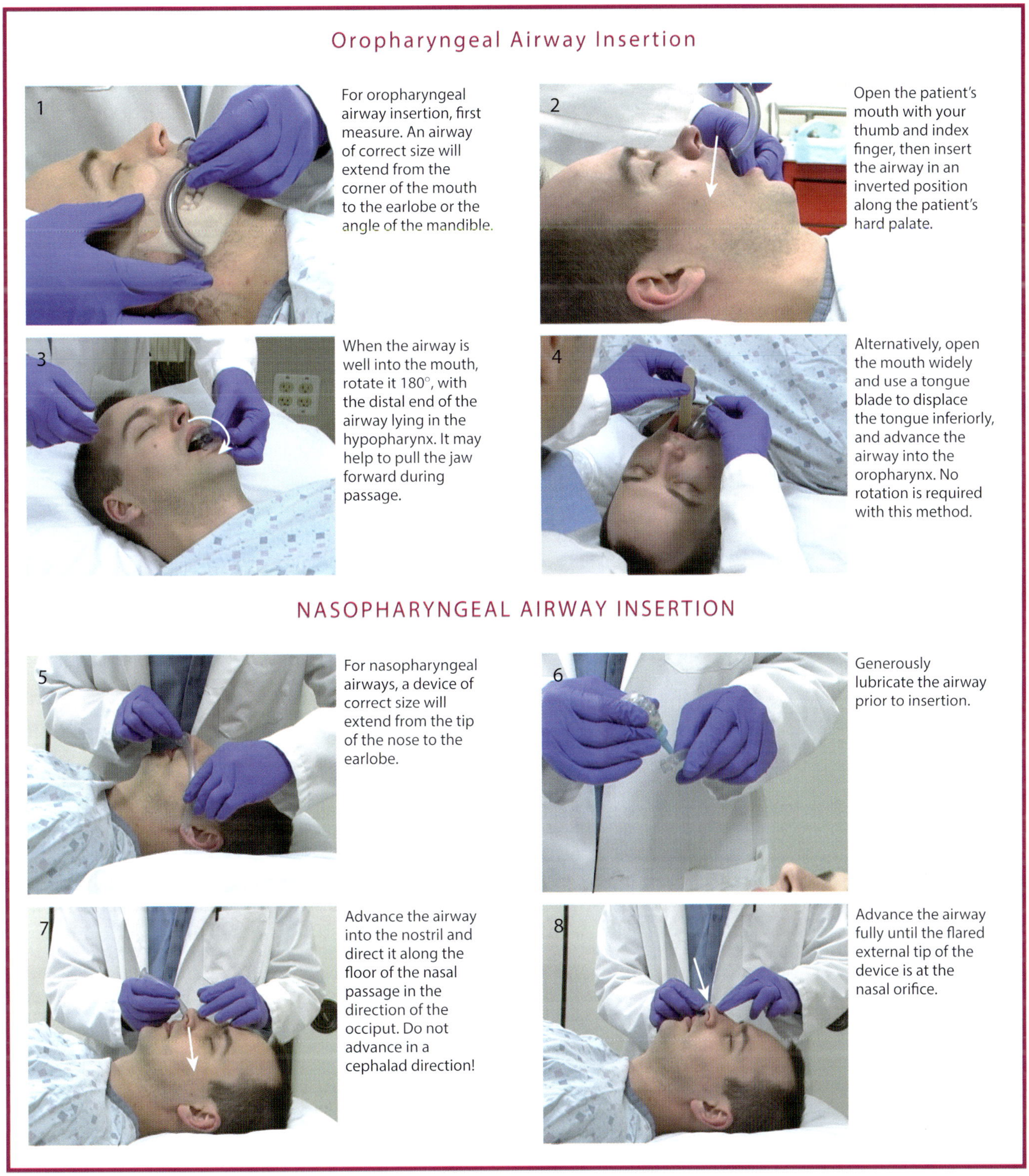

Fig. 3.7 Oropharyngeal and nasopharyngeal airway insertion.

Both oropharyngeal and nasopharyngeal airways provide airway patency similar to that achieved with the head-tilt/chin-lift maneuver. The nasal airway is better tolerated by semiconscious patients and is less likely to induce emesis in those with an intact gag reflex.

Complications

The nasopharyngeal airway may cause epistaxis and may be dangerous in patients with significant facial and basilar skull fractures. Semiconscious patients with nasopharyngeal airways may deteriorate and require intubation, so they should be monitored closely.

The oropharyngeal airway may induce vomiting when placed in patients with an intact gag reflex. It may also cause airway obstruction if the tongue is pushed against the posterior pharyngeal wall during insertion. The oropharyngeal airway should not be used as a definitive airway.

OXYGEN THERAPY

Adequate O_2 delivery depends on the inspired partial pressure of O_2, alveolar ventilation, pulmonary gas exchange, oxygen-carrying capacity of blood, and cardiac output (Video 3.3). The easiest factor to manipulate is the partial pressure of inspired O_2, which is accomplished by increasing the fraction of inspired oxygen (Fio_2) with supplemental O_2.

Indications and Contraindications

Resuscitate all patients in cardiac or respiratory arrest with 100% O_2. The most certain indication for supplemental O_2 is the presence of arterial hypoxemia, defined as an arterial oxygen partial pressure (Pao_2) lower than 60 mm Hg or arterial oxygen saturation (Sao_2) less than 90%.[55] Normal individuals will begin to experience memory loss at a Pao_2 of 45 mm Hg, and loss of consciousness occurs at a Pao_2 of 30 mm Hg.[56–58] Chronically hypoxemic patients can adapt and function with a Pao_2 of 50 mm Hg or lower.[59]

When tissue hypoxia is present or suspected, give O_2 therapy.[55,60] Shock states resulting from hemorrhage, vasodilatory states, low cardiac output, and obstructive lesions can all lead to tissue hypoxia and benefit from supplemental O_2. Whatever the cause of the shock state, administration of O_2 is indicated until the situation can be thoroughly evaluated and cause-specific therapy instituted. It is reasonable to administer O_2 to hypotensive patients and those with severe trauma until tissue hypoxia can definitively be excluded.[61]

Respiratory distress without documented arterial hypoxemia is a common indication for O_2 administration, although no evidence exists to support this practice.[61] Unless tracheal intubation is planned, respiratory distress without hypoxemia should generally not be considered an indication for oxygen supplementation.

Oxygen therapy is often recommended for acute myocardial infarction, but there is no difference in outcomes between patients receiving O_2 and those receiving room air after myocardial infarction.[62] A randomized trial of room air versus O_2 supplementation for patients with acute ST-elevation myocardial infarction demonstrated that patients who received O_2 had larger infarction size, as assessed by peak myocardial enzymes and cardiac magnetic resonance imaging at 6 months.[63] The AHA recommends O_2 in myocardial infarction only for patients with hypoxemia, signs of heart failure, shock, or respiratory distress.[64,65]

Although O_2 is routinely administered to acute stroke patients, there is no convincing evidence that this practice is beneficial without documented hypoxia, and it is not recommended by current guidelines.[66]

Administer 100% O_2 to patients with carbon monoxide poisoning. The half-life of carboxyhemoglobin is 4 to 5 hours in a patient breathing room air and can be decreased to approximately 1 hour by the administration of 100% O_2 by nonrebreather face mask at atmospheric pressure.[67]

There are no contraindications to O_2 therapy when a definite indication exists. The risks associated with hypoxemia are grave and undeniable. Never withhold oxygen therapy from a hypoxemic patient for fear of complications or clinical deterioration. Carbon dioxide retention is not a contraindication to O_2 therapy. Rather, it demands that the clinician administer O_2 carefully and recognize the potential for respiratory acidosis and clinical deterioration. Although the mechanism for the development of respiratory acidosis in patients with chronic obstructive pulmonary disease (COPD) who are administered O_2 is debated, its occurrence is not.[68,69] Therefore use caution when administering supplemental O_2 to hypoxic patients with arterial carbon dioxide pressure higher than 40 mm Hg, but do not withhold it.

Oxygen Administration During Cardiac Arrest and Neonatal Resuscitation

The AHA guidelines for CPR and emergency cardiovascular care address the potential harm of oxygen therapy and hyperoxemia following cardiac arrest and during neonatal resuscitation and provide the best recommendations. The recommendations are summarized in Box 3.1. Although it is still prudent to administer oxygen in the prehospital and ED setting, additional research may alter these recommendations. As a general guideline, fear of oxygen toxicity should not prevent the use of O_2 when there is an indication, and use the minimum concentration of O_2 necessary to achieve the therapeutic goals.

Oxygen Delivery Devices

A common misconception is that oxygen delivery devices can be cleanly separated into low-flow and high-flow categories. Almost any oxygen delivery device can be used across a wide range of flow rates. In fact, it is the source oxygen flow rate, not the device applied, that is the primary driver of the Fio_2 received by the patient.

Delivery of oxygen at low-flow rates provides gas flow that is less than the patient's inspiratory flow rate. The difference between the patient's inspiratory flow and the flow delivered by the device is met by a variable amount of room air being drawn into the system. Patients with normal respiratory rates and tidal volumes will require less outside air than those in respiratory distress, and therefore patients not in respiratory distress typically receive a higher Fio_2 than patients in respiratory distress, assuming equivalent supplemental oxygen flow rates. As a patient's inspiratory flow changes, so will the Fio_2 that they receive from a low-flow device.[70,71]

Delivery of high-flow oxygen, with rates that match or exceed the inspiratory flow of the patient (generally >30 L/min), provides a significantly higher Fio_2 than low-flow. High-flow oxygen can achieve Fio_2 values of more than 90%.

The prongs of a nasal cannula deliver a constant flow of O_2 that accumulates in the nasopharynx and provides a reservoir of oxygen-enriched air for inspiration. The Fio_2 delivered by nasal cannulas is determined by many factors, including the respiratory rate, tidal volume, pharyngeal geometry, and O_2 flow. Most importantly, at a constant O_2 flow rate, Fio_2 varies inversely with the respiratory rate.[72] Despite this limitation, nasal cannulas are very comfortable for patients and are the most common O_2 delivery device. They can be used with higher flow rates for brief periods of time and are uncomfortable to use in this manner, causing nasal dryness and irritation. Nasal cannula oxygen delivery is generally set to 2 to 4 L/min, which provides approximately 30% to 35% Fio_2.[72] Although it may seem intuitive, patients using a nasal cannula should be reminded that they should not smoke while oxygen is being delivered (Fig. 3.8).

Simple masks receive a constant flow of O_2 from the O_2 source and have multiple vent holes. During inspiration the

BOX 3.1 Recommendations for Oxygen Administration During Adult and Neonate Resuscitation: Excerpts From the Guidelines of the American Heart Association

OXYGEN SUPPLEMENTATION DURING CARDIAC ARREST

The goals of cardiopulmonary resuscitation are to restore energy to the heart so it can resume normal function and ensure adequate energy supply to the brain during resuscitation. Oxygen is vital to these goals, and during cardiac arrest, blood flow is the major limiting factor to adequate oxygen delivery to the heart and brain. Thus 100% Fio_2 should be administered during cardiac arrest for adults, children, and neonates to maximize oxygen delivery to vital organs.[141,146,230]

OVERVIEW OF POST–CARDIAC ARREST SUPPLEMENTAL OXYGEN FOR ADULTS AND CHILDREN[146,231,232]

Although 100% oxygen may have been used during initial resuscitation, clinicians should titrate inspired oxygen to the lowest level required to achieve an arterial oxygen saturation of ≥94%, to avoid potential oxygen toxicity. The goal oxygen saturation should be 94% to 99%. It is recognized that titration of inspired oxygen may not be possible immediately after out-of-hospital cardiac arrest until the patient is transported to the emergency department or, in the case of in-hospital arrest, the intensive care unit. The optimal Fio_2 during the immediate period after cardiac arrest is still debated. The beneficial effect of high Fio_2 on systemic oxygen delivery should be balanced with the deleterious effect of generating oxygen-derived free radicals during the reperfusion phase. Animal data suggest that ventilations with 100% oxygen (generating Pao_2 >350 mm Hg at 15 to 60 minutes after return of spontaneous circulation [ROSC]) increase brain lipid peroxidation, increase metabolic dysfunctions, increase neurologic degeneration, and worsen short-term functional outcome when compared with ventilation with room air or an inspired oxygen fraction titrated to a pulse oximeter reading between 94% and 99%. Data from human studies are mixed, with no clear evidence of harm or benefit from hyperoxia. There is no physiologic reason to expect that a Pao_2 >350 mm Hg is necessary or beneficial after cardiac arrest and very well may be harmful.

Once the circulation is restored, it is reasonable to use the highest available oxygen concentration until the oxyhemoglobin saturation or partial pressure of oxygen can be measured. As an arterial oxyhemoglobin saturation of 100% may correspond to a Pao_2 anywhere between ~80 mm Hg and 500 mm Hg, in general it is appropriate to wean Fio_2 when saturation is 100%. If the oxyhemoglobin saturation is 100%, it is reasonable to reduce the oxygen supplementation, provided that the oxyhemoglobin saturation can be maintained at ≥94%. The goal oxyhemoglobin saturation is 94% to 99%. Avoiding hypoxia is more important than avoiding hyperoxia.

ASSESSMENT OF OXYGEN NEED AND ADMINISTRATION OF OXYGEN IN THE NEONATE IMMEDIATELY AFTER BIRTH[230,233]

Oxyhemoglobin saturation may normally remain in the 70% to 80% range for several minutes following birth, thus resulting in the appearance of cyanosis during that time. Clinical assessment of skin color is a very poor indicator of oxyhemoglobin saturation during the immediate neonatal period and that lack of cyanosis appears to be a very poor measure of the state of oxygenation of an uncompromised baby following birth.

Optimal management of oxygen during neonatal resuscitation becomes particularly important because of the evidence that either insufficient or excessive oxygenation can be harmful to the newborn infant. Hypoxia and ischemia are known to result in injury to multiple organs. Conversely there is growing experimental evidence, as well as evidence from studies of babies receiving resuscitation, that adverse outcomes may result from even brief exposure to excessive oxygen during and following resuscitation. Two meta-analyses of several randomized controlled trials comparing neonatal resuscitation initiated with room air versus 100% oxygen showed increased survival when resuscitation was initiated with air.

It is recommended that the goal in babies being resuscitated at birth, whether born at term or preterm, should be an oxygen saturation value in the interquartile range of preductal saturations measured in healthy term babies following vaginal birth at sea level (see later). These targets may be achieved by initiating resuscitation with air or blended oxygen and titrating the oxygen concentration to achieve an Spo_2 in the target range using pulse oximetry. If the baby is bradycardic (heart rate <60 beats/min) after 90 seconds of resuscitation with a lower concentration of oxygen, oxygen concentration should be increased to 100% until recovery of a normal heart rate.

ASSESSMENT OF OXYGEN NEED AND ADMINISTRATION OF OXYGEN IN THE NEONATE

Targeted Preductal Spo_2 After Birth	
1 min	60%–65%
2 min	65%–70%
3 min	70%–75%
4 min	75%–80%
5 min	80%–85%
10 min	85%–95%

oxygen-enriched air that has accumulated in the mask, along with room air entrained through the vent holes, is inhaled. During expiration, 200 mL (the approximate volume of the mask) of exhaled gas is deposited in the mask, with the rest exiting through the vent holes. The continuous flow of O_2 then partially washes out the mask before the next inspiration. The mask itself provides the reservoir of oxygen-rich gas for inhalation. A complex interplay between mask volume, tidal volume, respiratory rate, and O_2 flow determines the Fio_2 delivered to the patient. At a flow rate of 10 L/min, Fio_2 is approximately 45% to 65% in healthy patients.[73] Notably, if the flow is increased to 30 L/min or higher, Fio_2 increases to 80% to 90%.[73] Fio_2 approximations at lower flow rates do not account for a patient in respiratory distress; as minute ventilation and inspiratory flow increase, Fio_2 will invariably decrease. This is also true for partial nonrebreather masks.

A partial nonrebreather mask incorporates a bag-type reservoir to increase the amount of O_2 available during inspiration, thereby requiring less outside air to be entrained. Non-rebreathing masks are similar to partial rebreathing masks and have a series of one-way valves. One valve lies between the mask and the reservoir and prevents exhaled gas from entering the reservoir. Two valves in the side of the mask permit exhalation while preventing the entry of outside air.

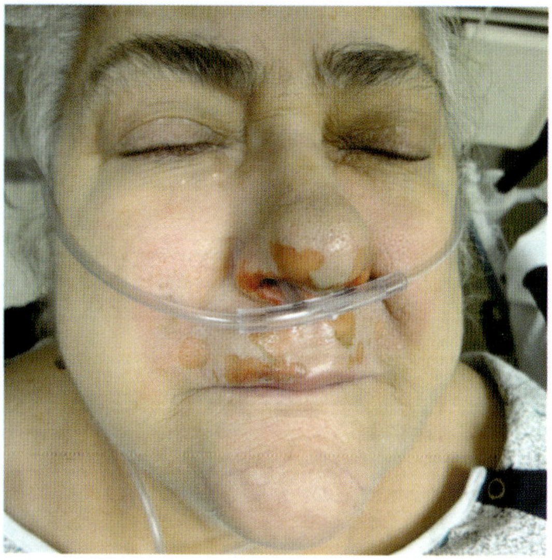

Fig. 3.8 This patient sustained serious facial burns and potential airway burns when she smoked a cigarette while oxygen was being delivered through a nasal cannula.

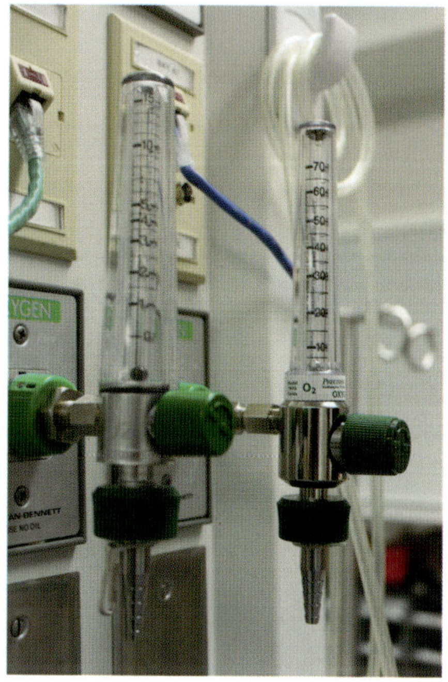

Fig. 3.9 A standard flow meter can measure flow up to 15 L/min but can usually achieve flow rates >40 L/min when fully opened to "flush"; the maximum possible flow rate is usually marked on the flow meter. Flow meters capable of precisely measuring flow up to 70 L/min are commercially available, which allow the clinician to deliver higher flow rates and thus higher Fio_2.

Though the exhalation ports may limit rebreathing of expired gas, room air still leaks avidly around the poorly sealed edges of the mask, especially if the patient's inspiratory flow is greater than the set flow rate. This outside air and the exhaled gas remaining in the mask dilute the O_2 from the reservoir and prevent the mask from providing 100% O_2. Oxygen flow to the mask should be sufficient to prevent collapse of the bag during inspiration. As with all oxygen devices that do not seal perfectly to the patient's face, the Fio_2 delivered varies with the patient's facial anatomy and respiratory pattern. Many clinicians have the misconception that a nonrebreathing mask with a source oxygen flow rate of 15 L/min can provide an Fio_2 near 100%. In practice, a nonrebreathing mask usually delivers an Fio_2 of approximately 50% when set at 15 L/min.[74,75] Fio_2 increases to 85% and higher when flow rates are set to >40 L/min.[74] Many clinicians (and most respiratory therapists) do not realize that higher oxygen flow rates can be achieved by simply dialing a standard flow meter to "flush" (the highest rate possible, achieved by rotating the knob until it will not rotate further) or replacing standard oxygen flow meters with flow meters capable of measuring flow up to 70 L/min, with flush capabilities of 90 L/min (Fig. 3.9).

The Venturi mask is a titratable oxygen delivery device that is widely available, though it is used more frequently in the inpatient and intensive care unit setting than in the ED (Fig. 3.10). It is important to understand that although Venturi masks are often referred to as *high-flow* systems, they cannot provide Fio_2 above 35%. The primary advantage of the Venturi mask system is that Fio_2 can be precisely controlled between 21% and 35% for patients who may not tolerate a higher or imprecise Fio_2. Room air is pulled into the system through entrainment ports and mixes with the O_2 provided from the O_2 source. The proportion of entrained air—and therefore Fio_2—is constant and determined by the velocity of the O_2 jet and the size of the entrainment ports. Because the total gas flow (O_2 plus air through the entrainment ports) meets or exceeds the patient's inspiratory flow rate, no additional entrainment of air occurs around the mask, thereby minimizing changes in Fio_2 as the patient's respiratory pattern changes.[70,71] The mask is continuously flushed by the

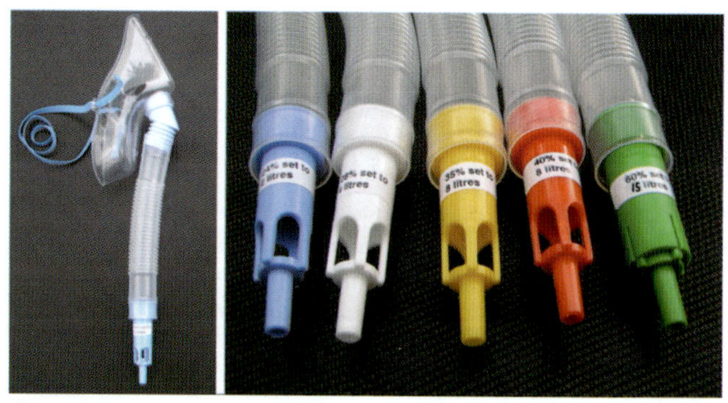

Fig. 3.10 The Venturi mask, also known as an air entrainment mask, delivers a known oxygen concentration to patients requiring controlled oxygen therapy. Venturi mask kits include multiple color-coded interchangeable oxygen dilution jets that are selected and placed in the base of the mask tubing to provide a specific Fio_2. Marked on each jet is the flow rate of wall oxygen required to deliver the specific Fio_2 associated with that diluter. For example, a blue jet provides 24% Fio_2 when 2 L/min is delivered from the wall oxygen source. There are stepwise increments, from the white jet providing 28% Fio_2 at 4 L/min, up to the green jet providing 60% Fio_2 at 15 L/min. (Courtesy Dr. Ronan O'Driscoll.)

high flow of gas, that prevents the accumulation of exhaled gas in the mask. Venturi masks are packaged with multiple inserts, each with a different size orifice for O_2 inflow. Fio_2 is determined by selecting the appropriate colored insert and O_2 flow rate according to the manufacturer's instructions. All Venturi mask settings and inserts provide a total gas flow of 30 L/min that matches the inspiratory flow rate of a resting adult. Importantly a patient in respiratory distress may have an inspiratory flow rate of 50 to 100 L/min.[71] If the patient's inspiratory flow rate exceeds the total gas flow delivered by the mask, additional air will be entrained around the mask, and inspired Fio_2 will decrease. This is especially true with masks rated above 35% Fio_2, that generally can only provide high Fio_2 if minimal room air is entrained around the edges of the mask. Caution should be used with masks rated above 35% in patients with respiratory distress because Fio_2 may be significantly reduced with high inspiratory flow rates.

High-flow nasal oxygen (HFNO) is the delivery of heated, humidified oxygen at high-flow rates (up to approximately 60 L/min) through wide-bore nasal cannulas. HFNO is hypothesized to deliver a higher Fio_2 than face mask oxygen because the nasopharynx acts as a natural reservoir that refills with oxygen after each breath,[76] though at high-flow rates face mask oxygen probably also fills the nasopharynx. HFNO requires three components: wide-bore nasal prongs, a humidifier, and a gas delivery device to control flow. Whereas HFNO requires additional equipment and a brief setup for each patient, it delivers very high Fio_2 and is better tolerated by patients than face mask oxygen and NIV.[74,77] At flow rates of 15 L/min, Fio_2 is 70% to 80%,[72] and at flow rates of 45 L/min, Fio_2 is 90% or higher.[74] These Fio_2 values remain relatively constant, even when the patient's mouth is open.[76] Commercially available HFNO systems typically use flow rates of 5 to 40 L/min and are capable of delivering an Fio_2 of close to 100%. HFNO is not well tolerated unless it is humidified, so commercially available systems (e.g., Vapotherm, Paykel Nasal High Flow, AquinOx) deliver oxygen with nearly 100% humidity. HFNO devices are popular in neonatal and pediatric intensive care units and are commonly used for respiratory support after extubation and for management of respiratory disease in neonates.[78,79]

HFNO has been demonstrated to increase tidal volumes and increase end-expiratory lung volumes after cardiac surgery[80] and was associated with lower rates of escalation to more invasive modes of ventilation in two ED studies.[81,82] A landmark trial that randomized patients with acute hypoxemic respiratory failure without hypercapnia to receive HFNO, face mask oxygen, or NIV found similar intubation rates but lower 90-day mortality in the HFNO group.[83] Though the results of this trial are not necessarily generalizable to ED patients, it does demonstrate that HFNO provides similar oxygenation support for patients with severe hypoxemia as compared to NIV. This makes HFNO a useful tool for patients who do not need immediate tracheal intubation and may be susceptible to mechanical ventilator–induced lung injury.

Procedure

In selecting the proper delivery device, consider the clinical condition of the patient and the amount of O_2 needed. Venturi systems should generally be used for patients who need precise control of Fio_2, such as COPD patients with chronic respiratory acidosis. Nasal cannulas and face masks set at lower flow rates are appropriate for patients who need supplemental O_2 and do not require precise control of Fio_2. Patients with significant hypoxemia, end-organ dysfunction, or respiratory distress require a higher Fio_2 delivery system.

Frequent clinical assessment and blood oxygen saturation (Spo_2) monitoring are needed in all patients receiving O_2 therapy. Equilibration of Sao_2 after changes in supplemental O_2 occurs within 5 minutes.[84] Fio_2 should be titrated to achieve therapeutic goals while minimizing the risk for complications. An Sao_2 of 90% to 95% ($Pao_2 \approx 60$ to 80 mm Hg) is an appropriate target for most patients receiving supplemental O_2.[61] Increases above these levels do not add appreciably to the O_2 content of blood and are unlikely to confer an additional benefit. One may exceed these parameters in patients with shock and end-organ dysfunction, and the added risk and small potential benefit should be considered on an individual basis.

An initial Fio_2 of 24% to 28% delivered by Venturi mask is indicated for patients with hypoxemia and chronic respiratory acidosis.[61,68] Periodic blood gas analysis or capnography is imperative for those at risk for respiratory acidosis.[85,86] In patients with COPD-associated hypercapnia, an Sao_2 of 90% ($Pao_2 \approx 60$ mm Hg) should be the goal of O_2 therapy.[85,86] Mechanical ventilation should be considered when oxygenation goals cannot be achieved without progressive respiratory acidosis.

Preoxygenation Prior to Tracheal Intubation

Preoxygenation prior to tracheal intubation is one of the most important aspects of emergency airway management and is a different concept than supplemental oxygenation. Whereas the goal of supplemental oxygenation is to maintain normoxemia, the goal of preoxygenation is to replace all nitrogen in the lungs with oxygen, thereby creating a reservoir of oxygen available to the body during the intubation process. Preoxygenation and oxygen therapy during apnea are discussed fully in Chapter 4.

Complications of Oxygen Therapy

Worsening of CO_2 retention leading to progressive respiratory acidosis and obtundation in patients with COPD is the complication most likely to be seen in the ED. This phenomenon is well documented and was first described by Barach in 1937.[87] It has been attributed to several mechanisms, including loss of hypoxic respiratory drive, ventilation-perfusion ($\dot{V}/\dot{Q}$) mismatch, and decreased hemoglobin affinity for CO_2 (Haldane effect). This avoidable complication is best prevented by administering O_2 to chronic CO_2 retainers only when there is an indication, administering it at the smallest effective dose, and carefully monitoring clinical, capnographic, and arterial blood gas parameters.

Exposing the brain and lung to excessive concentrations of O_2 can lead to toxicity and, in severe cases, can cause acute respiratory distress syndrome (ARDS). Injury to the pulmonary parenchyma is created by the formation of reactive oxygen species. Oxygen toxicity is of special concern in premature neonates, in whom prolonged hyperoxemia can lead to retinopathy. No data describe what concentration or duration of exposure to O_2 leads to toxicity, and presumably both these factors and individual patient characteristics determine the likelihood of toxicity. The benefits of O_2 therapy in the ED usually outweigh the risk for O_2 toxicity. Fear of toxicity should not prevent the use of O_2 when there is an indication and should encourage the clinician to use the minimum concentration of O_2 necessary to achieve therapeutic goals. High concentrations of O_2 are well tolerated over short periods and may be lifesaving.

In patients receiving high concentrations of supplemental O_2, nitrogen in the alveoli is largely replaced by O_2. If this O_2 is then absorbed into the blood faster than it can be replaced, the volume of the alveoli will decrease and absorptive atelectasis

Bag-Mask Ventilation

Indications

Initial ventilation technique in apneic patients
Rescue ventilation after failed intubation

Contraindications

Situations when application of a face mask is impossible (e.g., deforming facial trauma, thick beards)

Complications

Inability to ventilate
Gastric inflation

Equipment

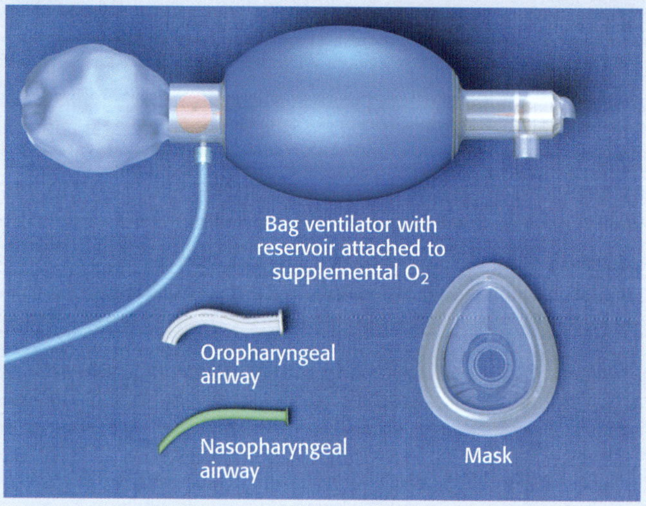

Review Box 3.2 Bag-mask ventilation: indications, contraindications, complications, and equipment

can occur. Airway obstruction potentiates this problem by preventing the rapid replacement of absorbed gas.

BAG-MASK VENTILATION

BMV is the single most important technique for emergency airway management (Review Box 2).[1,10,88] Bag-mask devices are widely available and are standard equipment in all patient care settings. Although the bag-mask method of ventilation appears to be simple, it can be difficult to perform correctly. BMV should only be used in apneic or nearly apneic patients. When a BMV device is used in spontaneously breathing patients an imperfect seal can be difficult to detect, and even if a perfect seal is present only room air might be delivered with many devices.[89] Good BMV skills are a prerequisite to more advanced methods of emergency airway management.[1] Manually opening the airway, properly positioning the head and neck, placing an oropharyngeal airway device, and achieving a tight face mask seal are the keys to good BMV.

Indications and Contraindications

BMV is the most common initial technique for ventilation of apneic patients and for rescue ventilation after failed intubation.[1,90] While BMV is relatively contraindicated in patients with a full stomach or unknown nil per os (NPO) status because of a higher risk for stomach inflation and subsequent aspiration, these are the patients for whom ED clinicians most commonly use BMV. In emergency situations the need for ventilation and oxygenation always takes priority over potential aspiration.[75]

The only contraindication to attempting BMV is when application of a face mask is impossible. It is often impossible to achieve an effective face mask seal on patients with significant deforming facial trauma and those with thick beards (Fig. 3.11). An extraglottic device, such as an LMA or King LT, is a better choice for initial ventilation in such patients.

Bag-Mask Ventilation Technique

Achieving adequate ventilation with a bag-mask device requires an open upper airway and a good mask seal. Overly aggressive BMV causes stomach inflation and increases the risk for aspiration. The goal is to achieve adequate gas exchange while keeping peak airway pressure low. Squeezing the bag forcefully creates high peak airway pressure and is more likely to inflate the stomach. Several studies have shown that increased tidal volume is associated with higher peak airway pressure and increased gastric inflation.[91–93] Decreased inspiratory time (faster bag squeeze) increases peak airway pressure and gastric inflation.[94,95] Therefore the best method of BMV is to provide a tidal volume of approximately 500 mL delivered over 1 to 1.5 seconds.[95] Using a ventilator (instead of a resuscitation bag) to provide the proper tidal volume and inspiratory time is an alternative to using a bag-valve device.[96] Effective ventilation and oxygenation should be judged by chest rise, breath sounds, SpO_2, and capnography.

A variety of mask configurations are available to facilitate a tight seal. The most common mask used in ED situations is a transparent disposable plastic mask with a high-volume, low-pressure cuff. This type of mask eliminates the need for an anatomically formed mask and can be used for a wide variety of patients with different facial features. Various mask sizes are available.

For a single rescuer, only one hand can be used to achieve the seal because the other must squeeze the bag. The rescuer must apply pressure anteriorly while simultaneously lifting the jaw forward. The thumb and index finger provide anterior pressure while the fifth and fourth fingers lift the jaw. The C-E clamp technique is often the most effective if an assistant is not available; the thumb and index finger form a "C" to provide anterior pressure over the mask, and the third, fourth, and fifth fingers form an "E" to lift the jaw (Fig. 3.12, steps 1 and 2). Generally, well-fitting intact dentures should be left in place to help ensure a better seal with the mask.

Laryngeal Mask Airway Insertion

Indications

Failed rapid-sequence intubation
Difficult bag-mask ventilation
Difficult intubation
Facial trauma
Obesity
Primary airway in cardiac arrest or use by emergency medical services

Contraindications

Limited mouth opening (<2 cm)
High airway pressure
Inadequate paralysis or sedation

Complications

Inability to ventilate (rare)
Inability to intubate
Aspiration (rare)

Equipment

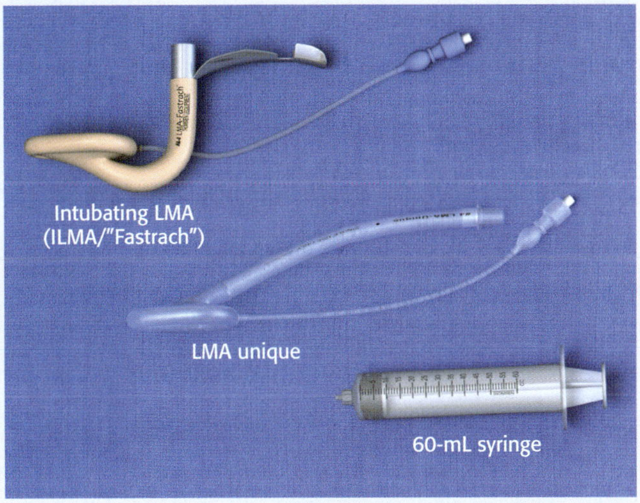

Review Box 3.3 Laryngeal mask airways: indications, contraindications, complications, and equipment.

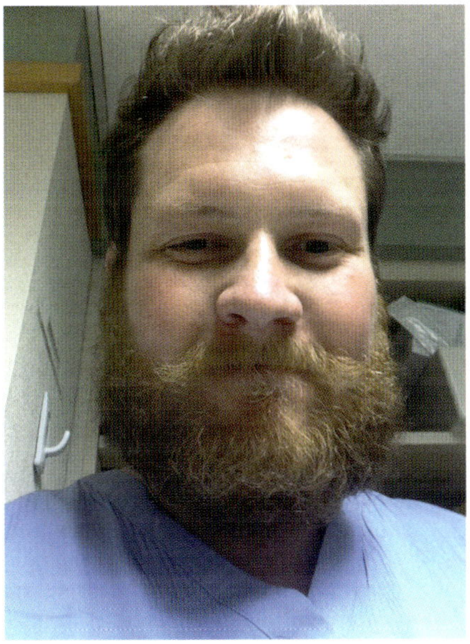

Fig. 3.11 Large beards and facial trauma make it difficult or impossible to obtain a tight seal against the face for bag-mask ventilation. For this patient, a laryngeal mask airway is probably the best first-line oxygenation device.

In the ED setting, it is best to hold the face mask with two hands and have an assistant squeeze the bag. If face mask ventilation is difficult, the most experienced clinician should hold the face mask while the less experienced clinician squeezes the bag.

There are two different methods for two-handed face mask control. The traditional technique is the double C-E method, where the thumb and index finger of both hands encircle the top of the mask (Fig. 3.12, step 3) and the third, fourth, and fifth fingers of both hands form an "E" to lift both sides of the mandible to meet the mask (Fig. 3.12, step 4). The problem with the double C-E technique is that it is difficult to perform a good jaw-thrust with the hands in this position.

The best two-handed method is to hold the mask in place with the thenar eminence of both hands (Fig. 3.12, step 5) and use the long fingers under the angle of the mandible to perform a jaw thrust while also pressing the mask firmly against the face (Fig. 3.12, step 6). This technique allows the operator to perform a good jaw lift (essentially a jaw thrust that creates mandibular protrusion—an "underbite") and creates a good mask seal with the strongest muscles of the hands (Fig. 3.13).[97,98] This method is best for patients with difficult mask ventilation, and it also allows inexperienced clinicians and those with small hands to do a better job with face mask ventilation.[98] Oropharyngeal or nasopharyngeal airways (or both) should be used whenever face mask ventilation is difficult, recognizing that a strong jaw lift may obviate need for their use.

All bag-mask devices should be attached to a supplemental O_2 source with a flow rate of 15 L/min or higher to avoid hypoxia. A significant problem with the bag-mask method is the low percentage of O_2 achieved with some reservoirs. The amount of O_2 delivered is dependent on the ventilatory rate, the volumes delivered during each breath, the O_2 flow rate into the ventilating bag, the filling time for reservoir bags, and the type of reservoir used. For adults, a bag-mask device should have an inspiratory valve, a 1500-mL bag reservoir, and one-way exhalation port to provide adequate oxygenation during use.[2] During positive pressure bagging to an apneic patient, 100% oxygen will be delivered regardless of the type of bag-mask device. During spontaneous breathing the configuration of the exhalation valve is of critical importance; bags without one-way exhalation port provide mostly room air during active inspiration.[89]

Pediatric bag-mask devices should have a minimum volume of 450 mL. Pediatric and larger bags may be used to ventilate infants with the proper mask size, and care must be maintained to administer only the volume necessary to effectively ventilate the infant. Avoid pop-off valves because the

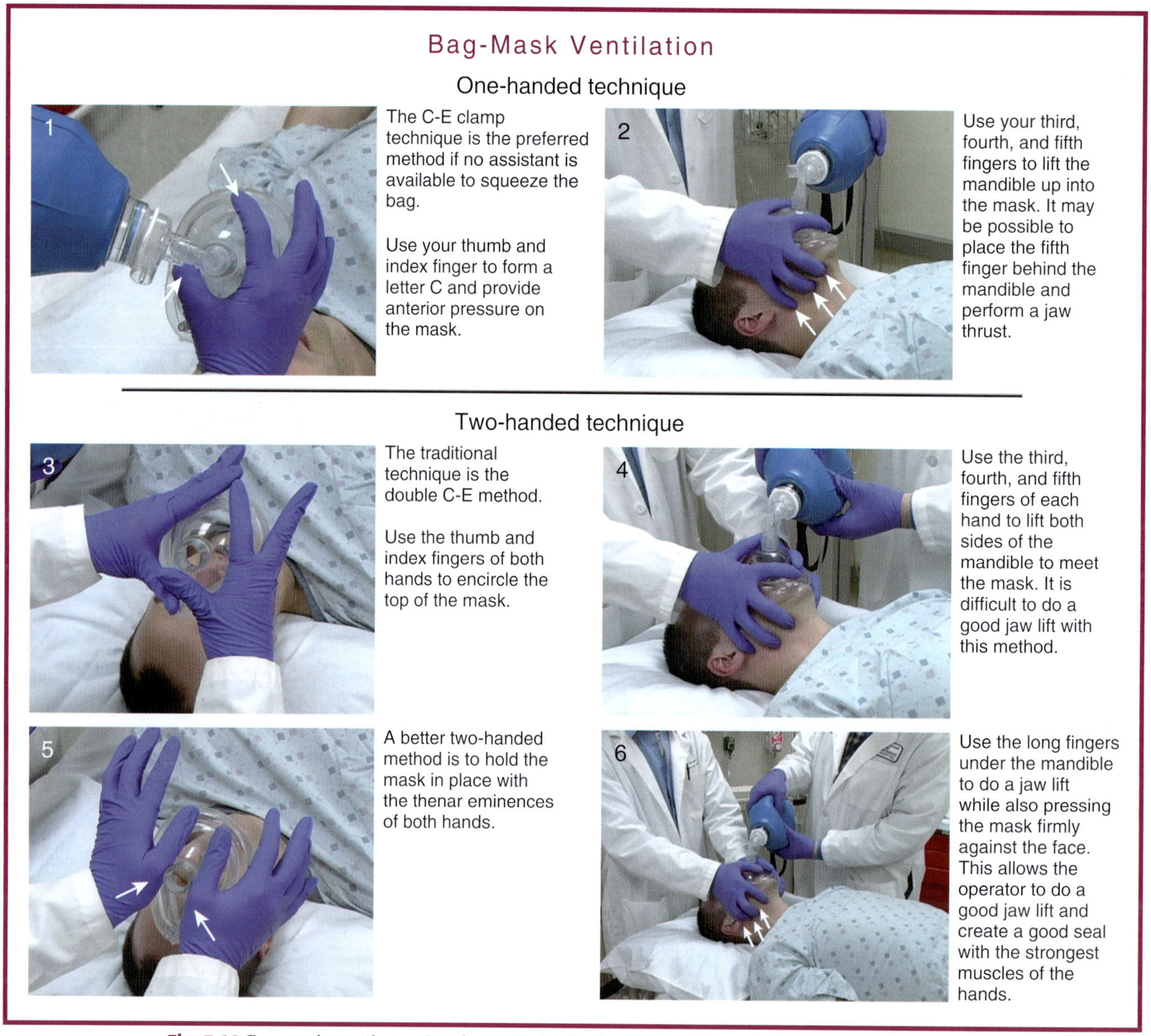

Fig. 3.12 Bag-mask ventilation. It is best to hold the face mask with two hands and have an assistant squeeze the bag. If face mask ventilation is difficult, the most experienced clinician should hold the mask while the less experienced clinician squeezes the bag.

airway pressure required for ventilation under emergency conditions can exceed the pressure of the valve.[99–101]

Previously it had been contended that mask ventilation could be made more difficult after administration of paralytic agents.[102] Many studies demonstrate that BMV after paralysis is generally easier and provides larger tidal volumes.[103–107] It is generally not necessary to test whether the patient can be successfully mask-ventilated before administration of paralytic agents, and it is prudent to assess for markers of difficult BMV (see Complications later).

BMV may be the best method of prehospital airway support in trauma patients and children. Murray and colleagues[108] performed a large retrospective study suggesting that patients with severe head injury had a higher risk for mortality if they were intubated in the prehospital setting. In the same year, Gausche and colleagues[109] reported that neurologic outcomes and ultimate survival rates after prehospital pediatric resuscitation with BMV by emergency medical service (EMS) clinicians were as good as those with tracheal intubation.

Some have advocated using pediatric resuscitation bags (~500 mL volume) for adult patients to minimize the risk of excessive ventilation.[93] Although this may be more relevant in stabilized intubated patients, there are no clinical studies to support this practice in the setting of BMV for nonintubated patients in emergency setting. This practice could result in inadequate tidal volumes because the volume delivered with BMV is often less than expected, especially when there is a mask leak or inexperienced operator.[110–112] Although low pressure and low tidal volume ventilation are appropriate for most patients who are in cardiac arrest or in the intensive care unit (ICU) after initial resuscitation, emergency and critical care clinicians manage patients with a wide variety of anatomic and physiologic derangements, and it is likely that some of them need higher ventilation pressure and volume when they are in extremis. There are no clinical studies on using pediatric resuscitation bags for adults with a wide variety of airway emergencies. Extrapolating data from intubated patients in the operating room setting or from manikin studies may be

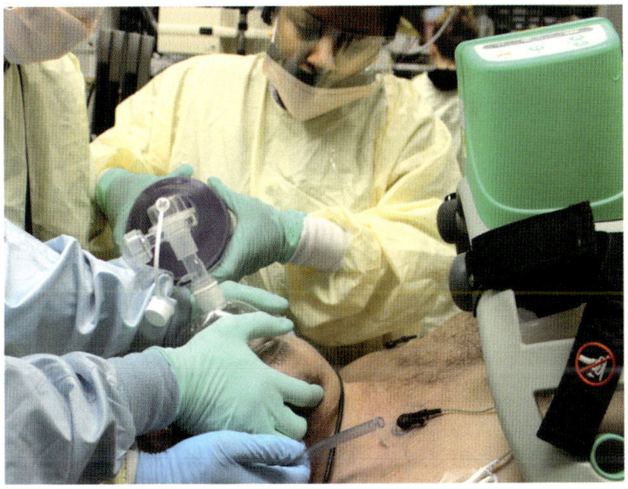

Fig. 3.13 A good example of bag-mask ventilation using the preferred two-handed technique. Using this method allows the strongest muscles of the hands to perform a jaw thrust, which pulls the face into the mask to create a seal.

misleading. Presently, it is safer to use adult-sized resuscitator bags and pay close attention to bagging technique.

Complications

The main complications of BMV are gastric inflation and inability to ventilate. Langeron and colleagues[113] performed a large prospective study of adults undergoing general anesthesia and reported a 5% incidence of difficult mask ventilation. The incidence is obviously much higher in the emergency setting. Risk factors for difficult BMV include presence of a beard, severe facial trauma, obesity, lack of teeth, age older than 55 years, history of snoring, short thyromental distance, limited mandibular protrusion, and decreased pulmonary compliance (severe asthma, COPD, ARDS, term pregnancy) (Box 3.2).[113–116] It may be best to paralyze patients who are not spontaneously breathing and still awake enough to interfere with BMV.

When mask ventilation is technically difficult, higher peak airway pressure is often required to provide adequate tidal volume. In these situations, gastric inflation is more likely and aspiration may occur. Be vigilant to recognize complications early and take corrective action. Even when BMV is easy and a good technique is used, some gastric distension will generally occur. Minor gastric distention should not be considered substandard in the setting of prolonged BMV. It may be reasonable to place an orogastric tube to decompress the stomach if bagging is prolonged or if there is obvious gastric distension.

Cricoid Pressure (Sellick Maneuver)

In 1961, Sellick described the use of cricoid pressure to prevent regurgitation during anesthesia, and this technique has since become known as the Sellick maneuver, though more properly termed cricoid pressure.[117] The purpose of this technique is to apply external force to the anterior cricoid ring to push the trachea posteriorly and compress the esophagus against the cervical vertebrae. In theory, cricoid pressure compresses the distensible upper esophagus but not the airway because the cricoid ring is fairly rigid.

BOX 3.2 Risk Factors for Difficult Mask Ventilation

Presence of a beard
Obesity
Lack of teeth
Age >55 years
History of snoring
Short thyromental distance
Limited mandibular protrusion

The proper technique for applying cricoid pressure is to place the thumb and middle finger on either side of the cricoid cartilage, with the index finger in the center anteriorly.[117] Apply 30 N (6.7 lb) of force to the cricoid cartilage in the posterior direction.[118,119] As a reference, approximately 40 N of digital force on the bridge of the nose will usually cause pain.[118]

There is no good evidence that cricoid pressure prevents esophageal regurgitation,[118,120] though it may prevent gastric inflation during BMV,[117,118,120–124] thereby reducing the risk for subsequent regurgitation and vomiting. Cricoid pressure has been demonstrated to reduce tidal volumes, increase peak inspiratory pressure, and prevent adequate air exchange when applied during BMV.[121,123–132] Cricoid pressure also decreases successful insertion of and intubation through LMAs.[133–140]

The routine use of cricoid pressure during BMV of patients in cardiac arrest is not recommended by the AHA guidelines for CPR and emergency cardiovascular care.[141] Cricoid pressure should be released immediately if there is any difficulty ventilating with a face mask in an emergency setting.[120] It is reasonable to release or relax cricoid pressure during insertion of an LMA or if ventilation with the LMA is difficult.[118,120,139] It may also be reasonable to release cricoid pressure during laryngoscopy and tracheal intubation (discussed in Chapter 4).

EXTRAGLOTTIC AIRWAY DEVICES

EGDs are devices that are blindly placed above or posterior to the larynx to allow rapid ventilation and oxygenation. These devices can provide rescue oxygenation and ventilation to a wide spectrum of patients and are especially useful for patients who are difficult or impossible to ventilate and oxygenate with a face mask (e.g., elevated BMI patients and those with large beards or significant facial trauma). In the emergency setting, EGDs can provide temporary rescue ventilation until tracheal intubation or a surgical airway can be performed. It is important to have at least one of these devices immediately available when managing emergency airways. EGDs can be divided into two groups, LMAs and retroglottic devices (King LT and others).

Laryngeal Mask Airways

The LMA consists of a hollow shaft or airway tube connected to an oval inflatable mask-like cuff designed to sit in the hypopharynx facing the glottis, with the tip at the esophageal inlet. The cuffed mask is designed to form a seal around the glottis when the device is placed properly. Some LMAs (LMA Fastrach and LMA Proseal; Teleflex) have handles that allow the operator to increase seal pressure by lifting the entire device toward the ceiling (Review Box 3.3). The first LMA, the LMA Classic (Teleflex) became available in 1988. Since then it has been used more than 200 million times and has been described in more than 2500 academic papers.[139,142] LMAs are widely considered to be essential adjuncts for rescue ventilation and difficult intubation,[143] can be inserted in less than 30 seconds, and provide effective ventilation in more than 98% of patients.[139] LMAs are primary rescue adjuncts in the difficult airway guidelines put forth by the American Society of Anesthesiologists[144] and the Difficult Airway Society in Europe.[145] Advanced Cardiac Life Support guidelines suggest that the LMA is a reasonable alternative to face mask ventilation.[141] Pediatric Advanced Life Support guidelines acknowledge the LMA as a backup device for difficult pediatric airways.[146] In anesthesia practice, LMAs are now used for a large percentage of cases in which an endotracheal tube may have been used in the past.

This chapter describes how to insert an intubating LMA (ILMA; LMA Fastrach) and use it for rescue ventilation. Chapter 4 expands on additional uses of the ILMA for tracheal intubation. The insertion and use of the nonintubating LMA Unique (the disposable version of the LMA Classic) and LMA Supreme (Teleflex) will also be described because they are inexpensive, disposable, well tested, and widely available, and their use is similar to EGDs made by other manufacturers.

Indications

Both ILMAs and nonintubating LMAs can be used in the "cannot intubate/cannot ventilate" scenario with high success rates and are useful when face mask ventilation is difficult because of a beard, massive facial trauma, or obesity (Fig. 3.14).

The ILMA should be the LMA of choice for emergency use. In the cannot intubate/cannot ventilate scenario, adequate ventilation with the ILMA is possible in nearly all cases and is more successful than the LMA.[5,139,147] In this scenario, ventilation with the ILMA is probably superior to BMV.[148] The ILMA can also be used as a primary ventilation and intubation device for patients with difficult airways[149] and is a reasonable alternative to BMV for reoxygenation after a failed tracheal intubation attempt. Tracheal intubation through the ILMA can be accomplished by using a blind technique or under endoscopic guidance (see Chapter 4 for tracheal intubation through the ILMA). Studies of difficult airway management with the ILMA show that almost all patients can be adequately ventilated with the ILMA and 94% to 99% can be intubated through the device.[5,139,150–158] In addition, for difficult airway management the ILMA is technically easier to use than the LMA. In the emergency setting, where obtaining a definitive airway (i.e., tracheal intubation) is the eventual goal, it is more practical to use an ILMA. In addition, the LMA Fastrach is the most widely used and well-studied ILMA and is easier to insert than the LMA Classic.[159–163] Finally, when the head is in the neutral position, the LMA Fastrach is more likely to allow successful ventilation than the LMA Classic during inline stabilization of the cervical spine.[164–166]

EGDs are especially useful in patients with difficult BMV caused by a beard, severe facial trauma, or obesity because none of these factors inhibits ILMA placement. When brisk bleeding above the glottis makes ventilation and intubation difficult, the ILMA can reduce aspiration of blood and facilitate blind or fiberoptic intubation. In patients requiring urgent cricothyrotomy, the ILMA can be used to counteract anterior neck pressure. In this capacity, the ILMA provides temporary ventilation and stabilizes the cervical spine during the surgical airway procedure.

Newer LMAs (and some ILMAs) feature a channel posterior to the airway that allows an orogastric tube to be placed into the stomach while the device is used for oxygenation and ventilation. This is particularly useful in patients with gastric distension after BMV, or as a primary device (instead of BMV) in neonates, infants, and children, because they are especially prone to gastric distension with face mask ventilation.

The LMA Classic (or single-use LMA Unique) is the most extensively tested LMA for children. It may provide a more secure and reliable means of ventilation than BMV.[4] The LMA allows adequate ventilation in 98% of adults with known difficult airways and in 90% to 95% of those with unexpectedly difficult airways.[139,167–170] It is also useful as a rescue device in difficult pediatric airways.[139] Two descriptive studies and 86 case reports describe use of the LMA for difficult pediatric airways.[139,171–177] In these reports, ventilation was adequate with the LMA in nearly all pediatric patients.[139,175,177,178] Case series and case reports also suggest that the LMA can provide an effective rescue airway during neonatal resuscitation if BMV and endotracheal (ET) intubation fail.[179]

Contraindications

The ILMA and LMA are contraindicated in patients with less than 2 cm of mouth opening because they require 2 cm of space between the upper and the lower incisors to be inserted. Any

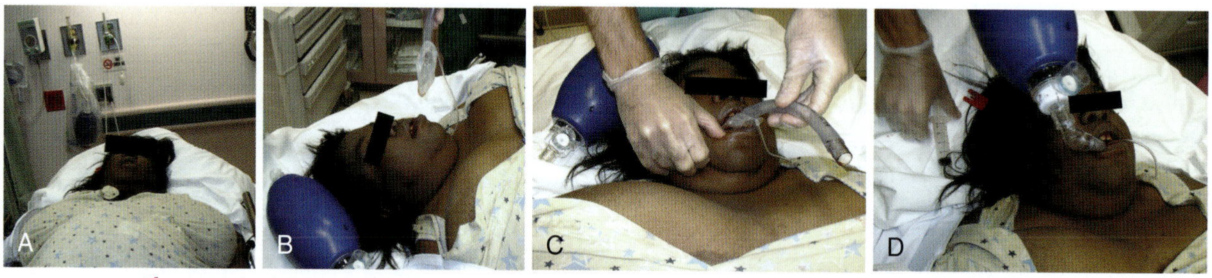

Fig. 3.14 (A) This patient with a markedly elevated body mass index was found asystolic by the emergency medical service. She could not be intubated in the field with multiple attempts and did not survive bag-mask resuscitation. This patient is a candidate for a laryngeal mask airway (LMA). (B–D) The LMA is inserted by depressing the jaw, introduced, advanced, inflated, and attached to a resuscitation bag. Postmortem ventilation with the LMA was very easy. In retrospect, the LMA device should have been the first airway adjunct chosen by the emergency medical service (and in the emergency department), totally bypassing attempts with other methods likely to fail.

LMA is relatively contraindicated in awake patients, especially those with a full stomach, because insertion of an LMA in an awake patient will cause coughing, gagging, or emesis. If an LMA is inserted when the patient is awake and the stomach is full, there is a high likelihood of emesis and aspiration. In the ED, an LMA should be used only if the patient is unconscious or after a paralytic agent has been given. Once an LMA is inserted and ventilation is established, the patient should not be allowed to wake up or gag. Consider giving a long-acting paralytic agent or multiple doses of succinylcholine after an LMA is placed and ventilation is adequate.

Types of LMAs

Several manufacturers now make LMAs as the patent on the LMA Classic expired in 2003. It is important to recognize that all LMAs are not the same.

There are four popular ILMAs. The LMA Fastrach has the most clinical use and research of all the ILMAs (Fig. 3.15A). Advantages include a handle that makes placement easier and allows the operator to lift up to improve the seal against the laryngeal inlet if needed. There is no gastric port that allows for gastric decompression. Blind intubation rates are significantly higher with the LMA Fastrach (Teleflex) compared with the Cook Gas Air-Q[180]; no adequate research has yet been performed comparing blind intubation rates to other devices. The Air-Q intubating laryngeal airway has four different models and is popular with some clinicians (Fig. 3.15B).

The iGel LMA (Intersurgical) features a thermoplastic elastomer cuff that does not need inflation (Fig. 3.15C).[181–190] A gastric channel is present to allow for gastric decompression using an orogastric tube, though this gastric channel is smaller compared with other extraglottic devices. The iGel has gained significant traction in the prehospital realm due to the cuff not needing inflation. The simplicity of the iGel may be a benefit in the prehospital setting, but there is little evidence to

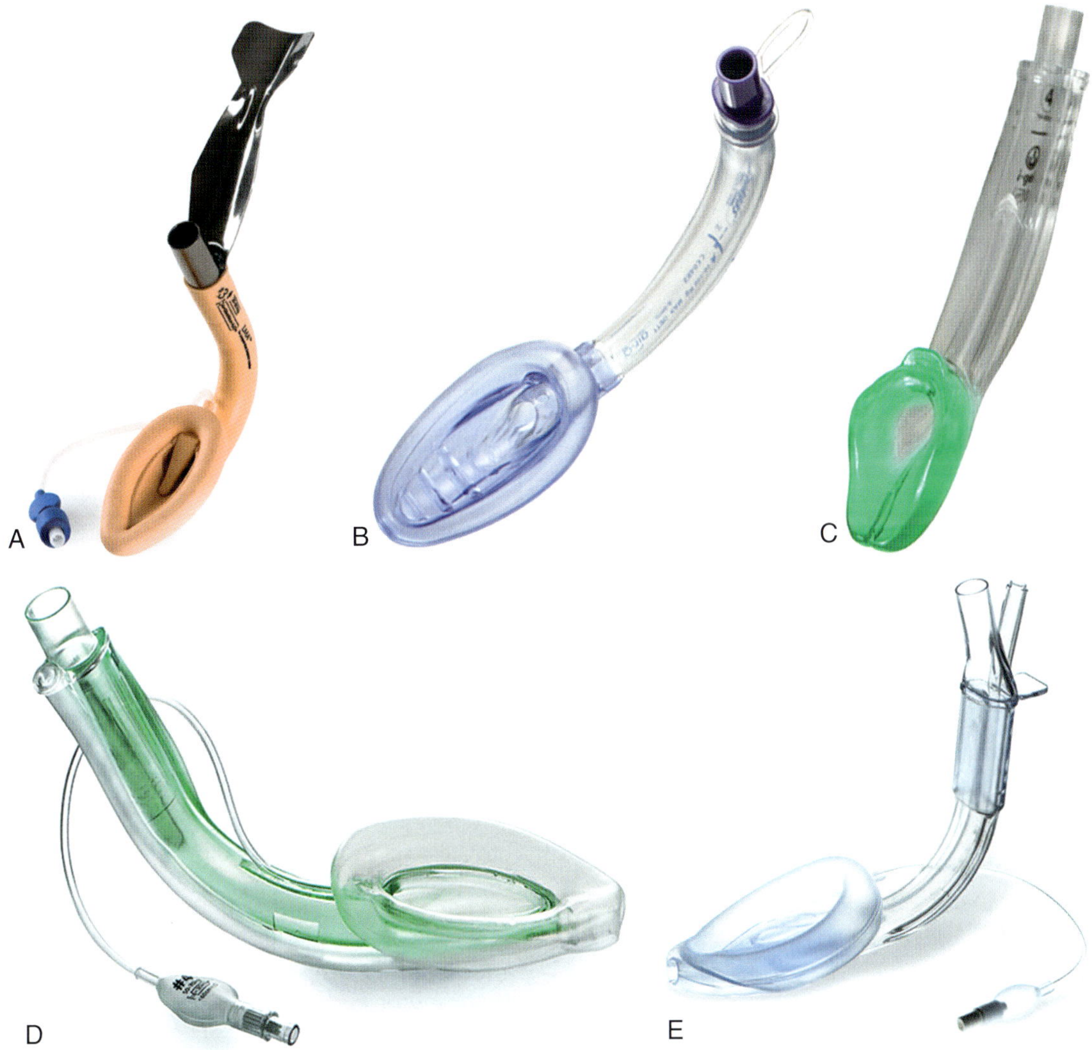

Fig. 3.15 Popular intubating laryngeal mask airways (LMAs) and the LMA Supreme (Teleflex). (A) LMA Fastrach (Teleflex), which has a handle that makes insertion easier and allows the operator to increase the seal pressure if needed, but has no gastric port. (B) Air-Q (Cook Gas LLC), which has four variations (disposable, reusable, noninflatable cuff, and blocker with gastric port). (C) IGel (Intersurgical), features a noninflatable cuff and gastric port. (D) Ambu AuraGain (Ambu), features a gastric port. (E) LMA Supreme, a nonintubating LMA with a rigid shape to make insertion easier and a gastric port.

support its superiority over other extraglottic devices in the ED setting.

The Ambu AuraGain is a newer ILMA with gastric access. In a small study of pediatric patients, the AuraGain demonstrated satisfactory clinical performance when compared to the LMA Supreme.[191] Similar results were found in a randomized study of spontaneously breathing anesthetized adults.[192] (Fig. 3.15D).

The LMA Supreme (Teleflex) is a redesign of the original LMA device (Fig. 3.15E) with slightly different mask shape that allows a better mask seal compared with prior models[193,194] (LMA Classic and LMA Unique) and a gastric evacuation channel. It features a firm curved shape and a bite block handle, so ease of insertion may be similar to that of the Fastrach, and it is available in all sizes from neonate to large adult.[195–204] This LMA does not facilitate tracheal intubation. The LMA Protector (Teleflex) is similar to the LMA Supreme and allows intubation using a flexible endoscope.

EDs should all stock some type of LMA. The brand and model are not of great importance, and consideration can be given for the ability to decompress the stomach and perform intubation through the device. These devices should be easily accessible during emergency airway management and all clinicians should be comfortable with their use.

TABLE 3.1 Laryngeal Mask Airway (LMA), Disposable LMA, and Intubating LMA Size Recommendations Based on Weight

WEIGHT (KG)	LMA	DISPOSABLE LMA	LMA FASTRACH[a]
<5	1	1	—
5–10	1.5	1.5	—
10–20	2	2	—
20–30	2.5	2.5	—
30–50	3	3	3
50–70	4	4	4
70–100	5	5	5
>100	6	—	—

[a]Note that the LMA Fastrach is only available for patients >30 kg; we suggest the Air-Q as an intubating LMA for pediatric patients.

TABLE 3.2 AirQ Size Recommendations Based on Weight

AirQ Size	Weight (kg)	Color	Max ETT Size (OD)
1	< 7		4.5
1.5	7–17		5.0
2	17–30		5.5
2.5	30–50		6.5
3.5	50–70		7.5
4.5	70–100		8.5

ETT, Endotracheal tube; *OD,* outer diameter.

Procedure

The insertion and use of the LMA Fastrach and LMA Classic will be described. Because insertion of all ILMAs and nonintubating LMAs follow similar steps, the procedure for the LMA Fastrach will be illustrative of steps for ILMAs and LMAs that have a rigid body or handle, and the LMA Classic will be illustrative for ILMAs and LMAs that are not rigid and do not utilize a handle.

Intubating LMAs

See Video 3.4. The first step is to select the appropriate size of ILMA, based on manufacturer's recommendations. The Fastrach ILMA is available in three sizes: size 3 for children weighing 30 kg to 50 kg, size 4 for small adults weighing 50 kg to 70 kg, and size 5 for adults weighing 70 kg to 100 kg (Tables 3.1 and 3.2). When there is doubt about which size is appropriate, it is probably better to use the larger size.

After choosing the correct ILMA, completely deflate the cuff while pushing it posteriorly so that it assumes a smooth wedge shape without any wrinkles (Fig. 3.16, step 1). Place a small amount of water-based lubricant onto the posterior surface of the ILMA just before insertion (Fig. 3.16, step 2). Open the patient's mouth and position the posterior mask tip so that it is flat against the hard palate, immediately posterior to the upper incisors (Fig. 3.16, step 3). Advance the airway straight into the mouth along the hard palate without rotation until the curved part of the airway tube is in contact with the patient's chin. Then rotate the ILMA completely into the hypopharynx by advancing it along its curved axis. Keep the posterior of the mask firmly applied to the soft palate and posterior pharynx until firm resistance is felt (Fig. 3.16, step 4). Cricoid pressure impedes proper placement of the ILMA, so briefly release cricoid pressure while the device is rotated into its final position, wedged into the proximal esophagus.[136,137,205] After insertion, the airway tube should emerge from the mouth directed somewhat caudally. Without holding the tube or handle, inflate the mask cuff (Fig. 3.16, step 5). The entire device will normally slide backward a bit when the cuff is inflated. Frequently, only half the maximum cuff volume is sufficient to obtain a good mask seal. Do not overinflate the cuff because this may make the seal worse. See the instruction manual for maximum cuff volumes. Attach a bag and ventilate the patient while using chest rise, breath sounds, and capnography to confirm adequate gas exchange. If bagging is easy and ventilation is good, the aperture of the ILMA is probably aligned correctly over the vocal cords.

If optimal ILMA placement is not accomplished initially, adjusting maneuvers can be attempted. The purpose of adjusting maneuvers is to align the aperture of the ILMA with the glottic opening. Proper positioning of the ILMA aperture with the glottic opening allows optimal ventilation and facilitates tracheal intubation. Before adjusting the ILMA, consider the patient's position and degree of relaxation because both may affect ILMA function. The ILMA works best in the neutral or sniffing position; cervical extension may interfere with proper placement. The patient should not react to ILMA placement with coughing or gagging because this may interfere with proper placement. Have a single operator perform the adjustment maneuvers by gripping the ILMA handle with

Intubating Laryngeal Mask Airway Insertion

1

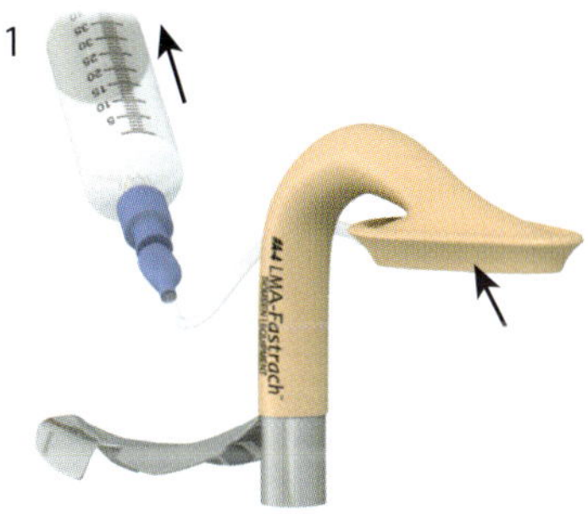

Completely deflate the cuff while pushing it posteriorly, so that it assumes a smooth wedge shape without any wrinkles.

2

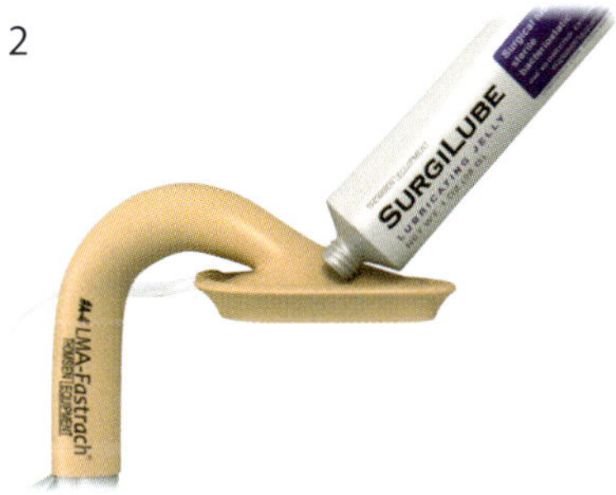

Place a small amount of water-based lubricant onto the posterior surface of the ILMA just before insertion.

3

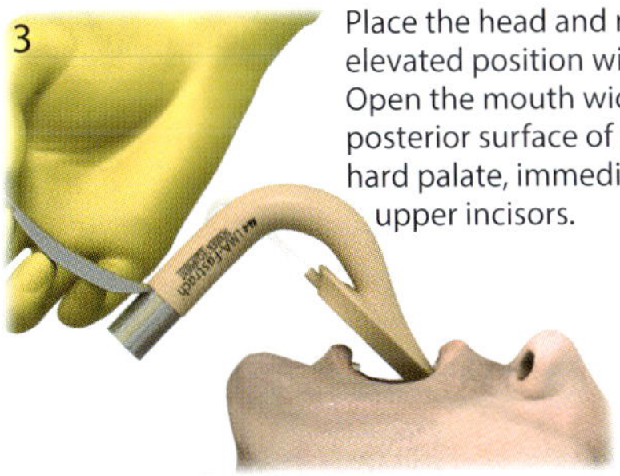

Place the head and neck in a slightly elevated position with minimal extension. Open the mouth widely and place the posterior surface of the device against the hard palate, immediately posterior to the upper incisors.

4

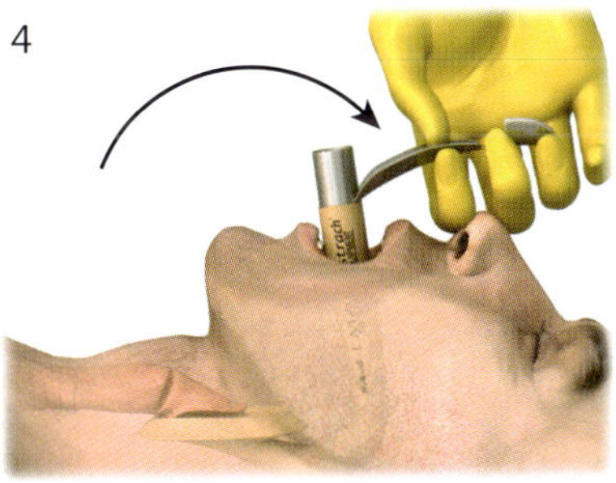

Advance the ILMA straight into the mouth until the curved part of the airway tube contacts the chin. Then, rotate the ILMA into the hypopharynx until firm resistance is felt. Release cricoid pressure during this step.

5

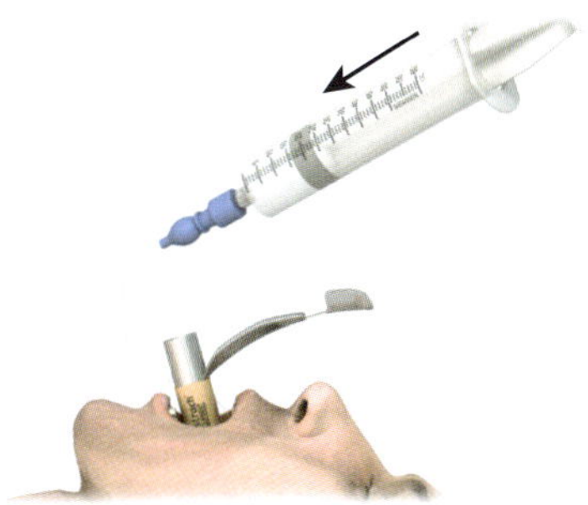

Let go of the handle and inflate the cuff. Initially inflate the cuff with only half of the maximum volume, and increase inflation as needed. Do not overinflate the cuff. (See product manual for maximum volumes.)

6

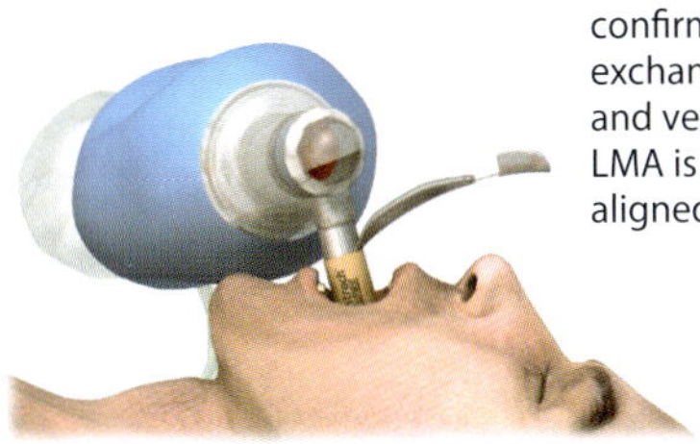

Attach a bag and ventilate the patient. Use chest rise, breath sounds, and capnography to confirm adequate gas exchange. If bagging is easy and ventilation is good, the LMA is probably correctly aligned over the glottis.

7

Chandy Maneuver Step 1

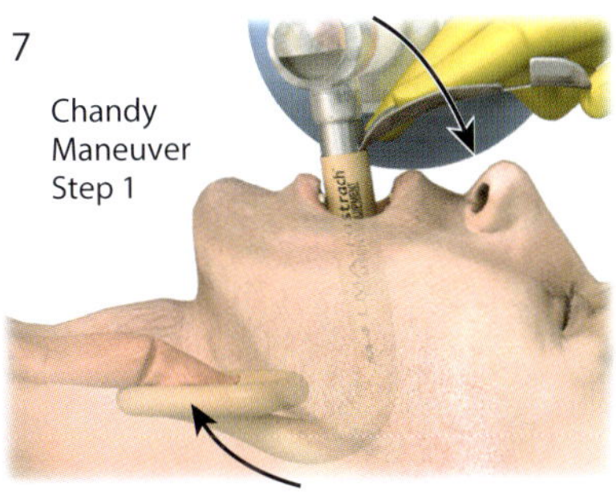

If adjustment is needed, try the Chandy maneuver. First, gently rotate the ILMA farther into the hypopharynx.

8

Chandy Maneuver Step 2

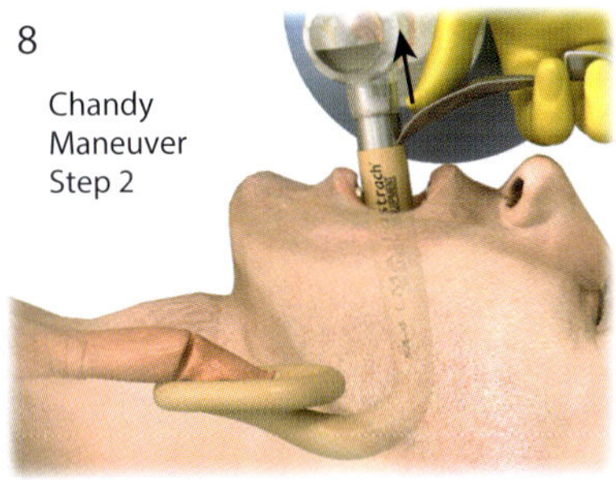

Next, lift the handle upwards, toward the ceiling above the patient's feet.

This manuever aligns the mask with the glottis and may provide for better ventilation.

9

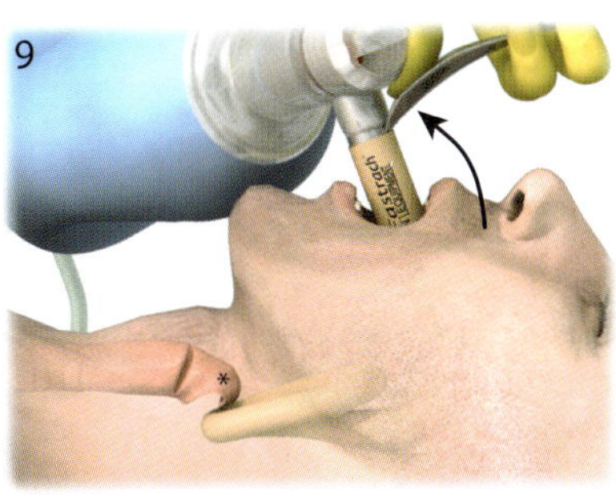

If these manuevers fail, the epiglottis may be folded down over the glottis (asterisk).

Perform the "up-down" manuever, by first rotating the ILMA out of the hypopharynx along its curvature about 5–6 cm.

10

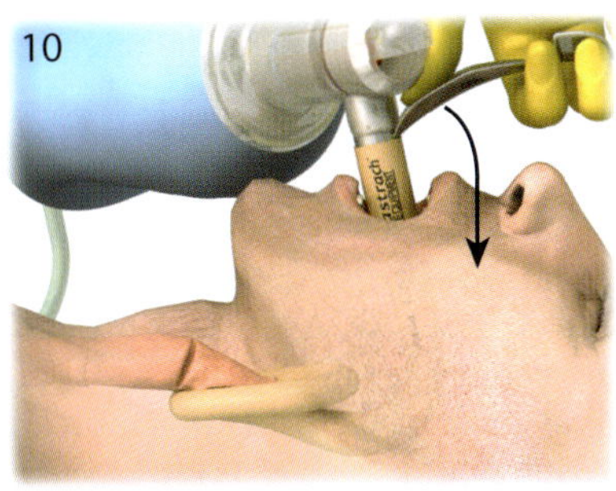

Next, slide the ILMA back into position while pressing it against the posterior pharynx.

(Note, the cuff should remain inflated during this maneuver.)

Fig. 3.16 Intubating laryngeal mask airway *(ILMA;* Fastrach, Teleflex) insertion.

one hand, in a "frying-pan" grip, and providing bag ventilation with the other hand. After each adjustment maneuver, assess the quality of bag ventilation and mask seal. Easy bag ventilation, good chest rise, and absence of an audible mask leak are indications of good ILMA alignment with the glottis (Fig. 3.16, step 6).

To adjust the position of the ILMA, first gently pull the handle toward you without rotation along the ILMA's curvature. Next, gently push the handle toward the patient's feet without rotating it. Finally, try the *Chandy maneuver*, which consists of gently rotating the ILMA farther into the hypopharynx and then lifting the handle toward the ceiling above the patient's feet (Fig. 3.16, steps 7 and 8). If these simple maneuvers do not result in adequate ventilation, consider the "up-down maneuver" (Fig. 3.16, steps 9 and 10). This technique is used to correct downfolding of the epiglottis, which is common with insertion of the ILMA and may interfere with ventilation or intubation. The up-down maneuver is accomplished by rotating the ILMA out of the hypopharynx along its curvature approximately 5 cm to 6 cm while the cuff remains inflated, and then sliding it back into position while pressing it against the posterior pharynx. Do not use excessive force when placing or adjusting the ILMA.

If adjusting maneuvers do not result in adequate ventilation, it is likely that the wrong size ILMA has been used. Incorrect ILMA size is more likely to be a problem if the device is too small; attempting insertion of a larger ILMA is a reasonable first approach. If another ILMA size is not available, external anterior neck manipulation or downward pressure may bring the glottis and ILMA cuff into proper alignment. If the size of the ILMA is not in question, consider completely removing and carefully reinserting the device (see Chapter 4 for intubation through the ILMA and ILMA removal).

Nonintubating LMAs

The following steps describe the use of the LMA Classic (or single-use LMA Unique), although these instructions will be similar for other LMAs that do not have a handle similar to the LMA Fastrach or LMA Supreme.

The first step is to select the appropriate size LMA. The LMA is available in a wide range of sizes, from size 1 for neonates weighing less than 5 kg to size 6 for adults weighing more than 100 kg. The disposable version is available in sizes 1 through 5, and not size 6. After selecting the proper size, completely deflate the LMA cuff while pushing it posteriorly so that it forms a smooth wedge shape without any wrinkles (Fig. 3.17, step 1). Place a small amount of water-based lubricant onto the posterior surface of the LMA just before insertion (Fig. 3.17, step 2). The best patient position for insertion of the LMA is the sniffing position, with the neck flexed and the head extended. The LMA may be inserted via two different techniques, depending on access to the patient. The most common method is the index finger insertion technique. This is accomplished by holding the LMA like a pen, with the index finger at the junction of the airway tube and the cuff (Fig. 3.17, step 3). Have an assistant open the patient's mouth and insert the LMA with the posterior tip pressed against the hard palate just behind the upper incisors (Fig. 3.17, step 4). Under direct vision, use the index finger to slide the LMA along the hard palate and into the oropharynx (Fig. 3.17, step 5). As the LMA is inserted farther, extend the index finger and push the posterior cuff along the soft palate and posterior pharynx. Exert counterpressure on the back of the patient's head during insertion. Continue to push the LMA into the hypopharynx until resistance is felt. Use the other hand to hold the proximal end of the LMA tube while removing your index finger from the patient's mouth (Fig. 3.17, step 6).

An alternative method is the thumb insertion technique. Use this technique when you have limited access to the patient from behind (see www.lmana.com for details). Hold the LMA with your thumb at the junction of the cuff and the airway tube. Place the mask against the hard palate under direct vision, as with the index finger technique. Use the thumb to push the LMA into the mouth along the palate and posterior pharynx. Hold the end of the airway tube with the other hand while removing your thumb from the patient's mouth.

After the LMA is fully inserted, let go of the proximal end of the airway tube and inflate the cuff enough to achieve a good seal over the glottis (Fig. 3.17, step 7). This may require only half the maximum cuff volume. Be careful to not over-inflate the LMA cuff (see the product packaging for maximal cuff volumes). Attach a bag and ventilate the patient, with chest rise, breath sounds, and capnography used to confirm adequate gas exchange (Fig. 3.17, step 8). If bagging is easy and ventilation is good, the aperture of the LMA is probably aligned correctly over the glottic opening. Proper positioning of the LMA aperture with the glottic opening allows optimal ventilation.

Several tips or techniques should be considered if LMA ventilation is inadequate. The best way to ensure proper ventilation is to optimize the insertion technique by carefully following the aforementioned directions. Position the patient's head and neck properly and ensure that the patient is deeply anesthetized or paralyzed. Listen for an audible cuff leak to make sure that a good mask seal has been achieved. Adjust the cuff volume if necessary to improve the mask seal and ensure optimal ventilation. Simply adding more air to the cuff will not necessarily improve the seal of the mask with the glottis. Cuff overinflation may cause a leak, and deflation with repositioning may improve the seal.

Sometimes adjusting the patient's head and neck position is easier than trying to change the position of the LMA. Move the patient into a better sniffing position or into the chin-to-chest position to see whether this improves the LMA cuff seal. If these positions do not help or are not possible, try a jaw-thrust or a chin-lift maneuver. Apply anterior neck pressure to help manipulate the glottis into improved contact with the LMA mask. This technique can be used in combination with any of the maneuvers just discussed.

If mask seal and ventilation are still not optimal after simple repositioning maneuvers, withdraw, advance, or rotate the LMA cuff. Another alternative is to completely remove and reinsert the LMA while paying careful attention to the details just described. If unsuccessful, change the size of the LMA. A larger LMA will usually improve ventilation even if it is more difficult to insert. It is much more common to need to increase the LMA size than to decrease it. Finally, consider using the ILMA, placing a King LT, or performing a surgical airway when ventilation with the LMA is not adequate.

Aftercare

If the LMA or ILMA will remain in place without tracheal intubation, either one can be secured like an endotracheal tube. Removal of the ILMA after tracheal intubation is easy, but more difficult than insertion of the device (see Chapter 4).

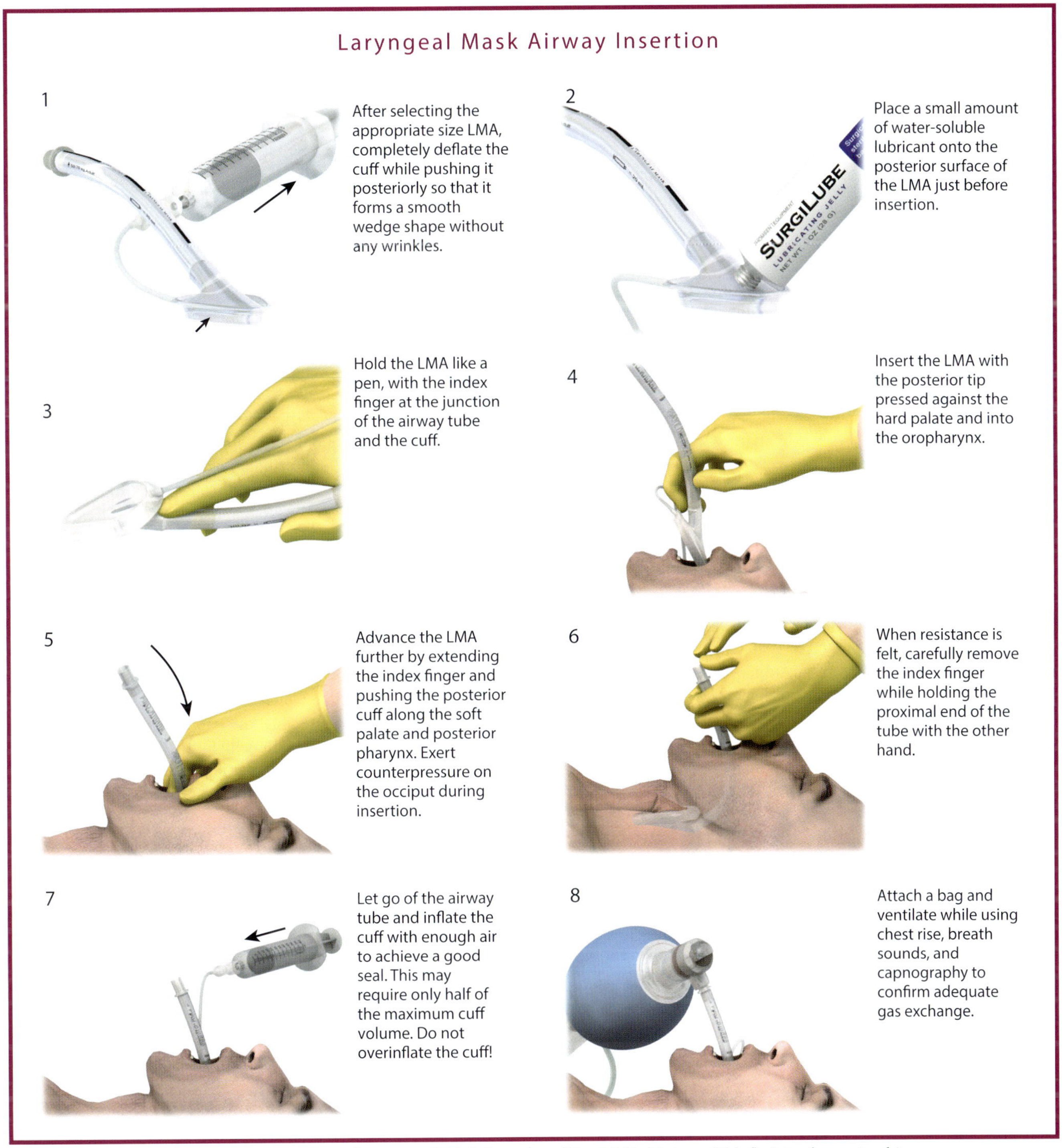

Fig. 3.17 Laryngeal mask airway *(LMA)* insertion. The LMA Unique (Teleflex) is shown in this sequence.

Complications

The most important complications associated with using the LMA are aspiration of gastric contents and hypoxia. The LMA does not fully protect against aspiration and may actually cause vomiting if the patient gags during placement of the device. In fasted anesthetized patients, the incidence of aspiration is very low, approximately 2 per 10,000 cases.[139] There are many descriptive studies and case reports of the use of an LMA for difficult airways with no mention of significant aspiration.[139] Although the risk for aspiration is surely higher than 2 per 10,000 when using the LMA in the ED, it probably results in less passive regurgitation gastric inflation compared to BMV.

Retroglottic Airway Devices

King LT

The King LT (King Airway-LTS-D EMS; King Systems) is a retroglottic device that functions similar to the esophageal-tracheal Combitube (see later). Like the Combitube, the LT is designed to isolate the glottic opening between an oropharyngeal cuff and an esophageal cuff (Review Box 3.4). Unlike

Retroglottic Airway Devices

Indications

Primary airway in the emergency medical services setting
Primary airway in cardiac arrest
Failed rapid-sequence intubation
Difficult bag-mask ventilation
Difficult intubation
Facial trauma
Obesity

Contraindications

Limited mouth opening
High airway pressure
Inadequate paralysis or sedation

Complications

Inability to ventilate
Aspiration (rare)
Specifically for the King LT device:
Tracheal placement
Tongue edema

Equipment

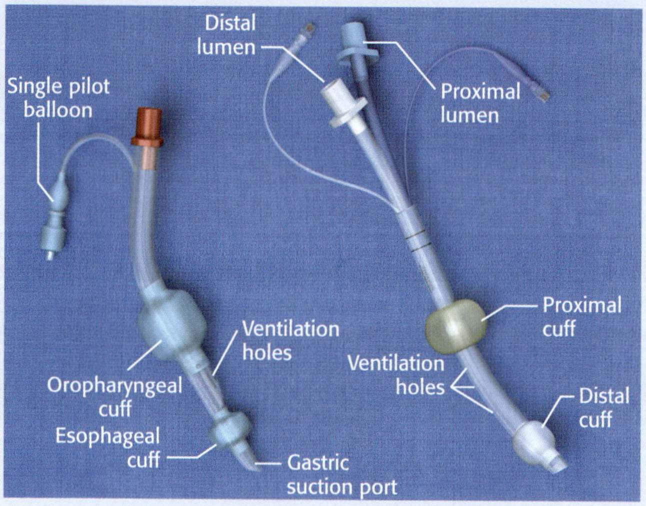

The King LTS-D *(left)* and the Combitube *(right)*.

Review Box 3.4 Retroglottic airway devices: indications, contraindications, complications, and equipment.

the Combitube, the King LT has only one airway lumen and a simplified cuff system, so both cuffs can be inflated from a single port. The literature regarding the King LT is confusing because many versions of the device have been clinically tested during the last decade. The latest disposable versions are the LT-D and the LTS-D. The LTS-D has an 18-Fr gastric suction port at the tip. The modern LTS-D has been available since 2004 and is also called the LTS II in some literature.[206,207]

The King LT is designed for blind placement and has a large proximal cuff and small distal cuff. The tip of the King LT is designed to be placed in the esophagus only. The shape of the King LT and the size of the tip in previous versions made it unlikely to be placed into the trachea.[208] The latest design of the LTS-D has a narrower tip and in one study had a 10% incidence of tracheal placement.[209] Most patients with tracheal placement of the LTS-D were still able to be adequately ventilated.[209]

Popularity of the LTS-D has grown rapidly in EMS systems, and it is now widely used by EMS agencies in the United States. Several studies have shown that the LTS-D has a high rate of successful ventilation in the operating room setting.[210–212] There are several case reports of the LT being used as a rescue device for the cannot intubate/cannot ventilate scenario and when placement of an LMA failed.[213,214] Some data suggest that the LTS-D may be useful in neonates and small infants when direct laryngoscopy fails,[215] though the smallest LT-D currently available in the United States is size 2 (patients 12 kg to 25 kg), and the smallest LTS-D is size 0 (patients <5 kg). In the EMS setting, the LT-D has a high success rate (95%) when used for ventilation of out-of-hospital cardiac arrest.[216] One study found a higher first-attempt success rate for paramedics using the King LT in cardiac arrest compared to ET intubation.[217] In addition, Frascone and colleagues found that the rate of successful insertion and ventilation with the LTS-D is essentially equivalent to that of standard tracheal intubation in the hands of paramedics.[218]

Indications and Contraindications

In the ED, the King LT is a good choice as a primary airway in patients who are unresponsive or in cardiac arrest. This is especially true in the uncontrolled prehospital environment. The King LT can be used in any emergency airway setting for rescue ventilation after failed BMV or failed intubation. In cases of failed intubation with an unexpectedly difficult airway, the King LT may be used to provide adequate ventilation and allow time for other methods of intubation or a controlled surgical airway.[208,219,220]

Because the King LT is a supraglottic airway and is designed to be placed blindly, it is relatively contraindicated in patients with obstruction of the upper airway by a foreign body and should not be used in patients with an intact gag reflex.

Placement of the King LT

See Video 3.5. The first step is to choose the proper size King LT. The LTS-D is available for patients of all ages, ranging from size 0 (<5 kg) to size 5 (patients taller than 6 feet).

After determining the appropriate size King LT, check the cuffs and then completely deflate them before placement. Lubricate the device with a water-based lubricant. The best patient position for insertion of the King LT is the sniffing position, and it can be placed with the head in the neutral position if necessary. Hold the LT at the connector with the dominant hand and hold the mouth open by grasping the chin with the nondominant hand. Introduce the tip of the device into the corner of the mouth while rotating the tube 45 to 90 degrees so that the blue orientation line on the tube is touching the corner of the mouth. Pass the tip of the device into the mouth and under the tongue. As the tip passes under the base of the tongue, rotate the tube back to the midline so that the blue orientation line faces the ceiling. Without exerting force, advance the King LT until the connector is aligned with the teeth. Inflate the cuffs with the minimum volume necessary to create a good seal (see the product brochure for maximum cuff volumes). While ventilating with a bag-valve system,

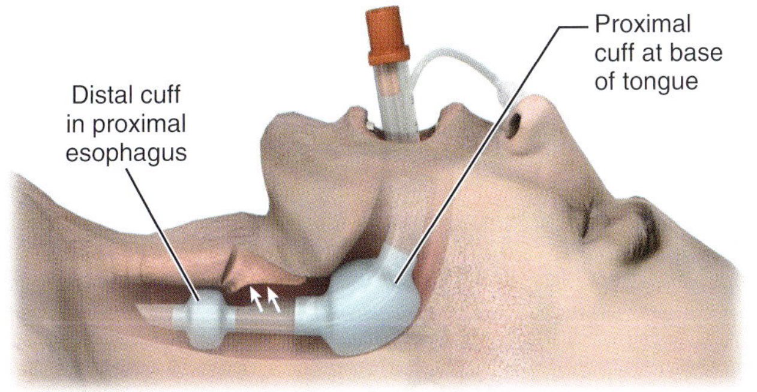

Fig. 3.18 King LTS-D. The device is properly placed posterior to the larynx, with the distal end in the proximal esophagus. The distal cuff is inflated in the proximal esophagus and the larger proximal cuff is inflated at the base of the tongue. The proximal portion of the tube is at the lip line and the distal aperture (between the cuffs) is aligned with the glottic opening; oxygen flow from the device to the glottis is depicted by the *arrows*.

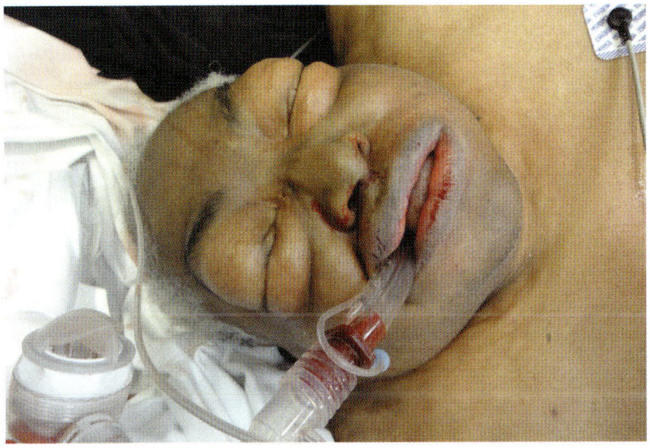

Fig. 3.19 Massive neck, periorbital, and facial edema following cardiopulmonary resuscitation with a King LT airway in place. The exact pathology was not determined but was thought to be a pharyngeal or esophageal perforation.

gently withdraw the King LT until ventilation becomes easy and free flowing. Confirm placement with chest rise, breath sounds, and capnography (Fig. 3.18).

Complications

It is hard to assess the complication rate of the King LT because the device has been modified several times in the last decade and there is no organized surveillance of out-of-hospital airway devices.[221] The current LT-D and LTS-D devices have been available since 2004. The LTS-D is referred to as the LTS II in some studies. The most serious complication is tracheal placement, which occurred in 10% of cases in one study and is probably significantly underappreciated and underreported.[209] Another complication that is not uncommon and certainly underreported is tongue edema. There is one case report of massive tongue edema occurring 3 hours after placement of the King LT,[222] and mild tongue edema is relatively common and not reported in the literature. Fig. 3.19 depicts probable pharyngeal or esophageal perforation, with massive subcutaneous neck and face emphysema following prehospital placement of a King LT. Because an autopsy was denied, the exact injury was never confirmed and may have been related to other interventions during resuscitation.

There is some concern that the large oropharyngeal balloon of the King LT might compress the carotid arteries and be detrimental in patients undergoing CPR, and currently this is only suggested in animal models[223]; no high-quality human research has been conducted to date, though one small study that reviewed computed tomography scans of the neck for 17 patients with extraglottic airway (EGAs) in place found no evidence of mechanical compression of the carotid arteries on image review.[224]

Combitube and EasyTube

The esophageal-tracheal Combitube (Nellcor) is a retroglottic airway device designed as a rescue device for difficult and emergency airways and can be placed blindly and rapidly.[225,226] The Combitube (Fig. 3.20) has two parallel lumens, a small distal cuff, and a large proximal cuff. When it is placed blindly the tip will end up in the esophagus in approximately 95% of cases and in the trachea in approximately 5%. The longer lumen or tube is used for ventilation when the tip is in the esophagus. It is perforated at the level of the pharynx and occluded at the distal end. The shorter lumen or tube is used for ventilation when the tip is in the trachea. It is open at the distal end, like a standard ET tube. The large proximal cuff or balloon is designed to occlude the pharynx by filling the space between the base of the tongue and the soft palate. The small distal cuff serves as a seal in either the esophagus or the trachea. Since the introduction of the King LT, the Combitube has essentially been replaced because the King LT requires a single inflation compared to the two required with a Combitube.

Placement of the Combitube

The Combitube is available in two sizes. The manufacturer recommends the smaller 37-Fr device for patients from 4 feet to 5 feet 6 inches tall and the larger 41-Fr device for patients taller than 5 feet 6 inches. Studies suggest that the smaller 37-Fr Combitube can be used safely in patients up to approximately 6 feet tall. The larger 41-Fr device is appropriate for patients taller than 6 feet.

To insert the Combitube, hold the device in the dominant hand and gently advance it caudally into the pharynx while grasping the tongue and jaw between the thumb and index finger of the nondominant hand. Pass the tube blindly along the tongue to a depth that places the printed rings on the proximal end of the tube between the patient's teeth and the alveolar ridge.[227] If resistance is met in the hypopharynx, remove the tube and bend it between the balloons for several seconds to facilitate insertion.[227] After insertion, fill the pharyngeal balloon with 100 mL of air and the distal cuff with 10 mL to 15 mL of air. The large pharyngeal balloon serves to securely seat the Combitube in the oropharynx and creates a closed system in the case of esophageal placement. Because approximately 95% of placements are esophageal, begin ventilation through the longer (blue) airway tube.[228]

Use chest rise, good breath sounds, and capnography, without gastric inflation, to confirm proper ventilation. Alternatively, use a Wee-type aspirator device on the shorter (clear) lumen to confirm that the tip is in the esophagus before ventilation through the longer (blue) lumen.[229] Inability to easily aspirate air confirms esophageal placement. Easy aspiration with the Wee-type device indicates tracheal positioning of

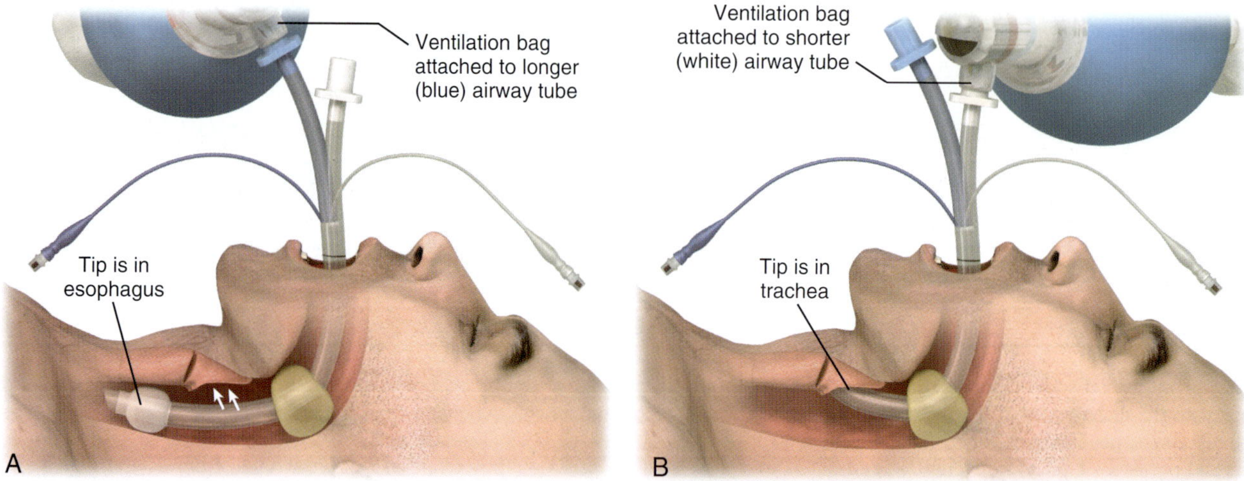

Fig. 3.20 Combitube. (A) Approximately 95% of placements are esophageal, so begin ventilation through the longer *(blue)* airway tube. Use chest rise, breath sounds, and capnography to assess for proper placement. When the distal tip is in the esophagus, ventilation occurs through the vent holes between the distal and proximal cuffs *(arrows)*. (B) If the tip of the Combitube is in the trachea, ventilation cannot be accomplished via the long *(blue)* airway tube. It is essential to recognize this quickly, and use the short *(white)* tube for ventilations.

the tube and requires changing the ventilation to the shorter (clear) tracheal lumen.

Complications

Inappropriate balloon inflation and incorrect Combitube placement can lead to air leaks during ventilation. The most common placement error is an improper insertion angle. Use a more caudal, longitudinal direction of insertion as opposed to an anteroposterior direction of insertion. The Combitube must also be maintained in the true midline position during insertion to avoid blind pockets in the supraglottic area, that can prevent passage of the tube.[228]

CONCLUSION

Good basic airway skills and the familiarity with and availability of proven rescue devices are the keys to emergency airway management. There are many techniques and devices that can be used to manage emergency airways. In difficult situations, clinicians will probably have the best success when basic skills are performed excellently.

REFERENCES AVAILABLE AT Elsevier eBooks+.

CHAPTER 4

Tracheal Intubation

Aaron E. Robinson, Brian E. Driver, and Robert F. Reardon

Tracheal intubation is often the pivotal procedure in the emergency management of critically ill patients. This procedure is just one part of airway management. The primary objective of airway management is to maintain adequate ventilation and oxygenation. Intubation only allows ventilation and oxygenation after the procedure is completed, not during the procedure.[1] Before a clinician gains tracheal intubation skills, they should have excellent basic airway management skills (see Chapter 3). Emergency clinicians should use intubation techniques that have a high likelihood of first-pass success, have the wisdom to recognize when a given approach has failed, and be able to quickly move to a different technique to ensure the patient receives adequate oxygenation. Emergency airway algorithms can help clinicians make difficult decisions in a timely manner (see Emergency Airway Algorithm section below).[2]

This chapter describes nearly every possible means of tracheal intubation, with emphasis on widely used techniques. The most common means of intubation in the emergency setting is rapid-sequence intubation (RSI), and this approach must be considered very carefully. If a difficult intubation is anticipated, awake intubation may be preferred. Although flexible endoscopic devices are commonly used for awake intubation, adequate topical anesthesia can allow for nearly any intubating technique to be used for awake intubation. Because many difficult airways cannot be predicted, it is essential to have a well-defined backup plan and appropriate resources. The intubating laryngeal mask airway (LMA Fastrach; Teleflex) is an ideal backup device for failed RSI because it provides ventilation and oxygenation and facilitates tracheal intubation in a high percentage of patients with failed RSI.[2]

GENERAL APPROACH TO EMERGENCY INTUBATION

See Videos 3.1 and 4.1 to 4.3. Preplanning is the key to successful emergency airway management. Clinicians should follow a clear, preconceived, practiced airway algorithm that uses readily available and familiar equipment and techniques. When encountering a difficult airway, it is more important to be comfortable with a few well-proven devices and techniques than to try new or unfamiliar devices.[2–4] It is essential to know when to abandon one approach and move on to the next. No single approach is mandated. The best technique is the one chosen by the clinician at the bedside based on one's individual experience and expertise given the specific clinical scenario—though some equipment, such as video laryngoscopy, will improve the chances of success.

A critical aspect of preparation is making sure that all essential equipment required to perform the airway maneuvers is immediately available and within easy access. This may be accomplished by wall-mounting essential equipment in the emergency department (ED) resuscitation room.[5] Alternatively, equipment can be placed in dedicated adult and pediatric airway carts or tackle boxes in an open, organized, and labeled manner, with the carts and boxes checked and stocked regularly (Fig. 4.1).[6] Essential equipment that is seldom used and is potentially lifesaving should be clearly identified and placed in an easily accessible location, such as a dedicated difficult airway cart. The importance of this concept cannot be overstated. Technical expertise cannot substitute for the lack of essential equipment. In airway management, failure has ominous consequences. Mental, physical, and equipment preparation maximizes the chance of success.

AIRWAY ANATOMY

An understanding of airway anatomy and its terminology is requisite for any discussion of airway management procedures (Fig. 4.2). The following terms are used frequently in this chapter.

- *Pharynx*: the upper part of the throat posterior to the nasal cavity, mouth, and larynx
  - *Nasopharynx*: base of the skull to the soft palate
  - *Oropharynx*: soft palate to the epiglottis
  - *Hypopharynx*: epiglottis to the cricoid ring (posteriorly), including the piriform sinus/recess/fossa
- *Piriform sinus/recess/fossa*: the pockets on both sides of the laryngeal inlet separated from the larynx by the aryepiglottic folds
- *Larynx*: the anterior structures of the throat (commonly called the voice box) from the tip of the epiglottis to the inferior border of the cricoid cartilage, including the laryngeal inlet
- *Laryngeal inlet*: the opening to the larynx bounded anterosuperiorly by the epiglottis, laterally by the aryepiglottic folds, and posteriorly by the arytenoid cartilage
- *Arytenoid/posterior cartilage*: the posterior aspect of the laryngeal inlet separating the glottis (anterior) from the esophagus (posterior)
  - *Corniculate cartilage*: the medial portion of the arytenoid/posterior cartilage
  - *Cuneiform cartilage*: the lateral prominence of the arytenoid/posterior cartilage
  - *Interarytenoid notch*: the notch between the posterior cartilage
- *Glottis*: the vocal apparatus, including the true and false cords and the glottic opening
- *Vallecula*: the space between the base of the tongue and the epiglottis
- *Median glossoepiglottic fold:* soft tissue fold connecting the base of the tongue and epiglottis
- *Hyoepiglottic ligament*: anterior midline ligament connecting the epiglottis to the hyoid bone (not visible to the intubator).

PREPARATION

Intubation is best accomplished with two operators, one to perform the intubation and the other to handle equipment, help with positioning, observe the patient and monitor, and keep track of time. Unfortunately, the ideal scenario and adequate time for preparation are not always available to the clinician, who makes calculated adjustments based on the situation at hand. Before intubating, it is preferable to take the following steps in chronologic order: (1) attach the necessary

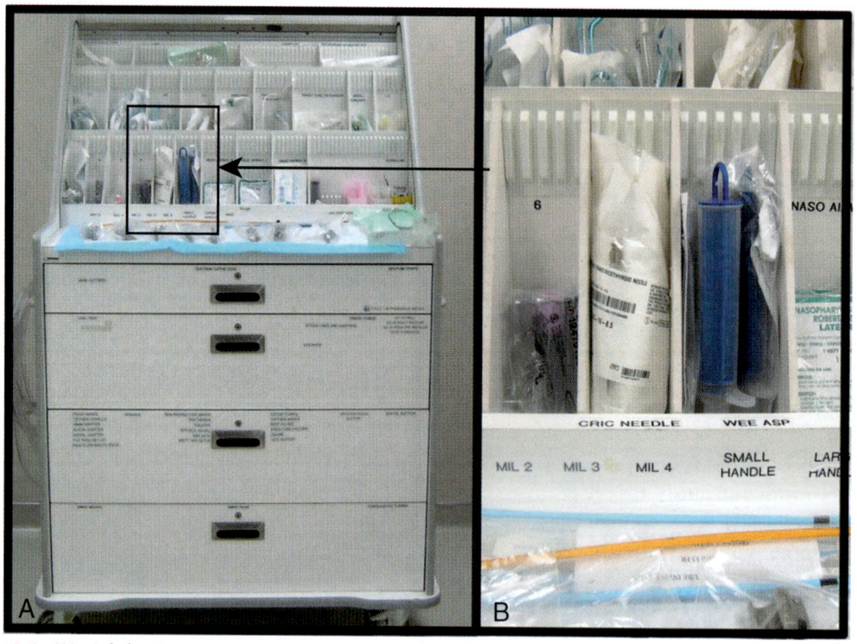

Fig. 4.1 (A) Adult airway cart. Equipment and materials are visible, labeled, and accessible. (B) Labeling is especially important because it lets you know what is missing. (Courtesy Dr. Ernest Ruiz, Department of Emergency Medicine, Hennepin County Medical Center, Minneapolis, MN.)

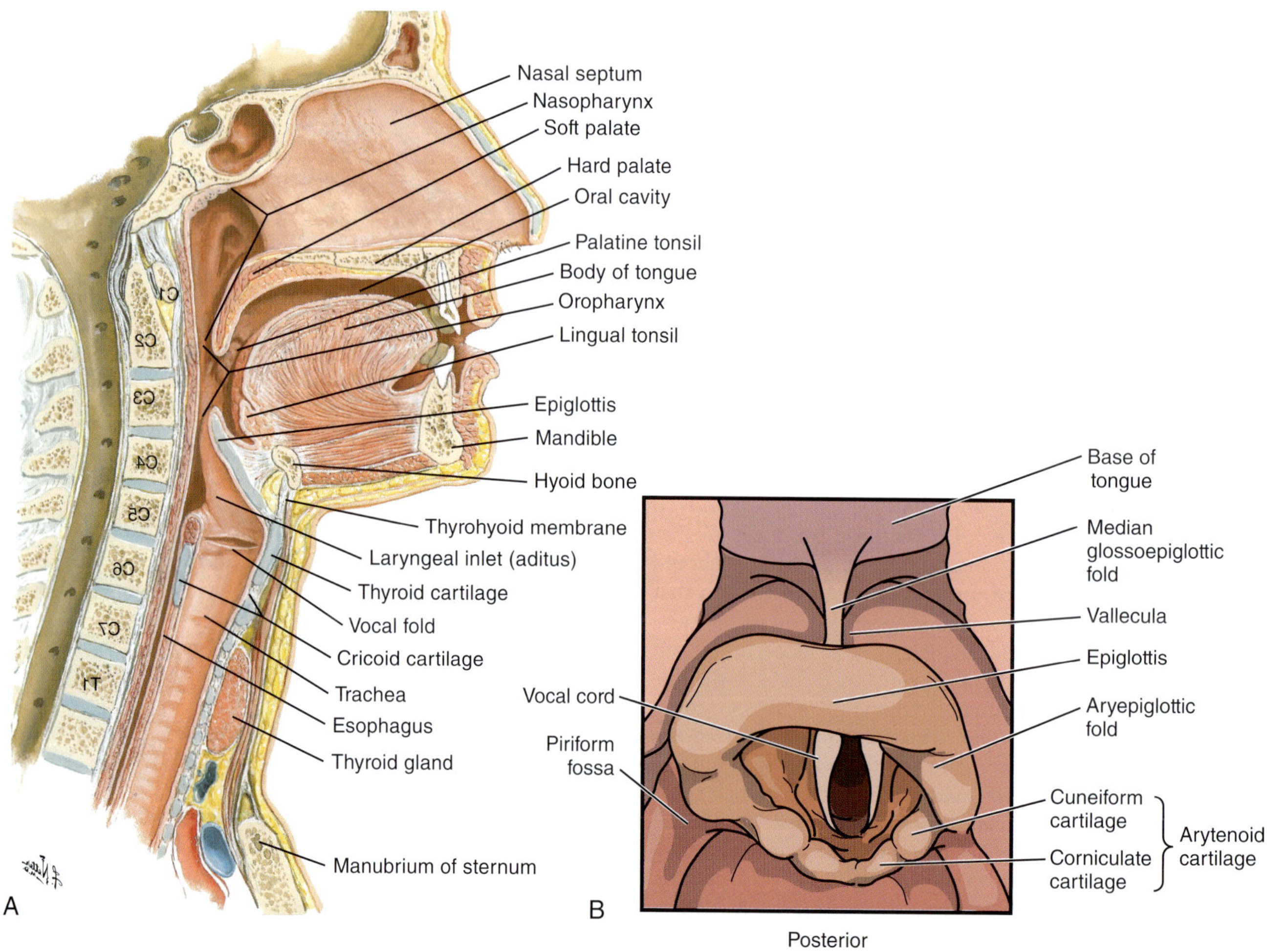

Fig. 4.2 (A) Anatomy of the upper airway. (B) View of the larynx, epiglottis, and vocal cords seen with a laryngoscope. The key to a successful intubation is identification of the vocal cords. (A, Netter illustration from www.netterimages.com. Elsevier, Inc. All rights reserved.)

monitoring devices and administer flush rate oxygen; (2) establish intravenous access; (3) draw up essential medications and label them; (4) confirm that the intubation equipment is available and functioning; (5) reassess oxygenation and maximize preoxygenation; (6) position the patient correctly; and (7) make sure that all team members are aware of the primary procedural approach and the most likely backup plan. In the haste of the moment, it is a common error to forget to preoxygenate or to position the patient optimally. Those omissions, or other simple steps such as failing to restrain the patient's hands or remove the patient's dentures or misplacing the suction tip, can seriously hamper the success of the procedure. Utilize universal precautions by wearing gloves, a gown, and eye and mouth protection.

The concept of using checklists to decrease medical errors and improve patient care has grown since a landmark article demonstrated decreased complications and mortality in surgical patients when checklists were utilized.[7] Timely and successful tracheal intubation, while minimizing hypoxemia and other complications, is paramount when caring for ill and injured patients who require intubation. Preintubation checklists can reduce cognitive load for the intubating physician by creating a framework for all emergency intubations. Checklists prompt clinicians to verify that all necessary equipment is available and functioning, to perform a standardized airway assessment, to execute optimal preoxygenation, and to develop an airway plan with patient-specific backups. The use of preintubation checklists has been shown to reduce periintubation complications in trauma patients.[8] An sample checklist is shown in Box 4.1.

BOX 4.1 Preintubation Checklists

PREARRIVAL

1. Bag-mask ventilation setup with oxygen running at >15 L/min
2. Suction connected and running
3. Laryngoscope functioning and ready; additional blade sizes easily available
4. Ready an endotracheal tube: check cuff. If using a bougie, prepare the bougie. If not using a bougie, insert stylet into the tube and form it into a "straight-to-cuff" shape with a 35-degree distal bend
5. Backup devices such as laryngeal mask airway or King laryngeal tube airway available and ready
6. Cricothyrotomy set located and readily available
7. End-tidal CO_2 detector ready

PREINTUBATION

1. Assess the airway: open mouth, examine neck mobility (unless the patient is immobilized), palpate anterior neck
2. Decide best approach: awake vs. rapid sequence intubation
3. Communicate intubation medication orders to nurses, including postintubation medications
4. Optimally position patient
5. Preoxygenate patient (usually with face mask oxygen at 60 L/min)
6. Apply nasal cannula at 10 to 15 L/min in preparation for apneic oxygenation
7. Discuss airway plan with entire team
8. Ensure functioning pulse oximeter
9. Ensure patient intravenous catheter
10. Ensure assistants are ready (nurses, respiratory therapists)

LT, *Laryngeal tube;* RSI, *Rapid-sequence intubation.*

PREOXYGENATION

Preoxygenation is one of the most important aspects of emergency airway management. The goal of preoxygenation is to replace all the nitrogen in the lungs with oxygen before the start of intubation attempts. This allows the lungs to act as an oxygen reservoir during the apneic period of RSI. This reservoir provides the intubator with additional time before the onset of hypoxemia and significantly increases the chance for successful intubation on the first attempt. It is not enough to achieve a peripheral oxygen saturation (Spo_2) value of 100% prior to intubation, because an Spo_2 of 100% does not correspond with complete removal of nitrogen and replacement of oxygen inside the lungs. Furthermore, partial pressure of arterial oxygen (Pao_2) at 100% Spo_2 can range from approximately 100 to 600 mm Hg. Failure to preoxygenate before RSI is often a critical factor when a straightforward emergency airway becomes an unexpected airway disaster. Those at greatest risk for rapid desaturation include pregnant, critically ill, pediatric patients as well as those with a high body mass index (BMI); these populations will benefit most from optimal preoxygenation.

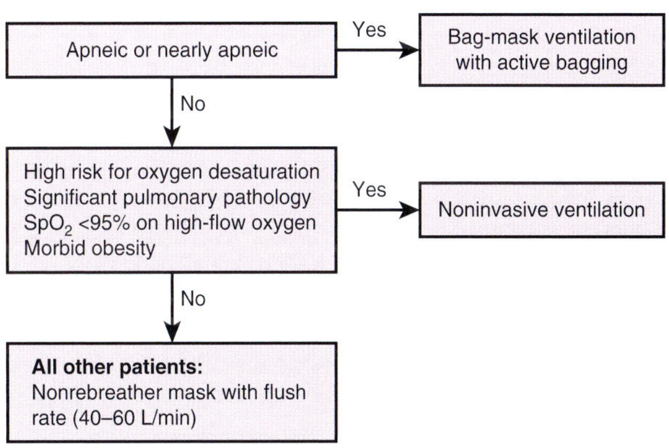

Fig. 4.3 A proposed algorithm for which preoxygenation method to use for an individual patient.

Preoxygenation Methods

See Video 4.4. Preoxygenation methods are simple and differ by patient. Fig. 4.3 shows a proposed algorithm for choosing a preoxygenation method for individual patients. In apneic or nearly apneic patients, preoxygenation can only be performed by bag-mask ventilation (BMV) with active squeezing of the bag (or, rarely, noninvasive ventilation). This is the only patient population that a bag-mask device should be used for preoxygenation, since bag-mask devices do not work well in spontaneously breathing patients.

Noninvasive ventilation (e.g., bilevel positive pressure ventilation [BiPAP]) should be used for patients at high risk of oxygen desaturation. The application of positive pressure can increase the volume of the pulmonary reservoir and improve preoxygenation.[9] Examples of patients who might benefit from noninvasive ventilation include those with significant pulmonary pathology, patients with morbid obesity, and those with an Spo_2 value <95% after administration of flush rate oxygen.

For all other patients—the majority of ED patients—preoxygenate by providing the maximal fraction of inspired oxygen (Fio_2) with a simple face mask or nonrebreather mask at flush rate.[10] The type of mask is less important than the oxygen flow rate[11]; at very high flow rates, the Fio_2 for any device usually exceeds 90%. At lower flow rates (<30 L/min), the Fio_2 will not be high enough for adequate preoxygenation,[12] so the oxygen flow rate should be at least 30 L/min. When using a standard oxygen flowmeter the highest (flush) rate can be accomplished by turning the knob counterclockwise until there is a hard stop. This provides flow much higher than the highest marked gradation, which is typically only 15 L/min. The maximal (flush) rate of the flowmeter is usually marked on the back side and is typically greater than 40 L/min. Oxygen flowmeters that can measure up to 70 L/min, with flush rates up to 90 L/min, are available (see Fig. 3.9). A flush rate greater than 40 L/min is typically sufficient for maximal preoxygenation. Providing flush rate oxygen eliminates nitrogen, washes out expired CO_2, fills the dead space of the nasopharynx and upper airway with oxygen, and compensates for any leak between the mask and the patient to avoid entrainment of room air during inspiration.[13] The importance of very high-flow oxygen (>40 L/min) administration during preoxygenation cannot be overemphasized. If a portable tank is being used for preoxygenation, such as in the prehospital or other environments where wall oxygen is not available, it is imperative to bypass the regulator on the portable tank if the regulator is not capable of reaching >40 L/min of flow.[14]

Unlike flush rate oxygen via face mask, BMV requires proper equipment and perfect technique to achieve adequate preoxygenation. Bags without one-way valves for both inhalation and exhalation will not function properly during spontaneous ventilation and will provide only room air.[15,16] Furthermore, unless flow rates are very high (>40 L/min) and continuous, the mask must be sealed perfectly to the patient's face (see Chapter 3 for proper technique).[17] If the seal is imperfect, room air will be entrained and Fio_2 will be close to that of room air.[18] This is analogous to holding a mask above a patient's face, which only provides oxygen content near that of room air. Because of the limitations associated with BMV, in spontaneously breathing patients, face masks with flush rate oxygen (>40 L/min) are the preferred oxygen delivery device for preoxygenation.

To augment oxygen delivery and prepare for apneic oxygenation (see following), apply a nasal cannula (at 15 L/min) to the patient during preoxygenation, in addition to other preoxygenation efforts.[19] Oxygen via a high-flow nasal cannula device (see Chapter 3 for details), if available, may also improve preoxygenation.[20]

Duration and Patient Positioning

Patients should receive preoxygenation for 3 to 5 minutes.[21] This permits nearly full replacement of nitrogen by oxygen within the lungs. If it is not possible to perform preoxygenation for 3 to 5 minutes prior to intubation, instruct the patient to take eight vital capacity breaths while delivering very high-flow oxygen to provide nearly the same result.[21,22] Many critically ill patients will not be able to take vital capacity breaths, so the preferred method is 3 to 5 minutes of tidal breathing. If possible, instruct the patient to exhale maximally before beginning preoxygenation.[23]

The preferred position for preoxygenation is head elevation of 20 to 25 degrees. This position minimizes atelectasis, decreases the pressure of the abdominal contents against the diaphragm, and allows the patient to continue taking deep breaths. In both adults with elevated BMIs[24,25] and adults with normal BMIs,[26,27] this position has been demonstrated to be advantageous for preoxygenation. For patients with spinal immobilization, the bed can be placed in 25 degrees of reverse Trendelenburg (head up) to achieve the same effect.[28]

Sedation for Preoxygenation

Sometimes patients who will benefit the most from preoxygenation are uncooperative because of delirium from hypoxia, hypercapnia, or other factors. Application of a face mask or noninvasive ventilation may be difficult or impossible. These patients may benefit from careful sedation without suppression of respirations, allowing for oxygenation with a face mask or for 2 to 3 minutes before administration of a paralytic agent; referred to as *delayed sequence intubation* (Video 4.5).

Ketamine (1 to 1.5 mg/kg by slow intravenous push) has been suggested for this technique.[9] Weingart and colleagues performed sedation for preoxygenation in 62 adults and demonstrated an increase in Spo_2 for most patients without any adverse events.[29] Because of the small sample size and because these patients were managed by experts in airway management and sedation, this technique is not necessarily generalizable to typical clinical practice. If a patient is sedated for preoxygenation, the clinician should be vigilant for respiratory depression, apnea, and airway obstruction and have all airway equipment available in case emergency control of the airway or breathing becomes necessary. In many cases, it may be safer to restrain the patient without sedation to facilitate preoxygenation.

Apneic Oxygenation During Intubation

See Video 4.6. Another method to delay desaturation during RSI is nasopharyngeal oxygen insufflation without ventilation, termed apneic oxygenation. Even in the absence of ventilation, oxygen is able to travel down the tracheobronchial tree to the alveoli and diffuse into the bloodstream, where it is consumed and converted into carbon dioxide. Oxygen diffuses across the alveoli much more readily than carbon dioxide, and oxygen and carbon dioxide have differences in gas solubility in blood, and because of the high affinity of hemoglobin for oxygen, more oxygen leaves the alveoli than carbon dioxide enters. This creates a pressure gradient that allows oxygen to travel from the nasopharynx to the alveoli and into the bloodstream.[9]

Studies have shown that providing oxygen therapy during apnea is much more beneficial than one might anticipate.[30–32] Multiple studies conducted in the operating room in patients with normal or markedly elevated BMIs have shown that oxygen administered nasally results in a significant delay in desaturation after the onset of apnea, with many subjects never developing hypoxemia even after 6 minutes of apnea.[30,32–34] The physiology of this technique is proven and sound.

Two randomized trials found no difference in the oxygen saturation nadir between patients who received and did not receive apneic oxygenation during intubation.[35,36] The most likely explanation is that the vast majority of patients who undergo tracheal intubation after sufficient preoxygenation have a relatively low risk of oxygen desaturation and are unlikely to have benefit from apneic oxygenation. If patients at high risk of oxygen desaturation or prolonged laryngoscopy were studied exclusively, the results might differ. Since it is not always known before intubation who will rapidly experience oxygen desaturation or have prolonged laryngoscopy, it seems reasonable to perform apneic oxygenation on all patients undergoing emergency intubation because the intervention is easy and cheap.

To perform apneic oxygenation, place a standard nasal cannula beneath the main preoxygenation device (face mask or bag-valve mask). End-tidal CO_2 nasal cannulas should be avoided because oxygen is administered through holes outside of the nose rather than through the prongs. If the patient is awake, limit the flow rate to 5 to 15 L/min during the preoxygenation phase because higher flow rates can be slightly uncomfortable. If the patient is comatose or unresponsive, set the nasal cannula to 15 L/min or higher when initially placed. When the preoxygenation device is removed for intubation, keep the nasal cannula in place. During intubation attempt, set the nasal cannula to at least 15 L/min. It may be beneficial to turn the oxygen flowmeter up as high as possible because higher flow rates have been shown to provide higher Fio_2.[37] If there is nasal obstruction, place a nasopharyngeal airway in one or both nares to facilitate oxygen delivery to the posterior nasopharynx. To optimize gas flow past the upper airway, position the patient for tracheal intubation and perform maneuvers to ensure upper airway patency (i.e., jaw thrust, head tilt/chin lift). Because conventional nasal cannula oxygen delivery is not humidified, apneic oxygenation at high flow rates will cause some desiccation of the nasopharynx, and this should not cause significant harm because of the short duration of this oxygen supplementation.

While apneic oxygenation likely provides some benefit in very hypoxemic patients, it should not be prioritized over good preoxygenation. It is much more important to adequately preoxygenate a patient, and this should not be compromised for apneic oxygenation. Apneic oxygenation should complement preoxygenation.

High-flow nasal cannula systems may be an even better method of apneic oxygenation and have been shown in an intensive care unit (ICU) study to be superior to simple nasal cannula, though both groups had low rates of hypoxemia.[20]

ASSESSING FOR A DIFFICULT AIRWAY

RSI is the near-simultaneous administration of a sedative and a neuromuscular blocking agent to facilitate tracheal intubation. After these medications are given the patient will be apneic and not able to breathe for themselves for at least several minutes. It is critical that the intubator assesses for anticipated difficulty before *every* tracheal intubation attempt. Failure to appreciate a difficult airway may cause implementation of an improper intubation plan that could lead to intubation failure, severe hypoxemia, and death.

Assessing for difficulty in the emergency setting is not as simple as learning scoring systems or mnemonics for markers of difficulty. Most of the literature on prediction of difficult laryngoscopy does not apply very well in the emergency setting. A study by Levitan and colleagues in 2004 showed that two-thirds of patients who were intubated in their ED via RSI could not be assessed with the most common difficult airway prediction tests (Mallampati scoring, measurement of thyromental distance, and neck mobility testing) because of altered mental status or cervical spine immobilization.[38] Even in the best circumstances, only approximately half the cases of difficult laryngoscopy can be predicted.[39,40] Many factors such as Mallampati scoring and measurement of the thyromental distance have not been found to accurately predict difficult laryngoscopy, especially in the emergency setting.[38,39,41,42] Only obvious anatomic and pathologic abnormalities and a history of difficult intubation are accurate predictors of difficult laryngoscopy.[38] The American Society of Anesthesiology Difficult Airway Guidelines state that "in patients with no gross upper airway pathology or anatomic anomaly, there is insufficient published evidence to evaluate the effect of a physical examination on predicting the presence of a difficult airway."[43,44] This does not mean that emergency clinicians should ignore factors known to be associated with difficult laryngoscopy, and these factors must be placed in perspective.

No examination finding alone can predict difficult laryngoscopy, and a combination of multiple factors makes difficulty more likely. The classic predictors of difficult intubation include a history of previous difficult intubation, prominent upper incisors, limited ability to extend at the atlanto-occipital joint,[45] poor visibility of pharyngeal structures when the patient extends the tongue (Mallampati classification or the tongue-pharyngeal ratio) (Fig. 4.4A),[46] limited ability to open the mouth (suggested by a space less than three fingerbreadths between the upper and lower incisors),[47] short thyromental distance (<6 cm from the thyroid notch to the chin with the neck in extension) (Fig. 4.4B),[48] and a limited direct laryngoscopic view of the laryngeal inlet (Fig. 4.5).[47] A relatively new test is the upper lip bite test, which has been shown in some studies to be more accurate and specific than older tests.[49–53] It is essentially a test of anterior mandibular mobility, and the less mobility the more difficult it is to intubate the patient. Upper lip bite criteria are as follows: class I, the lower incisors can bite the upper lip above the vermilion line; class II, the lower incisors can bite the upper lip below the vermilion line; and class III, the lower incisors cannot bite the upper lip.

Many of these predictors cannot be assessed in the emergency setting.[38] Some of the key predictors are apparent simply by observing the external appearance of the patient's head and neck. Patients with neck tumors, thermal or chemical burns, traumatic injuries involving the face and anterior aspect of the neck, angioedema, infection of pharyngeal and laryngeal soft tissues, or previous operations in or around the airway suggest a difficult intubation because distorted anatomy or secretions may compromise visualization of the vocal cords. Facial or skull fractures may further limit airway options by precluding nasotracheal (NT) intubation. Patients with ankylosing arthritis or developmental abnormalities such as a hypoplastic mandible or the large tongue of Down syndrome are difficult to intubate because neck rigidity and problems of tongue displacement can obscure visualization of the glottis.

Besides these obvious congenital and pathologic conditions, the presence of a short, thick neck is one of the more common predictors of a difficult airway. Such individuals are easily identifiable by observing the head and neck in profile. Obesity alone may not be an independent predictor of difficult intubation, and patients with elevated BMIs with large-circumference necks are likely to be difficult to intubate.[52] Facial hair can complicate a difficult airway by rendering BMV ineffective because of the lack of a good mask seal. One

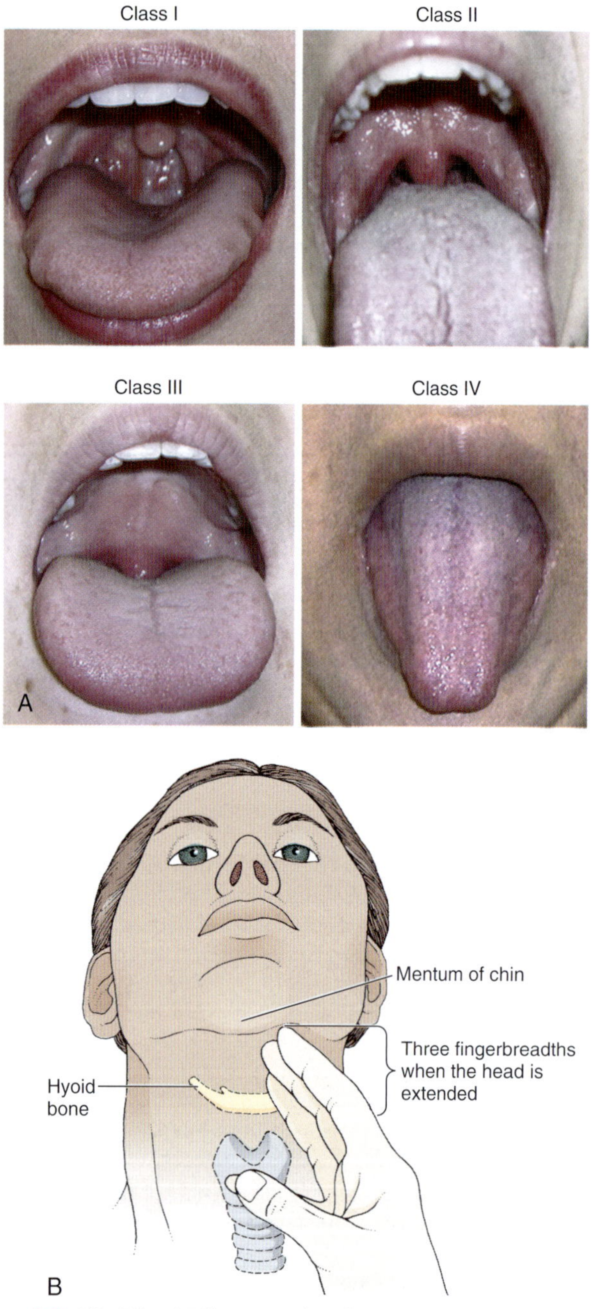

Fig. 4.4 (A) The Mallampati classification predicts intubation difficulty based on the visibility of intraoral structures. Classes III and IV predict difficult intubation. (B) A short thyromental distance (<6 cm or three fingerbreadths) when the head is extended predicts difficult intubation. (A, From Kryger MH. Sleep breathing disorders: examination of the patient with suspected sleep apnea. In: Kryger MH, ed. *Kryger Atlas of Clinical Sleep Medicine*. Elsevier; 2010.)

patient type that does not immediately stand out as a difficult intubation is a patient with an unusually long mandibulohyoid distance (the thyroid prominence appearing low in the neck) and a short mandibular ramus.[54] Visualization of the larynx is difficult because of the distance to the larynx and the relative hypopharyngeal location of the tongue.

Knowledge of the poor performance of difficult airway predictors should not make emergency clinicians more cavalier about using RSI; rather, it should create more concern. The solution is *not* to avoid RSI wholesale, because the use of neuromuscular blocking agents makes every intubation easier to some degree. The solution is to perform a focused airway assessment that will serve as a cognitive forcing strategy[55] and guide the clinician to plan and prepare for the airway intervention. At a minimum, the clinician should assess neck mobility (except in those with cervical immobilization) and mouth opening and consider whether there is any obstruction between the mouth and larynx. After the airway assessment, the clinician will determine whether to use RSI or keep the patient as awake as possible to preserve normal spontaneous breathing.

EMERGENCY AIRWAY DECISION-MAKING

The airway clinician must have many tools readily available to deal with an acutely compromised airway. It is important to be proficient in a number of different techniques and to tailor their use to the needs of the individual patient. Rescuers should practice potential scenarios before facing patients with a compromised airway. Failure to do so may lead to unnecessarily aggressive management in some situations or to irreversible hypoxic injury as a result of hesitation in others. Deciding who requires a definitive airway and who needs only supportive measures is a formidable task for even the most skilled clinician.

The following parameters should be assessed before the decision is made to establish a definitive airway:

- Adequacy of current ventilation
- Potential for hypoxia
- Airway patency
- Need for neuromuscular blockade (uncooperative, full stomach, teeth clenching)
- Cervical spine stability
- Safety of the technique and skill of the operator

Consideration of these factors should guide the clinician in deciding if tracheal intubation is necessary and in selecting the optimal technique. Choosing the initial approach is often straightforward. Difficulty arises precipitously when the initial approach fails. Time becomes critical as the risk for irreversible hypoxic injury and cardiac arrest rises. Anxiety then increases the potential for error. Forethought and practice are invaluable when managing these situations.

Clinicians who perform emergency intubation, especially RSI, must understand that oxygenation and ventilation, not tracheal intubation, are paramount when caring for critically ill patients. Patients who are hypoxic on arrival and those who develop hypoxia after a failed first intubation attempt need good BMV to restore oxygenation and keep them stable enough for further intubation attempts. The importance of BMV skill cannot be overstated (see Chapter 3), and mastery of this skill alleviates much of the anxiety associated with difficult emergency airways and improves the chance for successful RSI.[3] It is critically important to have an extraglottic device (EGD, also known as a supraglottic airway) immediately available during every RSI in the event that BMV is difficult or impossible. All clinicians who perform emergency intubation should be prepared to perform a surgical airway when intubation methods and backup ventilation techniques fail.

Decision to Perform Rapid-Sequence Intubation

RSI in anesthesia has evolved since the introduction of succinylcholine in 1951. RSI was initially used as an abbreviation

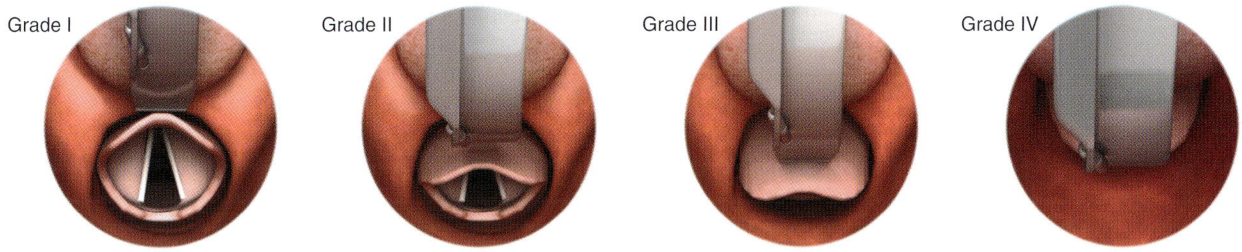

Fig. 4.5 Cormack and Lehane grading of laryngeal views during laryngoscopy. (A) Grade I. Most of the glottis is visible. (B) Grade II. The posterior aspect of the glottis is visible. (C) Grade III. Only the epiglottis is seen; no part of the laryngeal inlet is visible. (D) Grade IV. The epiglottis is not visible. Patients with grades I and II are usually easy to intubate with direct laryngoscopy, whereas those with grades III and IV are often difficult; the ability to see the arytenoid cartilage is the important difference.

for rapid-sequence induction and is now synonymous with rapid-sequence intubation. Initially, the main purpose of RSI was to decrease the risk for aspiration in patients with full stomachs who needed emergency intubation. RSI has now become the most common method of emergency airway management because paralysis facilitates optimal intubating conditions in critically ill patients.[56–60]

Emergency clinicians should not use RSI in a cavalier manner. When giving a paralytic agent, the clinician takes complete responsibility for airway maintenance, ventilation, and oxygenation of the patient. Consider one of many awake intubation (i.e., intubation without paralysis) options in patients with known or anticipated difficult airways (Box 4.2 and Video 4.7).

In the emergency setting, it is useful to think of difficult airways as opportunities for airway failure. The goal should be to avoid RSI in patients who cannot be intubated using direct or video laryngoscopy and cannot be ventilated with a bag-mask device. With modern airway equipment RSI is used in >95% of patients requiring intubation. RSI is the default technique unless significant difficulty with intubation and reoxygenation is anticipated.

Risk factors for difficult or impossible BMV have been well studied and include the presence of a beard, elevated BMI, lack of teeth, age older than 55 years, a history of snoring, short thyromental distance, and limited mandibular protrusion (see Box 3.2). It is also prudent to consider whether an EGD will be difficult to place because this is often the primary backup plan. RSI is contraindicated in patients who cannot be orally intubated, and it should usually be avoided in patients with laryngotracheal abnormalities caused by tumors, infection, edema, or a history of cervical radiation therapy.

If the clinician decides that RSI is not appropriate for a patient, there are many techniques that can be performed without paralysis (see Box 4.2). Flexible endoscopic intubation is a go-to procedure for most anesthesiologists and is also commonly performed by many emergency physicians (described later in the chapter). Direct and video laryngoscopy can also be performed without paralysis. If excellent topical anesthesia is achieved, some patients can be intubated without any sedation.

Ideal Versus Emergency Technique

The intubation plan that would be best in the ideal or elective situation is often not the best plan in the emergency setting. Consider the patient with rapidly increasing upper airway swelling due to anaphylaxis, causing impending complete airway obstruction. Because of predicted difficulty with direct and video laryngoscopy, some clinicians would not consider this patient a candidate for RSI. Other intubation strategies might have a higher chance of success if time was not a factor. The patient will likely develop complete airway obstruction, critical hypoxia, and death in the time required to set up and perform endoscopic nasal intubation. In this situation, the emergency clinician is "forced to act"[61] to complete timely tracheal intubation. The best course for this patient is likely RSI with modern video laryngoscopy equipment and a good backup plan, such as the LMA Fastrach (Teleflex), followed by a cricothyrotomy. There are many other scenarios in which the emergency airway plan is much different than the ideal airway plan, such as patients with multiple trauma who have several different life threats. In these patients, intubation often needs to be expedited so that other life threats can be addressed in a timely manner.

BOX 4.2 Intubation Methods for Emergency Airway Management

- Direct laryngoscopy
- Video laryngoscopy
- Video/optical laryngoscope with a tube channel
- Flexible Endoscope
- Intubating laryngeal mask airway
- Optical stylet
- Blind nasal
- Retrograde
- Cricothyrotomy

Failed Airways

A failed airway should be differentiated from a known or anticipated difficult airway. A patient is considered to have a failed airway in the following situations[62]: (1) inability to maintain oxygenation by BMV or EGD device; (2) failure of three or more intubation attempts by an experienced operator; and (3) failure of the first attempt in a "forced to act" situation.

If a patient has a failed airway, and oxygenation can be maintained, the clinician should attempt intubation by another method (e.g., flexible endoscopy, intubating LMA [ILMA], video laryngoscopy, surgical airway, and others); if a more experienced clinician is not already present, then one should be called for. This could be an emergency physician, paramedic, anesthesiologist, or any other clinician with significant airway expertise. If at any point there is failure of oxygenation, an EGD device should be placed while preparing for a cricothyrotomy. If the EGD device cannot oxygenate, a cricothyrotomy should be performed immediately.

Emergency Airway Algorithm

It is essential to appreciate the critical importance of having and communicating a clear backup plan when intubation with RSI fails.[38,63] This situation mandates the need for a preconceived algorithm that uses proven rescue techniques applicable to a broad range of clinical scenarios, such as the bougie (tracheal tube introducer) and the ILMA Fastrach.[2,64] The value of the bougie is indisputable, and it is clear that using the ILMA Fastrach after failed RSI has decreased the frequency of failed airways and the need for surgical intervention.[2,4,65–71] Because RSI is the "go-to" method for emergency intubation, clinicians must be prepared to perform a surgical airway when laryngoscopy, BMV, and backup devices fail.[2,72]

Critical decisions about how to maintain ventilation and oxygenation and when to use a different intubation approach are much easier when using a simple preconceived algorithm. The algorithm presented here is used in the Department of Emergency Medicine at Hennepin County Medical Center (Fig. 4.6). This algorithm is presented as an example. Individual clinicians and institutions should determine their own algorithms based on the availability of skills and resources. There are many similarities between this algorithm and those put forth by the American Society of Anesthesiologists and the Difficult Airway Society; our algorithm is simpler and more specific to emergency airway management.[44,73] Most published airway algorithms are not ideal for emergency airway management because they do not account for the conditions that are commonly encountered: patients with full stomachs who are critically ill and often uncooperative, and intubations that cannot be canceled if the airway is too difficult. Many algorithms resemble wish lists of equipment and skills that are simply not available

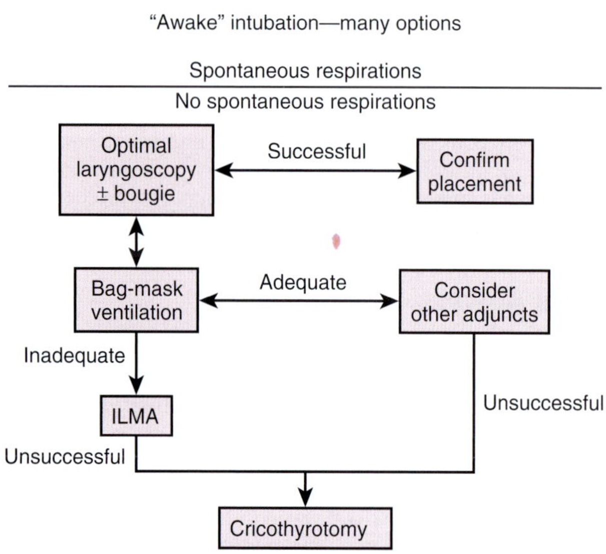

Fig. 4.6 Emergency airway management algorithm used at Hennepin County Medical Center. The end point of the algorithm is successful tracheal intubation. This algorithm is presented as an example. Individuals and institutions should formulate their own algorithms based on technical skills and the availability of resources. *ILMA*, Intubating laryngeal mask airway.

to many emergency airway clinicians. Our algorithm is based on the concept that oxygenation, not intubation, is the key.[1] It stresses well-proven concepts, procedures, and devices, and it is modeled after a simple algorithm developed by Combes and colleagues that was validated in a large prospective study.[2,66,71]

DIRECT LARYNGOSCOPY

See Videos 4.8 and 4.9. Direct laryngoscopy (DL) is a crucial skill even in the era of video laryngoscopy (Review Box 4.1).[74] Many experts believe that the ultimate intubation device is a Macintosh-shaped video laryngoscope, which allows simultaneous DL and video laryngoscopy. While the skill of DL itself remains valuable, it is difficult to think of indications for use of a direct laryngoscope blade without a camera in the ED. A Macintosh-shaped video laryngoscope allows the intubator to practice and perform DL with the option of looking at the video monitor if DL is more difficult than anticipated. The principles outlined below apply when using a DL-only device or when using a Macintosh-shaped video laryngoscope.

Indications and Contraindications

DL is indicated in any clinical situation in which a definitive emergency airway is necessary, including routine and difficult airways. Relative contraindications to DL include limited mouth opening, upper airway distortion or swelling, severe kyphosis, and copious blood or secretions.

Equipment

Laryngoscope

There are two basic blade designs for DL, curved (Macintosh) and straight (Miller) (Fig. 4.7). Each comes in various adult and pediatric blade sizes. Slight variations in laryngoscopic technique follow from the choice of blade design, and it is often a matter of personal preference. The tip of the straight blade goes under the epiglottis and lifts it directly, whereas the curved blade fits into the vallecula and indirectly lifts the epiglottis via engagement of the median glossoepiglottic fold and hyoepiglottic ligament to expose the larynx.

Each blade type has advantages and disadvantages. The straight blade is often a better choice in pediatric patients, in patients with an anterior larynx or a long floppy epiglottis, and in individuals whose larynx is fixed by scar tissue. It is less effective in patients with prominent upper teeth, and it is more likely to damage dentition. A straight blade may inadvertently be advanced into the esophagus and initially reveal unfamiliar anatomy until it is withdrawn. The blade has a light bulb at the tip, which may slightly limit vision. The wider, curved blades are helpful in keeping the tongue retracted from the field of vision and allowing more room for passing the tube through the oropharynx, and they are generally preferred for routine adult intubations. Aside from patient considerations, some clinicians prefer the curved blade because they find that it requires less forearm strength than the straight blade.

The illumination provided by the laryngoscope can make a big difference in the ability to visualize the laryngeal inlet. The importance of these factors is underappreciated, as demonstrated by Levitan et al.[75] in a survey of the Macintosh blades used in 17 Philadelphia EDs. It was found that only 24% of all blades provided the brightness necessary for fine inspection. This finding was largely explained by the fact that the majority of EDs used the A-Mac (American) as opposed to

Direct Laryngoscopy

Indications

Routine emergency intubation
Difficult airways

Contraindications

Limited mouth opening
Upper airway distortion or swelling
Kyphosis (extreme curvature of the upper back)
Copious blood or secretions

Complications

Hypoxic brain injury
Cardiac arrest
Aspiration
Upper airway trauma
Dental trauma

Equipment

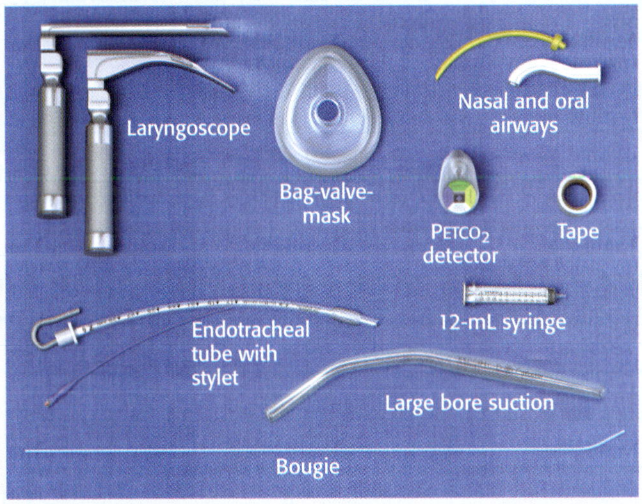

Review Box 4.1 Direct laryngoscopy: indications, contraindications, complications, and equipment.

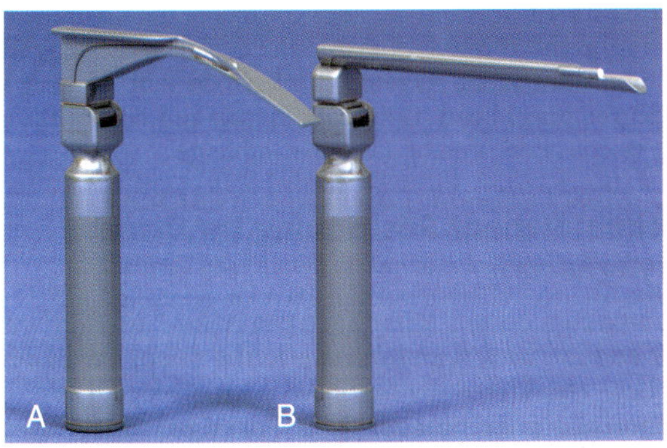

Fig. 4.7 (A) Macintosh (curved) and (B) Miller (straight) laryngoscope blades.

the clearly superior brightness design of the G-Mac (German) or the intermediate brightness of the E-Mac (English).

Tracheal Tubes

The standard adult endotracheal (ET) tube measures approximately 30 cm in length. Tube size is typically printed prominently on the tube and is based on the internal diameter (ID) and measured in millimeters. The range is 2.0 to 10.0 mm in increments of 0.5 mm. The outer tube diameter is 2 to 4 mm larger than the ID.[76] Tubes are also imprinted with a scale in centimeters that indicates the distance from a tube's distal tip.

Adult males can generally accept a 7.5- to 9.0-mm orotracheal tube, and females can usually be intubated with a 7.0- to 8.0-mm tube. Larger tubes are theoretically desirable because airway resistance increases as tube size decreases, and in practice, a 7.5-mm tube is adequate for almost all adults. In emergency intubations, particularly if a difficult intubation is anticipated, many clinicians choose a smaller tube and change to a larger tube later if indicated. Though generally an acceptable practice, this should be avoided in burn patients because swelling may prohibit subsequent tube placement. For nasal intubation, a slightly smaller (by 0.5 to 1.0 mm) tube may be easier to advance through the nasal passages.

Correct tube size is important in the pediatric population (Table 4.1). As tube size is based on the ID, a cuffed tube should generally be a half size (0.5 mm) smaller than an uncuffed tube. Historically, uncuffed tubes were used for children for fear of pressure-induced necrosis of the trachea from direct cuff pressure. The advent of low-pressure, high-volume cuffs has allowed cuffed tubes to be used in all ages of patients, including neonates. In a child, the smallest airway diameter is at the cricoid ring rather than at the vocal cords, as in adults. In children a tube may pass the cords but go no farther. If this should occur, the next smaller size tube should be passed. The American Heart Association (AHA) states that both cuffed and uncuffed tubes are acceptable for infants and children who are tracheally intubated.[77] If a cuffed tube is placed, careful attention must be paid to cuff pressures.

In children 2 years or older, the following formula is a highly accurate method for determining correct uncuffed and cuffed ET tube size:

$$\text{Uncuffed tube size (mm)} = [\text{age (years)}/4] + 4$$

$$\text{Cuffed tube size (mm)} = [\text{age (years)}/4] + 3$$

For most clinical situations, using the width of the nail of the patient's little (fifth) finger as a guide is sufficiently accurate and has been shown to be more precise than finger diameter (Fig. 4.8).[78] In order to reduce cognitive load during emergency situations,[79] it may be best to use a length-based tool to determine the appropriate size ET tube, tube depth, and other resuscitation measures.

A standard tracheal tube uses a high-volume, low-pressure cuff to avoid pressure necrosis of the tracheal lining. A clinical test for determining correct cuff inflation is to slowly inject air until no air leak is audible while the patient is receiving bag-tube ventilation. In adults, this usually occurs with 5 to 8 mL of air if the proper size tracheal tube has been selected. Many clinicians use the tension of the pilot balloon as a guide to cuff inflation. Slight compressibility with gentle external pressure

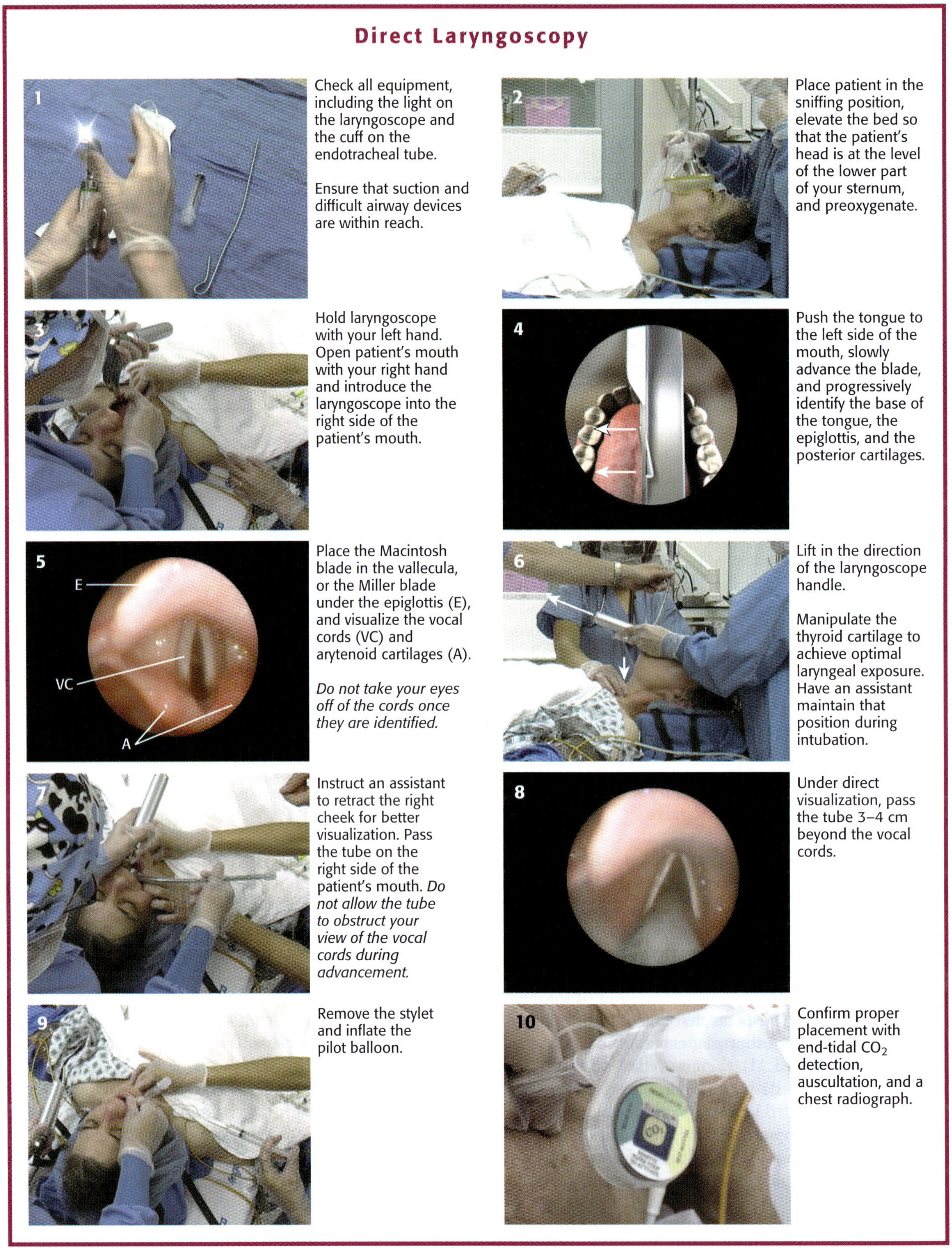

Fig. 4.11 Direct laryngoscopy.

Draw the patient's lower lip down with your right thumb, and introduce the tip of the laryngoscope into the right side of the patient's mouth (see Fig. 4.11, *step 3*). Slide the blade along the right side of the tongue while gradually displacing the tongue toward the left as you move the blade to the center of the mouth (see Fig. 4.11, *step 4*). If you initially place the blade in the middle of the tongue, it will fold over the lateral edge of the blade and obscure visualization of the airway. Placing the blade in the middle of the tongue and failing to move the tongue to the left are two common errors that prevent visualization of the vocal cords (Fig. 4.13). Recently some experts have questioned the utility of starting on the right side of the

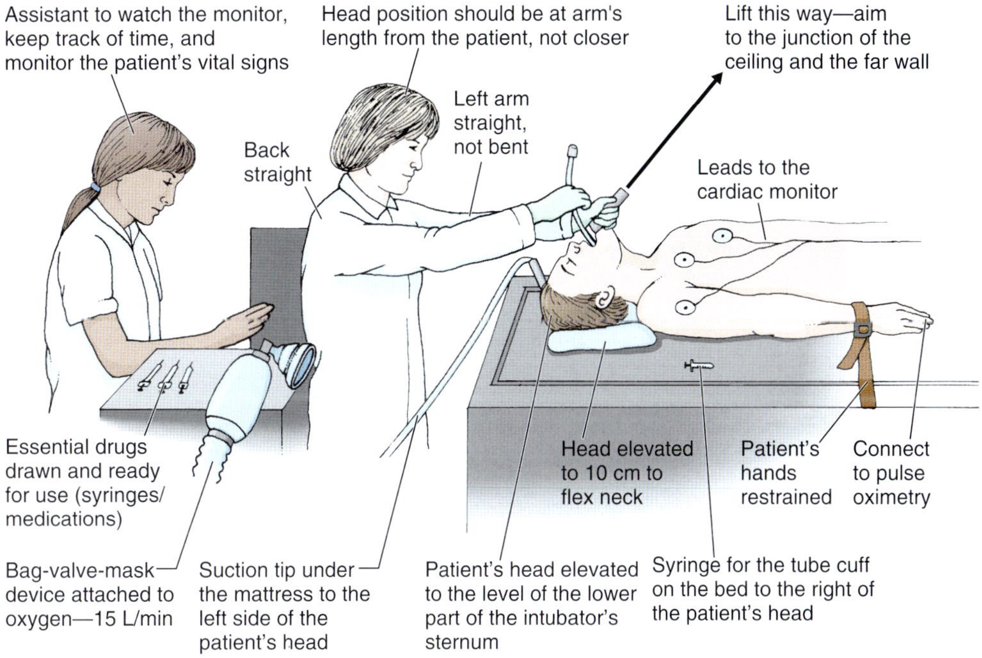

Fig. 4.12 Proper positioning of the clinician, patient, and assistant for tracheal intubation. The following points are demonstrated: the difficult airway cart is adjacent to the patient, the suction device is at the head of the bed, the patient is in the "sniffing position" with the occiput elevated and the clinician's right hand ready for additional adjustment if necessary, the bed is elevated and the clinician is at the appropriate distance from the patient, and the laryngoscope handle is angled at 45 degrees.

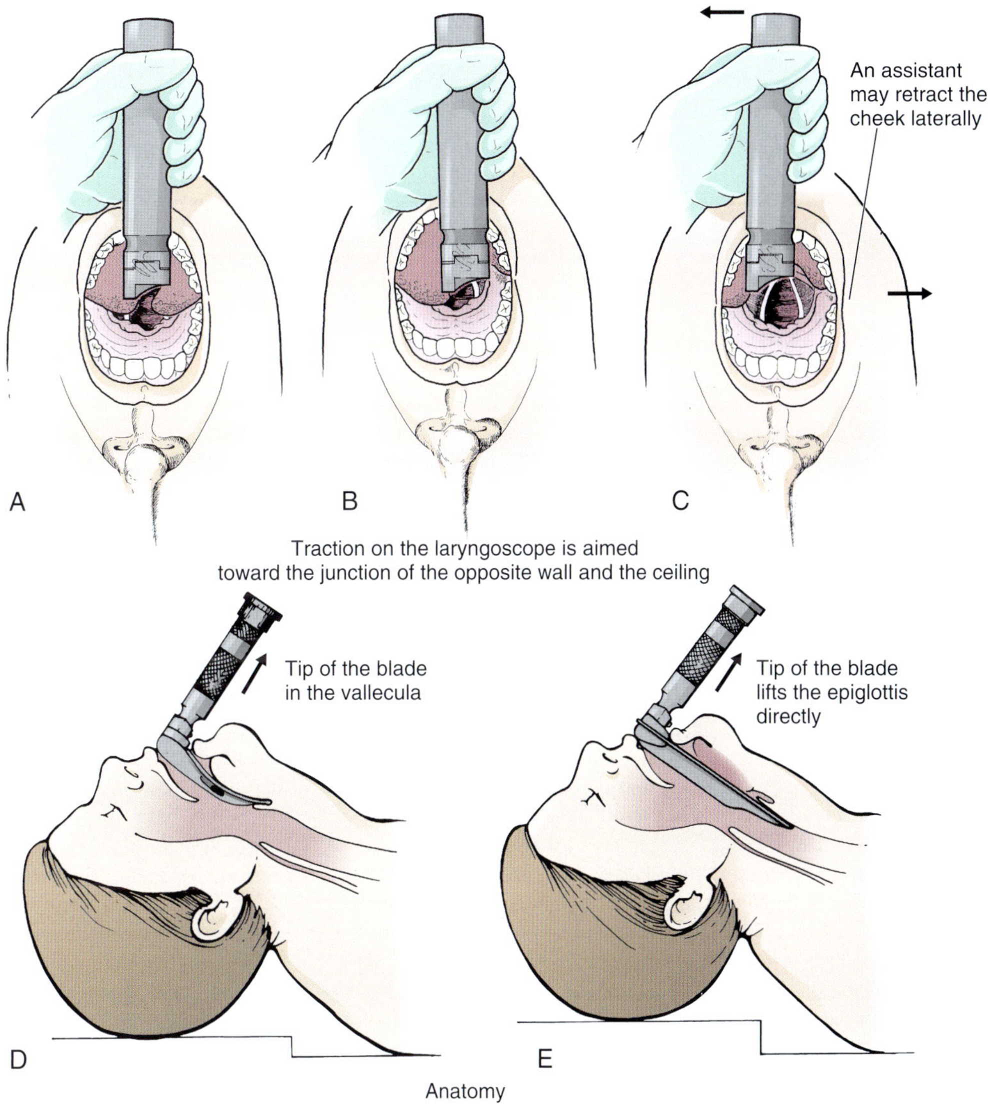

Fig. 4.13 Common problems encountered when using a laryngoscope. (A) The laryngoscope blade is under the middle of the tongue, with the sides of the tongue hanging down and obscuring the glottis. (B) The tongue is not pushed far enough to the left and is obscuring the glottis. (C) Correct blade position with the tongue elevated and to the left. (D) Use of the curved (Macintosh) laryngoscope blade. (E) Use of the straight (Miller) blade.

mouth and have begun using a midline approach from start to finish. A midline approach simplifies the procedure and helps assure that the distal tip of the blade ends up in the midline. Also, it is not as important to control the right side of the tongue when using a device that allows both DL and VL.

As you move the tip of the blade toward the base of the tongue, exert force along the axis of the laryngoscope handle by lifting upward and forward at a 45-degree angle (see Fig. 4.11, *step 6*). The direction of this force is critical because if the force is too horizontal or too vertical, poor visualization will result. Avoid bending the wrist because it can result in dental injury if the teeth are used as a fulcrum for the blade. Slowly advance the blade down the tongue, searching for the epiglottis. It may help to have an assistant retract the cheek laterally to further expose the laryngeal structures. Locating the epiglottis is a crucial step in laryngoscopy and has been termed *epiglottoscopy*.[98] The laryngeal inlet lies just distal and below the epiglottis.

The step after visualization of the epiglottis depends on which laryngoscope blade is being used. With the curved blade, place the tip into the vallecula, the space between the base of the tongue and the epiglottis (see Fig. 4.13D). Continued anterior elevation of the base of the tongue will partially lift the epiglottis. With the blade in the midline of the vallecula, engage the median glossoepiglottic fold and hyoepiglottic ligament with the tip of the blade to indirectly lift the epiglottis and expose the laryngeal inlet. If the tip of the blade is inserted too deeply into the vallecula, the epiglottis may be pushed down and obscure the glottis.[46] When using the straight blade, insert the tip under and slightly beyond the epiglottis and directly lift it up (see Fig. 4.13E). If the straight blade is placed too deeply, the entire larynx may be elevated anteriorly and out of the field of vision. Gradually withdraw the blade to allow the laryngeal inlet to drop down into view. If the blade is deep and posterior, the lack of recognizable structures indicates esophageal passage; gradually withdraw the blade to permit the laryngeal inlet to come into view.

Infants and Children

It is helpful to appreciate the anatomic differences between children and adults when intubating pediatric patients (Fig. 4.14 and Table 4.2). Children's proportionately larger heads naturally place them in the sniffing position, so a towel under the occiput is rarely necessary (Fig. 4.15). The large head of newborns can result in a posterior positioning of the larynx that prevents visualization of the vocal cords. A small towel under the infant's shoulders should correct this problem. This is not necessary in all children; rather, the goal of any positioning maneuvers should be alignment of the tragus with the anterior shoulder.

The head may also be floppy and may benefit from stabilization by an assistant. The child's increased tongue-to-oropharynx ratio and shorter neck hinder forward displacement of the tongue and, when coupled with a U-shaped epiglottis, can make visualization of the glottis difficult. DL in infants and young children is generally best performed with a straight blade: Miller size 0 for premature infants, size 1 for normal-sized infants, and size 2 for older children. The infant's larynx lies higher and relatively more anterior. If no laryngeal structures are visible after laryngeal pressure, gradually withdraw the blade. Inadvertent advancement of the blade into the esophagus is a common error.

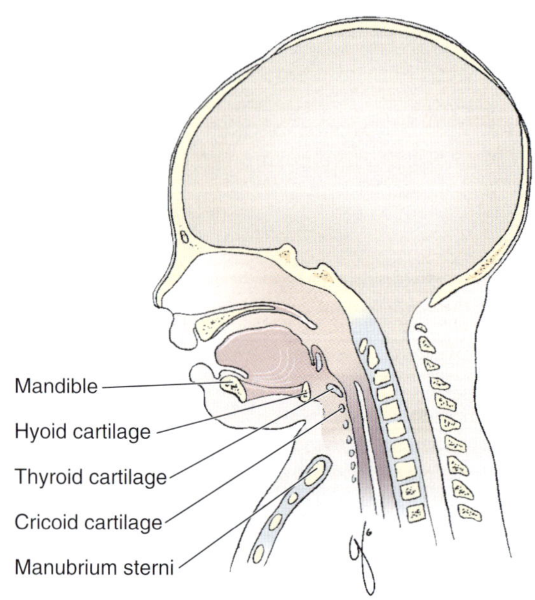

Fig. 4.14 Sagittal section of the neck of an infant. Note that in small children, the neck is shorter and the larynx is located more cephalad. (From Snell RS, Smith MS, eds. *Clinical Anatomy for Emergency Medicine*. Mosby-Year Book; 1993:16.)

Cricoid Pressure, ELM, Bimanual Laryngoscopy, and BURP

The differences between cricoid pressure, ELM, and backward, upward, rightward pressure (BURP) are often misunderstood. Cricoid pressure is the application of pressure at the anterior cricoid ring to displace it posteriorly to attempt to occlude the esophagus, with the intent of preventing regurgitation and aspiration; cricoid pressure is not intended to improve visualization during laryngoscopy. ELM is the application of pressure on the thyroid cartilage during laryngoscopy to help optimize visualization of the glottis. BURP is often the best combination of forces that need to be applied to the thyroid cartilage during ELM. Bimanual laryngoscopy refers to use of the right hand to perform ELM.

Cricoid Pressure

There is some good evidence that cricoid pressure (Sellick's maneuver) helps prevent gastric inflation during BMV,[99–104] though cricoid pressure during BMV reduces tidal volume, increases peak inspiratory pressure, and prevents good air exc hange.[100,102,103,105–112]

The only evidence suggesting that cricoid pressure prevents regurgitation during intubation consists of five cadaver studies,[104,113–116] one human study,[117] and some case reports,[118] collectively poor evidence by today's standards of evidence-based medical practice.[99,119] There are mixed data about the effects of cricoid pressure and laryngoscopic view,[120] and several studies have shown that it worsens visualization of the larynx.[121–123] A Cochrane review found insufficient evidence to support or refute the use of cricoid pressure during intubation.[124] There are many reports of significant regurgitation and aspiration regardless of the application of cricoid pressure.[125–128] Cricoid pressure also decreases successful insertion of and intubation through LMAs.[129–136] Despite the lack of evidence, many experts believe that Sellick's maneuver is critical during RSI.[137–140]

Because aspiration has dire consequences and cricoid pressure has traditionally been considered integral to patient

TABLE 4.2 Comparison of the Airway in Adults and Children

COMPARISON	CHILD	ADULT	CLINICAL CONSEQUENCES OR ADJUSTMENTS FOR CHILDREN
Head	Proportionately larger (up to approximately age 10 years)	Proportionately smaller	A child is naturally in the sniffing position when supine. Do not place a towel under the occiput; a child may benefit from elevation of the shoulders. The large head may be "floppy" and require the assistant to hold the head still during intubation.
Teeth	Easily knocked out	Stable unless decay or trauma is a factor	Teeth may be knocked out and aspirated or forced into trachea.
Tonsils or adenoids	Large and friable	Generally not a problem	Nasotracheal intubation in a child may cause excessive bleeding and is not recommended. Adenoid or tonsil tissue may plug the endotracheal tube or cause airway obstruction from aspiration.
Tongue	Relatively larger	Relatively smaller	The tongue is difficult to displace anteriorly in a child. Consider using a straight blade.
Larynx	Opposite C2-C3	Opposite C4-C6	A more superiorly located larynx or an "anterior" larynx is more difficult to visualize. Consider using a straight blade.
Epiglottis	U shaped, shorter, stiffer	Flatter, more flexible	The epiglottis is more difficult to manipulate in a child; it may fold down and obstruct the view with use of a curved blade. Consider using a straight blade.
Vocal cords	Concave upward; anterior attachment of the cords lower than posterior, thereby creating a slant	Horizontal	A concave shape does not affect intubation, but it may affect ventilation. For partial airway obstruction or to break laryngospasm, consider positive pressure ventilation with a jaw-lift maneuver to open the arytenoids. The anterior superior slant of the vocal cords may cause the endotracheal tube to hang up on the anterior commissure as it passes into the larynx. Rotate the tube 90 degrees counterclockwise. Overextension of the neck may cause partial airway obstruction as a result of airway collapse.
Length of the trachea	Relatively shorter	Relatively longer	A short trachea increases the likelihood of main stem bronchus intubation. Follow the formula for correct depth of placement (cm depth = 0.5 × age [years] + 12) measured from the corner of the mouth. The double black line on the endotracheal tube should pass just beyond the cords.
Airway diameter	Relatively smaller; smallest diameter at the cricoid ring	Relatively larger; smallest diameter between the vocal cords	Laryngoscope-induced trauma, edema, and foreign material will significantly alter the diameter of the airway. Be gentle. Extremes of flexion or extension may kink the airway. If trouble with bag-valve-mask ventilation occurs, reassess the degree of head flexion or extension. Cricoid pressure may cause complete airway obstruction. The endotracheal tube may pass through the cords but be too large to pass through the cricoid ring. If unable to pass into the trachea, use the next smaller tube.
Residual lung capacity	Relatively smaller	Relatively larger	A child becomes hypoxic more quickly than an adult does. Closely monitor O_2 saturation and avoid prolonged periods without ventilation.

safety during emergency airway management,[119] it is reasonable to apply cricoid pressure if it does not interfere with ventilation and intubation. There is significant evidence that it can interfere with ventilation and intubation, so it is best to apply cricoid pressure on a case-by-case basis with a full understanding of the benefits and drawbacks of cricoid pressure.[119] If cricoid pressure is utilized, it should be released immediately if there is any difficulty either intubating or ventilating a patient in an emergency setting.[108,119,128,141,142] Routine use of cricoid pressure during BMV of patients in cardiac arrest is not currently recommended in the AHA Guidelines for Cardiopulmonary Resuscitation and Emergency Cardiovascular Care.[143] It is reasonable to release or relax cricoid pressure during insertion of an LMA, during

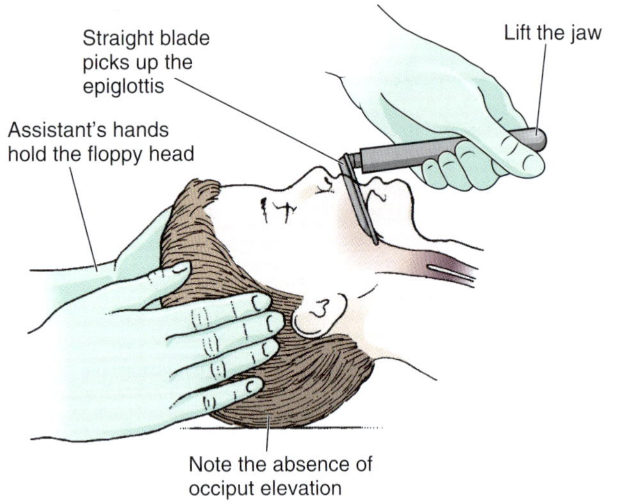

Fig. 4.15 Oral intubation in a child with a straight blade. The proportionately large floppy head of a child may present some difficulty, and an assistant may be required to hold the child's head straight.

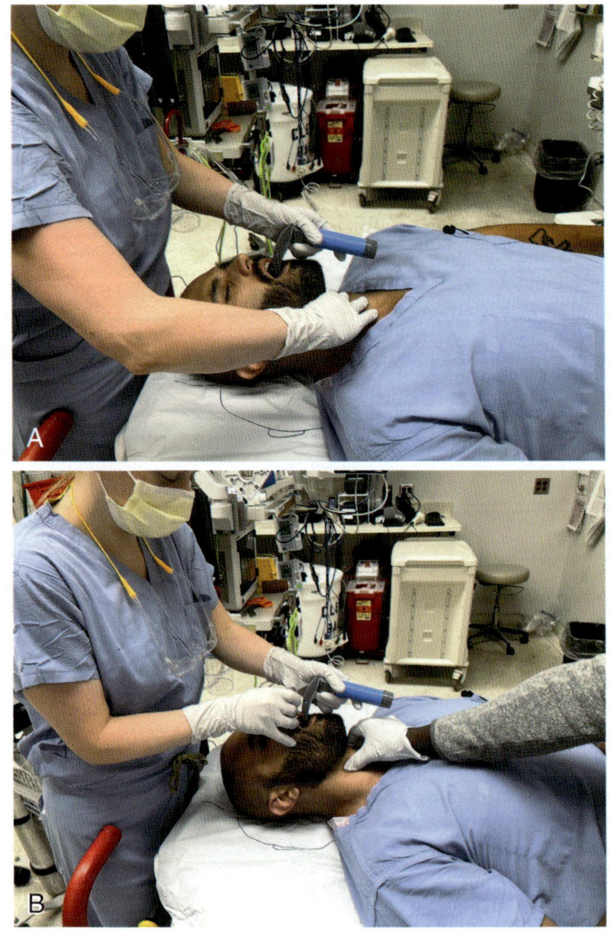

Fig. 4.16 External laryngeal manipulation (ELM) (or bimanual laryngoscopy). (A) ELM step 1. The laryngoscopist optimizes view of the larynx by reaching around to the patient's neck with the right hand and manipulating the thyroid cartilage while performing laryngoscopy. (B) ELM step 2. The assistant's hand replaces the laryngoscopist's hand on the anterior aspect of the neck and maintains the position of the larynx while the laryngoscopist places the tracheal tube.

intubation with an ILMA, or if ventilation with the LMA is difficult.[99,119,135]

Some authors believe that improper technique is to blame for the many reported failures of Sellick's maneuver.[99] The proper technique for applying Sellick's maneuver is to place the thumb and middle finger on either side of the cricoid cartilage and the index finger in the center anteriorly.[104] Apply 30 N (6.7 lb) of force to the cricoid cartilage in the posterior direction.[99,143] As a reference, approximately 40 N of digital force on the bridge of the nose will usually cause pain.[99]

ELM, Bimanual Laryngoscopy, and BURP

ELM is the application of pressure on the thyroid cartilage to improve the view of the larynx during laryngoscopy. Multiple studies have shown that ELM performed by the laryngoscopist (termed bimanual laryngoscopy) is superior to having an assistant apply anterior neck pressure.[122,144] Bimanual laryngoscopy is best because the direction and amount of force that will optimize laryngeal exposure are variable. BURP is sometimes optimal, though it often worsens the laryngoscopic view,[122] so it is best to move the larynx in a variety of directions to determine the optimal ELM. The best way to quickly apply a variety of different forces to the larynx to determine the optimal ELM is by manipulation of the larynx with the laryngoscopist's right hand (Fig. 4.16).[144]

Operator-directed posterior displacement of the larynx during laryngoscopy was described by Brunnings in 1912.[145] In 1993 Knill reported that having an assistant apply BURP to the cricoid or thyroid cartilage improved visualization of the glottis during two cases of difficult laryngoscopy.[146] In 1993 Takahata and coworkers performed a prospective study of 630 intubations and found that BURP produced better laryngeal exposure than just backward pressure in patients with difficult laryngoscopy.[147] A 2005 prospective crossover trial by Snider and colleagues found no benefit with routine application of the BURP maneuver.[148]

Studies by Benumof, Levitan, and colleagues have demonstrated that it is best to apply pressure on the thyroid cartilage (not the cricoid cartilage) and suggested that ELM should be applied by the laryngoscopist's right hand, not by an assistant.[122,144,149] They also found that the direction of force required for optimal ELM was not always upward and rightward and that the amount of backward pressure was variable.[122] In a 1996 study of 181 patients, Benumof and Cooper found that external manipulation was optimal when applied to the thyroid cartilage in 88% of patients and to the cricoid cartilage in only 11% of patients.[144] In a 2006 cadaveric study of 1530 laryngoscopies by 104 laryngoscopists, Levitan and associates found that bimanual laryngoscopy was more effective than both BURP and cricoid pressure for optimizing laryngeal exposure (Figs. 4.17 and 4.18; see also Fig. 4.16).[122] In addition, they found that cricoid pressure worsened the view of the larynx in 29% of cases and BURP worsened it in 35%.[122] In a 2002 study of eight first-year emergency medicine residents performing 271 intubations in an operating room setting, Levitan and colleagues found that bimanual laryngoscopy (ELM performed by the laryngoscopist) consistently improved laryngeal exposure by novice intubators.[149]

Bimanual laryngoscopy with ELM should be performed whenever the laryngeal view is not optimal after good laryngoscopic technique. To perform this procedure, the intubator applies posterior pressure on the thyroid cartilage. The force vector (right or left, upwards or downwards, and amount of

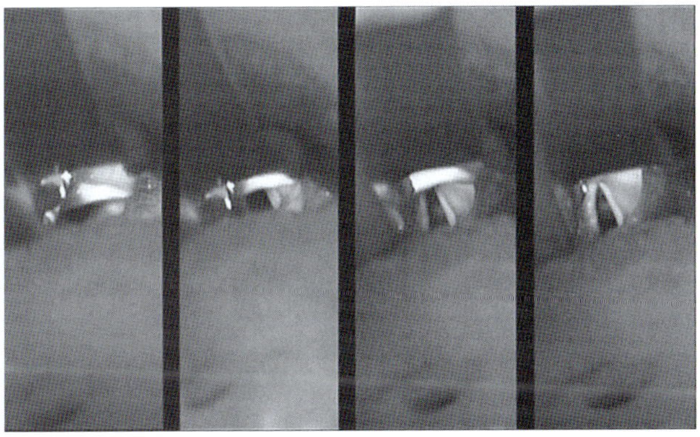

Fig. 4.17 The epiglottis is elevated and visualization of the vocal cords is improved by applying pressure on the hyoepiglottic ligament and external laryngeal manipulation. (Courtesy Richard M. Levitan, MD, Airway Cam Technologies, Inc., Wayne, PA.)

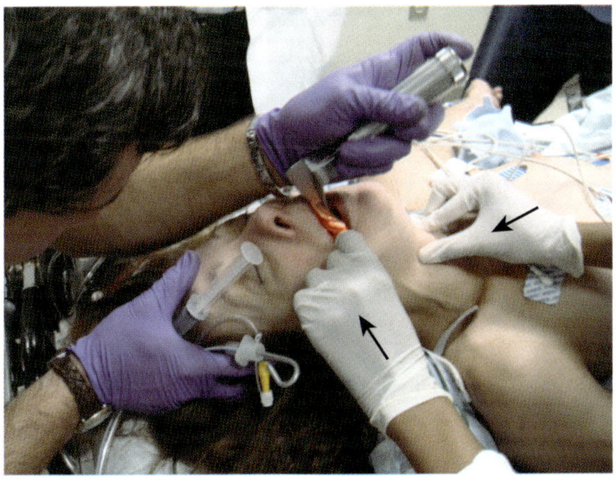

Fig. 4.18 Note the assistant manipulating the anterior part of the neck and retracting the cheek for better visualization.

posterior pressure) will vary from patient to patient, and the intubator should find the force vector that provides the best laryngeal view. Once this is established, an assistant applies the same force vector to the thyroid cartilage as the intubator removes pressure to free the hand in order to pass the tracheal tube. The assistant holds pressure while the intubator completes tracheal intubation.

Passing the Tube

Once the vocal cords have been visualized, the final step is to pass the tube through the vocal cords and into the trachea under direct vision. It is best to use either a tracheal tube introducer (bougie) or insert a malleable stylet.[64,150] If using a stylet, the best stylet shape is straight with a 35-degree hockey-stick bend at the proximal cuff ("straight-to-cuff"). In a 2006 study, Levitan and colleagues showed that stylet bend angles greater than 35 degrees made ET tube passage more difficult.[151]

Hold the tube in your right hand and introduce it from the right side of the patient's mouth. Lateral retraction of the cheek by an assistant may greatly aid overall visualization (see Fig. 4.18). Advance the tube toward the patient's larynx below the line of sight with the bend facing upward. When advanced in this manner, the tube does not obstruct the view of the larynx until the last possible moment before the tube enters the larynx. If the patient is not chemically paralyzed, pass the tube during inspiration, when the vocal cords are maximally open. It enters the trachea when the cuff disappears through the vocal cords. Advance the tube 3 to 4 cm beyond this point. It is not enough to see the tube approach the cords; watch the tube pass through the vocal cords to ensure tracheal placement. Directly observing the tube pass through the cords is the best way to immediately confirm correct placement. If part of the glottis is visualized and it is difficult to pass the tube, consider using a bougie (tracheal tube introducer).

Tracheal Tube Introducer (Bougie)

See Video 4.10. The bougie, though historically considered a rescue device or a device used for difficult airways, can also be used as a routine intubation device.[64,152] This adjunct is a long, thin, semirigid introducer that, with the aid of a laryngoscope, is passed through the laryngeal inlet and over which an ET tube is advanced through the cords and into the trachea. The technique, originally described more than 60 years ago by Macintosh,[153] was recommended for patients in whom visualizing the vocal cords was difficult. It has also been shown to be effective when the laryngeal inlet cannot be visualized at all.[154] It is the most common airway adjunct used in British EDs for complicated intubations.[155] Its efficacy has been demonstrated prospectively during difficult intubations in the operating room, as a pivotal component of a difficult airway algorithm in the operating room, and when compared with conventional laryngoscopy in the ED.[66,156,157] A recent single-center randomized controlled trial demonstrated significantly higher first attempt success with bougie over traditional stylet.[64] A follow-up multicenter randomized trial evaluating the same did not find the same difference when the operators were not used to bougie use.[152] Programs that have incorporated routine bougie use into airway bundles show substantial improvement in first attempt success.[158,159]

A variety of tracheal tube introducers are available today (Fig. 4.19). The original adjunct was called the gum elastic bougie, or simply "the bougie," and is currently available in a reusable form for both adult and pediatric patients (Eschmann Tracheal Tube Introducer; Portex Sims). The adult size comes in two forms: a 60-cm (15-Fr) version with a short, 40-degree hockey-stick curve at the end, and a straight one that is 70 cm. The adult version can accommodate a 5.5-mm ET tube. The pediatric version is 70 cm (10-Fr) and straight and can accommodate a 4.0-mm tube. A polyethylene introducer designed for single use is also available and comes only in the 60-cm version (Flextrach ET Tube Guide; Greenfield Medical Sourcing). A variation of this concept is the FROVA Introducer (Cook Critical Care), a plastic introducer with a similar profile to the others except that it has a hollow lumen through which the patient can be ventilated when an accompanying adapter is attached. The most commonly used bougie in recent randomized trials was manufactured by SunMed. Not all bougies are created equal. Many are too floppy and will not assist in difficult airways. The authors recommend bougies that are 70 cm as shorter bougies have slightly more difficulty in removal if they are advanced to the carina before tube passage.

Consider using a bougie for all intubations of critically ill adults and strongly consider its use when a difficult airway is anticipated and when visualization of the laryngeal inlet is limited. A trauma patient with cervical spine precautions is a typical example. The presence of blood and vomitus rarely prevents placement of the bougie into the trachea. Though there are anecdotes cautioning that the bougie causes iatrogenic injury that the ET tubes do not cause, data from 1800 patients in randomized trials show no difference in postintubation pneumothorax or tracheal injury.[64,152] Its safety record is impressive despite decades of use, reports of complications are rare, and it should be considered a safe airway adjunct.[160]

Shaping the introducer may not be necessary in many cases, and with difficult laryngeal views, create a 60-degree bend in the distal introducer (see Fig. 4.19D).[161] Ideally, tracheal tube introducer-assisted intubation is a two-person procedure (Fig. 4.20). As laryngoscopy begins, the assistant has both a styletted ET tube and bougie prepared and available. The intubator performs laryngoscopy in the normal fashion to obtain the best possible view of the larynx. If the cords are in full view, proceed with intubation using a styletted ET tube. If the view is suboptimal, an assistant can pass the tracheal tube introducer to the operator for placement anterior to the arytenoids and into the larynx. If only the epiglottis is visible, place the introducer, with a 60-degree distal bend, just under the epiglottis and direct it anteriorly. With the laryngoscope still in place and the introducer stabilized by the operator, the assistant slides the ET tube over the introducer. Pass the tube through the larynx. Just before entering the larynx, rotate the tube 90 degrees counterclockwise to avoid having the tip of the ET tube get caught on the laryngeal structures (Fig. 4.21).[80] Withdraw the laryngoscope and confirm proper tube placement. While securing the ET tube, ask the assistant to remove the introducer.

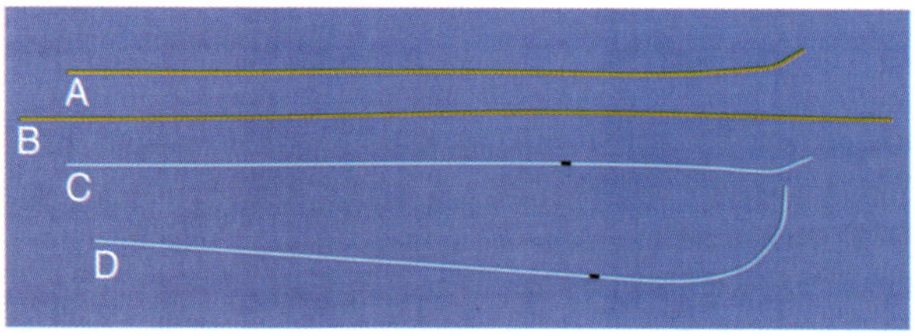

Fig. 4.19 Several types of tracheal tube introducers. The classic introducer, the gum elastic bougie (A) is reusable and comes in curved- and straight-tipped adult forms and a straight pediatric form. The straight bougies (B) are 70 cm long and the curved-tipped bougies are 60 cm long. The blue introducer (C; Flextrach ET Tube Guide; Greenfield Medical Sourcing) is polyethylene and designed for single use and comes only in a curved-tipped adult form (60 cm). (D) Create a 60-degree bend in the distal portion of the introducer if the laryngeal inlet cannot be seen on laryngoscopy.

There are a number of findings that confirm successful introducer placement. If any portion of the arytenoids is visible and the introducer was seen to pass anterior to them without resistance, the introducer is in the airway. Unlike seeing an ET tube "go through the cords" when in fact the laryngeal inlet may have been momentarily obscured by the tube or balloon, the smaller-caliber introducer does not obscure the view of the glottis and thus avoids this potential pitfall. In addition to better visual confirmation, successful passage is indicated, up to 90% of the time, by feeling clicks produced by the angled tip of the introducer as it strikes against the tracheal rings.[64,162] An assistant will also usually feel confirmatory movement in the airway if the anterior aspect of the neck is palpated. If there is still any question whether the introducer is in the airway, gently advance it at least 40 cm, at which point resistance should be felt as the introducer passes the carina and stops inside a main bronchus. If the bougie does not stop when advanced approximately 40 cm, the introducer is most likely in the esophagus. Withdraw it and reattempt placement.

Several technical points should be emphasized. The first is that it is important to create a curve in the distal portion of the introducer when the laryngeal inlet is not visible. It is a mistake to think that the factory-formed curve at the tip will be sufficient to access the glottis in these situations. Second, in some cases, the bougie will pass through the cords and will become lodged in the anterior trachea with an inability to advance. If this happens, withdraw slightly and rotate the bougie 90 degrees in either direction to move the curved tip. This will prevent the tip from striking the anterior trachea and allow the bougie to pass to the carina. Third, if there is difficulty passing an ET tube into the laryngeal inlet, this is most likely because the tip of the tube is caught on the

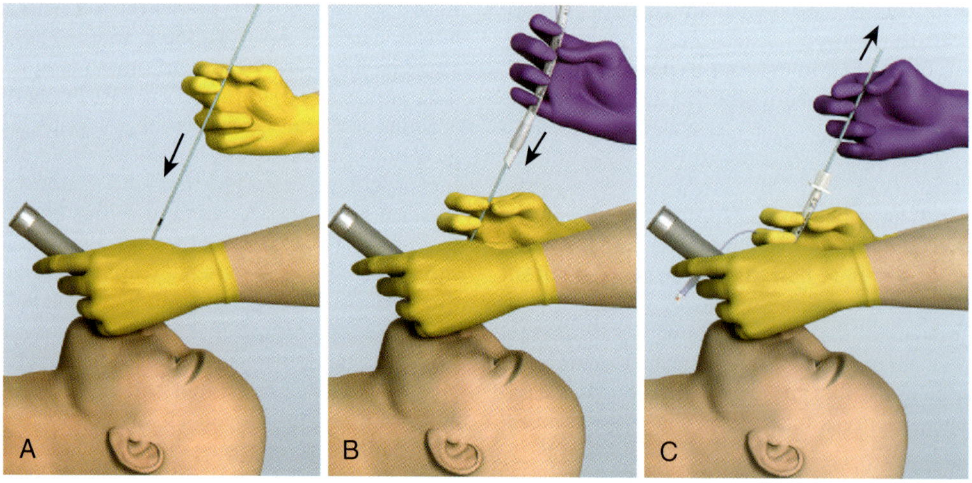

Fig. 4.20 Two-person tracheal tube introducer technique. The introducer is handed to the clinician after the best glottic view has been obtained. (A) The clinician places the introducer (the *black line* positioned at the teeth indicates the proper introducer depth to ensure stable positioning within the trachea while providing enough length to grasp the end of the introducer before passing the tube). (B) An assistant passes the tracheal tube over the introducer as the clinician holds the introducer steady. (C) The clinician passes the tracheal tube with a 90-degree counterclockwise rotation as the tube approaches the glottis, and the assistant withdraws the introducer.

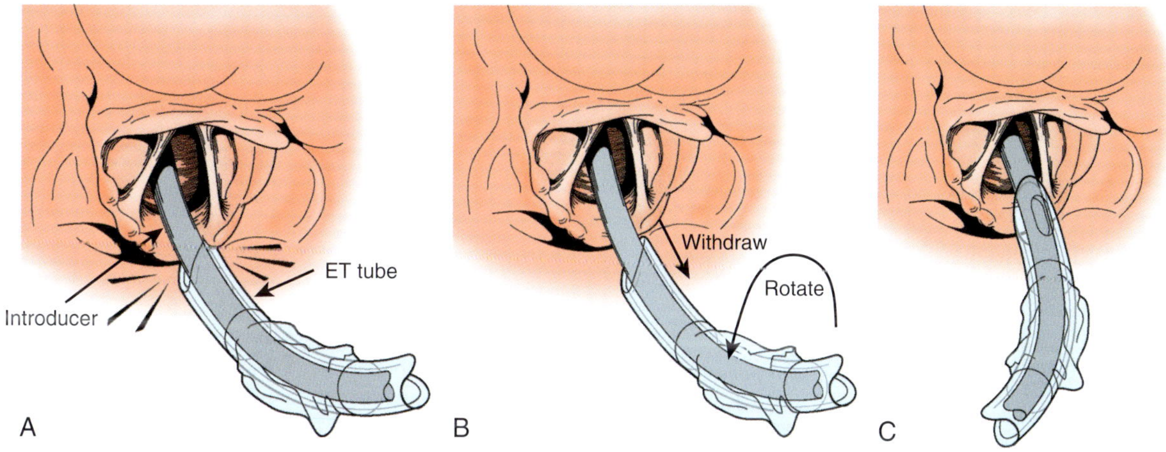

Fig. 4.21 A common cause of difficulty when railroading an endotracheal *(ET)* tube over a tracheal tube introducer. (A) The tip of the ET tube is caught on the right arytenoid as it is being railroaded over the introducer. (B) Corrective maneuvers: (1) withdrawal of the ET tube 2 cm to disengage the arytenoids and (2) counterclockwise 90-degree rotation of the ET tube to orient the bevel posteriorly. (C) The bevel of the ET tube is facing posteriorly and allows smooth passage through the glottis. (A–C, Courtesy Department of Emergency Medicine, Hennepin County Medical Center, Minneapolis, MN.)

right arytenoid cartilage. In this case, withdraw the tube 2 cm, rotate it 90 degrees counterclockwise, and advance it again (see Fig. 4.21). Fourth, although there may be some benefit to lubricating the distal end of the introducer, in emergency intubations, lubricating the full length of the introducer makes it slippery and hard to handle without conferring any obvious advantage. Lubricating the ET tube, conversely, remains critical for smooth passage through the vocal cords. Fifth, a common error when first using the tracheal tube introducer is to remove the laryngoscope before passing the ET tube over the introducer. This often results in difficulty placing the tube because it is displaced posteriorly by the weight of the pharyngeal soft tissues and gets hung up on the laryngeal structures. Reinsert the laryngoscope. Pull the tube back 2 cm to disengage the soft tissue. Rotate the tube 90 degrees counterclockwise and then readvance it. Sixth, in instances in which it is difficult to get the introducer sufficiently anterior to access the laryngeal inlet, make sure that the introducer enters from the side of the mouth and lines up with the operator's line of vision. If the introducer enters the mouth at a significant angle above this line, most often when the clinician is too close to the patient, it may be deflected posteriorly by the lip or intraoral structures and escape the attention of the operator. This creates the impression that the introducer is "too floppy."

In the prehospital setting, where assistance might not be available, the laryngoscope should be removed to mount the ET tube onto the introducer. Once the tube is on the introducer, reinsert the laryngoscope and advance the introducer through the glottic opening. Some clinicians prefer to keep the laryngoscope in place and instead pinch the bougie against the laryngoscope blade with their left hand. They then load the tube onto the bougie. Advance the ET tube while rotating it 90 degrees counterclockwise to ensure successful passage into the trachea. Mounting the tube onto the introducer to insert them as a unit is not advised because it is often difficult to direct the introducer into the laryngeal inlet as it moves within the ET tube.

Laryngospasm

If the patient is not paralyzed, laryngospasm, or persistent contraction of the adductor muscles of the vocal cords, may prevent passage of the tube. Pretreatment with topical lidocaine may decrease the likelihood of laryngospasm, though this is not routinely performed. After laryngospasm is noted, one option is to spray lidocaine (2% or 4%) directly onto the vocal cords. An infrequent and effective means of achieving tracheal anesthesia is transtracheal puncture and injection of 3 to 4 mL of lidocaine through the cricothyroid membrane. Laryngospasm is usually brief and often followed by a gasp. Be ready to pass the tube at this moment. Occasionally, the spasm is prolonged and needs to be disrupted with sustained anterior traction applied at the angles of the mandible, as in the jaw-thrust maneuver. Do not force the tube at any time because it could cause permanent damage to the vocal cords. Consider using a smaller tube. Prolonged, intense spasm may ultimately require muscle relaxation with a paralyzing drug (see Chapter 5). Pediatric patients are far more prone to laryngospasm than adults.[163] In a child, if vocal cord spasm prevents passage of the tube, a chest-thrust maneuver may momentarily open the passage and permit intubation.[164]

Positioning and Securing the Tube

Secure the ET tube in a position that minimizes both the chance of inadvertent, main stem endobronchial intubation and the risk for extubation. The tip should lie in the mid-trachea with room to accommodate neck movement. Because tube movement with both neck flexion and extension averages 2 cm,[165] the desired range of tip location is between 3 and 7 cm above the carina.

The average tracheal length is between 10 and 13 cm. In adults, the tip of the tube should ideally be 3 cm above the carina when the head and neck are in a neutral position. On a portable radiograph, the adult carina overlies the fifth, sixth, or seventh thoracic vertebral body. If the carina is not visible, it can be assumed that the tip of the tube is properly positioned if it is aligned with the third or fourth thoracic vertebra. In children, the carina is more cephalad than in adults, and it is consistently situated between T3 and T5. In children, T1 is the reference point for the tip of the ET tube.[166]

Estimate the proper depth of tube placement before radiographic confirmation by using the following formulas, in which length represents the distance from the tip of the tube to the upper incisors in children[167,168] and from the upper incisors[169] or the corner of the mouth[170] in adults:

Children: tracheal tube depth (cm) = [age (years) / 2] + 12
(or use length-based aid such as a Broselow tape)
Adults: females: tracheal tube depth (cm) = 21 cm;
males: tracheal tube depth (cm) = 23 cm

In adults, this method has been shown to be more reliable than auscultation in determining the correct depth of placement.[169] One can anticipate that tall male patients will often require deeper placement, to 24 or 25 cm, and that short females will often require a shallower placement of 19 or 20 cm.

Inflate the cuff to the point of minimal air leak with positive pressure ventilation. In an emergency intubation, inflate with 10 mL of air and adjust the inflation volume after the patient is stabilized.

After placement of the tracheal tube, confirm tracheal placement with end-tidal CO_2 and check that the depth is appropriate. With the tube in position and the cuff inflated, secure the tube in place. Attach commercial ET tube holders, adhesive tape, or umbilical (nonadhesive cloth) tape securely to the tube and around the patient's head (Figs. 4.22 and 4.23). Position the tube at the corner of the mouth, where the tongue is less likely to expel it. This position is also more comfortable for the patient and allows suctioning. A bite block or oral airway to prevent crimping of the ET tube or damage from biting is commonly incorporated into the system used to secure the tube.

Unintentional extubation can have disastrous consequences, particularly if the patient is difficult to intubate initially. Secure the ET tube immediately after correct placement has been confirmed. During transport, moving the intubated patient, or obtaining radiographs, designate one person to tend to the ET tube to avoid unplanned extubation. Inadequate sedation is another risk factor for unplanned extubation.[171] If long-acting paralytics have not been administered, consider sedation or physical restraints to prevent self-extubation by an agitated or confused patient.

Confirmation of Tracheal Tube Placement

See Video 4.11. The first step to confirm tracheal tube placement is to definitively see the tube pass through the vocal cords (Table 4.3). This is much easier when using a video laryngoscope. The very next step, before other clinical assessment, is to confirm tracheal location with end-tidal CO_2, which is more reliable than any clinical assessment.

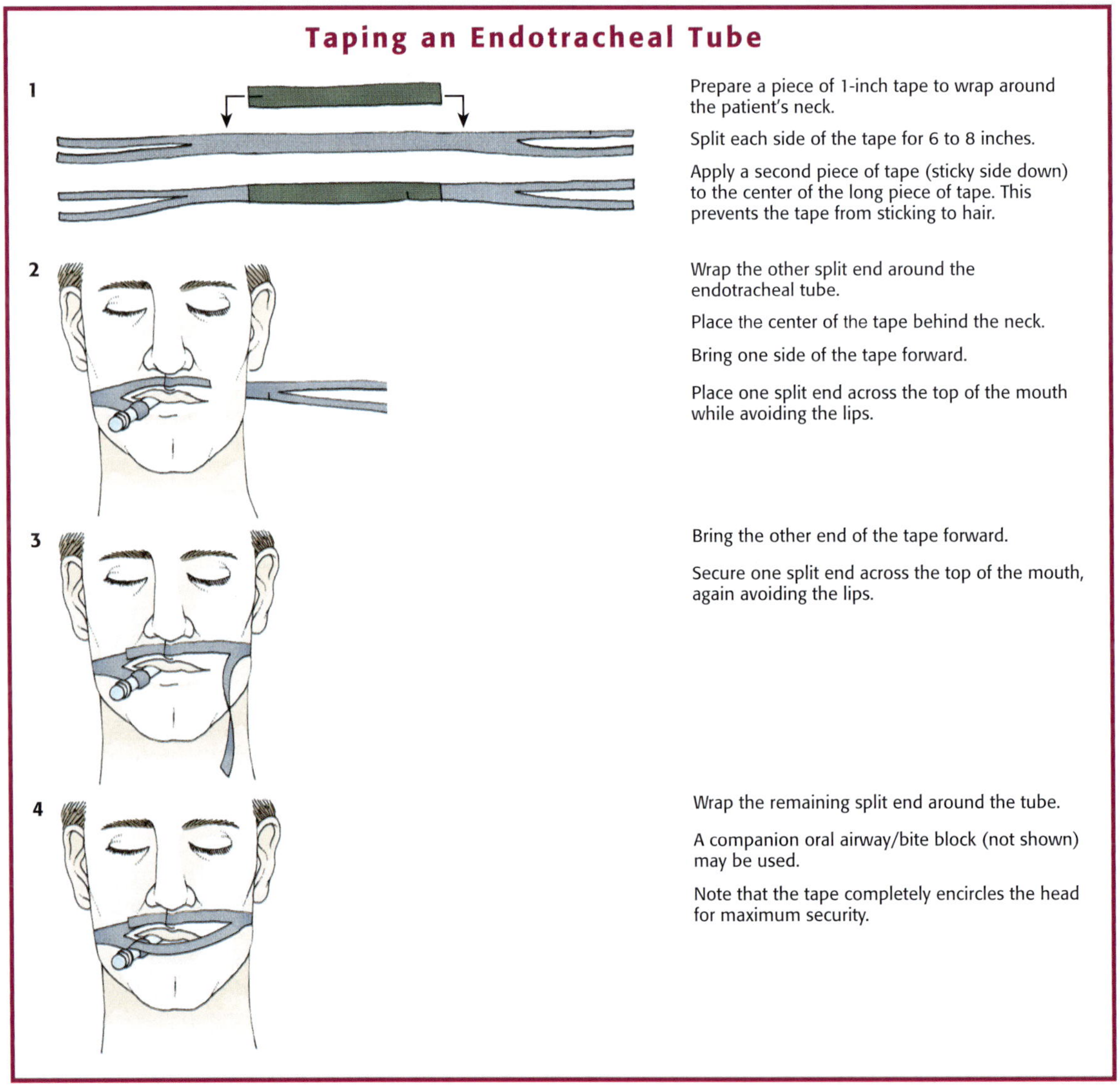

Fig. 4.22 Technique for taping an endotracheal tube. The method illustrated can be replaced by using a commercial holder or tracheostomy cloth tie. Avoid taping the lips.

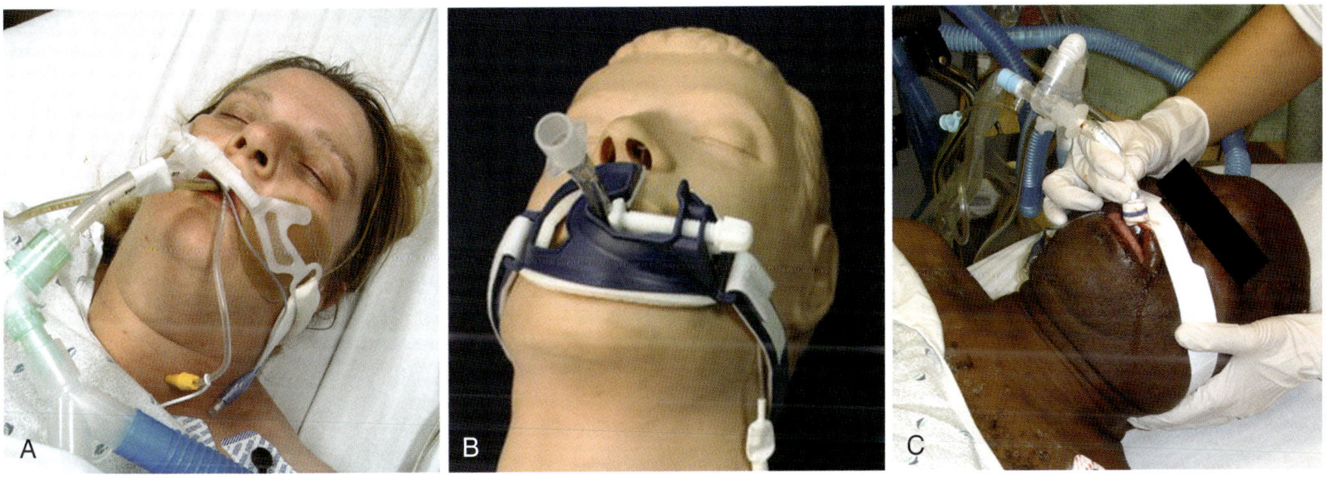

Fig. 4.23 (A) A commercial disposable tube holder is ideal and preferred to secure an endotracheal (ET) tube without the use of messy tape. (B) A plastic disposable ET holder firmly secures the ET tube with a small clamp. (C) When positioning a patient for transfer to another bed or for a chest radiograph, ensure the integrity of the ET tube by placing the right hand firmly against the right side of the face while holding the tube securely with the same hand. The other hand immobilizes the neck. (B, Courtesy Laerdal Medical, Wappingers Falls, NY.)

TABLE 4.3 Assessing Proper Tube Placement

TEST	INTERPRETATION
Observe the tube pass through the vocal cords	First step to ensure accurate placement; if in doubt, look again after intubation or have an experienced clinician look again
End-tidal CO_2 measurements	Gold standard for confirming placement. A good persistent waveform must be present to confirm. This can be misleading if the tube tip is just above the airway, which will also give a positive CO_2 reading
Auscultation of breath sounds over the chest	May be misleading, especially if only the midline is examined; listen in both axillae
Auscultation over the stomach	Not reliable, but gurgling may indicate esophageal placement
Condensation (fog) forms inside the tube with each breath	Not reliable to confirm tracheal placement
Observe the chest rise with positive pressure and fall with release	Not reliable whether observed or absent. May be absent in patients with a small tidal volume or severe bronchospasm
Chest radiograph	Not reliable for confirmation of tracheal placement. Cannot always differentiate between tracheal and esophageal placement. If known to be in the trachea by other measures, radiography can assess for proper depth of tube insertion
Aspiration technique	Tracheal location is confirmed (assuming patient ET tube) if 30–40 mL of air is aspirated without resistance; probable esophageal location if unable to aspirate the syringe easily or delayed bulb refill occurs; can be misleading with nasotracheal intubation if the tube has curled supraglottically. This should be used in conjunction with end-tidal CO_2.
Fiberoptic bronchoscope	Reliable if tracheal rings are seen down the endotracheal tube
Ultrasound detection of tracheal tube location	Appears to be reliable but not extensively studied. Should not be used as a sole confirmatory technique

If at any point there is uncertainty whether the tube is in the trachea or the esophagus (no capnography waveform), the tube position should be rechecked (if a laryngoscope is immediately available) or the tube should be removed and the patient should be ventilated using a bag-mask device, or an EGD. Tube removal is preferred, especially if the patient's oxygen saturation is falling. Even if the tube location is confirmed with laryngoscopy, evidence of adequate exhaled carbon dioxide must be sought. Waveform capnography is considered the gold standard for assuring that the patient is being ventilated, and it should be used whether ventilation is via BMV, an EGD, or an ET tube. It is crucial to ensure that the waveform capnographer is working properly, since it is the best objective evidence of patient ventilation, and loss of the capnography waveform is an emergency that requires immediate corrective action.

Clinical Assessment

Clinical assessments may be performed after the tube is visualized to pass between the vocal cords and after adequate waveform capnography is seen. Clinical assessment is of limited utility except to localize the tube in the trachea rather than in a mainstem bronchus. Absent or diminished breath sounds, any sound or vocalization from the patient, increased abdominal size, and gurgling sounds during ventilation are clinical signs of esophageal placement. Critically, esophageal placement is not always obvious. One may hear "normal" breath sounds if only the midline of the thorax is auscultated. The presence of condensation of the ET tube as a means of confirming tracheal placement may also be misleading. Blinded observers noted condensation of the ET tube during ventilation in 23 of 27 esophageal intubations in an animal model.[172] One way to clinically assess tracheal placement after several ventilations or during spontaneous respiration is to note whether air is felt or heard to exit through the tube. If tidal volume is adequate, the exit of air should be obvious. This technique should not be relied upon and should only be used in austere settings.

Asymmetric breath sounds indicate probable main stem bronchus intubation. Because of the angles of takeoff of the main bronchi and the fact that the carina lies to the left of the midline in adults, right main stem intubation is most common and is indicated by decreased breath sounds on the left side. When asymmetric sounds are heard, deflate the cuff and withdraw the tube until equal breath sounds are present. Bloch and coworkers[173] reported accurate pediatric tracheal positioning if after noting asymmetric breath sounds the tube is withdrawn a defined distance beyond the point at which equal breath sounds are first heard: 2 cm in children younger than 5 years and 3 cm in older children.

End-Tidal CO_2

End-tidal CO_2 detection is the best technique, in conjunction with visualizing the tube pass through the cords, to confirm tracheal placement of the ET tube. A high level of CO_2 in exhaled air is the physiologic basis for capnography and the principle on which end-tidal CO_2 pressure (P_{ETCO_2}) detectors were developed (see Chapter 2). Continuous waveform capnography is recommended by the AHA guidelines as the most reliable method of confirming and monitoring correct placement of an ET tube (class I, level of evidence [LOE]). This recommendation is based on multiple studies showing 100% accuracy of waveform capnography for detecting correct ET tube placement.[143] Continuous waveform capnography is accurate even in cardiac arrest and asthma. Patients with prolonged cardiac arrest will still have a typical square waveform and a low P_{ETCO_2} value. If a capnography waveform is not visualized, the explanation should *never* be due to the patient physiology. The cause should be presumed to be esophageal placement of the tube until proven otherwise.

When waveform capnography is not available, emergency clinicians may have to rely on colorimetric CO_2 indicators, that correspond to CO_2 levels flowing through the device when placed on the tracheal tube adapter (see Fig. 4.11, *step 10*). The typical device displays opposite colors (e.g., yellow and purple) to indicate low levels of CO_2 in esophageal gas versus the high levels of CO_2 exhaled from the respiratory tree. Handheld quantitative or semiquantitative electronic CO_2 monitors are also available. Eventually, all prehospital defibrillators will have advanced monitoring capability that includes capnography.

A multicenter study of a colorimetric device demonstrated an overall sensitivity of 80% and a specificity of 96%.[174] In patients with spontaneous circulation and an inflated tracheal tube cuff, the sensitivity and specificity were 100%. The poor sensitivity (69%) noted in patients in cardiac arrest was due to the fact that low exhaled CO_2 levels were seen with both very-low-flow states and esophageal intubation. The device must be used with caution in cardiac arrest victims. CO_2 levels return to normal after the return of spontaneous circulation. Colorimetric changes may be difficult to discern in situations with reduced lighting, and secretions can interfere with the change in color. Regardless of the monitoring device, patients should be ventilated for a minimum of six breaths before taking a reading. Recent ingestion of carbonated beverages can result in spuriously high CO_2 levels with esophageal intubation.[175] Colorimetric changes do not exclude supraglottic positioning of the tip of the ET tube. Adequate ventilation and oxygenation may be achieved in the supraglottic position, and there is still a risk for aspiration in the absence of a protected airway with the potential for further tube dislodgment. Glottic positioning may be difficult to detect clinically. The only signs may be persistent cuff leak or diminished chest rise with ventilation. Radiographic evidence or direct visualization confirms the diagnosis.[176]

Endoscopic Tube Confirmation

A flexible endoscope can be used to assess tube location. Passage of the scope through the tube with visualization of the tracheal rings and carina confirms ET placement and position within the trachea. The intubator should assess for tracheal rings, trachealis smooth muscle posteriorly, and should see the tip of the tube above the carina.

Esophageal Detector Device

An aspiration technique used to determine ET tube location was first described by Wee in 1988 and should be used in conjunction with detection of end-tidal CO_2 and not as a stand-alone technique.[177] The technique takes advantage of the difference in tracheal and esophageal resistance to collapse during aspiration to locate the tip of the tracheal tube. After intubation, attach a large syringe (e.g., Positube esophageal detector; Flotec) to the end of the ET tube and withdraw the plunger of the syringe. If the tube is placed in the trachea correctly, the plunger will pull back without resistance as air is aspirated from the lungs. If the tracheal tube is in the esophagus, resistance is felt when the plunger is withdrawn because the pliable walls of the esophagus collapse under the negative pressure and occlude the end of the tube. Another device that uses the same principle as syringe aspiration is the self-inflating bulb (e.g., Ellick device).

In the initial study conducted in an operating room, tube placement was identified correctly in 99 of 100 cases (51 esophageal, 48 tracheal).[177] The result was considered equivocal in the remaining case. That tube was removed and found to be nearly totally occluded with purulent secretions. Slight resistance was noted in one patient with right main stem intubation; the resistance decreased when the tube was pulled back. Before use, always check the esophageal detector device for air leaks. If any connections are loose, the leak may allow the syringe to be withdrawn easily, thereby mimicking tracheal location of the tube.

When using the aspiration technique, apply constant, slow aspiration to avoid occlusion of the tube from tracheal mucosa drawn up under the high negative pressure. If the tracheal tube is placed correctly, 30 to 40 mL of air can be aspirated without resistance. If air was initially aspirated and some resistance is then encountered, the tracheal tube should be pulled back between 0.5 and 1.0 cm and rotated 45 degrees. This takes the tube out of the bronchus if it has been placed too deeply and changes the orientation of the bevel if the tube has been temporarily occluded with tracheal mucosa. Air is easily aspirated if the tube was in the trachea, and repositioning it will make no difference if the tube was in the esophagus. The syringe aspiration technique can be used before or after ventilation of the patient. Inflation of the tube cuff has no effect on the reliability of the test.[178] This device is reliable, rapid, inexpensive, and easy to use.[178]

A squeeze-bulb aspirator is an alternative to the syringe technique. Attach the bulb to the ET tube and squeeze; if the tube is in the esophagus, it is accompanied by a flatus-like sound followed by absent or markedly delayed refilling. Insufflation of a tube in the trachea is silent with instantaneous refill. An early study with the Ellick evacuator bulb device reported that 82% of esophageal intubations were identified.[179] A later study using a slightly different bulb device (Respironics) found that all 45 esophageal intubations were detected.[180] The device is cheap, easy to use, and operated single-handedly in less than 5 seconds.[179] The bulb should not be used in freezing temperatures because of loss of elasticity. Confusion may occur if the esophageal tube is tested more than once because subsequent inflations may be silent. With repeated assessments, false-positive refilling of the bulb may occur as a result of instillation of air during the first attempt. This observation has led to a recommendation that the bulb be compressed before it is attached to the ET tube. Delayed, though complete refilling of the bulb may occur with bronchial tube placement or placement in the more pliable pediatric airway. The bulb suction modification of the aspiration technique has not been studied as thoroughly as the syringe technique.

A significant number of false positives occur with esophageal detection devices (the tube is correctly placed in the trachea, but the device suggests that it is in the esophagus). These patients almost uniformly have an elevated BMI. Endoscopic evaluation found that the tracheal wall was invaginated into the ET tube because of the negative pressure.[181] In such circumstances, if the intubation was felt to be successful, visually reconfirm that the ET tube is through the cords before removing the ET tube. Alternatively, if the patient has a perfusing rhythm and an exhaled CO_2 device is available, it should be used. To date, there has been one reported case of unrecognized esophageal intubation undetected by the syringe aspiration technique.[182] In this case, there was marked gastric distention from forceful BMV. The esophageal detection device is not reliable in confirming tracheal tube depth and position after intubation because easy aspiration of air will occur if the tip of the tube is located supraglottically (expired CO_2 will also be misleading).

Ultrasound Detection of Tracheal Tube Location

Sonographic sliding signs can also be used immediately after tracheal intubation is confirmed by waveform capnography to evaluate for main stem intubation before obtaining a chest radiograph.[183,184] Assuming there is no other underlying lung pathology, absence of sliding on the left after intubation indicates probable right main stem intubation. The ET tube can be withdrawn 2 cm, and sliding signs reassessed. This is especially helpful in pediatric patients, for whom right mainstem intubation is common.

There are preliminary data that ultrasound may be useful to confirm tracheal rather than esophageal tube location. Ultrasound may play a future role in confirming tracheal location of the ET tube location after intubation. All studies examining this study question are relatively small, and sensitivity ranges from 96% to 100% for confirming tracheal placement, whereas specificity (detecting esophageal intubation) ranges from 88% to 100%.[185–190] If the ET tube is in the trachea, acoustic shadowing is seen posterior to the anterior tracheal rings only. If the ET is in the esophagus, the esophagus is opened by the ET tube and shadowing is seen posterior to the anterior esophageal wall (as well as the trachea). This method relies on the esophagus being located in the paratracheal position; if the esophagus is directly posterior to the trachea, then detecting esophageal intubation is very difficult. This method may be useful if end-tidal CO_2 monitoring is not available.

Complications of Intubation

Failure to achieve adequate ventilation and oxygenation is the most serious complication of tracheal intubation. The potential for hypoxia exists just before intubation as more conservative oxygenation methods are attempted and then fail, during difficult intubation when ventilation is halted for an attempt at intubation, and after intubation if esophageal intubation goes undetected. Because irreversible cerebral anoxia occurs within minutes, conservative airway management maneuvers should be limited to 2 to 3 minutes; failure to achieve adequate oxygenation should lead to a quick intubation decision.

As a guide, limit intubation attempts to the amount of time that a single deep breath can be held by the patient. This is especially important in a child because the functional residual capacity of a child's lungs is less than that of an adult. Historically, the maximum recommended duration of an intubation attempt in an apneic patient has been 30 seconds, followed by a period of BMV before intubation is attempted again. Longer attempts at intubation are permissible when guided by accurate data from an oxygen saturation monitor because oxygen saturation may remain in the normal range for much longer in patients who have been preoxygenated. As a general rule, intubation attempts may continue if oxygen saturation is above 90% and should be interrupted for BMV when oxygen saturation drops below 90%.

Assessment of tube location is the top priority immediately after placement. The best assurance of tracheal placement is to first see the tube pass through the vocal cords and then to observe waveform capnography.

Though seldom associated with serious complications, unrecognized placement of the tip of the ET tube in the right main stem bronchus may cause hypoxia, atelectasis, pneumothorax, and unilateral pulmonary edema.[191] This can be mitigated by performing ultrasound immediately after intubation to check for bilateral sliding. Obtain a chest radiograph soon after intubation to confirm tube positioning approximately 5 cm above the carina in adults. Mainstem bronchus intubation was clinically unrecognized without a chest film in 7% of prehospital intubations in one study.[192] Persistent asymmetric breath sounds after correct tube positioning suggest unilateral pulmonary pathology (e.g., main stem bronchus obstruction, pneumothorax, hemothorax).

Prolonged efforts to intubate can also cause cardiac decompensation. Pharyngeal stimulation can produce bradycardia, especially in children, and atropine can be given to avoid this response. Bradycardia can also be caused by hypoxia or hypotension and this should be immediately recognized and corrected. Hypotension requiring intervention in the periintubation period occurs in approximately 10% to 15% of intubations.[193] If a patient is profoundly hypovolemic and does not need immediate intubation, it may be best to resuscitate with intravenous fluids prior to intubation to avoid worsening hypotension.

Generally, dentures are removed for intubation and kept in place for BMV. Check for loose or missing teeth before and after orotracheal intubation. Look for any avulsed teeth not found in the oral cavity on the postintubation chest film. Dental injury occurs in approximately 0.5% of intubations.[60] Laceration of the mucosa of the lips, especially the lower lip, may occur. Tracheal or bronchial injuries are rare and serious, usually occurring in infants and the elderly as a result of decreased tissue elasticity.[194]

Emesis with aspiration of gastric contents is a serious complication that can occur during intubation. Case reports of adult respiratory distress syndrome and chronic lung disease are thought to be due to aspiration of activated charcoal.[194,195] In patients who are obtunded or who are at high risk for seizures or vomiting, consider tracheal intubation before the rare administration of activated charcoal.

There are ongoing concerns that laryngosocpy may cause or worsen spinal cord injury in a patient with an unstable cervical spine injury. These concerns are essentially theoretical, with no credible data to prove or disprove a true effect. Many anesthesiologists prefer awake endoscopic intubation in this setting, and no data support one approach over another. A cadaveric study of intubation during fluoroscopy showed that DL with in-line immobilization in the setting of complete C4–5 ligamentous instability did not result in clinically significant movement.[196] The greatest degree of motion occurs at the atlanto-occipital junction and decreases with each sequential interspace, and studies of cervical spine instability at these higher levels have not been performed.[197] It can also be argued that cadaveric studies do not accurately depict the trauma setting, and this model is likely to remain the best available. Unless new information emerges regarding the risks of orotracheal intubation with DL, it appears to be a safe approach when performed in conjunction with in-line immobilization. The cervical collar should be removed for intubation, and cervical immobilization held manually by an assistant.

Intubation can be complicated by a persistent air leak. This is generally caused by failure of either the cuff or the pilot balloon or by positioning the cuff balloon between the vocal cords. If the cuff balloon is leaking, replace the tracheal tube (see Changing Tracheal Tubes section below). If the pilot balloon is determined to be leaking, this can usually be remedied without changing the tube.[198] An incompetent one-way balloon valve can be fixed by placing a stopcock in the inflating valve. Reinflate the cuff and shut off the stopcock to solve the problem. If the leak involves the pilot balloon or if the distal inflation tube has been inadvertently severed, cut off the defective part and slide a 20-gauge catheter into the inflation tube. Then connect the stopcock to the catheter, inflate the cuff, and close the stopcock.

Tracheal stricture used to be a significant late complication of long-term intubation with low-volume, high-pressure cuffs. The use of high-volume, low-pressure cuffs has markedly decreased the incidence of this complication.[199] Tubes with high-pressure cuffs are obsolete and should be avoided.

Conclusion

DL remains a core skill for emergency clinicians, though it should generally be performed using a video laryngoscope. With adequate preparation and emphasis on preoxygenation and positioning, it is usually successful. Once the patient is paralyzed, it becomes the clinician's supreme responsibility to ventilate, oxygenate, and protect the patient's airway. Mastery of laryngoscopy fulfills part of this obligation. Being prepared for failure and having a successful backup plan fulfills the remainder of this responsibility. The remainder of this chapter is devoted to adjuncts and alternatives to DL.

VIDEO AND OPTICAL LARYNGOSCOPES

See Videos 4.12–4.20. Video and optical laryngoscopes have transformed airway management (Review Box 4.2). These devices all use video, fiberoptics, or mirrors to visualize the larynx. They provide a better view of the glottis with less effort, and higher success rates are achieved in a shorter amount of learning time compared with DL. Macintosh-shaped video laryngoscopes (less commonly straight-blade video laryngoscopes) are designed to sweep the tongue aside and allow either a direct or video view of the larynx. Other devices, known as hyperangulated video laryngoscopes, are more curved and are designed to look around the curve of the tongue rather than lifting it or pushing it aside. The drawback of more angulated devices is that getting an excellent view of the vocal cords does not always correlate with easy intubation[200,201] because it can be difficult to manipulate the ET tube around the sharp curve of the blade. Adding a tube channel to the blade obviates the need to manipulate the ET tube around the sharp curve and may add other complexities.[200] Video laryngoscopes were historically expensive but are becoming more affordable, so cost is no longer a reason for an ED not to stock video laryngoscopes. Video laryngoscopy is associated with higher first-pass success rates compared with DL, especially in patients with known or suspected difficult airways.[202,203] Some experts recommend that video laryngoscopy be used for all emergency intubations.[204]

Video and optical laryngoscopes can be divided into three broad categories:

1. Video laryngoscopes with standard Macintosh blades (Storz C-MAC, GlideScope Titanium MAC, McGrath MAC, Venner A.P. Advance Mac Blade, PatCen OneScope Direct Blades).
2. Video laryngoscopes with angulated blades (GlideScope, McGrath X blade, Storz D-Blade, PatCen OneScope Hyperangulated Blades).
3. Video or optical laryngoscopes with a tube channel (Airtraq, Pentax AWS, KingVISION). (See the following sections for pictures and manufacturers of each device.)

Video Laryngoscopes With Standard Macintosh Blades

These devices have blades that are exactly the same or very similar to a standard English or German Macintosh direct

Video and Optical Laryngoscopy

Indications

Routine emergency intubation
Teaching of direct laryngoscopy skills to novices
Difficult airways
Failed direct laryngoscopy
Morbid obesity
Trauma patients with cervical spine immobilization

Contraindications

Limited mouth opening
Severe kyphosis
Copious blood or secretions

Complications

Dental trauma
Oropharyngeal trauma

Equipment

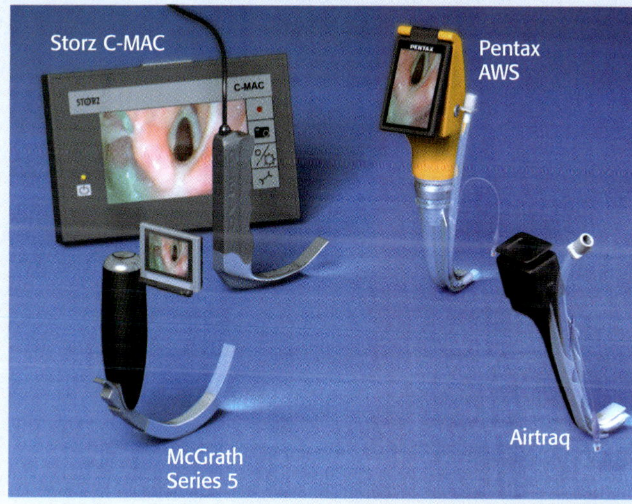

Ancillary equipment (endotracheal tubes, etc) not depicted

Review Box 4.2 Video laryngoscopy: indications, contraindications, complications, and equipment.

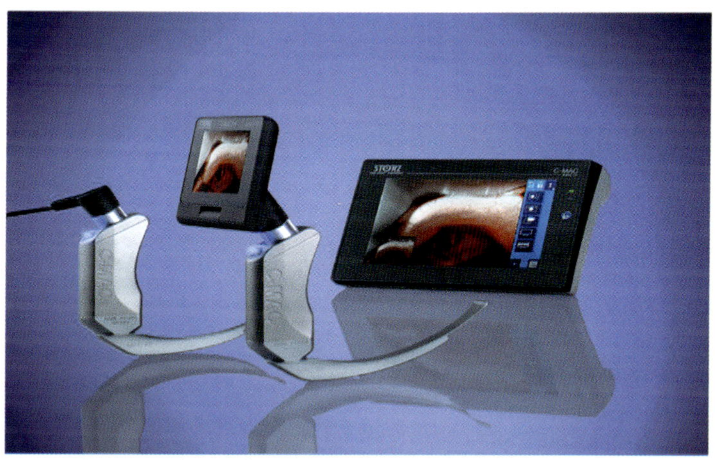

Fig. 4.24 The Karl Storz C-MAC video laryngoscope system.

laryngoscope. They all have a digital camera adjacent to the light source a few centimeters proximal to the tip. Each of these devices can be used for either conventional DL or video laryngoscopy. The Storz C-MAC (Karl Storz) is the only device in this group that has been sufficiently tested (Fig. 4.24).[96,205–212] The laryngeal view obtained on the video monitor is better than the direct view in essentially all patients.[206,207] The improved laryngeal view provided by the camera is especially helpful in patients with markedly elevated BMIs and in trauma patients who require cervical spine immobilization.[205,211]

Unlike other video laryngoscopy systems, those with Macintosh blades still allow direct visualization of airway structures even if blood or secretions obscure the camera view, or if there are any other camera malfunctions.[74] Though many cite blood or vomit as a reason to use DL rather than VL, multiple studies have shown that success with VL is higher than DL when body fluids are present in the mouth.[203,213] This is because the improved view is more important than the theoretical risk of the camera being obscured; this can be further mitigated by meticulous suctioning as the laryngoscope is inserted. The use of a video laryngoscopy system that still allows the ability to perform DL may be ideal for learning DL skills, as novices who learn intubation on a video laryngoscope system have higher success rates when performing DL.[93]

Background

The Storz Video Macintosh Laryngoscope was introduced into clinical practice by Kaplan et al. in 2002.[210] The latest version of this device, the Storz C-MAC, is smaller, more portable, and cheaper.[201] The C-MAC consists of a one-piece blade, a cable, and a monitor. It can record digital video or still images. This section will discuss the use of the Storz C-MAC because it is the most used and most tested video laryngoscopy system with a Macintosh blade. The procedure will be similar to other video laryngoscopy systems with a Macintosh blade. The GlideScope Titanium MAC (Verathon Medical), McGrath MAC (Fig. 4.25) and A.P. Advance Mac Blade

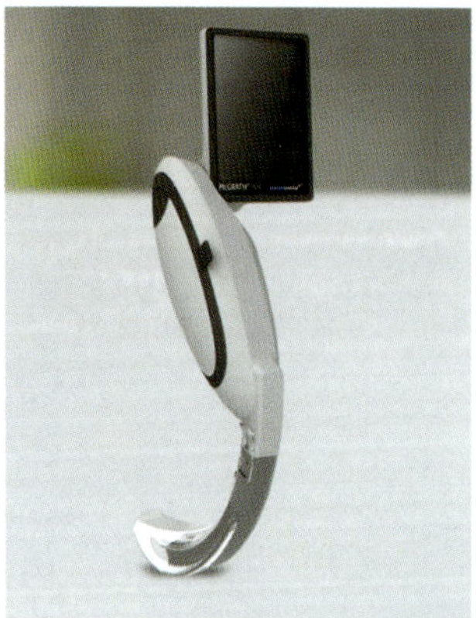

Fig. 4.25 The Medtronic McGrath MAC video laryngoscope.

(Venner Medical) function similarly and have different flange widths and light brightness.[214]

Indications

The C-MAC can be used for almost any orotracheal intubation attempt in an emergency setting. Since the C-MAC has the same shape as a traditional DL blade, the operator can intubate without looking at the screen (i.e., perform DL with a video laryngoscope). If intubation is difficult, the operator can view the screen without removing the blade. In a recent randomized trial of 1417 ED and ICU patients that showed video laryngoscopy to be vastly superior to DL, the Storz C-MAC with a Macintosh blade was the most commonly used device.[203]

The Storz C-MAC may be a good option for routine intubations at academic institutions that are teaching novice intubators. By viewing the video screen, the senior physician can teach laryngoscopy skills in real time while the learner performs DL. In 2008, Howard-Quijano and coauthors published a prospective, randomized, crossover study of 37 novice intubators (medical students and residents) who performed 222 intubations with the Storz Video Macintosh system.[96] The novice intubators performed only DL and were not allowed to see the video monitor in any case. Intubations were randomized so that either the instructors could see the video monitor or it was covered by a drape. Novice intubators were given 2 minutes to intubate before the instructor took over. When instructors were allowed to see the video monitor, the novice intubators had a 69% success rate and a 3% rate of esophageal intubation. When instructors were blinded to the video monitor, the novice intubators had a 55% success rate and a 17% rate of esophageal intubation.

Contraindications

Contraindications to the use of the C-MAC are rare. Like other video laryngoscopes, the lens on the video camera is susceptible to obscuration by secretions or blood. Unlike other video devices, the C-MAC facilitates direct visualization of anatomic structures.

Procedure

Much of the procedure for laryngoscopy with the C-MAC is similar to that for DL. When the tip of the Storz C-MAC is advanced into the vallecula, it gives an 80-degree-wide field of view and offers a panoramic view of the glottis. Moving slowly and using a progressive visualization technique to find the tongue, epiglottis, posterior cartilages, and vocal cords (as with DL) is the best approach to performing laryngoscopy with the C-MAC. A common novice error is to plunge the blade in too deep and then look for structures, rather than incrementally advancing down the tongue to find the epiglottis. The tip of the blade should be seated exactly between the tongue and epiglottis and should press against the median glossoepiglottic fold (Fig. 4.26), a midline structure easily visible with a video laryngoscope.[215]

Keep in mind that although the tip of the C-MAC is usually placed in the vallecula, it may help to directly lift the epiglottis with the tip of the blade if laryngoscopy is difficult; this is known as the *straight-blade technique*.[216]

Complications

A complication that may be encountered is blind passage of the ET tube into the mouth while fixating on the video monitor. This can result in damage to oral and pharyngeal structures.

Video Laryngoscopes With Angulated Blades

The GlideScope, McGrath X blade, and Storz D-Blade video laryngoscopes are similarly shaped devices that have sharply angulated, nonchanneled, and narrow-flanged blades.[200,201,217,218] All these devices have more extreme blade curvature with varying angulation of the blade tip with a digital camera a few centimeters proximal to the tip. These blades do not allow laryngoscopy by direct visualization. They are designed to follow the natural curvature of the upper airway and look around the tongue rather than displace it. Excellent visualization of the glottis is nearly always achieved when the distal tip of the blade is in or near the vallecula. Because the point of reference is from the location of the camera near the distal tip of these devices, they reliably provide a panoramic view of the larynx that cannot be achieved with DL. Use of these devices results in easy visualization of the larynx, even with inexperienced clinicians or difficult airway anatomy.[211,212,217,219–224] Maneuvering the ET tube around the severe angle of the blade and into the trachea is more difficult compared with systems with a Macintosh blade, creating problems.[200] In one large trial involving inexperienced GlideScope operators, the device was abandoned in 3.7% of intubations despite the fact that an excellent view of the glottis was achieved in most of these cases.[217]

Background

In 2001 the original GlideScope video laryngoscope became the first commercially available video laryngoscope. The first report of its use was in a case report of the management of a difficult airway.[225] GlideScope now offers reusable and single-use blades (Fig. 4.27). The GlideScope Titanium is the latest model. All GlideScope models have a lens antifog mechanism and digital recording capability. Though this section will discuss hyperangulated blades, current systems also offer blades with a Macintosh shape.

The McGrath portable video laryngoscope is another device with similar characteristics and is more compact. It became available in 2005, and the current model is called the McGrath X blade. The shape of the blade is very similar to that of the GlideScope, and it has a small video monitor (1.7 inches diagonally) on the end of the handle. It also has an adjustable-length, detachable metal blade (camera stick) that is covered by a disposable plastic blade during use, so no part of the handle or metal blade makes contact with the patient. It has no recording capability.

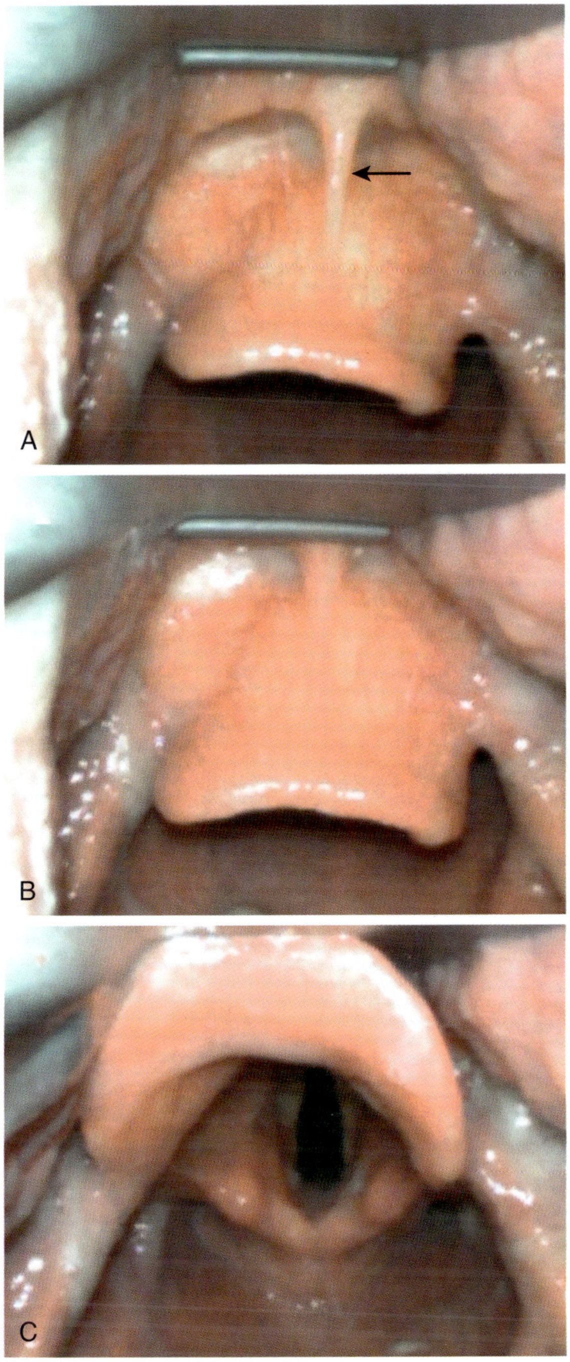

Fig. 4.26 (A) The intubator's view of the median glossoepiglottic fold (indicated by the *arrow*), a midline mucosal fold that connects the base of the tongue to the epiglottis, as the blade approaches the vallecula. (B) The blade begins to engage the fold, which helps indirectly lift the epiglottis. The intubator must place the tip of the blade deeply into the vallecula and ensure the tip is not too shallow (on the tongue) or too deep (on the epiglottis). (C) The laryngeal view after the epiglottis is lifted indirectly. (Courtesy Hennepin County Medical Center, Minneapolis, MN.)

The Storz D-Blade became available in 2010 and has a blade shape similar to that of the GlideScope. It is an optional blade for use with the Storz C-MAC system and has the same functionality as the other C-MAC blades and does not allow the option of direct visualization of the larynx. It was designed specifically for difficult intubations.

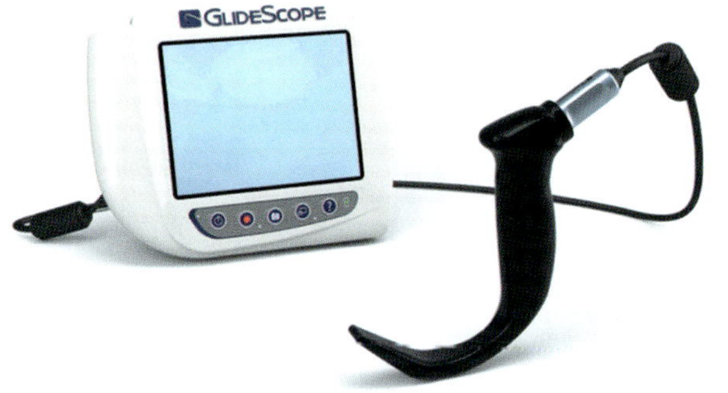

Fig. 4.27 The Verathon Medical GlideScope video laryngoscope system.

The GlideScope and its use are discussed as representative of this class of indirect video-assisted laryngoscopes with thin, sharply curved and unchanneled blades.

Indications

Like the C-MAC, video laryngoscopy systems with hyperangulated blades can also be used for routine intubations and have higher success rates than DL.[226,227] If DL fails, video laryngoscopy of either shape (Macintosh or hyperangulated) can be used.

A significant advantage of the more angulated video laryngoscopes compared with DL is that they can provide a good view of the larynx when the neck is in the neutral position. Not surprisingly, there are several small studies and case reports demonstrating that the GlideScope and McGrath provide good laryngoscopic views and a high rate of successful intubation in patients with cervical spine immobilization.[228–230] There is also a case report of a patient with severe ankylosing spondylitis who was easily intubated on the first attempt with the McGrath.[231] Whether hyperangulated video laryngoscopes are superior to Macintosh video laryngoscopes in this setting is not known. Macintosh-shaped video blades also perform very well in the setting of cervical immobilization.

There may be patients (estimated to be <1% of all intubations) in whom the larynx is so anterior that devices with a Macintosh blade are unable to adequately visualize the airway structures; hyperangulated blades may be especially useful in this situation.

Contraindications

Contraindications to using angulated video laryngoscopes are not well described in the literature. As with any video or optical device, blood or secretions on the lens may decrease visualization of the larynx. Fogging was a problem with older endoscopic devices, and this problem is rare with the newer video devices. Limited mouth opening (<2 cm) can make insertion of these devices more challenging, though they require less mouth opening than devices with Macintosh blades.[200] The biggest contraindication is lack of experience or absence of a rigid stylet or tracheal tube introducer to allow the operator to maneuver the ET tube around the sharp angle of the blade.[200]

Procedure and Technique

Grasp the video laryngoscope in the left hand and place it in the patient's mouth with the scissor technique. Under direct vision, not by viewing the screen, advance the blade through the oropharynx along the midline of the tongue (Fig. 4.28, *step 4*). Then look up at the monitor while continuing to advance

Video Laryngoscopy With a Hyperangulated Laryngoscope

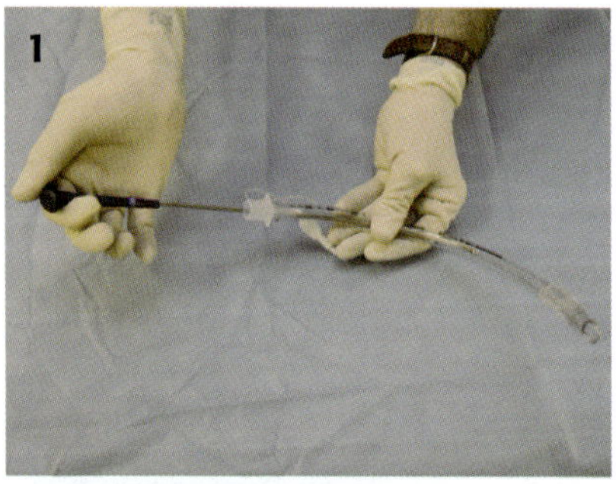

Prepare the endotracheal tube.

Depending on the system that you are using, insert a rigid stylet or preload the tube onto the device.

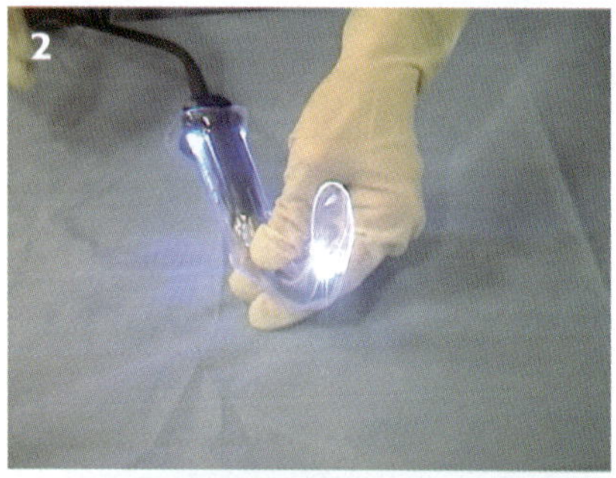

Check the rest of your equipment, including the light source and video monitor.

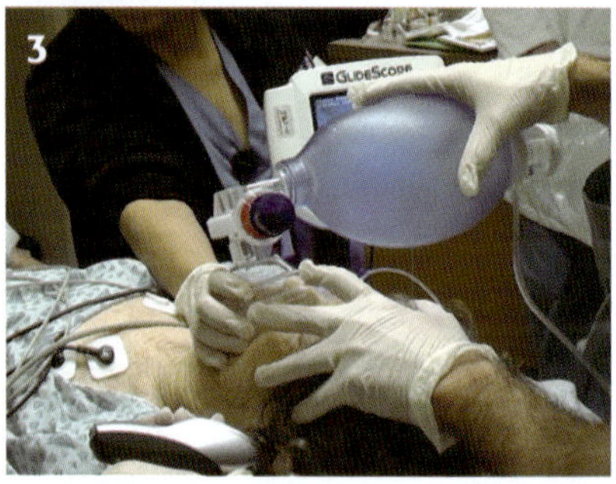

Preoxygenate and premedicate the patient as clinically indicated.

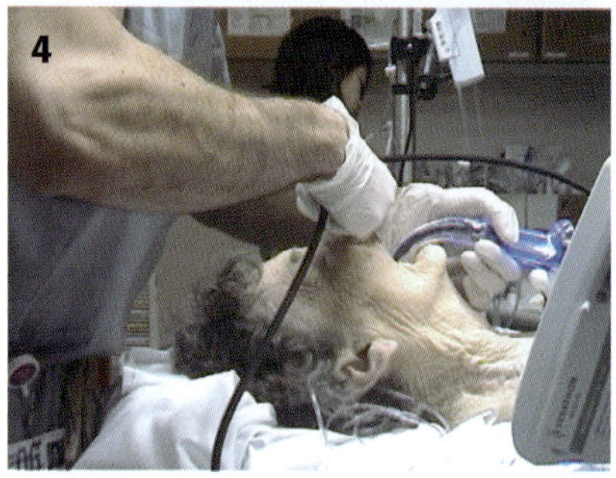

Place the blade into the mouth under direct visualization (don't look at the video monitor yet).

Keep the blade in the midline of the tongue throughout the procedure.

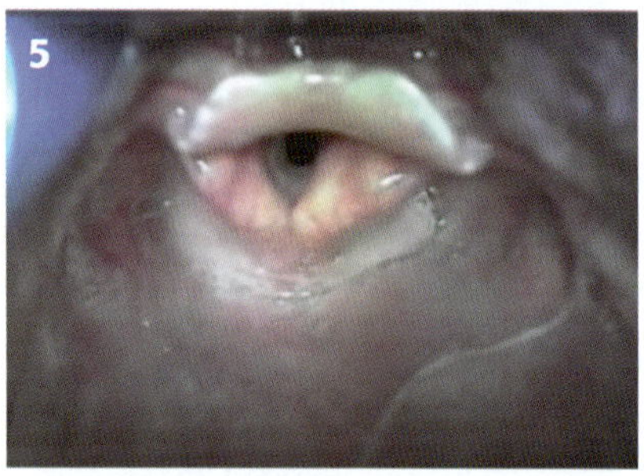

Slowly advance the blade, identifying the tongue and epiglottis.

Place the blade tip in or just proximal to the vallecula, and gently lift to obtain a panoramic view. A slightly restricted view eases tube passage.

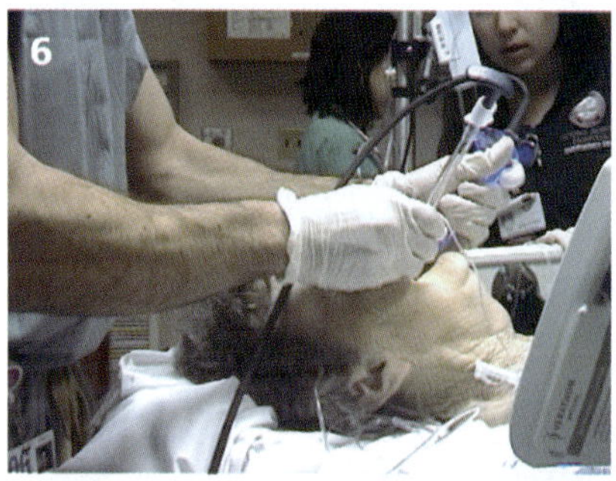

Under direct visualization (don't look at the monitor), pass the styleted tube through the mouth and into the posterior pharynx.

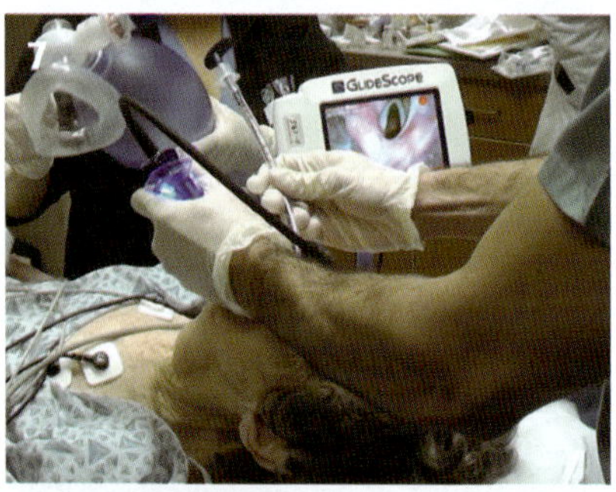

Look up at the video monitor and watch for the tip of the tube to appear.

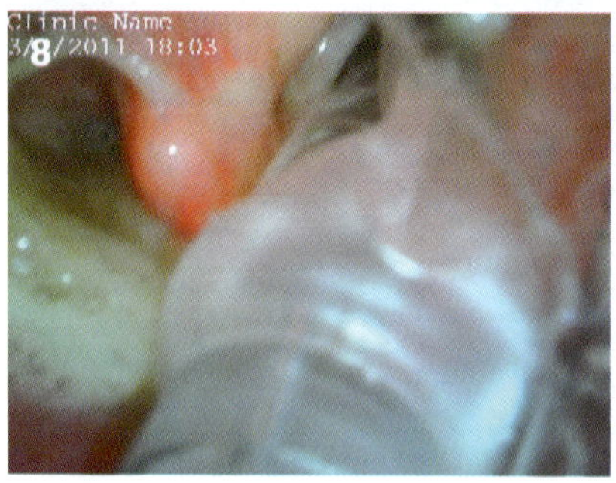

Direct the tube through the vocal cords under direct visualization on the video monitor.

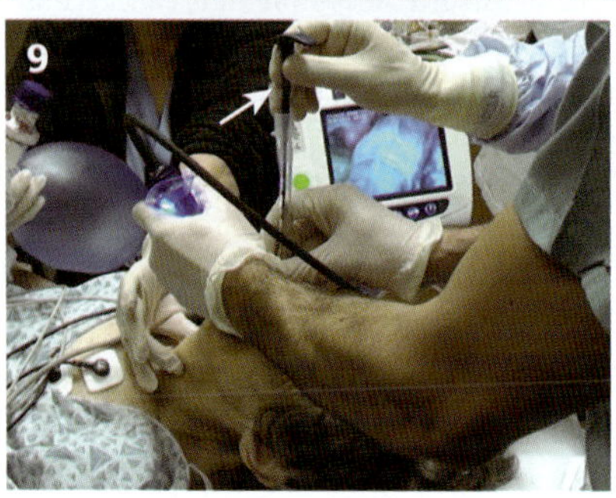

While the operator firmly secures the endotracheal tube, an assistant removes the stylet as the tube is passed through the vocal cords.

NOTE: This image sequence depicts video laryngoscopy using the GlideScope. The procedure sequence may vary with the use of other devices. Refer to text for additional information.

Be familiar with the equipment used at your institution prior to use.

Fig. 4.28 Video laryngoscopy with a hyperangulated video laryngoscope. Note that there are times when the operator *does not look at the screen* but rather uses direct vision (steps 4 and 6).

the blade down the midline of the tongue, progressively identifying the base of the tongue and the epiglottis. With a gentle lifting motion, place the tip of the blade in the vallecula or just before the vallecula. Elevate the epiglottis and expose the laryngeal inlet (see Fig. 4.28, *step 5*). The goal is not the best view. If you get the tip of the blade too close to the vocal cords, it may be difficult or impossible to pass the tube. The key to using hyperangulated laryngoscopes is to keep the tip of the blade back as far as possible, to obtain a panoramic/distant view of the vocal cords and surrounding structures. This approach allows easier tube placement and a higher first-pass success rate.[232] If the glottis is not well visualized, tilt the handle back slightly to enhance exposure. If needed, manipulate the neck externally to enhance visualization. If more exposure is required, place the tip of the blade under the epiglottis and gently lift and tilt back. Use a rigid steel GlideRite stylet, which has the same curve as the blade of the GlideScope, McGrath, and D-Blade. Alternatively, a malleable stylet with an aggressive distal bend or a similarly bent bougie may be acceptable, and these devices may fail if tube passage is challenging. Pass the ET tube through the oropharynx under direct vision until it passes under the curve of the blade, and then look for it on the monitor (see Fig. 4.28, *step 6*). Decrease the chance of soft tissue injury by carefully passing the ET tube along the side of the laryngoscope.[233] When the tip of the ET tube comes into view, direct it into the glottis and advance it to the appropriate depth (see Fig. 4.28, *step 8*). If a malleable stylet or bougie is used, it may be difficult to get the tube to go anterior enough. If a malleable stylet must be used, try introducing the tube from the right side of the patient and rotating it 90 degrees and vertically into a midline position behind the tongue. This will help the tip of the stylet maintain its shape as it passes through the oropharynx. Another option is to use a Parker Flex-It (Parker Medical) intubation stylet to direct the tip of the ET tube anteriorly.[217] The fixed steel (GlideRite) stylet should be withdrawn as the ET tube is passed through the vocal cords because the tip of the stylet will be essentially pointing toward the ceiling as it approaches the laryngeal inlet (see Fig. 4.28, *step 9*). The large knob on the proximal end of the GlideRite stylet is designed to be pushed up by the tip of the intubator's thumb, thus making ET tube advancement and stylet withdrawal a one-handed procedure.

Complications

Several relatively minor complications have been reported with use of the GlideScope. There are case reports of injury to the soft palate and tonsillar pillars, and two cases of puncture of the right palatopharyngeal arch, one requiring surgical repair.[233–235]

Summary

Video-assisted laryngoscopy is a major advancement in visualization of the laryngeal inlet. Macintosh video laryngoscopes achieve high success in the vast majority of patients undergoing emergency intubation while allowing for maintenance of DL skills. Given the challenges of tube delivery and the inability to perform DL, the role of hyperangulated blades in routine airway management is limited—though they are invaluable devices if intubation is not possible with a Macintosh-shaped video laryngoscope (<5% of intubation). The majority of intubation failures with a hyperangulated blade are due to an inability to pass the tube through the larynx despite excellent glottic views, even with use of a steel stylet.[200,217] Advancements need to be made in achieving tracheal intubation once the glottis is seen. The addition of a tube channel obviates the need to maneuver the ET tube around the sharp angle of the blade; channeled devices are described in the next section.

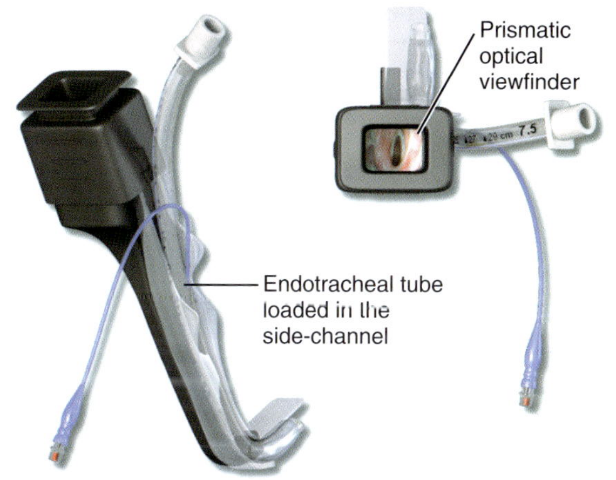

Fig. 4.29 Airtraq intubation device. The device pictured uses prisms and mirrors so that the larynx can be visualized via the eyepiece. A newer model features a video system with video out capability.

Video and Optical Laryngoscopes With a Tube Channel

Some devices allow indirect video or optical visualization of the larynx, providing a channeled blade to guide the ET tube through the vocal cords. They include the Airtraq (Fig. 4.29) (Prodol Meditec), the King Vision aBlade (Ambu), and Venner A.P. Advance Difficult Airway Blade (DAB) (Venner Medical). The ET tube is inserted into the channel before the device is placed in the airway, and the channel guides the ET tube into the trachea once the glottis is visualized. This design helps alleviate the most common problem associated with video and optical laryngoscopy: difficulty placing the ET tube despite an excellent view of the glottis.

All the channel-guided devices have the same curvature as the normal upper airway. They allow visualization of the glottis by looking around the tongue instead of trying to straighten the airway and push the tongue out of the way. They consistently provide a better view of the glottis and may lead to less airway trauma and hemodynamic stimulation compared with DL.[236–238] The concept of a laryngoscope shaped like the natural curvature of the upper airway and containing a channel to guide the ET tube is not new, and the addition of optics and video make this concept a reality.[238–241] The advantage of these devices is that they provide an excellent view of the glottis with little need for maneuvering, and they eliminate the requirement for the hand-eye coordination needed to pass the ET tube around an acute curve.[242–244]

Indications

Difficult intubation with DL is an indication for using a channel-guided optical or video device. They can also be used for routine intubation. The Airtraq and Pentax AWS have a high rate of success in patients with known or predicted difficult airways.[221,236,237] In 2009 a study by Asai and colleagues reported 270 patients with difficult airways by DL (grade III and IV views) and found that 268 of these patients (99.3%)

had good glottic visualization and were easily intubated with the Pentax AWS.[237] In a 2009 trial of patients with expected difficult airways, Malik and coworkers randomized 75 patients to DL, the Pentax AWS, or the GlideScope.[221] The rate of successful intubation was 84% with DL, 96% with the GlideScope, and 100% with the Pentax AWS.

These blades are particularly useful for difficult airways complicated by cervical spine immobilization and high BMI.[245–248] In 2007, Ndolo and coauthors published a study of 106 patients with markedly elevated BMIs who were randomized to intubation with DL or the Airtraq.[249] All patients randomized to the Airtraq were successfully intubated, and six patients in the DL group required rescue intubation with the Airtraq. In 2007, Maharaj published a study of 40 patients with cervical spine immobilization who were randomized to DL or the Airtraq.[247] All patients randomized to the Airtraq group were intubated on the first attempt and were intubated faster and with less difficulty than the DL group.

In 2008, Enomoto and associates studied 203 patients with manual in-line neck stabilization who required intubation.[246] They randomized these patients to intubation with DL or the Pentax AWS. The intubation success rate with DL was 89% versus 100% with the Pentax AWS. A similar study by Liu and coworkers in 2009 included 70 patients with manual in-line stabilization of the cervical spine and randomized them to intubation with the Pentax AWS or the GlideScope.[219] They reported a 100% rate of successful intubation with the Pentax AWS and 89% with the GlideScope. In addition, two studies used fluoroscopy to compare cervical spine motion during intubation with DL versus intubation with the Pentax AWS.[250,251] Both studies found that intubation with the Pentax AWS caused less movement of the upper cervical spine than DL.

The Airtraq is generally used during RSI and may also be used for awake intubation of patients with difficult airways.[252,253] When compared with DL, both the Airtraq and Pentax AWS consistently provide better visualization of the glottis and have a higher rate of successful intubation.[221,236,237,240,246] Two small studies and one large trial have shown that the Airtraq has a very high rate of success after failed DL.[4,236,240] In 2011 Amathieu and coauthors reported the results of a large prospective trial in which they used an algorithm that specified the use of the Airtraq as a backup for all cases of failed RSI with DL.[4] They had 28 patients who could not be intubated with DL after multiple attempts, including the use of a bougie. Intubation with the Airtraq was successful in 27 of 28 of these patients (97%), and the other patient was intubated with an ILMA.[4]

Contraindications

The greatest drawback of channeled video and optical devices is that copious amounts of blood or secretions can obscure the view. Because they do not allow a direct line of sight to the larynx, visualization and intubation are dependent on the video or optical image. If blood or fluid covers the tip of the lens, the image is obscured. This problem can be minimized by aggressively suctioning the hypopharynx before placing the device in the mouth.

Inability to open the mouth or severely limited mouth opening is a contraindication to using the channel-guided devices just described. If the patient's mouth opening is at least 2 cm, these devices can succeed in cases in which DL would be impossible. The normal adult-size Airtraq requires 18 mm of mouth opening, and the pediatric and infant sizes require 12.5 mm. The Pentax AWS requires approximately 20 mm of mouth opening.

Procedure

Before beginning the procedure check that you are using the correct size device, ensure that it is functioning properly, and choose the correct size ET tube for the device and the patient. Insert the ET tube into the channel of the device and advance it to the end of the channel while ensuring it is not advanced so far that it obscures the video or optical lens. Insert the tip of the blade into the mouth vertically so that the handle of the device is pointed toward the patient's feet. Rotate it into the pharynx and hypopharynx along the midline of the tongue until the tip is in the vallecula. If the glottis is not visualized immediately, try backing the blade out 1 to 2 cm and lift the device gently in the direction of the handle (toward the ceiling). A common mistake is to insert the blade too deep initially, which offers a narrower view of the glottis and may make intubation difficult. When the vocal cords are well visualized in the center of the video or optical image, advance the ET tube through the cords by sliding it forward within the channel. If the ET tube does not go through the cords, pull it back and realize that you need to adjust the position of the entire device to change the trajectory of the tube. If the tube tends to go posterior to the vocal cords, lift the device toward the ceiling and tip the handle back slightly (while avoiding contact with the upper teeth), and then advance the tube again. Alternatively, pass a bougie through the ET tube (or in the channel without an ET tube) and direct the curved tip up and through the vocal cords.

When using the Pentax AWS, it is important to know that the ET tube leaves the channel in line with the tip of the blade (more anterior than the Airtraq). Therefore when the tip of the AWS blade is in the vallecula, the tube often strikes the epiglottis when it is advanced. To avoid this problem, advance the tip of the AWS blade posterior to the epiglottis (as with straight-blade laryngoscopy) and lift the epiglottis out of the way before advancing the ET tube.

Dhonneur, Ndoko, and colleagues described alternative techniques for insertion of the Airtraq in patients with markedly elevated BMIs.[248,249] They rotate the device 90 to 180 degrees for initial insertion of the distal tip into the patient's mouth and then rotate it into the normal orientation (handle toward the patient's feet) before advancing it into the hypopharynx. This helps alleviate problems with the handle of the device striking the patient's chest during insertion.

Management After Intubation

A common mistake when using laryngoscopes with a tube channel is to quickly remove the laryngoscope after the ET tube is advanced into the trachea. Because the ET tube is already inside the trachea, it is best to attach a resuscitation bag and ventilate the patient. After giving several breaths, stabilizing oxygenation, and confirming tracheal placement with capnography, slowly and carefully remove the device while providing ongoing ventilation. It is appropriate to leave the laryngoscope in place for a few minutes after intubation to allow visual reconfirmation of proper tracheal placement, particularly if there is a problem with ventilation or oxygenation immediately following intubation. To remove the tube from the channel of these devices, hold the end of the ET tube firmly in the right hand and carefully wiggle the device to the left. When the tube slides out of the channel, slowly rotate the laryngoscope out of the patient's mouth. Reconfirm tracheal placement with capnography and adjust the depth of the ET tube as needed.

Complications

Because the blades of these devices are rigid and cannot be directly visualized after entering the mouth, they have potential for soft tissue damage. Complications of other video laryngoscopes are primarily a result of blind ET tube placement through the mouth and pharynx, and the tube channel devices eliminate this problem.

Intubating Laryngeal Mask Airways

ILMAs are unique devices because they are easy to insert, provide excellent ventilation and oxygenation (better than BMV), and also provide a reliable means of tracheal intubation (Review Box 4.3).[68,254–257] Many clinicians who have used the ILMA Fastrach in an emergency setting insist on having this device in their difficult airway tool kit.[2,66,70,256,258,259] It is impossible to overstate the value of this device for failed emergency RSI, and unlike other rescue devices, a large volume of data support its use in general and in the setting of failed RSI.[2,66,69–71,259–264] It has become the primary rescue device for failed RSI in many EDs.

There are many different LMAs and other EGDs on the market, and this can cause confusion. Although several EGDs (see Chapter 3) can be used for rescue ventilation or oxygenation, only the devices discussed here can also provide a reliable means of tracheal intubation. The Fastrach is the only device in this group that has been extensively tested and the only ILMA that can reliably facilitate blind intubation (without endoscopic guidance).[2,66,68,255–257,265–268]

Types of ILMAs

There are many popular ILMAs currently available (see Fig. 3.15). The LMA Fastrach (Teleflex) has been the most used and most studied ILMA. It has excellent blind intubation rates, much higher than the Air-Q (Cook Gas LLC)[265,266] or iGel (Intersurgical),[268,269] and there are numerous investigations detailing its success as a rescue device in difficult and failed airways. A unique feature of the Fastrach is the metal handle that makes insertion easier and enables lifting of the device to create a better seal against the glottis. There are also newer ILMA devices that show promise: the Air-Q, iGel, and AuraGain. Whereas the smallest Fastrach is size 3 (for children 30 to 50 kg), the other ILMAs are available in all sizes, including neonates less than 5 kg. The LMA Protector (Teleflex) is a recently released ILMA similar to the LMA Supreme and allows intubation using a flexible endoscope.

An important feature of newer ILMAs is gastric access channels, allowing placement of an orogastric tube through the gastric port and into the stomach with the ILMA in place. This is particularly useful in patients with distended stomachs after prolonged BMV, and in children who are more prone to gastric insufflation even with shorter BMV times. The Air-Q is available in several versions, one of which has a gastric port (Air-Q Blocker). The iGel and AuraGain both have gastric ports. The LMA Fastrach does not have gastric access.

Indications

ILMAs are indicated as an alternative to BMV or as a conduit for intubation of difficult airways.[261] In the cannot-intubate/cannot-ventilate scenario, it is a reliable rescue device. In this situation, adequate ventilation with the ILMA is possible in nearly all cases.[2,4,135,264] The ILMA is more successful for ventilation and intubation of difficult airways than the LMA Classic.[135] For inexperienced clinicians, ventilation with the ILMA is usually superior to face mask ventilation.[270]

The ILMA can also be used as a primary ventilation and intubation device in patients with difficult airways.[261] Studies of difficult airway management with the ILMA show that almost all patients can be adequately ventilated with the ILMA and 94% to 99% can be intubated through the dev ice.[2,66,68,70,135,255–257,261,264,271,272] Patients who are difficult to intubate by DL are often easy to intubate with the ILMA because many anatomic factors that cause difficult DL do not affect placement or function of the LMA Fastrach.[68,69]

The LMA Fastrach is especially useful in patients with difficult face mask ventilation because of a beard, severe facial

Intubating Laryngeal Mask Airway

Indications

Failed rapid-sequence intubation
Cannot-intubate/cannot-ventilate scenario
Difficult mask ventilation
Expected difficult intubation
Refractory hypoxemia despite preoxygenation

Contraindications

Unable to open mouth
Awake patient

Complications

Laryngeal or esophageal injury from blind intubation
Aspiration (rare)

Equipment

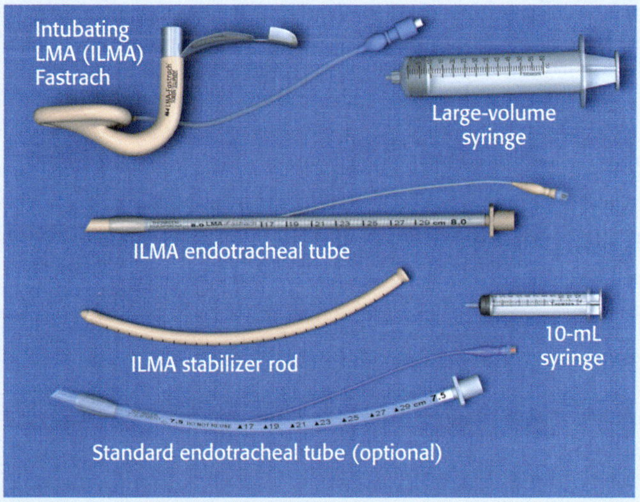

Review Box 4.3 Intubating laryngeal mask airway.

trauma, or obesity because none of these factors inhibit Fastrach placement. When brisk bleeding above the glottis makes ventilation and intubation difficult, the Fastrach can prevent aspiration of blood and facilitate blind or endoscopic intubation. In patients requiring urgent cricothyrotomy or percutaneous needle insertion into the trachea, the ILMA can be used to counteract anterior neck pressure. In this capacity, the Fastrach provides temporary ventilation and aids in stabilization of the cervical spine during the surgical airway procedure.

Contraindications

One limitation of the LMA Fastrach is that it cannot be used in infants and small children because the smallest size, a No. 3, is not suitable for patients smaller than 30 kg. Other ILMAs (or non-ILMAs) should be used in patients less than 30 kg. Other ILMAs require flexible endoscopic guidance for reliable tracheal intubation.

LMAs are contraindicated in patients with less than 2 cm of mouth opening. They are also relatively contraindicated in awake patients because of the high risk for emesis when the gag and airway reflexes are intact.

ILMAs can be successfully used in the setting of supraglottic swelling or anatomic distortion,[264,273] despite some assertions to the contrary.

Intubation Through the LMA Fastrach

The majority of intubations through the ILMA are performed blindly by using either the designated LMA ET tube or a standard ET tube. Regardless of the tube used, it is critical that the ILMA be optimally adjusted before attempting blind or flexible endoscopic intubation through the device.

The LMA ET tube, also known as the LMA Fastrach, is designed specifically for the ILMA. There are two versions of the LMA ET tube: a reusable and a single-use disposable. The reusable version is made of silicone and the single-use version is made of polyvinyl chloride (PVC). The specialized LMA ET tubes are soft and straight and have a midline-beveled tip. These features are designed to allow the LMA ET tubes to emerge from the ILMA mask at an acute angle and to minimize potential injury to the vocal cords and esophagus. The drawback of the specialized Fastrach ET tubes is that they have low-volume high-pressure cuffs, that could potentially cause ischemic damage to the trachea, and there are no clinical data on how long these tubes can remain in place.[274] Use of a standard ET tube for intubation through the LMA Fastrach has been well studied and is the current practice in many EDs.[264,275–277] Another option is to use a Parker Flex-Tip ET tube (Parker Medical) (see Fig. 4.9).[278]

Procedure and Technique for Blind Intubation

The LMA Fastrach is the only device that enables reliable tracheal intubation without the use of a flexible endoscope. If another ILMA is used, tracheal intubation has much lower success rates and, in general, blind intubation should not be attempted.

Before intubation through the LMA Fastrach, make sure that the patient is ventilating optimally through the device. Determine this by manually ventilating the patient while holding the ILMA handle with a "frying-pan" grip. If any resistance is felt, adjust the handle by slight rotation in the sagittal plane and then lift the entire device toward the ceiling (see the "Chandy maneuver," Fig. 4.30, *step 3*).

Before inserting the ET tube, lubricate it generously. Advance the ET tube with the curve opposite that of the LMA Fastrach curve (Fig. 4.30, *step 5*). When the tube has advanced to 15 cm, the tip will start to emerge from the LMA Fastrach mask. Just before advancing the tube, use the frying-pan grip and apply a slight anterior lift (not a tilt) to further align the aperture of the ILMA with the glottis (see second part of the Chandy maneuver, Fig. 4.30, *step 6*). Do not use a levering action. While holding the handle in this position, gently pass the tracheal tube to approximately 16.5 cm. In this position, the ET tube will push the epiglottic elevating bar up and may now come in contact with the larynx or esophagus. If cricoid pressure is being applied, decrease it because it may interfere with the passage of the ET tube through the glottis. If no resistance is encountered, advance the tube into the trachea until the tracheal tube adapter comes in contact with the proximal end of the ILMA tube (see Fig. 4.30, *step 7*). Do not use force when advancing the tube.

If the ET tube does not pass into the trachea easily, withdraw the ET tube to the 15-cm mark and readjust the position of the LMA Fastrach. If the tube meets resistance at approximately 17 cm, this may indicate a fully down-folded epiglottis or impaction of the tip of the tube against the anterior laryngeal wall. Rotating the tube may overcome impaction of the tip. To correct a down-folded epiglottis, remove the ET tube and perform the "up-down maneuver" by rotating the ILMA outward 5 to 6 cm without deflating the mask and then sliding it back into the hypopharynx (see Fig. 3.16, steps 9 and 10). If these maneuvers are unsuccessful, it is possible that the wrong size LMA Fastrach is being used. Additionally, blind intubation success varies between 80% and 100%, depending on the patient population and operator experience.[68,71,264,266,279–282] Consider using a flexible endoscope to guide intubation.

Once the LMA ET tube has passed into the trachea, inflate the tube cuff and attempt to ventilate the patient. Check for proper tube placement with an end-tidal CO_2. If the tube is in the trachea, deflate the cuff of the ILMA. There is no rush to remove the ILMA; it can remain in place for an hour or longer if more pressing patient care issues need to be addressed first.

Using a Standard Endotracheal Tube

Use of a standard ET tube is not recommended by the manufacturer, but it is a well-studied, common practice.[276,283,284] The manufacturer warns that using a standard ET tube may be associated with a greater likelihood of laryngeal trauma, and there are no known reports of such trauma in the literature, though there is a report of significant trauma with blind intubation through the LMA Fastrach causing esophageal perforation and subsequent death with use of the specialized LMA ET tube.[285] A laboratory study showed that a standard PVC ET tube exerts 7 to 10 times more pressure on distal structures than the silicone LMA ET tube, and the clinical relevance of this finding is unknown.[275,286] Some experts suggest warming the tip of a standard PVC ET tube (to soften it) before insertion through the LMA Fastrach.[276,283]

Because of the potential for injury with blind intubation through the ILMA, use endoscopic guidance if there is any difficulty. If using a standard ET tube, insert the ET tube with its curvature opposite the curvature of the LMA Fastrach tube (see Fig. 4.30, *step 5*). This allows the ET tube to exit the Fastrach at a less acute angle and facilitates advancement into the trachea.[262,283]

If intubation through the LMA Fastrach fails, the device can still be used to provide ventilation and oxygenation during

Endotracheal Intubation With the ILMA (Fastrach)

1

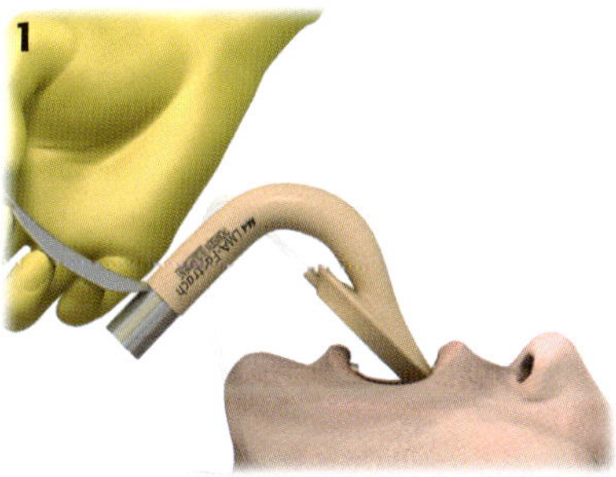

Insert the ILMA by sliding the posterior surface of the mask along the palate and posterior pharynx until firm resistance is felt (see Chapter 3).

2

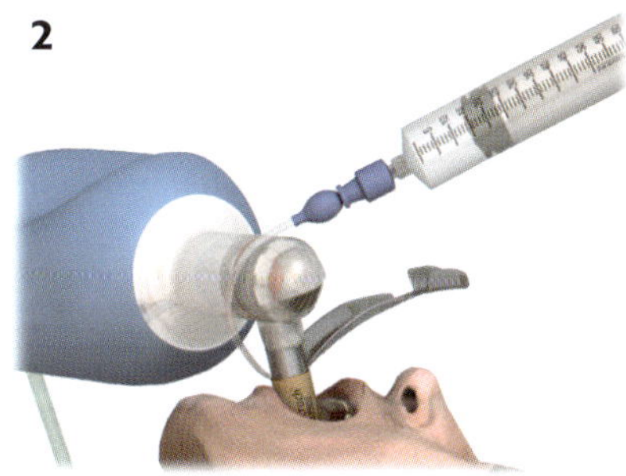

Inflate the ILMA cuff and begin ventilations through the device as you prepare for intubation.

3

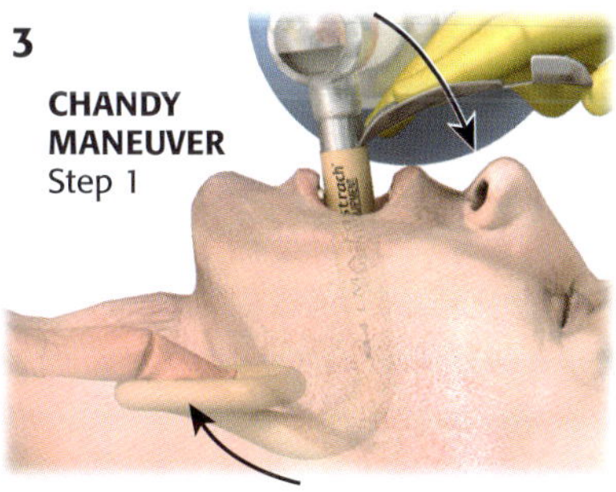

Rotate handle in the sagittal plane to move the cuff forward against the larynx.

This maneuver provides a good seal and optimal ventilations.

4

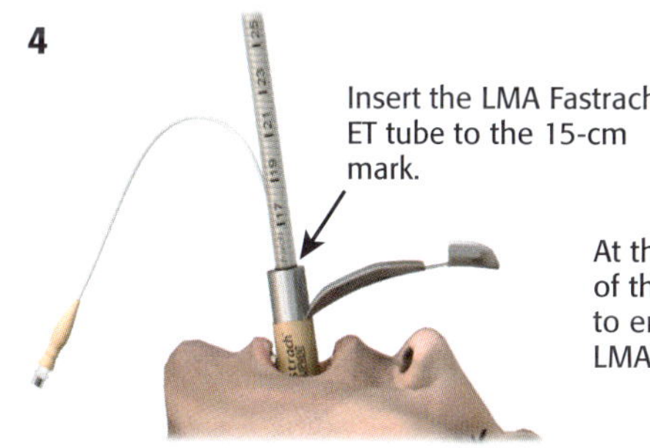

At this point, the tip of the tube will begin to emerge from the LMA.

5

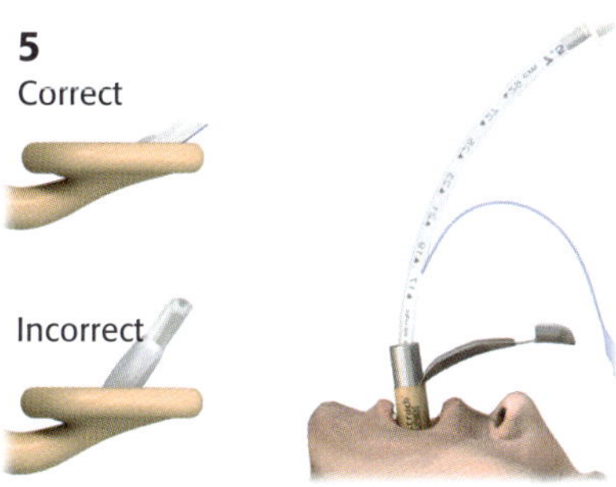

If using a standard ET tube, align the curve so that it is opposite of the LMA curve.

This allows the tube to exit the mask at an angle more conducive to tracheal entry.

6

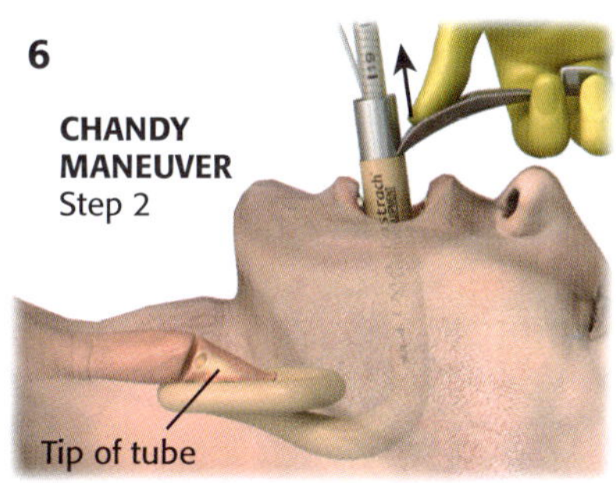

Prior to passing the tracheal tube, lift the handle anteriorly (not tilted) to better align the cuff and larynx for smooth ET tube passage.

7

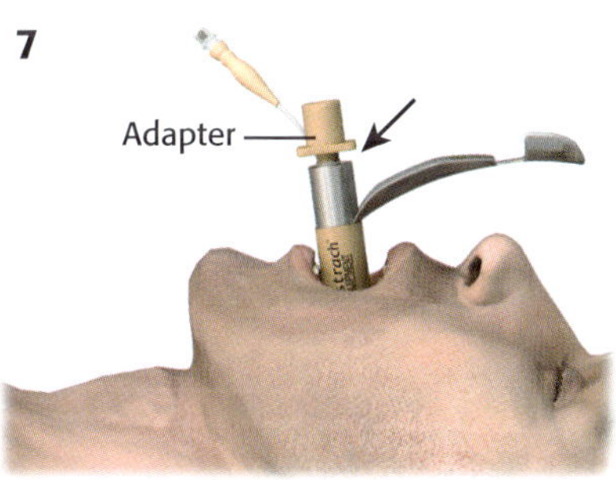

If no resistance is felt, advance the tube into the trachea until the adapter comes into contact with the ILMA airway tube.

Do not use force.

8

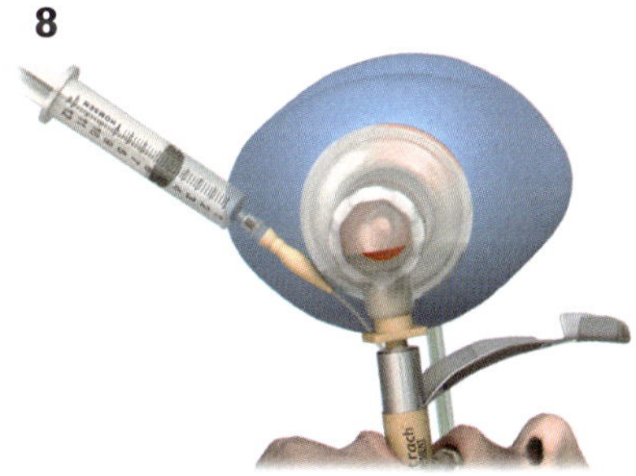

Inflate the ET tube cuff, ventilate, and check tube position with P_{ETCO_2}.

If the tube is properly positioned, deflate the LMA cuff.

9

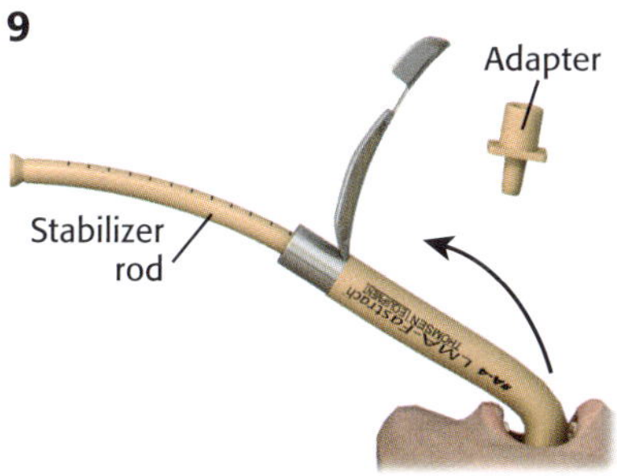

To remove the LMA, deflate the LMA cuff and remove the adapter from the tube.

Rotate the LMA out of the mouth while using the stabilizer rod to keep the tube in place.

10

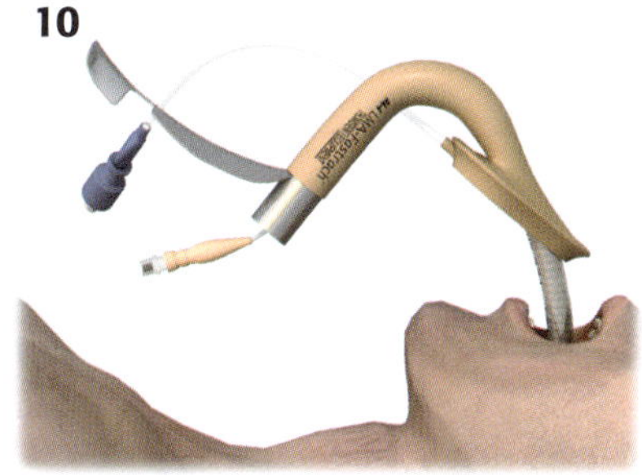

Remove the stabilizing rod when the mask is clear of the mouth, and complete removal of the LMA.

Reattach the adapter and resume ventilation.

Fig. 4.30 Endotracheal *(ET)* intubation with the intubating laryngeal mask airway *(ILMA)* (Fastrach; Teleflex).

more invasive airway procedures, such as retrograde intubation or cricothryotomy.[287]

Flexible Endoscopic Intubation Through ILMAs

A flexible bronchoscope can be used to verify the position of the larynx either before or during intubation. When intubating through the ILMA over an endoscope, a standard ET tube is sufficient and there is no reason to use the specialized LMA ET tube.

To use a flexible endoscope to intubate through the LMA Fastrach, first advance the ET tube through the ILMA Fastrach to 15 cm. At a 15-cm depth, the view through the endoscope should show the glottis beyond the epiglottic elevating bar. Advance the ET tube 1.5 cm before advancing the endoscope. This protects the camera elements from being damaged by the epiglottic elevating bar. The view at 16.5 cm should show the vocal cords and trachea. Advance the endoscope into the trachea and then pass the ET tube over the endoscope. If the vocal cords are not visualized immediately, check the tube depth and ensure it is not too deeply advanced.

An endoscope should be used to performing tracheal intubation through ILMAs other than the LMA Fastrach. Blind intubation may be possible but success is lower and is not recommended.[288–290] Using a tracheal tube introducer as a guide through an LMA is unlikely to be successful and is not recommended.[291,292] To use a flexible endoscope to intubate through other LMAs, the procedure is similar. First, place the ET tube approximately halfway to the opening in the laryngeal mask bowl. At this point, it may be useful to connect a swivel adapter to the ET tube adapter (Fig. 4.31) that will allow ongoing ventilation with the ability to place the flexible endoscope through the other port. If this step is performed, the cuff of the ET tube should be inflated during endoscopic intubation to minimize the air leak during ventilation. After the ET tube is placed halfway to the opening of the laryngeal mask bowl, the endoscope is introduced into the ET tube and advanced until the laryngeal inlet is visualized. Advance the endoscope into the trachea and then pass the ET tube over the endoscope. If the laryngeal inlet is not immediately visualized, the laryngeal mask should be repositioned before attempting intubation.

For children, the most common flexible bronchoscope has an outer diameter of 3.6 to 3.8 mm, which enables intubation of a 4.5 ET tube or larger. This allows intubation through an ILMA for children as small as 2 to 3 years old. Children younger than this should not be intubated through an ILMA, unless a smaller endoscope is used.

ILMA Removal After Intubation

To remove the ILMA, first deflate the cuff, if present (see Fig. 4.30, *step 8*), and be careful not to deflate the ET tube cuff. Start by removing the ET tube adapter. Then hold the proximal end of the ET tube in place while rotating the ILMA out of the hypopharynx. As the ILMA passes over the ET tube and out of the mouth, hold the ET tube in place with a stabilizer rod (see Fig. 4.30, *step 9*), without advancing the tube farther. If a stabilizer rod is not available, a second ET tube can also be used to aid in ILMA removal.[293] Some clinicians even prefer a second ET tube to the stabilizer rod because of its length. When the ET tube pilot balloon comes in contact with the stabilizer rod, remove the stabilizer rod to allow the pilot balloon to travel through the ILMA tube. Then reattach the ET adapter and resume ventilation. Adjust the depth of the ET tube as needed.

If the intubating clinician has never removed an ILMA after intubation, it is reasonable to leave the ILMA in place for a more experienced clinician to remove. The ILMA can be left in place for at least several hours with the cuffs deflated, and it can be left in place during interhospital transfer.

Complications When Intubating Through LMAs

Although most patients can be safely intubated blindly through the ILMA, there is a small chance of injury to the larynx or esophagus, especially with multiple blind attempts. There is one case report of a death caused by esophageal perforation during blind intubation through the ILMA. Consider using endoscopic guidance if blind intubation is difficult or if the clinician is inexperienced. Intubation through a non-ILMA is not recommended unless facilitated by an endoscope.

Summary

LMAs provide an excellent means of oxygenation and ventilation when face mask ventilation is difficult or impossible. In addition, ILMAs are particularly useful when managing patients who are difficult to intubate. By facilitating the management of difficult or failed ventilation and difficult or failed intubation, ILMAs are an indispensable component of the difficult airway algorithm.

FLEXIBLE ENDOSCOPIC INTUBATION

Flexible endoscopic intubation is a common technique used by anesthesiologists for known difficult airways (Review Box 4.4). Physicians who perform endoscopic intubations daily have a success rate of nearly 100% when using this technique for difficult intubations.[294] In the ED, with more difficult intubating conditions and less experienced operators, the success rate is 50% to 90%.[295–298] The most common reason cited for failure of flexible endoscopic intubation in the operating room is clinician inexperience.[299] In the ED, failure is most often attributed to poor visibility from blood, vomitus, and other secretions.[295–297] Mlinik and colleagues[297] found that successful ED endoscopic intubations averaged 2 minutes whereas failures averaged 8 minutes. They recommended consideration of alternative approaches if intubation attempts take more than 3 minutes.

Flexible endoscopic intubation is often the best method for intubating awake patients with a known difficult airway. It can be accomplished via the nasal or oral route and is typically better tolerated by awake patients than direct or video laryngoscopy. Endoscopic intubation usually provides excellent visualization of the airway and permits evaluation of the airway before placement of the tube. The infrequency of endoscopic intubation precludes mastery of this technique and is a potential drawback. Because of the uncommon use of a flexible endoscope for tracheal intubation,[60] clinicians are encouraged to learn and maintain this skill by performing bedside nasopharyngoscopy for patients with severe sore throat, new hoarseness, suspected foreign body, possible laryngeal injury after neck trauma, and in other cases when upper airway edema, obstruction, or pathology is suspected. One device that has been released in recent years is the

Flexible Endoscopic Intubation

Indications

Known or suspected difficult airway
Distorted airway anatomy
- Swelling
- Abscess/infection
- Morbid obesity
- Trauma
- Tumors/previous radiation therapy

Contraindications

Nasal approach
- Severe midface trauma
- Coagulopathy

Relative
- Active airway bleeding
- Vomiting

Complications

Hypoxia from prolonged intubation attempts
Vomiting
Laryngospasm
Soft tissue trauma

Equipment

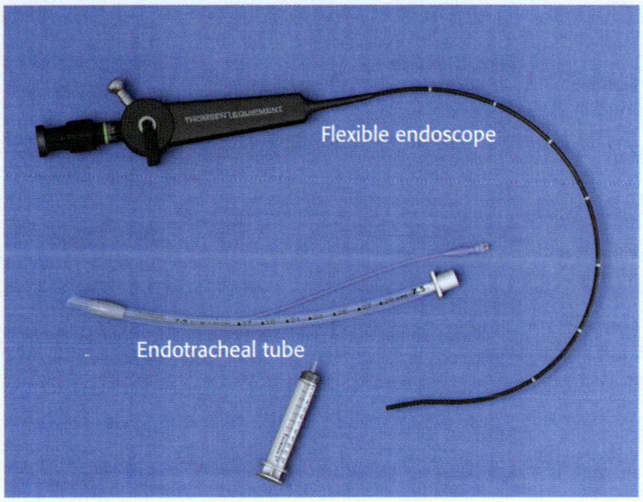

Review Box 4.4 Flexible endoscopic intubation.

Infrared Red Intubation System (IRRIS) (IntegraMedical), a simple device that is worn around the patient's neck and emits a bright infrared light through the cricothyroid membrane, allowing the clinician to visualize it during bronchoscopy and lead to faster intubation times. Devices such as this may aid clinicians with less experience with fiberoptic bronchoscopy or bronchoscopy with severe anatomical derangements.[300,301]

Expense has become less of an issue in recent years with the introduction of disposable endoscopes like the Ambu aScope. Disposable endoscopes are also available for both the Storz and GlideScope systems. Due to breakage of reusable bronchoscopes in the ED setting, disposable bronchoscopes are much more feasible. Nondisposable bronchoscopes tend to be costly and require routine maintenance and repair that adds significant cost. Single-use bronchoscopes avoid the cost of maintenance and repair.

Endoscopes are graded according to their external diameter, measured in millimeters. Endoscopes specifically designed for ET intubations are available from several companies (Pentax, Olympus, Machida, Storz, and Fujinon). A practical size for an intubating scope is approximately 3.5 to 5 mm. Although it is physically possible to pass an ET tube sized 0.5 mm larger over an endoscope, the fit is tight. As a rule, the ET tube should be approximately 1 mm larger than the intubating scope. The size of the working channel, the port that allows suction, administration of oxygen, and passage of fluid or catheters are also important when evaluating endoscopes. A working channel of approximately 2 mm is desirable to allow adequate suction of secretions; however, during endoscopic intubation, the working channel is used primarily for applying local anesthetic.

Older fiberoptic systems required the intubator to look into an eyepiece when performing intubation. Newer flexible endoscopic systems plug into a video monitor, enabling assistants and learners to visualize the airway anatomy; newer systems enable the intubator to maintain a more comfortable position while holding the endoscope and sheath properly.

Indications and Contraindications

Patients with known or suspected difficult airways are good candidates for awake or semi-awake endoscopic intubation. Patients with distorted airway anatomy, including swelling of the mouth or tongue, upper airway abscess or infection, morbid obesity, cervical spine injury, trismus, and penetrating and blunt neck trauma, are all good candidates for awake endoscopic intubation. Patients with laryngeal tumors, especially those with a history of radiation therapy encompassing the cervical region, may be impossible to intubate by any other nonsurgical method. An endoscope can also be helpful when assessing and intubating patients with airway obstruction from presumed foreign body aspiration. Flexible endoscopic intubation is best used as the initial approach to tracheal intubation, and it may be used as a rescue device when other methods fail.[273,302] Flexible endoscopic intubation can be performed through an ILMA or LMA after difficult ventilation or failed intubation.

Contraindications to the nasal approach are severe midface trauma and coagulopathy. Patients who are likely to receive thrombolytics should also be excluded. Although there are no clear contraindications to endoscopic orotracheal intubation, active airway bleeding, excessive oral sections, and vomiting are relative contraindications because successful endoscopic intubation is rarely achieved in these settings. Because of the time that must be expended preparing for and performing flexible endoscopic intubation, patients with impending airway closure from a dynamic process that is causing severe upper airway obstruction or swelling should have their airway secured by other means. Patients with multiple traumatic injuries are generally not good candidates for endoscopic

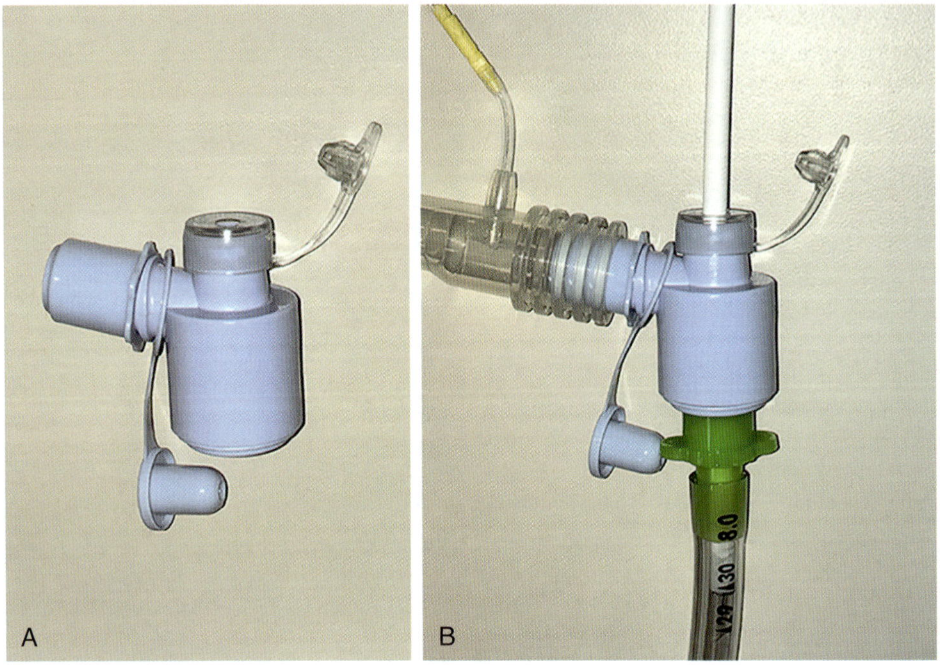

Fig. 4.31 Attaching a standard swivel adapter (A) to the end of the endotracheal (ET) tube during endoscopic intubation through the intubating laryngeal mask airway (ILMA) allows the patient to be ventilated during the entire procedure (B).

intubation because of the time-sensitive nature of their other injuries. Hypoxia despite attempts at oxygenation is another relative contraindication, especially if the intubator is inexperienced in flexible endoscopic intubation.

Procedure and Technique

Preparation and Anesthesia

Endoscopic intubation is performed for patients with difficult airways. The entire point of this procedure is for the patient to maintain normal airway reflexes and breathing. For this reason, sedation should be avoided, if possible. If necessary, small amounts of medications can be given for anxiolysis (e.g., 1 to 2 mg of midazolam). Ketamine can unpredictably cause dissociation and should be avoided as the ability for patients to follow commands makes the procedure substantially easier. If excellent topical anesthesia is achieved, parenteral sedation is sometimes unnecessary.

Proper preparation of the upper airway is crucial for successful awake or semi-awake endoscopic intubation. If time permits, administration of a drying agent such as glycopyrrolate 10 to 20 minutes before the procedure will reduce oral secretions and increase the effectiveness of topical anesthesia. Application of a vasoconstrictor such as oxymetazoline or phenylephrine is recommended to increase the caliber of the nasal passage and reduce the chance of epistaxis.

Topical anesthesia should be applied to the posterior oropharynx, hypopharynx, and larynx for all endoscopic intubations. If nasal intubation is planned, administer topical anesthesia to the selected naris.

Anesthesia of the Oropharynx and Larynx

Topical anesthesia should use either 4% or 5% lidocaine. Less potent lidocaine concentrations do not achieve dense anesthesia and should be avoided. Because topical lidocaine is not fully absorbed, the recommended maximum dose is 9 mg/kg of lean body weight,[303] which is higher than when injected subcutaneously. Lean body weight is about 80% of total body weight in patients with normal BMIs. The maximum dose of 9 mg/kg of lidocaine translates to about 12 mL of 4% lidocaine for a 70-kg patient of average height.

Deliver local anesthetic to the upper airway by one of several methods. Application of 4% or 5% lidocaine cream by "buttering" the base of the tongue is an effective technique to anesthetize the posterior tongue, vallecula, epiglottis, and laryngeal structures. The tongue is held in protrusion as the base of the tongue is buttered with 4% or 5% lidocaine cream using a tongue depressor. Because the patient is unable to swallow with a protruded tongue, the ointment warms, liquefies, and moves posteriorly and inferiorly to anesthetize the laryngeal structures. It is contended that the ointment also penetrates the mucosa to anesthetize the glossopharyngeal and superior laryngeal nerves.[304]

A flexible atomizer device that attaches to a standard syringe (Fig. 4.32) (LMA MADgic; Teleflex) can be used to accurately apply atomized 4% aqueous lidocaine to the posterior oropharynx and upper laryngeal structures; tracheal anesthesia can be accomplished by having the patient inspire as the medication is sprayed. Some laryngeal and tracheal anesthesia can be achieved by oral spray with a laryngeal tracheal anesthetic set, and this is probably less effective than other methods.

To properly anesthetize the perilaryngeal structures and avoid gagging during the procedure, a combination of lidocaine cream at the base of the tongue and atomizing lidocaine onto the larynx is required.

These steps are done before the procedure. Most patients will also require additional anesthesia to abolish sensation of the vocal cords and proximal trachea. This is achieved with administration of 4% aqueous lidocaine through the working channel of the endoscopic scope during the procedure via the "spray-as-you-go" technique. This technique requires an assistant to manage the syringe and lidocaine administration.

There are other historical methods of achieving laryngeal anesthesia, though they are not necessary and are of limited utility. Transcricothyroid injection of lidocaine achieves good anesthesia of the larynx and is invasive. Historically, nebulized lidocaine was used to attempt to achieve anesthesia, and this practice should be avoided. Nebulized medications travel readily into the lungs rather than onto oral mucosa.

Anesthesia of the Nasal Passage

Nasal anesthesia can be accomplished by several methods. A flexible atomizer (see Fig. 4.32) can be passed to the posterior nasopharynx, and then 4% aqueous lidocaine is sprayed as the patient sniffs. This is repeated several times as the flexible atomizer is slowly withdrawn. Alternatively, 4% lidocaine cream can be insufflated into the nare. In this method the clinician applies a pea-sized amount of cream onto their finger and inserts it into the patient's nasal vestibule. The patient vigorously sniffs to coat the nasal passage. This is repeated 3 to 5 times. Dense anesthesia is achieved with this method and is the authors' preferred approach for nasal anesthesia.

Patient Positioning and Endoscope Preparation

The optimal position of the neck is extension, as opposed to the slight cervical flexion desired when using DL. Extension allows better visualization of the glottis by elevating the epiglottis off the posterior pharyngeal wall. This is especially pertinent in a comatose patient who lacks the muscle tone necessary to maintain an open airway. If problems arise with the tongue and soft tissues falling back and obscuring the view of the endoscope, apply a jaw-lift maneuver or grasp the tongue and pull it forward and away from the soft palate and posterior pharyngeal wall. This also moves the epiglottis away from the posterior pharyngeal wall and facilitates exposure of the cords. Extend the head to accomplish the same objective.

Endoscopic intubation may be performed with the patient in the upright, semi-upright, or supine position. The upright and semi-upright positions help keep pharyngeal soft tissue from obstructing the airway. The upright position may be more familiar to emergency clinicians who are skilled at diagnostic nasopharyngoscopy. Stand facing the patient or at the patient's head, depending on personal preference.

The greatest impediment to successful endoscopic intubation is an inability to visualize the larynx because blood or secretions have covered the optical element and cannot be removed. Suction actively just before introduction of the endoscope. Application of a small amount of soap to the lens may decrease fogging. If the endoscope has a working channel, suction minor secretions through the suction port during the procedure. The camera can also be cleaned by pressing the lens against a moist mucosal surface or having the patient swallow. Whereas some advocate oxygen insufflation through the suction port to blow away secretions, defog the tip, and increase the inspired oxygen content, there are case reports of pulmonary barotrauma and gastric insufflation causing gastric rupture,[305–308] If oxygen insufflation is used to clear secretions, it should be used for a few seconds at a time. Supplemental oxygen can be administered separately, through the nose or mouth.

Nasal Approach

The nasal approach is believed by some to be easier than the oral approach because the angle of insertion allows better visualization of the larynx with minimal manipulation of the endoscope. In some patients, the mouth is not accessible at all because of trismus, swelling, or trauma (e.g., angioedema caused by an angiotensin-converting enzyme [ACE] inhibitor), so the nasal route may be the only option for endoscopic intubation (Fig. 4.33).

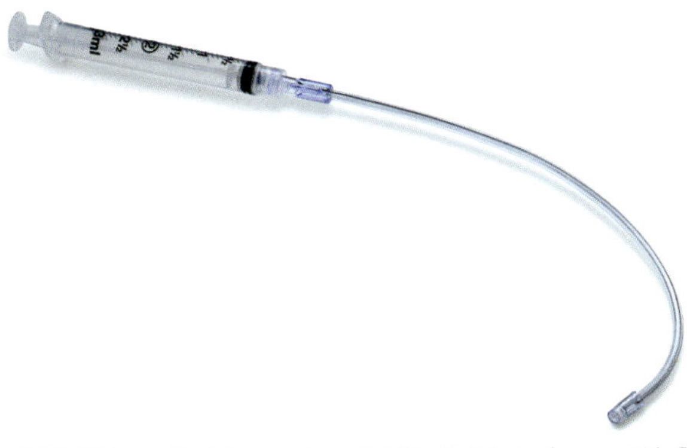

Fig. 4.32 This malleable atomizer (LMA MADgic device; Teleflex) allows topical anesthesia to be applied accurately to multiple areas.

Choose the most patent nostril. In a cooperative patient, determine this by simply occluding each nostril and asking the patient to identify the nostril that is easiest to breathe through. Identify the most patent nostril by direct vision or by gently inserting a gloved finger that is lubricated with viscous lidocaine into the nostrils. Once the nostril is selected, dilate the nasal passage by inserting your fifth finger and applying steady firm pressure. This will be relatively painless if dense anesthesia has been achieved. If this is painful, apply more lidocaine cream, wait a few minutes and try again. The fifth finger should be slowly advanced into the nasal cavity until approximately the level of the metacarpophalangeal joint (Fig. 4.34).

Next, place a well-lubricated ET tube in the nostril to a depth of approximately 12 to 14 cm before passing the scope through it. We have found that the best tube for nasal intubation is the Flex-Tip MicroLarygneal Endotracheal Tube (SunMed), which is available in sizes 4.0, 5.0, and 6.0 mm, and we use the 6.0 mm size for most adults. All SunMed Flex-Tip Microlarnygeal Tubes are 35 cm long, long enough even for the largest adult. This smaller size and Flex-tip design make the passage more comfortable while maintaining adequate tube length. Rather than advance the tube into the nose first, some operators prefer to mount the ET tube over the scope and first pass the scope through the nostril and then advance the tube over the scope (Fig. 4.35). Either sequence is acceptable. The advantage of first passing the tracheal tube through the nose is that it avoids the possibility of secretions covering the scope and positions the scope just above the laryngeal inlet. One disadvantage is that it may cause epistaxis, and, in some patients, the tube may not pass easily into the nasopharynx. If the tube will not pass into the nasopharynx, it is best to discover this at the beginning of the procedure rather than after the trachea has been intubated with the endoscope.

At an insertion depth of 12 to 14 cm, the ET tube should have advanced around the bend at the level of the nasopharynx. Now advance the endoscope into the ET tube. The laryngeal structures should be visible when the scope exits the distal end of the ET tube. If laryngeal structures are not immediately visualized, advance the endoscope and look for

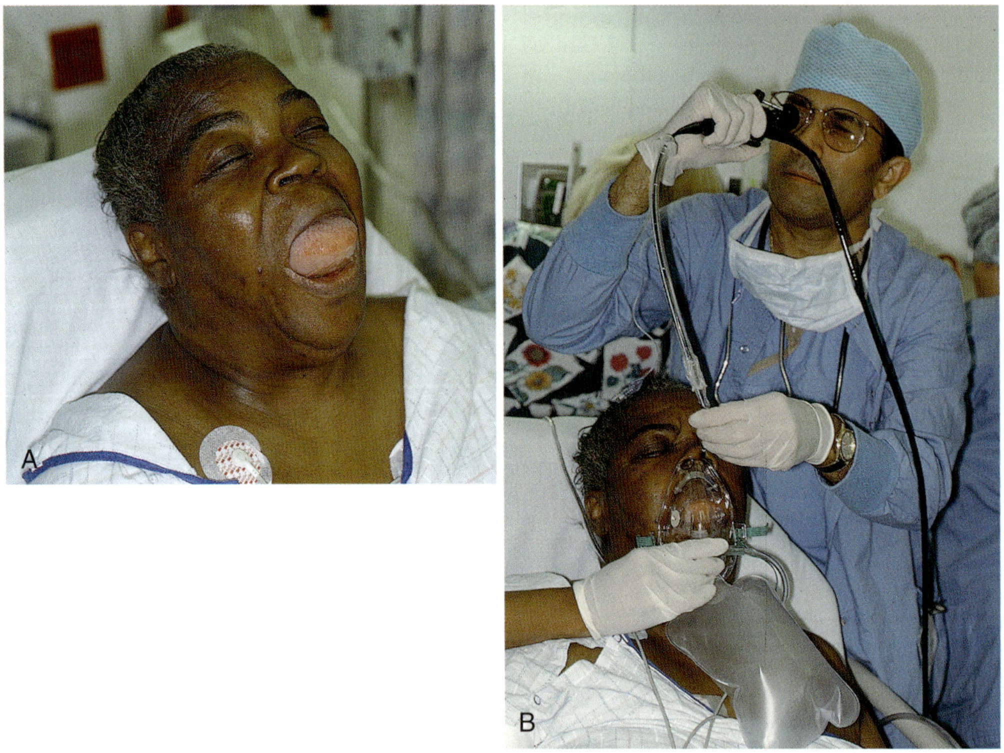

Fig. 4.33 (A) This patient with life-threatening angiotensin-converting enzyme inhibitor–induced angioedema is in severe distress, and oral intubation is impossible. This can be a lethal condition. (B) Endoscopic nasotracheal intubation is a good choice, but requires meticulous topical anesthesia. A surgical airway may be required. Note: In this case the tracheal tube was premounted on the scope before the scope was passed into the patient's nose. Alternatively, the tube may be first passed approximately 12 cm through the nose, and then the scope passed through the tube and into the trachea.

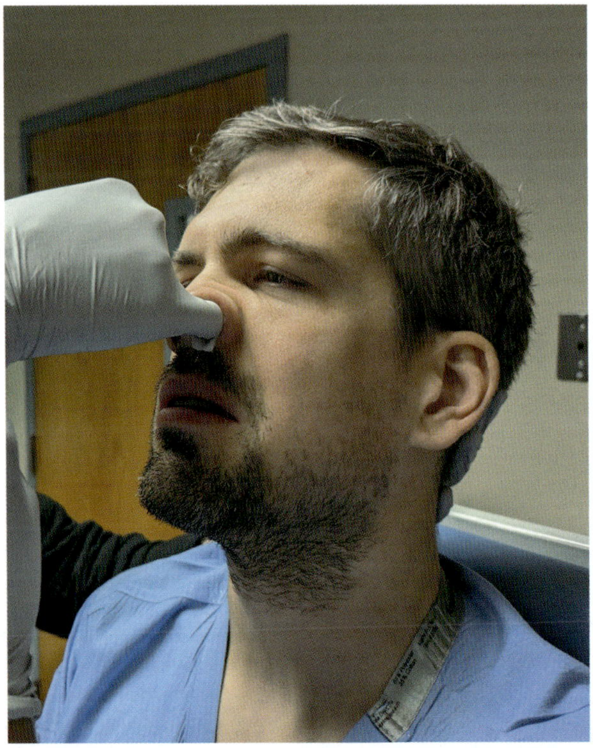

Fig. 4.34 The nare can be dilated by slowly advancing the pinky finger over 3 to 5 minutes to approximately the level of the metacarpophalangeal joint. Commercially available nasopharyngeal airways are collapsible and do not dilate nearly as well.

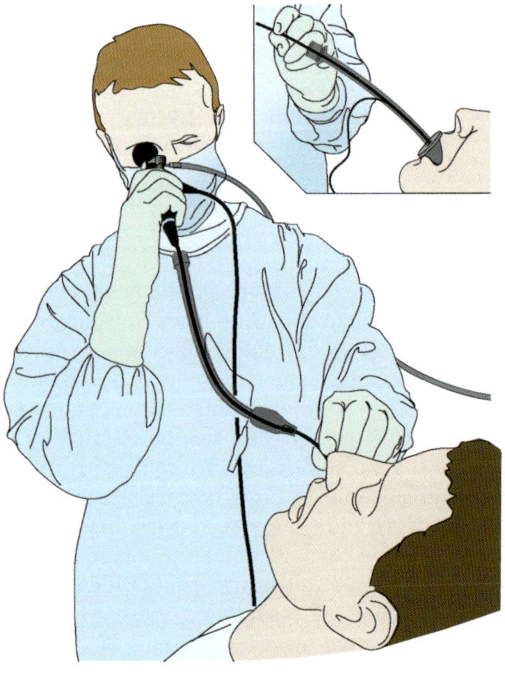

Fig. 4.35 Flexible endoscopic intubation, nasal approach. Note that the tracheal tube is first premounted on the scope. The fiberoptic scope enters the trachea and then serves as a guide over which the tracheal tube is passed. *Inset,* Use of an oral intubating airway via the oral approach. (Courtesy Department of Emergency Medicine, Hennepin County Medical Center, Minneapolis, MN.)

laryngeal structures. The epiglottis and vocal cords are seen with little or no manipulation of the tip of the endoscope in 90% of patients.[289] Advance the scope and keep the vocal cords in view by making frequent minor adjustments of the tip of the scope. If secretions are present or if the camera is covered with bodily fluids, ask the patient to swallow. This typically relieves the problem and dramatically improves the view. If there is persistent fogging or material on the camera lens, the tip of the camera can be touched to a mucosal surface, often clearing the lens.

Even with good anesthetic technique, the vocal cords and proximal trachea may not be fully anesthetized. To achieve complete anesthesia and ease tube passage, instill 1 to 2 mL of 4% aqueous lidocaine through the working channel of the endoscope with directed aim at the vocal cords while the patient inhales. The patient will cough. Wait 1 minute before proceeding to allow the lidocaine to take effect. Realize that the first injected mL of anesthetic will go into the channel and not into the patient, so you will depress the syringe for a total of 2 to 3 mL.

In a comatose or obtunded patient, the tongue and other soft tissues may obscure the view of the larynx. This can be alleviated by asking an assistant to pull the tongue forward or to apply a chin- or jaw-lift maneuver. Advance the scope through the larynx to the carina and pass the ET tube over the firmly held endoscope into the trachea. Remember that in adults, the average distance from the nares to the epiglottis is 16 to 17 cm. If the scope has been advanced much beyond this distance and the glottis is still not seen, the scope is probably in the esophagus.[309] If the scope meets resistance at approximately this same level and only a pink blur is visible, the tip of the scope is probably in a piriform sinus. Transillumination of the soft tissues may confirm this and indicate the necessary corrective maneuvers.

Once the scope has entered the trachea, difficulty advancing the ET tube may be encountered. The tip of the tube most commonly catches on the right arytenoid cartilage or vocal cord. To fix this, withdraw the tube 2 cm, rotate it counterclockwise 90 degrees, and readvance the tube (see Fig. 4.21).

Oral Approach

Oral endoscopic intubation is indicated when nasal intubation is contraindicated or oral intubation is preferred. Skilled endoscopists often find the oral approach just as easy as the nasal approach. For the less experienced, the oral approach may be more difficult because the path of the scope is less defined by the surrounding soft tissue and the tip of the scope is more likely to impinge on the base of the tongue or vallecula. Keeping the scope in the midline and elevating the soft tissue by pulling the tongue forward or applying the jaw-lift maneuver will minimize this difficulty. Because the oropharyngeal axis is not as well aligned with the larynx as the nasopharyngeal axis, more scope manipulation is required when using the oral approach.

The oral approach may be facilitated with the use of a specialized intubating oral airway (Fig. 4.36). These adjuncts resemble standard oropharyngeal airways and are longer with a specific design for endoscopic intubation. Though many exist the Williams Airway has been shown to offer a superior view and a slightly faster time to intubation than other airways.[310,311] The tip of this airway lies just above the laryngeal inlet and ensures midline positioning. Ensure that the patient is adequately anesthetized before the oral airway is placed to minimize gagging or emesis. The ET tube can be advanced to the distal tip of the oral airway before the oral airway is inserted, and then the scope passed through the ET tube. Alternatively, place a well-lubricated endoscope, premounted with an ET tube, through the well-positioned oral intubating airway. A key to using the Williams airway is to have an assistant carefully hold the device in the midline and work with the intubator to make minor adjustments to place the tip of the oral airway just above the laryngeal inlet. This is easier when using an endoscopic system with a video monitor, so that the intubator and assistant can both observe the camera image. Once the airway structures are visualized, advance the endoscope into the trachea (see Fig. 4.35, inset). Then advance the ET tube over the scope and into the trachea. This may require the same counterclockwise maneuver as described with the nasal approach. After successful intubation, the oral airway can be left in place as a bite block or may be removed over the ET tube after removal of the tube adapter. Some oral intubating airways can be removed from the mouth without disconnecting the ET tube adapter.

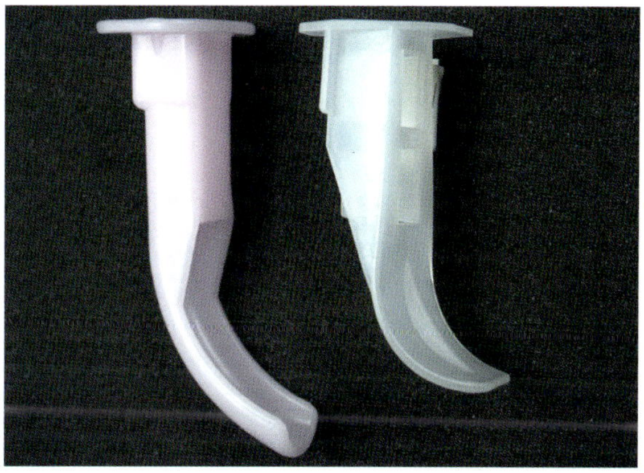

Fig. 4.36 Examples of oral intubating airways. The Williams Airway intubator (SunMed) *(left)* cradles the endotracheal (ET) tube in an open, curved guide, whereas the Ovassapian Fiberoptic Intubating Airway (Teleflex) *(right)* positions the ET tube on the posterior surface of the intubation airway.

An alternative, less practical, approach to the traditional oral endoscopic intubation for an anticipated difficult airway requires two clinicians. One performs DL or VL, places the tip of the endoscope under the epiglottis, and blindly advances it while the second clinician, holding the body of the scope, directs the tip of the scope through the cords (Fig. 4.37). Most patients who could be intubated with this technique can probably be intubated using video laryngoscopy with a well-curved bougie.

Endoscope Technique

Flexible endoscopic intubation will be more successful if proper technique is maintained. The scope body and endoscope controls are held in one hand, while the other hand stabilizes the sheath as it enters the ET tube or patient. The intubator directs motion in one plane (up or down) with the endoscope controls; to move perpendicular to that plane (right or left) the entire scope must be rotated. This is best accomplished by keeping the endoscopic sheath taut between the scope body and the point of entry into the patient, so that when the handle is rotated the entire scope (including the tip) rotates. If the sheath is not held taut, rotation of the handle will not cause rotation at the tip because of excessive slack in the sheath. Newer endoscope systems with video monitors make it easier to hold the endoscope and sheath properly (Fig. 4.38).

Complications

Complications of endoscopic orotracheal intubation include hypoxia from prolonged intubation attempts, emesis, and laryngospasm. Oxygen saturation monitoring should alert the clinician to hypoxia. Most complications seen with endoscopically guided NT intubation are associated with passing the ET tube through the nasopharynx. Epistaxis is the most common, followed by other nasopharyngeal injuries. A rare and potentially significant complication may result if, on blind advancement of the endoscope through the ET tube, the tip of the scope exits through Murphy's eye (the distal side port of the ET tube).[312] Attempts at passing the ET tube through the larynx will fail because the tip of the tube, now extending off the midline, will catch on the laryngeal structures.

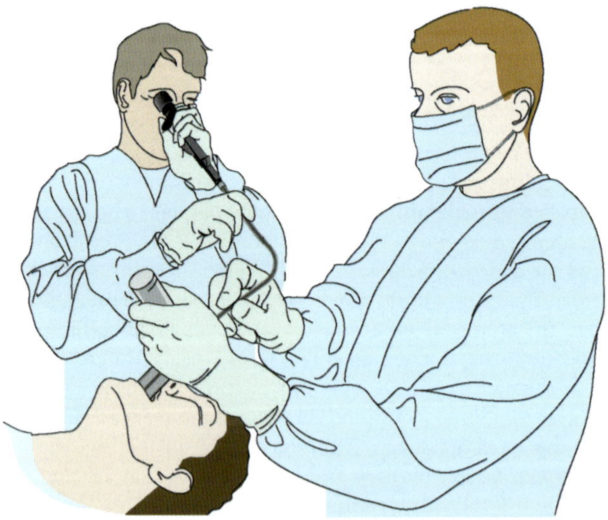

Fig. 4.37 Two-person fiberoptic intubation for difficult intubation. The laryngoscopist obtains the best hypopharyngeal exposure and directs the fiberoptic tip in the direction of the glottis. The second clinician, who manipulates the tip of the fiberoptic scope, directs the laryngoscopist to slowly advance the tip until it has successfully passed through the cords.

Summary

The primary advantages of endoscopic intubation are the ability to visualize upper airway abnormalities, to negotiate difficult airway anatomy, and to carefully perform tracheal intubation under visual guidance. Endoscopic intubation is noninvasive and well tolerated in fully awake patients if meticulous attention is paid to topical anesthesia. Its major limitation is poor visibility because of blood and secretions. If drying agents and suction cannot mitigate excessive secretions or blood, it is best to avoid endoscopic intubation. Procedural time can be another limitation. Endoscopic intubation requires more practice than many other methods of airway management, though this can be obtained in noncritically ill patients. Endoscopic intubation is more likely to be successful if used early in the management of a difficult airway rather than as a last resort after repeated failure with DL.

OPTICAL AND VIDEO INTUBATING STYLETS

A class of devices that incorporates optics or video into a semirigid metal or metal-reinforced stylet was introduced in the late 1990s. Intubating stylets are different from other video laryngoscopy devices in two important ways. First, they do not create potential space for tube passage like devices with blades. Second, they intubate the trachea directly. Intubating stylets remain popular with some anesthesiologists although are rarely used in emergency airway management with so many video laryngoscopy devices available.[60] If video laryngoscopy is available, the practicing emergency clinician can manage all airways *without* the use of these devices.

Intubating stylets can be used in conjunction with a laryngoscope or as stand-alone devices. They require laryngoscopic assistance in 8% to 20% of cases and are more successful when used in this way.[313,314] Visibility can be hampered by blood and secretions, and less so than with flexible endoscopy.[315] These devices are more intuitive and require less practice than flexible endoscopy. The Clarus Video System, Shikani Optical Stylet and Levitan FPS Scope (Clarus Medical) are examples of these malleable optical stylets (Fig. 4.39). The Bonfils Retromolar Intubation Fiberscope (Karl Storz) is rigid with structural and functional similarities to the Shikani. The distal end of the Bonfils has a fixed curve of 40 degrees, whereas the other scopes are malleable up to 120 degrees. The intubator

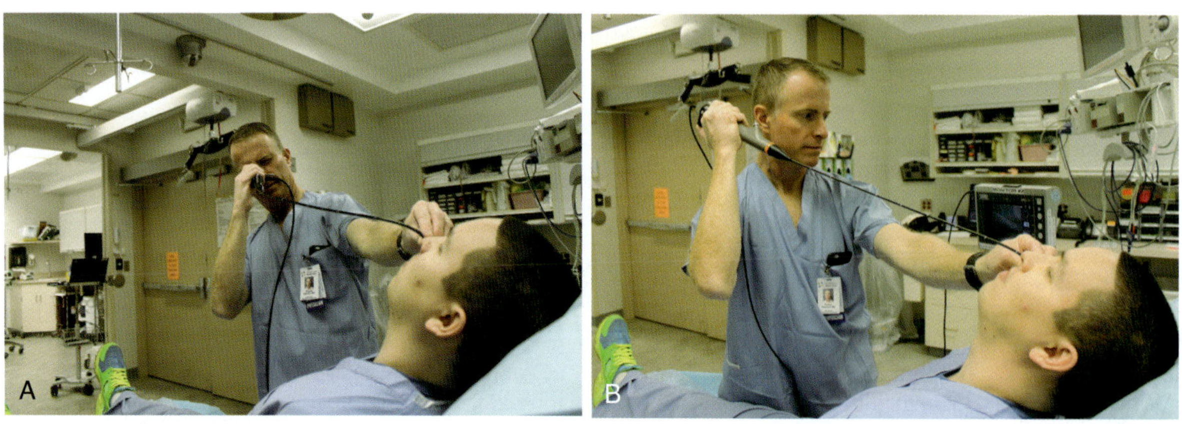

Fig. 4.38 The endoscopic sheath must be kept taut in order to successfully rotate the tip of the device. (A) This technique is difficult on older scopes that utilize an eyepiece. (B) Newer systems with a video monitor make it easier to manipulate the endoscope properly.

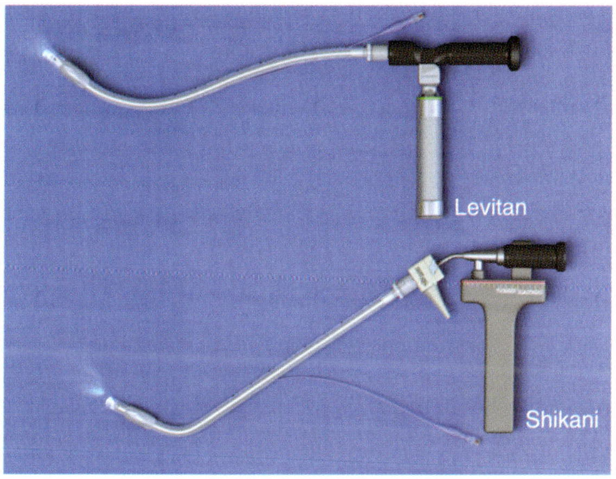

Fig. 4.39 Examples of semirigid fiberoptic stylets: the Clarus Medical Levitan *(top)* and Shikani *(bottom)*.

can look through an eyepiece or a video screen, depending on the model used.

Indications and Contraindications

Semirigid fiberoptic stylets are useful when the glottis cannot be readily seen and may be a useful adjunct for any difficult airway, especially if mouth opening is limited. A relative contraindication is the presence of significant blood or oral secretions.

Procedure and Technique

The semirigid fiberoptic stylet can be used with or without laryngoscopy. In either case, place the patient in the sniffing position. Load an ET tube onto a lightly lubricated stylet so that the ET tube extends 1 to 2 cm beyond the end of the stylet.

If the device is used alone, create an accentuated curve of between 70 and 80 degrees at the proximal aspect of the cuff of the tube so that it can negotiate the oropharynx. Suction the oropharynx well before attempting intubation. Grasp the mandible with the left hand. Next, raise the jaw to lift the tongue and epiglottis off the posterior hypopharyngeal wall. Ask an assistant to apply a jaw-thrust maneuver or grasp the tongue with gauze and retract it anteriorly. Place the device into the mouth, and while following the curve of the tongue, bring it up under the epiglottis with fiberoptic or video guidance. When the laryngeal inlet is visualized, direct the tip into the larynx. Advance the ET tube as you withdraw the stylet. If resistance is met while advancing the tube, the tip may be catching on the anterior larynx or trachea. Rotate the tube clockwise 120 degrees at the proximal end, which will result in a 90-degree rotation at the tip. With the bevel now anterior, allow the tube to advance without catching. It is important to remember that the direction of rotation of the ET tube is *clockwise* if resistance is encountered *after* going through the cords. For resistance encountered *before* the cords, such as with tracheal tube introducers, fiberoptic scopes, and NT intubation, rotate the tube *counterclockwise*.

If using the semirigid optical stylets with a laryngoscope, form the angle of the distal stylet less acute, at approximately 35 degrees. Introduce the device only after obtaining maximal visualization with the laryngoscope. If the epiglottis can be seen, advance the tip of the stylet just underneath it via direct vision. Be careful not to embed the tip of the ET tube in the supraglottic soft tissue because it will obscure visibility. At this point, guide the stylet-ET tube unit into the glottis and advance the tube off the stylet.

Summary

Semirigid fiberoptic stylets combine the features of direct and in DL and provide a valuable tool when approaching a difficult airway. They can be used alone or in conjunction with a laryngoscope. Although these devices function as intended, they do not offer any advantage over video laryngoscopes or flexible endoscopes and are generally not used by emergency clinicians.

Orotracheal Intubation With a King Laryngeal Tube or Combitube in Place

King LT (Ambu, Ballerup, Denmark) airways are used extensively in the prehospital setting because they can be placed quickly and provide reliable oxygenation and ventilation in the majority of patients. It is common for patients to arrive to the ED with a King LT (or Combitube [Covidien/Medtronic, Minneapolis, MN]) in place. Almost all patients will need to have it replaced with an ET tube at some point. Intubation through the King LT device is technically possible with fiberoptics or a bougie, but many who have tried this maneuver in clinical practice have been disappointed. The reason is that the aperture does not necessarily directly align with the glottis, even when the device is ventilating properly.[316] In one study, the glottis was visualized in only 51% of patients when a fiberscope was passed through the King LT.[317] The clinician has the choice of removing the functioning retroglottic airway before attempting intubation or leaving the device in place during intubation. An advantage of leaving the device in place is the maintenance of oxygenation and ventilation until just before the attempt begins, and the ability to reinflate the balloons and resume oxygenation immediately after a failed attempt, without having to replace the laryngeal tube (LT).

DL with the King LT in place is difficult. In contrast, video laryngoscopy usually allows excellent visualization of the glottis and placement of an ET tube while the King LT remains in place (with the balloons deflated) and is a reliable method of securing the airway with a LT in place.[318,319] This approach allows clinicians to avoid the risk of removing a functional airway in a patient who may be difficult to intubate (Fig. 4.40).

To perform this procedure, use a video laryngoscope to obtain a view of the large proximal balloon. Deflate the balloons. The glottis will usually come immediately into view. If it does not, optimize the view using the laryngoscope; small adjustments (rotation or slight retraction) of the LT may be needed. Pass a bougie into the airway, and then have an assistant place an ET tube onto the bougie; intubate the trachea as described previously. Inflate the ET tube and confirm placement. After the tube is known to be in the trachea and the patient is stable, remove the LT.

BLIND NASOTRACHEAL INTUBATION

See Video 4.21. Blind NT intubation can be one of the more technically demanding airway approaches, with the outcome being heavily dependent on the skill and experience of the clinician and a certain amount of luck. The primary advantage

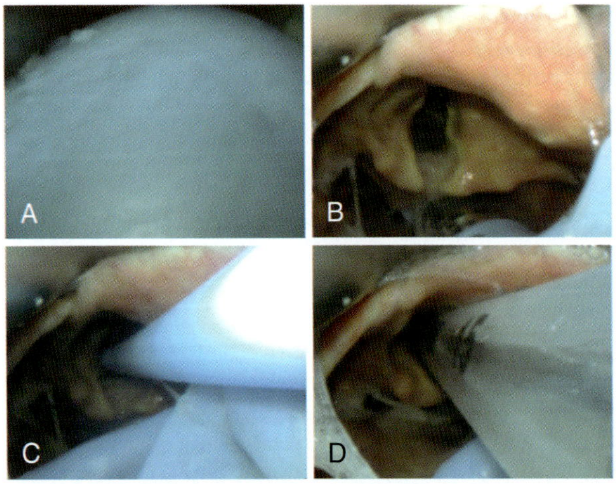

Fig. 4.40 Tracheal intubation around a King LT (Ambu) airway using video laryngoscopy. (A) The laryngoscope is placed in the mouth and advanced until the large balloon comes into view. (B) The balloon is deflated. Usually the glottis will immediately appear. If it does not, optimize the view by ensuring the laryngoscope blade is in the vallecula and engaged in the midline hyoepiglottic ligament. (C) Pass a bougie into the trachea. (D) The tube is passed over the bougie. After confirmation that the endotracheal tube is in the trachea, the King LT airway can be removed. If there is difficulty during the procedure, or if intubation is unsuccessful, inflate the King LT balloons and resume ventilation.

of the blind technique is that it minimizes neck movement and does not require mouth opening. In extenuating circumstances, it can be accomplished without an intravenous line.

NT intubation is technically more difficult than oral intubation and may have advantages in select circumstances. Blind NT intubation is possible with the patient in the sitting position, a distinct advantage when intubating a patient with congestive heart failure who cannot tolerate lying flat. In fact, patients in respiratory distress are the easiest to intubate blindly because their air hunger results in increased abduction of the vocal cords, facilitating entry of the tube into the trachea.

Indications and Contraindications

Patients requiring airway control who have spontaneous respirations can be considered for blind NT intubation. The typical patient is one with an anticipated difficult airway and persistently low oxygen saturation despite preoxygenation. Patients with severe chronic obstructive pulmonary disease (COPD) or asthma who have high airway pressures and may be difficult to ventilate with a face mask are another group to consider for NT intubation. Some other common examples of a difficult airway to consider for NT intubation are patients with short thick necks, trismus, or neck immobility. Other conditions that preclude successful orotracheal intubation include severe arthritis, fixed deformities of the cervical spine, or ACE inhibitor–induced angioedema. In the modern era, many of these patients may instead be intubated with awake flexible endoscopic intubation.

Apnea is the major contraindication to blind NT intubation because attempts to place the tube without respirations as a guide are futile. Avoid nasal intubation in patients with severe nasal or midface trauma. In the presence of a basilar skull fracture, an NT tube may inadvertently enter the cranial cavity.[320,321] Nasal intubation is also relatively contraindicated if the patient is taking anticoagulants, has a known coagulopathy, or has recently been or soon will be administered thrombolytics. Blind NT intubation should be avoided in patients with expanding neck hematomas and oropharyngeal trauma. If the patient has known abnormal glottic anatomy that would impede blind tube passage, other methods will probably be more successful. Patient combativeness, if not controlled with sedation, makes blind intubation difficult. Inability to open the mouth (such as a wired jaw) is a relative contraindication because emesis may be induced, and it may be impossible to clear the vomitus; endoscopic guidance may be preferred to reduce the risk of emesis. Exercise judgment in each individual case and be prepared to use neuromuscular blocking agents or to bypass the upper airway with a surgical technique if such a complication develops.

Procedure and Technique

Place the patient in the sniffing position with the proximal part of the neck slightly flexed and the head extended on the neck. Like endoscopic NT intubation, patient preparation is important. Apply phenylephrine drops, oxymetazoline (Afrin) spray, or 4% cocaine spray to both nares to dilate the nasal passages and reduce the risk of epistaxis. Topical anesthesia of the nares, oropharynx, hypopharynx, and larynx with lidocaine spray (4%) is also indicated if time permits (as described in the "Flexible Endoscopic Intubation" section of this chapter). Choose the most patent nostril. In a cooperative patient, simply occlude each nostril and ask the patient which naris is easier to breathe through. The most patent nostril can also be identified by direct vision or by gently inserting a gloved finger lubricated with viscous lidocaine into the nostrils. If time permits, dilate the nasal passage with a gloved pinky finger by slowly advancing to the metacarpophalangeal joint over 3 to 5 minutes.

After preparation of the nostril, insert a well-lubricated 7.0 ET tube along the floor of the nasal cavity. Do not direct the tube cephalad, as one might expect from the external nasal anatomy. Twist the tube gently to bypass any soft tissue obstruction in the nasal cavity. It is sometimes recommended that the tube's bevel be oriented toward the septum to avoid injury to the inferior turbinate. At 6 to 7 cm, one usually feels a "give" as the tube passes the nasal choana and negotiates the abrupt 90-degree curve required to enter the nasopharynx. This is the most painful and traumatic part of the procedure and must be done gently. If resistance persists despite continued gentle pressure and twisting of the tube, pass a suction catheter or endoscope down the tube and into the oropharynx to allow successful passage of the tube over the catheter.[322] If this attempt fails, try the other nostril. To avoid this difficulty from the outset, use a controllable-tip tracheal tube (Endotrol, Mallinckrodt Medical). The tube allows you to increase the flexion of the tube, thereby facilitating passage beyond this tight curve.

As the tube advances through the oropharynx and hypopharynx, it approaches the vocal cords, and breath sounds from the tube typically become louder. Fogging of the tube may also occur. At the point of maximal breath sounds, the tube is lying immediately in front of the laryngeal inlet. The tube is most easily advanced into the trachea during inspiration, when the vocal cords are maximally open. As the patient begins to breathe in, advance the tube in one smooth motion. If a cough reflex is present, the patient usually coughs and becomes stridulous during this maneuver, which suggests successful tracheal intubation. The absence of such a response should alert the clinician to probable esophageal passage. Remember that in adults, the average distance from the naris to the epiglottis is 16 to 17 cm; if the tube is advanced past this distance and is not in the trachea, it is probably in the esophagus. Once the tube is in the trachea, vocalization should cease. Persistent vocalizations suggest esophageal intubation. Breath sounds coming from the tube and tube fogging are other signs of correct ET tube placement. Reflex swallowing during blind NT intubation may direct the tube posteriorly toward the esophagus. If this occurs, direct conscious patients to stick out their tongue to inhibit swallowing and prevent consequent movement of the larynx. Application of laryngeal pressure may also help avoid esophageal passage.

After intubation, confirm tracheal placement with end-tidal CO_2 and administer sedation. Auscultate over both lungs while applying positive pressure ventilation. If only one lung is being ventilated, withdraw the tube until breath sounds are heard bilaterally. The optimum distance from the external nares to the tip of the tube is approximately 28 cm in males and 26 cm in females.[323] After verification of tracheal placement, inflate the cuff and secure the tube.

Technical Difficulties

The NT tube may slide smoothly through the hypopharynx and into the trachea on the first pass. Unfortunately, this is not always the case. In an operating room series, the first attempt was successful in less than 50% of instances.[324] When the initial pass is unsuccessful, there are four potential locations of the tip of the tube: anterior to the epiglottis in the vallecula, on the arytenoids or vocal cords, in a piriform sinus, or in the esophagus.

Observation and palpation of the soft tissues of the neck during attempted passage of the NT tube are helpful in finding the misplaced tube. Before reattempting placement, withdraw the tube slightly. Do not remove it from the nose because this will create additional trauma to the nasal soft tissues. If cervical spine injury is suspected, avoid any cervical maneuver that moves the neck significantly. To move the ET tube in relation to the laryngeal inlet, it is important to know how the tip of the ET tube responds to head movements. Flexion of the neck will move the tip posteriorly; extension of the neck will move the tip anteriorly; rotation of the neck to the right and left will move the tip of the tube contralateral to the direction of rotation. Based on the suspected location of the tip of the tube, the following methods will help achieve success when difficulties with tube placement are encountered.

Anterior to the Epiglottis

Difficulty advancing the tube beyond 15 cm or palpation of the tip of the tube anteriorly at the level of the hyoid bone suggests an impasse anterior to the epiglottis in the vallecula. Withdraw the tube 2 cm, decrease the degree of neck extension, and readvance the tube.

Arytenoid Cartilage and Vocal Cord

Contrary to the classic teaching,[325] studies have demonstrated a propensity for an NT tube, when placed through the right nares, to lie posteriorly and to the right as it approaches the larynx.[326,327] It is not surprising that the most common obstacles to advancement of the NT tube are the right arytenoid and the vocal cords. No data are available on common obstacles encountered if the tube is placed in the left nares. If the tube appears to be hanging up on firm cartilaginous tissue, withdraw the tube 2 cm, rotate it 90 degrees counterclockwise, and readvance it. This maneuver orients the bevel of the tube posteriorly and frequently results in successful passage (Fig. 4.41). When evaluated in the ED, this maneuver was successful 73% of the time.[328] Another technique is to pass a suction catheter down the tube. It will often pass through the larynx without difficulty, and the tube can then be advanced over the catheter (Fig. 4.42A).[329,330]

Piriform Sinus

Bulging of the neck lateral and superior to the larynx indicates tube location in a piriform sinus. Withdraw the tube 2 cm, rotate it slightly away from the bulge, and then readvance it. An alternative method is to tilt the patient's head toward the side of the misplacement and then reattempt placement.[331]

Esophageal Placement

Esophageal placement is indicated by a smooth passage of the tube and the loss of breath sounds through the tube. The larynx may be seen or felt to elevate as the tube passes under it. Assisted ventilation will usually produce gurgling sounds when the epigastrium is auscultated. Withdraw the tube until breath sounds are clearly heard, and reattempt passage while applying pressure to the cricoid. Increase extension of the head on the neck during placement. If attempts continue to result in esophageal misplacement, the following maneuver may result in successful tracheal intubation. From the precise point at which breath sounds are lost, withdraw the ET tube 1 cm and inflate the cuff with 15 mL of air. This results in elevation of the tube off the posterior pharyngeal wall and can help angle the tube toward the larynx. Advance the tube 2 cm. Continued breath sounds indicate a probable intralaryngeal location. At this point, deflate the cuff and advance the ET tube into the trachea (Fig. 4.42B–C). This technique may be particularly useful in patients with cervical spine injury because it requires no manipulation of the head or neck.[332] This maneuver, when used on the first pass in 20 patients in the operating room, was successful in 75% of cases.[324] This maneuver can also be combined with the passage of a suction catheter after inflation of the ET tube cuff. The suction catheter will often pass easily into the trachea; the cuff can be deflated and the tube advanced into the trachea.

If a controllable-tip ET tube (Endotrol) is used, flex the tip anteriorly to help avoid esophageal placement.[333] Remember

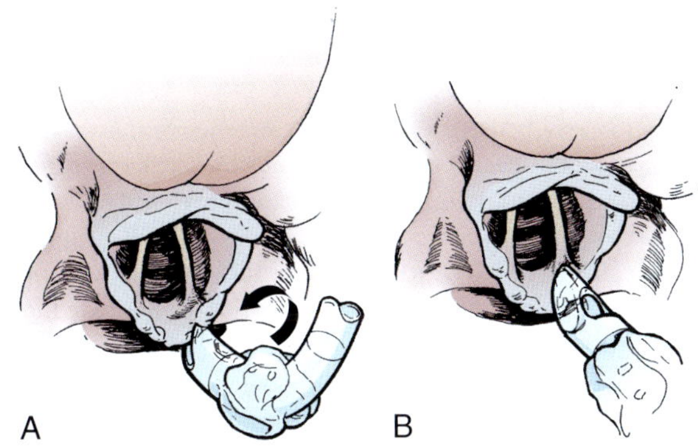

Fig. 4.41 A common problem with blind tracheal tube passage through the larynx. (A) The tip of the tube is caught on the arytenoid cartilage. (B) Rotation of tube 90 degrees counterclockwise orients the bevel of the tip posteriorly and allows passage into the larynx. (Courtesy Department of Emergency Medicine, Hennepin County Medical Center, Minneapolis, MN.)

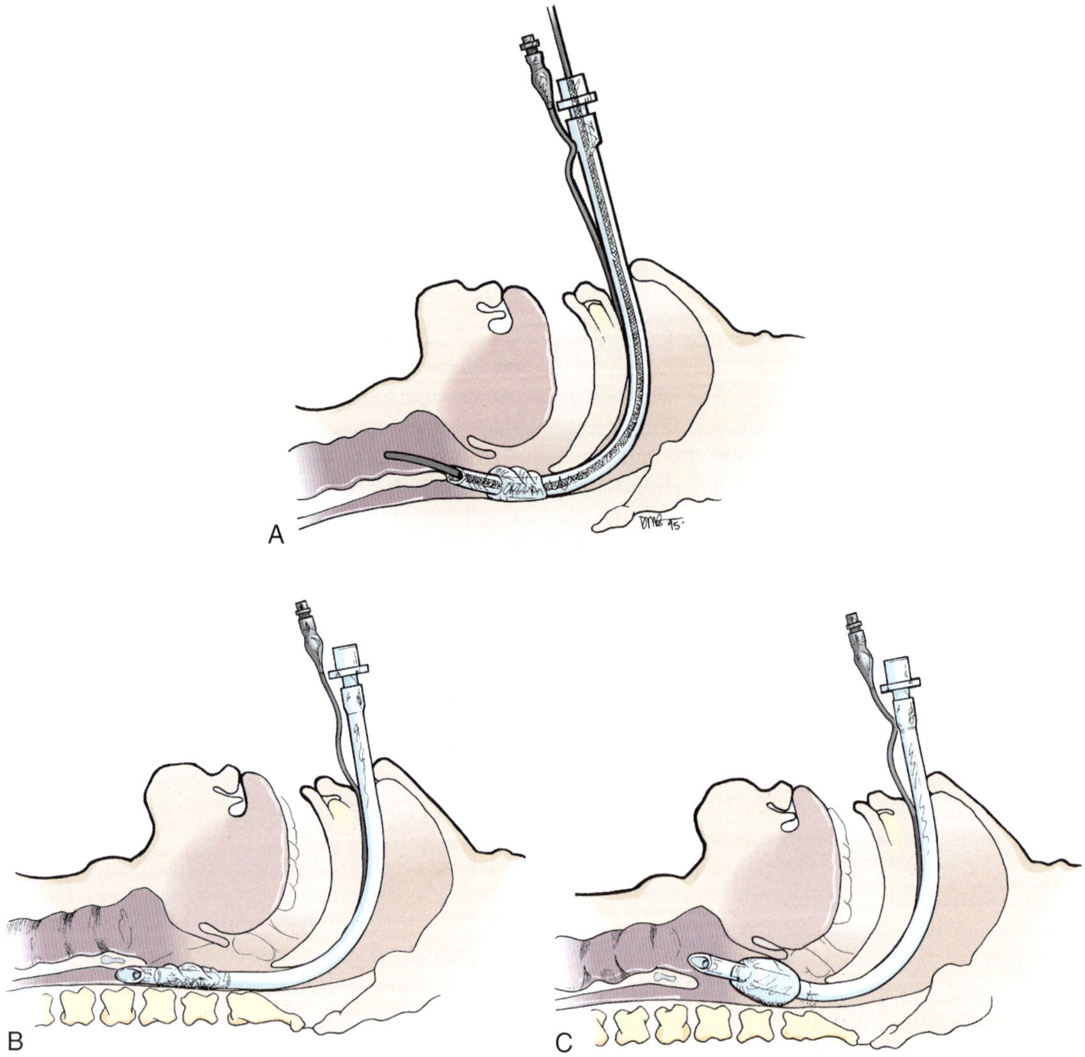

Fig. 4.42 Troubleshooting blind nasal intubation when the tube is near the glottic opening. (A) Use of suction catheter to aid in passage of a nasotracheal tube caught at the laryngeal inlet. The suction catheter is passed down the tracheal tube and into the trachea. The tracheal tube is then passed over the suction catheter, and the catheter is removed. (B) Inflating the tracheal tube cuff may help if the tube is placed posteriorly to the glottic opening. First, the tracheal tube is pulled back after passage through the esophagus. (C) Once breath sounds are heard, the cuff is inflated with 15 mL of air and readvanced into the laryngeal inlet. Once seated in the inlet, the cuff is deflated and the tube advanced into the trachea. (Courtesy Department of Emergency Medicine, Hennepin County Medical Center, Minneapolis, MN.)

that the tip is very responsive to pulling on the ring. A common mistake is exerting too much force on the ring, which can result in the tube curling up before the larynx and preventing advancement. There has been a case report of an Endotrol tube "kinking" at the point of sharpest curvature, causing difficulty with suctioning and problems with ventilation.[334] Another device that allows flexion of the distal ET tube is the Parker Flex-Tip stylet.

Laryngospasm

Laryngospasm is a common problem that arises when NT intubation is attempted. It is usually transient. Withdraw the tube slightly and wait for the patient's first gasp to advance the tube. This is frequently successful because the vocal cords are widely abducted during inhalation. Assess laryngeal anesthesia, and if topical and nebulized lidocaine have already been administered without success, consider transcricothyroid anesthesia (e.g., 2 mL of 4% lidocaine).[335] Occasionally, a jaw lift is necessary to break prolonged spasm. Another option is to use a smaller tube.

Complications

Epistaxis is the most common complication of blind NT intubation. Severe epistaxis was encountered in only 5 of 300 cases reported by Danzl and Thomas.[336] Tintinalli and Claffey[337] reported severe bleeding in 1 of 71 patients and less serious bleeding in 12 others. Bleeding is not usually a problem unless it provokes vomiting or aspiration and may be a serious potential problem in obtunded patients with trismus or a decreased gag reflex. Other immediate, less common complications include turbinate fracture, intracranial placement through a basilar skull fracture, retropharyngeal laceration or dissection, and delayed or unsuccessful placement.[320,338,339] Complications may be minimized by selecting a smaller tube and using a gentle technique.

Sinusitis in patients with an NT tube is common and can be an unrecognized cause of sepsis.[340] Rare and potentially fatal delayed complications include mediastinitis after retropharyngeal abscess[341] and massive pneumocephalus.[342]

Because most complications occur during tube advancement through the nasal passage and proximal nasopharynx, the complications of blind NT intubation and placement under direct vision are largely the same. Retropharyngeal laceration and esophageal intubation are more of a threat with blind placement techniques because they are more likely to go unrecognized.[337]

Summary

Blind NT intubation is rarely used in modern practice because of advances in emergency airway technology, and no modern algorithm includes its use. Its practice is most likely to be useful in austere settings, but it may be an effective and potentially lifesaving approach to a difficult airway.

DIGITAL INTUBATION

Digital intubation uses the index and middle fingers to blindly direct the ET tube into the larynx. It only has use in austere settings where BMV, EGDs, and surgical airway equipment are not available.

Indications and Contraindications

Digital intubation is indicated if someone requires definitive airway management and no other tools exist to manage the airway (e.g., laryngoscope, EGD, surgical airway equipment). If a patient can be ventilated with BMV or an extraglottic airway, or intubated by other means, digital intubation should not be performed. Digital intubation may be helpful in situations with abnormal patient positioning (e.g., in an extrication situation), or when standard intubation equipment is unavailable or malfunctioning, and no other approaches are possible. Contraindications are primarily precautions to protect the clinician. Digital intubation should not be attempted in any patient with a significant risk of biting.

Procedure and Technique

Place the patient's head and neck in the neutral position. Stand at the patient's right side, facing the patient. Introduce your left index and middle fingers into the right angle of the patient's mouth and slide them along the surface of the tongue until the epiglottis is felt. The tip of the epiglottis should be palpated 8 to 10 cm from the corner of the mouth in average adults. Use of a stylet in the tube is optional, and the largest reported series had good success without a stylet.[343] For a clinician with short fingers or a patient with an anterior larynx, a stylet is advantageous. If a stylet is used, place it in the tube and bend it into the form of an open J with the distal end terminating in a gentle hook. Introduce a lubricated tube from the patient's left side between the tongue and the rescuer's two fingers (Fig. 4.43). Cradle the tube between two fingers and guide the tip beneath the epiglottis. Apply gentle anterior pressure to direct the tube into the larynx. If the clinician has sufficiently long fingers, place them posterior to the arytenoids to act as a "backstop" for the tube, to both avoid esophageal passage and assist in laryngeal placement.[344] If a stylet has been used, withdraw it at this time while simultaneously advancing the tube. An alternative to using a stylet for directing the tube anteriorly is to select an ET tube with a controllable tip (Endotrol; Mallinckrodt Medical).

A variation of the technique of digital intubation has been described for intubating a newborn.[345] In this technique, only the index finger is used to guide the tube into the larynx. Bend the end of the tube and moisten both the tube and the finger with sterile water. Use the index finger of the nondominant hand to follow the tongue posteriorly and palpate the epiglottis and paired arytenoids. Use the thumb of the same hand to apply cricoid pressure and steady the larynx. Hold the ET tube in the dominant hand and advance it with the nondominant index finger used as a guide. The tube will encounter subtle resistance as it enters the trachea, and palpation of the tube through the trachea provides further confirmation of correct placement. A styletted tube, shaped in the form of a J, is usually desired until familiarity with the procedure is achieved.

Complications

The risk associated with esophageal intubation is always present, and the potential for esophageal misplacement is increased in comatose or cardiac arrest patients. If used in patients with a gag reflex, induction of emesis with aspiration is a risk. The greatest risk seems to be to the clinician, whose fingers may be bitten.

Summary

Most experience with digital intubation in adults has been prehospital use, and it can also be used in other austere settings. Video-assisted devices and EGDs have rendered digital intubation obsolete in other settings, and there is no good reason to use this technique if other airway equipment is available.

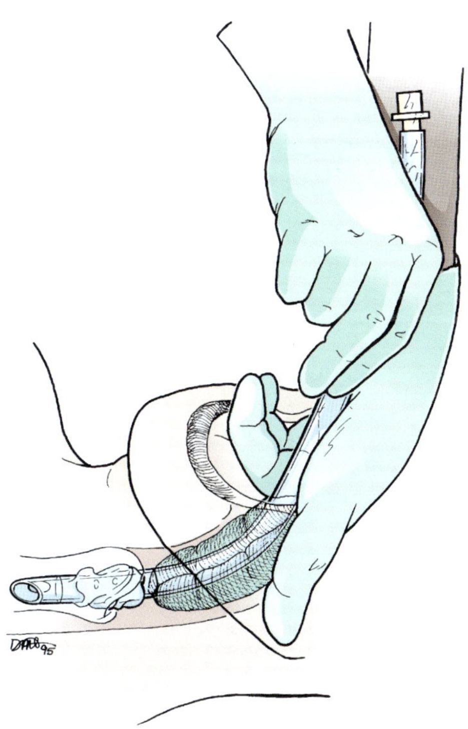

Fig. 4.43 Digital intubation. The tracheal tube is cradled between the index and middle fingers and guided into the glottic opening. (Courtesy Department of Emergency Medicine, Hennepin County Medical Center, Minneapolis, MN.)

Use of an EGD or performing a cricothyrotomy is probably preferable to blind intubation.

RETROGRADE INTUBATION

See Videos 4.22–4.24. Retrograde orotracheal intubation is a technique of guided ET intubation that involves the use of a wire or catheter placed percutaneously through the cricothyroid membrane or proximal trachea and exiting through the mouth or nose (Review Box 4.5). An ET tube is then passed over this guide and advanced through the vocal cords into the trachea. Introduced by Butler and Cirillo in 1960,[346] the technique has undergone several recent modifications that have enhanced its value as a means of establishing a definitive airway when more conventional techniques have failed. If the intubator does not have experience with this technique or does not have the necessary equipment, a cricothyrotomy should be performed.

Indications and Contraindications

Retrograde intubation is indicated when definitive airway control is required and less invasive methods have failed. Indications include trismus, ankylosis of the jaw or cervical spine, upper airway masses or swelling, unstable cervical spine injuries, and maxillofacial trauma.

It was used successfully in a 1-month-old with developmental abnormalities.[347] It can be particularly helpful in trauma patients with airway bleeding that prevents visualization of the glottis.[348]

Contraindications to retrograde intubation include the availability of a less invasive means of airway control and inability to open the mouth. If rapid control of the airway is needed, consider other alternate strategies including a cricothyrotomy because retrograde intubation takes several minutes to set up and perform.

Equipment

Materials include (1) local anesthetic and skin preparation material, (2) an 18-gauge needle, (3) a 60-cm epidural catheter-needle combination or an 80-cm (0.88-mm diameter) spring guidewire (J tip preferred), (4) a hemostat, (5) long forceps (e.g., Magill) for grasping the wire in the pharynx, (6) an ET tube of appropriate size, (7) a syringe for the tube cuff, and (8) material for securing the tube. A prepackaged alternative is the Cook Retrograde intubation set, which also contains a sheath.

Procedure and Technique

Locate the three important anatomic landmarks by palpation: hyoid bone, thyroid cartilage, and cricoid cartilage. Prepare the skin overlying the cricothyroid membrane and anesthetize it. Maintain a cephalad orientation of the needle bevel, and puncture the lower half of the cricothyroid membrane (Fig. 4.45). Alternatively, the needle puncture can be made below the cricoid ring into the trachea. The advantage of a lower puncture is that the needle entry site is further away from the glottic inlet and the sheath or ET tube is less likely to fall into the esophagus during the procedure.

After the needle has entered the trachea, direct the needle slightly cephalad. Aspirate air to confirm position of the tip of the needle within the lumen of the larynx.

Remove the syringe and pass the wire through the needle. Advance it until it is seen in the patient's mouth or until it exits the nose. A laryngoscope may facilitate this process. If the wire is found in the hypopharynx, grasp it with the Magill forceps and draw it out through the mouth. Remove the needle from the neck and secure the end of the wire at the puncture site with a hemostat. The next steps will depend on whether a plastic sheath, also referred to as an *obturator*, is available.

If no sheath is available, thread the oral end of the wire in through the ET tube side port (not the end of the tube) and advance it up the tube until it exits through the top. Threading the wire through the side port allows the tip of the tube to protrude 1 cm beyond the point at which the wire enters the larynx. Pull the wire taut and move it back and forth to ensure that no slack remains. Advance the ET tube over the wire until resistance is met. This is the most critical point in the procedure. Because retrograde intubation is a blind technique, it

Retrograde Intubation

Indications

Need for a definitive airway when other methods have failed
Trismus
Ankylosis of the jaw or cervical spine
Upper airway masses
Unstable cervical spine fractures
Maxillofacial trauma

Contraindications

Availability of less invasive means of airway control
Inability to open the mouth
Need for rapid airway control

Complications

Hemorrhage
Subcutaneous emphysema
Soft tissue infection
Failure to achieve intubation

Equipment

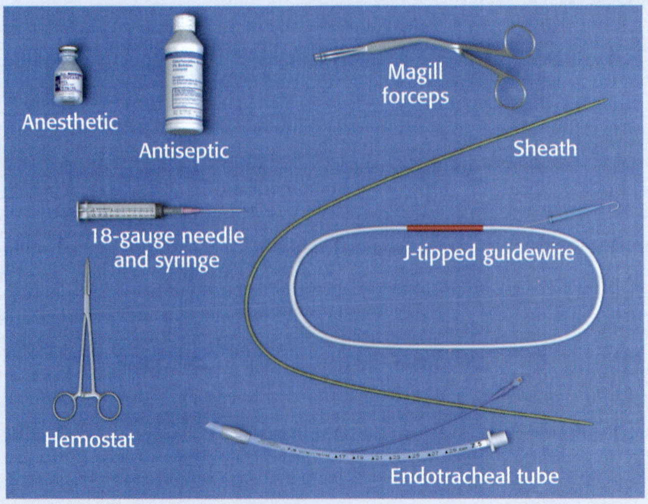

Review Box 4.5 Retrograde intubation.

may be difficult to determine whether the tube has entered the trachea or is impeded by more proximal structures. If the ET tube has successfully passed through the vocal cords and is being restricted by the guidewire as it traverses the anterior laryngeal wall, the clinician should feel some caudally directed tension on the wire at its laryngeal insertion point. If this does not occur, the tip of the ET tube may be proximal to the vocal cords, in the vallecula, in a piriform sinus, or abutting the narrow anterior aspect of the vocal cords. If in doubt, pull the tube back 2 cm, rotate it 90 degrees counterclockwise, and then readvance the tube. This will usually result in successful passage through the larynx.[309] When satisfied that the tube has entered the trachea, stabilize the tube and pull the guidewire out through the mouth. Some clinicians prefer to pull the guidewire through the neck to lessen the risk of tube dislodgement, though this creates the theoretical risk of soft tissue infection of the neck. Once the wire is removed, advance the tube farther into the trachea.

The classic method of retrograde intubation, as just described, is made easier with the addition of a plastic sheath that is passed antegrade over the wire until it meets resistance where the wire penetrates the laryngeal mucosa (Fig. 4.44).[349]

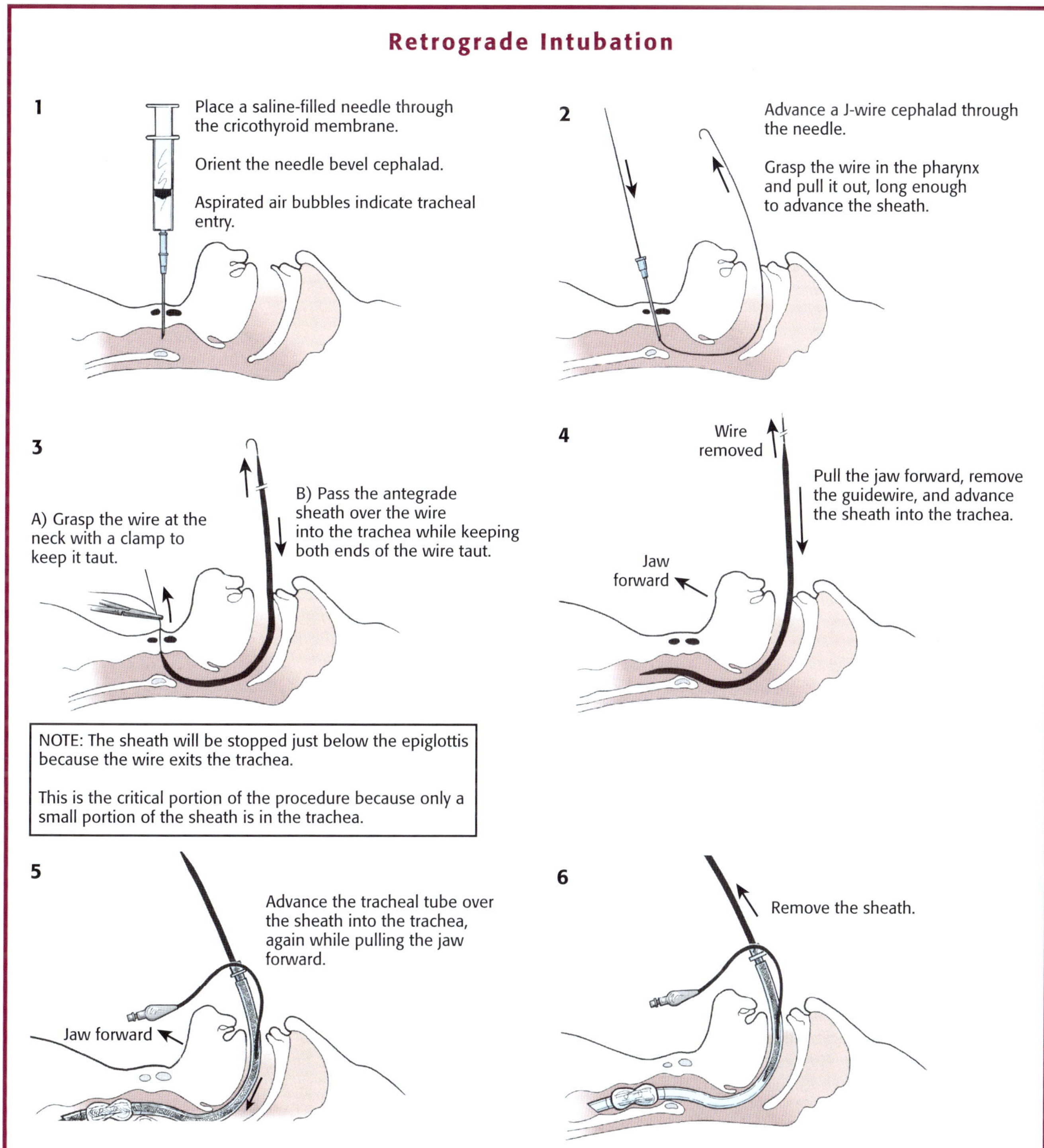

Fig. 4.44 Retrograde intubation using a guidewire and antegrade sheath. (Courtesy Department of Emergency Medicine, Hennepin County Medical Center, Minneapolis, MN.)

This sheath needs to be stiff enough to effectively guide an ET tube, yet small enough to easily pass through the vocal cords without impinging on any supraglottic or glottic structures.

If a sheath is available, after grasping the wire from the mouth, thread the plastic sheath over the wire until it comes to rest against the anterior laryngeal wall. Withdraw the wire from the mouth or neck and advance the sheath. Once the sheath is well within the trachea, pass the ET tube over the sheath. If any resistance at the arytenoids or vocal cords is encountered, pull the tube back 1 to 2 cm and rotate it 90 degrees counterclockwise. One advantage of the antegrade sheath is that it lies freely in the larynx, allowing more posterior passage through the widest distance between the cords. In contrast, the wire pulls the ET tube anteriorly toward the narrow commissure of the vocal cords and is more likely to result in impingement of the tube on the cords. In addition, use of the sheath permits unrestricted advancement of the ET tube, and a wire entering the larynx 1.0 to 1.5 cm below the vocal cords prevents the tube from advancing more than this distance before wire removal.

If no sheath is available, consider placing the needle inferiorly in the trachea, thereby increasing the distance that the ET tube can be advanced before being stopped by the wire.[350] This will decrease the likelihood of dislodging the tip of the ET tube when the guidewire is withdrawn.

Complications

The complications of retrograde intubation are largely related to puncture of the cricothyroid membrane (see Chapter 6). The potential for hemorrhage is minimized by taking care to puncture the cricothyroid membrane in its lower half to avoid the cricothyroid artery. Subcutaneous emphysema may occur, and it is of no clinical significance because no air is insufflated during this technique. A small incidence of soft tissue infection is reported with translaryngeal needle procedures.

Summary

Retrograde intubation is a technique that can achieve tracheal intubation in a patient who cannot be intubated by less aggressive means. It is more invasive than fiberoptic intubation and requires less skill. Retrograde intubation usually takes several minutes to complete,[344] and the patient can undergo BMV throughout much of the procedure. Its use has been minimized because modern algorithms rightly emphasize cricothyrotomy above retrograde intubation.

CHANGING TRACHEAL TUBES

A tracheal tube with a leaking cuff is a vexing problem, especially if the original intubation was difficult. A method of replacing the tube without losing control of the tracheal lumen is preferred. This can be achieved by passing a guide down the defective tube, withdrawing the tube while leaving the guide in place and introducing a new tube over the guide and into the trachea (Fig. 4.45).

A number of different guides have been described (e.g., simple nasogastric tubes, 18-Fr Salem sump tubes, feeding tubes), and they are poor substitutes for a bougie. Tracheal tube exchangers are also available and can be used successfully for tube exchange and are less stiff than a bougie. Bougies are generally easier to locate in the airway cart and intubators are more familiar with their use.

Advantages of using a bougie or tube exchanger include the following: they are long enough to allow deep placement within the airway while allowing easy exchange of the ET tubes, stiff enough to prevent dislodgment when the ET tube is introduced, and ready to use without modification.

Procedure and Technique

Before the procedure, sedate and restrain the patient properly. Preoxygenate the patient before placing the guide through the existing tube. Consider inserting a video laryngoscope to lift the tongue and soft tissues out of the way and visualize the tube exchange. Lubricate the guide and advance it into the defective tube so that it is well within the tracheal lumen (for adults, approximately 30 cm). Withdraw the defective tube over the guide and take care not to dislodge the guide when removing the tube. Slide the replacement tube over the guide and gently advance it into the trachea. At this juncture, it may be helpful to perform a jaw-thrust or chin-lift maneuver to facilitate passage through the pharynx. Resistance may be encountered at the laryngeal inlet or vocal cords. If this occurs, withdraw the tube 1 to 2 cm, rotate it 90 degrees counterclockwise, and readvance it. If there is any difficulty, visualize tube passage with a video laryngoscope. After the tube is visualized clearly in the trachea, remove the guide, inflate the cuff, and ventilate the patient. After correct placement has been verified, secure the new tube.

Complications are related to the time required to change the tube. A successfully performed procedure can be accomplished within 30 seconds. Laryngeal injury from forcing the exchange guide or the new ET tube can occur, and this can be mitigated by using lubricant and gentle pressure during the procedure.

An alternative method to exchange a defective tube is to use a video laryngoscope to obtain a view of the glottis (Fig. 4.46). A bougie is then passed into the airway adjacent to the tube so that both the defective tube and the bougie enter and occupy the trachea. Once it is confirmed that the bougie is definitively in the trachea (i.e., it lies between the arytenoid cartilages and the epiglottis), the defective tube is removed and a new tube is advanced over the bougie. The advantage of this technique is that ventilation can be maintained just up until removal of the defective tube.

PREVENTING UNPLANNED EXTUBATION

Unplanned extubation is undesirable and can be medically disastrous if unrecognized or if the medical condition requires immediate reintubation. Not all extubations can be prevented. They most often occur when patients suddenly pull out their own tube or during transport. It is not uncommon for a deceased patient to arrive at the medical examiner with a tube in an incorrect position that was dislodged during transit. Unplanned extubation is best prevented with the use of physical restraints, appropriate analgesia and sedation, and careful attention to the integrity of the ET tube position

Replacing a Malfunctioning Endotracheal Tube

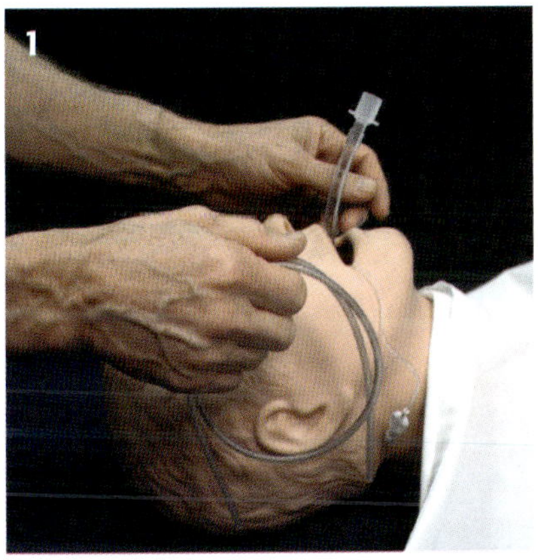

Preoxygenate and sedate the patient as clinically indicated.

The procedure here is demonstrated with an 80-mm TTX tube exchanger (Hudson Respiratory Care).

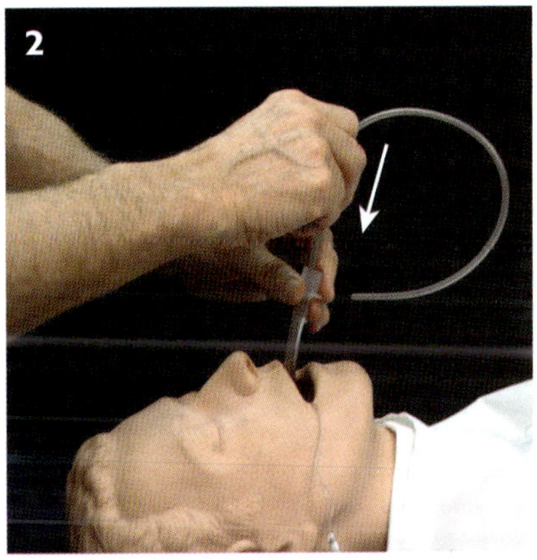

Pass the tube exchanger through the defective ET tube deep into the airway.

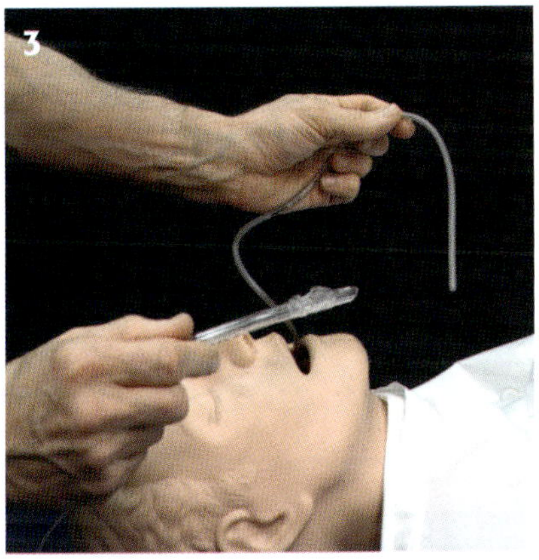

Remove the defective tube and leave the tube exchanger in place as a guiding stylet.

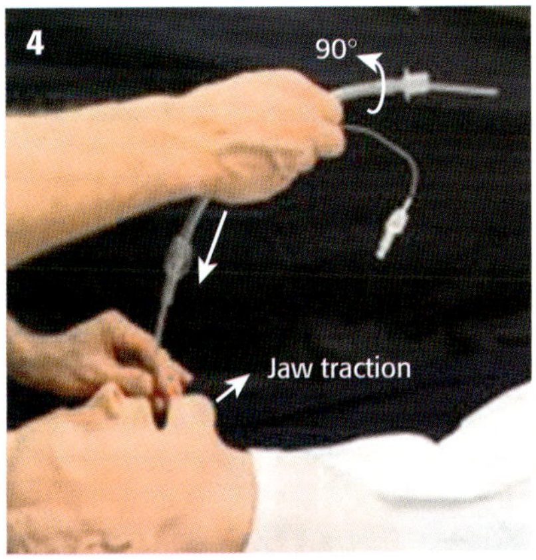

Pass a new ET tube over the tube exchanger and into the airway.

A 90° counterclockwise tube rotation and jaw traction will help the tube pass into the laryngeal inlet.

Use a laryngoscope to elevate soft tissues if necessary.

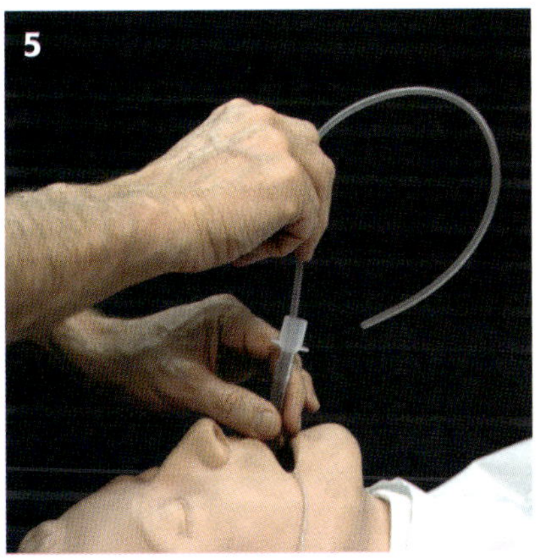

Place the ET tube into the trachea to the desired depth.

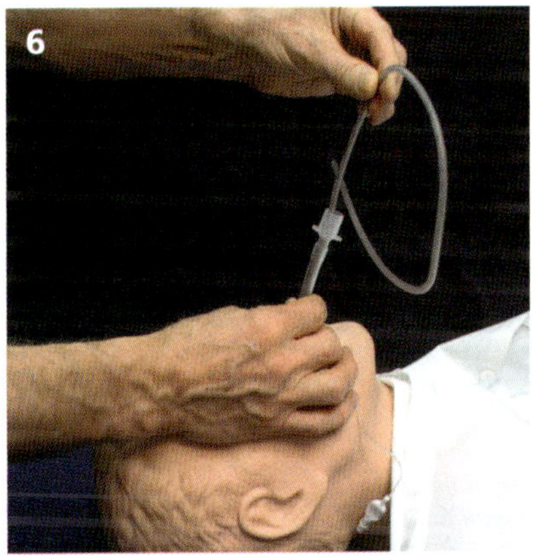

Remove the tube exchanger.

Confirm ET tube position.

Fig. 4.45 Replacing a malfunctioning endotracheal *(ET)* tube.

during procedures, such as positioning for postresuscitation chest radiographs or transfer to another bed.

CONCLUSION

Emergency airway management in critically ill or injured patients with acute airway compromise is one of the greatest challenges for clinicians. Although the definition of a difficult airway will change as our ability to visualize the laryngeal inlet continues to improve, the challenge of emergency airways will persist. Mastery of the basics of airway management and laryngoscopy, competency in a number of guided or indirect intubation techniques, and the ability to perform a surgical airway are all necessary skills for emergency airway management.

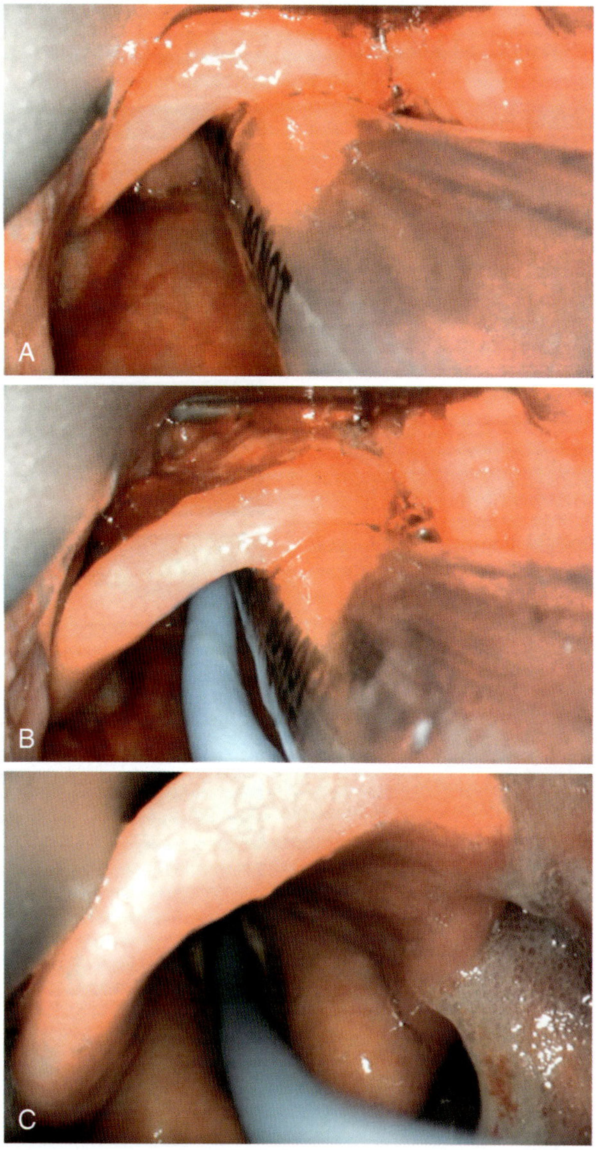

Fig. 4.46 An alternate method of exchanging a malfunctioning endotracheal tube that allows for continued ventilation during more of the procedure. (A) The malfunctioning tube and glottic opening are visualized with a video laryngoscope. (B) A bougie is passed into the airway next to the tube. When resistance is met at the level of the endotracheal tube cuff, deflate the cuff and remove the tube. Advance the bougie. (C) Now, just a bougie is in the trachea. Advance an endotracheal tube over the bougie into the trachea.

Mastery of technique, advance preparation of equipment, and experience in clinical decision-making are essential. Scenario visualization and advanced simulation models can provide an excellent means of practicing the difficult decision-making and technical maneuvers necessary for effective emergency airway management.

See Videos 4.1–4.21 for airway management procedures using various devices.

REFERENCES ARE AVAILABLE AT ELSEVIER EBOOKS+

CHAPTER 5

Pharmacologic Adjuncts to Intubation

Richard B. Schwartz, Daniel McCollum, and Ricaurte Solis

Endotracheal (ET) intubation in the emergency setting presents a challenge distinct from that associated with intubation of fasted, prescreened, and premedicated patients in the operating room (OR). Patients in the emergency department (ED) are frequently uncooperative, unstable, have medical problems, or have anatomic abnormalities that are unknown to the treating clinician. The ED clinician faces the challenge of quickly assessing and managing the patient's airway, within minutes and with scant data, while simultaneously diagnosing and managing other life-threatening problems.

In 1979 Taryle and colleagues[1] reported that complications occurred in more than half the patients intubated in a university hospital ED. They called for improved house officer training in ET intubation, including "more liberal use of the procedures and agents used in the OR, including sedatives and muscle relaxers."[1] Since this report, the use of neuromuscular blockade and rapid-sequence intubation (RSI) has become the standard for emergency medicine practice.[2,3]

In addition to RSI, emergency physicians now use airway devices such as video laryngoscopes, optical stylet, and flexible intubation video endoscopes to manage difficult and complex airways. In high-risk patients it is increasingly common for awake intubation techniques to be utilized.[4] This allows for the safe management of an emergent airway without the risk of completely eliminating the patient's airway reflexes or respiratory drive. A related approach that has been described as *delayed-sequence intubation* (DSI) has emerged in recent years.[5,6] This technique may be considered as procedural sedation to allow preoxygenation prior to intubation. Both awake intubation and DSI techniques have their own unique pharmacologic considerations. Clinicians must concentrate on the manual skills of airway management and also on selection of the appropriate drugs to achieve specific objectives. These objectives include (1) immediate airway control, including induction of unconsciousness and muscle paralysis as appropriate; (2) analgesia and sedation in awake patients; (3) minimization of the adverse physiologic effects of intubation, including systemic and intracranial hypertension; and (4) prevention of harm during the postintubation period, including inadequate sedation, hemodynamic instability, or oversedation.

This chapter reviews the mechanisms and strategic use of the drugs that are currently available to facilitate intubation in the ED.

OVERVIEW OF RAPID-SEQUENCE INTUBATION

The standard process for quickly intubating a patient in an emergency situation is referred to as *rapid-sequence intubation*. The steps in performing RSI are often described by the six "P's": preparation, preoxygenation, pretreatment, paralysis and induction, placement of the tube, and postintubation management (Fig. 5.1). This sequential technique of rapidly inducing unconsciousness (induction) combined with muscular paralysis to create optimal conditions for intubation has gained broad acceptance among ED clinicians. Often patients present with anatomical or physiological conditions that do not allow for the ideal scenario of RSI for tracheal intubation. RSI is the preferred method of emergency airway management for intubations that are not anticipated to be difficult. Awake techniques of intubation should be considered in high-risk patients with airways that are anticipated to be difficult.

Preparation occurs before and during preoxygenation. Assess the airway to determine the likelihood of a difficult intubation. Simultaneously, establish an intravenous (IV) line and connect the patient to cardiac, pulse oximetry, blood pressure, and end-tidal CO_2 monitors when available. Assemble all necessary drugs and equipment for intubation and the desired backup equipment for airway management.

Begin preoxygenation as soon as possible by administering 100% oxygen. The intent is to displace nitrogen from the lungs and replace it with an oxygen reserve that will last several minutes. Under optimal conditions in the OR setting, breathing 100% oxygen for 3 minutes has been demonstrated to maintain acceptable oxygen saturation for up to 8 minutes in previously healthy apneic individuals.[7] Another method is to give four vital capacity (maximal) breaths of 100% oxygen from a face mask, which can also maintain acceptable saturation for 6 minutes.[7] Comparable results may not be extrapolated to the ED setting because of differences in the underlying health and cooperation of the patient population. In the ED, The use of flush rate oxygen delivery through a nonrebreather mask has emerged as a rapid method of preoxygenation.[8] Preoxygenation may also be accomplished using noninvasive positive pressure ventilation or by adding a positive end-expiratory pressure (PEEP) valve to the bag-valve-mask (BVM) setup, especially in those patients with challenging oxygenation.[9]

A recent advance in preoxygenation of patients prior to intubation is the nasal oxygenation during efforts securing a tube (NO DESAT) technique.[10] In the NO DESAT or "apneic oxygenation" technique, a nasal cannula is placed underneath the nonrebreather face mask in spontaneously breathing patients or under the BVM device in patients who require ventilatory assistance. In awake patients, the nasal cannula can be comfortably set to 5 L/min of oxygen. After induction agents are given, this can be safely increased to 15 L/min of oxygen. The nasal cannula may be left on throughout the attempt to intubate, as it will not interfere with the ability to place an orotracheal tube. While there is recent evidence that NO DESAT may be associated with increased safe apnea time and improved first-pass success without hypoxemia during ET intubation in various clinical settings, robust outcome data specific to the ED are still pending.[11–15]

Pretreatment consists of the administration of medications to mitigate the potential untoward responses to intubation. Pretreatment during RSI usually occurs 2 to 5 minutes before induction of unconsciousness or muscular paralysis. The clinical utility of routine pretreatment to improve patient-oriented outcomes in ED RSI has been challenged.[16]

Paralysis and induction involve the induction of a state of unconsciousness with a sedative agent, followed immediately by muscle paralysis with a neuromuscular blocker (NMB). A protocol for ED-based RSI is summarized in Box 5.1.

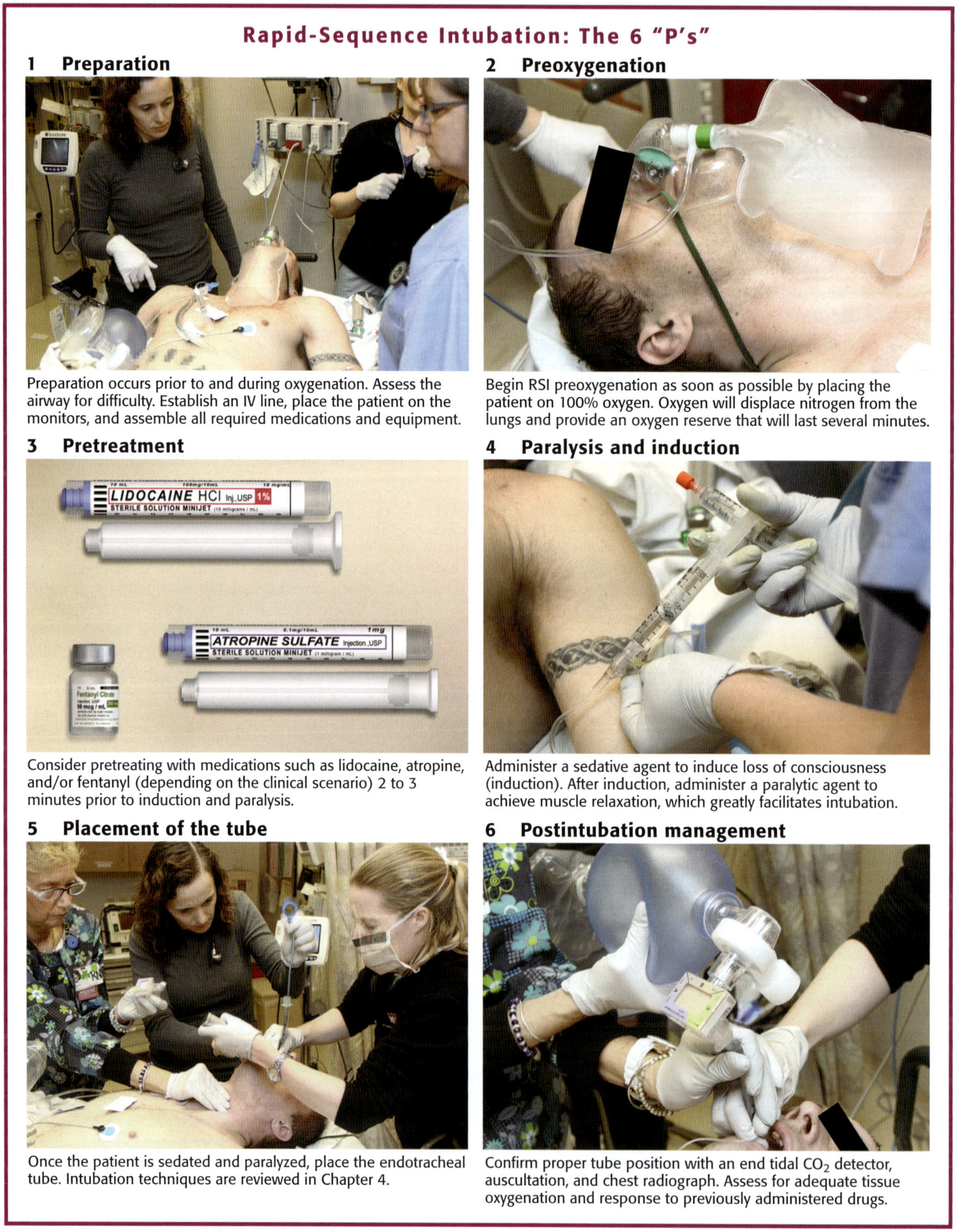

Fig. 5.1 The 6 "P's" of rapid-sequence intubation. *IV,* Intravenous; *RSI,* rapid-sequence intubation.

BOX 5.1 Rapid-Sequence Intubation Protocol

1. Preoxygenate (denitrogenate) the lungs by providing 100% oxygen by mask. Apply nasal cannula at high flow at this time if using nasal cannula for apneic oxygenation.
2. Assemble the equipment required:
   - Bag-valve mask device connected to an oxygen delivery system.
   - Suction with a Yankauer tip.
   - ET tube with an intact cuff, stylet, syringe, and tape.
   - Laryngoscope and blades, in working order.
   - Backup airway equipment.
3. Check to be sure that a functioning, secure intravenous line is in place.
4. Continuously monitor cardiac rhythm and oxygen saturation.
5. Premedicate as appropriate:
   - Fentanyl: 2 to 3 μg/kg given at a rate of 1 to 2 μg/kg per min intravenously.
   - Atropine: 0.02 mg/kg by intravenous push for children or adolescents.
   - Lidocaine: 1.5 to 2 mg/kg intravenously over a period of 30 to 60 seconds.
6. Induce anesthesia with one of the following agents administered intravenously: ketamine, etomidate, fentanyl, midazolam, or propofol.
7. Give succinylcholine, 1.5 mg/kg by intravenous push (use 2 mg/kg for infants and small children) or rocuronium 1.2 mg/kg.
8. Apnea, jaw relaxation, and/or decreased resistance to bag-mask ventilation (use only when oxygenation before rapid-sequence intubation cannot be optimized by spontaneous ventilation) indicates that the patient is sufficiently relaxed to proceed with intubation.
9. Perform ET intubation. If unable to intubate during the first 20-second attempt, stop and ventilate the patient with the bag-mask device for 30 to 60 seconds. Monitor pulse oximetry readings as a guide.
10. Treat bradycardia occurring during intubation with atropine, 0.5 mg by intravenous push (smaller dose for children; see item 5).
11. Once intubation is completed, inflate the cuff and confirm ET tube placement by auscultating for bilateral breath sounds and checking the pulse oximetry and capnography readings. Ultrasound for lung sliding on both sides may be a useful adjunct.
12. Secure the ET tube.

ET, *Endotracheal.*

ET intubation and RSI have also expanded beyond the ED into the prehospital setting. Prehospital RSI protocols use a sedative plus a paralytic for patients not in cardiac arrest, with success rates as high as 92% to 98%.[17–21] Without a full complement of medications, prehospital intubation becomes significantly more difficult, and success rates drop to approximately 60%.[22] Rates of misplaced ET tubes and complications by paramedics may be much higher than previously reported.[23,24] Studies indicate that outcomes may be worse for patients with traumatic brain injury intubated in the prehospital setting than in the ED.[25] For these reasons, many US-based prehospital systems have moved away from the use of RSI.

The technique for proper ET tube placement is discussed in Chapter 4. Postintubation monitoring should assess for proper tube placement, adequate tissue oxygenation, and response to previously administered drugs. After laryngoscopy, ensure ongoing analgesic and anxiolytic therapy.

PRETREATMENT: PREVENTING THE COMPLICATIONS OF INTUBATION

The process of tracheal intubation triggers various physiological responses, and efforts have been made to mitigate the negative effects caused by these responses. It is certain that intubation and adjunctive medications have the potential to alter reflexes, intracranial pressure (ICP), blood pressure, and pulse rate and may induce disturbances in cardiac rhythm. The actual clinical consequences of these commonly observed changes are largely unknown. Clinical experience suggests that most alterations in physiology occurring with ED intubation are transient, produce no long-term sequelae, and/or cannot easily be prevented. Prudent clinicians should consider potential adverse effects of intubation and be cognizant of methods to minimize them. Careful monitoring of postintubation conditions will guide specific interventions.

Overzealous attempts to suppress the physiologic responses that normally accompany airway manipulation may be counterproductive. It would be desirable to provide airway control under the best of circumstances and with the least amount of injury to the patient. The ideal approach to the physiologic responses to intubation is simply unknown. Most information has been extrapolated from experimental animal models or from the anesthesia experience and similar issues may not apply to the milieu of the ED experience. Avoiding periintubation hypotension, hypoxia, and acidosis is critically important, especially in patients with neurological injury.[26] Patients who theoretically would benefit the most from pretreatment medications are those who may be least able to tolerate any delay in securing a definitive airway. The following discussion serves as a general clinical guide to alterations in the physiologic response to intubation.

Pressor Response

The pressor response is a sympathetic reflex that occurs during laryngoscopy and intubation due to stimulation of the orolaryngopharynx. In addition to the ubiquitous sinus tachycardia, a number of dysrhythmias have been reported after intubation. They are primarily ventricular in origin and include ectopic beats, bigeminy, and short runs of ventricular tachycardia. No studies have established a direct relationship between the response and subsequent clinical deterioration in large patient populations. It is also unclear whether attenuation of the pressor response prevents dysrhythmias or electrocardiographic evidence of ischemia. It would be desirable to avoid sudden increases in heart rate or blood pressure in unstable patients with acute cardiac or vascular disease. It is unclear if outcomes are improved by attempting to mitigate the pressor response.[27]

Multiple medications have been evaluated to attempt to reduce the pressor response. Lidocaine has been the most extensively evaluated, and it has not been shown to improve outcomes.[27] A dose of 1.5 to 2 mg/kg may slightly reduce the heart rate or blood pressure increase caused by intubation.[28] One small trial demonstrated that nebulized tetracaine reduced increases in heart rate during intubation, and this is not commonly done in emergency practice.[29] Fentanyl dosed at 2 to 5 µg/kg is more likely to be effective at blunting the pressor response than lidocaine.[30,31] Fentanyl will be discussed in more detail later, in relation to its possible benefit in preventing increases in ICP.

Lidocaine and fentanyl are the drugs with the largest evidence base supporting their use to decrease the pressor response. Other drugs, including thiopental, sodium nitroprusside, labetalol, nitroglycerin, verapamil, nifedipine, clonidine, fentanyl, sufentanil, etomidate, magnesium, esmolol, and dexmedetomidine, have shown variable responses.[32–35] Due to the uncertainty of the benefit of any premedication in improving patient outcomes, these other medications cannot be recommended for routine use. In patients at very high risk for harm by transient increases in heart rate or hypertension (such as those experiencing hypertensive emergency or having an active myocardial infarction), it would be reasonable to consider fentanyl or lidocaine. There is a lack of literature to support improvement of patient-oriented outcomes, and it is also reasonable to not premedicate these patients.

Hypotension

A more pressing concern for most patients intubated in the ED is the importance of avoiding hypotension. Postintubation hemodynamic instability occurs in over 10% of emergency intubations.[36] Unlike the uncertainty regarding patient harm because of transient hypertension, transient hypotension is associated with poor patient outcomes.[37,38] This is of even higher concern in patients with known or suspected traumatic brain injury.[39]

Avoid hypotension by initiating adequate resuscitation prior to attempts at intubation. If the patient's clinical condition permits, pursue appropriate volume resuscitation with blood in actively bleeding patients and fluids in hypovolemic patients prior to intubation. A recent trial demonstrated the failure of routine fluid bolus prior to intubation to reduce cardiovascular collapse.[40] This should not discourage a clinician from administering fluids if clinically indicated in a hypovolemic patient, as these patients were excluded from this trial.

Even relatively hemodynamically stable drugs, such as etomidate, may contribute to hypotension in critically ill patients by reducing the endogenous catecholamine response.[41,42] The physiologic changes that contribute to hypotension following intubation include both the reduced venous return from positive pressure ventilation and the effects of medications given during intubation. It is a challenge to balance the need for airway control and the need to adequately resuscitate prior to intubation.

Once hypotension has occurred during or after intubation, the fastest way to correct this is with the use of vasopressors. If time permits clinically, it is advisable to start vasopressors prior to attempting to intubate if a patient is already hypotensive. Due to the logistics in setting up a vasopressor infusion through a pump, there has been recent increased attention to the use of push-dose vasopressors to treat periintubation hypotension (Box 5.2 and Fig. 5.2).[43–45] Push-dose pressors may be mixed at the bedside using local guidance and protocols; however, due to safety issues, we recommend using commercial or pharmacy preprepared ready-to-use syringes when available. Further details about how to mix a dilute solution of vasopressor for this purpose will be provided later. It is reasonable to give push-dose vasopressors through a peripheral IV line to avoid further delays in intubation by central line placement.[45]

BOX 5.2 How to Make Push-Dose Epinephrine Using Code Cart Epinephrine[a]

1. Gather materials: 10-mL syringe filled with saline, blunt-tip needle, and 10-mL syringe of 1 mg in 10-mL epinephrine from code cart (Fig. 5.2A).
2. Waste 1 mL of saline into sink (Fig. 5.2B). This will result in 9 mL of saline in a 10-mL syringe.
3. Draw up 1 mL of epinephrine (100 µg) from the code cart epinephrine into the 9 mL saline syringe using the blunt-tip needle. This creates a 10-µg/mL epinephrine solution (or 100 µg in 10-mL syringe) (Fig. 5.2C).
4. Shake vigorously after drawing a little air into syringe to evenly mix (Fig. 5.2D).
5. Clearly label syringe as epinephrine 10 µg/mL. This syringe must be clearly labeled to avoid unintentional bolus of 100 µg of epinephrine if someone mistook it for a regular saline flush (Fig. 5.2E).
6. Administer 1 mL to 2 mL (i.e., 10 µg to 20 µg) epinephrine every 2 to 5 minutes IV as needed for hypotension.

[a]*To minimize errors we recommend using commercially or pharmacy prepared push-dose products when available. Follow local institutional protocols if preparing medications at the bedside.*

Although current patient-oriented data on whether push-dose pressors improve outcomes in hypotensive patients are lacking, the clear harm of even transient hypotension makes the use of these agents a reasonable approach until additional data are generated. Care must be taken to avoid errors in mixing and administration of these potent vasoactive agents.[46]

Intracranial Hypertension

Stimulation of the respiratory tract by maneuvers such as laryngoscopy, tracheal intubation, and ET suctioning is commonly associated with a brief rise in ICP. The exact mechanism responsible for this rise is unknown. One potential mechanism is the coughing and gagging that frequently follow manipulation of the upper airway and subsequent transmission of intrathoracic pressure to the cerebral circulation. An alternative explanation is the release of catecholamines that accompanies laryngoscopy, which causes a rise in mean arterial pressure and cerebral perfusion pressure. A small rise in ICP has been reported after the administration of succinylcholine. The value of pretreatment with defasciculating doses of NMBs to prevent rises in ICP is unknown.[47]

Although the exact significance of a transient rise in ICP is not known, it is possible that it may be detrimental in patients with head trauma and/or intracranial hypertension. This theoretical harm comes from a possible reduction in cerebral blood flow if a rise in intracranial hypertension is not compensated for by a rise in systemic blood pressure. Several drugs, including lidocaine, succinylcholine, and the majority of anesthesia induction agents, have been studied to determine whether their use prevents this response. Many of the existing clinical data are not particularly relevant to the ED setting because they are derived from patients in various stages of general anesthesia, during which a wide variety of drug combinations and doses are utilized.

Good evidence suggests that deep general anesthesia prevents the rise in ICP associated with intubation. Depending on

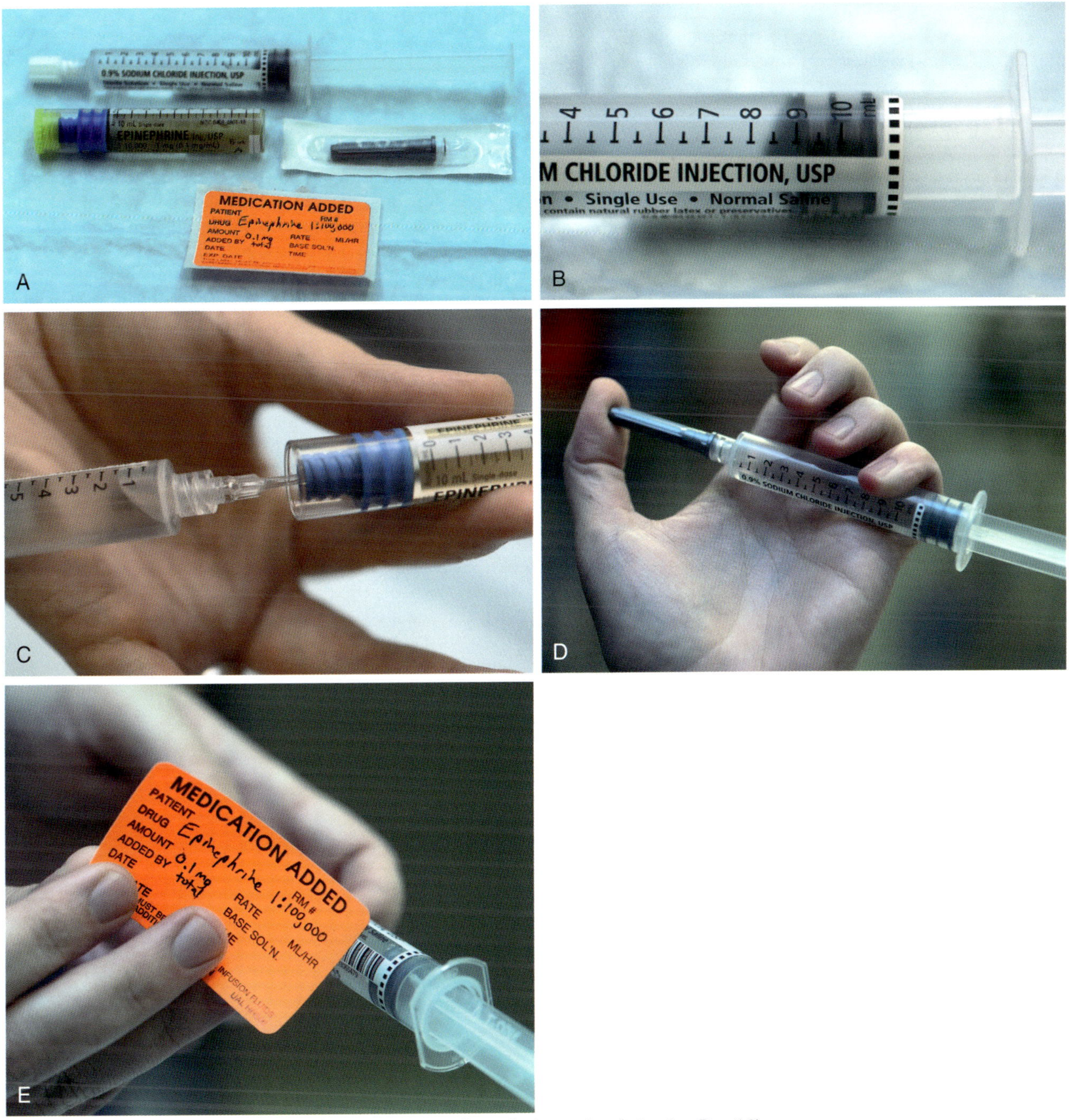

Fig. 5.2 How to make push-dose epinephrine (see Box 5.2).

the drug used, anesthesia may compromise cardiovascular performance and critically reduce cerebral blood flow.[48] The ideal anesthetic agents to facilitate intubation of patients with acute intracranial pathology may be those that have minimal effects on cardiovascular performance, such as etomidate or fentanyl. Etomidate has been demonstrated to prevent changes in both cerebral perfusion pressure and ICP after tracheal intubation of patients with space-occupying intracranial lesions.[49]

Fentanyl is perhaps the agent with the best evidence supporting its use in the prevention of increased ICP during intubation.[26,30,31] The dose is 2 to 5 µg/kg and is higher than dosages typically used for other indications of fentanyl. To be effective, this dose must be given well before intubation, preferably at least 3 minutes prior to intubation.[50]

Ketamine has been traditionally contraindicated in patients with head injuries, but this has come into question.[41,51] Whereas there may be minimal increases in ICP with ketamine, this effect is offset by a rise in systemic blood pressure. This appears to preserve cerebral blood flow and may in fact be cerebroprotective.[52,53] There are no current studies that have demonstrated poor patient outcomes due to the use of ketamine in critically ill patients.[54] See Box 5.3 for a sample protocol for the intubation of a head-injured adult patient.

Atropine for Prevention of Bradycardia

Bradycardia is not infrequent during intubation, especially in young children and neonates. Traditionally, premedication with atropine has been advocated to reduce the incidence of bradycardia.[55] A dose of 0.02 mg/kg (maximum of 0.5 mg in children) given intravenously is the standard dose for premedication. While there may be a slight decrease in the incidence of bradycardia with this medication, most studies cited to support premedication with atropine prior to RSI were undertaken in the OR setting and involved repeated doses of succinylcholine.[56] Patient-oriented outcomes have not been proven to benefit.[50,55] It is not unreasonable to use atropine only in response to bradycardia, as opposed to using it as a premedication.

BOX 5.3 Sample Protocol for Intubation of a Head-Injured Adult Patient[a]

1. Preoxygenate with 100% O_2 for 2 to 3 minutes.
2. Administer lidocaine, 1.5 to 2 mg/kg intravenously.
3. Sedate with fentanyl, 3 to 5 µg/kg.
4. Induce anesthesia with etomidate, 0.3 mg/kg.
5. Paralyze with succinylcholine, 1.5 mg/kg or rocuronium 1.2 mg/kg.
6. Perform intubation.
7. Maintain postintubation analgesia and sedation.
8. Maintain paralysis if indicated.

[a]*The benefit of this traditional protocol is unproved but can be supported if contraindications do not exist.*

Bronchospasm

Patients with reactive airway disease may have further bronchospasm during the process of intubation. Lidocaine has traditionally been used to decrease the incidence of bronchospasm in asthma patients who require intubation. A dose of 1.5 to 3 mg/kg given intravenously has been advocated.[27] This medication has not been proven to reduce the incidence of bronchospasm, but nebulized albuterol has shown some benefit.[57]

The clinical consequences of intubation-induced physiologic changes are not thoroughly understood currently. The role of drugs in preventing these changes is equally unclear. Despite this lack of data, it may be intuitively reasonable to attempt to protect patients at theoretical risk.

INDUCTION AGENTS

After premedication, a sedative agent is used to induce loss of consciousness. Numerous drugs are available in the ED to induce unconsciousness before intubation, including barbiturates, benzodiazepines, etomidate, ketamine, opiates, and propofol. The choice of a particular induction agent depends on the experience and training of the clinician, the patient's clinical status, drug characteristics, and institutional protocols (Box 5.4). Considerable evidence indicates that the selected sedative agent influences the quality of intubation conditions and the rapidity of their attainment. These effects persist even when paralytic agents are used. Commonly used drugs and their doses are summarized in Table 5.1.

BOX 5.4 Recommendations for Sedation of Patients Undergoing Rapid-Sequence Intubation in Specific Circumstances

The most appropriate medications for sedation before rapid-sequence intubation are based on evaluation of the clinical scenario, and no specific recommendations are appropriate for all circumstances. Different situations, too complex to list here, lend themselves to the use of certain agents (see text). There are no specific standards that must be followed, and the medical literature can be confusing, contradictory, or inadequate. The following conditions and sedation agent recommendations may guide the clinician. Note that appropriate paralytic drugs should also be used.

HEAD INJURY OR POTENTIALLY ELEVATED INTRACRANIAL PRESSURE

Pretreatment with the various medications described in the text are appropriate but of unproven value. Adequate cerebral perfusion pressure should be maintained to prevent secondary brain injury. Etomidate is traditionally suggested for induction of these patients, but ketamine is also likely to be safe in this population. For hypotensive patients, etomidate or ketamine may be used.

STATUS EPILEPTICUS

Propofol, ketamine, midazolam, or thiopental may be used for induction. Reduced doses should be used in the unusual circumstance of seizure with hypotension. Midazolam may be used for induction in those with adequate blood pressures.

HEMODYNAMICALLY STABLE PATIENT WITH SEVERE BRONCHOSPASM

Induction with ketamine or propofol is suggested. Etomidate and midazolam are acceptable alternatives. In hemodynamically unstable patients with severe bronchospasm, ketamine is suggested. Thiopental should not be used in these patients because it provokes release of histamine and can induce or exacerbate bronchospasm.

PATIENTS WITH CARDIOVASCULAR COMPROMISE

Both ketamine and etomidate are relatively hemodynamically stable. Both agents may be associated with a drop in blood pressure, with ketamine showing a slightly greater drop in blood pressure. Concerns over a possible association of etomidate with later mortality cause the authors to prefer ketamine over etomidate in this patient population. This is particularly true in patients with suspected sepsis. There is low quality evidence of this and more information is needed.

FOR AN "AWAKE LOOK" BEFORE INTUBATION OR DELAYED-SEQUENCE INTUBATION

Ketamine is suggested, but it may not be appropriate when these patients have cardiovascular disease or hypertension.

Adapted from Caro D, Walls RM, Grayzel J. Sedation or induction agents for rapid sequence intubation in adults. https://www.scribd.com/document/72424186/Sedation-or-Induction-Agents-for-Rapid-Sequence-ion-in-Adults.

TABLE 5.1 Recommended Anesthetic Dosing for Adult Rapid-Sequence Intubation and Clinical Considerations

DRUG[a]	IV DOSE	PREFERRED IN	AVOID IN
Thiopental	3–5 mg/kg	↑ ICP, SE	Hypotension, RAD
Methohexital	1–1.5 mg/kg	↑ ICP, SE	Hypotension, RAD
Fentanyl	5–15 µg/kg		Generally not used as sole induction agent in emergency medicine
Midazolam	0.1–0.3 mg/kg	SE	Hypotension
Ketamine	1–2 mg/kg	RAD, Hypotension	
Etomidate	0.3 mg/kg	Hypotension	Sepsis (unclear)
Propofol	2 mg/kg	↑ ICP, SE	Hypotension

[a]Any of these can drugs be used before the administration of a neuromuscular blocking agent to induce anesthesia (see text).
ICP, Intracranial pressure; *IV*, intravenous; *RAD*, reactive airway disease; *SE*, status epilepticus.

Ketamine

Unique among anesthetic agents, ketamine produces a dissociative anesthesia characterized by excellent analgesia and amnesia despite the appearance of wakefulness. As a drug that is potent and relatively safe with a rapid onset and brief duration of action, ketamine fits the profile of an agent that could be used effectively to facilitate intubation. Ketamine has been advocated for pharmacologic control of undifferentiated agitated and violent patients with hyperactive delirium syndrome with severe agitation. While ketamine does possess some pharmacologic properties that theoretically limit its use in selected circumstances, there is little evidence that this results in harm to patients.

Ketamine is a water- and lipid-soluble drug that rapidly penetrates the CNS. Like barbiturates, ketamine accumulates rapidly and then undergoes redistribution with subsequent degradation in the liver.[58] The recommended dose of ketamine before intubation is 1 to 2 mg/kg administered intravenously over a 1-minute period. Dissociative anesthesia occurs within 1 minute of completing the injection and lasts 5 to 10 minutes. A smaller additional dose (0.5 to 1 mg/kg) may be given 5 minutes after the initial dose if needed to maintain anesthesia. The intramuscular dose for intubation has not been well studied, and a suggested dose is 4 to 5 mg/kg. Onset of action occurs within 2 to 3 minutes. Because of its good vascularity, the anterior thigh muscle is theoretically the preferred site for administration. Due to larger drug volume needed for intramuscular dosing, the desired dose may need to be given via multiple intramuscular injections. Unlike other anesthetic agents that depress the reticular activating system, ketamine acts by interrupting association pathways between the thalamocortical and limbic systems. Characteristically the eyes remain open and patients exhibit spontaneous, though not purposeful, movements. Increases in blood pressure, heart rate, cardiac output, and myocardial oxygen consumption are seen and are most likely mediated through the CNS. In vitro studies indicate that ketamine is a myocardial depressant, and the CNS-mediated pressor effects generally mask the direct cardiac effects,[59,60] making it potentially useful in patients with hemorrhagic shock or hypotension. Compared to etomidate, there is a witnessed slight increase in postintubation hypotension in some studies.[61–63] It has been postulated that the myocardial depressant effects may dominate in critically ill patients, making ketamine less hemodynamically stable in this population. Respirations are initially rapid and shallow after ketamine administration, and they soon return to normal.[50]

Other features of ketamine anesthesia include increased skeletal muscle tone, preservation of the laryngeal and pharyngeal reflexes, hypersalivation, and relaxation of bronchial smooth muscle. Discussions continue regarding the appropriate role of ketamine in patients with head injury or potentially elevated ICP. Ketamine can potentially cause a rise in ICP through sympathetic stimulation, theoretically exacerbating the condition of patients with elevated ICP. Recent literature questions the degree that ketamine raises ICP,[64] with some studies actually showing a decrease in ICP following the administration of ketamine.[65] A 2009 trial demonstrated the safety of ketamine compared to etomidate in critically ill patients.[66] Ketamine may benefit patients with a neurologic injury by increasing cerebral perfusion pressure.[51]

Other studies suggest that ketamine does not interfere with cerebral metabolism or increase cerebral oxygen consumption and does not reduce regional glucose metabolism.[67] Ketamine can also offset any decrease in mean arterial pressure caused by fentanyl, a drug commonly used as part of RSI in patients with a head injury.[64] For similar reasons, some have advocated the addition of ketamine if propofol is to be used for induction. The resultant "ketofol" mixture is less likely to cause hypotension than propofol monotherapy.[68] The KEEP PACE trial demonstrated similar outcomes of ketofol to reduced dose etomidate.[69]

Overall, evidence suggesting that ketamine elevates ICP and results in harm is poor. Based on current evidence, it is reasonable to conclude that ketamine is an appropriate induction agent for RSI in patients with suspected ICP elevation and normal blood pressure or hypotension. In patients with hypertension and suspected ICP elevation, ketamine should be used with caution because of its tendency to further increase blood pressure. Patients with severe hypertension may be better served by using etomidate or propofol for induction.

A promising use of ketamine as an intubation adjunct has been in the setting of acute bronchospastic disease. Ketamine relaxes bronchial smooth muscle either directly through enhancement of sympathomimetic effects or indirectly through inhibition of vagal effects. Ketamine also increases bronchial secretions and may decrease the incidence of mucous plugging that is commonly seen in decompensating asthmatic patients.[70] Clinical reports have demonstrated a reduction in airway resistance and an increase in pulmonary compliance within minutes of ketamine administration[58] A recent systematic review, including a limited number of prospective studies with significant heterogeneity,[71] did not provide sufficient evidence to support the use of ketamine in refractory status asthmaticus. While it is crucial to conduct a large-scale prospective clinical trial before making any definite recommendations regarding its use in status asthmaticus, bronchospastic patients struggling to breathe and unable to tolerate oxygen masks or bronchodilators because of hypoxic encephalopathy may continue to breathe deeply and rapidly with ketamine anesthesia, allowing the maximum delivery of oxygen before a more elective intubation (Fig. 5.3).

A potential side effect that has raised some concern about the use of ketamine for RSI is its tendency to produce post-anesthesia emergence reactions, a characteristic that it shares with the structurally similar drug phencyclidine. The reemergence phenomenon, such as disturbing dreams as patients emerge from ketamine-induced anesthesia, is much less of a concern when the drug is used for RSI. In fact, there are no convincing data indicating that, when used for RSI, ketamine produces unpleasant reemergence reactions that are significant or common enough to limit its use for this purpose. One study found that although dreams occurred frequently following sedative doses of ketamine, they were generally pleasant and the frequency of reemergence phenomena and delirium was markedly reduced by the concomitant use of a benzodiazepine.[72] Rarely, reactions may be marked and distressing, with symptoms including floating sensations, dizziness, blurred vision, out-of-body experiences, and vivid dreams or nightmares. The true incidence of emergence reactions following RSI is unknown. Such reactions are less common in children than in adults and may be suppressed with benzodiazepines. Both diazepam and lorazepam appear to be useful in adults and the latter is more effective, most likely because of its enhanced amnestic effect. Midazolam is effective in adult patients at doses of 0.07 mg/kg[73] and may be the preferred agent because it has potent amnestic effects and a short duration of action. Studies in children have failed to show a reduction in the rate of emergence reactions in those treated with both ketamine and midazolam.[74,75] Much of the data on ketamine emergence comes from procedural sedation literature.

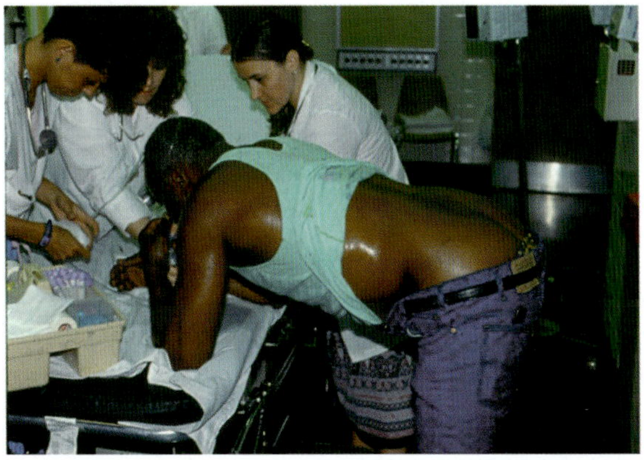

Fig. 5.3 This asthmatic is diaphoretic, confused, and agitated and cannot tolerate inhaled bronchodilators. He is about to suffer respiratory arrest and cannot be preoxygenated before intubation. Pulse oximetry shows an oxygen saturation of 82% to 84%. Ketamine is an ideal agent under these circumstances. Keeping him on the stretcher was difficult but within 60 seconds following intravenous administration of ketamine (100 mg), he stopped fighting but kept breathing rapidly. A nonrebreathing oxygen mask was tolerated and oxygen saturation rose to 98%, after which he was electively intubated under controlled preoxygenated conditions. A ketamine infusion (1 mg/kg per hour) was maintained for a few hours.

Emergence post-RSI may be masked by long-acting paralytics (e.g., rocuronium) and it is imperative to provide analgesia and sedation post-RSI while the patient remains paralyzed, regardless of the induction agent utilized.

Despite preservation of pharyngeal and laryngeal reflexes in patients sedated with ketamine, aspiration can still occur, and laryngospasm is a known, rare complication.[76] Ketamine does not relax skeletal muscles, and production of the desired intubating conditions requires the simultaneous administration of a paralytic agent, thereby removing all upper airway reflexes. Despite the possibility of aspiration, the use of ketamine is associated with very few airway complications. A study of over 1000 uses of ketamine for pediatric procedural sedation and analgesia revealed no cases of aspiration.[77] The use of ketamine without a paralytic is not recommended, as one study demonstrated a higher failure rate and increased complications with this approach.[78] Laryngospasm complicated 2% of all intubations in the same study.

Although rapid administration of IV ketamine during RSI typically does not pose a concern, boluses of rapidly administered ketamine may lead to brief and temporary apnea lasting approximately 30 seconds. To prevent this, it is recommended to administer IV ketamine slowly, at a rate of 100 mg/min. The physician should be prepared to promptly proceed with paralysis and intubation immediately after administering ketamine boluses.

Ketamine's excellent safety profile and preservation of respiratory drive make it an ideal agent for awake intubations or DSI.[6] This will be discussed further in later sections.

Etomidate

Etomidate is an ultrashort-acting nonbarbiturate hypnotic agent that has been used successfully as an anesthesia induction agent in Europe since the mid-1970s and in the United States since 1983. A significant benefit of etomidate in the emergency setting is its lack of cardiodepressant effects.[79,80] Several case series have now demonstrated its short-term safety and effective use in ED RSI.[81,82] Extensive experience with this agent now exists in both pediatric[83] and adult patients. Despite etomidate's efficacy during RSI, the uncertainty over a possible increase in mortality has caused the authors to prefer ketamine as an induction agent in most intubations.[84]

Etomidate is a carboxylated imidazole that is both water and lipid soluble. The drug reaches peak brain concentrations within 1 minute of IV infusion[85] and induces unconsciousness within 30 seconds of administration. Its effects last less than 10 minutes after a single bolus dose.[22] Redistribution of the drug is quite rapid, accounting for its short duration of action. Etomidate is rapidly hydrolyzed in the liver and plasma, forming an inactive metabolite excreted primarily in urine.[85] The recommended dose is 0.3 mg/kg via rapid IV bolus.[86] A lower incidence of postintubation hypotension is associated with a reduced (75%) dose of etomidate, with observation of more hypotension at doses higher than 0.3 mg/kg.[87] However, dose reduction may also be associated with a shorter sedation period highlighting the importance of providing prompt post-RSI analgesia and sedation when long-acting paralytics are used. There is virtually no accumulation of the drug, and anesthesia may be maintained through repeated doses. Etomidate should not be used as an infusion or in repeated bolus doses for maintenance of sedation after intubation in the ED.[88]

Etomidate acts on the CNS by stimulating γ-aminobutyric acid (GABA) receptors and depressing the reticular activating system. It produces electroencephalographic changes similar to those produced by barbiturates as patients pass rapidly through light to deep levels of surgical anesthesia. Because etomidate has no analgesic activity,[85] it should be used in conjunction with a parenteral analgesic when painful conditions are being treated, although it is most commonly used as a sole induction agent for intubation. Etomidate decreases cerebral oxygen consumption, cerebral blood flow, and ICP, appearing to have minimal effects on cerebral perfusion pressure.[49]

Etomidate is characterized by hemodynamic stability without significant changes in mean arterial pressure in most patients,[80–82] although a slightly increased heart rate may be observed.[88] Etomidate is suggested for induction of patients with significant cardiovascular disease requiring RSI. The hemodynamic stability that etomidate provides and the absence of induced hypertension may make it preferable to other sedatives in certain cases. While this hemodynamic stability persists even in patients with preexisting hypotension,[89] etomidate may still contribute to hypotension in critically ill patients by reducing the endogenous catecholamine response.[41,42] There is also concern for delayed hypotension associated with the use of etomidate in septic patients.[90]

The most common immediate side effects of etomidate are pain at the site of injection, nausea, vomiting, and common myoclonic jerks.[91] Pain on injection is reported in up to two-thirds of patients, although the clinical significance of this transient discomfort immediately prior to intubation is unclear. Patients may suddenly pull the arm where etomidate is being given, potentially compromising IV access during intubation. Securing the IV site and arm upon injection is recommended. Use of a large vein, simultaneous saline infusion, and opioid premedication can reduce the discomfort in appropriate situations.[92] Myoclonic activity has been reported in approximately one-third of cases and is believed to be caused by disinhibition of subcortical activity rather than CNS stimulation and does not represent seizure activity.[85] This sometimes dramatic effect is rarely seen during RSI as paralytics are given immediately after etomidate. Usually no treatment of myoclonus is necessary, and the effect is self-limiting. If persistent, an IV benzodiazepine may be administered. Etomidate need not be avoided in patients with seizure disorders, status epilepticus, head injury, or stroke.

Some degree of altered adrenal function has been demonstrated even after a single dose of etomidate.[93,94] The true clinical effect is unknown, and because the alteration in adrenal function appears to persist for 12 to 24 hours, there is theoretical concern about potential clinical consequences. Etomidate is a reversible inhibitor of 11β-hydroxylase, the enzyme that converts 11-deoxycortisol to cortisol. Although cortisol levels do not fall below the normal physiologic range, even a single induction dose of etomidate causes a measurable decrease in the level of circulating cortisol that occurs in response to the administration of exogenous adrenocorticotropic hormone (ACTH).

A sub-study of the Corticosteroid Therapy of Septic Shock (CORTICUS) trial evaluating the use of hydrocortisone in septic shock provided further evidence about the safety of etomidate use in patients with sepsis. There was a statistically significant increase in mortality (42.7% vs. 30.5%) for those who received etomidate.[95] Unfortunately, this effect was not diminished by the administration of hydrocortisone. In a separate study that compared etomidate with ketamine, a multicenter randomized trial of critically ill patients requiring emergency intubation found no significant difference in organ failure score, 28-day mortality, or intubating conditions between patients given etomidate for induction and those given ketamine.[66] Even though adrenal insufficiency occurred at a higher rate in the etomidate group (86%), it also developed in approximately 48% of patients receiving ketamine. A similar association of adrenal insufficiency was seen after a single dose in a surgical intensive care unit.[96]

Clinicians performing postintubation ACTH stimulation testing should be aware that the results may be affected by prior administration of etomidate. The empirical administration of glucocorticoids for the first 24 hours after a dose of etomidate has been given to patients with sepsis is not supported by outcome studies.[97]

The debate over the use of etomidate as an induction agent in those with known sepsis is unlikely to be definitively answered soon. It is not always immediately clear on arrival in the ED if patients who require intubation have sepsis. It is the recommendation of the authors that ketamine be considered in patients requiring intubation who have known sepsis. While the use of etomidate is not a violation of standard care, the favorable pharmacologic properties of ketamine make it a preferred induction agent for those with known sepsis.

Despite evidence that etomidate is at least as hemodynamically stable as ketamine, [62,63,98,99] there are data supporting an increase in mortality with etomidate. In one open-label randomized trial lower survival occurred in the etomidate arm during the first week of hospitalization.[100] However, this effect was not significant at 28 days. In older trials, a trend toward harm with etomidate has also been noted.[66]

Since a patient-oriented outcome such as mortality later in hospital stay is more important than a clinically oriented outcome such as postintubation hypotension, we recommend the use of ketamine as first-line for normotensive and hypotensive patients in the ED. Etomidate remains a valid alternative if ketamine is unavailable or for concerningly hypertensive patients, who remain an understudied patient population. This recommendation is based on limited information and is of low certainty.

Propofol

Propofol is a popular drug among anesthesiologists for OR-based induction and has potential ED use, especially in hypertensive patients.[101,102] Multiple reports have demonstrated the safety and efficacy of propofol for ED procedural sedation. Although some ED clinicians now routinely intubate with propofol, its role as an adjunct to intubation in the ED is undergoing evolution.[103] Propofol is an alkylphenol sedative-hypnotic used for induction and maintenance of general anesthesia. The drug has no analgesic activity and it exerts a powerful amnestic effect. Propofol tends to decrease vomiting through an unknown antiemetic effect. It produces dose-dependent depression of consciousness ranging from light sedation to coma. Propofol is a highly lipophilic, water-insoluble compound that undergoes rapid uptake by vascular tissues, including the brain, followed soon afterward by redistribution to muscle and fat. The drug is metabolized by the liver and excreted in urine.[104] After an IV induction dose of

2 mg/kg, unconsciousness occurs within 1 minute and lasts for 5 to 10 minutes. A smaller dose (1 to 1.5 mg/kg) is recommended in the elderly and when simultaneously administering other CNS depressants. Because propofol has a short duration of action and patients rapidly regain consciousness, repeat boluses are not a practical way to maintain a desired level of sedation after intubation has been completed.[104] Therefore a continuous infusion of 50 to 200 μg/kg per minute IV titrated to effect is preferred.

Propofol reduces airway resistance, making it a useful induction agent for patients with bronchospasm. Its neuroinhibitory effects make propofol a possible induction agent for patients with intracranial pathology, if they are hemodynamically stable. The propofol-induced decrease in mean arterial pressure, generally approximately 10 mm Hg, can reduce cerebral perfusion pressure, theoretically exacerbating CNS injury. As even transient hypotension has been associated with poor outcomes in critically ill patients, propofol should not be used if the patient is hypotensive or at high risk for hypotension.[37]

Propofol does not prolong the QT interval. Although the manufacturer lists egg or soybean allergy as a contraindication to the use of propofol, significant allergic reactions to the newer preparation of the drug are extremely rare. Evidence from 2016 suggests that there is no connection between propofol and egg, soy, or peanut allergy.[105]

Propofol suppresses sympathetic activity, thereby causing myocardial depression and peripheral vasodilation, particularly in the elderly or hypovolemic patients and when administered simultaneously with opioids. Hypotension can be minimized with appropriate fluid loading or with use of vasopressors. Due to an association with hypotension in trauma patients receiving this agent, we recommend against its routine use in trauma patients.[106] Propofol reduces cerebral blood flow and may cause mild CNS excitatory activity (e.g., myoclonus, tremors, hiccups) during induction. Propofol has been used in the treatment of status epilepticus,[107–110] and may be an attractive agent for induction of these patients. Pain on injection occurs commonly, even when the drug is infused slowly.[104] Pretreating the infusing vein with 1 mL of 1% lidocaine (10 mg) injected over a 30-second period or choosing a large antecubital vein will ameliorate this pain.

Propofol is a reasonable induction agent for RSI in the ED, especially if the patient is hypertensive or in status epilepticus. The safety of etomidate and ketamine is the main challenge to the routine use of propofol for intubation. Whereas propofol has an excellent record for stable patients in the OR and for procedural sedation,[50] the common side effect of hypotension precludes its use in many critically ill patients. Its short duration of action and ease of titration make it a more attractive agent for postintubation sedation than as a routine agent for induction. If not used for induction of RSI, a bolus (0.25 to 0.5 mg/kg) should be considered in select patients to achieve rapid sedation before starting a continuous infusion.

Benzodiazepines (Midazolam)

The benzodiazepines are a class of drugs characterized by anxiolytic, hypnotic, sedative, anticonvulsant, muscle relaxant, and amnestic effects. Several of these properties make the benzodiazepines appealing adjuvant agents for intubation, particularly when used in combination with opioids. It is important to remember that benzodiazepines do not have analgesic effects. Although they may produce excellent sedation and impair the patient's memory of an unpleasant experience, they will not prevent the pain associated with intubation. The high risk of hypotension in critically ill patients who receive both benzodiazepines and opiates limits this class for RSI induction in the ED.

Midazolam has replaced diazepam as a preoperative sedative agent, even in elderly patients.[111,112] When compared with diazepam, the primary advantages of midazolam include a twofold increase in potency, shorter half-life, and decreased potential for cardiorespiratory depression. Midazolam is water soluble in an acid medium and does not require suspension in propylene glycol like other benzodiazepines. It is rarely associated with phlebitis and can be given intramuscularly when a very rapid onset of action is not required. At physiologic pH, midazolam is lipophilic and rapidly accumulates in the CNS, with onset of sedation occurring in as little as 1 to 2 minutes. Outside the CNS it accumulates in fatty tissue and extensively binds to plasma, accounting for the paucity of non-CNS side effects. Its half-life of elimination is 1 to 4 hours and is dependent on release of the drug from adipose tissue and protein-binding sites. The period of sedation after a single IV dose is considerably shorter. Emergence from a 0.15-mg/kg dose occurs in 15 to 20 minutes.[112]

Clinical experience using midazolam with or without fentanyl for procedural sedation is considerable, and the authors prefer safer, more dependable agents such as ketamine or propofol. The recommended dose for moderate sedation with midazolam is 0.05 to 0.1 mg/kg given in 1-mg boluses and not exceeding 2.5 mg over a period of 2 minutes. Doses upward of 0.1 mg/kg are often needed to produce good conditions for intubation.[113,114]

The potential for adverse effects with midazolam is similar to that with other benzodiazepines. A small increase in heart rate is seen frequently, as is a small decrease in systolic blood pressure.[115] Changes in blood pressure may be exaggerated in the presence of hypovolemia.[116] An ED-based study reported a mean 10% decrease in systolic blood pressure, with 19% of intubated patients having systolic blood pressure lower than 90 mm Hg.[115] The cardiac index and coronary artery blood flow are not generally affected. In the prehospital setting, hypotension with midazolam was found to be dose related,[117] and it should be used cautiously in patients with hypovolemia or traumatic brain injury. Respiratory depression may occur even at standard doses, and it most often follows rapid administration of an excessive dose. Respiratory depression is also more likely to occur in debilitated or elderly patients and in those simultaneously receiving opioids. The effects of midazolam are rapidly reversed by administration of the benzodiazepine antagonist flumazenil. A study of various induction agents for ET intubation suggested that the use of midazolam alone for RSI may be associated with suboptimal intubating conditions and increased difficulty.[118] Other induction agents may be preferred over midazolam alone during RSI.

Whereas once a common agent for induction, midazolam cannot be recommended as a routine induction agent for intubation in the ED. At the doses required for consistent sedation, hypotension is very common. One study showed that 19% of those intubated with midazolam had hypotension.[118] The association of hypotension with poor outcomes[37] precludes the routine use of this medication. A possible exception to this is for patients in status epilepticus or in some overdose scenarios, additional research is needed in this area. Midazolam is a common agent for postintubation sedation, and it is more appropriate for this use than as an induction agent.

Opioids (Fentanyl)

Although any of several opioids administered intravenously could be used to induce unconsciousness, fentanyl has significant advantages over other opioid agents. A synthetic opioid, it has been widely used since its introduction in 1968. Its favorable pharmacologic properties include rapid serum clearance, high potency, and minimal release of histamine.[119–121] Fentanyl quickly crosses the blood-brain barrier and produces analgesia in as little as 1 to 2 minutes. Serum levels decline rapidly from peak concentrations because of extensive tissue uptake.[122,123] Unlike morphine, the brain concentration of fentanyl falls in conjunction with the serum level. The duration of analgesic action is 30 to 40 minutes, although at high doses a second peak of activity may be seen several hours later because of release of the bound drug from tissue stores. Fentanyl is approximately 50 to 100 times as potent as morphine.[124] This unique combination of potency and short half-life permits the administration of numerous small doses that can be titrated to the desired clinical effect. Like other opioids, fentanyl is competitively reversed with naloxone. Related agents include remifentanil, alfentanil, carfentanil, and sufentanil, and these synthetic opioids are not generally available in the ED setting.

The relative safety of fentanyl permits considerable latitude in dosing. When used as a primary anesthetic agent for major surgical procedures, doses ranging from 50 to 100 μg/kg produce minimal side effects.[125] Comparatively small doses produce sedation, and 3 to 5 μg/kg, given at a rate of 1 to 2 μg/kg per minute, is generally an effective analgesic dose. More rapid administration will cause greater depression of the level of consciousness. Mostert and colleagues[126] reported successful awake intubation in 99 of 103 patients who were administered an average cumulative dose of 3.7 μg/kg. Most of these patients were able to follow commands, and many recalled events surrounding the intubation. A small percentage could not be intubated, even after receiving 500 μg of fentanyl.

Larger doses, up to 25 μg/kg, may be needed to produce ideal intubating conditions, although if given rapidly, 10 μg/kg is usually adequate. Even this lower dose is more likely to produce unconsciousness than a lesser depth of sedation and it may cause a longer period of unresponsiveness than is desirable. It is preferable to use a lower dose of fentanyl (2 to 3 μg/kg) for analgesia combined with a paralytic agent (e.g., succinylcholine) to produce adequate muscle relaxation and a sedative (e.g., midazolam) to reduce anxiety and produce amnesia for the event. A recent study of remifentanil without use of NMBs showed worse performance than standard RSI with paralytics.[127]

Unlike other opioids, fentanyl causes little or no release of histamine, and its use is seldom associated with emesis or hypotension. It is probably safer than morphine and hydromorphone in hypovolemic patients. Fentanyl also has significantly fewer emetic effects than other opioids. Adverse effects that have been reported with fentanyl are few and primarily follow the rapid IV infusion of very large doses. Like other opioids, fentanyl may cause rigidity of the skeletal musculature, including the chest wall and diaphragm. Rigidity occurs with doses in excess of 15 μg/kg, and it has also been reported with doses as low as 10 μg/kg that may also be related to rapid administration.[126,128] The muscular rigidity may be prevented or treated with standard doses of succinylcholine or naloxone.[129] This rigidity is generally not a major concern during RSI due to the use of paralytics and may be observed during procedural sedation. The most common significant complication with fentanyl is respiratory depression, and it generally occurs when fentanyl is given in combination with other CNS depressants or in excessive amounts.[130,131]

Fentanyl appears to be a safe agent for use in the ED, and its main limitation as an induction agent is the variable patient response to the drug. Unlike ketamine and etomidate, the effect of a standard dose of fentanyl is unpredictable. This is especially true in patients who are not opioid naive. As mentioned previously, a small percentage of patients did not have adequate sedation despite doses of 500 μg, limiting its use as a sole induction agent. The main use of fentanyl in current practice is as a pretreatment drug to prevent increased ICP or elevated blood pressure. Fentanyl remains an excellent agent for analgesia following intubation and is a very reasonable agent to begin during the early stages of RSI.

NEUROMUSCULAR BLOCKING AGENTS

NMBs are used to achieve muscle relaxation for intubation. They permit complete airway control and greatly simplify visualization of the vocal cords. This is particularly important when intubation must be performed quickly under suboptimal circumstances. Sedatives may provide some muscle relaxation, and this requires rapid administration of large doses, which poses a risk for depression of the cardiovascular system. The combination of a paralytic agent and a sedative or analgesic agent is generally superior to the use of either agent alone. A 1999 report showed an 18% failure-to-intubate rate with a sedative alone versus a 0% failure rate for sedatives plus paralytics.[132] Procedural complication rates such as significant airway trauma and aspiration were also markedly higher in the group receiving sedation alone.

The only absolute contraindication to the use of NMBs is the inability to manage the airway once the patient becomes apneic. Though not absolutely contraindicated, it is considered inhumane to paralyze and intubate an alert patient. A sedative or an analgesic agent should always be administered simultaneously if the patient is able to perceive pain.

NMBs are classified as either depolarizing or nondepolarizing. Depolarizing agents mimic the action of acetylcholine (ACh) and produce sustained depolarization of the neuromuscular junction, during which time muscle contractions cannot occur. Nondepolarizing agents competitively block the action of ACh at the neuromuscular junction and prevent depolarization and therefore muscle contractions. Commonly used NMBs and their dosages and characteristics are listed in Table 5.2.

Succinylcholine

The standard depolarizing agent currently in use is succinylcholine.[133] It has a chemical structure similar to ACh and depolarizes the postjunctional neuromuscular membrane. Administration is followed by a brief period of muscle fasciculations that correspond to the initial membrane depolarization and muscle fiber activation. Unlike ACh, which is released in minute amounts and hydrolyzed in milliseconds, succinylcholine requires several minutes for breakdown to occur. During

TABLE 5.2 Commonly Used Neuromuscular Blocking Agents in Adults

AGENT	IV DOSE (mg/kg)	ONSET (min)	DURATION (min)
Succinylcholine	1.5	1	3–5
Pancuronium	0.1	2–5	60–180
Vecuronium	0.1	2–3	25–40
Atracurium	0.5	2–3	20–35
Mivacurium	0.15	2–3	15–20
Rocuronium	1.2	1–3	30–110

this time the neuromuscular junction remains depolarized, and the muscles relax, not contracting again until the neuromuscular end plate and adjacent sarcoplasmic reticulum return to the resting state and are again depolarized. Relaxation proceeds from the small, distal, rapidly moving muscles to the proximal, slowly moving muscles. The diaphragm is one of the last muscles to relax.

Succinylcholine is rapidly degraded in serum by the enzyme pseudocholinesterase, and the duration of action of a single dose is 5 to 10 minutes.[134] Relaxation may be maintained by repeated IV injections. Prolonged or repeated use of the drug enhances its vagal stimulatory effects, thereby resulting in bradycardia, hypotension, and other muscarinic effects. These effects may be seen even at normal doses, particularly in children.[135] For this reason, atropine pretreatment at a dose of 0.02 mg/kg has been recommended in the past by some experts for small children or for patients receiving multiple doses of succinylcholine, although the need and optimal dose are still in question.[135] Recent evidence shows a very low rate of bradycardia even in pediatric patients and the use of atropine or succinylcholine has no effect on the incidence of bradycardia during intubation.[136]

Repeated dosing with succinylcholine may produce a desensitization blockade and create a scenario in which the neuromuscular membrane returns to the resting state and becomes resistant to further depolarization by succinylcholine.[137,138] In general there is little need for repeated doses of succinylcholine if appropriately dosed the first time. If paralysis in excess of 5 to 10 minutes is desired, longer-acting, nondepolarizing agents such as rocuronium should be used.

The recommended dose of succinylcholine is 1 to 1.5 mg/kg given intravenously. Dosages at the upper end of this range are suggested to guarantee complete relaxation and avoid the need for repeated dosing. Dosage calculations should also be based on actual, not lean body mass because of alterations in both volume of distribution and pseudocholinesterase activity.[139] Neonates and infants require a slightly higher dose of succinylcholine (2 to 3 mg/kg intravenously) because of their higher volume of distribution.[88,140] It is crucial that succinylcholine be administered as a rapid bolus because slow administration may lead to incomplete relaxation. Use of a rapid 20-mL to 30-mL saline flush after IV administration may enhance its desired effect.

There are several potential adverse effects of the use of succinylcholine, ranging from minor to life-threatening. Muscle fasciculations accompany the initial depolarization of the neuromuscular membrane. Fasciculations are most prominent in muscular patients and create deep, aching muscle pain that may last for days.[141] It is unclear whether any regimen will totally prevent the succinylcholine-induced fasciculations (seen in 73% to 100% of patients) and myalgias (seen in 10% to 83% of patients), with varying effects reported after numerous interventions.[142] Interestingly, higher doses of succinylcholine may be associated with less myalgia. Traditionally, fasciculations have been prevented by the preadministration of a defasciculating dose (0.01 mg/kg) of pancuronium or vecuronium. The evidence available does not suggest that succinylcholine worsens outcomes in at-risk patients, nor does any evidence suggest that defasciculation improves outcomes in at-risk patients.[47]

A major consideration in the use' of succinylcholine is its propensity to cause hyperkalemia. This electrolyte disturbance is believed to occur secondary to asynchronous depolarization of muscle cells and resulting cellular injury. Elevation in serum potassium occurs in normal patients after standard doses but is generally clinically inconsequential, with increases of less than 0.5 mmol/L (mEq/L).[143] Increases in potassium are not prevented with defasciculating doses of nondepolarizing agents. Marked hyperkalemia is associated with increased extrajunctional muscle ACh receptors, which develop in patients with prolonged diseases of the neuromuscular system. Susceptibility may occur within as few as 5 to 7 days and persists indefinitely. In these cases, the hyperkalemic response may be as much as 5 mmol/L (mEq/L). Such conditions include late severe burns,[144] major muscle trauma,[145] spinal cord injury, muscular dystrophy, multiple sclerosis, and other upper motor neuron diseases[146,147] such as amyotrophic lateral sclerosis. These large elevations occur only in patients who have had significant tissue injury or muscle denervation for several days or weeks before the use of succinylcholine. Importantly, succinylcholine is not contraindicated in the initial management of patients with acute injuries, including burns, major crush injuries, and spinal cord injuries. Succinylcholine is also not contraindicated in normokalemic patients with renal failure because the magnitude of the rise in serum potassium is the same as in patients with normally functioning kidneys.[148] A retrospective review of the use of succinylcholine in 38 operative cases with moderate pre-RSI hyperkalemia (5.6 to 7.6 mmol/L) suggested that the risk for hyperkalemia-related complications may be lower than feared.[149] In a review of more than 41,000 intubations, 38 patients had hyperkalemia with a mean serum potassium level of 5.9 mmol/L, so Schow and colleagues[149] concluded that it is safe to administer succinylcholine to patients with a potassium level of 5.5 to 6.0 mEq/L.

Succinylcholine is best avoided (if other equally effective pharmacologic options such as rocuronium exist) in the setting of known or suspected preexisting hyperkalemia (e.g., renal failure patients not receiving regular dialysis or demonstrating a wide QRS complex). There is a higher risk of undiagnosed myopathies in pediatric patients, and succinylcholine remains a safe drug for most pediatric intubations.[140]

Malignant hyperthermia is a rare complication with an autosomal dominant inheritance pattern that is triggered by multiple anesthetic agents, including succinylcholine. Most provocative agents, such as halothane, are not used in the ED setting, and it is extremely rare for the ED physician to encounter this complication. It occurs in approximately 1 in

15,000 children and 1 in 50,000 adults.[150] The clinical syndrome consists of high fever, tachypnea, tachycardia, cardiac arrhythmias, hypoxia, acidosis, myoglobinuria, and impaired coagulation. In the recently paralyzed and intubated patient, rapidly rising $EtCO_2$ levels (>55 mm Hg) despite adequate minute ventilation may be the sign with the highest sensitivity and specificity. Unabated muscle contractions mediated by abnormal calcium channels are the physiologic basis for this condition.[151] Treatment includes aggressive cooling measures, volume replacement, and correction of hypoxia, as well as acid-base and electrolyte abnormalities. Dantrolene sodium, a direct-acting skeletal muscle relaxant, is thought to be effective in reducing the muscle hypermetabolism that causes the dramatic hyperpyrexia.[152] An associated abnormal response to succinylcholine is isolated masseter spasm,[153] and it can occur in isolation or portend the subsequent development of malignant hyperthermia. Though rare, it has been reported in the emergency medicine literature.[154] In this condition, forcible sustained contraction of the masseter muscles occurs and prevents mouth opening and oral intubation. Management is controversial, with recommendations ranging from use of a BVM, securing a surgical airway until the contraction abates, to attempting to suppress the contractions through administration of a nondepolarizing NMB. A case report of an ED patient with masseter spasm during RSI described successful management with the use of a nondepolarizing NMB (vecuronium).[155] Unlike routine cases in the OR, most ED patients require definitive airway management and cannot be allowed to simply have the succinylcholine wear off. With the limited evidence available on the management of this rare condition, it is the authors' recommendation that rocuronium be used to treat masseter spasm attributed to succinylcholine.

Prolonged paralysis after the administration of succinylcholine may occur in clinical conditions that result in decreased pseudocholinesterase levels and subsequent decreased metabolism of succinylcholine. Physiologic states associated with this condition include hepatic disease, anemia, renal failure, organophosphate poisoning, pregnancy, chronic cocaine use, advanced age, bronchogenic carcinoma, and connective tissue disorders. Patients with these conditions experience a twofold to threefold increase in the duration of apnea.[156] Patients with cocaine intoxication may also experience prolonged muscle relaxation because cocaine is competitively metabolized by the cholinesterases. An inherited deficiency of pseudocholinesterase is also present in approximately 0.03% of the population and can lead to prolonged paralysis from the administration of succinylcholine.[152] The prolonged duration of paralysis for these patients is likely to be of little clinical significance for the majority of ED patients, as the vast majority of patients intubated in the ED are not ready for extubation shortly afterward and are unlikely to be harmed by slightly prolonged paralysis.

Succinylcholine can also result in an increase in ICP, and the magnitude and significance of the increase in ICP remains controversial.[157,158] Several investigators have reported increases in the range of 5 to 10 mm Hg, and other researchers have shown no increase. There is no evidence of neurologic deterioration associated with these transient elevations in ICP. Mechanisms that have been proposed to explain the elevated ICP include: (1) a direct effect of fasciculations, (2) an increase in cortical electrical activity with a resultant increase in cerebral blood flow and blood volume, and (3) sympathetic postganglionic stimulation. Limited studies have been performed to evaluate the significance of this rise in ICP in a brain-injured human patient population. These studies have shown no significant change in electroencephalographic activity or ICP with succinylcholine, and the small size of the studies limits the ability to draw conclusions about clinical outcomes.[140,159,160]

Questions concerning the safety of succinylcholine in the setting of acute intracranial pathology do not have clear answers. The drug has been used widely and successfully in this setting and its continued use is supported by this experience. The very real risk for airway compromise and secondary cerebral insult because of hypoxia from delayed or failed intubation must always be weighed against the theoretical harmful effects. Succinylcholine, despite its many potential side effects, is currently the most frequently used agent for neuromuscular blockade with RSI because of its rapid onset and offset and reliable muscle relaxation characteristics.

Nondepolarizing Agents

Nondepolarizing agents act in a competitive manner to block the effects of ACh at the neuromuscular junction. Drugs in this class include pancuronium, atracurium, vecuronium, mivacurium, and rocuronium. These drugs, particularly the intermediate-acting agents, have fewer side effects than succinylcholine and they have the potential for reversal. They generally have a longer onset and duration of action than succinylcholine. Rocuronium has arisen as a popular competitor to succinylcholine, with fewer contraindications. Knowledge of appropriate nondepolarizing NMBs is important for situations when succinylcholine may be contraindicated or unavailable.

Because nondepolarizing agents act competitively at neuromuscular junction receptors, increasing the concentration of ACh may reverse their effects. Cholinesterase inhibitors such as neostigmine or edrophonium may be used and will not be effective until some spontaneous signs of reversal are seen. The concept of reversal is of limited clinical importance in the ED with rare exceptions, such as performance of a neurologic examination on a previously paralyzed patient. When reversal is required, neostigmine, 0.02 to 0.04 mg/kg, is given by slow IV push. An additional dose of 0.01 to 0.02 mg/kg may be given in 5 minutes if reversal is incomplete, and the total dose should not exceed 5 mg in adults. Atropine, 0.01 mg/kg (with a minimum dose of 0.1 mg in children and a maximum dose of 1 mg in adults), should be given concurrently with neostigmine to block its systemic cholinergic effects.[161–163]

Another potential reversing agent, sugammadex, binds directly to the aminosteroid NMB rather than to cholinesterases.[164] For reversal of shallow or profound neuromuscular blockade, 2 or 4 mg/kg intravenously, respectively, is recommended. The most concerning risk with this medication is anaphylaxis.[165,166] Unfortunately, no studies other than case reports currently address its use in emergency situations. It is not in wide use in the emergency setting.

A study by Lee and colleagues[167] demonstrated that rocuronium with sugammadex administration leads to faster recovery than succinylcholine after neuromuscular blockade. Whereas the rocuronium/sugammadex arm recovered faster than the succinylcholine arm, sugammadex still took several minutes to reverse many patients. This may be unacceptable in a "cannot-intubate/cannot-oxygenate" situation. A case report of sugammadex use in a cannot-intubate/cannot-oxygenate situation showed that despite partial reversal of paralysis, a tracheostomy was still required.[168] The availability of this reversal agent for use in the ED does not change the need to be prepared for a surgical airway if required. The high cost of this medication will also make it cost prohibitive for many EDs.[169] The use of sugammadex in cases where emergency airway management has been unsuccessful or complications arise is not supported by current evidence.[170] Additionally, caution should be exercised if giving larger doses of sugammadex (e.g., 16 mg/kg for immediate rocuronium reversal) as rocuronium may not be effective for the next 24 hours.

Intermediate-Acting Agents: Vecuronium, Atracurium, Mivacurium, and Rocuronium

Vecuronium and atracurium are intermediate-acting agents with an onset of action of approximately 3 minutes and a duration of action of 30 minutes. Mivacurium has an onset of action of 2 to 3 minutes and a duration of action of 15 to 20 minutes. Rocuronium has an onset of action of 1 to 1.5 minutes and a duration of action of 20 to 75 minutes (longer in geriatric patients). These drugs have minimal cardiovascular effects, cause little release of histamine (with the exception of mivacurium),[140] and lack cumulative effects.[171]

The recommended doses of vecuronium, atracurium, mivacurium, and rocuronium are listed in Table 5.2. Use of larger doses hastens the onset of action and prolongs the period of paralysis.

Rocuronium, a structural analogue of vecuronium, is emerging as a desirable alternative agent for RSI when succinylcholine is contraindicated. At a dose of 1.2 mg/kg, rocuronium consistently provides good to excellent intubating conditions within 1 minute of administration. Its duration of action is dose dependent and ranges from 20 to 75 minutes.[172,173] Smaller anesthesia and ED-based studies have demonstrated its clinical utility and safety in RSI protocols.[172,174,175] Rocuronium creates appropriate intubating conditions faster than vecuronium,[173] making rocuronium the nondepolarizing agent of choice for RSI in the ED. The onset of rocuronium may be hastened by a priming dose of rocuronium, pretreatment with ephedrine, or pretreatment with magnesium.[176] These interventions reduced time to onset by 21 seconds, 22 seconds, and 28 seconds. The clinical benefit of this in emergency medicine is unknown and likely to be small in most patients.

A 2015 Cochrane analysis including 37 studies compared rocuronium to succinylcholine for RSI. It revealed slightly superior intubating conditions with succinylcholine when compared to rocuronium. Once limited to studies that only utilized 1.2 mg/kg rocuronium, this difference disappeared. It is the authors' recommendation that 1.2 mg/kg of rocuronium be used as the routine dose of this medication.

There is increasing focus on the phenomenon of patients being aware during paralysis. Two recent studies demonstrated that while rare, awareness does occur in patients intubated in the ED.[177,178] There was an association between the use of rocuronium and awareness of paralysis in one study and a trend in the other. It is known that patients receiving rocuronium have longer delays to sedation initiation than those receiving succinylcholine.[179]

Teams caring for patients intubated with rocuronium must recognize its prolonged paralysis. For instance, if etomidate is administered as induction with rocuronium as a paralytic, without prompt post-RSI analgesia and sedation, patients will appear sedated for up to an hour due to paralysis. When etomidate's effects dissipate (after 5 minutes), patients may awaken but will be unable to express discomfort due to skeletal muscle paralysis. This may lead to hemodynamic and psychological complications such as tachycardia, hypertension, and long-term posttraumatic stress disorder (PTSD).[177]

There is insufficient information to clearly demonstrate whether succinylcholine or rocuronium is the superior paralytic for RSI in the ED. Succinylcholine has a much shorter duration and has a much longer list of contraindications. EDs frequently receive undifferentiated patients in respiratory failure requiring immediate airway management, often before a full medical history can be obtained or initial potassium level has been assessed. As mentioned previously, it is far from clear how harmful the transient elevation in potassium is for patients requiring RSI.[149] Rocuronium has much cleaner pharmacology and a much longer duration of action. Neither the short duration of succinylcholine nor the availability of reversal agents for rocuronium are major benefits to using one agent over the other, as definitive airway management will be required in the vast majority of ED cases.[168]

The cleaner pharmacology and lack of contraindications have caused some to call for rocuronium to be the first-line paralytic for RSI.[180] Concerns about succinylcholine remain mostly theoretical, as harm has not been demonstrated in multiple trials.[181,182] There is even evidence that succinylcholine provides better intubating conditions with faster intubation time, and this study was done with a lower dose of 0.6 mg/kg of rocuronium.[183] Further randomized trials would certainly be welcome due to the frequency of RSI, and there currently is no strong evidence of improvement of patient-oriented outcomes with rocuronium and a possibility that succinylcholine is superior.

The authors have no strong preference for succinylcholine or rocuronium in the majority of patients. We avoid the use of succinylcholine in patients with known end-stage renal disease and rarely encounter the other contraindications to succinylcholine. Rocuronium is an excellent agent, and we are concerned by the frequency of awareness of paralysis and delays to sedation associated with its use. Providers using rocuronium must be certain that sedation is started very soon after intubation or even prior to it. Those practicing in environments that cannot guarantee early sedation should avoid use of rocuronium where possible. Both agents have their merits and emergency physicians should become comfortable using both agents.

THE "AWAKE LOOK" EVALUATION OF THE AIRWAY BEFORE RSI

In selected patients, conditions may exist that preclude the immediate use of RSI, and the more prudent approach would be to thoroughly assess for airway anatomy and intubation needs as well as potential difficulties and complications before proceeding with full induction and paralysis. Consideration should be given to directly visualizing the larynx while the patient is awake or minimally sedated when there are significant concerns about the clinician's ability to secure the airway and take over the patient's oxygenation and ventilation quickly and effectively. This approach, referred to as a "sedated look" or "awake look," is used when the clinician suspects a difficult intubation. By conducting a thorough airway assessment, the clinician can anticipate and identify potential difficulties and determine the most suitable techniques and equipment for successful intubation. This approach may enhance patient safety, improve the chances of successful airway management, and may minimize complications during RSI in patients with a potentially anatomically or physiologically difficult airway. Examples are significantly elevated body mass index (BMI) patients, patients with significant angioedema or smoke inhalation, and patients with preexisting hypoxemia or acidosis who may not tolerate apnea without rapidly decompensating. This technique allows the patient to maintain respiratory drive during assessment of the airway and allows the clinician to verify that the laryngeal structures are indeed visible and accessible before committing to induction and paralysis. This approach is distinct from the practice of intubation with sedation alone or nonparalytic RSI, in which the patient receives a full induction dose of a sedative agent and no neuromuscular blocking agent. This older practice may create a vulnerable and compromised patient in whom intubating conditions are then problematic.[184]

Traditionally in the OR, topical anesthesia (e.g., atomized 4% lidocaine) either with or without anxiolysis, analgesia and/or mild-moderate sedation has been used to allow a view into the airway while enabling the patient to maintain respiratory drive and protective airway reflexes. Although more research is needed to determine which medications are best for awake or sedated looks in the ED, ketamine may be ideal in this circumstance, allowing the patient to maintain respiratory drive while providing analgesia, amnesia, and sedation. Ketamine's analgesic properties may allow it to be used as the sole agent in patients with a bloody traumatized airway, for which topical anesthesia is unlikely to work effectively. Other options are discussed in the following section.

AWAKE TRACHEAL INTUBATION

An alternative to induction of unconsciousness in patients requiring intubation is the use of local anesthetic and sedative agents in conscious patients. The availability of relatively effective and safe induction agents made this a less attractive alternative in the past, and these techniques of awake tracheal intubation (ATI) may be desirable in specific patients, such as for flexible intubating videoscope or fiberoptic intubation of a predicted difficult airway. Difficult airway prediction can be notoriously unreliable,[185] and there are certain features that may identify patients who may require ATI. These features include, but are not limited to:

- Patients with abnormal head and neck anatomy and/or pathology, such as trauma, malignancy, previous surgery, congenital malformation, or radiotherapy
- Reduced mouth opening or tongue obstruction
- Limited neck mobility
- Obstructive sleep apnea
- Elevated BMI
- Progressive airway compromise
- Predicted difficult physiology: preexisting hypoxemia, acidosis, or hemodynamic compromise

In these patients, ATI offers a number of potential advantages over RSI. The natural airway is maintained along with spontaneous respiration and a degree of protection from aspiration, and physiologic compromise due to induction agents and apnea is avoided. The use of adequate topical anesthesia and sedative and/or analgesic agents to produce a state of anxiolysis or mild to moderate sedation are the principal components needed for awake intubation.

Thomas[186] likened standard laryngoscopy in an awake patient to the "mouth being held open with a wrench." Awake nasotracheal intubation and flexible video or fiberoptic intubation can also be an extremely unpleasant experience. The upper airway is richly innervated by sensory branches of the 5th, 7th, 9th, and 10th cranial nerves. In addition to pain fibers, there are stretch receptors that stimulate the coughing and gagging reflexes with even minor airway manipulation. It is essential that adequate anesthesia and analgesia be provided before intubation in all but the most extreme circumstances. Treatment options include topical application of anesthetic agents to the pharyngeal and tracheal mucosa and IV infusion of analgesic or sedative agents.

Local or topical anesthesia techniques may be used in patients who are awake, either in place of or as a supplement to IV analgesia or sedation. They are particularly useful as adjuncts to nasotracheal and fiberoptic intubation and may also facilitate video laryngoscopy.[187,188] Occasionally, the time required to achieve good topical anesthesia may limit the usefulness of these techniques in emergency situations. Before proceeding with ATI, the clinician should generally consider whether the patient is so unstable or the airway sufficiently difficult such as to warrant proceeding straight to a surgical airway.

Topical anesthesia may be achieved by direct application, by cricothyroid membrane puncture, or by inhalation of an atomized or nebulized anesthetic.

Direct Application of Topical Anesthetics

Achieving anesthesia of the nasal, oral, and pharyngeal mucosa is a relatively simple procedure that involves the use of commonly available agents such as lidocaine or a combination such as 14% benzocaine, 2% butamben, and 2% tetracaine. Achieving anesthesia of the hypopharynx is more difficult because optimal results require application of the anesthetic to the epiglottis and vocal cords.

Lidocaine, the most commonly used local anesthetic agent for airway topicalization, offers several theoretical safety advantages compared with other agents. Its favorable cardiovascular and systemic toxicity risk profile makes it a preferred choice in airway topicalization. It is essential to carefully monitor lidocaine doses to prevent potential toxicity. Studies have indicated that toxic plasma concentrations or clinical signs of toxicity can occur when lidocaine doses exceed the range of 6.0 to 9.3 mg/kg of lean body weight.[189] The Difficult Airway Society Guidelines[190] recommend not to exceed a maximum dose of topical lidocaine of 9 mg/kg lean body weight.

If time allows, administer an anticholinergic agent, such as glycopyrrolate, at a dose of 5 μg/kg (0.2 to 0.4 mg in an adult patient) IV or IM to help reduce airway secretions. Preferably, administer this medication 15 minutes prior to intubation for maximal effect, although some effects take place within 7 minutes.[191] It is important to attempt to dry the airway with suction and gauze, as glycopyrrolate will only reduce additional secretions and will not remove existing moisture. A dry airway will make topical anesthetics more effective.

Begin this procedure by spraying the tongue and pharynx with a topical agent. Atomization devices are available that attach to air or oxygen supply, have a directional tip (e.g., EZ-100m, Alcove Medical, Inc.; EZ-Spray SMR;

Pulmodyne, Inc.), and are designed for the rapid anesthetization of patients using aqueous or viscous medications or solutions (Fig. 5.4). Atomization devices that attach to standard syringes (e.g., Mucosal Atomization Device [MAD]; Wolfe Tory Medical, Inc.) can also provide effective drug dispersal without a forceful spray (Fig. 5.5). The more forceful pressurized canister sprays commonly provoke a cough reflex. After allowing at least 2 to 3 minutes to achieve numbing of the tongue and pharynx, spray the epiglottis and vocal cords with the atomizer. A malleable extension tube allows the tip of the MAD to pass around the base of the tongue, thereby permitting direct spraying of the epiglottis and vocal cords, while the directional tip of the EZ-100 allows for a similar function. This is generally well tolerated. Lidocaine will have an onset of anesthetic effect within 2 minutes, which peaks at 2 to 5 minutes postapplication and will continue to have an effect for 14 to 15 minutes.[192] An alternative method is to visualize the epiglottis and vocal cords with a laryngoscope and directly spray them with the anesthetic agent. The use of a laryngoscope to visualize the vocal cords is much more stimulating to the patient and often not well tolerated. Some authors have demonstrated awake oral intubation using Macintosh direct or standard-geometry video laryngoscopy facilitated with topical anesthetic agents directly applied in the distribution of the glossopharyngeal nerve, in the posterior third of the tongue.

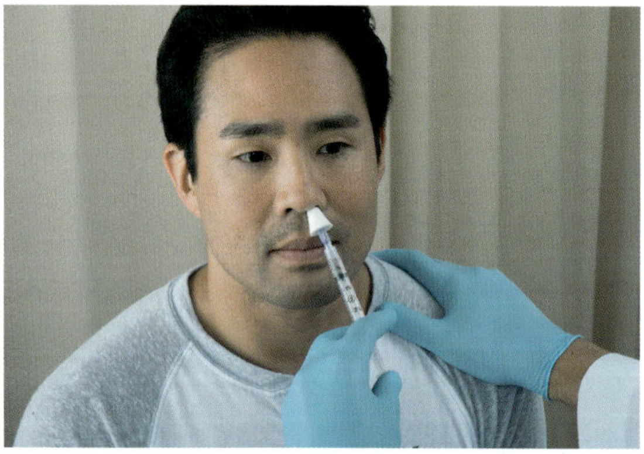

Fig. 5.4 The Mucosal Atomization Device. (Courtesy Teleflex. Copyright 2025 Teleflex Incorporated. All rights reserved.)

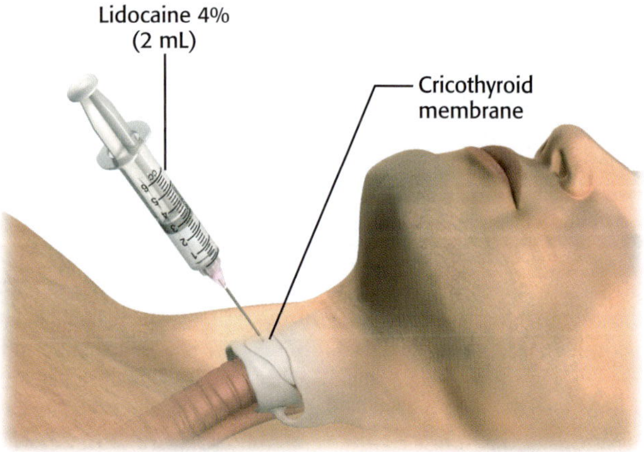

Fig. 5.5 Cricothyroid membrane puncture. Prepare the skin with an antiseptic and then puncture the cricothyroid membrane in the midline. Advance the needle until air can be aspirated and then rapidly inject 2 mL of 4% lidocaine. Alternatively, 3 mL to 4 mL of 2% lidocaine can be used.

The awake, compliant patient can be directed to "gargle and spit" liquid 4% lidocaine, or 5% lidocaine ointment can be applied with a tongue depressor.[193] Another alternative is percutaneous injection of an anesthetic agent into the trachea at the level of the cricothyroid membrane.[194,195]

Cricothyroid Membrane Puncture

Direct application of topical anesthetics to the subglottic region can also be achieved through cricothyroid membrane puncture (Fig. 5.5). In this procedure, identify the cricothyroid membrane immediately below the thyroid cartilage. After antiseptic skin preparation, puncture the overlying tissue and membrane with a 22-gauge needle in the midline and just above the superior border of the cricoid cartilage. Take care to maintain the needle in the midline at all times to avoid injury to the recurrent laryngeal nerve. Advance the needle until air can be aspirated, indicating placement of the needle in the trachea. Inject a 2-mL volume of 4% lidocaine rapidly. If the 4% concentration is not available, use 3 mL to 4 mL of 1% to 2% lidocaine. Typically, this will precipitate a cough and distribute the anesthetic over the upper part of the trachea, vocal cords, and epiglottis. Whereas more invasive than the other described techniques, intratracheal injection may provide superior local anesthesia,[196,197] and there is limited evidence comparing different techniques.

Nebulized Anesthesia

Nebulized anesthesia is a simple and painless technique that can be used to facilitate awake intubation when the patient's condition is stable enough to permit a several-minute delay. Deliver the anesthetic via a standard nebulizer and face mask connected to an oxygen source that delivers 4 to 8 L/min. It is critical that the oxygen source not be set to the high-flow rate commonly used to nebulize medications such as albuterol. Doing so will anesthetize the lungs without properly anesthetizing the vocal cords. Nebulize a 4-mL volume of a 4% lidocaine solution over a period of approximately 5 minutes. Bourke and colleagues[198] reported achieving consistently good topical anesthesia with this technique, although their patients were often premedicated with combinations of opioids and sedatives. This technique has been successfully used in pediatric patients.[199] Parkes and colleagues[200] demonstrated that the plasma levels of lidocaine following nebulized lidocaine for awake intubation were detectable, and far below the toxic threshold. Further evidence of the effectiveness and safety of this procedure has been found through its use in decreasing the pain of placing nasogastric tubes.[201]

Sedation for Awake Intubation

Many patients can be intubated while awake with adequate topical anesthesia, and anxiolysis with mild to moderate sedation may be helpful for selected patients. The use of propofol in low doses (0.2 to 0.3 mg/kg) may be helpful, and exercise caution because propofol can cause hypotension in critically ill patients despite using a low dosage.

A newer sedative agent, dexmedetomidine (an α_2-adrenoreceptor agonist), has been described for use in awake intubation.[202–206] Dexmedetomidine produces sedation and anxiolysis with minimal respiratory depression. Patients become sleepy and, if stimulated, can easily be aroused and are generally cooperative. These properties make it seem like an ideal agent for awake intubation, and its use is limited in emergencies by a requisite 10-minute loading dose followed by a maintenance infusion. Future studies will be needed before this medication can be recommended for use in the ED.

The sedative that is most conducive to awake intubation in the ED is ketamine. It preserves spontaneous respirations, does not generally cause hypotension, and can safely provide a deep level of sedation. Ketamine's tendency to cause increased airway secretions may be partially corrected with glycopyrrolate or atropine, and there are rather limited data on the need to use an anticholinergic.[207] Ketamine may be used at subdissociative doses (<0.3 mg/kg) if adequate topical anesthesia has been obtained. It may alternatively be used at dissociative doses (>1 mg/kg) and theoretically can cause more side effects. An attempt to appropriately anesthetize the airway is important as ketamine preserves airway reflexes. Ketamine's safety profile makes it a good choice for sedation in awake intubations. The clinician should be prepared for possible laryngospasm during the use of a scope with ketamine. Whereas no cases of this have been reported,[204] preparedness for transition to a surgical airway or traditional RSI is essential.

Delayed-Sequence Intubation

Some patients may be unable to tolerate adequate preoxygenation prior to an initial attempt to intubate. DSI is a technique used to safely manage the airway in certain clinical scenarios where traditional RSI may not be feasible or safe. DSI involves the administration of a dissociative anesthetic, typically ketamine, to achieve an adequate level of sedation and oxygenation before proceeding with intubation.

DSI has been described as procedural sedation for the procedure of preoxygenation.[6] The primary goal of DSI is to optimize the patient's preoxygenation and reduce the risk of periintubation hypoxia, which can be particularly critical in patients with compromised respiratory function or difficult airways. By providing a period of preoxygenation and allowing the patient to reach a state of deeper sedation, DSI aims to improve oxygenation and minimize the risk of desaturation during the subsequent intubation procedure.

While the decision to proceed with DSI should be based on individual patient assessment and clinical judgment, some specific patient populations may potentially benefit from DSI:

- Agitated or combative patients: DSI can help achieve sedation and calmness in patients who are agitated or uncooperative, allowing for preoxygenation and a safer intubation process.
- Patients with severe respiratory distress: DSI may be considered in patients experiencing severe respiratory distress, allowing for adequate preoxygenation and optimization of their oxygenation status before intubation.
- Patients with difficult airways: Individuals with anticipated difficult airways, such as those with abnormal anatomy, prior surgeries, or pathologic airway changes, may benefit from DSI. It provides an opportunity for careful airway assessment, appropriate preparation, and optimization of conditions for successful intubation.
- Patients at risk of periintubation hypoxia: DSI can be valuable in patients with a high risk of desaturation during the intubation process, such as those with limited oxygen reserves, significant shunt physiology, or a high oxygen consumption rate.

Ketamine is given at 1 mg/kg IV to provide sedation. This allows the patient to tolerate preoxygenation with any appropriate combination of high-flow nasal cannula, BVM (preferably with PEEP valve), nonrebreather mask, or noninvasive ventilator. Once adequately preoxygenated, the patient's airway may be managed by intubation with a direct laryngoscope, video laryngoscope, or fiberoptic scope after neuromuscular blockade. It is important to note, however, that during DSI, the clinician must be prepared for immediate intubation as ketamine still has the potential risk to precipitate laryngospasm or apnea.[208] Maintaining a state of readiness for prompt conversion to RSI and intubation is crucial to manage any adverse events that may arise during DSI.

Evidence for improved patient-oriented outcomes, such as mortality or periintubation hypoxia, specifically related to DSI with ketamine, is limited. DSI is a relatively new concept, and robust, high-quality studies specifically evaluating its impact on these outcomes are currently lacking. Most of the available evidence comes from case reports, retrospective studies, and observational data.[209–211] In a prehospital study, a care bundle including DSI with ketamine was associated with lower rates of periintubation hypoxia than standard out-of-hospital RSI.[212] Additionally, a recent small randomized controlled trial (RCT) showed a significantly lower incidence of periintubation hypoxia and improved first-pass success.[213]

CONCLUSION

There have been many major advances in the pharmacologic adjuncts to intubation in the ED. There has been an increasing deemphasis on the importance of premedications prior to intubation. The importance of avoiding hypotension and hypoxia has caused far less focus on the use of lidocaine, fentanyl, or other medications prior to intubation. Ketamine has now joined etomidate as a first-line induction agent, with many providers using it almost exclusively. Rocuronium has emerged as the nondepolarizing paralytic of choice in most EDs in recent years, and succinylcholine remains an excellent choice. An increased emphasis on awake intubations and the new concept of DSI have further expanded the use of topical anesthetics and ketamine to assist in difficult airways. A mastery of the pharmacology of drugs used to intubate remains a critical skill for all providers who see critically ill patients.

ACKNOWLEDGMENTS

The editors and authors wish to acknowledge the contribution of Laura R. Hopson and Greene Shepherd to this chapter in previous editions.

REFERENCES ARE AVAILABLE AT ELSEVIER EBOOKS+

CHAPTER 6

Cricothyrotomy and Percutaneous Translaryngeal Ventilation

Randy B. Hebert and Daniel Thomas

INTRODUCTION

Few clinical scenarios are as critical as when a patient's airway cannot be controlled with traditional endotracheal (ET) intubation. When ET intubation has failed or is contraindicated, cricothyrotomy is often the procedure of last resort. The conditions accompanying an airway emergency are often stressful and chaotic and require the emergency department (ED) physician to be intimately familiar with surgical options. Rescue surgical airway procedures occur infrequently in the ED, with approximately half performed in the setting of acute trauma.[1] Cricothyrotomy is rarely required,[2–6] and the incidence of surgical airways has been decreasing since the advent of adjunctive intubation techniques.[7,8] The incorporation of rescue devices such as a gum elastic bougie or extraglottic device may be contributing to this trend.[1] Surgical cricothyrotomy occurs at a similar rate as several other high-acuity procedures like cardiac pacing and lateral canthotomy. The infrequency of these suggests that emergency clinicians may need ongoing training beyond clinical experience alone to maintain competency.[9]

Both surgical cricothyrotomy and needle cricothyrotomy entail puncture of the cricothyroid membrane through the overlying skin to gain access to the airway. *Surgical cricothyrotomy* is a procedure in which an incision is made in the cricothyroid membrane and a tracheostomy tube or modified ET tube is placed into the airway to ventilate the patient. *Tracheostomy* differs from cricothyrotomy in that the incision is made between two of the tracheal rings. *Needle cricothyrotomy* refers to insertion of a catheter via percutaneous needle puncture of the cricothyroid membrane to allow *percutaneous translaryngeal ventilation* (PTLV). The term *transtracheal jet ventilation* is often used interchangeably with PTLV in conjunction with needle cricothyrotomy, but PTLV is more accurate because the cricothyroid membrane is part of the larynx and not the trachea. PTLV is sometimes provided by bag insufflation instead of jet ventilation. The term *jet ventilation* can refer to low-frequency jet ventilation with oxygen from a wall source, as opposed to high-frequency jet ventilation from a dedicated jet ventilator.

ANATOMY

The central structure of importance is the cricothyroid membrane, an elastic membrane located anteriorly and midline in the neck. The membrane is bordered superiorly by the thyroid cartilage and inferiorly by the cricoid cartilage. The lateral aspects of the cricothyroid membrane are partially covered by the cricothyroid muscles, and the central triangular portion is subcutaneous, making it an ideal location to access the airway.

Identify the cricothyroid membrane by locating the prominent thyroid cartilage superior to it. The thyroid cartilage consists of two lateral laminae that join at an acute angle in the midline to form the laryngeal prominence. Commonly known as the *Adam's apple*, this structure is more pronounced in males. The internal aspect of the anterior body of the thyroid cartilage provides the attachment for the vocal ligaments. Superior to the thyroid cartilage and connecting it to the hyoid bone is the thyroid membrane, which allows passage of the superior laryngeal vessels and the internal branch of the superior laryngeal nerve through its laterally located foramina.

The cricoid cartilage forms the inferior border of the cricothyroid membrane and is the only completely circumferential cartilaginous structure of the larynx. It is composed of a broad posterior segment that tapers laterally to form a narrow anterior arch. The tracheal rings descend inferior to the cricoid cartilage.

Identify the cricothyroid membrane between the previously mentioned structures as a shallow depression measuring approximately 6 to 8 mm longitudinally and 30 mm transversely.[10] If the depression is obscured by excessive soft tissue or swelling, estimate the location of the cricothyroid membrane at approximately 2 to 3 cm inferior to the laryngeal prominence or four fingerbreadths above the sternal notch.[11] Digital palpation alone may not always accurately locate the cricothyroid membrane.[12–14]

The area overlying and immediately adjacent to the cricothyroid membrane is relatively avascular and free of other significant anatomic structures. The cricothyroid arteries branch from the superior thyroid arteries and may form a small anastomotic arch traversing the superior aspect of the cricothyroid membrane. The external branch of the superior laryngeal nerve runs along the lateral aspect of the larynx and innervates the cricothyroid muscles inferior to the membrane. The isthmus of the thyroid gland most often overlies the second and third tracheal rings, although an aberrant pyramidal lobe of the gland may extend just superior to the cricothyroid membrane. The anterior attachments of the vocal cord structures are protected by the thyroid cartilage[15,16] (Fig. 6.1).

In children, the larynx is positioned more superiorly than in adults.[17] There is also more overlap between the thyroid cartilage and the cricoid cartilage, making the cricoid membrane proportionally smaller[18] (Fig. 6.2).

SURGICAL CRICOTHYROTOMY

Indications and Contraindications

The chief indication for surgical cricothyrotomy is an inability to secure the airway with less invasive techniques in a patient with impending or ongoing hypoxia.[19]

Surgical cricothyrotomy, like any invasive procedure, is associated with significant complications and should not be attempted until less invasive measures have failed. No simple algorithm fits all cases. When time and the clinical situation allow, it may be appropriate to attempt to intubate multiple times with traditional laryngoscopy or to try alternative intubation techniques. Emergency decisions are subject to controversy, differing on a case-by-case analysis, and alternatives to cricothyrotomy include bag-valve-mask ventilation, the gum elastic bougie, and laryngeal mask airways. At some point, further attempts at intubation become futile and the benefits of a surgical airway outweigh the risks associated with ongoing hypoxia.[20]

When approaching a patient with a compromised airway, the clinician must have a clear potential algorithm in mind with a well-defined plan that shifts the airway approach from laryngoscopy to alternative techniques, and then to cricothyrotomy.[21] The first step in deciding whether cricothyrotomy is indicated is anticipating a possible difficult intubation.[22]

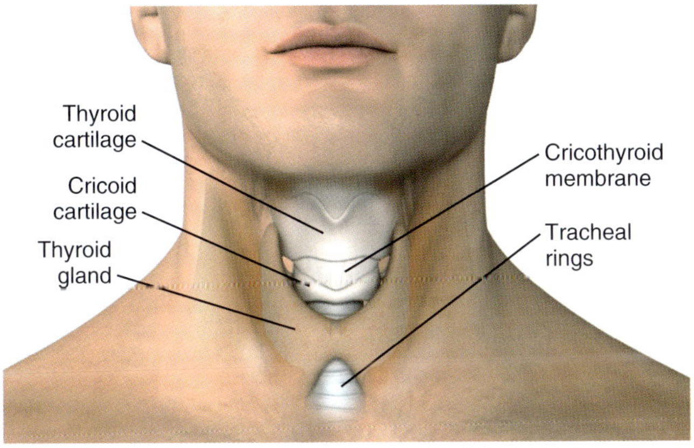

Fig. 6.1 Normal adult larynx. Note position and configuration of the cricothyroid membrane.

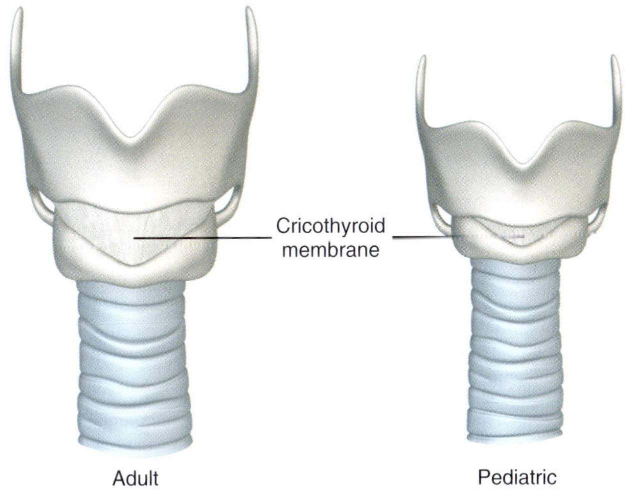

Fig. 6.2 Adult larynx compared with a pediatric larynx.

Cricothyrotomy

Indications

Inability to maintain >90% saturation between intubation attempts or after three attempts

Inability to bag-mask-valve ventilate the patient between intubation attempts or after three attempts

Multiple attempts at endotracheal intubation fail to secure the airway after failed rescue maneuvers (e.g., gum elastic bougie intubation, intubating laryngeal mask airway)

Contraindications

Age younger than 5–12 years (depending on the source)

Tracheal transection, fracture, or obstruction below the cricothyroid membrane

Complications

Acute

- Bleeding
- Tube malposition
- Bronchial intubation
- Laryngotracheal injury
- Tension pneumothorax
- Tube obstruction

Late

- Subjective voice changes
- Difficulty swallowing
- Infections
- Persistent shortness of breath
- Persistent stoma
- Subglottic or glottic stenosis

Equipment

Traditional surgical cricothyrotomy

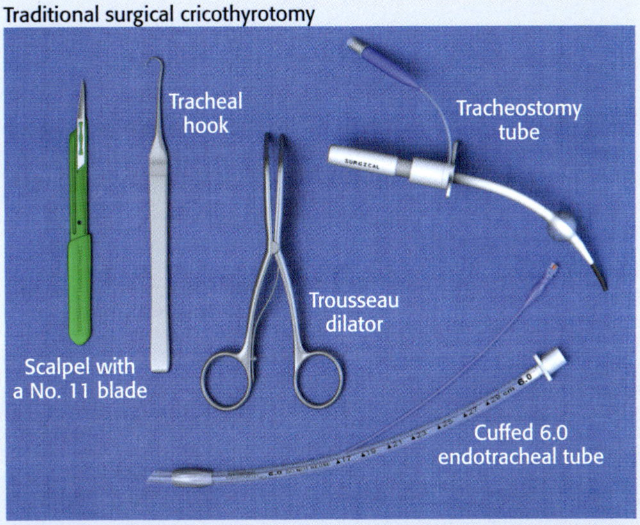

Melker technique

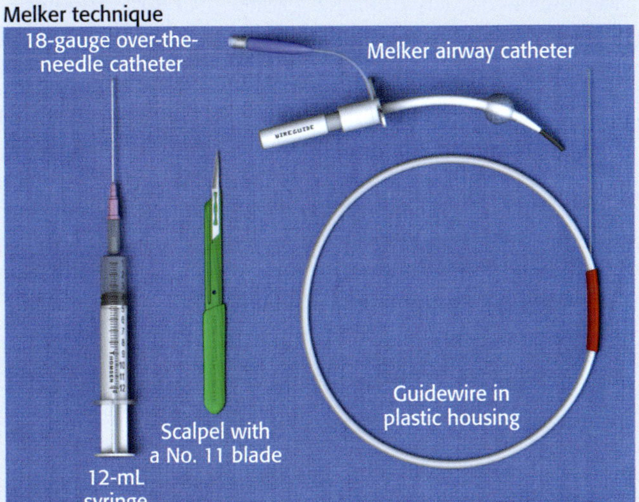

Review Box 6.1 Cricothyrotomy: indications, contraindications, complications, and equipment.

BOX 6.1 Clinical Indicators of a Difficult Airway

High Mallampati score
High LEMON score
Thyroid-to-hyoid distance <2 fingerbreadths
Obesity
Large incisors
Limited neck mobility
Airway obstruction (partial or complete)

- Nontraumatic
  - Oropharyngeal edema
  - Laryngospasm
  - Mass effect (cancer, tumor, polyp, web, or other mass)
- Traumatic
  - Oropharyngeal edema
  - Foreign body obstruction
  - Laryngospasm
  - Obstruction secondary to a mass effect or displacement
  - Stenosis

Modified from Soyuncu S. Determination of difficult intubation in the ED. Ann J Emerg Med *2009;8:905.*

Several studies in the anesthesia and emergency medicine literature have attempted to identify predictors of a difficult airway. The Mallampati score and the modified LEMON score are examples of bedside assessment tools that can be used in an attempt to predict a difficult intubation[23–26] These prediction tools have limited value in critically ill ED patients and do not obviate the need to prepare for a difficult airway.[27] Additional indicators of a difficult airway include obesity, oropharyngeal edema, hemorrhage, and laryngospasm[28–31] (Box 6.1). In anticipation of a failed airway, it may be reasonable to mark the cricothyroid membrane using ultrasound guidance to prepare for the possibility of a cricothyrotomy.[32]

Cricothyrotomy is indicated when a difficult airway becomes a "failed airway." Various algorithms have been designed to define a failed airway. The American Society of Anesthesiologists suggests defining a failed airway as an inability to maintain oxygen saturation greater than 90%, signs of inadequate ventilation (cyanosis, absent breath sounds, hemodynamic instability) with positive pressure bag-mask ventilation, or more than three failed attempts at ET intubation or failure to intubate after 10 minutes by an experienced operator.[33] As more rescue airway adjunctive devices become available, it is reasonable to continue beyond three attempts at ET intubation if adequate ventilation and oxygen saturation greater than 90% can be maintained.[34]

Because of the anatomic differences between children and adults, including a smaller cricothyroid membrane and a rostral, funnel-shaped, and more compliant pediatric larynx, surgical cricothyrotomy has been contraindicated in infants and young children. The exact age at which surgical cricothyrotomy can be performed is controversial and not well defined. Various references list the lower age limit from 5 years[35] to 10 years[36] or 12 years.[37] The advanced cardiac life support and pediatric advanced life support define an infant airway as age up to 1 year and a child airway as age 1 to 8 years.

Some authors also identify tracheal transection or low tracheal obstruction (below the cricoid) as absolute contraindications to cricothyrotomy because of the need to secure the airway below the injury.[38]

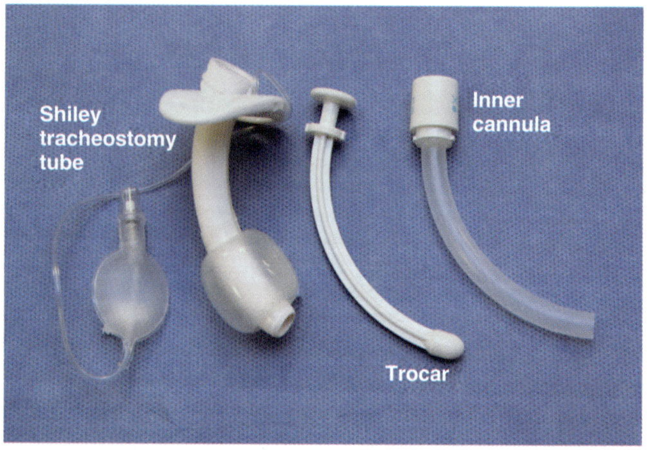

Fig. 6.3 Standard Shiley tracheostomy tube with removable obturator and inner cannula.

Equipment

The equipment necessary to perform a traditional surgical cricothyrotomy includes a scalpel with a No. 11 blade, a Trousseau dilator, a tracheal hook, and a tracheostomy tube or modified ET tube (see Review Box 6.1). In addition, the sterile tray may include a syringe and lidocaine with epinephrine for local anesthesia, sterile drapes or towels, antiseptic preparation solution, 4 × 4-cm sterile gauze, scissors, hemostats, and suture material. Familiarity with the dimensions of several standard tracheostomy and ET tubes is essential when selecting the appropriate size for surgical airways. Cuffed tracheostomy tubes are recommended, and they come in various sizes. Shiley tracheostomy tubes are commonly available in most EDs. The No. 4 tube has an inner diameter (ID) of 5.0 mm and an outer diameter (OD) of 9.4 mm, and the No. 6 tube has an ID of 6.4 mm and an OD of 10.8 mm. Shiley tracheostomy tubes have three parts: a cuffed outer cannula, a removable inner cannula, and a removable obturator that is solid and removed after insertion (Fig. 6.3). ET tubes are often used temporarily in place of a tracheostomy tube. With respect to ID, ET tube OD can vary with the manufacturer. As an example, the Mallinckrodt TaperGuard Evac Endotracheal Tube with IDs of 6.0 and 8.0 mm have ODs of 9.0 and 11.8 mm, respectively.[39] Although a No. 11 scalpel blade is most commonly used, a No. 20 or a No. 10 blade is recommended in some variations of the technique. Commercially available kits include the Melker Cricothyrotomy Kit (Cook Critical Care) for percutaneous cricothyrotomy, which uses the Seldinger technique to insert a cuffed or uncuffed airway catheter.

Procedure

Positioning plays a critical role in success, and the ideal patient position may be impossible because of clinical parameters. For example, hypoxic patients often cannot recline. Ketamine anesthesia does not suppress the respiratory drive and may aid in patient cooperation and positioning. Ketamine is theoretically the superior agent to facilitate the procedure. When feasible, use the supine position with the neck exposed. Unless the patient has a known or suspected cervical spine injury, hyperextend the neck to more readily identify the landmarks.

Surgical cricothyrotomy can safely and successfully be performed with minimal cervical spine movement.[40] Preoxygenate the patient by bag-mask ventilation. Prepare the skin of the anterior aspect of the neck with antiseptic solution and create a sterile field with the use of drapes or towels. If the patient is awake or responding to pain, give a subcutaneous and translaryngeal injection of lidocaine with epinephrine as a local anesthetic. Test the integrity of the balloon on the tracheostomy or ET tube by inflating it with 10 ml of air. Wear sterile gloves and take standard precautions by wearing a mask, goggles, and gown. Some preparatory steps may be omitted depending on the urgency of the procedure.

Traditional Technique

The "traditional" (open) cricothyrotomy technique (Fig. 6.4) has changed little since the original description of elective cricothyroidotomy by Brantigan and Grow in 1976.[41] McGill and colleagues[42] described the addition of a tracheal hook for emergency cricothyrotomy in 1982. In a follow-up report in 1989, Erlandson and colleagues[43] emphasized the importance of making an initial vertical skin incision and using a relatively small (No. 4 Shiley) tracheal tube. These modifications have generally been accepted and are commonly described as part of the traditional technique.[44]

Prepare the tracheostomy tube by testing the balloon, removing the inner cannula, and inserting the solid white obturator. If right hand dominant, stand at the bedside on the patient's right side. Stabilize the larynx with the nondominant hand by grasping both sides of the lateral thyroid cartilage with the thumb and middle finger. Palpate the depression over the cricothyroid membrane with the index finger. Control the larynx throughout the procedure by stabilizing it in this manner (see Fig. 6.4, *step 1*). Accurate localization of the cricothyroid membrane by landmark palpation may be variable.[13] In shorter patients, those with an increased body mass index, or in patients with neck swelling, these landmarks may be even more difficult to identify by palpation alone.[45,46] If the laryngeal landmarks are not easily identifiable, bedside ultrasonography has been shown to assist in identifying the cricothyroid membrane, and decrease injuries to the larynx and trachea.[47–49] (Fig. 6.5).

The use of ultrasound with regard to facilitating procedures is not new to emergency medicine and cricothyroidotomy is no exception. Ultrasound has been shown to markedly increase the accuracy with which providers correctly identify the cricothyroid membrane compared with external palpation alone, especially in patients with challenging anatomy.[50–52] Proficiency in the technique is easily attainable.[53] Ultrasound is not without its downsides; its use is associated with significantly increased procedure completion time and may not contribute to overall increased success rate.[54]

While holding the scalpel with a No. 11 blade in the dominant hand, make an approximately 2- to 3-cm *vertical incision* through the skin and subcutaneous tissue (see Fig. 6.4, *step 2*). With the index finger of the nondominant hand, palpate the cricothyroid membrane through the incision. It is important to understand that the remainder of the procedure should be performed by palpation of the anatomy, not visualization, because bleeding may obscure the field and there is no time to delay while trying to achieve hemostasis. If the cricothyroid membrane cannot be palpated, extend the initial incision superiorly and inferiorly and try to palpate again. Using the stabilizing nondominant index finger as a guide, make a *horizontal* incision of less than 1.0 cm in length through the cricothyroid membrane (see Fig. 6.4, *step 3*). Note that the skin incision is vertical and the membrane incision is horizontal. Place the nondominant index finger into the stoma momentarily and exchange the scalpel for the tracheal hook.[55]

Using the dominant hand, place the tracheal hook into the opening in the cricothyroid membrane. Rotate the handle cephalad while grasping the inferior border of the thyroid cartilage with it. Ask an assistant to provide upward traction or provide traction yourself by passing the handle of the hook to the nondominant hand (see Fig. 6.4, *step 4*). Use the tracheal hook to stabilize the larynx and keep it in place throughout the remainder of the procedure.

With the dominant hand, place the tips of the Trousseau dilator into the opening in the membrane with the spreading action oriented initially in the longitudinal or vertical plane so that the handle is facing horizontal or perpendicular to the direction of the neck (see Fig. 6.4, *step 5*). This instrument works the opposite to that of most ordinary instruments, such as hemostats. Squeezing the handles opens rather than closes the blades. This can be confusing the first time you use it, and it is worth practicing before you need it in an emergency. If this instrument is not available in an emergency, Mayo scissors, a hemostat, or even the blunt end of a scalpel handle can be used to dilate the incision in the cricothyroid membrane.[56]

Dilate the incision vertically with the Trousseau dilator. Hold the handles of the Trousseau dilator with the nondominant hand and rotate the handle 90 degrees until the handle is vertical or parallel to the neck (see Fig. 6.4, *step 6*). If the dilator is left horizontal, the blades of the dilator may impede passage of the tracheostomy tube into the trachea. While holding the dilator with the nondominant hand, take the tube in the dominant hand and insert it between the blades of the dilator until the flanges rest against the skin of the neck (see Fig. 6.4, *step 7*). Keep the thumb on the obturator throughout the procedure. Carefully remove the Trousseau dilator (see Fig. 6.4, *step 8*). Remove the obturator and insert the inner cannula. Inflate the balloon (see Fig. 6.4, *step 9*). Remove the tracheal hook while being especially careful to not puncture the cuff.[57,58]

If a tracheostomy tube is not available or if there is difficulty placing the tracheostomy tube into the opening in the cricothyroid membrane, try using a 6-0 cuffed ET tube cut to a shorter length. The ID/OD ratios of tracheostomy tubes are comparable to those of ET tubes. Use of a gum elastic may facilitate and even hasten placement of an ET tube through the cricothyroid membrane into the trachea.[59] The advantage of using the bougie is that you can get immediate confirmation that the device is inside the trachea because of the "washboard" vibration that the curved tip makes as it contacts the tracheal rings.[60] Modify the ET tube by cutting the distal end and replacing the adapter to the cut end (Fig. 6.6). Be careful not to cut the pilot balloon or inflation port. If the ET tube is shortened, it is less likely to kink once it is attached to a ventilator. Advance the ET tube only approximately 5 cm from the tip to avoid main stem intubation. Keep in mind that standard ET tubes do not have centimeter markings at the distal end. Inserting the ET tube so that the distal cuff is approximately 2 cm beyond the cricothyroid membrane usually ensures proper placement (Fig. 6.6).

Confirm proper placement in the same manner as with ET tube placement: end-tidal CO_2, bilateral chest movement, and breath sounds. Secure the tracheostomy tube with a circumferential tie around the neck or with sutures (see Fig. 6.4 *step 10*). Verify placement with a postprocedure portable chest radiograph.

SURGICAL CRICOTHYROTOMY: TRADITIONAL TECHNIQUE

1

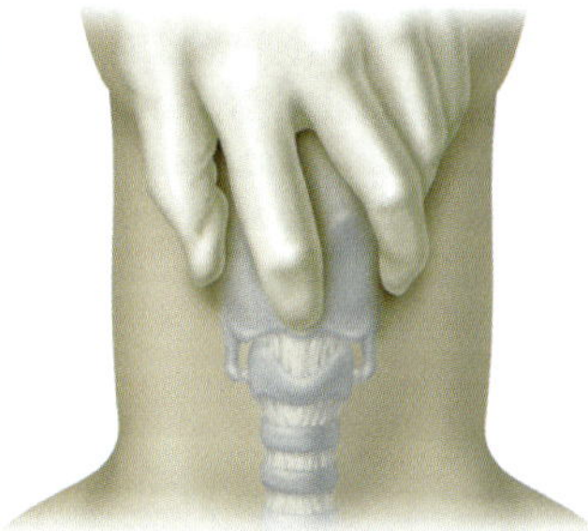

Extend the neck whenever possible for better access to the trachea. Immobilize the larynx with your nondominant hand and palpate the cricothyroid membrane with your index finger.

2

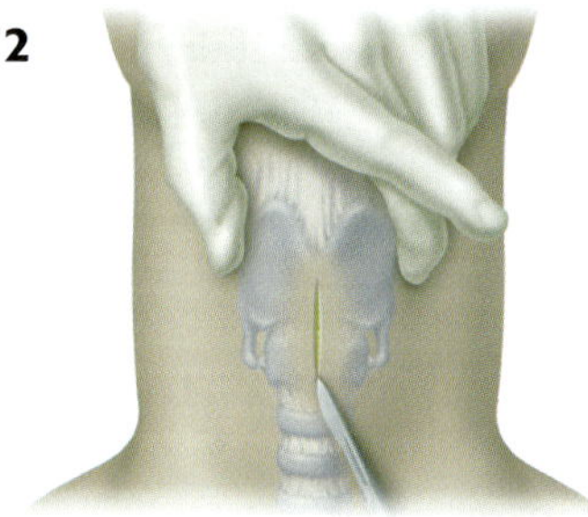

Make a 3- to 5-cm *vertical* midline incision through the skin and subcutaneous tissues.

Palpate the membrane through the skin to confirm the anatomy.

3

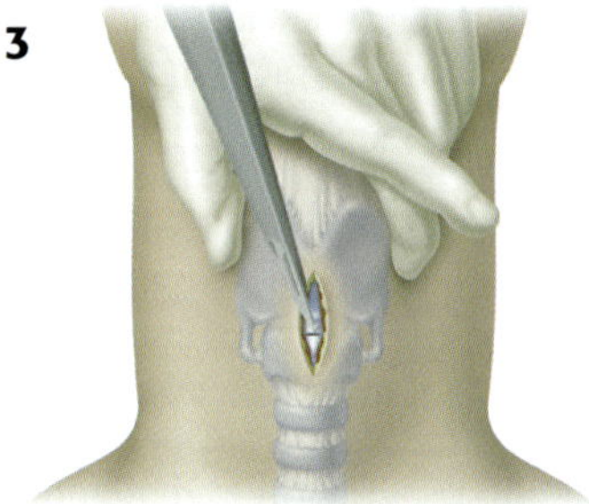

Make a <1-cm *horizontal* incision through the cricothyroid membrane. *Note that the skin incision is vertical, but the membrane incision is horizontal.*

4

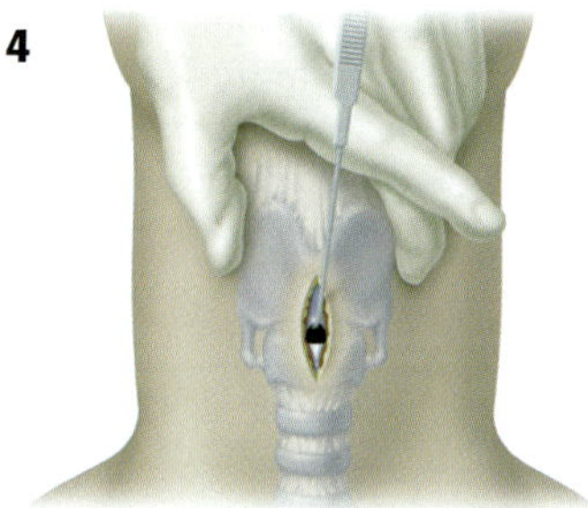

Insert the tracheal hook in the opening of the membrane, and rotate it cephalad, while grasping the inferior border of the thyroid cartilage. Ask an assistant to provide upward traction on the hook.

5

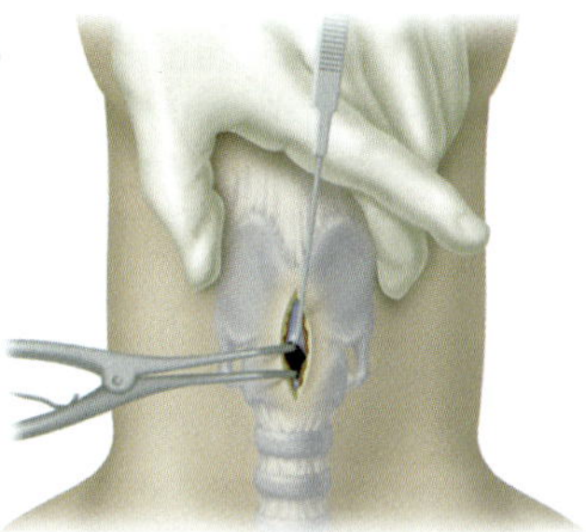

Place the tips of the Trousseau dilator into the opening in the membrane and spread in the longitudinal (vertical) plane.

6

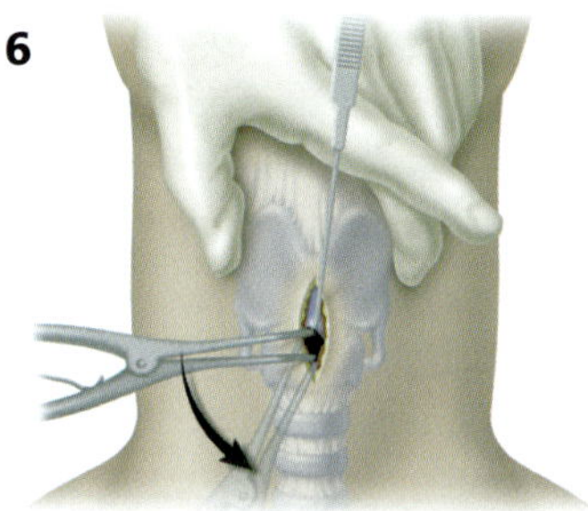

Rotate the handle 90° until the handle is vertical or parallel to the neck.

7

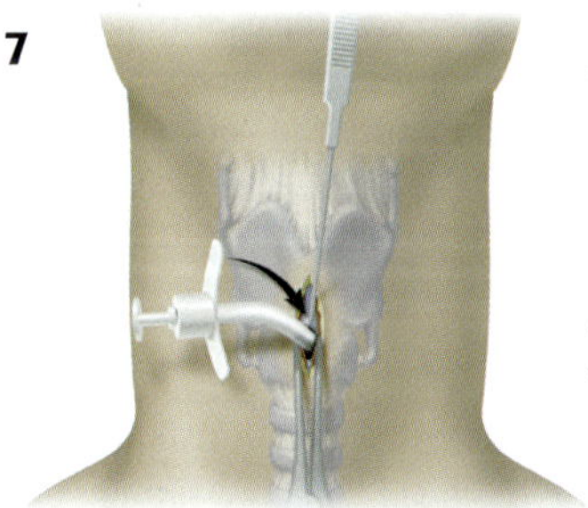

Insert the tube between the blades of the dilator until the flanges rest against the skin of the neck.

Keep your thumb on the obturator during tube insertion.

8

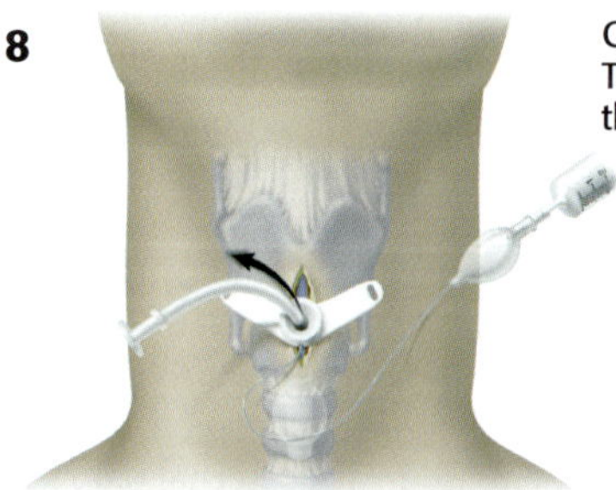

Carefully remove the Trousseau dilator and the obturator.

9

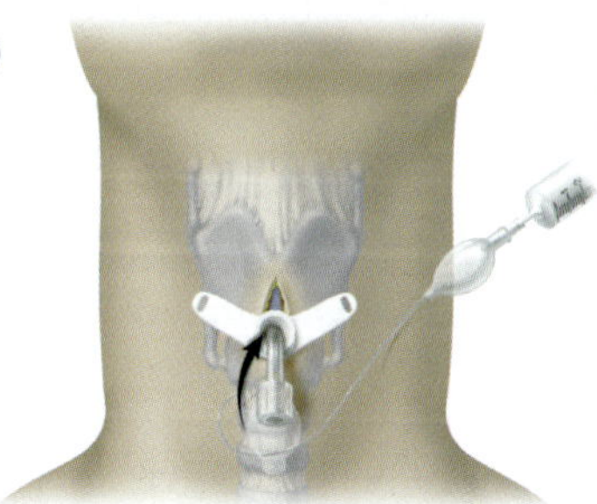

Replace the inner cannula of the tracheostomy tube and inflate the balloon.

10

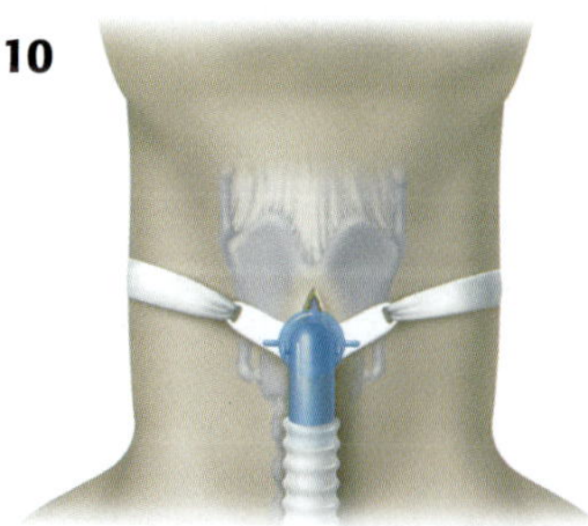

Ventilate and confirm tube position by auscultation and end-tidal CO_2.

Secure the tube in place.

Fig. 6.4 Surgical cricothyrotomy: traditional technique. (Adapted from Custalow CB. *Color Atlas of Emergency Department Procedure*. Saunders; 2005.)

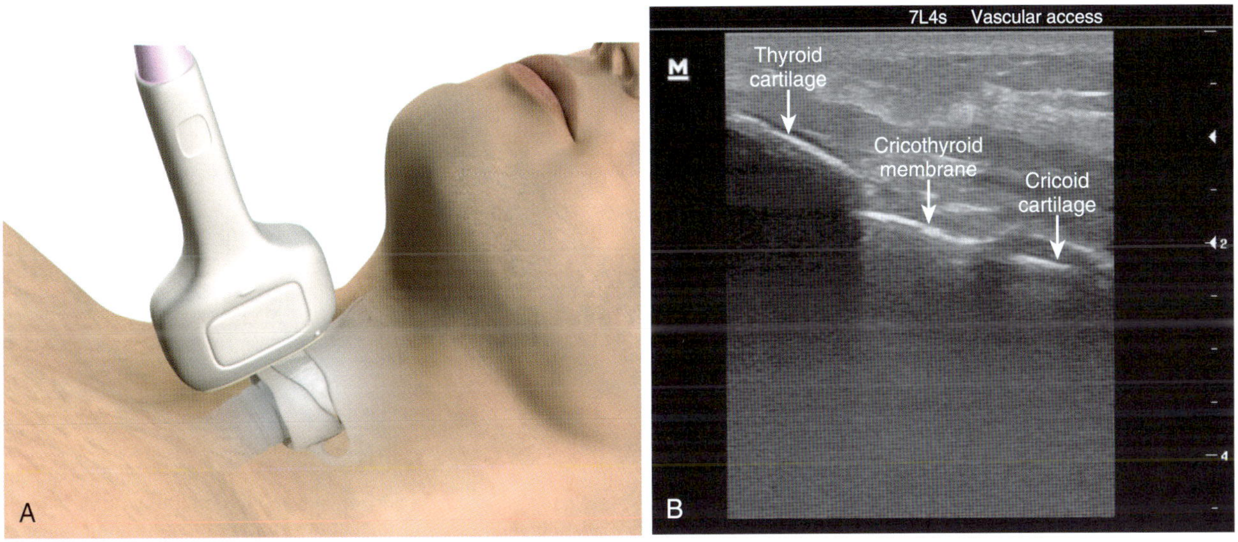

Fig. 6.5 (A) As an option, use the linear ultrasound probe to locate the cricothyroid membrane. (B) Ultrasound image of the cricothyroid membrane in the sagittal plane. (B, From Mallin M, Curtis K, Dawson M, et al. Accuracy of ultrasound-guided marking of the cricothyroid membrane before simulated failed intubation. *Am J Emerg Med.* 2014;32:61.)

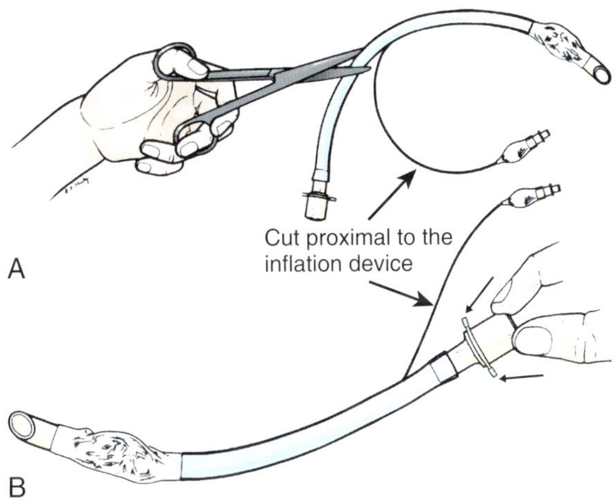

Fig. 6.6 (A) Modify the standard endotracheal (ET) tube for use in surgical cricothyrotomy as a temporary alternative to a tracheostomy tube. Cut the proximal end of the ET tube but be careful to not cut the balloon inflation apparatus. (B) Replace the adapter on the cut end of the tube.

Rapid Four-Step Technique (Brofeldt)

See Video 6.1. Brofeldt and colleagues[61] developed a rapid four-step technique (RFST) to decrease the amount of time required to establish an airway and reduce complications of hypoxia. It combines aspects of traditional cricothyroidotomy and ET intubation. If right handed, stand at the bedside to the patient's left. Palpate the depression over the cricothyroid membrane with the nondominant hand (Fig. 6.7, *step 1*). With the dominant hand, make a single horizontal stab incision with a No. 20 scalpel blade approximately 1.5 cm in length through the skin, subcutaneous tissue, and cricothyroid membrane (see Fig. 6.7, *step 2*). With the scalpel blade as a guide, pick up the cricoid cartilage with the tracheal hook and provide traction in the caudal direction to stabilize the trachea (see Fig. 6.7, *step 3*). Place a No. 4 cuffed tracheostomy tube or a 6-0 cuffed ET tube through the opening (see Fig. 6.7, *step 4*).

Because this technique omits dilating the stoma with the Trousseau dilator, it may be more difficult to pass a tracheostomy tube. A gum elastic bougie, using the Seldinger technique, may assist in this step[61] (Videos 6.2–6.4).

There is evidence that use of a bougie as a routine part of this procedure increases successful placement of the tube.[62,63] Bair and colleagues[64] modified this technique further by introducing a new device called a *Bair Claw* to replace the tracheal hook. The technique is similar to the four-step method except for positioning the operator at the head of the bed instead of the patient's side and the use of a double-hook device rather than a single hook. By replacing the single hook with the double hook, they found a decrease in the incidence of cricoid ring fractures in cadavers (Fig. 6.8).

This method has been further simplified, using ultrasound to localize the cricothyroid membrane. Then a single horizontal laceration is made, again through the skin, subcutaneous tissue, and cricothyroid membrane. The scalpel is turned 90 degrees to allow passage of a gum elastic bougie, over which an ET tube is passed.[65] Care should be taken when turning the scalpel 90 degrees so as to make sure no other structures (or the operator) are lacerated.

Melker Percutaneous Cricothyrotomy Technique

The Melker Cricothyrotomy Kit is a prepackaged commercial kit for use with the Seldinger technique to place a tracheostomy tube over a guidewire. The kit comes supplied with a 6-ml syringe, an 18-gauge needle with an overlying tetrafluoroethylene (TFE) catheter (the TFE catheter is not included in some kits), a guidewire, a tapered dilator, and a Melker airway catheter in lieu of a tracheostomy tube.[66] Similar to retrograde intubation or needle cricothyrotomy with PTLV, the cricothyroid membrane must be easy to identify because no initial skin incision will be made. Anatomic distortion will make locating the cricothyroid membrane with a needle more difficult.

Preparation for this technique is similar to that for the other techniques. Positioned at the patient's left, palpate the cricothyroid membrane with the nondominant hand. With

SURGICAL CRICOTHYROTOMY: RAPID FOUR-STEP TECHNIQUE

1

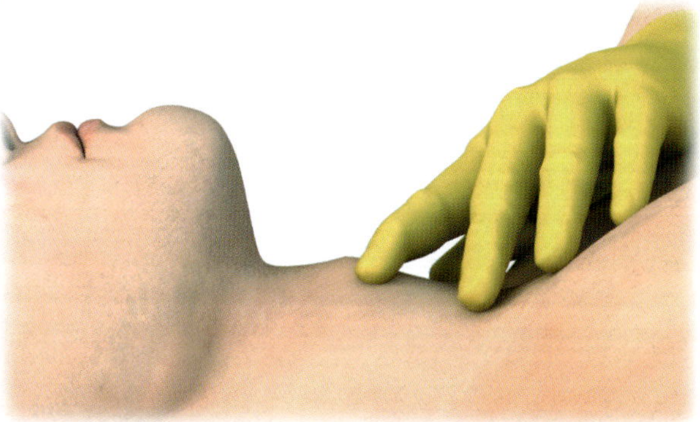

If possible, extend the neck to better expose the trachea. Palpate the depression over the cricothyroid membrane with your nondominant hand.

2

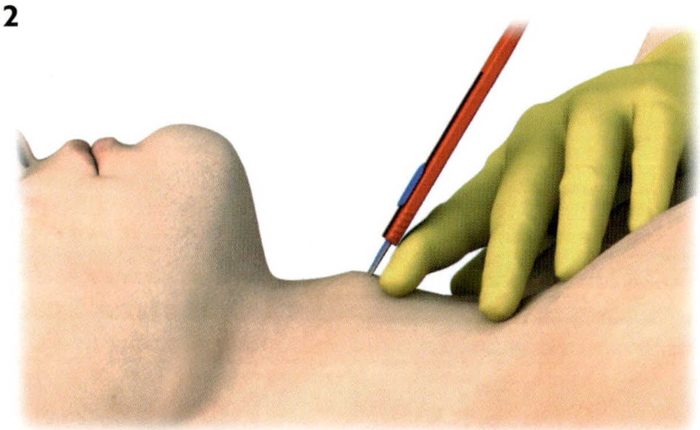

Make a 1.5-cm single horizontal stab incision through the skin, subcutaneous tissue, and cricothyroid membrane.

3

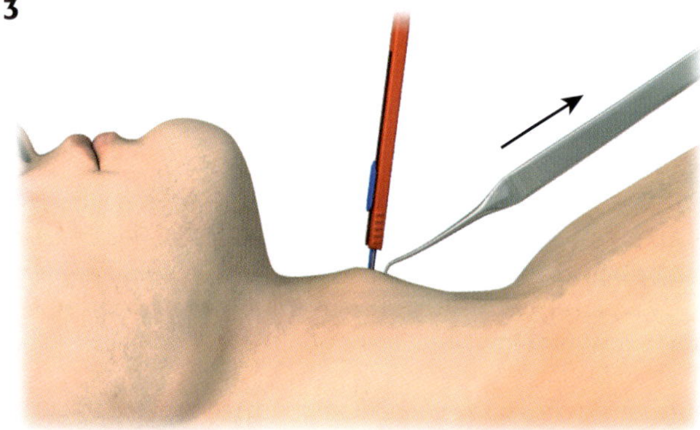

Using the scalpel blade as a guide, pick up the cricoid cartilage with the tracheal hook and provide traction in the caudal direction to stabilize the trachea.

4

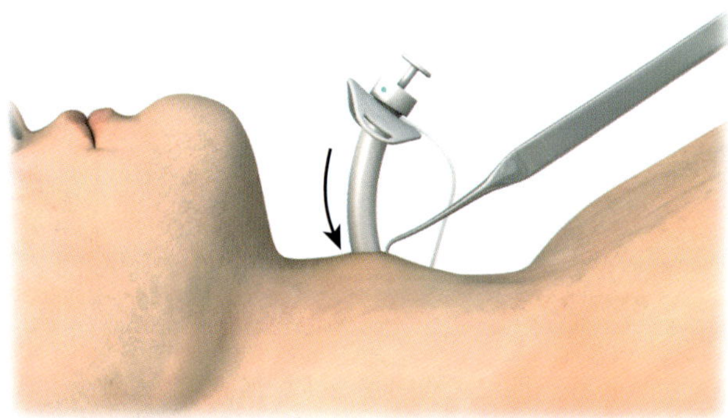

Place a No. 4 cuffed tracheostomy tube or a 6.0 cuffed endotracheal tube through the opening.

Fig. 6.7 Surgical cricothyrotomy: rapid four-step technique. Extension of the neck (if clinically feasible) facilitates the procedure. (Adapted from Brofeldt BT, Panacek EA, Richards JR. An easy cricothyrotomy approach: the rapid four step technique. *Acad Emerg Med.* 1996;3:1060.)

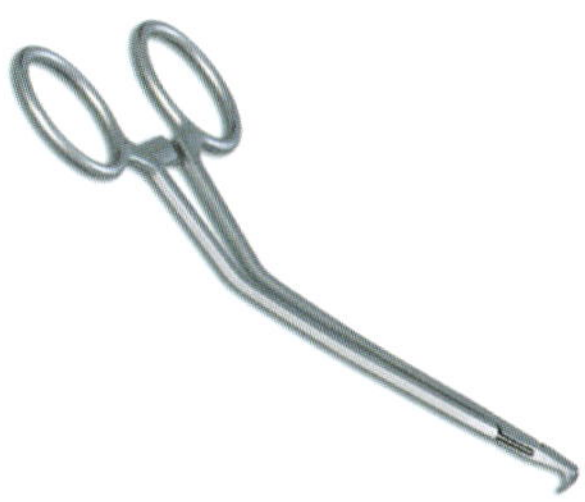

Fig. 6.8 Bair Claw.

the dominant hand, attach the needle to the syringe and insert it through the cricothyroid membrane pointing caudally at a 45-degree angle relative to the skin surface (Fig. 6.9, *step 1*). Be careful not to advance the needle too far because this may result in perforation of the posterior aspect of the trachea. To help recognize when the trachea has been entered, place a small amount of saline in the syringe before the procedure. Apply gentle negative pressure while advancing the syringe. When the membrane is pierced and the trachea is entered, air will be aspirated into the syringe and air bubbles will appear in the saline.

When the needle is in the trachea, pull the syringe and needle back and advance the flexible TFE catheter through the distal end of the trachea to its hub. If the needle does not have an overlying catheter, leave the needle in place and remove the syringe. Thread the guidewire through the needle or the catheter (see Fig. 6.9, *step 2*). Once the guidewire is placed securely in the trachea, remove the needle or catheter. With a disposable No. 15 scalpel, make a small incision in the skin at the point of guidewire entry to facilitate passage of the dilator and airway catheter (see Fig. 6.9, *step 3*).

Place the gray-tipped dilator into the airway catheter and thread it over the wire as one unit (see Fig. 6.9, *step 4*). Once it is through the skin and into the trachea, advance the airway catheter to its hub until it is flush against the neck. Remove the guidewire and dilator. Confirm placement in the trachea by standard methods. Secure the kit in place with "trach tape."

Complications

Surgical cricothyrotomy is performed infrequently and usually under circumstances that are inherently chaotic. These patients often have confounding medical issues, with high

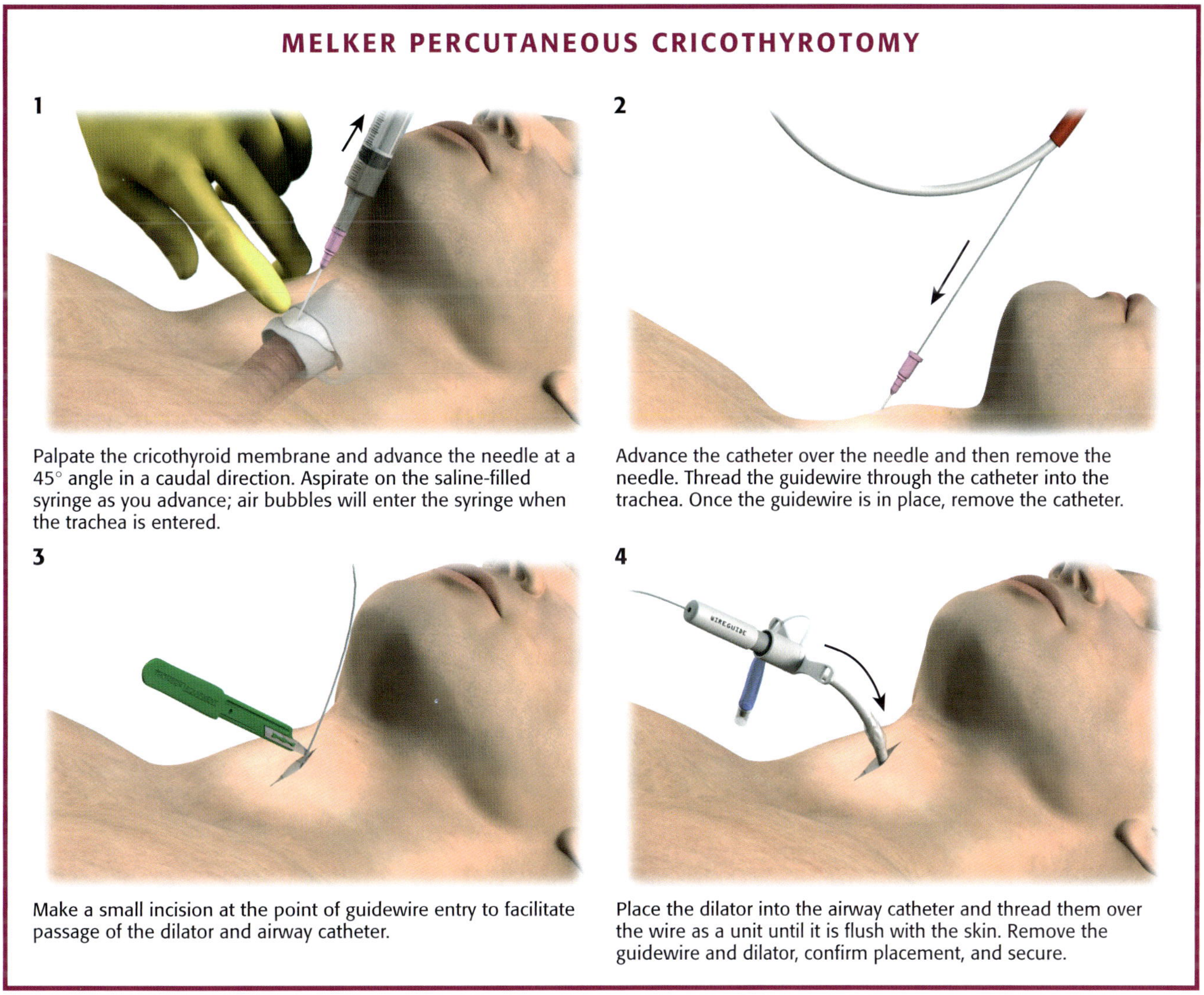

Fig. 6.9 Melker percutaneous cricothyrotomy. As with other cricothyrotomy techniques, extension of the neck (if clinically feasible) exposes the trachea and facilitates the procedure.

morbidity and mortality rates. Evaluation of short- and long-term complications in this population is difficult.[67]

Surgical cricothyrotomy has been studied to assess the periprocedure and short-term complications that occur with significant frequency. Acute complication rates have been reported to be between 8.7%[68] and 40%.[43] The most frequent complications are uncontrollable bleeding and misplacement of the tube.[42,69] Most bleeding is from small superficial vessels that can be controlled, and significant bleeding can also occur as a result of the procedure. The cricoid arteries branch from the superior thyroid arteries and anastomose at the anterior superior aspect of the cricothyroid membrane. The laterally running superior thyroid arteries are more often damaged when the initial incision is broad and horizontal. To prevent hemorrhage from these vessels, make the initial skin incision longitudinal as in the traditional technique and maintain careful awareness of the landmarks.[70] When making the horizontal incision in the cricothyroid membrane, avoid the cricoid artery by incising the membrane at its inferior aspect. Misplacement or malposition of the tracheostomy or ET tube during cricothyrotomy is a common complication as well.[71] If the opening in the cricothyroid membrane is not carefully stabilized during the procedure, the tube may inadvertently be inserted into subcutaneous tissue. This complication can be recognized by the presence of subcutaneous emphysema when attempting to ventilate the patient. It is essential to recognize this immediately to prevent the development of hypoxia and obliteration of anatomic landmarks. Failure to detect end-tidal CO_2 and absence of breath sounds by auscultation should alert the physician to a misplaced tube. If suspected, remove the tube and reassess the airway.

Many other occult complications have been reported less frequently or have been described in case reports, such as main stem bronchial intubation,[72] laryngotracheal injury,[73] tension pneumothorax,[74] and obstruction of the tracheostomy tube with blood or secretions.[75] One case of retrograde pharyngeal intubation has been reported.[76] (Box 6.2)

Chevalier Jackson's 1921 report highlighted the concern that subglottic stenosis was a major and frequent complication of cricothyrotomy.[77] It was later refuted by Brantigan and Grow's 1976 study,[41] which reported not only an overall complication rate of just 6.1% but also no occurrence of chronic subglottic stenosis as a long-term complication. Since the publication of this latter report, numerous other studies have

BOX 6.2 Complications of Surgical Cricothyrotomy

ACUTE COMPLICATIONS

- More common
  - Bleeding
  - Malposition of the tube
- Less common
  - Bronchial intubation
  - Laryngotracheal injury
  - Tension pneumothorax
  - Obstruction of the tube

LATE COMPLICATIONS

- More common
  - Subjective voice changes
  - Difficulty swallowing
  - Infections
  - Persistent shortness of breath
  - Persistent stoma
- Infrequent
  - Subglottic or glottic stenosis

corroborated their findings that chronic subglottic stenosis is an infrequent long-term complication of surgical cricothyrotomy.[78] Factors that increase the likelihood of development of subglottic stenosis include concurrent laryngotracheal pathology, prolonged time until decannulation, old age, and diabetes.[79,80]

Long-term complications resulting in "minor airway problems" have been reported more frequently than subglottic stenosis.[81] Of these complications, subjective voice change is the most frequently reported.[82] Other reported complications include difficulty swallowing, subjective shortness of breath, wound infections, and "noisy breathing."[83]

When comparing cricothyrotomies to tracheostomies, it appears that airway stenosis is the most common long-term complication, albeit occurring at low rates, in both procedures. Additionally, the incidence of bleeding, subglottic stenosis, and other complications were similar among patients undergoing emergency cricothyroidotomy or tracheostomy.[84,85]

To decrease the morbidity and mortality associated with prolonged hypoxia and other factors inherent in an airway emergency, attempts have been made to determine which technique is superior with regard to complication rate and time needed to secure the airway. When comparing the RFST with the traditional five-step technique, one study found an increased incidence of cricoid ring fracture when the single hook was used for caudal traction on the cricoid cartilage and concluded that the traditional technique produced a lower complication rate.[73] Another study in which the same two techniques were performed by inexperienced medical students and residents on human cadavers concluded that the single-hook RFST was executed significantly faster than the traditional technique.[55] They noted that there were more complications with the RFST and that the difference in complication rates failed to reach statistical significance. A later study revisited this comparison and replaced the single hook in the RFST with the double-hooked Bair Claw. The revised study showed that the airway could be secured faster with the RFST and that the complication rate was comparable.[86] Use of the Bair Claw with the RFST did not cause any fractures of the cricoid cartilage and showed an overall lower complication rate than with the traditional technique.[87]

Some studies show no difference in time to ventilation or complication rate when the traditional technique is compared with the Seldinger technique.[88] Some studies report that the surgical method is faster than the Seldinger method,[89–94] whereas others conclude the opposite.[95,96]

Many complications of cricothyrotomy are relatively minor in comparison to those caused by prolonged hypoxia. Be aware of these potential complications and prepare for them, and do not delay performing the procedure due to fear of complications. Reduce complication rates by maintaining a sterile field and being familiar with the techniques and anatomy.

When deciding which surgical cricothyrotomy technique to use, consider the advantages and disadvantages of each technique, the clinical scenario, availability of equipment, and comfort and familiarity with each individual technique.

Success Rate

Success rates for ET intubation in the ED are quite high. The reported first-pass success rate is 83%, and 99% of all intubations are successful in three or fewer attempts. The "rescue" cricothyrotomy rate is reported to be just 0.3% according to the National Emergency Airway Registry.[4] A study including more than 6000 trauma patients similarly reported a 0.3% cricothyrotomy rate in those requiring airway management within the first hour after arrival.[97] In pediatric patients, the first-pass attempt success rate for all ED intubators is 85%, with rescue cricothyrotomy performed less than 1% of the time.[98]

Although the reported success rate for cricothyrotomy has been quite high (89% to 100%) in most studies,[31,42,43,67,75,87,99] one study found only a 62.5% success rate.[100] In a community hospital setting, the rather optimistic success rate reported from trauma centers probably cannot be duplicated. In one ED study, the incidence of failed cricothyrotomy (e.g., tube misplacement into the pretracheal space or failed attempts) was 3.6%,[87] with earlier ED studies being between 7.9% and 10%.[42,43] In a cadaver model, the first-time performance of cricothyrotomy by intensive care unit clinicians, versus standard surgical cricothyrotomy with the Seldinger technique, resulted in successful tracheal placement in only 70% with the standard technique and 60% with the Seldinger technique.[88] In an animal model, paramedics had a 90.9% success rate with a percutaneous technique and a 100% success rate with the open surgical technique.[89]

PERCUTANEOUS TRANSLARYNGEAL VENTILATION

PTLV (Review Box 6.2) is a procedure in which oxygen is delivered through a 12- to 14-gauge catheter inserted through the cricothyroid membrane via needle cricothyrotomy. Needle cricothyrotomy does not differ greatly from the Seldinger technique variation of surgical cricothyrotomy. Administration of oxygen through the percutaneous translaryngeal catheter is by bag insufflation for pediatric patients younger than 5 years, and by a high-flow source for older children and adults. The methods for controlling jet ventilation have evolved over recent years. The initial use of continuous oxygen flow provided adequate oxygenation and no ventilation.[101] The

Percutaneous Translaryngeal Ventilation

Indications

Similar to surgical cricothyrotomy
Failed attempts at endotracheal intubation with an inability to bag-mask ventilate to an oxygen saturation >90%
Airway obstruction above the level of the cricothyroid membrane
Securing a failed airway in infants and children

Contraindications

Ability to secure the airway through less invasive means
Laryngeal transection or fracture

Complications

Associated with needle placement
- Subcutaneous emphysema
- Kinking of the catheter
- Bleeding
- Malposition of the catheter
- Posterior tracheal wall perforation
- Pneumothorax

Associated with ventilation
- Barotrauma, pneumothorax, pneumomediastinum
- Hypercapnia, respiratory acidosis

Equipment

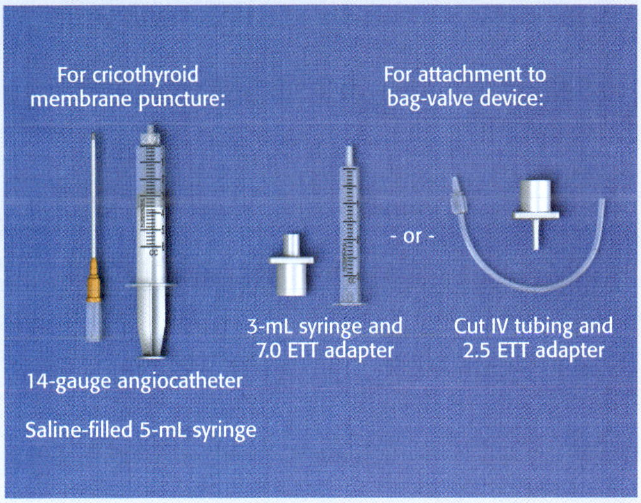

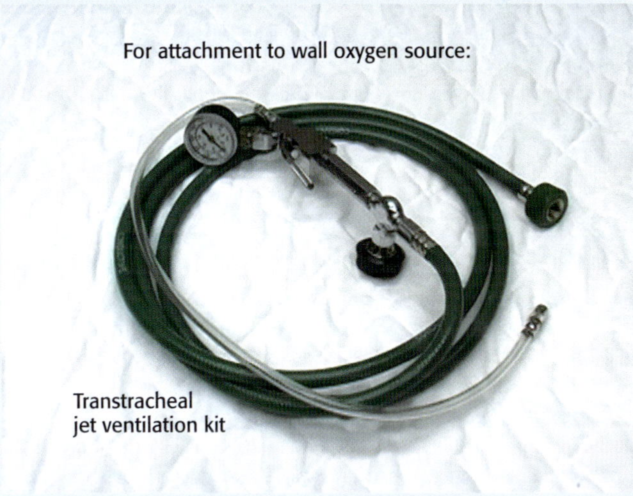

Review Box 6.2 Percutaneous translaryngeal ventilation: indications, contraindications, complications, and equipment.

technique has evolved so that shorter bursts of oxygen are followed by a longer passive exhalation to resemble a more physiologic respiratory state.

Indications and Contraindications

The indications for and contraindications to needle cricothyrotomy with PTLV are similar to those for surgical cricothyrotomy. Indications include failed attempts at ET intubation, inability to bag-mask ventilate to an oxygen saturation greater than 90%, or airway obstruction above the level of the cricothyroid membrane. Based on the operator's experience, needle cricothyrotomy may be relatively indicated over surgical cricothyrotomy in adult patients. Much of the otolaryngology literature supports the use of PTLV as a means of nonemergency ventilation during head and neck surgery because the smaller ventilation catheter provides a relatively unobstructed field in which to work.[102] In an emergency airway situation, needle cricothyrotomy may successfully allow time to establish an airway via surgical cricothyrotomy[103] or the ET route.[104] Case reports describe PTLV to be preemptively indicated over the more invasive surgical cricothyrotomy when ET intubation has failed as a result of copious oropharyngeal secretions, bleeding, or anticipated difficult ET intubation otherwise.[105,106] Providing temporary ventilation through the needle catheter may allow sufficient time to clear the upper airway of secretions or obstructions and give the operator more time to establish ET intubation.[107,108]

Surgical cricothyrotomy is contraindicated in infants and young children. The contraindication arises from the fact that the cricothyroid membrane is too small to insert a tracheostomy tube and there is a significant risk for injury to surrounding structures. Needle cricothyrotomy is the preferred method of securing the airway in failed airway situations in infants and young children.[109]

An absolute contraindication to needle cricothyrotomy is the ability to secure the airway without difficulty through less invasive means.[110] Similar to surgical cricothyrotomy, needle

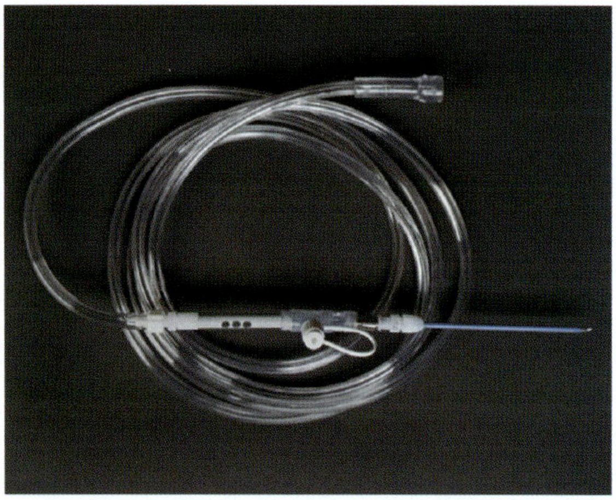

Fig. 6.10 ENK oxygen flow modulator set available as separate kit. (Courtesy Cook Critical Care, Bloomington, IN.)

cricothyrotomy is contraindicated in cases of laryngotracheal transection or fracture because the airway needs to be established below this level.[38] It has been suggested that in cases of complete upper airway obstruction, needle cricothyrotomy is relatively contraindicated in comparison to surgical cricothyrotomy. This concern, which is debatable, is due to the fact that the PTLV catheter theoretically does not permit adequate expiration volumes and results in hypercapnia and barotrauma.[111]

Equipment

The essential material needed for PTLV includes a needle with an overlying catheter, oxygen tubing, an oxygen source with a means of regulating the pressure, and a means to connect them together.

Commercial kits are available, and a standard 12- or 14-gauge Angiocath attached to a 3- or 5-mL syringe can be used to make the puncture through the cricothyroid membrane. The catheter can be left in place to serve as the conduit for oxygen delivery. The larger the diameter of the catheter, the greater the oxygen flow, depending on the method of oxygen delivery.[112] Commercial catheters, such as wire-coiled nonkinking catheters and fenestrated catheters, are available as part of prearranged kits (Fig. 6.10). Larger-caliber, 3.0 to 4.0 mm-ID percutaneous tracheal catheter devices are also available.

There are two different basic means and therefore armories of equipment to choose from to deliver oxygen through the transtracheal catheter. One method uses a standard ventilation bag to supply oxygen through the catheter. This requires the constant effort of manual bag insufflation as long as the patient is being oxygenated and ventilated. Attach the bag to the adapter of a 7.0-mm ET tube and insert it into the back of a plungerless 3-mL syringe connected to the translaryngeal catheter (Fig. 6.11). Alternatively, attach the bag directly to the catheter with the adapter of a 3.5-mm pediatric ET tube.[113] An inherent problem with this setup is the rigidity of the system. Although the translaryngeal catheter itself is flexible, there is no flexibility from the hub of the catheter to the bag. Slight movements of the bag relative to the patient may cause dislodgment of the catheter. To ameliorate this obstacle, connect standard intravenous infusion tubing directly to the translaryngeal catheter and attach the distal cut end of a 2.5-mm ET tube to the bag.

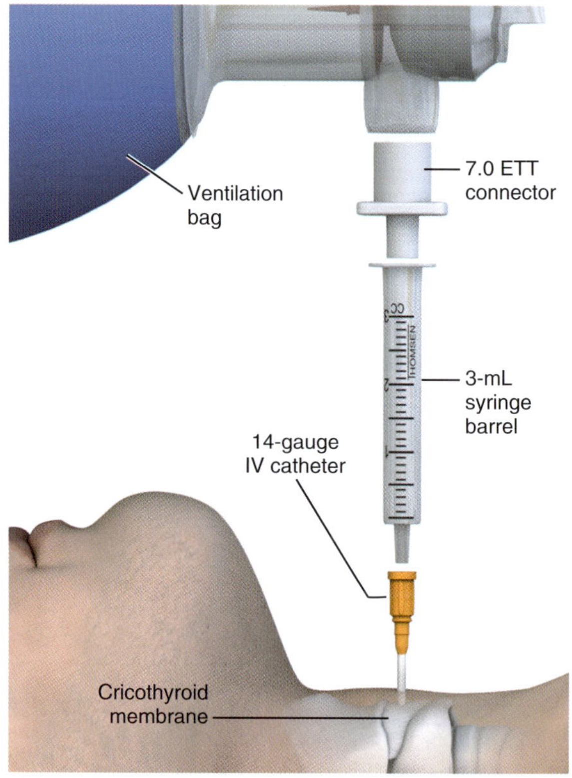

Fig. 6.11 Homemade ventilation setup for transtracheal catheter ventilation using a ventilation bag, a standard endotracheal tube adapter, a 3-mL syringe, and a 14-gauge angiocatheter. *ETT*, Endotracheal tube; *IV*, intravenous.

In an alternative method, oxygen can be supplied from a standard 50 psi wall source, connecting the high-pressure oxygen tubing to the wall source. Then secure the oxygen tubing to a manual on/off valve that is attached to the hub of the catheter. The on/off valve controls the inspiratory-to-expiratory ratio. This valve may be a trigger that is pushed down and released, the third arm of a three-way stopcock open to the atmosphere (Fig. 6.12), or holes placed at the end of the oxygen tubing. A pressure gauge connected to a hand-triggered jet injector may also be used to control the amount of air pressure reaching the catheter. This value can be titrated from 20 to 50 psi in adults and 5 to 30 psi in children, using chest rise as an indicator of adequate ventilation[114,115] (Fig. 6.13). Commercial kits are available that contain prepackaged systems already assembled. Otherwise, assemble the apparatus in the ED. In an emergency, it is unlikely that one would be able to assemble an apparatus for PTLV from individual components in a timely manner. If a prepackaged PTLV kit is not available, prepare the appropriate components from the ED ahead of time and place them with other airway supplies for easy access.

Assemble additional materials such as antiseptic preparation solution, sterile drapes, sterile gauze, and suture material or trach tape in the kit.

Procedure

As with the surgical cricothyrotomy technique, place the patient in the supine position with the neck exposed. Prepare the skin of the anterior aspect of the neck. Wear appropriate protective equipment, including sterile gloves, gown,

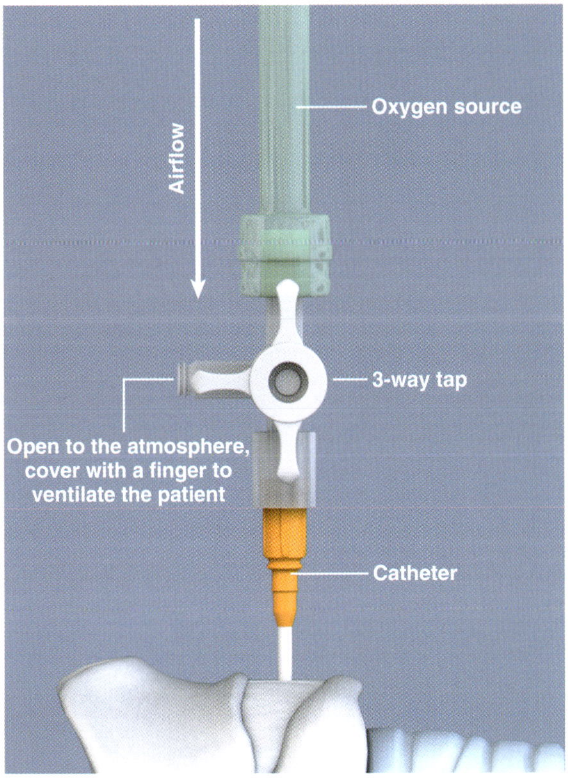

Fig. 6.12 Three-way stopcock connecting the oxygen tubing to the hub of the catheter with the third arm open to the atmosphere.

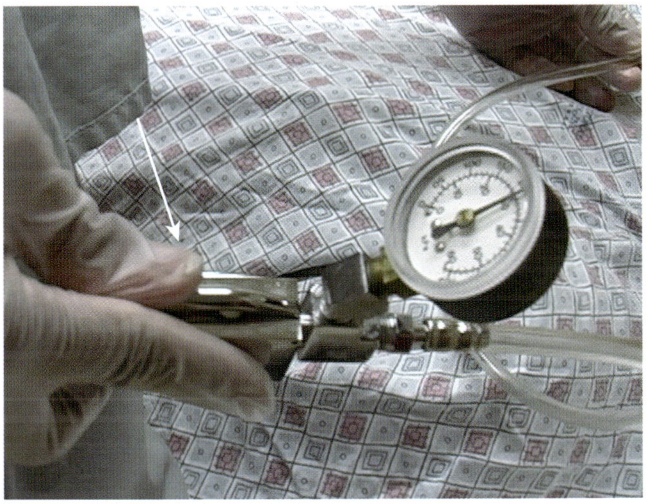

Fig. 6.13 Hand-triggered jet injector. Depressing the lever with the thumb *(arrow)* delivers oxygen to the patient.

protective eyewear, and a face shield. Hyperextend the patient's neck unless a suspected cervical spine injury prohibits it. Infiltrate the skin with local anesthetic.

Similar to the needle insertion technique used for guidewire-assisted surgical cricothyrotomy, while positioned at the patient's left, locate the cricothyroid membrane with the nondominant hand. Locate the thyroid cartilage and cricoid cartilage and palpate the cricothyroid membrane in the depression between the two while keeping in mind that this depression will be proportionately smaller in children (Fig. 6.14, *step 1*). Similar to the open technique, ultrasound has been shown to improve localization of the membrane.[116,117]

Attach a 12- to 14-gauge angiocatheter to a 3- or 5-mL syringe filled with 1 to 2 mL of saline or lidocaine. Once the cricothyroid membrane has been located, insert the needle through the overlying skin, subcutaneous tissue, and membrane directed at a 30- to 45-degree angle caudally (see Fig. 6.14, *step 2*). While doing so, aspirate gently with the syringe. The cricothyroid membrane has been pierced and the airway entered when air bubbles are seen in the fluid or there is an increase in the ease of air aspiration (see Fig. 6.14, *step 3*). Once through the membrane, hold the needle in place, advance the catheter to the hub, and then remove the needle (see Fig. 6.14, *steps 4* and *5*). Hold the catheter by hand until the oxygen supply is connected and appropriate placement is confirmed (see Fig. 6.14, *step 6*). Make sure that the hub of the catheter is flush against the skin to avoid an air leak and then secure it with a circumferential tie around the neck. To prevent the tube from being dislodged, keep one hand on the hub of the catheter until the entire procedure is completed and the airway is secured.

Oxygen can be supplied to the catheter through several different conduits. With the resuscitation bag setup, manually ventilate the lungs through the catheter by squeezing and releasing the bag. When coupled with a 14-gauge angiocatheter, ventilation with a resuscitation bag produces low maximal tidal volumes, approximately 100 mL per 1 second of inspiratory time in one study.[118] Children, especially those younger than 5 years, have small total lung capacities and need smaller tidal volumes. In these cases, use the bag instead of the jet ventilator. To use this setup, control the volume of air inspired and adjust it breath by breath based on chest wall motion, pulse oximetry, and capnography. This method is not appropriate for adults because the operator cannot provide adequate tidal volumes and allow enough time for exhalation.[119,120]

If using high-flow oxygen supplied from a wall source, attach the oxygen tubing to the wall source and secure the distal end of the tubing apparatus to the hub of the translaryngeal catheter. The flow rate recommended for children is 1 L/min per year of age, with titration upward in increments of 1 L/min based on chest wall movement.[121] Most wall-mounted oxygen flow meters have a maximum flow rate marked at 15 L/min. Pressures generated at this flow rate have been shown to be inadequate to sustain ventilation in adults.[122,123] To provide the additional pressure necessary to ventilate an adult, open the oxygen flow meter to full output, which will allow a flow of 30 to 60 L/min.[124] Ventilate the patient by alternating between allowing and inhibiting airflow through the catheter. This is done by occluding and then releasing the hole or holes if using a stopcock or the ENK oxygen flow modulator (Cook Medical) or by pushing and releasing a trigger if using this type of modulator. Watch for chest wall rise and fall, and make sure to allow enough time for exhalation before the next cycle. A pressure gauge, if attached, can help guide inspiration time.

Complications

Complications reported with needle cricothyrotomy are similar to those associated with surgical cricothyrotomy: bleeding, misplacement of the catheter, subcutaneous emphysema, and pneumothorax.[125,126] Complications more specific to needle cricothyrotomy include catheter kinking and perforation of the posterior aspect of the trachea.[127,128] It is noted that with the rapid increase in ultrasound utilization, one study out of Anesthesia and Critical Care found that US improves

PERCUTANEOUS TRANSLARYNGEAL VENTILATION

1

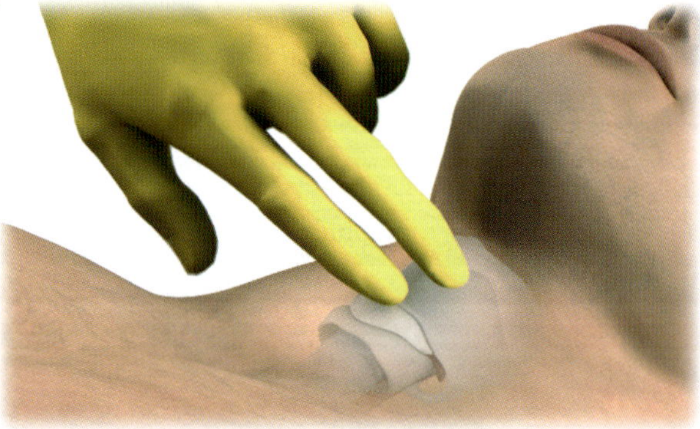

Hyperextend the patient's neck if possible. Locate the cricothyroid membrane with your nondominant hand.

2

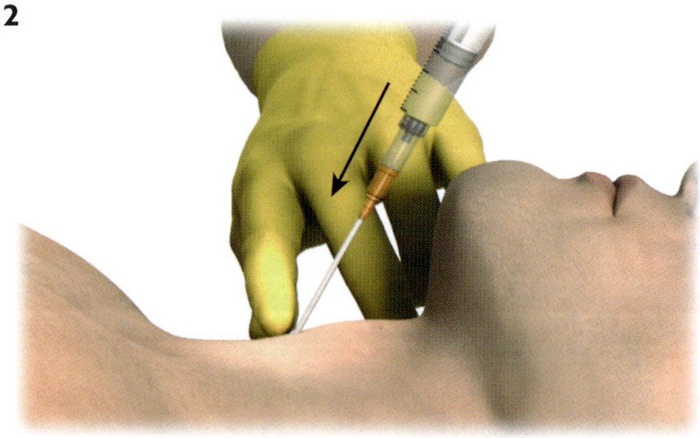

Attach a 14-gauge angiocatheter to a saline-filled syringe. Insert the needle through the skin, subcutaneous tissue, and membrane directed at a 30° to 45° angle caudally.

3

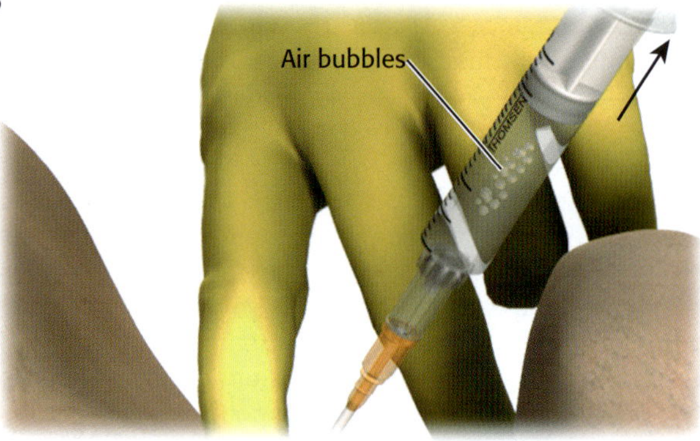

Aspirate the syringe as you advance the needle; air bubbles will be seen in the syringe when the trachea is entered.

4

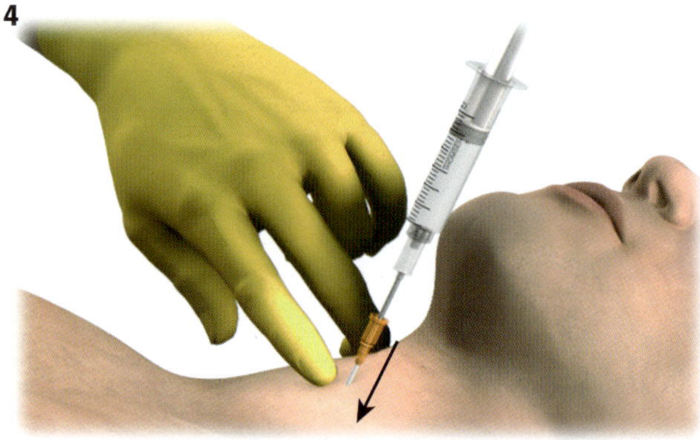

Once the trachea is entered, advance the catheter over the needle until the hub is flush with the skin.

5

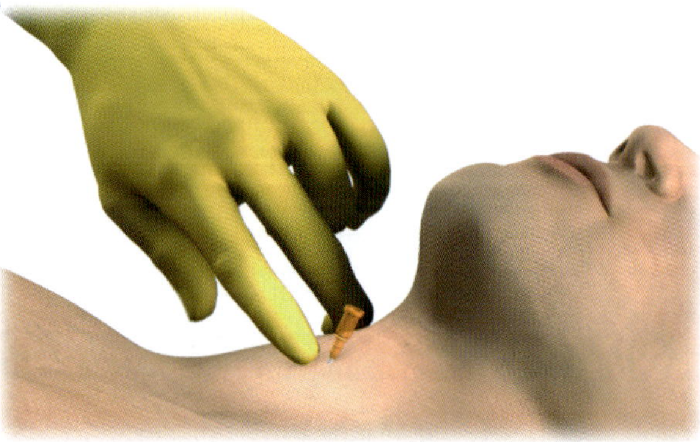

Remove the needle.

6

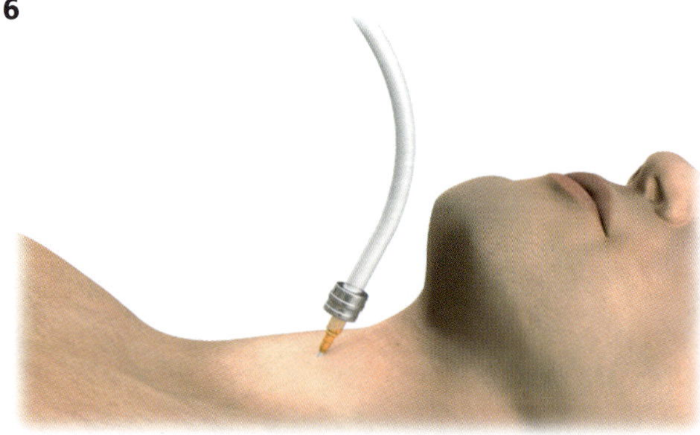

Attach the oxygen supply and begin to ventilate the patient.

Fig. 6.14 Percutaneous translaryngeal ventilation.

percutaneous needle cricothyrotomy success in the novice anesthesia provider compared with the landmark technique alone.[92]

One would assume that a translaryngeally placed catheter would not afford any airway protection against aspiration because the diameter of the catheter is not nearly large enough to occlude the lumen of the trachea. A few studies, though, have shown a decreased rate of aspiration in dogs that were ventilated with PTLV versus control animals that were not ventilated, thus suggesting some airway protection with this mode of ventilation.[129,130]

The potential complications more specific to PTLV than to ventilation through a tracheostomy tube stem from the idea that, especially in cases of complete upper airway obstruction, egress of inspired gas is limited through the relatively small translaryngeal catheter. It has been reported that PTLV inevitably causes retention of CO_2 in adults. This leads to poor ventilation despite adequate oxygenation. This assumption

BOX 6.3 Complications of Percutaneous Translaryngeal Jet Ventilation

COMPLICATIONS ASSOCIATED WITH NEEDLE PLACEMENT

- Subcutaneous emphysema
- Kinking of the catheter
- Bleeding
- Malposition of the catheter
- Posterior tracheal wall perforation
- Pneumothorax

COMPLICATIONS ASSOCIATED WITH VENTILATION

- Barotrauma (more common with complete upper airway obstruction)
- Pneumothorax
- Pneumomediastinum
- Hypercapnia, respiratory acidosis

may be a remnant of earlier oxygenation techniques in which continuous low-flow "apneic oxygenation" was used without ventilation.[101] Many animal studies have shown that adequate ventilation, normal blood pH, and normal arterial CO_2 partial pressure can be maintained with PTLV for 30 or even 60 minutes.[131,132] Factors that seem to improve ventilation are increased expiratory time and a high-flow oxygen source.[133,134] Even with partial or nearly complete oropharyngeal obstruction, adequate ventilation has been achieved.[135,136] Unfortunately, none of these studies looked at ventilation for extended periods. Barotrauma is a significant risk associated with PTLV and occurs when upper airway obstruction prevents air from being exhaled. This causes an increase in lung volume and pressure and leads to lung injury.[137,138] Using a lower respiratory rate and the ENK oxygen flow modulator versus the Manujet (Mainline Medical, Inc.), decreases pulmonary pressure, theoretically reducing the likelihood of barotrauma.[139] The ENK oxygen flow modulator may also be superior to a three-way stopcock for similar reasons.[140] The Ventrain device (Armstrong Medical Ltd) (Video 6.5), which allows more rapid expiration, has also been shown to have improved minute ventilation, peak airway pressures, and decreased hemodynamic depression compared with previous methods when studied in animal models, simulators, and based on a few pediatric case reports.[141–143] Use of a bidirectional valve or an expiratory ventilation assistance ejector device has been shown to improve ventilation dynamics and decrease the complications associated with PTLV in patients with complete upper airway obstruction (Box 6.3).[144,145] There is also a correlation between cricothyroidotomy needle length and posterior tracheal wall injury.[146]

CONCLUSION

The majority of crash airway scenarios are controlled successfully with ET intubation. The development of airway aids such as the gum elastic bougie, laryngeal mask airway, and fibroscopic laryngoscope has increasingly obviated the need to convert efforts to an invasive surgical technique. Nevertheless, situations arise when an airway cannot be secured with one of these aids or the patient cannot be ventilated via bag-mask-valve ventilation. In these situations, a surgical approach is indicated.

Researchers have attempted to delineate which method of gaining emergency airway access is superior by comparing all techniques across the spectrum from traditional surgical cricothyrotomy to needle cricothyrotomy to commercially available kits such as the QuickTrach (Teleflex Medical). Given the variety of equipment and techniques to choose from and the advantages and disadvantages reported about each throughout the literature, it would be difficult for an inexperienced physician to know which to choose in a critical situation. As most physicians do not perform this procedure during residency on a living patient, and only approximately 68% do so on a recently deceased patient, familiarity with available methods and equipment is paramount.[147] Aside from being familiar with the equipment available in the ED, research shows that physicians at all levels of training have increased success rates when they are exposed to simulated situations before an actual airway emergency.[148]

REFERENCES ARE AVAILABLE AT ELSEVIER EBOOKS+

CHAPTER 7

Tracheostomy Care

John C. Greenwood and Michael E. Winters

INTRODUCTION

Placement of a tracheostomy tube is a common procedure in critically ill patients. Common indications for this procedure include upper airway obstruction, head or neck trauma, and prolonged respiratory failure.[1,2] Approximately one-fourth of patients in the intensive care unit (ICU) will require a tracheostomy tube for prolonged respiratory support or weaning from mechanical ventilation.[3] The recent COVID-19 pandemic caused a significant increase in the incidence of acute respiratory distress syndrome and need for prolonged mechanical ventilation, which has also led a dramatic increase in the number of tracheostomy patients worldwide.[4] Advances in health care allow many patients with tracheostomies to live at home or in other relatively low-technology environments such as rehabilitation facilities and nursing homes. Tracheostomy care is often provided by a variety of caregivers, including family members, home health care nurses, and patient care technicians.[5,6]

Patients with tracheostomies are seen in EDs for a variety of tracheostomy-related concerns.[7] Many emergency clinicians will have minimal experience with such patients, and it should be emphasized that complications or problems with tracheostomies often require specialty consultation in the ED to be fully evaluated or definitively remedied.

Common complaints include difficulty breathing as a result of tube obstruction, tube displacement, or equipment failure; poor oxygenation from infection or altered patient anatomy; and bleeding. In some cases, complications can be life threatening. Emergency clinicians must be knowledgeable regarding the evaluation and management of patients with tracheostomies. This chapter reviews the relevant tracheal anatomy and essential equipment for tracheostomy management in the ED, discusses pertinent tracheostomy care, provides a systematic approach to the evaluation and management of selected complications, and identifies high-risk patient populations.

BACKGROUND

Most tracheostomies are performed electively. For elective tracheostomies, the surgical site is between the first and second or the second and third tracheal rings. With an open, or surgical, tracheostomy, the anterior aspect of the trachea is generally left sutured to the skin until the tract matures, approximately 4 to 5 days after the procedure. Percutaneous dilational tracheostomy has become the preferred technique for many ICU patients. It can be performed at the bedside and eliminates the risks associated with transporting critically ill patients to an operating room. Postoperative complications vary and depend on the timing and insertion technique (Box 7.1). Sixteen to twenty percent of patients experience early complications, while 6% to 8% experience late complications.[8] Although elective and emergency tracheostomies are generally performed with the same technique, the complication rate associated with emergency procedures may be higher than the rate for elective tracheostomies.[9,10]

TRACHEAL ANATOMY AND PHYSIOLOGY

The lower respiratory tract begins at the vocal cords. Inferior to the vocal cords lies the cricoid cartilage, encasing the 1.5- to 2-cm subglottic space. Inferior to the cricoid cartilage is the trachea (Fig. 7.1). The typical adult trachea is 10 to 12 cm in length. The anterior and lateral walls of the trachea are supported by 18 to 22 incomplete cartilaginous rings. A fibromuscular sheet lying anterior to the esophagus completes the posterior wall. The interior diameter of the adult trachea is 12 to 25 mm, and it is lined with mucosa covered by respiratory epithelium. Blood is supplied to the trachea by branches of the inferior thyroid, innominate (brachiocephalic), bronchial, and subclavian arteries. Critically, the innominate artery (IA) lies in close proximity to the tracheostomy stoma. From its origin at the aortic arch, the IA courses between the sternum and the anterior aspect of the trachea and veers right at the sternomanubrial joint. The location of the IA is important because erosion of the anterior tracheal wall can lead to life-threatening bleeding. The recurrent laryngeal nerve innervates the intrinsic laryngeal muscles and mucosa below the vocal cords. Efferent vagal fibers stimulate bronchoconstriction, mucosal secretions, and vasodilation. Efferent sympathetic fibers of the pulmonary plexus stimulate tracheal bronchodilation and vasoconstriction.

The upper airway, including the oropharynx and nasal passages, filters particulate matter, humidifies inspired air, and aids in the expectoration of secretions. These functions are reduced in patients with a tracheostomy.[9] Placement of a tracheostomy bypasses upper airway humidification and can lead to the formation of thick, dry secretions. In the absence of humidification, squamous metaplasia and chronic inflammatory changes develop in the trachea.[11] Bronchoconstriction resulting in reduced airflow can occur if the inspired air temperature is below room temperature. Normal mucociliary clearance is also impaired because of the increased viscosity of respiratory secretions.

The tracheostomy procedure weakens the anterior tracheal wall and blunts the normal cough mechanism, an important component for clearance of secretions by the trachea. Normally, the epiglottis and vocal cords close to trap air in the lungs and raise intrathoracic pressure before a cough. Patients with a tracheostomy tube are generally unable to generate sufficient pressure to initiate a strong cough and facilitate airway clearance.[12] Muscle wasting and decreased immune response as the result of prolonged illness also increase the risk of complications.

EVALUATION OF TRACHEOSTOMY PATIENTS

Every ED patient with a tracheostomy who has a respiratory complaint or a complaint related to the tracheostomy should be thoroughly evaluated. Begin the primary assessment with a review of the patient's vital signs and evaluation of the airway. Examine the tracheostomy tube for signs of dislodgement, obstruction, or fracture. Next, assess the patient's respiratory status. If the patient is receiving mechanical ventilation on arrival and is in acute distress, remove the patient from the ventilator, perform manual ventilation with a bag-valve-mask

BOX 7.1 Complications of Tracheostomy

EARLY COMPLICATIONS (DAYS TO WEEKS)

Hemorrhage—postoperative
Tube dislodgement or obstruction
Subcutaneous emphysema
Soft tissue infection
Pneumothorax, pneumomediastinum

LATE COMPLICATIONS (>3 WEEKS)

Tracheal stenosis or tracheal malacia (granulation tissue)
Tube dislodgement or obstruction
Equipment failure
Tracheoinnominate artery fistula
Tracheoesophageal fistula
Infection—pneumonia, aspiration

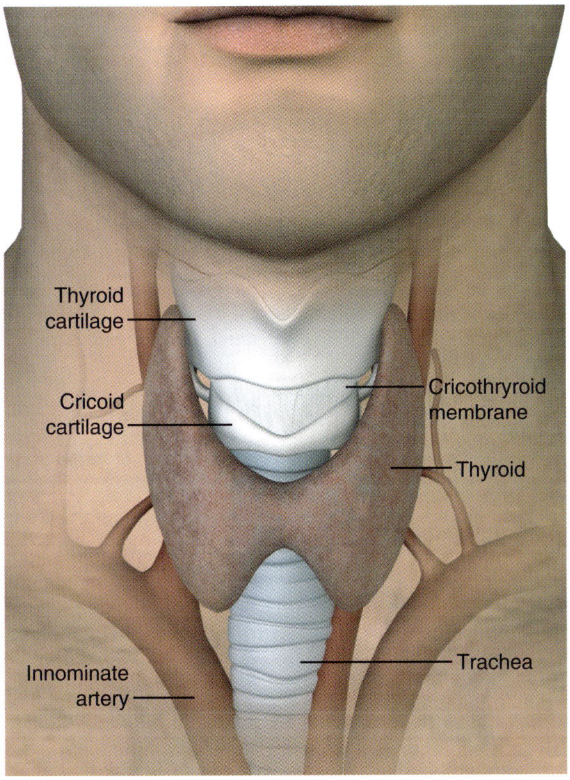

Fig. 7.1 Normal tracheal anatomy.

device, and auscultate for breath sounds. Initiate continuous cardiac monitoring, pulse oximetry, and capnography, if available, in all tracheostomy patients in respiratory distress.

In the history of the present illness, include the indications for placement of a tracheostomy, the length of time from placement to arrival at the ED, and any previous complications. Investigate for any previous bleeding complications, anatomical concerns, and whether a permanent tracheostomy or decannulation of the tracheostomy is anticipated. Ask whether there have been any recent changes in ventilator settings or tracheostomy care, including increased oxygen use, increased suctioning, equipment failure, or changes in equipment.

After the primary assessment and focused history, perform a thorough physical examination to differentiate between

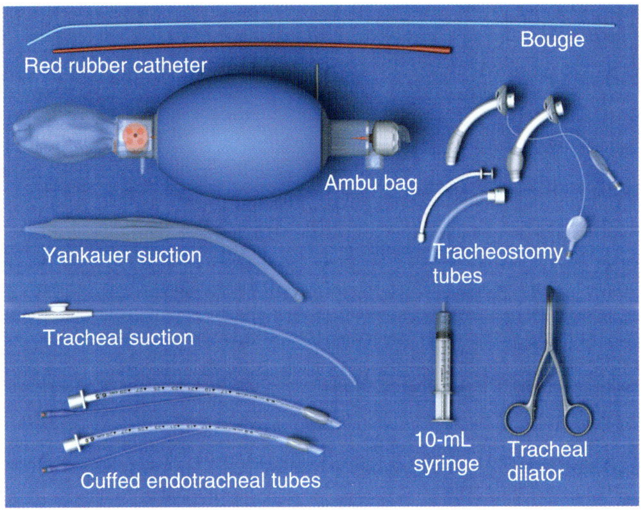

Fig. 7.2 Suggested equipment for tracheostomy care.

tracheostomy complications and other causes of the patient's respiratory complaint. The differential diagnosis may include pneumonia, exacerbation of chronic obstructive pulmonary disease, congestive heart failure, pulmonary embolism, pneumothorax, and acute coronary syndrome. During the secondary evaluation, evaluate the patient's stoma for signs of bleeding, infection, or skin breakdown. Make a note of the specific type and model of equipment, in the event that a replacement tube is needed. Important tracheostomy tube-related information is usually found on the flanges of the tracheostomy itself.

GENERAL EQUIPMENT FOR TRACHEOSTOMY PATIENTS

Before performing any procedure on the tracheostomy tube, it is important that the emergency clinician ensure that essential equipment is readily available at the patient's bedside. These items are shown in Fig. 7.2 and Video 7.1. Adequate preparation is crucial in preventing a poor outcome should complications arise. Most of this equipment can be placed in a designated airway box that can easily be accessed within the room or ED.

ROUTINE TRACHEOSTOMY MAINTENANCE

Routine tracheostomy maintenance involves (1) regular cleaning of the tube, (2) frequent stomal care, and (3) periodic monitoring of cuff pressure. There are many different types of tracheostomy tubes, and the focus of this section is on the most commonly used tracheostomies with a removable inner cannula (Fig. 7.3A). Regular cleaning of the tracheostomy tube and inner cannula can prevent the accumulation of dried secretions. Lack of cleaning and maintenance of the inner cannula is the primary cause of tube obstruction (see Fig. 7.3B). Under normal circumstances the inner cannula should be in place. It sits snugly within the tracheostomy tube and can easily be removed without disturbing the tube itself. The inner cannula should be cleaned daily. Soak it in a half-strength hydrogen peroxide solution for 10 to 15 minutes and remove encrustations with a soft-bristle tracheostomy brush.[13] Clean dried debris and blood from the tracheostomy tube flanges as well. To prevent damage to the tracheal mucosa, rinse all airway

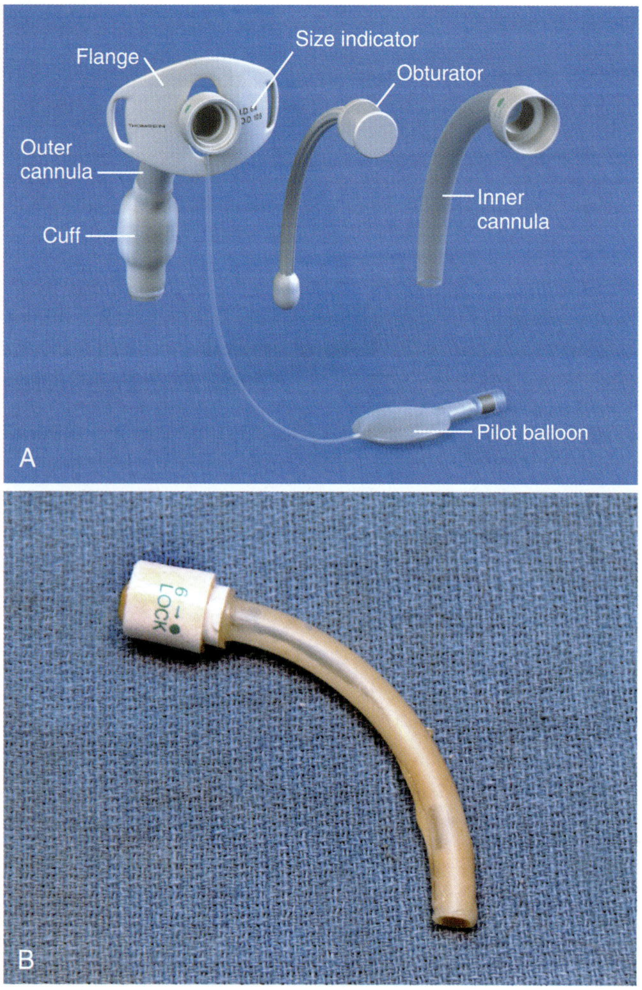

Fig. 7.3 Shiley tracheostomy tube. (A) The obturator is placed inside the tube (while the inner cannula is removed) to facilitate insertion through the stoma. The inner cannula must be inserted into the tube to ventilate the patient. (B) The inner cannula should always be in place and removed only for daily cleaning. An inner cannula clogged with mucus and debris, as seen in this figure, is the most common cause of respiratory distress in patients in the emergency department.

equipment with sterile saline before reinsertion. Important stomal wound care includes changing contaminated tube ties, cleaning the tube flanges regularly, and using precut tracheostomy gauze. Loose fibers from hand-cut gauze may irritate the stomal site and increase inflammatory changes.[12]

The tracheostomy cuff provides a tight seal to allow positive pressure ventilation and prevent aspiration. Cuff pressure should ideally be maintained below 25 mm Hg.[14] Overinflation is common and can cause disastrous injury to the tracheal wall and mucosa and lead to tracheomalacia, tracheal stenosis, or the development of a fistula between surrounding anatomic structures.[15] It is a good practice to regularly check and document cuff pressure with a handheld pressure manometer to document inflation volumes. If an air leak occurs at the maximum recommended cuff pressure, the tube may have become dislodged or the patient may have developed an anatomical complication, such as tracheal dilation, secondary to prolonged tracheal wall pressure from the tracheostomy balloon.

It is essential that adequate air humidification be provided to patients with a tracheostomy. Inadequate humidification can result in obstruction of the tube from thick secretions,

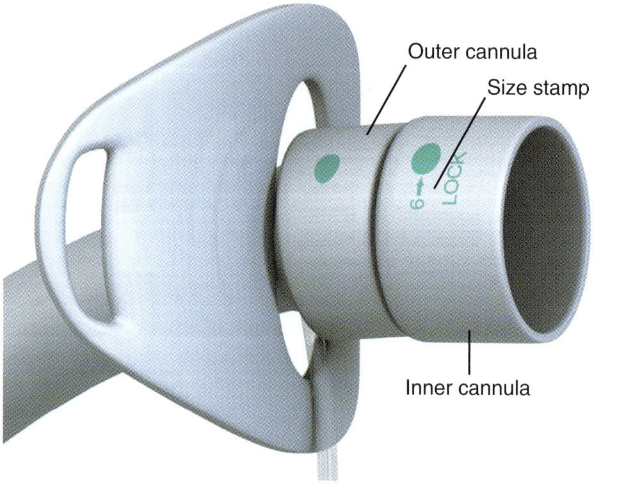

Fig. 7.4 Close-up of a Shiley tracheostomy tube. Note that only the *inner* cannula has a 15-mm adapter that will accept an Ambu bag or a ventilator; the *outer* cannula will not. The inner cannula MUST be in place to ventilate the patient.

sputum retention, keratinization or ulceration of the tracheal mucosa, and impaired gas exchange caused by lung atelectasis. Ambulatory patients and those who require low-flow oxygen can be fitted with a heat-moisture exchanger that attaches to the external opening of the tracheostomy tube. Patients receiving long-term ventilation or high-flow oxygen often require an in-line humidification system.

VENTILATING TRACHEOSTOMY PATIENTS

To properly ventilate ED patients with a tracheostomy, it is important to determine the make, model, and type of tube (Fig. 7.4). For proper positive pressure ventilation, the tracheostomy must have a pilot balloon, and a 15-mm tube/Ambu bag or ventilator tube adapter is required to connect to the tube itself or to the end of the inner cannula. If the patient requires manual or mechanical ventilation and the tracheostomy tube is not suitable for ventilatory support, immediately replace it with a similarly sized, cuffed tracheostomy tube or a temporary 6-0 cuffed endotracheal (ET) tube for ventilation. If exchanging the tracheostomy tube for an equivalent size ET tube, it is important recognizing there will be a significant length of the ET tube that is outside of the patient.

TRACHEAL SUCTIONING

Tracheal suctioning is required to remove secretions or aspirated material from the upper airway in patients whose cough is impaired or in whom an artificial airway is in place. Tracheal suctioning can be performed through an ET tube, a tracheostomy tube, a minitracheostomy placed in the cricothyroid membrane, or the nasopharynx. The indications, equipment, procedure, and complications are similar for each technique.

Indications

The primary indications for tracheal suctioning are to remove secretions, enhance oxygenation, or obtain samples of lower respiratory tract secretions for diagnostic tests. In the ED, tracheal suctioning should be performed to enhance oxygenation in any tracheostomy patient in respiratory distress. In addition, tracheal suctioning should be performed when the patient has coarse rales, rhonchi, or tubular breath sounds; acute or worsening dyspnea; or arterial oxygen desaturation. It is important to emphasize that tracheal suctioning should be performed only when it is clinically indicated; frequent, routine suctioning is not recommended.[16,17] There are no absolute contraindications to tracheal suctioning. Relative contraindications include severe bronchospasm, persistently elevated intracranial pressure (ICP), and hemodynamic instability that may be exacerbated by suctioning.[18] Bronchodilators, sedatives, and paralytics may alleviate these symptoms.

Equipment

A suction catheter and vacuum system, open or closed, is required to perform tracheal suctioning (Fig. 7.5). It is recommended that the diameter of the suction catheter be no larger than half the inner diameter of the tracheostomy tube.[19,20] The size of the suction catheter in French gauge (Fr) can be calculated as follows:

$$\text{Size (Fr)} = 2 \times (\text{size of the tracheostomy tube} - 2)$$

For example, a 7-0 tracheostomy tube will require a 10-Fr suction catheter because 2 × (7 – 2) = 10 Fr. If the catheter is too small, it will not remove excess secretions adequately. If the catheter is too large, it can obstruct airflow during insertion and cause alveolar collapse with resultant hypoxemia.

In adults, the suction catheter should be inserted only 10 to 15 cm, depending on the length of the tracheostomy tube. The goal of suctioning is to remove secretions only from the proximal airways. *Shallow suctioning* occurs when the catheter is placed just beyond the hub of the tracheostomy tube to remove proximal secretions. *Premeasured suctioning* occurs when a catheter is inserted such that the distal side ports are beyond the caudal end of the tracheostomy tube. *Deep suctioning* occurs when the suction catheter is advanced until resistance is met. It is used for clearing excess secretions in the lower airways.[17] Deep suctioning has not been shown to be more beneficial than shallow suctioning and should not be performed routinely because it might damage the mucosal epithelium and lead to an increase in granulation tissue.[20,21]

A number of suction catheter tips have been designed to maximize removal of secretions without causing mucosal injury. Tips may have a single or multiple side ports proximal to the distal tip. Directional or Coude tip catheters are available for selective suctioning of the main stem bronchi.

In-line suction catheters are often preferred and have a sterile sheath attached to ventilator tubing. This prevents the suction catheter from being contaminated by contact with the outside environment and allows tracheal suctioning to be performed without interrupting ventilatory support. The vacuum should be set to the lowest possible pressure to reduce

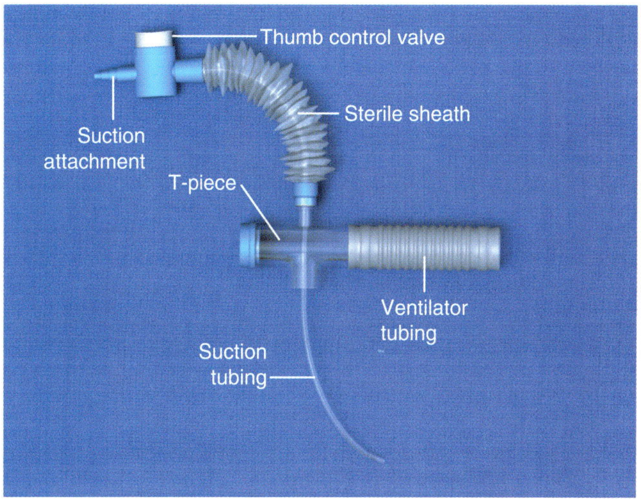

Fig. 7.5 Closed-system suction catheter.

Tracheostomy Suctioning

Indications

Removal of excess secretions
Worsening dyspnea
Decreased oxygenation in the presence of rales, rhonchi, or tubular breath sounds
Arterial oxygen desaturation
Respiratory distress

Contraindications

Absolute
- None

Relative
- Severe bronchospasm
- Persistently elevated intracranial pressure

Complications

Hypoxemia	Atelectasis
Increased intracranial pressure	Mucosal injury
Dysrhythmias	Bleeding
Patient agitation	Infection/tracheitis

Equipment

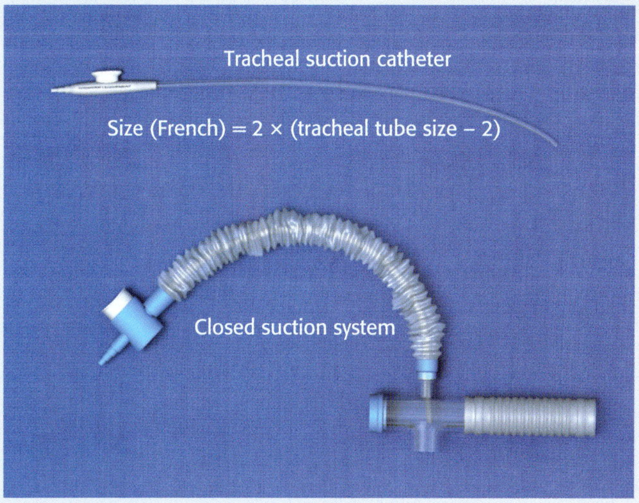

Review Box 7.1 Tracheal suctioning: indications, contraindications, complications, and equipment.

atelectasis. Vacuum pressure should not exceed 80 mm Hg in infants or 150 mm Hg in adults.[22]

Procedure and Technique

Before tracheal suctioning, continuous pulse oximetry, cardiac monitoring, and continuous capnography, if available, should be initiated (Fig. 7.6, *step 1*). Awake and alert patients should be sitting upright with their head in a neutral position. For mechanically ventilated patients, the head of the bed should be elevated to 30 degrees to improve respiratory mechanics. Aseptic technique should be used throughout all suctioning procedures to prevent the introduction of bacteria. Backup airway equipment should be readily available (see Fig. 7.2). Preoxygenate the patient for at least 30 to 60 seconds. For mechanically ventilated patients, increase the fraction of inspired oxygen (FiO_2) to 100%. For nonventilated patients, provide 10 to 15 L of high-flow oxygen. Humidify the air before suctioning to reduce the viscosity of respiratory secretions. Routine instillation of normal saline has not been shown to provide regular clinical benefit and is no longer recommended.[22,23]

Once the patient has been adequately preoxygenated, insert the suction catheter through the inner cannula in situ (see Fig. 7.6, *step 2*). If the carina is irritated during deep suctioning, a vigorous cough reflex will be activated. After reaching the desired depth, withdraw the suction catheter 1 to 2 cm and then apply suction while slowly removing the catheter (see Fig. 7.6, *steps 3* and *4*). Gently rotate the catheter as it is withdrawn to facilitate removal of secretions. The duration of suctioning should not exceed 10 to 15 seconds.

Monitor the patient throughout the procedure for signs of cardiac dysrhythmia, hypoxemia, or a rise in end-tidal CO_2. Immediately stop suctioning if any of these signs develop (see section on "Complications of Suctioning"). If marked respiratory distress is presumed to be secondary to significant tracheal obstruction, continue with expeditious suctioning to remove the obstruction (see section on "Obstruction and Complications from Tube Changes").

Complications of Suctioning

Complications that occur during or after suctioning are relatively common and can result in significant morbidity. Most complications can be anticipated and simple maneuvers can reduce their incidence and severity.

Hypoxemia from suctioning may cause increased ICP, dysrhythmias, or even death. In neonates, hypoxia during

TRACHEAL SUCTIONING

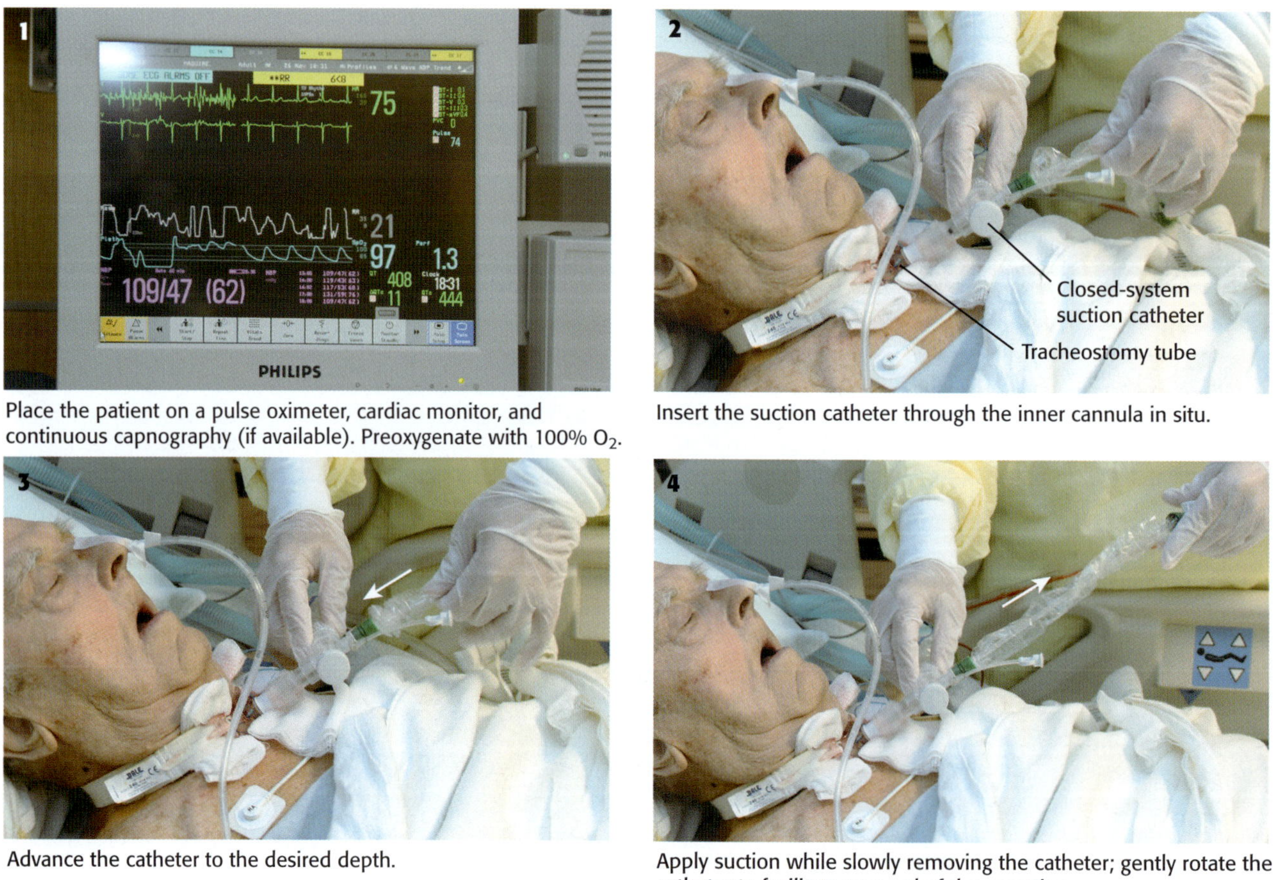

1. Place the patient on a pulse oximeter, cardiac monitor, and continuous capnography (if available). Preoxygenate with 100% O_2.
2. Insert the suction catheter through the inner cannula in situ.
3. Advance the catheter to the desired depth.
4. Apply suction while slowly removing the catheter; gently rotate the catheter to facilitate removal of the secretions.

Fig. 7.6 Tracheal suctioning.

suctioning may contribute to spontaneous intracerebral hemorrhage.[24] A number of factors contribute to suctioning-related hypoxemia, including interruption of mechanical ventilation, aspiration of air from the respiratory tract, and suctioning-related atelectasis.[25] Use in-line suction catheters for ventilator-dependent patients to allow continuous oxygen delivery and positive pressure ventilation. Select the catheter size carefully to reduce the evacuation of airway gases during suctioning and help prevent atelectasis. Limit the duration of suctioning to 10 to 15 seconds and perform no more than three passes in succession. Measurement of arterial oxygen saturation may not be sufficient to assess hypoxia after suctioning. Oxygen consumption increases during suctioning despite insignificant changes in oxygen saturation. This increase in oxygen consumption is more prevalent in patients who possess a vigorous cough, are agitated, or resist suctioning.[26]

Dysrhythmias associated with suctioning may be caused by hypoxia, increased myocardial oxygen consumption, vagal stimulation, hypoventilation, or catecholamine release. Vagal stimulation caused by suctioning can cause bradycardia and hypotension.[27] Bradycardia in the setting of hypoxia potentiates ventricular dysrhythmias, including ventricular fibrillation. Nebulized or intravenous atropine is recommended for bradycardia and can be used as pretreatment in patients at risk for bradycardia, particularly infants. Sympathetic stimulation may occur as a result of hypoxia, pain, or stress of the procedure. Pain medications, anxiolytics, and preparation of the patient for the procedure may blunt the sympathetic response. Suctioning should be stopped immediately if a dysrhythmia develops.

Increases in ICP during suctioning are well documented.[28–30] Tracheostomy suctioning can induce a strong cough reflex, which is thought to contribute to the increased ICP by raising intrathoracic pressure, reducing cerebral perfusion pressure, and increasing systemic blood pressure. In susceptible patients, increases in ICP can lead to devastating outcomes.[24,29,31] If there is concern that increases in ICP could harm the patient, several preventive steps should be taken before initiating tracheal suctioning. The most important interventions are providing adequate sedation and maximizing oxygenation.[18] Hyperventilation before and between passes of the suction catheter can transiently lower ICP by reducing systemic CO_2.[29] One minute before suctioning, hyperventilate the patient by increasing the respiratory rate to approximately 30 breaths/min. If not heavily sedated, most patients will cough vigorously when suctioned. Lidocaine can be instilled into the trachea to blunt the cough reflex, thereby preventing an increase in ICP. To anesthetize the trachea locally, instill 1 to 1.5 mg of 2% lidocaine into the tracheostomy tube. After administering the medication, prepare the patient for suctioning by ensuring that sedation and oxygenation are adequate. After 10 minutes to allow the lidocaine to produce its local effect, begin tracheal suctioning. This method has been shown to prevent increases in ICP and changes in cerebral hemodynamics.[32]

Atelectasis can occur when airway gases are suctioned too rapidly. To reduce this complication, choose a suction catheter that is less than half the inner diameter of the tracheostomy tube and minimize the duration and suction pressure. Atelectasis can be minimized by using a closed suction system and providing positive end-expiratory pressure after suctioning.[33] Hyperventilation should not be performed routinely to resolve suction-related atelectasis.[25]

Mucosal injury is a common complication of tracheal suctioning. Invagination of the mucosa into the side ports of the catheter occurs during suctioning and causes the tracheal mucosa to become denuded, edematous, and predisposed to bleeding. Mucosal damage also interferes with mucociliary transport. Tracheitis can occur due to frequent or improperly performed suctioning.

Minitracheostomy Suctioning Procedure

The minitracheostomy (*minitrach*) is a device that was designed to improve tracheal hygiene in patients with intact cough reflexes, normal ventilatory function, and vocalization. The minitrach serves as a small port solely for suctioning secretions. Commonly, a 4-mm indwelling cuffless cannula is inserted through the cricothyroid membrane into the trachea. Patients who are suctioned through a minitrach are at lower risk for gagging and aspiration because they are able to maintain laryngeal and glottic function.[34] The minitrach device is seldomly used in children because they have smaller airway diameters.

The technique used to suction through a minitrach is the same as that for tracheal suctioning. The smaller port size may require that smaller catheters be used. Most patients with minitrachs are decannulated before discharge from the ICU and are rarely seen in EDs.

CHANGING A TRACHEOSTOMY TUBE

Indications

See Videos 7.2–7.4. Maturation of the tracheostomy tract is generally completed by postoperative day 7.[35] Most ED patients with a tracheostomy are seen after the stomal tract has matured, so routine changes of the tracheostomy tube can be done safely in the ED.[36] Indications for exchange of the tracheostomy tube include cuff rupture or leak, leakage around the tube caused by tracheomalacia, other changes in tracheal anatomy causing difficulties with positive pressure ventilation, complete or partial tube occlusion, and conversion to an alternative tube style.[37] There are no absolute contraindications to exchanging a tracheostomy tube in the ED, as long as the stomal tract has matured. Before undertaking the exchange, consider whether further tissue trauma or hemorrhage might occur or whether anatomic abnormalities could make the exchange difficult.[37]

There is conflicting evidence on how frequently tracheostomy tubes should be changed.[38] Do not perform tube changes on a predetermined schedule, but rather as the patient's clinical condition dictates. There is some evidence that tubes left in place longer than 3 months are at higher risk for infection.[39] Most manufacturers recommend that tracheostomy tubes be changed approximately 30 days after placement.

Equipment

When changing a tracheostomy tube, familiarize yourself with the resources and equipment available in the ED. Keep the equipment readily available, if not at the patient's bedside. The necessary equipment is depicted in Fig. 7.2.

Tracheostomy tubes are most commonly made from synthetic material such as plastic or metal. Plastic tubes are either polyvinyl chloride, which softens at body temperature, or

Changing a Tracheostomy Tube

Indications
Complete or partial tube obstruction
Mechanical failure
- Peritubal leak
- Cuff rupture

Conversion to an alternative tube style (only with a mature stomal tract)

Contraindications
Absolute: None
Relative: Tracheostomy placement <7 days earlier

Complications
Hemorrhage
False passage
Obstruction
Prolonged procedure time
Tract closure
Hypoxia
Subcutaneous emphysema
Aspiration

Equipment
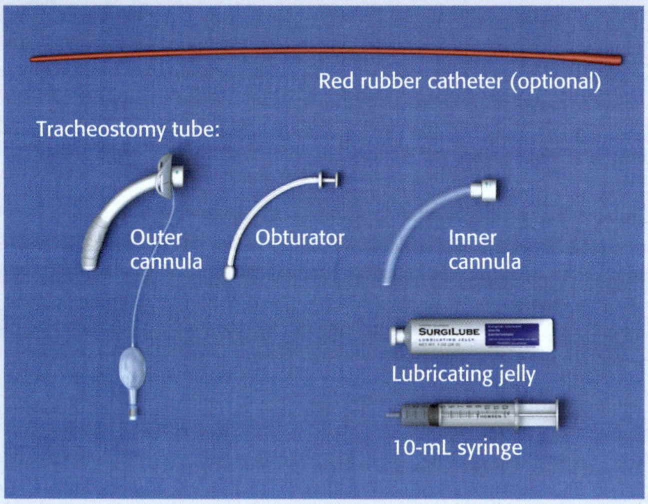

Review Box 7.2 Changing a tracheostomy tube: indications, contraindications, complications, and equipment.

TABLE 7.1 Common Tracheostomy Tube Sizes With Dimensions

Portex Cuffed BLUselect Tracheostomy Tubes				Shiley Tracheostomy Tubes[a]			
TUBE SIZE (mm) AND COLOR CODE	INTERNAL DIAMETER (mm)	OUTER DIAMETER (mm)	LENGTH (mm)	TUBE SIZE (JACKSON)	INTERNAL DIAMETER (mm)	OUTER DIAMETER (mm)	LENGTH (mm)
6.0 (pink)	6.0	9.2	64.5	4	6.5	9.4	62
7.0 (green)	7.0	10.5	70.0	6	7.5	10.8	74
8.0 (gray)	8.0	11.9	75.5	8	8.0	12.2	79
9.0 (blue)	9.0	13.3	81.0	10	10.0	13.8	79
10.0 (yellow)	10.0	14.0	87.5				

[a]Shiley also offers tracheostomy tubes with both distal and proximal (relative to the cuff) extended lengths for patients with large necks or other abnormal anatomy.
DIC, Disposable inner cannula.

silicon, which is naturally soft and unaffected by temperature. Metal tubes are constructed of silver or stainless steel and lack both a cuff and a 15-mm connector to attachment to a ventilator or Ambu bag.

Sizing

To determine the appropriate size of a replacement tube, consider the internal diameter (ID), outside diameter (OD), length, and curvature of the tube. The Chevalier Jackson sizing system indicates the length and tapering of the OD. This sizing method applies to metal tubes and most Shiley dual-cannula tracheostomy tubes. Table 7.1 lists common tracheostomy tubes and their dimensions. For dual-cannula tracheostomy tubes, the inner cannula has a 15-mm connection for a ventilator. The tracheostomy outer diameter is a critical measurement when considering a replacement tube. Note that tracheostomy tubes with the same ID can have very different ODs and lengths. Consider the pretracheal distance before selecting a replacement tube of the appropriate size for patients with increased body mass index (BMI) (see the section on "Special Populations").

Single-cannula tracheostomy tubes are sized by the ID of the tube at its smallest dimension. The size of the tube is usually stamped on the flange. Before changing a tube, have the appropriate size of tube at the bedside along with tubes that are one or two sizes smaller. As a rule of thumb, most females can accommodate a tube with an OD of 10 mm, and most males can accommodate a tube with an OD of 11 mm.[14] Table 7.1 lists the most commonly recommended tracheostomy tube sizes.

Components

Most tracheostomy tubes have three standard components: an outer cannula, an obturator, and an inner cannula (see Fig. 7.3A). The outer cannula is the permanent portion of the tracheostomy tube and should not be removed unless a tube change is needed. Attached to the outer cannula is a flange on either side with eyelets used to secure the tube with tracheostomy ties that loop around the patient's neck. The obturator is a white rounded or cone-shaped object that is used to facilitate insertion of the tube. When the obturator is inserted into the outer cannula, it extends several millimeters beyond the distal end of the tube.

Tracheostomy tubes can be cuffed or uncuffed. Cuffed tracheostomy tubes are used for patients on long-term mechanical ventilation and those at risk for aspiration. Cuffed tubes also prevent loss of volume during positive pressure ventilation while preventing air leaks across the vocal cords. Speech is not possible for patients with a cuffed tube. Most tubes have a high-volume, low-pressure cuff that reduces mucosal injury and the risk for tracheal erosion, stenosis, and aspiration.[40,41] Inflate the tracheostomy cuff and deflate it by attaching a syringe to the Luer-Lok port at the proximal end of the pilot balloon and either injecting or removing approximately 10 mL of air. Determine cuff pressure by connecting the Luer-Lok port to a handheld manometer.

Uncuffed and metal tubes are used in patients with adequate ventilatory effort who are alert and at low risk for aspiration. Depending on the size of the tracheostomy tube and how much of the tracheal diameter is filled by the tube itself, the patient may be able to speak. Air must be able to bypass the tube and be transmitted across the vocal cords. Digital occlusion of the tracheostomy tube or the use of specialized speaking valves can occlude expired air from the tracheostomy and facilitate voice production. Fenestrated tubes also allow air to be transmitted across the vocal cords. The fenestrations are generally located at the superior, posterior arch of the tube and can also be found on the inner cannula in some models.

During tracheostomy weaning, tracheal buttons can be used to maintain patency of the stoma in patients who do not require mechanical ventilation. They can be retained permanently if decannulation is not possible. Tracheal buttons have a hollow outer cannula and a solid inner cannula and extend from the outer skin into the tracheal lumen. Tracheal buttons can become displaced into the tracheal lumen if they are not tethered correctly and may become clogged with secretions.[42] Tracheostomy tubes may have a speaking valve, such as the Passy-Muir or the Shiley Phonate (Mallinckrodt Medical). These devices generally clip or twist onto the 15-mm coupling of the tracheostomy tube or inner cannula. Remove the speaking valve before changing the tracheostomy tube.

General Good Practices for Airway Exchange and Aerosol Generating Procedures

Airway management procedures including tube replacement, laryngoscopy, bronchoscopy, administration of nebulized medications, and tracheostomy care are generally considered high-risk procedures that can increase the risk of infection to healthcare providers from viral containing droplets.[43] As learned during the COVID-19 pandemic, it is paramount that healthcare workers take proper precautions to avoid healthcare-associated transmission of infectious diseases. Evidence-based methods to reduce preventable exposures include proper personal protective equipment, use of negative pressure rooms, and minimizing aerosol generating procedures if there is a concern for high-risk respiratory infections.[44]

Procedure

It is essential to ensure that all airway equipment is at the patient's bedside before performing the tube exchange. In addition to having airway equipment ready, place the patient on continuous pulse oximetry, cardiac monitoring, and capnography, if available, to confirm tube placement. Identify the tracheostomy tube model and determine its size. Have this size and two other tubes that are one or two sizes smaller in the event that tube replacement is difficult. Inspect all equipment for proper function, the tracheostomy tube cuff for air leaks, and the obturator for ease of insertion and removal (Fig. 7.7, *step 1*). Coat the replacement tracheostomy tube with a water-based lubricant (see Fig. 7.7, *step 2*).

Place the patient in a semirecumbent position with the neck slightly extended to ensure proper alignment of the external stoma and the tracheostomy tract. Do not flex the neck because this may misalign the tissues and make tube replacement more difficult. Remove the old tracheostomy dressing and clean the stomal site. If breathing spontaneously and off mechanical ventilation preoxygenate the patient by placing a non-rebreather oxygen mask over the tracheostomy site for 3 minutes and then suction the oropharynx. If the patient is ventilator dependent, increase the FIO_2 to 100% for at least 1 minute before beginning the tube exchange to ensure adequate oxygenation. If needed, provide the patient with soft restraints or anxiolytic medication to improve compliance with the procedure.

The tracheostomy tube can be changed by either of two methods. If the tracheostomy tract is well matured, the tube can be exchanged with an obturator. If two experienced providers are available, one can be responsible for deflating the cuff and removing the old tube while the other inserts the new device. To remove the old tracheostomy tube, first deflate the cuff completely (if present) (see Fig. 7.7, *step 3*). Remove the existing tube with an "out-then-down" movement while the patient exhales (see Fig. 7.7, *step 4*). Next, with the obturator in place, insert the new tube into the stoma at a 90-degree angle to the cervical axis (see Fig. 7.7, *step 5*). Next, gently rotate the tube downward in a fluid, sweeping motion so the external flange is flush against the neck. If necessary, use a tracheal hook to hold the stoma open. Remove the solid obturator immediately, insert the hollow internal cannula, inflate the cuff, return the patient's head to the neutral position, and secure the external flange (see Fig. 7.7, *steps 6* to *8*).

The second technique involves exchanging the tube with a modified Seldinger technique using a red rubber catheter, nasogastric tube, gum elastic bougie, or fiberoptic nasopharyngeal scope (Fig. 7.8).[14,45] This technique is preferable if the tracheostomy tract is not well defined or if there is concern that tube exchange could be difficult. Using a nasopharyngeal scope can also confirm placement by way of direct visualization. To exchange a tracheostomy tube with this method, first premeasure the distance needed to extend the

CHANGING A TRACHEOSTOMY TUBE

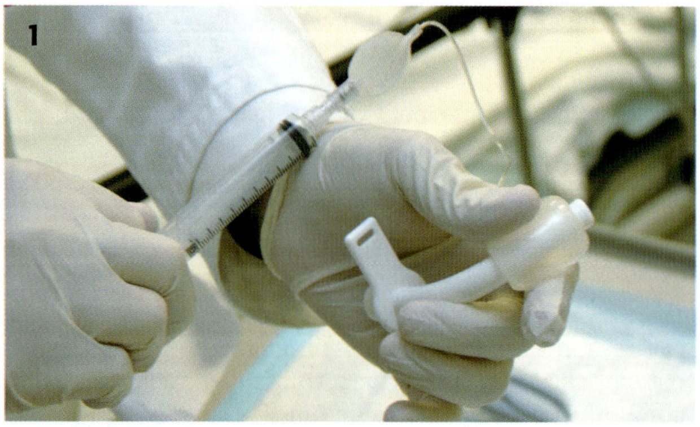

Inspect the tube for proper function; check for a cuff leak.

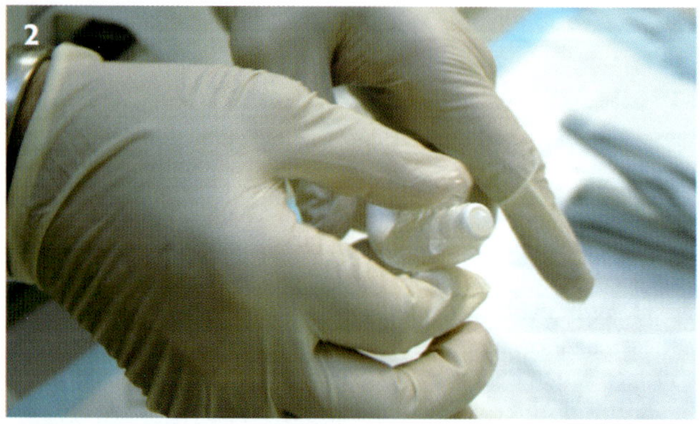

Apply a water-based lubricant to the tube.

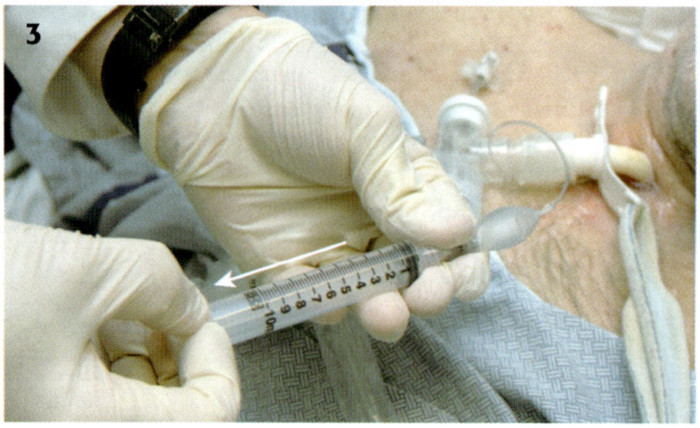

Deflate the cuff on the old tube completely.

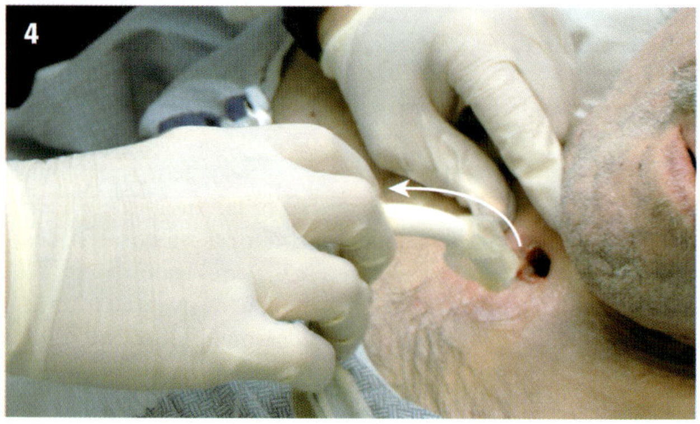

Remove the old tube during exhalation.

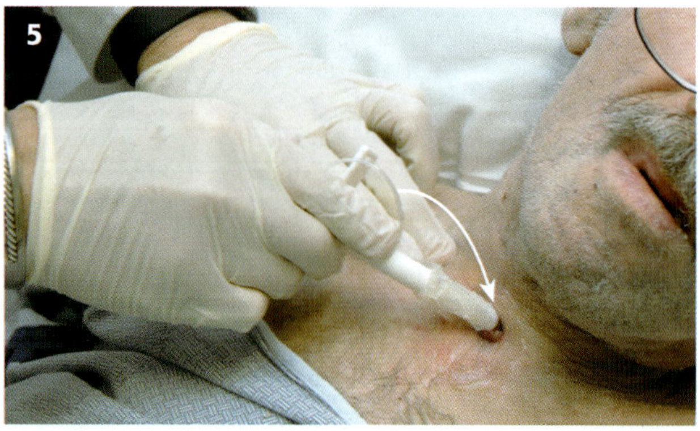

Insert the new tube (with the obturator in place) into the stoma at a 90-degree angle; push the tube downward in a fluid, sweeping motion.

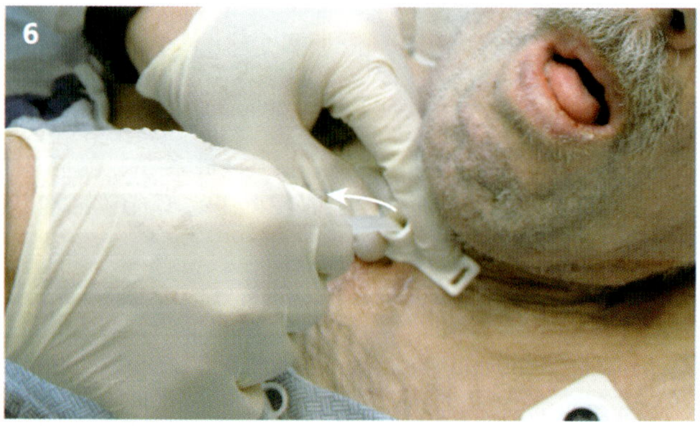

Remove the obturator, and insert the inner cannula.

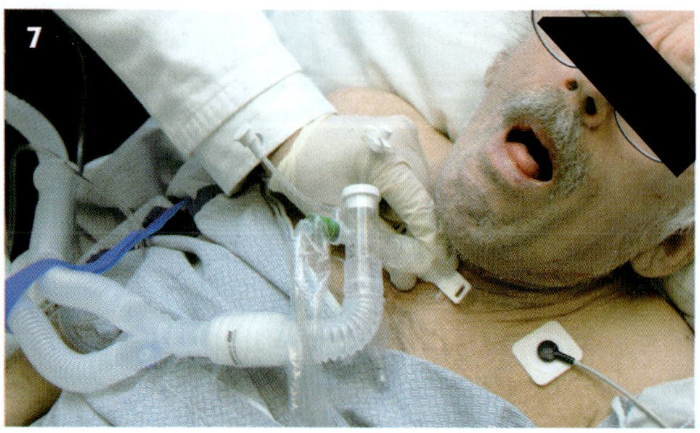

Attach the ventilator to the tracheostomy tube.

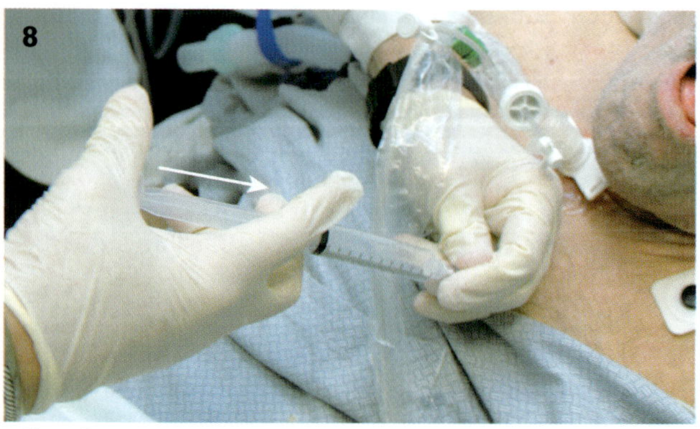

Inflate the cuff.

Fig. 7.7 Changing a tracheostomy tube. Maintain the neck in the same position (slightly extended) for removal and insertion so that the tract is not lost. If the tube is already out, and the specifics of the tract are unknown, extending the neck to align the stoma with the tissue tract is the first best position for tube replacement.

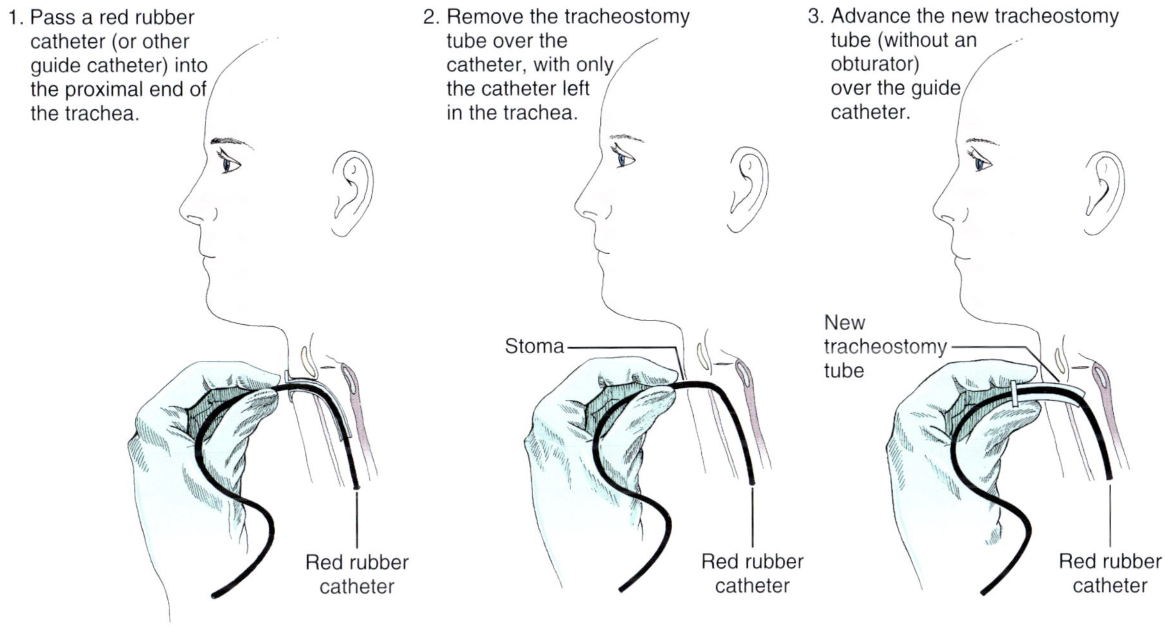

Fig. 7.8 Changing a tracheostomy tube over a guide catheter.

guidewire device beyond the distal tip of the old tracheostomy tube. Advance the guide to the premeasured distance, deflate the cuff, and remove the tube as described previously. Next, without the obturator in place, advance the new device over the guide until it is seated securely in the trachea. Remove the guide and secure the new tube. Weinmann and Bander developed a modified Seldinger technique involving the use of an airway exchange catheter to allow jet or bag ventilation into the trachea during tube exchange. This adjunct delivers intratracheal oxygen and is helpful if hypoxemia is likely to occur.[37]

Confirm proper placement of the tube within the trachea with one of several possible techniques. Traditionally, the patient is ventilated and correct tube placement confirmed by observation of equal chest rise and auscultation of bilateral breath sounds. Although both signs are important to confirm correct placement, quantitative waveform capnography is now a class I American Heart Association recommendation for confirmation of proper airway placement.[46] Multiple studies have shown capnography to be a highly sensitive tool for confirming correct placement of airway devices.[47,48] Correct tube placement can also be confirmed by direct visualization of the intraluminal tracheal rings with a fiberoptic scope.

COMPLICATIONS OF TRACHEOSTOMY

Complications related to tracheostomy placement are common and sometimes life threatening. This section addresses the emergency development of late postoperative complications (occurring more than 3 weeks after the operation). Patients with immediate and early postoperative complications are usually still hospitalized and are less likely to be seen in the ED.[49] Late postoperative tracheostomy complications encountered in ED patients include obstruction, dislodgement, equipment failure, infection, anatomic disruption, and hemorrhage. Management of the patient varies depending on the type of complication that the patient is experiencing. Rapid recognition of the problem is paramount and can drastically affect the outcome.

Obstruction and Complications From Tube Changes

See Video 7.5. Obstruction of the tracheostomy tube is a common complication and can occur at the external opening of the tube, within the inner cannula, or at the distal end of the outer cannula. In one review, 30% of ED visits for respiratory distress were due to an obstructed tube.[36] Obstruction is caused most commonly by dried respiratory secretions and, less often, by blood, aspirated material, or granulation tissue. Recent literature specific to patients with recent COVID-19 found tenacious secretions and bleeding as a cause for tracheostomy obstruction.[43] The obstructing object may act as a ball valve and allow air to enter and restricts expiration. Such obstruction is easily remedied in the ED by removing the inner cannula and then cleaning and replacing it.

Preparation

First, assess the patient's airway for patency and respiratory status. Place the patient on a cardiorespiratory monitor, a pulse oximeter, and continuous capnography. Gather appropriate airway equipment at the bedside. Be sure to have a large-bore suction catheter available in case the appropriate size of catheter is inadequate. Examine the tracheostomy tube to see whether the inner cannula is obstructed or has any obvious external obstruction.

Interventions

Administer high-flow oxygen and encourage patients who can breathe spontaneously to cough. Manually remove any obstruction seen at the external tracheal tube opening. If there is no obvious external obstruction, remove the inner cannula and suction the secretions. Inspect the inner cannula and remove any obstructing objects. If the patient's tracheostomy does not have an inner cannula, suction the tracheostomy tube to remove obstructing plugs. Thick secretions can be loosened in a *critically ill* patient by instilling normal saline into the tracheostomy tube, and this is no longer recommended for routine suctioning.[23]

If the obstruction persists, evaluate the distal tip of the tracheostomy tube. First, deflate the tracheostomy cuff and supply high-flow oxygen via face mask if the patient is breathing spontaneously or via a bag-valve-mask device if the patient is unable to breathe without assistance. *Note that if the tracheostomy cuff is inflated, you will not be able to provide supplemental oxygen or ventilatory support through the oropharynx.* If the patient is still in respiratory distress despite these interventions, remove the outer tube and replace it. If these maneuvers are ineffective, consider more distal causes of airway obstruction, such as granulation tissue, a mass, or a clot. Be sure to have a surgical airway kit and a fiberoptic bronchoscope or nasopharyngoscope available at the patient's bedside.

Dislodgement

Displacement of the tracheal tube is a serious complication that can have a disastrous outcome if not recognized and corrected quickly. Patients at highest risk for poor outcomes from a dislodged tube are those who have an increased BMI, who have recently inserted or changed tubes, who have anatomic abnormalities, and who are difficult to ventilate or were difficult to intubate in the past.[50–52] Evidence of tube dislodgement is usually obvious. Signs and symptoms include hypoxemia, agitation, respiratory distress, altered mental status, subcutaneous emphysema, and high airway pressure. Dislodgement can occur during patient transfers, when traction is placed on the tube, or when the tube is manipulated for bag-valve-mask ventilation or ventilator tube connection. If a tracheostomy tube is too long, it can become displaced inferiorly, which causes the tip to either abut the mucosal wall of the trachea or obstruct it at the level of the carina.

It is important to know when and why the tracheostomy was placed because such information will influence evaluation and management of the patient.[53] If a tracheostomy tube becomes dislodged within the first 7 days after initial placement, the stoma can close rapidly and make reinsertion difficult (Video 7.5). Blind, forceful attempts at reinsertion of the tracheostomy tube in the early postoperative period can result in the creation of a false passage and possible respiratory arrest. If accidental decannulation occurs before the tract has time to form, orotracheal intubation is the safest approach in the ED, unless the patient has had a laryngectomy (see section on "Special Populations"). Reinsertion of the tracheostomy tube is possible; however, the patient will most likely require ET intubation to secure the airway. Patients with abnormal neck anatomy or other causes of a "difficult airway" may not benefit from reinsertion in the ED. In these cases, the procedure may need to be performed in the operating room. Seek emergency surgical consultation for complicated cases.

Preparation

As for all patients with tracheostomy complications, begin with a quick primary assessment and place the patient on appropriate monitoring devices. Continuous waveform capnography can be invaluable in determining whether the tracheostomy tube is placed properly. Absence of a waveform or end-tidal CO_2 partial pressure less than 10 mm Hg is an indication that the airway device has become dislodged or was placed inappropriately.[54] It is essential to have advanced airway equipment at the bedside, including two replacement tracheostomy tubes (each with an inner cannula). A fiberoptic nasopharyngeal scope or bronchoscope, if available, can be helpful. Position the patient with the neck in extension to maximize alignment of the stoma and trachea. Neck flexion can cause downward displacement of the tube by as much as 3 to 4 cm.[55]

Interventions

First, determine that the tube flanges rest snugly at the skin. If the tracheostomy tube appears to be minimally displaced, attempt to reposition the tube by gentle manipulation. If the tracheostomy tube is completely dislodged or no waveform is present on capnography, tube replacement should be attempted.

If the tracheostomy stoma was created less than 7 days earlier, be prepared to orally intubate the patient. First, cut any flange sutures and remove the tracheostomy tube (Fig. 7.9). If the patient is stable, attempt to reinsert the tracheostomy tube with the assistance of a gum elastic bougie or fiberoptic scope.[14] If the patient is unstable and there is a concern the tracheostomy site cannot be used to reinsert an airway, cut the flange sutures, remove the tracheostomy tube, and orally intubate the patient.

If the tracheostomy stoma was created 7 to 30 days earlier, remove the tube and any other cause of obstruction from the stoma. If the patient can ventilate independently, allow the patient to oxygenate and then reinsert the tube when ready. If the patient is unstable, occlude the stoma with moist gauze or other occlusive device and provide oropharyngeal bag-valve-mask ventilation. Once the patient is stabilized, replace the tracheostomy tube. If a replacement tube is not available, check the outer diameter of the tracheostomy tube, and

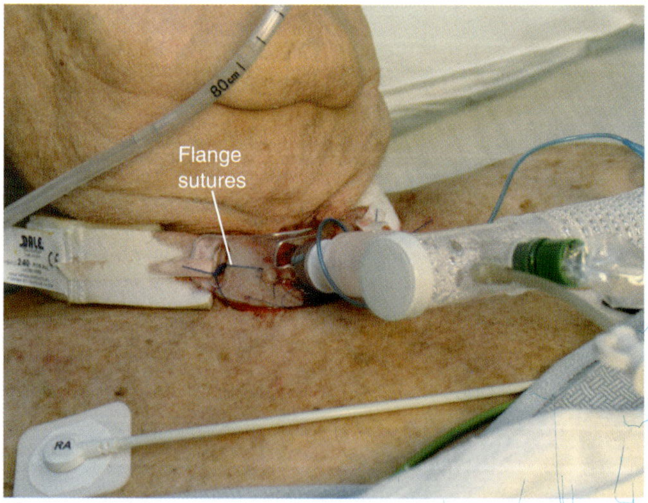

Fig. 7.9 Newly inserted tracheostomy tube. Replacement under emergency conditions can be difficult, particularly if the event occurs soon after the tube is initially placed and before a tract has formed (usually approximately 5 days after the procedure). Blind forceful attempts at reinsertion in this circumstance can be associated with the creation of a false passage and respiratory arrest. Orotracheal intubation is another option for accidental decannulation occurring before tract formation. In patients with surgical tracheostomies, traction on stay sutures placed circumferentially around the tracheal rings (which are generally cut long and often taped to the anterior chest wall—not shown here) will facilitate reintubation.

insert a cuffed ET tube of equal size (or at minimum, 6-0) as a substitute.

If the tracheostomy is more than 30 days old, the tube may not need to be replaced. If the patient is unstable, prepare as described for reinsertion or ET intubation. If the patient is stable and ventilating spontaneously without any signs of distress, contact the appropriate specialty care clinician to discuss the need for emergency reinsertion.

Once the tube is reinserted, confirm correct placement with auscultation and waveform capnography. Tube position can also be confirmed by direct visualization with a fiberoptic scope.

False Passage

A false lumen can be created during replacement of a tracheal tube or during repositioning of a dislodged tube. Patients with an increased BMI are at high risk for false passage because of their redundant neck tissue (see section on "Special Populations"). Subcutaneous air, crepitus, or distortion of anterior neck landmarks may indicate placement of the tracheostomy tube into a false passage. Absence of a waveform on capnography confirms misplacement of the tracheostomy tube. Abdominal distention after bag-valve-mask ventilation may indicate placement of the tracheal tube through a tracheoesophageal fistula (TEF). If a false passage is suspected, remove and replace the tracheostomy tube expeditiously.

Equipment Failure

Fracture

Tracheostomy tubes do not fracture frequently. When fractures do occur, they are most often located at the juncture of the flange and the tube connection.[56,57] A fractured tube fragment may migrate inferiorly and obstruct the tracheal lumen. Patients may have acute respiratory complaints such as cough, dyspnea, choking, or wheezing. Prolonged retention of a foreign body can result in chronic respiratory symptoms such as wheezing, coughing, or recurrent bouts of pneumonia or bronchiectasis. To manage this problem, replace the tube if possible and arrange bronchoscopy for retrieval of the tube fragment.

Tracheal Cuff Complications

Complications related to the tracheal tube cuff include perforation that results in a poor seal and increased risk for aspiration; overinflation that causes pressure on or impingement of the esophageal lumen; and distention of the cuff distal to the tracheal tube that results in obstruction of the tracheal tube opening. During the COVID-19 pandemic, tracheostomy cuff hyperinflation to avoid any air leak was not uncommon in patients who are COVID-19 positive, increasing the risk of progressive tracheomalacia, fistula, and injury.[58] Mucosal injury is less common since the use of low-pressure cuffs has become standard practice. Pain with ventilation or swallowing, inadequate oxygenation, or the presence of gastric secretions in the tracheostomy tube may indicate cuff problems. Verify inflation pressure with a manometer (target range, 18 to 25 mm Hg) and appropriate cuff position. Replacement of the tube is indicated if the symptoms persist.

Infection

Patients who require long-term tracheostomy and mechanical ventilation are at high risk for nosocomial pneumonia, ventilator-associated pneumonia (VAP), and tracheobronchitis. In general, the frequency of infection increases with the duration of mechanical ventilation, and the risk for infection is highest in the first week following intubation. Nonventilated tracheostomy patients are also at increased risk for pneumonia, tracheobronchitis, stomal infections, and other soft tissue infections.

Risk factors for systemic infection include impairment of host defenses and exposure to large numbers of bacteria that bypass the upper airway defense systems. In healthy patients, the upper respiratory tract is colonized by normal oropharyngeal flora. In tracheostomy patients, the normal flora can be replaced by virulent pathogens such as enteric gram-negative bacteria.[59] The organisms most commonly cultured from tracheostomy stomas and tubes are *Pseudomonas aeruginosa*, *Acinetobacter*, and *Staphylococcus aureus*.[60] Colonization rates are high in these patients, even in the absence of systemic infection. The tracheostomy tube bypasses the natural protective barriers of the upper airway. Suctioning a colonized tracheostomy tube can introduce bacteria into the lower respiratory tract.

Ventilator-associated tracheobronchitis (VAT) is the result of colonization of the upper airway and can eventually progress to VAP.[57] Patients with VAT have fever, production of purulent sputum, and positive respiratory cultures and no evidence of a new infiltrate on chest radiography. VAT is frequently caused by multidrug-resistant organisms. When choosing antimicrobial therapy, consider recent hospitalizations, previous infections, recent antibiotic use, and the hospital's antibiogram.

Tracheostomy patients requiring long-term mechanical ventilation are also at risk for VAP. These patients are similar to those with VAT, except that they have an infiltrate on chest radiography. A common cause of VAP is aspiration. Patients become predisposed to aspiration if they have altered neurologic function, have an abnormal swallowing mechanism, or are mechanically ventilated and kept in the supine position for a prolonged time. Some degree of aspiration occurs in 33% to 61% of all tracheostomy patients.[61,62] To reduce the risk for aspiration, keep patients requiring mechanical ventilation in a semirecumbent position. It is generally recommended that 30 to 45 degrees is adequate to reduce the risk for VAP.[63–65]

Stomal infections and cellulitis are also common.[36] The bacteria cultured most frequently from patients with tracheostomy-related cellulitis are *S. aureus*, *Pseudomonas* species, and *Monilia*. Consider *Candida albicans* infection in patients previously treated with antibiotics and those who have an underlying immunocompromised state. Peristomal cellulitis can usually be treated with good wound care and oral antibiotics. The most dangerous complications from cellulitis are mediastinitis, mediastinal abscess, necrotizing fasciitis, and paratracheal abscess. Consider these complications in patients who have pain with breathing, pain with swallowing, or signs of systemic infection. Strongly consider a deep neck infection in diabetic patients.[66] β-Hemolytic streptococci or coagulase-positive staphylococci are the cause in 90% of patients with craniocervical necrotizing fasciitis.[67] Sputum samples, obtained via tracheal suctioning, should be analyzed when infectious complications are suspected. Radiologic studies, namely, a chest radiograph, cervical computed tomography (CT), and chest CT, should be ordered as indicated.

Antimicrobial treatment in the ED should cover the most common organisms for the suspected site of tracheostomy-related infection. Broad-spectrum systemic antimicrobials, along with adjuvant aerosol therapy, should be given urgently to high-risk patients.[68]

Tracheal Stenosis and Tracheomalacia

Tracheal stenosis and tracheomalacia are late complications of a tracheostomy, often presenting weeks to months after decannulation. Its overall incidence is unknown, and clinically significant stenosis has been estimated to develop in 10% of all tracheostomy patients.[69] Tracheal stenosis occurs most often at the level of the stoma and can develop proximal (suprastomal) or distal to the stoma as a result of a poorly fitting tube or cuff, or from prolonged ET intubation prior to tracheostomy. Pressure on the tracheal lumen from the tube or cuff can cause epithelial destruction, tracheitis, ulceration, persistent inflammation, and subsequent stenosis. Stenosis at the stoma can occur from rigid tube systems with excessive motion and pressure points. Symptoms become evident when the tracheal diameter is narrowed by 50% to 60%.[70] Stridor typically occurs when the tracheal lumen is narrower than 5 mm.[55] Respiratory symptoms such as cough, retained secretions, and progressive dyspnea with exertion are indications of clinically significant stenosis.

Tracheomalacia is weakening of the tracheal cartilage from pressure necrosis and results in luminal widening. A loose tracheostomy tube with excessive mobility can cause air leaks or tracheal collapse (Fig. 7.10). Patients with significant tracheomalacia experience tracheal collapse on expiration. This can result in air trapping and retained respiratory secretions. Pediatric patients are less able to tolerate cartilaginous weakening and tracheomalacia.

Interventions

Relief of respiratory compromise is problematic because a high-grade stenosis may make ET intubation difficult or impossible. To treat a patient with respiratory distress secondary to tracheal stenosis, first attempt to improve ventilation by elevating the head of the bed and placing the patient on high-flow humidified oxygen. Nebulized bronchodilators, racemic epinephrine, and heliox may also be helpful. Extracorporeal membrane oxygenation can be considered in high-risk patients prior to hemodynamic or respiratory collapse. Keep a cricothyrotomy kit readily available in the event that ET intubation is impossible, recognizing the level of obstruction may be beyond the level of the cricothyroid membrane. Tracheal stenosis can be diagnosed definitively by visualization with a flexible fiberoptic scope. A CT scan of the patient's neck can be helpful in determining the level and grade of stenosis. Treatment of tracheal stenosis involves operative dilation or resection of granulomatous tissue in the operating room.

Tracheoesophageal Fistula

TEF is an uncommon, late complication of tracheostomy. It occurs in 1% of tracheostomy patients as a result of injury to the posterior tracheal wall.[71] Early TEF can occur if a puncture wound or small laceration is made in the anterior esophageal wall during placement of the tracheostomy. The most common cause of a TEF is a poorly fitted tracheostomy tube or an overinflated cuff.[71] Injury to the esophageal mucosa from a nasogastric or orogastric tube can also cause a TEF.

Most patients with a TEF have increased secretions, recurrent pneumonia, or aspiration of gastric contents while receiving mechanical ventilation. The most frequent sign of a TEF is cough after swallowing. A persistent cuff leak or abdominal distention may also indicate a TEF. The clinician may be able to auscultate breath sounds over the lung fields and the epigastrium simultaneously, and this finding is unreliable. Bronchoscopy, barium esophagography, or mediastinal CT can aid in making the diagnosis.

Interventions

Once a TEF is diagnosed, the immediate goal should be to reduce the amount of tracheal and pulmonary soilage by inflating a cuff below the level of the fistula. If the current tracheostomy tube is not long enough to allow placement of a cuff distal to the TEF, exchange it with a longer tracheostomy tube or an ET tube. An orogastric or nasogastric tube can also be inserted to prevent gastric contents from further contaminating the respiratory tract. Early consultation with an otolaryngologist or thoracic surgeon is appropriate because the definitive treatment is surgical.[71] Antibiotics that target gram-negative, gram-positive, and anaerobic organisms should be initiated if there is a suspicion for pneumonia. TEF

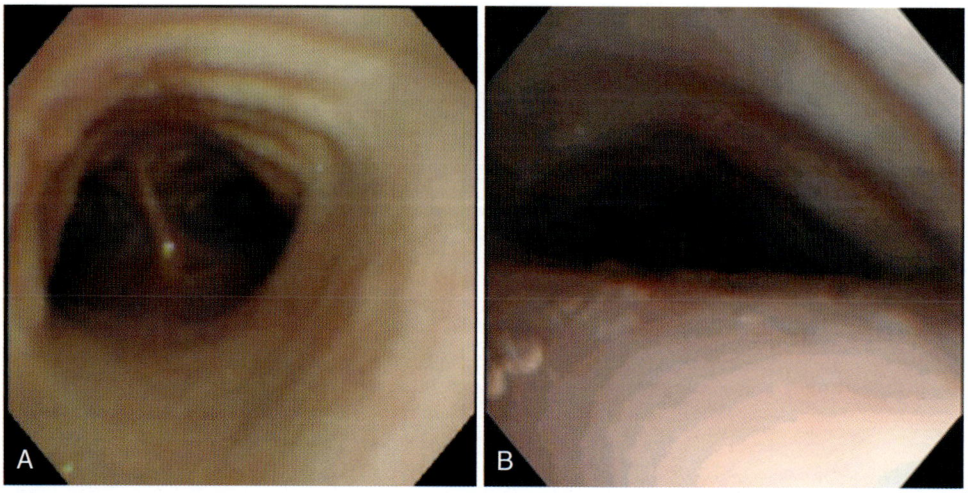

Fig. 7.10 (A–B) Tracheomalacia. (From Patterson AG, Cooper JD, eds. *Pearson's Thoracic and Esophageal Surgery*. Elsevier; 2008.)

is not usually an immediately life-threatening complication, and tube exchange can be performed in conjunction with the surgical team.

Bleeding

Major Bleeding

See Video 7.6. Major bleeding is one of the most feared complications of tracheostomy. A history of bleeding or minor bleeding that has stopped spontaneously cannot automatically be attributed to minor irritation or skin erosion. It may not be possible to fully evaluate bleeding from a tracheostomy site in the ED without consultation or specialized equipment such as a fiberoptic endoscope. Sources of bleeding include pharmacologic anticoagulation, thyroid vessels, anterior jugular veins, brachiocephalic (innominate) artery, carotid artery, and aortic arch.[72,73] Bleeding from esophageal or gastric sources may occur if a TEF is present or if the patient has aspirated blood. Erosion of a major vessel from the cuff or tip of the tube is responsible for 10% of all tracheostomy hemorrhages and is a devastating complication. The IA is the vessel most commonly involved.[74]

A tracheoinnominate artery fistula (TIF) is a late complication of tracheostomy that usually occurs within the first 4 weeks after insertion, and it can happen at any time.[11,75] The mortality rate associated with a TIF approaches 100%.[76] The anatomic proximity of the IA to the trachea places it at higher risk for fistulization if the anterior tracheal wall is injured. The vessel crosses from left to right as it moves superiorly and lies immediately anterior to the trachea at the level of the superior thoracic inlet. Risk factors for TIF include placement of the stoma below the third tracheal ring, caudal migration of the tracheal tube, and the presence of a cephalad-coursing IA.

A single episode of hemoptysis or tracheal bleeding may be the only warning sign of a TIF. Any amount of bleeding or hemoptysis exceeding 10 mL within 48 hours after placement of the tube should be considered a "sentinel bleed" and an indication that a fatal hemorrhage may be imminent. Some patients report only a new cough or retrosternal pain.[77] Presume that a history or evidence of 10 mL or more of blood is from an arterial source.

Preparation

When evaluating a patient with a suspected TIF, place advanced airway equipment at the bedside. Emergency surgical consultation is mandatory. Position the patient with the head of the bed elevated and the neck in slight extension. Secure adequate intravenous access, obtain type and crossmatched blood, and prepare the patient to go to the operating room. In addition to the equipment noted in Fig. 7.2, have a scalpel with a No. 10 or 11 blade and a 50-mL syringe at the bedside.

Interventions

If the patient is stable, an attempt to visualize the bleeding site with direct visualization using a fiberoptic scope should be performed. Look for evidence of bleeding on the anterior tracheal wall at or below the sternal notch. If significant tracheal bleeding or an unstable clot is present, remove the fiberoptic scope and hyperinflate the tracheostomy tube cuff with the 50-mL syringe to compress the artery against the posterior sternal wall. Inflate the balloon slowly to prevent rupture of the cuff. Depending on the make and model of the tube, inflating the cuff with the entire 50 mL may not be possible. If a TIF has been caused by cuff erosion, this procedure should tamponade the bleeding. If the patient's tracheostomy tube does not have a cuff, replace it with a cuffed ET or tracheostomy tube.

If cuff hyperinflation is unsuccessful, the TIF may be located at or beyond the distal tip of the tracheostomy tube. In this circumstance, the current tracheostomy tube must be removed and replaced with either an oral ET tube or an ET tube inserted through the stoma.

Position the cuff of the ET tube below the stoma at the level of the upper part of the sternum and hyperinflate it. If the patient continues to bleed despite this maneuver, apply digital pressure through the tracheal stoma to compress the anterior tracheal wall against the sternum. Digital pressure is considered a reliable technique to stop hemorrhage and can provide control of bleeding during transport to the operating room, and patients may not be able to be ventilated while holding manual pressure (Fig. 7.11). Extension of the stoma with a vertical incision to the jugular notch may be necessary if the provider cannot reach the TIF through the original stoma. The clinician should be careful not to damage surrounding vasculature when making the incision.

Minor Bleeding

All bleeding from a tracheostomy site must be evaluated for a potentially life-threatening event. Seemingly minor or self-limited bleeding may be a harbinger of subsequent severe hemorrhage. Sentinel hemorrhages frequently precede massive bleeding. Consider endoscopic examination for complete evaluation unless a superficial bleeding site is confirmed.

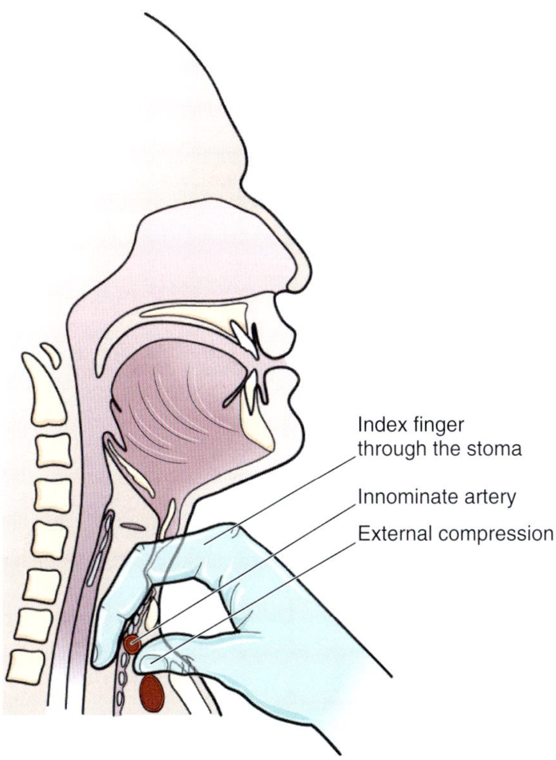

Fig. 7.11 Technique to attempt to control innominate artery bleeding by digital compression. Any bleeding from a tracheostomy site can portend subsequent massive hemorrhage and should be carefully evaluated. Bleeding from erosion into the anteriorly positioned innominate artery is catastrophic.

Minor bleeding is most likely the result of irritated granulation tissue and is usually confined to the skin surrounding the stoma. Bloody secretions from the tracheostomy tube may represent tracheitis, bleeding running down from the skin or thyroid, or superficial tracheal ulceration from tracheal suctioning or tracheal tube pressure.

Examine the stoma site and tube first in an attempt to locate the source and quantify the volume of blood loss. If the source of bleeding is within the stoma or from within the trachea, remove the tracheostomy tube if it was placed more than 7 days before the current event. Visualize the tracheal lumen, proximal end of the trachea, and inner stoma with a nasopharyngoscope or a small pediatric laryngoscope. It is important to differentiate superficial erosions from active bleeding. Do not attempt to remove clots in the trachea because this may increase the rate of hemorrhage. Consider obtaining a basic metabolic panel, complete blood count, and coagulation studies to evaluate for other factors complicating bleeding, such as uremia, thrombocytopenia, or coagulopathy.

Preparation

Prepare patients with minor tracheostomy bleeding in the same way that you would those with major bleeding. Gather the appropriate airway equipment at the bedside. In addition to the standard equipment shown in Fig. 7.2, obtain the following:

- Sterile gauze
- Sterile saline for irrigation
- 22-gauge needle with syringe
- 1% lidocaine with 1:100,000 epinephrine
- Topical hemostatic agents (e.g., Surgicel)
- Suture kit with suturing material
- Electrocauterization or chemical cauterization supplies, if available

Interventions

For external or stomal bleeding, begin with local irrigation to find the source of the bleeding. Most incisional or stomal bleeding can be stopped by applying direct pressure for 3 to 5 minutes. Application of absorbable hemostatic material may improve the outcome of direct pressure application. If an external bleeding site continues to ooze, consider adjunctive treatment. Options include injecting 0.5 to 1.0 mL of lidocaine with epinephrine near the source, placing a single suture for hemostasis, or using cauterization. Last, replace the tracheostomy tube. Following tube replacement, suction carefully to confirm resolution of the bleeding and to identify secondary sources of bleeding.

If stomal bleeding or intratracheal sites do not account for the bleeding, consider other causes. Placement of a nasogastric tube will help in the identification of gastrointestinal bleeding. Examine the nasopharynx and oropharynx for bleeding sources. If the patient has undergone radiation therapy, examine the area above the level of the tracheostomy stoma, where mucosal injury secondary to radiation damage may be the cause of blood in the tracheal secretions.

TRANSESOPHAGEAL PUNCTURE FOR VOICE RESTORATION

Transesophageal puncture (TEP) has become one of the most widely used and accepted techniques for voice rehabilitation. Developed in the 1980s, it can be performed as a primary or secondary procedure after laryngectomy or other pharyngeal surgeries. A puncture site is created through the anterior esophagus and posterior tracheal wall, where the TEP prosthesis is later inserted. The mucosa in segments of the pharyngeal esophagus vibrates in response to airflow, thereby creating speech.

Complications

Operative and immediate postoperative complications of TEP are infrequent.[78] Long-term complications include stomal stenosis, aspiration of the prosthesis, fistula leakage, TEP necrosis, and swallowing impairment. Reported infectious complications associated with TEP include deep neck abscess, aspiration pneumonia, and cervical cellulitis.[77]

The emergency care provider should be aware of the most common complications, a few that are life threatening. Accumulation of thick or inspissated secretions or food above the TEP can cause upper airway obstruction. Prosthesis dislodgement, occlusion, or erosion secondary to infection should be considered in all patients with acute changes in voice production or decreased ability to speak. Esophageal edema causing dysphagia and loss of TEP speech has been reported and should be differentiated from other causes of esophageal obstruction.[79]

When evaluating patients with a TEP, review the medical records, assess airway and esophageal patency, and determine whether the patient has experienced changes or difficulty in voice production. In stable patients, management of prosthesis complications should be referred to a specialist, most commonly an otolaryngologist.

TRANSTRACHEAL OXYGEN DELIVERY SYSTEMS

Low-flow oxygen is prescribed for patients who have adequate ventilatory function and chronic hypoxia. Many patients with chronic obstructive pulmonary disease, pulmonary fibrosis, sleep apnea, lung cancer, and α_1-antitrypsin deficiency are candidates for outpatient use of supplemental oxygen.[80,81] Traditionally, supplemental oxygen has been delivered by nasal cannula. Although nasal cannula oxygenation is easy to administer, it has several side effects, including drying of the nasal mucosa, epistaxis, ear discomfort, contact dermatitis from the oxygen tubing, and dry throat. Use of a nasal cannula is inefficient because it delivers oxygen only during inspiration and the oxygen must traverse the anatomic dead space of the nares and hypopharynx.

Transtracheal oxygen (TTO) delivery systems enhance the efficiency of oxygenation by administering oxygen directly to the lower respiratory tract. These systems reduce complications, improve patient comfort, and increase compliance.[82] Oxygen is delivered through all phases of the respiratory cycle and directly into the trachea, thereby bypassing dead spaces in the upper airway. As a result, the required oxygen flow rate is commonly reduced by at least 50%.[82] Gas mixture in the distal end of the trachea is more effective in eliminating CO_2. Clinically, TTO systems usually reduce the patient's work of breathing and exertional dyspnea. Physiologic benefits include reduced erythrocytosis, decreased pulmonary vascular resistance, improved cor pulmonale, improved arterial oxygen tension, and increased exercise capacity.[83]

TTO catheters are small tubes that deliver oxygen directly to the lumen of the trachea. The catheter is held in place by a subcutaneous tract and is inserted into the lower part of the trachea. Low-flow oxygen (2 to 10 L/min) is supplied directly to the trachea by a narrow (7- to 11-Fr) catheter. Typically, an 11-cm catheter sits in the trachea with its tip 1 to 2 cm above the carina. It can have a single or multiple distal ports for oxygen flow. The catheter is held in place by a thin band or necklace through two openings in the flange.

The surgical procedure is often done in an outpatient setting with the patient under local anesthesia. Initially, a small stent is placed percutaneously into the anterior aspect of the neck; it is then replaced with a TTO catheter in 1 to 2 weeks after the tract matures. Dislodgement of the catheter during this time can result in closure of the tract within a matter of minutes. Once the tracheocutaneous fistula has epithelialized, the catheter may be inserted. Early catheter changes should be done in the clinician's office via a modified Seldinger technique if the integrity of the stoma is questionable. After the tract has fully matured, most patients can change their catheter at home.

Regular maintenance includes cleaning and changing the TTO catheter. One milliliter of sterile saline is instilled into the catheter, and a cleaning rod is inserted as far as possible. The cleaning rod is inserted and extracted three times to remove secretions and encrustations from the lumen of the catheter. Catheters are usually changed according to the manufacturer's recommendations, from twice daily to once every 2 weeks. The stoma should be cleaned twice each day and inspected thoroughly for signs of infection. All patients should be given supplemental oxygen by nasal cannula during catheter maintenance procedures. Adequate humidification, cleaning, and systemic hydration will help reduce the incidence of mucous blockage.

Early complications (developing within 3 weeks after the procedure) occur in approximately 30% of patients and include bleeding, infection, pneumothorax, costochondritis, and dislodgement (that can be caused by coughing).[81,84] Pneumomediastinum and sudden death have been reported as possible, yet rare complications.[85] Late complications occur in approximately 40% of patients and include mucous plugging, bleeding, infection, and hemoptysis.[83] A mucous ball is an accumulation of inspissated mucus that adheres to the outer surface of the TTO catheter tip. It can cause coughing, wheezing, and dyspnea. Life-threatening airway obstruction resulting from the formation of a large mucous ball has been reported.[86]

Dyspnea or increased coughing may indicate that the TTO catheter is obstructed by a mucous ball, that the tube is kinked, or that the tip of the catheter is positioned cephalad to the stoma. Obstruction within the catheter tubing may cause a whistling sound from the oxygen tank humidifier. Always examine the patient for signs of subcutaneous air and catheter dislodgement.

If routine broad-spectrum antibiotics are used by the patient for a chronic infection, *Candida* infections can develop at the stoma. Such infections are more common in patients receiving systemic antibiotics, long-term corticosteroids, or patients with diabetes. Tracheal chondritis may result from bacterial infection of the cartilage. Many patients with chondritis have a deep, indurated, nonfluctuant lump around the tract that may be tender to palpation. A 3-week course of an oral antibiotic that specifically covers *S. aureus* should be prescribed as treatment.

Interventions

If obstruction is suspected while the patient is in the ED, clean and replace the catheter. If the stoma tract has not healed or appears to be infected, change the catheter via a modified Seldinger technique. Use a water-soluble lubricant for the catheter change. If changing the catheter does not relieve the obstruction and the patient's airway is intact, encourage the patient to perform maneuvers that raise intrathoracic pressure to increase the force of the cough. Ask the patient to sit upright, hold a pillow to the abdomen, and cough forcefully after three deep inspirations. This maneuver may help mobilize secretions or small mucous plugs in the airway. Dyspnea and coughing should lessen with effective removal of the obstruction.

Manage minor bleeding at the catheter site with gauze packing or cauterization. If significant bleeding is identified or suspected, consult a specialist on an emergency basis and manage the airway definitively as clinically indicated (see section on "Major Bleeding"). Manage skin and pulmonary infections with the techniques discussed for tracheostomy care.

Stents

Tracheal stenosis and tracheomalacia are known complications of artificial airways. Management options include surgery and placement of silicone stents in the trachea. Patients who have had their tracheostomy tubes successfully decannulated may need stents if symptomatic stenosis or tracheomalacia occurs. Indications for and complications of tracheal stents are beyond the scope of this chapter, and the clinician should be aware of the possibility that these indwelling devices may be present in patients who have undergone head and neck surgery or previous tracheostomies.[51,87]

SPECIAL POPULATIONS

Patients With Increased Body Mass Index

The prevalence of patients with increased BMI (≥30) and those with markedly increased BMI (≥40) has risen dramatically over the past few decades.[88,89] Obesity increases the patient's risk for cardiovascular and metabolic comorbidities, and patients with increased BMI have a higher risk for ventilatory dysfunction secondary to altered respiratory mechanics.[90] Lung compliance, functional residual capacity, and expiratory reserve volume in these patients are reduced exponentially in relation to BMI.[91,92] As weight increases, vital capacity and total lung capacity decrease. Ultimately, these patients have decreased pulmonary reserve, which can cause a rapid onset of hypoxia if they become critically ill.

Patients with markedly increased BMI are particularly at risk for life-threatening complications related to tracheostomy.[93] Tube obstruction and accidental dislodgement appear to be more common in these patients. Dislodgement is specifically associated with increased rates of morbidity and mortality.[52] Delayed recognition of tube dislodgement because of abnormal neck anatomy accounts for nearly 30% of tracheostomy-related deaths in this population.

Preparation

For the management of a patient with increased BMI with a tracheostomy-related complaint, it is important to have all advanced airway equipment at the bedside (see Fig. 7.2). In addition to standard equipment, attempt to obtain an extra-long or adjustable-flange tracheostomy tube to span the elongated pretracheal distance that is common in these patients.[94] In these patients, standard tracheostomy tubes may be too short proximal to the cuff and have a higher risk for malposition.

In addition to standard monitoring, use continuous capnography, if available, to prevent delay in the recognition of tube dislodgement.[52] Physical signs, such as reduced breath sounds and subcutaneous air, may be more difficult to recognize in patients with increased BMI. Fiberoptic bronchoscopy may be needed to confirm correct tube placement. The patient should be positioned with the neck in slight extension, and the head of the bed should be elevated to approximately 30 degrees.

Interventions

Approach patients with increased BMI with the same protocols outlined previously in this chapter for the applicable complication. If the tube is obstructed, deflation of the tracheostomy cuff may not be sufficient to allow adequate ventilation because of external compression caused by abnormal neck anatomy and soft tissues. If tube dislodgement is suspected, tracheostomy replacement over a fiberoptic bronchoscope or oral ET intubation may be preferred over blind reinsertion due to the increased risk for false passage.[93] Tube placement should be confirmed with end-tidal CO_2 measurement.

Laryngectomy Patients

It is important to distinguish the patient with a routine tracheostomy from the patient with a laryngectomy as this could potentially limit the ability to provide ventilation by way of the upper airway. A patient who has undergone a total laryngectomy no longer has an upper airway that is in continuity with the lungs. A patient with a partial laryngectomy will have a contiguous upper and lower airway, and interventions by way of the upper airway may be limited.

The basic principles of emergency tracheostomy care still apply to the laryngectomy patient, and it is critical to recognize that a patient with a total laryngectomy cannot be resuscitated with traditional oxygenation and ventilation techniques, such as oropharyngeal bag-valve-mask ventilation and face mask oxygenation. Interventions should be made by way of the laryngectomy stoma rather than the upper airway. Partial laryngectomy patients should also be ventilated through their stoma, and their mouth and nose should be kept closed to avoid air escape.

Interventions

Should a patient with a laryngectomy need positive pressure ventilation, there are a few important steps to consider prior to inserting a cuffed tracheostomy or ET tube through the stoma. First, it is important to inspect the laryngectomy stoma for any mechanical obstruction. Suction the stoma to make sure it is clear of excessive secretions or mucous plugs. Stoma buttons should be removed, whereas tracheoesophageal speaking valves may be left in place as long as they are not displaced.

External ventilation with a pediatric face mask or laryngeal mask airway can be performed.[95] A standard cuffed tracheostomy tube may be placed to facilitate mechanical ventilation. If inserting an ET tube, it is important that the provider avoid advancing it too far as this can lead to main stem bronchus intubation. The approximate distance between the skin of the stoma and the carina is approximately 6 cm.[96]

Pediatrics

Most considerations for pediatric patients follow adult guidelines and are discussed in the appropriate sections of this chapter, and some specific considerations should be mentioned. The tracheostomy-related mortality rate in pediatric patients ranges from 0.5% to 6%.[97] The main causes of death are accidental dislodgement and obstruction of the tracheostomy tube.[98] Complication rates are highest in patients requiring tracheostomy for airway obstruction. In comparison, patients with central nervous system disorders, respiratory distress syndrome, and congenital heart disorders are less likely to experience complications.[20]

Equipment

When replacing a tracheostomy tube in a child, always have at least two tracheostomy tubes available: the current size and a size smaller. Pediatric tubes generally have a much smaller diameter than adult tracheostomy tubes, and many of them do not have an inner cannula. Pediatric tracheostomy tubes rarely have inflatable cuffs, except for those used for certain special indications.[99] Suction catheters, a bag-valve-mask device, ET tubes, resuscitation medication, and equipment appropriate for the pediatric population should be available when treating pediatric tracheostomy patients. Continuous capnography may detect certain tracheostomy complications and is recommended.[100]

Sizing

Pediatric tracheostomy tubes share most of the same components as the tubes used in adults. The inner and outer diameters of the tracheostomy tube are stamped on the outer cannula flange, and that information should guide the clinician's choice of replacement tubes. Recommended tube sizes according to age are listed in Table 7.2. Age guidelines can be helpful, although they may not be reliable in pediatric patients

TABLE 7.2 Tracheostomy Tube Sizes Based on Patient Age

AGE	SIZE	INNER DIAMETER (mm)	OUTER DIAMETER (mm)
Premature	00	3.1	4.5
Newborn–3 months	0	3.4	5.0
3–10 months	1	3.7	5.5
10–12 months	2	4.1	6.0
13–24 months	3	4.8	7.0
2–9 years	4	5.0	8.5
10–11 years	6	7.0	10
≥12 years	8 10	8.5 9.0	12.0 13.0

Adapted from Mullins JB, Templer JW, Kong J, et al. Airway resistance and work of breathing in tracheostomy tubes. *Laryngoscope*. 1993;103:1367.

because of complex medical problems. Premature infants may be small for their age and weight, thus making estimation of tube size more difficult.

Like ET tubes, tracheostomy tubes are sized by the tube's ID. When the tracheostomy tube is seated correctly in a pediatric patient, it should extend at least 2 cm beyond the stoma and no closer than 1 to 2 cm above the carina. Its curvature should be such that when the tube is placed appropriately, the distal portion of the tube is concentric and collinear with the trachea. After replacing a tracheostomy tube, confirm its position by auscultating breath sounds, using capnography, and confirming the location of the distal tip with a chest radiograph.

Cuff

The general rule that cuffed tracheostomy tubes should not be used in patients younger than 6 years is under a great deal of debate and does not universally apply to tracheostomy patients. If a patient requires high-pressure ventilation or only nocturnal ventilation or is at risk for aspiration, a cuffed tube may be appropriate. Cuffed tubes are also used in patients with a tracheal anomaly. Replacement of these tubes should ensure that the individual's anatomic and physiologic needs are met.

Cuff pressure recommendations for pediatric patients are less than 20 cm H_2O.[101] With few exceptions, low-pressure, high-volume cuffs should be used.

Humidifiers

Humidifiers for pediatric tracheostomy tubes attach to the external port. Some humidifiers have lithium-coated moisture exchangers. Systemic absorption of lithium is unlikely to cause clinical symptoms in adults and may be a consideration in children. Use humidifiers regularly to keep secretions loose and help prevent obstruction of the tube.[102]

Suctioning

Suctioning recommendations in pediatric patients support the use of a premeasured suction catheter to reduce the rate of mucosal irritation and to limit the development of granulation tissue. The premeasured technique uses an exact depth of insertion, which reduces epithelial damage if the catheter is inserted too deeply and inadequate suctioning if the catheter is not inserted deeply enough. Depth of insertion can be estimated by measuring a similar tube before inserting the suction catheter. In children with fenestrated tracheostomy tubes, suction catheters may accidentally go through the fenestrations and cause mucosal irritation. If this happens repeatedly, granulation tissue may develop at the site.[102]

Complications

Pediatric tracheostomy complications are similar to those in the adult population. Their incidence is estimated to be between 5% and 49%.[97] Late complications most likely to be seen in the ED include obstruction, dislodgement, bleeding, pneumothorax, infection, pneumomediastinum, TEF, and TIF. Chronic respiratory complications include tracheomalacia, tracheal stenosis, vocal cord paralysis, and vocal cord fusion.

Granuloma formation is common in pediatric patients. It often occurs in the tracheal lumen either at the superior margin of the tracheostomy or at the level of the tip of the tube. The development of granulation tissue is the result of persistent mucosal irritation and inflammation. Any patient with a clinically significant granuloma should be evaluated by a pediatric specialist for definitive care.

Pneumomediastinum and pneumothorax are generally thought to be early complications of tracheostomy, and they should always be considered in a pediatric tracheostomy patient. In children, the pleural apices rise higher than in adults and can even extend into the lower part of the neck. These complications can be caused by a dislodged tube positioned in a false passage or a malpositioned tube that causes an increase in intrathoracic pressure.[98]

The most common bacterial species that colonize pediatric tracheostomies are *P. aeruginosa* and *S. aureus*. As in adults, colonization does not require treatment unless signs of acute infection are present.[98] Suprastomal collapse of the anterior tracheal wall is very common in pediatric patients and can cause air trapping. A tracheostomy tube that places excessive pressure on the tracheal rings will cause inflammation, chondritis, and weakening of the cartilaginous rings. Significant collapse can hamper subsequent decannulation success.

Management of major bleeding in pediatric patients follows the same recommendations given for adults. The smaller stoma size may prevent the application of digital pressure to the site of hemorrhage. If the clinician is unable to reach the source of the bleeding, expeditious ET intubation followed by cuff overinflation may temporize the bleeding until the patient can be taken to the operating room.

CONCLUSION

A tracheostomy emergency can be one of the most high-risk scenarios in the ED. The emergency clinician must be well prepared for a variety of tracheostomy complications and should approach the patient in an organized, stepwise fashion so that interventions can be initiated in a timely fashion. Often specialty consultation in the ED is required to fully assess or treat complications. Tube dislodgement and obstruction are common and associated with an extremely high mortality rate, especially in patients with increased BMI. Always ensure correct tube position, have backup airway equipment readily available, and obtain surgical support early if the patient needs to go to the operating room.

REFERENCES ARE AVAILABLE AT ELSEVIER EBOOKS+

CHAPTER 8

Mechanical Ventilation

Kara Ward and Jairo Santanilla

INTRODUCTION

Mechanical ventilation (MV) is an important tool for resuscitation of critically ill patients in the emergency department (ED). It is vital that ED practitioners have a thorough understanding of the basics of MV, knowing when to apply these principles and how to support patients in respiratory or cardiac failure. Hospital overcrowding has led to a delay in transfer of mechanically ventilated patients out of the ED, and ventilator management often falls on the emergency medicine physician. In addition, during nights and weekends in some facilities, the ED physician may be called on to troubleshoot or stabilize mechanically ventilated patients in the intensive care unit (ICU). The traditional view of MV as a prescription that fits virtually all patients equally should be discarded as a gross misunderstanding of pulmonary pathophysiology. Increasing evidence has shown that the mechanism of lung ventilation by MV may be as deleterious as it is helpful.[1] Because patients remain in the ED while mechanically ventilated, ED clinicians should embrace the established paradigm of pulmonary-protective MV strategies as a cornerstone of overall patient care.

BASIC PHYSIOLOGY

Understanding basic pulmonary physiology is essential to understanding how to initiate MV. This ensures that the method of gas delivery meshes with the patient's underlying physiology to avoid ventilator-induced lung injury and other deleterious complications.

Minute Volume and Alveolar Ventilation

The volume of air that moves in and out of a patient's lungs per minute is termed *minute volume* ($\dot{V}_E$). $\dot{V}_E$ is the product of tidal volume (VT) and respiratory frequency or rate (f): Normal $\dot{V}_E$ is 7 to 10 L/min. VT can be further broken down into alveolar volume (VA) and dead space volume (VDS):

$$Vt = Va + Vds$$

In healthy young persons, the anatomic dead space is accounted for by the trachea and the larger airways and is approximately 2.2 mL/kg lean body weight. In disease states, in addition to the anatomic dead space, there is a variable amount of "pathologic" dead space, corresponding to ventilated alveoli and respiratory bronchioles that are not adequately perfused. The sum of anatomic and pathologic dead space is often referred to as *physiologic dead space*.

Alveolar minute ventilation ($\dot{V}_A$) is the product of rate times VT minus dead space: $\dot{V}_A$ and the rate of CO_2 production by the body determine the partial pressure of CO_2 in the alveoli ($PACO_2$), which is approximately equal to systemic arterial CO_2 tension.

Volume-Pressure Relationship

Volume and pressure are related for a given respiratory system. A given volume (V) will create a certain pressure (P) relative to the compliance (C) of the respiratory system. The respiratory system consists of the ventilator tubing, endotracheal (ET) tube, trachea, airways, lung parenchyma, chest wall, and diaphragm tension. For example, a 500-mL volume will create a certain pressure based on the compliance of the respiratory system. Increasing the volume will increase the pressure in the system. Decreasing the volume will result in lower pressure. Decreasing the compliance (i.e., making the system "stiffer") will increase the pressure in the system. Increasing the compliance will decrease the pressure in the system. Using a balloon as an example, the more deflated the balloon is, the easier it is to inflate and distend. The more inflated, the less likely it can be inflated further, reflecting less compliance. Another way to think of compliance is a thicker balloon is harder to inflate (low compliance) and the thinner balloon is easier to inflate (high compliance).

$$P = V / C$$

Conversely, this relationship also holds for volume. For example, a pressure of 20 cm H_2O will create a certain volume based on the compliance of the system. Increasing pressure will result in a higher volume. Decreasing pressure will result in a lower volume. Decreasing compliance will result in a lower volume. Increasing compliance will result in a higher volume.

$$V = P \times C$$

Airway Pressures

Plateau Pressure

Plateau pressure is measured at the end of inspiration with a short breath-hold (Fig. 8.1). This would be the pressure in the balloon/system when fully inflated and the end of the balloon would be sealed. At this point, no airflow should be occurring. This is considered a static pressure. By understanding the aforementioned volume-pressure relationship, one can easily deduce how plateau pressure is inversely related to respiratory system compliance and directly related to volume. Anything that decreases compliance will increase plateau pressure. Increasing compliance will decrease plateau pressure. Decreasing volume will decrease plateau pressure (a major tenet in lung-protective ventilation).

Peak Airway Pressure

Peak airway pressure is derived during inspiration and incorporates airflow. In the balloon analogy, this is the pressure required to inflate the balloon and is a dynamic measure. Because there is air movement during this measurement, it is considered a dynamic pressure. It reflects the dynamic compliance of the entire respiratory system and incorporates static compliance and airflow. Peak airway pressure can never be lower than plateau pressure. In addition, because its main distinction is that it incorporates airflow, peak pressure is reflective of the resistance to airflow. Anything that decreases compliance or increases resistance to airflow will increase

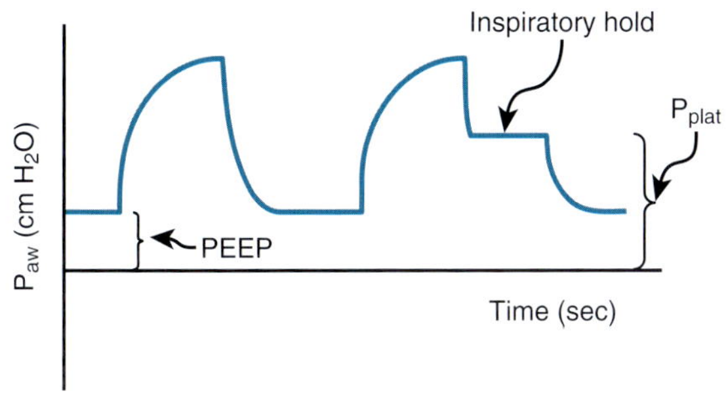

Fig. 8.1 Schematic of a pressure-time curve showing an inspiratory breath-hold and subsequent plateau pressure (P_{plat}) measurement. P_{aw}, Airway pressure; *PEEP*, positive end-expiratory pressure.

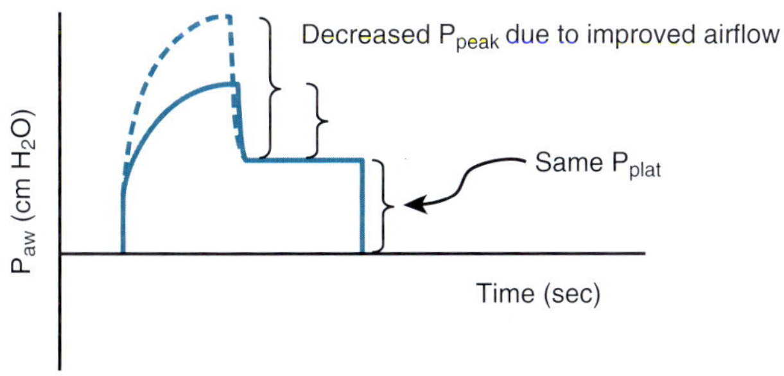

Fig. 8.2 Schematic of two superimposed pressure-time curves showing an isolated decrease in peak inspiratory pressure (P_{peak}) with no change in plateau pressure (P_{plat}) as airflow resistance improves. P_{aw}, Airway pressure.

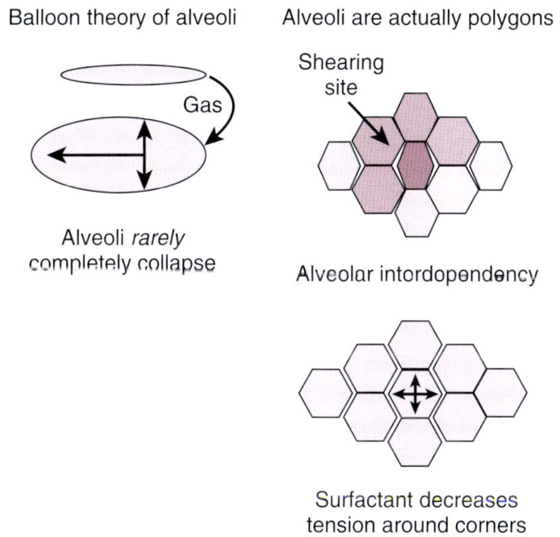

Fig. 8.3 Alveolar interdependence. Note that alveoli are not round in shape; instead, they are polygons. Polygons have corners and may have two opposing surfaces that may adhere to one another via surface tension. Surfactant works to reduce this surface tension and allow alveoli to open with reduced shear stress at the junction of closed and open alveoli. Alveoli are connected via the pores of Kohn. These pores allow opening alveoli to pull a relatively closed alveolus open while equalizing pressure between adjacent alveoli. The central alveolus on the right is fairly closed in the upper part of the diagram, but it is pulled open by its neighbors as they expand and accept gas.

peak airway pressure. Increasing compliance or decreasing resistance to airflow will decrease peak airway pressure.

A physiologically appropriate means of detecting and monitoring bronchospasm is the peak-plateau gradient. A normal gradient is less than 4 cm H_2O pressure, and elevated values indicate increased airway resistance. The efficacy of treatment with β_2-agonists, steroids, intravenous magnesium, or diuresis may be assessed by monitoring the changes in this gradient (Fig. 8.2).

Positive End-Expiratory Pressure

Positive end-expiratory pressure (PEEP) is the pressure in the airway at the end of exhalation. PEEP helps keep the large noncartilaginously supported airways and the smaller alveoli open to prevent collapse, atelectasis, and ensuing hypoxia. The ventilation required to compensate for this triad commonly worsens lung compliance and is associated with ventilator-induced lung injury. Progressive increases in PEEP result in elevations in both total lung pressure and total lung volume. For example, serial elevations in PEEP often result in increased plateau pressure and elevated functional residual capacity (FRC; i.e., lung volume).

Extrinsic PEEP

When discussing MV and PEEP, most often authors are referring to extrinsic PEEP ($PEEP_e$). This is also referred to as applied PEEP. It is the PEEP that is extrinsically applied by the ventilator. When PEEP is used without a subscript in this chapter, it refers to $PEEP_e$. The useful PEEP range is from 3 to 20 cm H_2O.[2] PEEP is used to increase FRC and move the zero pressure point of each alveolar unit more proximally in the airway, preventing early alveolar collapse.[3] By so doing, PEEP increases the available number of alveolar units that can participate in gas exchange. The primary effect of PEEP on gas exchange is improvement in oxygenation, not removal of CO_2. CO_2 clearance is rather efficient and will be well preserved, even in hypoxic situations. By opening one alveolar unit, the tendency of adjacent units is to open as well (i.e., alveolar codependency) (Fig. 8.3).[4] Excessive PEEP will compromise hemodynamics. There are two primary questions to ask when using PEEP to augment oxygenation: (1) What is the "optimal PEEP?" and (2) Is the current amount of PEEP compromising the patient's hemodynamics?

PEEP is not without untoward side effects, and increased levels of PEEP can lead to lung injury and hemodynamic compromise.[5] Increased intrathoracic pressure can result in cardiac compression and collapse, principally of the right atrium. It is imperative that the patient be adequately volume-resuscitated because preload depletion compounds this problem. Desired levels of PEEP simply may not be possible because of deleterious effects on cardiac output.

Optimal PEEP can be determined in several ways. One is to increase PEEP until there are no longer increases in partial pressure of oxygen (Po_2). This method may result in several untoward events. First, oxygen tension may increase steadily, and carbon dioxide pressure (Pco_2) may increase as a result of alveolar overdistention. With overdistention, alveolar pressure may exceed pulmonary arteriolar pressure and actually decrease pulmonary blood flow and clearance of CO_2. Second, alveolar overdistention may increase total intrathoracic pressure and result in diminished venous return and cardiac output. Third, decreased venous return may cause cerebral venous hypertension. The optimal PEEP for one organ system may be deleterious for another. For example, the optimal PEEP for ideal oxygenation may be the worst PEEP for cerebral venous drainage.

An alternative is to increase PEEP until a complication of PEEP occurs (e.g., elevation in Pco_2, hypotension) and then

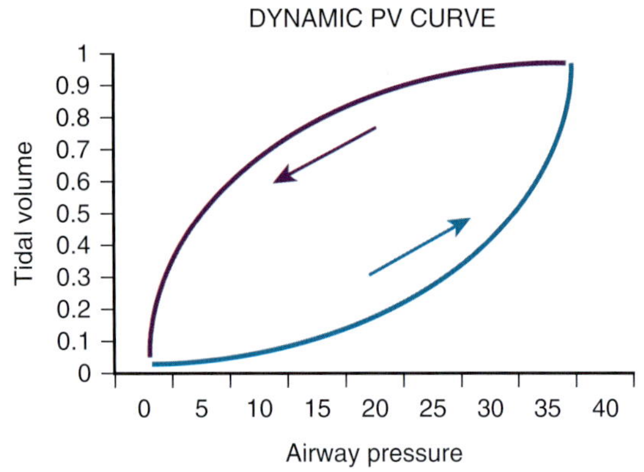

Fig. 8.4 Dynamic pressure-volume *(PV)* loop. Note that as soon as pressure is delivered to the airway, there is an increase in measured tidal volume. The *lower arrow* denotes inspiration and the *upper arrow* indicates exhalation. This indicates that the airways are open and do not need to be forced open by increasing the pressure in the airway. If this latter case were true, the PV loop would initially be flat along the *x*-axis.

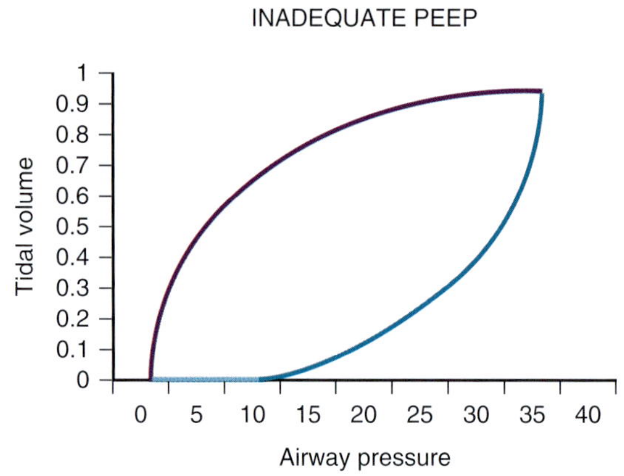

Fig. 8.5 Inadequate positive end-expiratory pressure *(PEEP)* and the pressure-volume loop. Compare this curve with that in Fig. 8.4. Note that the loop is initially flat *(lower segment)* along the *x*-axis. Once airway pressure is high enough to open the alveolar units, each increase in airway pressure is matched by a corresponding increase in tidal volume.

reduce PEEP if needed (inability to tolerate hypercapnia) or expand the patient's intravascular volume to combat the decreased venous return.

Another excellent method of determining the optimal PEEP is guided by assessing changes in plateau pressure with changes in PEEP. As PEEP is increased from a minimal level, the patient's peak airway pressure and plateau pressure will increase by the amount of $PEEP_e$. When the optimal PEEP for the lung units is achieved, plateau pressure will no longer increase. As the lung is optimally recruited, peak and plateau pressure may decrease because more volume of lung is available to receive a set VT. Once this level is exceeded, there will be further increases in plateau pressure beyond the incremental increase in PEEP as the units overdistend. The clinician must readily identify the plateau in this plateau pressure trend. The same relationship may be displayed graphically in the dynamic pressure-volume loop (Fig. 8.4). The lower limb of the loop represents the pressure required to open the alveolar units.[6,7] In the absence of PEEP (or inadequate PEEP), this limb is prolonged and flattened and has an inflection point far to the right of the origin of the loop (Fig. 8.5). As PEEP is progressively increased, the inflection point travels to the left. When the optimal PEEP is achieved, there will be a rapid upstroke of the loop because the vast majority of the functional lung units are already open and ready to be ventilated (see Fig. 8.4). This strategy is known as the *open lung model* of MV.[6]

Irrespective of what technique is used, it is widely agreed that plateau pressure should not exceed 30 cm H_2O. If respiratory system compliance is so low that plateau pressure exceeds 30 cm H_2O, either PEEP or VT has to be decreased. If this is not possible because of either recalcitrant hypoxia or acidosis, rescue therapies may need to be used (see the section "ALI and ARDS").

Intrinsic PEEP

Intrinsic PEEP ($PEEP_i$) is additional pressure that is generated within the airways from trapped gas that should have been exhaled and for various reasons (commonly obstruction to exhalation such as in chronic obstructive pulmonary disease [COPD]) was not. $PEEP_i$ is also referred to as auto-PEEP,

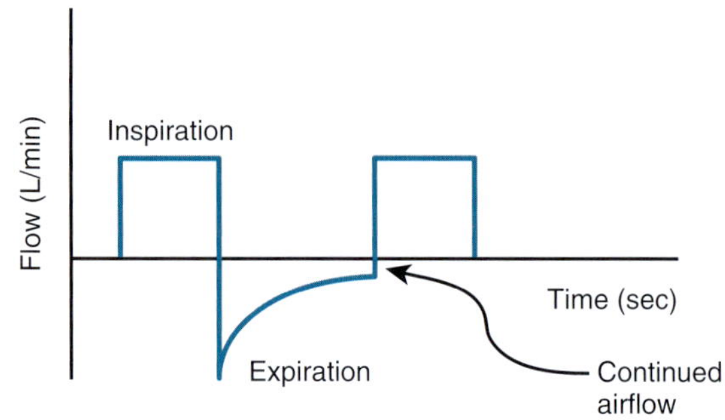

Fig. 8.6 Schematic of a flow-time curve showing potential air trapping. Note that full exhalation has not occurred before initiation of the next breath. This is seen by the fact that flow has not reached zero when the next breath is given. A square waveform is being used in this example. Continuation of this state can lead to intrinsic positive end-expiratory pressure.

dynamic hyperinflation, and breath stacking. For the remainder of this chapter, it will be referred to as $PEEP_i$.

$PEEP_i$ can cause hemodynamic instability secondary to decreased venous return, similar to high levels of PEEP.[7] $PEEP_i$ may be detected in two ways: (1) evaluation of the flow-time trace or (2) disconnection of the patient from the ventilator and listening for additional exhaled airflow after an exhalation should have occurred.[6] The flow-time trace will demonstrate that the exhalation is not yet completed before the next breath has been initiated (Fig. 8.6).[8] A common way of overcoming PEEPi is to allow for more time for exhalation by decreasing the respiratory rate.

Indications for MV

There are wide-ranging reasons for patients to require MV in the ED, and there are no absolute contraindications. Many time-honored indications for invasive ventilation are now identified as appropriate indications for noninvasive ventilation and are addressed later. Indications for MV range from loss of normal airway anatomy (edema, direct or indirect trauma, burns, infection), loss of protective airway mechanisms (intoxicants, brain injury, stroke), inability to ventilate, inability to oxygenate, or the expected clinical course. Indications for ET intubation may be separated into several categories—emergency, urgent, delayed, and elective—based on the immediacy of establishing a definitive airway.

EQUIPMENT—STANDARD OPTIONS

Perhaps one of the most confusing aspects of MV is the plethora of terms and acronyms that are used. Understanding the basic terminology helps clarify this subject. The following discussion explores machine features and settings. Regardless of which ventilator is used, a limited number of standard features are common to each (Fig. 8.7).

Set Respiratory Rate

Most ventilators allow the clinician to set a respiratory rate. The respiratory rate and actual VT determine a patient's minute ventilation. Patients intubated for airway protection because of trauma or toxicosis often do well with a normal minute ventilation. Initially setting the respiratory rate at 10 to 14 breaths/min and VT at 7 to 8 mL/kg ideal body weight (IBW) is usually sufficient. Adjustments can be made based on arterial blood gas (ABG) analysis, end-tidal CO_2, or venous blood gas and pulse oximetry. Patients who are septic or have severe acidosis often require a higher minute ventilation. Respiratory rates can be increased, as can VT, and volumes higher than 10 mL/kg IBW should not be used because of the risk of inducing ventilator-associated lung injury. In special scenarios such as acute lung injury (ALI) and acute respiratory distress syndrome (ARDS), initial VT values should be lowered to 6 mL/kg IBW within 2 hours of intubation. Some of these specific scenarios are discussed later.

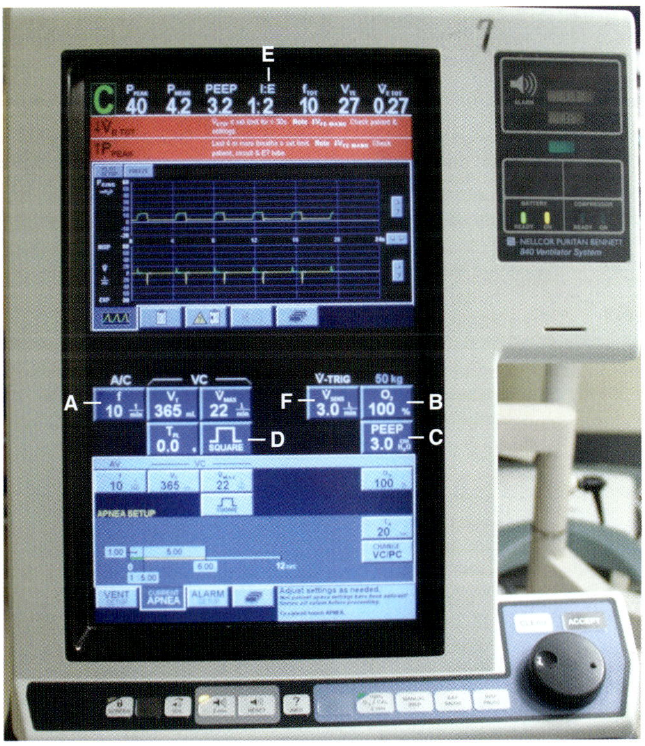

Fig. 8.7 The Nellcor Puritan Bennett 840 Ventilator system. Selected features common to all ventilators include the respiratory rate *(A)*, fraction of inspired oxygen (Fio_2) *(B)*, positive end-expiratory pressure *(PEEP)* *(C)*, waveform *(D)*, inspiratory-to-expiratory ratio *(I:E)* *(E)*, and trigger *(F)*.

Fraction of Inspired Oxygen

All ventilators can deliver an adjustable fraction of inspired oxygen (Fio_2). Recommendations are to set it initially at 1.0 because the act of transitioning from negative pressure ventilation (normal physiologic breathing) to positive pressure ventilation (PPV) may unpredictably alter ventilation-perfusion ($\dot{V}/\dot{Q}$) matching. Although initially an Fio_2 of 100% is optimal, it is beneficial to quickly titrate Fio_2 down because of the risk for oxygen toxicity and formation of oxygen free radicals. Make adjustments based on ABG analysis or pulse oximetry, with a goal of keeping arterial Po_2 higher than 60 mm Hg or arterial oxygen saturation (Sao_2) at 88% to 92% to avoid potential oxygen toxicity. These adjustments may be accomplished in the ICU rather than the ED, after the entire clinical scenario can be analyzed and all interventions are appropriately adjusted. Importantly, if there is a delay in transfer to the ICU, adjustments should be made in the ED.

PEEP

$PEEP_e$ is typically set at 5 to 8 cm H_2O. Most patients should be started at a PEEP of 5 cm H_2O, which is considered a physiologic level to overcome the ventilator system. It is used to offset the gradual loss of FRC in supine, mechanically ventilated patients. PEEP can be increased by 2 cm H_2O every 10 to 15 minutes as needed or tolerated by patients who remain hypoxic or faster in a deteriorating patient. The initial goal is to reduce Fio_2 to nontoxic levels. This goal is coming under increasing scrutiny as new information challenges the time frame and concept of O_2-induced lung injury at Fio_2 levels greater than 0.6.[9] Exercise care when using PEEP levels higher than 8 cm H_2O in the setting of elevated intracranial pressure (ICP),[10] unilateral lung processes, hypotension, hypovolemia, or pulmonary embolism. High PEEP can potentially lead to hypotension as it increases intrathoracic pressure and decreases venous return and subsequently, cardiac output.

Flow Rate

The flow rate is the speed, in liters per minute, that the ventilator is delivering gas. It is found in volume-targeted modes, and not pressure-targeted modes. The flow rate is typically set at 60 L/min, meaning that a set VT will be delivered at that speed. Patients wanting higher flow rates will not receive them and may display air hunger. Increase flow rates to deliver the set volume faster, shortening the inspiratory time (thereby increasing the inspiratory-to-expiratory [I/E] time ratio).

Waveform

The waveform determines how the ventilator delivers the flow of gas. It is traditionally set to a "decelerating waveform" in an effort to optimize recruitment, accounting for different time constants in the lung.

Decelerating (Ramp)

Once the maximal inspiratory flow is reached, the rate of gas delivery immediately begins to slow in a preprogrammed fashion. When compared with the square waveform, longer time is spent in inhalation to deliver the set VT or achieve the target pressure, allowing for improved oxygenation. This waveform also achieves lower peak airway pressure and higher mean airway pressure.

Square

Once the maximal inspiratory flow rate (IFR) is achieved, gas flow is constant until the set volume is delivered. When that point is reached, gas flow is terminated. This waveform is best for patients with asthma, COPD, and head injury because gas delivered with this waveform allows a longer expiratory time (T_e), thereby increasing the I/E time ratio and lowering mean airway pressure. The longer T_e is beneficial for patients with restrictive airway diseases such as asthma or COPD. Spending a longer time in exhalation allows improved venous drainage from the brain and greater loss of trapped VT. The drawback with this waveform is increased peak airway pressure, which often requires lower VT. This can lead to inadequate alveolar recruitment in patients with ALI.

I/E Time Ratio

The ratio of inspiratory time (the time that it takes to take a breath) to expiratory time (the time that it takes to exhale a breath) is automatically reported in some modes, whereas in others it is dialed in.

The normal I/E ratio in a spontaneously breathing, nonintubated patient is 1:4.[11] Intubated patients commonly achieve I/E ratios of 1:2. Shorter ratios may lead to decreased exhalation by compromising T_e. In its extreme form, inverse ratio ventilation (IRV), the normal pattern of breathing is reversed. A longer time is spent in inhalation to allow more time for oxygenation and alveolar recruitment. The decrease in T_e can lead to air trapping, elevated mean airway pressure, and rising PCO_2. These problems lead to hypercapnia, respiratory acidosis, and $PEEP_i$[12] (Fig. 8.8).

Trigger

The trigger is the aspect that initiates a machine-generated breath. The trigger can be set to detect either a pressure or a flow gradient. It should be set so that the patient can trigger the ventilator without great effort.

Sensitivity

This refers to the sensitivity of the trigger. If the trigger is set too high (not sensitive enough), the work of breathing incurred by the patient can be substantial. Some providers have been known to set the sensitivity at a high level if the patient is markedly overbreathing the set rate. This is not recommended because it causes an undue increase in the work of breathing. Many ventilators are set to a pressure trigger with a sensitivity of 1 to 3 cm H_2O.[13] If the sensitivity is set too low (too sensitive), the ventilator can "auto-trigger" (inappropriate initiation of machine-generated breaths) because of oscillating water in the ventilator tubing, hyperdynamic heartbeats, or patient movement.

MODES OF VENTILATION

Once some of the standard features are understood, the next step is determining the ventilator's target. Most ventilators can be set to achieve spontaneous breathing, volume-targeted ventilation, pressure-targeted ventilation, or some combination. In volume-targeted ventilation, the ventilator is set to reach a determined volume regardless of the pressure required to do so. Pressure-targeted modes are set to reach a determined pressure regardless of the volume generated. Dual modes combine the benefits of both strategies (Fig. 8.9).

Spontaneous Breathing

Spontaneously breathing patients can be supported on the ventilator by pressure support ventilation (PSV). In this mode, the ventilator provides a supplemental inspiratory pressure to each of the patient-generated breaths. The clinician sets FIO_2 and PEEP. The patient dictates the respiratory rate and generates the desired flow rate. The applied pressure is turned off once the flow decreases to a predetermined percentage. VT is dictated by the pressure support given, patient effort, and compliance of the respiratory system. There is no set

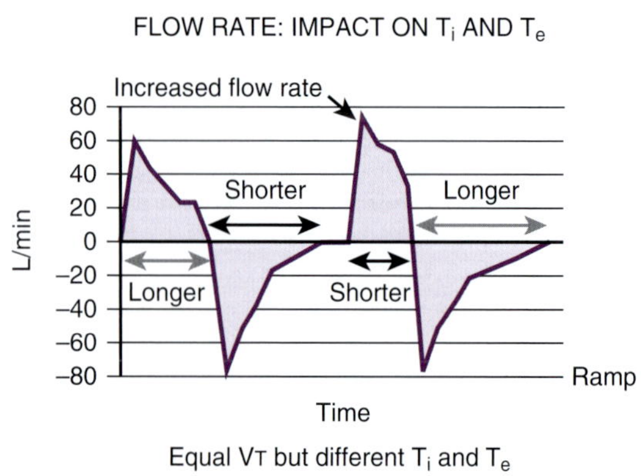

Fig. 8.8 Effect of flow rate on inspiratory *(T_i)* and expiratory *(T_e)* time. Note that as the flow rate changes, there are corresponding alterations in the effective times for inspiration and exhalation. Deflections above the *x*-axis (time) indicate inspiration, and those below indicate exhalation. The tidal volume *(VT)* delivered for each cycle is the same, but T_i and T_e are different.

Initial Ventilator Settings for Standard Patient

VCV: AC, RR 10–14, VT 7–8 mL/kg IBW, PEEP 5, FIO_2 100%
Flow rate 60 L/min, decelerating waveform

PCV: AC, RR 12–16, pressure high 20, PEEP 5, FIO_2 100%
- Monitor size of VT obtained with this pressure, adjust pressure to obtain a VT around 7–8 mL/kg IBW

- SIMV can be picked for either VCV or PCV. If SIMV is picked, add PSV at a sufficient level to obtain an adequate VT

- Adjust FIO_2 based on PO_x or PaO_2
- Adjust PEEP based on hypoxia
- Adjust minute ventilation based on blood pH (remember that on AC, decreasing the RR does not change minute ventilation in a patient breathing over the set rate)

Fig. 8.9 Initial ventilator settings for standard patients. *AC,* Assist/control mode; *FIO_2,* fraction of inspired oxygen; *IBW,* ideal body weight; *PaO_2,* partial pressure of O_2; *PEEP,* positive end-expiratory pressure; *PCV,* pressure-cycled ventilation; *PO_x,* pulse oximeter; *PSV,* pressure support ventilation; *RR,* respiratory rate; *SIMV,* synchronized intermittent mandatory ventilation; *VCV,* volume-cycled ventilation; *VT,* tidal volume.

respiratory rate, although most modern ventilators have a backup apnea rate.

Volume-Cycled Ventilation

Volume-cycled ventilation (VCV) may also be termed volume-limited, volume-control, volume-assist, or volume-targeted ventilation. Volume-targeted modes are the most commonly used and the most familiar mode of MV in adults. As its name implies, "volume"—in this case VT—is the ventilator's targeted parameter. With this target, the ventilator seeks to deliver a preset amount of gas. The ventilator will generate the necessary driving pressure to reach this "target." In addition to VT, the clinician sets the desired respiratory rate, FIO_2, and PEEP. It should be noted that other important aspects of the mechanical ventilator can be controlled in this setting, such as waveform (decelerating or square), I:E ratio, flow rate, trigger, and sensitivity.

The time of gas flow is determined by the set volume, flow rate, and waveform of gas delivery. When the set volume is reached, gas flow is terminated and expiration passively begins. An advantage is that VCV delivers a reliable volume, and it does not take into account dynamic changes in lung compliance, that may alter the ability of the lung to deliver gas in gas-exchanging alveoli.

Pressure-Cycled Ventilation

Pressure-cycled ventilation (PCV) may also be termed pressure-limited, pressure-control, pressure-assist, or pressure-targeted ventilation. As its name implies, "pressure" is the ventilator's targeted parameter. The ventilator will generate an inspiratory pressure that has been set by the clinician. With this target, the ventilator alters gas flow to achieve and maintain a preset airway pressure for the duration of a preset inspiratory time (T_i). Gas flow is terminated when the preset pressure is achieved. The volume delivered is determined by the compliance of the patient's respiratory system, airway resistance, T_i, and the pressure target. In addition, the clinician sets the desired PEEP, respiratory rate, FIO_2, T_i, I:E ratio, and trigger mode. Pressure is maintained with a variable or intermittent flow rate for the set T_i. In the setting of hypoxemia, T_i may be increased quite precisely to increase mean airway pressure and oxygenation. This strategy is much more difficult, if not impossible, to manipulate with VCV.

An advantage of PCV is that airway pressure is tightly managed to limit or eliminate alveolar overdistention and to reduce ventilator-induced lung injury.[14] It should be noted that the clinician does not control waveform or peak inspiratory flow. Patients can generate their desired flow rate and thus reduce air hunger. Pressure-targeted modes, growing in popularity, might have better pressure distribution, improved dissemination of airway pressure, and greater distribution of ventilation.[14]

One problem with PCV is that the volume received by the patient is potentially variable. Any change in system compliance or resistance (or both) will affect the VT generated. For example, if the patient bites on the ET tube or a mucous plug develops, the set pressure that was generating an adequate volume will no longer do so. In contrast, a sudden increase in system compliance might result in the generation of VT that may be considerably larger than desired. Instead of the traditional pressure alarm limits, one must adjust and be cognizant of VT and minute ventilation alarm settings. Uncertainties such as these have led many clinicians to favor volume-targeted strategies or dual-controlled strategies in the acute care setting.

Modes of Ventilation Commonly Used in the ED

Assist/control (AC) and synchronized intermittent mandatory ventilation (SIMV) are the ventilation modes most commonly used in the ED. Both are acceptable, and no data have demonstrated a better outcome with either mode. Other modes are also acceptable based on clinician preference.

AC Ventilation

Here, ventilator-initiated breaths, known as *machine breaths* (i.e., control breaths), are provided at a preset rate. Every breath is fully supported by the ventilator, whether the breath is initiated by the patient or the ventilator. The clinician sets the base ventilation rate, and if the patient tries to breathe faster than the set rate, additional breaths can be initiated by the patient, known as *spontaneous breaths* (i.e., assist breaths). A potential downside is inappropriate hyperventilation.

AC modes may be either volume or pressure cycled. Both assist breaths and control breaths will reach the set target, be it a set volume (in a volume-targeted mode) or a set pressure (in a pressure-targeted mode). In VCV, the spontaneous breath receives the same *VT* that is set for the machine breath. In PCV, the spontaneous breath receives the same *pressure* that is set for the machine breath. To be more specific, in the *volume-targeted mode*, the clinician sets VT, as well as the IFR, flow waveform, sensitivity to the patient's respiratory effort (i.e., trigger), and the basal ventilatory rate. In the *pressure-targeted mode*, the clinician determines the basal ventilatory rate and how sensitive the ventilator will be to the patient's inspiratory effort and also selects pressure levels and T_i. In this mode, VT is not set by the ventilator and is dependent on the compliance of the lung and chest wall and airway pressure. This helps avoid pressure-induced lung injury, and a specific VT is not guaranteed.

For the patient to trigger the ventilator and initiate flow for a spontaneous breath, mean airway pressure must decrease by a preset amount below PEEP if set on a pressure trigger or flow to be generated if set on a flow trigger. The amount necessary to open the inflow valve is the sensitivity setting.

Caution should be exercised *to avoid auto-PEEP* (also known as breath stacking) when using volume-targeted AC modes. Because each mechanically delivered breath is given at full VT, patients with a high actual respiratory rate on AC may not have sufficient time to completely exhale between breaths. This results in progressive air trapping, that leads to an increase in auto-PEEP ($PEEP_i$) (see Fig. 8.6). This is of particular clinical concern in patients with asthma, in whom auto-PEEP can significantly reduce cardiac output and even promote cardiovascular collapse/arrest.

SIMV

SIMV provides breaths at a preset rate (machine breath), similar to the AC mode. The patient can initiate an additional spontaneous breath between the mandated or preset number of ventilator-supported breaths. Such spontaneous breaths above the preset ventilatory rate are not supported by the ventilator, and the patient receives only a spontaneous VT that reflects the depth and time spent in the patient-controlled inspiration. For each of these nonmandatory (i.e., spontaneous) breaths, the patient has a high work of breathing. SIMV is typically partnered with PSV to aid in spontaneous breathing support and to overcome the intrinsic resistance associated with MV. This mode was initially recommended by those who thought that, as a patient's need for mechanical ventilatory support decreased, the set respiratory rate could be decreased and the patient "weaned" to PSV alone and ensuing extubation. Subsequent data have shown that this method of liberation actually increases the number of ventilator days.[15] The synchronized version of intermittent MV allows the ventilator to attempt to coordinate spontaneous and machine breaths to prevent it from delivering a scheduled breath on top of a spontaneous breath or during exhalation after a spontaneous breath. This could lead to elevated mean airway pressure, alveolar overdistention, and biotrauma.[16]

Both volume-targeted ventilation and pressure-targeted ventilation modes can be set to either an AC or SIMV mode to achieve the desired minute ventilation. In a chemically paralyzed patient with no intrinsic respiratory drive, AC and SIMV look virtually identical. Both will reach their target (volume or pressure) at the set rate. If a patient triggers the ventilator at a rate greater than the set rate, these two strategies diverge. In AC, each breath above the set respiratory rate will result in a full mechanically supported breath to reach either the set volume or pressure target. In SIMV, the ventilator will give only the set number of breaths that the clinician has selected. Each additional breath will require the patient to generate a spontaneous V_T without mechanical assistance. This patient-generated breath must overcome any resistance caused by the artificial airway and ventilator circuitry. Pressure support should be added to SIMV for patient-generated breaths to reduce any increase in the work of breathing related to the resistance imposed by the ventilator circuit and ET tube.

Advanced Modes of MV

Dual-Control Modes

Advanced modes of MV use a closed-loop ventilator logic that combines the features of volume- and pressure-targeted ventilation (Box 8.1). This is commonly called pressure regular volume control (PRVC). These modes automatically alter control variables, either breath to breath or within a breath, to ensure a minimum V_T or minute ventilation.[17] Detailed explanation of these modes is beyond the scope of this chapter. If these modes are encountered, one should discuss options with a respiratory therapist and critical care medicine specialist.

Other Modes

High-Frequency Ventilation

High-frequency ventilation (HFV) attempts to achieve adequate gas exchange by using asymmetric velocity profiles when combining very high respiratory rates with V_T levels that are smaller than the volume of anatomic dead space. It is used more commonly in neonates and infants with neonatal respiratory failure. There has been renewed interest in using HFV in adult patients with ALI or ARDS under the rationale that the small V_T may cause less ventilator-associated lung injury. More trials are necessary to determine whether HFV can improve mortality outcomes in these patients.[18]

BOX 8.1 Advanced Modes of Mechanical Ventilation

BREATH TO BREATH

Pressure-regulated volume control (PRVC)
Auto flow
Volume control plus (VC+)
Adaptive pressure ventilation (APV)
Variable-pressure control (VPC)

WITHIN A BREATH

Volume-assured pressure support ventilation (VAPSV)
Pressure augmentation

OTHER

High-frequency ventilation (HFV)
Airway pressure release ventilation (APRV)
Bilevel
Proportional assist ventilation

Airway Pressure Release Ventilation and Bilevel Ventilation

Both these modes are proprietary names yet function in essentially the same manner. The clinician sets a pressure high, a pressure low, and a time at each level (time high and time low). Although at first glance this appears to be similar to PCV, it differs markedly in that the majority of time is spent at pressure high with brief periods at pressure low. The patient typically spends 4 to 6 seconds in time high. Pressure high may be as high as 40 cm H_2O or greater. Ventilation occurs during the release from pressure high to pressure low. Time low is typically 0.2 to 0.8 seconds in restrictive lung disease and 0.8 to 1.5 seconds in obstructive lung disease. It is probably prudent to start at 0.8 and titrate to meet individual patient requirements. Time low is also referred to as the release phase.[19] The long time that high-level pressure is maintained achieves oxygenation, and the short release period achieves clearance of CO_2 (Fig. 8.10). The long time at high-level pressure results in substantial recruitment of alveoli from markedly different regional time constants at rather low gas flow rates. The establishment of $PEEP_i$ by the short release time enhances oxygenation. CO_2 clearance is aided by recruitment of the patient's lung at close to total lung capacity. Elastic recoil creates large-volume gas flow during the release period.

In a paralyzed patient, airway pressure release ventilation and bilevel ventilation (APRV/Bilevel) are identical to pressure-targeted IRV. For these reasons, some have described this mode as *inverse ratio ventilation*. A major difference between APRV/Bilevel and IRV is that IRV typically requires chemical paralysis or heavy sedation. APRV/Bilevel is a fundamentally different mode from cyclic ventilation. This mode allows the patient to spontaneously breathe during all phases of the cycle, making it relatively more comfortable and reducing the level of sedation or paralysis needed. This mode is enabled to succeed by having a floating valve that is responsive to the patient's needs, regardless of the location within the respiratory cycle. The patient is allowed to breathe in or out during the pressure high phase and during the release phase. Accordingly, the sequence is

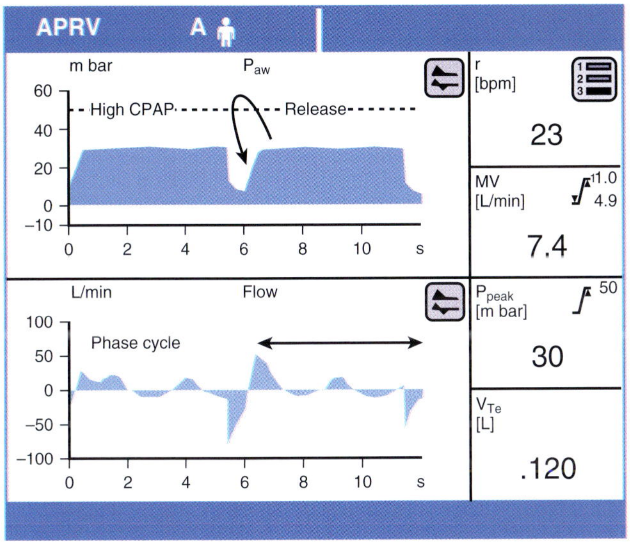

Fig. 8.10 Airway pressure release ventilation *(APRV)*—airway pressure-time and flow-time traces. Note that peak airway pressure (P_{aw} high) is maintained for a long period. This phase establishes oxygenation (T_{high}). There is a short period of release when most CO_2 is cleared (T_{low}). The bottom trace indicates flow over time. The combined time for T_{high} and T_{low} is known as a *phase cycle*. Note that the number of phase cycles is not the respiratory rate because patients breathe within the entirety of T_{high}. As the release phase is initiated, the flow rate is identified as negative and is of a high rate (here, ≈7.5 L/min), consistent with significant alveolar recruitment. During the high continuous positive airway pressure *(CPAP)* phase, the patient is allowed to exhale (negative deflections on the flow-time trace). Thus APRV is quite dissimilar from traditional cyclic ventilation. This unique mode is made possible by a floating valve system. *MV,* Mechanical ventilation; P_{peak}, peak inspiratory pressure; V_{Te}, exhaled tidal volume.

called a *phase cycle*. There is no set T_i or T_e and no readily identifiable respiratory rate in the traditional sense. During the pressure high phase, patients may exhale 50 to 200 mL or more of gas as the lung volume becomes full of gas. This is not a full exhalation, and the release of excess gas should not be counted as a breath. APRV has been used successfully for neonatal, pediatric, and adult forms of respiratory failure. It is considered an alternative open lung model approach to MV.[19]

Given the spontaneous nature of the mode, there should be virtually no need for continuous infusion of neuromuscular blocking drugs in patients placed on this mode of ventilation. This may result in a shorter length of ICU stay and a reduced incidence of prolonged neuromuscular blockade syndrome. The need for sedatives is reduced because patients are more comfortable on this spontaneous mode than on cyclic ventilation.[20] APRV/Bilevel has gained popularity in patients with hypoxemic respiratory failure because it improves oxygenation by optimizing alveolar recruitment and $\dot{V}/\dot{Q}$ matching.[21]

A common mistake with this mode is setting the time low too long. This essentially mimics a pressure-targeted SIMV strategy. Transport of patients on APRV with pressure high greater than 20 cm H_2O should occur with the patient attached to the ventilator instead of being hand-ventilated.[22] Hand ventilation is unable to match the manner of gas delivery and pressure dynamics that the patient requires. Attempts at hand ventilation, even with an appropriately set PEEP valve, are frequently complicated by unexpected hypoxemia and hemodynamic instability.

Noninvasive Positive Pressure Ventilation

See Videos 8.1 and 8.2. Noninvasive ventilation is defined as the provision of ventilatory assistance without an invasive artificial airway. Noninvasive ventilators consist of both negative and positive pressure ventilators. Because negative pressure ventilation is so rarely used today, our discussion is limited to PPV.

Before the 1960s, the use of negative pressure ventilation in the form of a tank ventilator (the "iron lung") was the most common form of MV outside the anesthesia suite. It was not until the 1952 polio epidemic in Copenhagen that anesthesiologist Bjorn Ibsen showed that he could improve the survival of patients with respiratory paralysis by using invasive PPV.

Nonetheless, negative pressure or "iron lungs" were the mainstay of ventilatory support for patients with chronic respiratory failure until as late as the mid-1980s. In the early 1980s, nasal continuous positive airway pressure (CPAP) was introduced to treat obstructive sleep apnea. These tightly fitting masks proved to be an effective means of assisting ventilation, and noninvasive positive pressure ventilation (NPPV) quickly displaced traditional negative pressure ventilation as the treatment of choice for chronic respiratory failure in patients with neuromuscular and chest wall deformities. Current NPPV devices are able to provide a set respiratory rate, set V_T, and set F_{IO_2}. The use of NPPV has also been integrated into the acute inpatient setting, where it is now used to treat acute respiratory failure.[23]

Definitions

The current literature uses different definitions for NPPV. Although some authors use NPPV as an umbrella term that includes CPAP and bilevel positive airway pressure, more recently, authors have used the term NPPV as synonymous with bilevel and consider CPAP a separate entity. The terms NPPV and noninvasive intermittent positive pressure ventilation (NIPPV) are often used interchangeably with bilevel.

As its name suggests, CPAP supplies continuous positive pressure via a tightly fitting face mask (Fig. 8.11). CPAP can very simply be thought of like PEEP. NPPV or bilevel provides an inspiratory positive airway pressure (IPAP) in addition to end-expiratory positive airway pressure (EPAP), and breaths are usually triggered by the patient (Fig. 8.12). On many such devices, backup rates may be set that deliver bilevel pressure, even if patients fail to initiate a breath.

Rationale for Using NPPV

The most important advantage of NPPV is avoiding the complications associated with invasive MV. It has been well documented that invasive MV increases the incidence of airway and lung injury and augments the risk for nosocomial pneumonia. NPPV avoids these complications by keeping the upper airway defense mechanisms intact and allows the patient to retain the ability to eat, clear secretions, and communicate normally when NPPV is used intermittently (NIPPV).[23] NPPV has the potential to reduce the mortality of a selected group of patients with acute respiratory failure and may shorten hospital stays, thereby reducing cost. Specific to the ED, appropriate initiation of NPPV may avoid unnecessary intubation

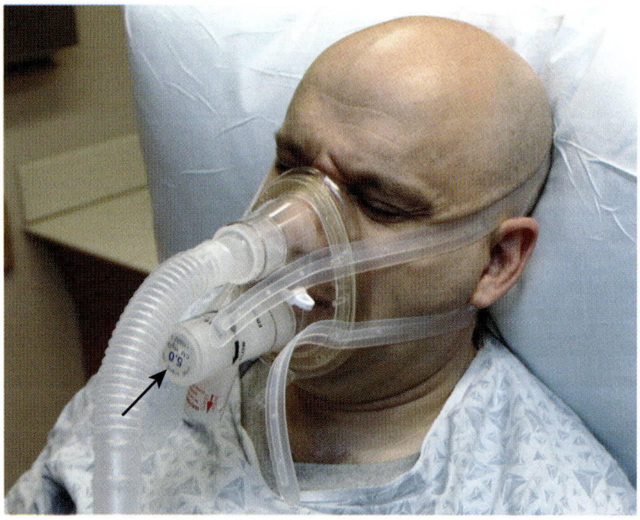

Fig. 8.11 Continuous positive airway pressure (CPAP) mask (Vital Signs, Inc.). The device shown provides continuous positive airway pressure and is run simply by attaching the mask tubing to a wall oxygen source. The amount of CPAP delivered can be adjusted by changing the threshold resistor valve *(arrow)*.

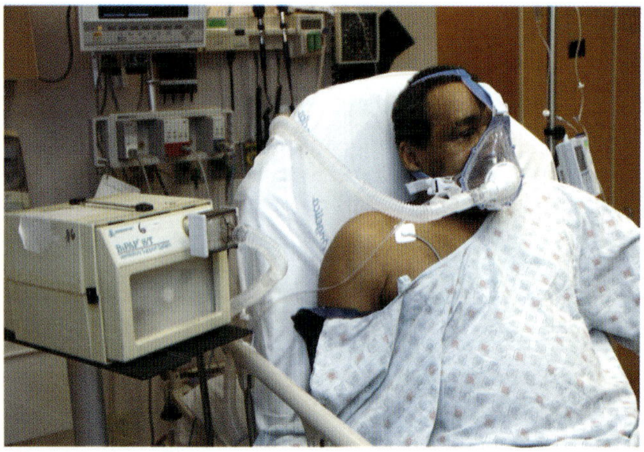

Fig. 8.12 Bilevel positive airway pressure (BiPAP) S/T noninvasive ventilation system (Philips Respironics, Inc.). Adjustable parameters include inspiratory positive airway pressure, expiratory positive airway pressure, and breaths per minute. Both BiPAP and continuous positive airway pressure are used to support ventilation in patients with decompensated congestive heart failure, chronic obstructive pulmonary disease, pneumonia, and asthma, but neither mode has a clear benefit over the other.

of certain patients, hence reducing ICU admission, lowering cost, decreasing complications, and improving mortality.

Pathophysiologic Effects of NPPV

CPAP increases alveolar recruitment and size, thereby enhancing the area available for gas exchange, and improves the $\dot{V}/\dot{Q}$ relationship. The term CPAP is synonymous with $PEEP_e$ and bilevel EPAP. It can also negate the effects of $PEEP_i$. In patients with dynamic hyperinflation (such as asthma or COPD), an escalating $PEEP_i$ increases the magnitude of the drop in airway pressure that the patient must generate to trigger a breath. This causes increased work of breathing for the patient. Careful application of $PEEP_e$ can reduce this gradient and decrease the patient's work of breathing. PPV also creates an increase in intrathoracic pressure. This causes preload to decrease as a result of diminished venous return and also decreases transmural pressure, which reduces afterload.[24]

In NPPV, IPAP is similar to pressure support and, when combined with EPAP, further augments alveolar ventilation, thereby allowing some rest of the respiratory muscles during the inspiratory phase (Box 8.2).

BOX 8.2 Indications for Initiating Noninvasive Positive Pressure Ventilation

- Exacerbation of chronic obstructive pulmonary disease
- Exacerbation of congestive heart failure and cardiogenic pulmonary edema
- Exacerbation of asthma
- Immunocompromised patients
- Hypoxemic respiratory failure
- Do-not-resuscitate/do-not-intubate advance directive

Acute Exacerbation of COPD

Numerous studies have shown that NPPV can reduce the need for intubation, length of hospital stay, and in-hospital mortality in patients with acute exacerbations of COPD.[25,26] NPPV should be initiated early and along with standard medical therapy. If it is started late, after the failure of medical treatment, the benefits conferred by NPPV (hospital mortality, length of ICU stay, number of days on the ventilator, overall complications) are eliminated.[27] Early implementation of NPPV in patients seen in the ED with an acute exacerbation of COPD and without contraindications should be considered the standard of care.

Acute Cardiogenic Pulmonary Edema

CPAP has been shown to produce a reduction in the rate of intubation and a trend toward decreasing mortality.[28] CPAP and NPPV both reduce the risk of intubation in the ED.[29] An early article described an increased rate of acute myocardial infarction in patients with acute cardiogenic pulmonary edema treated with NPPV,[30] and several subsequent trials have refuted this increased risk for myocardial infarction.

Hypoxemic Respiratory Failure

Although some of the literature suggests that NPPV may be beneficial in the setting of acute hypoxemic respiratory failure, doubt still exists. A large multicenter trial of NPPV in patients with acute hypoxemic respiratory failure that excludes patients with cardiogenic pulmonary edema and COPD may help clarify the use of NPPV in this setting.

NPPV has been used increasingly in the ICU for hypoxemic respiratory failure. It can be considered for patients who are hemodynamically stable with single-organ (i.e., pulmonary) failure, and extremely close monitoring is required.

Immunosuppressed Patients

When faced with a severely immunosuppressed patient with acute hypoxemic respiratory failure in the ED, early initiation of NPPV may be beneficial in avoiding the serious complications of ET intubation. NPPV can keep upper airway defenses intact and minimize the risk for ventilator-associated pneumonia, which is universally fatal in these patients.[31] NPPV has been shown to be associated with a lower rate of ET intubation, shorter ICU stay, and lower ICU mortality. In-house mortality did not differ significantly.[32]

"Do-Not-Intubate/Do-Not-Resuscitate" Patients

In do-not-intubate/do-not-resuscitate (DNI/DNR) patients willing to undergo NPPV, success would be measured by improved ventilation, oxygenation, and comfort. NPPV can provide support for the patient while the underlying cause of the respiratory failure is being treated. NPPV should be discontinued if it is not producing the desired response, or if the patient is unable to tolerate this therapy. In these circumstances, it should be a joint decision between the health care team, the patient, and the family to limit NPPV and transition toward comfort measures.

In patients who have chosen to forego any life-sustaining therapy and are receiving comfort care measures, NPPV might be used as a form of palliative care in an attempt to reduce the associated dyspnea. In this circumstance, the use of NPPV is considered successful if it alleviates the patient's symptoms. If it causes any discomfort to the patient, it should be discontinued. This use of NPPV is controversial, and no studies have assessed the benefits of NPPV in these patients.[33] Another use of NPPV in patients who have chosen comfort care measures is a time-limited trial to achieve the goal of survival until the arrival of family and friends. In this situation, NPPV would be used to provide life support until friends and family can achieve closure.

Even if a patient with a known DNI advance directive arrives at the ED with acute respiratory failure of reversible etiology, it can be beneficial to discuss the use of NPPV with the patient and family. In this situation, communication about the expectations and goals of care is of utmost importance.

Initiation of NPPV

There is no standard approach to the initiation of NPPV. Different methods have been used in clinical trials, and these methods have never been compared. There are two main strategies: a high-low approach and a low-high approach (Fig. 8.13).

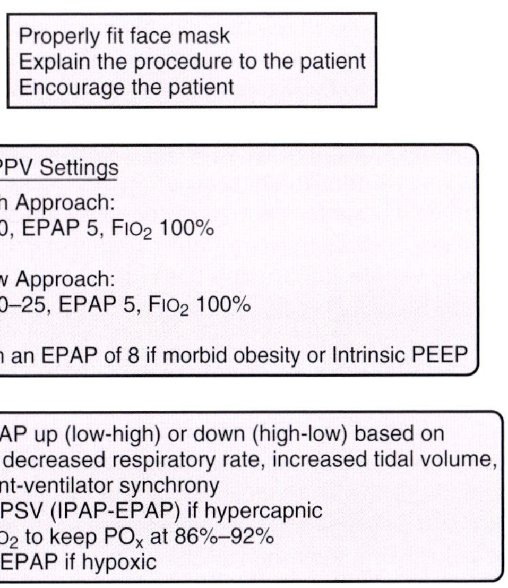

Fig. 8.13 Initiation of noninvasive positive pressure ventilation (*NPPV*). *EPAP,* End-expiratory positive airway pressure; F_{IO_2}, fraction of inspired oxygen; *IPAP,* inspiratory positive airway pressure; *PEEP,* positive end-expiratory pressure; PO_x, pulse oximeter; *PSV,* pressure support ventilation.

Emphasis should be placed on the importance of close follow-up of patients in whom NPPV is started in the ED. It is important to serially assess patient response as soon as 30 minutes after the initiation of NPPV. Those who are persistently tachypneic and acidemic should be considered for intubation sooner rather than later. It is imperative to closely observe patients for deterioration. ABGs should be checked within 1 to 2 hours after initiation of NPPV to assess treatment success or failure. Patients who do not improve clinically should be considered for intubation.

Cautions With the Use of NPPV

Most studies involving NPPV have excluded patients who were hemodynamically unstable, had an altered level of consciousness, or were unable to protect their airway. This was based on the concern that a depressed sensorium would predispose the patient to aspiration. The International Consensus Conference in Intensive Care Medicine on Noninvasive Positive Pressure Ventilation in Acute Respiratory Failure held in April 2000 considered the presence of severe encephalopathy, as manifested by a Glasgow Coma Scale score lower than 10, to be a contraindication to NPPV.[34]

Other accepted contraindications to NPPV are listed in Box 8.3.

Recently, studies have looked specifically at the use of NPPV in patients with hypercapnic coma secondary to acute respiratory failure. This was based on the observation that some DNI patients who declined intubation had successful outcomes with NPPV therapy despite their initial comatose state. Diaz and colleagues conducted an observational study and found that success rates were comparable between the comatose and noncomatose groups.[35] Scala and coworkers performed two studies, both showing that NPPV could be used successfully in treating patients with exacerbations of COPD and hypercapnic encephalopathy. Their 2007 study showed that the performance of NPPV by an experienced team led to similar short- and long-term survival, fewer nosocomial infections, and shorter durations of hospitalization than in patients who underwent MV.[36,37] Of note, these studies were conducted in the ICU[35] or specialized respiratory care units[37] with a nursing ratio of at least 1:3. The patients were very closely monitored by staff while they received NPPV. This high nursing-to-patient ratio may not be feasible in a busy ED.

The other key point in these studies was the rapid improvement in neurologic status that occurred 1 to 2 hours after the initiation of NPPV. The importance of close monitoring of patients in whom NPPV is started is crucial in identifying those who will fail this therapy.

BOX 8.3 Contraindications to Noninvasive Positive Pressure Ventilation

Impending cardiovascular collapse or respiratory arrest
Severe upper gastrointestinal bleeding
Facial surgery, trauma, or deformity limiting placement of the mask
Upper airway obstruction
Inability to cooperate or protect the airway, altered mental status
Inability to clear respiratory secretions
High risk for aspiration

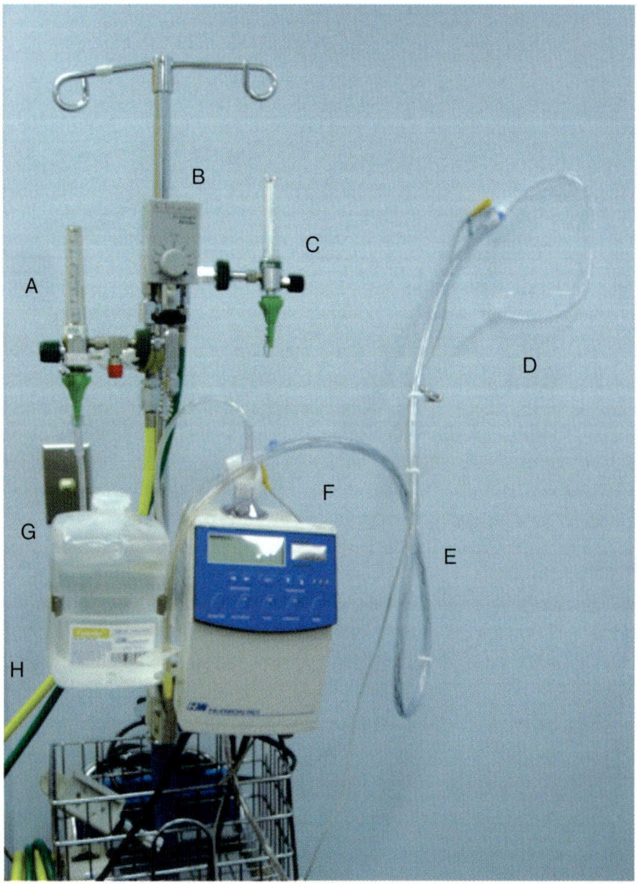

Fig. 8.14 High-flow nasal cannula system. *A*, High-flow flow meter; *B*, oxygen blender; *C*, low-flow flow meter; *D*, nasal cannula; *E*, low compliance, heated-wire circuit; *F*, high-flow humidifier; *G*, water reservoir; *H*, air/O_2 supply. (From Yeow ME, Santanilla JI. Noninvasive positive pressure ventilation in the emergency department. *Emerg Med Clin North Am.* 2008;26:835-847.)

High-Flow Nasal Cannula

The high-flow nasal cannula (HFNC) is a relatively new oxygen delivery system. A conventional nasal cannula uses a low-flow system and at higher flow (>6 L/min) can cause nasal dryness, epistaxis, and patient discomfort. The HFNC system (Fig. 8.14) is a novel device that combines oxygen, pressurized air, and warm humidification to deliver via nasal cannula a tolerable flow of up to 40 L/min or 60 L/min depending on the device. F_{IO_2} and flow rates can be adjusted. With higher flow, less room-air entrainment occurs, and the higher flow rates help match the dyspneic patient's increased minute ventilation.

Its use has been studied more extensively for neonatal respiratory care, where ongoing studies suggest that HFNC may be as effective as nasal CPAP in preterm neonates.[38] One study looked at the effect of HFNC on exercise performance in adults with COPD.[39] Studies have shown that HFNC use in hypoxic respiratory failure can decrease the incidence of intubation without having an effect on mortality.[40] HFNC has been used with increasing frequency with success for hypoxic patients and should be considered as a mode of treatment.

Conclusions

NPPV has been shown to work well in patients with reversible conditions and acts as a bridge while allowing medical therapy (e.g., bronchodilators, steroids, diuretics) to take effect, thereby potentially avoiding the need for ET intubation. Those with less reversible causes of their acute respiratory failure (ARDS, pneumonia) may be less likely to respond. With careful patient selection, NPPV can be safely initiated in the ED, give time for medical treatment to work, and potentially avoid ICU admission. Patients being considered for intubation should be evaluated for the potential use of NPPV.

Close monitoring and follow-up of patients placed on NPPV is crucial in determining whether the therapy has been successful or whether further intervention is needed. In EDs in which the staff has been adequately trained, selected patients, even those in a hypercapnic coma, can be considered for a short trial of NPPV. Extreme diligence in monitoring these patients must be used, and if improvement is not seen in 1 to 2 hours, intubation should not be delayed.

NEUROMUSCULAR BLOCKADE/PARALYZING AGENT FOR MECHANICALLY VENTILATED PATIENTS

The short-term administration of paralyzing agents, in combination with sedation and analgesia, for mechanically ventilated patients in the ED is appropriate to improve patient-ventilator synchrony, enhance gas exchange, diminish the risk for barotrauma, decrease muscle oxygen consumption, facilitate brief procedures, and prevent movement in patients with elevated ICP. Importantly, neuromuscular blocking agents (NMBAs) have no sedative, amnestic, or analgesic properties, and all patients administered such an agent must receive concomitant sedation and analgesia.

The long-term use of chemical paralysis in the ICU has greatly diminished because of prolonged recovery secondary to drug and metabolite accumulation. Cases of prolonged paralysis, also known as critical illness myopathy, postparalysis syndrome, polyneuropathy of critical illness, and acute quadriplegic myopathy syndrome, lead to protracted ICU stays.[40] In the ICU, daily discontinuation of NMBAs for a few hours or avoiding their use entirely has been recommended to potentially decrease the incidence of these conditions. When clinically feasible, it is advisable to stop administration of the NMBA in the ED and reassess the need for continued paralysis.

A number of drugs are available, and the nondepolarizing agents vecuronium and pancuronium are the most commonly prescribed agents for short-term paralysis in the ED.[41] Both are given by intermittent bolus administration as needed. Continuous infusion, though potentially useful, is rarely indicated in the ED. Nondepolarizing NMBAs can be reversed by neostigmine at a dose of 0.035 to 0.07 mg/kg.

Vecuronium has an intermediate duration of action with a half-life of 80 to 90 minutes, slightly longer in the elderly, and not affected by renal or hepatic failure. Vecuronium, compared with pancuronium, has minimal adverse cardiovascular effects and is the drug of choice for patients with cardiovascular disease or hemodynamic instability. The dose for intermittent bolus administration is 0.1 mg/kg.

Pancuronium is long acting with a half-life of 100 to 130 minutes. Its duration of action is prolonged in patients with renal or hepatic failure. There is a moderate risk for adverse cardiovascular effects associated with pancuronium, such as tachycardia, hypertension, and increased cardiac output

BOX 8.4 Common Sedatives and Analgesics Used With Mechanical Ventilation

SEDATIVES

Propofol, 5–80 μg/kg per minute
Dexmedetomidine, 0.2–1.5 μg/kg per hour
Lorazepam, 1–5 mg IV prn; infusion at 0.5–7 mg/h if multiple doses required
Midazolam, 1–6 mg IV prn
Haloperidol, 2–10 mg IV every 20–30 minutes until stable, then 25% of the loading dose q6h prn
Remifentanil infusion: 0.025–0.2 μg/kg per hour (no bolus used, provides both sedation and analgesia)

ANALGESICS

Fentanyl, 25–100 μg IV q 15–30 minutes prn
Hydromorphone, 0.2–1 mg IV prn
Morphine, 2–5 mg IV prn
Fentanyl infusion: 50–200 μg/h if more than 2–3 boluses per hour of above agents are needed

q, *Every;* prn, *as needed.*

secondary to vagal blockade. The dose for intermittent bolus administration is 0.05 to 0.1 mg/kg.

SEDATION

See Box 8.4 for common sedatives and analgesics. It is recommended that only the minimal amount needed to achieve patient comfort be used. Sedation should be targeted to a specific sedation scale (such as the Richmond Agitation Sedation Scale). Agents with a quick offset are preferable to improve spontaneous awakening and for breathing trials once the patient is a candidate for extubation. Benzodiazepines should be avoided if possible. Intubation and MV are uncomfortable. If paralyzing drugs are used for neuromuscular blockade, it is imperative to provide aggressive sedation because pain and anxiety in paralyzed patients cannot be evaluated. It is prudent to conclude that a paralyzed ventilated patient is awake and can hear and feel unless sedated.

SPECIFIC DISEASE PROCESSES

Asthma and COPD (Fig. 8.15)

As asthma and COPD treatment (β-agonists, steroids) take effect, peak pressure will begin to lower, the peak expiratory flow rate should increase, and the expiration flow time should shorten (Fig. 8.16). It is necessary to adequately sedate these patients because their hypercapnic state is a powerful stimulus to breathe rapidly. Opiates such as fentanyl and sedatives such as propofol and ketamine have gained increased roles in these patients. Occasionally, one will be required to chemically weaken these patients with the use of paralytics to keep their respiratory rate and expiratory time controlled. Paralysis cannot be avoided in some cases, and this should be a final option with the understanding that the side effects of steroids and paralytics can be quite devastating[42,43]. In the ICU, paralysis is commonly titrated to an effect monitored by a peripheral nerve monitor applied over the ulnar nerve or other peripheral nerve distribution.[44] No blockade results in four twitches of the adductor pollicis muscle caused by four supramaximal triggering stimuli; complete blockade yields no response to the same trigger. A common goal of blockade is to use enough of the agent to result in two twitches out of a "train of four." A peripheral nerve monitor is not commonly used in the ED and is not a standard intervention during resuscitation and interim ED care.

Peri-intubation

Monitor the rate of BVM ventilation
Provide an IVF bolus
Consider ketamine as an induction agent if available
$NaHCO_3$ bolus if known to have a pH <7 before RSI

Initial Ventilator Settings

Volume targeted (VCV), AC, RR 8–10, V_T 6 mL/kg IBW, PEEP 5, F_{IO_2} 100%
Flow rate 80 L/min, square waveform
- These strategies may worsen hypercapnia (termed permissive hypercapnia) because of a decrease in minute ventilation and is tolerated if pH >7.15
- $NaHCO_3$ infusion or the administration of THAM (tris[hydroxymethyl] aminomethane) may be required to keep arterial pH above 7.15 to 7.20

After Intubation

Adequate sedation and analgesia; consider the use of propofol, ketamine, or opiates
Monitor flow-time curves and pressure-time curves
Follow peak pressure and plateau pressure
Consider chemical weakening as a last resort (goal TOF 2–4)
Consider heliox if available

Fig. 8.15 Initial ventilator settings for exacerbation of asthma. *AC,* Assist/control mode; *BVM,* bag-valve-mask ventilation; F_{IO_2}, fraction of inspired oxygen; *IBW,* ideal body weight; *IVF,* intravenous fluid; $NaHCO_3$, sodium bicarbonate; *PEEP,* positive end-expiratory pressure; *RR,* respiratory rate; *RSI,* rapid-sequence induction; *THAM,* tris(hydroxymethyl)aminomethane; *TOF,* train of four; *VCV,* volume-cycled ventilation; V_T, tidal volume.

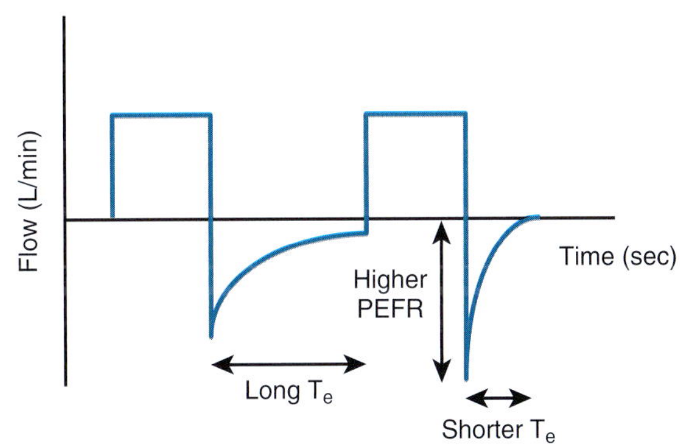

Fig. 8.16 Schematic of a flow-time curve showing improvement in an obstructive process. Note that the peak expiratory flow rate *(PEFR)* increases and the expiratory time (T_e) decreases with improvement and flow reaches zero before the next breath is given.

Valuable information can be gained from flow-time curves and pressure-time curves. Improvement (see Fig. 8.16) or worsening of airway obstruction and air trapping (see Fig. 8.6) can often be evident in these curves before becoming clinically apparent. In ideal situations, $PEEP_i$ can be measured with an end-expiratory hold. This measurement is often inconsistent, difficult to obtain, and changes dynamically with therapy. Some authors have recommended that $PEEP_e$ be applied at 80% of the measured $PEEP_i$.[45] Because of the difficulty in accurately measuring $PEEP_i$ and the potential hazard of adding too much $PEEP_e$,[46] others have suggested that it should be set at 50% of the measured $PEEP_i$. If $PEEP_i$ becomes severe enough, it will affect plateau pressure. Current recommendations for obstructive airway disease are to keep plateau pressure below 35 cm H_2O,[47,48] and many clinicians follow the ALI/ARDS recommendations and maintain plateau pressure at less than 30 cm H_2O.

$PEEP_e$ can be used to decrease some of the negative pressure that the patient has to generate to initiate a breath. For example, a patient with a $PEEP_i$ of 10 cm H_2O and a set pressure trigger of −2 cm H_2O (and no applied PEEP) has to generate an alveolar pressure of 12 cm H_2O to produce a breath. Adding a $PEEP_e$ of 5 cm H_2O means that the ventilator will trigger a breath when alveolar pressure is 3 cm H_2O. The patient has to generate a decrease of only 7 cm H_2O (instead of 12 cm H_2O), thereby reducing the inspiratory effort required.

Though seemingly counterintuitive, decreasing the respiratory rate and VT in a critically ill asthmatic may be beneficial and result in an acceptable elevation in Pco_2, termed permissive hypercapnia.[50] It may not be advisable to meet arbitrary Pco_2 levels in a ventilated asthmatic and rather concentrate on maintaining acceptable oxygenation (Po_2 > 60 mm Hg, Sao_2 of 88% to 92%) while minimizing $PEEP_i$ and optimizing plateau pressure.

If cardiovascular collapse occurs in a ventilated asthmatic with either pulseless electrical activity or sudden hypotension, a first step in troubleshooting is to remove the patient from the ventilator. This is both a diagnostic and a therapeutic maneuver for air trapping. Some clinicians also advocate fluid loading and rapid and deep chest compressions while the patient is disconnected from the ventilator to expel the excess volumes of air trapped by prior aggressive ventilation (Fig. 8.17).[51] Tension pneumothorax must also be considered (see later).

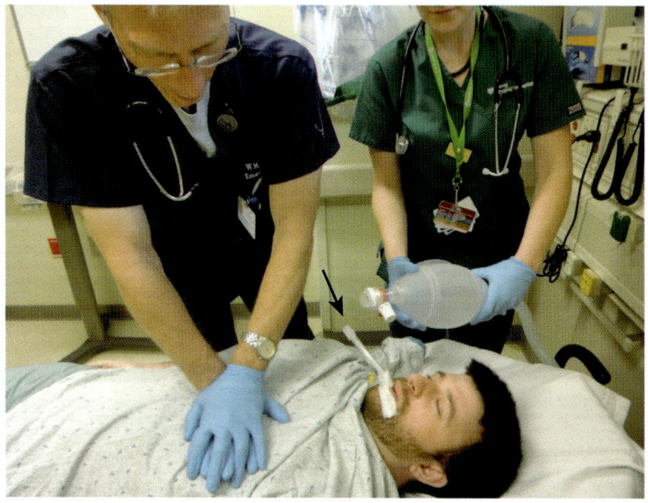

Fig. 8.17 The crashing asthmatic. Once a struggling asthmatic is intubated, the temptation is to rapidly hyperventilate with deep breaths, but this may cause cardiovascular collapse because of exacerbating previous auto–positive end-expiratory pressure (PEEP)/breath stacking. A hyperinflated asthmatic lung severely diminishes venous return, which leads to a marked decrease in cardiac output, even pulseless electrical activity. If a recently intubated asthmatic suffers these consequences, stop ventilating the patient entirely *(arrow)*, compress the chest until no more air is exhaled, and then continue ventilating as per discussion in text. Acceptable permissive hypercapnia may ensue.

ALI/ARDS/Diffuse lung injury initial ventilator settings
VCV, AC, RR 20, VT 8 mL/kg IBW, PEEP 8, Fio_2 100%
Titrate Fio_2 and PEEP based on oxygenation (goal Pao_2 ≥≈60, Po_x 88%–92%). An ARDSNet PEEP table is helpful
Titrate VT down to 6 mL/kg IBW over the first 2 hours (may need to increase RR if minute ventilation is not adequate to keep pH >7.2)

Monitor plateau pressures (keep below 30)
- If >30, incrementally lower VT to 4 mL/kg IBW

Monitor blood pH
- Permissive hypercapnia expected and tolerated at pH >7.2
- $NaCO_3$ infusion may be required to keep pH 7.15 to 7.20
- Continuous renal replacement therapy may be required if patient is oliguric/anuric and markedly acidotic

Insert a central venous catheter:
If not in shock, follow a fluid conservation strategy

Fig. 8.18 Initial ventilator settings for acute lung injury *(ALI)*, acute respiratory distress syndrome *(ARDS)*, and diffuse lung injury. *AC*, Assist/control mode; *Fio_2*, fraction of inspired oxygen; *IBW*, ideal body weight; *$NaHCO_3$*, sodium bicarbonate; *Pao_2*, partial pressure of O_2; *PEEP*, positive end-expiratory pressure; *PO_x*, pulse oximeter; *RR*, respiratory rate; *THAM*, tris(hydroxymethyl)aminomethane; *VCV*, volume-cycled ventilation; *VT*, tidal volume.

ALI and ARDS

Initial ventilator settings for patients with ALI and ARDS can be found in Fig. 8.18.

Efforts should be made while the patient is in the ED to decrease VT down to 6 mL/kg IBW, as recent data have shown that settings made in the ED are more likely continued in the ICU. Forty-one percent of patients never received recommended settings during hospitalization.[52] Fuller and colleagues also showed that lung-protective ventilation was used only 47% of the time in patients with ARDS in the ED.[53]

A common finding in lung-protective ventilation is the occurrence of patient-ventilator dyssynchrony. This is thought to be due to the patient wanting a higher flow rate than the ventilator is providing while on a volume-targeted strategy. This occasionally leads to double or triple cycling of the ventilator. It should be noted that in this situation the patient is actually receiving a higher VT and not benefiting from lung-protective ventilation. Sedation needs to be optimized, and at times different modes, such as pressure-targeted modes, may be attempted. Temporarily weakening the patient with paralytics may be considered.

There are several areas of uncertainty with MV in patients with ALI or ARDS. Patients with traumatic brain injury, intracranial hemorrhage, fulminant hepatic failure, and elevated ICP in whom ARDS develops must be managed carefully because lung-protective ventilation may induce hypercapnia. Acutely, this may lead to cerebral vasodilation and an increase in ICP. There is little evidence to support the recommendation for any particular rescue therapy in patients with severe refractory hypoxia, such as recruitment maneuvers, high-dose albuterol, IRV, HFV, prone ventilation, and extracorporeal membrane oxygenation. In dire circumstances, these modalities may be used on the basis of clinician preference, expertise, and consultation with a critical care specialist as soon as possible. The PROSEVA trial showed that prone positioning for patients with a P:F ratio <150 has a large survival benefit.[54]

Lessons Learned in COVID

Patients with moderate to severe COVID-19 often developed severe or refractory hypoxia. Throughout the pandemic, the approach to this hypoxia evolved as studies and information were shared. Initially, patients were intubated early and it was found that those who were intubated earlier had an overall higher mortality. This generated a renewed interest in utilizing noninvasive forms of respiratory support. The RECOVERY-RS trial compared the use of CPAP, HFNC, or conventional oxygen therapy and showed a trend toward decreased intubation and decreased mortality in the group using the noninvasive techniques. In addition, the HIFLo-COVID Trial comparing HFNC with conventional oxygen therapy also showed a reduction in intubation in the HFNC group. Further studies are needed to confirm these data, and it is reasonable to use a noninvasive strategy for the hypoxemic COVID-19 patient. In addition, prone positioning for the severely hypoxic COVID-19 patient became standard of care.

COMPLICATIONS OF MV

Though necessary to sustain life, MV is associated with a number of pathophysiologic derangements that can lead to morbidity and mortality, including pulmonary barotrauma, ventilator-associated lung injury, hemodynamic compromise, $PEEP_i$, and elevated ICP.

Pneumothorax

Pneumothorax that is not associated with trauma in a mechanically ventilated patient typically stems from alveolar overdistention (continuous or episodic) and leads to alveolar rupture and escape of gas into the pleural space.[52] In patients receiving PPV, it is wise to drain the pleural space to prevent a simple pneumothorax from progressing to tension pneumothorax with hemodynamic compromise. Loculated pneumothoraces may be successfully drained percutaneously under ultrasound (US) or computed tomography (CT) guidance. Successful drainage of air space disease leads to enhanced liberation from MV.[53] Pneumothorax or tension pneumothorax may also result from aggressive bag-valve-mask ventilation. Patients with intrinsic lung disease such as COPD or asthma are more prone to the development of pneumothorax than the average patient.[55]

A simple pneumothorax can be drained by surgical tube thoracostomy with a small-bore tube (24 Fr), a commercially available pneumothorax kit (Arrow [Teleflex, Morrisville, NC]), or a pigtail catheter placed into the pleural space via the Seldinger technique (see Chapter 10). Each of these catheters should be placed into a chest drainage collection unit that incorporates a water seal chamber and variable suction control. Treat persistent air leaks initially with continuous suction (usually suction at 20 cm H_2O) to evacuate the pleural space and promote coaptation of the visceral and parietal pleurae. Reduce suction and place the chest tube on the water seal only after resolution of any air leak. Remove the chest tube directly from the water seal if no pneumothorax is apparent on a chest film or after a test period of tube clamping and subsequent radiographic evaluation. The author favors a 4-hour period of clamping because recurrent pneumothorax is easier to treat by unclamping a tube than by placing a new one. Not all patients with a pneumothorax require invasive techniques to evacuate air from the pleural space. It is important to recognize that small pneumothoraces, occurring in *spontaneously breathing patients* (i.e., negative pressure ventilation), may be reevaluated in 4 to 6 hours with a repeated chest radiograph and drained only if they are expanding. This option is *not* advised for patients who are on any form of PPV because a simple pneumothorax can rapidly become a tension pneumothorax with subsequent development of hypotension and death. Tension pneumothoraces may be recognized by tachycardia, hypotension, elevated peak airway pressure (if mechanically ventilated, tachypnea if not), jugular venous distention, thoracic resonance by percussion *on* the affected side, diminished or absent breath sounds *on* the affected side, and tracheal deviation *away from* the affected side. Because not all signs or symptoms are present in all patients, treatment should be dictated by the patient's clinical condition.

Loculated pneumothoraces or fluid collections develop in certain patients. If the collections are either single or immediately adjacent to one another and readily identified, they may be drained under US guidance at the bedside.[56] Loculations are frequently in inaccessible areas or are difficult to image with US. CT scanning of the thorax can provide precise anatomic definition of the presence and number of loculated collections and be used as a guide for the interventional radiologist. Successful treatment involving CT-guided drainage of loculated pleural collections (air and fluid) to assist in weaning of patients from mechanical ventilator support has been reported.[53]

Ventilator-Induced Lung Injury

There are several causes of ventilator-induced lung injury, including biotrauma, volutrauma, barotrauma, and atelectasis-related trauma. *Biotrauma* refers to the self-sustaining process of lung injury from MV that follows alveolar overdistention or rupture, alveolar hypoperfusion, and repetitive shear stress across alveolar walls. Originally, this problem was thought to be caused by too much pressure (barotrauma).[57] Current principles hold that elevated airway pressure is a straightforward reflection of excess volume delivered to a lung that cannot accept excess gas (i.e., in volutrauma, excess volume is delivered).[58] Lung injury is an inhomogeneous process with areas of normal lung immediately adjacent to diseased and injured segments.[59] The healthy and compliant segments with shorter regional time constants will readily accept gas, and their neighbors with reduced compliance and longer regional time constants will not. The end result is overdistention of the compliant segments, alveolar injury, liberation of inflammatory cytokines and chemokines, activation of endothelin and arachidonic acid pathways, and the expression of adhesion molecules along the vascular endothelium.[60] This leads to infiltration of inflammatory cells, release of destructive lysosomal enzymes, and induction of toxic oxygen metabolites. Avoiding this inflammatory cascade is an intelligent means of protecting a patient's lungs from volume-pressure–induced lung injury. Such a notion has given rise to lung-protective ventilator strategies based on low-VT ventilation (6 mL/kg IBW) and low plateau pressure (<30 cm H_2O).[61] Several studies have reported the development within hours of ventilator-induced lung injury in patients with normal lungs who were ventilated with larger VT (12 mL/kg).[62–66] Current recommendations are for all MV to be conducted with lower VT than the once-standard 12 to 15 mL/kg. Patients with abnormal lungs (interstitial lung disease, lung resection, severe pneumonia, edema) or the presence of an ALI risk factor (sepsis, aspiration, transfusion) should be ventilated at a VT of 6 mL/kg IBW. These patients may initially be markedly acidotic and may require starting VT at 8 mL/kg IBW and titrating down to 6 mL/kg IBW within 2 hours. Those with normal lungs and no ALI risk factors should be started at a VT of less than 10 mL/kg IBW.[66]

Hemodynamic Compromise

In all circumstances, the volume of venous return exactly matches the volume of cardiac output. Any process that impedes venous return will decrease the available volume that establishes cardiac output. For patients receiving PPV, each gas delivery increases intrathoracic pressure, and exhalation decreases that pressure. Venous return principally occurs during exhalation. If the ventilator settings lead to increased intrathoracic pressure during exhalation, venous return will be reduced. Variables that can lead to this circumstance are increased PEEP, auto-PEEP, and IRV. Venous return depends on a relatively negative pressure within the thoracic cavity and also relies on a sufficient amount of time for flow into the thoracic vasculature and right side of the heart. Significantly high respiratory rates may compromise venous return. An additional untoward side effect of impaired venous return is cerebral venous hypertension from impeded venous drainage. Because of the absence of valves between the cerebral parenchyma and the right atrium, increased pressure on the right atrium reduces cerebral venous flow and may contribute to cerebral ischemia in patients with traumatic brain injury or stroke, especially in those with compromised systemic hemodynamics. These patients are prone to watershed infarction, and cerebral venous hypertension may increase this risk.

Intrinsic PEEP

Maneuvers directed at elimination of $PEEP_i$ result in a decrease in inspiratory time and an increase in expiratory time. Decreasing the respiratory rate and VT and increasing the IFR effectively accomplish this goal. Frequently, this cannot be achieved without sedation and possibly requires the addition of pharmacologic paralysis.

Difficulty Triggering the Ventilator

To trigger a ventilator, a patient must cause either a drop in pressure or an increase in airflow at the proximal airway, depending on the type of settings used. The magnitude of change required to trigger the ventilator is adjusted by setting the sensitivity, usually in the range of −1 to −2 cm H_2O below the level of $PEEP_e$. Patient difficulty triggering the ventilator is often hard to detect. When it becomes obvious by physical examination that the patient is using the accessory muscles of respiration to trigger the ventilator, the problem may be severe. The condition can be detected earlier by inspecting the pressure-volume time curve on the ventilator display, if available. A large negative deflection at the beginning of inhalation suggests that ventilator sensitivity needs to be increased.

More commonly, high $PEEP_i$ is the cause. The patient must first lower intrathoracic pressure enough to overcome $PEEP_i$ before airway pressure can drop to the threshold sensitivity. The solution to this problem is to raise $PEEP_e$ to a level half to three quarters of $PEEP_i$, which allows the patient to perform less work to trigger each inhalation. This process mandates frequent reassessment of $PEEP_i$ and manipulation of the ventilator during this dynamic period.

Auto-Cycling

Auto-cycling refers to a phenomenon when the ventilator set in AC mode begins to rapidly trigger without the patient initiating respiration. The cause is usually vacillations in airway pressure that the ventilator "interprets" as patient effort. Tremors, shivering, voluntary motion, convulsions, and oscillating water in the ventilator circuit are all potential causes. Auto-cycling should prompt immediate disconnection from the ventilator circuit and ventilation with a bag-valve device until the problem is resolved.

Rapid Breathing

When attempting to ventilate a patient with an obstructive process, the goal is to eliminate $PEEP_i$. Permissive hypercapnia is best achieved at low respiratory rates, understanding that hypercapnia is a powerful stimulus to breathe. This can typically be quelled with a combination of sedation with high-dose opiates, ketamine, or propofol. Neuromuscular blockade should be considered a last resort, undertaken only after careful consideration of the risk of prolonged paralysis and potential development of neuropathy in critical illness. If undertaken, the goal should be to weaken the patient sufficiently to inhibit dyssynchrony with the ventilator. Other common causes of rapid breathing include sepsis, pulmonary embolism, pregnancy, hepatic encephalopathy, intracranial hypertension, stroke, hemorrhage, and hypercapnia.

Outstripping the Ventilator and Double Cycling (Table 8.1)

Hypercapnia will develop in patients receiving low-VT ventilation for ARDS or for an obstructive process and generate an increased respiratory drive. Outstripping the ventilator refers to the patient's effort to draw a higher VT than set while in a volume-targeted mode. This can be detected by observing the exhaled VT or by finding a negative deflection at the end of inhalation on the pressure-volume time plot. Double cycling occurs when the patient desires a larger VT than is set and continues to inspire despite the delivery of a breath. The ventilator will then provide a second breath almost immediately after the first. This is especially problematic because the actual VT delivered is twice the set volume. As with controlling rapid breathing, the solution is sedation and analgesia, particularly with opiates. Switching to a pressure-targeted mode or increasing the set VT may alleviate this issue.

Straining Over the Ventilator

Straining over the ventilator indicates that the patient on a volume-targeted mode is attempting to inhale at a flow rate in

TABLE 8.1 Ventilator Troubleshooting

PROBLEM	SIGNS	SOLUTIONS
Overstripping	Higher exhaled V_T than set Negative deflection at end of inhalation	Increase V_T Sedation Pressure control
Double cycling	Sustained inspiratory effort beyond time In pressure control: increasing V_T Volume control: increase V_T and airway pressure	Increase V_T Sedation Increasing E time
Straining over the vent	Trying to take a bigger flow than offered	Increase flow rate, change to pressure control, sedation

V_T, Tidal volume.

excess of the set IFR. On the pressure-volume time plot, the rise in pressure during inhalation will be concave rather than convex. Potential solutions are to raise the IFR, switch to a pressure-targeted mode or PSV, or use sedation and analgesia.

Coughing

Coughing is a common problem that arises from increased secretions, airway foreign body (ET tube), or an underlying pulmonary disease process. Coughing can lead to autocycling, poor patient comfort, dislodgment of the ET tube, and rarely airway injury. Accurate placement of the ET tube above the carina should be confirmed. Suctioning and provision of warmed, humidified air are often helpful. If these simple measures fail to provide relief, aerosolized or ET-tube–administered lidocaine or suppression with opiates may increase patient comfort.

Equipment Failure

Whenever a patient decompensates while undergoing MV, consideration should be given to equipment failure as the primary cause. Interruption of the oxygen supply, erroneous settings, disconnected ventilator circuitry, and obstructed tubes are all potential culprits. Immediate action should include disconnection from the ventilator and bag ventilation with 100% O_2. The mnemonic made popular by the American Heart Association Pediatric Advanced Life Support Course is useful for recalling the causes of unexpected decompensation: DOPE (*D*islodgment of the ET tube, *O*bstruction of the tube, *P*neumothorax, and *E*quipment failure). Confirmation of ET tube placement, suctioning via the ET catheter, auscultation, chest radiography, and equipment troubleshooting are necessary actions.

TROUBLESHOOTING

Critically ill patients are encountered in the ED every day. Some of them required intubation in the prehospital setting, whereas others are intubated on arrival or during ED evaluation. After their airway has been secured and their condition stabilized, patients may remain in the ED because of a lack of critical care beds. In some hospitals, a dedicated intensivist will take charge of these patients, and in others, this type of coverage may not be available. Acute complications or deterioration must often be handled by the emergency physician.

This section provides a framework for managing crashing, mechanically ventilated patients. The information provided will assist the practitioner in determining whether the patient's condition is related to the underlying pathology that necessitated MV or whether it is being caused by MV itself.

Determine Hemodynamic Stability

The initial step in managing a crashing ventilated patient is to determine the patient's hemodynamic stability. A ventilated patient is, by definition, critically ill. The patient can fall anywhere on the spectrum from being ventilated for airway protection, with normal vital signs, blood pressure, and oxygen saturation, to being ventilated and in cardiac arrest. Determining where the patient is on this spectrum, including assessment for hypotension and hypoxia, will dictate how much time that the practitioner has to implement rescue strategies. In addition, it is important to anticipate the patient's clinical course. The approach to a patient who is intubated for hypoxia stemming from pneumonia and whose blood pressure and oxygenation gradually trend down over a period of hours or days is different from the approach to a patient who is declining over a span of minutes (Fig. 8.19).

As a general rule, the following evaluation should be performed on patients with new unexplained hypotension (systolic blood pressure [SBP] < 90 mm Hg), new unexplained hypoxia (Sao_2 < 90%), or a new marked change in vital signs (a drop in SBP by more than 20 mm Hg or a drop in Sao_2 by more than 10%) within an hour. Patients with *stable* SBP between 80 and 90 mm Hg and Sao_2 between 80% and 90% should be evaluated expeditiously in the hope of halting the decline. Those with SBP lower than 80 mm Hg or Sao_2 less than 80%, and those who continue to decline rapidly, should be evaluated emergently, with consideration given to entering the cardiac arrest/near-arrest algorithm. These values are arbitrary demarcation points and do not take precedence over bedside clinical judgment.

Cardiac Arrest and Near-Arrest Patients

Time is of the essence in a patient with cardiac arrest or near arrest. Advanced cardiac life support should be implemented quickly, and there are some key points to remember in a ventilated patient in cardiac arrest or one who becomes acutely hemodynamically unstable. The ED practitioner should develop a stepwise approach in this situation. During each step, the practitioner should "look, listen, and feel" to run through the differential diagnosis.

During stabilization of these patients, it is important to keep in mind the original pathology that necessitated intubation. Sudden decompensation in an asthmatic is a common example of physician intervention worsening the scenario unless the pathophysiology of the arrest is appreciated (see Fig. 8.17). A crashing ventilated patient may simply be worsening from the primary pathology. A multitrauma patient may have an intrathoracic or intraabdominal catastrophe, and a septic patient may be deteriorating clinically from the lack of source control.

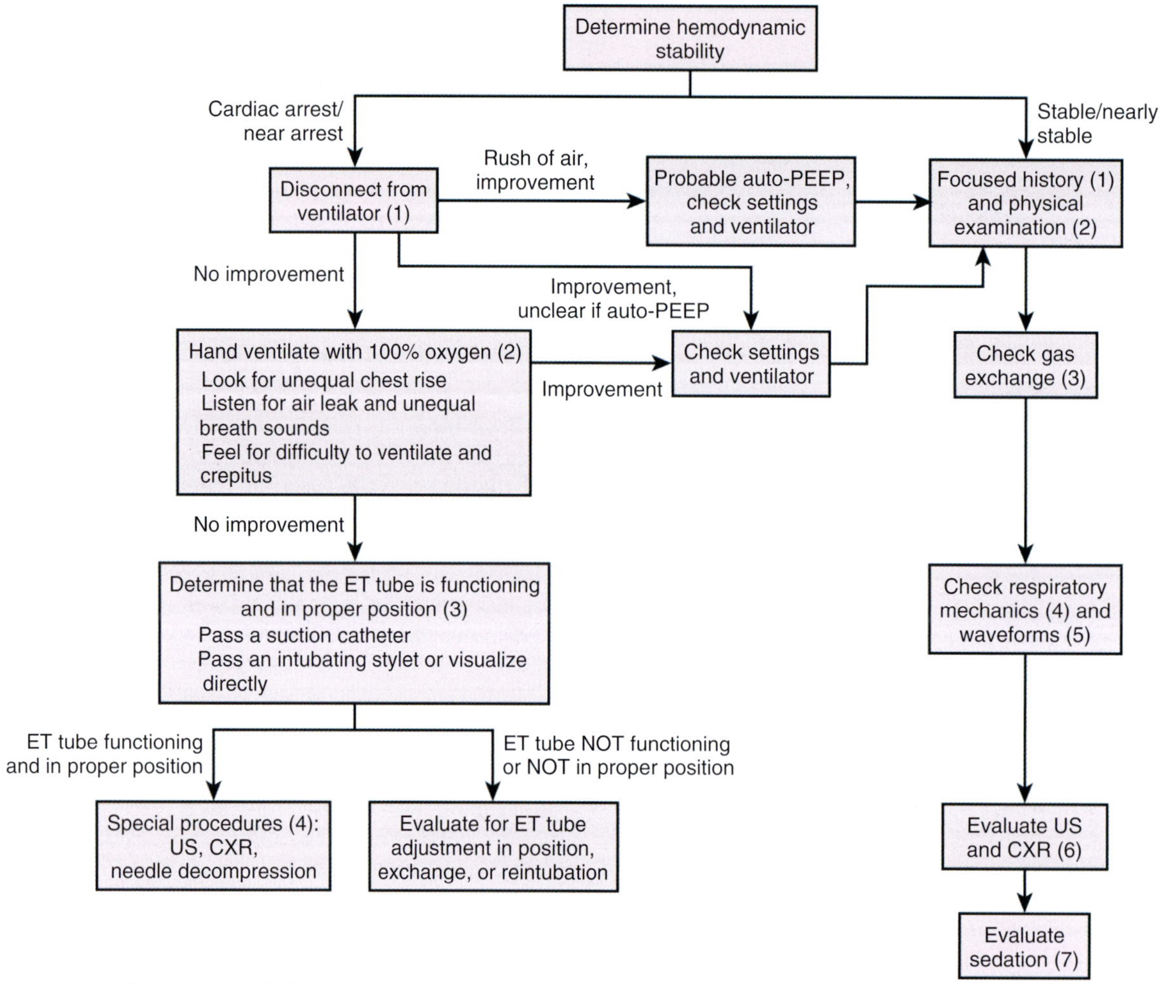

Fig. 8.19 Troubleshooting algorithm for respiratory distress and hemodynamic instability in critically ill ventilated patients. *CXR*, Chest x-ray; *ET*, endotracheal; *PEEP*, positive end-expiratory pressure; *US*, ultrasound.

It is also important to determine and address special circumstances that the ventilator can precipitate, the most significant of which are tension pneumothorax and severe auto-PEEP. Tension pneumothorax can lead to marked hypotension as a result of decreased cardiac output and marked hypoxia from $\dot{V}/\dot{Q}$ mismatch.[65] Auto-PEEP (also referred to as $PEEP_i$, breath stacking, or dynamic hyperinflation) is caused by trapped volume in the pulmonary system. If severe enough, it will eventually lead to increased intrathoracic pressure. This can cause hypotension and decreased cardiac output from decreased venous return and marked hypoxia from $\dot{V}/\dot{Q}$ mismatch.[66]

In critically ill ventilated patients with respiratory distress who are hemodynamically unstable, the following steps will assist the ED physician in determining the cause of the decompensation.

Step 1: Disconnect the Patient From the Ventilator

This is perhaps the easiest step to perform. It can be both diagnostic and therapeutic in a crashing ventilated patient. A quick rush of air or prolonged expiration of trapped air from the ET tube can be diagnostic of ventilator-induced auto-PEEP. A few seconds of observation can determine whether this entity is present. Return of hemodynamic stability implies that the maneuver was successful.

Patients undergoing cardiopulmonary resuscitation (CPR) should not be connected to a ventilator. The variations in intrathoracic pressure caused by CPR will trigger ventilator breaths at high rates if set on AC mode. Patients treated with inhaled nitric oxide (iNO) should not be removed from iNO abruptly, and effort should be made to quickly establish this supply through the bag-valve system. In addition, care should be taken when disconnecting patients who are on high PEEP, such as those with ARDS. When disconnecting the ventilator, it is important to address auto-PEEP because derecruitment can occur and hypoxia may be worsened. Once auto-PEEP has been ruled out, PEEP valves may be used to maintain PEEP levels and avoid derecruitment. PEEP valves may be problematic in a markedly hypotensive patient. They may increase intrathoracic pressure and decrease venous return.

Step 2: Breathing—Hand-Ventilate With 100% Oxygen

Ensure that 100% oxygen is being delivered and limit the respiratory rate to 8 to 10 breaths/min. Particular attention should be paid to the delivery of hand ventilation. Inadvertent rates as high as 40 breaths/min are often used in codes.[67,68] Excessive rates will increase intrathoracic pressure and lead to a decrease in venous return and cardiac output.[69] Look at both sides of the chest to determine whether there is equal chest rise. Unequal chest rise can signify main stem intubation, pneumothorax, or a mucous plug. Listen for air escaping from the mouth or nose (a sign of an air leak). Listen over the epigastric area and in both axillae. Decreased breath sounds may provide clues regarding main stem intubation, pneumothorax, or an atelectatic lung. Feel for subcutaneous crepitus (a sign of pneumothorax) and assess for difficulty in hand ventilating (a sign of low dynamic or static respiratory system compliance).

Step 3: Airway—Determine That the ET Tube Is Functioning and in the Proper Position

The ET tube functions by providing a conduit to the lower part of the trachea. The cuff creates a seal between it and the inner wall of the trachea. To determine whether the ET tube is functioning properly, pass the suction catheter and listen for an air leak (Fig. 8.20). Easy passage of the suction catheter does not guarantee that the ET tube is in the trachea because the catheter may be passing down the esophagus. If it is difficult or not possible to pass the suction catheter, the ET tube is either dislodged or obstructed. Attempt to correct this by repositioning the head in the case of a twisted or bent ET tube or inserting a bite block if the patient is biting on the tube. Dislodged or obstructed ET tubes require reintubation. Patients with dislodged ET tubes should be treated as difficult intubations because unplanned extubations are notorious for causing trauma to the glottis and for creating vocal cord edema.[70]

In a cardiac arrest or near-arrest patient, the best choice for determining that the ET tube is in the proper position is direct visualization of the ET tube passing through the cords. This step is often omitted in a crashing ventilated patient because

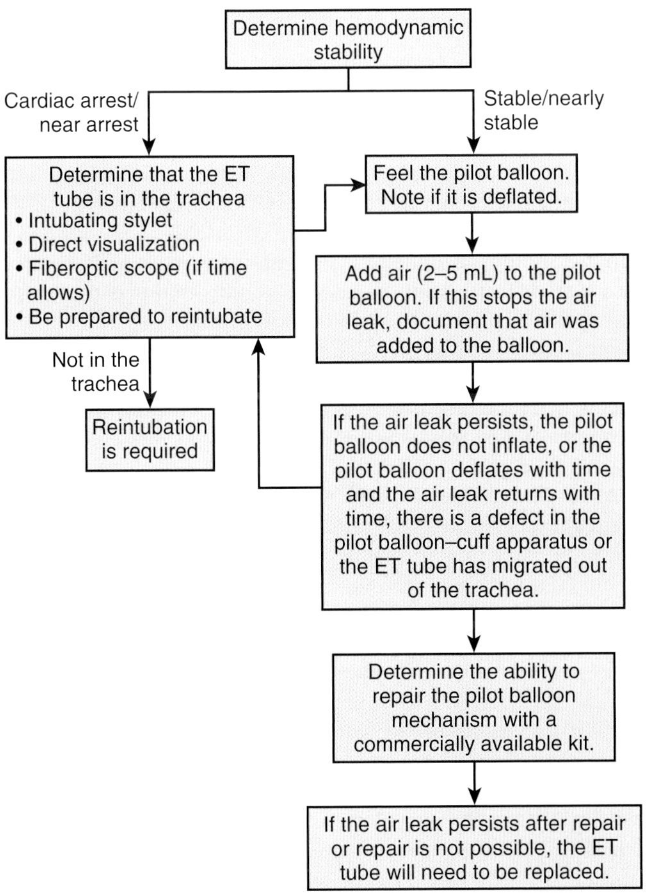

Fig. 8.20 Troubleshooting an air leak. *ET*, Endotracheal.

of the belief that the ET tube has not migrated. Unfortunately, unrecognized ET tube migration can occur during routine care of a critically ill patient. Patients are frequently moved in and out of emergency medical service vehicles, transferred to and from stretchers for imaging studies, and turned for procedures or bathing, all of which are capable of dislodging the tube. This visualization step can be performed while providing ventilation by hand.

Other simple techniques may be used to confirm that the ET tube is in the trachea. Direct visualization of the carina with a fiberoptic scope is an option, understanding that this device is not typically readily available to the ED practitioner. Another quick and readily available technique is to pass an intubating stylet (gum elastic bougie or Eschmann introducer).[71] The stylet is passed gently through the ET tube. If resistance is met at 30 cm, the ET tube is most likely in the trachea. If the stylet passes beyond 35 cm without resistance, the ET tube is probably in the esophagus. If resistance is met too soon, the intubating stylet may be catching on the ET tube.

At least one of these techniques to determine proper positioning should be used early enough in the resuscitation to correct any airway issues. In addition, proper positioning should be confirmed before simply removing the ET tube and reintubation, particularly if the patient is deemed to have a difficult airway (unless it is glaringly evident that the patient is extubated).

Step 4: Special Procedures

If the patient is still in cardiac arrest or near arrest after being disconnected from the ventilator, ensuring proper placement of the ET tube, and hand ventilating with 100% oxygen, a clinical decision will be required regarding needle decompression of the chest. If time permits, a focused history from the bedside nurse, respiratory therapist, or paramedic and a focused physical examination will indicate which side of the chest to decompress. In addition, depending on the urgency of the situation, bedside US and chest radiography may be used. Bedside US has been shown to exclude pneumothorax in the presence of "lung slide." This is depicted in M-mode as the "seashore sign" (Fig. 8.21) and, in its absence, as the "stratosphere sign/bar code sign" (Fig. 8.22).[72–74]

At times, the clinical situation does not allow imaging studies, and the focused history and physical examination may not be helpful. In these cases, needle decompression of both sides of the chest should be considered if other more likely causes of acute decompensation are not found. It is important to remember that chest tube placement is required in patients after needle decompression.[75–77]

Stable and Nearly Stable Patients

If the patient is deemed stable or near stable or quickly regains stability after disconnection from the ventilator and ventilation by hand, the event should be approached in a systematic manner. The patient should be placed on 100% oxygen during this evaluation.

Step 1: Obtain a Focused History

A focused history should be obtained from the practitioners most involved in the patient's care (bedside nurse, respiratory therapist, resident, paramedic). Valuable information includes the indication for intubation, difficulty of the intubation,

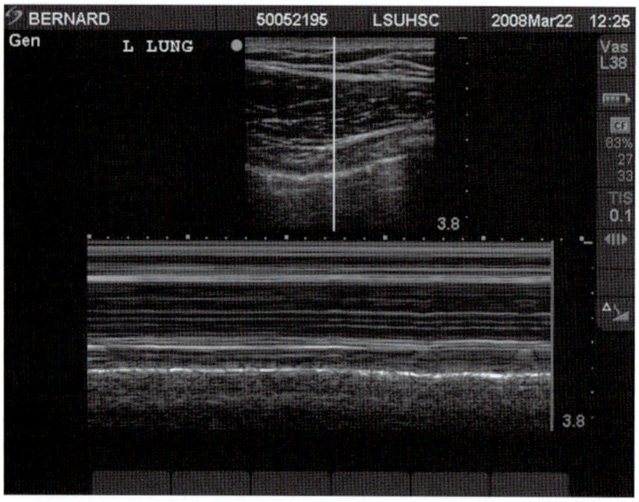

Fig. 8.21 Ultrasound image of a lung slide ("seashore sign") in M-mode. This patient does not have a pneumothorax.

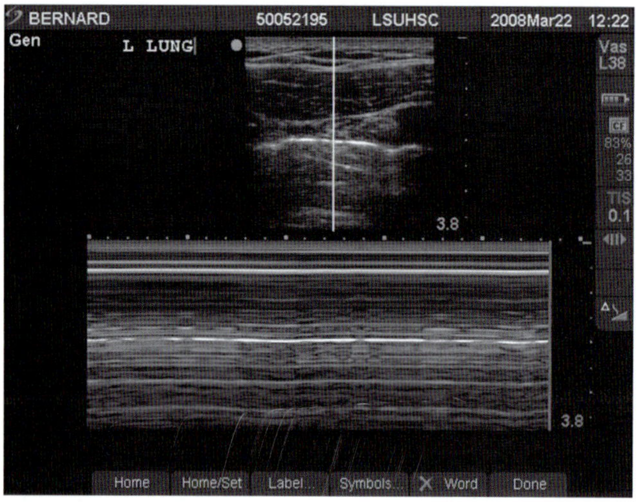

Fig. 8.22 Ultrasound image of the "bar code" sign in M-mode, indicative of pneumothorax. See the Ultrasound Box in Chapter 10 for additional details.

depth of the ET tube, ventilator settings, and recent procedures or moves (central line insertion; chest tube placement; removal or transition to a water seal; thoracentesis; ET tube manipulation; transport off the stretcher; rotation for cleaning, a procedure, or chest radiography).

Step 2: Perform a Focused Physical Examination

Take a general survey of the patient. Observe for agitation, attempts to pull at the ET tube and lines, gasping for breath (the patient will have the mouth open and appear dyspneic), and tearing of the eyes.

Airway

Look at the ET tube and determine if it has migrated from its previous position. It is possible that the ET tube has migrated out of the trachea or into a main bronchus. Adjust if necessary. Listen for escaping air (an air leak) from the mouth or nose (see Fig. 8.20). This typically signifies that the tube has lost its seal with the trachea and occurs with extubation or cuff failure. Feel the pilot balloon. If it is deflated, the cuff is deflated. Add air to the pilot balloon. If this stops the air leak, make a note that air was added to the balloon. If the pilot balloon does not inflate or deflates over time, there is a defect in the pilot balloon-cuff apparatus, and the ET tube will probably need to be exchanged. Occasionally, it may be possible to repair the pilot balloon mechanism with commercially available kits. This is a good option for patients who are difficult to intubate.

Determine that the ET tube is functioning properly by passing the suction catheter. If it is difficult or not possible to pass the suction catheter, the ET tube is either dislodged or obstructed. Attempt to correct by repositioning the head in the case of a twisted or bent ET tube or inserting a bite block if the patient is biting on the tube. Dislodged or obstructed ET tubes require reintubation.

Determine that the ET tube is in proper position if at any point in the evaluation it is suspected that extubation has occurred. Any of the techniques discussed in the previous section may be used.

Breathing

Look at both sides of the chest to determine whether there is equal chest rise. Unequal chest rise can signify main stem intubation, pneumothorax, or a mucous plug. Look at the ventilator tubing and determine whether there is an oscillating water collection. Listen for air escaping from the mouth or nose (a sign of an air leak). Listen over the epigastric area and in both axillae. Decreased breath sounds may provide clues regarding main stem intubation, pneumothorax, or an atelectatic lung. Feel for subcutaneous crepitus (a sign of pneumothorax).

Circulation

Check for pulses and cycle the blood pressure cuff frequently. If the patient has an arterial line, make sure that the transducer is level. Determine the need for a fluid bolus or vasopressors.

Step 3: Assess Gas Exchange

Hypoxia can be diagnosed with pulse oximetry if the waveform is reliable. The waveform should not be highly variable and the frequency of the waveform should match the heart rate on the cardiac monitor. In a few instances, such as carbon monoxide poisoning, pulse oximetry is not reliable.[78] In these cases or if the pulse oximeter is not picking it up, an ABG sample should be obtained. Patients with a partial pressure of O_2 (Pao_2)/Fio_2 ratio of less than 200 should be evaluated for ARDS. Those with a ratio between 200 and 300 should be evaluated for ALI.[79] A lung-protective strategy should be implemented in those determined to have ALI or ARDS (see Fig. 8.18).[80] Hypoventilation cannot be identified with pulse oximetry. ABG analysis is beneficial in this event.

Step 4: Check Respiratory Mechanics

Determine whether peak pressure and plateau pressure have changed from their previous values. These values should be obtained on volume-targeted modes. Airway pressure is a function of volume and respiratory system compliance. The respiratory system incorporates the ventilator circuit, ET tube, trachea, bronchi, pulmonary parenchyma, and chest wall. A set volume with a set system compliance results in a specific pressure. Peak pressure is a function of volume, resistance to airflow, and respiratory system compliance. Plateau pressure is obtained during an inspiratory pause, thus eliminating airflow, and therefore reflects only respiratory system compliance. An isolated increase in peak pressure is indicative of increased resistance to airflow. An isolated increase in plateau pressure is indicative of a decrease in respiratory system compliance. Note that plateau pressure can never be higher than peak pressure and that if plateau pressure rises, so will peak pressure. It is important to keep in mind the Δ relationship (peak pressure − plateau pressure). These measurements assume a comfortable patient, and peak pressure and plateau pressure values are not reliable in an agitated patient.[81,82]

Step 5: Observe Ventilator Waveforms

The two most helpful ventilator waveforms are the flow-time curve and the pressure-time curve. The flow-time curve can be used to detect air trapping. The pressure-time curve can be used to determine plateau pressure with an inspiratory hold (see Fig. 8.1).

A notching in the pressure-time curve during inspiration can signify air hunger. In this situation, the patient desires a higher flow rate than the ventilator is delivering. It is commonly seen in volume-targeted modes. Increasing the flow rate will often alleviate this phenomenon. Another solution is to change to a pressure-targeted mode.

Double cycling can also be seen on ventilator waveforms. This occurs when the patient desires a higher V_T than the ventilator is set to deliver. The patient is still inspiring when the first breath has finished cycling and the ventilator immediately gives a second mechanical breath. This is frequently seen with low-V_T ventilation, which is used in patients with ARDS and status asthmaticus. It is important to recognize because the actual V_T being provided is essentially twice the set V_T. This has important ramifications for patients with ARDS and obstructive processes such as asthma and COPD, for whom the goal is lower V_T. Typically, improved sedation with emphasis on blunting the respiratory drive with opiates alleviates double cycling. Other adjustments that may prove helpful are increasing the flow rate, increasing V_T by 1 mL/kg of predicted body weight up to 8 mL/kg, or changing from a volume-targeted mode to a pressure-targeted mode.

Step 6: Imaging Studies—Chest Radiograph and Bedside US

Evaluate the chest radiograph for ET tube position, main stem intubation, lung atelectasis, pneumothorax, and a worsening parenchymal process. Bedside US, if available, is typically quicker in evaluating for pneumothorax, and it will be less accurate in providing information on the location of the ET tube, lung atelectasis, or parenchymal processes (see Figs. 8.21 and 8.22).

Step 7: Evaluate Sedation

Patients requiring MV often need sedation and analgesia to make the ET tube and ventilation tolerable. Rarely, some patients, such as those with drug overdoses or traumatic head injuries, may not require any sedation. Others may tolerate intubation well while almost fully awake. The majority of patients require some form of sedation or analgesia. Note that a plethora of non–MV-associated conditions, such as unrecognized bladder obstruction, alcohol or drug withdrawal, occult fractures, compartment syndrome, or bowel ischemia, can cause significant agitation that can mistakenly be attributed to the stress of intubation and ventilation.

Selection of agents should be based on the desired effect. If a patient appears agitated, sedative-hypnotics should be used. Such drugs include propofol, dexmedetomidine, benzodiazepines, and haloperidol. It is important to note that these agents do not provide an analgesic component. If a patient is being given adequate sedative doses and still appears agitated, consider pain as a cause. Typical opiates that can be used are fentanyl, hydromorphone, and morphine. A remifentanil infusion is ultrashort acting and can provide both sedation and analgesia. Remifentanil does not accumulate in patients with renal or hepatic insufficiency. Ideally, prompt reversal of analgesia and sedation should be seen on discontinuation. Remifentanil is an alternative to fentanyl for patients requiring frequent neurologic assessment or those with multiorgan failure.

The goal of sedation and anesthesia in ventilated patients who are not being evaluated for extubation is one in which the patient will arouse with gentle stimulation and will return to a sedated state when left alone. Patients who are being sedated and require deep stimulation to get a response are oversedated.

Patients who display air hunger and have a high respiratory rate can be given a trial of opiates to relieve their symptoms. Proper sedation and analgesia are paramount in patients being treated with a strategy that allows or permits hypercapnia, such as those with status asthmaticus, and in patients being treated with lung-protective strategies, such as those with ARDS. Hypercapnia is a powerful stimulus to the respiratory drive, and opiates are often required to control respiratory rates. Patients who tend to be difficult to control (besides those with status asthmaticus and ARDS) include patients with hepatic encephalopathy or intracranial processes such as a mass effect or hemorrhage. Chemical weakening with intermittently dosed paralytics may be required if patients have undergone a good trial of sedation, analgesia, and ventilator changes and are still markedly tachypneic. Careful consideration should be given before this step because prolonged paralysis has been implicated in critical illness polyneuropathy.[83,84] In addition, expert consultation should be obtained before prolonged paralysis of a neurosurgical patient. The goal in chemical paralysis in these patients is to weaken them enough to control their interaction with the ventilator. Usually, this does not require a full dose of the paralytic.

Hemodynamic instability in mechanically ventilated and sedated patients may be a result of medications because sedatives and analgesics can precipitate or worsen hypotension. As a general rule, continuous infusions should be withheld in these cases. Patients who are hypoxic and agitated and not hypotensive may benefit from improved sedation. It is possible that their pulmonary status is so tenuous that they are agitated from the hypoxia and their condition is worsened by the oxygen consumption caused by their agitation. Patients who are agitated and hypotensive may respond well to a low-dose benzodiazepine and opiate if the agitation is a precipitant of hypotension. In all these cases, it is imperative to determine whether sedation is a factor in the decompensation. Chemical paralysis should be reserved as a final option. It is important to remember that without continuous electroencephalographic recordings, seizure activity cannot be monitored if the patient is paralyzed.

SPECIAL SCENARIOS

Two special scenarios should be mentioned. One is a crashing intubated pediatric patient and the second is a patient with a tracheostomy. The approach described earlier can be used in pediatric patients, and there are a few caveats that may improve the approach. The first is to recognize that migration of the ET tube is common with small movements of the head and neck. A simple solution is to use a cervical collar for immobilization, limiting neck movement. Second, small ET tubes are sometimes uncuffed and do not have a pilot balloon. Air leaks in this scenario should prompt the clinician to consider that the ET tube is either dislodged or too small. Finally, specialized equipment such as intubating stylets and fiberoptic scopes are typically not available in pediatric sizes.

Important questions that have ramifications in the care of a crashing ventilated patient with a tracheostomy are the following: (1) Does the patient have a laryngectomy? (2) Why does the patient have a tracheostomy? and (3) How old is the tracheostomy? These are important because patients with a laryngectomy cannot be intubated orally, patients with a tracheostomy secondary to anatomic considerations or difficult or failed airways may be difficult to intubate orally, and the tract in a patient with a recent tracheostomy (less than a week old) may not have matured enough to safely reintroduce a tracheostomy tube.

LIBERATION FROM THE VENTILATOR

Occasionally, patients can be considered for extubation while still in the ED. Before extubating a patient, several questions should be answered in the affirmative (Fig. 8.23). The most important question is: "Has the reason the patient was intubated in the first place been resolved?" Patients who were difficult intubations or required multiple attempts should have a planned extubation. It may be prudent to allow the edema from a traumatic intubation to subside.

Once these screening questions have been answered in the affirmative, one should perform an awakening trial followed by a spontaneous breathing trial. Extubation should be considered if the patient does not fail the breathing trial.

For patients intubated for exacerbation of COPD, NPPV should be considered. For patients with COPD who failed a spontaneous breathing trial, extubating to NPPV decreases mortality, hospital length of stay, the incidence of ventilator-associated pneumonia, and the total duration of MV.[85]

CONCLUSION

Mechanically ventilated patients are typically the most critically ill patients that the ED practitioner will manage. The underlying disease process that required intubation is typically life-threatening. When patients become unstable, the physician should take a stepwise approach toward determining whether the patient is deteriorating because of the underlying disease process or because of interaction with the ventilator. It is hoped that the approach presented here will assist practitioners with a framework to evaluate and stabilize crashing ventilated patients. It is important to remember that the intubated patient will undergo dynamic changes during their treatment process and need to be frequently reevaluated. For further information, Wood and Winters present an up-to-date review of the care of ventilated patients in the ED and evaluation of potential problems.[86]

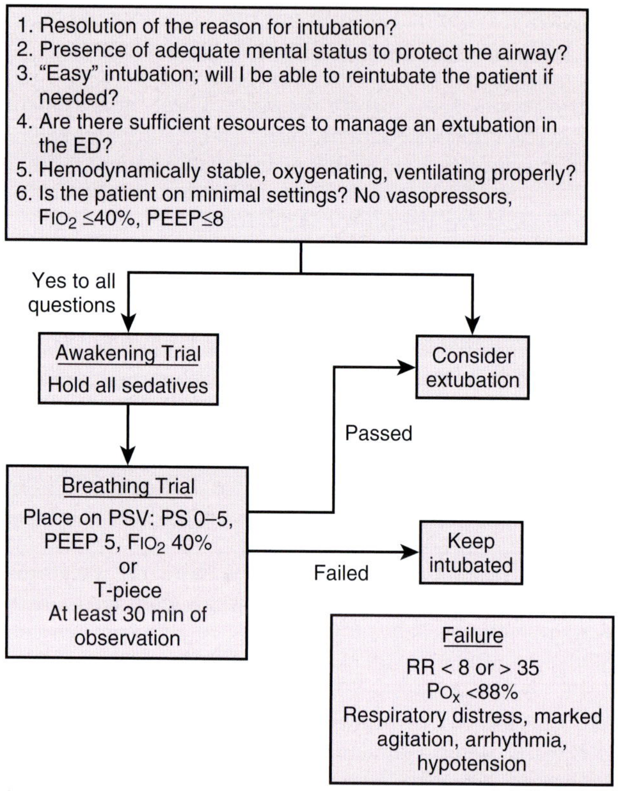

Fig. 8.23 Liberation from ventilator. *ED*, Emergency department; *FIO₂*, fraction of inspired oxygen; *PEEP*, positive end-expiratory pressure; *PO_x*, pulse oximeter; *PSV*, pressure support ventilation; *RR*, respiratory rate.

REFERENCES ARE AVAILABLE AT Elsevier eBooks+

CHAPTER 9

Thoracentesis

Barbara K. Blok

Thoracentesis is a percutaneous procedure during which a needle is inserted into the pleural space to remove fluid for diagnostic or therapeutic purposes. When performed using ultrasound (US) guidance, thoracentesis has a low rate of complications.

ANATOMY

The thoracic cavity is lined by thin serous membranes: the visceral pleura, which wraps around the lungs, and the parietal pleura, which lines the inner surface of the thoracic cavities and meets the visceral pleura at the root of the lungs in the mediastinum. The space between these two linings is called the *pleural space*. Each pleural membrane is comprised of a superficial mesothelial cell layer and an underlying connective tissue layer containing systemic capillary beds. These membranes are leaky, allowing for easy movement of both fluid and protein. In the healthy state, the hydrostatic pressure of the systemic capillaries produces a small net movement of fluid across both pleurae into the low-pressure pleural space.[1] This fluid is removed primarily via lymphatic stomata found in the parietal pleura. Normally there is a small amount of fluid, estimated at 0.26 mL/kg of body mass, present in the pleural space.[2] An excess amount of fluid in the pleural space is termed *pleural effusion*.

Because the lymphatic system can remove 20 times more pleural fluid than its basal rate,[3] it is believed that in most instances, the development of a pleural effusion requires both an increase in fluid entry into the pleural space and a decrease in its removal.

ETIOLOGY OF PLEURAL EFFUSIONS

The most common causes of pleural effusion in adults are congestive heart failure (CHF), pneumonia, malignancy, and pulmonary embolism (PE).[1,4] The most common cause in children is pneumonia, followed by heart failure, and malignancy.[5,6] Pleural effusions can be classified as either transudates or exudates. Distinguishing between transudates and exudates narrows the differential diagnosis and directs management and therapy. A comprehensive list of causes can be found in Box 9.1. The most common are discussed in the following sections.

Transudates: Overwhelming the System

Transudates are caused by either an increase in intravascular hydrostatic pressure or a decrease in intravascular oncotic pressure. This generates an increased fluid flow into the pleural space across noninjured capillary beds. These effusions are typically straw-colored and serous with very low cellular and protein content.

The most common cause of a transudate is CHF. The increased pulmonary and systemic capillary hydrostatic pressure in patients with CHF results in a net fluid flow across the pleurae and into the pleural space. In addition, elevated systemic venous pressure decreases lymphatic flow out of the thorax. Any process that causes compromised left ventricular outflow can result in a pleural effusion, including myocardial infarction, cardiomyopathy, and valvular disease. These effusions are typically small and bilateral with larger effusions on the right (Fig. 9.1).[7] Large effusions or those with a high degree of asymmetry should raise suspicion for another cause.

In patients with advanced cirrhosis and portal hypertension, ascitic fluid can pass through the diaphragm into the lung through preexisting micro defects. Termed hepatic hydrothorax, these cirrhosis-related effusions are typically right-sided and reaccumulate quickly after drainage.[8]

Renal disease may also lead to transudative pleural effusion. Examples include the hypoalbuminemic state of patients with nephrotic syndrome, intraabdominal fluid associated with peritoneal dialysis, or retroperitoneal fluid with obstructive uropathy.

Exudates: Pathology of Tissues, Destroying the System

Exudates are caused by pleural inflammation, increased pleural membrane permeability, or lymphatic obstruction. More than 90% of exudative effusions are due to malignancy, pneumonia, PE, and gastrointestinal diseases (e.g., pancreatitis, esophageal perforation).[1] In patients from regions with high prevalence of tuberculosis (TB), this should be considered in the differential for exudative effusion.[9] These pathologic processes produce high pleural fluid protein and/or lactate dehydrogenase (LDH) content.

The primary mechanism of cancer-related pleural effusion is obstruction of pleural lymphatic outflow, either via damage to lymphatic stomata or more distal involvement of the mediastinal lymph nodes. Other mechanisms include metastases to the pleurae, increasing capillary permeability, and obstruction of the thoracic duct with consequent chylothorax.

A pleural effusion associated with pneumonia or a lung abscess is termed a parapneumonic effusion. In the first, or exudative, stage of parapneumonic effusion, an increase in pulmonary interstitial fluid leads to flow of sterile fluid and inflammatory cells across the visceral pleura into the pleural space. When the infection and resultant inflammation continue unchecked, there is increased capillary permeability with bacterial and additional inflammatory cell transfer to the pleural space, causing the parapneumonic effusion to become complicated. This worsening pleural space inflammation results in the deposition of fibrin on the pleural surfaces with the formation of loculations which ultimately can result in a tough outer layer that encases the lung. Because complicated parapneumonic effusions are associated with longer hospital stays and increased morbidity, early identification and diagnostic evaluation of a parapneumonic effusion is essential.[10]

A pleural effusion develops in up to 40% of those with PE.[11–13] Therefore when the cause of the effusion is unclear, PE should be strongly considered. The effusions associated with PE are often too small to require thoracentesis. They are usually exudative, probably resulting from ischemia and infarction-induced increases in pulmonary capillary permeability.

BOX 9.1 Causes of Pleural Effusion

TRANSUDATES

Most Common

- Congestive heart failure
- Cirrhosis

Less Common

- Nephrotic syndrome
- Peritoneal dialysis
- Pulmonary hypertension
- Acute atelectasis
- Urinothorax

Rare (Usually Exudate)

- Myxedema
- Malignancy
- Pulmonary embolism
- Sarcoidosis
- Central venous occlusion
- Pericardial disease

EXUDATES

Most Common

- Malignancy
- Pneumonia
- Pulmonary embolism
- Tuberculosis (high-prevalence region)

Less Common

- Post–myocardial infarction
- Post–coronary artery bypass graft
- Trauma
- Esophageal perforation
- Pancreatitis
- Intraabdominal abscess
- Myxedema
- Connective tissue disease
- Drug induced
- Chylothorax
- Asbestosis
- Sarcoidosis
- Uremia
- Endometriosis
- Meigs syndrome
- Ovarian hyperstimulation syndrome
- Radiation therapy

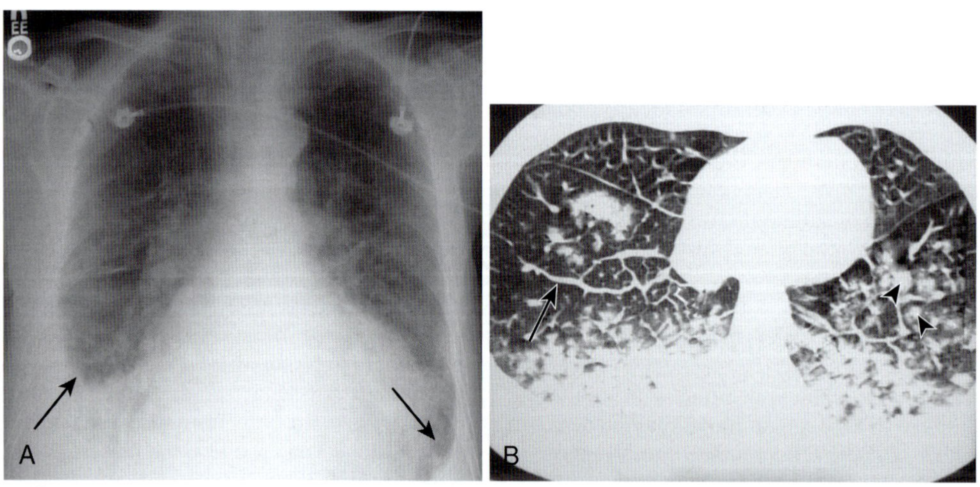

Fig. 9.1 Effusion from congestive heart failure. (A) A frontal chest radiograph in a patient with pulmonary edema shows cardiomegaly, bilateral pleural effusions *(arrows)*, and central interstitial thickening, including Kerley's A-lines. Note that the right effusion is slightly larger than the left effusion. (B) High-resolution computed tomography scan in a patient with pulmonary edema shows interstitial edema with bilateral, basilar, centrilobular ground-glass opacity nodules *(arrowheads)* and smooth interlobular septal thickening *(arrow)*. Bilateral pleural effusions are also present. (Courtesy Michael B. Gotway, MD, Department of Radiology, University of California, San Francisco.)

Traumatic Effusions: Acute and Catastrophic Destruction of the System

Effusions can also result from significant injuries that allow nonphysiologic material to enter the pleural space. Esophageal rupture can result from forceful vomiting, as in the case of Boerhaave's syndrome, or from instrumentation, as in the case of endoscopy, gastroesophageal balloon tamponade tube placement, or rigid nasogastric tube placement. Hemothorax can result from traumatic injuries, cannulation of the subclavian vein or artery, PE, or aortic aneurysm rupture. Chylothorax develops from acute disruption of the thoracic duct, usually in the setting of trauma or malignancy. These effusions are often large-volume collections that accumulate over a short period and rapidly compromise both oxygenation and circulation.

CLINICAL PRESENTATION

Symptoms of small pleural effusions are usually representative of the underlying disease process and not the effusion itself. An effusion greater than 300 mL may cause symptoms on its own, usually dyspnea, chest pain, or cough. The dyspnea from a larger pleural effusion is typically the result of impaired chest wall and diaphragm movement and not decreased oxygenation or lung function.[14] Chest pain may be dull and aching from the effusion itself or pleuritic from localized irritation of the parietal pleura, which has abundant nerve fibers. Cough is usually attributed to bronchial irritation from compression of the lung parenchyma. Patients occasionally present in extremis from a large pleural effusion that is compressing the heart and causing tamponade physiology with cardiovascular compromise.[15]

There are numerous described physical exam findings for pleural effusion, but these may be difficult to appreciate in the emergency department (ED) environment depending on the acuity of the patient and the ambient noise (Box 9.2). Dullness to percussion and decreased tactile fremitus over the effusion have been shown to be the most useful physical examination findings on systematic review.[16] Percussion over the effusion produces a characteristic dull resonance, which shifts when the patient changes position if the fluid is free flowing. Placing the flat hand over the patient's back while the patient says the word "toy" or the phrase "blue moon" will demonstrate a reduced or absent fremitus because the fluid separates the lung from the thoracic wall and absorbs vibrations from the lung.

RADIOLOGIC DIAGNOSIS

Chest Radiograph

Because pleural fluid is denser than air-filled lung, a free-flowing effusion will first accumulate in the most dependent parts of the thoracic cavity: the subpulmonic space and the lateral costophrenic sulcus. Pleural effusions are usually visible on an upright chest radiograph if 200 to 250 mL of fluid is present. A lateral radiograph may reveal an effusion of 50 to 75 mL.

The earliest recognized sign of a pleural effusion on an upright chest radiograph is blunting of the lateral costophrenic angle, which may be seen on either the frontal or the lateral view (Fig. 9.2). With a larger free-flowing effusion, the pleural fluid appears as a meniscus that curves downward toward the mediastinum in the frontal view and appears "lowest" midway through the thoracic cavity on the lateral view (Fig. 9.3). The presence of

BOX 9.2 Examination Findings in Pleural Effusion

- Decreased chest wall excursion
- Bulging intercostal spaces
- Egophony at superior border of effusion
- Diminished breath sounds
- Dullness to percussion
- Decreased tactile fremitus
- Pleural friction rub

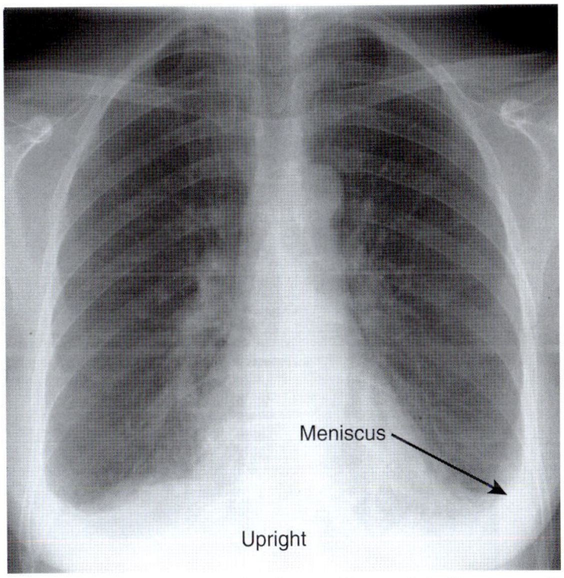

Fig. 9.2 Posteroanterior upright chest radiograph indicating a pleural effusion with a bilateral meniscus *(arrow)* at the costophrenic angles. The pleural effusion has a curvilinear upper margin concave to the lung and is higher laterally than medially.

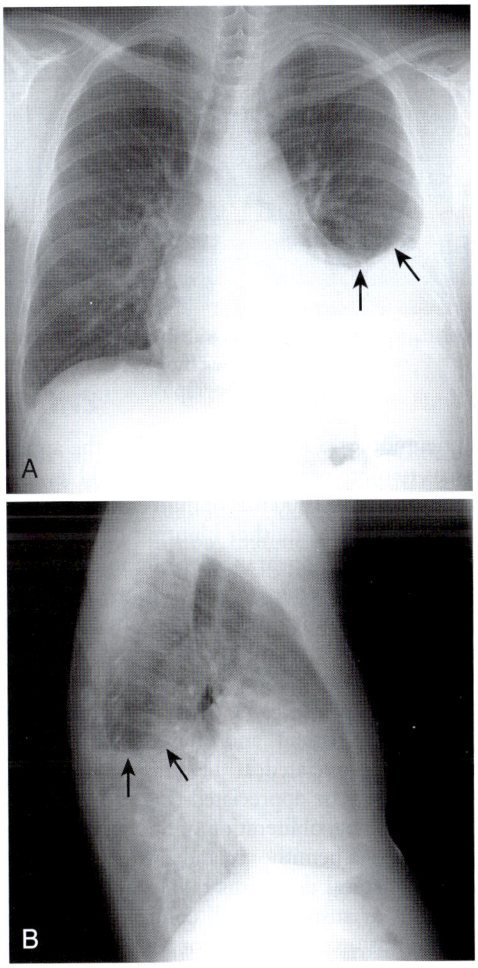

Fig. 9.3 Left-sided pleural effusion seen on (A) posteroanterior and (B) lateral radiographs. The meniscus can be visualized on both views *(arrows)*.

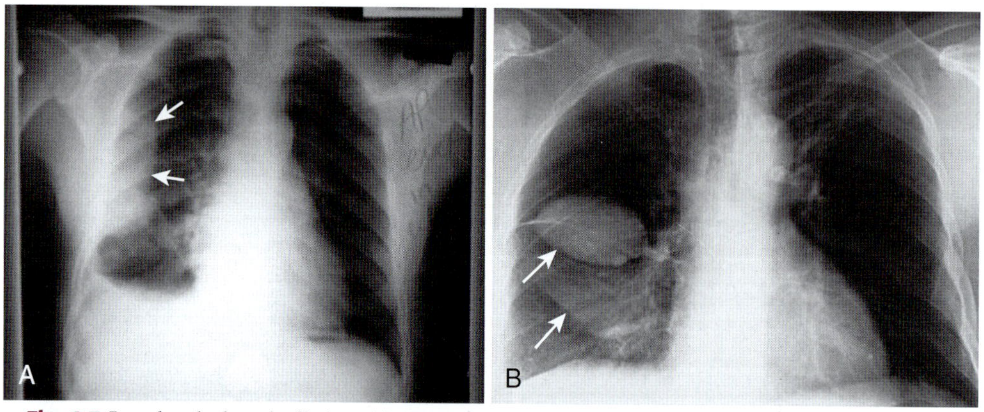

Fig. 9.7 Loculated pleural effusion. (A) A posteroanterior radiograph demonstrates the D-shaped appearance of a right-sided loculated pleural effusion *(arrows)* in the midchest region. (B) Occasionally, pleural effusions *(arrows)* may become loculated in the fissures.

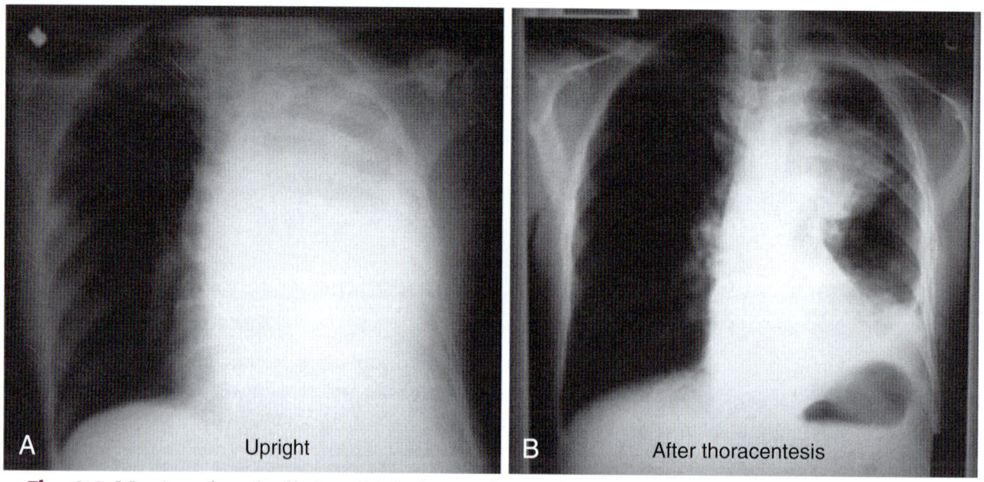

Fig. 9.8 Massive pleural effusion (A) before and (B) after thoracentesis. Notice the underlying mass that is seen following thoracentesis. A computed tomography scan would have prospectively confirmed this radiograph.

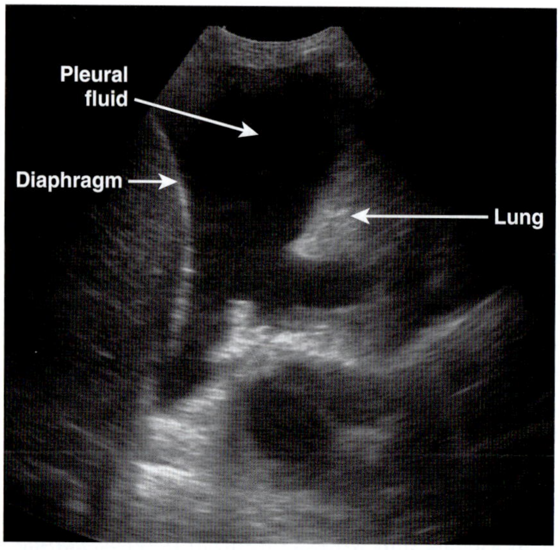

Fig. 9.9 Ultrasound image of a patient with a large right-sided pleural effusion. Note the dark appearance of the pleural effusion with a free-floating lung. Ultrasound is also useful for identifying the diaphragm *(at right)* and the top of the effusion *(at left)*. (From Thomsen T, Setnik G, eds. *Procedures Consult—Emergency Medicine Module*. Elsevier; 2008.)

is another relative contraindication, but the risk associated with these abnormalities can be virtually eliminated with the use of US guidance.[24,26–28] US guidance should also be used for loculated effusions to mitigate the risk of pneumothorax, and in patients undergoing mechanical ventilation because of a theoretical increased risk of tension pneumothorax.

TECHNIQUE

See Videos 9.1 and 9.2. Thoracentesis is usually an elective procedure. Before starting the procedure, obtain and document informed consent according to hospital policy. Follow sterile technique throughout the entire procedure to avoid introduction of infection.

Equipment

The specific device used for thoracentesis depends on the type of procedure, hospital availability, and provider experience. For diagnostic purposes in which a small volume of fluid is being withdrawn, a 2-inch 22-gauge needle for patient with small to normal body habitus or a 22-gauge spinal needle for larger patients can be used. For therapeutic procedures, placing a small French (6–14F) pigtail thoracic drainage catheter via the

Seldinger technique avoids prolonged insertion of a needle in the pleural space while large volumes of fluid are being removed and allows for easier use of real-time US-guided needle placement for a single provider than traditional over-the-needle thoracentesis catheters. The smallest French pigtail catheter available should be used. Commercial over-the-needle thoracentesis catheters have built-in safety features which may include a blunt spring-loaded safety cannula that extends beyond the sharp needle tip once the pleural space is entered to protect the lung from puncture, a one-way valve that prevents air entry into the catheter during removal of the needle, and a built-in side port for drainage of fluid (Fig. 9.10). These over-the-needle catheters, however, require stabilization of the needle with the nondominant hand, eliminating the ability for a single provider to preform real-time US-guided needle placement to enhance patient safety. It is important to familiarize yourself with the features of the pigtail and thoracentesis catheters available in your institution and utilize the most familiar device.

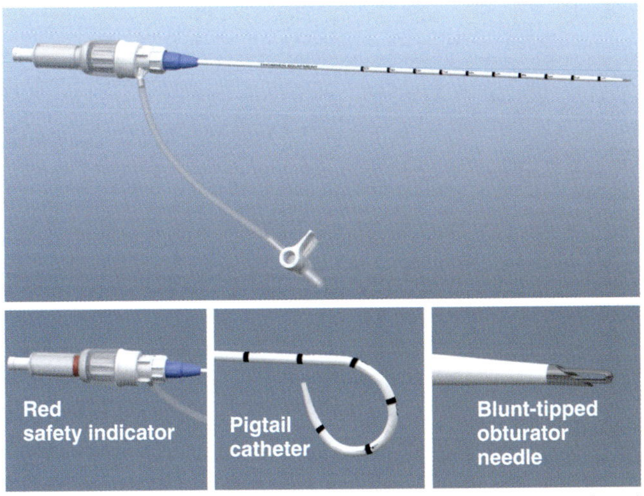

Fig. 9.10 The Safe-T-Centesis needle, which is available in a prepackaged kit. Safety features of this device include a blunt-tipped obturator needle, a color-changing indicator, a pigtail catheter, and an attached three-way valve. The blunt-tipped obturator retracts with pressure, exposing the sharp needle tip. This causes the color in the device to change from white to red. Once the pleural space is entered and there is no longer pressure on the tip, the spring-loaded obturator covers the sharp needle tip, preventing damage to the lung. This will cause the color to revert to white. Devices from other manufacturers have similar features.

Gather all the necessary equipment before the procedure; see Review Box 9.1 for a list of recommended equipment. If the procedure is for diagnostic reasons, remember to draw and send peripheral blood to the laboratory for serum protein and LDH measurement. Keep atropine available at the bedside in case the patient has a vagal reaction during the procedure. Monitor oxygen saturation by pulse oximetry and administer supplemental oxygen as needed.

Patient Position and Site of Entry

Fig. 9.11 illustrates various patient positions for thoracentesis. Upright positioning is desired for draining most pleural effusions. For this position, have the patient sit upright on the edge of the bed with arms extended on a bedside table or Mayo stand (Fig. 9.12). If the effusion is sufficiently large, allow the patient to lean forward slightly. Locate the height of the effusion and the level of the diaphragm using US (Fig. 9.13 and Ultrasound Box). The site of entry should be one to two intercostal spaces below the highest level of the effusion in the posterior axillary line (Fig. 9.14). In all cases, the level of needle entry must be above the ninth rib as the risk for diaphragmatic, hepatic, or splenic injury increases with entry below this level. Needle entry should also be a minimum of 7 cm lateral to the spinous process to avoid risk for arterial injury and hemothorax as the intercostal artery runs more centrally and is tortuous when it first enters the intercostal space at the spine.[29–32] More than 1 cm of fluid thickness should

Thoracentesis

Indications

Suspected pleural space infection
New effusion without a clear clinical diagnosis
Relief of dyspnea associated with a large effusion

Contraindications

Absolute
None
Relative
Severe clotting abnormality
Infection or herpes zoster at selected site

Complications

Pneumothorax	Reexpansion pulmonary edema
Cough	Air embolism
Infection	Catheter fragment in the pleural space
Hemothorax	Intraabdominal hemorrhage

List of equipment:

Bedside ultrasound
Skin cleanser
Sterile drape
Gauze
1% Lidocaine
25-Gauge needle
22-Gauge needle
Two 10-mL syringes
60-mL syringe
Sterile syringe cap
Occlusive dressing
Blood culture bottle

If large volume:
Pigtail or over-the-needle catheter
Collection bag
Three-way stopcock
Scalpel

Review Box 9.1 Thoracentesis: indications, contraindications, complications, and equipment.

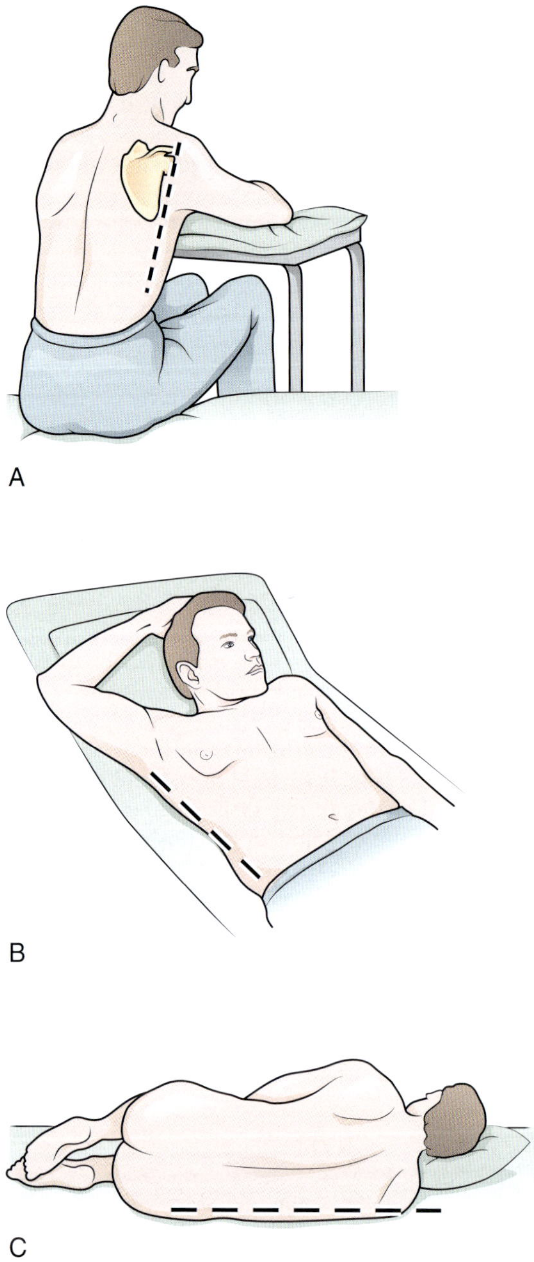

Fig. 9.11 (A–C) Various patient positions for thoracentesis. Note the posterior axillary line when the patient is sitting upright. Thoracentesis should be performed a minimum of 7 cm lateral to the spinous process to decrease risk of trauma to the neurovascular bundle.

be present on US at the selected site. Mark your entry site using a skin marker. If the patient is too ill to sit upright, perform the procedure with the patient supine with the head of bed elevated as much as possible. Alternatively, position the patient in the lateral decubitus position, with the side of the effusion down and the back at the edge of the bed. For both alternative patient positions, the site of entry should be the posterior axillary line. Determine the fluid level and thickness by bedside US and make sure the selected site is above the ninth rib. A time-out should be performed immediately before the procedure to verify the correct patient, procedure, and site.

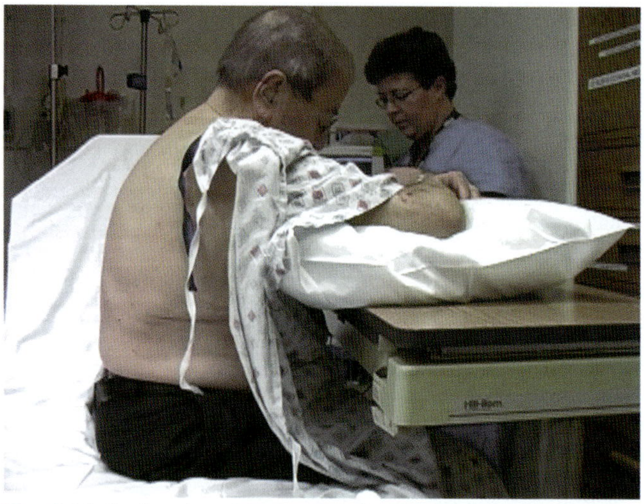

Fig. 9.12 Preferred positioning for thoracentesis by the posterior approach is with the patient sitting upright and leaning over an adjacent Mayo stand.

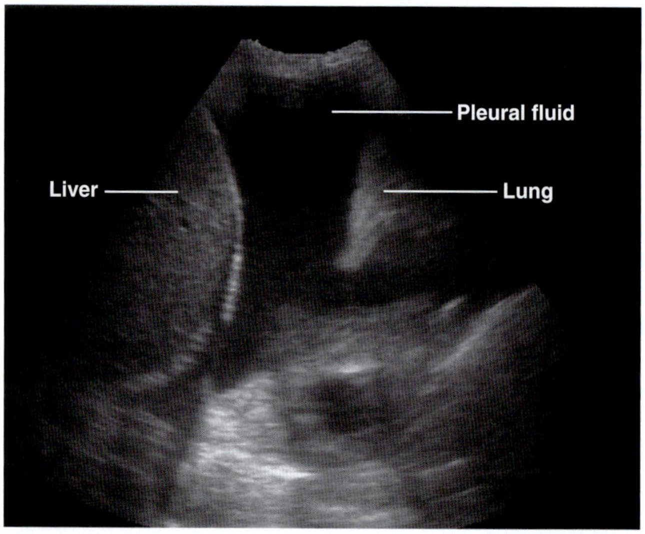

Fig. 9.13 Ultrasound image of a right-sided pleural effusion. Ultrasound can be used during the procedure itself if a sterile probe cover is used. This enables the operator to view the tip of the needle entering the effusion and to thus avoid vital structures such as the lung or diaphragm. Note the superior, inferior, and medial landmarks that are used during the procedure itself.

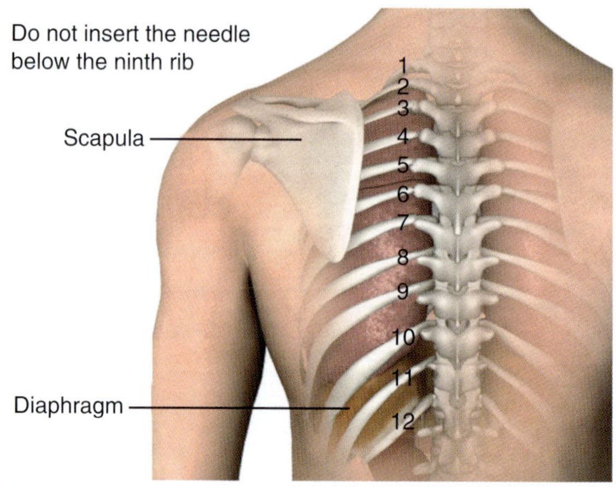

Fig. 9.14 The inferior tip of the scapula is at the seventh rib. Do not insert the thoracentesis needle below the ninth rib. (From Thomsen T, Setnik G, eds. *Procedures Consult—Emergency Medicine Module.* Elsevier Inc. 2008. All rights reserved.)

ULTRASOUND: Thoracentesis

by Christine Butts, MD

Ultrasound is an excellent tool for both identifying and directing the aspiration of pleural effusions. It can be used to "mark the spot" for thoracentesis, screen for intercostal vessels at the aspiration site, and directly guide the procedure.

Equipment

A 3.5- to 5-mHz transducer will reliably identify most pleural effusions. A higher-frequency transducer should be used when direct visualization of the procedure is desired.

Interpretation of Images

A normal lung is filled with air and will typically appear as a hazy gray area when viewed by ultrasound (Fig. 9.US1). Reverberation or comet tail artifacts may also be seen (Fig. 9.US2). When pleural fluid is present, it will typically be seen in the most dependent area of the thorax, typically in the recesses above the diaphragm. Pleural fluid will appear as anechoic (black) collections of varying size (Fig. 9.US3). Depending on the consistency of the fluid, it may appear heterogeneous, with areas of lighter gray representing more solid components (such as clotted blood).

Procedure and Technique

Once a pleural effusion is known or suspected to be present, scan the area over the posterior aspect of the thorax with a low-frequency transducer (Fig. 9.US4). Identifying the abdominal organs (e.g., kidney, liver, spleen) and diaphragm first will often help orient the sonographer (Fig. 9.US5). Assess the recess superior to the diaphragm for the presence and size of the effusion. If the procedure is to be performed blindly, mark a location several rib spaces above the diaphragm to avoid any possible intraabdominal injury. Using color Doppler with probe oriented in the intercostal space, sweep the intercostal space at the selected site looking for flow indicating the presence of an intercostal artery or vein.[33] If flow is present, repeat the above steps to identify a needle insertion site more lateral and perform the color Doppler sweep for intercostal vessels. If there is no evidence for intercostal vessels, the procedure can then proceed in the usual fashion. If the procedure is to be performed under direct ultrasound guidance, cover the high-frequency transducer with a sterile sheath. Once the field has been prepared, use the sterile transducer held in a longitudinal direction at the previously marked site to locate the fluid pocket. At this

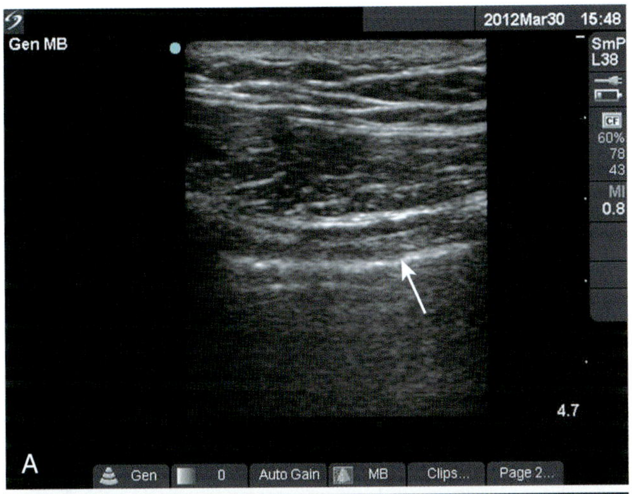

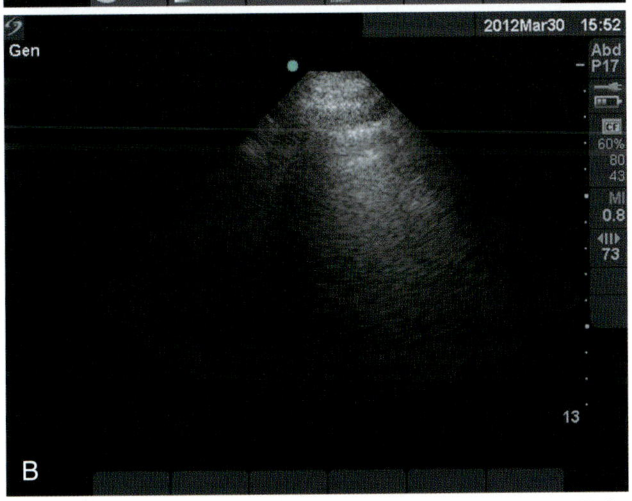

Fig. 9.US1 Ultrasound images of a normal lung. (A) High-frequency image. In this view, the pleura can be seen as a brightly echogenic *(white)* horizontal line deep to the ribs and corresponding rib shadows *(arrow)*. (B) Low frequency. In this image, less of the pleura is visible. However, abnormalities such as effusions may be recognized more easily.

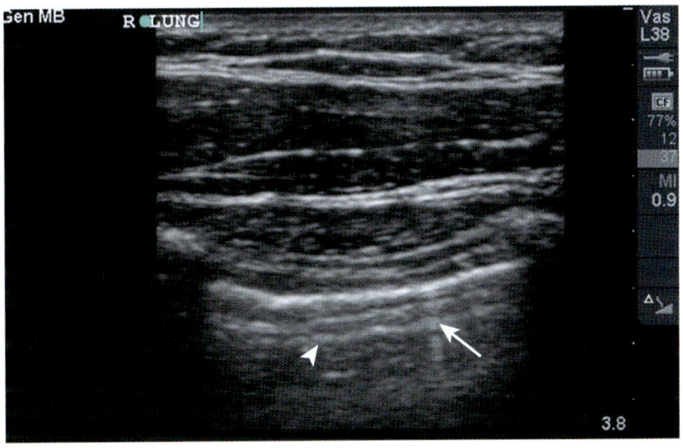

Fig. 9.US2 This image demonstrates two key artifacts seen in a normal lung. As with the previous image, the pleura is recognized as a hyperechoic horizontal line deep to the ribs *(at far right and left)*. A comet tail, or a small vertical line, can be seen extending deep to the pleura *(arrow)*. This is a normal artifact created by the pleura. A-lines, or a series of horizontal lines extending deep to the pleura, can also be seen *(arrowhead)*. These artifacts are created by reverberation and may be seen in a normal aerated lung.

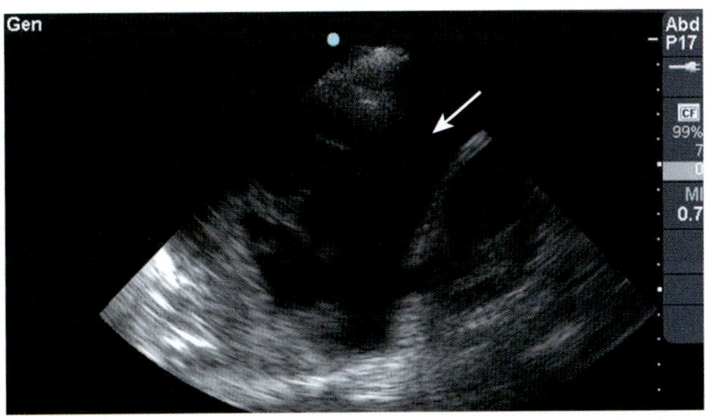

Fig. 9.US3 Large pleural effusion seen on ultrasound with a low-frequency transducer. In this longitudinal image, the thorax is seen on the left side of the image, and a large anechoic *(black)* fluid collection can also be seen *(arrow)*. Within the thorax the lung can be seen as the hypoechoic *(dark gray)* mass on the left of the image.

Continued

ULTRASOUND: Thoracentesis—cont'd

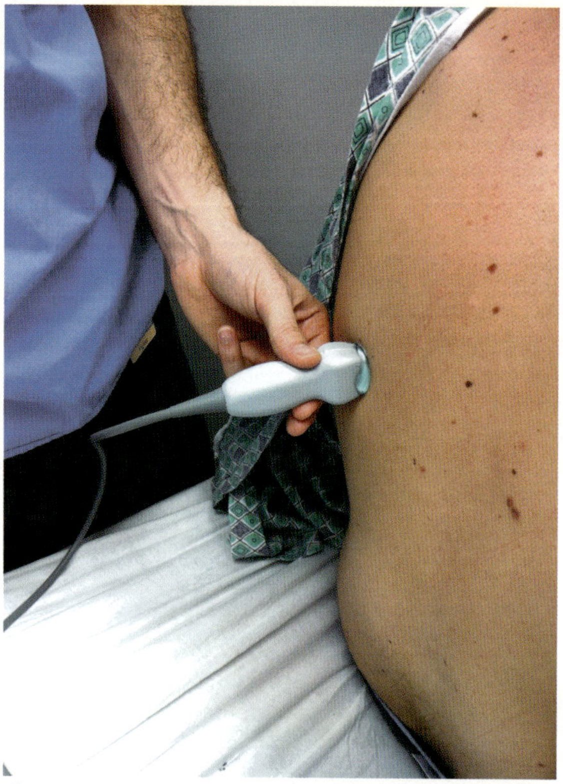

Fig. 9.US4 Placement of the ultrasound transducer over the posterior of the thorax to identify a pleural effusion.

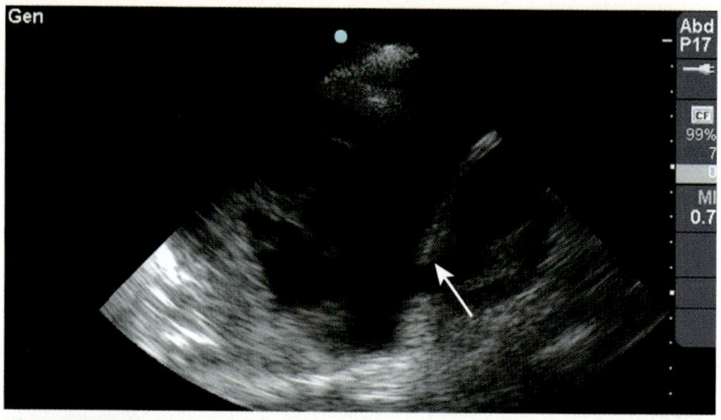

Fig. 9.US5 Longitudinal image of the lower part of the thorax and upper part of the abdomen demonstrating a large pleural effusion. The *bright white* (hyperechoic) *line* arcing over the kidney *(arrow)* is the diaphragm, which is an important landmark in planning the location of aspiration.

time, introduce the needle alongside the center of the transducer and visualize the needle as it enters the pleural space and the effusion (see Chapter 67 for more on direct needle guidance).

Complications

Most complications occur when the sonographer incorrectly interprets the image or the anatomy. Special care should be taken during the initial evaluation to identify the diaphragm and to direct any attempts at aspiration superior to this point to avoid injury to the abdominal cavity. Effusions that are loculated may not be gravity dependent and may be found in varying areas of the thorax.

Anesthesia and Pleural Fluid Localization

Once you have used US to identify and mark the entry site and the skin has been sterilized and draped, create a skin wheal at the upper edge of the rib just below the marked entry site using 1% or 2% lidocaine and a 25-gauge needle. Use the upper edge of the rib as the needle insertion site to minimize accidental trauma to the intercostal artery typically located along the inferior margin of each rib. Next, a 22-gauge needle can be used to anesthetize the deeper tissues. Holding the needle perpendicular to the chest wall will help to avoid inadvertent trauma to the intercostal artery. With each 1 mm to 2 mm of needle advancement, aspirate and then infiltrate the tissues with 1 mL to 2 mL of anesthetic. While the aspiration-infiltration process is continued, "walk" the needle above the superior edge of the rib and advance it through the intercostal space until the pleural space is entered (Fig. 9.15). On entering the pleural space, a pop may be felt. Aspirate fluid to ensure that the pleural space has been reached. Once fluid is aspirated, withdraw the needle slightly and infiltrate a small amount of lidocaine to anesthetize the parietal pleura. Finally, grasp the needle just proximal to the skin with the thumb and index finger and withdraw it. This allows measurement of the proper depth of penetration needed during subsequent needle insertion. If no fluid is encountered (dry tap) in the setting of a free-flowing pleural effusion, the needle is too short or the site chosen is too high or too low. If air bubbles are encountered, the chosen sight is likely too high. For both of these scenarios, as long as the patient has no new symptoms to suggest pneumothorax or intraabdominal injury, reevaluate the fluid level using sterile US guidance and reattempt fluid localization.

Needle Aspiration Technique for Diagnostic Thoracentesis

Once the tissue has been anesthetized and pleural fluid localization has been completed, reenter the pleural space with a 22-gauge needle attached to a 10-mL syringe, using real-time US guidance to visualize the needle entering the pleural space (see Ultrasound box). Once fluid is aspirated, halt advancement of the needle. Stabilizing the needle with the nondominant hand, remove the 10-mL syringe, covering the exposed hub of the needle with your finger to prevent air entry into the pleural space, and replace it with a 60-mL syringe. Aspirate 50 mL of fluid. Once aspiration is complete, instruct the patient to exhale fully, and then withdraw the needle.

Pigtail Thoracic Drainage Catheter Placement

After the tissue is anesthetized, and pleural fluid localization has been completed, insert the guide needle attached to a 10-mL syringe and walk the needle over the rib through the anesthetized area and into the pleural space while applying gentle negative pressure with the syringe. Real-time US guidance should be used to visualize the needle during insertion into the pleural

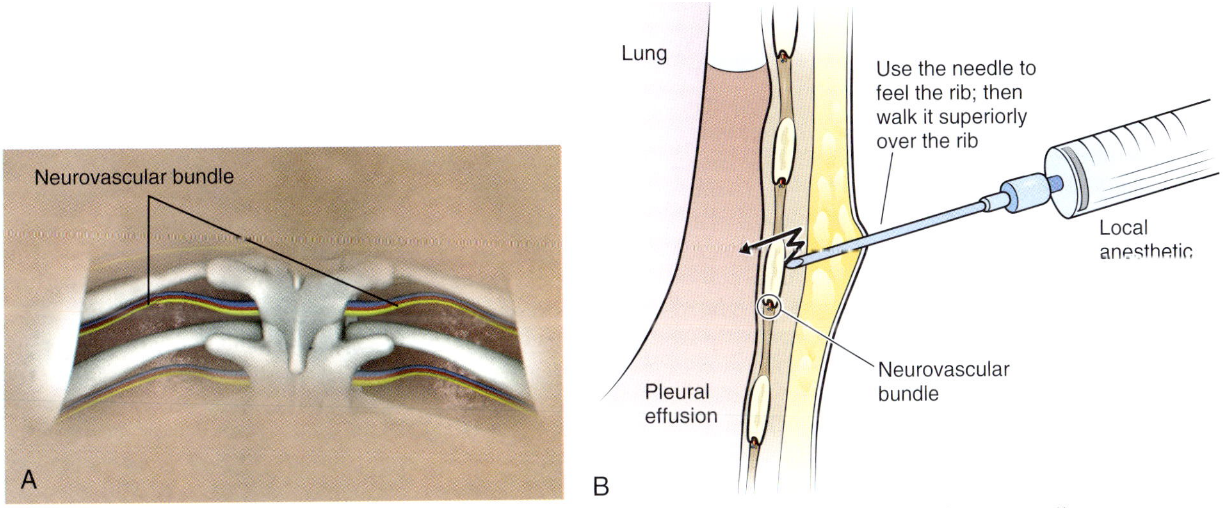

Fig. 9.15 (A) Anatomy of the neurovascular bundle. The intercostal nerve, artery, and vein typically run inferior to the rib. (B) The proper approach mandates walking the needle up and over the rib to avoid these vital structures. (From Thomsen T, Setnik G, eds. *Procedures Consult—Emergency Medicine Module*. Elsevier; 2008.)

space. Once fluid is aspirated, halt advancement of the needle. Stabilizing the needle with the nondominant hand, remove the syringe and cover the exposed hub of the needle with your finger to prevent air entry into the pleural space. Feed the guidewire through the needle and into the pleural space. Remove the needle while stabilizing the guidewire to keep it in the pleural space. While continuing to stabilize the guidewire, thread the dilator over the guidewire and insert it just enough to dilate the soft tissue, then remove it. Depending on the size of the catheter, a small incision in the skin with a No. 11 blade at the base of the wire may be required to allow passage of the catheter through the skin. Thread the catheter over the guidewire and into the pleural space, assuring constant control of the guidewire by holding it at all times. Once inserted fully, remove the guidewire and cover the exposed hub of the catheter with your finger to prevent entry of air into the pleural space. Attach a 3-way stopcock with a 60-mL syringe into the catheter hub. The lever should be closed to the unused stopcock port. Aspirate fluid with the syringe for diagnostic studies, then close the lever to the patient. Now connect the tubing of a sterile collection bag to the stopcock side port. Alternate syringe aspiration with expelling fluid from the syringe, through the tubing, and into the bag. Alternatively, you can use gravity to drain the pleural fluid by placing the tubing-connected sterile collection bag 3 or more feet below the catheter insertion site with the stopcock closed to the syringe which you can then remove. The use of vacuum bottles is controversial with evidence supporting a greater incidence of both complications and patient discomfort with their use and only 3 minutes of time savings over manual syringe aspiration for 1500 mL of fluid removal.[34] Always turn the stopcock lever off to the patient when changing collection devices. Stop the procedure when 1500 mL of fluid is removed or if the patient develops persistent cough, chest pain, or worsening shortness of breath raising concern for complication. The recommended maximum of 1500 mL is to avoid significantly negative pleural pressures, which has been associated with both symptomatic hypovolemia and the potentially fatal complication of reexpansion pulmonary edema.[35,36] Once aspiration is complete, instruct the patient to exhale fully, and then withdraw the catheter.

Over-the-Needle Catheter Insertion Technique for Therapeutic Thoracentesis

There are numerous over-the-needle catheters available, each with varying types and degrees of safety features. Here we will discuss performing the procedure with the most basic needle-catheter. Familiarize yourself with the features present on the device at your institution prior to initiating the procedure.

After anesthetizing the tissue and completing pleural fluid localization, use a scalpel to pierce the skin at the needle insertion site. This will ease the entry of the catheter through the skin. Attach the thoracentesis catheter to a 10-mL syringe. Mark the depth of the pleural space determined from the anesthetic needle by gently grasping the shaft of the needle-catheter unit with the index finger and thumb of the nondominant hand. This stabilizes the device and controls the advance. Walk the needle-catheter unit over the rib through the anesthetized area and into the pleural space while applying gentle negative pressure with the syringe. When fluid is encountered, angle the needle-catheter unit slightly caudally. While holding the needle steady, twist the catheter to break its seal and advance it into the pleural space. Withdraw the needle and immediately cover the exposed hub of the catheter with your finger to prevent air entry into the pleural space if the commercial device does not have a self-sealing valve feature. Next, attach a three-way stopcock with 60-mL syringe into the catheter hub. The lever should be closed to the unused stopcock port. Aspirate fluid with the syringe for diagnostic studies, then close the lever to the patient. Now connect the tubing of a sterile collection bag to the stopcock side port. Alternate syringe aspiration with expelling fluid from the syringe, through the tubing, and into the bag. Alternatively, you can use gravity to drain the pleural fluid by placing the tubing-connected sterile collection bag 3 or more feet below the catheter insertion site with the stopcock closed to the syringe which you can then remove. The use of vacuum bottles is controversial with evidence supporting a greater incidence of both complications and patient discomfort with their use and only 3 minutes of time savings over manual syringe aspiration for 1500 mL of fluid removal.[34] Turn the stopcock lever off to the patient when changing collection devices. Stop the procedure when 1500 mL of fluid is removed or if the patient develops persistent cough, chest pain, or worsening shortness of breath raising concern for complication. The recommended maximum of 1500 mL is to avoid significantly negative pleural pressures, which have been associated with both symptomatic hypovolemia and the potentially fatal complication of reexpansion pulmonary edema.[35,36] Once aspiration is complete, instruct the patient to exhale fully, and then withdraw the catheter. Commercial thoracentesis catheters with safety features can simplify the procedure. Most have a self-sealing valve that obviates the need to cover the catheter hub with your finger as the needle is removed, and a built-in side port that allows fluid collection without a three-way stopcock (see Fig. 9.10).

PEDIATRIC PATIENTS

The indications for and contraindications to performing thoracentesis are much the same in children as in adults. Positioning is similar but will likely require an assistant to hold the patient and prevent movement. Sedation may be helpful when respiratory distress is minimal. Determine the effusion level by examination and bedside US. Make sure that the needle insertion site is not lower than the ninth rib. The smallest possible needle, pigtail catheter, or over-the-needle catheter device is recommended.

POSTPROCEDURE EVALUATION

Routine chest radiography or lung US should be reserved for patients who have new symptoms during thoracentesis that do not resolve upon completion of the procedure or if the procedure was difficult, required multiple needle passes, or resulted in aspiration of air.[37,38] Notably, the postprocedure radiograph rarely shows new findings that aid in identifying the cause of the effusion, such as an underlying mass or infiltrate[39] (Fig. 9.16).

PLEURAL FLUID ANALYSIS

Pleural fluid should be analyzed in an organized and thoughtful manner based on clinical suspicion for a disease process. In all cases send fluid for LDH, protein, glucose, differential cell count, Gram stain and culture, and cytology.[38] Many laboratories are comfortable performing all required tests from the initial 60-mL syringe, so dividing the specimens into individual tubes at the bedside is often unnecessary. Analyze the fluid within 4 hours when possible, but results remain accurate for much longer if the sample is refrigerated at 4°C.[40] Exceptions include using an anticoagulant-containing tube (e.g., lavender top) for differential cell count to prevent clumping of cells, inoculating aerobic and anaerobic blood culture bottles in addition to standard fluid culture to increase the yield of identifiable organisms, and transferring samples for pleural fluid pH immediately to a blood gas syringe, placing it on ice, and analyzing it within 1 hour to prevent falsely high pH measurements.[41] Because of differences in laboratory preference, consult your individual laboratory for its policies on specimen collection and delivery.

Visual Inspection

Identifying a cause based on pleural fluid appearance alone is inaccurate, but certain findings are suggestive. The presence of blood suggests trauma, malignancy, pulmonary infarction, or pneumonia. White or milky fluid suggests the presence of lipids. Purulent, malodorous fluid indicates empyema. Pleural effusion containing food particles is highly suggestive of esophageal rupture.

Distinguishing Transudate From Exudate: Light's Criteria

The first step in the evaluation of pleural fluid is the categorization of the fluid as exudative or transudative. Exudates are caused by pleural inflammation, increased pleural membrane permeability, or lymphatic obstruction and therefore contain high levels of LDH and protein. Light and colleagues

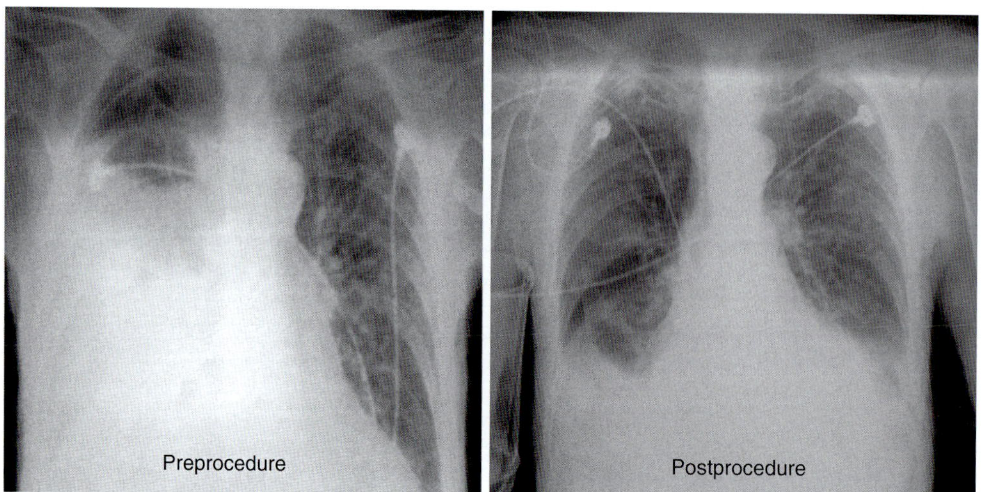

Fig. 9.16 Chest radiographs before and after thoracentesis. Postprocedure films are not always routine but should be performed if air was aspirated during drainage or in patients who are at risk for adhesions, have new symptoms during thoracentesis that do not resolve upon completion of the procedure, require multiple needle passes, or are mechanically ventilated.

published criteria for distinguishing transudates from exudates in 1972 based on measurements of serum and pleural fluid protein and LDH.[42] The value for LDH was subsequently changed to accommodate variations in assay conditions. These criteria have since become known as Light's criteria (Box 9.3). Because Light's criteria have very high sensitivity but lower specificity, it may misclassify up to 25% of transudates. An exception to using Light's criteria for differentiating transudates from exudates is in the setting of diuretic-treated CHF, as diuretic use has been shown to increase pleural fluid protein and LDH concentrations, thus making the transudative fluid appear exudative by Light's criteria. Other criteria for differentiating exudate from transudate should be used in this setting (Box 9.4).[4,43,44]

Once the fluid is classified as transudative, no further fluid analysis is required, and therapy is directed at the underlying cause of the effusion (e.g., CHF, cirrhosis, nephrotic syndrome).

The presence of an undifferentiated exudative effusion, however, requires more extensive fluid evaluation.

Evaluation of Exudates

For all undifferentiated exudates, pleural fluid evaluation should include differential cell count, glucose, Gram stain and culture, and cytologic examination at a minimum (Table 9.1). Add pleural fluid hematocrit if the fluid appears bloody. Add pleural fluid pH for all parapneumonic effusions or when pleural infection is suspected. Clinical suspicion for an underlying disease process should guide additional fluid assessment.

Differential Cell Count

Exudates typically have a pleural fluid white blood cell count greater than 1000 cells/mm^3, and counts may reach levels higher than 100,000 cells mm^3, most commonly with parapneumonic effusions. The differential cell count can be useful in identifying the cause of an exudative effusion. A predominance of neutrophils indicates an acute process, such as pneumonia or pulmonary infarction. A predominance of lymphocytes is consistent with a more chronic pleural process, such as malignancy or TB. Eosinophil counts greater than 10% often have no clear etiology but have traditionally been associated with blood or air in the pleural space.

BOX 9.3 Transudate Versus Exudate: Light's Criteria

If at least one of the following three criteria is present, the fluid is virtually always an exudate; if none is present, the fluid is virtually always a transudate:

- Pleural fluid: serum protein ratio >0.5
- Pleural fluid lactate LDH level greater than two-thirds the upper limit of the serum reference range
- Pleural fluid: serum LDH ratio >0.6

LDH, *Lactate dehydrogenase.*

BOX 9.4 Separating Exudate From Transudate in the Diuretic-Treated CHF Patient

The effusion is likely a transudate if one of the following is present:

- Serum albumin minus pleural albumin >1.2 g/dL
- Pleural fluid N-terminal pro-brain natriuretic peptide >1500 pg/mL

CHF, *Congestive heart failure.*

Glucose

The concentration of glucose in exudates is extremely variable and, in general, does not correlate with any specific disease process. Routine measurement of pleural fluid glucose for exudative effusions is recommended because a low glucose concentration (<60 mg/dL) narrows the differential diagnosis to complicated parapneumonic effusion, malignancy, TB, rheumatoid effusion, and the uncommonly seen paragonimiasis or eosinophilic granulomatosis with polyangiitis.[1] Keep in mind, however, that these diagnoses are not excluded by a high or normal pleural fluid glucose.

Culture

If bacterial infection is a consideration, culture the pleural fluid by both bedside inoculation of blood culture bottles and standard laboratory culture. The addition of blood culture bottles increases the overall yield of identifiable pathogens in parapneumonic effusions by 20%, from a baseline of 40% yield with standard laboratory culture alone.[45] As little as 2 mL of fluid can be used in each bottle without affecting the results.

Cytology

Perform cytologic analysis on all undiagnosed effusions or when malignancy is suspected. The sensitivity for diagnosing pleural malignancy hovers at approximately 55%, regardless of whether small or large (>50 mL) volumes are analyzed.[46]

Pleural Fluid Hematocrit

In general, the presence or absence of red blood cells is not useful in determining the cause of effusion and it takes only a small amount of blood to impart a blood-tinged appearance. A grossly bloody effusion is suggestive of trauma, malignancy, or pulmonary infarction. A pleural fluid hematocrit of greater than 50% of the peripheral hematocrit is indicative of hemothorax and often requires tube thoracostomy.

Pleural Fluid pH

A pleural fluid pH <7.30 indicates pleural inflammation which can be seen in myriad conditions. Pleural fluid pH should be sent in all cases of parapneumonic effusion (see following section) to determine if the effusion is complicated requiring further therapeutic intervention (see "Complications").

Parapneumonic Effusion

Patients with suspected parapneumonic effusions warrant rapid evaluation and outcome risk assessment based on pleural anatomy, pleural fluid bacteriology, and pleural fluid chemistry.[47] All patients with parapneumonic effusions require at least diagnostic thoracentesis with the goal of identifying those with complicated parapneumonic effusions. Indications for tube thoracostomy or other surgical procedure include

TABLE 9.1 Exudates: Evaluation of an Undiagnosed Exudative Effusion

PLEURAL FLUID ASSAY	RESULT	PROBABLE DIAGNOSIS (DIFFERENTIAL DIAGNOSIS)
Standard Testing: Perform on All Exudative Effusions		
Differential Cell Count		
WBC count	>10,000 cells/mm^3	Parapneumonic effusion (pancreatitis, collagen vascular disease)
Neutrophils	>50%	Acute pleural process (infection, PE)
Lymphocytes	>50%	Chronic pleural process (malignancy, chronic TB)
Eosinophils	>10%	Air or blood in the pleural space (numerous other causes)
Cytology	Abnormal cells	Malignancy
Glucose	<60 mg/dL	Complicated parapneumonic effusion, (malignancy, TB, rheumatoid arthritis eosinophilic granulomatosis with polyangiitis, paragnomiasis)
Gram stain and culture	Presence of organism	Pleural space infection
Selective Testing: Order if High Clinical Suspicion for Diagnosis		
Adenosine deaminase[a]	>40 IU/L	TB (lymphoma, empyema)
Albumin	Serum albumin-pleural albumin >1.2 g/L	Congestive heart failure if diuretic treated
Amylase	Pleural fluid amylase >serum amylase	Pancreatitis, esophageal rupture, malignancy
Cholesterol	>45 mg/dL	Exudative effusions (inaccurate alone)
Creatinine (with serum measurement)[b]	Pleural fluid creatinine >serum creatinine	Urinothorax
N-terminal pro–brain natriuretic peptide[c]	≥1500 pg/mL	Congestive heart failure
pH	<7.2	Complicated parapneumonic effusion (collagen vascular disease, esophageal rupture, malignancy, TB)
Pleural fluid hematocrit	>50% of peripheral hematocrit	Hemothorax (trauma, malignancy, PE)
Triglycerides[d]	>110 mg/dL (>50 if fasting or malnourished)	Chylothorax (intrathoracic TPN infusion)

[a]Porcel JM, Esquerda A, Bielsa S. Diagnostic performance of adenosine deaminase activity in pleural fluid: a single-center experience with over 2100 consecutive patients. *Eur J Intern Med*. 2010;21(5):419-423; Light RW. Update on tuberculous pleural effusion. *Respirology* 2010;15(3):451-458.
[b]Garcia-Pachon E, Padilla-Navas I. Urinothorax. Case report and review of the literature with emphasis on biochemical diagnosis. *Respiration* 2004;71:533-536.
[c]Porcel JM. Utilization of B-type natriuretic peptide and NT-proBNP in the diagnosis of pleural effusions due to heart failure. *Curr Opin Pulm Med*. 2011;17(4):215-219.
[d]Maldonado F, Hawkins FJ, Daniels CE et al. Pleural fluid characteristics of chylothorax. *Mayo Clin Proc*. 2009;84(2):129-133.
PE, Pulmonary embolism; *TB*, tuberculosis; *TPN*, total parenteral nutrition; *WBC*, white blood cell.

large or loculated effusions, pleural thickening on CT, aspiration of frank pus (empyema), positive Gram stain or culture, pleural fluid pH <7.20, pleural fluid glucose <40 mg/dL, and pleural fluid LDH >1000 IU/L (Box 9.5).[48]

COMPLICATIONS

Pneumothorax

Pneumothorax is the most frequently reported complication of thoracentesis. US guidance has been shown to decrease this complication rate from approximately 6% to 1%.[20,21,23,49] Procedure and patient-related factors that appear to contribute to pneumothorax include an inexperienced operator, lack of US use, multiple needle attempts, >1500 mL fluid removal, and a low BMI.[22,23,50] Recent studies show no increased risk in patients who are mechanically ventilated.[22]

Pneumothorax Ex Vacuo

Pneumothorax ex vacuo is a form of pneumothorax that occurs when the lung is unable to reexpand during therapeutic thoracentesis due to the presence of an endobronchial lesion or other structural pathology.[51] Negative pleural pressures created in this scenario cause a transient passage of air from the lung to the pleural space. It is a likely explanation for pneumothorax occurring after a seemingly uncomplicated therapeutic thoracentesis.

BOX 9.5 Indications for Surgical Management of Parapneumonic Effusions

Effusion >50% of the hemithorax
Loculated effusion
Pleural thickening seen on a computed tomography scan
Aspiration of frank pus (empyema)
Positive Gram stain or culture of pleural fluid
Pleural fluid pH <7.2
Pleural fluid glucose <40 mg/dL
Pleural fluid LDH >1000 IU/L

LDH, *lactate dehydrogenase.*

Cough

Cough is typically considered a minor complication that results only in patient discomfort, though it can be a harbinger of a pneumothorax or reexpansion pulmonary edema. Terminate the procedure if persistent coughing occurs.

Uncommon Serious Complications

Less common, but serious complications include hemothorax, splenic rupture, abdominal hemorrhage, unilateral pulmonary edema, infection, air embolism, and fragmentation of the catheter in the pleural space.

Hemothorax is typically caused by intercostal artery laceration. It should be suspected with rapid reaccumulation of pleural fluid or by a change in the patient's vital signs during or after the procedure. The risk of hemothorax is decreased by using US to scan the intercostal space, choosing a lateral insertion site, and inserting the needle directly above the rib.[31,52] Other causes include laceration of the lung, diaphragmatic, or internal mammary vessels. Hemothorax requires immediate surgical consultation, thoracostomy tube placement, and close monitoring of hemodynamics with resuscitation as needed.

Puncture of the spleen or liver through the diaphragm may result in a localized organ hematoma or, more seriously, hemoperitoneum. Clinically, this is suspected when the needle pass does not yield fluid (dry tap) and is followed by the patient's complaint of abdominal pain. If this diagnosis is suspected, appropriate resuscitation is the initial treatment, followed by abdominal CT imaging with contrast, when possible. If the patient is hemodynamically unstable, obtain bedside FAST (focused assessment with sonography) US and immediate surgical consultation.

Reexpansion pulmonary edema is a complication associated with rapid reexpansion of the lung and negative pleural pressures during thoracentesis. Symptoms include dyspnea, tachypnea, tachycardia, cough, and frothy sputum. It is believed that this problem can be avoided by discontinuing the procedure when pleural pressure is greater than −20 mm Hg, which is unlikely to occur until after 1500 mL of fluid has been acutely removed.[35,36] As pleural pressure is rarely measured in the ED, 1500 mL of fluid is considered to be the maximum amount that can be safely withdrawn at one time.

REFERENCES ARE AVAILABLE AT Elsevier eBooks+

CHAPTER 10

Tube Thoracostomy

Asa Matthew Margolis and Thomas D. Kirsch

Tube thoracostomy is used to evacuate an abnormal accumulation of fluid or air from the pleural space and can be performed on an elective, urgent, or emergent basis. Abnormal accumulations can result from a spontaneous or traumatic pneumothorax, traumatic hemothorax, malignancy, infection (empyema), or lymph (chylothorax). The first modern methods to evacuate the contents of the pleural space were developed in the 19th century, but these techniques did not become widespread until 1918 when they were used to treat postinfluenza empyema. Military experience demonstrated that thoracic drainage combined with antiseptics and antibiotics reduced mortality related to thoracic trauma from 62.5% during the Civil War to 24.6% in World War I and 12% in World War II.[1]

PATHOPHYSIOLOGY

The lung is surrounded by two layers, the parietal pleura, which lines the interior of the chest wall, and the visceral pleura, which covers the lungs. The potential space between is the *pleural space*, which usually contains a thin layer of lubricating fluid. A small negative pressure within the pleural space helps keep the lung inflated and the two layers closely apposed. With inspiration, chest expansion increases negative intrathoracic pressure and leads to lung inflation. If the pleural space is disrupted air, blood, or other fluid can accumulate between the two layers of the pleura. The result is that the pressure gradient associated with normal respiration is compromised and can lead to the "collapse" of the lung. As the amount of fluid or air increases respiratory function worsens leading to symptoms of dyspnea, often with pleuritic chest pain and anxiety. The degree of respiratory compromise depends on the volume of fluid or air in the pleural space, the patient's age, baseline pulmonary status, and the integrity of the chest wall. The hallmark of tension physiology is impaired ventricular filling and subsequent decrease in cardiac output manifesting as hypotension and reduced ventilation, leading to obstructive shock and cardiovascular collapse, if untreated. This is due to a progressive accumulation of air or fluid in the pleural space, ultimately leading to a mass effect on intrathoracic structures, including heart compression.

Pneumothorax

A pneumothorax is the presence of air in the pleural space and results in the loss of the normal negative pressure (Fig. 10.1). Air can enter the pleural space from outside of the chest wall from a penetrating injury ("open pneumothorax") or internally from a ruptured lung bleb, rib fracture, or damaged trachea ("closed pneumothorax"). Iatrogenic injuries from needle procedures such as subclavian venous cannulation, transthoracic biopsy, thoracentesis, or noninvasive procedures such as positive pressure ventilation (PPV) or cardiopulmonary resuscitation can also cause pneumothoraces (Fig. 10.2).

Spontaneous (Closed) Pneumothorax

Spontaneous pneumothorax is caused by the rupture of a subpleural lung bleb with little or no trauma. It can be categorized as either primary or secondary based on underlying lung disease. *Primary spontaneous pneumothorax* (PSP) occurs in young people without overt lung disease. The typical patient with a PSP is a tall, thin, 20- to 40-year-old male smoker (Fig. 10.3). *Secondary spontaneous pneumothoraces* (SSPs) occur in patients with underlying lung or pleural disease including emphysema, chronic bronchitis, asthma, Marfan's syndrome, infection, and neoplasm. SSPs are more common than PSPs. Additionally, the morbidity, mortality, and long-term complications associated with pneumothorax are increased in patients with underlying lung disease.[2,3] Rarely, spontaneous pneumothorax may be bilateral, and even more uncommon, a spontaneous pneumothorax may progress to tension pneumothorax resulting in a potentially life-threatening condition. PSPs may be managed by selective observation with or without oxygen therapy, or aspirated. SSPs usually require a tube or catheter (e.g., pigtail) thoracostomy.

Patients who have had one spontaneous pneumothorax have a 30% to 50% chance of recurrence within 2 years, and after the second pneumothorax, there is a 50% to 80% chance of developing a third.

Traumatic Closed Pneumothorax

A traumatic closed pneumothorax usually occurs from a rib fracture that penetrates the lung but can also occur when an alveolus or bleb ruptures after blunt trauma or from an iatrogenic procedure. The air leak from a closed pneumothorax is generally self-limited but can, in rare cases, progress to a tension pneumothorax. A pneumothorax may also develop in patients with asthma or emphysema from the high pressure required for ventilation, which could lead to a tension pneumothorax.

Traumatic Open Pneumothorax

An open pneumothorax occurs when the chest wall is penetrated and the negative intrapleural pressure is lost. Each breath can increase intrapleural pressure especially if the diameter of the chest wound is greater than the diameter of the trachea. With each respiration, air moves preferentially through the chest wall opening rather than down the trachea, limiting meaningful ventilation of the involved lung.

Tension Pneumothorax

An open pneumothorax can occasionally manifest as a tension pneumothorax, a life-threatening condition requiring immediate intervention. A tension pneumothorax occurs when an injury creates a one-way "flap valve" in the chest wall that allows air into the pleural space with inspiration but then closes with expiration and traps the air (Fig. 10.4). The progressive accumulation of air in the pleural space leads to ipsilateral complete lung collapse and then impingement on the mediastinum with a shift of the heart toward the uninvolved side. This restricts ventricular filling and subsequently decreases cardiac output. The severe disruption in respiratory and cardiac function can lead to hypotension and reduced oxygenation (hypoxia) and ventilation (CO_2 retention) and eventually to cardiopulmonary collapse.

A tension pneumothorax is usually caused by penetrating chest injuries but can also result from a fracture of the trachea or bronchi, a ruptured esophagus, the presence of a

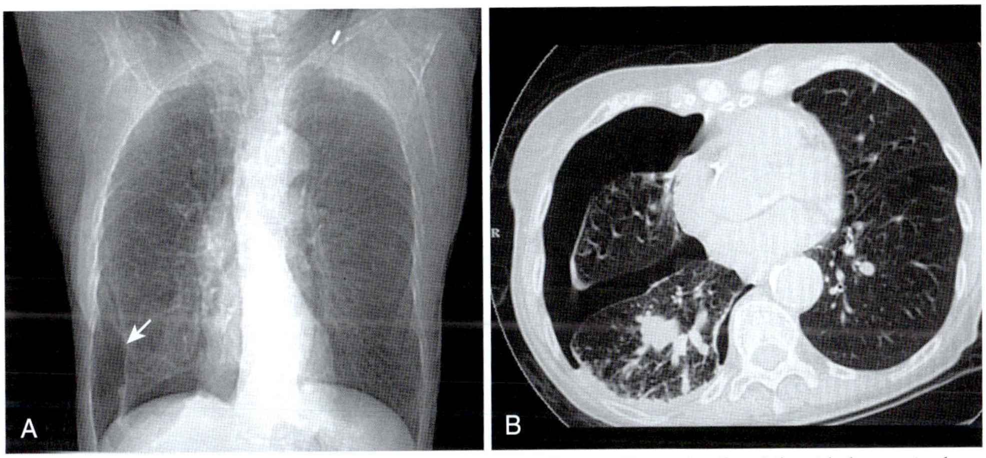

Fig. 10.1 Pneumothorax (PTX). (A) Anteroposterior chest radiograph of a right-sided, seemingly small, simple PTX. Note the absence of peripheral lung markings on the right side and the distinct line indicating the edge of the collapsed lung *(arrow)*. Although this appears to be a small PTX, it produced significant dyspnea in this patient with chronic obstructive pulmonary disease and required a chest tube. (B) Computed tomography scan showing the extent of the collapse. Adhesions kept part of the lung expanded.

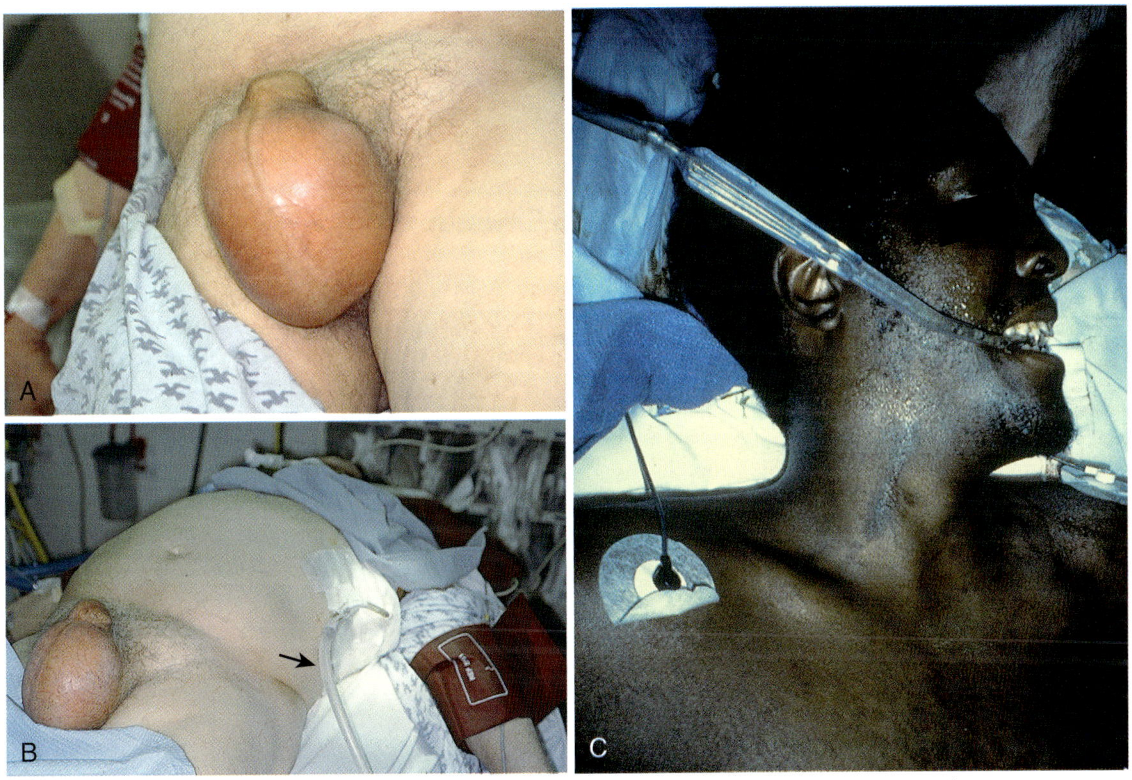

Fig. 10.2 (A) After successful cardiopulmonary resuscitation and intubation, this patient began to deteriorate, with a precipitous drop in blood pressure and decreasing oxygen saturation. Marked subcutaneous air was noted in the scrotum and abdominal wall, but there was little air in the chest wall tissue. The subcutaneous air from a pneumothorax and positive pressure ventilations created by the resuscitation had curiously tracked via abdominal wall tissue planes, a distinctly unusual place for air to accumulate. Usually, subcutaneous air is felt around the chest tube insertion site, neck, and chest wall. (B) A chest tube *(arrow)* quickly reversed the decompensation from the pneumothorax. (C) This patient experienced respiratory arrest from heroin injected into a neck vein (note the extensive scar). After bag-mask resuscitation, the respiratory depression returned, and the blood pressure dropped precipitously. He was unresponsive to naloxone and was very difficult to ventilate. He had a small pneumothorax from a nick in the lung from the neck injection. The positive pressure ventilations produced a tension pneumothorax.

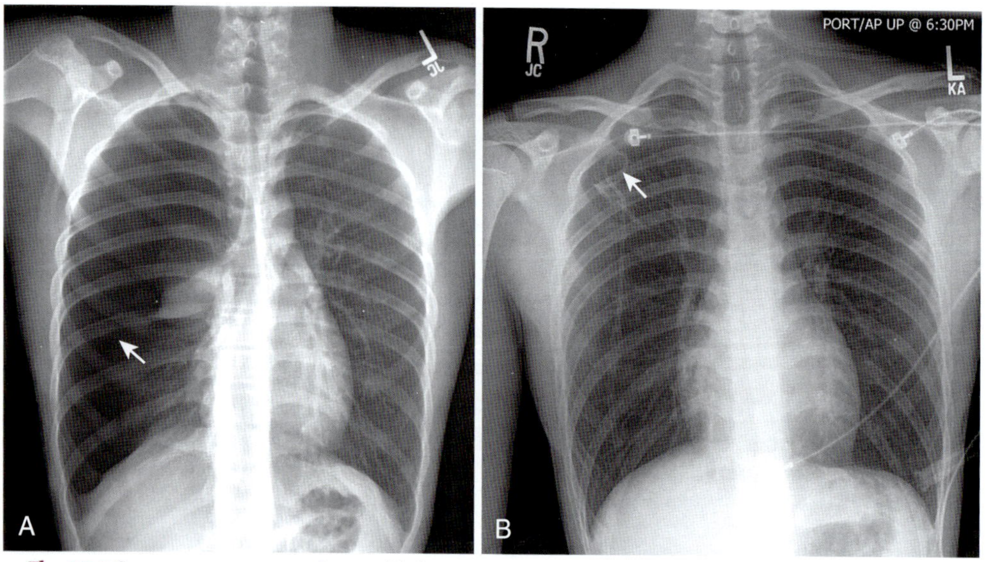

Fig. 10.3 Spontaneous pneumothorax. (A) Spontaneous pneumothorax in a young male patient. There is a nearly total collapse of the right lung, and lung markings are absent lateral to the visible pleural reflection *(arrow)*. Note also the slight deviation of the mediastinum to the contralateral side. (B) The patient was treated with a pigtail catheter inserted in the second intercostal space in the midclavicular line *(arrow)*. Note that the lung has reexpanded, and the mediastinum has shifted back to the midline.

dressing over an open pneumothorax, and PPV. Patients with chest or lung injuries treated with PPV are at much greater risk for developing a tension pneumothorax. Consequently, any patient with a penetrating thoracic injury (even without immediate evidence of a hemothorax or pneumothorax) should be considered for a chest tube before mechanical ventilation.

Hemothorax

Hemothorax is an accumulation of blood in the pleural space caused by an injury to the heart, great vessels, vessels of the lungs, mediastinum, or chest wall. Bleeding from the lung parenchyma is usually low pressure, self-limited, and ceases with the insertion of a chest tube. However, bleeding from an intercostal artery, a pulmonary artery, or the internal mammary artery can be profuse and potentially require surgical intervention.

Empyemas and Effusions

An empyema is an accumulation of pus in the pleural space, usually from a parapneumonic infectious effusion (Fig. 10.5). An empyema can also be caused by violation of the thoracic space during surgical procedures (e.g., tube thoracostomy), trauma, and esophageal perforation. The microbiology of complicated pleural effusions and empyema varies with the source of infection, route of acquisition, local epidemiology, site of acquisition (community vs. hospital-acquired), and patient-specific risk factors. Parapneumonic pleural space infections typically result as complications of community-acquired pneumonia or aspiration pneumonia. Those associated with community-acquired pneumonia tend to be caused by the pyogenic bacteria that cause community-acquired pneumonia (e.g., *Streptococcus pneumonia* and *Staphylococcus aureus*). In contrast, those associated with aspiration pneumonia tend to be polymicrobial and caused by oral streptococci and anaerobes. The list of pathogens associated with nonparapneumonic pleural space infections is more extensive and varies by source.[4,5]

Chylothorax

Chylothorax results from injury to the thoracic duct during central line placement, operative injury, or chest trauma. Primary thoracic duct injury is usually asymptomatic because the chyle initially collects extrapleurally and may not begin to fill the pleural cavity for 2 to 10 days. As the fluid accumulates, respiratory symptoms slowly develop. The chest radiograph or ultrasound demonstrates a pleural effusion and the diagnosis is made when thoracentesis reveals a milky fluid with a high fat and lymphocyte content and 4 to 5 g/dL of protein. Definitive treatment is either repeated thoracentesis or tube thoracostomy combined with parenteral alimentation until the volume of chyle decreases.

DIAGNOSIS

Symptoms

The symptoms of patients with abnormal collections in the pleural space range widely depending on the size of the pneumothorax, the rapidity of accumulation, the patient's age, and the presence of comorbidities, especially underlying lung disease. Specific symptoms range from mild dyspnea with exertion and pleuritic chest pain to hypotension or severe dyspnea, especially in those patients with tension pneumothorax. The signs and symptoms do not always correlate well with the size or cause of the collapsed lung or the amount of fluid in the pleural space. With a spontaneous pneumothorax, patients can complain of the sudden onset of sharp, pleuritic chest pain, shoulder pain, or both. Sixty percent of patients experience dyspnea, and 12% have a mild cough. Dyspnea and anxiety are more common in older patients.

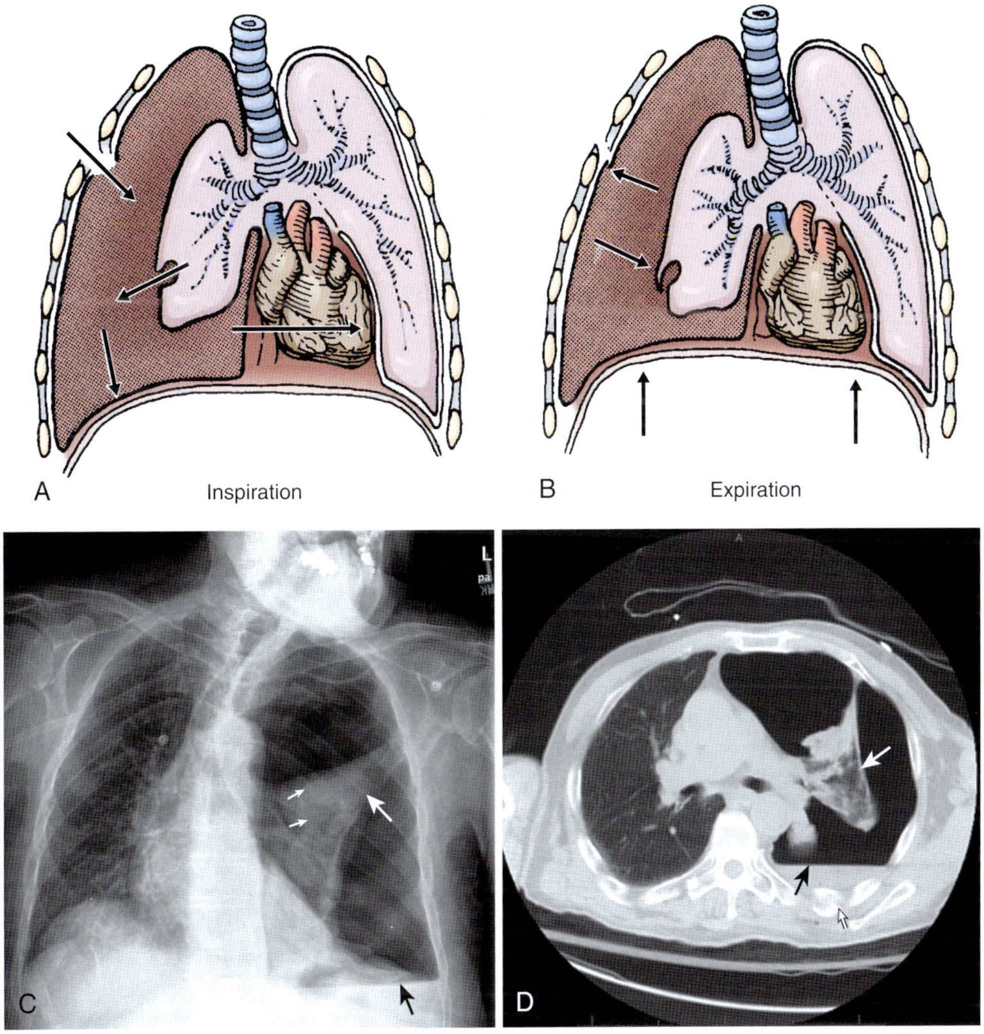

Fig. 10.4 Traumatic tension pneumothorax. (A–B) Pathophysiology of a tension pneumothorax. During inspiration, air enters the pleural space through a one-way valve either from the outside or the lung itself. The injury/valve closes on expiration, trapping an increasing air volume in the pleural space. Eventually, the mediastinum shifts, compromising cardiac filling and, ultimately, cardiac output. (C) This elderly patient sustained a tension hemopneumothorax after slipping and falling on ice. The left hemithorax is very dark (radiolucent) because of the total collapse of the left lung *(large white arrow)*. Note the dramatic shift of the mediastinum to the right, indicative of tension. Multiple posterior rib fractures are present but are difficult to appreciate on this film *(small white arrows)*. The air-fluid level *(black arrow)* indicates the presence of air in addition to fluid (blood) in the pleural cavity. (D) Computed tomography scan of the same patient.

Tension pneumothorax must be considered in patients with sudden or severe respiratory or cardiac deterioration with hypotension and in intubated patients who become difficult to ventilate. Signs of tension pneumothorax include increased airway pressure, hypotension, or elevated central venous and pulmonary artery pressure. Severe dyspnea, restlessness, agitation, and a feeling of impending doom can develop rapidly in conscious patients with tension pneumothorax. Initially, these patients may be only tachycardic and tachypneic but can quickly become hypotensive.

The symptoms of hemothorax can be similar to those of pneumothorax but may be accompanied by hypotension due to exsanguination as blood accumulates in the pleural space. The onset of symptoms with effusions is usually much more gradual, with increasing shortness of breath and dyspnea on exertion occurring for days to weeks.

Physical Examination

Unstable Patients

During the initial phase of resuscitation (airway, breathing, circulation, disability), consider the diagnosis of pneumothorax in patients who are tachycardic, hypotensive, and dyspneic. These symptoms are not specific, as similar ones occur with pulmonary embolism, pericardial tamponade, large pleural effusion, and severe multilobar pneumonia. Serial examinations are critical as a tension pneumothorax may develop subtly over time. Use "look, listen, and feel" as your guideline. Observe the exposed chest wall for asymmetric chest expansion and the neck and forehead veins for distention. Venous distension may be present even when the patient is hypotensive. The trachea may be deviated away from the side of the pneumothorax. Percuss the chest wall for hyperresonance on the affected side and palpate for the

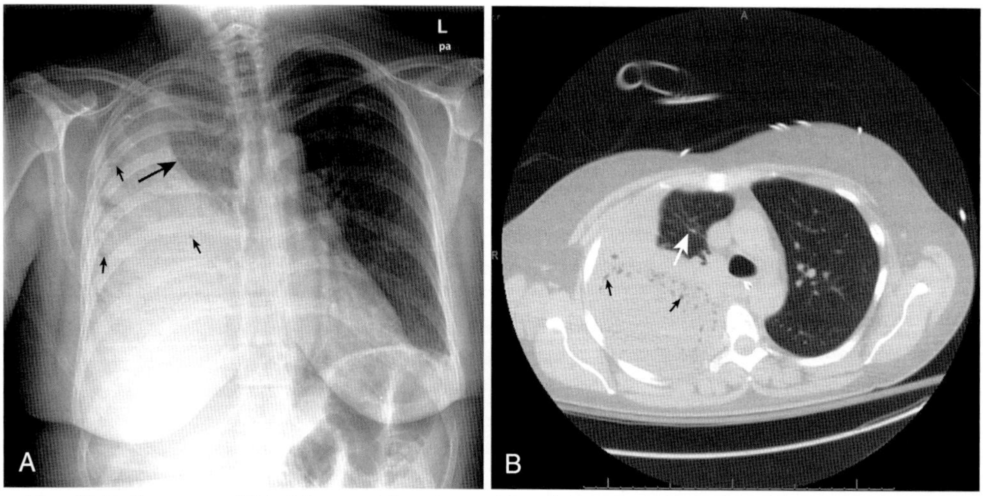

Fig. 10.5 Empyema. This 34-year-old patient with a history of alcoholism had a fever, cough, pleuritic chest pain, and hypoxia. (A) Posteroanterior chest radiograph demonstrating nearly total opacification of the right hemithorax. The presence of a meniscus *(large arrow)* suggests a pleural effusion. However, small lucent areas *(small arrows)* can be seen throughout the opacity, which may represent air bronchograms in the consolidated lung parenchyma. Thus a computed tomography (CT) scan was performed. (B) The CT revealed the almost total collapse of the right lung with only a small portion of the apex remaining inflated *(white arrow)*. The massive pleural fluid collection with gas bubbles throughout *(black arrows)* suggests a pyogenic empyema. A tube thoracostomy drained more than 1700 mL of purulent fluid. Fluid cultures grew *Streptococcus anginosus*.

crispy crunch of subcutaneous emphysema. Auscultation may demonstrate diminished breath sounds on the injured side. A recent meta analysis evaluating the diagnostic accuracy of lung auscultation in adult patients with acute respiratory pathology demonstrates low sensitivity and an acceptable specificity.[6] Pulsus paradoxus (diminished pulse or blood pressure during inspiration) may be evident. An early sign of tension pneumothorax for intubated patients is increased peak airway pressure. Additionally, poor compliance may be noted when providing respiratory support by bagging.

In injured patients with apnea, hypotension, or cardiopulmonary arrest, diagnose and treat a presumptive tension pneumothorax by immediate needle thoracostomy, simple thoracostomy (incision with scalpel and penetration directly into the thoracic cavity with clap or finger), or tube decompression thoracotomy. Do not take the time to obtain and review a radiograph because delay can increase morbidity and mortality. Confirm the diagnosis of tension pneumothorax after decompression by rapid improvement in vital signs and a rush of air.

Stable Patients

In more stable patients, the findings on physical examination are less sensitive, and a chest radiograph, ultrasound, or computed tomography (CT) scan is usually necessary for diagnosis. Physical findings may include unilaterally decreased breath sounds, tachypnea, tachycardia, decreased tactile fremitus, increased resonance with percussion, or subcutaneous emphysema. Patients with a pneumothorax involving less than 20% of the hemithorax will often have completely normal findings on chest examination, including equal breath sounds (Fig. 10.6).

Pleural fluid collections are difficult to detect by physical examination, particularly with less than 500 mL of fluid in the pleural space. Physical examination may reveal diminished breath sounds, dullness on percussion, egophony, and decreased tactile fremitus on the involved side. Parapneumonic effusions and empyemas are often accompanied by fever, cough, chest pain, dyspnea, and purulent sputum (see Fig. 10.5). Fever often develops in patients with an indwelling chest tube and empyema. The pleural fluid drainage may become copious and purulent, and respiratory symptoms may worsen.

Radiography

Plain Radiographs

A chest radiograph is an essential tool for diagnosing a pneumothorax in stable patients. In unstable patients with a potential tension pneumothorax, the diagnosis should be made clinically, but in rare cases, a portable radiograph may be obtained in the resuscitation room if a clinician carefully monitors the patient. Bedside ultrasound is a beneficial diagnostic modality in these peristable patients. The best plain radiographs for detecting hemothorax or pneumothorax are traditional upright inspiratory posteroanterior and lateral chest radiographs. Diagnostic sensitivity is not increased with an expiratory upright chest radiograph. Upright is preferable to a supine chest radiograph, particularly for a hemothorax, because even with large amounts of blood, there may only be slight differences in the density of the lung fields as the blood may layer out evenly. Approximately 200 mL pleural fluid needs to be present for blunting of a costophrenic angle to be visible on a lateral chest radiograph while literature has shown lateral decubitus radiograph with the affected side down can identify an effusion of approximately 15 mL (Fig. 10.7).[7] If CT is not available, other valuable views to aid diagnosis include a bilateral decubitus chest radiograph, with the pneumothorax expected to be seen on the side away from the table (upward) as gravity pulls the affected lung down, but a pleural effusion or hemothorax, will be better seen on the side toward the table (downward).

On a chest radiograph, the partially collapsed lung of a pneumothorax appears as a visceral pleural line with no pulmonary markings beyond (see Figs. 10.1, 10.3, 10.6, and

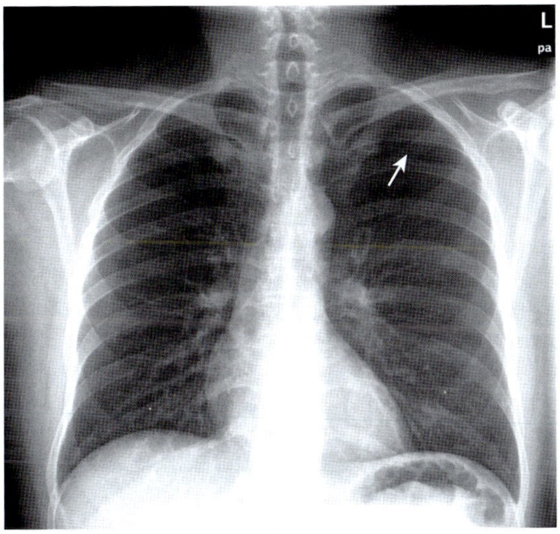

Fig. 10.6 Smaller pneumothoraces such as this (note the faintly visible pleural reflection *[arrow]*, absence of lung markings at the left apex, and relative crowding of vessels at the left hilum) are challenging to see on radiographs and almost impossible to identify by physical examination. Patients with a pneumothorax of less than 20% will often have completely normal findings on chest examination, including equal breath sounds.

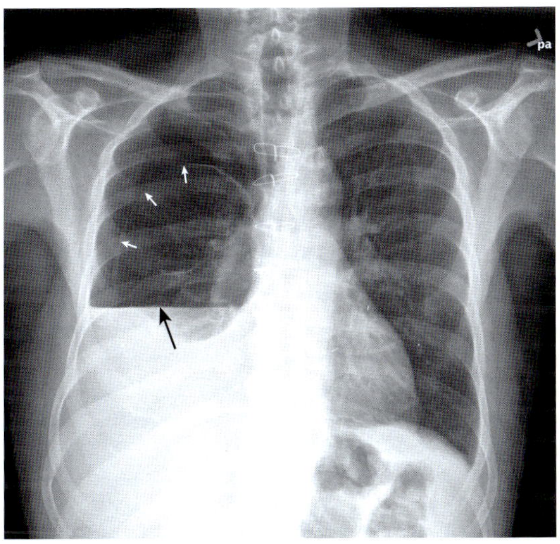

Fig. 10.7 Hydropneumothorax. This radiograph is an excellent example of a hydropneumothorax. When accumulated fluid in the chest cavity is seen as a straight line on a radiograph (an air-fluid level *[black arrow]*) with no meniscus up the side, air must be present in the pleural space. In this patient, the pneumothorax is readily visualized, with no lung markings seen laterally or superior to the pleural reflection *(white arrows)*.

10.7). Large blebs, the scapular border, skin folds, or indwelling lines can all be mistaken for a pneumothorax, but a CT scan may quickly confirm the presence of a pneumothorax (Fig. 10.8). Other radiographic findings include hyperlucency of the affected hemithorax, a double diaphragm contour, increased visibility of the inferior cardiac border, better visualization of pericardial fat at the cardiac apex, and possibly a depressed diaphragm. If subcutaneous air is found on the chest radiograph of a patient with blunt chest trauma, assume that the air came from an injured lung and that a pneumothorax exists until proven otherwise. It is difficult to predict the size of a pneumothorax on plain radiographs; a CT scan is more accurate. With a tension pneumothorax, the chest radiograph reveals lung collapse, a depressed hemidiaphragm on the affected side, and a shift of the mediastinum and trachea to the opposite side (see Fig. 10.4). Keep in mind, with a bilateral pneumothorax, a mediastinal shift may not be seen.

Thoracic Computed Tomography

CT scans can detect a pneumothorax that is not easily visible on a plain radiograph and are much more sensitive than plain radiographs in detecting hemothorax and chylothorax. They are also more accurate for identifying the cause and estimating a pneumothorax's size and other characteristics (see Figs. 10.1, 10.4, and 10.8). A CT scan may be helpful when the diagnosis is unclear or when looking for small amounts of pleural fluid. CT scans are particularly helpful in determining whether an empyema is loculated or draining successfully.

Approximately 10% of trauma patients with normal findings on a chest radiograph will demonstrate a small hemothorax or pneumothorax on a CT scan.[7–9] The clinical significance of a small, previously undetected occult injury is probably not great, and it has been suggested that they may be left untreated and simply observed in otherwise stable patients. Some patients with a pneumothorax seen only on CT may also safely undergo PPV without placing a chest tube.[9]

An extensive evaluation is not usually recommended for the first episode of a small primary pneumothorax. When patients have recurrent spontaneous pneumothoraces, further evaluation, including for surgical treatment, are more often indicated. The underlying lung pathology of a patient with a spontaneous pneumothorax is best initially evaluated with CT. Frequently, this is followed by diagnostic or therapeutic visual inspection of the lung and pleural space by fiberoptic thoracoscopy.[9a]

Ultrasound

Thoracic ultrasound is a valuable bedside tool to assess the lung fields and pleural space rapidly, diagnose pleural and lung parenchymal abnormalities, and guide pleural-based procedures including thoracentesis with or without catheter insertion and evaluation of placement for chest tube. Ultrasound is an integral part of the evaluation of thoracic and lung pathology in a variety of situations, including patients with chest trauma, evaluation for postprocedural iatrogenic pneumothorax, patients presenting with undifferentiated shortness of breath, hypoxia, or chest pain, and following chest tube placement to assess resolution of pneumothorax. Thoracic ultrasound has several advantages over standard chest radiographic imaging, including the absence of radiation, portability, and the ability to perform dynamic imaging. Several studies indicate that thoracic ultrasound may be superior to conventional chest radiograph in the detection of pneumothorax[10–13] and is considered superior for detecting and characterizing pleural effusion.[14] Additionally, bedside thoracic ultrasound can help differentiate between consolidation, atelectasis, and effusion, all of which can appear as an opacity or "white out" on a chest radiograph.[15] Ultrasound can also help evaluate chest wall pathology. More importantly, thoracic ultrasound is beneficial for guiding pleural procedures to mitigate the risk of complications, particularly in the presence of pleural adhesions from prior infections, pleurodesis, or pulmonary surgery.[16]

ULTRASOUND: Recognizing Pneumothorax

A high-frequency transducer should be used to evaluate for pneumothorax. In a supine patient, the transducer should be placed on the anterior chest wall in the midclavicular line at approximately the second to third intercostal space (Fig. 10.US1). The probe indicator should be pointed cephalad and moved progressively toward the lateral chest.[17] Adjust the depth of the image until the ribs are seen as brightly echogenic (white) arcs with acoustic shadows behind. The pleural line is just deep to the ribs and is seen as a horizontal, echogenic line (Fig. 10.US2).

Air moves to the least dependent portion of the lung; therefore the radiographic appearance of a pneumothorax depends upon the patient's position. When x-ray is performed in the upright position, the pneumothorax can be appreciated in the apical or apicolateral position. Alternatively, when the patient is in the supine position, pleural gas accumulates anteriorly and in a subpulmonic location. It is estimated that approximately 500 mL of air in the pleural space is needed for x-ray-based detection of pneumothorax in the supine position; another reason why ultrasound is more useful in detecting smaller pneumothoraces. The evaluation of pneumothorax should focus on looking for the presence of four sonographic artifact signs: lung sliding, B-lines, the lung pulse, the lung point sign, and include M-mode sonography.

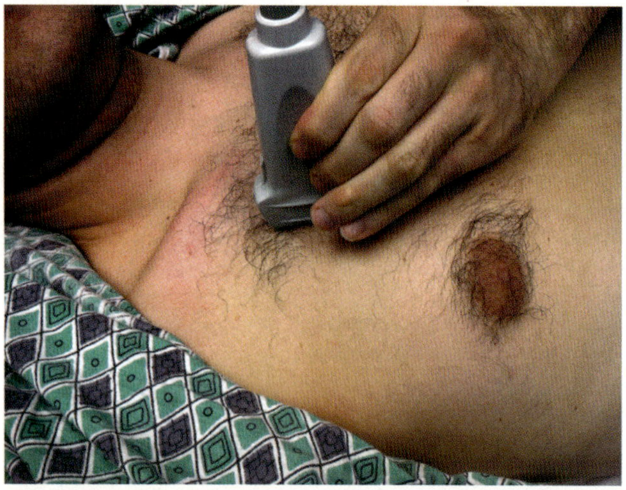

Fig. 10.US1 Proper positioning of the probe for evaluation of pneumothorax.

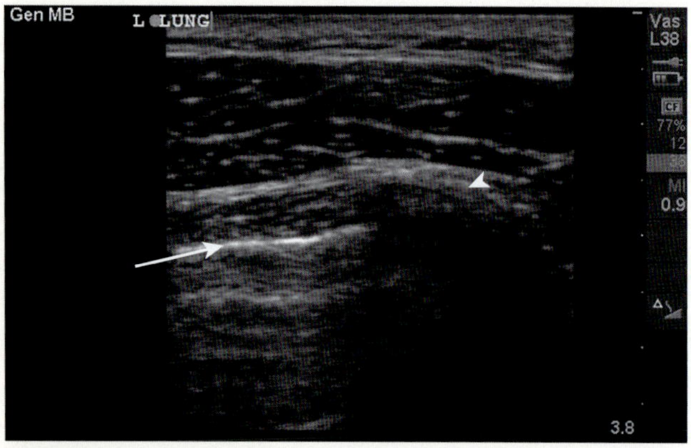

Fig. 10.US2 Ultrasound image of the pleura as seen with a high-frequency transducer. The pleura is a hyperechoic *(white)* line *(arrow)* that normally moves back and forth with respiration. Identifying the rib, along with its accompanying shadow *(arrowhead)*, often aids in identifying the pleura because it will lie immediately below the rib.

Lung Sliding

In a normal lung, the visceral and parietal pleural layers slide past each other as the lungs expand when the patient breathes. This is referred to as the "slide sign." When this interface is disrupted (such as by a pneumothorax), the sliding is lost, and the pleural line does not change with respiration. Although the slide sign carries significant sensitivity for ruling out a pneumothorax, other secondary confirmatory findings should also be sought.[1]

B-Lines (Comet Tail Artifacts)

Two main types of lung artifacts caused by air-tissue interfaces are common: A-lines and B-lines.[18] Horizontal artifacts, or A-lines, are echogenic lines between rib shadows observed in normal lungs. B-lines arise at the border between aerated and compressed lungs. They are often described as comet tail artifacts and are characteristic in that they spread to the edge of the screen without fading, move synchronously with the lung during respiration, and tend to erase A-lines (Fig. 10.US3). Patients with a pneumothorax lack comet tails because the normal pleural interface is disrupted.

Lung Point Sign

The lung point sign is the most specific sonographic sign for pneumothorax and occurs when the lung intermittently comes into contact with the chest wall during inspiration. This represents the edge of the pneumothorax. The presence of a lung point is 100% specific for ruling in pneumothorax.[19]

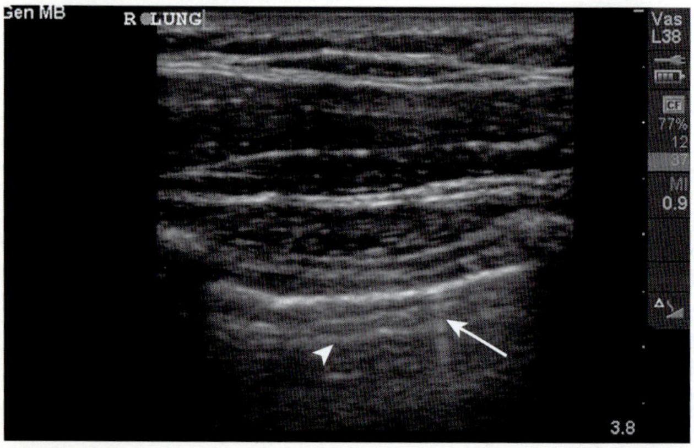

Fig. 10.US3 This image demonstrates two key artifacts seen in a normal lung. The pleura is the hyperechoic horizontal line deep to the ribs (at the *far right and left* of the image). A comet tail (a small vertical line) is seen extending deep to the pleura *(arrow)*. This is a normal artifact created by the pleura, and its presence aids in ruling out a pneumothorax. A-lines, or a series of horizontal lines extending deep to the pleura, can also be seen *(arrowhead)*. These artifacts may be seen both in normal lungs and in the presence of pneumothorax.

Continued

ULTRASOUND: Recognizing Pneumothorax—cont'd

Lung Pulse

Lung pulse describes the vertical movement of the pleural line synchronous to the cardiac rhythm and is caused by the transmission of heartbeats through the lung.[17] The presence of lung pulse indicates that the lung is fully inflated at the site of probe placement on the chest wall, so there is no pneumothorax present at that examination site. The absence of lung pulse indicates the possibility of pneumothorax, but there are also other causes for its absence.

Motion mode (M-mode) may also be used to identify a pneumothorax. M-mode is used to evaluate objects in motion and plots a linear representation of motion on the screen. An upward deflection represents objects moving toward the surface (or the transducer). A downward deflection represents those that move away. A solid line represents immobile objects. When a healthy patient breathes, the pleura slides back and forth. Because this motion is neither toward nor away from the transducer but instead is parallel, the motion is seen as a series of hazy lines deep to the pleura. The immobile overlying soft tissue is seen as a series of clear, flat lines. This typical appearance is called the *seashore* sign (Fig. 10.US4). The M-mode tracing in patients with a pneumothorax demonstrates clear, flat lines throughout the frame, referred to as the *stratosphere* or *bar code* sign (Fig. 10.US5).

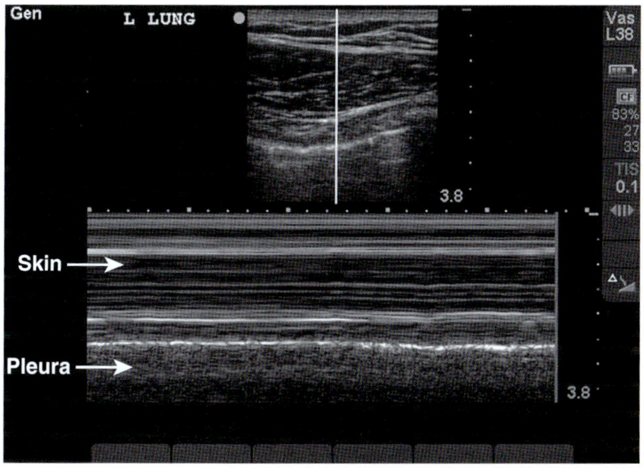

Fig. 10.US4 Seashore sign in a normal lung. This M-mode image shows the movement of the pleura. The solid lines at the top of the image represent the immobile skin, soft tissue, and muscle. The hazy lines at the bottom of the image represent the back-and-forth movement of the normal pleura.

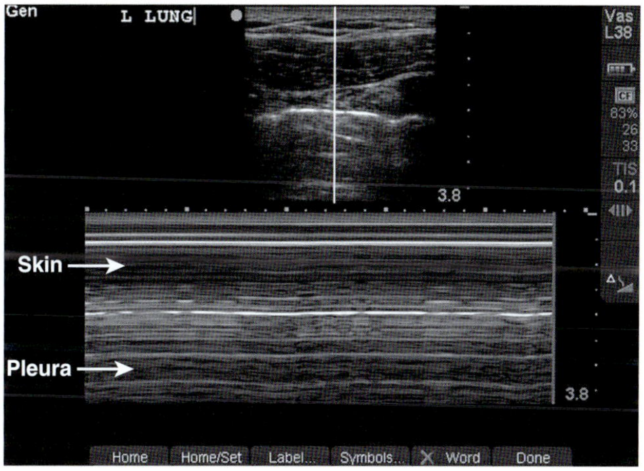

Fig. 10.US5 Bar code sign consistent with a pneumothorax. This M-mode image shows the lack of movement of the pleura. Unlike the previous image, the solid lines can be seen to continue past the point of the pleural line. There is no movement is seen in this image because a pneumothorax causes the pleura to appear stationary.

Ultrasound-guided thoracentesis, with or without subsequent catheter placement, can be performed by static or dynamic technique. The static technique involves identifying the structure (or vessel), marking the insertion area on the skin, and then proceeding without visual aid. When using the dynamic technique, visualize the needle in real-time throughout the insertion process. Placement of tube thoracostomy is typically performed by static ultrasound technique to identify the intercostal spaces, pleura, and effusion, as well as the best angle of approach. The examiner may also observe diaphragmatic excursion through several respiratory cycles to choose a location sufficiently above the diaphragm to avoid a laceration. The skin is then marked, the probe removed, and the procedure is carried out the same way as during landmark thoracentesis or tube thoracostomy.

INDICATIONS FOR TUBE THORACOSTOMY

Pneumothorax

The approach to treating a pneumothorax depends on its cause (spontaneous vs. traumatic), the patient (age, comorbidities), and severity (stable, unstable). Treatment should address several fundamental issues: (1) removal of air, (2) preventing further air accumulation, (3) healing the injury that caused the initial accumulation, (4) promoting lung reexpansion, and (5) preventing or limiting reoccurrences.[20]

Spontaneous Pneumothorax

In 2001 the American College of Chest Physicians developed guidelines for managing primary and SSP that have not yet been updated (Box 10.1).[21]

Chest tube placement is probably unnecessary in healthy patients with small primary spontaneous or isolated small traumatic pneumothoraces in the absence of respiratory compromise or concomitant injuries or when PPV will not be required. With no intervention, a small pneumothorax will resolve over days to weeks. Supplemental oxygen may speed the process of lung reexpansion by increasing the rate of pleural air absorption. Some trials recommend conservative management (observation) or aspiration of first-time PSPs. These approaches result in similar outcomes as traditional tube thoracostomy but have fewer complications, shorter hospital stays, and lower costs.[22–25] Newer trials provide modest evidence that conservative management of PSP was noninferior to interventional management, with a lower risk of serious adverse events.[26] The management of

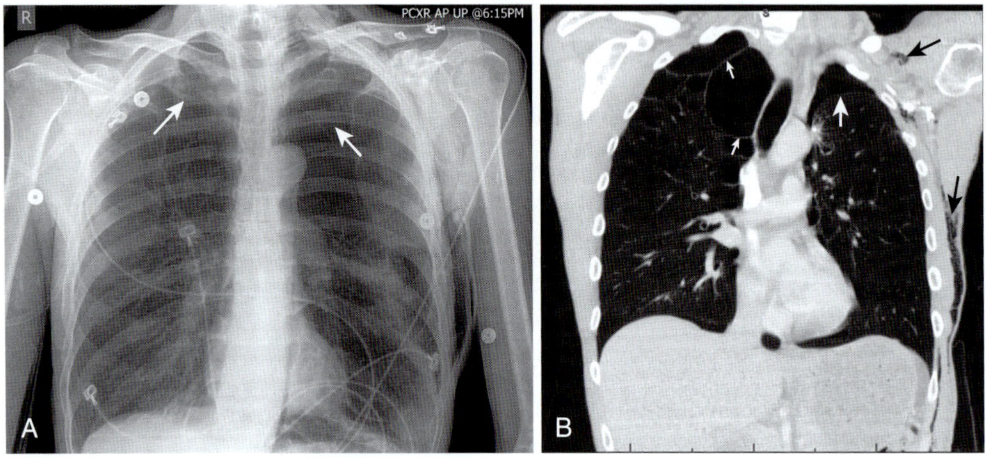

Fig. 10.8 Pneumothorax and bullous emphysema. This patient had a history of severe chronic obstructive pulmonary disease and arrived at the emergency department in respiratory distress. (A) On the chest radiograph, both apices are relatively radiolucent, and faint lines that are not clearly blebs or pleural reflections *(arrows)* are visible coursing through. (B) A computed tomography (CT) scan was defines the pathology in detail. The right apex has no pneumothorax but rather large blebs *(small white arrows)*. A pleural reflection on the left is clearly visible *(large white arrow)*, indicating pneumothorax. Subcutaneous air is also noted in the thoracic soft tissues *(black arrows)*, thus further supporting the diagnosis of pneumothorax. (This finding is also evident on the chest radiography but was overlooked in the initial interpretation.)

BOX 10.1 Guidelines of the American College of Chest Physicians for the Management of Primary and Secondary Spontaneous Pneumothoraces

PRIMARY SPONTANEOUS PNEUMOTHORAX (NO UNDERLYING LUNG DISEASE)

A clinically stable patient must have all of the following: respiratory rate lower than 24 breaths/min, heart rate higher than 60 beats/min or less than 120 beats/min, normal blood pressure, room air O_2 saturation higher than 90%, and the ability to speak in whole sentences between breaths.

CLINICALLY STABLE PATIENTS WITH SMALL PNEUMOTHORACES (<3 CM APEX-TO-CUPOLA DISTANCE)

Clinically stable patients with small pneumothoraces (PTXs) should be observed in the emergency department (ED) for 3 to 6 hours and be discharged home if a repeated chest radiograph excludes progression of the PTX (good consensus). Patients should be provided with careful instructions for follow-up within 12 hours to 2 days, depending on the circumstances. A chest radiograph should be obtained at the follow-up appointment to document resolution of the PTX. Patients may be admitted for observation if they live distant from emergency services or follow-up care is considered unreliable (good consensus). Simple aspiration of the PTX or insertion of a chest tube is not appropriate for most patients (good consensus) unless the PTX enlarges. The presence of symptoms for longer than 24 hours does not alter the treatment recommendations.

CLINICALLY STABLE PATIENTS WITH LARGE PNEUMOTHORACES (≥3 CM APEX-TO-CUPOLA DISTANCE)

Clinically stable patients with large PTXs should undergo a procedure to reexpand the lung and should be hospitalized in most instances (very good consensus). The lung should be reexpanded by using a small-bore catheter (≤14 Fr) or placement of a 16- to 22-Fr chest tube (good consensus). Catheters or tubes may be attached either to a Heimlich valve (good consensus) or to a water seal device (good consensus) and may be left in place until the lung expands against the chest wall and any air leaks have resolved. If the lung fails to reexpand quickly, suction should be applied to a water seal device. Alternatively, suction may be applied immediately after placement of a chest tube in all patients managed with a water seal system (some consensus).

Reliable patients who are unwilling to undergo hospitalization may be discharged home from the ED with a small-bore catheter attached to a Heimlich valve if the lung reexpanded after the removal of pleural air (good consensus). Follow-up should be arranged within 2 days. The presence of symptoms for longer than 24 hours does not alter management recommendations.

SECONDARY SPONTANEOUS PNEUMOTHORAX

Clinically Stable Patients With Small Pneumothoraces

Clinically stable patients with small PTXs should be hospitalized (good consensus). Patients should not be managed in the ED with observation or simple aspiration without hospitalization (very good consensus). Hospitalized patients may be observed (good consensus) or treated with a chest tube (some consensus), depending on the extent of their symptoms and the course of their PTX. Some of the panel members argued against observation alone because of a report of deaths with this approach. Patients should not be referred for thoracoscopy without prior stabilization (very good consensus). The presence of symptoms for longer than 24 hours did not alter the panel members' recommendations.

Clinically Stable Patients With Large Pneumothoraces

Clinically stable patients with large PTXs should undergo placement of a chest tube to reexpand the lung and should be hospitalized (very good consensus). Patients should not be referred for thoracoscopy without prior stabilization with a chest tube (very good consensus). The presence of symptoms for longer than 24 hours did not alter the panel members' recommendations.

This is meant to be a guide; clinical judgment should always be used.
From Baumann MH, Strange C, Heffner JE, et al. Management of spontaneous pneumothorax: an American College of Chest Physicians Delphi consensus statement. Chest. *2001;119:590-602.*

adolescent and young adult PSP is varied. Best practices exist to optimize some aspects of care. Further prospective studies are needed to better determine optimal timing of operative intervention, the most effective operation, and management of recurrence after observation, tube thoracostomy, or operative intervention.

There is currently little consensus regarding the management for children with PSP.[27,28] Variability in adult guidelines and lack of pediatric-specific protocols illustrate the need to establish evidence-based management algorithms for children. In patients with a simple pneumothorax, prolonged suction is rarely required, and the tube can be attached to a Heimlich valve or underwater seal.[29–31]

Because SSPs occur in older patients with underlying diseases and have a higher risk of complications and recurrence, they are generally managed by tube or catheter thoracostomy and hospital admission. In 2020 the British Thoracic Society recommended a tiered approach: inpatient observation if the SSP is <1 cm at the hilum; needle aspiration (14 to 16 gauge) and observation if the pneumothorax is 1 to 2 cm at the hilum; tube thoracostomy (<14 Fr) if the patient is unstable, breathless, if the pneumothorax is >2 cm at the hilum, or >1 cm after an attempted aspiration. As all interventions require inpatient observation, surgical consultation is recommended.

Some pneumothoraces require operative intervention. Surgery may be recommended for a first pneumothorax in the following situations: life-threatening tension pneumothorax, massive air leaks with incomplete reexpansion, an air leak persisting 4 days after a second tube placement, associated hemothorax with complications, identifiable bullous disease, or failure of easy reexpansion in patients with cystic fibrosis. Studies have shown excellent short- and long-term outcomes after video-assisted thoracoscopic treatment (VATS) of PSP and SSP, with lower recurrence rates than after other treatment modalities. However, VATS continues to have a higher complication rate than tube or catheter thoracostomy, with 4.6% of patients with spontaneous pneumothorax experiencing serious side effects due to the procedure.[32,33]

Traumatic Pneumothorax

In patients with traumatic causes, the urgency and type of treatment depend primarily on the stability of the patient. A hypotensive patient with a tension pneumothorax requires immediate decompression before a chest tube (Fig 10.9), whereas a patient with normal vital signs and a small pneumothorax may be observed initially. Needle or simple thoracostomy is only a temporary solution that requires an ipsilateral tube thoracostomy for definitive treatment. Other factors that modify treatment include the patient's age, the size of the pneumothorax, whether bilateral pneumothoraces are present, and whether the current episode represents a recurrence.

Because of the risk of a tension pneumothorax, a chest tube should be considered in all patients with a penetrating chest injury if PPV is used or if they will be transported a long distance for definitive care. However, CT scans of trauma patients have demonstrated that many patients with small pneumothoraces not detected by standard radiographs can safely undergo PPV with close observation for signs of tension pneumothorax.[9]

Hemothorax

Tube thoracostomy is the treatment for hemothorax and is used to monitor the amount and rapidity of blood output to determine the need for additional interventions, including VATS or open thoracotomy. Approximately three-fourths of patients with a traumatic hemothorax can be managed by tube thoracostomy and volume replacement alone. The remaining patients will require immediate or delayed elective thoracotomy. The indications for surgery after an acute hemothorax vary somewhat between authors but are summarized in Box 10.2. Early administration of blood replacement is recommended for patients with a massive hemothorax (>2000 mL) because they are often associated with continuing hemorrhage. VATS can locate and stop the bleeding, evacuate blood clots, and break down adhesions for patients with active blood loss but stable hemodynamics.

Empyema

Empyema treatment depends on the infection's severity and the patient's underlying condition. Patients with an empyema require admission, so interventions are usually directed by the inpatient services. Some patients with empyema can be treated with serial thoracenteses, but most need continuous drainage with a chest tube (see Fig. 10.5). Thoracoscopic decortication represents definitive therapy for severe cases. The diagnosis of an empyema may be made in the emergency department when a thoracentesis finds thick pus, positive Gram stain, fluid glucose level lower than 60 mg/dL, pH less than 7.20, or elevated lactate dehydrogenase. Once an empyema is detected, definitive therapy should not be delayed because the fluid can quickly become loculated. Generally, the chest tube is left in place until the pleural drainage fluid becomes clear yellow and accumulates less than 150 mL in 24 hours. An empyema that fails to resolve on chest radiography within 48 hours requires a chest CT and careful review of antibiotic choice. A Cochrane review compared the surgical option of VATS with chest tube drainage of pleural empyema and found no difference in mortality or complications between the groups. However, early VATS reduced the hospital length of stay.[34]

CONTRAINDICATIONS

There are no absolute contraindications to tube thoracostomy for unstable trauma patients with a pneumothorax or hemothorax. In critical patients, the placement of a chest tube is often performed empirically. In stable patients, relative contraindications include anatomic problems such as multiple pleural adhesions, emphysematous blebs, or scarring. Coagulopathic patients should be evaluated for clotting factors and platelet replacement before any invasive procedure.

TREATMENT

Treatment of a Possible Tension Pneumothorax in an Unstable Patient

See Videos 10.1 and 10.2. Immediate chest decompression must be considered in all injured patients with unexplained hypotension or tachypnea, particularly those with penetrating chest injuries. The goal is to open the pleural space quickly, allowing any accumulated air to escape and decompress the chest cavity. This can be accomplished with a scalpel and clamp, as is done at the beginning stages of a thoracostomy (Fig. 10.9), or more commonly, decompression can be achieved with a large-bore needle/angiocatheter combination

Emergency Pleural Decompression

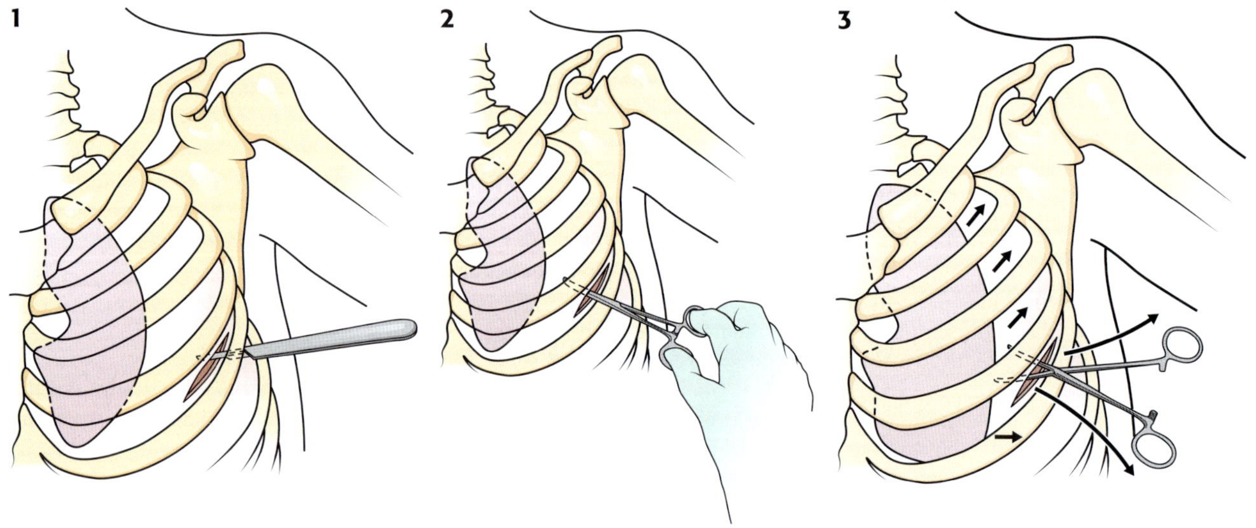

1. Use a No. 10 scalpel to make a deep incision in the skin and subcutaneous tissue over the fourth or fifth rib in the anterior axillary line.
2. Insert a long closed Kelly clamp over the top of the rib, and stab into the pleural space. A "pop" is usually felt.
3. Once the Kelly clamp is in the pleural space, open it widely to create a rent in the parietal pleura. Air should immediately vent. Insert a chest tube.

Fig. 10.9 Emergency pleural decompression. During resuscitation of a patient with a tension pneumothorax, there may be no time for a chest tube and needle decompression may not be effective. Under these circumstances, the pleural cavity can be vented in seconds. This assumes that the patient is intubated.

BOX 10.2 Indications for Surgery After Tube Thoracostomy Based on Results of the Thoracostomy

- Massive hemothorax, >1000 mL to 1500 mL initial drainage
- Continued bleeding
  - >300 to 500 mL in the first hour
  - >200 mL/h for the first 3 or more hours
- Increasing size of the hemothorax on a chest film
- Persistent hemothorax after two functioning tubes are placed
- Clotted hemothorax
- Large air leak preventing effective ventilation
- Persistent air leak after placement of a second tube or inability to fully expand the lung

This is meant to be a guide; clinical judgment should always be used.

(minimum of 16 gauge) (Fig. 10.10). There are two landmarks used for this procedure, the second or third intercostal space midclavicular line and the fourth or fifth intercostal space midaxillary line. Studies of both prehospital and hospital providers have demonstrated that though landmarks can be described, they are not always accurately identified. Cadaver studies have shown improved success in reaching the thoracic cavity when the fourth or fifth intercostal space midaxillary line is used instead of the second intercostal space midclavicular line in adult patients. Advanced trauma life support (ATLS) now recommends this location for needle decompression in adult patients.[35] The needle should be inserted on the side with the pneumothorax and immediately above the rib to avoid the neurovascular bundle. If the primary site for decompression is inaccessible or unsuccessful, the secondary

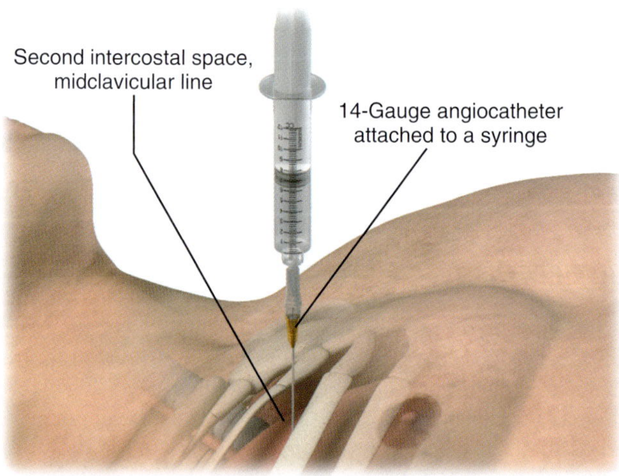

Fig. 10.10 Needle decompression. Use a large-bore needle/catheter combination to puncture the parietal pleura and establish the presence of fluid or air in the pleural space. The needle can be placed anywhere in the pleural space, but traditionally at the same sites used for tube thoracostomy: the anterior second intercostal space in the midclavicular line or the anterior axillary line in the fourth or fifth interspace. Introduce the needle directly over the rib to avoid neurovascular injury. The needle is then withdrawn while leaving the catheter behind to create a simple open pneumothorax. The procedure can be done with or without the syringe attached to the catheter. This is only a temporary solution, and a chest tube must also be inserted.

site should be chosen. Remove the needle, but leave the angiocatheter in place to create a simple pneumothorax. Regardless of whether needle decompression improves the patient's vital signs, a chest tube should be immediately placed following the decompression. If the needle decompression is ineffective, an open thoracostomy can be started, even without the immediate availability of a chest tube, to help create an exit for the air so that the patient's respiratory and cardiovascular functions can normalize.

Prehospital Treatment

Needle decompression thoracostomy may be used in the prehospital setting when a patient with a suspected pneumothorax rapidly deteriorates or is initially seen in extremis. The primary site for needle decompression thoracostomy is the fourth or fifth intercostal space at the midaxillary line. If no change in the patient's status, a second attempt at decompression should be attempted at the secondary site of the second intercostal space in the midclavicular line. In such cases, attach the needle (or catheter) to a one-way (Heimlich) valve, or even a flutter valve (fashioned from the fingers of a surgical glove) so that the air can continue to escape during expiration but cannot enter during inspiration.

There is concern raised in the literature regarding the effectiveness of needle thoracostomy.[36–38] As a result, some out-of-hospital agencies have implemented emergency medical services protocols enabling paramedics to perform simple (incision with scalpel and penetration directly into the thoracic cavity with clamp or finger) thoracostomy in patients with high clinical suspicion of tension pneumothorax. One study found that finger thoracostomy was frequently performed by intensive care flight paramedics and was associated with a lower rate of significant complications than needle thoracostomy.[39,40]

When a patient has an open chest wound in the prehospital setting, a three-sided occlusive dressing over the wound acts one-way valve to prevent a tension pneumothorax while providing wound protection. This dressing allows air to escape during expiration but prevents air from entering the chest cavity during inspiration. A simple method is to tape down only three sides of a sterile dressing, such as petrolatum-impregnated gauze, that extends 6 to 8 cm beyond the wound in all directions. Additionally, multiple commercially available vented and nonvented chest seals can be applied over the wound. In the case of the nonvented chest seal, the provider may need to release or "burp" the chest seal if the patient demonstrates signs or symptoms again consistent with a tension pneumothorax after they were successfully needle decompressed.

Emergency Department Treatment

Equipment

The standard instruments for a tube thoracostomy tray are listed in Box 10.3 and depicted in Review Box 10.1. The most basic needs are a scalpel, a large (Kelly) clamp, and the thoracostomy tube.

Thoracostomy tubes are clear plastic tubes of various diameters that are open at both ends (Fig. 10.11). There is a radiopaque strip along the length of the tube that is interrupted by a series of holes along the distal length of the tube. The strip allows visualization of the tube's location on the postprocedure radiograph and ensures that the side ports are within the pleural cavity. Tubes come in various sizes and materials to best suit the patient's clinical needs, with smaller tubes used for smaller pneumothoraces and larger tubes for hemothorax and empyema. They are generally measured by the internal diameter of the tube in French units (one increment of the French scale is equal to a one-third-millimeter diameter). Generally, a 20-Fr or larger tube is considered large-bore, and those less than 20 French are considered small-bore.[41] Pigtail catheters, whose curled tip prevents dislodgement, are a common type of small-bore chest tube.[42] Large-bore tubes are usually used to treat significant traumatic pneumothoraces, hemothoraces, and viscous disease processes such as complex exudative effusions and empyemas, while small-bore tubes are used for a simple pneumothorax or empyema and transudative pleural effusions. Small-bore chest tubes are associated with less pain for the patient, fewer complications, shorter drainage duration, and reduced hospital length of stay. For pediatric patients, 14-, 16-, 20-, and 24-Fr tubes are adequate.

BOX 10.3 Recommended Equipment for Tube Thoracostomy

PROCEDURE
Sterile drapes
10- to 20-mL syringe and assorted needles (for local anesthesia)
Local anesthetic (1% to 2% lidocaine)
Antiseptic solution
Scalpel with a No. 10 blade
Large clamps (Kelly)
Needle holder
Chest tubes (size appropriate)
No. 0-0 or 1-0 silk or similar suture
Forceps
Straight (suture) scissors
Large, curved (Mayo) scissors
Soft arm restraints

DRAINAGE SYSTEM AND TUBING
Drainage apparatus with sterile water for the water seal
Hard plastic serrated connectors
Sterile tubing

DRESSING
Petrolatum gauze or similar occlusive dressing
Gauze or similar pads
Adhesive tape—cloth backed
Tincture of benzoin

Since the advent of common pleural drainage techniques in the early 20th century, physicians have preferred large-bore tubes inserted via blunt dissection for thoracic drainage and decompression. This preference for tubes greater than 16 Fr in diameter was mainly born of concern for fibrin blockage, inadequate drainage capability, and the perception of frequent dislodgement of small-bore tubes. To date, no large, high-quality randomized clinical trials have compared the use of large- versus small-bore tubes, but a recent meta-analysis has found numerous benefits to using small-bore tubes in certain circumstances.[43] Review of the available data suggests that the blockage and dislodgement rate is similar with large- and small-bore tubes and that drainage capability is comparable in all but the most extreme circumstances.[44–47] Another study has shown that large-bore tube placement is associated with significantly more pain and slightly increased rates of empyema.[48]

Review articles have attempted to establish rough guidelines for small-bore tube use. The literature suggests that

Tube Thoracostomy

Indications

Spontaneous and traumatic pneumothorax
Hemothorax
Empyema
Patients with penetrating chest trauma undergoing positive pressure ventilation or long-distance transport

Contraindications

Absolute
None
Relative
Presence of multiple pleural adhesions
Presence of emphysematous blebs
Coagulopathy

Complications

Infection
Laceration of an intercostal vessel
Pulmonary injury
Intraabdominal or solid organ tube placement
Failure of reexpansion of pneumothorax
Reexpansion pulmonary edema

Equipment

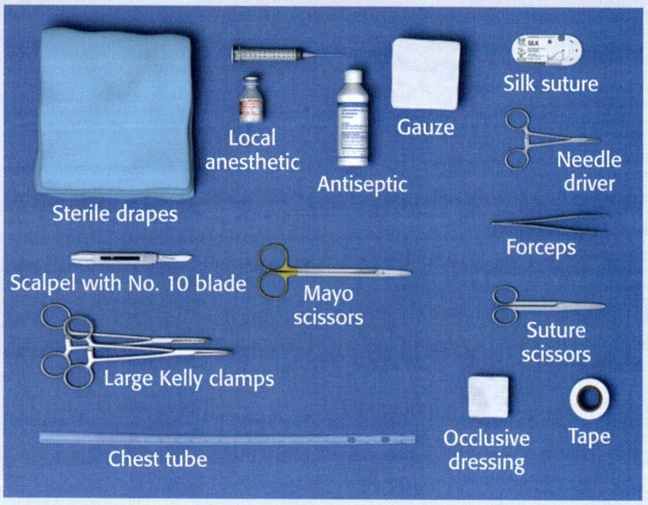

Review Box 10.1 Tube thoracostomy: indications, contraindications, complications, and equipment.

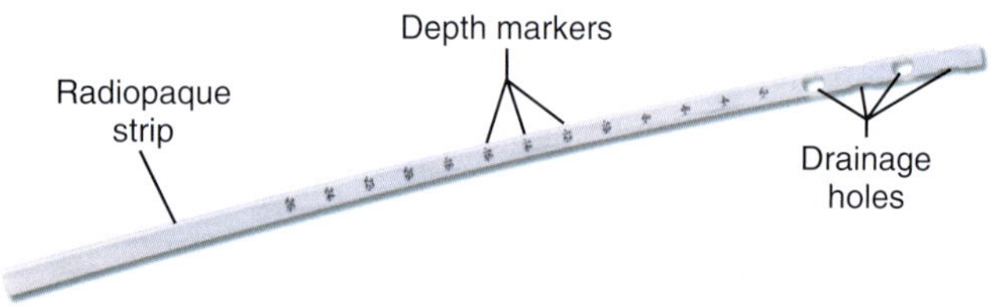

Fig. 10.11 Thoracostomy tube. Chest tubes have radiopaque lines that are interrupted by drainage holes. To ensure the tube is deep enough, all gaps in the line must be within the pleural cavity on the radiograph.

patients with malignant effusion, simple pneumothorax without penetrating injury, a suspected air leak, and those with simple or complex parapneumonic effusions are good candidates for small-bore tubes. Patients with empyema, penetrating injury, traumatic hemothorax, or complex pneumothorax, and those on mechanical ventilation require large-bore tubes because of the potential for large-volume air leaks in such patients and the need for rapid evacuation of the pleural space.[49,50] However, emerging trauma literature suggests that small-bore (14-Fr) percutaneous catheters are equally as effective as 28- to 32-Fr tubes in their ability to drain traumatic hemothorax with no difference in complication rates. Ultimately, the clinician should consider multiple factors when deciding on the type of chest tube, including the patient's underlying pathology and clinical status, patient comfort, simplicity of the procedure, desired outcome, and potential complications.

Procedure

See Videos 10.3 and 10.4. Conduct the procedure as sterilely as possible and wear a gown, glove, mask, and goggles. When feasible, obtain consent.

Tube Insertion Site

Insert the tube over the top of the rib rather than near the bottom to avoid the neurovascular structures on the inferior aspect of the ribs. The most common location for a chest tube is the midaxillary to the anterior axillary line, usually in the fourth or fifth intercostal space (Fig. 10.12). The ideal insertion point is through an external landmark space known as the triangle of safety. The space is bordered by the edge of the latissimus dorsi muscle, pectoralis major muscle, the base of the axilla, and transverse to the nipple line or inframammary fold at or above the fifth intercostal space.[51] This approach is cosmetically preferable and better tolerated than the anterior chest wall approach in the second intercostal space of the midclavicular line. The fifth intercostal space is approximately at the level of the nipple or the inferior scapular border in most patients, although the position of the female breast mass leads to variance. To avoid penetrating the abdominal cavity, choose a more superior insertion site because the external landmarks can be misleading. An important point to consider is that the diaphragm of a supine patient not taking a deep breath is much higher than expected.

Hold the tube next to the chest wall with the tip of the tube at the level of the clavicle to estimate the distance that the tube needs to be advanced from the incision site to the apex of the lung. Place a clamp on the tube to mark the

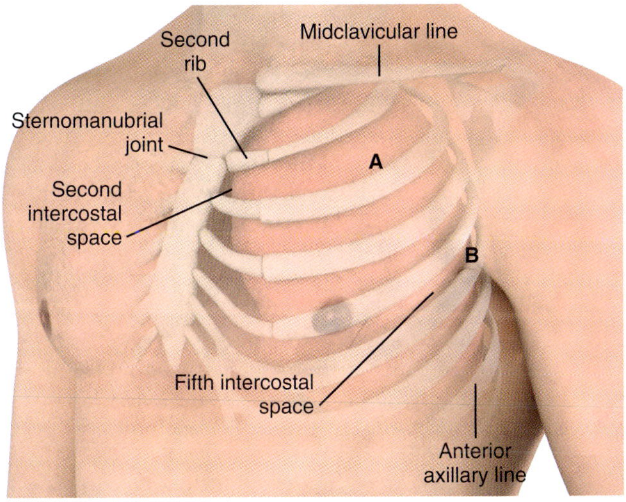

Fig. 10.12 Entry sites for tube thoracostomy. The second intercostal space in the midclavicular line is the preferred site for needle aspiration or catheter insertion *(A)*. To find the second intercostal space, palpate the sternomanubrial joint where the second rib articulates. The second intercostal space is below this rib. The fourth or fifth intercostal space, midaxillary to anterior axillary line (posterolateral to the pectoralis muscle and breast tissue), is preferred for a chest tube *(B)*. The fifth intercostal space is usually at the level of the nipple. The breast may need to be retracted by an assistant to identify landmarks and avoid low placement.

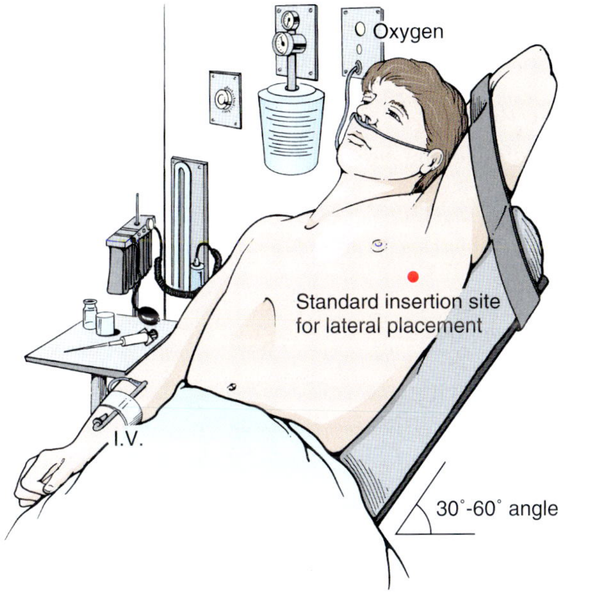

Fig. 10.13 To insert a chest tube, position the patient semierect with the ipsilateral arm abducted as far as possible and preferably restrained. Supplemental oxygen and monitoring are recommended.

maximum length that the tube should be inserted to prevent the tube from advancing too far. Confirm that the last drainage hole is within the pleural space at the level of the insertion site to ensure that the tube has been advanced sufficiently far. In patients with a largely elevated body mass index, failing to advance the tube far enough is common, with the last hole left in fatty tissue rather than in the pleural space.

Patient Preparation

If indicated clinically, start oxygenating and monitoring the patient continuously with cardiac and pulse oximetry. When possible, elevate the head of the bed 30 to 60 degrees (Fig. 10.13) to lower the diaphragm and decrease the risk of injury to the diaphragm, spleen, and liver. Abduct the arm on the affected side, place it over the patient's head, and restrain it. To facilitate, explain the process to the patient in detail, if conditions are appropriate, and use an assistant to help hold the patient and offer comforting support. Clean the skin with a standard surgical scrub and drape the field sterilely.

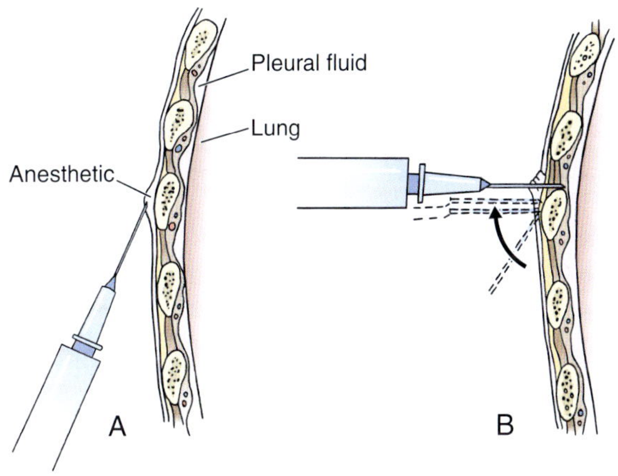

Fig. 10.14 Local anesthesia is essential to reduce the pain of inserting a chest tube. Infiltrate the skin, the entire track of the tube, and the pleura with a generous amount of local anesthetic. (A) The anesthetic is first infiltrated over the rib at the incision site. (B) The needle is then advanced slowly over the top of the rib while intermittently infiltrating and aspirating until the pleura is breached and air or fluid is withdrawn. Inject the anesthetic liberally (maximum of 5 mg/kg of lidocaine) to cover the pleural lining. (Based on Hughes WT, Buescher ES. *Pediatric Procedures*. 2nd ed. Saunders; 1980:234.)

Anesthesia

Preprocedure Anesthesia

Tube thoracostomy can be extremely painful, so consider giving parenteral analgesics or procedural sedation to stable patients before starting the procedure. A common problem is inadequate systemic analgesia and local anesthesia. Use generous local anesthesia, such as up to 4 mg/kg of locally injected 1% lidocaine with or without epinephrine. Slowly inject local anesthetic over the superior aspect of the rib, through the muscle, periosteum, and parietal pleura, and along the entire anticipated tract of the tube (Fig. 10.14). Intermittently aspirate for air or fluid with the needle to find the pleural cavity. If air or fluid is not found, consider changing the insertion site. Use of ultrasound can help assure proper tube placement.

Procedural Anesthesia

During the procedure, an additional local anesthetic injection (1% lidocaine) can be administered just before bluntly penetrating through the tough parietal pleura with the large Kelly clamp, which is often the most painful part of the procedure.

Postprocedure Anesthesia

Use parenteral analgesic agents as needed to control pain. In a stable patient, some advocate for administering local anesthetic through the tube into the pleural space to reduce pain caused by the tube rubbing against the pleura.[52]

Insertion

Avoid muscle and breast tissue when making the incision. A common problem is that the skin incision is too short to create and maintain an adequate tract to insert the thoracostomy tube. Ensure the incision is no less than 3 to 5 cm long (Fig. 10.15, *step 1*). Make a transverse incision through the skin and subcutaneous tissue with a No. 10 blade over the rib. Some authors advocate making the initial skin incision at a location one rib lower than the intended intercostal space through which the tube will enter, followed by "tunneling" the tube under the skin and up over the next rib. This is theoretically done to prevent air leaks, but no good evidence supports this practice. It is more common to make the incision at the intended location so that there is a straight path to the pleural cavity over the appropriate rib. This avoids the problem of losing the entrance point or increasing damage to the soft tissues, both issues that are particularly problematic in patients with an elevated body mass index. After the incision, insert a large Kelly clamp to push and spread the deeper tissues. Bluntly dissect a tract over the rib while avoiding the intercostal vessels and nerve on the inferior margin of each rib (Fig. 10.16; see also Fig. 10.15, *step 2*). Continue dissecting through the subcutaneous tissue, the three muscular layers of the intercostal space (i.e., the external intercostal muscle, the internal intercostal muscle, and the innermost intercostal muscle), and transthoracic fascia until the clamp reaches the parietal pleural. When attempting to enter the fifth intercostal space, it is important to dissect not perpendicular to the chest wall but generally posterior and apical; the direction that most tubes should be placed. Dissecting perpendicular to the chest wall and into the fifth intercostal space can lead to the tube heading directly into the oblique fissure and then being entrapped by the subsequently expanded lung, rendering the tube ineffective after lung reexpansion. Firm resistance will usually be felt when the tough parietal pleura is met. Close the clamp and push it forward with strong pressure to penetrate the pleura and enter the cavity, considerable force may be needed. To prevent the clamp from penetrating too deeply, hold the clamp a few centimeters distal to the incision and rest the tip against the pleura before pushing through (Fig. 10.17). Penetrating the pleura is usually the most painful portion of the procedure, so consider injecting extra anesthetic or analgesic before pushing through. A palpable pop may be felt upon entering the pleural cavity, followed by a rush of air or fluid. With only the tip of the clamp in the pleural cavity, spread the clamp to make an adequate hole in the pleura and then withdraw it (see Fig. 10.15, *step 3*). Make the opening in the parietal pleura wide enough to comfortably insert both a finger and the tube, but avoid a larger pleural opening to reduce the risk of an air leak (Fig. 10.18).

Another common problem occurs at this point as the dissected tract and pleural opening can be lost when the clamp is withdrawn. To prevent this, slide a sterile gloved finger over the clamp and into the pleura before removing the clamp (Fig. 10.19). This is done to define the tract further, verify that the pleura has been entered, and ensure that no solid organs have been penetrated. Whenever possible, leave the finger in the pleural space, make a 360-degree sweep to verify the correct space, feel for adhesions, and ensure the thoracostomy tract is not lost (see Fig. 10.15, *step 4*). Pass the tube over, under, or beside the finger into the pleural space, with the fingertip being used to guide the course of the tube (Fig. 10.20). This step allows the clinician to feel the tube passing into the pleural cavity, avoids subcutaneous dissection by the tube, and enhances proper direction of the tube. Pass the tube alone or hold on to a large curved clamp with the tip of the tube protruding beyond the end of the clamp (Fig. 10.21; see also Fig. 10.15, *step 5*). Typically, the tube should pass with little resistance. If resistance is met, the tube may not be in the pleural cavity and instead is passing subcutaneously, is in a fissure, or is abutting against the mediastinum (Fig. 10.22). Still using the finger that remains in the pleural space, direct the tube posteriorly, medially, and superiorly until the last hole of the tube is clearly in the thorax, the marker clamp that was previously attached touches the chest wall, or resistance is felt (see Fig. 10.15, *step 6*). Ensure that all the holes in the tube are within the pleural space. Rotate the tube 360 degrees to reduce the likelihood of kinking.

Attach the tube to the previously assembled water seal or suction before releasing the clamp. Ask the patient to cough and look for bubbles in the water seal chamber to check the system's patency.

In cases in which there may be broken ribs or significant resistance, some authors recommend the use of a bougie to ensure that the thoracostomy tract (that was formed by the Kelly clamp and the inserted finger) is not lost. After confirmation of the correct space by finger sweep, insert the bougie while the finger is in the pleural space and direct it posteriorly, medially, and superiorly. Measuring the bougie before the procedure and marking the bougie with an appropriate marking pin can help the operator identify the correct distance for advancement. Once the operator is satisfied that the bougie is in the proper place, the chest tube can then be inserted over it. As with most modified Seldinger techniques, the bougie must be secured by one hand at all times, and the tube must be advanced to its correct depth over the bougie while the bougie remains stationary (Video 10.5).

Confirmation of Tube Placement

There are many ways to confirm the position of the tube. Slide a finger along the tube to verify it has entered the pleural cavity. Look for condensation inside the tube and listen for air movement, which is audible during respirations. Observe the free flow of blood or fluid. Check to be sure that the tube rotates freely after insertion. A chest radiograph is used for the definitive assessment of tube placement (Fig. 10.23). If the tube and the most proximal hole are not entirely within the pleural space, and if the field has remained sterile, advance the tube. If the tube is kinked, dysfunctional, or the sterile field has been lost and advancement is required, place a new tube in a sterile fashion through the same tract. If the tube has been advanced too far, simply withdraw it to the correct depth.

Securing the Tube

See Video 10.6. Once the position of the tube has been verified with a radiograph, secure it. There are numerous methods to do so. The usual method is to sew the tube to the skin with large 0-0 or 1-0 silk sutures. Nylon sutures are also acceptable but must be tied tightly, or they will slip on the surface of the tube. One common method is a "stay" suture,

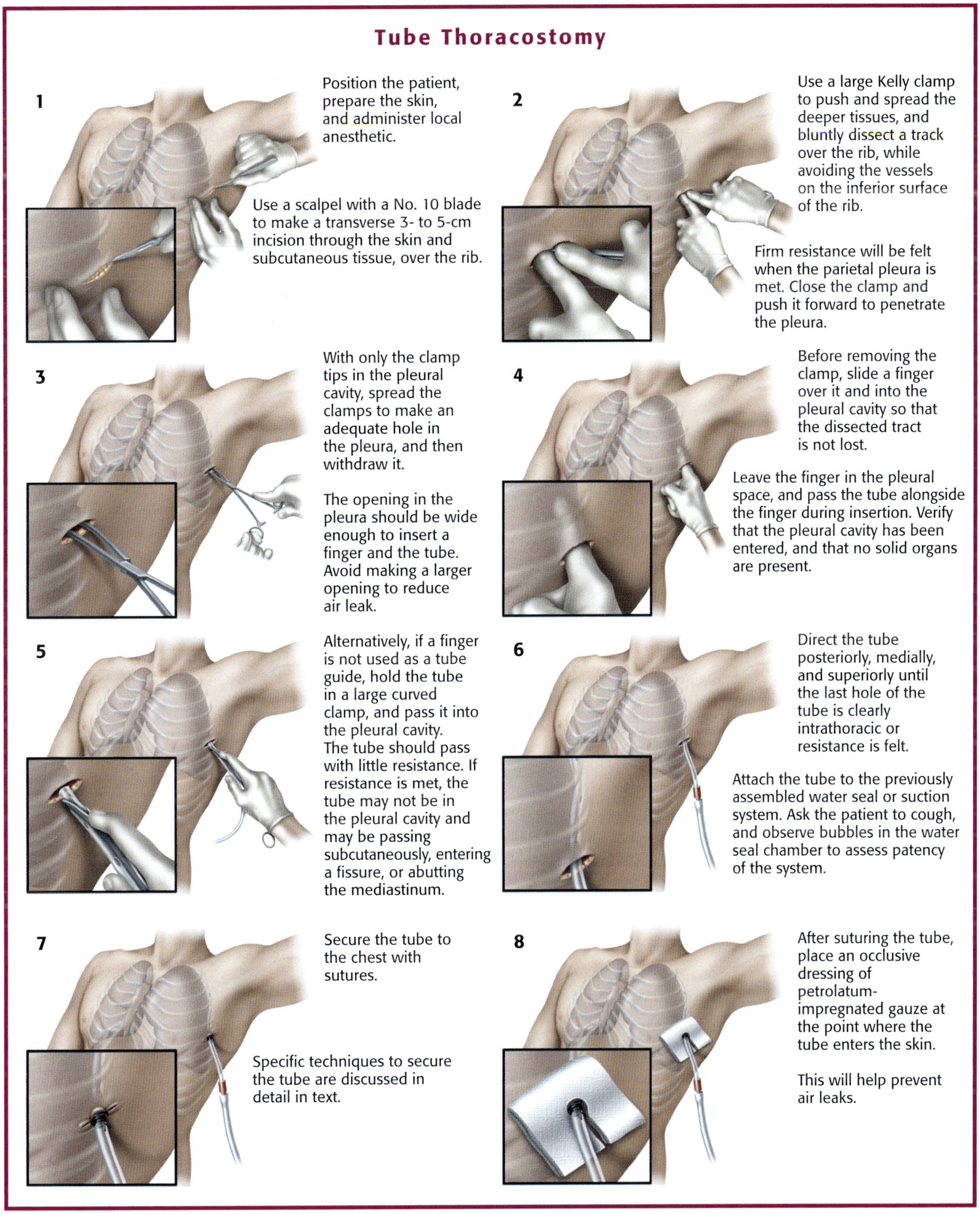

Fig. 10.15 Tube thoracostomy. (From Custalow CB. *Color Atlas of Emergency Department Procedures*. Saunders; 2005.)

in which the same suture that closes the skin incision is used to hold the tube (Fig. 10.24, *plate 1*). After this suture is used to close the skin incision, wrap the ends tightly and repeatedly around the chest tube and tie it securely. Tie the sutures tightly enough to indent the chest tube slightly and avoid slippage. Use additional simple sutures to close the skin incision as needed.

Another optional suture technique can help close the skin around the tube and completely close the incision once the chest tube is removed. To do this, place a *horizontal mattress suture* approximately 1 cm across the incision on either side of the tube, essentially encircling it (see Fig. 10.24, *plate 2*). Secure it with a simple knot that can easily be untied so that it can be opened and retied to close the incision after removing the tube.

After suturing the tube in place, apply an occlusive dressing of petrolatum-impregnated gauze around the tube where it enters the skin to help reduce air leaks. Cover the skin with two or more gauze pads with a Y-shaped cut from the middle of one side to the center (see Fig. 10.24, *plate 3*). Secure this dressing with wide (8 cm to 9 cm) cloth or elastic adhesive tape, with or without benzoin.

Use approximately 10 to 12 cm of tape split into three pieces, extending halfway along its length. Place the two outside pieces on the skin on either side of the tube site, and wrap the center section tightly around the tube (see Fig. 10.24, *plate 4*). Repeat this with a second piece of tape placed at a 180-degree angle to the first. In addition, securely tape the tube connections. To further secure the tube, use tape to create a loop or stalk by wrapping it around it. Then press the tape together for 1 to 2 cm before applying the tape to the chest wall (see Fig. 10.24, *plate 5*).

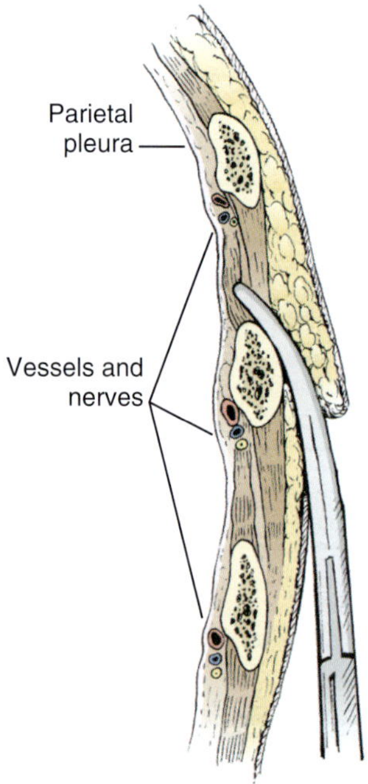

Fig. 10.16 Direct the Kelly clamp over the top of the rib to avoid the intercostal neurovascular bundle that courses under the rib above. Do not use excessive tunneling. (From Millikan JS, Moore EE, Steiner E. Complications of tube thoracostomy for acute trauma. *Am J Surg.* 1980;140:739.)

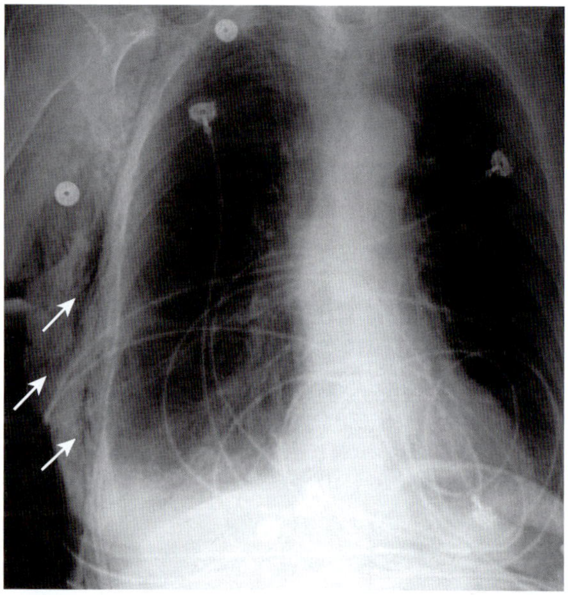

Fig. 10.18 Right-sided subcutaneous emphysema after chest tube placement secondary to making too large a hole in the pleura with a subsequent air leak *(arrows)*. This is usually benign and self-limited but can become problematic if the patient receives positive pressure ventilation. It is essential to make the right-sized pleural hole initially because there is no way to close the pleura.

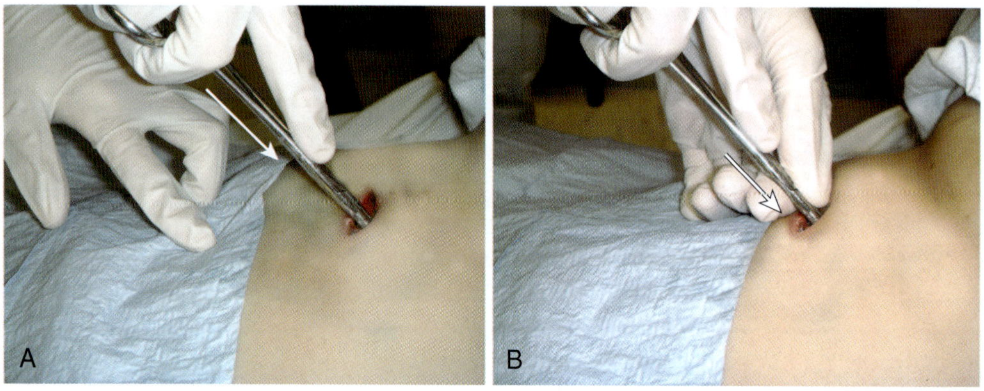

Fig. 10.17 (A–B) Use the right hand to push the clamp through the pleura *(white arrows)*. Firmly encircle the midportion of the clamp with the fingers of the left hand to serve as a safety stop measure to avoid penetrating too deeply.

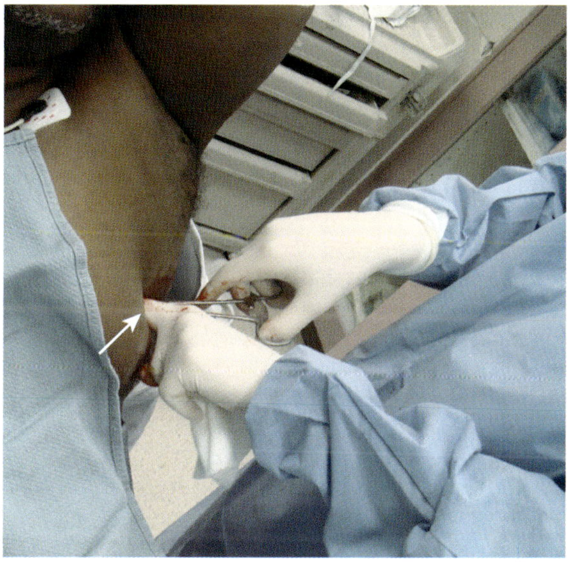

Fig. 10.19 After puncturing the pleural lining and spreading with the clamp, slide a gloved finger over the clamp to ensure that the pleural space has been reached *(white arrow)* and no solid underlying masses are present. Then withdraw the clamp but keep the finger inside the thoracostomy tract. Use the finger to guide the chest tube to ensure entry into the pleural cavity.

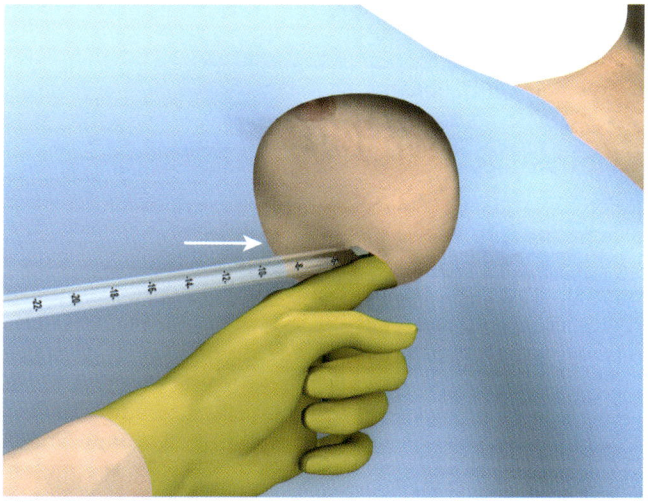

Fig. 10.20 Leave your finger in the pleural space and use it to guide the course of the tube *(arrow)*.

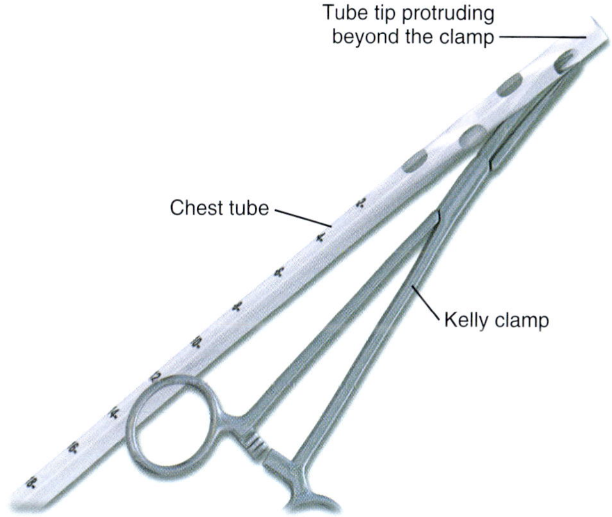

Fig. 10.21 Hold the tube with the tip of the tube protruding beyond the end of the clamp to reduce the risk of pulmonary injury.

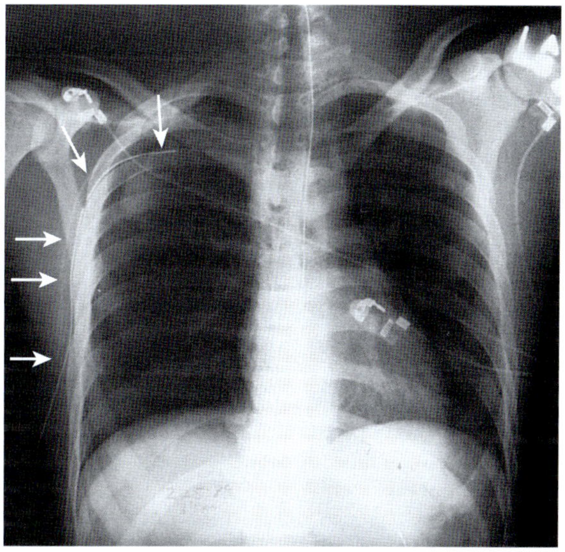

Fig. 10.22 Subcutaneous placement of a chest tube *(arrows)* can occur because the tube can dissect through tissue planes with relative ease. The radiograph may erroneously "confirm" intrapleural placement despite the tube being subcutaneous throughout its entire course. However, there would be no air fogging the tube with respirations. A computed tomography scan would identify improper placement.

Drainage and Suction Systems

Once placed, chest tubes are usually attached to a pleural drainage unit and set to active suction or to water seal (off suction). A basic understanding of chest tube drainage systems is necessary to prevent life-threatening complications associated with their use. All drainage systems have two essential components: a one-way valve to allow air or fluid to drain out of the pleural space without letting air back into the pleural space and a suction mechanism to increase the drainage rate. The simplest drainage device is just a one-way valve without suction. This can be accomplished with a water seal or a flutter (Heimlich) valve attached to the end of the chest tube (Fig. 10.25). Normal respiration and coughing are often sufficient to create the pressure necessary to remove excess air from the pleural space and allow the lung to expand. The Heimlich valve does not require suction and can be used for outpatient therapy.

A one-bottle system is the simplest but rarely used in modern healthcare. With a one-bottle system, the intrapleural fluid or air exits under a small amount of water. It collects in a single reservoir and mixes with the water (Fig. 10.26A). The water above the tube acts as a seal because it is too heavy to be drawn back into the chest. For drainage to occur, intrathoracic pressure must be greater than the water pressure at the distal end of the immersed tube. The height of the water above the exit port of the tubing determines this pressure. When the height is too great (the tube is too deep in the water), even coughing may not raise intrapleural pressure sufficiently to drain the chest. Place the collecting bottle below the patient, usually on the floor, to prevent inspiration from generating

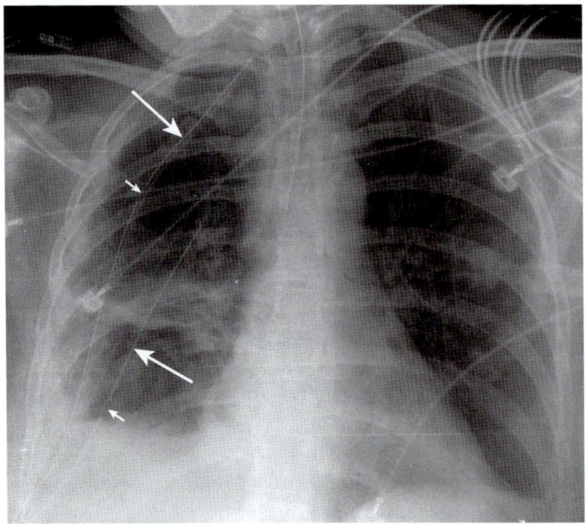

Fig. 10.23 A chest radiograph to assess chest tube placement. This patient has two chest tubes in place, and the radiopaque marking white lines on the tubes *(large arrows)* are readily visible. Chest tubes have radiopaque lines that are interrupted by drainage holes *(small arrows)*. To ensure the tube is deep enough, all gaps in the line must be within the pleural cavity on the radiograph.

enough negative pressure to pull the contents of the collection bottle into the chest cavity.

The suction device should have a high suction flow (≥20 L/min) and be able to keep the suction constant. The amount of suction in the chest tube depends on the depth of water in the water seal reservoir, not on the suction from the wall valve. When negative pressure from the suction source exceeds the depth of the water in the chamber, air enters from the top of the third tube and causes continuous bubbling (see Fig. 10.26B). This prevents a further increase in pressure in the chest tube. The wall suction dial can be turned down until only occasional bubbling can be detected. Vigorous bubbling does not equate with more suction.

Many commercial, enclosed systems are available that essentially combine a two-bottle method that can be connected to suction but with the addition of an "air leak chamber" (see Fig. 10.26C). Bubbling in this chamber indicates the presence of an air leak, usually from the drainage system itself due to a loose tube connection. If bubbling is present, check the drainage system, tube, and connectors for any problems or loose connections. If the leak continues, check whether all the holes of the chest tube are within the thorax. If the bubbling continues after these steps, the air leak may be due to a large hole in the lung parenchyma, usually seen only with expiration or with coughing. A continuous air leak or a leak during inspiration indicates a more extensive and possibly more significant lung injury.[53] Surgical intervention is indicated if an air leak persists for more than 72 hours or the lung is not entirely reexpanded.

The drainage reservoir must remain below the level of the chest to prevent the fluid in the collection system from reentering the chest. Place the reservoir on the floor or hang it from the edge of the bed. Simple respirations do not generate enough negative intrathoracic pressure to pull the water in the reservoir up to the height of the chest if the reservoir is kept on the floor and the patient is either sitting or lying at standard chair or bed height. The tubing should be long enough so that the reservoir can be kept below the level of the patient but not long enough to cause it to form dependent loops of fluid or kinks. Dependent loops collect fluid and create an additional water seal that, if large enough, can require greater intrapleural pressure to drain. A tension pneumothorax may result if these pressures become high enough (15 to 25 cm H_2O).

When the drainage system is functioning properly, the height of the fluid level in the drainage tube fluctuates with inspiration and expiration. The absence of respiratory fluctuation or a decrease in drainage may indicate that the system is blocked or that the lung is fully expanded. If the tube is blocked, the chest tube, collecting tubing, or both can be changed or *stripped* to dislodge clots. Replacing the tube is a complicated process associated with risks, but the stripping procedure is controversial because of the concern that the potentially high negative pressure from the procedure could damage lung tissue.[54] For stripping, clamp the tube proximally, progressively compress it distally, and then release it to allow the tube to spring open. The sudden increase in negative pressure may extract clots and fluid from a more proximal location.

Stripping a chest tube is not without potential negative consequence, as it may significantly increase negative intrathoracic pressures that could cause harm (e.g., tissue entrapment, increased bleeding, left ventricular dysfunction), thereby further impairing patients' recovery.[55] Perform occlusive chest tube clamping only with close monitoring because a tension pneumothorax can result in rare cases. Patients with chest tubes in place are best transported with a Heimlich valve or water seal only, not with the tube clamped.

Prophylactic Antibiotics

Posttraumatic empyema and pneumonia are potential complications of tube thoracostomy, and prophylactic antibiotics have been advocated to decrease the incidence of these infections. The term presumptive antibiotics has been suggested rather than prophylactic antibiotics to more accurately reflect the fact that antibiotics are given soon after injury rather than *before*, as typically occurs prior to an operative procedure. The practice of administering presumptive antibiotics to decrease the incidence of infectious complications in tube thoracostomy is controversial. The Eastern Association for the Surgery of Trauma (EAST) Practice Management Guidelines Work Group revised their initial guidelines recommending using first-generation cephalosporins during the first 24 hours for patients undergoing chest tube drainage for hemothorax. They currently report insufficient published evidence to support any recommendation for or against using presumptive antibiotics to reduce the incidence of empyema or pneumonia in tube thoracostomy for traumatic hemopneumothorax. The routine practice of presumptive antibiotics in tube thoracostomy for chest trauma will most likely remain controversial until a large, randomized, controlled trial can be performed.[56]

Tube Removal

Emergency clinicians rarely remove chest tubes. The usual indication for removal of a chest tube is after a chest radiograph demonstrates complete resolution of the pneumothorax and there is no evidence of an ongoing air leak. Before removal, discontinue suction and establish a water seal.

Securing a Thoracostomy Tube

1

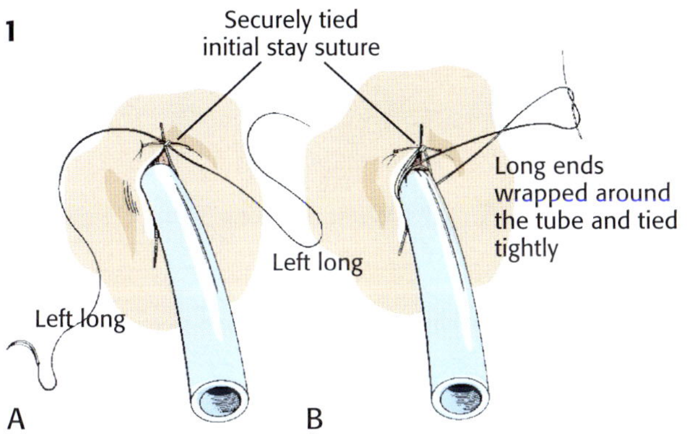

A, To secure the tube, first close the skin incision with a "stay" suture near the tube. **B**, Tie the knot securely and leave the suture ends long for wrapping around and tying the tube. Wrap the suture tightly at least twice around the tube, enough to indent the tube slightly, and tie securely.

2

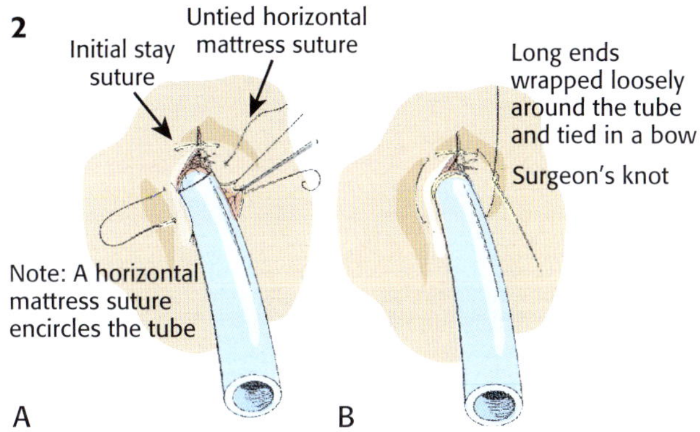

Another method to close the wound and secure the tube is with a horizontal mattress suture combined with a stay suture. **A**, A horizontal mattress suture is placed on either side (above and below) of the tube and held only with a surgeon's knot. **B**, The loose ends are also wrapped around the tube and tied loosely in a bow to identify the suture. This suture will be untied and used to close the skin incision after removal of the tube.

3

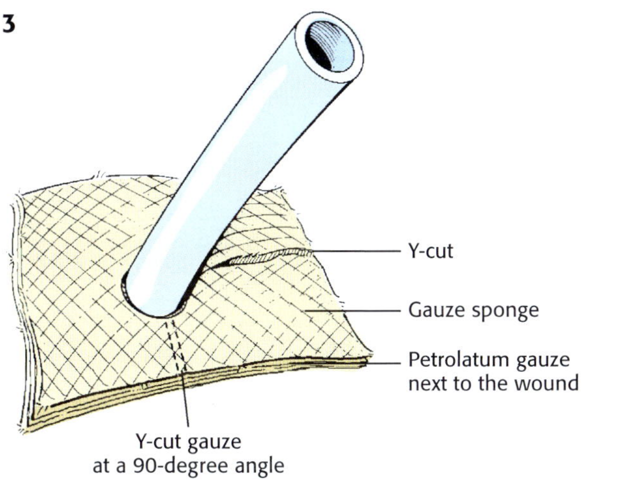

To dress the wound and reduce the risk for air leaks, an occlusive dressing should be applied. First wrap the base of the tube at the skin incision with a petroleum-impregnated dressing. A two-layer dressing of gauze sponges with a Y-shaped cut centered at the tube is shown. Place the second layer at a 90-degree angle to the first.

4

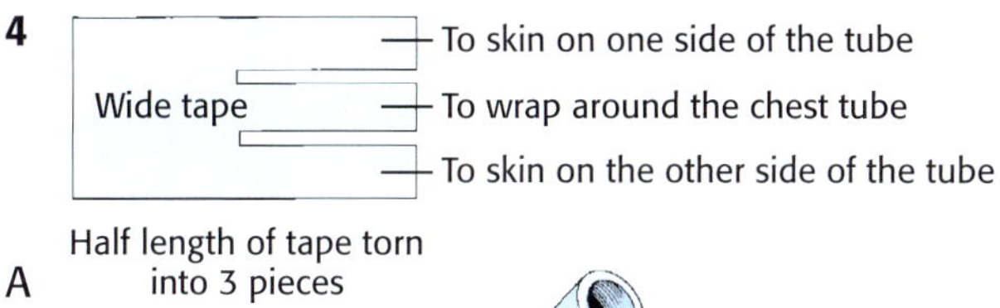

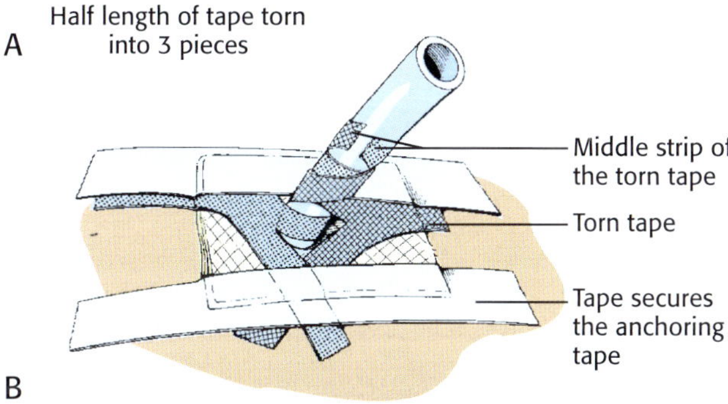

One method to further secure the tube is to use wide, split cloth tape. **A**, The distal half of a 15- to 20-cm-long, wide piece of tape is longitudinally split into three pieces. The two outside pieces are placed on the skin on either side of the tube, and the center strip is wrapped around the chest tube itself. **B**, This process may be repeated with a similar piece of tape placed at a 90-degree angle. The tape is securely anchored to the skin (benzoin is optional, but the skin must be clean and dry), and the torn tape is wrapped around the tube. Each anchoring piece is covered by another piece of tape.

5

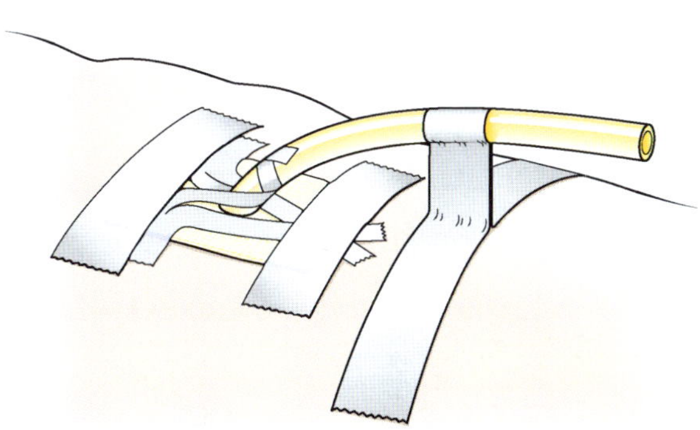

The tube can be further secured with an additional anchor system farther down on the tube. Wrap a 20- to 25-cm piece of tape or elastic, adhesive dressing around the tube and seal at least 3 cm of the tape together on the side of the tube nearest the chest wall. Spread the remaining tape against the dry skin of the chest wall and secure with additional tape.

Fig. 10.24 Methods of securing a thoracostomy tube.

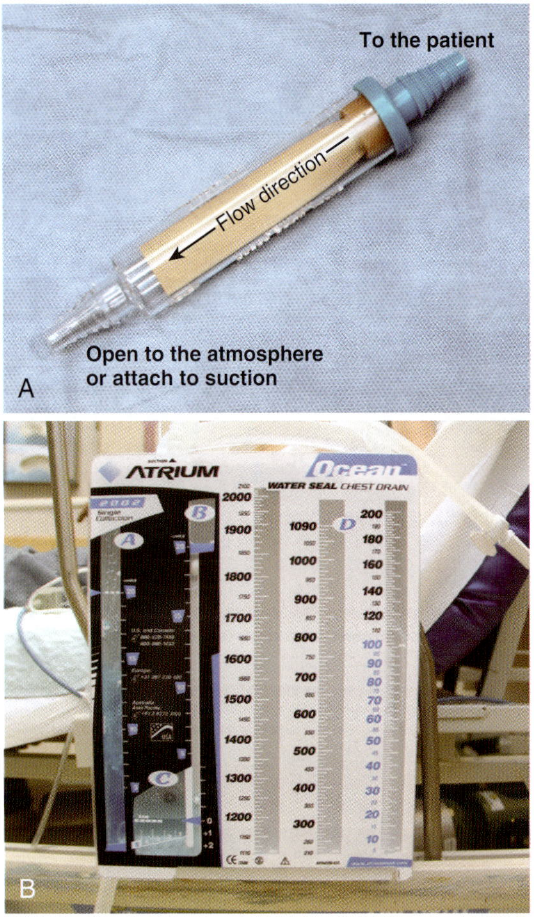

Fig. 10.25 Pleural drainage devices. (A) A one-way Heimlich valve alone is often sufficient to treat a pneumothorax, but not for a hemothorax. (B) Disposable water seal chest drain set.

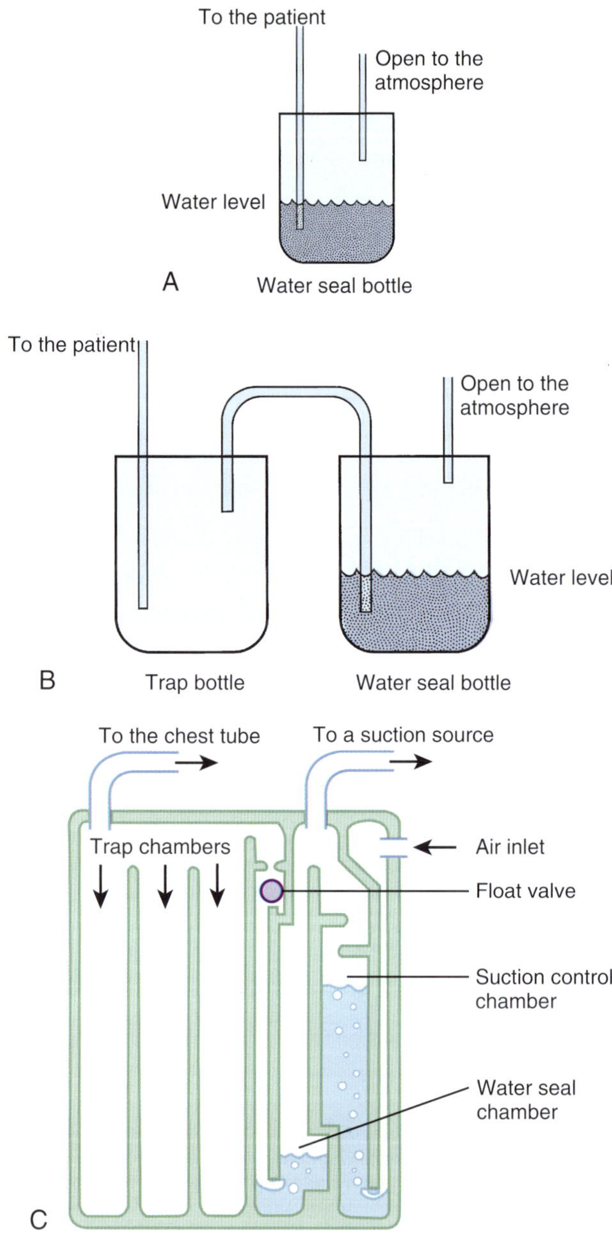

Fig. 10.26 (A) A single-bottle (water seal) collection device. (B) A two-bottle system. The trap reservoir proximal to the water seal keeps the accumulating drainage from affecting the water seal pressure. (C) This has now been replaced by a disposable system that mimics the two-bottle system. (Courtesy Thora Klex System, Davol, Inc., Warwick, RI.)

To remove the chest tube, ask the patient to sit upright at approximately a 45-degree angle. Use sterile technique, clean the skin, and drape the insertion site. Suturing equipment is needed to close the wound after the tube is removed, except when a purse-string suture was placed at the time of insertion, which requires only sterile scissors to cut the suture. Keep additional equipment available to reinsert a chest tube if the lung collapses. Prepare a petrolatum- or antibiotic-impregnated gauze dressing to cover the wound.

If a purse-string suture was to secure the tube, loosen it and prepare it for closing the wound. Cut the skin loop of the suture holding the tube to the skin and remove it from the skin. Timing the chest tube removal with the respiratory cycle has been debated. One recommendation is to remove the tube at the end of expiration during a Valsalva maneuver, corresponding to the time when the difference between the atmospheric and pleural pressure is at its lowest.[57] Alternatively, other studies emphasized the importance of a Valsalva maneuver during tube removal regardless of the respiratory phase. Pull the tube out in one swift motion. Quickly tie the purse-string suture or suture the wound closed, and then cover it with an occlusive dressing. If a purse-string suture was not used, suture the skin as quickly as possible after removing the tube. Observe the patient for 2 to 6 hours and obtain a chest radiograph before discharge. Any increase in symptoms requires prompt reevaluation. After 48 hours, the patient may remove the dressing. Sutures should be removed in 7 to 10 days.

OTHER TECHNIQUES

Initial management of stable patients who present with PSP depends upon the size of the pneumothorax, associated symptoms, and whether the event is a first or a recurrent event. Management of an SSP adds the additional consideration of underlying pathology. Treatment options include observation alone, observation with oxygen, simple aspiration, and tube or catheter thoracostomy.

Clinical stable patients with first episode of PSP that is small (≤3 cm at the apex or ≤2 cm at the hilum) can be considered for observation with or without supplemental oxygen and be discharged if clinically appropriate pending reassessment. The rationale for this approach comes from data from a trial that suggest many patients in this category improve with this strategy without an invasive procedure for the removal of air.[58] Patients with the first occurrence of a large PSP may have treatment options that include aspiration, chest tube with or without an ambulatory device, or observation. Choosing among these options depends on the severity of symptoms and local expertise.

Aspiration can be considered in clinically stable patients with a PSP. Some authors recommend catheter rather than needle aspiration using equipment available in most commercial thoracentesis kits since needle aspiration alone may increase the risk of perforating the visceral pleural membrane and perpetuate the pneumothorax. Studies that support aspiration in patients with a first PSP rather than tube or catheter thoracostomy are largely observational or small randomized trials that report efficacy rates ranging from 30% to 80%, shorter hospital stays, and fewer complications with aspiration.[59–62] For patients with SSP, the procedure for aspirating air is similar to that described in patients with PSP except the threshold for admission following aspiration and/or the threshold for catheter or tube thoracostomy should be lower since the likelihood of failed aspiration is higher.

Clinically stable patients with PSP and failed observation or aspiration, patients who are unstable due to pneumothorax, and patients with recurrent PSP should have a tube or catheter thoracostomy placed and be admitted. Choosing between tube or catheter thoracostomy at this point is often at the clinician's discretion and available expertise. However, catheters are being increasingly used since they are easy to place, less painful, and as effective for the drainage of air as tube thoracostomy.

Most clinically stable patients with an SSP should be treated with catheter or tube thoracostomy based upon the rationale that compared with PSP, patients with SSP have underlying lung disease that increases the likelihood of failure of aspiration, a prolonged air leak, and the development of tension pneumothorax.[63] In general, chest tube or catheter thoracostomy is preferred over simple aspiration for drainage of air in patients with SSP because it is more likely to be successful.[64] However, exceptions may exist. For example, for patients with a small SSP and who are asymptomatic or have minimal symptoms, treating with observation and supplemental oxygen and/or aspiration may be appropriate. The threshold to admit the patients should be low. Progression of symptoms or an enlarging pneumothorax is an indication for pleural drainage.

Guidewire Technique for Catheter Aspiration

See Videos 10.7 to 10.11. Catheters designed specifically for aspirating a pneumothorax are made of flexible, thrombosis-resistant radiopaque material with multiple distal side ports to reduce the risk of occlusion. Commercially available small-bore catheter systems are ideal for this procedure.

The catheters are placed via a standard "over-the-wire" (Seldinger) technique. Either standard location (the midaxillary to anterior axillary line at the fourth or fifth intercostal space or the midclavicular line at the second intercostal space) can be used, but the latter is more common.

Place the patient in a semi-upright position. Using sterile technique, clean the skin with an antiseptic solution and drape the area. Infiltrate lidocaine locally and deeply for anesthesia. Advance the guide needle in a straight line at a 60-degree angle cephalad over the top of the rib (Figs. 10.27 and 10.28). Be careful to create a straight tract, or it will be difficult to advance the floppy catheter (tunneling up and over the rib cannot be used). When the pleural space is identified by intermittent aspiration, halt the advancement of the needle. Use your hand to stabilize the needle against the chest wall and feed the guidewire through it and into the pleural space. Remove the needle while stabilizing the guidewire to keep it in the pleural space. Make a small incision in the skin with a No. 11 blade scalpel at the base of the wire to allow passage of the catheter through the skin. Some systems use a dilator over the wire to open the path through the soft tissue. Thread the minicatheter over the guidewire and into the pleural space. Advance the catheter through the subcutaneous tissue with a twisting motion. Remove the wire and dilator while leaving the catheter in the pleural space. Secure the catheter to the skin with a suture and dress the incision site. Suction may be needed for a few days, depending on the size of the pneumothorax. If the catheter becomes clogged with mucus or blood, inject sterile saline through the device to clear it.

To aspirate the pneumothorax, attach a three-way stopcock to the catheter and slowly aspirate air with a 60-mL syringe until resistance is felt. Several aspirations may be required to remove all the air. Gentle wall suction can also be used. Then take a chest radiograph to determine if the lung has fully reexpanded. If a residual pneumothorax is present, attempt further aspirations. If the residual pneumothorax persists and air cannot be aspirated, the catheter may be kinked or blocked with soft tissue. To relieve the blockage, place the patient in the full upright position and have the patient cough or take a deep breath. Alternatively, rotate or twist the catheter gently to straighten the kink.

TUBE THORACOSTOMY IN PEDIATRIC PATIENTS

See Videos 10.12 and 10.13. Pneumothoraces can occur in the neonatal population. They are often associated with resuscitative measures (such as mechanical ventilation) for meconium aspiration or prematurity. For the rest of the pediatric population, trauma is the most common cause. A pneumothorax will develop in approximately one-third of children with thoracic trauma. As in adults, physical examination of newborns and infants with pneumothorax can be highly variable, thus necessitating the use of a chest radiograph for diagnosis. Ideally, use both anteroposterior and cross-table lateral radiographs because small pneumothoraces may be seen only on the lateral view. A chest CT is more sensitive and specific in the evaluation of pneumothorax.

Tube thoracostomy is the treatment of choice for a symptomatic pneumothorax in infants. When signs of tension pneumothorax are present, immediately aspirate with a plastic catheter-over-the-needle device. Small pneumothoraces (<20% of the hemithorax) in relatively asymptomatic infants (e.g., those without other problems who do not require positive airway pressure) can be observed.

The technique of tube thoracostomy in pediatric patients is essentially the same as that in adults, but the body size and small spaces between the ribs make the procedure more difficult. The tube size increases with the patient's weight, starting with 8- to 10-Fr catheters for premature infants (Table 10.1).

Catheter Aspiration of Pneumothorax: Seldinger Technique

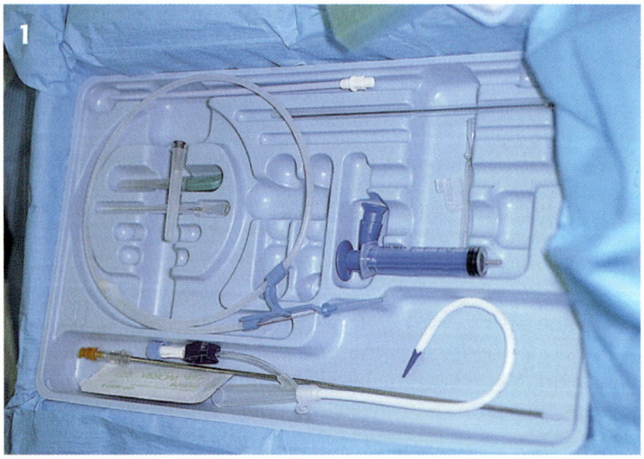

The Seldinger-type catheter kit contains a pigtail catheter and all necessary equipment, including local anesthesia, introducing needle and syringe, scalpel, guidewire, and dilator.

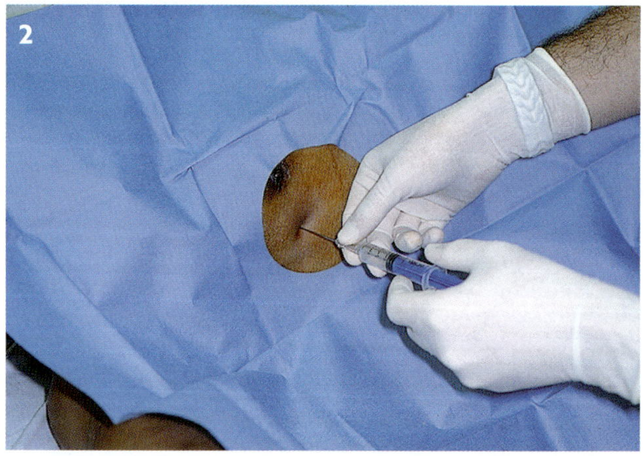

After generous local anesthesia, advance the introducing syringe in a straight line over the top of the fifth rib until air is aspirated. Unless a straight tract is created, it will be difficult to advance the floppy catheter, and a tunneling approach cannot be used.

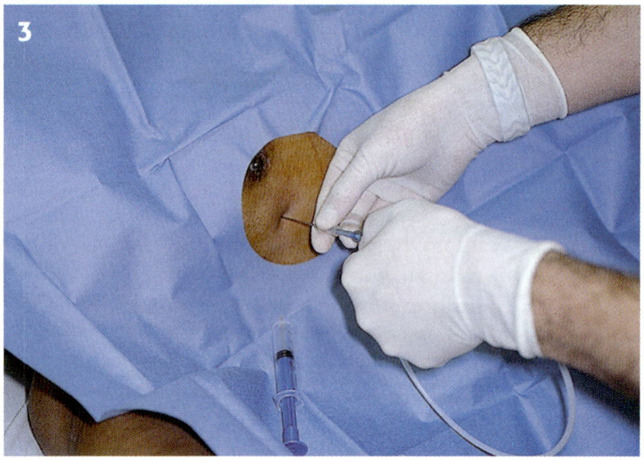

Advance the guidewire through the introducing needle into the pleural space, and then remove the needle. The procedural steps are analogous to initiating a central venous catheter via the Seldinger technique.

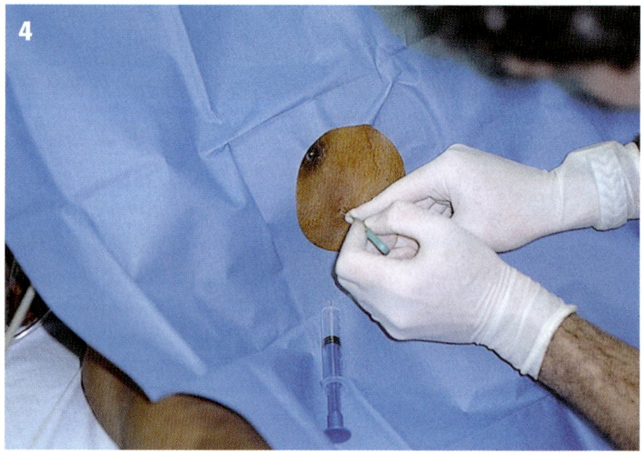

Puncture the skin at the site of wire insertion with a scalpel. Make the incision large enough to accept the dilator and pigtail catheter.

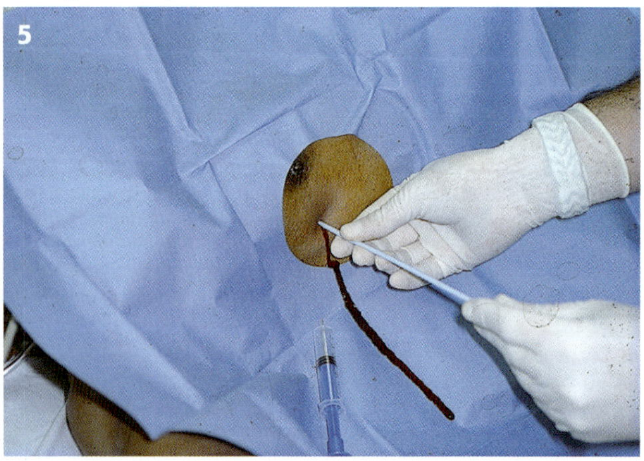

Advance the dilator over the wire to create a tract for the catheter. Remove the dilator while leaving the wire in place. Again, this is analogous to establishing a central venous line.

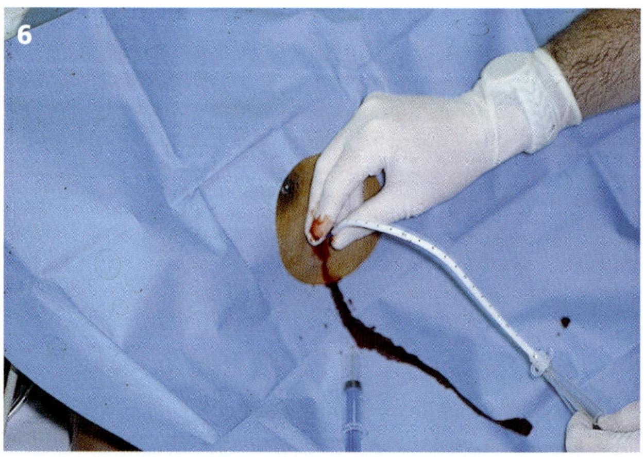

Advance the pigtail catheter over the wire through the dilated tract. It will assume its pigtail configuration when it is in the pleural space. A twisting motion may be needed to advance the catheter through subcutaneous tissue. Advance the catheter to the hilt and secure to suction. This catheter may be removed after a period of observation, or the suction may be maintained for a few days.

Fig. 10.27 Aspiration of a pneumothorax with an Arrow 14-Fr Percutaneous Cavity Drainage Catheterization Kit (Teleflex). This 23-cm pigtail multi-hole catheter is ideal for such purposes. Air can be aspirated from the catheter with a syringe, or the catheter can be attached to suction or a Heimlich valve. This catheter is not used for ventilated patients, those with continuing air leaks, or those with a hemothorax. It is ideal for stable patients who have a primary spontaneous pneumothorax or minor injury (such as induced by intravenous drug use, minor blunt trauma, or insertion of a central venous catheter).

Aspiration of Pneumothorax: Catheter-Over-the-Needle Technique

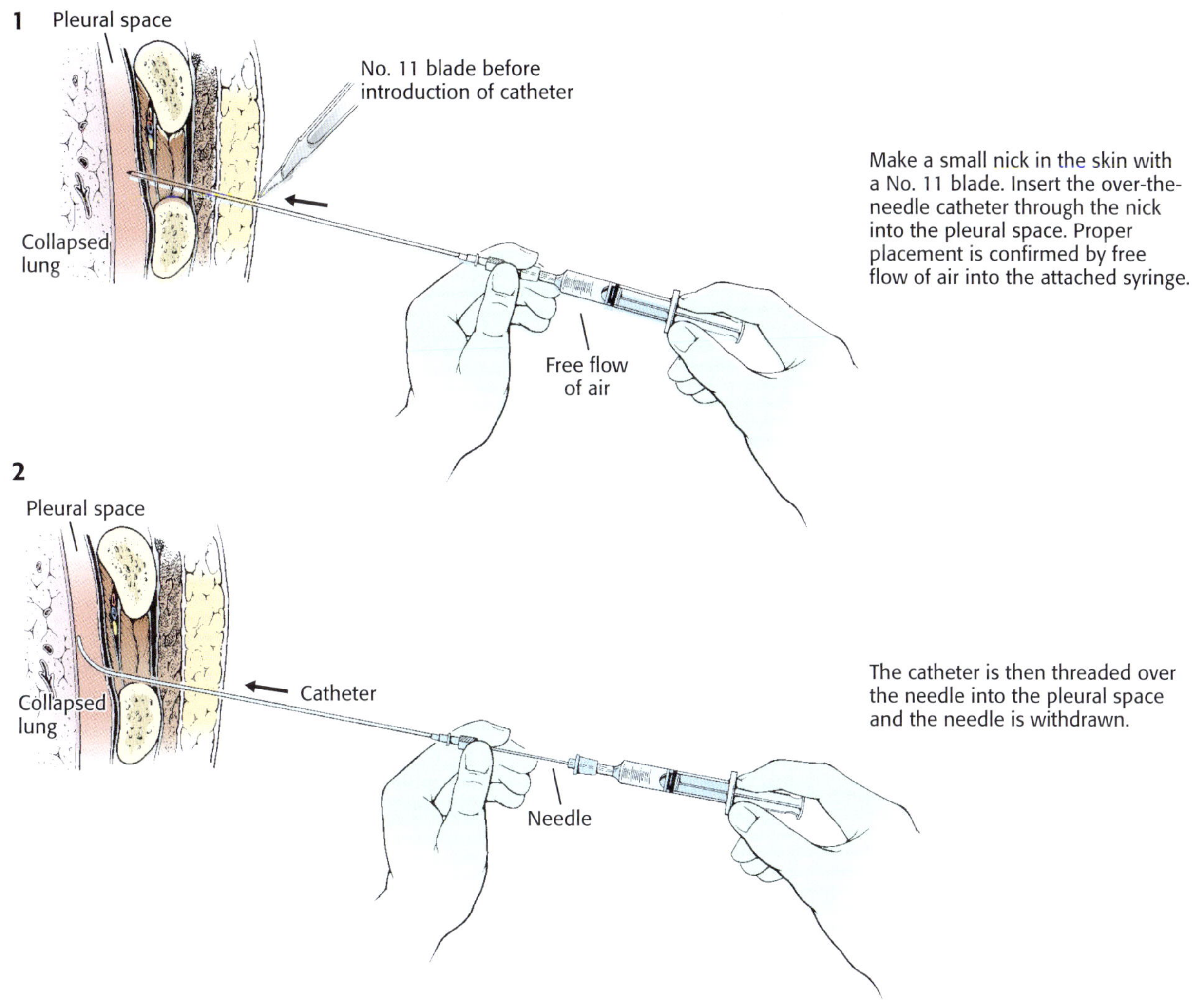

Fig. 10.28 Catheter-over-the-needle technique for aspiration of a pneumothorax.

Because of the risk of future breast deformities, avoid the midclavicular approach. Instead, use the anterior axillary line through the fifth intercostal space for newborns and infants.[65]

COMPLICATIONS

The complication rates associated with tube thoracostomy are variable and have been reported to be as high as 40%.[66–68] The variability is likely due to a lack of a universally accepted way to categorize complications. One proposed method uses the following categories: insertional, positional, removal, malfunction, and infectious.[69] The most common complications include infection, laceration of an intercostal vessel, laceration of the lung, and intraabdominal or solid organ placement of the chest tube (Boxes 10.4 and 10.5). Local infection at the insertion site is common and often related to the emergency nature of the procedure. Subcutaneous emphysema is a frequent, usually benign complication that is self-limited and generally caused by an excessively large opening in the pleura. The development of palpable subcutaneous air is another complication of chest tube placement or the inciting incident. It is usually limited to the insertion site but can become massive with PPV in a patient with continued air leak or an occluded tube. Intercostal arteries or veins may be lacerated, but this can be minimized by using blunt dissection and carefully directing the tube immediately above the rib. The tube may adequately tamponade such bleeding. If the bleeding persists, extend the incision to ligate the bleeding vessel. If the bleeding continues, consult a thoracic surgeon.

Failure of a pneumothorax to reexpand may be due to a mechanical air leak, but it may also indicate a bronchopleural fistula, a continued parenchymal lung leak, or a bronchial injury. Tension pneumothorax can occur if a blockage in the drainage system at any point is associated with an ongoing air leak from the lung. Insertion of a new tube or placement of a second tube may be indicated if the first tube is not functioning. In general, if the patient is deteriorating and their chest tube is not working correctly, quickly replace it or insert another. Manipulating the tube by pushing it deeper into the chest cavity increases the risk of infection.

TABLE 10.1 Approximate Pediatric Chest Tube Size by Weight

WEIGHT (kg)	CHEST TUBE (Fr)
<3	8–10
3–5	10–12
6–10	12–16
11–15	17–22
16–20	22–26
21–30	26–32
>30	32–40

BOX 10.4 Physical Complications of Tube Thoracostomy

INFECTION
Pneumonia
Empyema
Local infection of the incision
Osteomyelitis
Necrotizing fasciitis

PHYSIOLOGIC
Allergic reactions to the surgical preparation or anesthesia
Pulmonary atelectasis
Reexpansion pulmonary edema
Reexpansion hypotension

INJURIES: BLEEDING
Local incision hematoma
Intercostal artery or vein laceration
Internal mammary artery laceration (with midclavicular line placement)
Pulmonary vein or artery injury
Great-vessel injury

INJURIES TO SOLID ORGANS OR NERVES
Lung, liver, spleen, diaphragm, stomach, colon; long thoracic nerve, intercostal nerve

MISCELLANEOUS
Subcutaneous or mediastinal emphysema
Persistent pneumothorax
Retained hemothorax
Recurrence of pneumothorax after removal of the chest tube

BOX 10.5 Mechanical Complications of Tube Thoracostomy

MECHANICAL PROBLEMS
Dislodgement of the chest tube from the chest wall
Incorrect tube position
Subcutaneous placement
Intraabdominal placement

AIR LEAKS
Leaks within the drainage system (tubing or drainage device)
Last tube port not within the pleural space
Leaks from a skin site

BLOCKED DRAINAGE
Flow of drainage contents into the chest from elevation of the drainage bottles
Kinked chest tube or drainage tubes
Occlusion of the tube by clots

Re-expansion pulmonary edema is a rare but potentially fatal complication of thoracentesis and usually occurs unilaterally after rapid re-expansion of a collapsed lung. This ranges from mild to severe, but fatalities have been reported.[70] The onset ranges from shortly after reexpansion to hours later. Reexpansion pulmonary edema is more common when a pneumothorax has been present for at least 3 to 4 days, but the time frame is variable. The proposed mechanisms include anoxic damage to the alveolar-capillary basement membrane, loss of surfactant, or rapid fluid shifts. Treatment is supportive with noninvasive PPV and mechanical ventilatory support occasionally required.

CONCLUSION

Treatment of an abnormal accumulation of fluid and/or air from the pleural space depends on many factors and includes observation with or without supplemental oxygen, aspiration, small- and large-bore tube thoracostomies, catheter thoracostomy, and surgical interventions such as VATS. This can be done on an elective, urgent, or emergent basis based on the patient's underlying pathology and clinical stability. Chest tubes reestablish the negative intrathoracic pressure, allowing the lung to reexpand and restore physiologic oxygenation, ventilation, and cardiac output. With advances in technology and ongoing focus on less invasive procedures, the management of pleural conditions will continue to evolve. It is incumbent on the clinician to be proficient with multiple approaches and strategies to managing pleural conditions as well as the associated complications and benefits to help achieve the most optimal patient outcome.

EFERENCES ARE AVAILABLE AT Elsevier eBooks+

SECTION III

Cardiac Procedures

CHAPTER 11

Techniques for Supraventricular Tachycardias

Steven Lai and Scott R. Votey

INTRODUCTION

Supraventricular tachycardias (SVTs) refer to cardiac rhythms of more than 100 beats/minute, originating outside of the ventricles and above the bundle of His. These include sinus tachycardia, junctional tachycardia, reentrant tachycardias, multifocal atrial tachycardia (MAT), atrial fibrillation (AF), and atrial flutter (Fig. 11.1). SVTs are a common cause of emergency department (ED) visits and can cause significant patient discomfort and distress.

Patients experiencing an SVT most commonly complain of palpitations and dizziness, but may present with a wide range of signs and symptoms, including syncope and cardiac arrest. Chest pain is another common complaint, but not all chest pain in this situation indicates myocardial ischemia. Other symptoms arising from the dysrhythmia, such as nausea and diaphoresis, may also overlap with those of myocardial ischemia. Symptoms of tachycardias depend on the hemodynamic consequences of the rate and rhythm, with those patients who are experiencing hypoperfusion presenting with severe symptoms, such as syncope, chest pain, or cardiac arrest. Hypotension and poor perfusion are more typically dependent on the heart rate produced by any tachycardia than they are on the source of tachycardia. In some cases, patients presenting with ventricular tachycardia (VT) can be relatively stable and a patient with an extremely rapid SVT may be unstable. Decisions must be guided principally by the clinical presentation and exact rhythm identification should be subservient to the goal of prompt appropriate management.

The acute and chronic management of tachycardias differ importantly. Acute management focuses on stabilization and typically involves emergent administration of intravenous (IV) medications or external electrical cardioversion, while chronic management increasingly relies on more advanced interventions beyond the scope of emergency medicine. This chapter focuses on the acute management of SVTs (Box 11.1). A discussion of the treatment of VT and ventricular fibrillation (VF) is provided in Chapter 12.

TACHYCARDIA PATHOPHYSIOLOGY

Under normal circumstances, the sinoatrial (SA) node is the pacemaker for the heart. Depolarization is initiated in the SA node, and the impulse is conducted through the atrium to the atrioventricular (AV) node. Atrial depolarization corresponds to the P wave on the ECG. Conduction to the ventricles is slowed in the AV node, which provides a measure of protection against hemodynamically unstable SVTs. The normal slowing in the AV node is seen on the ECG as the PR interval. After the impulse traverses the AV node, it is conducted first down the His bundle, followed by the left and right bundle branches, and then dispersed to the ventricular myocardium via the Purkinje fibers. Ventricular depolarization corresponds to the QRS wave on the ECG. Normal impulse conduction produces a narrow QRS complex. It therefore follows that a narrow QRS complex is supraventricular in origin, while a wide QRS complex is either a ventricular origin or involves abnormal conduction (either due to structural causes, such as bundle branch or fascicular blocks, or toxic-metabolic causes, such as hyperkalemia or sodium-channel blockade).

Tachycardias can be generated from any focus in the heart, because essentially all myocardial tissue has intrinsic pacemaker activity. There are two principal mechanisms by which tachycardias arise: reentry and enhanced automaticity. Reentry is a phenomenon in which an initial depolarizing impulse travels a closed-loop path that returns cyclically to its point of origin and, in doing so, generates a regular, sustained tachydysrhythmia. The requirements for a reentrant tachydysrhythmia are: (1) a closed-loop conduction path; (2) slower conduction and prolonged refractoriness in one limb of the loop; (3) propagation of the initiating impulse down the faster limb of the loop, with antegrade conduction down the slower limb blocked; and (4) retrograde excitation of the initially blocked slower limb, returning the impulse to its point of origin, where depolarization is reinitiated (Fig. 11.2). A premature beat is the typical precipitant, and repetition of this cycle sustains the dysrhythmia.

Enhanced automaticity is an increase in the rate of the spontaneous depolarization of myocardial cells above their electrical threshold. Sinus tachycardia is the physiologic response to enhanced automaticity of the SA node. When enhanced automaticity results in more rapid depolarization of extra-nodal myocardial cells, these foci can produce ectopic tachycardias. Examples include paroxysmal atrial tachycardia (PAT) and junctional tachycardia. Enhanced automaticity often occurs as a result of increased sympathetic tone

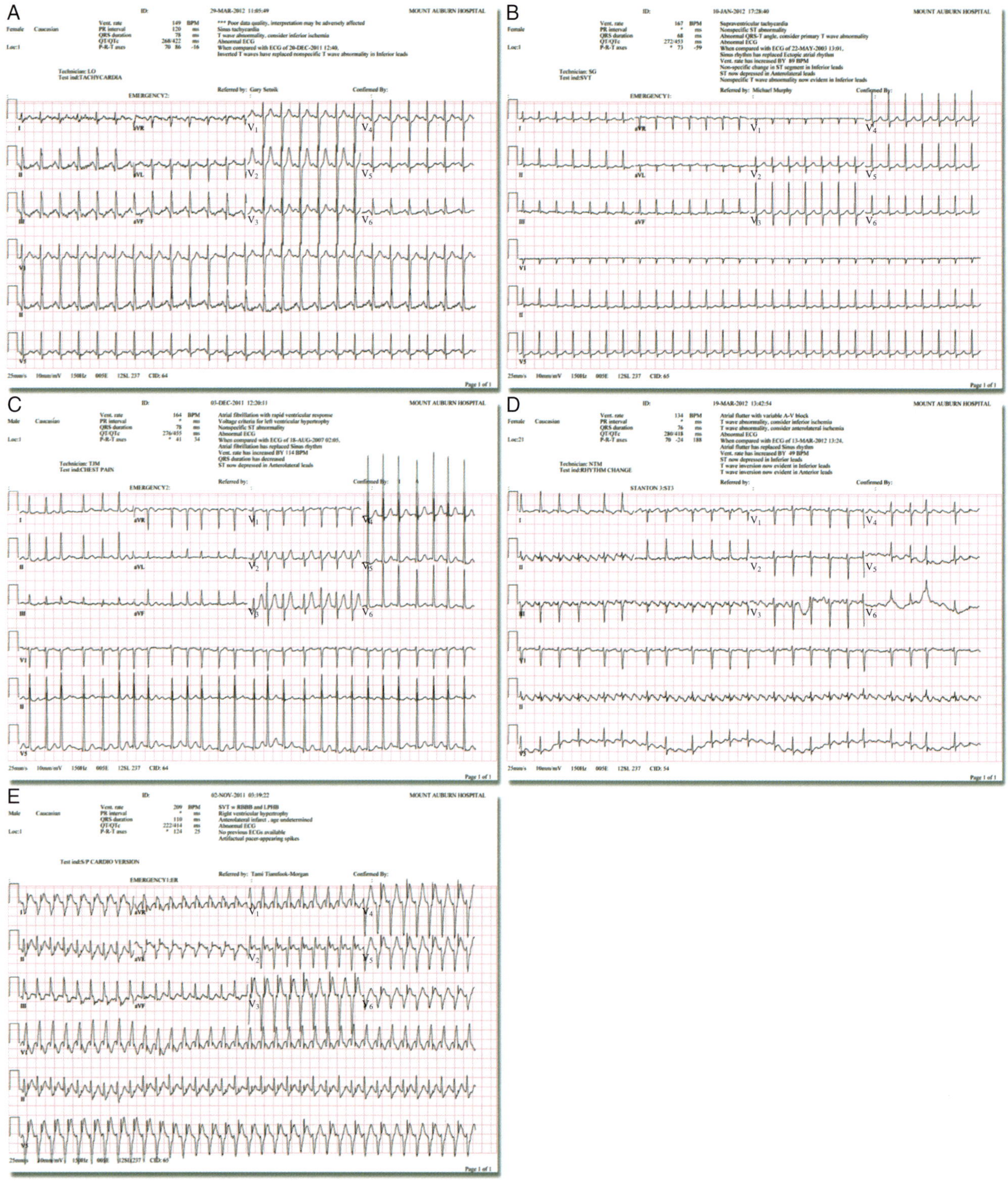

Fig. 11.1 Tachydysrhythmias. (A) Sinus tachycardia. (B) Supraventricular tachycardia (SVT). (C) Atrial fibrillation. (D) Atrial flutter. (E) SVT with aberrancy.

(e.g., with fever, thyrotoxicosis, or sympathomimetic overdose). Treatment of these dysrhythmias generally should be directed at removing the underlying stressor.

EVALUATION

In the ED, where diagnostic data are often limited and the patient's condition warrants prompt action, tachycardias are most successfully managed using an algorithmic diagnostic and therapeutic schema that is easily remembered and applied.

Step 1. Be Prepared for a Cardiopulmonary Arrest

Any patient experiencing a tachydysrhythmia is at risk for deterioration, because of the tachycardia or its treatment. Be prepared for a cardiopulmonary resuscitation by having advanced airway equipment and a defibrillator at the bedside. The patient should be placed on a cardiac monitor, and adequate intravenous access should be obtained. Pads for cardioversion should be placed on the patient in preparation for the possibility that their rhythm deteriorates to pulseless VT or VF, which would require immediate defibrillation and initiation of chest compressions.

Step 2. Determine Stability

Determine what hemodynamic effect the rhythm is having on the patient. In this context, unstable is defined as a heart rate and blood pressure inadequate to maintain vital organ perfusion and function, generally manifested clinically by significant chest pain, dyspnea, altered mental status, syncope, or hypotension. Categorizing a patient as stable or unstable is complicated by the innumerable gradations on the continuum from asymptomatic health to cardiopulmonary arrest. Altered mental status, signs of systemic hypoperfusion, or presumed ischemic chest pain with or without ECG changes of ischemia are convincing evidence of instability. Electrical cardioversion should be used to treat unstable patients with any tachycardia except sinus tachycardia and MAT. Stability is subject to change on a minute-to-minute basis, and therapy must be adjusted accordingly.

Blood pressure is one of the most commonly used determinants of patient stability. It is important to remember that arbitrary blood pressure cutoffs for defining stable or unstable do not consider the patient's baseline blood pressure. A systolic blood pressure of 90 mm Hg is of far more concern in a hypertensive patient over 65 years of age than in a healthy 20-year-old. In general, heart rates of less than 150 beats/min are less prone to cause hemodynamic instability. However, those patients with certain structural heart abnormalities (e.g., mitral stenosis), pulmonary hypertension, or diastolic heart failure may tolerate SVTs poorly even with lower heart rates.

After clinical stability is assessed, the ECG should be rapidly and systematically evaluated. Although most therapeutic decisions can be made on the basis of a rhythm strip, it is prudent to obtain a 12-lead ECG as soon as it is feasible. A 12-lead ECG can help determine if myocardial ischemia is present and can aid in differentiating among tachycardias, especially between sinus tachycardia and other regular SVTs. If a patient is unstable due to monomorphic VT or another tachydysrhythmia (aside from pulseless VT and VF above), perform synchronized cardioversion utilizing procedural sedation if possible. It is prudent to ensure the device is not syncing on the T wave to avoid a R-on-T phenomenon, potentially inducing VF. Unstable polymorphic VT may require defibrillation if cardioversion is not possible due to a very rapid rate.

BOX 11.1 Diagnostic and Therapeutic Approaches to Supraventricular Tachycardias

VAGAL MANEUVERS

Carotid sinus massage
Pressure on the carotid sinus

Valsalva Technique

Forced expiration of air against a closed glottis
Apneic facial exposure to cold water ("cold water diving reflex")
Immersion of the face into cold water

Oculocardiac Reflex

The trigeminovagal reflex initiated by pressure on the eyeball

PHARMACOLOGIC AGENTS

Adenosine
Calcium channel blockers (verapamil, diltiazem)
β-Blockers, including esmolol
Digoxin
Amiodarone
Procainamide

CARDIOVERSION

Administration of a synchronized shock

Step 3. Determine the Rate

The more extreme the ventricular rate, the more likely the patient is to become unstable. Sinus tachycardia rarely exceeds

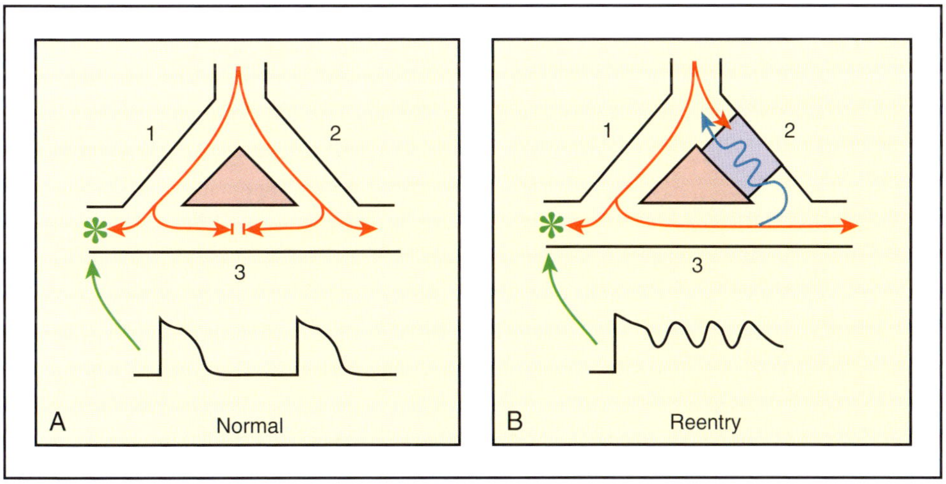

Fig. 11.2 Cardiac conduction in supraventricular tachycardia. (A) Normal depolarization down paths *1* and *2* that will "extinguish" or "cancel out" at point *3*. Normal depolarization/repolarization and conductance. (B) Reentrant pathway. *1*, Normal conduction; *2*, delayed/slowed conduction with unidirectional block; *3*, normal conduction pathway.

160 to 180 beats/min in adults. Although SVTs typically have rates slower than 180 beats/min, they can be faster in young people and in the presence of a bypass tract. VT is not slowed by passage through the AV node and can thus be much faster (250 to 300 beats/min) but is usually less than 220 beats/min.

Step 4. Determine the QRS Complex Width

When emergency cardioversion is not required, subsequent decisions can be based on the duration of the QRS complex. In an adult, a QRS width of greater than 0.12 ms is considered "wide." In many adults with a wide-complex tachycardia, the QRS duration is substantially greater than 0.12 ms. In children, the QRS duration is age dependent, but any QRS duration >0.10 ms is considered wide. It is usually possible to determine if a rhythm is wide or narrow from a rhythm strip alone, but if there is uncertainty, the widest QRS complex in the 12-lead ECG should be used as the measure.

Narrow-complex tachycardias can be assumed to be supraventricular. Wide-complex tachycardias are the result of any of three distinct pathophysiologic processes:

1. The rhythm originates in the ventricle and does not use the normal conduction pathway.
2. The origin of the tachycardia is supraventricular, but there is a block of the normal conduction pathway below the AV node (bundle-branch block [BBB]), often referred to as "aberrancy."
3. The origin of the tachycardia is supraventricular, but there is an accessory conduction pathway that bypasses the normal conduction pathway.

With rare exceptions, a wide-complex tachycardia should be treated as VT for three reasons: (1) VT is the most common cause of a wide-complex tachycardia; (2) despite the existence of diagnostic criteria, VT cannot be reliably distinguished from SVT with aberrancy in the clinical setting, and treating VT as SVT can be fatal (although treating SVT as VT is not harmful); and (3) even if the tachycardia has a supraventricular origin, there may be an associated bypass tract, in which case, some standard SVT treatments (e.g., verapamil) are contraindicated. It is never safe to assume that a wide-complex tachycardia is caused by aberrancy. It is more likely to be VT with increasing age, cardiac history, and increasing QRS duration.

Step 5. Assess the Regularity of the RR Intervals

An irregular narrow-complex tachycardia is usually caused by AF, although it can occasionally be caused by MAT or atrial flutter with variable AV block. Because VT is usually regular except during the first few beats, an irregular wide-complex tachycardia should also raise the suspicion of AF with a BBB (AF-BBB) or a bypass tract. Distinguishing which patients have AF with a bypass tract is important because the treatment of choice for these patients is cardioversion, even if they are stable. Although this differentiation can be difficult, two characteristics are helpful. In contrast to patients with AF-BBB, patients with AF with a bypass tract may have (1) very rapid conduction, with some RR complexes intervals equivalent to >250 beats/min, and (2) bizarre morphology QRS complexes resulting from fusion and partial fusion of beats from normal AV and bypass-tract conduction. At very high rates, the heart rate may appear to be regular (e.g., "pseudo-regularization") and utilizing calipers or marching out the beats may be helpful.[1]

Step 6. Determine the Presence or Absence of P Waves

Determine whether P waves are present, their morphologic characteristics, whether they are regular, and how they are related to the QRS complexes. Regular uniform P waves preceding the QRS complex help distinguish sinus tachycardia from other SVTs. A normal P-wave axis is one with an upright P wave in leads I, II, and aVF and negative in aVR. This axis strongly suggests the atrial activity is coming from the SA node and is indeed sinus in nature. Although similar P waves may be present with the much rarer PAT, an abnormal P-wave axis or morphology should alert one to the ectopic origin of that rhythm. An irregular narrow QRS-complex rhythm with more than three P-wave morphologies is indicative of MAT. One should, in addition, look for the regular sawtooth deflections of the ECG baseline that characterize atrial flutter waves. If no P waves are seen, these may instead be replaced by flutter or fibrillation waves, which are generally best seen in the inferior and right-sided precordial leads. If it is unclear whether there are P waves or fibrillation waves present, comparison to P-wave morphology in prior ECGs (if available), or obtaining a Lewis Lead ECG may be helpful. There are multiple described methods of Lewis lead placement.[2–4] A common way is moving the right arm (RA) electrode to the manubrium, the left arm (LA) electrode to the fifth intercostal margin/right sternal border, the left leg (LL) electrode over the right lower costal margin, and keeping the right leg (RL) electrode in standard position on the RL. Monitoring lead I or II will monitor the increased amplitude of any hidden P waves. Increasing the calibration from 10 to 20 mm/mV and/or paper speed from 25 to 50 mm/s can also further amplify the atrial activity (Fig. 11.3).

Application of this schema organizes tachycardias into four major categories based on the ECG appearance, with the additional distinction of clinically stable or unstable. The four categories are (1) narrow complex, regular, P waves present or absent; (2) narrow complex, irregular, P waves present or absent; (3) wide complex, regular, no P waves; and (4) wide complex, irregular, no P waves. Generally, each of the specific dysrhythmias that fall into each of these categories is treated in the same fashion, thus the simplicity of the approach. Occasionally, unstable patients need treatment initiated before analysis of the rhythm can be completed. In addition, once the rhythm is stabilized, the patient may require additional pharmacologic treatment to prevent recurrent dysrhythmias.

DIFFERENTIAL DIAGNOSIS AND ED MANAGEMENT

Narrow-Complex Tachycardias

Tables 11.1 and 11.2 outline the pharmacologic and electrical therapy for patients presenting with a wide variety of tachycardias. Table 11.3 summarizes a simplified differential and approach for tachydysrhythmias.

Narrow Complex, Regular, P Waves Present

Sinus tachycardia makes up the overwhelming majority of these cases. The tachycardia is generally a normal physiologic response to physical, emotional, or pharmacologic stressors. Generally, therapy for sinus tachycardia should be directed at the rhythm's underlying cause rather than at

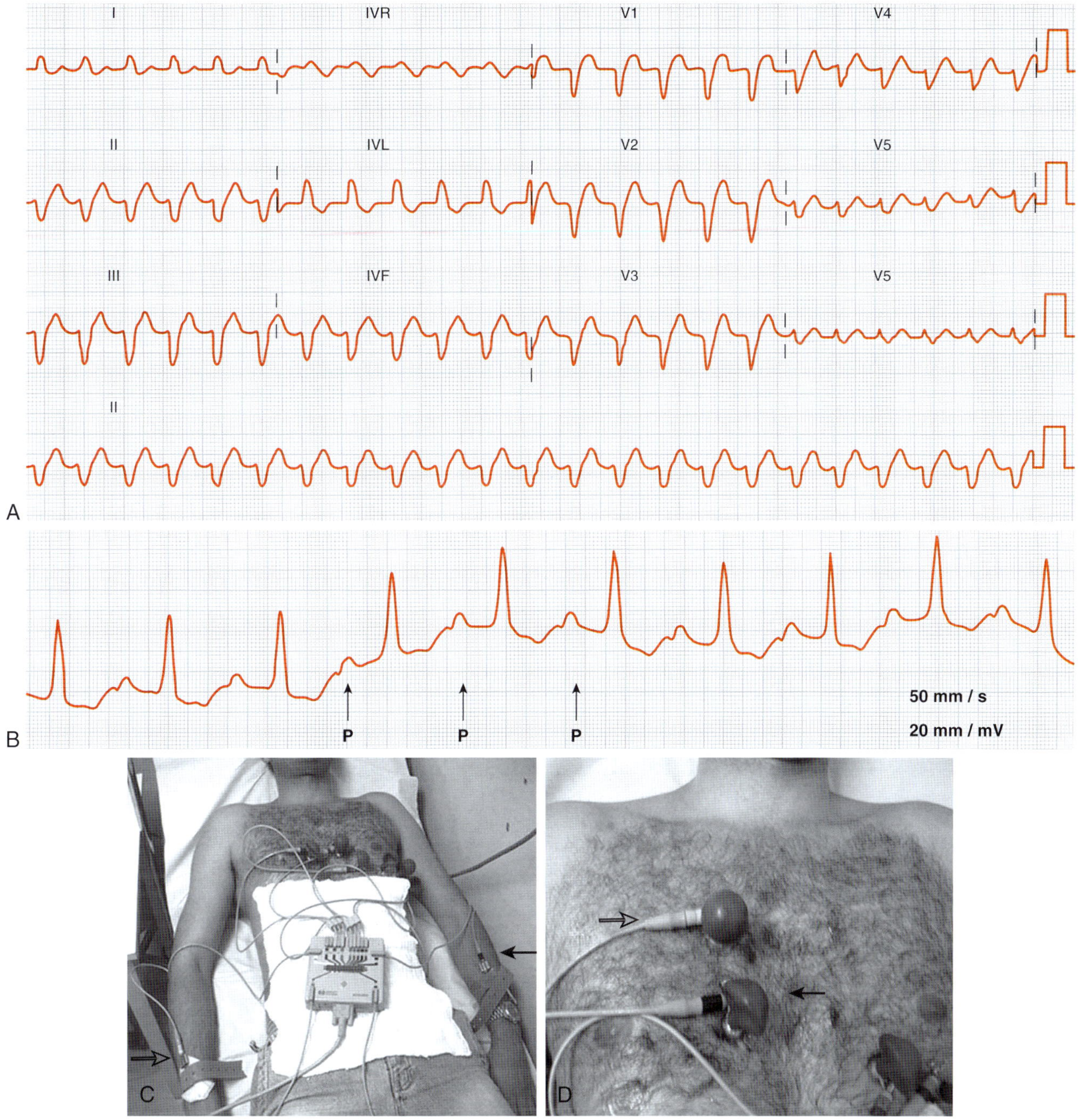

Fig. 11.3 Lewis lead in wide-complex tachycardia. (A) 12-lead ECG showing a wide QRS tachycardia. (B) Lead I strip: Lewis lead obtained with a paper speed of 50 mm/s and twice normal calibration at 20 mm/mV. Regular P waves can now be clearly identified. (C) Conventional right *(open arrow)* and left *(solid arrow)* arm electrodes. (D) The same electrodes positioned in the second *(open arrow)* and fourth *(solid arrow)* intercostal position to obtain Lewis lead. (From Rodrigues de Holanda-Miranda W, Furtado FM, Luciano PM, Pazin-Filho A. Lewis lead enhances atrial activity detection in wide QRS tachycardia. *J Emerg Med*. 2012;43(2):e97-e99.)

the rhythm itself, but there are a few conditions in which pharmacologic slowing of sinus tachycardia is beneficial. For example, administering β-blockers is important in thyroid storm to counteract the adverse consequences of excessive sympathetic drive.

PAT is a rare alternative diagnosis for regular narrow-complex tachycardias with P waves. PAT arises from enhanced automaticity in a nonsinus atrial focus. It is usually precipitated by prior atrial surgery, fever, drug toxicity, hyperthyroidism, or electrolyte or acid-base disturbances. PAT is generally regular and may have normal or abnormal P-wave morphology. As with sinus tachycardia therapy should be directed at the underlying cause with consideration of administering β-blockers in select cases.

Narrow Complex, Regular, No P Waves

The differential diagnosis includes paroxysmal supraventricular tachycardia (PSVT) and atrial flutter with a consistent AV block. Generally, all these reentrant rhythms are treated in the same way with blockade of the AV node (Fig. 11.4).

TABLE 11.1 Selected Drugs for Supraventricular Tachycardias

DRUG	DOSAGE	CONTRAINDICATIONS	SIDE EFFECTS	COMMENTS
Adenosine	6 mg IV rapid push, followed by a saline flush Repeated doses of 12 or 18 mg may be used	• Known VT • AV node block • AF with WPW syndrome • Caution in severe asthma	• Hypotension; transient • Prolonged AV block (rare) • Chest pain • Flushing	Reduce dose in patients taking carbamazepine or dipyridamole (start at 3 mg), heart transplant patient, or administration via central line (start at 1–2 mg)
Amiodarone	150 mg over 10 min; 1 mg/min for 6 h; 0.5-mg/min maintenance infusion; 150-mg boluses for breakthrough VT/VF. 300 mg IV push in pulseless VT or VF	• AV block • Renal failure	• Hypotension • Bradycardia • AV block • Torsade de Pointes	Amiodarone has many side effects when given chronically but not acutely
Metoprolol	5 mg IV over 1–2 min; repeated every 5 min up to 15 mg if required.	• Asthma/COPD • Hypotension • AF with WPW syndrome • AV node block • Decompensated heart failure	• Hypotension • High-degree AV block • Bradycardia • Bronchospasm	Secondary choice for most tachycardias because of negative inotropic effects. Atenolol is dosed identically
Diltiazem	5–10 mg IV slowly for AF, repeated to total of 50 mg in first 30 min, if required. This may be followed by an infusion of 5–15 mg/h to maintain rate control.	• Regular wide-complex tachycardias/suspicion of VT • AV node block • Hypotension • Digoxin toxicity • AF in WPW syndrome • Age <2 years • Caution with left ventricular ejection fraction <40%	• Hypotension • High-degree AV block • Bradycardia	Contraindicated for AF when patient known to have EF <40% given its potential to exacerbate HF
Esmolol	0.5 mg/kg bolus over 1 min; followed by 0.1–0.3 mg/kg per minute infusion titrated to effect	• As for other β-blockers	• Hypotension • High degree • AV block • Bradycardia	A very short half-life makes this a good choice when it is unclear whether the patient can tolerate β-blockers
Lidocaine	1 mg/kg IV, repeated at 0.5–0.75 mg/kg IV to a total of 3 mg/kg, if required. Infusion of 1–4 mg/min	• AF (increases AV conduction)	• Seizures, confusion, lethargy, but only in overdose • Bradycardia • Asystole	Used for stable VT, but efficacy is poor. May reduce recurrent VT/VF but not helpful for primary prophylaxis
Magnesium	2–4 g IV over 5 min Infusion of 1–2 g/h	• AV block • AF with WPW syndrome • Renal failure (infusion) or oliguria	• Hypotension • Flushing • Respiratory muscle weakness • Bradycardia, and asystole with high doses	Patients with infusions running should be checked every few hours to determine respiratory status and reflexes. Decreasing reflexes suggest magnesium toxicity, and infusion should be stopped

Continued

TABLE 11.1 Selected Drugs for Supraventricular Tachycardias—cont'd

DRUG	DOSAGE	CONTRAINDICATIONS	SIDE EFFECTS	COMMENTS
Procainamide	10–17 mg/kg loading at no more than 50 mg/min Infusion of 1-4 mg/min	• Hypotension (relative contraindication)	• Hypotension; give IV fluids and slow rate of infusion • QRS widening • QT prolongation	Effective in SVT with aberrancy. Reduces conduction though accessory pathways but may increase conduction through the AV node
Verapamil	5–10 mg IV at over 5 min for PSVT	• As for diltiazem	As for diltiazem	May cause more hypotension than diltiazem. Not extensively studied in patients with congestive heart failure

AF, Atrial fibrillation; *AV,* atrioventricular; *COPD,* chronic obstructive pulmonary disease; *IV,* intravenous; *PSVT,* paroxysmal supraventricular tachycardia.

TABLE 11.2 Electrical Therapy of Tachycardias

RHYTHM	BIPHASIC DOSE (J)	NOTES
PSVT	50–100	Synchronized
Atrial flutter	50	Synchronized
Atrial fibrillation	50–200	Synchronized
Ventricular tachycardia	120–200	Synchronized
Torsade de pointes	200	Unsynchronized (defibrillation)
Wide-complex AF	50–200	Synchronized
Ventricular fibrillation	200	Unsynchronized (defibrillation)

PSVT, Paroxysmal supraventricular tachycardia.

Paroxysmal Supraventricular Tachycardia

PSVT makes up the majority of cases in this category. The two main types of PSVT are atrioventricular nodal reentrant tachycardia (AVNRT) and atrioventricular reentrant tachycardia (AVRT), the differentiation of which is not important in the ED. Paroxysmal SVT refers to a clinical syndrome in which there is a sudden onset and abrupt termination of tachycardia. Females are twice as likely as males to develop PSVT, with older patients having approximately a fivefold increase in risk compared with those under 65 years old.[5–7] Lone SVT is a clinical syndrome of PSVT without any known cardiovascular risk factors. Patients with lone SVT tend to be younger, have higher heart rates, and have a higher proportion of AVNRT. This accounts for almost half of all females who present with SVT, but only about 10% of males.[8–12]

Patients with PSVT who have signs of end-organ hypoperfusion should be cardioverted; more than 90% convert with small doses of electrical energy (≤50 J). Pharmacologic treatment of PSVT is directed at blockade of the AV node. Vagal maneuvers may be tried first: carotid sinus massage, the Valsalva maneuver, or the modified Valsalva maneuver, which has been shown in one randomized controlled trial to be superior to traditional Valsalva in the conversion of SVT.[13] Cold water facial immersion may be attempted in infants or young children too young to be coached to perform the other maneuvers. Because many patients with recurrent PSVT are familiar with vagal maneuvers, they often present for treatment only when these maneuvers have failed; therefore these maneuvers are only occasionally effective in the ED.

If vagal maneuvers fail or are contraindicated, pharmacologic treatment options include adenosine or calcium channel blockers (e.g., verapamil, diltiazem) and β-blockers. Intravenous adenosine, because of its brief duration of action and resultant lack of sustained hemodynamic effect, is the drug of choice (Videos 11.1–11.3). The recommended initial dosage of adenosine is a rapid 6-mg bolus quickly followed by a saline flush. If there is no response in 1 to 2 minutes, a 12-mg dose can be administered in the same manner. The use of doses of adenosine upward of 24 mg as a bolus has been reported in the literature, but is only marginally more effective than 12 mg.[14,15] It is important that the drug be given as a rapid bolus to achieve high levels in the heart. Adenosine is degraded so rapidly in plasma that the most proximal IV access possible (usually an antecubital vein) is desired. Dosing should be reduced by half if adenosine is given centrally, such as via a port-a-cath, PICC line, or central line.

There are a variety of alternative methods to administer adenosine (Fig. 11.5). Proposed methods include utilizing a three-way stopcock with the adenosine syringe connected to one port and a 10-mL saline flush to the other. After adenosine is pushed, the valve is turned, and the saline flush administered rapidly. Another method utilizes mixing the adenosine and normal saline in a 20-mL syringe allowing a single rapid IV push and obviating the need for switching between two syringes or a three-way stopcock.[16–25] Adenosine may cause sensation of chest pain, shortness of breath, and a metallic taste in the mouth in as many as half of patients.

In the absence of contraindications to calcium channel blockers (hypotension, congestive heart failure, SA or AV nodal disease, or the previous use of IV β-blockers), verapamil is a safe and effective therapy for SVT.[26] Substantial data,

TABLE 11.3 Simplified Differential and Approach of Tachydysrhythmias

	DIFFERENTIAL	GENERAL APPROACH	GENERAL TREATMENT
Narrow regular	Sinus tachycardia SVT (AVNRT/OAVRT) Atrial flutter 2:1 conduction	Evaluate for presence of P waves as well as rate and variability	Treat underlying cause Vagal maneuvers Adenosine AV nodal blockers
Narrow irregular	MAT AF Atrial flutter with variable block	Consider if AF is primary or secondary to an underlying process	Treat underlying cause versus rate/ rhythm control
Wide regular	VT SVT + conduction abnormality Hyperkalemia	Assume VT if in doubt Consider empiric calcium gluconate if potassium level not available	Electrical cardioversion versus medical therapy
Wide irregular	Polymorphic VT AF with aberrancy AF + WPW Hyperkalemia	Avoid AV nodal blockers unless identical morphology to baseline ECG Consider empiric calcium gluconate if potassium level not available	Electrical cardioversion if unstable. Electrical cardioversion is also treatment of choice for AF + WPW. Magnesium for TdP. Consider procainamide or amiodarone for AF with aberrancy (if known)

AF, Atrial fibrillation; *AV,* atrioventricular; *AVNRT,* atrioventricular nodal reentrant tachycardia; *MAT,* multifocal atrial tachycardia; *OAVRT,* orthodromic atrioventricular reciprocating tachycardia; *SVT,* supraventricular tachycardias; *TdP,* Torsades de pointes, *VF,* ventricular fibrillation; *WPW,* Wolff-Parkinson-White [syndrome].

Effects of Carotid Sinus Massage on Various Arrhythmias

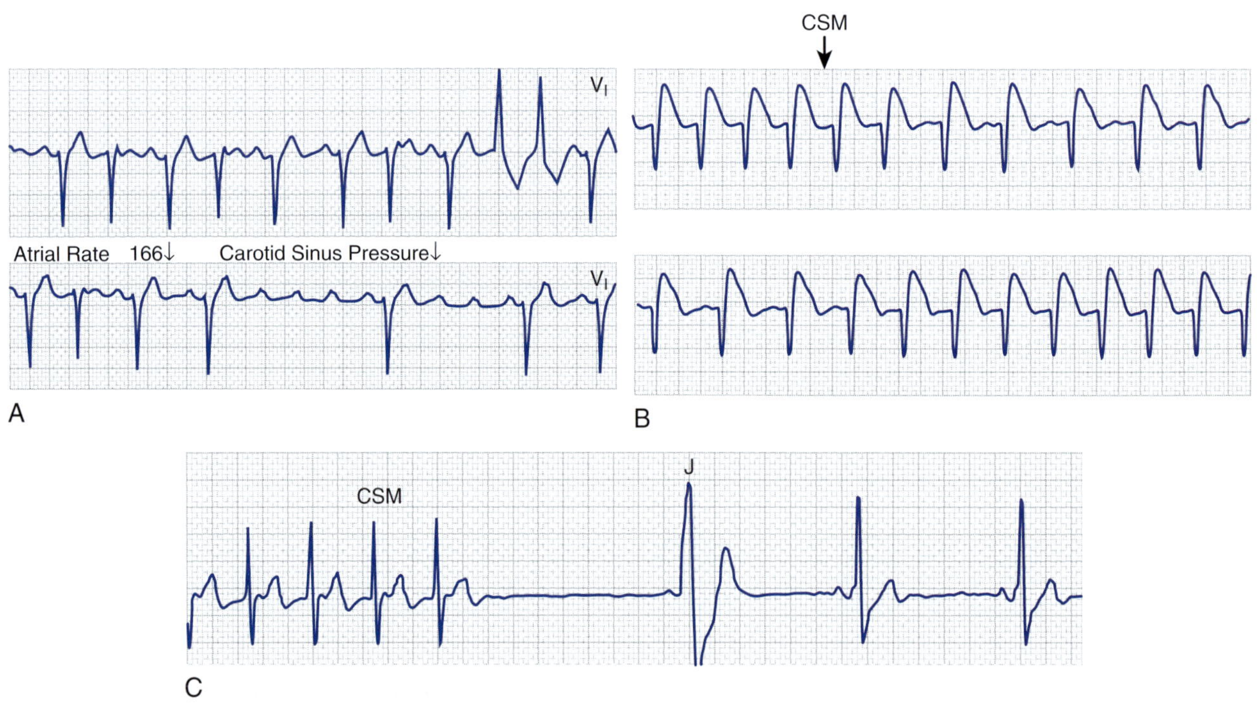

Fig. 11.4 (A) Paroxysmal atrial tachycardia with variable block. Carotid sinus massage *(CSM)* uncovers P waves hidden in the ventricular complex. The upper strip resembles atrial flutter or atrial fibrillation with ventricular ectopic beats. The lower strip shows paroxysmal atrial tachycardia with variable block at an atrial rate of 166 beats/min. (B) Sinus tachycardia. The sinus P wave is obscured within the descending limb of the T wave. CSM transiently slows the sinus rate and exposes the P wave. The rate then increases. The strips are continuous. (C) Paroxysmal atrial tachycardia. CSM abolishes the dysrhythmia and results in a period of sinus suppression with a junctional *(J)* escape beat. Prolonged periods of asystole may produce anxiety in physicians waiting for the resumption of a sinus pacemaker.

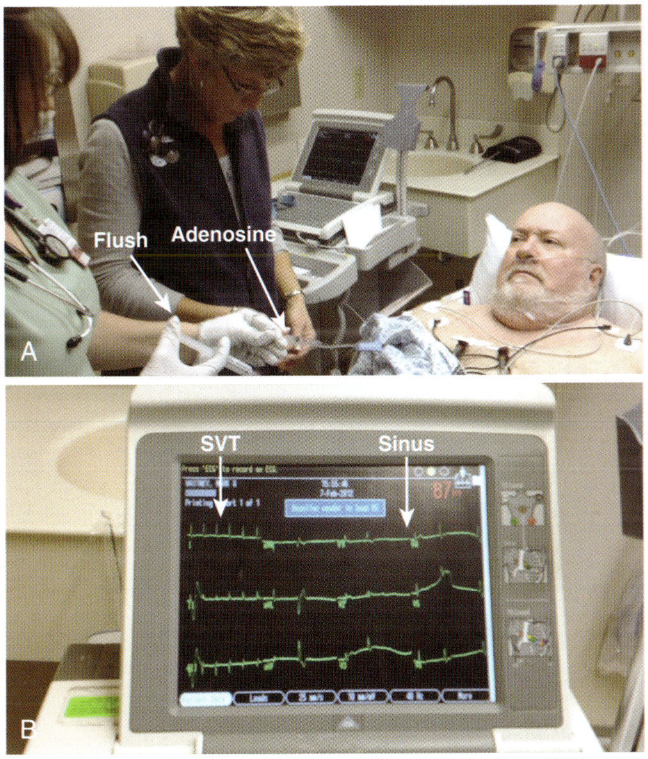

Fig. 11.5 Treatment of supraventricular tachycardia *(SVT)* with adenosine. (A) Because of its ultrashort half-life (<10 s), adenosine must be given rapidly, followed by a 20-mL saline flush. (B) Adenosine slows conduction through the atrioventricular node, thereby effectively converting SVT (left side of the screen) to sinus rhythm (right side of the screen).

including a large Cochrane review, suggest equivalent rates of conversion with verapamil versus adenosine, fewer minor adverse effects such as chest pain, and no difference in hypotension when used in patients without contraindications.[27] Verapamil can be administered via bolus dosing of 2.5 to 5 mg IV over 2 minutes, repeated as needed every 20 minutes up to a maximum dose of 20 mg, or an infusion of 20 mg at 1 mg/min until SVT termination. Slow infusion seems to be associated with less hypotension than bolus dosing. Many pediatric cardiologists consider it unsafe to use verapamil in children younger than 1 year of age and exclusively use adenosine in this age group.

Diltiazem is a safe and effective alternative to verapamil. The standard initial dose is a 10-mg IV bolus, and most patients convert to sinus rhythm within about 2 minutes. Incremental doses up to a total of 50 mg in the first 30 minutes are usually successful in patients unresponsive to the initial dose.

AVNRT is a common tachydysrhythmia in pregnancy, and vagal maneuvers and adenosine are first-line therapy. If pharmacologic treatments fail or are contraindicated, synchronized cardioversion is an alternative treatment option (see Table 11.1).

Atrial Flutter

Atrial flutter is a macro-reentrant arrhythmia in which the circular current flow produces characteristic "sawtooth" waves without an isoelectric baseline, best seen in leads V1 and II, III, and aVF (see Fig. 11.1D). Atrial rates between 260 and 300 beats/min are typical, and the most common AV block of 2:1 produces ventricular rates of approximately 150 beats/min. Variable AV block can cause an irregular narrow-complex rhythm (Fig. 11.6).

Although the diagnosis of atrial flutter is often fairly easy, some patients with flutter at first glance appear to be in other rhythms. If sawtooth flutter waves are not clearly discernable and the diagnosis is uncertain, vagal maneuvers or adenosine can be useful in distinguishing between atrial flutter and PSVT. Vagal maneuvers can sometimes transiently slow conduction though the AV node enough to decrease the ventricular rate and thereby reveal hidden flutter waves (if they are present). Adenosine, however, is particularly effective in this regard. Although useful diagnostically, such transient AV nodal blockade rarely results in cardioversion and neither vagal maneuvers nor adenosine have any further role in the treatment of atrial flutter.

The ED management of atrial flutter is similar to that of AF. Therapeutic options are electrical or chemical cardioversion versus rate control (see section on "Atrial Fibrillation"). The decision of which modality to use must be made in the context of many factors: clinical stability, patient comorbidities, and associated stroke risk, since atrial flutter carries a similar risk of stroke and many patients in atrial flutter also experience AF.

Many authorities advocate electrical cardioversion given the high electro-sensitivity of atrial flutter with most patients converting with doses of 30 to 50 J. Despite the efficacy of electrical cardioversion, chemical cardioversion has advocates. As with AF, amiodarone and procainamide are currently commonly used agents in the ED. Rate control is also a viable option with calcium channel blockers (verapamil and diltiazem), β-blockers (metoprolol and esmolol), and digoxin capable of slowing the ventricular response in atrial flutter.

The atrial activity in flutter is typically much faster than the ventricular response, and procainamide can increase the conduction through the AV node from 2:1 or 3:1 to 1:1, causing hemodynamic deterioration. This potential complication can be avoided by slowing the ventricular rate before administering procainamide.

Since atrial flutter may increase the risk of systemic embolization, and since many patients with atrial flutter also have AF, anticoagulation is generally recommended in patients with atrial flutter in a similar manner as for AF (see section on "Atrial Fibrillation" for risk assessment and anticoagulation recommendations).

Narrow Complex, Irregular, P Waves Present

Multifocal Atrial Tachycardia

MAT is characterized by P waves of at least three different morphologies and changing PR intervals with an isoelectric baseline and is an uncommon cause of irregularly irregular SVT. Because MAT originates in the atria, it is associated with narrow QRS complexes, except in the presence of underlying BBB. MAT occurs primarily in patients with chronic lung disease, and within this group, MAT was most common in patients with high or toxic levels of theophylline.[28–30] As the use of methylxanthines for the treatment of lung disease has declined, so has the incidence of MAT. Although MAT is seldom life-threatening, it has been shown to be a poor prognostic sign when developed during acute illness. Treating MAT involves treatment of the underlying condition. The ability to control it, however, can provide symptomatic benefit. Rhythm control using various antiarrhythmics has not been shown to be effective, though there are some data showing magnesium may be effective. Rate control using verapamil is the primary management strategy recommended. β-Blockers are probably less effective and should be used with caution in MAT associated with chronic obstructive pulmonary disease (COPD). Electrical cardioversion is not useful in MAT.

Narrow Complex, Irregular, No P Waves

An irregular narrow-complex tachycardia is almost invariably AF or atrial flutter with variable block (see Fig. 11.1C–D). Occasionally, the P waves of MAT are overlooked, and that rhythm is confused with AF.

Atrial Fibrillation

AF is the most common arrhythmia in adults and remains the most common arrhythmia treated in the ED and intensive care unit (ICU).[31,32] AF is marked by rapid disorganized atrial activation, often accompanied by rapid ventricular response (RVR). ED management of AF is complex due to the heterogeneity of patients and their clinical presentations.[33] When choosing therapy, it is important to consider the ventricular response rate, hemodynamic consequences, duration of AF, and presence of underlying heart disease. It is also important to consider the history and the precipitant of the patient's presentation because the patient with chronic AF who develops an acute illness may be managed differently than a patient who developed new-onset AF (NOAF) secondary to a physiologic stressor (e.g., sepsis or pulmonary embolism). Common causes of NOAF can be found in Box 11.2.

In the majority of patients presenting with AF and RVR, the tachycardia itself (which profoundly decreases the time available for diastolic filling of the ventricles as well as coronary artery perfusion), rather than the loss of atrial systole, is responsible for the hemodynamic consequences. Patients with hypertrophic cardiomyopathy as well as other patients with significant diastolic dysfunction are an exception, because their stiff ventricles fill slowly, and they thus rely on active atrial systole for an inordinate proportion of their end-diastolic ventricular volume. Consider the possibility of an accessory tract (e.g., AF plus Wolff-Parkinson-White [WPW] syndrome) if the heart rate is over 200 beats/min.

At the other extreme, a slow ventricular response in new-onset AF is worrisome unless the patient is already taking medications that slow conduction in the AV node. Such patients may have AV node dysfunction, are rarely unstable, and often need to be admitted for pacemaker consideration. Attempted cardioversion may lead to asystole or prolonged bradycardia and should be avoided.

BOX 11.2 Common Causes of New-Onset Atrial Fibrillation

Electrolyte abnormalities (e.g., hypokalemia and hypomagnesemia)
Myocardial ischemia
Sepsis
Hypovolemia or fluid overload
Thyrotoxicosis
Toxicology/medications
- Alcohol (e.g., "Holiday heart syndrome")
- Substance use (e.g., cocaine, amphetamines, methamphetamine)
- Beta-agonists (e.g., norepinephrine, epinephrine, dobutamine)
- Theophylline

Adrenergic states
- Alcohol withdrawal
- Pain, agitation

Neurologic disorders (e.g., intracranial hemorrhage, ischemic stroke)
Respiratory failure
- Pulmonary embolism
- Pneumonia, COPD, hypoxemia, hypercapnia

AF, *Atrial fibrillation;* COPD, *chronic obstructive pulmonary disease.*

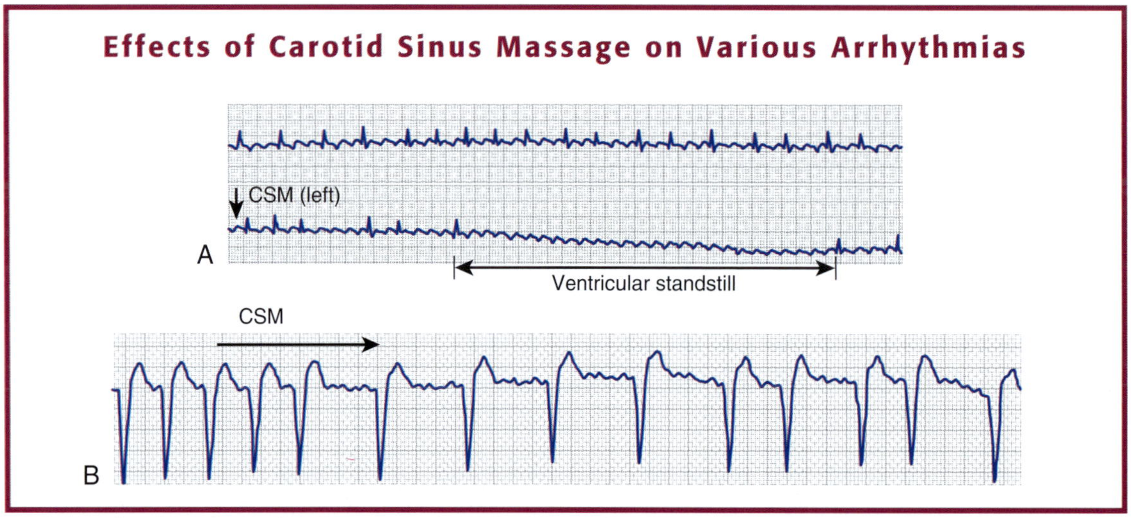

Fig. 11.6 (A) Atrial flutter. Carotid sinus massage *(CSM) (down arrow)* produces marked slowing of the ventricular rate in atrial flutter. Note the obvious flutter waves with an atrial rate of 300 and a long period of ventricular standstill. The strips are continuous. (B) Atrial fibrillation. CSM slows the ventricular response transiently, and thus the fibrillating baseline is revealed. The ventricular rate subsequently accelerates.

Many patients seen in the ED with AF, particularly in circumstances in which AF is an incidental finding, have chronic AF, are taking medications for rate control, and are hemodynamically stable. Digitalis has long been used for chronic rate control. Cardioversion in patients taking digoxin is a risk because of the potential for asystole. If cardioversion is required because of extreme hemodynamic compromise, it should initially be attempted at lower energy levels, such as 50 J. The calcium channel blockers diltiazem or verapamil, or a β-blocker are preferred to digoxin for chronic rate control because these agents control rate not only at rest but also during exercise.[34] Patients with acute or chronic AF should be admitted to the hospital if they have signs of hemodynamic decompensation that requires cardioversion or if hemodynamic effects and RVR are not easily controlled.

Anticoagulation is an important management issue for patients with AF. Not only are patients with AF at risk for systemic embolization, but evidence suggests that even shorter periods of AF may carry a risk of embolization, particularly following conversion to sinus rhythm, regardless of whether cardioversion is electrical or pharmacologic. Recent guidelines suggest that any patient with nonvalvular AF, i.e., without mechanical valve or moderate or severe mitral stenosis, be anticoagulated based on stroke risk using the $CHADS_2VASC$ score (Table 11.4).[35] Patients with a score of 2 or greater require long-term anticoagulation, whether the AF is paroxysmal, persistent, or permanent. Even if accurate, a history of a brief duration of AF may fail to preclude the possibility of embolization caused by intraatrial clot formation during the period of atrial standstill that can follow conversion to sinus rhythm. For this reason, some authorities say that in the absence of contraindications, AF less than 48 hours duration should be anticoagulated prior to electrical or chemical cardioversion, and for 3 weeks before and 4 weeks after conversion to sinus rhythm. Other strategies involve risk stratification based on known risk factors for clot formation and a selective approach to anticoagulation in acute AF. A caveat remains in the critically ill patient with NOAF, where the risks of anticoagulation have to be weighed against the potential benefits. While the decision has to be tailored to each individual case, there is some evidence that anticoagulation for AF secondary to critical illness may increase the bleeding risk without reducing the incidence of stroke.[31,36–38] In the absence of contraindications, most notably chronic kidney disease and the presence of a mechanical valve, non–vitamin K oral anticoagulants (NOACs) are recommended as first-line therapy for nonvalvular AF. Several trials have showed either noninferiority or superiority of these medications over warfarin, and they have the added benefit of not requiring frequent laboratory monitoring.[39]

On the other hand, studies of transesophageal echocardiography (TEE) used to rule out an intraatrial thrombus prior to conversion of AF suggest that a negative TEE reduces the risk of embolization enough to obviate the need for anticoagulation before cardioversion. Of course, if it is necessary because of hemodynamic instability, cardioversion should never be withheld.

For stable patients presenting with AF of >48 hours' duration with RVR, treatment is directed at slowing the ventricular rate while conversion to sinus rhythm is a secondary consideration. Chronic AF is generally a strong indicator for rate control strategy because AF leads to electrical remodeling overtime, making it harder to convert to a sinus rhythm. Prior to initiating rate control therapy, it is important to consider what is precipitating the RVR. Just as an acute physiologic stress will increase catecholamine levels and result in sinus tachycardia in patients with a healthy heart, elevated catecholamines may precipitate an acute paroxysm of AF with RVR in a patient with an at-risk heart or induce RVR in a patient with chronic AF. Consequently, an older patient with a history of chronic AF presenting with a fever, tachycardia, and evidence of sepsis is better treated with IV fluids, antibiotics, and antipyretics than with pharmacotherapy directed at rate control. Some of these patients may benefit from a mild compensatory tachycardia, and aggressively lowering the heart rate down to a "normal range" (less than 100 beats/min) can be harmful.

TABLE 11.4 $CHA_2DS\text{-}VASc_2$ Score for Stroke Risk in Atrial Fibrillation

LETTER	RISK FACTOR	SCORE
C	Congestive heart failure	1
H	Hypertension	1
A2	Age ≥75	2
D	Diabetes mellitus	1
S2	Prior TIA/stroke/ embolism	2
V	Vascular disease	1
A	Age 65–74	1
S	Sex (female)	1
	MALES	**FEMALES**
$CHA_2DS\text{-}VASc_2$ score 0	Not recommended	Not recommended
$CHA_2DS\text{-}VASc_2$ score 1	Consider	Not recommended
$CHA_2DS\text{-}VASc_2$ score 2	Recommended	Consider
$CHA_2DS\text{-}VASc_2$ score ≥3	Recommended	Recommended

2019 AHA/ACC/HRS focused update on the 2014 guideline for the management of patients with atrial fibrillation. *TIA*, transient ischemic attack.

Diltiazem and metoprolol are the two most commonly used rate control medications in the ED. In stable patients, diltiazem is typically given at a dose of 0.1 to 0.25 mg/kg IV over 2 minutes, repeated as necessary every 5 minutes to a total dose of 60 mg. Following bolus injection, rate control can be maintained with an IV infusion of 5 to 15 mg/h. Although occasionally used to mitigate the hypotensive effects of diltiazem, IV calcium preparations are not supported by the literature in this regard. Diltiazem may be given to patients with AF-RVR and congestive heart failure, though caution should be used. It should, however, be avoided in patients with digoxin toxicity. Metoprolol can be given in doses of 2.5 to 5 mg IV, repeated every 5 to 10 minutes to a maximum dose of 15 mg. Once rate control is achieved, initiation of oral β-blocker therapy is indicated if the patient is hemodynamically stable. β-blockers are contraindicated in patients with active wheezing from reactive airway disease. There is some evidence that diltiazem is more effective than metoprolol at achieving rate control in the first 30 minutes with no increase in adverse events.[40,41] The literature however remains conflicted regarding diltiazem's ultimate comparative efficacy. Notably, in many patients with AF who are critically ill, the dysrhythmia is precipitated by increased sympathetic tone. Rate control with β-blockers may be more efficacious among these patients.[42–48] Patients who are refractory to adequate rate control should be reevaluated for any occult underlying process contributing to increased sympathetic tone. Transition to another agent may be indicated, but it is generally prudent to avoid combining intravenous β-blockers and calcium channel blockers because overlapping these agents may lead to hypotension.

Alternative rate control agents include digoxin, amiodarone, and magnesium. Digoxin may be given as 0.5 mg IV or orally, followed by 0.25 mg, 4 and 8 hours later. Use of digoxin in the emergency setting is rarely recommended due to the delay in action (several hours) and the fact that it works via the vagal pathway and thus is less effective at controlling catecholamine-mediated AF-RVR. Digoxin may have a role in rate control in patients with chronic AF and heart failure with reduced ejection fraction (given its ability to reduce heart rate while simultaneously functioning as a positive inotrope), particularly if immediate control of tachycardia is not necessary and if the patient has adequate renal function. Amiodarone can also be useful for rate control, particularly in a patient with hypotension or left ventricular (LV) dysfunction, but it can lead to undesired cardioversion to sinus rhythm. The loading dose is generally 150-mg bolus, followed by an infusion at 1 mg/min. Infusion may subsequently be converted to oral administration after 24 hours. There is evidence that IV magnesium has reasonable efficacy for reduction in heart rate and rhythm control in AF, with an excellent safety profile. Although magnesium is rarely used alone for these indications, it may augment the efficacy of other antiarrhythmic agents and electrical cardioversion.[49–53]

Aside from considering pharmacotherapy for the critically ill patient with AF, addressing the underlying etiology remains key. Often times, uncontrolled AF is a manifestation of concurrent sepsis, PE, thyrotoxicosis, or other causes of shock and anchoring on AF as the cause of the patient's hemodynamic instability can be detrimental. Optimization of fluid status (e.g., diuresis if the patient is volume overloaded, which can cause atrial dilation, or volume administration if the patient is overtly hypovolemic), treating pain or withdrawal (which can drive sympathetic tone and precipitate AF), addressing hypoxemia or respiratory distress, and repleting electrolyte deficiencies (particularly hypokalemia and hypomagnesemia) may attenuate AF.

The ED management of stable patients with recent onset AF or flutter recent onset AF has evolved in the past decade. recent onset AF, defined as <48 hours of symptoms, has many causes ranging from benign to life-threatening. It has long been standard practice to admit patients with recent onset AF to evaluate the possibility of serious underlying disease (e.g., acute myocardial infarction, mitral valve disease, pulmonary embolism, thyrotoxicosis, or drug effect) as its cause. However, 80% to 95% of stable patients with recent onset AF. do not prove to have an acutely critical etiology, and those who do almost always have other worrisome clinical findings in addition to the dysrhythmia itself. Given the drive for cost-effective resource utilization and the emerging data, consideration may be given to discharging a reliable, hemodynamically stable, recent onset AF patient with no indications of serious underlying etiology, and prompt outpatient follow-up.

A second key management decision is intertwined with the decision to admit or discharge the patient with recent onset AF—whether to attempt cardioversion to sinus rhythm in the ED or merely control the ventricular response rate.

Rate control and admission are appropriate for high-risk, but stable patients with recent onset AF. Rate control followed by discharge home on an oral rate control agent and, if indicated, anticoagulation, may be appropriate for low-risk patients for whom prompt follow-up can be arranged. The target heart rate for outpatients is generally regarded to be less than 110 beats/min (based on the results of the RACE II trial).[54] This management strategy is being used with increasing frequency in the era of cost containment and many EDs have instituted rapid follow-up protocols in concert with cardiology.

In support of cardioversion and subsequent discharge of patients with recent onset AF are several ED-based studies demonstrating a high success rate of cardioversion and an extremely low risk of mortality or stroke. In the largest prospective study of ED cardioversion of recent onset AF patients, the authors observed no cases of stroke in over 600 patients discharged from the ED,[55] albeit in a short follow-up period. However, this does not exclude the possibility that some subgroups of patients may benefit from one strategy over the other.

Pharmacologic agents that have been the subject of at least limited testing in the cardioversion of recent onset AF include amiodarone, clonidine, dofetilide, flecainide, ibutilide, magnesium, procainamide, propafenone, and sotalol. Rates of successful cardioversion and adverse effects vary. Of these medications, procainamide has been more extensively studied for the cardioversion of recent onset AF. Procainamide has a 50% to 58% effectiveness rate, a relatively rapid onset (median time to cardioversion about 1 hour) and an acceptable safety profile when used in the ED.[56,57] It should be noted that the spontaneous conversion rate of recent onset AF patients seen in the ED is high, reaching 60% at 24 hours and 80% at 48 hours.

With the widespread adoption of safe and effective procedural sedation in the ED elective synchronized electrical cardioversion of recent onset AF has emerged as a viable therapeutic option. Often utilized following failed chemical cardioversion, success rates for electrical cardioversion are greater than 90% in selected patients with or without a preceding attempt at chemical conversion and have demonstrated a favorable safety profile.[55]

Because of concerns about thromboembolic stroke, patient selection is important if either chemical or electrical cardioversion is to be attempted in the ED. Patients with AF >48 hours or of uncertain duration, and those at high risk of stroke (including a mechanical valve, rheumatic heart disease, prior stroke, and congestive heart failure) should not undergo elective ED cardioversion. To further reduce the risk of stroke, some centers perform TEE before elective cardioversion of recent onset AF. In patients being discharged from the ED after rate or rhythm control, anticoagulation, if not already instituted, is recommended according to the $CHADS_2VASC$ score (see Table 11.4).[35] Bleeding risk may be assessed using the HAS-BLED (hypertension, abnormal renal/liver function, stroke, bleeding history or predisposition, labile international normalized ratio [INR], age ≥65 years, drugs/alcohol concomitantly) score, which has been validated and predicts bleeding complications in patients receiving anticoagulation for AF (Table 11.5).[58,59]

In summary, the choice of rate versus rhythm control and admission versus discharge of recent onset AF patients from the ED can be guided by evidence-based algorithms, local standards, and careful patient selection. There is increasing evidence that discharge home following rate or rhythm control, is safe, effective, and resource-sparing. Overall, both strategies are generally reasonable, and it remains important to tailor your treatment decision to institutional guidance, and patient specifics and preference.

The therapy for unstable patients with AF and RVR is one of the most challenging situations in all of dysrhythmia management. Many of these patients have baseline decreased ventricular function, are resistant to cardioversion, and may have an underlying condition producing their shock or hypoperfusion. With ventricular rates less than 150 beats/min, it is vital to seek other etiologies for hypotension such as hypovolemia, bleeding, or sepsis, and these entities should be addressed. If adequate perfusion or blood pressure cannot be achieved and the rate remains high, electrical cardioversion is recommended. The current American Heart Association (AHA) advanced cardiac life support (ACLS) recommendation is to cardiovert with a 120 to 200 J biphasic shock. Electrical cardioversion, even if initially successful, may fail as a strategy for the management of AF in critically ill patients because many will revert back to AF. Consider multimodal therapy adding synergistic agents, such as an antiarrhythmic and magnesium, to electrical cardioversion.[60]

Alternatively, amiodarone has been used in unstable AF in a number of small case series, and in one randomized trial, it was found to be inferior to magnesium.[61] Amiodarone slows ventricular rate and marginally increases the frequency of conversion to sinus rhythm. As with electrical cardioversion, if a critically ill patient is successfully cardioverted with amiodarone, administering ongoing amiodarone therapy may reduce the incidence of reversion to AF.[62]

In some cases, the cautious use of a vasopressor may be required to maintain blood pressure. Given that atrial contraction does not recover rapidly after conversion to sinus rhythm, cardioversion can be considered essentially a rapid form of rate control. The seriousness of this clinical situation cannot be overemphasized, and no therapy is without significant risk. All patients in whom recent onset AF cannot be verified are at risk of embolization and should receive prompt anticoagulation after conversion to sinus rhythm unless contraindicated.

TABLE 11.5A HAS-BLED Score

LETTER	RISK FACTOR	SCORE
H	Hypertension[a]	1
A	Abnormal renal or liver function (1 point each)[b]	1 or 2
S	Stroke	1
B	Bleeding	1
L	Labile international normalized ratio (INR)[c]	1
E	>65 Years old	1
D	Drugs or alcohol (1 point each)[d]	1 or 2

[a]Uncontrolled, >160 mm Hg systolic.
[b]Dialysis, transplant, serum creatinine >2.26 mg/dL or >200 µmol/L *or* cirrhosis or bilirubin >2× normal with aspartate aminotransferase/alanine aminotransferase/alkaline phosphatase >3× normal.
[c]Unstable/high INRs, time in therapeutic range <60%.
[d]Medication usage predisposing to bleeding (e.g., aspirin, clopidogrel, nonsteroidal antiinflammatory drugs) *or* ≥8 drinks/week.

TABLE 11.5B

HAS-BLED SCORE	BLEEDS PER 100 PATIENT-YEARS[a]	RISK OF MAJOR BLEEDING[b]	RECOMMENDATION
0	1.13	0.9%	Anticoagulation should be considered
1	1.02	3.4%	
2	1.88	4.1%	Anticoagulation can be considered
3	3.74	5.8%	
4	8.70	8.9%	Alternatives to anticoagulation should be considered
5[c]	12.5	9.1%	

[a]Adapted from Pisters R, Lane DA, Nieuwlaat R, de Vos CB, Crijns HJ, Lip GY. A novel user-friendly score (HAS-BLED) to assess 1-year risk of major bleeding in patients with atrial fibrillation: the Euro Heart Survey. *Chest*. 2010;138(5):1093-1100. https://doi.org/10.1378/chest.10-0134.
[b]Adapted from Lip GY, Frison L, Halperin JL, Lane DA. Comparative validation of a novel risk score for predicting bleeding risk in anticoagulated patients with atrial fibrillation: the HAS-BLED (Hypertension, Abnormal Renal/Liver Function, Stroke, Bleeding History or Predisposition, Labile INR, Elderly, Drugs/Alcohol Concomitantly) score. *J Am Coll Cardiol*. 2011;57(2):173-180. https://doi.org/10.1016/j.jacc.2010.09.024.
[c]Scores greater than 5 were too rare to determine risk, but are likely over 10%.

Wide-Complex Tachycardias

Wide Complex, Regular, No P Waves

Diagnostic possibilities include monomorphic VT (see Chapter 12), PSVT with aberrancy (BBB), and the antidromic SVT of WPW syndrome. When in doubt, the clinician should always consider regular, wide-complex tachycardia to be VT or hyperkalemia until proven otherwise. Several clinical and ECG criteria have been devised to enable clinicians to distinguish between VT and SVT with aberrancy. Useful ECG indicators that make VT more likely include fusion and capture beats, and the presence of AV dissociation. However, none of the established criteria have ever been shown to yield more than 90% sensitive, and though they may be useful to rule in VT, they are inadequate to rule out VT. Importantly, clinical features such as age greater than 35 years old and a history of heart disease portend a high likelihood of VT. Thus drugs contraindicated in VT (e.g., verapamil) are dangerous when used to treat wide-complex tachycardia. Adenosine may be used to treat regular wide-complex tachycardia of uncertain etiology, because it is probably safe (if only very rarely effective) in VT and will convert most episodes of PSVT. Similarly, current guidelines do not comment on the use of vagal maneuvers in this setting, but these maneuvers can generally be employed for situations where adenosine is indicated.[63–65] Most experts recommend electrical cardioversion as first-line therapy when treating undifferentiated regular wide-complex tachycardia.

PSVT can manifest with wide QRS complexes when BBB (either underlying or rate-related) is present. The duration of the QRS complex in this circumstance is not likely to exceed 0.14 second, and heart rates usually range between 130 and 200 beats/min. Nevertheless, it is virtually impossible to be certain that a wide-complex tachycardia represents PSVT with BBB, rather than VT and therapy should almost never be based on this assumption.

Wide Complex, Irregular, No P Waves

Diagnostic possibilities include AF-BBB, AF with the WPW syndrome, polymorphic VT of which torsade de pointes is a subset, and VF.

Wide-Complex Atrial Fibrillation

A few patients with AF present with wide QRS complexes caused by an underlying or rate-related BBB or by the WPW syndrome. In the presence of known underlying BBB, treatment can be similar to that for routine narrow-complex AF (e.g., cardioversion for severely unstable patients and diltiazem for rate control in stable patients).

Patients with rate-related BBB often demonstrate both wide complexes (in beats that follow short RR intervals) and narrow complexes (in beats that follow longer RR intervals), but patients with AF and the WPW syndrome may also have both wide and narrow QRS complexes, depending on the conduction path followed by each depolarization. It is critical to recognize this latter entity because agents that slow conduction through the AV node are absolutely contraindicated.

In WPW, the presence of rapidly conducting accessory pathways predisposes to a number of dysrhythmias, of which AF is the most dangerous. AF generates atrial impulses at 300 to 600 per minute. The accessory pathways of WPW syndrome, which bypass the AV node and its protective slowing, conduct impulses to the ventricle at rates exceeding 250 beats/min. The ventricle will fail or undergo fibrillation if these excessively rapid atrial impulses are conducted for more than a short period. Many patients are aware that they have WPW syndrome. Among patients who give no history of WPW syndrome, the possibility should be considered when the irregular rhythm is wide and very fast (>200 beats/min), the QRS complexes are variable and bizarre, and the R-R intervals are very short (200 to 250 ms). Morphology can vary with different beats and some beats may be fusion complexes if the AV node and the accessory pathway fire at a similar time.

Drugs that impair the AV node (e.g., adenosine, calcium channel blockers, β-blockers, and digitalis) are contraindicated in WPW syndrome with wide-complex AF, as they can increase the speed of conduction through the bypass tract. More importantly, relative blockade of the AV node causes preferential conduction through the bypass tract, thereby resulting in much higher ventricular response rates that can deteriorate into VF. Amiodarone should also be used with caution in these patients as it also has AV nodal blocking properties and may have similar potential to increase conduction down the bypass tract and increase the ventricular rate.[46,65] For patients who are hemodynamically stable, intravenous procainamide may be an option for preexcited AF given its effect on atrial and ventricular myocardium without AV nodal blocking effect.[57,66] As termination of AF and control of the ventricular response remains the primary therapeutic goal for preexcited AF, even in the absence of acute hemodynamic deterioration, patients with WPW syndrome-related AF are best treated with electrical cardioversion.

Polymorphic Ventricular Tachycardia and Ventricular Fibrillation (see Chapter 12)

Vagal Maneuvers

Vagal maneuvers refer to nonpharmacologic, physical interventions performed by the clinician, with the goal of increasing vagal parasympathetic tone, potentially slowing or terminating an SVT (Table 11.6).[67–73] They are often utilized as a first-line effort to abort episodes of stable SVT. Classic vagal maneuvers include the Valsalva maneuver, carotid sinus massage, cold water facial immersion, and ocular pressure. Ocular pressure is no longer recommended due to its potential harm.[65] Less commonly used maneuvers described in the literature but not discussed here include stimulation of the gag reflex, applied abdominal pressure, lying backwards, headstands, and utilizing devices to provide resistance to exhalation.[74,75] Vagal maneuvers may also be utilized diagnostically, as an alternative to adenosine, in settings in which slowing conduction in the SA or AV node could provide useful information. When used early in appropriately selected patients presenting with AVNRT, vagal maneuvers have a 20% to 40% success rate of conversion back to sinus rhythm. This may be higher with patients in AVRT or SVT associated with a bypass tract.[76–78]

Prior to performing a vagal maneuver, it is recommended that the patient be placed on a continuous cardiac monitor and reliable IV access should be in place. The provider should also have cardioversion and appropriate antiarrhythmic medications available as the next step in treatment if the vagal maneuvers are unsuccessful. No guidelines currently exist regarding the appropriate number of attempts of vagal maneuvers prior to initiating other therapies, although most providers will try a maximum of two to three attempts.

Valsalva Maneuver. The Valsalva maneuver consists of a variety of techniques designed to increase intrathoracic and intraabdominal pressure, resulting in stimulation of the aortic and carotid baroreceptors, causing an increase in vagal input into the AV node. Most versions of the maneuver involve forced exhalation against a closed glottis or bearing down as though to defecate for 15 to 30 seconds, creating an intrathoracic pressure of at least 30 to 40 mm Hg.[67,71] While the maneuver was classically performed with the patient in a semirecumbent position, the most recent SVT guidelines recommend that the Valsalva maneuver be performed in the supine position.[79,80]

The REVERT postural modification of the Valsalva maneuver (Video 11.4) demonstrated a higher rate of conversion to sinus rhythm when compared to a standard Valsalva control group (Valsalva for 15 seconds while sitting at 45 degrees with no postural changes)[13] (Fig. 11.7) and appears to have a higher success rate in terminating SVT and maintaining rhythm compared to carotid sinus massage.[76] The modified technique involves performing a Valsalva strain maneuver (e.g., forceful exhalation against a closed glottis) for 15 seconds while sitting at 45 degrees. Subsequently, the patient is laid supine with a passive leg raise for 15 seconds immediately after the strain phase. This can be repeated once if unsuccessful.

Cold Water Facial Immersion. See Video 11.5. Cold water facial immersion utilizes the human dive reflex and may be particularly useful in children who are often unable to cooperate in performing a Valsalva maneuver. There are limited data regarding the efficacy of this maneuver, but the optimal conditions to increase vagal tone require complete facial immersion or coverage by a cold pack 10°C or cooler for 30 to 40 seconds.[80a] Conversion to sinus rhythm generally occurs after 15 to 35 seconds. This procedure can be self-administered and is noninvasive. Cold water facial immersion is generally safe; however, there are several case reports of subcutaneous fat necrosis in pediatric patients following recurrent or prolonged use. This can be

TABLE 11.6 Nonpharmacologic Treatment of Stable SVT

VAGAL MANEUVER	TECHNIQUE	CONTRAINDICATIONS	COMPLICATIONS
Valsalva maneuver	• Vagal stimulation via increasing intrathoracic and intraabdominal pressure. • Most versions involve forcing air out from a closed glottis and/or simultaneously bearing down for 15–30 s. • Variations include supine or Trendelenburg positioning, passive leg raise, and applied abdominal pressure. • Higher rates of conversion occurred with the REVERT postural modification.[13] • Success rate 20-40% in appropriately selected patients	• Clinically unstable • Uncooperative or unable to follow commands and perform Valsalva • Dyspneic or tachypnea preventing Valsalva	
Carotid sinus massage (CSM)	• Application of steady pressure over the carotid sinus for 5–10 s • Can be performed in conjunction with Valsalva maneuver • The mean changes in bradycardia with CSM are generally less than those obtained with the Valsalva maneuver or cold water facial immersion	• Presence of carotid bruit • Recent CVA or MI • Diffuse or advanced CAD • Digoxin use	• CSM carries a very small risk of TIA and stroke (ranging from 0% to 0.9%). Assessment for a carotid bruit is unreliable for predicting these events • Case reports of cervicomediastinal hematoma, VF and VT
Cold water facial immersion	• Utilizes human dive reflex • Little data regarding efficacy • Generally used in children where effectively performing the Valsalva maneuver is often difficult • Eliciting maximal vagal tone may require complete facial immersion or coverage by a cold pack (10°C or colder) for a duration of 30–40 s		• Prolonged utilization or recurrent use can lead to subcutaneous fat necrosis

Note that unstable SVT is a contraindication for all of the above maneuvers.
CAD, Coronary artery disease; *CVA*, cerebrovascular incident; *MI*, myocardial infarction; *SVT*, supraventricular tachycardia; *TIA*, transient ischemic attack; *VF*, ventricular fibrillation; *VT*, ventricular tachycardia.

avoided by shorter application periods, application to less fatty areas of the face, and use of a cloth barrier.[81,82]

The vagal response and mean changes in bradycardia are generally greater with the Valsalva maneuver and cold water facial immersion as compared to carotid sinus massage.[83–87]

Carotid Sinus Massage CSM is a bedside vagal maneuver involving digital pressure on the richly innervated carotid sinus and its baroreceptor (Fig. 11.8). The patient should generally be relaxed and supine. Steady pressure is applied over the carotid sinus for 5-10 seconds and can be repeated if there is no response after a minute. Pressure on the carotid sinus may be steady or undulating in intensity; the force, however, must not occlude the carotid artery (Fig. 11.9). CSM can be performed in tandem with a Valsalva maneuver and/or passive leg raise. Initial application of pressure on the patient's right carotid bulb is preferred as there may be greater cardioinhibitory effect on this side (Table 11.7).

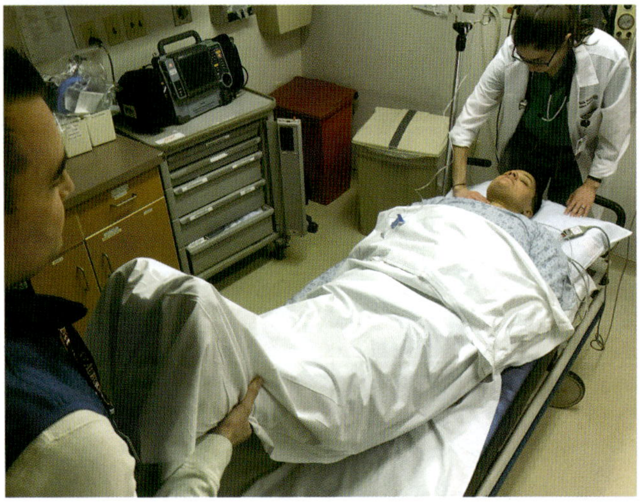

Fig. 11.7 Passively raising the patient's legs during Valsalva or carotid sinus massage is recommended and may increase the probability of successful conversion.

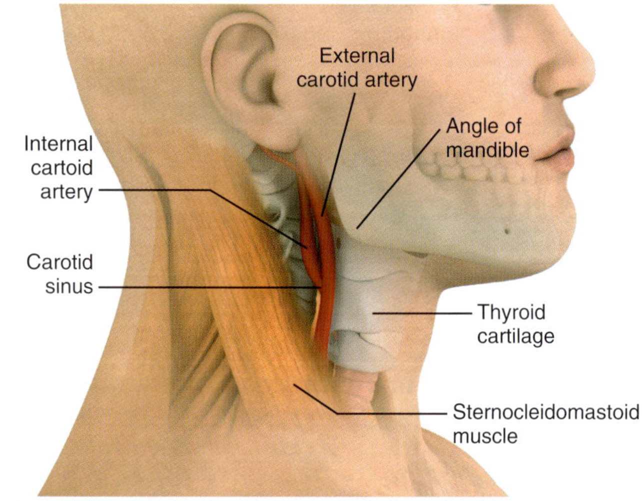

Fig. 11.8 The carotid sinus. This baroreceptor is found just below the angle of the mandible at the upper level of the thyroid cartilage, anterior to the sternocleidomastoid muscle.

Carotid Sinus Massage

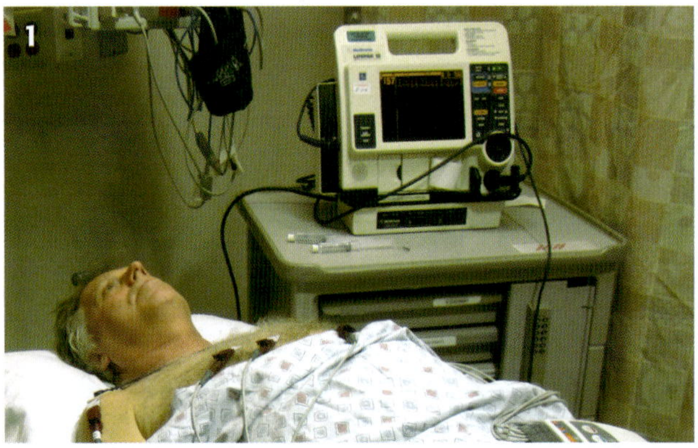

Prior to carotid sinus massage, place the patient on a cardiac monitor, initiate an IV line, and have antiarrhythmic medications and a defibrillator ready.

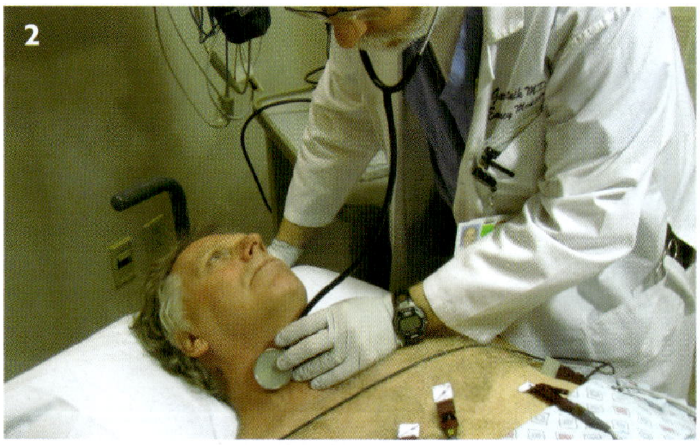

Auscultate for carotid bruits on both sides of the neck. The presence of a bruit is a contraindication to massage.

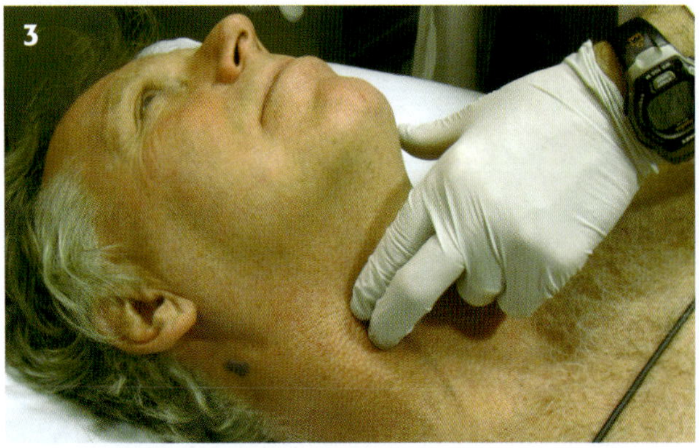

With the patient's head tilted backward and slightly to the opposite side, palpate the carotid pulse just below the angle of the mandible at the upper level of the thyroid cartilage and anterior to the sternocleidomastoid muscle. Once the pulsation is identified, use the fingertips to administer CSM for 5 seconds in a posteromedial direction, aiming toward the vertebral column.

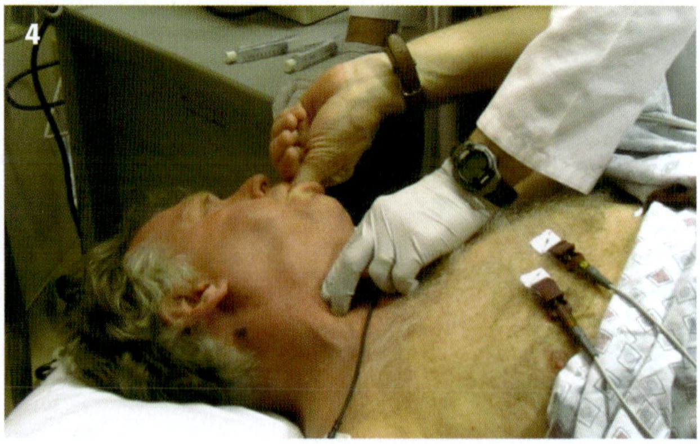

If the initial massage is unsuccessful, repeat after 1 minute. The opposite side may be massaged in similar fashion.

Simultaneous vagal maneuvers may also be beneficial, such as the Valsalva maneuver depicted here, as might repeated massage after the administration of calcium channel or β-blockers.

Fig. 11.9 Carotid sinus massage. *CSM*, Carotid sinus massage; *IV*, intravenous.

TABLE 11.7 Ventricular Response to Vagal Maneuvers

TYPE OF ARRHYTHMIA	ATRIAL RATE (BEATS/MIN)	RESPONSE TO VAGAL MANEUVERS
Sinus tachycardia	>100–180	Slowing with return to the former rate on release; appearance of diagnostic P waves
AV nodal reentry	150–250	Termination or no effect
Atrial flutter	250–350	Slowing with return to the former rate on release; increasing AV block; flutter persists
Atrial fibrillation	400–600	Slowing with persistence of a gross irregular rate on release; increasing AV block; fibrillation persists
Atrial tachycardia	150–250	Abrupt slowing with return to a normal sinus rhythm on release; tachycardia often persists
AV junctional rhythm	40–100	None; ± slowing
Reciprocal tachycardia using accessory (WPW) pathways	150–250	Abrupt slowing; termination or no effect; may unmask WPW
Ventricular tachycardia	60–100	None; may unmask AV dissociation
Digitalis toxicity–induced arrhythmias	Variable	Do not attempt CSM

AV, Atrioventricular; *CSM*, carotid sinus massage; *WPW*, Wolff-Parkinson-White [syndrome].
Adapted from Braunwald E, ed. *Heart Disease: A Textbook of Cardiovascular Medicine*. 6th ed. Saunders; 2001:642.

Simultaneous bilateral CSM is absolutely contraindicated because the cerebral circulation may be severely compromised. It is also advised that the provider auscultate for carotid bruits on both sides of the neck prior to performing CSM as the presence of a bruit is a contraindication to the procedure. Ultimately, CSM carries a very small but documented risk of stroke, thought to be secondary to traumatic rupture of atherosclerotic plaques in the carotid artery. Rates of carotid massage resulting in transient ischemic attack (TIA) and stroke is generally low, ranging from 0% to 0.9%. While age, by itself, is not a contraindication to CSM, older individuals are more likely to have carotid artery disease and may experience transient and, very rarely, permanent neurologic or visual symptoms after CSM. A recent cerebral infarction is another contraindication because even a marginal reduction in cerebral blood flow may produce further infarction. CSM should also be avoided in patients with known recent myocardial infarction due to higher risk for VT or VF. Other complications resulting from CSM described in case reports include cervicomediastinal hematoma leading to airway compromise, non-fatal VF and VT, and fatal VF.[88–99] While rare, these potentially serious complications should be balanced against the relatively low-to-moderate efficacy of CSM.

CONCLUSION

The availability of safe and effective medications to treat supraventricular tachycardias has given emergency clinicians a powerful armamentarium to be used in their management. Improvements in procedural sedation have also made electrical cardioversion a more accepted alternative. Both have resulted in a diminished role for vagal maneuvers. Nonetheless, vagal maneuvers are occasionally useful diagnostically, and therapeutically principally in the setting of PSVT.

REFERENCES ARE AVAILABLE AT Elsevier eBooks+

CHAPTER 12

Cardioversion and Defibrillation

Jeremy Lacocque

INTRODUCTION

Cardioversion and defibrillation are emergency procedures performed to terminate arrhythmias. Cardioversion is distinguished from defibrillation by synchronization with the ventricular depolarization for delivery of the electrical current. Defibrillation is used for arrhythmias such as ventricular fibrillation (VF) and pulseless ventricular tachycardia (VT), commonly found in victims of sudden cardiac arrest (SCA) (Review Box 12.1).

PRINCIPLES OF RESUSCITATION

The clinical approach to cardiac resuscitation is an evolving and dynamic endeavor, and guidelines are frequently updated. The most recent American Heart Association (AHA) guidelines, released in 2020 (with focused updates in 2023 on poisoning), recognize that out-of-hospital cardiac arrest (OHCA) survival rates have plateaued since 2012 and emphasize enhanced algorithms, early cardiopulmonary resuscitation (CPR), early epinephrine use, audio feedback and using $EtCO_2$ to guide efforts.[1–4]

DEFIBRILLATION: INDICATIONS

The most effective treatment of VF and pulseless VT in their early phase is defibrillation,[5–7] which generally becomes less effective the longer it is delayed—for every minute the heart is in VF without treatment, survival decreases by 7% to 10%.[8,9] (Fig. 12.1A–B). The integration of high-quality CPR (see Chapter 17) with defibrillation, when appropriate, increases the chance for successful defibrillation and survival from SCA.[10] When defibrillation is performed early and with high-quality CPR, return of spontaneous circulation (ROSC) rates are as high as 74% in human studies.[11] Other dysrhythmias, which may also be encountered in patients with SCA, such as pulseless electrical activity (PEA) and asystole, are not discussed in this chapter given that cardioversion and defibrillation are not effective treatments for them (Fig. 12.2).

Immediate defibrillation is indicated as soon as VF or pulseless VT is diagnosed. If unsuccessful, CPR should be initiated or continued and interruptions should be minimized. Defibrillation should occur during rhythm/pulse checks. Once defibrillation has been initiated, a cycle of CPR should be administered after defibrillation given delays in recovery of sufficient cardiac contractility.

If VF or VT is present in a trauma patient, the priority is to treat reversible traumatic causes, such as hypovolemia from blood loss or ventricular rupture. CPR and defibrillation are less likely to have an effect without first prioritizing other interventions and may ultimately prove to be of little value.

Defibrillation and Cardioversion

Indications

Defibrillation
- Ventricular fibrillation
- Pulseless ventricular tachycardia

Cardioversion (usually reserved for unstable rhythms)
- Ventricular tachycardia with a pulse
- Supraventricular tachycardia
- Atrial fibrillation
- Atrial flutter

Contraindications

Defibrillation
- Presence of a pulse
- Asystole or pulseless electrical activity
- Obvious signs of death
- Valid do-not-resuscitate order

Cardioversion
- Arrhythmias due to digitalis toxicity
- Sinus tachycardia

Complications
- Chest wall burns
- Shock of a health care worker
- Myocardial tissue injury

Equipment

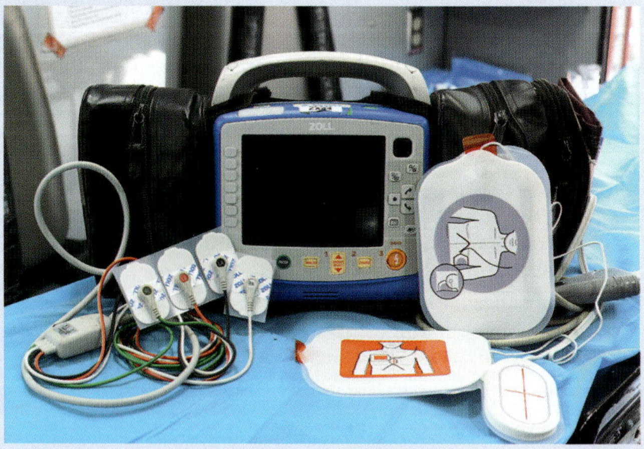

Cardiac monitor/defibrillator

Review Box 12.1 Defibrillation and cardioversion: indications, contraindications, and equipment.

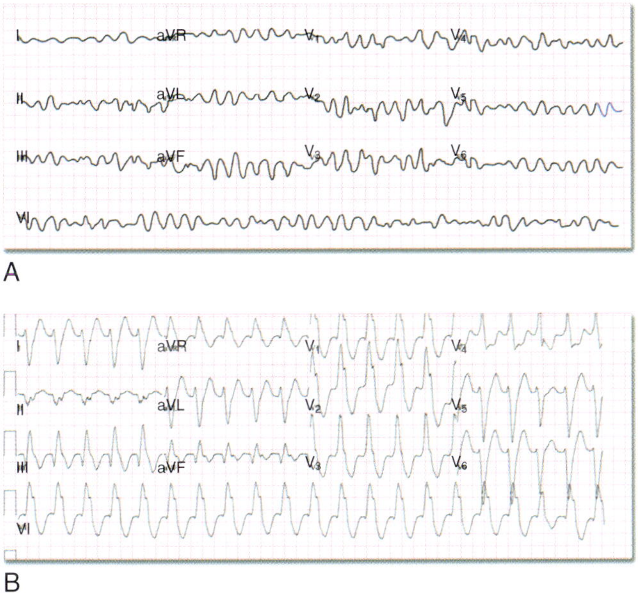

Fig. 12.1 Ventricular dysrhythmias. (A) Ventricular fibrillation. (B) Ventricular tachycardia.

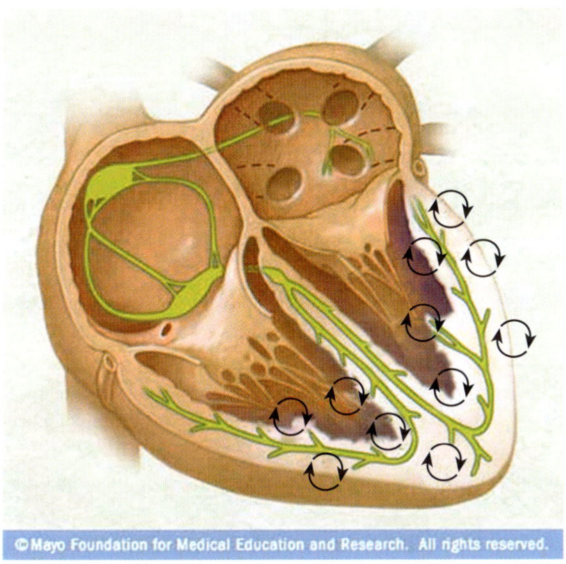

Fig. 12.2 During ventricular fibrillation, chaotic electromechanical activity prevents the ventricle from ejecting blood into the circulation. Defibrillation passes a therapeutic burst of current through the myocardium and terminates this activity.

Finally, if the patient with VF or pulseless VT is pregnant, treatment remains mostly unchanged. The initial primary intervention should be relief of aortocaval compression by left lateral uterine displacement to maximize venous return. Resuscitative hysterotomy, covered in Chapter 57), should also be performed within 5 minutes of maternal arrest to relieve aortocaval compression by the uterofetoplacental unit as well.

DEFIBRILLATION: CONTRAINDICATIONS

When evaluating the rhythm of a patient, if there is any doubt or confusion regarding the type of rhythm present, check multiple leads.

Absolute contraindications to defibrillation include presence of a pulse, clear medical futility of the procedure, or a valid do-not-resuscitate order. To ensure that asystole is indeed present before abandoning the possibility of defibrillation, especially if termination of resuscitation is being considered, be certain to check in more than one lead. Point-of-care ultrasound may also be useful to determine cardiac contractility. A potentially explosive environment is a relative contraindication to defibrillation.[12]

Findings or conditions that are *not* contraindications to delivery of an electrical impulse include medication-releasing patches (e.g., nitroglycerin, contraceptive hormones, antihypertensive agents, smoking cessation adjuncts, analgesics) even when metal containing, metallic piercings, or implantable cardiac devices such as pacemakers or implantable cardiac defibrillators (ICDs). Modify the placement of the electrodes or paddles to avoid contact with the medication patch, piercing, or automatic ICD (AICD). If the patient is stable, one can remove the piercings or medication patches with a gloved hand before cardioversion or defibrillation to avoid reduction of current to the myocardium, current arcing, sparks, or other complications.

Pregnancy at any stage is not a contraindication to cardioversion or defibrillation.[12]

Complications

Complications of defibrillation include soft tissue injury, myocardial injury, and cardiac dysrhythmias. AICDs that fire while a patient is conscious, either because of recognition of true VF or VT or in error, can cause discomfort and psychological sequelae. Use of AEDs in public access defibrillation programs has not been reported to have produced any significant mishaps or adverse outcomes.[13]

PATHOPHYSIOLOGY

The electrical impulse for myocardial contraction normally originates spontaneously in the sinoatrial (SA) node and spreads through the atria, which causes it to contract. As the impulse arrives at the atrioventricular (AV) node, it undergoes decremental conduction in which the electrical impulse is slowed down as the atria contract and "preload" the ventricles. Subsequently, the impulse activates the bundle of His and Purkinje fibers, which then cause ventricular contraction via excitation-contraction coupling. The electrical events precede the mechanical events. As the original impulse from the SA node travels through the atria and into the ventricles, various action potentials are generated regionally. The summation of all these action potentials produces the characteristic electrocardiographic (ECG) tracing PQRST (Figs. 12.3 and 12.4). The ECG tracing is a graphic representation of the electrical activity that induces the mechanical activity of systole. Systole occurs as a result of excitation-contraction coupling. As the ion channels reset, the myocytes return to the resting membrane and diastole occurs. Each "cardiac cycle" lasts approximately 300 ms. During each cardiac cycle, there are two key periods: the absolute and relative refractory periods (Fig. 12.5). During the absolute refractory period, the myocytes do not respond to excitatory stimuli because the channels are in full operation. During the relative refractory period, the myocytes can be stimulated with an impulse that is proportionately larger than usual as more and more ion channels reset.

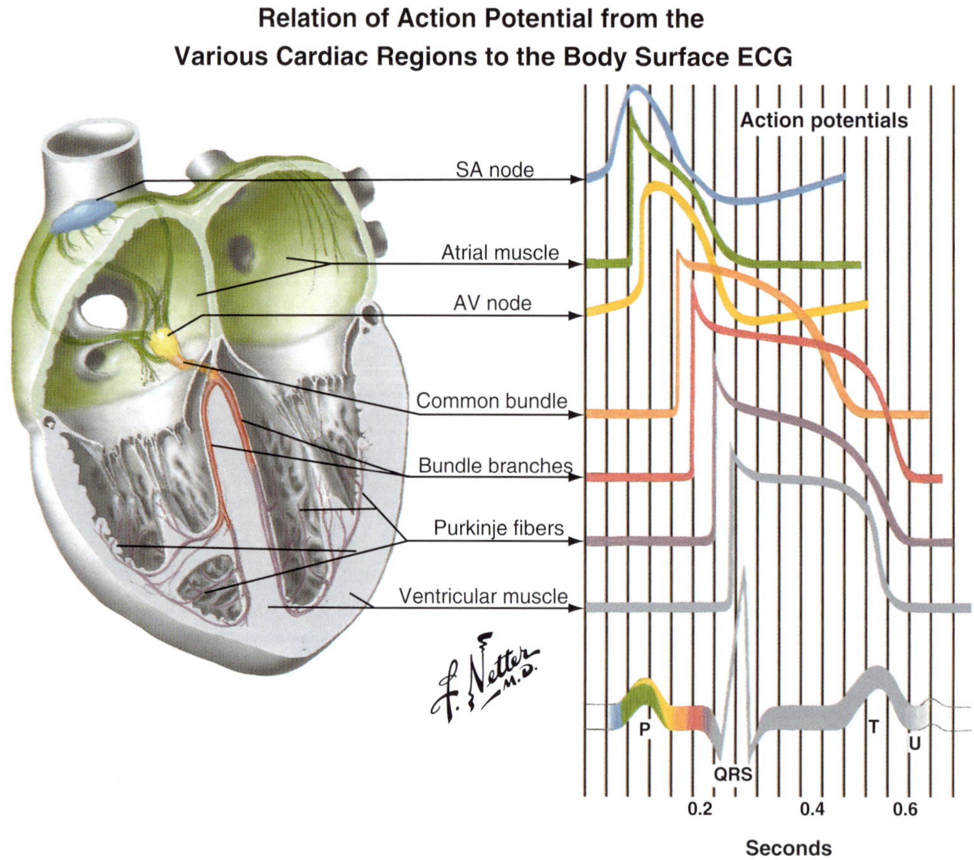

Fig. 12.3 Regional action potentials and electrocardiographic correlation. *AV*, Atrioventricular; *SA*, sinoatrial. (Netter illustration from https://www.netterimages.com. Elsevier Inc. All rights reserved.)

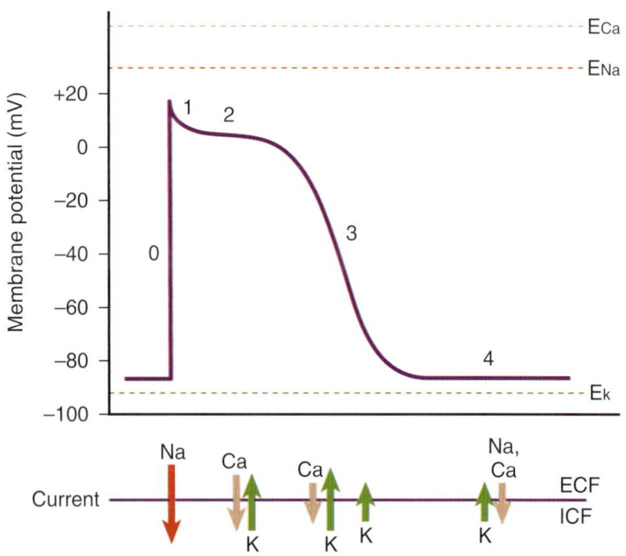

Fig. 12.4 Cardiac action potential is a result of ion flux across the cell membrane. *ECF*, Extracellular fluid; *ICF*, intracellular fluid. (Adapted from Costanzo LS. *Physiology*. 4th ed. Saunders; 2009.)

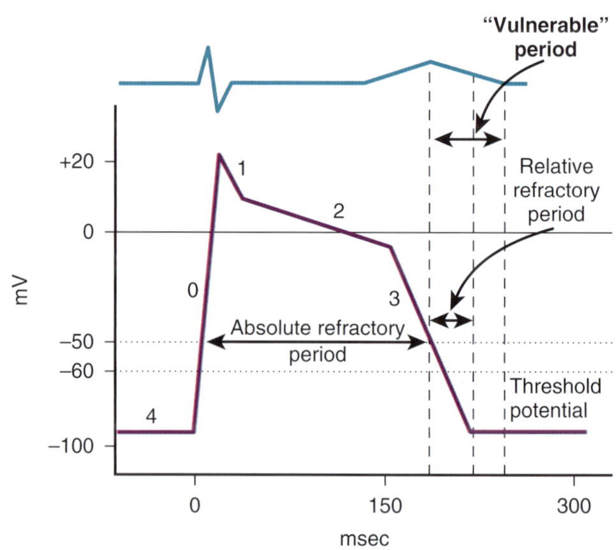

Fig. 12.5 Absolute and relative refractory periods.

Even with an ROSC, prearrest cardiac output may not be reached due to injury or transient myocardial dysfunction, known as "stunning." Cardiogenic shock, and recurrence of cardiac arrest, can be common depending on the extent of injury to the heart from the arrest and its etiology, resulting in consideration of the need for early use of intravenous pressors and/or cardiac catheterization.

Cardiopulmonary Resuscitation

Fig. 12.6 shows the AHA adult cardiac arrest algorithm. If it can be accomplished without distracting from CPR, place the

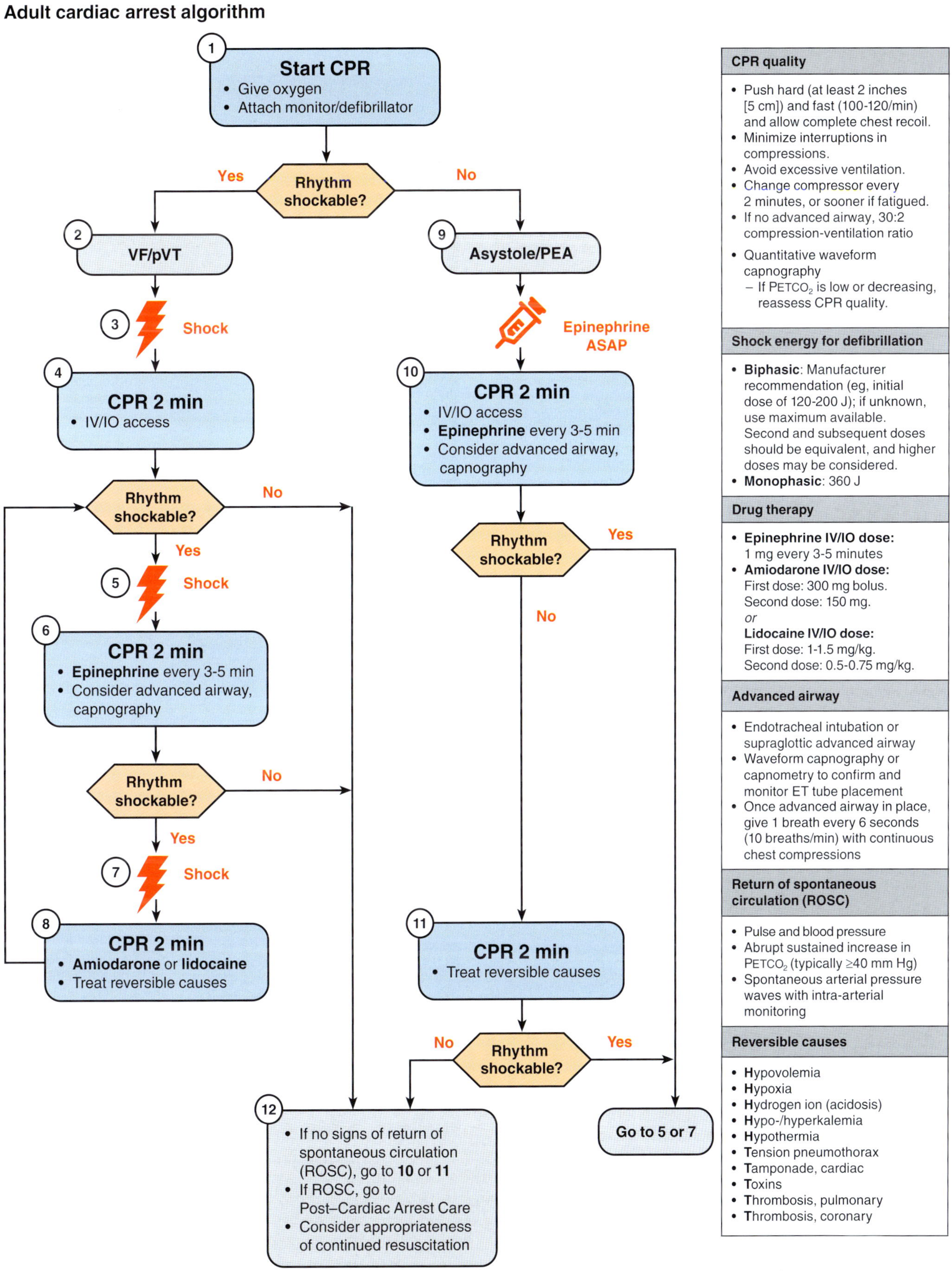

Fig. 12.6 Adult cardiac arrest algorithm. *CPR*, Cardiopulmonary resuscitation; *ET*, endotracheal; *IO*, intraosseous; *IV*, intravenous; *PEA*, pulseless electrical activity; *P_{ETCO_2}*, end-tidal CO_2 pressure; *VF*, ventricular fibrillation; *pVT*, pulseless ventricular tachycardia. (From *Circulation*. 2020;142:S469–S523. Copyright 2020 American Heart Association.)

DEFIBRILLATION

1

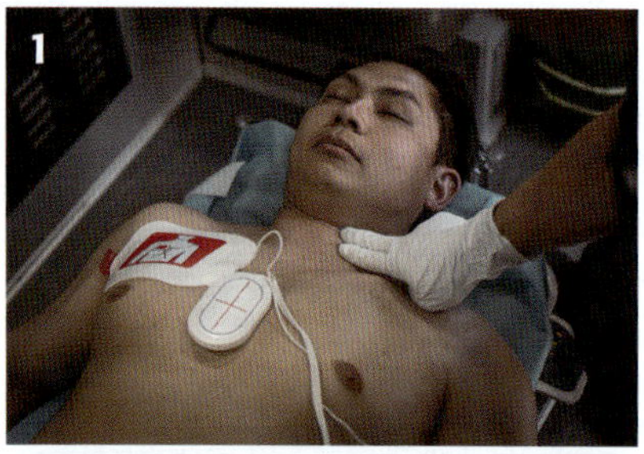

Assess patient responsiveness, breathing, and circulation. Check for a pulse for <10 seconds. Call for help and have the code cart delivered to the bedside.

2

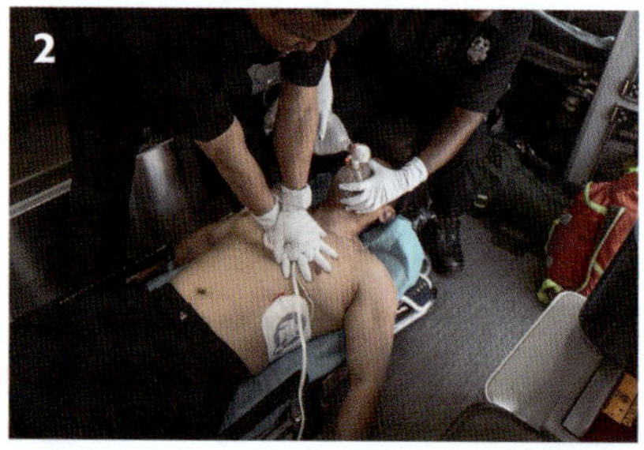

If there is no pulse, begin CPR at a rate of >100 compressions per minute with a ratio of 30 compressions to 2 ventilations. Avoid interruptions in CPR, PUSH HARD, and PUSH FAST.

3

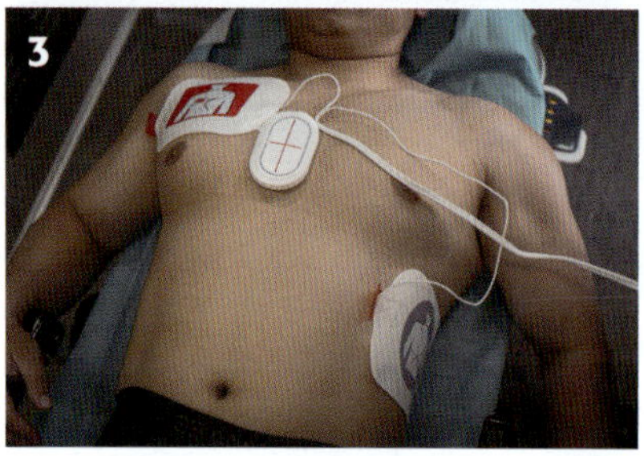

Apply the electrodes to the patient's chest. Place the sternal electrode below the clavicle, to the right of the sternum. Place the apical electrode in the midaxillary line at the fifth intercostal space.

4

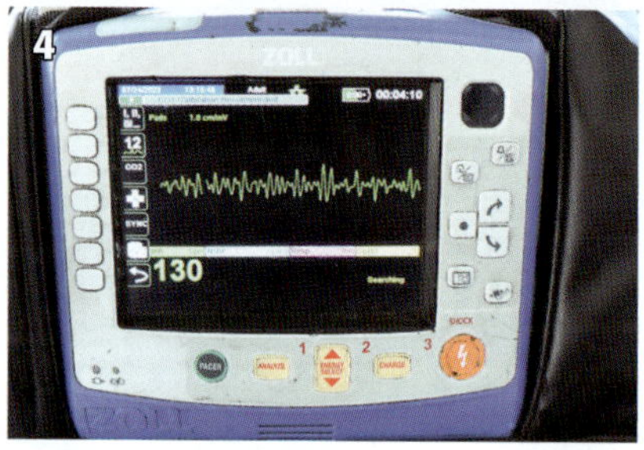

Check the rhythm on the monitor. If there is a shockable rhythm (i.e., VF or pulseless VT), prepare for immediate defibrillation.

5

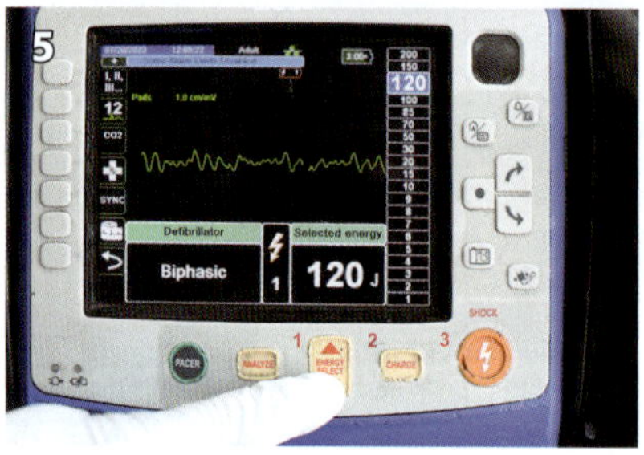

Select the appropriate energy for the initial shock. For biphasic defibrillators, a default energy of 200 J is appropriate (see text for details). For monophasic machines, use 360 J. Make sure that "SYNC" is turned *off.*

6

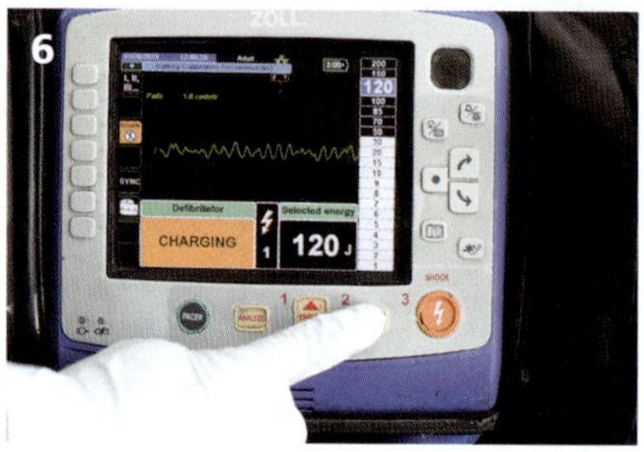

Once the energy has been selected and the decision to defibrillate confirmed, press the "CHARGE" button on the defibrillator.

7

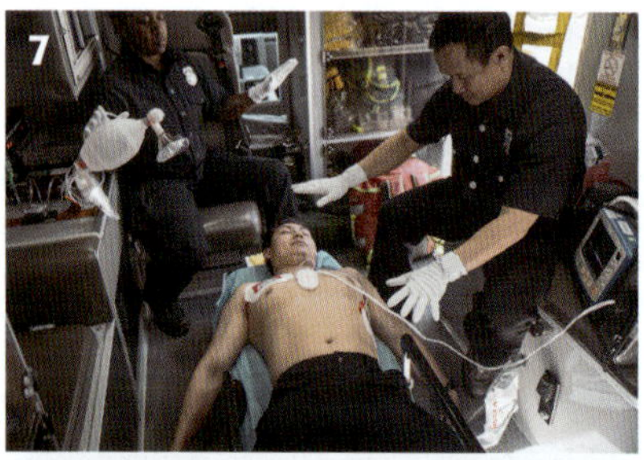

As the "CHARGE" button is depressed, loudly announce "I'm clear, you're clear, everybody's clear!" and make sure that no caregivers are in contact with the patient.

8

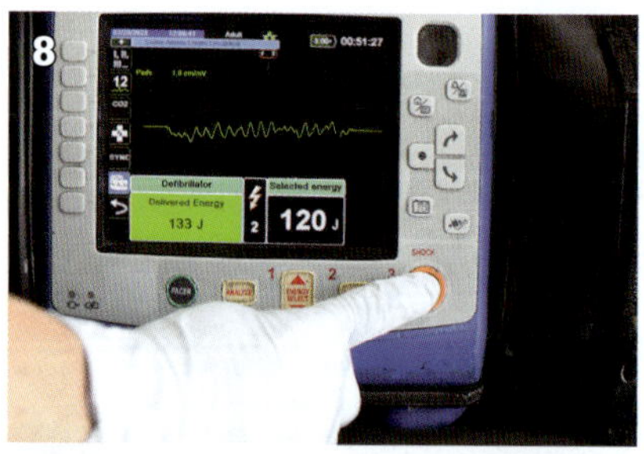

Check once again to make sure that everyone is clear, and then depress the "SHOCK" button to defibrillate the patient.

9

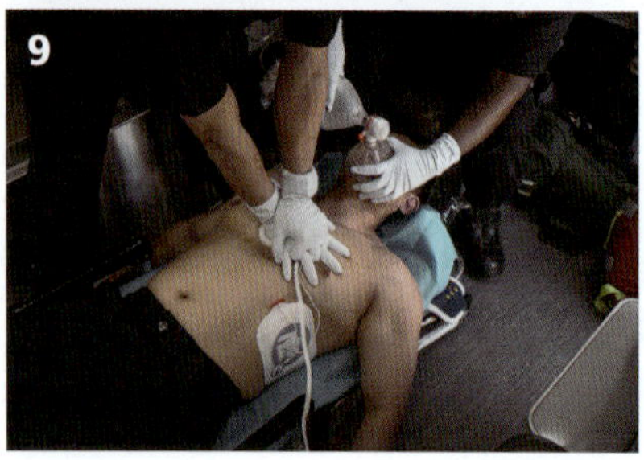

Resume CPR *immediately* and continue for 5 cycles/ 2 minutes. Additional interventions such as IV/IO access and airway management may be pursued but should not interfere with continuous CPR.

10

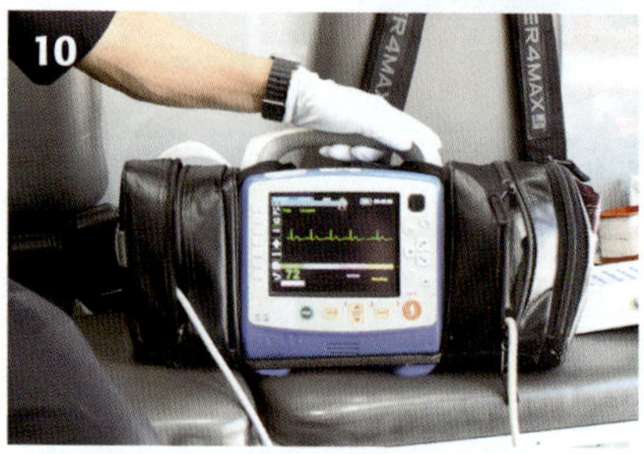

After 2 minutes of CPR, reassess the patient and the rhythm. Refer to the text and algorithms in this chapter for additional information.

Fig. 12.7 Defibrillation. *CPR,* Cardiopulmonary resuscitation; *IO,* intraosseous; *IV,* intravenous; *VF,* ventricular fibrillation; *VT,* ventricular tachycardia.

patient on the monitor, place defibrillation pads on the patient, and establish IV access. Attempt to palpate the carotid pulse (<10 seconds; Fig. 12.7, *step 1*). If no pulse is present, begin a sequence of 30 chest compressions followed by 2 ventilations/ breaths (Fig. 12.7, *step 2*). This should continue uninterrupted for 2 minutes. The hands should remain on the lower half of the sternum and compress it at least 2 inches (5 cm) at a rate of 100 to 120 compressions/min. Watch for full chest recoil to allow adequate ventricular filling and do not lean on the chest before the next compression. When the defibrillator or automated external defibrillator (AED) arrives, continue the 30:2 ratio of compressions to ventilations during CPR, attach the patient to the defibrillator via pads applied to the patient's chest, and initiate the rhythm check (Fig. 12.7, *step 3*). Every attempt should be made to minimize interruption of compressions. If the resuscitation occurs in a health care setting (first responder or in a hospital), the above should be done while also obtaining vascular access for blood draw and medication administration, securing the airway, and working to identify and treat reversible causes of the arrest. In some settings, a mechanical compression device may be available. These devices are common in the prehospital setting and can relieve responders of compressions to focus on other priorities. Notably, mechanical compressions can continue being delivered even during defibrillation.

Rhythm Assessment

Once the defibrillator is at the patient's side, turn on the defibrillator/monitor and place electrodes on the patient's chest using the multifunctional electrode pads that can acquire ECG signals and be used concomitantly to defibrillate the patient.

The correct position for placement of the adhesive pads is illustrated in Fig. 12.8. Frequently, the pads are labeled with a diagram as a guide to placing the electrodes on the chest wall. Place the sternal electrode just below the clavicle and just to the right of the sternum. Place the apical electrode in the midaxillary line around the fifth or sixth intercostal space. The pads can also be placed in an anterior-posterior fashion. Once the electrodes or pads are in position, set the selector dial or switch on the defibrillator monitor to the appropriate position to acquire the ECG signal from the input source. In addition, adjust the controls for gain of the ECG signal to increase the sensitivity or gain of the ECG amplifier to ensure that fine VF is not interpreted as asystole. As the ECG rhythm appears on the monitor, make a diagnosis of the type of rhythm or lack thereof (Fig. 12.7, *step 4*). If a shockable rhythm such as VF or pulseless VT is present, defibrillation is indicated. Proceed to select the appropriate energy level for the anticipated defibrillation.

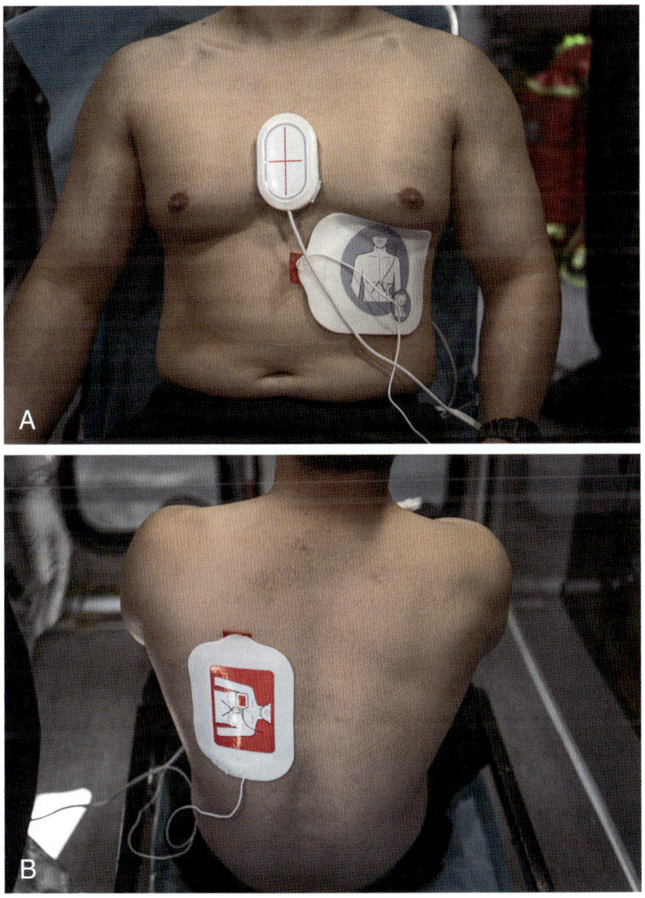

Fig. 12.8 Electrode positioning for defibrillation. Anterior-posterior placement. Place the anterior pad just to the left of the sternum (A) and the posterior pad directly behind it (B), approximating the position of the heart.

Energy Selection

Defibrillators should be set to an energy level of 120 J to 200 J for biphasic defibrillators (most common) (Fig. 12.7, *step 5*). Monophasic defibrillators are less common but still in use and have a maximum shock of 360 J. For patients in VF or pulseless VT, AHA guidelines recommend using the maximum energy allowable by the machine. Second and subsequent doses should be at equivalent levels. Additionally, some evidence supports dual sequential defibrillation, where two defibrillators are used one after the other (within one second) to terminate refractory VF. Despite some supporting evidence, the 2020 AHA guidelines do not yet support it and were released before this particular study was published in the *New England Journal of Medicine* (Video 12.1).[14]

Mode Selection

In VF or pulseless VT, the defibrillator should be set to the unsynchronized mode. Most defibrillators default into the unsynchronized "defibrillation" mode between shocks. If in the synchronized mode, the defibrillator may not discharge when the shock buttons are depressed because it is triggered by identification and tracking of the QRS complex, which is not present in VF.

Defibrillation

See Video 12.2. Continue CPR until the defibrillator is charged and ready to defibrillate. Waiting to initiate a charge until after or during the pulse check after VF or VT can unnecessarily prolong the pause in CPR. Once the energy level has been selected and the defibrillator is charged, clear the patient for defibrillation by loudly stating "I'm clear, you're clear, everybody's clear," and then activate the button to deliver the shock (Fig. 12.7, *steps 6 and 7*). This will be followed by a perceptible whole-body muscle twitch in the patient. If no obvious response or twitch of the patient is seen, check the defibrillator controls to make sure that the mode is set to unsynchronized and the pads are properly connected.

Once the shock has been delivered (Fig. 12.7, *step 8*), immediately resume resuscitation with chest compressions (Fig. 12.7, *step 9*) and continue for approximately five cycles of 30:2 compressions to ventilations, or approximately 2 minutes of CPR until the next rhythm and pulse check (Fig. 12.7, *step 10*). This facilitates the transition from SCA to ROSC after the heart has been stunned by the defibrillation and may not be functioning at optimal contractility for a few minutes after the shock while also minimizing pauses if ROSC is not achieved.

Subsequent shocks should be at higher energy within the 120 J to 200 J range.

Automated External Defibrillator Application

The availability of AEDs (Fig. 12.9) or semiautomated defibrillators has increased, typically in public areas like airports, gyms, schools, and noncritical care sections of hospitals. Although AEDs are designed for lay public use, application of these devices may also occur in the clinical setting. As in the algorithm, assess the patient, summon help, and apply the AED. Operation of the AED is guided by voice and occasionally visual prompts. Turn the device on, apply the patient electrodes in the appropriate positions, analyze the rhythm, and deliver a shock if a shockable rhythm is present. The AED will determine the rhythm and choose the energy level. Unfortunately, while AEDs are often available, their use by the public is low. Public education and dispatcher prearrival instructions are therefore key in the chain of survival.

PEDIATRIC DEFIBRILLATION

Cardiac arrest in infants and children is most often secondary to respiratory failure. SCA due to VF and pulseless VT is much less likely to occur in children than in adults; however, 5% to 15% of pediatric and adolescent SCA events demonstrate VF in the prehospital setting. In in-hospital arrests, a 20% occurrence of VF is reported at some point during the resuscitation. As in adults, rapid intervention and defibrillation improve outcomes from SCA. Causes of SCA, VF, and pulseless VT are more diverse in pediatric patients.[15] Cardiac arrest is not usually a result of a primary cardiac issue. Therefore the approach to resuscitation of a pediatric patient in VF or pulseless VT may differ depending on the cause of the arrest.

Similar to adults, pediatric patients with rhythms who received defibrillation for documented VF have been reported to have a higher survival-to-discharge rate than do children who sustained asystole or PEA.[16] Therefore there is a similar indication for early defibrillation in the pediatric population.

The procedure for pediatric defibrillation is similar to the algorithm for adult defibrillation (Fig. 12.10). These guidelines do not apply to children younger than 1 year. For children younger than 1 year, evidence is limited on efficacy of defibrillation and a manual defibrillator should also be used in lieu of an AED to ensure proper energy dosing. The pediatric resuscitation guidelines incorporated findings from a comprehensive review of the data.[17]

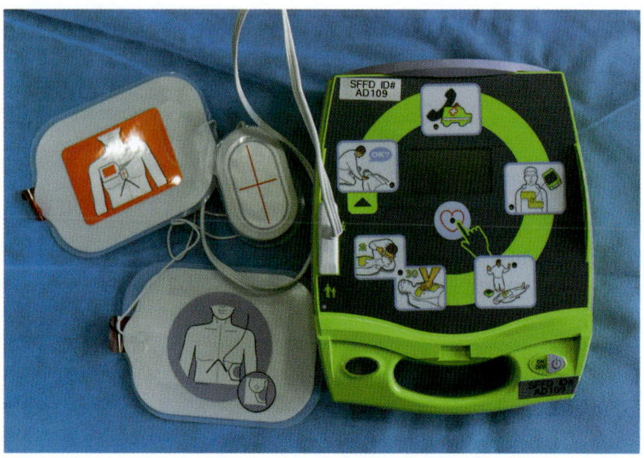

Fig. 12.9 Automated external defibrillator.

To perform pediatric defibrillation, a defibrillator monitor capable of adjustments in energy appropriate for children is needed. If an AED is to be used, it should have an energy attenuator for adjusting the energy to the appropriate level for a child (Fig. 12.11A). Pads should also be the appropriate size that will not overlap (see Fig. 12.11C). If the attenuator and pediatric pads are not available, the adult sized may be used, ensuring the pads do not overlap.

Choose an optimal pad size—the largest surface area possible without direct electrode-to-electrode contact—which will decrease transthoracic impedance and enhance defibrillation.[18] To accomplish this, use infant pads for children weighing less than 25 kg. In children who weigh more than 25 kg (mean age, 8 years), use adult pads.[18]

Apply the pads firmly to the chest, one to the right of the sternum, just below the clavicle, and the other to the left of the left nipple, over the ribs and the apex of the heart (see Fig. 12.7, *step 3*). Another option is to place one pad just to the left of the sternum and the other over the back so that they approximate the position of the heart (see Fig. 12.8).

No recommendations for the use of a defibrillator or AED in children younger than 1 year have been provided as of this writing.[19] A pediatric energy dose attenuator (see Fig. 12.11A) should be used to prevent the delivery of too much current to the myocardium. If a pediatric dose attenuator is not immediately available, an adult AED may be used, ensuring the pads do not overlap.

An energy level of 2 to 4 J/kg should be used. If a second defibrillation is indicated, 4 J/kg should be used. Subsequent shocks can be increased, but should not exceed 10 J/kg or the maximum adult dose.[1,16] Before defibrillation, check to make sure that the defibrillator is set to the unsynchronized mode. Most defibrillators default into the unsynchronized mode between shocks.

Cardioversion: Indications

Cardioversion is appropriate for all supraventricular arrhythmias as well as VT with a pulse. Neither irregularity (i.e., atrial fibrillation) nor QRS complex width affects the choice of cardioversion versus defibrillation. Cardioversion, rather than defibrillation, is indicated even in the unstable patient as long as there is a pulse. The shock in cardioversion is timed to occur during the R wave, the refractory period of the cardiac cycle. This is accomplished by setting the defibrillator to synchronized mode (Videos 12.1–12.3). The dosages for cardioversion typically start lower than defibrillation. Failure to set the defibrillator controls to "synchronized" can result in an "R on T" phenomenon, with a depolarizing stimulus delivered during the T wave, a period of repolarization, potentially resulting in VF.[20]

Cardioversion: Contraindications

Cardioversion is contraindicated in situations with tachydysrhythmias that are known to be caused by digitalis toxicity, as well as a known sinus tachycardia. Dysrhythmias caused by enhanced automaticity will *not* be terminated by uniformly depolarizing myocardial tissue because a homogeneous depolarization state already exists. Enhanced automaticity is the cause of most cases of digitalis toxicity–induced dysrhythmia,

Pediatric cardiac arrest algorithm

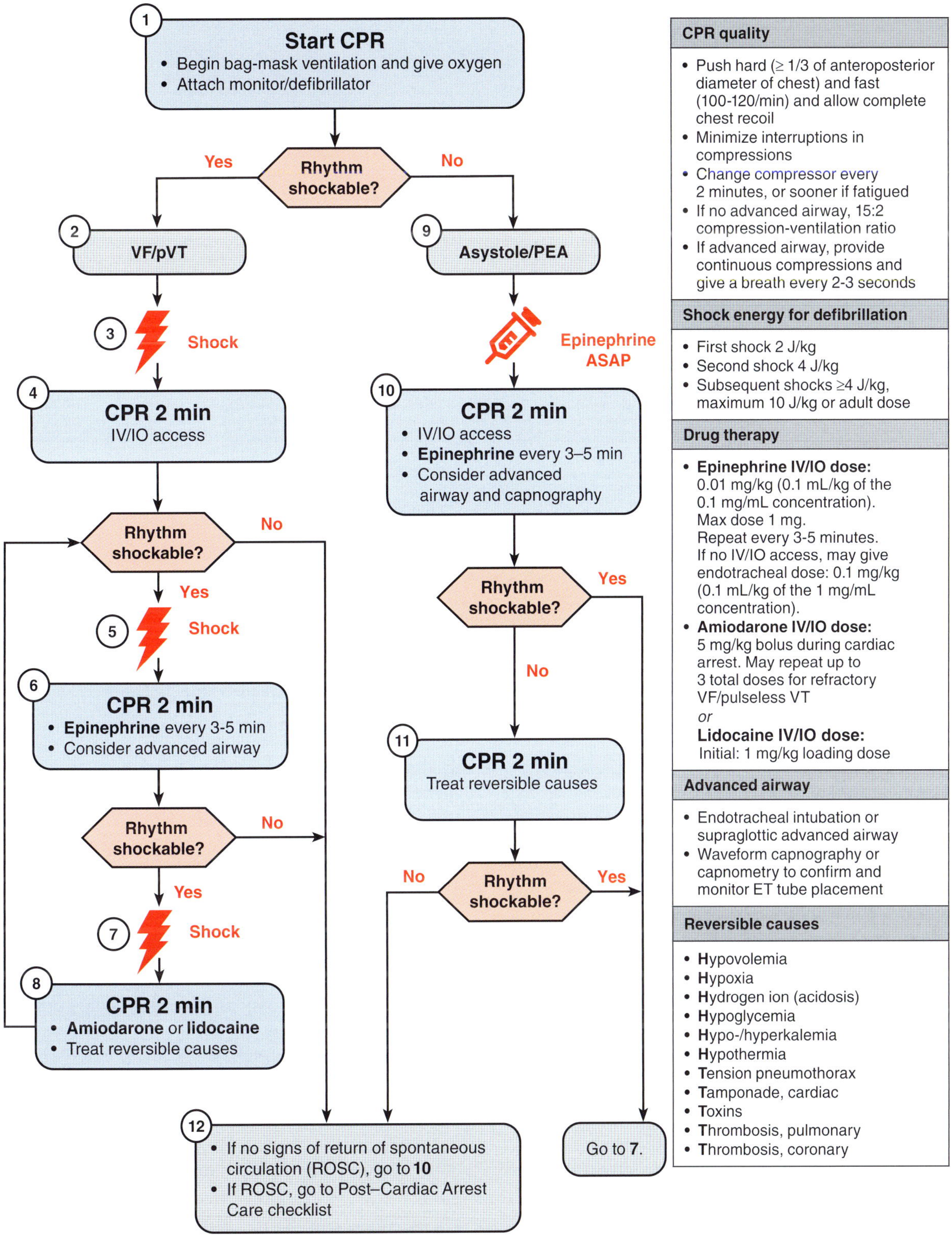

Fig. 12.10 Pediatric defibrillation algorithm. *CPR,* Cardiopulmonary resuscitation; *ET,* endotracheal; *IO,* intraosseous; *IV,* intravenous; *PEA,* pulseless electrical activity; P_{ETCO_2}, end-tidal CO_2 pressure; *VF,* ventricular fibrillation; *pVT,* pulseless ventricular tachycardia. (From *Circulation*. 2020;142:S469–S523. Copyright 2020 American Heart Association.)

sinus tachycardia, and multifocal atrial tachycardia. Although cardioversion will not work in these cases, medications that suppress automaticity, including potassium and magnesium, may be useful. In digoxin toxicity, not only is cardioversion ineffective, but it is also associated with a higher incidence of postshock VT and VF.[21] However, in a patient with a therapeutic digoxin level, the risk associated with cardioversion is now thought to be no different from that of other patients.

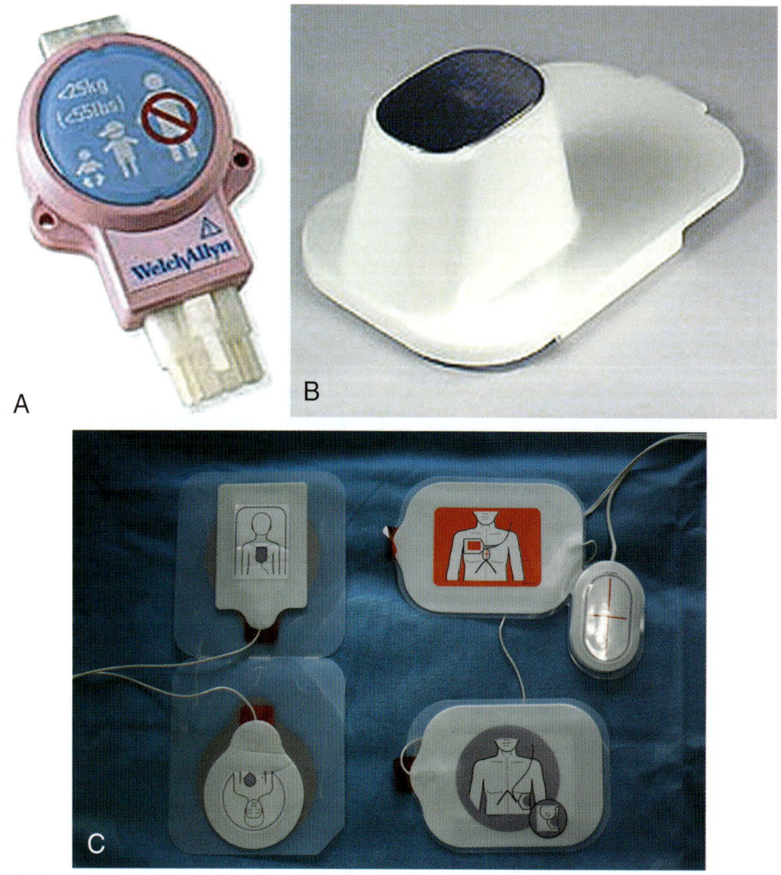

Fig. 12.11 Pediatric defibrillation equipment. (A) Pediatric energy attenuator for the automated external defibrillator. (B) Pediatric quick-look electrode paddle adapters. (C) Pediatric adhesive electrode pads.

Digoxin is still generally withheld for 24 hours before cardioversion as a precaution against inadvertently elevated levels.

A pitfall in selection of patients for cardioversion includes misdiagnosis of sinus tachycardia, especially at fast rates when the P wave is buried in the T wave. This may mimic SVT when the QRS complex is narrow, or VT when the QRS is wide from baseline bundle branch block or aberrancy.

Cardioversion: Complications

These are similar to those that occur with defibrillation. Complications are dose-related and may involve the airway, heart, or chest wall, or they may be psychological. Hypoxia may develop in patients if sedation is excessive or the airway becomes compromised. Ideally, a dedicated clinician such as a respiratory therapist (RN) or a second physician should be placed in charge of monitoring the patient's airway during the procedure. Routine supplemental oxygen is suggested for all patients undergoing sedation and should be used in conjunction with end-tidal CO_2.

Chest wall burns resulting from electrical arcing are generally superficial partial-thickness burns, although deep partial-thickness burns have occurred.[22] While much less common than when paddles were routinely used, they can still occur when pads are placed over medication patches or ointments, especially those containing nitroglycerin, because electrical discharge may cause ignition and result in chest burns.[23]

Cardiac complications after cardioversion are proportionate to the energy dose delivered. In the moderate energy levels used most commonly, the hemodynamic effects are small. At higher energy levels, however, complications include dysrhythmias, hypotension, and rarely, pulmonary edema, which may occur several hours after the countershock. The dysrhythmias occurring after high-dose (200 J) DC shocks include VT and VF, bradycardia, and AV block, in addition to transient and sustained asystole.[23] Sustained VT or VF was reported following 7 of 99 shocks in a study of patients undergoing electrophysiologic study and requiring cardioversion for VT, VF, or AF. These episodes occurred only in patients with prior VT or VF. Patients with ischemia or known coronary artery disease appear to be at much higher risk for significant postshock bradycardia, with rate support pacing being required after 13 of 99 shocks in the aforementioned study. Therefore the proclivity for dysrhythmias is greater with high-dose cardioversion of an ischemic heart. In addition, there is the risk of a shock delivered during the repolarization phase resulting in degeneration into VF and the need for immediate defibrillation.

Cardioversion: Procedure

See Video 12.3. The critical components of preparation for cardioversion are IV access, airway management equipment, drugs for sedation, monitoring, and cardiac monitor/defibrillator (cardioverter) (Fig. 12.12, *step 1*). Fig. 12.13 shows the AHA adult tachycardia with a pulse algorithm.

Secure IV access is essential for delivery of sedatives, antidysrhythmics, fluids, and possibly paralytic agents. Although many of these drugs are not used routinely, if they are needed,

CARDIOVERSION

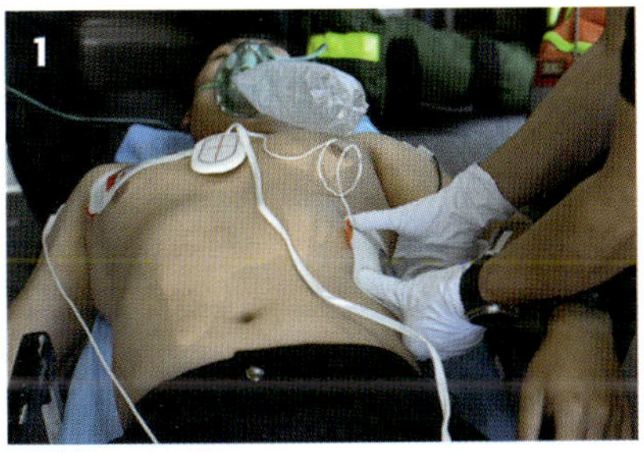

1 Obtain IV access, administer oxygen, and place the patient on cardiac, pulse oximetry, and end-tidal CO_2 monitors. Anticipate and prepare sedative and antidysrhythmic medications.

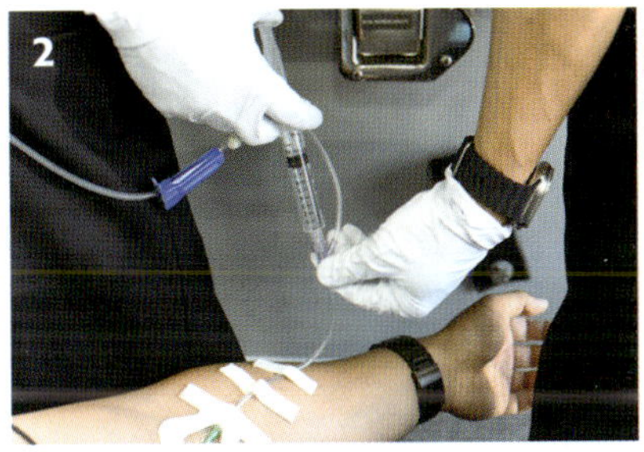

2 Administer procedural sedation if time and the clinical scenario permit.

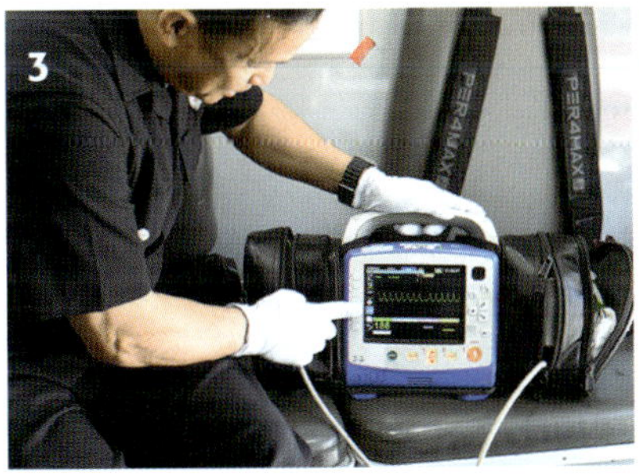

3 Push the "SYNC" button to select the synchronized mode. Check to see that the machine is correctly identifying the R wave of the complexes (*arrow*).

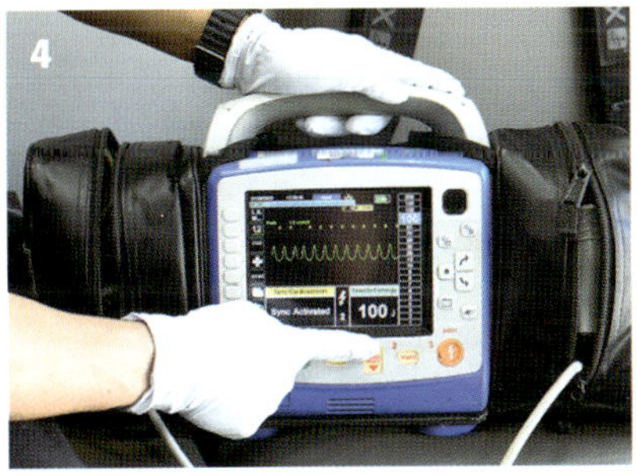

4 Select the appropriate energy level. This will depend on the rhythm being cardioverted. See text and the cardioversion algorithm for details.

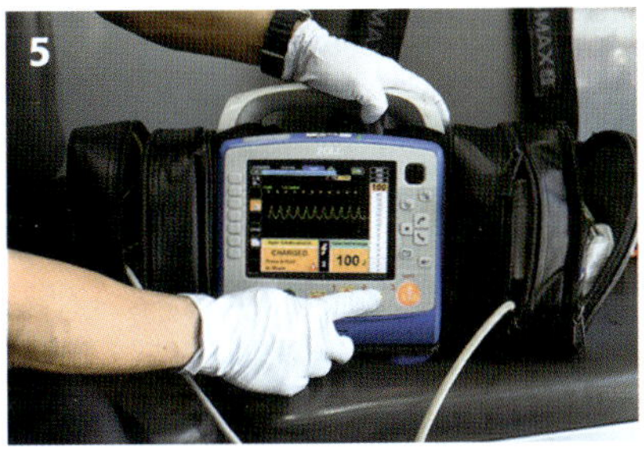

5 Once the energy has been selected and the decision to cardiovert confirmed, press the "CHARGE" button on the defibrillator.

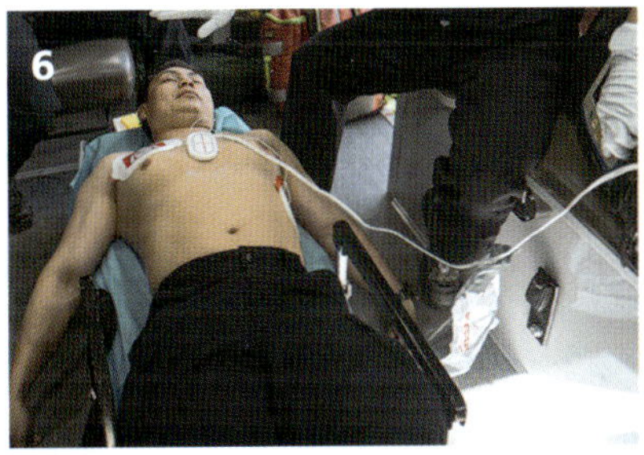

6 As the "CHARGE" button is depressed, loudly announce "I'm clear, you're clear, everybody's clear!" and make sure that no caregivers are in contact with the patient.

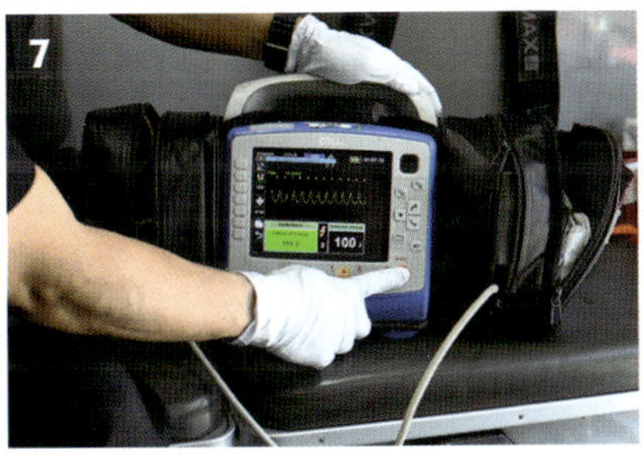

7 Check once again to make sure that everyone is clear, and then depress the "SHOCK" button to cardiovert the patient.

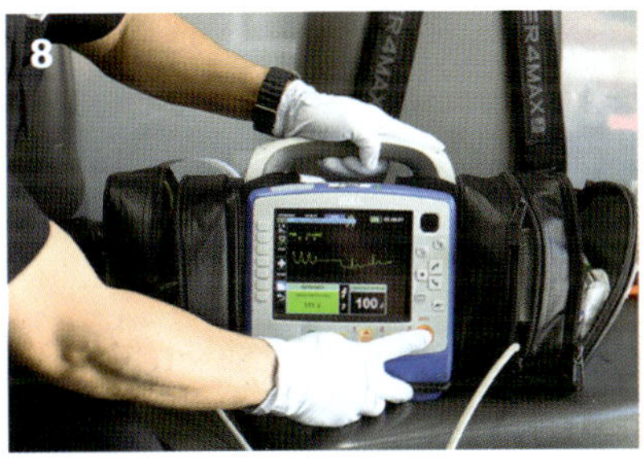

8 After delivery of the energy, reassess the patient and heart rhythm.

Fig. 12.12 Cardioversion.

timing is likely to be critical. At least one, and preferably two, large-bore IV catheters should be inserted and confirmed to flush and draw prior to beginning the procedure. An IV at, or proximal to, the patient's antecubital area can ensure efficacy of adenosine, if needed at any point.

A significant and preventable complication of procedures involving sedation is hypoventilation leading to hypercarbia and hypoxia. Airway management equipment includes a working IV, suction, bag-valve-mask (BVM) apparatus, oxygen, and appropriately sized laryngoscope and endotracheal tube or supraglottic airway. If available, a respiratory therapist should be at the patient's bedside as well. A pulse oximeter, cardiac monitor, 12-lead ECG equipment and $EtCO_2$ monitoring are essential as well. A rising $EtCO_2$ level will be an early clue to hypoventilation secondary to sedation because oxygen saturation may remain normal for several minutes, especially if the patient is receiving supplemental oxygen.

Sedative medications should be ready for use in labeled syringes, along with prefilled saline syringes for flushing the catheter. Antidysrhythmic medications for ventricular dysrhythmias (e.g., amiodarone, lidocaine) and for unexpected bradycardia (e.g., atropine) should be readily accessible as well.

Preprocedure

If time permits, correction of lab or vital sign abnormalities may increase the likelihood that cardioversion is successful. At a minimum, hypoxia should be corrected with supplemental oxygen, taking care to not mask hypoxia from hypoventilation. If a patient has metabolic acidosis,

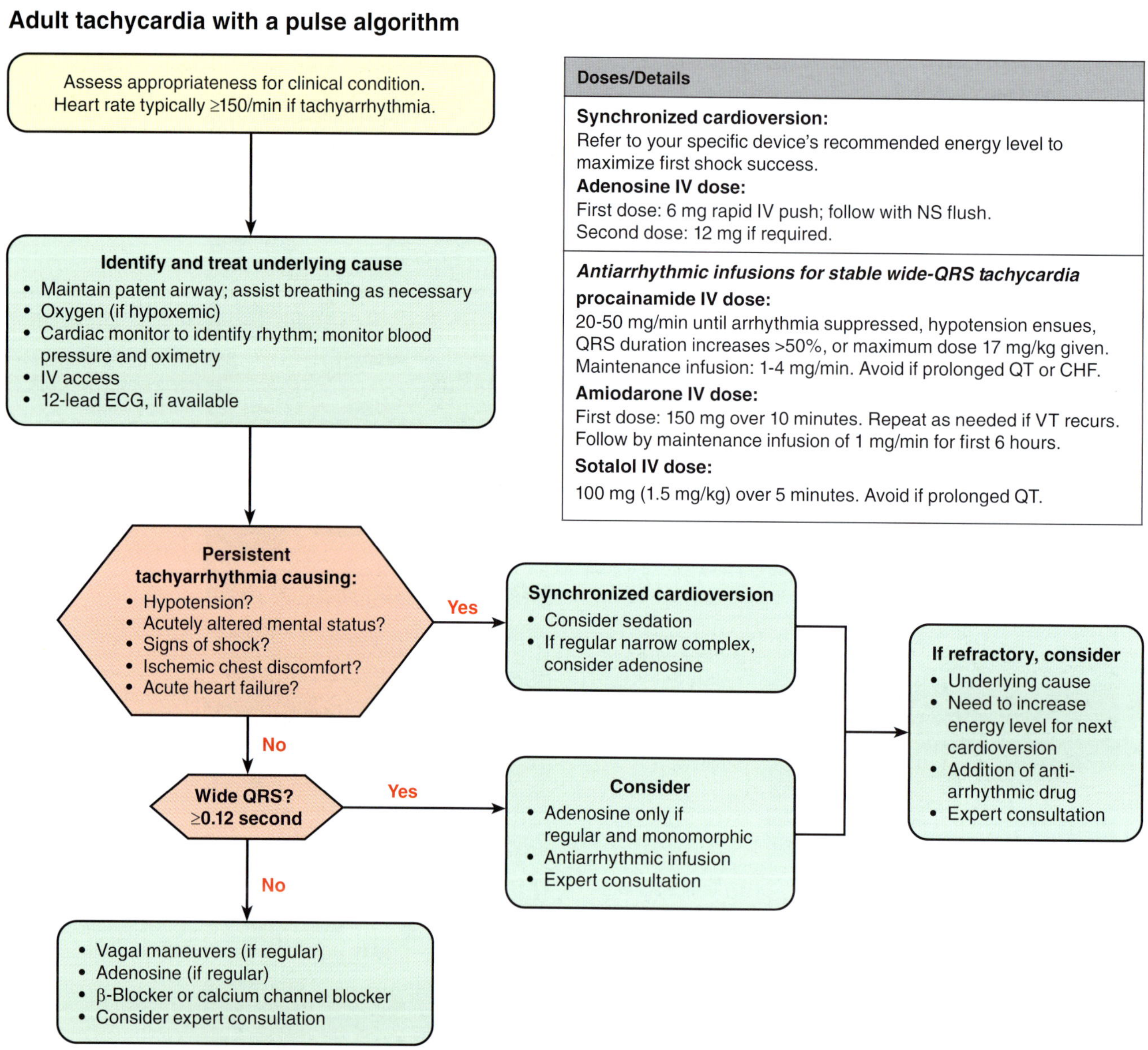

Fig. 12.13 Cardioversion algorithm. *CHF,* Congestive heart failure; *ECG,* Electrocardiogram; *IV,* intravenous; *NS,* normal saline.

compensatory hyperventilation after endotracheal intubation may be indicated before cardioversion. When possible, respiratory acidosis should be treated before the use of sedative drugs. Repleting potassium and magnesium in patients with hypokalemia and hypomagnesemia should also be a priority.

Sedation

Cardioversion without sedation is extremely painful and terrifying. Patients must be adequately sedated before its use (Fig. 12.12, *step 2*). Patients who are not adequately sedated may experience extreme anxiety, fear and even posttraumatic stress disorder (PTSD).[24] Several IV medications are available for sedation of patients before cardioversion, including etomidate (0.15 mg/kg), midazolam (0.05–0.1 mg/kg), and propofol (0.5–1.0 mg/kg). In addition, IV ketamine (1 mg/kg), with or without a benzodiazepine or slightly reduced-dose propofol, may be administered (Table 12.1).

Midazolam is probably the most commonly used agent, with induction occurring approximately 2 minutes after a dose of approximately 0.05 to 0.1 mg/kg. Although induction with midazolam takes slightly longer than with the other medications, its amnestic properties are an advantage. Ketamine is less likely to cause hypotension compared to other sedatives and best preserves the respiratory drive, although on very rare occasions it can cause laryngospasm. The other sedative medications listed are more likely to cause hypotension and decrease the respiratory drive but can be effective when used with proper caution and preparation.

In elderly patients, the pharmacodynamics and kinetics are altered by coexisting illness and polypharmacy rather than by any intrinsic effect of old age.[25] Drug doses should be reduced in these patients.

In general, anesthetic agents should be given slowly over a period of 30 seconds to a minute, depending on the medication that is administered. Administering the agent too quickly

TABLE 12.1 Commonly Available Intravenous Medications Used for Sedation in Cardioversion[a]

DRUG	DOSE	COMMENTS
Midazolam	0.05–0.1 mg/kg	Most commonly used Sedation occurs in approximately 2 min Potential for a small drop in blood pressure
Etomidate	0.15 mg/kg	Potential for mild drop in blood pressure Painful IV infusion
Propofol	1.5 mg/kg	Potential for a small drop in blood pressure Painful IV infusion
Fentanyl	1 µg/kg	An opiate Added for more sedation Can cause respiratory depression, especially with concurrent benzodiazepine use
Ketamine	1.5 mg/kg	Less likely to cause hypotension, preserves respiratory drive May be combined with reduced-dose propofol (0.5 mg/kg) or a full-dose benzodiazepine

[a]See also Chapter 33.
IV, Intravenous.

may result in worse side effects, such as hypotension and hypoventilation; administering it too slowly may not allow blood levels to reach a therapeutic range if the agent has a rapid rate of metabolism. The procedure can begin once the patient has reached a level of deep sedation; they should not be arousable to voice and may need ventilatory support.

Cardioverter Use

Selection of the synchronized or unsynchronized mode is the next critical step (Fig. 12.12, *step 3*). In the synchronized mode, the cardioverter searches for a large positive or negative deflection, which it interprets as the R or S wave. It then automatically discharges an electric current that lasts less than 4 ms, thereby avoiding the vulnerable period during repolarization when VF can easily be induced. Once the cardioverter is set to synchronize, a brief delay will occur after the button is pushed for discharge as the machine searches for an R wave. This delay may be disconcerting to an unaware operator.

If concern exists about whether the R wave is large enough to trigger the electrical discharge, the clinician can place the lubricated paddles together and press the discharge button. Firing should occur after a brief delay. When the R- or S-wave deflection is too small to trigger firing, change the lead that the monitor is reading or move the arm leads closer to the chest. If there is no R or S wave to sense, as in VF, the cardioverter will not fire. Always turn off "synchronization" if VF is noted.

Electrode positioning is the same as for defibrillation. Safety is a key concern in the performance of cardioversion. The operator must announce "all clear" and give staff a chance to move away from the bed before cardioversion. Care must be taken to clean up spills of saline or other liquid because they may create a conductive path to a staff person at the bedside.

The amount of energy required for cardioversion varies with the type of dysrhythmia, the degree of metabolic derangement, and the configuration and thickness of the chest wall (Fig. 12.12, *step 4*). Obese patients may require a higher energy level for cardioversion, and the anteroposterior pad position is sometimes more effective in these patients. If patients are shocked while in the expiratory phase of their respiratory cycle, energy requirements may also be lower.

Cardioversion can also be considered in hemodynamically stable patients in VT. It is safe, effective, and quicker than chemical cardioversion. Cardioversion can be attempted before or after a trial of chemical cardioversion should be synchronized. To confirm the machine has synchronized correctly to the R wave, while in synchronized mode, there should be SYNC markers on the screen that align with the R wave. If the initial attempts at electrical cardioversion are unsuccessful, the energy level should be gradually increased, until a perfusing rhythm is restored. If subsequent attempts are still unsuccessful, additional antiarrhythmic medications can be added, or further efforts to diagnose and treat the underlying cause should be made. Immediately after conversion of VT, antiarrhythmic medications should be given to prevent recurrence.

Pediatric Cardioversion

Pediatric cardioversion is similar to adult cardioversion. As described previously, the purpose of the procedure is to depolarize the myocytes completely at the most opportune time, during the peak of the R wave so that VF is not precipitated, and allow a slower perfusing rhythm to resume. However, the energy levels for pediatric cardioversion are different from those for adults. In the pediatric procedure, the initial recommended energy dose is 0.5 to 1 J/kg with the defibrillator in the synchronized mode. If needed, repeated cardioversion may be attempted at 2 J/kg, again while the defibrillator is in the synchronized mode. Remember to resynchronize the defibrillator after each cardioversion attempt and look for the appropriate markers on the monitor to ensure that the current is delivered at the appropriate phase of the cardiac cycle. If medication is needed, amiodarone at a dose of 5 mg/kg intravenously over a 20- to 60-minute period or procainamide at a dose of 15 mg/kg over 30- to 60-minute period can be used (do not give these drugs together).

ACKNOWLEDGMENT

The editors and author would like to acknowledge the significant contributions to this chapter in previous editions by Steven Gazak, MD, William Burdick, MD, Jerris R. Hedges, MD, Michael Greenberg, MD, and John Krimm, DO, Bohdan M. Minczak, MD, and Glenn W. Laub, MD. We also thank the San Francisco Fire Department for their assistance with the images in Figs. 12.1, 12.7, 12.8, and 12.12.

REFERENCES ARE AVAILABLE AT Elsevier eBooks+

CHAPTER 13

Assessment of Implantable Cardiac Devices

Robert T. Gerhardt and Steven G. Schauer

Patients with implanted pacemakers, automatic implantable cardioverter defibrillators (AICDs), or implantable loop monitors are commonly seen in the emergency department (ED). Fortunately, the increased reliability of these devices has precluded a marked increase in patients with emergencies related to device malfunction, but due to the complexity of their underlying conditions, they will present with issues directly or indirectly related to their device. Pacemaker complications are not uncommon, with rates ranging from 4.8% to 7.5%.[1] Many pacemakers fail within the first year. AICD complication rates, including inadvertent shocks, occur in up to 34% of patients with the device. Complications are often highest among recipients of upgraded or revised cardiac resynchronization therapy (CRT) devices.[2]

The basic evaluation and treatment of patients with cardiac complaints are not substantially different in patients with pacemakers, AICDs, and CRTs than in those without; however, a general knowledge of the range of problems, complications, and techniques for evaluating or inactivating these devices is important for emergency clinicians. These devices are complicated and emergency physicians are not expected to be experts in all complications; therefore appropriate consultation is often necessary depending on the clinical situation.

PACEMAKER CHARACTERISTICS

In essence a pacemaker consists of an electrical pulse–generating device and a lead system that senses intrinsic cardiac signals and then delivers a pulse. The pulse generator is hermetically sealed with a lithium-based battery device that weighs approximately 30 g and has an anticipated lifetime of 7 to 12 years. A semiconductor chip serves as the device's central processing unit. The generator is connected to sensing and pacing electrodes that are inserted into various locations in the heart, depending on the configuration of the pacemaker. Newer models are programmable for rate, output, sensitivity, refractory period, and modes of response. They can be reprogrammed noninvasively after implantation, via radiotelemetric or other wireless technologies.

Pacemakers are classified according to a standard five-letter code developed by the North American Society of Pacing and Electrophysiology/British Pacing and Electrophysiology Group (Table 13.1). Known as the NBG code, it consists of five positions or digits. The first letter designates the chamber that receives the pacing current; the second, the sensing chamber; and the third, the pacemaker's response to sensing. The fourth letter refers to the pacemaker's rate modulation and programmability, and the fifth describes the pacemaker's ability to provide an antitachycardia function. Whereas standard pacemakers generally do not have an antitachycardia function, AICDs do have this capability and overdrive pacing is the device's first response to tachycardia. In normal practice, only the first three letters are used to describe the pacemaker (e.g., VVI or DDD).

Pacemaker wires are embedded in plastic catheters. The terminal electrodes, which may be unipolar or bipolar, travel from the generator unit to the heart via the venous system. In a unipolar system, the lead electrode functions as the negatively charged cathode, and the pulse generator case acts as the positively charged anode into which electrons flow to complete the circuit. The pulse generator casing must remain in contact with tissue and be uninsulated for pacing to occur. In the case of bipolar systems, both electrodes are located within the heart. The cathode is at the tip of the lead, and the anode is a ring electrode roughly 2 cm proximal to the tip. Bipolar leads are thicker, draw more current than unipolar leads, and are commonly preferred because of several advantages, including a decreased likelihood of pacer inhibition which may result from extraneous signals, and decreased susceptibility to interference by electromagnetic fields. Pacer spikes are more apparent on electrocardiograms (ECGs) performed on a patient with a unipolar pacemaker than those done on patients with a bipolar pacemaker because the pulse generator acts as the anode and is located on the chest wall (Fig. 13.1).

The typical entry point for inserting the leads is the central venous system, which is generally accessed via the subclavian or cephalic vein. The terminal electrodes are placed either in the right ventricle or in both the right ventricle and the atrium under fluoroscopic guidance. Proper lead placement, sensing, and pacing thresholds are assessed with ECGs. The typical radiographic appearances of implanted pacemakers and implantable cardioverter defibrillators to include an example of lead fracture are depicted in Fig. 13.2A–E.

The pacemaker is typically programmed to pace at a rate of 60 to 80 beats/min. A significantly different rate usually indicates malfunction. When the battery is low, the rate generally begins to drop and gets slower as the battery fades. Sensing of intracardiac electrical activity is a combination of recognizing the characteristic waveforms of P waves or QRS complexes while discriminating them from T waves or external interfering signals, such as muscle activity or movement. The pacing electrical stimulus is a triphasic wave consisting of an intrinsic deflection, far-field potential, and an injury current, which typically delivers a current of 0.1 to 20.0 mA for 2 ms at 15 V.

Pacemakers have a reed switch that may be closed by placing a magnet over the generator externally on the chest wall; this inactivates the sensing mechanism of the pacemaker, which then reverts to an asynchronous rate termed the *magnet rate*. Essentially, the magnet turns the demand pacemaker into a fixed-rate pacemaker. The magnet rate is usually, but not always, the same as the programmed rate.

Several innovations in rate regulation have been incorporated into some pacemakers. When present, the hysteresis feature causes pacing to be triggered at a rate greater than the intrinsic heart rate. When the hysteresis feature is used in a single-chamber ventricular pacemaker, it is designed to maintain atrioventricular (AV) synchrony at rates that are lower than what would be normal for a ventricular-paced rhythm (60 to 80 beats/min) alone. To illustrate, were the hysteresis feature of the pacemaker set at 50 beats/min, an intrinsic rate lower than 50 beats/min would trigger ventricular pacing, and rates above 50 beats/min would be tolerated so long as AV synchrony was maintained. Unlike a standard ventricular pacemaker, the hysteresis feature would be set to offer a

TABLE 13.1 North American Society of Pacing and Electrophysiology/British Pacing and Electrophysiology Group Generic Pacemaker Code (NBG Code)

I: Chamber Paced	II: Chamber Sensed	III: Response to Sensing	IV: Rate Modulation and Programmability	V: Antitachycardia Features
0—None	0—None	0—None	0—None	0—None
A—Atrium	A—Atrium	I—Inhibited	I—Inhibited	P—Antitachycardic pacing
V—Ventricle	V—Ventricle	T—Triggered	M—Multiple	S—Shock
D—Dual	D—Dual	D—Dual	C—Communicating	D—Dual
			R—Rate modulation	

ventricular pacing rate at a significantly higher rate (e.g., 70 beats/min or greater) once the intrinsic rate dropped below the hysteresis threshold.

Rate modulation by sensor-mediated methods is an additional feature triggered and mediated by a sensed response to various physiologic stimuli. The primary application for this rate modulation feature is in patients with pacemakers who continue to engage in vigorous physical activity. When present, the rate regulation feature is engaged and modulated through motion sensors installed within a pulse generator device, with a corresponding increase or decrease in the pacing rate depending on the degree of motion sensed by the pacemaker device. Other physiologic sensors that may be installed as part of the pacemaker system include those designed to sense minute ventilation, the QT interval, temperature, venous oxygen saturation, and right ventricular contractions. The latter sensors generally require that additional leads be placed.

CRT, also known as *biventricular pacing*, may improve left ventricular function, and thus cardiac output, by restoring left ventricular synchrony.[3] This is used primarily in patients with dilated cardiomyopathy and widened QRS complex, which can result from the presence of a left bundle branch block. In addition to a conventional right ventricular endocardial lead, CRT also employs a coronary sinus lead for left ventricular pacing. A right atrial lead may also be included.

AICD Characteristics

The basic components of an AICD, including sensing electrodes, defibrillation electrodes, and a pulse generator (Fig. 13.3), can be seen on a chest radiograph. Transvenous electrodes have obviated the previous need for surgical placement. They are inserted into the pectoralis muscle. Many transvenous systems consist of a single lead containing a distal sensing electrode and one or more defibrillation electrodes in the right atrium and ventricle.[4] Leads are inserted through the subclavian, axillary, or cephalic vein into the right ventricular apex. The left side is preferred because of a smoother venous route to the heart and a more favorable shocking vector.[4] In an effort to improve the efficiency of defibrillation, an additional defibrillation coil may be used.[4] Various placements of AICDs are demonstrated in Fig. 13.4.

The pulse generator has a battery, voltage converters and resistors, capacitors to store charge, microprocessors and integrated circuits to control analysis of the rhythm and delivery of therapy, memory chips to store electrographic data, and a telemetry module.[4] Although a pacemaker can draw the voltage required for function from its component battery, the energy needed for defibrillation requires a battery that is prohibitively large. To circumvent this problem, an AICD contains a capacitor that maximizes the voltage required by transferring energy from the battery before discharge. To achieve the energy required, AICDs use capacitors that are charged over a period of 3 to 10 seconds by the battery and then release this energy rapidly for defibrillation.[4] The maximal output is 30 J in most units and 45 J in higher-energy units. This energy is high enough that a discharge is obvious and often distressing to the patient.

Most AICDs use a system in which the pulse generator is part of the shocking circuit, often described as a "can" technology, and most of them have a dual-coil lead with a proximal coil in the superior vena cava and a distal coil in the right ventricle.[4] Current flows in a three-dimensional configuration from the distal coil to both the proximal coil and the generator.[4] This dispersion of the electrical field increases the likelihood of depolarizing the entire myocardium at once, thereby leading to successful defibrillation.[4]

AICDs may have the same programming capabilities as pacemakers and can be single chambered, dual chambered, or used with the aforementioned CRT.[3] Single-chamber devices have only a right ventricular lead. They often have difficulty identifying atrial arrhythmias, which can result in inappropriate defibrillation of atrial tachycardias. Dual-chamber AICDs have right atrial and right ventricular leads and improved ability to discriminate rhythms. In most studies, dual devices have been found to offer improved discrimination between ventricular and supraventricular arrhythmias, thus decreasing inappropriate shocks resulting from rapid supraventricular rhythms or physiologic sinus tachycardia.[4] Of AICDs implanted annually 27% are single chamber, 32% dual chamber, and 41% are CRT systems.[5] In patients requiring both AICD and pacemaker functions, a single device that can perform both functions is placed.

AICDs use a combination of antitachycardia pacing, low-energy cardioversion, defibrillation, and bradycardic pacing in a combination also known as *tiered therapy*, which obviates the need for unnecessary energy requirements. They are programmed with specific algorithms that identify and treat specific rhythms. Ventricular arrhythmias may initially be converted (or undergo attempts at conversion) with antitachycardiac pacing as opposed to immediate defibrillation. This *overdrive pacing* may terminate the rhythm without the need

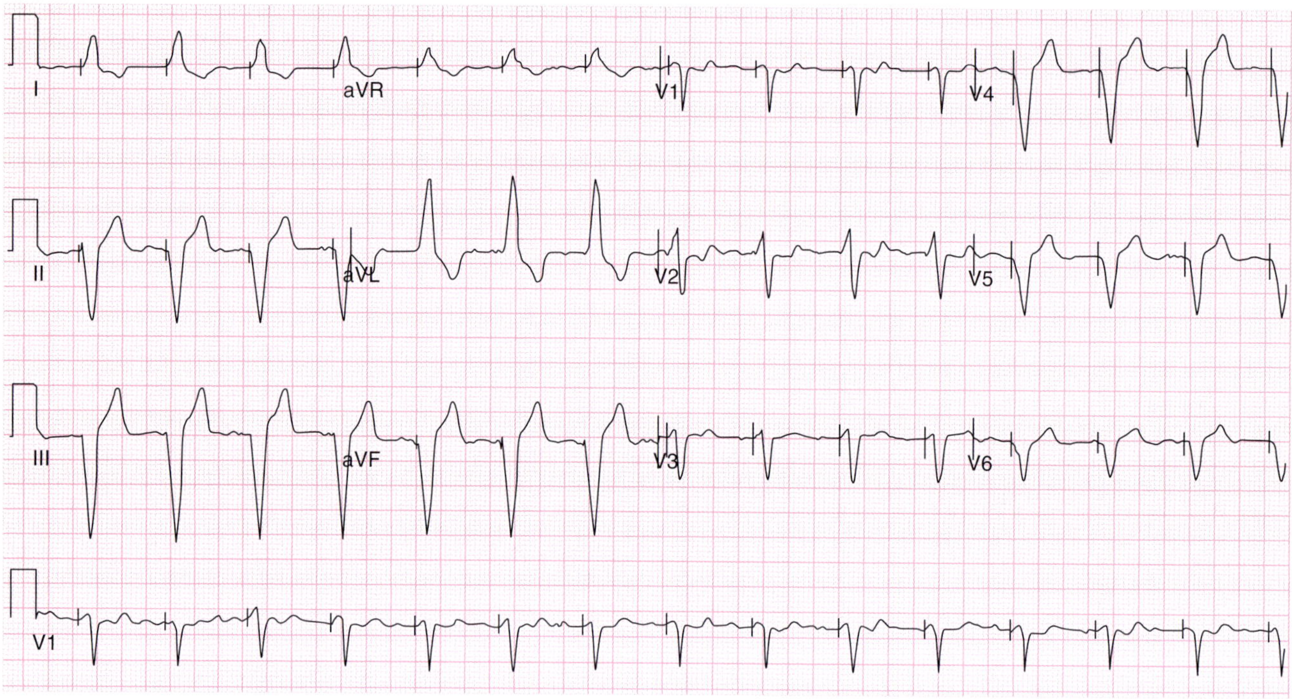

A

Vent. rate	84	BPM	Electronic ventricular pacemaker
PR interval	204	ms	
QRS duration	128	ms	
QT/QTc	406/479	ms	
P-R-T axes	* -58	91	

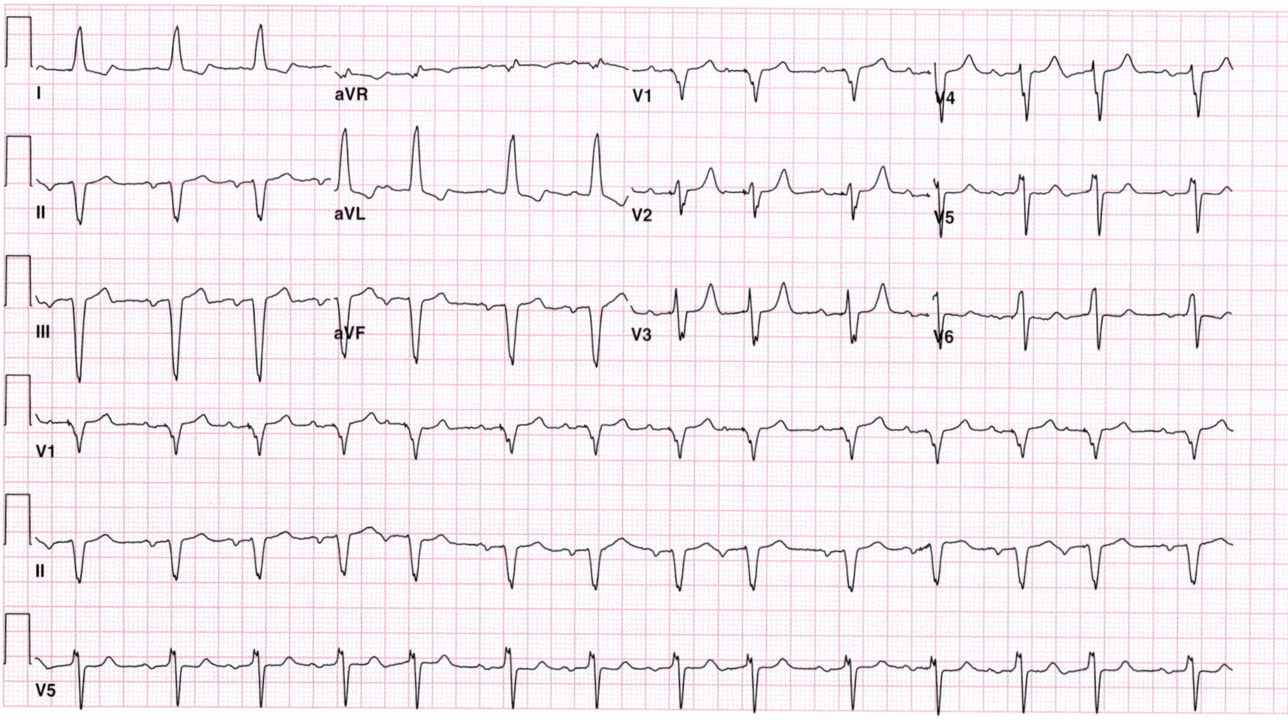

B

Fig. 13.1 (A) ECG in a patient with a pacemaker with unipolar leads. Note that the pacer spikes are obvious in almost all leads, whereas in a bipolar system (B), the pacer spikes are barely visible blips, most noticeable in leads V_1 to V_3 just before the QRS complex.

for electrical defibrillation in up to 90% of events. It is most successful for terminating monomorphic ventricular tachycardia (VT) with a rate of less than 200 beats/min. Overdrive pacing is better tolerated by patients than cardioversion and reduces the risk for inducing atrial fibrillation. These events may be silent, not felt by the patient, and discovered only by interrogating the device.

If unsuccessful, the next intervention may be low-energy cardioversion (<5 J). The device may be programmed to very low levels of electricity that are better tolerated by the patient.

This works best for ventricular rates higher than 150 and lower than 240 beats/min. This may be followed by a high-energy defibrillation. Traditionally, the energy level of the first shock is set at least 10 J above the threshold of the last defibrillation measured. If the first shock fails a backup shock may be required, but this may induce or aggravate ventricular arrhythmias (see the later section on "Pacemaker-Mediated Tachycardia"). Unlike the proarrhythmic effects of medication, these arrhythmias are almost never fatal, although they may be associated with increased morbidity. Currently used biphasic waveforms have improved defibrillation thresholds.

Complications associated with AICDs that have antibradycardiac pacing algorithms include a tendency toward oversensing, increased current drain, potential detection problems, and an increased incidence of hardware and software design problems. At the time of insertion, the amount of energy required for various AICD functions, such as the defibrillation threshold, is determined for any given patient, and output

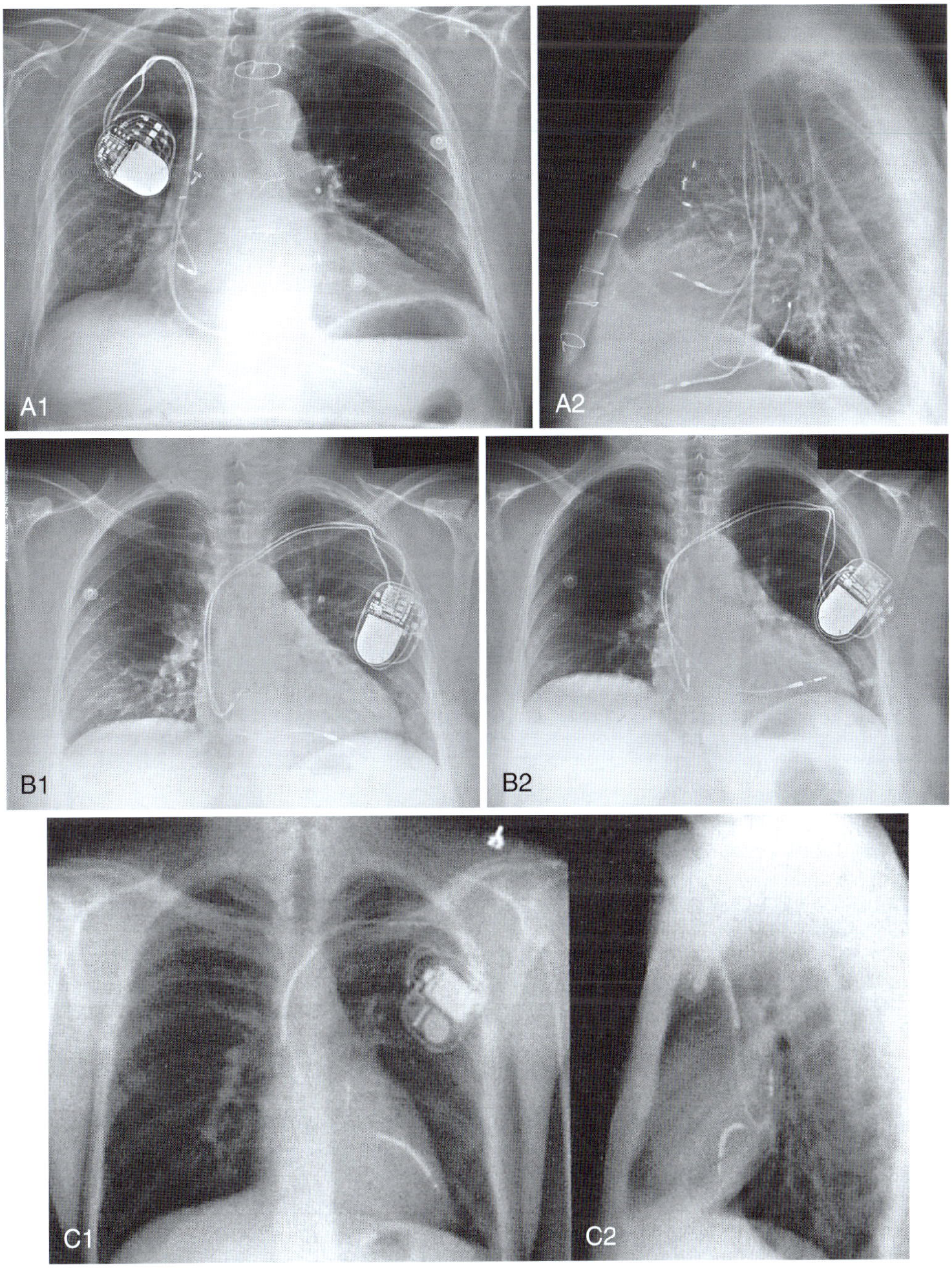

Fig. 13.2 (A) Various radiographs of an implanted pacemaker and automatic implantable cardioverter defibrillator showing battery and lead wires. Posteroanterior (PA; A1) and lateral (A2) chest radiographs demonstrate a biventricular pacing system. There are three leads—the first is positioned in the right atrium, the second is in the right ventricular apex, and the third courses posteriorly in the coronary sinus and into the posterolateral cardiac vein. (B) PA chest radiographs of a dual-chamber pacemaker. (B1) The ventricular lead is passing through an atrial septal defect into the left ventricle. (B2) The lead is repositioned in the right ventricular apex. (C) A dual-chamber implantable cardioverter defibrillator with active fixation leads has been implanted via a transvenous approach to place the atrial lead in the systemic venous atrium and the ventricular lead across the baffle into the morphologic left ventricle.

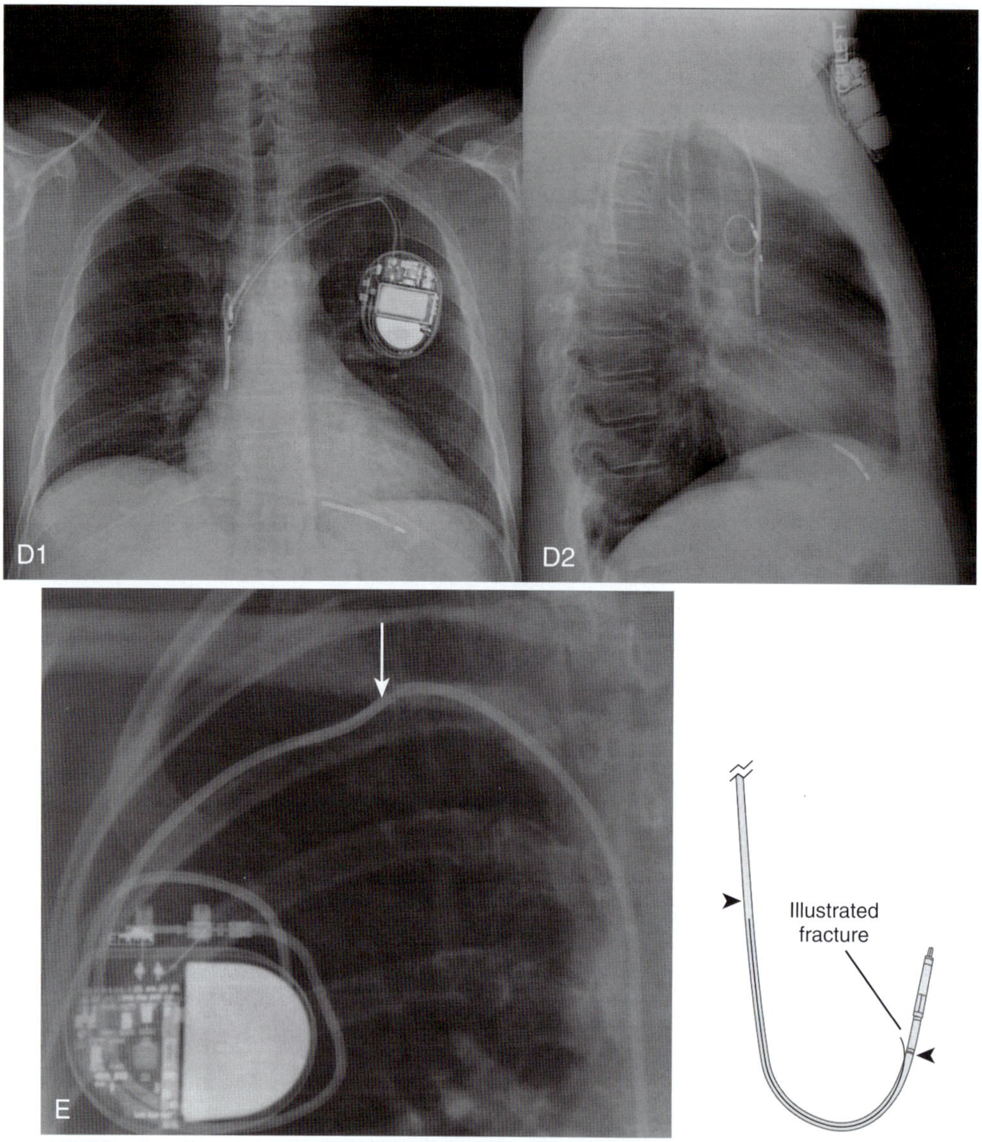

Fig. 13.2, cont'd (D) PA chest radiograph of a patient with a dual-chamber pacemaker. (D1) The atrial lead, originally positioned in the right atrial appendage, is clearly no longer positioned in the right atrial appendage. A lateral view (D2) also shows definite dislodgement of the atrial lead. (E) Close-up view of a portion of the PA chest radiograph of a patient with a single-chamber pacemaker. The lead has fractured (a subtle finding) at the point where it passes below the clavicle *(arrow)*. The device showed intermittent ventricular failure to capture and intermittent failure to output on the ventricular lead. Impedance was intermittently measured at more than 9999 Ω. *Inset*, Diagram of the fracture site. (E inset, Courtesy Telectronics Pacing Systems, Englewood, CO.)

and sensing functions can be adjusted by reprogramming as needed.

In 2012 the Food and Drug Administration approved the use of a subcutaneous defibrillator. This consists of a subcutaneous lead with a shock coil flanked by two sensing electrodes; this coil is tunneled along the parasternal margin from the pulse generator that is implanted in a subcutaneous pocket. It is placed by anatomic landmarks and, as such, no fluoroscopy is required.[6] It delivers an 80-J biphasic shock across the precordium. Fig. 13.5 depicts a radiograph of a patient with a subcutaneous defibrillator.

The subcutaneous implantable device may be an alternative to patients who have difficult vascular access or who are at risk for transvenous complications. These could include the pediatric populations, patients with congenital disease, complicated vascular anatomy, patients at high risk for infection, or patients on dialysis.[7,8] The notable limitation of the subcutaneous internal defibrillator when compared with conventional devices is the inability to provide long-term bradycardia pacing or antitachycardiac pacing.[8] Patients who need resynchronization therapy are also unsuitable candidates.[9]

IMPLANTABLE LOOP MONITORS

Unlike the aforementioned devices, implantable loop monitors are specifically designed for diagnostic purposes only. Patients who are under evaluation for occasional episodes of syncope (generally under one per month) or other forms of symptomatic bradycardia are the most common patients to receive these devices. Implantable monitors have gained in popularity because they are able to operate for durations up to 3 years, and do not require active patient participation.[10]

INDICATIONS FOR PLACEMENT OF IMPLANTABLE PACEMAKERS AND AICDS

The most common indication for placement of a cardiac pacemaker is for the treatment of symptomatic bradydysrhythmias.[3] Roughly 50% of pacemakers are placed in such patients for the treatment of sinus node dysfunction (sick sinus syndrome). Other diagnoses include symptomatic sinus bradycardia, atrial fibrillation with a slow ventricular response, high-grade AV block (including Mobitz type II and third-degree AV block), tachycardia-bradycardia syndrome, chronotropic incompetence, and selected prolonged QT syndromes. Though not classified as absolute indications, pacemakers are sometimes placed for the treatment of severe refractory neurocardiogenic syncope, paroxysmal atrial fibrillation, and hypertrophic or dilated cardiomyopathy.

CRT is a primary approach for patients with severe diastolic dysfunction and a low left ventricular ejection fraction (LVEF).[3] Commonly such patients manifest low-grade AV blocks and left bundle branch block. The resultant delay in left ventricular conduction often results in corresponding biomechanical delays in ventricular contraction, which in turn cause a further decrement in cardiac output and worsening congestive heart failure. Such prolongation may occur in as many as 33% of patients with advanced heart failure. This electromechanical dyssynchrony has been associated with increased risk for sudden cardiac death.[11]

CRT comprises atrial-synchronized, biventricular pacemaking, which overcomes the atrial and ventricular blocks while optimizing both preload and LVEF.[3] Clinical trials and systematic reviews have confirmed the efficacy of CRT, with decrements in mortality of 22% to 30%, in addition to improved LVEF and quality of life.[11] Mortality rates have also improved as experience with CRT has increased, as lower mortality has been seen in patients with CRT implanted from 2015–17 than in patients implanted in 2012–14 and 2009–11.[12] In certain population subgroups, CRT with a defibrillator may have increased long-term survival over CRT with pacemaker only.[13,14]

AICD technology is used principally for both primary and secondary prevention in patients at risk for sudden death. Primary prevention is an attempt to avoid a potentially malignant ventricular arrhythmia in patients identified as being at high risk. Secondary prevention is for patients who have already had a ventricular arrhythmia and are at risk for further events. In addition, AICDs are implanted for a number of other congenital or familial cardiac conditions.

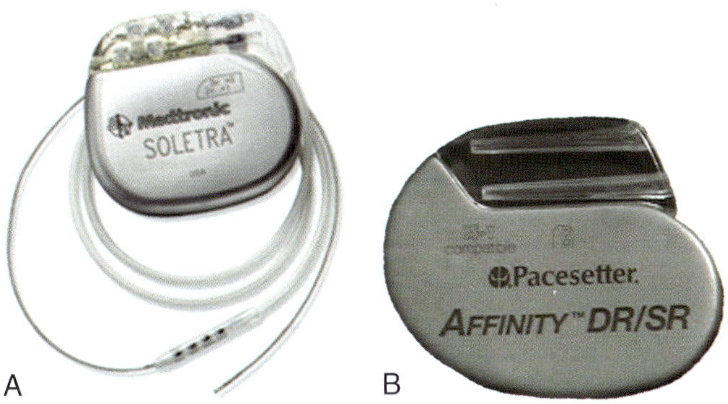

Fig. 13.3 (A) Automatic implantable cardioverter defibrillator (SOLETRA). (B) Implantable pacemaker. (A, Courtesy Medtronic, Inc., Minneapolis, MN.)

Ventricular Assist Devices

As the management of heart failure continues to evolve, emergency physicians will encounter patients who have surgically implanted mechanical circulatory support devices (MCSD), also referred to as ventricular assist devices (VADs).[15] VADs are implanted pumps used to assist a failing ventricle.[16] Although they have been used in the right ventricle and for biventricular support, they are primarily used as a left ventricular assist device or LVAD. The first-generation of these devices utilized a pulsatile flow pump, but these are no longer in use. The modern LVADs provide continuous flow using axial flow or centrifugal pumps. These devices are smaller and more durable, with higher energy efficiency than the first-generation models.[17]

The LVAD consists of an inflow cannula that is placed in the apical part of the ventricle and allows blood to flow to a pump. The pump is attached to the outflow cannula, which is placed in the ascending aorta. The device is connected through a percutaneous lead or driveline to batteries located outside

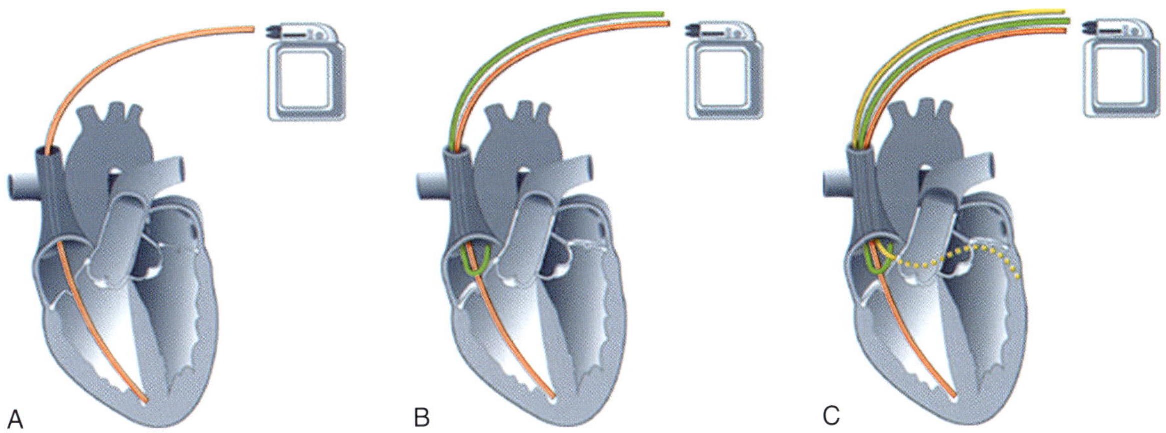

Fig. 13.4 Diagrammatic demonstration of various automatic implantable cardioverter defibrillator (AICD) configurations. (A) Single-chamber AICD. (B) Dual-chamber AICD. (C) Biventricular AICD.

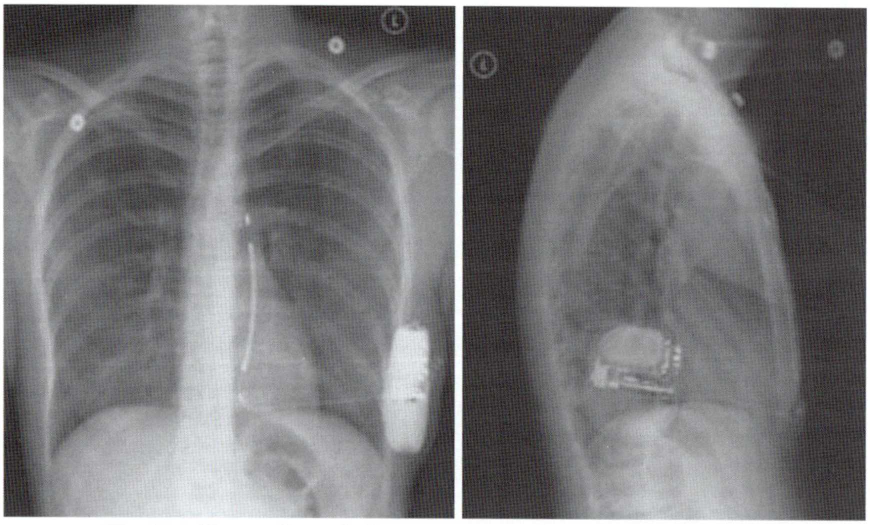

Fig. 13.5 Chest radiograph demonstrating a subcutaneous defibrillator.

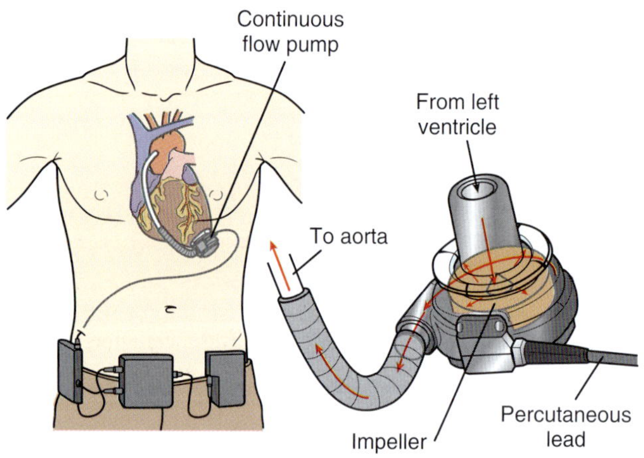

Fig. 13.6 HeartWare left ventricular device basic components and function.

the body along with a device controller. Figs. 13.6 and 13.7 demonstrate the components of a left ventricular device. They are provided with backup batteries and a charging system.

Indications for Placement of LVADs

Patients with advanced heart failure (stage D) have severe and persistent symptoms of heart failure, severe cardiac dysfunction, recurrent hospitalizations, and severe impairment of exercise capacity despite goal-directed medical therapy (GDMT).[18] Of the estimated 150,000 to 200,000 patients with advanced heart failure, roughly 2200 undergo heart transplantation annually.[19] The rest have the options of continuing GDMT, LVAD placement, or palliative care.

Initially used as a bridge to heart transplantation, LVADs are now also being used as a bridge to candidacy for heart transplantation (i.e. time to manage other comorbid conditions such as pulmonary hypertension or obesity), bridge to recovery of heart function (such as in patients with myocarditis), and for permanent (destination) therapy.[3] Survival for patients with LVADs has continued to improve despite increasing patient acuity. Median survival improved from 46.5 months to 54.6 months when comparing patients with LVADs placed from 2010 to 2014 to those placed from 2015 to 2019.[20]

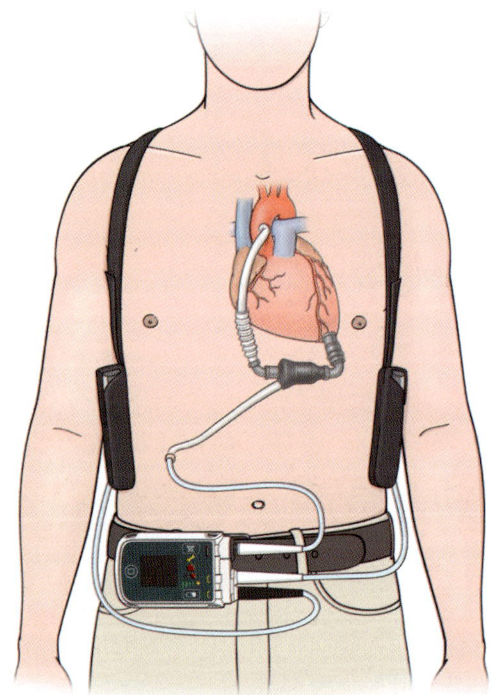

Fig. 13.7 The HeartMate II continuous flow device receives blood from the left ventricular apex and returns to the ascending aorta. The pump is connected with a percutaneous lead to an eternal controller and batteries worn by the patient.

CLINICAL EVALUATION OF PATIENTS WITH IMPLANTED PACEMAKERS, AICDS, AND LVADS

History

Although patients who go to the ED because of implantable pacemaker–related issues may have one or more of several complaints, those with AICD-related issues are generally seen because their device has discharged. They will often describe a sensation of being kicked or punched in the chest, and the sensation is not subtle. In fact, some patients live in fear of the shock after having experienced it previously, and this is one reason for removal of the device. Ask the patient about the number of discharges and associated symptoms, including chest pain, shortness of breath, lightheadedness, palpitations, syncope, extremity edema (raising concern for congestive heart failure or lower extremity deep vein thrombosis), or dyspnea on exertion. In addition, elicit general symptoms such as fever, chills, nausea, or vomiting, which could be indicative of infection, especially in the setting of a recently placed device (less than 8 weeks postprocedure). Inquire about medication history. Ask about the specific implanted device that they possess. Most pacemaker and AICD patients should have an identification card on their person that will identify the manufacturer, model number, lead system, and a 24-hour emergency contact number. Sophisticated information and the prior electrical events and settings of the device can be ascertained in the ED by simply placing an external interrogating device over the unit.

When a patient with an LVAD arrives in the ED, the provider should identify who the patient's cardiologist and cardiothoracic surgeon are. In most instances contact should be made with these providers and the patient may need to be transferred to a center with expertise in these devices. They are usually provided with a card to carry that contains key contact information. In addition to the key history questions previously listed for patients with AICDs, it is important to inquire about bleeding, as most patients with LVADs are on anticoagulants.

Physical Examination

First, assess for airway patency, adequate ventilation, and cardiovascular status. The patient's mental status may also be an important clue to the severity of the symptoms. Perform an appropriate physical examination with emphasis on examining the heart and lung to seek murmurs, pericardial friction rubs, and evidence of pulmonary effusion or other abnormalities. Inspect the pacemaker, AICD site, or LVAD driveline site for erythema or edema. Palpate the skin for evidence of obvious lead abnormalities. Examine the extremities for evidence of edema or erythema.

There are several unique characteristics to consider in patients with LVADs. On physical examination, the provider should listen to the chest to determine if an audible "hum" is present. Patients typically lack a palpable pulse given the device's continuous flow and because their cardiac function at baseline is poor, but some patients with LVADs may still have some preserved cardiac function that generates a weak pulse. The blood pressure should be obtained by using a Doppler on either the radial or brachial artery. Inflate the cuff until you cannot hear flow. The cuff pressure should then be released, listening for the presence of flow.[21] There is some degree of controversy about whether this is mean arterial pressure (MAP) or systolic pressure, however.[22,23] When in doubt, an arterial line would be the most accurate method to identify MAP. MAP is usually kept between 70 and 90 mm Hg.[11] Pulse oximetry may also be unreliable, and a true measurement should be obtained with an arterial blood gas or arterial line, if needed. A capillary refill of more than 2 seconds indicates hypotension in the setting of an LVAD and may be used as a surrogate marker.

The LVAD machine should be evaluated as part of the usual physical examination as well. This includes flow which should be between 4 and 7 L/min, similar to a normal cardiac output. The LVAD battery level should also be noted and if there is a concern it can be plugged into a standard outlet during the evaluation. Finally, check to make sure the power is not significantly higher or lower than the normal range of 4 to 6 W.

Emergency Department Pacemaker Interrogation

Traditionally, evaluation of implanted devices required the participation of specially trained staff primarily because the equipment used to interrogate the device could also be used to reprogram it. Such personnel are not readily available outside of routine working hours, and in more rural EDs, may not be available at all.

The major manufacturers of these devices (Abbott/St. Jude, Biotronik, Boston Scientific, Medtronic) have deployed "read-only" interrogation systems that were originally designed to allow patients to perform remote monitoring of their devices at home. The technology has become widespread, and it is now feasible for ED staff to interrogate them in a timely and efficient manner.[24,25]

The first step is to identify the patient's device. As noted above, a chest x-ray (CXR) can be helpful in identifying the device if the patient does not have their wallet card. A comprehensive algorithm, CaRDIA-X has been developed that can assist with identification from a CXR through a manual process that compares various characteristics of different devices.[26] This algorithm has also been incorporated into several smartphone or web-based applications.[27,28]

Given that read-only interrogation equipment cannot reprogram an implanted device, one study specifically assessed the safety of using brand-mismatched remote interrogators.[29] The authors were unable to identify any instances of reprogramming or other misadventure related to using mismatched equipment and they concluded that such mismatched interrogation was unlikely to result in any adverse effects. Accordingly, this suggests that when the manufacturer of a specific implanted device cannot be readily identified, a safe and efficient practice would be to serially attempt to interrogate the device with different brand-specific equipment until a match was confirmed and the interrogation was successful.[29] Further experience is needed to endorse this as a standard practice.

Radiography

The imaging modality of choice, at least initially, in a patient with complaints related to an implanted pacemaker or AICD is the plain chest radiograph. If the patient's hemodynamic stability is in question, a portable anteroposterior film is appropriate. In addition to the standard cardiac, pulmonary, vascular, and skeletal evaluation, this study will probably confirm the location of the pulse generator case, as well as the current location of any leads. Survey the radiograph for evidence of lead fracture or displacement (see Fig. 13.2E). Compare with previous chest films. If the patient does not have a device identification card in immediate possession, take an overpenetrated radiograph to look for a radiopaque marker identifying the model type. Fig. 13.8 demonstrates a radiograph of a patient with an LVAD.

Ultrasound is especially useful in the early evaluation of an LVAD patient, in particular for noting the sizes of the left

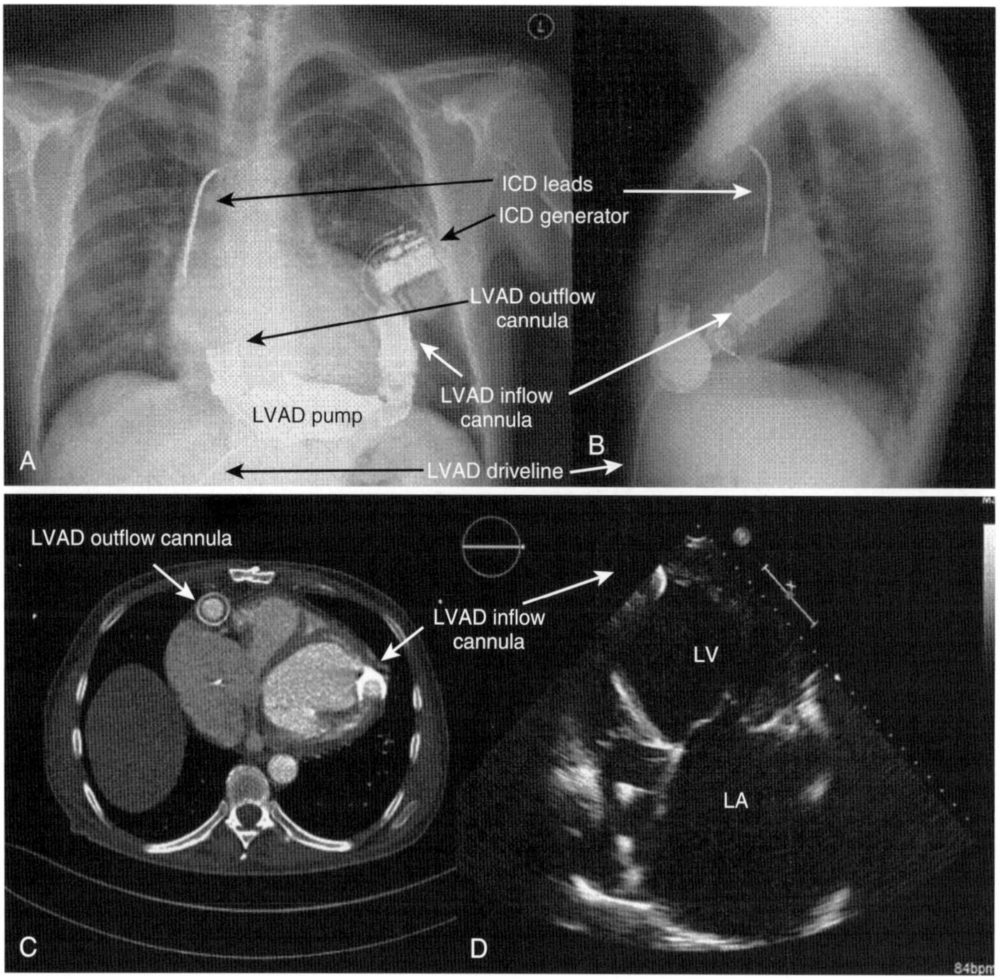

Fig. 13.8 HeartMate II model of left ventricular assist device (LVAD) appearance in (A) posterior-anterior and (B) lateral chest x-ray, (C) computerized tomography, and (D) ultrasound examination. *ICD*, Implantable cardioverter defibrillator; *LV*, left ventricle; *LA*, left atrium.

ventricle (LV) and right ventricle (RV), which can help determine the cause of an LVAD complication.

Electrocardiography

Perform an ECG to seek evidence of pacing, ectopy, and ST-segment or T-wave abnormalities. A comparison ECG may be helpful. If an AICD shock has been delivered, the shock itself can cause transient electrocardiographic changes, and waiting for several minutes to repeat the ECG may identify whether the changes are caused by the discharge or an ongoing disease process.

It can be difficult to evaluate an ECG obtained from a patient with an LVAD due to a high amount of artifact produced by the LVAD. In order to reduce the artifact and analyze the underlying rhythm, the ECG operator can adjust the low-pass filter threshold from the usual 150 Hz to 20 Hz. It is also important to reset the settings to their normal values after obtaining the ECG so that subsequent ECGs obtained in the ED are unaffected.

Cardiopulmonary Resuscitation, ACLS Interventions, and External Cardiac Defibrillation in Patients With Implanted Pacemakers, AICDs, or LVADs

In general, advanced cardiac life support (ACLS) interventions may be performed safely and effectively in patients with pacemakers and AICDs when indicated. Cardiopulmonary resuscitation (CPR) can usually be performed in standard fashion. If an AICD is present, rescuers may notice mild electrical shocks while performing CPR; these shocks are harmless to the rescuer and can be reduced if wearing gloves. If the AICD shocks are impeding rescuer performance of CPR, or if supraventricular tachycardias are noted during resuscitation, disable the AICD by applying a magnet over the corner of the device from which the leads emerge. This location is generally found easily by palpation but may be located blindly by slowly relocating the magnet until AICD activity ceases.

External cardiac defibrillation may be performed safely in patients with pacemakers and AICDs with the standard expected efficacy; however, it is recommended that external paddles or defibrillator pads be placed at a location approximately 10 cm distant from the pulse generator if possible. A transcutaneous cardiac pacemaker may also be used in similar fashion with a recommendation that the pacing pads be placed in anatomically appropriate locations but preferably at a distance of 10 cm from the pulse generator.

Placing the external defibrillation or transcutaneous pacemaker pads in an anteroposterior configuration is advised because this configuration may circumvent energy shunting and shielding. Every attempt should be made to avoid application of the defibrillators directly over the device. Use of the lowest possible energy setting for cardioversion or defibrillation is recommended. If available, biphasic cardioverter defibrillators are further suggested. In the event of successful resuscitation and return of spontaneous circulation, the pacemaker or AICD should be interrogated expeditiously by a cardiologist or electrophysiologist to ensure that no damage was sustained as a result of the resuscitation effort.

Regarding pharmacologic adjuncts, amiodarone has been reported to be more effective for the treatment of potentially lethal arrhythmias in the setting of implanted devices. Antiarrhythmic medications may be required for a resistant malignant rhythm when the AICD is functioning properly, but the arrhythmia persists (Fig. 13.9G).

Several additional considerations are unique to the setting of ACLS in patients with a pacemaker or AICD. In cases of acute myocardial infarction involving areas of the myocardium in contact with the pacemaker leads, the implanted pacemaker may experience operative failure. Therefore maintain a high level of suspicion for the potential requirement for supplemental transcutaneous or transvenous cardiac pacing.

LVAD patients who go into cardiac arrest offer some unique challenges. As noted earlier, every attempt should be made to contact the patient's LVAD team during the initial evaluation. Evaluate the patient's perfusion by assessing the MAP, mental status, skin color, temperature, and capillary refill, and end-tidal CO_2 if an advanced airway is in place. If the patient has signs of poor perfusion, ensure all external LVAD connections are maintained, that the battery is charged or connected to a power source, and the machine has an audible hum. If the LVAD is working correctly or has a problem that cannot be rapidly corrected and the patient has signs of poor perfusion with a low MAP, begin CPR and follow the standard ACLS algorithms. The American Heart Association (AHA) recommends starting CPR if the MAP is less than 50 though different sources recommend different MAPs.[30] VT or ventricular fibrillation (VF) with a normal or abnormal mental status should still be corrected as persistent VT/VF can lead to worsening RV failure and decompensation.

The lack of peripheral pulses also makes the use of ACLS problematic, but a pulse check should be included in the ACLS algorithm given some patients may have a palpable pulse. There has been concern that standard CPR may dislodge the cannula or damage the unit's outflow conduit, but there have also been reports that this is not as harmful as previously thought, and sources agree that CPR is indicated in the case of arrest.[31,32] There was also a report of an emergency physician who replaced the driveline connections in a patient who had cut the wires resulting in subsequent resumption of the pump function.[33]

In the postresuscitation setting involving a patient with an implanted pacemaker or AICD, it is important to maintain a higher index of suspicion for device lead fracture or disruption resulting from CPR. This may be checked with a plain radiograph. Finally, in the postresuscitation phase, the clinician should closely watch for the development of pneumothorax, hemothorax, pericardial effusion, or other pathophysiologic processes that could adversely affect the function of the implanted device.

COMPLICATIONS AND MALFUNCTION OF IMPLANTED PACEMAKERS

See Video 13.1. Complications associated with pacemakers are listed in Box 13.1. In addition, patients with previously implanted and otherwise stable pacemakers may experience complications related to direct or indirect trauma affecting the pulse generator or leads. Major complications of pacemaker placement or those caused by subsequent injuries that the emergency clinician might encounter include: local or systemic infections resulting from pacemaker placement, thrombophlebitis involving the transvenous route of the pacemaker leads, a venous thromboembolic event, pneumothorax or hemothorax, pericarditis, air embolism, localized hematoma interfering with pacemaker operation or sensing, lead dislodgement, cardiac perforation, hemopericardium with possible progression to cardiac tamponade, and development of the phenomenon known as *pacemaker syndrome*. This condition is often seen in patients with single-chamber ventricular pacemakers who have an underlying component of congestive heart failure. It is believed to be a consequence of the loss of AV synchrony resulting from ventricular pacing, and may be manifested as vertigo, syncope, hypotension, and signs specific to the exacerbation of congestive heart failure.

In addition to the complications associated with initial pacemaker placement, malfunctions of these devices may occur in the short-, intermediate-, and long-term phases of their functional life spans. Most malfunctions result from one or a combination of three primary problems: failure of the pace generator to provide output, failure to capture, or failure to sense the intrinsic cardiac rhythm.

Pacemaker Output Failure

Pacemaker generator output failure is present when no pacing spike is noted on the ECG despite an indication for pacing. This condition may result from battery failure, fracture or loss of insulation in the pacer leads, oversensing of extraneous signals resulting in pacer inhibition, disconnection of the leads from the pacer generator, or in the case of a dual-chamber pacer, erroneous sensing of the pacemaker's atrial signal by a ventricular sensor. The latter phenomenon is commonly referred to as *crosstalk*.

Given most pacemakers are implanted for the treatment of an underlying bradycardia condition, initial clinical management of patients with pacer output failure will usually focus on pharmacologic management aimed at restoring an acceptable intrinsic heart rate. Subsequently, a transcutaneous or transvenous pacemaker may be required to ensure stabilization of the patient. This can be placed even in the setting of an implanted pacemaker. Once stabilization has been accomplished, further ED management should include a thorough secondary survey, 12-lead electrocardiography and continuous cardiovascular monitoring, portable chest radiograph to assess the condition of the pacemaker leads and identify related pathology, and any other pertinent diagnostic studies. At this point the clinician should seek to identify the type and model of the pacemaker and should consult an available cardiologist or electrophysiologist. Final disposition of the patient depends on the results of the stabilization, diagnostic studies, and cardiology consultation, and admission is often required.

Failure-to-Capture

In the case of failure-to-capture, pacemaker spikes are present on the ECG. However, some or all the spikes are not followed by atrial or ventricular complexes as appropriate for the pacemaker model in question. Failure-to-capture may result from: deterioration of lead insulation; fracture or dislodgement of

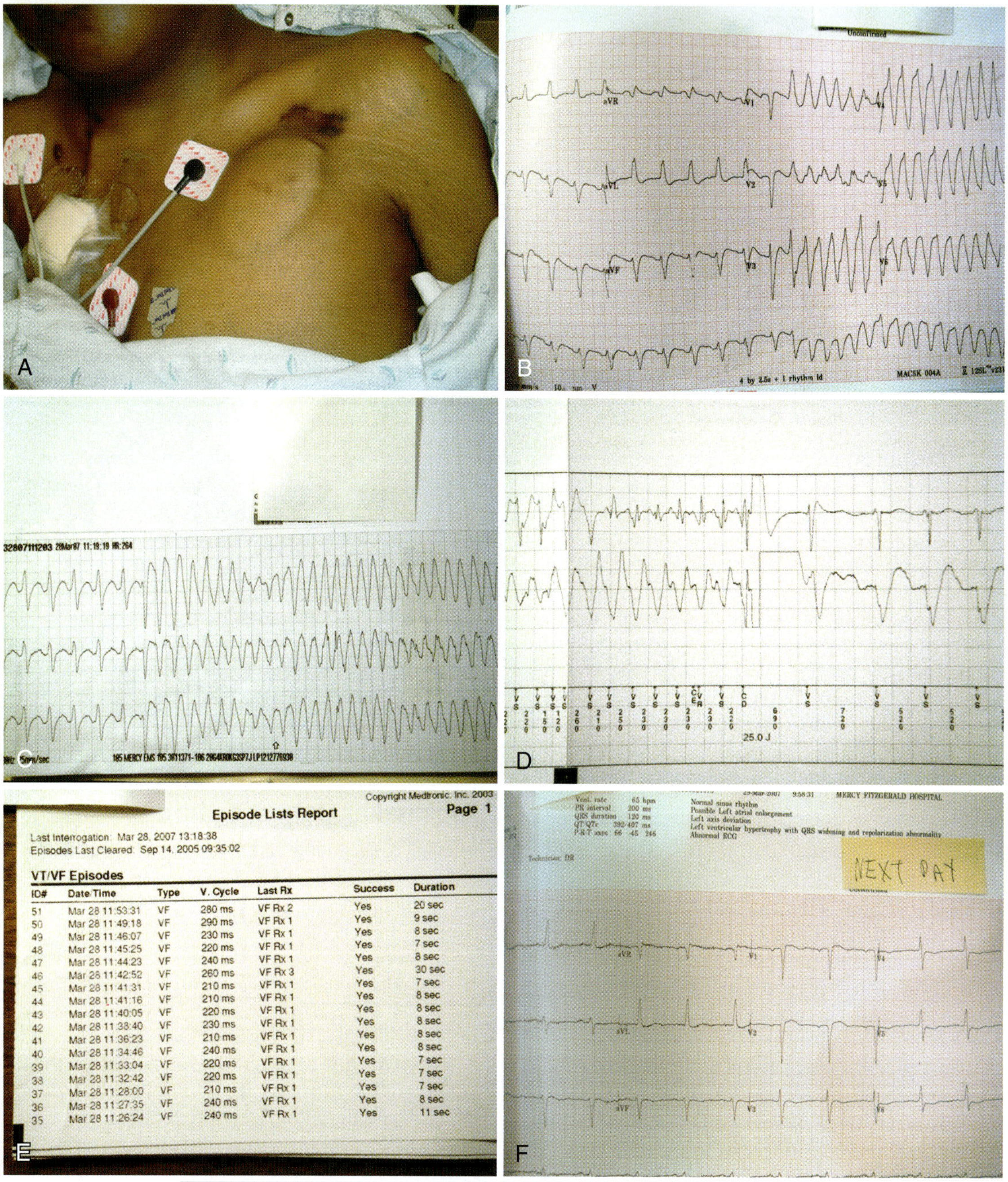

Therapy for AICD-Resistant Ventricular Tachycardia

- Correct electrolyte derangements
- Sedation and/or pain control for ongoing discomfort
- Procainamide, 30 mg/min until 17 mg/kg;
- Amiodarone, 150 mg over 10 minutes, followed by an infusion at 1 mg/min for 6 hours, then 0.5 mg/min for 18 hours;
- Lidocaine, 1-1.5 mg/kg, repeat 0.5-0.75 mg/kg every 5-10 minutes to a maximum of 3 mg/kg;
- Propranolol, 1-3 mg every 5 minutes up to a total of 5 mg in combination with another antiarrhythmic;
- Esmolol, 500 mcg/kg bolus, then 50-100 mcg/kg/min;
- Magnesium sulfate, 2 g over 15 minutes, may repeat an additional dose

G

Fig. 13.9 (A) Patient with an automatic implantable cardioverter defibrillator (AICD) who experienced multiple discharges from an AICD because of recurrent ventricular tachycardia (VT). (B) Electrocardiogram (ECG) of VT in the presence of an underlying tachycardia as the possible cause. (C) A rhythm strip demonstrates persistent polymorphic (torsades de pointes) VT. (D) After attempts at overdrive pacing failed, the AICD appropriately discharges with temporary termination of VT. (E) Interrogation of the device uncovers a history of more than 20 episodes of recurrent VT within 30 minutes. *This patient was terrified of a subsequent shock because he could sense the VT and knew of the impending shock. In addition to antiarrhythmic medication, a quiet dark room and aggressive sedation are suggested to reduce catecholamine levels.* (F) ECG after medical therapy with multiple medications, including magnesium. *Metoprolol seemed to be the deciding factor in terminating the VT in this case.* (G) Current suggested medical therapy for VT in the presence of an appropriately functioning AICD.

BOX 13.1 Complications of Permanent Pacemakers

FAILURE TO PACE (NO PACEMAKER ACTIVITY PRESENT)

Lead fracture
Lead disconnection
Battery depletion
Component failure
Oversensing
External interference

FAILURE TO SENSE (CONSTANT PACEMAKER SPIKES DESPITE ONGOING INTRINSIC CARDIAC ELECTRICAL ACTIVITY)

Lead dislodgement
Lead fracture
Fibrosis around the tip of the lead
Battery depletion
Pacer in asynchronous mode
External interference
Low-amplitude intracardiac signal

FAILURE TO CAPTURE (PACEMAKER SPIKES BUT NO SUBSEQUENT CARDIAC ACTIVITY)

Lead dislodgement, including perforation
Lead fracture
Lead disconnection
Poor lead position
Fibrosis around the tip of the lead
Battery depletion
Metabolic abnormalities
Medications

INAPPROPRIATE PACEMAKER RATE (RUNAWAY PACEMAKER)

Pacemaker reentrant tachycardia
Resetting from external interference
Battery depletion

OTHER

Infections: pocket, wires
Lead displacement: cardiac perforation, tamponade, pericarditis, vascular perforation
Vascular complications: thrombosis, superior vena cava syndrome
Psychiatric: anxiety, panic attacks

the leads; electrolyte disturbances, including hyperkalemia or hypocalcemia; a new condition requiring an elevated pacing threshold; acid-base disturbance; direct damage to the myocardium, which is in contact with the pacer lead's tip (such as myocardial infarction or direct trauma); or dysfunction of the microcircuitry of the pulse generator. In addition, flecainide, a class IC antiarrhythmic medication, has been identified as an acute cause of the rise in ventricular capture thresholds in patients with implanted pacemakers. Likewise, all class I antiarrhythmic agents (sodium channel antagonists) may affect pacer capture thresholds and should therefore be identified as potential etiologic agents in patients experiencing failure to capture.

Failure-to-Sense

Failure of an implanted cardiac pacemaker to sense the patient's intrinsic cardiac rhythm may be subdivided into conditions related to oversensing or undersensing. *Oversensing* is present when the pacemaker erroneously identifies extrinsic electrical signals, such as those from skeletal muscle potentials or electromagnetic interference (EMI), and is inhibited from delivering an appropriate pacemaker pulse. For additional information on extrinsic EMI, refer to the section on Electromagnetic Interference and Implantable Devices later in this chapter.

Management of pacemaker failure-to-sense will be driven largely by the patient's clinical condition. The evaluation should be based on the history and physical examination findings, as well as bedside diagnostics. In the event of symptomatic bradycardia, placement of a magnet over the pacemaker pulse generator may be indicated because this maneuver will usually place the pacemaker in an asynchronous ventricular pacing mode and thereby restore a stable and regular paced ventricular rhythm while a consulting cardiologist or electrophysiologist is summoned.

Undersensing is said to occur when the pacemaker fails to identify intrinsic cardiac depolarization and delivers a pacing signal. This condition may result from damage or dislodgement of the pacemaker leads, myocardial infarction, direct cardiac trauma, failure of the pacemaker's power source, and even the application of a magnet. Initial ED management of this condition is like that performed in the case of oversensing. Magnet placement may also be appropriate in this setting because it will restore a stable, regular, and normal cardiac rhythm until the pacemaker and its leads may be more thoroughly examined. It may also be used as a temporary diagnostic maneuver.

Runaway Pacemaker Syndrome

This condition is seen almost exclusively in older pacemaker models particularly as they approach the end of their battery life, or when the pulse generator is damaged by exposure to radiation or direct impact. The hallmark of runaway pacemaker syndrome is uncontrolled tachycardia resulting in ventricular rates approaching 300 to 400 beats/min. In addition to initial attempts at stabilization, magnet placement may be attempted. However, this is often ineffective. If the patient is hemodynamically unstable in the setting of runaway pacemaker syndrome, it may be necessary to disconnect the pulse generator. To do this, identify the location of the pacer leads by physical examination or a portable chest radiograph. Dissect through the skin and subcutaneous tissue and then sever the leads with a wire cutter or similar tool.

Pacemaker-Mediated Tachycardia

In some circumstances patients with implanted pacemakers or AICDs may be seen in the ED because of symptomatic tachycardias resulting specifically as a complication of their pacemaker devices. This condition, referred to as *pacemaker-mediated tachycardia*, and alternatively as *pacemaker-induced tachycardia*, results most often from one of three clinical scenarios. In patients with dual-chamber pacemakers, one of the pacemaker leads may function as a pathway for either anterograde or retrograde conduction and result in what is referred to as *endless loop syndrome* and thus a tachycardic arrhythmia, which may often become hemodynamically unstable. In general, patients with endless loop syndrome will not have a ventricular rate greater than the maximum tracking rate of the pacemaker device. Consequently, this condition will rarely be manifested as hemodynamic instability. One caveat, however, is that patients with underlying coronary artery disease and endless loop syndrome may experience coronary ischemia. In such a case or in a patient who is hemodynamically unstable because of the increased ventricular rate, application of a magnet will terminate the syndrome in most cases. Once stabilized, this condition may be prevented or at least mitigated by reprogramming of the pacemaker's atrial sensor lead by an electrophysiologist.

A second scenario in patients with dual-chamber pacemakers occurs under the circumstance in which the patient experiences an intrinsic atrial tachycardia, at which point the implanted pacemaker begins to continuously discharge at its maximum preprogrammed ventricular rate. This condition may continue until the underlying atrial tachycardia is terminated by intervention.

A third instance of pacemaker-mediated tachycardia occurs in patients with AICD units that have backup antibradycardia pacing capability. It appears that if this pacemaker feature is switched on in such patients and an ectopic ventricular stimulus is delivered after a sudden pause in the intrinsic ventricular depolarization cycle, a ventricular tachyarrhythmia may be triggered.

DIAGNOSIS OF ACUTE MYOCARDIAL INFARCTION IN THE PRESENCE OF A PACED CARDIAC RHYTHM

Patients undergoing active ventricular pacing from an implanted pacemaker device without CRT will normally have ECGs that resemble a left bundle branch block pattern. As a result, electrocardiographic diagnosis of acute ischemic changes is equally challenging in both populations. Sgarbossa and colleagues published a series of criteria in 1996 that offer some utility in the interpretation of ECGs in patients with active ventricular pacing in whom acute coronary syndromes are suspected and can be applied in the setting of a pacemaker. Subsequently, Smith et al. modified criterion three, substituting an absolute discordant ST elevation of 5 mm or more with proportionally excessive discordant ST elevation in any lead, as defined by an ST/S ratio of equal to or more than 0.25.[34] More recently, Dodd, et al reported the results of a multicenter registry study confirming the superiority of the modified Sgarbossa criteria as well as extending criterion b of the modified Sgarbossa criteria regarding concordant ST depression to include any of the precordial leads from V_1 to V_6.[35] An ECG only needs to have one lead meet one of the modified Sgarbossa criteria to be considered positive for acute coronary occlusion. These criteria are depicted in Table 13.2.

TABLE 13.2 Criteria for Electrocardiographic Diagnosis of Acute Myocardial Infarction in the Setting of a Ventricular-Paced Rhythm

MODIFIED SGARBOSSA CRITERIA FOR PACED RHYTHMS	LEADS
Concordant ST-segment elevation >1 mm	Any lead
Concordant ST-segment depression >1 mm	V_1 to V_6 only
Discordant ST-segment elevations with ST/S ratio >25%	Any lead

The ST/S ratio is calculated by measuring the magnitude of the ST-segment deflection from baseline and dividing by the total magnitude of the S segment measured from baseline. If this is greater than 0.25, modified Sgarbossa criterion C is positive.

AUTOMATIC IMPLANTABLE CARDIOVERTER DEFIBRILLATORS: UNIQUE MALFUNCTIONS

Issues with sensing problems, lead migration, and battery failure are similar to pacemaker complications, and most occur within 3 months after implantation. Some data show that a dual-chamber device is associated with a higher risk of device-related complications but a similar 1-year mortality compared to a single-chamber device.[36] A large meta-analysis put the incidence of in-hospital adverse events between 2.8% and 3.6%.[37] Complications related to the insertion include cardiac injury, lead dislodgement, infection, hemorrhage, and pneumothorax. A potential malfunction unique to AICDs is inappropriate defibrillation or lack of defibrillation of the device.

The AICD may not terminate ventricular arrhythmias, which may or may not be the result of malfunction of the device. AICD malfunction may be a result of battery depletion, component failure, failure-to-sense, or lead malfunction. Failure to cardiovert or defibrillate occurring in the setting of a functioning AICD system may be caused by inappropriate cutoff rates, failure to satisfy multiple detection criteria, completion and exhaustion of therapies, and cross-inhibition by a separate pacemaker. The advent of AV or dual-chamber AICD devices has improved the sensitivity of detecting arrhythmias and thus prevents the delivery of inappropriate shocks. The AICD may also be unable to terminate ventricular arrhythmias in the case of refractory VT/VF or *electrical storm*. This phenomenon occurs when three or more shocks are delivered in a 24-hour period, occurs in 10% to 20% of AICD patients, and constitutes a medical emergency. Management of refractory VT/VF is discussed in Chapter 12.

Inappropriate AICD-delivered shocks occur in 20% to 25% of patients and are the most common adverse events observed in AICD patients. The main causes are atrial arrhythmias, sinus tachycardia, nonsustained VT, or lead fracture, or EMI. Multiple shocks may be a manifestation of inefficient termination of tachycardia, such as inappropriately low-energy delivery at the first shock, increased defibrillation thresholds, and migration or dislodgement of the defibrillation lead system, or failure of the defibrillator system. Shocks that occur every few minutes may suggest that recurring ventricular tachyarrhythmias are being terminated appropriately (see Fig. 13.9).

AICD discharges in the setting of chest pain may be a result of myocardial ischemia–induced tachyarrhythmias. As noted earlier, any electrocardiographic abnormalities noted immediately after shocks should be interpreted with caution because ST elevation or depression can occur immediately after a shock in the absence of ischemia. If the patient receives shocks in association with chest pain, ischemia is suggested, but other causes, including hypokalemia, hypomagnesemia, drug-induced proarrhythmia, or drugs that can prolong the QT interval (such as phenothiazines), should also be considered as underlying causes.

BOX 13.2 Outcome of Automatic Implantable Cardioverter Defibrillator Placement: Estimated Events Over a 5-Year Period After Placement for Current Criteria[a]

For every 100 patients in whom an AICD is placed:

- 30 patients will die anyway because of underlying disease.
- 7–8 patients will be saved by AICD.
- 10–20 will have a shock delivered that is not needed.
- 5–15 will have an ICD complication.

The rest will not experience the device firing.
Some will ask to have it removed to allow natural death.

[a]*Left ventricular ejection fraction less than 30% to 35% and anticipated survival with good functional capacity beyond 1 year.*
AICD, *Automatic implantable cardioverter defibrillator;* ICD, *implantable cardioverter defibrillator.*

In some settings the AICD may fail to sense sustained VT or VF. Such failure may be caused by an intrinsic arrhythmia rate below the programmed detection rate, usually because of concurrent pharmacologic therapy. If the patient is hemodynamically stable, it may be advantageous for the cardiologist to interrogate the pacer before initiating further antiarrhythmic therapy. If unsuccessful or if the patient is experiencing a nonperfusing ventricular arrhythmia, other pharmacologic interventions include procainamide or amiodarone. Box 13.2 depicts the outcome of AICD placement in a general population.

Subcutaneous defibrillators have some of the same complications as the venous AICDs including hematoma, infection, lead displacement, and inappropriate shocks.

LVAD Complications

In patients with LVAD, infection is the second most common cause of death after cardiac failure.[38] VAD infections can be divided into three categories: VAD-specific infections including the pump, pocket, and driveline; VAD-related infections such as bloodstream infections, endocarditis, and mediastinitis; and non-VAD infections.[39] Infections can involve any portion of the LVAD, including the surgical site, pocket, pump, and most commonly the driveline, which goes from internal to external. The patient may have nonspecific symptoms or have fever, localized erythema, or wound drainage. Infections occur most commonly within the first 3 months of device implantation with the risk of severe infection and sepsis peaking at 1 month.[40] Most infections are caused by gram-positive organisms such as *Staphylococcus aureus*. *Enterococcus* is also common, as are gram-negative organisms, most commonly *Pseudomonas*. Treatment includes broad-spectrum antibiotics, though localized infection may be treated for gram-positives alone. LVAD-associated endocarditis has a high mortality rate,[41] and can range from minimal symptoms to fever and systemic emboli in a presentation similar to prosthetic valve endocarditis.

Given that most patients are on both antiplatelet therapy and anticoagulant therapy, bleeding is another frequent adverse event in LVAD patients. The increase in bleeding susceptibility is thought to be related to the development of acquired von Willebrand syndrome secondary to shearing forces through the LVAD.[42] Second- and third-generation LVADs have also led to nonsurgical gastrointestinal (GI) bleeding secondary to arterial venous malformations. It is thought that reduced pulse pressure from continuous infusion results in hypoperfusion of the gastrointestinal mucosa and neovascularization, which, with friable vessels, is prone to bleeding.[42] These patients need endoscopy and possibly anticoagulation reversal with the use of fresh frozen plasma, prothrombin complex concentrates, or specific antagonists depending on the agent used. Providers should discuss reversal with the patient's LVAD team whenever possible, and non-life-threatening bleeding can likely be managed successfully without reversal. In the case of life-threatening bleeding such as intracranial hemorrhage, reversal of anticoagulation should be strongly considered.

A suction event is a specific LVAD complication that can occur in the setting of hypovolemia due to infection, bleeding, GI losses, or poor oral (PO) intake, or can occur due to RV failure. This causes crowding of the LVAD's inflow cannula due to collapse of the LV free wall, further decreasing cardiac output. A suction event can lead to arrhythmias and initial intervention includes IV fluids if the suction event is thought to be caused by hypovolemia and slowing down the LV rate to allow for adequate filling.

LVAD thrombosis is a potentially devastating complication occurring in 2% to 13% of continuous flow LVAD patients.[43] Thrombosis can occur throughout the device resulting in thromboembolic stroke, thromboembolism, and LVAD malfunction and failure, resulting in life-threatening hemodynamic impairment, cardiogenic shock, and death. The patient may have very mild and nonspecific symptoms such as tea-colored urine or symptoms as severe as decompensated heart failure. Useful laboratory tests include coagulation studies and tests for hemolysis to include a urinalysis and lactate dehydrogenase (a level of three times normal indicates hemolysis).[42] CXR may reveal malposition of the outflow cannula and chest CT angiography may diagnose inflow malposition or outflow obstruction.[44] These patients need to be urgently transferred to a center with mechanical support because the definitive therapy is removal of the device and cardiac transplantation.[43]

Dysrhythmias are a common problem in patients with advanced stages of cardiomyopathy, but patients are also at risk from placement of the device. Atrial arrhythmias should be treated in the same manner as the heart failure population by initially controlling the rate with β-blockers or calcium-channel blockers.[45] LVAD patients are also at risk for ventricular arrhythmias and most of them will have an AICD in place before their placement. Patients with persistent ventricular arrhythmias, despite the AICD discharges, may require IV β-blockers in addition to reprogramming the device.[46]

Resuscitation of these patients can be challenging given their sensitivity to both preload and afterload. A decrease in systemic volume may result in a suction event and subsequent clinical deterioration.[47] Uncontrolled increase in MAP higher than 90 mm may reduce LVAD outflow, cardiac output, and distal perfusion. These patients are at risk for cerebral vascular events and should be treated promptly with afterload-reducing medications.[21,23]

As noted earlier, ultrasound can be helpful in differentiating between LVAD complications. If the RV and LV both appear small, the patient is more likely to be hypovolemic, with infection or bleeding as likely causes. Consider pulmonary hypertension, a pulmonary embolism, or acute coronary syndrome if the RV is large and the LV is small. Finally, a large RV and large LV can suggest hypervolemia, hypertension, or pump thrombosis.

Pacemaker and AICD Response to Magnet Placement

In the clinical setting, placement of a magnet over the pulse generator of a pacemaker is a technique that can be used either diagnostically or therapeutically by the emergency clinician. Application of a magnet is used to suspend antitachyarrhythmia detection and therapy of an AICD without changing pacing mode, or to produce asynchronous (fixed-rate) pacing of a pacemaker. Hence, a magnet may change a demand pacemaker (synchronous) to a fixed-rate (asynchronous) pacemaker. However, it is important to note that each pacemaker is programmed to respond in a specific fashion to a magnet as determined by the manufacturer. The response to magnet placement may not only vary by manufacturer, but also by model and by the particular mode in which the pacemaker is currently operating. Some devices (Boston Scientific, St. Jude, Biotronik devices) may be programmed to disable the magnet function and hence not respond to magnet application. Some leadless pacemakers do not initiate asynchronous pacing in response to a magnet application. In most cases manufacturers set the asynchronous (fixed-rate) baseline pacing rate in a range approximating 70 beats/min. An indicator of aging of the pacemaker and weakening of the battery is that this asynchronous baseline pacing rate will decrease over time as the battery approaches the point at which replacement is required.

With these provisions in mind, there are standard responses that the provider might expect to see in most circumstances. In the case of single-chamber ventricular pacemakers, the response will most likely be asynchronous pacing (V00). In the case of dual-chamber pacemakers, placement of a magnet usually results in dual-chamber asynchronous pacing (D00). In either case, it is important for the clinician to note that placement of a magnet over the pacemaker pulse generator will not turn the pacemaker off.

Placing a magnet over any of the currently available AICD models will temporarily disable tachyarrhythmia intervention (Fig. 13.10). An ECG should be obtained before and after magnet placement for comparison (Fig. 13.11). Most commercially available pacer magnets are 7 cm in size and can be used with most implantable devices. The magnetic field closes a reed switch in the generator circuit that will disable recognition of tachyarrhythmias and subsequent firing of the device. There may be a variety of tones (continuous, intermittent, or silent) during activation or inactivation with the magnet,

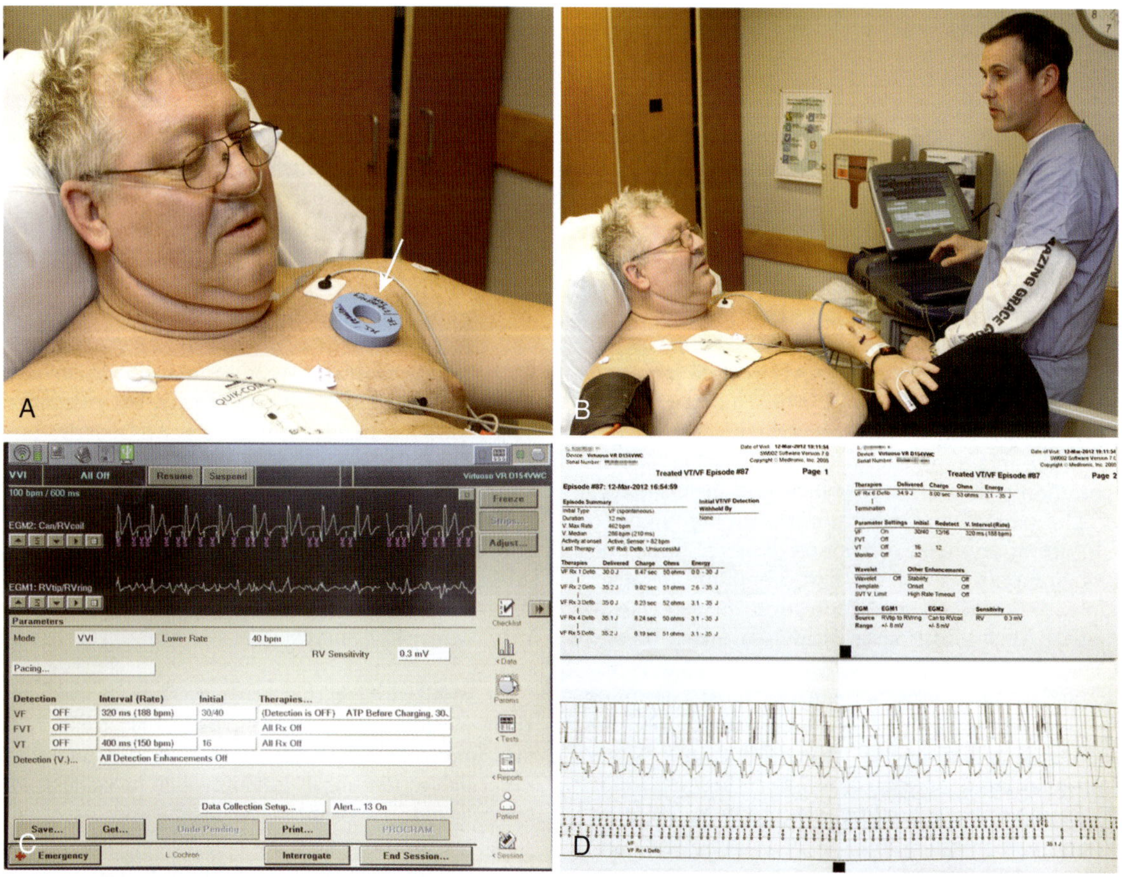

Fig. 13.10 (A) This patient experienced 13 discharges of his automatic implantable cardioverter defibrillator over the course of 1 hour. In the emergency department, he was noted to have a discharge while in sinus rhythm, and a magnet *(arrow)* was placed over the device to deactivate it. (B) An electrophysiology specialist came to the emergency department to interrogate the device. Note that newer devices can communicate wirelessly. (C–D) Interrogation and intracardiac electrocardiograms were consistent with fracture of the right ventricular lead. The device was deactivated and replaced shortly thereafter.

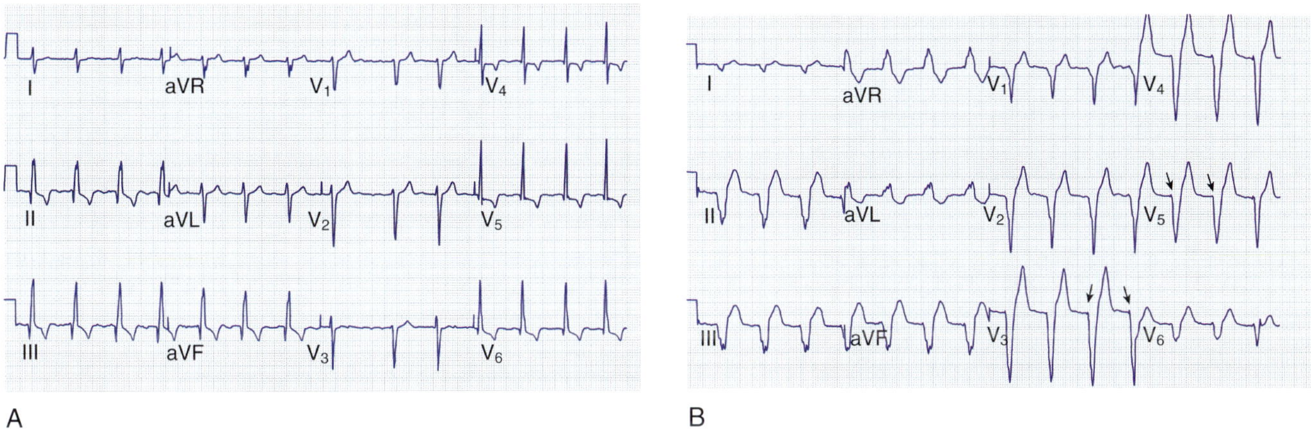

Fig. 13.11 (A) Electrocardiogram (ECG) of a patient with a nonfiring pacemaker. The intrinsic cardiac rate is 80 beats/min, and no pacemaker activity is seen. (B) ECG of the same patient with a magnet applied over the pacemaker, which produced a paced rhythm. Pacer spikes are evident *(arrows)*, and the magnet rate is 85 beats/min. Note the left bundle branch bundle typical of a pacer lead in the right ventricle.

which are dependent on the manufacturer. Some devices may be programmed to not respond at all. After the desired effect is obtained, the magnet should be secured to maintain inactivation.

Pacemaker and AICD patients should carry an identification card that includes information regarding manufacturer, model type, and lead system, in addition to a 24-hour emergency number to allow rapid identification of the model when it is necessary to inactivate the device. In lieu of the availability of a device identification card, the general type, polarity, and number of ventricles involved with the implanted device may be inferred accurately by viewing an overpenetrated anteroposterior chest radiograph.

If a patient with an AICD has a ventricular arrhythmia, the assumption should be made that the device is inoperable and standard ACLS protocols should be used to stabilize the patient.

In some patients with an increased body mass index or those with heavily developed chest wall musculature, the magnetic field emitted by a single magnet device may not be strong enough to elicit the desired effect on the implanted device. In such cases the clinician may find greater efficacy by using two magnets, one on top of the other.

Use of a Magnet for AICD

A patient who is experiencing inappropriate AICD discharges in the ED can be treated by inactivation of the device with a magnet. If the patient is experiencing recurrent rhythms that require activation of the AICD, do not inactivate the device because it is functioning as required.

Technique

The method for inactivating an AICD device is outlined in Box 13.3. The orientation of the device in the abdominal pocket should be determined, with the lead connections normally being cephalad. A ring magnet is then placed over the corner adjacent to the lead connections (usually the upper right-hand corner of the device). A series of beeping tones will sound that correspond to the sensed QRS complexes. In the absence of organized QRS activity, random beeps will sound. When the magnet is left in place for 30 seconds, a continuous beep is heard. This indicates that the AICD is inactivated. The magnet should then be removed, and the AICD will remain inactivated. The AICD may be reactivated by applying the magnet for 30 seconds and removing it when the steady beep changes to intermittent beeping. Note that unlike a pacemaker, in which a magnet will turn a demand pacemaker to a fixed-rate pacemaker, a magnet will not affect the pacing function of an AICD.

BOX 13.3 Method for Inactivation of an Automatic Implantable Cardioverter Defibrillator

1. Determine the orientation of the device in the abdominal pocket radiographically or by palpation.
2. Place a ring magnet over the upper right-hand corner of the device.
3. A beeping tone will sound that corresponds to the sensing of QRS complexes.
4. Leave the magnet in place for at least 30 seconds.
5. When the beeping changes to a continuous tone, the device is inactivated.
6. Remove the magnet.

"Twiddler" Syndrome

In some cases, patients with implantable pacemakers choose to "twiddle" with the device: they manipulate the pulse generator case within its physiologic pocket under the skin in the chest.[3] Note that a generator may also be placed in the abdominal wall (Fig. 13.12). This practice of twiddling may result in coiling, dislodgement, or disconnection of the pacemaker leads (Fig. 13.13). It may even lead to actual displacement of the pulse generator case. At a minimum, it may result in physical discomfort and may, in fact, precipitate cardiac arrhythmias or other complications local to the site of pacemaker placement. After initial stabilization of the complaint, these patients may require readjustment or replacement of their pacemaker

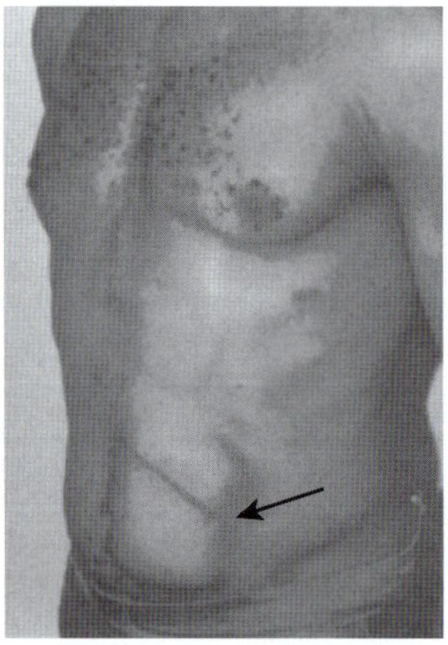

Fig. 13.12 Pacemakers and automatic implantable cardioverter defibrillators may be implanted in the abdominal wall, in addition to the more common pectoralis muscle.

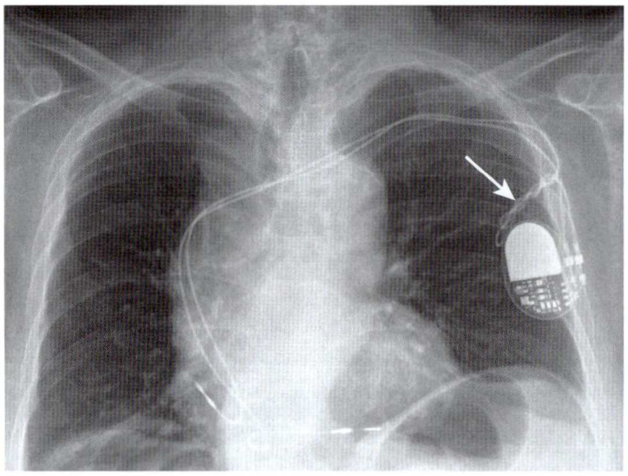

Fig. 13.13 Twiddler syndrome. Note the twisting of the pacemaker leads as they exit the device *(arrow)*. This twisting is a direct result of the patient "twiddling" with the device and may result in dislodgement or disconnection of the pacemaker leads.

devices. As part of their care, pacemaker patients should be educated to avoid manipulating their pacemakers.

Mental Health Issues Related to Implanted Pacemakers and AICDs

Patients with these devices may manifest several anxiety-related complications including adjustment disorder, panic attacks, depression, imaginary shock, PTSD, and as end-of-life approaches, defibrillator dependence.[48] These patients may benefit from psychiatric referral either as an outpatient or as part of the admission evaluation if applicable.[49] The conditions may be severe enough that the device is removed by patient request.

Implantable Pacemaker and AICD Recalls

Since 1990 more than 60 device or lead advisories have been announced, affecting more than one million device patients.[50] These advisories were issued as a result of unanticipated failure of devices identified after release of the product and widespread clinical use.[51] A systematic review of studies from 2015 evaluating pacemaker malfunctioning concluded this continued to be an issue.[52] The decision to remove a device is complex, and there has been difficulty reaching consensus on the optimal management of patients with these recalled devices. The decision to replace them should be multifactorial and take into consideration the estimated malfunction rate of the device, anticipated consequences of failure of the device, the individual center's procedural risk for complications resulting from generator replacement, and patient preferences and desired level of risk tolerance. This discussion is generally outside the scope of care in the ED and would involve the patient's cardiac care team.

Electromagnetic Interference and Implantable Devices

Given the plethora of new technologies there is always concern about the interaction of EMI with pacemakers and AICDs. The sources of EMI comprise a significant spectrum and may involve radiated and conducted sources.

The most common response of implanted devices to EMI is inappropriate inhibition or triggering of pacemaker stimuli, reversion to asynchronous pacing, and spurious detection of tachyarrhythmias by the AICD. Reprogramming of operating parameters and permanent damage to the circuitry of the device or the electrode-tissue interface can also occur but are much less frequent. Additional adverse effects that may occur include inhibition of bradycardia pacing, inadvertent delivery of a shock, or antitachycardia pacing.

The use of hermetic shielding in metal cases, filtering, interference rejection circuits, and bipolar sensing have helped mitigate most of this interference.[53] Nonetheless, the clinician should be familiar with common sources of EMI that may affect pacemakers and AICDs.[54,55]

It has been estimated that patients with pacemakers and AICDs have a 50% to 75% chance of developing an indication for magnetic resonance imaging (MRI) over the lifetime of the device.[55] Historically, MRIs have been strongly contraindicated unless the benefits of imaging far outweigh the risk.[56] Because many of the newer pacemakers are MRI-compatible, the MRI staff can assess the compatibility based on manufacturer provided information.[57]

Several caveats will help to avoid the deleterious effects of EMI on implantable devices. Cell phones should not be kept in a pocket over the device. When in use they should be held at least 6 inches away from the device. When hands-free headphones are used, these devices should be placed in the ear opposite the implanted pacemaker or AICD. In addition, patients should be advised not to linger in theft detection areas or airport metal detectors; however, brief exposures are safe. Box 13.4 identifies different devices and the corresponding potential EMI that can occur with pacemakers and AICDs.

Out-of-Hospital Discharge of AICD

Patients are told to adhere to standard advice defining an appropriate response to out-of-hospital discharges of the AICD (Box 13.5). However, many come to the ED for evaluation after every shock. There is no standard ED intervention mandated by historical information, and clinical decisions are made on an individual basis corresponding to the current scenario. Options include prolonged ED observation, consultation, cardiac monitoring, laboratory testing (such as electrolytes and cardiac enzymes), or interrogation.

BOX 13.4 Sources of Electromagnetic Interference and Its Potential Effects on Implanted Pacemakers and Automatic Implantable Cardioverter Defibrillators

GENERALLY THOUGHT TO BE SAFE WITH EMI

Copy machines
Electric blankets
Household appliances (microwaves, washer/dryer)
DVD/CD players, TVs
Personal computers
Remote controls
Heating pads

SOME EVIDENCE OF INTERACTION

Cell phones
Induction ovens
Power toothbrushes
Battery-powered, cordless power tools
Arc welding equipment
Chain saws
Drills
Hedge clippers
Lawn mowers
Leaf blowers
Snow blowers
High-voltage lines
Theft detection systems
Airport scanners/metal detectors

AVOID BECAUSE OF INTERACTION

Electrolysis
MRI
Jackhammers

MEDICAL DEVICES REQUIRING CAUTION

Electrocautery (especially unipolar) equipment
High-energy radiation sources
TENS units
MRI scanners
Body fat–measuring scales
Diathermy equipment
Electrolysis equipment
Spinal cord stimulators
Direct current external cardioversion/defibrillation equipment
Radiofrequency catheter ablation equipment
Lithotripsy equipment

SAFE MEDICAL DEVICES

CT scanners
Dental drills
Diagnostic x-ray machines
Electrocardiography equipment
Ultrasound equipment

CT, *Computed tomography;* EMI, *electromagnetic interference;* MRI, *magnetic resonance imaging;* TENS, *transcutaneous electrical nerve stimulation.*

BOX 13.5 Follow-up of Patients With an AICD

Follow-up assessments of patients with an AICD are made on a routine basis, every 3 to 6 months, and when discharge of the device occurs. Analysis of any previous clinical event and testing of defibrillation function are readily accomplished. Internet-based remote follow-up systems may replace some office follow-up. Follow-up can occur remotely with vendor-specific equipment to interrogate and upload data. Remote follow-up, however, permits only device interrogation and retrieval of diagnostic data, not threshold testing or reprogramming. Device interrogation includes the following:

- Determination of pacing and sensing thresholds.
- Analysis of recorded episodes of arrhythmia detection and AICD activation, including pacing and delivered shocks. Data include the date and time of each episode and a stored electrocardiogram from the event.
- Battery status.

DEFIBRILLATOR DISCHARGE

An appropriate shock is delivered in approximately 50% of patients by 2 years after implantation. Patients may not sense antitachycardic (overdrive) pacing to terminate arrhythmias. Not all episodes of defibrillator discharge require immediate medical evaluation, although many patients go to the ED immediately. Patients with a first shock may be seen on an urgent or elective basis to ascertain the specifics of the event and to determine whether the device is functioning properly. Discharges that are accompanied by changes in cognition (syncope, seizure, or loss of consciousness) require ED evaluation.

Per guidelines, patients who have had a single AICD discharge with immediate return to baseline clinical status and no associated symptoms (e.g., chest pain, shortness of breath, lightheadedness) may have the device interrogated within 1 to 2 days.

Delivery of frequent shocks or clusters of shocks is either appropriate (because of recurrent VT) or inappropriate (because of atrial fibrillation, supraventricular tachycardia, or device malfunction). Such patients generally require emergency evaluation and hospital admission to determine the cause. Additional therapy (such as an antiarrhythmic drug or catheter ablation) may be required.

AICD, *Automatic implantable cardioverter defibrillator;* ED, *emergency department;* VT, *ventricular tachycardia.*

Disposition Criteria

In most cases, patients seen in the ED with pacemaker complications or malfunctions will be symptomatic. Accordingly, and regardless of the clinical requirement for admission, they will probably require device interrogation and possible recalibration or replacement by a cardiologist. In most cases this will be accomplished during hospital admission; however, as more device-interrogation tools become available to emergency physicians, the ability to disposition them home when appropriate will likely increase.[1]

Regarding AICD malfunctions and disposition, patients who have had a single shock and no other specific complaints or comorbidity may be discharged with follow-up in 24 to 48 hours.[1] Patients with symptoms concerning for ischemia, potentially lethal arrhythmias, or symptomatic illness will likely require admission. Patients who have had multiple shocks will need admission for observation and interrogation of their AICD device. Interrogation reveals significant information about the device such as why it fired, the rhythm history, and an accurate assessment of the underlying problem.

REFERENCES ARE AVAILABLE AT Elsevier eBooks+

CHAPTER 14

Basic Electrocardiographic Techniques

Joshua S. Easter, William J. Brady, and Theodore C. Chan

INTRODUCTION

The electrocardiogram (ECG) is a graphic recording of the electrical activity of the heart. Normally the heart generates an electrical signal from the sinoatrial node in the right atrium that is conducted through the atria and ventricles. The standard ECG records this electrical activity through surface electrodes placed on the skin. The appearance of the electrical activity depends on the type and location of the recording electrode. Developed over 100 years ago, the ECG remains a critical initial diagnostic tool for the evaluation of patients presenting with chest pain, dyspnea, syncope, cardiac arrest, and toxicologic exposures. Standard electrocardiography machines are small, self-contained, and portable, thus allowing them to be used in virtually any setting. High-quality acquisition of ECGs is crucial, as improperly performed ECGs can lead to misdiagnoses and improper treatments.

INDICATIONS

The most frequent indication for electrocardiography in the emergency department (ED) is the presence of chest pain; other common indications are described in Table 14.1. The benefits of the ECG are myriad; it can help establish a diagnosis, select appropriate therapy, determine the response to treatment, assist in correct disposition of the patient, and help predict risk for both cardiovascular complications and death. In particular, it is crucial in establishing the presence of a ST-elevation myocardial infarction (STEMI) in a timely fashion, which improves morbidity and mortality.[1] The American Heart Association recommends patients with signs or symptoms concerning for myocardial infarction (MI) undergo ECG testing and interpretation in the prehospital setting when possible or within 10 minutes of arrival to the ED (Fig. 14.1). Despite significant emphasis on timely ECG acquisition, approximately 13% of patients with STEMI do not undergo ECG within 10 minutes of arrival.[1] Delays are more common for patients who are female, Black, non-English speaking, diabetic, or patients presenting with chief complaints that are not chest pain.[2] Various consensus protocols exist to promote timely ECG acquisition, particularly among diverse patients presenting with atypical symptoms; Table 14.2 depicts a sample protocol. Ideally the ECG is acquired while the patient is being triaged. Protocols tend to maximize sensitivity at the expense of specificity.[3] While the ECG itself is inexpensive, these protocols can have profound downstream financial and clinical consequences, as abnormal ECGs may prompt further unnecessary testing.[4] Moreover, ECGs require timely interpretation by clinicians, which leads to numerous interruptions in patient care.[5] In the future artificial intelligence that incorporates interpretation of the ECG, patient's presenting chief concerns and risk factors might improve diagnostic accuracy of triage and the initial ECG.[6–8] In the meantime, a liberal approach to ECG acquisition seems appropriate given the high morbidity associated with delays in recognition of STEMI.

When the initial ECG shows STEMI, it is impactful; however, it often is normal or shows non–ST-elevation changes, such as ST-segment depression, T-wave inversions, flat T waves, or pseudo-normalization of T waves. These nondiagnostic ECG findings have a sensitivity for acute MI (AMI) of only approximately 55%, and therefore cannot rule out myocardial ischemia. Bundle branch block, left ventricular hypertrophy, and ventricular pacing often obscure findings of ischemia, limiting sensitivity. The negative predictive value of a normal ECG is greater, but it still misses 3% to 10% of MIs.[9] In patients with concerning presentations and normal or non–ST-elevation changes on their initial ECGs, acquisition of serial ECGs improves sensitivity.[10] When there is high concern for STEMI but the initial ECG is nondiagnostic, the American Heart Association (AHA) recommends acquiring ECGs at 5- to 10-min intervals to improve sensitivity and mitigate potential delays in diagnosis.[11]

Abnormal ECG findings can often be nonspecific. Comparison to prior ECGs can improve specificity, as findings present on ECGs prior to the current presentation are less likely to represent acute ischemia, although an unchanged ECG also cannot completely rule out acute coronary syndrome (ACS). For patients at high risk, continuous ST-segment monitoring may improve early detection of ischemia.[12] A repeat ECG is also useful if symptoms recur or the patient's clinical situation changes.

The initial 12-lead ECG obtained in the ED can also be an important tool for the determination of cardiovascular risk and patient disposition. Brush et al. found that high-risk ECG features were associated with more frequent MIs and life-threatening complications (e.g., ventricular fibrillation, heart block, etc.) during hospital admission (Table 14.3).[13] Combining low-risk ECG features and clinical characteristics may identify patients at low risk of ACS, who do not require further testing.[14]

BASIC EQUIPMENT

12-Lead Electrocardiogram

Although there is variability, most ECGs in use today are three-channel recorders with computer memory. Such multichannel systems, which record electrical events in several leads concurrently, offer advantages over the antiquated single-channel recorder systems as follows: capturing transient events on multiple leads simultaneously; banking the data in computer memory for storage, comparison, and transmission; and allowing presentation of data on a single sheet of paper. The electrocardiographic tracing is printed in a standardized manner on standardized paper by the electrocardiograph, which has default settings regarding the speed at which the paper moves through the machine, in addition to the amplitude of the deflections to be made on the tracing (Fig. 14.2A). Electrocardiographic paper is divided into a grid with a series of horizontal and vertical lines; the thin lines are 1 mm apart, and the thick lines are separated by 5 mm. At the standard paper speed of 25

TABLE 14.1 Potential Indications for ECG Acquisition in the ED

Symptoms	Chest pain Dyspnea Syncope or lightheadedness Palpitations
Physical examination	Extreme tachycardia Bradycardia Irregular heart rhythm
Differential diagnosis	Acute coronary syndrome Pulmonary embolism Toxic ingestion Myocarditis Pericarditis Electrolyte abnormalities Arrhythmia Cardiac arrest

ECG, Electrocardiogram; *ED*, emergency department.

mm/s, each vertical thin line thus represents 0.04 seconds (or 40 ms), and the thick vertical lines correspond to 0.20 seconds (or 200 ms).

The standard ECG includes 12 leads derived from 10 electrodes placed on the patient; each is color-coded and represented by a two-character abbreviation (Table 14.4; see also Fig. 14.2B). Distinction is made between the terms *lead* and *electrode* with the former referring to the electrical view or perspective and the latter the actual wire attached to the patient. Placement of limb leads includes the left and right arms (LA and RA, respectively) and the left and right legs (LL and RL, respectively). Caution is advised with anatomic placement of the leads; incorrect lead placement produces electrocardiographic findings which can mimic illness with resultant unnecessary clinical interventions and further diagnostic testing (see subsequent section on "Electrode Misplacement and Misconnection").

Anatomy

The standard 12-lead ECG depicts cardiac electrical activity from 12 points of view (i.e., leads), that can be grouped according to planar orientation into limb, precordial, and augmented leads. Six leads (I, II, III, aVR, aVL, and aVF) are oriented in the frontal (i.e., coronal) plane and are derived from the four limb electrodes. The six *precordial leads* (V_1, V_2, V_3, V_4, V_5, and V_6) are oriented in the horizontal (i.e., transverse) plane. Leads I, II, and III are termed *limb leads* and are bipolar in that they record the potential difference between two electrodes (Fig. 14.3). The fourth electrode located on the right leg serves as an electrical ground. The positive poles of these bipolar leads lie to the left and inferior, a position approximating the major vector forces of the normal heart from the SA node toward the apex of the heart. This early convention was established so that the tracing would feature primarily upright complexes. In contrast, *augmented leads* aVR, aVL, and aVF are unipolar leads with the positive electrode located at the respective extremities. These augmented leads serve to fill the "electrical gaps" between leads I, II, and III. Lead aVR stands alone with a polarity and resultant orientation opposite that of the other limb and augmented leads because its positive electrode is located in the opposite direction (superior and to the right) of the major vector force of the normal heart (inferior and to the left). Thus its complexes usually appear "opposite" in direction from the other leads.

Merging of the vector axes of the limb and augmented leads around a central axis yields a hexaxial system representing cardiac electrical activity in the frontal plane (Fig. 14.4). The six precordial leads, oriented in the horizontal plane, represent six unipolar electrodes with vector positivity oriented toward the chest surface and the central terminal of the hexaxial system serving as a negative pole. In contrast to the frontal-plane leads, the angles between each of the precordial leads in the horizontal plane are not equal. They can vary depending on electrode placement and body habitus.

PROCEDURE

Standard Electrode Placement

The four limb electrodes are conventionally placed on the extremities as follows: RA on the right wrist, LA on the left wrist, RL on the right ankle, and LL on the left ankle. The precordial electrodes should be placed as follows: V_1—right sternal border, fourth intercostal space; V_2—left sternal border, fourth intercostal space; V_3—midway between V_2 and V_4; V_4—left midclavicular line, fifth intercostal space; V_5—left anterior axillary line, same horizontal level as V_4; and V_6—left midaxillary line, same horizontal level as V_4 and V_5 (Fig. 14.5). Note that V_4 to V_6 are placed at the same horizontal level and not all in the fifth intercostal space. If V_5 and V_6 are situated in the intercostal space rather than on the same horizontal level as V_4, they are superiorly displaced as the ribs curve around the side of the thorax.

Intercostal space number can be determined by first palpating the sternal angle (angle of Louis), which is the junction of the manubrium and body of the sternum (see Fig. 14.5). This transverse bony ridge is located about 5 cm caudal from the sternal notch in adults. Immediately lateral and inferior to it is the second intercostal space; two spaces farther down lie the fourth intercostal space, where V_1 and V_2 should be placed. Precordial electrode placement should not be approximated because as little as 1 to 2 cm of electrode displacement can result in significant morphologic alteration in the precordial QRS complexes.[15,16] For females, appropriate positioning may require displacement of the breast to apply electrodes for V_4-V_6.

Most commonly, errors occur in the positioning of V_1 and V_2 followed by V_5 and V_6. For example, in one study, the correct position of V_1 was identified by 49% of nurses, 31% of noncardiology physicians, and 16% of cardiologists.[17] This error in lead placement likely stems from challenges identifying the second intercostal space. It typically cannot be directly visualized and relies on palpation, which can be particularly difficult in patients with large body habitus.

Misplacement of precordial electrodes has significant implications. It may lead to falsely concerning findings, such as T-wave inversions, ST-segment shifts, Q waves, and morphologies similar to Brugada syndrome. Minor changes in the position of the precordial leads will alter the ECG tracing, so

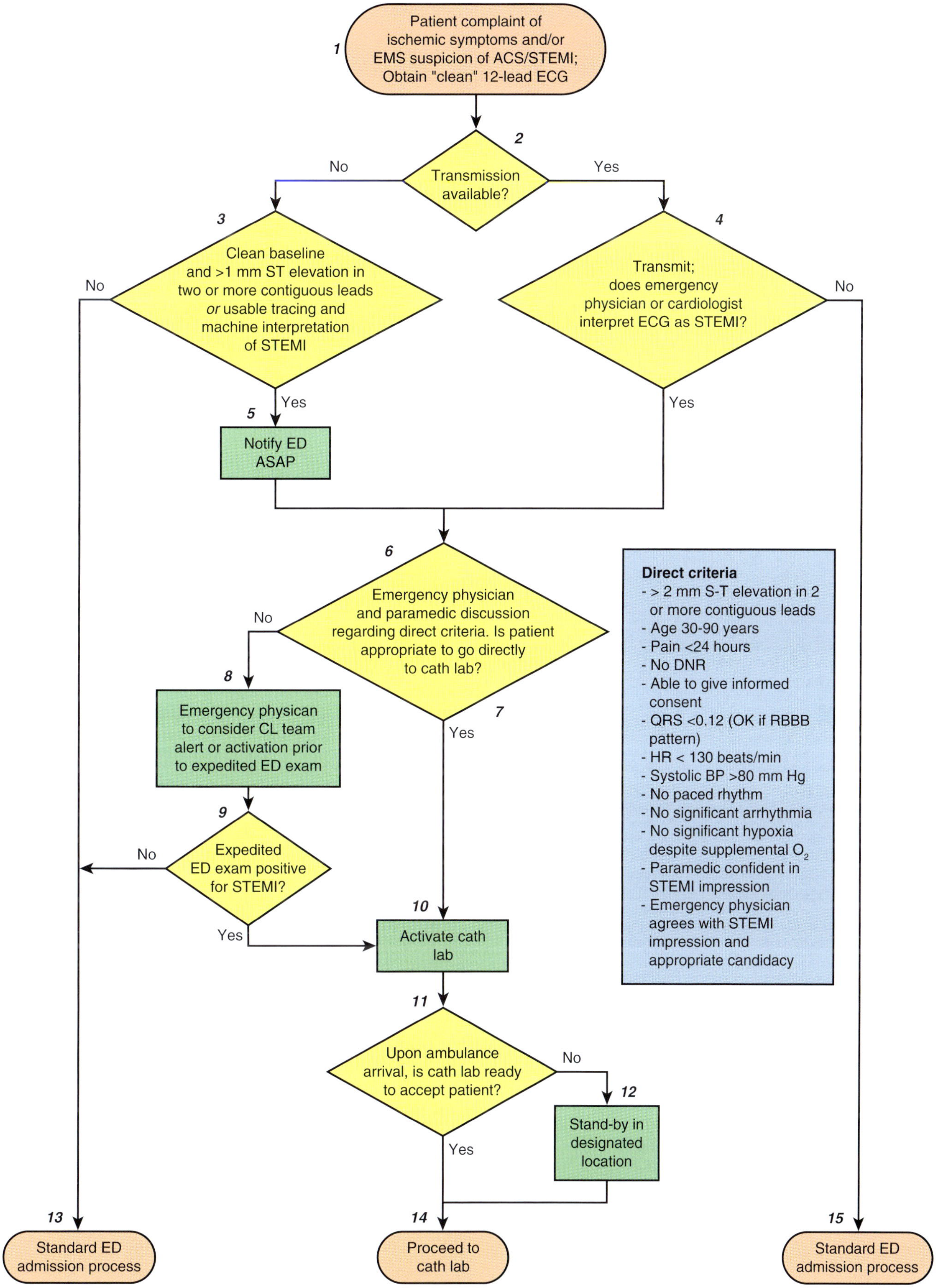

Fig. 14.1 American Heart Association Prehospital Activation of Hospital Resources (PreAct) STEMI algorithm. *ACS*, Acute coronary syndrome; *CL*, catheterization lab; *DNR*, do not resuscitate; *ECG*, electrocardiogram; *ED*, emergency department; *HR*, heart rate; *RBBB*, right bundle branch block; STEMI, ST-elevation myocardial infarction.

it is important to keep the adhesive leads in place throughout the ED stay so that lead placement is identical during serial ECG comparisons. Misplacement has been associated with prolonged ED stay, unnecessary diagnostic testing, and potentially expensive and risky treatments that are not indicated.

Modified Electrode Placement

More proximal placement of limb electrodes may be necessary (e.g., amputation, severe injuries) or be attempted to minimize motion artifact. The Mason-Likar lead position entails placing the electrodes on the torso; arm electrodes are located in the infraclavicular fossae medial to the insertion of the deltoid, while the left electrode is located midway between the costal margin and the iliac crest in the left anterior axillary line. This configuration is commonly utilized for treadmill testing or monitoring ST segments during thrombolytic administration. This configuration is easier to acquire and reduces limb artifact. However, it also tends to shift the axis vertically and may mask as much as half of ST deviations in the lateral leads and Q waves in the inferior leads.[18] Therefore this modified lead placement should not be the typical approach in the ED. In particular, placement of the LA electrode on the clavicle appears to have a large effect on the ECG and should be avoided, except when necessary.[18] It is also helpful to denote on the ECG if torso leads are employed and to repeat the ECG with standard lead placement, if the clinical presentation is concerning or worrisome abnormalities are visualized on the ECG.[19,20]

TABLE 14.2 Sample Protocol of Indications for ECG Acquisition Less Than 10 Minutes After ED Arrival to Screen for STEMI

AGE	INDICATION
<30 years	Chest pain with recent cocaine use
	Chest pain with congenital heart disease
	Chest pain with prior stent placement or surgery
>30 years	Nontraumatic chest pain
	Shortness of breath
	Nontraumatic arm or jaw pain
	Dizzy or near syncope
	Palpitations
>50 years	Nausea
	Upper abdominal pain
	Weakness

The protocol also recommends ECG acquisition for any patient where clinician has concern for a cardiac etiology for their presentation.
ECG, Electrocardiogram; *ED*, emergency department; *STEMI*, ST-elevation myocardial infarction.
Adapted from Wang YC, Chen KW, Tsai BY, et al. Implementation of an all-day artificial intelligence-based triage system to accelerate door-to-balloon times. *Mayo Clin Proc*. 2022;97:2291–2303 and Fakhri Y, Andersson H, Gregg RE, et al. Diagnostic performance of a new ECG algorithm for reducing false positive cases in patients suspected acute coronary syndrome. *J Electrocardiol*. 2021;69:60–64.

An alternative electrode configuration is the Lund system, in which the arm electrodes are placed laterally on the LA and RA at the level of the axillary folds, and the leg electrodes are positioned laterally on the greater femoral trochanters. Similar to the Mason-Likar configuration, this approach mitigates motion artifact from the limbs. The Lund system has been found to more directly approximate the electrocardiographic recordings obtained with conventional positioning compared to the Mason-Likar configuration.[15,21]

If the patient's body habitus or pathologic process precludes placement of a precordial electrode in the ideal location, it can be placed within the radius of the width of one interspace of the recommended position, with appropriate notation on the tracing. If the situation demands further displacement, it is recommended that the lead be omitted, with appropriate documentation on the tracing.[19] Placement of precordial leads on the breast may be preferred by females but also might distort the tracing.[22,23]

Preformatted lead placement is used by some clinicians. The quality of the resultant ECG tracing is excellent, with lower rates of artifact and minimal impact on standard electrocardiographic structures.[24] These preformatted lead placement systems are more expensive, however, as compared to standard lead placement wiring.[25]

Pediatric Electrode Placement

The heart occupies a larger proportion of the chest in a child than an adult and the right ventricle is dominant in children

TABLE 14.3 Prognostic Value of Initial ECG Findings

	HIGH RISK	LOW RISK	+LR (95% CI)
ECG finding	ST elevation[a] ST depression[a] T-wave inversion[a] LVH LBBB Paced	Normal ECG Nonspecific ST/T wave changes Unchanged from prior ECG	
Myocardial infarction	57%	15%	4 (2.6–5.5)
Life-threatening complication	14%	1%	23 (3.2–167)
Mortality	10%	0%	17 (2.3–120)

[a]Changes present in anatomic pattern concerning for ischemia or strain.
+LR, Positive likelihood ratio; *CI*, confidence interval; *ECG*, electrocardiogram; *LBBB*, left bundle branch block; *LVH*, left ventricular hypertrophy.
Data from Fakhri Y, Andersson H, Gregg RE, et al. Diagnostic performance of a new ECG algorithm for reducing false positive cases in patients suspected acute coronary syndrome. *J Electrocardiol*. 2021;69:60–64.

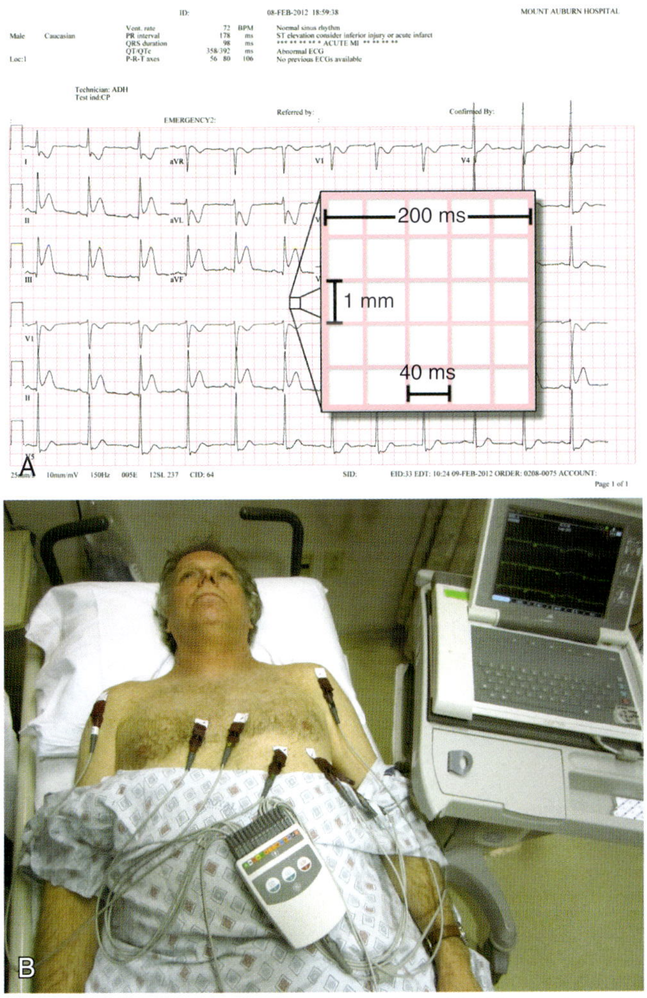

Fig. 14.2 Standard electrocardiographic (ECG) tracing. By convention, the thick lines are 5 mm apart, and the thin lines (barely visible on this reproduction) are 1 mm apart. At the standard paper speed of 25 mm/s, each vertical thin line represents 0.04 seconds (40 ms) and each vertical thick line represents 0.20 seconds (200 ms). The *inset* represents one "big box," which is outlined by thick lines 5 mm apart. (B) Standard 12-lead ECG machine. Note the color coding of the leads.

TABLE 14.4 Conventional Electrodes for the 12-Lead ECG

LOCATION	NOTATION	COLOR
Right arm	RA	White
Left arm	LA	Black
Left leg	LL	Red
Right leg	RL	Green
Precordial leads	V_1	Brown/red
	V_2	Brown/yellow
	V_3	Brown/green
	V_4	Brown/blue
	V_5	Brown/orange
	V_6	Brown/violet

ECG, electrocardiogram.

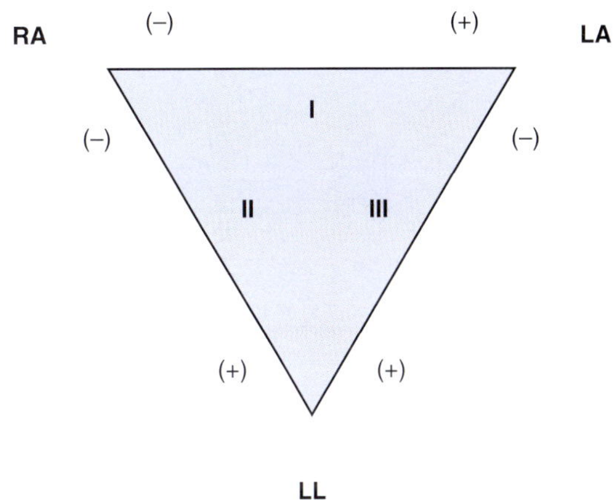

Fig. 14.3 Bipolar limb leads. Leads I, II, and III are shown as a triangle, known as *Einthoven's triangle*. Left arm *(LA)*, right arm *(RA)*, and left leg *(LL)* placement is shown. Orient these bipolar leads so that the positive poles lie inferiorly and to the left (given that the bottom apex of the triangle is directed toward the left leg), as does the major electrical vector of the heart.

under 3 years. Until puberty, additional right-sided leads aid in visualizing the entire heart. Leads V_4R and V_3R are mirror images of their left-sided counterparts (see section on "Additional Leads" later in this chapter). Various guidelines suggest omitting V_3 when V_4R is obtained. In infants less than 1 year of age, an additional electrode, V_7, should be placed in the left posterior axillary line on the same horizontal level as V_4. The chest of an infant may not accommodate all the precordial electrodes; in such cases, the following array is recommended: V_3R or V_4R, V_1, V_3, and V_6. Limb electrode placement is the same as in adults. Distraction with movies, stickers, and bubbles can help minimize artifact from movement in active children.

PREPARATION

Given the potential ramifications of a poorly obtained ECG, the individual performing the ECG should have adequate training and have undergone assessment to ensure they can appropriately obtain an ECG. They should explain their role and explain the purpose and steps of the procedure to the patient. They should inform the patient that it may require a modicum of disrobing but otherwise, there are limited risks, primarily a transient rash at the site of electrode placement. Overall, the test is brief and painless. Informed consent should be obtained and is typically performed verbally. Confirmation of the patient's identity is paramount, including ensuring the identifying information printed on the ECG matches the patient.

Patients should remove any clothing that restricts access to electrode placement and can be covered after electrodes are placed and the leads are attached. If possible, a chaperone should be at bedside with the individual performing the ECG. Patients should be positioned horizontally to 45 degrees with their limbs supported to reduce muscle tension and potential artifact. Acquisition in an upright position may alter ST morphology.[26] The skin may require preparation with cleaning or

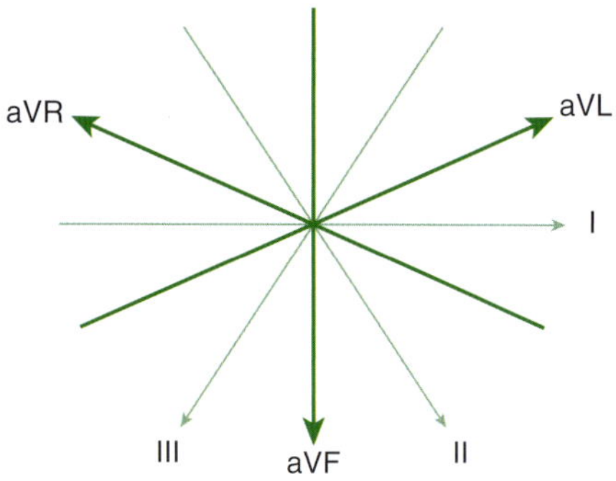

Fig. 14.4 Hexaxial system of limb and augmented leads in the frontal plane. Each lead is separated by 30 degrees in this frontal-plane representation of the limb and augmented leads. Augmented leads, which begin with "a," are shown in bold. *Arrows* denote positive polarity. Note that the inferior leads (II, III, aVF) logically lie at the bottom of this figure and the lateral leads (I, aVL) lie on the left side of the figure, where the lateral aspect of the heart is located if this were superimposed on a patient.

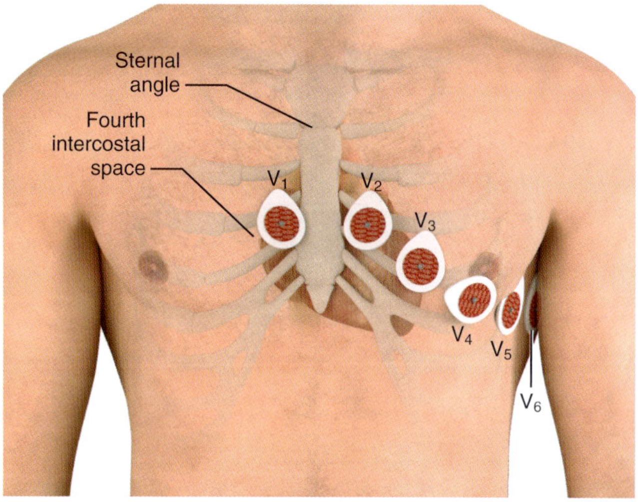

Fig. 14.5 Normal precordial (V_1–V_6) lead placement for the standard 12-lead electrocardiogram. If multiple or repeated electrocardiographic tracings are anticipated, mark the original lead placements on the patient's chest wall or leave stick-on leads in place after the electrocardiographic wires are removed.

shaving of chest hair to ensure adherence of the electrode and mitigate skin to electrode impedance.

FEATURES OF THE ECG

Information Provided by the Computer

In addition to the patient demographic data entered by the operator, the tracing will often feature computations regarding rate, intervals, and axes along the top of the paper. On some tracings, a computer-generated interpretation, or "reading," will also be displayed at the top of the tracing. Unlike the printed ECG reviewed by the clinician that displays only a 2.5-second sample of each lead, the computer has access to the full 10 seconds of each lead. Most computer programs craft a representative wave for each lead by creating a median wave from all visualized beats. In contrast, a clinician tends to review each beat individually and determine if it is relevant. Unlike clinicians, the computer typically does not incorporate

TABLE 14.5 Common Errors Associated With Computer Interpretation of ECGs

CHALLENGE	COMPUTER MISINTERPRETATION
Recognizing pacemaker spikes	Infarction, bundle branch block, conduction delay
Identifying P waves	Atrial fibrillation, missed AV block
Distinguishing T waves from P waves	Double counting the heart rate
Accurately determining end of T wave	QT prolongation
Appreciating early repolarization or pericarditis	STEMI

AV, Atrioventricular; *ECG*, electrocardiogram; *STEMI*, ST-elevation myocardial infarction.

corroborating evidence, including age, sex, and prior ECGs. Finally, the computer program also struggles with improperly obtained ECGs, as it often cannot recognize limb lead reversal.

As a result, computer interpretations are incorrect in approximately 10% of ECGs, including clinically significant misinterpretations.[27] The computer often misses more subtle findings suggestive of dysrhythmias or MIs (Table14.5).[28,29] For example, the computer often struggles to detect low amplitude or morphologically distinct P waves that may be obscured by T waves or baseline artifact leading to an incorrect interpretation of atrial fibrillation. Alternatively, when baseline artifact is construed as P waves, the computer might interpret an ECG as atrial fibrillation when the patient is in fact in sinus rhythm.[30] The computer may also miss atrioventricular (AV) block, as it misses P waves obscured by ST segments or T waves. Computer interpretations tend to overestimate the QT interval by 30 to 40 ms due to difficulty identifying the termination of flat T waves. Interestingly the computer also might miss a prolonged QT interval in nearly half of patients.[31] As pacemakers have evolved to reduce their electrical voltage in order to reduce the battery load, pacemaker spikes have gotten smaller and harder for computers to detect. This may lead to misinterpretation of a pacemaker rhythm as a left bundle branch block or infarction. Finally, the computer also often struggles with MI, with the frequency of false-positive interpretation varying from 0% to 42% and false-negative from 22% to 42%.[32] The computer often misconstrues ST-segment elevations resulting from early repolarization, pericarditis, or bundle branch blocks as representing infarction. Interestingly, novel artificial intelligence programs have shown promise, e.g., in recognizing early repolarization[33] and identifying signs of atrial fibrillation, including in patients presenting in sinus rhythm.[34]

Regardless of the computer program, currently there is a sufficiently high frequency of computer misinterpretation that all ECGs should also be over-read by an experienced clinician. Per AHA guidelines, this includes clinician interpretation prior to initiation of a STEMI protocol.[35] The properly trained and experienced clinician provides more accurate

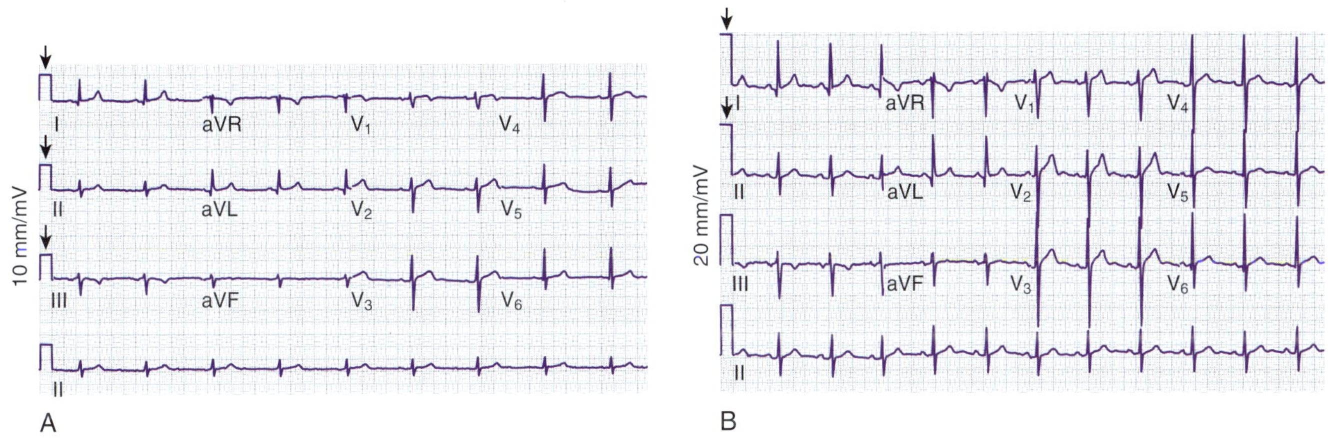

Fig. 14.6 (A) Normal 10-mm/mV calibration. Note the box-shaped mark to the left of the complexes *(arrows)*; this is a graphic representation of the calibration for the tracing. Routinely note this parameter before interpretation of the electrocardiogram (ECG). Note the change in part B. (B) Abnormal 20-mm/mV calibration. The calibration in this tracing was (inexplicably and unexpectedly) changed to 20 mm/mV by the computer, not by the operator. When compared with a baseline ECG it appeared that voltage criteria had developed for left ventricular hypertrophy and ST-segment elevation. A was recorded minutes later with correction of calibration to the standard 10 mm/mV and was unchanged from baseline tracings.

electrocardiographic interpretation, as compared with the machine's computer algorithm.

Adjustable Features

A notation of electrocardiographic paper speed (in millimeters per second), calibration (in millimeters per millivolt), and the frequency response (in hertz) is displayed, usually in the left lower corner of the recording. *Paper speed* is usually set at a default of 25 mm/s such that one ECG page will show 10 seconds of the cardiac cycle. It may be manipulated for purposes of deciphering a dysrhythmia, as described later (see section on "Alteration in Amplitude and Paper Speed").

Calibration, or standardization, refers to the voltage/amplitude of the waveforms on the tracing. It is usually set at a default value of 10 mm/mV and is graphically depicted by a plateau-shaped waveform that appears at the extreme left side of the tracing, in front of the first complex (Fig. 14.6A). This calibration can be modified by the operator or by the computer itself, as was the case in Fig. 14.6B, in which the patient appeared to have acquired voltage criteria for left ventricular hypertrophy when in reality the tracing was unchanged from his baseline (see Fig. 14.6A). Increasing the calibration to 20 mm/mV will increase the size of the complexes and is helpful when trying to decipher P-wave morphology (Fig. 14.7). Decreasing the calibration to 5 mm/mV is helpful in cases in which the amplitude of the QRS complex (usually in the precordial leads) is so large that it encroaches on those of adjacent leads. If unintended and unrecognized, reducing the calibration voltage can lead to concern for a pericardial effusion based on the low amplitudes.

Increasing the paper speed to double the standard to 50 mm/s has the effect of artificially slowing the rhythm. Each box on the ECG then represents 20 ms instead of 40 ms. This technique is most advantageous when assessing patients with marked atrial or ventricular tachycardia. Increasing the paper speed exaggerates any existing irregularity (such as in atrial fibrillation) and can improve recognition of smaller deflections, such as P waves, in the presence of a significant tachycardia. Faster paper speeds also make it possible to measure short electrocardiographic intervals (such as PR or R-R) more accurately (Fig. 14.8). Diagnostic accuracy of narrow-complex tachycardias improves when clinicians analyze ECGs recorded at the faster 50 mm/s paper speed, as opposed to a standard 12-lead ECG.[36] Waveforms will appear prolonged at the higher paper speed and thus could lead to inaccurate diagnosis of atrial enlargement, AV block, bundle branch block, or a prolonged QT interval.

ADDITIONAL ELECTROCARDIOGRAPHIC LEADS

While not necessary for all patients undergoing ECG, additional ECG leads may be used in the evaluation of a patient with possible ACS. These leads can be considered in a patient with a presentation consistent with ACS yet demonstrating an unrevealing or nondiagnostic 12-lead ECG. These additional leads include posterior leads (V_7, V_8, and V_9), right ventricular leads (especially V_4R), and procedural leads (transvenous pacemaker wire placement and pericardiocentesis). They are particularly useful in detecting right ventricular and posterior MIs, as the standard 12-lead ECG does not assess these areas directly, producing delays in diagnosis and potential reperfusion.[37] The standard ECG coupled with the posterior leads constitutes the 15-lead ECG.

Posterior and Right Ventricular Leads

Several different investigations have explored the use of the 15-lead ECG incorporating posterior and right-sided electrodes.[38–40] In a study of all ED patients with chest pain, Brady and associates[40] reported that the 15-lead ECG provided a more accurate description of myocardial injury in patients with AMI, yet failed to alter rates of diagnosis or use of reperfusion therapies or to change disposition locations. In contrast, a recent observational study of patients with chest pain undergoing 15-lead ECG found in 15% of cases the MI was detected only with the additional leads.

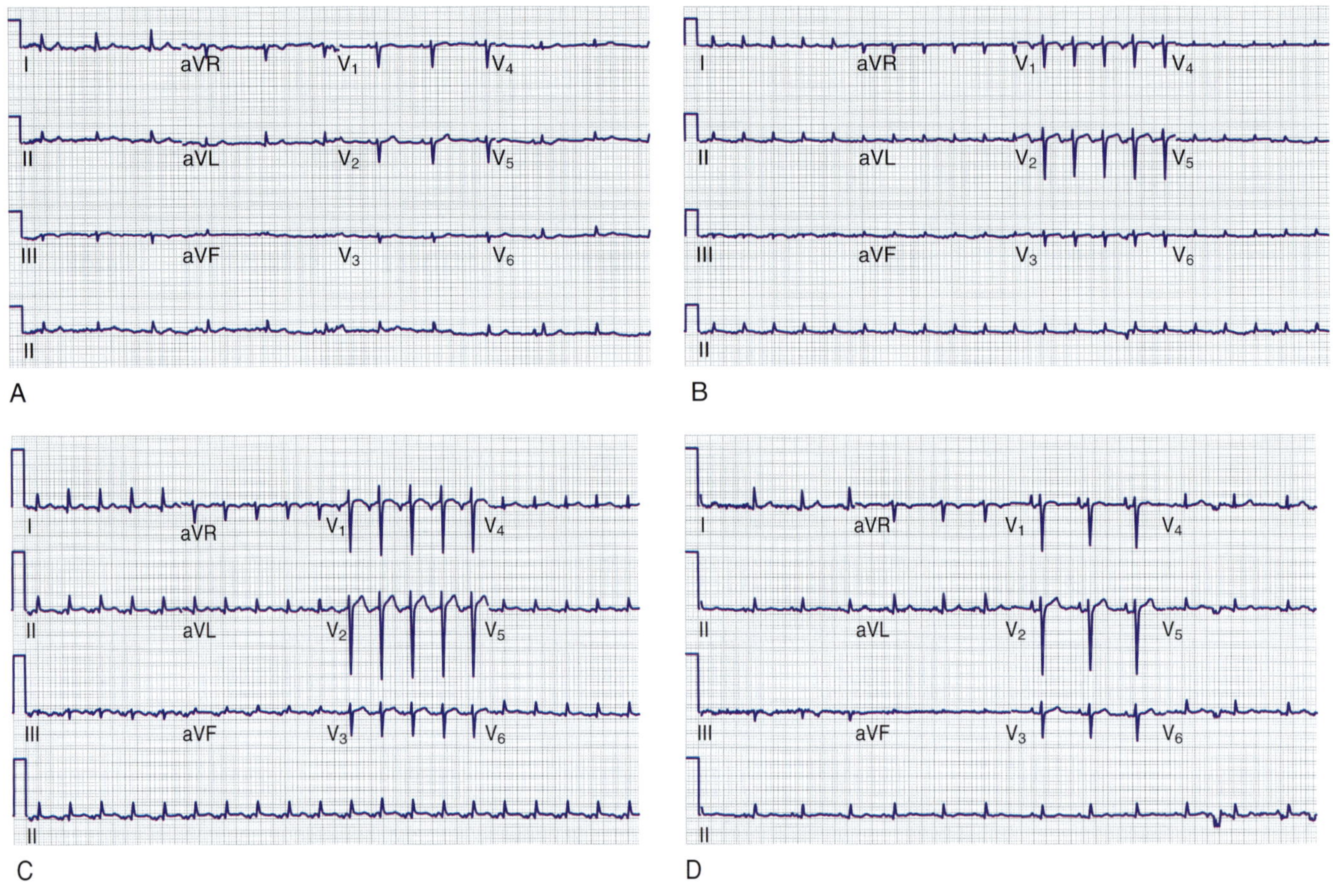

Fig. 14.7 (A) Baseline electrocardiogram (ECG) of a patient before the development of an abnormal rhythm (10 mm/mV). Note the P-wave morphologies, especially in leads I, II, and V_1. (B) ECG during ectopic atrial tachycardia (10 mm/mV). Note the change in P-wave morphology, especially in lead V_1. (C) ECG during ectopic atrial tachycardia (20 mm/mV). The P waves are now easier to see in all leads. (D) ECG after reversion to a normal atrial focus (20 mm/mV). Contrast these accentuated P waves with those in part C.

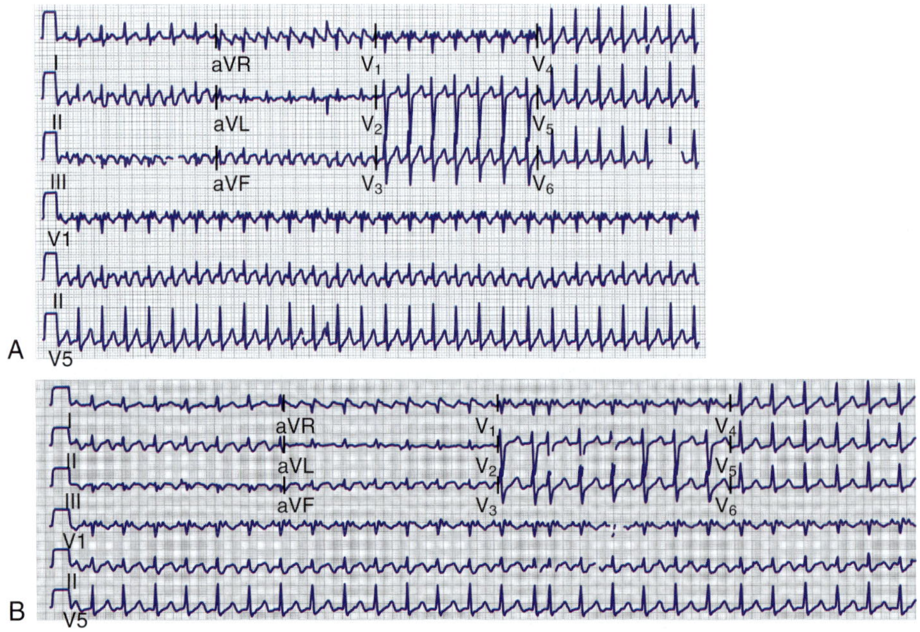

Fig. 14.8 (A) Electrocardiogram (ECG) with tachycardia at normal paper speed (25 mm/s). Because of the rapid rate, the actual P waves are difficult to discern, thus making determination of the rhythm difficult. The computerized interpretation is sinus tachycardia with a first-degree atrioventricular (AV) block. (B) ECG with tachycardia at double paper speed (50 mm/s). With increased paper speed, atrial P-wave activity is accentuated, and atrial flutter with a 2:1 AV block is demonstrated. Carotid sinus massage may have slowed the rhythm and also revealed P waves.

This detection led to initiation of reperfusion therapy.[41] In the diagnosis of posterior AMI, leads V_8 and V_9 are superior to reliance on detecting the reciprocal ST-segment depression seen in leads V_1 to V_3. Potential indications for 15-lead ECGs in patients with suspected ACS are outlined in Table 14.6.

The posterior electrodes V_8 and V_9 are placed on the patient's back in the same horizontal plane as V_6; V_8 is placed at the tip of the left scapula and V_9 in an intermediate position between lead V_8 and the left paraspinal muscles. An additional electrode, V_7, may also be used and is placed on the posterior axillary line equidistant from electrode V_8 (Fig. 14.9). The degree of ST-segment elevation in the posterior leads is often less pronounced than the ST-segment elevation seen in the standard 12 leads in patients with STEMI. This diminution in posterior lead ST-segment elevation results from both the relatively greater distance of these leads from the posterior surface of the heart and the presence of air and soft tissue between the epicardium and the electrocardiographic electrodes. It has been suggested that the threshold criterion for intervention be lowered from the standard 1 mm of ST-segment elevation to 0.5 mm when evaluating the posterior leads for STEMI.[42]

The right ventricular electrocardiographic electrodes are placed across the right side of the chest in a mirror image of the standard left-sided electrodes and are labeled V_1R to V_6R; alternatively, RV_1 to RV_6 is another commonly used nomenclature for this electrode distribution (Fig.14.10). Lead V_4R (right fifth intercostal space, midclavicular line) is the most useful lead for detecting ST-segment elevation associated with right ventricular infarction and may be used solely for the evaluation of possible right ventricular infarction. The ST-segment elevation that occurs in association with right ventricular infarction is frequently quite subtle because of the relatively small muscle mass of the right ventricle; at other times the ST-segment elevation is quite prominent, similar in appearance to the ST-segment changes seen with the standard 12 leads (Fig. 14.11). Depending on the ECG computer, it will be important to label any 12-lead ECG with alternative leads (particularly RV leads) as such to avoid any confusion in terms of interpretation at that time or comparison in the future.

TABLE 14.6 Potential Indications for Posterior or Right Ventricular Electrodes

Posterior leads	ST-segment depressions in V_1–V_3; may be deep (>2 mm) and flat/horizontal
	Prominent R waves in V_1–V_3 (>30 ms)
	Upright T waves in V_1–V_3
	R wave larger than S wave in V_2–V_3
Right-sided leads	ST-segment elevation inferiorly
	ST-segment elevation in III > II
	ST-segment elevation in V_1
	ST depression in V_2 or V_3

Invasive Procedural Leads for Pacing or Pericardiocentesis

Patients with severely compromising bradydysrhythmia may require a transvenous pacemaker. In such instances, it may be necessary to place the pacing wire without the benefit of fluoroscopy. The recommendation is to advance the wire under electrocardiographic guidance with the patient connected to the limb leads of a grounded electrocardiographic machine and the pacing wire connected to the V lead (see Chapter 15). As the electrode enters the superior vena cava and high right atrium, the P wave and QRS complex will be negative. While traversing the atrium, the P wave and QRS complex

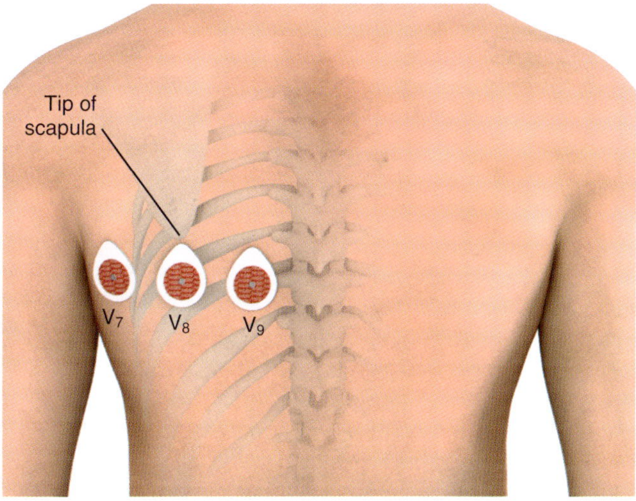

Fig. 14.9 Posterior lead placement. Place leads V_7, V_8, and V_9 on the same horizontal plane as V_6, with V_7 at the posterior axillary line, V_8 at the tip of the left scapula, and V_9 near the border of the left paraspinal muscles.

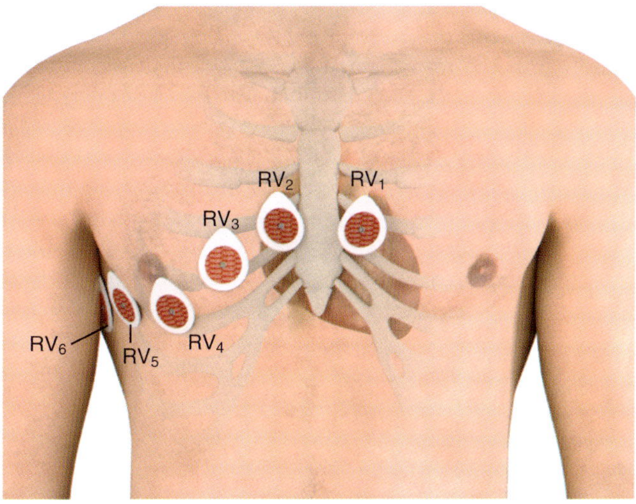

Fig. 14.10 Right-sided lead placement. Place right-sided leads V_1R to V_6R on the chest as a mirror image of the standard precordial leads. This alteration in lead placement is used to investigate the possibility of a right-sided acute myocardial infarction that may not be appreciated with normal lead placement.

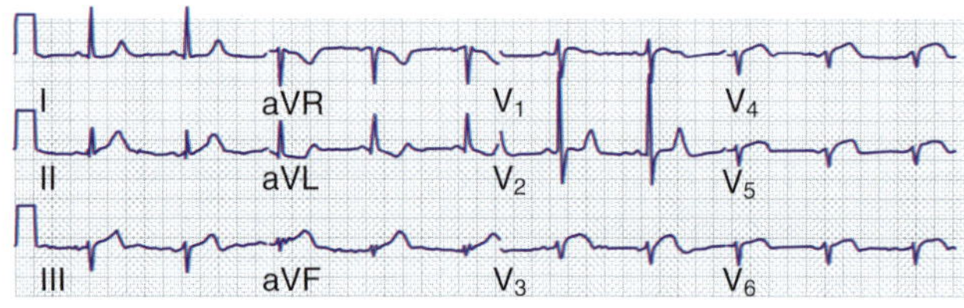

Fig. 14.11 Right-sided precordial leads. This alteration in lead placement is used to investigate the possibility of a right-sided acute myocardial infarction (MI) that may not be appreciated with normal lead placement. This tracing displays the right-sided precordial leads in an elderly male with chest pain, and they are consistent with acute coronary syndrome. There is ST-segment elevation that is somewhat subtle in the inferior leads (II, III, and aVF), which together with the reciprocal ST-segment depression seen in lead aVL is consistent with a diagnosis of acute inferior MI. Leads V_1 to V_6 are in actuality leads V_1R to V_6R—right-sided precordial leads. The convex upward ST-segment elevation seen in leads V_3R to V_6R is indicative of concomitant right ventricular infarction. This patient was found to have a subtotal proximal occlusive lesion of his right coronary artery at cardiac catheterization.

will become positive, and the latter will become larger as the ventricle is approached. If a balloon-tipped flotation catheter is used, deflate the balloon once it is in the right ventricle. Next, advance it until contact is made with the endocardium and the ventricle is captured. Ventricular wall contact will be indicated by marked ST-segment elevation. (see Chapter 15 for additional information on this procedure).

For patients undergoing urgent pericardiocentesis, an electrocardiographic lead may be placed on the syringe needle to aid in correct positioning of the catheter in the pericardial space through monitoring of the ST segments while the needle is inserted. A sudden appearance of ST-segment elevation indicates that the needle has moved too far internally (i.e., beyond the pericardial space) and has contacted the epicardium. (See Chapter 16 for additional information on this procedure.) Notably, bedside ultrasound guidance has largely supplanted electrocardiographic assisted placement and is associated with less complications.

PREHOSPITAL ECG

Early treatment, primarily reperfusion therapy, is an important goal in the management of ACS, particularly STEMI. Early treatment is made possible by early STEMI diagnosis, which is achieved by prompt application of the diagnostic tools, namely the 12-lead ECG. The AHA recommends early acquisition of prehospital ECGs. Emergency medical services (EMS) have systems and strategies that optimize STEMI care including early application of the ECG (and potentially electronic transmission of the ECG to the hospital prior to arrival), which has been shown to reduce the time to initiation of reperfusion therapy.[35] The prehospital ECG can also impact EMS management, allowing selection of appropriate therapies, transport modality, and destination facility.

Many studies have demonstrated benefits of prehospital ECGs in decreasing door-to-fibrinolytic treatment and door-to-percutaneous coronary intervention (PCI) times in patients with STEMI.[43,44] Other studies have shown even further reductions in time to revascularization when cardiac catheterization laboratories are activated prior to patient arrival at the hospital with various protocols recommending transport directly to the catheterization lab (Fig. 14.1).[43–45]

The early acquisition, interpretation, and transmission of a prehospital ECG can dramatically decrease the time to treatment for a patient with ACS, particularly STEMI. Importantly, this reduction in time to management is seen in urban, suburban, and rural settings, regardless of the transport time or type of reperfusion strategy selected for the particular patient. Notably, prehospital activation of hospital resources for the treatment of a potential STEMI intermittently (11% to 16% of cases) results in inappropriate activation and marshaling of resources. This inappropriate prehospital activation most commonly arises from misinterpretation of the ECG, typically from STEMI mimics.[46,47] Interpretation of the ECG and confirmation of the need for activation of resources to manage the STEMI by a physician may reduce the frequency of false-positive activations and improve mortality.[46]

The minimal prolongation in EMS scene time arising from ECG acquisition is acceptable considering the vital information provided by the ECG and its impact on overall time-to-therapy considerations. The prehospital ECG can be obtained within as little as 2 to 3 minutes; furthermore, it can be obtained while en route to the hospital. The significant reduction in time to definitive therapy for STEMI compensates for any small transport delay.

ALTERNATIVE TECHNIQUES FOR ASSESSMENT OF RHYTHM

Electrocardiographic rhythm assessment depends on a clear signal of both atrial and ventricular electrical activity over a period. Although continuous 12-lead electrocardiographic rhythm monitoring has the advantage of recording cardiac activity over multiple leads (thus maximizing atrial and ventricular monitoring), it is often impractical. Acquisition of a standard 12-lead ECG often fails to detect the abnormal rhythm. For example, screening with a 12-lead ECG for detection of atrial fibrillation is not superior to pulse palpation.

Identification of the cardiac rhythm on an ECG can be difficult in some clinical settings. Rapid atrial or ventricular rates, especially those above 150 beats/min, often lead to simultaneous or nearly simultaneous deflections that can alter the usual waveforms or cause smaller deflections to be buried within larger ones (such as P waves buried within the QRS complex). In addition, rapid rates result in smaller, narrower waveforms, which makes visual recognition on the ECG challenging. Finally, assessment of atrial activity in general is more difficult because of the smaller electrical impulse and resulting electrocardiographic waveform generated by the atria.

Lead V_1 is generally considered the most appropriate lead for detecting the P wave, followed by lead II. In a study of 62 measurements in 28 patients, lead V_1 demonstrated the tallest P wave 53% of the time, followed by lead II (29%), lead I (7%), and lead III (3%).[48] A number of alternative techniques have been developed to improve assessment of rhythm, including alterations in the standard 12-lead ECG, as well as the addition of nonstandard leads to monitor cardiac and, in particular, atrial rhythm activity.

Alternative Leads

Assessment of rhythm often requires electrocardiographic monitoring over a longer and continuous period, and the 12-lead ECG might miss dysrhythmias. A number of alternative

TABLE 14.7 Alternative Leads for Assessment of Rhythm

Lead I[a]	RA = negative electrode	LA = positive electrode
Lead II[a]	RA = negative electrode	LL = positive electrode
Lead III[a]	LA = negative electrode	LL = positive electrode
Alternative lead	Negative electrode position	Positive electrode position
Lewis[b]	Right second costochondral junction	Right fourth intercostal space, 1 inch right of the sternum
Drury	Second right costochondral junction, center of the sternum	Seventh right costal cartilage, inferior angle of the scapula 2 inches right of the spine
Schoenwald	Third intercostal space along the right sternal border, third intercostal space along the R sternal border	Left leg, right arm
Lu	First intercostal space directly above V_1	Approximately 3 inches directly below V_4
Vertical sternal ("Barker leads")	Below the suprasternal notch at the manubrium	Xiphoid process
MCL_1	Left shoulder (1 cm inferior to the left midclavicle)	V_1 (fourth intercostal space, right sternal border)
MCL_6	Left shoulder (1 cm inferior to the left midclavicle)	V_6 (≈sixth rib, midaxillary line)

[a]First, set the electrocardiographic machine to record the rhythm strip with this lead. If the recording rhythm strip is lead I, the RA wire becomes the negative electrode, which is placed as noted in the table, and the LA wire becomes the positive electrode, which is placed as noted in the table. If lead II or lead III is the lead that is set to record the rhythm strip, the positive and negative electrodes will vary.
[b]Example: One way to record the Lewis lead is to set the electrocardiographic machine to record lead I, use the RA wire as the negative electrode, and place it in the right second costochondral junction. Use the LA wire as the positive electrode and place it in the right fourth intercostal space, 1 inch to the right of the sternum. The Lewis lead may also be recorded on lead II and lead III, but the wires that serve as the positive and negative electrodes will vary.
LA, Left arm; *LL*, left leg; *RA*, right arm; *RL*, right leg.

lead systems requiring fewer electrodes have been described that allow for improved assessment of rhythm. Many of these systems use the limb bipolar leads (RA, LA, LL) in alternative positions over the chest. Leads I, II, or III are then recorded depending on the positions of the positive and negative electrodes. Although various alternative leads provide additional information to the clinician, there are no standard guidelines mandating the use of any alternative leads in the ED. They are more commonly utilized outside of the ED.

Alternative positioning of leads may enhance detection of dysrhythmias (Table 14.7 and Fig. 14.12). With Lewis leads, the RA lead is placed over the right second costochondral junction, whereas the LL lead is placed in the right fourth intercostal space 1 inch to the right of the sternum, with the LA and RL leads left in their usual positions. It is particularly helpful in identifying P waves during wide-complex tachycardias.

Alternatively, with the vertical sternal "Barker" lead configuration, the positive electrode (i.e., LL) is placed at the xiphoid process and the negative electrode (i.e., RA) is placed just below the suprasternal notch on the manubrium. This may produce a larger P wave (in lead II as shown in Table 14.7) than other lead configurations. In addition, the vertical sternal electrodes are placed over bone, which may reduce artifact caused by muscle activity on recordings (see Fig. 14.12).

With limb-precordium leads, a sequential pattern of bipolar leads are placed on the chest in combination with the original

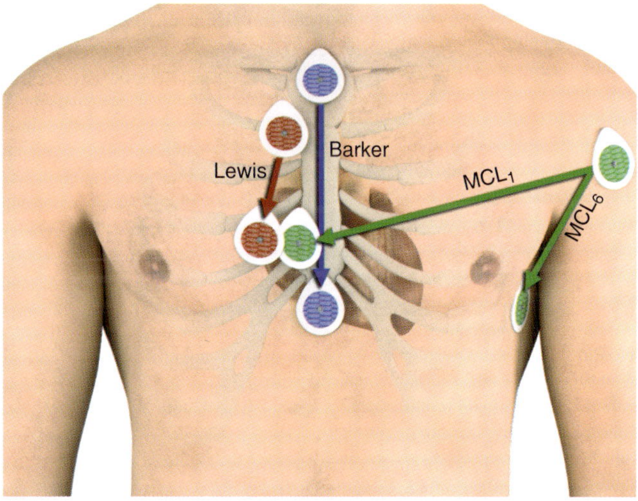

Fig. 14.12 Alternative leads. Three of the more commonly used alternative lead strategies for clarification of the atrial rhythm (Lewis leads *[red]*, vertical sternal or Barker leads *[blue]*, and modified bipolar chest lead 1 *[MCL_1]*) and monitoring of the ST-T wave *(MCL_6)* are shown. For the Lewis leads, designed to further evaluate for atrial fibrillation, the right arm lead was placed over the right second costochondral junction, whereas the left leg lead was placed in the right fourth intercostal space 1 inch to the right of the sternum, with the left arm and right leg leads left in their usual positions. See text for further explanation of other leads.

Einthoven limb leads. In this system, standard limb leads are placed on the patient. The RA electrode is then repositioned sequentially at the fourth intercostal space just to the right of the sternum, the fourth intercostal space just to the left of the sternum (low parasternal), the first intercostal space just to the left of the sternum, and the first intercostal space just to the right of the sternum (high parasternal). During this sequential mapping, tracings are recorded for leads I and II until atrial activity is identified.

Modified bipolar chest leads (MCLs) are the most commonly used leads for monitoring cardiac rhythm (i.e., telemetry). The positive electrode is placed on the chest at a precordial position (V) concordant with the MCL desired (e.g., the V_1 position for MCL_1). The negative electrode is placed on the left shoulder. On standard electrocardiographic machines, the LA electrode is placed at V_1, RA at the left shoulder, LL at V_6, and RL at a remote location on the chest to serve as ground. Lead I would then reflect MCL_1 and lead II, MCL_6. MCL_1 may be useful in distinguishing atrial activity; MCL_5 and MCL_6 more commonly in monitoring of the ST-T wave; and both MCL_1 and MCL_6 in evaluating wide-complex tachycardias (see Fig. 14.12).[49]

Esophageal Leads

Both unipolar and bipolar esophageal leads have been developed. The electrode, which is connected to the ECG by thin wires, is either swallowed or passed through the nares into the esophagus. Once in the esophagus, the location of the electrode is determined either by fluoroscopy or by making a series of low to high esophageal recordings. The position of the electrode in the esophagus is adjusted by slowly pulling the electrode wire out the nares or mouth. In normal adults, leads E_{15-25} (the electrode is located in the esophagus 15 to 25 cm from the nares) generally records atrial activity; E_{25-35}, activity of the AV groove; and E_{40-50}, activity of the left ventricular posterior surface. The esophageal lead should be recorded through lead channel I simultaneously with lead channel II and the other surface channels. Because of its posterior location, this lead is often superior in detecting atrial deflections and recording the activity of the posterior surface of the left ventricle.

Smartwatches

Over the last decade, wearable devices, such as smartwatches, have become commonplace. While many watches rely on a photoplethysmography signal to detect irregular pulses, technology has advanced to allow many to record real-time single-channel electrocardiograms. Most smartwatches employ an opportunistic, intermittent sampling strategy rather than continuously monitoring the pulse. In a study of over 400,000 patients, when the smartwatch reported an irregular pulse, slightly over one-third of these patients had atrial fibrillation on a subsequent ECG patch recording.[50] Notably, the absence of atrial fibrillation on their subsequent patch recording did not necessarily mean the smartwatch finding was erroneous, as atrial fibrillation is often paroxysmal. When the patient had an ECG patch in place at the time of the reported irregular pulse from their smartwatch, there was concordance of 84% between the smartwatch and ECG patch. While the study was not designed to assess sensitivity, the smartwatch detected atrial fibrillation in only 56% of patients who identified it with other modalities. Smartwatches perform similarly in the detection of other

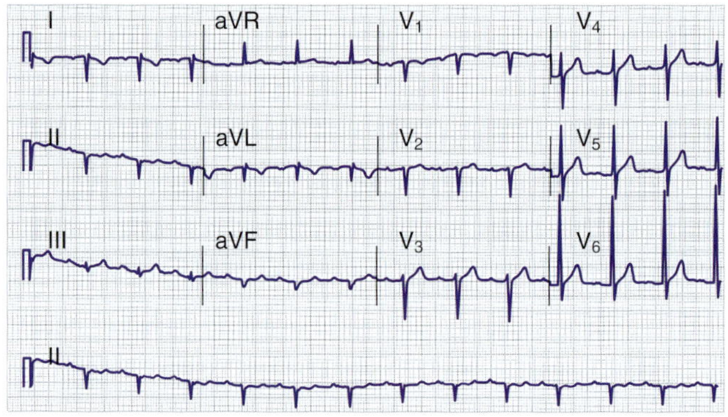

Fig. 14.13 Arm electrode reversal (left arm ↔ right arm). The most common of limb electrode reversals, the clues lie in leads I and aVR. Lead I features a negative P wave, as well as a principally negative QRS complex and T wave. This could suggest dextrocardia, but the precordial leads demonstrate a normal transition, which is not consistent with dextrocardia. Note also the unusual appearance of aVR in this tracing.

arrhythmias. In the future, smartwatches may also be able to detect myocardial ischemia; a small study showed high concordance between a multiple-channel ECG obtained via a smartwatch and standard ECG for ST-segment elevations and nonspecific ECG findings.[51]

ELECTRODE MISPLACEMENT AND MISCONNECTION

Limb Electrode Reversal

Although the limb electrodes are not often misplaced, the cables that link them to the ECG are at times improperly connected, resulting in artifact that appears as false-positive "electrocardiographic changes." A multitude of possibilities for misconnection of the limb electrodes exists; the most likely are summarized below. Many are recognizable without comparison to an old ECG, while others require comparison. The incidence of electrode reversal in the ED has not been quantified, but it has been observed to occur in an intensive care unit setting in 4% to 5% of tracings.[52,53]

Easily Recognizable Without an Old ECG

The most common of all misconnections is reversal of the LA and RA electrodes[49] (Fig. 14.13). The hallmark is a negative P wave and a primarily negative QRS complex in lead I and potentially also in aVL, which creates a right or extreme axis deviation (depending on the principal vector of the QRS complex in lead aVF).

Dextrocardia or situs inversus is also possible with negative P waves and Q waves in leads I and aVL. However, with dextrocardia, there will be progressive diminution in QRS amplitude as the eye moves from lead V_1 (right sided) toward lead V_6 (left sided). Moreover, lead aVR is actually aVL in this circumstance, and thus lead aVR may feature both an upright P wave and QRS complex; the former does not occur in normal sinus rhythm, and the latter is clinically unusual as the QRS vectors in leads aVR and V_6 are usually opposite unless the heart has a superior frontal-plane axis.[43]

A further clue to arm electrode reversal is the resultant discrepancy in the major QRS vectors of leads I and V_6. Because the vectors of these two leads are leftward, the QRS complexes are expected to point in similar directions when the ECG is performed properly. These two leads will feature discordant QRS vectors when the arm electrodes are reversed (see Fig. 14.13). A prominent Q wave in lead I could also represent an infarct of the superior aspect of the left ventricular wall. However, in contrast to limb reversal, P waves in lead I remain upright.

Transposition of the RA and LL cables is also easily recognized; all leads are flipped in comparison to the usual patterns with the exception of aVL, which is unchanged.[54,55] Anytime that the RL electrode is transposed with another extremity lead, one of the limb leads will appear isoelectric as virtually a straight line. This might be misattributed to a disconnected electrode; however, such a disconnection would impact all leads using this electrode, not just one lead. The most common example is RA/RL reversal, which causes a nearly flat line in lead II (Fig. 14.14). An exception to this rule is if the leg electrodes are reversed (RL ↔ LL), in which case the ECG is virtually identical to one with correct placement of the limb electrodes. Reversal of the leg electrodes is largely insignificant in that the potentials at the LL and RL are essentially the same.

Not Easily Recognizable Without an Old ECG

One limb electrode reversal that is not readily recognizable without comparison to a previous tracing is transposition of the LA and LL electrodes. This causes transposition of lead I with lead II on the tracing in addition to lead aVL with aVF. In effect, two inferior leads (II and aVF) have become the lateral leads (I and aVL) and vice versa, thus making this misconnection difficult to detect at times without a baseline ECG for comparison. Furthermore, lead III will be upside down

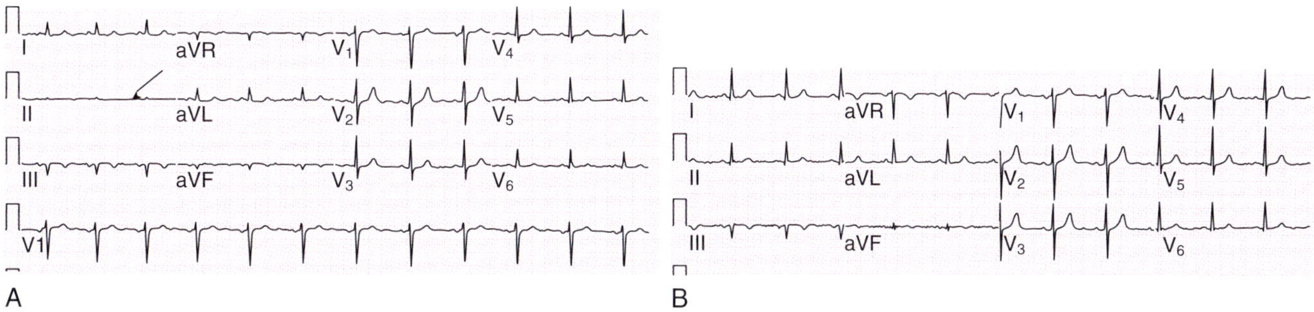

Fig. 14.14 Right-sided electrode reversal (right arm ↔ right leg). (A) In this tracing, the nearly flat line in lead II *(arrow)* suggests that the right leg electrode has been switched with the right arm electrode. The trivial voltage in lead II reflects the expected lack of potential difference between the two legs (the right leg electrode is in the right arm position; lead II normally runs from the right arm to the left leg, but now it effectively runs from the right leg to the left leg). (B) The second tracing was acquired with correct electrode placement.

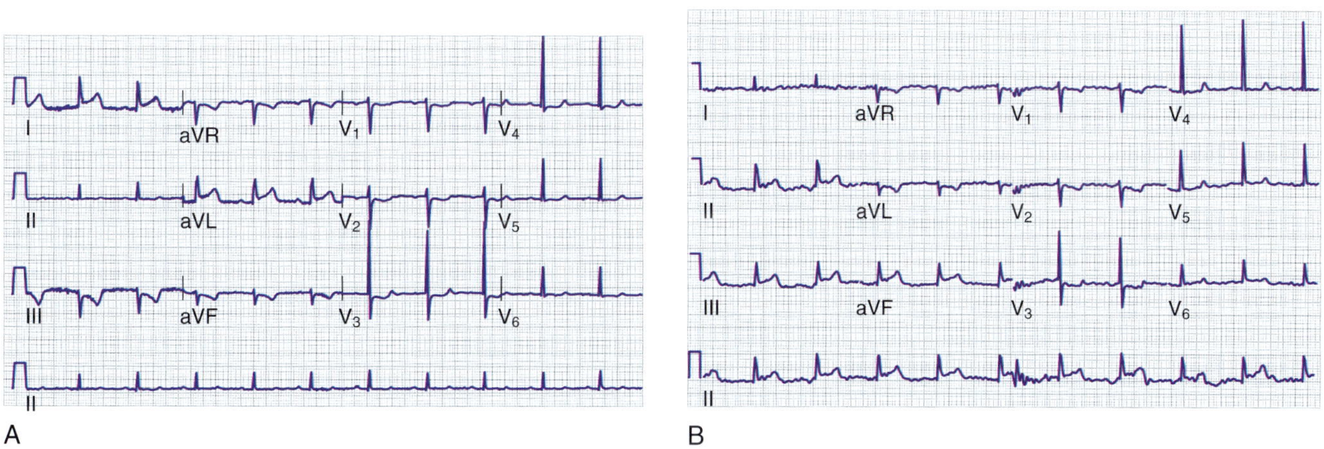

Fig. 14.15 (A) Left-sided limb electrode reversal (left arm [LA] ↔ left leg [LL]). A patient with a history consistent with acute coronary syndrome was brought to the emergency department after this electrocardiogram was recorded in a clinic. Leads I and aVL suggest an acute high lateral infarction, but surprisingly there are no corresponding changes in leads V_5 and V_6. The deep T-wave inversions in III and aVF were at first thought to be inferior ischemia or reciprocal changes (see also B). (B) Correction of electrode reversal (LA ↔ LL). After the electrodes were reconnected, this tracing reveals an acute inferior wall myocardial infarction (MI) and deep T-wave inversion in aVL, a harbinger of acute inferior MI. In comparing this tracing with that in part A note the following: lead I ↔ lead II, lead aVL ↔ aVF, and lead III is inverted. Thus inferior changes become lateral, and lateral changes become inferior, the hallmark of LA ↔ LL reversal.

(although a negative QRS complex in lead III is not unusual), and aVR will be unchanged (Fig. 14.15). Suspect LA/LL reversal when comparing two ECGs with changes that do not make clinical sense; if the P-QRS-T-wave morphologies in lead III in the two tracings are mirror opposites, repeat the ECG with close attention to correct electrode connection. Clues to limb electrode reversal are summarized in Table14.8.

Precordial Electrode Misplacement and Misconnection

Unlike the limb electrodes, the precordial electrodes are more prone to misplacement, especially when variations in body habitus (e.g., obesity, breast tissue, pectus excavatum, chronic lung disease) make proper electrode placement more difficult. This may cause some variability in the amplitude and morphology of the complexes in the precordial leads. However, these changes are not usually grossly abnormal and therefore can be difficult to detect. Variation often becomes evident when comparing the current tracing with an old ECG. In such cases, it is useful to go to the bedside and examine where the electrodes were positioned relative to the recommended placement (see section on "Electrode Placement" earlier in this chapter). One cannot ensure, however, that the baseline ECG was done with proper electrode placement. When comparing the precordial leads on the current ECG with a baseline tracing, ST-segment and T-wave changes should be viewed in the context of the relative morphologies of the associated QRS complexes. If a marked difference is noted between the two tracings in the amplitude or polarity of the QRS complex in a given precordial lead—the R/S ratio for that QRS complex—the corresponding ST-T-wave changes may be the result of variability in electrode placement, although cardiac ischemia cannot be completely excluded as the cause.

Misconnection of the precordial cables is usually easy to detect. The expected progression of P-, QRS-, and T-wave morphologies across the precordium will be disrupted (Fig. 14.16). An abrupt change in wave morphology evolution—followed by a seeming return to normalcy in the next lead—is a good clue to misconnection of the precordial electrodes.

TABLE 14.8 Clues to Improper Limb Electrode Connections[57]

REVERSED LEADS	NEED OLD ECG FOR DETECTION?	KEY FINDINGS
LA ↔ RA	No	P-QRS-T waves upside down in lead I precordial leads normal (not dextrocardia)
LA ↔ LL	Yes	III upside down from baseline I ↔ II, aVL ↔ aVF, no change in aVR
LA ↔ RL	No	III is a straight line
RA ↔ LL	No	P-QRS-T waves upside down in all leads except aVL
RA ↔ RL	No	II is a straight line
LL ↔ RL	Cannot detect change	Looks like normal electrode placement
LA ↔ LL + RA ↔ RL	No	I is a straight line, aVL and aVR are the same polarity and amplitude, and II is upside down III

LA, Left arm; *LL*, left leg; *RA*, right arm; *RL*, right leg.

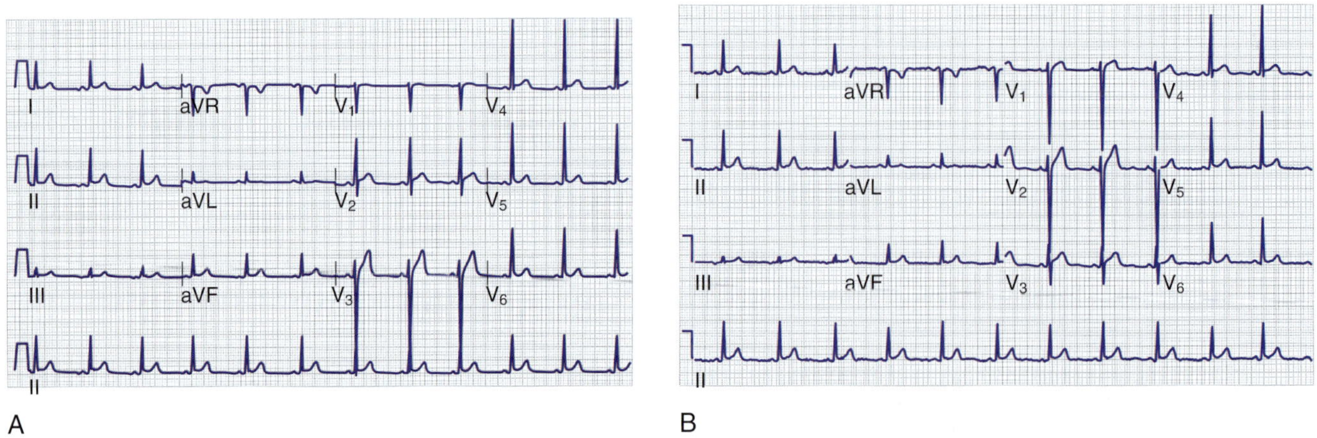

Fig. 14.16 (A and B) Precordial electrode reversal ($V_2 \leftrightarrow V_3$). Note that the usual precordial progression of R-wave growth in leads V_2 and V_3 is disrupted in the tracing displayed in part A. (B) Return to a normal V_3 transition zone.

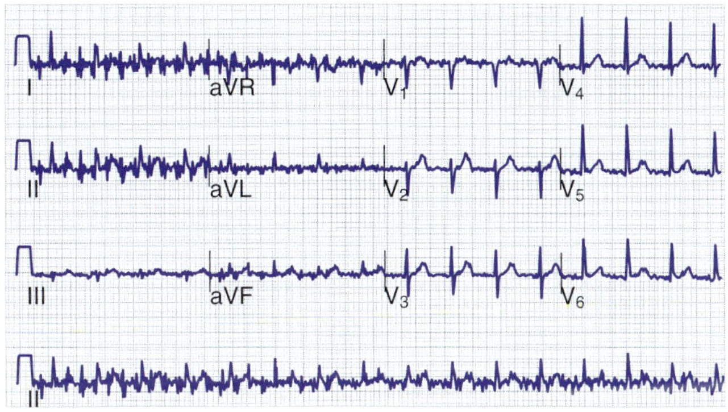

Fig. 14.17 Artifact secondary to a physiologic cause. The patient's monitor was alarming because of a perceived heart rate greater than 200 beats/min, and the computerized alert system called this ventricular tachycardia. The patient, who had Parkinson disease, was without complaint. The electrocardiogram demonstrates a marked artifact that is giving the appearance of atrial flutter in lead V_1.

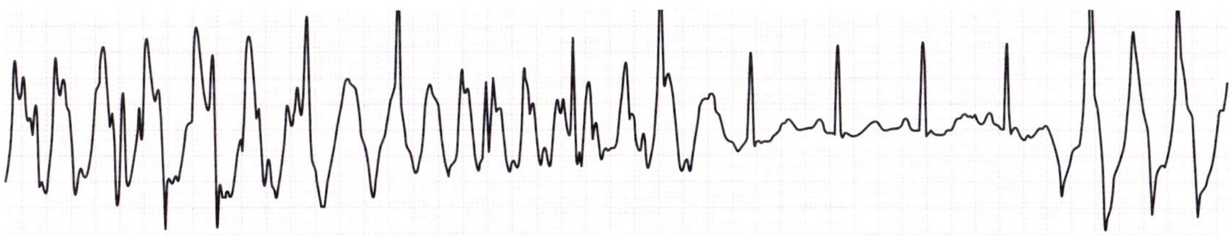

Fig. 14.18 Artifact secondary to rigors. This tracing features a pseudodysrhythmia. The intrinsic RR interval can be traced back through the "dysrhythmia" and reveals an underlying sinus rhythm. As a clue to the artifact, the patient was clinically stable and asymptomatic during the event, except for his rigors.

ARTIFACT

Electrocardiographic artifact is commonly encountered yet not always easy to recognize. Failure to identify it can lead to misdiagnoses of arrhythmias or MIs. Artifact arises from signals external to the patient's heart and can be attributed to either physiologic (internal) or nonphysiologic (external) sources. The former includes muscle activity, patient motion, and poor electrode contact with the skin. Tremors, hiccups, and shivering may produce frequent, narrow spikes on the tracing and simulate atrial and ventricular dysrhythmias (Fig. 14.17). In particular, the ECG manifestation from the frequency of Parkinsonian tremor (5 Hz) closely resembles atrial flutter. A wandering baseline featuring wide undulations in addition to other "noise" on the ECG can often be traced to patient movement and high skin impedance, which leads to inadequate contact of the electrode with the skin. Minimizing skin impedance and artifact may be achieved by (1) avoiding electrode placement over bony prominences, major muscles, or pulsating arteries; (2) clipping rather than shaving thick hair at electrode sites; and (3) cleaning, and most importantly, drying the skin surface before reapplying the electrode with additional electrode gel. Placement of a heavy towel on the extremity can mitigate artifact from tremor.

Nonphysiologic artifact is most often caused by 60-Hz electrical interference, which is ascribable to various other sources of alternating current near the patient. This will be manifested as a wide, indistinct isoelectric baseline. Electrocardiographic artifact should be considered when the clinical picture indicates stability, coincident procedures are in progress (e.g., hemodialysis, blood warmer, bronchoscopy), or devices are in use (e.g., nerve stimulators).[55] In these scenarios, the ECG can be repeated after the procedure is completed or when patients are able to turn off nonessential devices that are in use. Notably, left ventricular assist devices (LVADs) often render the ECG uninterpretable due to the high-frequency artifact created by the motor in the device. Adjusting the ECG low-pass filter from 150 Hz to 20-40 Hz can improve the interpretability of the ECG for patients with LVADs. Other sources of nonphysiologic artifact include those attributable to the monitoring equipment: loose connections, broken monitor cables, and mechanical issues with the machine (e.g., broken stylus, uneven paper transport). The 60-Hz artifact caused by electrical current interference can be minimized by straightening the lead wires so that they are parallel to the patient's body in the long axis.

Differentiation of artifact from true electrocardiographic abnormality is intuitively important; moreover, clinical consequences have been reported that are directly attributable to confusion of artifact with disease. Unnecessary treatment and procedures—including cardiac catheterization, electrophysiologic testing, and even implantation of a pacemaker and an automatic defibrillator—have been reported.[56] Characteristics that may aid in differentiating artifact from dysrhythmia include the absence of hemodynamic instability during the event (or even absence of any symptoms), normal QRS complexes occurring during the "dysrhythmia," instability of the baseline on the tracing during and immediately after the "dysrhythmic" event, association with body movement, and observance of "notches" amid the complexes of the pseudodysrhythmia that "march out" with the normal QRS complexes that precede and follow the disturbance (Fig. 14.18).[57,58] Often artifact can be distinguished from true arrhythmia, because the artifact-induced anomaly will not be present in all leads visualized on the ECG. Similarly, recognition that ST elevation is not present consistently in all beats of a lead suggests it is likely arising from artifact and not ischemia.

CHAPTER 15

Emergency Cardiac Pacing

Kenny Vinh Banh

The purpose of cardiac pacing is to restore or ensure effective cardiac depolarization. Emergency cardiac pacing may be instituted either prophylactically or therapeutically. Prophylactic indications include patients with a high risk for atrioventricular (AV) block. Therapeutic indications include symptomatic bradyarrhythmias and need for overdrive pacing. Pacing for asystole has very minimal success, but it has been used for this condition. Several approaches to pacing can be taken, including transcutaneous, transvenous, transthoracic, epicardial, endocardial, and esophageal. Transcutaneous and transvenous pacemakers are the two techniques most commonly used in the emergency department (ED). Because it can be instituted quickly and noninvasively, transcutaneous pacing (TCP) is the technique of choice in the ED when time is of the essence. Transvenous pacing (TVP) should be reserved for patients who require prolonged pacing or have a very high (>30%) risk for heart block. TCP is generally a temporizing measure that may precede transvenous cardiac pacing. Although it is not an expectation that all emergency clinicians will be adept at placing temporary transvenous cardiac pacemakers, many have mastered the techniques and are often the only clinicians available to perform this lifesaving procedure.

BACKGROUND

In 1872 Duchenne de Boulogne reported successful resuscitation of a child by attaching one electrode to a limb while a second electrode was rhythmically touched to the precordium of the thorax.[1] Successful overdrive pacing of the human heart with a precordial electrode was reported by von Ziemssen in 1882.[2]

In 1952 Zoll introduced the first practical means of TCP. Using a ground electrode attached to the skin and a subcutaneous needle electrode over the precordium, he reported successful resuscitation of two patients in ventricular standstill.[3] One patient was paced for 5 days and subsequently discharged from the hospital. Zoll later introduced a machine that delivered impulses lasting 2 ms through 3-cm diameter metal paddles pressed firmly against the anterior chest wall. This device was the first commercial transcutaneous cardiac pacemaker. During the 1950s, both Zoll and coworkers and Leatham and colleagues demonstrated the effectiveness of TCP in patients with bradycardia and asystole.[4–7] Leatham and colleagues used larger electrodes (4 × 6 cm) and a longer pulse duration (20 ms) to successfully pace two patients with bradydysrhythmias.[7]

Until the late 1950s TCP was the only clinically accepted method of cardiac pacing. The original technique involving bare metal electrodes had adverse effects, including local tissue burns, muscle contraction, and severe pain.[3,7] With the development of the first implantable pacemakers from 1958 to 1960, and the improvement in transvenous electrodes during the early 1960s, TCP was rapidly discarded.[8]

Refinements in electrode size and pulse characteristics led to the reintroduction of TCP into clinical practice.[9,10] Increasing the pulse duration from 2 to 20 ms or longer was found to decrease the current output required for cardiac capture.[11,12] Longer impulse durations also make induction of ventricular fibrillation less likely.[11] Electrodes with a larger surface area (80 cm^2 to 100 cm^2) decrease the current density at the underlying skin and therefore decrease pain and the possibility of tissue burns.[9]

Indications for Cardiac Pacing

The purpose of cardiac pacing is to stimulate effective cardiac depolarization. In most cases the specific indications for cardiac pacing are clear; however, some areas are still controversial. The decision to pace on an emergency basis requires knowledge of the presence or absence of hemodynamic compromise, the cause of the rhythm disturbance, the status of the AV conduction system, and the type of dysrhythmia. Hemodynamic compromise is suggested by hypotension, anginal chest pain, pulmonary edema, or evidence of decreased cerebral perfusion. The clinician caring for the patient is in the best position to decide on pacing. Controversy exists throughout the literature, and this discussion is not meant to set a standard of care for individual circumstances.

In general, the indications can be grouped into those that cause either tachycardias or bradycardias (Review Box 15.1). TCP has become the mainstay of emergency cardiac pacing and is often used pending placement of a transvenous catheter or to determine whether potentially terminal bradyasystolic rhythms will respond to pacing.

Bradycardias

Sinus Node Dysfunction

Sinus node dysfunction may be manifested as sinus arrest, tachybrady (sick sinus) syndrome, or sinus bradycardia. Although symptomatic sinus node dysfunction is a common indication for elective permanent pacing, it is seldom cause for emergency pacemaker insertion.

Seventeen percent of patients with acute myocardial infarction (AMI) will experience sinus bradycardia.[13] It occurs more frequently with inferior than with anterior infarction and has a relatively good prognosis when accompanied by a hemodynamically tolerable escape rhythm. However, sinus bradycardia is not a benign rhythm in this situation; it has a mortality rate of 2% with inferior infarction and 9% with anterior infarction.[14] Sinus node dysfunction frequently responds to medical therapy but requires prompt pacing if such therapy fails.

Asystolic Arrest

TVP in an asystolic or bradyasystolic patient has little value and is not recommended.[15] In a study of 13 patients who had a cardiac arrest, capture of the myocardium was noted in 4 patients, but there were no survivors.[16] TVP alone may also not be effective for postcountershock pulseless bradyarrhythmias.[17] This failure of pacing has likewise been demonstrated with transcutaneous pacemakers, thus suggesting that failure of effective pacing is primarily related to the state of the myocardial tissue.[16] Cardiac pacing may be used as a last-ditch effort in bradyasystolic patients but is rarely

Transvenous Cardiac Pacing

Indications

Bradycardias

- Symptomatic sinus node dysfunction
- Second- and third-degree heart block
- Atrial fibrillation with a slow ventricular response
- With myocardial infarction: new left bundle branch block, bifasicular block, alternating bundle branch block
- Malfunction of an implanted pacemaker

Tachycardias

- Supraventricular dysrhythmias
- Ventricular dysrhythmias

Contraindications

- Prosthetic tricuspid valve
- Severe hypothermia

Complications

- Inadvertent arterial puncture
- Venous thrombosis/thrombophlebitis
- Pneumothorax/other anatomic injury
- Ventricular arrhythmia
- Misplacement of the pacing catheter
- Myocardial/pericardial perforation
- Entanglement of the pacing catheter

Equipment

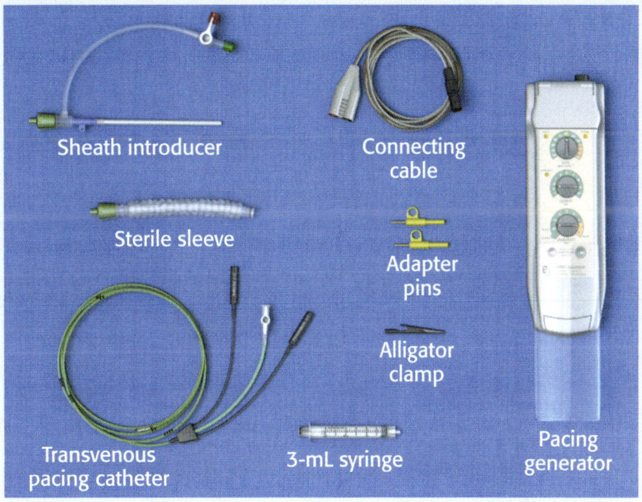

The contents of a typical transvenous pacemaker kit are shown here. Additional equipment required for insertion of the sheath introducer is reviewed in Chapter 22. Individual kits may vary by manufacturer; be familiar with the equipment available at your institution before performing the procedure.

Review Box 15.1 Transvenous cardiac pacing: indications, contraindications, complications, and equipment.

successful and is not considered standard practice. Early pacing (within the first 10 minutes) is essential when done for this purpose if success is to be achieved[18–20] (see later in this section). Most importantly, given the continued emphasis on the importance of maximizing chest compressions during cardiopulmonary resuscitation (CPR), interrupting CPR to institute emergency pacing is not recommended.[21]

Atrioventricular Block

AV block is the classic indication for pacemaker therapy. In symptomatic patients without myocardial infarction (MI) and in asymptomatic patients with a ventricular rate lower than 40 beats/min, pacemaker therapy is indicated.[22]

In patients with AMI, 15% to 19% progress to heart block: first-degree block develops in approximately 8%, second-degree block in 5%, and third-degree block in 6%.[23] First-degree block progresses to high-grade AV block or third-degree block 30% of the time, and second-degree block progresses to high-grade AV block or third-degree block approximately 33% of the time.[24]

AV block occurring during anterior infarction is believed to result from diffuse ischemia in the septum and infranodal conduction tissue. Because these patients tend to progress to high-degree block without warning, a pacemaker is often placed prophylactically.

During inferior infarction, early septal ischemia is the exception and typically block develops sequentially from first-degree to Mobitz type I second-degree and then to third-degree AV block. These conduction abnormalities frequently result in hemodynamically tolerable escape rhythms because of sparing of the bundle branches. A hemodynamically unstable patient who is unresponsive to medical therapy should be paced promptly. Whether and when stable patients should be paced is unclear, but placing a transcutaneous pacer is one option that can be attempted before placing a TVP catheter.

Trauma

Pacing is not a standard intervention in traumatic cardiac arrest, but in selected cases, it may be considered. Several rhythm and conduction disturbances have been documented in patients with nonpenetrating chest trauma. In these patients, traumatic injury to the specialized conduction system may predispose to life-threatening dysrhythmias and blocks that can be treated by cardiac pacing.[25]

Hypovolemia and hypotension can cause ischemia of conduction tissue and cardiac dysfunction.[26] Marked bradyarrhythmias that persist even after vigorous volume replacement may rarely respond to cardiac pacing in patients with such trauma.[27]

Bundle Branch Block and Ischemia

Bundle branch block occurring in AMI is associated with a higher mortality rate and a greater incidence of third-degree heart block than is an uncomplicated infarction. Atkins and colleagues noted that 18% of patients with MI had a bundle branch block.[28] Of these patients, complete heart block developed in 43% who had right bundle branch block (RBBB) and left-axis deviation, in 17% who had left bundle branch block (LBBB), in 19% who had left anterior hemiblock, and in 6% who had no conduction block. The investigators concluded that RBBB with left-axis deviation should be paced prophylactically.

A study by Hindman and associates confirmed the natural history of bundle branch block during MI.[29] In their study, the presence or absence of first-degree AV block, the type of bundle branch block, and the age of the block (new versus old) were used to determine the relative risk for progression to type II second-degree or third-degree block (Table 15.1). Because of the increased risk, consider pacing for the following conduction blocks: new-onset LBBB, RBBB with left-axis deviation or other bifascicular block, and alternating bundle branch block.[29]

Most of the studies investigating temporary pacing in the setting of AMI were done in the era before the use of thrombolytic agents or percutaneous coronary intervention. Nonetheless, whereas modern treatment of AMI has reduced the frequency of emergency transvenous pacemaker insertion, the indications are essentially unchanged and it remains a potentially lifesaving intervention.[30,31]

TABLE 15.1 Influence of Different Variables on the Risk for High-Degree Atrioventricular Block in Patients With Bundle Branch Block During Myocardial Infarction

PATIENTS	PROGRESSING TO HIGH-DEGREE AVB (%)
Infarct location	
Anterior	25
Indeterminate	12
Inferior or posterior	20
PR interval	
>0.20 s	25
≤0.20 s	19
Type of BBB	
LBBB	13
RBBB	14
RBBB + LAFB	27
RBBB + LPFB	29
ABBB	44
Onset of BBB	
Definitely old	13
Possibly new	25
Probably new	26
Definitely new	23

ABBB, Alternating bundle branch block; *AVB*, atrioventricular block; *BBB*, bundle branch block; *LAFB*, left anterior fascicular hemiblock; *LBBB*, left bundle branch block; *LPFB*, left posterior fascicular hemiblock; *RBBB*, right bundle branch block. From Hindman MC, Wagner GS, JaRo M, et al. The clinical significance of bundle branch block complicating acute myocardial infarction. 2. Indications of temporary and permanent pacemaker insertion. *Circulation*. 1978;58:690.

Tachycardias

Hemodynamically compromising tachycardias are usually treated with medications or electrical cardioversion. Supraventricular dysrhythmias, with the exception of atrial fibrillation, respond well to atrial pacing. By "overdrive" pacing the atria at rates 10 to 20 beats/min faster than the underlying rhythm, the atria become entrained, and when the rate is slowed the rhythm frequently returns to normal sinus. A similar procedure is done for ventricular dysrhythmias.[32] Overdrive pacing is especially useful for arrhythmias with recurrent prolonged QT intervals, such as those seen with quinidine toxicity or torsades de pointes.[33] TVP is also useful in patients with digitalis-induced dysrhythmias, in whom direct current cardioversion may be dangerous, or in patients in whom there is further concern about myocardial depression with drugs.[34]

Drug-Induced Dysrhythmias

Significant dysrhythmias can be caused by excessive therapeutic medication (often in combination therapy) and overdose of cardioactive medications. Because these drugs have direct effects on cells of the myocardial pacemaker and conduction system, cardiac pacing is usually of little therapeutic value. Both bradycardias and tachycardias may result. Tachycardic rhythms from amphetamines, cocaine, anticholinergics, cyclic antidepressants, theophylline, and other drugs do not benefit from cardiac pacing. Drug-induced torsades de pointes may theoretically be overdriven by pacing, but data on this technique are lacking. Any drug that affects the central nervous system (e.g., opiates, sedative-hypnotics, clonidine) may produce bradycardia. Uncommon causes of toxin-induced bradycardia include organophosphate poisoning, various cholinergic drugs, ciguatera poisoning, and rarely, plant toxins. Cardiac pacing is not used for bradycardias from these sources; rather, the underlying central nervous system depression is addressed.

Severe bradycardia and heart block often accompany overdose of digitalis preparations, β-adrenergic blockers, and calcium channel blockers. Although intuitively attractive, cardiac pacing is not generally effective for serious toxin-induced bradycardias, even though there have been rare case reports of success.[35–38] In β-blocker overdose, pacing may increase the heart rate but rarely benefits blood pressure or cardiac output. Worsening of blood pressure may occur as a result of loss of atrial contractions with ventricular pacing. Likewise, calcium channel blocker overdose and digitalis-induced bradycardia and heart block rarely benefit from cardiac pacing. Pharmacologic interventions, such as digoxin-specific Fab, glucagon, calcium, high-dose insulin, inotropic medications, and vasopressors, remain the mainstay in the treatment of drug-induced dysrhythmias. Given the lack of success of pacing, possible downsides, and the greater effectiveness of specific antidotes, it is not standard to routinely attempt transvenous cardiac pacing in the setting of drug overdose. However, as a last resort, cardiac pacing can be supported.[39]

Contraindications for Cardiac Pacing

If known, the presence of a prosthetic tricuspid valve is generally considered to be an absolute contraindication to transvenous cardiac pacing.[40] In addition, severe hypothermia will occasionally result in ventricular fibrillation when pacing is attempted. Because ventricular fibrillation under these conditions is difficult to convert, caution is advised when considering pacing severely hypothermic and bradycardic patients. Rapid and careful rewarming is often recommended first, followed by pacing if the patient's condition does not improve.

Specific Indications for Transcutaneous Pacing

TCP is the fastest and easiest method of emergency pacing. This technique is useful for initial stabilization of patients in the ED who require emergency pacing while arrangements or decisions about transvenous pacemaker insertion are being made. The equipment is readily mastered, the procedure is fast, and it is minimally invasive.[10,41] Refinements in equipment have made TCP the emergency pacing procedure of choice. TCP is also widely used in the prehospital environment, as well as in the hospital in the cardiac catheterization laboratory, operating room, intensive care units, and on general medical floors.[42–44] The technique may be preferable to TVP in patients who have received thrombolytic agents or other anticoagulants. No central venous puncture, with the attendant risk of hemorrhage, is required. Limited experience suggests that TCP may also be useful in the treatment of refractory tachydysrhythmias by overdrive pacing.[45–50] Although small pediatric electrodes for TCP have been developed, experience with pediatric TCP has been limited.[51–53]

This technique is temporary and is indicated for short intervals as a bridge until TVP can be initiated or the underlying cause of the bradydysrhythmia (e.g., hyperkalemia,[41] drug overdose) can be reversed.[54]

Delay from the onset of arrest to the initiation of pacing is a major problem that limits the usefulness of TCP in prehospital care. Hedges and associates reported that the everyday availability of pacing increased the number of patients who underwent pacing within 10 minutes of hemodynamic decompensation and also increased long-term patient survival.[20] Prehospital pacing may be most useful in the treatment of patients with a hemodynamically significant bradycardia who have not yet progressed to cardiac arrest (e.g., heart block in the setting of AMI) or in patients who arrest after the arrival of prehospital providers.[19,20]

In conscious patients with hemodynamically stable bradycardia, TCP may not be necessary. It is reasonable to attach electrodes to such patients and to leave the pacemaker in standby mode against the possibility of hemodynamic deterioration while further efforts at treatment of the patient's underlying disorder are being made. This approach has been used successfully in patients with new heart block in the setting of cardiac ischemia.[55] Generally, when a transvenous pacemaker becomes available it is preferred because of better patient tolerance.

Sedation/Analgesia

Most patients cannot tolerate TCP for prolonged periods because they will sense each depolarization spike. Hence, TCP is often rapidly replaced by TVP. Standard sedatives (such as benzodiazepines) and opioids (such as morphine) should be administered as needed to control anxiety and discomfort.

Equipment

Since their reintroduction, transcutaneous pacemakers have undergone rapid evolution and are now standard equipment in most EDs, as well as in other hospital settings and the prehospital environment. The pacemakers introduced in the early 1980s tended to be asynchronous devices with a limited selection of rate and output parameters. Units introduced more recently have demand mode pacing and more output options and are often combined with a defibrillator in a single unit. Combined defibrillator pacers offer advantages in cost, ease, and rapidity of use when compared with stand-alone devices. An example of a combined unit is shown in Review Box 15.2.

Transcutaneous Cardiac Pacing

Indications

General indications are identical to those for transvenous pacing (see Review Box 15.1)
Initial stabilization of patients requiring pacing while arrangements for transvenous pacing are being made
Pacing in various environments (prehospital, hospital ward, etc.)
Pacing in patients treated with thrombolytics or other anticoagulants

Contraindications

No absolute contraindications

Complications

Failure to recognize the presence of underlying treatable ventricular fibrillation
Induction of ventricular fibrillation (rare)
Soft tissue discomfort

Equipment

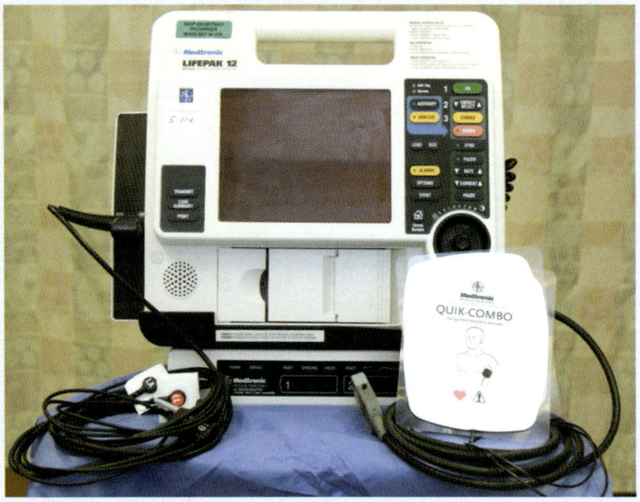

Review Box 15.2 Transcutaneous cardiac pacing: indications, contraindications, complications, and equipment.

All transcutaneous pacemakers have similar basic features. Most allow operation in either a fixed-rate (asynchronous) or a demand mode (VVI). Most allow rate selection in a range from 30 to 200 beats/min. Current output is usually adjustable from 0 mA to 200 mA. If an ECG monitor is not an integral part of the unit, an output adapter to a separate monitor is required to "blank" the large electrical spike from the pacemaker impulse and allow interpretation of the much smaller ECG complex. Without blanking protection, the standard ECG machine is swamped by the pacemaker spike and is uninterpretable. This could be disastrous because the large pacing artifacts can mask treatable ventricular fibrillation (Fig. 15.1). Pulse durations on available units vary from 20 ms to 40 ms and are not adjustable by the operator.

Two sets of patient electrodes are usually required for the operation of the device. One set of standard ECG electrodes is used for monitoring. The much larger pacing electrodes deliver electrical impulses for pacing. Newer combined defibrillator-pacemakers can use a single set of electrodes for ECG monitoring, pacing, and defibrillation. This approach makes the device simpler to use, although the ECG waveform and analysis may be suboptimal. Provisions are generally made for separate ECG monitoring electrodes for use as desired by the operator.

Along with the widespread use of TCP come problems arising from lack of standardization of equipment. Pacing electrodes placed on a patient before arrival at the hospital may be incompatible with the transcutaneous pacemaker used in the ED, and likewise, the equipment in the ED may differ from inpatient units. Efforts should be made to establish a single standard for pacing electrode connectors within an institution and out to the prehospital environment if possible.

To facilitate rapid setup, the pacing electrodes should be connected to the pacemaker at all times. With conventional packaging, the leads are inside the packet with the pads, which means that the packet must be opened to allow connection to the pacing unit. However, exposure to air causes the electrodes to dry out and lose their conductivity, thus requiring continual replacement of the unused electrodes. Newer packaging leaves the connectors outside the packet, thus allowing connection to the pacemaker while preserving the shelf life of the pacing electrodes.

Technique

See Videos 15.1 and 15.2.

Pad Placement

The pacing electrodes are self-adhesive. The anteroposterior positioning shown in Fig. 15.2 is more likely to capture

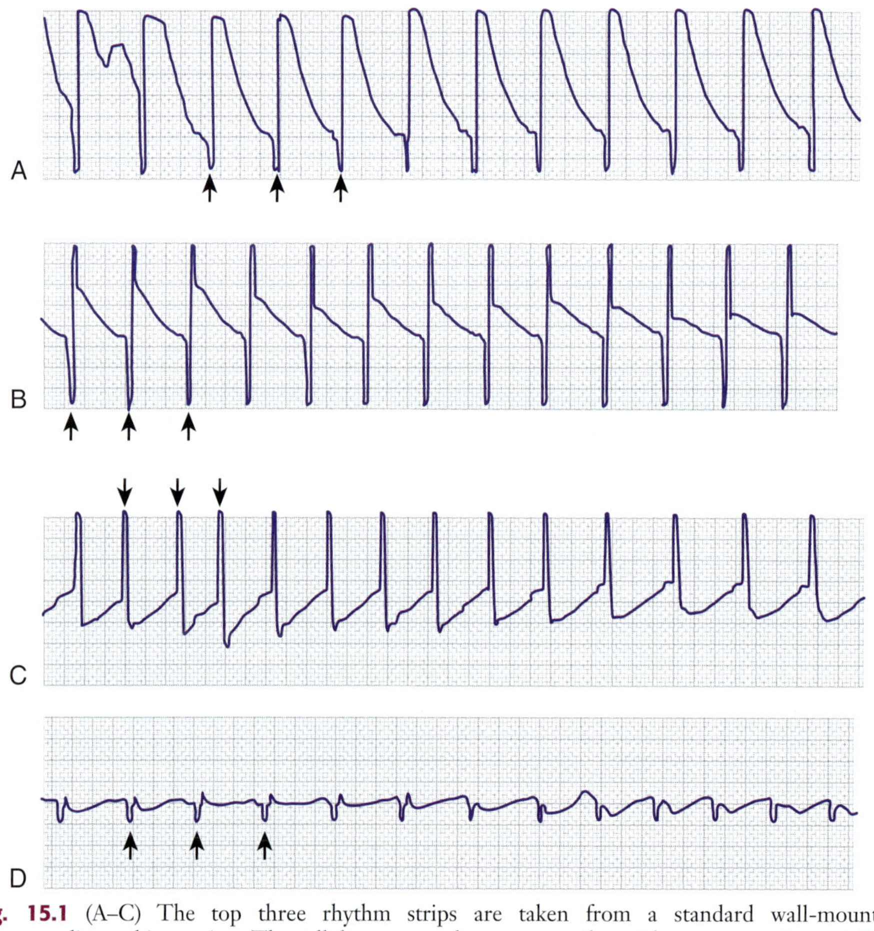

Fig. 15.1 (A–C) The top three rhythm strips are taken from a standard wall-mounted electrocardiographic monitor. They all demonstrate large pacer spikes without capture *(arrows)*. The underlying rhythm cannot be determined and could be treatable ventricular fibrillation. (D) The bottom rhythm strip demonstrates a tracing on the same patient with the external pacer monitor (special dampening). Note that the pacing spikes are much smaller, and it is easy to see that the underlying rhythm is asystole, without pacer capture. The presence of a T wave after the QRS complex is a good indicator of ventricular capture.

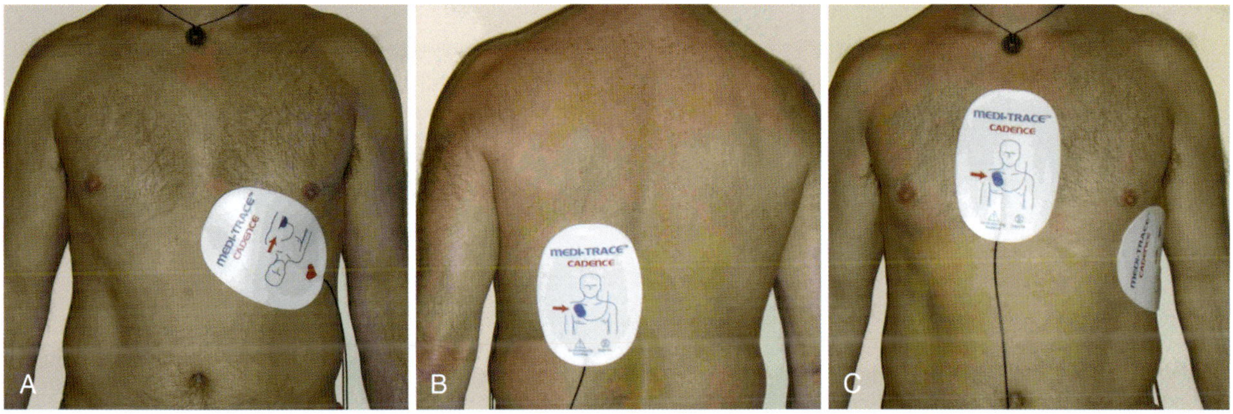

Fig. 15.2 Correct placement of transcutaneous pacemaker electrodes. (A–B) Anteroposterior positions. (C) Anterolateral positions (see text).

than anterolateral pad placement.[56] Take care to avoid placing the electrodes over an implanted pacemaker or defibrillator. Remove any transdermal drug delivery patches if they are in the way. Remove excessive hair if time permits. Place the anterior electrode (cathode or negative electrode) as close as possible to the point of maximal impulse on the left anterior chest wall. Place the second electrode directly posterior to the anterior electrode (see Fig.15.2A–B). The posterior electrode serves as the ground. An alternative arrangement for the pacing electrodes is shown in Fig. 15.2C. On people with breast tissue, place the electrode beneath the tissue and against the chest wall. Because data regarding optimum electrode placement are scarce, selection can be based on the clinician's preference and the patient's habitus.[57,58] Nonetheless, suboptimal capture as a result of poor electrode placement may be rectified with a small change in electrode position. Although the polarity of the electrodes does not appear to be important for defibrillation, at least one study has indicated that it may be important for pacing.[59] The electrodes are labeled by the manufacturer to indicate which one should be placed over the precordium, and it is prudent to observe this recommendation. ECG electrodes (if used) are placed on the chest wall or limbs, or both, as required and connected to the instrument cable. Some clinicians prophylactically apply pacing electrodes to all critically ill patients with bradycardia to facilitate immediate TCP should decompensation occur.

There is little risk for electrical injury to health care providers during TCP. The power delivered during each impulse is less than 1/1000 of that delivered during defibrillation.[60] Chest compressions (CPR) can be administered directly over the insulated electrodes while pacing.[61] Inadvertent contact with the active pacing surface results in only a mild shock.

Pacing Bradycardic Rhythms

To initiate TCP, apply the pacing electrodes and activate the device (Fig. 15.3, *steps 1 and 2*). Slowly increase the output from minimal settings until capture is achieved (see Fig. 15.3, *step 4*). Rate and current (output) selections are adjustable. Generally, a heart rate of 60 to 70 beats/min will maintain adequate blood pressure (by blood pressure cuff or arterial catheter) and cerebral perfusion.

Assess electrical capture by monitoring the ECG tracing on the filtered monitor of the pacing unit (see Fig. 15.3, *steps 5 and 6*). Assess mechanical capture by palpating the pulse. Because of muscular contractions triggered by the pacer, carotid pulses may be difficult to assess, so palpating the femoral pulse may be easier. Additionally, bedside US may prove useful in determining ventricular capture.[62,63] Ideally, continue pacing at an output level just above the threshold of initial electrical capture to minimize discomfort. One study involving 16 normal male volunteers who were paced without sedation noted cardiac capture at a mean current of 54 mA (range, 42 to 60 mA).[64] Most volunteers could tolerate pacing at their capture threshold; only one participant required discontinuation of pacing at 60 mA because of intolerable pain. Heller and coworkers compared subjective pain perception and capture thresholds in 10 volunteers paced with five different transcutaneous pacers.[65] Capture rates (40% to 80%), thresholds (66.5 to 104 mA), and subjective discomfort varied from pacemaker to pacemaker.

Failure to capture with TCP may be related to electrode placement or patient size. Patients with barrel-shaped chests and large amounts of intrathoracic air conduct electricity poorly and may prove refractory to capture. In one study, the scarring associated with thoracotomy was found to nearly double the pacing threshold.[66] A large pericardial effusion or tamponade will also increase the output required for capture.[67] Failure to electrically capture with a transcutaneous device in these settings is an indication to consider immediate placement of a transvenous pacer.

Patients who are conscious or who regain consciousness during TCP will experience discomfort because of muscle contraction.[55,64,65] Analgesia with incremental doses of an opioid agent, sedation with a benzodiazepine compound, or both, will make this discomfort tolerable until TVP can be instituted.

Overdrive Pacing

Overdrive pacing of ventricular tachycardia or paroxysmal supraventricular tachycardia is performed in patients who are stable enough to tolerate the brief delay associated with the preparation needed for this technique.[45–50] Few data exist on the efficacy or use of this procedure in the ED. As explained earlier, sedate the patient and place pacing and monitoring electrode pads, then initiate brief trains (6 to 10 beats) of asynchronous pacing. Set the pacer rate at approximately 20 to 60 pulses/min greater than the dysrhythmia rate.[68] Generally, an impulse rate of 200 pulses/min is used for ventricular

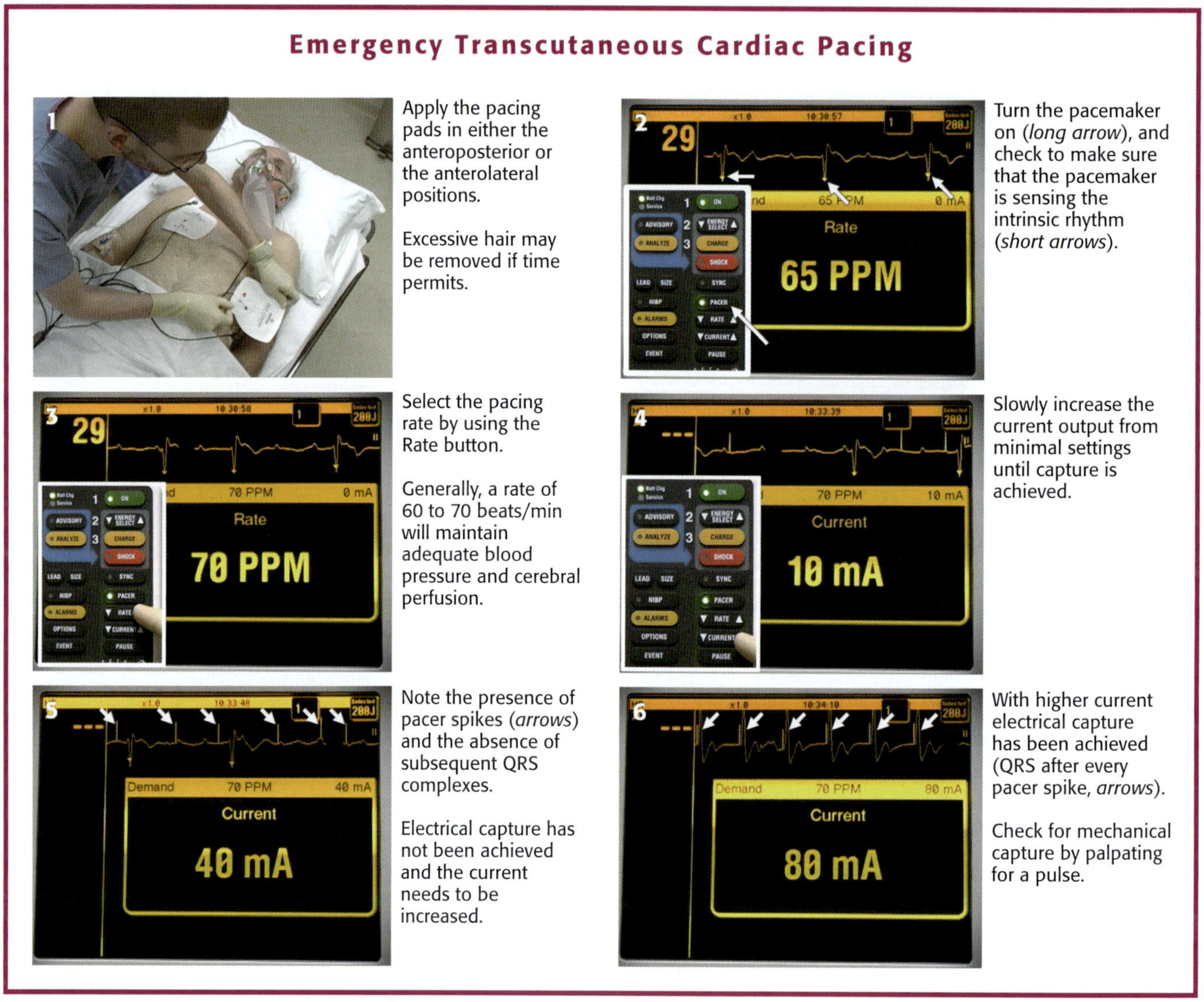

Fig. 15.3 Emergency transcutaneous cardiac pacing.

tachycardias (the rate is usually 150 to 180 beats/min), and a rate of 240 to 280 pulses/min is used for paroxysmal supraventricular tachycardias (the rate is commonly 200 to 250 beats/min).

Because rhythm acceleration is possible during overdrive pacing, it is essential to keep resuscitation equipment, including a defibrillator, at the bedside.

Complications

The major potential complication of TCP is failure to recognize the presence of underlying treatable ventricular fibrillation. This complication is primarily due to the size of the pacing artifact on the ECG screen, a technical problem inherent in systems without appropriate dampening circuitry.

A rare complication of TCP is induction of ventricular fibrillation. Studies of fibrillation thresholds using large precordial electrodes have shown that the longer impulse durations used in modern devices seem to decrease the chance of inducing ventricular fibrillation with TCP. Nonetheless, asynchronous TCP for tachydysrhythmias has been associated with acceleration in rhythm and the development of ventricular fibrillation.[48]

If the patient has an implanted cardioverter defibrillator that is not delivering effective pacing, disable the defibrillator by placing a magnet over it prior to initiating TCP. Failure to do so may trigger the device to administer an unnecessary shock to the patient.[69]

Studies looking at prolonged TCP in humans have not been extensive. Zoll and colleagues reported 25 humans paced for up to 108 hours with impulses of 20-ms duration.[6] Pacer-induced dysrhythmias did not occur. Leatham and colleagues paced one patient for 68 hours with impulses 20 ms in duration.[7] The patient died 2 days after pacing was discontinued. Pathologic examination revealed no evidence of pacer-induced myocardial damage. Madsen and colleagues paced 10 healthy volunteers at threshold for 30 minutes and found no enzyme or echocardiographic abnormalities.[70] TCP appears unlikely to produce cardiac injury with short-term use in the ED.

Soft tissue discomfort with potential injury may still occur with current transcutaneous pacemakers. Most patients are able to tolerate the discomfort, especially after sedation and analgesia, which should be routine. Nonetheless, prolonged use may still induce local cutaneous injury, particularly in pediatric patients because of the use of smaller electrodes.[71,72]

Patients who cannot tolerate TCP or who will need long-term pacing are candidates for TVP.

EMERGENCY TRANSVENOUS CARDIAC PACING

The transvenous method of endocardial pacing is commonly used and is both safe and effective. In skilled hands, the semi-floating transvenous catheter is successfully placed under electrocardiographic (ECG) guidance in 80% of patients.[73] The technique can be performed in less than 20 minutes in 72% of patients and in less than 5 minutes in 30%. However, in some instances, anatomic, logistic, and hemodynamic impediments can prohibit successful pacing by even the most skilled clinician. As with other medical procedures, it should not be performed without a thorough understanding of its indications, contraindications, and complications.[74]

As with all procedures, there is a chance of failure. This may be because the condition is not amenable to pacing (e.g., asystole, drug overdose) or because of technical difficulties inherent with the procedure.

Background

In 1951 Callaghan and Bigelow first used the transvenous approach to stimulate asystolic hearts in hypothermic dogs.[75] Furman and Robinson demonstrated the transvenous endocardial approach in humans in 1958.[76] They treated two patients with complete heart block and Adams-Stokes seizures, thus reconfirming that low-voltage pacing could completely control myocardial depolarization. Other early clinical studies also demonstrated the utility of TVP.[77] Fluoroscopic guidance was used for placement of the pacing catheter in all these studies.

In 1964 Vogel and coworkers demonstrated the use of a flexible catheter passed without fluoroscopic guidance for intracardiac electrocardiography.[78] One year later, Kimball and Killip used this technique to insert endocardial pacemakers at the bedside.[79] They noted technical problems in 20% of their patients, including intermittent capture, difficulty passing the catheter, and catheter knotting. During the same year, Harris and colleagues confirmed the ease and speed with which this procedure could be accomplished.[80]

Before 1965 all intracardiac pacing was done asynchronously, which meant that the pacing catheter could cause electrical stimulation during any phase of the cardiac cycle. Asynchronous pacing frequently resulted in the pacemaker firing during the vulnerable period of an intrinsic depolarization; this occasionally caused ventricular tachycardia or fibrillation. In 1967 a demand pacemaker generator that sensed intrinsic depolarizations and inhibited the pacemaker for a predetermined period was used successfully by Zuckerman and associates in six patients.[81] Since then there has been steady progress in the design and functionality of pacemakers. Table 15.2 summarizes the four-letter code that is used to describe modern pacemakers (there is a fifth letter for combined pacemaker-cardioverter/defibrillators). The most commonly used emergency transvenous pacemaker is represented by the code VVI: the ventricle is paced, the ventricle is sensed, and when a native impulse is sensed, the pacemaker is inhibited. Dual-chamber pacing (DDD or DDDR) is the preferred methodology for permanent pacing but is rarely used on an emergency basis because of the increased complexity of the procedure.

Rosenberg and coworkers introduced an improved pacing catheter known as the Elecath semifloating pacing wire.[73] The Elecath was stiffer than the Flexon steel wire electrode that was in prevailing use. Rosenberg and coworkers[73] achieved pacing in 72% of their patients with an average procedure time of 18 minutes. They also noted that 30% of their patients were paced in 5 minutes or less. In 1970 Swan and Ganz introduced the technique of heart catheterization with a flow-directed balloon-tipped catheter.[82] Schnitzler and colleagues successfully used this method for placement of a right ventricular pacemaker in 15 of 17 patients.[83]

In 1981 Lang and associates compared bedside use of the flow-directed balloon-tipped catheter with insertion of a semirigid electrode catheter in 111 perfusing patients.[84] These researchers found a significantly shorter insertion time (6 minutes 45 seconds vs. 13 minutes 30 seconds), a lower incidence of serious arrhythmias (1.5% vs. 20.4%), and a lower incidence of catheter displacement (13.4% vs. 32%) with the balloon-tipped catheter. They concluded that the balloon-tipped catheter was the method of choice for temporary TVP.

Although placing temporary transvenous pacemakers has long been considered a core skill in the ED, it has not been well studied. Birkhahn and coworkers retrospectively compared the experience of emergency physicians with that of cardiologists in placing transvenous pacemakers under ECG guidance.[85] They reported a 13% risk for major complications in both groups of specialists. They concluded that pacemaker placement by emergency physicians under ECG

TABLE 15.2 Four-Letter Pacemaker Code

FIRST LETTER	SECOND LETTER	THIRD LETTER	FOURTH LETTER
Chamber paced	Chamber sensed	Sensing response	Programmability
A = Atrium	A = Atrium	T = Triggered	P = Simple
V = Ventricle	V = Ventricle	I = Inhibited	M = Multiprogrammable
D = Dual	D = Dual	D = Dual (A triggered and V inhibited)	R = Rate adaptive
O = None	O = None	O = None	C = Communicating O = None

guidance without fluoroscopy had success and complication rates that were comparable with those of their cardiology colleagues. In a retrospective review of 43 ED patients in whom emergency transvenous pacemaker placement was attempted, there was a 95% success rate and no immediate or delayed complications.[86]

Equipment

Several items are required to insert a transvenous pacemaker adequately. Like most special procedures, a prearranged tray is convenient. The usual components required to insert a transvenous cardiac pacemaker are depicted in Review Box 15.1.

Pacing Generator

Many different pacing generators are available, but in general, they all have the same basic features. The controls will frequently have a locking feature or cover to prevent the generator from being switched off or reprogrammed inadvertently. An amperage control allows the operator to vary the amount of electrical current delivered to the myocardium, usually 0.1 to 20 mA. Increasing the setting increases the output and improves the likelihood of capture. The pacing control mode is determined by adjusting the gain setting for the sensing function of the generator. By increasing the sensitivity, one can convert the unit from a fixed-rate (asynchronous mode) to a demand (synchronous mode) pacemaker. The typical pacing generator has a sensitivity setting that ranges from approximately 0.5 mV to 20 mV. The voltage setting represents the minimum strength of the electrical signal that the pacer is able to detect. Decreasing the setting increases the sensitivity and improves the likelihood of sensing myocardial depolarization. In the fixed-rate mode, the unit fires despite the underlying intrinsic rhythm; that is, the unit does not sense any intrinsic electrical activity. In the full-demand mode, however, the pacemaker senses the underlying ventricular depolarizations, and the unit does not fire as long as the patient's ventricular rate is equal to or faster than the set rate of the pacing generator. A sensing indicator meter and a rate control knob are also present.

Temporary pacing generators are battery operated, and thus it is always good practice to install a fresh battery whenever pacing is anticipated. An example of a pacing generator is shown in Fig. 15.4.

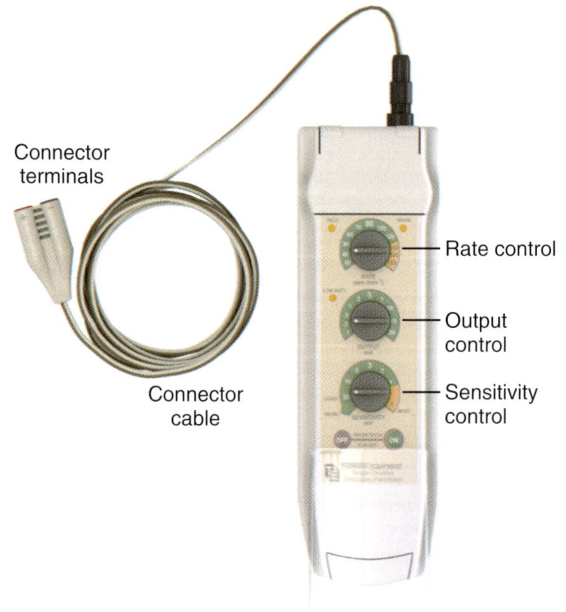

Fig. 15.4 Pacemaker energy source: controls and connections.

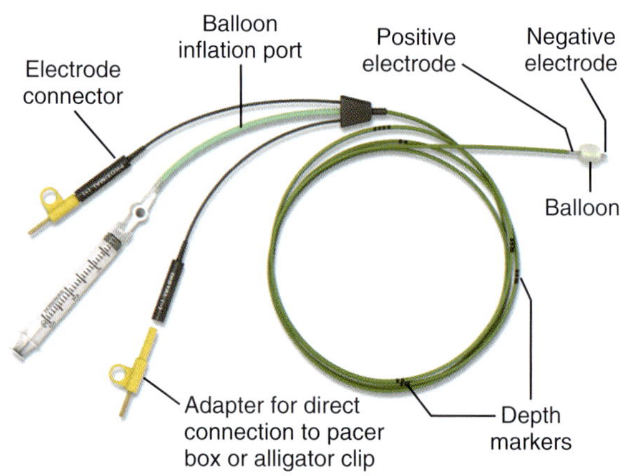

Fig. 15.5 Balloon-tipped pacing catheter.

Pacing Catheters and Electrodes

Several sizes and brands of pacing catheters are available. In general, most range from 3 Fr to 5 Fr in size and are approximately 100 cm in length. Lines are marked along the catheter surface at approximately 10-cm intervals and can be used to estimate catheter position during insertion. Pacing catheters differ with respect to their stiffness, electrode configurations, floating characteristics, and other qualities. For emergency pacing, the semifloating bipolar electrode catheter with a balloon tip is used most frequently (Fig. 15.5). The balloon holds approximately 1.5 mL of air, and the air injection port has a locking lever to secure balloon expansion. Before insertion, check the balloon for leakage of air by inflating and immersing it in sterile water. The presence of an air leak is noted by a stream of bubbles rising to the surface of the water. An inflated balloon helps the catheter "float" into the heart, even in low-flow states, but is not advantageous in cardiac arrest.

For all practical purposes, temporary TVP is accomplished with a bipolar pacing catheter. The terms unipolar and bipolar refer to the number of electrodes in contact with the portion of the heart that is to be stimulated. All pacemaker systems must have both a positive (anode) and a negative (cathode) electrode; hence, all stimulation is bipolar. In the typical bipolar catheter used for temporary TVP, the cathode (stimulating electrode) is at the tip of the pacing catheter. The anode is located 1 cm to 2 cm proximal to the tip, and a balloon or an insulated wire separates the two electrodes. The distinction between unipolar and bipolar pacing catheters is that a bipolar catheter has both electrodes in relatively close proximity to the catheter and both may contact the endocardium. In a bipolar catheter, the electrodes are usually stainless steel or platinum rings that encircle the pacing catheter. When properly positioned, both electrodes will be within the right ventricle so that a field of electrical excitation is set up between the electrodes. With a bipolar catheter, the cathode does not need to be in direct contact with the endocardium for pacing to occur, although it is preferable to have direct contact.

A unipolar system is also effective but is used infrequently for temporary TVP. In a unipolar system, the cathode is at the tip of the pacing catheter and the anode is located in one of three places: in the pacing generator itself, more proximally on the catheter (outside the ventricle), or on the patient's chest. A bipolar system may be converted to a unipolar system by simply disconnecting the positive proximal connection of the bipolar catheter from the pacing generator and running a new wire from the positive (pacing generator) terminal to the patient's chest wall. Such a conversion may be required in the unlikely event of failure of one lead of the bipolar system.

ECG Machine and Monitoring

An ECG machine can be used to record the heart's inherent electrical activity during the insertion of the pacer and to aid in localization of the tip of the catheter without fluoroscopy. The ECG machine must be well grounded to prevent leakage of alternating current, which can cause ventricular fibrillation. Such leakage should be suspected if interference of 50 to 60 cycles per second (Hz) is noted on the ECG tracing.

The ECG machine should be placed in a manner that allows easy visibility of the rhythm during insertion. One method is to place the machine near the level of the patient's midthorax, facing the operator, on either side of the patient as logistics and operator preference allow (Fig. 15.6). Note that the operator stands at the head of the patient during passage of the catheter through the internal jugular or subclavian vein and at the midabdomen for insertion through the femoral or brachiocephalic vein. Newer patient monitors may be equipped with suitable ECG connections to allow their use in place of a stand-alone ECG machine. Because these patients will already be attached to a monitor, it may prove convenient to use the same piece of equipment to assist in insertion of the pacemaker.

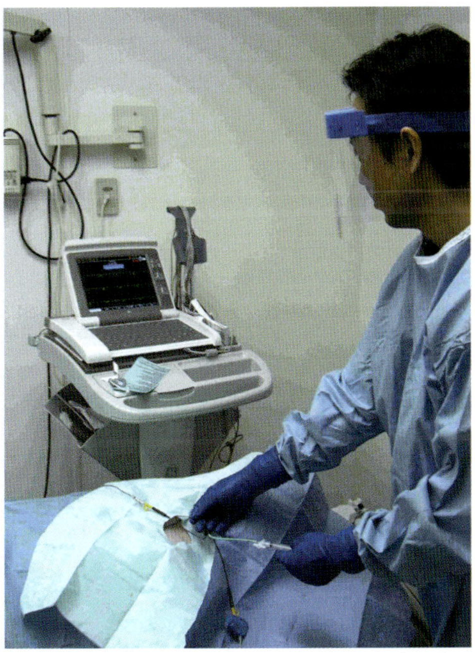

Fig. 15.6 Position of operator and electrocardiographic device during insertion of a pacemaker catheter through the left subclavian vein (a preferred site).

Introducer Sheath

An introducer set or sheath is required for venous access (see Chapter 22). Some pacing catheters are prepackaged with the appropriate equipment, whereas others require a separate set. The introducer set is used to enhance passage of the pacing catheter through the skin, subcutaneous tissue, and vessel wall. The sheath must be larger than the pacing catheter to allow it to pass. The size of the pacing catheter refers to its outside diameter, whereas the size of the introducer refers to its inside diameter. Thus a 5-Fr pacing catheter will fit through a 5-Fr introducer. Introducer sheaths are available with a perforated elastic seal covering the opening through which the pacing catheter is passed (pacer port). The seal allows the catheter to be manipulated while preventing blood from escaping or air from entering the vein. A side port allows the sheath to be used for central venous access. A makeshift sheath can be fashioned with an appropriately sized intravenous (IV) catheter. For a 3-Fr balloon-tipped catheter, a 14-gauge 1.5- to 2-inch IV catheter is suitable. A 4-Fr balloon-tipped catheter will also fit through a 14-gauge catheter or needle. However, without a seal over the hub, blood will leak from the end of the IV catheter.

Overall, the key to success with this procedure is preparation. In a typical ED, there are often a variety of vascular access kits and devices, but only some will work well for passing a pacing catheter. It is imperative that one examine all the components of the tray before starting the procedure to ensure that all wires, sheaths, dilators, and syringes fit as expected. Ideally, all the equipment and accessories needed for emergency pacemaker insertion should be kept together in a designated location.

Procedure

See Videos 15.3 and 15.4. A checklist for the preparation and initial setup of a pacing generator is shown in Box 15.1. It may be useful to have a copy of this checklist or a similar list stored with the pacemaker, to have on hand in emergency situations.

BOX 15.1 Checklist for a Temporary Transvenous Pacing Generator[a]

- Insert a new battery.
- Turn the pacemaker ON.
- Set the RATE (80 beats/min), OUTPUT (5 mA), and SENSITIVITY (3 mV).[b]
- Connect the patient cable to the pacemaker.
- Open both connector terminals on the patient cable.
- Insert the PROXIMAL (+) pin of the pacing catheter into the POSITIVE (+) connector terminal on the patient cable.
- Tighten the connection firmly.
- Use alligator clips to connect the DISTAL (–) pin of the pacing catheter to lead V_1 of the electrocardiographic machine.
- When the catheter is in position, remove the DISTAL (–) pin from V_1 and insert it into the NEGATIVE (–) connector terminal on the patient cable.
- Tighten the connection firmly.

[a]*Adjust pacemaker settings as needed to achieve proper capture and sensitivity (see text).*

[b]*Guidelines only. Follow the recommendations of the device's manufacturer if different.*

TABLE 15.3 Advantages and Disadvantages of Pacemaker Placement Sites

VENOUS CHANNELS	ADVANTAGES	DISADVANTAGES
Brachial	Very safe route Vessel easily accessible, either by cutdown or a percutaneous approach Compressible	Often requires a cutdown Easily displaced and poor patient mobility Not reusable if a cutdown technique is performed The catheter is more difficult to advance than in central or larger vessels
Subclavian	Direct access to the right side of the heart (especially via the left subclavian) Rapid insertion time Good patient mobility	Pneumothorax and other intrathoracic trauma are possible Noncompressible
Femoral	Direct access to the right side of the heart Rapid insertion time Compressible	Increased incidence of thrombophlebitis Can be dislodged by leg movement Poor patient mobility Infection
Internal jugular	Direct access to the right side of the heart (especially via the right internal jugular) Rapid insertion time Compressible	Possible carotid artery puncture Dislodgment with movement of the head Thrombophlebitis

Patient Preparation

Patient instruction is an extremely important aspect of any procedure. Frequently, there is not enough time to give patients a detailed explanation or to obtain written informed consent. Nonetheless, sufficient information should be provided so that the patient feels at ease. It is always prudent to obtain and document informed consent from the patient, if possible, before any invasive procedure or to document that the circumstances did not allow informed consent. Patients should be assured that they will feel no discomfort after the venipuncture site has been anesthetized and that they will feel better when the catheter is in place and is functional. Continued reassurance is required during the procedure because patients are usually facing away from the operator and their faces are often covered; thus they may be unsure of what is occurring. Sedation and analgesia should be considered when appropriate.

All operators should wear surgical masks, caps, gloves, and gowns to decrease the risk for infection before catheter placement. Patients should be prepared and draped in the usual sterile fashion. This aseptic precaution should also be explained to the patient.

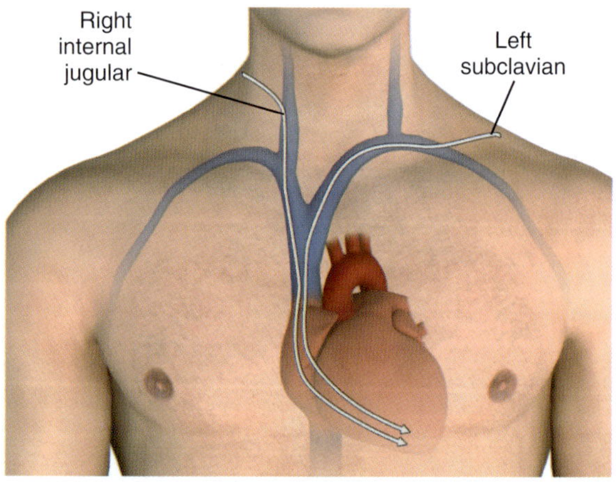

Fig. 15.7 The right internal jugular and left subclavian veins have the straightest anatomic pathway to the right ventricle and are generally preferred for temporary transvenous pacing.

Site Selection

The four venous channels that provide easy access to the right ventricle are the brachial, subclavian, femoral, and internal jugular veins (Table 15.3). The route selected is often one of personal or institutional preference. The right internal jugular and left subclavian veins have the straightest anatomic pathway to the right ventricle and are generally preferred for temporary TVP (Fig. 15.7). Some centers may prefer right internal jugular placement to keep the left subclavian open for future permanent pacemaker placement.

The subclavian vein can be accessed through both an infraclavicular and a supraclavicular approach; the infraclavicular approach is most commonly reported for all temporary transvenous pacemaker insertions. This route is preferred because of its easy accessibility, close proximity to the heart, and ease in catheter maintenance and stability. The supraclavicular approach has been described in the literature for several years and has gained popularity among some clinicians. The left subclavian vein is preferred because of the less acute angle traversed than with the right-sided approach, but either side may be used.[87,88]

The internal jugular approach may also be used. In this case, the right internal jugular vein is preferred because of the direct line to the superior vena cava. Problems with this approach include dislodgment of the pacemaker with movement of the head, puncture of the carotid artery, and thrombophlebitis.

During CPR, use of the right internal jugular vein and the left subclavian vein for pacemaker insertion has been demonstrated to result in the highest rates of proper placement in the right ventricle.[89] The right internal jugular vein is the more direct route of the two and may be the most appropriate site.

Femoral veins, like neck veins, are compressible and easily catheterized. Problems include easy dislodgment, infection, and increased risk for thrombophlebitis.[90,91]

Brachial vein catheterization is easy to perform but results in a high incidence of infection and vessel thrombosis.[92] In addition, the catheter is easily dislodged with arm motion. This approach is seldom used in the emergency setting.

Although the left subclavian and right internal jugular veins are the preferred routes for access, in emergency situations clinicians should use the approach with which they are most experienced to minimize the time spent cannulating the vein and to reduce the potential for complications from the venipuncture.

Skin Preparation and Venous Access

Clean the skin over the venipuncture site twice with an antiseptic solution such as chlorhexidine or povidone-iodine. Prepare a wide area because of the tendency for guidewires and catheters to spring from the hands of an unsuspecting operator. Similarly, drape widely in the standard manner to maintain a sterile field and to allow clear visibility of the venipuncture site.

The infraclavicular approach is used in this chapter to illustrate venous access, although the mechanics are generally the same as for other vascular approaches.

Occasionally, a patient who already has a central venous line in place requires emergency placement of a pacing catheter. An existing central venous pressure (CVP) line can be used to place the pacing catheter if the lumen of the catheter is large enough to accept a guidewire. Withdraw the CVP line 3 cm to 5 cm to expose an area of sterile tubing. Transect the tubing through a sterile area while holding it firmly at skin level. Pass a guidewire through the tubing, and then withdraw the tubing so that only the wire is left in the vein. Never release the guidewire and the tubing because embolization may result.

With the guidewire in place, pass a dilator and introducer sheath together over the guidewire, as is done in the Seldinger technique. Remove the dilator and guidewire and pass the pacing catheter through the introducer sheath (Fig. 15.8, *step 1*). One key additional step to help preserve sterility while manipulating the pacing catheter is to attach an extensible sleeve on the end of the introducer before inserting the pacing catheter (see Fig. 15.8, *steps 1 and 6*). In this way, the pacing catheter can be advanced and withdrawn multiple times without fear of contamination.

Bedside ultrasound (US) can be useful as an aid in securing central venous access, and its use in the setting of emergency TVP has been reported.[93,94]

Pacemaker Placement

Emergency Blind Passage

In an emergency, a transvenous pacemaker wire can be advanced blindly. Attach the pacer wire to the pacemaker energy source and turn it on at a rate of 80 beats/min, output at 20 mA of current, and set the asynchronous (fixed-rate) mode. After the wire is blindly advanced to 15 to 20 cm depth (two hash marks on the wire) inflate the pacing wire balloon and advance the pacing wire while viewing the patient's cardiac monitor. When capture is seen on the ECG monitor by observing a pacer spike followed by QRS ST-segment elevation, the pacing wire is in the proper position. Deflate the balloon and secure the pacing wire at the skin.

When time permits, or if the blind passage procedure is not successful, the procedure can be done under US and/or ECG guidance, both of which are described subsequently.

Ultrasound Guidance

Ultrasound is an important tool to assist in the placement of emergency transvenous pacing catheters.[95–97] US may also help demonstrate whether mechanical capture has been achieved. The advantages of US over fluoroscopy are no exposure to ionizing radiation, lower rates of complications, and faster times to pacemaker insertion.[98,99] US guidance can be used in place of or in conjunction with ECG guidance (Ultrasound Box).

Electrocardiographic Guidance

Connect the patient to the limb leads of an ECG machine and turn the indicator to record the chest (V) lead.

With newer ECG machines, the pacemaker may be attached to any of the V leads (usually V_1 or V_5) that are displayed during rhythm monitoring. The distal terminal of the pacing catheter (the cathode or lead marked "negative", "–.", or "distal") must be connected to the V lead of the ECG machine by a male-to-male connector or by an insulated wire with an alligator clip on each end. Some prepackaged kits contain an alligator clamp that can be connected to the lead with an adapter pin (Fig. 15.8, *step 2*). The pacing catheter is thus an exploring electrode that creates a unipolar electrode for intracardiac ECG recording. The ECG tracing recorded from the electrode tip localizes the position of the tip of the pacing electrode. Because the tracing on the ECG machine may be slightly delayed, advancement of the catheter after initial insertion must be evaluated carefully. Insert the catheter 15 to 20 cm so the tip is safely in the central venous system and inflate the balloon with air (Fig. 15.8, *step 3*). The inflation port should be locked and the syringe left attached.

Advance the pacing catheter both quickly and smoothly. Monitor the ECG V lead and observe the P wave and QRS complex to ascertain the location of the tip of the pacing catheter (Fig. 15.8, *step 4*). Use of electrocardiography to guide placement of a pacing catheter is based on two concepts. First, the complex will vary in size depending on which chamber is entered. For example, when the tip of the pacing catheter is in the atrium, one will see large P waves, often larger than the corresponding QRS complex. Second, the sum of the electrical forces will be negative if the depolarization is moving away from the catheter tip and positive if the depolarization is moving toward the catheter tip. Therefore if the tip of the catheter is above the atrium, both the P wave and QRS complex will be negative (i.e., the electrical forces of a normally beating heart will be moving away from the catheter tip). As the tip progresses inferiorly in the atrium, the P wave will become isoelectric (biphasic) and will eventually become positive as the wave of atrial depolarization advances toward the tip of the catheter. The ECG tracing resembles an aVR lead initially when in the left subclavian vein (Fig. 15.9A) or the midportion of the superior vena cava (Fig. 15.9B). At the high right atrial level, both the P wave and QRS complex are negative. The P wave is larger than the QRS complex and is deeply inverted (Fig. 15.9C–D). As the center of the atrium is approached, the P wave becomes larger and biphasic (Fig. 15.9E). As the catheter approaches

Emergency Transvenous Cardiac Pacing

1

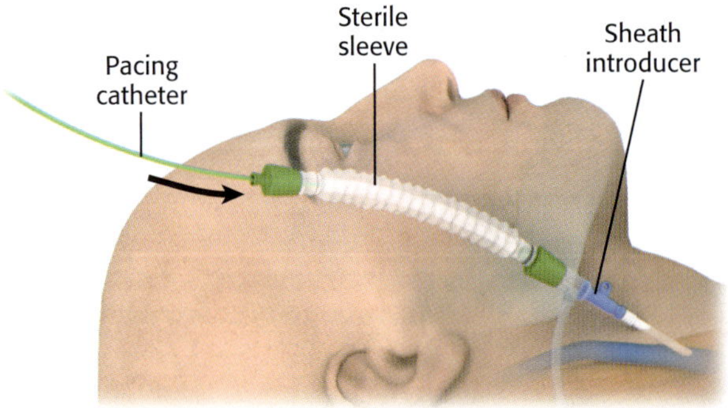

Establish a sheath introducer in the selected vein. Attach the still-compressed sterile sleeve to the introducer hub. Check the balloon for integrity and then advance the catheter into the sleeve. (Full sterile drapes should be used but are not depicted here.)

2

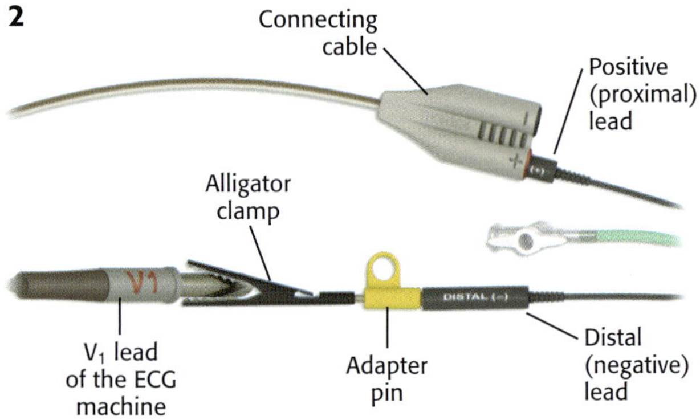

Instruct an assistant to make the following nonsterile connections. Attach the proximal (+) lead to the positive terminal of the connecting cable and the distal (–) lead to the V_1 lead of an ECG machine with an alligator clamp. (Alternatively, an insulated wire with an alligator clip on each end may be used.)

3

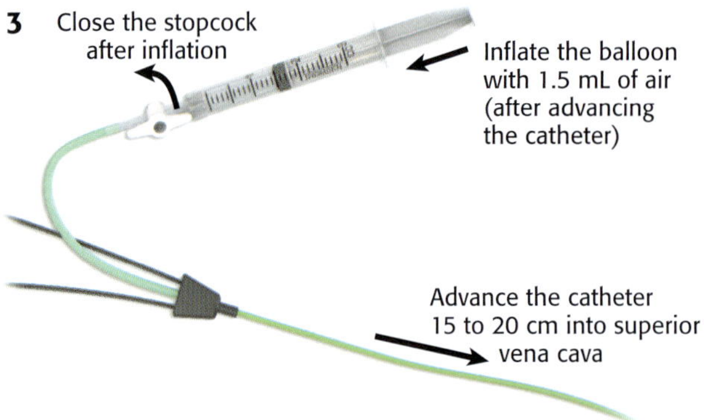

Advance the catheter approximately 15 to 20 cm so that the tip lies within the superior vena cava. Then inflate the balloon with 1.5 mL of air. Close the stopcock valve to keep the balloon inflated.

4

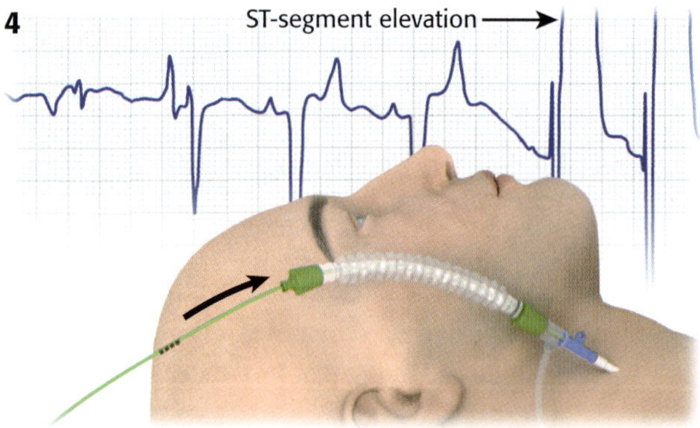

Advance the pacing catheter quickly and smoothly. Monitor the V lead on the electrocardiogram to ascertain the location of the tip of the pacing catheter. The P wave and QRS complex will vary in size depending on which chamber the tip is in, and the sum of the electrical forces will be negative if depolarization is moving away from the catheter tip and positive if depolarization is moving toward it. ST-segment elevation will occur when the tip contacts the endocardium.

5

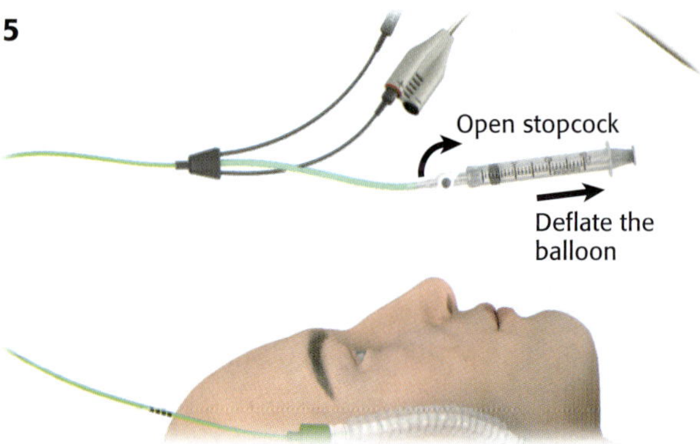

When the pacing catheter is in the desired position, deflate the balloon by unlocking the stopcock and allow the syringe to spontaneously refill with air.

6

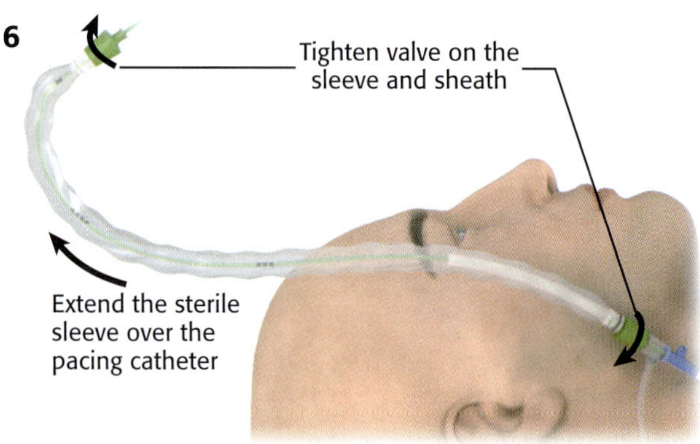

Extend the sterile sleeve so that it fully covers the pacing catheter. If your sheath and sleeve have valves, close them by turning clockwise to keep the wire and sleeve in place.

Fig. 15.8 Emergency transvenous cardiac pacing. Note that by attaching the pacing catheter to the electrocardiographic (ECG) machine *(step 2)* and observing the V_1 ECG tracing, the negative lead now becomes an exploring lead that tells the operator the position of the tip of the pacing catheter in the body (see Fig. 15.9).

Continued

Emergency Transvenous Cardiac Pacing, CONTINUED

7

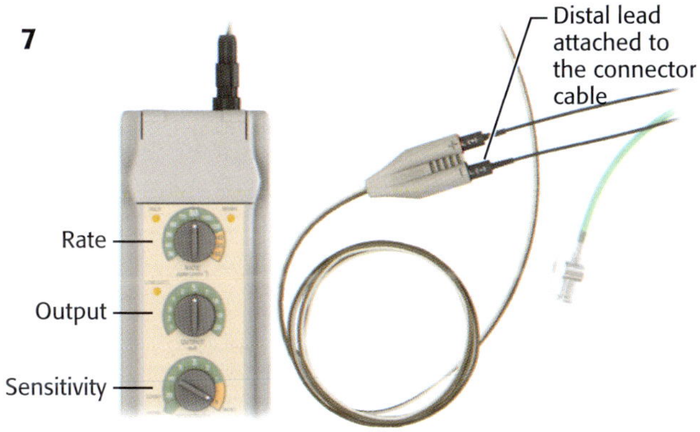

Disconnect the catheter's distal (negative) lead from the ECG machine and attach it to the energy soure via the connector cable. Set the rate to 80 beats/min, the output to 5 mA, and the sensitivity to full-demand mode (most sensitivity), and turn the pacer on.

8

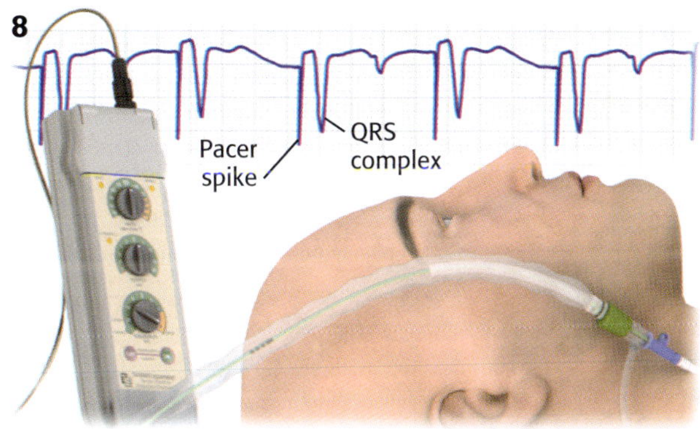

Assess for electrical capture by looking for a QRS complex to follow each pacer spike on the ECG monitor. Assess for mechanical capture by checking for a palpable pulse that equals the pacemaker rate. Reposition the catheter if needed.

9

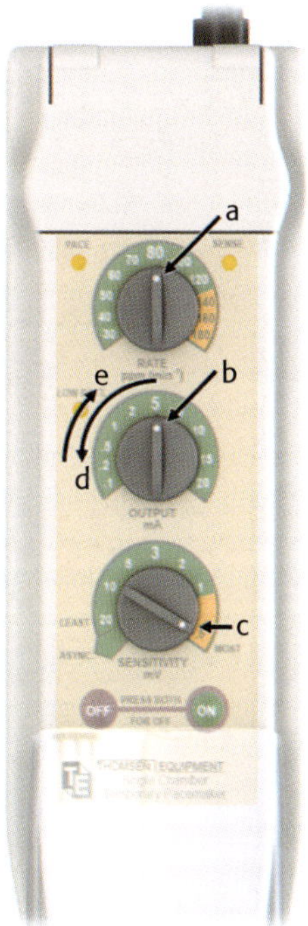

Testing Threshold

a. Set rate to 80 beats/min.
b. Set output to 5 mA.
c. Set sensitivity to maximum.
d. Reduce output slowly until capture is lost. This output is the threshold.
e. Increase output to 2.5 times the threshold to ensure consistency of capture (usually 2 to 3 mA).

10

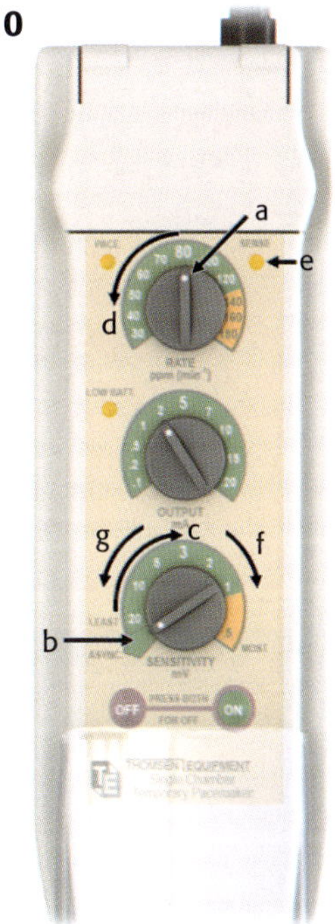

Testing Sensing

a. Set the rate at 10 beats/min greater than intrinsic rhythm.
b. Place the pacemaker in asynchronous mode (minimum sensitivity) and ensure that there is complete capture.
c. Adjust the sensitivity to midposition (approx. 3 mV).
d. Decrease the rate until pacing is suppressed by the intrinsic rhythm.
e. Check that the sensing indicator signals each time that a native beat is sensed.
f. If the pacer fails to sense an intrinsic rhythm, increase the sensitivity.
g. If the pacer oversenses (e.g., triggered by P or T waves or artifact), decrease the sensitivity.
h. Once the sensitivity threshold is determined, set the millivoltage to half that value.

Fig. 15.8, cont'd

the lower atrium (Fig. 15.9F), the P wave becomes smaller and upright. The QRS complex is fairly normal. When striking the right atrial wall, an injury pattern with a P-Ta segment is seen (Fig. 15.9G). As the electrode passes through the tricuspid valve, the P wave becomes smaller and the QRS complex becomes larger (Fig. 15.9H). Placement in the inferior vena cava may be recognized by a change in the morphology of the P wave and a decrease in the amplitude of both the P wave and the QRS complex (Fig. 15.9I).

Once the pacing catheter is in the desired position, deflate the balloon by unlocking the port, observe that the syringe refills with air spontaneously, and then remove the syringe (Fig. 15.8, *step 5*). Avoid drawing back on the syringe because this may rupture the balloon. If the syringe does not refill spontaneously, the balloon might be ruptured. Do not inflate the balloon. Withdraw the pacing catheter, and check the balloon for leaks. If a leak is found, use a new pacing catheter.

After successful passage of the catheter into the right ventricle, advance the tip until contact is made with the endocardial wall. When this occurs, the QRS segment will show ST-segment elevation (Fig. 15.9J). Ideally, the tip of the

ULTRASOUND: Transvenous Cardiac Pacing

by Christine Butts, MD

Using ultrasound to guide placement of a transvenous pacemaker (TVP) gives the physician the advantage of direct visualization of the tip of the pacemaker and the ability to directly maneuver it into the correct position to obtain capture. Although placement of a TVP is a relatively rare procedure in the emergency department, the use of ultrasound has been described to facilitate the procedure.[1,2] Ultrasound can also be used to evaluate placement in cases in which blind attempts at TVP are unsuccessful. Additionally, ultrasound is useful in achieving the central venous access necessary to introduce the pacemaker.

Equipment

A low-frequency (2 mHz to 5 mHz) transducer offers the optimum depth to evaluate the heart. A phased-array or microconvex transducer is ideal for this purpose because its small footprint enables the sonographer to "see" between the patient's ribs. In the absence of a phased-array or microconvex transducer, a curvilinear transducer may be adequate. Although insertion of a TVP is a sterile procedure, the transducer does not need to be sterile if it is used away from the field. If the transducer will be used near or on the field, it can be placed inside a sterile cover or a sterile glove.

Image Interpretation

The subxiphoid view of the heart is the optimum view for this procedure (Fig. 15.US1). It enables the operator to view all four chambers of the heart at once. The subxiphoid view is obtained by placing the transducer just inferior to the xiphoid process with the indicator pointing toward the patient's right side (Fig. 15.US2). A hand should be placed on top of the transducer to enable the sonographer to push downward into the epigastric area. The transducer can then be aimed toward the left side of the chest until the four-chambered view of the heart is seen. In this view, the left lobe of the liver is seen at the top of the image. Deep to this is the heart, with the right atrium and ventricle abutting the liver.

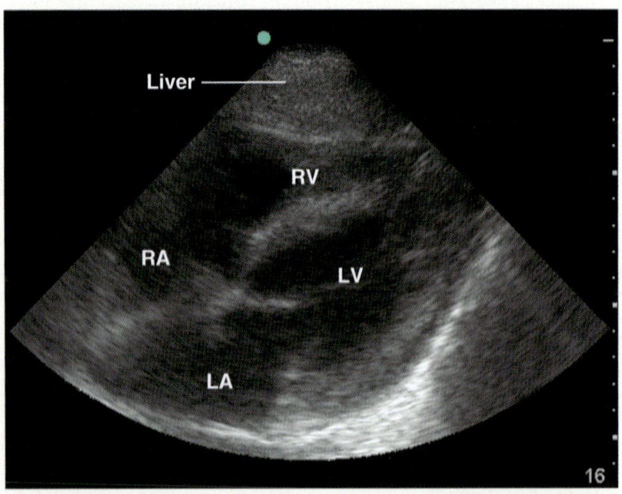

Fig. 15.US1 Ultrasound subxiphoid image of the heart. In this ultrasound the liver is seen at the top of the image. The heart is seen below, with the right ventricle *(RV)*, right atrium *(RA)*, and left atrium *(LA)* abutting the left lobe of the liver. The left ventricle *(LV)* and atria are deep to the right side at the bottom of the image.

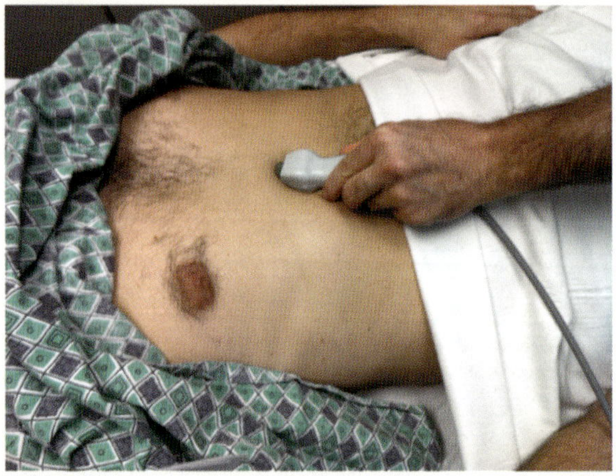

Fig. 15.US2 Placement of the ultrasound transducer to obtain a subxiphoid image of the heart.

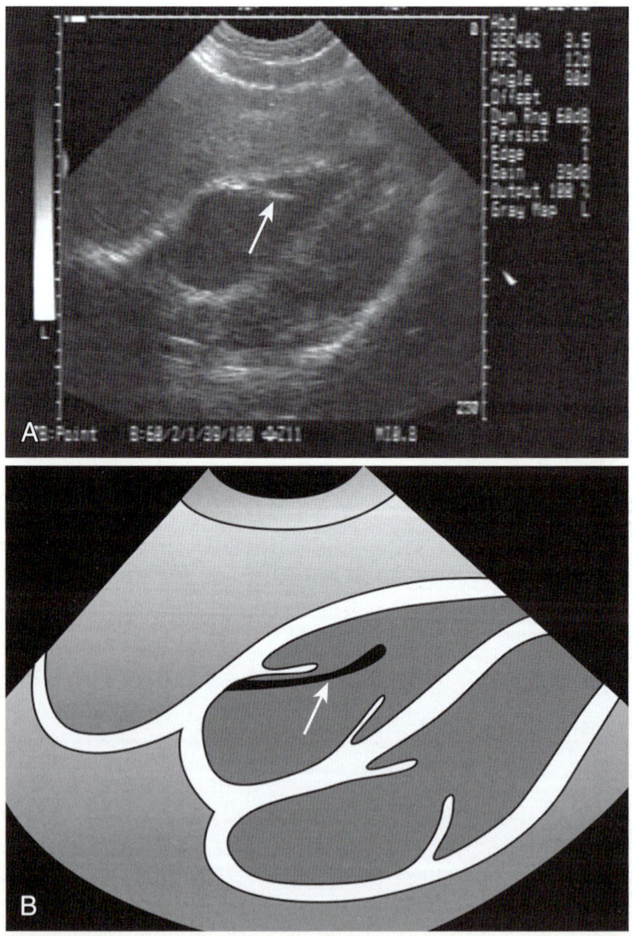

Fig. 15.US3 Pacing wire within the right ventricle *(arrows)*. (A) Sonographic image. (B) Schematic representation. The right ventricle is seen through the subxiphoid window, which provides excellent views of the heart without interfering with placement of the pacemaker line. The pacemaker wire is seen as a brightly echogenic structure within the right ventricle.

Continued

ULTRASOUND: Transvenous Cardiac Pacing—cont'd

Procedure and Technique

To guide the placement of the TVPM, the procedure should begin in the usual fashion (as described earlier). Once the pacer wire has been inserted, the sonographer should begin observing the right atrium. The wire will appear as a hyperechoic (white) linear echo as it enters the right atrium and it can be seen to advance in real time (Fig. 15.US3). The wire should be followed as it enters the right ventricle. This can be observed simultaneously with the electrical readings on the monitor. Capture of the pacemaker can be confirmed by visualization of coordinated, rhythmic contractions of the myocardium at the set rate. The monitor can also be evaluated for signs of electrical capture.

REFERENCES

1. Aguilera P, Durham B, Riley D. Emergency transvenous cardiac pacing placement using ultrasound guidance. *Ann Emerg Med*. 2000;36:224-227.
2. Macedo W, Sturmann K, Kim JM, et al. Ultrasonographic guidance of transvenous pacemaker insertion in the emergency department. *J Emerg Med*. 1999;17:491-496.

catheter should be lodged in the trabeculae at the apex of the right ventricle; however, pacing may also be successful if the catheter is in various other positions within the ventricle or outflow tract.

If the pacer enters the pulmonary artery outflow tract, the P wave again becomes negative, and the QRS amplitude diminishes (Fig. 15.9K). If the catheter is in the pulmonary artery, withdraw the pacing catheter into the right ventricle and readvance it. Sometimes a clockwise or counterclockwise twist of the catheter will redirect its path in a more favorable direction. If catheter-induced ectopy develops, withdraw the catheter slightly until the ectopy stops, and then readvance it. Once ventricular endocardial contact is made, disconnect the catheter from the ECG machine and connect the distal lead to the negative terminal on the pacing generator (Fig. 15.8, *step 7*). Set the pacing generator at a rate of 80 or 10 beats/min faster than the underlying ventricular rhythm, whichever is higher. Select the full-demand mode with an output of approximately 5 mA. Then turn on the pacing generator.

Assess the patient for electrical and mechanical capture. Electrical capture will be manifested on the ECG monitor as a pacer spike followed by a QRS complex (Fig. 15.8, *step 8*). If a pacer spike is seen but no QRS follows, capture is not occurring. Mechanical capture means that a pacer spike with its corresponding QRS triggers a myocardial contraction. This can be assessed by checking that a palpable pulse is present and equal to the rate set on the pacemaker. If complete capture does not occur or if it is intermittent, the pacer will need to be repositioned. When proper capture occurs, assess the pacer for optimal positioning. This is done by testing the thresholds for pacing and sensing, and by physical examination, electrocardiography, and chest radiography.

Catheter Placement in Low-Flow States

If cardiac output is too low to float a pacing catheter or if the patient is in extremis, there may not be enough time to advance a pacing catheter via the previously described techniques. Such a situation would be asystole or complete heart block with malignant ventricular escape rhythms (although one can make a case for TCP in such conditions). In such emergency situations, connect the pacing catheter to the energy source, turn the output to the maximum amperage, and select the asynchronous mode (see earlier section on "Emergency Blind Passage"). Advance the catheter blindly in the hope that it will enter the right ventricle and pacing will be accomplished. Rotate, advance, withdraw, or otherwise manipulate the pacing catheter according to clinical response. The right internal jugular approach is the most practical access route in this situation.

Testing Threshold

The threshold is the minimum current necessary to obtain capture. Ideally, it is less than 1.0 mA, and usually it is between 0.3 and 0.7 mA. If the threshold is in this ideal range, good contact with the endocardium can be presumed.

To determine the threshold, set the pacing generator to maximum sensitivity (full-demand mode) at 5-mA output and a rate of approximately 80 beats/min (or at least 10 beats/min greater than the patient's intrinsic rate) (Fig. 15.8, *step 9*). Reduce the current (output) slowly until capture is lost. This current is the threshold. Carry out this maneuver two or three times to ensure that this value is consistent. Increase the amperage to 2.5 times the threshold to ensure consistency of capture (usually between 2 and 3 mA).

Testing Sensing

Test the sensing function in patients who have underlying rhythms. Set the rate at approximately 10 beats/min greater than the endogenous rhythm, place the pacemaker in asynchronous mode (minimum sensitivity, which is the maximum setting on the sensitivity voltage control), and ensure that there is complete capture (Fig. 15.8, *step 10*). Then adjust the sensitivity control to its midposition or approximately 3 mV and gradually decrease the rate until pacing is suppressed by the patient's intrinsic rhythm. The sensing indicator on the pacing generator should signal each time a native beat is sensed and should be in synchrony with each QRS complex on the ECG monitor. If the pacer fails to sense the intrinsic rhythm, increase the sensitivity (decrease the millivolts) until the pacer is suppressed. Conversely, if the sensing indicator is triggered by P or T waves or by artifact, decrease the sensitivity until only the QRS complex is sensed. Once the sensitivity threshold is determined, set the millivoltage to approximately half that value.

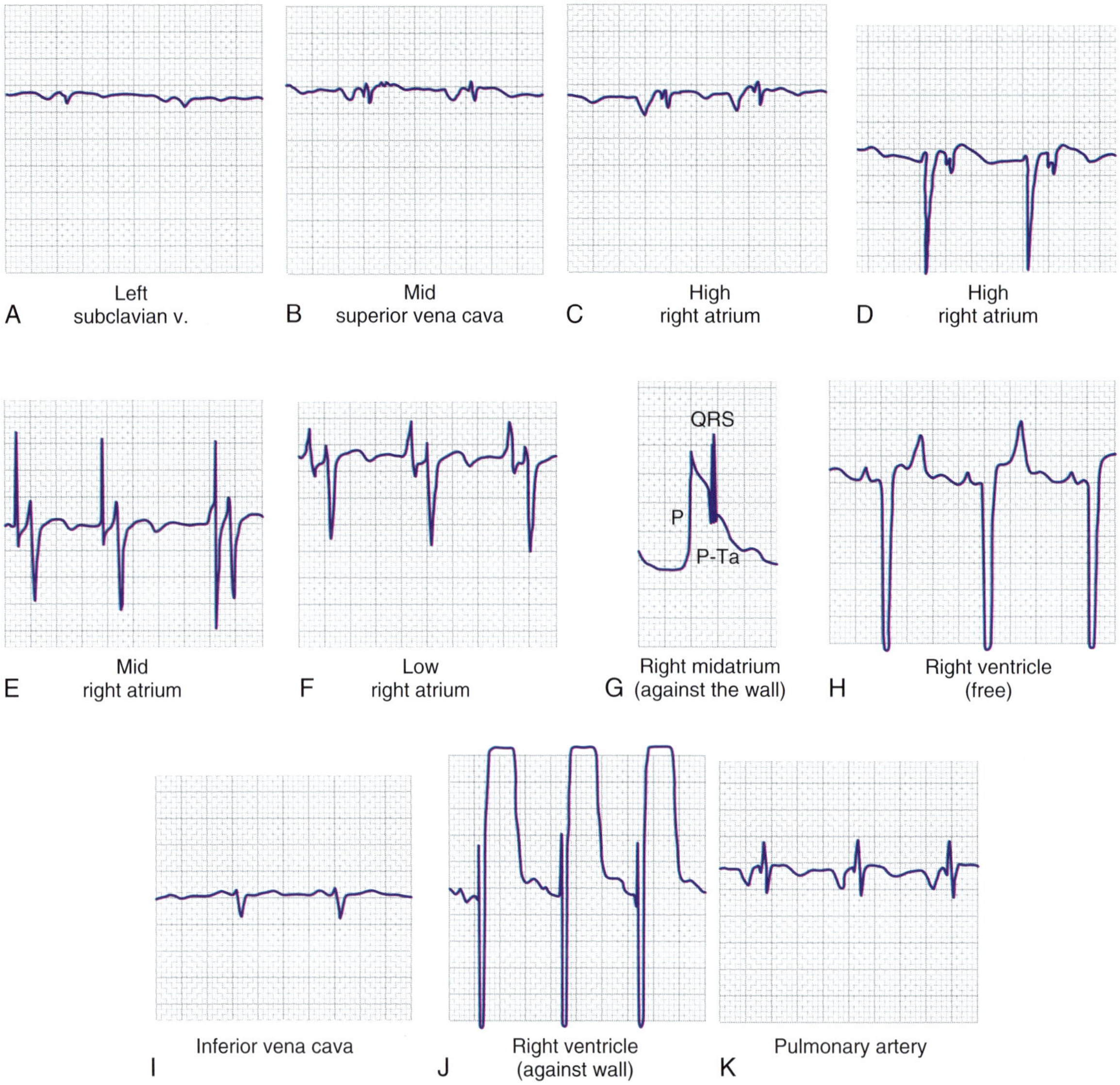

Fig. 15.9 For pacemaker placement with electrocardiographic (ECG) guidance, connect the patient to the limb leads of an ECG machine, and turn the indicator to record the chest (V) lead. With newer ECG machines, the pacemaker may be attached to any of the V leads (usually V_1 or V_5) that are displayed during rhythm monitoring. The distal terminal of the pacing catheter (the cathode or lead marked "negative", "–." or "distal") must be connected to the V lead of the ECG machine by a male-to-male connector or by an insulated wire with an alligator clip on each end. As one advances the pacing catheter and records the ECG complex that is obtained from the distal electrode (the exploring lead), the location of the tip of the pacing wire can be ascertained. (A–C) Left subclavian vein, mid superior vena cava, and high right atrium, respectively. (D) With the tip of the pacer in the high right atrium, above the sinoatrial node, the P waves are large and negative which indicates that the cardiac forces are moving away from the tip of the catheter. (E) Mid right atrium. (F) With the exploring electrode in the low right atrium the P waves are now positive because the sinus depolarization is now coming toward the tip of the electrode. (G) Right midatrium. (H) With the recording electrode tip free in the right ventricle positive P waves and large QRS complexes are seen. (I) Inferior vena cava. (J) When lodged against the ventricular wall, the current of injury denotes proper pacer tip placement. (K) Pulmonary artery. (A–F and H–K, From Bing OH, McDowell JW, Hantman J, et al. Pacemaker placement by electrocardiographic monitoring. *N Engl J Med*. 1972;287:651. G, From Goldberger E. *Treatment of Cardiac Emergencies*. 3rd ed. Mosby; 1982:252.)

Securing and Final Assessment

After the pacemaker's position has been tested for electrical accuracy, it must be secured in place. If a sealed introducer sheath was used, the hub should be fixed firmly to the skin with suture (e.g., 4-0 nylon or silk). A fastening suture should be sewn to the skin and the hub tied securely in place. If a plain introducer was used, withdraw it to prevent leakage and suture the catheter in place. In either case, coil the excess pacing catheter and secure it in a sterile manner underneath a large sterile dressing. Assess pacemaker function again, and take a chest film to ensure proper positioning. Ideal positioning of the pacing catheter is at the apex of the right ventricle (Fig. 15.10).

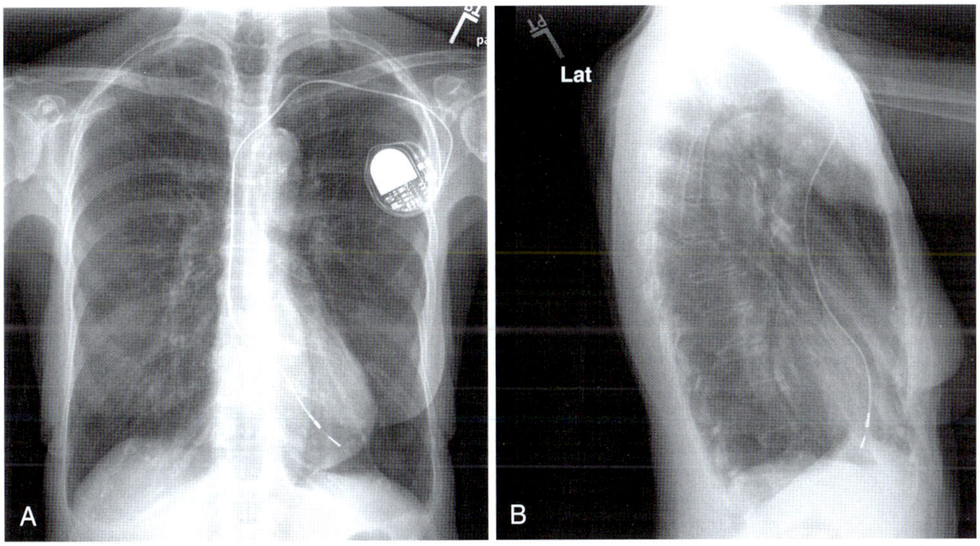

Fig. 15.10 (A) Normal pacemaker position in the apex of the right ventricle on posteroanterior chest film and (B) lateral chest film.

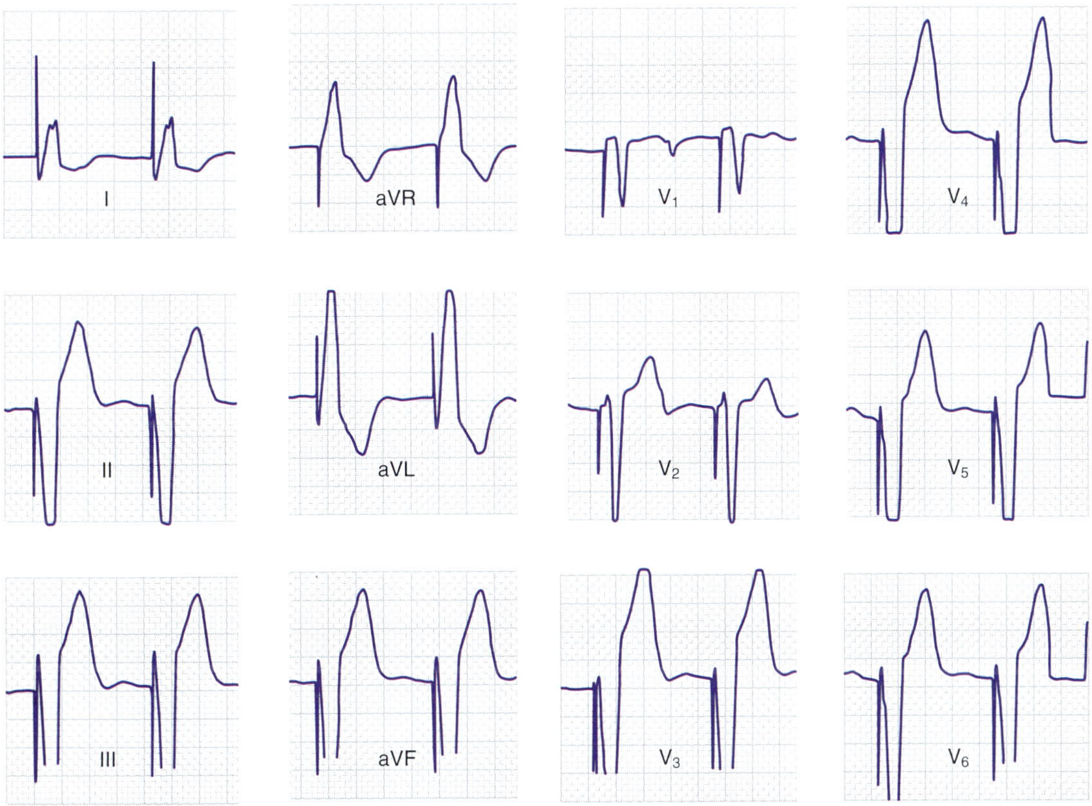

Fig. 15.11 Electrocardiographic pattern of a right ventricular pacemaker.

A 12-lead ECG tracing should be obtained after placement of the transvenous pacemaker. If the catheter is within the right ventricle, an LBBB pattern with left-axis deviation should be evident in paced beats (Fig. 15.11). If an RBBB pattern is noted, coronary sinus placement or left ventricular pacing secondary to septal penetration should be suspected (Fig. 15.12).

With a properly functioning ventricular pacemaker, large cannon waves may be noted on inspection of the venous pulsations at the neck. When the pacemaker achieves ventricular capture, there may be times when the atria contract against a closed tricuspid valve and a cannon wave results. On auscultation of the heart, a slight murmur may be evident, secondary to tricuspid insufficiency as a result of the catheter interfering with the tricuspid valve apparatus.[100] Following each pacemaker impulse, a clicking sound may be heard during expiration; this is believed to represent either intercostal or diaphragmatic muscular contractions caused by the pacemaker.[101] Note that this can also be a sign of cardiac perforation.[102] On auscultation of the second heart sound,

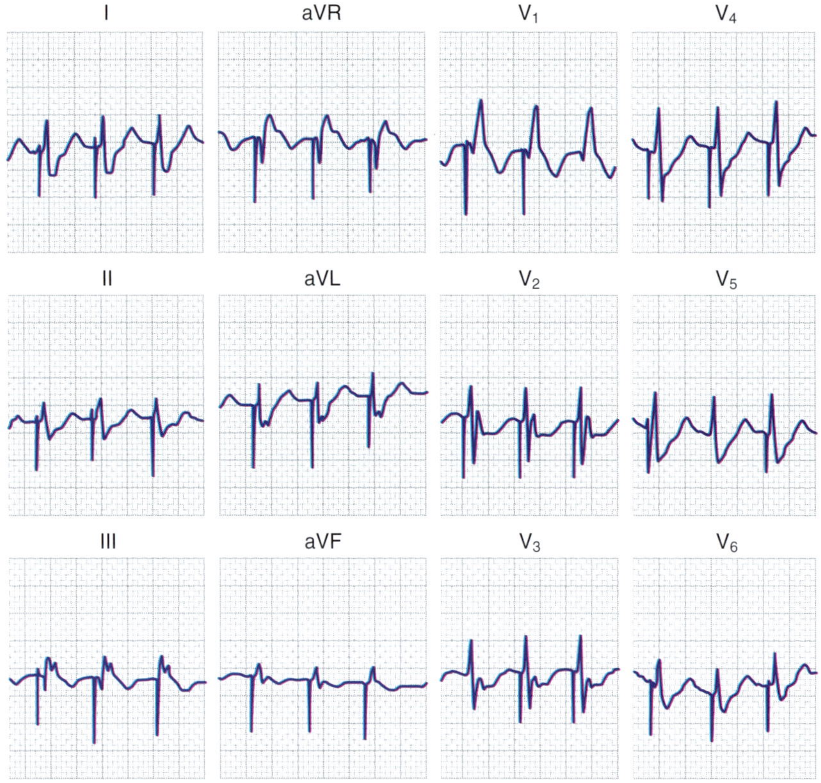

Fig. 15.12 Coronary sinus pacing. Note the paced right bundle branch block pattern.

paradoxical splitting may be noted. This represents a delay in closure of the aortic valve because of delayed left ventricular depolarization.

As in any procedure, assess the patient for improvement in clinical status. Evaluate vital signs, mentation, congestive symptoms, and urinary output. In addition, look for complications secondary to the procedure and treat as needed.

Complications

The complications associated with emergency transvenous cardiac pacing are numerous and represent a compendium of those related to central venous catheterization,[85,103] those related to right-sided heart catheterization, and those unique to the pacing catheter itself. Overall rates of adverse events using modern flexible, balloon-tipped catheters are in the range of 20%.[85,104] However, the majority of complications are a result of obtaining venous access, and when US guidance is used the rate is markedly decreased.[105]

Problems Related to Central Venous Catheterization

Inadvertent arterial puncture is a well-known complication of the percutaneous approach to the venous system.[105] This problem is usually recognized quickly because of the rapid return of arterial blood. Firm compression over the puncture site will almost always result in hemostasis in 5 minutes or less.

Venous thrombosis and thrombophlebitis are also potential problems with central venous catheterization. Thrombophlebitis, which occurs early after insertion, is an uncommon complication. Thrombosis of the innominate vein is also a rare problem, with pulmonary embolism being an even more uncommon event.[106] Femoral vein thrombosis, however, appears to be a much more common event associated with femoral vein catheterization.[90,107] Studies using noninvasive techniques have shown a 37% incidence of femoral vein thrombosis, with 55% of these patients having evidence of pulmonary embolism on ventilation-perfusion scans.[107] At least one study suggests that the use of low-dose enoxaparin is safe and effective in reducing pacemaker-related femoral vein thrombosis.[108]

Pneumothorax is consistently a problem with the various approaches to the veins at the base of the neck. The decision to place a chest tube in patients with this complication depends on the extent of the air leak and the clinical status of the patient. In addition, laceration of the subclavian vein with hemothorax,[109] laceration of the thoracic duct with chylothorax, air embolism, wound infections, pneumomediastinum, hydromediastinum, hemomediastinum,[110] phrenic nerve injury,[111] and fracture of the guidewire with embolization[112,113] are all potential complications.[33,109]

Complications of Right-Sided Heart Catheterization

A frequent complication of the pacing catheter is dysrhythmia, with premature ventricular contractions being a common occurrence. One study noted a 1.5% incidence of serious dysrhythmias with a balloon-tipped catheter inserted under ECG guidance.[84] Another study noted a 6% incidence of ventricular tachycardia during insertion.[90] An ischemic heart is more prone to dysrhythmias than a nonischemic heart.[114] Therapy for catheter-induced ectopy during insertion involves repositioning the catheter in the ventricle. This usually stops the ectopy; however, if after repeated attempts it is found that the catheter cannot be passed without ectopy, myocardial suppressant therapy may be used to desensitize the myocardium.

Misplacement of the pacing catheter has been well studied. Passage of the catheter into the pulmonary artery can be

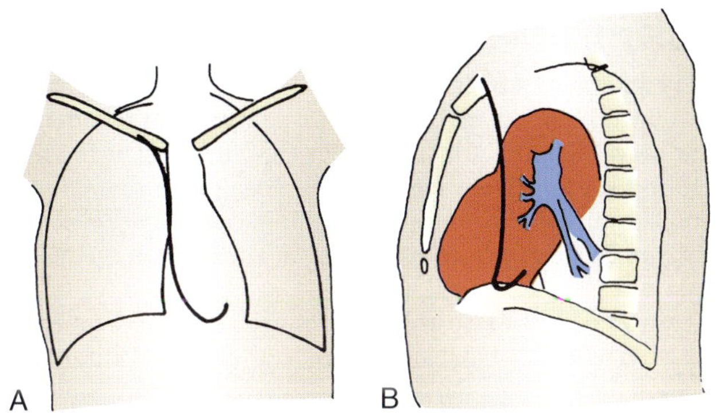

Fig. 15.13 Coronary sinus position. (A) Posteroanterior view. (B) Lateral view. Normally, the tip of the catheter should point anteriorly toward the apex of the heart. With coronary sinus placement, the tip is displaced posteriorly and several centimeters from the sternum. (A–B, From Goldberger E. *Treatment of Cardiac Emergencies*. 3rd ed. Mosby; 1982.)

diagnosed electrocardiographically by observing the return of an inverted P wave and a decrease in the voltage of the QRS complex. Misplacement in the coronary sinus may occur and should be suspected in patients in whom a paced RBBB pattern on the electrocardiogram is seen with right ventricular pacing (see Fig. 15.12). Rarely, an RBBB pattern can be seen with a normal right ventricular position; therefore all RBBB patterns do not represent coronary sinus pacing.[115] Further evidence of coronary sinus location can be obtained by viewing the lateral chest film. Normally the tip of the catheter should point anteriorly toward the apex of the heart; however, with placement in the coronary sinus, the tip of the catheter is displaced posteriorly and several centimeters away from the sternum (Fig. 15.13). Other potential forms of misplacement include left ventricular pacing through an atrial or ventricular septal defect, septal puncture, extraluminal insertion, and arterial insertion.[116]

Perforation of the ventricle is a well-described complication that can result in loss of capture,[117] hemopericardium, and tamponade.[118,119] Reported symptoms and signs of this problem include chest pain, pericardial friction rub, and diaphragmatic or chest wall muscular pacing.[120] At least one case of a postpericardiotomy-like syndrome and two cases of endocardial friction rub have been reported without perforation[121,122]

Pericardial perforation is suggested radiographically when the pacing catheter is outside or abuts the cardiac silhouette and is not in proper position within the right ventricular cavity (Fig. 15.14).[123] ECG clues include a change in the QRS complex and T-wave axis or failure to properly sense. In suspected cases, a two-dimensional echocardiogram usually demonstrates the catheter's extracardiac position. Simply pulling the catheter back and repositioning it in the right ventricle can usually treat uncomplicated perforation.

During insertion of a temporary pacing catheter when a nonfunctioning permanent catheter is in place, there is a small risk of entanglement or knotting.[124] This potential also exists with other central lines and pulmonary artery catheters. Even without the presence of other lines, the pacing catheter can become knotted.[125] Frequently, these lines can be untangled under fluoroscopy with the use of specialized catheters.

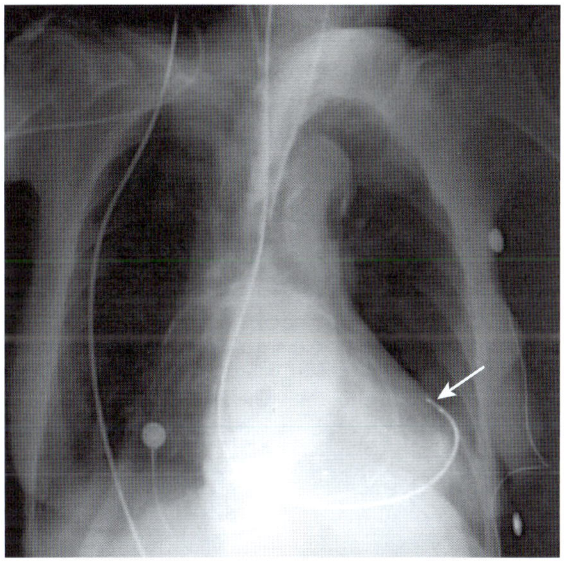

Fig. 15.14 A pacing catheter tip *(arrow)* that is outside or abuts the cardiac silhouette and is not properly positioned within the right ventricular cavity suggests myocardial perforation. (From Tarver RD, Gillespie KR. The misplaced tube. *Emerg Med Clin North Am*. 1988;20:97.)

Local and systemic infection,[92] balloon rupture, pulmonary infarction,[126] phrenic nerve pacing,[127] and rupture of the chordae tendineae are also potential complications.

Complications of the Pacing Electrode

Complications related to the pacing electrode can be separated into three groups: mechanical, organic, and electrical.

Mechanical failures include displacement, fracture of the catheter, and loose leads. Displacement can result in intermittent or complete loss of capture or improper sensing, malignant dysrhythmias, diaphragmatic pacing, or perforation. Displacement should be suspected with changes in amplitude, with changes of greater than 90 degrees in vector, or with a change in threshold.[128] Frequently, catheter fractures may be detected by careful review of the chest film or may be suspected because of a change in the sensing threshold. As with displacement, catheter fractures may result in intermittent or complete loss of capture.

Organic causes of pacemaker failure result in changes in the threshold or sensing function.[129] Progressive inflammation, fibrosis, and thrombosis may result in more than doubling of the original threshold.[130] However, this process takes several weeks and is of no concern in the setting of pacemaker placement in the ED.

Electrical problems with pacing in the past have included failure of the pacemaker generator, dysrhythmias, and outside interference. Modern devices are extremely reliable and resistant to outside interference. Although ventricular tachycardia and ventricular fibrillation have been reported to result from pacemakers, these dysrhythmias are rare. Therefore patients with such dysrhythmias should be evaluated for a non–pacemaker-induced cause.[131] Defibrillation and cardioversion are safe in patients who have temporary pacemakers.

REFERENCES ARE AVAILABLE AT Elsevier eBooks+

CHAPTER 16

Pericardiocentesis

Semhar Z. Tewelde and Rohit Menon

DEFINITION

Pericardial effusion, the accumulation of fluid within the pericardial space, arises from various causes. When fluid volume reaches a critical threshold, it elevates pericardial pressure, impairs cardiac filling, and leads to circulatory insufficiency. This condition is termed pericardial tamponade. If compensatory mechanisms fail, obstructive shock develops, culminating in cardiac arrest without immediate intervention. Fluid removal remains the definitive treatment to stabilize hemodynamics at this stage.

ANATOMY AND PHYSIOLOGY

Pericardium and Pericardial Space

The pericardium is an avascular, fibroelastic, two-layered sac that surrounds the heart.[1] The visceral pericardium is a single-cell layer that adheres to the epicardium. The outer parietal pericardium is richly innervated often causes retrosternal chest pain when inflamed.[2] The pericardial space is the potential space in between these two layers and normally contains up to 50 mL of plasma ultrafiltrate, which acts as a lubricant and shock absorber. The pericardium is not essential to life but has multiple functions. It maintains pressure-volume relations, limits heart displacement, modulates hemodynamics and contractility, and acts as a mechanical barrier to infection.[3]

The pericardium, though tense, possesses elasticity that restricts excessive cardiac dilation during diastole while supporting and enhancing atrial and ventricular mechanical interactions during systole.[4] This semielastic nature enables the accommodation of up to 80 to 120 mL of acute pericardial fluid accumulation over hours to days without significantly increasing intrapericardial pressure, represented by the flat portion of the pericardial pressure-volume curve (Fig. 16.1).[5,6] Beyond this threshold, even minor additions (20 to 40 mL) can double intrapericardial pressure transitioning to the steep portion of the pressure-volume curve (Fig. 16.1) causing cardiac tamponade. Clinical tamponade generally manifests when intrapericardial pressures reach 15 to 20 mm Hg.[7]

Slow and chronic accumulation of pericardial fluid over weeks to months allows the pericardium to stretch circumferentially, accommodating upwards of 1-2 liters of fluid with minimal alteration in intrapericardial pressure. This gradual adaptation prevents significant hemodynamic compromise, and may present asymptomatically. No specific pericardial volume predicts the hemodynamic consequences of an effusion; rapid rates of accumulation are more likely to overwhelm the pericardium's ability to stretch, leading to tamponade.

Pathophysiology of Pericardial Tamponade

To generate an effective stroke volume, the left ventricle (LV) must be filled during diastole, a process largely dependent on sufficient right ventricular (RV) filling. During normal inspiration, negative intrathoracic pressure increases venous return and promotes RV filling, causing the chamber to dilate secondary to a reduction in the tension in the RV free wall.

Elevated intrapericardial pressure in early tamponade restricts RV expansion, which affects LV filling due to ventricular interdependence. This is the physiological phenomenon where the function and filling of one ventricle directly influence the function and filling of the other ventricle due to their shared common pericardial sac and interventricular septum. To accommodate RV filling, the interventricular septum bows abnormally into the LV, reducing its diastolic volume. LV filling, stroke volume, and ultimately distal tissue perfusion are reduced.[8] LV filling is also reduced by the collapse of right-sided structures. After a critical volume is reached on the pressure-volume curve (see Fig. 16.1), the intrapericardial pressure is transmitted to the inferior vena cava (IVC) and right atrium. These thin-walled structures then become compressed and reduce filling of the RV.

The atria and pulmonary circulation, being lower-pressure systems, are also vulnerable to rising intrapericardial pressure (Fig. 16.2). Late in tamponade, a "pressure plateau" occurs in which right atrial pressure, RV diastolic pressure, pulmonary artery diastolic pressure, and pulmonary capillary wedge pressure are virtually identical. This equalization of chamber pressure leads to a reduction in venous return and the echocardiographic hallmark of tamponade: diastolic collapse of the RV. At this point, hemodynamic collapse is imminent, with severe hypotension, and potentially pulseless electrical activity (PEA) developing. Unless intrapericardial pressure is decreased immediately, cardiac arrest will ensue.[9]

Compensatory Mechanisms and Pericardiocentesis

Early in tamponade, the sympathetic nervous system compensates by increasing heart rate, arterial vasoconstriction to sustain mean arterial pressure, and venoconstriction to preserve venous and atrioventricular filling gradients. These compensatory mechanisms are usually effective in maintaining adequate cardiac output.[8]

Compensatory mechanisms also preserve normal cardiac contractility and myocardial perfusion.[10,11] When the pericardial pressure overwhelms the compensatory mechanisms, coronary perfusion pressure is reduced, leading to myocardial ischemia, systolic dysfunction, and ultimately a reduction in cardiac output. Experimental induction of severe tamponade demonstrated microscopic ischemic cardiac injury.[12] Lactic acidosis caused by reduced cardiac output and systemic hypoperfusion, further impairs cardiac contractility and output.[9]

Pericardiocentesis reverses the pathophysiologic processes improving cardiac output. Interestingly, the pressure-volume relationship of the pericardial space demonstrates hysteresis. This means withdrawing a certain quantity of fluid reduces

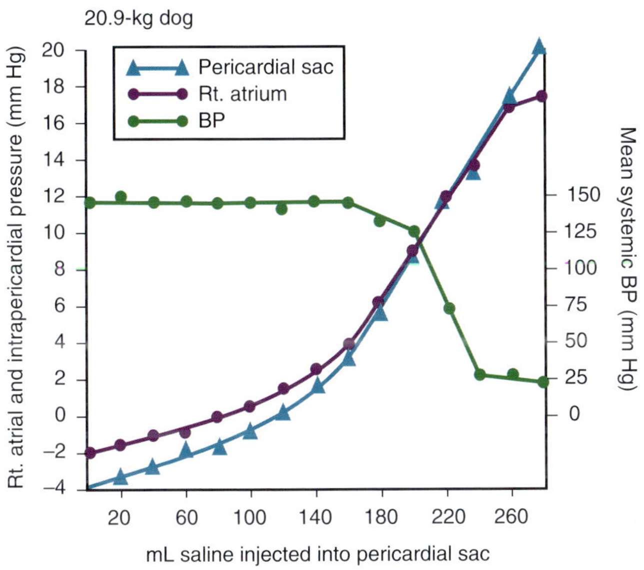

Fig. 16.1 Production of cardiac tamponade by injection of saline into the pericardial sac. The pericardial space can accommodate the acute introduction of 80 to 120 mL of fluid without a significant increase in pericardial pressure, but with approximately 200 mL of saline, pressure increases steeply and rapidly (within minutes) and blood pressure *(BP)* drops. Once critical volumes are reached, very small increases cause significant hemodynamic compromise. *Rt*, Right. (From Fowler NO. Physiology of cardiac tamponade and pulsus paradoxus. II: physiological, circulatory, and pharmacological responses in cardiac tamponade. *Mod Concepts Cardiovasc Dis*. 1978;47:116. Reproduced by permission of the American Heart Association, Inc.)

intrapericardial pressure more effectively than adding the same volume increases it. This phenomenon highlights the pericardium's semi-elastic properties and its ability to adapt during fluid accumulation. This effect, however, is not universal and may vary among patients and in various disease states (Fig. 16.3).[13]

Special Considerations in Patients With Pericardial Effusion and Tamponade

Positive pressure ventilation, such as mechanical ventilation, typically reduces venous return to the right heart by increasing intrathoracic pressure. In tamponade, where right-sided filling is already impaired, this effect can exacerbate hemodynamic instability.[14] Therefore positive pressure ventilation should be avoided in patients with known or suspected tamponade unless it is absolutely necessary.

Low-pressure pericardial tamponade is defined as a hemodynamically significant effusion with an intrapericardial pressure that is lower than expected.[15] This category of tamponade occurs in patients with subacute or chronic effusions, but present with a superimposed hypovolemia (e.g., associated with long-term diuretic use, dehydration, or excessive dialysis).[16] The diagnosis may be challenging as classic symptoms, such as distended neck veins, may be absent.[17] Ultrasound is most helpful in making the diagnosis in these patients. Fluid boluses can temporarily stabilize hemodynamics while preparing for definitive treatment, such as pericardial decompression.

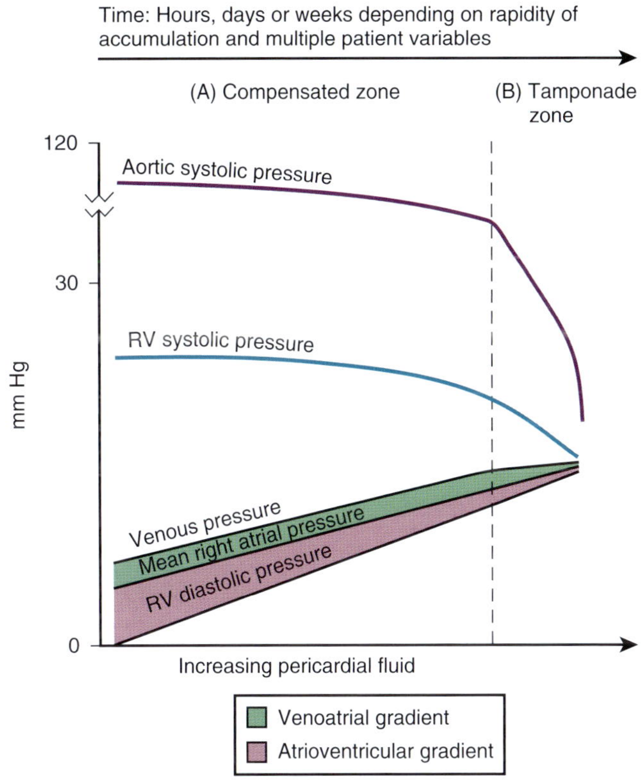

Fig. 16.2 Summary of physiologic changes in tamponade. Note the initial slow changes, then the rapid decrease in systolic pressures once critical pericardial volume and pressure are reached. *RV*, Right ventricle. (From Shoemaker WC, Carey JS, Yao ST et al. Hemodynamic monitoring for physiological evaluation, diagnosis, and therapy of acute hemopericardial tamponade from penetrating wounds. *J Trauma*. 1973;13:363; and Spodick D. Acute cardiac tamponade: pathologic physiology, diagnosis, and management. *Prog Cardiovasc Dis*. 1967;10:65.)

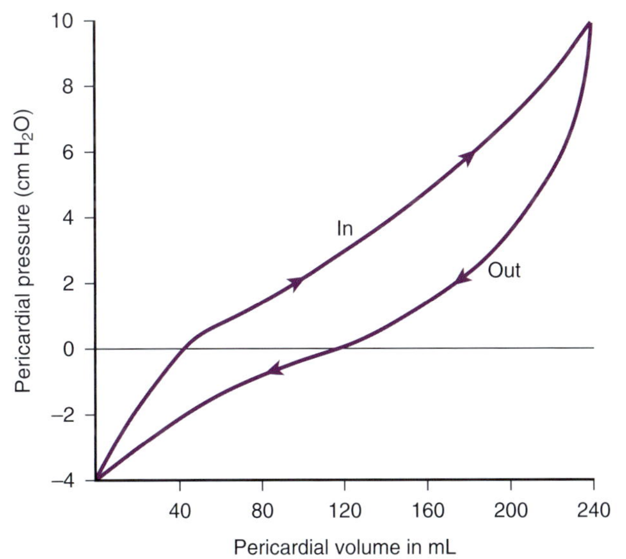

Fig. 16.3 Relationship of intrapericardial pressure to volume of pericardial fluid. Pressure drops rapidly when a small amount of fluid is removed, hence the initial significant benefit of pericardiocentesis. (From Pories W, Gaudiani V. Cardiac tamponade. *Surg Clin North Am*. 1975;55:573.)

EPIDEMIOLOGY

The major categories of pericardial effusion include infection, inflammation, malignancy, trauma, and metabolic abnormalities. Pericardial effusions may also arise from aortic disease, connective tissue disease, or idiopathic causes. Determining the incidence of specific pericardial effusion types is challenging due to variations in patient populations, local epidemiology, and diagnostic protocols. The prevalence of a chronic effusion is also difficult to ascertain because it is often asymptomatic and underreported. For instance, the Framingham study identified extra echocardiographic spaces in 6.5% of participants. Prevalence ranged from less than 1% in individuals in their 20s and 30s to more than 15% in those over 80 years old.[18]

CAUSES OF PERICARDIAL EFFUSION

Acute Hemopericardium

Acute hemopericardium, or rapid accumulation of blood in the pericardial space, can result from either traumatic or non-traumatic causes. (Box 16.1). This condition is particularly dangerous because the semielastic pericardium cannot accommodate sudden increases in pericardial fluid leading to rapid clinical deterioration. Diagnosis can be challenging, as early imaging, such as chest radiography, may not reveal pericardial enlargement. Common causes include trauma, such as penetrating cardiac injuries or blunt force, and non-traumatic events like aortic dissection extending into the pericardium. Immediate recognition and intervention are critical to prevent hemodynamic collapse.

Traumatic Hemopericardium

Penetrating Trauma

Penetrating cardiac trauma can be caused by external forces or internal forces. Cardiac perforation can lead to rapid clinical deterioration and PEA.

External cardiac puncture is often associated with stab wounds or gunshot injuries. Tamponade develops in nearly 70% of penetrating cardiac injuries and as high as 90% of patients with cardiac stab wounds.[19] Stab wounds are thought to cause tamponade more frequently because if the pericardial injury is small, it can reseal and trap blood within the pericardial space, whereas a gunshot typically produces large myocardial and pericardial wounds that allow continuous drainage into the mediastinal and pleural space. Clinical deterioration is usually secondary to hypovolemia. Penetrating cardiac injuries are an uncommon presentation at most hospitals, estimated as less than 10 cases per year due to only 6% of patients reaching the hospital alive.[20] Any penetrating injury to the chest, back, or upper part of the abdomen may injure the pericardium and cause tamponade.

Internal penetrating trauma is typically caused by invasive diagnostic or therapeutic procedures. Hemopericardium results from puncturing a cardiac chamber, a coronary artery, or a great vessel (e.g., the superior vena cava). Pericardiocentesis itself (treatment of a pericardial effusion) can cause hemopericardium if a coronary vessel or the myocardium is injured during the procedure. The procedures most often associated with this injury are valve replacement surgeries, percutaneous cardiac interventions, cardiac ablation therapy, and implantation of cardiac pacemakers. Cardiac tamponade is a complication of many other interventions including but not limited to perihiatal surgery, laparoscopic antireflux surgery, graft fixation, helical tack, and, most commonly, mechanical hernia repair with the primary mechanism being injury through the diaphragmatic dome.[21]

Internal jugular and subclavian venous catheters are commonly inserted in the emergency department (ED). In rare cases, hemopericardium results from perforation of the superior vena cava, right atrium, or RV. The incidence ranges from 0.0001% to nearly 1.5% and the signs and symptoms can arise within a few minutes or up to 5 months after placement. Thirty-six percent of tamponade cases occurred within the first day, and 82% occurred within the first week. Mechanisms include direct trauma at the time of insertion, catheter migration, and mechanical or chemical erosion.[22] Although this complication seldom occurs, it should always be considered when a patient experiences sudden hemodynamic deterioration or symptoms of chest or epigastric pain following an invasive procedure.

Blunt Trauma

Blunt trauma to the chest can occur from sudden deceleration causing compression of internal organs between the sternum and spine or an explosive force, where a pressure wave can cause disruption of the local tissue or blood vessels.[23] Major blunt chest trauma can cause hemopericardium with or without obvious signs of injury, from rupture of a cardiac chamber or, less commonly, damage to a coronary artery. Tamponade often occurs with as little as 200 mL of fluid. In certain cases where hemopneumopericardium occurs, a "bruit de Moulin" splashing murmur may be auscultated.[24] Direct impact and increased intraabdominal pressures can cause pericardial injuries such as cardiac evisceration or herniation with high mortality rates, while the deceleration mechanism can cause aortic injuries resulting in tamponade. Tamponade caused by ventricular rupture is more frequent and rapid than atrial rupture due to its lower compliance and the lower atrial pressures.[23]

Chest compressions during cardiopulmonary resuscitation (CPR) can also cause hemopericardium from broken ribs or bleeding intercostal vessels.[25] Hemopericardium following CPR has been described in case reports but is unlikely to be significant, much less to cause tamponade.[26,27]

Atraumatic Hemopericardium

Spontaneous hemopericardium, or atraumatic hemopericardium, is often challenging to diagnose due to its subtle presentation and lack of obvious clinical findings. Maintain a high index of suspicion for this condition in patients with risk factorssuch as anticoagulant use, malignancy, or tuberculosis within endemic areas.

Bleeding diathesis is an important cause of spontaneous hemopericardium and may be associated with the use of anticoagulants, although most recent data are limited to case series.[28–31] Direct oral anticoagulants are reported to have an incidence of pericardial bleeding of 0.02%.[32] Patients who have undergone cardiac surgery are at increased risk because of the anticoagulative effects of the cardiopulmonary bypass machine and medications started postoperatively (e.g., clopidogrel, warfarin). The incidence of cardiac tamponade for open heart surgery are reported to be 0.8% to 0.9%; however, this may increase as high as 4.3% in valvular surgery.[33] Fortunately, tamponade is generally detected in the postoperative period prior to discharge and is usually

BOX 16.1 Causes of Pericardial Effusion

NEOPLASM
Mesothelioma
Lung
Breast
Melanoma
Lymphoma

PERICARDITIS
Radiation related (especially after Hodgkin's disease)
Viral
Bacterial
- *Staphylococcus*
- *Pneumococcus*
- *Haemophilus*

Fungal
Tuberculosis
Amebiasis
Toxoplasmosis
Idiopathic

CONNECTIVE TISSUE DISEASE
Systemic lupus erythematosus
Scleroderma
Rheumatoid arthritis
Acute rheumatic fever

METABOLIC DISORDERS
Myxedema
Uremia
Cholesterol pericarditis
Bleeding diatheses

CARDIAC DISEASE
Acute myocardial infarction
Dissecting aortic aneurysm
Congestive heart failure
Coronary aneurysm

DRUGS
Hydralazine
Phenytoin
Anticoagulants
Procainamide
Minoxidil
Doxorubicin
Daunorubicin
Bleomycin

TRAUMA
Blunt
- Major trauma
- Closed-chest cardiopulmonary resuscitation

Penetrating
- Major penetrating trauma

Intracardiac injections
Transthoracic and transvenous pacing wires
Pericardiocentesis
Cardiac catheterization
Central venous catheters

MISCELLANEOUS
Serum sickness
Chylous effusion
Löffler syndrome
Reiter syndrome
Behçet syndrome
Pancreatitis
Postpericardiotomy
Amyloidosis
Ascites

Data from Guberman BA, Fowler NO, Engel PJ et al. Cardiac tamponade in medical patients. Circulation. *1981;64:633; and Pories WJ, Caudiani VA. Cardiac tamponade.* Surg Clin North Am *1975;55:573.*

prevented by the intraoperative placement of mediastinal or pericardial drains.

Hemopericardium can occur as a complication of myocardial infarction (MI) and is associated with significant morbidity and mortality. Early after a transmural MI (1 to 3 days), necrotic myocardial tissue can cause inflammation of the overlying pericardium, leading to the development of an effusion. In later stages, typically weeks after the MI, autoimmune pericarditis—commonly referred to as Dressler's syndrome—can result in pericardial effusion. Improved reperfusion techniques have drastically reduced the incidence of post-MI pericarditis and effusion diagnosed by echocardiography and clinical findings; however, recent advances in imaging reveal that early global pericardial enhancement can be seen on cardiac MRI about 1 week after, in more than three out of four ST-segment elevation acute MI (STEMI) cases. The clinical significance of this is unclear.[34]

Ascending aortic dissection is a catastrophic condition that can rapidly result in hemopericardium and tamponade. The dissection may expand in a retrograde fashion by extending to the base of the aorta and into the pericardial sac. Diagnosing aortic dissection can be particularly challenging and often requires advanced imaging, such as bedside ultrasound or computed tomography (CT).[35] The most common risk factors for aortic dissection include hypertension, atherosclerosis, previous cardiac surgery, collagen vascular disease such as Marfan syndrome, iatrogenic cause, and the use of sympathomimetics drugs such as cocaine.[36]

Ventricular free-wall rupture is a rapidly fatal cause of acute hemopericardium that can occur after MI leading to cardiac failure and shock. This complication, estimated to occur in up to 0.52% of acute MI (AMI), is less common today than in the past secondary to improved revascularization techniques, better therapeutic medications, and faster intervention times (shorter door-to-balloon times) for coronary ischemia.[37] Mortality has also improved with prompt recognition and intervention.[38] Prognosis is grim once tamponade occurs.

Nonhemorrhagic Effusions

Nonhemorrhagic pericardial effusions usually accumulate slower than acute hemopericardium over a period of weeks to months. Chronic fluid accumulation allows the pericardium to stretch circumferentially and accommodate upwards of 1 to 2 L of fluid without any hemodynamic compromise.[39] Effusions that grow slowly allow the circulatory system to adapt to increased intrapericardial pressure, thereby further maintaining hemodynamic stability. Asymptomatic patients with moderate to large effusions may not need emergency pericardiocentesis, in contrast to patients with acute hemopericardium.[40,41]

Nonhemorrhagic effusions have several causes (see Box 16.1), and may not be obvious during the initial evaluation without diagnostic pericardiocentesis. Common causes of nonhemorrhagic effusions are discussed in the following sections.

Idiopathic Effusions

Idiopathic pericardial effusions are often suspected to have a viral etiology, even when specific pathogens are not identified. Commonly implicated viruses include Coxsackievirus, echovirus, and other enteroviruses, which can cause pericardial inflammation and effusion. Idiopathic pericardial effusions may be asymptomatic or present as pericarditis.[42] These effusions are often labeled *idiopathic* because the diagnosis cannot be made noninvasively, based on the history, physical examination, or serum testing, and the risk associated with diagnostic pericardiocentesis often outweighs the risk of observation.[43] There has been a longstanding recommendation to drain large idiopathic effusions based on data reporting that one-third of patients with large effusions will eventually progress to tamponade; however, recent investigations have noted a much smaller percentage and higher event-free survival with conservative management.[44]

Neoplastic Effusion

Tumors of the pericardium or myocardium may cause nonhemorrhagic effusions. Primary cardiac tumors are less common (0.001% to 0.003%) than metastases from another site (2% to 18%), but either may cause a malignant effusion.[45] Although no malignancy preferentially metastasizes to the heart, certain tumors commonly involve the heart when they metastasize; frequently implicated are melanoma, lymphoma, leukemia, and carcinoma of the lung, breast, and esophagus, most of which are clinically silent compared to their primary source.[46]

The classic signs and symptoms of tamponade (e.g., chest pain and dyspnea) may not be obvious with malignant tamponade. When present, they may be mistakenly attributed to the underlying malignancy. Screening patients with malignancy for pericardial effusion with ultrasound in the relevant clinical scenario may be beneficial.

Radiation

Pericardial effusions secondary to radiation-induced pericarditis can develop acutely during radiation therapy or may be delayed for years. Risk factors include the radiation dose, duration of exposure, and age of the patient. Patients treated with radiation for lymphoma disease have the highest association of radiation-induced pericarditis and subsequent effusions.[47] These effusions can be serous, hemorrhagic, or fibrinous.[48]

Congestive Heart Failure

Congestive heart failure (CHF) is a cause of pericardial effusion. Diagnosis may be difficult because of overlapping signs and symptoms with exacerbations of CHF (e.g., chest pain or dyspnea). 12% to 20% of patients with CHF have a coexisting pericardial effusion, further adding to diagnostic complexity.[49] Fortunately, treatment of CHF-associated pericardial effusion does not differ from that for an effusion from other causes: treat the underlying cause unless the patient has evidence of hemodynamic compromise.

HIV-Associated Effusions

HIV can cause nonhemorrhagic pericardial effusion and tamponade. Previous incidence has been reported to be approximately 11% in patients with HIV infection or acquired immunodeficiency syndrome. At least one modern post–combination antiretroviral (cART) therapy study found 0.25% of patients to have pericardial effusion by echocardiography.[50]

HIV-related effusions have been attributed to bacterial (e.g., *Staphylococcus aureus*), viral (e.g., cytomegalovirus), fungal (*Cryptococcus neoformans*), and mycobacterial causes (e.g., tuberculosis, the most common cause of HIV-related effusions worldwide). Kaposi sarcoma and lymphoma can cause noninfectious pericardial effusions in HIV patients.[51]

Renal Failure and Uremia

Pericardial effusion is known to develop in patients with end-stage renal disease although the extent is unclear. Various studies cite the incidence to be 12% to 44%. Many factors such as dialysis efficiency, nutritional status, and comorbid conditions can affect these data.[52] In many cases, effusions secondary to renal failure can be managed solely with aggressive dialysis without pericardiocentesis. Any sign of hemodynamic compromise, however, warrants strong consideration of pericardiocentesis.

Hypothyroidism

Pericardial effusions associated with hypothyroidism are typically characterized by a high protein content secondary to increased permeability of epicardial vessels and decreased lymphatic drainage. These effusions are often large but patients are rarely symptomatic due to the slow rate of accumulation, which allows the pericardium to stretch and adapt.[53] The incidence is reported at 3% to 6%. Tamponade and pretamponade as a presentation are rare.[54] Medically managing the underlying hypothyroidism often reverses the effusion without the need for pericardiocentesis.

SARS-CoV-2

Patients with COVID-19 have been shown to have serosanguinous, serous, and hemorrhagic pericardial effusion. This is often a rare and delayed finding but can be seen across the spectrum from the outpatient setting to the intensive care unit.[55] Children who have had COVID-19 can experience postexposure multisystem inflammatory syndrome in children (MIS-C), which includes cardiovascular complications such as pericardial effusion.[56]

Special Considerations in Pericardial Disease

Pericardial tamponade is classically described as being secondary to circumferential effusion, which causes a generalized increase in pericardial pressure and compression of multiple cardiac chambers. Loculated effusions (caused by a local hematoma or an infectious process) or pericardial adhesions (from previous inflammation) can lead to tamponade by compressing one or more cardiac chambers and thus reducing both cardiac filling and cardiac output.

Constrictive pericarditis occurs following chronic pericardial inflammation, infection, or mediastinal irradiation. These processes cause scarring, fibrosis, or calcification, and the pericardium eventually becomes a nonelastic and "constrictive" sac around the heart. Myocardial relaxation and cardiac filling are impaired, and diastolic dysfunction ensues. Constrictive pericarditis patients can infrequently present with comparable clinical features and have similar echocardiogram and even MRI findings that may only be discerned by more invasive testing such as cardiac catheterization.[57]

Effusive-constrictive pericarditis is defined by the presence of both pericardial effusion and pericardial constriction. It may be quite difficult to differentiate between effusive-constrictive pericarditis and pericardial tamponade in stable patients because both are associated with effusions. Fortunately, distinguishing between these diagnoses is less important in hemodynamically unstable patients given identical management.[58]

Pneumopericardium is an interesting, though rare cause of cardiac tamponade. It is most associated with trauma, either blunt or sharp, but is also associated with pneumothorax caused by barotrauma (e.g., mechanical ventilation), acute asthma exacerbations, iatrogenic factors (e.g., thoracocentesis, thoracic surgery, endotracheal intubation), fistulous communications with other air containing structures, foreign body aspiration, forceful emesis and toxins such as cocaine inhalation and chlorine gas exposure.[59]

DIAGNOSING CARDIAC TAMPONADE

Diagnosing cardiac tamponade requires a combination of clinical assessment, imaging, and hemodynamic evaluation. The initial clinical findings may be vague and nonspecific sometimes alluding even experienced clinicians. Chest pain and dyspnea may be ascribed to alternative differentials delaying diagnosis until incidentally found on imaging or hemodynamic changes occur.

The clinical presentation of tamponade in trauma patients can be masked by hypovolemia or other injuries, making diagnosis challenging. In hemodynamically unstable patients, there must be a low threshold to employ ultrasound imaging and therapeutic interventions to avoid subsequent rapid clinical deterioration and cardiac arrest.

Once a pericardial effusion is suspected (or diagnosed), the next step is to determine its size and hemodynamic significance and presence of underlying or associated diseases.[48] Specific therapies will hinge on this information and is discussed in the following sections.

History: Patient Profile and Symptoms

The historical features of pericardial effusions are nonspecific and the diagnosis may easily be overlooked. There are even multiple case reports where abdominal pain was found to be the primary symptom of tamponade.[60] A detailed patient history is essential for identifying the underlying cause of pericardial effusion or tamponade. Key elements of the history include recent illness, trauma, medical procedures, and chronic conditions such as malignancy, autoimmune diseases, or renal failure. Medication use, particularly anticoagulants, should also be assessed, as these can predispose patients to hemorrhagic effusion. Common symptoms of pericardial effusion are nonspecific and may include chest discomfort, dyspnea, fatigue, and orthopnea. In tamponade, symptoms are often more severe and may include lightheadedness, syncope, or altered mental status. Patients may report a sensation of fullness or pressure in the chest, and symptoms often worsen in a supine position. Subtle signs such as low-grade fever, weight loss, or night sweats may suggest an infectious or malignant etiology. Box 16.2 lists important details to be ascertained from the history when pericardial effusion is suspected.[61]

Physical Examination

Physical examination of patients with pericardial effusion (e.g., displaced point of maximal impulse, muffled heart sounds) lacks sensitivity and specificity. If the history suggests pericardial effusion, the physical examination should focus on determining the underlying cause to guide definitive diagnostic testing. Ironically, many pericardial effusions are not diagnosed from the history or findings on physical examination but are found incidentally during the evaluation for other diseases.

In 1935 Beck characterized the physical manifestations of tamponade with two triads, one for chronic and one for acute tamponade.[62] Beck's chronic triad consists of increased central venous pressure (CVP) (i.e., distended neck veins), ascites, and a small, quiet heart. *Beck's triad* is a classic description of acute cardiac compression, which includes increased CVP, decreased arterial pressure, and muffled heart sounds.[63,64] Additional studies have found that the sensitivity of one finding of Beck's triad was 50%, whereas the sensitivity of having all three was only as high as 19%.[65] The utility of this triad is further limited because all three signs are usually observed shortly before cardiac arrest.

It would be clinically desirable to identify patients in early tamponade, before hemodynamic collapse. Unfortunately, findings on physical examination in early tamponade are nonspecific and may be indistinguishable from those of other critical diseases such as septic shockor right heart failure.[48] Patients initially seen in late tamponade also have nonspecific findings. They may be agitated, panic-stricken, confused, uncooperative, restless, cyanotic, diaphoretic, acutely dyspneic, or hemodynamically unstable. Such patients should undergo a brief and focused physical examination followed by a rapid hemodynamic assessment with bedside ultrasound as the time between initial evaluation and full arrest may be brief.

Additional findings on physical examination associated with tamponade are described later. A more comprehensive list is presented in Box 16.3.

Vital Sign Abnormalities

There are three sequential stages that are typically described to reflect the natural history of acute tamponade (Table 16.1).[66] The time course within each stage varies from patient to patient. Some patients are stable within a given stage for hours, whereas others proceed through all three stages and develop cardiac arrest within minutes.[9,66] Grade I tamponade is characterized by normal blood pressure and cardiac output with an increase in the heart rate and CVP (measured invasively with a central venous catheter). Grade II tamponade is defined by normal or slightly reduced blood pressure; CVP and the heart rate remain increased. Grade III tamponade is identified on the basis of Beck's triad: hypotension, tachycardia, and elevated CVP.

BOX 16.2 Information to Obtain From Patients When Pericardial Effusion Is Suspected

ONSET AND DURATION OF SYMPTOMS

Acute

Trauma
Recent cardiac surgery
Recent myocardial infarction
Acute aortic dissection
Recent diagnostic or therapeutic intervention (e.g., catheterization)
Recent upper thoracic vascular procedure (e.g., hemodialysis catheter, central line, peripherally inserted central catheter line, Mediport)
Recent placement of a pacemaker or automatic implantable cardioverter-defibrillator

Subacute/Chronic

Metabolic (e.g., uremia)
Endocrine (e.g., hypothyroidism)
Infectious
- Viral (e.g., human immunodeficiency virus)
- Bacterial (e.g., *Staphylococcus*)
- Fungal (e.g., *Aspergillus*)

Neoplastic
- Primary cardiac
- Metastatic

Autoimmune disorders (e.g., lupus)
Inflammatory
- Vasculitis

MEDICAL/SURGICAL HISTORY

Autoimmune disorders
- Lupus
- Mixed connective tissue disease
- Vasculitis

Endocrine disease
- Hypothyroidism
- Ovarian hyperstimulation syndrome

Metabolic diseases
- End-stage renal disease and uremia
- Thyroid disorders
- Coagulopathies

Artificial cardiac valves
- Anticoagulation medications
- Risk for myocarditis

Cardiac disease
- Anticoagulation medications
- Pericarditis
- Aneurysm

Recent placement of a vascular catheter
Recent cardiac surgery
Recent cardiac intervention
Recent thoracic radiation

MEDICATIONS

Anticoagulants and Antiplatelet Agents
Antiarrhythmic
- Procainamide (drug-induced lupus)

Tuberculosis therapy
- Isoniazid (drug-induced lupus)

COMMON SYMPTOMS

Altered mental status, confusion
Fatigue
Dizziness, light-headedness
Orthostatic changes
Exercise intolerance
Hoarseness
Hiccups
Fever
Chills
Chest pain
- Substernal
- Pleuritic
- Positional

Scapular pain (phrenic nerve irritation)
Palpitations
Cough
Dyspnea
Myalgia
Arthralgia

It is estimated that tachycardia occurs in 65% to 88% of patients with pericardial tamponade. The physiologic purpose of tachycardia is to maintain normal cardiac output despite reductions in stroke volume from worsening tamponade. Exceptions to the pairing of tachycardia with tamponade usually relate to conduction system disease or the concomitant use of certain medications (e.g., β-blockers).[63]

Adding to the diagnostic complexity, not all patients in tamponade have a reduction in blood pressure. Multiple studies have shown that patients ranges and averages have been well over 100 mm Hg and that the sensitivity of hypotension is poor, between 24% and 38%. Several tamponade patients were also found to be hypertensive (27% to 43%) with elevated blood pressure likely due to circulating catecholamines. These patients were previously hypertensive and paradoxically had reduced systolic blood pressure following pericardiocentesis.

Studies have limited data on tachypnea during tamponade. There are estimates that it is present in 80% of patients and that the average patient presenting to the ED in tamponade will have a respiratory rate of 21. Tachypnea could very well be blunted in the case of respiratory muscle fatigue.[63]

Pulsus Paradoxus

Pulsus paradoxus, an exaggerated drop in systolic blood pressure of more than 10 mm Hg during inspiration, is a hallmark clinical sign of cardiac tamponade. This phenomenon occurs due to the impaired filling of the left ventricle during inspiration, as increased venous return to the right ventricle causes the interventricular septum to shift, reducing left ventricular stroke volume. (Fig. 16.4A). While highly suggestive of tamponade, pulsus paradoxus can also be seen in other conditions: RV infarction, restrictive cardiomyopathy, cardiac compression from iatrogenic surgery obesity or pectus excavatum,

BOX 16.3 Physical Examination Findings Suggestive of Pericardial Effusion or Tamponade

VITAL SIGNS

Normal vital signs
Tachycardia (tamponade)
Hypotension (tamponade)
Narrow pulse pressure
Pulsus paradoxus
Fever (if the cause is infectious or neoplastic)

APPEARANCE

Normal appearance
Anxiety
Sense of impending doom
Diaphoretic
Cold and clammy
Pallor
Altered mental status, confusion

NECK

Supraclavicular retractions
Distended neck veins (may be flat with hypotension)

CARDIOVASCULAR

Normal findings on examination
Tachycardia
Increased pain with a supine position, relieved by leaning forward
Muted, distant heart sounds
Pericardial friction rub (inflammatory pericarditis)
Displaced point of maximal impulse
Increased cardiac borders with percussion
Distended neck veins
Auscultatory dullness along the left scapular area

PULMONARY

Telegraphic speech
Respiratory distress
Supraclavicular retractions, abdominal breathing
Cough
Hoarseness
Clear breath sounds (may distinguish tamponade from congestive heart failure)

ABDOMINAL

Hepatomegaly
Splenomegaly

SKIN

Cool extremities
Clammy extremities
Dilated head and scalp veins
Peripheral edema

pulmonary diseases such as severe asthma, chronic obstructive pulmonary disease (COPD), pulmonary embolism, tension pneumothorax, and large pleural effusions. Pulsus paradoxus can also be found in volvulus of the stomach, diaphragmatic hernia, and thoracic outlet syndrome, although nonpericardial disease will have both a systolic and diastolic drop in blood pressures upon inspiration, whereas pericardial disease will have a drop in mainly the systolic pressure with minimal effect on the diastolic pressure.[67,68]

Pulsus paradoxus is measured with a manual sphygmomanometer and stethoscope. The cuff should be inflated until Korotkoff sounds are absent. The first sound will be heard during expiration and the second sound will be heard during both inspiration and expiration. The variation of these two systolic pressures is the measurement. Of note, this measurement should only be conducted with the patient's normal respirations. The patient should not be taking large tidal volumes or having any prolonged expirations, more than their usual pattern.

In pericardial effusion, pulsus paradoxus has a sensitivity greater than 80% for cardiac tamponade. There are several conditions where cardiac tamponade may occur without pulsus paradoxus: intracardiac shunt or valvular insufficiency, elevated ventricular diastolic pressures (severe systemic hypertension, aortic stenosis, cor pulmonale), aortic dissection, and hypovolemia.[68]

Measuring pulsus paradoxus can be time consuming and challenging in patients who are tachycardic, tachypneic, or hypotensive. Other methods have been described including noting the respiratory variation on pulse oximetry waveforms or arterial line tracings.[67,69] When managing unstable patients, bedside ultrasound can especially be useful in measuring respiratory variation in transvalvular flows.[70]

Neck Vein Distention and Elevated CVP

Neck vein distention (a surrogate for measuring CVP) occurs late in tamponade, when right-sided chambers (e.g., the RV) collapse. Neck vein distention may be obvious on examination (Fig. 16.5A), but visualization of such distention is less accurate than measuring CVP by central venous catheter or evaluation of the IVC with ultrasound (Table 16.2). Patients with significant tamponade typically have a CVP of 12 cm H_2O or higher. Finally, although initial CVP readings are useful and diagnostic when grossly elevated (e.g., 20 to 30 cm H_2O), upward trends in CVP can be a more sensitive diagnostic tool.[71]

Overreliance on increased CVP and venous distention should be avoided because they do not always indicate tamponade. For example, increased intrathoracic pressure (as induced by positive pressure ventilation or Valsalva maneuvers) increases CVP and causes neck vein distention even without pericardial effusion. Conversely, hypovolemic patients may have reduced CVP and no neck vein distention despite having clinical tamponade. The absence of distended neck veins may also result from severe venoconstriction secondary to intrinsic sympathetic discharge, vasopressor use, or severe hypovolemia.

Diagnostic Testing

Diagnostic testing should be initiated when pericardial effusion or tamponade is suspected. Definitive diagnosis requires imaging, which may be done by CT but preferably is done by cardiac ultrasound (see Fig. 16.5B). Bedside ultrasound is the fastest and most reliable diagnostic tool because it is noninvasive, does not emit radiation, and can be performed at the bedside without transporting unstable patients outside the ED.

As discussed previously, pericardial effusions are occasionally discovered incidentally during evaluation for other disorders. For example, a chest radiograph and ECG

TABLE 16.1 Shoemaker System of Grading Cardiac Tamponade

GRADE	PERICARDIAL VOLUME (mL)	CARDIAC INDEX	STROKE INDEX	MEAN ARTERIAL PRESSURE	CENTRAL VENOUS PRESSURE	HEART RATE	BECK'S TRIAD
I	<200	Normal or ↑	Normal or ↓	Normal	↑	↑	Venous distention, hypotension, muffled heart sounds usually not present
II	≥200	↓	↓	Normal or ↓	↑ (≤12 cm H_2O)	↑	May or may not be present
III	>200	↓↓	↓↓	↓↓	↑↑ (30–40 cm H_2O)	↑	Usually present

From Shoemaker WC, Carey SJ, Yao ST et al. Hemodynamic monitoring for physiologic evaluation, diagnosis, and therapy of acute hemopericardial tamponade from penetrating wounds. *J Trauma*. 1973;13:36.

performed on a patient being assessed for acute coronary syndrome (ACS) may suggest findings of a large pericardial effusion. If the clinical context supports pericardial effusion as the primary diagnosis rather than ACS, further workup for the effusion should be ordered. If neither diagnosis is more likely than the other, dual workups may be necessary.

Chest Radiography

Chest radiographs are not diagnostically useful in patients with acute traumatic tamponade because the pericardium does not have sufficient time to change size or shape (see section on "Pathophysiology of Pericardial Tamponade"). Radiographs, however, may reveal other associated findings such as hemothorax, bullets in the thorax, or even pneumopericardium. Chest radiography may also be helpful when other diagnoses have clinical findings similar to those of pericardial effusion. For example, a dyspneic patient with a clear chest film may be less likely to have decompensated heart failure than tamponade.

In patients with chronic pericardial effusions, chest films often demonstrate an enlarged, saclike, "water-bottle" cardiac shadow or a pleural effusion (see Fig. 16.5C). Unfortunately, it is difficult to differentiate a large effusion from myocardial enlargement as radiographs demonstrate only the cardiac silhouette and not the physiologic differences between these two diagnoses.

Electrocardiography

Pericardial effusion secondary to acute pericarditis is suspected on the basis of typical changes on the ECG. Pericarditis has four stages: (1) diffuse ST-segment elevation with PR depression, (2) ST- and PR-segment normalization, (3) diffuse T-wave inversion, and (4) normalization of T waves.[2]

The four most commonly described electrocardiographic findings in pericardial effusion are tachycardia, PR depression, low-voltage QRS complexes, and electrical alternans. Tachycardia is thought to be seen in 47% to 88% of ECGs with pericardial tamponade. PR-segment depression is defined as depression of 1 mV or greater in at least one lead other than aVR. This is seen much less commonly at 18%. Low-voltage QRS complexes (most frequently associated with moderate to large effusions) are defined by a QRS complex with an amplitude of 5 mm or less across all limb leads. Alternatively, low-voltage QRS complexes can be identified by a sum of 10 mm or less for all precordial lead QRS amplitudes. Low voltages have been described in ECGs between 22% and 56% of the time in patients with pericardial tamponade. Electrical alternans is a beat-to-beat alternation in QRS axis caused by the pendulum motion of the heart within the fluid-filled pericardial sac. It has been observed between 3% and 21% of tamponade patients. Electrical alternans of P waves and QRS complexes (i.e., total electrical alternans) is a rare finding but, when seen, is pathognomonic of tamponade (see Fig. 16.6). Other notable ECG features seen in tamponade are the presence of ST-segment elevation (18% to 30%) and atrial arrhythmias (0% to 9%).[63] This is particularly important when considering antiplatelet or anticoagulation as these therapies could precipitate hemorrhagic tamponade if erroneously administered to the incorrect patient.

Electrocardiography has acceptable specificity but poor sensitivity in diagnosing pericardial tamponade. In a study of patients with pericardial tamponade, low-voltage criteria had a sensitivity of 64% to 69% while the specificity was 95% to 99%. PR depression had a sensitivity of 12% and specificity of 100%, electrical alternans had a sensitivity of 5% and specificity of 100% and sinus tachycardia had a sensitivity of 69% and specificity of 80%. Therefore an ECG cannot be used as a screening tool for diagnostic tamponade; however, has value as an additional test in the appropriate clinical circumstance[72] (Fig. 16.6).

Echocardiography

Cardiac tamponade is one of the conditions that can cause unexplained hypotension. The RUSH (rapid ultrasound in unexplained hypotension) approach using bedside ultrasound can rapidly make the diagnosis and allow the clinician to intervene using pericardiocentesis (Video 16.1).

Echocardiography is the best tool for diagnosing pericardial effusion or tamponade (Figs. 16.7–16.9 and the Ultrasound Box). It not only demonstrates the presence of a pericardial effusion, but can also detect hemodynamic abnormalities. Ultrasonography (used interchangeably with *echocardiography* from here on) has the advantage that it is noninvasive, portable for use at the patient's bedside, and involves no ionizing radiation.[9] Echocardiography is a very sensitive and specific tool for the diagnosis of pericardial effusion and tamponade, and its use in diagnosing pericardial effusions has been endorsed by several academic societies.[63]

ULTRASOUND: Pericardiocentesis

by Christine Butts, MD

Pericardiocentesis has traditionally been performed blindly. This approach was associated with a low success rate and a high rate of complications, such as inadvertent puncture of the lung, ventricle, or epicardial vessels.[1] Using ultrasound to both diagnose and guide pericardiocentesis has resulted in increased success rates, as well as a lower rate of complications.[2,3]

Bedside ultrasound may additionally allow the emergency physician to make a rapid diagnosis of pericardial effusion. Evidence of impending cardiac tamponade, including RV collapse and distention of the IVC, can also be identified.

Equipment

The pericardium should be imaged with a low-frequency (2 to 4 mHz) transducer to achieve adequate depth. A phased-array or microconvex transducer is preferred for its smaller footprint, which enables the sonographer to image between the ribs. However, a curvilinear transducer may be used if that is what is available.

Image Interpretation

The initial step in the procedure is to evaluate the pericardium in multiple windows. This will allow identification and characterization of the effusion, as well as planning of the best approach for drainage. This chapter focuses primarily on the views most commonly used in this procedure, the subxiphoid and parasternal.

The subxiphoid view is best known to most emergency physicians as part of the focused abdominal sonography in trauma (FAST) examination. This view provides a four-chamber view of the heart and uses the left lobe of the liver as an acoustic window. To obtain this view, the transducer is placed just inferior to the xiphoid process in the midline. The indicator faces the patient's right side (Fig. 16.US1). To obtain the best image possible, it is best to place the hand over the transducer and press down into the epigastric area. The transducer can then be aimed toward the left side of the chest until the heart comes into view. The depth may need to be adjusted to view all four chambers of the heart, as well as the pericardium.

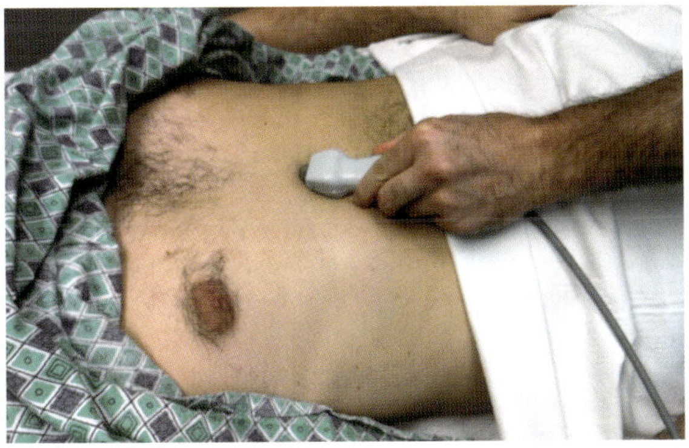

Fig. 16.US1 Placement of the ultrasound transducer to obtain a subxiphoid image of the heart.

In this view, the left lobe of the liver can be seen at the top of the image. Deep to the liver, a four-chambered view of the heart should be seen, surrounded by the brightly white (hyperechoic) border of the pericardium (Fig. 16.US2). The RV will abut the liver, with the LV located deeper into the body. A pericardial effusion can be identified as an black (anechoic) or dark grey (hypoechoic) collection between the heart and pericardium (Fig. 16.US3). Although fluid will typically collect at the most gravity-dependent area, loculated collections may not follow this rule.

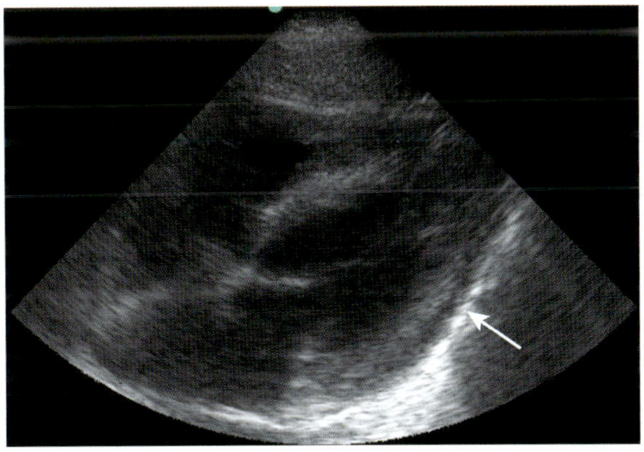

Fig. 16.US2 Normal subxiphoid view of the heart seen with ultrasound. The pericardium *(arrow)* can be identified as a bright white (hyperechoic) outline, typically best seen at the inferior aspect of the heart. The pericardium should directly abut the heart, as seen in this image.

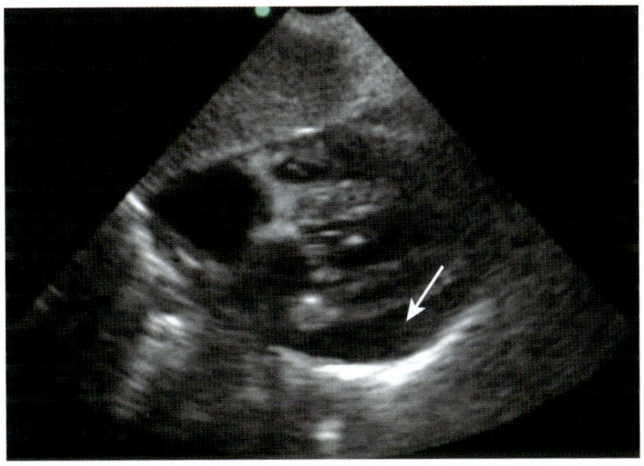

Fig. 16.US3 Subxiphoid view demonstrating a pericardial effusion. When comparing this image with the normal view, a black (anechoic) fluid collection *(arrow)* can be seen between the pericardium and the left ventricle.

The parasternal view is obtained by placing the transducer to the left of the patient's sternum in the fourth to fifth intercostal space. The indicator should be pointing toward the patient's right shoulder (Fig. 16.US4). Slight adjustments in angle may be needed to obtain the best image of the heart. If the patient's hemodynamic status allows, placing the patient in a left lateral decubitus position may improve this view by moving the heart closer to the anterior chest wall and displacing the air-filled lungs.

Continued

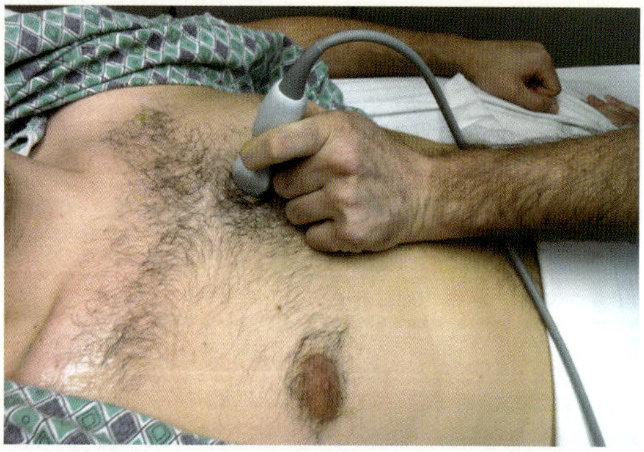

Fig. 16.US4 Placement of the ultrasound transducer to obtain a parasternal long-axis view of the heart.

The parasternal view will demonstrate the left atrium, LV, and a small portion of the RV (Fig. 16.US5). The pericardium can be seen as an echogenic (white) border surrounding the heart. As in the subxiphoid view, an effusion will appear as an anechoic (black) or hypoechoic (dark gray) collection between the heart and pericardium (Fig. 16.US6).

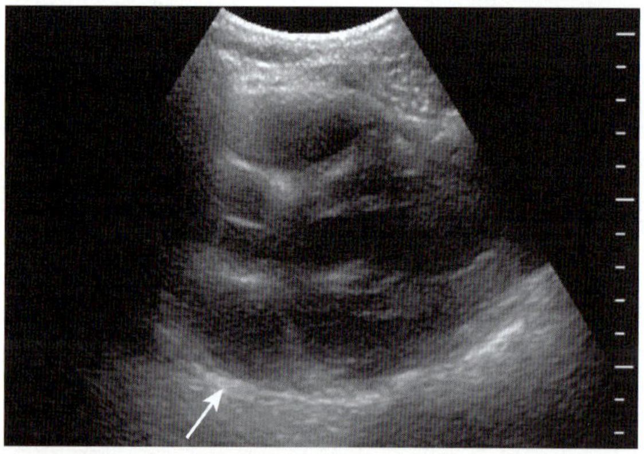

Fig. 16.US5 Normal parasternal long-axis view of the heart. The pericardium can be seen as a bright white (hyperechoic) outline surrounding the heart *(arrow)*. As with the subxiphoid image, the pericardium should directly abut the heart with no intervening fluid.

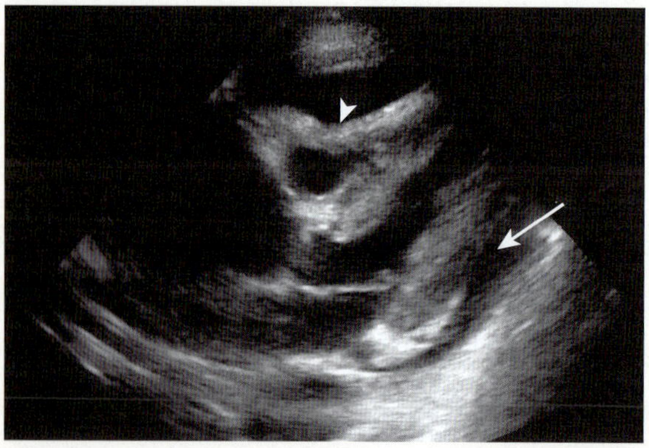

Fig. 16.US6 Parasternal long-axis view demonstrating a pericardial effusion. An anechoic *(black)* fluid collection can be seen on the right of the image *(arrow)*, between the left ventricle and the pericardium. The right ventricle, at the top of the image *(arrowhead)*, can be seen to "bow" inward from the pressure exerted by the effusion. This finding, right ventricular collapse, indicates that the effusion is causing hemodynamic compromise.

Procedure and Technique

Once the views have been evaluated and an effusion has been identified, evaluate the pericardium in multiple views to determine the best area to attempt pericardiocentesis. Tsang and colleagues described the procedure for ultrasound-guided pericardiocentesis in detail in 1998.[4] Ideally, the procedure should be attempted at the site at which the largest fluid collection is closest to the skin surface. Typically, the anterior chest wall is preferred because of its proximity to the pericardium and the absence of vital interfering structures such as the liver. The air-filled lung creates a scatter artifact that does not allow the ultrasound beam to pass. Therefore if the heart and pericardium can be viewed clearly, avoidance of the lung can be ensured. The sonographer should also attempt to approximate and avoid the location of the internal mammary artery, which lies 3 to 5 cm lateral to the sternum. Once the optimal site is identified, the practitioner should place the needle in a trajectory that follows that of the ultrasound beam. Sterilize the field. Anesthetize the area to be traversed with local anesthetic. Place the ultrasound transducer in a sterile covering. Take care to not reposition the patient after initial assessment because this will alter the position and trajectory. Use a 16-gauge catheter with a retractable needle to minimize potential injury to the underlying structures. After the field is prepared, attach the catheter to a syringe. Advance the needle in the predetermined location along the predetermined trajectory. This can be done blindly or can be guided directly by the transducer. Apply gentle continuous pressure to the syringe until the pericardial space is entered and fluid is obtained.

If there is any question of whether the needle tip is in the pericardial space, inject agitated saline through the catheter under direct ultrasound guidance. This will allow analysis of the location of the needle tip. Prepare saline echocardiographic contrast medium by using two 5-mL syringes, one with saline and the other with air, connected via a three-way stopcock to the needle catheter sheath. Saline in one syringe is rapidly injected between the syringes and then injected into the sheath once it is agitated. Entrance of the agitated saline into the pericardial space will appear sonographically as a brightly echogenic area.

Complications

Complications may occur when a pericardial effusion is misdiagnosed. The most common factor causing misdiagnosis is the presence of a fat pad anterior to the heart. Unless the effusion is loculated, it should lie within the most dependent portion of the heart and should be circumferential, depending on its size. Considering these factors and evaluating the pericardium in multiple views will aid in decreasing this misdiagnosis. Additionally, take care when performing pericardiocentesis in stable patients, particularly when the effusion is small. Smaller effusions may be more difficult to access and therefore lead to increased complications.

REFERENCES

1. Salem K, Mulji A, Lonn E. Echocardiographically guided pericardiocentesis—the gold standard for the management of pericardial effusion and cardiac tamponade. *Can J Cardiol.* 1999;15:1251–1255.
2. Tsang TS, El-Najdawi EK, Seward JB, et al. Percutaneous echocardiographically guided pericardiocentesis in pediatric patients: evaluation of safety and efficacy. *J Am Soc Echocardiogr.* 1998;11:1072–1077.
3. Vayre F, Lardoux H, Pezzano M, et al. Subxiphoid pericardiocentesis guided by contrast two-dimensional echocardiography in cardiac tamponade: experience of 110 consecutive patients. *Eur J Echocardiogr.* 2000;1:66–71.
4. Tsang TS, Freeman WK, Sinak LJ, et al. Echocardiographically guided pericardiocentesis: evolution and state-of-the-art technique. *Mayo Clin Proc.* 1998;73:647–652.

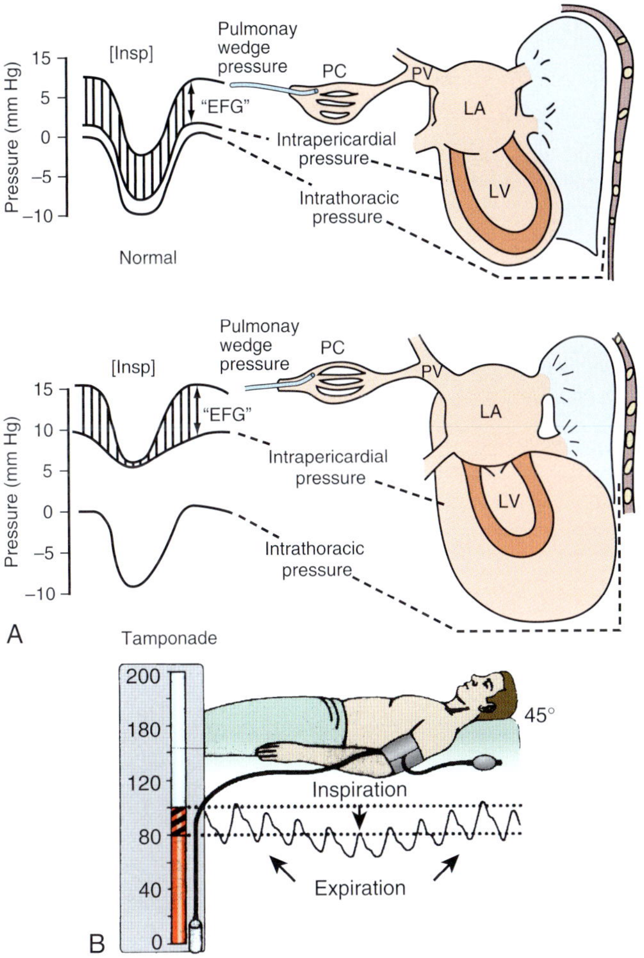

Fig. 16.4 Pulsus paradoxus to diagnose pericardial tamponade. (A) *Top*, The normal situation in which changes in intrathoracic pressure are transmitted to both the pericardial sac and the pulmonary veins. The effective filling gradient *(EFG)* changes only slightly during respiration. *Bottom*, Cardiac tamponade in which changes in intrathoracic pressure are transmitted to the pulmonary veins but not to the pericardial sac. The EFG falls during inspiration *(Insp)*. (B) Normally, systolic blood pressure drops slightly during Insp. To assess for pulsus paradoxus, have the patient breathe normally while lying at a 45-degree angle. Inflate the blood pressure cuff well above systolic pressure and slowly deflate it. When the pulse is first heard only during expiration, this is the upper value. Deflate the cuff until the pulse is heard during both inspiration and expiration; this is the lower value. A difference of more than 10 mm Hg between the two values indicates pulsus paradoxus. *LA*, Left atrium; *LV*, left ventricle; *PC*, pulmonary capillaries; *PV*, pulmonary veins. (A, Adapted from Sharp JT, Bunnell IL, Holand JF et al. Hemodynamics during induced cardiac tamponade in man. *Am J Med*. 1960;25:640.)

Diagnosing Pericardial Effusions and Tamponade

Fluid found within the pericardial space is not always pathologic as it normally holds 15 to 50 mL of fluid. Small effusions may be clinically insignificant. The sonographer/clinician should exercise caution to not over-read an effusion, particularly when the patient is hemodynamically stable. Small effusions typically contain 50 to 100 mL with an echo-free space less than 10 mm in thickness between the visceral and parietal pericardium. Moderate effusions typically contain 100 to 500 mL with 10 to 20 mm of echo-free space. Large effusions contain more than 500 mL and have an echo-free space greater than 20 mm. Moderate and large effusions tend to have a more evenly distributed echo-free space seen circumferentially around the heart.[73] A loculated pericardial effusion can present in an atypical location and may be more difficult to appreciate compared to the nonloculated types described previously.

Once a pericardial effusion is discovered, the next step is to evaluate the patient for evidence of hemodynamic compromise. Echocardiographic signs include (1) early diastolic collapse of the RV, (2) systolic right atrial collapse, (3) plethoric IVC, and (4) respirophasic variation in mitral and tricuspid inflow velocities.

RV diastolic collapse occurs when the intracardiac pressure no longer exceeds the pericardial pressure. It has a specificity of 75% to 90% and a sensitivity of 48% to 60%. This feature can be identified in all four basic cardiac views. The right atrium is at its lowest pressure immediately after late diastole when relaxing and the collapse during systole can be one of the earliest findings of tamponade. Systolic right atrial collapse has specificities that range from 33% to 100% and sensitivities that range from 50% to 100% as tamponade progresses. This is best visualized in the apical four-chamber and subxiphoid views. Absence of either right atrial or RV collapse carries a negative predictive value of 90%.[63]

As obstructive physiology progresses, blood often backs up into the IVC. A plethoric IVC has a sensitivity of 95% to 97%. The specificity is approximately 40% and can be found in heart failure and other pulmonary processes as well as when the patient is undergoing positive pressure ventilation. A more advanced measurement is obtaining inflow variations at the mitral and tricuspid valves. Similar to the physiology of pulsus paradoxus physiology described earlier, the blood flow through the mitral and tricuspid valves varies significantly with inspiration and expiration. The view can best be obtained in the apical four-chamber view. A pulse wave Doppler gate is placed between the tips of the valve leaflets of the RV or the LV during diastole. The peaks during expiration (the tallest peak) and inspiration (the shortest peak) can be compared. Tamponade physiology often creates a 25% decrease in mitral valve variation and a 40% increase in tricuspid valve variation. Usually this variation is approximately 10% without tamponade.[63]

The presence of any of these signs should alert the clinician to the possibility of hemodynamic instability. Obtain expert consultation if there is any uncertainty about the ultrasound findings.

Limitations of Ultrasound

Ultrasound is the best diagnostic tool for pericardial effusion and tamponade, but great care must be taken when it is used as the only diagnostic modality. In a postoperative series of cardiac surgery patients, 60% of loculated effusions causing tamponade were missed on transthoracic echocardiography but were visualized with transesophageal echocardiography.[74]

There are several false-positive findings for a pericardial effusion on ultrasound. Examples include pericardial thickening, large pleural effusions, atelectasis, and mediastinal lesions.[75] Epicardial (or anterior) fat pads can also be misinterpreted as pericardial effusions, although several details help distinguish between the two entities. First, epicardial fat pads tend to occur anteriorly, unlike circumferential effusions, which occur posteriorly. If a fat pad is suspected, multiple ultrasound views should be obtained to rule out a posterior effusion. Second, the echocardiographic appearance of an

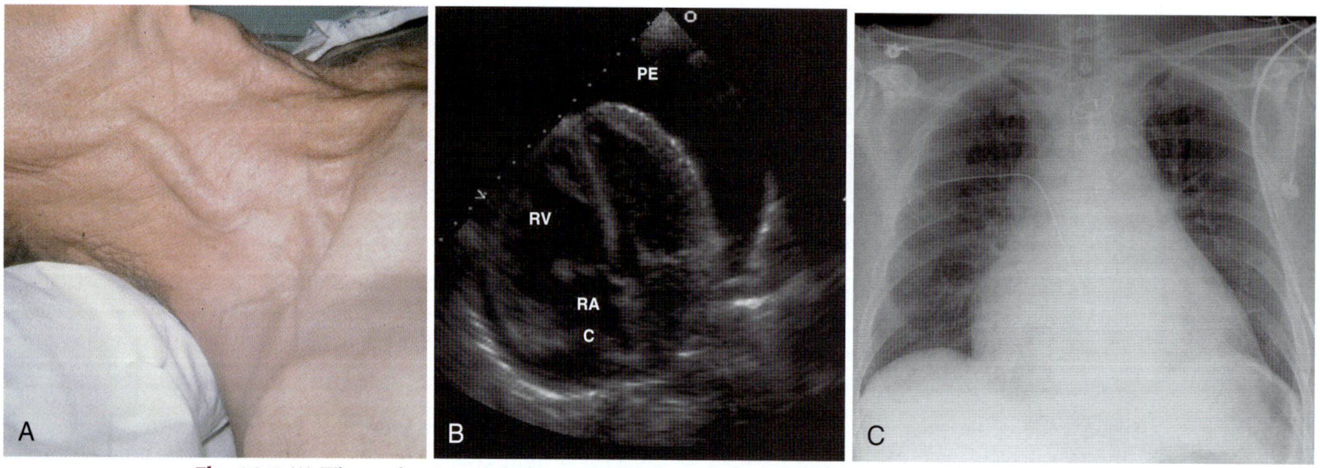

Fig. 16.5 (A) The neck veins might be markedly distended with cardiac tamponade, but this finding is not universal, especially in patients with hypovolemic trauma. (B) Ultrasound. An apical view of a large pericardial effusion in early ventricular diastole reveals marked right atrial collapse. (C) Chest radiograph showing an enlarged, globular cardiac silhouette (water-bottle heart) in a patient with tamponade caused by a malignant effusion. The chest film has minimal value in diagnosing tamponade but is usually abnormal when significant *chronic* effusions are present. *C*, Collapsed segment of the right atrial wall; *PE*, pericardial effusion; *RA*, right atrium; *RV*, right ventricle.

TABLE 16.2 Noninvasive Estimation of Right Atrial Pressure With Ultrasound

DIAMETER (CM) OF INFERIOR VENA CAVA	CHANGE IN DIAMETER WITH RESPIRATION	ESTIMATED RIGHT ATRIAL PRESSURE (MM HG)
Normal (<2.1)	Decrease >50%	~3 (normal, 0–5)
Dilated (<2.1)	Decrease <50%	~8 (intermediate, 5–10)
Dilated (>2.1)	Decrease >50%	~8 (intermediate, 5–10)
Dilated (>2.1)	Decrease <50%	>15 (high, 10–20)

Based on Rudski LG, Lai WW, Afilalo J et al. Guidelines for the echocardiographic assessment of the right heart in adults: a report from the American Society of Echocardiography endorsed by the European Association of Echocardiography, a registered branch of the European Society of Cardiology, and the Canadian Society of Echocardiography. *J Am Soc Echocardiogr*. 2010;23:685.

ELECTRICAL ALTERNANS IN PERICARDIAL TAMPONADE

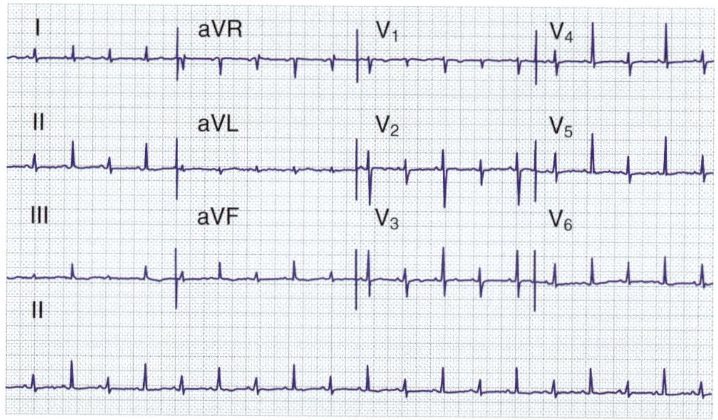

Fig. 16.6 Electrical alternans may develop in patients with pericardial effusion and cardiac tamponade. Notice the beat-to-beat alternation in the voltage in the P-QRS-T axis; this is caused by the periodic swinging motion of the heart in a large pericardial effusion. Relatively low QRS voltage and sinus tachycardia are also present. Overall, the electrocardiogram has low sensitivity for pericardial effusion and tamponade. Note that electrical alternans may be more evident in the V leads.

epicardial fat pad is isoechoic and homogeneous. This differs from blood in the pericardial space, which may look like fronds of clot waving within an anechoic pericardial space. Third, an epicardial fat pad does not alter hemodynamics as tamponade does; it should not cause diastolic collapse of the RV free wall, dilation of the IVC, or any signs indicating hemodynamic compromise. After careful examination, if doubt still exists regarding the presence of an effusion, hemodynamically stable patients should have a formal echocardiogram; consider CT scan if an echocardiogram is not available.

CT Scan

CT may be the only diagnostic option at institutions where ultrasound or formal echocardiography is not available in the ED. It is also helpful when concomitant diseases of the lung or mediastinum are considered. CT can demonstrate dilated hepatic veins, a plethoric IVC, and interventricular septal bowing.[76] This modality is less desirable than bedside ultrasound because it requires patients to be transported to the radiology suite and does not provide as much information on how the effusion is affecting hemodynamics. Thus patient safety and cardiopulmonary stability must be considered before the decision is made to transport the patient. Unstable patients should never be transported until they are fully stabilized.

For stable patients, CT is effective in defining the presence, severity, and extent of pericardial effusions (i.e., circumferential versus loculated). In certain circumstances, it even provides a more definitive diagnosis than echocardiography does because it may reveal the type of pericardial fluid (by differences in tissue density) and pericardial disease (e.g., constrictive pericarditis).[77] In one series of eight equivocal echocardiograms

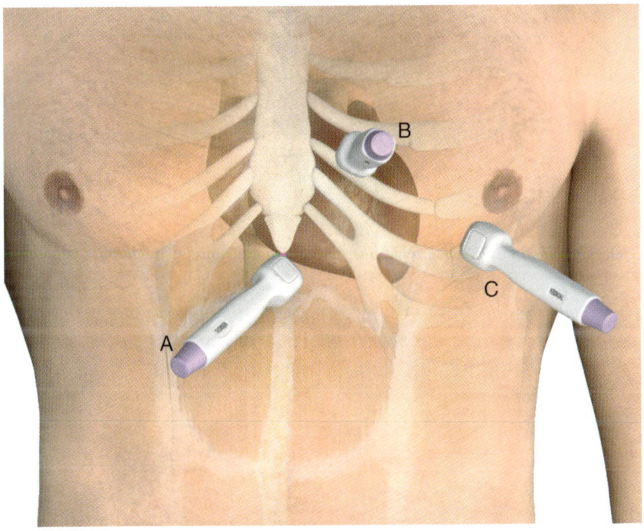

Fig. 16.7 Areas of the chest to obtain basic echocardiographic windows: *A*, subxiphoid (subcostal) view; *B*, parasternal view; *C*, apical four-chamber view.

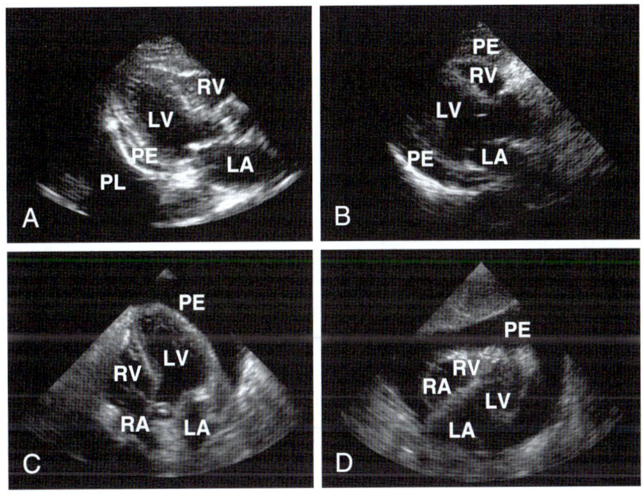

Fig. 16.9 Examples of pericardial effusion. (A) Small pericardial effusion (parasternal long-axis view). (B) Moderate pericardial effusion (parasternal long-axis view). (C) Large pericardial effusion (apical four-chamber view). (D) Large pericardial effusion (subcostal/subxiphoid view). *LA*, Left atrium; *LV*, left ventricle; *PE*, pericardial effusion; *PL*, pleural effusion; *RA*, right atrium; *RV*, right ventricle.

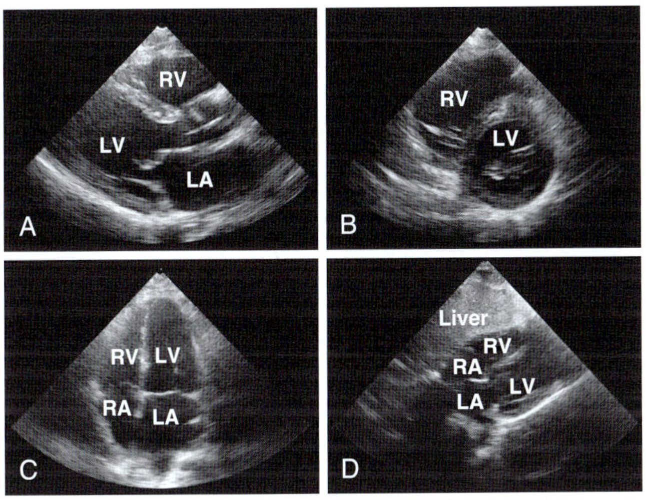

Fig. 16.8 Normal echocardiographic views. (A) Parasternal long-axis view. (B) Parasternal short-axis view. (C) Apical four-chamber view. (D) Subxiphoid (subcostal) view. *LA*, Left atrium; *LV*, left ventricle; *RA*, right atrium; *RV*, right ventricle.

evaluated by follow-up CT, two patients thought to have pericardial effusion by ultrasonography were found to have pleural effusions, and another was found to have an epicardial lipoma. Additionally, CT identified three patients with loculated pericardial effusions that had been missed by ultrasonography and two patients with hemopericardium.[78] Another study showed that pericardial effusion volume calculated by echocardiography correlated better with actual volume drained from a pericardial effusion than effusion volume calculated by CT.[79] It has also been shown that CT may overestimate the volume of a pericardial effusion compared to echocardiography.[80]

Treating Pericardial Effusions and Tamponade

Treatment of pericardial effusions in the ED depends on the degree of hemodynamic compromise. Patients with stable effusions should be treated supportively while the underlying cause (known or suspected) is addressed. For example, stable patients with pericardial effusions secondary to uremia may best be treated with dialysis, observation, and serial echocardiograms.[81] Even when the diagnosis is unknown, there may be no need to perform emergency pericardiocentesis if the effusion is small to moderate and has no effect on hemodynamics. Deferring diagnostic pericardiocentesis to the inpatient setting may be preferred because the cardiac catheterization laboratory or operating room is a more sterile and controlled environment than the ED.[48]

Patients with evidence of tamponade need urgent pericardiocentesis. Even those with early tamponade who are stable can decompensate quickly with little warning. Fluid boluses may improve hemodynamics temporarily, especially in patients with concomitant hypovolemia.[43] Administration of a vasopressor is a temporizing measure and should be initiated while preparing for emergency pericardiocentesis. Finally, positive pressure ventilation should be avoided as, it can lead to hemodynamic collapse secondary to changes in intrathoracic pressure.

INDICATIONS FOR PERICARDIOCENTESIS

There are two indications for pericardiocentesis: (1) to diagnose the presence and cause of a pericardial effusion (diagnostic pericardiocentesis) and (2) to relieve tamponade (therapeutic pericardiocentesis). Diagnostic pericardiocentesis is an elective procedure. It is ideally performed under visual guidance (e.g., ultrasound or fluoroscopy). Therapeutic pericardiocentesis may be an urgent or emergent procedure based on patient hemodynamics. In the semistable patient, ultrasound guidance should be utilized for pericardial fluid aspiration; however, in the case of cardiovascular collapse or cardiac arrest, a blind approach may be warranted.

Diagnostic Pericardiocentesis

Multimodal imaging including CT, cardiac MRI, and positron emission tomography (PET)/CT are being increasingly utilized in the diagnosis of pericardial disorders. Pericardial drainage is recommended in cases of overt or near tamponade and suspected bacterial or neoplastic etiologies. Following an assessment of c-reactive protein (CRP) and treating any associated diseases, it is then used to provide diagnostic utility for chronic (>3 months) effusions.[44] Recovery of pericardial fluid to assess for tumor, autoimmune, and biochemical markers in addition to bacterial and viral cultures with Gram stain can be valuable in making the diagnosis. Measurement of pericardial fluid pH can point towards inflammatory etiology as inflammatory fluid is significantly more acidotic than noninflammatory fluid.

The diagnostic accuracy of pericardiocentesis is variable, and certain diagnoses are unlikely to be made from pericardial fluid. In one large series, fluid samples were obtained in 90% of aspirations, but the specific cause was determined from only 24% of those specimens. Another series demonstrated false-negative cytologic results in certain cases of lymphoma and mesothelioma.[82] When a biopsy is obtained, it is often during implementation of a subxiphoid pericardiotomy (pericardial window).

A pericardial window is typically employed to obtain both pericardial fluid and a pericardial biopsy specimen, because once a tissue sample is obtained, a definitive diagnosis is much more likely. It is reserved for those with recurring episodes of tamponade.[83] This procedure can be performed safely in the operating suite without general anesthesia. In a prospective series of 57 patients who underwent subxiphoid pericardiotomy, a definitive diagnosis was obtained in 36%, a probable diagnosis in 40%, a possible diagnosis in 16%, and no diagnosis in 7%. It is uncertain whether this technique is safer than ultrasound-guided pericardiocentesis, but published reports show low rates of complications in experienced hands.[84]

Larger effusions and effusions associated with clinical signs of pericarditis are more likely to be yield a diagnosis.[84] Unfortunately, the only methods of making definitive diagnosis are pericardial fluid aspiration with analysis and pericardial biopsy.

Diagnostic pericardiocentesis has limited utility for hemopericardium secondary to traumatic causes. If blood is present with clots, it may be difficult to aspirate. If there is uncertainty about the presence of tamponade, the FAST examination rapidly and noninvasively identifies pericardial fluid.

Therapeutic Pericardiocentesis

The ultrasonographic finding of a large pericardial effusion (>20 mm) in a stable patient should lead to early cardiology or cardiothoracic surgery consultation for percutaneous drainage or placement of a pericardial window. Patients with a pericardial effusion who remain hypotensive despite fluid resuscitation require urgent therapeutic drainage. The decision to wait for consultants is best made by the emergency physician at the bedside and should be based on clinical judgment. Until recently, few algorithms existed to assist in the risk stratification of patients with pericardial effusions and who should undergo emergency versus delayed pericardiocentesis. In 2012, Halpern and colleagues introduced a scoring system based on effusion size, echocardiography derangements, and clinical criteria.[85] Similarly, Ristic and colleagues in 2014 created a system incorporating etiology, clinical factors, and diagnostic imaging.[86] Such tools can aid the emergency physician in identifying who would benefit most from ED pericardiocentesis and who could await consultant recommendations (Fig. 16.10).

For patients in extremis, pericardiocentesis should be performed immediately even if consultation is unavailable. The clinician who performs the procedure should be the one who is most experienced in both sonography and pericardial fluid aspiration.

Tamponade of Uncertain Cause: Pulseless Electrical Activity

A major indication for emergency pericardiocentesis is a patient in cardiac arrest with PEA. Always consider cardiac tamponade in the differential diagnosis for PEA, especially if jugular venous pressure is elevated or a pericardial effusion is demonstrated on ultrasound. In a series of 20 patients with PEA, 3 had tamponade and another 5 had some degree of pericardial effusion.[87] In this setting, blind (i.e., landmark method), ECG-guided, or ultrasound-guided pericardiocentesis can be lifesaving.

Tamponade Caused by Nonhemorrhagic Effusions

Most nonhemorrhagic effusions are liquid. They can be drained by pericardiocentesis with a small needle or by a catheter left in the pericardial space. Removal of even a small amount of fluid can cause immediate and dramatic improvement in blood pressure and cardiac output.

If aspiration with small-needle pericardiocentesis fails, the patient may have a purulent, malignant, or loculated effusion. Placement of a pericardial catheter is more useful in the long-term management of these patients. In Krikorian and Hancock's series, 24% of patients were managed successfully with a single pericardiocentesis procedure, but 37% needed multiple aspirations or an indwelling catheter (39% required surgical drainage and 55% of these patients had traumatic hemopericardium). Therefore if time and patient stability permit, consider pericardiocentesis with a catheter to reduce the necessity for repeated aspirations.[82]

Patients with renal failure and tamponade require urgent pericardiocentesis. Without signs of tamponade, these patients may be better managed by dialysis. In one series, 63% of renal failure patients were managed successfully with only dialysis.[82] Consultation with specialists is advised when there is no evidence of hemodynamic collapse but pericardial drainage is still being considered.

An algorithm for the urgent management of nonhemorrhagic cardiac tamponade is presented in Fig. 16.11.

Pericardiocentesis in Patients With Hemorrhagic Tamponade

For hemorrhagic tamponade, pericardiocentesis is rarely the definitive treatment. Aspiration of a small quantity of fluid may cause a dramatic improvement in hemodynamics, but pericardial clots can prevent adequate drainage, causing reaccumulation of blood. Patients with traumatic pericardial hemorrhage ultimately require thoracotomy to explore and repair the cardiac injury. Pericardiocentesis simply delays this definitive procedure. A study investigating traumatic cardiac injury found that all patients who underwent surgery within 2 hours of the injury survived but the mortality rate was higher in patients who experienced longer operating room delays.[88]

Sugg and associates documented a 43% mortality rate when pericardiocentesis was the sole treatment of traumatic

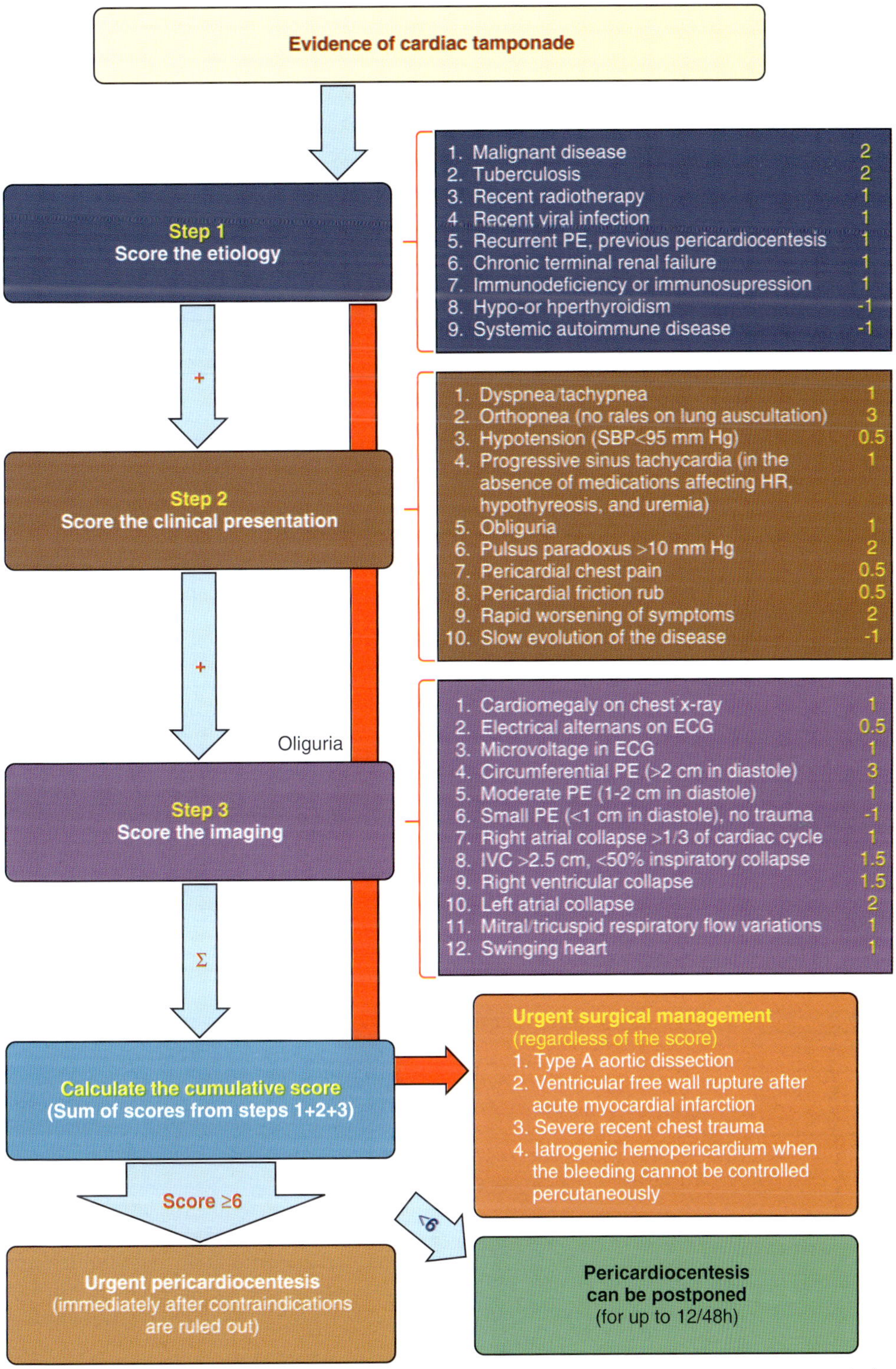

Fig. 16.10 Three-step scoring system to triage patients requiring urgent percutaneous or surgical drainage of pericardial effusion. Diagnosis of cardiac tamponade is based on clinical symptoms, signs, and echo findings. Total score ≥6 indicates urgent pericardiocentesis. *HR*, Heart rate; *IVC*, inferior vena cava; *PE*, pulmonary embolism; *SBP*, systolic blood pressure. (From Ristic A, Imazio M, Adler Y et al. Triage strategy for urgent management of cardiac tamponade: a position statement of the European Society of Cardiology Working Group on Myocardial and Pericardial Diseases. *Eur Heart J*. 2014;35:2279. Oxford University Press.)

tamponade, as compared with 16% in those who also underwent surgical intervention.[89] All patients managed by pericardiocentesis had repairable wounds at autopsy, thus suggesting that in this population, operative repair is preferable. The number of deaths from stab wounds has been decreasing over time, and this is in part due to a shift in trauma philosophy in which early thoracotomy is supported rather than repeated pericardiocentesis.

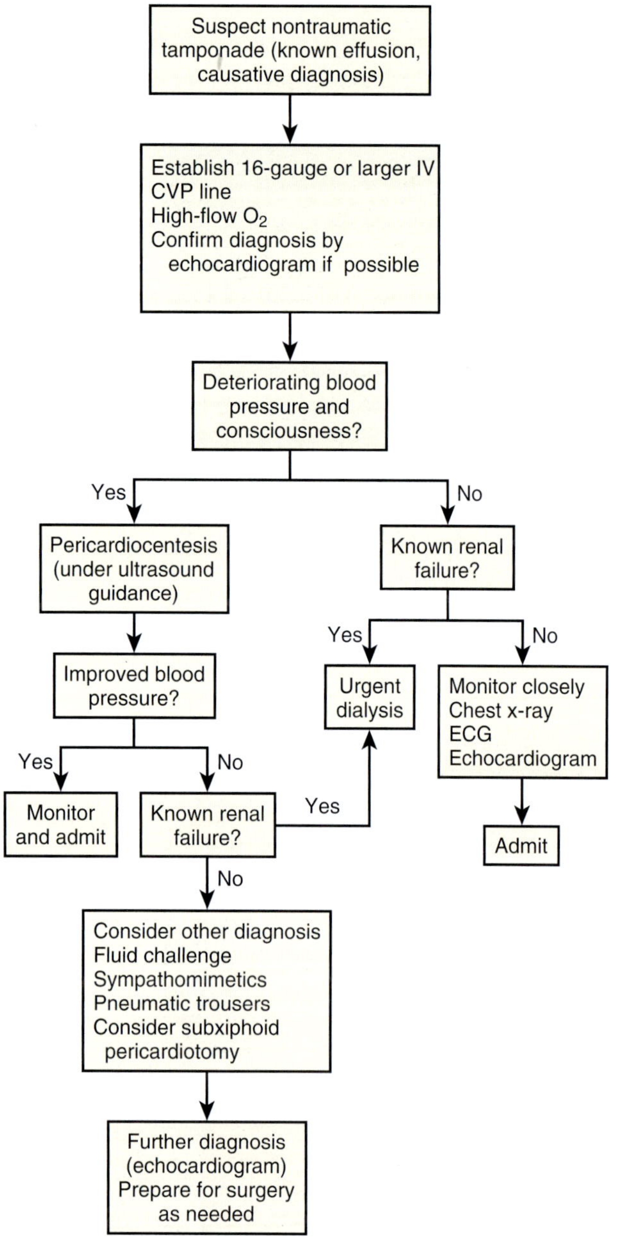

Fig. 16.11 Management of nontraumatic cardiac tamponade. *CVP*, Central venous pressure; *ECG*, electrocardiogram; *IV*, intravenous line.

In the austere setting where no surgeon is immediately available and hemopericardium is identified on FAST exam, pericardiocentesis can serve as a lifesaving bridge until definitive surgical intervention is arranged (Fig. 16.12). A study of penetrating trauma patients with tamponade found that preoperative pericardiocentesis decreased the mortality rate from 25% to 11%.[90]

CONTRAINDICATIONS

There are no absolute contraindications to pericardiocentesis in hemodynamically unstable patients. Relative contraindications to pericardiocentesis include coagulopathy, previous thoracoabdominal surgery, the presence of prosthetic heart valves, pacemakers, or cardiac devices, inability to visualize the effusion with ultrasound during the procedure, and situations

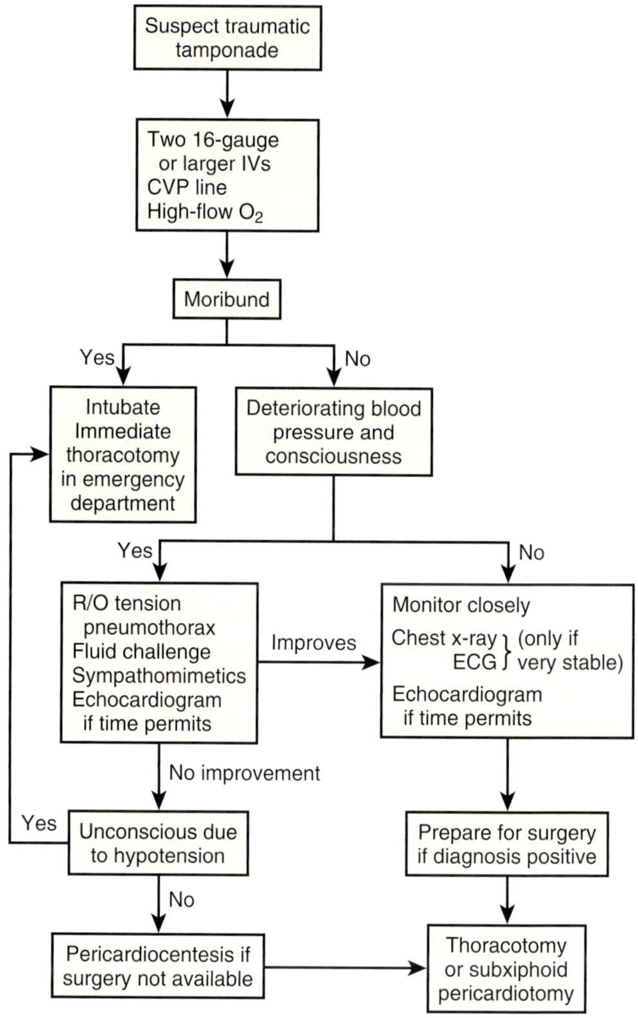

Fig. 16.12 Management of traumatic cardiac tamponade. *CVP*, Central venous pressure; *ECG*, electrocardiogram; *IVs*, intravenous lines; *R/O*, rule out.

in which better treatment modalities are immediately available (e.g., thoracotomy for trauma patients).

Ideally, pericardiocentesis is performed in the cardiac catheterization laboratory under fluoroscopic or echocardiographic guidance. With the advent of bedside ultrasound and immediate visualization of large pericardial effusions, pericardiocentesis is being performed in the ED more frequently. Ultrasound can accurately identify the area of the heart with the greatest fluid accumulation and clarify its relationship to the body wall.[91] This allows the physician to choose an entry site and angle of penetration with the greatest likelihood of obtaining fluid while avoiding vital structures.

OVERVIEW OF TECHNIQUES AND EQUIPMENT

In an urgent situation (e.g., PEA arrest) with no adjunctive equipment available, pericardiocentesis can be performed with minimal equipment. Use a long 18-gauge or 16-gauge spinal needle attached to a 10-mL syringe to withdraw fluid from the pericardial sac. Although the procedure can be done with these two simple devices, access to several others would be beneficial during the procedure. Of all the components, the most essential is an ultrasound machine, which first is used to determine whether a pericardial effusion is present and then assists in accurate needle placement. Ideally, use a probe with a small footprint and a frequency of 2 MHz to 4 MHz. If this type of probe is not available, use a 2- to 3.5-MHz curvilinear probe in the subxiphoid view, which will also provide excellent images of the heart.

Before the introduction of real-time sonography to guide needle placement, electrocardiographic monitoring was used to indicate appropriate needle placement. This is done by connecting the electrocardiographic machine to one of the precordial leads (e.g., V_1). That precordial lead is then attached to the portion of the spinal needle closest to the syringe with an alligator clamp (Fig. 16.13). The precordial lead can then be used as a rhythm strip to monitor the needle tip continuously.

Other tools that are desirable for urgent pericardiocentesis can be found easily in the ED or in a pericardiocentesis kit (see Review Box 16.1): a finder needle, Seldinger wire, dilator, flexible catheter guide, 6- to 8-Fr pigtail catheter, plastic drainage tube, extra syringes, sterile hat, gown, gloves, and drape, and local anesthetic.

PROCEDURE

Temporizing Measures

Cardiac tamponade is an emergency that requires urgent therapy. Therapy typically consists of either pericardial drainage by needle aspiration or placement of a pericardial window. These procedures are not classically performed in an ED, so temporizing methods are the mainstay of therapy unless the patient is unstable (e.g., in PEA arrest). If pericardial tamponade is traumatic, blood should be considered before crystalloids. The most common therapeutic procedures used as temporizing measures in the setting of tamponade are intravascular volume expansion with crystalloids and administration of vasopressors or inotropes. Fluid resuscitation does have the theoretical risk of pulmonary edema and compression of the left-sided chambers. Unless the patient is hypovolemic, volume expansion greater than 500 mL should be used with caution.[63]

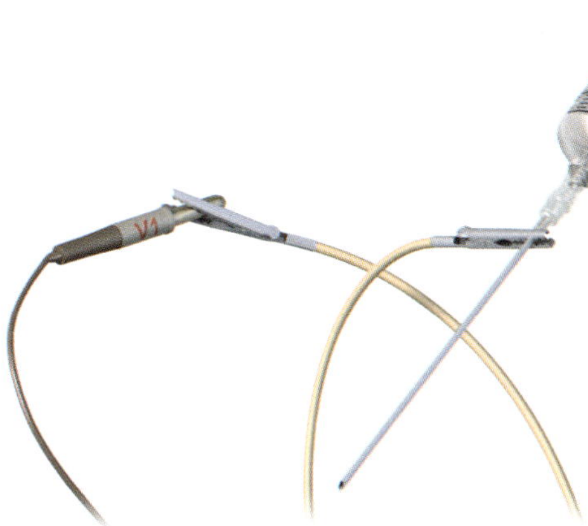

Fig. 16.13 For emergency pericardiocentesis, a long 18-gauge spinal needle is connected to a V lead of an electrocardiographic machine via a cable with alligator clips.

Pericardiocentesis

Indications

Diagnostic

Determining the cause of pericardial effusion

Therapeutic

Shock/hemodynamic instability

Cardiac arrest, pulseless electrical activity

Contraindications

Absolute

None (if hypotension or hypoperfusion is evident or if the patient is in cardiac arrest)

Relative

Coagulopathy

Prosthetic heart valve

Pacemakers and cardiac devices

Lack of direct visualization (e.g., ultrasound) during the procedure

Traumatic pericardium (thoracotomy preferred)

Equipment

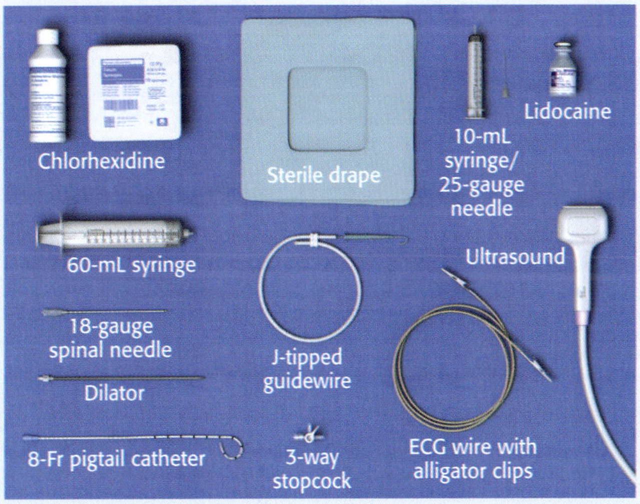

Complications

Dysrhythmias
Intra-abdominal injury (e.g., liver injury)
Air embolism
Fluid reaccumulation
Hemothorax
Pneumothorax
Pneumopericardium
Costochondritis
Suppurative pericarditis
Coronary artery injury (puncture or laceration)
Internal mammary artery injury
Intercostal vessel or nerve injury
Atrial or ventricular puncture or laceration

Review Box 16.1 Pericardiocentesis: indications, contraindications, complications, and equipment.

Norepinephrine, isoproterenol, dopamine, and dobutamine have all been evaluated as the vasopressor or inotropes of choice in patients with cardiac tamponade. Norepinephrine and isoproterenol increased cardiac output in animal models of tamponade, but failed to increase it in humans.[92,93] Dopamine and dobutamine increased cardiac output and improved hemodynamics in the setting of tamponade. Any of these agents may be beneficial as a temporizing agent only, but theoretically, dobutamine is preferable because of its greater β-adrenergic activity.[93] Dobutamine may need to be accompanied or preceded by another vasopressor especially in the hypotensive patient given its vasodilatory properties. Patients who are on a β-blocker and are exhibiting inappropriately normal range heart may benefit from a chronotrope such as epinephrine to counteract the effects of the β-blocker.

Preparation

Before preparing for pericardiocentesis, place all resuscitation equipment at the bedside in anticipation of clinical deterioration. Most patients undergoing pericardiocentesis in the ED have already experienced hemodynamic collapse and are lying supine. If the patient is able to cooperate, elevate the chest 30 to 45 degrees to bring the heart closer to the chest wall. Sedation of stuporous patients is typically forgone because of the risk for further hemodynamic collapse. If the patient is awake and undergoing the procedure without obvious hemodynamic compromise, short-acting medications (e.g., ketamine, midazolam, or fentanyl) are preferred.

Every effort should be made to ensure aseptic technique. Prepare the chest and upper part of the abdomen with a chlorhexidine-based solution. Drape the patient and ensure that all care providers involved in the procedure are wearing a sterile hat, mask, gown, and gloves. If the patient is awake, anesthetize the skin and the proposed route with 1% lidocaine (see Review Box 16.1). Because the pericardium is extremely sensitive, it should be anesthetized.[94]

The approach to pericardiocentesis depends on the clinical status of the patient, the availability of ultrasound, and the distribution of pericardial fluid. Pericardial fluid is not always distributed circumferentially in the pericardial sac, so ultrasound can quickly identify the maximal effusion pocket and demarcate the appropriate site for needle placement. Pericardiocentesis with ultrasound guidance is currently the safest and most reliable method for the diagnosis and treatment of pericardial effusion and tamponade.[91] There are various studies that each support the parasternal long axis, apical four-chamber and subxiphoid approaches. Many studies have suggested the parasternal and apical approaches have less complications than the subxiphoid approach, later described. The best option is often the site where the visualized pocket is clearest, largest, and shallowest.[63] Before the advent of ultrasound guidance, the subxiphoid approach (discussed later in this chapter) was the preferred method of pericardiocentesis. It is still used frequently during cardiac arrest and when ultrasound is not readily available.

ECG Monitoring

If ultrasound is not readily available to guide needle placement, electrocardiographic monitoring can serve as a useful adjunct. Electrocardiographic monitoring is used to prevent puncture of the ventricle. When using this method, an assistant is essential to ensure sterile technique, observe for dysrhythmias, and make sure that the electrocardiographic machine is functioning properly.

After all equipment is sterile, attach an alligator clip from one of the precordial leads (e.g., V_1) as in FIg. 16.13 to the distal end of the spinal needle. Record a rhythm strip of this lead (the "exploring electrode") continuously. Advance the needle through the skin while remembering that any contact with the epicardium will cause a current-of-injury pattern that can be seen on the ECG. Typically, this is represented as a wide-complex premature ventricular contraction with an elevated ST segment (Fig. 16.14). When a current-of-injury pattern is seen, the needle is probably touching the epicardium. Withdraw it several millimeters to prevent laceration of the myocardium or coronary vessels. After slight withdrawal, the needle should be within the pericardial space. Aspirate any fluid, but watch for changes on the ECG. Electrocardiographic monitoring is not infallible: if the patient has an abnormal myocardium from conditions such as a previous MI or the formation of scar tissue, no current-of-injury pattern will be generated on the rhythm strip. This method is more difficult to do under sterile conditions and has been largely replaced by other image-guided methods.

Ultrasound-Guided Pericardiocentesis

See Video 16.2. Pericardiocentesis has traditionally been performed blindly. This approach was associated with a low success rate and a high rate of complications, such as inadvertent puncture of the lung, ventricle, or epicardial vessels. Using ultrasound to both diagnose and guide pericardiocentesis has resulted in increased success rates, as well as a lower rate of complications. The techniques are described in the Ultrasound Box.

Subxiphoid/Subcostal Approach

As mentioned earlier, the traditional blind subxiphoid approach can still be used for pericardiocentesis in the ED (e.g., for patients in cardiac arrest and when ultrasound is not available). The technique is performed as follows: introduce the needle 1 cm inferior to the left xiphocostal angle at a 30-degree angle to the skin (Fig. 16.15). Because the heart is an anterior structure, angles greater than 45 degrees may lacerate the liver or stomach. Aim toward the left shoulder and advance the needle slowly while continuously maintaining negative pressure on the syringe to aspirate any fluid. Aspirate with an "in-and-out" vector only, not "side-to-side," which may lacerate tissue. If no fluid is aspirated, withdraw the needle completely and redirect it in a deeper posterior trajectory.

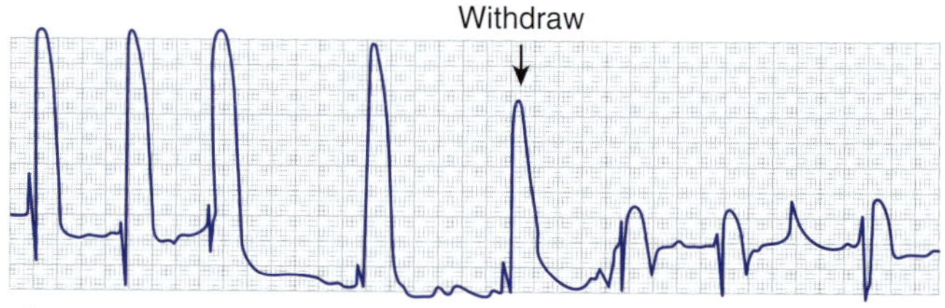

Fig. 16.14 Current-of-injury. There is an obvious change in the electrocardiogram when the pericardiocentesis needle touches the epicardium. Following slight withdrawal *(arrow)*, the ST-segment elevation diminishes. This is best seen when the needle is directly attached to the electrocardiographic V lead.

PERICARDIOCENTESIS (SUBXIPHOID APPROACH)

1

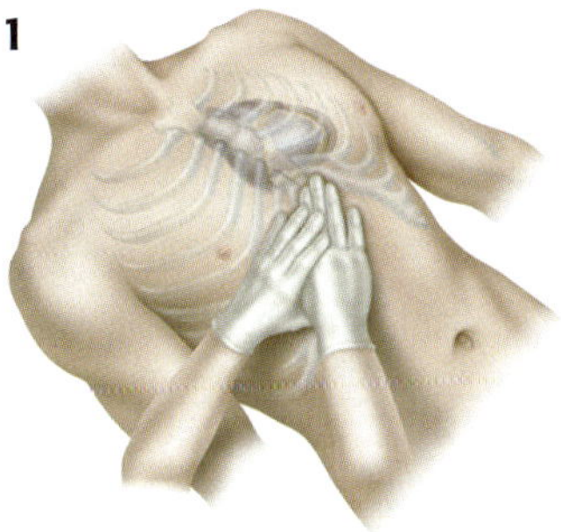

Examine the patient and identify the xiphoid process and the costal margin.

Prepare the area with antiseptic and administer local anesthetic.

2

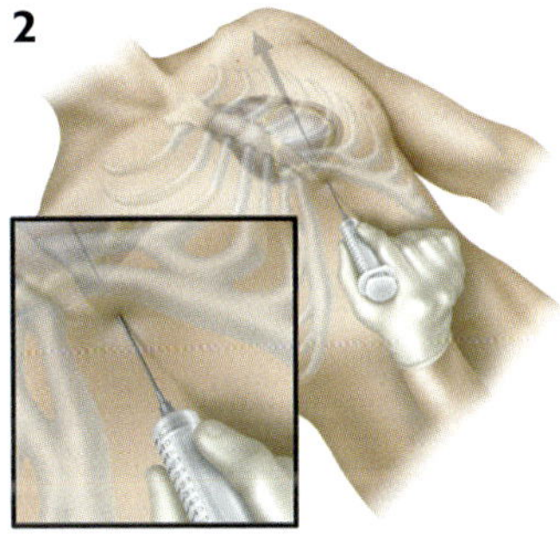

Introduce the needle 1 cm inferior to the left xiphocostal angle at a 30-degree angle to the skin.

Aim toward the left shoulder.

3

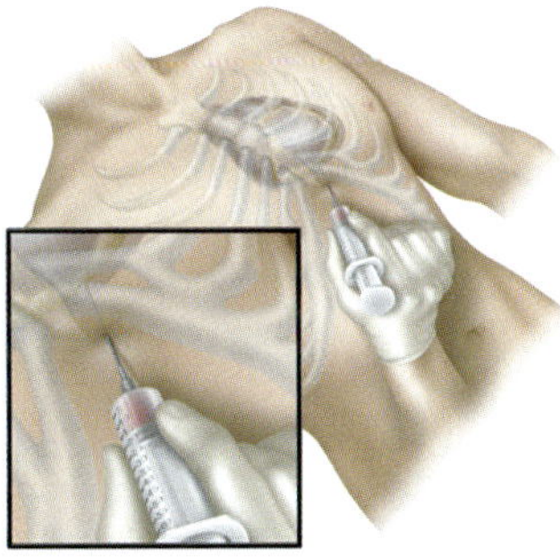

Aspirate during needle advancement and monitor for fluid return.

Stop advancing once fluid is returned.

4

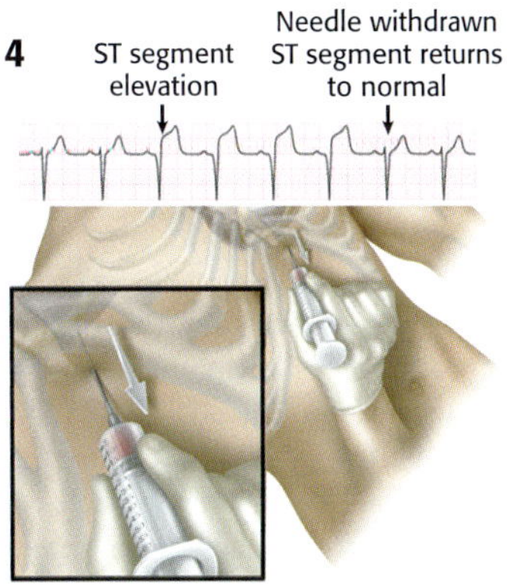

If using electrocardiographic monitoring, observe for current of injury during needle advancement, which indicates epicardial contact. If this occurs, withdraw the needle slightly.

5

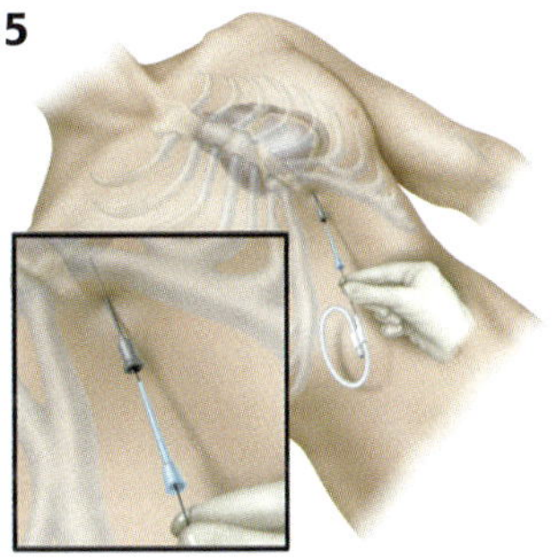

Advance a J-tipped guidewire through the needle and into the pericardium.

6

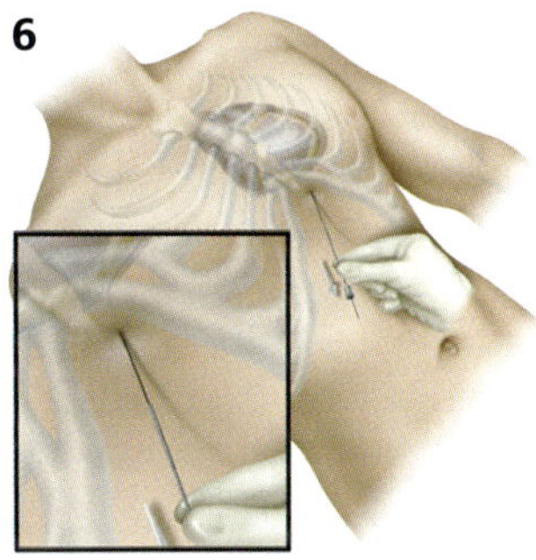

Remove the needle, while leaving the guidewire in place in the pericardium.

7

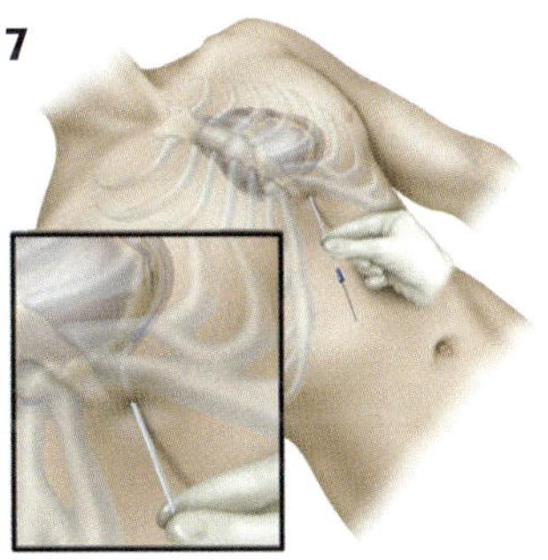

Advance a 6- to 8-Fr dilator over the wire and then remove the dilator.

8

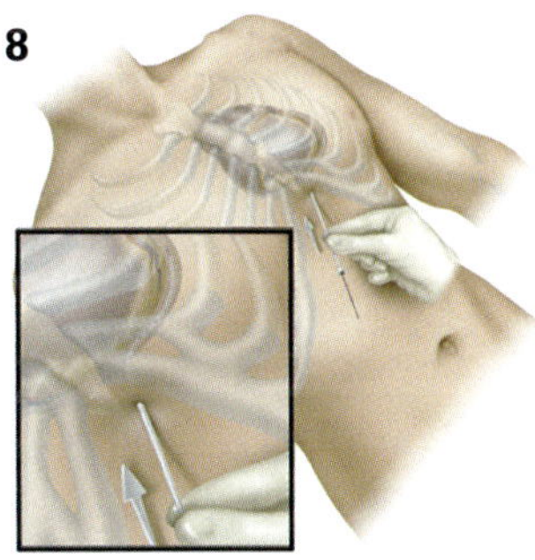

Advance a 6- to 8-Fr pigtail catheter over the wire and into the pericardium.

9

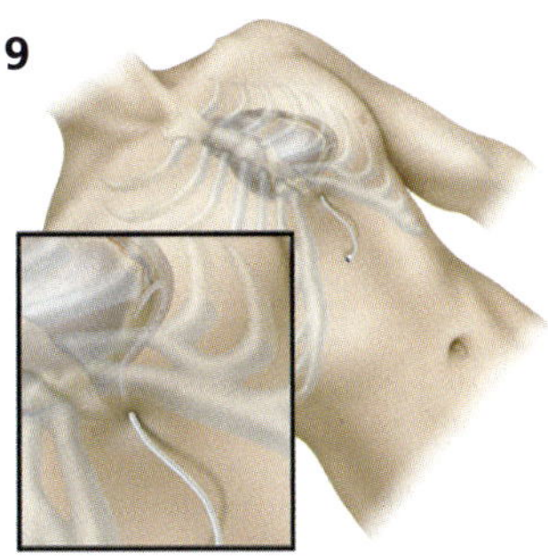

Remove the wire and drain the pericardial fluid.

Fig. 16.15 Pericardiocentesis (preferred subxiphoid approach). (From Custalow CB. *Color Atlas of Emergency Department Procedures*. Saunders; 2005:123.)

If no fluid is aspirated after redirecting the needle, withdraw the needle and redirect it, working from the patient's left to right, until it is aimed at the right shoulder. The subxiphoid approach often has the longest distance the needle has to traverse (5.6 cm), nearly double the other approaches. It does have less chance to cause a pneumothorax and may be better in cardiac arrest with ongoing compressions.[63]

Apical Approach

The apical approach is occasionally used as an alternative to the subcostal approach to drain a pericardial effusion when ultrasound is available. Use ultrasound to identify the largest area of the apical effusion (Fig. 16.16A) or simply feel for the apex. If the apex cannot be palpated, it typically lies within the area of cardiac dullness, often between the fifth, sixth, or seventh intercostal space, between the midclavicular and midaxillary lines. Introduce the needle 1 cm lateral to and into the intercostal space below the apical heartbeat. Advance the needle over the cephalad border of the rib and aim it toward the right shoulder to avoid the neurovascular bundle located caudal to the rib space. This area is close to the lingula and the left pleural space, thus making pneumothorax a frequent complication. Theoretically, this technique is used because the coronary vessels are small at the apex and the structure most likely to be entered is the thick-walled LV, which is more likely to seal off after ventricular injury. The apical approach may also be useful when there is a significantly larger posterior pericardial effusion to target compared to the anterior side.

Parasternal Approach

The parasternal approach is an alternative approach to the previously described techniques. First, identify the largest area of the parasternal effusion on ultrasound if possible. If ultrasound is not available or if the effusion is not clearly identified on the ultrasound image, proceed by introducing the needle 1 cm lateral to the sternal border at the left fifth or sixth intercostal interspace. Advance the needle over the cephalad border of the rib to avoid the neurovascular bundle on the caudal aspect of the rib. Avoid going too far laterally from the sternal border because of potential injury to the internal mammary artery.[95] Occasionally, a right parasternal approach may be used when ultrasound predicts superior access to an effusion from this direction.

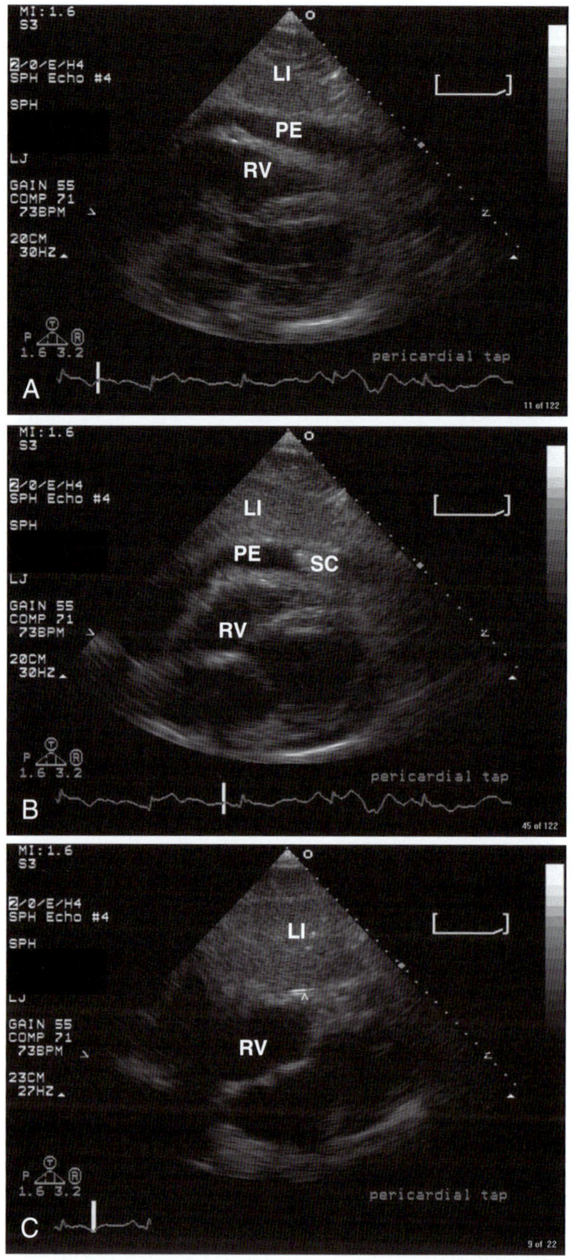

Fig. 16.16 Placement of a pigtail catheter in the pericardial space under ultrasound assistance: subcostal view of a small but hemodynamically significant pericardial effusion during pericardiocentesis. (A) The effusion. (B) After the injection of approximately 0.1 mL of agitated saline through the pericardiocentesis needle to confirm its position in the pericardial space. (C) The shaft of the pigtail catheter (*arrowhead*, two discrete parallel echogenic lines reflect the catheter walls; the echo-free area represents the catheter lumen) lying in the pericardial space after the majority of fluid has been drained. *LI*, Liver; *PE*, pericardial effusion; *RV*, right ventricle; *SC*, saline contrast.

Procedure and Technique

Confirm the trajectory and depth of the needle before puncturing the skin. Be aware that repositioning the patient alters the position of the heart and pericardial sac within the chest, so reassessment will be necessary. Prepare the skin antiseptically and place a sterile cover over the ultrasound probe. If time permits, anesthetize the selected area with 1% lidocaine, using the superior border of the adjacent rib as a landmark. Select an 18-gauge spinal needle. Ideally, the needle should have a sheath that allows it to be withdrawn after the pericardial space is entered. This helps avoid injury to the heart and other vital structures. Attach a saline-filled syringe to the needle, and gently aspirate while slowly advancing the needle. Keep the ultrasound probe on the chest wall, immediately adjacent to the aspiration site.

Once the pericardial space is entered, inject agitated saline to confirm needle placement, particularly if the pericardial fluid is grossly bloody or if there is any question about needle position (see Fig. 16.16B). Prepare a saline echocardiographic contrast medium by using two 5-mL syringes, one with saline and the other with air. Connect them via a three-way stopcock to the needle and catheter. Rapidly inject saline between the syringes and then inject it into the sheath. Monitor the entrance of the agitated saline into the pericardial space sonographically—it appears as a brightly echogenic stream. If the use of agitated saline proves to be inconclusive or suboptimal, use an echocardiographic contrast agent (e.g., Definity) as a safe and successful alternative.[96,97] Contrast agents contain gas microbubbles, which markedly enhance the fluid echo by introducing multiple liquid-gas interfaces. Inject this solution as a bolus. If the contrast material clears immediately after administration (as occurs with agitated saline) or persists temporarily within the cardiac chambers, an intracardiac location is suggested.

Fluid Aspiration and Evaluation

Removal of even a small amount of pericardial fluid (e.g., 30 to 50 mL) usually results in either return of spontaneous circulation or hemodynamic improvement. Consider placement of a temporary pericardial drain not only to ensure rapid access into the pericardial sac but also to allow more fluid to be removed quickly if hemodynamic collapse recurs. A temporary drain can be placed via any approach with the Seldinger technique, described in Chapter 22. If a pericardiocentesis kit is not available, a central venous catheter or pigtail catheter kit can be used. Ensure the catheter length is substantially greater than the distance from the skin to the pericardial fluid, especially if using the subxiphoid approach. If drainage of pericardial fluid becomes sluggish, flush the catheter with a heparinized saline solution to ensure patency of the lumen.[94]

Aspiration of blood during pericardiocentesis raises the possibility of cardiac puncture. Blood retrieved from the ventricle usually clots faster than bloody fluid aspirated from the pericardium. In general, hemorrhagic pericardial effusions have local fibrinolytic activity, which prevents clot formation. If the bleeding is brisk enough, however, blood may still clot and does not necessarily point toward ventricular puncture. The hematocrit of pericardial fluid should always be lower than that of a sample from the systemic vascular system, except in patients with aortic dissection or acute myocardial rupture. These circumstances aside, a hematocrit value similar to that for systemic blood should raise concern for an intracardiac needle location. Several other simple laboratory tests can differentiate normal from abnormal pericardial fluid, but they require the availability of a centrifuge system and time. Under normal conditions, pericardial fluid is less than 50 mL in volume and clear to pale yellow in color with no red or white blood cells, inflammatory markers, bacteria, or cancer cells and with a glucose concentration similar to that of blood.

Immediately following the procedure, obtain a chest film to ensure the absence of pneumothorax and free air under the diaphragm. Place the patient on continuous cardiac monitoring for at least 24 hours and watch for signs of reaccumulating fluid or iatrogenic complications. Repeating the ultrasound examination within 24 hours is recommended. Diagnostic evaluation of nonhemorrhagic fluid is similar to that for pleural fluid (see Chapter 9).

COMPLICATIONS

Emergency physicians often perform pericardiocentesis under duress on a patient in PEA arrest. Many also perform the technique blindly because they have little or no time to gather adjunctive assistance or tools. It is critical for the emergency physician to be aware of both the traditional and contemporary methods of performing the procedure and the complications that can be associated with these methods (see Review Box 16.1).

With the advent of ultrasound- and CT-guided pericardiocentesis, the complication rate has been greatly reduced. Major complication rates can be as low as 0.3% to 3.9% and minor complications 0.4% to 20%.[91] Earlier studies of blind pericardiocentesis documented morbidity rates of 20% to 40% and mortality rates as high as 6%.[98] Because pericardiocentesis is performed in moribund patients, the likelihood of cardiac arrest and death is high. However, they are not usually a direct complication of pericardiocentesis but of poor cardiopulmonary reserve. Cardiac arrest and death are rarely associated with echocardiographically guided pericardiocentesis.

One of the most frequent complications is a dry tap, especially when a blind approach is used. A dry tap is often caused by blockage of the needle with clotted blood or a skin plug. With the parasternal approach, the needle can become blocked by vigorous probing of the anterior costal cartilage. The problem can be solved by repositioning or irrigating the needle, which allows the effusion to be aspirated unless it is loculated.

Preventricular contractions are frequently noted after the needle enters the pericardial sac; however, no serious dysrhythmias resulting in hemodynamic compromise have been mentioned in the literature. Dysrhythmias are not common. Krikorian and Hancock reported one episode of ventricular tachycardia and several "hypotensive vasovagal reactions" that were associated with bradycardia and responded to atropine and fluid loading.[82] Duvernoy and associates reported one case of ventricular tachycardia and one case of atrial fibrillation in 352 procedures.[99] Maggiolini and coworkers reported transient third-degree heart block in a single patient.[100]

Pericardiocentesis can cause damage to surrounding structures. The traditional subxiphoid approach carries a risk for liver laceration, colon or stomach perforation and irritation to the diaphragm or phrenic nerve. The parasternal and apical approaches have been documented as causing pneumothorax and pneumopericardium in several case series, but without any clinical consequence (Fig. 16.17).[91] The pneumothoraces were treated with 100% oxygen or thoracostomy. There have also been infrequent reports of pneumopericardium after removal

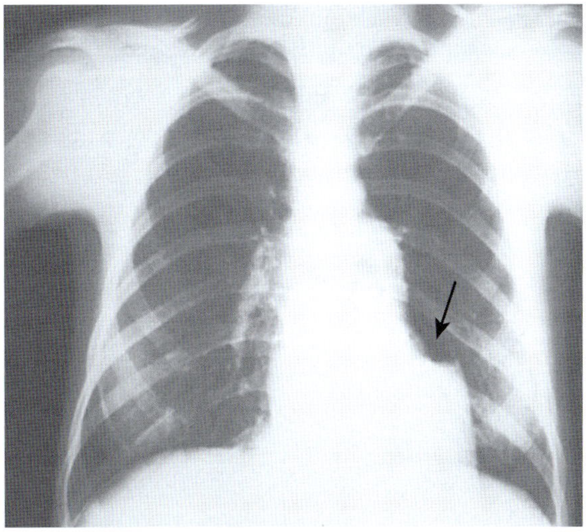

Fig. 16.17 Air-fluid level *(arrow)* in the pericardial space immediately after pericardiocentesis. A minor pneumopericardium is inconsequential; a larger collection may cause tamponade.

of a pericardiocentesis catheter. The cause of the pneumopericardium is thought to be the formation of a bronchopericardial fistula, but the exact mechanism is unclear. The mortality rate associated with tension pneumopericardium is approximately 50%, so consider pneumopericardium when patients complain of dyspnea and hypotension after removal of their catheter.[101,102]

Very few studies have reported ventricular or coronary vessel laceration during pericardiocentesis. These complications occur more frequently during blind or electrocardiographically guided procedures. Most cardiac perforations occur in the RV, but punctures in the LV and atria have also been reported. When these perforations occur, they tend to be silent and result in hemopericardium and death. In patients taking anticoagulants, it is important to check coagulation factors and monitor them closely after pericardiocentesis because hemopericardium could develop just from the procedure itself.

In the series compiled by Krikorian and Hancock, hemopericardium developed in 13 of 123 patients as a result of pericardiocentesis, one as a result of a lacerated coronary artery. One patient died of a punctured ventricle. Surgical control was necessary in four patients in whom tamponade developed, whereas it did not develop in eight patients with hemopericardium, and they were managed conservatively.[82] Guberman and colleagues reported three lacerations of the RV in 46 patients; one was fatal.[40] Wong and colleagues found five punctures of the RV, four in patients with nonproductive pericardiocentesis, but none caused any adverse sequelae.[103] In their series of 352 procedures, Duvernoy and associates reported 23 penetrations. In two cases, both the RV and LV had been perforated, and in all other cases, the RV had been entered.[99]

Researchers differ in their opinions regarding the adverse effects of ventricular puncture. Most ventricular punctures involve the lower aspect of the RV. The wall of the RV is thin and therefore vulnerable to laceration. However, pressure in the RV is low, so a puncture should cause little bleeding. In a series of patients who underwent ultrasound-directed pericardiocentesis, ventricular puncture occurred in 1.5% but was without consequence.[104] In another study, laceration of the RV occurred in one patient despite the use of echocardiography; it resulted in tamponade and necessitated emergency surgery.[105] Of the 23 perforations in the series by Duvernoy and associates, three were considered major complications (two patients required thoracotomy). LV pseudoaneurysm typically occurs as a complication of MI. It is rarely seen after surgery, trauma, or infection. Rare cases of severe LV pseudoaneurysm after pericardiocentesis have been reported.[106,107]

Even when pericardiocentesis has induced no physical injury, adverse events have been documented. Most have to do with the fact that during pericardiocentesis the stroke volume of the previously collapsed RV increases 75% after the first 200 mL of fluid is removed.[8] In general, this increase in stroke volume is greater initially than that demonstrated by the LV. This imbalance can cause significant consequences for both RV and LV function. Three of six patients in whom large effusions were removed by pericardiocentesis experienced RV dilation and overload, abnormal septal motion, and either no increase or a decrease in the RV ejection fraction.[108] These patients subsequently and slowly returned to normal hemodynamic status.

Pulmonary edema following pericardiocentesis has also been reported, presumably caused by a sudden increase in venous return to the LV when peripheral vascular resistance is still high from compensatory catecholamine secretion.[109–112] Supporting evidence for this explanation is that RV stroke volume increases more than LV stroke volume after relief of tamponade.[11] Circulatory collapse with persistently low arterial blood pressure has been reported in a patient from whom 700 mL of clear fluid was drained at a rate of 100 mL/min.[113]

The previously described case of pulmonary edema may now be known as pericardial decompression syndrome (PDS). It was first described in 1983, but only became more prominent in the 2010s. PDS is a rare life-threatening complication following drainage of tamponade that is not entirely well understood. It is thought that rapid relief of pressure and increase of pulmonary venous return contributes to acute onset heart failure. The presentation is paradoxical worsening of a patient's hemodynamics, but the onset can range from immediately occurring to up to 48 hours after the pericardiocentesis. Treatment options may include inotropic support, aggressive heart failure support including pressors, diuretics, and even intraaortic balloon pump. PDS can rarely even develop with as little as 450 mL. Many authors recommend that the pericardial drainage rate not exceed 50 mL/min, and other experts recommend even stopping the initial drainage when hemodynamics improve and only allowing slower gradual decompression once the myocardium has adapted to the changes in filling pressures.[109,114,115]

ACKNOWLEDGMENTS

The editors and authors acknowledge the contributions of Richard J. Harper to this chapter in previous editions. Linda J. Kesselring, MS, ELS, from the Department of Emergency Medicine at the University of Maryland School of Medicine, copyedited the manuscript for the previous edition.

REFERENCES ARE AVAILABLE AT Elsevier eBooks+

CHAPTER 17

Cardiopulmonary Resuscitation and Artificial Perfusion During Cardiac Arrest

Benjamin S. Abella, Susan R. Wilcox, and Lance B. Becker

Cardiopulmonary resuscitation (CPR) can be lifesaving for a patient in cardiac arrest, particularly in conjunction with other therapies such as defibrillation or delivery of medications. In several large clinical studies, data have shown that prompt delivery of CPR serves as an important predictor of successful outcome and increases the chance of survival by up to twofold.[1,2] Each minute without treatment, however, is associated with a 10% to 15% decrease in the probability of survival.[3,4]

The quality of CPR is an important technical issue and has a direct effect on patient outcome. For example, shallow chest compressions (<2 cm depth in adult CPR) have an adverse impact both on the success of defibrillation and eventual survival.[5,6] Because of these and related data, emphasis has recently been placed on improving the quality of CPR, and such priority has been codified in consensus CPR guidelines promulgated by the American Heart Association. These guidelines are formulated through a formalized data evaluation process and are updated every 5 years.[7]

Worrisome data have shown that the quality of CPR during actual resuscitation is endemically poor.[8,9] Specifically, chest compressions are often administered too slowly with inadequate depth. In addition, pauses in chest compressions are too long, and hyperventilation of arrest patients is common. These deficiencies may be due to a variety of factors, including infrequent training, lack of awareness of the quality of CPR during resuscitation, and inadequate team performance during resuscitation efforts.[10]

CONVENTIONAL CPR

Although CPR is widely taught to health care personnel and reassessed periodically, the importance of high-quality CPR cannot be stressed enough. High-quality CPR immediately before defibrillation increases the chance of successful restoration of circulation.[5,11] Consensus opinion, based on a growing foundation of clinical data, is that early CPR and defibrillation (when appropriate) have a significant impact on patient survival and recovery.[12–14] Quality chest compressions also increase the efficacy of drugs administered during resuscitation, whereas inadequate circulation leads to minimal effects from peripherally delivered drugs.[15] Hyperventilation is also widely prevalent and dramatically compromises hemodynamics. In animal studies, hyperventilation leads to reduced survival from arrest. In this section, we review the key procedural aspects of manual CPR.

Compressions

The 2020 resuscitation guidelines emphasize the importance of quality chest compressions[7] by recommending that clinicians focus on maintaining proper chest compression depth and rate. Compress the sternum to a depth of between 2.0 and 2.4 inches with a rate of between 100 and 120 compressions/min. Box 17.1 provides a summary of procedural recommendations for CPR. If possible, place a backboard under the victim to ensure appropriate thoracic compression. In addition, adjust the height of the bed or have the rescuer stand on top of a stepstool so that the entire weight of the rescuer above the waist is directed onto the patient's sternum (Fig. 17.1A and Video 17.1). This enhances the depth of compressions and helps prevent leaning on the patient's chest between compressions, which is another key deficiency that has been widely observed. Extend the arms fully and place them perpendicular to the patient's chest while making sure to pull away from the chest sufficiently between compressions to allow full chest recoil. Rotate rescuers aggressively (approximately every 2 to 3 minutes) to avoid deteriorating quality of compressions due to exhaustion. Properly delivered compressions are highly fatiguing, and rescuer bravado often interferes with the realization of declining CPR quality over time.

Minimize pauses in chest compressions because even short pauses have profound effects on coronary perfusion pressure and outcomes.[16] As stated earlier, long pauses in chest compressions before delivery of a shock are associated with failure of defibrillation.[5] Do not stop CPR to deliver medications because the drugs can be administered at the same time as the compressions. Keep pauses in chest compressions to a minimum (e.g., for procedures such as intubation or pulse checks).

Ventilations

Deliver ventilations at a rate of 8 to 10 breaths/min (see Fig. 17.1B). Hyperventilation (e.g., ventilation rates greater than 30 per minute) is common during resuscitation. To prevent unwittingly hyperventilating the patient, one practical technique is to ask the rescuer who is providing ventilations to remove their hand completely off the bag-valve-mask apparatus between ventilations. The team leader should be vigilant in the observation of delivery of ventilations and should be ready to verbally prompt rescuers to ventilate the patient at the appropriate rate if hyperventilation is performed.

Pediatric CPR

There are slight differences between adult and pediatric CPR. An arrest in a pediatric patient is much more likely to have been the result of respiratory compromise. Chest compressions to ventilation ratio should be 30:2 with one provider at a rate between 100 and 120 per minute. The ratio changes to 15:2 with two rescuers, emphasizing more frequent ventilations for a potential respiratory cause of arrest. Additionally, if the child does have a pulse but at a rate less than 60 beats/min despite adequate ventilation and oxygenation, CPR should be initiated. Compress the lower half of the sternum while avoiding the xiphoid process. Compress the chest to at least one-third the anterior-posterior diameter of the chest, or approximately 1.5 inches in infants or 2 inches in children. If an adequate pulse is present, breaths should be delivered at a rate of 20 to 30 breaths/min. Similarly, if an advanced airway is present in a child without an adequate pulse, breaths should be delivered at a rate of 20 to 30 breaths/min).

BOX 17.1 Key Procedural Elements of Manual CPR

COMPRESSIONS

Between 100 and 120 compressions/min
Depth of between 2.0 and 2.4 inches/compression
Allow full chest recoil between compressions
Minimize pauses in compressions

VENTILATIONS

8–10 ventilations/min (avoid hyperventilation)
Minimize pauses in chest compression for intubation
Use of continuous capnography recommended for intubated patients

CPR, *Cardiopulmonary resuscitation.*

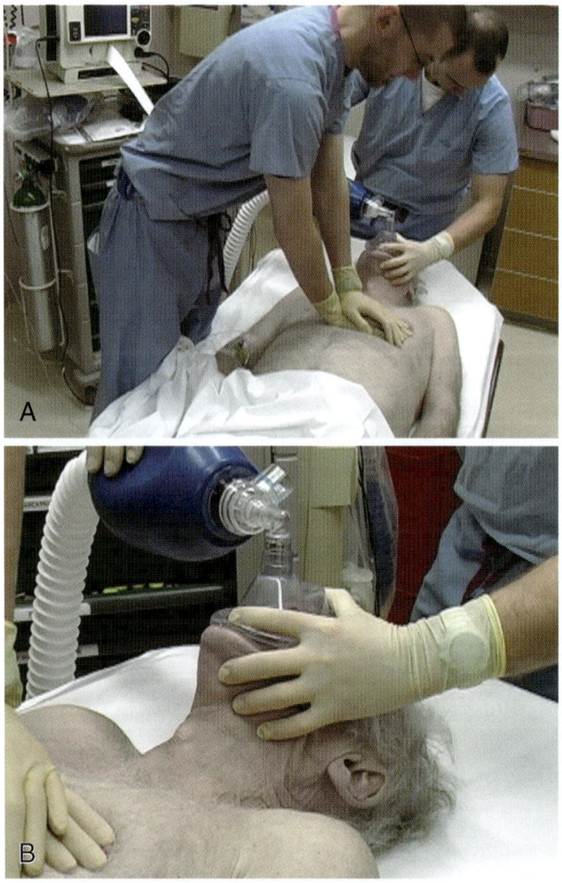

Fig. 17.1 Conventional cardiopulmonary resuscitation (CPR). Note that no alternative technique or device in routine use has consistently been shown to be superior to conventional CPR. (A) Compress the sternum to a depth between 2.0 and 2.4 inches at a rate between 100 and 120 compressions/min. Better CPR can be achieved by having the rescuer stand on a stepstool during compressions, rotating rescuers every 2 to 3 minutes, and minimizing pauses. (B) Deliver ventilations at a rate of 8 to 10 breaths/min. Avoid hyperventilation during resuscitation.

Pulse Checks

Pulse checks are generally performed too frequently during resuscitation efforts and take too much time. If a pulse cannot be readily felt within seconds, return to chest compressions as soon as possible. It is the responsibility of the team leader or code timer to ensure pulse checks take no longer than 10 seconds. Attempt pulse detection at the location of the carotid or femoral artery because peripheral pulse checks during profound shock or cardiac arrest states are notoriously unreliable. Frequently, a "pulse" can be detected during CPR itself; this phenomenon is often due to venous back pressure during compressions and does not indicate that compressions should be stopped, nor does it necessarily suggest that the compressions are of adequate quality.

Manual palpation of a pulse can be difficult due to several factors including patient's body habitus, environmental stress, time limitations, and assessor experience.[17] Adjuncts such as a femoral arterial line or a Doppler ultrasound (US) can be helpful to determine the presence of a pulse. When compared to the gold standard of an arterial line, one study found that US was significantly more accurate than manual palpation for detecting any pulse. Doppler US was used to determine the peak systolic velocity (PSV) through the femoral artery, with PSV values above 20 cm/s correlating with systolic blood pressure ≥60 mm Hg. This is of the utmost importance because the management strategy will change once the patient has achieved return of spontaneous circulation (ROSC).[17] While arterial lines are useful in this stage of a resuscitation, they may be difficult to place due to need for other interventions, access to the patient, ongoing compressions, and small arterial caliber due to low circulating volume.

Recent work has suggested a potential role for transesophageal echocardiography (TEE) during CPR to assess for blood flow and pulse restoration; future work will be required to validate whether this approach is appropriate for broad implementation.[18]

Monitoring end-tidal CO_2 pressure (P_{ETCO_2}) also affords an opportunity to detect a pulse during CPR, and other work has suggested that P_{ETCO_2} can even be potentially used to monitor efficacy of CPR to generate blood flow before ROSC.[19] During ongoing resuscitation of a pulseless patient, capnography will generally remain low (often less than 20 mm Hg), which is indicative of low blood flow. If the patient achieves ROSC, a sharp increase in the P_{ETCO_2} value (usually greater than 25 to 30 mm Hg) is consistent with return of adequate perfusion.[20]

Leadership and Teamwork

See Videos 17.2–17.4. Cardiac arrest resuscitations are often crowded, chaotic episodes filled with stress and anxiety during both prehospital and in-hospital resuscitation events. To maximize calm and efficiency and to ensure quality of care, establish a team protocol. Designate someone to be the leader of the resuscitation, and make sure that all participants are clearly aware of this designation; the team leader should explicitly identify themselves as such to the team and give loud and clear verbal directions during resuscitation efforts. The designated team leader should be responsible for monitoring the rhythm, for giving orders to initiate and terminate chest compressions, and for delivery of drugs and other therapies. The team leader should be situated either at the head of the bed or at a place where they can direct the resuscitation. It is important that the team leader does not actually perform compressions, ventilations, or other specific procedures unless absolutely necessary because they must maintain situational awareness and direct efforts of the entire team. As most rescuers are unable to detect when their own quality of compressions is diminishing, the team leader must observe CPR closely and order rescuer rotations throughout the duration of the resuscitation.[21,22]

Important Option for Layperson CPR: Chest Compression CPR

Chest compression–only CPR (CC-CPR) has been shown in a number of investigations to be as effective as standard CPR in resuscitation efforts initiated by members of the lay public.[23,24] Give compressions at a rate between 100 and 120 per minute, as with conventional CPR with interposed ventilations. CC-CPR can also be done for pediatric patients and infants in cardiac arrest.

Because of its simplicity, CC-CPR minimizes pauses in chest compressions while maintaining proper rate and depth. Lay rescuers in the community may be less experienced with standard CPR and uncomfortable with the performance of mouth-to-mouth resuscitation. The simplicity of CC-CPR makes it relatively easy for first responders to initiate resuscitation efforts and for emergency medical dispatchers to guide lay rescuers remotely. Starting in 2010, and affirmed in 2020, the American Heart Association guidelines have shifted emphasis from "ABC" (airway, breathing, compressions) to "CAB" (compressions, airway, breathing) for lay rescuers. Their endorsement of "hands-only CPR" (a synonym for CC-CPR) educational programs reflects additional evidence that a focus on chest compressions during CPR may lead to an increase in bystander CPR, as well as improvements in patient outcomes.[25] Investigations have shown that CC-CPR is associated with improved survival of patients with out-of-hospital cardiac arrest (OHCA) when performed by lay bystanders. A period of CC-CPR before intubation and rhythm evaluation also improves outcomes when used by emergency medical service (EMS) personnel.[26,27] Many community training programs have moved toward CC-CPR training as a default, and EMS agencies are increasingly emphasizing the importance of compressions over early intubation, as the latter often results in long compression pauses.

ADJUNCTS TO IMPROVE THE QUALITY OF CPR

Numerous techniques and adjunctive devices have been investigated in attempts to improve long-term survival rates with CPR. Data are conflicting and contrary, and as of this writing, no alternative technique or device in routine use has consistently been shown to be superior to conventional CPR. Unless breakthrough technology or new information on the parameters affecting the outcome of CPR emerge, this admonition will probably endure. Nonetheless, a variety of technologies have been developed to improve the quality of CPR. Some of these tools directly improve chest compressions, whereas others are less direct and aim to improve human performance or enhance hemodynamics during the delivery of chest compressions. This section describes some of these promising, intuitively useful, yet still unproven techniques.

Active Compression-Decompression CPR

Active compression-decompression CPR (ACD-CPR) is a variant of CPR in which the passive relaxation phase of CPR is converted into an active phase by means of a handheld or mechanical suction device, which can theoretically improve both myocardial and cerebral circulation when compared with traditional CPR.[28,29] However, data on these devices are mixed; there have been studies on OHCA using this technique that did not find any improvements in either initial outcome or survival to discharge, and as with many devices, there are instances when its application is impractical.[30,31] More recent data agree that ACD-CPR does not appear to improve outcomes compared with standard CPR and little research is ongoing in this area.[32]

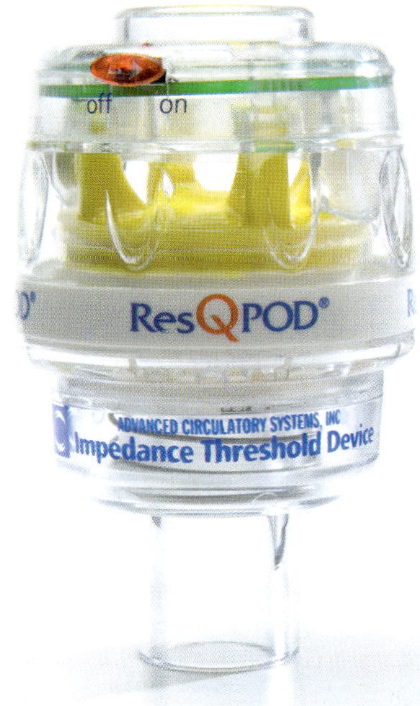

Fig. 17.2 Impedance threshold device (ITD). The ITD is placed in-line between the mask or endotracheal tube and the bag-valve apparatus. This is the Res-Q-Pod; the flashing light indicator is used to time the respiratory rate. (Courtesy Advanced Circulatory Systems, Inc., Roseville, MN.)

Impedance Threshold Device

The impedance threshold device (ITD) optimizes chest compression hemodynamics via manipulation of intrathoracic pressure.[33] During resuscitation, the ITD, placed between the endotracheal tube and the bag-valve apparatus (Fig. 17.2), prevents air from entering the thorax during recoil of the chest wall after each compression by generating a small but hemodynamically significant negative pressure within the chest. In laboratory studies, this negative pressure enhances venous return to the heart and results in increased cardiac output with each subsequent chest compression.

Numerous studies and clinical trials using one particular model of ITD (Res-Q-Pod; Advanced Circulatory Systems, Inc.) have demonstrated improved hemodynamics during CPR.[33,34] However, the findings from randomized controlled trials of ITD use in patients with OHCA have offered opposing data, thus suggesting that there is not a significant improvement in patient outcomes when these devices have been used.[35]

Monitoring and Feedback Devices

Emphasis on CPR quality and minimizing interruptions has spurred the development of devices to monitor the quality of chest compressions and ventilations and then provide audio or visual prompts to improve performance. These devices aim to improve human delivery of CPR and, unlike ACD-CPR or the ITD, do not enhance hemodynamics or patient physiology directly.

One method of monitoring chest compressions involves placing a relatively small external device on the patient's sternum and performing chest compressions on top of the device (Fig. 17.3). The device measures the quality of compressions via a force detector or accelerometer (or both) that determines the rate and depth of chest compressions. Different versions of these CPR quality–monitoring and feedback devices are on the market. Some are incorporated into defibrillators (MRx-QCPR; Philips Healthcare; R series with Real CPR Help, Zoll Medical Corp.), whereas others are stand-alone devices applied to the chest. A systematic review and meta-analysis of 17,600 cases found use of feedback devices improved chest compression depth and increased ROSC for patients experiencing in-hospital cardiac arrest (IHCA) but failed to show increased ROSC for patients presenting after OHCA or an increase in survival to hospital discharge.[36]

Mechanical CPR Devices

The adjuncts described previously all rely on human performance of CPR. Another general approach to improve CPR quality is to provide compressions via a mechanical device that is independent of human fatigue or vagaries in performance. Such tools have been introduced in previous decades but fell out of favor because of unwieldy design and other practical considerations.

A newer generation of devices has brought the notion of mechanical CPR back to active consideration. One such device uses a "load-distributing compression band" (Autopulse; Zoll Medical Corp.). The Autopulse device works via a wide band that is attached to a backboard and battery-powered motor and is placed across the torso. Through cycles of constriction and relaxation, the band compresses the chest in a circumferential manner at a fixed rate and depth consistent with resuscitation guidelines. In this fashion, pauses are also minimized by eliminating rescuer switching. Such devices have a unique role in OHCA because compressions can be delivered while transporting a patient downstairs or into an ambulance.

Studies to determine the efficacy of the Autopulse have had mixed results. Although initial smaller investigations appeared promising, a large multicenter randomized trial was stopped early because patients in the manual CPR arm had survival equivalent to those receiving care via the Autopulse, with a trend toward worse outcomes in the Autopulse group.[37]

A separate nonrandomized trial showed a marked improvement in survival when using the device.[38] A 2007 randomized trial in Europe demonstrated the utility and feasibility of automated compression devices (in this case the Autopulse) in the resuscitation of OHCA patients.[39] A 2015 pragmatic trial in the United Kingdom, evaluating a mechanical CPR device known as LUCAS (Physio-control), demonstrated equivalency between mechanical CPR and traditional manual CPR.[40] The LUCAS device (Fig. 17.4 and Video 17.5), in contrast to the band mechanism of the Autopulse, uses a piston/suction cup to compress the anterior aspect of the chest, much like during manual CPR, with the suction cup providing some degree of active compression-decompression, as described earlier in this chapter.

Additional studies comparing mechanical CPR to conventional CPR continue to show no difference in several key areas including rates of ROSC in nontraumatic OHCA patients[41] and rates of ROSC, survival to hospital discharge, or survival with a good neurological outcome at 6 months for IHCA patients.[42] One systematic review and meta-analysis of the use of mechanical CPR for IHCA demonstrated improved hospital or 30-day survival and short-term survival though quality of evidence was very low.[43] This lack of improved outcomes may in part be related to a higher rate of compression-induced injuries from mechanical compression than from manual compression, including posterior rib fractures, and heart and liver lesions.[44]

Despite this lack of demonstrated improved outcomes, there are potential benefits that may be difficult to measure regarding the use of mechanical compression devices. For example, during the COVID-19 pandemic, these devices allowed fewer providers to be in the room during a resuscitation, and thus potentially fewer providers exposed to the

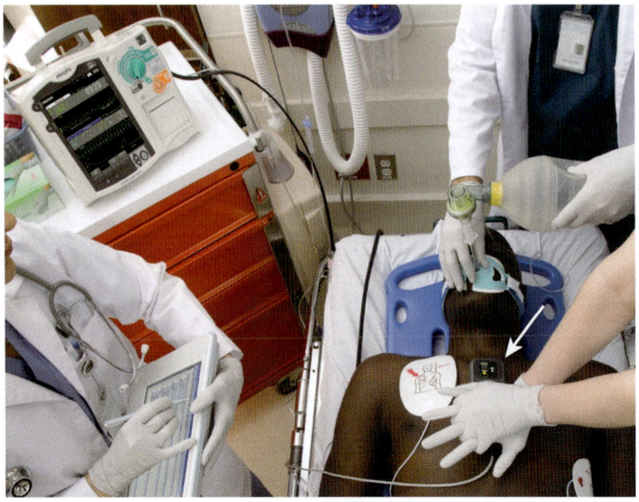

Fig. 17.3 Cardiopulmonary resuscitation–sensing defibrillator. The chest compression pad with force detector and accelerometer is indicated *(arrow)*. Several such devices are currently marketed; this is the MRx-QCPR. (Courtesy Philips Healthcare, Andover, MA.)

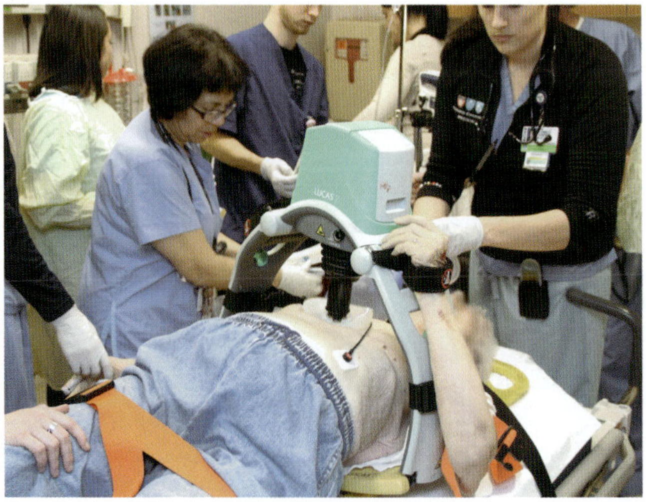

Fig. 17.4 The LUCAS-2 mechanical cardiopulmonary resuscitation device. (Courtesy Physio-control, Redmond, WA.)

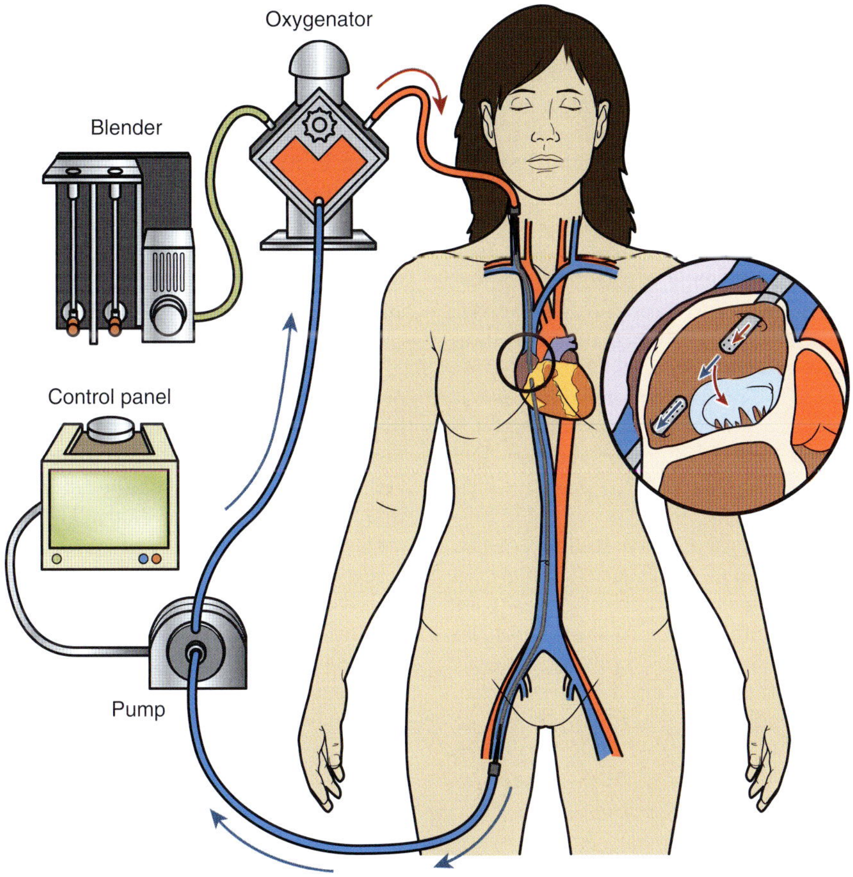

Fig. 17.5 Extracorporeal cardiopulmonary resuscitation (ECPR). Venous blood is withdrawn from a central vein *(blue arrows)*, pumped through an oxygenator, and reinfused into a central vein *(red arrow)*. Further research is required in this experimental procedure, which may benefit a select cohort of patients in cardiac arrest. Currently, ECPR is restricted to institutions that have access to the highly trained personnel and equipment required to execute this complex procedure. (Modified from Abrams D, Combes A, Brodie D. Extracorporeal membrane oxygenation in cardiopulmonary disease in adults. *J Am Coll Cardiol.* 2014;63(25 Pt A):2769-2778.)

virus.[45] These providers who are no longer needed for manual CPR are thus available to provide care for other patients in the hospital, which can be especially useful in resource-limited settings.

To highlight an intriguing opportunity available with mechanical CPR devices, there has been much discussion about the potential utility of these tools in clinical situations in which coronary angiography might be performed concurrently with ongoing resuscitation efforts.[46,47] If clinical evidence suggests a major coronary event as the cause of the arrest, mechanical devices could be used to perform high-quality, continuous chest compressions as percutaneous coronary intervention is being performed. Case studies have demonstrated the feasibility of using the LUCAS device during intraarrest coronary angiography with good patient outcomes,[48,49] but additional data will be necessary to draw clearer conclusions about clinical practices and patient outcomes in these situations.

Extracorporeal CPR

Extracorporeal membrane oxygenation (ECMO) can be employed when traditional CPR fails, in a technique called extracorporeal CPR or ECPR. ECPR is an important and growing consideration for patients with refractory cardiac arrest. The goal of ECPR is to restore perfusion promptly, minimize ischemic organ damage including anoxic brain injury, and allow time for treatment of the underlying etiology of arrest.

See Video 17.6. However, ECPR is a resource-intensive intervention requiring substantial advanced planning and collaboration. Health care teams with ECPR programs should consider both OHCA as well as patients who arrest in the emergency department (ED) (IHCA) and plan for each patient population.

Patient Selection

The optimal patient population to benefit from ECPR after OHCA has not been clearly delineated, but a number of groups have proposed guidelines for ECPR implementation.[50–52] Each ECPR center will have its own specified criteria based upon its patient population, resources, and health care system, but generally, the patients who will benefit most are those who are aged 18 to 75 years, with witnessed cardiac arrest and bystander CPR, ventricular fibrillation or pulseless ventricular tachycardia as the presenting rhythm, a transport time to an ECPR center of less than 30 minutes, and the ability to be cannulated within 60 minutes since the time of arrest.[52,53] The goal of selecting a patient for ECPR is to cannulate patients before irreversible organ damage occurs, but not cannulate those who would otherwise have prompt ROSC and survive without the risks of ECMO cannulation. Guidelines recommend calling for ECMO after 10 to 20 minutes of ongoing arrest, with a goal of cannulating as soon as possible once the decision is made.[50] One recent study found that only 4% of patients with OHCA would be clinical candidates for ECPR.[54]

The few patients who are eligible for ECPR may see a significant individual benefit. A recent randomized control trial of ECPR versus conventional advanced cardiac life support (ACLS) care, the ARREST trial, was stopped early for significantly improved survival in the ECPR arm after enrolling only 30 patients.[53] Six of 14 patients receiving ECPR (43%) survived to discharge, and all had good functional outcomes at 6 months. This was compared with one survivor in the ACLS arm (7%), who had a poor functional outcome and had died by the 3-month evaluation (hazard ratio for cumulative survival: 0.16, 95% confidence interval [CI] 0.06 to 0.41; log-rank test $P < .0001$) Nonetheless, the positive findings of this trial have not been easily replicated. A systematic review of ECPR found substantial heterogeneity, including two prior randomized trials without benefit.[52,55,56] However, these trials enrolled different patient populations, limiting generalizability. The observational studies reviewed had the same limitations. An international study of The Extracorporeal Life Support Organization's (ELSO) registry of OHCA patients treated with ECPR found survival to hospital discharge was 27.6% (95% CI 22.1% to 34.0%).[57]

Procedure

Once a patient is determined to be an ECPR candidate, high-quality CPR should be continued without pulse checks, unless the patient shows signs of life. A mechanical CPR device may assist in consistent CPR delivery, allowing clinicians to perform other aspects of the procedure. The ACLS team leader should continue to guide appropriate ACLS care, and a separate provider should be the cannulator. Femoral cannulation, either unilateral or bilateral, is appropriate in most instances. Once the patient is cannulated and ECMO flow is slowly increased up to 3 L/min, CPR should be held.[50] The team should anticipate reducing vasopressor and inotrope infusions with the initiation of ECMO.

A right radial arterial line should be placed, if not already present. Frequent blood gas measurements are essential to follow oxygen and carbon dioxide levels, targeting normal values for both. The sweep gas on the ECMO circuit will oxygenate the blood and remove CO_2. Dropping the CO_2 precipitously can be hazardous and should be avoided. Patients should be taken to the cardiac catheterization lab from the ED after cannulation unless a noncardiac cause of arrest is found. Patients should also have a head CT, as well as CT scans of the chest, abdomen, and pelvis to evaluate for organ injury from CPR that may complicate anticoagulation from ECMO.

MONITORING DURING CPR

Overview of CPR

Despite extensive research and attempts to alter the outcome of cardiac arrest, it is discouraging to realize that at present, there are no reliable clinical criteria that clinicians can use to assess the efficacy of CPR. Although P_{ETCO_2} serves as an indicator of the cardiac output produced by chest compressions and may indicate ROSC, there is little other technology available to provide real-time feedback on the effectiveness of CPR. Pulse oximetry is not helpful during arrest. Early defibrillation has been linked to better survival rates, but no medications have been shown to improve neurologically intact survival from cardiac arrest. Despite the widespread use of epinephrine and several studies of vasopressin, no placebo-controlled study has shown that any medication or vasopressor given routinely during human cardiac arrest (for any initial arrest rhythm) increases the rate of long-term survival after cardiac arrest.

Arterial blood gas monitoring during cardiac arrest is not a reliable indicator of the severity of tissue hypoxemia, hypercapnia (and therefore the adequacy of ventilation during CPR), or tissue acidosis. Current evidence in patients with ventricular fibrillation neither supports nor refutes the routine use of intravenous fluids. There is no evidence that any antiarrhythmic drug given routinely during human cardiac arrest increases survival to hospital discharge. There is insufficient evidence to recommend for or against the routine use of fibrinolysis for cardiac arrest.

No blood testing is considered routine or standard during the initial stages of cardiopulmonary arrest, although early serum potassium and blood glucose monitoring is prudent if resuscitation is successful.

Capnography

Capnography measures respiratory CO_2, which is delivered to the lungs and expelled during exhalation (Fig. 17.6). The highest CO_2 levels occur at the end of each exhalation, called P_{ETCO_2}. During cardiac arrest, P_{ETCO_2} falls abruptly at the onset of cardiac arrest, increases during the delivery of effective CPR, and returns to physiologic levels after ROSC. P_{ETCO_2} correlates with cardiac output under low-flow states such as CPR.[58] Because of this relationship with cardiac output, P_{ETCO_2} has been regarded as a probable indicator of the quality of CPR. During effective CPR in animal trials, P_{ETCO_2} positively correlates with cardiac output, coronary perfusion pressure, efficacy of cardiac compression, ROSC, and even survival. Research is currently being done to further understand the use of P_{ETCO_2} during CPR. At the other end of the spectrum, P_{ETCO_2} could be useful in determining when to terminate resuscitation efforts.[59]

Although capnography is a common method of confirming correct endotracheal tube placement, it has also been regarded as a potential method of measuring hemodynamics and perfusion during cardiac arrest, as well as for determining the outcome of resuscitation efforts (specifically, detection of ROSC). The 2020 resuscitation guidelines recommend continuous waveform capnography for all intubated patients during resuscitation efforts.[7]

Ultrasound Monitoring

With advances in ultrasound equipment, properly trained users can portably and accurately monitor cardiac function in real time. Studies have demonstrated that trained physicians can assess cardiac function and obtain adequate images rapidly by using the parasternal and subcostal approaches to standard echocardiography in the cardiac arrest setting.[60] However, it is important to note that use of ultrasound during CPR has

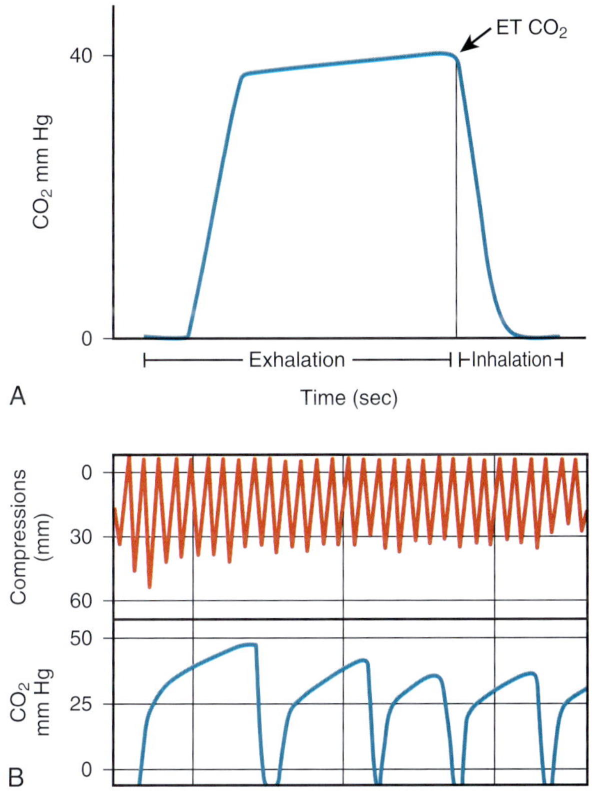

Fig. 17.6 Waveform capnography during cardiac arrest. (A) $PETCO_2$: diagram showing a typical ventilation cycle and CO_2 waveform. The point that represents $PETCO_2$ is marked with an *arrow*. (B) $PETCO_2$ recording during cardiopulmonary resuscitation. This image demonstrates the use of capnography during ongoing resuscitation. The chest compression waveform is shown in red *(top panel)*, and the $PETCO_2$ waveform is shown in blue *(bottom panel)*. *ET CO_2*, End-tidal CO_2.

been shown to lead to significantly longer pauses between chest compressions and its use should not interfere with the performance of high-quality CPR.[61] As mentioned previously, the team leader or code timer should ensure pauses between compressions are no longer than 10 seconds. Ultrasound use to detect a pulse is described in the "Pulse Checks" section.

Preparation for an incoming arrest should include placing an ultrasound nearby in anticipation of its use for assessment during CPR and to aid with any procedure that may need to be performed during resuscitation. In order to minimize interruptions during CPR, it is imperative the operator has a clear goal in mind when planning to ultrasound during a pulse check. The Cardiac Arrest Sonographic Assessment (CASA) protocol recommends the code timer count the seconds of each pause out loud while performing three different exams with one exam done per pulse check. During the first pulse check, evaluate for cardiac tamponade, then for right heart strain during the second pulse check, and finally for cardiac activity during the third pulse check.[62]

Finally, there is ongoing research on the use of transcranial Doppler ultrasound to determine the prognosis after cardiac arrest. One preliminary study concluded that patients with severely disabling or fatal outcomes could be identified within the first 24 hours with this method.[63] Other current research has shown potential for TEE as an assessment modality during CPR; TEE can identify potential arrest culprits (e.g., intracardiac thrombus, pulmonary embolism) and can be used to assess the efficacy of hand position during manual CPR.[18]

CONCLUSION

Physicians and other health care workers have been performing CPR for more than 60 years, but only since the 1990s has the full importance of the quality of CPR become apparent through an evidence-based approach. Chest compressions and ventilations appear to be deceptively easy for the newly trained, but in fact they are highly complex skills and are difficult to perform well under stress. New technologies have been developed to assist in delivery of CPR, and use of these tools may improve the ability to save lives from cardiac arrest in the coming years.

REFERENCES ARE AVAILABLE AT Elsevier eBooks+

CHAPTER 18

Resuscitative Thoracotomy

Russell F. Jones and Emanuel P. Rivers

In the United States, unintentional injury is the leading cause of death in people aged 1 through 44.[1] Blunt trauma accounts for the majority of injury mortality overall, but in urban settings penetrating trauma, including firearm-related injuries, accounts for an increased proportion of trauma deaths. In 2020 more than 45,000 firearm-related deaths occurred in the United States,[2] with many patients arriving at the emergency department (ED) in extremis. Severe traumatic injuries can be associated with a high mortality rate. However, on rare occasions, an aggressive approach involving the use of ED thoracotomy (EDT) leads to survival in patients with impending or recent traumatic arrest. EDT is a highly invasive intervention performed outside the operating room and often in the absence of trained cardiothoracic or trauma surgeons. Though supported as a potential lifesaving procedure, EDT is not a mandated standard of care nor a procedure that is expected to be performed in most EDs. The first successful thoracotomy was reported more than 100 years ago, and the first EDT was reported in 1966.[3] Since then, multiple studies have reported outcomes, indications, techniques, and risks associated with the procedure. In 2003 the National Association of EMS Physicians Standards and Clinical Practice Committee and the American College of Surgeons Committee on Trauma (ACSCOT) proposed specific guidelines for EDT.[4] Since then, several other consensus guidelines have been published attempting to identify ideal candidates for EDT.[5,6]

Given the circumstances surrounding the procedure and the associated injuries, few patients survive. The poor overall survival rates, however, should not discourage performance of the procedure in the correct setting and when appropriate surgical backup is available for definitive care.

EDT is not a simple procedure. Identifying specific structures within a chest cavity filled with blood, coupled with a collapsed lung and an injured heart and major vessels, can be formidable. Localizing the injuries that can be reversed quickly and safely is even more difficult.

This chapter focuses on three major objectives: (1) identifying possible indications for and contraindications to EDT, (2) describing the technical aspects of the procedure and adjunctive maneuvers to repair specific injuries, and (3) recognizing the associated risks and complications.

Because of the controversies surrounding EDT, every institution should have guidelines for its appropriate use. An institutional plan for chest wound management and postprocedural care should also be established with the service that will provide backup when members of the surgical team cannot be on site at the time of resuscitation. Debate regarding who should perform EDT is not necessary because everyone who is licensed to perform resuscitative thoracotomy should be trained, competent, and prepared for the technical and initial critical care aspects of patient management. Patient care needs in the event of successful resuscitation should be considered in advance and the surgical and intensive care teams notified so that they can mobilize the appropriate supplies, equipment, and personnel.

INDICATIONS AND CONTRAINDICATIONS

In the ED, the vast majority of thoracotomies are performed on penetrating trauma patients in cardiac arrest. Beall and coworkers initially proposed EDT for the treatment of penetrating cardiac injuries in 1966.[3] Since then it has been expanded to include extrathoracic injuries, blunt trauma, and nontraumatic pathology. Studies show wide variation in survival rates and outcomes. Taking 50 years of collective EDT data into account, the survival rate of patients undergoing EDT for blunt trauma is nearly 2%, whereas that for penetrating trauma is nearly 10%,[5] but these survival rates depend on many variables and are not applicable to every situation. There is a paucity of data concerning survival rates in patients with EDT performed for nontraumatic causes, and it is not recommended that this procedure be regularly used in these settings.

Make the decision to perform EDT quickly based on whether the patient is likely to benefit from the procedure, has a reasonable chance of survival, and cannot tolerate a delay in operative intervention. In addition, consider the risks associated with performing the procedure. Trauma researchers have identified several factors that are considered crucial when determining who will benefit from EDT (Box 18.1).

The first assessment is made in the prehospital setting, where determination of the mechanism of injury and the presence or absence of a pulse is critical. Multiple guidelines recommend against EDT in patients without a pulse, blunt traumatic mechanisms, and without signs of life.[4–6] Such patients do not survive, regardless of the intervention. In one of the largest EDT series to date, Branney and coworkers[7] reviewed 868 consecutive patients over a 23-year period. They found that no blunt trauma patients survived EDT when they had no vital signs in the field. In 2000 Rhee and colleagues[8] examined 4620 cases of EDT from 24 studies over a 25-year period. The overall survival rate after blunt trauma was just 1.4%, which led to EDT falling out of favor for this indication. Recent articles, however, have challenged the idea of limiting EDT to those in cardiac arrest from penetrating injury only.[5,6,9–11]

The survival rate of pulseless trauma patients sustaining penetrating injury is significantly higher than that of blunt trauma patients. Several penetrating injury subtypes have been studied as follows: firearm injuries, stab wounds, and penetrating explosive injuries. Thoracic stab wounds consistently show the highest rates of survival after EDT.[5,7,12–14] This is theoretically because of the decreased amount of tissue damage related to the weapon and the ability to quickly identify anatomic structures and injuries. Penetrating firearm injuries are more likely to result in death because of increased tissue damage from the missile and concussive surrounding forces. Patients with firearm injuries are more likely to have multiple wounds, and the depth of penetration is increased in comparison to stab wounds. One published cohort of combat casualties from explosive penetrating injuries reported comparable survival rates to those after firearm-related penetrating injuries.[14]

The location of the penetrating injury helps determine the futility of EDT. A trend toward increased survival rates in patients with thoracic injuries was found in historical

BOX 18.1 Factors Used to Determine Which Patients May Benefit From EDT

Mechanism of injury
Location of injury
Initial cardiac rhythm
Resuscitation (cardiopulmonary) time
Signs of life

data.[4,5,14–23] Isolated cardiac wounds have the highest survival rate after EDT, with approximately 17% of patients surviving the procedure.[5] Penetrating abdominal injuries have beneficial outcomes when EDT is performed to cross-clamp the aorta, with survival rates in the midteens.[7,14,24,25] Extremity injuries rarely require EDT because the use of a tourniquet can control the hemorrhaging until the patient can be transported to the operating room. When EDT is used for traumatic extremity exsanguination survival rates range from 10% to 25%.[14] Patients in cardiac arrest associated with head injuries, especially those with open cranial wounds, have dismal survival rates and are considered poor candidates for further resuscitative efforts, including EDT.[5,9]

The type of cardiac electrical activity can be helpful in determining who may benefit from EDT. Battistella and colleagues[26] reviewed 604 patients undergoing cardiopulmonary resuscitation (CPR) for traumatic cardiopulmonary arrest and found that of the 212 patients who were in asystole, none survived. Fulton and associates[27] found that of patients in traumatic arrest, survival was improved when the patients exhibited ventricular fibrillation, ventricular tachycardia, or pulseless electrical activity rather than asystole or an idioventricular rhythm. In another study of EDT for traumatic arrest, asystole, idioventricular rhythm, or severe bradycardia was indicative of poor outcomes or an unsalvageable patient.[4]

The duration of pulselessness prior to EDT has traditionally been used as a decision point. With traumatic injury, survival rates and meaningful neurologic outcomes diminish as the duration of CPR increases. The traditional dogma is that any trauma patient who has undergone CPR for longer than 15 minutes has an exceedingly dismal survival rate and further resuscitation should be considered futile.[4,6,12,13,27–30] Guidelines from 2013 have questioned the 15-minute dogma and consensus timing on futility of the procedure remains elusive.[5,31]

Perhaps the most critical determinant of the appropriateness of EDT is whether the patient demonstrates "signs of life." Signs of life are objective physiologic parameters that are present in patients who survive EDT. They include pupillary response, extremity movement, cardiac electrical activity, measurable or palpable blood pressure, spontaneous ventilation, or the presence of a carotid pulse. The presence of one or more of these indicators has been associated with good neurologic outcomes and increased rates of survival.[3–11,32,33]

Although survival remains the ultimate gauge of the effectiveness of EDT, it is also essential to consider quality of life, especially neurologic function of the patient. It is somewhat surprising that survivors of EDT generally have good neurologic outcomes. Rhee and colleagues[8] reported that 280 of 303 (92.4%) patients discharged after EDT were neurologically intact. It is not possible to accurately predict which patients are likely to survive intact, but the study by Branney and coworkers[7] demonstrated that all survivors with full neurologic recovery had respiratory effort at the scene, and 75% still had respiratory effort on arrival at the ED. The presence or absence of a palpable pulse was not an absolute prognostic indicator in this study. The first 24 hours after EDT rapidly demonstrates which patients are likely to become long-term survivors. Baker and associates[16] showed that with 168 emergency thoracotomies for mixed trauma, most patients with fatal injuries died within 24 hours. Of patients surviving the first 24 hours, 80% (33 of 41) lived and were discharged from the hospital. Full neurologic recovery occurred in 90% of these survivors. Overall only 2.4% (4 of 168) remained severely disabled or in a persistent vegetative state. Guidelines from 2015 show that 90% of penetrating trauma patients surviving EDT were neurologically intact on discharge, although this rate falls to near 60% in blunt trauma.[5]

Cardiac Injuries: Penetrating

Sixty percent to 80% of cardiac stab wounds result in pericardial effusion regardless of the presence of shock.[34] Tamponade can occur if the wound is smaller than 1 cm in size, depending on which chamber is involved. Wounds larger than 1 cm usually continue to bleed regardless of which chamber is involved. Low-pressure atrial wounds generally form a thrombus before tamponade develops. The thicker-walled left ventricle may spontaneously seal stab wounds up to 1 cm in length. As little as 60 to 100 mL of blood acutely filling the pericardium will impede diastolic filling, reduce stroke volume, decrease cardiac output, and increase release of catecholamine. Catecholamine release may mask the severity of illness because it maintains blood pressure through an increase in peripheral vascular resistance. In penetrating cardiac injury, the right ventricle is the chamber most likely to be involved because of its anterior location, followed by the left ventricle and the atria.[35,36]

The progression from compensated cardiac function to uncompensated tamponade can be sudden and profound. Although one may suspect tamponade based on well-described signs, clinical diagnosis of pericardial tamponade in an unstable trauma patient is difficult because of the combined effect of hemorrhagic and cardiogenic shock. The classic signs of Beck's triad (distended neck veins, hypotension, and muffled heart sounds) described in 1926[37] have limited diagnostic value for acute penetrating cardiac trauma.[38] The most reliable signs of tamponade are elevated central venous pressure, hypotension, and tachycardia.

The advent of ultrasound and the focused assessment with sonography in trauma (FAST) examination has improved the diagnosis of pericardial effusion and tamponade. Findings indicative of tamponade include the presence of pericardial fluid with right atrial or ventricular collapse during diastole (Fig. 18.1). FAST is a rapid bedside screening examination used to detect hemopericardium and hemoperitoneum and is now important in the evaluation of unstable trauma patients.[39,40] A systematic review and meta-analysis of 75 studies with 24,350 patients reported 91% sensitivity and 94% specificity in detecting pericardial fluid and 74% sensitivity and 98% specificity detecting peritoneal fluid in trauma patients.[41] Ultrasound can have false-negative results when pericardial fluid from a cardiac injury decompresses into the thoracic cavity through a wound in the pericardium.[42] A 2015 study by Inaba and colleagues showed a high sensitivity and

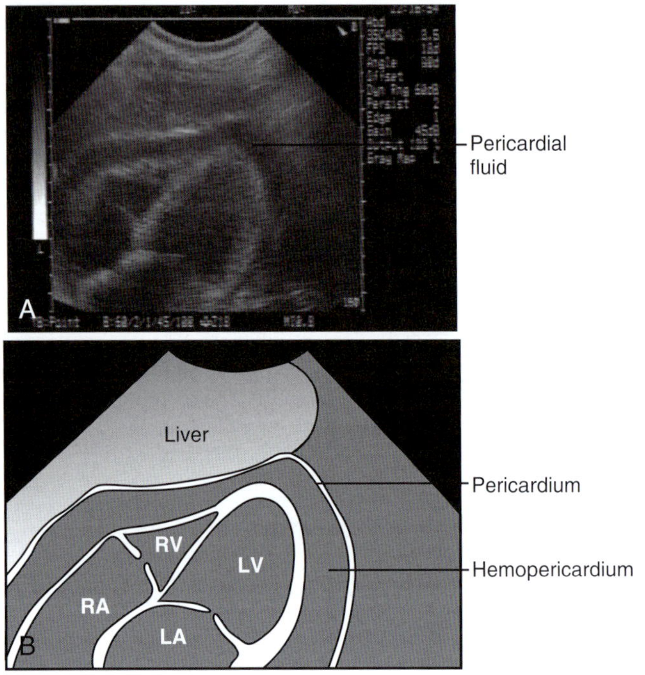

Fig. 18.1 (A) Bedside ultrasound demonstrating the hemopericardium. (B) Schematic of the chambers of the heart, the pericardium, and the hemopericardium as seen on ultrasound. *LA*, Left atrium; *LV*, left ventricle; *RA*, right atrium; *RV*, right ventricle.

negative predictive value of FAST exam in determining which patients will not benefit from EDT.[43] In this study the likelihood of survival if pericardial fluid and cardiac motion were both absent was zero.

After EDT for penetrating cardiac wounds, survival is also related to the mechanism of injury. Patients with stab wounds fare better than do patients with gunshot wounds. Rhee and colleagues[8] noted that 16.8% of patients with stab wounds survived to hospital discharge after EDT. Branney and coworkers[7] reported a 29% survival rate in stab wound patients with tamponade, and a 15% survival rate in those without tamponade.

In contrast, gunshot wounds are often large injuries unable to seal themselves; tamponade occurs in only 20%. Patients with penetrating cardiac injuries from gunshot wounds are more likely to present with profoundly compromised hemodynamics. In addition, the increasing prevalence of larger-caliber weapons has made it more difficult to resuscitate patients with gunshot wounds to the chest. Of 112 patients with gunshot wounds to the heart,[7] only 2% survived neurologically intact.

Cardiac Injuries: Blunt

Blunt trauma to the heart can range from minor contusion to cardiac rupture. The most common cause of death after nonpenetrating cardiac injuries is myocardial rupture, and in approximately 25% of such patients, the ascending aorta is ruptured simultaneously.[34] Branney and coworkers[7] observed a 2% survival rate in blunt trauma patients resuscitated with EDT. Those who survived had vital signs present in the field. The poor outcomes associated with this type of injury are a result of the poor cardiac function caused by myocardial contusion, even if the hemorrhage has been treated.

Pulmonary Injuries

Pulmonary injuries can be divided into three types: parenchymal, tracheobronchial, and large vessel. Parenchymal and tracheobronchial injuries rarely require EDT because they are either rapidly fatal or treated initially by tube thoracostomy. Tracheobronchial injury is more common in blunt than in penetrating trauma. Bertelsen and Howitz[44] reviewed 1128 patients at autopsy and found only three to have this injury. The airway is usually maintained, even with complete transection. The stiff tracheobronchial cartilage tends to hold the lumen open, and the paratracheal and parabronchial fasciae preserve the relationship of the proximal to distal bronchi. Ninety percent of tracheobronchial tears occur within 2.5 cm of the carina and most commonly involve the main stem bronchi. Complete division of the trachea is extremely rare. Depending on the size and location of the injury, patients may have massive hemoptysis, airway obstruction, pneumomediastinum, pneumothorax, or tension pneumothorax. Massive subcutaneous emphysema and pneumomediastinum are usually seen, although up to 10% of patients with this injury have no abnormal findings on the initial radiograph.[45] If hemorrhage is profuse or if the site of the injury can be determined, use of a bifid endotracheal tube or unilateral intubation of a main stem bronchus will help secure the airway.

Lacerations of the lung parenchyma that are not accompanied by injury to major vessels generally respond to tube thoracostomy. If the initial chest tube drainage is more than 1,500 mL or if there is persistent hypotension or cardiac arrest, consider immediate thoracotomy. For pulmonary injuries, survival after EDT is also related to the mechanism of injury. Branney and coworkers[7] reported a 17% survival rate after pulmonary stab wounds, 3% after gunshot wounds, and 5% after blunt trauma.

Air Embolism

Air embolism is a complication of pulmonary parenchymal injuries that may require immediate thoracotomy if the patient is hemodynamically unstable. The development of air embolism after penetrating injuries of the lung is often insidious, and the diagnosis is usually made at the time of thoracotomy.[46] Preoperative and postmortem diagnosis of air embolism is difficult, and it is likely that most air emboli are not detected. Air embolism is confirmed at thoracotomy by needle aspiration of a foamy air-blood mixture from the left or right ventricle or by visualization of air within the coronary arteries.

Air embolism may appear in either the right or the left side of the circulatory system. Involvement of the right side of the circulation is referred to as *venous* or *pulmonary* air embolism. Generally, venous air is well tolerated, but death can occur when the volume of air reaches 5 to 8 mL/kg. The rate at which air moves into the circulation and the body's position are important determinants of the volume that can be tolerated. If the body's position allows dispersion of air into the peripheral circulation, more air can be tolerated, although the damage to peripheral structures and end-organs can be extensive. Rapid death usually results from obstruction of the right ventricle or the pulmonary outflow tract. Injuries to the vena cava or the right ventricle can also create portals of entry into the right circulatory system.

Air embolism involving the left side of the circulatory system is referred to as *arterial* or *systemic* air embolism. The lethal volume depends on the organs to which it is distributed. As little as 0.5 mL of air in the left anterior descending coronary artery can lead to ventricular fibrillation. Two milliliters of air injected into the cerebral circulation can be fatal. The formation of traumatic bronchovenous fistulas creates potential entry points for air to move into the left side of the circulatory system. The only requirement is the formation of an air-blood gradient conducive to the inward movement of air. Although lowered intravascular pressure from hemorrhage is a risk factor, the most important element in all reports of air embolism has been the use of positive pressure ventilation.[47]

In a review of 447 cases of major thoracic trauma, Yee and coworkers[48] found adequate chart data to suggest the diagnosis of air embolism in 61 patients. Approximately 25% of patients with air embolism have blunt trauma, with associated lung injury secondary to multiple rib fractures or hilar disruption. The overall mortality is higher than 50%.

The diagnosis of air embolism is easily overlooked because the signs and symptoms are similar to those of hypovolemic shock. Two valuable signs that are present in 36% of patients are hemoptysis and the occurrence of cardiac arrest *after intubation and ventilation*. The development of focal neurologic changes, seizures, or central nervous system dysfunction in the absence of head injury is also suggestive of the diagnosis.[49] Overall, the diagnosis is subtle and must be considered when there is no evidence of the more common causes of extremis in a trauma patient.

Blunt and Penetrating Abdominal Injury

In the setting of penetrating abdominal injury, thoracotomy with cross-clamping of the thoracic aorta has been advocated as a means of controlling hemorrhage, redistributing blood flow to the brain and heart, and reducing blood loss below the diaphragm. Unfortunately, aortic cross-clamping can also have detrimental effects. Kralovich and colleagues[50] studied the hemodynamic consequences of aortic occlusion in a swine model of hemorrhagic arrest. There was no difference between groups in return of spontaneous circulation; however, the occluded aorta group experienced statistically greater impairments in left ventricular function and systemic oxygen utilization in the postresuscitation period. Branney and coworkers[7] found that 8 of 76 patients undergoing EDT for *penetrating abdominal injury* survived neurologically intact. More recently, Seamon and colleagues[25] achieved a 16% survival rate with good neurologic outcomes (8 of 50 patients) when EDT was used before laparotomy for abdominal exsanguination from trauma. Of note, none of the survivors in this study were in cardiac arrest at the time of EDT, but they did have severe hemorrhagic shock, and six of the eight had unmeasurable blood pressure. The resurgence of resuscitative endovascular balloon occlusion of the aorta (REBOA) has changed many institutional trauma algorithms dealing with exsanguinating abdominal and pelvic hemorrhage.[51] Current recommendations suggest that EDT be performed judiciously in patients with abdominal trauma as an adjunct to definitive repair of the abdominal injury.

Open-Chest Resuscitation for Nontraumatic Arrest

Paradis and associates[52] found that humans need a minimal coronary perfusion pressure (CPP) of 15 mm Hg to achieve return of spontaneous circulation. Although a CPP of 15 mm Hg does not guarantee return of spontaneous circulation, there is 100% failure of resuscitation if CPP is below this level. It has been shown in a limited number of human studies that open-chest cardiac massage (OCCM) produces a higher mean cardiac index (1.31 vs. 0.6 L/min per square meter)[53] and mean CPP (32.6 vs. 7.3 mm Hg)[54] when compared to closed-chest CPR. Animal models suggest not only improved hemodynamic parameters, but also a possible increase in 24-hour survival rates,[55] but neurologic outcomes are unknown, and the American Heart Association guidelines for CPR do not promote the regular use of OCCM in patients with out-of-hospital cardiac arrest (OHCA).Nontraumatic Hypothermic Cardiac Arrest

Another small study reviewed 11 cases of cardiac arrest in the setting of hypothermia, 7 of whom underwent EDT with OCCM and mediastinal rewarming. EDT with mediastinal irrigation can produce core rewarming rates as fast as 8°C/h, with the heart and lungs preferentially being rewarmed first.[56] Mediastinal irrigation involves heating sterile saline in a microwave oven to 40°C, then pouring it slowly over the heart and into the thorax. Although five patients survived with good neurologic outcome, there are no data demonstrating better outcomes in hypothermic arrest treated with OCCM than with closed-chest CPR. Other methods of core rewarming, such as cardiopulmonary bypass or extracorporeal membrane oxygenation, are more rapid while others are less rapid but do not carry the morbidity of EDT and may be just as effective.

EQUIPMENT

Carefully select the instruments to be included in the EDT equipment tray. See Review Box 18.1 for a complete list.

PROCEDURE

See Videos 18.1 and 18.2.

Preliminary Considerations

All trauma patients arriving at the ED with hypotension must be assumed to be hypovolemic and should be treated accordingly. Rapidly exclude other causes as well, including tension pneumothorax, cardiac tamponade, air embolism, and neurogenic or cardiogenic shock. A useful algorithmic overview of the approach to chest trauma is presented in Fig. 18.2. The use of autotransfusion, if available, has several benefits, but its use is not widespread or considered standard.[57]

Airway Control

Intubate the patient orotracheally, if possible, but be aware that access to the thoracic organs, surgical repairs, or surgical procedures may be hampered by frequent inflations of the left lung. If necessary, selectively intubate the right lung by blindly advancing a standard single-lumen endotracheal tube to a depth of 30 cm (measured from the corner of the mouth) in adult patients.[58] Although the left lung and the right upper lobe are not ventilated with the tracheal tube in this position, both animal studies and data from humans suggest that selective right lung ventilation provides adequate oxygenation and ventilation for at least 60 minutes.[58] With the left lung deflated

Resuscitative Thoracotomy

Indications
Trauma victims with severe refractory instability or cardiac arrest
Nontraumatic hypothermic cardiac arrest

Contraindications
Blunt trauma cardiac arrest patients without signs of life
Trauma patients with obvious non-survivable injuries
Initial rhythm of asystole without signs of life
Signs of prolonged arrest including lividity or rigor

Complications
Phrenic nerve injury
Coronary artery injury
Infection
Injury/disease transmission to health care worker

Equipment

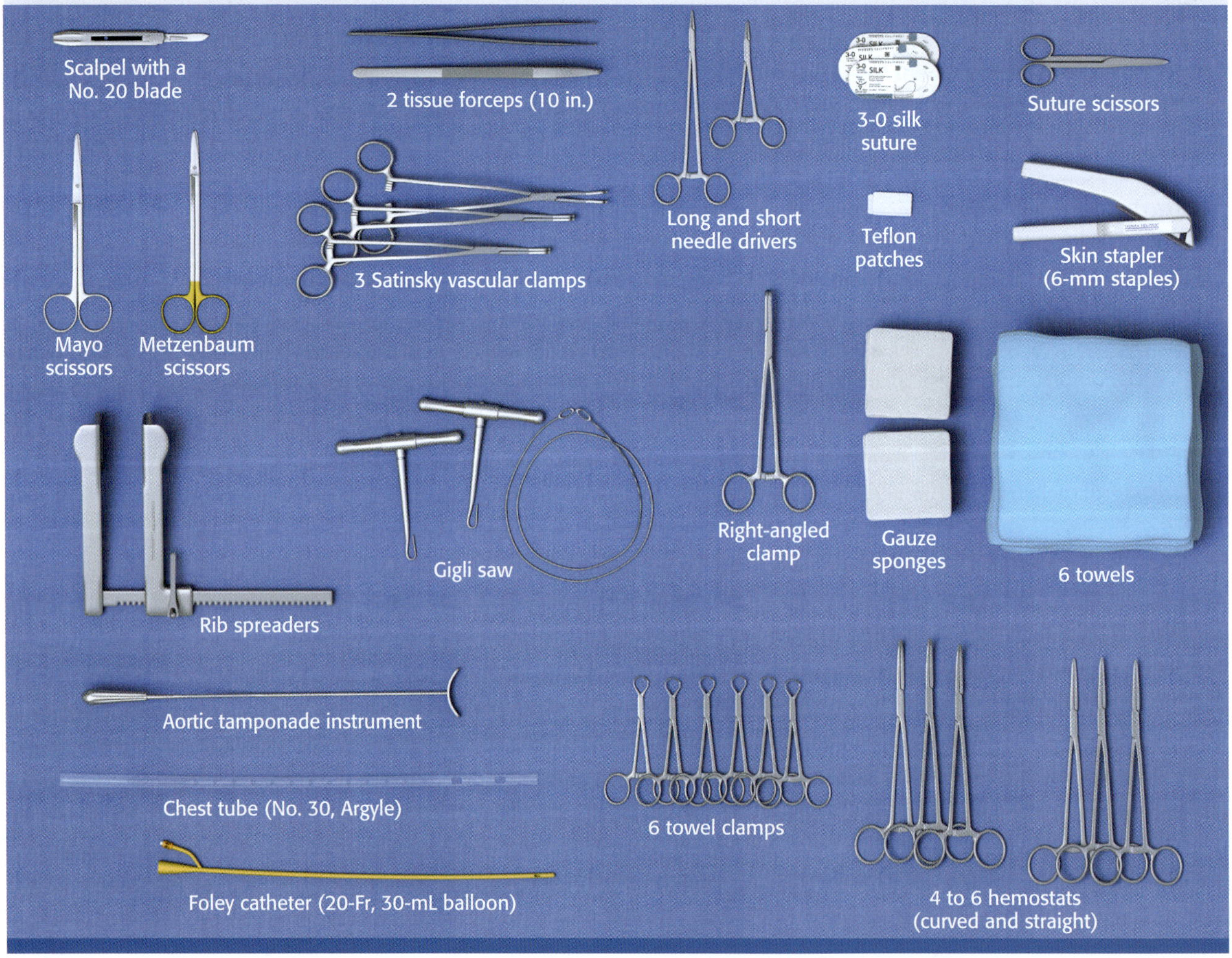

Review Box 18.1 Resuscitative thoracotomy: indications, contraindications, equipment, and complications.

one can expedite thoracotomy by maximizing space in the left thoracic cavity. Keep in mind that extending the thoracotomy into the right thoracic cavity may necessitate switching to bilateral lung ventilation or left lung ventilation to allow maximum right thoracic exposure.

Anesthesia and Amnesia

Comatose patients undergoing resuscitation may regain consciousness during successful EDT, but this awareness may not be apparent if they are still pharmacologically paralyzed. Anticipate and recognize this phenomenon and administer adequate analgesic, amnestic, and muscle-relaxing agents to a ventilated patient who may also be in shock. No specific regimen has been studied, but ketamine appears to be an ideal agent to use in the ED. It is prudent to administer anesthetic agents routinely if a paralyzed patient demonstrates perfusion during resuscitation. This is not only humane but decreases systemic oxygen consumption.

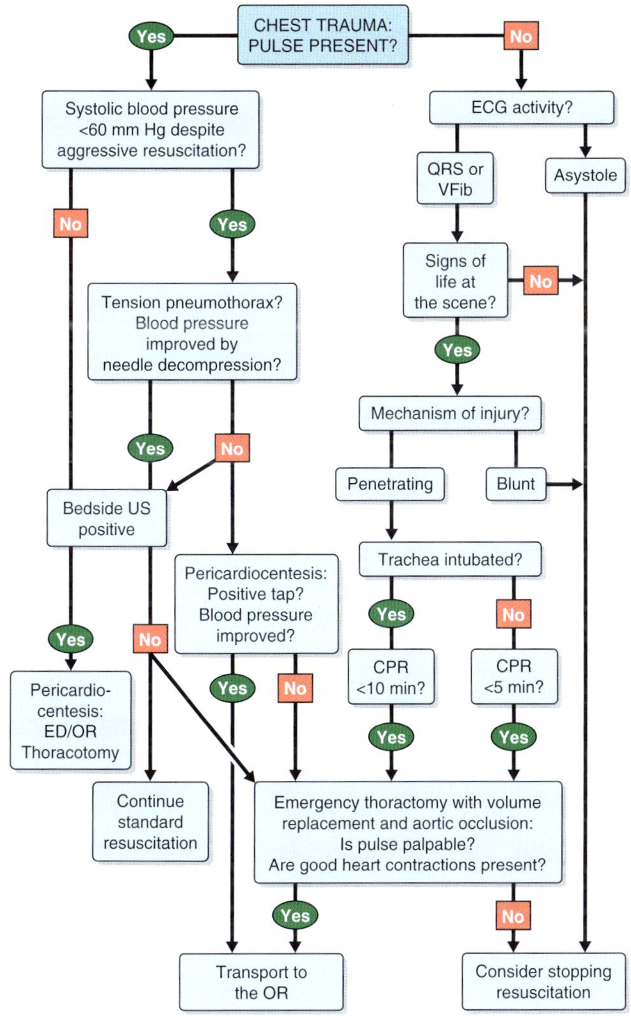

Fig. 18.2 Algorithmic approach to chest trauma. Pulseless blunt trauma management is controversial with some data supporting stopping resuscitation immediately, whereas recent data recommend emergency department *(ED)* thoracotomy if cardiopulmonary resuscitation (CPR) has been ongoing less than 5 minutes. *ECG*, Electrocardiogram; *OR*, operating room; *QRS*, organized electrical activity; *TAP*, pericardial tap yielding blood; *US*, ultrasonography; *VFib*, ventricular fibrillation.

Anterolateral Thoracotomy Incision

Manually ventilate the patient during the procedure. Ask an assistant to pass a nasogastric tube, which helps differentiate the esophagus from the aorta, but do not allow this procedure to delay thoracotomy. If CPR is being performed, ask an assistant to continue closed-chest compressions up to the point of making the initial incision. Take universal precautions to avoid blood exposure and use a suction catheter to minimize contact with blood. Sterile gloves (consider double-glove protection), gown, mask with an eye shield, and an operative surgical cap are recommended for the procedure.

Prepare the skin of the left anterior aspect of the chest with antiseptic if readily available. Wedge towels or sheets under the left posterior part of the chest and place the patient's left arm above the head (Fig. 18.3A). On the left side of the chest, make an anterolateral incision at the fourth to fifth intercostal space with a No. 20 blade scalpel (Fig. 18.4, *step 1*). Do not take the time to count ribs; simply estimate the location to be just beneath the nipple in patients without breast tissue, and at the inframammary fold in patients with breast tissue (see Fig. 18.3). It is important to establish wide exposure by beginning the incision on the right side of the sternum and extending the skin incision past the posterior axillary line. Beginning here will save time if the right side of the chest needs to be opened as well. Inadequate exposure, rib fractures, and additional delays occur when the skin incision is too limited. With the first sweep of the scalpel, separate skin, subcutaneous fat, and the superficial portions of the pectoralis and serratus muscles.

Cut the intercostal muscles with scissors to expose the thoracic cavity (see Fig. 18.4, *step 2*). Use scissors to divide the intercostal muscles because the risk for lung laceration is greater when a scalpel is used. Make the incision just over the top of the rib to avoid the intercostal neurovascular bundle. Just before opening the pleura, stop ventilations momentarily. This will allow the lung to collapse away from the chest wall. Should the internal mammary artery be transected during the procedure, hemorrhage is generally minimal until after perfusion is reestablished, at which time bleeding may be profuse. If actively bleeding, the internal mammary artery should be ligated or clamped. Do not forget to address the internal mammary artery if perfusion is reestablished because this can be a source of significant bleeding.[33]

After entering the pleural cavity, gain good exposure. Karmy-Jones and associates[59] found that 20% of their patients undergoing EDT via the anterolateral approach needed to have the initial incision extended. To gain better exposure first use your hands to open the chest cavity. Then place a Finochietto retractor (rib spreader) between the ribs with the handle and the ratchet bar directed downward toward the axilla (see Fig. 18.4, *step 5*). If the retractor were to be placed with the handle up, the ratchet bar would prevent extension of the incision into the right side of the chest. Ribs may be broken during spreading, so be careful to not get cut on the sharp bone edges. If massive hemothorax is encountered, remove the clots manually, suction out the blood, and use towels to absorb any blood spilling from the chest. If the site of injury is to the right of the heart and cannot be reached, extend the incision into the right side of the chest with a Gigli saw, Liebsche knife, sternal osteotome, or standard trauma shears. Before performing EDT it would be prudent to familiarize oneself with the instruments included in the EDT tray, but do not take the time for this during an actual case.

Pericardiotomy

For a patient in cardiac arrest, if there is no other obvious injury in the chest and the myocardium cannot be visualized, open the pericardium. It may be difficult to definitively rule out pericardial tamponade by visual inspection alone. If in doubt, use forceps to elevate a portion of pericardium and carefully incise it to assess for hemopericardium.

If you are confident that there is no pericardial tamponade, leave the pericardial sac closed while you address other life-threatening injuries. Opening the pericardium increases the risk for complications such as delay in the onset of cardiac compressions, damage to the myocardium or coronary vessels, or cutting of the left phrenic nerve. Previous pericardial disease may also have caused adhesions, and if you attempt to separate these adhesions rapidly, you can tear the atria or right ventricular wall. The incidence of traumatic rupture of the atria or the right ventricle during massage is greater when the pericardium is open. Furthermore, with an intact pericardium

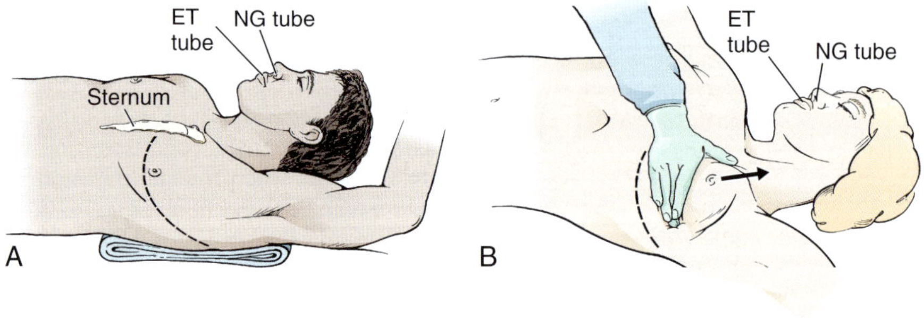

Fig. 18.3 Left anterolateral thoracotomy. (A) Place several towels or sandbags under the left scapula and raise the arm above the head. The patient should be intubated. Insert a nasogastric *(NG)* tube to differentiate the esophagus from the aorta. Make a left anterolateral submammary incision. (B) *Dashes* indicate the incision site in the inframammary fold in patients with breast tissue. *ET,* Endotracheal.

pressure is distributed over a larger area, and the pericardial fluid seldom allows compressing fingers to remain in one spot for a prolonged period.

Perform pericardiotomy if tamponade is present or suspected. This procedure is performed anterior and parallel to the left phrenic nerve (see Fig. 18.4, *step 6*). Begin the incision near the diaphragm to avoid injury to the coronary arteries. Lift the pericardial sac with toothed forceps, and use scissors to make a small hole. Extend the incision with scissors in a cephalad direction along the anterior aspect of the pericardium. Extend the incision so that it reaches from the apex of the heart to the root of the aorta. When the pericardium is under tension, it may be difficult to grasp the pericardium with forceps. In this case, use sharp, straight Mayo scissors to divide the pericardium by layers. If the heart is in arrest, speed is important, so use sharp scissors to "catch" the pericardium and start the pericardiotomy. To do this procedure, hold the point of the scissors almost parallel to the surface of the heart and use enough pressure to create a wrinkle in the pericardium to puncture it as the scissors move forward. Apply moderate pressure to puncture the fibrous pericardium. Be cautious because if the point of the scissors is unnecessarily angled toward the heart, the sudden "give" that occurs when you open the pericardium may result in laceration of the myocardium. Remove clots of blood from the pericardial sac with a sweeping motion using your gloved hand, sterile lap sponges, or gauze pads. If cardiac repair or cardiac compressions are needed, deliver the heart from the pericardial sac. To do this, place your right hand through the pericardial incision and encircle the heart, pull it into the left side of the chest, and place the pericardial sac behind the heart.

Internal Cardiac Defibrillation

It is not uncommon to encounter cardiac dysrhythmias during EDT resuscitative efforts. Recommendations for internal defibrillation are the same as those for external defibrillation: ventricular fibrillation and tachycardia without pulses are immediate indications for defibrillation. With an open chest, internal defibrillation is the procedure of choice.

To perform internal defibrillation, place the *internal paddles* on the anterior and posterior aspects of the heart. The current is delivered through the circular tips of the paddles onto the surface of the heart. There is decreased electrical impedance with direct myocardial contact, and as a result less energy is needed than with standard defibrillation (typically 10 to 50 J). If internal paddles are not available, perform defibrillation in the usual manner with external paddles or electrodes.

Direct Cardiac Compressions

Three techniques for cardiac compression have been described: one-handed compression, one-handed sternal compression, and two-handed (bimanual) compression (Fig. 18.5). To perform the one-handed compression method, place your thumb over the left ventricle, the opposing fingers over the right ventricle, and your palm over the apex of the heart. To perform one-handed sternal compression, hold your fingers flat. Keep the fingers tightly together to form a flat surface over the left ventricle and compress the heart up against the sternum with your fingers. To perform two-handed compression, cup the left hand and place it over the right ventricle. Hold the fingers of the right hand tightly together to form a flat surface supporting the left ventricle. Push the flat surface of your right-hand fingers to compress the heart against the cupped surface of the left hand. The bimanual technique has been shown to be consistently superior.[60]

A difference of opinion exists regarding the optimal rate at which the heart should be compressed. Some recommend a rate of 50 to 60 compressions/min; however, no physiologic data support such a recommendation. American Heart Association guidelines for closed-chest CPR recommend a rate of at least 100 compressions/min. It is conceivable that this would also apply to OCCM.

It is important to remember the following points while performing cardiac compression:

1. Use the entire palmar surface of the fingers. Avoid fingertip pressure.
2. For each method, adjust the force of compression so that it is perpendicular to the plane of the septum. The anterior descending coronary artery is located over the interventricular septum, making this a helpful landmark to orient your hand properly.
3. Position your fingers so that the coronary arteries will not be occluded.
4. Venous filling of the heart is especially sensitive to changes in position. Maintain a relatively normal anatomic position of the heart to prevent kinking of the vena cava and pulmonary veins. Do not angle the heart more than 30 degrees into the left side of the chest.
5. It is essential to completely relax the heart between compressions to allow it to refill completely.

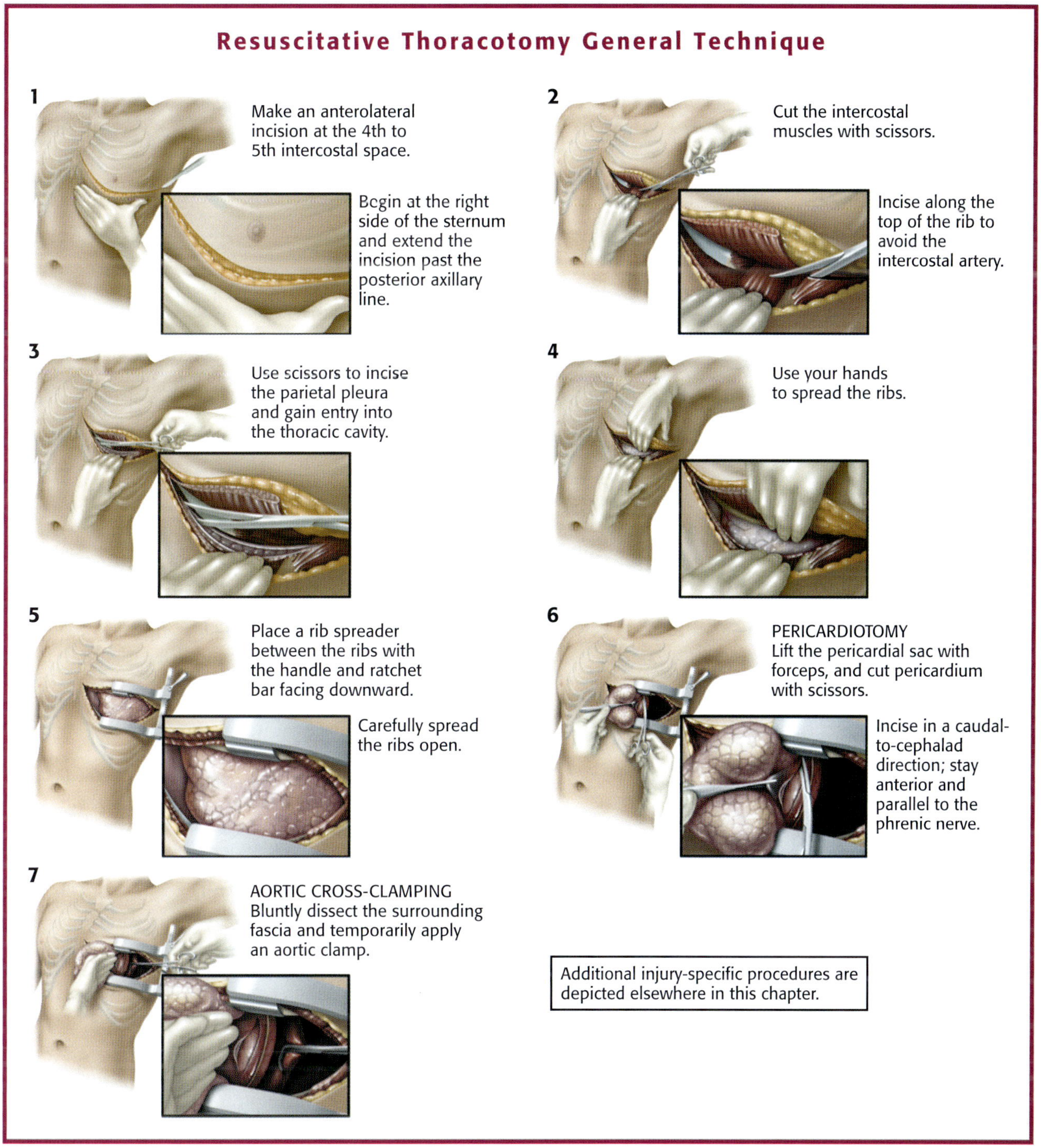

Fig. 18.4 Resuscitative thoracotomy, general technique. (From Custalow CB. *Color Atlas of Emergency Department Procedures*. Saunders; 2005.)

Control of Hemorrhagic Cardiac Wounds

To partially control active bleeding from a ventricular wound, place one finger over the wound and use the other hand to stabilize the beating heart. This maneuver buys time while you begin to repair the injury and continue with resuscitation. If the heart is not beating, you may perform closure of the injury before resuscitation and defibrillation, although this is controversial. If you elect to repair the injury before attempting to restart the heart, perform intermittent cardiac massage. Surgical staples can be used to close a ventricular wound and are an extremely rapid method for controlling hemorrhage (Fig. 18.6).[61] This technique is particularly useful with large or multiple lacerations. Another advantage is that stapling does not expose the operator to the risk associated with needlestick. Macho and coworkers[62] reported a 93% success rate in temporarily controlling hemorrhage in 28 patients (33 lacerations) with penetrating injuries to both the atria and ventricles by using a standard skin stapler with wide (6-mm) staples placed at 5-mm intervals (Auto-Suture 35W, US Surgical Corp.). The rotating long neck of the Ethicon Proximate Quantum Skin Stapler (Model PQW-35, Ethicon, Inc.) is helpful in obtaining proper orientation of the staples during

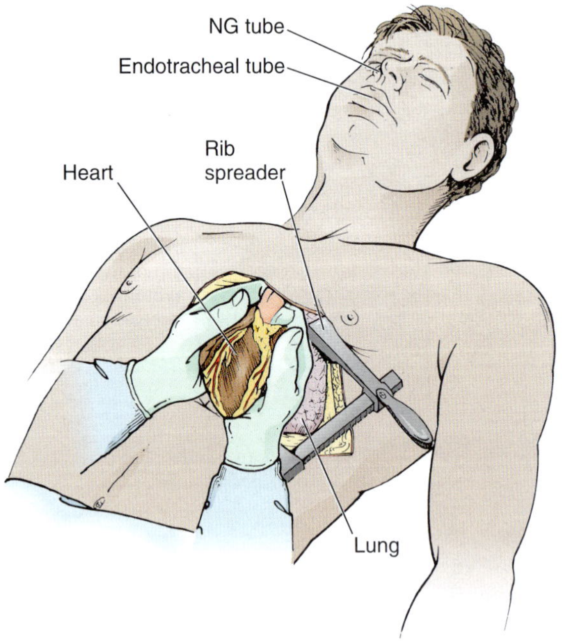

Fig. 18.5 Two-handed method of cardiac massage. Compress the ventricles toward the interventricular septum. Note how the hands flank the left anterior descending artery, which overlies the septum. Avoid using excessive fingertip pressure or lifting the heart, which slows ventricular filling by distorting the soft atrial-caval junction. *NG*, Nasogastric.

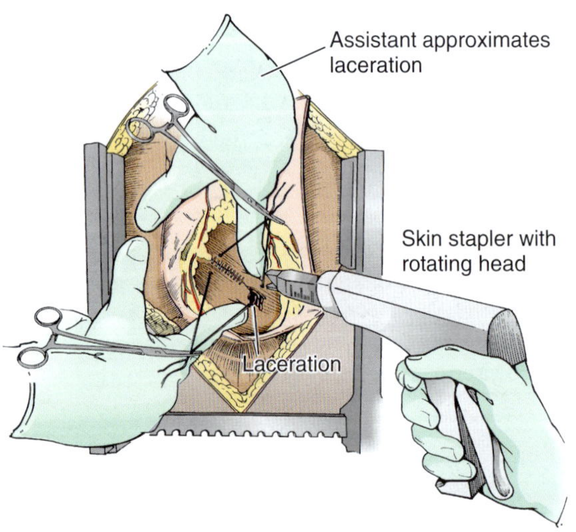

Fig. 18.6 Technique of cardiac stapling to temporarily control hemorrhage. Ask an assistant to approximate the tissues with fingertip pressure, or as illustrated, use two half-horizontal sutures to approximate the wound edges and reduce bleeding. Use a skin stapler with wide (6-mm) staples and place them 5 mm apart. This technique may be used for atrial and ventricular lacerations. After stabilizing the patient's condition, revise the wound in the operating room.

placement. The staples can be left in place and reinforced or replaced on further exploration in the operating room.

Alternatively, repair the wound by placing several horizontal mattress sutures under the tamponading finger (Fig. 18.7). Polypropylene 2-0 or 3-0 monofilament (Prolene) suture is recommended for cardiac repair, but nonabsorbable silk can also be used. Avoid smaller sutures and nylon sutures. If multiple sutures are needed, lay them all in place before they are tied. This allows you to attain equal distribution of wound tension, which prevents tearing of the myocardium.[63] Alternatively, pass the suture underneath, over, and through Teflon pledgets to prevent the suture from cutting through the myocardium. Pledgets are especially important for reinforcement when the myocardium has been weakened by the blast effect of a bullet,[64] or when suturing the thinner-walled atria or right ventricle. An alternative to Teflon pledgets is to use small rectangles of pericardial tissue cut from the opened pericardium.

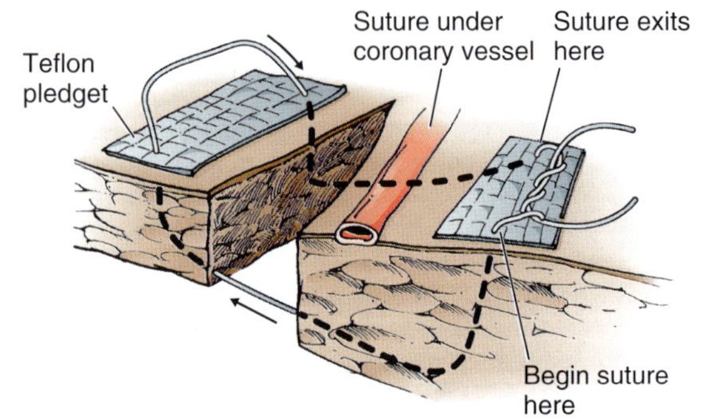

Fig. 18.7 Technique of cardiac suture repair. Place multiple horizontal mattress sutures 6 mm from the edge of the wound before tying. Close the wound just enough to stop the bleeding. Use Teflon pledgets on the cardiac surface, and pass all surface sutures through these reinforcements. Sutures come from underneath, lie over, then pass back through the pledgets. Closure without pledgets incurs the risk of sutures ripping through the contracting myocardium. Similarly, the use of simple vertical sutures should be discouraged because of the risk for suture dissection through the myocardium. For repairs near a coronary artery, take care to pass the suture under the artery. Note that rectangles of pericardial tissue may be substituted for ready-made Teflon pledgets.

For large wounds that cannot be controlled with pressure, place an incomplete horizontal mattress suture on either side of the wound (Fig. 18.8). Cross the free ends to stop the bleeding. Then the actual reparative sutures can be placed accurately. It must be stressed that suturing the myocardium requires good technique. Excessive tension may tear the myocardium and aggravate the situation. Keys to success include using appropriately sized suture, obtaining a generous "bite" with the needle, and applying only enough tension to control the bleeding.

If exsanguinating hemorrhage is not controlled by the aforementioned methods, temporarily occlude inflow to the heart. Apply inflow occlusion intermittently for 60 to 90 seconds. During occlusion, the heart shrinks, hemorrhage is controlled, and you can place sutures in a decompressed injury. Two techniques that are useful are vascular clamping of the superior and inferior vena cava for partial inflow occlusion,[65] and the Sauerbruch grip (Fig. 18.9).[66] The Sauerbruch grip can be performed quickly with the added advantage of cradling and stabilizing the heart while you repair the wounds over either the ventricle or the left atrium. It involves occlusion of the vena cava between the ring and middle fingers of the left hand to create partial occlusion of inflow. The Sauerbruch grip will interfere only with the repair of wounds involving the right atrium.

Another technique for temporarily controlling hemorrhage is to insert a Foley catheter (20 Fr with a 30-mL balloon) through a wound.[67] After inserting the catheter, inflate the balloon, clamp the catheter to prevent air embolism, and

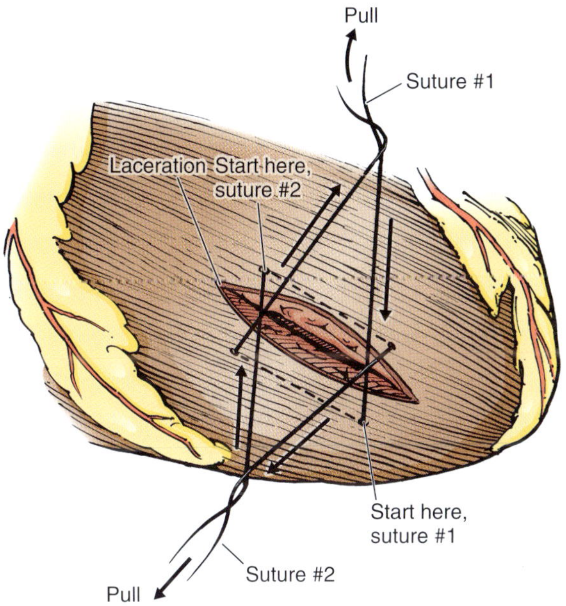

Fig. 18.8 Control of hemorrhage with two widely placed incomplete mattress sutures. Ask an assistant to cross two half-horizontal sutures to bring the wound edges into apposition. By controlling the hemorrhage in this manner, the assistant's hands are outside the operative field and the edges of the wound are fully exposed. This facilitates more orderly closure of the wound. After the wound is repaired, the sutures may be either removed or tied to each other.

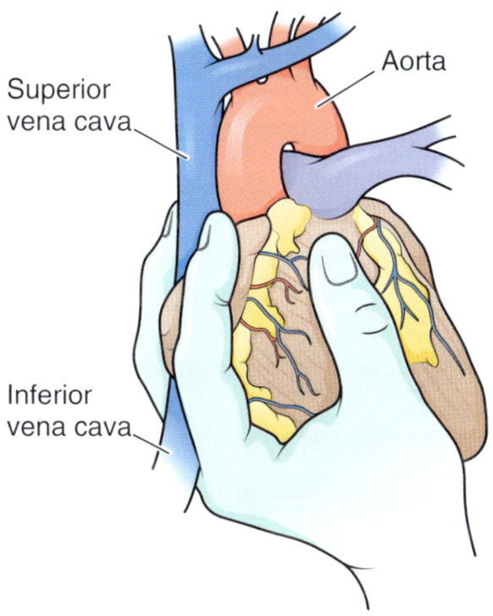

Fig. 18.9 The Sauerbruch maneuver is the method of choice for reducing heavy bleeding from cardiac wounds. Occlusion of venous inflow is achieved by using the first and second, or second and third fingers as a clamp.

apply gentle traction (Fig. 18.10). Apply enough traction to slow the bleeding and provide an acceptable level to visualize and repair the wound. Excessive traction can pull the catheter out and enlarge the wound. The balloon will effectively occlude the wound internally. Use a purse-string suture to close the wound. When repairing the wound be careful with the suture needle because it can easily rupture the balloon. Temporarily pushing the balloon into the ventricular lumen during passage of the needle can be done to avoid this complication. Use normal saline when inflating the balloon because using air could result in air embolism if the suture needle ruptures the balloon.

Foley catheters have several advantages over other methods for controlling cardiac wounds. With the digital method, your fingertip will often slip if there is a strong heartbeat, you cannot visualize the wound during repair, and digital pressure significantly interferes with cardiac massage. Intermittent total venous inflow occlusion is an effective method of controlling bleeding and decompressing the heart, but such control will be at the expense of poor cardiac output. Attempting to elevate the heart for control and repair of posterior cardiac wounds often results in cardiac arrest by reducing both venous and arterial flow. With posterior injuries use of a Foley catheter does not require continued viewing after initial placement. If bleeding can be controlled, repairs in this location should await full-volume expansion or cardiopulmonary bypass.[68] Regardless of location the most valuable feature of the Foley catheter is that you can control hemorrhage without interfering with cardiac compression. The catheter can also be used for infusion of fluids (see Fig. 18.10B).[69]

To initially manage wounds of the atria, use partial-occlusion clamps (Fig. 18.11). Because of the thin structure and instability of the atrial wall, you will not be able to effectively stop bleeding with digital pressure. Injuries near the cavoatrial junction are not amenable to clamping; in this location, use a Foley catheter to tamponade the wound.[67] Be careful not to obstruct atrial filling with the inflated balloon. Skin staples may also be used for closure of atrial wounds.[62]

Wounds of the septa, valves, and coronary arteries require definitive repair in the operating suite. Hemorrhage from a coronary artery can generally be controlled with digital pressure. Avoid ligation of a coronary artery whenever possible.

Control of Hemorrhagic Great-Vessel Wounds

Wounds of the great vessels can be controlled with digital pressure or partial-occlusion clamps. If desired, close small aortic wounds with 3-0 Prolene suture.[70] To prevent exsanguinating hemorrhage from the left subclavian artery, try to cross-clamp the intrathoracic portion of the artery. Cross-clamping of the right subclavian artery is very difficult. For injuries to this vessel, use laparotomy pads for compression in the apex of the pleura from below and the supraclavicular fossa from above (Fig. 18.12) to prevent further bleeding as the patient is stabilized and moved to the operating suite.[61]

Aortic Cross-Clamping

For persistent hypotension (systolic blood pressure [SBP] <70 mm Hg) after thoracotomy and pericardiotomy, perform temporary occlusion of the descending thoracic aorta. This maneuver can maintain myocardial and cerebral perfusion (Fig. 18.13; see also Fig. 18.4, *step* 7), although Kravolich and colleagues[50] suggested that the benefit of significant improvement in CPP may be overstated. When the aorta has been injured by blunt trauma, selective clamping is necessary (Fig. 18.14). Aortic occlusion has a limited role in controlling hemorrhage below the diaphragm. In patients with a tense abdomen and massive hemoperitoneum, aortic cross-clamping is beneficial when applied just before laparotomy.[25]

The aorta can be very difficult to identify in an ED, especially when collapsed as a result of exsanguination. It is situated immediately anterior to the vertebrae and actually lies on the vertebral bodies themselves. The esophagus lies anterior and slightly medial to the aorta. Passing a nasogastric tube

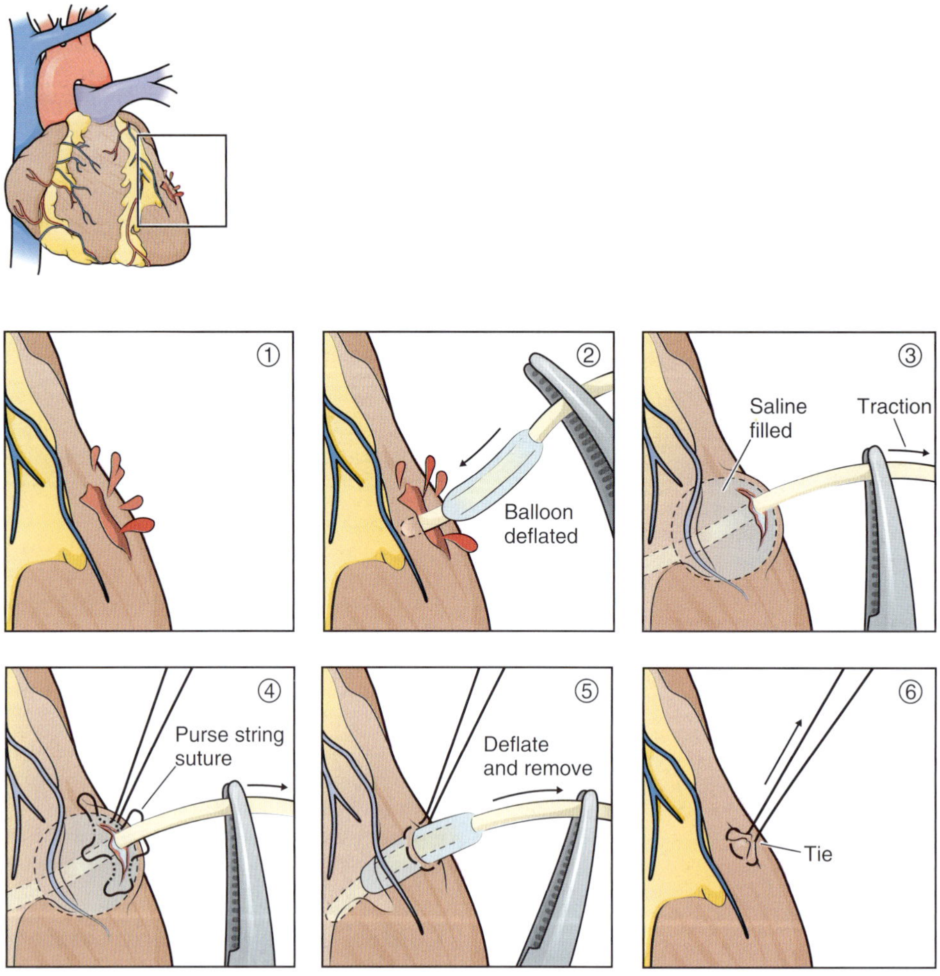

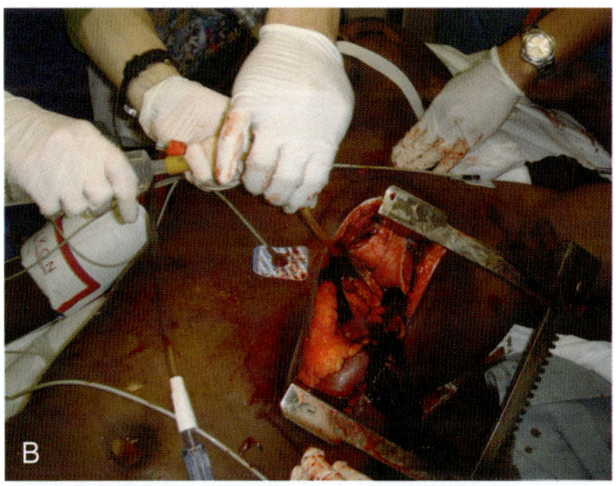

Fig. 18.10 (A) Serial illustration. Gentle traction on an inflated Foley catheter may control hemorrhage and allow repair. Inflate the balloon with saline while taking care to not rupture the balloon with the suture needle. This technique is particularly useful for injuries to the inferior cavoatrial junction, for posterior wounds, and during cardiac massage. Volume loading can be achieved by infusion of blood or crystalloid solution through the lumen of the catheter. Take care to avoid an air embolus through the lumen of the catheter during placement. (B) Foley catheter in an atrial stab wound. Keep gentle traction on an inflated balloon and inject saline directly into the heart via the catheter. Note how difficult it is to identify structures in the chest cavity. The heart is collapsed and not beating, which makes even this organ hard to find. The aorta could not be isolated before stopping resuscitation efforts.

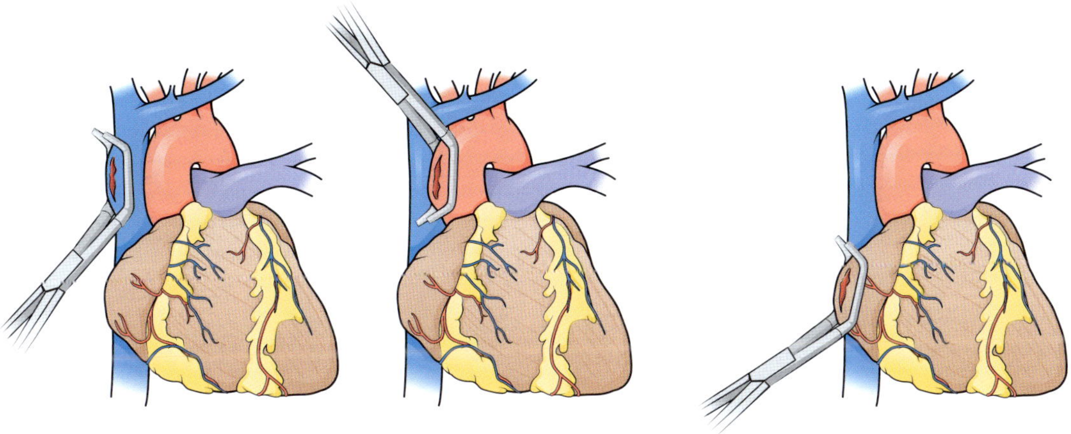

Fig. 18.11 Use a partial-occlusion clamp in different locations for control of bleeding and subsequent repair.

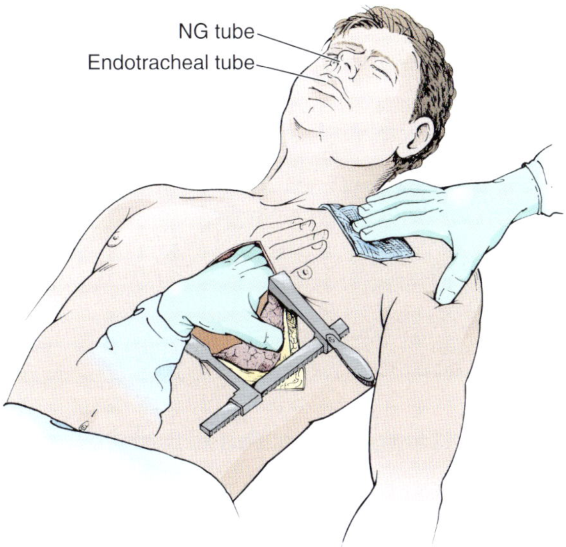

Fig. 18.12 Cross-clamping for control of subclavian bleeding is difficult and time-consuming. Compression with laparotomy pads in the apical pleura from below and the supraclavicular fossa from above will control hemorrhage while the patient's condition is stabilized and the patient is transported to the operating room. *NG*, Nasogastric.

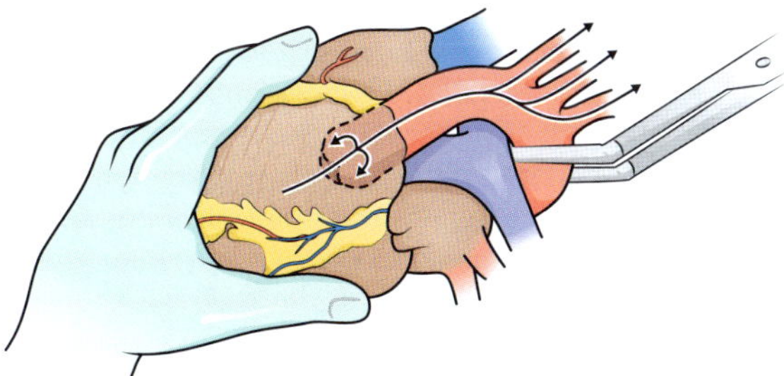

Fig. 18.13 Manual cardiac massage and cross-clamping of the aorta can be used to increase coronary and cerebral perfusion selectively.

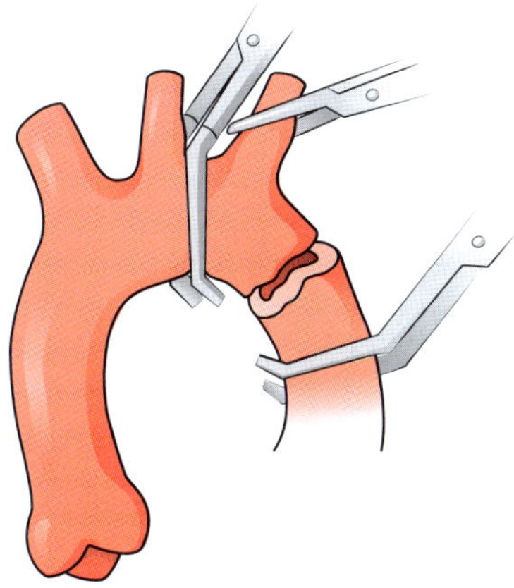

Fig. 18.14 Traumatic rupture of the aorta is usually a fatal injury. Three clamps are required for control. Backbleeding will occur if fewer than three clamps are used.

from above may help in identifying the esophagus. To expose the descending aorta, ask an assistant to retract the left lung in a superomedial direction. To achieve adequate exposure, it is sometimes necessary to divide the inferior pulmonary ligament (be careful not to injure the inferior pulmonary vein). Identify the aorta by advancing the fingers of the left hand along the thoracic cage toward the vertebral column. Open the mediastinal pleura and bluntly dissect the aorta away from the esophagus anteriorly and the prevertebral fascia posteriorly before clamping. To locate the aorta, use a DeBakey aortic clamp or a curved Kelly clamp for blunt dissection, and spread the pleura open above and below the aorta (Fig. 18.15). Alternatively, if excessive hemorrhage limits direct visualization, bluntly dissect with the thumb and fingertips. Separate the aorta from the esophagus, which lies medially and slightly anteriorly. It may be difficult to separate the esophagus from the aorta by feel in a hypotensive or cardiac arrest situation. When the aorta is completely isolated, use the index finger of the left hand to flex around the vessel and apply a large Satinsky or DeBakey vascular clamp with the right hand. Check brachial blood pressure immediately after the occlusion. If systolic pressure is higher than 120 mm Hg, slowly release the clamp and adjust it to maintain a systolic pressure of less than 120 mm Hg.[24]

Given the need for timely intervention, the simplest and most desirable approach to aortic occlusion is to have an assistant digitally compress it or use the aortic tamponade instrument (Fig. 18.16). The aortic tamponade instrument, however, may be applied blindly to the vertebral column and permits safe, quick, and complete aortic occlusion.[71] This technique

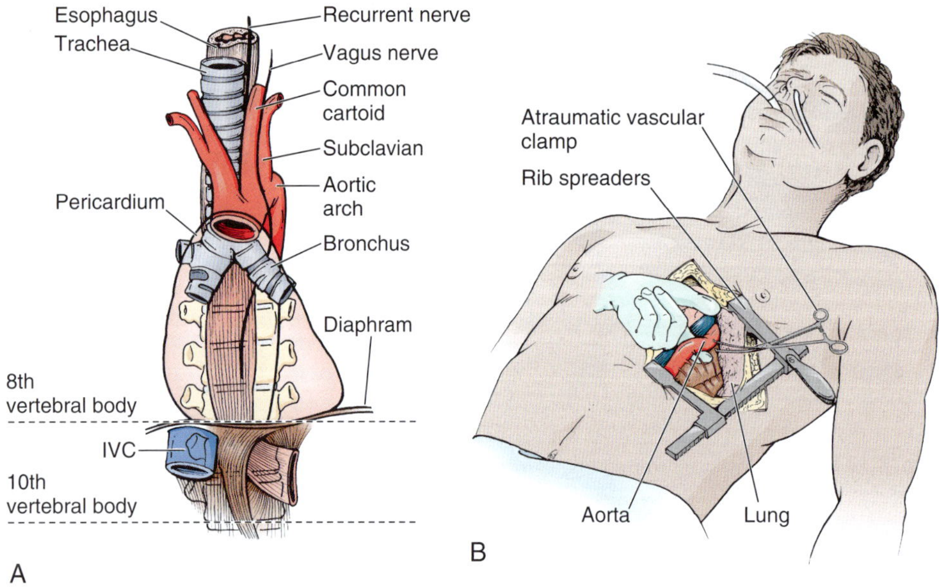

Fig. 18.15 Identification of the aorta is very difficult during emergency department thoracotomy. (A) If possible, first pass a nasogastric tube to help identify the esophagus. The aorta is in the posterior mediastinum, directly anterior to the vertebral bodies. The esophagus is anterior and slightly medial to the aorta. In the lower part of the thorax, both are covered on the anterolateral surface by the mediastinal pleura, which must be dissected before isolating the aorta for cross-clamping. (B) Aortic cross-clamping. Using blunt dissection, spread the pleura above and below the aorta. Fully mobilize the vessel and clearly separate the esophagus before clamping. The aorta is the more posterior structure and is in contact with the vertebral bodies.

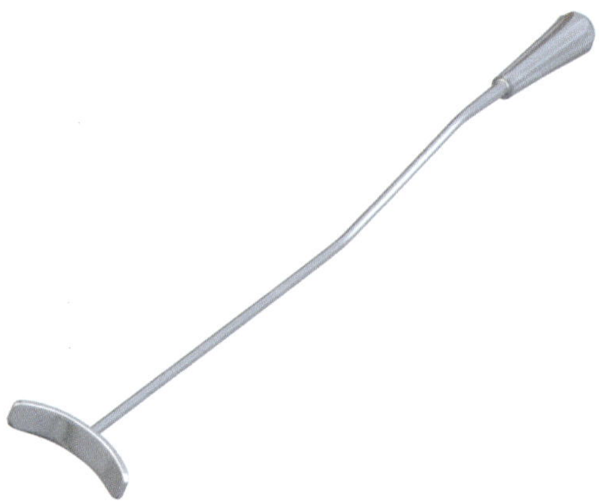

Fig. 18.16 Use of a Conn aortic compressor is an excellent method for aortic occlusion because it is fast, does not interfere with the operative field, and is associated with minimal risk for injury. Alternatively, direct digital occlusion can be used, but this technique is more awkward.

may be most prudent when isolation of the aorta is difficult. The instrument's unique shape allows it to remain in place and to provide atraumatic occlusion with little interference in the operative field when compared with digital compression. The degree of occlusion can be varied by the amount of pressure exerted by the operator.

Potential complications of aortic cross-clamping include ischemia of the spinal cord, liver, bowels, and kidneys. In addition, iatrogenic injury to the aorta and the esophagus may occur. Fortunately, these complications are infrequent. The metabolic penalty of aortic cross-clamping becomes exponential when occlusion time exceeds 30 minutes.[72] Whenever possible, unclamp the aorta for 30 to 60 seconds every 10 minutes to increase distal perfusion. Perform final release of the aorta gradually.

Control of Hemorrhagic Pulmonary Wounds

Central lung injury with massive bleeding must be controlled expeditiously. First, briefly stop ventilation or selectively intubate the contralateral, nonbleeding lung if not already done. If simple measures are insufficient, either of two maneuvers can be used to stop the hemorrhage. The first is to guide a tangential occlusion clamp across the pulmonary hilum to cut off blood flow to the hemorrhaging lung.[73] Clamping may be difficult due to the presence of the rigid bronchus, limiting hemorrhage control.

Another option is the pulmonary hilum twist which does not require any special tools. First, divide the inferior pulmonary ligament to the level of the inferior pulmonary vein without injuring the vein. Then, rotate the lower lobe anteriorly over the upper lobe 180 degrees and place laparotomy packs at the base and apex of the lung to prevent untwisting. Definitive management includes a pneumonectomy once hemodynamics are stabilized. Both techniques can be used on the right or left lung and, if successful, can control hemorrhage as well as prevent air embolism.[74]

Management of Air Embolism

In those at risk for air embolism spontaneous ventilation is preferred. It is essential that the source of the air embolism be controlled rapidly. Place the patient immediately in the Trendelenburg (head-down) position to minimize cerebral involvement and direct the air emboli to less critical organs. If the chest injury is unilateral, consider isolating the injured lung by selectively intubating the contralateral lung. If this is unsuccessful, perform a left anterolateral thoracotomy. Flood the exposed thorax with sterile saline and look for bloody froth created during positive pressure ventilation to identify peripheral bronchovenous fistulas. Carry out a quick search for hilar injuries. If the source of the air embolism is not readily apparent, perform a contralateral thoracotomy. Once the bronchovenous communication is controlled, use a needle to aspirate the residual air that commonly remains in the left ventricle and the aorta. If the patient is hypotensive, consider cross-clamping the aorta. Be aware, though, that cross-clamping the aorta before controlling bronchovenous fistulas and removing residual air may result in further dissemination of air to the heart and brain.

Air emboli traverse capillary beds if the blood pressure is high enough. After controlling the bronchovenous fistula, produce a brief period of proximal aortic hypertension by cross-clamping the descending aorta. Maintain systemic arterial pressure with adequate fluid resuscitation. Vasopressors such as dopamine, epinephrine, or norepinephrine may be required to increase systemic pressure and facilitate the passage of air bubbles from left to right.[75]

Maintain left atrial pressure at a high level. Keep the ventilator inspiratory pressure as low as possible and use 100% oxygen to facilitate diffusion of nitrogen from emboli. Consider high-frequency ventilation, which allows the use of small volumes and has been used successfully in individual patients. The most important adjunctive therapy is hyperbaric oxygen. Although it is best to begin treatment within 6 hours of the traumatic insult, there are cases of success and improvement when hyperbaric oxygen has been started even 36 hours after injury.[76]

INTERPRETATION AND HEMODYNAMIC MONITORING

Use SBP after the first 30 minutes of resuscitation as a decision point for further treatment. A report of EDT for blunt and penetrating trauma demonstrated a relationship between blood pressure at 30 minutes and the eventual outcome.[77] Of the 146 cases reviewed, 45 patients (31%) were transferred to the operating room after initial resuscitation and aortic cross-clamping when necessary. For patients who survived with full neurologic recovery, the average SBP after the first 30 minutes of resuscitation was 110 mm Hg. In those who were long-term survivors but had significant brain damage, the average SBP was 85 mm Hg. No patients survived when mean SBP was lower than 70 mm Hg. Transfer of these patients to the operating room for definitive repair of these mortal wounds would be futile.

EDT IN CHILDREN

Trauma is the leading cause of death and morbidity in children older than 1 year.[1] Just as with adults, improved transportation of injured children to the hospital has resulted in the survival of more patients who would have been pronounced dead at the scene. Although the role of EDT has been reviewed extensively in the adult population, experience and data in the pediatric population are limited. One systematic review of 319 children who underwent EDT found similar survival rates in children and adults with about 2% survival in those who sustained blunt trauma and 13% survival in those who sustained penetrating trauma. Overall survival was 7%.[78–80] Anatomic injury patterns showed a higher proportion of blunt trauma and of concomitant head injuries in the pediatric population. Rates of survival below age 15 are very poor. Expert consensus based on a systematic review recommended EDT for traumatic pediatric patients with similar indications to those in adults discussed earlier in this chapter. A conditional recommendation was made to allow for provider discretion in performing EDT in pediatric patients who presented with signs of life after blunt injury if emergency adjuncts indicated an intrathoracic injury with low suspicion for severe TBI. EDT was not recommended for any pediatric trauma patient presenting without signs of life.[78]

COMPLICATIONS

A variety of significant complications occur in patients surviving EDT, but most of them are related to the primary injury rather than the thoracotomy. Techniques to avoid iatrogenic complications include noting the position of the left phrenic nerve and coronary arteries during EDT. Surprisingly, serious infections are uncommon. Patients receiving antibiotics during or immediately after the procedure have a low rate of infectious complications. Standard antibiotic regimens targeting skin flora are recommended, but should not delay the procedure.[81] As a general rule, excessive attention to antiseptic skin preparation should be avoided because it may delay performance of the procedure.[82]

Another potentially serious complication of EDT is injury or transmission of disease to health care workers. In an emotionally charged environment in which many clinicians are attempting to perform a lifesaving procedure under difficult conditions, it is easy for sharp objects to cause injury. In one large study of 305 EDTs with 1,360 participants (attendings, trainees, nurses, and other ED staff) Nunn and colleagues found that the majority of exposures during EDT were sustained by trainees injured by scalpels, fractured bone (Fig. 18.17), needles, and scissors.[83] One urban ED found the seroprevalence of human immunodeficiency virus (HIV) in trauma patients to be 2.2%.[84] Another found that 9.4% of patients with penetrating trauma were positive for anti-HIV (1.2%), HBsAg (0.6%), or anti-HCV (7.6%).[85] Hepatitis C is now the most common viral hepatitis seen in health care workers since the advent of the hepatitis B vaccine. The risk for seroconversion after occupational exposure to HIV is estimated to be 0.3% for needlestick and as high as 4.5% for deep injury.[86] Hepatitis C seroconversion rates after occupational exposure are estimated to be between 1.8% and 10%.[86] One study found that each personal protective equipment (PPE) item utilized during EDT correlated with a 34% decreased risk of occupational exposure.[83] Keep the risk for exposure to staff in mind, and rigorously follow universal precautions. Although EDT must be performed rapidly to be of value to the patient, excessive haste is not warranted if it threatens the health of members of the medical team.

RESUSCITATIVE ENDOVASCULAR BALLOON OCCLUSION OF THE AORTA (REBOA)

In the correct clinical context, REBOA can be a more rapid and less invasive method than thoracotomy for obtaining

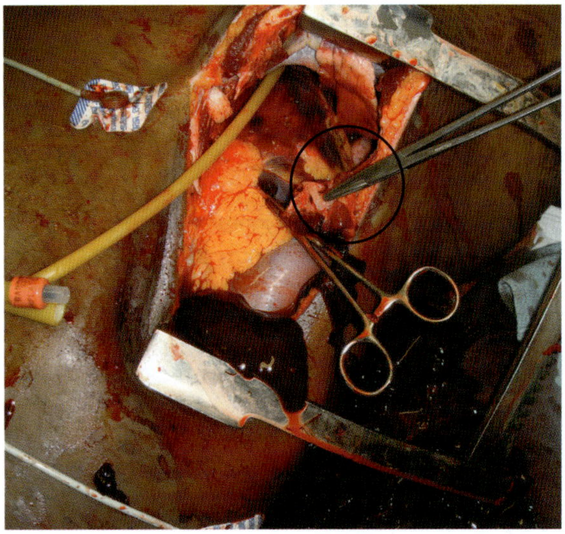

Fig. 18.17 Note the sharp edges of this rib (indicated by the *circled* clamp), which was fractured during unsuccessful emergency department thoracotomy. Health care workers may be exposed to blood-borne diseases (e.g., human immunodeficiency virus, hepatitis) if sharp objects puncture the gloves and skin.

hemorrhage control.[87] It is thought that REBOA increases perfusion to the brain and heart, decreases transfusion needs, and decreases the drug distribution volume of vasoactive medications, increasing their efficacy by occluding the distal portion of the aorta during a resuscitation. It may also stimulate aortic baroreceptors and activate the parasympathetic nervous system which could decrease rates of ventricular fibrillation.[88]

REBOA is not a definitive hemorrhage control device. Except in the very rare circumstance, REBOA should only be placed at an institution where a surgeon can rapidly obtain hemorrhage control in the operating room and deflate the balloon soon after placement.[87]

In practice, REBOA is placed by providers from several different specialties. One study comparing REBOA outcomes between surgeons and nonsurgeons (emergency physicians, radiologists, anesthetists) did find a significant difference in mortality (44.5% for surgeons vs. 62% for nonsurgeons). However, this study also found a significant difference in patient age (34 for surgeons and 58 for nonsurgeons) and injury severity score (32 for surgeons and 41 for nonsurgeons, where a higher score indicates a more severely injured patient). This study did not find a difference in time to balloon inflation or in potential complication rate.[89]

Another study found that high- or medium-volume REBOA centers had improved outcomes compared to low-volume REBOA centers, where high- or medium-volume centers had lower mean SBP at deployment, faster placement and lower overall mortality.[90]

It is unclear if REBOA improves patient outcomes. It has been shown that REBOA consistently improves SBP, in one study by a mean of 53 mm Hg.[91] However, in a study of patients randomized to REBOA plus standard of care verses standard of care alone, all-cause mortality was higher in the REBOA group than the standard of care group. Another study comparing REBOA to thoracotomy for patients presenting with noncompressible torso hemorrhage below the diaphragm found a similar 24-hour mortality between the groups, but the time to aortic occlusion was significantly longer in the REBOA group.[88]

Anatomy

The balloon can be inflated in either zone 1 or zone 3 of the aorta (Fig. 18.18). Zone 1 is approximately 20 cm in length and extends from the left subclavian artery to the celiac artery. Zone 2 is approximately 3 cm and is the no-occlusion zone from the celiac artery to the more caudal renal artery. Finally, zone 3 is approximately 10 cm in length, measuring from the more caudal renal artery to the aortic bifurcation. Zone 1 occlusion is used if the patient is found to have a positive FAST ultrasound for intraabdominal fluid. Zone 3 is more typically used for hemorrhage related to pelvic fractures.

It is generally recommended that balloon occlusion occur in zone 1 for no longer than 30 minutes, and no longer than 60 minutes in zone 3. The total occlusion time should be as short as possible until definitive hemorrhage control can be achieved. Some studies suggest this time can be lengthened by using a partial REBOA (pREBOA) strategy where the balloon is not fully inflated or inflation is titratable, allowing some blood flow past the occlusion to perfuse vital organs. Early data suggest fewer complications, better hemodynamic responses, and longer occlusion time, with comparable mortality.[93]

The access site for this procedure is the common femoral artery distal to the inguinal ligament. In case reports, REBOA has been deployed using alternate access sites such as brachial, axillary, and carotid arteries for various indications, but these sites are not commonly used in practice.[91]

Indications and Contraindications

As more studies are performed and best practices are identified, indications and contraindications are expected to change. The below is a broad overview of when this procedure should be performed based on current recommendations.[87,91–96] Institutions should develop a formal REBOA protocol that involves the relevant specialties as to when to perform aortic balloon occlusion.

REBOA can be performed in patients presenting to the hospital with life-threatening hemorrhage below the diaphragm, who are unresponsive or only transiently responsive to resuscitation.[87] While the most common indication in the ED will be traumatic abdominopelvic hemorrhage or hemorrhage from ruptured AAA, it has also been used for patients with postpartum hemorrhage, upper GI hemorrhage, and pelvic hemorrhage during pelvis or sacral tumor surgery.[91,92]

There is also ongoing research into use of REBOA for nontraumatic OHCA. While use of REBOA did help achieve return of spontaneous circulation (ROSC) in four out of five study patients, all patients in this small study rearrested after deflation of balloon.[94]

There is no universally accepted blood pressure cutoff under which REBOA should not be performed. One study suggested an SBP between 60 and 80 mm Hg as ideal for REBOA placement, with mortality >50% below 60 mm Hg.[95]

REBOA is contraindicated if there is evidence of trauma above the diaphragm such as severe head trauma, blunt cardiac injury, thoracic aortic injury, penetrating neck or chest trauma, pericardial tamponade, or pneumothorax.[96] It should also not be performed if patients have inaccessible femoral

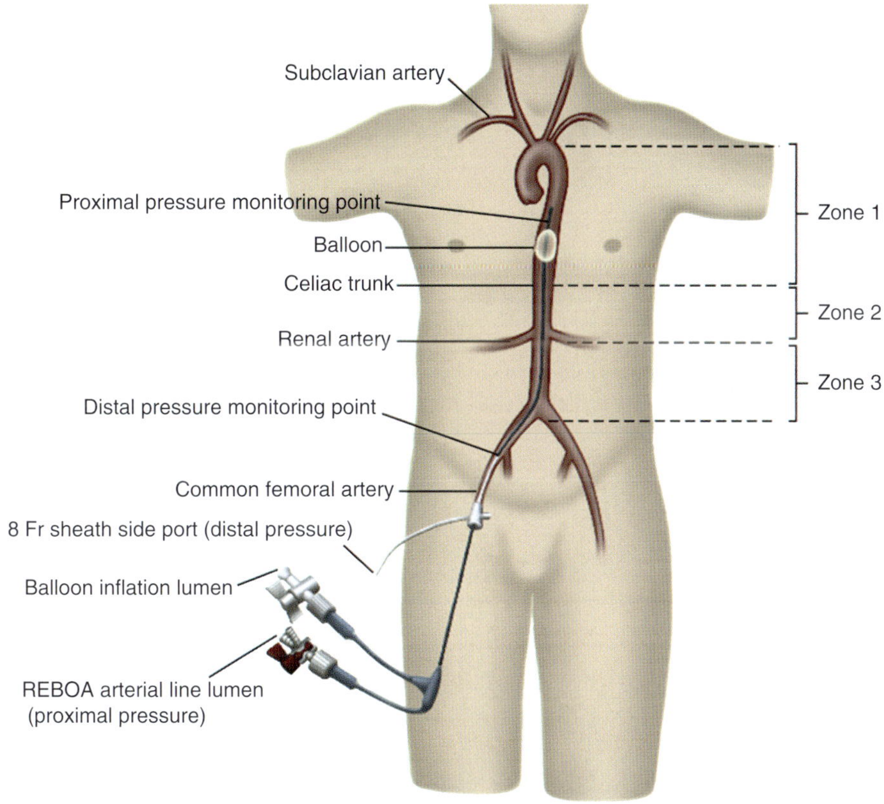

Fig. 18.18 Diagram of key anatomy and equipment for resuscitative endovascular balloon occlusion of the aorta *(REBOA)*. (From Parsons HM, Wood A, Milne A. Resuscitative endovascular balloon occlusion of the aorta. *BJA Educ.* 2022;22(11):412-415.)

vessels due to pelvic distortion from trauma. REBOA is relatively contraindicated in patients with prolonged cardiac arrest due to exsanguination (greater than 10 minutes) and in those unlikely to survive the procedure due to comorbidities. There is little research into REBOA use in the pediatric or geriatric populations, and currently, no guidelines exist regarding its use in these populations.[96]

Procedure

Kits may differ between institutions (Fig. 18.19), and it is imperative the proceduralist be familiar with their institutional kit before attempting REBOA placement. It is helpful to have an assistant during the procedure who can help with the "big three" of REBOA placement: (1) monitoring the patient's MAP, (2) maintenance of wire, sheath, and balloon position, and (3) maintenance of occlusion.[97]

Initial access is generally gained through placement of a femoral arterial line via the Seldinger technique, ideally with the use of an ultrasound. This access will need to be upsized in order to introduce the larger sheath that enables REBOA catheter placement. If a patient appears stable upon arrival but has high likelihood of decompensation and need for REBOA, an arterial line can be placed while the patient is stable to aid with more rapid placement of REBOA should the need arise. Though the common 18-gauge femoral arterial line can be used, they are flimsy and wire passage may be difficult. If available, a 5- or 7-Fr catheter is preferred.

Ideally, sterility is maintained throughout placement of REBOA, but the need for ongoing resuscitation may take priority depending on the patient's condition. The proceduralist should wear full PPE during this procedure and use their best judgment when preparing and draping the patient as per local protocol.

Remove the arterial line over a wire that is at least twice its length. Increase the incision size at the skin with a scalpel, then pass a large sheath over the wire. This sheath can range in size from 7 to 12 Fr depending on the kit and is likely to have an inner dilator in place. There should also be a three-way stopcock attached to the end of the sheath that is "off" to the side port. Depending on the kit, this step may need to be repeated in order to upsize to a sheath large enough to accommodate the balloon catheter.

Once the large sheath is in place, measure the long (typically 180 cm) guidewire on the patient's body from the insertion point to the xiphoid process and mark the distance on the guidewire. Then measure and mark the ideal insertion distance for the catheter. If the goal of the occlusion is zone 1, measure from the insertion site to above the xiphoid. For zone 3, measure from insertion site to just above the umbilicus.

Insert the large guidewire to the desired distance and remove the inner dilator if present. The assistant should hold the guidewire against the patient's leg to ensure it does not move once in the desired location. If the wire floats further in, it can damage cerebral or coronary vessels, and it may limit the operator's ability to place the catheter if it is pushed out.

Finally, insert the catheter over the long guidewire through the sheath to the previously marked distance. Some catheters have radiopaque markers on or near the balloon. If the goal is zone 1 of the aorta, a radiograph should show the markers between T4 and L1 (Fig. 18.20). If zone 3 is the goal, the

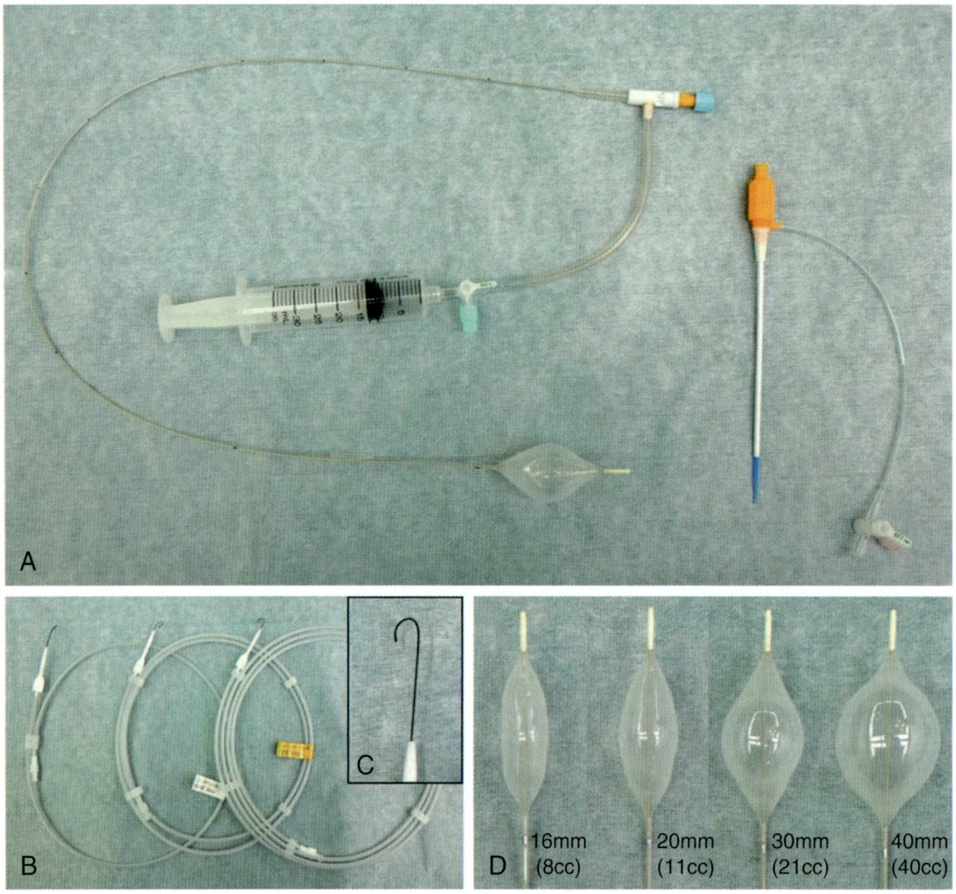

Fig. 18.19 This low-profile resuscitative endovascular balloon occlusion of the aorta (REBOA) device (Rescue Balloon; Tokai Medical Products Inc.) is an over-the-wire balloon catheter with a double lumen. This device is an all-in-one package that includes a 19-gauge puncture needle (Seldinger type), a 30-mL syringe, a 0.035-inch sheath guide wire (80 cm), a J-shaped (C) 0.025-inch balloon catheter guide wire (145 cm, for the femoral approach; 240 cm, for the brachial approach), a 7-Fr sheath (11 cm), a dilator, and a balloon catheter (insertable length, 80 cm), reinforced by an internal stiff wire stylet (A–B). The balloon is made of polyurethane and has high compliance (balloon length, 60 mm; diameter, 16 mm [8 mL of internal fluid] to 40 mm [40 mL]; the internal fluid of the balloon is normal saline or a dilute contrast medium) (D). (From Shoji T, Tarui T, Igarashi T et al. Resuscitative endovascular balloon occlusion of the aorta using a low-profile device is easy and safe for emergency physicians in cases of life-threatening hemorrhage. *J Emerg Med*. 2018;54(4):410-418, 2017.)

markers should be between L2 and L4. Remove the long guidewire once the catheter is in place.

Again, an assistant should be charged with maintaining the position of the catheter after placement. Inflate the balloon with a 50:50 mixture of sterile saline and iodinated contrast. The viscosity of pure contrast is too high for the balloon and may make removal difficult. Be careful not to overinflate the balloon. Several markers can be used to identify the ideal inflation volume including disappearance of the contralateral femoral pulse, a large increase in the SBP, moderate resistance with inflation, or change in shape of the edges of the balloon seen on radiographs from convex to parallel. The latter is more commonly seen when using fluoroscopy, which is typically unavailable in the ED. Ultrasound may also be used to evaluate arterial flow distal to the occlusion. The volume needed to fully occlude the aorta will differ between patients but can be between 10 and 25 mL. Typically, more volume is needed to fully occlude zone 1 than zone 3.

Once the aorta has been occluded, turn the three-way stopcock toward the balloon to maintain inflation and record the time of occlusion, insertion distance of the balloon, volume inserted into the balloon, and blood pressure change. Suture the catheter into place; most kits come with a catheter clamp that can aid with securing the line and suturing it to the skin. Place an occlusive dressing over the access site. Obtain a radiograph to confirm positioning and expedite the patient to the operating room or interventional radiology suite.[97]

Reboa Removal

Though typically not performed in the ED, if REBOA placement for other indications (such as nontraumatic OHCA) becomes more prevalent, it will be important for EM providers to have knowledge of its removal.

It is important to do these steps slowly and again use an assistant who can maintain position of the catheter. As the balloon is deflated, anticipate hypotension, acidosis, and washout of metabolic byproducts as perfusion returns to the rest of the body. Resuscitate as needed and consider multiple rounds of deflation and inflation.[97]

Remove the balloon then the sheath and hold pressure on the access site for at least 10 minutes. Consider vascular surgery

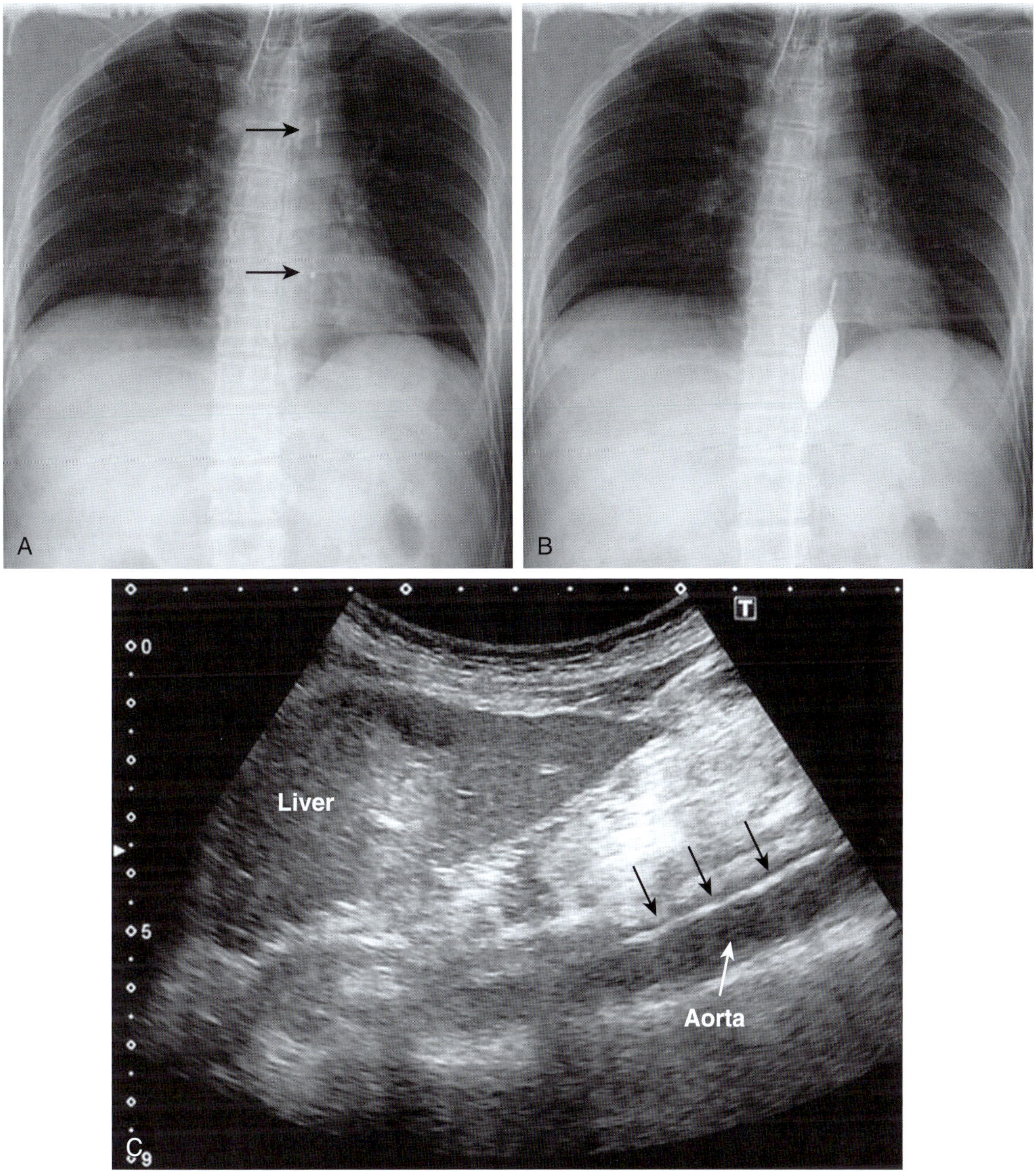

Fig. 18.20 This low-profile resuscitative endovascular balloon occlusion of the aorta (REBOA) device (Rescue Balloon; Tokai Medical Products Inc.) has two radiopacity markers on the catheter tip *(white arrow)* to confirm the position of the balloon catheter by fluoroscopy or portable radiography. (A) The catheter before the inflation of the balloon. (B) The catheter in zone I after the inflation of the balloon with contrast agent. (C) Ultrasonography image by long-axis subxiphoid view shows that the guide wire *(black arrows)* is inside the supraceliac aorta. (From Shoji T, Tarui T, Igarashi T. Resuscitative endovascular balloon occlusion of the aorta using a low-profile device is easy and safe for emergency physicians in cases of life-threatening hemorrhage. *J Emerg Med.* 2018;54(4):410-418.)

consultation for arteriotomy repair if bleeding is not sufficiently controlled with pressure. Frequent reassessment of lower extremity perfusion should be performed over the following 24 hours.[97]

Complications

There are myriad complications that can occur as a result of placement of REBOA. Delays in access can lead to delays in definitive hemorrhage control and death. Prolonged occlusion of the aorta can have fatal complications due to prolonged organ ischemia or lead to spinal cord injury due to hypoperfusion.[87]

Arterial injury can occur as a result of femoral access or direct injury to the aorta at the site of balloon insertion. Injury types include dissections, pseudoaneurysms, thrombosis, and embolization, which can lead to extremity ischemia, compartment syndrome, limb loss, and death.[87,93] Lower limb ischemia was shown to be the most prevalent complication with an incidence of 16% (range 4.0% to 52.6%).[93] The iliac vessels can also be damaged if the balloon is dilated within their lumen. A smaller diameter sheath (<8 Fr) has been associated with fewer limb complications.[89,96]

Reperfusion injury should be anticipated as the balloon is deflated and blood flow returns to the previously nonperfused region of the body. Large electrolyte shifts, coagulopathy, and systemic inflammatory response occur that can lead to acute kidney injury, myocardial infarction, acute respiratory distress syndrome, sepsis, gastrointestinal complications, and multisystem organ failure, among others. Of these, acute kidney failure was the most common, with an incidence ranging from 5.6% to 46.0%. Various studies report widely variable mortality rates ranging from 29% to 88%.[87,93]

ACKNOWLEDGMENT

The editors and authors acknowledge the contributions of Robert L. Bartlett, MD, and Michael E. Boczar, MD, to this chapter in previous editions.

REFERENCES ARE AVAILABLE AT Elsevier eBooks+

SECTION IV

Vascular Techniques and Volume Support

CHAPTER 19

Pediatric Vascular Access and Blood Sampling Techniques

Genevieve Santillanes and Ilene Claudius

Obtaining vascular access and blood samples in an infant or child can challenge and frustrate even the most skilled emergency clinician and can be especially challenging in children who are dehydrated or in shock. Resuscitation of critically ill and injured children should not be delayed for lack of vascular access; intraosseous (IO) access is the preferred technique if peripheral vascular access cannot be rapidly obtained. This chapter reviews the basic principles and techniques of blood sampling and placement of IO lines, peripheral and central intravenous (IV) and intraarterial catheters in infants and children, including the use of umbilical catheters in neonates. Rehydration techniques are also reviewed. Emergency cutdown is a very rarely required, but occasionally useful, method of obtaining vascular access, and a section of this chapter is devoted to cutdown techniques.

PATIENT PREPARATION AND RESTRAINT

Fear and anticipation of procedural pain can make the hospital experience traumatic for anyone and certainly for children. Before beginning any painful procedure in a stable child, explain the procedure and the reasons it is necessary to the parents. For children capable of understanding, explain the procedure in developmentally appropriate language before starting and before each successive step. Parents should generally be present during emergency department (ED) procedures.[1] Parental presence is generally comforting to children, and children with a parent present have been shown to demonstrate less stress during procedures.[2,3] Nonpharmacologic techniques such as music, toys, or being held by a parent may further reduce children's distress during attempts at vascular access.[4,5] Many applications for smart phones, including some that produce "bubbles" for the child to "pop" on the screen are excellent and typically available distractions. While parents can assist by holding their child in a comfort position or distracting with songs or conversation, parents should not be asked to restrain an extremity or restrain their child on the gurney.

The success of blood sampling or obtaining vascular access depends in part on proper positioning and restraint of the patient. In most cases this requires the assistance of at least one other staff person and immobilization of the extremity a joint above and below the intended insertion site. Young infants are at risk of hypothermia if disrobed and exposed during prolonged attempts at venipuncture or vessel cannulation, especially if their perfusion is compromised due to sepsis or hypovolemic shock. Consider overhead lights, warm blankets, or other warming modalities to prevent accidental hypothermia in vulnerable patients. Furthermore, there is some evidence that radiant warmth is effective as an analgesic for minor procedures in newborns.[6]

Anesthesia

Many products are available to decrease the pain associated with vascular access. Do not delay IV access in critically ill or injured children to use these medications or devices, but consider use in stable patients. These medications and products are discussed in more detail in Chapter 29. Options include vapocoolants, topical and subcutaneous anesthetics, and vibrating devices. Orally administered sucrose solution has been demonstrated to decrease the pain response in young infants during procedures.[7,8] Procedural sedation is commonly used during central venous and arterial cannulation in children (Chapter 33).

BLOOD SAMPLING TECHNIQUES

Capillary Blood Sampling

Indications and Contraindications

Capillary blood sampling is frequently used to obtain blood samples from young infants. In children and adults, capillary blood samples are most commonly obtained from the fingertip, but the distance from the skin to bone is often insufficient in young infants to perform fingerstick blood draws. Consequently, the heel is the preferred location for capillary blood draws in infants under 6 to 12 months of age. Heel sticks are more painful than venipuncture but are useful in the event of difficult access or when "arterialized" samples are needed for blood gas analysis.[9] Heel stick blood sampling is useful when repeated measurements such as blood glucose or serial hemoglobins are needed. If a sufficient volume is obtained, blood from a capillary sample can also be sent for other routine laboratory studies.

Avoid sampling from an area of local inflammation or hematoma. Avoid repetitive sampling from the same site because it may induce inflammation and subsequent scarring. In general, heel stick sampling is not ideal for blood gas analysis when the infant is hypotensive, the heel is markedly bruised, or there is evidence of peripheral vasoconstriction.

Equipment and Setup

Use a lancet or automated disposable incision device designed for infant heel sticks to perform this procedure. Perform blood collection with either heparinized capillary tubes or pediatric micro blood collection tubes (e.g., Microtainer, Becton Dickinson) with a collector attachment.

Technique

The heel stick method of capillary blood sampling will be described, but capillary blood samples can also be obtained from a digit or earlobe if there is sufficient soft tissue (Fig. 19.1). The soft tissue is thickest on the medial and lateral portions of the heel, so the puncture should occur on the medial or lateral aspect, avoiding the central portion of the heel. If previous heel sticks have been performed, avoid previous puncture sites. Prewarm the foot by wrapping it in a warm cloth or a heat pack for 5 minutes to produce hyperemia and enhance blood flow. Immobilize the foot in a dependent position with one hand. First, cleanse the heel with antiseptic solution and allow it to dry. Next, puncture the skin with the lancet. Avoid squeezing the foot because it may inhibit capillary filling, decreasing blood flow. Furthermore, squeezing may lead to hemolysis of the sample. If blood does not flow freely, another puncture may be required.

Wipe away the first small drop of blood with gauze and allow a second drop to form. Place a capillary tube in the drop of blood and invert the proximal end of the tube to allow it to fill by capillary action. Fill the capillary tube until blood reaches the demarcation line on the tube. Avoid over- or underfilling the tube. If micro blood collection tubes are used, hold the tube at an angle of 30 to 45 degrees from the surface of the puncture site. Touch the collector end of the tube to the drop of blood and allow the blood to drain into the tube. Gently tap the tube to facilitate flow to the bottom. Once filled, seal the tube with the accompanying cap. After an adequate specimen is obtained, apply a dry dressing to the puncture site.

When a heel stick is performed for an arterialized blood sample, use the same technique, but take care not to introduce ambient air into the sample. Place the tip of the tube as near the puncture site as possible to minimize exposure of the blood to environmental oxygen. Fill the tube as completely as possible and avoid collecting air in the tube. When the tube is full, occlude the free end with a gloved finger to prevent the entry of air, and cap both ends. Excessive squeezing of the foot may artificially lower the partial pressure of oxygen (Po_2).

Complications

When performed properly, heel sticks are associated with a very low incidence of complications. Use an automatic incision device to prevent lacerations. Rare complications include infection, scarring, and calcified nodules.

Interpretation

Studies have demonstrated a good correlation between arterial and capillary specimens for determining pH and partial pressure of carbon dioxide (Pco_2) in hemodynamically stable patients.[10] However, the determination of Po_2 is not reliable when performed on blood obtained by capillary sampling.

Venipuncture

Indications and Contraindications

Venipuncture is used to obtain larger quantities of blood from infants and children and to obtain blood for culture. When collecting blood for culture, prepare the area of venipuncture with an appropriate antiseptic solution and allow the skin to dry. Wash off the cleanser promptly after blood has been collected because antiseptic solutions can irritate infant skin.

Equipment and Setup

A small-gauge butterfly or straight needle with a syringe is generally preferred for specimen collection in infants and young children because the negative pressure generated by standard specimen collection tubes (e.g., Vacutainer, Becton Dickinson) may collapse small veins. A 3-mL or 5-mL syringe is less likely than a 10-mL syringe to result in collapse of small veins. Many clinicians find that it is easier to control needle position with a butterfly needle rather than a straight needle. If other access is not available, the butterfly needle may also serve as a temporary infusion line after an adequate amount of blood is obtained. A 23-gauge butterfly needle will generally suffice for venipuncture, regardless of patient size.

Technique

As in adults, the usual site for venipuncture in infants and children is the antecubital fossa. However, any easily visible or palpable peripheral vein that will not be needed for IV cannulation may be used. Veins on the hands, feet, or scalp are frequently visible in young children (Fig. 19.2). Imaging devices (e.g., ultrasound, transillumination, or infrared devices) may also be used to locate and identify veins for venipuncture. These devices are discussed later in this chapter (see section on "Vascular Line Placement: Venous and Arterial").

Assemble all necessary equipment, especially needles, out of sight of the child and have equipment within easy reach before beginning. Ask an assistant to help immobilize the patient when drawing blood from infants and small children. If an extremity vein is to be used, apply a tourniquet proximal to the selected vein. In small infants a rubber band can be used as a tourniquet. Be sure that the tourniquet is not so tight that it impedes arterial filling.

Cleanse the area surrounding the chosen site of skin penetration with antiseptic solution and allow it to dry. Apply slight distal traction to the skin to immobilize the vein. Insert the needle quickly through the skin and advance it slowly into the vein at an angle of approximately 30 degrees with the bevel facing up (Fig. 19.3). Successful vessel penetration is heralded by a flashback, or flow, of blood into the needle hub or butterfly tubing. Apply gentle suction by slowly withdrawing the plunger of the syringe. If the required amount of blood is greater than the capacity of the attached syringe, pinch off the tubing, remove the filled syringe, attach a new syringe, and apply gentle suction again after releasing the pinched tubing. Remove the tourniquet. After the required amount of blood is withdrawn, remove the needle and apply a sterile dressing and direct pressure to the puncture site.

Although peripheral sites for venous blood sampling are preferable in infants, the external jugular and femoral veins may also be used for venipuncture during resuscitation or when peripheral sites are inadequate. The external jugular vein lies in a line from the angle of the jaw to the middle of the clavicle and is usually visible on the surface of the skin (Fig. 19.4). When the infant is crying, this vein is more prominent.

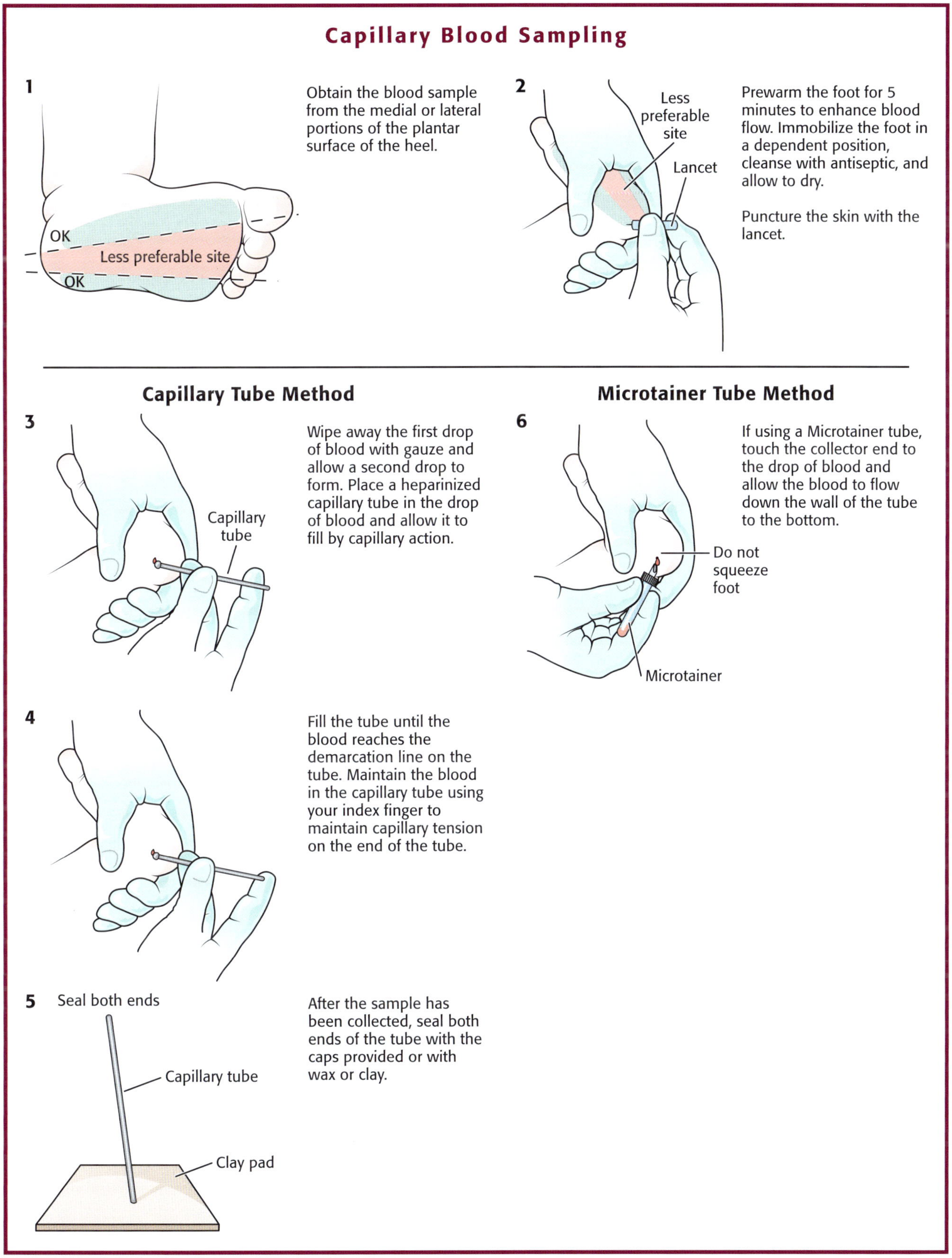

Fig. 19.1 Capillary blood sampling: capillary tube and Microtainer tube methods.

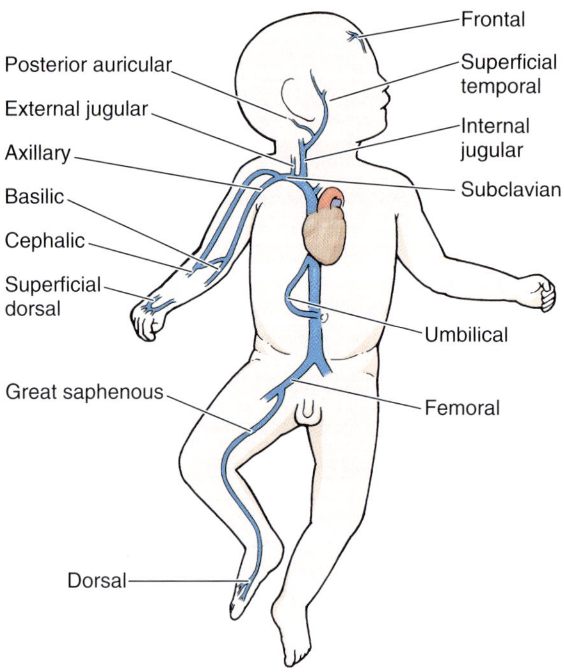

Fig. 19.2 Venous access sites in neonates and young infants. If venous access is unavailable, arterial blood may be used for most laboratory tests, including blood cultures.

Venipuncture Using a Butterfly Needle

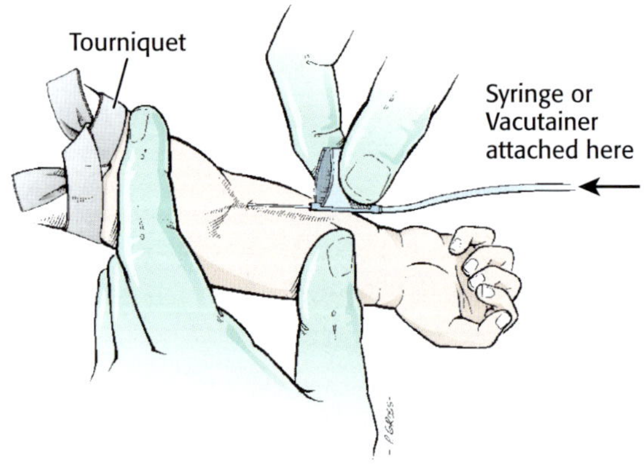

Apply a tourniquet and cleanse the skin. Maintain slight distal traction and quickly enter the vein at an angle of approximately 30 degrees. Often two people are required–one to hold the arm and insert the needle and the other to aspirate the blood. Once blood is obtained, the butterfly needle may be used as an infusion site.

Fig. 19.3 Venipuncture using a butterfly needle.

Ask an assistant to restrain the infant in a supine position with the head and neck extended over the edge of the bed. Alternatively, place a towel roll or pillow under the child's shoulders. Turn the head approximately 40 to 70 degrees from the midline. Cleanse the skin surrounding the area to be punctured with alcohol or another antiseptic solution. Apply finger pressure just above the clavicle to help distend the jugular vein. Use a 21- to 25-gauge straight needle or a 21- to 25-gauge butterfly needle attached to a syringe. Puncture the skin and then advance the needle slowly until the jugular vein is entered and a flashback of blood is observed. Keep the syringe connected to the needle at all times to maintain constant negative pressure and avoid air embolism. After the necessary blood is obtained, withdraw the needle and apply slight pressure to the vessel. Place the child in an upright position if possible after the needle is removed, and hold pressure over the puncture site for 3 to 5 minutes. Observe the puncture site closely afterward to identify any persistent bleeding.

In most patients, the femoral vein lies medial to the femoral artery and inferior to the inguinal ligament (Fig. 19.5A). Ask an assistant to position the patient's hips in mild abduction and extension while you palpate the artery. Identify its location by placing a mark on the skin just superior to the femoral triangle. If available, use ultrasound to assess the position of the femoral vessels. Prepare the femoral triangle with alcohol or another antiseptic agent. Use a povidone-iodine or chlorhexidine scrub when obtaining blood for culture. Puncture the skin and then direct the needle or catheter toward the umbilicus at a 30- to 45-degree angle to the skin and just medial to the pulsation of the femoral artery (see Fig. 19.5B). Apply constant slight negative pressure on the syringe constantly throughout insertion. After the needle enters the femoral vein, withdraw the desired blood samples. Afterward, remove the needle or catheter unless an IV catheter for venous access is desired in this location. Apply pressure over the puncture site in the femoral triangle for a minimum of 5 minutes. Observe closely for persistent bleeding.

Scalp veins can be very useful for venous sampling in small infants when other options are not readily available.

Complications

Complications of venipuncture include hematoma formation, arterial puncture, local infection, injury to adjacent structures, and phlebitis. Serious complications are uncommon. Use special care when attempting to puncture the external jugular or femoral vein. Inadvertent deep puncture in the neck can injure the carotid artery, vagus nerve, phrenic nerve, or the apex of the lung. The femoral artery or nerve can be injured during puncture of the area around the femoral triangle. Fortunately, these injuries are unlikely when proper technique is used.

Arterial Blood Sampling

Indications and Contraindications

Arterial blood sampling is most often indicated to obtain an arterial blood gas (ABG) analysis. All blood gas parameters except Po_2 are generally accurate from capillary and venous blood samples, so consider whether arterial blood samples are necessary. Arterial blood may be drawn for routine laboratory analysis or blood culture if venous blood is difficult to obtain. Avoid puncture of an artery if the overlying skin is infected, burned, or otherwise damaged. In addition, consider the presence of adequate collateral circulation and any potential coagulation disorders.

Equipment and Setup

For arterial puncture in infants and children, a small-gauge butterfly needle is preferable to a needle and syringe. A 23-gauge butterfly needle is used most often, although a 25-gauge butterfly needle may be preferable in newborns. Some clinicians prefer to use a 25-gauge needle connected to a syringe, but a butterfly allows better control of the needle while an

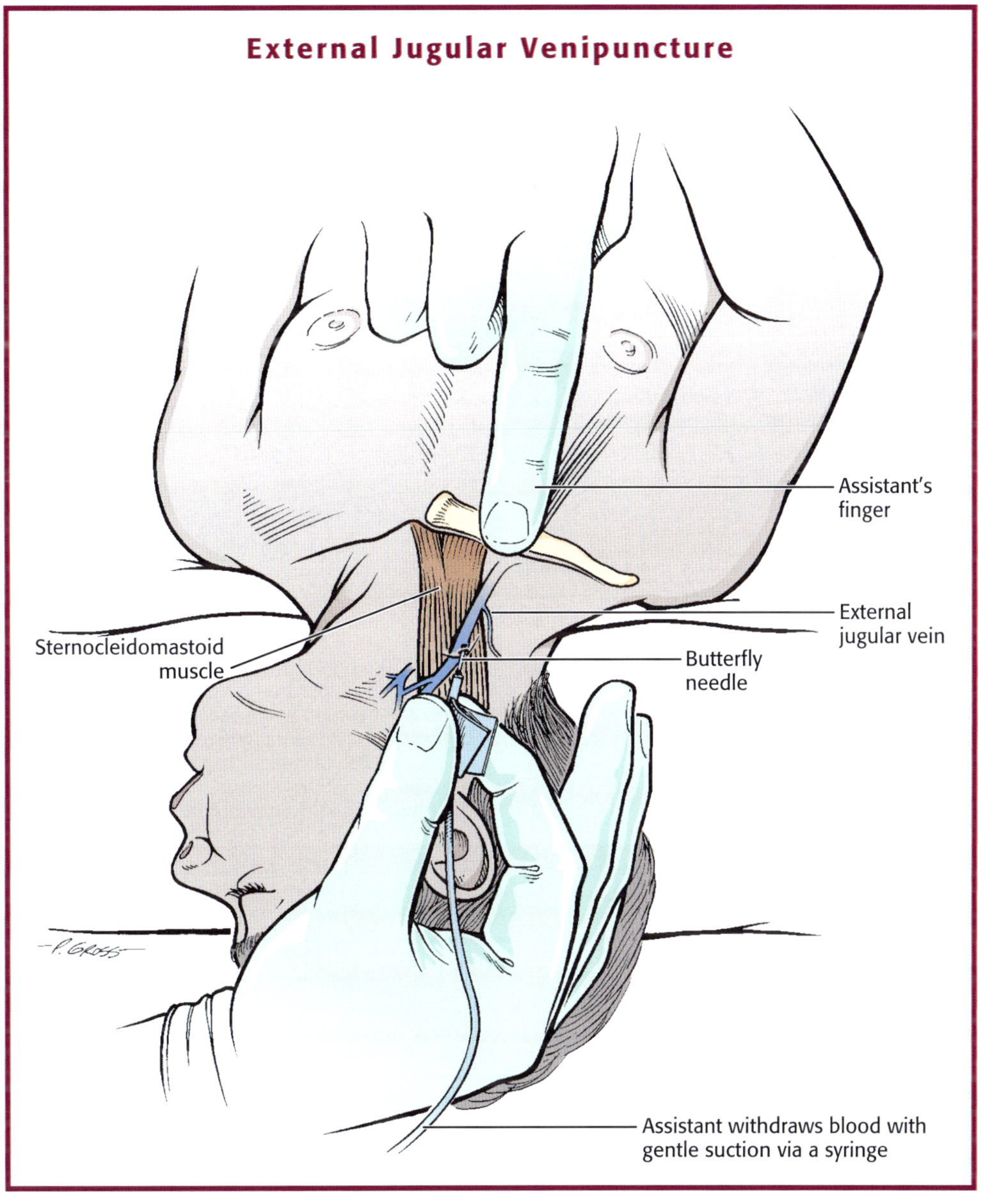

Fig. 19.4 External jugular venipuncture. A syringe or a butterfly needle may be used. Venous distention is aided when an assistant's finger occludes the vein or when the infant cries. The neck is extended, either over the side of the bed or by placing a rolled towel under the shoulders. This procedure requires two people.

assistant aspirates the syringe. This technique may also permit a larger volume of blood to be withdrawn.

Technique

Potential sites for arterial blood sampling include the radial, brachial, dorsalis pedis, and posterior tibial arteries. In newborn infants the umbilical arteries are also available. The radial artery has several advantages and is the most commonly used artery for blood sampling. First, its location makes it easy to palpate and puncture (Fig. 19.6A and B). The ulnar artery can be more difficult to locate. Second, no vein or nerve is immediately adjacent to the radial artery, minimizing the risk of obtaining venous blood or damaging a nerve. Another advantage of the radial artery is the presence of good collateral circulation from the ulnar artery. Limit use of the ulnar artery to preserve collateral circulation to the hand. The brachial and femoral arteries should be avoided due to insufficient collateral circulation.

Because the radial artery is used most frequently to obtain percutaneous arterial blood samples, the technique for radial artery puncture will be described. (See Chapter 20 for a discussion of the Allen test and the effect of heparin on arterial blood sampling.)

Hold the patient's wrist and hand in your nondominant hand (Fig. 19.6B). Hold the hand fully supinated with the wrist slightly extended (i.e., dorsiflexed). Palpate the arterial pulsation just proximal to the transverse wrist creases. Overextension of the wrist can cause loss of the arterial pulse during palpation. Make a small indentation in the skin with a fingernail to mark the insertion site. Cleanse the area with antiseptic and allow the skin to dry. The topical anesthetic options discussed previously may be used if the clinical situation permits. Puncture the skin with the needle at a 30- to 45-degree angle, advancing the needle slowly until the radial artery is punctured or resistance (bone) is met (Fig. 19.7). In young infants,

Femoral Venipuncture

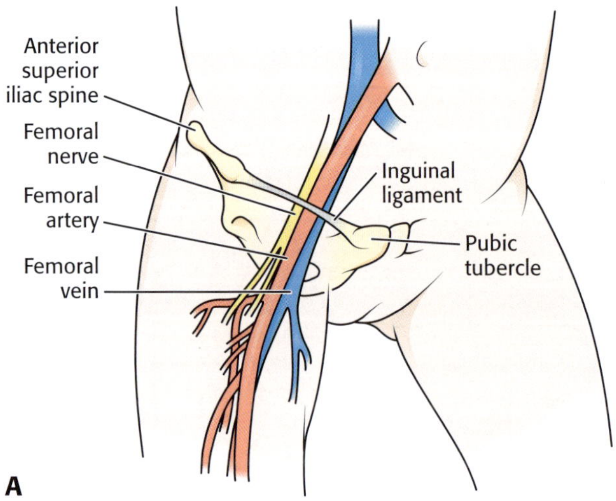

A

The femoral vein lies medial (in most patients) to the femoral artery and inferior to the inguinal ligament.

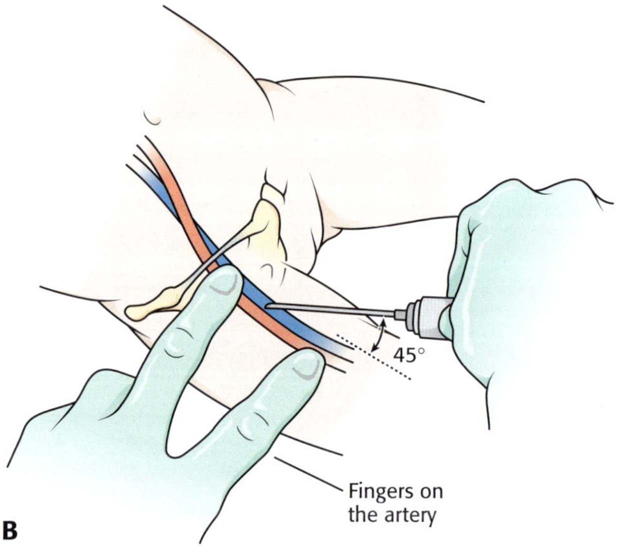

B

Position the hips in mild abduction and extension. Palpate the artery just superior to the femoral triangle. Puncture the skin and direct the needle toward the umbilicus at a 30- to 45-degree angle to the skin while remaining just medial to the femoral artery pulsation. Maintain slight constant negative pressure throughout the insertion. Apply pressure for a minimum of 5 minutes after the procedure and monitor for bleeding.

Fig. 19.5 Femoral venipuncture. (A) Anatomy. (B) Technique.

Radial Arterial Blood Sampling

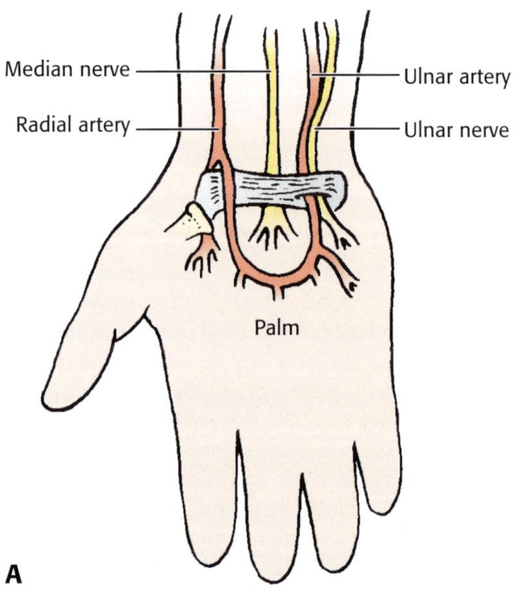

A

The radial artery is preferred for sampling procedures. Its superficial location is easy to palpate and puncture, and there are no immediately adjacent nerves or veins that may be injured or accidentally punctured.

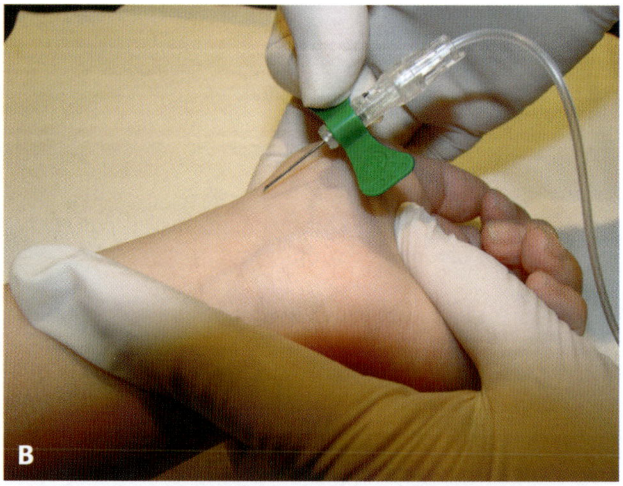

B

Hold the wrist in a position of supination and slight extension. Insert the needle at a 30- to 45-degree angle while applying continuous, gentle suction with the plunger. Advance the needle until the radial artery is punctured and blood is returned or until resistance is met(see Fig. 19.7).

Fig. 19.6 Radial arterial blood sampling. (A) Anatomy. (B) Technique.

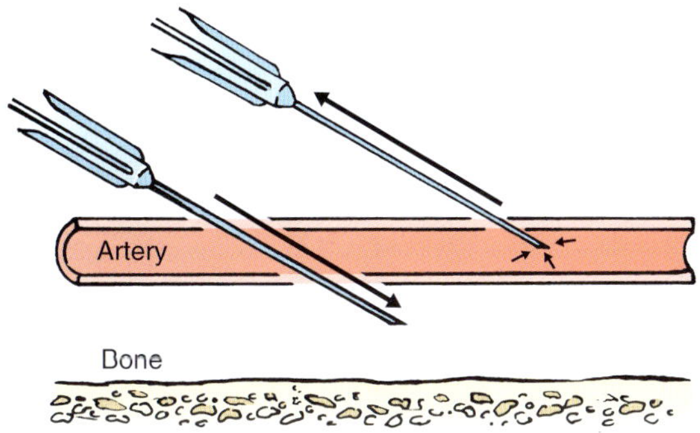

Fig. 19.7 Resistance met during passage of the blood gas needle usually indicates contact with bone. The needle should be withdrawn slowly. If the needle has traversed both walls of the artery, blood will be obtained as the needle is slowly withdrawn into the arterial lumen.

some clinicians prefer to have an assistant provide continuous, very gentle suction by pulling back on the plunger as the needle is advanced. Avoid stronger suction which can collapse the artery. Pulsating or rapidly flowing blood that appears in the hub of the needle indicates that the radial artery has been punctured. Some clinicians prefer to advance a butterfly needle without an attached syringe and attach the syringe only after blood return is noted.

If there is no blood return with the initial puncture, withdraw the needle slowly, watching for blood return. Both walls of the artery may have been punctured and the needle tip may reenter the lumen of the artery on withdrawal. If there is no blood return, withdraw the needle slowly to the point at which only the distal tip of the needle remains beneath the skin. Repeat the procedure after checking the location of the pulse and reorienting the needle. After the desired amount of blood is obtained, remove the needle and apply pressure for 5 minutes or longer to prevent hematoma formation.

Complications

Complications of radial artery puncture include infection, hematoma, arterial spasm, tendon injury, and nerve damage. With proper technique, however, the complication rate is extremely low. If the infant starts to cry before blood is obtained, the Po_2 and Pco_2 values may not reflect the infant's true steady state.

VASCULAR LINE PLACEMENT: VENOUS AND ARTERIAL

Intravascular lines are indicated when ongoing access to the venous or arterial circulation is necessary. If the clinical situation permits, consider using local anesthetics or procedural sedation.

Peripheral Venous Catheterization: Percutaneous

Indications and Contraindications

In general, peripheral IV lines are indicated when the patient is unable to attain medical and nutritional goals with enteral therapy. These lines are used to provide fluids for resuscitation and maintenance needs and for the administration of medications.

Equipment and Setup

Over-the-needle catheters are the mainstay of peripheral venous catheterization. These thin-walled, flexible catheters range in size from 10 to 24 gauge. Larger-diameter catheters allow more rapid administration of fluids in emergency situations but may decrease the success of cannulation in young children with small veins. In general, use the smallest-gauge catheter that is appropriate for the clinical situation. For infants, a 22- to 24-gauge catheter is generally appropriate.

Prepare tape ahead of time to secure the catheter and place strips of tape in a location that will be easily accessible once the catheter is in place. T-connector extension tubing facilitates blood collection and makes flushing the catheter easier, especially while taping and securing the IV line. It also allows dressing changes without disturbing the IV insertion site.

Use either a homemade or commercially available device to protect the IV site from a child's movements and attempts to remove the line. An arm or leg board appropriate for the size of the child provides stabilization of the extremity after insertion. In active infants and children, wrapping the immobilized extremity in gauze or a disposable diaper can further protect the IV from being pulled out. Macro drip tubing and liter bags are not appropriate for use in infants and young children because they can result in the inadvertent infusion of large amounts of fluid. An infusion pump is an ideal way of limiting fluid infusion while keeping the vein open.

Vein Imaging Devices

A variety of imaging modalities, including ultrasound, transillumination, and infrared technologies, can be used to help locate peripheral veins for cannulation. In adults, ultrasound has been demonstrated to improve the success rate of IV cannulation.[11] The data are more limited in pediatric patients, but ultrasound does appear to improve both first-pass and overall success rate.[12]

Transillumination devices work by shining a bright light through the area to be cannulated, causing the veins to contrast with surrounding tissue, making them easier to locate. Data are mixed on success rates with transilluminator devices with some data showing improved success rates and some data showing decreased success rates compared to traditional visualization and palpation.[13–15] Newer vein imaging technology, available as VeinViewer (Christie Medical Holdings), AccuVein, NextVein, Vasculuminator (WeLLDesign) and others, uses near-infrared technology to project an enhanced image of the subcutaneous veins onto the patient's skin. Theoretically, knowledge of the location of the venous valves and the course of the vessel can assist the clinician in selecting the best area to be cannulated. However, multiple studies have not demonstrated improved overall success rates in obtaining IV access.[16–23]

Technique

Fig. 19.2 shows sites available for placement of a peripheral IV line. The most common sites chosen for IV insertion in infants and children are the superficial veins of the dorsum of the hand, the antecubital fossa and the dorsum of the foot (Video 19.1). In small infants, scalp veins are also common sites of IV placement. The veins on the dorsum of the hand are relatively straight and are easily stabilized because they lie flat on the metacarpals. If the hand is chosen, take the child's hand preference into consideration and avoid the dominant hand or hand used for thumb sucking whenever possible. Veins in the antecubital fossa (cephalic and basilic veins) are easily accessible; however, the angulation across the fossa can make advancement of the catheter difficult. Tributaries of the dorsal venous

Peripheral Intravenous Catheterization

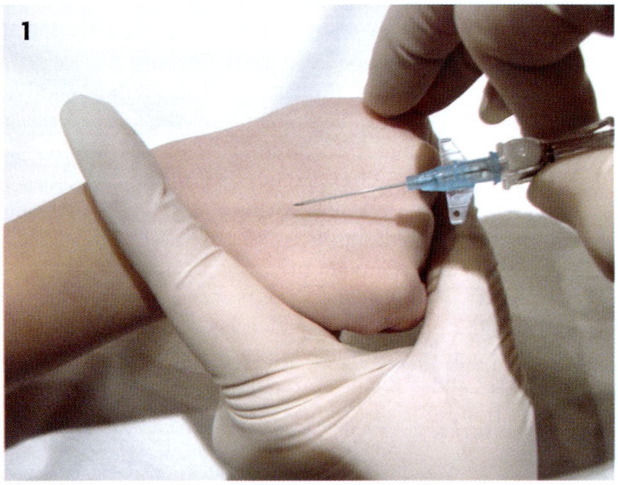

Direct the catheter at a 10-to 20-degree angle toward the insertion site and advance until blood return is seen in the catheter and hub. Advance the catheter over the needle and into the vein.

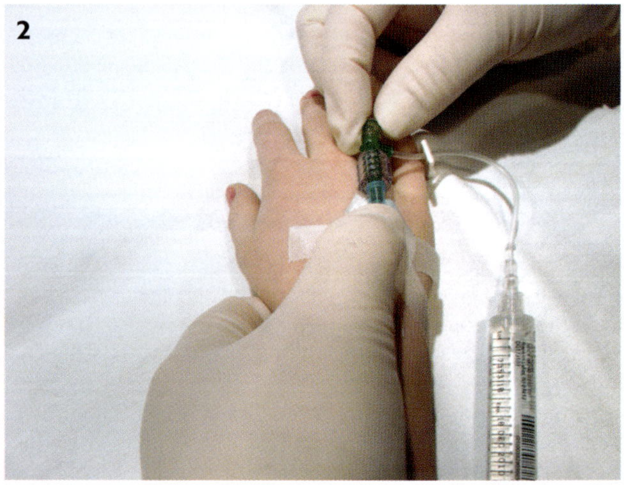

Remove the needle, and attach the T-extension set to the catheter hub. Flush with saline, and secure the catheter to the skin with tape.

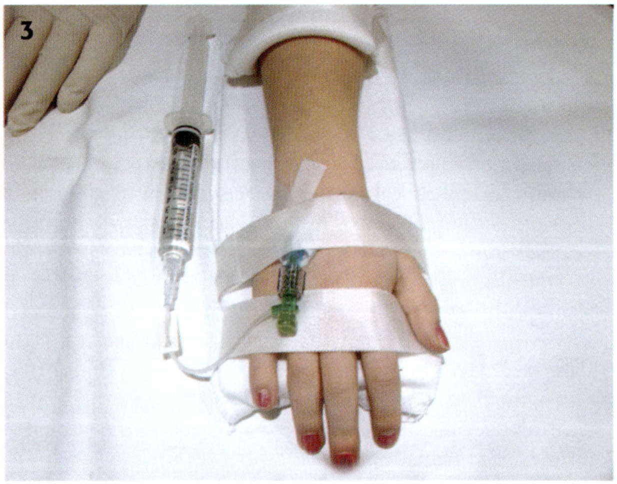

Secure the hand and forearm to an arm board.

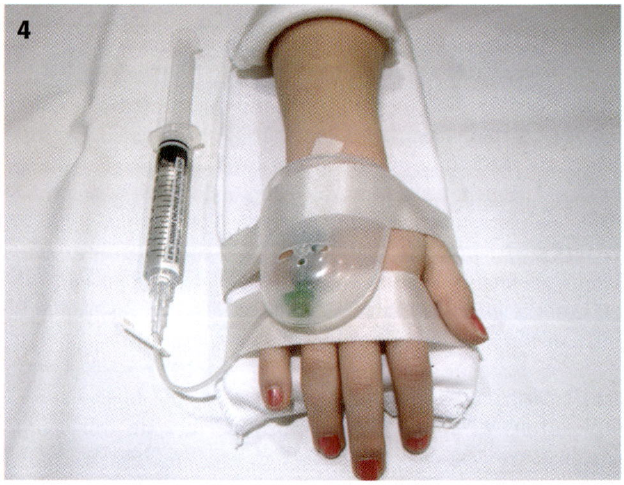

Cover the insertion site with the plastic wrapper from the extension set for additional protection.

Fig. 19.8 Pediatric peripheral intravenous catheterization. (See Fig. 21.6 for additional details on proper intravenous technique.)

arch on the dorsum of the foot, like those on the dorsum of the hand, are relatively straight, and the extremity is easily immobilized after insertion. Because indwelling catheters in this location prevent mobility, consider using this site only in patients who are not ambulatory or after attempts at other sites have been unsuccessful. If peripherally inserted central venous catheter (PICC) placement may be required during the hospitalization, avoid PICC insertion sites if possible.

With few exceptions, the same techniques used for IV insertion in adults may be used in infants and children, especially in the veins of the distal ends of the extremities. If an extremity location is chosen, place a tourniquet proximal to the planned site of insertion. If time allows, warming the extremity to vasodilate the surface veins can facilitate IV cannulation. Flush the tubing of the T-extension set before venipuncture with a sterile IV solution, such as normal saline (NS), to prevent air embolism. Direct the IV catheter through the skin at a 10- to 20-degree angle and slowly advance it until blood return is noted (Fig. 19.8, *step 1*). Next, advance the catheter over the needle and into the vein. Retract the needle and connect the IV line to the hub of the catheter by means of a T-extension set (Fig. 19.8, *step 2*). After 1 mL of saline has been flushed through the line, inspect the site for swelling, which may indicate infiltration. If an artery is entered during placement of the needle and fluid is infused, blanching will occur in the area. If this happens, remove the IV catheter, maintain slight pressure for 5 minutes, and repeat the procedure at another site.

Secure the catheter to the skin with a piece of tape passed over the catheter hub and skin. Place a second thin strip of tape adhesive side up and slip it under the catheter hub. Cross it over the catheter hub in a V shape (see Fig. 19.8, *step 2*). Tearing a piece of tape lengthwise so it is half the width of standard tape facilitates securing the IV in a V shape. After securing the catheter with tape, cover the entire area with a transparent sterile dressing such as Tegaderm or OpSite. Loop back the tubing of the T-extension set, place a piece of tape midway over the tubing, and secure it to the skin. This ensures that the IV tubing will not be accidentally dislodged if it is suddenly pulled. Securely tape the hand and forearm to an arm board for immobilization (Fig. 19.8, *step 3*). Occasionally, the flow rate of the infusion may depend on the position of the catheter, especially if the catheter spans a joint or the tip abuts a venous valve. Adjust the hand position or catheter with strategically placed sterile gauze or withdraw the catheter slightly to remedy the problem.

Obtain blood specimens just after IV insertion. If the IV line has been flushed, the initial blood draw will be diluted. To prevent dilution, withdraw 5 mL of blood from the catheter before collecting the samples. Next, remove the syringe. Connect the T-extension tubing to the IV infusion tubing, and set the infusion pump at the desired rate. Send blood for culture only if the skin was cleaned with an appropriate antiseptic before insertion of the IV catheter.

If a butterfly infusion set is used, grasp the wings of the butterfly between the thumb and forefinger and introduce the needle beneath the skin approximately 0.5 cm distal to the anticipated site of vein entrance (Fig. 19.9, *step 1*). Advance the needle slowly toward the vessel until blood appears in the tubing, which indicates that the vessel has been entered. Next, remove the tourniquet if one was used. Flush the needle with 0.5 to 2 mL of IV fluid, such as NS, to ensure that the needle is properly in place within the vein. If infiltration occurs, as noted by a subcutaneous bump, remove the IV line and repeat the process at another site.

After the wings are secured, tape the tubing of the butterfly set in a loop so that it is not pulled inadvertently. Place a wisp of cotton under the wings of the butterfly if the flow rate of the infusion is affected by the position of the catheter. Tape a small medication cup over the wings and the needle to protect the IV line (Fig. 19.9, *step 2*). Connect the tubing of the butterfly set to the tubing from the IV system. It is preferable to use standard over-the-needle IV catheters whenever possible, whether for extremity or scalp IV lines, because they are less likely to infiltrate and will last longer. However, a small butterfly needle that can be inserted temporarily until additional access is obtained is sometimes the only option short of IO access.

Technique with Ultrasound Guidance (See also Chapter 67)

There are multiple techniques described for ultrasound-guided IV access.[24,25] In children, visualizing the vein to be cannulated in the short axis is often preferred due to the small diameter of the vessels. First, use the high-frequency linear array ultrasound probe with the smallest footprint possible to identify the best vessel to cannulate and identify any surrounding structures to avoid. Forearm, saphenous, basilic, or cephalic veins are commonly cannulated vessels. Find a vessel with a sufficient diameter and identify the straightest segment to cannulate. In adults, long catheters are commonly used to place ultrasound-guided IVs in deep veins. However, long 22- and 24-gauge catheters are not commonly stocked, so ensure that the vessel is superficial enough to be cannulated with the available catheter.

The technique of dynamic needle tip positioning in the short-axis view will be described. Visualize the vessel to be cannulated in short axis (cross-sectional view of the vessel) with the vessel in the center of the screen. Puncture the skin at a 30- to 45-degree angle and then find the needle tip with the ultrasound by sliding the probe up toward the puncture site. Once the needle tip is identified, move the ultrasound probe 1 mm proximally. Advance the needle until it is again seen on the screen, then advance the ultrasound probe another 1 mm and repeat these steps until the needle tip is visualized puncturing the vessel. At this point, decrease the angle of insertion,

Scalp Vein Intravenous Catheterization

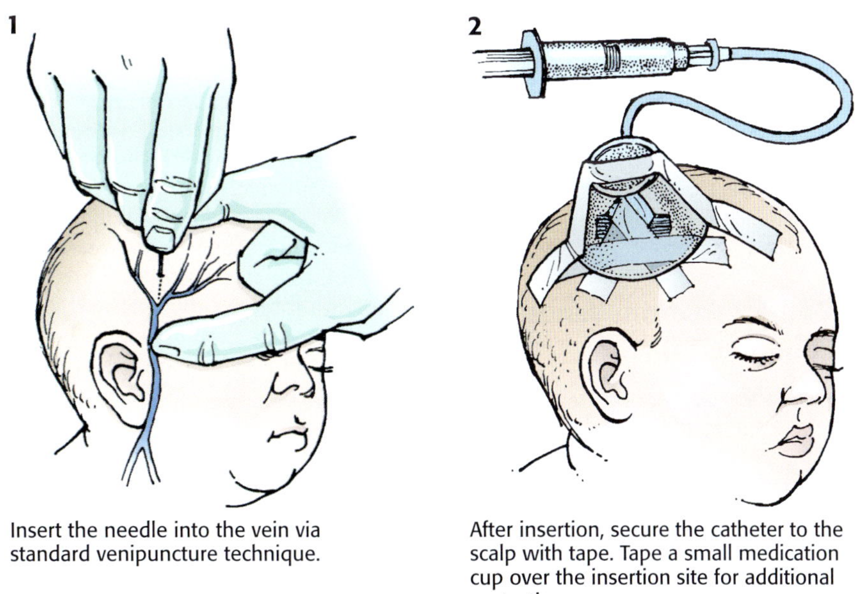

Fig 19.9 Scalp vein intravenous catheterization using a butterfly needle.

and continue sequentially advancing the probe, then needle tip, and ensure that the catheter (and not just the tip of the needle) is in the vessel before advancing the catheter into the vessel. Thoroughly clean the ultrasound gel off the skin and secure the IV as described earlier (see Video 21.1).

External Jugular Venous Catheterization

The external jugular vein is superficial and easily visible. It can be used when other attempts at peripheral IV access have been unsuccessful but can be difficult to access if airway or other procedures are occurring simultaneously. As with all other procedures, external jugular access should be discussed with parents if the clinical situation allows because parents may understandably have fears about a needle being placed in their child's neck.

Technique. The external jugular vein is most often entered with a standard over-the-needle IV catheter. The vein lies in a line from the angle of the jaw to the middle of the clavicle and is usually visible on the surface of the skin. It is more prominent when the child is crying or in Trendelenburg position. Ask an assistant to restrain the patient in a supine position with the head and neck extended and a towel roll placed under the shoulders. Turn the head approximately 40 to 70 degrees from the midline and away from the side to be punctured (see Fig. 19.4). Cleanse the skin surrounding the area to be punctured with alcohol (or another antiseptic solution). If time allows, infiltrate the overlying skin with 1% lidocaine. Place a finger just above the clavicle to distend the jugular vein.

Puncture the skin approximately one-half to two-thirds of the distance from the angle of the jaw to the clavicle. Advance the needle slowly until the jugular vein is entered. Once there is a flash in the needle hub, advance the catheter into the vein. Attach preflushed extension tubing or a syringe and obtain blood samples. Take particular care to avoid introducing air to prevent air embolism. Secure the catheter in place and apply a sterile occlusive dressing.

Complications

Serious complications of peripheral IV lines and IV fluid therapy are rare. Complications include infection, phlebitis, inadvertent arterial puncture, injection of sclerosing agents into the subcutaneous space with resultant necrosis of the skin (especially in small infants), pneumothorax, air embolism, and administration of inappropriate volumes of fluid. Puncture of the apex of the lung leading to pneumothorax is possible with external jugular puncture if the needle is inserted too far. Attention to antiseptic procedures during insertion and maintenance of the IV system decreases the risk of infection.

Peripheral Venous Catheterization: Venous Cutdown (See Also Chapter 23)

Indications and Contraindications

Peripheral venous cutdown is rarely performed in the ED because IO access is rapid and safe. Even in experienced hands, a saphenous vein cutdown may take more than 10 minutes and is associated with a higher rate of infection than other routes of vascular access. Nevertheless, if peripheral venous, central venous, or IO access cannot be obtained, venous cutdown may provide an alternative means of emergency venous access. Contraindications to peripheral venous cutdown are major trauma to the extremity, vascular injury of the extremity proximal to the intended site of cutdown, or soft tissue infection of the intended incision site. A coagulation disorder is a relative contraindication.

Equipment and Setup

Successful venous catheterization via cutdown in infants and small children requires an assistant, good lighting, and a selection of standard IV catheters or silastic catheters prefilled with NS. Sterile instruments may be available in a "cutdown tray" or can be individually assembled. Assemble regular and mosquito hemostats, fine forceps, a vein dilator, a vein lifter, silk suture, a needle driver, and fine scissors or a scalpel.

Technique

Exposure and cannulation of the saphenous vein are discussed (Fig. 19.10). The same principles apply when cutdown is performed on most peripheral veins. Begin with complete immobilization of the thigh, leg, ankle, and foot by taping them to a padded leg board. Attach this board in turn to the table or bed where the procedure is being performed (see Fig. 19.10, *step 1*). Prepare the area around the medial malleolus with antiseptic solution and drape it with sterile towels. Infiltrate 1% lidocaine in an area approximately 1 cm proximal and 1 cm anterior to the medial malleolus. No major nerves or tendons accompany the saphenous vein in this location.

Place a tourniquet proximally on the leg and make a transverse skin incision (usually approximately 2 cm in length) in the anesthetized area. Insert a small mosquito hemostat into the wound with the concavity of the clamp upward. Using the tip of the hemostat, "scoop up" all tissue lying against the bone (see Fig. 19.10, *step 2*). This will invariably lift the vein out of the wound along with the surrounding tissue. Use fine forceps or a mosquito hemostat to separate and remove all nonvenous structures so that only the saphenous vein is left tented over the hemostat (see Fig. 19.10, *step 3*). To avoid injury to the vein during dissection, spread the ends of the hemostat parallel to the direction of the vein, never transversely.

Pass two 4-0 silk sutures under the vein. Place one distally to stabilize the vein, and place the other proximal to the intended site of venipuncture. The distal suture may be tied, but if left untied it can still be used for stabilization of the vein and to occlude blood flow by applying gentle traction. Removing the untied distal suture after cannulation of the vein may allow subsequent recannulation after eventual catheter removal. Once the vein is isolated, either place a catheter surgically through a venotomy or cannulate the vein directly with a standard IV catheter. If venotomy is chosen, use fine scissors or a scalpel blade to make an oblique or V-shaped incision in the anterior wall of the vein between the sutures (see Fig. 19.10, *step 4*). Grasp the silastic catheter (prefilled with saline solution) with forceps and advance it 2 to 3 cm into the vein (see Fig. 19.10, *steps 5 and 6*). This is usually the most difficult and time-consuming portion of the procedure. Use a vein dilator, an L-shaped lifter, or a forceps to hold the venotomy incision open (see Fig. 19.10, *steps 7 and 8*). Pull downward on the distal tie to provide countertraction and stabilize the vein during advancement of the catheter. Remove the tourniquet and tie the proximal suture around the vein with the catheter inside. Take care to avoid tying the suture so tightly that it occludes the catheter. If the distal suture was tied, tie the free ends of the suture around the catheter to provide additional stability. If the distal suture was not tied, remove it at this point. Tie the proximal suture to secure the catheter, but leave the ends long

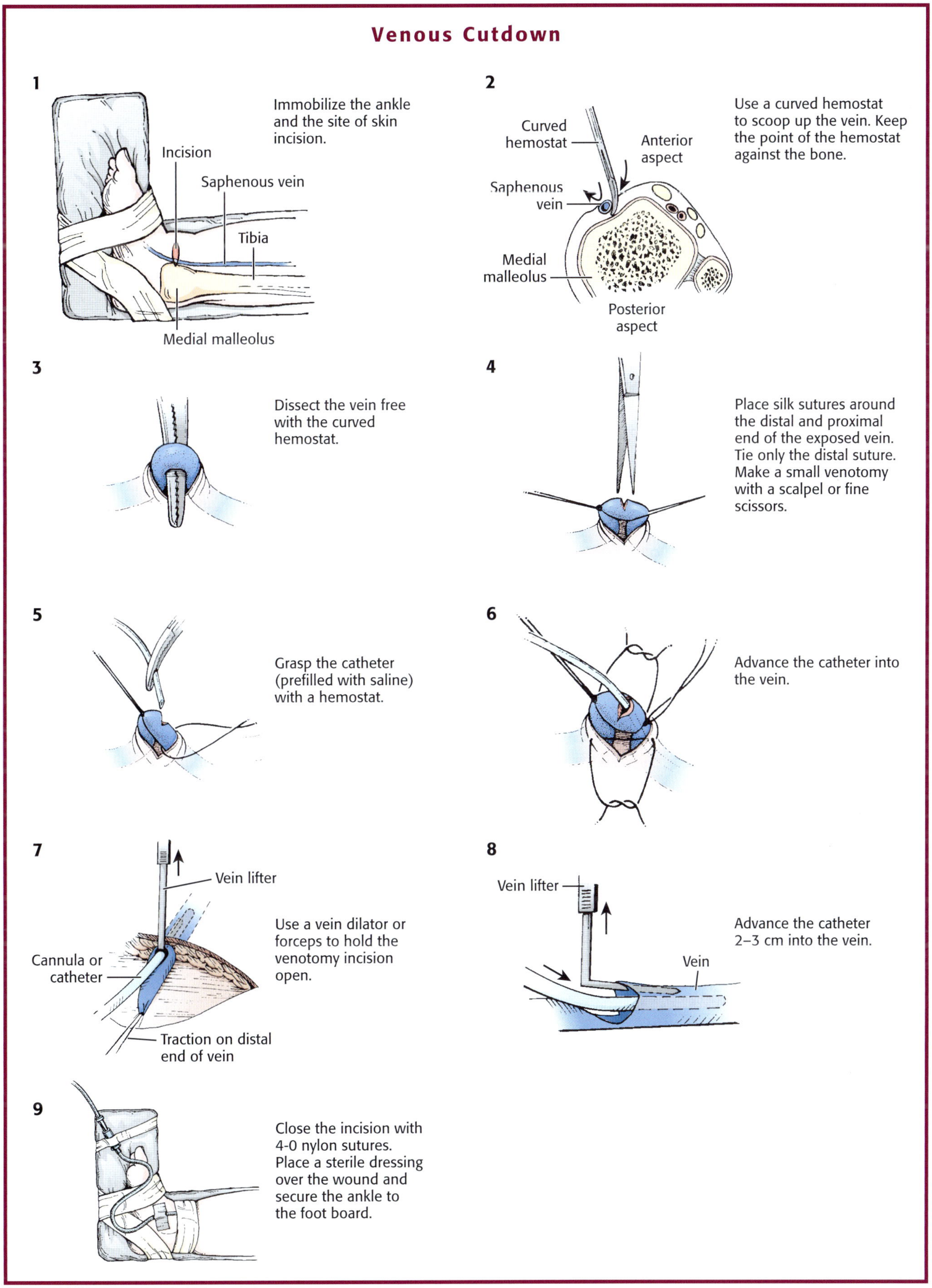

Fig. 19.10 Venous cutdown (saphenous vein). (From Suratt PM, Gibson RS. *Manual of Medical Procedures*. Mosby; 1982.)

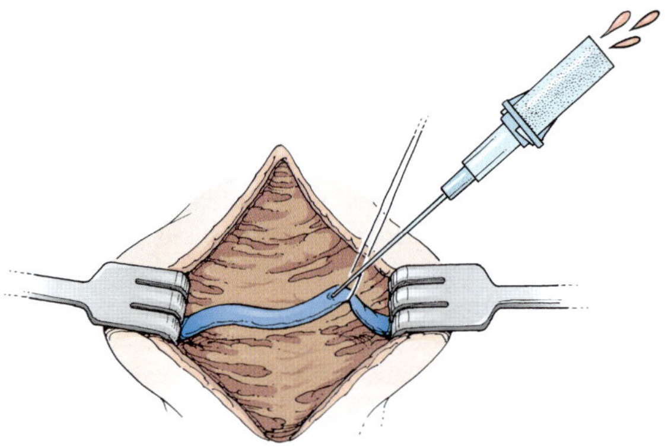

Fig. 19.11 The "mini-cutdown" procedure using a standard intravenous catheter-over-the-needle system is technically easier than a full cutdown and may be preferred in an emergency.

enough so that the suture can later be removed. This allows recannulation once the catheter is removed.

Alternatively, direct cannulation of the vein may be achieved more rapidly and, unlike venotomy, may preserve the vein for future cannulation. If direct cannulation is chosen, isolate and immobilize the vein, using a standard IV catheter to directly cannulate the vein. Essentially a percutaneous catheter insertion technique is used to catheterize a directly visualized vein (Fig. 19.11).

Continued infusion of IV fluids through the catheter from an attached syringe will ensure patency. Orient the catheter into one corner of the incision and close the incision with interrupted 4-0 nylon suture. Secure the skin suture around the IV catheter to hold the catheter in place. Control bleeding with direct pressure. Place antibiotic ointment over the wound and apply a sterile occlusive dressing. Connect the IV tubing and tape it securely to the foot board to prevent inadvertent removal of the catheter (see Fig. 19.10, *step 9*).

When cared for properly catheters can remain in place for as long as 7 to 10 days, but generally it is best to replace the catheter and insert it into another site after 3 to 4 days. Remove the catheter at the first sign of infiltration or infection. See Chapter 23 for more information on venous cutdown techniques.

Complications

In addition to the problems with percutaneous catheter placement that were discussed previously, venous cutdown can result in wound infection and thromboembolism. Adjacent structures may be injured during the incision and subsequent blunt dissection. Extravasation may result if the vein is not ligated. Light pressure on the closed wound will generally prevent continued extravasation.

Central Venous Catheterization: Percutaneous

Indications and Contraindications

Central venous cannulation is an option in the ED when peripheral venous access is limited or unachievable. In young children central line placement can almost always be delayed until after initial stabilization. Central venous lines have traditionally been used for hemodynamic monitoring, but with the use of point-of-care ultrasound in the ED and a more clinical and lab-based approach to monitoring of sepsis, this is a less common indication. While central venous access is preferred for infusion of sclerosing and long-term vasoactive medications, pediatric sepsis guidelines state that vasoactive infusions can be started via IO or peripheral venous lines, often obviating the need for central line placement in the ED.[26]

TABLE 19.1 Pediatric Central Line Sizes

AGE (Years)	WEIGHT (kg)	CATHETER SIZE (Fr)
<1	<10	3.0
1–5	10–20	4.0
6–10	20–32	5.0
11 +	32 +	6.0

This table serves as a guide for approximate sizes. Sizes may need to be adjusted based on the individual child.

Simulation can improve provider confidence and time to insertion.[27] The Agency for Healthcare Research and Quality has identified the use of ultrasound guidance for placement of central venous catheters as an important patient safety practice.[28] Use of ultrasound for central line placement increases success and decreases complications. [29–32] If ultrasound is utilized, single-use gel should be applied to the probe, then covered with a sterile sleeve. (See Chapter 22 for more information on ultrasound-guided central line placement.)

Contraindications to percutaneous placement of central venous catheters include local infection or burns at the insertion site; vascular insufficiency of an extremity; or obstruction or compression of the access veins by tumor, abnormal vessels, hematoma, or thrombus. Caution should be used in patients with uncorrected coagulopathies or with malformations or deformations distorting vascular anatomy. Attempts at central venous access should not result in a delay in medication and fluid administration during resuscitation efforts, but if a central line is in place, medications should be given centrally rather than peripherally.[33]

Equipment and Setup

Commercially available kits are convenient because they contain most of the items needed for the procedure. The catheters in these kits are typically made of a silicone elastomer, polyvinyl chloride, or polyethylene; some are available with an antimicrobial coating, which may reduce infection rates. Catheter length is variable and one- to three-lumen catheters are available. Rapid volume replacement, as in the case of severe dehydration or acute blood loss from trauma, is best achieved by inserting a short, large-bore catheter for the initial resuscitation and stabilization. Table 19.1 lists approximate central line sizes by age and weight.

Other necessary equipment includes antiseptic solution, gauze pads, sterile drapes, gowns, sterile gloves, caps, masks, syringes (3, 5, and 10 mL), sterile transparent skin coverings, Luer-Lok three-way stopcocks, 0.25% to 1% lidocaine, flush solution (10 units heparin/mL NS), and IV tubing with a T-connector extension. Depending on the vein to be accessed, restraint of the extremity, pelvis, or head may require a padded support, an assistant, or both.

Technique

Young patients should ideally be sedated, or if that is not possible, well restrained, to minimize movement during the procedure. Local anesthesia should be administered prior to central line placement. Equipment should be placed in an easily accessible location to minimize the need to reach or move while inserting the catheter. All catheter lumens should be preflushed with saline and clamped before beginning the procedure.

Strict sterile precautions with cap, gown, mask, and sterile drapes should be used when placing all but the most emergent central lines to decrease the risk of catheter-associated bloodstream infections. The skin should be cleaned with chlorhexidine in preparation for the procedure unless there is a specific contraindication to chlorhexadine.[34,35] In this case, betadine may be used.

Percutaneous placement of central venous catheters can be accomplished with either a guidewire (Seldinger) technique or an over-the-needle catheter. It can be difficult to thread a guidewire in young children; one technique to maximize the chance of placing a usable catheter is to use the over-the-needle catheter from the central line kit for the initial puncture in lieu of the needle alone. Once the vein is accessed and the needle removed, the catheter can be left in place for initial resuscitation or the guidewire can be advanced through the catheter. If the guidewire can be threaded into the vein, the catheter can then be removed, the skin dilated, and the longer central catheter can be placed over the wire. If the guidewire cannot be advanced sufficiently through the catheter, remove the guidewire and leave the catheter in place for venous access. The catheter-over-the-needle technique can be used in the femoral, subclavian, or internal jugular (IJ) veins.

When the guidewire technique is used, either through a needle or catheter, always gently pass the wire. The wire should not meet resistance. If resistance to passage of the wire is encountered, remove it to assess the needle's position within the vessel. If resistance to removal of the wire is encountered, do not force the guidewire out through the needle, as it can shear off a portion of the guidewire. In these situations, the wire and needle may need to be removed together and the procedure restarted, unless an appropriate wire position can be verified via ultrasound and the needle removed. Throughout the procedure, make certain that a portion of the wire is visible and that the operator maintains control of the wire to prevent inadvertent passage of the entirety of the wire into the vein. Occlude the hub of the open finder needle or catheter with a sterile gloved finger when the wire is not in place to prevent excessive blood loss or air embolism.

Once the wire is in place and the catheter or needle removed, make a small incision (1 to 2 mm) with a No. 11 scalpel blade in the skin at the wire's entry point to allow passage of the dilator (Fig. 19.12, *step 2*) and the catheter itself. When making the incision, point the sharp edge of the blade away from the wire. When using a multilumen catheter, as is commonly used in small children, advance the dilator gently over the wire and then remove the dilator. Then advance the catheter over the wire and into the vein (see Fig. 19.12, *step 3*). Remove the wire. When using a Cordis, the line and dilator are introduced together and then dilator and wire are removed simultaneously. Withdraw blood from the catheter ports and then flush them with a sterile saline solution. Secure the catheter or Cordis to the skin with silk or nylon sutures (see Fig. 19.12, *step 4*). Place a sterile, transparent, and impermeable dressing over the exit site.

Femoral Catheterization

Femoral venous catheterization is the central venous access route most commonly used in infants and children in emergency situations (Fig. 19.12). The anatomy is fairly straightforward and the femoral arterial pulse provides a good landmark for femoral venous catheterization. The femoral site is advantageous because the risk of mechanical complications is low. In the event of inadvertent arterial puncture or venous laceration, hemostasis can be achieved by the application of direct pressure. Femoral vein catheterization does not carry any risk for hemothorax or pneumothorax. An advantage is that placement of a femoral catheter is less likely to interfere with other resuscitative procedures than placement of a subclavian or IJ catheter.

Technique. Restrain the child adequately to permit exposure of the inguinal region. Use an introducer needle with or without a syringe to enter the femoral vein. If using landmarks rather than ultrasound to locate the vein, palpate the femoral artery with one finger, and puncture the skin just medial to the artery. Ultrasound can also be used to identify the femoral vein and determine the location of the femoral artery. Enter the skin at a 30- to 45-degree angle approximately 1 cm below the inguinal ligament. Direct the needle in a line toward the umbilicus. When the vein is accessed, follow the steps outlined in central line technique above to complete the procedure.

Note that during cardiopulmonary resuscitation (CPR), palpable pulsations or Doppler tones in the femoral vein may be detected. Hence, if the vein is not found medial to the pulsations, consider catheterization of the pulsating vessel during CPR as a last resort when other options for vascular access or drug delivery are unavailable. Alternatively, ultrasound can be used to locate the femoral vein.

Internal Jugular Venous Catheterization

The IJ veins lie within the carotid sheath along with the carotid artery and vagus nerve. The lower part of the vein lies within the triangle formed by the sternal and clavicular heads of the sternocleidomastoid muscle and then becomes more lateral and anterior to the artery as it joins the subclavian vein. The right IJ vein is preferred over the left because the IJ, the innominate vein, and the superior vena cava form a nearly straight line into the right atrium and pneumothorax rates appear to be lower.[36] Placement of IJ venous access may not be possible when other critical procedures are occurring and it is not possible if the patient is in a cervical spine immobilization device.

Technique. Three approaches to IJ catheterization are possible (including the anterior, median or central, and posterior approaches, as discussed in Chapter 22). The median or central approach is described here. Use of ultrasound to guide cannulation of the IJ vein appears to improve success rates (see Chapters 22 and 67).[37] Position the child supine with the head rotated 30 degrees to the contralateral side. The Trendelenburg position will distend the vein. For the medial or central approach, use the apex of the angle formed by the sternal and clavicular heads of the sternocleidomastoid muscle as the puncture site. If a line were drawn from the mastoid process to the sternal notch, the apex of the angle formed by the two muscular heads would fall approximately along the middle third of that line. Introduce a needle attached to a syringe at the apex of the triangle at an angle of 30 degrees downward and toward the ipsilateral nipple (Fig. 19.13). Advance the needle slowly until the jugular vein is entered. Keep the syringe connected to the needle at all times to maintain constant

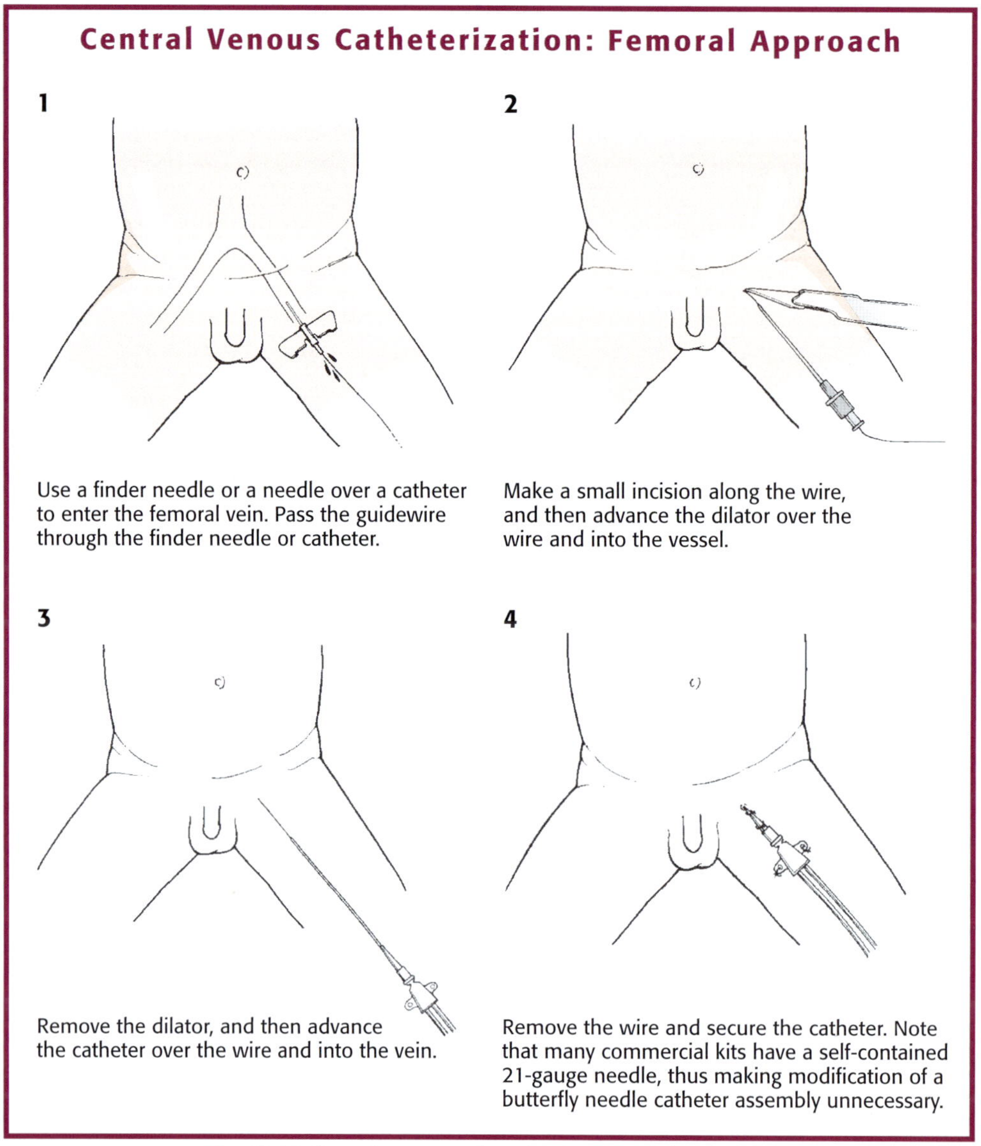

Fig. 19.12 Central venous catheterization: femoral approach.

negative pressure and avoid air embolism. After blood flow is obtained, remove the syringe and place a finger over the hub of the needle. Insert a guidewire following the technique described above. Confirm proper location of the catheter and rule out pneumothorax with a chest radiograph.

If ultrasound is used, it can be helpful in identifying the position of the carotid artery and minimize the chance of accidental puncture. Although the right IJ is typically larger, patients can be identified who have a larger left IJ. Beginning with a short-axis view to identify the carotid and assess the diameter of the IJ, then switching to long axis to confirm wire placement is recommended.[38]

Subclavian Venous Catheterization

The subclavian vein is used less frequently for central venous access in children than in adults (see Fig. 19.13). The technique is more difficult in pediatric patients because of the smaller size of the vessel, as well as a more cephalad location under the clavicles.

Technique. The approach to the vein is more lateral in children than in adults. The infraclavicular approach is described. Place a towel roll under the shoulders when possible. The right side is preferred because the dome of the lung is more cephalad on the left side. The needle insertion site is at the distal third of the clavicle in the depression created between the deltoid and the pectoralis major muscles.

Introduce the finder needle bevel up and advance it slowly while applying negative pressure with the attached syringe. Keep the syringe and needle parallel to the frontal plane. Direct the needle medially and slightly cephalad, beneath the clavicle toward the posterior aspect of the sternal end of the clavicle (i.e., toward a fingertip placed in the sternal notch). Advance the needle until blood return is obtained. Turn the syringe so that the bevel of the needle points caudad to direct the guidewire to the superior vena cava. Remove the syringe from the needle and insert the wire during a positive pressure breath or natural exhalation. Remove the needle and introduce the catheter over the wire via the Seldinger technique, as previously described. The cardiac monitor may show a rhythm disturbance if the wire is advanced too far. Remove the wire and secure the catheter in place with sutures and apply a sterile, occlusive dressing. Perform auscultation of bilateral breath sounds and obtain a chest radiograph to confirm proper

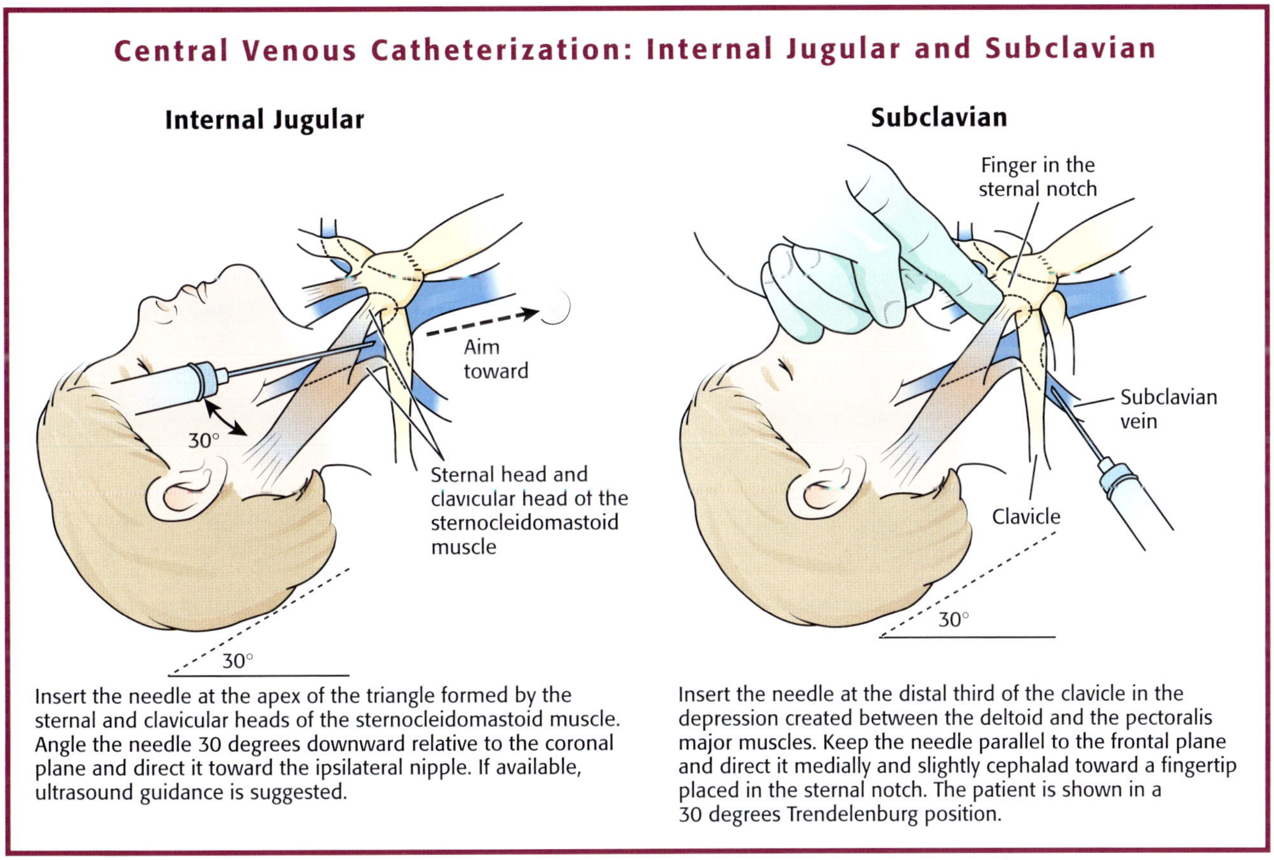

Fig. 19.13 Central venous catheterization: internal jugular and subclavian approaches.

positioning of the catheter in the superior vena cava and to rule out procedural complications such as pneumothorax or hemothorax.

In a small study, there was no difference between supraclavicular and infraclavicular placement of subclavian lines in infants, though supraclavicular placement is a rarely used technique in young children.[39] Another small study exploring the utility of a supraclavicular approach informed by ultrasound with the 13-6 MHz 25-mm linear array probe placed in the right supraclavicular region showed a 90% success rate if a full venous view was achieved (compared with 41% if a suboptimal view was seen). This was done by placing the probe at the level of the cricoid cartilage to achieve a cross-sectional view, then moving caudally to visualize the subclavian-IJ junction, and rotating medially to find the brachiocephalic vein as it courses next to the pleura. The needle was then inserted close to the long axis of the probe.[40]

Complications

Infection, thrombosis, and arterial puncture are the major risks associated with central venous catheters. The risks of pneumothorax and hemothorax are approximately 2% and 1%, respectively, with subclavian catheter placement.[35] Pneumothorax is a less frequent complication of IJ catheter insertion. Other complications include accidental displacement, phlebitis, hemorrhage, hematoma, dysrhythmia, air embolism, vascular obstruction or perforation, right atrial perforation, catheter fracture and localized edema. Central line–associated bloodstream infection occurs in approximately 1.57 per 1000 device days, with higher rates in transplant and hematology/oncology patients, as well as patients with multiple episodes of the central line being accessed.[41] Literature is mixed on femoral location as a significant contributor to infection.[42–46] Sterile technique on placement and utilization of central lines, as well as daily review of necessity and prompt removal minimize risk of catheter-associated bloodstream infections.

Emergency Vascular Access

Vascular access is a key component of any resuscitation to allow the administration of fluid and medications and to obtain blood samples. However, achieving venous access during pediatric resuscitation can challenge even the most seasoned clinician, not infrequently requiring 10 or more minutes. Children who are successfully resuscitated have vascular access achieved significantly sooner than those not resuscitated. Emergency IV access is most prolonged in children younger than 2 years, the age group in which the majority of cardiopulmonary arrests occur.

For these reasons, clinicians should obtain IO access in critical patients if IV access is not established quickly, rather than delay treatment with attempts to place peripheral or central venous catheters (see Chapter 25).[33] IO lines are easily and rapidly placed, can accept any drug given parenterally in similar doses, and are likely underused in many EDs.[47] If no IV or IO line is available, certain drugs can be given via the endotracheal tube (see Chapter 26) while attempts at venous access are initiated. However, endotracheal drug administration has been shown to be less efficacious than IV administration in adults, and this route of administration should be used only when no alternatives are available. Recently, intranasal medications have been shown useful for specific conditions such as fentanyl for pain or midazolam for seizures. Placement of an

IJ, subclavian, or femoral line can prove time-consuming[48] and is thus discouraged in the initial resuscitation of the unstable patient. Umbilical and IO lines are effective alternatives.

Umbilical Vein Catheterization

Indications and Contraindications

The primary indication for umbilical vein catheterization is the need to access the vascular system for emergency resuscitation and stabilization of neonates. It may also be used for exchange transfusions and short-term central venous access in newborns. The umbilical vein may remain patent for up to 2 weeks after birth. In neonates who require emergency access in the ED, a peripheral vein would be preferable, but attempting to cannulate one of the umbilical vessels could be lifesaving. Omphalitis, omphalocele, gastroschisis, and peritonitis are all contraindications to access of the umbilical artery or vein.

Equipment and Setup

Place the infant beneath a radiant warmer because keeping the infant warm during the procedure is critical. Restrain the extremities. Wear a mask, cap, gown, and sterile gloves. For umbilical lines anticipated to be maintained for a long period of time, depth of insertion is important and should be assessed before the procedure. For emergent lines, the depth of insertion will be no more than 4 to 5 cm. An umbilical line or sterile feeding tube can be used.

Technique

Hold the umbilical stump upright and scrub the cord with a bactericidal solution. Avoid pooling of liquid at the infant's side because this may be associated with blistering of the skin under a radiant warmer. Drape the umbilical area in sterile fashion with the infant's head left exposed for observation (Video 19.2).

Place a loop of umbilical tape or a purse-string suture at the junction of the skin and the cord to provide hemostasis and to anchor the line after placement (Fig. 19.14, *step 1*). Cut the cord with a scalpel approximately 1 cm from the skin (often less in infants who are not newly born), and identify the vessels. There are two arteries and one vein in the umbilicus. The vein is usually located at 12 o'clock and has a thin wall and large lumen. It may continue to bleed after cutting. The two arteries have thicker walls and smaller lumens. Constriction reduces bleeding after the arterial vessels are cut. Occasionally, a persistent urachus may be mistaken for the umbilical vein, but the presence of urine in the urachus may help correctly identify that structure.

Flush the catheter (3.5 Fr [preterm infants] to 5.0 Fr [term infants]) with heparinized saline and attach it to a three-way stopcock. Place the catheter into the lumen of the umbilical vein and advance it gently (Fig. 19.14, *step 2*). An umbilical vein line can be placed in a fashion that is intended either for emergency use or for more chronic use. In an emergency case, advance the catheter only 1 to 2 cm beyond the point at which good blood return is obtained. This is usually only 4 to 5 cm in a term-sized infant. Beyond this distance, the umbilical vein branches, and a catheter inserted further can enter a branch of the portal vein within the liver (as evidenced by resistance at 5 to 10 cm). Infusion of medications into a catheter in the portal vein can result in liver necrosis. In an emergent case, a line placed no greater than 5 cm into the patient can be used without confirmatory radiographs. If used for more than a brief period of time, the line can migrate, so depth of insertion should be reassessed periodically.[49]

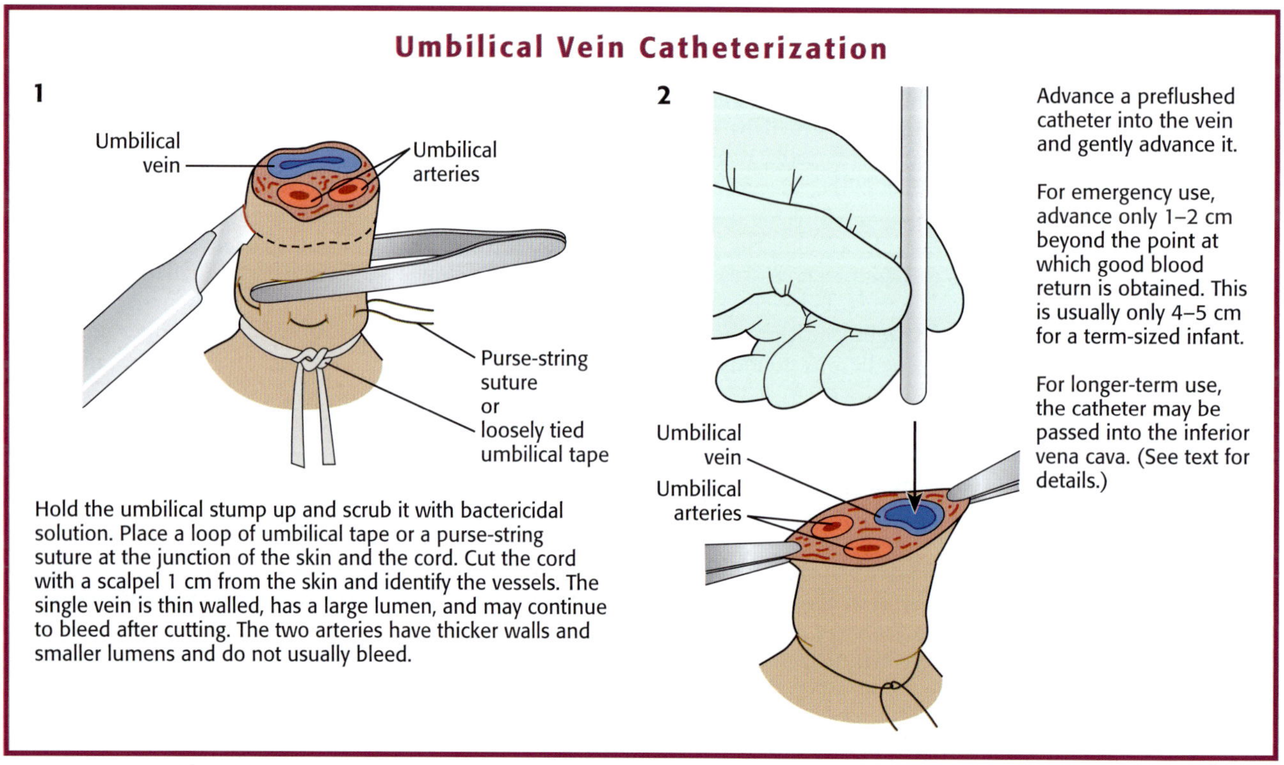

Fig. 19.14 Umbilical vein catheterization. (From Zaoutis L, Chiang V. *Comprehensive Pediatric Hospital Medicine.* Elsevier; 2007.)

If the patient does not require emergent access and a more enduring line is desired for blood draws, monitoring central venous pressure or infusion of medications, high concentrations of glucose (>10%), IV fluids, and hyperalimentation solutions, then the line is instead inserted 10 to 12 cm in a term-sized infant to reach the inferior vena cava (IVC). Because of the potential for placement into the portal vein and resultant complications, radiographs are required prior to usage to confirm placement into the IVC. Note that an umbilical venous catheter will proceed directly cephalad (without making a downward loop) until it passes through the ductus venosus (Fig. 19.15). Some practitioners use standardized graphs to estimate the length of insertion for these lines. Such graphs are based on the shoulder-to-umbilicus length (Fig. 19.16A). Shoulder-to-umbilicus length is the perpendicular line measured from the tip of the shoulder to the horizontal level of the umbilicus. Formulas based on birth weight, such as (1.5 × birth weight in kg) + 5.5 cm, can further guide placement.[50] Ultrasound may be helpful in helping guide placement, though is not currently gold standard for determining successful placement or location.[51–53]

Air embolism may occur at the time of catheter removal if the infant generates sufficient negative intrathoracic pressure (as during crying) and causes air to be drawn into the patent umbilical vein. Therefore, caution must be used during removal of the catheter to ensure that the vein is promptly occluded (by tightening a purse-string suture or applying pressure on or just cephalad to the umbilicus). This will also help to secure the catheter in place. Another method described for securing the catheter is to use an umbilical clamp.[54] Additionally, the catheter can be taped to abdomen with an H-frame of tape demonstrates taping of an umbilical artery line; an umbilical venous line can be taped similarly).

An alternative method has been described. In this method, maintain the clamp on the umbilical cord, then make a cut proximally in the amniotic membrane over the umbilical vein and bluntly dissect through Wharton's jelly down to the vein. At this point, place a catheter into the umbilical vein through this site. The remainder of the procedure is identical to the

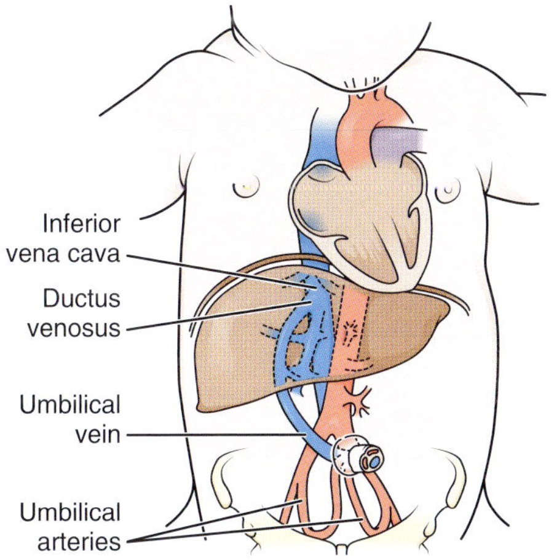

Fig. 19.15 An umbilical venous catheter will proceed directly cephalad (without making a downward loop) until it passes through the ductus venosus.

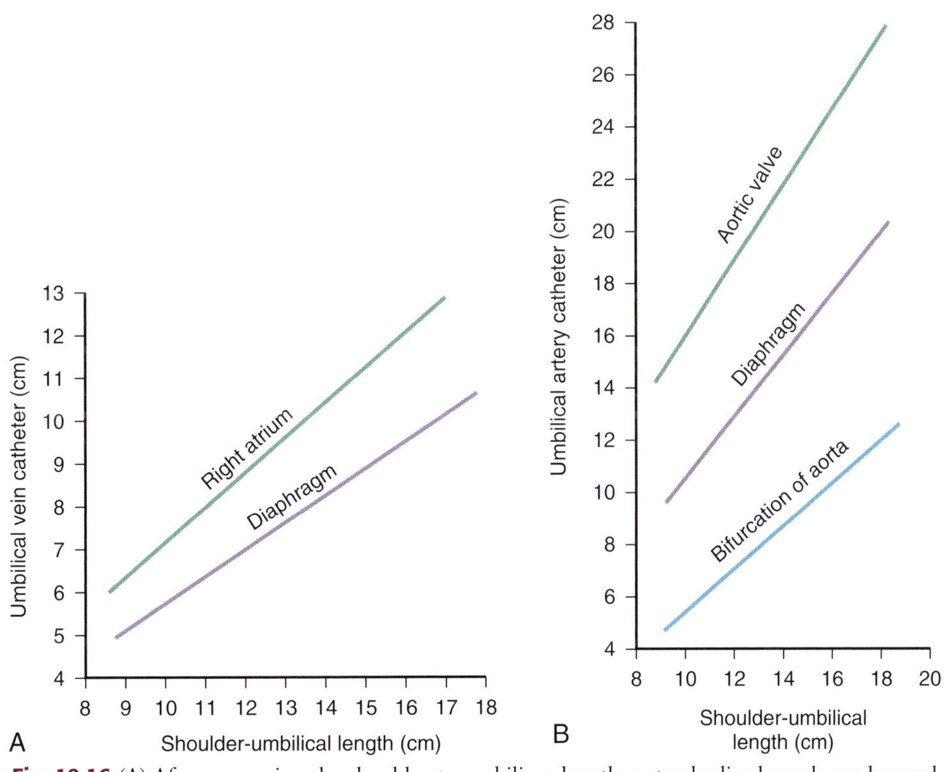

Fig. 19.16 (A) After measuring the shoulder-to-umbilicus length, a standardized graph can be used to determine the appropriate length of the umbilical venous catheter, or (B) the umbilical arterial catheter. The venous catheter should be inserted into the inferior vena cava below the level of the right atrium. The appropriate length of the arterial catheter depends on whether a "high" or "low" line is desired (see text for explanation). (From The Johns Hopkins Hospital, Nechyba C, Gunn VL. *The Harriet Lane Handbook: A Manual for Pediatric House Officers*, 16th ed. Mosby; 2002.)

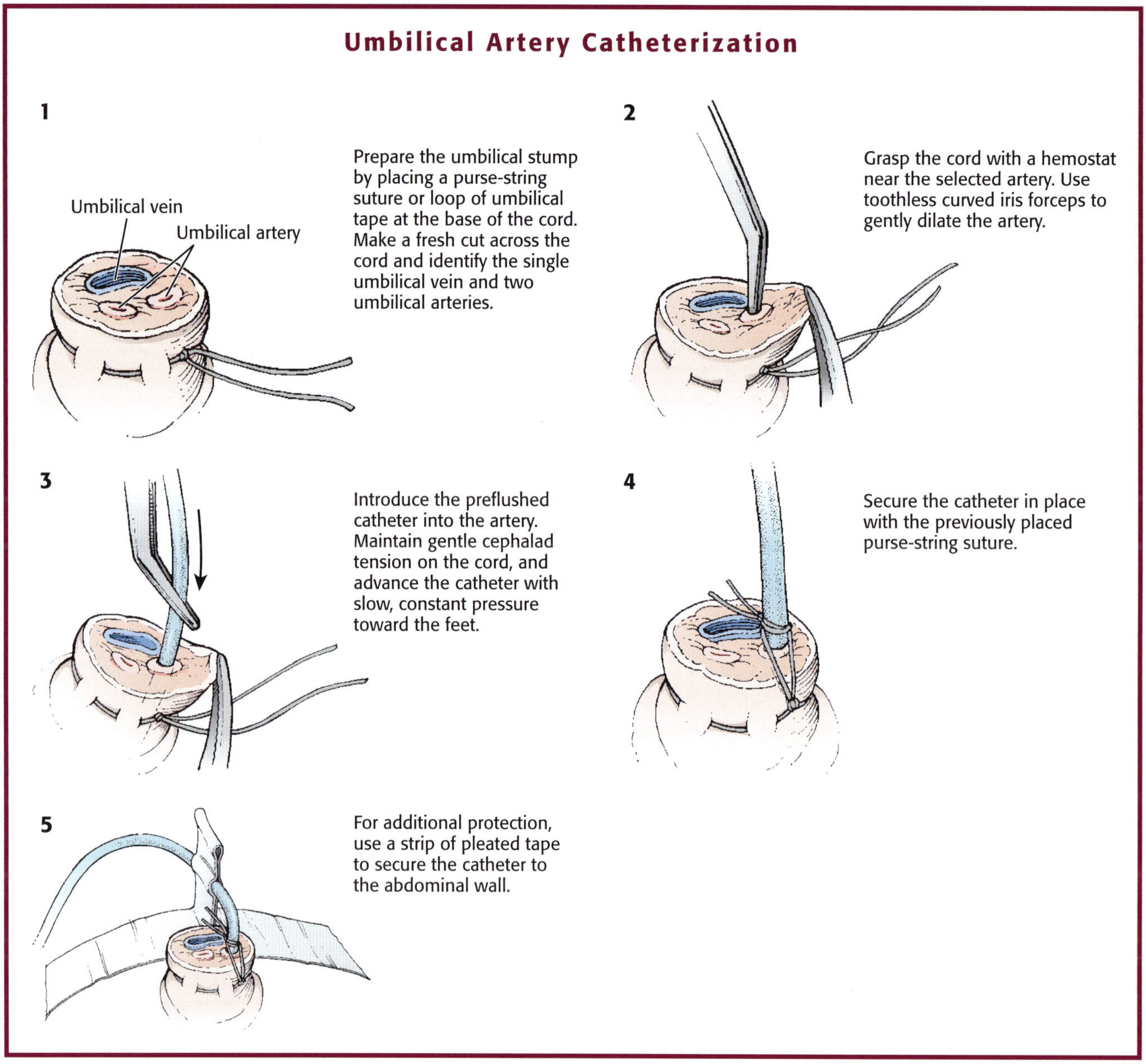

Fig. 19.17 Umbilical artery catheterization.

standard technique. This option may be attractive in situations where transecting the cord proximal to the site of the clamp is not possible or not desired.[55] Use of a 14-gauge angiocatheter with the needle removed has been described, and may be an option if an umbilical line or feeding tube is not readily available.[56]

Complications

Complications of umbilical venous catheters include hemorrhage, infection, injection of sclerosing substances into the liver (resulting in hepatic necrosis), air embolism, catheter tip embolism and resultant ischemia (including myocardial infarction), liver hematoma, arrhythmias, effusions, malplacement, and vessel perforation,[57–59] at a rate of 13.4%.[60] Studies suggest that umbilical venous catheters have thrombosis rate lower than femoral catheters,[61] and an infection rate comparable to femoral venous catheters or PICC lines.[62] Patients with a long catheter duration or prematurity have a higher risk of complications.[63]

Umbilical Artery Catheterization

Indications and Contraindications

Umbilical artery catheterization is a useful procedure in the care of newborn infants who require frequent monitoring of ABGs and arterial blood pressure, fluid and medication administration, exchange transfusions, and some interventional procedures.[64] Either one of the two umbilical arteries may be cannulated for resuscitation purposes, but an umbilical vein is generally technically easier to cannulate and may be preferred in an emergency. These arteries can typically be accessed up to 7 days after birth.[65] This is not typically a procedure that is required in the emergency setting. Contraindications include those described in umbilical venous access, as well as necrotizing enterocolitis.

Equipment and Setup

The equipment required for umbilical artery catheterization is identical to that used for umbilical venous catheterization. Additional equipment needed for continuous arterial pressure monitoring and infusion should be readily available. Estimate the catheter length needed before starting the procedure. Do this by using a standard graph (Fig. 19.16B) or a birth weight regression formula.

Technique

The technique of umbilical artery catheterization is similar to that described for umbilical vein catheterization in the preceding section. After the umbilical arteries have been located (Fig. 19.17, *step 1*), grasp the cord with a curved hemostat near the selected artery. Ask an assistant to use two hemostats to grasp each side of the cord and slightly evert the edges to aid in exposure of the arteries. Alternatively, a suture placed through the wall of the vessel and part of cord can be used to elevate the vessel for cannulation.[66] Using curved iris forceps without teeth, gently dilate the artery (Fig. 19.17, *step 2*). Sometimes, repeated passes of the forceps are required because the umbilical artery can spasm and make the procedure difficult. Attach an umbilical catheter or feeding tube to a three-way stopcock and flush it with a sterile heparinized solution. Introduce the catheter into the dilated artery (Fig. 19.17, *step 3*). Use a 3.5-Fr catheter for infants weighing less than 2 kg. For those weighing 2 kg or more, a 3.5-Fr or 5-Fr catheter can be used, depending on artery size.

When the catheter is being inserted, place gentle tension on the cord in a cephalad direction, and advance the catheter with slow, constant pressure toward the feet. Resistance is occasionally felt at 1 to 2 cm. Overcome this with gentle, sustained pressure. On the other hand, if the catheter passes 4 to 5 cm and then meets resistance, this generally indicates that a "false passage" through the vessel wall has occurred, with the catheter curving caudad. Occasionally, one may bypass the perforation by reattempting catheterization with a larger catheter.

Acceptable positions of umbilical artery catheters are between T6 and T9 ("high line") and between L3 and L5, just above the aortic bifurcation ("low line"), as confirmed by radiograph. High lines are associated with a lower incidence of thrombotic complications.[67] Graphs and formulas can be used to estimate the proper catheter length for insertion at both the high and low positions (see Fig. 19.16B), but confirm placement with a radiograph. These formulas may not be as accurate in babies at the extremes of weight. The formula (4 × birth weight in kg) + 7 cm, accurately predicts high-line location 83% of the time.[68] Once sterile technique is broken, do not advance the line. Therefore it is preferable to position the catheter too high and to withdraw it as necessary according to postinsertion radiographs. The anticipated course of the catheter is proceeding from the umbilicus down toward the pelvis, making an acute turn into the internal iliac artery, continuing toward the head into the bifurcation of the aorta, and then moving up the aorta slightly to the left of the vertebral column (Fig. 19.18). After it has been properly positioned, tie the catheter with the previously placed suture and tape it to the abdominal wall (see Fig. 19.17, *steps 4 and 5*).

Complications

Complications of umbilical artery catheterization include hemorrhage, infection, thromboembolic phenomena (especially involving the kidneys, gastrointestinal tract, and lower

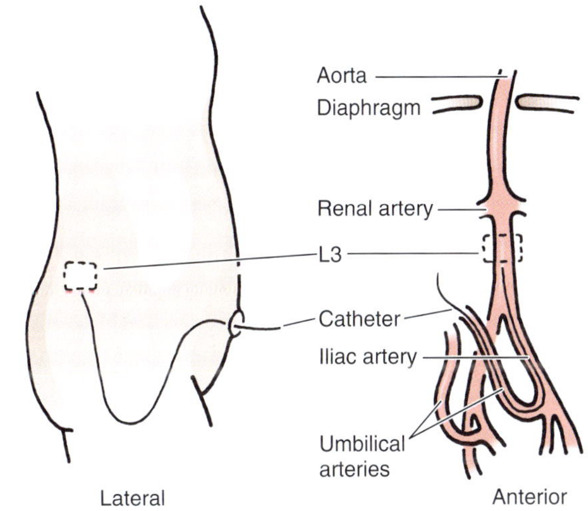

Fig. 19.18 The umbilical artery catheter makes a loop downward before heading cephalad (schematic drawing of a radiograph interpretation).

extremities), aortic thrombosis, aortic aneurysm/dissection, vasospasm, air embolism, vessel perforation, peritoneal perforation, nerve lesions, hypertension or renal failure from renal artery obstruction and complications of occlusion of the mesenteric arteries causing bowel ischemia, infarction and necrotizing enterocolitis.[69–73] If placed too high, the catheter position can be responsible for refractory hypoglycemia.

If the catheter becomes plugged or fails to function properly, or if there is blanching or discoloration of the buttocks, heels, or toes, remove the catheter at once. Umbilical arteries are most easily cannulated in the first few hours of life but may provide a viable vascular route as late as 5 to 7 days after birth.

Intraosseous Catheterization (See Also Chapter 25)

Compared to other forms of access, the IO line is rapid, cost-effective, and has a high success rate.[74] In the simulation setting, IO lines were placed an average of 46 seconds more quickly than umbilical lines without a significant difference in adverse events for neonatal resuscitations.[75] Success rates are typically around 92%[76] with less success in neonates, likely due to the small size of the marrow cavity. In spite of this, IO lines have not been associated with increased survival rates in cardiac arrest patients; in fact, there are some data suggesting decreased survival.[77] This delivery system makes use of the venous sinusoids in the medullary cavity of the long bones to infuse fluids, medications, and blood products into the venous system. Potential sites include the flat portion of the proximal tibia (1 cm medial and 1 fingerbreadth below the tibial tuberosity), distal femur, medial malleolus (2 cm above), humeral head, distal radius, and ulna. The sternum is a potential IO site; however, its use is not recommended with most modern drill sets. In growing children, care must be taken to avoid the growth plate.[65]

Indications and Contraindications

IO access is recommended when peripheral access cannot be obtained safely at a pace that matches the illness of the child. Because the fluid can extravasate into the surrounding tissue causing a compartment syndrome, IO access should be avoided in a bone that is fractured or in which an IO line has been attempted within the previous 24 hours.[78] A proximal vascular injury, bony or overlying infection, and osteogenesis imperfecta are also contraindications. Typically, the duration of use of an IO line is limited to 24 hours.[79]

Equipment and Setup

IO access can be achieved with the use of manual or mechanical puncture. The mechanical options include spring-loaded devices and reusable drills. In infants and children, both are successful, with more time required for manual insertion.[80] If a reusable drill is used, different sized needles are available depending on the weight and habitus of the patient. Needle options for the EZ-IO (Teleflex) include pink 15-mm (3 to 39 kg), blue 25-mm (>40 kg), and yellow 45-mm (>40 kg with excess subcutaneous tissue) needles. Typically, the pink needles are used for pediatric patients receiving tibial IO lines; however, consideration should be given to use of a longer needle if the line penetrates more soft tissue (e.g., femoral IO).

Technique

All IO lines should be performed with sterile technique. The proximal tibia (2 fingerbreadths caudal and 1 fingerbreadth medial to the lower pole of the patella) is preferred in children. Alternatively, the distal femur (midline and 2 to 3 cm above the superior pole of the patella) or the humeral head at the greater tubercle) are options. The proximal humerus allows for flow rates comparable to the tibia, but can be difficult in children <7 years due to the ossification center in that area not forming until 5 years of age. After sterile preparation, the needle is held at a 90-degree angle to the bone and inserted. If a manual IO needle is used, a rotary motion will ease passage through the bone, whereas the drills are held stationary, and perform the rotary motion independent of the operator. A slight "give" or "pop" signifies that the needle is through the first cortex and into the medullary space. It is imperative to stop at that point to prevent penetration out of the bone into the soft tissue. The needle should stand unassisted if it is firmly implanted in the bone. Often bone marrow can be aspirated to confirm placement, and to send for laboratory analysis. If labs are drawn, hemoglobin/hematocrit, glucose, blood urea nitrogen (BUN), creatinine, chloride, and albumin are reliable. Catheters are provided with some needles. The line should be flushed with 5 to 10 mL of saline while the provider's hand is on the patient's calf (or area surrounding the medullary space used) to confirm that fluid is not extravasating into the soft tissue.

In an awake patient, administration of preservative-free lidocaine (typically, lidocaine intended for IV use in arrhythmias) prior to the initiation of fluid can mitigate the pain associated with distension of the medullary cavity. The usual lidocaine dose in adults is 20 to 50 mg, and in children 0.5 mg/kg. Maximum gravity flow rates of 20 mL/min and pressure-driven rates of 40 mL/min are achievable, and standard resuscitation medications, including vasopressors, glucose, and blood products, can be infused.[65] Pushing fluid via a syringe or the use of a pressure bag may be necessary to allow an acceptable rate of delivery in a critically ill patient. Most commercial drill-based IO needles come with materials to secure the needle once inserted. For those that do not, a simple solution is to surround the needle and proximal tubing with a small inverted paper cup with the bottom removed and the cup taped to the leg (Fig. 19.19) if a device to secure the line is not included with the device.

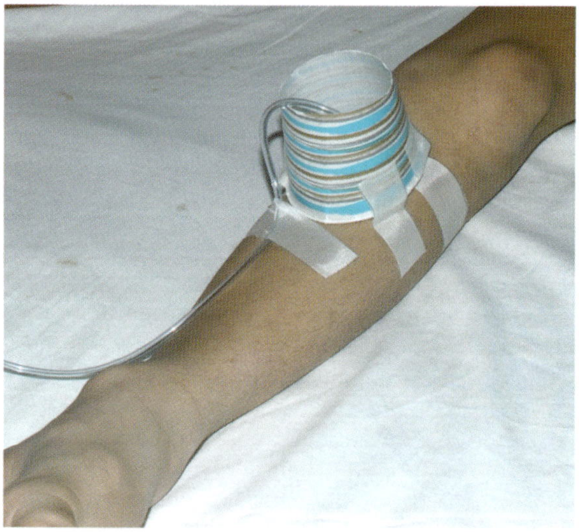

Fig. 19.19 Intraosseous line protected by a paper cup.

Complications

Complications of IO access are rare,[81] and include cellulitis, osteomyelitis, bony fracture, fat or bone marrow embolism, and extravasation of fluid into the extraosseous tissue leading to compartment syndrome.[50] When minor complications, like dermal abrasion or dislodgement, are included, complication rates are 7% to 20% for manual placement and 0% to 26% for drill placement.[76,82] If both cortices of a bone have been penetrated and fluid extravasates, a new bone must be selected. Depending on the amount of fluid that has extravasated, monitoring for compartment syndrome may be indicated. Clearly, use of the sternum may be associated with additional risks, due to the potential for trauma if both cortices of the sternum are penetrated.

Percutaneous Arterial Catheterization

Indications and Contraindications

Despite the growing use of noninvasive devices for monitoring transcutaneous oxygen and carbon dioxide, percutaneous peripheral artery catheterization may be indicated when there is a need for frequent blood gas sampling, continuous monitoring of arterial blood pressure, or both. However, mounting evidence supports minimizing the frequency of ABG sampling; therefore, this is not an intervention that should be considered mandatory in the intubated intensive care unit patient.[83–86] Arteries used for peripheral catheters in infants and children include the radial, ulnar, femoral, dorsalis pedis, and posterior tibial arteries. If preductal blood gas values are required, the right radial artery is used. This procedure is rarely performed in the ED.

Peripheral arterial catheterization is contraindicated when: (1) adequate peripheral artery samples can be obtained by percutaneous puncture, (2) the circulation of the extremity to be catheterized is compromised, (3) occlusion of the vessel to be catheterized compromises perfusion of the extremity, (4) there is an ongoing bleeding diathesis, (5) localized infection or inflammation overlies the artery to be cannulated, (6) intensive monitoring of line function is not available, or (7) vascular grafts are present in the extremity.

Equipment and Setup

The equipment needed for arterial catheterization is essentially the same as that required for percutaneous peripheral

Radial Artery Catheterization

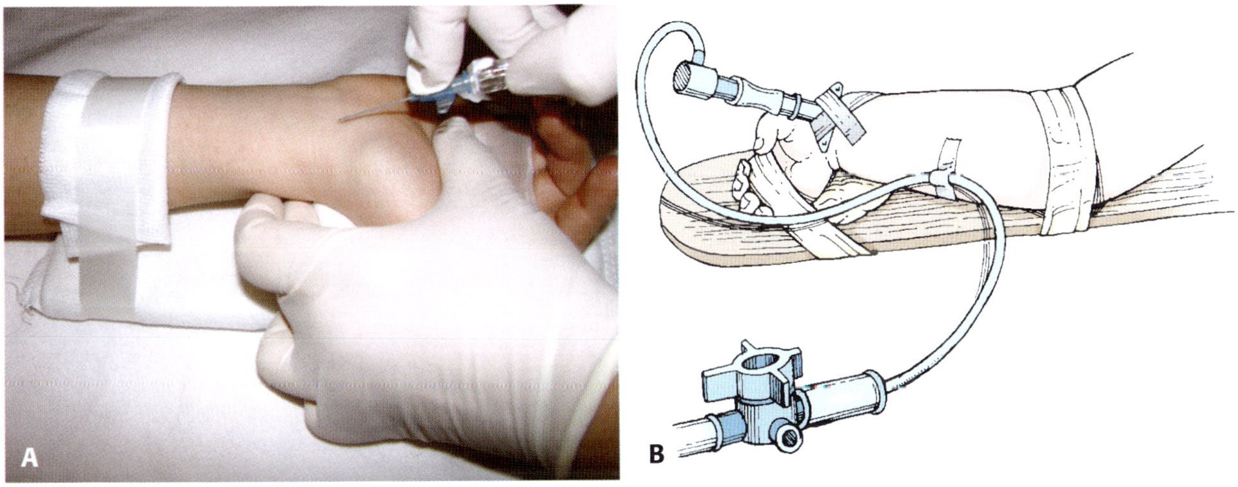

Introduce the catheter assembly into the radial artery through the skin at a 10- to 20-degree angle. This is a smaller angle than that used for simple arterial puncture.

One technique of taping the arterial catheter. The arm board should be well padded and secured.

Fig. 19.20 Radial artery catheterization. (See Fig. 20.5 for additional details on this technique.)

venous catheterization. Some centers use commercially available arterial line kits, which come with all the necessary supplies and equipment. Alternatively, standard 22- or 24-gauge over-the-needle IV catheters, a T-piece connector, and a three-way stopcock can be used. Connect the T-piece and the stopcock and then fill them with NS solution. Prepare an infusion pump with heparinized saline.

Technique

Perform the procedure with good lighting and an adequate work area and monitor the infant's heart rate and respiratory rate closely. Palpate the radial artery proximal to the transverse wrist crease on the palmar surface of the wrist, medial to the styloid process of the radius. The ulnar artery is occasionally larger than the radial in children, and can be attempted as well.[87] Before the procedure, compress the artery and observe the hand and fingers for change in color. If blanching or cyanosis is noted (indicating poor collateral circulation), do not perform catheterization. If locating the artery by palpation is difficult, a transillumination device, Doppler probe, or ultrasound may be helpful. Use of ultrasound improves success rate over Doppler alone.[88–90] A small body of data indicates that local use of topical or subcutaneous lidocaine may facilitate placement of a peripheral arterial catheter.[91]

Secure the infant's or child's hand and lower part of the forearm to an arm board, with the wrist dorsiflexed 45 to 60 degrees by placing a roll of gauze underneath it. Take care to leave the fingers exposed to allow assessment of the peripheral circulation. Palpate the radial artery at the point of maximal impulse and mark it by making a gentle indentation with a gloved fingernail. Prepare the area over the radial artery with povidone-iodine or another antiseptic solution and wash it with alcohol. Use a topical or local anesthetic (such as 1% lidocaine without epinephrine), or both, at the planned insertion site. Insert the catheter with the needle through the skin just proximal to the transverse wrist crease at a 10- to 20-degree angle (Fig. 19.20A). With the bevel of the needle facing proximally, advance the catheter slowly until blood appears in the catheter hub, which signifies puncture of the anterior arterial wall. Slowly advance the catheter until blood appears in the needle and then carefully lower the angle of the needle to approximately 10 degrees. Slowly advance the catheter over the needle and into the lumen of the artery. Remove the needle. Attach the stopcock and T-piece connector to the catheter hub. Open the stopcock to the syringe to confirm return of pulsatile blood. Flush it with 0.5 mL of heparinized solution very gently to clear the catheter and observe the fingers and the hand for evidence of blanching or cyanosis.

Kits are available to allow placement of an arterial line using the Seldinger technique. With this method, after the artery is accessed with the needle, insert a guidewire and remove the needle over the guidewire. Make a small incision in the skin at the base of the guidewire and then insert the catheter over the guidewire to the hub. Remove the guidewire. If there is resistance when the guidewire is inserted, remove the guidewire and attempt an alternate site. Sterile preparation and care of the catheter mirror standard technique.

Fix the catheter to the skin with a thin piece of tape. With the adhesive side up, place the tape under the catheter hub and cross it over the catheter in a V shape. Pass a second piece of tape around and over the catheter hub to fix it to the wrist (see Fig. 19.20B). Add a transparent sterile dressing such as Tegaderm or OpSite for an additional layer of security and protection. Use a small piece of tape to attach the T-piece connector to the wrist area or to the splint. Be sure that the fingers are easily visible.

Use only heparinized NS or half NS for infusion. Do not infuse medications, blood, blood products, amino acid solutions, IV fat solutions, or hypertonic solutions through the catheter. Remove the catheter if there is evidence of blanching or cyanosis, if it is impossible to withdraw blood from the catheter, or if it becomes difficult to flush the catheter.

Complications

Complications, which have been reported with every type of arterial catheter, include hemorrhage, thrombosis, spasm, infection, scars, air embolism, retrograde blood flow, transient elevation in blood pressure with rapid (<1 second) infusion, arteriovenous fistula formation, and nerve or tendon sheath damage. There is the potential for loss of digits, an entire extremity, or large areas of skin, and perfusion must be carefully monitored. Additionally, concerns regarding the type of flush used in the arterial line and the impact on results of blood samples drawn from that line must not be underestimated. Normoglycemic patients have received insulin therapy based on falsely elevated glucose readings in samples taken from an arterial line flushed with dextrose-containing fluid.[92,93] When decannulating the artery, apply pressure over the site for 3 to 5 minutes following removal to minimize bleeding.

REHYDRATION TECHNIQUES IN INFANTS AND CHILDREN

Approach to Dehydration

The literature on clinical assessment of the degree of dehydration in children with acute gastroenteritis is inconsistent. Physician gestalt alone typically performs poorly, with a reported sensitivity of 42%.[94] Parental report of symptoms associated with dehydration (emesis, diarrhea, poor fluid intake, decreased urine output, weak cry, sunken fontanelle, sunken eyes, decreased tears, dry mouth, and cool extremities) is sensitive, but not specific. Table 19.2 presents a more thorough list of the signs, symptoms, and definitions of mild, moderate, and severe dehydration. Different dehydration scales exist to improve assessment, with a wide range of accuracy. A 2015 paper suggests a simpler model in which sunken eyes, decreased skin elasticity, weak radial pulse, and general appearance are used, with two factors being predictive of at least 5% dehydration and three or four factors predictive of 10% dehydration.[95] A popular assessment tool, the Clinical Dehydration Scale, also uses four features for assessment: general appearance, eyes, mucous membranes, and tears, with scores for each ranging from 0 to 2.[96] Point-of-care ultrasound demonstrating an IVC to aortic diameter ratio of 0.8 or less can also be predictive of dehydration.[97]

Oral Rehydration

Oral rehydration therapy (ORT) has been shown to be equivalent to IV therapy in children with acute gastroenteritis in terms of rehydration, subsequent diarrheal episodes, and the development of sodium abnormalities.[98] Failure rates are 4% to 4.9%[99] as compared with 1.3% for IV therapy, and use of ORT can avoid the need for IV hydration in 24 of every 25 patients.[100] This is the modality of choice for rehydration of a mildly to moderately dehydrated infant or child aged 1 month or older. Oral rehydration solutions (ORSs) come in a number of commercial forms (World Health Organization rehydration salts, Enfalyte [Mead Johnson Nutrition], Pedialyte or Rehydralyte [Abbott], CeraLyte [Cera Products]). The ideal composition is 50 mEq/L of sodium, 25 g/L of dextrose, and 30 mEq/L of bicarbonate,[101] and a solution can be made at home with five cups of water, eight teaspoons of sugar, and one teaspoon of salt. Dilute apple juice instead of ORS has been shown effective for rehydration of mildly dehydrated patients, resulting in fewer treatment failures,[102] and carrying a substantially lower cost than commercial electrolyte solution.[103] The target volume is 50 to 100 mL/kg over a period of 2 to 4 hours. Typically, this is started with a spoon, cup, or syringe delivering 5 mL to children younger than 2 years and 10 mL to children older than 2 years every 5 minutes and then increasing volumes slowly as tolerated (Fig. 19.21). Vomiting

TABLE 19.2 Estimating Dehydration

DEHYDRATION	SYMPTOMS	SIGNS	FLUID LOST IN INFANTS	FLUID LOST IN OLDER CHILDREN	TREATMENT
Mild	Thirsty	Slightly dry mucous membranes	50 mL/kg	3%–5% total fluid	ORS, 50–100 mL/kg over a 2- to 4-h period Consider other methods if not tolerated No laboratory studies
Moderate	Decreased urine output Absent tears	Tachycardia Capillary refill >2 s Dry mucous membranes Weak pulse Abnormal respirations Sunken eyes	100 mL/kg	6%–9% total fluid	ORS, 50–100 mL/kg over a 2- to 4-h period Consider other methods if not tolerated No laboratory studies
Severe	Abnormal mental status, lethargy	Abnormal skin turgor Sunken fontanelle Hypotension	150 mL/kg	>9% total fluid	20–60 mL/kg of NS by IV bolus Serum chemistries

IV, Intravenous; *NS,* normal saline; *ORS,* oral rehydration solution.

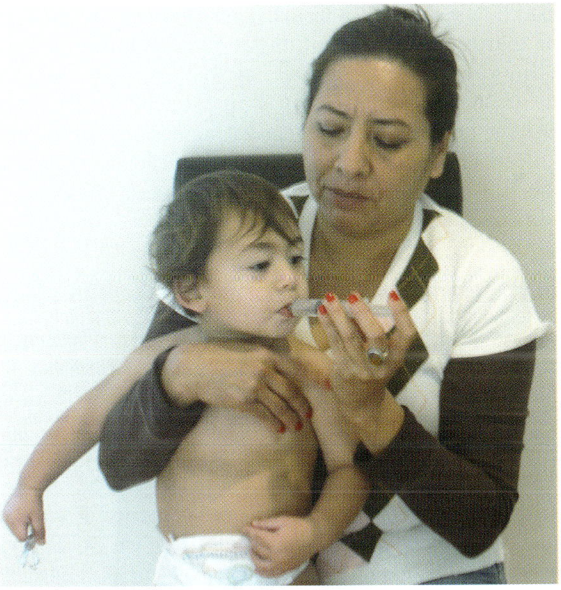

Fig. 19.21 Oral rehydration with a syringe. The parent is instructed on the technique in the emergency department.

is not a contraindication to attempting ORT because children can typically tolerate these small volumes. Some practitioners fear accompanying electrolyte abnormalities; however, hypernatremic dehydration responds well to ORT. Delayed capillary refill and higher degree of dehydration portend a risk of oral rehydration failure.[104]

Oral rehydration can be facilitated with the use of an antiemetic. Ondansetron has been shown to decrease ED vomiting (number needed to treat [NNT] = 5), decrease the need for IV hydration (NNT = 5), and possibly decrease the need for admission (NNT = 14),[105] with a 50% decrease in IV fluid requirement in young children not responding to a first attempt at oral hydration.[106] These results have been substantiated in a primary care setting as well.[107] In addition to being considered safer in children, ondansetron appears to outperform other antiemetics for cessation of emesis.[108] Ondansetron is administered at a dose of 0.15 mg/kg in the form of syrup or oral dissolving tablets, which can be repeated if the child vomits within 15 minutes. An alternative, simplified dosing regimen is to give 2 mg for children 8 to 15 kg, 4 mg for children 15 to 30 kg, and 8 mg for children greater than 30 kg. Oral rehydration should be initiated 15 to 30 minutes after administration of ondansetron.[109] Most oral ondansetron studies include children 6 months and older, but several studies using IV ondansetron have included infants as young as 1 month, and it is Food and Drug Administration (FDA) approved for postoperative nausea and vomiting down to 1 month of age. Concern regarding the possibility of ondansetron delaying the identification of more pathologic diagnoses is likely unfounded. Literature on the impact of ondansetron on return ED visits within 72 hours is mixed, and it has previously been shown that antiemetic therapy does not mask alternative diagnoses.[110–112] Recently, a newer article identified a higher hospitalization risk in repeat visitors who had been given ondansetron on the first visit (43.8% vs. 28.5%), with the 5 of 89 patients receiving a serious diagnosis on admission all treated with ondansetron on the first visit.[113] It does not seem to impact outcomes following ED discharge.[114] Outpatient prescriptions for ondansetron do not affect recidivism or readmission rates, though data are sparse and a larger trial is currently underway looking at multidose ondansetron protocols.[115]

Ondansetron has received attention for its ability to prolong the QT interval, and rare but serious arrhythmias noted in pediatric patients.[116] In children, a single dose of oral ondansetron has not been shown to cause concerning QTc prolongation nor potentially fatal arrhythmias.[117] A single IV dose appears safe as well.[118,119] It may contribute to mild and self-limited diarrhea.[109] Other antiemetics and antimotility agents are not recommended by the American Academy of Pediatrics for use in children younger than 5 years, and they have a high incidence of side effects. There is an FDA "boxed warning" against the use of promethazine in children younger than 2 years and a strong recommendation against its use even in older children. For patients with diarrhea, the antisecretory agent racecadotril is used in several European countries in conjunction with ORS, with a favorable treatment and adverse event profile.[120]

Laboratory Tests

The American Academy of Pediatrics recommends electrolyte testing in patients with severe dehydration, those who need IV rehydration, or children with moderate dehydration and findings on the history or physical examination inconsistent with straightforward diarrheal episodes. A prospective study of patients 2 months to 9 years of age, in whom parenteral rehydration was deemed required on clinical grounds, demonstrated a 48% rate of laboratory abnormalities, 10.4% of which changed treatment management. More than 9% of their patients had hypoglycemia, so it is recommended to obtain a glucose level urgently, as well as electrolytes when feasible, in patients who require IV rehydration.[121] It is difficult to provide recommendations regarding the management of low bicarbonate because the level has been found to correlate poorly with the need for admission and unscheduled revisit rate in some studies,[122,123] whereas it correlates well in others.[124] One paper even demonstrated more normal bicarbonate values were correlated with earlier discharge but also with increased rates of ED return.[125] Urine specific gravity tends to lag behind the child's hydration status and is particularly unreliable in infants younger than 1 year. BUN levels are also poorly sensitive in young children,[101] but significant elevations in these levels and in creatinine may be specific.[126] Children hospitalized for gastroenteritis can have rates of acute kidney injury up to 25%, but this is a specific population not representative of undifferentiated ED patients.[127] Serum ketones have been shown in one study to correlate with clinical dehydration scores.[128] $ETCO_2$ has been evaluated for its utility in assessing dehydration, and is a poor predictor.[129] In summary, the decision for admission in patients with gastroenteritis should primarily be a clinical one, without emphasis on laboratories. Hypoglycemia has been identified in up to 9% to 15% of young children with gastroenteritis in some studies, so assessment of glucose in children with persistent abnormalities of mental status is reasonable.[130,131]

Parenteral Rehydration

Obtaining IV access is covered elsewhere in this section. If parenteral administration of fluids is deemed appropriate, standard therapy involves 20-mL/kg boluses of NS or balanced solution (e.g., lactated Ringer) infused over a 60-minute period each until normalization of pulse, perfusion, and mental status occurs, with balanced solutions improving serum bicarbonate more effectively.[132] Recent literature has demonstrated comparable efficacy of rapid rehydration protocols involving the administration of 50 to 60 mL/kg over a 60-minute period in otherwise healthy children,[133–136] though it may paradoxically lengthen time to discharge. Adverse events were minimal in these studies; however, they were not entirely powered to ensure safety.[137] There are no clear contraindications to this strategy, though some suggest employing it in patients over 3 months of age without substantial electrolyte disorders.[138] In cases where an aberrancy of sodium is identified, unless proven to be acute, rehydration should occur more slowly (beyond correction of shock), ideally over 24 to 48 hours. There are some recommendations for the addition of dextrose to bolus fluids for normoglycemic patients as well.[138] This practice seemed safe and decreased ketone levels, but did not significantly decrease the admission rate.[139,140]

Children who have received parenteral fluids and subsequently tolerated oral fluids can typically be discharged home from the ED, although an unscheduled revisit rate of 16% has been reported.[141] If the child requires admission for continuance of maintenance fluids, isotonic saline with dextrose is recommended because of a documented 17% to 45% risk for hyponatremia with the use of hypotonic fluid.[142–144] The amount of maintenance fluid is calculated as 100 mL/kg for the first 10 kg of body weight, 50 mL/kg for 10 to 20 kg of body weight, and 20 mL/kg for the remaining body weight in a 24-hour period. For example, a 50-kg child would require (100 mL × 10 kg) + (50 mL × 10 kg) + (20 mL × 30 kg) divided evenly over 24 hours.

For malnourished children with potential sepsis, there is recent evidence to suggest some caution with fluid administration. There are few trials examining this issue in dehydration from acute gastroenteritis, but no data to support restrictive fluid protocols in this setting.[145]

Nasogastric Tube Rehydration

Nasogastric (NG) rehydration is a potentially effective, safe, and cost-effective alternative to parenteral rehydration in children who refuse to take fluids orally in the quantity required for rehydration. In settings with fewer resources, NG hydration has been shown to be effective for severe dehydration as well,[146] and internationally it is used for that indication.[147] NG rehydration is a recommended form of rehydration by European Society for Paediatric Gastroenterology, Hepatology and Nutrition.[148] NG rehydration is accomplished by placement of an NG tube, with a 5-Fr feeding tube typically being adequate for children younger than 3 years. For comfort, the use of topical anesthetic or nebulized lidocaine (5 mg/kg diluted in NS) before insertion is recommended. A bolus of 50 mL/kg of electrolyte solution (e.g., Pedialyte) is administered by continuous infusion via an enteral feeding pump over a 3-hour period. Twenty-four-hour rehydration regimens (50 to 100 mL/kg for the first 10 kg of body weight and then 25 to 50 mL/kg for the remaining body weight) have also been proposed but seem to have equivalent outcomes to more rapid rehydration protocols.[149] Unscheduled revisit rates are not significantly different compared with patients who have received IV rehydration. No study has evaluated the use of frequent, small boluses; however, experience with ORT would indicate that 5- to 10-mL parent-administered syringe boluses to equal 50 mL/kg would be an option in the event that a pump for continuous administration is unavailable. In other contexts, enteral fluid has been compared to IV fluid for hospitalized children with bronchiolitis,[150] yielding equivalent lengths of stay with an increase in insertion success, decrease in complications,[151,152] and lower cost.[153] This has been proven reasonable in even youngest infants under 2 months.[154]

Subcutaneous Rehydration

Subcutaneous rehydration therapy, also known as hypodermoclysis, is an option in children with mild to moderate dehydration in whom IV or IO access is not available or feasible. Its utility as a bridge to facilitating commencement of IV hydration in severely dehydrated children has been postulated, but not studied. Although the potential has been recognized since the early 1900s, the hyaluronan-containing intercellular matrix of subcutaneous tissue prevents easy delivery and absorption of large quantities of fluid, and the previous preparations of hyaluronidase (enzymes that hydrolyze hyaluronan) were animal based and allergenic. More recently, a recombinant formulation of human hyaluronidase, HuPH20 (Hylenex, Halozyme Therapeutics), has become available, thus making this technique more accessible. Its primary utility has been in geriatric and hospice patients requiring hydration, but several studies have substantiated its safety and efficacy in pediatric patients as young as 2 months, with mean volumes delivered comparable to IV hydration. In assessing recidivism, pediatric patients treated with subcutaneous hydration and discharged from the ED had an unscheduled revisit rate comparable to those receiving IV hydration.[155] The cost-effectiveness profile is advantageous when compared with equivalent IV therapy, with children below 3 years of age representing the most difficult cases for IV access and, thus, the greatest cost savings.[156]

After sterile preparation, a 22- or 24-gauge angiocatheter or 25-gauge butterfly needle is inserted at a 30- to 45-degree angle to the hub into subcutaneous tissue. After placement of a small piece of gauze under the hub of the catheter to maintain the angle, it is secured with a sterile occlusive dressing. Although the interscapular area is often used, the thigh, abdomen (left iliac fossa), chest, and upper part of the arm are also options.[157] If possible, an area with a pinchable fat fold of 1 inch should be selected. The catheter should be aspirated for absence of blood return. A 150-unit dose of hyaluronidase is injected through the catheter, and the fluid infusion is started. Typically, isotonic fluids such as 0.9% NS are used. Mean fluid infusion rates are highly variable in adults and range in children from 18.9 mL/kg over the first hour to 38.4 mL/kg for a 4-hour infusion.[158] An eventual infusion rate of approximately 20 mL/kg per hour should be selected and titrated down if the infusion pump indicates occlusion. Because the hyaluronidase requires approximately 15 minutes to take full effect, some providers prefer to start more slowly and titrate upward.[159] Initially, an erythematous swelling may appear at the infusion site (Fig. 19.22), but it will decrease in size after 5 minutes and disappear 1 to 2 hours after cessation of the fluid infusion. Some pain may occur at the infusion site. Suggestions for troubleshooting subcutaneous infusion problems can be found in Table 19.3. Maximal diffusion of fluid into the IV compartment occurs in 1 hour. An injection of hyaluronidase allows subcutaneous infiltration for 48 hours, and maintenance fluids, including those containing dextrose and

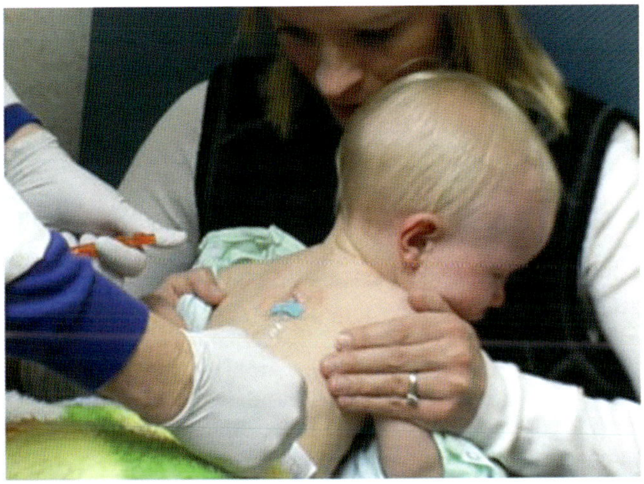

Fig. 19.22 Subcutaneous rehydration with normal swelling 5 minutes after beginning the infusion. (Courtesy Dr. Corburn Allen.)

TABLE 19.3 Troubleshooting Subcutaneous Rehydration Complications

PROBLEM	ACTION
The catheter becomes dislodged	Restart in the same area without an additional dose of hyaluronidase[99]
The infusion pump indicates occlusion	Slow the infusion rate by 10 mL/h
The area becomes firm, indurated, and painful	Administer an additional dose of hyaluronidase
The child does not respond to outpatient therapy	Continue infusion of fluid through the catheter for 48 h as maintenance

potassium, can be infused through the catheter after the bolus if required.

Subcutaneous rehydration is not recommended in patients with signs of shock, coagulation deficits, gross edema, significant electrolyte abnormalities (sodium >150 mEq/L or <130 mEq/L), or no intact skin sites (e.g., massive burns). The most common adverse events reported are redness, swelling, or bruising at the infusion site. Potassium-containing solutions may be painful. Allergic reactions have not been reported with the newer formulation of hyaluronidase, and skin infections are rare. However, when compared to IV hydration, subcutaneous hydration is either equivalent or superior.[160]

Discharge

Commonly held beliefs that include avoidance of dairy products, need for formula change or overdilution of formula with water, gut rest for 24 hours or longer, and the BRAT diet (bananas, rice, applesauce, toast) are not supported by the literature in most cases. Once rehydration has been achieved, returning to a normal diet is suggested as soon as possible, with continued replacement of ongoing losses with an ORS or potentially dilute juice. Continuation of breastfeeding is encouraged and routine use of lactose-free diets seems of little benefit.

Most children seen in the ED with acute dehydration will be corrected and discharged home. Admission criteria include inadequate care at home or inability to follow return precautions, inability to take or failure of rehydration with ORT, concern for more serious pathology, severe dehydration, sodium levels outside of 131 to 149 mmol/L range and neonatal dehydration. Infants <3500 g, patient with altered sensorium, those with chronic relevant illness, patients with persistent bloody diarrhea, and those with failure to thrive should also be considered for admission.

A recent follow-up study utilizing a phone call at 1 week following careful discharge teaching showed complete improvement in 86% of patients, with the majority improving by 24 to 48 hours from the visit.[125] Factors that predict development of moderate to severe dehydration following discharge in infants under 2 years of age are younger age, frequency of vomiting, increasing dehydration severity at the ED visit, prior ED visit for same episode of acute gastroenteritis, administration of intravenous fluid at ED visit.[161] These patients should be followed more closely following discharge.

Return to school or day care 48 hours after the last episode of diarrhea or emesis is a reasonable recommendation.

REFERENCES ARE AVAILABLE AT Elsevier eBooks+

CHAPTER 20

Arterial Puncture and Cannulation

Erick Eiting and Caroline W. Burmon

Arterial puncture is the most accurate blood sampling technique for true arterial blood gas (ABG) and acid-base determination. Intraarterial cannulation with continuous blood pressure measurement remains an accepted standard in critically ill patients. Though noninvasive technologies have greatly improved in their accuracy, intraarterial monitoring of blood pressure may in some situations better reflect the force of systemic perfusion than noninvasive monitoring. Arterial monitoring is also one of the most important determinants of cardiac work. However, invasive monitoring requires specific expertise and technical support that may be a limitation in its implementation versus noninvasive monitoring.

INDICATIONS AND CONTRAINDICATIONS

Indications for and contraindications to arterial puncture and cannulation are listed in Review Box 20.1. The use of arterial lines for continuous monitoring is generally reserved for the intensive care setting but may be initiated in the emergency department (ED). The indications for placement of an arterial line fall into two major categories[1]:

1. *Repetitive and direct arterial blood sampling:* Arterial catheter access removes the need for multiple arterial punctures and allows either repeated sampling or placement of sensors for continuous monitoring of blood gas and other chemistry values.
2. *Continuous real-time monitoring of blood pressure and cardiac function:* Catheter access allows superior monitoring and moment-to-moment detection of changes in systemic perfusion. As such, intraoperative and intensive care unit (ICU) management is often facilitated by placement of an arterial line. Some patients with critical pathologies like severe burns, dialysis grafts or shunts, or with physical limitations such as morbid obesity may need ongoing monitoring of perfusion that is best served by arterial catheterization.

Although acute respiratory decompensation and metabolic emergencies are the most common reasons for ABG sampling, all blood tests performed on venous blood may also be performed on arterial blood. Patients with moderate respiratory decompensation may be managed without arterial puncture by using continuous, noninvasive pulse oximetry, end-tidal or transcutaneous carbon dioxide monitoring, as well as venous sampling for carbon dioxide, carboxyhemoglobin, and methemoglobin, or any combination thereof.[2] Nonetheless, a role still exists for arterial blood sampling. The initial correlation between venous acid-base values and arterial values is often important in critical illness to set a baseline or verify a trend. Some authors use ABG sampling in the initial evaluation of critically ill trauma patients.[3] Vasoactive drugs (e.g., nitroprusside and norepinephrine) are best administered in conjunction with continuous monitoring of arterial pressure to guide titration. The response of trauma and post–cardiac arrest patients to acute resuscitative efforts may also be more easily monitored with the use of arterial catheterization.

Few contraindications to arterial puncture exist and none are absolute. For example, after thrombolysis, arterial cannulation should be performed only if it will provide essential data that cannot be obtained by other methods. If absolutely necessary, a single arterial puncture of the readily compressible radial artery may be preferred. Arterial puncture can be performed safely in patients who are anticoagulated or who have other coagulopathies but should be undertaken with extreme caution in patients with severe disseminated coagulopathies.

There are reports of patients with bleeding complications who have required transfusions, and some patients have experienced compression neuropathies secondary to hematomas at the puncture site. Repeated arterial sampling in such patients should be accomplished by insertion of an indwelling cannula to minimize trauma to the arterial wall.

The presence of severe arteriosclerosis, with or without diminution in flow, is a relative contraindication to arterial puncture. In hemodynamically unstable patients with advanced cardiovascular disease, the benefits of invasive monitoring may nonetheless outweigh its risks. Consider an alternative site if an isolated, decreased palpable pulse or bruit is felt over the site selected. Additionally, consider an alternative site if there is evidence of decreased or absent collateral flow in areas where flow normally exists, such as in Raynaud's syndrome or an abnormal result on the modified Allen test (discussed later in the section on "Techniques"). Avoid puncturing a specific arterial site when infection, burn, or other damage to cutaneous defenses exists in the overlying skin and similar for a surgical shunt.

Arterial Versus Venous Analysis

Arterial sampling has been the traditional approach to evaluating acid-base abnormalities in critically ill patients, especially those being maintained on a ventilator. In most ED settings, however, venous blood gas analysis will suffice. Studies have demonstrated that analysis of venous blood (especially central venous blood) for pH, bicarbonate, lactate, base excess, and carbon dioxide pressure (Pco_2) are within 95% limits of agreement with arterial sampling and can safely supplant it.[4,5] On the other hand, arterial blood sampling is still required for accurate analysis of oxygen pressure (Po_2).[6–8]

EQUIPMENT: ARTERIAL PUNCTURE

Arterial Puncture With a Needle/Syringe

To obtain a single sample of arterial blood by the percutaneous method, attach a 3-mL syringe (preferred and most common) to a needle. Select the needle size based on puncture location and patient size and age. For an adult, use a 20-gauge, 2.5-inch needle for a femoral sample and a 22-gauge, 1.25-inch needle for a radial artery puncture. For pediatric arterial sampling, use a needle with a slightly shorter length in the range of 22 to 24 gauge at the same sites as in adults.

Precoated blood gas plastic syringes (with dry lithium heparin) are commonly used and allow a longer shelf life and ready use (Fig. 20.1). Such devices are designed to minimize sampling error as a result of heparin. If necessary, prepare a regular syringe with 1 or 2 mL of a heparinized saline solution

Arterial Puncture and Cannulation

Indications

Blood gas sampling
Continuous pressure monitoring
Need for frequent blood sampling
Major surgery involving fluid shifts/blood loss
Hypothermia (induced or environmental)
Diagnostic angiography
Therapeutic embolization

Contraindications

Strict	*Relative*
Inadequate circulation	Previous surgery in the area
Raynaud syndrome	Anticoagulation/coagulopathy
Buerger disease	Skin infection at the site
Full-thickness burns	Atherosclerosis
	Inadequate collateral flow
	Partial-thickness burns

Complications

Hematoma formation
Infection
Bleeding
Ischemia
Thrombosis/embolism
Arteriovenous fistula formation
Pseudoaneurysm formation

Equipment

Arterial Puncture

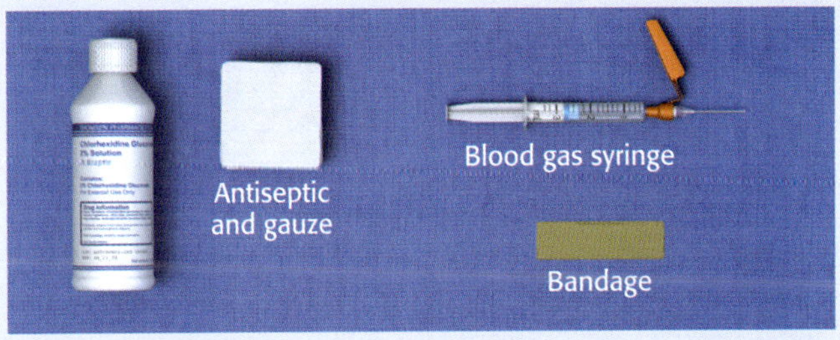

Arterial Cannulation

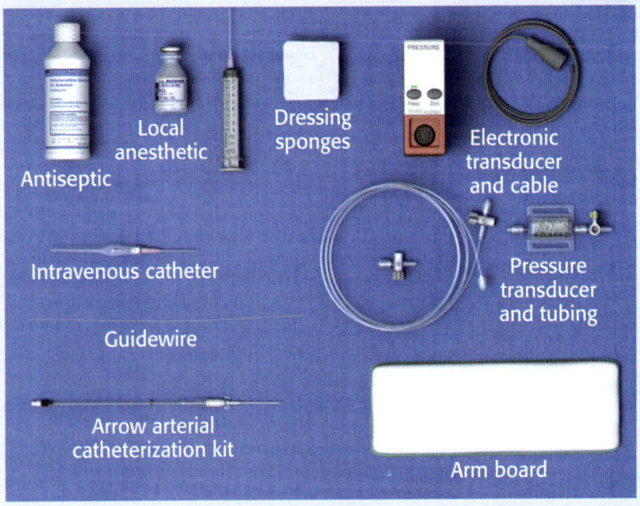

(Not shown: bag of normal saline, pressure infuser)

Review Box 20.1 Arterial puncture and cannulation: indications, contraindications, complications, and equipment.

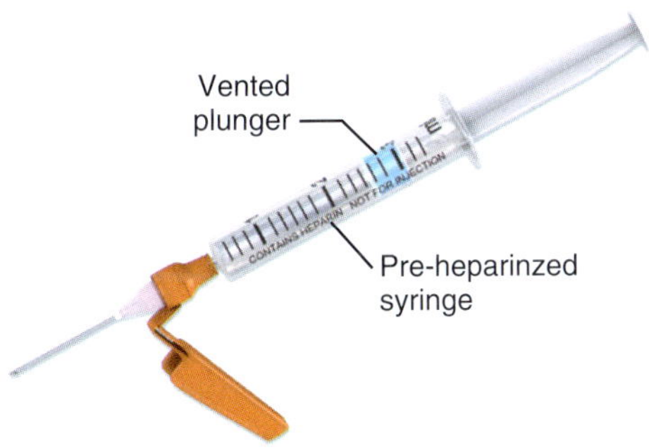

Fig. 20.1 Arterial blood gas syringe. This device is precoated with dry lithium heparin. Additionally, the plunger is vented, which allows air in the syringe to escape through the plunger as the sample is collected. To use this type of syringe, pull back the plunger to the desired volume before arterial puncture. When the needle enters the artery, blood will fill the syringe spontaneously—there is no need to pull back on the plunger.

(1000 international units [IU]/mL) drawn into the syringe to coat the barrel and needle. Fully eject the heparin through the needle immediately before skin puncture to minimize heparin-related errors. Although the syringe may appear devoid of heparin, enough heparin remains in the needle and syringe to provide anticoagulation. Even dry heparin may produce abnormalities in ABG results because of a heparin-induced dilutional effect.

The latest blood gas and chemistry analyzers require only 0.2 mL of whole blood for accuracy, and some point-of-care devices can perform analyses on single drops of blood. However, sample sizes of less than 1.0 mL of blood aspirated into heparin-coated syringes may result in a heparin-related error on ABG values.

Stored heparin solution has higher Po_2 and lower Pco_2 values than blood does. Proper technique with dry lithium heparin–prefilled syringes or full ejection of excess heparin will prevent such problems if more than 2 mL of blood is collected. A falsely low Pco_2 is the most clinically significant change caused by excess heparin. Neither Po_2 nor pH levels are significantly altered by the addition of heparin in most instances, although a slight increase in Po_2 and a minimal decrease in pH may occur if high concentrations of heparin (25,000 IU/mL) are used. If 2 to 3 mL of blood is collected, heparin-related effects are likely to be clinically inconsequential.

Continuous Monitoring via Arterial Catheter

The fluid-filled recording systems used with arterial cannulation can have a great influence on the accuracy of

BOX 20.1 Equipment for Insertion and Maintenance of an Indwelling Arterial Cannula

Antiseptic solution
1% lidocaine (without epinephrine); usually 2 to 3 mL delivered by a 25- to 27-gauge needle is required for adequate anesthesia of the cannulation site
10- × 10-cm dressing sponges
Arm board for brachial, radial, or ulnar cannulation
Appropriately sized intravenous catheters
Syringes (3 and 5 mL for anesthesia, 5 mL for aspiration)
Pressure tubing
Two three-way stopcocks
Pressure transducer
Connecting wire
Monitor display
500- to 1000-mL bag of normal saline
Pressure blood infuser set up with a continuous flush device

ADDITIONAL EQUIPMENT REQUIRED FOR THE CUTDOWN INSERTION TECHNIQUE

Scalpel blade (No. 11)
Tissue spreader, self-retaining
Two hemostats
2-0 silk ties, multiple
2-0 silk suture with a straight needle
Needle driver with a 2-0 nylon skin needle

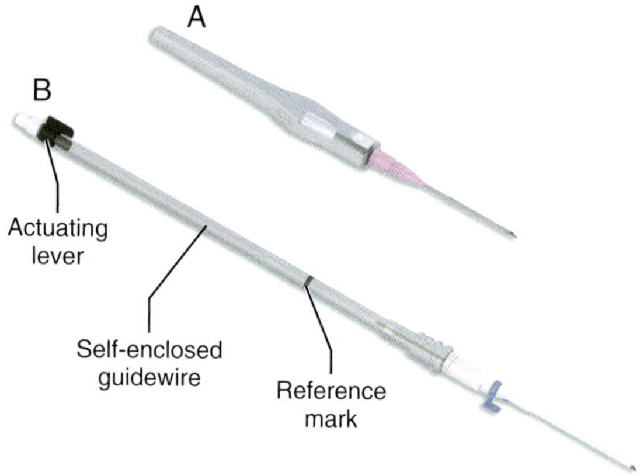

Fig. 20.2 Catheters for arterial cannulation. (A) Standard intravenous catheter. Use 20 gauge for the radial artery and 16 or 18 gauge for the femoral artery. (B) Arrow arterial catheterization kit. This device has a self-enclosed guidewire that is advanced into the artery by moving the actuating lever forward. When the lever reaches the reference mark on the barrel of the device, the tip of the guidewire is at the opening of the needle lumen. (Courtesy Arrow International, Reading, PA.)

pressure measurements. The frequency responses of tubing, transducers, and other components of the monitoring system influence the accuracy of systolic and diastolic pressure measurement. Failure to recognize recording system artifacts will lead to errors in interpretation of the pressure.

Various catheter types have demonstrated similar frequency-response characteristics, but some have different complication rates. Teflon catheters may carry an increased rate of thrombosis. Another contributing element leading to thrombosis is catheter diameter; the incidence of thrombosis is inversely related to the ratio of vessel lumen to catheter diameter. Thus the risk for thrombosis increases as the diameter of the catheter decreases. The incidence of thrombosis also increases with increased duration of catheter placement. In contrast, a higher risk for thrombosis was seen in the femoral artery than in the radial artery in a study involving a pediatric population.[9] Catheters coated with a combination of chlorhexidine and silver sulfadiazine have produced lower infection rates.[10]

Preparation for Arterial Cannulation

Box 20.1 lists the usual equipment for arterial cannulation, although most of prepackaged kits contain the supplies needed (see also Review Box 20.1). Shorter catheters are ideal for peripheral artery cannulation, whereas use of a longer catheter and the Seldinger technique is preferable for the femoral artery.

For arterial cannulation in adults, use a 16- to 18-gauge catheter for the femoral artery and a 20-gauge catheter for the radial artery (Fig. 20.2). Small children and infants require a 22- to 24-gauge catheter, which may need to be inserted percutaneously via the Seldinger technique or through a femoral cutdown. Based on patient size, older pediatric patients usually require 20- to 22-gauge catheters.

The tubing that connects the catheter to the pressure transducer has a significant effect on accuracy of the monitoring system. The higher the frequency response of the entire system, the more accurate the determination of systolic and diastolic pressure; however, artifact also becomes more of a problem.[1] Use stiff, low-capacitance plastic tubing for arterial catheterization and monitoring. Place the electronic pressure transducer connection as close as possible to the patient and zero it appropriately as the frequency response of a tube is inversely related to its length.

The pressure wave produced with each contraction is transmitted from the artery through the catheter and connecting tubing to a measuring device. The arterial fluid wave is received by an electromechanical transducer that changes the mechanical pressure wave into an electrical signal that can be displayed on the monitor. The most basic technique for obtaining blood pressure values involves the use of a simple manometer. This system can be assembled quickly if materials are available.

A continuous method of flushing the pressure tubing is required to maintain patency of the catheter lumen during intraarterial pressure monitoring. A three-way stopcock through which the tubing is intermittently flushed with saline (a minimum of every 15 to 30 minutes) is a simple and effective method. Continuous flush devices push a set amount of fluid (usually 2 to 3 mL/h) through the line. A typical monitoring system that includes this device is shown in Fig. 20.3. The pressure transducer must be mounted at the level of the patient's heart. Current pressure-monitoring setups include not only built-in

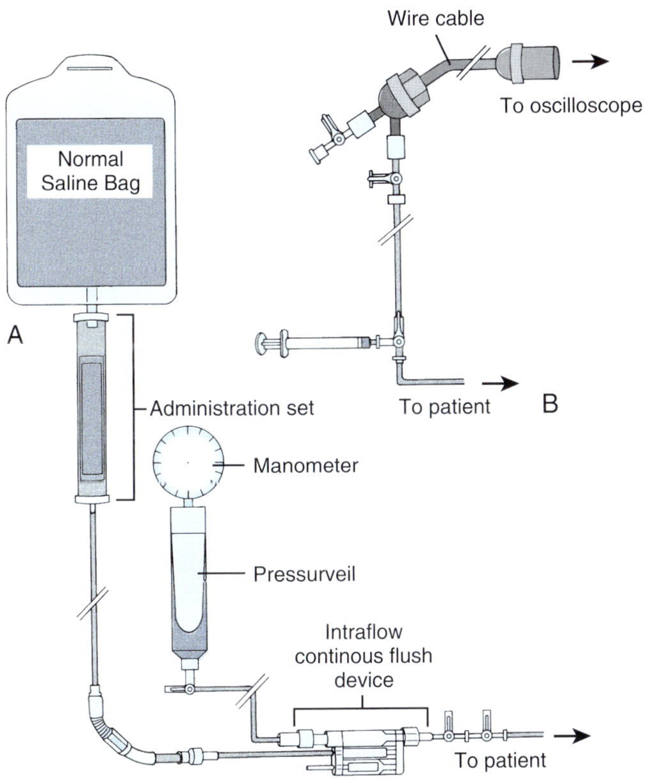

Fig. 20.3 Arterial pressure–monitoring systems. (A) System for continuous flushing. A 1-L bag of normal saline is pressurized to 250–300 mm Hg with a metered blood pump (not shown). The continuous flush device is set to deliver 3 mL/h of saline. A mechanical pressure transducer is depicted. The transducer device is a sterile, inexpensive, fully assembled monitor that can be used during patient transfer. Alternatively, the electronic transducer depicted in B may be used. (B) System for manual flush. A saline flush solution can be injected manually through a syringe at the proximal or distal port. The transducer dome should be maintained at the level of the patient's heart. (From Beal JM, ed. *Critical Care for Surgical Patients.* Macmillan; 1982.)

stopcocks but also in-line flushing plungers to facilitate clearance of blood after sampling.

Intravascular transducers were initially seen as an improvement over the external electromechanical transducers in use since the mid-1970s. Many of the numerous brands are fragile, temperature sensitive, of variable quality, and more difficult to place in vessels than catheters are. Despite anecdotal reports of fibrin deposition on these devices, no increased incidence of thrombus formation has been noted. The most important advantages of intravascular transducers are the ability to continuously monitor ABG values and to eliminate potential errors induced by catheters, stopcocks, and connecting tubing.

SITE SELECTION

The radial, brachial, and femoral arteries are the sites most often punctured for blood gas sampling in adults. Pediatric sites commonly used for arterial puncture include arteries in the foot and the umbilical artery in newborns.

When an artery is cannulated for longer-term use, there is a risk of complete loss of blood flow through a vessel as a result of intraluminal thrombosis. This is important when choosing a site for arterial puncture. Because the most frequent complication of arterial catheterization is bleeding, the ability to control hemorrhage must also be considered. For these reasons, the radial and femoral arteries are favored because of their good collateral blood flow and ease of compression in case of hemorrhage. Patient comfort and nursing care concerns should also be considered when selecting the site.

TECHNIQUES

Arterial Puncture

See Videos 20.1 to 20.6. Palpate the arterial pulse to ascertain the location of the vessel and prepare the overlying skin with an antiseptic solution (Fig. 20.4, *step 1*). Anesthetize the patient's skin with a wheal of local anesthetic (e.g., 1% lidocaine without epinephrine) through a small needle (25 or 27 gauge) (Fig. 20.4, *step 2*). If local anesthesia is to be given, take care to use only a small amount because a large wheal may obscure the pulse. If the patient is in extremis or unresponsive to pain in the area to be punctured, anesthetic infiltration may be omitted.

Isolate the arterial pulsation with the index and middle fingers of the gloved, nondominant hand and identify the course of the vessel. Puncture the skin through the anesthetic wheal, immediately distal to the palpated pulse under the index finger (Fig. 20.4, *step 3*). Hold the syringe like a dart with the bevel up and the syringe kept in view so that blood flow can be seen immediately. Advance the needle slowly toward the pulsating vessel at an approximately 30-degree angle. A larger angle is required to puncture the deeper femoral artery. Once the needle enters the arterial lumen, allow the syringe plunger to rise with the arterial pressure on its own to discriminate between arterial and venous sampling (Fig. 20.4, *step 4*). As soon as blood flows, stop advancing the needle and allow the syringe to fill. If no blood flow is obtained or if bone has been hit, withdraw the needle slowly because both walls of the vessel may have been punctured and the lumen may be entered as the needle is withdrawn. Redirect the needle only when the needle has been retracted to a location just deep to the dermis. After at least 1 to 2 mL of blood has been obtained, remove the needle from the artery. Apply firm pressure at the puncture site for 3 to 5 minutes (Fig. 20.4, *step 5*). If the patient is anticoagulated or has a coagulopathy, 10 to 15 minutes of pressure may be required).

Use of ultrasound is rapidly becoming a standard in procedures involving central vascular access. The same ultrasound-guided techniques are also being applied to arterial cannulation (Ultrasound Box). Shiloh and colleagues reported 71% improvement in the likelihood of success at the first attempt when using ultrasound guidance.[11] Vascular Doppler can also be used to improve success rates. Hold the probe over the artery just proximal to the puncture site. An important indication of vessel identification is the loss of audible pulsations with compression.[12]

Arterial Puncture (Radial Artery)

1

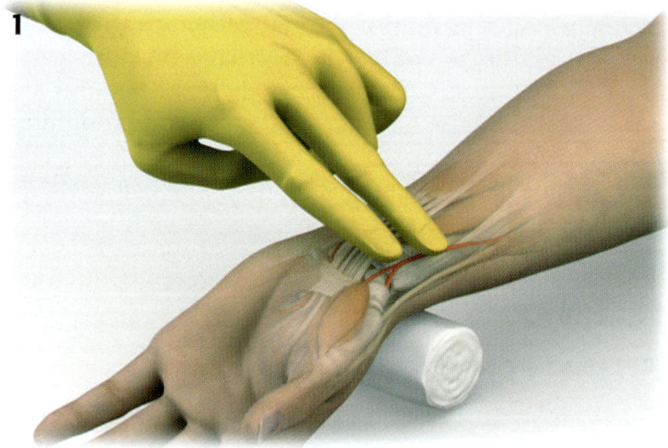

Position the wrist in slight dorsiflexion, cleanse the skin with antiseptic solution, and palpate the radial pulse.

2

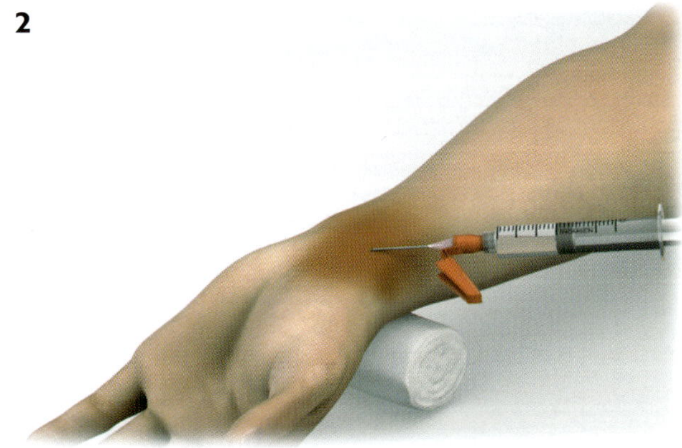

Optionally, place a small wheal of local anesthetic (e.g., 1% lidocaine without epinephrine) over the entry site. Avoid placing too large of a wheal, which may obscure the artery.

3

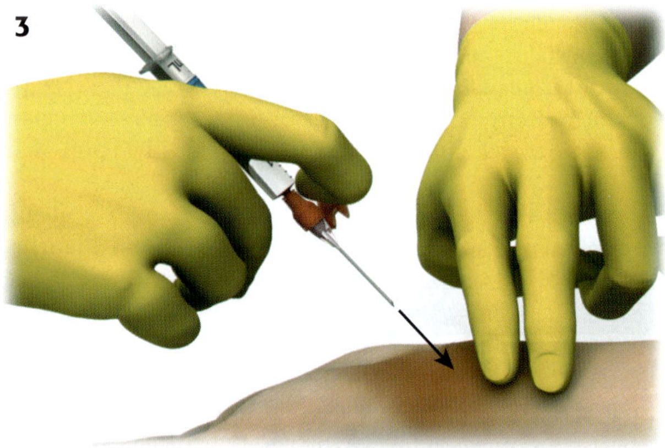

Hold the syringe in your hand like a dart, with the bevel up. Palpate the artery with the index and middle fingers of your other hand. Puncture the skin distal to your finger, and slowly advance the needle at a 30-degree angle toward the pulsating vessel.

4

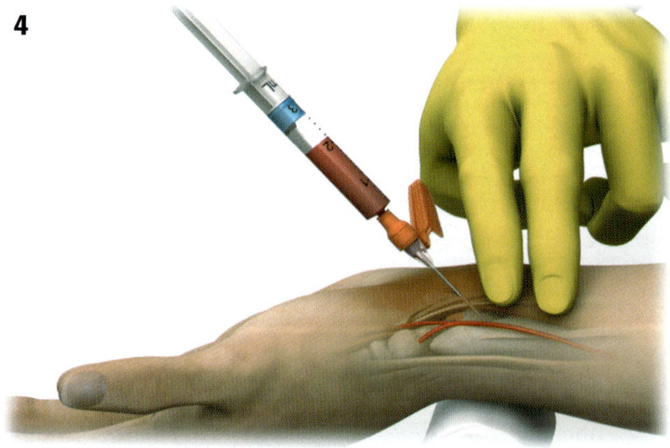

As soon as blood flows, stop advancing the needle. Allow the syringe to fill on its own. If bone is encountered, withdraw slowly because both vessel walls may have been penetrated and the lumen may be entered as the needle is withdrawn.

5

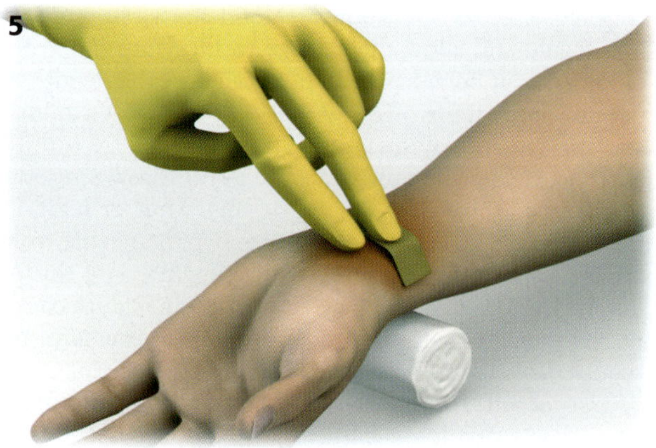

Remove the needle from the artery after the syringe has filled. Apply a bandage and firm pressure to the puncture site for a minimum of 3 to 5 minutes.

6

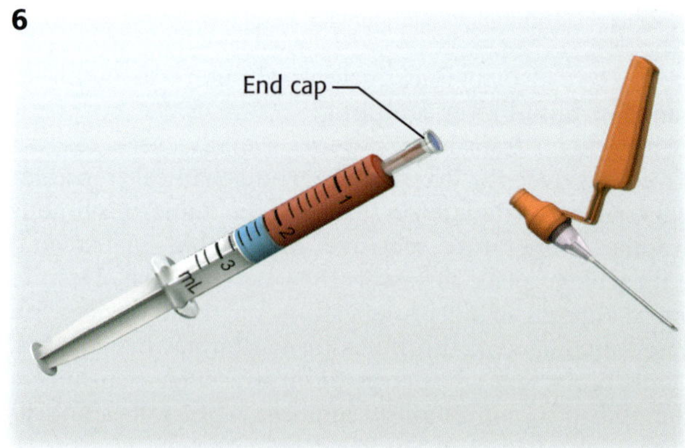

Remove all air from the syringe by holding it upward, gently tapping it, and depressing the plunger. Attach the end cap to the syringe to maintain anaerobic conditions, and submit the sample to the laboratory.

Fig. 20.4 Arterial puncture (radial artery).

ULTRASOUND: Arterial Puncture

by Christine Butts, MD

Ultrasound can be used with great success in the placement of peripheral and central intravenous lines, and it can also be used for the placement of arterial catheters.

First, identify the target vessel with ultrasound. Use a high-frequency transducer (10 to 12 mHz) to ensure proper resolution. The target vessel is typically easiest to identify in the transverse plane (with the indicator pointing toward the patient's right side) (Fig. 20.US1). Arteries usually appear as rounded structures with thick walls, as opposed to veins that are ovoid. Depending on the size of the vessel, pulsations may be noted in the arteries. Application of color flow Doppler to a suspected artery will frequently demonstrate a pattern of pulsatile flow (Fig. 20.US2). Although arteries are usually thought to resist collapse from outside pressure (such as from applying pressure with the overlying transducer), smaller arteries in the periphery may show some degree of collapse.

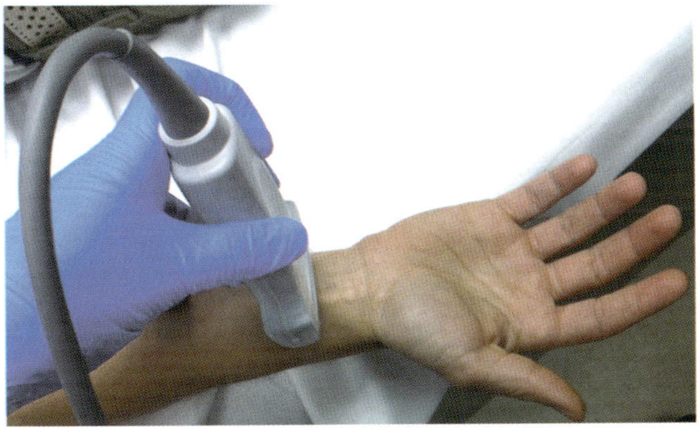

Fig. 20.US1 Placement of the transducer over the distal end of the arm in the transverse plane to localize the radial artery.

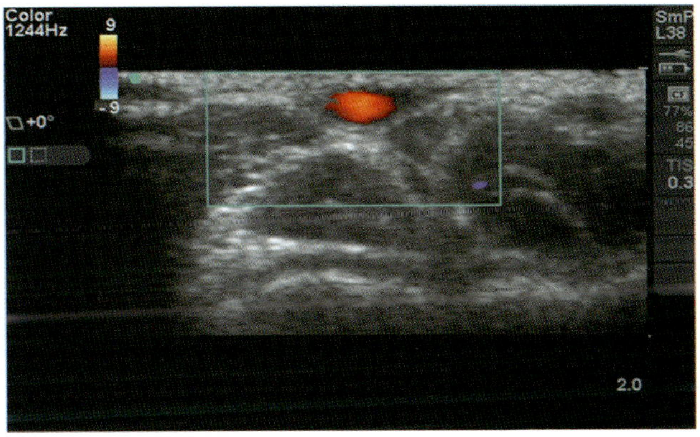

Fig. 20.US2 Image of the radial artery with color flow. Applying color flow will enable the operator to correctly identify the artery.

Once the vessel has been identified, ultrasound can also be used to directly guide cannulation. Sterile technique should be maintained, particularly when accessing central arteries such as the femoral artery. A full description of the technique of ultrasound-guided venous access can be found in both the general ultrasound chapter (Chapter 67) and the central venous access chapter (Chapter 22) in this textbook. The principles of these procedures also apply to arterial cannulation, although a few points should be emphasized. When guiding access to the radial artery, a transverse approach is typically used because the vessel is small and difficult to visualize in the longitudinal approach. Additionally, it may be difficult to keep the image of the longitudinal vessel centered on the screen, especially when one physician is directing both the ultrasound and the needle.

Proper handling of the sample and rapid analysis are very important. When the needle is withdrawn, expel any air bubbles present in the syringe to avoid a false elevation in Po_2. Remove the air neatly and easily by tapping the inverted syringe (needle pointing upward) to force any air to the top; then carefully and slowly depress the syringe plunger to push out the remaining air (Fig. 20.4, *step 6*). A gauze pad or alcohol wipe may be used to collect any excess blood expelled with the syringe held upright and the plunger side down. Remove the needle and cap the syringe to ensure anaerobic conditions. Alternatively, many of the commercially available ABG kits come with an air bubble removal device (Filter-Pro [Smiths Medical]) that allows the clinician to expel air bubbles from the sample and reduce potential exposure from the blood product.

Air in the sample can significantly increase Po_2 (mean increase, 11 mm Hg) after 20 minutes of storage, even if kept at 4°C. pH and Pco_2 are not significantly altered by air bubbles if the blood is stored at 4°C for 20 minutes and no significant deterioration has occurred. If blood is stored at room temperature for longer than 20 minutes, Pco_2 will increase and the pH will decrease, probably as a result of leukocyte metabolism. In a stored sample, Po_2 varies to such an extent that the change is unpredictable for chemical interpretation at 30 minutes, regardless of the storage method. High leukocyte or platelet counts, such as those seen in leukemic patients, may shorten acceptable storage intervals. ABG samples should be kept on ice and analyzed within 15 to 20 minutes. Samples that cannot be analyzed within this time frame should be considered unreliable.

PERCUTANEOUS TECHNIQUE FOR ARTERIAL CANNULATION

Direct Over-the-Needle Catheter Cannulation

Placement of an angiocatheter directly into an arterial lumen in a manner similar to placement of an intravenous catheter is the most practiced and simplest method but is not always successful because of technical difficulties. The only routine site for this technique is the radial artery. Use of a catheter over a guidewire, also described as the Seldinger technique, is strongly advised at most other sites.

Take time to ensure proper alignment of the desired site. Delays, complications, and inability to successfully cannulate an artery often occur as a result of failure to properly prepare the desired site and involved limb. An important preparatory step is to ensure that the target limb is secured flat and not rotated; any rotation could result in the desired artery being shifted from the expected anatomic position, making it more difficult to cannulate. For example, to adequately prepare the radial artery, immobilize the wrist and hand in mild dorsiflexion with some padding for support underneath the wrist (Fig. 20.5, *step 1*). Prepare the skin

Arterial Cannulation: Over-the-Needle Catheter Technique

1

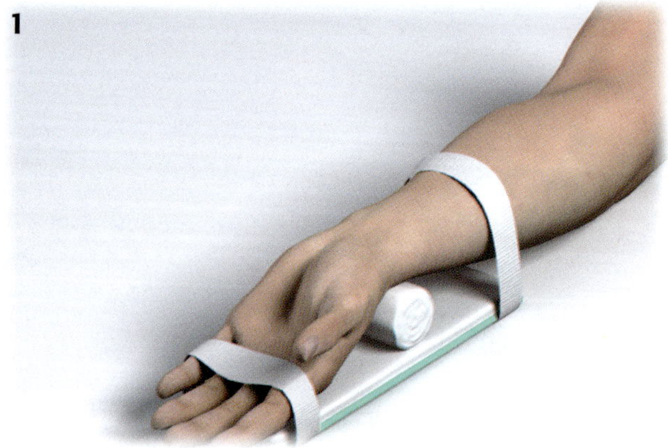

Immobilize the hand and wrist in mild dorsiflexion on a padded arm board. Prepare the skin with antiseptic, anesthetize, and apply a sterile drape.

2

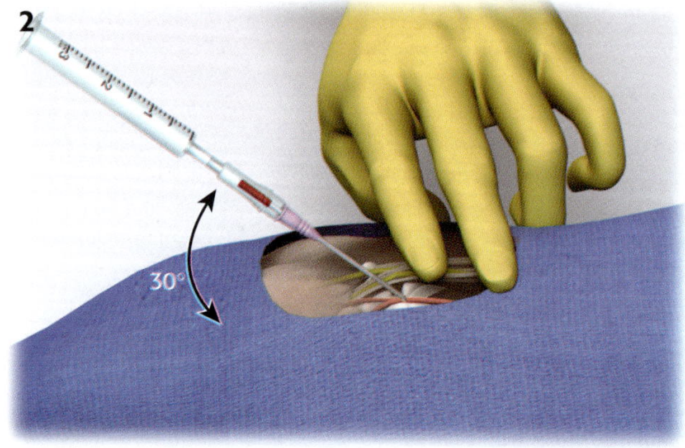

Advance the needle into the artery at a 30- to 45-degree angle to the skin. Confirm arterial puncture by observing a flash into the needle hub.

3

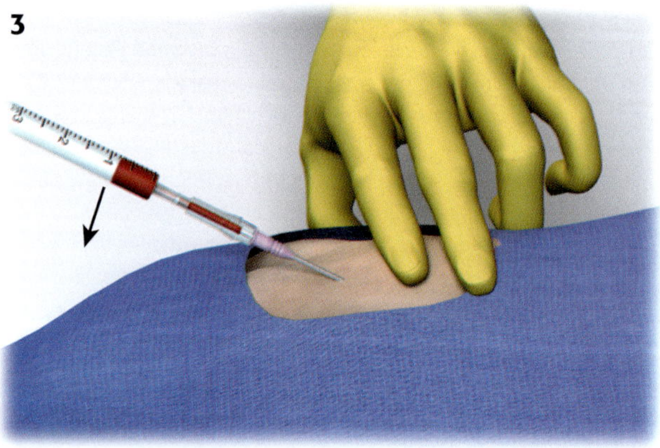

Lower the angiocatheter and advance it 2 mm forward to ensure that the tip has cannulated the vessel. Confirm proper placement by observing continuous arterial blood return.

4

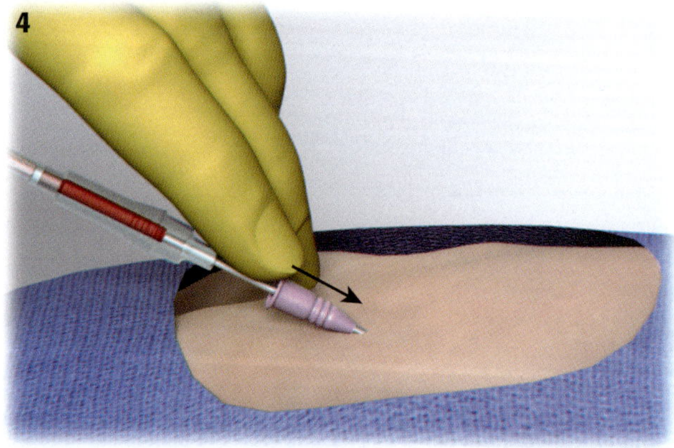

Carefully advance the catheter over the needle and into the artery. Do not force the catheter; if it fails to easily thread, it has not properly entered the vessel lumen. (See text for troubleshooting tips.)

5

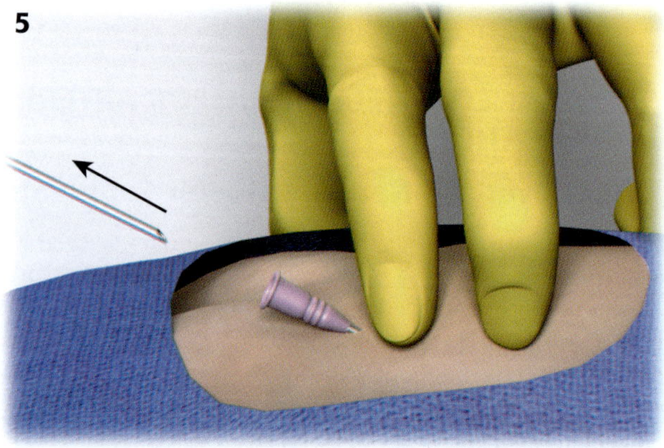

Tamponade over the artery proximal to the tip of the catheter (to prevent blood loss), and remove the needle.

6

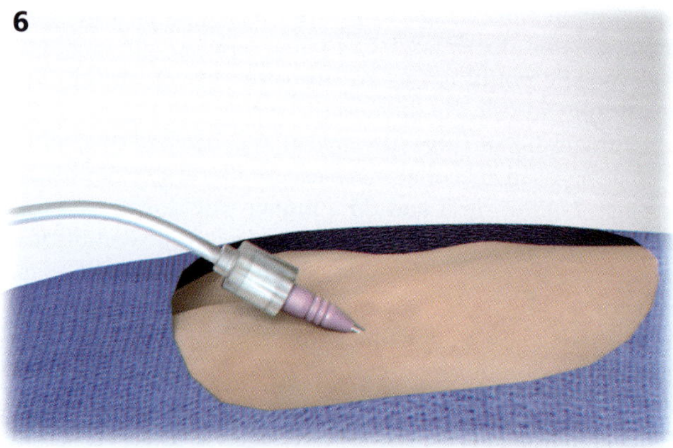

Attach the tubing from the pressure transducer to the catheter. Suture the catheter hub to the skin and cover with a sterile dressing, such as Tegaderm.

Fig. 20.5 Arterial cannulation: over-the-needle catheter technique. Note that in this example the angiocatheter *does not have a safety mechanism* such as a retracting needle. This allows a syringe to be attached to the back of the hub as a blood reservoir. Such angiocatheters may be difficult to find in some institutions.

with sterile technique. Inject local anesthetic with a 25-gauge or smaller needle to achieve sufficient infiltration and to ensure a painless procedure. Subcutaneous infiltration of lidocaine or a similar anesthetic may also reduce vessel spasm at the time of arterial puncture.

Check the catheter assembly for proper movement and function. Alternatively, a 3-mL syringe with the plunger removed can be used as a blood reservoir. Advance the catheter toward the palpated artery at a comfortable angle for the operator, generally 30 to 45 degrees from the skin (Fig. 20.5, *step 2*). Make a small incision with a No. 11 scalpel blade or a larger-bore needle to eliminate the problem of damage to the catheter from kinking on the skin. The tip of the needle may be perceived to pierce the artery, but successful puncture is confirmed by identifying a "flash" of arterial blood flow into the needle hub and reservoir. As the needle-catheter assembly advances through the skin toward the artery, the initial flash of arterial blood is obtained by the needle alone, which protrudes beyond the catheter. For this reason, the needle-catheter assembly should be lowered and advanced 2 mm forward to ensure that the tip of the catheter has cannulated the vessel, along with the needle (Fig. 20.5, *step 3*). The position of the catheter within the vessel lumen is confirmed by continuous return of arterial blood. The catheter alone can now be advanced with care over the needle and into the artery (Fig. 20.5, *step 4*). If the catheter fails to thread, it has not properly entered the vessel lumen and should not be forced to advance without confirmation of placement by active blood return.

When successful blood flow into the needle-catheter assembly has ceased, it may have pierced the backside of the arterial wall and may no longer be in the artery. If double puncture has occurred and blood has ceased to flow into the collection reservoir, do not remove the entire needle-catheter assembly. Instead, simply retract the needle slightly to determine whether blood flow into the catheter can be reestablished. If blood flow occurs, gently advance the catheter. If not, slowly withdraw the catheter until pulsatile blood flow reappears and then advance the catheter into the artery.

Once the catheter is fully advanced into the vessel lumen, maintain occlusive pressure on the proximal end of the artery to limit blood loss, and then remove the needle (Fig. 20.5, *step 5*). Next attach narrow-bore, low-compliance pressure tubing to the catheter (Fig. 20.5, *step 6*). Securely suture the apparatus to the wrist, and then apply an appropriate sterile dressing.

Ultrasound guidance is now routinely used for both peripheral and central venous access and can also assist with arterial cannulation (see Ultrasound Box). Ultrasound-guided radial artery cannulation is associated with an increased first attempt success rate, fewer attempts prior to success, and a lower incidence of hematoma formation compared to the traditional method of palpation. As with all procedures, this is dependent on the training and experience of the proceduralist.

With B-mode ultrasound, visualize the targeted artery in real time by using a 7.5- to 10-MHz linear array transducer. Differentiate the target artery from the adjacent vein by its pulsatility and noncompressibility under mild pressure by the transducer. Use color Doppler to further distinguish between arteries and veins. Either transverse or longitudinal views can be applied during arterial cannulation, but the transverse view is often more useful in smaller arteries. Once the catheter has entered the artery and it is confirmed by blood flow, place the ultrasound transducer on the field to free up the nondominant hand.[13,14]

The number of attempts and additional arterial punctures increases the size of the developing hematoma and the risk for vessel wall damage, thrombosis, and even loss of arterial flow through the vessel. Despite the added trauma, there is no reported increase in complications when both walls, rather than one, are punctured in a single cannulation attempt.[15]

Guidewire Techniques for Arterial Cannulation

A modified Seldinger technique can often rescue a failed direct cannulation attempt with an over-the-needle catheter (Fig. 20.6). If the catheter has been placed in the arterial lumen with successful blood return, pass a properly sized guidewire through the catheter and into the artery. Advance the catheter over the guidewire and fully into the vessel. Stiffer guidewires, unlike most prepackaged ones, do not have a softer, more flexible end tip and the vessel wall may be damaged or even perforated with excessive force. Alternatively, catheter sets are available with an attachable, catheter-contained, wire stylet that permits a modified Seldinger technique for placement of the catheter. The over-the-needle catheter follows the self-contained guidewire during cannulation. Numerous commercially available sets feature styles of guidewire and reservoir attachments that are different from an over-the-needle catheter assembly. Many resemble the Arrow Arterial Catheterization Kit (Arrow International) (Fig. 20.7; see also Fig. 20.2). These kits are very practical for smaller vessels, especially the radial, brachial, and axillary arteries, and have excellent success rates for first-time placement.

Seldinger Technique

Overall success rates with the Seldinger, guidewire-directed technique are superior to those with direct arterial cannulation. A few available kits are designed specifically for cannulation of larger arteries, but single-lumen venous catheters with guidewires may be used if catheter size and length are appropriate for specific arteries (see the following section for guidelines). The guidewire technique should be used initially for critical patients.

Place the needle percutaneously into the arterial lumen, as described previously. Then place a guidewire through the needle into the vessel lumen, and remove the needle. Thread the catheter over the wire, and pull the wire out. Although most kits have vessel dilators caution is advised, especially with larger catheter sizes. Dilate the tract only and not the artery to avoid unnecessary blood loss and excessive arterial injury.

Cutdown Technique for Arterial Cannulation

The cutdown technique is rarely used, but in certain circumstances it may be performed to obtain arterial access. With the increasing use of ultrasound-assisted catheter placement, this technique is rarely required. Perform cannulation after direct visualization of the vessel. A cutdown can be performed on any artery but is most commonly reserved for distal lower limb arteries and, rarely, the brachial artery. After a site has been selected, prepare the overlying skin with an antiseptic solution. Using sterile technique, inject local anesthetic solution subcutaneously in a horizontal line 2 to 3 cm long and perpendicular to the artery. Omit this step if the patient is unconscious or otherwise anesthetized at the cutdown site.

Arterial Cannulation: Guidewire Technique

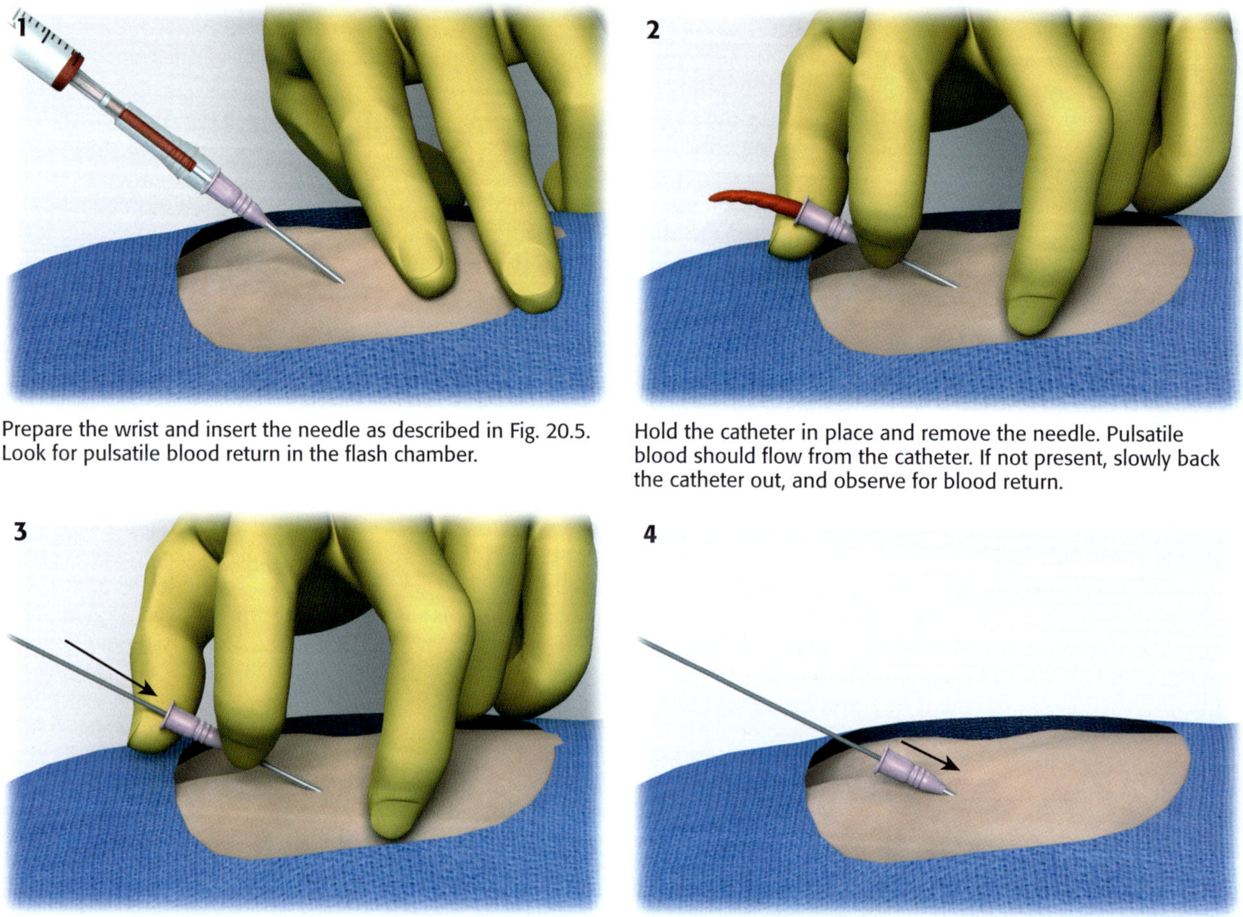

Prepare the wrist and insert the needle as described in Fig. 20.5. Look for pulsatile blood return in the flash chamber.

Hold the catheter in place and remove the needle. Pulsatile blood should flow from the catheter. If not present, slowly back the catheter out, and observe for blood return.

Insert the guidewire through the catheter. It should advance freely and easily into the vessel. Do not force it.

Advance the catheter over the wire and into the artery. Remove the wire, attach the catheter hub to the transducer tubing, and secure it to the skin.

Fig. 20.6 Arterial cannulation: guidewire technique.

Use a No. 10 or 15 scalpel blade to incise the skin along the anesthetic wheal. Spread the underlying tissues parallel to the artery with a mosquito hemostat. Palpate the pulse repeatedly throughout the procedure to ensure proper positioning. Once the surrounding soft tissue has been retracted and after exposing approximately 1 cm of the artery, isolate the artery by passing two silk sutures underneath it with the hemostat. Strip away only enough perivascular tissue to expose the artery. Perivascular tissue will help limit bleeding at the time of catheter removal. Introduce an over-the-needle catheter device, such as the kind used in the percutaneous method, and introduce it through the skin just distal to the incision. Advance it into the surgical site (Fig. 20.8). Alternatively, use a modified Seldinger guidewire setup to catheterize the artery. Puncture the arterial wall with the tip of the needle, and thread the catheter into the vessel lumen. When this has been accomplished, remove the two silk sutures, which have only been used to control the vessel, and close the skin incision. Do not tie off the artery the way that a vein is tied off during a venous cutdown. Apply firm pressure over the cutdown site, as used after arterial puncture. If pressure is not applied, separation of the soft tissues during the procedure may allow considerable hemorrhage into the tissue.

Local Puncture Site and Catheter Care

Once the catheter has been placed successfully, advance it until the hub is in contact with the skin. Secure the catheter by fastening it to the skin with suture material. Silk (2-0) or nylon (4-0) sutures provide good anchoring. To accomplish this, take a moderate bite of skin with the needle, and tie a knot in the suture while leaving both tails of the suture long. Avoid pinching the skin too tightly. Tie the loose ends of the suture around the catheter at its hub. Then after laying two ties, place a second set of knots on the back portion without occluding the lumen by constriction (Fig. 20.9).

Another option to secure these lines is to apply commercially available sutureless securement devices. According to one study, sutured lines are associated with a 10% rate of catheter-related bloodstream infection. In comparison, lines that were secured with a sutureless method had an infection rate of less than 1% and eliminated the potential for accidental needlestick from suturing.[16]

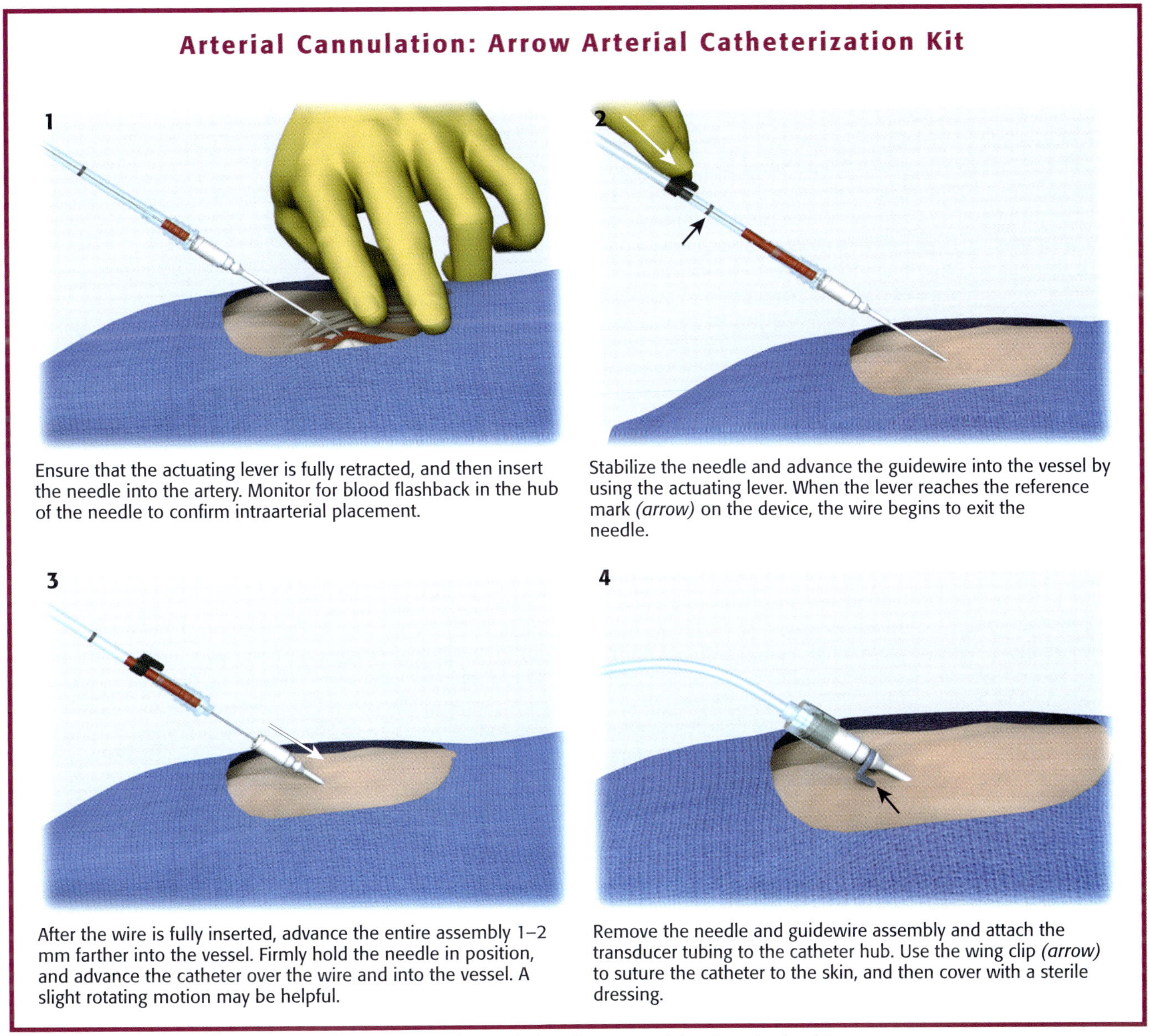

Fig. 20.7 Arterial cannulation: Arrow arterial catheterization kit.

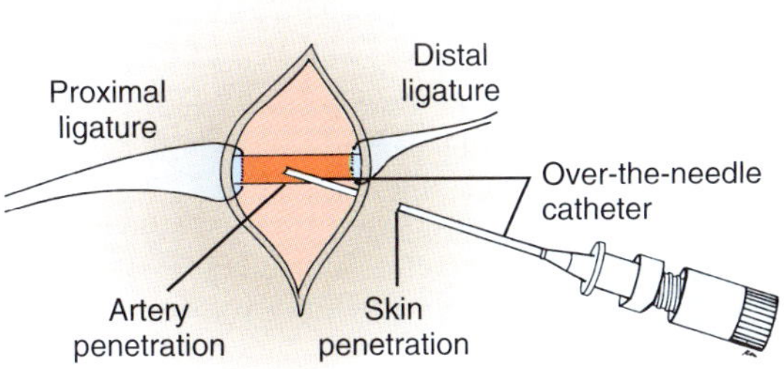

Fig. 20.8 Placement of an arterial line using the cutdown technique. Note that the catheter enters the surgical wound percutaneously to minimize entry of bacteria into the healing wound and permit better stabilization of the catheter. Entry of the catheter into the vessel is more parallel to the vessel than illustrated. Ligatures are only used to *temporarily* isolate the artery and to control bleeding. *The artery should not be tied off.* The catheter is secured by suturing the hub to the skin.

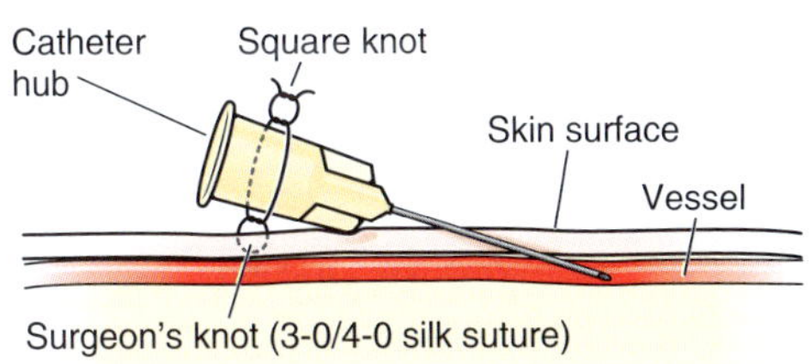

Fig. 20.9 A technique for securing a vascular catheter to adjacent skin.

After tying the catheter in place, apply a self-adhesive dressing over the area. Certain transparent dressings containing chlorhexidine gluconate can slow the colonization of bacteria.[17] Further secure the catheter and its connecting tubing with sterile sponges and adhesive tape. Make sure that all tubing connections are tight and secure. If the tubing becomes disconnected inadvertently, the patient can exsanguinate rapidly.

Fluid-Pressurized Systems

When successful arterial cannulation has been performed, attach the catheter to a pressurized fluid-filled system. A three-way stopcock can be interposed between the patient and the transducer for blood gas sampling and to allow flushing of the system. Flushing can be periodic or continuous at a rate of 3 to 4 mL/h through a continuous-flow device. Most institutions use normal saline in place of heparinized solution to maintain patency. Use of a heparinized flush solution in pressurized arterial lines may result in greater long-term accuracy of pressure monitoring, but no real difference in catheter blockage has been reported, and this approach avoids heparin-related complications such as drug incompatibility, thrombosis, local tissue damage, and hemorrhage.[18] For short-term setups as in the ED, saline is sufficient.

Blood samples are obtained easily from the arterial catheter system. Attach a syringe to the three-way stopcock and aspirate and discard the blood to clear the line. Short lengths of tubing between the catheter and the aspiration port minimize the necessary discard volume. A reasonable approach is to aspirate 4 to 5 mL for a tubing length of 91 cm (36 inches), and for a tubing length of 213 cm (84 inches), aspirate 8 mL. Attach a second syringe that has been heparinized, and aspirate 3 mL of blood to send for ABG analysis. If the blood is to be used for other tests, the second syringe does not need to be heparinized. Self-contained, nondetachable, blood sample withdrawing systems allow less blood wasting for sampling. Flush the stopcock and line to avoid clotting.

SELECTION OF ARTERIES FOR CANNULATION

Radial and Ulnar Arteries

The radial artery is most frequently used for prolonged cannulation. Widespread collateral flow is present in the wrist because of two major palmar anastomoses known as arches (Fig. 20.10). The superficial palmar arch lies between the aponeurosis palmaris and the tendons of the flexor digitorum sublimis. The arch is formed mainly by the terminal ulnar artery and the superficial palmar branch of the radial artery. The other major communication of these two vessels, the deep palmar arch, is formed by connections of the terminal radial artery with the deep palmar branches of the ulnar artery. Some collateral flow is almost always present at the wrist

Before attempting radial artery cannulation, the adequacy of collateral flow to the hand may be assessed by performing a bedside examination called the Allen test. This examination was originally described by E.V. Allen in 1929 and is used to assess arterial stenosis in the hands of patients with thromboangiitis obliterans. This test identifies patients at increased risk for ischemic complications from radial artery catheterization. The modified Allen test is performed as follows: occlude both the radial and ulnar arteries with digital pressure and then ask the patient to tightly clench the fist repeatedly to exsanguinate the hand. Then open the hand and release the occlusion of the ulnar artery only (Fig. 20.11). After 2 minutes, repeat the test in the same manner with release of the radial artery only. Rubor should return rapidly to the hand following the release of pressure from either vessel.

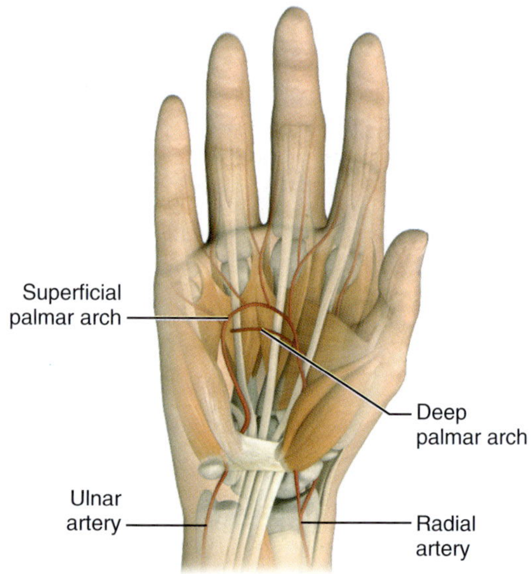

Fig. 20.10 Arterial anatomy of the hand and wrist.

An abnormal (positive) Allen test result, suggestive of inadequate collateralization, is the continued presence of pallor 5 to 15 seconds after release of the radial artery.[3] If return of color takes longer than 5 to 10 seconds, do not perform radial artery puncture. Be careful to avoid overextension of the hand with wide separation of the digits, which may compress the palmar arches between fascial planes and yield a false-positive result. Time permitting, performance of some variation of the Allen test is desirable before ulnar or radial puncture, especially for prolonged cannulation. This test is not mandatory or standard for one-time radial artery puncture for blood gas sampling. Moreover, there have been reports of ischemic sequelae after cannulation even after a normal Allen test result and others that have found no ischemic complications following radial artery catheterization and abnormal results on the Allen test. Although there are no guarantees against digital ischemia after radial artery cannulation, the finding of an abnormal Allen test result should be documented and lead one to search for an alternative site for the procedure.

At the wrist, the radial artery rests on the flexor digitorum superficialis muscle, the flexor pollicis longus muscle, the pronator quadratus muscle, and the radius bone. Isolate the pulsation of the artery on the palmar surface of the wrist. The radial artery is more superficial as it moves closer to the wrist. In this location, it provides a more consistent site for cannulation because of its fixation and decreased mobility. Dorsiflexing the wrist at approximately a 45-degree angle over a towel or sandbag and fixing the wrist to an arm board will also help isolate the artery.[19] This degree of preparation should be considered standard when time for setup permits (see Fig. 20.5, *step 1*).[15]

Antegrade radial artery cannulation may be accomplished in infants and children when the radial arteries are obstructed and retrograde blood flow is observed during a failed cutdown attempt at standard retrograde arterial cannulation. In addition, displacement of perivascular interstitial fluid in neonates and bright light make the course of the artery visible. Then, under direct vision, cannulation of the artery becomes as easy as venous cannulation.[20] Doppler ultrasound on selected patients with poor peripheral pulses may also

The Allen Test

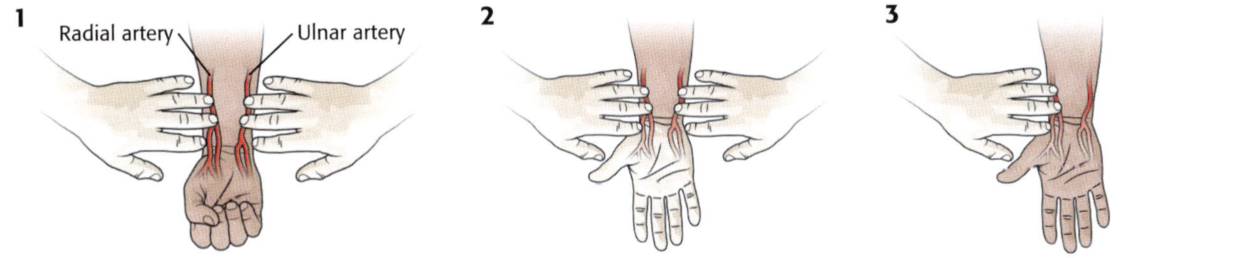

1. Compress both the radial and ulnar arteries to occlude arterial flow, and instruct the patient to repeatedly make a tight fist to squeeze venous blood out of the hand. Alternatively, the hand may be squeezed first and then the arteries occluded.

2. Instruct the patient to relax the hand and extend the fingers. Carefully observe the hand—it should be blanched.

3. Release the ulnar artery and observe the hand for return of rubor, which signifies good flow in the ulnar artery. If filling does not occur within 5 to 10 seconds, radial artery cannulation should not be done. If brisk filling occurs, repeat the test with release of the radial artery to assess radial artery patency. If both the radial and ulnar arteries demonstrate patency, the wrist may be used for arterial cannulation.

Fig. 20.11 Allen test. Before puncturing the radial artery for cannulation, it is important to identify a competent ulnar artery should injury to the radial artery occur. This is not generally required, nor standard, for a single arterial puncture. (Adapted from Schwartz GR, ed. *Principles and Practice of Emergency Medicine*. Saunders; 1978:354.)

facilitate percutaneous radial artery cannulation and minimize the number of punctures needed for placement.

The ulnar artery is seldom used because its smaller size makes it more difficult to puncture than the radial artery. At the wrist, the ulnar artery runs along the palmar margin of the flexor carpi ulnaris in the space between it and the flexor digitorum sublimis. Use caution because the artery runs next to the ulnar nerve as both pass into the hand just radial to the pisiform bone. Minimize any potential injury by approaching the ulnar artery from the radial side.[21] Make the ulnar artery more accessible with dorsiflexion of the wrist.

Brachial Artery

Although it appears safe for arterial puncture, the brachial artery does not have the anatomic benefit of the collateral circulation that is found in the wrist. The brachial artery begins as the continuation of the axillary artery and ends at the head of the radius, where it splits into the ulnar and radial arteries. The preferred puncture site of the brachial artery is in or just proximal to the antecubital fossa. In this region, the artery lies on top of the brachialis muscle and enters the fossa underneath the bicipital aponeurosis with the median nerve, and on the medial side of the artery (Fig. 20.12). Both the radial and the axillary arteries are preferred over the brachial artery in the upper extremity. With the brachial artery, there is increased risk for ischemic complications from the reduction in collateral circulation, as well as the need to maintain the arm in extension for puncture and prolonged cannulation. A longer catheter (10 cm) is required for the brachial artery so that sufficient length is available to traverse the elbow joint.

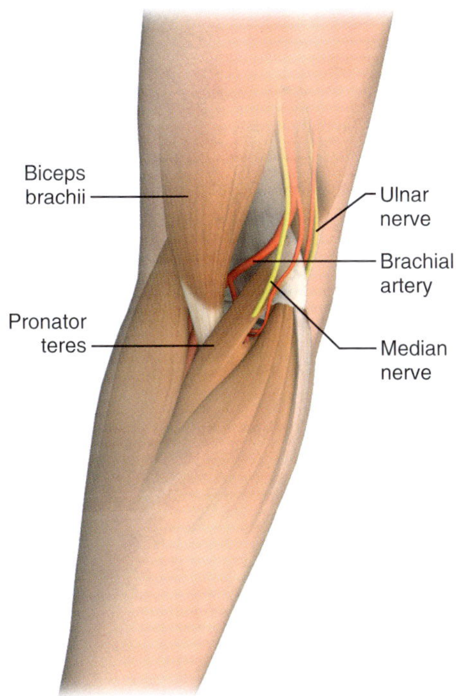

Fig. 20.12 Brachial artery anatomy.

Dorsalis Pedis Artery

The dorsalis pedis artery continues from the anterior tibial artery and runs from approximately midway between the malleoli to the posterior end of the first metatarsal space, where it forms the dorsal metatarsal and deep plantar arteries. The lateral plantar artery, a branch of the posterior tibial artery, passes obliquely across the foot to the base of the fifth metatarsal. The plantar arch is completed at the point where the lateral plantar artery joins the deep plantar artery between the first and second metatarsals. On the dorsum of the foot, the dorsalis pedis artery lies in the subcutaneous tissue parallel

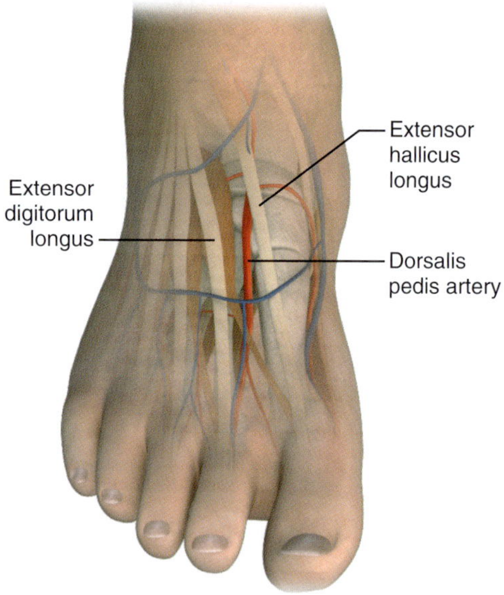

Fig. 20.13 Dorsalis pedis artery anatomy.

to the extensor hallucis longus tendon and between it and the extensor digitorum longus (Fig. 20.13).

Cannulate the artery in the midfoot region. Although this vessel is amenable to cutdown, the vascular anatomy of the foot is quite variable. This is of no consequence if a pulse can be palpated. Although the dorsal pedis and posterior tibial arteries form similar collateral foot circulation as in the hand, the nature of advancing vascular disease makes this a more difficult cannulation, with higher complication rates than in the wrist. This site has its major utility in pediatric monitoring cases. Attempts to predetermine collateral flow with a modified Allen test using the posterior tibial and dorsalis pedis arteries is not as easily performed in the foot as in the hand, nor are there good data to prove its validity. Monitoring problems also exist with this artery.

Femoral Artery

The femoral artery is the second most commonly used vessel for arterial cannulation. Based on its ease of cannulation and low record of complications, it has been called the vessel of choice for arterial access.[22] Along with the axillary artery, the femoral artery more closely resembles aortic pressure waveforms than those from any other peripheral site. The femoral artery is the direct continuation of the iliac artery and enters the thigh after passing below the inguinal ligament. Arterial puncture should occur distal to the ligament to prevent hemorrhage into the pelvis or peritoneum. The artery is generally easily palpated midway between the pubic symphysis and the anterior superior iliac spine. The advantage of cannulating the artery at a site just distal to the inguinal ligament is that the artery can be compressed against the femoral head. Cannulation becomes more difficult the more distal the puncture site is from the inguinal ligament because the femoral artery splits into the superficial femoral and the deep femoral arteries. These arteries, especially the deep femoral, can be challenging to compress if bleeding needs to be controlled. One method of locating an appropriate arterial puncture site is to place the thumb and fifth finger on the pubis symphysis and the anterior iliac spine and locate the artery underneath the middle knuckle. When puncturing this vessel, be careful to

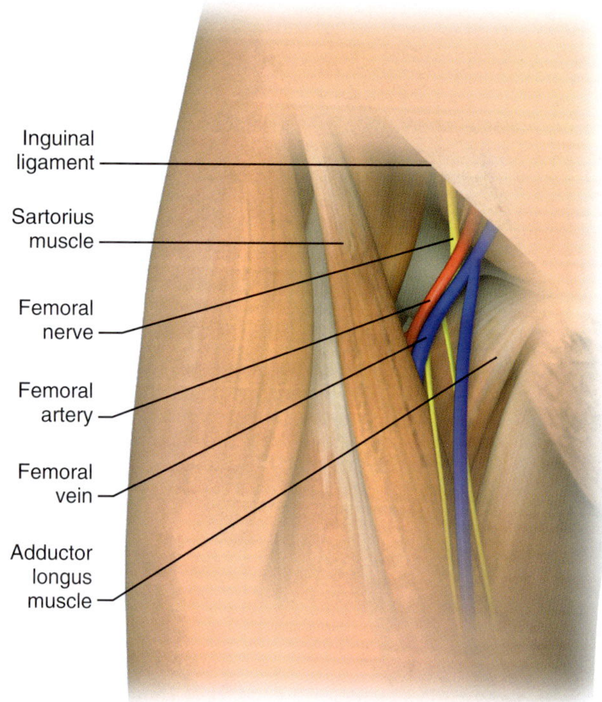

Fig. 20.14 Femoral artery anatomy.

avoid the femoral nerve and vein, which form the lateral and medial borders, respectively (Fig. 20.14).

A longer, larger-diameter catheter is required for accurate monitoring of the femoral artery because of its size and the relatively greater depth at which it lies. Only the Seldinger technique is recommended for this site, which enables placement of a 15- to 20-cm plastic catheter for prolonged monitoring. Avoid using catheter-through-the-needle or over-the-needle devices because of the vessel's distance beneath the skin. Leakage around the catheter can occur with these devices as a result of the high arterial pressure and the loose fit of the cannula in the hole in the vessel wall. Regardless of the device used, enter the skin with the needle at an angle of approximately 45 degrees instead of the usual 15 to 20 degrees.

The extremely large ratio of arterial diameter to catheter diameter is thought to reduce the incidence of thrombosis, particularly total occlusion. However, occlusion has been reported with femoral cannulation for monitoring purposes. A commonly perceived disadvantage of this site is the increased possibility of bacterial contamination because of its proximity to the warm, moist groin and perineum; however, there are not good data to support this. The femoral area is inconvenient for any patient who is awake and mobile or for a patient who is able to sit in a chair. If the patient is that mobile, reconsider the risk-benefit ratio of invasive monitoring. Despite theoretical difficulties, some hospitals use femoral arterial lines almost exclusively, and the ICU nursing staff is often more comfortable caring for these lines than those at other sites.

Umbilical and Temporal Arteries

In neonates, arterial access can be accomplished for a short time through the umbilical artery (see Chapter 19). After this artery closes, the temporal artery provides a safe alternative. Use the cutdown method with a 22-gauge catheter after the artery's course has been traced with an ultrasonic flow detector. Because of the increasing accuracy of ear oximeters and the use of capillary blood gas samples for determination of pH, prolonged arterial cannulation has become less frequent during infant care.

COMPLICATIONS OF ARTERIAL CANNULATION

Arterial cannulation is safe when care is taken to avoid complications. Most can be avoided by adhering to a few simple principles. Reported clinical sequelae of arterial puncture and cannulation range from simple hematomas to life-threatening infections and exsanguination. In addition, ischemia, arteriovenous fistula, and pseudoaneurysm formation are possible. The incidence of complications varies with the site selected, the method of cannulation, and the clinician's level of skill and experience.

It is difficult to compare complication rates at various sites because most published studies have primarily used only the radial artery. No studies have compared the approach and complication rates of arterial catheters in the ED with those placed in the ICU or operating room. In a large study spanning 24 months, 2119 ICU patients had arterial catheters placed at admission: 52% at the radial site and 45% at the femoral site. The most common complication was vascular insufficiency (4%), followed by bleeding (2.1%) and infection (0.6%). No difference was reported in infection rates at femoral versus radial sites.[23] There are reports of complications from arterial puncture for procedures unrelated to cannulation, such as arteriography or simple puncture for blood sampling as routinely performed in the ED.

Hematoma formation at the puncture site is common. Bruising is usually of minimal clinical significance, but leakage can be dangerous when it occurs around the catheter or from the puncture site after the catheter is removed (Fig. 20.15). Compression neuropathies requiring surgical decompression have been reported after arterial puncture secondary to hematoma formation.[24,25] The large amount of soft tissue surrounding the femoral artery makes bleeding in this area difficult to control. Large hematomas can occur after femoral artery catheterization. Though uncommon, a clinician should be aware of the potential development of a retroperitoneal hematoma following femoral artery cannulation. Suspect this complication in patients in whom hypovolemic shock with a falling hematocrit develops following the procedure.[26] Another serious complication is the formation of a pseudoaneurysm as the walls of the punctured artery fail to seal properly. Although most pseudoaneurysms can be managed conservatively, they are susceptible to both rupture and infection. Several treatment options are now available, and identification of a pseudoaneurysm should prompt referral to a vascular surgeon.[27,28] More commonly, hematomas are painful, slow to resolve, and prone to infection. Multiple-site punctures and inadequate pressure applied for insufficient time account for most hematomas. Multiple punctures can be avoided in most instances by experienced operators and the use of ultrasound-aided techniques.

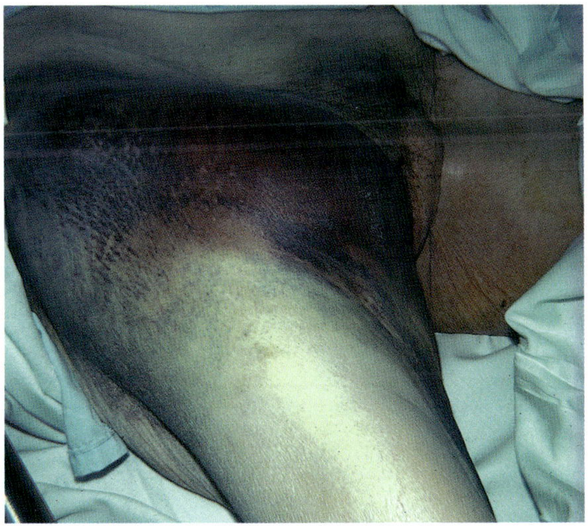

Fig. 20.15 Right groin hemorrhage with resulting hematoma 3 days after iatrogenic injury. The injury resulted from a failed attempt to place a right femoral artery catheter via the Seldinger technique. Inadequate pressure after the procedure resulted in bleeding from the artery.

Thrombotic occlusion after radial arterial cannulation occurs commonly in infants and small children; however, ischemia from occlusion is rare because of collateral blood supply from the ulnar artery. Insertion sites closest to the bend of the wrist increase the chance of maintaining patency. Nonpatency is four times more likely with insertion at sites 3 cm or more proximal to the bend in the wrist.[29] Serious complications after radial artery cannulation are extremely rare in the absence of contributing factors such as preexisting vasospastic arterial disease, previous arterial injury, protracted shock, high-dose vasopressor administration, prolonged cannulation, or infection.

Prevention of bleeding complications can be accomplished with frequent careful inspection of the puncture site and the use of prolonged compression after removal of the catheter or needle. Maintain firm pressure for 10 minutes or longer after removing a peripheral artery catheter and longer after femoral cannulation or if the patient has received anticoagulants. Five minutes of pressure is sufficient after puncture for a blood gas sample in an individual with normal coagulation. Exsanguination may occur if the arterial line apparatus becomes disconnected. This is more common in an obtunded or combative patient, and restraints may be required for patients with indwelling arterial cannulas. Exsanguination should not occur if tight connections are maintained throughout the system and if frequent, careful inspections of both the circuit and the patient are made.

Meticulous attention to aseptic technique is necessary during insertion and catheter maintenance to minimize the risk for catheter-related infections.[30] Serious infections rarely complicate arterial cannulation. Simple interventions can reduce the risk for serious catheter-related infection. Evidence supports the use of full-barrier precautions during catheter insertion, specialized nursing care, and newer-generation catheters with antiseptic hubs or antimicrobial agent–impregnated catheters. The incidence of catheter-related infections increases with prolonged cannulation. Catheters placed via sterile technique have an extremely low rate of infection in the first 96 hours after placement.

Most infections begin locally at the puncture site and remain localized, although systemic sepsis has been reported. The radial and femoral sites have a similar incidence of complications, but axillary cannulation seems to have a much higher incidence of infection (although no large studies of cannulation at this site exist). Arterial cannulas are more prone to infectious complications than other vascular catheters. Many mechanisms have been proposed for this increased incidence. The arterial pressure–monitoring system usually consists of a long column of fairly stagnant fluid and is subject to frequent manipulation. The sampling stopcock is a site of frequent bacterial contamination.

The risk for infection also increases as the duration of cannulation is prolonged. Older studies recommend that catheters be changed after 4 days if continued monitoring is necessary. However, the risk for noninfectious complications increases with more frequent catheter and site changes. Therefore daily evaluation of the site is advised, and catheter change should not be mandatory until 7 to 8 days if the site remains clean.

The current standard is a clean, nonocclusive, dry dressing. An antibiotic- or silver-impregnated catheter is recommended for long-term placement.

Thrombosis of the vessel in which the cannula is placed is another frequently encountered problem. The incidence of thrombosis varies with the method used to determine the presence of clots. Angiographic studies show deposition of fibrin on 100% of catheters left in place for longer than 1 day, although clinical evidence of ischemia secondary to occlusion by such thrombi is seen in less than 1% of cases in most studies.[31] Most reports of nonangiographic catheterization involve the radial artery. Larger catheter sizes, trauma during cannulation, and the presence of atherosclerosis have all been postulated to increase the incidence of thrombosis; however, conflicting studies abound.

Arterial spasm after puncture (usually following multiple attempts) can predispose to thrombus formation and can even lead to ischemic changes without fibrin deposition. Successful reversal of spasm with intraarterial lidocaine, reserpine, and phentolamine has been reported, but no good studies of their efficacy in this clinical situation have been published.

Thrombosis can be minimized by decreasing the duration of catheterization and proper flushing. Surgical embolectomy or thrombectomy is rarely required because the smaller vessels that are most likely to occlude usually have good collateral circulation. The larger femoral artery, which has poor collateralization, rarely occludes with catheterization when used for monitoring purposes.

A few less common complications are easily prevented. One that occurs only with the percutaneous catheter-through-the-needle method is catheter embolization. Once the catheter has been placed through the needle, it should never be pulled back because the end of the catheter may be sheared off by the sharp needle bevel. If this complication occurs, surgical removal of the tip of the catheter is necessary.

One feared complication of indwelling radial and brachial arterial catheters is the occurrence of a cerebrovascular accident secondary to embolization from flushing of the catheters. Cerebral embolization can be prevented with the use of continuous flush systems (3 mL/h) and by ensuring the integrity of the tubing and transducer systems to prevent entry of air. In addition, small volumes (<2 mL) of intermittent flush solution should be used.

Once the monitoring system is set up, manipulate it as little as possible. Perform any handling with aseptic technique. Change the tubing and other fluid-filled devices every 48 hours, and insert catheters into a vessel that provides the largest vessel-to-catheter ratio as possible.

If these principles are followed and the patient and system are carefully inspected at frequent intervals, complications of arterial puncture and cannulation can be minimized.

INTERPRETATION

An indwelling arterial catheter provides continuous blood pressure monitoring. The trend of a patient's pressure facilitates assessment of the effect of various therapeutic interventions. The absolute systolic and diastolic pressure measured will vary at different catheter sites, with higher peak systolic pressures measured at the periphery. The pressure will also be higher when measured at the distal end of the lower limb. A wide variance between direct arterial pressure and the pressure measured with a standard pneumatic cuff will always exist in some patients. Oscillometric blood pressure measurement can significantly underestimate arterial blood pressure.[32] For this reason, regularly compare a cuff pressure with that obtained via invasive monitoring. Moreover, a change in their relationship may be the first indication of difficulty with the direct measuring system.

Waveform analysis may also provide an early indication of thrombosis in the arterial catheter. Many variables affect the waveform, including cardiac valvular disease and arteriosclerosis. Waveforms may vary tremendously among patients, but after an adequate monitoring system has been established, a change in an individual's pressure wave is usually indicative of thrombosis or a malfunction in the monitoring system. A change in waveform may also indicate a change in the patient's cardiovascular status, such as a papillary muscle rupture. Before making a therapeutic decision based on an electronically generated number, recheck the patient's blood pressure with a pneumatic cuff. This device is less fallible than the electromechanical system.

Radial systolic arterial pressure poorly estimates the actual ascending aortic pressure, with more than 50% of cases reporting a difference in values of 10 to 35 mm Hg. Mean arterial pressure and diastolic pressure, in contrast, are closer to aortic values. Longer catheters have also been used successfully from radial sites to more accurately reflect central aortic pressure for cardiac surgery patients.[33]

An indwelling arterial cannula can provide valuable information about the hemodynamic status of a patient (through continuous pressure monitoring) and about the patient's respiratory and metabolic status (through intermittent sampling for ABG analysis and other blood tests). The Pco_2 and pH of the blood can be used to define four major groups of metabolic derangement: respiratory acidosis or alkalosis and metabolic acidosis or alkalosis. However, rarely will a disorder be strictly classified into one of these groups.

Adequacy of blood oxygenation can be determined from the measured Po_2 of arterial blood and the known concentration of oxygen that the patient is inspiring. To avoid iatrogenic complications of intensive care, one must be certain that the data are from an arterial sample that has been properly analyzed before basing one's treatment decisions on the numbers obtained. Not uncommonly, a venous sample is interpreted as though it were arterial. Furthermore, false readings may result if the sample is not free of air bubbles, not promptly chilled, or not analyzed within 20 to 30 minutes. Though still controversial, blood gas values that are not corrected for body temperature appear to be more appropriate for guiding therapy in hypothermic patients.[34,35]

CONCLUSION

As intensive care knowledge grows and technology develops, cannulation of the arterial system may decrease in frequency. Oximeters can determine the quality of blood oxygenation transcutaneously and are becoming more accurate and sophisticated. Electronic sphygmomanometers are being refined for continuous indirect blood pressure monitoring. As these devices improve and noninvasive sampling methods for clinically relevant electrolytes and physiologic markers are refined, the indwelling arterial cannula may in time become considered overly invasive. Despite improvements in noninvasive monitoring devices, the current need for frequent blood sampling for chemical and hematologic analysis remains an indication for its use in selected critically ill patients. Overzealous blood gas analysis may lead to iatrogenic anemia in the ICU. Multiple reports have documented the advantages of limiting frequent blood sampling.[36–38]

Arterial puncture and cannulation are invaluable aids to the emergency and critical care clinician. Long-term catheterization is a safe procedure when the catheter is placed, maintained, and removed with care. The radial artery is the most favored location for puncture, but as more experience is gained and reported with femoral artery catheterization, the latter has become a more frequently used site. Selection of either site is associated with a low complication rate and should be determined by the skill of the clinician, the nursing team, and the relative convenience and comfort of the patient. Ultrasound guidance for arterial catheter placement is becoming the standard and should be considered in every instance to reduce the need for multiple puncture attempts.

ACKNOWLEDGMENT

The author acknowledges the work of Drs. Dave Milzman, Tim Janchar, and Hyung T. Kim, who were authors of this chapter in previous editions.

REFERENCES ARE AVAILABLE AT Elsevier eBooks+

CHAPTER 21

Peripheral Intravenous Access

Bonnie L. Kaplan and Shan W. Liu

INTRODUCTION

Intravenous (IV) access is a mainstay of modern medicine. IV cannulation is a procedure performed by a wide array of healthcare professionals, including physicians, nurses, physician assistants, phlebotomists, and emergency medical technicians. In the emergency department (ED), uncomplicated peripheral venous access is usually secured by a nurse or technician. In the United States, more than 200 million peripheral IV catheters are placed in patients each year as vascular access for the administration of medications and fluids and the sampling of blood for analysis. IV access can usually be accomplished in less than 5 minutes. Despite their growing number, dedicated IV teams are very costly and not always cost effective, but in cases of difficult peripheral IV access, this resource may save time for ED staff.[1,2] Moreover, in the ED setting, multiple providers may be called on to obtain IV access, thus making it an essential skill for both emergency physicians and nurses to master. Subtleties in technique are important and can be improved with practice; newer technologies such as ultrasound can assist providers in placing IV lines in even the most challenging situations.

HISTORICAL PERSPECTIVE

Bloodletting, or bleeding, dates to the time of Hippocrates. The ancient technique consisted of tying a bandage around the arm to distend the forearm veins, opening a vein with a sharp knife, and collecting the blood into a basin. In the Middle Ages, this was performed by barber-surgeons. In 1656, Sir Christopher Wren injected opium into dogs intravenously with a quill and bladder, thereby becoming the father of modern IV therapy.[3] Blood transfusions also date back to the mid-1600s. The French physician Jean Denis is credited with the first successful transfusion by giving lamb's blood to a 15-year-old boy.[4,5]

Originally, 16- to 18-gauge indwelling steel needles were used for IV infusions. In the 1950s the Rochester needle was introduced, which was a resinous catheter on the outside of a steel introducer needle. Because of increased comfort and mobility, plastic catheters have replaced indwelling metal needles and are now almost universal.

INDICATIONS AND CONTRAINDICATIONS

Obtaining timely and adequate vascular access is a top priority during any resuscitation. In patients with normal perfusion, differences in delivery times for injections centrally versus peripherally are minimal. During cardiopulmonary resuscitation (CPR), however, medications have been shown to reach the central circulation faster with central access than with peripheral venous access. A change in outcome, though, has not been demonstrated with the central administration of advanced cardiac life support drugs; hence, peripheral IV cannulation is the procedure of choice even during CPR because of the speed, ease, and safety with which it can often be accomplished. In less critically ill patients, the role of IV therapy is more often debated and access is ultimately unnecessary in a large proportion of patients in whom it is obtained.[6] In broad terms, IV access or therapy is needed in patients for whom IV medications are required or when oral therapy is inadequate (e.g., severe shock states), contraindicated (e.g., surgical emergencies), or impossible (e.g., intractable vomiting). Saline or heparin locks are preferable when IV medications are needed and there are limited foreseeable fluid requirements. Saline locks cost less than a full IV fluid and tubing assembly and are especially helpful when vascular access is needed suddenly. Access to the catheter requires irrigation with a separate syringe and flush.

A peripheral IV central catheter (PICC) shares the attributes of both central and peripheral venous IV lines. A PICC is composed of a thin tube of biocompatible material with an attachment hub. It is inserted percutaneously, under ultrasound guidance by a dedicated PICC team, into a peripheral vein and then advanced into a large central vein, followed by radiographic confirmation of placement. PICCs are suitable for long-term vascular access for blood sampling, infusion of antibiotics and hyperosmolar solutions such as total parenteral nutrition, and infusion of certain chemotherapeutic agents.

A midline catheter is another peripheral IV option. It is inserted in a larger vessel than for a standard peripheral IV (basilic, cephalic, or median vein in the antecubital fossa). Typically, an 8- to 12-cm-long catheter is used for adults with ultrasound guidance. After insertion, the catheter is advanced until the distal tip rests in the upper arm right below the axillary line. While this line is typically suitable for 14 days of use, it can be an alternative option for patients with difficult access or ones needing longer term therapy.[7] When compared to PICCs, one study found they had fewer associated bloodstream infections and occlusions, with a very similar number of thrombotic events.[8]

Peripheral IV lines should not be placed in extremities with massive edema, burns, sclerosis, phlebitis, or thrombosis due to risk for extravasation or suboptimal volume flow. Avoid placing an IV line in extremities on the same side as radical mastectomies, though they can be used when an urgent condition exists and other peripheral access is not possible. When feasible, cannulation at infected sites, such as through an area of cellulitis, and extremities with shunts or fistulas should be avoided because it may cause bacteremia or thrombosis. If possible, do not cannulate a vein over or distal to a recent fracture site on an extremity (Fig. 21.1). Veins that drain from an area affected by trauma or major vascular disruption (e.g., distal to a ruptured aorta) are also suboptimal because fluid or medications may not be delivered to the circulatory system.

Blood samples for laboratory analysis are usually drawn before IV cannulation to avoid contamination with IV fluid or medication. However, studies have shown that accurate basic electrolyte and hematologic values can be obtained with peripheral IV lines when infusions are shut off for at least 2 minutes, at least 5 mL of blood is wasted, and all tubes are completely filled to avoid inaccurate bicarbonate readings.[9] By adopting these techniques, one can reduce the number of peripheral needlesticks, minimize trauma to, or sclerosis of, the vein, and improve patient satisfaction.

ULTRASOUND GUIDANCE AND TRANSILLUMINATION

Ultrasound can assist in the placement of peripheral lines. For IV placements that have been designated "difficult" after a certain number of attempts by nursing staff, use of ultrasound guidance increases the success rate and decreases the number of attempts necessary for successful cannulation in both adult and pediatric patients.[10–12] One 2016 randomized controlled trial showed that ultrasound guidance is particularly helpful in patients with perceived difficult access. The caliber of the vein identified on ultrasound is predictive of its ability to be cannulated. If no vessel is identified, cannulation is not usually possible.[14,15] An additional issue with ultrasound-guided peripheral IV lines is their longevity. One study highlighted the high premature failure rate of ultrasound-guided peripheral lines.[16] Ongoing studies are evaluating this concern. It is likely related to the depth of the veins being cannulated, the length and type of catheter used, and the angle of the catheter through soft tissue.

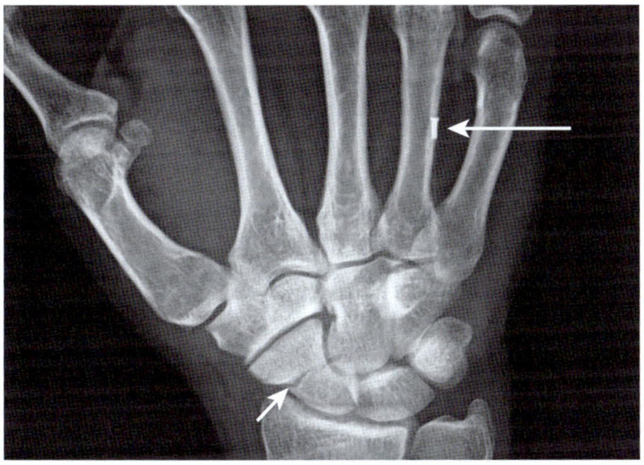

Fig. 21.1 Do not place peripheral intravenous (IV) access *(long arrow)* near or distal to a fracture in an extremity *(short arrow)*. In this case an IV line for pain medication was placed before obtaining the radiograph. The scaphoid fracture was not suspected and the opposite arm had difficult access.

Other devices transilluminate the veins to increase their visibility. This appears to be especially helpful in infants, though little evidence exists evaluating their utility. One 2012 study showed an increase in successful first-attempt rates in pediatric patients with difficult peripheral access.[17] As emergency providers have become more comfortable with these advancing technologies, ultrasound-guided and illumination-assisted insertion of peripheral lines have increased (Videos 21.1–21.7).

ANATOMY

The success of cannulation depends on familiarity with the vascular anatomy of the extremities. In the upper extremity, the veins of the hands are drained by the metacarpal and dorsal veins, which connect to form the dorsal venous arch (Fig. 21.2). These sites are excellent for IV therapy and comfortably accommodate 22- and 20-gauge catheters. The venous supply of the wrist and forearm consists of the basilic vein, which courses along the ulnar portion of the posterior aspect of the forearm. It is often ignored because of its location but can easily be accessed if the patient's forearm is flexed and the clinician stands at the head of the patient. On the radial side of the forearm, the cephalic vein is commonly known as the *intern vein*. Readily accessible, this vein can accommodate 22- to 16-gauge catheters. The median veins of the forearm course through the middle of the forearm, and the accessory cephalic veins on the radial aspect of the forearm are easily stabilized and accessible.

The antecubital veins consist of the medial cubital, basilic, and cephalic veins; these are often selected for catheters or blood drawing. IV placement here is easy, but mobility of the arm is restricted once the catheter is in place. The larger veins above the antecubital space, the cephalic and basilic veins, are often more difficult to see but can often be accessed relatively easily if necessary.

The relevant lower extremity venous anatomy starts with the dorsal digital veins, which become the dorsal metatarsal veins and form the dorsal venous arch. The arch ultimately

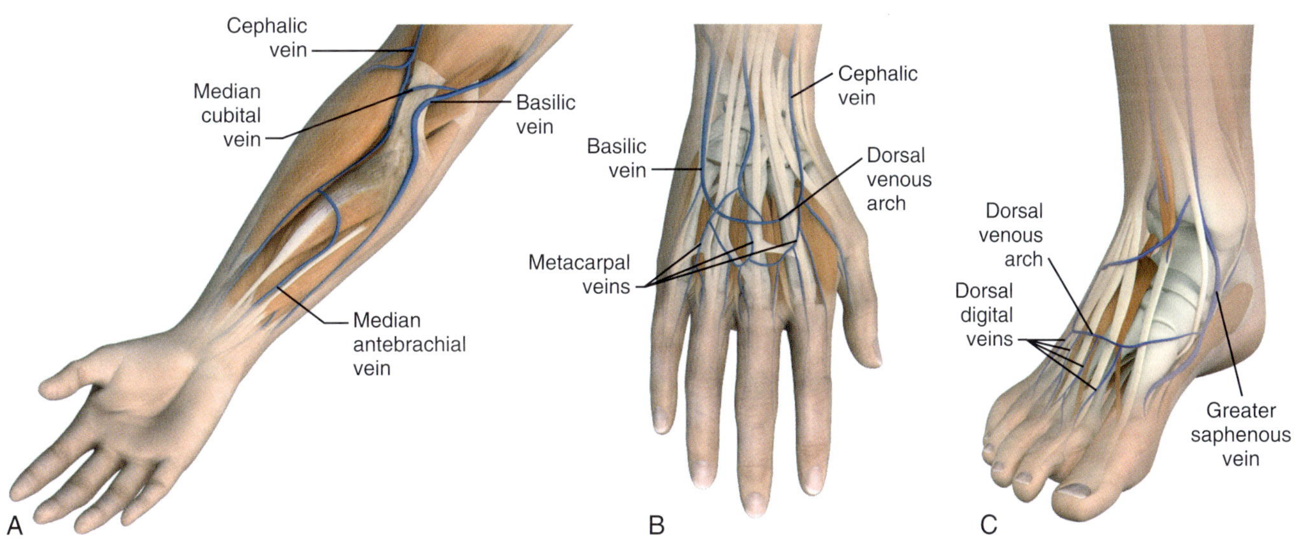

Fig. 21.2 (A–C) Anatomy of extremity veins for peripheral intravenous cannulation.

ULTRASOUND: Peripheral Intravenous Access

by Christine Butts, MD

Ultrasound-guided access is indicated when standard placement is difficult. This may include patients with no palpable or visible peripheral veins, history of intravenous drug use or multiple previous peripheral lines causing scarring or thrombosis, obesity, or previous surgeries causing distortion of the anatomy. Use of ultrasound to achieve peripheral intravenous access has been found to increase the rate of success, decrease both the time to placement and the number of attempts, and increase overall patient satisfaction.[1] Nursing use of ultrasound to guide peripheral intravenous access has also shown to improve success and decrease complications.[2]

There are two methods by which ultrasound may be used to access peripheral veins. In the first method, ultrasound is used to simply evaluate the underlying anatomy. Frequently, veins are present superficially but cannot be seen or palpated from the surface of the skin. Apply the transducer to rapidly locate an ideal vein and cannulate it "blindly" in the typical fashion. The second method calls for ultrasound to be used to directly guide venous access. This method may be most practical when the veins are deeper within the tissues or adjacent to other important structures.

Use a high-frequency (7.5- to 10-mHz) transducer to obtain the necessary resolution for evaluating the anatomy. Typically, for peripheral venous access, a sterile field is not necessary. However, it is important to clean the area with alcohol or chlorhexidine solution before the procedure. Use universal precautions. Apply a tourniquet when appropriate to assist in distending the veins and to make them easier to identify.

Multiple peripheral vessels are available for ultrasound-guided access. The basilic vein lies on the ulnar aspect of the forearm and the cephalic vein can be found on the radial aspect (Fig. 21.US1). The larger median cubital vein represents the junction of these two veins and lies in the antecubital fossa (Fig. 21.US2). The deep brachial vein is found on the median aspect of the distal end of the arm in the bicipital groove (Fig. 21.US3). The external jugular vein is found superficially in the neck and runs diagonally across the sternocleidomastoid muscle.

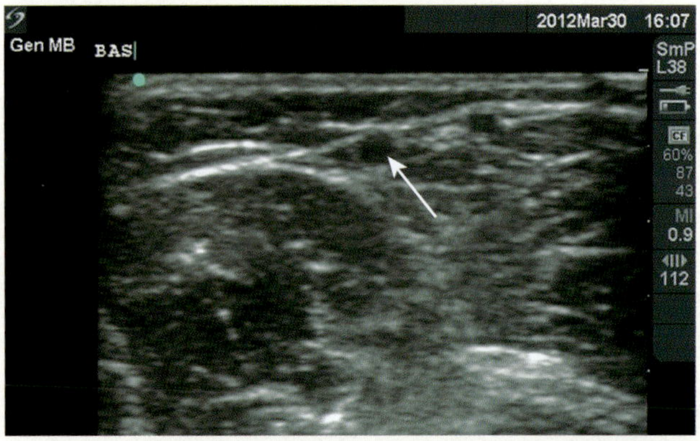

Fig. 21.US1 Ultrasound image of the basilic vein *(arrow)*.

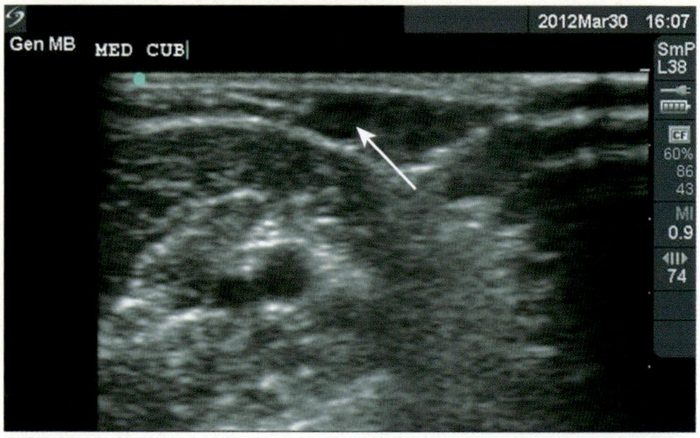

Fig. 21.US2 Ultrasound image of the median cubital vein *(arrow)*.

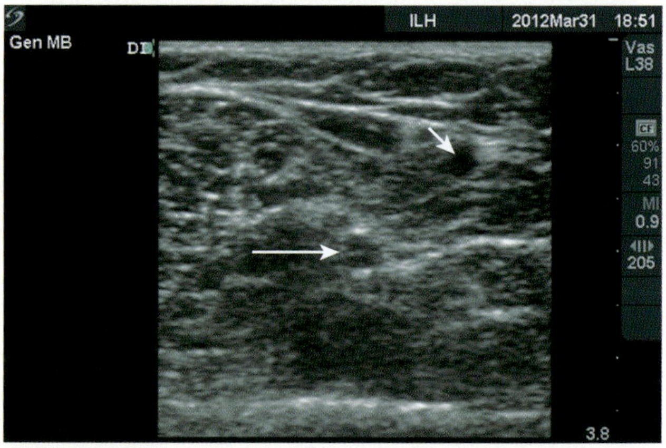

Fig. 21.US3 Ultrasound image of the deep brachial vein *(large arrow)*. Another smaller vein can be seen more superficially to the right of the image *(small arrow)*.

Distinguishing the artery from the vein may prove more challenging than with central vessels. Peripheral veins and arteries are smaller, and even arteries may collapse with pressure. Evaluate the veins before application of the tourniquet. Veins should collapse easily and in fact may collapse from only the pressure of applying the transducer to the skin. Placing the heel of the operator's hand on the patient's arm and then applying the transducer may decrease this effect. Arteries can be further identified by evaluating the Doppler flow pattern of the vessel. Even small arteries will have a biphasic, pulsatile flow pattern versus the steady low-amplitude venous pattern. Finally, venous augmentation can be used for confirmation. Color flow imaging is used over the vessel in question. Squeezing the arm distal to the area should cause a temporary flush of flow in the vein (Fig. 21.US4). The artery should not show any change in its typical pulsatile flow.

Continued

ULTRASOUND: Peripheral Intravenous Access—cont'd

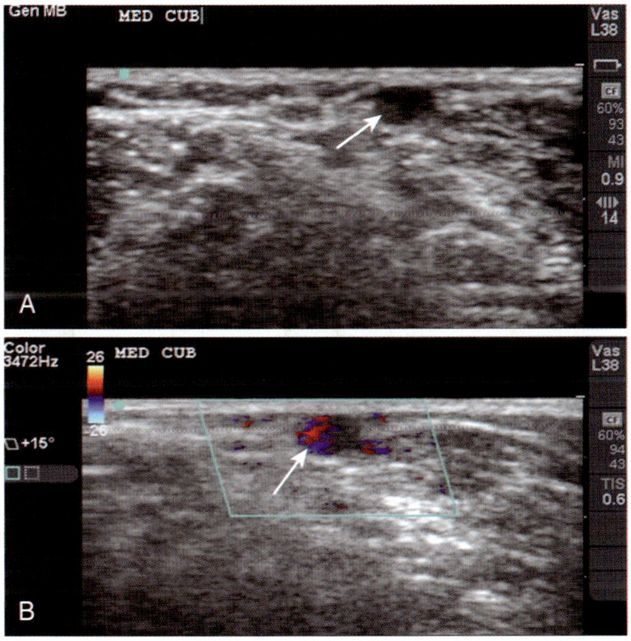

Fig. 21.US4 Demonstration of venous augmentation. (A) Ultrasound view of a suspected vein *(arrow)*. (B) Once the wrist is lightly squeezed, adding color Doppler flow to the area will demonstrate a "flush" of color within the vessel *(arrow)*.

Once a location for cannulation has been chosen, scan the relevant area to locate the desired vessel. Once the vein has been identified, the cannulation procedure is identical for all peripheral veins. A transverse, or short-axis, approach is universally used because of the small size of the peripheral veins. Center the transducer over the target vessel. The depth of the image on-screen should be decreased as much as possible so the best image is obtained. A blunt object (e.g., a fingertip) is applied over the center of the transducer to ensure that the vessel in question is centered. Then introduce the needle at a 45-degree angle slightly back from the transducer (Fig. 21.US5). Once the tip of the needle is identified on-screen, advance it toward the vessel. Watch the catheter closely for a flash of blood. Once the flash is obtained, set the ultrasound aside and continue the procedure in the typical fashion.

A pitfall that may frustrate the sonographer is kinking or difficulty threading or advancing the catheter once a flash has been obtained. This frequently occurs in deeper vessels, such as the deep brachial. Using a longer, stiffer catheter (e.g., 1.75-inch Arrow twin catheter [Teleflex] or the longer catheter from the Arrow arterial line kit) may help reduce this problem.

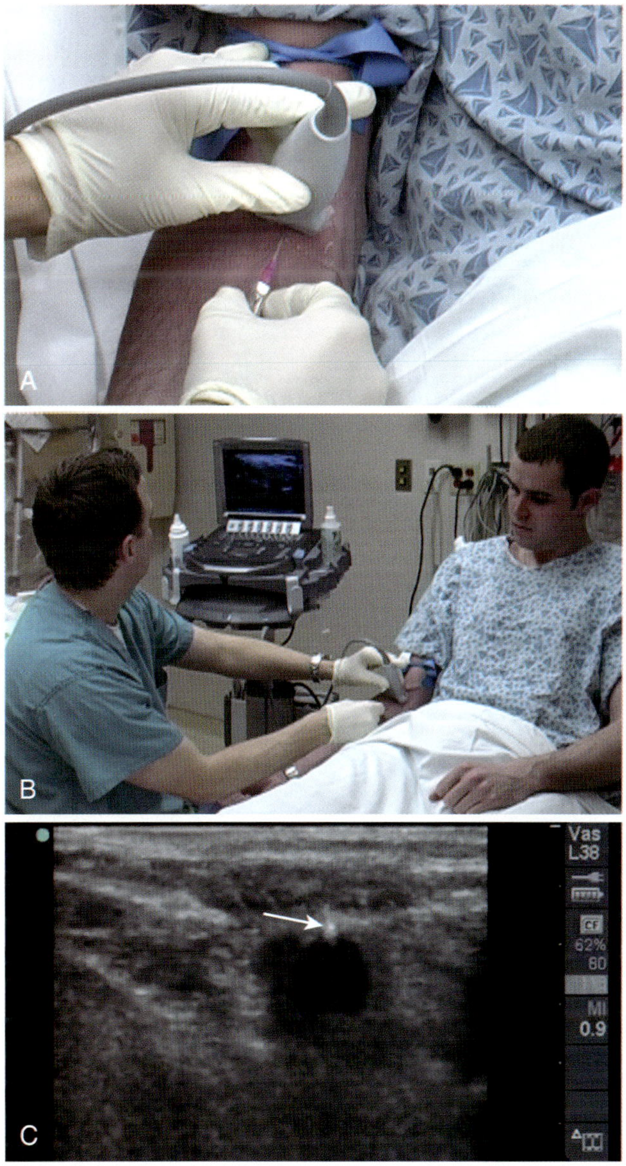

Fig. 21.US5 (A) Introduce the needle at a 45-degree angle, slightly back from the transducer. (B) Identify the tip of the needle on-screen. (C) Advance the tip of the needle *(arrow)* toward the vessel.

REFERENCES

1. Costantino T, Parikh AK, Satz WA, Fojtik JP. Ultrasonography-guided peripheral intravenous access versus traditional approaches in patients with difficult intravenous access. *Ann Emerg Med.* 2005;46:456–461.
2. Brannam L, Blaivas M, Lyon M, Flake M. Emergency nurses' utilization of ultrasound guidance for placement of peripheral intravenous lines in difficult-access patients. *Acad Emerg Med.* 2004;11:1361–1363.

splits into the great saphenous vein, which travels up the medial aspect of the ankle, and the small saphenous vein, which courses laterally up the opposite side. These are the vascular structures most easily accessible for IV therapy.

The external jugular vein is formed below the ear and behind the angle of the mandible (Fig. 21.3). It then passes downward and obliquely across the sternocleidomastoid and under the middle of the clavicle to join the subclavian vein. It is important to note the presence of valves in the external jugular, usually approximately 4 cm above the clavicle, because they can impede IV function.[18]

PREPARATION

Safety

Universal precautions should be applied to all patients, especially in emergency care settings, where the risk for exposure to blood is increased and the infection status of patients is largely unknown. Newer catheter devices have emerged that prevent inadvertent needle injuries (Fig. 21.4). The ProtectIV Safety IV Catheter System (Smiths Medical) has a protective sleeve that encases the sharp stylet as it is retracted from the catheter. The needle of the Insyte Autoguard Shielded IV Catheter (Becton Dickinson) is instantly encased inside a tamper-resistant safety barrel by pressing an activation button. The Saf-T-Intima IV catheter (Becton,Dickinson), Punctur-Guard Safety Winged Set (Gaven Medical), Vacutainer Safety-Lok (Becton Dickinson), Shamrock safety winged needle (Smiths Medical), and Angel Wing Safety Needle systems (Medtronic) are all types of winged safety devices with shields that advance over the needle to prevent its exposure.[3]

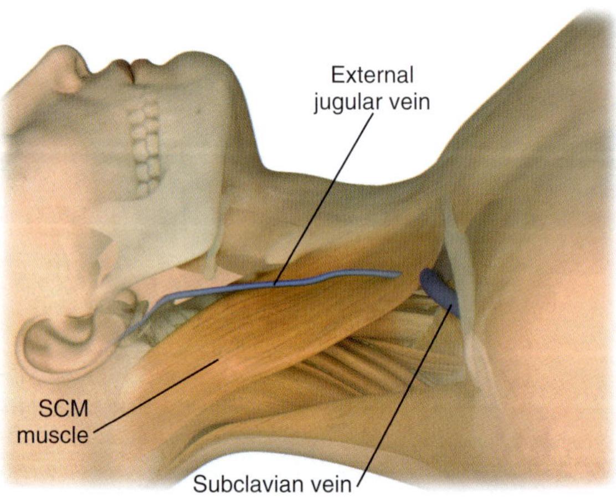

Fig. 21.3 External jugular anatomy. *SCM*, Sternocleidomastoid.

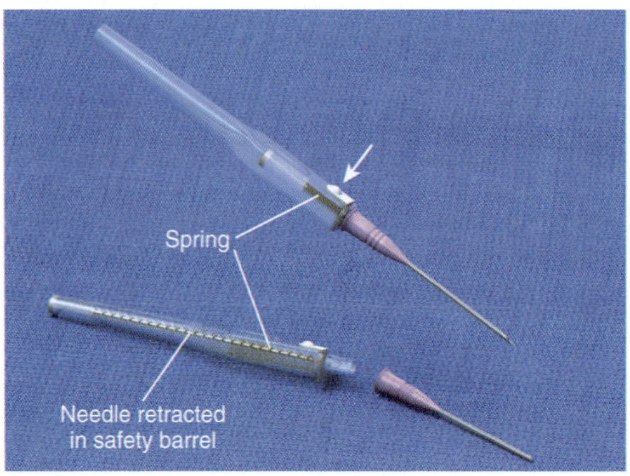

Fig. 21.4 Intravenous catheter safety device. When the activation button is depressed *(arrow)*, the spring is released and the needle is retracted into the safety barrel.

Choosing the Catheter Gauge

See Video 21.8. The specific gauge of catheter to use depends on the clinical scenario (Fig. 21.5). The narrowest catheter typically used in adults is a 22 gauge, which is sufficient for the routine administration of maintenance fluids and antibiotics. A 20 or 18 gauge is necessary for the administration of blood products, and a 16-gauge needle is preferred in resuscitation settings when large amounts of fluid must be given quickly. A second IV line at a different location allows additional IV therapy and also acts as a backup line in critical resuscitations. An 18-gauge catheter in the antecubital fossa is the standard device for IV contrast–enhanced computed tomography (CT) studies such as pulmonary CT angiogram.

Appropriate Site

Site selection depends largely on the expected duration of IV therapy, the patient's activity level, and the condition of the extremities. When choosing a location to initiate IV access, the best place to start is the hand and then advance cephalad as necessary. Hand veins are appropriate for 22-gauge catheters. Cephalic, accessory, or basilic veins are ideal for larger-bore IV lines. Avoid veins that are not resilient and feel hard or cordlike because they may be thrombosed. Deep, percutaneous antecubital venipuncture and external jugular vein cannulation are also options in patients with difficult veins or those who may need IV access quickly. The lower extremity veins can also be useful locations, especially in pediatric patients. In patients who have undergone radical mastectomy, avoid the arm on the same side as the surgery because IVs may impair circulation, affect flow, or lead to edema and other complications.[12] Scalp veins are commonly used in neonates.

Adjuncts for Finding a Vein

Patients often have nonvisible and nonpalpable veins. A common method of increasing venous distention is to ask patients

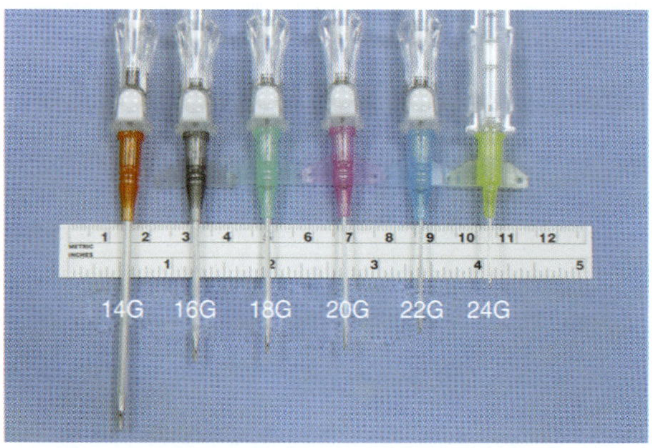

Fig. 21.5 Various gauges of intravenous catheters. Needles are sized according to gauge, from large to small (14 to 24 gauge).

to open and close their fist. Lowering the arm below the level of the heart can also increase venous distention. Light tapping can likewise be effective, although heavy tapping may cause the vein to spasm. If these methods are inadequate, heat packs can be applied for 10 to 20 minutes to increase venous engorgement. This is particularly useful in the pediatric population.[3]

Nitroglycerin ointment applied to the hands of patients with small-caliber veins can increase the diameter of the vein and increase the rate of successful first-attempt cannulation. Once the tourniquet is applied to the wrist, apply a quarter inch of 2% nitroglycerin to a 2.5-cm^2 area, leave it on for 2 minutes, and then rub it off. Nitroglycerin alone can have adverse effects in neonates and premature babies, however. The combination of topical nitroglycerin with local anesthetics has been shown to increase success and decrease the pain of cannulation in children 1 to 11 years old.[19] This technique is contraindicated in hypotensive patients.

Anesthesia

Though sometimes time-consuming, local anesthesia at the site should be considered part of routine care. Local anesthesia significantly decreases pain before cannulation. Anesthetics such as lidocaine or bupivacaine may be instilled just beneath the skin at the site of planned cannulation through a tuberculin (1-mL) syringe equipped with a 27- or smaller-gauge needle. Adding bicarbonate (e.g., buffered lidocaine), warming the solution to room temperature, instilling the solution slowly, and distracting the patient during injection all contribute to reducing pain.[20] In both the pediatric and adult population, 2.5 g of EMLA (eutectic mixture of local anesthetics) can be applied topically over the site.[3] Its main disadvantage is slow onset, with as long as an hour needed for induction of anesthesia before cannulation. Other options include ethyl chloride topical spray, which temporarily numbs the skin, and oral sucrose in infants.[21]

Intraveous Assembly

Review Box 21.1 itemizes the materials necessary for IV cannulation. The procedure is detailed in Fig. 21.6. The first step is to prepare the IV fluids and tubing. Remove the cap from the IV tubing and the tab from the IV bag. Clamp the IV tubing shut and insert the spiked end into the IV fluid bag. Pinch the drip chamber and fill it halfway. Open the clamp slightly to flush the IV tubing. If saline locks are being used, flush them similarly before cannulation. To do this, attach the lock to a saline-filled syringe and push saline through it.

Inspection and Positioning

After collecting and preparing the equipment and supplies, palpate the veins. Position the patient comfortably on a flat surface. Place a 1-inch-wide tourniquet on the upper part of the patient's arm or forearm and pull it sufficiently tight to impede venous flow but not tight enough to compromise arterial flow. After placement of the tourniquet, palpate the veins with the index and middle finger of one's nondominant hand. The veins are soft, elastic, resilient, and pulseless.

Cannulation

After performing hand hygiene, don gloves (nonsterile is adequate), and clean the injection site with iodine, alcohol, or both. If using alcohol, allow it to dry on the surface of the skin. Stabilize the vein without contaminating the prepared site. One

Peripheral Intravenous Access

Indications

Venous blood sampling
Intravenous fluid infusion
Intravenous medication infusion
Blood transfusion
Intravenous contrast infusion

Contraindications

Extremity with significant edema, burns, sclerosis, phlebitis, or thrombosis
Ipsilateral radical mastectomy or fistula
Overlying cellulitis

Complications

Early	*Late*
Bruising	Phlebitis
Infiltration	Infection
Air embolism	Nerve damage
	Thrombosis

Equipment

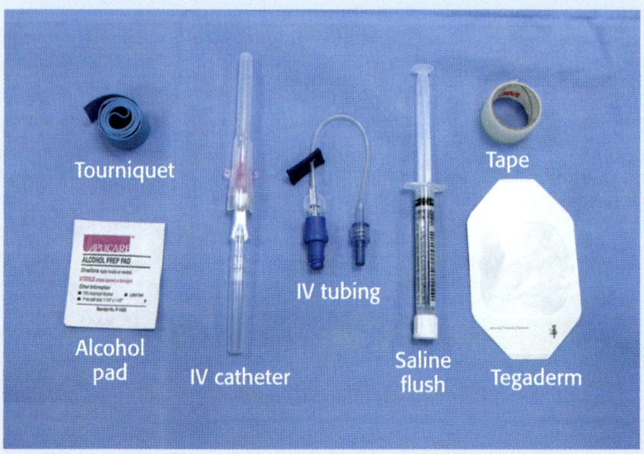

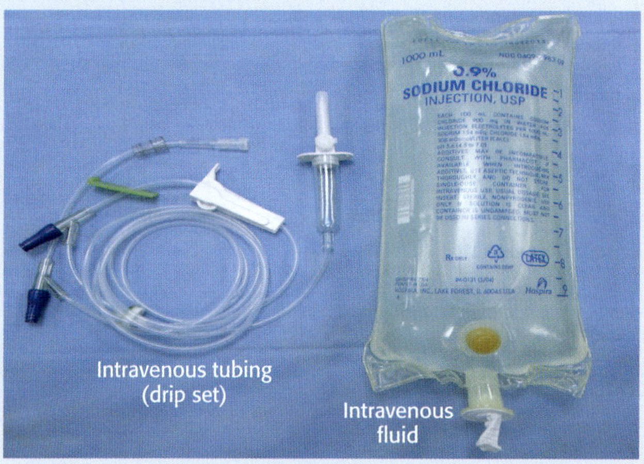

Review Box 21.1 Peripheral intravenous access: indications, contraindications, complications, and equipment.

Peripheral Intravenous Access

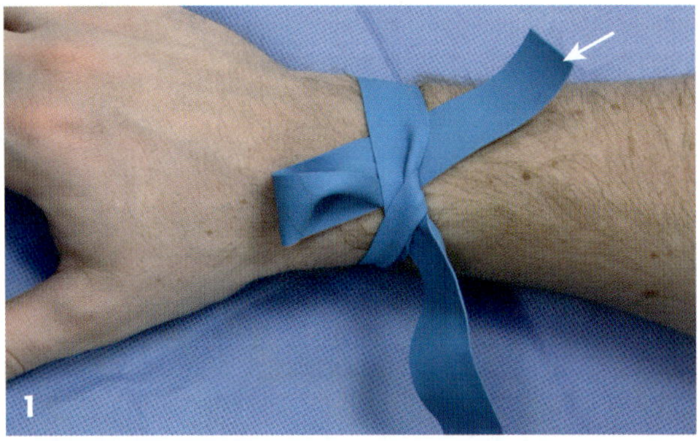

Apply tourniquet to arm.

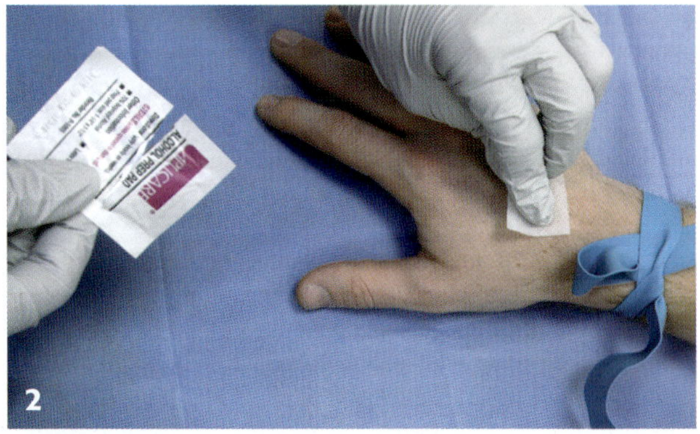

Prepare the insertion site with an alcohol pad.

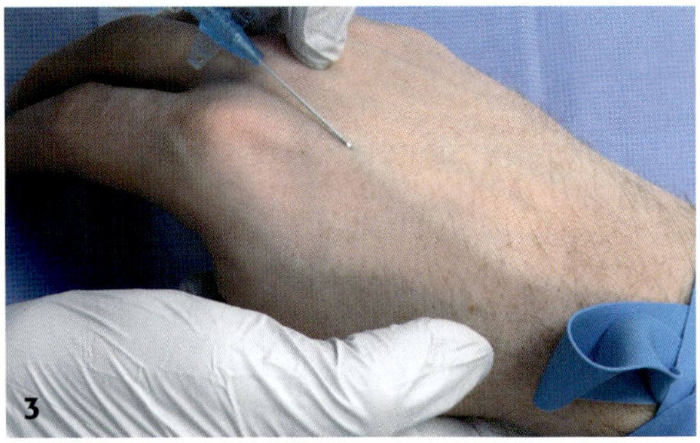

Insert the IV catheter with the bevel facing upward.

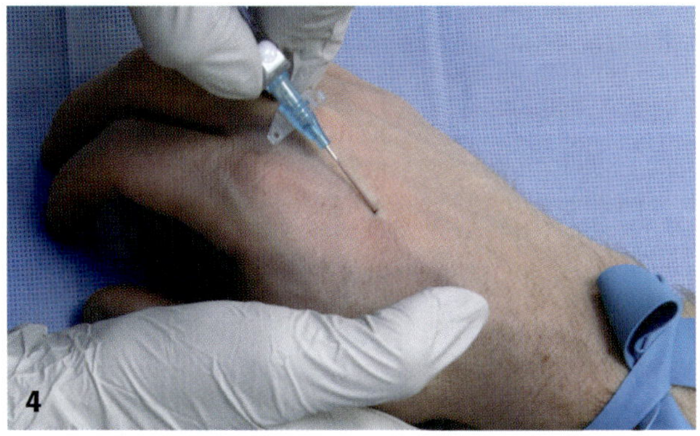

Advance the needle until a flash of blood is seen.

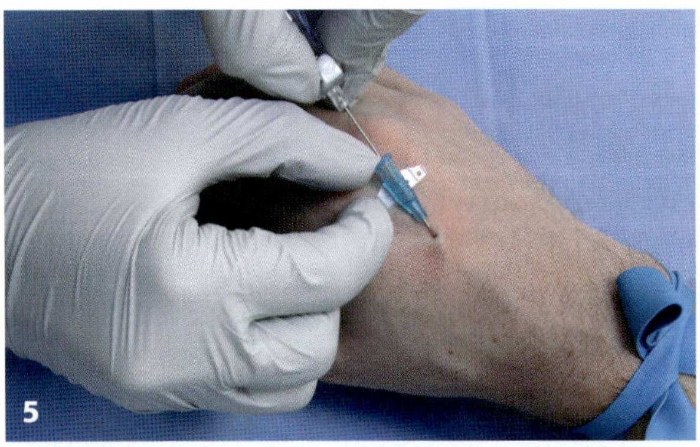

Advance the catheter over the needle until flush with the skin.

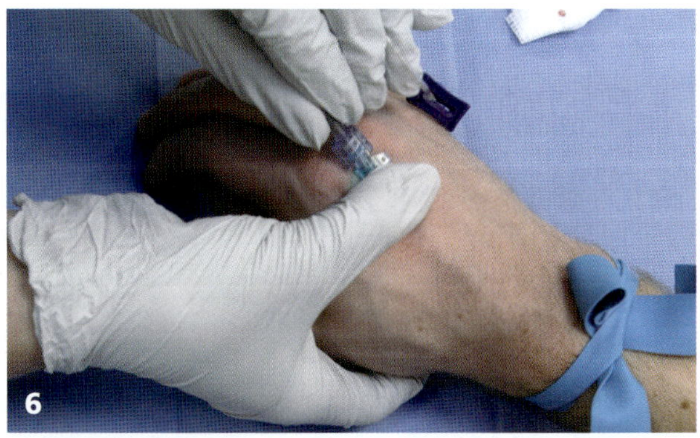

Attach the preflushed saline lock.

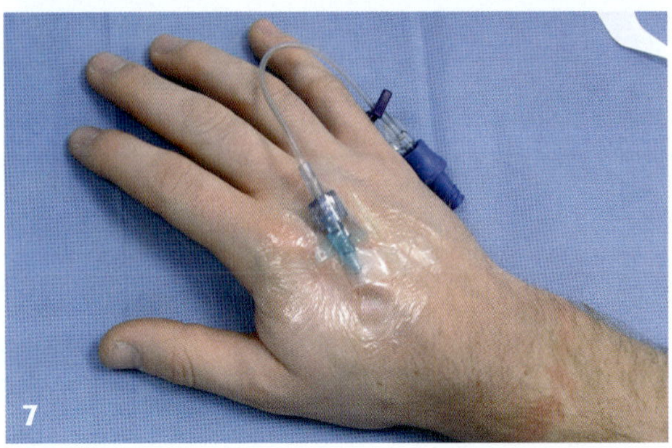

Cover the insertion site with Tegaderm (or similar) dressing.

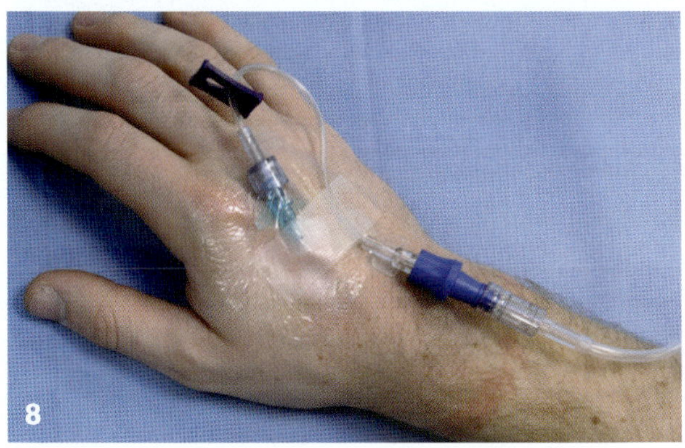

Attach IV tubing to the saline lock for IV fluid administration.

Fig. 21.6 Peripheral intravenous *(IV)* access. IV lines placed in the dorsum of the hand are associated with the lowest infection rates from venous cannulation.

method is to position one's thumb alongside the vein and pull down while the index finger is positioned more cephalad and pulls upward. Take the angiocatheter between the thumb and forefinger of the dominant hand. With the bevel up, angle the angiocatheter 10 to 30 degrees between the catheter and the vein and parallel to the vein. Puncture the vein. Once a flash of blood is seen, advance the catheter several millimeters more to ensure that the catheter has entered the vein and not just the wall. Avoid advancing too far and puncturing the posterior wall. Loosen the stylet and advance only the catheter. Use the fingers that were anchoring the vein to occlude the vein at the tip of the catheter to prevent extravasation of blood from the angiocatheter. Remove the needle; connect the saline lock, IV lining, or syringe for phlebotomy; and release the tourniquet.

Cannulation of the external jugular vein deserves a special note (Fig. 21.7). In patients with otherwise limited peripheral access, it can be cannulated as follows. Place patient in the Trendelenburg position to fill the external jugular vein. Rotate the head to the opposite side and prepare the area as described earlier. Take the cannula and align it in the direction of the vein with the point aiming toward the ipsilateral shoulder. Puncture midway between the angle of the jaw and the midclavicular line while lightly compressing the vein with the free finger above the clavicle. Proceed as described previously for cannulation.

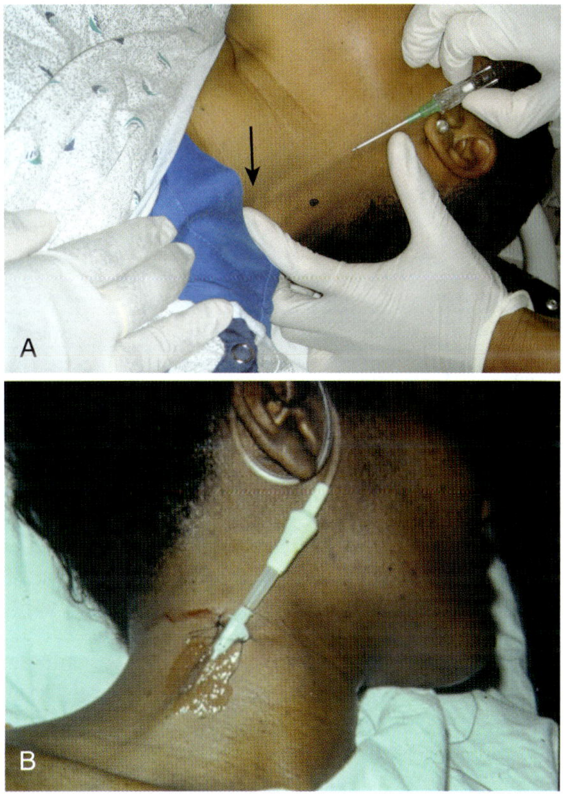

Fig. 21.7 External jugular vein cannulation. (A) Note that traction on the vein is applied with the thumb of the nondominant hand while the index finger tamponades the vessel *(arrow)* (essentially serving as a tourniquet) near the clavicle. Flow is dependent on neck position. (B) Intravenous catheters may be sutured in place for stability. The Trendelenburg position and a Valsalva maneuver can facilitate cannulation.

Anchoring the Device

After the IV cannula has been connected to the saline lock or IV tubing, anchor the device (see Fig. 21.6). Use a half-inch-wide strip of tape, adhesive side up, under the hub of the catheter and fold it over in a bow-shaped manner. This will secure the catheter and prevent lateral movement. Clear polyurethane dressings can also be used with or instead of tape. Saline locks can be connected to needleless hubs to prevent accidental needle injury. Then secure the loose saline lock or IV tubing with tape to prevent accidental dislodgement. Connect the IV tubing to the angiocatheter and anchor it. Alternatively, use a commercially available securing device. Sign and date the dressings to ensure timely dressing changes. As an option, topical antibiotics or iodophor ointment may be applied to the insertion site to prevent infection, though the efficacy of doing so is unproven.

Maintaining Patency

An important component of IV care is maintaining patency with frequent flushing. Heparin solutions have previously been used to flush catheters and maintain patency, but heparin can cause problems such as hemorrhage. Saline flushes are as effective as heparin in maintaining patency and preventing phlebitis but do not carry the risks of bleeding or heparin-induced thrombocytopenia.

Dressing

It is not cost effective to continually redress peripheral venous catheters at periodic intervals. Sterile gauze or transparent, semipermeable, polyurethane dressings can be left in place until removal of the catheter, as long as the site is regularly evaluated. Securing techniques that use proprietary devices, such as the StatLock IV (Bard Access Systems), a sterile, adhesive-backed anchor, and distal male Luer-tip extensions, may reduce complications by decreasing mobility and risk of dislodgement. Commonly used topical antimicrobial ointments have not been consistently proven to reduce the rate of peripheral catheter–related infection but have been associated with increased rates of antimicrobial resistance and *Candida* colonization. Such ointments are not harmful in the ED, but their routine use is not supported.

Percutaneous Brachial Vein Cannulation

Brachial vein cannulation is an option when attempts at peripheral IV access have failed or are contraindicated and may obviate the need for central venous access or surgical cutdown. Complications include brachial artery puncture, hematoma, and transitory paresthesias.

To cannulate the brachial vein, palpate the brachial artery in the antecubital fossa. Prepare the site in the usual manner and apply a tourniquet above the antecubital space. At a point immediately medial or lateral to the pulse, insert an angiocatheter with an attached syringe and advance it at a 45-degree angle while maintaining suction on the syringe. After entrance into the vein, continue 2 to 3 mm further to ensure cannulation. Advance the catheter and remove the needle as usual.[16]

COMPLICATIONS

Although IV placement is a common procedure, it is not without complications. Fortunately, morbidity is rarely

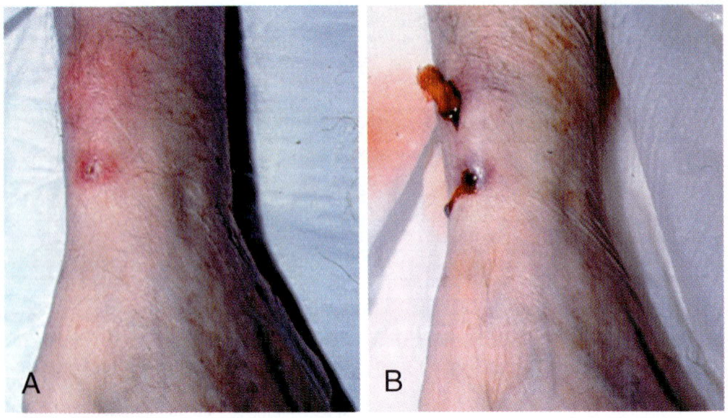

Fig. 21.8 (A) Suppurative phlebitis from a peripheral intravenous line. (B) After incising and cleaning the infected subcutaneous tract, a gauze pack was placed for 24 hours and oral antibiotics were given with good results.

severe. Phlebitis, infiltration, infection, nerve damage, air embolism, bruising, and thrombosis are the most common complications and rarely cause significant morbidity or fatality.

Phlebitis is a common complication after IV cannulation and is described as the presence of a palpable cord accompanied by warmth, erythema, tenderness, and induration over the involved vein (Fig. 21.8). Phlebitis necessitates removal of the catheter and replacement on another extremity. Avoiding IV placement in the lower extremities (where there is more often stagnant blood flow) and across joints (where motion traumatizes the venous wall) minimizes the incidence of IV catheter–related phlebitis.[3] Other causes of phlebitis include IV infusion of potassium chloride, certain antibiotics (vancomycin, erythromycin), many cytotoxic chemotherapy agents, phenytoin, and any hyperosmolar solution (e.g., 50% dextrose solution). The role of in-line filters to prevent phlebitis is controversial. Particulates from reconstituted medications, degradation products, precipitates, glass from vials, and other foreign debris may all play a part in post infusion phlebitis. In-line filters may therefore play a role in preventing phlebitis, but given their cost, risk of clogging, and paucity of evidence that they improve outcomes, these filters have not become routine.

Even with the most pristine technique, there is approximately a 0.5% incidence of catheter-related bloodstream infection with peripheral IV catheters. IV devices facilitate infection by damaging epithelial barriers and thereby providing microorganisms direct access to the bloodstream. The risk for infection with peripheral venous catheters is higher in the lower extremity than in the upper extremity and higher in the wrist or upper part of the arm than in the hand. A common infectious complication of peripheral IV access is self-limited cellulitis. It is generally safe to use peripheral IV lines for up to 72 hours before they are relocated. With rates of clinically significant bacteremia lower than 0.5%, some argue that routine replacement of catheters is now no longer needed. Nonetheless, infection can be a costly and potentially significant complication of IV therapy. Suppurative thrombophlebitis is extremely rare. It most frequently occurs in patients with thermal injury and long-term or lower extremity cannulation. Local signs of inflammation or suppuration are often absent and can occur 2 to 10 days after removal of the catheter. Treatment is immediate surgical excision of the entire length of the involved vein and tributaries. Though rare with peripheral IV catheters, intravascular device–related bloodstream infection may be an unrecognized cause of nosocomial infection. Peripheral IV catheters are most often associated with staphylococcal and candidal species. Infectious complications can be reduced significantly by hand washing, wearing gloves, preparing the site with iodine, and monitoring the site for signs of infection.[3]

Bruising is a common complication of IV therapy. Contrary to popular belief, flexing of the elbow after venipuncture does not prevent bruising in the antecubital site. Applying direct pressure immediately after decannulation is the most useful technique to prevent bruising.

Tissue or interstitial infiltration occurs when the catheter is dislodged from the vein during infusion. It is a common and usually relatively minor complication of IV therapy. Extravasation of certain infusions, such as hypertonic solutions, vasopressors, or chemotherapeutic agents, however, poses a significant risk for necrosis and skin sloughing when infiltration and extravasation occur. In extreme cases, skin grafting may be required.[3] For extravasation of dopamine or epinephrine, local injection of antidotes such as phentolamine may be used to reverse the tissue damage.

Nerve injury is rare after IV cannulation. Any peripheral nerve is potentially vulnerable to a needle-induced injury, and sequelae can range from a minor motor or sensory abnormality to complete paralysis. Nerve damage may be due to direct injury by the needle, intraneural microvascular damage from hematomas, or toxic effects of the agent injected. The first symptoms are usually pain, numbness, or paresthesias. Pain may persist for years and can be debilitating. Fortunately, most simple procedures do not result in nerve injury because nerves tend to roll or slide away from a needle. Like all procedures, knowledge of the relevant anatomy is essential. Should a patient complain of numbness or severe pain after a needle puncture, stop the injection immediately.

Thrombosis and subsequent pulmonary embolism (PE) have sometimes been associated with centrally placed IV catheters. Though rare, thrombosis followed by clinically significant PE may occur in patients with peripheral IV lines if saline locks are not flushed or IV fluids run dry. Should this occur, aspirate the line. If the return fluid appears bloody, discard the syringe and then gently flush the saline lock and resume the infusion. If there is no bloody aspirate, use 2 to 3 mL of saline to gently flush the line. If resistance is encountered, stop flushing immediately because there is a risk for development of an embolism. Attempt IV insertion at another site.

Venous air embolism is another significant, though exceedingly rare, complication of peripheral IV access. Symptoms include chest pain, shortness of breath, sudden vascular collapse, cyanosis, and hypotension. If air embolism is suspected, place the patient in the left lateral decubitus Trendelenburg position. Invasive maneuvers include aspiration of air through a central venous catheter and even thoracotomy with direct aspiration from the heart. This complication can be prevented by eliminating air from the IV tubing before initiating therapy and not allowing IV lines to run dry.[3] If air bubbles are present in an IV line, tap the tubing while holding it taut to allow the air to escape to the top. Similarly, curl the tubing around a pen or syringe to accomplish the same goal. If the air is near a Y-connector, one can use a needle and syringe to directly remove it. If all else fails and there is air between the Y-connector and the patient, disconnect the tubing and flush it.

Recommendations of the Centers for Disease Control and Prevention for IV catheter care to prevent complications are as follows:

1. In adults, use an upper-extremity site for catheter insertion. Replace a catheter inserted in a lower extremity site to an upper-extremity site as soon as possible.
2. In pediatric patients, the upper or lower extremities or the scalp (in neonates or young infants) can be used as the catheter insertion site.
3. Perform hand hygiene procedures, either by washing hands with conventional soap and water or with alcohol-based hand rubs (ABHRs). Hand hygiene should be performed before and after palpating catheter insertion sites as well as before and after inserting, replacing, accessing, repairing, or dressing an intravascular catheter. Palpation of the insertion site should not be performed after the application of antiseptic, unless aseptic technique is maintained.
4. Wear clean gloves, rather than sterile gloves, for the insertion of peripheral intravascular catheters, if the access site is not touched after the application of skin antiseptics.
5. Prepare clean skin with an antiseptic (70% alcohol, tincture of iodine, an iodophor or chlorhexidine gluconate) before peripheral venous catheter insertion.
6. There is no need to replace peripheral catheters more frequently than every 72 to 96 hours to reduce risk of infection and phlebitis in adults.
7. Replace peripheral catheters in children only when clinically indicated.[22]

EXTRAVASATION OF MEDICATIONS AND VASOPRESSORS

Usually, infiltration of a vein is a relatively minor and common complication of IV therapy if only sterile fluid extravasates, even in large amounts. This often occurs when the catheter is dislodged from the vein during infusion. However, if the infusions consist of hypertonic substances, vasopressors, or chemotherapeutics, there is a significant risk for skin sloughing when infiltration and extravasation occur (Box 21.1). Pain at the infusion site or the alarm sounding on an infusion pump device requires inspection of the infusion site for extravasation. In extreme cases, grafting may be required for skin sloughing (Fig. 21.9).[1] If dopamine, phenylephrine (Neo-Synephrine [Hospira, Inc., Lake Forest, IL]), or norepinephrine extravasate, phentolamine may be used as an antidote to prevent ischemia locally; its use is encouraged as soon as extravasation is identified. Reversal of ischemia with phentolamine is a common technique, but its ability to totally reverse or prevent skin sloughing is not absolute. However, if infiltration of these vasopressors occurs, the authors suggest that it be used. There are few downsides to this intervention, although hypotension is a theoretical side effect because phentolamine is an α-adrenergic antagonist. To inject phentolamine, place 5 mg in a vial and dilute with equal parts of saline (final form: 5 mg in 2 mL). For large areas, use two vials with the contents of each vial injected 10 minutes apart through a 25- to 27-gauge needle or a tuberculin syringe. If the IV line is still in place, inject approximately 1 mL of phentolamine through the catheter before it is removed; however, the IV line is often removed before this can be done. The entire area of skin blanching, or suspected area of extravasation, is injected with multiple small aliquots of the solution, approximately 0.25 to 0.5 mL each. The procedure may be repeated in 2 to 4 hours. Hyaluronidase is probably benign

BOX 21.1 Medications and Solutions That May Cause Tissue Injury When Extravasation Occurs in a Peripheral Vein[a]

Aminophylline
Calcium chloride 10%
Carmustine
Chlordiazepoxide
Colchicine
Crystalline amino acids 4.25%/dextrose 10%
Crystalline amino acids 4.25%/dextrose 25%
Dactinomycin
Daunorubicin
Dextrose 10%
Dextrose 50% in water
Diazepam
Dobutamine
Dopamine
Doxorubicin
Epinephrine
Ethyl alcohol
Mechlorethamine
Metaraminol
Mithramycin
Mitomycin
Nafcillin
Neo-Synephrine
Nitroglycerin
Norepinephrine
Parenteral nutrition solutions
Phenytoin[b]
Potassium solutions
Propylene glycol
Renografin-60
Sodium bicarbonate 8.4%
Sodium thiopental
Tetracycline
Vasopressin
Vinblastine
Vincristine
Vindesine

[a]Many medications and intravenous solutions will cause pain and occasionally skin sloughing if significant amounts extravasate into soft tissues. Thus, any complaint of pain during infusion or signs of tissue swelling should prompt an investigation for extravasation. Most extravasations have no specific therapy, so prevention is the only option. Phentolamine, injected subcutaneously to reverse vasoconstriction, is the most common technique, but its efficacy has not been well studied.

[b]Use a maximum concentration of 2 mg/mL of saline or fosphenytoin solution to minimize this risk.

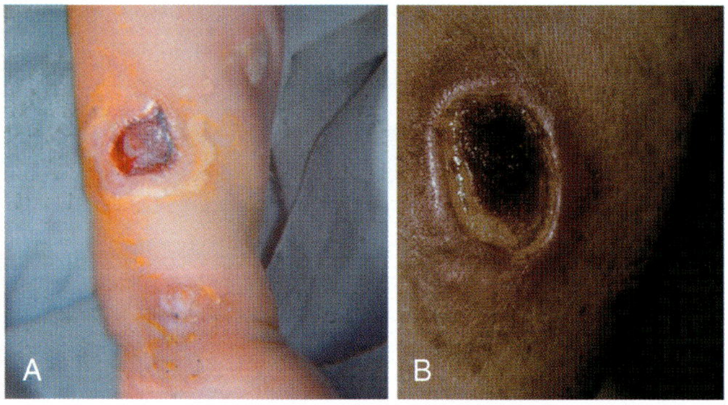

Fig. 21.9 (A) Infiltration of calcium chloride in an infant. Once this occurs, there is no treatment except debridement and possible skin grafting. Calcium gluconate will not cause such a reaction. Extravasation of hypertonic dextrose, phenytoin, and vasoconstrictors or vasopressors will cause similar necrosis. (B) Full-thickness tissue injury from doxorubicin extravasation, not obvious until 7 to 10 days after the infusion.

and has been suggested in the past to ameliorate some effects of extravasation of other solutions. Though it has been a common suggestion, its efficacy has not been well established, and the product is not readily available. Ice and heat have varying effects in counteracting fluid extravasation. Extravasation of IV contrast material is discussed in Chapter 36.

Extravasation of chemotherapy solutions is particularly common and can produce full-thickness tissue sloughing. The patient may complain of pain and burning at the time of infusion, but skin sloughing may be delayed for many days. Table 21.1 lists possible antidotes and dosages for chemotherapy-induced extravasation injury. Results of these interventions vary.

Injury from extravasation of phenytoin can be minimized or avoided by using dilute solutions, no more than a 2-mg/mL concentration (1 g in 500 mL saline), or by using fosphenytoin instead of phenytoin. When possible, use calcium gluconate, not calcium chloride, in a peripheral IV line.

TABLE 21.1 Possible Antidotes for Extravasated Chemotherapeutic Agents[a]

CHEMOTHERAPEUTIC AGENT	ANTIDOTE	DOSE
Anthracycline	Dexrazoxane hydrochloride[b]	First dose, inject the equivalent of 500 mg dexrazoxane intravenously over 1–2 h, second dose at 24 h, and third dose at 48 h.
Mechlorethamine	Sodium thiosulfate	Multiple subcutaneous injections in and around the area of extravasation with a 25-gauge needle: 4 mL of 10% sodium thiosulfate + 6 mL water.
Vinca alkaloids (vincristine, vinblastine, and vinorelbine)	Hyaluronidase	Inject subcutaneously in and around the area of extravasation with a 25-gauge needle: 150 units (1 mL). For vinca alkaloids, apply local hot compresses.
Doxorubicin	Granulocyte-macrophage colony-stimulating factor[c]	Inject subcutaneously in and around the area of extravasation with a 25-gauge needle.
Doxorubicin, daunorubicin, and mitomycin	Dimethyl sulfoxide (free radical scavenger)	Apply a 50%–70% solution topically qid for 14 days. Leave uncovered.
Mitomycin	Pyridoxine[c]	Inject subcutaneously in and around the area of extravasation with a 25-gauge needle.
Nonspecific	Saline	Inject subcutaneously in and around the area of extravasation with a 25-gauge needle.
Nonspecific	Corticosteroids[d]	Inject subcutaneously in and around the area of extravasation with a 25-gauge needle: hydrocortisone, 500 mg diluted in 500 mL saline.

[a]Many of these interventions are anecdotal and none are guaranteed to reverse or ameliorate tissue injury. Controversy surrounds the actual benefit, and no randomized prospective trials have been conducted for many of the suggested regimens. Also consider elevation and surgical debridement when necessary.
[b]Approved by the US Food and Drug Administration for this indication.
[c]Not well studied, theoretical benefit.
[d]Results are variable; injury is not an inflammatory reaction.
qid, Every 4 hours.

The bottom line is that most extravasated chemotherapy and other agents have no specific antidote or reversal agents to alter the final outcome. At most extravasation sites it may be best to avoid the empirical use of suggested treatments such as sodium bicarbonate, sodium thiosulfate, heparin, calcium gluconate, magnesium sulfate, lidocaine, cimetidine, diphenhydramine, and other chemical substances that are believed to inactivate drugs and reduce toxic effects on cells. In some experimental settings, these substances have made the necrosis and ulceration worse.

REFERENCES ARE AVAILABLE AT Elsevier eBooks+

CHAPTER 22

Central Venous Catheterization

George Willis and Brian Parker

INTRODUCTION

Central venous catheter (CVC) insertion is a procedure that remains a mainstay of resuscitation both in the emergency department (ED) and intensive care unit. CVCs allow several capabilities for providers in the care of critically ill patients including placement of devices such as transvenous pacemakers, rapid infusion of fluid, and administration of selected medications that require reliable central venous access. Central venous access is most commonly obtained through the subclavian vein (SV), internal jugular (IJ) vein, or femoral vein (FV) as these central veins are easily accessible utilizing identifiable landmarks. The use of bedside ultrasonography has increased when performing this procedure so that now it is recognized as the standard of care to perform with real-time ultrasound guidance. Ultrasound-guided central venous catheterization has been shown to be safer with reduced complications, greater success, and overall cost savings. There are several methods to obtaining central venous access and this chapter will discuss those that should be practiced and mastered by anyone caring for critically ill patients in the ED.

ANATOMY

Subclavian Vein Anatomy

The SV starts at the proximal end of the axillary vein at the outer edge of the first rib. The axillary vein drains the larger veins of the arm, the brachial, basilic, and cephalic veins. On the other end, the IJ vein combines with the SV to become the brachiocephalic or innominate vein, which empties into the superior vena cava (SVC). The SV when fully dilated is around 1 to 2 cm in diameter, has a length of around 3 to 5 cm, and is valveless. The SV courses under the clavicle until it reaches the junction of the medial third of the bone where it crosses to a posterior position. The costoclavicular ligament lies anterior and inferior to the SV, and the fascia contiguous to this ligament invests the vessel. As with most veins, the subclavian artery (SA) lies in close proximity to the SV. However, the SA lies posterior to the vein and, during most of its course, is separated by the anterior scalene muscle. Other structures proximate to the SV include the thoracic duct (only in proximity to the left SV), the phrenic nerve (which lies near the junction of the SV and IJ vein), and, most importantly, the apex of the lung. The apex of the lung is more cephalad on the left than on the right, but both are susceptible to overpenetration of a needle (Fig. 22.1).

Internal Jugular Vein Anatomy

The IJ vein arises from the combination of venous sinuses in the skull. The sinuses, namely the inferior petrosal sinus and the sigmoid sinus, exit the jugular foramen at the base of the skull and combine to form the IJ. The IJ passes under the clavicle and joins with the SV to form the innominate or brachiocephalic vein. The IJ is the largest vein in the head and neck region.[1] The carotid artery runs concurrently with the IJ in the carotid sheath along with the vagus nerve. The carotid artery typically courses medial and posterior to the IJ in the neck, although there is significant variation in this anatomy. The position of the IJ can differ on either side of the neck, with some studies showing the left IJ lying more anteromedial compared to the right IJ which is more commonly anterolateral.[2,3] Additionally, head rotation has been shown to vary the location as well with excessive rotation causing significant displacement of the IJ.[2,4]

Anatomic landmarks for locating the IJ vein include the sternal notch, the medial third of the clavicle, and the sternocleidomastoid muscle (SCM). The two heads of the SCM and the clavicle form a triangle that is key to understanding the underlying vascular anatomy. The IJ vein can be located at the apex of the triangle as it courses along the medial head of the SCM and occupies a position in the middle of the triangle at the level of the clavicle before it joins the SV and forms the innominate vein. At the level of the thyroid cartilage, the IJ vein can be found just deep to the SCM.

Generally, the right IJ vein is bigger than the left IJ vein because of its closer proximity to the SV and the right atrium. The IJ vein can be pulsatile when visualized in the neck, but, in contrast to the aorta, these pulsations are not palpable. When visualized, however, the presence of venous pulsations can give an indication of patency of the IJ vein to the right atrium. The IJ vein also changes size with respiration. Because of the negative intrathoracic pressure at end-inspiration, blood in the IJ vein is drawn into the right atrium and the negative intravascular pressure causes the diameter of the IJ vein to shrink. In contrast, at end-expiration the increased intrathoracic pressure will limit return of blood to the right atrium and the diameter of the IJ vein will increase. Another unique characteristic of the IJ vein is its distensibility. The IJ vein will enlarge when pressure in the vein is increased, such as when flow of blood back to the right atrium is obstructed, as with thrombosis. This distensibility can be advantageous for the placement of central venous access. Use of a head-down (Trendelenburg) position or a Valsalva maneuver will increase the diameter of the IJ vein and thereby increase the likelihood of successful venipuncture (Fig. 22.2).

Femoral Vein Anatomy

The FV begins at the adductor canal (also known as Hunter's canal) and ends at the inferior margin of the inguinal ligament, where it becomes the external iliac vein. It is contained within the femoral triangle (inguinal ligament, medial border of the adductor longus, and lateral border of the sartorius muscle). On the medial side, the FV is adjacent to lymphatic vessels, while medially, the FV courses with the femoral artery. Lateral to the femoral artery lies the femoral nerve. These relationships from lateral to medial can be remembered with the mnemonic NAVEL (nerve, artery, vein, empty space, lymphatics). As the femoral artery and vein course distally down the leg within the femoral sheath, their side-by-side relationship frequently rotates such that the femoral artery may lie on top of the vein. When using landmark techniques to access the FV, it is safest to limit puncture approaches to as close as possible to and below the inguinal ligament (Fig. 22.3).

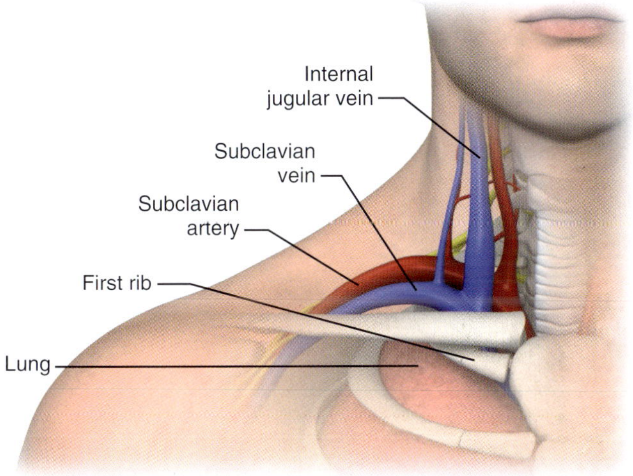

Fig. 22.1 Subclavian vein anatomy. The subclavian vein runs parallel to the clavicle and anterior to the subclavian artery. The cupula of the lung lies just caudad to these structures. If the introducer needle is kept almost parallel to the clavicle, the artery and lung should not be encountered.

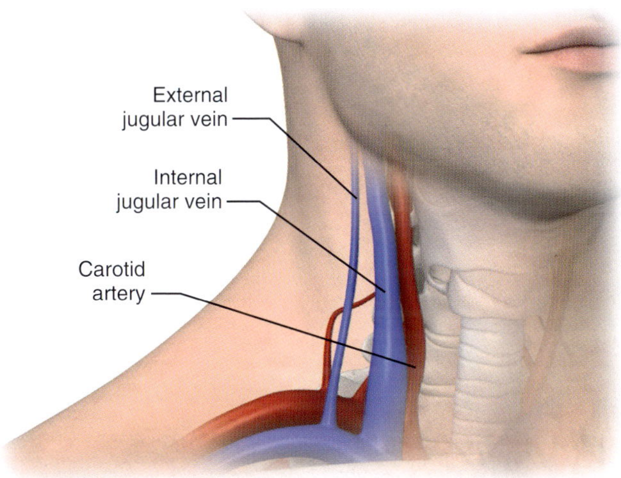

Fig. 22.2 Internal jugular anatomy. The internal jugular vein runs parallel and lateral to the carotid artery but lies almost directly above the carotid artery at the level of the clavicle.

INDICATIONS

As with performing any procedure, considerations for risk versus benefit must be weighed. There are two main indications for central venous cannulation. The first is for the administration of a medication with significant adverse effects if delivered for a prolonged period through a peripheral vein. The second is to provide venous accesses in patients with limited peripheral access (see Review Box 22.1 for indications for central venous access). Once the decision to access a central vein is made, a decision must be made on which central vein should be cannulated.

Infusion of Vasoactive and Concentrated Solutions

Central venous access for infusion of appropriate medications is probably the most common indication. Vasoactive medications, such as vasopressors and inotropes, are very commonly administered via central venous access as they provide direct access to the central circulation and the heart. Prior to recent years, vasoactive medications were contraindicated to be given via peripheral vein due to reports of increased phlebitis and sclerosis leading to tissue necrosis, especially if there was extravasation of the vasoactive medication into the skin. However, recent literature has shown that vasoactive agents at low doses and infusion rates can be initiated via reliable large-bore peripheral vein access while central venous access is obtained.[5–7] Any central venous access site is acceptable for the administration of vasoactive agents.

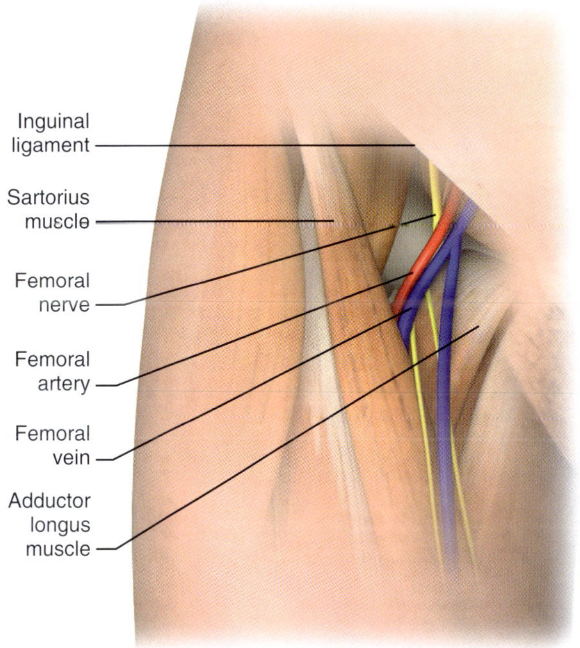

Fig. 22.3 Femoral vein anatomy. The femoral vital structures are located in the femoral triangle: inguinal ligament superiorly, sartorius muscle laterally, and adductor longus muscle medially. The triangle can be remembered by the mnemonic SAIL (sartorius, adductor longus, and inguinal ligament). Note the femoral structures from lateral to medial: nerve, artery, vein, empty canal, and lymphatics (mnemonic: NAVEL). The femoral vein lies medial to the femoral artery. *Important anatomic note:* at sites more distal to the inguinal ligament, the vein lies directly above the artery.

Other medications that are commonly given through central venous access include hyperosmolar medications. Hyperosmolar solutions or medications have the potential to cause thrombophlebitis if given through peripheral access. Examples of hyperosmolar solutions include potassium chloride (>40 mmol/L), hypertonic saline, 10% calcium chloride, chemotherapeutic agents, and acidifying solutions such as ammonium chloride. Similar to vasoactive agents, any central venous access site is acceptable for the administration of hyperosmolar medications.

Lastly, hyperalimentation with parenteral nutrition is safe and reliable via central venous access. Use of the infraclavicular subclavian technique is preferred since it frees the patient's extremities and neck.

Delivery of High-Flow Fluid Boluses and Blood Products

In patients who are hypotensive and severely volume-depleted and/or hypothermic, rapid infusion of IV fluids or blood products has been shown to be beneficial. Commercial systems

Central Venous Catheterization

Indications
Central venous pressure monitoring
High-volume/flow resuscitation
Emergency venous access
Inability to obtain peripheral venous access
Repetitive blood sampling
Administering hyperalimentation, caustic agents, or other concentrated fluids
Insertion of transvenous cardiac pacemakers
Hemodialysis or plasmapheresis
Insertion of pulmonary artery catheters

Relative Contraindications
Infection over the placement site
Distortion of landmarks by trauma or congenital anomalies
Coagulopathies, including anticoagulation and thrombolytic therapy
Pathologic conditions, including superior vena cava syndrome
Current venous thrombosis in the target vessel
Prior vessel injury or procedures
Morbid obesity
Uncooperative patients

Equipment (contents of a typical central venous catheterization kit)

Complications
Arterial puncture and hematoma
Pneumothorax (subclavian and internal jugular approach)
Hemothorax (subclavian and internal jugular approach)
Vessel injury
Air embolism
Cardiac dysrhythmia
Nerve injury
Infection
Thrombosis
Catheter misplacement

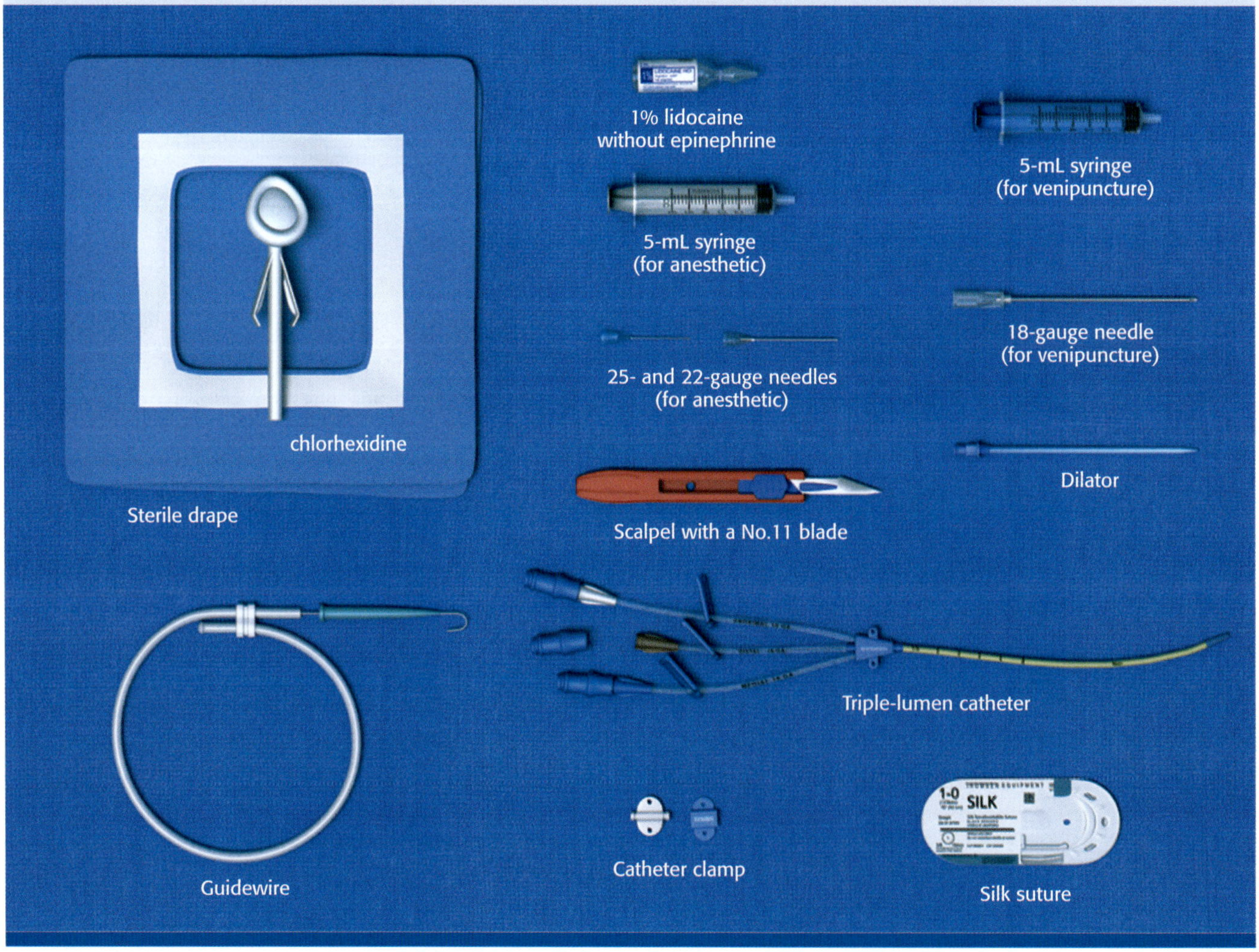

Review Box 22.1 Central venous catheterization: indications, contraindications, complications, and equipment.

exist to warm such rapid high-volume infusions to prevent hypothermia. The use of large-bore CVCs permits infusion rates up to 1500 mL/min. The Level 1 Rapid Infuser (Smiths Medical) and the Belmont FMS 2000 (Belmont Instrument Corporation) are examples of modern systems with rapid infusion rates.[9] Short large-caliber peripheral catheters can be as effective as central access if sufficiently large extremity veins can be cannulated.

Emergency Venous Access and Inability to Achieve Peripheral Access

There are circumstances when rapid venous access is required to administer time-critical medications. The predictable anatomic locations of the SV and FV and the speed with which they can be cannulated have prompted their use in cardiac arrest and other emergency situations. Intraosseous needle placement (see Chapter 25) has been shown to be faster, safer, and associated with less complications and should be utilized until a CVC can be safely placed.[10,11]

Additionally, even in noncritical circumstances, obtaining peripheral venous access can be difficult. Patients with a history of IV drug use, major burns, chronic disease, dehydration, those with an increased body mass index, and those who require long-term access may have inadequate peripheral veins easily accessible for IV insertion. Central venous cannulation may be indicated as the only means of obtaining venous access in these patients, even under nonemergency conditions.[12] More recently with the use of ultrasound, deep brachial, axillary, and basilic vein cannulation may be attempted before central venous catheterization and has been shown to decrease the use of central venous access insertion in patients with difficult access.[13–15] This approach avoids the complications that can be associated with central venous access.

Insertion of Invasive Devices

Invasive devices that perform either invasive hemodynamic monitoring or intracardiac activity are usually placed via central venous access. These devices include pulmonary artery catheters, transvenous pacemakers, cardiac catheterization, pulmonary angiography, and hemodialysis.[16,17] This may include patients with pulmonary hypertension and patients who may be in cardiogenic shock.[18,19] Hemodialysis catheters, such as the Uldall and Quinton devices, can be inserted into any of the central circulation veins. Extra caution should be applied during their insertion, possibly under ultrasound or fluoroscopic guidance, as they are stiffer catheters and can damage vital structures surrounding the insertion point.

Central Venous Pressure Monitoring and Oximetry

CVP monitoring can be performed through placement of an SV or IJ catheter. Monitoring the CVP has limited indications but might include assessment of response to fluid resuscitation and assessment for intrathoracic large vessel or cardiac obstructions. Evidence shows that the CVP can be affected by several factors and that it was a not a reliable marker of true intravascular volume. Additionally, there is very little evidence to support central venous oxygen saturation, although consultants will occasionally ask for blood gas samples to be obtained from CVC catheters.

Routine Serial Blood Drawing

The potential complications of CVCs make them inappropriate solely for routine blood sampling. However, lines already in place may be used for this purpose if they are properly cleared of IV fluid. A 20-cm, 16-gauge catheter contains 0.3 mL of fluid, so at least this much must be withdrawn to avoid dilution of blood samples. Interposition of a three-way stopcock in the IV tubing simplifies access and is an acceptable method for sampling blood in the intensive care setting, regardless of the IV site.

Additionally, serial lactate levels may help guide early goal-directed resuscitation. Arterial and central venous lactate correlate closely more than 96% of the time, whereas peripheral venous lactate and arterial lactate correlate only 87% of the time.[20]

CONTRAINDICATIONS

Each access to the different central veins has its own indications and contraindications. General contraindications to the various techniques of central venous access are presented in Review Box 22.1, while Table 22.1 lists the general advantages and disadvantages with each approach. Most contraindications listed are relative and should be viewed in the context of the patient's overall condition, urgency of need, and availability of alternative options for vascular access. Placement of a CVC through clearly infected skin is an absolute contraindication. Allergies to the composition of a catheter or to chemicals impregnated in a catheter are another strong contraindication. Use of catheters with teratogenic chemicals should be avoided in pregnant patients. Perhaps the only true absolute contraindication is insertion of catheters impregnated with antibiotics (most commonly tetracycline, rifampin, or chlorhexidine) if the patient has a serious allergy to the drug or is pregnant, as the impregnated antibiotics are commonly teratogenic.[21] In those circumstances, using a nonantibiotic-impregnated catheter is recommended. Local cellulitis and distorted local anatomy or landmarks preventing safe insertion are relative contraindications to any access route and an alternative site should be sought.

One of the more commonly encountered impediments to CVC placement is in patients with an elevated body mass index.[22] Surface landmarks in the neck are often obscured, and an abdominal pannus can block the femoral access site and consequently require deeper insertions and steeper angles. An ultrasound-guided IJ or femoral approach is safer under these circumstances.[22]

Insertion of another catheter on the same side as a preexisting one risks the complication of entrapment or inadvertent puncture of the preexisting catheter.[23]

Uncooperative patients are another factor to consider as patients who are moving during the procedure increase the risk for complications, forcing the clinician to have to consider sedation to facilitate placement. In this circumstance, it is sometimes better to sedate and intubate critically ill patients before attempting central venous catheterization. Other relative contraindications include conditions predisposing to sclerosis, vessel stenosis, or thrombosis of the central veins, such

TABLE 22.1 Advantages and Disadvantages of Central Venous Access Techniques

TECHNIQUE	ADVANTAGES	DISADVANTAGES
IJ	• Good external landmarks • Improved success with ultrasound • Less risk for pneumothorax than with SV access • Can recognize and control bleeding • Malposition of the catheter is rare • Almost a straight course to the superior vena cava on the right side • Carotid artery easily identified	• More difficult and inconvenient to secure • Possibly higher risk for thrombosis than with SV access • Higher risk of arterial puncture
Femoral	• Good external landmarks • Useful alternative with coagulopathy	• Difficult to secure in ambulatory patients • Higher risk for thrombus
SV, infraclavicular	• Good external landmarks • Can be done blind or with ultrasound	• Unable to compress bleeding vessels • Higher risk of pneumothorax
SV, supraclavicular	• Good external landmarks • Practical method of inserting a central line in cardiorespiratory arrest • Can be done blind or with ultrasound	• Unable to compress bleeding vessels

IJ, internal jugular; *SV*, subclavian vein.

as vasculitis, previous long-term cannulation, or illicit IV drug use via any of the deep venous systems.

Coagulopathy or thrombocytopenia is a frequent concern surrounding insertion of a CVC, with the overall risk for clinically significant hemorrhage in these patients approximating 2%.[24] Transfusion of fresh frozen plasma and/or platelets is commonly thought to correct any existing coagulopathy. However, a 2005 review concluded that if good technique is used, correction of coagulopathy is not generally required before or during the procedure.[25] Mumtaz and coworkers found that even in thrombocytopenic patients (platelet count <50 × 10^9/L), bleeding complications occurred approximately 3% of the time and were limited to bleeding at the insertion site; these complications were managed with additional sutures.[26] Additionally, van Baarle and colleagues discovered that platelet transfusion in thrombocytopenic patients did not significantly improve the bleeding complications.[27] Although the occasional patient may require a blood transfusion or replacement of clotting factors if a hemorrhagic complication arises, prophylactic correction of an abnormal international normalized ratio (INR) or platelet count before the procedure is not routinely necessary.[25,27] Risk can be further reduced in coagulopathic patients with the use of ultrasound-guided placement techniques and by choosing a site that has a compressible vessel if the option exists.[28–33] No studies exist examining complications in medically anticoagulated patients, although the complications in these patients would be expected to be similar to other patients with clotting abnormalities.

Contraindications to the SV Approach

SV access is relatively contraindicated in patients who have previously or recently undergone surgery or sustained trauma involving the clavicle, the first rib, or the subclavian vessels; those with previous radiation therapy involving the clavicular area; those with significant chest wall deformities; and those with marked cachexia or obesity. Patients with unilateral deformities not associated with pneumothorax (e.g., fractured clavicle) should have the opposite side chosen for placement of the catheter. Subclavian venipuncture is not contraindicated in patients with penetrating thoracic wounds unless the injuries are known or suspected to involve the subclavian vessels or SVC. Generally, cannulate the vein on the same side as the chest wound to avoid the possibility of bilateral pneumothoraces. When (preexisting) SV injury is suspected, cannulate on the opposite side. Exercise greater caution when placing a CVC in the SV in coagulopathic patients because this vessel is not compressible. Formerly, subclavian venipuncture was not recommended for use in small children, but in experienced hands it has been demonstrated to be safe.[34–36]

Contraindications to the IJ Approach

IJ access is relatively contraindicated in patients with neck trauma complicated by swelling or any other anatomic distortion at the intended site of IJ venipuncture. Likewise, the presence of a cervical collar is problematic. Although bleeding disorders are relative contraindications to central venous cannulation, the ultrasound-guided IJ approach is preferred over the SV route because the IJ site is compressible. However, prolonged compression of the artery to control bleeding could impair the cerebral circulation if collateral blood flow is compromised. In a study by Oguzkurt and colleagues, only minor bleeding complications occurred in less than 2% of patients after ultrasound-guided IJ vein catheterization.[37] In the setting of severe bleeding diatheses, the ultrasound-guided femoral approach is an acceptable alternative. Ultrasound-guided IJ vein catheter placement is preferred in patients with abnormal anatomy from previous IJ vein trauma, small IJ vessels, and morbid obesity. Additionally, thrombosis in the vessel, another contraindication as the clot can be dislodged and travel downstream leading to thromboembolic conditions, can be visualized with ultrasound. Historically, carotid artery disease (obstruction or atherosclerotic plaque) is a relative contraindication to IJ vein cannulation because inadvertent puncture or manipulation of the artery could dislodge a plaque. If a preceding SV catheterization has been unsuccessful, the ipsilateral IJ route is generally preferred for a subsequent attempt. In this manner, bilateral iatrogenic complications can be avoided.

Contraindications to the Femoral Approach

Contraindications to femoral cannulation include known or suspected intraabdominal hemorrhage or injury to the pelvis, groin, iliac vessels, or inferior vena cava (IVC). Additionally, avoid the femoral approach when known or suspected deep venous thrombosis is present. Ultrasound-guided catheterization of the FV during CPR is more successful, and it is less likely to incur inadvertent arterial puncture than the standard landmark-oriented approach.[38] However, the functionality of a femoral line during CPR in adults may be limited by the low-flow state through the abdomen limiting the ability of medications to reach the heart.

PROCEDURE

CVC insertion is relatively straightforward. It involves the Seldinger (guidewire) technique, in which a thin-walled needle or catheter is used to introduce a guidewire into the vessel lumen, which holds a tract in place over which the catheter can be inserted directly into the vessel. This technique is illustrated in Fig. 22.9. To obtain vascular access, insert a small needle into the intended vessel. Once the introducer needle is positioned within the lumen of the vessel, thread a guidewire through the needle and into the vessel lumen and then remove the needle. Alternatively, a catheter over the needle can be used to introduce the wire. The guidewire, now within the vessel, serves as a guide over which the catheter is inserted. Although the Seldinger technique involves several steps, it can be performed quickly once mastered. More importantly, this technique broadens the application of central venous cannulation by permitting the insertion of standard infusion catheters, multilumen catheters, large-bore rapid infusion systems, introducer devices, hemodialysis devices, and even peripheral cardiopulmonary bypass cannulas. Given this flexibility, the use of Seldinger-type systems is advantageous despite their greater cost.

Ultrasound guidance has revolutionized the insertion of CVCs. Landmark-based approaches to central venous cannulation have been associated with a higher risk of complications than cannulation using ultrasound.[29,33,39–41] Additionally, ultrasound guidance increases first-attempt success rate and decreases needle to vein time. As with all anatomic structures in the human body, veins are highly variable in their location. Not surprisingly, research has demonstrated that the ability to see the internal structure's location and proximity to other structures greatly increases the safety and success rate while decreasing the time required to perform the procedure.[29,30,38] Many hospitals now require the use of ultrasound guidance for the placement of all CVCs.

Equipment

See Video 22.1. Before any procedure, preparation and organization of all equipment ahead of time are imperative. The basic materials required for central venous cannulation are shown in Review Box 22.1 and are discussed here in further detail. Most CVCs come in a kit prepackaged with most of the materials necessary to maintain a sterile environment for the procedure to be performed, including sterile drapes and personal protective equipment. Additionally, it is recommended that additional equipment in additional sizes is stored in a readily accessible storage room or, even better, in a dedicated cart for central lines. This is a part of the "bundling" practice that has been shown to reduce the search for supplies, improve compliance with full-barrier technique, and subsequently decrease catheter-related infections.[42–47] While the use of these bundles has been shown to be effective, the use of them varies across hospital systems and is at least partially dependent on resources available.[46,48] Maximum sterile barrier precautions with cap, face mask, sterile gown, and sterile gloves should be used at all times during insertion of CVCs.[49,50]

Ultrasound

See Video 22.2. As discussed before, the use of ultrasound during insertion of CVC has largely supplanted landmark-based approaches, especially with IJ and FV site approaches. Historically, many clinicians preferred to first locate the position of a central vein with a small exploratory or "finder" needle rather than directly cannulating the vein with a larger needle to accommodate a guidewire or catheter. Ultrasound-guided CVC placement allows the provider to survey the anatomy before the procedure, guide insertion of the needle into the correct vessel, and confirm placement of the wire and catheter in the vessel (see Ultrasound Box).[3,31,38,40,41] When utilizing ultrasound, it is important to use a sterile ultrasound probe cover to further maintain the sterile environment. There are commercially available probe covers for this purpose.

Needle

Virtually any needle or catheter can be used to introduce a guidewire into a vessel, but there are advantages to using needles specifically designed for passage of a guidewire. These needles must be large enough to accommodate the guidewire yet be as small as possible to minimize bleeding complications. The introducer needles provided with CVC kits or introducer devices are usually thin walled to maximize lumen size relative to the overall needle diameter. If a needle that is not thin walled is used, choose a size that is one gauge smaller (larger bore) than that listed in Table 22.2. If unsure, simply test the equipment first to ensure compatibility.

Standard needles may have a uniformly straight-bore lumen throughout their length. A wire passing into a straight needle may encounter an obstacle at the proximal end. The proximal end of a Seldinger needle incorporates a funnel-shaped taper that guides the wire directly into the needle (Fig. 22.4). It is advisable to use a non–Luer-Lok or slip-tip type of syringe because the added twisting that is required to remove a Luer-Lok syringe from the introducer needle may dislodge a tenuously placed needle. Safety syringe systems exist that permit passage of the wire without removal of the aspirating syringe by using a central tunnel in the barrel. This device incorporates a hollow syringe through which the guidewire can pass directly into the introducing needle without detachment. It also reduces the risk for air embolism, which can occur when the needle is open to air. It is not uncommon for the wire to

TABLE 22.2 Needle Sizes for Venous and Arterial Catheters[a]

STANDARD FULL-LENGTH COIL GUIDEWIRE CATHETER SIZE (Fr)	NEEDLE GAUGE[b]
3	21
4–4.5	20
5–6.0	20–19
6–8.5	19–18

[a]Any size of catheter from 3.0 to 8.5 Fr may be introduced with a 22-gauge needle if a solid wire (e.g., Cor-Flex) is used.

[b]All needle gauges are for thin-walled needles only, the type supplied in central line kits.

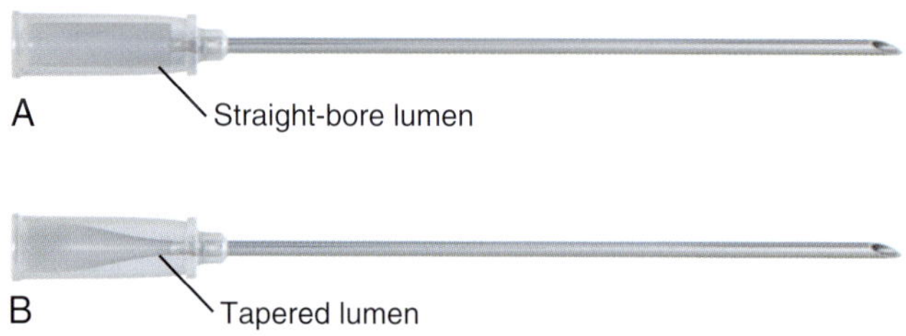

Fig. 22.4 Introducing needles. (A) Ordinary needle with a straight-bore lumen. (B) Seldinger needle with a tapered lumen, which allows easy entry of the guidewire.

become snagged at the junction of the safety syringe and the needle hub. In this case, simply remove the syringe and insert the wire directly.

Additionally, some CVC kits come with an angiocatheter. This combines a finder needle and a catheter than can be inserted into the vessel, leaving just the catheter in place. This catheter can then accommodate the guidewire eliminating the problems that can arise when using the needle alone. The disadvantages of the catheter include that it is thin-walled and is prone to kink if inserted at a sharp angle, which can sometimes make the guidewire difficult to insert.

Guidewire

Two basic types of guidewires are used for central line placement: straight and J-shaped. Straight guidewires are for use in vessels with a linear configuration, whereas J-shaped guidewires are for use in tortuous vessels. Both guidewires have essentially the same internal design (Fig. 22.5). The flexibility of the guidewire is the result of a stainless-steel coil or helix that forms the bulk of the guidewire. Within the central lumen of the helix is a straight central core wire, called a mandrel, that adds rigidity to the steel coil. The mandrel is usually fixed at one end of the helix and terminates between 0.5 and 3.0 cm from the other end to create a flexible or floppy tip. Guidewires are also available with two flexible ends, one straight and the other J-shaped. The flexible end of the guidewire allows it to flex on contact with the wall of a vessel. If the contact is tangential, as with an infraclavicular approach to the SV, a straight guidewire is generally preferred. If the angle is more acute, as with an external jugular approach to the SV, or if the vessel is particularly tortuous or valves must be traversed, a J-shaped guidewire may be used. The more rounded leading

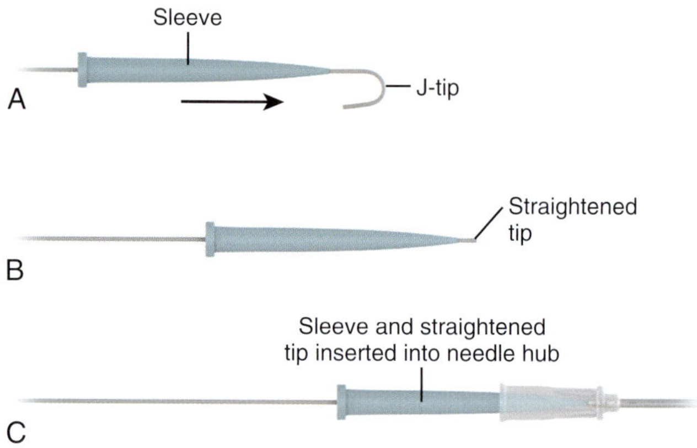

Fig. 22.5 J-wire. (A) Plastic sleeve in the retracted position demonstrating the J-tip. (B) Plastic sleeve advanced to straighten the curve for easy introduction into the needle hub. (C) Plastic sleeve inserted into needle hub. In an emergency, take care to not misplace or throw the sleeve away. Without it, placing the J-wire into the hub of the needle is very difficult. Some wires may have a "soft-tipped" straight end on the opposite end of the wire. These wires are engineered to be flexible (to avoid vessel injury) and may be used if there is difficulty passing the J-end.

edge of the J-shaped guidewire provides a broader surface to manipulate within the vessel and decreases the risk for perforation. This is especially advantageous when attempting to thread a guidewire through a vessel with valves. Many guidewires also contain a straight safety wire that runs parallel to the mandrel to keep the wire from kinking or shearing.

The standard size for guidewires is 0.025 to 0.035 inch (0.064 to 0.089 cm) in diameter, which permits introduction through an 18-gauge thin-walled needle or catheter. A modification of this standard guidewire uses a bare mandrel with the flexible coil soldered to its end. This construction provides a guidewire with a diameter of just 0.018 inch (0.047 cm) but with the same rigidity as the larger guidewires. The manufacturer states that such a guidewire can be introduced through a 22-gauge thin-walled needle yet still guide an 8.5-Fr catheter (Micropuncture introducer sets and trays with Cor-Flex wire guides, Cook Critical Care). Most guidewires are marked with indicators on the wire to indicate distance. This is to ensure that the operator is able to ascertain how much guidewire is inside the patient. They are demarcated in increments of 10 cm, with each distance of 10 cm demarcated by the multiple of 10 (one line indicates 10 cm, two lines indicate 20 cm, etc.).

It is important to note that guidewires are delicate and are prone to bend, kink, unwind, or very rarely, knot.[51] A force of 4 to 6 lb may cause a guidewire to rupture. Guidewires should thread easily and smoothly and never be forced; the worst complications of CVC placement are associated with the application of excessive force across parts of the apparatus that are not threading smoothly. If a guidewire is not passing easily, withdraw the guidewire and the introducer needle as a single unit. Embolization of portions of the guidewire is possible, and sharp defects in the guidewire may perforate vessel walls (Fig. 22.6). If one encounters a good flash of blood but cannot readily manipulate the guidewire, this may indicate that the outer wire coils are entrapped against the proximal sharp edge of the needle bevel. Guidewires should be inspected for small defects such as kinks, sharp ends, or spurs before use and especially after a failed attempt. Guidewires may be threaded

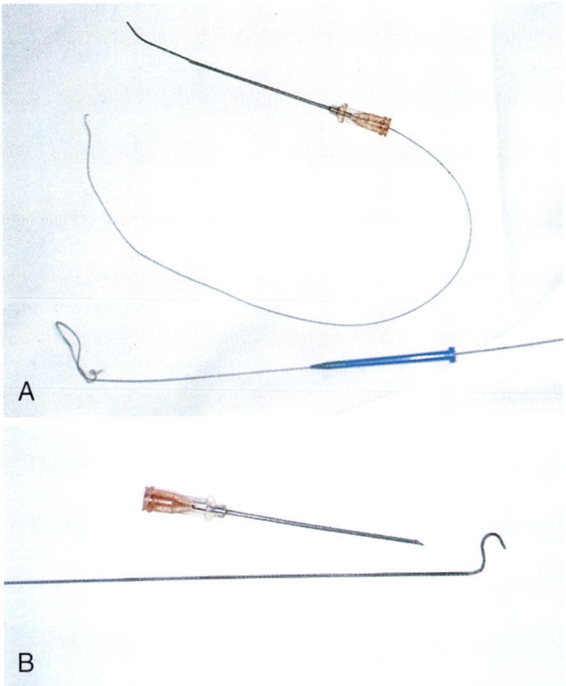

Fig. 22.6 (A–B) Although newer guidewires are more resistant to shearing, if a guidewire will not advance, withdraw both the needle and the wire in one motion. These pictures demonstrate a permanently deformed guidewire that could not be advanced. Withdrawing the wire with the indwelling introducer needle in place within a vessel may shear off a portion of the wire and result in systemic embolization.

into the introducer needle hub more easily by using the plastic sleeve attached to the guidewire, as shown in Fig. 22.5C.

Dilators

CVC kits come equipped with a rigid tissue dilator. This device is used to dilate the soft tissue surrounding the vessel for easier guidance of the catheter through the soft tissue and into the vessel. The device has a thicker wall to prevent bending when being inserted into the soft tissue but also a narrow lumen to allow passage over the guidewire without allowing the guidewire to kink inside the dilator. The end of the dilator tapers to allow easier passage into the tissue as well as more gradual dilation without destruction of the overlying tissue. The dilator is intended to be inserted about one-third to one-half of its length into the soft tissue with the intent to dilate the soft tissue and not the vessel itself. As the dilator is inserted into the tissue, it is important to periodically ascertain if the guidewire remains freely mobile within the dilator lumen by simply moving the guidewire back and forth within the dilator. Despite its rigidity and thicker walls, dilators can still kink, usually at the tapered tip, and can even bend the guidewire inside of it; both usually occur due to inadequate skin incision around the guidewire. Any misshapen dilators and/or guidewires should be removed as a single unit to prevent potential unwinding or rupture of the guidewire.

Catheters

There are several different catheter and introducer devices that have been developed by different manufacturers and each

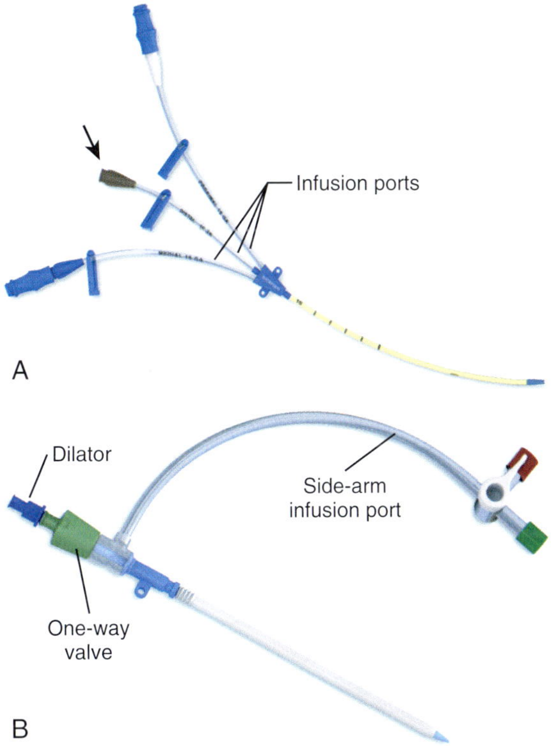

Fig. 22.7 (A) Triple-lumen catheter. The catheter ports are used for infusion of fluids, administration of medications, and monitoring of central venous pressure and are typically labeled as proximal, medial, and distal. The distal or brown port, typically 16 gauge, facilitates passage of the guidewire. Note that the end cap of the distal port *(arrow)* must be removed before insertion to allow passage of the guidewire. (B) Sheath introducer. This large-bore device (8.5 Fr) is used as an introduction catheter for devices such as Swan-Ganz catheters and transvenous pacemakers. Note that the dilator must be placed through the catheter before the device is inserted into the patient.

kit may vary in its method of insertion. In general, one can place single-, double-, and triple-lumen catheters by sliding the catheter directly over a guidewire into the intended vessel (Fig. 22.7A). Larger catheters or devices without lumens can be introduced with a sheath-introducer system. Over-the-needle catheters can be introduced once intravascular placement is attained.

The Desilets-Hoffman type sheath introducer became available in 1965 to aid in arteriography procedures that require many catheter changes. This sheath-introducer device is commonly but incorrectly called a "Cordis," which is a proprietary trade name. The sheath-introducer unit includes two parts, an inner dilator, and an outer sheath, as shown in Fig. 22.7B. The dilator is rigid with a narrow lumen to accommodate the guidewire. It is longer and thinner than its sheath and has a tapered end that dilates the subcutaneous tissue and vessel defect created by the needle. The sheath (or introducer catheter when used as a cannula for inserting Swan-Ganz catheters, transvenous pacemakers, or other devices) has a blunt end and is simply a large-diameter catheter.

Many modifications of the sheath exist, such as side arms and diaphragms to aid in the placement of devices without lumens. Care must be taken when using side-arm sets for rapid administration of fluid because some catheters are 8.5 Fr in diameter but have only a 5-Fr side arm. Some sets have a "single-lumen infusion catheter," which performs the same function but is more easily secured to the sheath introducer. Selection of the appropriate diameter of introducer catheter should correspond to the indication for placement of a CVC. Generally, an 8.5-Fr catheter is used to facilitate placement of a Swan-Ganz catheter and a 6.0-Fr catheter is used to facilitate transvenous placement of a pacemaker. If the introducer catheter is larger than required to support the intraluminal device, a leak may develop at the diaphragm insertion point. Adjustable diaphragms are present on many introducers that allow the operator to tighten down the proximal end of the diaphragm to prevent leaks.

Additionally, there are single and multi-port CVCs that are not intended for device placement. The primary indication for these devices is the infusion of medications, intravenous fluids, and/or blood products as well as aspiration of blood to measure central serum levels, such as central venous oxygen saturation. These devices always have a central distal lumen that corresponds with the central port on the other end. Any additional ports that a device has correspond to a lumen that exits to the side of the distal lumen. Importantly, these lumens are all independent and separate and do not communicate with each other within the catheter allowing no intermixing of substances within the lumens of the catheter. Furthermore, because of their distal tip location in the central venous circulation, these devices can be modified to allow the measurement of CVP. Special catheters have been developed to prevent bacterial contamination and line sepsis. These catheters are impregnated with either antiseptics (silver sulfadiazine and chlorhexidine) or antibiotics (minocycline, rifampin, or cefazolin) to reduce bacterial colonization and microbial growth. The use of these antibiotic-impregnated catheters has been shown to decrease the incidence of central line–associated bloodstream infections (CLABSI) in both adults and pediatrics.[21,52–55] Heparin-coated catheters are also available that prevent fibronectin binding, thereby inhibiting the formation of bacterial biofilm on the catheter's surface. These catheters can decrease catheter-associated infection (CAI) significantly and are cost-effective. They should be avoided in patients with a history of heparin-induced thrombocytopenia.[56,57] Minocycline- and rifampin-impregnated catheters are currently considered to be the most effective and have largely supplanted heparin-coated catheters.[21,55] Other interventions that decrease central line infections include the use of full sterile barrier precautions, skin preparation with chlorhexidine solution, and placement by experienced physicians.[43–45,48,58–61]

TECHNIQUE

Preprocedure Preparation

See Video 22.3. When possible, discuss the procedure with the patient and obtain informed consent. Patient positioning on the bed varies depending on the vessel selected for access. If available, perform an ultrasound survey to identify the patient's anatomy, ensure vessel patency, and confirm the puncture site (Fig. 22.8). Ultrasound-guided CVC placement has been shown to decrease procedure times, as well as complication rates.[29,32,33,38,40,41] Additionally, compliance with a central line bundling policy has been shown to significantly decrease central line–associated bloodstream infections (CLABSIs).[43–45,48] Prepare and drape the puncture site while maintaining sterile technique, and observe universal precautions throughout the procedure (Fig. 22.9, *steps 1 and 2*). Personal protective

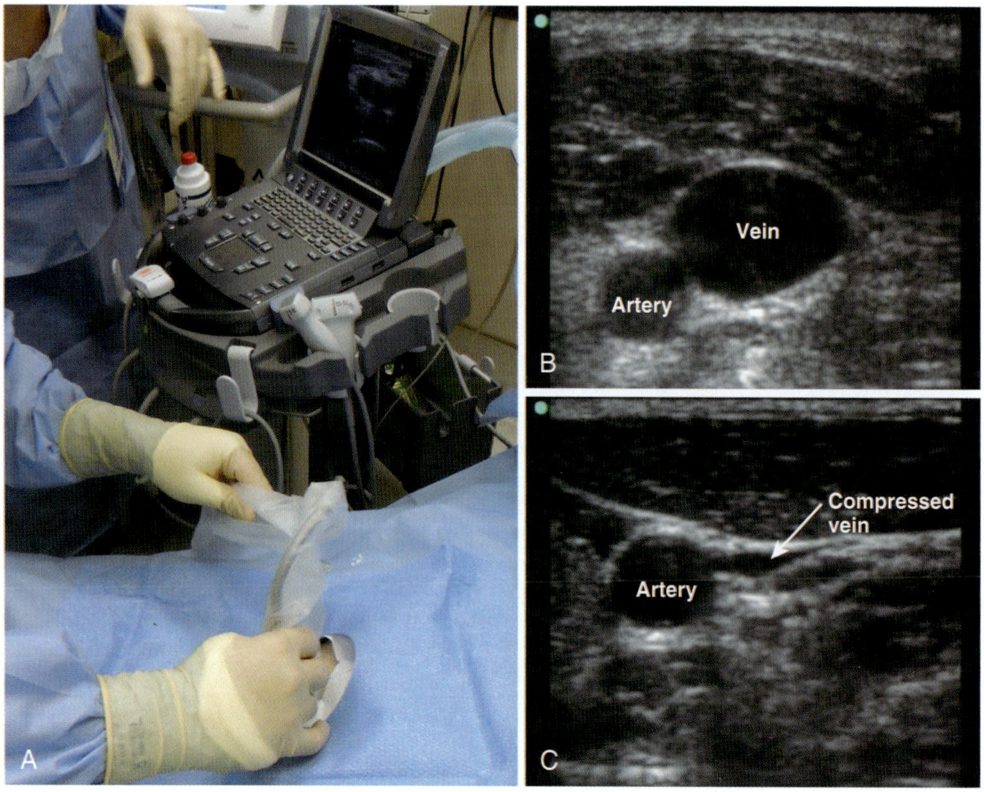

Fig. 22.8 (A) Ultrasound survey. Perform an ultrasound survey to identify the anatomy before beginning the procedure. (B) Cross-sectional view of the artery and noncompressed vein. (C) Cross-sectional view of the artery and compressed vein.

Central Venous Catheterization (Internal Jugular Approach)

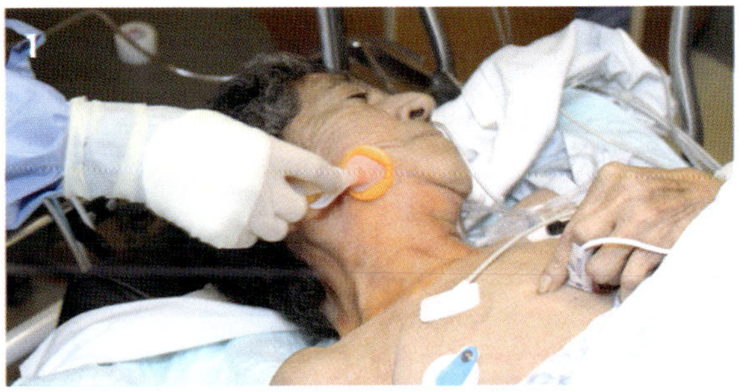

Prepare the area with chlorhexidine solution. A gown, surgical cap, mask, eye protection, and sterile gloves should be worn throughout the procedure.

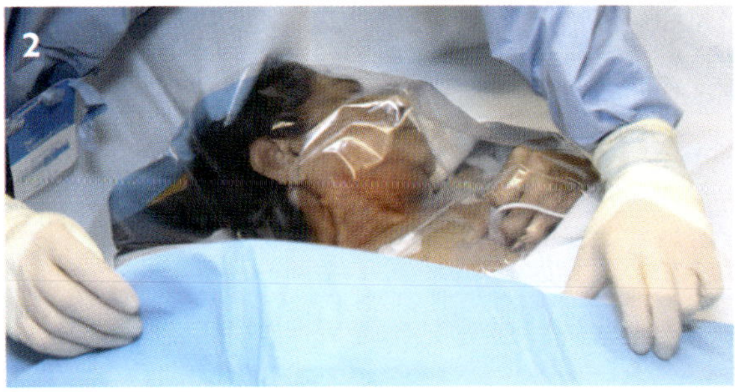

Apply a full-body, sterile drape. Meticulous attention must be paid to sterile technique to avoid iatrogenic infection.

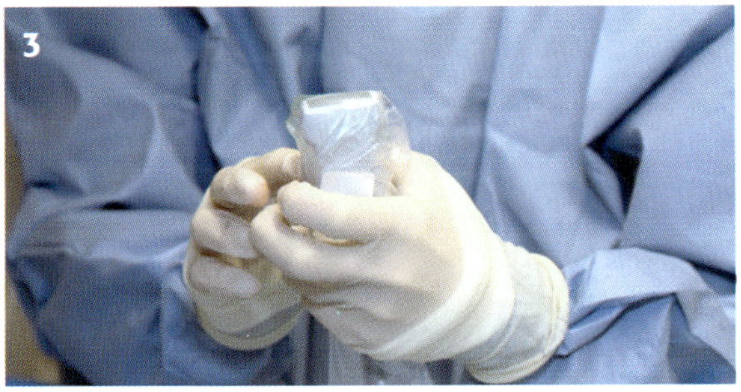

Insert the ultrasound probe into a sterile sheath and use sterile ultrasound gel during the procedure. Enlist the help of an assistant in patient preparation and maintenance of sterility.

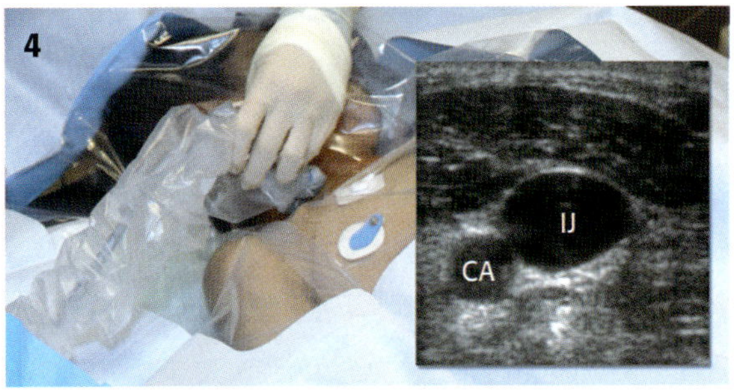

Identify the anatomic structures with ultrasound. The internal jugular vein (*IJ*) and carotid artery (*CA*) must be clearly distinguished from each other (see text for more details).

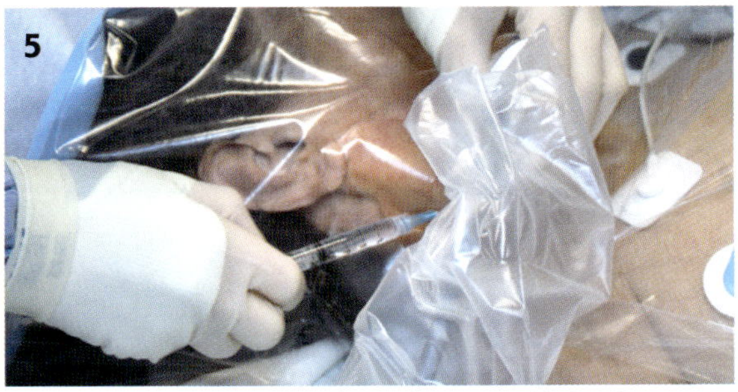

Anesthetize the tissues overlying the vein with local anesthetic. Here, the operator is using ultrasound guidance to ensure a proper entry site.

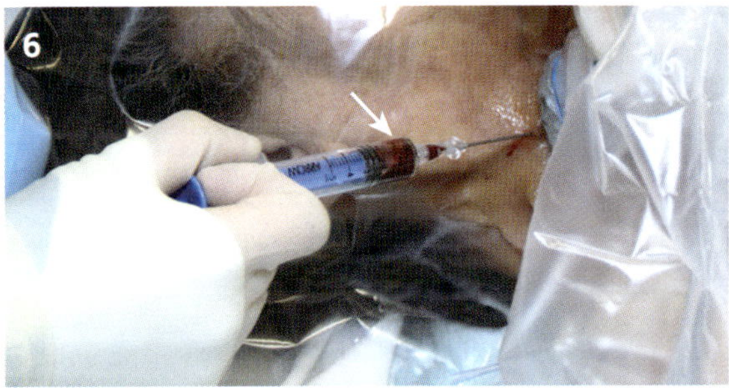

Insert the needle and syringe while slowly advancing and applying negative pressure to the plunger. Follow the needle trajectory with ultrasound until the vein is entered and blood enters the syringe *(arrow)*.

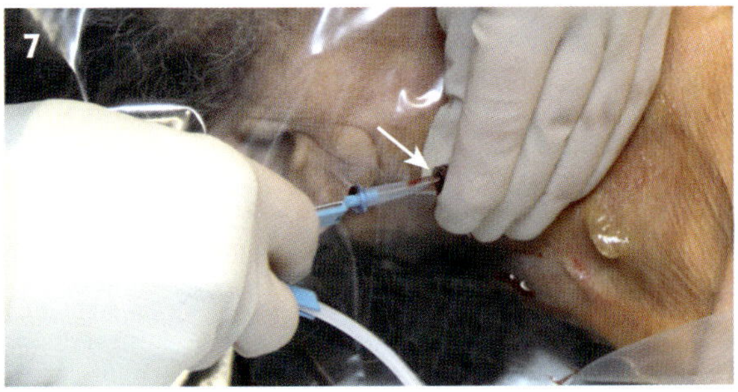

Remove the syringe and advance the guidewire through the needle. Use the straightener *(arrow)* to facilitate entry of the J-wire into the hub. NEVER FORCE THE WIRE!

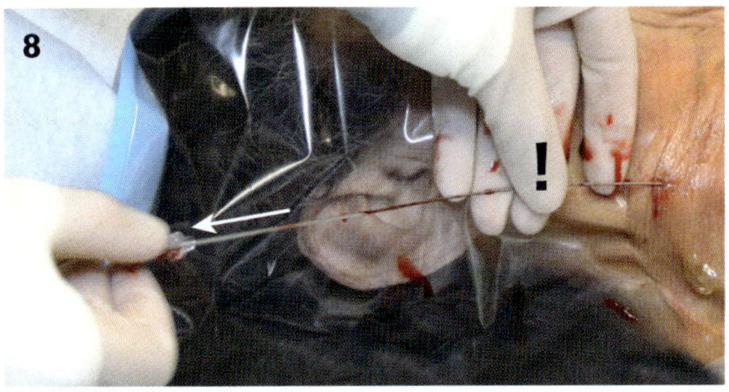

Once the wire has been inserted to the appropriate depth (see text for details), remove the needle *(arrow)*. It is *essential* to *always* maintain a grip on the wire throughout the procedure *(!)*.

Fig. 22.9 Ultrasound-guided internal jugular central venous catheterization.

Continued

Central Venous Catheterization (Internal Jugular Approach)

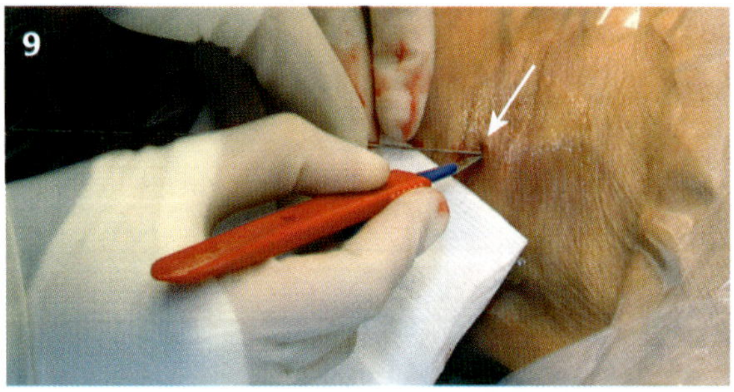

Make an incision at the site of the wire to facilitate dilator and catheter passage. Make the incision the width of the catheter and extend it completely through the dermis.

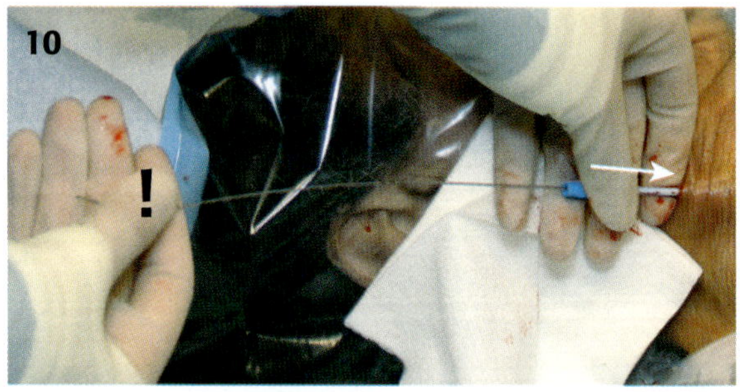

Thread the dilator over the guidewire. The wire must *always* be protruding from the end of the dilator and firmly in your grasp *(!)*. Advance the dilator several centimeters into the vessel and then remove.

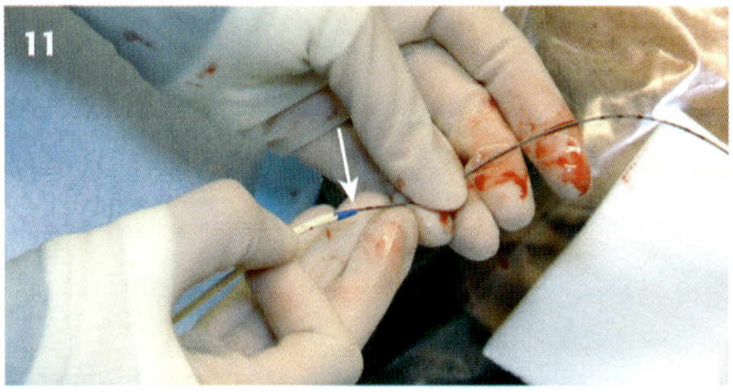

Advance the catheter over the wire. It can be difficult to align the two pieces; hold the very end of the catheter and the wire to make this step easier.

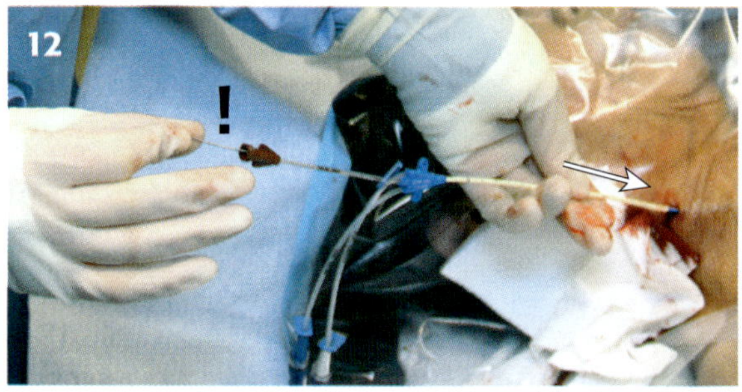

Advance the catheter into the vessel. The guidewire will emerge from the distal port. It is essential that the guidewire protrudes from the hub and is grasped before catheter advancement *(!)*.

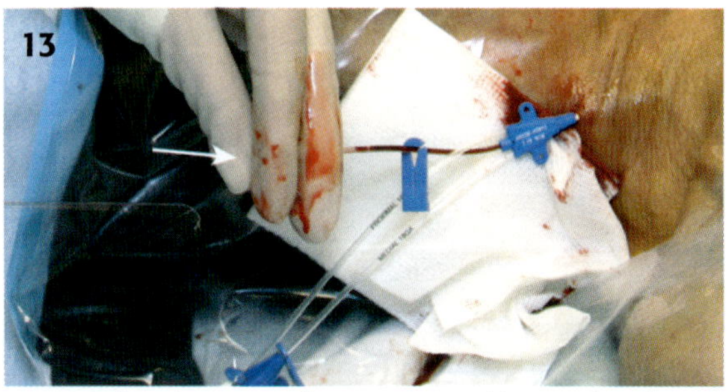

Remove the wire. Cover the open port with your thumb *(arrow)* until the end cap is screwed on.

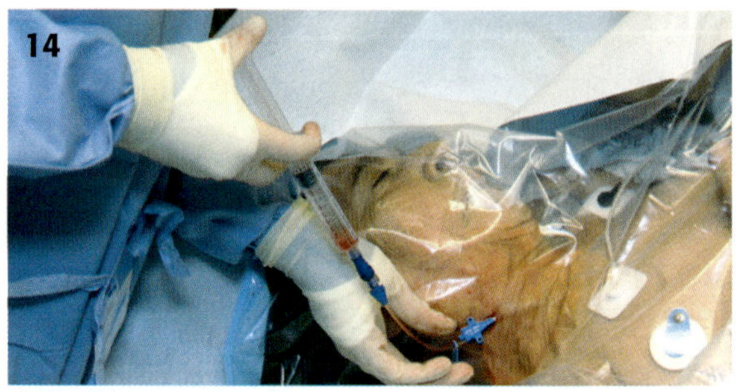

Flush all ports with saline.

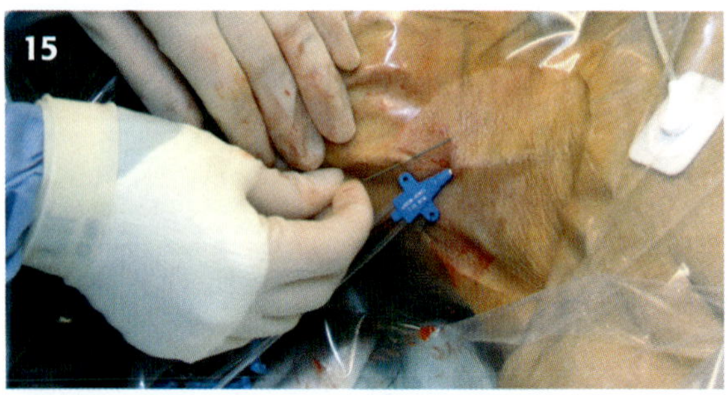

Suture the catheter into place using nonabsorbable silk sutures. Several knots should be made to secure the line. Avoid making knots that place excessive pressure on the skin.

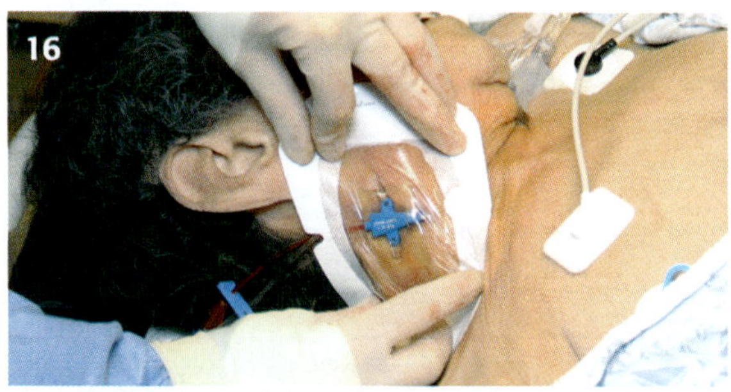

Clean the area around the catheter insertion site with chlorhexidine. Place a simple dressing, avoiding excessive amounts of gauze and tape.

Fig. 22.9, cont'd

equipment including a gown, surgical cap, mask, eye protection, and sterile gloves should be worn throughout the procedure when possible. When performing ultrasound-guided placement of a CVC, ensure that a sterile transducer sheath and sterile transducer gel are used during the procedure (see Fig. 22.9, *step 3*). An assistant will prove valuable assistance in patient preparation, maintenance of sterility, and handling of the equipment.

Guidewire Placement With the Seldinger Technique

See Videos 22.4–22.12. When preparing to perform an ultrasound-guided CVC procedure, it is useful to perform an ultrasound survey of the site to evaluate the target vein, surrounding structures, and venipuncture location, as shown in Fig. 22.8. Veins can easily be distinguished from the nearby artery by applying external pressure with the transducer, as the veins collapse completely with pressure and the arteries do not usually collapse. Occasionally, the vein does not collapse with pressure. If this occurs, a thrombus may be present in the vein, or the structure has been misidentified. If a suspected vein does not collapse with pressure, it is not an appropriate vessel for cannulation. If available, Doppler functions may also be helpful in the differentiation of veins and arteries. The IJ vein may be seen collapsing spontaneously during the inspiratory phase of the respiratory cycle. Select a venipuncture location where branching of the vein will allow the shortest path of the needle, will not obstruct passage of the catheter, and will not allow inadvertent puncture of other vital anatomic structures. (See Chapter 66 for additional information and descriptions of the ultrasound technique.)

Prepare the catheter for insertion by flushing each lumen with sterile normal saline. This ensures the patency of each lumen as well as removes all air from the lumen. Most CVC kits contain an anesthetic such as lidocaine or bupivacaine, which should be used to anesthetize the skin and underlying structures to minimize patient discomfort during the procedure (see Fig. 22.9, *step 5*). Attach a small syringe to an introducing needle that is large enough to accommodate the guidewire. Insert the needle and syringe together. Slowly advance the needle into the vein and apply steady negative pressure on the syringe (see Fig. 22.9, *step 6*). It is important to always maintain negative pressure on the syringe once the needle enters the skin. This allows the operator to have tactile confirmation of the needle entering a vessel or a non-vessel structure, such as the apex of the lung. Importantly, any aspiration of air should be interpreted as an increased likelihood of pneumothorax and the procedure should be aborted until confirmatory imaging is obtained. When performing ultrasound-guided CVC placement, follow the needle trajectory in the soft tissue and observe penetration of the vessel. If the tip of the needle is not visualized at all times with ultrasound, the needle may be passed into structures other than the vein. The key concept in using ultrasound guidance for venous access is to visualize the tip of the needle at all times during cannulation (Figs. 22.10 and 22.11). Once the tip of the needle enters the vessel lumen, blood will be aspirated freely. Stabilize the needle hub to prevent movement of the needle and displacement of the tip from the vessel while the syringe is removed. This action is the most associated with failure to pass a wire after the vein has initially been entered. The need to disconnect the syringe can be eliminated by use of the Arrow Safety Syringe (Teleflex), which has a lumen through the syringe through which the guidewire can be inserted. After removing the syringe, cap the needle hub with your thumb before passing the guidewire to minimize the potential for air embolism.

Alternatively, a catheter-over-the-needle device may be used to cannulate the vein. This technique can be used without the need of the syringe if a longitudinal US view is used, similar to that for placement of a peripheral venous catheter (Fig 22.11).

Confirm that the blood flow is nonpulsatile. It is possible to assess this primarily with the syringe while aspirating upon entering the vessel by visualizing the color of the blood aspirated as well as visualizing the rapidity the blood is aspirated. However, it should be confirmed when the syringe is removed by visualizing those same characteristics as the blood flows freely from the needle. Bright red pulsatile blood is very suggestive of arterial puncture. Be aware that in shock states or marked arterial desaturation, dark, nonpulsatile blood does not rule out arterial cannulation. If there are concerns about possible arterial puncture, either remove the introducer needle and draw a sample for blood gas analysis from the needle to compare with an arterial blood gas sample or insert an 18-gauge single-lumen catheter over the wire and into the vessel because this step does not require the use of a dilator. The catheter can then be connected to a pressure transducer to confirm the presence of venous waveforms and venous pressure.

Introduce the flexible end of the guidewire into the hub of the needle (see Fig. 22.9, *step 7*). It may be easier to introduce

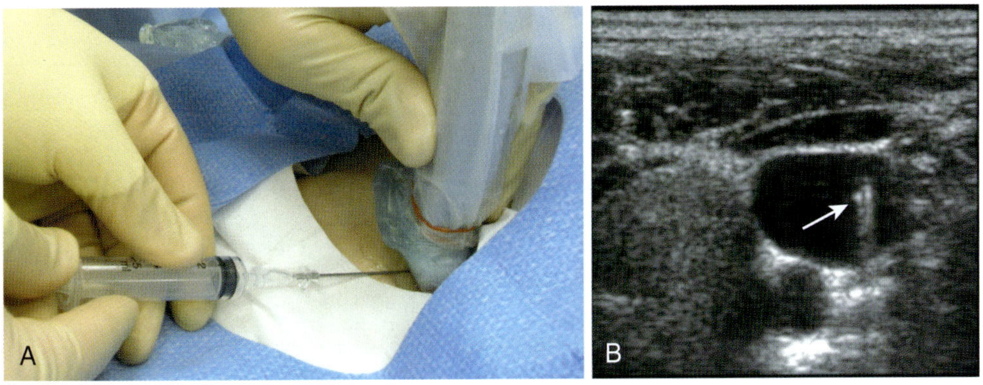

Fig. 22.10 (A) Ultrasound-guided insertion of the introducer needle. (B) Cross-sectional ultrasound image of the needle *(arrow)* within the vessel.

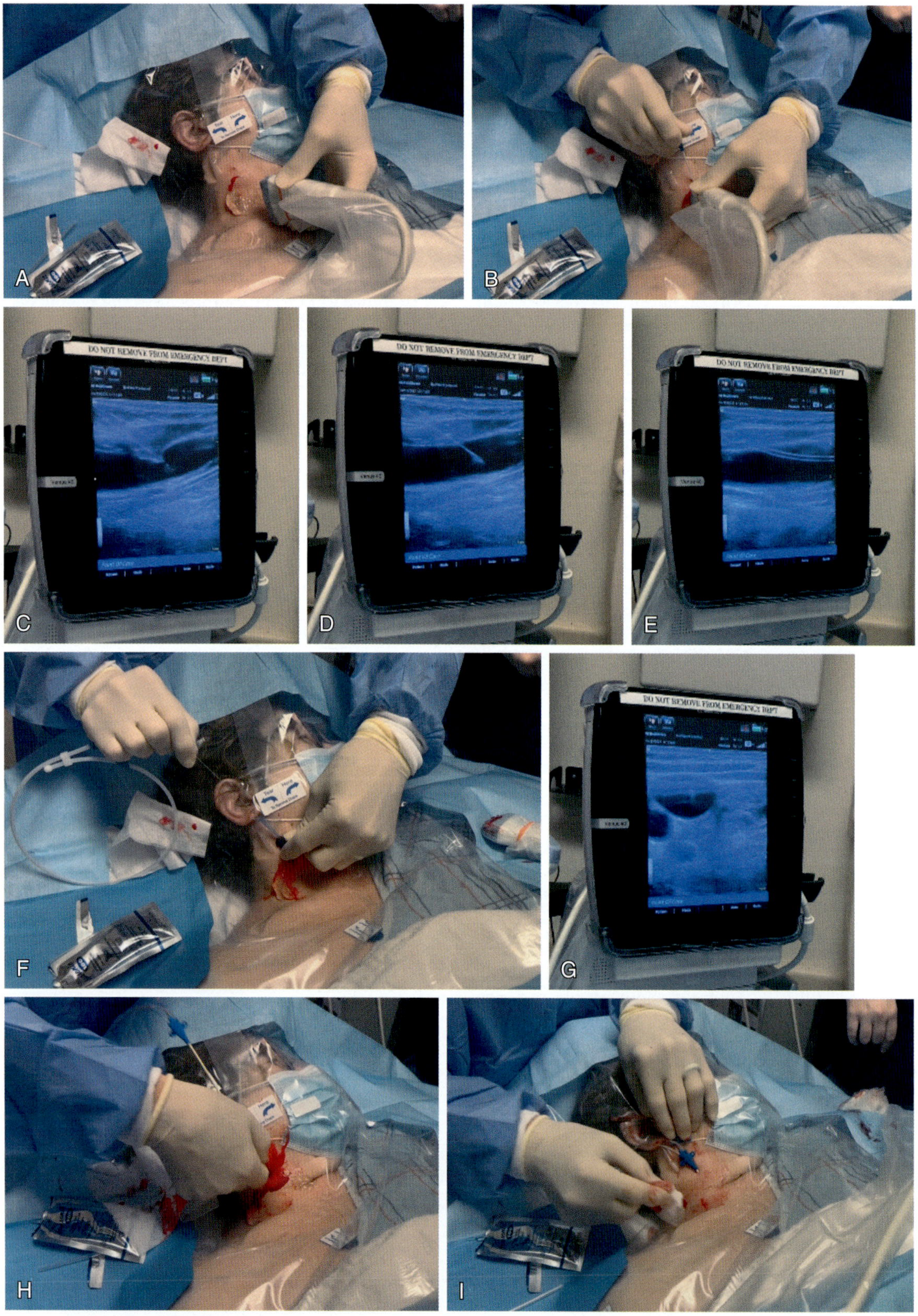

Fig. 22.11 (A) Identifying internal jugular (IJ) vein with ultrasound probe (US) in longitudinal view. (B) Making skin incision in line with IJ vein. (C) Inserting needle with catheter through skin incision under direct US vision. Needle with catheter tenting IJ just prior to entry. (D) Needle with catheter visualized in IJ vein. (E) Catheter visualized in vein after advanced off of needle. (F) Guide wire being advanced through catheter into vein. (G) Guide wire visualized in vein. (H–I) Triple-lumen catheter being advanced into vein.

the J-wire by advancing the plastic sleeve contained in the kit onto the floppy end of the wire to straighten the J-shape. This straightened end is then introduced into the needle hub. The guidewire should thread smoothly through the needle into the vessel without resistance. Do not force the wire if resistance is encountered but remove it from the needle and reattach the syringe to aspirate blood and reconfirm intravascular needle placement. It is important for the wire to slip easily from the needle during removal. If resistance to removal of the wire is felt, the wire and needle should be removed as a single unit to prevent shearing of the wire and resultant wire embolism. It has been recommended by some that no guidewire that is stuck should ever be withdrawn through the introducing needle.[62] Although there are no clinical data to support this recommendation and newer guidewires are stronger and more resistant to shearing, it represents the safest course of action. The recommendation to remove the needle and guidewire as a unit is sometimes disregarded because of reluctance to abandon a potentially successful venipuncture. The clinician performing the procedure must use both caution and good judgment to determine the best course of action but should not withdraw the guidewire against resistance. Manipulation of the guidewire within an introducer needle should be done only with standard coil guidewires. Solid wires (e.g., Cor-Flex Wire Guides) have a small lip at the point at which the flexible coil is soldered to the guidewire. This lip can become caught on the edge of the tip of the needle and shear off the coil portion of the guidewire. Solid wires must thread freely on the first attempt, or the entire guidewire and needle assembly must be removed. Keep backup guidewires on hand. All of these complications can be avoided if a catheter, rather than a needle, is used to introduce the guide wire (Fig. 22.11).

Occasionally, a guidewire must be teased into the vessel; rotating the wire or needle often helps in difficult placements. If the wire does not thread easily, pull back slightly on the needle itself just before advancing the wire. This helps if the opening of the needle is abutting the vessel's inner wall and blocking entry of the wire or if the vein is compressed by introduction of the needle. Changing wire tips from a straight wire to a J-wire or vice versa may also solve an advancement problem. If the inner lumen of a vessel is smaller than the diameter of the J, the wire will be prevented from returning to its natural shape and the spring in the coil will generate resistance. Any advantages of a J-wire will be negated if the wire fails to regain its intended shape. In this instance, it should be possible to introduce a straight tip without a problem. Alternatively, if the angle of entry of the needle into the vessel is more acute than suspected, a straight wire may not be able to bend appropriately, as it encounters the vessel's far wall. A J-tipped wire may be used and threaded in such a manner that the wire resumes its J-shape away from the far wall. All these maneuvers are performed with gentle free motions of the wire within the needle. If at any time the wire cannot be advanced freely, suspect improper placement and reevaluate the attempt.

If the guidewire threads easily, advance the guidewire until at least one-quarter of the wire is within the vessel. The further into the vessel the wire extends, the more stable its location when the catheter is introduced. However, advancing the guidewire too far may result in ventricular ectopy secondary to endocardial irritation, myocardial puncture leading to tamponade, or entanglement in a previously placed pacemaker, internal defibrillator, or IVC filter. In both the left and right IJ vein and infraclavicular SV approaches, fluoroscopic study during passage of the guidewire has determined the mean distance from skin to the SVC-atrial junction to be 18 cm.[62] This distance has been recommended as the greatest depth of guidewire insertion for these approaches, although this may be adjusted due to patient factors such as body habitus or height. The distance indicators on the guidewire, if present, can be helpful in determining how much guidewire is inside the patient.

Patients should be connected to cardiac monitoring prior to CVC insertion to evaluate for any potential ventricular dysrhythmias. Any increase in premature ventricular contractions or a new ventricular dysrhythmia should be interpreted as evidence that the guidewire is inserted too far and should be remedied by withdrawing the wire until the rhythm reverts to baseline. Usually, the procedure can be continued after a moment, with care taken to not readvance the wire. Persistent ventricular dysrhythmias require standard advanced cardiac life support treatment and consideration of a new vascular approach.

Occasionally, a wire threads easily past the tip of the needle and then suddenly will not advance farther. If the introducer needle demonstrated free return of blood at the time of wire entry and the initial advancement of the wire met no resistance, the two options are to halt the procedure or seek confirmation of the wire position. The guidewire within the lumen of the vessel can be visualized and confirmed via cross-sectional and longitudinal views on ultrasound. Alternatively, the needle may be removed, the wire fixed in place with a sterile hemostat, and a radiograph taken to confirm the position of the wire.[51,62] A freely advancing wire may suddenly stop once it is well within a vessel if the vessel makes an unsuspected bend, is mechanically obstructed, such as a thrombosis, or is being compressed or deviated by another structure, such as a bone or muscle. This seems especially common with the infraclavicular approach to the SV and can sometimes be remedied by a more lateral approach.

Sheath Unit and Catheter Placement

Once the guidewire is placed into the vessel, remove the needle in preparation for passage of the catheter (see Fig. 22.9, *step 8*). Proper positioning of the guidewire within the vessel lumen can be confirmed by cross-sectional and longitudinal ultrasound imaging (Fig. 22.12).[41,63,64] This can be done at any point while inserting the wire to ensure that the correct vessel has been cannulated and that puncture of the posterior wall has not occurred. This technique can also be useful when resistance is encountered while feeding the guidewire. A small skin incision is required at the site of the wire to widen the opening (see Fig. 22.9, *step 9*). Make the incision approximately the width of the catheter to be introduced and extend it completely through the dermis. Take caution to not incise the guidewire; this can be avoided by pointing the blade edge *away* from the guidewire when incising the skin. Alternatively, if US guidance is being used, the skin incision may be made first and the needle introduced through the incision. This avoids the problem of trying to make the skin incision directly on the guide wire, which can be a challenge if there is blood at the point of the skin puncture (Fig. 22.11).

When placing soft multiple-lumen catheters, the tissue must be dilated with the tissue dilator from the skin to the vessel before placement of the catheter. Thread the guidewire

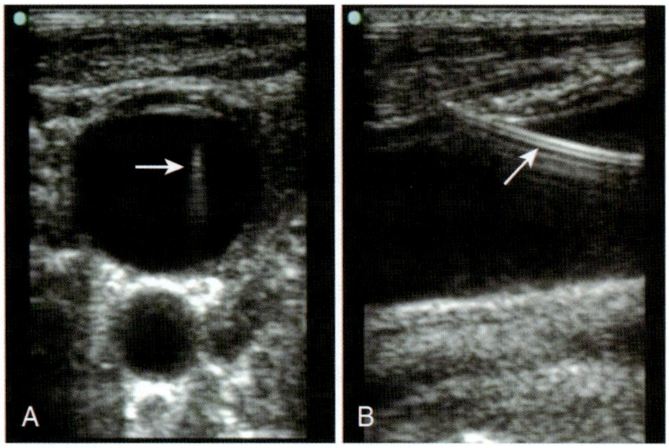

Fig. 22.12 (A–B) Cross-sectional and longitudinal ultrasound images demonstrating a guidewire *(arrows)* in the lumen of the targeted vein.

through the distal opening of the rigid dilator until it extends through the proximal end of the dilator (see Fig. 22.9, *step 10*). The guidewire must always be visibly protruding from the end of the dilator or catheter during insertion to avoid inadvertent advancement of the guidewire into the circulation and potential loss of the wire. While maintaining control of the guidewire proximally, thread the dilator over the wire into the skin with a twisting motion. Advance the rigid dilator only a few centimeters into the vessel and then remove it. Once the dilator is removed, thread the soft catheter into position over the wire. Placement of multiple-lumen catheters requires identification of the distal lumen and its corresponding hub. Find the distal lumen at the very tip of the catheter. The corresponding hub is usually labeled "distal" by the manufacturer. If there is any confusion, inject a small amount of sterile saline through each hub until it is observed exiting the distal lumen. Once the distal hub is identified, remove its cover cap to allow passage of the guidewire. Place the catheter by threading the guidewire into the distal lumen and advancing it until it protrudes from the identified hub (see Fig. 22.9, *step 11*). It is imperative that the guidewire protrude from the catheter hub and that it be firmly grasped as the guidewire and catheter are advanced. If the wire does not protrude from the proximal end of the catheter, advance the guidewire backward through the catheter at the skin entry point until it protrudes enough to be grasped. While maintaining control of the guidewire proximally, advance the catheter forward into the vessel to the desired catheter insertion length (see Fig. 22.9, *step 12*). Ultrasonography can be used to verify proper catheter placement.[39,65] After insertion of the catheter, the wire must be removed (see Fig. 22.9, *step 13*) and the catheter must be anchored to the skin with sutures. When removing the wire from a catheter it must slip out easily. If any resistance is met, remove both the wire and the catheter as a single unit and reattempt the procedure. A common cause of a "stuck wire" is a small piece of adipose tissue wedged between the wire and the lumen of the catheter. Avoid this problem by creating a deep enough skin nick and adequate dilation of the tract before inserting the catheter. Making the skin incision first avoids this problem.

When placing a single-lumen, Desilets-Hoffman sheath–introducer system, the dilator and larger single-lumen catheter are inserted simultaneously as a dilator-sheath unit. The dilator-sheath unit must first be assembled by inserting the dilator through the catheter's diaphragm (Fig. 22.13, *step 2*). When assembled correctly, the dilator snaps into place within the lumen of the sheath and protrudes several centimeters from the distal end of the catheter.

After successful guidewire placement and after the skin incision is made, thread the dilator-sheath assembly over the wire (see Fig. 22.13, *step 3*). It is imperative that the guidewire protrude from the proximal end of the dilator-sheath assembly and that it be firmly grasped as the wire and unit is advanced. If the wire does not protrude from the proximal end of the assembly, advance the wire back through the dilator-sheath assembly at the skin entry point until it protrudes out of the port of the dilator enough to be grasped. While maintaining control of the guidewire proximally, advance the assembly through the skin with a twisting motion until it is within the vessel. Grasp the unit at the junction of the sheath and dilator. This prevents the thinner sheath from kinking or bending at the tip or from bunching up at the coupler end. Keep the assembly intact and advance it through the skin to the hub. Once the catheter is placed, remove the wire and dilator from the sheath simultaneously (see Fig. 22.13, *step 4*). When removing the wire and dilator, the dilator must "unsnap" from the sheath unit and the wire must slip out easily. Once the single-lumen sheath–introducer catheter is placed correctly, it may be used to facilitate the placement of additional intraluminal devices such as a pulmonary artery catheter, transvenous cardiac pacemaker, or an additional multiple-lumen catheter. At times, critically ill patients who require initial large-volume resuscitation will later require multiple medications and therapies that dictate the need for a multiple-lumen catheter. An alternative method of placing a multiple-lumen catheter is to thread the catheter through a standard Desilets-Hoffman sheath–introducer system.

It is important to consider the depth of insertion of the catheter. The proper depth of catheter insertion is site-specific when using the IJ or SV approach, and complications can arise if overinsertion occurs. The length of the catheter with the femoral approach does not commonly result in problems due to its distance from the myocardium. Traditionally, clinicians could use the Peres formula to estimate the catheter length needed based upon the patient's height. However, there are several studies that demonstrate the use of the Peres formula is inaccurate, especially in patients with increased body mass index, and can lead to overinsertion.[66–69] Therefore preprocedural landmark-based estimation and postprocedural imaging are the most accurate methods of accurately positioning the catheter tip.

After successful CVC placement, the catheter should be anchored to the skin with sutures (see Fig. 22.9, *step 15*). Each port should be immediately capped, checked again for patency by aspirating blood, and then flushed with a saline solution (see Fig. 22.9, *step 14*). The catheter insertion site should be dressed appropriately, and all sharp implements disposed of in appropriate receptacles (see Fig. 22.9, *step 16*).

Replacement of Existing Catheters

In addition to placing new catheters, clinicians may use the guidewire technique to exchange existing catheters. Many patients with CVCs are seriously ill and will require subsequent monitoring of pulmonary artery wedge pressure, placement of a transvenous pacemaker, or insertion of a different catheter. Initially, there were concerns about an increased incidence of bacteremia. However, there are several studies that

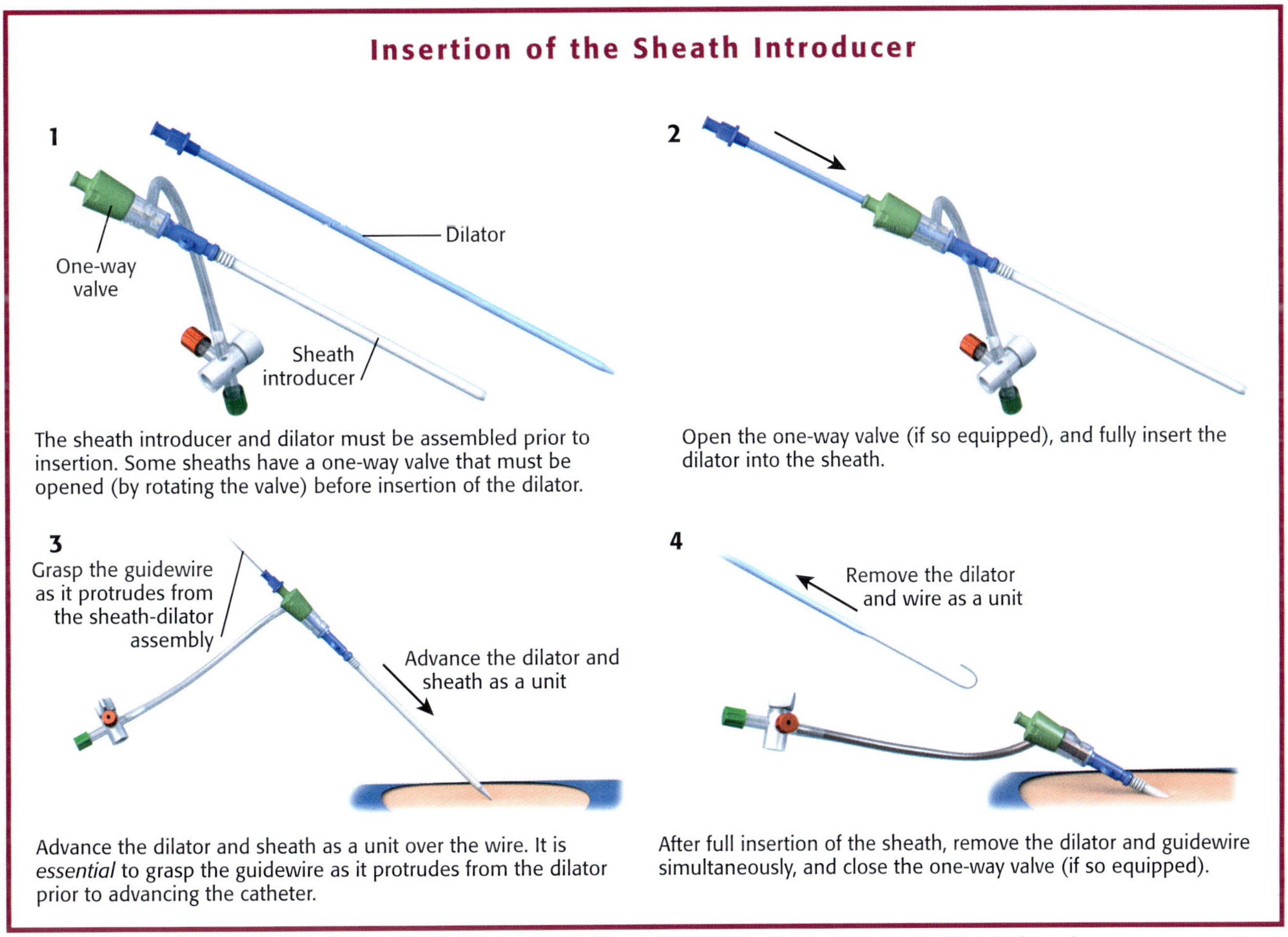

Fig. 22.13 Insertion of the sheath introducer. Insertion of a sheath introducer varies slightly from that for a triple-lumen catheter—the dilator and the catheter are inserted simultaneously, as depicted. The remainder of the steps are analogous to those in Fig. 22.9. Once inserted, sheath introducers facilitate the placement of devices such as pulmonary artery catheters and transvenous pacemakers.

show an equivocal rate of complications, including bacteremia, along with the additional benefit of saving other venous access sites and lack of a need to perform new venipuncture.[70–72] The CVC that is initially inserted should have a lumen large enough to accept a guidewire and facilitate conversion to a different catheter. Clinicians may use the guidewire technique to change a single-lumen CVC to a triple-lumen catheter or a sheath-introducer set. Not all commercially available CVCs will accept a guidewire.

Replacement of an existing catheter begins with selecting a guidewire longer than either of the devices to be exchanged. Use meticulous aseptic technique.[70–72] Insert the guidewire into the existing CVC until a few centimeters of wire protrudes from the proximal end. With one hand holding the wire securely, remove the catheter and wire as a single unit until the tip of the catheter just clears the patient's skin. Grasp the wire at the point where it exits the skin and only then release the wire at the other end. Then slide the catheter off the wire and insert the new device in the normal fashion. Exercise caution with this technique because catheter embolization can occur, especially if a catheter is cut to allow use of a shorter guidewire for the exchange.

Over-the-Needle Technique

An optional method for cannulation of a central vein is to place an over-the-needle catheter percutaneously. Over-the-needle devices (e.g., Angiocath, Becton Dickinson) use a tapered plastic catheter that passes through the vessel wall into the lumen, with the tip of the needle being used as a guide. There are advantages with this system. The catheter does not pass through a sharp needle and there is less risk of shearing and resultant catheter embolization. Additionally, the hole made by the needle in the vessel wall is smaller than the catheter, thus producing a tighter seal. Lastly, these procedures are quickly performed as the steps involving the guidewire are eliminated.[73] The IJ vein and SV via the supraclavicular approach are the most popular and appropriate approaches for this technique. These devices may be useful when rapid central venous access is required (e.g., in cardiac arrest). These catheters are not suitable for high-volume fluid resuscitation, and they are too small for passage of a pacemaker lead. Once the clinical situation stabilizes, exchange this device for a larger central catheter via the Seldinger technique, which is able to be performed through the catheter.[74]

Prepare the skin with chlorhexidine solution. Use a longer peripheral-type catheter (such as a 16-gauge, 5¼-inch angiocatheter) in an adult. Smaller-diameter devices, such as 20-gauge catheters, may be easier to pass but provide slower infusion rates. Attach the needle to a syringe and slowly advance it into the vein with steady negative pressure applied to the syringe. This may be difficult because of the longer length of the needle relative to the catheter. When using bedside ultrasound, follow the trajectory of the needle into the soft tissues and visualize penetration of the vessel. With over-the-needle catheters, the needle extends a few millimeters past the tip of the catheter. Return of blood will be obtained when the tip of the needle is in the vein, although the catheter may still remain outside the lumen. If the needle is withdrawn before the catheter is advanced, the tip of the catheter will remain outside the vein. It is therefore important to advance the needle a few millimeters after the venous flash is seen and then hold it steadily while advancing the catheter into the vein. Secure the catheter and verify its placement, as detailed later in this chapter.

SITE SELECTION

Subclavian Approaches

Subclavian venipuncture is the most frequently used means of achieving central venous access. The infraclavicular SV approach was the first popular means of central venous access and has been used widely for nearly half a century. It is useful in many clinical situations and relatively easy to learn. It is often the best approach in trauma because a cervical collar can interfere with the IJ technique. The supraclavicular SV approach may be preferable during CPR because it minimizes physical interference in chest compressions and airway management. In addition, the supraclavicular SV technique has been performed in the sitting position in patients with severe orthopnea. The SV route is associated with highest risk of pneumothorax. Historically, the SV route was associated with a decreased risk of CLABSI. However, studies are showing that the more experienced the provider and maintaining strict sterile technique equates to low rates of CLABSI and relatively similar rates of infection between the sites.[75–77] Finally, the left SV provides a more direct route to the SVC and is the preferred site for pacemaker placement.

IJ Approach

The IJ vein provides an excellent site for placement of a CVC. Historically, the IJ approach had the highest rate of complication compared to the SV or the FV approach. However, ultrasound and its common use in this approach has led to a significant decrease in complication rates that make it comparable to the other sites.[78,79] Despite its potential complications, the IJ vein is, in many cases, preferred over other options for central venous access. In contrast to the SV, arterial punctures are easier to control because direct pressure can be used, and the incidence of pneumothorax is lower. Hematoma formation is easier to diagnose because of the close proximity of the IJ vein to the skin. In addition, the right IJ vein provides a straight anatomic path to the SVC and right atrium. This is advantageous for passage of catheters or internal pacemaker wires to the heart. Disadvantages of IJ vein cannulation over other sites include a relatively high carotid artery puncture rate and poor landmarks in edematous patients or those with increased body mass index; however, these complications have largely decreased with the use of ultrasound.[79,80]

The IJ technique is useful for routine central venous access and for emergency venous access during CPR because the site is removed from the area of chest compressions. Catheter malposition is more frequent in the SV but can still occur in the IJ.[79,81–83] There is a decreased risk of pneumothorax with the IJ approach compared to the SV approach, but again, the risk is still present with the IJ approach, although very low.[79,84] Although there may be a slight difference in complications between the two routes, in the absence of specific contraindications clinicians should use the technique with which they are most familiar.

Femoral Approach

Historically, the FV approach was reserved for emergent access due to its association with higher rates of complications, specifically CLABSI. However, as stated before, that increased risk has been mostly negated with bundles and maintaining sterile technique.[76,77] The relatively simple and superficial anatomy surrounding the FV affords a rapid approach to the central venous system and avoids many of the more significant complications associated with cannulation of the IJ vein and the SV. Other indications for ED femoral cannulation include emergency cardiopulmonary bypass for resuscitation purposes, charcoal hemoperfusion for severe drug overdoses, and dialysis access. The femoral area is less congested with monitoring and airway equipment than the head and neck area, and conscious patients who are still bedridden may turn their head and use their arms more freely without moving the central line.

SPECIFIC VESSEL ACCESS TECHNIQUES

If SV or IJ vein approaches are planned, prepare the skin in the area, including puncture sites for both the infraclavicular and supraclavicular SV and IJ vein approaches. The most commonly used skin antiseptic is chlorhexidine gluconate (CHG). Importantly, CHG is applied back and forth over the area as opposed to betadine, which is applied in concentrically expanding circles. By prepping both sites, this permits the clinician to change the site after an unsuccessful attempt without repeating the preparation or having to obtain an interval chest radiograph. Prepare the area, including the ipsilateral anterior aspect of the neck, the supraclavicular fossa, and the anterior chest wall 3 cm to 5 cm past the midline and the same distance above the nipple line. Prepare for femoral access by applying chlorhexidine to cover an area the breadth of and extending 10 cm above and below the inguinal ligament.

Each approach to central venous cannulation is described separately in the following sections. As with any invasive procedure, briefly describe the procedure to awake patients, and restate each step as it is about to be performed. After descriptions of the common approaches to the central veins, puncture site care, verification of placement, and other adjuncts to the procedure are summarized.

Infraclavicular Subclavian Approach

Descriptions of subclavian venipuncture often focus unduly on angles and landmarks. Indeed, recent studies have demonstrated that some traditional positioning maneuvers may hinder successful cannulation efforts.

Positioning

Place the patient supine on the stretcher with the head in a neutral position and the arm adducted at the side. Some authors have advocated various shoulder-, back-, head-, and arm-positioning maneuvers, but they take extra time and the help of an assistant and are often not helpful.[85–88]

We believe that the best position for almost all infraclavicular SV attempts is the neutral shoulder position with the arm adducted.[86,87] Turning the head ipsilaterally has been shown to be helpful by increasing the cross-sectional area of the vessel in adults and children, but it is certainly not required if cervical injuries are suspected.[86,89,90]

Placing the patient in a moderate Trendelenburg position (10 to 20 degrees) decreases the risk for air embolism.[91] The claim that this position distends the vein is controversial, but it may do so to a small favorable degree.[86,92] If the Trendelenburg position is impractical, the SV approach is probably less affected than the IJ vein approach when resorting to a neutral or even an upright position.

Placing a pillow under the back is commonly recommended to make the clavicle more prominent, but as the shoulder falls backward, the space between the clavicle and the first rib narrows, thus making the SV less accessible. Therefore the use of a pillow is no longer recommended. Furthermore, significant compression of the subclavian vessels between these bony structures occurs as the shoulders retract, which can cause a "pinch off" of the catheter as it slides through the SV between the clavicle and the first rib. There are case reports of "pinch off syndrome" with some serious complications, including fracture and subsequent embolization of the catheter.[93–95]

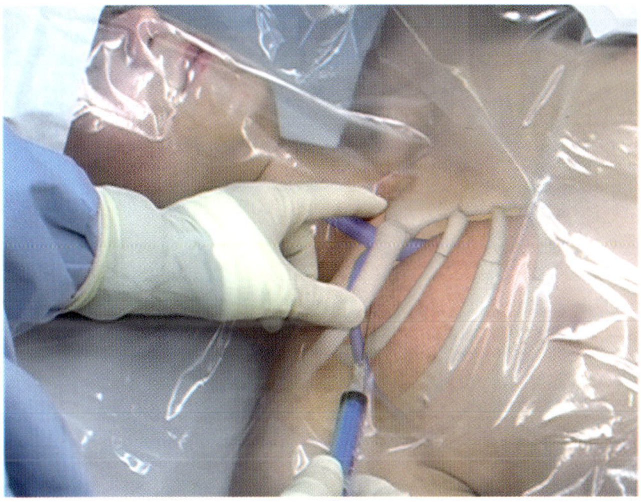

Fig. 22.14 Infraclavicular subclavian approach. Place your index finger in the suprasternal notch and your thumb at the costoclavicular junction; these landmarks will serve as reference points for the direction that the needle should travel. Orient the bevel of the needle inferomedially and aim the needle above and posterior to your index finger. Note: to avoid puncturing the lung or the subclavian artery, once the needle tip is under the clavicle keep the needle parallel to the clavicle, NOT directed posteriorly.

Venipuncture Site

The right SV is usually selected first because of the lower pleural dome on the right and the need to avoid the left-sided thoracic duct. The more direct route between the left SV and the SVC is a theoretical advantage of left-sided subclavian venipuncture; however, there is no higher incidence of catheter malposition when the right infraclavicular SV approach is used. In conscious patients, anesthetize the point of needle entry with 1% lidocaine. If possible, infiltrate the periosteum of the clavicle, found by touching the bone with the needle, to make the procedure less painful. Opinions vary regarding the best point of needle entry, more so than for the IJ or femoral approaches. The junction of the middle and medial thirds of the clavicle is the usual landmark for the SV approach. Inserting the needle 1 cm lateral to this landmark results in venipuncture because, further medially, the vein lies just posterior to the clavicle and above the first rib, which acts as a barrier to penetration of the pleura. This protective effect is theoretically diminished when a more lateral location is chosen. However, when approaching the vein more medially, some clinicians have difficulty puncturing the SV, dilating the tissues, and passing the J-wire. Other recommended sites of approach include lateral and inferior to the junction of the clavicle and the first rib, with the needle aimed at this junction, and entry at the site of a small tubercle in the medial aspect of the deltopectoral groove.

Needle Orientation

Orient the bevel of the needle inferomedially to direct the wire toward the innominate vein rather than toward the opposite vessel wall or up into the IJ vein. Align the bevel of the needle with the markings on the barrel of the syringe to permit awareness of bevel orientation after skin puncture.

Before inserting the needle, place your left index finger in the suprasternal notch and your thumb at the costoclavicular junction (Fig. 22.14). These landmarks serve as reference points for the direction that the needle should travel. Aim the needle immediately above and posterior to your index finger. Watch for vessel entry, signaled by flashback of dark venous blood, which usually occurs at a depth of 3 cm to 4 cm. If the tip of the needle is truly intraluminal, there will be free-flowing blood. Return of pulsatile flow signifies arterial puncture and the needle should be withdrawn immediately. A single arterial puncture without laceration rarely causes serious harm. Using this technique eliminates the need to measure angles, to "walk" the clavicle, or to concentrate excessively on maintaining the needle parallel to the chest wall. Avoid using sweeping motions of the tip of the needle to prevent unseen injuries.

Unsuccessful Attempts

Cannulation of the SV may not succeed on the first attempt. It is reasonable to try again, but, after three or four unsuccessful attempts, it is wise to move to a different anatomic approach or to allow a colleague to attempt the procedure. Use a new setup each time that blood is obtained because clots and tissue will clog the needle and mislead the clinician even if the vein has been entered successfully on subsequent attempts. If several attempts are made, inform the admitting clinician or anesthesiologist so that proper precautions are taken to identify subsequent complications. It is advisable to obtain radiographs of the chest even after unsuccessful attempts. If the initial puncture site was placed properly, use the same needle hole for subsequent attempts, if possible, for aesthetic reasons. If the SV route is unsuccessful on one side, attempt IJ vein catheterization on the same side rather than SV cannulation on the opposite side to avoid bilateral complications.

Supraclavicular Subclavian Approach

Positioning

The goal of the supraclavicular SV technique is to puncture the SV in its superior aspect as it joins the IJ vein. Insert the needle above and behind the clavicle, lateral to the clavicular head of the SCM muscle. Advance it in an avascular plane while directing it away from the SA and the dome of the pleura (Fig. 22.15). The right side is preferred because of the lower

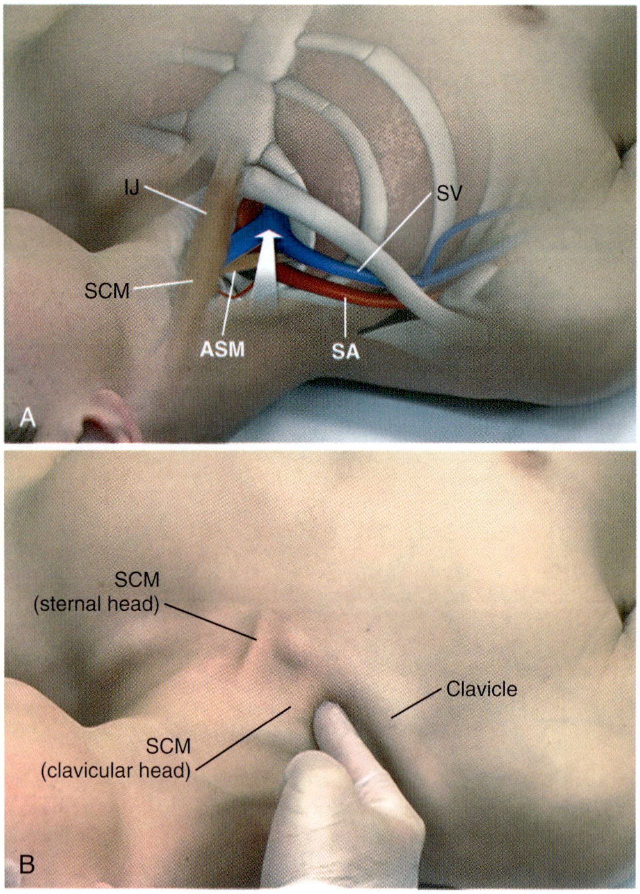

Fig. 22.15 Supraclavicular subclavian approach. (A) Anatomy. As the subclavian vein passes over the first rib, it is separated from the subclavian artery by the anterior scalene muscle. The dome of the pleura is posterolateral to the confluence of the great veins. (B) Approach. Insert the needle 1 cm posterior to the clavicle and 1 cm lateral to the clavicular head of the sternocleidomastoid muscle such that the angle made by the clavicle and lateral border of the muscle is bisected. The needle traverses an avascular plane and punctures the junction of the SV and IJ veins behind the sternoclavicular joint. The right side is preferred because of a direct route to the superior vena cava and absence of the thoracic duct. The needle is directed 45 degrees from the sagittal plane and 10 to 15 degrees upward from the horizontal plane and aimed toward the contralateral nipple. Note that the vein is just posterior to the clavicle at this juncture. *Arrow*, Needle target; *ASM*, anterior scalene muscle; *IJ*, internal jugular; *SA*, subclavian artery; *SCM*, sternocleidomastoid muscle; *SV*, subclavian vein.

pleural dome, its more direct route to the SVC, and location of the thoracic duct on the left side.

Needle Orientation

After the area of the supraclavicular fossa has been prepared and draped, identify a point 1 cm lateral to the clavicular head of the SCM and 1 cm posterior to the clavicle. Alternatively, use the junction of the middle and medial thirds of the clavicle as the landmark for needle entry. Anesthetize the area with 1% lidocaine. If a 3-cm-long needle is used for anesthesia, it may also be used to locate the vessel in a relatively atraumatic manner. The SV can almost always be located with this needle because of its superficial location and the absence of bony structures in the path of the needle. Advance a CVC kit needle along the path of the scout needle. Apply gentle negative pressure with an attached syringe.

When seeking the SV, aim the needle so that it bisects the clavicosternomastoid angle and the tip points just caudal to the contralateral nipple. Orient the bevel medially to prevent the catheter from getting trapped against the inferior vessel wall. Point the tip of the needle 10 degrees above the horizontal. Successful vessel puncture generally occurs at a depth of 2 cm to 3 cm.

Subclavian Ultrasound Technique

Typically, puncture of the SV occurs at the point where the vein is coursing deep to the clavicle and has been performed almost exclusively using a landmark-based approach. Approaches with ultrasound had proven difficult as visualization of the SV can be challenging at this location because of interference with the overlying bone. Consequently, the vein is more accessible to ultrasound the more lateral and further away from the clavicle it gets. Hence, access to the SV typically occurs lateral to the curve of the clavicle bone, in the proximal axillary vein. As the vein moves laterally, it becomes deeper and further away from the skin, with the mean depth from the skin increasing from 1.9 cm to 3.1 cm. Additionally, the distance from the rib cage to the vein increases from 1 cm to 2 cm. The arteriovenous distance also increases from 0.3 cm to 0.8 cm and there is less overlap of the artery and vein.[96] Because the vein is not in close proximity to the clavicle, if a hematoma develops, manual pressure can be used to stop the bleeding. Furthermore, the axillary vein is farther from the chest wall and pleural surface, thus decreasing the possibility of pleural injury and subsequent pneumothorax. In clinical studies, using the ultrasound for axillary vein cannulation has resulted in higher first-stick success rate, higher success rates, and decreased rates of pneumothorax.[97–100] Despite the use of ultrasound, however, the catheter malposition rate and the rate of arterial sticks was at least equivalent compared to the SV landmark-based approach.[97,98]

IJ Approach

Positioning

Position is critical for maximizing the success of cannulation of the IJ vein. Place the patient in a supine position with the head down and turned approximately 15 to 30 degrees away from the IJ vein to be cannulated. Rotate the head slightly away from the site of insertion. Rotating the head more than 40 degrees has been shown to increase the risk for overlapping the carotid artery over the IJ vein.[101,102] Occasionally, placing a towel roll under the scapula helps extend the neck and accentuate the landmarks. Stand at the head of the bed with all equipment within easy reach. This may involve moving the bed to the center of the room to allow a table or work surface to be placed at the head of the bed.

Ask the patient to perform a Valsalva maneuver just before inserting the needle to increase the diameter of the IJ vein. Alternatively, the patient can be asked to hum. Trendelenburg positioning, the Valsalva maneuver, and humming all increase the area of the vessel by approximately 30% to 50%.[103,104] If the patient is unable to cooperate, coordinate the insertion with respiration because the IJ vein is at its largest diameter just before inspiration. In intubated patients this relationship is reversed because mechanical ventilation increases intrathoracic pressure at end-inspiration.

Venipuncture Site

The right IJ vein provides a more direct route to the right atrium for transvenous pacing. The left IJ vein is often more tortuous, and catheters must negotiate two 90-degree turns at the junction of the left IJ vein with the SV and at the junction of the SV with the SVC. However, if the right IJ vein is obstructed or scarred by previous access, the left IJ vein may be accessed with the same technique. Of note, the right IJ vein has been observed to be larger than the left IJ vein in 72% of normal adults.[105] Therefore the R IJ is the preferred approach.

Aspirate before injecting anesthetic so that it is not injected into the carotid artery or IJ vein. Once infiltration is completed, use the needle to locate the IJ vein by aspirating blood into the syringe. Note the depth and angle of needle entry and use this as a mental guide to finding the IJ vein with the introducer needle. The operator may choose from three approaches: central, posterior, and anterior (Fig. 22.16).

Central Approach

This approach is favored by some who believe that the incidence of cannulation of the carotid artery is decreased.[105] It is also the approach used when utilizing ultrasound for insertion. First, palpate and identify the triangle formed by the clavicle and the sternal and clavicular heads of the SCM. Use a marking pen or a local anesthetic skin wheal to mark the lateral border of the carotid pulse and perform all subsequent needle punctures lateral to this point.

When using the scout needle technique, attach a 22-gauge, 3-cm needle to a 5- to 10-mL syringe. Insert the needle near the apex of the triangle and direct it caudally at an angle of 30 to 40 degrees to the skin. Direct the needle initially parallel and slightly lateral to the course of the carotid artery. Estimate the course of the IJ vein by placing three fingers lightly over the course of the carotid artery as it runs parallel to the vein, using the fingers as a guide for needle placement. The vein consistently lies just lateral to the carotid artery, albeit often minimally so. Prolonged deep palpation of the carotid artery may decrease the size of the vein, so use the three-finger technique lightly to identify the course of the artery.

Posterior and Anterior Approaches

The use of ultrasound has largely made these two approaches obsolete as ultrasound use has resulted in less complications. However, in the event an ultrasound is not available for use, knowledge of these two approaches gives the clinician an alternative approach to the more commonly used central approach.

In the posterior approach, make the puncture at the posterior (lateral) edge of the lateral or clavicular head of the SCM, approximately midway between its origin at the mastoid process and its insertion at the clavicle. The external jugular vein courses in this area and can be used as a landmark, with the puncture occurring where the external jugular vein crosses the posterolateral border of the SCM. Be careful to not strike the external jugular vein. Advance the needle toward the suprasternal notch, just under the belly of the SCM, at an angle of approximately 45 degrees to the transverse plane. During advancement of the needle, apply pressure to the SCM, as if attempting to lift the body of the muscle. The vein is usually reached at a depth of 7 cm in an average-sized adult. Because the posterior approach occurs higher in the neck, there is less risk for hemothorax, pneumothorax, or carotid puncture.[106]

In the anterior approach, needle puncture occurs along the anterior or medial edge of the SCM approximately two to three fingerbreadths above the clavicle. Insert the needle at an angle of 30 to 45 degrees toward the ipsilateral nipple, away from the carotid pulse. If cannulation is unsuccessful, withdraw the needle to the skin and redirect it slightly toward the carotid artery. The anterior approach is associated with increased risk of pneumothorax and inadvertent carotid puncture.

Once the approach is chosen, slowly advance the needle toward the IJ vein. Create gentle negative pressure with the syringe while advancing the needle. Once blood is seen, stop advancing the syringe. Remove the syringe from the needle to determine whether the vessel is pulsatile. Be careful not to allow negative intrapleural pressure to draw air into the venous system through the open needle. Because the tip of the introducer needle is beveled, lateral motions of the needle tip may cause lacerations of the deep structures of the neck. It is therefore very important to remove the needle from the neck completely before any redirection of the needle.

Once cannulation of the IJ vein has been confirmed, remove the syringe from the needle and place a gloved digit over the needle hub to prevent air embolism. Insert a guidewire through the needle into the IJ vein and place the catheter using the Seldinger technique. Once the wire is inserted into the IJ vein, reduce the angle to the skin to make the needle nearly parallel to the vein. This allows a greater chance of directing the wire toward the heart. Do not let the guidewire extend into the right atrium. The average distance from the insertion site to the junction of the SVC and right atrium is 16 ± 2 cm for the right IJ vein and 19 ± 2 cm for the left IJ vein. The spring wires supplied in kits are often much longer, up to 60 cm in length. If the full length of the wire is inserted, the wire could enter the right atrium or ventricle and cause myocardial irritability and subsequent dysrhythmias. Monitor cardiac rhythm during insertion of the spring wire to detect cardiac irritability. The distance that the catheter is introduced depends on the distance from the site of introduction to the junction of the SVC and right atrium. This distance will be shorter with the right IJ vein than with the left IJ vein.

IJ Ultrasound Technique

Cannulation of the IJ vein is an optimal location for the use of ultrasound guidance. There is adequate access to visualize the vein but also other important structures, especially the carotid artery. Even with novice users of ultrasound for IJ vein cannulation, first-attempt success is significantly increased when compared to the blind landmark technique.[40,107] Use of ultrasound for placement of central lines in the IJ vein has also been shown to decrease overall catheter placement failures, reduce complications, and decrease the need for multiple catheter placement attempts in comparison to the standard landmark placement technique.[4,37,98] The primary reason for the increased success rate is the variation in anatomy of the IJ vein relative to the carotid artery. The anatomy of the IJ vein has been shown to be aberrant in a small number of cases.[4,108] Furthermore, the IJ vein may be unusually small (i.e., <0.5 cm) in a minority of patients. The IJ vein is thrombosed in up to 8% of some patient populations and preprocedural screening with ultrasound was shown to decrease the number of attempts.[109,110]

With the use of ultrasound there is no need for reliance on normal anatomy for cannulation. Therefore the IJ vein may

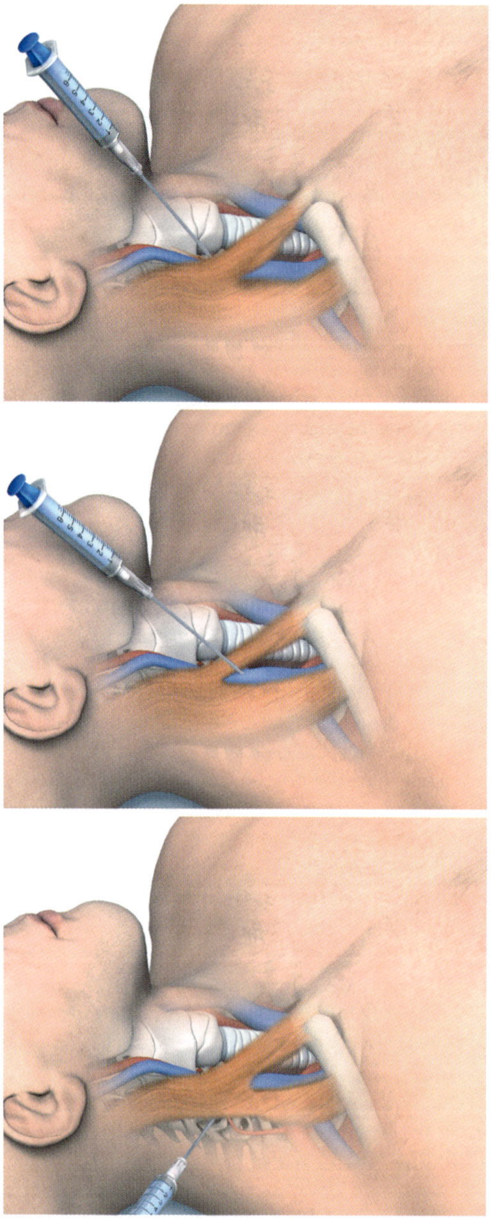

Fig. 22.16 Approaches to the internal jugular vein. *IJ*, Internal jugular; *SCM*, sternocleidomastoid.

be cannulated despite abnormal anatomy. Hence, cannulation may occur at the apex of the triangle, near the base at the junction with the innominate vein, or anywhere in between.

Femoral Approach

Positioning and Needle Orientation

Place the patient in the supine position for the FV approach. This approach does not require any special positioning or tilting of the bed. Fully expose and thoroughly cleanse the area with a soapy washcloth or surgical scrub brush to remove obvious soiling, which may be more common at this site. Next, prepare the skin at the site broadly with chlorhexidine, including the anterior superior iliac spine laterally and superiorly, extending to the midline, and continuing 10 to 15 cm below the inguinal ligament. If the patient has a urethral catheter, tape it to the contralateral leg. In a patient with an increased body mass index, have an assistant retract the abdominal pannus manually or secure it with wide tape.

After the instillation of local anesthetic, introduce the needle at a 45-degree angle in a cephalic direction approximately 1 cm medial to this point and toward the umbilicus (Fig. 22.17). Palpate the femoral pulse two fingerbreadths beneath the inguinal ligament. Note that while palpating the artery, pressure from the operator's fingers can compress the adjacent vein and impede cannulation. Avoid this anatomic distortion by releasing digital pressure while keeping the fingers on the skin to serve as a visual reference to the underlying anatomy. The depth of the needle required to reach the vein varies with body habitus, but in thin adults, the vein is quite superficial and is usually reached at a depth of approximately 2 to 3 cm, so advance the needle slowly. Return of dark, nonpulsatile blood signals successful venous penetration.

Although using the femoral arterial pulse as a guide is ideal, it may not be palpable in a hypotensive patient or one with an increased body mass index.

A more detailed understanding of the femoral landmarks can be used to guide cannulation attempts. On all but the

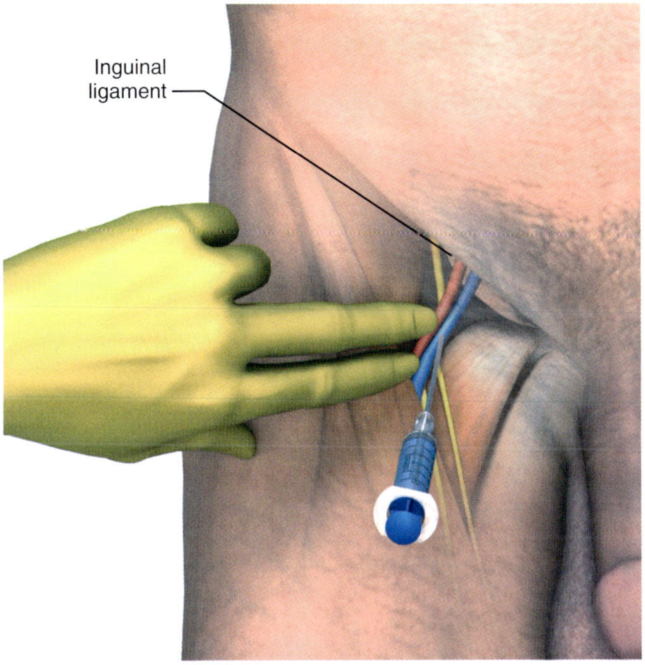

Fig. 22.17 Femoral approach. Palpate the femoral artery two fingerbreadths beneath the inguinal ligament. Keep the fingers on the artery to aid the femoral vein cannulation and to avoid the femoral artery. Introduce the needle at a 45-degree angle in a cephalic direction 1 cm medial to this point and toward the umbilicus. Importantly, more distally the vein lies over the artery, so place the catheter near the inguinal ligament, or use ultrasound guidance.

most severely injured trauma patients with a disrupted pelvis (in which case a femoral approach would be contraindicated), the anterior superior iliac spine and the midpoint of the pubic symphysis are easily palpated. The line between these two bony references describes the inguinal ligament. When this line is divided into thirds, the femoral artery should underlie the junction of the medial and middle thirds. The FV will lie approximately one fingerbreadth medial to this point. Alternatively, the vascular anatomy of the region can be evaluated, and the line placed via ultrasound guidance.

Venipuncture

During advancement of the needle, always maintain gentle negative pressure on the syringe while the needle is under the skin. Direct the needle posteriorly and advance it until the vein is entered, as identified by a flash of dark, nonpulsatile blood. If the vessel is penetrated when the syringe is not being aspirated, the flash of blood may be seen only as the needle is being withdrawn. The FV lies just medial to the femoral artery at the level of the inguinal ligament. It is closer to the artery than many clinicians appreciate. As the vein progresses distally in the leg, it runs closer to and almost behind the femoral artery.

Femoral Ultrasound Technique

Cannulation of the FV under ultrasound guidance is very similar to that for the IJ vein. Using ultrasound is associated with decreased complications and faster success rates compared to landmark-based approaches.[40,41] Using ultrasound, the common FV, its junction with the saphenous vein, and the branches of the common FV (i.e., the superficial and deep FVs) are easily identified. Additionally, other structures surrounding the vein are easily identifiable, especially the femoral artery and FV. Typically, placement of the catheter should occur proximal to the bifurcation of the common FV and preferably proximal to the junction with the saphenous vein.

ANCHORING THE CENTRAL LINE

After the CVC is placed, it will need to be anchored in place by one of three techniques: StatLock (Bard Medical), suture, or staple (Fig. 22.18). The StatLock may not hold well in patients with oily skin but is excellent for older patients with thin skin. For suturing, one will need the sterile, nonabsorbable suture material (usually 2-0 silk) provided in the CVC kit. The straight suture needles found in many sets are awkward for many clinicians, so a curved needle with a driver may be helpful. To avoid a needlestick with the straight needle, pass the blunt end of the needle through the anchoring devices and pull the suture forward manually. Place the suture in the skin approximately a half centimeter from the catheter to anchor the central line in place. Several knots should be made to secure the line. Avoid making knots that place excessive pressure on the skin because this can lead to difficulty removing the knots and necrosis. Loose knots can lead to migration of the catheter and loss of access. Stapling a central line into place can be just as effective as suturing; however, the staples tend to fall out after a few days.

Dressing

Clean the area around the catheter insertion site with chlorhexidine, and then use a clear dressing (e.g., Tegaderm, 3M) to cover up the insertion site of the catheter once secured (see Fig. 22.9, *step 16*). Apply a chlorhexidine patch (Biopatch, Ethicon) at the site where the catheter enters the skin (see Fig. 22.18E–F). Tegaderm also makes a CHG IV securement dressing that eliminates the need for the patch as it has a chlorhexidine gel on the underside of the adhesive dressing. Because dressings are inspected and changed periodically, place a simple dressing and avoid excessive amounts of gauze and tape. Take care to protect the skin against maceration.

Assessing Line Placement

See Video 22.13. Check all tubing and connections for tightness to prevent air embolism, loss of fluid, or bleeding. Before infusing IV fluids, lower the IV fluid reservoir to below the level of the patient's right atrium and check the line for backflow of blood. Free backflow of blood is suggestive but not diagnostic of intravascular placement. Backflow could occur from a hematoma or hemothorax if the catheter is free in the pleural space. A pulsatile blood column may be noted if the catheter has been inadvertently placed in an artery. Less pronounced pulsations might also occur if the catheter is advanced too far and reaches the right atrium or ventricle. In addition, pulsations may be noted with changes in intrathoracic pressure as a result of respirations, although these pulsations should occur at a much slower rate than the arterial pulse. A transducer can be applied to the CVC to determine if the catheter lies in the artery or vein. A final method of checking intravascular placement is to attach a syringe directly to the catheter hub and aspirate venous blood. It is also advisable to ensure that the catheter is easily flushed with a saline solution. This carries the additional benefit of removing air

ULTRASOUND: Central Venous Catheterization

by Christine Butts, MD

IJ Vein

When evaluating the IJ vein, the transducer (7.5 to 20 MHz) should be initially placed over the right or left side of the neck to evaluate the anatomy. An ideal initial location to begin is at the apex of the triangle formed by the two heads of the subclavian muscle (Fig. 22.US1). Placing the transducer over this area in the transverse orientation will enable the vessels to be located in cross section, where they can best be evaluated. The internal carotid artery and IJ vein will be seen as paired structures with anechoic central areas (Fig. 22.US2). The position of one relative to the other can be variable, but typically the IJ vein lies lateral and superficial to the carotid artery. Several characteristics of the IJ vein serve to distinguish it from the carotid artery. The IJ vein is typically more oval in shape, or even triangular, versus the rounded shape of the carotid artery, is thinner walled, and will compress with gentle pressure. Additionally, the size of the IJ vein will change with respiration and should be seen to increase in size with a Valsalva maneuver.

Complications can be reduced by several methods. First, ensure that the target vessel is indeed the vein and not the artery. Variant anatomy or variations in volume status (either depletion or overload) may make the vessels difficult to distinguish from one another. Confirmation should be attempted by noting multiple characteristics of the vessel (compressibility, shape, anatomic location, etc.). Once the vessel has been confirmed as the vein, the operator must take great care to ensure that the position of the tip of the needle is apparent at all times. Most complications occur when the tip of the needle is deeper or more medial than the operator realizes, thus placing it in proximity to other structures (e.g., lung, carotid artery). An extensive discussion of each approach can be found in the basic ultrasound chapter (see Chapter 66), and each approach has its drawbacks in determining position. In the transverse method, the angle of approach can be difficult to ascertain and cause the tip of the needle to be deeper than the operator realizes. Additionally, the tip of the needle may be difficult to follow. In the longitudinal approach, the medial to lateral orientation of the needle can be difficult to appreciate. Additionally, slight movements of the transducer may result in loss of the appropriate image. A combination of these two, or an oblique approach, may minimize these difficulties.

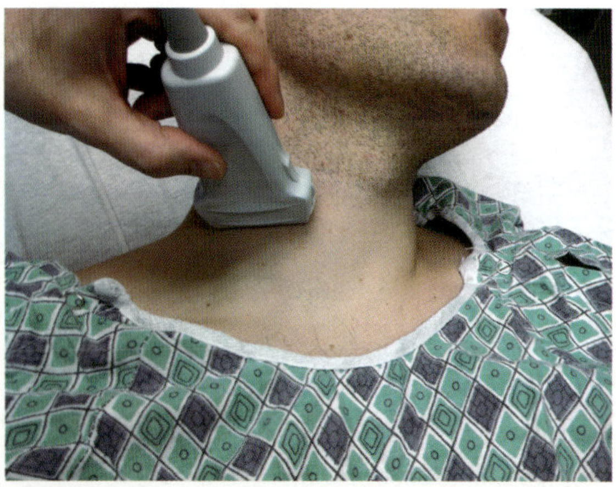

Fig. 22.US1 Placement of the ultrasound transducer at the apex of the triangle formed by the heads of the sternocleidomastoid.

Femoral Vein

The femoral artery and vein lie together with the femoral nerve within a common sheath. They can be found at the level of the inguinal crease on the medial aspect of the thigh. Palpating the femoral pulse will also aid in localizing the vascular bundle. The transducer (7.5 to 10 MHz) should be placed in a transverse or slightly oblique orientation overlying this area. Slightly rotating the thigh externally may facilitate this step. Classically, the artery is described to lie lateral to the vein. However, this is often not the case and multiple variations may be noted. The femoral artery and vein will appear as rounded anechoic structures (Fig. 22.US3). The FV can be recognized by

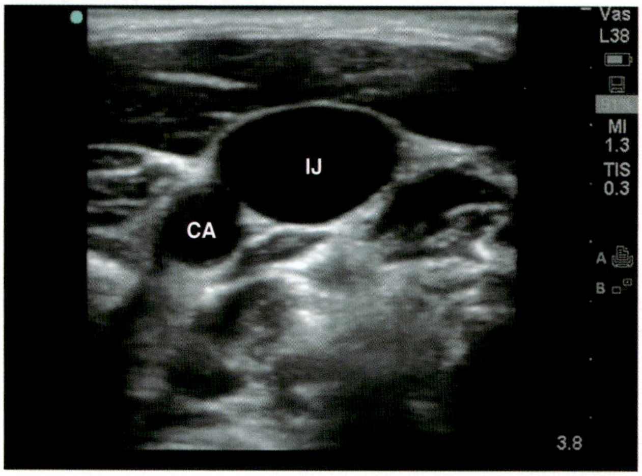

Fig. 22.US2 Transverse image of the carotid artery and internal jugular *(IJ)* vein. The IJ vein can be recognized by its oval or triangular shape and its thinner walls, and it will collapse with light pressure. Although both are rounded and contain anechoic *(black)* fluid, the IJ vein is slightly larger and more oval in shape. Though not evident in this image, slight pressure will cause collapse of the IJ vein. *CA*, Carotid artery.

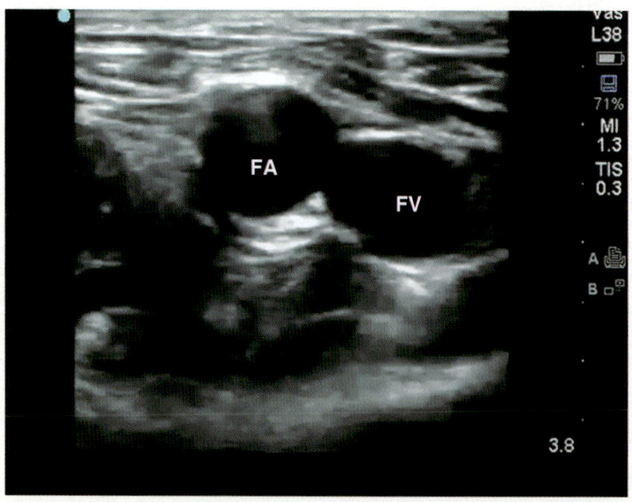

Fig. 22.US3 Transverse image of the femoral artery and femoral vein. Similar to vessels in the neck, the femoral vein is more oval or triangular in shape. Though not evident in this image, slight pressure will cause collapse of the vessel. *FA*, Femoral artery; *FV*, femoral vein.

Continued

ULTRASOUND: Central Venous Catheterization—cont'd

its thinner walls and slightly more oval shape, and it will collapse with gentle pressure. It will also typically increase in size when the lower part of the leg is squeezed. The vascular bundle may need to be followed inferiorly or superiorly to determine the most optimal location for puncture.

Complications can be reduced by several methods. First, ensure that the target vessel is indeed the vein and not the artery. Variant anatomy or variations in volume status (either depletion or overload) may make the vessels difficult to distinguish from one another. Confirmation should be attempted by noting multiple characteristics of the vessel (compressibility, shape, anatomic location, etc.). Once the vessel has been confirmed as the vein, the operator must take great care to ensure that the position of the tip of the needle is apparent at all times. The tip of the needle may be difficult to follow in the transverse approach and result in an inadvertent puncture of the posterior wall of the vessel. When the artery lies deep to the vein, arterial puncture or cannulation may result. In the longitudinal approach, the medial to lateral position of the needle may be difficult to appreciate and result in accidental arterial puncture. The oblique approach may minimize these difficulties.

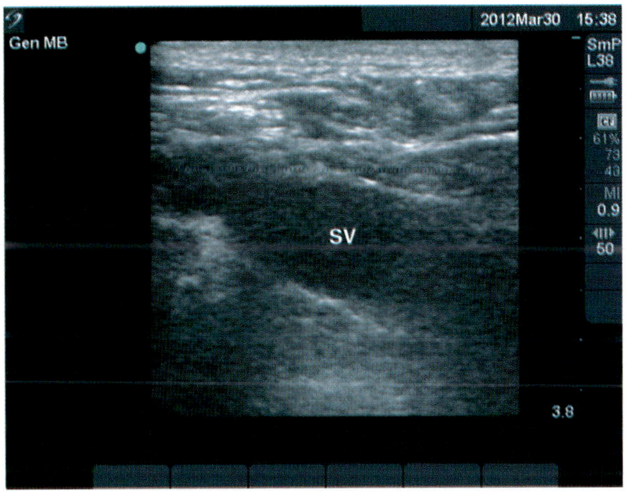

Fig. 22.US5 Long-axis view of the subclavian vein. The subclavian artery, not seen in this image, will be seen as a similar-appearing vessel deep to the vein. Color flow and Doppler can be used to distinguish between the two vessels. *SV,* Subclavian vein.

Subclavian Vein

The subclavian vessels can be imaged from either a supraclavicular or an infraclavicular approach. For the supraclavicular approach, the transducer (7.5 to 10 MHz) is placed along the long axis of the clavicle on the superior aspect (Fig. 22.US4). It should be angled downward. In this view, the vessels should be seen in their long axis (Fig. 22.US5). The vein can be identified by its variation with respiration and change in size with the Valsalva maneuver. The vein can also be followed to identify the junction with the IJ vein, thereby offering further confirmation. In the infraclavicular approach, the transducer is placed beneath the clavicle at its most lateral aspect, in a sagittal or slightly oblique orientation, following the position of the clavicle (Fig. 22.US6). In this view, the vessels will be seen in cross section or a slightly oblique plane (Fig. 22.US7). The pleura may also be seen deep to the vessels as an echogenic vertical line that slides back and forth with respiration.

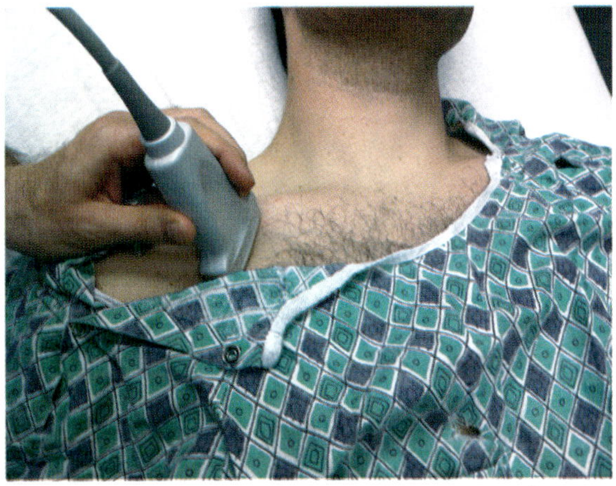

Fig. 22.US6 Placement of the ultrasound transducer inferior to the clavicle to enable visualization of the subclavian vessels in short axis. A sagittal (shown) or slightly oblique orientation should be used.

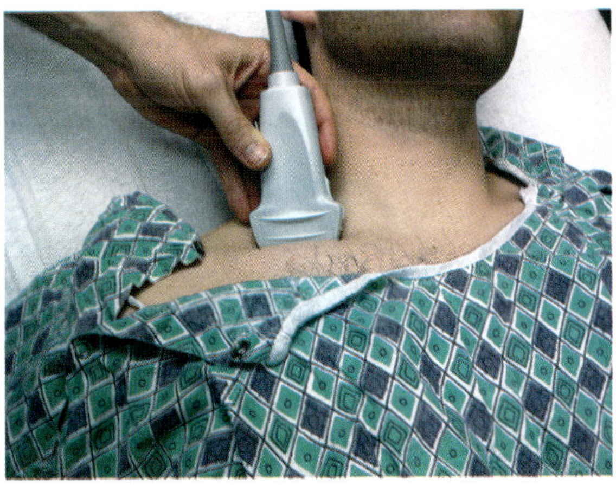

Fig. 22.US4 Placement of the ultrasound transducer superior to the clavicle to enable visualization of the subclavian vessels in the long axis.

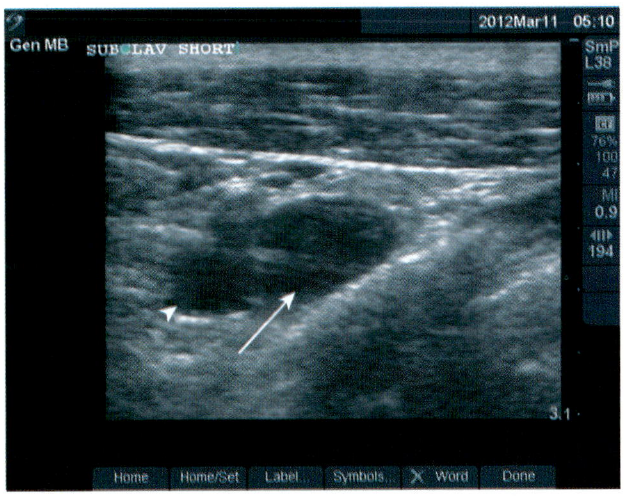

Fig. 22.US7 Short-axis view of the subclavian artery *(arrowhead)* and vein *(arrow)* as seen from the inferior aspect of the clavicle.

ULTRASOUND: Central Venous Catheterization—cont'd

A longitudinal approach should be used in which the needle is introduced from the end of the transducer in either the infraclavicular or the supraclavicular approaches. This will enable a shallow angle to be used and thereby minimize the chance of damaging deeper structures such as the lung. Once a flash of blood has been obtained, the ultrasound transducer can be set aside, and the procedure continued as described previously.

The SA and SV lie in close opposition to the pleura, so pneumothorax is a more common complication. Using a long-axis approach (in which the needle is introduced from the end of the transducer rather than from the middle) offers the advantage of visualizing the entirety of the needle in its course toward the vein. A shallow angle can be used, and the relationship of the needle to the pleura can also be appreciated.

Securing a Central Venous Catheter

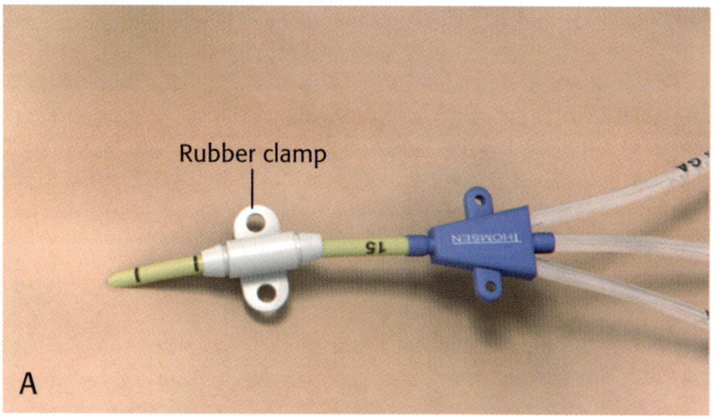

A white rubber clamp is provided to secure the catheter when the full length is not needed. Twist open the pliable clamp and place it over the catheter at a site a few centimeters from the insertion site.

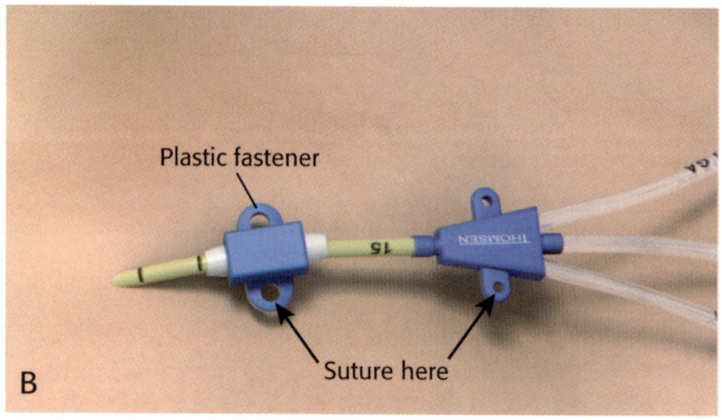

The rubber clamp is covered with a blue plastic fastener, and both the clamp and fastener are sutured to the skin to secure the catheter. The hub of the catheter is also sutured to the skin.

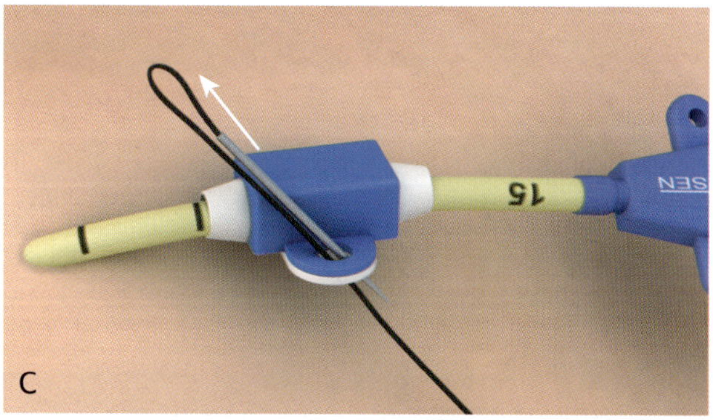

To avoid a needlestick, the blunt end of the needle is used to pass the suture through the holes of the fastening devices.

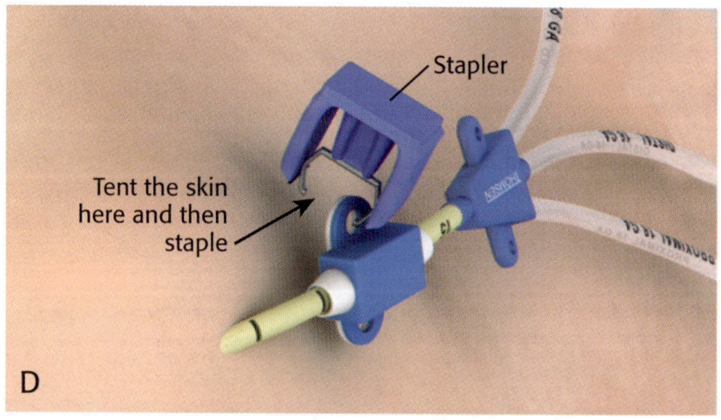

Alternatively, skin staples may be used. Tent the skin and pass the staples through the anchoring eyes.

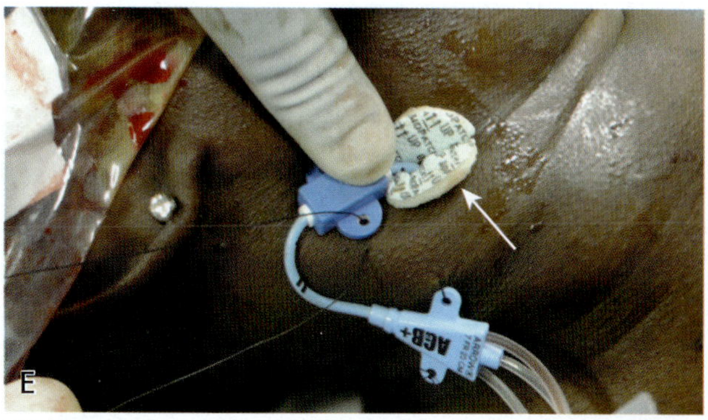

This Biopatch is a chlorhexidine-containing hydrophilic covering placed at the site where the catheter enters the skin to deliver local antisepsis for 7 days.

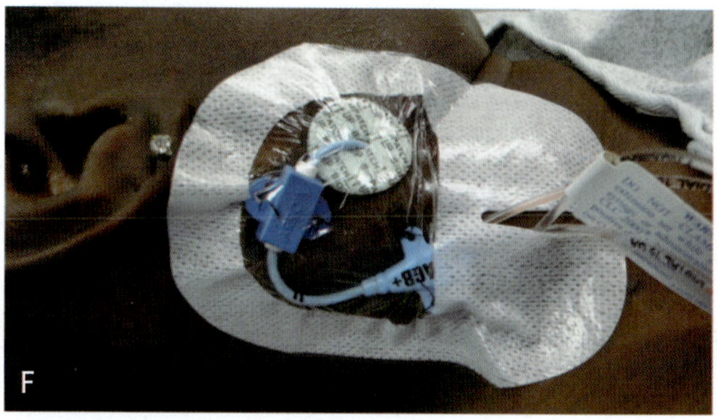

A simple Tegaderm clear covering is then applied.

Fig. 22.18 Methods to secure a central venous triple-lumen catheter.

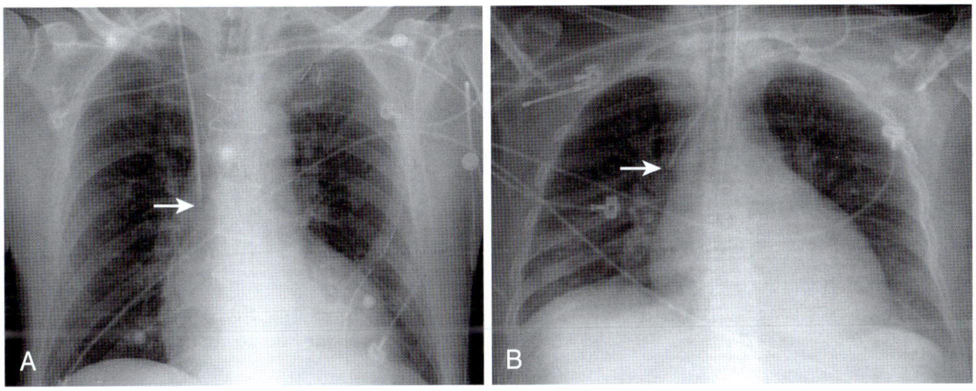

Fig. 22.19 Chest radiographs obtained after placement of (A) right internal jugular central venous catheter and (B) left subclavian central venous catheter. The tips of the catheters are appropriately placed in the superior vena cava *(arrows)*. The tip should not lie within the right atrium or the right ventricle.

from the system. Radiographs are also always indicated to verify catheter location and assess for potential complications, except after routine femoral line placements.

Imaging

Following placement of lines involving puncture of the neck or thorax, listen to the lungs to detect any inequality of lung sounds suggestive of a pneumothorax or hemothorax. Obtain a chest film as soon as possible to check for hemothorax, pneumothorax, and the position of the tip of the catheter (Fig. 22.19). Because small amounts of fluid or air may layer out parallel to the radiographic plate with the patient in the supine position, take the film in the upright or semi-upright position whenever possible. In ill patients, a rotated or oblique projection on a chest radiograph may be obtained, and the clinician may be confused about the proper position of the catheter. In such cases, repeat the radiograph. A misplaced catheter tip is usually obvious on a properly positioned standard posteroanterior chest radiograph (Fig. 22.20), but occasionally, injection of contrast material may be required. For example, a catheter in one of the internal thoracic veins may simply appear more lateral than expected, but because of the close proximity of these veins and the SVC, malposition may not be appreciated by this subtle finding. Misplaced catheters should be repositioned or replaced. Attention should also be given to the possibility of a retained guidewire. Although this complication is rare, if not specifically considered it can be overlooked by both clinicians and radiologists.[111,112]

Routine postprocedure radiographs are commonly used to evaluate placement of the catheter to ensure it is in correct position. However, there is also literature that ultrasound is an acceptable alternative for confirmation of placement and ruling out clinically relevant complications so as to not delay utilizing the catheter while waiting for radiographs to be obtained.[39,65] The operator can visualize the catheter in the vessel with ultrasound as well as evaluate for pneumothorax by looking in the lung windows for ultrasonographic signs of pneumothorax. Additionally, the operator can confirm relative placement by evaluating the right atrium and ventricle with an apical four-chamber view and either visualizing the catheter tip or injecting saline through the central port and looking for bubbles in the ventricle.[65]

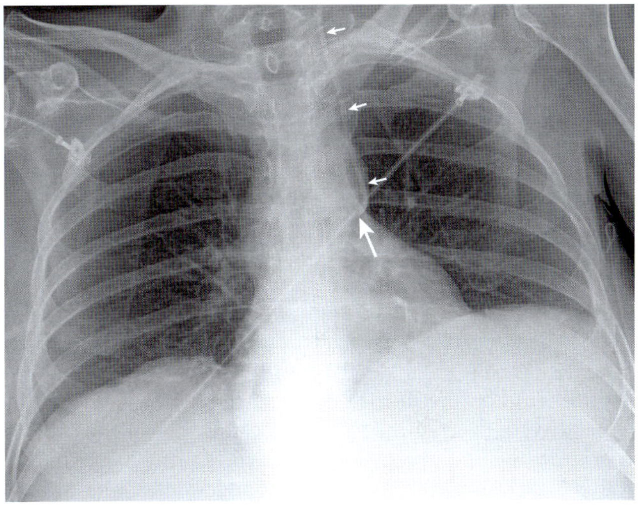

Fig. 22.20 Chest radiograph obtained after left internal jugular catheterization. Note that the course of the catheter *(small arrows)* does not cross the midline and that the tip *(large arrow)* projects to the left of the midline near the aortic arch. Although the catheter may have been located intravascularly in a venous anatomic variant, it was decided to remove this line and replace it with a new catheter.

SPECIAL CONSIDERATIONS FOR OTHER VESSELS

External Jugular Vein Approach

Central venous catheterization via the external jugular vein is time consuming and often difficult. The difficulty in converting an external jugular catheter into a CVC frequently renders it a lower-yield clinical procedure. Use of the external jugular vein for achieving central venous access requires that a guidewire be used. After cannulation of the vein and intraluminal placement of the guidewire, advance the guidewire into the thorax by rotating and manipulating the tip into the central venous circulation. Advancement of the guidewire is the most difficult and time-consuming portion of the procedure, and the time requirement limits the usefulness of this technique in an emergency. A small-radius J-tipped wire, a distended vessel lumen, and exaggeration of patient head tilt, coupled with skin traction, may facilitate successful passage of the guidewire. Partially withdrawing the wire and twisting it 180 degrees before readvancing the tip may also be helpful.

Basilic and Cephalic Approaches

Passing a catheter into the central circulation is difficult via the basilic and cephalic routes, and failure is common. Insertion of a peripheral IV central catheter (PICC) through these routes is often performed by specialized teams and is less suitable for emergency indications. The cephalic vein may terminate inches above the antecubital fossa or bifurcate before entering the axillary vein and send a branch to the external jugular vein. The cephalic vein may also enter the axillary vein at a right angle, thereby defeating any attempt to pass the catheter centrally. Furthermore, both the basilic and the cephalic systems contain valves that may impede catheterization. A flexible catheter is introduced into the basilic vein until the tip is judged to be proximal to the junction of the cephalic and basilic veins and distal to the junction of the IJ vein with the innominate vein. The wire stylet is withdrawn 18 cm, and the catheter is advanced slowly 1 cm at a time, with 2 seconds allowed between each 1-cm insertion. The natural flexibility of Bard catheters contributed to negotiation into the SVC when the patient was upright. This time-consuming technique is contraindicated when the patient cannot tolerate an upright position.

The basilic and cephalic venous systems are entered through the large veins in the antecubital fossa. Placement of a tourniquet aids venous distention and initial venous puncture. When veins are not visible, they may be identified with bedside ultrasound (as described in Chapter 66). The basilic vein, located on the medial aspect of the antecubital fossa, is generally larger than the radially located cephalic vein. Furthermore, the basilic vein usually provides a more direct route for passage into the axillary vein, SV, and SVC.

A much more useful technique is the use of a midline. Midlines are peripherally inserted into the basilic or cephalic vein and the tip of the catheter ends in the axillary vein. They are anywhere between 8 cm and 25 cm long and can be single- or double-lumened. While not technically a central line, it is associated with decreased bloodstream infection rates compared with PICC lines and is a fast and easily accessible line that can be used in lieu of a central line with less risk of complications.[113,114]

Vascular Access in Cardiac Arrest

Immediate vascular access is required for resuscitation during cardiac arrest. Intraosseous access is a reasonable alternative to central venous access as flow rates and medication delivery are adequate. Femoral CVCs are often used in this setting. The infraclavicular SV approach is also commonly used during cardiac arrest if logistics permit. The intuitive rationale for femoral CVC placement has been that much of the resuscitation activity, including chest compressions, occurs on the thorax, thus limiting the clinician's ability to safely place a higher line. Blind femoral central line insertions during arrest are less than optimal. Blood flow across the abdomen in an adult in cardiac arrest can limit the utility of medication administration from femoral catheters. The increasingly available intraosseous placement systems and bedside ultrasonography are commonly used to supplant such blind CVC placements during cardiac arrest and other emergencies that require immediate vascular access.

CVP Measurement

See Video 22.14. CVP measurement has been used as a guide for determination of volume status, fluid requirements, and investigation of tamponade, although its reliability has never been clearly established.[114a–114d] Advancements in our knowledge of complex hemodynamics (particularly during sepsis) and improvements in noninvasive dynamic imaging (ultrasound) have largely supplanted CVP monitoring in the critical care environment.[114e–114f]

Physiology

CVP values are determined by a complex interaction of intravascular volume, right atrial and ventricular function, venomotor tone, and intrathoracic pressures.[114a,114f] To measure CVP, the tip of a pressure-monitoring catheter is inserted into any of the great systemic veins of the thorax or into the right atrium.[114d,114g,114h] The catheter may be connected to a simple manometer or to an electronic pressure transducer (Figs. 22.21 and 22.22). Electronic transducers may be connected to monitors in the same format as arterial pressure lines or through self-contained autocalibrating transducers. If using a manometer, the zero point of the manometer should be at the level of the right ventricle. The same position should be used for the electronic transducer. CVP measurements only reflect the physiology of the right side of the vasculature. To measure left-sided pressures a pulmonary capillary wedge pressure (PCWP) is required.

In spontaneously breathing patients, readings should be taken at the end of a normal inspiration. If the patient is receiving positive pressure ventilation, the changes in CVP during the respiratory cycle are reversed and readings are recorded at the end of expiration.

Readings should be taken only after accurate placement of the catheter tip has been established. To ensure optimal measurement, place the patient in the supine position. Whenever the patient is repositioned, take care to ensure that the transducer has been recalibrated to reflect the new position of the patient.

Since the observed value of the CVP is of limited value, it is the delta in these measurements that is most useful in the management of a critically ill patient. The changes that occur in response to fluid administration or blood losses or those following administration of medications are more useful than individual static readings. Interpret the specific CVP values with respect to the entire clinical picture remembering that the changes in the CVP are more important than the initial reading.

Interpretation of CVP Measurement

Ranges of normal CVP measurements:

- Low: <6 cm H_2O
- Normal: 6 to 12 cm H_2O
- High: >12 cm H_2O

In the late stages of pregnancy (30 to 42 weeks), the CVP is physiologically elevated, and normal readings are 5 cm H_2O to 8 cm H_2O higher. A CVP reading of less than 6 cm H_2O is consistent with low right atrial pressure and reflects a decrease in the return of blood volume to the right heart. This may

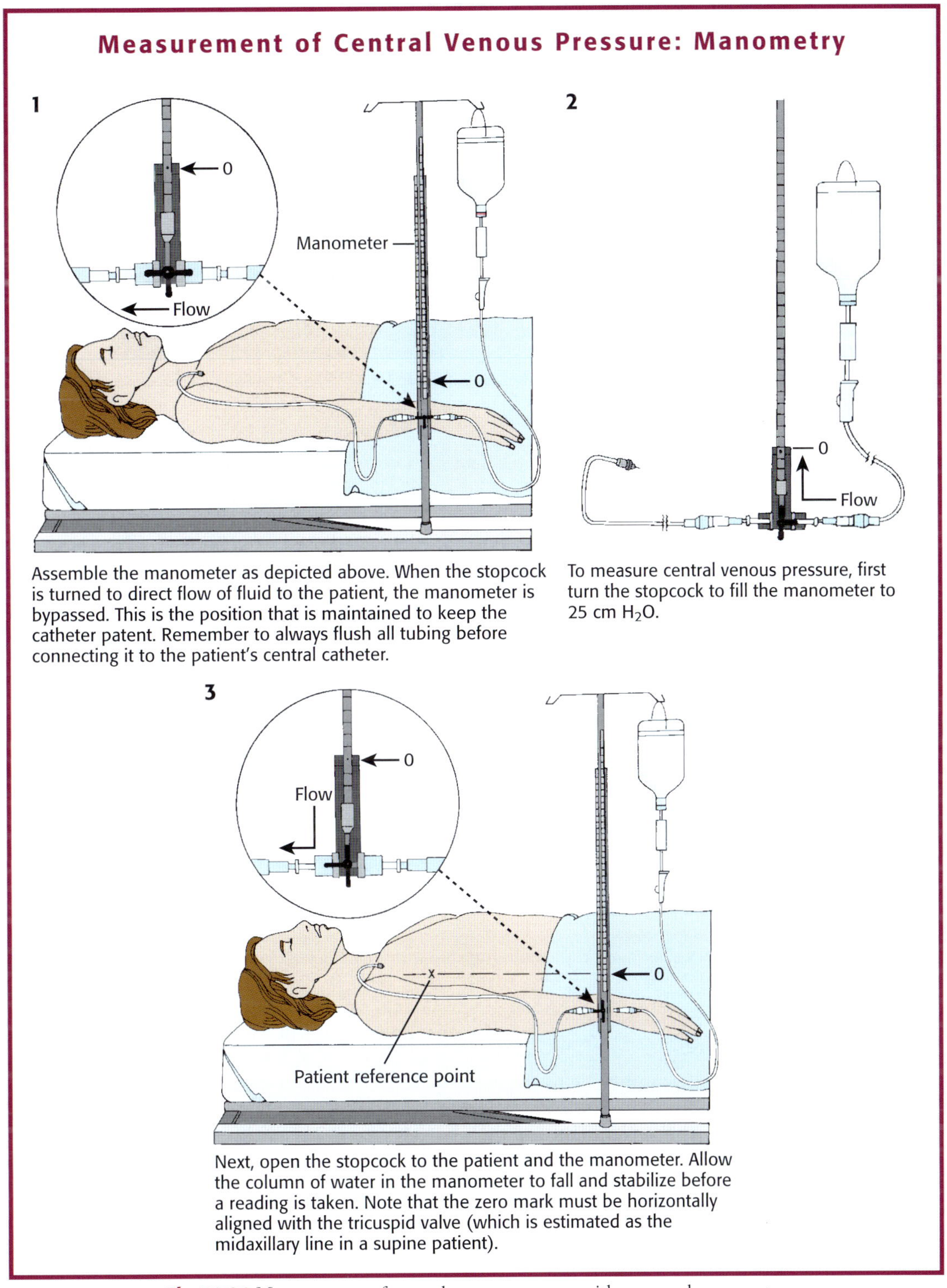

Fig. 22.21 Measurement of central venous pressure with a manual manometer.

indicate that the patient requires additional fluid or blood. A low CVP reading is also obtained when vasomotor tone is decreased, as with sepsis, spinal cord injury, or other forms of sympathetic interruption.

A CVP reading falling within a normal range must be viewed in relation to the clinical scenario. A reading higher than 12 cm H_2O indicates that the heart is not effectively circulating the volume presented to it. This may occur in a normovolemic patient with underlying cardiac disease, such as left ventricular hypertrophy (with associated poor ventricular compliance), or in a volume-overloaded patient with a normal heart. High CVP can also be related to variables other than pump failure, such as pericardial tamponade, restrictive pericarditis, pulmonary stenosis, tricuspid regurgitation, pulmonary hypertension, and pulmonary embolism.[124]

Changes in blood volume, vessel tone, and cardiac function may occur alone or in combination with one another; therefore it is possible to have a normal or elevated CVP in the presence of normovolemia, hypovolemia, and hypervolemia.[114d,114h]

Measurement of Central Venous Pressure: Transducer

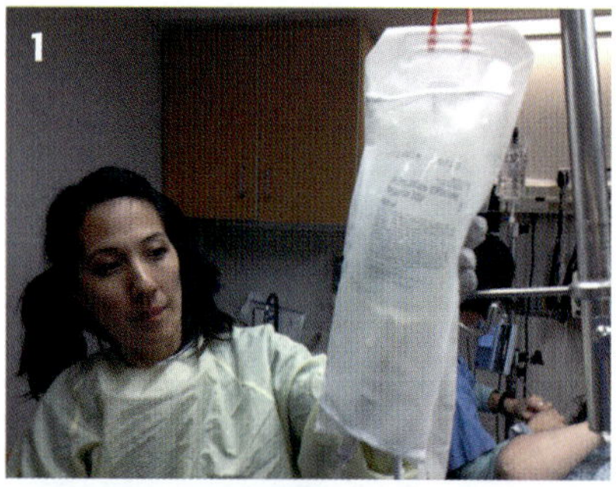

Insert a bag of normal saline into a pressure bag and inflate to the recommended pressure (usually 300 mm Hg).

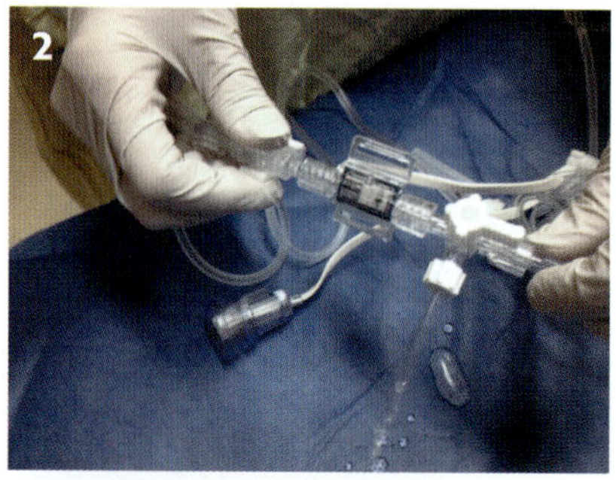

Flush all air bubbles from the system by opening the stopcock and running saline through the line. Any air left in the system will cause erroneous central venous pressure readings. Take care to not flush air into the patient.

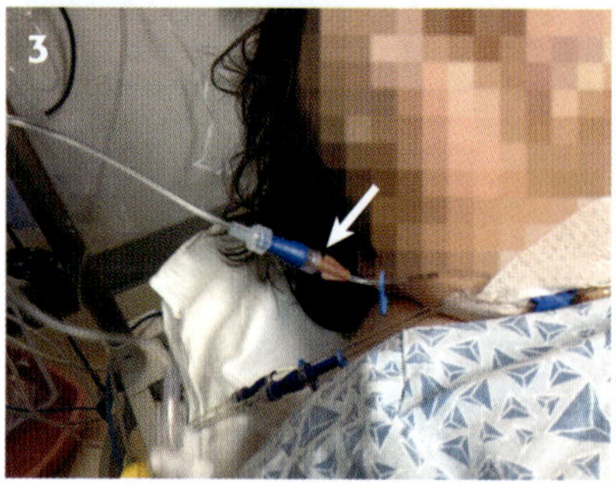

Connect the flushed transducer tubing to the patient's central line *(arrow).*

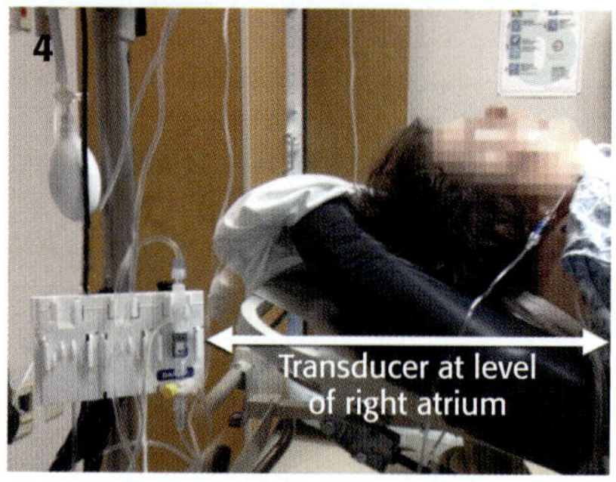

Mount the transducer at the level of the patient's right atrium. This level can be approximated on the skin surface as a point at the midaxillary line and fourth intercostal space.

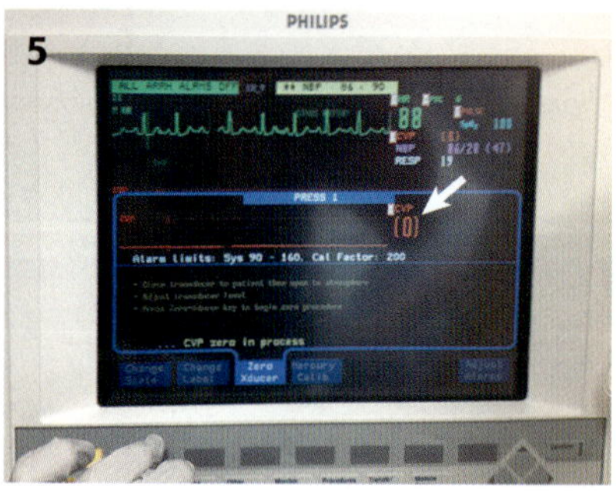

Adjust the stopcock so that the transducer is open to air, and zero the system *(arrow)*. The exact process for the zeroing procedure will vary by the equipment manufacturer.

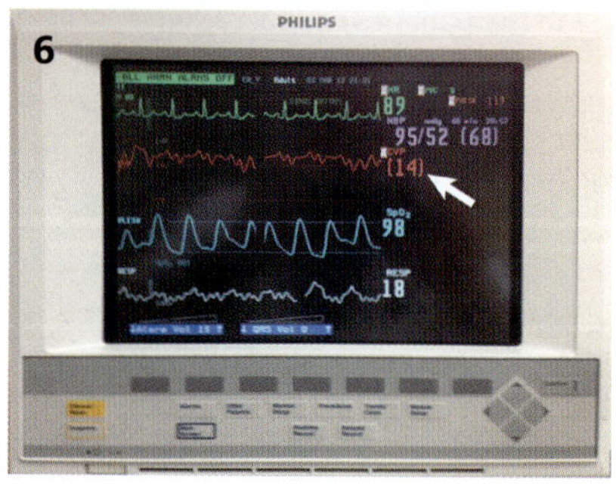

Finally, set the stopcock so that it is open to the transducer and the central venous catheter. Observe for a venous waveform and central venous pressure reading on the monitor *(arrow).*

Fig. 22.22 Measurement of central venous pressure with a traditional electronic transducer.

Fluid Challenge

Monitoring CVP may be helpful as a practical guide to fluid therapy.[114a,114h-114k] Serial CVP measurements provide a fairly reliable indication of the capability of the right side of the heart to accept an additional fluid load. Although PCWP is a more sensitive index of left heart's fluid needs, repeated measurements of CVP can nonetheless provide useful information.

A fluid challenge can help assess both volume deficits and pump failure.[114k] Generally, fluid boluses of 250 to 500 mL of crystalloid are administered sequentially and CVP is measured 10 minutes after each bolus. Repeat the fluid challenge until measurements indicate that adequate volume expansion has occurred. Discontinue the fluid challenge as soon as hemodynamic signs of shock are reversed or signs of cardiac incompetence are evident.

Cardiac Tamponade

In cardiac tamponade, pericardial pressure rises to equal right ventricular end-diastolic pressure. The pericardial pressure encountered in pericardial tamponade characteristically produces an elevated CVP.[114c] The degree of elevation in CVP is variable, and one must interpret measurements cautiously; CVP readings in the range of 16 to 18 cm H_2O are typically seen with acute tamponade, but elevations of up to 30 cm H_2O may be encountered. The precise CVP reading is often lower than one might intuitively expect, and it is not uncommon to encounter tamponade with a CVP of 10 to 12 cm H_2O. A normal or even low CVP reading may be seen if the tamponade is associated with significant hypovolemia. An excessive rise in CVP after fluid challenge may be more important than a single reading in the diagnosis of pericardial tamponade. Additionally, physician-operated point-of-care ultrasound has proven to be exceptionally sensitive for visualizing tamponade physiology when pericardial pressures have begun to impair right ventricular filling.[114l]

Excessive straining, positive pressure ventilation, agitation, inflation of pneumatic antishock garments, and tension pneumothorax may all increase intrathoracic pressure, produce a high CVP reading, and erroneously suggest the diagnosis of pericardial tamponade.

BOX 22.1 Complications of Central Venous Access

GENERAL

Mechanical

Puncture of an adjacent artery
Hematoma formation
Air embolus
Pneumothorax
Pericardial tamponade
Catheter embolus
Arteriovenous fistula
Mural thrombus formation
Large-vein obstruction
Dysrhythmias
Catheter knotting
Catheter malposition

Infectious

Bloodstream infection
Generalized sepsis
Septic arthritis
Osteomyelitis
Cellulitis at the insertion site

Thrombotic

Pulmonary embolism
Venous thrombosis

SV AND IJ APPROACHES

Pulmonary

Pneumothorax
Hemothorax
Hydrothorax
Chylothorax
Neck hematoma and tracheal obstruction
Endotracheal cuff perforation
Tracheal perforation

Neurologic

Phrenic nerve injury
Brachial plexus injury
Cerebral infarct

FEMORAL APPROACH

Intraabdominal

Bowel perforation
Psoas abscess
Bladder perforation

IJ, *Internal jugular;* SV, *subclavian vein.*

COMPLICATIONS

The medical literature is replete with reports of CVC complications. Understanding the pathophysiology surrounding CVC complications helps clinicians anticipate, recognize, and manage complications should they arise and better educate patients and their families during the informed consent process.

More than 15% of patients who receive CVCs experience some type of complication, and complications occur despite pristine technique.[59,78] This percentage is not surprising in view of the close proximity of vital structures, the complexity of patients' medical conditions, and the exigent circumstances under which many of these procedures are often performed. Common complications and the different approaches are summarized in Box 22.1 and can generally be categorized as mechanical, infectious, and thrombotic. Key complications and injuries by approach are discussed in the following sections.

One retrospective review of all central catheters placed in a hospital (SV, IJ, and FV lines) reported a mechanical complication rate of 5.9% per CVC placed.[78] Complications were defined as pneumothorax, hematoma, line misplacement, hemothorax, or any duration-limited issue with the CVC (including infection or thrombosis) that required an inpatient consultation. In general, failure and complication rates increase as the number of percutaneous punctures increases. Historically, operator skill and experience have reliably predicted complication or success rates.[59] It has previously been reported that clinicians who have placed more than 50 CVCs have less than half the complication rates of those who have fewer than 50 attempts.[59]

Published complication rates vary in the literature and can now be classified according to whether ultrasound guidance was used during the procedure (Table 22.3).[37] Studies have demonstrated that ultrasound-guided CVC placement techniques have improved success rates, reduced complication rates, and decreased time needed to perform the procedure.[29,30,37] As a result, ultrasound guidance for CVC placement is recommended by the US Department of Health and Human Services as well as professional medical societies. Reports by the Agency for Healthcare Research and Quality (AHRQ) list ultrasound guidance for central vein cannulation as one of its most highly rated and most evidence-based safety practices.[126]

Mechanical Complications

Redirection of Misplaced Catheters

Improper catheter tip position occurs commonly. It has been reported that only 71% of SV catheters are located in the SVC on the initial chest film. Complications of improper positioning include hydrothorax, hemothorax, ascites, chest wall abscess, embolization to the pleural space, and chest pain. More commonly, improper location is associated with poor flow caused by kinking. An unusual complication attributable to improper tip position is cerebral infarction, which can occur following inadvertent cannulation of the SA.

Misdirection or inappropriate positioning of the tip of a CVC, when promptly recognized and corrected, is an inconsequential complication. Loop formation, lodging in small neck veins, tips directed caudally, and innominate vein position are common problems. Reposition misplaced catheters as soon as logistically possible. If the catheter is being used for fluid resuscitation, the malposition may be tolerated for some time. If vasopressors or medications are infused, proper positioning of the tip of the catheter is more critical. Several options are available to remedy malpositioning. One strategy is to insert a 2-Fr Fogarty catheter through the lumen of the central line and advance it 3 cm beyond the tip. Withdraw the entire assembly until only the Fogarty catheter is in the vein. Inject 1 mL of air into the balloon and advance the Fogarty catheter. It is hoped that blood flow will direct the assembly into the SVC. Deflate the balloon and advance the central line over the Fogarty catheter, which is then withdrawn.

Another anecdotal strategy is to withdraw the catheter until only the distal tip remains in the cannulated vessel. This measurement is best appreciated by comparing the length of the indwelling catheter with another unused catheter. The clinician then simply readvances the catheter in the hope that it becomes properly positioned. Other manipulations with guidewires have been suggested, but reinsertion with another puncture is often required for the misplaced catheter to be positioned properly. This approach also decreases the risk for infection by avoiding the introduction of bacteria into the vessel from any nonsterile segment of the CVC.

TABLE 22.3 Frequency of Mechanical Complications With and Without Ultrasound Guidance

	Without Ultrasound			With Ultrasound		
COMPLICATION	IJ	SV	FEMORAL	IJ	SV	FEMORAL
Arterial puncture	6.3%–10.6%	3.1%–14%	9.0%–15.0%	1.6%	2%	1.8%
Hematoma	<0.1%–8.4%	1.2%–2.1%	3.8%–7.2%	0.4%	0%	3.6%
Hemothorax	1.7%	0.4%–0.6%	NA	0%	NA	NA
Pneumothorax	<0.1%–2.4%	1.5%–3.1%	NA	0%	0%	NA

IJ, Internal jugular; *NA*, not applicable; *SV*, subclavian vein.
Data from references 28, 31, 40, and 62.

Arterial Puncture and Hematoma

The most commonly reported mechanical complications, especially with IJ and FV approaches, are arterial puncture and hematoma. Inadvertent arterial puncture and hematoma formation are usually easily recognized and controlled with simple compression. Rarely, an artery is lacerated to such an extent that bleeding is significant and operative repair is necessary. Even more rare but also more ominous is when the artery is either dilated and/or is cannulated with the catheter. These often result in significant morbidity and mortality with some patients requiring operative repair, some experiencing strokes, and some resulting in death.[127] In cases where the artery was dilated or cannulated with the catheter, a vascular surgeon should be consulted for management. The optimal situation when arterial puncture occurs is to recognize it *before* dilation with the tissue dilator. In cardiac arrest, low-flow, or shock states, arterial puncture may not be obvious, and arterial cannulation and intraarterial infusions have occurred. When systolic blood pressure rises, arterial pulsations become more obvious. In critically ill patients, however, this complication may escape detection for some time. It has been reported that ultrasound-guided placement of IJ CVCs decreases the rate of arterial puncture to as low as 0.1%.[37,79] Additionally, ultrasound was found to decrease the incidence of clinically significant hematoma formation as well.[40]

Although central venous access procedures may be performed safely in patients with bleeding disorders without antecedent correction of the coagulopathy, caution is strongly urged. Areas amenable to arterial compression (i.e., IJ or FV) are preferred in these patients. Studies have shown that although there is increased bleeding risk, there are no significant differences between clinically significant bleeding in patients with coagulopathy compared to those without coagulopathy nor does prophylactic use of fresh frozen plasma confer any additional benefit.[128,129] Similarly, patients who were found to be thrombocytopenic were not associated with increased bleeding risk and prophylactic platelet transfusions were not found to confer any benefit.[27] The majority of thrombocytopenic and coagulopathic patients who experience bleeding complications are limited to oozing around the insertion site and hematoma formation. Most bleeding complications can be managed with direct compression and, if that fails, a small suture to staunch bleeding, taking care not to puncture the catheter when placing the suture.

Pneumothorax and Other Thoracic Mechanical Complications

Pneumothorax occurs in up to 6% of subclavian venipunctures and can also occur with the IJ approach (Fig. 22.23A).[59] Clinical clues of a possible pneumothorax include aspiration of air when inserting the needle, complaints of chest pain or shortness of breath, or clinical signs of hemodynamic instability that suddenly occur while performing the procedure. Initially, the importance of this complication was minimized, but reports of fatalities caused by tension pneumothorax, bilateral pneumothoraces, and combined hemopneumothorax followed.[115] One would expect a higher incidence of pneumothorax if the procedure is performed during CPR or positive pressure ventilation. A small pneumothorax can quickly become a life-threatening tension pneumothorax with positive pressure ventilation. Treatment of a catheter-induced pneumothorax is controversial, but not all patients will require formal tube thoracostomy. Some authors have reported that many stable outpatients exhibiting a pneumothorax after insertion of a CVC can be managed successfully by observation alone (60% in one series) or catheter (pigtail/Heimlich valve) aspiration, with large tube thoracostomy being reserved for refractory cases or emergency settings.[116] Critically ill patients or those undergoing mechanical ventilation are more likely to require invasive treatment for a catheter-induced pneumothorax.

Hemothorax may occur after laceration of the SV or SA, puncture of the pulmonary artery, or intrathoracic infusion of blood (see Fig. 22.23B). Hydrothorax occurs as a result of infusion of IV fluid through the catheter into the pleural space. Hydromediastinum is also possible. These are rarely serious complications, but fatalities have been reported. Surgical repair is occasionally required. Arteriovenous fistula formation has also been reported.[117] Additional pulmonary complications include esophageal, tracheal, and endotracheal cuff perforation.[118]

Air Embolism

Air embolism is a very rare, but potentially life-threatening complication of central venous cannulation. Undoubtedly, minor and clinically inconsequential amounts of air enter the venous circulation during many cannulation procedures. Maintaining constant occlusion (with the operator's finger) on all needles that are located in central veins can minimize this occurrence. A 14-gauge needle can transmit 100 mL of air per second with a 5 cm H_2O pressure difference across the

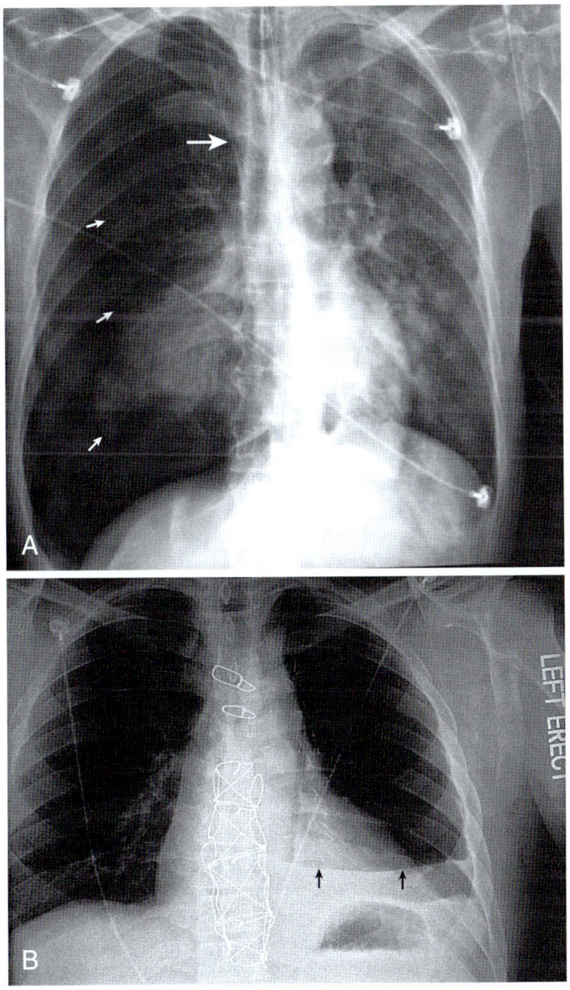

Fig. 22.23 Pneumothorax and hemothorax. A chest radiograph should be taken routinely to assess the position of a central venous catheter introduced via the subclavian or internal jugular route. This confirms placement of the catheter. Chest radiography can also show potential complications of the procedure. (A) Large right pneumothorax after right internal jugular catheterization. The catheter is still in place *(large arrow)*, and the absence of lung markings on the right and the pleural reflection *(small arrows)* are readily apparent. (B) Left hydropneumothorax after left subclavian venipuncture (the catheter was removed before this radiograph). Note the straight line of fluid (air-fluid level, *black arrows*) and no meniscus, indicating that a pneumothorax must also be present. The edge of the partially collapsed lung is difficult to appreciate. No clinician can place central venous catheters and fail to have at least some complications that are inherent to the procedure, regardless of even flawless technique.

needle.[91] Air embolism may occur if the line is open to air during catheterization or if it subsequently becomes disconnected. The recommended treatment is to place the patient in the left lateral decubitus position to relieve air bubble occlusion of the right ventricular outflow tract.[91] If this is unsuccessful, aspiration with the catheter advanced into the right ventricle has been advocated.[91] Emergency thoracotomy to aspirate air (see Chapter 18) and cardiothoracic surgical consultation may also be warranted.

Guidewire Complications

Retained guidewires and guidewire embolizations are another mechanical complication. Most retained guidewires are discovered on postprocedure radiographs after the procedure is completed. There is a positive association with guidewire retention and lack of experience according to one study in the UK, with 88% of cases with a retained guidewire being performed by trainee doctors.[119] These events are reported as sentinel events with a lot of hospitals moving toward putting initiatives in place to prevent this complication. One of the easiest methods to prevent this complication is to never let go of the wire when placing the CVC. The most common step when the guidewire is lost is upon placing the catheter over the guidewire and threading the catheter into the vein, often forgetting to feed the guidewire retrograde to grab the guidewire on the other side. Remembering to always hold on to the guidewire until the catheter is in place will often avoid any retained guidewires. Additionally, being sure to remember the number of guidewires used (in cases of guidewire malfunction) will also help prevent this complication.

Catheter or wire embolization resulting from shearing of a through-the-needle catheter by the tip of the needle is a serious and generally avoidable complication. Embolization can occur when the catheter or wire is withdrawn through the needle or if the guard is not properly secured. Adverse events after embolization include arrhythmias, venous thrombosis, endocarditis, myocardial perforation, and pulmonary embolism.[62,95] Transvenous retrieval techniques by interventional radiology are usually attempted, followed by open surgery if unsuccessful.[62,93,94] Entire guidewires may also embolize to the general circulation if the tip is not constantly secured by the operator throughout the procedure. Initiatives by national safety bodies such as the National Quality Forum in the United States have focused on reducing the incidence of retained wires by classifying them as "never" events that require mandatory reporting in many states.

Placement Complications

Delayed perforation of the myocardium is rare, but it can be a fatal complication of central venous catheterization by any route.[120,121] The presumed mechanism is prolonged contact of the rigid catheter with the beating myocardium. The catheter perforates the myocardial wall and causes tamponade either by bleeding from the involved chamber or by infusion of IV fluid into the pericardium. The right atrium is involved more commonly than the right ventricle.[120] All clinicians who insert such catheters or care for such patients should be aware of this deadly complication, which results in profound deterioration with hypotension, shortness of breath, and shock. Emergency echocardiography, pericardiocentesis, and operative intervention by a thoracic surgeon may all be required for salvage of the patient. This can also occur with misplacement of the CVC in the pericardiophrenic vein.[122,123] Fortunately, this complication is preventable by using a postinsertion chest film to confirm the position of the tip of the catheter and retracting the catheter if the tip is within the cardiac silhouette.

Catheter knotting or kinking may occur if the catheter is forced or repositioned or if an excessively long catheter is used.[51,124] The most common result of kinking is poor flow of IV fluids, although rare complications from thrombosis to as severe as SVC obstruction have been seen.

Neurologic complications are extremely rare and presumably caused by direct trauma from the needle during venipuncture or hyperosmolar medications being infused around

Central Venous Pressure Measurement

Indications

Acute circulatory failure
Anticipated massive blood transfusion or fluid replacement therapy
Cautious fluid replacement in patients with compromised cardiovascular status
Suspected cardiac tamponade
Fluid resuscitation during goal-directed therapy for severe sepsis

Contraindications

Other resuscitative interventions that take priority over central venous access and central venous pressure setup
Large vegetations on the tricuspid valve
Superior vena cava syndrome
Right atrial tumor or thrombus

Complications

Faulty central venous pressure readings:
- Increased intrathoracic pressure (ventilator, straining, coughing)
- Failure to calibrate or zero the transducer
- Malposition of the tip of the catheter
- Obstruction of the catheter
- Air bubbles in the circuit
- Readings during the wrong phase of ventilation
- Vasopressors (presumed)

Equipment

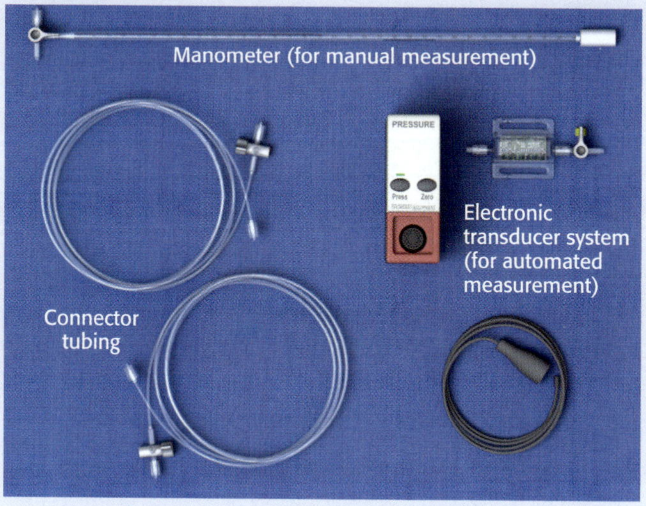

Review Box 22.2 Central venous pressure measurement: indications, contraindications, complications, and equipment.

the nerves. Brachial plexus palsy and phrenic nerve injury with paralysis of the hemidiaphragm have been reported.[125,130] Malposition can lead to thrombosis or infusion of hypertonic medications into the IJ vein which may result in a variety of neurologic complications from retrograde perfusion of intracranial vessels.[131] Again, this complication can be easily avoided by inspecting a postprocedure radiograph to confirm proper placement prior to utilization of a newly placed catheter.

Infectious Complications

Infectious complications can range from local cellulitis to frank bacteremia and can progress further to septic emboli. The incidence of infectious complications varies from 0% to 25% and is associated with higher hospital costs.[132] The frequency with which infectious complications occur is directly related to the attention given to aseptic technique during insertion and aftercare of the catheter. Femoral venous catheterization was thought to carry a greater risk for infection than subclavian catheterization. However, more recent literature has shown that the infectious risk is similar amongst the three access sites as long as strict sterile technique is followed.[75,76] Ultrasound-guided IJ CVC placement has resulted in a decrease in the rates of CLABSIs.[41,109] The exact mechanism by which ultrasound-guided CVC placement results in a lower risk for infection is unclear; it may be related to a reduced number of skin punctures. Organisms most commonly recovered from colonized femoral catheters are coagulase-negative staphylococci, Enterobacteriaceae, *Enterococcus* species, and *Pseudomonas aeruginosa* with a higher incidence of multidrug resistant organisms in more recent years.[133]

CVCs cause an estimated 80,000 CLABSIs and are implicated in up to 28,000 deaths per year in patients in the intensive care unit.[42,60] The average cost has been estimated at $2.3 billion annually.[60,132] The Centers for Disease Control and Prevention has recommended that central line bundling policies should be implemented to significantly decrease the incidence of CLABSI.[46,60] This bundling policy includes five evidence-based interventions: (1) hand washing, (2) maximal barrier precautions, (3) chlorhexidine skin antisepsis, (4) optimal catheter site selection with avoidance of the FV if possible, and (5) daily review of the necessity for the line and prompt removal of unnecessary lines.[46,61]

Thrombotic Complications

Thrombosis and thrombophlebitis are significant risks associated with placement of a CVC. The risk for catheter-related thrombosis is directly related to the site of access. In one trial, catheter-related thrombosis was reported in about 2.2% of patients who had a CVC placed and no significant difference comparing location, which differs from earlier data where FV had higher risk of thrombosis.[78] For SV and IJ CVCs, it is important to determine that the tip of the catheter rests in the SVC. Thrombi may form secondary to prolonged contact of the catheter against the vascular endothelium. The clinical importance of these thrombi remains unclear; however, any thrombosis has the potential to embolize. Moreover, catheter-related thrombosis is a cause of SVC obstruction syndrome.[134,135]

Site-Specific Complications

Subclavian Approaches

Although both approaches to the SV are relatively safe, the infraclavicular SV approach is more likely to be associated with complications. Two randomized, prospective comparisons of supraclavicular SV and infraclavicular SV puncture showed that complication rates were higher in the infraclavicular group.[136,137] The most significant complications are pneumothorax and puncture of the SA. Adherence to the techniques recommended for supraclavicular SV puncture decreases the risk for these complications because the needle is directed away from the pleural dome and SA. The relatively superficial location of the vein when approached from above the clavicle (1.5 to 3.5 cm) lessens the risk for puncture or laceration of deep structures. Additionally, the utilization of ultrasound will decrease the incidence of these complications.

IJ Approach

Many complications of IJ vein cannulation are similar to those of SV access, although the risk of arterial puncture is higher, and the risk of pneumothorax is lower with the IJ approach. The incidence of complications appears to be higher with use of the left IJ vein than with the right.[3] One common complication unique to the IJ approach is a localized hematoma in the neck.[138] With the IJ approach, pressure can easily be maintained on the area of swelling, and most hematomas will resolve spontaneously. If puncture of the carotid artery is recognized and treated with compression, it rarely causes significant morbidity in the absence of marked atherosclerotic disease, although arteriovenous fistulas may occur after IJ vein puncture.[121] Several neurologic complications unique to the IJ site of venipuncture have also been reported as a result of hematomas or direct injury. Such complications include damage to the phrenic nerves, iatrogenic Horner's syndrome, trauma to the brachial plexus, and even passage of a catheter into the thecal space of the spinal canal.[130] If the carotid artery is punctured, one may again attempt IJ vein or SV cannulation on the same side after appropriate, prolonged (15- to 20-minute) compression.

Femoral Approach

Because vital structures in the neck and chest are not at risk, complications of FV cannulation are generally less severe than those of other routes for central venous access. The most common immediate complications involve bleeding from damage to either the femoral artery or the FV (Fig. 22.24). This can usually be managed with 10 to 15 minutes of direct pressure. Extra care should be taken in anticoagulated patients or after the administration of thrombolytic agents. In extreme cases when hemostasis cannot be achieved through direct pressure, a vascular surgeon should be consulted.

The peritoneum can also be violated with resultant perforation of the bowel. Bowel penetration is especially likely if the patient has a femoral hernia. Injury to the bowel is usually minimal and unlikely to require specific treatment. Nonetheless, the potential bacterial contamination of the femoral puncture site can pose a significant problem. Aspiration of air during placement of a femoral line necessitates removal of the catheter and reinsertion at another site. Other complications include muscular abscesses, infection of the hip joint, damage to the femoral nerve, and puncture of the bladder. Risk for these outcomes can be mitigated by strict aseptic technique, thorough assessment of landmarks, careful control of the needle's depth, and the use of bedside ultrasound.

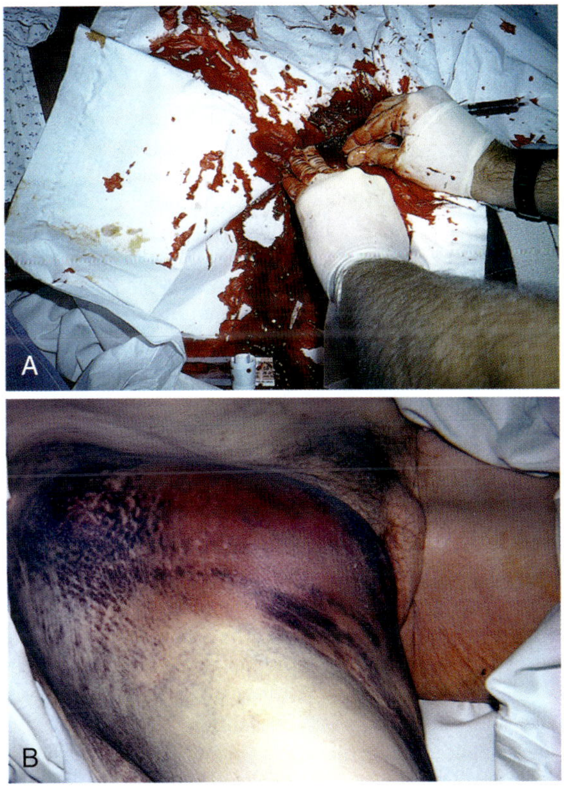

Fig. 22.24 A femoral vein catheter is more prone to deep vein thrombosis than a subclavian or internal jugular line, but it is a standard access route in the emergency department. Strict attention to sterile technique and limiting use to a few days will negate most of the negatives of this approach. (A) Significant hemorrhage can occur after puncture of the femoral artery, but this area is readily compressed. The femoral route may be the approach of choice in a patient with an inadvertently placed arterial catheter who requires a central line. (B) Bleeding from an inadvertently placed arterial catheter that was removed without adequate pressure in an anticoagulated patient.

TRAINING AND SIMULATION

CVC placement and ultrasound guidance techniques have a relatively steep learning curve. Simulation has been shown to increase success rates and decrease complications in both adult and pediatric patients.[139,140] Simulation is recommended by the AHRQ to teach these techniques.[115] Simulation training is independently associated with higher rates of correct needle insertion on the first attempt, as well as with higher successful CVC placement rates.[139,140] There are many simulation models that can be used. Kendall and Faragher described a phantom model as an easy, inexpensive method for ultrasound-guided CVC placement training.[141]

REFERENCES ARE AVAILABLE AT Elsevier eBooks+

CHAPTER 23

Venous Cutdown

Bárbara Lara and Pablo Aguilera

Management of critically ill or injured patients requires immediate and adequate vascular access to provide rapid infusion of crystalloid or blood products. Venous cutdown, a time-honored surgical technique, has largely been replaced by alternative methods of obtaining venous access, including intraosseous lines, the Seldinger technique, and ultrasound-guided central and peripheral venous cannulation.[1,2] Nonetheless, venous cutdown still has a role as an emergency method of achieving vascular access when other techniques and equipment are unavailable, particularly in settings with limited resources.

First described by Keeley in 1940 and Kirkham in 1945,[2,3] venous cutdown offered an alternative to venipuncture in patients with shock. Percutaneous vascular access may be infeasible in a pulseless, hypovolemic, or anatomically scarred patient. With a thorough understanding of the anatomy, the procedure, and its potential complications, this mechanically simple procedure can be performed effectively.[4]

INDICATIONS

Venous cutdown may be used as an alternative to venipuncture for patients in need of vascular access when less invasive options have been exhausted or are not available. Patients with severe shock, asystole, or pulseless electrical activity will lack palpable femoral pulses, thus making percutaneous femoral vein catheterization more difficult. Surface landmarks may be obscured and veins may be unusable in intravenous (IV) drug users, extensively injured, or severely burned patients, and those with severe extremity contractures or congenital deformities, making attempts at percutaneous venous cannulation complicated or even impossible. Venous cutdown (Video 23.1) and intraosseous routes (see Chapter 25) are both viable options in such scenarios.

Children

Venipuncture in small children poses a challenge in even the healthiest of patients, let alone those in extremis. The distal saphenous vein at the ankle is often recommended for venous cutdown in children given its large diameter and anatomic predictability at this location.[5,6]

Hypovolemic Shock

Initially popularized during the Vietnam War for rapid transfusion, venous cutdown has since been used for resuscitation of patients with profound hypovolemia. The flow rate of saline through a standard IV extension set cut to a length of 28 cm (12 inches) and inserted directly into the vein is 15% to 30% greater than through a 5-cm, 14-gauge catheter. This difference is larger if pressure is applied to the system. Moreover, the improvement in flow rate through large-bore lines is greater for blood than for crystalloid solutions because the viscous characteristics of blood impede its passage through small-bore tubing.[7] A unit of blood can be transfused in as little as 3 minutes through IV extension tubing inserted directly into the vein.

CONTRAINDICATIONS

Venous cutdown is contraindicated when less invasive alternatives exist and when performing the procedure would cause excessive delay.[8]

Absolute contraindications include major blunt or penetrating trauma involving the extremity on which the procedure is to be performed. Relative contraindications include vascular injury proximal to the cutdown site, overlying soft tissue infection, coagulopathies, compromised host defense mechanisms, and impaired wound healing. Other considerations include any previous saphenous vein harvest for coronary artery bypass or other vascular surgery proximal to the anticipated cutdown site. The indications for venous cutdown should be weighed against these potential complications.[7]

ANATOMY AND SELECTION OF THE SITE

Knowledge of the relevant anatomy is imperative for success. Veins in both the upper and lower extremities may be used. The size and accessibility of the target vessel, along with the clinician's experience and training, are the principal factors in selection of the site. There are four primary locations at which venous cutdown is performed: the great saphenous vein distally at the ankle and proximally at the thigh, the basilic vein above the elbow, and the cephalic vein below it. Brachial vein cutdown is no longer recommended as an emergency venous access route because of its time-consuming dissection and risk for neurovascular injury.

Great Saphenous Vein

The great saphenous vein is the longest vein in the body, and it runs subcutaneously throughout much of its course (Fig. 23.1). It is most easily accessible at the ankle but may also be cannulated below the knee and below the femoral triangle. The great saphenous vein begins just anterior to the medial malleolus where it is a continuation of the medial marginal vein of the foot. The vein crosses 1 cm anterior to the medial malleolus and, together with the saphenous nerve, ascends along the anteromedial aspect of the leg. The saphenous nerve at this level is of relatively little clinical significance, for if transected, it causes sensory loss in only a small area along the medial aspect of the foot. At the ankle, the vessel can be exposed with minimal blunt dissection. The vein's superficial, predictable, and isolated location has made the distal saphenous vein the traditional pediatric cutdown site.[5]

In the thigh the saphenous vein begins on the medial aspect of the knee and crosses anterolaterally as it ascends toward the femoral triangle. Approximately 4 cm below the inguinal ligament and 3 cm lateral to the pubic tubercle, the saphenous vein dips through the fossa ovalis, where it penetrates the femoral sheath and joins the femoral vein. The saphenous vein is easily isolated from the surrounding fat at this site because of its large caliber (4 to 5 mm in outside diameter) and superficial relationship to the femoral sheath (Fig. 23.2). Also lying anteromedially in the thigh is the lateral femoral cutaneous vein, which has a smaller diameter and lies lateral to the great saphenous vein.[9] The saphenous vein at the thigh is a preferred site for

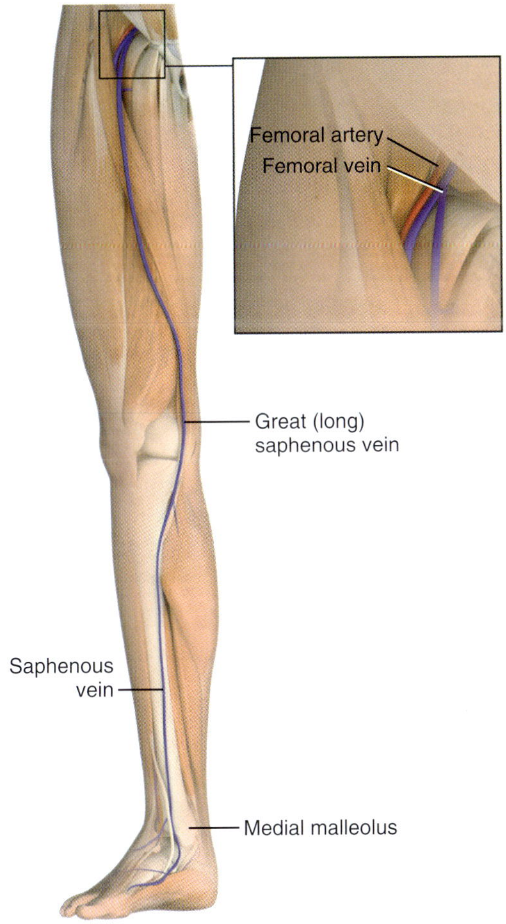

Fig. 23.1 Superficial veins of the lower limb.

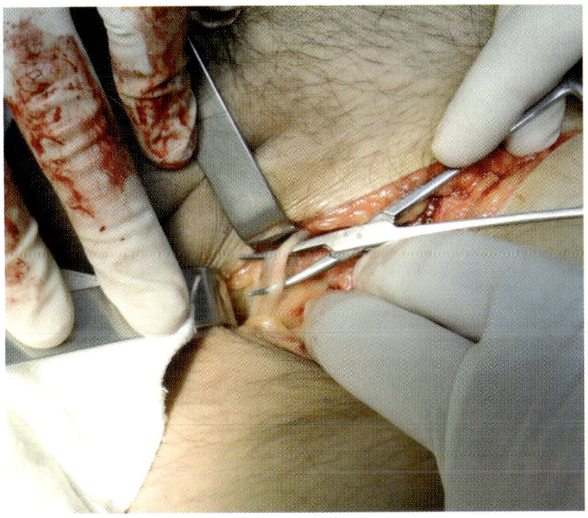

Fig. 23.2 Subcutaneous dissection in the proximal part of the thigh. The saphenous vein is easily distinguished from surrounding fat with blunt dissection. The hemostat is under the vein. (Courtesy Pablo Aguilera, MD, Hospital Dr. Sótero del Río, Santiago, Chile.)

cutdown given its large diameter and ease of accessibility. An 8.5-Fr catheter is easily introduced at this level and is ideal for rapid infusion of crystalloid or blood during resuscitation.

Basilic Vein

The basilic vein is a preferred site for venous cutdown in the upper extremity because of its predictable anatomic location. The size of this vein enables it to be located easily, even in hypotensive or hypovolemic patients. Superficially at this level there are no important associated structures, but the brachial artery and the median nerve are found deep to the basilic vein.

Veins of the dorsal venous network of the hand unite to form the cephalic and basilic veins, which travel along the radial and ulnar sides of the forearm, respectively (Fig. 23.3). At the midforearm level, the basilic vein crosses anterolaterally and then courses ventrally at the medial epicondyle. The medial cubital vein crosses over from the radial side of the arm to join the basilic vein just above the medial epicondyle. The basilic vein then continues proximally, where it occupies a superficial position between the biceps and pronator teres muscle. In this segment it lies in close proximity to the medial cutaneous nerve, which supplies sensation to the ulnar side of the forearm. At approximately midway in the upper part of the arm, the basilic vein perforates the deep fascia, where it joins the brachial vein and continues on into the axillary vein.[9]

The basilic vein is consistently found at the antecubital fossa, 2 cm above and 2 to 3 cm lateral to the medial epicondyle, on the anterior surface of the upper part of the arm. It is exposed through a transverse incision on the medial aspect of the proximal antecubital fossa. It is this predictability in anatomic location that makes the basilic vein an ideal site for venous cutdown in the upper extremity.

Cephalic Vein

This cephalic vein begins on the radial aspect of the wrist, crosses anteromedially, and ascends toward the antecubital fossa. In the forearm, it lies in close association with the lateral cutaneous nerve, which supplies sensory innervation to the radial aspect of the forearm (Fig. 23.3). In the antecubital fossa, it lies subcutaneously and just lateral to the midline. It is at this level where the median cubital vein connects to the cephalic and basilic veins. The cephalic vein then ascends in the upper part of the arm over the lateral aspect of the biceps muscle and through the deltopectoral groove. Just below the clavicle, it pierces the clavipectoral fascia, becomes a deep structure, and enters the axillary vein.[9]

Venous cutdown is easily performed on the cephalic vein because of its large diameter and superficial location. In the forearm, it is important to avoid the lateral cutaneous nerve. A preferred location is in the antecubital fossa at the distal flexor crease. Cutdown on the cephalic vein at the wrist has also been reported, but the thin skin overlying the vein at this level usually permits simple percutaneous cannulation when the vein is available for cannulation.[10] The cephalic vein may also be entered in the deltopectoral groove. However, the slightly deeper position and possible interference with the performance of other procedures make this approach more difficult.

EQUIPMENT

The material required to perform a formal venous cutdown is shown in Review Box 23.1. Perhaps the most important piece of equipment and the most difficult to find is the vein dilator/lifter, a plastic device with a 90-degree angle that is used to facilitate entrance of a catheter into the cut vein. For pediatric patients, use a warming table, or radiant warmer, and a padded extremity board.

Choose a catheter based on the desired function of the venous line. When central venous pressure (CVP) needs to be

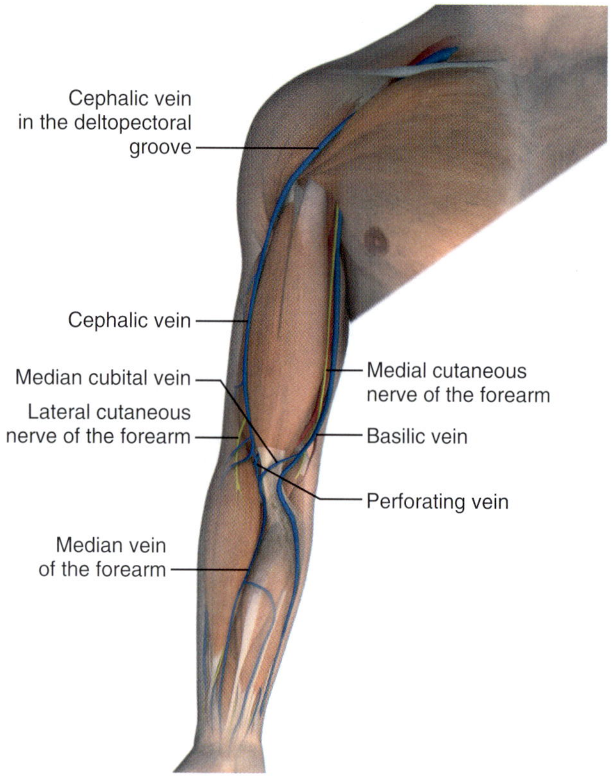

Fig. 23.3 Veins of the upper limb.

monitored, choose a catheter long enough to reach the superior vena cava. Approximate this distance by aligning the catheter over the chest with the tip at the level of the manubrial-sternal junction. The average distance from the antecubital fossa to the superior vena cava is 54 cm in adult males. Lumen size is relatively unimportant when the line is inserted for monitoring CVP or to infuse drugs, but it is a critical factor in the treatment of hypovolemia. Short, large-bore catheters are preferred when fluid must be delivered rapidly. Silastic catheters, IV plastic tubing, or 5- or 8-Fr pediatric feeding tubes may be used as infusion catheters in older children and adults.

eTables 23.1–23.3 list the flow rates of various fluids through some commonly used catheter systems. It is essential to know the relative flow rates if maximal benefit is to be obtained from the time spent performing the cutdown. Excellent flow rates can be achieved by threading IV tubing directly into the vein or by using a 5-cm, 10-gauge IV catheter. Cut sterile tubing to the appropriate length and leave a slight bevel on the end to facilitate cannulation of the opened vein.

eTABLE 23.1 Comparative Average Flow Rates (mL/min) for Tap Water
CAN BE FOUND ON ELSEVIER EBOOKS+

eTABLE 23.2 Comparative Average Flow Rates (mL/min, 200-mm Hg Pressure) for Red Blood Cells
CAN BE FOUND ON ELSEVIER EBOOKS+

Venous Cutdown

Indications

As an alternative to venipuncture in critically ill patients in need of vascular access and in whom venipuncture may be difficult:
- Shock
- Asystole or pulseless electrical activity
- Sclerosed veins of intravenous drug users
- Extensive burn or other injury
- Small children

Contraindications

Absolute:
- When less invasive options exist for venous access
- Major blunt or penetrating trauma at proposed cutdown site

Relative:
- Overlying soft tissue infection
- Bleeding diasthesis
- Immunocompromise
- Extremity injuries proximal to the site

Complications

Transection of the vein
Transection of the artery
Bleeding
Hematoma
Phlebitis
Sepsis
Thrombus formation
Injury to surrounding structures

Equipment

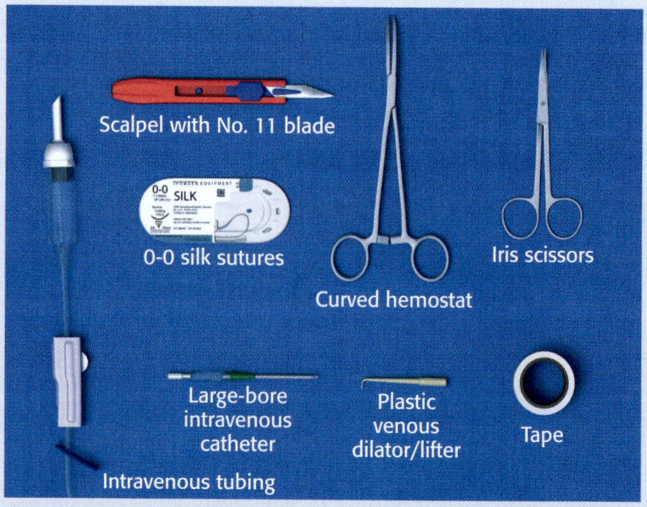

Review Box 23.1 Venous cutdown: indications, contraindications, complications, and equipment.

eTABLE 23.3 Comparative Average Flow Rates (mL/min)
CAN BE FOUND ON ELSEVIER EBOOKS+

TECHNIQUE

See Videos 23.1 and 23.2. Experienced clinicians may perform a cutdown relatively quickly depending on the vascular status of the patient. However, the lack of experience with this procedure among current practitioners leads to much longer access times for this technique.

The technique of venous cutdown is essentially the same regardless of the vessel cannulated (Fig. 23.4).[11,12] Prepare the skin around the incisional area with an antiseptic solution and then cover it with sterile drapes. Place a tourniquet proximal to the cutdown site to help visualize the vein. For children, immobilize the lower part of the leg or elbow (depending on the cutdown site) on a padded board before beginning the procedure.

In conscious patients, apply a local anesthetic before the procedure. Make a skin incision perpendicular to the course of the vein. A longitudinal incision, even though it decreases the risk of transecting neurovascular structures, may not provide sufficient exposure. Incise the skin through all its layers until subcutaneous fat bulges through the incision. Very carefully dissect the subcutaneous tissues bluntly by spreading them gently with a curved hemostat parallel to the course of the vein and with the tips pointed downward. This is the most difficult and delicate portion of the procedure and may damage the vein and render it unable to be cannulated. Bleeding, however, is usually minimal unless the vein is nicked. Use a tissue spreader or a self-retaining retractor, if needed, to provide a wider field. Isolate the vein from the adjacent tissue and mobilize it for 1 to 3 cm.

For the standard venous cutdown technique, after mobilizing the vein, use a hemostat to pass proximal and distal silk ties under the vein for stabilization (Fig. 23.5).

Tie the distal ligature after initial placement, but leave the ends long for maneuvering the vein. This will sacrifice the vein for future blood return. As an option, use traction on the distal suture to control the vein, but do not tie it off. Leave the proximal ligature untied to maneuver the vein for insertion of the catheter or tubing and control of backbleeding (by lifting the sutures). Elevate the vein with a hemostat and stretch it flat. This provides good visualization, controls the vessel, and limits bleeding when the vessel is incised. Alternatively, place gentle traction on the proximal tie to control oozing around the puncture site. Using a No. 11 scalpel blade or a pair of iris scissors, incise through one-third to one-half the diameter of the vein at a 45-degree angle. If the incision is too small, the catheter may pass into a false channel in the adventitia. Conversely, if the incision is too large, the vein may tear completely and retract from the field buried within tissue.[13] If desired, make a longitudinal incision in the vein to avoid transecting the vessel, but realize that this technique makes it more difficult to identify the lumen. Be aware that some bleeding will normally occur after the vein has merely been nicked on the surface. To perform a mini-cutdown at this point, puncture the vein with an IV catheter and introducer needle and do not make an incision in the vein. Alternatively, a Seldinger technique may be used and a wire introducer wire can be placed into the lumen of the nicked vein.[14]

Before introducing the cannula into the vein, make a bevel in the cannula at a 45-degree angle. This is unnecessary if the cannula has a tapered tip. Make the bevel short, but be careful to not make it sharp to avoid piercing the posterior wall or otherwise damaging the vein. If using the rounded tip of a feeding tube, it may be more difficult to introduce but can be advanced less traumatically. If using an IV cannula, introduce it directly through the skin incision or through a separate stab incision.

Threading the catheter into the vein is often the most difficult and time-consuming portion of the procedure. Difficulty threading has several causes. The lumen may have been incorrectly identified, or a false passage into the adventitia may have been created. This can be difficult to recognize because a catheter can easily pass between layers of the vessel wall and never reach the lumen of the vein. Other causes include penetrating the posterior vessel wall, getting stuck in a valve, or using a catheter that is too large to cannulate the vein.

Use of a plastic venous dilator can help identify and elevate the vessel lumen. Thread the small, pointed tip of the dilator into the vein to expose the lumen before advancing the tip of the catheter. Alternatively, bend a sterile 20-gauge needle at a 90-degree angle to serve as a venous dilator or elevator. A vein dilator is useful for very small veins, such as in pediatric cutdowns, but is generally unnecessary in adults. To thread large catheters in adults, grasp the proximal edge of the vessel with small forceps or a mosquito hemostat. Apply countertraction and advance the catheter (Fig. 23.6). Never force a catheter that will not advance easily.

Once the catheter is advanced into the lumen, backbleed any air from the cannula and connect it to IV tubing. Tie the proximal ligature around both the vessel and the cannula (Fig 23.7). If the distal suture has not been tied, remove it. If it has been tied, cut the ends of the suture near the knot. Remove the tourniquet, affix the catheter to the skin, and close the incision. Apply antibiotic ointment at the point where the catheter passes through the skin, and dress the wound. In an emergency situation one may delay skin closure if necessary and simply wrap the wound with sterile dressing. Loop the IV tubing under the outer layers of the dressing to minimize the risk of pulling the cannula out if the external IV line is inadvertently tugged.

Mini-Cutdown

The mini-cutdown is an alternative method designed to preserve the vein and bypass the time-consuming step of inserting a catheter into the vein. It is preferred if time is limited. Basically, a deep vein is cannulated through an incision under direct vision with a standard peripheral IV catheter. Use a skin incision and blunt dissection to locate the vessel. Once identified, puncture the vein under direct vision with a percutaneous venous catheter. Introduce the needle through either the skin incision or a separate stab incision. If an over-the-needle device (e.g., Angiocath [Becton Dickinson], Medicut [Medtronic]) is used, withdraw the needle and discard it. With a through-the-needle device, thread the cannula into the vein and withdraw the needle to the surface of the skin (Fig. 23.8). Place a guard on the tip of the needle, fix the catheter device to the skin, and close the incision. The mini-cutdown method eliminates the need for tying or cutting the vein, thereby permitting repeated catheterization. Venipuncture is easier and uses the same equipment as percutaneous venous cannulation. A simple skin

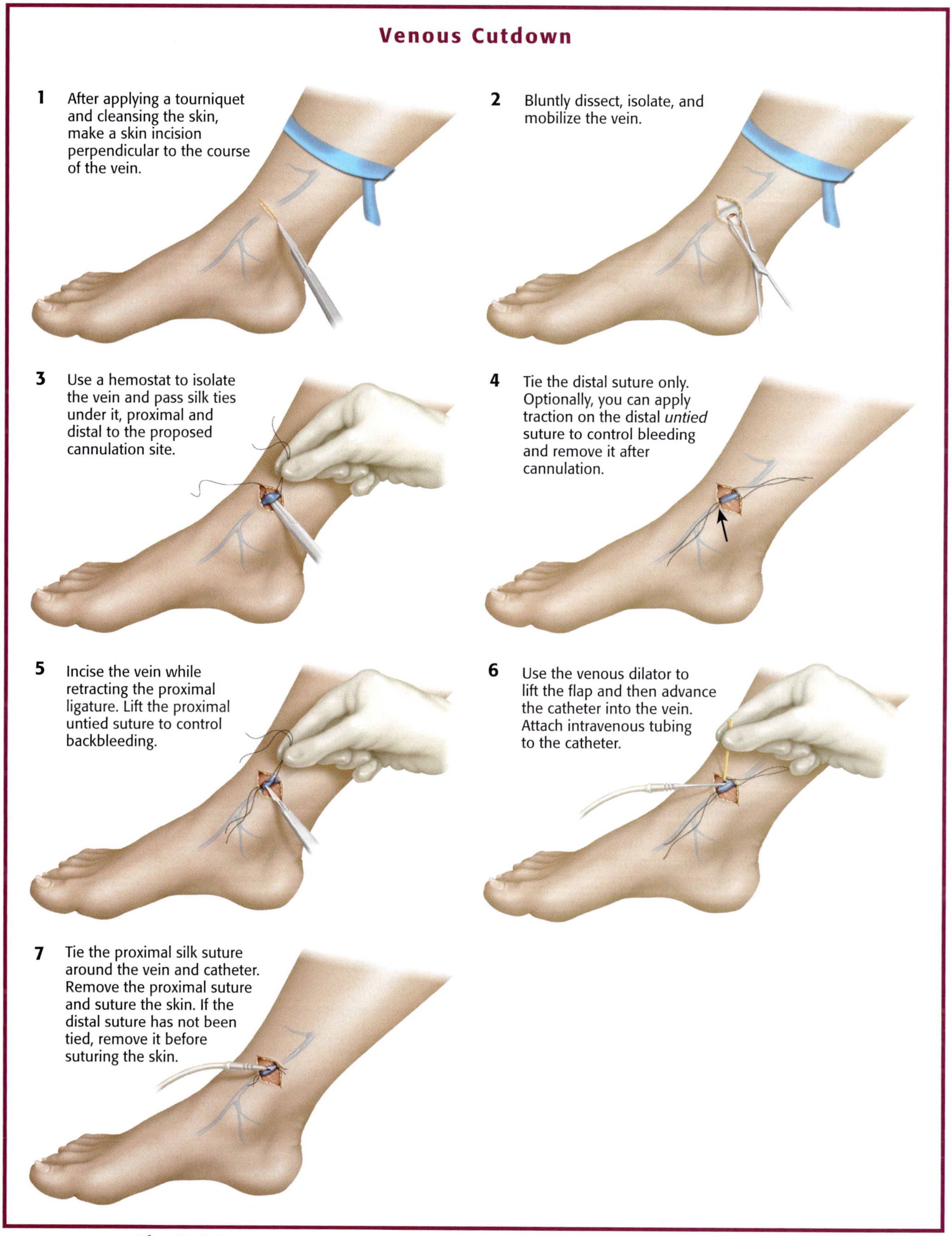

Fig. 23.4 Venous cutdown. (Adapted from Custalow CB. *Color Atlas of Emergency Department Procedures*. Saunders; 2005.)

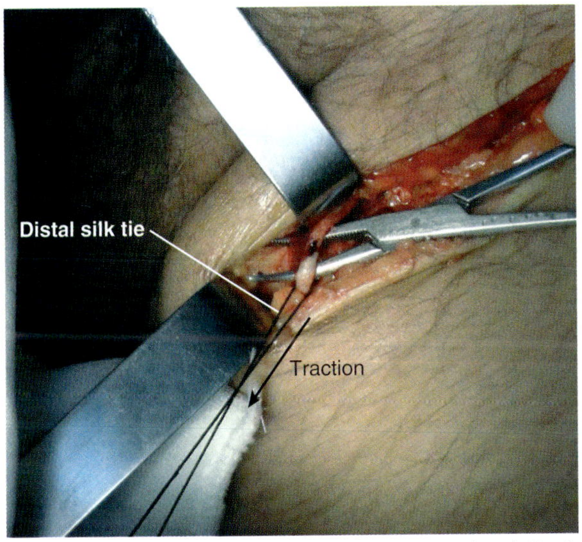

Fig. 23.5 With the assistance of a hemostat, proximal and distal silk ties may be placed under the vein for stabilization. Above, a distal tie is placed under the great saphenous vein at the thigh to aid in stabilizing the vein during cannulation. Traction on this suture will occlude blood flow and minimize bleeding during catheterization of the vein. Traction on the proximal suture will also control backbleeding (proximal suture not shown here). Note that a small incision has been made in the vein to accept a catheter, but traction *(arrow)* on the distal suture prevents bleeding. Once the catheter is in place, the distal suture is usually tied. (Courtesy Pablo Aguilera, MD, Hospital Dr. Sótero del Río, Santiago, Chile.)

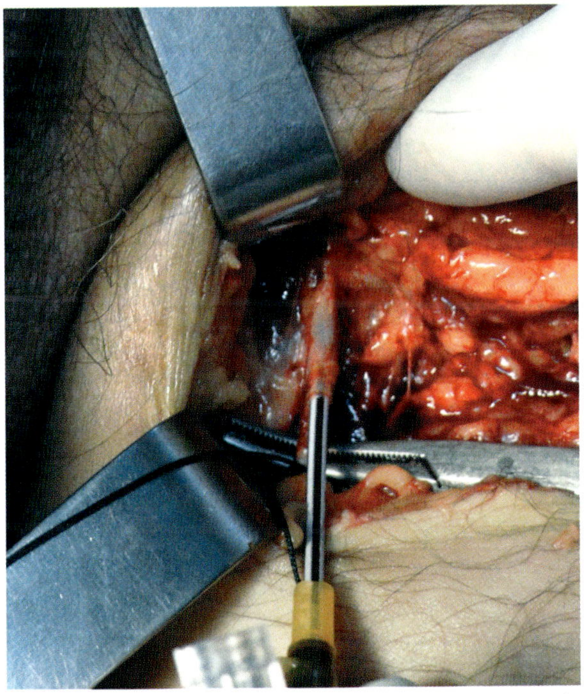

Fig. 23.6 Advancement of the standard intravenous catheter under direct vision through the great saphenous vein at the thigh. The distal suture is tied, thereby sacrificing the vein for further use. The proximal suture is not yet secured around the catheter. (Courtesy Pablo Aguilera, MD, Hospital Dr. Sótero del Río, Santiago, Chile.)

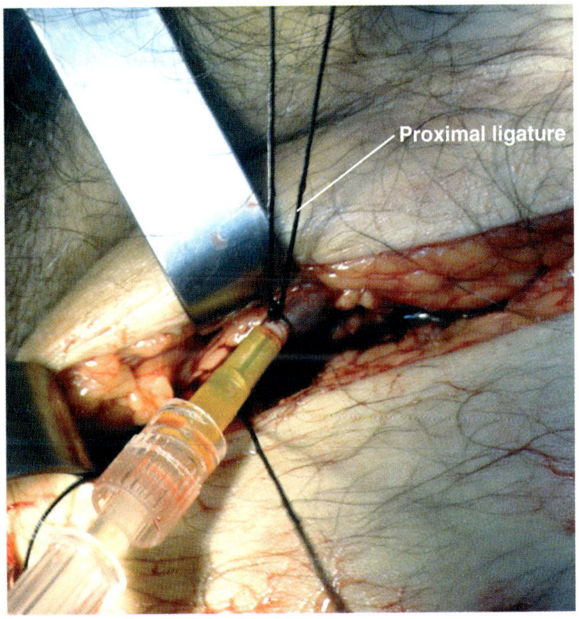

Fig. 23.7 Once the catheter is inserted into the lumen of the vein, tie the proximal ligature around both the vessel and the cannula. (Courtesy Pablo Aguilera, MD, Hospital Dr. Sótero del Río, Santiago, Chile.)

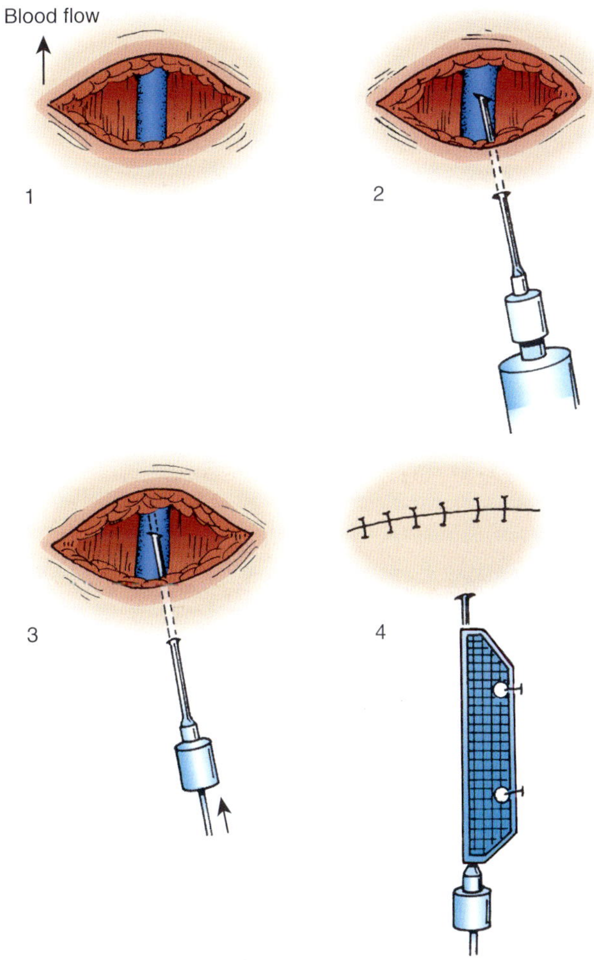

Fig. 23.8 The mini-cutdown technique is an alternative to the venous cutdown method. The vein is cannulated under direct vision with standard percutaneous catheters. A separate entry site (shown) may be used, or the vein can be cannulated through the skin incision. Note that the vein is not tied off with this technique. A standard Angiocath (Becton Dickinson) intravenous set may also be used instead of the through-the-needle catheter shown here.

incision may also permit direct visualization of veins in an obese patient and facilitate standard percutaneous venipuncture.

Modified Cutdown Technique

Shockley described a further modification in which a guidewire, dilator, and sheath system are inserted after standard cutdown and venotomy.[14] To perform this modification set up the guidewire, dilator, and sheath system before making the skin incision. Once the vein has been incised, insert the end of the guidewire followed by the dilator and sheath. Remove the wire and dilator while leaving the sheath. Ligatures are not usually needed with this technique. These authors found that when performed by novices, this technique saved more than 2 minutes in comparison to the standard technique. Moreover, in the event of a transection there was an increased vein salvage rate. To remove catheters inserted by cutdown, cut the skin stitches holding the catheter in place and then withdraw the catheter. Control backbleeding from the proximal venous end by applying a simple pressure dressing.

COMPLICATIONS

Complications of venous cutdown include local hematoma, infection, sepsis, phlebitis, embolization, wound dehiscence, and injury to associated structures. An indirect but significant complication is deterioration of an unstable patient during a time-consuming attempt at cutdown. Documentation of complications and their frequency in the literature has been sparse. Infectious complications may result from the introduction of pathogens during placement of the line, transcutaneous invasion along the course of the cannula, or deposition of blood-borne organisms on the tip of the catheter. Adherence to sterile technique will decrease the possibility of a procedure-related infection. Unfortunately, this is not always possible in the midst of a critical resuscitation. That said, a clear correlation exists between the incidence of infectious complications and the length of time that a catheter is left in place.[13,15] Early catheter removal is a key factor in the prevention of both phlebitis and the infectious complications of venous cutdown. This is especially true of lines inserted during emergency resuscitative treatment. Such lines should be removed as soon as the patient's condition permits and alternative access routes are in place. Proper attention to details of the surgical technique will limit the occurrence of minor complications such as local hematoma, abscess, and wound dehiscence. One can avoid injury to associated structures by selecting a site where the vein is well isolated, and the physician feels most comfortable performing the procedure.

ACKNOWLEDGMENT

The authors and editors sincerely thank Veronica Vasquez, Patricia Lanter, and Justin Williams for their contributions to this chapter in previous editions.

REFERENCES ARE AVAILABLE AT Elsevier eBooks+

CHAPTER 24

Indwelling Vascular Access Devices: Emergency Access and Management

Marc Thomas Bartman, Rebecca Teague, Diann M. Krywko, and Jeanhyong Park

Indwelling vascular access devices (IVADs) provide routes for short- and long-term infusion of antibiotics, hyperalimentation fluids, chemotherapeutic agents, blood products, analgesics, and anesthetic agents. In addition, they provide access for lifesaving procedures such as hemodialysis (HD) and plasmapheresis. As of 2017, nearly 746,557 patients (with approximately 20,000 new cases per year) were receiving HD therapy, with greater than 8 million central venous catheters (CVCs) being placed yearly in patients in the United States.[1,2] For the purpose of this chapter, all implanted devices and intermediate- to long-term catheters for vascular access are considered IVADs. Arteriovenous (AV) fistulas and AV grafts are included because of their similarities to IVADs.

HISTORICAL PERSPECTIVE

The first documented CVC was placed by Werner Frossmann in 1929.[3] Dr. Frossmann placed a ureteric catheter in his right antecubital vein and under fluoroscopy advanced it into his right ventricle. Following this publication, the body of literature began to rapidly grow. Most notably, Aubaniac in 1952 and Yoffa in 1965 described the utilization of the subclavian vein for central access.[4] A major advancement that led to the widespread use of CVC was the development of Silastic (polymerized silica rubber) by Dow Corning in 1948. This biocompatible material is an ideal substrate for intravenous (IV) catheters because it is chemically inert, antithrombogenic, rigid at room temperature, and pliable at body temperature. In 1973, Broviac and coworkers used this material to develop an indwelling right atrial (RA) catheter for total parenteral nutrition (TPN).[5] In 1979, Hickman and colleagues reported their experience with a catheter that could be used for blood products and drug therapy in bone marrow transplant recipients.[6] A totally implantable vascular access device (TIVAD) was described by Fortner and Pahnke in 1976.[7] Since that time, TIVADs have become a mainstay of treatment in oncology patients, improving quality of life by allowing less painful IV access and permitting unrestricted mobility.

Temporary access for HD via an external AV shunt was pioneered by both Quinton and Scribner and their coworkers in 1960.[8,9] This original shunt was composed of a loop of tubing lying on the volar aspect of the forearm that connected the radial artery to a wrist vein. Although it provided effective dialysis, it was associated with a high rate of infection, thrombosis, and restriction of patient activity. Brescia and colleagues then introduced the peripheral subcutaneous autogenous AV fistula in 1966.[10] This Brescia-Cimino internal fistula used a side-to-side anastomosis to connect the radial artery to the cephalic vein in the nondominant hand. Erben and associates described the routine use of percutaneous cannulation of the subclavian vein for HD in 1969.[11] Finally, in 1979, Uldall and coworkers reported the development of a single-needle, subclavian HD catheter.[12]

INDWELLING VASCULAR ACCESS DEVICES

IVADs are typically chosen based on the type of therapy and the estimated duration. Once the appropriate catheter is selected the smallest size and least invasive method of insertion is chosen to decrease the risk of complications.[13] Long-term IVADs consist of cuffed, tunneled RA catheters, and implantable ports. Medium-term IVADs include midline catheters (lasting weeks) and peripherally inserted central catheter (PICC) lines (lasting months). Short-term devices (see Chapters 21 and 22) include short peripheral IV, subcutaneous, percutaneous, and nontunneled central catheters. Additional IVADs include those used for dialysis, in addition to AV fistulas and grafts.

Cuffed, Tunneled RA Catheters

Several cuffed, tunneled RA catheters are available (Fig. 24.1A). The Broviac (Bard Peripheral Vascular) is an all-Silastic, single-lumen catheter, with a 1.0-mm internal diameter (ID). It is 90 cm long with a thin intravascular segment (55 cm). The Hickman (Bard), also a Silastic catheter, has a 1.6-mm ID. It allows more frequent blood sampling without jeopardizing luminal patency.[14] Single-, double-, and triple-lumen variations exist. Hemocath/Permacath has the largest bore of the RA catheters, with an ID of 2.2 mm. Quinton Instrument Company manufactures these catheters for HD, plasmapheresis, long-term nutritional support, and pain control. The main advantage of these catheters is that they can be used immediately as a bridge to longer-term devices. They are not recommended for long-term access in patients undergoing dialysis if an AV fistula or graft is possible, as long-term dialysis with tunneled catheters has been associated with an increased risk for death, a five- to tenfold increase in the risk for infection, and a decreased likelihood of adequate dialysis.[15]

RA catheters are typically inserted nonemergently in an operating room or interventional radiology suite. The device is introduced via the arm, upper anterior chest wall, or neck, and tunneled subcutaneously to enter the superior vena cava (SVC) system via the cephalic, subclavian, internal, or external jugular vein (Fig. 24.2), advancing the distal tip of the flexible catheter to the distal SVC or into the mid-RA area. The subcutaneous tunnel isolates the venous puncture site from the skin and decreases the potential for bacterial contamination. Dacron cuffs (one near the venous entrance site and one near the skin exit site) anchor the catheter and are believed to inhibit colonization of the SVC by skin organisms.[16] Advantages of an RA catheter include ease of insertion and use, minimal interference with patient activity, low incidence of major complications or unintended dislodgment, ease of removal, and potential repair via a kit. Disadvantages include the need for regular maintenance and the potential for unacceptable cosmesis.

Groshong Catheter

In contrast to the Broviac and Hickman catheters, the Groshong catheter has slit-like openings just proximal to the end

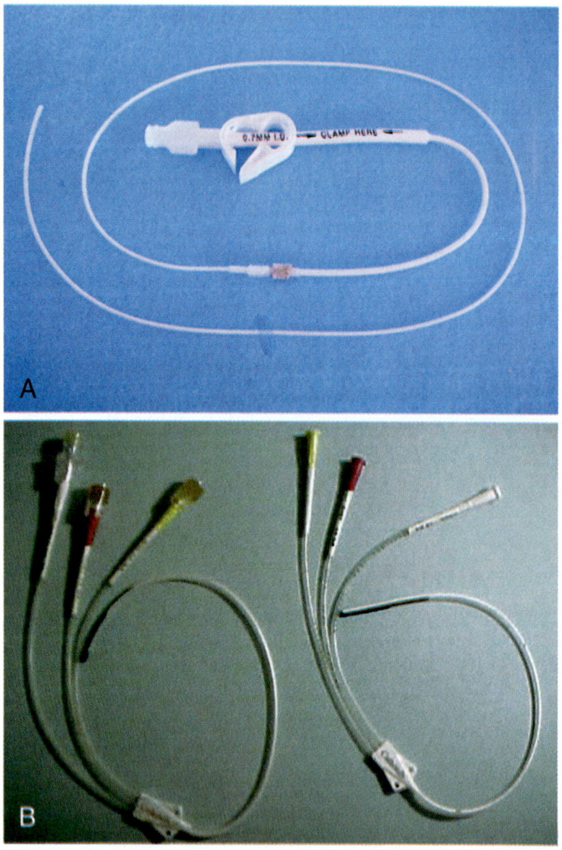

Fig. 24.1 (A) Broviac (Bard) Pediatric 4.2-French Single-Lumen CV Catheter with SureCuff Tissue Ingrowth Cuff and VitaCuff Antimicrobial Cuff. (B) The Groshong (Bard) catheter has a valve to prevent backbleeding.

of the intravascular portion of the catheter (Fig. 24.1B). This functions as a one-way valve to stop backbleeding and prevents air entry and embolism from the negative intrathoracic pressure. This feature obviates the need to use a heparin lock (saline may be used). In addition, external catheter clamping is not necessary. Disadvantages are its high cost and requirement for pressurized infusion systems.[17]

Totally Implantable Vascular Access Devices/ Ports

Since 1983, implanted ports have become the mainstay for long-term cancer therapy. TIVADs are tunneled RA catheters, featuring a subcutaneous titanium or plastic portal with a self-sealing septum (Fig. 24.3) that may be accessed by puncturing a specially designed needle (90-degree angled Huber needle) through intact skin (Fig. 24.4). Cosmetically, they are superior to external tunneled catheters, require less maintenance, and afford patients greater freedom of movement and activities, such as swimming or bathing.

TIVADs may be inserted on an outpatient basis under local anesthesia via a subcutaneous tunnel or open cutdown. The cutdown technique offers potential speed (mean placement time, 15 minutes), safety (negligible risk for pneumothorax), and avoidance of early and late complications.[18] Preferred placement is in the nondominant arm, with the portal in the upper part of the arm or chest, unless a vein is occluded or radiation therapy is planned on that side

Disadvantages of this type of device include increased cost, the need for a specific noncoring, small gauge (20 to 22), Huber

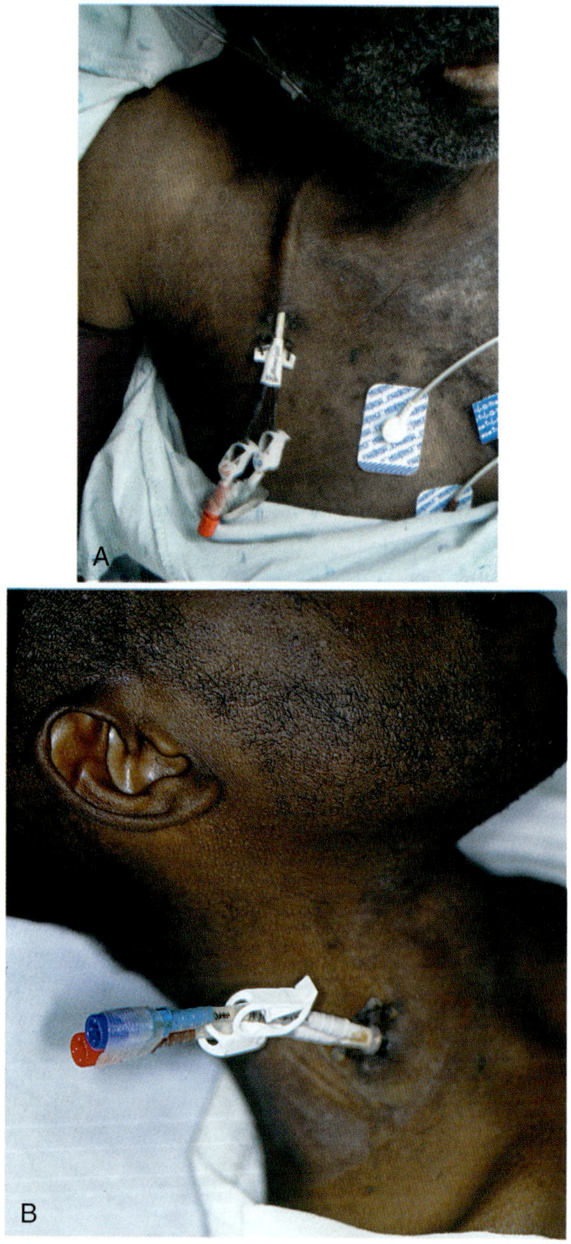

Fig. 24.2 (A) Subclavian-placed catheter with a subcutaneous tunnel. (B) Quinton dialysis catheter in the right internal jugular vein, often used for emergency dialysis or as a bridge until a dialysis fistula or graft is ready for use (i.e., when it matures).

access needle, which limits fluid infusion rates.[17] While previously TIVADs did not have the capability to withstand the pressure required for computed tomography contrast power injection, many newer ports are now rated for this capability. For example, PowerPort by Bard is an implantable port that allows for power injections required for contrast-enhanced computed tomography angiogram scans. If the patient does not have the implanted device–identifying card, a radiograph can be obtained to reveal the radiopaque titanium identifier with radiolucent "CT" letters on the bottom surface.

Peripherally Inserted Central Catheters (Nontunneled, Noncuffed)

Peripherally inserted central catheter (PICC) lines are used in patients in need of prolonged IV therapy. Such therapies include antibiotics, IV fluids, chemotherapy, TPN, and

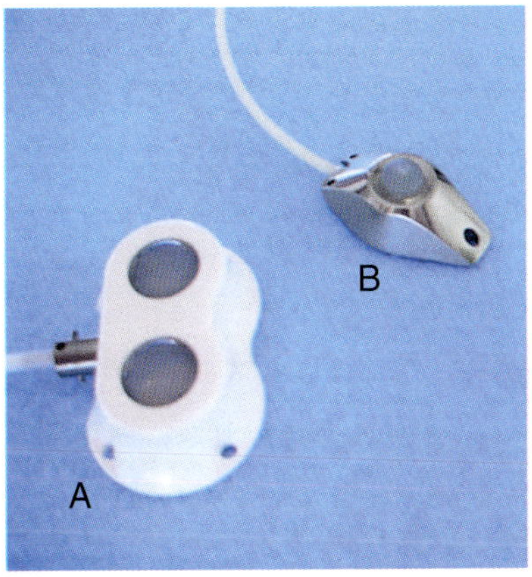

Fig. 24.3 (A) Port-A-Cath (Deltec, Inc.) double-lumen port (for chest placement). (B) Port-A-Cath single-lumen port (for upper extremity placement). The Port-A-Cath system is accessed by inserting a Huber needle through the skin into the portal septum.

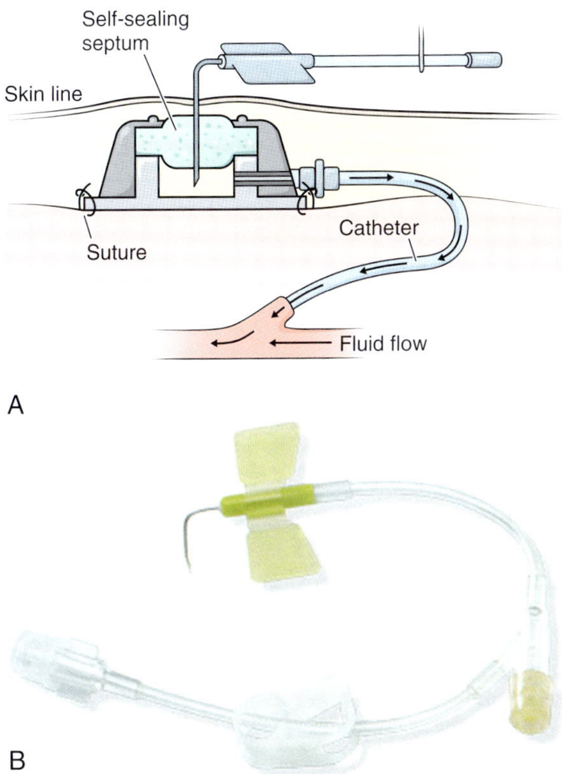

Fig. 24.4 (A) Port-A-Cath system (Deltec, Inc.). This device is subcutaneous and accessed with a Huber needle introduced through the skin into the portal septum. (B) The Huber needle is used to access the septum. Always use sterile technique.

delivery of medications that are irritating to peripheral vessels. PICCs (Fig. 24.5) are made of two substances, either polyurethane (Intracath) or silicone (Intrasil), are radiopaque, and measure 50 cm to 60 cm in length, with an outside diameter of 2 Fr to 7 Fr. The catheter may have a single- or double-lumen configuration and can be open- or close-ended or valved (e.g., Groshong). An open-ended PICC cannot prevent feedback of blood into the catheter and therefore must be flushed one or more times daily with heparinized saline. The Groshong valve reduces backup of blood into the catheter and therefore requires flushing as infrequently as once a week.

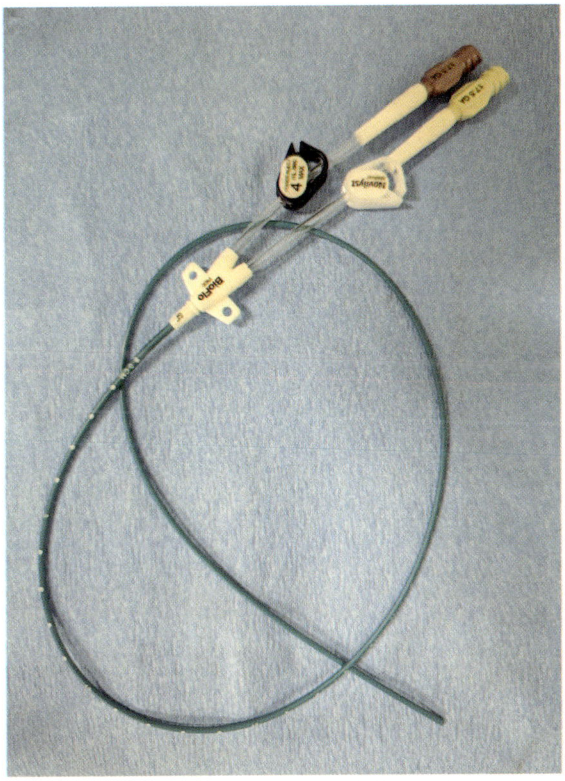

Fig. 24.5 The double-lumen percutaneously inserted central catheter (5.0 Fr, 18 gauge) is placed in the arm with the tip of the catheter in the superior vena cava. Shorter, 20-cm versions (not shown) look similar but terminate in the axillary vein and are termed midline peripheral catheters.

Selection of the device should be based on the number of lumens necessary for therapy. Selection of the access site depends on many factors including: the suitability of target vessels, body habitus, handedness, ability to manage self-care, comorbid conditions, desired infusion rate, number and compatibility of concurrent infusions, infusate characteristics, and the estimated duration of therapy. Infusate that is hyperosmolar (e.g., TPN) or vesicant requires rapid dilution. Accordingly, the tip must be in the SVC, where the estimated blood flow rate is 2000 mL/min. PICC lines are most frequently placed in the superficial veins proximal to the antecubital fossa (usually the basilic or cephalic vein) (Fig. 24.6). However, they may also be placed via a transhepatic or translumbar approach when the SVC is thrombosed or occluded.[19]

Advantages of PICC lines include usefulness in a wide variety of clinical situations, ease of placement, and ease of use and maintenance. They do not require surgical insertion and may be placed in an outpatient setting. A PICC line is an excellent vehicle for medium- to long-term IV therapy. With proper care, PICCs can remain in place for long periods, even months to years.[20] To remove a PICC line, simply withdraw it from the vein, and apply pressure and a sterile bandage.

Midline Peripheral Catheters

Midline catheters are often confused with PICC lines (Fig. 24.7). They are also placed peripherally in the superficial veins of the antecubital fossa or upper part of the forearm. They differ from PICCs in that they are peripheral, not central catheters. Midlines are typically shorter (20 cm), with

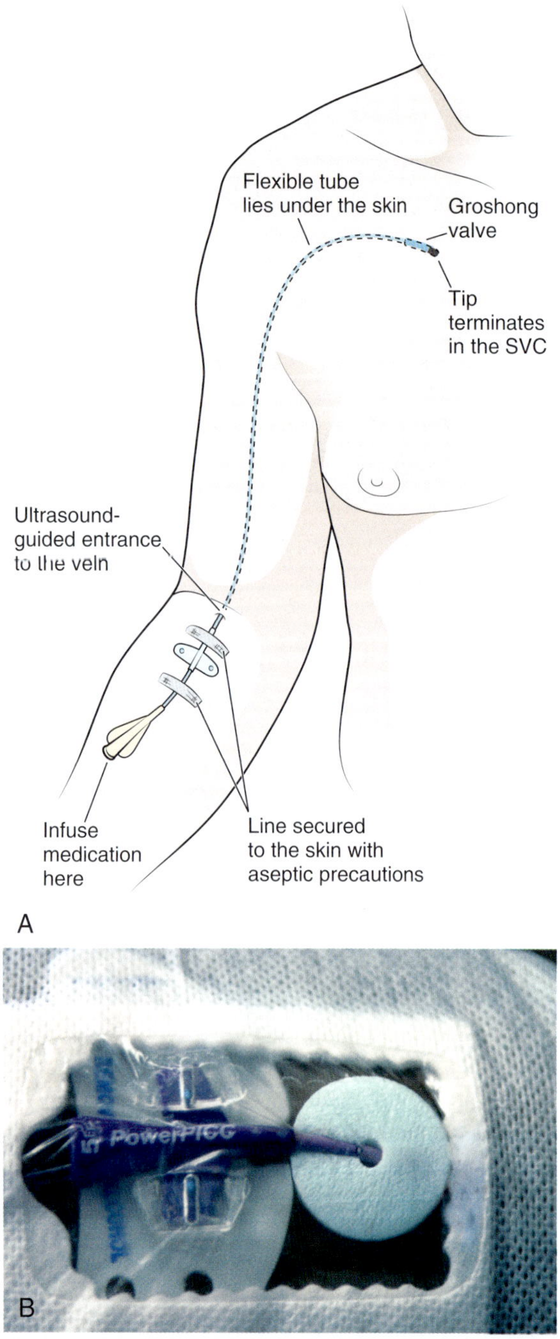

Fig. 24.6 (A) Percutaneously inserted central catheter (PICC) line placement in the upper extremity with the internal catheter tip at the superior vena cava (SVC). (B) Most PICC lines are used for outpatient therapy, such as prolonged antibiotic therapy, so proper aseptic technique at the catheter site is essential.

the tip terminating near the axillary vein. Placement above the axillary vein results in a higher risk for thrombosis. They are designed for short- to medium-term use, a shorter period than with a PICC. Because midline catheters do not enter the central circulation with high flow, delivery of medication and infusion types are limited, and routine blood withdrawal is not recommended. Differentiating between these two catheters in situ may be difficult because their outward appearance is similar. Obtaining a radiograph for visualization of tip placement will help in determining catheter type; PICC tip near SVC, midline catheter tip in arm when properly positioned.

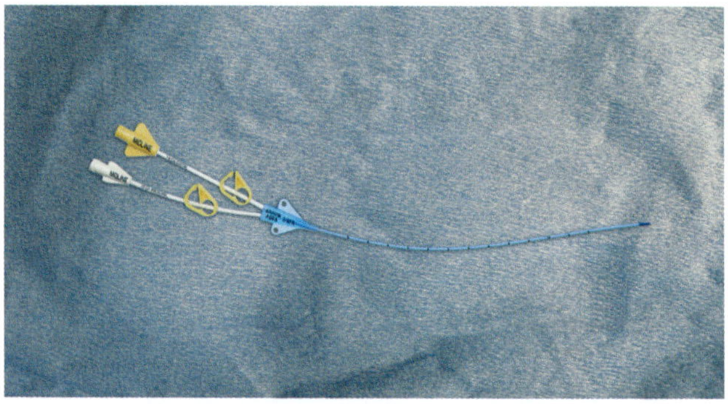

Fig. 24.7 Midline peripheral catheters are shorter than PICC lines, usually 20 cm. They are placed in similar areas as PICC lines but midline catheters terminate in the axillary vein.

Hemodialysis IVADs

Maintaining vascular access is a major issue faced by all patients with end-stage kidney disease undergoing HD. From the moment that the first access is created, an ongoing process starts that will end with loss of all access sites if the patient survives long enough.[21] Clinical practice guidelines of the National Kidney Foundation–Disease Outcomes Quality Initiative (NKF-DOQI) recommend early construction of an AV fistula and avoidance of catheters for permanent or prolonged vascular access, except in rare circumstances where AV graft or fistula formation is not feasible because of a lack of acceptable anatomic sites or limited life expectancy of the patient.[22] However, close to 70% of patients in the United States begin dialysis with a central catheter because a well-developed AV fistula is not available at the time of the initial catheter requirement.[23]

Temporary Dialysis Catheters

Temporary vascular access catheters (Fig. 24.8) are used for emergent HD or for temporary HD access if a more permanent dialysis route (AV fistula or graft) is not available, or has recently been placed and not yet matured. The advantage of tunneled catheters is the ability to provide immediate access or temporary access while a more permanent structure matures, but this carries an increased long-term risk for infection, dysfunction, and central venous stenosis. Most bacteremia episodes in patients undergoing HD are caused by HD catheters, with an approximate 20% to 25% risk over the average duration of use.

These large-bore catheters allow the necessary blood flow rate of 300 mL/min for HD, with two ports, one to deliver the patient's blood to the dialysis machine, and another to return the blood to the patient's circulation (see Fig. 24.2B). These catheters are placed in a central vein, either the internal jugular, femoral, or subclavian. The right internal jugular approach is preferred, even if permanent access is to be created on the right side, because it has the lowest thrombosis rate. The NKF-DOQI recommends avoiding the subclavian vein unless no other options exist, or the ipsilateral arm has no more permanent access sites. For patient comfort, a special 180-degree catheter can be used (Fig. 24.9). There are two avenues to place this catheter: percutaneous or surgical. Emergency percutaneous placement may be performed by the emergency clinician at the bedside. Using sterile technique and after injection of a local anesthetic, the catheter is inserted

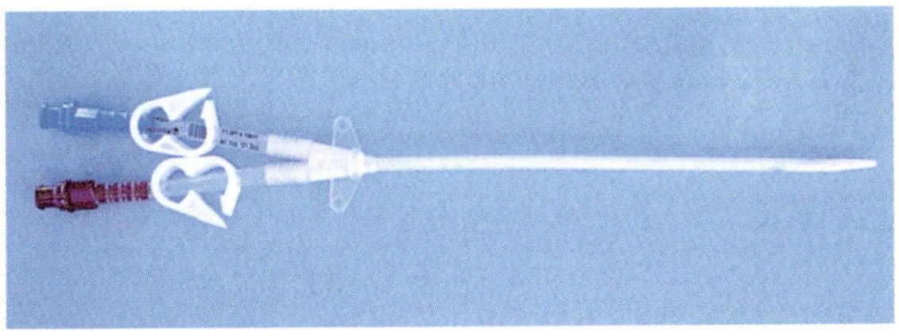

Fig. 24.8 Mahurkar 11.5 Fr × 16 cm double-lumen catheter (Medtronic) for temporary hemodialysis, apheresis, and infusion.

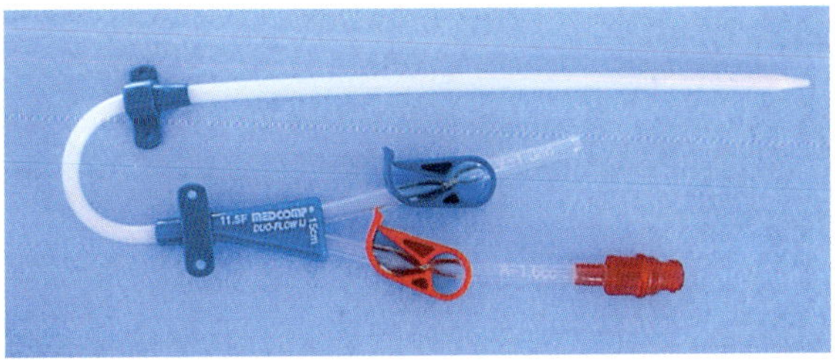

Fig. 24.9 MedComp (Medical Components, Inc.) Duo-Flow Internal Jugular Vascular Catheter (11.5 Fr × 15 cm). The angle of the catheter makes it more comfortable for the patient.

via the same procedure for placing a central line into one of the central veins.

The surgical technique uses a slightly larger catheter (Quinton, Hickman) and is performed in the operating room under local anesthesia, with or without general sedation. This catheter is placed in much the same fashion as the tunneled RA catheters described previously. Surgically implanted catheters are preferred if more than temporary use is anticipated because the risk for infection is decreased and they can be used for a longer time.

Chronic HD Vascular Access

The goal of chronic HD vascular access is to provide safe, effective, and repeated facilitated access to the circulation. The three principal types of access are native AV fistulas, synthetic grafts, and double-lumen tunneled cuffed catheters (described previously). Fistulas and grafts are collectively termed shunts. It may be difficult to distinguish a fistula from a graft by gross inspection alone. Clues to identification include shape and location. Fistulas tend to be more tortuous and serpentine, whereas synthetic grafts are straighter or C-shaped. Grafts are rarely placed in the forearm, which is the preferred site for fistulas. Grafts feel like a hard tube compared to the spongy, pulsatile feeling of a fistula.

HD access types differ in failure rates, patency, complications, and other morbidity. Both grafts and fistulas are subject to vascular perturbation and integrity issues from the high flow rates and repeated access. Fistulas, subjected to bulging of the vessel walls, may form a true aneurysm. Dilated veins in a fistula can simulate an aneurysm. Grafts are subject to pseudoaneurysms when there is a breach in the integrity of the graft, and they are more likely to rupture. Both types of vascular deformities can rupture. Multiple defects may require replacement access.

Both fistulas and grafts must mature before they can be used for HD, a process that may take several weeks to several months. HD is often performed via a temporary dialysis catheter during this time. A patient who presents to the emergency department (ED) with both a catheter and a shunt likely has a nonfunctioning fistula or graft, or an access site that is still immature.

Complications common to both fistulas and grafts are thrombosis, infection, steal syndrome, venous hypertension, bleeding, seromas, and aneurysms (Fig. 24.10). Overall, grafts are more likely to experience infection and thrombosis requiring thrombectomy or require other types of access intervention.

Arteriovenous Fistulas

AV fistulas are surgically constructed by anastomosing an artery to a vein (see Fig. 24.10). Various configurations are possible, but AV fistulas are typically an end-to-side, vein-to-artery anastomosis. The radial cephalic (Brescia-Cimino) fistula in the forearm is the most frequently used (Fig. 24.11), with the brachial-cephalic, brachial-basilic, and rarely the proximal part of the thigh being alternatives. A new minimally invasive endovascular approach has been developed for AV fistula creation utilizing a radiofrequency magnetic catheter-based system. Benefits of this procedure include quicker recovery time, decreased fistula maturation time, increased rates of primary patency and a decreased need for intervention during the maturation process.[24]

Over time, the venous portion of the shunt is subjected to high pressure, and the fistula becomes arterialized (hypertrophied and dilated), which renders it suitable for repeated vascular access. The minimum time for fistula maturation is at least 1 month, much longer than required for graft maturation. Full epithelialization of the shunt does not occur for 3 to 6 months, thus necessitating anticipatory placement as renal function worsens.

AV fistulas are the preferred means of vascular access for HD over grafts because of superior long-term patency and lower thrombotic and infectious complication rates. Fistulas have a 23% rate of primary failure, defined as being unable to provide reliable access because of early thrombosis or failure to mature.[25] However, once a fistula matures, long-term patency is high (69% of AV fistulas vs. 37% of AV grafts at 5 years), with low infection rates relative to grafts.[26]

Historically, however, the percentage of patients with AV fistulas fell well below the recommended goal, with most patients receiving AV grafts or long-term vascular access catheters. In recent years there has been a concerted effort to increase the utilization of AV fistulas, most notably the NKF's Fistula First Breakthrough Initiative.[27] The most recent data from the Dialysis Outcomes and Practice Patterns Study (DOPPS) show that, from 2002 to 2011, AV fistula use in the United States nearly doubled (32% to 62%), and AV graft use fell by more than 50%.[28]

Arteriovenous Grafts

If a forearm fistula cannot be constructed or has failed, an AV bridge graft using a donor vein or synthetic material is a well-accepted alternative. AV grafts can be cannulated earlier than fistulas, often within weeks of placement. Several synthetic materials are used for grafts. Polytetrafluoroethylene is most used, taking 3 weeks to mature. There are products available that can be accessed within 24 hours of placement. A standard graft is 6 mm to 8 mm in diameter with multiple possible configurations (Fig. 24.12). They are usually positioned in a U-shaped subcutaneous tunnel in the forearm. The graft

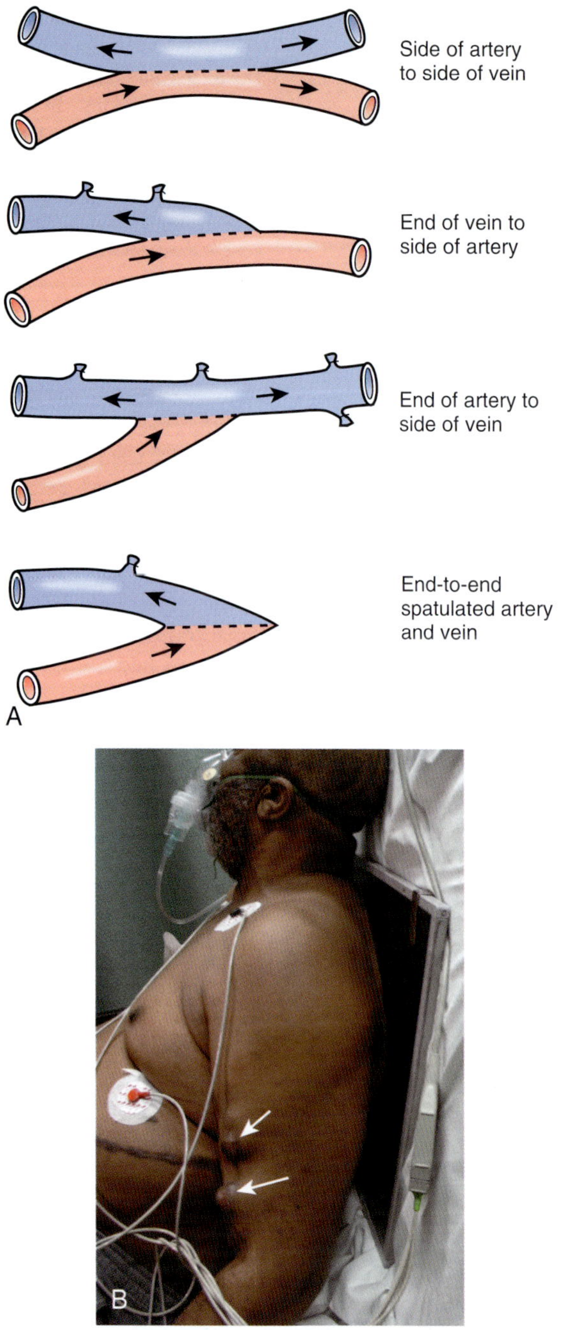

Fig. 24.10 (A) Various possible anastomotic configurations between the artery and vein for autogenous fistula formation. A thrill should be palpated if this fistula is functioning. (B) Older dialysis fistula. Fistulas can develop multiple aneurysms *(arrows)* from multiple time use. It may be difficult to distinguish a fistula from a graft by merely looking at the site. (A, Adapted from Ozeran RS. Construction and care of external arteriovenous shunts. In: Wilson SE, Owens ML, eds. *Vascular Access Surgery.* Mosby–Year Book; 1980.)

is attached by end-to-side anastomoses to the brachial artery and antecubital vein. If no suitable antecubital vein is available, a straight bridge graft between the brachial artery and either the axillary or the basilic vein is often used. A jump graft between opposite extremities with creation of a loop across the chest or anastomosis of the axillary artery to the iliac vein is possible, when all other sites have been exhausted.

When compared with AV fistulas, AV grafts have a significantly higher incidence of thrombosis, infection, pseudoaneurysm formation, and limb loss. The risk for infection with HD

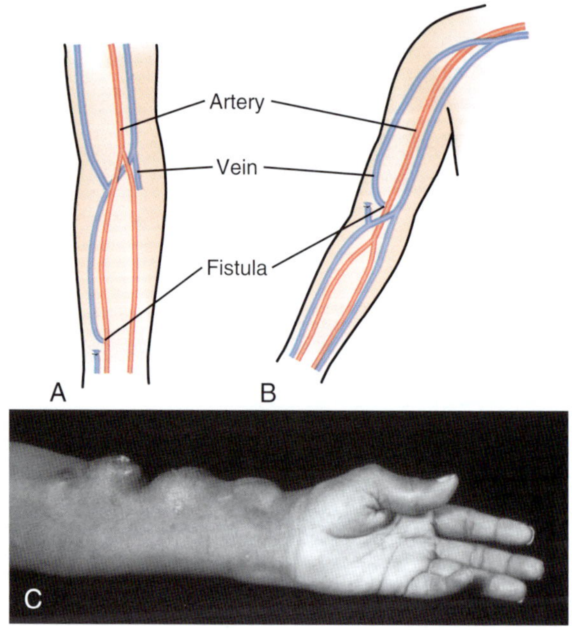

Fig. 24.11 Arteriovenous fistula. (A) Brescia-Cimino (radial-cephalic) fistula performed at the level of the wrist. (B) Brachial-cephalic fistula performed proximal to the antecubital fossa. (C) Multiple asymptomatic pseudoaneurysms resulting several years after creation of an autogenous wrist (Brescia-Cimino) arteriovenous fistula. (B, Adapted from Rutherford RB, ed. *Vascular Surgery*. 5th ed. Saunders; 2001.)

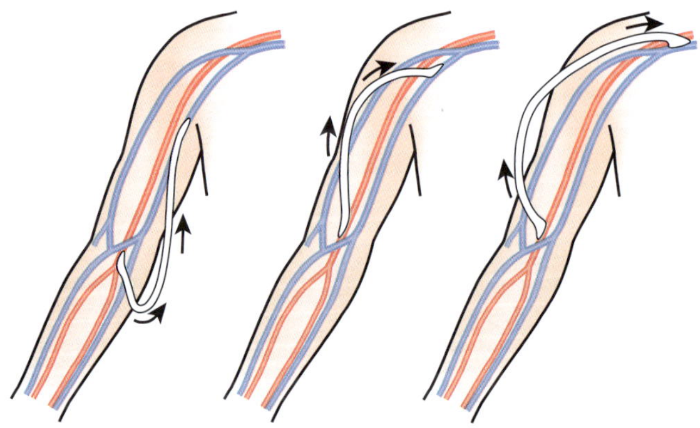

Fig. 24.12 Three possible graft configurations for jump grafts in which standard sites have been used. Note the typical C shape of the graft. (Adapted from Tilney NL, Lazarus JM, eds. *Surgical Care of the Patient with Renal Failure.* Saunders; 1982; as shown in Haisch CE. Chronic vascular and peritoneal access. In: Davis JH, Sheldon GF, eds. *Clinical Surgery.* Mosby;1995.)

grafts is approximately 10% over prolonged use and 1% with HD fistulas.[24] Graft infection requires complete excision to eradicate an infection of the foreign material, whereas fistula infections may resolve with IV antibiotic use. AV grafts have a low primary patency rate (31% at 1 year according to one study).[29] However, they have a low incidence of aneurysm formation and are comparatively easy to revise. The estimated life span of an AV graft in clinical practice is often less than 2 years.

ACCESSING IVADs IN THE ED

When IV access is required in patients with IVADs, standard methods of peripheral access should be attempted first to preserve the life span of the device and avoid complications.

However, IVADs, AV fistulas, and grafts may be accessed as a last resort in emergency situations for phlebotomy and infusion of medications and fluids. Because of the complications of infection and catheter malfunction, dislodgment, and fracture, only personnel with the requisite knowledge and skill should access IVADs if feasible. When IVADs are accessed, ensure antiseptic preparation and sterile technique throughout the procedure (Video 24.1). Assuming that proper access methods are used to prevent infection, the greatest risk is sludging in the catheter with resultant occlusion.

Accessing Long-Term Venous Access Catheters

To access the catheter (except for Groshong catheters, which have backflow valve protection), first clamp it to prevent air embolism prior to removing the cap. Patients usually carry their own clamps, but a hemostat will suffice in an emergency. In this case, wrap tape around the teeth of the hemostat to prevent tube damage. After sterile preparation, remove the cap of the catheter and withdraw any mobile clots with a syringe. Remove approximately 3 mL to 5 mL of blood and then attach a 10-mL syringe to a single-dose vial of sterile normal saline. Smaller syringes generate greater amounts of pressure for infusion, which can lead to increased intraluminal pressure and rupture of the catheter. To accomplish phlebotomy, attach a separate syringe to remove the desired amount of blood. If clots are withdrawn again, continue withdrawing blood until it is clot free.[29]

On completion of either blood withdrawal or medication infusion, inject 3 to 4 mL of saline utilizing a new 10-mL syringe to flush, verify backflow before all subsequent procedures, and then inject heparin according to hospital protocol, which may vary depending on the type of catheter used. Clamp the line and reposition the cap. Do not inject larger amounts because it can systemically heparinize the patient, and always confirm concentration and dosing protocols, especially in children.[26]

Groshong catheters need not be flushed with heparin but instead may be flushed briskly with 5 to 10 mL of saline. Multilumen central catheters have one port for each lumen, so access each one in the same manner. Perform phlebotomy through the proximal lumen to prevent mixing with medications being delivered through the other ports. Deliver IV infusions in similar fashion and inject a normal saline flush between medications. Following the procedure, flush with heparin through each port. More pronounced infusion might be necessary to ensure the patency of Groshong catheters.[29]

Do not administer medications concurrently that are known to be incompatible when mixed (e.g., calcium and bicarbonate), even through separate ports of multilumen catheters. Deliver a 5-mL normal saline flush between medications with a 10-mL syringe.

Accessing TIVADs

The procedure for accessing TIVADs is unique as these devices are not external. Instead, a circular reservoir (cylinder) lies subcutaneously on the anterior chest wall. First, palpate the cylinder, feeling for an elevated, compressible diaphragm (or two if double lumen) and then prepare the overlying skin with antiseptic solution. Fill a 10-mL syringe with normal saline and attach it to connecting tubing. Attach the connecting tubing to a 19- to 22-gauge, 90-degree tapered (Huber) needle. The Huber needle is a specialized needle designed for use with TIVADs to prevent damage to the portal septum. It has a 90-degree bend with a slightly curved tip and the opening on the side rather than on the end. Most importantly, the Huber is a noncoring needle. This avoids damage to the Silastic septum and allows up to 2000 punctures. Do not access the TIVAD with a standard needle unless an arrest is in progress and a Huber needle is not immediately available. Apply a clamp to the connecting tubing whenever the system is open. Expel the air and insert the Huber needle through the septum of the reservoir. Insert the needle slowly and steadily through the diaphragm until it contacts the back of the reservoir. Be aware that although incomplete perforation of the septum will block flow, substantial pressure may also damage the back of the device and bend the tip of the needle. Remove the clamp slowly and inject 5 mL of solution to ensure patency. If patency is not easily demonstrated, consider using alteplase (recombinant tissue plasminogen activator) as a fibrinolytic agent for catheter occlusion.[30] Thirty-minute dwell protocols for alteplase have been shown to be efficient and safe when compared to the longer dwell protocols.[31]

Once the solution has been injected, apply gentle negative pressure to demonstrate backflow of blood. Stabilize the Huber needle by building a 4 × 4 inch gauze pad about the needle and further reinforce it with 2.54-cm (1-inch) silk tape. Remove 8 to 9 mL of blood with a separate syringe, waste it, and then perform phlebotomy through the extension tubing. If necessary, deliver IV solutions through extension tubing, but remember that the rate of flow will be limited by the smaller radius of the Huber needle. Deliver a 5-mL sterile normal saline flush between medications. Complete the procedure with a heparin flush and remove the Huber needle.[29]

Accessing AV Fistulas, Grafts, and HD Catheters

AV fistulas, grafts, and temporary dialysis catheters are placed in patients who require HD, and they represent the sole access for that purpose. Consequently, routine use of these sites for phlebotomy and fluid administration is strongly discouraged. In fact, venipuncture in the same extremity as a patent AV shunt is not recommended, except for the veins in the dorsum of the ipsilateral hand. However, when standard IV access cannot be obtained under emergency circumstances, fistulas, grafts, and catheters may all be used to administer lifesaving IV solutions and medications (Fig. 24.13). The option to access these sites is based on clinical judgment by the clinician. If possible, ascertain patency of the fistula by noting a bruit and palpable thrill, although these signs may not be appreciable if the patient is in extremis.

Prepare the area overlying the fistula with antiseptic solution and access the fistula with the smallest gauge needle that is appropriate. Puncture 1 cm to 2 cm from the end of the anastomosis nearest the venous side and avoid aneurysmal sites.[32] Access AV grafts similarly by placing the smallest needle possible in the catheter and bridging the arterial and venous circulations. Apply local pressure for at least 5 minutes after the procedure is completed and monitor subsequently for hemorrhage.

Access HD catheters in much the same way that multilumen central catheters are accessed. After aseptic technique, remove fluids through the retaining cap on each arm. Up to

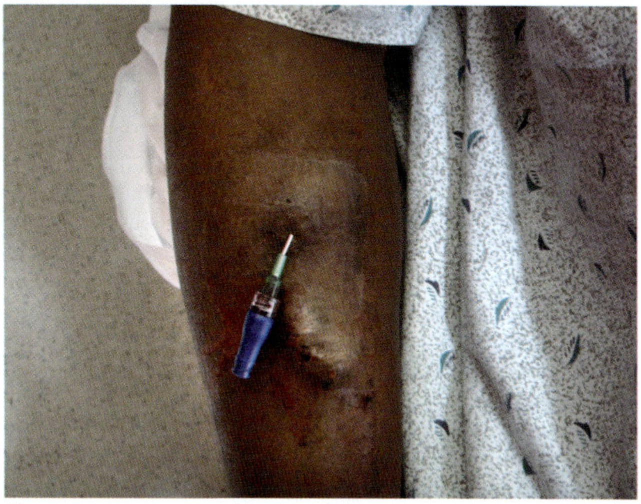

Fig. 24.13 For resuscitation or delivery of advanced cardiac life support drugs, a venous catheter may be used to access a shunt, but otherwise avoid this whenever possible.

5000 units of heparin are present within the two lumens, thus it is imperative to aspirate before administering fluid or medications. After use, flush each catheter arm with 10 mL of normal saline and instill heparin per institutional protocol.

COMPLICATIONS OF IVADs

IVADs are commonplace and patients with these devices are seen in the ED on a regular basis. Given a complication rate of 7.2% to 32.1%,[33] it is essential that emergency clinicians be aware of these complications and their management. The risk for complications associated with an IVAD is dependent on several factors including: the type of catheter, underlying patient pathology and anatomy, the site chosen for placement, and the experience of health care workers obtaining access and caring for the device.[34]

Complications of IVADs include (1) infection, (2) coagulation and hemorrhage abnormalities, (3) malfunction, and (4) miscellaneous problems (Box 24.1).

BOX 24.1 Complications of Indwelling Vascular Access Devices

INFECTION

Skin/exit site
Reservoir/pocket
Tunnel
Catheter tip/lumen
Sepsis

MALFUNCTION

Occlusion
Failure of delivery of medication
Failure to infuse/withdraw
Pinch-off syndrome
Steal syndrome
Malposition
False aneurysms
Catheter dislodgment

COAGULATION/HEMORRHAGE

Thrombosis
Phlebitis
Deep venous thrombosis
Fibrin sheath
Bleeding
Local puncture site
Arterial bleeding
Excess heparinization

MISCELLANEOUS

Embolism
- Air
- Thrombus
- Catheter fragment

Arrhythmias
Cutaneous Dacron cuff erosion
High output cardiac failure
Precipitants

Infection

Infection is the most common complication leading to removal of IVADs and potentially the most serious. Infection can also result in shunt thrombosis, rupture, or massive hemorrhage. It is estimated that more than 250,000 cases of nosocomial IVAD-related bacteremia occur annually in the United States with an associated mortality rate greater than 10%.[35] Infectious complications include endocarditis, septic arthritis, pulmonary emboli, osteomyelitis, and spinal epidural abscess. The definitions of IVAD-related infections are not uniform, which makes it difficult to compare the results of various investigations. However, it is generally agreed that risk factors for infection include the site of insertion, duration of catheter placement, type of catheter, and patient factors. Most studies show a lower incidence of infection for TIVADs than for external systems, presumably because of lack of direct access by cutaneous organisms. Rates of IVAD infection tend to be highest in the first 3 months after insertion, with skin flora being most common.[36,37] The rate of infection decreases significantly and reaches a plateau after 5 to 6 months.[37]

Clinical findings are unreliable in the diagnosis of infection secondary to IVADs. Fever, rigors, and an elevated white blood cell count are nonspecific, whereas purulent drainage at the insertion site is specific but not sensitive. Therefore evaluation beyond physical examination alone is essential when infection is suspected, including Gram stain and culture of purulent material at the site, blood cultures, and culture of catheter segments. In addition, echocardiography is indicated if valvular vegetations are suspected by blood cultures positive for *Staphylococcus aureus*, persistent bacteremia or fungemia after removal of the catheter, or lack of clinical improvement despite treatment.

If there is a clinical concern for a catheter-related infection, draw two sets of blood for culture, with one set through the catheter itself (if clinically appropriate; no overlying cellulitis, etc.) and one from a peripheral site. Positive blood cultures for *S. aureus*, coagulase-negative staphylococci, or *Candida* species, in the appropriate patient setting and in the absence of another identifiable source of infection, should increase suspicion for catheter-related bloodstream infection.[36] Similarly, if cultures drawn from the IVAD become positive 2 or more hours before peripherally drawn cultures, it suggests the patient has a catheter-related bloodstream infection.[38] Infusate-related bloodstream infection is uncommon and defined as isolation of the same organism from both the infusate and separate percutaneous blood cultures, along with no other source of infection. When this diagnosis is suggested, cultures of the infusate should be performed in addition to catheter and peripheral blood cultures.[36]

When a catheter-related infection is suspected, an important management decision is required to determine whether to remove the catheter. Removal is recommended in patients who have a catheter placed solely for short-term use. In patients with long-term catheters, removal of the catheter is advised in the setting of severe sepsis, suppurative thrombophlebitis, endocarditis, or persistent positive blood cultures (longer than 72 hours) while on appropriate antibiotics. For patients who require long-term vascular access for survival or have no other vascular access options, salvage of the catheter may be attempted in consultation with infection disease and other specialists. If the decision is made to leave the catheter in place, obtain repeated blood cultures and remove the catheter promptly if they remain positive following 72 hours of appropriate antibiotic therapy[39] or in cases of *S. aureus*, *Pseudomonas*, or fungi. [40]

If an IVAD is removed, determination of the offending organism may be made by culturing a portion of the catheter. Place the catheter in a sterile container and send it to the laboratory for culture, sensitivity, and Gram stain. The most widely used laboratory technique for the clinical diagnosis of catheter-related infection is the semiquantitative method, in which a segment of the catheter is rolled across the surface of an agar plate and colony-forming units (CFUs) are counted after incubation overnight. Quantitative culture of the catheter segment requires either flushing the segment with broth or vortexing in broth, followed by serial dilutions and surface plating on blood agar. A yield of 15 CFUs or more from a catheter by semiquantitative culture or a yield of 102 or more from a catheter by quantitative culture with accompanying signs of local or systemic infection is indicative of a catheter-related infection.[36]

The process of HD requires several connections to the HD catheter, thereby increasing the risk for infection. The rate of bacteremia in HD patients attributed to the vascular access site varies from 48% to 73%. The incidence is highest when central venous dialysis catheters are used, whereas native AV fistulas carry the lowest risk for infection.[41] As with other IVADs, if infection is suspected, initiate empirical antibiotic therapy based on epidemiologic and patient factors, followed by narrowed-spectrum therapy after isolation and determination of sensitivities. The most common infecting organism is *S. aureus*.

Antimicrobial Therapy

Pending the results of culture, the initial choice of an antibiotic is empirical and depends on the clinical setting, site of infection, type of device, host factors (e.g., immunocompromised state), severity of illness, and whether the device has been left in situ. If an IVAD-related bloodstream infection is suspected, vancomycin should be initiated empirically as coagulase-negative *Staphylococcus* is the most common infectious organism and the prevalence of methicillin-resistant *S. aureus* continues to increase.[42] This should be followed by a semisynthetic penicillin or other appropriate antibiotics as guided by sensitivity studies. If the patient is severely ill, septic, in an immunocompromised state, or has a femoral catheter in place, additional coverage for gram-negative bacilli should be initiated.[42] Institute a third-generation cephalosporin unless the organism is extended-spectrum β-lactamase positive, in which case a carbapenem is more appropriate.[43] If there is concern for *P. aeruginosa* (male sex, advanced age, HD, solid organ transplant, cancer, heart disease, immunodeficiency, chronic ventilator dependence, diabetes mellitus, and chronic obstructive airway disease)[44] initiate therapy with a fourth-generation cephalosporin (e.g., cefepime) or piperacillin/tazobactam, with or without an aminoglycoside.

In addition to bacterial pathogens, fungemia should be suspected in septic patients who are receiving TPN; those with prolonged use of antibiotics; those with a history of a hematologic malignancy, or a bone marrow or solid organ transplant; or if a femoral catheter is in place.[42] If fungemia is suspected or confirmed, initiate an antifungal medication and remove the catheter. An echinocandin medication (e.g., micafungin, caspofungin) is the recommended empirical treatment of suspected fungal infection.[43]

Although there are no compelling data to specify a duration of antibiotic therapy, expert recommendation is to treat *S. aureus* infection for 14 days, gram-negative bacilli for 7 to 14 days, and candidal infection with antifungal therapy for 14 days after the first negative blood culture. Complicated infections (e.g., those with suppurative thrombophlebitis, endocarditis, or other similar infections) require 4 to 6 weeks of antibiotic treatment.[43]

If an exit site infection is suspected, any drainage from the site should be cultured in addition to obtaining blood cultures. For uncomplicated exit site infections (those lacking signs of systemic infection, positive blood cultures, or purulence) initial treatment consists of topical antimicrobials. If the infection does not resolve with topical antimicrobials, systemic antibiotics should be administered, and consideration given to removing the catheter. Patients with a tunnel infection or port abscess should have the catheter removed and receive systemic antibiotics for 7 to 10 days.[43]

If the IVAD is retained, consider antibiotic lock therapy (ALT). ALT is a therapeutic option if the goal is to salvage the catheter. Most infections in tunneled catheters originate in the hub and spread to the catheter lumen. A biofilm can form and make eradication of the organism difficult because systemic antibiotics cannot achieve therapeutic levels there. ALT involves filling the catheter hub and lumen with a higher concentration of antibiotics and leaving them in place for extended periods. It is recommended that dwell times not exceed 48 hours before reinstilling the antibiotic solution. [43,45] Dwell time should not exceed 24 hours for femoral catheters. ALT should always be used in conjunction with systemic antibiotics, and the recommended duration of treatment is 7 to 14 days. [43]

Prophylactic Measures

Antibiotic Prophylaxis During Initial Line Insertion

Prophylaxis with antibiotics during central line insertion has not demonstrated a benefit in reducing catheter-related bloodstream infections. The Centers for Disease Control and Prevention (CDC) guidelines recommend against giving antibiotics prophylactically because it is an independent risk factor for the acquisition of resistant pathogens.[46–48] In a more recent review of antibiotics in interventional radiology, routine antibiotic prophylaxis prior to vascular access device insertion was again not recommended.[49] Rather than using antibiotic prophylaxis, emphasis should be placed on interventions designed to discourage the emergence of antimicrobial resistance such as maximal barrier precautions.[50]

Impregnated Catheters

Using antimicrobial- or antiseptic-impregnated catheters or silver-impregnated collagen cuffs may be an effective intervention to reduce IVAD-related bloodstream infection. A 2013 meta-analysis favored impregnated catheters in reducing catheter-related bloodstream infections (CRBSIs), but it was acknowledged that the overall methodology of the studies included was poor.[50] A 2020 review of surface modification agents for vascular devices showed that some impregnated catheters show promise of reducing CRBSI from pathogenic bacteria; further studies are needed to confirm their ability and safety.[51] Nonetheless, the CDC currently recommends the use of these devices if the catheter is anticipated to remain in place for more than 5 days and if the institution's CRBSI rate is not decreasing after implementation of a comprehensive strategy to reduce catheter-associated infections.[48]

Lock Solution

Antibiotic antimicrobial lock solutions (AMLs) and nonantibiotic AMLs have been developed to try to reduce CRBSI rates in dialysis patients. AMLs such as gentamicin, sodium citrate, taurolidine, ethanol, and citrate-methylene blue-propylparaben (C-MB-P) have been previously studied. Despite some studies suggesting these lock solutions can reduce CRBSI rates, the CDC does not recommend using AMLs unless a patient has a history of multiple CRBSIs due to higher costs and risk of microbial resistance.[52,53]

Caps and Hubs

Caps and hubs have been developed to also reduce CRBSI rates. Most commercially available caps contain nonantibiotic antimicrobial agents such as chlorhexidine or isopropyl alcohol to kill microbes at the ports of IVADs.[53] Due to the relatively low cost and effectiveness of these hub and cap devices, they are usually changed at the treatment centers three times a week for these patients.[54]

Catheter Exit Site Interventions

Usage of chlorhexidine-impregnated dressings has been shown to markedly reduce CRBSI rates. Since a 2017 update to the CDC guideline for strategies for prevention of catheter-related infections, chlorhexidine-impregnated sponge dressings have become the standard of care to protect nontunneled catheter sites in place of usage of antibiotic ointments due to increasing concern for the emergence of resistant organisms (Fig. 24.14).[53,54]

Routine Line Changing

Due to increased risk for infections and other complications, routine changing of IVADs is not recommended. Cobb and coworkers found that replacement of IVADs every 3 days did not prevent infection and that doing so over a guidewire actually increased the risk for bloodstream infection.[55] In some patients with limited venous access or extensive thrombosis, catheter exchange over a guidewire is considered a salvage option if required.[56]

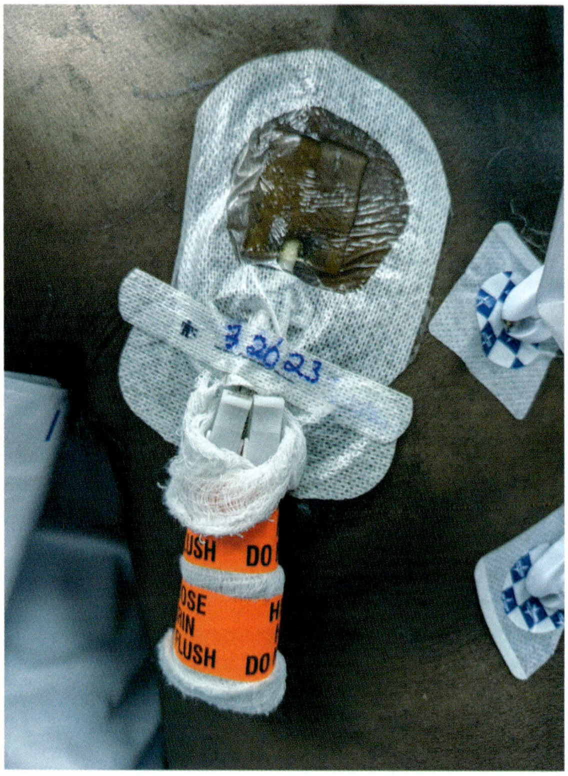

Fig. 24.14 Chlorhexidine-impregnated dressing placed at catheter exit sites have been shown to decrease infection rates.

Catheter Occlusion

Occlusion of the catheter or low flow can be caused by the following: improper positioning (Fig. 24.15), kinking, or compression of the catheter; intraluminal thrombi; extraluminal thrombi; fibrin deposits at the tip of the catheter; or intraluminal precipitation of infusate.

Pinch-off syndrome occurs when the vascular device (most often a PICC) is compressed between the clavicle and the first rib. It is manifested clinically as difficulty injecting that is related to posture.[57] Due to this "pinch-off" syndrome, subclavian vein insertion of these devices should be avoided.[58] Overzealous withdrawal of the syringe will collapse the catheter and cause occlusion. Chest radiographs may reveal scalloping of the catheter.

Maneuvers to facilitate flow of a potentially occluded catheter include the Valsalva maneuver, the reverse Trendelenburg position, slight tension on the catheter, placement of the catheter more laterally, IV hydration, and extension of the arms above the head.[59] If these measures are unsuccessful, the occlusion may be caused by clot formation.

Thrombus Formation

Thrombus formation may occur within the vascular walls or within the catheter (Fig. 24.16) (Video 24.2). It has been estimated that 4.5%to 53% of IVADs are associated with deep venous thrombosis (DVT).[60] The majority of these thrombi are asymptomatic. The incidence of clinically overt DVT has been found to range from 0.3% to 28.3%, with most studies finding the incidence to be less than 5%. After the first 2 weeks, the most common dysfunction of IVADs is caused by thrombosis.[61]

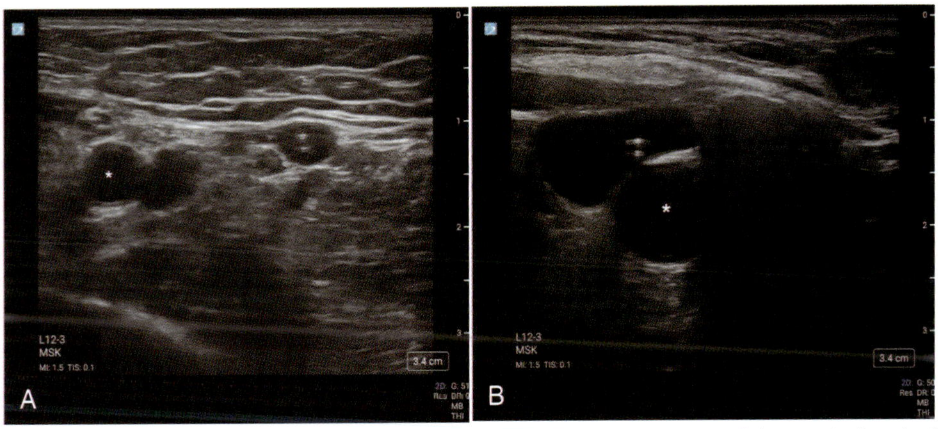

Fig. 24.15 Point-of-care ultrasound images showing improper positioning of the terminal end of a percutaneously inserted central catheter in the right internal jugular. (A) Catheter visualized in the basilic vein. *Asterisk* indicates brachial artery. (B) Distal end of catheter visualized in the internal jugular vein. *Asterisk* indicates carotid artery.

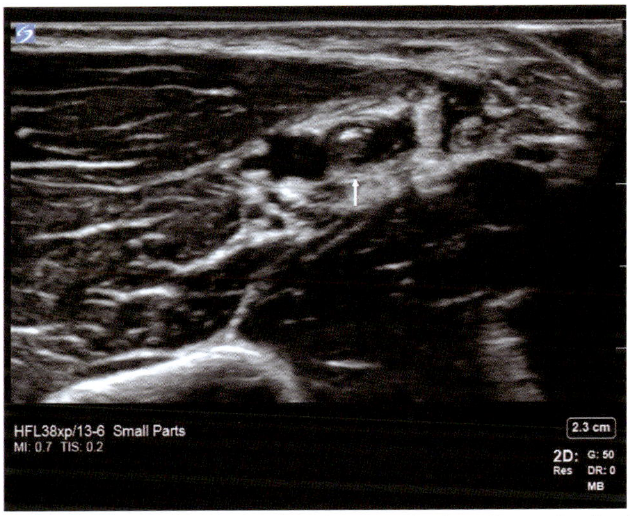

Fig. 24.16 Point-of-care ultrasound image of a thrombus at the distal end of a midline (see Video 24.2).

Risk factors for catheter-related DVT include the composition, diameter, and position of the IVAD; elevated intraluminal pressure; turbulent blood flow; vascular calcification; and endothelial injury.[61,62] Catheter material plays a role in rates of thrombosis as silicone catheters have a lower rate of IVAD-related DVT than do polyurethane, polyethylene, or Teflon-coated catheters. Other material advances such as nitric oxide-releasing or heparin-releasing catheter surface modifications have been developed to decrease thrombosis.[63] A catheter with a smaller external diameter has a lower incidence of DVT.[64] Incorrect placement of the IVAD in the SVC, as opposed to the junction of the SVC and RA, results in a higher incidence of catheter-related DVT.[65]

Clinicians should be familiar with local institutional recommendations for thrombolysis in the setting of recent IVAD occlusion attributed to a fibrin plug. Admission and consultation are usually required. Maneuvers to address clotted or occluded catheters are not a standard ED procedure but may be performed under proper circumstances and according to local guidelines. Alteplase has been shown to be both effective and safe in treating CVC occlusions caused by a clot.[66] If attempted, first withdraw any mobile clot by aspiration with a syringe. Instill 2 mL of alteplase (1 mg/mL) and allow it to dwell for up to 120 minutes. If it remains occluded, the dose may be repeated once.

Most HD access (fistula/graft) failures are related to thrombosis (60% to 85%), with greater than 90% of these thrombi associated with venous outflow stenosis.[67] Histologically, hyperplasia of the endothelium and fibromuscular vessel wall occurs. This may continue to the point of complete occlusion and prevent infusion or aspiration from the access site. Early detection may be enhanced by maintaining a high index of suspicion and noting prolonged bleeding after withdrawal of the cannula. HD access sites are routinely surveilled and monitored at treatment centers. Clinically, an absence of a thrill or change in the bruit on examination indicates occlusion of the fistula or graft (Fig. 24.17). Prompt consultation with a vascular surgeon or interventional radiology for declotting of the thrombosed access and correction of any underlying stenosis is indicated.[68] Percutaneous thrombolysis via interventional radiology has a high success rate of HD access recovery.[69]

Embolization

Serious but uncommon complications of IVAD use include air emboli, catheter fragment emboli, septic emboli, and thrombotic emboli.[59,70,71] Air embolism can occur when the lumen of the catheter is left open to air, or the catheter is fractured, perforated, or cut. The three-way valve in the Groshong catheter prevents this complication. Be careful to maintain a closed system by clamping the catheter appropriately to prevent delivery of air into the venous circulation. Should the externalized portion of a catheter be damaged, immediately place an appropriate clamp (see section on "Accessing IVADs in the ED") between the damaged portion and the skin.[72] Consider air embolism if an open or damaged catheter is found in association with tachypnea and hypotension.[73] Place the patient in a left lateral decubitus and Trendelenburg position to reduce ventricular outflow obstruction by air pockets. Initiate supportive measures, including high-flow oxygen. If this is unsuccessful, aspiration with the catheter advanced into the right ventricle may be attempted. Cardiothoracic surgery consultation and emergency thoracotomy to aspirate air (see

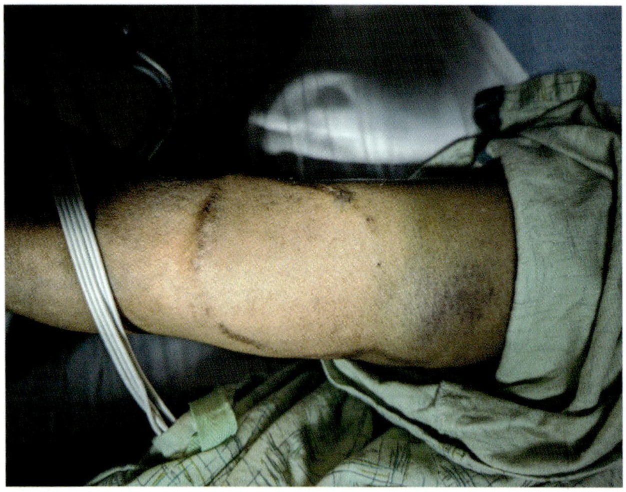

Fig. 24.17 In addition to the absence of a thrill or bruit, subtle signs of arteriovenous graft thrombosis include ecchymosis around the site.

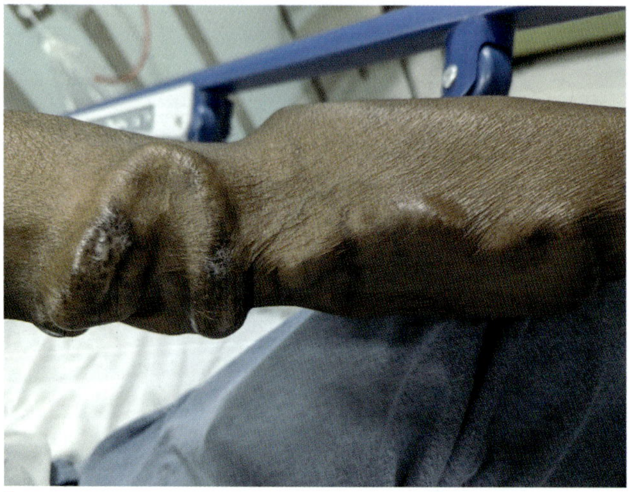

Fig. 24.18 Because of repeated access and high venous pressure, the integrity of the shunt vessel can be compromised. Pseudoaneurysms form in a synthetic graft and are covered with skin. True aneurysms form in a fistula from bulging of the entire vessel. Both can rupture. A tortuous vein under pressure can mimic an aneurysm.

Chapter 18) may be warranted. Hyperbaric oxygen therapy, when available, should also be considered.

Embolization of a catheter fragment is a potentially life-threatening complication that can cause acute dyspnea, palpitations, atypical chest pain, hypoxia, and atrial fibrillation. As with any foreign body, embolus sequelae include sepsis, lung abscess, dysrhythmias, vascular or cardiac perforation, and sudden death. Catheter fragments may be identified radiographically, or potentially by ultrasonography, and may be removed either surgically or by intravascular retrieval methods.[74,75]

Embolization of thrombi with potentially lethal sequelae may occur during routine flushing and injection of solutions through the catheter. A 2014 meta-analysis showed that when catheters were flushed with heparin or urokinase, there was a 10% to 15% rate of thromboembolism. However, when comparing different types of flushes such as heparin, urokinase, lepirudin, vitamin C, or normal saline, there was no significant difference of occlusion and thromboembolism.[76] In another 2014 meta-analysis studying thrombosis related to PICC lines, the incidence of thromboembolism was found to be 8.1% with resultant incidence of pulmonary embolism of 1.3% despite DVT prophylaxis.[77]

Hemorrhagic Complications

Bleeding may occur with any IVAD or AV shunt and is a potentially fatal complication. The mortality rate from vascular access hemorrhage is estimated to be under 1 episode per 1000 patient-years on HD.[78] Major bleeding for new AV shunts (<6 months) is approximately 4% to 4.5%.[79] Bleeding from vascular access sites is often related to mechanical trauma, transient or preexisting thrombocytopenia, uremia or drug-induced platelet dysfunction, and infection. Repeated cannulation of the fistula or graft weakens the wall of the device. Many fistulas will develop aneurysms from repeated use; synthetic grafts can develop pseudoaneurysms from frequent punctures (Fig. 24.18).

Severe life-threatening hemorrhage from this high-pressure system may occur and necessitates rapid control. The primary goal is to control bleeding and prevent exsanguination; however, care should be taken to minimize damage to the IVAD that would prevent future use. Use full universal precautions, including eye protective gear, as there is an increased risk for communicable disease in this patient population (5% for hepatitis C virus, 1.5% for HIV in the United States).[80,81] Once the bleeding stops, observe the patient for a minimum of 2 hours for evidence of rebleeding and to detect shunt thrombosis.

Treatment of hemorrhage can be divided into mechanical modalities and correction of coagulopathy.

Mechanical Treatment of Hemorrhage

Literature addressing acute hemorrhage in patients with IVADs is sparse. Many of the techniques discussed are anecdotal examples used by emergency clinicians, nephrologists, and vascular surgeons informally polled at our institutions. Individual institutional guidelines, techniques, and preferences may vary; therefore, discussion with consultants is recommended when possible.

Approach to Bleeding Complications

It is important to identify the specific bleeding site, which is challenging when hemorrhage is massive (Fig. 24.19). This is most easily accomplished by (1) applying concomitant digital pressure over the feeding and draining vessels of the shunt above and below the bleeding site (see Fig. 24.22), or (2) applying a pneumatic blood pressure cuff or tourniquet proximal and distal to the bleeding site.

The most easily controlled bleeding is typically that occurring immediately after dialysis, when the bleeding is from dialysis access puncture sites. Spontaneous bleeding between dialysis treatments often signifies more serious problems, such as infection, or mechanical problems with the access site. High pressure from venous stenosis secondary to long-term dialysis complicates the control of bleeding (Fig. 24.20).

Direct Pressure

Once the site of bleeding is found, begin management of bleeding with direct pressure. Always use sterile technique to lessen the chance of infecting a bleeding shunt. With gloved hands, apply direct pressure with fingers and a sterile gauze bandage. For bleeding AV fistulas and grafts

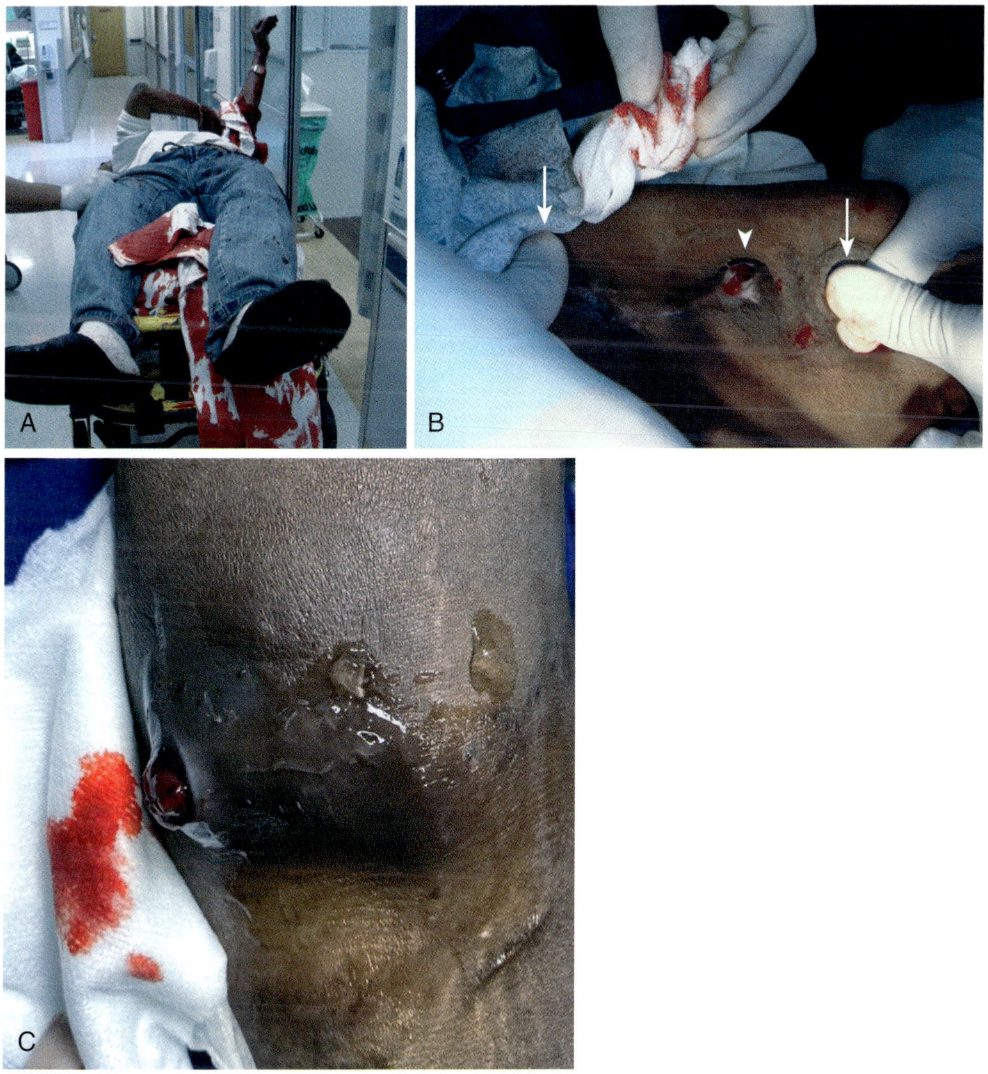

Fig. 24.19 (A) Spontaneous rupture of this fistula resulted in massive hemorrhage and hypovolemic shock. Failure to put direct pressure over the bleeding site, as indicated in B, exacerbated the blood loss. (B) This infected pseudoaneurysm *(arrowhead)* precipitated the spontaneous massive hemorrhage seen in A. The actual graft is exposed. Note that control of bleeding to identify the compromised site is achieved by firm digital pressure on the vessels on both sides of the rupture *(arrows)*. Infected grafts must be replaced. Infected fistulas may be salvaged with antibiotics. (C) Bleeding of a shunt can also signal thrombosis of a major vein.

secondary to cannulation, apply pressure focally over the site of cannulation. For tunneled catheters, apply pressure over the site of vascular entry of the catheter, not the subcutaneous exit site. Note that this is not possible with subclavian IVADs. Hold the pressure for a minimum of 5 minutes and then reevaluate for hemostasis. Holding direct pressure for extended periods or maintaining more diffuse pressure may cause thrombosis and ultimate shunt failure (a known and unfortunate risk). Wrapping the site with an elastic bandage for a few minutes is acceptable, but longer application in this broad manner may lead to the entire graft clotting.

Dialysis Clamps

Special self-retaining dialysis clamps may be applied over a specific bleeding site (Fig. 24.21). Be careful that the clamp does not slip off the bleeding site because the surface area of the clamp is small. Place sterile gauze or topical thrombin-impregnated gauze under the clamp. Ten to fifteen minutes may be required to stop the bleeding. It is best to avoid frequent checks during the first 5 to 8 minutes to avoid disrupting hemostasis.

Thrombogenic and Dermal Adhesive Agents

If venous oozing fails to stop with direct pressure, oxidized cellulose hemostatic agents (Surgicel [Ethicon], PushBan [Nipro]), chitosan polysaccharide dressings (HemCon, Greer), or a skin adhesive such as 2-octyl-cyanoacrylate (Dermabond, Ethicon) may be used to achieve hemostasis.[82] Apply topical hemostatic agents directly over the site of bleeding and hold them in place with gloved hands and a gauze bandage or clamp. If utilizing a skin adhesive, ensure that the bleeding site is free of blood (proximal and distal pressure on the shunt) and dry for the adhesive to bind.[83] After achieving hemostasis, the patient should be observed for one hour to ensure rebleeding does not occur.

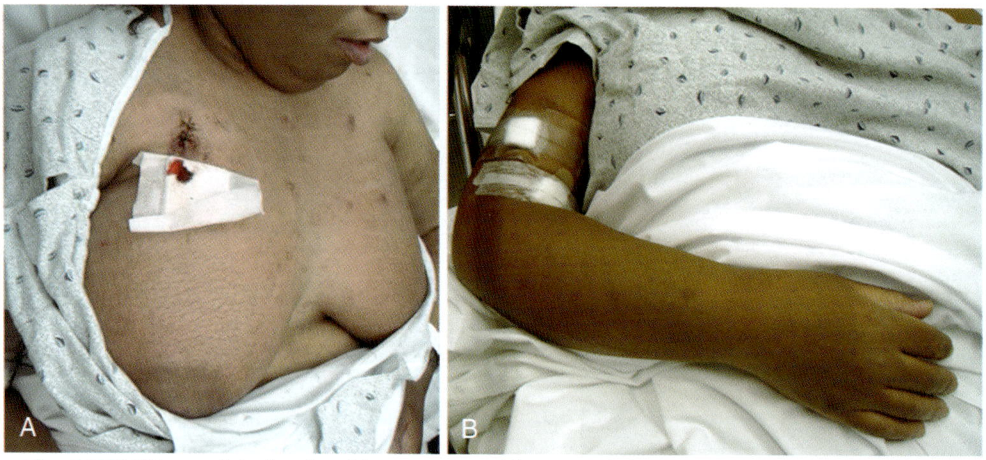

Fig. 24.20 Edema of the hand and breast occurred because of the high venous pressure of chronic venous stenosis secondary to long-term hemodialysis. (A) Obstruction of the innominate vein or superior vena cava may cause breast and face swelling, and sometimes headaches because of intracranial hypertension. This may be difficult to differentiate from thrombosis. Anticoagulation will not help this unfortunate patient. Surgical revision to divert blood flow into a patent vein is sometimes possible to restore unobstructed flow. (B) Arm edema may also be a sign of shunt infection.

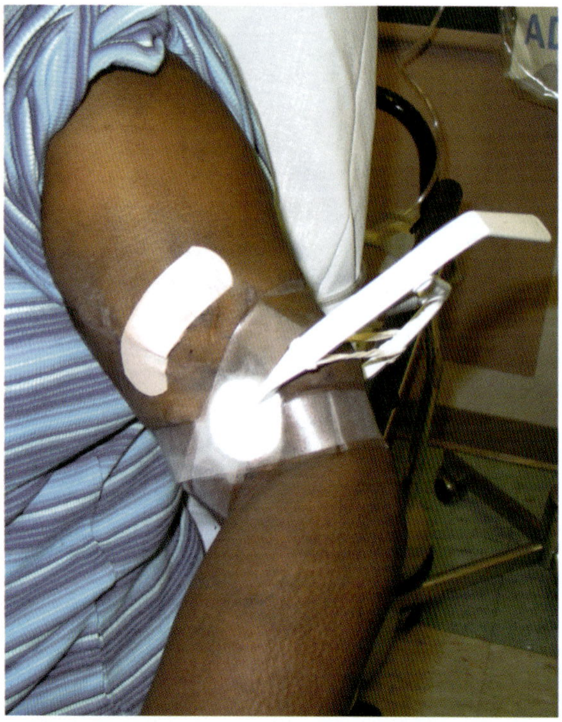

Fig. 24.21 Bleeding from a dialysis graft or fistula can be massive because of the high pressure. This dialysis graft clamp with sterile gauze (option: impregnate the gauze with topical thrombin) is kept in place for approximately 10 minutes. Other options for a bleeding graft are discussed in text. Bleeding after dialysis is related to needle size and the degree of anticoagulation, but prolonged bleeding may signal outflow stenosis, infection, or skin atrophy and the need for evaluation of the shunt.

Vasoconstrictive Agents

Subcutaneous injection of 2 to 4 mL of lidocaine 1% with epinephrine 1:100,000 to form a wheal around the site may decrease bleeding by both vasoconstriction and local pressure. This may be used in conjunction with chemical cautery.

Chemical Cautery

Silver nitrate ($AgNO_3$), a mildly caustic and hemostatic agent, may stop residual bleeding. The agent needs to be protected from light until just before use. When ready, remove the wooden stick from the container and black plastic wrap and gently apply the gray-tipped end directly on the site. Do not apply it aggressively because this can result in dissolution or dislodgement of the formed clot.

Once the bleeding is controlled, rebleeding is infrequent. It is prudent to observe the patient for 1 hour and have the patient walk around and use the arm gently to ensure that bleeding will not recur when discharged. If no bleeding recurs, discharge is appropriate unless precluded by other conditions.

Suture

If direct pressure and previously mentioned techniques fail to achieve hemostasis, suturing may be necessary (Video 24.3). Inject the bleeding site subcutaneously with lidocaine 1% with epinephrine 1:100,000. Place a figure-of-eight or horizontal mattress suture with 4-0 nonabsorbable polypropylene or nylon (noncutting needle) at the site of bleeding (Fig. 24.22). The noncutting needle is very important to prevent further damage to the shunt. Be careful to suture as superficially as possible to prevent damage to the underlying graft or fistula (Video 24.4). The patient may require a venogram for evaluation of shunt patency before use. The sutures will require removal in 2 to 4 days and should have follow-up with their vascular surgeon prior to vascular use to ensure patency.

Perchik Button

A vascular control button, such as the Perchik Button, can assist the emergency physician in rapid control of hemorrhage after HD access. Additionally, this tool reduces the rate of superficial tissue damage and increases the ability to easily remove sutures.[84] The vascular access buttons are most often used for dialysis care. It has the added benefit of decreasing stenosis and thrombosis with grafts and fistulas.[85]

When utilizing the Perchik Button, use sterile technique. Apply the button over the access site, flat side down. Feed the

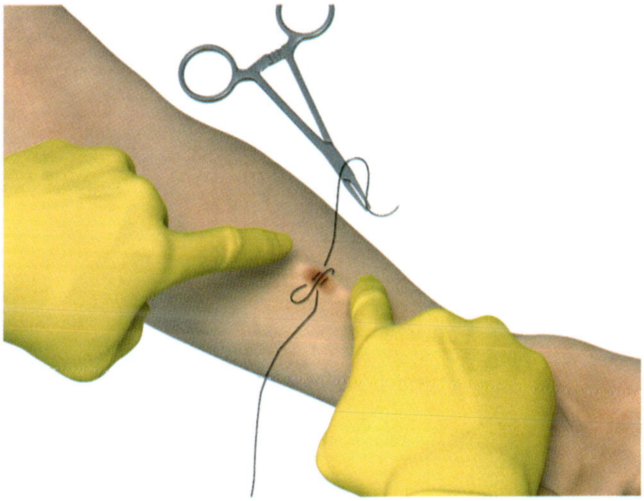

Fig. 24.22 To suture a bleeding dialysis shunt, instruct an assistant to apply proximal and distal pressure to stem the flow of blood and then inject the site with lidocaine with epinephrine. Place a figure-of-eight (shown) or horizontal mattress suture as superficially as possible to prevent damage to the underlying graft or fistula.

suture ends through the holes on the button. Secure tails with the secured knot over the crevice on the top of the Perchik Button (Video 24.5). If a Perchik button is not available, a regular 2-hole or 4-hole button (one which is normally used on clothing) may be used in its place. This device can be left in place for a short period of time. For example, it may be removed at the next dialysis session. When removing the button, scissors or scalpels should always be guided with the cutting edge of the blade pointing upwards beneath the suture knot. If using a scalpel, draw the blade up through the knot while moving the cutting edge away from the patient.[85]

Woggle Technique

Should an emergency physician encounter continuous bleeding after catheter insertion, temporary direct pressure should be applied to achieve hemostasis. If this fails, a technique utilized by interventional radiologists may be considered. The Woggle technique is completed by placing a suture through the skin and guiding a curved noncutting needle underneath the catheter and back through the skin. It is important to ensure that your noncutting needle passes underneath the catheter when placing the suture to avoid damage to the catheter. Ensuring to leave tails on both ends of the suture, remove the needle and pull the ends of the sutures up and away from the patient. Twist the suture and maneuver both ends of suture through a standard three-way stopcock ensuring that the side port is turned to the open position. Push the stopcock against the skin and then turn the lever on the stopcock causing it to apply pressure against the area of hemorrhage (Video 24.6). Bleeding should be controlled with adequate pressure. Secure the device and reassess the bleeding after 15 to 30 minutes by rotating the stopcock in reverse. If bleeding resumes, rotate the stopcock again in the original manner for an additional 15 to 30 minutes and reassess.[86] Once bleeding is resolved, the suture can be pulled out after opening the stopcock. This technique can also be used for bleeding AV shunts. However, for this purpose, the suture is not passed under the shunt, but rather superficially to provide direct pressure on the site of bleeding (this is essentially an easily removed figure-of-eight technique described earlier). The advantage is that if bleeding is persistent after a check, the three-way stopcock can be secured again without having to reapply sutures.

Correction of Coagulopathy

Control of hemorrhage may require treatment of an underlying coagulopathy. HD patients are generally considered to be at increased risk for bleeding because of uremic platelet dysfunction. The incidence of major bleeding in these patients is increased with the concomitant use of anticoagulant medications.[87] Perform laboratory testing for evaluation as follows: complete blood count, blood urea nitrogen, prothrombin time, international normalized ratio (INR), partial thromboplastin time, and other tests depending on the patient's medical history or presenting signs. The only lab abnormality may be the bleeding time, which does not result immediately. Consult nephrology, vascular surgery, or both (if possible) before reversing therapeutic anticoagulation given the potential for shunt thrombosis as well as the need for close follow-up.

Uremic Platelet Dysfunction

If platelet dysfunction is suspected because of uremia, administer desmopressin (DDAVP]) or cryoprecipitate to control the hemorrhage.[88] Adult dosing of DDAVP to control uremic bleeding is 0.3 µg/kg intravenously as a single dose diluted in 50mL 0.9% saline administered over 15--30 min that may be repeated if needed. Onset occurs in 1 to 2 hours, and its duration is 6 to 8 hours after a single dose.[89] Disadvantages include high cost and adverse reactions, including anaphylaxis, hyponatremia, and thrombotic events (rare). Use of DDAVP may be most appropriate if the platelet count and standard coagulation profile is otherwise normal.

Heparin-Associated Coagulopathy

Heparin is routinely administered during dialysis, and although there is no standardized dosing there are common regimens, which include providing an initial bolus (25 to 30 IU/kg) followed by intermittent, lower dose boluses (500 to 2000 IU) or an initial bolus followed by a continuous infusion.[90] Heparin is usually stopped approximately 1 hour before the end of dialysis, and hence heparin-related bleeding is unusual in the ED. If uncontrollable bleeding occurs in the context of recent heparin use (within 48 hours), reversal of heparin's effect with protamine sulfate may be necessary. Administering 1 mg of protamine sulfate will effectively reverse the anticoagulant effect of 100 units of unfractionated heparin. Protamine is less efficacious in the reversal of low-molecular-weight heparins. Nonetheless, current recommendations are to administer 1 mg of protamine for every 1 mg of low-molecular-weight heparin that the patient received not exceeding 50 mg total.[91]

Warfarin and Other Anticoagulant-Associated Coagulopathy

The use of warfarin and direct oral anticoagulants (DOACs) predisposes patients to potentially serious bleeding complications. In an actively bleeding patient on warfarin with an elevated INR, immediate reversal of the medication's effect can be achieved with fresh frozen plasma or prothrombin complex concentrates (PCCs). PCCs have the advantage of requiring less total volume to achieve reversal of anticoagulation and therefore less risk for volume overload.[92] Vitamin

K should also be considered for reversal, following warfarin-associated bleeding guidelines. DOACs may require specific reversal agents or PCCs depending on the type. Risk of clotting exacerbation versus the benefit of reversal should always be considered before systemic anticoagulation reversal.

Catheter Displacement or Malposition

The catheter should be firmly secured with sutures, sterile tape strips (with care taken to avoid direct contact with the catheter itself), or specific manufactured devices.[93] Even with these measures disruption of placement may still occur. With regard to TIVADs, malposition of the intravascular portion may occur as a result of incorrect initial positioning or secondarily from forceful flushing, neck flexion, obesity, severe coughing, emesis, or upper extremity movement. Malposition of the port body may occur intentionally or by unintentional manipulation of the port (Twiddler's syndrome). Obtain a computed tomography scan of the chest to diagnose this condition. Surgical intervention is usually necessary.[94]

Catheter Fracture

Fracture of an IVAD can occur either subcutaneously or in the externalized portion.[95] While it may take place with certain physical activities that involve repetitive and excessive motion such as golfing, swimming, and weightlifting, most fractures occur during insertion or removal.[96] Subcutaneous fractures cause pain and swelling and require removal of the line. Fractures in the externalized portion may be repaired with commercially available kits and do not always require replacement. In rare cases, fractured parts of IVADs can embolize and cause complications, which will require surgical or endovascular intervention.[97]

Steal Syndrome

Vascular steal syndrome is an uncommon but serious complication of AV shunts, which is difficult to predict and may lead to access failure or distal extremity ischemia.[98] It occurs because of preferential flow through the low-resistance fistula at the expense of the distal circulation. The syndrome is manifested by classic arterial insufficiency symptoms with exacerbation during dialysis: pain, pallor, numbness, motor weakness, and diminished or absent pulses distal to the shunt.[99] Steal syndrome must be differentiated from diabetic or uremic neuropathy because it may lead to the development of irreversible neuromuscular dysfunction, tissue necrosis, and amputation. Prompt recognition and correction of hand ischemia leads to increased salvage and use of functioning shunts. Steal syndrome usually requires ligation of the AV access with placement of a new access device in the opposite extremity.

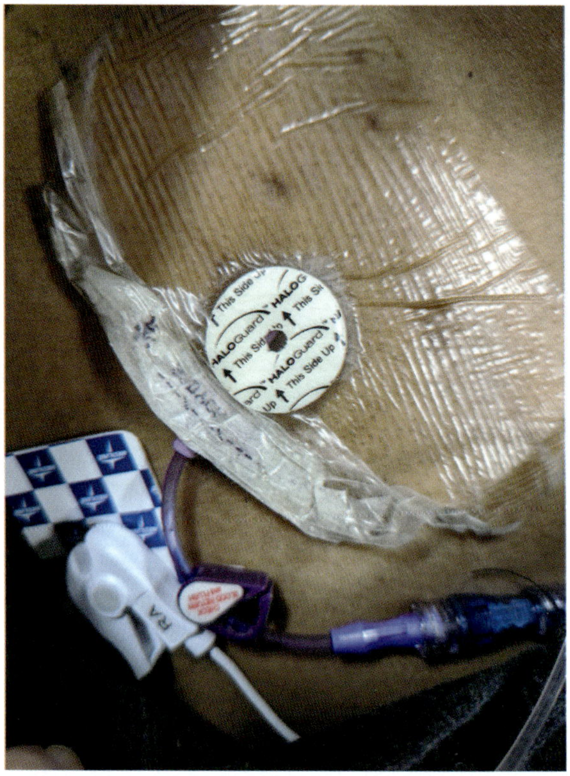

Fig. 24.23 It can be difficult for patients to keep their indwelling vascular access device exit site properly maintained. If you notice a catheter site that is improperly dressed, as in this example, make extra effort to redress the site in proper sterile fashion.

AFTERCARE INSTRUCTIONS

ED providers should be familiar with and be able to instruct the patient regarding proper catheter care to prolong the device's lifetime, and to decrease morbidity and mortality.[100] Patients may bathe and swim normally after maturation of AV shunts or TIVADs; they should avoid direct pressure on the reservoir and report bruising or bleeding immediately. Long-term venous access catheters and multilumen catheters should be dressed in sterile fashion (Fig. 24.23) and observed daily for bleeding and signs of infection, including fever, pain, redness, swelling, and purulent drainage. IVADs should be gently flushed on a routine basis, per instructions given when they are placed.[101] Heparin flushes are essential to prevent thrombosis. Tunneled (e.g., Hickman) and nontunneled (e.g., PICC) catheters require flushing twice weekly. TIVADs require flushing with heparin every 4 weeks and after use. Generally, Groshong catheters are flushed with 5 mL of saline once weekly. Mahurkar and Uldall catheters are flushed during dialysis. Mahurkar catheters are also used for apheresis, in which case they are treated three times a week with normal saline and heparin, as outlined earlier. As many different practice variations exist, concentration and volume of heparin should always be confirmed with institutional protocols (especially in pediatric patients). Patients should not allow phlebotomy or infusion into an extremity with an IVAD, with the exception of phlebotomy in the ipsilateral dorsum of the hand. Blood pressure measurement should be avoided in an extremity containing an AV shunt. Finally, practice sterile technique, use care in handling, and avoid use unless an emergent situation requires access of the IVAD.

ACKNOWLEDGMENT

We gratefully acknowledge the photo/video submissions from Al Sacchetti, MD, Earl "Quinn" Cummings, MD, and Kaitlyn Pereira, MD. We also acknowledge the work of the authors of this chapter in previous editions of this text.

REFERENCES ARE AVAILABLE AT Elsevier eBooks+

CHAPTER 25

Intraosseous Infusion

Kenneth Deitch

Establishing vascular access in critically ill and injured patients is central to the practice of emergency medicine. Moreover, placing an intravenous (IV) catheter in an acutely ill child can be one of the most challenging and frustrating procedures that a clinician can be called on to perform. Children have small peripheral vessels that collapse during shock, and their higher proportion of body fat makes visualization and palpation of peripheral vessels difficult. These factors often result in prolonged attempts and high failure rates.

In a review of vascular access success rates in children in cardiac arrest, the average time needed to establish percutaneous peripheral IV access was 7.9 ± 4.2 minutes, with only a 17% success rate.[1] Some authors advocate the use of central venous lines in children, but such lines are also difficult to place and are associated with risk for arterial injury, infection, and pneumothorax. Alternative routes of drug administration, such as the endotracheal and rectal routes, are not reliable in patients in shock or cardiac arrest.[2]

Peripheral IV access can also be difficult in adults, including those with an elevated body mass index, have burn injuries, are volume-depleted, or are in shock.[3] This difficulty is compounded in the prehospital or military setting, where environmental factors and the need for rapid transport can challenge even the most skilled practitioners.[4]

Intraosseous (IO) access can provide rapid, lifesaving intravascular access in challenging environments and in both pediatric and adult patients. All drugs and fluids that are delivered through a peripheral or central venous line can also be administered through an IO cannula. Drug and fluid dosing is the same as for IV administration. The serum concentrations and onset of action of IO-administered medications during cardiopulmonary resuscitation (CPR) are comparable to those achieved with IV administration. Per animal studies, the IO route is as effective as central venous administration and may be superior to the peripheral IV route during cardiac arrest.

The American Heart Association, the American Academy of Pediatrics, and the American College of Surgeons all recommend IO access in children in emergency situations when IV access is not immediately possible.[5,6] The latest edition of the advanced trauma life support course of the American College of Surgeons also notes that IO access using specially designed equipment is an important option in adult trauma patients.[5] IO access is often faster than IV access, and the success rate after failed IV attempts is high. In a retrospective study of pediatric cardiac arrest patients, time to IO access was significantly shorter than time to IV access.[7] In a similar review of intravascular access during pediatric cardiac arrest, Brunette and Fischer[1] noted that when compared with central venous access and venous cutdown, IO access and IV access were faster, and the success rate for IO access was 83% versus 17% for IV access. IO access can also be a rapid and successful technique in adults.[8] IO success rates are twice as high as IV line placement in critical trauma patients who do not have a measurable blood pressure and IO access should have priority over IV placement.[9] Because of their success under difficult battlefield conditions, the US military has adopted the use of IO infusion devices.[5]

IO access is not always successful. In a 5-year review of prehospital IO needle placement, success rates were higher in children younger than 3 years (85%) than in older children or adults (50%).[7] The main causes of failure were errors in identification of landmarks and bending of the needles. Better needle design and new devices have helped overcome problems with bone penetration (see later section on "Equipment and Setup").

IO needle insertion has been shown by multiple studies to have high success rates when placed by physicians, nurses, and paramedics in multiple populations including adults, and children, animals, as well as simulation model studies.[10,11] Despite its ease of use and high success rates, IO access is underutilized.[12] Barriers to the use of IO insertion include a lack of confidence in the indications for IO access and the belief that nurses do not have familiarity with IO access and care.[13] For IO access to serve as a useful and efficacious lifesaving tool, the entire health care team should optimally be educated on the process. Only small case series have been conducted to attempt to increase training and comfort levels in establishing IO access.[14] A few studies have attempted to draw stress correlations between individual and team performances. They have shown those who are more confident and less stressed perform better in establishing IO access.[14] Emergency medical service (EMS) personnel, medical providers, and nursing staff should be trained on the speed, ease of use, and ability to infuse mediations or fluids via IO access.

HISTORICAL PERSPECTIVE

One of the earliest references describing the IO route is attributed to Drinker and colleagues,[15] who examined the circulation of the sternum in 1922 and suggested it as a site for transfusion. The route was not used clinically until 1934 when Josefson,[16] a Swedish clinician, injected liver concentrate into the sternum of 12 adult patients with pernicious anemia and reported that all 12 improved. Subsequently, the technique became widespread in Scandinavian countries. In 1944 British physician Hamilton Bailey[17] described the utility of sternal IO access in blackout conditions in London during World War II.

In 1940, the technique was introduced to American clinicians by Tocantins and associates,[18–20] who described a series of animal and clinical studies demonstrating that fluid is rapidly transported from the medullary cavity of long bones to the heart. They recommended using the manubrium in older children and adults and the upper part of the tibia or lower part of the femur in children 3 years or younger. Over the next two decades, thousands of cases of IO infusion of blood, crystalloid substances, and drugs were reported.[21–25] The procedure was more commonly used in children because of the difficulty in achieving other forms of IV access. Nevertheless, during the 1940s IO infusion was also used extensively in adults, and a sternal puncture kit for bone marrow infusion was a common component of emergency medical supplies during World War II.[4,26] This resulted in more than 4000 reported cases of successful IO access in wounded soldiers.[25] During this time relatively few complications were reported despite the fact that the needles were often left in place for 24 to 48 hours. In 1947

Heinild and coworkers[23] reviewed 982 cases of IO infusion and reported only 18 failures and 5 cases of osteomyelitis. None of the cases of osteomyelitis occurred in patients who received isotonic solutions.

With the introduction of plastic catheters and improved cannulation techniques, the need for IO infusion as an alternative route for IV access diminished, and the technique was all but abandoned. In the mid-1980s James Orlowski brought about a renaissance in the use of IO access for pediatric resuscitation. While traveling through India during a cholera epidemic, he observed emergency health care workers using IO access to deliver fluids and medications. In 1984 he wrote an editorial, "My Kingdom for an Intravenous Line,"[26] in which he advocated the use of IO access during pediatric resuscitation. After Orlowski's editorial, others began promoting the use of IO access to allow rapid drug delivery during CPR in children.[1,27,28] In 1988 IO techniques were adopted by the American Heart Association and included in the pediatric advanced life support guidelines.[6] Since then the technique has become widespread throughout the United States and is recognized as an accepted alternative to IV access in pediatric emergencies, and, increasingly, in neonatal and adult emergencies. In addition, the safety, ease, and effectiveness of the technique have led to its use in prehospital emergency care.[7,29–32]

ANATOMY AND PHYSIOLOGY

Long bones are richly vascular structures with a dynamic circulation. They can accept large volumes of fluid and rapidly transporting fluid or drugs to the central circulation. The bone, like most organs, is supplied by a major artery (nutrient artery). The artery pierces the cortex and divides into ascending and descending branches, which further subdivide into arterioles that pierce the endosteal surface of the stratum compactum to become capillaries. The capillaries drain into medullary venous sinusoids throughout the medullary space, which in turn drain into a central venous channel (Fig. 25.1). The medullary sinusoids accept fluid and drugs during IO infusion and serve as a route for transport to the central venous channel, which exits the bone as nutrient and emissary veins.[33] The medullary cavity thus functions as a rigid, noncollapsible vein, even in the presence of profound shock or cardiopulmonary arrest.[34] Radiographic studies have demonstrated that radiopaque dye spreads only a few centimeters in the medullary space before being transported to the venous system.[35]

Almost every drug and fluid commonly used during resuscitation has been reported upon in clinical and preclinical IO studies. Essentially, all medications and fluids that might be delivered via a venous line can also be

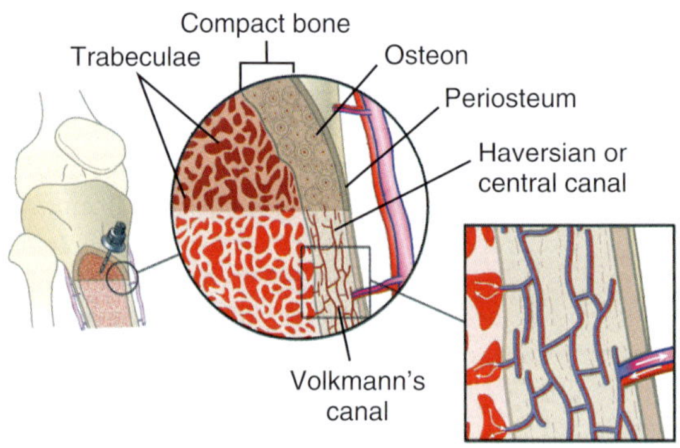

Fig. 25.1 Vascular anatomy of a long bone with an intraosseous needle in place.

Intraosseus Infusion

Indications

Emergency intravascular access when other methods have failed
Cardiac arrest in infants and young children
Military applications
Obtaining blood for laboratory evaluation

Contraindications

Osteoporosis and osteogenesis imperfecta
Fractured bone
Prior use of same bone for IO infusion
Cellulitis or burn overlaying insertion site

Complications

Technical difficulties	*Soft tissue and bony complications*
Over-penetration	Infection
Incomplete penetration	Bony inflammatory reaction
Needle obstruction	Skin sloughing
Fluid extravasation	Compartment syndrome
	Epiphyseal injury
	Fat embolism
	Pain with infusion

Equipment

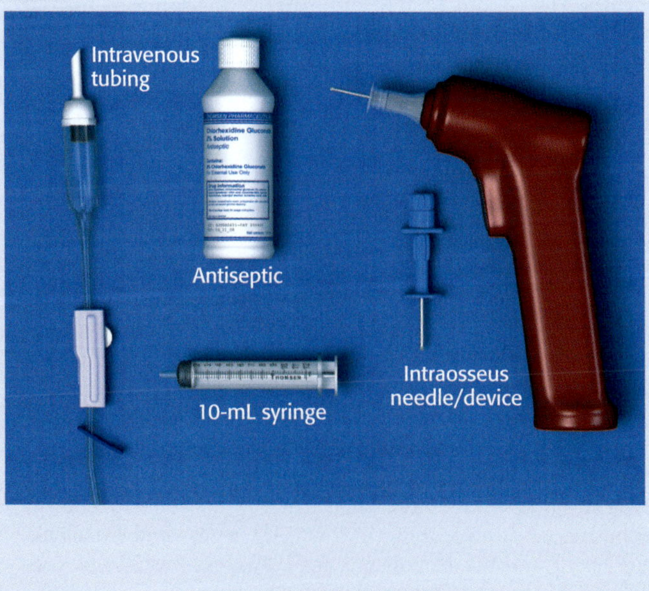

Review Box 25.1 Intraosseous infusion: indications, contraindications, complications, and equipment.

BOX 25.1 Medications and Fluids That Can Be Administered Intraosseously

MEDICATIONS

Adenosine
Antibiotics
Antitoxins
Anesthetic agents
Atracurium besylate
Atropine
Calcium chloride
Calcium gluconate
Contrast media
Dexamethasone
Diazepam
Diazoxide
Digoxin
Dobutamine
Dopamine
Ephedrine
Epinephrine
Heparin
Insulin
Levarterenol
Lidocaine
Lorazepam
Mannitol
Morphine
Naloxone
Pancuronium
Phenobarbital
Phenytoin
Propranolol
Sodium bicarbonate
Succinylcholine
Thiopental
Vecuronium

FLUIDS

Crystalloids

Dextrose solutions
Sodium chloride solutions
Lactated Ringer's solution

Colloids

Blood and blood products
Packed red blood cells
Plasma

Data from Getschman SJ, Dietrich AM, Franklin WH, Allen HD. Intraosseous adenosine. As effective as peripheral or central venous administration? Arch Pediatr Adolesc Med. *1994;148:616-619; and Sawyer RW, Bodai BI, Blaisdell FW, McCourt MM. The current status of intraosseous infusion.* J Am Coll Surg. *1994;179:353-360.*

administered through the IO route. Dosing of IO medications and fluids is the same as for IV administration. Medications and fluids that have been administered through IO infusion are listed in Box 25.1. Crystalloid infusion studies in animals have demonstrated that infusion rates of 10 to 17 mL/min may be achieved with gravity infusion and rates as high as 42 mL/min with pressure infusion.[36–38] In a swine model of hemorrhagic shock, Neufeld and colleagues found that the IO delivery rate of crystalloid was similar to peripheral and central venous administration.[37] IO crystalloid infusions have also been shown to produce a significant increase in blood pressure in a hemorrhagic shock model in rabbits.[38] In small animals (7 kg to 8 kg), the size of the marrow cavity is the rate-limiting factor, whereas in larger animals (12 kg to 15 kg), the size of the needle determines the flow.[39,40] Blood under pressure can be infused approximately two-thirds as fast as crystalloid fluids.[39] However, in a swine model evaluating IO infusion for mild therapeutic hypothermia, IO infusion of ice-cold saline was not as efficacious as IV infusion.[41]

Comparisons of IO and IV infusion of drugs have demonstrated that the drugs reach the central circulation by both routes in similar concentrations and at the same time.[20,42] This holds true even during CPR, during which sodium bicarbonate has been shown to provide greater buffering capacity when administered by the IO route than by the peripheral IV route.[43] Early IO access and infusion of epinephrine improved 24-hour survival in a swine model of ventricular fibrillation versus delayed IV administration.[44] IO infusion of iodinated computed tomographic contrast material has also been reported as being successful,[45] as has scorpion antivenin.[46] In a porcine model of septic shock, IO and IV infusions had similar peak concentrations.[47] IO infusion of intralipid reversed bupivacaine toxicity in a rat model.[48] Cyanide toxicity reversal with hydroxocobalamin has been shown to be equally efficacious between the IO and IV routes in a porcine model.[49] IO administration has been successfully used for rapid sequence intubation.[50] IO injection of iodinated computed tomography contrast agent in an adult blunt trauma patient has also been shown to be successful.[51]

Voelckel and associates demonstrated that bone marrow blood flow responds to both the physiologic stress of hemorrhagic shock and vasopressors given during resuscitation after hypovolemic cardiac arrest in dogs.[42] After successful resuscitation, bone marrow blood flow decreased after high-dose epinephrine but was maintained after high-dose vasopressin. These findings in animal models suggest the need for pressurized IO infusion techniques during hemorrhagic shock and certain drug therapies.

INDICATIONS

When children or adults need immediate resuscitation and IV access cannot be achieved quickly or reliably, the IO route provides a rapid and effective means of administering drugs, fluid, and blood (Review Box 25.1). Once the patient has been stabilized, percutaneous peripheral or central intravascular access may be achieved.

Obtaining venous access can be a difficult task even under the best circumstances. This difficulty is compounded during high-stress situations or low-flow states such as cardiac arrest. Studies have shown that IO devices provide a rapid and effective means of fluid and drug administration during pediatric CPR.[1] This is also true during resuscitation of critically injured infants and children in whom IO infusion of blood, colloids, or crystalloids (or any combination thereof) may be lifesaving. IO infusion is also beneficial in the management of children with other medical conditions, including those with respiratory distress, neurologic insults, dehydration, and sepsis.[52–54] The widespread use of IO devices has led to improved prehospital vascular access and a marked reduction in critical transport with failed vascular access.[55]

IO access is not commonly used in infants, but it is recommended as an alternative for medication and crystalloid administration when venous access is not readily obtained.[56] IO infusion has been used with success in both premature and term infants.[57–59] In one study, 30 IO lines were placed in 20 preterm and 7 full-term neonates with a variety of illnesses (e.g., respiratory distress syndrome, perinatal asphyxia, congenital cardiac anomalies) in whom conventional venous access had failed.[60] All survived resuscitation with no long-term effects from IO line placement. Gestational age ranged from 32 to 41 weeks and birth weight ranged from 515 g to 4050 g.[60] In 2000 Abe and coworkers reported on the speed and ease of establishing newborn emergency vascular access by using turkey bones and plastic infant legs to simulate IO access and fresh umbilical cord to simulate umbilical venous catheterization.[59] They demonstrated that for individuals who do not perform newborn resuscitation frequently, IO placement was easier and quicker than umbilical venous catheterization. A comparison of umbilical venous versus IO access in a simulated model of neonatal resuscitation showed that IO access was faster with no difference in error rate or perceived difference in ease of use.[60]

IO infusion is also indicated for adult patients in whom attempts at peripheral or central venous access have been unsuccessful. This may include adult patients with burns, trauma, shock, dehydration, or status epilepticus.[61] IO placement for resuscitation has been shown to be significantly faster than central line placement, with a significantly lower failure rate.[62] Multiple sites including the iliac crest, femur, proximal and distal ends of the tibia, humeral head, radius, clavicle, and calcaneus may be used.[63–66] Of these, the tibia may be less desirable because red marrow is replaced by less vascular yellow marrow or fat by the fifth year of life. In contrast, the sternum has been advocated as the best site to establish IO access in adults because it is large and flat and can readily be located.[67] In addition, the sternum's cortical bone is thin (1 mm to 2 mm) and the marrow space relatively uniform (6 mm to 11 mm).[68]

There has also been renewed interest in IO access by the US military. In addition to logistic constraints that limit the volume of isotonic crystalloid fluids available to resuscitate injured soldiers, hypotension, environmental and tactical conditions, and the presence of mass casualties can lead to excessive delay in obtaining vascular access.[4] The Army Institute for Research has compared several IO infusion devices, including the FAST-1 IO Infusion System (Teleflex), the Bone Injection Gun (BIG; PerSys Medical), the Sur-Fast hand-driven threaded needle (Cook Critical Care), and the Jamshidi straight needle (Allegiance Health Care).[62] Success rates with these devices were similar (94% to 97%), and all were inserted in less than 2 minutes. The participants rated no individual device as being significantly better than the others. It was concluded that each device was easy to master and could be used appropriately during special operations when IV access could not be accomplished.[62] The US Army Committee on the Tactical Combat Casualty Care (TCCC) guidelines (2010) recommends using IO infusion in any resuscitation scenario in which IV access is not obtainable.[69]

In addition to serving as a route for fluid administration, the IO needle may be used to obtain blood for typing, crossmatching, and determining blood chemistry in the marrow cavity. Serum electrolyte, blood urea nitrogen, creatinine, glucose, and calcium levels are very similar to those in samples obtained from an IO aspirate.[70–72] Blood gas values obtained from the IO site were similar to those obtained from central venous sites during steady and low-flow states in one animal model.[73] Brickman and colleagues[74] demonstrated that bone marrow aspirates obtained from an IO needle in the iliac crest could be used reliably to type and screen blood for transfusion. Animal studies have shown expected values for blood gases, creatinine, sodium, and creatinine kinase in stable and hemorrhagic swine models, but lactate and glucose values vary.[75] Potassium values seem to be generally higher in IO samples compared with arterial and venous values in several studies.[76] Blood typing is accurate even after blood transfusion through an IO device in a patient in shock, allowing type and crossing to be performed even after emergent transfusion.[77] A complete blood cell count may not be reliable because it reflects the marrow cell count rather than the cell count in the peripheral circulation. Furthermore, the aspirated blood usually clots within seconds, even if placed in a tube that contains heparin.

CONTRAINDICATIONS

Relatively few contraindications to IO infusion exist. Osteoporosis and osteogenesis imperfecta are associated with a high potential for fracture. Therefore, unless absolutely necessary, the procedure should be avoided when these diagnoses are known. A fractured bone should be avoided because as fluid is infused, it increases intramedullary pressure and forces fluid to extravasate at the fracture site. This may slow the healing process, cause nonunion of the bone, or lead to a compartment syndrome. A similar extravasation of fluid can occur through recent IO puncture sites placed in the same bone. Hence, recent use of the same bone for IO infusion represents a relative contraindication to IO line placement. Needle insertion through areas of cellulitis, infection, or burns should also be avoided. Patients with right-to-left intracardiac shunts (e.g., tetralogy of Fallot, pulmonary atresia) may be at higher risk for fat or bone marrow embolization.[78,79]

EQUIPMENT AND SETUP

The following is a review of products currently available for IO infusion. Information regarding the use of these products is limited, and few prospective studies have compared IO needles or devices in clinical practice. Until more information becomes available, practitioners are encouraged to review the products available and choose those that best meet their needs.

IO Needles (Fig. 25.2)

Needles used for IO access range in size from 13- to 20-gauge and must be sturdy enough to penetrate bone without bending or breaking. They must also be long enough to reach the marrow cavity. Standard needles used for drawing blood or administering medications are not adequate for IO infusions; they are not sturdy enough to penetrate bone and do not have a stylet to prevent bone from plugging the lumen. A cadaver study of IO puncture suggested that nonstyletted needles (2.5-cm, 18-gauge phlebotomy needles and 7.6-cm, 14-gauge IV needles) enter the marrow space successfully only approximately half the time.[80] In the past, an 18-gauge spinal needle was commonly used in children younger than 12 to 18 months. This needle, although readily available in most emergency departments (EDs), often bends, is too long for rapid infusion of fluid, and has a greater risk for occlusion from clotted blood.[81] Very small butterfly needles have been used with success in preterm infants.[82]

Bone Marrow Aspiration Needle

Bone marrow aspiration needles can be used if needles specifically designed for IO access are not available. These needles

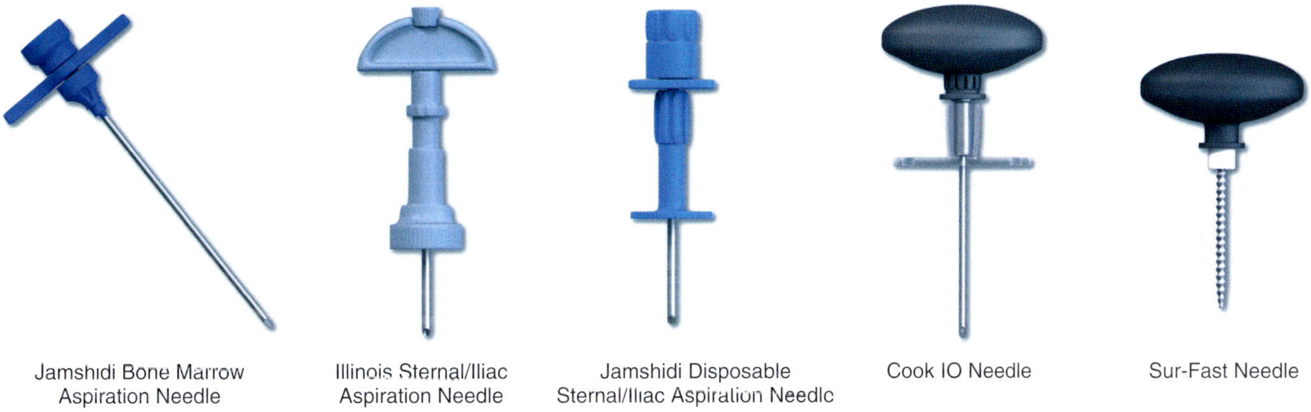

Fig. 25.2 Various intraosseous needles.

are large enough (16 gauge) to be used in older children and adults and are suitable for rapid administration of fluid.

Illinois Sternal/Iliac Aspiration Needle

The Illinois Sternal/Iliac Aspiration Needle (Monojet, Sherwood Medical) was designed for bone marrow aspiration but can be used for IO infusion. The needle is available in both 16- and 18-gauge. It has an adjustable plastic sleeve to prevent the needle from penetrating through the opposite bony cortex. However, its long shaft and poorly designed handle make it prone to dislodgement during transport and other procedures.

Jamshidi Disposable Sternal/Iliac Aspiration Needle

Like the Illinois Sternal/Iliac Aspiration Needle, the Jamshidi Disposable Sternal/Iliac Aspiration Needle (Cardinal Health) was designed for bone marrow aspiration, but it has a shorter shaft and smaller handle, which makes it easier to use. It comes in either 15- or 18-gauge and features an adjustable plastic sleeve to prevent overpenetration. Once inserted the needle protrudes approximately 2 inches from the skin, which increases the risk for accidental dislodgement. In a study using a turkey bone model participants rated the Jamshidi needle easier to use than the Cook IO needle.[83]

Cook IO Needle

The Cook IO needle (Cook Critical Care) is specifically designed for IO insertion and infusion. It comes in a variety of sizes from 18- to 14-gauge and can be inserted to a depth of 3 cm to 4 cm. It has a detachable handle, which reduces the risk of it being dislodged, and a depth marker to help ensure proper placement.

Sur-Fast Needle

The Sur-Fast needle (Cook Critical Care) is also specifically designed for IO insertion and infusion. It has a threaded shaft that helps secure the needle in the bone and a detachable handle that may be reused with multiple needles. In a study by Jun and associates,[84] the Sur-Fast IO needle had a success rate similar to that of a standard bone marrow aspiration needle.

IO Devices

FAST-1 Intraosseous Infusion System (Fig. 25.3)

The FAST-1 Intraosseous Infusion System (Teleflex) uses an impact-driven device designed for sternal placement only. The FAST-1 has been used successfully by both military and prehospital care providers.[62,85] In one prehospital study, flow rates of 80 and 150 mL/min were obtained by using gravity and a pressure bag, respectively.[86] In a prospective prehospital evaluation, the mean time to successful placement was 67 seconds.[87] The device has a series of stabilizing probes that help maintain good contact with the sternum and serve as the depth control mechanism for insertion of the needle. These probes use the surface of the manubrium rather than the patient's skin to ensure the proper depth of insertion. Once the device is positioned against the sternum, additional pressure triggers the release of a hollow needle into the medullary space. The needle comes preconnected to IV tubing. The handle is automatically released from the stylet and infusion tubing once the needle has met its preset depth. Removal of the needle requires a threaded tool provided with the device. The FAST-1 is larger and heavier than other IO devices and once triggered cannot be reused.

Bone Injection Gun

The BIG (PerSys Medical) is another spring-loaded, impact-driven device that comes in both pediatric and adult sizes (Fig. 25.4). Like the FAST-1 system, this device is designed for single use only. An advantage of the BIG is the ability to adjust the depth of insertion, which allows it to be used at different sites (e.g., tibia, humerus). However, if the device is not carefully stabilized before and during insertion, incorrect placement can occur. In addition, there is the potential for operator and patient injury if the device is accidentally triggered or mistargeted.[87] In a prospective, prehospital setting the BIG device was shown to have a 71% success rate in children and a 73% success rate in adults.[88] In another prehospital study, 91% of 181 patients had successful insertion on the first attempt.[89]

EZ-IO Device (Fig. 25.5)

The EZ-IO device (Teleflex) is a handheld, battery-powered device that drills an IO needle to the appropriate depth in the IO space. The EZ-IO device allows the operator to control the pressure or force used during insertion.[90] Placement can be achieved in less than 10 seconds in the vast majority of patients, with first-time successful insertion rates ranging from 77% to 97%.[90–93] In the United States, the EZ-IO has been approved for use at

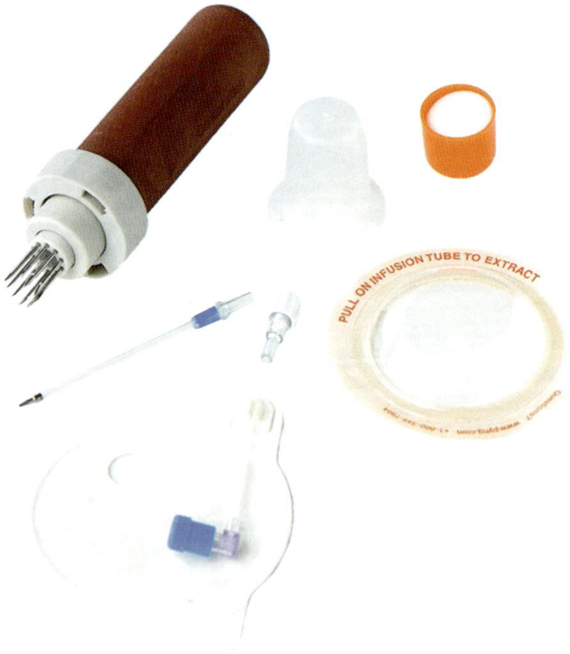

Fig. 25.3 FAST-1 intraosseous infusion system. (Courtesy Teleflex, Morrisville, NC.)

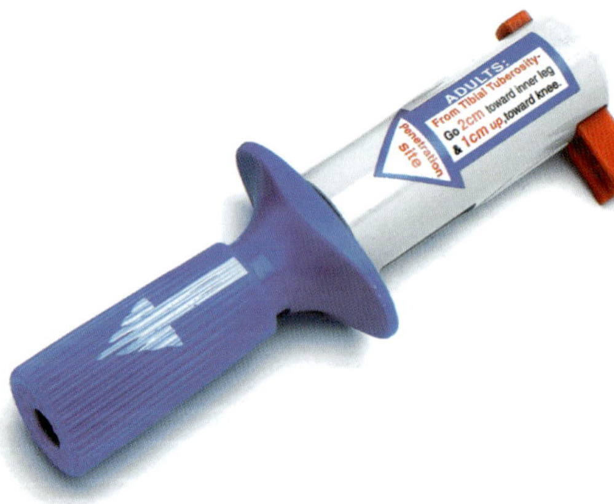

Fig. 25.4 Bone injection gun. (Courtesy PerSys Medical, Houston, TX.)

two anatomical sites, the proximal tibia and the humeral head.[34] The EZ-IO has been shown to have a first-pass success rate in the prehospital setting of 84% to 92%.[94] The limitation of this device is cost and the inability to replace the drill battery.

NIO Device

The New Intraosseous (NIO) device (PerSys Medical) is a Food and Drug Administration (FDA)-approved device that is spring-loaded and used primarily for tibial insertion (Fig. 25.6). It can also be used in the humerus. It is lightweight, does not require batteries, and is a self-contained unit designed for single use and ease of deployment. There is some early published evidence that suggests that it has comparable successful deployment rates for both tibial and humeral placement as the EZ-IO.

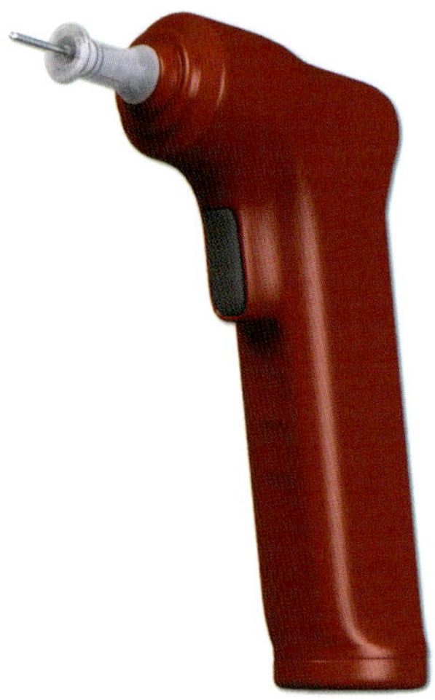

Fig. 25.5 EZ-IO device. (Courtesy Teleflex, Morrisville, NC.)

Comparative Trials Between Devices

The effectiveness, speed, and complication rates of manually placed versus mechanical drill-assisted IO catheters by emergency medicine resident physicians were compared in a 2013 study.[95] The mechanical placement was shown to be significantly faster (3.66 vs. 33.57 seconds, $P = .01$), the Jamshidi 15G needle, the FAST-1, and the BIG were compared in a helicopter-based emergency service system. In this randomized controlled trial, the Jamshidi needle and the FAST-1 had similar success and complication rates. However, the Jamshidi needle was placed significantly faster than the FAST-1. Frascone and colleagues conducted two sequential prospective nonrandomized trials to compare the FAST-1 with the EZ-IO, both in the prehospital setting. Of 178 IO insertions evaluated, 64 of the 89 FAST-1 insertions were successful as were 78 of the 89 EZ-IO insertions (72% vs. 87%). During the 5-year study period, 11 technical complications were recorded with the EZ-IO and 25 with the FAST-1. There were no differences in provider comfort or provider assessed device performance between the two devices. The BIG has also been compared to the EZ-IO in the adult population in two randomized trials. Twenty patients were treated with the BIG and 20 with the EZ-IO, with success rates in the first attempt of 85% and 90%. Mean procedure time was 2.2 min ± 1.0 for the BIG, versus 1.8 min ± 0.9 for the EZ-IO. Five technical problems were reported with the BIG, none with the EZ-IO. In five patients who were treated with the BIG, the stylet became stuck within the cannula and could only be removed with a clamp.[63] In a large multiyear retrospective analysis of a trauma database, rates of success on first attempt were significantly higher with the EZ-IO compared with the manual needle and the BIG. Overall success rates were 50% with the manual needle, 55% with the BIG, and 96% with the EZ-IO.[96]

Simulation Studies Comparing Devices

In a simulation cadaver model laboratory with US military providers, four IO devices were compared: the FAST-1, the BIG, the hand-driven threaded Sur-Fast needle, and the Jamshidi needle. High success rates were recorded for all four devices (94% to 97%), but the BIG had the fastest placement time. In another randomized crossover study, the BIG and the EZ-IO were tested on a turkey bone model. Study results showed that the EZ-IO had a one-attempt success rate of 96.5% (28/29)

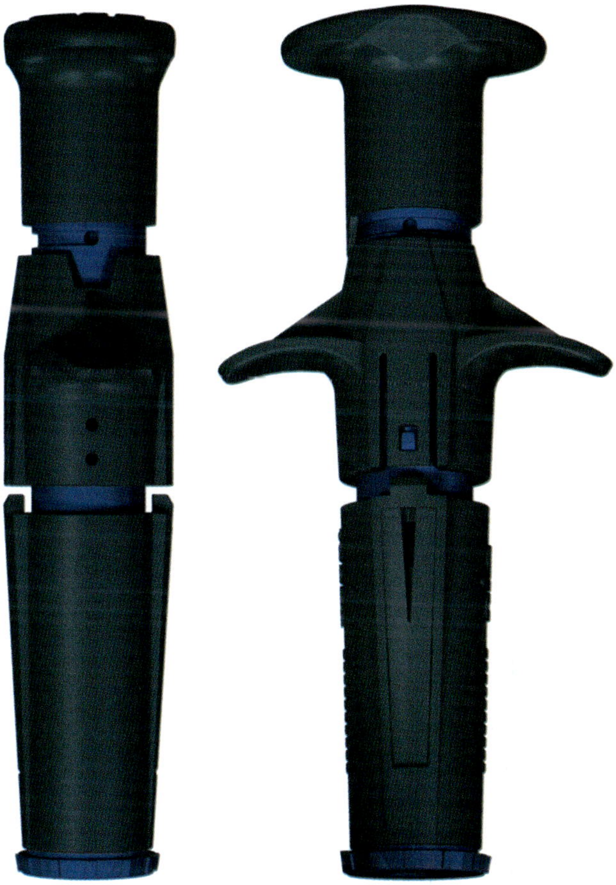

Fig. 25.6 NIO device (PerSys Medical, Houston, TX).

compared to 65.5% (19/29) for the BIG, and that nearly 70% of the study subjects chose the EZ-IO as their preferred device. Six technical complications were reported with BIG, none with the EZ-IO.[97] In another study, using a cat cadaver model, the EZ-IO, the BIG, and the Jamshidi manual needle were compared. This study showed a higher success rate with the EZ-IO than the other two devices (96% vs. 75% and 88%, respectively).[98] In another simulation study using paramedics, the BIG had the highest success at first pass (91%), versus the EZ-IO (82%) and the Jamshidi needle (47%).[99]

PROCEDURE

Sites for IO Needle Placement

The patient's age and size are the two most important factors when choosing the best site for needle penetration. In infants and children younger than 6 years, the proximal end of the tibia is the preferred site, followed by the distal ends of the tibia and femur. Other sites such as the clavicle and humerus have been used, but neither has gained popularity. In adults, the distal part of the tibia has been the most common site for IO access. However, with the introduction of spring-loaded and drill devices, IO locations once reserved only for children are now also potential sites in adults. In addition, the FAST-1 system makes the sternum a simple and effective location for IO access in adults.[91]

Proximal Tibia

The tibia is a large bone with a thin layer of overlying subcutaneous tissue that allows landmarks to be palpated readily. Insertion here does not interfere with airway management or CPR. This is one of the most common infusion sites. On the proximal end of the tibia, the broad, flat, anteromedial surface is used, and the tibial tuberosity serves as a landmark. The site of IO cannulation is approximately 1 cm to 3 cm (2 finger widths) below the tuberosity (Fig. 25.7A). This location is far enough away from the growth plate to prevent damage, but it is in an area where the bone is still soft enough to allow easy penetration with the needle. In adults, penetrating the thick bone in the proximal end of the tibia is much more difficult and requires a 13- to 16-gauge needle. A spring-loaded device such as the BIG or a battery-powered drill such as the EZ-IO can make penetration much easier and allows the use of smaller-gauge needles. In a comparison of first-attempt success between tibial and humeral IO insertion during out-of-hospital cardiac arrest, tibial placement was significantly more successful (90%) than humeral placement (60%) with a lower rate of needle dislodgement.[100]

Distal Tibia

The distal end of the tibia, although a preferred site in adults, may also be used in children.[81,101] The cortex of the bone and the overlying tissue are both thin. The site of needle insertion is the medial surface at the junction of the medial malleolus and the shaft of the tibia, posterior to the greater saphenous vein (see Fig. 25.7B). The needle is inserted perpendicular to the long axis of the bone or 10 to 15 degrees cephalad to avoid the growth plate.[102]

Distal Femur

The distal portion of the femur is occasionally used as an alternative site in children, but because of thick overlying muscle and soft tissue it is more difficult to palpate bony landmarks (see Fig. 25.7C). If chosen, the needle should be inserted 2 cm to 3 cm above the femoral condyles in the midline and directed cephalad at an angle of 10 to 15 degrees from the vertical.[103]

Humerus

See Videos 25.1, 25.2. The proximal end of the humerus is an option for IO access that is well tolerated and easily accessed. The proximity of the greater tubercle of the humerus to the heart provides rapid infusion of medication and fluid into the general circulation. The humerus has been shown to be an effective site relative to peripheral or central access in a prospective resuscitation model.[103,104] A study evaluating flow rates through all three sites in a porcine model showed that the proximal humerus had almost double the flow rate than either the tibial or distal femur site.[105] In a retrospective study in a prehospital setting of cardiac arrest, IO insertion into the humerus had a higher success rate than into the proximal tibia.[100] However, in another study first-pass success for humeral placement in a paramedic performed prehospital population during cardiac arrest was over 90%.[106] The patient's arm should be placed such that the hand is resting on the patient's umbilicus, with some adduction. Medial rotation of the humerus will allow better identification of the proximal humeral head. The humerus is most easily palpated at the insertion point for the deltoid muscle, between the biceps and triceps muscles. This point is approximately midway along the length of the arm. Palpation of the bone requires pressure because of overlying structures. The surgical neck can be located by palpating up the length of the humerus until the clinician feels a notch or groove. The appropriate insertion

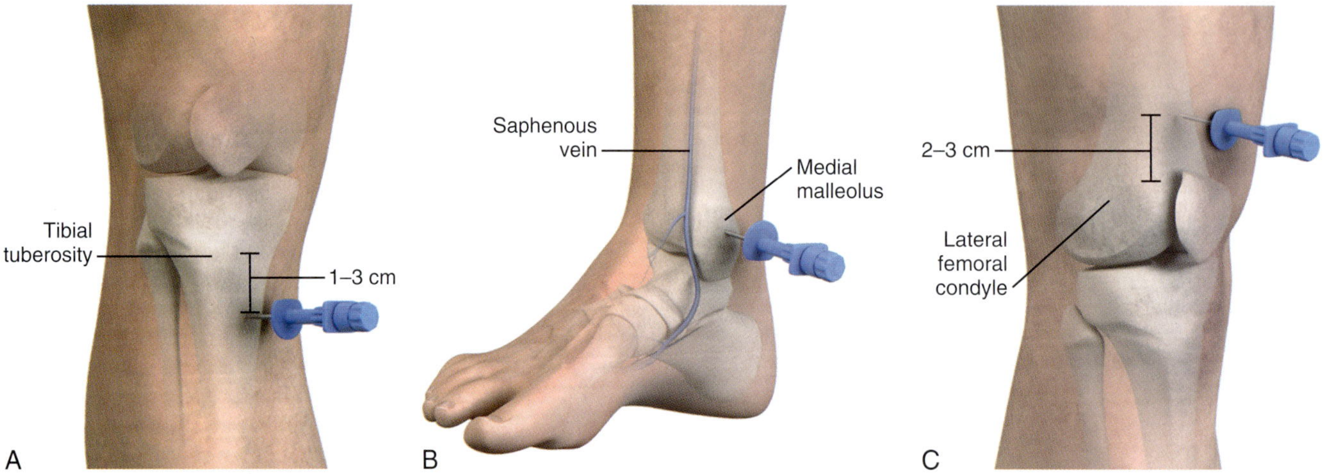

Fig. 25.7 Intraosseous (IO) insertion sites. (A) Proximal tibia. Insert the IO needle 1 cm to 3 cm distal to the tibial tuberosity and over the medial aspect of the tibia. Direct the bevel of the needle away from the joint space. (B) Distal tibia. Insert the IO needle on the medial surface of the distal end of the tibia at the junction of the medial malleolus and the shaft of the tibia, posterior to the greater saphenous vein. Direct the needle cephalad, away from the growth plate. (C) Distal femur. Insert the IO needle 2 cm to 3 cm above the femoral condyles in the midline and directed cephalad away from the growth plate.

site is approximately 1 cm above the surgical neck for most adults (see Fig. 25.12). A study evaluating the humeral head approach during tactical situations was shown to have a 96% first-pass success rate using an EZ-IO, and a 90% success rate using a manual driver.[107]

Sternum

The sternum has several advantages over peripheral bones but is rarely used in the ED. Its advantages include a large, relatively flat body that can be readily located; retention of a high proportion of red marrow, which allows rapid transfer of infused fluids and drugs to the central circulation; and thinner, more uniform cortical bone overlying a relatively uniform marrow space. In addition, the sternum is less likely to be fractured in major trauma.[85] Introduction of the FAST-1 System, which allows safe and effective penetration of the sternum, has led to increased use and popularity of sternal IO insertion in adults.

Other Sites

Other sites, including the clavicle and calcaneus, can be used as alternatives, but these sites are less popular.

Site Preparation

To prepare the proximal end of the tibia or distal end of the femur for IO insertion, place a small support such as a towel roll behind the knee. Cleanse all insertion sites with chlorhexidine, povidone-iodine, or an alcohol-based antibacterial solution. If the patient is conscious, anesthetize the skin and periosteum.

Manual Needle Insertion

See Fig. 25.8. Before insertion stabilize the site with the free hand (i.e., the hand not holding the IO needle) and use it to identify the landmarks. For example, during the proximal tibia insertion, stabilize the proximal end of the tibia with the thumb and index finger of the free hand and use them to palpate the tibial tuberosity (the main bony landmark for proximal tibia insertion). During insertion avoid injury to this hand by keeping it out of the plane of insertion and clear of the puncture site. Direct the IO needle perpendicular (90 degrees) to the bone's long axis and slightly caudad (60 to 75 degrees). Directing the needle slightly caudad helps avoid penetration of the growth plate. Advance the needle with a twisting or rotating motion (but not a rocking motion) to drive it into the bone and to puncture the cortex. Once the cortex has been penetrated, there will be a sudden decrease in bony resistance and a "crunchy" feeling as the needle enters the marrow cavity. Penetration of the inner cortex usually occurs at a depth of approximately 1 cm.

Aspirate for blood or marrow contents (or both) to confirm correct placement; however, aspiration may not always produce blood even with a properly placed IO needle. Other signs of correct placement include the needle's ability to remain upright without support and to have free-flowing fluid without signs of extravasation into surrounding tissue. Note that some resistance to flushing is expected because the bone marrow is not distensible.[108,109]

Once proper placement is confirmed, secure the needle and tubing with tape. Fasten the leg to an appropriately sized leg board to further stabilize a lower extremity insertion site in infants and small children. Protect the needle from accidental dislodgement by cutting the bottom out of a plastic cup and taping and bandaging the cup in place over the device. Commercially made shields are also available for this purpose. Remove the IO needle as soon as IV access has been secured and apply a sterile dressing over the site. Control excessive bleeding by applying direct pressure over the site for 5 minutes.[110]

USE OF SPECIFIC IO DEVICES

FAST-1

See Fig. 25.9. The FAST-1 device (Teleflex) was designed specifically to penetrate the sternum.[68,111] It is prepackaged

Manual Intraosseous Needle Insertion

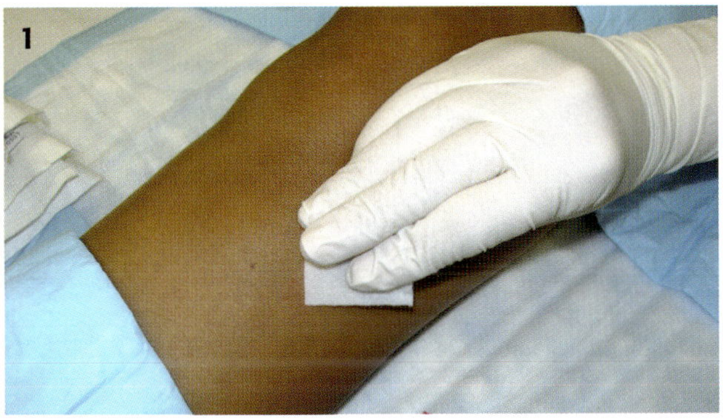

Cleanse the skin with antiseptic.

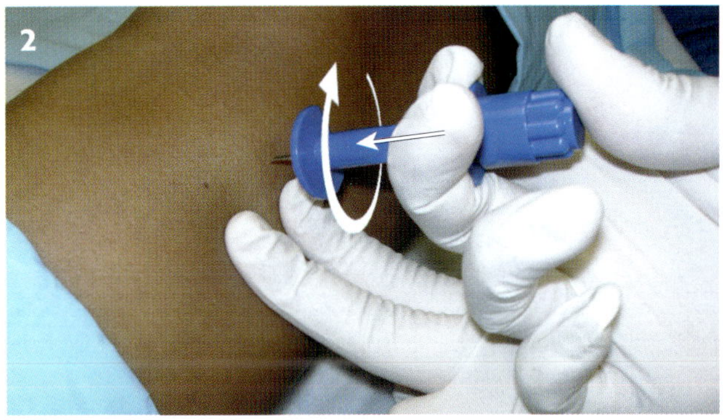

Stabilize the leg and identify the tibial tuberosity with your free hand. Insert the needle perpendicular or slightly caudad with a twisting or rotating motion.

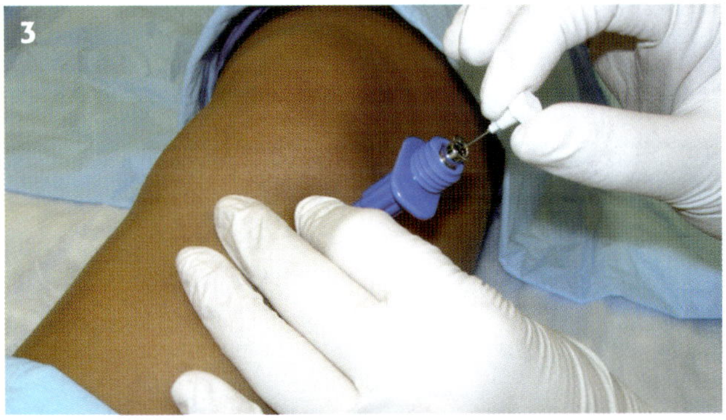

Remove the stylet once the cortex is penetrated (feel for a decrease in resistance and a "crunchy" feeling).

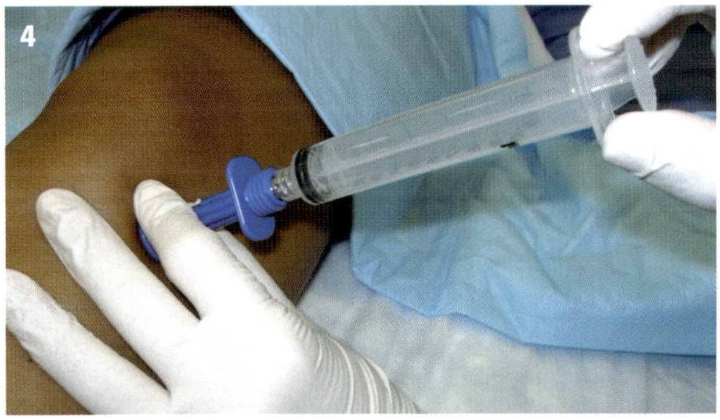

Aspirate blood and/or marrow to confirm the correct position. If the patient is awake, very slowly infuse 2–5 mL of 2% lidocaine a few minutes prior to infusion. Flush the needle with 10 mL of saline to prime the infusion.

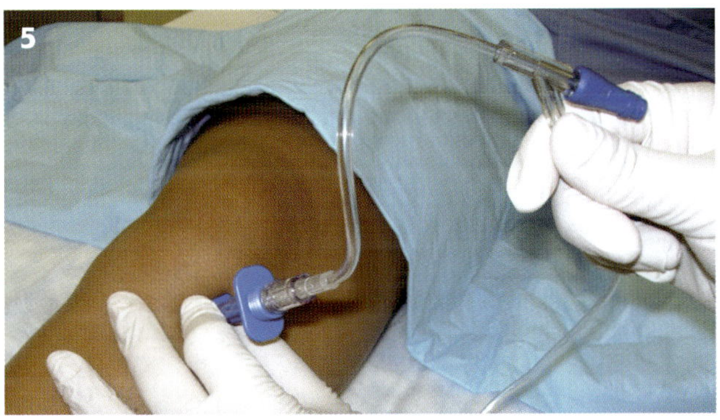

Connect the IV tubing to the needle.

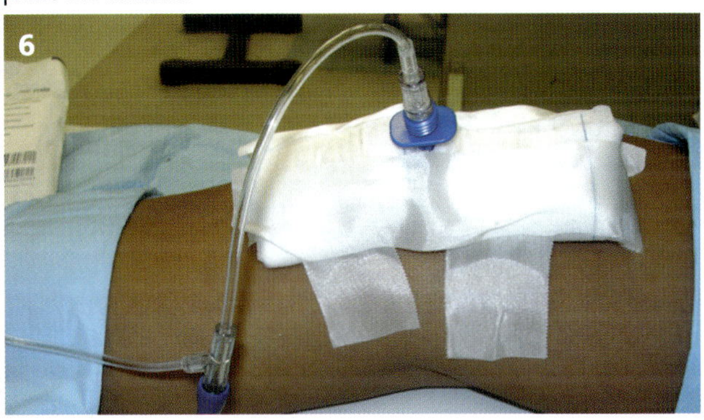

Secure the IO needle in place with tape.

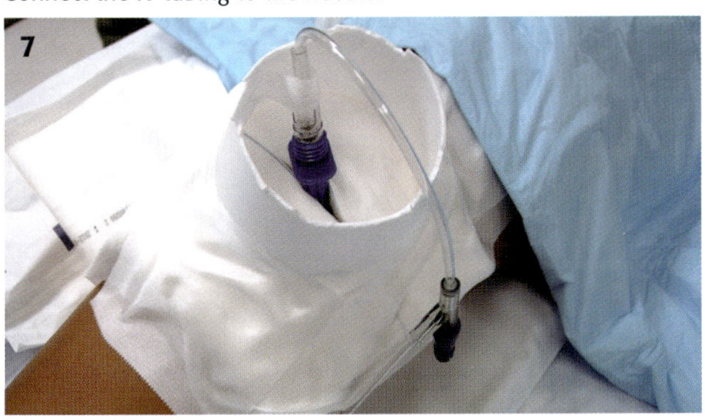

Protect the needle from dislodgement with a plastic cup in which the bottom has been cut out, and then tape and bandage if in place over the needle.

Fig. 25.8 Manual intraosseous (IO) needle insertion. *IV*, Intravenous.

FAST-1 Intraosseous Device

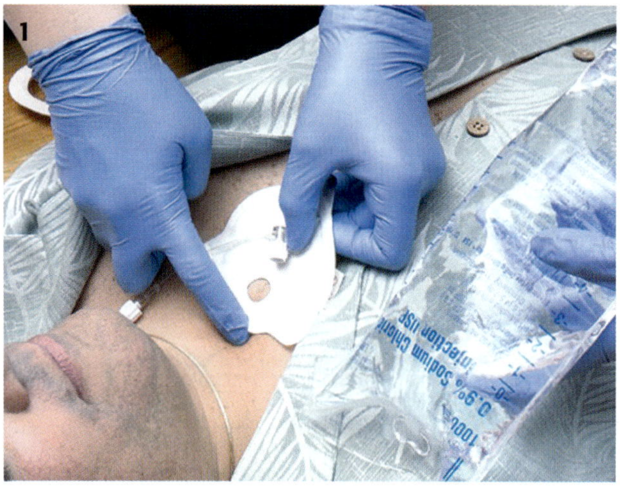

Cleanse the overlying skin with antiseptic and then place the adhesive target patch over the midline of the manubrium; the target hole should be approximately 1.5 cm below the sternal notch.

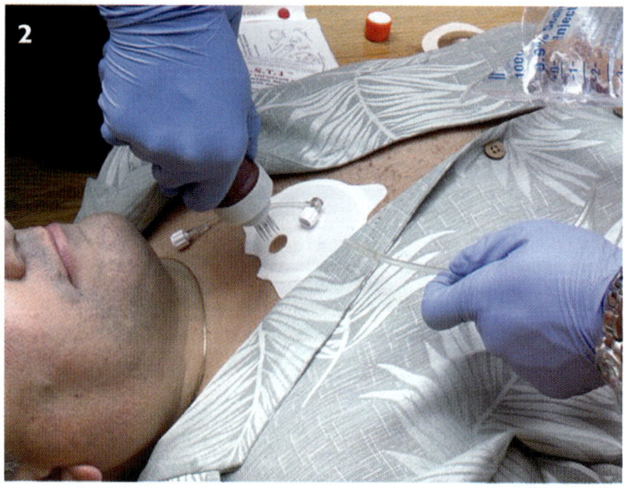

Place the introducer in the center of the target zone. Apply pressure to the handle to release the needle. The central IO needle will advance to the cortex-medullary junction.

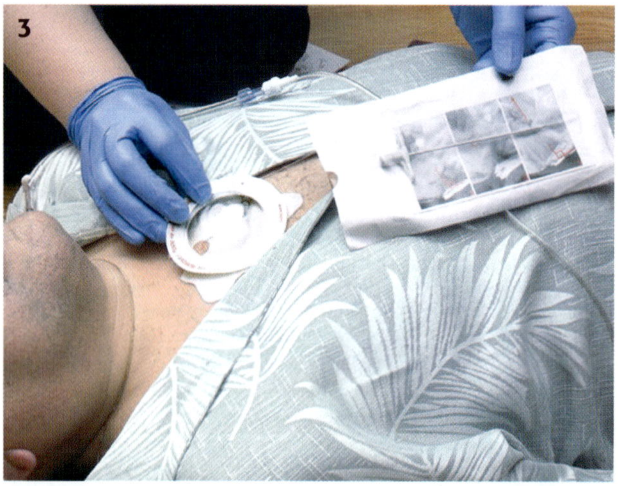

Attach the plastic dome to the target patch to secure the tube in place.

Fig. 25.9 Insertion of the FAST-1 intraosseous device (Teleflex, Morrisville, NC).

with alcohol and iodine and comes with a protective dressing to hold the device in place. It also includes a threaded-tip remover for easy removal of the metal tip and infusion tubing.

After disinfecting the skin site over the sternum, place the target patch over the midline of the manubrium with the hole in the middle of the target approximately 1.5 cm below the sternal notch. Next, place the FAST-1 introducer in the center of the target zone. The introducer has a "bone cluster" of needles that form a circle. These needles "sense" the cortex of the sternum and help ensure proper needle depth. Once the introducer is in position over the target zone, apply pressure to the handle to release the inner needle located in the center of the bone cluster. This needle has a small metal tip that is preconnected to plastic infusion tubing. After release, the central IO needle will advance 5 mm beyond the circular cluster of needles, stop at the bony cortex, and position the metal tip at the cortex-medullary junction. At this point withdraw the handle so that only the plastic infusion tube is left protruding from the insertion site. Marrow aspiration and rapid flow of fluid help verify the appropriate position. Attach the plastic dome to the target patch via Velcro fasteners and secure the tubing in place. Removal of the infusion tube requires the use of a threaded-tip remover, which is included. The tube can also be removed by directly pulling it; however, the metal tip is sometimes left behind and must be extracted through a small incision.[67]

BIG

See Fig. 25.10. The BIG (PerSys Medical) incorporates a loaded spring to facilitate penetration of the bone (see instruction video at https://persysmedical.com/products/vascular-access/bone-injection-gun-adult/). To adjust the depth of insertion, remove the safety pin from one end and turn the other end clockwise or counterclockwise to reduce or increase needle depth, respectively. Place the BIG firmly against the skin perpendicular or slightly caudad to the long axis of the bone. Fire the gun by applying palmar force on the back of the unit and pulling on the flanges with the middle and ring

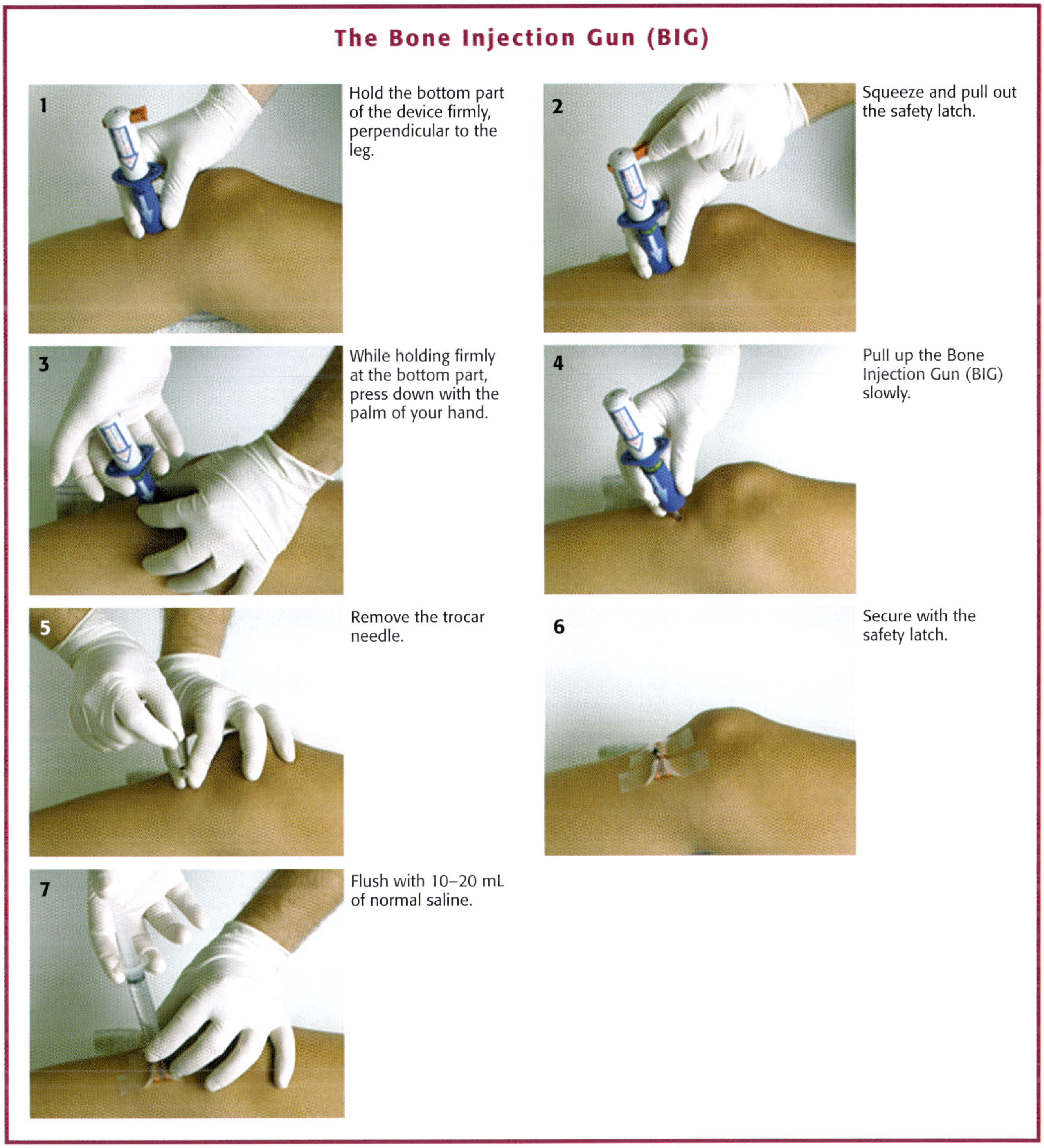

Fig. 25.10 Use of the bone injection gun (PerSys Medical, Houston, TX).

fingers. Confirm placement by aspirating marrow, flushing with the same syringe, and observing flow through the IV tubing. Slide the slotted safety pin into the needle to maintain stability. To remove the needle, rotate it back and forth using the small clamps provided with the unit. Dress the site in a manner determined by the care provider.

EZ-IO Needle

See Figs. 25.11 and 25.12 and Videos 25.3–25.8. This battery-operated "drill" can drive the IO needle through thick bone with relative ease. The EZ-IO kit comes with a battery-operated drill and an IO needle with a stylet. The EZ-IO AD (adult) comes with a 15-gauge, 25-mm IO needle for use in patients heavier than 40 kg, and the EZ-IO PD (pediatric) comes with a 15-gauge, 15-mm needle for use in patients lighter than 39 kg. To operate the drill, insert the needle into the driver tip and make sure that it is securely seated onto the drill. Remove the safety cap from the needle and position the drill perpendicular (or slightly caudad) to the insertion site. While applying gentle pressure, squeeze the trigger to penetrate the skin. When the tip of the needle comes in contact

EZ-IO Intraosseous Device

1

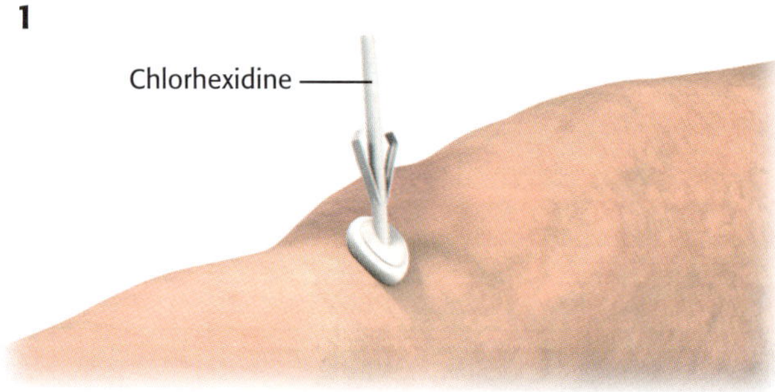

Cleanse the site with an antiseptic agent per institutional protocol.

2

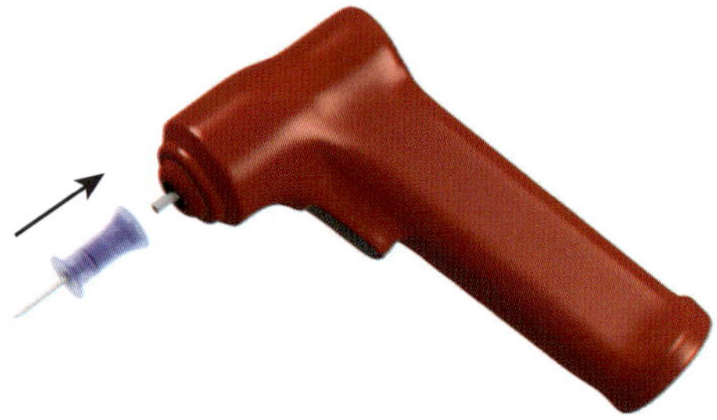

Connect the appropriate needle set to the driver (pink 15 mm = patients 3–39 kg; blue 25 mm = patients > 40 kg; yellow 45 mm = proximal humerus, patients with excessive tissue over the site).

3

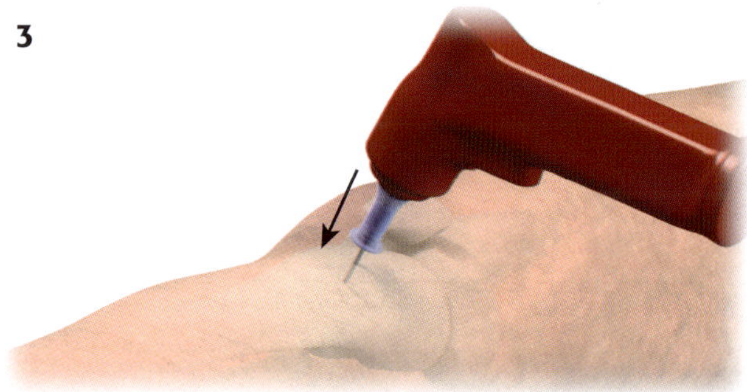

Position the driver at the insertion site with the needle at a 90-degree angle to the surface of the bone. Gently pierce the skin with the needle set and advance needle *without using the trigger yet*, until the needle set tip touches the bone.

4

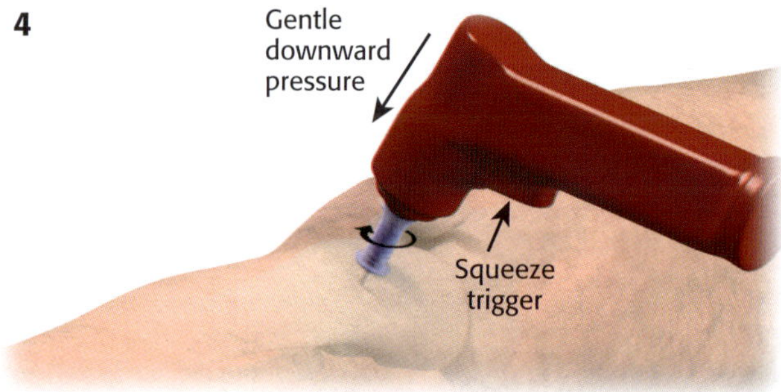

Penetrate the bone cortex by now squeezing the driver's trigger and applying gentle, consistent, steady downward pressure. Allow the driver to do the work.

5

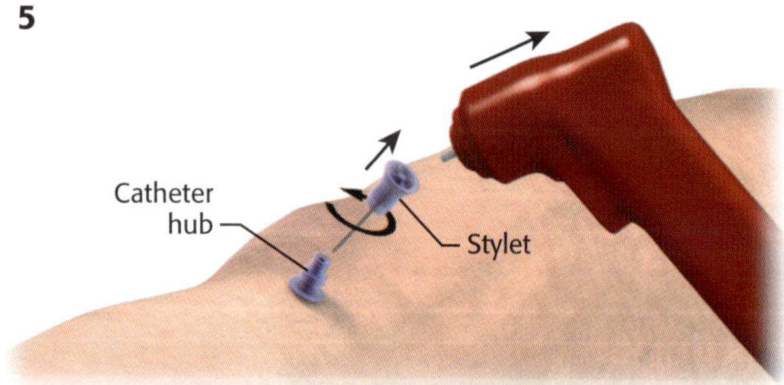

Remove the power driver from the needle set while stabilizing the catheter hub, and then remove the stylet by turning it counterclockwise.

6

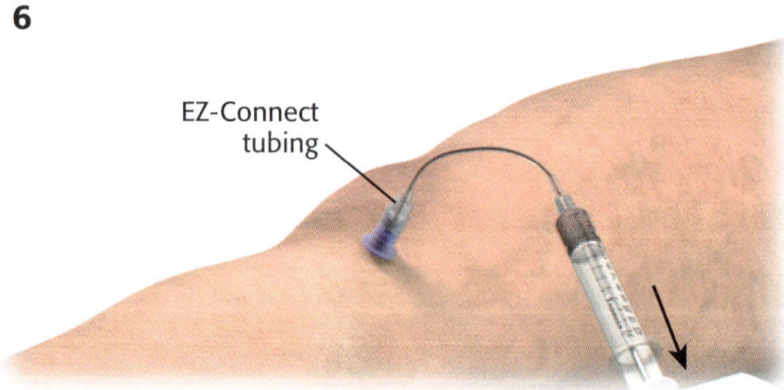

Attach the EZ-Connect tubing to the Luer-Lok adapter on the catheter hub. Confirm placement by aspirating blood and/or marrow contents.

7

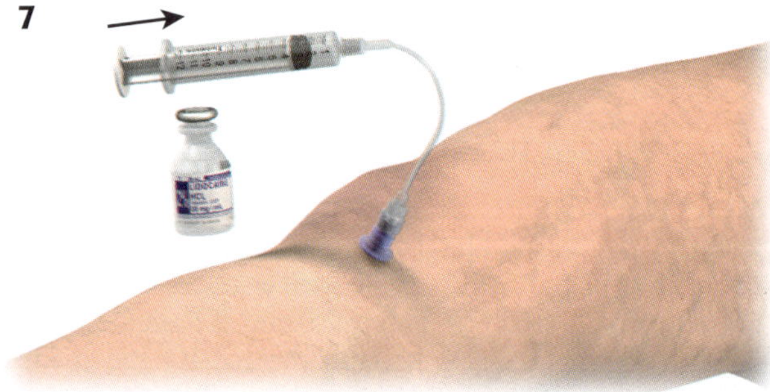

If the patient is responsive to pain, consider *slowly* administering plain 2% lidocaine for anesthetic effect *before* flushing with 10 mL of saline. Begin the infusion with a pressure bag.

8

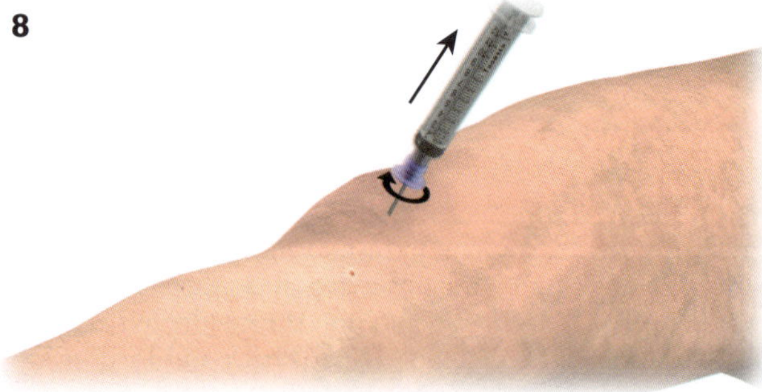

Remove the device within 24 hours. Connect a sterile Luer-Lok syringe to the catheter hub, and rotate clockwise while pulling straight up. Avoid rocking the needle on removal.

Fig. 25.11 Use of the EZ-IO device (Teleflex, Morrisville, NC).

EZ-IO Proximal Humerus Insertion

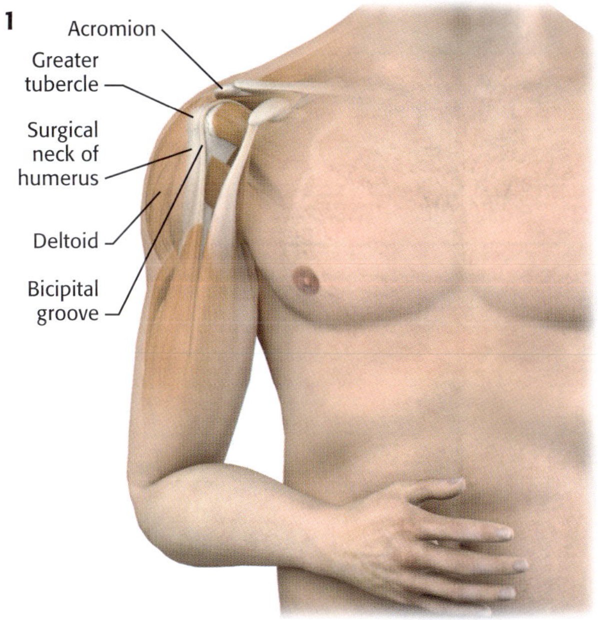

Position the patient with the arm adducted and the hand over the umbilicus. This results in internal rotation of the humerus and shifts the greater tubercle to a more anterior position. Identify the greater tubercle of the humerus (firm pressure may be required because of overlying structures such as the deltoid). Identify the surgical neck of the humerus by palpating up the humerus until a "notch" or "groove" is felt.

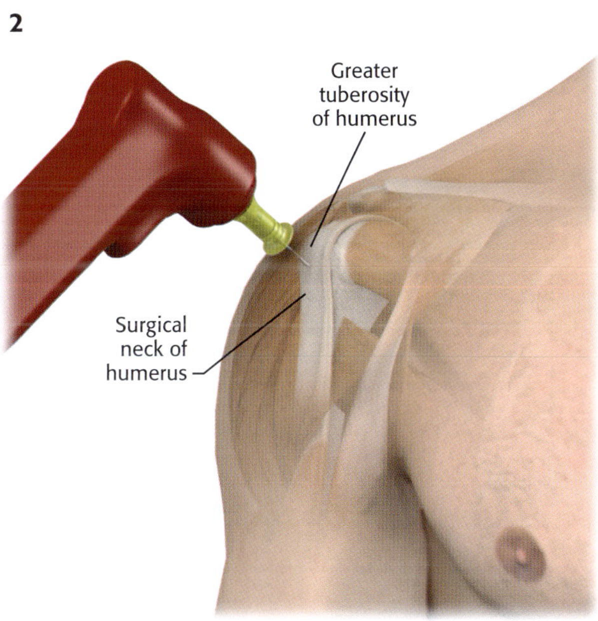

The appropriate insertion site is 1 cm superior to the surgical neck for most adults. Use the yellow 45-mm needle set. The process of EZ-IO insertion and removal at the humerus site is identical to that described in Fig. 25.11.

Fig. 25.12 EZ-IO (Teleflex, Morrisville, NC) proximal humeral insertion.

with the bone, at least 5 mm of the IO catheter should be visible. If not, the overlying soft tissue may be too deep for the needle to enter the marrow cavity. To penetrate the bone, continue to squeeze the trigger while applying steady downward pressure until a sudden "give" or "pop" occurs, which signals entry into the medullary space. Too much pressure on the device can cause the drill to stall and prevent the needle from penetrating the cortex.

After entry into the marrow cavity, attach the EZ-Connect extension set provided with the EZ-IO kit and aspirate blood and bone marrow contents to confirm correct placement. Once catheter placement has been checked, fluids or medications can be infused. Avoid attaching syringes and IV tubing directly to the IO needle because this can enlarge the hole in the cortex and result in extravasation of fluid. Secure the tubing with tape and cover the area with an appropriate dressing. (See instruction video at https://www.teleflex.com/usa/en/product-areas/emergency-medicine/intraosseous-access/arrow-ez-io-system/index.html/.)

NIO Needle

See Fig. 25.13 and Video 25.9. Place the device approximately 2 cm medial and 1 cm proximal to the tibial tuberosity. Unlock the NIO by rotating the cap 90 degrees in either direction. Place the dominant hand over the cap and press the device against the patient. While pressing down on the device with the palm, pull trigger wings upwards with fingers. Gently pull the NIO up in a rotating motion while holding the needle stabilizer against the insertion site. Continue holding the needle stabilizer in place and pull up the stylet to remove. (See instruction video at: https://persysmedical.com/products/vascular-access/nio-adult/.)

COMPLICATIONS

Technical Difficulties

Technical difficulties are the most common complications, but they decrease as familiarity with the technique increases (Fig. 25.14). The most common mistake is to place excessive pressure on the needle during insertion and force it entirely through the bone and out the other side (Fig. 25.15). Minimize this risk by using appropriate landmarks and keeping the needle perpendicular to the long axis of the bone. In addition, hold the needle with the index finger approximately 1 cm from the bevel. When this finger touches the skin, the needle should be in the marrow cavity and no further pressure needs to be applied. Some IO needles have a mark 1 cm from the bevel (e.g., Cook IO needle), whereas others have a special guide or mechanism to ensure proper insertion and depth of penetration (e.g., Illinois Sternal/Iliac Aspiration Needle). If available, use of these adjuncts will also help prevent overpenetration.

At times the needle appears to be in the marrow cavity, but blood or bone marrow cannot be aspirated, and fluids do not flow freely. This may follow incomplete penetration of the

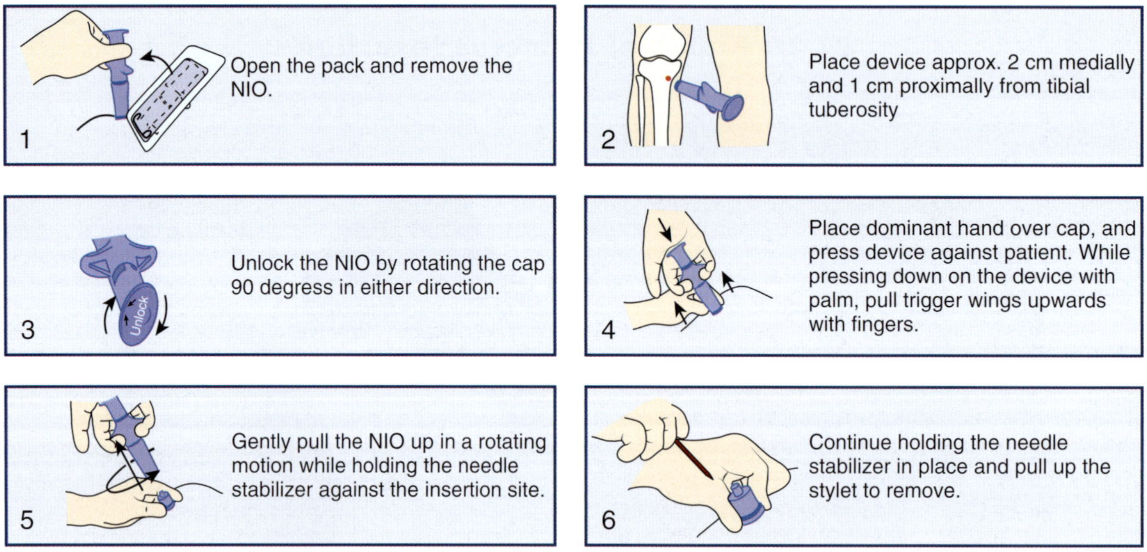

Fig. 25.13 Use of the NIO device (PerSys Medical, Houston, TX).

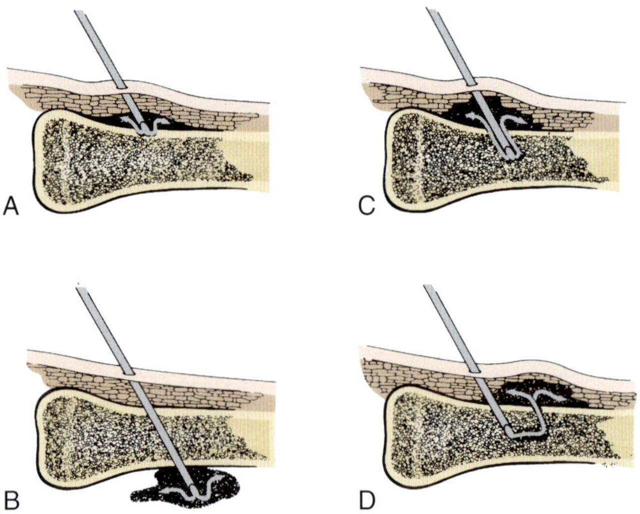

Fig. 25.14 Possible problems encountered with intraosseous infusion. (A) Incomplete penetration of the bony cortex. (B) Penetration of the posterior cortex. (C) Fluid escaping around the needle through the puncture site. (D) Fluid leaking through a nearby previous cortical puncture site.

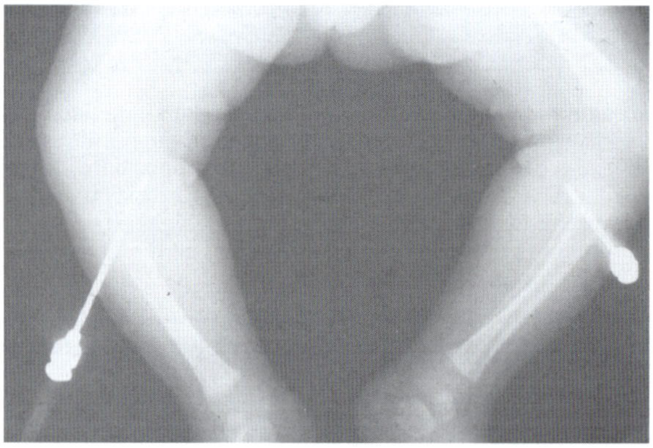

Fig. 25.15 Radiograph of bilaterally misplaced intraosseous needles with penetration through the posterior tibial cortices.

bone or overpenetration into the opposite cortex. Incomplete penetration usually results in extravasation of fluids and can be corrected by replacing the stylet and slowly advancing the needle until successful aspiration of marrow contents and free flow of fluids occur. Penetration into the opposite cortex generally results in little or no flow. If overpenetration is suspected, pull the needle back 1 mm to 2 mm and check for free flow of fluids.

To ensure flow, rapidly inject 10 mL of saline into the marrow. This is a painful procedure in awake patients, but failure to initially flush the compartment is a common reason for inadequate flow. A pressurized bag system is suggested if large volumes of fluid are administered. Flush each dose of medication with 3 mL to 5 mL of saline. Fluids that initially flowed freely may stop flowing if the needle becomes clogged by blood clots or bone spicules. Flush the needle frequently with 3 mL to 5 mL of saline to help avoid this problem. If none of these maneuvers results in free flow of fluid, remove the needle and attempt insertion in the opposite extremity or another site. This helps avoid fluid extravasation through the hole that is left after removing the needle.

Extravasation of fluid is less common but may be associated with a number of adverse events.[111,112] Extravasation may be caused by fluids being infused under excessive pressure and with prolonged use of an IO site.[113] As noted previously, extravasation may also result from incomplete needle penetration or penetration through the opposite cortex. Even when an IO needle has been positioned properly, fluid can leak out through holes made by previous IO attempts or through an insertion site that was made too large by "rocking" during insertion or from an improperly secured needle that becomes loose with movement.[111–115] Interestingly, the type of needle used does not appear to influence extravasation rates.[116] Regardless of the cause, if extravasation occurs, remove the needle quickly and apply pressure to the site. If left unchecked, extravasation can lead to several adverse events (see following section). In addition, though not directly harmful, extravasation of fluid through multiple cortical defects from previous IO attempts has been associated with lower serum levels of infused drugs.[117]

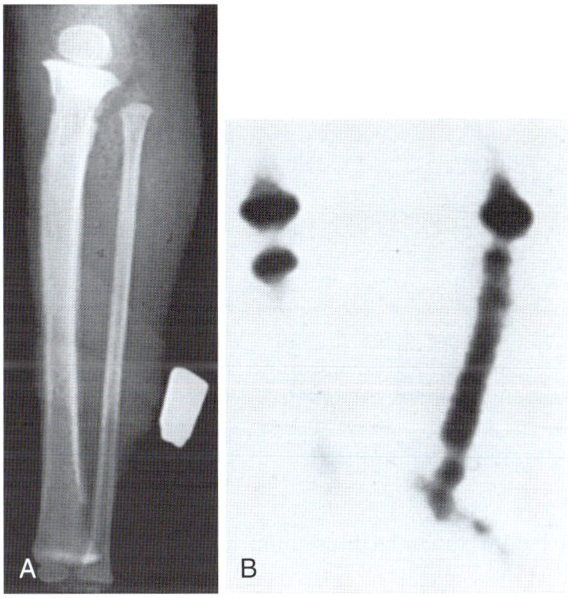

Fig. 25.16 (A) Radiograph and (B) bone scan of the tibia demonstrating an inflammatory reaction 4 days after the patient received intraosseous phenytoin and phenobarbital. The periosteum is elevated along the length of the bone and is mimicking osteomyelitis on the plain film and the bone scan. Diagnosis of osteomyelitis requires either clinical evidence of infectious toxicity or positive cultures (blood or periosteal aspirate).

Soft Tissue and Bony Complications

Infection

In the past, concerns about infection led clinicians to shy away from using the IO route. Although the potential for infection is real, its actual incidence is low. A literature review of more than 4000 cases from 1942 to 1977 found a 0.6% infection rate.[3] Although most of the affected access sites were not placed under emergency conditions, the needles were often left in place for 1 to 2 days, thus increasing the likelihood of infection. A survey of more than 1000 US and foreign medical schools found that the incidence of infection for IO needles placed in emergency conditions was less than 3%.[118] The most common infection is cellulitis at the puncture site, which usually responds well to antibiotics. Osteomyelitis is less common but also usually responds well to antibiotics. Heinild and coworkers[23] reported 3 cases of osteomyelitis in 25 patients who received infusions of undiluted 50% dextrose in water. More recently, Platt and coworkers[119] reported a case of fungal osteomyelitis and sepsis secondary to an IO infusion device. A case of tibial osteomyelitis with IO abscess has also been reported.[120]

In addition to infection, inflammatory reactions of the bone may be seen. Such reactions are most common when hypertonic or sclerosing agents are used and may produce an elevation of the periosteum on plain radiographs or a positive bone scan (Fig. 25.16). Unlike patients with osteomyelitis from bacteria, a child with a sterile inflammatory reaction should not appear ill. One hypertonic sclerosing drug that may be used during cardiac arrest is sodium bicarbonate. Heinild and coworkers[23] reported 78 cases of bicarbonate infusion with no complications. Animal studies have reported a decrease in cellularity with edema and destruction of some cells, but these changes are temporary and resolve completely in a few weeks.[121–124] A case of systemic fibrinolysis through IO vascular access in a patient with ST-elevation myocardial infarction has also been reported.[125]

Skin Sloughing

Skin sloughing and myonecrosis have been reported secondary to extravasation of infused fluids and medications.[124] This occurs if fluid or drugs extravasate from the puncture site into the surrounding tissue. When drugs such as calcium chloride, epinephrine, and sodium bicarbonate are infused, be careful to prevent dislodgement of the needle and extravasation into tissue. In addition, it is best to infuse such drugs only by gravity because infusion under pressure increases the risk for extravasation.

Compartment Syndrome

Compartment syndrome may occur when fluids leak out of the bone into a closed compartment such as the anterior or deep posterior compartment of the lower leg.[126–129] The risk for compartment syndrome can be reduced by carefully placing and securing the IO needle, limiting the number of attempts in the same bone, and removing the needle once IV access has been obtained. In addition, it is prudent to check the insertion site frequently, especially when fluids are being infused under pressure.

Epiphyseal Injuries

Injury to the growth plate and subsequent developmental abnormalities of the bone are ongoing concerns with the IO route. Regardless, these fears are largely unsupported in the available literature. In fact, there have been no reports of growth plate damage or permanent abnormalities of the bone. Two animal studies specifically examined damage to the epiphysis. Sodium bicarbonate was injected directly into the epiphysis and no radiologic evidence of epiphyseal injury was found.[130,131] In addition, two prospective radiologic analyses failed to identify any growth abnormalities 1 year after tibial IO insertion.[132,133] By pointing the needle away from the joint space and using the previously mentioned landmarks for insertion, the risk for epiphyseal injury is remote.

Whereas growth plate abnormalities appear to be very rare, tibial fractures have been reported after IO placement.[134] Hence, it is appropriate to take follow-up radiographs of patients who have undergone IO needle attempts or placement. Cortical defects may be seen on radiographs for up to 40 days after injection.[135]

Fat Embolism

Fat embolism is another potential complication of IO insertion.[3,81] However, this condition is rare and has been reported only in adult patients.[71] Animal studies have found no changes in blood gases during IO infusion and limited evidence of fat globule collections in the lungs.[78,79] In a swine cardiac arrest model, there was no difference in the risk for fat emboli in pigs that had an IO line inserted versus those receiving IV medications.[136,137] Because the marrow in infants and children is primarily hematopoietic, this potential complication is unlikely to occur in this population.

Pain With Infusion

Most patients undergoing IO infusion will not be in a condition to sense pain, but infusion into the bone marrow is painful. Slowly infusing 1 mL to 2 mL of 2%

preservative-free lidocaine (0.5 mg/kg in children, not to exceed adult dose [40 mg or 2 mL]), over 1 minute before flushing and infusion of medications and fluids, has been suggested to relieve pain in awake patients. The duration of analgesic effect is approximately 1 hour and may be repeated as needed. Caution should be exercised with repeat dosing and maximum weight-based limits of local anesthetics. Systemic opioids are also helpful. Medications intended to remain in the medullary space, such as local anesthetics, must be injected very slowly until the desired anesthetic effect is achieved. A 2010 study suggests that lidocaine is efficacious in attenuating the pain related to IO infusion.[138]

TRAINING

Procedural training can be performed on simulation models, animal bones (e.g., chicken or turkey legs), or cadavers. IO insertion techniques are part of the curriculum of the pediatric advanced life support, advanced pediatric life support, and advanced trauma life support courses. Training typically consists of an hour of didactics followed by a hands-on session. Novice users have achieved success rates of 93% to 97% for manual and battery-powered IO placement in a variety of simulated settings.[5,14,28,44,54,61,88,139-141] Battery-powered IO placement has also been shown to have high success rates after training.

DURATION OF USE

IO cannulation is used for temporary vascular access and should be replaced with a venous line as soon as possible. IO cannulation may be left in place during transport and for up to 24 hours, but local edema, infiltration, and an increased risk for osteomyelitis are seen after 24 hours.

ACKNOWLEDGMENT

The author sincerely thanks Rachael Stanley, MD, for her contribution to this chapter in previous editions.

REFERENCES ARE AVAILABLE AT Elsevier eBooks+

CHAPTER 26

Alternative Methods of Drug Administration

Solomon Behar

ENDOTRACHEAL ADMINISTRATION OF MEDICATION

Certain drugs can be delivered to the central circulation by way of the endotracheal (ET) tube. Because the efficacy of ET medication administration is not clear,[1] this method is best reserved for situations in which a patient's condition warrants immediate pharmacologic intervention but more conventional means of drug delivery, such as intravenous (IV) and intraosseous (IO), are not readily available. Such circumstances may arise in the prehospital or cardiac arrest setting. Knowledge of the appropriate drugs and dosages that can be delivered by this route may be useful (Review Box 26.1).

Recommendations for ET Drug Delivery

ET drug delivery is not the delivery method of choice if other routes are available. The American Heart Association (AHA) recommends that if IV access is not available, IO access should be obtained.[2] The 2020 AHA cardiopulmonary resuscitation (CPR) guidelines only advise using ET epinephrine in neonates if no other access is available and have no specific recommendations for ET epinephrine use in adults or children.[3–14]

Appropriate Dose

Much of the existing literature is controversial regarding proper dosing of ET medications.[11,15–19] The ET dose of a medication should be at least equal to the IV dose of the same drug when given for the same indication, but most studies agree that higher doses are needed when administering drugs via the ET route. For advanced cardiac life support (ACLS) medications in adults, an ET dose that is 2 to 2.5 times the usual IV dose is used.[2,20–22] Studies using both normotensive and cardiac arrest canine models have shown that epinephrine doses of 0.01 mg/kg administered via ET produced serum levels approximately one-tenth of that produced when the same dose is given intravenously.[10,23,24] These studies suggested increasing the ET epinephrine dose to 0.05 to 0.1 mg/kg for the 1 mg/mL concentration of epinephrine and are the basis for the 2020 AHA neonatal recommendations.[14] One notable exception of epinephrine ET concentration is in the neonatal population (the first month of life) in which the AHA recommends using the 0.1 mg/mL (not 1 mg/mL that is used in pediatric patients and adults).[25]

ET drug delivery is associated with a "depot" effect, with ET drugs being "stored" and released slowly over time, similar to a continuous IV drip. This presumably occurs as a result of local vasoconstriction and lymphatic storage of the drug[9] or pooling in lung tissue because of poor lung perfusion.[26] With ET epinephrine use, the depot effect can produce postresuscitative dysrhythmias, hypertension, and tachycardia together with resultant increased myocardial oxygen demand. Given these conflicting data, it seems reasonable in adults to start with a dose 2.0 to 2.5 times the usual IV dose.

Volume for a Single Dose

For ET drugs, the AHA previously recommended a total volume of 10 mL in adults,[2] 5 mL in pediatric patients,[13] and 1 mL in neonates.[14] Animal and human studies demonstrate that diluting medications in higher volumes of liquid increases

Endotracheal Medication Administration

Indications
Cardiac arrest with no peripheral or intraosseous access

Contraindications
Peripheral or intraosseous access

Complications
Depot effect of drug
Transient hypoxemia
Loss of catheter or needle down endotracheal tube

Equipment

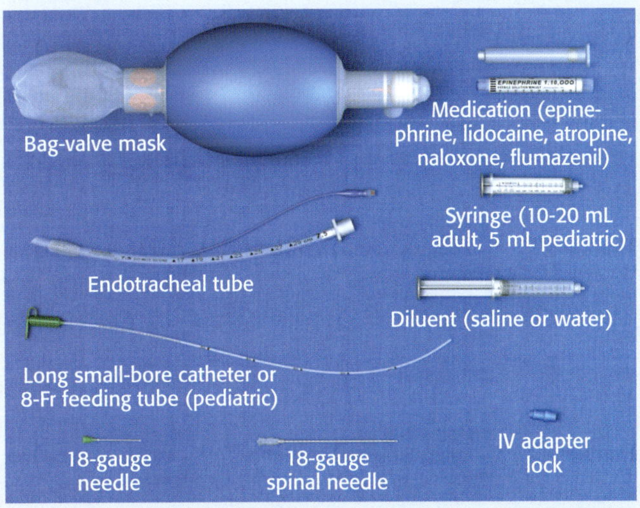

Review Box 26.1 Endotracheal medication administration: indications, contraindications, complications, and equipment. Gloves, mask, and eye protection are also necessary equipment for endotracheal medication administration. See text for further explanation on medication.

blood levels of the drug but at the expense of decreases in partial pressure of arterial oxygen (Pao_2).[27–30] Data and volume recommendations in the setting of multiple doses of the drug are lacking. It may be difficult or impossible to limit the total volume of the drug solution to 10 mL when using prefilled syringes in adolescents or adults. Prefilled syringes of epinephrine contain 1 mg in 10 mL. Giving 2.5 times the IV/IO dose would require the administration of 20 mL to 25 mL. Higher epinephrine concentration is recommended (i.e., 1 mg/mL) and further diluting to a total volume of 5 mL to 10 mL; however, the higher concentration of epinephrine may not be readily available. Likewise, prefilled syringes of atropine contain 1 mg in 10 mL (0.1 mg/mL). Prefilled syringes of lidocaine contain 20 mg/mL (100 mg/5 mL). A dose of 2 to 2.5 times the IV/IO dose could easily amount to 20 mL or more total volume in an adult patient.

Appropriate Diluent

Both normal saline and sterile water may be used as diluents for ET drug administration, but it remains unclear which is preferred. Normal saline may produce less pulmonary dysfunction than sterile water, but sterile water appears to deliver a greater amount of drug than when the drug is mixed in normal saline.[28,29,31,32]

Technique for ET Drug Delivery

Techniques for ET drug administration include direct instillation into the proximal end of the ET tube, administration via a catheter that extends just beyond the distal tip of the ET tube, deep endobronchial administration using a longer catheter, administration via ET tube monitoring ports, administration with equipment developed specifically for ET atomized drugs, and injection through the side of the ET tube with a needle. Several studies have indicated that the use of a catheter or feeding tube may not be needed to enhance the drug's effectiveness,[33,34] including neonates.[35] In studies of patients with normal perfusion, some support "deep bronchial" ET drug administration, whereas others do not.[36–38] Some[17,21] suggest that drug absorption with direct instillation into the ET tube is inconsistent during cardiopulmonary arrest, and one study found no difference in plasma epinephrine levels when epinephrine was instilled during apnea versus instillation during the ventilator inspiratory cycle.[39] Considering the conflicting studies, employing a catheter for deep pulmonary delivery is a viable option, but in the absence of a catheter, direct injection into the ET tube is also an acceptable alternative.

Effects of Hypoxia, Hypotension, and Cardiopulmonary Arrest

Despite concerns that medications might not be absorbed in states of hypoxia or low blood flow, the data available reveal the opposite to be true. In a hemorrhagic shock model, Mace[40] demonstrated that higher plasma lidocaine levels were obtained via the ET route during shock than during nonshock states. In a lamb model, when epinephrine was administered endotracheally, higher plasma epinephrine levels were achieved during hypoxia-induced low pulmonary blood flow than during baseline, normal pulmonary blood flow.[41] Finally, plasma lidocaine levels rose earlier when lidocaine was administered endotracheally to dogs that were hypoxemic than to dogs that were not.[42]

Indications

ET drug therapy is indicated when emergency pharmacologic intervention is needed and other access, either IV or IO, is not available. Specific indications for the delivery of a drug endotracheally are the same as those for IV and IO administration. However, only a limited number of emergency drugs can be given safely by the ET route. Medications that are appropriate for ET administration based on animal and human studies include epinephrine,[9,11,43] atropine,[44–46] lidocaine,[37,42,47] and naloxone.[12,48] Diazepam has also been used,[49,50] but with the possibility of a medication- (or diluent)-induced pneumonitis.[51] The AHA has removed diazepam from its list of medications that can be given safely via the ET route.

Experimental studies of vasopressin,[52,53] midazolam,[54] flumazenil,[55] and propranolol,[44] in animal models suggest that these medications may also be administered endotracheally, but no clinical studies in humans have been conducted to verify these findings. As midazolam is approved for intramuscular (IM) use, it seems unlikely that ET administration would be frequently used. Palmer et al.[55] demonstrated that therapeutic blood levels of flumazenil were obtained within 1 minute after ET delivery of 1 mg of the drug diluted in 10 mL of saline, which is 10 times the recommended IV dose of 0.1- to 0.2-mg aliquots.

Contraindications

At present, the only true contraindication to the ET delivery of an appropriate drug is the presence of another form of access to the systemic circulation. Specific medications have been shown to be ineffective or unsafe when given via the ET route. Sodium bicarbonate and amiodarone have direct deleterious effects on the lungs.[56,57] Bretylium and isoproterenol have not been shown to attain adequate serum levels despite high ET doses given.[45,58]

Procedure

The procedure of choice is one that will deliver the medication to the patient in the least amount of time. Secure the ET tube before instilling medications endotracheally to prevent the tube from being expelled if the patient coughs. Inflate the cuff of the tube, if present.

Direct Instillation Into the ET Tube

While the patient is being ventilated, draw up the desired drug into a syringe (or use a prefilled syringe) (Fig. 26.1, *step 1*). Dilute the drug to a final volume of 10 mL (adults), 5 mL (children), or 1 mL (neonates) with normal saline or distilled water. Attach an 18- or 19-gauge needle. Some authors recommend using an 8.9-cm (3.5-inch) spinal needle. If using a prefilled syringe, draw up an appropriate volume of diluent in a second syringe so that the total instillation volume (drug plus diluent) equals 10 mL (adults), 5 mL (children), or 1 mL (neonates). Attach an 18- or 19-gauge needle, which will be used to flush the ET tube after instillation of the drug.

Interrupt the connection between the proximal end of the ET tube and the bag ventilation device. Insert the needle of the syringe into the proximal opening of the ET tube (see Fig. 26.1, *step 2*). Hold the proximal end of the needle with one hand to prevent loss of the needle into the tube. Inject

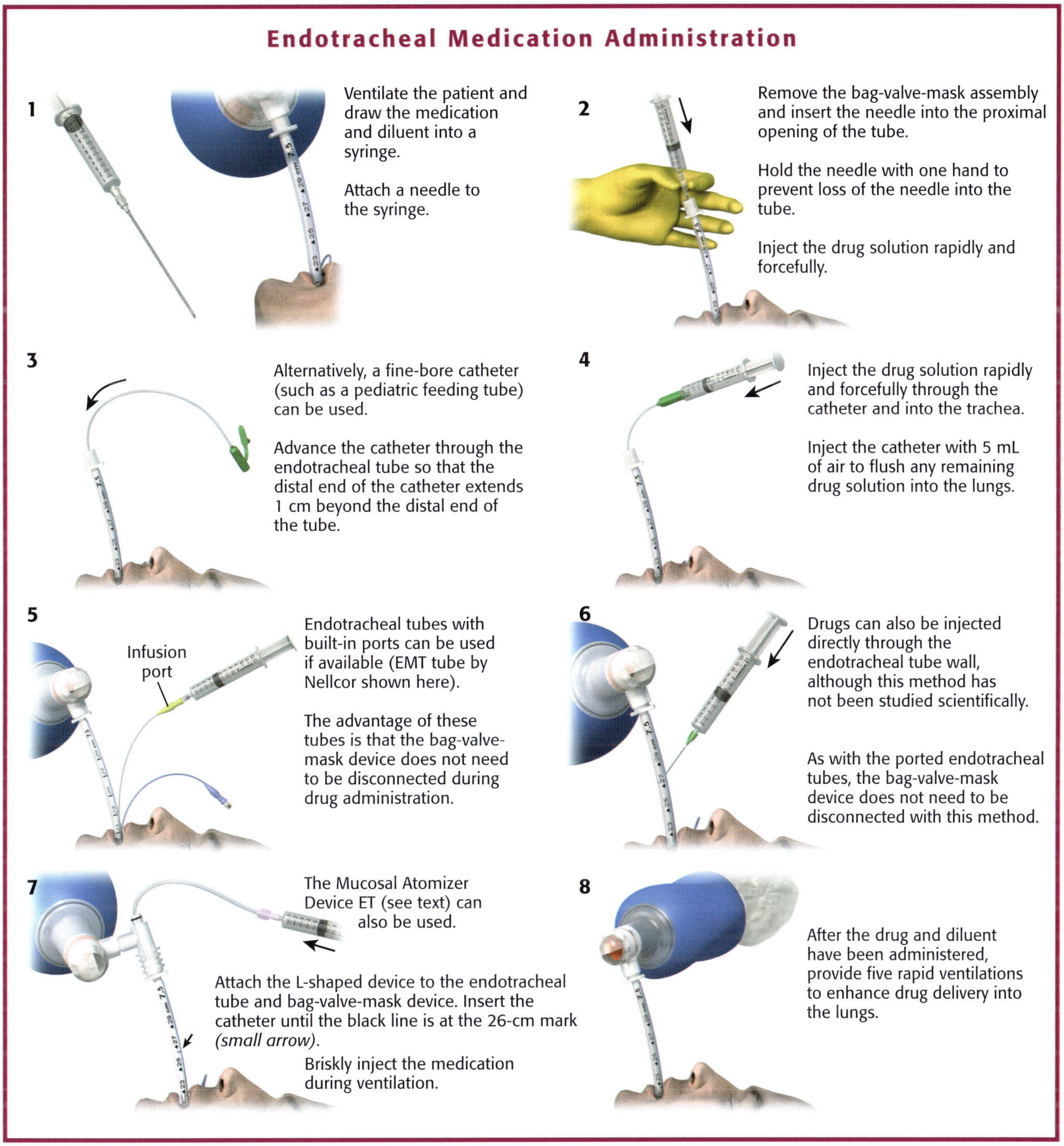

Fig. 26.1 Endotracheal administration of medication.

the drug solution rapidly and forcefully. If using a prefilled syringe, flush the tube immediately with the diluent in a second syringe. If the patient makes an effort to cough, place a thumb over the opening of the ET tube to prevent expulsion of the solution. Reattach the bag ventilation device and deliver five rapid insufflations.

Use of a Catheter

Draw the plunger back to add 5 mL of air to the liquid in the syringe. If the drug to be delivered is in a prefilled syringe, place an IV adapter lock on the catheter if necessary to accommodate the syringe needle or needleless tip. Attach the syringe to the catheter at this time or once the catheter has been placed within the ET tube. In addition, draw up the appropriate volume of diluent (normal saline or distilled water) plus 5 mL air into a second syringe to flush the catheter after instillation of the drug from the prefilled syringe. The air flush presumably forces out any medication adhering to the walls of the catheter's lumen. Rehan and colleagues[35] determined that, when using a catheter in a neonatal model, more medication was delivered with an additional air flush than without an air flush.

Disconnect the proximal end of the ET tube from the bag ventilation device. Place the catheter into the lumen of the ET tube in such a manner that the distal end of the catheter extends approximately 1 cm beyond the distal end of the ET tube (see Fig. 26.1, *step 3*). Hold the proximal ends of the catheter and ET tube at all times during the procedure. If it has not already been done, attach the syringe to the catheter. Inject the drug solution rapidly and forcefully through the catheter into the trachea followed by the 5 mL of air needed to flush the catheter of any remaining drug solution (see Fig. 26.1, *step 4*). If using a prefilled syringe, use the second syringe to promptly flush with the diluent and air. Immediately remove the syringe and catheter from the ET tube. Reconnect the bag ventilation device with supplemental oxygen to the ET tube and deliver five rapid ventilations.

Injection Through the Wall of the ET Tube

This method of drug delivery has not yet been evaluated scientifically but has been used clinically.[59,60] As with ET tubes with drug delivery lumens, this technique requires no interruption of the connection between the bag ventilation device and the ET tube (see Fig. 26.1, *step 6*). Placing an IV adapter lock on the needle allows it to be left inserted in the ET tube for use with additional medications.[60]

Use of the ET Atomizer

The Mucosal Atomizer Device-Endotracheal Tube (Teleflex) is an L-shaped port that attaches to both the ventilator bag and the ET tube (Fig. 26.2; see also Fig. 26.1, *step 7*). A catheter is inserted into the adapter and a mark is aligned at the 26-cm line of the ET tube. The catheter is then locked into place in the adapter. The L shape allows ventilation of the patient to be uninterrupted while medication is administered via the catheter and atomized into the patient's lung mucosa at the distal tip that protrudes from the end of the ET tube. This device can be used only with ET tubes 7.0 mm or larger and longer than 28 cm.

Complications

Reported complications of ET drug therapy are rare, in part because of the infrequent use of this technique. Because most patients who receive ET drug therapy are in cardiopulmonary arrest or are otherwise critically ill, it is difficult to ascertain whether an adverse outcome is the result of the therapy.

With regard to the techniques of ET drug administration, no serious complications have been reported. A theoretical complication is loss of a needle or catheter down the ET tube, which can be prevented by holding the catheter or needle while instilling the drug.

After ET drug administration, the well-described systemic effects of drugs administered in emergency situations may produce adverse effects. Administration of epinephrine during CPR has been noted in case reports to produce prolonged hypertension, tachycardia, and arrhythmias after the return of a perfusing rhythm.[11,23] It appears that these side effects are related to the depot effect, in which larger doses of drugs administered endotracheally are released slowly over time. In addition to epinephrine, atropine and lidocaine also exhibit a depot effect when administered endotracheally.[56] No serious long-term sequelae, however, have been reported to result from this effect.

A potential concern with ET drug therapy is a transient decrease in arterial oxygen content during or after drug delivery. If total volumes are maintained between 5 mL and 10 mL in adults, the effect on pulmonary function appears to be minimal. Supplemental oxygen should always be administered to improve oxygenation and offset any transient drop in arterial oxygen content that might develop.

One unusual complication of ET epinephrine is that, during CPR, some of the instilled medication may be expelled and enter the eye. This will produce a fixed dilated pupil, simulating brain death or, if unilateral, brain herniation.

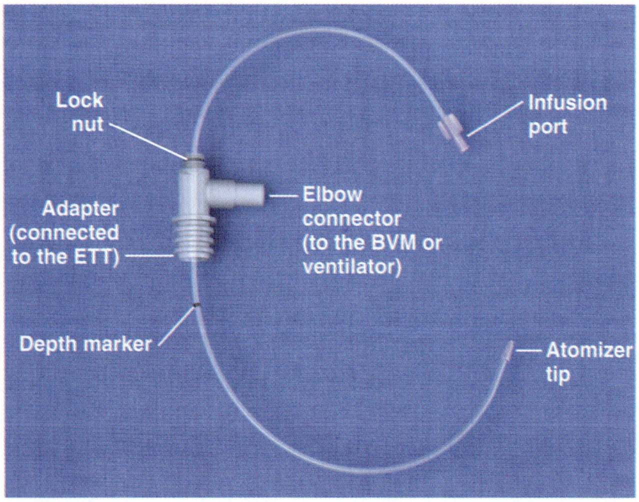

Fig. 26.2 The mucosal atomizer device-endotracheal tube. The L-shaped port attaches to both the bag-valve-mask device *(BVM)* and endotracheal tube *(ETT)* and allows uninterrupted ventilation during drug administration. The catheter should be inserted until the black depth marker is at the 26-cm mark on the ETT.

INTRANASAL ADMINISTRATION OF MEDICATION

See Videos 26.1–26.5.

Anatomy and Physiology

The human nasal cavity is a convenient and readily available site to deliver medications. In adults, it has a volume of 15 mL to 20 mL and a total surface area of approximately 150 cm^2.[61] The nasal cavity is divided into two mostly symmetric halves by the nasal septum. Each half consists of four anatomically and histologically distinct regions: the vestibule, atrium, and the respiratory and olfactory regions (Fig. 26.3). The respiratory and olfactory regions are areas of high vascularity and good permeability. The respiratory region has the largest surface area at approximately 130 cm^2.[62] Blood flow in the nasal mucosa is higher, per cubic centimeter, than in muscle, brain, or liver tissue.[63]

The olfactory mucosa has been theorized to have a direct connection to the brain and bypasses the first-pass metabolism of orally administered medications.[64,65] Drugs that can be delivered via the nasal mucosa are generally small in molecular weight, stable, and lipophilic.[66]

Indications and Contraindications

The IN route may be very useful in circumstances where placing an IV line is not possible or practical and an oral medication is refused. This is especially true in patients at the extremes of age. Thus knowledge of this painless, needleless

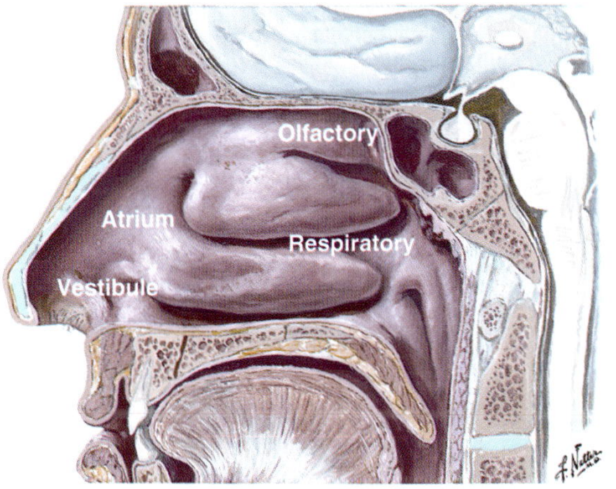

Fig. 26.3 Regions of the nasal cavity.(Netter illustration from www.netterimages.com. Elsevier Inc. All rights reserved.)

route of drug administration is important for practicing emergency physicians. IN administration of medication has been used for more than 30 years.[67] Drugs used routinely in the emergency department (ED) that have been studied intranasally include the opioid antagonist naloxone, the benzodiazepine midazolam, the sedative-hypnotic ketamine, the opioids fentanyl and sufentanil, and most recently, the α2-agonist sedative dexmedetomidine. Most of these studies have focused on the pediatric patient population as an alternative to IV medication. The patient does not need to be developmentally able to "sniff" in order to enjoy the benefits of IN medication, but only to have the mucosal surface coated in the medication, making its use in the very young patient feasible.

Opioid Overdose

In November 2015 the FDA approved IN naloxone for use in opioid overdose.[68] The 2015 AHA ACLS guidelines support its use in "a patient with known or suspected opioid overdose who has a definite pulse but no normal breathing or only gasping (i.e., a respiratory arrest), in addition to providing standard BLS (basic life support) care".[69] IN naloxone at a dose of 2 mg was shown to be as effective as IV naloxone in patients with known or suspected opioid overdose.[70] Patients receiving IN naloxone had an increase in the respiratory rate that was statistically equivalent to that with IV naloxone. IN naloxone was shown to reduce the need to initiate an IV line in opioid overdose patients.[71] Using the IN approach can help reduce the risk for needlestick injuries in the prehospital setting, especially in high-risk patient population. Nebulized naloxone has also been used to treat opioid intoxication in nonapneic patients.

Seizures

In pediatric patients with seizures, midazolam (0.2 mg/kg) delivered intranasally was found to have a more rapid onset of seizure cessation compared with rectal diazepam.[72] IN midazolam is now used in both the prehospital setting and the ED to deliver midazolam until an IV line can be initiated. A systematic review and meta-analysis comparing non-IV midazolam (IN, buccal, IM routes) and per rectum (PR) diazepam showed non-IV midazolam is similar to rectal diazepam in terminating early status epilepticus.[73] In a network analysis, IN midazolam was better than buccal midazolam, sublingual lorazepam, PR diazepam, and IM midazolam at stopping seizures at 10 minutes, and for seizures lasting more than 1 hour.[74]

Sedation

IN midazolam (0.3 mg/kg) compared favorably against buccal and oral routes of midazolam use in children requiring procedural sedation, exhibiting a faster onset of sedation, achieving adequate sedation in a greater proportion of patients, and more parent satisfactions.[75] IN midazolam has equivalent efficacy to IV midazolam for sedation during simple laceration repairs in children.[76] The acidity of midazolam can cause nasal mucosa irritation, especially when administered as drops, but premedication with intranasal lidocaine may reduce this irritation.[77,78]

Ketamine (5 mg/kg) in combination with midazolam (0.3 mg/kg) administered intranasally has been used as an anesthesia induction agent with a rapid onset of sedation. Compared with IN midazolam (0.2 mg/kg) as a premedication agent, IN ketamine (5 mg/kg) had a longer time to onset and was associated with more side effects than midazolam.[79] One small study of 30 pediatric patients requiring laceration repair found a dose of 6 mg/kg of IN ketamine provided adequate sedation to repair 77% of that small cohort.[80]

For dissociative levels of sedation, doses of 7 to 9 mg/kg of IN ketamine[78,79] have been necessary to attain this state. The volume of medication required to reach these higher doses often exceeds the nasal cavity capacity to absorb the medication, rendering IN ketamine for dissociative sedation impractical.

Dexmedetomidine, an α2-agonist with sedative, anxiolytic, and analgesic properties can be given intranasally (2 to 4 µg/kg) to sedate children for nonpainful procedures.[80–96] Dexmedetomidine has been combined with ketamine, so-called "ketodex" (2 µg/kg dexmedetomidine with 1 mg/kg ketamine) IN or with buccal midazolam (0.2 mg/kg midazolam with 3 µg/kg dexmedetomidine) in order to complete nonpainful procedures, such as echocardiogram, advanced imaging,[97,98] and dental procedures.[99] Further study is needed to determine the ideal dosage of these combination medications.

Dexmedetomidine monotherapy is not ideal for painful procedures. In one phase II dose ranging study, 3 to 4 µg/kg resulted in adequate sedation in only ~60% of pediatric patients requiring simple laceration repair.[100] Onset of action is 10 to 25 minutes and its duration of action is 40 to 100 minutes (measured as ability to be discharged). Overall side effects are rare (bradycardia and hypotension), and dexmedetomidine has little effect on respiratory drive. There is a case report of vasovagal syncope and bradycardia in an 11-year-old child who had received IN dexmedetomidine at a dose of 2.4 µg/kg.[101]

Pain Management

Fentanyl is widely used for the management of acute pain. IN fentanyl has desirable pharmacokinetics in the treatment of acute pain.[102,103] Foster and colleagues demonstrated that in adults, IN fentanyl (75 to 200 µg) had comparable pain reduction with IV fentanyl.[103]

IN fentanyl analgesia has been shown to be comparable to IV morphine with a similar side effect profile.[104] IN fentanyl can be used in patients prior to initiating an IV line or as a noninvasive alternative to IV or IM injections. Onset of action of IN fentanyl is 2 to 5 minutes, lasting ~60 minutes. Pediatric dosing is usually given at a range of 1 to 3 µg/kg.[103–111] One case report describes IN fentanyl stopping a blue "tet spell" in a cyanotic infant with Tetralogy of Fallot.[112]

Combination IN therapy using sufentanil (0.5 μg/kg) and ketamine (0.5 mg/kg) has also been described.[113] IN Ketamine (1 to 1.5 mg/kg) seems to be a promising candidate in a role as an opiate sparing pain medication in children.[114] Among adult patients, an average dose of 1 mg/kg of IN ketamine reduced acute pain in just over one half of patients.[115] Adult dosing of IN ketamine has not been well studied.

Contraindications

There are no absolute contraindications to the intranasal administration of medication except for medication allergy. Abnormal nasal anatomy or increased mucous production may reduce absorption and necessitate repeated dosing.[66]

Equipment

The only equipment necessary is the desired medication, a needle to draw the medication from the vial, a syringe, and an atomizing device if available (Review Box 26.2).

Procedure

Two methods to deliver drugs to the nasal mucosa can be used: drops or aerosol. Nasal drops require a cooperative patient and correct positioning to enhance drug delivery. Atomization of medication is much preferred to drops, in that much of the drug is lost to the environment by dripping out the nose or into the throat and then swallowed.[116,117] This can result in metabolism of the drug in the liver through first-pass metabolism. Nasal atomization has been found to be the optimal method of enhancing mucosal coverage and increasing plasma concentrations of IN medications.[61,116,117] Regardless of the method, the relatively small volume of the nasal cavity limits the volume of medication to approximately 1 mL per naris. If the volume is greater than 1 mL, split the dose and instill half into each naris. Use concentrated forms of medications to decrease the overall volume.[66]

Nasal Drops

Draw up the appropriate dose and volume of medication. Position the patient properly to enhance delivery to the mucosa and prevent runoff or swallowing. Instill the drops slowly to prevent runoff.

One position is to place the patient on the back with the head down and nose pointing up. Slowly instill the drops into each naris along the nasal septum and allow the medication to flow into the turbinates. A second position is the lateral decubitus position with the head angled downward. Use pillows or towels to elevate the body at the shoulders if necessary. Instill the drops into the naris that is "up" so that the medication runs along the nasal septum and turbinates. An alternative, though more uncomfortable position is to place the patient on the knees with the head down and the vertex parallel to the bed, essentially in a position similar to starting a forward roll. Instill the medication against the septum and let it flow to the turbinates.[116,117]

Nasal Atomization

Many commercial devices are available for home and outpatient use to deliver medications intranasally. The Mucosal Atomization Device (Teleflex) is small, easy to use, and attaches to nearly any syringe (Fig. 26.4). Atomization of midazolam was found to achieve higher plasma concentrations than nebulized midazolam.[118] Atomization results in very fine particles that distribute over the mucosal surface enhancing absorption.

Draw up an appropriate volume of medication into a syringe with an additional amount to accommodate for the dead space of the device (0.1 mL). Insert the device approximately 0.25 inch to 0.5 inch into the vestibule. Rapidly depress the plunger. If the total volume is greater than 1 mL, repeat this in the other naris (Fig. 26.5).

Intranasal Medication Administration

Indications

Pain relief
Anxiolysis/sedation
Seizure control
Narcotic overdose

Contraindications

Abnormal nasal anatomy
Nasal trauma

Complications

Side effects of the specific medication
Local nasal irritation
For epinephrine: Fixed dilated pupil(s) if expelled into eye(s) during CPR

Equipment

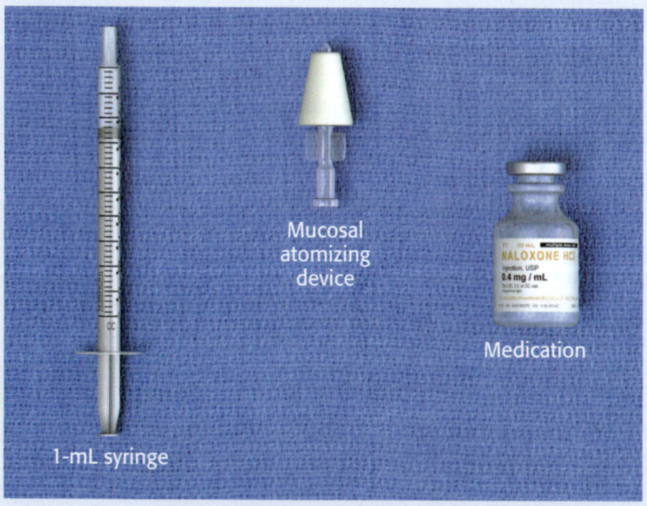

Review Box 26.2 Intranasal medication administration: indications, contraindications, complications, and equipment.

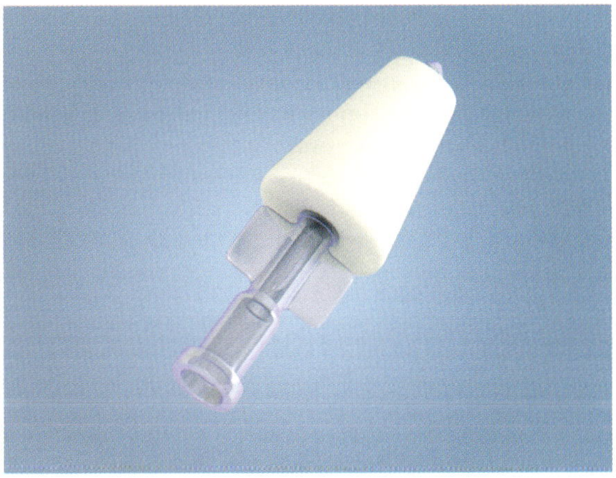

Fig. 26.4 Mucosal atomization device.

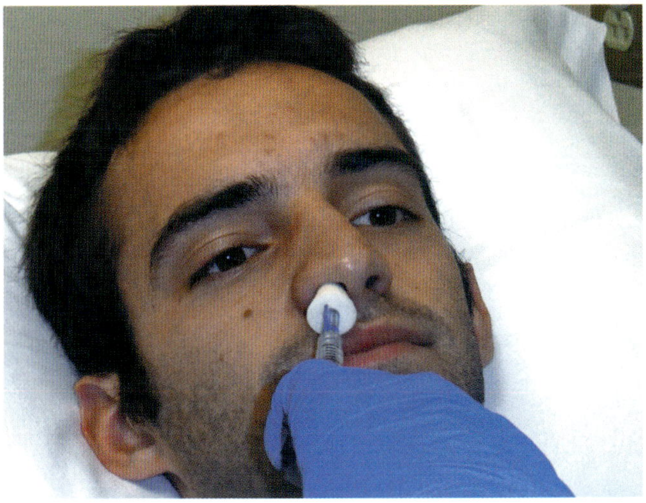

Fig. 26.5 Insert the device approximately 1 cm into the vestibule and rapidly depress the plunger. If the total volume is greater than 1 mL, repeat in the other naris.

An obvious advantage of an atomizer is that proper positioning is less necessary and the medication is instilled rapidly. This can result in less runoff and requires less cooperation from the patient.

Complications

Aside from the side effects of the medications (allergy, nausea, apnea, etc.), there are few to no complications when using IN medications. As mentioned previously, midazolam has been noted to cause short-term local irritation.

NEBULIZED ADMINISTRATION OF MEDICATION

Anatomy and Physiology

A nebulized medication is delivered through a nebulizer, a device that converts liquid medication into a fine mist that can be inhaled into the lungs (and oral/nasal mucosa). Once the misted medication reaches the lungs, it gets deposited on the airway surfaces and is absorbed into the bloodstream through the thin membranes in the alveoli. From there, it can be transported throughout the body to exert its therapeutic effects. Traditionally, its use was limited to β-agonists and other medications for use in asthma and other chronic obstructive pulmonary diseases, but newer indications have increased the scope of use of this route of administration.

Opiate Overdose: Nebulized Naloxone

Naloxone has been administered via nebulization to reverse opioid intoxication.[119] The potential benefit of nebulized naloxone is that IV access is not required. The reversal effect may be continued as long as the nebulizer is used, and there may be a more gradual, but often not complete, reversal of opioid intoxication. Additionally, nebulized naloxone may offer the advantage of gradual reversal avoiding abrupt awakening and resultant agitation. Nevertheless, limited data support nebulized naloxone. Weber and colleagues[120] reported success with nebulized naloxone in approximately 80% of spontaneously breathing patients with suspected opioid intoxication when paramedics administered the medication. The procedure is only applicable to *nonapneic* patients and can be used by both prehospital and ED clinicians. Empirical dosing is 2 to 4 mg of naloxone in 3 mL of saline, delivered by an oxygen driven nebulizer is the most common method described. Rescue IN, IM, or IV naloxone should be available for those not responding appropriately.

Anxiolysis/Sedation: Nebulized Dexmedetomidine

Dexmedetomidine at a dose of 2 to 2.5 μg/kg inhaled has been used to obtain anxiolysis, with low rates of postsedation nausea/vomiting.[121]

Bleeding: Nebulized Tranexamic Acid

Tranexamic acid (TXA) is an antifibrinolytic drug that functions by blocking the binding of plasmin to the fibrin clot, the mesh-like structure that holds the clot together. By inhibiting the action of plasmin, TXA helps to maintain the stability and integrity of the clot, preventing its premature breakdown. Nebulized TXA has been used in cases of hemoptysis[122] and in patients with pulmonary hemorrhage (including patients taking oral anticoagulants).[123–126] Small studies and case reports show promise of nebulized TXA controlling postoperative tonsillectomy bleeding.[127–131]

Dosing of TXA ranges are reported to be 250 mg (for children <25 kg) to 500 to 1000 mg for older children and adults. Optimal dosing of inhaled TXA is unknown. Nebulized TXA does not seem to carry the same risks of thromboembolic events or seizures as the IV form of the medication.[132–134]

Contraindications

Nebulized therapies do not work in apneic patients (though they can be bagged into a ventilation circuit) and are generally less effective in hypoventilating patients.

Equipment

A nebulizer machine with a reservoir to place the liquid medication and a mouthpiece or (in children) an appropriate size mask to fit over the nose and mouth of the patient and tubing to deliver the medication from the nebulizer to the mouthpiece/mask is required.

Procedure

Preparation: The medication in liquid form is measured and placed into the nebulizer device reservoir.

Nebulization: The nebulizer device contains a small compressor that generates compressed air or ultrasonic vibrations. This energy source converts the liquid medication into a mist by creating small droplets. The mist is then released into a chamber or cup of the nebulizer.

Inhalation: The person using the nebulizer places the mouthpiece or mask over their nose and mouth, creating a seal. They then breathe in the misted medication. As they inhale, the medication is carried deep into the lungs, targeting the airways and lung tissues.

Complications

Aside from the side effects of the medications (e.g., allergy, nausea, apnea), there are rarely complications when using nebulized medications.

SUBLINGUAL ADMINISTRATION OF MEDICATION

The sublingual route is an appealing method of administration in patients unable or refusing to take medications by other routes. It does require a cooperative patient and can be used in most pediatric patients over the age of 2 years. Drug absorption from the sublingual route occurs directly from the mucosal tissue into the blood stream avoiding first-pass metabolism by the liver. Orally dissolving tablets (ODT) are often given in sublingual space; however, ODT tablets are designed to break into small residues that can be easily swallowed. ODT preparations are generally not absorbed from mucosal surfaces (e.g., ondansetron) and must be swallowed. An ODT preparation is not synonymous with sublingual absorption.

Indications

Psychosis/Agitation

Recently, a sublingual preparation of dexmedetomidine was approved by the FDA for treatment of agitation associated with schizophrenia or bipolar disorder. The drug is available as a 180 µg or 120 µg sublingual film. In clinical trials, significant reduction in agitation was observed 20 minutes after administration that persisted for up to 2 hours.[134a] Risks of sublingual dexmedetomidine are similar to IV preparation of the drug (e.g., bradycardia/hypotension). When considering use of a recently approved medication cost of the drug should be considered (in 2023 one film average wholesale price was ~$130).

Lorazepam is a benzodiazepine reliably absorbed from oral mucosa. Historically, lorazepam has been used for the treatment of anxiety and agitation by sublingual administration, potentially offering a faster onset of action compared with oral administration.[134b] Recent studies have also shown sublingual lorazepam as an abortive intervention in patients with prolonged seizures.[134c] In patients with anxiety and agitation in the ED who are cooperative, or who cannot tolerate oral medications due to nausea or vomiting, sublingual administration of lorazepam may be considered.

Asenapine is a second-generation antipsychotic indicated for the treatment of schizophrenia and acute mania associated with bipolar I disorder. The usual dose is 5 to 10 mg administered sublingually with initial onset of effect around 15 minutes and maximal effect around 2 hours.[135]

Common side effects include drowsiness and oral hypoesthesia.

RECTAL ADMINISTRATION OF MEDICATION

Medications may be administered rectally when other preferable routes are not available. This most often occurs when IV access is impractical or impossible, the medication is not suitable for IM administration, or other nonparenteral routes are unavailable or less desirable. In these situations, rectal administration may offer an alternative method of drug delivery. The major drawback to rectal drug administration is unpredictable and often erratic drug absorption.

Drug absorption from the rectum is a simple diffusion process across the lipid membrane. In general, the rate of absorption rises with increasing lipid solubility of the drug and, when applicable, with increased rate of drug release from its carrier (e.g., time to liquefaction of suppository preparations). Other factors affecting transmucosal rectal absorption include the volume of liquid, concentration of the drug, length of the rectal catheter (i.e., site of rectal drug delivery), presence of stool in the rectal vault, pH of the rectal contents, rectal retention of the drug or drugs administered, and differences in venous drainage within the rectosigmoid region.[27]

Anatomy and Physiology

The rectum is the terminal portion of the large intestine; it begins at the confluence of the three taeniae coli of the sigmoid colon and ends at the anal canal. In adults, the anal canal is approximately 5 cm in length and the rectum is approximately 10 cm to 15 cm in length. In children, the size of the rectum varies with age (Table 26.1).

The rectum has two main routes of venous drainage. The superior rectal vein drains into the portal circulation (by way of the inferior mesenteric vein), whereas the middle and inferior rectal veins drain into the caval system (by way of the inferior iliac vein). This pattern of venous drainage has a significant impact on the peak serum concentrations achieved by rectally administered drugs. Drugs administered high in the rectum (the area drained by the superior rectal vein) are carried directly to the liver via the portal vein and are subject to first-pass metabolism. In contrast, drugs administered low in the rectum are delivered systemically into the inferior vena cava, thereby avoiding first-pass elimination in the liver.

Indications and Contraindications

Rectal drug administration is indicated when more desirable routes are unavailable or impractical. For example, IV access in small children may be very difficult to obtain and frightening to the child. In these situations, the option of rectal administration may outweigh the benefits of IV drug delivery. Patients who refuse parenteral drug administration may also benefit from rectal delivery, as will those with nausea and vomiting or an inability to swallow.

Rectal Administration Of Medication

Indications

Drug administration when more desirable routes are unavailable or impractical:
- Children frightened of intravenous catheterization
- Patients who refuse parenteral drug administration
- Patients with nausea/vomiting or inability to swallow

Contraindications

Immunosuppression
Severe thrombocytopenia or coagulopathy
Active gastrointestinal bleeding
Diarrhea
Chronic anorectal problems (fissures, hemorrhoids, fistulas. etc.)

Complications

Erractic absorption
- Delayed, prolonged, or unusually rapid

Local trauma
Pain

Equipment

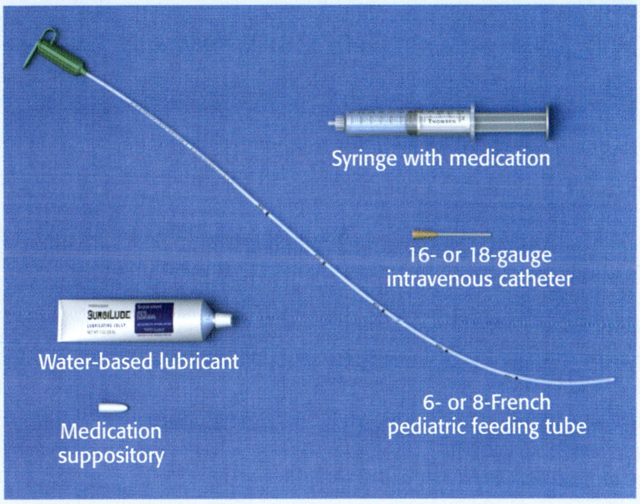

Review Box 26.3 Rectal medication administration: indications, contraindications, complications, and equipment.

TABLE 26.1 Age-Related Changes in Rectal Dimensions

AGE	DIAMETER (cm)	LENGTH (cm)	VOLUME (mL)	LENGTH TO INSERT CATHETER (cm)
1 month	1.5	3	7	1.5
3 months	3.0	6	42	3
1 year	3.5	7	67	3.5
2 years	4.0	8	100	4
6 years	4.5	9	143	4.5
10 years	5.0	12	235	6

From Smith S, Sharkey I, Campbell D. Guidelines for rectal administration of anticonvulsant medication in children. *Pediatr Perinatal Drug Ther*. 2001;4:140-147.

There are few, if any, absolute contraindications to rectal drug administration. Rectal administration should be avoided in immunosuppressed patients, in whom even minimal trauma could lead to bacteremia, and in patients with severe thrombocytopenia or coagulopathy to avoid difficult-to-control bleeding.[27,136] Patients with active lower gastrointestinal bleeding and those with severe diarrhea are not generally candidates for rectal drug administration. Finally, patients with a variety of acute or chronic anorectal problems such as fissures, hemorrhoids, perianal abscesses, or fistulas may not tolerate rectal drug administration.

Equipment (Review Box 26.3)

For medications in suppository form, a water-soluble lubricant will reduce the discomfort associated with insertion. For liquid and gel formulations, use an appropriately sized syringe attached to a small (e.g., 6- or 8-Fr) rubber feeding tube or an 18- or 16-gauge plastic IV catheter with the needle removed. A specialized rectal catheter, the Macy Catheter (Hospi Corp) (Fig. 26.6), is a device that offers a rectal route for administration of medications or fluids via rectal mucosal absorption. The catheter is a thin silicone tube 14-Fr in diameter with a 15-mL balloon at the tip, sized to allow secure retention, yet also provide for ready elimination in the event of need for defecation. It features multiple exit ports for fluid and medication passage, and an internal one-way check valve to prevent backflow of fluids.[137]

Procedure

Suppositories

Place adults and large children in a lateral recumbent position on the stretcher or examination table. Flex the upper leg at the knee and hip, but keep the lower leg extended. Infants, because of their small size, can be placed in almost any position. Place the lubricated suppository at the rectal opening and gently push it into the rectum toward the umbilicus until the gloved index finger has been inserted approximately 7.5 cm in adults, 3.5 cm in children, or 1.5 cm in infants (see Table 26.1). To help prevent expulsion of the suppository, do not allow the patient to get up for approximately 10 to 15 minutes after insertion.

Most suppositories have an apex at one end (pointed end) and taper to a blunt base at the other end. For ease of insertion, manufacturers recommend inserting the tapered end first. However, in 1991 Abd-El-Maeboud and colleagues found that inserting suppositories blunt end first resulted in greater retention within the rectum and a lower expulsion rate.[138] Nonetheless, these findings have not been corroborated and have been challenged by nursing educators as insufficient evidence on which to base clinical practice.[139]

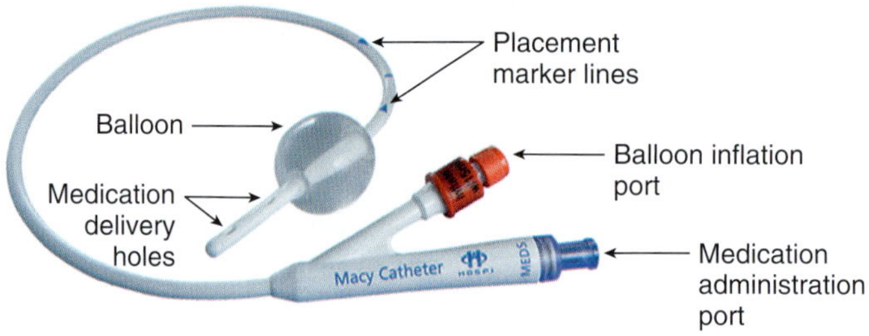

Fig. 26.6 Macy rectal catheter. (Courtesy Hospi Corporation.)

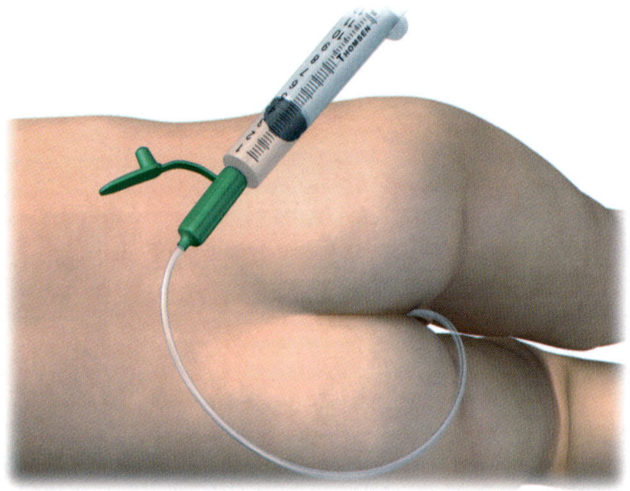

Fig. 26.7 Pediatric rectal administration of medication via a pediatric feeding tube.

Liquids and Gels

Position the patient as described for insertion of a suppository. Draw up the desired dose of medication into an appropriately sized syringe attached to a 6- or 8-Fr rubber feeding tube (adults and large children) or an 18- or 16-gauge IV catheter (infants and small children) with the needle removed (Fig. 26.7). The goal is to deposit the drug in the low to mid-portion of the rectum to avoid first-pass elimination by the liver. For adults, insert the rubber feeding tube approximately 7.5 cm to 10.0 cm and slowly inject the drug. In children, catheter depth varies with age (see Table 26.1). When administering rectal medication to infants and young children, be sure to squeeze the buttock cheeks closed after withdrawing the catheter to prevent expulsion of the medication. A 3-inch piece of tape placed across the buttocks also works well and frees the clinician to perform other duties.

Medications

A variety of medications can be administered rectally. In emergency medicine practice, the most common medications given rectally are analgesics and antipyretics, sedative-hypnotic agents, anticonvulsants, and antiemetics.

Analgesics and Antipyretics

Acetaminophen is frequently administered rectally in children for both fever and pain. Common reasons for rectal administration include refusal to take the medication orally, vomiting, and altered mental status. Acetaminophen is commercially available in suppository form and is easy to obtain and administer. Studies comparing oral and rectal administration of acetaminophen have demonstrated equal antipyretic effectiveness.[140,141] Rectal dosing of acetaminophen is the same as oral dosing (Table 26.2).

Though not commonly administered rectally, aspirin, nonsteroidal antiinflammatory drugs (NSAIDs) including indomethacin and diclofenac (diclofenac suppositories are not available in the United States), and morphine also come in rectal formulations and can be very useful in a variety of ED encounters. For example, aspirin is commonly administered rectally to adults with symptoms of a transient ischemic attack, an acute stroke, or an acute coronary syndrome who may have an impaired swallowing mechanism or are too unstable to take medications orally. Like acetaminophen, the oral and rectal doses of aspirin are similar (see Table 26.2). Rectal NSAIDs and morphine may be an alternative for patients discharged from the ED who require ongoing analgesia but cannot tolerate oral medications.[142–146] Rectal doses of indomethacin and morphine are shown in Table 26.2.

Sedative-Hypnotic Agents

Sedative-hypnotic agents, including midazolam, methohexital, and thiopental, may be administered rectally in children requiring sedation in the ED.[147–150] This occurs most often in pediatric patients in whom IV access may be problematic or for procedures that require only minimal sedation in conjunction with the use of local anesthetics. Rectal administration of methohexital is particularly useful for nonpainful procedures such as sedating children before advanced imaging studies. The major drawback of rectal administration is an inability to titrate these medications to the desired level of sedation.

The rectal doses of midazolam and methohexital in children are 0.25 to 0.5 mg/kg and 25 mg/kg (see Table 26.2). For pain control, one study found the combination of rectal ketamine (5 to 7 mg/kg) combined with intranasal dexmedetomidine (1 to 2 μg/kg) to provide adequate pain control for burn patients undergoing painful dressing changes.[151]

Antiseizure Medications

Antiseizure medications are generally administered orally, IM, or intravenously in the ED. However, in outpatient settings, patient families are at times instructed to administer seizure abortive medications rectally.[152] Studies have demonstrated that diazepam, because of its high lipid solubility, is rapidly absorbed from the rectum and can quickly halt seizures.[152,153]

Diazepam is commercially available in a gel formulation that is preloaded in a rectal delivery system. However, the undiluted parenteral formulation can also be used. The preloaded rectal delivery system is available for both pediatric and adult use. The adult device contains 4 mL (20 mg) of diazepam gel and has a 6-cm tip for rectal administration. This device is designed to deliver set doses of 12.5, 15, 17.5, and 20

TABLE 26.2 Drugs Commonly Administered Rectally in the Emergency Department

DRUG	RECTAL DOSE/FREQUENCY	ONSET[a]	DURATION	COMMENTS
Analgesics/Antipyretics				
Acetaminophen	Adults: 325–650 mg every 4–6 h or 1000 mg every 6–8 h (max, 4 g/day) Children: 10–20 mg/kg every 4–6 h (not to exceed 5 doses per day, maximum dose 75 mg/kg per day not to exceed 1625 mg/day)	~1 h	~4–6 h	Studies have demonstrated equal antipyretic efficacy with rectal and oral administration of acetaminophen
Aspirin	Adults: 300–600 mg every 4–6 h (max, 4 g/day) Children: 10–15 mg/kg every 4–6 h (max, 90 mg/kg per day or 4 g/day, whichever is lesser)	~1 h	4–6 h	Contraindications are the same as for oral administration (e.g., children with chickenpox or recent flulike symptoms)
Indomethacin	Adults: 25–50 mg per dose every 8–12 h (max, 200 mg/day)	~30 min	4–6 h	Indocin suppositories only come in 50-mg doses, which may exceed non–adult-sized pediatric dosing needs
Morphine	Adults: 10 mg every 4 h as needed	~30–60 min	~3–7 h	Rectal absorption may vary widely; not FDA approved for use in children
Sedative Hypnotics				
Midazolam	Children: 0.25–0.5 mg/kg as a one-time dose	~10–30 min	~60–90 min	Because these drugs cannot be titrated when given rectally, close monitoring for oversedation is mandatory
Methohexital	Children: 25 mg/kg as a one-time dose	~5–15 min	~45–60 min	Prepare a solution of methohexital for rectal administration by adding 5 mL of sterile water or saline to a 500-mg vial and mix well
Anticonvulsants				
Diazepam	Children and adults: 0.2–0.5 mg/kg as a one-time dose (maximum 20 mg/dose)	~2–10 min	~60–120 min	Dosing guidelines are for status epilepticus; products available in 2.5-, 10-, and 20-mg syringes
Antiemetics				
Prochlorperazine	Adults: 25 mg every 12 h as needed	~60 min	3–12 h	Central nervous system effects similar to those with other routes of administration for both prochlorperazine and promethazine
Promethazine	Adults: 12.5–25 mg every 4–6 h Children >2 years: 0.25–0.5 mg/kg per dose every 4–6 h (maximum 25 mg/dose)	~60 min	4–12 h	

[a]The onset of action of rectally administered medications may vary widely because of erratic absorption and first-pass elimination in the liver.

mg of diazepam. Two pediatric devices are available: one contains 0.5 mL of a 5-mg/mL gel, and the other contains 2 mL of a 5-mg/mL gel. The latter is designed to deliver set doses of 5, 7.5, and 10 mg of diazepam. Both pediatric devices have a 4.4-cm tip for rectal administration. The recommended dose of diazepam rectal gel for treating actively seizing children and those in status epilepticus is 0.2 to 0.5 mg/kg (depending on age); the adult dose is 10 to 20 mg as a single dose (see Table 26.2).

Antiemetics

Antiemetics are frequently used in the ED for patients with nausea and vomiting. In most cases, these medications are given intravenously. Oral dissolving tablets (ODT) antiemetics such as ondansetron have largely replaced the use of rectal antiemetics as this route is preferred by most patients. However, for patients with mild symptoms who do not otherwise require IV access and for discharged patients expected to have ongoing nausea and vomiting (e.g., patients with viral gastroenteritis), rectal administration is an alternative. Rectal administration may also be used as the initial treatment of ED patients with active vomiting in whom IV access will be delayed and ODT antiemetics have failed.

Historically, the two most common antiemetics administered rectally in the ED are prochlorperazine and promethazine. Both come in suppository formulations, which makes rectal administration easy. Prochlorperazine requires a higher dose when given rectally, whereas promethazine dosing is the same regardless of the route of administration (see Table 26.2).

Complications

Complications specific to rectal administration include erratic absorption and local trauma. Absorption of a rectally administered drug may be delayed or prolonged, or uptake may be almost as rapid as though the agent were administered intravenously.[27] Unusually rapid absorption resulted in the death of a 7.5-month-old child receiving rectal morphine for postoperative pain.[154] In addition to erratic absorption, peak serum concentrations may vary considerably depending on how much of the drug undergoes first-pass elimination in the liver. These factors make rectal drug administration less desirable in most cases when parenteral administration is possible.

Insertion of a suppository or catheter into the rectum may cause mild pain and mucosal irritation, which is usually well tolerated by most patients. Similarly, bleeding from local trauma is usually of no clinical consequence, except in patients with a clinically significant coagulopathy or severe thrombocytopenia.[136] Development of a perianal or perirectal abscess is a theoretical concern in neutropenic patients, and thus rectal drug administration is best avoided in such patients.

Transdermal Administration of Medication

Anatomy and Physiology

Intact skin offers a large surface area to absorb medications for a variety of indications including pain control, local anesthesia, and blood pressure control. Transdermal medications work by direct absorption through the epidermis. Transdermal medications bypass first-pass metabolism by the liver and often minimize the side effects of systemic medications.

Indications and Contraindication

In emergency medicine, transdermal medications are used most commonly for topical anesthesia for painful procedures, pain from minor burns, exposures such as rhus dermatitis (topical anesthetics), for emergent vasodilatory effects in angina pectoris (nitroglycerin), and for treatment of cannabis hyperemesis syndrome (capsaicin). Contraindications include allergy to a medication or component of the patch or cream being used, or underlying skin conditions (e.g., atopic dermatitis, psoriasis, icthyosis), which could make medication absorption unreliable or worsen the skin condition. Most transdermal medications are designed to be applied to intact skin.

Equipment

Sterile gauze, and water or alcohol swab, skin occlusive dressing.

Procedure

Clean and disinfect area of skin onto which the patch or topical medication will be applied with plain water or alcohol swab. Unless otherwise stated by the manufacturer, apply the medication only to intact skin. Institutionally compounded topical lidocaine/epinephrine/tetracaine liquid or gel can be used on open wounds. Once applied, topical treatments may remain better in the location you applied it by placing an occlusive dressing over the area. Patches containing medications do not need occlusive dressings.

Medications

Nitroglycerin

Nitroglycerin 2% can be applied to the chest as an ointment and acts as a vasodilator reducing cardiac preload from venous dilation and oxygen demand to the heart. Time to effect is usually 15 to 30 minutes.[155] Topical nitroglycerin also can be used to treat pain from anal fissures.[156,157]

Lidocaine and Other Combination Topical Anesthetics

Lidocaine-based topical products may be used to relieve pain in minor injuries and are commonly used for laceration repair.[158] Eutectic mixture of local anesthetics (EMLA) cream (lidocaine and prilocaine) is a widely used topical anesthetic for intact skin that reaches a maximal depth of anesthesia of 3 mm after a 60-minute application, and 5 mm after a 120-minute application. Lidocaine 4% or 5% cream has similar efficacy and a shorter onset of action (15 to 40 minutes). Both work by reversibly blocking nerve conduction of the dermal free ends of afferent nociceptive pain fibers near their site of administration. A combination of lidocaine 4%, epinephrine (0.1%), and tetracaine (0.5%) (aka "LET") mixed as a gel can be applied to open wounds for local anesthesia before suture repair. After 15 to 30 minutes, a ring of pallor around the wound edges will alert the clinician that anesthesia has been achieved. Avoid applying LET (which contains epinephrine) to end-arteriolar structures such as fingertips, nose tips, and penis.

Opioids

Use of opioid patches such as fentanyl and buprenorphine are generally not indicated for emergent use in acute pain given the delay of onset of analgesia (12 hours to onset of pain relief). Furthermore, precise titration and conversion of patches are necessary, accounting for the patient's chronic opioid usage and tolerance, rendering these interventions impractical in emergency medicine.

Capsaicin

Topical capsaicin cream applied to the abdomen has shown some benefit as an opioid-sparing treatment in patients with cannabis hyperemesis syndrome.[159,160]

Complications

The main complications of transdermal medications are skin irritation, burning, or itching related to a contact or allergic dermatitis from contents in the cream or patch. Topical lidocaine overdoses can result in seizures,[161] methemoglobinemia, arrhythmias, and even death.[162] Maximum recommended dose (by age and weight) of EMLA is shown in Table 26.3. Topical capsaicin exposures to the eye can result in eye pain.

OTHER ALTERNATE ROUTES OF ADMINISTRATION OF MEDICATION

There is a limited but growing body of evidence demonstrating the benefits of rehydration of patients (usually the elderly[163–165] or very young[166,167]) in the ED using a subcutaneous route called "hypodermoclysis" (Box 26.1). Historically, hypodermoclysis in humans was used in the elderly in nonemergency situations for rehydration. The advent of human

TABLE 26.3 Maximum Dose of EMLA Cream

Newborns 0–2 months	Up to 1 g and 10 cm^2 for 1 h
Infants 3–11 months	Up to 2 g and 20 cm^2 for 1 h
Toddlers and children 1–5 years	Up to 10 g and 100 cm^2 for 1–5 h
Children 6–11 years	Up to 20 g and 200 cm^2 for 1–5 h

From EMLA package insert https://www.ema.europa.eu/en/documents/referral/emla-cream-article-30-referral-annex-iii_en.pdf.

BOX 26.1 Subcutaneous Hydration (Hypodermoclysis)

INDICATIONS

Moderate dehydration with difficult IV access

CONTRAINDICATIONS

Severe dehydration, hypovolemic shock, overlying cellulitis at insertion site

COMPLICATIONS

Pain, swelling with infusion
Cellulitis at IV site (rare)

EQUIPMENT

IV fluid bag with tubing
Small-gauge butterfly needle (21-gauge or higher)
Hyaluronidase
Lidocaine 1%
Gloves
Alcohol swabs or povidone-iodine solution
Occlusive dressing

recombinant hyaluronidase has made it possible to give faster rates of IV fluid infusion making its use in the ED feasible. The most common practical use of this method is in the setting of dehydration when IV access is unobtainable, though theoretically, medications may also be given via this route. Potential advantages of subcutaneous rehydration compared with IV rehydration are that it expedites and simplifies parenteral access, requires fewer staff resources, and is potentially less distressing to parents and patients.[166]

Anatomy and Physiology

Hypodermoclysis uses human recombinant hyaluronidase to break up hyaluronan, a mucopolysaccharide found in the intercellular matrix of connective tissue that normally prevents flow of fluids across the subcutaneous layer of tissue. This transiently increases permeability of the connective tissue matrix, allowing movement of subcutaneously administered fluids (and medications) into the surrounding tissues, with subsequent systemic absorption via the capillary beds.

Indications and Contraindications

Subcutaneous hydration is indicated in moderately dehydrated patients in whom IV access is not easily obtainable, and in whom enteral routes (oral [PO]/nasogastric [NG]) of rehydration have failed. This method should not be employed in severely dehydrated patients in hypovolemic shock, where IO or central venous access should be considered. Do not use hypodermoclysis if an enteral route (PO, NG) is tolerated.

Equipment

An IV solution bag, a tube with a drip chamber, a small-gauge (21 or smaller) long-tube butterfly needle, povidone-iodine solution or alcohol skin preparation, and a sterile occlusive dressing.

Procedure

Hypodermoclysis sites include the abdomen, upper chest, above the breast, over an intercostal space and the intrascapular area, the lateral thighs, the abdomen, and the outer aspect of the upper arm (Fig. 26.8). In uncooperative adult patients or pediatric patients, the intrascapular site may be preferred to avoid dislodgment of the setup by the patient (Fig. 26.9). Assemble fluid and tubing. Prime line with selected fluid and 150 units of hyaluronidase. Swab the site with povidone-iodine skin or alcohol preparation solution. Inject local anesthetic into insertion site. Pinching the skin between fingers, insert a 21-gauge (or smaller) needle, bevel up, into subcutaneous tissue at a 45- to 60-degree angle. Administer 150 units of human recombinant hyaluronidase into the subcutaneous space. Secure needle and tubing with occlusive dressing. Adjust fluid drip rate as desired.

REFERENCES ARE AVAILABLE AT Elsevier eBooks+

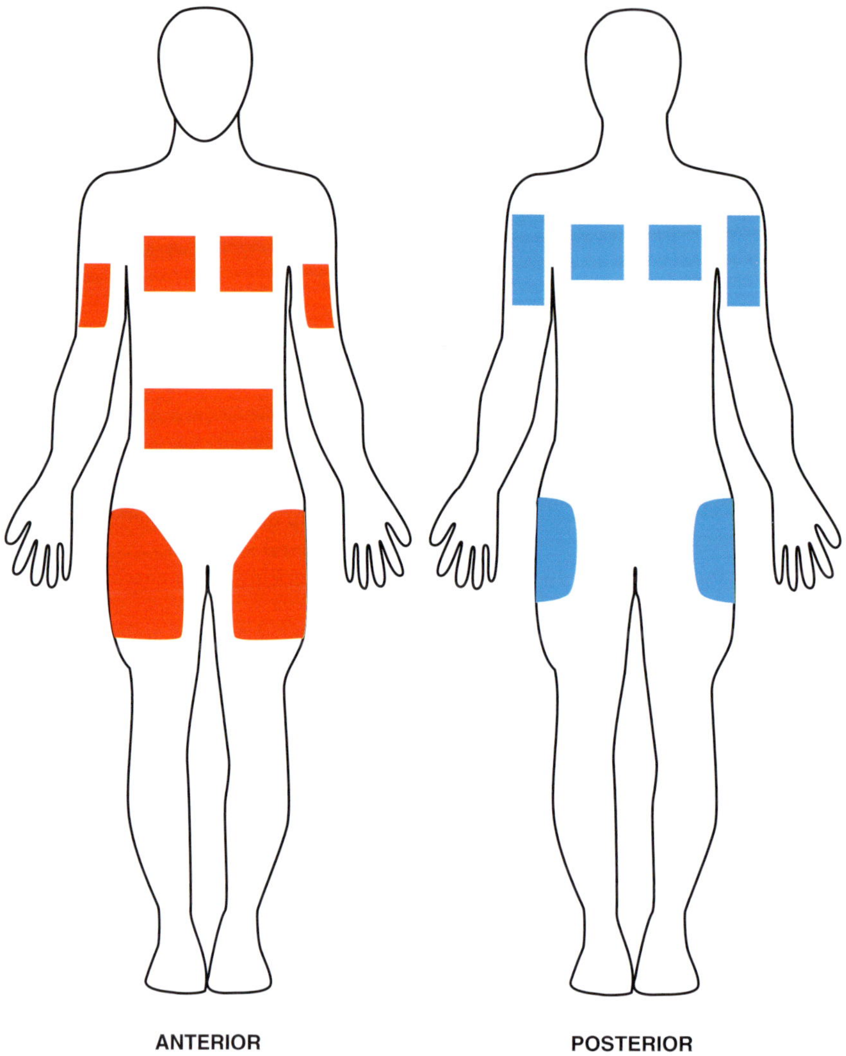

Fig. 26.8 Anatomic sites usable for hypodermoclysis. (From Bruno VG. Hypodermoclysis: a literature review to assist in clinical practice. *Einstein.* 2015;13(1):122-128.)

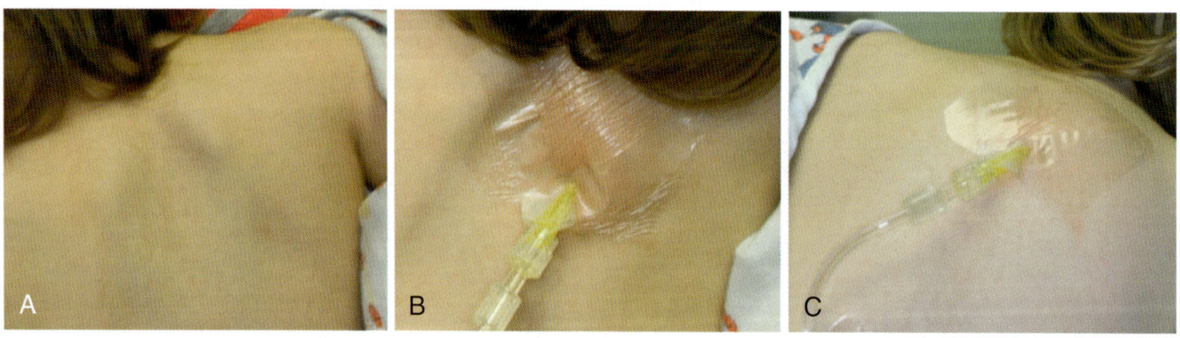

Fig. 26.9 Appearance of interscapular hypodermoclysis in a child: (A) prior to infusion, (B) 4 minutes after infusion, and (C) 44 minutes after infusion. (From Allen CH, Etzwiler LS, Miller MK et al. Recombinant human hyaluronidase-enabled subcutaneous pediatric rehydration. *Pediatrics.* 2009;124(5):e858-e867.)

CHAPTER 27

Autotransfusion

Chad M. Bleske, Mark J. Neavyn, and Margarita E. Pena

INTRODUCTION

Autologous blood transfusion, or autotransfusion, is the collection and reinfusion of a patient's own blood for volume replacement.[1] Preoperative blood banking and intraoperative cell salvage techniques have increased in a multitude of surgical specialties.[2–7] Autotransfusion in the emergency department (ED) is usually limited to patients with severe, traumatic hemothorax and clinically significant blood loss.

Autotransfusion is usually performed in trauma centers or in EDs with high trauma volume. Though not a uniform standard of care for emergency clinicians, it is applicable to any ED. As the procedure requires familiarity with the equipment, continuing education, and quality control, it would be counterproductive to institute the procedure in a hospital that has a low trauma census or in a setting of infrequent use, creating staff education challenges. Clinicians practicing in more austere environments with a paucity of clinical resources, such as low-resource settings, combat, and disaster zones, may find that the benefits of autotransfusion outweigh the risks.[8–11]

BACKGROUND

Reports of autotransfusion can be found as early as 1818 when Dr. James Blundell, an English practitioner, reinfused shed blood after witnessing a female exsanguinate from uterine hemorrhage.[12] In 1886 Duncan published the first known human account of autotransfusion in which he reinfused shed blood in a patient with a traumatic amputation without any notable ill effects.[13] In 1917 Elmendorf published a description of the first case of autotransfusion in a patient with traumatic hemothorax.[14]

The discovery of ABO blood typing at the turn of the century and the institution of blood banks in the 1930s led to the almost exclusive use of allogeneic (homologous) blood up to

Autotransfusion

Indications

Hemothorax containing >1500 mL
Hemothorax with an immediate need for transfusion and insufficient allogeneic blood available
Hemothorax with an urgent need for blood and the patient's religious beliefs prohibit the use of banked blood

Contraindications

Coagulopathy or disseminated intravascular cougulation
Possibility of malignant cells in the salvaged blood
Active infection
Gross contamination of pleural blood from gastrointestinal contents

Complications

Hematologic
- Decreased platelet count
- Decreased fibrinogen level
- Increased fibrin split products
- Prolonged prothrombin time
- Prolonged partial thromboplastin time
- Red blood cell hemolysis
- Elevated plasma free hemoglobin
- Decreased hematocrit

Nonhematologic
- Bacteremia
- Sepsis
- Microembolism
- Air embolism
- Renal insufficiency

Equipment

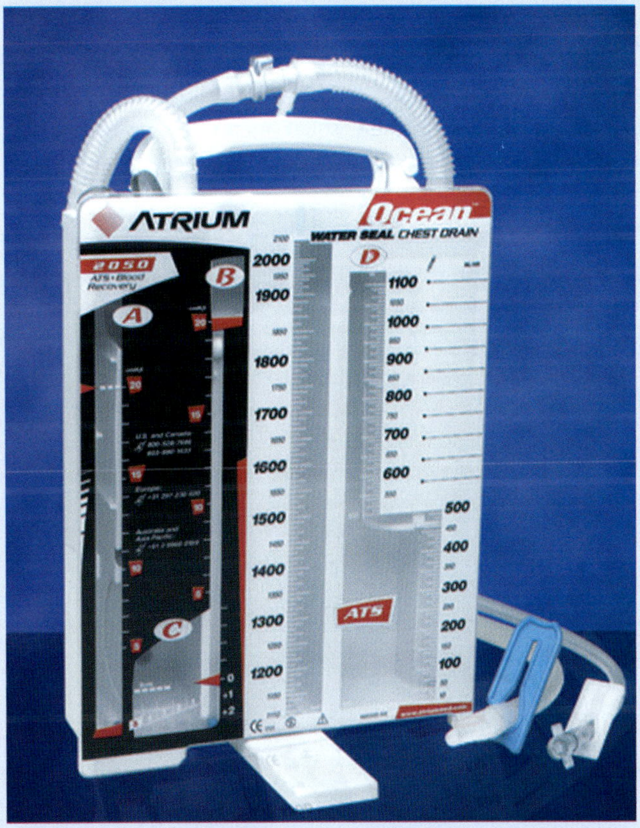

Chest drainage and autotransfusion system (Atrium Ocean ATS).

Review Box 27.1 Autotransfusion: indications, contraindications, complications, and equipment.

and following World War II. During the 1960s and 1970s, cardiopulmonary bypass surgery and combat trauma experience during the Vietnam War generated extensive data regarding intraoperative retrieval of large quantities of blood for reinfusion.[15,16] This revitalized interest, coupled with increased experience in surgical, trauma, and combat situations initiated a new era in autotransfusion.

ANATOMY

Hemothorax refers to a collection of blood within the pleural space. Severe hemorrhage is more often associated with laceration of vessels on the inside of the chest wall, such as the internal mammary and intercostal arteries. Blunt and penetrating trauma are by far the most common causes of hemothorax. Spontaneous hemothorax can occur secondary to intrathoracic malignancy,[17] pulmonary infarction, bullous emphysema, virulent pulmonary or mediastinal infection, vascular malformation, and endometriosis of the pleura (catamenial).[18]

PATHOPHYSIOLOGY

The pathophysiologic sequelae of hemothorax include both hemodynamic instability and respiratory compromise. The pleural cavity can accommodate more than 50% of the total blood volume, so clinically significant intrathoracic blood loss can occur with minimal external signs of bleeding. The clinician should suspect hemothorax in the setting of chest trauma with clinical signs of hypovolemia. Physical examination may demonstrate decreased breath sounds and reduced tactile fremitus. Imaging during the initial resuscitation period is usually limited to supine chest radiographs, which may show haziness in the affected lung field as blood layers in the posterior pleural space (Fig. 27.1). Ultrasound is also useful in the initial evaluation of hemothorax, and recent studies suggest it is more sensitive than a chest x-ray for detection of a hemothorax (Fig. 27.2).[19–21]

ADVANTAGES

Shed blood from traumatic hemothorax is immediately available for rapid transfusion. The blood is normothermic and compatible, avoiding the risk of immune-mediated and blood type incompatibility reactions, allergic reaction, or infection from transfusion transmissible diseases. There are numerous transfusion transmissible diseases, including viruses such as human immunodeficiency virus (HIV) and hepatitis, bacteria, parasites, and most recently reported, the prion disease variant Creutzfeldt-Jakob disease.[22–24] Although the risk for transfusion transmissible diseases has decreased dramatically in developed countries, it is still very problematic worldwide.[25–27] Immunologic transfusion reactions and posttransfusion sepsis continue to be risks as well.[28] In trauma patients, allogeneic transfusions have been shown to be an independent risk factor for infection, which may be dose dependent and independently associated with increased morbidity and mortality.[29–34] In patients whose religious convictions (e.g., Jehovah's Witness) prohibit transfusions with homologous blood, reinfusion of autologous blood that does not involve blood storage may be an acceptable alternative.[35]

A 2015 multicenter study by Rhee and colleagues[36] compared outcomes in 136 patients receiving autotransfused blood from a traumatic hemothorax to an equal number receiving only allogeneic transfusions. There was no difference between the groups in mortality or in-hospital complications (sepsis, disseminated intravascular coagulation [DIC], acute lung injury, or renal insufficiency). Despite its retrospective design, this study offers support for the practice of autotransfusion based on patient-oriented outcomes.

Autologous blood provides societal benefits by preserving the limited stores of banked blood and reducing the cost of medical care.[37,38] Adias and colleagues compared the direct cost of banked blood with the cost of autologous blood transfusion and found substantial savings with autotransfusion.[39] A recent UK consensus document by the Association of Anaesthetists of updated guidelines on cell salvage for perioperative blood conservation in 2018 recommended wider use of cell salvage and universal availability in hospitals performing major surgery.[40]

The use of autotransfusion in low-resource settings may help improve outcomes in traumatic injuries when blood transfusion is necessary. Safe and sufficient blood products are often unavailable or limited. Two recent studies by Palmqvist et al. and Sjöholm et al. found that autotransfusion in low-resource settings is not widely established due to bottlenecks such as the lack of low-tech autotransfusion devices and insufficient knowledge and experience of doing autotransfusion.[41,42]

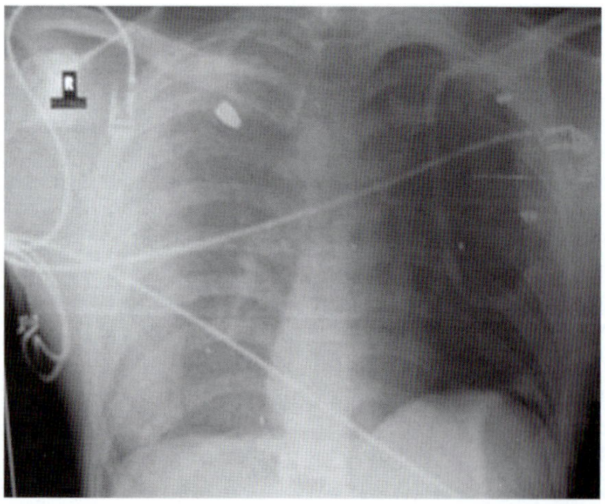

Fig. 27.1 Hemothorax secondary to a gunshot wound. Note the haziness over the right hemithorax with the bullet seen in the right upper lobe. In this supine radiograph, the volume of the hemothorax may not be fully appreciated. (From Marx JA. *Rosen's Emergency Medicine*. 7th ed. Mosby; 2009.)

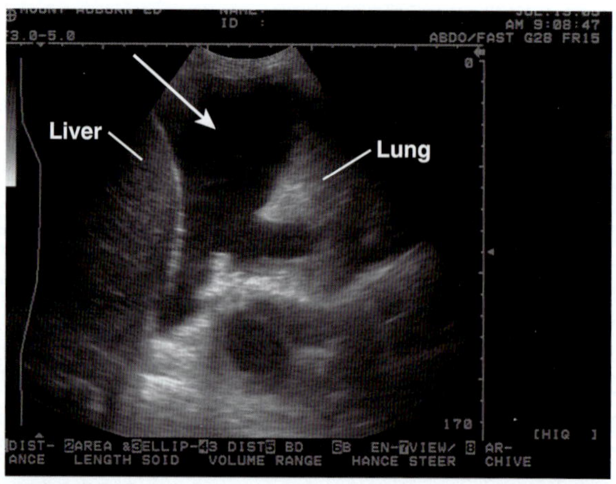

Fig. 27.2 Ultrasonographic appearance of hemothorax. Blood in the pleural cavity appears anechoic *(arrow)* and is easily seen interspersed between the collapsed lung and diaphragm.

BOX 27.1 Advantages of Autotransfusion

- Immediately available—no delay in crossmatching and no storage required
- Blood compatibility and allergic reaction not an issue
- Autologous blood usually normothermic
- No risk for transfusion transmissible disease
- No risk for hypocalcemia or hyperkalemia[55]
- Decreased risk for acute respiratory distress syndrome
- Higher levels of 2,3-diphosphoglycerate than in banked red blood cells[80]
- Decreased use of banked blood; more available for subsequent patients in need[38]
- Decreased cost of medical care[37,38]
- May be acceptable to religions opposed to homologous blood transfusions[44]
- May be a valuable alternative to banked blood in developing countries where infected donor blood is a problem

Developing specific protocols or simple low-tech devices may improve the usage of autotransfusion in low-resource settings.

Box 27.1 summarizes the advantages of autotransfusion.

INDICATIONS

In general, all patients sustaining severe trauma, whether blunt or penetrating, should be considered potential candidates for autotransfusion. Several categories of patients for whom emergency autotransfusion is suitable have been described and are summarized in Review Box 27.1. Reul and associates described the ideal autotransfusion candidate as a patient with blunt or penetrating trauma and hemothorax consisting of 1500 mL or more of blood.[43] Other patients who may benefit include those with an immediate need for transfusion for whom insufficient homologous blood is available (because of a shortage or a difficult crossmatch) and those whose religious convictions prohibit homologous transfusion.[44]

CONTRAINDICATIONS

In some situations, emergency autotransfusion may pose more risk than benefit. Coagulopathy and DIC are important contraindications.[8,45] Others include active infection, gross contamination, and the possibility of malignant cells in the salvaged blood.[46] With direct autotransfusion of pleural blood through a microfilter, the risk of reinfusing tumor cells is unknown. Work using perioperative cell salvage suggests that the risk for dissemination of malignant disease is minimal.[47] Concerns regarding gross contamination from concomitant gastrointestinal tract injury have also been disputed.[48]

More recent studies on contamination involving cell salvage systems that incorporates a cell-washing step are favorable.[49,50] Notably, the randomized control trial by Bowley et al. of 44 patients with penetrating abdominal trauma found that the 21 patients who underwent intraoperative cell salvage required less allogenic blood without increasing postoperative infection rates or mortality.[49] In a 2014 study by Caliste et al. of 179 patients with full-thickness hollow viscus injury due to blunt or penetrating abdominal trauma found that the 71 patients who received emergent autotransfusion and banked blood had no evidence of worsened outcome compared with the 108 patients who received only banked blood products.[51] Most recently in a retrospective cohort study of 185 trauma patients with full-thickness hollow viscus injury present on laparotomy by Lilienstein et al., the use of autotransfusion in enteric-contaminated laparotomy fields was not associated with increased blood bank use, mortality attributed to sepsis, overall mortality, or complications.[52] Nonetheless, the current consensus is that exsanguinating hemorrhage without available homologous blood is the only acceptable indication for autotransfusion when there is recognized intestinal contamination[53] and concurrent use of systemic antibiotics is adv ised.[8,9,49,50,53,54]

EQUIPMENT AND MATERIAL

Autotransfusion should be performed within 4 to 6 hours from the time of injury,[55,56] although it has been performed after this period in combat situations without significant complications.[8,50]

Tube thoracostomy, typically using size 32-Fr to 40-Fr chest tube, is the treatment of choice for traumatic hemothorax. Pigtail catheters have emerged as an alternative to traditional chest tubes for treatment of pneumothorax,[57] and there is also evidence for their use in the treatment of traumatic hemothorax.[58] A recent multicenter prospective randomized control study by Kulvatunyu et al. of 119 trauma patients with traumatic hemothorax found that 14-Fr pigtail catheters were as effective as traditional 28-Fr to 32-Fr chest tubes in terms of drainage capability without a difference in complications and better tolerated.[59] Patients who were hemodynamically unstable requiring emergent tube placement were excluded.

Blood Filters

In-line filtration is used routinely during reinfusion of blood products to reduce the danger of microembolization and resultant pulmonary insufficiency.[1,55,56] The relationship between the presence of microaggregates and the development of acute respiratory distress syndrome is controversial. Most investigators advise the use of a micropore filter with pore size recommendations ranging from 20 μm to 170 μm.[60,61] The majority of investigators believe that a pore size of 40 μm minimizes the risk for microembolization without undue elevation in filtration pressure.[43,62,63] The manufacturers of the commercial devices discussed in this chapter also recommend at least a 40-μm filter size.[2]

Vacuum Suction

The level of vacuum suction should be limited to minimize hemolysis of red blood cells.[63] The precise level at which clinically significant hemolysis occurs is uncertain, and there is wide variation (5 mm Hg to 100 mm Hg) in recommendations.[43,64–66] Several commercial products recommend a starting vacuum pressure of 20 mm Hg.[67]

Anticoagulation

Blood retrieved from the pleural and abdominal cavities frequently will not clot because it is devoid of fibrinogen.[68] This is believed to be because moderate rates of bleeding allow time for defibrination by contact with the serosal surfaces and by mechanical agitation from respiratory and cardiac movement. For this reason, some recommend simple reinfusion through a filter without any anticoagulant.[16,60,65,69] Wounds of the great vessels may bleed at a rate that allows coagulable blood to enter the collection reservoir and clot the entire system.[63,65,66] In the ED setting where autotransfusion is indicated for rapid blood loss, anticoagulation is recommended.

The use of heparin as an anticoagulant in trauma patients is not recommended by the manufacturers of autotransfusion devices.[67] Heparin anticoagulation is possible. Local heparinization of the tubing and reservoir may lead to the formation of platelet microaggregates on the filter and in the line, as well as increase the risk for systemic heparinization.[43,70]

Citrate compounds, an alternative to heparin, are frequently recommended for autotransfusion.[45] Citrates bind with the calcium ion and prevent conversion of protein fibrinogen into insoluble fibrin, which would cause the blood to clot. Because citrate binds only with calcium, it anticoagulates just the blood in which it is dissolved. Once the anticoagulated blood is infused, citrate is rapidly metabolized by the liver. Early studies used acid citrate dextrose (ACD).[55] More recently, citrate phosphate dextrose (CPD) has been used because it necessitates less volume as an anticoagulant and results in less acidosis than ACD.[43,71] Rarely, excessive use of CPD can cause cardiac dysrhythmias.[43] Use of insufficient or outdated CPD may result in clotting of collected blood. Baldan and colleagues described the use of simple autotransfusion in more than 200 patients with penetrating chest injuries and recommended using half-dose CPD adenine solution.[9] Although anticoagulant therapy and dosage recommendations are at the discretion of the physician, commercially available devices do offer some general guidelines (Table 27.1).

TABLE 27.1 ACD-A and CPD Dosage Recommendations

BLOOD VOLUME EXPECTED	FOR 1:7, ADD THIS AMOUNT OF ACD-A	FOR 1:20, ADD THIS AMOUNT OF ACD-A
ACD-A Dosage Recommendations[a] (Ratio of ACD-A to Blood)		
Low = 140–250 mL; incremental volume over 250 mL	20–35 mL; 1 mL for each 100 mL of collected blood	7–12 mL; 5 mL for each 100 mL of blood collected
Medium = 250–500 mL	40–70 mL	12.5–25 mL
High = 500–1000 mL	70–140 mL	25–50 mL

CPD dosage recommendations: Anticoagulant CPD solution can be added at the discretion of the physician at a control dosage of 14 mL of CPD solution to 100 mL of blood collected (70 mL CPD/500 mL blood).

[a]Dosage ratios are approximate. Note that 35 mL of ACD-A provides a 1:7 ratio of ACD-A to blood for low volume and a 1:20 ratio for high-volume blood and may be a good starting point if it is unclear how much blood will accumulate.

ACD-A, Acid citrate dextrose anticoagulant; *CPD*, citrate phosphate dextrose.

From *A Personal Guide to Managing Chest Drainage Autotransfusion*. Atrium Medical Corporation. http://www.atriummed.com/PDF/Red%20Handbook.pdf

Historical Techniques Using Standard ED Equipment

Before purpose-built systems were available, autotransfusion was possible by using common items available in most EDs. These techniques have not been as widely tested and are more appropriate for use in dire situations, such as may occur in a disaster or on the battlefield.[9]

Symbas described a simplified collecting system involving a standard chest tube bottle.[72] More than 400 patients were autotransfused via this method with no adverse effects attributable to the procedure. After insertion of a chest tube, blood was collected into a standard bottle containing 400 mL of normal saline, with suction maintained at 12 mm Hg to 16 mm Hg. The blood collected in the chest bottle can be reinfused in one of two possible ways, either directly from the collected bottle of blood or after transferring the blood to a sterile blood bag (Fig. 27.3). Improvements on his historical technique, such as the addition of anticoagulants and blood filters, should be considered.

Autotransfusion Units

All the commercially available autotransfusion systems (ATSs) are based on the same three-stage system (called the *three-bottle system*) for collection of pleural fluid. (Fig. 27.4). Currently used devices incorporate the three-bottle system into one unit. Stage 1 is the collection of pleural fluid (blood). Stage 2 is the water seal stage, in which water acts as a one-way valve (water seal) that allows air to be sucked out of the pleural space and not leak back in. Stage 3 is the suction control stage, which is essentially a safety stage. If the degree of suction suddenly increases beyond the set point, the system will pull air from the atmosphere instead of inappropriately increasing suction in the pleural cavity. Historically, water is frequently used in the suction control stage.

The disadvantage of using water in stages 2 or 3 is that if the device is knocked over, loss of the water seal and spillage of water from the suction control stage can occur. Newer designs have solved this problem, and two systems currently available do not use water (Atrium Express [Atrium Medical Corporation] and Pleur-evac Sahara [Teleflex]). These newer devices use a one-way valve instead of a water seal in stage 2 and a pressure regulator instead of water in the suction control stage (stage 3).

To collect blood for autotransfusion, a collection bag can be connected beforehand in series with the chest drainage system. With this arrangement, blood goes from the patient to the blood collection bag to the chest drainage system. When the blood bag is filled, it is removed and replaced with a new blood collection bag. If the bag overfills, the fluid will spill into the usual chest fluid collection system. Eventually, when no more blood needs to be autotransfused, the blood collection bag is taken out of the series and the chest tube drainage system functions as usual. Because blood goes directly into the blood collection bag, anticoagulant needs to be added to the blood collection bag before the blood flows into it.

Blood may also be drawn directly from a chest drainage system. Some devices have an additional port at the bottom called an ATS access line. This is referred to as a self-filling ATS. Not all devices permit withdrawal of blood directly from

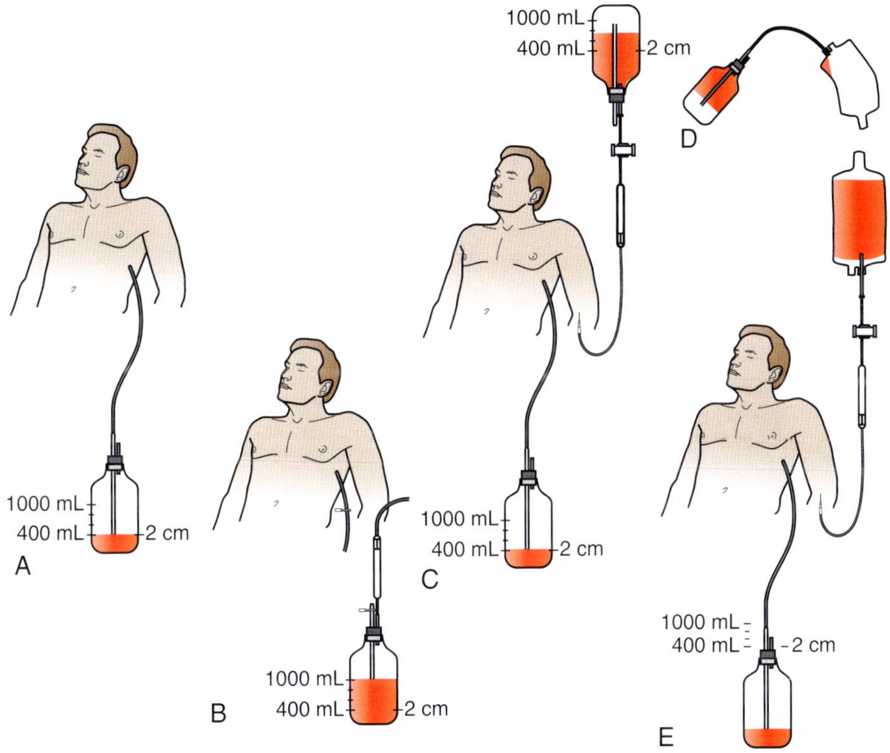

Fig. 27.3 Historical technique of autotransfusion for traumatic hemothorax. (A) Blood is collected into a sterile blood collection bottle with 400 mL of normal saline. (B) After blood is collected, the chest tube is disconnected from the collection bottle. (C) Blood is infused directly from the blood collection bottle while a new chest tube drainage bottle is connected to the chest tube, or (D) blood collected from the chest tube is transferred into a sterile blood bag. (E) Blood transferred into the blood bag is infused into the patient. (From Symbas PN. Extraoperative autotransfusion from hemothorax, *Surgery*. 1978;84:722.)

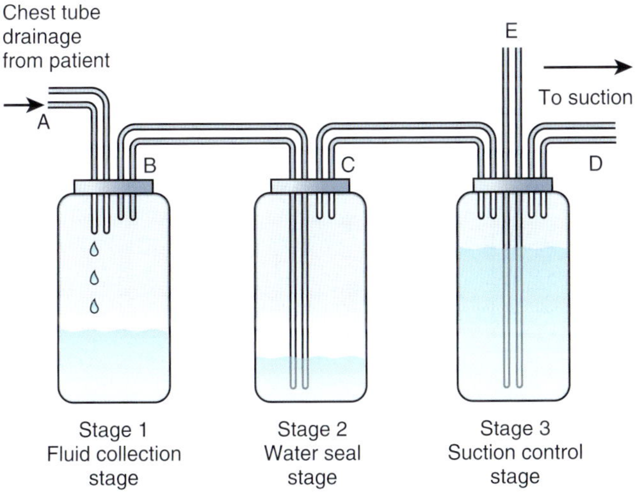

Fig. 27.4 Three-bottle chest drainage system. *A*, From the patient's chest tube. *B*, Connection to a water seal bottle (stage 2). *C*, Connection to the suction control bottle. *D*, Connection to suction. *E*, Vent tube for suction control.

the chest drainage system. In devices without this option, any blood that goes into the chest drainage system is not available for transfusion. The advantage of the ATS access line is that autotransfusion need not be anticipated before the chest tube collection system is connected to the chest tube. Because blood first goes to the collection chamber of the chest drainage device, anticoagulant needs to be added to the collection chamber before blood enters it.

Some models allow these chest drainage systems to be connected directly to the patient to provide continuous autotransfusion. In this setup, a blood filter with intravenous (IV) blood tubing is hooked up to an IV infusion pump. The blood can be continuously reinfused as it collects in the chest drainage system; it goes from the blood collection chamber out the ATS access line and is pumped into the patient with an IV infusion pump in a closed system (Fig. 27.5). Other models offer continuous infusion directly from a blood collection bag and not the chest drainage device. The blood simply goes from the chest tube into the blood collection bag, and a port on the bag is accessed to return the blood back to the patient.

PROCEDURE FOR AUTOTRANSFUSION

Whether in-line, self-filling, or continuous techniques are chosen depends on the chest tube drainage system used. Some systems allow more than one technique to collect blood for autotransfusion. The specific port locations and connections may vary slightly among the different designs, and the general concepts are relatively universal. See Figs. 27.6 and 27.7 for a description of several different systems from Atrium and Pleur-evac.

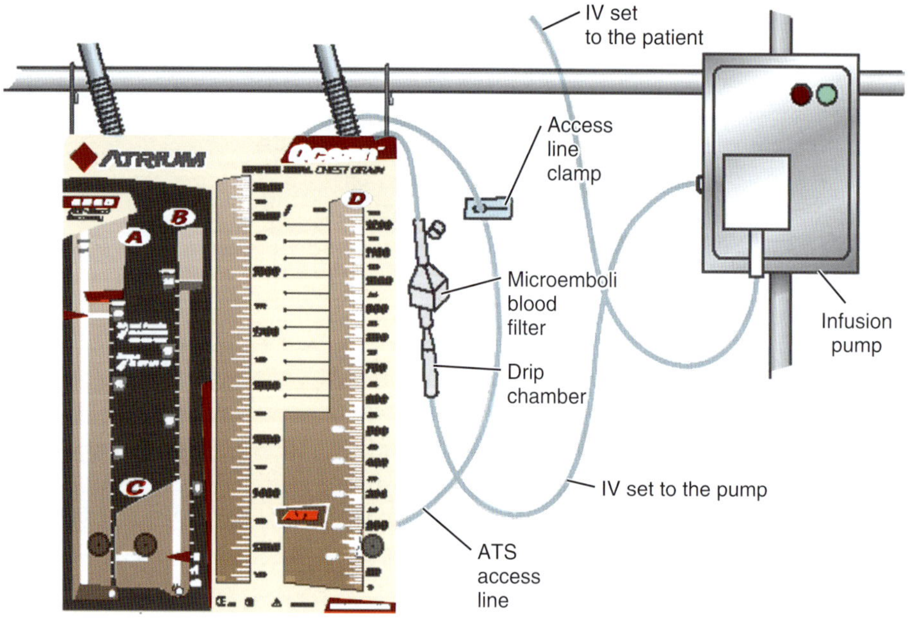

Fig. 27.5 Continuous autotransfusion. Blood is continuously reinfused into the patient as it collects in the chest drainage system. *ATS*, Autotransfusion system; *IV*, intravenous. (Courtesy Atrium Medical Corporation.)

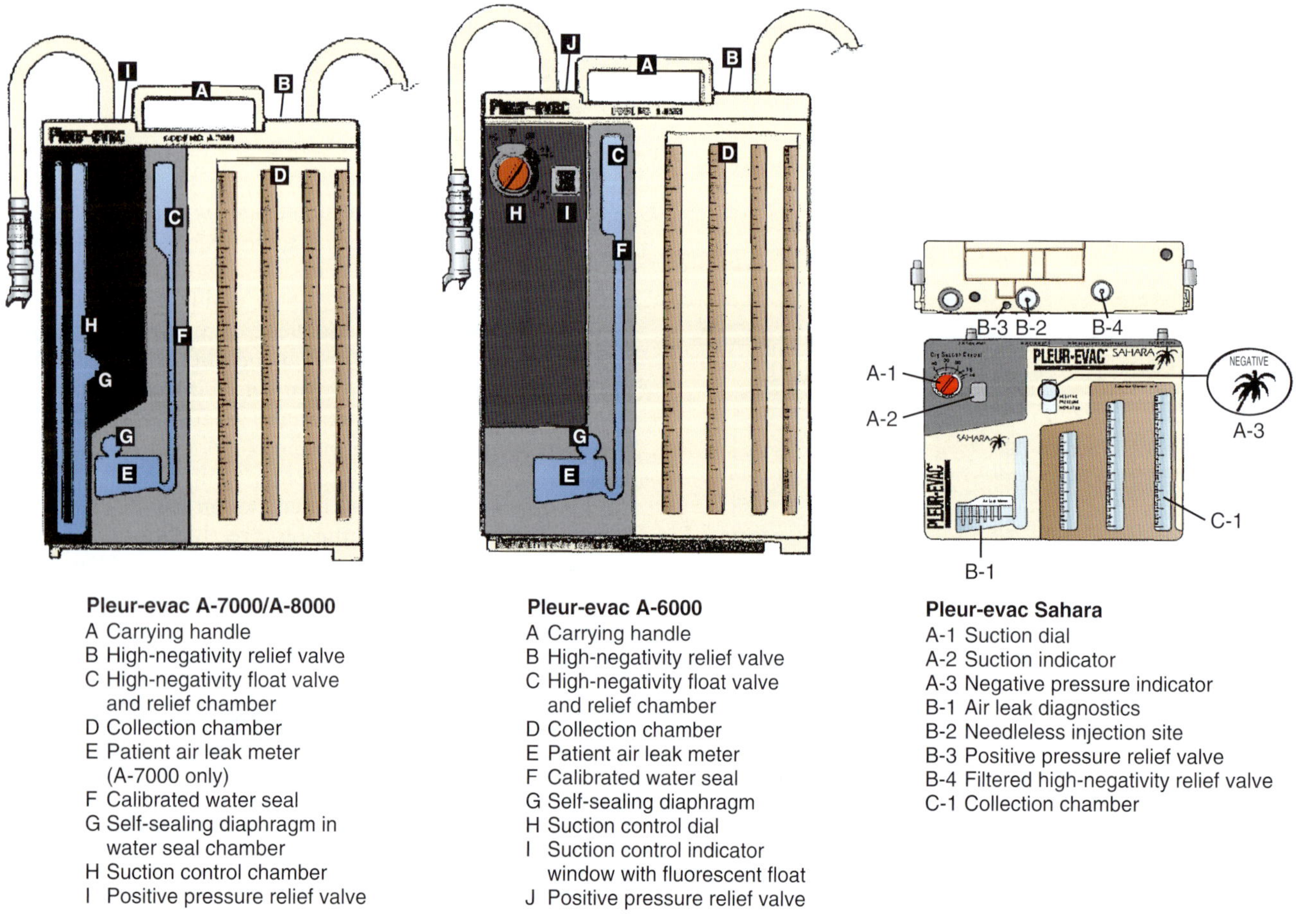

Fig. 27.6 Pleur-evac chest drainage systems. (Courtesy Teleflex Medical.)

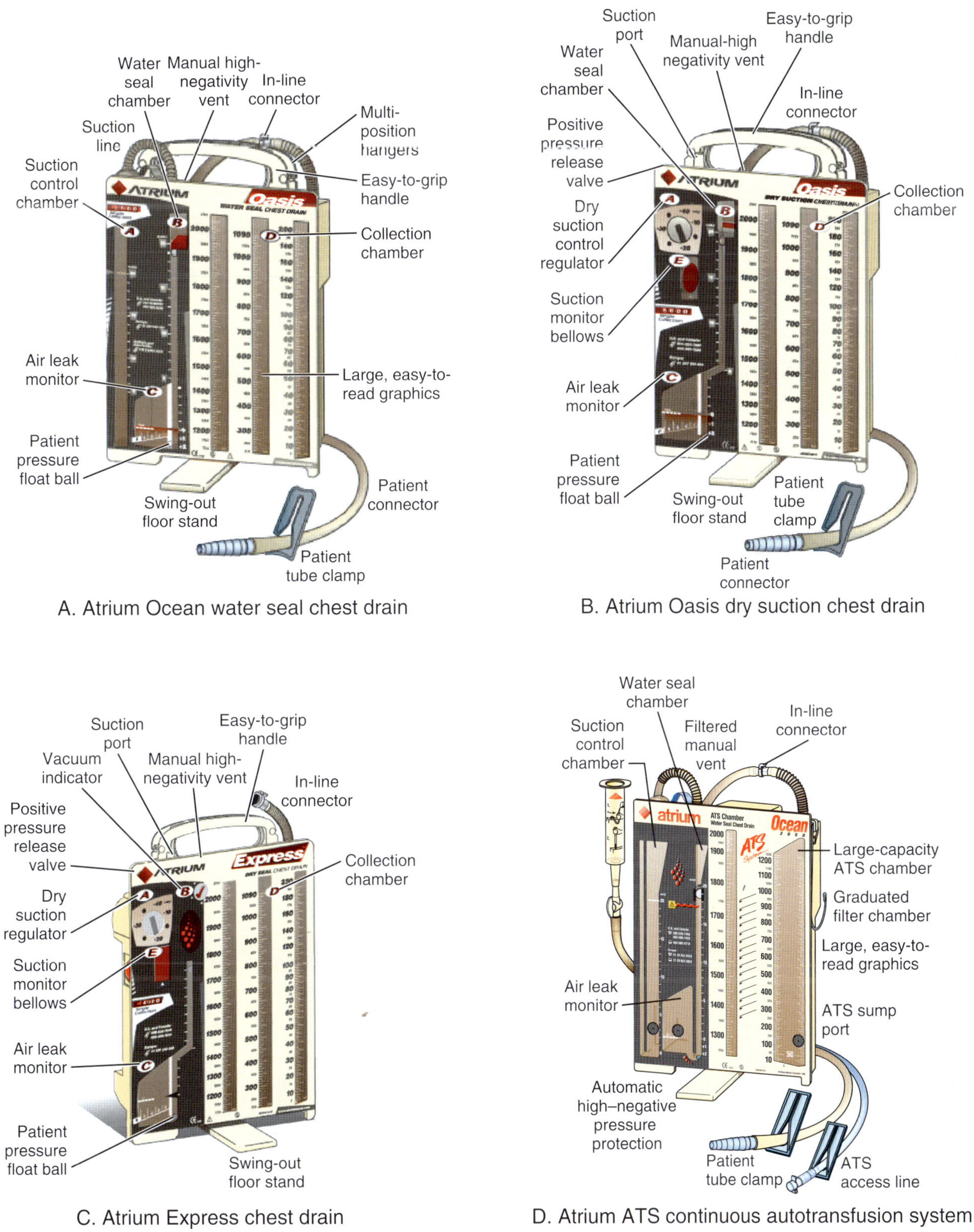

Fig. 27.7 Atrium chest drainage systems. *ATS*, Autotransfusion system. (Courtesy Atrium Medical Corporation.)

The procedure described here is for in-line blood collection and infusion using the Atrium Ocean model; all Atrium models have similar connectors. The procedure using Pleur-evac systems is also similar (Video 27.1)[73]

In-Line Autotransfusion Blood Collection and Infusion Procedure (Fig. 27.8)

1. Place the autotransfusion blood bag onto the chest drain via the attached flexible hanger.
2. Close both autotransfusion blood bag clamps and remove the protective caps over the autotransfusion bag connectors.
3. Close the patient's chest tube clamp.
4. Separate the connectors between the patient's chest tube and the Ocean chest drain by depressing the connector lock.
5. Insert the male patient chest tube connector into the female autotransfusion bag connector.
6. Insert the male autotransfusion bag connector into the female Ocean chest drain connector.

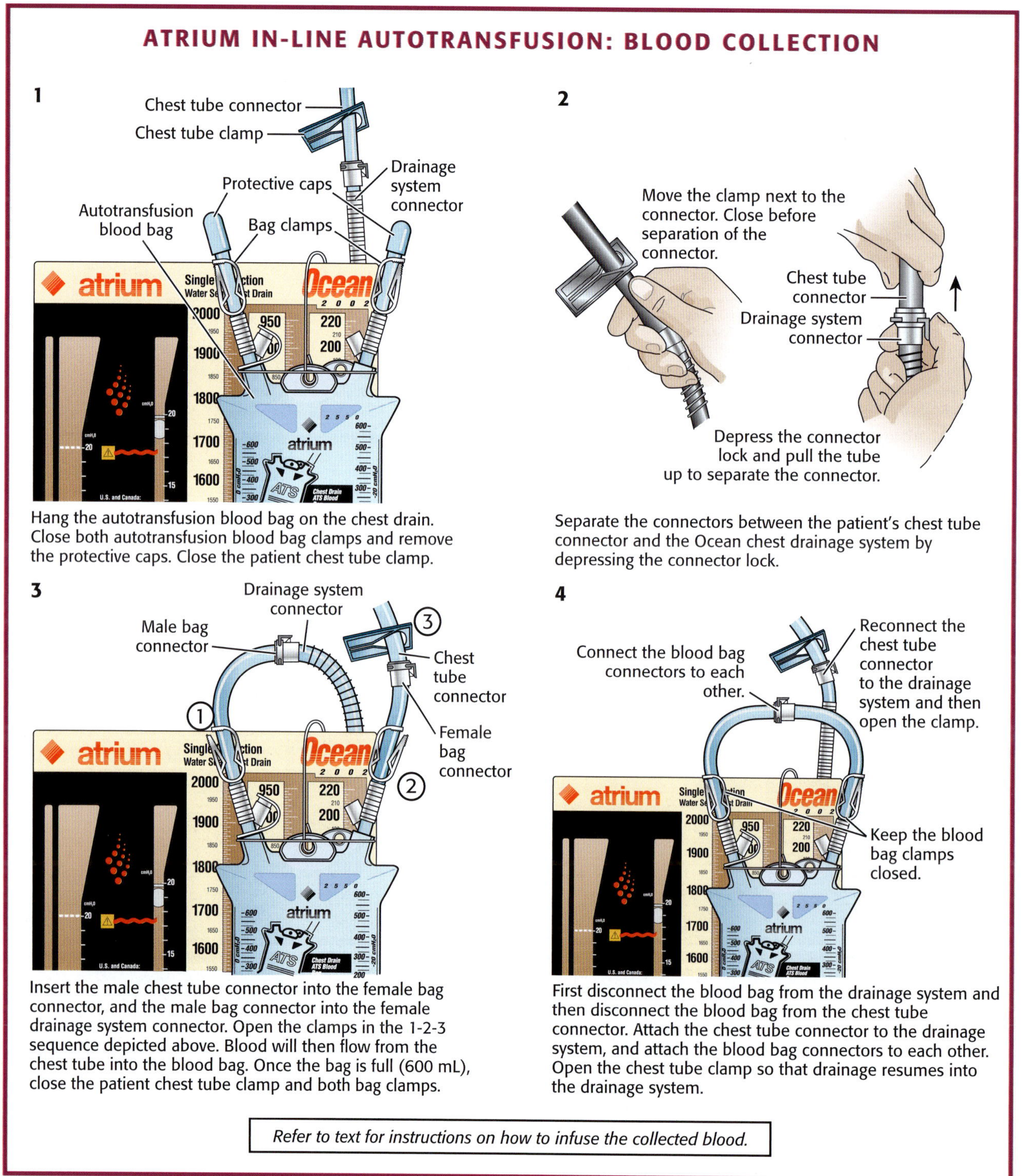

Fig. 27.8 Atrium in-line autotransfusion: blood collection. (Courtesy Atrium Medical Corporation.)

7. Open the clamps in the following order:
   a. Open the autotransfusion bag clamp going to the Ocean chest drain.
   b. Open the autotransfusion bag clamp going to the patient's chest tube.
   c. Open the patient's chest tube clamp to resume drainage. (Blood will then flow from the patient's chest tube into the autotransfusion blood bag.)
8. When the blood bag is filled (600 mL maximum), close the patient's chest tube clamp and both autotransfusion blood bag clamps.
9. First, disconnect the autotransfusion blood bag connection with the Ocean chest drain connection.
10. Disconnect the autotransfusion blood bag from the patient's chest tube connector.
11. Insert the male patient chest tube connector into the female Ocean chest drain connector.
12. Open the patient's chest tube clamp, so that drainage may resume into the Ocean chest drain device.
13. Connect the male and female autotransfusion bag connectors to each other.
14. Connect and preprime the blood filter and the IV blood tubing with sterile saline (spike the blood tubing into the filter).
15. Invert the autotransfusion bag so that the spike port at the bottom points upward.
16. Remove the tethered cap with sterile technique.
17. Insert the saline-primed filter spike into the autotransfusion bag spike port with a firm twisting motion.
18. Return the autotransfusion bag to an upright position and place it on a standard IV pole.
19. Open the filtered air vent located on top of the autotransfusion bag before opening the IV tubing clamp.
20. Evacuate all the remaining air from the IV line and attach it to the patient to begin the infusion.
21. For gravity infusion, leave the air vent at the top of the autotransfusion bag open.
22. For pressure infuser application, the filtered air vent must remain closed (the maximum ATS bag infuser pressure is 150 mm Hg).

COMPLICATIONS

In general, complications from autotransfusion are clinically insignificant if proper technique is followed. Complications may be categorized as hematologic and nonhematologic.

Hematologic Complications

The degree that autotransfusion contributes to the development or exacerbation of coagulopathy in an actively bleeding patient has still not been conclusively determined.[74]

Broadie and coworkers found that blood collected from trauma patients during thoracotomy or laparotomy had markedly elevated prothrombin, partial thromboplastin, and thrombin times, as well as absent fibrinogen.[68] Salhanick and associates found that there was a statistically significant increase in proinflammatory cytokines such as interleukin (IL)-6, IL-8, tumor necrosis factor-α (TNFα), and other markers in shed pleural blood from traumatic hemothorax.[75] Schmidt and partners found that while the mediastinal blood shed during coronary artery bypass graft patients was high in in IL-6, autotransfusion of this blood did not cause measurable elevations in plasma levels of IL-6.[76] The dilemma is that severely injured trauma patients who are candidates for autotransfusion are more likely to have other independent risk factors for coagulopathy and being in a proinflammatory state, such as hypothermia and acidosis. Horst and colleagues studied 154 trauma patients who underwent intraoperative autotransfusion and found that patients who received more than 15 units of autologous blood or more than 50 units of combined autologous and banked blood were coagulopathic and also more severely injured, hypothermic, and acidotic.[77] Although coagulation test abnormalities following the infusion of salvaged blood have been interpreted as evidence of DIC, these changes are probably the result of infusion of fibrin degradation products and do not represent consumptive coagulopathy.[78] In general, even though coagulopathy should be anticipated, it has not proved to be clinically important when volumes of autotransfused blood remain below 1500 mL to 2000 mL in adult patients.[79] When reinfused volumes exceed 3500 mL, laboratory evidence of dilutional coagulopathy may become evident.[61] When volumes of autotransfused blood are greater than the patient's total blood volume, animal studies suggest that the risk for a true consumptive coagulopathy is increased.[80]

Recommendations regarding the volume of autologous blood that should trigger the infusion of plasma or platelets range from 25% of the total blood volume (approximately 1250 mL in a 70-kg adult) to 3500 mL[61,81] (Box 27.2). Others advise reliance on laboratory tests and clinical findings rather than a volume-based protocol.[71] Prudent clinical judgment dictates application of the more liberal guidelines for replacement therapy in patients with extensive hepatic injury, intractable shock, or ongoing loss requiring immediate surgical intervention.

Hemolysis occurs with autotransfusion, in part because of prolonged exposure of cells to the serosa of the traumatized body cavities.[82] Hemolysis also results from mechanical damage during collection and reinfusion or from excessive exposure to air-fluid interfaces.[43] The hematocrit falls in direct proportion to the quantity of blood transfused, with the average decline being 10% to 20%.[43,72] Nontraumatized red blood cell survival has been reported to be normal in all cases studied.[16,61]

BOX 27.2 General Autotransfusion Information

- Use each liner bag only once.
- Insert a new filter for each autotransfusion bag used.
- To minimize risk for bacterial overgrowth, blood collected must be reinfused within 6 hours from the time of injury.[a]
- After reinfusing a total of 3500 mL (approximately 7 units) of autologous blood, it has been suggested that 1 unit of fresh frozen plasma be given for every 2 units (approximately 1000 mL) of autotransfused blood.[43]
- If some or all the collected blood becomes clotted in the liner bag, the blood should be discarded.
- To reduce the risk for air embolism, remove all the air from the bag with the collected blood before hanging it for reinfusion.[82]

[a]*The American Association of Blood Banks suggests no more than a 6-hour shelf life between collection and reinfusion.[56] The age of blood collected should be calculated from time of injury. Blood reinfused after this time should be considered hazardous.*

Nonhematologic Complications

The theoretical risk for sepsis after the administration of potentially contaminated blood always exists within the nonsterile environment of the typical ED. Experience has shown this risk to be minimal after autotransfusion from an isolated hemothorax, and there is no evidence suggesting that routine prophylaxis with systemic antibiotics is beneficial.[55] Collected blood is generally transfused as soon as the collection bag is full. The American Association of Blood Banks guidelines allow a 6-hour interval between collection and reinfusion.[56] The age of collected blood should be calculated from the time of injury (see Box 27.2). Blood reinfused after this 6-hour period should be considered potentially hazardous.

The risk for microemboli secondary to platelet aggregation and fat emboli has largely been eliminated by the use of micropore filters.[61,64] During reinfusion of collected blood, there is usually a mild increase in screen filtration pressure, indicative of the formation of microemboli trapped by the filter.[64] There has been no clinical evidence of pulmonary insufficiency or elevation of the alveolar-arterial oxygen gradient that might be attributed to the passage of microemboli beyond micropore filter systems.[43]

As with all IV infusions, improper technique, such as applying pressure to air-containing systems, may lead to air embolism. This uncommon and potentially fatal complication has been associated with ATSs that use automated roller pump units in which the aspirate reservoir was inadvertently allowed to run dry.[55,83,84] Air embolism with gravity or with a manually assisted technique is rare.

Infusion of large quantities of unwashed blood that contains hemolyzed red blood cells may contribute to renal failure, particularly in patients with preexisting renal insufficiency.[46] Elevated plasma-free hemoglobin is a consistent finding in patients who have undergone autotransfusion.[43,70,72] In the past, it was believed that elevated levels of free hemoglobin following hemolytic transfusion reactions caused renal failure by its precipitation and obstruction of renal tubules. More recent evidence suggests that the mechanism in this setting is independent of free hemoglobin and is the result of an antigen-antibody–induced intravascular coagulation that when compounded by vasoconstriction and hypotension, leads to renal ischemia.[85] Even though renal failure as a direct consequence of autotransfusion has not been reported, transient elevations in serum creatinine do occur. In the presence of shock and systemic acidosis, acute tubular necrosis remains a potential complication.[32,86] The clinician must weigh the urgency of blood transfusion against the timely availability of an alternative source.

RESOURCES

Brief educational videos are available online for Atrium products at https://www2.getinge.com/us/education/chest-drain-education/ and show in detail the step-by-step processes to initiate autotransfusion with their devices. They also have a 24-hour help line to assist with any questions during the setup or use of their devices (800-528-7486). Pleur-evac has some limited information available online (http://www.teleflexmedical.com) and can be contacted during regular business hours (866-246-6990).

REFERENCES ARE AVAILABLE AT Elsevier eBooks+

CHAPTER 28

Transfusion Therapy: Blood and Blood Products

Christopher E. San Miguel, Kimberly Bambach, and Colin G. Kaide

INTRODUCTION

Transfusion of blood components (red cells, white cells, platelets, whole plasma, or plasma fractions) is commonplace in the emergency department (ED). In 2015 11.4 million blood units of packed red blood cells (PRBCs) were transfused along with 2.7 million plasma units and 2 million platelet units.[1] Although acute hemorrhage is the most common emergency indication for blood transfusion, more nonemergency transfusions and blood component therapy now occur in the ED linked to the general migration of health care away from inpatient settings. Technical advances have made component therapy directed at specific acute and chronic pathologic conditions practical, safe, and affordable.

BACKGROUND

RBC Antigens and Antibodies

The first documented transfusion took place in the early 1600s, and sporadic advancement in transfusion medicine occurred over the next three centuries, mainly dabbling in cross-species whole blood transfusions. It was not until the early 1900s that the Austrian Karl Landsteiner found that an individual's serum reacted with the red cells of some and not all other individuals, thereby discovering the red cell antigen-antibody system.

RBC membranes contain a series of glycoprotein moieties, or antigens, that give the cell an individual identity. Two different genetically determined antigens, type A and type B, occur on the cell surface. Any individual may have one, both, or neither of these antigens. Because the type A and type B antigens on the surface of the cell make the RBC susceptible to agglutination, these antigens are termed agglutinogens. The presence or absence of agglutinogens is the basis for the ABO blood group classification, and the blood types are named accordingly as A, B, or AB. Blood type O contains neither the A nor the B agglutinogen.

Within the first year of life, antibodies begin to form against the standard red cell agglutinogens that are not present in the individual patient. These agglutinins are γ-globulins of the immunoglobulin (Ig) M and IgG types and are probably produced by exposure to agglutinogens in food, bacteria, or exogenous substances other than blood transfusions. In the absence of type A agglutinogens (blood types B and O), anti-A antibodies, or agglutinins, spontaneously develop in the plasma. Similarly, in the absence of type B agglutinogens (blood types A and O), anti-B antibodies develop. When both A and B agglutinogens are present (blood type AB), no agglutinins are formed. Blood groups and their genotypes and constituent agglutinogens and agglutinins are shown in Fig. 28.1.

The reaction between red cell antigens and the corresponding agglutinins results in red cell destruction when noncompatible blood types are mixed. As many as 300 different red cell antigens have been identified, and clinically the A and B antigens are most important. Severe, potentially fatal agglutination can occur with the first transfusion of ABO-incompatible blood.

The Rh system is clinically significant because there is a chance that transfusion of Rh-positive PRBCs to a Rh-negative patient will result in the formation of anti-Rh antibodies. These antibodies can trigger severe hemolysis following a second exposure to the Rh antigen. Of the 40 antigens in the Rh system, D is the most antigenic, and others can also stimulate the production of antibodies in recipients lacking the antigen, complicating future transfusions. This is most significant for females of childbearing age. If a Rh-negative female is exposed to Rh-positive PRBCs and develops anti-Rh antibodies, future pregnancies with Rh-positive fetuses are at risk of developing hemolytic disease of the newborn. This occurs when the anti-Rh antibodies cross the placental barrier and induce hemolysis of the fetal RBCs.

Other antigen systems in which antibodies could potentially cause hemolytic reactions are the Kell (K and k alleles), Duffy (Fy^a and Fy^b), Kidd (Jk^a and Jk^b), and MNS (M and N and closely linked S and s) systems. These antigen systems are rarely of clinical importance in transfusion therapy, except in certain patient populations who may require repeated transfusions, such as those with sickle cell anemia.

Collection and Storage of Blood Products

Whole blood is collected from donors into 500-mL plastic bags containing 63 mL of citrate-phosphate-dextrose with a resultant hematocrit of 35% to 40%. Immediately after collection, sophisticated techniques permit separation of the whole blood into various components and fractions. Blood components such as fresh frozen plasma (FFP), PRBCs, granulocytes, and platelets are prepared from a single donor, separated, and transfused as single units. Minor blood fractions, including albumin, γ-globulin, cryoprecipitate, fibrinogen, and sometimes platelets, are often pooled from multiple donors. Within 24 hours of collection, untreated blood is essentially devoid of normally functioning platelets and some clotting factors, especially the labile factors V and VIII. Separation into individual components permits specialized storage and transfusion techniques designed to optimize the survival and availability of each component.

As is true of whole blood, PRBCs can be stored for up to 21 days, although newer preservatives such as ADSOL (adenine, dextrose, saline, mannitol, and water) may allow 49-day storage. Red cell viability decreases approximately 1% per day. Storage of blood contributes to a variety of other derangements or "storage lesions." Cell metabolism continues during storage and causes a mild acidosis. This acidosis is buffered effectively by the bicarbonate derived from the metabolism of citrate, assuming normal hepatic function in the recipient. Even with massive transfusions, acidosis is more often the result of disruption of normal physiologic function than the storage of blood products themselves. Levels of 2,3-DPG decrease during storage, thereby shifting the oxygen-hemoglobin dissociation curve to the left. This shift is of small clinical significance because 2,3-DPG levels are usually normal in transfusion recipients

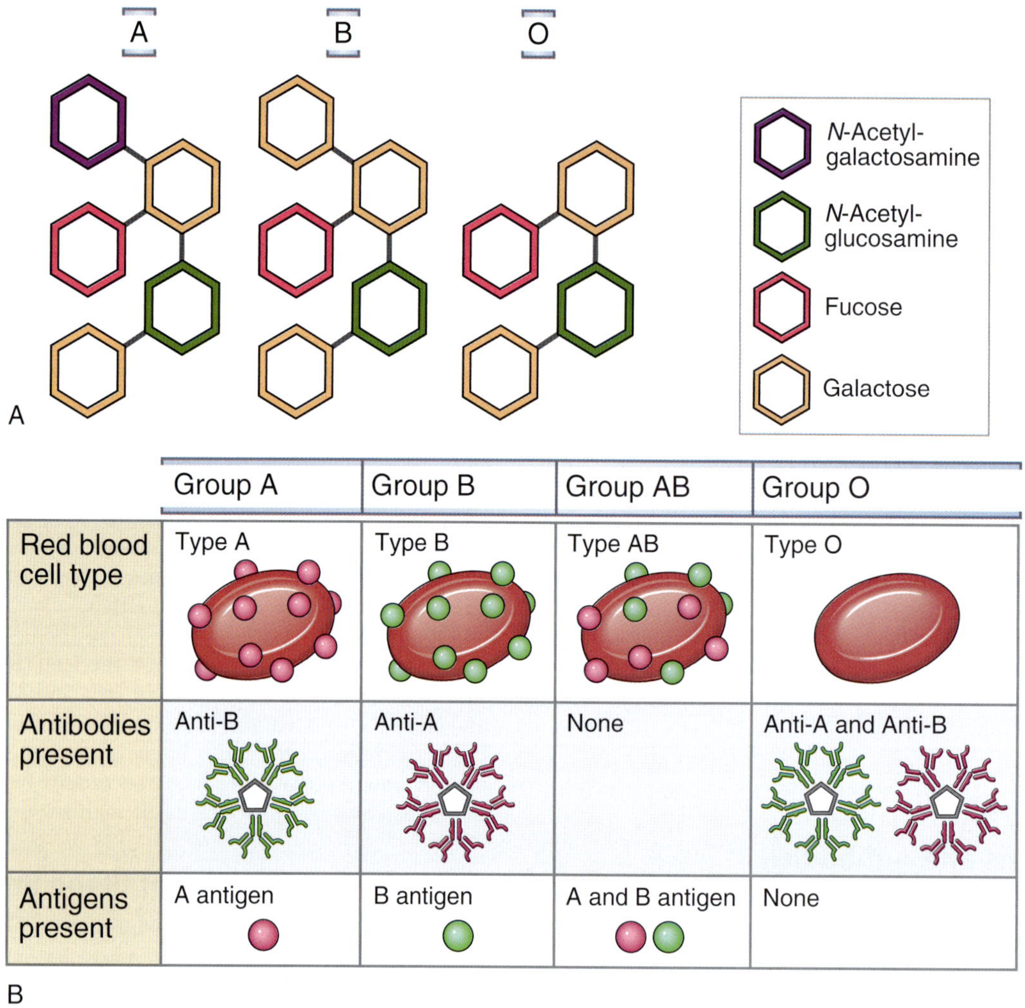

Fig. 28.1 Overview or red blood cell ABO grouping. (From Abbas AK, Lichtman AH, Pillai S, eds. Transplantation immunology. In: *Cellular and Molecular Immunology*. 9th ed. Elsevier; 2018.)

within 24 hours of infusion. Potassium commonly leaks from red cells during storage because of a less efficient sodium-potassium adenosine triphosphatase–dependent pump. Most of the potassium is either absorbed by the remaining blood cells, excreted by the kidneys, or shifted back into the cells as a result of the alkalosis produced by metabolism of citrate in the preservative. Hyperkalemia may be of particular importance in newborns and patients with renal impairment.

PRETRANSFUSION CONSIDERATIONS

Ordering Blood

When it has been decided that a patient needs a transfusion and the patient's condition is stable enough, ask the patient about any previous transfusion reactions and whether the patient abides by any religious or cultural prohibitions to transfusion. A "type and hold" or "type and screen" (no crossmatch) request alerts the blood bank to the possibility that a blood product may be required for the patient so that appropriate units can be acquired and kept on hand. A type and screen reports the patient's ABO and Rh blood type. It also screens the patient's blood for major anti-RBC antibodies. Ordering a "type and crossmatch" implies that the decision has already been made to administer a transfusion. A crossmatch procedure takes 45 minutes and restricts a unit of blood to a specific patient. In this procedure, the patient's blood is matched with a compatible donor blood product based on the type and screen results. The donor's and patient's blood are then mixed and observed for agglutination that would indicate incompatibility. This is sometimes carried out by an electronic crossmatch, which does not physically mix the blood. This method is more efficient and less sensitive for transfusion reaction. Therefore any patient with a history of transfusion reaction should have their blood physically crossmatched prior to receiving a transfusion. In general, a type and crossmatch should be ordered if the emergency physician (EP) anticipates transfusing blood in the ED, and a type and screen should be ordered if the need for a blood transfusion is still unknown or likely to occur later in the patient's hospitalization. If the patient is hemodynamically unstable secondary to hemorrhage and/or anemia, it is appropriate to administer type O– or O+ (if not a female of childbearing age) PRBCs while awaiting type specific blood products.

Be sure to draw and transport blood according to your local blood bank's policies and procedures. This is often a strictly regimented process designed to minimize clerical errors and resultant patient harm events. The individual blood components are discussed in the following sections. A summary of

TABLE 28.1 Summary and Dosage of Blood Products

BLOOD COMPONENT	DOSE	NOTES	EXPECTED RESULTS
Packed red blood cells	1 unit = 250 mL	• ABO and Rh compatibility is preferred but in an emergency can give O– to females of childbearing age and O– or O+ to all others • Almost always leukocyte reduced • Washed, irradiated, and CMV-negative preparations available	Each unit should raise the hemoglobin 1 g/dL and the hematocrit by 3%
Platelets	≈1 unit/10 kg 1 apheresis pack or a 6 (4)-pack of pooled platelets	• ABO and Rh compatibility is preferred but in an emergency is not necessary • 30–50 mL/unit ≈180–300 mL/6-pack • Available in 5–15 min • 3× the usual dose is required to reverse clopidogrel and ASA • The duration of platelet life is severely diminished with ITP	Each unit should raise the platelet count by 5000–10,000, so a 6-pack or 1 apheresis unit should raise the count by 30,000–60,000
Fresh frozen plasma	15 mL/kg or ≈1000 mL or 4 units in a 70-kg patient	• ABO compatibility is desirable but not required in an emergency, and Rh compatibility is never required • 200–250 mL/bag • Available in 45–60 min • Should begin with 4 units minimum to correct an elevated INR • Not possible to get an INR <1.5 with FFP	Each unit raises all coagulation factors by 2%–3% in average-sized adults.
Cryoprecipitate	10–20 bags, depending on the indication	• ABO compatibility is desirable but not required in an emergency, and Rh compatibility is never required • Hypofibrinogenemia <100 mg/dL: give 10 bags, 15–20 mL/bag • Fibrinolytic-induced bleeding: give 10–12 bags • Factor VIII deficiency when specific factor therapy is not available: 1 bag/5 kg • Available in 20 min	With fibrinolytic-induced bleeding, recommended doses may help correct bleeding. In factor VIII deficiency, the recommended dose will raise factor VIII to 50% of normal.

ASA, Acetylsalicylic acid; *CMV*, cytomegalovirus; *FFP*, fresh frozen plasma; *INR*, international normalized ratio; *ITP*, idiopathic thrombocytopenic purpura.

the dosages and characteristics of each component is provided in Table 28.1.

Blood Products

Whole Blood

See Videos 28.1–28.3. The normal blood volume of a healthy adult and healthy child is approximately 70 mL/kg and 80 mL/kg, respectively. The military experience with using whole blood dates back to World War I where type-specific, cross-matched blood was used in combat.[2] Whole blood transfusion has not traditionally been as popular in the civilian population, and renewed interest has brought its use to some trauma centers. Stored whole blood (SWB) can be preserved for 21 days at 1°C to 6°C. The use of citrate-phosphate-dextrose adenine (CPDA-1) at 1°C to 6°C can increase that time to 35 days. Whole blood older than 2 weeks may require the addition of fresher whole blood or supplemental platelets to avoid contributing to coagulopathy.[2] SWB is more concentrated than when a 1:1:1 ratio of PRBCs, plasma, and platelet are transfused with an average hematocrit and platelet count of 35% to 38% and 150 to 200 K/μL versus 29% and 90 K/μL for the balanced ratio component strategy.

Outcomes when using SWB are at least as good as component (RBC + plasma + platelet) therapy in hemorrhaging patients. We recommend the use of whole blood when available. The argument for using SWB early in the resuscitation process can be summarized as follows.[3–7]

- SWB provides a physiologic balance of blood components that are simultaneously transfused.
- A smaller volume of anticoagulant/preservative solution is transfused with SWB.
- Platelet function in SWB may be significantly enhanced compared with component therapy.
- Higher levels of hemostatic factors are delivered with SWB.

- Fibrinogen delivery is higher when utilizing SWB, as FFP does not deliver significant amounts of fibrinogen.
- Hemolytic transfusion reaction rate in SWB is low (about 1:120,000); therefore transfusions are generally safe and confer fewer donor exposures compared with component therapy (Chapter 27), occurring in 1:1:1 protocols.
- Administration of all components together in one unit can improve the time to complete a transfusion.
- Errors associated with transfusion of type-specific blood can be minimized.

Autotransfusion using blood from the thorax after trauma is safe and effective. This strategy has numerous advantages including immediate availability, blood compatibility, elimination of donor-to-patient disease transmission, lower risk of circulatory overload, and fewer direct complications related to the transfusion itself, such as hyperkalemia, hypothermia, hypocalcemia, or metabolic acidosis.

Packed Red Blood Cells

PRBCs are prepared by centrifugation and removal of most of the plasma from citrated whole blood. One unit of PRBCs contains the same red cell mass as one unit of whole blood at approximately half the volume and twice the hematocrit (55% to 80%) in 250 mL of volume. One unit of PRBCs raises the hematocrit approximately 3% in an adult or increases the hemoglobin level of a 70-kg individual by 1 g/dL. In children, there is an approximate rise in hematocrit of 1% for each 1 mL/kg of packed cells. For example, if 5 mL/kg of PRBCs is transfused, the hematocrit will rise by approximately 5%. Actual changes depend on the state of hydration and the rate of bleeding. Because most of the plasma has been removed, PRBCs cause fewer transfusion and allergic reactions than SWB.

PRBCs contain less sodium, potassium, ammonia, citrate, hydrogen ions, and antigenic protein than SWB. This may offer advantages in patients with reduced cardiovascular, renal, or hepatic function. The rate of urticaria is still relatively high at 1% to 3% of transfusions, and the incidence of adverse reactions to packed cells is approximately one-third of that noted with SWB. The benefit of increased hemoglobin must be weighed against the potential for volume, electrolyte, and acid-base imbalances following PRBC administration. In cases of massive transfusion (>10 units), there is a significant risk for metabolic and respiratory acidosis, as well as hypocalcemia, that can reach life-threatening levels. Although underlying illness or injury obviously plays a major role in the cause of death, the overall mortality of patients requiring massive PRBC transfusions is approximately 60%.

Transfusion of PRBCs is indicated to provide additional oxygen-carrying capacity and expansion of volume. Packed cells are most commonly used to treat acute hemorrhage and anemia that is not amenable to nutritional correction. When treating acute hemorrhage, PRBCs are usually given (1) if the hemoglobin level falls below established critical levels for that particular patient population (see the section on "Transfusion Indications and Thresholds"); (2) after rapid crystalloid infusion fails to restore normal vital signs; or (3) concurrently with crystalloid infusion in the treatment of obvious life-threatening blood loss.[8]

Specially prepared or screened types of red cells are listed in the following sections. Their mechanisms and indications for use are summarized in Table 28.2.

Washed RBCs

After centrifugation, red cells can be washed to further remove leukocytes, platelets, microaggregates, and plasma proteins. Washing reduces the titer of anti-A and anti-B, thereby permitting safer transfusion of type O PRBCs into non-O recipients. This process also removes many allergens, thereby

TABLE 28.2 Indications for the Use of Specialty Red Blood Cells for Transfusion

SPECIALTY BLOOD PRODUCT	MECHANISM	INDICATIONS
Irradiated	Irradiation destroys WBCs thereby reducing the risk of transfusion-related graft-versus-host disease.	• Neonates • Patients with hematologic malignancies • Stem cell–transplant patients • Directed donations from family members • HLA-matched platelets • Patients with cellular immune deficiency
Washed	Washing with saline removes proteins and plasma, thereby reducing the risk of allergic reactions.	• Recipients with a history of severe allergic transfusion reactions • IgA-deficient patients • Paroxysmal nocturnal hemoglobinuria
Leukocyte reduced	Filtering removes 99.99% of leukocytes.	• Multiple-transfused patients • Multiparous females • Cancer patients undergoing chemotherapy Becoming standard to leukocyte reduce all PRBC units
CMV seronegative	CMV and EBV testing is performed on the blood.	• Seronegative patients who are currently pregnant • Premature or low–birth-weight infants • Bone marrow or organ transplant recipients • Immunosuppressed patients

CMV, Cytomegalovirus; *EBV,* Epstein-Barr virus; *HLA,* human leukocyte antigen; *IgA,* immunoglobulin A; *PRBCs,* packed red blood cells.

making it a desirable preparation for patients who have had recurrent allergic-type reactions to transfusions.

Leukocyte-Reduced RBCs

Leukocyte-reduced blood products contain less than 5 × 10^6 leukocytes/unit, whereas standard RBC units contain 1 to 3 × 10^9 leukocytes. Reduction can be performed at the time of collection, in the transfusion laboratory, or at the bedside during transfusion. Leukocyte filters can reduce the number of white blood cells (WBCs) by 99.99%. Leukocyte-reduced products are used to decrease the likelihood of febrile reactions, immunization to leukocytes, and transmission of disease. Currently, approximately 95% of the US blood supply is leuko-reduced. Several groups advocate the use of 100% leukocyte-reduced blood products because of the many adverse transfusion reactions that are associated with leukocytes. Non–leukocyte-reduced products are virtually the exclusive method of transmission of several viruses, including human T-lymphotropic viruses 1 and 2, Epstein-Barr virus (EBV), and cytomegalovirus (CMV). Additionally, they help reactivate and disseminate CMV and human immunodeficiency virus (HIV). Increased rates of bacterial contamination and postoperative and line infections have been associated with the use of non–leukocyte-reduced products. Leukocytes lead to human leukocyte antigen (HLA) alloimmunization, which results in increased graft rejection and platelet refractoriness.

Irradiated RBCs

Blood products can be irradiated to reduce the risk for graft-versus-host disease (GVHD) in susceptible patients. GVHD occurs in 1 in 1 million transfusions and has a 90% mortality rate.[9] The populations that should receive irradiated RBCs generally include immunocompromised patients or patients who have a close HLA match to the donor, as occurs in the case of a directed donation. Irradiation does shorten the life of the PRBCs.

CMV-Negative Blood

Because CMV is endemic worldwide, most donated blood is CMV positive. Even after an acute infection with CMV cleared, it remains present in leukocytes. CMV testing can identify units of PRBCs that are free of the virus and safe to transfuse in at-risk populations.

Platelet Concentrates

Platelet concentrates are prepared by rapid centrifugation of platelet-rich plasma. Platelets are obtained by single-donor apheresis or from pooled random-donor whole blood units. Platelets obtained by single-donor apheresis have the advantage of exposing the recipient to only one donor. This reduces the risk for exposure to many different donors and confers a lower risk for transfusion-transmitted disease and other complications. HLA-matched platelets may be used when HLA antibodies develop due to repeated, random-donor platelet transfusions. Platelet concentrates contain most of the platelets from one unit of blood in 30 mL to 50 mL of plasma.

Confusion sometimes arises when ordering platelets. Platelets are typically ordered by the "pack." Many institutions use a "six-pack" composed of six individual units of platelets. While some institutions use a four-pack, a four- to six-pack of random-donor units delivers approximately the same number of platelets as a single-donor apheresis unit. Unfortunately, some hospitals also refer to the four- or six-pack as a unit. It is important to become familiar with the blood bank terminology at your hospital. For this discussion, the term *unit* is used to describe individual units and not a four- or six-pack.

One individual unit of random-donor platelet concentrate raises the platelet count by 5000 to 10,000/mm^3. The usual adult dose is one random-donor unit for every 10 kg of body weight. In an average adult, this works out as approximately six to eight units of platelet concentrate. Therefore six units (or one six-pack) or one single-donor apheresis unit given to a normal-sized adult should increase the platelet count by approximately 50,000/mm^3. If there is no evidence of platelet consumption, this transfusion should be adequate for 3 to 5 days. In cases of severe platelet consumption, transfusion may be required every 6 to 24 hours. Platelet concentrates are viable for 5 days when kept at room temperature and gently agitated at intermittent periods or when kept in motion. They should not be refrigerated.

Crossmatching is unnecessary for platelet transfusion, and the donor and the recipient should be ABO and Rh compatible. Note that platelet concentrates contain enough RBCs to sensitize a Rh-negative individual. In an emergent situation, if ABO-compatible platelets are not available, unmatched platelets can be transfused. This will reduce the number of platelets available from the transfusion and otherwise does not cause the same hemolytic reaction that is expected with an incompatible red cell transfusion.

Fresh Frozen Plasma

FFP is prepared by separating plasma from the cellular components of single-donor whole blood, followed by rapid freezing and storage at 18°C or lower. Freezing preserves the soluble coagulation factors of the contact activation (intrinsic) and tissue factor (extrinsic) clotting systems, including the labile factors V and VIII. FFP also contains fibrinogen, though not as much as cryoprecipitate does. Plasma stored for 3 months retains approximately 60% of the normal factor VIII activity and has a shelf life of up to 1 year. Thawed solvent- or detergent-treated plasma stored at 4°C for 6 days still contains sufficient coagulant activity of factors II, V, VII, VIII, IX, XI, and XII; fibrinogen; antithrombin; protein C; and von Willebrand factor (vWF) antigen and can be safely administered. Ideally, transfused plasma should be compatible with the recipient's ABO group. Rh compatibility is not considered essential. Each unit of FFP has a volume of approximately 200 mL to 250 mL. The international normalized ratio (INR) of a unit of FFP is approximately 1.5. Transfusion of even very large amounts of FFP into a patient with an elevated INR will not correct the INR to below 1.5. It is not clinically useful to give FFP to patients with an INR lower than 1.7.

Cryoprecipitate

Cryoprecipitate is prepared from single-donor plasma by gradual thawing of rapidly frozen plasma. This process causes precipitation of proteins rich in fibrinogen and factor VIII. Each unit of cryoprecipitate typically yields 100 mg to 250 mg of fibrinogen, 80 to 100 units of factor VIII, and 50 mg to 60 mg of fibronectin. Cryoprecipitate is a plasma product and therefore requires ABO compatibility (see earlier discussion in the section on "Fresh Frozen Plasma"). The volume of each bag unit is approximately 15 mL to 18 mL.

Factor VII

Activated recombinant factor VII (rFVIIa) is a DNA product that is structurally similar to human serum factor VIIa. It has been approved by the FDA for the prevention and treatment of bleeding in patients with hemophilia A or B who have inhibitors to factors VIII and IX, as well as prevention and treatment of bleeding in patients with congenital factor VII deficiency. It works by binding to the surface of activated platelets, which activate factor X by using the tissue factor pathway (formerly known as the extrinsic pathway). This obviates the need for either factor VIII or IX. Activated factor X then complexes with factor Va, which leads to thrombin burst and clot formation. Factor VII has a half-life of 2.7 hours. A thromboembolic rate of 1% to 2% has been reported.

The use of rFVIIa for the prevention and treatment of bleeding in patients without hemophilia, (including trauma patients and patients with intracranial hemorrhage) denoted an increased arterial clot risk while failing to show a mortality benefit and is not generally recommended. This recommendation also applies to bleeding associated with vitamin K antagonists (warfarin).

Factor VIII

Factor VIII can be produced by isolation from human plasma or produced by recombinant technology. Since the gene for production of factor VIII was discovered in 1984, recombinant factor VIII has become the agent of choice in hemophilia. It is inherently safer, lacking any chance of viral transmission and can be produced and delivered in virtually unlimited quantities, making it more cost-effective and plentiful. Factor products are either standard duration or longer-lasting recombinant factor VIII preparations. Although longer-acting products are more expensive, they have the advantage of less frequent dosing translating into ease of use and possibly improved compliance. There are currently three plasma-derived factor VIII concentrates that contain adequate amounts of vWF to be effective in treating von Willebrand disease.

Administration of one unit of factor VIII concentrate per kilogram of body weight should increase factor VIII activity by 2%. The dosage should be individualized according to the severity of bleeding, the known deficiency of factor VIII activity, and the presence of factor VIII antibodies. Factor VIII levels should be increased to 20% to 40% of normal levels for minor bleeding (e.g., small joint), 40% to 60% for moderate bleeding (e.g., large joint, neck, oral cavity), and 60% to 100% for life-threatening bleeding (e.g., intracranial, intraabdominal, pharyngeal).

Antibodies develop in up to 15% of factor VIII recipients. rFVIIa and factor VIII inhibitor-bypassing activity (FEIBA) have proved to be very useful and effective hemostatic agents when inhibitors are present. Patients with factor VIII antibodies may also be on a drug called emicizumab (Hemlibra). This is a bispecific antibody that reacts with factor IX and factor X, obviating the need for factor VIII to be present to allow coagulation to proceed. Patients on emicizumab who are bleeding will still need factor replacement.

Factor IX

Factor IX is indicated for the treatment of bleeding episodes in hemophilia B patients with a severe deficiency of factor IX. Like factor VIII, factor IX can be obtained from human blood or artificially by a recombinant process. Although factor IX obtained from human blood is treated to eliminate viruses, there is a very small, and not zero risk of viral transmission. The recombinant version of factor IX product does not contain virus. Both appear to be equally effective in the treatment of hemophilia B.[10]

Administration of 1 unit/kg body weight will increase the factor IX concentration by approximately 1%. High levels of factor IX are not required to control bleeding. Levels should be increased to 15% to 25% of normal for mild to moderate bleeding and to 25% to 50% for more serious bleeding or before major surgery.

Prothrombin Complex Concentrate

Prothrombin complex concentrate (PCC) (also known as factor IX complex) is a plasma-derived concentrate of nonactivated clotting factors II, VII, IX, and X. These preparations undergo a process of viral inactivation to reduce the risk for viral transmission. Some PCC products also contain protein C and protein S. These are added to balance the procoagulant effect of the concentrated clotting factors. The product is called Kcentra (CSL Behring) in the United States and Beriplex P/N (CSL Behring) in Europe.[11]

In the ED, PCCs can play a very important role in the reversal of anticoagulation from warfarin (see hereafter). One concern with these preparations is a possible prothrombotic effect. Two more recent reviews comparing four-factor PCCs to FFP in the reversal of warfarin-induced coagulopathy found similar rates of thrombotic events in both groups.[12,13]

Activated Prothrombin Complex Concentrate (Factor VIII Inhibitor-Bypassing Activity)

Factor VIII inhibitor-bypassing activity (FEIBA) is a product derived from pooled human plasma that contains factors II, IX, and X, each mainly nonactivated, and factor VII mainly in the activated form. It promotes coagulation, bypassing the need for factors VIII and IX. FEIBA is used to treat bleeding episodes in hemophilic patients with antibodies to factor VIII and is generally efficacious in this role. It has been used as an alternative to PCC for the reversal of vitamin K antagonists. Adverse reactions include headache, fever, chills, flushing, nausea, vomiting, and an occasional allergic reaction. The risk for thrombotic complications exists, especially in patients with liver and heart disease or those who are pregnant or breastfeeding.

Transfusion Indications and Thresholds

Packed Red Blood Cells

PRBCs are a precious commodity. Guidelines to limit transfusions to those that are absolutely necessary have set transfusion thresholds or "triggers." In 2016 the AABB (formerly known as the American Association of Blood Banks), published a clinical practice guideline regarding red blood cell transfusion. The guideline suggests a restrictive transfusion strategy and a hemoglobin treatment threshold of 7 g/dL for most stable hospitalized patients. They suggest a threshold of 8 g/dL in patients undergoing orthopedic surgery, cardiac surgery, or with preexisting cardiovascular disease.[14]

More recently, in a study of patients with acute upper gastrointestinal (GI) bleeding, Villanueva and colleagues found that using a transfusion threshold of 7 versus 9 g/dL resulted in decreased incidence of further bleeding, decreased adverse events, and increased survival at 6 weeks.[15] The decision to transfuse RBCs requires clinical judgment balancing adequate tissue perfusion and hemostasis.[16] Particularly close attention should be paid to the subset of patients at risk for coronary ischemia, with more liberal triggers possibly being applied to these patients. No single criterion should be used as an indication for red cell component therapy. Multiple factors related to the patient's clinical status and oxygen delivery needs should be considered. Current practice focuses on the needs of the individual patient. We recommend transfusion with ongoing signs of inadequate perfusion, such as elevated serum lactate level, altered mental status, or decreased urinary output. Hemoglobin level in acute hemorrhage can be misleading and should not exclusively be used to guide acute management. A recent study of trauma patients demonstrated that a hemoglobin level of 11.8 g/dL or below on arrival to the hospital was only 88% sensitive for predicting significant hemorrhage.[17]

The judicious and restricted administration of PRBCs appears to be clinically founded in the majority of patients. By implementing a restrictive transfusion strategy, the probability of a patient requiring blood can be decreased by 42% and the volume of PRBCs transfused can be decreased by 0.93 units per patient.

MASSIVE TRANSFUSION

Massive transfusion is loosely defined. In the 1970s it was considered to be the transfusion of more than 10 units of blood to an adult, equivalent to one blood volume, within 24 hours. Historically, massive transfusion was associated with dismal survival rates (<10%). As blood banking technology and storage methods have improved, the mortality associated with massive transfusions has decreased significantly. There is no clear physiologic threshold to define a massive transfusion, and a more practical and efficacious application of the concept is the transfusion of three units of PRBCs over an hour or the use of four components over 30 minutes. Acute blood loss involves more than just the loss of red cells, so physiologically it makes sense to replace all components of blood after more than a few units of PRBCs have been transfused. Massive transfusion protocols (MTP) are variable and most trauma centers use a ratio of 1:1:1 (PRBCs:FFP:platelets). This is initiated when more than three units of PRBCs are used. MTP should be considered when large and ongoing blood loss is anticipated.

The use of thromboelastography (TEG) or rotational thromboelastometry (ROTEM) has been studied to better predict which blood components may be helpful in normalizing coagulation. A 2015 systematic review was unable to show that TEG/ROTEM was superior to standard coagulation studies although it does alter transfusion patterns.[18] Another study in trauma patients compared transfusion guided by TEG to transfusion based on standard coagulation parameters and showed a higher mortality in the conventional group.[19] While promising, further study is needed to clarify the role of routine TEG/ROTEM in trauma care.

Platelet Concentrates

In 2015 the AABB published a clinical practice guideline concerning the general transfusion of platelets. Transfusion in adults should be done for platelet counts less than 10 K/μL given the risk of spontaneous hemorrhage. For patients undergoing central venous catheter placement, consideration of transfusion is recommended below 20 K/μL. Patients undergoing lumbar puncture and nonneuroaxial surgery should be considered for transfusion below 50 K/μL. It is generally recommended that active hemorrhage be treated by platelet transfusion if the platelet count is lower than 50,000/mm^3, and prophylactic transfusion may be withheld safely until the count is lower than 20,000/mm^3.[20]

Patients with idiopathic thrombocytopenic purpura (ITP) may be severely thrombocytopenic. Despite low platelet counts in ITP, it is uncommon to see spontaneous bleeding. Because of the presence of antiplatelet antibodies in these patients, transfused platelets may last only a short time (minutes to hours) before being removed from the circulation. Nonetheless, patients with ITP and life-threatening bleeding or severe head trauma should be given platelets at two to three times the normal dose.[21]

Platelet transfusion should be avoided in patients with thrombotic thrombocytopenic purpura (TTP), a rare microangiopathic hemolytic anemia, because platelets will result in further microemboli. TTP may be suspected in patients with both anemia and thrombocytopenia, but not leukopenia. Clinical features often include fluctuating neurologic symptoms and signs, jaundice, renal dysfunction, and fever. Laboratory confirmation includes the identification of intravascular hemolysis on a peripheral blood smear (e.g., schistocytes), as well as other laboratory evidence of hemolysis. Treatment consists of plasma exchange, although emergency treatment may begin with an infusion of FFP.[22]

Platelet transfusion is generally not recommended in patients with heparin-induced thrombocytopenia (HIT), although it may be indicated in cases of severe bleeding.[23] Platelet transfusion seems logical in patients on antiplatelet agents with intracranial hemorrhage; however, transfusion has not been shown to be helpful and led to increased mortality according to the PATCH trial (Platelet Transfusions for Intracerebral Hemorrhage).[24]

Fresh Frozen Plasma

Because each unit of FFP increases levels of all coagulation factors by 2% to 3% in an average-sized adult, it is useful in clinical scenarios involving depletion of clotting factors. FFP may also be valuable in patients with hereditary or acquired clotting abnormalities, such as a deficiency of factor II, V, VII, X, XI, or XIII; von Willebrand syndrome; hemophilia A (factor VIII deficiency); hemophilia B (factor IX deficiency); or hypofibrinogenemia. Because of the large volume of FFP that is generally required, its effectiveness is limited in these inherited diseases with severe clotting abnormalities. Specific factor replacement, when available, is always preferred over FFP.

FFP is also indicated for clotting factor deficiencies resulting from massive blood replacement. Pathologic hemorrhage after massive transfusions is often caused by thrombocytopenia rather than by a depletion of clotting factors. More aggressive FFP replacement formulas are becoming commonplace, rather than the accepted one unit of FFP for every five to six units of PRBCs.

It is appropriate to use FFP to treat the acquired deficiency of multiple factors, such as seen in patients with severe liver disease, disseminated intravascular coagulation (DIC), or vitamin K depletion, and for plasma exchange in those with TTP or hemolytic-uremic syndrome. FFP is not appropriate for volume expansion or enhancement of wound healing.

The use of FFP has also recently been described in the treatment of angiotensin-converting enzyme (ACE) inhibitor–induced angioedema, as FFP contains c1-inhibitor and kininase II enzymes. Case reports and series suggest that the administration of two units of FFP may lead to significant reduction of edema within 2 to 4 hours.[25]

Cryoprecipitate

Cryoprecipitate is indicated for the treatment of patients with fibrinogen deficiency, congenital afibrinogenemia, dysfibrinogenemia, and factor XIII deficiency and in some patients with hemophilia A or von Willebrand disease. It can also be used as a second-line treatment to correct a deficiency in coagulation factor VIII (in hemophilia A) when factor VIII concentrates are not readily available. Because cryoprecipitate contains no factor IX, it is of no value in the treatment of factor IX deficiency (hemophilia B).

Mild deficiencies in factor VIII are defined as 10% to 30% of normal activity and severe deficiencies as less than 3% of normal activity. When treating bleeding, the goal depends on the site and severity of hemorrhage, and in general one should aim for at least 50% of normal factor VIII activity. For life-threatening hemorrhage, aim for 100% activity. The amount of cryoprecipitate required to correct coagulation defects ranges from 10 to 20 units/kg for minor bleeding, such as hemarthrosis, to 50 units/kg for control of bleeding in surgery or trauma. Guide specific replacement by laboratory assay of factor VIII activity. The half-life of factor VIII in plasma is 8 to 12 hours.

One bag of cryoprecipitate per 5 kg of body weight will raise the recipient's factor VIII level to approximately 50% of normal. In a 70-kg patient, this equals 14 bags. The large number of units that must be given increases the chance of exposure to blood-borne diseases. Factor VIII concentrate is a better choice because of improved methods of viral inactivation and the availability of factor VIII prepared with recombinant DNA technology.

The vWF in cryoprecipitate degrades during storage, thus leading to variable amounts in each bag. It can be used for life-threatening bleeding in patients with von Willebrand disease and only when the proper preparations of concentrated vWF are not available.

Cryoprecipitate may be required to correct significant hypofibrinogenemia (<100 mg/dL). A typical adult dose of approximately 10 bags of cryoprecipitate raises the fibrinogen level by up to 1 g/L (60 to 100 mg/dL). In cases of severe bleeding after the use of a fibrinolytic agent such as tissue plasminogen activator, cryoprecipitate can be used to help control the bleeding. A consensus on dosing has not been reached, and many sources recommend between 10 and 12 bags.

Blood Product Shortages

Unfortunately, lifesaving blood products are frequently in short supply. In January of 2022 the American Red Cross declared an unprecedented national blood crisis due to the shortage of available blood products.[26] This shortage was precipitated by US supply chain instability during the omicron variant surge of the COVID-19 pandemic. Shortages of blood may require more restrictive transfusion practices, with consideration for evidence-based, equitable, and ethical distribution of blood products.[27,28] Emergency physicians are uniquely positioned for responsible stewardship of this precious resource.

Reversal of Anticoagulation

Warfarin-Induced Coagulopathy: Reversal Strategies

Elevated INRs may be encountered incidentally or in patients with trauma or serious medical conditions. Guides to approaching and treating such patients are found in Table 28.3. Reflex reversal of an elevated INR should be avoided, especially in the absence of bleeding. Even minor bleeding can be tolerated in lieu of losing the beneficial effects of anticoagulation in selected patients (e.g., those with mechanical heart valves, left ventricular assist devices [LVADs], or active clots). In the presence of significant trauma or serious hemorrhage, any warfarin effect should be reversed.

TABLE 28.3 Indications for Reversal of Supratherapeutic INR Levels

CONDITION	ACTION
INR above the therapeutic range but <5.0 and no bleeding	Lower or omit the dose, monitor more frequently, and resume at a lower dose when the INR is therapeutic; if only minimally above the therapeutic range, dose reduction may or may not be required.
INR ≥5.0 but ≤10 and no significant bleeding	Omit the next 1 or 2 doses, monitor more frequently, and resume at a lower dose when the INR is in a therapeutic range. Consider the use of vitamin K, 1–2.5 mg orally, particularly if at increased risk for bleeding. Note that INR correction with vitamin K in this situation may result in prolonged warfarin resistance for the next 3–5 days.
INR >10 and no significant bleeding	Hold warfarin therapy and give a higher dose of vitamin K (5–10 mg orally) with the expectation that the INR will be reduced substantially in 24–48 h. Monitor more frequently and use additional vitamin K if necessary. Resume therapy at a lower dose when the INR is therapeutic.
Serious or life-threatening bleeding at any elevation of INR	Hold warfarin therapy and give vitamin K (10 mg by slow intravenous infusion), and four-factor prothrombin complex concentrate or fresh frozen plasma.

INR, International normalized ratio.
Adapted from Holbrook A, Schulman S, Witt DM et al. Evidence-based management of anticoagulant therapy: antithrombotic therapy and prevention of thrombosis 9th edition: American College of Chest Physicians evidence-based clinical practice guidelines. *Chest*. 2012;141:e152S-184S, 2012.

Warfarin works as a vitamin K antagonist by inhibiting vitamin K epoxide reductase, decreasing available vitamin K, and thereby blocking synthesis of the active forms of the vitamin K–dependent coagulation factors II, VII, IX, and X, along with proteins S and C. The factors that are made under the influence of warfarin are biologically inactive. Over a few days, the body's remaining stores of active factors are used up and replaced by the inactive forms creating a coagulopathy. Because protein S and C synthesis is relatively quickly blocked, the antithrombotic effect of these proteins is likewise curtailed, creating a transient hypercoagulable state while the warfarin is slowly developing its anticoagulation effects.

There are two parts to warfarin reversal: sustained reversal via the administration of vitamin K and "immediate" reversal using agents described in the following section.

Vitamin K_1 (Phytonadione)

The first step in the reversal of warfarin is to replete active vitamin K by administering vitamin K according to the recommended dosing and route guidelines outlined in Table 28.4. This provides a sustained reversal effect. Vitamin K can be given either orally or intravenously. Oral use is universally safe and should be used when possible. Although IV administration of vitamin K has been implicated in anaphylactoid-like systemic reactions, the incidence of these reactions is very small (3/10,000) and should not preclude its use when the oral route is unavailable.[29] Additionally, administration of the IV dose over at least 20 minutes may help to mitigate such reactions. Some institutions may elect to extend default administration times to 30 to 60 minutes as a further precautionary measure. The best treatment for a systemic reaction to intravenous administration of vitamin K is unknown, and general supportive measures for anaphylactoid reactions seem to work well.[29] Because of erratic absorption patterns, subcutaneous administration of vitamin K is not recommended.

Reduction in the INR begins within 1 to 2 hours when vitamin K is given intravenously, with peak effects seen in 12 to 14 hours. Oral doses generally have an onset of effect in 6 to 10 hours, with a peak effect in 24 to 48 hours. Correction to within the normal range is generally achieved in these time frames if hepatic function is normal and a sufficiently large dose is given. Reversal of anticoagulation with vitamin K can be sustained for several days, making reanticoagulation with warfarin difficult. This is often referred to as *warfarin resistance*. This situation can happen with a patient on warfarin who has an artificial valve or an LVAD and has an acute GI bleed. Temporary reversal of anticoagulation may be necessary awaiting definitive correction of the GI bleeding source, followed by the rapid reintroduction of anticoagulation to protect the valve or LVAD. In these cases, it may be desirable to withhold the vitamin K while attempting to achieve a short term reversal with FFP or PCC.

Prothrombin Complex Concentrates

The next step in the rapid correction of an elevated INR is to replace the missing clotting factors (II, VII, XI, and X). Traditionally, FFP has been used for this purpose. FFP is effective but requires a significant volume and takes time to thaw and prepare for administration. PCCs have largely replaced FFP to reverse undesirable warfarin effects. Studies have demonstrated the effectiveness of PCCs in normalizing elevated INRs within 15 minutes after administration without the complication of excessive volume or a delay in time to administration.

Studies comparing the use of PCCs and FFP have failed to show significant benefits in survival.[30] The rapidity of administration, low volume required, and quick correction of the INR are compelling reasons to choose PCCs over FFP when managing an acutely bleeding patient. A recent comparison of four-factor PCCs to FFP has shown that the risk of inappropriate thrombosis is roughly the same.[31]

TABLE 28.4 Summary and Dosage of Reversal Agents for Warfarin[a]

AGENT	DOSE	NOTES
Vitamin K	1–10 mg PO or IV	• SC delivery is no longer used • Reduction in the INR begins within 1–2 h when given IV with peak effects seen in 12–14 h • Oral doses generally have onset of effect in 6–10 h with a peak effect in 24–48 h
Prothrombin complex concentrate Three-factor (Profilnine), four-factor (Kcentra[b])	Strategy 1: INR- and weight-based dosing • INR 2–4: 25 IU/kg IV • INR ≥4-6: 35 IU/kg IV • INR >6: 50 IU/kg IV Strategy 2: INR-based dosing • INR <5: 500 IU IV • INR ≥5: 1000 IU IV Strategy 3: Fixed dose • All 1500 IU IV	• Multiple dosing strategies • INR-based dosing is most effective with three-factor preparations • Absolute dosing strategies should not be used with three-factor PCCs • Any of the three strategies can be used with four-factor PCCs • The authors' institution uses strategy 1: weight- and INR-based dosing
Fresh frozen plasma (FFP)	10–15 mL/kg (minimum starting dose of 4 units)	• Reversal requires the administration of a large volume • Takes longer to prepare than PCC
aPCC (FEIBA)	INR <5: 500 units IV INR >5: 1000 units IV	• May be more thrombogenic than nonactivated PCC and should be reserved for use when four-factor PCC is not available

[a]Most of the dosing is off-label and is derived from various studies using these agents for unapproved conditions. Other dosing regimens may exist.
[b]FDA approved for the reversal of warfarin-related bleeding.
aPCC, Activated prothrombin complex concentrate; *FEIBA*, factor VIII inhibitor-bypassing activity; *INR*, international normalized ratio; *IU*, International Unit; *IV*, intravenous; *PCC*, prothrombin complex concentrate; *PO*, oral; *SC*, subcutaneous.

Fresh Frozen Plasma

FFP in doses of 10 to 15 mL/kg (with a minimum starting dose of four units) seems to effectively reverse coagulopathy, as measured by a decreasing INR. Issues related to volume expansion and the time required to obtain FFP have been discussed earlier. If PCCs are not readily available, FFP should be administered as quickly as possible in the coagulopathic, bleeding patient. Good judgment must be used when deciding to wait for the type and crossmatch, thawing, and administration of FFP in a critically sick, bleeding patient who requires transfer to another facility that can provide definitive treatment for the source of bleeding.

Factor VIII Inhibitor Bypass Activity

FEIBA has also been studied as a potential reversal strategy for warfarin-induced bleeding. One study found FEIBA to be effective. FEIBA should only be considered when a four-factor PCC and FFP are not available. Dosing of agents used to reverse warfarin can be found in Table 28.4. A comparison of PCC, activated PCC (aPCC), and FFP is provided in Table 28.5.

Reversal of the Direct Anticoagulants

Direct Factor II Inhibitors (Dabigatran)

Although dabigatran is removed by dialysis, such an intervention is rarely practical in an acutely bleeding patient. Idarucizumab (PraxBind), a monoclonal antibody fragment to dabigatran, was introduced in the fall of 2015. It has an affinity for dabigatran that is 350 times higher than that of thrombin.[32] In a phase I trial of healthy volunteers, idarucizumab rapidly and effectively corrected abnormal coagulation test results without significant adverse events.[33] In a 2015 uncontrolled trial of patients on dabigatran with a serious bleeding event or the need for an urgent procedure, idarucizumab reversed the effects of dabigatran in minutes in 88% to 98% of the patients studied. Importantly, the effectiveness of idarucizumab in this study was measured by reversal of abnormal clotting parameters, not by clinical cessation of bleeding.[32] There is currently no evidence that the reversal of dabigatran with idarucizumab will lead to improved patient outcomes. Notwithstanding, in the absence of a specific and clearly safe alternative, patients on dabigatran with life-threatening bleeding should be considered potential candidates for idarucizumab treatment. The recommended dose of idarucizumab is 5 g. The fibrinogen level should be checked in patients with dabigatran-associated bleeding. If fibrinogen is less than 200 mg/dL, two pools of cryoprecipitate should be given in addition to the idarucizumab.

Direct Factor Xa Inhibitors (Rivaroxaban, Apixaban, Edoxaban)

A variety of strategies using rFVIIa, PCC, and FEIBA have been tried in the treatment of these patients. Two strategies are currently employed to reverse anticoagulation on Xa inhibitors. The recommended first strategy is to use a specific antidote.

Approved for use in 2018, coagulation factor Xa (recombinant) inactivated-zhzo (also known as andexanet alfa) (Andexxa), is a recombinant decoy factor Xa molecule. It works by binding to circulating Xa inhibitors. It is approved for bleeding patients on apixaban and rivaroxaban. Although it will theoretically work on any agent that binds to Xa (edoxaban, betrixaban, fondaparinux, and enoxaparin), it is only FDA approved for apixaban and rivaroxaban. The onset of action of andexanet alfa when measuring anti-Xa activity as a surrogate marker is about 2 minutes, and the effect persists during the 2-hour infusion. Thrombin generation was restored to baseline in 100% of the patients.[34] Since coagulation rapidly resumes when the inhibitor is removed, the duration of infusion is thought to be adequate to accomplish appropriate clotting.[35] The risk of thrombotic events with the use of andexanet alfa was as high as 10% in one study, and no thrombotic episodes occurred after oral anticoagulation restart.[36] The ongoing Annexa-I study comparing Andexxa to usual care was stopped early because the efficacy endpoint was met, demonstrating improved control of bleeding compared with usual care.

The second strategy that is recommended when andexanet alfa is not available, is to use four-factor PCC. Theoretically the addition of coagulation factors II, VII, IX, and X could potentially overwhelm a circulating Xa inhibitor. Large studies comparing PCC to andexanet alfa are still lacking, and

TABLE 28.5 Comparison of Reversal Agents

REVERSAL AGENTS	ADVANTAGES	DISADVANTAGES
Kcentra (four-factor PCC)	• Onset within 10 min • Low risk for viral contamination • Effectively and immediately decreases INR	• Clotting events have been reported. • Duration of 12–24 h may be an advantage or disadvantage. The coadministration of vitamin K will prevent a rebound of anticoagulation. • There is no significant evidence that the use of PCCs is more effective than FFP or that it improves clinical outcomes.
Activated PCC (FEIBA)	• Onset within 10 min • Effective and rapid lowering of an elevated INR	• May be more thrombogenic than nonactivated PCCs • There is no significant evidence that the use of PCCs (activated or nonactivated) is more effective than FFP or that they improve clinical outcomes.
FFP	• Cost: approximately $65/unit: 70-kg adult = $273 • Clinician familiarity • Universal Availability	• High volume of fluid may be required • Slow onset • Frozen—must be thawed over a 30-min period • Risk for TRALI

smaller studies show similar results using either strategy with a slight advantage for andexanet alfa.[37,38] The risks and benefits must be thoroughly weighed when choosing to reverse anticoagulation with agents that could cause thrombosis. Dosing for agents used to reverse bleeding in patients on Xa Inhibitors can be found in Table 28.6.

ACTIVE TRANSFUSION CONSIDERATIONS

Blood Request Forms

Proper identification of the patient and the intended unit of blood is critical. Transfusion of an incorrect unit is a potentially fatal error. Most transfusion reactions are attributable to clerical error, and the vast majority of such errors occur at the bedside (e.g., not in the blood bank). Just before administering the blood, the nurse or clinician (or both) must check the identity of the numbered labels. In addition, the blood bank laboratory slip must identify the patient by name and number and contain the identification number of the unit of blood.

Blood Products for Jehovah's Witnesses

There are approximately 1.2 million Jehovah's Witnesses in the United States. Based on the belief that the Bible prohibits blood or blood product transfusion (Acts 15:28–29), Jehovah's Witnesses are taught that it is against God's will to accept transfusions of whole blood, packed cells, WBCs, platelets, plasma, or autologous blood. Since 1961, willing acceptance of a blood transfusion by an unrepentant member can lead to congregational disciplinary actions, including *disfellowshipping*, a term for formal expulsion and shunning. Some members may permit the infusion of albumin, clotting factor solutions, plasma expanders, or intraoperative autotransfusion. Although no guidelines for the administration of blood products to Jehovah's Witnesses are absolute, certain recommendations can be made.

Even though a transfusion may be necessary to save a patient's life and would otherwise be considered standard of care, administration of blood or blood products in the face of refusal can legally be considered battery. In an awake and otherwise competent adult, courts have ruled that clinicians cannot be held liable if they comply with a patient's directive and withhold lifesaving blood administration after refusal of transfusion when specific and detailed information of the consequences of such an omission in treatment are provided.

The issue becomes clouded when patients are incompetent, unconscious, or minors. In the absence of specific directives to the contrary and in the setting of a true medical emergency, it is prudent to administer blood products to patients who are unconscious, judged to be incompetent adults, or minors. Explicit documentation of the intent of the clinician to preserve life attempts to contact surrogate decision makers, the emergent nature of the condition, and clarification of the patient's mental competence should be included in the clinician's documentation.

The most complicated scenario is perhaps when a surrogate decision-maker declines a blood transfusion for the patient. The individual clinician should quickly escalate this matter to hospital administration and legal teams. Particularly in the setting of caring for a minor, emergency legal assistance (e.g., court orders, appointment of a temporary guardian) can be sought with rapid judicial resolution.

When caring for patients who decline transfusions, various clinical techniques to maximize oxygen delivery and minimize oxygen consumption should be used. Examples include

TABLE 28.6 Summary and Dosage of Reversal Agents for Xa Inhibitors

AGENT	DOSE	NOTES
Andexanet (Andexxa)	• The low-dose regimen consists of a 400-mg IV bolus given at a rate of 30 mg/min, followed by a 2-hour IV infusion at a rate of 4 mg/min • The high dose is an 800-mg IV bolus given at a rate of 30 mg/min, followed by a 2-hour IV infusion given at a rate of 8 mg/min	• Rivaroxaban with last dose ≤10 mg regardless of timing of last dose = low-dose regimen • Rivaroxaban with last dose >10 mg or unknown, with last dose <8 hours = high-dose regimen • Rivaroxaban with last dose >10 mg or unknown, with last dose ≥8 hours = low-dose regimen • Apixaban with last dose ≤5 mg regardless of timing of last dose = low-dose regimen • Apixaban with last dose >5 mg or unknown, with last dose <8 h = high-dose regimen • Apixaban with last dose >5 mg or unknown, with last dose ≥8 h = Low-dose regimen • Only approved for reversing rivaroxaban and apixaban, but theoretically should work with any Xa Inhibitor
Four-Factor PCC (Kcentra)	• 25–50 units/kg	• Not to exceed 5000 units • Repeat doses beyond 50 units/kg not recommended • Off-label use
aPCC (FEIBA)	• 25–100 units/kg • 25 units/kg is used by many institutions for this specific indication	• If still clinically significant bleeding, consider redosing, but no sooner than 6 h

aPCC, Activated prothrombin complex concentrate; *FDA*, Food and Drug Administration; *FEIBA*, factor VIII inhibitor-bypassing activity; *PCC*, prothrombin complex concentrate.

From Momin JH, Candidate P, Hughes GJ. Andexanet alfa (Andexxa) for the reversal of direct oral anticoagulants. *P T*. 2019;44(9):530-549.

limited blood drawing, the use of high-dose erythropoietin and nutritional support with aggressive iron supplementation, hypothermia, volume expansion, sedation, oxygen, and the use of synthetic hemoglobin substitutes. Hyperbaric oxygen therapy can dissolve sufficient oxygen to sustain life in the absence of hemoglobin and may be another option when blood cannot be used. It can be used in a pulsed fashion (3 to 4 h/day) to reduce the oxygen debt until hemoglobin can rise to adequate levels.

Administration of Blood Products

Intravenous Transfusions

Do not open a unit of blood unless a free-flowing IV access line has been established in a large-bore vein. During an active resuscitation, use a 14- to 16-gauge IV catheter, if possible, both to minimize hemolysis and to ensure rapid infusion of fluid for the treatment of hypovolemia or hypotension. When a large quantity of blood must be given rapidly, administer it by means of a high-flow infusion system if possible. The purpose of a large-bore infusion line is defeated if blood is piggybacked with an 18- to 20-gauge needle through a side port in the infusion tubing. For a less emergent transfusion, blood may be given through a smaller lumen. Combining hemodilution (250 mL of saline with one unit of PRBCs) and pressurization can safely increase the flow rate through 20- and 22-gauge catheters severalfold. No significant hemolysis occurs when small (21-, 23-, 25-, and 27-gauge) short needles are used for the transfusion of fresh blood or packed cells in infants and children and when the maximum rate of infusion is less than 100 mL/h. For rapid infusion, connect the blood administration tubing directly to the infusion catheter. Monitor the infusion site for infiltration, infection, or local reactions.

If the patient already has a suitable IV line in place, flush the system with a solution of normal saline before administering the blood. Do not use other IV fluids because of the risk for hemolysis or aggregation (e.g., with 5% dextrose in water). Do not place any medications in the unit of blood or infusion line for the same reasons.

Errors associated with blood transfusions have serious consequences and frequently result in severe transfusion reactions and death. The Joint Commission on Accreditation of Healthcare Organizations has set forth guidelines to reduce these errors, including the following:

- Training personnel in procedures and recognition of reactions.
- Redesigning methods to identify patients, attain patient and blood verification, gain consent, and process multiple samples. It was strongly suggested that room numbers be discontinued as a method of identifying patients and use of a unique identification band be considered for patients receiving blood.
- Enhancing technical and computer support of the process.
- Discontinuing the use of refrigerators for multiple blood units.

Many EDs have moved to a two-nurse mandate for checking patient and blood unit identities before administration. As the risk for infectious complications associated with transfusion medicine gradually declines, medical errors have supplanted them as the most serious cause of transfusion mishaps.

Intraosseous Transfusions

Although IV administration is by far the most common route of blood and blood component therapy, intraosseous (IO) administration is safe and effective. Administration rates via an IO route are generally slower (on average 21 versus 35 mL/min by the IV route) and appear to be metabolically and hemodynamically equivalent. In animal models, no evidence of fat embolism and lung or kidney inflammation was noted after IO-PRBC infusion. Administration of IO liposome-encapsulated hemoglobin (one of the forms of hemoglobin-based oxygen carriers [HBOC] therapy) is also effective and may have additional advantages over the IV route. Similarly, limited studies on the administration of other blood products via the IO route have been promising.

Filters

Infuse all blood and blood products through an appropriate filter, such as those supplied in-line in blood administration tubing sets. In the past, filtration was required merely to keep the IV line from becoming blocked by clots. Adverse consequences from infusing unfiltered blood products have since been recognized. Debris consisting of clots and aggregates of fibrin, WBCs, platelets, and intertwined RBCs (ranging in size from 15 μm to 200 μm) accumulates progressively during the storage of blood. The usual filter, made of a single layer of plastic with multiple 170-μm pores, traps larger particles and allows the rapid infusion of 2 to 3 units of blood before flow is obstructed. Purified components of blood plasma can be safely administered through a filter with pores as fine as 5 μm.

It has been suggested that microaggregates of debris that can pass through a 170-μm filter may contribute to the syndrome of "shock lung" seen after the transfusion of many blood units in patients with severe trauma and hemorrhage. Some clinicians recommend using a microaggregate blood infusion filter with a mesh pore size of 40 μm when multiple units of blood are administered to trauma patients, patients with compromised pulmonary function, and neonates. Microaggregate filters tend to become blocked, impede the rate of infusion more quickly, and are not commonly required in the emergency setting. A significant number of platelets are removed by microaggregate filters, and some clinicians advise against using these filters when platelet packs are infused. Others believe that although platelets are removed with the microaggregate filters, the trapped platelets can be removed with a saline flush without any significant loss. Replace standard filters after 2 to 3 units of blood product have been administered. Change microaggregate filters after each unit.

Rate of Infusion

One unit of whole blood can be safely administered to a hypotensive patient at a rate of at least 20 mL/kg per hour. In the setting of hypovolemic shock and continued hemorrhage, there is no limit to the transfusion rate. Multiple units may be transfused simultaneously, even under pressure. Use of a rapid transfuser device can assist in the rapid administration and warming of blood. In stable patients, administer one unit of whole blood (500 mL) over approximately a 2-hour period (3 to 4 mL/kg per hour). After this time RBCs begin to lose metabolic activity. The unit of blood, which is an excellent culture medium, is likely to become contaminated if bacteria and fungi are allowed to grow at room temperature. Give packed cells at approximately the same rate. Give plasma products more rapidly; in a patient without cardiovascular compromise, administer FFP at a rate faster than 15 to 20 min/unit because the coagulant activity begins to deteriorate rapidly after thawing. In patients with severe anemia and congestive heart failure, administer a rapidly acting diuretic, such as furosemide at the onset of transfusion to prevent circulatory overload.

If a transfusion of blood must be interrupted or delayed for any reason, return the remainder of the blood unit to the blood bank. Refrigerators in the ED or on the hospital unit should not be used to store blood products unless they are specifically equipped and authorized to do so.

For patients in hemorrhagic shock, administer blood through two large-bore catheters, at different sites if necessary. Usually, gravity provides a sufficient pressure gradient if the unit is raised above the patient to increase the rate of infusion when the clamps are wide open. Using a pressure pump makes the infusion quicker. Do not use a standard sphygmomanometer cuff wrapped around a unit of blood to create increased infusion pressure because the nonuniform application of pressure could burst the plastic bag containing the blood component.

If desired, dilute PRBCs with normal saline (0.9% without dextrose) before infusion simply by opening the clamps on the upper tubes of the Y-infusion set and leaving the lower (recipient end) clamps closed. Although it is generally agreed that lactated Ringer's (LR) solution should not be mixed with blood because of possible clot formation, multiple studies have challenged this belief and results have shown that small amounts of LR solution (up to 150 mL) are safe in the clinical setting. Furthermore, larger volumes of LR solution have not been found to produce microaggregate clots in laboratory settings when using AS-3–preserved PRBCs, a typical additive nutritive solution containing sodium chloride, sodium citrate, sodium phosphate, citric acid, dextrose, and adenine.

Diluting blood, while increasing its volume, will allow more rapid infusion by decreasing blood viscosity, which is dependent on hematocrit. Alternatively, add approximately 200 mL of normal saline directly to the bag of PRBCs to bring the hematocrit in the blood bag to approximately 45%.

Rewarming

Blood is stored at approximately 4°C to maintain cellular integrity and prevent the growth of microorganisms. Blood products usually passively warm to 10°C by the time that they are administered to the patient unless administered under pressure. The adverse effects of hypothermia on cardiac conduction and flow rates are evident when rapid administration of a large volume of blood is performed without prewarming.

Various mechanisms have been used to warm blood to 35°C to 37°C. An ideal blood warmer should allow liberal flow rates while preventing thermal hemolysis of blood cells. Commonly used devices include those with bath coils that allow a plastic tube to reside in a closely regulated warm water bath and dry heat devices that allow blood to circulate through flat, thin bags sandwiched between aluminum blocks that contain electric heating elements. Both devices have relatively low flow rates and suboptimal thermal clearance.[6] Immersion of blood bags in warm water baths is safe and also considered imprecise and slow. Despite some evidence of their safety, the use of microwave heating devices is not recommended by the Association of Blood Banks because of concerns of hemolysis. PRBCs should not be heated above 50°C because significant hemolysis can be seen starting at 51°C.

Rapid mixture warming is a promising alternative technique. Mix the unit of whole blood with an equal amount of normal saline that has been preheated to 60°C to 70°C. Once mixed, administer the product to the patient; this gives a resultant delivery temperature of approximately 35°C. This technique combines dilution of blood product and warming into one step. Regardless of the rewarming technique used, warming refrigerated blood to body temperature decreases its viscosity twofold to threefold and avoids venous spasm, thus facilitating transfusion.

Monitoring

During the first part of the transfusion of any blood product, carefully monitor the patient for evidence of a transfusion reaction. Look for signs and symptoms such as hives, chills, diarrhea, fever, pruritus, flushing, abdominal or back pain, tightness in the chest or throat, and respiratory distress. A potentially life-threatening acute hemolytic transfusion reaction in a patient who has previously received transfusions may differ clinically from a minor allergic reaction only by its effects on the patient's pulse and blood pressure. Transfusion reactions are discussed in the next session.

On completion of a transfusion, make an entry in the patient's record to indicate the type and volume of the transfusion and the presence or absence of any reaction. The progress note, the transfusion record sheet, or the transfusion laboratory slip can be used for this purpose and should be signed and dated by the clinician, in accordance with hospital policies. Hemoglobin can be checked for response 15 minutes after the completion of the transfusion. Be sure to emphasize to the patient and family how critically important any blood transfusion is to the patient's care.

POSTTRANSFUSION CONSIDERATIONS

Infectious Complications of Transfusions

Though rare, transmission of infectious diseases may be the transfusion-related complication most well-known and feared by the public. Historically, a wide variety of infectious diseases have been reportedly transmitted via blood transfusion, and modern screening methods have sharply reduced the frequency of these adverse events.

Bacterial Transmission

Concern over the direct transmission of bacteria is responsible for the practice of completing transfusions within 4 hours and returning unused blood products to the blood bank refrigerator for future use only if they have been unrefrigerated for less than 30 minutes. The refrigeration and the standard citrate preservative kill most bacteria. Bacterial culture-positive transfusion reactions (BCPTRs) have recently been defined as a reaction occurring in the setting of a positive blood culture from the transfused blood product, the recipient, or from both. These reactions were analyzed for both imputability and against stricter CDC criteria. Cases with high imputability that met the CDC criteria were defined as septic transfusion reactions (STR). In a recent study, 688,514 transfusions over an 8-year period were analyzed for transfusion reactions. A total of 18 (0.003%) BCPTRs were reported, and of these 18 incidents, 7 (0.001%) were classified as STR. In total, there was only a single fatality and two additional cases considered life-threatening that were associated with a BCPTR. Platelets were the blood product most frequently associated with bacterial transmission, accounting for 83% and 85% of the BCPTRs and STRs, respectively.[39] As a result of previous studies showing this association with platelet transfusions, bacterial screening of platelet products has been mandatory since 2004.

A STR should be considered in any patient who develops a fever during or shortly after a transfusion. Fever is defined by the American Association of Blood Banks as a temperature higher than 38°C and a 1°C rise above pretransfusion temperature. It can be difficult to distinguish an STR from the much more common febrile nonhemolytic transfusion reaction (FNHTR) and hemolytic transfusion reaction. Other vital sign abnormalities, such as tachycardia and hypotension, indicate a more serious reaction than FNHTR as does a 2°C or greater rise in temperature. Signs of hemolysis are indicative of a hemolytic transfusion reaction, and they may not be present early in the course of the reaction. Consequently, any patient receiving a transfusion who develops a fever that does not meet the criteria for a FNHTR or has acute hemodynamic collapse without another clear explanation should be evaluated and treated for both a potential STR and a hemolytic transfusion reaction until clarity is provided by the subsequent laboratory work up.

As with any transfusion reaction, the first step in managing a STR is to stop the transfusion. The remaining blood product should be returned to the lab so that a gram stain and culture can be collected. Blood cultures should also be drawn from the patient. In cases of hemodynamic compromise or high suspicion for STR, antibiotics should be empirically started. The antibiotic regimen should provide a broad coverage of both gram-positive and gram-negative bacteria. Hemodynamics should be supported with fluid administration and vasopressors as in any other case of septic shock.

Viral Transmission

Viruses are the organisms most likely to be transmitted by transfusion and are the agents with the greatest potential to cause serious disease. They include CMV, EBV, HIV, West Nile virus (WNV), and the hepatitis viruses. It is unlikely for any of these pathogens to cause immediate problems after receiving the blood transfusion. Therefore it most important for the EPs to understand the risk of transmission when obtaining informed consent for transfusion.

The testing of all blood products for hepatitis B virus (HBV), hepatitis C virus (HCV), and HIV is mandatory. These screening tests all have very high sensitivities. A 2020 study, examining the past 10 years of blood donations at the American Red Cross concluded that the risk of receiving a blood product with HIV was one in 2.3 million. Similarly, the risks of exposure to HCV and HBC were one in 2.6 million and 1 in 1.5 million.[40]

CMV is endemic throughout the world and for most people does not cause significant illness. CMV is a significant teratogen and can cause severe disease in organ transplant recipients. The commonplace, leukocyte-reduction preparation of packed red cells, essentially reduces the transmission risk of this virus to zero as the dormant virus is found in the host leukocytes. For high-risk groups such as seronegative pregnant patients, intrauterine transfusions, premature or low–birth-weight infants, and organ transplant patients, donor blood should be tested for CMV and only transfused if negative.

Transfusion Reactions

Transfusion reactions can be divided into two phases: acute and chronic. The vast majority of transfusion reactions occur proximate to or concurrently with the administration of the blood product. If the ED is the site for a nonemergency transfusion and the patient is otherwise stable enough for discharge, it is a common practice for the patient to be released shortly after the transfusion is completed.

Acute Reactions

A key step in the treatment of any acute transfusion reaction is to stop the transfusion. Any decompensation, development of a new symptom, or change in vital signs should prompt the clinician to pause the transfusion. If the reaction is severe, the remaining blood product and its tubing should be returned to the blood bank for subsequent testing. The blood bank should be made aware of any suspicion the clinician has for a transfusion reaction. A simplified algorithm for evaluating and treating acute transfusion reactions is presented in Fig. 28.2.

Allergic Reactions

The most common manifestation of a minor allergic transfusion reaction is urticarial, while wheezing and angioedema have also been observed. The allergic response is usually triggered by the reaction of host antibodies to donor plasma proteins. For minor allergic reactions, the transfusion should be stopped, and the blood not necessarily returned to the blood bank. Treatment is the same as for other allergic reactions and includes antihistamines and corticosteroids. For mild reactions limited to skin findings, the transfusion can be resumed once the patient responds to the symptomatic treatment.

Anaphylactic Reactions

The reported incidence of transfusion-associated anaphylaxis is 1 in 20,000 to 50,000. The exact trigger in the blood product is unknown in most cases of transfusion-related anaphylaxis, and it has been described in IgA-deficient patients who have developed anti-IgA antibodies of the IgE class. Manifestations of an anaphylactic transfusion reaction can include shock, hypotension, angioedema, dyspnea, bronchospasm, urticaria, and laryngospasm. The symptoms are typically rapid in onset and begin within seconds to minutes of starting the transfusion. As with all cases of anaphylaxis, the mainstays of treatment are limiting exposure to the allergen (stopping the transfusion) and administering intramuscular (IM) or subcutaneous epinephrine. Supportive treatment with fluids, antihistamine, and corticosteroids are also commonly given. If a transfusion is still required, the patient needs to be pretreated with corticosteroids and antihistamines 30 to 60 minutes before the transfusion. In addition, the patient should receive no further blood products from that particular donor. Alternatively, or in addition, plasma can be treated with solvent/detergent and cellular products can be washed to limit the introduction of potential allergens.

Febrile (Nonhemolytic) Reactions

A FNHTR is defined as an increase in temperature of 1°C or higher during or within 6 hours of the transfusion without another medical explanation. The mechanism for this type of reaction is attributed to an interaction between recipient antibodies, donor leukocytes, and a release of cytokines that occurs due to damage of some donor RBCs that occurs during storage. Although a FNHTR is not life-threatening, it is difficult to distinguish from more serious transfusion reactions. All patients who experience a fever attributable to a transfusion

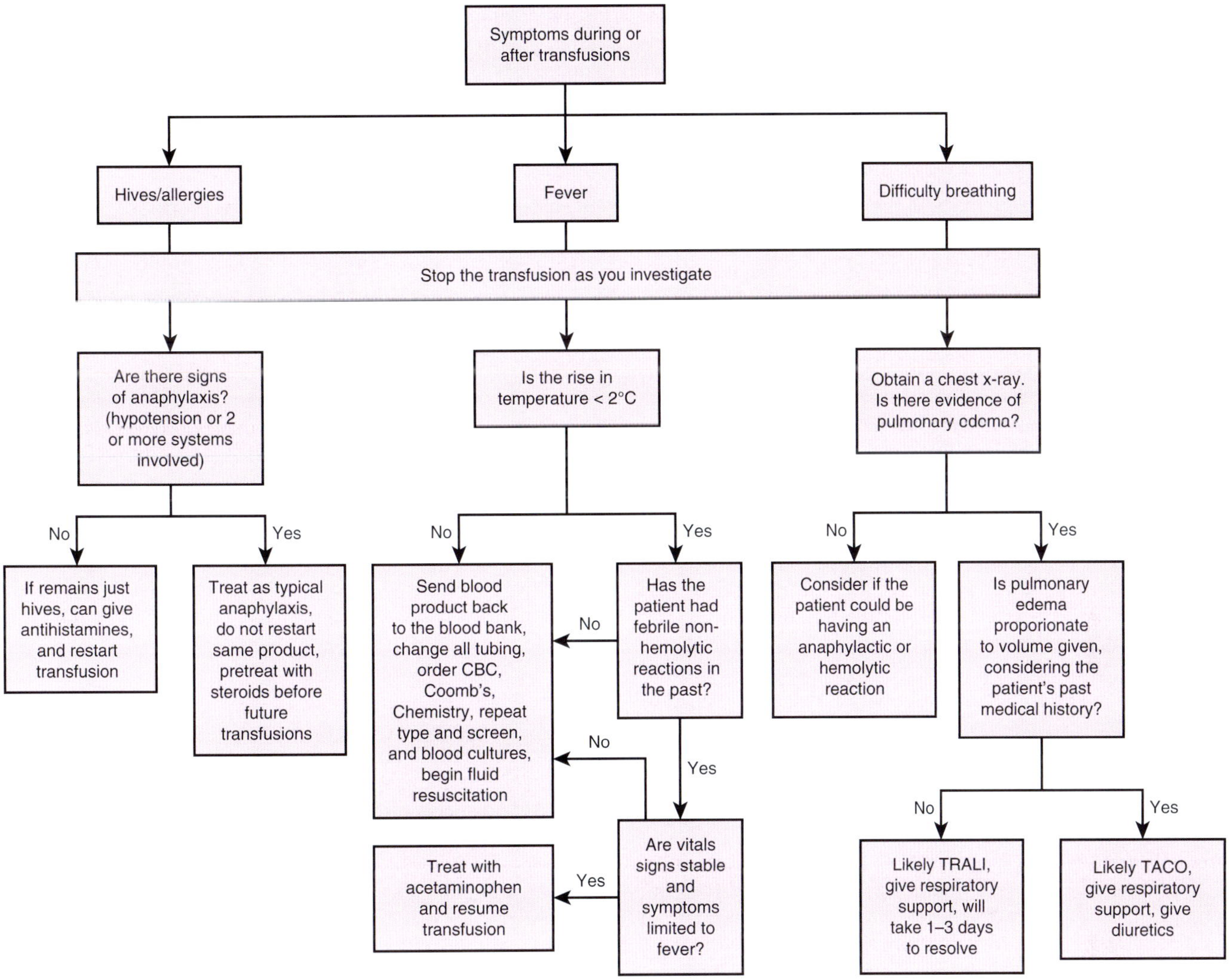

Fig. 28.2 Algorithm for treating transfusion reactions. *CBC,* Complete blood count; *TACO,* transfusion-associated circulatory overload; *TRALI,* transfusion-related acute lung injury. (From Walls RM, Hockberger RS, Gausche-Hill M et al. Blood and blood components. In *Rosen's Emergency Medicine: Concepts and Clinical Practice*. Elsevier; 2003.)

for the first time must be treated as an acute hemolytic reaction until proven otherwise.

The transfusion should be stopped, the product returned to the blood bank, hemolysis labs should be drawn from the patient (direct antiglobulin test [DAT], plasma-free hemoglobin level, complete blood count [CBC], chemistry, haptoglobin, lactate dehydrogenase [LDH], bilirubin, PT/PTT, D-dimer, fibrinogen, and a repeat type and crossmatch), and the patient should be monitored closely for the development of any additional symptoms or hemodynamic instability. The fever can be treated with acetaminophen or nonsteroidal anti-inflammatory drugs. If the patient develops any vital sign instability, a rise in temperature greater than 2°C, or any additional symptoms, treatment for a hemolytic transfusion reaction should be initiated (see following section). If the patient's condition remains stable and the hemolysis labs return negative, a new transfusion with a new blood product can be started.

If a patient has a known history of FNHTR, and they develop a mild fever during a subsequent transfusion, the transfusion may be continued as long there is vital sign stability, the temperature does not rise more than 2°C, and they do not exhibit any other symptoms. Pretreatment with acetaminophen may help to prevent FNHTR in these patients.

Acute Hemolytic Reactions

An acute hemolytic reaction is usually the result of donor-recipient major ABO incompatibility. This is most commonly the result of blood product misassignment related to clerical error. Hemolytic transfusion reactions are estimated to occur once per every 70,000 blood units transfused. The most recent data from 2010 to 2019 showed a significant decline in the incidence of acute hemolytic reaction fatalities from ABO incompatibility, reporting a rate of 1 per every 1.74 million units transfused.[41]

When incompatible blood is given, the result may range widely from no effect to death. If the recipient does not have antibodies (naturally occurring or acquired) directed against the foreign RBC antigen received, there will be no immediate reaction. Antibodies to the infused blood may develop within weeks, limiting the safety of subsequent transfusions from the same donor or same antigenic type. If the recipient's serum has preformed antibodies directed against the donor RBCs (e.g., an incompatibility in the major crossmatch), the recipient will begin to hemolyze the donor cells within seconds or minutes. In most cases of major crossmatch reactions, RBCs of the donor blood are agglutinated and hemolyzed. It is rare for transfused blood to produce agglutination of the recipient's cells because the plasma portion of the donor blood becomes diluted by the plasma of the recipient. This reduces the titer of the infused agglutinins to a level too low to cause significant agglutination. Because the recipient's plasma is not diluted to any significant degree, the recipient's agglutinins can react with donor PRBCs.

The end result of antigen-antibody incompatibility is red cell hemolysis. Occasionally this occurs immediately, and more often the cells first agglutinate. They are then trapped in small vessels and become phagocytized over a period of hours to days and release hemoglobin into the circulatory system. Clinical manifestations of acute hemolysis include chills, fever, tachycardia, abdominal pain, back pain, hypotension, fainting, and a feeling of "impending doom." Derived from the liberation of intracellular material associated with hemolysis, vasoactive substances may cause hypotension and shock; other substances may precipitate DIC and high-output cardiac failure. Acute renal failure may also result. Symptoms may start immediately and the effect of agglutination and hemolysis is additive, so the symptoms progressively worsen and can take up to 24 hours to fully manifest. The presence of hemoglobinemia and hemoglobinuria is essential in making the diagnosis. A decrease in hematocrit and haptoglobin or an increase in lactate dehydrogenase may also be seen.

Treatment of an acute hemolytic reaction begins with immediate cessation of the transfusion. The blood bank should be alerted immediately in the event that two blood products were switched and another patient may soon be at risk. The remaining blood product and tubing should be sent to the blood bank for further testing. Vigorous crystalloid fluid therapy should be initiated with the goal of maintaining a urine output of 1 to 2 mL/kg per hour. Hemodialysis is sometimes utilized to treat the hyperkalemia that results from the hemolysis, or the renal failure caused by DIC. Recipient blood should be sent for a DAT, plasma-free hemoglobin level, CBC, chemistry, haptoglobin, LDH, bilirubin, prothrombin time (PT)/partial thromboplastin time (PTT), d-dimer, fibrinogen, and a repeat type and crossmatch. Urine should be tested for free hemoglobin. Vasopressors and diuretics are sometimes utilized to augment this urinary output. The diagnosis is confirmed by the detection of free hemoglobin in the recipient's blood or urine and a positive Coombs' test posttransfusion samples.

Transfusion-Related Acute Lung Injury

Transfusion-related acute lung injury (TRALI) refers to noncardiogenic pulmonary edema occurring during or shortly after the transfusion of blood products. A leading cause of transfusion-related mortality and morbidity, TRALI has been reported to occur in about 1 in 60,000 transfusions and accounts for 29% of all transfusion-related deaths.

The exact pathophysiology of TRALI remains unknown. It is theorized to be an immune-mediated reaction between donor and recipient. This ultimately leads to increased pulmonary capillary permeability, allowing for high protein fluid to leak into the alveoli. Initial symptoms include respiratory distress, hypoxia, hypotension, fever, and bilateral pulmonary edema. The spectrum of TRALI can also include much milder reactions. The treatment of TRALI is supportive and includes supplemental oxygen, noninvasive positive pressure ventilation, endotracheal intubation, and cardiovascular support as necessary. Diuresis and corticosteroids are not effective. Of course, if the blood product is still transfusing it should be stopped. It is safe to initiate a transfusion from a different donor.

Transfusion-Associated Circulatory Overload

Transfusion-associated circulatory overload (TACO) is volume overload after transfusion that is proportional to the volume transfused. Risk factors for developing TACO include preexisting heart disease (e.g., CHF), significant renal insufficiency, and extremes of age. The development of TACO is not entirely explained by the volume of blood products given. Although the pathophysiology is not entirely understood, a two-hit hypothesis for the development of TACO is the prevailing theory. The first hit is preexisting, volume incompliance, and the second hit is the composition of the fluid given (PRBCs vs. crystalloid solutions). In both animal models and human studies, subjects with underlying heart or renal dysfunction that received blood transfusions were more likely to develop pulmonary edema from increased hydrostatic pressure when compared with healthy subjects who received the same volume and type of blood transfusions. This was also reflected in those subjects with underlying heart or renal dysfunction who received the same volume of crystalloid solution.[42]

TACO appears to develop in about 1% of transfused patients, and this number may underestimate the true incidence since many cases spontaneously resolve with diuresis. There is no specific test or single criteria to definitively diagnose TACO, and it should be considered in any patient who develops pulmonary edema during or shortly after a blood transfusion. Management of TACO is similar to other causes of volume overload. The transfusion (if ongoing) should be stopped, and diuretics should be administered. Theoretically, nitroglycerine would have similar effect in TACO as in any other volume overload situation and can be started at 50 to 100 µg/min IV and titrated to reduce afterload. Patients with increased work of breathing greatly benefit from noninvasive intermittent positive pressure ventilation (NIPPV) that will drive fluid back into the intravascular space. If the patient develops intractable symptoms, intubation and mechanical ventilation may be required. In future transfusions, the rate of transfusion may be slowed, and prophylactic diuretics can be given to decrease the risk of another episode of TACO.

Chronic Reactions

Graft-Versus-Host Disease

GVHD is a transfusion complication most commonly associated with allogeneic hematopoietic cell transfusions. It can occur whenever immunologically competent lymphocytes are transfused, especially in immunocompromised hosts. Donor lymphocytes engraft in the recipient and then attack host tissue. Symptoms are typically observed 7 to 14 days after the transfusion and include fever, rash, and diarrhea. Hepatitis and marrow aplasia also occur. GVHD is often fatal; failure of the host's marrow leads to overwhelming infection or bleeding. The use of gamma-irradiated cellular components prevents this complication by making the donor lymphocytes incapable of proliferating.

REFERENCES ARE AVAILABLE AT Elsevier eBooks+.

SECTION V

Anesthetic and Analgesic Techniques

CHAPTER 29

Local and Topical Anesthesia

Douglas L. McGee

Local anesthetic agents are important tools used in the everyday practice of emergency medicine. This chapter describes the mechanism of action, the nuances of clinical use, and the adverse reactions to anesthetics that are commonly used in the emergency department (ED). Detailed technical guidance for the performance of topical and infiltrative local anesthesia is provided.

BACKGROUND

The first local anesthetic was cocaine, an alkaloid in the leaves of the *Erythroxylon coca* shrub from the Andes Mountains. Early Incan society used cocaine for invasive procedures, including cranial trephination. In 1884 Koller[1] used topical cocaine in the eye and was credited with the introduction of local anesthesia into clinical practice. In the same year, Zenfel used a topical solution of alcohol and cocaine to anesthetize the eardrum, and Hall[2] introduced the drug into dentistry. In 1885 Halsted[3] demonstrated that cocaine blocked nerve transmission, thereby laying the foundation for nerve block anesthesia. The search for alternatives to cocaine led to synthesis of the benzoic acid ester derivatives and the amide anesthetics used today. It was not until the 1960s that detailed understanding of the physiochemical properties, mechanism of action, pharmacokinetics, and toxicity of these agents emerged.

PHARMACOLOGY AND PHYSIOLOGY

Chemical Structure and Physiochemical Properties

Most useful local anesthetic agents share a basic chemical structure:

Aromatic segment—Intermediate chain—Hydrophilic segment

Subtle variations in this basic structure determine each agent's main physiochemical properties: the negative log of dissociation constant (pK_a), the partition coefficient (a measurement of lipid solubility), and the degree of protein binding. Each of these properties determines the drug's potency, onset, and duration of action. However, physiochemical properties are not the sole determinant of clinical activity; other factors influence the drug's effect. The intermediate chain between the aromatic and the hydrophilic segments is either an amino-ester or an amino-amide; these chemical structures form the basis for the two main classifications of local anesthetics. Common ester-type agents include procaine, chloroprocaine, cocaine, and tetracaine. Common amide-type agents include articaine, lidocaine, mepivacaine, prilocaine, bupivacaine, and etidocaine. Different biochemical pathways metabolize each class. Esters are hydrolyzed by plasma pseudocholinesterase. Cocaine, an ester, is also partly metabolized by N-demethylation and nonenzymatic hydrolysis. Individuals with pseudocholinesterase deficiency may have a greater potential for cocaine toxicity if large doses are used, although this has not been an issue when cocaine is used clinically as an anesthetic. Amides are metabolized in the liver by enzymatic degradation. Local anesthetics are poorly soluble weak bases combined with hydrogen chloride to produce the salt of a weak acid. In solution, the salt exists both as uncharged molecules (nonionized) and as positively charged cations (ionized). The nonionized form is lipid soluble, which enables it to diffuse through tissues and across nerve membranes. The ratio of nonionized to ionized forms depends on the pH of the medium (vial solution or tissue milieu) and on the pK_a of the specific agent. The pK_a is the pH in which 50% of the solution is in the uncharged form and 50% is in the charged form. When the pH of the solution or tissue is less than the pK_a, more of the drug is ionized. When the pH increases, more of the drug is in the nonionized form. Because the nonionized form of drug can diffuse through tissues and nerves, manipulating the pH of the solution can alter a drug's diffusion properties.

Local anesthetics are available in single-dose vials or ampules and in multidose vials, with and without epinephrine. Most solutions have a pH higher than 5. Multidose vials contain methylparaben (MPB), an antibacterial preservative. Local anesthetics premixed with epinephrine also contain an antioxidant (sodium bisulfite or sodium metabisulfite) to prevent deactivation of the vasoconstrictor. These solutions must be adjusted to a more acidic pH, approximately 3.5 to 4.0, to maintain the stability of epinephrine and its antioxidant. These properties as they relate to the amide group are depicted in Table 29.1.

Nerve Structure and Impulse Transmission

Functional and Structural Components of a Peripheral Nerve

The functional nerve unit includes the nerve axon and its surrounding Schwann cell sheath. The Schwann cell (Fig. 29.1)

TABLE 29.1 pH and Additives of Amide Local Anesthetics

SOLUTION CONTENT	pH (RANGE)	PRESERVATIVE (METHYLPARABEN)	ANTIOXIDANT
Plain, single dose	4.5–6.5	–	–
Plain, multidose	4.5–6.5	+	–
Commercial epinephrine, single dose	3.5–4.0	–	+
Commercial epinephrine, multidose	3.5–4.0	+	+
Prepared epinephrine, single dose	4.5–6.5	–	–

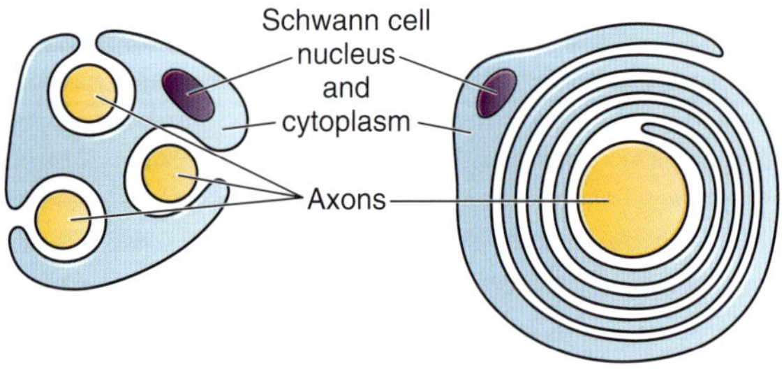

Fig. 29.1 Schwann cell sheath of unmyelinated *(left)* and myelinated *(right)* nerve fibers. (From Wildsmith JAW. Peripheral nerve and local anesthetic drugs. *Br J Anaesth* 1986;58:692.)

may surround several unmyelinated axons or a single myelinated nerve fiber and form a myelin sheath. Junctions between sheaths along the axon, called *nodes of Ranvier*, contain sodium channels necessary for depolarization. As myelin sheath thickness increases from autonomic to sensory to motor fibers, the nodes of Ranvier are spaced farther apart. The most important structure affecting transmission of nerve impulses is the axon membrane (Fig. 29.2). The membrane consists of a double layer of phospholipids into which are embedded protein molecules that serve as channels containing pores for the movement of ions in and out of the cell. Most pores have a filter, or gate, that controls ion-specific movement and a sensory mechanism that opens or closes the gate. Bundles of nerve fibers (Fig. 29.3) are embedded in the endoneurium, which is made of collagen fibrils, and they are surrounded by a cellular layer, the perineurium. The perineurium functions as a diffusion barrier and maintains the composition of extracellular fluid around the nerve fibers. Surrounding the entire structure is the outer layer of a peripheral nerve, the epineurium, which is composed of areolar connective tissue.

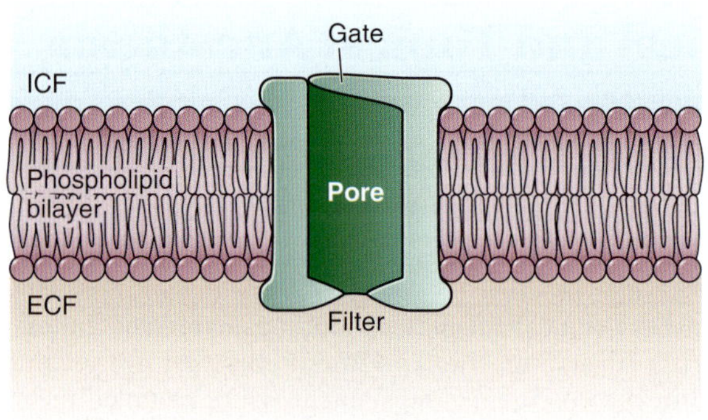

Fig. 29.2 Axon membrane. *ECF*, Extracellular fluid; *ICF*, intracellular fluid. (From Wildsmith JAW. Peripheral nerve and local anesthetic drugs. *Br J Anaesth*. 1986;58:692.)

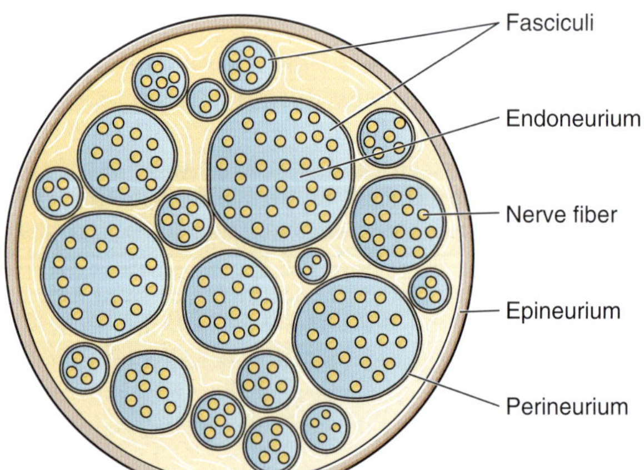

Fig. 29.3 Cross section of a peripheral nerve. (From Wildsmith JAW. Peripheral nerve and local anesthetic drugs. *Br J Anaesth*. 1986;58:692.)

Nerve Impulse and Transmission

The inside of a nerve fiber, or axoplasm, is negative (–70 mV) at rest in comparison to the outside. This resting potential is the net result of the differences in ionic concentration on each side of the axonal membrane and the forces that tend to maintain that difference. Specifically, there is a surplus of sodium extracellularly and potassium intracellularly. The sodium channel is closed, thereby preventing these ions from moving along their concentration gradient (out → in). Although potassium can leave the cell to follow its concentration gradient (in → out), the need to maintain electrical neutrality inside the cell prevents it from doing so completely. Potassium is in equilibrium between the concentration gradient and the electrochemical gradient, thus creating the negative resting potential.

The sodium channel opens when a nerve is stimulated. Sodium ions enter slowly at first until a critical threshold is reached. They then enter the cell rapidly, along the electrochemical and concentration gradients, and cause depolarization. The influx of sodium is halted when the membrane potential reaches +20 mV, but potassium continues to move out of the cell and repolarizes it until the resting potential is reached. When the excitation process has been completed and the nerve cell is electrically quiet, the relative excess of sodium inside the cell and potassium outside the cell is readjusted by the adenosine triphosphate–dependent sodium-potassium pump.

Depolarization of a portion of the nerve causes a current to flow along the adjacent nerve fiber. This current makes the membrane potential less negative and actuates the sensor to open the next sodium channel. The action potential cycle is repeated, thereby propagating the impulse. Nerve conduction is essentially unidirectional because the sodium channel is not only closed but inactivated as well, and delayed closure of specific potassium channels prevents the critical threshold from being reached in the segment just depolarized. Impulses travel continuously down the axon in unmyelinated nerve fibers. In myelinated fibers, current flows from node to node and depolarizes intervening segments at once. This saltatory conduction causes a faster rate of impulse transmission in myelinated fibers.

Mechanism of Action

How local anesthetic agents block nerve conduction depends on the active form of the agent and the specific physiologic and cellular activity.

Active Form

Anesthetic solutions contain uncharged and charged forms. The concentration of the uncharged form increases in more alkaline milieus. Only this uncharged lipid-soluble form can cross tissue and membrane barriers. Once the uncharged drug is through a barrier, it reequilibrates into uncharged and charged forms in a proportion dependent on the prevailing pH. Because local anesthetics are more effective in alkaline solutions, it was originally thought that the uncharged form was responsible for conduction blockade. Alkaline solutions are currently believed to be more effective because of increased penetration through tissue barriers, but it is the cationic charged form that is responsible for the actual neuronal blockade.

Physiologic and Cellular Basis for Neuronal Blockade

Prevention of sodium influx across the nerve membrane forms the physiologic basis for conduction blockade. Local anesthetics slow sodium influx, thereby decreasing the rate of rise and amplitude of depolarization. If sufficient anesthetic is present and the firing threshold is not reached, the action potential is not formed. With no action potential, no impulse is transmitted and conduction is blocked, which results in local anesthesia.

How anesthetic agents prevent sodium influx is still not completely understood. It is believed that the cationic charged form blocks the action potential from inside the membrane; the agent enters the sodium channel from the axoplasmic side and binds to a receptor.[4,5] This "specific receptor" theory is well accepted and is considered the predominant mechanism in preventing influx of sodium. However, this theory cannot account for the action of benzocaine and other neutral compounds or the uncharged base forms of the common local anesthetics.

In summary, when a local anesthetic (other than benzocaine) surrounds the perineurium, it equilibrates into its uncharged and charged forms based on tissue pH and pK_a. In a more alkaline environment, a greater proportion of the uncharged form is present. The uncharged lipid-soluble form penetrates tissue, nerve sheath, and nerve membrane to gain access to the axoplasm and reequilibrates into both charged and uncharged forms. The charged form enters the sodium channel, decreases movement of sodium into the cell, and halts nerve transmission. The uncharged base is also involved in sodium channel blockade, but the exact nature of this mechanism is unknown.

Activity Profile During Neuronal Blockade

A local anesthetic's onset, potency, duration, and ability to produce a differential blockade in mixed nerves are a function of its physiochemical properties, the physiologic environment, and to some extent, manipulation by the clinician.

Onset of Action

The pK_a of an anesthetic is the primary physiochemical factor that determines its onset of action. Increased tissue penetration and a shortened onset of action are found in drugs with a lower pK_a because more of the lipid-soluble uncharged form is present (Tables 29.2 and 29.3). Although in isolated nerve fibers the onset of action directly parallels pK_a, other physiochemical factors also influence drug activity. For example, prilocaine and lidocaine have the same pK_a, but lidocaine's onset is faster because of its enhanced ability to penetrate through nonnerve tissue.

The site of administration also influences the onset of action. Onset times are prolonged as the amount of interspersed tissue or the size of the nerve sheath increases because of the greater distance that the agent must travel to reach its receptor. The pattern of onset for large nerves is determined by the structural arrangement of its fibers. Peripheral (mantle) fibers are blocked before core fibers. Because mantle fibers innervate more proximal regions, nerve blockade proceeds in a proximal to distal progression.

Adding sodium bicarbonate to raise the pH of the anesthetic solution (a technique that decreases pain on injection) yields a higher concentration of the uncharged lipid-soluble form and decreases onset time. Increasing the total dose by using a higher concentration of the same volume or a greater volume of the same concentration also shortens onset time.

TABLE 29.2 Activity Profile With a Primary Physiochemical Determinant

AGENT	ONSET: pK_a	POTENCY: LIPID SOLUBILITY	DURATION: PROTEIN BINDING
Tetracaine	Slow	8	Long
Procaine	Slow	1	Short
Chloroprocaine	Fast	1	Short
Lidocaine	Fast	2	Moderate
Mepivacaine	Fast	2	Moderate
Prilocaine	Fast	2	Moderate
Bupivacaine	Moderate	8	Long
Etidocaine	Fast	4–6	Long

TABLE 29.3 Physiochemical Properties of Selected Local Anesthetics

AGENT	TYPE	SITE OF METABOLISM	pK^a	LIPID SOLUBILITY (PARTITION COEFFICIENT)	PROTEIN BINDING (%)
Tetracaine	Ester	Plasma	8.5	High (4.1)	76
Procaine	Ester	Plasma	8.9	Low (0.02)	6
Chloroprocaine	Ester	Plasma	8.7	Low (0.14)	—
Lidocaine	Amide	Liver	7.9	Medium (2.9)	64
Mepivacaine	Amide	Liver	7.6	Medium (0.8)	78
Prilocaine	Amide	Liver	7.9	Medium (0.9)	55
Bupivacaine	Amide	Liver	8.1	High (27.5)	95
Etidocaine	Amide	Liver	7.7	High (141.0)	94

Note: a common way to remember the class of anesthetic (amide versus ester) is that all amides have the letter "i" appearing twice in the generic name. The others are esters. Cocaine, not listed in this table, is also an ester.

For most procedures performed in the ED, the time of onset of most agents is short enough that manipulation to achieve shorter times is unnecessary.

Potency

The lipid solubility of an anesthetic is a primary physicochemical factor determining potency. The drug's partition coefficient, not the concentration of the lipid-soluble form determined by the pK_a or pH, confers its lipid solubility. Because the nerve membrane is lipid, lipophilic anesthetics pass more easily into the cell and few molecules are needed to block conduction (see Tables 29.2 and 29.3).

The degree of vasodilation produced by the anesthetic also affects potency because vasodilation promotes vascular absorption, thereby reducing the amount of locally available drug. Lidocaine is more lipid soluble than prilocaine or mepivacaine, but it produces more vasodilation. Although lidocaine is twice as potent as prilocaine or mepivacaine in vitro, it is equipotent in vivo. Though not a primary reason for its use, epinephrine increases the depth of anesthesia by producing vasoconstriction and making more molecules available to the nerve. Drugs more readily absorbed by fat have reduced potency. Increased concentration also increases potency. Choosing an anesthetic for its potency is not usually necessary for any given site because the commercially available concentration of an agent may be manipulated to make most drugs equianesthetic. For example, lidocaine, being one-fourth as potent as bupivacaine, is usually used at four times the concentration (1% to 2% vs. 0.25% to 0.5%, respectively). For different sites and techniques, different concentrations and volumes of a given agent are needed to produce adequate blockade.

Duration

The degree of protein binding of an anesthetic primarily determines its duration of action. Agents that bind more tightly to the protein receptor remain in the sodium channel longer (see Tables 29.2 and 29.3). Like potency, the duration of action is reduced by the vasodilation produced by local anesthetics. Prilocaine, which is less protein-bound than lidocaine, has a longer duration of action because of its lesser degree of vasodilation. The duration of action also varies with the mode of administration. It is shorter when agents are applied topically.

The duration of action may be prolonged by several methods. Increasing the dose, usually by increasing the concentration, prolongs the duration to limits imposed by toxic effects. Raising the pH of the anesthetic solution has also been shown to prolong duration.[6,7] The most practical way to increase duration is to use solutions that contain epinephrine.[8] Epinephrine causes vasoconstriction, decreases systemic absorption, and allows more drug to reach the nerve. The effect of epinephrine varies according to the agent. Anesthetics that intrinsically produce more vasodilation (e.g., procaine, lidocaine, mepivacaine) benefit more from epinephrine's vasoconstrictive action. The long-acting, highly lipid-soluble agents (e.g., bupivacaine, etidocaine) are less affected because they are substantially taken up by extradural fat and released slowly. In fact, lidocaine with epinephrine may be effective for as long as bupivacaine without epinephrine. Generally, most ED procedures can be accomplished quickly before the anesthesia wears off regardless of which drug is selected. Choose agents with a long duration of action when the procedure is lengthy or if postoperative analgesia is desired.

TOPICAL ANESTHESIA

Local anesthetic agents may be applied topically to mucous membranes, intact skin, and open wounds. There are sufficient differences among these sites to merit a separate discussion of each one. Topical anesthesia of the eye is discussed in Chapter 63.

Mucous Membranes

Agents and Uses

Effective anesthesia of the intact mucous membranes (not intact skin) of the nose, mouth, throat, tracheobronchial tree, esophagus, and genitourinary tract may be provided by several anesthetics (Box 29.1). Tetracaine, lidocaine, and cocaine are the most effective commonly used agents (Table 29.4 and Box 29.1). Benzocaine (14% to 20%) is commonly used for intraoral or pharyngeal anesthesia (Fig. 29.4). The anesthesia produced is superficial and does not relieve pain that originates from submucosal structures. The onset of action may be slow, which limits its usefulness in urgent situations (such as passing a nasogastric tube). Agents applied topically can be absorbed systemically, and concentrated topical agents can cause toxicity.

Tetracaine solution is an effective and potent topical agent with a relatively long duration of action. It is used in concentrations from 0.25% to 1% with a recommended maximum adult dose of 20 mg. In overdose, it has the disadvantage of severe cardiovascular toxicity without any preceding central nervous system (CNS) stimulatory phase.

Lidocaine is also an effective topical agent that is marketed in a variety of forms (solutions, jellies, and ointments) and concentrations (2% to 10%). The 10% form is most effective, and minimal topical anesthesia is achieved with less potent concentrations. Lidocaine is commonly used as the 2% viscous solution prescribed for inflamed or irritated mucous membranes of the mouth and pharynx. Patient misuse of viscous lidocaine, by repeated self-administration, can lead to serious toxicity. Topical lidocaine provides an adequate duration for most procedures, with the maximum safe dose being 250 mg to 300 mg.

Cocaine is an effective, but potentially toxic topical agent that is applied to the mucous membranes of the upper respiratory tract. Although it is an ester, hepatic metabolism occurs, as does hydrolysis by plasma pseudocholinesterase. Absorption is enhanced in the presence of inflammation. Cocaine is the only anesthetic that produces vasoconstriction at clinically useful concentrations, hence its popularity for treating epistaxis. This major advantage is offset by its susceptibility to abuse and toxic potential. The toxic effects are due to direct stimulation of the CNS and blockade of norepinephrine reuptake in the peripheral nervous system. Cocaine should not be administered to patients who are sensitive to exogenous catecholamines or who are taking monoamine oxidase (MAO) inhibitor antidepressants. Clinical manifestations of toxicity include CNS excitement, seizures, and hyperthermia. Central and peripheral effects of hypertension, tachycardia, and ventricular arrhythmias may also be seen. Acute myocardial infarction has been reported after topical application.[9] Cocaine is commonly used as a 4% solution with a maximum safe dose of 200 mg (2 to 3 mg/kg). A 10% solution is available, but this concentration adds little to the topical effect while enhancing the potential for toxicity. Coronary vasoconstriction may occur with doses as low as 2 mg/kg applied to the nasal mucosa. Although the clinical

BOX 29.1 Common Local and Topical Anesthetics Used in the ED

- Benzocaine spray will produce transient anesthesia of the mucous membranes. Rarely, it can precipitate methemoglobinemia in standard doses.
- EMLA cream (lidocaine and prilocaine) will produce anesthesia of intact skin, but it must be in place for approximately 60 minutes to provide significant benefit.
- ELA-Max, now known as LMX4, is another topical lidocaine preparation with a more rapid onset of action.
- "Magic mouthwash" contains equal parts of diphenhydramine elixir, aluminum-magnesium hydroxide antacid suspension, and 2% viscous lidocaine. It is swished, held in the mouth for 1 to 2 minutes, and expectorated.
- Lidocaine (2%) may be used intraorally, but repeated use may produce systemic toxicity, especially in children. Each 5-mL teaspoon contains 100 mg of lidocaine. It should not be swallowed but, instead, expectorated after holding it in the mouth for a few minutes. Viscous lidocaine is not useful for acute pharyngitis.

ED, *Emergency department;* EMLA, *eutectic mixture of local anesthetics.*

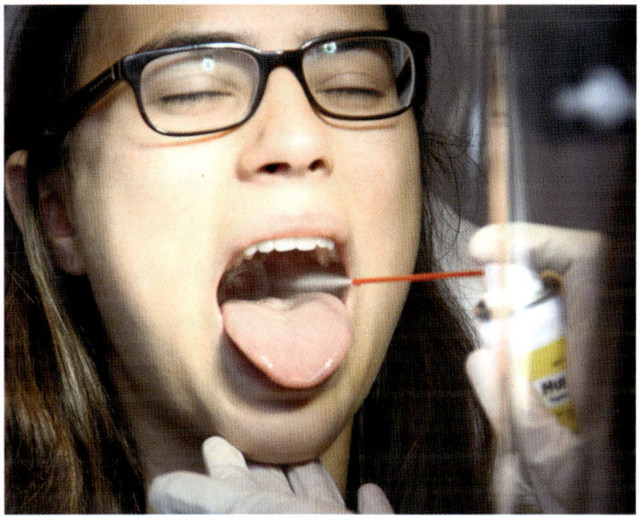

Fig. 29.4 Topical anesthetics can provide effective anesthesia of intact mucous membranes. Here, Hurricaine spray (benzocaine 20%) is used before incision and drainage of a peritonsillar abscess. A rare side effect of topical benzocaine is methemoglobinemia.

TABLE 29.4 Practical Agents for ED Use: Mucosal Application

		Maximum Dosage[a]			
AGENT	USUAL CONCENTRATION (%)	ADULT (mg)	PEDIATRIC (mg/kg)	ONSET (min)	DURATION (min)
Tetracaine	0.5	20	0.75	3–8	30–60
Lidocaine	2–4	250–300[b]	3–4[b]	2–5	15–45
Cocaine[c]	4	200	1–2[b]	2–5	30–45

[a]These are conservative figures; see text for explanations.
[b]The lower dosage should be used for a maximum safe dose when feasible.
[c]The 10% cocaine solution is best avoided because of minimal additional clinical benefit and the potential for coronary vasoconstriction in patients with coronary artery disease.
ED, Emergency department.

effect of this vasoconstriction is usually benign and without electrocardiographic changes, topical cocaine should be used cautiously in patients with known or suspected coronary artery disease. Dyclonine offers advantages over other topical anesthetic agents. It is a ketone derivative without an ester or amide linkage and may be used in patients who are allergic to common anesthetics. Extensive experience with the topical preparation has shown it to be effective and safe.[10] Dyclonine is marketed in 0.5% and 1% solutions, often in sore throat preparations, with a maximum adult recommended dose of 300 mg.

Benzocaine is an ester that is marketed in its neutral form in 14% to 20% preparations (see Fig. 29.4). Its low water solubility prevents significant penetration of the mucous membranes, thus reducing systemic toxicity if applied to intact mucosa. However, it is not a potent anesthetic and has a brief duration of action. It is more allergenic than other topical agents. Benzocaine is usually dispensed in an admixture with other therapeutic ingredients and is clinically effective only at relatively high (>14%) concentrations. Benzocaine is available as a nonprescription gel and liquid (6.3% to 20%) and is used for a variety of maladies, including ear pain, mouth pain, and teething, although the Food and Drug Administration (FDA) recommends against the use of benzocaine in children under age 2 years. Dentists commonly use it to produce mucosal anesthesia before intraoral nerve blocks (see Chapter 30). Adriani and Zepernick[10] recommended this agent for lubricating catheters, airways, endotracheal tubes, and laryngoscopes and reported only one adverse reaction (methemoglobinemia) in their experience with approximately 150,000 patients. Methemoglobinemia occurs rarely after standard doses of benzocaine sprays used in endoscopic or dental procedures procedures.[11,12] Another topical preparation is a combination of lidocaine, prilocaine, and tetracaine, especially useful for dental mucosa anesthesia. Topical gel mixtures of 2.5% lidocaine and 2.5% prilocaine (eutectic mixture of local anesthetics [EMLA]) are commonly used on intact skin but have also been used on mucous membranes. EMLA is more effective than 20% benzocaine when applied to the oral mucosa before needle injection for dental anesthesia. One study demonstrated that pain was reduced more quickly with EMLA than with benzocaine when applied to the buccal mucosa.[13]

As with infiltrated anesthesia, toxic reactions to topically applied anesthetics correlate with the peak blood levels achieved and not necessarily with the dose administered. Systemic absorption of a topical agent is more rapid, with a higher level being achieved than with the same dose given by infiltration. The total dose of a topical anesthetic should be considerably less than that used for infiltration at a given site. Fractionating the total dose into three portions administered over a period of several minutes effectively reduces peak blood levels. Inadvertent suppression of the gag reflex, combined with difficulty swallowing, may lead to aspiration, an important potential adverse reaction to topical anesthesia of the nose, mouth, and pharynx. Infections from drug solutions in multidose vials for topical anesthesia of the larynx and trachea have not been substantiated.

Technique and Precautions

A commonly used "magic mouthwash" for the topical treatment of painful gingivostomatitis in children is often prescribed by emergency clinicians and pediatricians. There has been little scientific study of the preparation and it is not available commercially, but it has been used safely for decades. It consists of equal parts viscous lidocaine (2%), aluminum-magnesium hydroxide suspension (e.g., Maalox) as a binder, and diphenhydramine elixir. Corticosteroids or nystatin is often added when the mixture is used to treat chemotherapy-induced mucositis.[14] However, a 2004 review found no evidence that magic mouthwash is effective in treating this condition.[15] The creamy mixture is swished around the mouth and expectorated, or painted on specific lesions with a cotton swab. Packing an area with a cotton ball soaked with this mixture is another option. Repeated doses or swallowing of the elixir can produce systemic toxicity, so careful instruction should be given to limit the use of the solution to every few hours. This combination would be theoretically less toxic than simply using topical lidocaine.

Emergency clinicians often prescribe 2% viscous lidocaine (20 mg/mL) for patients with pharyngitis, stomatitis, dental pain, or other inflammatory or irritative lesions in the oropharynx. Although this intervention is widely used and generally safe, the common misconception that topical anesthesia is totally innocuous may result in poor patient instructions and serious consequences. Topical lidocaine is helpful for painful mouth lesions but is of little practical value for acute pharyngitis, for which systemic analgesics are usually a better option. Seizures and death from topical lidocaine have been reported when excessive repeated doses have been administered.[16,17] Toxic blood levels may occur because the anesthetic effect of viscous lidocaine lasts for only 30 to 60 minutes and patients with recurrent pain may either ignore or be ignorant of the safe dosing interval of 3 hours and medicate themselves more frequently. Patients tend to increase each dose to obtain greater relief, and inflammation may increase systemic absorption. In addition, painful oral lesions may last for several days. Ice is as effective as 5% lidocaine gel applied to mucous membranes before intraoral injections.[18]

Children are at higher risk for the rare toxicity of oral lidocaine. When compared with adults, children may exhibit increased lidocaine absorption, decreased clearance, and a longer half-life.[19] Continued medication use allows lidocaine and its major metabolites monoethylglycinexylidide (MEGX) and glycinexylidide (GX) to accumulate. Both MEGX and GX are produced from the hepatic metabolism of lidocaine and are excreted in urine. They possess anesthetic and antiarrhythmic activity and have the potential for CNS toxicity. Although these metabolites are less potent than lidocaine, their elimination half-lives are considerably longer. Several investigators regard MEGX and GX to be the cause of CNS toxicity with prolonged topical use of lidocaine.[17] The length of time that viscous lidocaine is retained in the mouth and whether the excess is expectorated or swallowed also affect the blood level produced. Expectorating the medication after swishing it in the mouth produces much lower blood levels than when it is swallowed. It seems logical that the most hazardous mode of administration would be to retain the solution in the mouth "until absorbed."

Clearly explain the proper way to use viscous lidocaine and inform patients not to dose themselves ad libitum. Note that a 2% solution contains 20 mg/mL, or 100 mg per standard teaspoon (5 mL). The recommended maximum adult dose is 300 mg (15 mL of a 2% solution) no more frequently than every 3 hours. When possible, instruct the patient to decrease the dose by using direct cotton swab application. When gargled or swished in the mouth, limit application time to 1 to 2 minutes and instruct the patient to expectorate excess solution.

Limit use to 2 or 3 days, especially if swallowing the solution is necessary to obtain relief. Prescribe lower doses for patients at risk for decreased clearance (see later section on "Systemic Toxic Reactions"). Doses for children are prescribed at 3 mg/kg. Because infants cannot expectorate well, do not use viscous lidocaine for minor oral irritation and teething. Administering lidocaine to ease the discomfort of teething in infants is strongly discouraged; lidocaine provided for painful mouth ulcers does not improve oral intake in children as is commonly believed.[20,21]

Recommend that no food be eaten for 1 hour after application because anesthesia of the oropharynx can interfere with swallowing and cause aspiration. Special note should be made of the over-the-counter availability of benzocaine, commonly used for toothaches and teething. A gel or liquid is available in 6.3% to 20% formulations. When used repeatedly in the oral cavity on irritated tissue, systemic toxicity, including methemoglobinemia, may occur.

Lidocaine 4% solution can be atomized with a standard nebulizer device commonly used for delivering asthma medications and inhaled by the patient before insertion of a nasogastric tube. This method effectively anesthetizes the nasopharyngeal and oropharyngeal tissues, thereby easing the pain of tube insertion.[22,23] Lidocaine (4%) and cocaine (4%) atomized by a single-use mucosal atomizer, compared with lidocaine gel (4%), demonstrated equal reductions in nasal pain scores during the insertion of a nasogastric tube in healthy study participants, although they indicated that overall discomfort was less with lidocaine gel injected into the nose.[24] Atomized lidocaine applied to the airway mucosa is occasionally used to facilitate awake oral intubation, though bilateral superior laryngeal and transtracheal recurrent laryngeal nerve blocks are more effective and allow for faster intubation.[25] When applied to the airway to facilitate intubation, atomized lidocaine should not exceed 9 mg/kg of lean body mass.[26]

Intact Skin

Agents and Uses

The stratum corneum provides a cutaneous barrier that prevents the commonly marketed aqueous solutions (acid salts) from producing anesthesia, but saturated solutions of the bases of local anesthetics are effective on intact skin. When applied topically to abraded skin, most anesthetic agents produce peak blood levels similar to those resulting from infiltration in 6 to 10 minutes.

Lidocaine Cream and Patch

In 1974 Lubens and coworkers[27] used 30% lidocaine cream, saturated on a gauze pad and adherent to an elastic patch, for a myriad of procedures including minor operative procedures (e.g., excision of lesions, incision, and drainage of abscesses), lumbar puncture, venipuncture, and allergy testing. Today, lidocaine is available in 5% and 4% patches and remains one of the most commonly used topical compounds. Recent literature regarding its effectiveness, however, has been mixed. In a study by Cheng, a lidocaine patch applied at the site of rib fractures in patients taking oral pain medication decreased pain scores when compared with a placebo patch.[28] Lidocaine patches applied over rib fractures reduced opiate use but did not reduce hospital length of stay or pulmonary complications.[29] In contrast, a meta-analysis of 251 patients in five trials compared lidocaine patches with placebo patches for acute or postoperative pain, but failed to conclusively demonstrate that a lidocaine patch decreased pain intensity, reduced opioid consumption, or reduced hospital length of stay.[30] Lidocaine patches are often prescribed or purchased over the counter for musculoskeletal neck and low back pain. Clinical trials do not suggest that patients benefit from lidocaine patches applied to the site of pain but considering their low toxicity, lidocaine patches used for neck or back pain may be useful when opiates, nonsteroidal antiinflammatory agents, or other modalities must be avoided.[31,32]

EMLA Cream, ELA-Max, and Tetracaine Base Patch

Various topical anesthetics have been suggested to decrease the pain of venipuncture or injections and to provide topical anesthesia for painful skin abrasions and lesions. These agents have been studied extensively and are safe, but they are not practical in many ED settings because of their slow onset of action and inadequate efficacy. Tetracaine base is available as a solution, a gel, and a patch preparation. It is effective in crossing the lipid-rich barrier of the stratum corneum because it is highly lipophilic. EMLA was approved in the United States in 1992. It contains 2.5% lidocaine and 2.5% prilocaine in a unique oil-and-water emulsion, yielding 5% EMLA. The mild lipophilic and hydrophilic properties of the component drugs are greatly increased when mixed together, thereby allowing absorption through intact skin. ELA-Max and ELA-Max5, now known as LMX 4 and LMX 5, respectively (Ferndale Laboratories Inc), are topical lidocaine anesthetic creams with a more rapid onset of action than EMLA cream. ELA-Max is a 4% concentration, and 5% ELA-Max is marketed as an anorectal cream that may benefit patients undergoing painful rectal procedures. Neither product has prilocaine, as is found in EMLA cream, and neither has US FDA approval for pain relief before painful injections or intravenous (IV) insertion, but both have such potential.[33]

Tetracaine base seems to offer the advantage of being able to achieve effective anesthesia with a shorter application time and a longer duration.[34] For tetracaine and EMLA preparations, onset, depth of anesthesia, duration, and blood levels vary directly with application time, use on thinner or inflamed skin, and larger doses.[35] These preparations exhibit a reservoir effect.[36] The drug is deposited in the stratum corneum and continues to diffuse along its concentration gradient, even after it is removed from the skin.

Tetracaine base, lidocaine cream, and EMLA can be useful in the ED for providing anesthesia for many procedures: venous cannulation, venipuncture, or any needle insertion, including preinfiltration anesthesia and lumbar puncture; a variety of minor surgical procedures; and anesthetizing the tympanic membrane and external auditory canal. EMLA has also been used effectively for debridement of ulcers.[37] EMLA cream applied to wound edges prior to local wound infiltration with 1% lidocaine decreased the pain of laceration repair compared with infiltrative anesthesia alone.[38]

EMLA and 5% lidocaine cream are equally effective in reducing the pain of IV insertion in many studies.[39] Luhmann and colleagues[40] demonstrated that 5% lidocaine cream applied for 30 minutes under an occlusive dressing was as effective as infiltrated buffered lidocaine before IV catheter insertion in children. EMLA does not appear to reduce the pain of venipuncture in infants or lumbar puncture in adults compared with placebo.[41,42]

Obviously, infiltrative administration of buffered lidocaine requires skin puncture, but its onset of anesthesia is almost immediate. When time is not an issue, topical creams may be an acceptable alternative to infiltrated anesthesia or no anesthesia at all. Approximately a 60-minute interval after application is required for these preparations to provide optimal topical analgesia to the intact skin for such procedures as venipuncture. Early cutaneous placement of these agents (e.g., over common IV sites while the patient is being triaged) is important for practical ED use.

Ethyl Chloride and Trichloromonofluoromethane and Dichlorodifluoromethane (Fluori-Methane) Sprays

These topical agents are often used for limited skin incisions (e.g., drainage of small abscesses), trigger point injections, joint aspiration, or injection of bursitis or tendinitis. These agents evaporate quickly from the skin and cool it to the point of freezing. Anesthesia is effective and immediate, but drawbacks include its short duration (only up to 1 minute), potential pain on thawing, and possibly lowered resistance to infection and delayed healing. Highly volatile ethyl chloride spray is flammable. Ethyl chloride has been studied in both children and adults to reduce the pain of venipuncture, but the results are mixed.[43–45] Given their short duration of action and the time needed to perform pediatric venipuncture, these preparations have limited use for this purpose when EMLA cream may be a better alternative.[46] Vapocoolant spray applied before digital block reduces the pain of needle puncture and infiltration.[47]

Technique

Lidocaine Cream

Topical lidocaine cream is saturated on a gauze pad that is adherent to an elastic patch and placed over the area to be injected or incised.[27] The high concentration of anesthetic and an occlusive patch are needed to achieve effective skin penetration. The duration of action varies with the application time. A 45-minute application time is needed for most procedures. To achieve a topical anesthetic duration of 30 minutes, a 2-hour application is necessary. This cream is not currently commercially available in the United States.

Tetracaine Base Patch and EMLA Cream

Because both agents demonstrate a reservoir effect, anesthesia may increase or begin many minutes after removal of the drug. A precise description of application times and duration is not possible. Tetracaine base requires a minimum of 20 to 30 minutes of application time to produce several hours of anesthesia. EMLA requires an application time of 1 to 2 hours for a reported duration of 30 minutes to several hours. Occlusive dressings seem to increase penetration of EMLA whenever the cream is used. Patches are more convenient and cause no loss of effectiveness.

EMLA dosing is based on the amount of cream applied, not on the amount of anesthetic. Each gram of EMLA cream contains 25 mg of lidocaine and 25 mg of prilocaine. Dosages are given in grams of cream, not milligrams of anesthetic. In general, apply EMLA as a thick layer over intact skin under an occlusive dressing for approximately 1 hour before a procedure. Application of a thick layer approximates to 1 to 2 g/10 cm^2. For minor procedures such as needle insertions, apply 2.5 g of EMLA over 20 to 25 cm^2 for at least 1 hour. For more painful procedures, apply approximately 2 g of cream per 10 cm^2 for at least 2 hours. The maximum application area (MAA) determines the appropriate total dose applied. Base the MAA on the patient's weight as follows: 5 to 10 kg, MAA = 20 cm^2; 10 to 20 kg, MAA = 100 cm^2; more than 20 kg, MAA = 200 cm^2.

Ethyl Chloride and Fluori-Methane Sprays

Collect all the equipment required and make all preparations needed to immediately perform the desired procedure. Invert the bottle 25 cm from the skin and spray a stream along the proposed incision site until the area turns white and hard. Make the incision or local anesthetic injection immediately or during actual spraying of the agent for optimal results because the effect is fleeting. Some clinicians use these vapocoolant sprays to decrease the pain of injection of a more traditional local anesthetic such as lidocaine.

Iontophoresis

Anesthetic agents may be drawn into the skin without needles by electrical current applied through electrodes in a process called *iontophoresis*. Lidocaine with epinephrine administered via iontophoresis provides adequate anesthesia before venipuncture in pediatric patients and is superior to EMLA in providing cutaneous anesthesia.[48–51] Iontophoresis is not widely used in emergency medicine but may be another alternative to applied anesthetic agents. Lidocaine and dexamethasone delivered by iontophoresis for soft tissue injuries in the ED provided greater pain reduction and reduced utilization of ibuprofen when compared with ibuprofen alone.[52]

Microneedle Pretreatment

Recently developed technology known as microneedle pretreatment may improve the efficacy of cutaneously applied topical anesthetics. A functional microarray of fine needles painlessly perforates the stratum corneum to facilitate the penetration of applied medications without using traditional needle injections. A 2010 study demonstrated that perforation of the skin of healthy volunteers with a microneedle to which dyclonine was applied resulted in decreased time to anesthesia and a greater degree of pain reduction than did application of dyclonine to nonperforated skin.[53] Microneedling followed by the application of EMLA prior to facial laser resurfacing, and lidocaine 2.5%/prilocaine 2.5% prior to full face fractional microneedling for atrophic acne scars was superior to either topical anesthetic applied alone.[54,55] This emerging technology may improve the practical application of anesthetics to intact skin in the ED.

Jet Injection

Jet injection of anesthetic through intact skin may overcome some of the limitations imposed by the cutaneous application of anesthetics without needle infiltration. A jet injector is a device containing carbon dioxide gas that rapidly forces a plunger to expel the drug through a small orifice applied over intact skin. Medication penetrates the epidermis to a depth of 5 mm to 8 mm in 0.2 seconds and causes the drug to be rapidly dispersed through the skin. Safety is improved because no needles are used to penetrate the skin. Several studies have demonstrated that jet injection of anesthetics provides more rapid anesthesia than topical application of anesthetic agents and is preferred by patients over no anesthesia at all for painful procedures such as laceration repair, lumbar puncture, IV insertion, and arterial blood gas sampling.[56–60]

Complications

General adverse reactions to anesthetic agents are discussed in the later "Complications" section in this chapter.

Tetracaine leads to low blood concentration after proper use. In one study, cutaneous erythema developed at the site of application in approximately 25% of patients.[36] This vasodilatory effect may actually be an advantage when starting IV lines or performing venipuncture. EMLA has a higher rate of local skin reactions, they are mild and transient, with disappearance 1 to 2 hours after removal of the cream. Despite the reported successful use of EMLA cream on skin ulcers, Hansson and associates[37] and Powell and coworkers[61] described an increase in bacterial growth, infection, and inflammation when used in experimental wounds. Methemoglobinemia resulting from the metabolites of prilocaine may occur with EMLA.[35] The risk for clinically significant methemoglobinemia seems remote when EMLA is used properly. It is contraindicated in any infant younger than 3 months and in infants between 3 and 12 months of age who are currently taking methemoglobinemia-inducing drugs (nitrites, sulfonamides, antimalarials, phenobarbital, and acetaminophen). The risk for adverse effects is increased in patients with anemia, respiratory or cardiovascular disease, and deficiencies in glucose-6-phosphate dehydrogenase or methemoglobin reductase. Prolonged inhalation of ethyl chloride spray may produce general anesthesia, coma, or cardiorespiratory arrest. Ethyl chloride is also flammable, thus precluding its use with electrocautery.

Topically applied anesthetics are often covered with an occlusive dressing to contain the medication. Covering the medication with an occlusive dressing may dramatically increase drug absorption and metabolites. Oni and associates demonstrated that 4% lidocaine cream applied to volunteers with an occlusive dressing resulted in three times the level of serum lidocaine and double the level of MEGX when the same dose was applied to volunteers without occlusion.[62] Use caution when occluding topical anesthetics over intact skin because markedly elevated serum levels of the drug may be reached.

Lacerations

Background

In 1980 Pryor and colleagues[63] reported their experience with a topical anesthetic solution (tetracaine-adrenaline-cocaine [TAC]) for wound repair. The original formula, used in most subsequent studies, consists of a solution of 0.5% tetracaine, 1:2000 epinephrine (adrenaline), and 11.8% cocaine. Traditionally, anesthesia is produced by firmly applying a solution-saturated gauze pad or cotton ball directly to the laceration for 10 minutes. The resulting loss of cutaneous sensation is centered on the area of application. Gel formulations of topical wound anesthesia (TWA) with alternative mixtures of agents promise to improve the ease and safety of topical anesthetic solutions for wound repair in the ED. Advantages of TWA include painless application, no distortion of wound margins, good hemostasis, and good patient and parental acceptance in the pediatric age group.

Indications and Contraindications

Use of TWA is generally restricted to young children with wounds less than 5 cm in length, in whom the delay in application of an anesthetic is acceptable and proper application can be ensured (Fig. 29.5). TWA containing vasoconstricting agents is not generally used in structures without a collateral

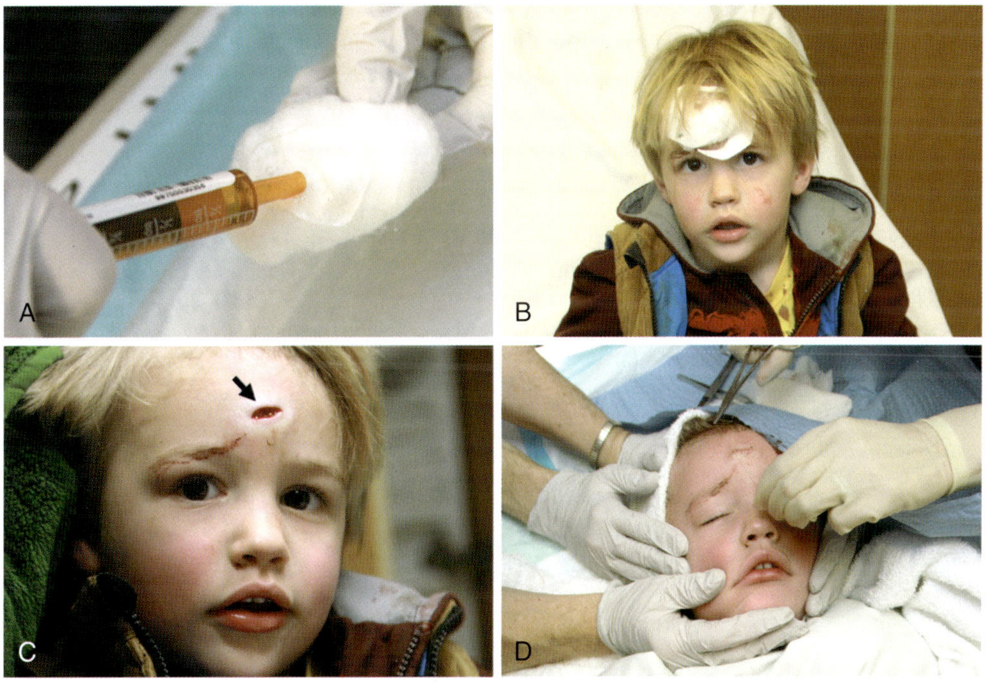

Fig. 29.5 Topical wound anesthesia. (A) The topical anesthetic (in this case, lidocaine-epinephrine-tetracaine gel) is applied to a cotton ball or gauze pad. (B) The anesthetic is held in place with an occlusive dressing such as Tegaderm. (C) After a 30-minute application period, vasoconstriction of local tissue can be readily observed *(arrow)*, and effective anesthesia has been achieved. (D) Local wound repair, including additional infiltrative anesthesia if necessary, can proceed with little if any patient discomfort.

blood supply (e.g., digits, tip of the nose, pinna of the ear, penis), although there is no evidence that this is unsafe. When some wound preparation is desired before anesthesia, remove large debris and clotted blood to allow the appropriate application of TWA and then finish wound preparation once the wound is properly anesthetized.

TWA appears to be less effective on the trunk and extremities than on the face and scalp and less effective than lidocaine infiltration in these areas. The 10- to 20-minute onset time may be unacceptable in a busy ED.[64] Two other often mentioned drawbacks may be more theoretical than real. Vasoconstrictor-induced higher infection rates (see the later section on "Complications") have not been clearly demonstrated. The argument that the necessary 10-minute application period is time-consuming and takes valuable nursing time is partially offset by using the child's caretaker or adhesive paper tape alone to hold the solution in place. It is not necessary for anyone to "hold" the medicine in place when gel is used.

Some EDs still stock topical anesthetic gels that contain cocaine. Cocaine use is complex because of cost and federal regulations requiring storage in a locked cabinet and maintenance of separate written records of its use. In view of the evidence that mixtures without cocaine are efficacious, avoid the potential complications related to cocaine and do not have the potential for abuse that cocaine does, the practicality of cocaine-containing TWA has also been questioned.[65]

Agents and Effectiveness

TAC and Related Mixtures

Three clinical trials directly compared TAC with infiltrated lidocaine. Without specifying wound location, Pryor's group[63] found equal anesthetic effect. Complete anesthesia with TAC was achieved in 82% to 86% of patients as compared with 83% to 92% for subcutaneous lidocaine. The remaining patients obtained partial anesthesia. Hegenbarth and associates[66] and Anderson and coworkers[67] demonstrated results similar to those of Pryor's group.[63] Hegenbarth and associates found TAC to be equal to lidocaine only on the face and scalp and inferior to it at other locations. In contrast, other studies have confirmed excellent rates of effectiveness, especially on the face and scalp.[68–72] TAC is more effective than its component drugs alone. On the face and scalp, TAC was found to be superior to tetracaine alone, although on nonfacial areas, both produced equally poor results.[68] TAC was found to be more effective than cocaine alone and more effective than a tetracaine-epinephrine solution in the same dosage ratio.[70,73]

In 1990 Bonadio and Wagner[71] showed that an epinephrine-cocaine solution (1:2000 epinephrine and 11.8% cocaine) was equal to TAC in effectiveness. Bonadio and Wagner[69] also found that half-strength TAC (0.25% tetracaine, 1:4000 epinephrine, 5.9% cocaine) achieved excellent results in patients with dermal lacerations of the face, lip, and scalp. Smith and Barry[74] compared three strengths of TAC and found equal effectiveness among them; they recommended the lowest-strength cocaine formulation (1% tetracaine, 1:4000 epinephrine, 4% cocaine). Ernst and colleagues[75] found similar effectiveness to TAC when a slightly different lidocaine-epinephrine-tetracaine (LET) solution (4% lidocaine, 1:2000 epinephrine, 1% tetracaine) was used.

TAC has also been compared with EMLA when placed in a wound for 60 minutes before wound repair. In a study of 32 wounds, supplemental anesthesia was required less often with EMLA.[76]

The non–cocaine-containing formulations are generally considered less toxic and have advantages in terms of reduced cost and avoidance of controlled substance requirements during storage.

LET and Related Solutions

Many variations of mixtures that do not contain cocaine have been studied; these include LET, lidocaine-epinephrine, tetracaine-phenylephrine, tetracaine-lidocaine-phenylephrine, bupivacaine-norepinephrine, and prilocaine-phenylephrine. Schilling and associates[77] found that a LET solution (4% lidocaine, 1:1000 epinephrine, 0.5% tetracaine) was as effective as TAC. LET gel preparations are at least as effective as LET solutions.[78] Singer and Stark[79] determined that EMLA or LET gel placed in a wound on initial evaluation and before infiltration with lidocaine reduced the pain of infiltration, thereby allowing an essentially painless injection of lidocaine. Gauze soaked with lidocaine 2% without vasoconstrictive agents placed in a wound was not effective in eliminating the need for infiltrative anesthesia prior to suturing.[80] EMLA, typically used on intact skin, provides anesthesia comparable to LET when applied to wounds.[81]

Technique and Dosage

Because the topical mixtures noted earlier (especially TAC) are not innocuous anesthetics, pay close attention to the technique of application and the recommended maximum dose. There is no uniformly accepted application technique, composition of components, or concentration of components.

Generally, apply topical solutions such as TWA to the wound in a gravity-dependent position and carefully fill the wound cavity. After 3 minutes, place a single 2 × 2 cm gauze pad or cotton ball saturated with TWA on the wound. Tape or hold the pad firmly in place for 15 to 20 minutes. The person holding the gauze should wear latex examination gloves to minimize the risk for cutaneous absorption of the solution. The average dose of TWA mixture for most wounds is 2 mL.

Gaufberg and coauthors[82] described "sequential layer application" (SLA) of topical lidocaine with epinephrine (TLE) to deeper wounds that might not typically be amenable to the use of TWA. Cotton soaked with TLE was applied to the wound surface and 2 mm of surrounding skin for 10 to 15 minutes and then removed. A second similarly soaked piece of cotton was packed deeper into the wound for 10 to 15 minutes. Deep wounds were treated with a third piece of TLE-soaked cotton placed deeper into the wound. Anesthesia was presumed when 3 mm or more of pallor was seen on all wound margins. The group receiving lidocaine by SLA was compared with a group receiving infiltrated 2% buffered lidocaine with epinephrine. Both groups experienced a similar degree of anesthesia during suturing. Mean time to anesthesia with SLA was 29 minutes versus 5 minutes for the infiltration group. Despite the longer time in the SLA group, the authors argued that the additional time is worthwhile because the painful injection, risk for hollow-bore needle injury, and tissue distortion with infiltration were eliminated. If time permits, the SLA technique may be useful for wounds that would have otherwise required infiltrated anesthesia.

Hegenbarth and associates[66] estimated the maximum safe dose of full-strength TAC to be 0.09 mL/kg based on the known maximal safe dose of infiltrated tetracaine, the mucosal application of cocaine, and an estimate of absorption of solution onto the applicator. The key to safety is to avoid TAC on mucosal surfaces or areas in which sniffing or swallowing may accidentally occur. Topical mucosal anesthesia is discussed elsewhere in this chapter.

Prepare an epinephrine-cocaine gel by adding 0.15 g of methylcellulose to 1.5 mL of epinephrine-cocaine solution. Stir the mixture thoroughly for a minute or two until a gel consistency is obtained. After sterile preparation, place the wound in a gravity-dependent position and apply the gel with a cotton-tipped swab to coat the entire wound cavity and margins. Allow the wound to stand for 15 to 20 minutes and thoroughly wash the wound cavity to remove the gel. In Bonadio and Wagner's study,[72] the average dose used was 0.35 mL of gel containing only 40 mg of cocaine. Again, other agents are equally efficacious and safer; select these over cocaine-containing mixtures whenever possible.

Complications

Most adverse events associated with TWA occur with mixtures that contain cocaine. Lidocaine toxicity is a well-recognized, adverse event when higher doses are used (see later section on "Systemic Toxic Reactions"), but lidocaine toxicity has not been reported with TWA mixtures.

Mucosal application may rarely lead to significant systemic toxicity; fatalities have been reported after application. Even after nonmucosal TAC use, cocaine levels appear in the blood and cocaine metabolites appear in the urine in the majority of patients,[83,84] but tetracaine does not. Gel formulations of TAC tend to stay in the wound and thus reduce the risk of solution runoff onto mucosal surfaces. There is no need to use a gauze pad to apply the medication in a gel formulation or to hold it in place. Because the entire applied dose will stay in the wound, a lower dose can be used. Gel also provides more uniform application to tissues, which improves the anesthetic effect. In tissues containing end-arteries, ischemia caused by vasoconstrictors may occur. Avoid TAC on the digits, the tip of the nose, the penis, and the pinna of the ear. Use TAC with caution on patients with coronary artery disease, uncontrolled hypertension, seizures, or peripheral vascular disease. Patients with decreased plasma cholinesterase levels are theoretically at increased risk for systemic toxic effects, but this potential risk is of little clinical concern.

INFILTRATION ANESTHESIA

Background

Injection of an anesthetic agent directly into tissue before surgical manipulation is known as *infiltration anesthesia* (Fig. 29.6). Field block anesthesia is also considered a form of infiltration anesthesia, particularly as the agents, concentrations, and recommended maximum dosages are the same. To create a field block, inject a field of anesthetic around the operative site. Make the injection proximal to or surrounding the area that you plan to manipulate. Combine infiltrative anesthesia with procedural sedation (see Chapter 33) to reduce anxiety or motion.

Indications and Contraindications

Infiltration anesthesia is indicated when good operative conditions can be obtained with this technique. It may be used for the majority of minor surgical procedures, such as excision of skin lesions and suturing of wounds. Infiltration anesthesia is considered quicker and safer than nerve block and general anesthesia. Local infiltration can provide hemostasis, both by direct distention of tissue and by the concurrent use of epinephrine.

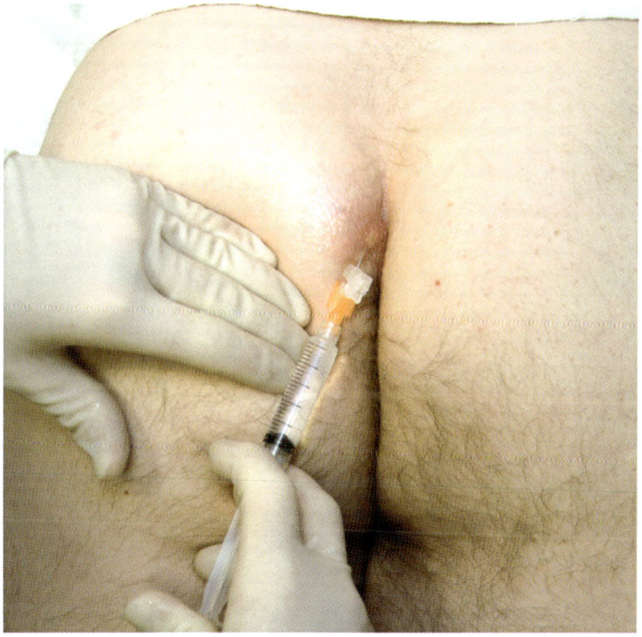

Fig. 29.6 Infiltration anesthesia for incision and drainage of a pilonidal abscess. Minimize pain by using a small needle (ideally 30-gauge if injecting through intact skin or 25- to 27-gauge if going through the cut edges of a wound), buffering the anesthetic with sodium bicarbonate, warming the anesthetic to body temperature, and injecting slowly in the subdermal plane.

A disadvantage of local infiltration over nerve blocks is that a relatively large dose of the drug is needed to anesthetize a relatively small area. For extensive wounds, the amount of anesthetic required may risk systemic toxicity. The maximum allowable volume can be increased by adding epinephrine, using a lower concentration of the anesthetic agent, or both (Table 29.5). When large volumes are anticipated and a nerve block is anatomically feasible, the nerve block is preferred. Avoid using infiltration for large procedures in small children and in apprehensive patients, especially those with previous adverse reactions to the medications (whether vasovagal or otherwise). Local infiltration distorts the tissues that will be incised or repaired, which makes it undesirable in areas requiring precise anatomic alignment (e.g., some lip repairs).

Choice of Agent

The local anesthetic agents most frequently used for infiltration are 0.5% to 1% lidocaine, 0.5% to 1% procaine, and 0.25% bupivacaine (Table 29.6). Higher concentrations are of no additional benefit. Lidocaine is most commonly used because of its excellent activity profile, low allergenicity, low toxicity, user familiarity, and ready availability. Procaine is useful for patients who are allergic to amide anesthetics. Some clinicians prefer bupivacaine because of its prolonged duration. Bupivacaine may also be preferred when postoperative analgesia is desired, for prolonged procedures, for dental anesthesia, or even for short procedures that may be interrupted in a busy ED.

A comparison of equianesthetic doses of lidocaine and bupivacaine for infiltration anesthesia (Table 29.7) revealed that the duration of action is the major difference between the two agents. For the majority of ED procedures, it is not necessary to extend the duration of anesthesia beyond 1 hour, which makes plain lidocaine a logical anesthetic choice. However, patients experience a moderate amount of pain after repair of a laceration when the lidocaine wears off in approximately 1 hour.[85] Bupivacaine reduces the pain after repair of lacerations for at least 6 hours. This benefit of a prolonged duration of anesthesia must be weighed against the hazards of injury to the mucous membranes or an unprotected limb or the annoyance of prolonged numbness in patients who have undergone simple surgical procedures.

A prolonged duration of anesthesia can also be achieved by adding epinephrine, sodium bicarbonate, or both to lidocaine. Epinephrine provides excellent wound hemostasis and slows systemic absorption. This latter property decreases the peak blood level, reduces the potential for a toxic reaction, and allows a greater volume of agent to be used for extensive lacerations. The major disadvantage of epinephrine is theoretical damage to host defenses, but it is clinically inconsequential (Box 29.2). Bicarbonate added to the anesthetic just before injection decreases the pain of administration. Bupivacaine, if used with due caution, is safe and easy to use. The deciding factors are many, but some logical choices are as follows:

- For a wound with excessive bleeding, use lidocaine with epinephrine and sodium bicarbonate.
- For an apprehensive patient, use lidocaine with sodium bicarbonate.

TABLE 29.5 Maximum Allowable Volume (Adults)

AGENT	CONCENTRATION (%)	MAXIMUM[a] SAFE DOSE (mg)	MAXIMUM VOLUME (mL)
Lidocaine	0.5 (5 mg/mL)[b]	300	60
	1 (10 mg/mL)	300	30
Bupivacaine[c]	0.25 (2.5 mg/mL)	175	70
Lidocaine-epinephrine[d]	0.5 (5 mg/mL)	500	100
	1 (10 mg/mL)	500	50
Bupivacaine-epinephrine	0.25 (2.5 mg/mL)	225	90

[a]These are quite conservative figures for infiltration anesthesia; see text for explanation.
[b]Also see Table 29.9. A 0.5% solution is 0.5 g/100 mL = 500 mg/100 mL = 5 mg/mL. A 1% solution is 1 g/100 mL = 1000 mg/100 mL = 10 mg/mL.
[c]Some physicians recommend 400 mg as the maximum safe dose for bupivacaine.
[d]Caution with total epinephrine content; for example 1:100,000 is 10 μg/mL of epinephrine and 100 mL will yield 1000 μg or 1 mg of epinephrine.

TABLE 29.6 Practical Agents for Emergency Department Use: Local Infiltration

AGENT	USUAL CONCENTRATION (%)	Maximum Dosage[a,b] ADULT (mg)	PEDIATRIC (mg/kg)	ONSET (min)	DURATION[c]
Procaine	0.5–1.0	500[d] (600)	7 (9)	2–5	15–45 min
Lidocaine	0.5–1.0	300 (500)	4.5 (7)[e]	2–5	1–2 h
Bupivacaine	0.25	175 (225)	2 (3)[f]	2–5	4–8 h

[a]These are quite conservative figures; see text for explanation.
[b]The higher maximum dose for solutions containing epinephrine appears in parentheses.
[c]These values are for the agent alone; they can be extended considerably with the addition of epinephrine.
[d]Some authorities recommend up to 1000 mg or 14 mg/kg for procaine.
[e]Some authorities recommend up to 7 mg/kg of plain lidocaine in children older than 1 year.
[f]Because of lack of clinical trial experience, drug companies do not recommend the use of bupivacaine in children younger than 12 years, but bupivacaine is commonly used without problems in children.

TABLE 29.7 Comparison of 1% Lidocaine and 0.25% Bupivacaine: Infiltration Anesthesia

	LIDOCAINE	BUPIVACAINE	ADVANTAGE
Onset	2–5 min	2–5 min	Equal
Effectiveness (equianesthetic dose)	Excellent	Excellent	Equal
Duration	1–2 h	4–6 h	Bupivacaine
Infection potential	No	No	Equal
Administration pain	Less	More	Lidocaine
Maximum volume[a]—plain lidocaine	Less	More	Bupivacaine
Maximum volume—epinephrine	Less	More	Bupivacaine
Toxic potential	Less cardiotoxic; equal CNS	More cardiotoxic; equal CNS	Lidocaine

[a]See Table 29.6 for volume and concentration comparison.
CNS, Central nervous system.

BOX 29.2 Epinephrine Use

ADVANTAGES

- Prolongs the duration
- Provides hemostasis
- Slows absorption:
  - Decreases the agent's toxic potential
  - Allows an increased dose
- Increases the level of blockade

DISADVANTAGES

- Impairs host defenses—increases the incidence of infection[a]
- Delays wound healing[a]
- Do not use for:
  - Areas supplied by end-arteries
  - Patients "sensitive" to catecholamines
- Toxicity—catecholamine reaction[b]

[a] *Based on laboratory studies and is of unknown clinical importance.*
[b] *For example, in patients taking monoamine oxidase inhibitors.*

- For anticipated prolonged postprocedure pain, use bupivacaine.

Equipment

The pain of injection is reduced with the use of small-gauge needles. Ideally, a 30-gauge needle is used if the injection is made through skin. If the injection is made through the cut edges of the wound, a 25- to 27-gauge needle suffices. A small-gauge needle slows the rate of injection and reduces the rate and pain of tissue distention. A 10-mL syringe is recommended both for its ease of handling and for the slow rate of injection that it allows.

Technique

Once an agent has been chosen, proper administration technique minimizes pain, prevents spread of bacteria, and avoids intravascular injection. Buffering, temperature manipulation, and careful infiltration also reduce the pain of injection.

Buffering

Raising the pH of an anesthetic by adding sodium bicarbonate decreases pain dramatically, whereas lowering the pH by adding epinephrine increases pain. Buffering is the best way to reduce the pain of local anesthetic injections, and its routine use is highly recommended. It is probable that pH is not the sole factor in producing pain because the pain produced by various agents does not correlate strictly with the pH. Sodium bicarbonate probably works by increasing the ratio of nonionized to ionized molecules, which either renders the pain receptors less sensitive or causes more rapid diffusion of solution into the nerve and a shorter time to the onset of anesthesia.

To alkalinize lidocaine, add 1 mL of sodium bicarbonate (8.4%, 1 mmol/mL) to every 10 mL of anesthetic solution. As the pH of the solution is raised, the anesthetic becomes unstable and has a decreased shelf life. It was initially recommended that buffered lidocaine be prepared just before use to avoid precipitation and degradation, but buffered lidocaine retains its effectiveness for 1 week and refrigeration may further increase its shelf life.[86,87] Bicarbonate may be combined with plain lidocaine for both infiltrative anesthesia[88,89] and digital nerve blocks.[90] In one volunteer study, sodium bicarbonate was effectively combined with lidocaine and epinephrine.[87]

Sodium bicarbonate can be added to bupivacaine, but the solution tends to precipitate as the pH rises. The clinical effect of such precipitation is unclear, but if it occurs, it is prudent to use another solution prepared with less buffer. Precipitation varies directly with the concentration of bupivacaine and the time since mixture.[91] Cheney and coworkers[92] showed that 0.05 mL of 8.4% sodium bicarbonate (measured in a tuberculin syringe) could be mixed with 10 mL of 0.5% bupivacaine without precipitation. The goal of using bupivacaine is to prolong the duration of anesthesia; this effect can also be accomplished somewhat by using buffered lidocaine (plain or with epinephrine).

In view of the amount of published literature demonstrating that adding sodium bicarbonate to lidocaine before infiltrative anesthesia reduces the pain of injection without adverse effects, buffering lidocaine should be considered, factoring in that this technique leads to significant waste of unused bicarbonate.

Temperature Manipulation

Warming an anesthetic to body temperature (37°C to 42°C) reduces the pain of infiltration,[93–95] but warming may not reduce injection pain as much as buffering with sodium bicarbonate does. Bartfield and colleagues[96] found that lidocaine warmed to 38.9°C was more painful than room temperature buffered lidocaine during intradermal injection. Brogan and associates,[97] using lidocaine warmed to 37°C, found the warmed lidocaine and room temperature buffered lidocaine to be equivalent during wound infiltration. Neither study found a synergistic effect with combined warming and buffering. Martin and coworkers[98] found that warmed (37°C) lidocaine was no less painful than buffered lidocaine. Anesthetic solutions can be warmed in a baby food warmer with thermostat temperature control or in an IV solution warmer. Warming is not believed to adversely affect the shelf life of the local anesthetic.

Locally cooling the area to be infiltrated may provide additional pain relief. Leff and colleagues[99] demonstrated that patients receiving local infiltrative anesthesia for repair of an inguinal hernia had less pain when the incision area was cooled before infiltration. Patients were randomized into two groups and had a 1000-mL bag of saline placed over the inguinal area for 5 minutes. One group used saline bags at room temperature, the other group used saline bags cooled to 4°C. A significant decrease in pain perception was found in the group in which the inguinal area was cooled before lidocaine infiltration. Cooling of wounds in the ED before infiltration has not been studied.

Injection

The pain from injection of local anesthetics is primarily a result of skin puncture (which can be minimized with small-gauge needles) and subcutaneous injection. Although patients fear the needle, there is little perceived pain merely from the needle's presence in subcutaneous tissue. Place the injection in subdermal tissue to minimize needle puncture pain and the tissue distention that occurs with intradermal placement. Place the needle "up to the hub" and inject while withdrawing along the just-created subdermal tunnel to minimize tissue distention. After an initial injection, instead of totally withdrawing the needle from the tissue, redirect it along another path to lessen the number of skin punctures. Slowly inject the smallest volume necessary to reduce pain. Hamelin and coworkers demonstrated that blinded volunteers receiving digital nerve block with 2 mL of lidocaine and epinephrine (1:100,000) experienced less pain when the solution was injected over 60 seconds rather than over 8 seconds.[100]

Because the patient barely feels a needle placed subcutaneously and skin puncture is often quite painful, make all wound injections through the wound edge and not through the skin (Fig. 29.7).[101,102] Spread of infection beyond the wound margin has not been demonstrated clinically with this technique. Some clinicians choose to inject the anesthetic through intact skin in patients with a grossly contaminated wound. Bierman[103] described a technique of patient distraction by applying light pressure to alternate sides of the wound with one's fingers and repeated ambiguous questioning about feeling the light pressure rather than the ongoing wound injection. Ask school-aged children to count backward or "say your ABCs" to distract them during injection. Inject 1% lidocaine through intact skin with the needle bevel facing upward because this is less painful than injecting with the needle bevel facing downward.[104]

To prevent a systemic toxic reaction, avoid giving an intravascular injection. For infiltration anesthesia with a small-gauge needle, however, aspiration is usually unnecessary unless the injection is deeper than the subcutaneous area or the area to be injected contains many large vessels.

SPECIAL CONSIDERATIONS

Hematoma Block

Hematoma block (Videos 29.1–29.3) has been used for many years to provide anesthesia for fracture reduction, particularly of the distal end of the forearm and hand (Fig. 29.8). Its popularity has waned somewhat because of the fear (unproven and theoretical) of introducing infection at the fracture site and its limited efficacy. Although several studies have shown hematoma block to be safe, the anesthesia that it provides is not as good as that provided by a Bier block (see Chapter 32). Nevertheless, there are several reasons to consider this technique.[105,106] The procedure is simple and quick to perform and does not require additional personnel. There is no need to wait for an anesthesiologist. A lower dose of the anesthetic agent is required for a hematoma block than for a Bier block (see Chapter 32). A hematoma block is particularly useful when a Bier block and general anesthesia are contraindicated.

Prepare the skin over the fracture site with antiseptic solution and insert the needle into the hematoma, as confirmed by aspirating blood. Slowly inject 5 to 15 mL of

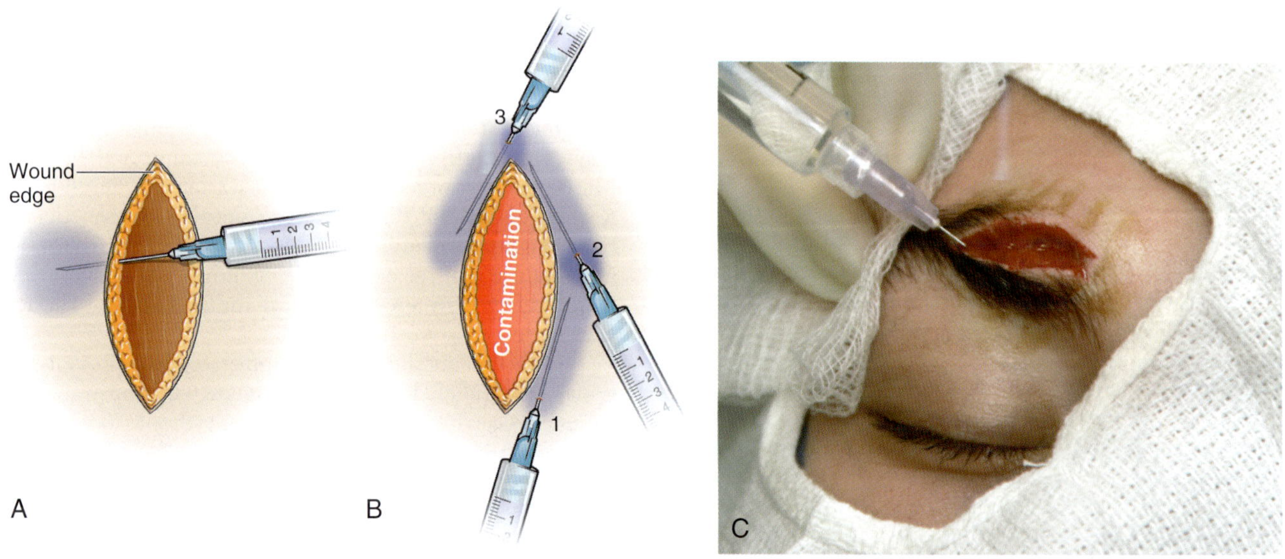

Fig. 29.7 (A) Except in the setting of gross contamination, wounds should be anesthetized by inserting the needle through the cut edges, not through the intact skin. Patients often will not feel a 25-gauge or smaller needle passed into subcutaneous tissue when it is advanced slowly through the cut edge. However, pain generally occurs with distention of tissue by the anesthetic, and hence injection should be slow and deliberate. (B) If a wound is grossly contaminated, the anesthetic may be introduced through the intact skin. The operator should limit the number of needlesticks. The needle is first introduced at a point in line with the wound and beyond the wound edge *(1)*, and while the anesthetic is slowly injected, the needle is advanced to include one entire side of the wound (if possible) to a point well past the opposite end of the wound. If the needle is not long enough to encompass the entire wound, the skin is painlessly punctured at a midway point that has already been anesthetized *(2)*. The other side may be anesthetized by passing the needle through the area already infiltrated by the first injection *(3)* to make the skin puncture painless. A 3.8-cm (1.5-inch) 27-gauge needle is a good choice. (C) Inject local anesthetic through subcutaneous tissue, not intact skin.

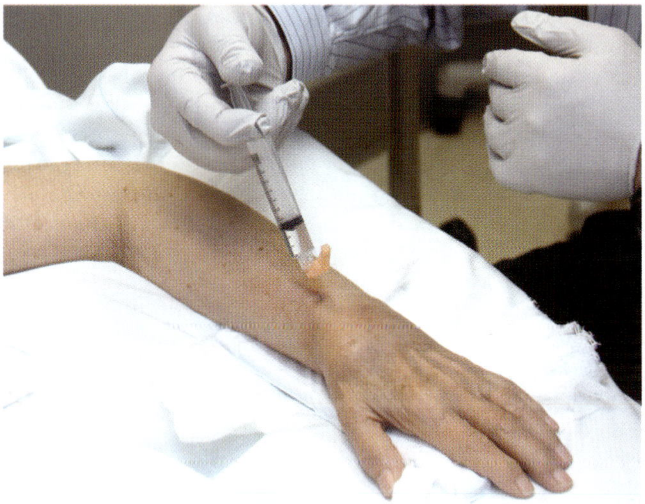

Fig. 29.8 Hematoma block. This technique is useful for reducing fractures of the distal end of the forearm and hand. Here, it is being used before reduction of a distal radius (Colles) fracture. To perform the block, slowly inject 5 mL to 15 mL of plain 1% lidocaine into the fracture cavity and around the adjacent periosteum. It may require 10–15 minutes for anesthesia to occur.

plain 1% lidocaine or 5 to 10 mL of plain 2% lidocaine into the fracture cavity and around the adjacent periosteum. Larger fractures require larger volumes of local anesthetic. Adequate anesthesia occurs in approximately 5 to 10 minutes and may last for several hours. A common error is to attempt the procedure too soon after injection. Do not perform this procedure through dirty skin or with open fractures.

Intraarticular Anesthesia and Analgesia

Findings from the history and physical examination of an acutely traumatized joint, such as the knee, often underestimate the severity of the injury. Instillation of 5 mL of 1% lidocaine after joint aspiration may help relieve pain and facilitate an examination, but its use is not routinely recommended.[107] As spasm and apprehension are often not relieved by local anesthesia, the information gained from this maneuver does not usually influence the ED treatment plan. Intraarticular anesthesia of the knee has no effect on gait pattern or joint proprioception.[108] Postprocedure weight bearing may be allowed without fear of producing or increasing injury if otherwise indicated. Intraarticular anesthesia may enhance elbow use after aspiration of a hemarthrosis associated with a radial head fracture.[109] The technique of administration is analogous to arthrocentesis (see Chapter 55). Intraarticular lidocaine has been effective in facilitating reduction of a shoulder dislocation. Animal experiments have demonstrated chondrotoxicity when local anesthetics are continuously infused into a joint.[110,111] Although continuous joint infusion of anesthetic may be harmful when used in a postoperative setting, there is no evidence that a single injection of intraarticular anesthetic in the ED is harmful.

Morphine may be injected directly into joints for postoperative pain relief and potentially provide prolonged analgesia after reduction of fractures. Theoretically, there are local opioid receptors in joints that are capable of being stimulated by rather small doses of morphine to provide relief for up to 24 hours with a single dose. There may also be some systemic absorption of the intraarticular morphine that contributes to analgesia, but adverse systemic opioid effects are not seen with this technique. Data are sparse on the exact mechanism and optimal doses. A period of 3 to 6 hours may be required for analgesia to reach its maximum effect. In a systematic review, Gupta and colleagues concluded that postoperative intraarticular morphine injected into the knee joint at doses of 2 mg to 4 mg provides analgesia for up to 24 hours.[112] There is a wide variability in efficacy, which may be dose related. Though studied primarily for postoperative use after knee surgery, a similar concept may be intuitively applied to traumatic joint pain, but this has not been studied adequately.

Intrapleural Anesthesia

Indications

Intrapleural anesthesia introduces a local anesthetic into the pleural space (i.e., between the parietal and visceral pleura) through an epidural catheter. The anesthetic can also be introduced through a previously placed chest tube. The technique can provide relief for several conditions, primarily postthoracotomy pain, postcholecystectomy pain, and most importantly for emergency clinicians, posttraumatic chest pain (e.g., rib fractures, pneumothorax, hemothorax). This procedure is not only useful for pain relief but also facilitates turning, coughing, and deep breathing. Several studies have demonstrated improved respiratory mechanics when intrapleural anesthesia is used.[113,114] Though not unanimous, most studies show that intrapleural anesthesia is effective in providing analgesia.[115,116] Concern has been raised that intrapleural anesthesia may create a level of anesthesia below the umbilicus and make posttraumatic abdominal examinations unreliable. Until this issue is clarified, it seems prudent to rule out intraabdominal injury before intrapleural anesthesia is used.[117]

Technique

If a chest tube is in place, it is preferable to inject anesthetic into the pleural space through the chest tube. Clamp the tube for 10 to 15 minutes to allow the anesthetic to diffuse. When the tube cannot be taken off suction or if no tube is present, inject the local anesthetic percutaneously.[118] With the patient in the lateral position (with the affected side up), place a 16-gauge Tuohy needle 8 to 10 cm from the posterior midline in the eighth intercostal space. Angle the needle 30 to 40 degrees with respect to the skin and aim medially, with the bevel up and directed just above the rib. After perforating the posterior intercostal membrane (felt as a distinct resistance), remove the stylet and attach a well-wetted, air-filled glass syringe to the Tuohy needle. Advance the needle until it enters the pleural space, which is denoted by the plunger being drawn down the syringe as a result of the negative pressure created during inspiration. Remove the syringe and introduce an epidural catheter 5 cm to 6 cm into the pleural space. Remove the Tuohy needle, obtain a chest radiograph to confirm proper position, and secure the catheter.

The most commonly used anesthetic and dose is 20 mL (0.3 mL/kg) of 0.5% bupivacaine. A dose repeated every 8 hours is safe and effective.[119] Alternatively, infuse 0.25% bupivacaine at 0.1 to 0.2 mL/kg per hour after a bolus has been administered.[113] The solution presumably diffuses from the pleural space "back" through the parietal pleura and the intercostal muscle to reach the intercostal spaces, where it blocks the intercostal nerves. The level of anesthesia can extend from T2 to T12 and involve the skin, chest, abdominal wall, and potentially the viscera if the visceral afferent fibers are blocked at the sympathetic chain in the paravertebral gutter.

Though not yet a consistently proven or a completely standardized technique, intrapleural anesthesia offers promise for patients and is a valuable procedure for the emergency clinician to master.

COMPLICATIONS

Local Anesthetic Effect on Wounds

Wound Healing

Local anesthetics produce cytotoxic effects on cell structure and function in a dose- and time-related manner. These effects, at doses well below those used clinically, involve fibroblasts more than nervous tissue. Local anesthetics impair mitochondrial function and fibroblast proliferation and hasten apoptosis in vitro; the clinical relevance of these effects to the ED use of local anesthetics is likely to be minimal.[120,121] Collagen synthesis is inhibited by lidocaine and bupivacaine.[122] Morris and Tracey[123] found that lidocaine in increasing concentrations progressively reduces the tensile strength of wounds. Epinephrine added to 1% and 2% concentrations of lidocaine further reduced tensile strength, but when epinephrine was added to distilled water or to 0.5% lidocaine, it had little effect. Several conclusions may be clinically relevant. Although it may delay the onset of anesthesia, 0.5% lidocaine solution, without epinephrine, may be best for maintaining wound strength.

Eriksson and associates[124] found that lidocaine reduces the inflammatory response in wounds by decreasing the number of white cells and their metabolic activity. Although an inflammatory response may be beneficial in a contaminated wound, it can be detrimental in a sterile wound because of tissue toxicity created by the release of superoxide anions, lysosomal enzymes, thromboxanes, leukotrienes, and interleukins. The clinical relevance of this is unknown. None of the concerns mentioned earlier should prohibit the use of standard anesthetics or epinephrine when their use is otherwise indicated.

Wound Infection

Though not generally appreciated, it has long been known that local anesthetics possess antimicrobial activity in vitro. Lidocaine and procaine demonstrate concentration-dependent inhibition of culture growth of most gram-negative organisms.[125–127] Gram-positive isolates are also significantly affected by lidocaine and, to a lesser extent, by procaine. Lidocaine inhibits the growth of common nosocomial pathogens, including *Enterococcus faecalis*, *Escherichia coli*, *Pseudomonas aeruginosa*, and several strains of methicillin-resistant *Staphylococcus aureus* and vancomycin-resistant enterococci.[127] Administering anesthetics before obtaining material for culture, including injecting a joint before arthrocentesis, may give false-negative culture results. To avoid this problem, if possible, inject the skin at the injection site and along the needle tract but not into the actual joint space until after a synovial fluid specimen has been obtained for culture. Berg and coworkers[128] demonstrated that lidocaine administered before tissue biopsy of chronic wounds did not affect the culture results when the exposure time before culture was less than 2 hours. This effect is also significant when anesthetic ointments are applied before culture. EMLA cream applied before culture demonstrates powerful antimicrobial properties.[128] Furthermore, it has been shown that adding sodium bicarbonate to lidocaine greatly enhances its inhibitory effect on bacteria.[129] Although local anesthetics can interfere with culture testing, several studies have shown that local anesthetics, by themselves, do not appear to alter the incidence of wound infection.[130,131]

Epinephrine appears to exert a deleterious effect on host defenses, at least in animal models. Studies of infiltrated and topically applied epinephrine solutions in contaminated animal wounds show an increased potential for infection.[130,131] Epinephrine-induced vasoconstriction may contribute to tissue hypoxia, slow the killing of *S. aureus* by leukocytes, and reduce leukocyte migration into the tissue.[132] Most clinical studies using topical anesthetics with vasoconstrictor properties (e.g., TAC mixtures) do not demonstrate a significant rise in infection rates.[63,66,67,72] The concerns mentioned earlier should not prohibit the use of epinephrine for wound preparation when its use is otherwise appropriate.

Local Injuries

Injury may result from the direct application of an anesthetic agent to a nerve or from passage of a needle through soft tissue structures. Factors implicated in transient or persistent neuropathy include acidic solutions, additives, the agent itself, needle trauma, compression from hematomas, and inadvertent injection of neurolytic agents. Born[133] described a series of 49 wrist and metacarpal blocks with bupivacaine in which significant neuropathy developed in eight patients. He postulated that damage occurred from trapping the drug in a confined space and recommended that whenever bupivacaine is used in this situation, it should be low in concentration and volume. Infection, hematomas, and broken needles are other local problems that can be avoided by using proper technique. Erroneous needle placement can also produce complications such as pneumothorax during a brachial plexus or intercostal block.

Use of Epinephrine With Local Anesthetics

Epinephrine in conjunction with local anesthetics prolongs the duration of anesthesia and produces a temporary hemostatic effect, but its inclusion in digital block solutions has traditionally been discouraged because of the belief that it can lead to ischemia and necrosis. Areas of special concern include the digits, penis, tip of the nose, and earlobe. Although tissue ischemia and sloughing have been reported with concentrations of 1:20,000, current practice involves concentrations in the range of 1:100,000 to 1:200,000 and the use of submaximal doses. Several authors suggest that epinephrine-containing solutions can be safely injected into the fingers without adverse sequelae.[134–137]

A study of more than 3000 cases of elective injection of low-dose epinephrine (≤1:100,000) into the hand and fingers failed to identify a single case of digital tissue loss, and phentolamine was not required to reverse vasoconstriction.[134] Of 1111 procedures reported by Chowdhry and coauthors[138] involving digital blocks with 1% lidocaine plus epinephrine (1:100,000) at a dose ranging between 0.5 mL and 10 mL (average, 4.3 mL), no patient in the epinephrine group exhibited digital ischemia or experienced nerve injuries or unusually delayed wound healing. Current data support the use of epinephrine, when correctly applied, for the performance of digital blocks of the fingers and toes.

The use of phentolamine, which produces postsynaptic α-adrenergic blockade, is recommended for clinically significant vasoconstrictor-induced tissue ischemia. This medication is usually given by local infiltration, in the area where epinephrine has been injected, at a dose of 0.5 mg to 5.0 mg diluted 1:1 with saline. If local infiltration is ineffective because of tension within a tissue compartment or if the area of vasoconstriction is large, give phentolamine by the intraarterial route.[139]

Systemic Toxic Reactions

Although systemic toxic reactions occur in only 0.1% to 0.4% of patients after the administration of local anesthetics, they are the most frequent serious adverse reactions encountered (Table 29.8).[140] After the administration of a local anesthetic, some of the drug reaches its intended target and some is absorbed quickly into the systemic circulation. Peak blood levels are generally produced within 30 minutes. Many vagal reactions, nonspecific anxiety reactions, and sensitivity to preservatives have been attributed to "allergies" or to systemic toxicity to local anesthetics. Patients may also demonstrate systemic reactions to hidden allergens that may mimic a systemic reaction, such as anaphylactic reactions to the latex in surgical gloves.

High Blood Levels

Systemic toxic reactions result from high blood levels of local anesthetic. Several factors are important in producing high blood levels, including the site and mode of administration, rate of administration, dose and concentration, addition of epinephrine, specific drug, clearance, maximum safe dosage, and inadvertent intravascular injection.

Site and Mode of Administration

In comparing the routes of administration for a given dose, the intravascular route produces the highest levels, followed by topical mucosal application and then infiltration. The more vascular the site, the more systemic absorption that occurs and the higher the level obtained. The following blocks are arranged in decreasing order of systemic absorption: intercostal, caudal, epidural, brachial plexus, and subcutaneous. It follows that the site of administration is an important variable in determining the safe dose of an anesthetic. For example, 400 mg of lidocaine may produce a nontoxic blood level with subcutaneous abdominal wall infiltration but produce a toxic level when used for an intercostal nerve block.

Rate of Administration

A more rapid IV injection will produce a higher blood level than a slower injection. A single topical application leads to a higher level than a dose that is fractionated over time.

Dose and Concentration

The larger the total dose, the higher the peak blood level. It is uncertain whether increasing the concentration while maintaining the total dose by decreasing the volume affects the serum level.

Addition of Epinephrine

Epinephrine produces vasoconstriction and reduces systemic absorption, thereby resulting in lower peak blood

TABLE 29.8 Differentiating Systemic Adverse Reactions

FINDINGS	TOXIC REACTIONS	ALLERGY	VASOVAGAL	EXCESS CATECHOLAMINES, ANXIETY[a] (ENDOGENOUS), VASOCONSTRICTOR (EXOGENOUS)
Relatively specific signs and symptoms	Metallic taste Tongue numbness Drowsiness Nystagmus Slurred speech Seizures[b] Coma Respiratory arrest[b]	Acute rhinitis Pruritus[b] Dermatitis Urticaria[b] Facial swelling Laryngospasm Bronchospasm[b]	Syncope[b,c]	Headache Hypertension[b] Palpitations Apprehension[b,d]
Overlapping signs and symptoms	Paresthesia Light-headedness Tinnitus Tremor Tachypnea Tachycardia (early) Bradycardia[b] Hypotension[b] Cardiac arrest	Light-headedness Tachycardia[b] Hypotension[b] Cardiac arrest Nausea and vomiting Dyspnea	Light-headedness Tinnitus Tachypnea Tachycardia (early) Bradycardia[b] Hypotension[b] Diaphoresis	Paresthesia[b] Light-headedness[b] Tremor Tachypnea[b] Tachycardia[b] Nausea and vomiting Dyspnea Diaphoresis

[a]Anxiety reaction, including hyperventilation syndrome.
[b]Denotes common and significant reactions.
[c]Vasovagal syncope occurs with the patient upright; any loss of consciousness in the recumbent position implies a severe toxic or anaphylactic reaction.
[d]Although apprehension is classically associated with anxiety and vasoconstrictor reactions, milder toxic and allergic reactions may cause patient apprehension.

levels. Occasionally, the apprehension, tachycardia, or palpitations induced by epinephrine can be incorrectly interpreted by both the clinician and patient as an "allergic" reaction.

Specific Drugs

The more potent agents are more toxic on a milligram-to-milligram basis. Because anesthetics are used in equipotent doses (e.g., 1 mg of bupivacaine vs. 4 mg of lidocaine), they are approximately equitoxic. The blood levels achieved by a particular agent depend on the agent's absorption, distribution, and clearance from the circulation. Agents with high lipid solubility and lower protein binding (etidocaine > bupivacaine > lidocaine > mepivacaine) tend to become sequestered in tissue and have slower absorption and lower blood levels. Agents with a greater volume of distribution or faster clearance (etidocaine > lidocaine > mepivacaine > bupivacaine) also produce lower blood levels. Together, these effects produce margins of safety for each anesthetic, with etidocaine having the greatest safety margin, followed by bupivacaine, which is equal to or better than lidocaine.

Esters are difficult to measure in blood because of their rapid hydrolysis by pseudocholinesterase. As a group, toxicity is inversely proportional to the rate of hydrolysis. Tetracaine is slowly hydrolyzed and is most toxic. Chloroprocaine is quickly hydrolyzed and is the least toxic. Procaine falls between the two.

Clearance

The liver metabolizes amides, with the clearance rate being a function of hepatic blood flow and the extraction capacity of the liver. Decreased hepatic blood flow, produced by norepinephrine, propranolol, or general anesthesia, slows clearance, and potentially raises drug blood levels. Decreased drug extraction, associated with congestive heart failure, cirrhosis, or hypothermia, may produce a higher blood level. Hypovolemia, which decreases hepatic flow, does not raise blood levels because it causes an offsetting decrease in absorption.

Decreased clearance of esters and an increased risk for toxicity occur in patients with either low levels or an atypical form of pseudocholinesterase. Low levels occur in various disease states, including severe liver disease and renal failure, and in pregnancy. Atypical pseudocholinesterase is an inherited trait, and its presence reduces the hydrolysis rate of procaine to a greater extent than low levels do.

There are significant differences between pediatric and adult drug distribution and metabolism. Neonates exhibit both reduced levels of pseudocholinesterase and reduced hepatic metabolism, thus increasing the risk for toxicity. In older children, the effects of increased hepatic metabolism and a relatively larger volume of distribution increase their tolerance for higher doses.

Because lidocaine is metabolized in the liver by cytochrome P-450 enzymes, drugs that inhibit these enzymes may slow lidocaine clearance and increase the risk for lidocaine toxicity. Although the effect of ciprofloxacin and erythromycin on infiltrated lidocaine has not been studied, these drugs decrease the metabolism of lidocaine and increase the concentration of its major metabolites when lidocaine is injected intravenously.[141–143] The clinical effect of this previously discussed phenomenon is unknown and probably of little consequence in ED wound care.

Maximum Safe Dosage

The maximum safe dose of a drug may be defined as the dose that produces a blood level of the drug just below the toxic level (Table 29.9). One maximum dose of an anesthetic agent appropriate for all patients and all conditions cannot be stated. A maximum safe dose cannot be based solely on the weight of a patient. In an adult, peak blood levels do not correlate well with weight because the volume of drug distribution is relatively constant.[144,145] As an approximation, Arthur and McNicol[146] recommended that maximum dosages for children be based on weight. Plain lidocaine may be used in doses of up to 4.5 mg/kg, and the addition of epinephrine allows a maximum dose of 7 mg/kg. Bupivacaine is not recommended for children younger than 12 years, although it is commonly used without adverse consequences. Furthermore, the dose should be modified according to the site and mode of administration.

Maximum safe doses as stated on package inserts should be used only as guidelines because most of them are derived from animal experiments and are based on absorption data only. Levels vary with the site of administration, use of a vasoconstrictor, and to some extent, the health of the patient. Levels may be exceeded safely when the drug is administered accurately. Drugs may be toxic even within the "safe range" when inadvertently injected intravenously.

Inadvertent Intravascular Injection

Most toxic reactions are caused by inadvertent intravascular injection of anesthetics whose doses were calculated for their intended extravascular sites. For example, lidocaine 300 mg is a safely infiltrated dose that would probably cause toxicity if directly injected into the bloodstream.

Anesthetics that are injected intravascularly must pass through the lungs before they reach other organs. Lung tissue sequesters a significant amount of drug, which lowers the arterial blood concentration. Anesthetics that bypass the lungs, in cases of inadvertent injection into the carotid or vertebral arteries or in patients with intracardiac right-to-left shunts, can produce CNS toxicity at low doses. Intraarterial injections into subcutaneous end-arteries about the head or neck are capable of retrograde flow into the cerebral circulation if the injection pressure exceeds arterial pressure. Because the blood volume in the brain is only approximately 30 mL at any given moment, even 1 mg of lidocaine injected into the carotid artery can theoretically produce toxic concentrations. Patients with low cardiac output or hypovolemia and preferential cerebral blood flow may experience enhanced CNS toxicity.

Host Factors

Four factors tend to lower the body's systemic tolerance to local anesthetic agents: hypoxia, acid-base status, protein binding, and concomitant drug use.

Hypoxia

It was initially thought that an overdose of a local anesthetic produces CNS stimulation and subsequent intracellular hypoxia, which then became the key precipitant for all toxic manifestations of the drug. It is now known that hypoxia may enhance anesthetic toxicity but is not the primary factor.

Acid-Base Status

Although studies of metabolic alkalosis have produced conflicting results, acidosis, particularly respiratory acidosis, can

TABLE 29.9 Calculation of Anesthetic Doses[a]

- Anesthetic solutions are marketed with the drug concentration expressed as a percentage (e.g., bupivacaine 0.25%, lidocaine 1%). To ascertain the strength of a solution in milligrams per milliliter, consider the following: A 1% solution is prepared by dissolving 1 g of drug in 100 mL of solution; therefore 1 g/100 mL = 1000 mg/100 mL = 10 mg/mL.
- Note: To calculate the strength from the percentage quickly, simply move the decimal point one place to the right, as follows:

0.25% = 2.5 mg/mL	e.g., bupivacaine
0.5% = 5 mg/mL	e.g., tetracaine
1% = 10 mg/mL	e.g., lidocaine
2% = 20 mg/mL	e.g., viscous lidocaine
4% = 40 mg/mL	e.g., cocaine
5% = 50 mg/mL	e.g., lidocaine ointment
20% = 200 mg/mL	e.g., benzocaine

- When combined in an anesthetic solution, epinephrine is usually in a 1:100,000 or a 1:200,000 dilution. For example:
  1:100,000 concentration of epinephrine = 1 g/100,000 mL = 1000 mg/100,000 mL = 1 mg /100 mL or 0.01 mg/mL.
  1 mL of 1:1000 epinephrine = 1 mg.
  0.1 mL of 1:1000 epinephrine in 10 mL of anesthetic solution = 1:100,000 dilution = 0.01 mg/mL.
  0.1 mL of 1:1000 epinephrine in 20 mL of anesthetic solution = 1:200,000 dilution = 0.005 mg/mL.
- Some examples detailing epinephrine content:

	1:100,000	1:200,000
5 mL	0.050 mg	0.025 mg
10 mL	0.100 mg	0.050 mg
20 mL	0.200 mg	0.100 mg

- Therefore 50 mL of 1% lidocaine with epinephrine 1:200,000 contains 500 mg of lidocaine and 0.25 mg of epinephrine.

[a]We caution against mixing epinephrine and local anesthetics at the bedside. Use commercially available products whenever available.

increase toxicity. The elevated CO_2 produced by respiratory acidosis crosses the blood-brain barrier, where it may act directly on the receptor and indirectly by lowering intracellular pH. The lower pH causes more of the drug to ionize, thereby furthering the block in the sodium channel and increasing the potential for toxicity.

Protein Binding

The concentration of unbound drug relates more closely to toxic effects than does the total drug concentration (bound plus unbound) as measured in the blood. The amount of α-acid glycoprotein (AAG), the major plasma protein responsible for binding local anesthetics, is considerably decreased in neonates in comparison to adults. Arthur and McNicol[146] implied that the low AAG levels in neonates are responsible for the increased toxic potential. Tucker and colleagues[147] listed several disease states that alter AAG levels and protein binding but questioned whether they lead to changes in free drug concentration in vivo.

Concomitant Drugs

For years, barbiturates were used to prevent and treat local anesthesia–induced seizures. Barbiturates were found to worsen anesthetic-induced apnea and cardiovascular depression. CNS depressants are used with caution when concern exists for local anesthetic toxicity. CNS stimulants have been shown to increase anesthetic-induced excitability and are avoided. Mixtures of local anesthetics have an additive effect on toxicity. If two drugs are used at half strength, they produce the same degree of toxicity as though each were used alone at normal strength. As discussed previously, drugs that slow metabolism by inhibiting hepatic enzymes may increase the risk for toxicity.

Recognition of CNS Toxicity

The earliest manifestation of systemic toxicity is CNS stimulation resulting from blockade of inhibitory synapses. CNS depression follows and is produced by direct depression of the medulla, although hypoxia may play a role. The signs and symptoms are dose related. Potential signs and symptoms of CNS toxicity, in progressing order, are numbness of the tongue, light-headedness, tinnitus, visual disturbances, muscle twitching, convulsions, coma, and apnea. Drowsiness, commonly seen with lower doses of lidocaine, is not associated with bupivacaine or etidocaine. Tetracaine may produce apnea or cardiovascular toxicity without CNS manifestations.

Recognition of Cardiovascular Toxicity

Moderate blood concentrations of local anesthetics produce slight increases in cardiac output, heart rate, and arterial pressure because of the effects of direct peripheral vasodilation and CNS stimulation. At concentrations generally well above CNS toxicity levels, local anesthetics cause direct myocardial depression, hypotension, and bradycardia, perhaps leading to cardiovascular collapse. These agents also slow electrical conduction and lead to reentry phenomena and various supraventricular and potentially lethal ventricular dysrhythmias, especially with bupivacaine and etidocaine.

Prevention of Toxicity

Knowledge of factors contributing to toxicity guides preventive measures. Avoid esters in patients with an atypical form or a quantitative deficiency of pseudocholinesterase. Use amides with caution in patients with severe liver disease or congestive heart failure. Pay attention to maximum safe dosages based on the site, technique, use of epinephrine, and patient status. Add epinephrine when possible to decrease the rate of drug absorption at vascular sites. Reduce the drug concentration by saline dilution to increase the volume for administration when a large area must be infiltrated. Frequently aspirate in areas of high vascularity, even though a negative aspiration may not prevent IV administration.[148] Slow infiltration is safer and less painful.

Treatment of Systemic Toxicity

Local anesthetics should not be administered without the ability to recognize and treat a toxic reaction, including having all necessary equipment and drugs readily available and being knowledgeable in their use. Despite taking all possible precautions, toxic reactions still occur, and close observation of the patient allows early detection and treatment.

Providing proper oxygenation and ventilation at the earliest sign of a reaction is the cornerstone of treatment. Encourage patients who are alert to moderately hyperventilate to lower the pressure of carbon dioxide (PCO_2) and raise the seizure threshold. Intubation with high-flow oxygen and hyperventilation is performed for patients who cannot adequately ventilate. Initiate IV access and monitor vital signs and cardiac rhythm closely.

Seizures are generally self-limited but are treated if they persist or prevent adequate ventilation. Because respiratory depression secondary to toxicity may follow, low-dose lorazepam or an ultrashort-acting barbiturate (thiopental or sodium methohexital) is preferred. Intubate the patient to ensure an effective airway and prevent further lactic acidosis if the seizures persist. If toxicity is caused by an ester, especially if there is an associated pseudocholinesterase problem, succinylcholine will compete with the anesthetic for the pseudocholinesterase and may increase the toxicity of both compounds.

Treat hypotension and bradycardia with fluids, leg elevation, α- and β-agonists (epinephrine, ephedrine, or dopamine), or atropine as the need dictates. Of note, local anesthetic systemic toxicity guidelines recommend lower doses of epinephrine (i.e., starting with 1 μg/kg).

Intravenous Lipid Emulsion

Animal studies, case reports/small series, and personal opinion have advocated the use of 20% lipid emulsion intravenously as a remarkable antidote to resuscitate bupivacaine- and mepivacaine-related cardiac arrest, a situation that is usually fatal (see https://lipidrescue.com).[149,150] Rosenblatt and associates[151] described the IV injection of 100 mL of 20% lipid emulsion (formulation used for hyperalimentation) followed by an infusion (0.5 mL/kg per minute over a 2-hour period) and related this intervention to successful resuscitation in a scenario that appeared hopeless. Picard[152] considers lipid emulsion a "crucial antidote" that should be available when local anesthetics are used for peripheral nerve blocks. A large collaborative workgroup of leading toxicologists recommends lipid emulsion infusion during cardiac arrest associated with bupivacaine but strikes a neutral posture for cardiac arrest due to other local anesthetics.[153] Lipid emulsion therapy is typically administered intravenously but bupivacaine-induced toxicity is reversed in rats when lipid emulsion is administered by the intraosseous route.[154] Intraosseous infusion may be a reasonable alternative to IV infusion when IV access is not available, though this route of administration in humans is of unproven benefit. Lipid emulsion therapy in otherwise hopeless situations of cardiac arrest secondary to local anesthetic overdose is supported (Box 29.3). American Society of Regional Anesthesia and Pain Medicine (ASRA) recommends rapid identification of local anesthetic systemic toxicity and prompt treatment with lipid emulsion. ASRA provide a practical checklist that can be adopted in areas where local anesthetics are given in the ED.[154a]

Allergic Reactions

Allergenic Agents

True allergic reactions are rare and account for only 1% to 2% of all adverse reactions, but they are important to recognize because of their serious potential. Ester solutions (procaine, tetracaine) that produce the metabolite para-aminobenzoic acid (PABA) account for the majority of these reactions. Amide solutions (lidocaine, bupivacaine) are rarely involved, and usually the preservative MPB, which is structurally similar to PABA, is responsible. Although pure esters and pure amides do not cross-react, amides may appear to do so if multidose vials containing MPB are used. Patients may manifest an allergic response on first contact with a local anesthetic because of previous sensitization to these agents. MPB is found in creams, ointments, and various cosmetics, and PABA is an ingredient in many sunscreen preparations. Patients who are latex sensitive may have an allergic reaction incorrectly attributed to the local anesthetic.

BOX 29.3 Strategies for Lipid Emulsion Rescue Therapy in Patients With Severe Local Anesthetic Systemic Toxicity[a]

- Intravenous lipid emulsion (ILE) is available as a 20% fat emulsion.
- Patient weight ≥70 kg: Bolus 100 mL IV over 2–3 min and infuse 250 mL over 15–20 min.
- If patient remains unstable, repeat bolus and double the infusion.
- Patient weight <70 kg: Bolus 1.5 mL/kg over 2–3 minutes and infuse 0.25 mL/kg per min for 15–20 min.
- If patient remains unstable, repeat bolus and double the infusion.

[a]*Continue other resuscitative efforts, including cardiopulmonary resuscitation.*
From Neal JM, Neal EJ, Weinberg GL. American Society of Regional Anesthesia and Pain Medicine Local Anesthetic Systemic Toxicity checklist: 2020 version. Reg Anesth Pain Med. *2021;46(1):81-82.*

Cell-mediated delayed reactions manifesting as dermatitis are rare; it is immediate hypersensitivity that most concerns the emergency clinician. A spectrum of signs and symptoms may occur, from rhinitis and mild urticaria to bronchospasm, upper airway edema, or anaphylactic shock. Onset may be immediate and occur even during administration of the agent. Treat anaphylaxis in the usual manner.

The more frequent problem facing emergency clinicians is a patient who claims to have a past history of allergy to local anesthetics. Most patients assume that any adverse reaction to a local anesthetic procedure is an allergy. Because allergy is rarely the cause, a careful history, and a review of previous records, if available, are crucial in evaluating these patients. Procaine was commonly used in dentistry, and many patients who experienced many types of reactions in the dentist's office, rarely true allergy, state they are allergic to Novocaine. Procaine is no longer used in dental practice, but it is the local anesthetic in intramuscular penicillin preparations (procaine penicillin G).

Attempts to uncover the actual cause of the past reaction and the specific agent involved are often fruitless. Ask about the exact signs and symptoms, technique of administration, amount of drug used, and how the patient was treated. If an allergic reaction cannot be ruled out and the drug previously used is known, use an agent from the other class (whether amide or ester). Lidocaine from a dental cartridge does not contain MPB, and if this were the allergenic source, an ester agent could be used. However, if lidocaine from a multidose vial is implicated, do not use an ester because MPB may cross-react with PABA. In this case, it may be safer to use an amide without MPB or to choose an alternative (see later). In most cases, the allergen is an ester, and the patient can safely be given an amide without MPB. Single-dose ampules of 1% lidocaine without MPB, readily obtainable from a resuscitation cart, can be used for this purpose.

Uncertainty often exists regarding the specific agent involved, and the clinician must choose an alternative approach to local anesthesia. If the wounds are extensive and the risk is acceptable, procedural sedation (see Chapter 33) or general anesthesia may be used. Conversely, if minimal pain is expected and the procedure is short (e.g., one or two sutures or staples in the scalp), no anesthesia may be required. These methods may be useful, but the degree of anesthesia produced is frequently not sufficient. Antihistamines injected into a wound have been used successfully for many years and represent a good alternative. Local anesthetic efficacy is found in varying degrees with all antihistamines. Ketamine anesthesia may be a useful alternative in some situations and is commonly used in children.

Diphenhydramine and Benzyl Alcohol

Several studies have demonstrated that 1% diphenhydramine is as effective as 1% lidocaine for infiltrative anesthesia.[155–157] As long as diphenhydramine is not used at concentrations greater than 1%, potential problems of skin necrosis or significant sedation are rare. Dilute the standard 5% parenteral form to a 1% concentration for subcutaneous injection (1 mL of drug to 4 mL of saline). The duration of action of diphenhydramine is shorter than that of lidocaine but appears to be adequate for most procedures. The injection pain of diphenhydramine exceeds that of lidocaine but can be diminished by reducing the concentration to 0.5%. At this lower concentration, the effectiveness of this agent on facial wounds is lost.[158] The addition of epinephrine to 0.5% diphenhydramine results in a more painful solution with a shorter duration of action than a standard buffered lidocaine with epinephrine solution.[159] Benzyl alcohol (0.9%) with epinephrine (1:100,000) compares favorably with diphenhydramine as an effective local anesthetic. This appears to be a useful alternative to diphenhydramine when lidocaine cannot be used but is of shorter duration than diphenhydramine.[160–162]

Skin Testing

Skin testing and progressive subcutaneous challenge doses deserve special mention because they appear to be logical and well-studied approaches. However, intradermal skin testing with local anesthetics is controversial and often of no practical benefit in the ED. False-positive results are frequently produced by local release of histamine in response to needle trauma, tissue distention, or preservatives in the solution.[163] In addition, a high incidence of false-negative results can occur. It is questionable whether these low-molecular-weight drugs or their allergenic metabolites are ever capable of eliciting positive responses.[164] Other disadvantages of skin testing include its time-consuming nature and potential hazard when even minute traces of an allergen may precipitate a serious reaction. Subcutaneous challenge testing in graduating doses has been advocated and may well eliminate many false responses, but it does not eliminate the problems of time and hazard. Swanson,[165] recognizing that allergy to pure lidocaine is extremely rare, recommended 0.1 mL as a single intradermal skin test. Although his approach eliminates the time disadvantage, intradermal placement can still produce false responses. It would seem more reasonable to give this test dose subcutaneously while exercising due caution in the unlikely event that a patient exhibits a serious reaction.

Summary of Anesthetic "Allergy" Management

Generally speaking, the optimal approach to a patient with a presumed anesthetic allergy is to determine the specific anesthetic agent associated with a presumed allergic reaction and then use a preservative-free agent from the other class (see earlier discussion). If the agent is unknown, use an antihistamine or give 0.1 mL of preservative-free lidocaine as a subcutaneous test dose and proceed with the full dose if no reaction occurs within 30 minutes. Given the studies mentioned earlier, prudent choices would seem to be diphenhydramine or benzyl alcohol. Epinephrine (1:100,000) can be added to both these drugs to prolong the duration of action.

Catecholamine Reactions

Anxiety and vasoconstrictor (epinephrine) reactions are discussed together because each produces similar manifestations caused by elevated catecholamine levels. These relatively common disorders are difficult to distinguish from each other and are not generally serious.

Excess catecholamine levels produce tachycardia, palpitations, hypertension, apprehension, tremulousness, diaphoresis, tachypnea, pallor, and on occasion, anginal chest pain. Thus catecholamine excess may resemble the CNS stimulation phase of local anesthetic toxicity.

Catecholamine reactions are not usually caused solely by exogenous epinephrine because if it is used in its optimal concentration (1:200,000), the maximum safe dose (0.25 mg) is rarely exceeded. However, many patients produce significant endogenous catecholamines because of anxiety about the anesthetic approach or upcoming procedure. In this case, even the addition of small amounts of epinephrine could trigger a catecholamine reaction. Therefore patient preparation includes

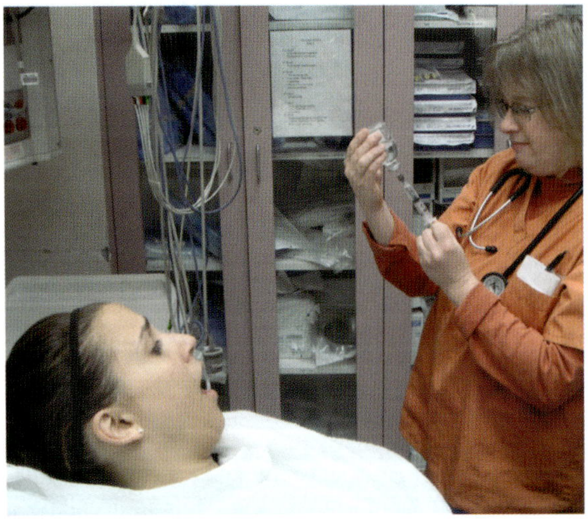

Fig. 29.9 Drawing up local anesthetic with a syringe and needle in front of the patient may lead to anxiety and a vasovagal reaction. Avoid this potential complication by simply performing this task out of view of the patient.

proper explanation and reassurance to decrease anxiety. Exercise caution with patients who have hyperthyroidism, hypertension, or atherosclerotic cardiovascular disease, although these conditions do not contraindicate the judicious use of epinephrine-containing anesthetics. Do not give epinephrine-containing anesthetics to patients taking MAO inhibitors.

Treatment of a catecholamine reaction includes stopping further drug administration, observing the patient closely, and administering α- or β-antagonists or benzodiazepine agents, if necessary, to combat severe reactions.

Special mention should be noted regarding mixing of epinephrine with local anesthetics at the bedside. Mixing errors and inadvertent administration of high doses of epinephrine have resulted in patient harm and death, especially in perioperative settings. Epinephrine dosing can be confusing and conversion from milligrams per milliliter to ratio expressions is error prone. We advise to use commercially available epinephrine-containing local anesthetic products whenever available.

Vasovagal Reactions

It is not standard to monitor patients (cardiac, pulse oximetry) during routine local anesthesia procedures. Vasovagal reactions are, however, common, especially in dental procedures (reported incidence, 2% to 3%), during which the patient is generally in an upright position. To limit vasovagal reactions related to local anesthesia in the ED, do not draw up medication in a syringe in front of the patient, and inject only when the patient is supine (Figs. 29.9 and 29.10). The patient initially experiences anxiety when a triggering event, commonly the sight or sensation of needle insertion, causes loss of sympathetic tone and an increase in vagal tone. The resultant hypotension and bradycardia may lead to syncope. Address the patient's anxiety and administer the injections with the patient recumbent as useful preventive measures. Cardiac monitoring may help identify the onset of vagally induced bradycardia when suggested by the past history. Lay the patient supine and elevate the legs. Rarely, atropine is required. Should a patient lose consciousness while in a recumbent position, consider diagnoses other than vasovagal syncope, although significant bradycardia and even complete heart block may accompany a vagal reaction in a supine patient.

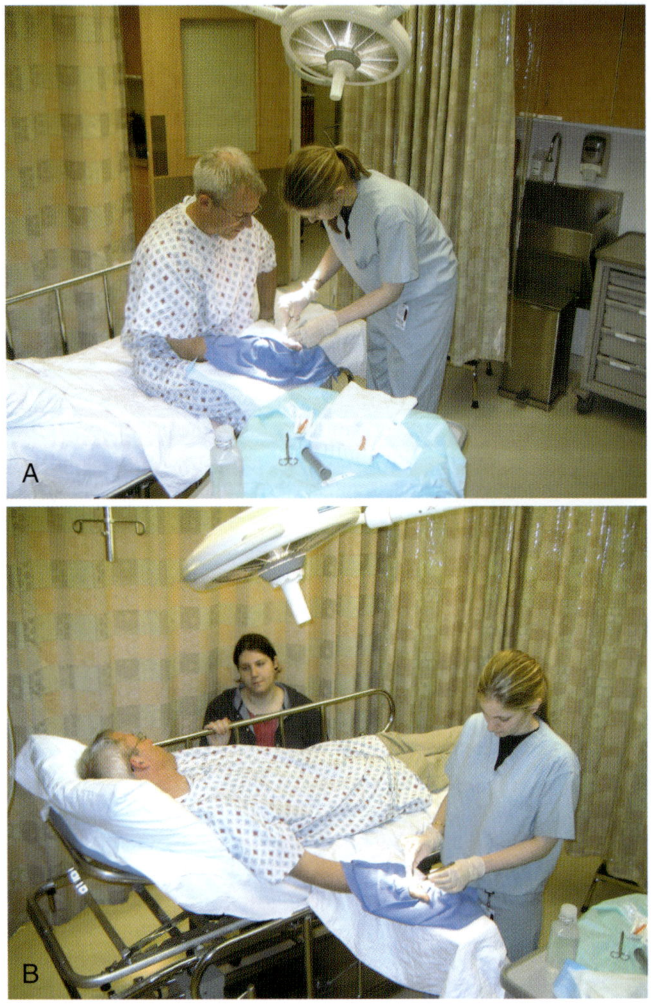

Fig. 29.10 (A) What is wrong in this picture? Almost everything! The patient is sitting upright and directly observing the procedure. This may lead to a vasovagal event, and should he fall from the bed, significant injury may occur. Additional problems include improper positioning of the overhead light (behind the physician's back), lack of privacy (open curtain and door), equipment tray placed too far away, and a hunched-over posture of the physician. (B) A much better approach. Note that the patient is supine, the bed is raised, the light and equipment tray are in a better position, the curtain is closed, and a family member is present (but sitting to avoid a "bystander vagal event") to distract the patient during the procedure. The clinician could also be seated for comfort.

SUMMARY

Emergency medicine cannot be practiced without the use of local anesthetic agents. Their effectiveness when applied topically or by infiltration makes them extremely adaptable to many clinical circumstances. A working knowledge of commonly used agents is necessary to ensure the safe administration of these medications. Aim specific efforts at maximizing the drugs' anesthetic effects while minimizing the pain of administration and risk for toxicity.

REFERENCES ARE AVAILABLE AT Elsevier eBooks+

CHAPTER 30

Regional Anesthesia of the Head and Neck

Ryan M. Spangler and Michael K. Abraham

Emergency physicians encounter patients with dental pain, facial lacerations, and other injuries of the head on a regular basis. The assessment of these injuries can be both time-consuming and painful. Thankfully, regional anesthesia for these conditions is easy to instill, reliable, and safe. Techniques such as nerve blocks can be used for patient comfort during repair of lacerations of the face, ear, forehead, and, particularly, the lips. A block avoids direct infiltration into the actual laceration, which preserves the anatomy in these delicate areas and thus allows better cosmetic repair.

Nerve blocks can also be used to give patients with dental pain almost immediate relief. They can be used to treat dentalgia caused by infection, fracture, or dry socket. They decrease the need for narcotic drugs. The ability of an emergency physician to master these blocks leads to fast and efficient patient care as well as improved patient satisfaction (Table 30.1).

ANATOMY OF THE TRIGEMINAL NERVE (CRANIAL NERVE V)

Sensation to the face and head region is supplied primarily by cranial nerve V (CN V), which is also known as the trigeminal nerve, due to its three large branches: V_1, the ophthalmic nerve; V_2, the maxillary nerve; and V_3, the mandibular nerve (Fig. 30.1A). This is the largest of the 12 cranial nerves, originating at the upper portion of the pons. CN V contains motor neural fibers that control the muscles of mastication. This chapter focuses on its sensory function (Fig. 30.1B).

The ophthalmic nerve, V_1, courses through the cavernous sinus and exits through the supraorbital fissure. It then gives off three branches: the frontal, lacrimal, and nasociliary (Fig. 30.1C). These nerves and their branches innervate the eye, orbit, forehead, and portions of the nose.[1]

The maxillary nerve, V_2, exits through the foramen rotundum and gives off several branches, including the infraorbital nerve and the posterior, middle, and anterior superior alveolar nerves (ASANs) (see Fig. 30.1C). These nerves innervate the face, lip, maxillary teeth, and mucosa.[1]

The mandibular nerve, V_3, exits through the foramen ovale into the infratemporal fossa. It then splits into many branches that supply the dura and muscles of mastication (motor function), as well as the buccal branch and the auriculotemporal, lingual, and inferior alveolar branches (see Fig. 30.1C). These branches supply sensation to the skin on the side of the head, the auricle of the ear, the tongue, the mucosa and skin of the cheek, the mandibular teeth, and the lower lip.[1]

EQUIPMENT FOR FACIAL NERVE BLOCKS

The equipment needed to perform facial nerve blocks is very minimal and should be available in any emergency department (ED) (Review Box 30.1). Medications include common anesthetics such as lidocaine or bupivacaine, with or without epinephrine. The practitioner should always be aware of the maximum doses of anesthetic agents being utilized, although most blocks will require much less than the maximum dosing. Bupivacaine can be beneficial due to its longer duration of action (up to 7 hours) than lidocaine (1 to 2 hours), especially if the procedure goal is sustained pain control. The longer duration is less beneficial if the goal is to anesthetize for a short procedure, such as laceration repair. Less commonly used medications in the ED, such as articaine, may have some allure, as the increased lipid solubility reduces any concern for systemic toxicity.[2] However, this medication is rarely available in the ED and its benefit may be more obvious in cases of longer procedures requiring repeated dosing of anesthetic, a rarity in the ED setting. Standard 25- to 27-gauge needles are recommended. Using a smaller needle can lead to false-negative aspiration in the case of an arterial puncture. Some of the equipment listed in Review Box 30.1 might not be necessary for all blocks, and some can be substituted. For instance, a tongue depressor is recommended for use as a retractor, but any other acceptable instrument or even a finger can be used for this purpose. As with the other aspects of emergency medicine, ultrasound can be used to facilitate procedural anesthesia.

GENERAL RECOMMENDATIONS

Some general recommendations apply to nearly all types of blocks (Fig. 30.2). These procedures have very few contraindications. One of them involves infected tissue: the needle should never be inserted through infected tissue because this approach could result in inoculation of deep tissue with bacteria. In addition, patients with an allergy to the anesthetic agent should not undergo these procedures unless an alternative agent is available. Although not an absolute contraindication, coagulopathy might present a higher risk for hematoma and bleeding complications, so, as for any procedure, the risks should be considered and might outweigh the benefits. As direct oral anticoagulants become more common, one must always inquire about current medications as these can pose a bleeding risk.

When performing many of these blocks, inserting the needle with the bevel facing toward the bone allows the anesthetic to be injected as close to the nerve or bone as possible and increases the likelihood that the procedure will be successful. During and after injection, particularly when working in areas near the lip, slight exterior pressure and massage not only help the anesthetic diffuse to its target but also help prevent ballooning of the lip or facial tissue. Finally, it is generally recommended that the full length of the needle should not be inserted into the mucosa when performing an intraoral injection, so that it can be retrieved if it breaks.

Application of a topical anesthetic before insertion of the needle is not a necessary step prior to inducing any of the intraoral blocks, but it can increase patient comfort (Fig. 30.3). To apply a topical anesthetic, first dry the tissue with gauze and then apply a topical mucosal anesthetic, for instance, viscous lidocaine. Another technique is to soak a piece of gauze with the anesthetic and then place it over the dry mucosa. Spray anesthetics such as cetacaine are popular and effective alternatives to lidocaine-soaked gauze.

TABLE 30.1 Nerve Blocks and Indications

NERVED BLOCKED OR AREA INJECTED	AREA ANESTHETIZED
Supraperiosteal infiltration	Individual teeth
Posterior superior alveolar nerve	Second and third molars and partial anesthesia of first molar
Middle superior alveolar nerve	First and second premolars, as well as partial anesthesia of first molar
Anterior superior alveolar nerve	Central incisor to the canine
Infraorbital nerve	Midface region, skin of lateral nose, lower eyelid, and MSA and ASA regions
Inferior alveolar nerve	All ipsilateral mandibular teeth, lower lip, and chin
Mental nerve	Mucosa and skin of lower lip and chin
Scalp block	Skin of the scalp within the blocked area
Greater and lesser occipital nerve	Occipital region of the scalp
Ophthalmic nerve	Skin of the forehead and scalp (as far back as lambdoid suture), upper eyelid

ASA, Anterior superior alveolar; *MSA*, middle superior alveolar.

Supraperiosteal Injection

Indication

Supraperiosteal injection is generally used to achieve anesthesia of individual maxillary teeth, but it can be used for any tooth. This block works well if the anesthesia is needed for only one or two teeth, and it can be very helpful to alleviate pain associated with a simple toothache. As noted previously, care should be taken to avoid inserting the needle through any infected tissue.

Anatomy

The nerves for each individual tooth enter at the apex of that tooth and are protected by the bone supporting the tooth. Supraperiosteal injection is designed to anesthetize a single tooth (Fig. 30.4A).

Approach

Begin by applying a topical anesthetic, as previously described. Once the anesthetic has had time to take effect, retract the lip until the tissues are taut (down and out for maxillary teeth and up and out for mandibular teeth). Insert the needle at the mucobuccal fold, with the bevel facing the tooth. The needle needs to be inserted only a few millimeters (Fig. 30.4B). Intraarterial injection is unlikely in this block, but you should aspirate prior to slowly injecting 1 mL or 2 mL of anesthetic. Apply slight pressure and massage as previously discussed. Because the anesthetic needs to penetrate the bone, a few minutes are needed for anesthesia to occur.

Complications

Complications with this injection are very rare. The risk of inoculating deeper tissues with bacteria is possible if the injection goes through infected tissue. Anesthesia can fail if the injection is too high, too low, or too far away from the nerve.

Posterior Superior Alveolar Nerve Block

Indication

The posterior superior alveolar nerve (PSAN) block can be used to provide anesthesia for the first through the third maxillary molars. However, it is likely that only partial anesthesia of the first molar will be achieved due to its innervation with accessory nerves, particularly at the mesiobuccal root of this molar.

Anatomy

The PSAN branches from the maxillary branch of the trigeminal nerve and travels inferiorly just before the maxillary nerve enters the infraorbital groove. The nerve descends along the posterior lateral portion of the maxillary tuberosity and gives off branches to the second, third, and partially the first maxillary molars (Fig. 30.5A).

Approach

Two techniques for creating a PSAN block have been well described in the literature. The traditional method begins similar to the other blocks, that is, by applying a topical anesthetic to the mucosa. The insertion point for the needle is just distal to the root of the second molar, at the height of the mucobuccal fold (Fig. 30.5B). For this block, because of the posterior and medial location of the nerve complex, insert the needle in an upward, inward, and posterior direction (toward the maxillary tuberosity), approximately 45 degrees in each direction.[3] Ultimately, the needle should be inserted approximately 15 mm and certainly no more than 25 mm. The operator should not feel any resistance while inserting the needle and should not encounter bone. If resistance or bone is felt, withdraw the needle to the bevel and then redirect it. Once the appropriate depth is reached, aspirate, and, if negative, slowly inject 1 mL to 3 mL of anesthetic.

The second technique involves a curved 24-mm needle, to approach the posterior maxillary surface. Again, anesthetize the mucosa with a topical anesthetic. The insertion point for the needle is more posterior than the traditional approach, just distal to the third molar, at the corner of the posterior lateral portion of the maxilla and directed along the posterior maxilla. Insert the needle 10 to 12 mm from the initial insertion point along the posterior wall of the maxilla and orient it just slightly medially. After aspirating, inject 1 to 3 mL of lidocaine.[4]

In a study of 200 patients undergoing extraction of the second and third molars, Thangavelu and colleagues achieved successful anesthesia with the curved needle technique in all cases at 10 minutes, with no complications.[4] In contrast, after a randomized, controlled comparison of the straight-needle and bent-needle techniques, Singla and Alexander concluded that use of a straight needle was more successful in achieving anesthesia.[3]

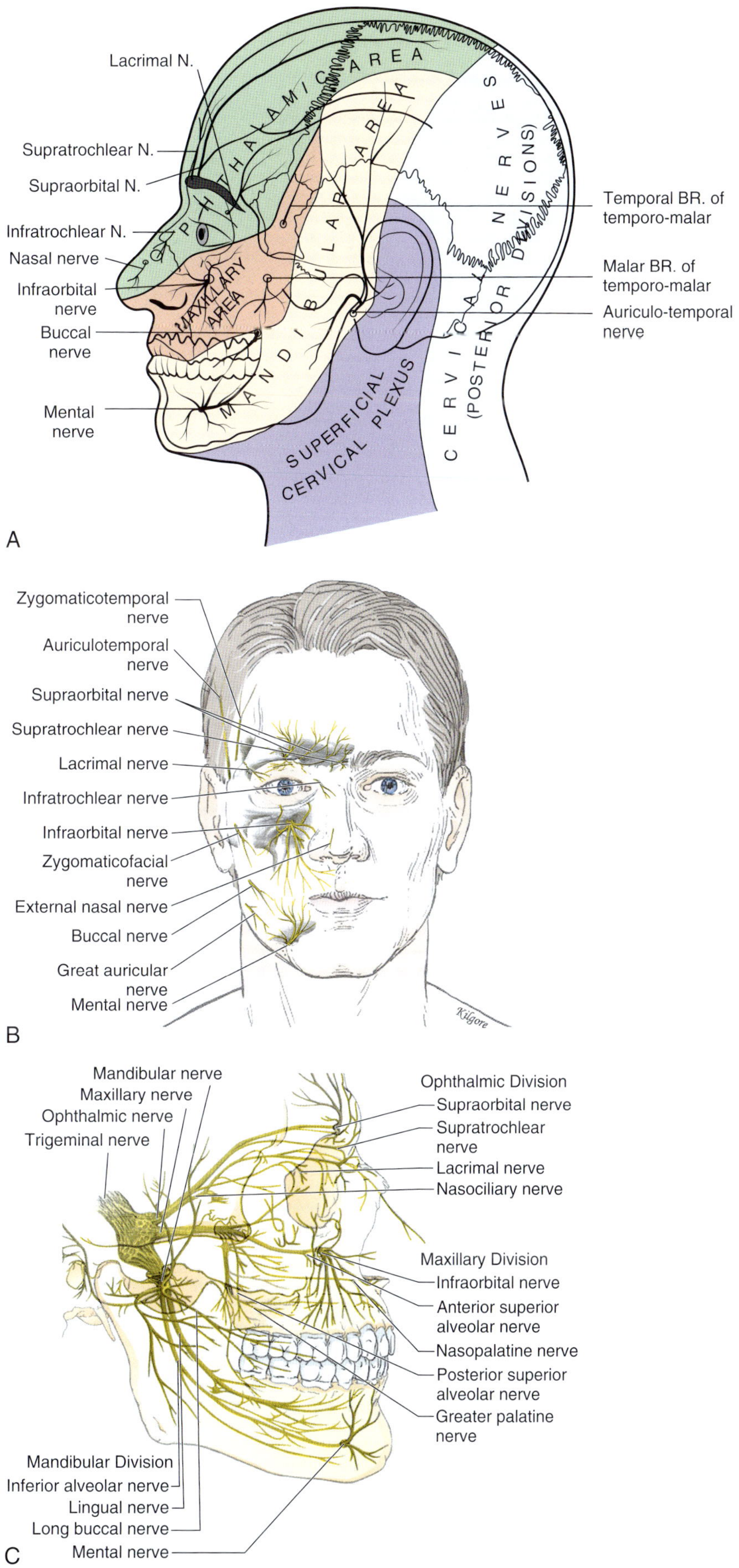

Fig. 30.1 (A) Distribution of the areas innervated by the three major branches of the trigeminal nerve. (B) Cutaneous branches of the trigeminal nerve and their exit points from the skull. (C) Branches of the trigeminal nerve. *BR*, Branch; *n*, nerve. (A, From Carter HV, Gray H, Anatomy of the human body 1918. In: *Gray's Anatomy*, Plate 784. B–C, Adapted from Eriksson E, ed. *Illustrated Handbook in Local Anesthesia*. Saunders; 1980.)

Regional Anesthesia of the Head and Neck

Indications
Anesthesia of the teeth for dental pain
Anesthesia of the soft tissues of the face

Contraindications
Lack of patient cooperation
Inability to perform the procedure without passing through an infected area
Anticoagulated patients (e.g., warfarin)

Complications
Local anesthetic toxicity if maximum amounts are exceeded
Failure to obtain anesthesia
Allergy to local anesthetic
Infection extending to the deep spaces of the head and neck because of injecting through an infected area
Hematoma
Failure to aspirate blood
Intravascular injection of epinephrine
Needle breakage (rare)
Needlestick of the operator

Equipment

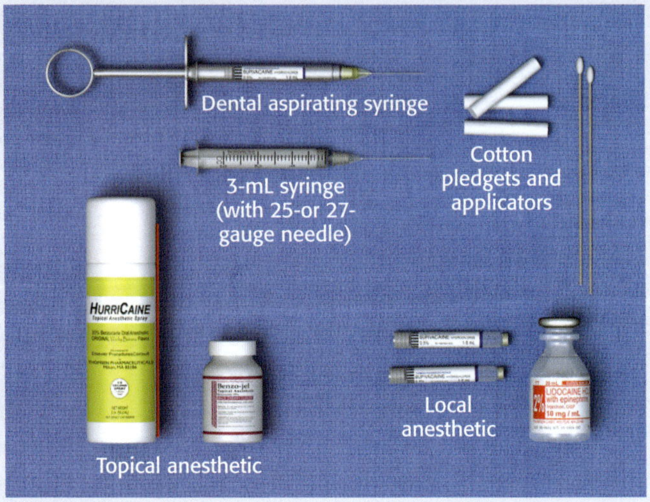

Review Box 30.1 Regional anesthesia of the head and neck: indications, contraindications, complications, and equipment.

Head and Neck Regional Anesthesia: General Technique

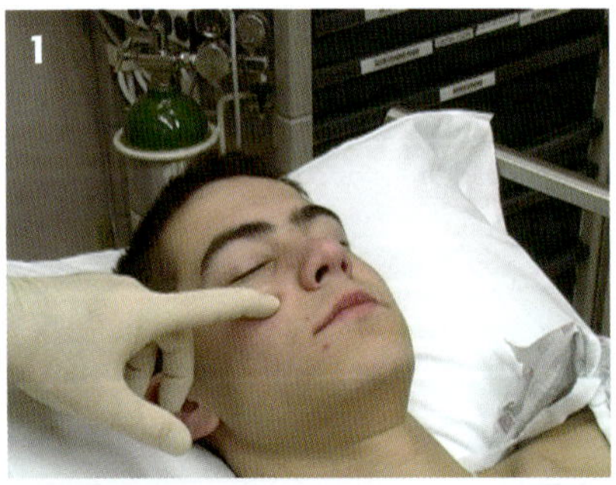

Confirm relevant local anatomy (in this example, the infraorbital nerve block is depicted).

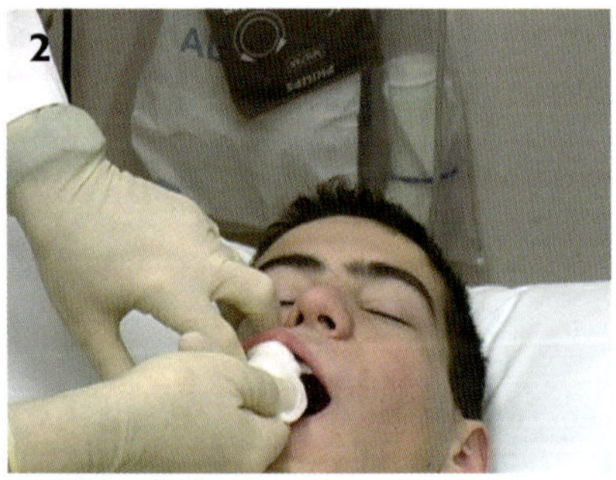

Retract the lip and dry the mucous membranes with gauze or a cotton pledget.

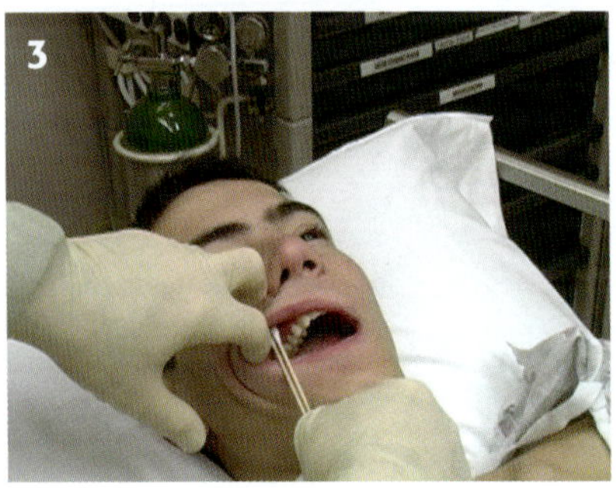

Apply a topical anesthetic, such as Benzo-Jel, on a cotton-tipped applicator (shown here), or use Hurricaine spray (not depicted).

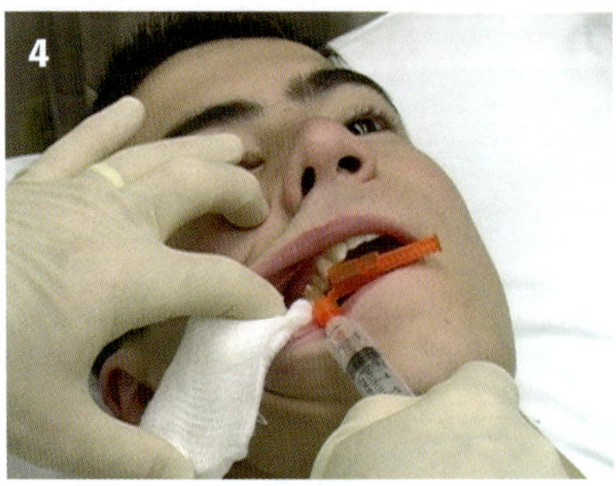

Insert the needle, aspirate the syringe to exclude intravascular placement, and then inject the appropriate amount of local anesthetic (usually about 2 mL).

Fig. 30.2 Head and neck regional anesthesia: general technique depicting the infraorbital nerve block.

Complications
Diplopia and a presentation resembling Horner syndrome (ptosis, enophthalmos, miosis), thought to be caused by diffusion of the anesthetic superiorly and medially to the orbital nerves, were reported in a case series.[5] Isolated fourth cranial nerve (trochlear) palsy has also been reported and seems to be very rare.[6] All these complications were temporary. Visual disturbances are uncomfortable and disturbing for patients but do not appear to be permanent.

The pterygoid plexus can be damaged by a needle that is too long; therefore the use of shorter needles is recommended. Based on a literature review, Singla and Alexander

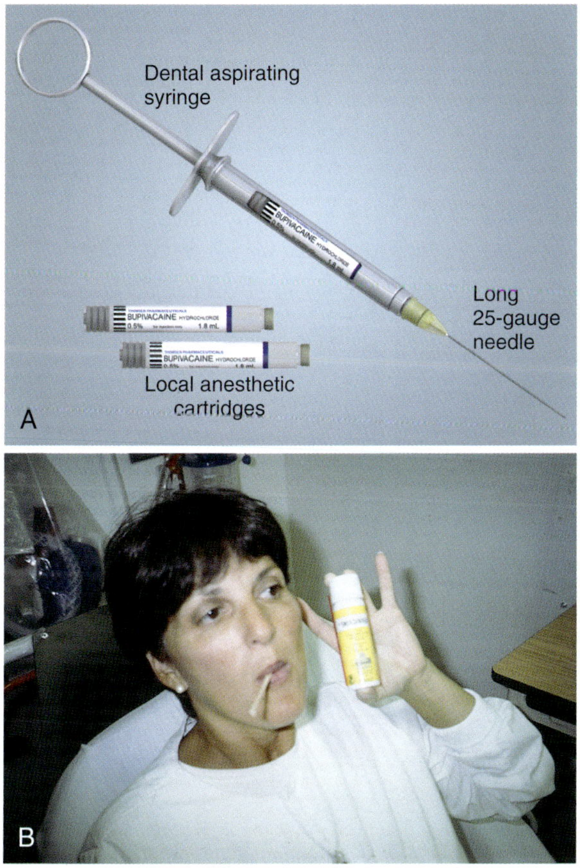

Fig. 30.3 (A) Local anesthesia: basic setup for intraoral application using an aspirating dental syringe. (B) Topical mucosal anesthesia can make the injection nearly painless. Swab the gauze-dried mucosa with the topical agent or have the patient hold cotton swabs soaked in the agent, and wait for 1 to 3 minutes.

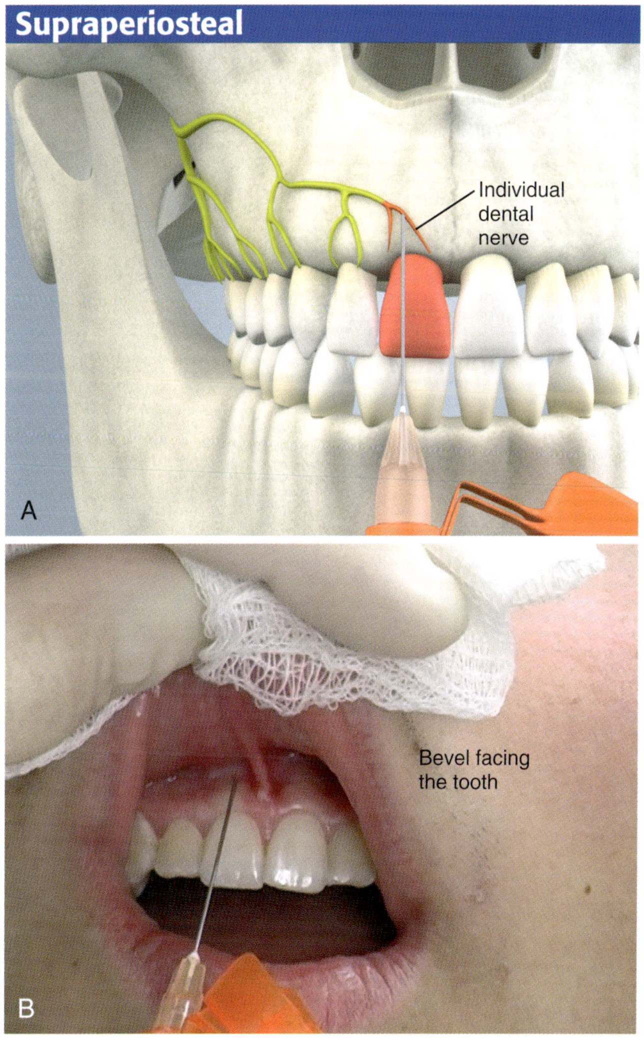

Fig. 30.4 Supraperiosteal nerve block for anesthesia of an individual anterior tooth. (A) Anatomy and distribution. (B) Technique for supraperiosteal injection. Anesthetic should be deposited next to the periosteum, with the bevel of the needle facing the bone.

recommended insertion to approximately 15 mm; however, this is lower than many recommendations and up to 25 mm, no deeper, may be required. The further the needle is inserted, the greater the risk of complications.[3]

Middle Superior Alveolar Nerve Block

Indication

The middle superior alveolar nerve (MSAN) block can be used to anesthetize the lateral upper lip and the first and second premolars simultaneously, as well as the mesiobuccal root of the first molar. This technique can be especially useful if the lateral lip is not anesthetized by an infraorbital nerve block.

Anatomy

The MSAN descends posteriorly to anteriorly along the lateral maxillary wall as an extension of the maxillary nerve. The landmark needed for this procedure is the junction between the first molar and the second premolar (Fig. 30.6A). A subset of patients has an anatomic variant in which the MSAN does not exist.[1]

Approach

Begin as you would for any of the other intraoral block procedures, by applying topical anesthetic. Retract the upper lip and pull the tissues taut. Direct the needle toward the intersection of the first molar and the second premolar at the mucobuccal fold and insert it 5 to 10 mm at a 45-degree angle posteriorly, with the bevel facing the bone, in an effort to place as much anesthetic near the nerve as possible (Fig. 30.6B). Slowly inject 1 to 3 mL of anesthetic while massaging the tissue.

Complications

Complications of this procedure are few: they are the same complications inherent to all procedures, such as bleeding. Because this is an area with low vascularity, hematoma formation and arterial aspiration are rare. For patients with the anatomic variation of absence of the MSAN, this block will obviously fail, so an infraorbital nerve block, an ASAN block, or a PSAN block will be necessary, depending on the region needing anesthesia.

Anterior Superior Alveolar Nerve Block

Indication

Depending on the area of injury or pain, multiple areas of the maxilla might require anesthesia. If anesthesia from the central incisor to the canine is required, the ASAN can be blocked.

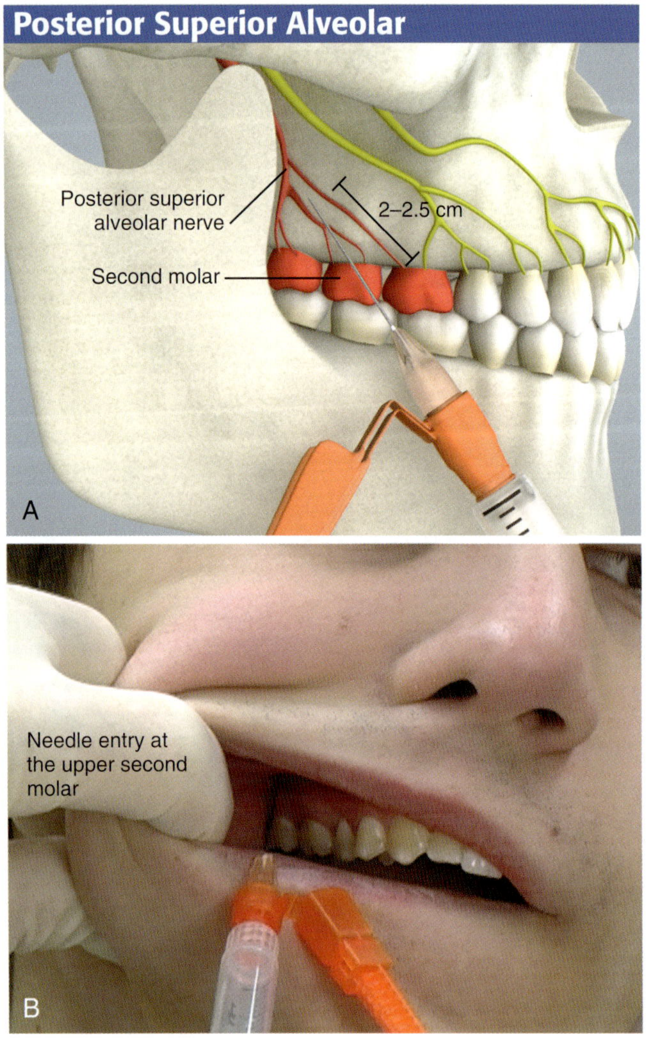

Fig. 30.5 Posterior superior alveolar nerve block for anesthesia of the upper posterior molars. (A) Anatomy and distribution. (B) Technique. Insert the needle at the upper second molar and direct it upward, inward, and backward to the maxillary tuberosity, 15–25 mm.

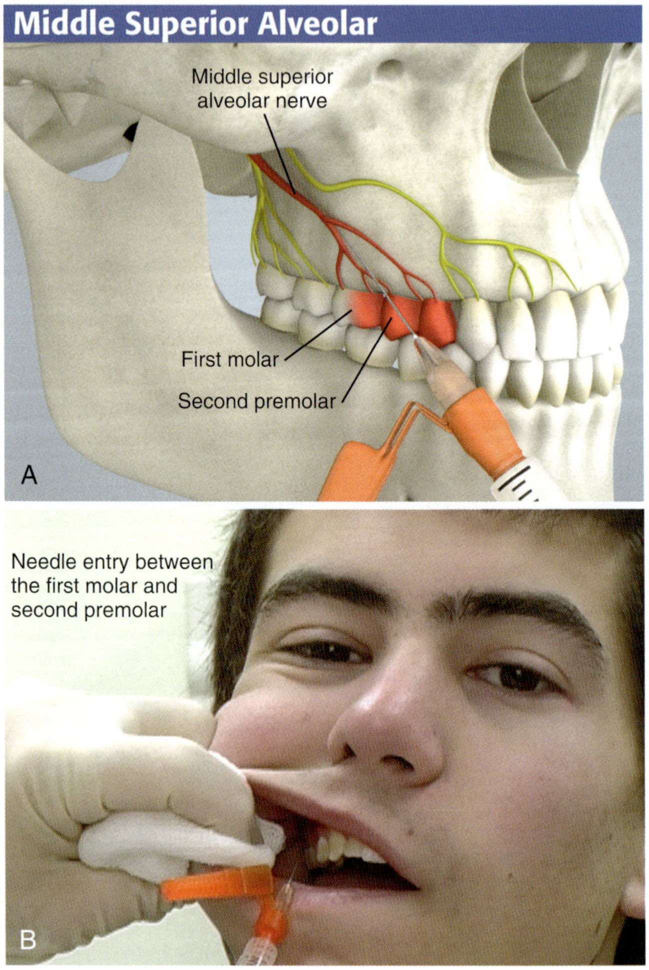

Fig. 30.6 Middle superior alveolar nerve block for anesthesia of the upper middle teeth. (A) Anatomy and distribution. (B) Technique. Insert the needle between the second premolar and the first molar, directing it at a 45-degree angle. For an alternative similar nerve block, see Fig. 30.8.

Anatomy

The ASAN is a distal branch from the infraorbital nerve. As the infraorbital nerve travels down the anterior maxilla, it gives off the ASAN, which travels to innervate the area from the central incisors to the canine of the ipsilateral side. The landmark needed is the apex of the canine (Fig. 30.7A).

Technique

Begin by applying a topical anesthetic, as for the blocks described previously. Then, at the height of the mucosal reflection toward the apex of the canine, insert the needle at a 45-degree angle, to a depth of 5 mm (Fig. 30.7B). Inject 1 to 2 mL of anesthetic slowly.

Complications

Complications associated with this procedure are rare, unless the needle is inserted too far. The infraorbital nerve could be blocked, depending on the final depth of the needle. The block could be unsuccessful if the needle insertion is too superficial for the anesthetic to reach the nerve.

Anterior Middle Superior Alveolar Block

Indications

This approach is indicated when anesthesia is needed from the central incisor to the bicuspid. It can be used for greater palatine anesthesia as well as nasopalatine, anterior superior alveolar (ASA), and middle superior alveolar (MSA) nerve coverage, with the goal of avoiding multiple injections and avoiding anesthetizing the lip unnecessarily by incidental infiltration of anesthetic into the surrounding soft tissue.

This block uses the palatal nutrient pores to distribute anesthesia through the palate to the ASA and the MSA simultaneously. Small pores in the palate allow diffusion of the anesthetic after injection into the palate.

Approach

All the blocks described earlier in this chapter began on the buccal surfaces to anesthetize the maxillary teeth. The injection for the anterior middle superior alveolar block is placed through the hard palate at the intersection of an imaginary line dividing the premolars at a point halfway between the midpalatine crest and the free gingival margin (Fig. 30.8).[7] The anesthetic must be injected very slowly—no faster than

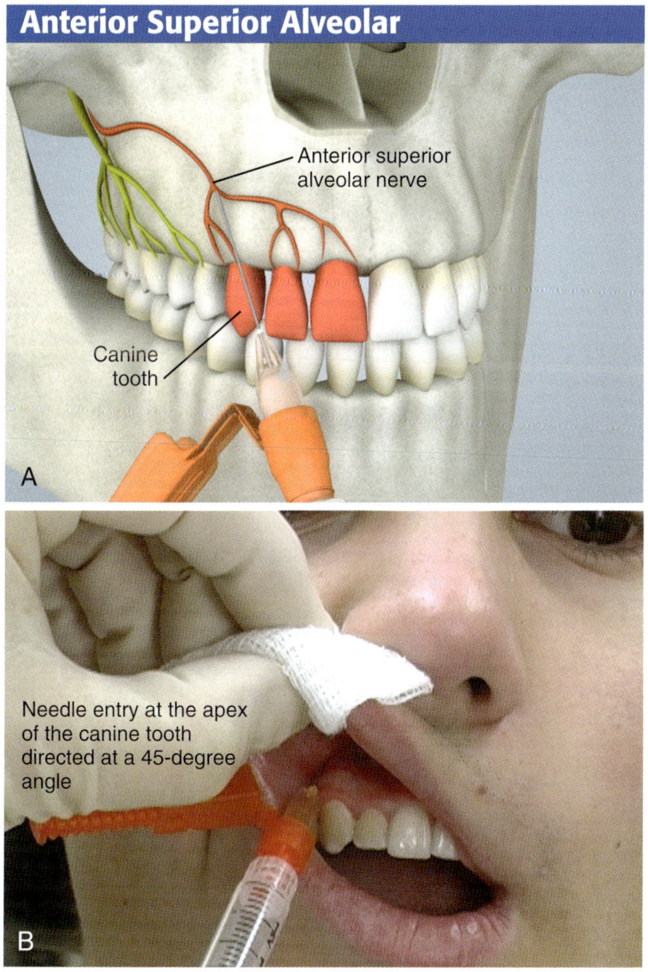

Fig. 30.7 Anterior superior alveolar nerve block for anesthesia of the front teeth. (A) Anatomy and distribution. (B) Technique. Insert the needle at the apex of a canine tooth and direct it at a 45-degree angle.

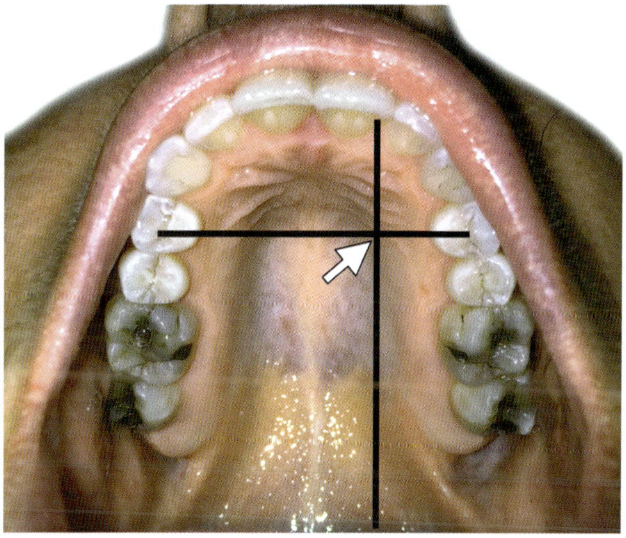

Fig. 30.8 For the anterior middle superior alveolar nerve block, inject anesthetic through the hard palate at the intersection of an imaginary line dividing the premolars at a point halfway between the mid-palantine crest and the free gingival margin *(arrow)*.

0.5 mL/min for 4 to 5 minutes—to avoid pain and discomfort and to allow diffusion. Lee and colleagues found that computer-assisted delivery of the anesthetic was more successful than the traditional clinician-controlled approach, due to the slow pace that is necessary.[8]

Complications

Few complications are associated with this injection because of low vascularity in the area involved. The main challenges presented by this approach are pain, the time needed for the injection, and the time until the block takes effect. As noted previously, Lee and colleagues had greater success with computer-assisted delivery of the anesthetic (which is not available in most EDs) than with administration by a clinician, but failure rates were still high for both techniques, suggesting that this block is not reliable for inducing anesthesia.[8]

Infraorbital Nerve Block

See Video 30.1.

Indications

The ability to induce an infraorbital nerve block is a necessary skill for an emergency medicine provider. This block can be achieved with an intraoral or extraoral approach. It anesthetizes the midface from the lateral upper lip to the lower eyelid, including the nasal skin but not the mucosa (Fig. 30.9A). This block is helpful in wound care and abscess drainage.

Anatomy

The infraorbital nerve is the terminal branch of the mandibular branch of the trigeminal nerve. The second division exits the cranium from the foramen rotundum and ultimately enters the face through the infraorbital canal. The infraorbital foramen is located on the inferior border of the infraorbital ridge on a vertical (sagittal) line with the pupil when the patient stares straight ahead (Fig. 30.9B). The middle and superior alveolar nerves are also in close proximity to the main trunk of the infraorbital nerve near the foramen.

Intraoral Approach

Due to the location of the foramen, an intraoral approach is preferred. Provide local anesthetic to the buccal and gingival mucosa, as previously described. Place one finger extraorally on the foramen. This has two purposes: it gives the practitioner a tangible feeling of the needle, and the pressure will help direct the deposited anesthetic from pushing upward into the lower eyelid. Retract the cheek and enter the mucosa above the second premolar. Aim the needle toward the infraorbital foramen, approximately 2 cm from the mucosal surface, taking care not to enter the foramen (Fig. 30.9C). Once the needle is in the proper position, inject 2 to 3 mL of anesthetic and gently massage the tissue overlying the area to promote distribution of the anesthetic. The alternative method is to perform a field block, which is less precise and anesthetizes a larger area. This technique can be used if the patient has no palpable landmarks or if a wider area of anesthesia is necessary.

Extraoral Approach

The infraorbital foramen can also be approached from an extraoral route (Fig. 30.10). This approach requires external preparation of the skin. Use the same landmarks as those used to locate the infraorbital foramen as described in the intraoral approach. The needle can be felt as it passes through the skin, the subcutaneous tissue, and the quadratus labii superioris muscle. After injection, firmly massage the infiltrated tissue

Infraorbital—Intraoral Approach

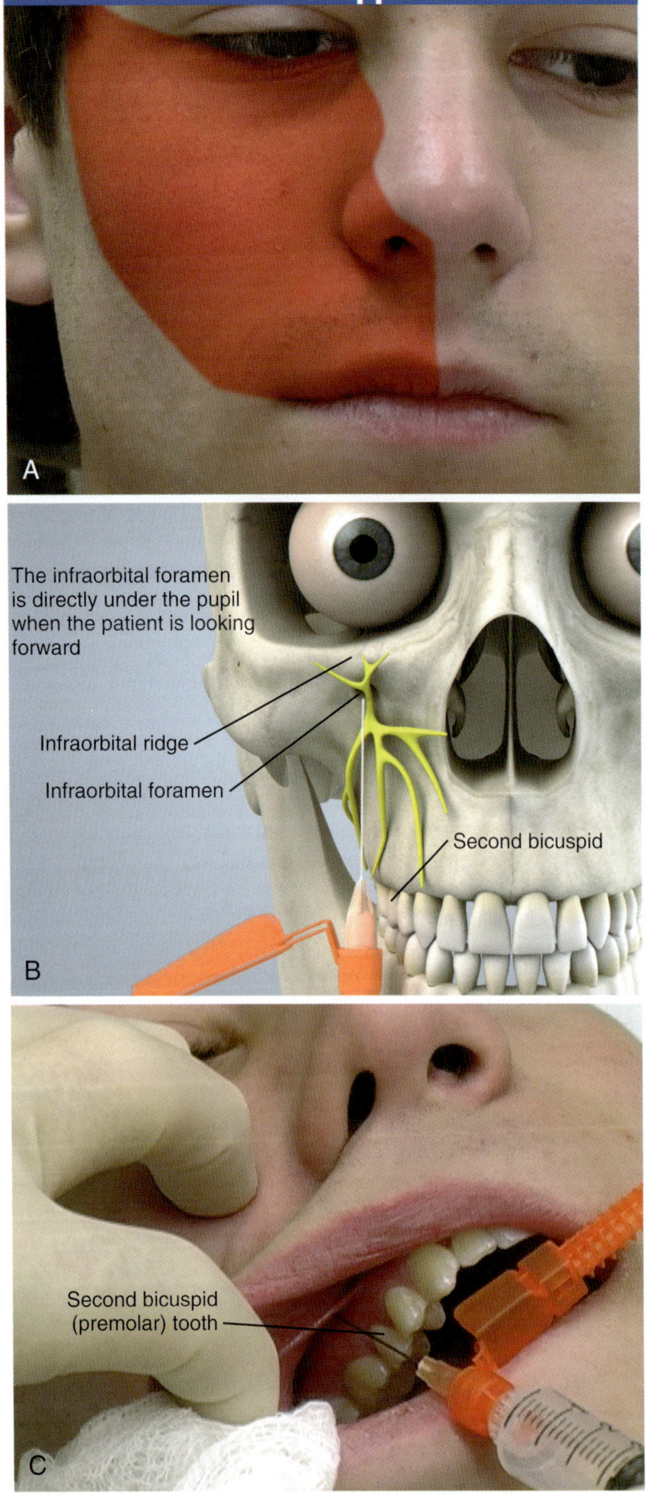

Fig. 30.9 Infraorbital nerve block. (A) Distribution. (B) Anatomy. (C) Insert the needle directly above and parallel to the upper second premolar toward the infraorbital foramen. Placing a finger over the foramen helps to direct and determine the depth of insertion.

for 10 to 15 seconds. It is usually visibly swollen. Place a finger under the eye to limit edema.

Complications

If the needle is angled posteriorly, it might enter and anesthetize the orbit. The risk of such positioning can be limited by

Infraorbital—External Approach

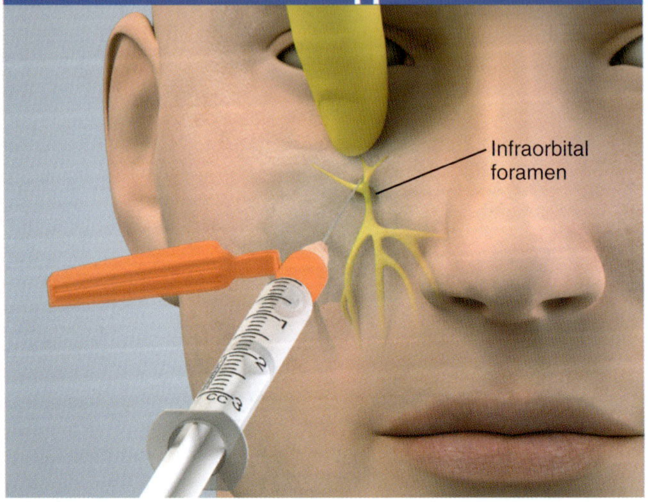

Fig. 30.10 Infraorbital nerve block, external approach. While injecting, place a finger under the eyelid to minimize lid swelling.

placing the finger on the foramen and palpating the needle below the orbital rim. Injection into, as opposed to near, the foramen can cause neuropraxia. Be careful not to anesthetize the facial artery and vein, which could lie on either side of the nerve. Do not use epinephrine, as its injection would cause vasoconstriction of the facial artery. If severe blanching occurs, apply warm compresses to the patient's face immediately.

Inferior Alveolar Nerve Block

See Video 30.2. Regional anesthesia of the inferior alveolar nerve (IAN) should be in every emergency provider's armamentarium. Dental complaints have been the cause of an increasing number of ED visits. If the pain or an injury involves the mandibular teeth or the lower lip and chin, the IAN block will be a useful tool. Examples of its application are for facial or dental trauma, dry socket, periapical abscess, and pericoronitis. The IAN block provides anesthesia to all the teeth on that side of the mandible and desensitizes the lower lip and chin via blockade of the mental nerve. The IAN can be anesthetized using the classic approach, the Gow-Gates technique, or Akinosi-Vazirani methods.

Anatomy

The IAN is the largest of the branches of the mandibular nerve (V_3). It provides sensation to all the lower teeth and lip; the central incisors, lateral incisors, and the buccal aspect of the molar teeth may also receive sensory innervation. The nerve descends, covered by the external pterygoid muscle, and passes between the ramus of the mandible and the sphenomandibular ligament to enter the mandibular canal. It is accompanied by the inferior alveolar artery and vein, proceeds along the mandibular canal, and innervates the teeth. At the mental foramen, the nerve bifurcates into an incisive branch, which continues forward to supply the anterior teeth. It gives off a side branch, the mental nerve, which exits from the mental foramen to supply the skin.

Approach

The patient can be seated either in a chair or upright with the head firmly against the back of the stretcher, so that when the mouth is opened, the body of the mandible is parallel to the floor. The easiest approach for the provider is with the patient seated or slightly reclined. Depending on the practitioner's handedness and comfort level, the best approach is to be positioned on the contralateral, or opposite, side of the nerve you are trying to block, as this will give better visual access to the targeted area. The best approach to regional anesthesia is to use a topical anesthetic over the approach area to increase patient compliance. Place a gauze pad soaked with topical lidocaine in the area of the IAN while preparing the rest of the supplies, or use a cotton swab with viscous lidocaine. Despite the use of topical anesthesia, be ready for an unexpected quick jerk of the head when an anxious patient first feels the needle.

To begin the technique, palpate the retromolar fossa with the index finger or thumb. With this maneuver, the greatest depth of the anterior border of the ramus of the mandible (the coronoid notch) can be identified (Fig. 30.11A). With your thumb in the patient's mouth, resting in the retromolar fossa, and your index finger placed externally behind the ramus at the same height as the thumb, retract the tissues toward the buccal (cheek) side, and then visually locate the pterygomandibular triangle (Fig. 30.11C). This technique also moves your finger safely away from the tip of the needle.

When topical anesthesia has been achieved, hold the syringe parallel to the occlusal surfaces of the teeth, angled so that its barrel lies between the first and second premolars on the opposite side of the mandible (Fig. 30.11B). Failing to achieve the required angle is the most common reason for failure of this nerve block. If a large-barrel syringe is used, the corner of the mouth might hamper efforts to obtain the proper angle; therefore a 5- or 10-mL syringe with a 25-gauge needle should be sufficient. If achieving the necessary angle is difficult, carefully bend the 25-gauge needle approximately 30 degrees (Fig. 30.12). This modification presents the risk of needle fracture and its inherent risks; an alternative is to use one of the other blocks described in the following sections. Puncture inside the pterygomandibular triangle at a point 1 cm above the occlusal surface of the molars. If the needle enters too low (e.g., at the level of the teeth), the anesthetic will be deposited over the bony canal and prominence (lingula) that house the mandibular nerve and not over the nerve itself.

The needle can be felt as it passes through the ligaments and the muscles covering the internal surface of the mandible. Stop when the needle has reached bone, which signifies contact with the posterior wall of the mandibular sulcus. You must feel bone with the needle. Failure to do so generally results from directing the needle toward the parotid gland (too far posteriorly) rather than toward the inner aspect of the mandible, which will anesthetize portions of the facial nerve. Withdraw the needle slightly and aspirate. Deposit approximately 1 to 2 mL of the anesthetic. If the needle position is suboptimal 3 to 4 mL could be required. In children, the angulation is not parallel to the occlusal surfaces of the teeth, so the barrel of the syringe should be held slightly higher because the mandibular foramen is lower.

One of the benefits of an IAN block is its ability to affect the other nerves in relative proximity. For example, one can anesthetize the lingual nerve, which innervates the anterior two thirds of the tongue, by placing several drops of anesthetic solution in that area while slowly withdrawing the syringe and needle. This technique consistently blocks the lingual nerve because of the proximity of the two nerves. The area that is

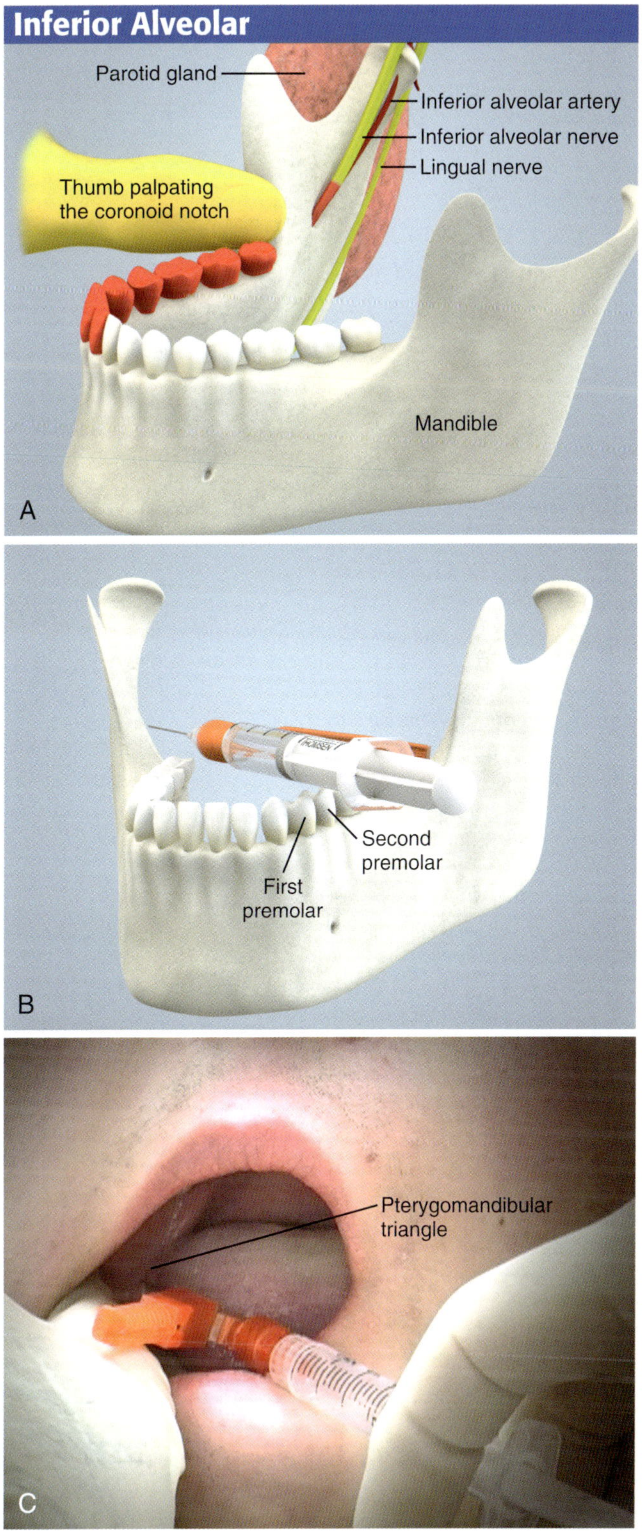

Fig. 30.11 Inferior alveolar nerve block for anesthesia of all the lower teeth on one side. (A) Anatomy and distribution. Identify the anterior border of the mandibular ramus (coronoid notch) with the thumb. (B) Approach. (C) Technique. Also see Fig. 30.12.

anesthetized can also be extended by blocking the long buccal nerve by injecting 0.5 mL of anesthetic just distal and buccal to the last mandibular molar. Supplementing the IAN block with both lingual and buccal nerve blocks helps anesthetize any aberrant fibers that are innervating the teeth. Shortly after a successful injection, the patient will report tingling in

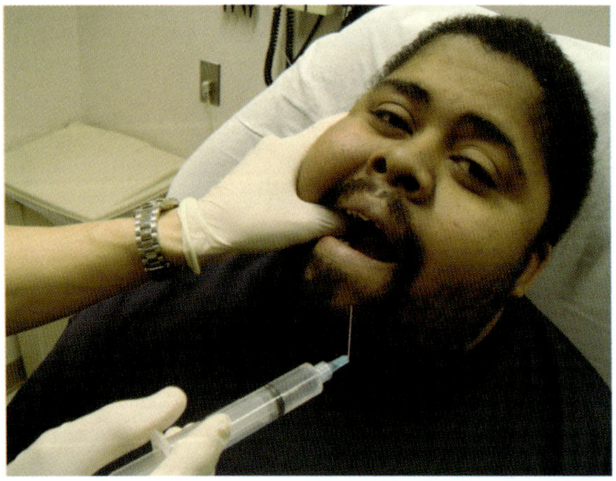

Fig. 30.12 To compensate for difficulty in obtaining the correct approach with a straight needle for the inferior alveolar nerve block, bend a 25-gauge, 1.5-inch needle with the needle guard.

the lower lip; however, 3 to 5 minutes is usually required to achieve complete anesthesia. An additional adjunct that has been described in the anesthesia literature is using point-of-care ultrasound to aid in the success of the IAN block.

Ultrasound guidance for blocking the IAN has been reported in dental literature to treat trismus in case reports.[9,10] Cadaveric studies have demonstrated the possibility of IAN anesthesia via infiltration of the pterygomandibular space as well.[11] However, studies involving emergency medicine patients and indications are lacking at this time.

Complications

This nerve block reportedly has a 15% to 20% failure rate. As with any block, the complications are mainly related to deposition of the anesthetic in inadvertent areas; for the IAN block, misplacement most commonly affects the parotid gland, anesthetizing the facial nerve. This is a relatively benign complication that causes temporary facial paralysis (similar to Bell palsy). It affects the orbicularis oculi muscle, making the patient unable to close the eyelid. Should this occur, protect the eye with an eye patch or tape until the local anesthetic has worn off (2 to 3 hours for 1% lidocaine). The duration of this complication is elongated to 3 to 6 hours if anesthesia is induced with bupivacaine (perhaps longer if it is used in combination with epinephrine).

Gow-Gates Block

Because the IAN block is frequently unsuccessful, other techniques have been developed to facilitate anesthesia in this region. The Gow-Gates and Akinosi-Vazirani techniques for regional anesthesia can augment or replace the IAN block. Introduced in the 1970s, the Gow-Gates mandibular block is an acceptable technique for achieving mandibular anesthesia, especially if traditional approaches fail (Fig. 30.13A).[12] It involves the deposition of anesthetic at the lateral aspect of the anterior condylar head, in an attempt to anesthetize the trunk of the mandibular branch of the trigeminal nerve as it exits the foramen ovale (Fig. 30.13B).

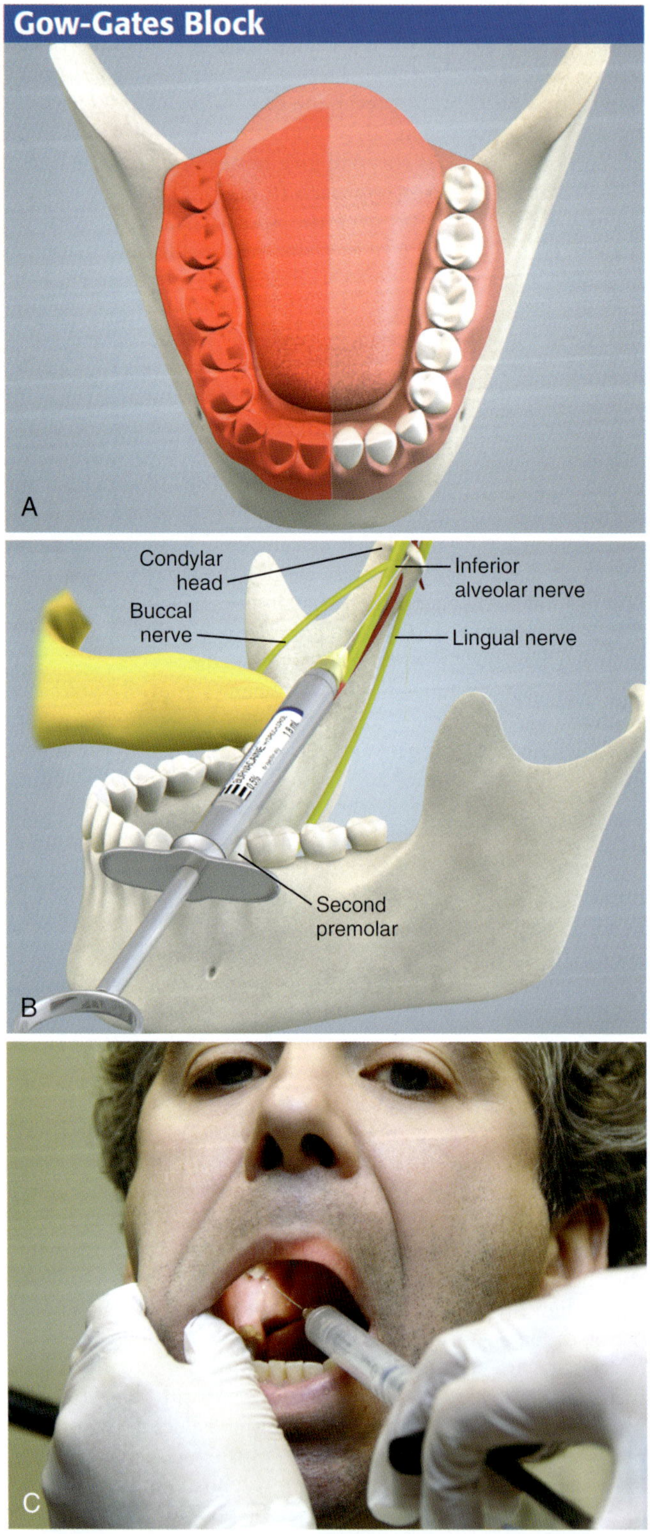

Fig. 30.13 Gow-Gates block. (A) Distribution. (B) Anatomy and approach. Angle the needle from the opposite premolar toward the condylar head. (C) Technique. Note the angle across and up toward the condylar head. Placing a finger at the condylar head can help to identify landmarks. (Adapted from Norton NS. Mandibular injections. In *Netter's Head and Neck Anatomy for Dentistry*. Elsevier; 2007:572-574.)

Approach

The key to this technique is patient compliance because the patient has to be able to open their mouth wide enough to allow the angle of approach that is necessary to achieve this block (Fig. 30.13C). The optimal plane is parallel to an imaginary line drawn from the corner of the mouth to the intratragal notch. This is different from the plane used with the classic IAN block. Place a finger inferior to the tragus of the ear as the landmark for the lateral aspect of the anterior

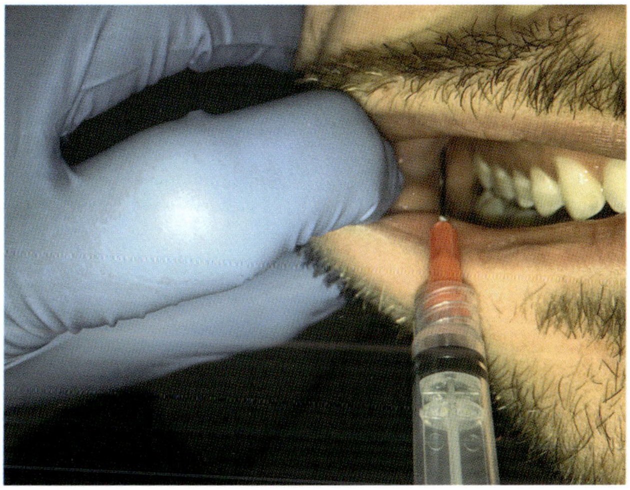

Fig. 30.14 General approach to the Akinosi-Vazirani nerve block technique.

condyle (which is now sitting at the eminence). Insert the needle opposite the second molar with the barrel of the syringe between the opposite lower premolars and the corner of the mouth (similar to the inferior alveolar approach). With this plane maintained, advance the needle until it reaches the condylar neck. The goal is to head below the insertion of the lateral pterygoid muscle, and it uses extraoral landmarks (tragus of the ear and corner of the mouth).[13] Withdraw the needle, aspirate, and inject 1 to 2 mL of anesthetic.[12,13]

Complications

The positive vascular aspiration rate with the Gow-Gates procedure is reported to be 1.6%, compared with 3.5% to 22% for the conventional IAN block technique.[7] If the needle is directed more toward the medial aspect of the anterior condylar process, it will be in the proximity of the pterygoid plexus of veins and the sympathetic plexus of the internal carotid artery. If the sympathetic plexus is anesthetized, the patient will experience a temporary version of Horner syndrome.

Akinosi-Vazirani Block

The Akinosi-Vazirani block can be used to anesthetize the IAN, including its mental and lingular nerve branches. A benefit of this block is that it can be performed when the patient's mouth is closed. This can be very helpful for the emergency physician because the condition necessitating the block can cause trismus, so opening the mouth wide enough for the classic or Gow-Gates techniques might not be possible.

Approach

With the patient's mouth closed, retract the buccal surface from the teeth, which will allow palpation of the bony landmarks. The main difference with this procedure and the IAN or Gow-Gates block centers on the fact that you do not want to hit bone with the needle; instead, you are aiming for the pterygomandibular space. The syringe should be positioned at the height of the gingival junction of the maxillary teeth and parallel to the occlusal surfaces of the teeth (Fig. 30.14). If bone is contacted, simply redirect the needle slightly toward the teeth, which should allow you to enter the desired space. The temporalis muscle is also in this area, and care should be taken to not inject the anesthetic into it.

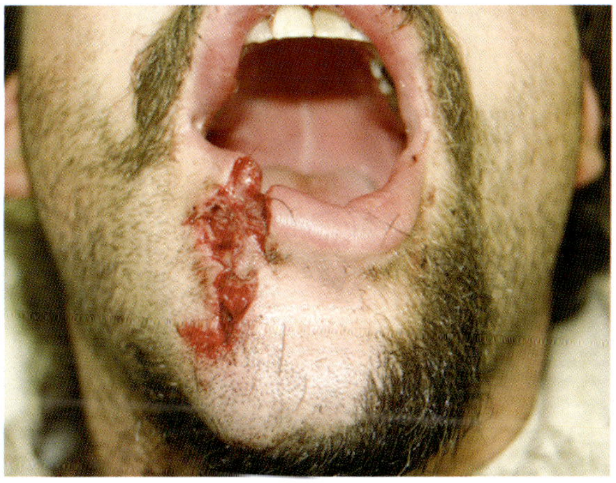

Fig. 30.15 A mental nerve block is ideal for a complicated lower lip laceration, because it will not distort the local tissue or the vermilion border. See Fig. 30.16.

Mental Nerve Block

See Videos 30.3 and 30.4. The mental nerve block is an easy and useful form of regional anesthesia and should be considered for all lower lip laceration repairs, especially those involving the vermilion border (Fig. 30.15). The mental nerve can be blocked with a complete IAN block or alone where it exits the mental foramen. An intraoral or extraoral approach can be used. An isolated block of the mental nerve is achieved by infiltrating local anesthetic where the nerve exits its bony foramen on the mandibular surface.

Anatomy

The mental nerve is a continuation of the IAN and innervates the mucosa and skin of the lower lip on the ipsilateral side of the mandible, with limited crossover of midline fibers. The nerve emerges from the mental foramen below the second premolar (Fig. 30.16A–B). Generally, the foramen will be just medial to the pupil of the eye (when the patient stares straight ahead) along a sagittal plane.

Approaches

Like the infraorbital nerve, the mental nerve block can be performed via an intraoral or extraoral approach. As the area being anesthetized is very sensitive and limiting scarring is a priority, the intraoral approach should be used when possible. Before using either approach, identify the mental foramen by palpation approximately 1 cm inferior and anterior to the second premolar. As with the IAN block, packing a gauze pad soaked in viscous lidocaine into the gingival sulcus while preparing the remainder of the supplies is a good way to ensure topical anesthesia. Approach the mental foramen at approximately a 45-degree angle with a 1.3 cm (0.5 inch), 25- or 27-gauge needle on a 3-mL syringe, and infiltrate the area adjacent to the foramen with 1 to 2 mL of local anesthetic (Fig. 30.16C). Avoid inserting the needle into the mental nerve foramen because the injection of liquid into that site can produce neuropraxia. Infiltrate around the foramen to provide anesthesia of the lower lip and soft tissue of the chin. For lacerations over the midline of the lip, administer anesthetic over the mental foramina bilaterally. This practice anesthetizes the crossover fibers and will ensure midline anesthesia.

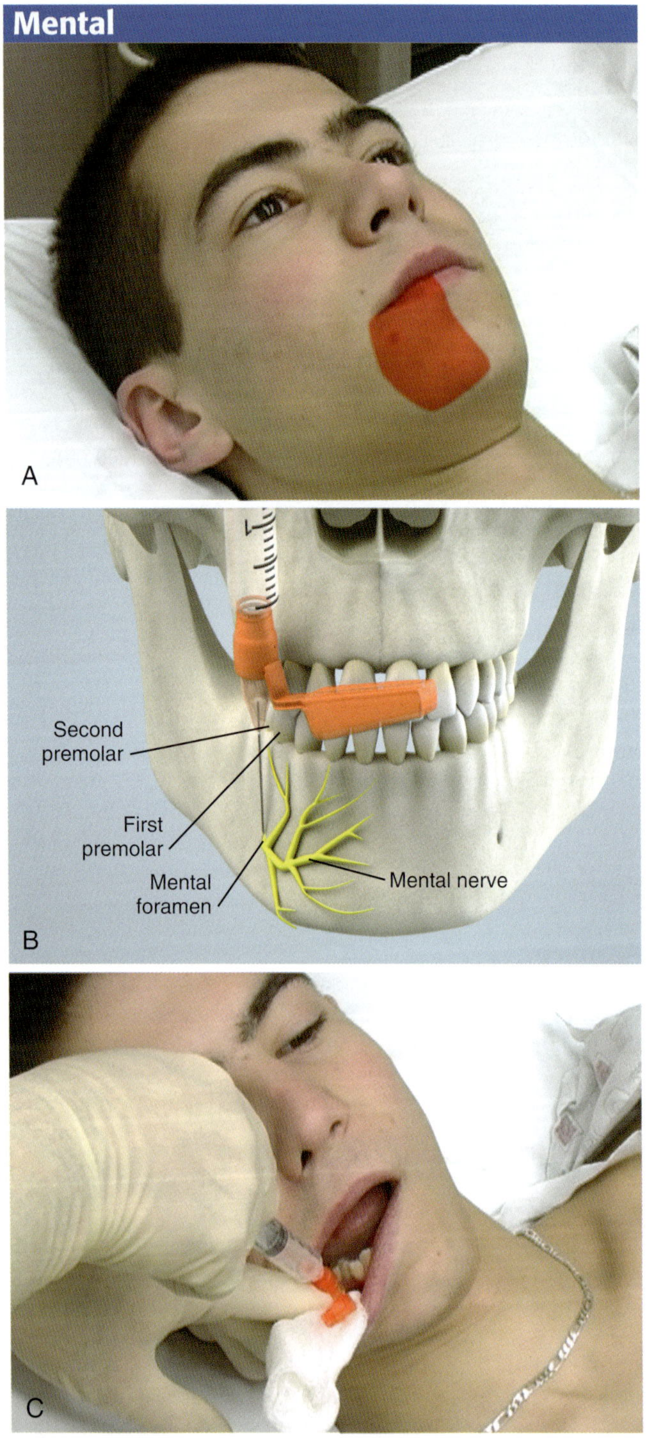

Fig. 30.16 Mental nerve block. (A) Distribution. (B) Anatomy and approach. The mental foramen is found inferior to the second premolar. (C) Technique. Insert the needle toward the mandibular foramen, inferior to the second premolar. Palpate the mental foramen with a finger, if necessary, to aid needle direction and depth, but keep the finger well away from the needle.

Complications

The main complication of the mental nerve block stems from damaging the mental nerve where it exits the foramen, by direct needle trauma or pressure from the injection, causing neuropraxia.

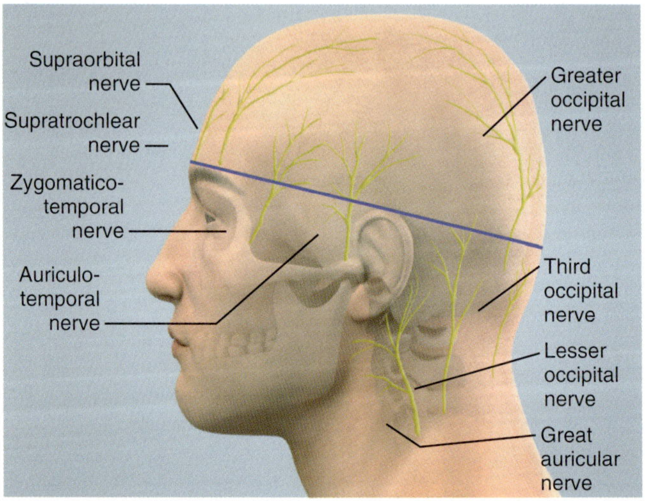

Fig. 30.17 Origin of the sensory nerve supply to the scalp. Nerves above the *blue line* become superficial and converge toward the vertex of the scalp.

Scalp Anesthesia

Scalp blocks provide surgical anesthesia for repair of lacerations, drainage of superficial abscesses, and exploration and debridement of wounds. In general, the larger nerves innervating the scalp are blocked best when they are induced near the exit of the nerve from the skull. This is because the nerves branch and spread superficially very quickly, so it becomes difficult to achieve regional anesthesia.

Anatomy

As shown in Fig. 30.17, the scalp receives its nerve supply from branches of the trigeminal nerve (CN V) and the cervical plexus. The forehead is supplied by the supraorbital and supratrochlear nerves, both of which are branches of the ophthalmic division of the trigeminal nerve. The temporal region receives its nerve supply from the zygomaticotemporal nerve (a V_2 branch nerve) and the temporomandibular and auriculotemporal nerves (V_3 branch nerves). The posterior aspect of the scalp is innervated by the great auricular and the greater, lesser, and least (third) occipital nerves. The nerves that supply the posterior aspect of the scalp originate from the cervical plexus.

Topographically, the nerves and vessels of the scalp are located in the subcutaneous tissue above the epicranial aponeurosis (Fig. 30.18). From this level, they divide into small branches that extend to the deeper layers (epicranium and periosteum).[14] The scalp is a very vascular structure, so take care to provide hemostasis with vasoconstrictive agents while simultaneously monitoring the systemic effects of the chosen agents.

Approaches

A complete scalp block can be accomplished by individually blocking each nerve that supplies the scalp, but this approach is time-consuming, difficult, and rarely necessary. Because the nerves on the scalp are located superficially, especially above the eyebrows to the vertex of the skull, a local anesthetic can be used around the wound's edges in most cases. Injection of local anesthetic to deeper levels is necessary only if bone is to be removed. Injection of a local anesthetic only in the deeper

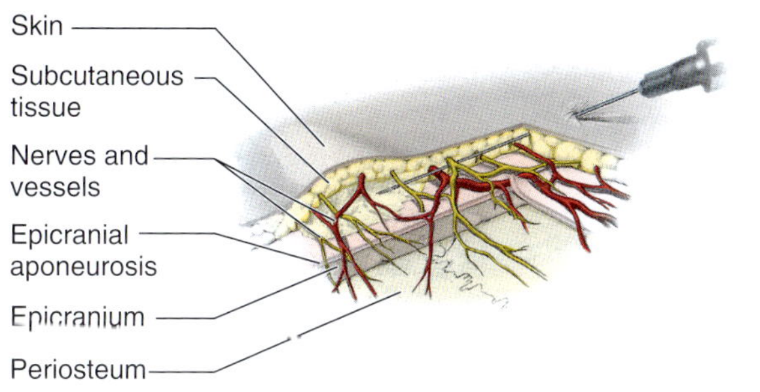

Fig. 30.18 Topographic anatomy of the scalp. Generously infiltrating this area in a fanlike motion will block multiple sensory nerves.

layers without subcutaneous infiltration results in an unsuccessful block and a greater amount of bleeding during surgical intervention.

In preparation for the procedure, clip hair or use sterile petroleum gel to slick hair away from the injured area. Prepare the skin with an antiseptic solution and raise a skin wheal at any point along the skin with a 1.3 cm (0.5 inch), 25-gauge needle. Insert a 7.6 cm (3 inch), 22-gauge needle through the skin wheal and into the subcutaneous tissue. Advance it along the scalp circumferentially to surround the wound. Inject 0.5% to 1% lidocaine or 0.125% to 0.25% bupivacaine with epinephrine (1:200,000). Use a local anesthetic with epinephrine, unless contraindicated, to provide vasoconstriction and prevent excessive blood loss and absorption of local anesthetic. The total dose of the local anesthetic should not exceed the recommended dose for that particular agent. The first 10 to 15 minutes after the injection is the most critical period to monitor for local anesthetic toxicity.

Greater and Lesser Occipital Nerve Block

This relatively simple block may be useful in the ED for treating occipital neuralgia various headaches including tension and migraine headaches. For occipital neuritis, a long-acting corticosteroid such as methylprednisolone (20 to 40 mg) can be combined with a local anesthetic.

Anatomy

The posterior aspect of the head is supplied by the posterior rami of the cervical nerves. Two important branches of these nerves are the greater and lesser occipital nerves. The greater occipital nerve becomes superficial on each side at the inferior border of the obliquus capitis inferior muscle and runs superiorly toward the vertex over this muscle. The nerve is located medial to the occipital artery. The lesser occipital nerve is located approximately 2.5 to 3.5 cm lateral and 1 to 2 cm caudal to the greater occipital nerve (Fig. 30.19A).

Approach

It is not usually necessary to shave or clip the scalp before performing greater and lesser occipital nerve blocks. The greater occipital nerve is best blocked at the nuchal line, which extends from the middle of the external occipital protuberance to the mastoid process. The nuchal line is located between the insertion sites of the trapezius muscle and the semispinalis muscles. At this site, the greater occipital nerve is just medial to the occipital artery.

First, palpate the occipital artery. Next, attach a 3.8-cm, 23- to 25-gauge needle to a syringe containing 5 mL of local

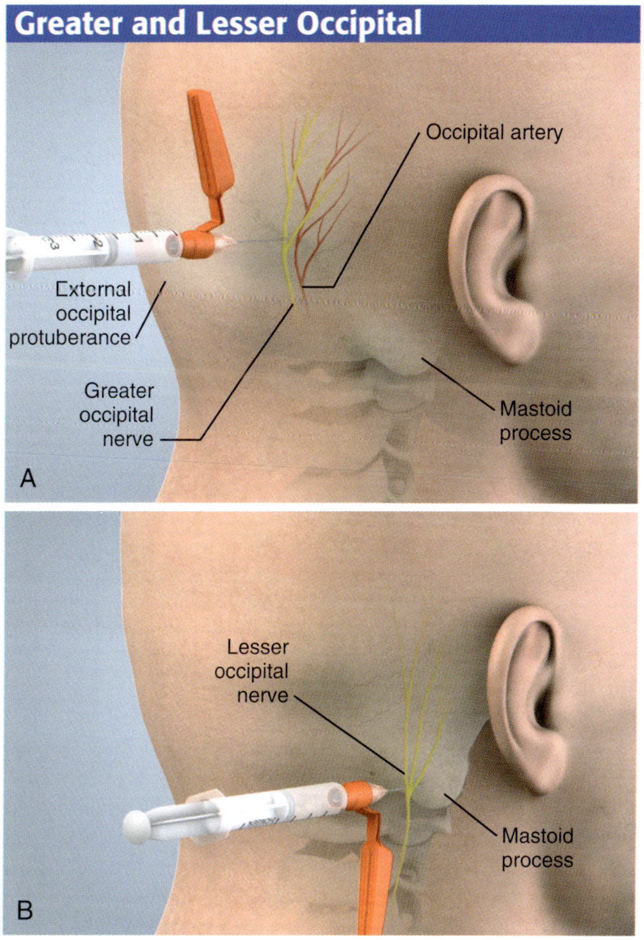

Fig. 30.19 Occipital nerve blocks. (A) Block the greater occipital nerve on a line 3 cm lateral to the external occipital protuberance and the base of the occipital bone. (B) Block the lesser occipital nerve by injection of 2 to 3 mL of anesthetic solution along the posterior border of the mastoid process of the temporal bone.

anesthetic. Insert the needle into the skin (Fig. 30.19B). After obtaining paresthesia at the vertex, inject 5 mL of local anesthetic solution. Block the lesser occipital nerve with a fanlike injection of a local anesthetic solution, 2.5 to 3.5 cm lateral and 1 cm caudal to the point described for the greater occipital nerve.

This procedure is not usually associated with any complications. Intraarterial injections can be avoided by careful aspiration.

Ultrasound guidance has been described to administer a greater occipital nerve block. When treating occipital neuralgia or cervicogenic headache with local anesthetic and steroid injection, outcomes at 4 weeks were improved with ultrasound techniques. This approach utilizes a slightly lower target, at the C2 level compared with the landmark-based technique. The user should identify the transverse process of C2, followed identification of the GON deep to the semispinalis capitis and superficial to the obliquus capitis inferior muscles. In-line imaging of the needle can be used to deposit anesthetic with or without corticosteroid surrounding the nerve.[15]

Ophthalmic (V_1) Nerve Block

The lateral and medial branches of the supraorbital, supratrochlear, and infratrochlear nerves can be blocked by

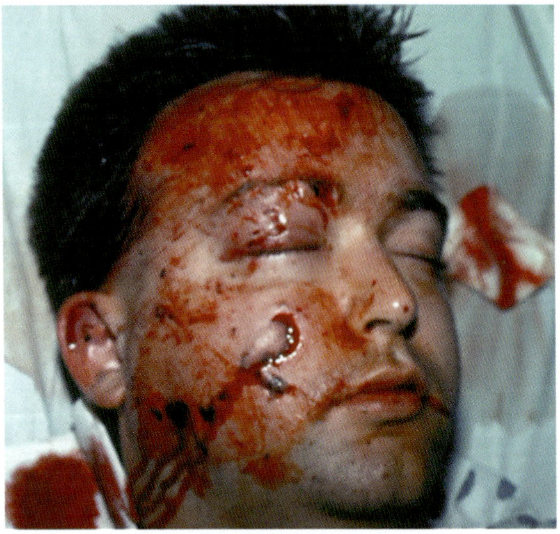

Fig. 30.20 An ophthalmic (V_1) nerve block (supraorbital and supratrochlear nerves) would be ideal for this patient with extensive forehead and upper eyelid lacerations from a windshield injury, and for exploration for foreign bodies. Additionally, an infraorbital (V_2) block could be used to provide anesthesia for repair of the maxillary laceration.

percutaneous local injection at the point where they emerge from the superior aspect of the orbit. Anesthesia of the forehead and scalp is achieved as far posteriorly as the lambdoid suture. This block can be used for debridement or topical treatment of burns or abrasions and for delicate lacerations of the upper eyelid. It is also ideal for removing small pieces of glass embedded in the forehead from a windshield injury (Fig. 30.20). Although this block is used infrequently, it is easily performed and not associated with serious side effects. It should be considered when anesthesia of the forehead or the anterior aspect of the scalp is desired.

Anatomy

The subtle supraorbital notch, which is in line with the pupil (when the patient is staring straight ahead), can be palpated along the superior orbital rim (Fig. 30.21B). This landmark is the site of injection for blockade of the supraorbital nerves. The supratrochlear nerve is found 0.5 cm to 1.0 cm medial to the notch. This nerve innervates the midline and should be blocked bilaterally for wounds or procedures that require midline anesthesia. The infratrochlear nerve is not usually blocked but is found in the most medial aspect of the superior orbital rim.

Approach

See Video 30.5. With the patient in the supine position, hold a finger or a roll of gauze firmly under the orbital rim to avoid ballooning of anesthetic into the upper eyelid and raise a skin wheal over the lateral border of the upper orbital ridge. This should be approximately 0.5 cm from the supraorbital notch. Extend a 3.8-cm, 23- to 25-gauge needle attached to a syringe containing 5 mL of local anesthetic. Inject 1 mL to 3 mL of anesthetic in the area medial to the supraorbital notch (Fig. 30.21C) and continue to withdraw the needle. Place another 1 to 2 mL of anesthetic in the area of the supraorbital notch as well. This effectively places a line of anesthetic solution along the orbital rim laterally to medially to ensure a block of all the branches of the ophthalmic nerve. Paresthesia in the form of an electric shock sensation over the forehead indicates a successful block.

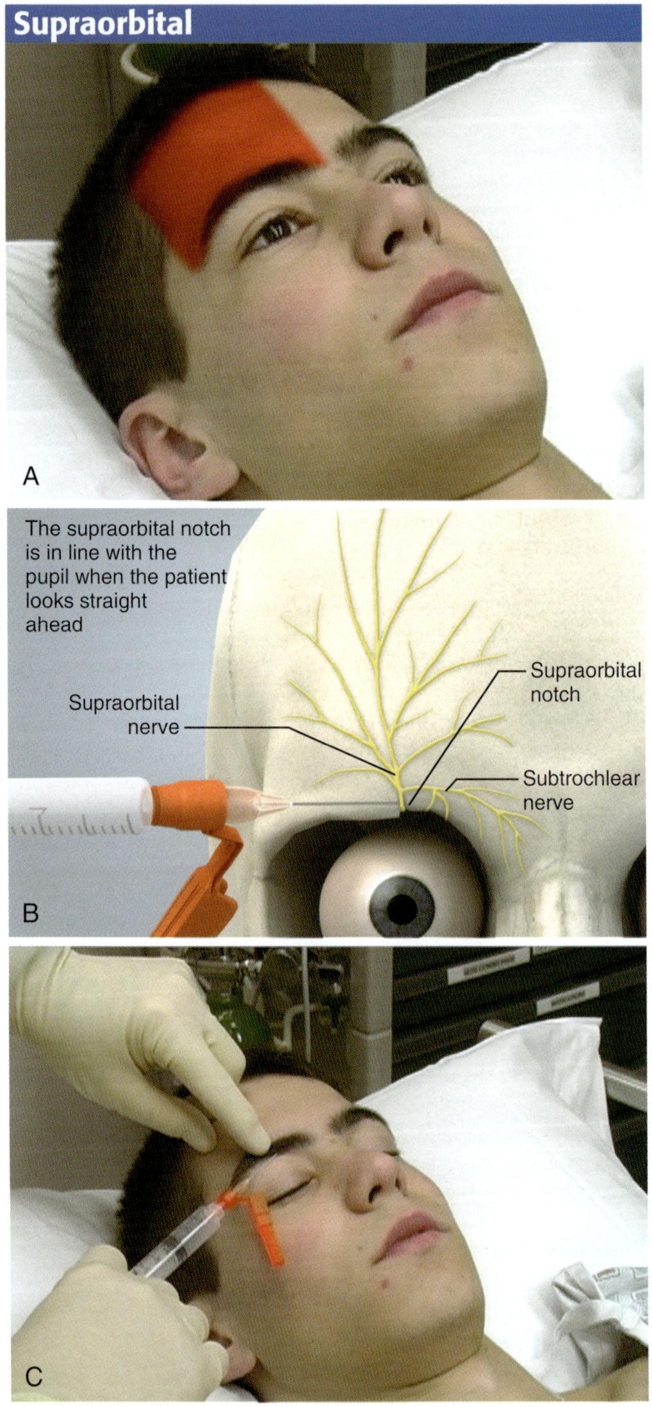

Fig. 30.21 Supraorbital/supratrochlear nerve block, branches of V_1. (A) Distribution. (B) Anatomy and approach. (C) Technique. Insert the needle laterally and advance medially to include the supratrochlear nerve. Aspirate and then inject while withdrawing the needle across the canal. Extra anesthetic can be inserted directly over the supraorbital notch. Placing a finger inferiorly to the orbital rim can prevent eyelid swelling, and aid in landmark identification. This nerve block will include the upper eyelid.

Complications

Hematoma formation or swelling of the eyelid may occur but requires only local pressure to limit expansion.

Occasionally, ecchymosis of the periorbital region will appear the next day, and the patient should be warned of this possibility.

CONCLUSION

Nerve blocks about the head and neck are relatively painless when induced carefully and slowly after topical mucosal anesthesia (for intraoral approaches) or local skin anesthesia (for extraoral blocks and approaches). They can alleviate patient apprehension, minimize wound margin misalignment, and contribute to better patient outcomes. The blocks should be considered in all cooperative patients who require regional anesthesia in the head and neck.

ACKNOWLEDGMENTS

We thank James T. Amsterdam and Kevin P. Kilgore for writing the original chapter and developing many of the images. We thank Linda J. Kesselring, MS, ELS, for her copyediting, formatting, and organization.

REFERENCES ARE AVAILABLE AT Elsevier eBooks+

CHAPTER 31

Regional Anesthesia of the Thorax and Extremities

Robert Allen and Thomas Mailhot

INTRODUCTION

Regional anesthesia is the process of blocking targeted peripheral nerves to anesthetize a specific part of the body. Emergency medicine providers are commonly tasked with providing safe and effective analgesia for a wide variety of conditions. However, the recent opioid epidemic has highlighted the need to limit opiate usage and find alternative methods of analgesia. It is against this backdrop that emergency physicians have increasingly incorporated regional anesthesia into clinical practice, so much so that in 2021 the American College of Emergency Physicians identified nerve blocks as a core skill for emergency physicians.[1]

Most of the key principles of regional anesthesia remain unchanged from prior editions. This chapter is not an exhaustive list of all possible nerve blocks and techniques; however, we chose to highlight the more commonly performed nerve blocks in current practice. As regional anesthesia is a rapidly expanding field, there are new blocks and techniques that we omit but may be highlighted in future editions when they are more widely adopted.

The growing use of point-of-care ultrasound (POCUS) has expanded into regional anesthesia. Subsequently, a noticeable change from the prior edition is that many nerve blocks previously described by landmark techniques have been replaced by an ultrasound-first technique. In addition to added safety and efficacy, the use of POCUS in regional anesthesia has made previously daunting blocks more accessible. We hope this chapter serves as a helpful primer for those wishing to get started or as a reference for those hoping to refresh their knowledge and skills.

GENERAL CONCEPTS

Indications

For most lacerations and injuries seen in the emergency department (ED), local infiltrative anesthesia is adequate and more efficient than using a nerve block (see Chapter 29). However, there are multiple scenarios in which a peripheral nerve block may be advantageous:

- Optimizing cosmesis: Peripheral nerve blocks may be preferred for laceration repairs in which local infiltrative anesthesia may distort the tissue, compromising cosmetically ideal closures (e.g., digital or facial lacerations).
- Avoiding toxic doses of anesthetic: Large, multiple, or complex lacerations may require a higher volume of local anesthetic that could exceed the maximum recommended dose. Peripheral nerve blocks typically require a smaller volume of local anesthetic and can anesthetize a larger surface area.
- Reducing systemic analgesics: Regional anesthesia can be used as part of multimodal analgesia for a range of painful conditions (e.g., multiple rib fractures, hip fractures) in order to reduce the number of systemic medications and their associated complications.
- As an alternative to procedural sedation: Strategic use of regional anesthesia can avoid the need for procedural sedation (e.g., shoulder dislocation).
- Eliminating the need for operative repair: Complex laceration repair or incision and drainage that may otherwise require general anesthesia in the operating room can be done at the bedside aided by the use of regional anesthesia. In addition to avoiding hospitalization and its associated costs, this may be desirable in patients with comorbidities or a higher risk of complications from general anesthesia.

Preparation

A brief history, including drug allergies (particularly to local anesthetics), medications, and systemic illnesses, should be taken from the patient. Peripheral vascular, heart, and liver disease may increase the risk for complications, so their presence should be noted. The procedure should be explained to the patient, noting the likelihood of pain on needle insertion, paresthesia, and possible complications.

Equipment

In general, supplies needed for nerve blocks include gloves, skin antiseptic (e.g., chlorhexidine), an appropriately sized syringe, an 18-gauge needle for drawing up anesthetic, and a nerve block needle (see later).

For large-volume blocks or blocks near vascular structures, cardiac monitoring equipment and advanced cardiac life support supplies including a defibrillator should be on hand. Lipid emulsion should be readily available as an antidote for local anesthetic toxicity (see Appendix II).

Needle Choice

Specially designed needles for nerve blocks exist; however, these are more expensive than standard needles and less likely to be available in a typical ED. In general, noncutting needles (e.g., Sprotte) are ideal to decrease the risk of iatrogenic nerve damage. The gauge and length of the needle should be selected based on the patient's body size and habitus, as well as the block being performed (Tables 31.1–31.3). For more superficial nerve targets, the shortest needle should be chosen (e.g., 1.5 inch) to reach the target and avoid iatrogenic injury. Longer needles (e.g., 3.5 inch) may be required for deeper nerve targets. Thinner needles (e.g., 25 gauge) minimize the pain of injection and are well suited for blocks of superficial nerves. However, when using ultrasound guidance for nerve blocks, the desire to use a thin needle must be balanced against the need to visualize the needle with ultrasound, as smaller needles may be more difficult to locate.

Choice of Anesthetic

Factors influencing the choice of anesthetic agents for nerve blocks are similar to those for local infiltration (see Chapter 29). When choosing a local anesthetic, consider the indication for the desired nerve block. For example, a local anesthetic with a longer duration of action (e.g., bupivacaine or ropivacaine) may be desired for fractures or other traumatic injuries, which continue to be painful long after the ED visit. Conversely, lidocaine with its shorter half-life is ideal for simple procedures including foreign body removal and laceration repair. Additive agents such as bicarbonate may be considered to buffer the anesthetic to lessen the pain of infiltration (see Chapter 29).[2] Other additives such as steroids (e.g., dexamethasone) have also been suggested to extend the duration of analgesia.[3] Traditionally, the addition of epinephrine has been discouraged for areas at risk of end-organ damage (e.g., digital blocks). However, the validity of this dogma has been questioned (see section on "Traditional Digital Block of the Toe").[4]

In general the minimum amount of anesthetic should be used to achieve the desired effect. Typically the concentration of local anesthetic is less important than the volume of anesthetic. For example, for compartment blocks in which blockade of multiple nerves is desired, a large volume of lower concentration anesthetic may be desired. Care should be taken to avoid exceeding the maximum safe recommended dose, factoring in age, weight, and comorbidities (e.g., hepatic or renal dysfunction, heart failure, pregnancy). When larger volumes of anesthetic are required but would risk potential toxicity, the vial of local anesthetic may be diluted 50:50 with saline to halve the concentration of anesthetic, in this way preserving

TABLE 31.1 Recommended Anesthetic Volumes and Needle Choices for Thoracic Nerve Blocks

NERVE BLOCK	VOLUME (mL)	NEEDLE (Gauge + Length)
Serratus anterior plane block	20–30	20–22 gauge, 3.5 inch
Erector spinae plane block	20–30	20–22 gauge, 3.5 inch
Superficial cervical plexus block	2–15	25 gauge, 1.5 inch

Volumes of anesthetic and needle gauge/length may be adjusted as appropriate for the patient's body size and habitus as well as availability of supplies.

TABLE 31.2 Recommended Anesthetic Volumes and Needle Choices for Upper Extremity Nerve Blocks

NERVE BLOCK	VOLUME (mL)	NEEDLE (Gauge + Length)
Interscalene brachial plexus block	10–30	22 gauge, 1.5 inch
Supraclavicular brachial plexus block	20–30	22 gauge, 1.5 inch
Forearm nerve blocks (ulnar, median, radial nerve)	3–5 mL per nerve	21 or 25 gauge, 1.5 inch
Ulnar nerve block (wrist)	3–5	25 gauge, 1.5 inch
Median nerve block (wrist)	3–5	25 gauge, 1.5 inch
Radial nerve block (wrist)	2–5	25 gauge, 1.5 inch
Digital nerve block (dorsal approach)	2–4	25 gauge, 1.5 inch
Digital nerve block (volar approaches)	1–3.5	25 gauge, 1.5 inch

Volumes of anesthetic and needle gauge/length may be adjusted as appropriate for the patient's body size and habitus as well as availability of supplies.

TABLE 31.3 Recommended Anesthetic Volumes and Needle Choices for Lower Extremity Nerve Blocks

NERVE BLOCK	VOLUME (mL)	NEEDLE (Gauge + Length)
Femoral nerve/3-in-1 block	20–30	20–22 gauge, 3.5 inch
Fascia iliaca compartment block	20–40	20–22 gauge, 3.5 inch
Popliteal sciatic nerve block	20–30	20–22 gauge, 3.5 inch
Saphenous nerve block (mid-thigh)	5–10	22–25 gauge, 1.5 inch
Posterior tibial nerve block (ankle)	3–5 (landmark based) 5–7 (US guided)	25 gauge, 1.5 inch
Deep peroneal nerve block (ankle)	3-5 (landmark based) 2–4 (US guided)	25 gauge, 1.5 inch
Superficial peroneal nerve block (ankle)	4–10	25 gauge, 1.5 inch
Sural nerve block (ankle)	3–5 (landmark based) 2–4 (US guided)	25 gauge, 1.5 inch
Saphenous nerve block (ankle)	3–5	25 gauge, 1.5 inch

Volumes of anesthetic and needle gauge/length may be adjusted as appropriate for the patient's body size and habitus as well as availability of supplies. *US*, ultrasound.

enough volume for the block to be effective. Ropivacaine may be considered as a substitute for bupivacaine as it is considered to lessen the risk of local anesthetic toxicity; however, its use may be limited by cost and availability.[5]

General Technique

The technique of performing a nerve block involves a lot of commonalities regardless of the specific nerve being targeted. To avoid repetition throughout the text, these universal recommendations are laid out in the following section and are applicable to all nerve blocks unless otherwise noted.

Before Performing a Nerve Block

- Perform and document a focused neurological exam on the affected region. This is important as a rare but serious complication of regional anesthesia is nerve injury.
- Confirm that your planned block is appropriate for the patient and there are no contraindications. Depending on the nerve block and the indication, it may be appropriate to discuss with involved consultants that they have no objection to the nerve block.
- Ensure that all necessary monitoring equipment and medications are available at the bedside. Continuous cardiac monitoring is not required for peripheral nerve blocks using small volumes of anesthetic. Larger volume blocks and those near large blood vessels (e.g., femoral) are at higher risk of complications such as local anesthetic systemic toxicity (LAST), and continuous cardiac monitoring and intravenous access are recommended.
- Consider obtaining informed consent for blocks with more than minimal risk of complications.

While Performing the Block

- Position the patient in an optimal fashion to expose the target area and maximize the chances of successful blockade.
- If using ultrasound, position the ultrasound on the opposite side of the patient so that the monitor is directly in front of you (Fig. 31.1).
- Clean the affected area with skin antiseptic. Allow the antiseptic solution to dry fully to achieve its maximal antibacterial effect. Sterile technique (e.g., drapes, sterile gloves) is generally not required.
- Whenever feasible, and for larger volume and deeper blocks, consider using the two-person technique (Fig. 31.2). This approach allows for greater fine motor control and for controlled injection of local anesthetic. If using connecting tubing, ensure that both the tubing and needle are flushed with saline solution to prevent injecting air, as even small volumes of air will disrupt attempts to visualize the anatomy with ultrasound.
- Aspirate the plunger of the syringe prior to injecting anesthetic to avoid accidental intravascular injection.
- Consider hydrodissection if appropriate using saline to better visualize the nerve target.

After the Block Has Been Performed

- Document in the medical record that you performed the block. Include the date and time of the procedure, the local anesthetic, and its volume. Record if the block was successful in its desired effect, as well as any complications.

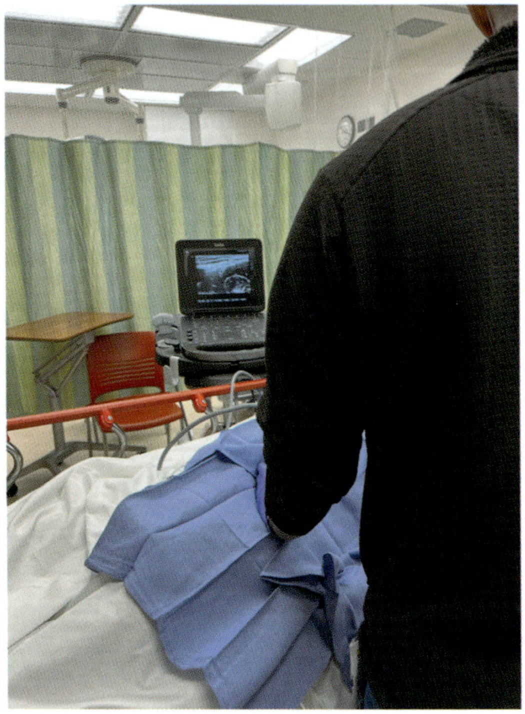

Fig. 31.1 Placing the ultrasound machine on the opposite side of the patient allows for better comfort and visualization while performing a nerve block.

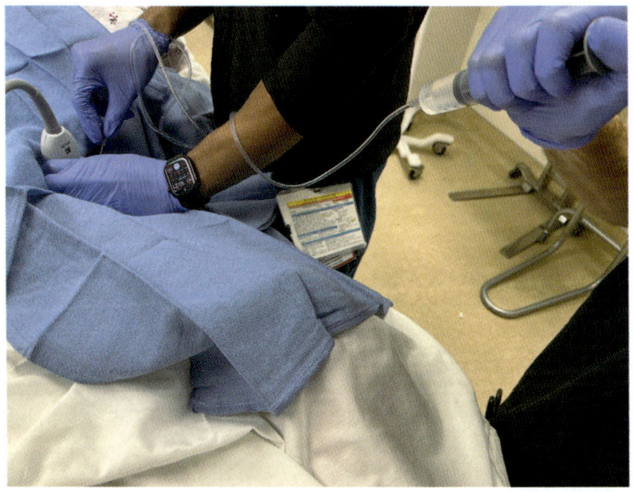

Fig. 31.2 Two-person technique allows for greater dexterity: the first operator holds the ultrasound probe with their nondominant hand and the needle with their dominant hand. The second operator injects local anesthetic from the syringe attached to the needle via connection tubing.

- If using a higher volume block, monitor the patient for up to 30 minutes for signs and symptoms of LAST (see the section on "Complications and Precautions").

Injecting the Anesthetic

Strive to ensure that the anesthetic agent is not inadvertently injected into a vessel or nerve bundle. In practice, a misplaced intravascular injection is usually of minimal consequence, but small amounts of epinephrine may cause systemic symptoms such as tachycardia or anxiety, while local anesthetic may precipitate LAST. Intraarterial injection theoretically is more dangerous than intravenous injection. Either way, aspirate the syringe to check for blood before injection.

Nerve bundle injection has the potential to cause nonspecific nerve injury. Severe pain or paresthesia during injection or resistance to depressing the plunger suggests the possibility of intraneural placement of the needle. If any of these problems occur, immediately stop injecting and reposition the needle.

The onset and duration of anesthesia are both greatly influenced by how close the injected anesthetic is to the nerve. Onset occurs within a few minutes if the anesthetic is in immediate proximity to the nerve. Onset takes longer or may not occur at all if the anesthetic must diffuse more than 2 to 3 mm, which underscores the importance of accurately targeting the nerve.

More anesthetic is required if it must diffuse a long distance to the nerve. A range of suggested volumes of anesthetic is given with each nerve block description and summarized in Tables 31.1–31.3. In general, blocks performed with ultrasound guidance allow for a smaller volume of anesthetic due to the ability to position the anesthesia in immediate proximity to the nerve. If a block appears to have been unsuccessful, one option is to repeat the block, administering additional local anesthetic. Before doing so, ensure that the soft tissue can accommodate additional anesthetic volume and that the toxic thresholds of anesthesia are recalculated. The difference between a successful and an unsuccessful block may be merely an additional 2 mL of anesthetic.

With most blocks, the onset of anesthesia occurs in 2 to 15 minutes, depending on the distance that the anesthetic must diffuse to the nerve and the type of anesthetic used. Wait 30 minutes before deciding that a block is unsuccessful.

Ultrasound

See Videos 31.1–31.3. POCUS has been a standard part of training for emergency physicians since 2001[6]; however, it is only more recently that ultrasound has been advocated for use with regional anesthesia. The American College of Emergency Physicians published a policy statement in 2021 endorsing the use of ultrasound-guided nerve blocks.[1] Prior to the adoption of ultrasound, nerve blocks were performed blindly using landmark guidance with or without neurostimulation. However, multiple studies have consistently shown that ultrasound improves efficacy, efficiency, and safety compared with the blind approach.[1,7–10] Additionally, the use of ultrasound has allowed nerve blocks that were not typically attempted in the ED to become feasible.

Position the ultrasound machine on the opposite side of the patient, in a direct line of sight of the operator (see Fig. 31.1). Maintaining a straight line between the operator, needle, targeted nerve, and ultrasound screen minimizes the need for the operator to turn their head, thus preventing undesired shoulder and arm movements with the attendant risk of inadvertently moving the needle away from its intended location.

Needle-based procedures using ultrasound can be performed using an "in-plane" or "out-of-plane" approach (see Chapter 67) (Fig. 31.3). With an in-plane approach, the needle is introduced in the same plane as the ultrasound transducer (along its long axis) such that the entire needle can be visualized as it approaches its target, and structures that must be avoided can easily be avoided. In contrast, with an out-of-plane technique, the plane of the needle is perpendicular to the plane of the ultrasound beam, allowing only a tiny portion of the needle (ideally the needle tip) to be visible at any one time. With an out-of-plane approach, it can be difficult to ensure the needle is correctly positioned and has not traversed

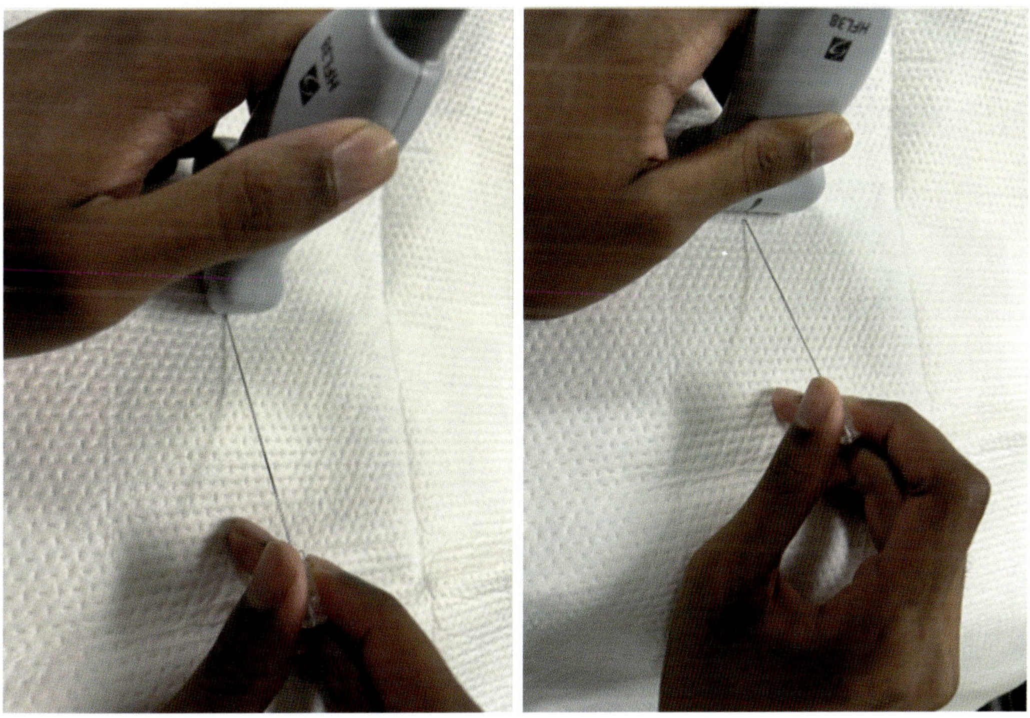

Fig. 31.3 *Left*, In-plane technique in which the needle is parallel to the long axis of the ultrasound (US) probe. *Right*, Out-of-plane technique in which the needle is held perpendicular to the long axis of the US probe.

important structures enroute to the nerve. Therefore, whenever possible, an in-plane approach is preferred for nerve blocks. However, this is not always feasible for a given nerve block due to variations in individual anatomy.

Ultrasound offers the clinician the opportunity to see precisely where the anesthetic is injected in relation to the nerve. In general, a successful nerve block is heralded by the appearance of a halo of anesthetic encircling the nerve (Fig. 31.4). Achieving this can be difficult, as various layers of soft tissue and fascia may compartmentalize the injectate and prevent it from contacting the nerve itself. By carefully injecting small aliquots (0.1 mL) of saline as the needle is slowly advanced toward the target, the operator can "hydrodissect" through tissue planes until proximity to the target is achieved. At this point, the nerve is bathed in the desired volume of local anesthetic in a circumferential pattern.

Complications and Precautions

Complications may result from peripheral nerve blocks but are rare in clinical practice. General precautions include measures to minimize nerve injury, intravascular injection, and systemic toxicity. The adoption of ultrasound-guided nerve blocks has decreased but not eliminated the incidence of complications compared with blind techniques.[11] Potential complications unique to certain blocks will be covered later in the respective nerve block sections.

Nerve Injury

Studies from anesthesia literature suggest that post-block neurologic symptoms are transient with less than 1% lasting longer than 6 months.[12] The exact cause of nerve injury related to peripheral nerve blockade is unknown. Direct intraneural injection has been postulated as a cause of nerve dysfunction following nerve blocks, but studies have shown that permanent nerve damage is uncommon even with intraneural injection.[13,14] An alternate theory is that nerve injury may be related to the injection pressure. It is therefore recommended to minimize the risk of complications related to intraneural injection by avoiding high injection pressures.[15,16]

Vascular Injury

Complications related to iatrogenic vascular injury (hematoma) and accidental intravascular injection of local anesthetic are rare and can be reduced with use of ultrasound.[17] Care should be taken to aspirate prior to injecting to avoid accidental intravascular injection. Furthermore, carefully weigh the risks and benefits of nerve blocks in individuals on blood thinners and those with abnormal coagulation and platelet function.

Local Anesthetic Systemic Toxicity

The deadliest and most feared complication of regional anesthesia is LAST. LAST classically presents as a spectrum of symptoms that begin shortly after injection of local anesthetic. Symptoms typically progress from mild symptoms such as perioral paresthesias to more severe neurologic sequelae (e.g., seizures, altered mental status), followed by cardiac complications (e.g., arrhythmias, hemodynamic instability) and subsequent cardiac arrest. However, patients may present with delayed symptoms or symptoms that do not follow the usual progression.[18] Early recognition allows for prompt treatment and improved outcomes. Treatment is largely supportive; however, patients presenting with life-threatening symptoms warrant consideration for early lipid emulsion therapy and venoarterial extracorporeal membrane oxygenation (VA-ECMO).

Despite the increase in the use of peripheral nerve blocks, the incidence of major complications from LAST has decreased over the past decade.[19,20] Reasons may include a greater recognition and earlier treatment of LAST and increased use of ultrasound.[11] While the incidence of LAST has decreased, the risk still exists and proper precautions should be undertaken. Furthermore, data on the incidence of LAST largely come from anesthesiology literature; given that anesthesiologists routinely perform peripheral nerve blocks and are well versed in recognition and avoidance of LAST, it is possible that emergency physicians (with more sporadic use of nerve blocks) might have a higher rate of complications. Multiple risk factors for LAST exist, including extremes of age, pregnancy, chronic conditions affecting

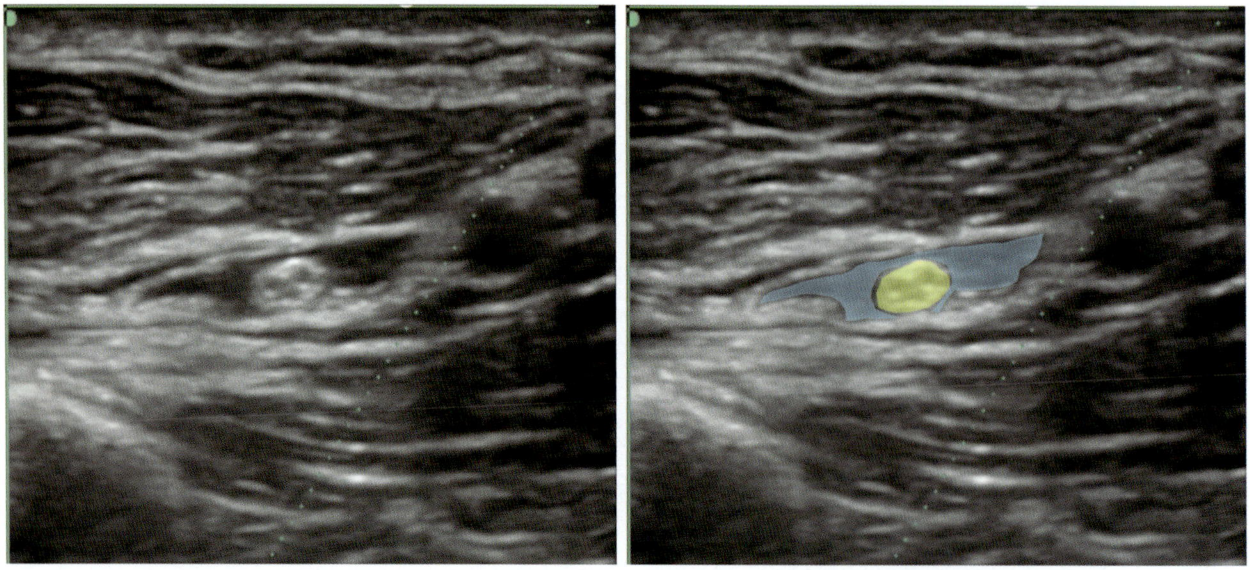

Fig. 31.4 Unlabeled and labeled ultrasound images showing a "halo" of local anesthetic *(blue)* encircling the ulnar nerve *(yellow)* in the mid-forearm, highly predictive of a successful block.

local anesthetic clearance (severe heart failure, renal or hepatic insufficiency), nerve block sites with higher rates of absorption, and large volumes of local anesthetic. As a general precaution, the minimum amount of local anesthetic should be used to achieve the desired effect. Other precautions include using ultrasound when indicated (see the following sections), injecting slowly to monitor for early signs and symptoms of LAST, and always aspirating before injecting local anesthetic. Any patient about to receive a block that poses a theoretical risk of LAST should have intravenous access, cardiac monitoring, and frequent assessments for early signs and symptoms of LAST. Appropriate resuscitative equipment and medications including lipid emulsion should be readily available.

THORACIC NERVE BLOCKS

The past decade has seen an increased utility of regional anesthesia of the thorax in the ED, spurred in part by the discovery and development of novel plane blocks. In this section, we describe three such blocks, which hold a myriad of uses for ED patients.

Previous editions of this chapter suggested the use of intercostal nerve blocks for analgesia of rib fracture-related pain. However, in our experience, this block is not routinely performed in the ED, perhaps secondary to the nonminimal risk of pneumothorax and the rise of alternative peripheral nerve blocks that may be safer and more efficacious.

Serratus Anterior Plane Block

Anatomy

The lateral cutaneous branches of the thoracic intercostal nerves lie in a fascial plane delineated by the latissimus dorsi muscle superficially and the deeper serratus anterior muscle. Beneath the serratus anterior muscle, the ribs and intercostal muscles are superficial to the pleural space.

Indications

The serratus anterior plane block (SAPB) was initially described in anesthesia literature in the perioperative management in breast surgery.[21] A successful block anesthetizes the lateral cutaneous branch of the thoracic intercostal nerve which provides sensory innervation to the anterolateral hemithorax (Fig. 31.5). Recent studies have demonstrated that SAPB is safe and effective for treating rib fracture-related pain in the ED.[22,23] Other potential indications include analgesia related to tube thoracostomy and even for herpes zoster neuralgia.[22]

Technique

The block is best performed with the patient either supine or in the lateral decubitus position with the targeted side facing up. A high-frequency linear (HFL) ultrasound probe is then positioned in the coronal or oblique plane in the midaxilla along the fifth rib (Fig. 31.6). A 20- to 22-gauge needle, with sufficient length (e.g., 3.5 inch) should be used. Using an in-plane approach, the needle is inserted to the depth of

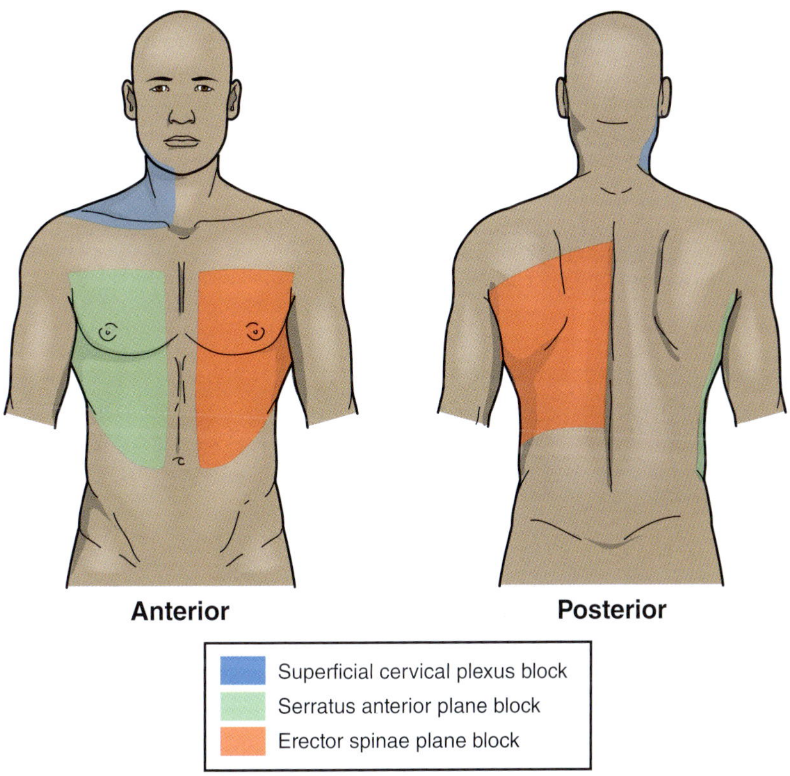

Fig. 31.5 Diagram showing areas of anesthesia provided by the superficial cervical plexus block, serratus anterior plane block, and erector spinae plane block. The superficial cervical plexus provides sensory loss spanning from the lower auricle of the ear to the clavicle. The serratus anterior plane block provides sensory loss to the anterior, lateral, and posterior hemithorax between approximately T2 and T9. The erector spinae plane block provides sensory loss to the anterior, lateral, and posterior hemithorax up to six dermatomes away from the level of the block.

the fascial layer between the serratus anterior and the latissimus dorsi muscles. Alternatively, the needle can be inserted deep to the serratus anterior muscle and superficial to the rib, using the rib as a target for the needle (Fig. 31.7). The deeper approach carries a higher theoretical risk of pneumothorax, but with the added benefit of a slightly larger area of sensory loss.[21] Inject approximately 20 to 30 mL of local anesthetic.

Complications and Precautions

Pneumothorax is a potential complication that can be avoided by using ultrasound and by targeting the more superficial plane.

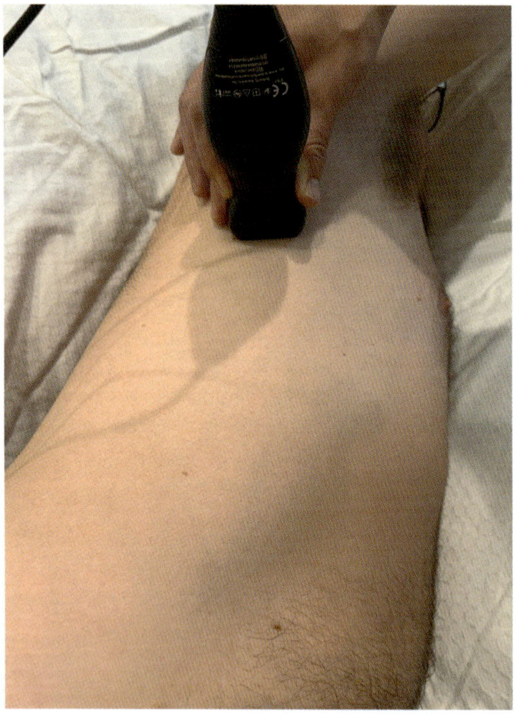

Fig. 31.6 The serratus anterior plane block is performed with the patient lying in a lateral decubitus (or upright) position with the ipsilateral arm abducted over their head. A linear, high-frequency ultrasound probe is placed in the transverse or coronal plane in the mid-axilla along the fifth rib.

Erector Spinae Plane Block

Anatomy

The erector spinae muscles run longitudinally along the length of the spine. Thoracic spinal nerves branch into the dorsal and ventral rami after exiting the intervertebral foramina. The dorsal rami travel posteriorly through the erector spinae muscles dividing into lateral and medial branches. The medial branches provide sensory innervation to the skin of the back. The ventral rami becomes the intercostal nerves, which divide into anterior cutaneous and lateral cutaneous branches that provide sensory innervation to the anterior and lateral aspects of the hemithorax, respectively.[24]

Indications

Cadaveric studies demonstrate that the erector spinae plane block (ESPB) allows for the spread of local anesthetic to both dorsal and ventral rami of the thoracic nerve, providing sensory blockade of the posterior, lateral, and anterior hemithorax (see Fig. 31.5).[24] Like the SAPB, the ESPB can be performed in the ED to provide analgesia for rib fractures; however, it has the added theoretical advantage of providing analgesia for posterior rib fractures as well.[24] Other indications in the ED include tube thoracostomy, herpes zoster,[25,26] and renal colic.[27,28]

Technique

The block is performed with the patient lying prone, in the lateral decubitus position, or in an upright position. Place a HFL ultrasound transducer in a cephalocaudal orientation on the ipsilateral side at the desired sensory level (Fig. 31.8). Slide the ultrasound probe laterally and medially until the transverse process is visualized. Correct placement can be confirmed by differentiating the transverse process from the posterior rib, which is more rounded in appearance and further lateral. A 20- to 22-gauge needle, with sufficient length (e.g., 3.5 inch) should be used. The needle is inserted in-plane, typically from a cephalad to caudal direction and approximately 20 to 30 mL of local anesthetic is injected just superficial to the transverse vertebral process. Correct needle placement will demonstrate the erector spinae muscles elevating off the transverse process (Fig. 31.9). Local anesthetic should spread cephalad and caudad across multiple vertebrae, providing sensory blockade across multiple levels.

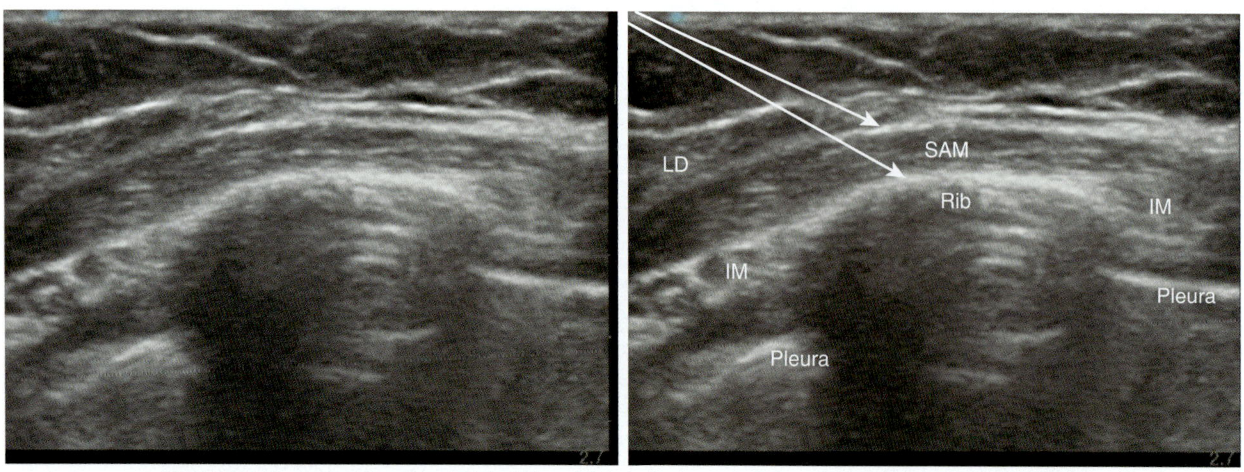

Fig. 31.7 Ultrasound images (unlabeled and labeled) demonstrating the anatomy of the serratus anterior plane block; the probe marker is lateral. The two *arrows* indicate the typical needle trajectories that target either deep or superficial to the serratus anterior muscle *(SAM)*. *IM*, Intercostal muscle; *LD*, latissimus dorsi muscle.

Complications and Precautions

If performing an ESPB for herpes zoster-mediated pain, the procedure should be moved 1 to 2 levels either superiorly or inferiorly to avoid needle insertion through vesicles.[25,26]

Superficial Cervical Plexus

Anatomy

The superficial cervical plexus (SCP) originates from the anterior rami of the C1-C4 spinal nerves before branching into greater auricular, lesser occipital, transverse cervical, and suprascapular nerves.[29] At the posterolateral border of the sternocleidomastoid (SCM) muscle, the SCP runs deep to the SCM and superficial to the levator scapulae and middle scalene muscles. Importantly, the prevertebral fascia divides the SCP from the deeper cervical plexus.

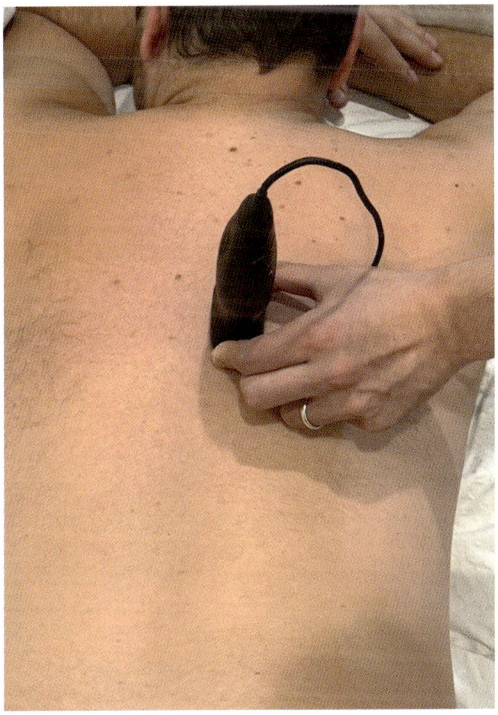

Fig. 31.8 The erector spinae plane block is performed with the patient lying in a prone, lateral decubitus, or upright position. A linear ultrasound transducer is placed in a cephalocaudal orientation on the ipsilateral side at the desired sensory level.

Indications

Successful blockade of the SCP provides anesthesia to the anterolateral aspect of the neck, ear, clavicle, and shoulder (see Fig. 31.5). Indications for a SCP block include neck laceration repair, clavicular fracture, and placement of an internal jugular catheter.[29] There have no randomized controlled trials studying the SCP block; however, a prospective observational study found a reduction in pain scores for ED patients with cervical pain, clavicle fractures, acromioclavicular joint injuries, radicular pain, and rotator cuff disorders after the block.[30]

Technique

The patient is positioned in the supine position with the head rotated to the contralateral side to expose the landmarks. With the ultrasound in the transverse orientation at the level of the thyroid cartilage (Fig. 31.10), the SCM is located superficial to the internal jugular vein and carotid artery. The probe is then slid laterally to identify the fascial plane deep to the SCM muscle and superficial to the levator scapula muscle (Fig. 31.11). A 25-gauge, short (e.g., 5 cm) needle is then inserted from lateral to medial using an in-plane technique. Once positioned within the fascial plane, 2 to 15 mL of local anesthetic is injected to target the SCP.

Complications and Precautions

Potential complications can result from accidental puncture of the internal jugular vein or carotid artery. This is best avoided by using ultrasound to visualize the needle tip at all times. Spread of the anesthetic can cause inadvertent blockade to deeper surrounding nerves including the brachial plexus, phrenic nerve, recurrent laryngeal nerve, and deep cervical plexus.[29] This rarely results in paralysis of the diaphragm (from phrenic nerve blockade) and transient hoarseness (from

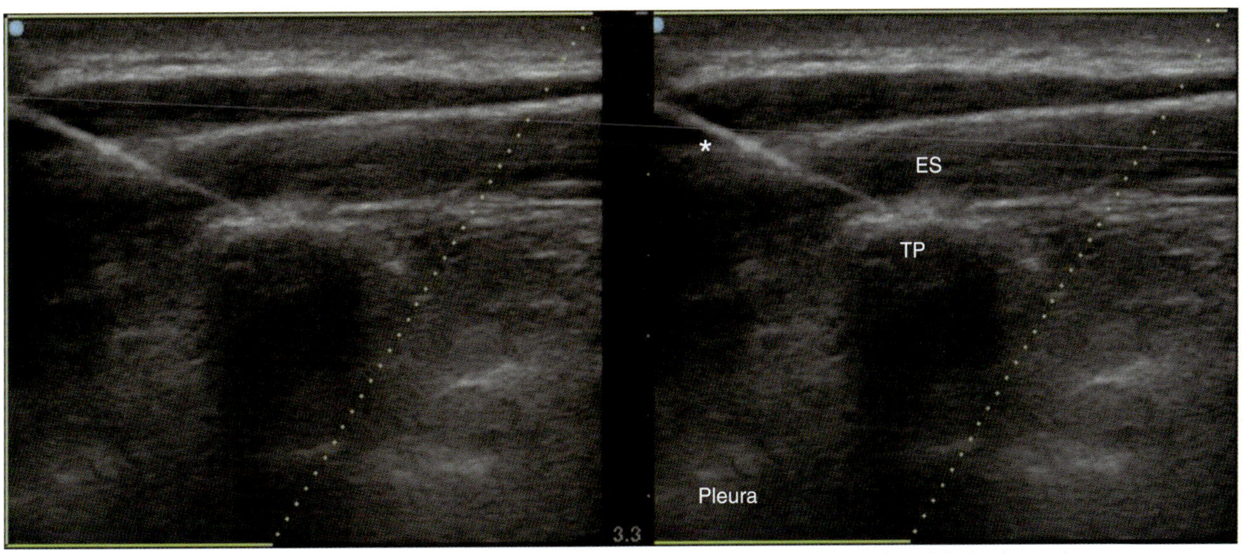

Fig. 31.9 Ultrasound images (unlabeled and labeled) of the erector spinae plane block; the probe marker is cephalad. The needle *(asterisk)* is inserted in-plane from cephalad to caudal and targets the plane deep to the erector spinae muscle *(ES)* and superficial to the transverse process *(TP)*.

recurrent laryngeal blockade).[30] A case of transient Horner syndrome has been described after performing a SCP block.[31]

UPPER EXTREMITY NERVE BLOCKS

See Videos 31.4 and 31.5. Hand and arm injuries are common in the ED, and therefore the need to provide anesthesia to control pain and facilitate procedures for these injuries is great. Local infiltration of anesthetic is an option that may be limited by the volume of anesthesia required (e.g., in cases of extensive lacerations), or for injuries of the palm where the spread of local anesthesia is limited by fibrous septa. Major joint dislocations (shoulder and elbow) of the upper extremity that might otherwise require procedural sedation can also be treated by nerve blocks.

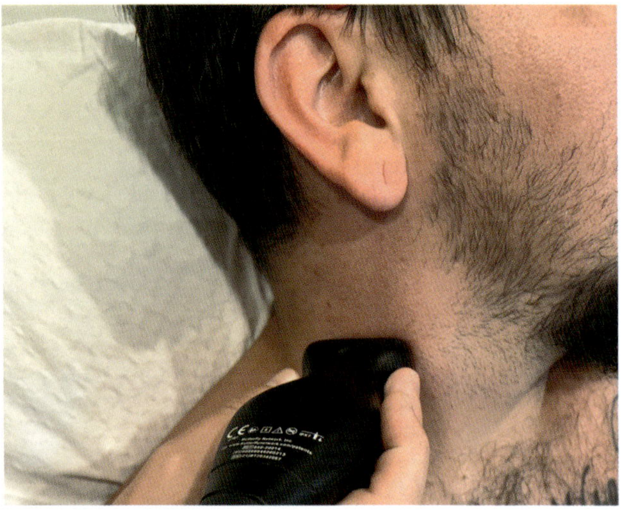

Fig. 31.10 The patient is positioned in the supine position with the head rotated to the contralateral side. A linear, high-frequency ultrasound probe is placed in the transverse orientation at the level of the thyroid cartilage.

Interscalene Brachial Plexus

See Video 31.6.

Anatomy

The targets of the interscalene brachial plexus are the C5, C6, and C7 nerve roots. C5 and C6 lie between the anterior and middle scalene muscles, while the C7 root is located inferiorly. Superficial landmarks include the SCM muscle, the SCP, and the prevertebral plexus. Importantly, the phrenic nerve lies just superficial to the anterior scalene muscle and is commonly blocked with the interscalene brachial plexus block.

Indications

The interscalene brachial plexus block anesthetizes nerve roots C5–C7 providing anesthesia to the shoulder and lateral aspect of the arm (Fig. 31.12). Indications for the block in the ED include shoulder dislocation (eliminating the need for procedural sedation), humerus fractures, and laceration repair or incision and drainage over the deltoid. When compared with procedural sedation for shoulder reduction, the interscalene brachial plexus block has been shown to reduce ED length of stay and healthcare provider one-on-one time.[32]

Technique

The procedure is performed by positioning the patient in a supine or upright position with the head rotated to the contralateral side (Fig. 31.13). Place a HFL ultrasound transducer in the transverse position at the level of the thyroid cartilage, observing the internal jugular vein and carotid artery deep to the SCM. Slide the transducer laterally to identify the anterior and middle scalene muscles. The C5, C6, and C7 roots of the interscalene brachial plexus appear

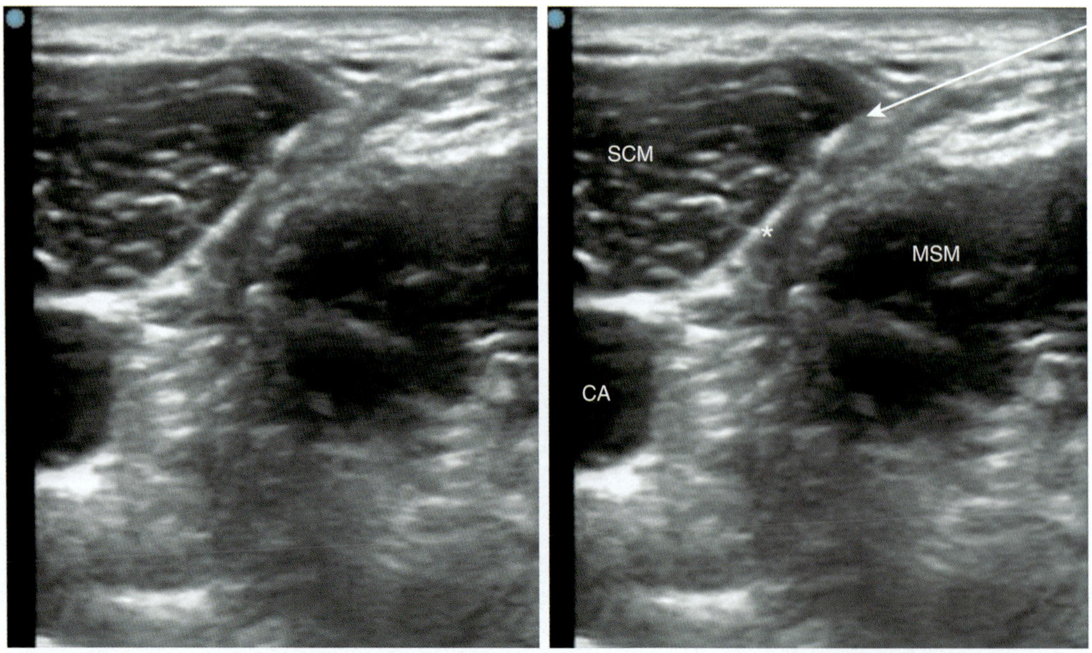

Fig. 31.11 Ultrasound images (unlabeled and labeled) showing anatomy of the superficial cervical plexus *(asterisk)* block; probe marker is medial. The *arrow* indicates the typical needle trajectory for a superficial cervical plexus block just deep to the posterolateral border of the sternocleidomastoid muscle *(SCM)*. *CA*, Carotid artery; *MSM*, middle scalene muscle.

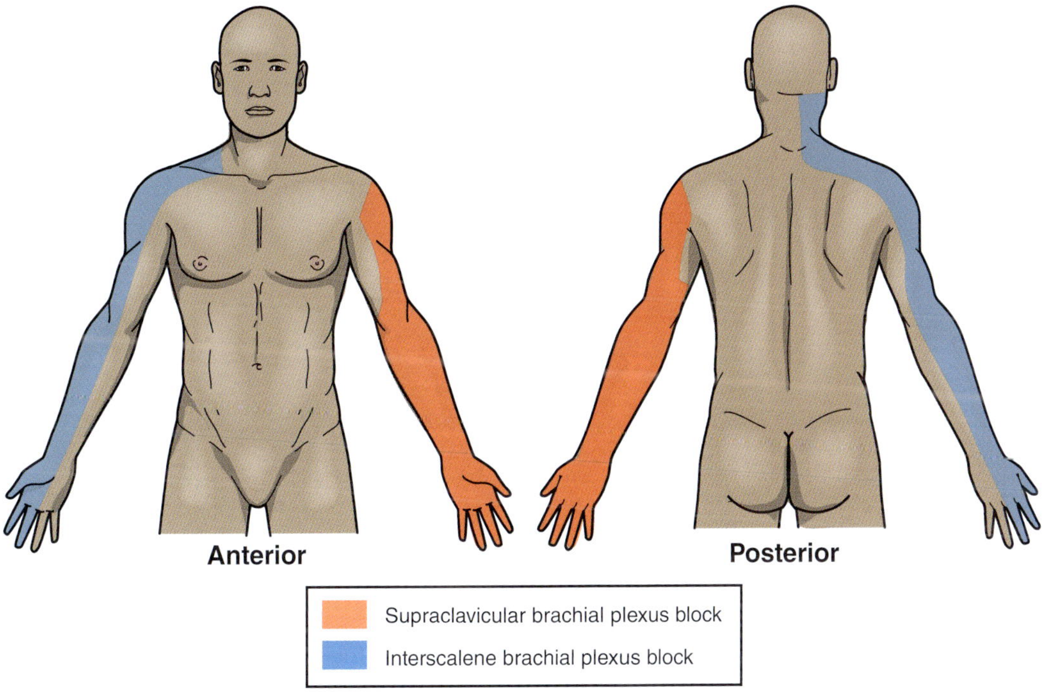

Fig. 31.12 Distribution of anesthesia for upper extremity nerve blocks. The interscalene brachial plexus block provides sensory loss to the shoulder and lateral aspect of the arm. The supraclavicular brachial plexus block provides sensory loss to the lateral aspect of the arm.

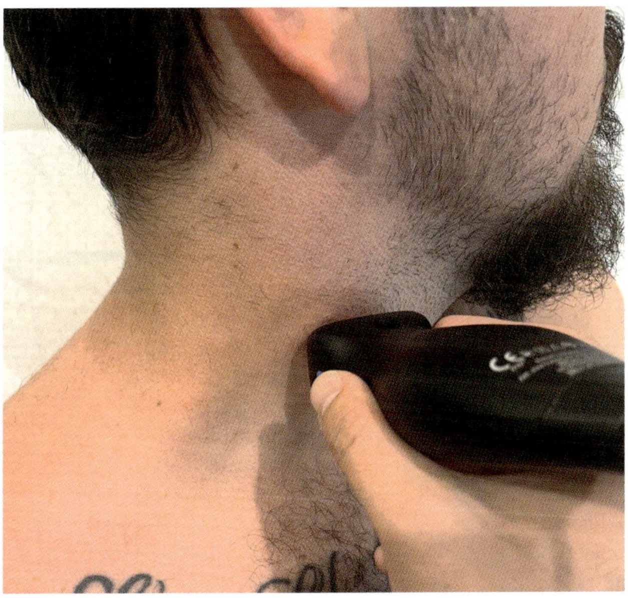

Fig. 31.13 The patient is positioned in the supine or upright position with the head rotated to the contralateral side. A linear ultrasound probe is placed in the transverse position, over the medial border of the sternocleidomastoid muscle at the level of the thyroid cartilage.

as a vertically stacked series of hypoechoic circular structures located between the anterior and middle scalene muscles (Fig. 31.14). Using in-plane visualization, insert a 22-gauge, 1.5-inch needle from lateral to medial, injecting a total of 10 to 30 mL of local anesthetic around the nerve roots to achieve the desired effect.

Complications and Precautions

Blockade of the interscalene brachial plexus reliably causes temporary ipsilateral phrenic nerve dysfunction and diaphragmatic paralysis. In patients with known preexisting lung disease (e.g., COPD), contralateral phrenic nerve dysfunction, or those at risk of respiratory compromise, extreme caution should be used before attempting this block. Pneumothorax can also occur because of accidental puncture of the pleura. The use of ultrasound guidance can minimize the risk of pneumothorax and can be used post-procedurally to assess for pneumothorax (see Chapter 68).

Supraclavicular Brachial Plexus

Anatomy

At the level of the clavicle, the brachial plexus divides into the upper, middle, and lower trunks. The upper trunk contains the C5 and C6 roots, the middle trunk contains the C7 root, and the lower trunk contains C8 and T1 roots. The brachial plexus is contained within a connective tissue nerve sheath. The first rib and lung pleura lie deep to the lower trunk of the brachial plexus.

Indications

The supraclavicular brachial plexus block is an alternate method of anesthetizing the brachial plexus, slightly distal to the interscalene approach. Like the interscalene approach, the supraclavicular brachial plexus block provides anesthesia to the arm and can be used for upper extremity fractures as well as anesthesia for skin and soft tissue repair, including in the deltoid region (see Fig. 31.12). Compared with the interscalene approach, the ultrasound anatomy for a supraclavicular brachial plexus block is easy to identify, making this a safe and efficacious block to perform in the ED. A small prospective randomized study in the ED comparing the supraclavicular brachial plexus block to procedural sedation for upper extremity injuries found that patients who received the block had a shorter length of stay.[33]

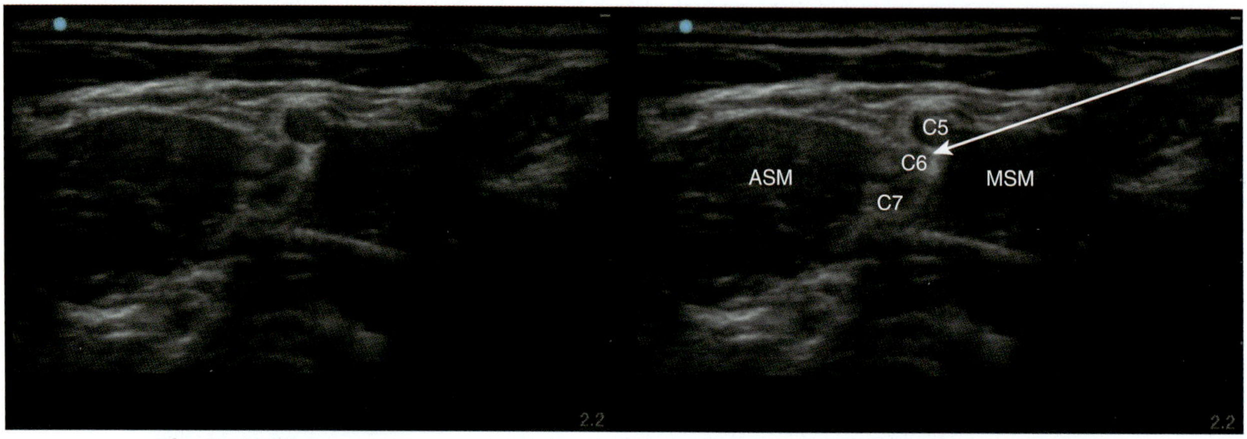

Fig. 31.14 Ultrasound images (unlabeled and labeled) showing the anatomy of the interscalene brachial plexus block; the probe marker is lateral. Roots C5–C7 lie between the anterior *(ASM)* and middle scalene muscles. The *arrow* indicates the typical needle trajectory in-plane coming from lateral to medial, through the middle scalene muscle and targeting the space between roots C5 and C6. *CA*, Carotid artery; *MSM*, middle scalene muscle.

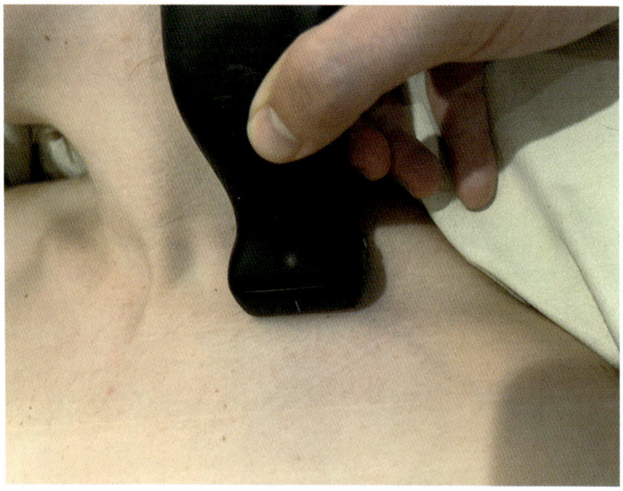

Fig. 31.15 The patient is positioned in the supine or upright position with the head rotated to the contralateral side. A linear ultrasound probe is placed parallel and superior to the mid-shaft of the clavicle.

Technique

To perform the block, the patient is positioned either in the supine or upright position with the head rotated to the contralateral side. A HFL ultrasound transducer is oriented parallel and superior to the mid-shaft of the clavicle (Fig. 31.15). The brachial plexus is identified just lateral to the subclavian artery, which in turn lies just lateral to the SCM muscle (Fig. 31.16). The first rib lies posterior to the neurovascular bundle and provides a safeguard against accidental puncture of the adjacent lung pleura. Color Doppler can be used to detect blood vessels within the brachial sheath, such as the dorsal scapular artery. Coming from a lateral approach with in-plane visualization, use approximately 20 to 30 mL of local anesthetic around the brachial plexus. Note, to anesthetize all three trunks, the needle may need to be repositioned between the trunks during the block.

Complications

Pneumothorax is a potential complication given the proximity of the pleura to the target of the block. The use of ultrasound guidance can minimize the risk of pneumothorax.

Nerve Blocks of the Forearm and Wrist

See Video 31.7. Sensation to the hand is provided by three peripheral nerves: the median, ulnar, and radial nerves, and their branches. While it is possible to block each of these nerves in a variety of locations, most commonly these blocks are performed in the volar mid-forearm ("forearm nerve block") or at the level of the wrist ("wrist block"). In general, a more proximal block (e.g., forearm) will produce anesthesia via fewer needle entries and redirections because a proximal block can be done before the nerve has given off its various sensory branches. Balanced against this is the fact that more proximal blocks will also produce more motor weakness from the unintended blockade of motor branches. With respect to forearm and wrist blocks, the difference is not likely to be clinically relevant since the bulk of gross motor function of the hand is supplied by forearm musculature which is innervated proximal to the location of these nerve blocks.

The radial, ulnar, and median nerves supply cutaneous and osseous sensation to the hand, and these nerves can be blocked, singly or in combination, in either the forearm or at the wrist, to provide anesthesia for a variety of conditions, including hand fractures and dislocations, lacerations and other soft tissue injuries, foreign body removal, and peripheral neuropathic pain.[34–39] Awareness of the sensory distribution of each peripheral nerve will enable the operator to choose the appropriate nerve(s) to block (Fig. 31.17).

In the forearm, ultrasound easily identifies the nerves to facilitate a forearm nerve block. In the wrist, each nerve courses in a predictable location with respect to surface anatomy, such that anatomical landmarks may be used to produce a reliable wrist block. Nevertheless, forearm nerve blocks using ultrasound have been shown to have greater success than landmark-based wrist blocks.[40] Wrist blocks have similar effectiveness to local infiltration at the site of injury, but may require fewer needle insertions to achieve anesthesia.[41]

Knowledge of the course of these peripheral nerves in the anatomical area where the block will be performed is an essential prerequisite to obtaining a successful nerve block. We will discuss each nerve individually, proceeding from proximal (forearm) to distal (wrist).

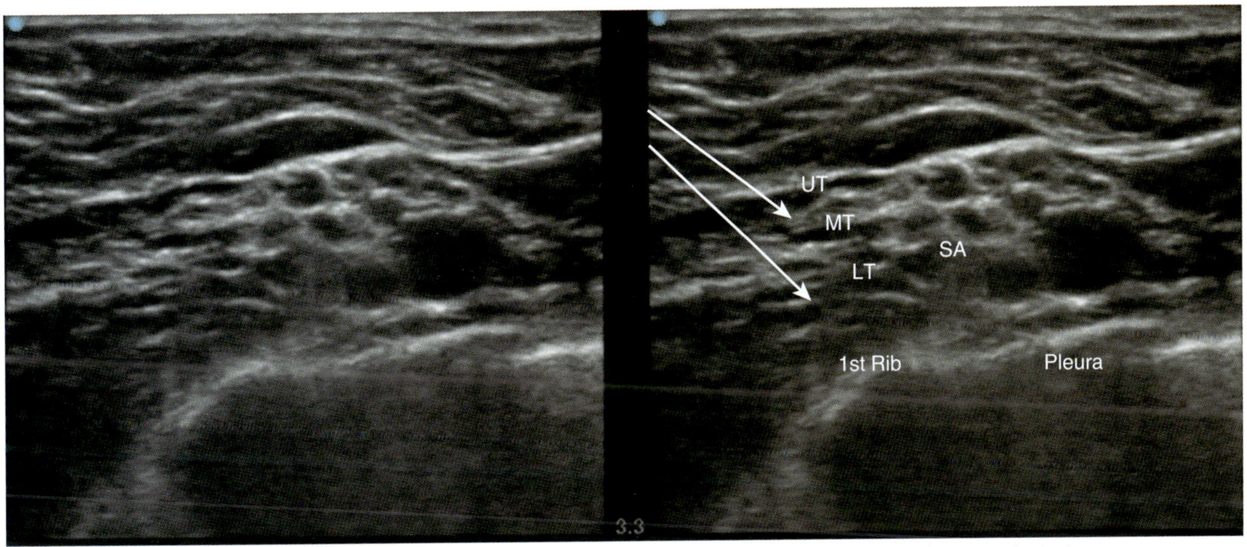

Fig. 31.16 Ultrasound images (unlabeled and labeled) showing the anatomy of the supraclavicular brachial plexus; the probe marker is lateral. The *arrows* indicate the typical needle trajectories in-plane coming from lateral to medial, targeting the space between the (1) upper *(UT)* and middle trunks *(MT)* and (2) the lower trunk *(LT)*. *SA*, Subclavian artery.

Median Nerve

See Video 31.8.

Anatomy

See Fig. 31.18. Upon entering the forearm, the median nerve initially accompanies the ulnar artery before the latter heads medially to travel with the ulnar nerve. By the time it has reached the mid-forearm, the median nerve lies between two volar muscle groups: the flexor digitorum superficialis (FDS) and flexor digitorum profundus (FDP) (Fig. 31.19).

As it approaches the wrist and assumes a more superficial location, the median nerve is situated between the palmaris longus and flexor carpi radialis tendons. It first gives rise to a *palmar cutaneous branch*, which exits from the radial side of the median nerve an average of 4 cm to 8 cm proximal to the volar wrist crease.[42] The palmar cutaneous branch of the median nerve crosses the wrist outside the carpal tunnel and supplies sensation to the lateral (radial) surface of the palm.

After passing through the carpal tunnel, the median nerve gives rise to the *palmar digital branch*, which innervates the palmar surface and nail beds of the lateral (radial) 3½ digits.

Because of the early sensory (palmar cutaneous) branch, it is beneficial to block the median nerve some distance before the carpal tunnel to obtain a block of both cutaneous sensory branches.

Technique: Median Nerve Block at the Forearm

Place a HFL ultrasound transducer in a transverse plane at the mid-forearm (Fig. 31.20) and identify the hypoechoic FDS and FDP muscles, separated by a fascial plane running horizontally on the screen. The median nerve is a hyperechoic, oval structure with a honeycomb appearance (Fig. 31.21). Fanning the probe will cause the nerve to alternate between hypoechoic and hyperechoic due to changes in the beam angle relative to the nerve (see Chapter 68). When the beam angle is perpendicular to the nerve, it will be easiest to identify (hyperechoic) and block. Use an in-plane approach, directing the needle to an area immediately adjacent to the median nerve, with the goal of obtaining spread of anesthesia around the nerve. A total of 3 to 5 mL of local anesthetic is used.

Technique: Median Nerve Block at the Wrist

To block the median nerve at the level of the wrist, first identify the palmaris longus and flexor carpi radialis tendons. The palmaris longus tendon, which may be unilaterally or bilaterally absent in a small percentage of the population, can be more easily palpated by asking the patient to flex the wrist while opposing the small finger and thumb (Fig. 31.22). The flexor carpi radialis tendon lies just lateral (radial) to the palmaris longus tendon. It becomes more prominent when the wrist is flexed and radially deviated. Insert the needle at a 45-degree angle between these two tendons approximately 2.5 cm proximal to the wrist crease with the needle directed distally (Fig. 31.23A). Advance the needle approximately 3 to 5 mm, or until a pop is felt indicating entry into the appropriate fascial plane. Inject a total of 3 to 5 mL of local anesthetic. Alternatively, inject perpendicular to the skin at the proximal wrist crease up to 1 cm deep (Fig. 31.24).

Ulnar Nerve

See Video 31.9.

Anatomy

See Fig. 31.18. In the proximal forearm, the ulnar nerve is located deep to the flexor carpi ulnaris muscle. It is soon joined by the ulnar artery in the mid-forearm and both continue distally (see Fig. 31.19). *The ulnar nerve is ulnar to the ulnar artery*. Approximately 5 cm proximal to the wrist, the ulnar nerve branches into a *dorsal cutaneous branch* (sensory to the small finger and ulnar aspect of the ring finger) which runs along the ulnar posterior wrist.[43]

The ulnar nerve then continues as the *palmar branch* (sensory to the medial palm), crossing the wrist lateral to the pisiform bone and flexor carpi ulnaris tendon, and lying medial

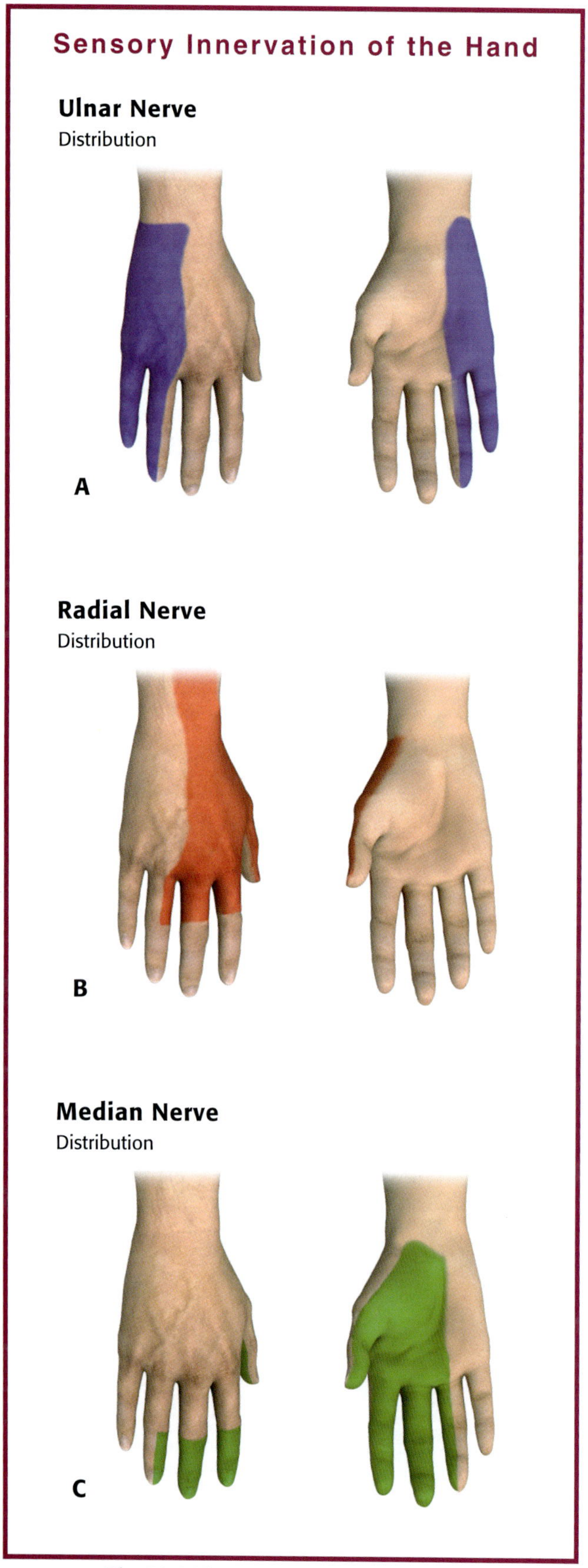

Fig. 31.17 Sensory innervation of the hand.

to the ulnar artery (see Fig. 31.24). Blocking the ulnar nerve at the mid-forearm is proximal to this bifurcation, allowing for complete anesthesia in the ulnar distribution with a single injection.

Technique: Ulnar Nerve Block at the Forearm

Place a HFL ultrasound transducer in a transverse plane at the volar wrist to identify the ulnar artery. Center the ulnar artery on the screen and slide the transducer proximally toward the mid-forearm (see Fig. 31.20). The ulnar nerve is a comet tail–shaped hyperechoic structure with a honeycomb appearance just medial (ulnar) to the artery (Fig. 31.25). The nerve gets slightly larger as the probe slides from the wrist to the mid-forearm. The optimal location to perform the block is roughly between the proximal one-third and middle one-third of the forearm.[44] In this location, the nerve is more superficial and somewhat separate from the artery. Using an in-plane approach, direct the needle from medial to lateral, aiming to bathe the nerve in local anesthetic. Approximately 3 to 5 mL of local anesthetic are sufficient.

Since the ulnar nerve is in a medial position in the forearm, and one approaches the block using a medial-to-lateral needle insertion, this poses an ergonomic challenge if the patient has their arms at their sides: the operator must position themself in-between the patient's body and the patient's arm to perform this block. This obstacle can be overcome by having the patient's arm abducted to 90 degrees or more, thus freeing up space for the operator to position themself. Alternatively, the patient can flex at the elbow, allowing the operator to advance the needle more comfortably while facing the patient.

Technique: Ulnar Nerve Block at the Wrist

Identify the tendon of the flexor carpi ulnaris muscle, palpable immediately proximal to the pisiform bone. Ask the patient to flex and ulnar deviate the wrist to make this tendon more prominent.

Insert a needle perpendicular to the skin in a coronal plane, just proximal to the pisiform bone and underneath the flexor carpi ulnaris tendon (see Fig. 31.23C). Advance the needle to a depth of no more than 0.5 cm to 1 cm and inject a total of 3 mL to 5 mL of local anesthetic.

To cover the dorsal cutaneous branch, insert the needle in a subcutaneous plane on the dorsal wrist, aiming just beyond the ulnar styloid. As the needle is slowly withdrawn, inject an additional 5 mL to 6 mL of local anesthetic as a subcutaneous wheal.[45]

Radial Nerve

Anatomy

See Fig. 31.18. Upon entering the forearm, the radial nerve divides into a deep motor branch (posterior interosseous nerve) and the *superficial branch*, a sensory nerve that provides cutaneous innervation to the dorsum of the hand. A radial nerve block at the forearm or further distally targets only the superficial (sensory) branch, leaving motor function intact.

In the mid-forearm, the superficial branch of the radial nerve runs adjacent to the radial artery (see Fig. 31.19). *The radial nerve is radial to the radial artery*. By the time it reaches the distal forearm and wrist, the radial nerve diverges from the artery and heads dorsally, passing in the subcutaneous tissue of the anatomic snuffbox before innervating most of the dorsal hand, including the web space between thumb and index finger (see Fig. 31.24).[46]

Technique: Radial Nerve Block at the Forearm

Place a HFL ultrasound transducer in a transverse plane at the volar wrist to identify the radial artery. Center the radial artery on the screen and slide the transducer proximally toward the mid-forearm (see Fig. 31.20), paying

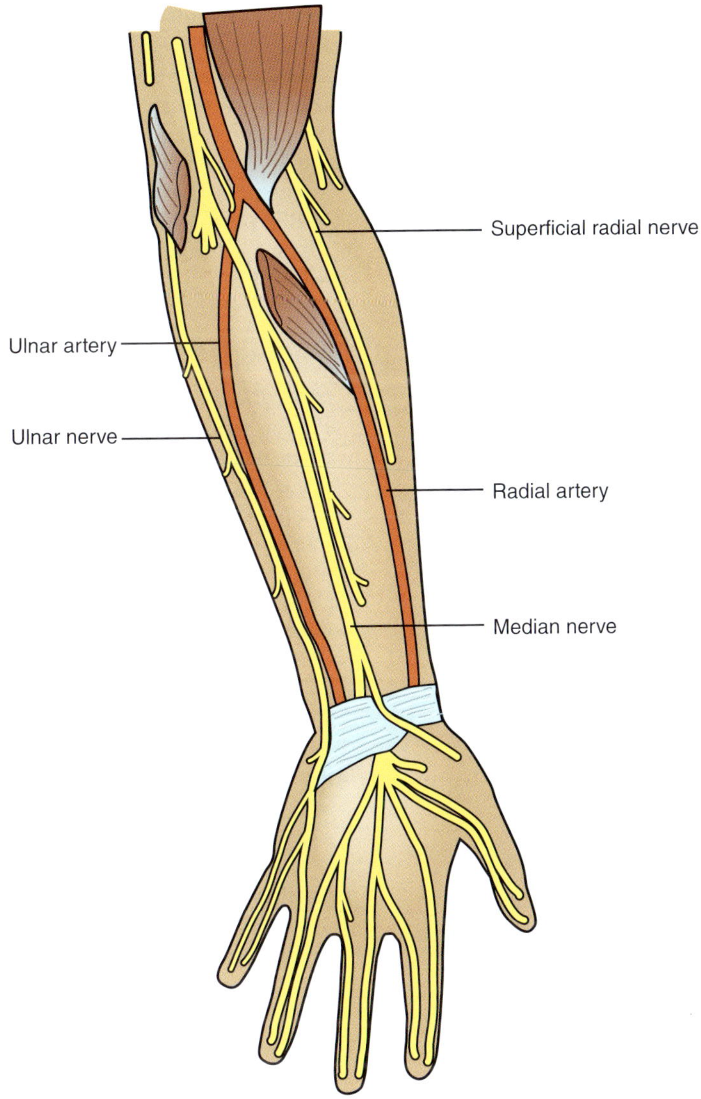

Fig. 31.18 Peripheral nerves of the forearm and wrist.

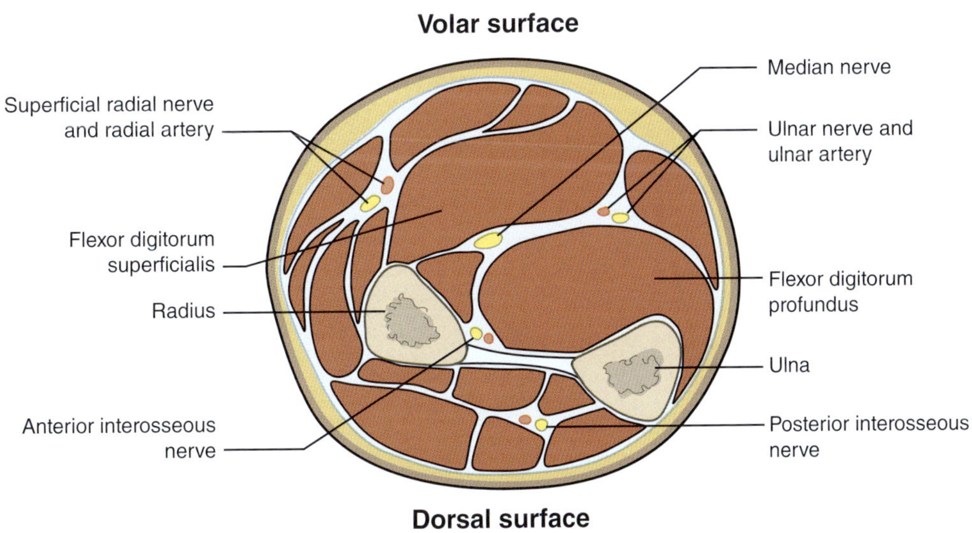

Fig. 31.19 Cross-sectional anatomy of the mid-forearm showing location of the peripheral nerves to the hand.

attention to the lateral (radial) aspect of the artery. As the probe is moved proximally, the radial nerve appears as a hyperechoic structure immediately radial to the artery with characteristic honeycomb pattern in a comet tail shape (Fig. 31.26). Using an in-plane approach, direct the needle from lateral to medial, aiming to bathe the nerve in local anesthetic. Approximately 3 to 5 mL of local anesthetic is sufficient.

Technique: Radial Nerve Block at the Wrist

The area of intended local anesthetic deposition is near the proximal border of the anatomic snuffbox, which can be assessed by abducting the patient's thumb to identify its borders: extensor pollicis longus (medial) and extensor pollicis brevis (lateral) (Fig. 31.27).[47] Insert a needle approximately 3 cm proximal to the radial styloid just lateral to the radial artery pulsation and inject 2 to 5 mL of local anesthetic. Next, direct the needle in a subcutaneous plane angling dorsally, and inject 5 to 6 mL of local anesthetic in a wheal as the needle is withdrawn (see Fig. 31.23B).[45,48] When performing a radial nerve block at the wrist, be careful not to puncture the radial artery or the superficially located cephalic vein.

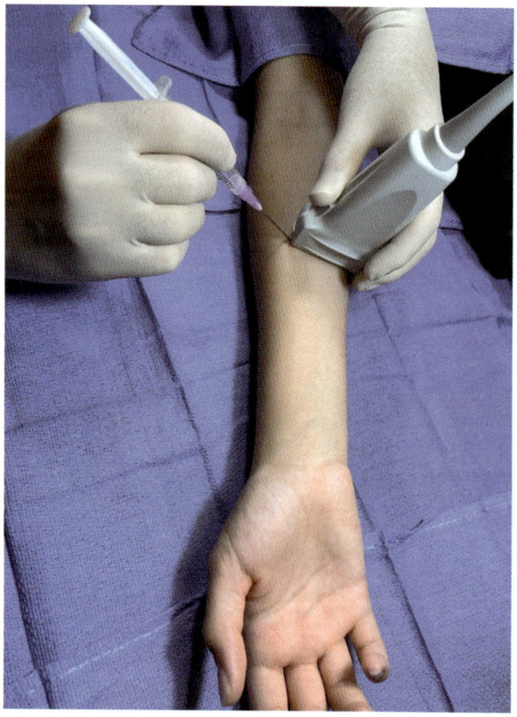

Fig. 31.20 Ultrasound probe placement for forearm nerve blocks. Blocks are performed at the mid-to-proximal forearm. The exact position of the probe will vary depending on the nerve being targeted.

Digital Nerve Blocks of the Hand

Indications

Finger maladies including lacerations, crush injuries, fractures, dislocations, foreign bodies, and infections are common occurrences in the ED; therefore anesthesia to the finger is frequently required, both for pain control as well as to facilitate procedures. Local infiltration of anesthetic into an injured finger may be problematic for many reasons. First, due to abundant nerve endings (especially at the tip of the finger), injections may be extremely painful. Additionally, the small size of a finger limits its ability to accommodate additional volume from local infiltration, particularly if the finger is already swollen due to injury. The finger pad contains fibrous septa oriented perpendicular to the underlying bone that limit the spread of local anesthetic. Furthermore, injecting fluid into a small space may distort tissue and render it challenging to repair.

Anatomy

Anesthesia to the finger can be accomplished quite readily by means of a digital nerve block (DNB). Innervation to the finger is supplied via four digital nerves, including two each on the ulnar and radial aspects of the finger (palmar/volar and dorsal respectively) (Fig. 31.28). The palmar nerves are located roughly at 4 o'clock and 8 o'clock, and the dorsal nerves are found at 2 o'clock and 10 o'clock. Blocking these nerves will provide complete anesthesia for any procedure on the finger, and will also relieve pain from an injury occurring to the phalanges or soft tissues of the finger (Fig. 31.29).[41]

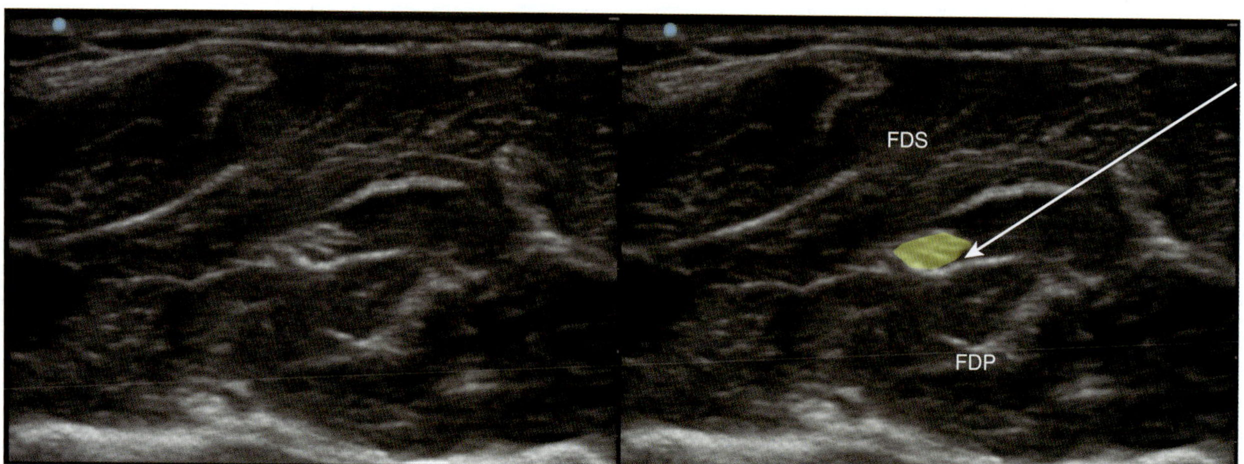

Fig. 31.21 Ultrasound images (unlabeled and labeled) showing median nerve anatomy in the volar mid-forearm. The median nerve *(yellow)* lies between two flexor muscles. The *arrow* indicates the typical needle trajectory for a forearm median nerve block. *FDS*, Flexor digitorum superficialis; *FDP*, flexor digitorum profundus.

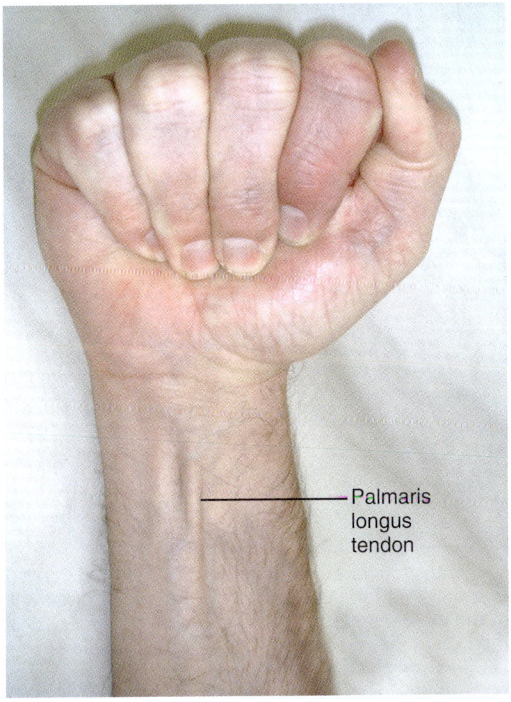

Fig. 31.22 Flexing the wrist with the thumb and small finger opposed will accentuate the appearance of palmaris longus tendon.

Technique

Several methods of DNB have been described, and the choice of which type of block to perform will be influenced by the patient's injury and provider familiarity with the various block techniques. Each technique is described separately in the following sections.

Complications and Precautions

A recent meta-analysis compared the efficacy of three of these techniques: the traditional dorsal DNB, the transthecal palmar DNB, and the subcutaneous palmar DNB. Time to onset of anesthesia, patient perception of pain during the injection, and failure to achieve complete anesthesia (requiring rescue injections) were similar for all three techniques.[49] The palmar techniques (transthecal and subcutaneous) are more likely to provide inadequate anesthesia to the dorsal aspect of the proximal phalanx, so injuries in this area are best approached with a traditional dorsal DNB.[50–52] For other locations of pain or injury, given that the palmar approaches to DNB involve one injection rather than two, it seems reasonable to use these approaches barring other factors.

Historically, it has been recommended to avoid lidocaine with epinephrine when performing a digital block for fear of provoking an excessive degree of vasoconstriction, resulting in digital necrosis. Recent reviews of the literature find no evidence of an adverse effect of lidocaine plus epinephrine in typical, low-dose (i.e., 1:100,000 to 1:200,000) concentrations for DNBs. However, there is a paucity of studies involving patients with poor peripheral circulation, thus limiting the ability to draw conclusions regarding the use of epinephrine combined with local anesthetic for this patient population.[4,53] Until further data are available, it seems prudent to avoid the use of epinephrine when performing digital blocks in patients with impaired circulation unless there are compelling reasons to use it. If there is concern for finger ischemia after performing a DNB, treatment options include warm water immersion, topical nitroglycerin, and phentolamine (see Chapter 29).

"Traditional" Dorsal Digital Nerve Block

The traditional dorsal technique involves injections at the ulnar and radial aspect of the finger. With the patient's hand positioned palm down on a flat surface, insert a small (e.g., 25-gauge) needle starting at either the 10 o'clock or 2 o'clock positions on the dorsal aspect of the finger at the base of the proximal phalanx (approximately 2 mm to 3 mm lateral to the midline) just distal to the metacarpophalangeal (MCP) joint. Directing the needle alongside the proximal phalanx and aiming toward the palmar aspect of the hand, enter the web space. Inject 0.5 to 1 mL of local anesthetic initially for the dorsal digital nerve, then an additional 0.5 mL to 1 mL as the needle is advanced and then withdrawn to anesthetize the volar digital nerve. Repeat this process on the opposite side of the finger so that both the ulnar and radial sides of the finger have been injected (Fig. 31.30A).

A variation on this technique involves redirecting the needle 90 degrees after the first injection is complete but before withdrawing the needle completely. In this way, the second needle puncture site can be anesthetized prior to being punctured, potentially making the procedure more tolerable (see Fig. 31.30B).

An advantage of this approach includes providing better anesthesia to the dorsal aspect of the thumb and fingers than the volar approaches to DNB.[54] Although the block is generally well tolerated, this version of the DNB does require two injections rather than a single-needle puncture, therefore it might be less preferred by needle-phobic patients. There is also a risk of neurovascular injury with the tip of the needle.

Transthecal Volar Digital Nerve Block

See Video 31.10. The transthecal technique uses a single injection at the volar surface of the base of the finger to enter the flexor tendon sheath with the tip of the needle, allowing local anesthetic to diffuse along the flexor tendon sheath to reach the distal-most aspect of the finger. Anesthetic diffuses throughout the finger including along the digital nerves. Various versions of this technique have been described, differing in their choice of anatomic landmarks and depth of needle insertion (see Fig. 31.31C).

In the original description of this technique, the flexor tendon of the finger to be anesthetized is palpated as it glides over the metacarpal head in the distal palm. At this point, the needle is inserted through the skin until a difference in resistance alerts the operator that the needle has entered the tendon sheath, at which point local anesthetic is infused. If the operator has overshot and the needle tip lies within the tendon, resistance to flow will signal the operator to slowly withdraw the needle until anesthesia can easily be administered.[55]

A subsequent modification simplified the technique by using surface landmarks only. According to this method, the needle enters the skin in the palmar midline of the finger at the palmar digital crease. The needle is directed through both flexor tendons until contact with bone is made. At this point, the needle is slowly withdrawn while gentle pressure is applied to the syringe plunger. Easy flow of local anesthetic heralds a successful placement of local anesthetic in the tendon sheath; any resistance

Nerve Blocks at the Wrist

Median Nerve

Distribution

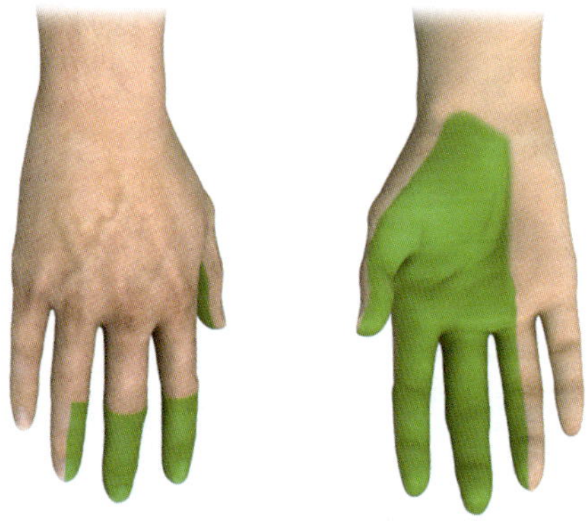

A

Anatomy and Technique

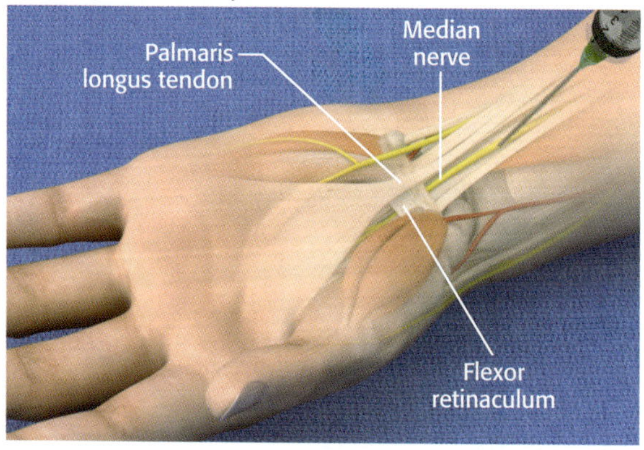

Locate the palmaris longus tendon and the adjacent (lateral) flexor carpi radialis tendon. At a point approximately 2.5 cm proximal to the wrist crease, insert a needle at 45 degrees between the two tendons. Feel for a "pop" as the needle enters the correct fascial plane (3-5 mm deep), then inject 3-5 mL of anesthetic.

Radial Nerve

Distribution

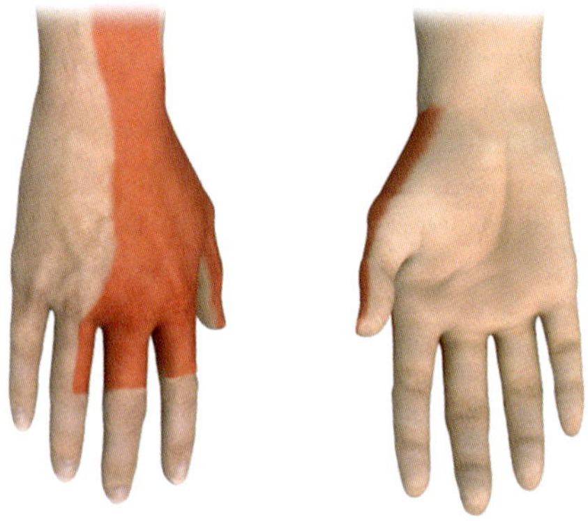

B

Anatomy and Technique

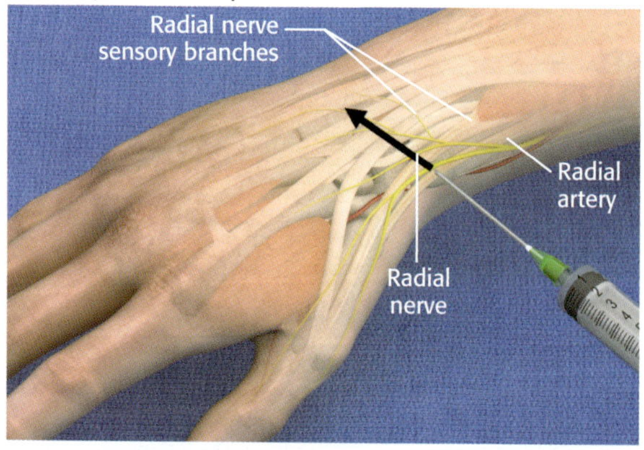

First inject 2 to 5 mL of anesthetic immediately lateral to the radial artery at the level of the proximal palmar crease (not shown). Then inject another 5 to 6 mL from the initial injection point to the dorsal midline.

Ulnar Nerve

Distribution

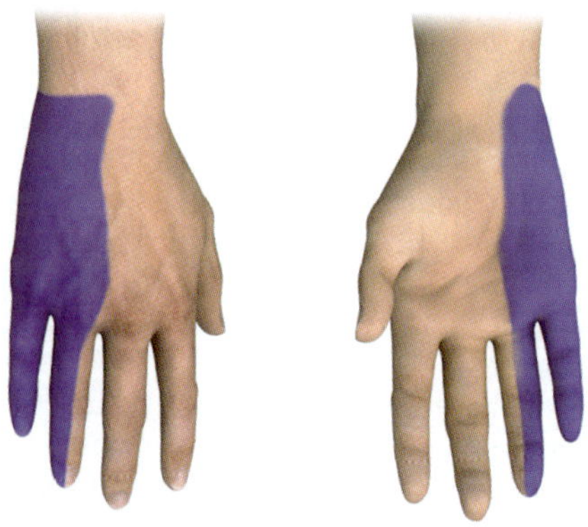

C

Anatomy and Technique

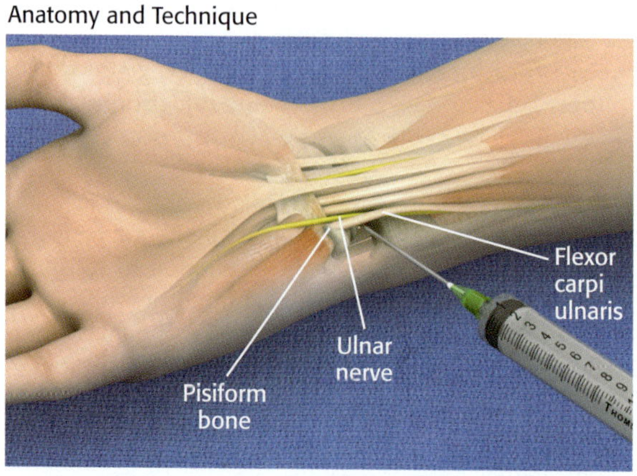

Insert the needle on the ulnar aspect of the wrist at the proximal palmar crease, under the flexor carpi ulnaris tendon. Inject 3 to 5 mL of anesthetic. Next, deposit 5 to 6 mL of anesthetic from the lateral border of the flexor carpi ulnaris to the dorsal midline (not shown).

Fig. 31.23 Landmark-guided wrist block for (A) median nerve, (B) radial nerve, and (C) ulnar nerve.

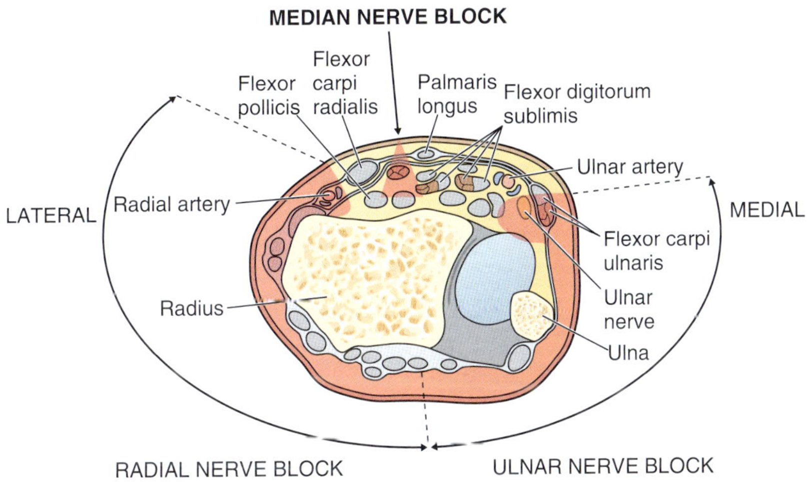

Fig. 31.24 Cross-sectional anatomy at the wrist demonstrating peripheral nerves to the hand. A complete wrist block will result in a horseshoe-shaped deposition of local anesthetic to block these nerves and their branches.

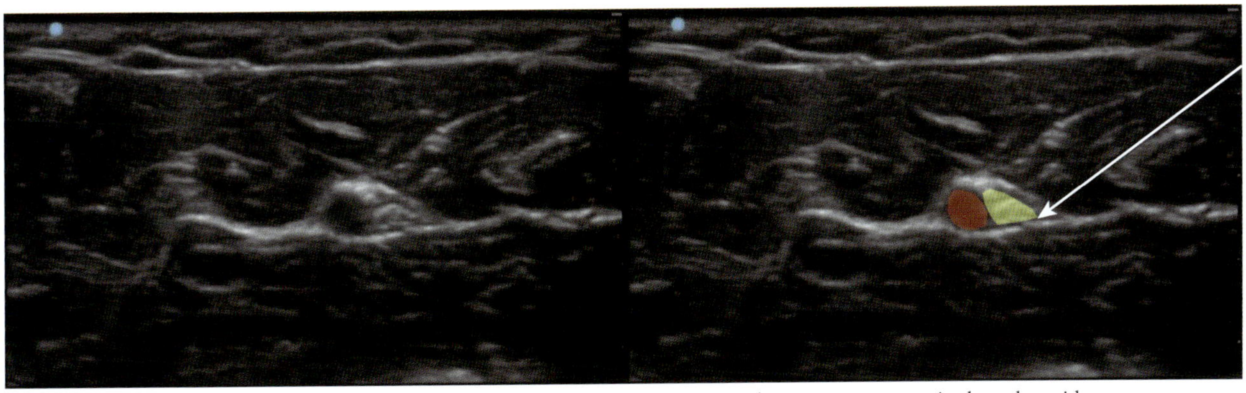

Fig. 31.25 Ultrasound images (unlabeled and labeled) showing ulnar nerve anatomy in the volar mid-forearm; probe marker is lateral. The ulnar nerve *(yellow)* is ulnar, or medial, to the ulnar artery *(red)*. The *arrow* indicates the typical needle trajectory for a forearm ulnar nerve block, approaching the nerve from the side opposite the artery.

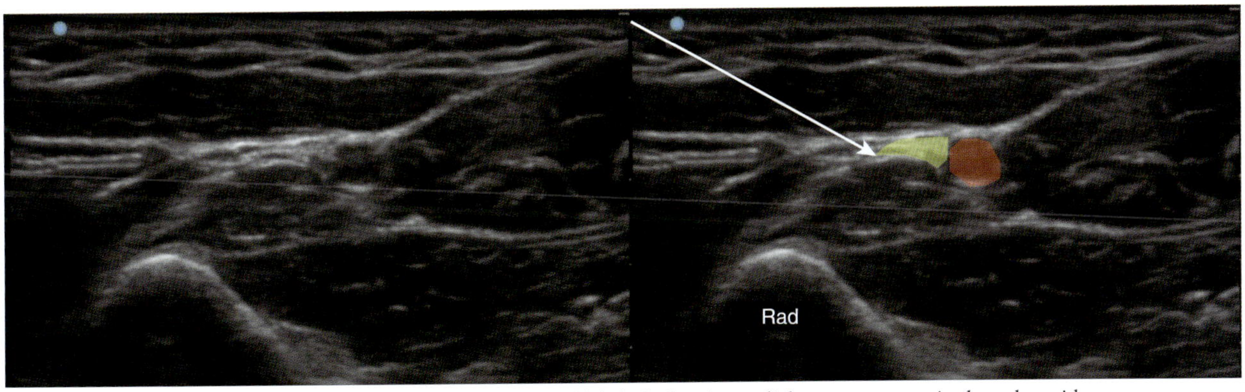

Fig. 31.26 Ultrasound images (unlabeled and labeled) showing radial nerve anatomy in the volar mid-forearm. The radial nerve *(yellow)* is radial, or lateral, to the radial artery *(red)*. The *arrow* indicates the typical needle trajectory for a forearm radial nerve block, approaching the nerve from the side opposite the artery. *Rad*, Radius.

to flow implies that the needle is either in contact with bone or within the tendon itself, rather than in the tendon sheath.[56]

In either scenario, begin by supinating the patient's hand. Avoid using force to inject anesthetic, as resistance to flow with even low pressure on the syringe plunger may indicate that the needle tip is within the flexor tendon rather than in the tendon sheath. A total volume of 2 mL of anesthetic is injected.[57] In children, smaller volumes (1 to 1.5 mL) have been reported.[58]

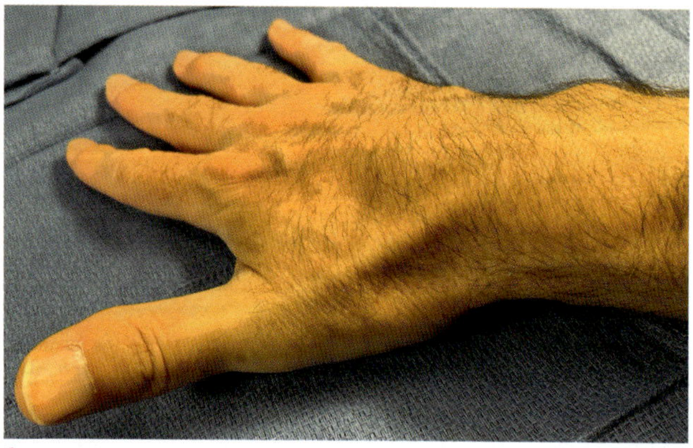

Fig. 31.27 The anatomic snuffbox, useful as a landmark to determine the location of the sensory branches of the radial nerve on the dorsum of the hand.

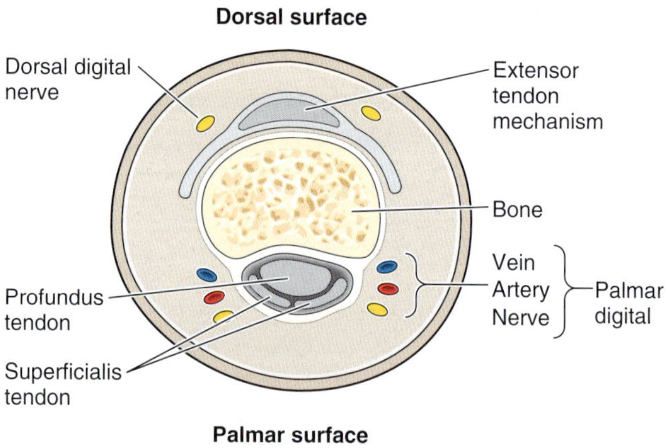

Fig. 31.28 Digital nerves as seen in cross section. Note the presence of two palmar (volar) and two dorsal nerves.

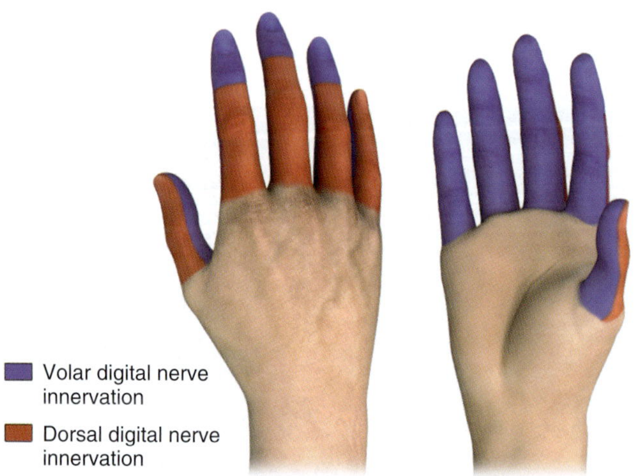

Fig. 31.29 Sensory innervation of the digital nerves. The palmar (volar) nerves also innervate the dorsal nail bed and distal phalanx.

Advantages of this approach include a single injection, a lower total volume of anesthetic, and a more rapid onset of anesthesia (approximately 3 to 4 minutes).[55] There is no risk of damage to the neurovascular bundle with this method; however, there is a potential risk of mechanical injury to the flexor tendon.

Volar Subcutaneous Digital Nerve Block

A further modification to the transthecal volar DNB is known as the volar subcutaneous block. It is like the transthecal approach in that the injection site is volar. However, rather than entering the flexor tendon sheath, the goal is to infiltrate the subcutaneous soft tissues superficial to the tendon sheath with local anesthetic. The anesthetic will then diffuse to anesthetize the digital nerves, particularly on the palmar side.[59]

Using a small-gauge needle, enter the skin at either the palmar digital crease at the base of the finger[59] or the volar aspect of the proximal phalanx.[60] Inject between 2 and 3.5 mL of anesthetic slowly into the subcutaneous space, superficial to the flexor tendon sheath (see Fig. 31.31D). Similar volumes were used in a pediatric series.[61] When larger volumes (approaching 3.5 mL) of anesthesia are used, the subcutaneous tissue of both the volar and dorsal surfaces of the base of the finger will feel moderately distended.[54,60]

Just as with the transthecal approach, this block may be better tolerated than the traditional dorsal block which requires two injections, and it poses no risk to the neurovascular bundle or the flexor tendon. In addition, some clinicians consider the volar subcutaneous block easier to perform than the traditional dorsal technique.[54] However, this method of DNB may be insufficient for injuries to the proximal dorsal finger, which are not always well anesthetized by this technique.[51,52,59]

Other Considerations

In the needle-phobic patient, other adjunct measures while performing a DNB might be considered. Vapocoolant spray may reduce pain associated with both needle entry and injection of anesthetic.[62] A jet injector (e.g., J-tip) to deliver anesthesia may also be useful in select patients to reduce the pain of injection while still delivering adequate anesthesia.[63]

LOWER EXTREMITY NERVE BLOCKS

The lumbosacral plexus and its branches, chief among them the femoral and sciatic nerves, innervate the leg and are targets for regional anesthesia for a variety of painful conditions seen in the ED. As ultrasound becomes more ubiquitous, several ultrasound-guided blocks are now well within the scope of emergency physicians, along with the traditional landmark-based blocks that also make up this section.

Hip fractures are of particular importance, as nerve blocks have become recognized as a safe and effective way to provide analgesia while decreasing or eliminating opioid use. A Cochrane review found that in addition to lower pain scores, patients who received nerve block for hip fractures were less likely to have an acute confusional state or develop a chest infection.[64]

Femoral Nerve Block

Anatomy

The femoral nerve lies lateral to the femoral artery and vein at the level of the femoral crease. The femoral nerve is located deep to two fascial planes: a superficial fascia lata, and a deeper layer, the fascia iliaca, which invests the iliopsoas muscle. Although the fascia iliaca contains the femoral nerve, the femoral artery and vein lie outside of this fascial plane. The sartorius muscle is superficial to the femoral nerve.

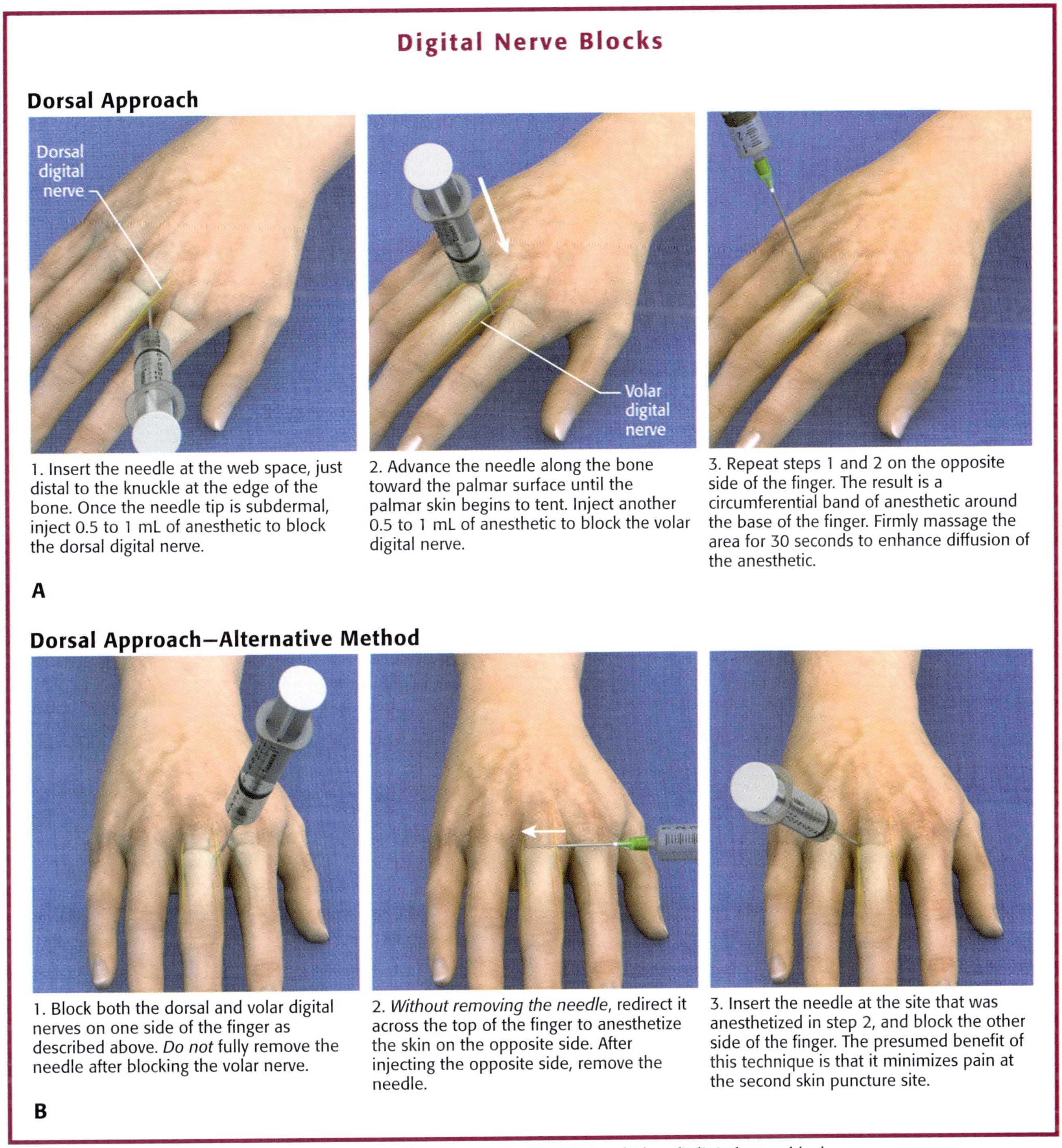

Fig. 31.30 Two methods of performing a traditional (dorsal) digital nerve block.

Indications

Femoral nerve block has shown to be feasible and effective for the management of hip and femoral fractures in the ED (Fig. 31.32). This block can be done by a landmark approach; however, this has fallen out of favor with the widespread adoption of ultrasound. An ED study of patients undergoing femoral nerve block found that the ultrasound approach allowed for faster pain relief than the landmark approach.[65]

Technique

To perform the block, the patient should be in a supine position. Using a high-frequency, linear transducer, the femoral nerve can be found by positioning the probe in a transverse orientation in the medial third of the femoral crease (Fig. 31.33). Coming from a lateral approach, 20 mL to 30 mL of local anesthetic should be injected around the femoral nerve (Fig. 31.34). Because the femoral nerve lies deep to the fascia iliaca, the needle tip must pierce this fascial layer for the block to be effective.

The three-in-one block is a variation of the femoral nerve block. A larger volume of local anesthetic, typically 25 mL to 30 ml, is injected at the same location as a femoral nerve block. The additional local anesthetic is theorized to track along the fascial sheath and block the obturator and lateral femoral cutaneous nerves in addition to the femoral nerve. Human cadaveric studies have rebuked this theory and suggest that the obturator nerve is not reliably blocked.[66] We include this

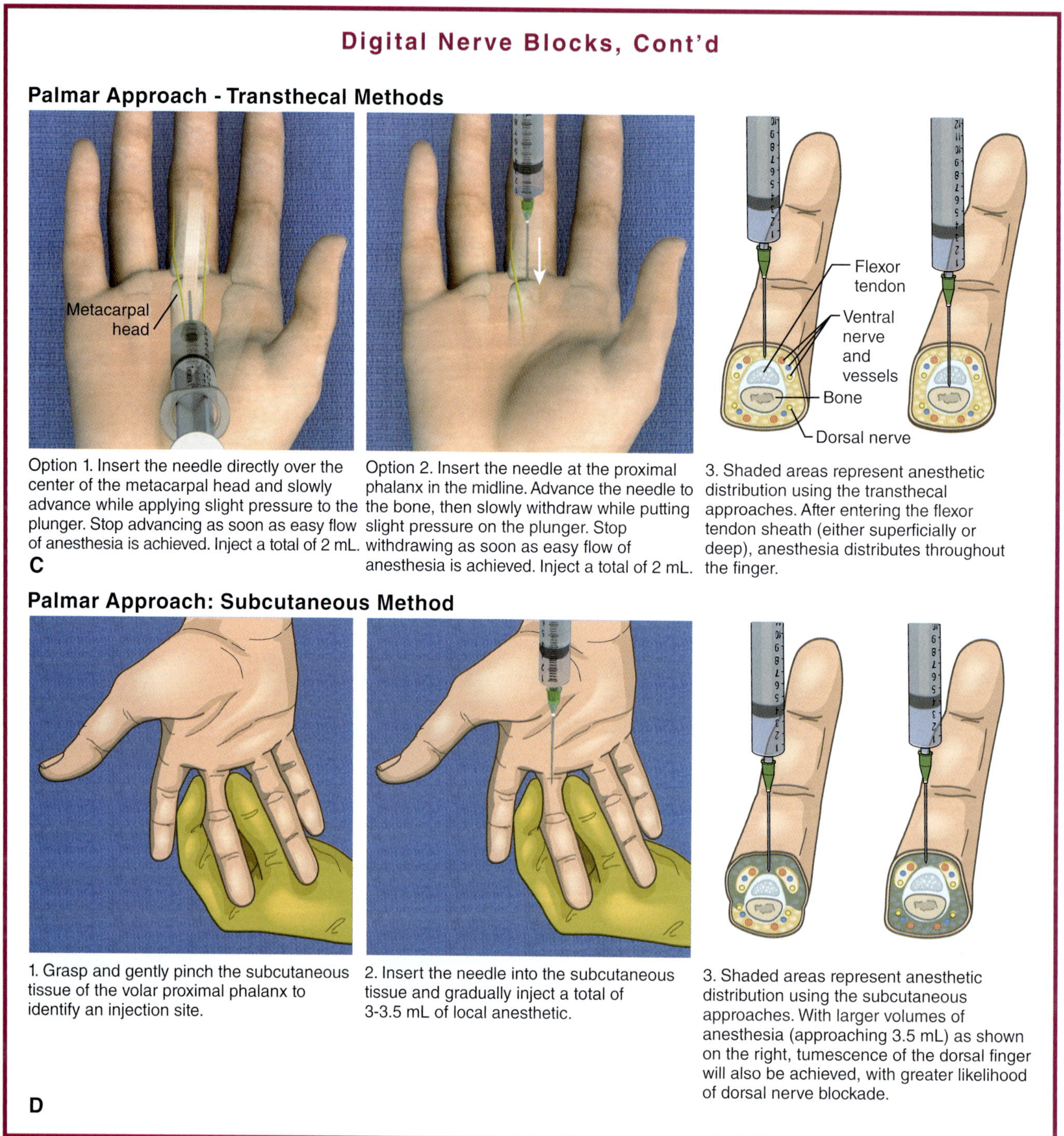

Fig. 31.31 Digital nerve block performed via a palmar injection, including (C) transthecal methods and (D) subcutaneous approaches.

block for thoroughness but agree with Moore who suggests that this block is a misnomer, and should be referred to instead as a femoral nerve block.[67]

Fascia Iliaca Compartment Block

See Videos 31.11 and 31.12.

Anatomy

The fascia iliaca is bound by the iliopsoas muscle deep and the sartorius muscle superficially. The femoral, lateral femoral cutaneous, and obturator nerves all lie within the fascia iliaca.

Indications

The fascia iliaca compartment block (FICB) is commonly performed in the ED, primarily for the management of hip fractures.[68] The FICB may be chosen over a femoral nerve block to anesthetize two other nerves that may contribute to analgesia: the lateral cutaneous femoral nerve and the obturator nerve (see Fig. 31.32). Prior randomized controlled trials have demonstrated that both adult and pediatric patients receiving a FICB have less pain and require fewer opiates.[69,70] Other indications include patellar fracture, proximal tibia fracture, and management of lacerations and abscesses of the anterior thigh.

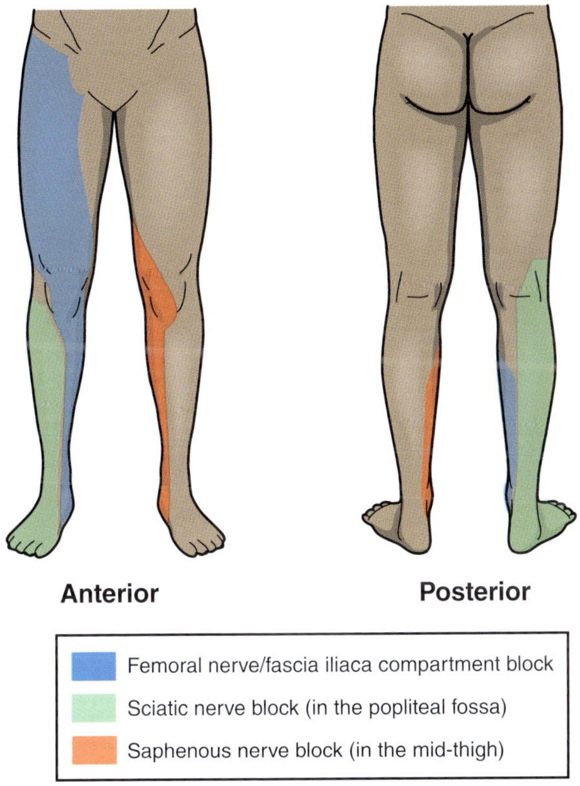

Fig. 31.32 Distribution of anesthesia for select lower extremity nerve blocks.

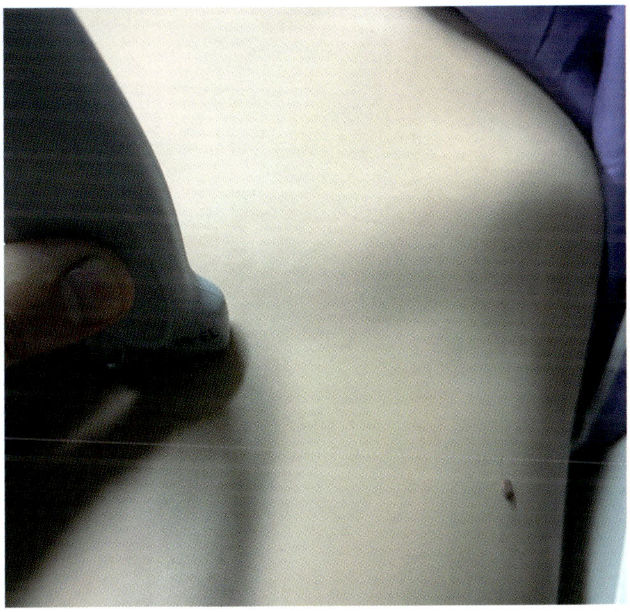

Fig. 31.33 To perform a femoral nerve block, place the patient in the supine position. A linear ultrasound probe is placed parallel to and in the medial third of the femoral crease.

Technique

This block has historically been performed without ultrasound; however, the use of ultrasound has been shown to increase the success rate.[10] Given both theoretical and real-world evidence of the advantages of ultrasound guidance, we only describe the ultrasound technique in this edition.

We prefer the infrainguinal approach which is performed with the patient lying supine. A HFL ultrasound probe is placed in a transverse orientation in the medial one-third of the femoral crease (see Fig. 31.33). The target fascial plane is identified deep to the sartorius muscle and superficial to the iliopsoas muscle; the femoral nerve, artery, and vein will be medial to the target area. Insert the needle using an in-plane approach from lateral to medial (Fig. 31.35). If using a blunt-tipped needle, the practitioner may feel two "pops" as first the fascia lata and then the fascia iliaca are transected. A total of 20 mL to 40 mL of local anesthetic is injected. A successful block occurs when the injectate causes the sartorius and iliopsoas muscles to separate from the fascial plane.

Sciatic Nerve Block (Popliteal Fossa)

See Videos 31.13 and 31.14.

Anatomy

The sciatic nerve and its branches supply most of the sensation to the leg, except for a small area of the medial leg, ankle, and foot (Fig. 31.32). The sciatic nerve is formed from the L4–S3 nerve roots of the lumbosacral plexus and travels posteriorly in the thigh, branching into the tibial and common peroneal nerves at the proximal aspect of the popliteal fossa. The sciatic nerve and branches are surrounded by a common nerve sheath.[71,72] Due to its superficial location in the popliteal fossa, the sciatic nerve can be readily visualized with ultrasound here to perform a nerve block.

Indications

Published uses in the ED for the sciatic block include ankle and foot fractures and dislocations, lacerations, and extensive soft tissue procedures such as removal of multiple ingrown toenails.[73–76]

Technique

Place the patient in the prone or lateral decubitus position (Fig. 31.36). However, injured patients may be unable to adjust positions; therefore the leg may need to be elevated and supported by an assistant to perform the block.[77,78]

A HFL ultrasound transducer is adequate for most patients, but a curvilinear transducer may be necessary for patients with larger body habitus. With the transducer positioned posteriorly in an axial plane in the popliteal fossa, the popliteal artery and vein can be identified (Fig. 31.37). The tibial nerve will be seen superficial, and slightly lateral to the popliteal vein, which lies superficial to the popliteal artery. Sliding the transducer proximally while maintaining a view of the tibial nerve allows a second nerve (the common peroneal nerve) to be identified, appearing lateral to the tibial nerve. As the transducer is moved more proximal still, these two nerves will eventually merge, forming the sciatic nerve (Fig. 31.38). The nerve can be blocked at or just inferior to the bifurcation.

To determine the optimal location for the popliteal sciatic nerve block, several studies have compared a single injection proximal to sciatic nerve bifurcation to two injections distal to the bifurcation.[79,80] While the injections targeting a post-bifurcation location were shown to produce slightly quicker onset of anesthesia, these differences are small (approximately 10 minutes faster) and therefore not likely to be clinically relevant.[81]

Insert a spinal needle using an in-plane approach from lateral to medial, directing the needle tip to an area at or near the confluence of the common peroneal and tibial nerves. The goal is to perform a subparaneural injection (into the nerve

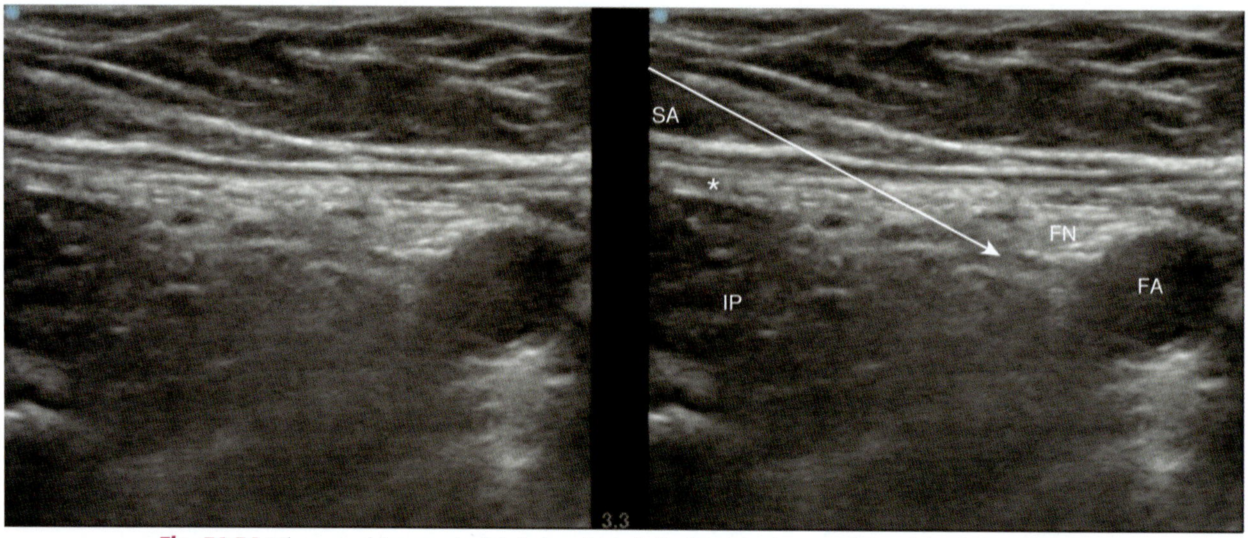

Fig. 31.34 Ultrasound images (unlabeled and labeled) showing the anatomy of the femoral nerve *(FN)*; probe marker is lateral. The *arrow* indicates the typical needle trajectory in-plane coming from lateral to medial, targeting the femoral nerve, which lies within the fascia iliaca *(asterisk)* which separates the sartorius *(SA)* and the iliopsoas *(IP)* muscles. The femoral artery *(FA)* is medial to the femoral nerve.

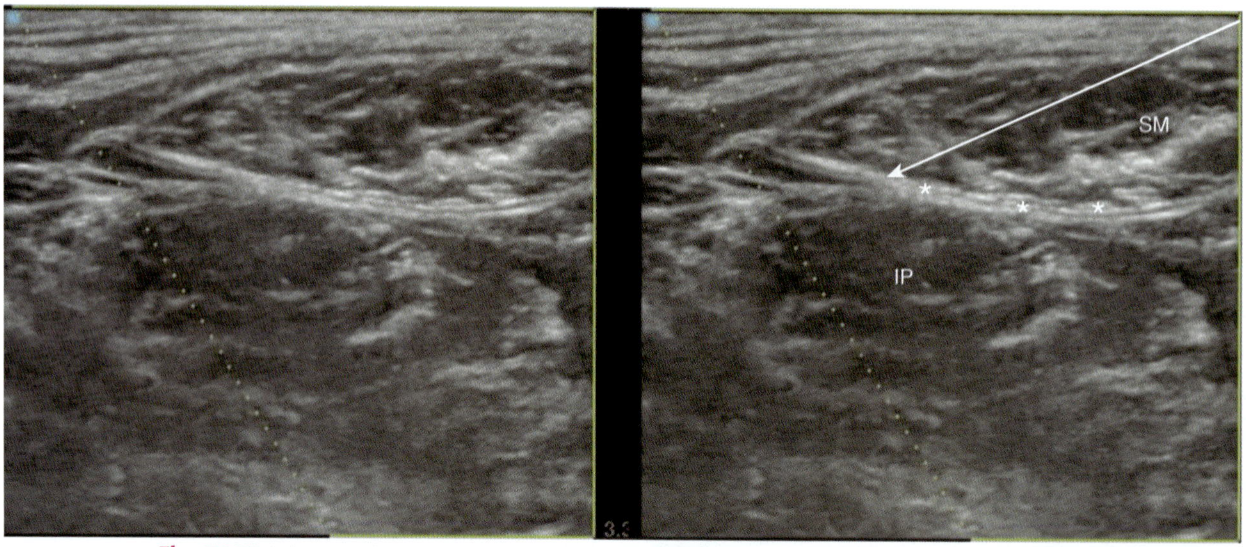

Fig. 31.35 Ultrasound images (unlabeled and labeled) showing the anatomy of the fascia iliaca *(asterisk)*; probe marker is lateral. The *arrow* indicates the typical needle trajectory in-plane coming from lateral to medial, targeting the fascia iliaca, deep to the sartorius muscle *(SM)* and superficial to the iliopsoas muscle *(IP)*.

sheath, but outside the actual nerve) to allow anesthesia to spread proximally and produce full anesthesia.[82] Inject 20 to 30 mL of local anesthetic, aiming to achieve circumferential spread of the anesthesia around both branches of the sciatic nerve.[72]

Saphenous Nerve Block (Mid-Thigh)

Anatomy

The saphenous nerve is a purely sensory, terminal branch of the femoral nerve originating in the thigh where it gives off branches to the knee, before continuing medially to the leg and foot. Although most of the sensation to the foot and ankle derives from the sciatic nerve and its branches, the saphenous nerve innervates an area of skin along the medial ankle and foot as well as the medial aspect of the tibia (see Fig. 31.32). Therefore to achieve complete anesthesia of foot and ankle, both the sciatic and the saphenous nerves must be blocked.

In the upper mid-thigh, the saphenous nerve travels lateral to the femoral artery, eventually crossing anteromedially at the level of the adductor canal. Below the knee, the saphenous nerve continues along the medial leg, accompanying the lesser saphenous vein until crossing the ankle. The saphenous nerve can be blocked along its course via a variety of ultrasound-guided approaches. In this section, we describe an ultrasound-guided approach to saphenous nerve block in the mid-thigh, which takes advantage of readily visualized vascular structures to facilitate correct needle placement.[83]

Indications

In addition to surgical procedures, saphenous nerve blockade has been used for ankle fracture or dislocation reduction, foreign body removal, abscess incision and drainage, and knee osteoarthritis.[84,85]

Technique

The patient is ideally positioned supine with the leg slightly abducted and externally rotated (Fig. 31.39). Place a HFL ultrasound transducer in a transverse plane at the mid to distal thigh, identifying the femoral artery and vein. The saphenous nerve may be seen as a hyperechoic structure either just lateral or anteromedial to the femoral artery (depending on how proximal or distal the probe is positioned), but the nerve may not be apparent until after local anesthesia has been injected (Fig. 31.40). The neurovascular bundle (femoral artery/vein and saphenous nerve) is surrounded by a fibromuscular compartment known as the adductor canal, which is bordered by the sartorius muscle anteromedially, the vastus medialis muscle laterally, and the adductor longus muscle posteriorly. Slide the transducer distally along the femoral artery until the artery dives deep, then move the probe back proximally (approximately 2 cm) to perform the block.[86] Insert a needle using an in-plane technique, injecting 5 mL to 10 mL of local anesthetic around the nerve to achieve the desired effect. Using larger volumes of anesthetic risks producing partial motor blockade of the quadriceps muscle (because local anesthetic tracks proximally within the adductor canal blocking the nerve to the vastus medialis muscle).[87]

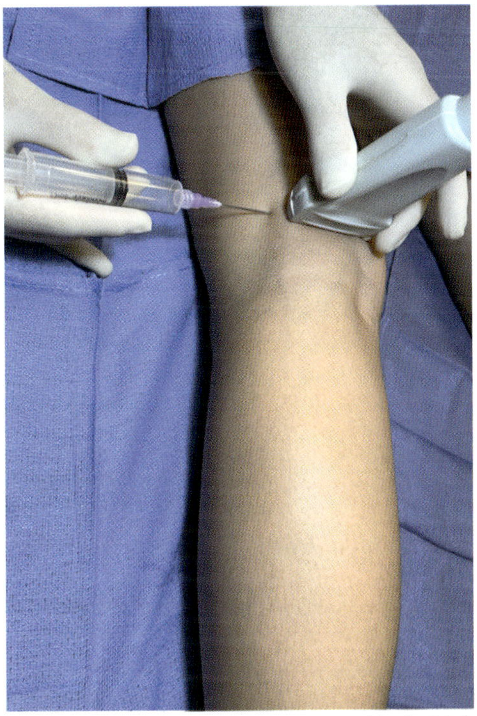

Fig. 31.36 Probe position for a sciatic nerve block. If the patient is unable to lie prone or in lateral decubitus, the leg may also be supported by an assistant and the popliteal fossa accessed posteriorly.

Nerve Blocks of the Ankle

Sensory innervation to the foot is supplied by five peripheral nerves which originate from the terminal branches of the sciatic nerve (superficial and deep peroneal, posterior tibial, and sural nerves) and femoral nerve (saphenous nerve). These five nerves can be blocked at the level of the ankle to produce anesthesia to the foot. Because most of the motor function of the foot is supplied by musculature originating in the calf, an ankle block provides primarily sensory blockade. The decision of which nerve(s) to block is determined by the nature of the injury or painful condition being treated, and knowledge of the sensory distributions of each of these nerves is a prerequisite to performing regional anesthesia of the foot (Fig. 31.41).

Indications

Some of the many reported indications for ankle blocks in the ED include laceration exploration and repair, foreign body removal (especially on the plantar surface of the foot), incision and drainage of foot wounds, calcaneus fractures, and frostbite injuries to the foot.[88–90]

Technique

A landmark-based approach can be used to perform a complete (five-nerve) ankle block with good success.[91] For the three nerves located in the superficial tissue (superficial

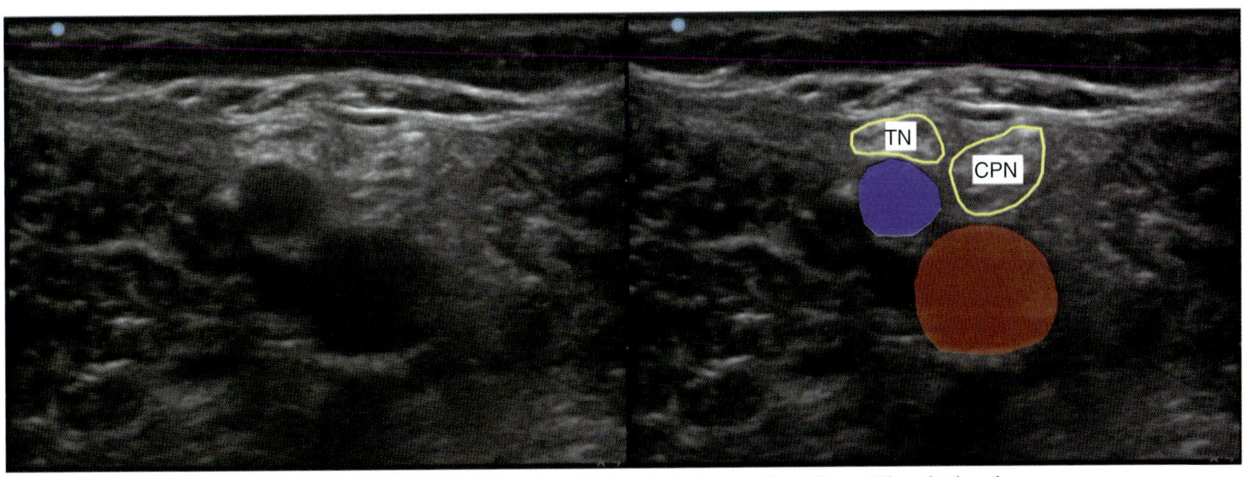

Fig. 31.37 Ultrasound images (unlabeled and labeled) in the popliteal fossa. The tibial and common peroneal nerves (outlined in *yellow*) are seen in close proximity, just superficial to the underlying popliteal vein *(blue)* and popliteal artery *(red)*. *CPN*, Common peroneal nerve; *TN*, tibial nerve.

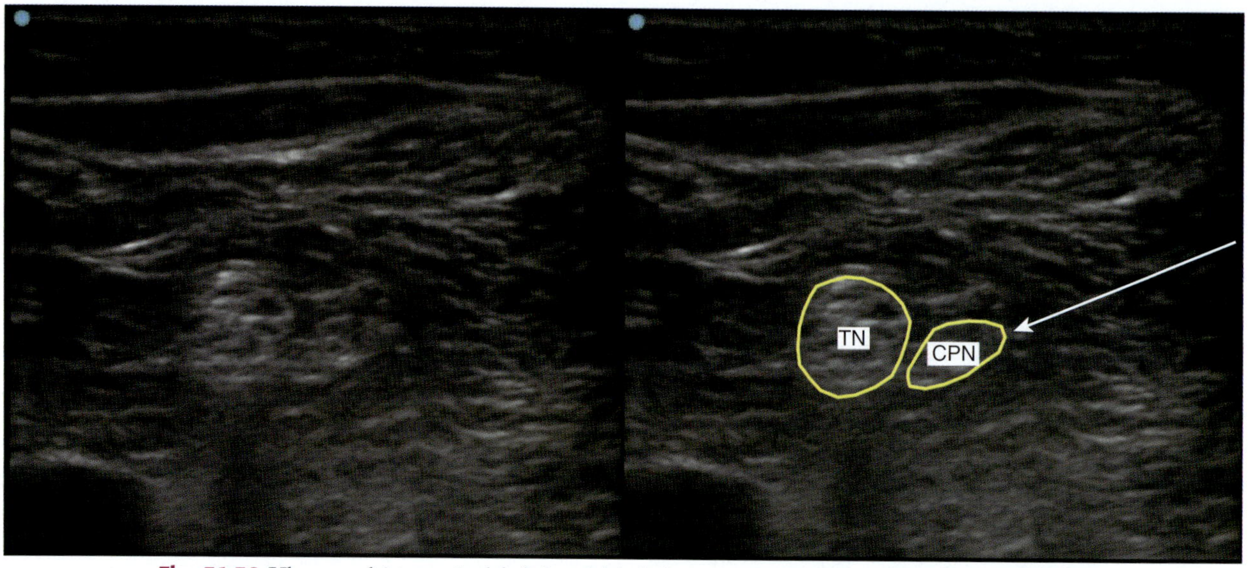

Fig. 31.38 Ultrasound images (unlabeled and labeled) at the apex of the popliteal fossa showing the sciatic nerve as it bifurcates into tibial nerve *(TN, outlined)* and common peroneal nerve *(CPN, outlined)*. An *arrow* shows a typical needle trajectory to perform the sciatic nerve block in the popliteal fossa.

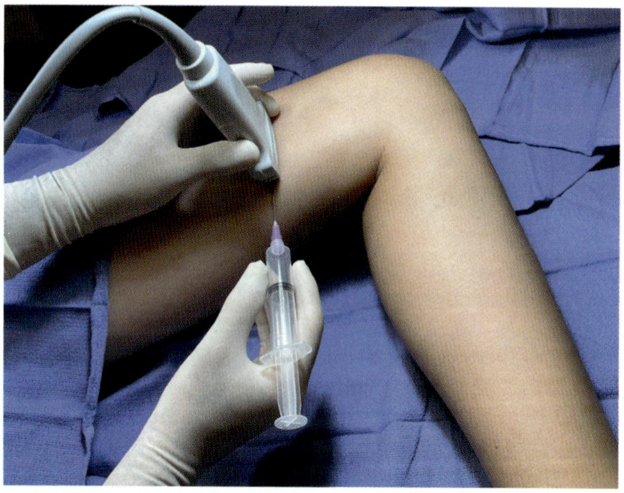

Fig. 31.39 Probe position to locate the saphenous nerve in the thigh.

peroneal, saphenous, and sural nerves), a subcutaneous, landmark-based approach often suffices. The techniques for the individual nerve blocks are described in the following sections. If performing these blocks as part of a complete ankle block, these techniques may be combined in a single block resulting in the deposition of local anesthetic in a horseshoe-shaped pattern around the medial, anterior, and lateral ankle (Fig. 31.42). Ultrasound guidance is not typically used for these nerve blocks as they are readily performed using a subcutaneous landmark technique. Furthermore, these nerves are often difficult to identify on ultrasound due to their smaller size, lack of easily visible arteries adjacent to them, and division into smaller branches by the time of their arrival at the ankle.

The remaining two nerves (deep peroneal and posterior tibial nerves) are located more deeply and are therefore suitable to an ultrasound-guided approach (as well as the landmark-based approach). Compared with using landmarks, ultrasound guidance results in a higher success rate for complete ankle blocks[92] as well as posterior tibial nerve blocks,[93,94] but not necessarily for deep peroneal nerve blocks.[95] Ultrasound guidance also permits a smaller volume of local anesthetic to be used compared with the landmark approach (16 vs. 30 mL in one study, with similar outcomes in the immediate post-block time period).[96] Here we describe both landmark-based as well as ultrasound-guided techniques.

Superficial Peroneal Nerve (Ankle)

Anatomy

The superficial peroneal (fibular) nerve divides into two or more superficial branches in the lower leg before crossing over the dorsal ankle into the foot. The superficial peroneal nerve provides cutaneous innervation to most of the dorsal foot. The nerve and its branches are in the subcutaneous tissue superficial to the extensor retinaculum.

Technique: Superficial Peroneal Nerve Block (Landmark Based)

See Fig. 31.43A. Draw a line between the medial and lateral malleolus. Insert a needle in a subcutaneous tissue plane starting at the extensor hallucis longus (EHL) tendon and directing the needle toward the lateral malleolus. Advance the needle slowly, injecting small aliquots of local anesthetic as the needle is advanced along the dorsum of the ankle. A total of 4 to 10 mL of local anesthetic will be used.

Saphenous Nerve (Ankle)

Anatomy

The saphenous nerve is the only nerve to the foot that originates from the femoral nerve rather than the sciatic nerve. It supplies cutaneous sensation to the medial ankle and foot to a variable degree, as far as the first metatarsal in some cases.[97,98] In the leg, the nerve courses in a subcutaneous plane down the medial side of the leg posterior to the greater saphenous vein. A few centimeters above the medial malleolus, the saphenous nerve branches into an anterior and posterior branch which course near the medial malleolus.

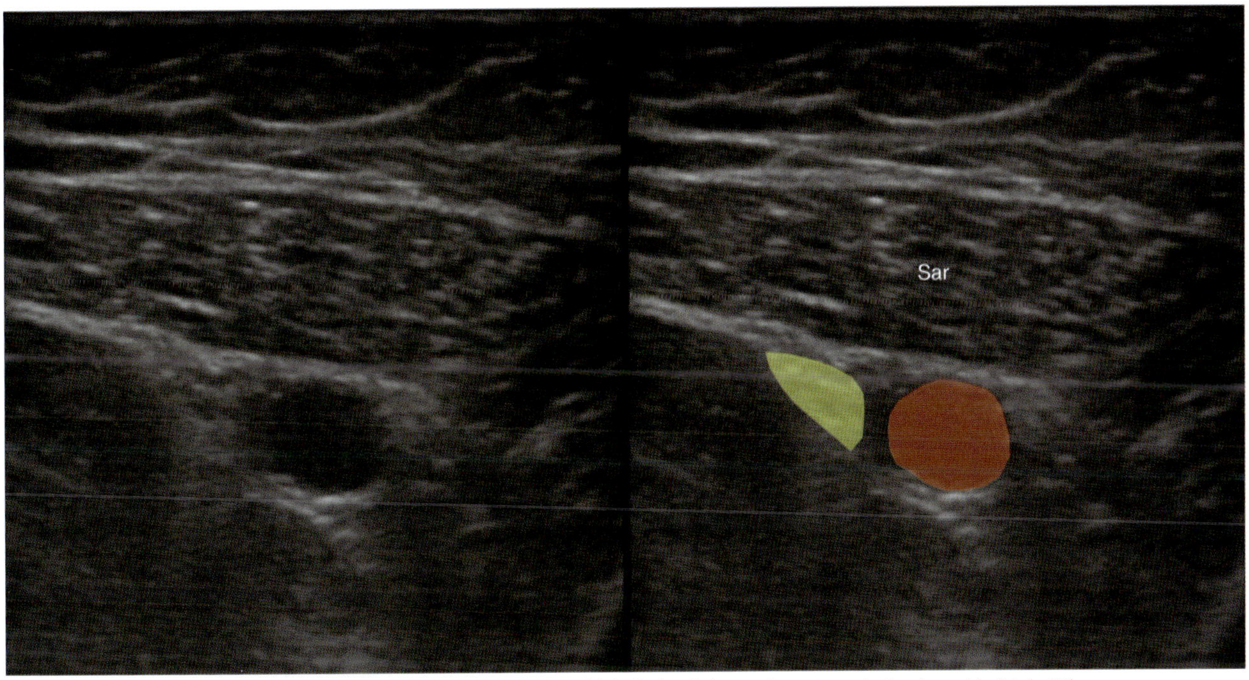

Fig. 31.40 Ultrasound images (unlabeled and labeled) of the saphenous vein in the mid-thigh. The femoral artery *(red)* is adjacent to the saphenous nerve *(yellow)*. *Sar,* Sartorius muscle.

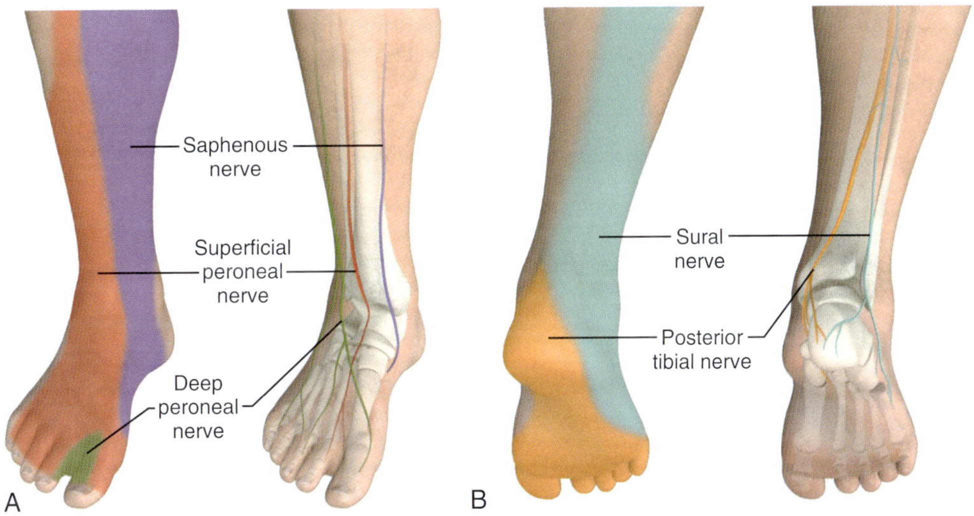

Fig. 31.41 Sensory distribution to the foot is supplied by five peripheral nerves.

Technique: Saphenous Nerve Block (Landmark Based)

See Fig. 31.43B. Using a line drawn between the medial and lateral malleolus, inject in a subcutaneous plane between the tibialis anterior tendon and the skin overlying the medial malleolus. A total of 3 to 5 mL of local anesthetic will be used. Take care not to inadvertently inject local anesthetic into the greater saphenous vein when approaching the medial malleolus.

Sural Nerve Block (Ankle)

Anatomy

The sural nerve is formed from branches of the sciatic nerve in the distal calf. It travels near the lesser saphenous vein, entering the foot in the subcutaneous tissue posterior to the lateral malleolus.[99] The sural nerve is a purely sensory nerve, innervating the lateral ankle and foot.

Technique: Sural Nerve Block (Landmark Based)

See Fig. 31.43C. Using a line drawn between the top of the lateral malleolus and the Achilles tendon, insert a needle in the subcutaneous plane, entering the skin just lateral to the edge of the Achilles tendon and directed toward the lateral malleolus. Inject a total of 3 to 5 mL along a subcutaneous wheal.

Technique: Sural Nerve Block (Ultrasound Guided)

Ultrasound can be used to facilitate a sural nerve block at the ankle, with some authors reporting superior results compared with the landmark-based approach.[100] Although the nerve itself may be difficult to visualize, the proximity of the sural nerve to the lesser saphenous vein provides a convenient landmark with which to identify a target for injection.

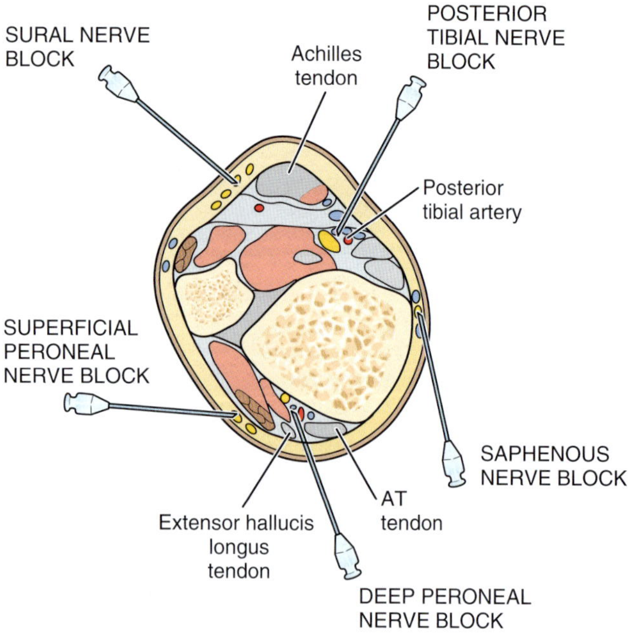

Fig. 31.42 Cross-sectional anatomy of the ankle illustrating the position of the peripheral nerves to the foot relative to adjacent landmarks. A complete, landmark-based ankle block will produce anesthesia deposited in a horseshoe-shaped distribution around the ankle at the level of the malleoli. *AT*, Anterior tibialis.

Placing a HFL ultrasound transducer in transverse orientation at the lateral malleolus, identify the lesser saphenous vein as an oval, easily compressible vein located in the subcutaneous tissue just posterior to the lateral malleolus and anterior to the Achilles tendon. A venipuncture tourniquet may accentuate the saphenous vein, making it easier to identify. Inject 1 to 2 mL of local anesthetic on either side of the vein with the goal of surrounding the vein on both sides with local anesthetic.

Deep Peroneal Nerve

Anatomy

The deep peroneal (fibular) nerve innervates the first dorsal web space cutaneously (i.e., between the great toe and second toe), as well as the dorsal surface of the foot bones. At the ankle, the deep peroneal nerve runs lateral to the anterior tibial artery along the surface of the anterior tibia. The nerve is lateral to the EHL and tibialis anterior tendons, and medial to the extensor digitorum longus tendon.

Technique: Deep peroneal Nerve Block (Landmark Based)

See Fig. 31.44D. Identify the EHL and extensor digitorum longus tendons by having the patient dorsiflex the great toe (EHL) and remaining toes (EDL). Approximately 1 cm above the malleoli, insert the needle beneath the medial border of the EHL tendon and advance the needle laterally until contact with the tibia is made, then withdraw slightly. Inject a total of 3 to 5 mL of local anesthetic here. When performing this block, be careful not to puncture the anterior tibial artery.

Technique: Deep Peroneal Nerve Block (Ultrasound Guided)

Place a HFL transducer in a transverse plane across the distal tibia at or near a line drawn between the malleoli (Fig. 31.45). The anterior tibial artery is a pulsatile structure located immediately anterior to the tibia. Use of color flow Doppler may help to identify the artery (Fig. 31.46), and one or more veins may be also seen on either side of the artery. The deep peroneal nerve is located lateral to the artery (Fig. 31.47) but may be difficult to visualize. If the nerve is seen, inject 3 mL to 4 mL of local anesthetic circumferentially around the nerve. In the event the nerve is not well visualized, inject 1 to 2 mL on either side of the artery.

Posterior Tibial Nerve

See Video 31.15.

Anatomy

The posterior tibial nerve innervates most of the cutaneous surface of the plantar foot, as well as the plantar surface of the bones of the foot. The posterior tibial nerve runs posterior to the posterior tibial artery and divides into a calcaneal branch and plantar branches in variable locations at or near the ankle.

Technique: Posterior Tibial Nerve (Landmark Based)

See Fig. 31.44E. Palpate the posterior tibial artery posterior to the medial malleolus. Direct the needle posterior to the arterial pulsations, 1 cm proximal to the medial malleolus, and at a point midway between the medial malleolus and the Achilles tendon. Advance the needle perpendicular to the skin for approximately 1 cm (or until making contact with bone), then inject 3 mL to 5 mL of local anesthetic. The injection may be performed either with a single-needle approach, or by using a fan-like distribution (directing the needle in multiple directions successively) to increase the chance of the anesthetic being placed near the nerve. Given that this is a blind approach, there is some risk of arterial puncture, which will necessarily increase with each redirection of the needle.

Technique: Posterior Tibial Nerve (Ultrasound Guided)

Position the patient in lateral decubitus position with the foot to be anesthetized toward the bed; the patient's other leg should be moved out of the operator's way. Place a HFL ultrasound transducer in a transverse plane over the medial malleolus (Fig. 31.48). Tendons and neurovascular structures can be identified sequentially posterior to the medial malleolus using the mnemonic Tom (*t*ibialis posterior tendon), Dick (flexor *d*igitorum tendon), ANd (tibial *a*rtery and tibial *n*erve) Harry (flexor *h*allucis longus tendon). One or more posterior tibial veins may also be seen adjacent to the posterior tibial artery; these can be distinguished from the artery by their easy compressibility and lack of pulsations. After the artery has been identified, the nerve will be recognized near the artery (Fig. 31.49). Slide the transducer approximately 5 cm proximal on the leg, maintaining a visual of the posterior tibial nerve (Fig. 31.50). A total of 5 to 7 mL of local anesthetic is used to surround the nerve. Injecting at this level will enable blockade of both the plantar branch and the calcaneal branch.

Digital Nerve Blocks of the Foot

Indications

Anesthesia of the toes may be required for patients with painful infections and injuries of the toes, including fractures, dislocations, nail bed injuries, ingrown toenails, and abscesses. Local infiltration of anesthetic in the toes is suboptimal due to limited space in the soft tissues for the volumes of anesthesia required. Additionally, fibrous septa present on the

Superficial Nerve Blocks of the Ankle

Superficial Peroneal

Distribution

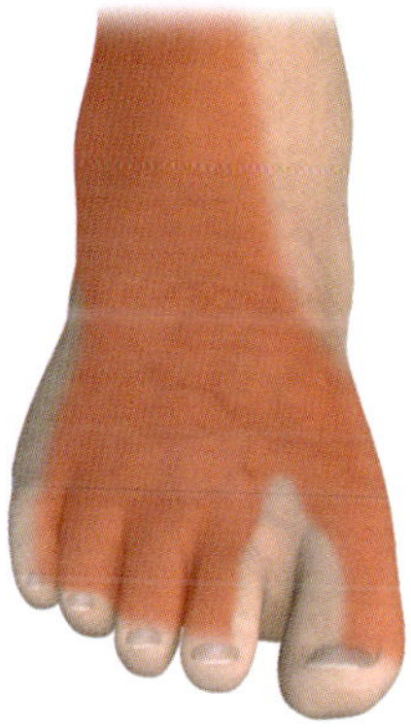

A

Anatomy and Technique

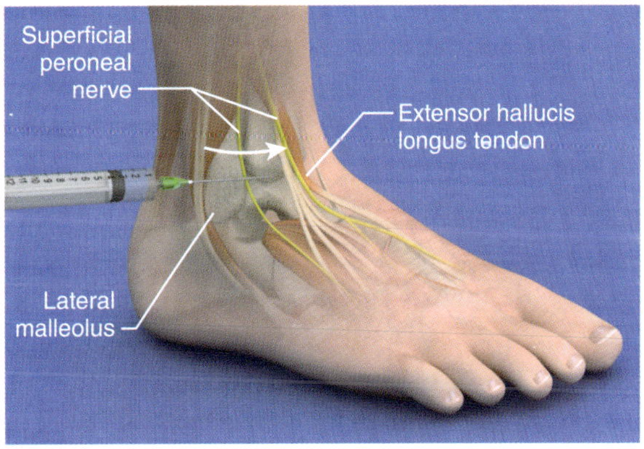

Palpate the extensor hallucis longus tendon and the lateral malleolus. Inject 4 to 10 mL of anesthetic subcutaneously in a band between the tendon and the malleolus.

Saphenous

Distribution

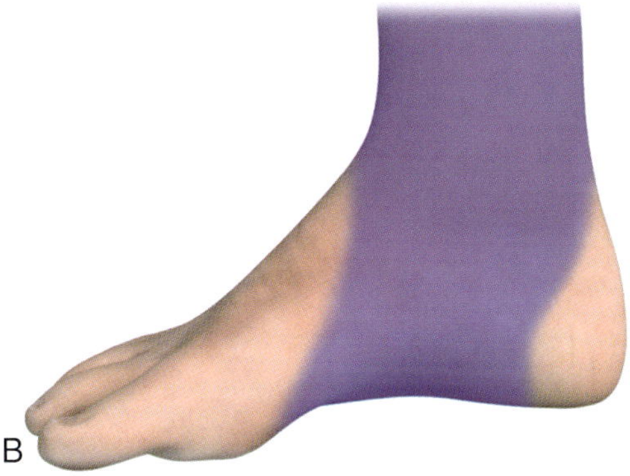

B

Anatomy and Technique

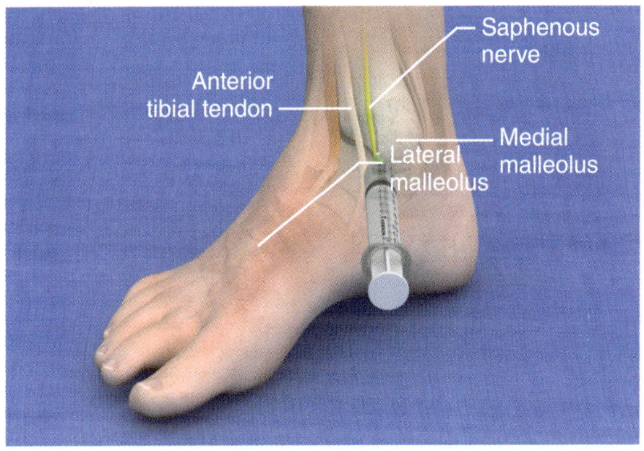

At the level of the malleoli, inject in a subcutaneous plane between the tibialis anterior tendon and the skin overlying the medial malleolus. A total of 3-5 mL of local anesthetic will be used in a subcutaneous wheal.

Sural

Distribution

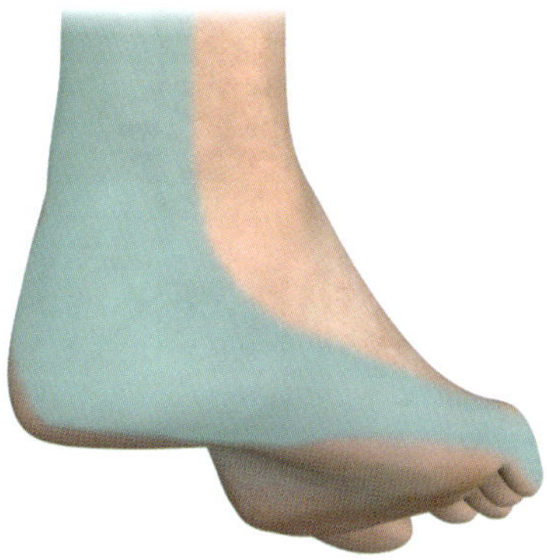

C

Anatomy and Technique

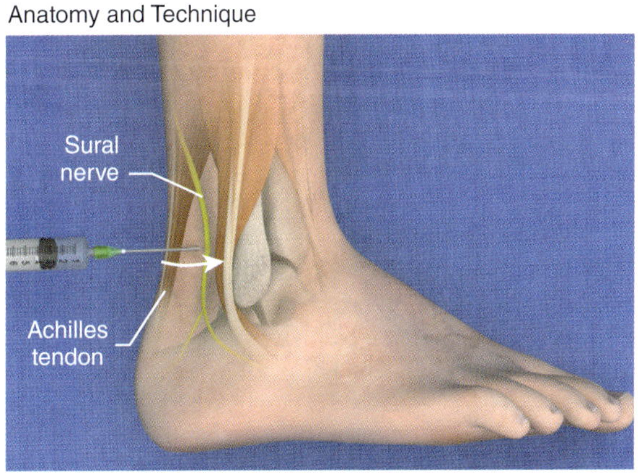

Palpate the Achilles tendon and lateral malleolus. Inject 3 to 5 mL of anesthetic subcutaneously in a band between the Achilles tendon and lateral malleolus, about 1 cm superior to the malleolus.

Fig. 31.43 Landmark-based approach to superficial nerve blocks of the ankle.

Deep Nerve Blocks of the Ankle

Deep Peroneal

Distribution

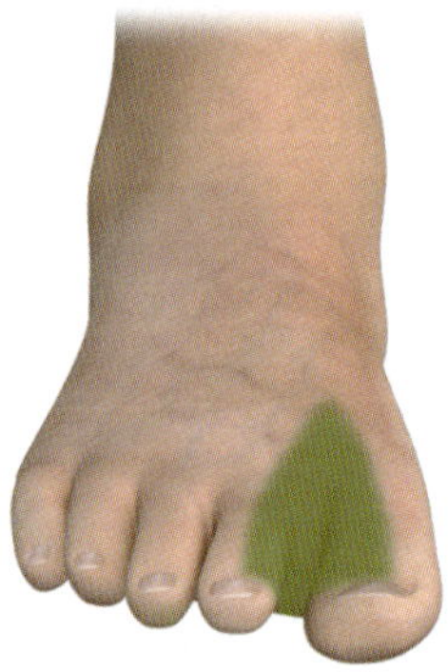

D

Anatomy and Technique

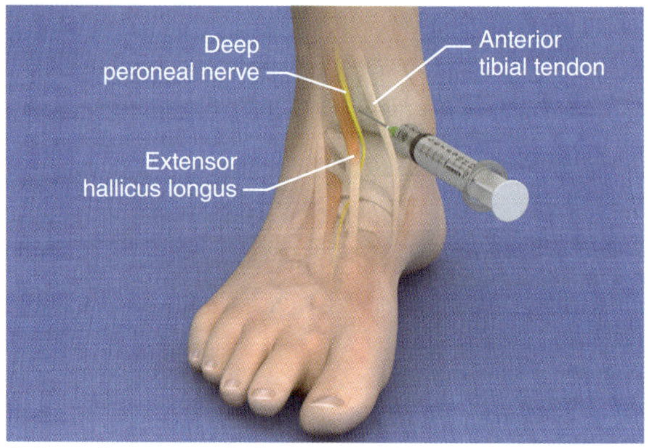

Palpate the extensor hallucis longus (EHL) and anterior tibial tendons while the patient dorsiflexes the foot and big toe. Insert the needle at a level 1 cm superior to the medial malleolus, and direct it laterally under the EHL tendon until it strikes the tibia. Inject 3 to 5 mL of anesthetic.

Posterior Tibial

Distribution

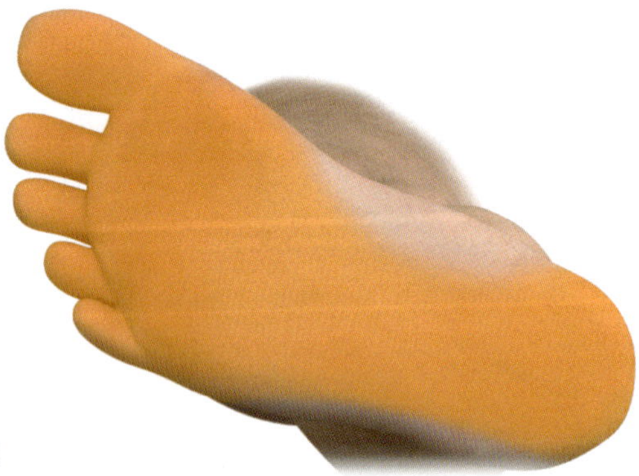

E

Anatomy and Technique

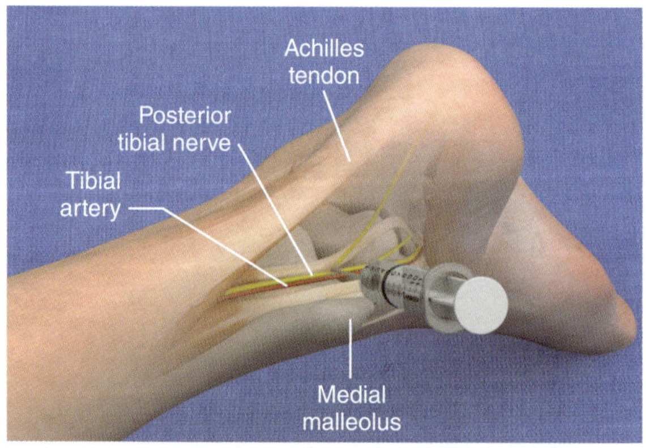

Palpate the tibial artery posterior to the medial malleolus. Insert the needle 1 cm superior to this point, perpendicular to the skin. At a depth of 1 cm, inject 3 to 5 mL of anesthetic. See text for additional details.

Fig. 31.44 Landmark-based approach to deep nerve blocks of the ankle.

plantar surface of the toes prevents anesthesia from spreading, limiting its effectiveness. DNBs avoid these complications, allowing for complete anesthesia to the toe without distorting tissue landmarks.

Anatomy

Innervation of the toes is analogous to that of the fingers. Two dorsal digital nerves (located at 2 o'clock and 10 o'clock) originate from the superficial and deep peroneal nerves. Two plantar digital nerves (at 4 o'clock and 8 o'clock) are extensions of the sural and posterior tibial nerves. The dorsal digital nerves run near the dorsal digital arteries in a neurovascular bundle.

Technique

Despite the anatomical similarity with the hand, there is a relative paucity of data regarding DNBs of the toe compared with DNBs of the fingers. Several approaches to performing a toe block have been described, differing in terms of location (metatarsal, web space, proximal phalanx, or a combination), number of needle insertions (1 vs. 2 or more), and needle trajectory (vertical, horizontal, and/or oblique). No clear consensus has emerged as to which method is best.

Blocks done at the metatarsal and web space levels have more subcutaneous soft tissue and can accommodate larger volume of injectate (with less pain) than blocks at the proximal phalanx, where subcutaneous tissue is thin and high volumes might result in tissue ischemia.[101] Nerve locations are less predictable at the metatarsal level, however.

Needle insertions on the plantar surface are more painful than dorsal injections due to the higher concentration of nerve endings, and the provider should take this into account when contemplating an injection on the plantar surface of the foot. The plantar skin is also much thicker than on the dorsal toe, requiring more force to penetrate the subcutaneous space.

Topical anesthesia (eutectic mixture of local anesthetics [EMLA] cream) to lessen the pain of a digital block of the toe has been studied, unfortunately with mixed results.[102,103]

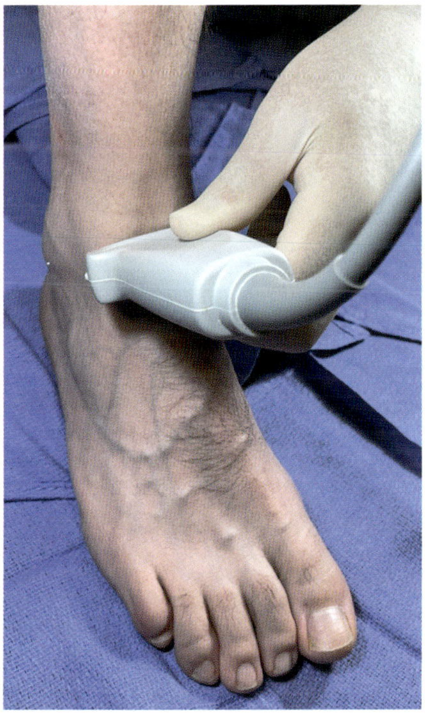

Fig. 31.45 Ultrasound probe positioning to identify the deep peroneal nerve at the ankle.

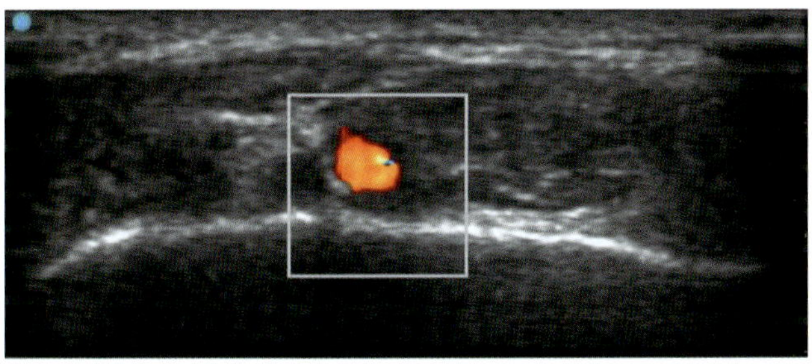

Fig. 31.46 Using color Doppler *(white box)* to identify the tibial artery *(red)*. The tibial artery lies just medial to the deep peroneal nerve (not seen here). If the nerve cannot be seen, 1 to 2 mL of local anesthetic may be injected on either side of the artery.

Traditional Digital Block of the Toe

This technique involves two needle insertions on the dorsal toe overlying the proximal phalanx. First the needle is inserted on the dorsomedial aspect of the toe just beyond the web space. A total of 1 mL of local anesthetic is injected as the needle slowly advances in a dorsal to plantar direction. This procedure is then repeated on the lateral aspect of the toe (see Fig. 31.51A).

Because patients tend to experience greater pain with more rapid injections of anesthesia, a modification of this approach was studied in which the initial injection consisted of 0.2 mL instead of 1 mL. After waiting for 2 minutes while leaving the needle in place, the same injection was repeated with the remaining 0.8 mL of local anesthetic. Patients reported reduced pain with this two-stage version of the digital block.[104]

A further variation of this technique is sometimes referred to as an "H-block" due to the path that the needle takes, evoking the letter H (see Fig. 31.51B). This variation involves two needle insertions and is described here at the level of the proximal phalanx; however, it can also be done at the web space level. Two sites for needle puncture are identified on the dorsal surface of the proximal phalanx, one on the lateral side and the other on the medial side. Choosing one of the injection sites, insert the needle in an anterior-posterior (dorsal-plantar) direction, keeping the needle to the side of the phalanx. Inject a total of 2 mL of local anesthetic along this line. Next withdraw the needle almost all the way, until the bevel of the needle is in the subcutaneous tissue. Redirect the needle 90 degrees aiming across the dorsum of the toe toward the other injection site. Dorsiflex the toe and advance the needle across the toe and beneath the extensor tendon, injecting another 1 mL of local anesthetic. After removing the needle, reinsert at the second injection site in an anterior-posterior direction (toward the plantar surface), again keeping the needle to the side of the bone and injecting a total of 2 mL of local anesthetic along the way.[105] Anesthesia will be deposited on three of the four sides of the toe in this block.

V-Block

Only one needle insertion is required for the V-block, and as implied by its name, the trajectory of the needle will resemble the letter V (see Fig. 31.51C). Begin by identifying a single site for needle insertion along the dorsal surface of the proximal phalanx in the sagittal midline of the toe. Pinch the dorsal skin overlying the proximal phalanx and inject 1 mL of local anesthetic into the subcutaneous tissue overlying the extensor tendon. Next, without removing the needle, angle 45 degrees medially and slightly proximally, with an overall needle trajectory toward the plantar

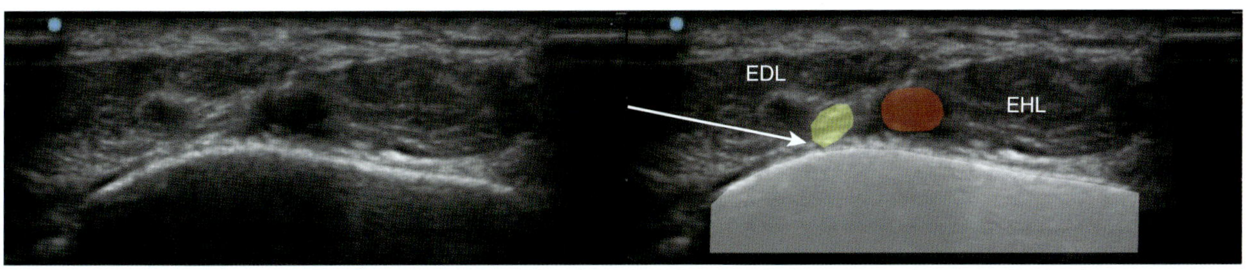

Fig. 31.47 Ultrasound images (unlabeled and labeled) showing the deep peroneal nerve at the distal tibia just proximal to the ankle joint. The deep peroneal nerve *(yellow)* is lateral to the tibial artery *(red)*, and immediately in front of the underlying tibia *(gray)*. An *arrow* shows the typical trajectory of a needle entering from lateral to medial (opposite the artery). *EDL*, extensor digitorum longus; *EHL*, extensor hallucis longus.

surface. After advancing the needle along this line, inject 1 mL of local anesthetic. While slowly withdrawing the needle along this path, continue injecting another 1 mL, but do not completely remove the needle. Finally, angle the needle 45 degrees lateral in the same manner as before, injecting another 1 mL on the plantar aspect of the needle insertion and an additional 1 mL while withdrawing the needle completely.[106]

One study compared the H-block and V-block techniques and found similar efficacy.[105] Since the V-block only requires a single-needle insertion, it may be better tolerated by patients.

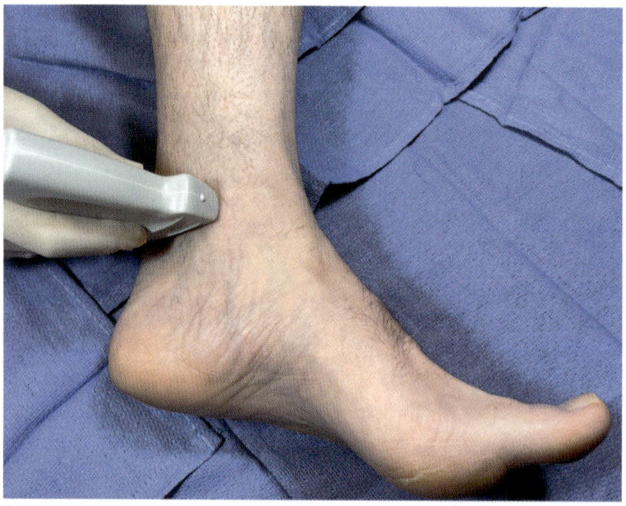

Fig. 31.48 Ultrasound probe placement to identify the posterior tibial nerve behind the medial malleolus.

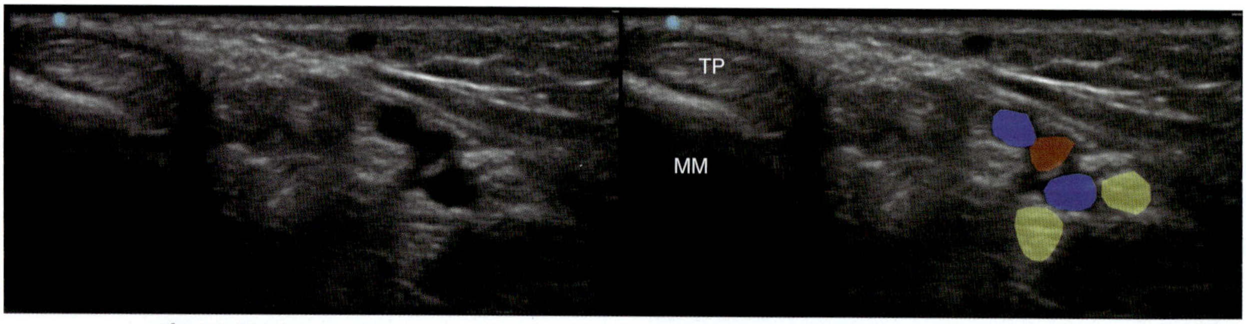

Fig. 31.49 Ultrasound images (unlabeled and labeled) showing posterior tibial nerve anatomy at the ankle. The posterior tibial nerve *(yellow)* is adjacent to the posterior tibial artery *(red)* and veins *(blue)* and is split at this level. *MM*, Medial malleolus; *TP*, tibialis posterior tendon.

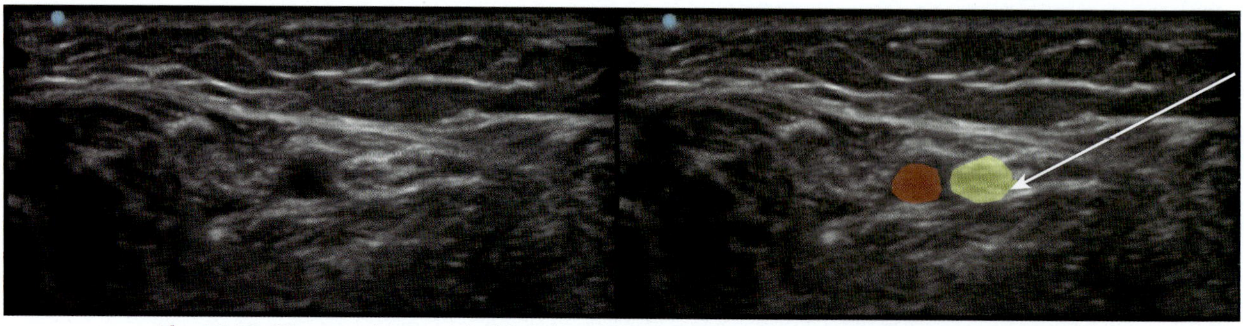

Fig. 31.50 Ultrasound images (unlabeled and labeled) showing posterior tibial nerve anatomy approximately 5 cm proximal to the malleolus. The posterior tibial nerve *(yellow)* is blocked at this level, with the needle *(arrow)* entering opposite the posterior tibial artery *(red)*.

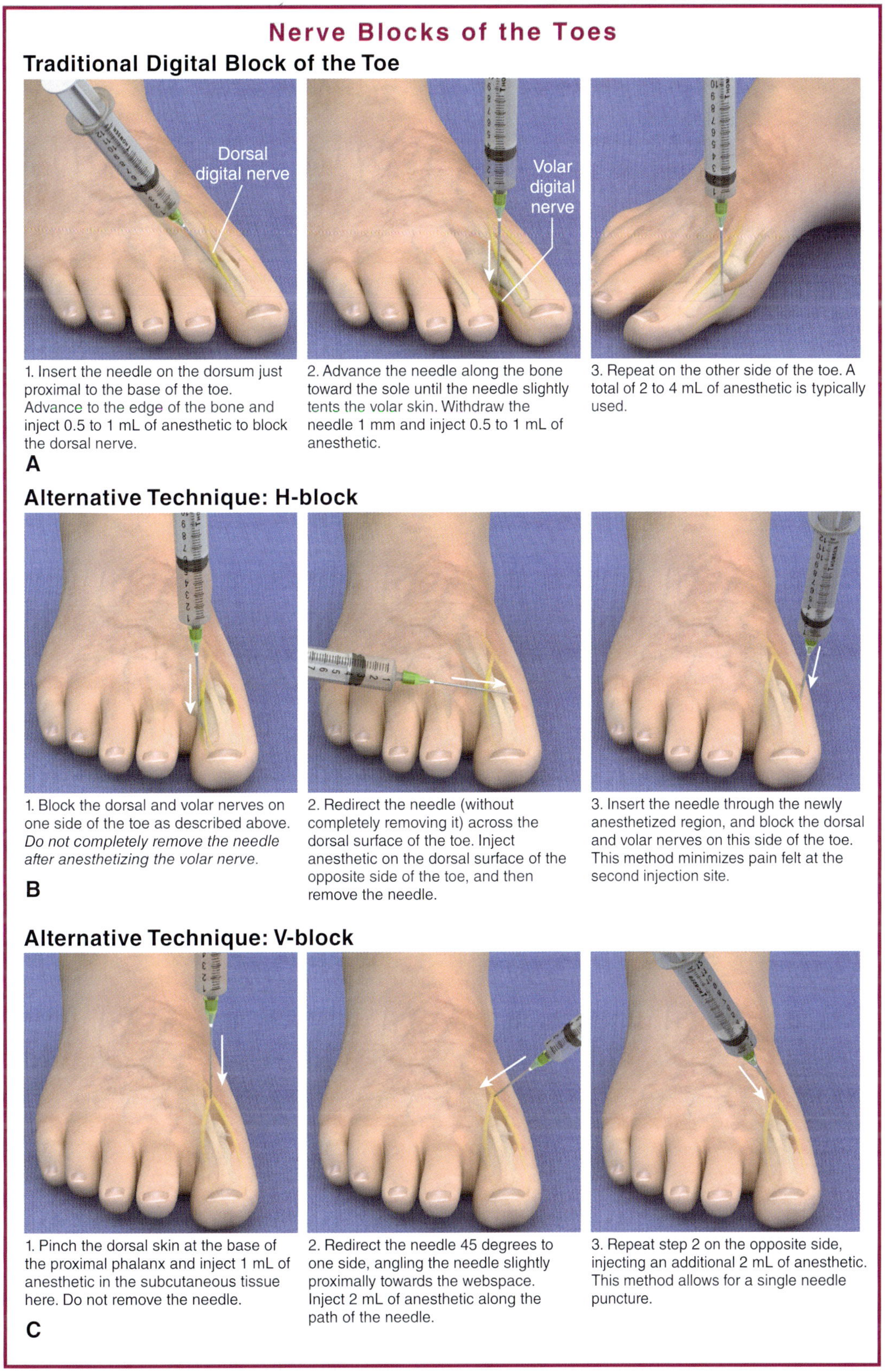

Fig. 31.51 Three different methods of performing digital nerve block of the toe. (A) Traditional method. (B) "H" block variation. (C) "V" block utilizing a single injection.

Complications

Both blocks described, as well as other related techniques, have the potential to injure the neurovascular bundle, so caution is advised. Blocks at the level of the metacarpal bones can accept higher volumes of anesthesia than more distal blocks, but nerve locations are less predictable here.

REFERENCES ARE AVAILABLE AT Elsevier eBooks+

CHAPTER 32

Intravenous Regional Anesthesia

Angelica Loza-Gomez and Salvador Rios

INTRODUCTION

Clinical use of intravenous regional anesthesia (IVRA) has been well established as a simple and safe anesthetic technique for short surgical procedures of the upper and lower extremities.[1,2] Though historically relegated to the operating room, the procedure is also readily applicable to outpatient use. Because of its reliability, safety, and ease of use, it is now commonly used in the emergency department (ED) and clinic. In the ED, the technique provides quick and complete anesthesia, muscle relaxation, and a bloodless operating field. The procedure is free from the troublesome side effects associated with other regional blocks, such as the axillary block. The procedure is easily mastered and has a very low failure rate; consistently good results can be expected. Although not a standard requirement of ED personnel, this technique can be safely used by trained ED clinicians, including physician assistants and nurse practitioners, and does not have to be administered by an anesthesiologist.[2] The first practical use of analgesia associated with the intravenous (IV) injection of a local anesthetic agent was described by August Gustav Bier in 1908,[3] a technique now referred to as the *Bier block* (Video 32.1).[4] Although the procedure has been in existence for many years, the need for special equipment and a safe anesthetic agent limited its use. However, the Bier block has now gained wide acceptance as a safe and effective procedure. In this chapter, the technique, indications, and complications are discussed according to their application in the ED.

INDICATIONS AND CONTRAINDICATIONS

Indications for IVRA include any procedure on the arm or leg that requires operating anesthesia, muscle relaxation, or a bloodless field, such as reduction of fractures and dislocations, repair of major lacerations, removal of foreign bodies, debridement of burns, and drainage of infection (Fig. 32.1). IVRA is commonly used for extremity surgery, such as carpal tunnel surgery or tendon repair. The procedure may be carried out on any patient of any age who is able to cooperate with the clinician.

The only absolute contraindications are allergy to the anesthetic agent and uncontrolled hypertension. Relative contraindications include severe Raynaud disease, Buerger disease, or a crushed or already hypoxic extremity in which further transient ischemia would be detrimental. Homozygous sickle cell disease is a theoretical contraindication, but few data exist on the treatment of patients with this condition. IVRA is best used for procedures requiring no more than 60 to 90 minutes of tourniquet time. Continuous cardiac or blood pressure monitoring is not required but is recommended for unexpected complications. The judicious use of procedural sedation may facilitate the use of IVRA in an anxious or transiently uncooperative patient.

EQUIPMENT

The equipment required for IVRA consists of the following (Review Box 32.1 and Fig. 32.2):

- 1% lidocaine (Xylocaine [commercial preparations with preservatives are commonly used; 0.5% is also available]), *without epinephrine*, to be diluted to a 0.5% solution. (Note: 1% lidocaine = 10 mg/mL; hence 1 mL of 1% lidocaine = 10 mg.)
- Sterile saline solution as a diluent
- 60-mL syringe
- 18-gauge needle
- Pneumatic tourniquet (single or double cuff) such as the Zimmer ATS 2000 Automatic Tourniquet System (Figs. 32.2 and 32.3) (Note: Do not use a standard blood pressure cuff.)
- IV catheters (20 or 22 gauge) or a 21-gauge butterfly needle
- Esmarch bandage
- 500 mL of 5% dextrose in water (D_5W) and IV extension tubing (optional)

PROCEDURE

The procedure should be explained to the patient in advance and consent documented. Premedication with midazolam (Versed), diazepam (Valium), or an opioid (e.g., morphine, fentanyl) is recommended as pain may occur from pneumatic pressure insufflation. The procedure should not be done on patients who are persistently uncooperative, intoxicated, or obtunded or who have had a previous reaction to a local anesthetic.

As a precaution, establish a second IV in the upper extremity (opposite the upper extremity block). While not mandatory, the authors recommend placing the patient on continuous cardiac and peripheral oxygen saturation (SpO_2) monitoring and performing regular blood pressure checks throughout the procedure. Standard resuscitation medications, airway adjuncts, and intravenous fluids should be readily available.[5]

While the patient is being prepared, keep the lidocaine solution ready, but withhold it until the injured extremity is exsanguinated and the cuff is in place and inflated, as discussed later. The standard dose of lidocaine for the arm is 3 mg/kg. Inject it as a 0.5% solution (1% lidocaine mixed with equal parts sterile saline in a 60-mL syringe). Hence, for a 70-kg patient, infuse 210 mg of lidocaine (21 mL of 1% lidocaine) mixed with 21 mL of saline for a total volume in the infusing syringe of 42 mL of 0.5% lidocaine. Farrell et al. described a procedure termed the *minidose Bier block* in which 1.5 mg/kg of lidocaine is used and reported a 95% success rate.[6] This lower dose may decrease the incidence of central nervous system side effects and is more desirable in the ED setting. Additional lidocaine may be infused if the initial dose is inadequate. Do not use lidocaine with epinephrine. Plain lidocaine is also available as a 0.5% solution and can therefore be used directly to avoid diluting the stronger solution. Some prefer preservative-free lidocaine, but most clinicians use standard lidocaine with preservatives.

Apply a pneumatic tourniquet with cotton padding (to prevent ecchymosis) under the cuff proximal to the pathology.

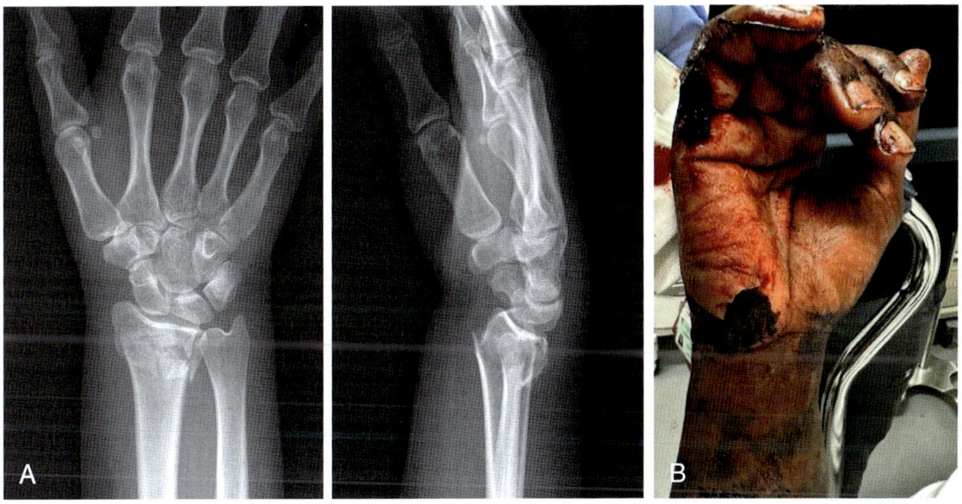

Fig. 32.1 Intravenous regional anesthesia can be used in the emergency department for any procedure on an extremity that requires anesthesia, muscle relaxation, or control of hemorrhage, such as closed reduction of displaced distal radius fracture (A) or complex laceration (B).

Intravenous Regional Anesthesia

Indications

Procedures of the arm or leg that require operating anesthesia, muscle relaxation, or a bloodless field:

- Reduction of fractures and dislocations
- Repair of major lacerations
- Removal of foreign bodies
- Débridement of burns
- Drainage of infection

Contraindications

Absolute

- Allergy to anesthetic agent
- Uncontrolled hypertension

Relative

- Severe Raynaud disease
- Buerger disease
- Crushed or hypoxic extremity
- Procedures taking >90 minutes

Complications

- Lidocaine allergy (rare)
- Lidocaine toxicity
- Thrombophlebitis
- Tissue extravasation of anesthetic agent

Equipment

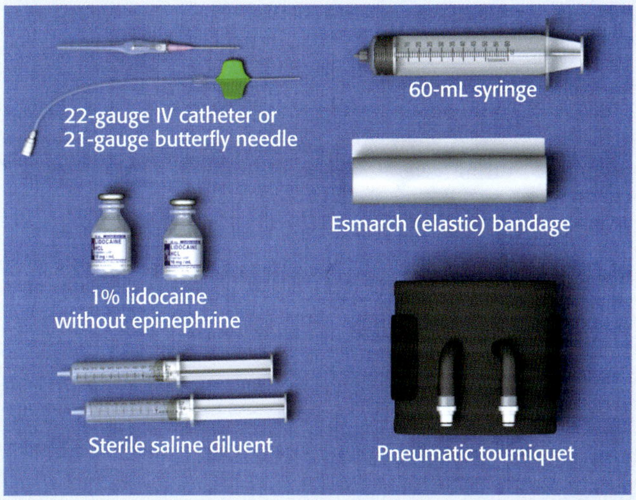

Review Box 32.1 Intravenous regional anesthesia: indications, contraindications, complications, and equipment. A double-cuff tourniquet is shown. Not shown is a device required to provide continuous cuff pressure (see Fig. 32.2). *Do not use a standard blood pressure cuff.*

It is strongly advised to not use a regular blood pressure cuff because these cuffs often leak or rupture and are not designed to withstand high pressure for any length of time. A specially designed portable double-cuff pneumatic system, such as that marketed by Zimmer Corporation, is ideal and preferred by the authors.

Premix the anesthetic and saline solution in the syringe. Insert a plastic catheter or a metal butterfly needle in a superficial vein as close to the pathologic site as possible, and securely tape it in place (Fig. 32.3, *step 1*). It is usually desirable to use a vein on the dorsum of the hand, but importantly, the injection site should be at least 10 cm distal to the tourniquet to avoid injection of anesthetic proximal to or under the tourniquet. Keep the hub on the catheter to avoid backbleeding, or attach the syringe to the butterfly tubing. This catheter will be the route of injection of the anesthetic agent. Anesthesia from a fingertip-to-elbow direction seems to occur irrespective of the site of infusion of the anesthetic, but selecting an injection location near the site of pathology may provide more rapid anesthesia at a lower dosage.

Next, passively exsanguinate the extremity to allow the anesthetic agent to fill the drained vascular system. Simple elevation of the extremity for a few minutes may be adequate, but wrapping the extremity in a distal-to-proximal direction

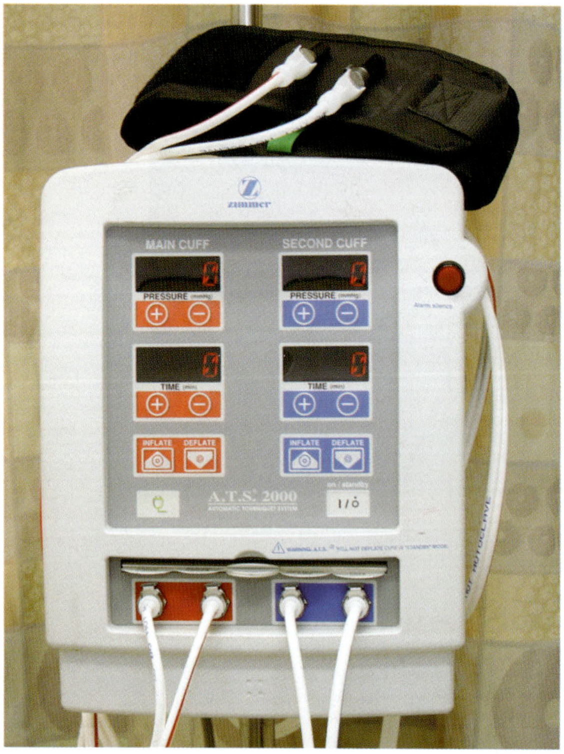

Fig. 32.2 A digital-controlled double-cuff system by Zimmer allows safe intravenous regional anesthesia and the ability to lessen pain from the arterial tourniquet.

with an elastic or Esmarch bandage, while being careful to not dislodge the infusion needle, significantly enhances exsanguination (Fig. 32.3, *step 2*). Wrapping may be painful, so this step can be eliminated if it causes too much anxiety for the patient. If the wrapping procedure is not done, the extremity should be elevated for at least 5 minutes as this has been shown to be equally as efficacious at exsanguinating the extremity.[7] During the wrapping procedure, take care to not dislodge or infiltrate the infusion catheter.

With the extremity still elevated or wrapped, inflate the tourniquet to 250 mm Hg or 100 mm Hg above systolic pressure (Fig. 32.3, *steps 3–4*). In a child, inflate the tourniquet to 50 mm Hg above systolic pressure. In the leg, inflate cuff pressure to 300 mm Hg or approximately twice the systolic pressure measured in the arms. Place the arm (or leg) by the patient's side, and remove the elastic exsanguination bandage (Fig. 32.3, *step 5*).

With the tourniquet now inflated, slowly inject the 0.5% lidocaine solution into the infusion catheter at the calculated dose (Fig. 32.3, *step 6*). Note that the solution is placed in the arm in which the circulation is blocked, not in the precautionary keep-open IV line on the unaffected side. At this point, blotchy areas of erythema may appear on the skin. This is not an adverse reaction to the anesthetic agent but merely the result of residual blood being displaced from the vascular compartment, and it indicates success of the procedure.

In 3 to 5 minutes, the patient will experience paresthesia or warmth beginning in the fingertips and traveling proximally, with final anesthesia occurring above the elbow, to the level of the tourniquet. Complete anesthesia ensues in 10 to 20 minutes, followed by muscle relaxation. Note that adequate analgesia may exist even if the patient can still sense touch and position and has some motor function. If the "minidose" technique (initial dose of 1.5 mg/kg of lidocaine) does not provide adequate anesthesia, infuse an additional 0.5 to 1 mg/kg of diluted lidocaine at this time. As an example, for a 70-kg patient, an additional 0.5 mg/kg of lidocaine equals 35 mg lidocaine (3.5 mL of 1% lidocaine), and when the 1% lidocaine is diluted equally with saline, the final volume of the additional 0.5% lidocaine is 7 mL. Additional lidocaine was required in 7% of cases in one series in which the minidose regimen was used.[6] The clinician should be patient, however, and wait a full 15 minutes before infusing additional lidocaine. Alternatively, if analgesia is slow or inadequate, an extra 10 mL to 20 mL of *saline* solution may be injected to supplement the total volume of solution to enhance the effect. Do not exceed a 3-mg/kg total dose of lidocaine. For obese patients, a maximum of 300 mg of lidocaine is suggested for the arm and no more than 400 mg for the leg. Data for very obese patients do not exist. Next, withdraw the infusing needle and tightly tape the puncture site to prevent extravasation of the anesthetic agent. Perform the surgical procedure or manipulation, including postreduction radiographs and casting or bandaging (Fig. 32.3, *step 7*).

On completion of the procedure, deflation of the tourniquet should be *cycled* to prevent a bolus effect of any lidocaine that may remain in the intravascular compartment. Deflate the cuff for 5 seconds and reinflate it for 1 to 2 minutes (Fig. 32.3, *step 8*). Repeat this action two or three times.

If the tourniquet has been in place for less than 30 minutes, an increase in transient lidocaine-related side effects may be seen if cycled deflation has not been used because adequate tissue fixation of the lidocaine has probably not occurred. This may result in a higher peak plasma lidocaine level, with increased side effects. If the surgical procedure is completed rapidly and the 3-mg/kg limit of lidocaine has been infused, the tourniquet should remain inflated until 20 to 30 minutes has elapsed, and only then should it be deflated via the cycling technique. It is reasonable to use a 20-minute cutoff if the minidose technique is used or a total of 200 mg or less of lidocaine has been administered because this dose is equal to a commonly administered antiarrhythmic IV bolus.

Sensation returns quickly when the tourniquet is removed, and in 5 to 10 minutes the extremity returns to its preanesthetic level of sensation and function. Many patients describe a transient intense tingling sensation after cuff deflation. If the procedure takes longer than 20 or 30 minutes, many patients complain of pain from the tourniquet because it is not inflated over an anesthetized area. Use of a double-cuff tourniquet may alleviate the problem of pain under the cuff. A wide tourniquet cuff (14 cm) is less painful than a narrow tourniquet (7 cm) when the cuff is inflated 10 mm Hg above loss of the arterial pulse.[8] The reason for pain under the tourniquet is unknown, but this can be a limiting factor because most patients begin to feel significant discomfort after 30 minutes if only a single cuff is used. Tourniquet pain can be significantly reduced, and tourniquet time extended by adding ketorolac to the lidocaine anesthesia.

In the *preferred* double-cuff system, two separate tourniquets are placed side by side on the extremity (Figs. 32.2 and 32.4). One is termed the *proximal cuff* and the other the *distal cuff*. The proximal cuff is inflated at the beginning of the procedure, and anesthesia is obtained under the deflated distal cuff. When the patient begins to feel pain under the proximal cuff, the distal cuff is first inflated over an already anesthetized area, and the pain-producing proximal cuff is then deflated.

Intravenous Regional Anesthesia

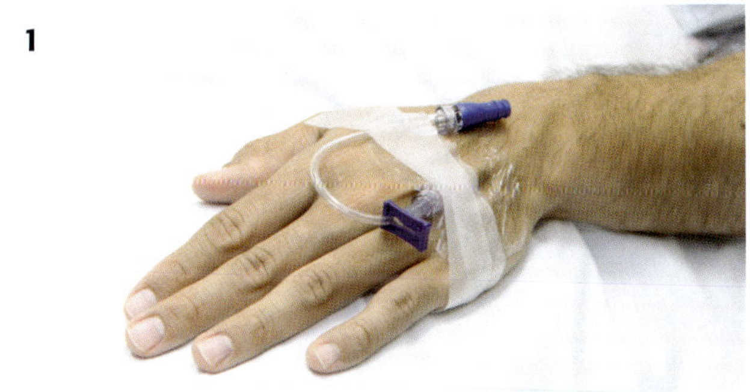

Place an IV catheter or butterfly needle as close to the pathologic site as possible. The site should be at least 10 cm distal to the tourniquet. A dorsal hand vein is ideal.

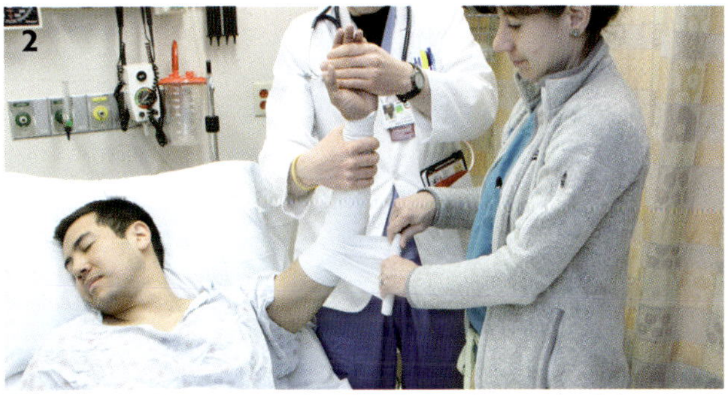

Exsanguinate the extremity by elevating and wrapping it in a distal-to-proximal fashion. Here, an Esmarch bandage is being used.

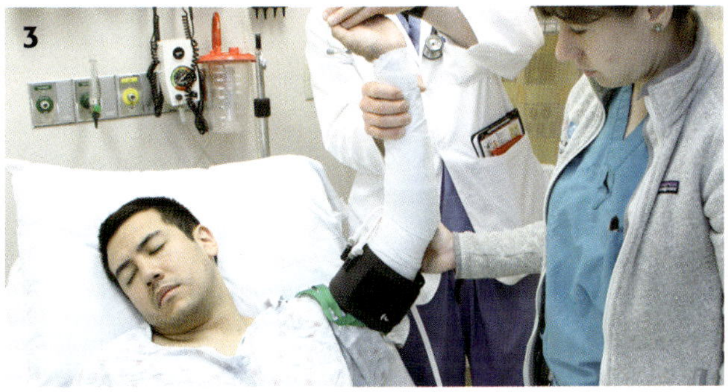

Apply the tourniquet to the patient's arm.

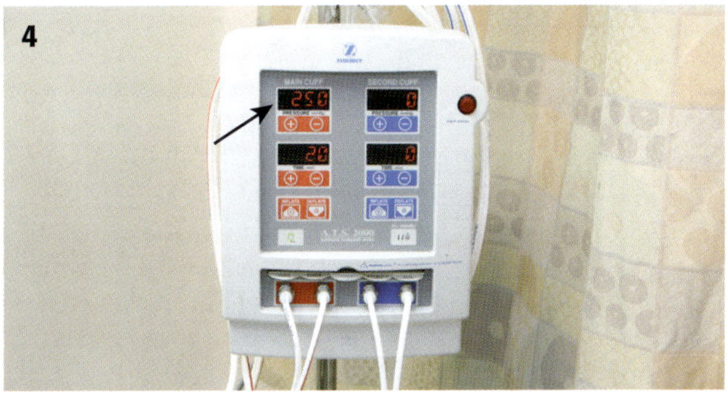

Inflate the tourniquet to 250 mm Hg or 100 mm Hg above systolic pressure. In the leg, inflate the cuff to 300 mm Hg or twice the systolic pressure measured in the arm.

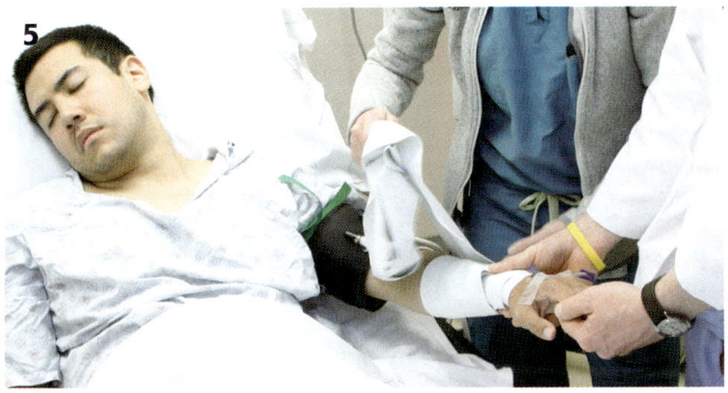

Place the patient's arm by his side and remove the Esmarch bandage. The tourniquet remains inflated.

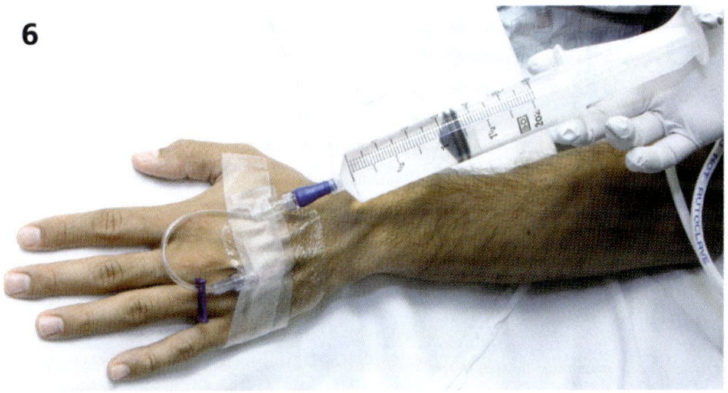

Slowly inject the 0.5% lidocaine solution into the infusion catheter at the calculated dose. See text for details and dosing information.

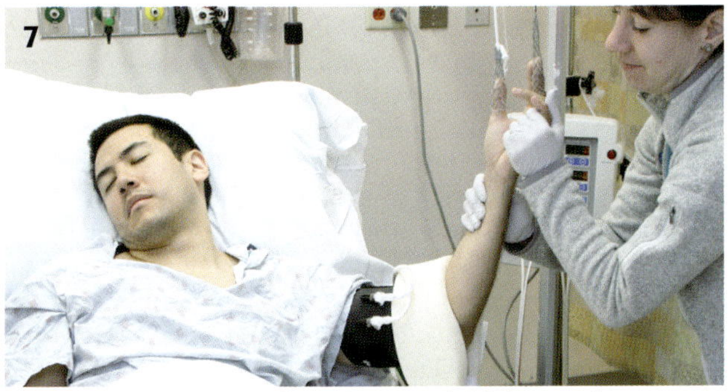

Remove the infusing needle/catheter, and tightly tape the puncture site to prevent extravasation of the anesthetic agent. Perform the procedure, including postreduction films and casting.

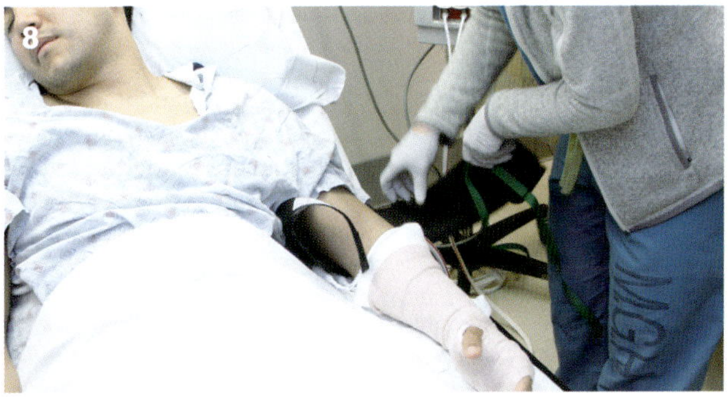

Once the procedure is complete, deflate the tourniquet in a cycling fashion (deflate for 5 seconds, reinflate for 1 to 2 minutes) 2 or 3 times. Then remove the tourniquet.

Fig. 32.3 Intravenous regional anesthesia. The procedure depicted demonstrates the use of a single tourniquet; refer to the text for details regarding the use of a double tourniquet.

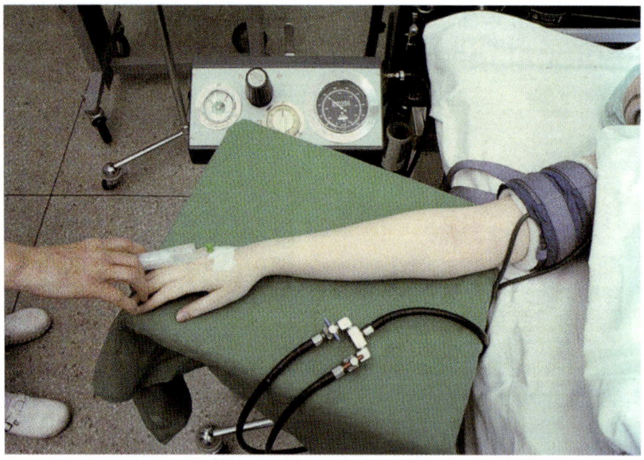

Fig. 32.4 Intravenous regional anesthesia. The preferred double-cuff tourniquet is shown as two tourniquets side by side on the extremity. (From https://commons.wikimedia.org/wiki/File:Venadaxili_regional_anesteziya.jpg.)

One must be certain to inflate the distal cuff before the proximal cuff is released; otherwise, the anesthetic will rapidly diffuse into the general circulation.

After 45 to 60 minutes of observation, the patient may be discharged. Observation time depends on the use of other medications, procedural difficulties, and overall assessment of the patient. There are no standard or specific postprocedural instructions, but precautions like those given for procedural sedation are reasonable. Driving is best prohibited for 6 to 8 hours, and the patient should leave with a responsible adult. Delayed complications from lidocaine have not been reported.

MECHANISM OF ACTION

Some of the anesthesia is undoubtedly related to the ischemia produced by the tourniquet, but most of the anesthesia is secondary to the anesthetic agent itself. Although the exact mechanism by which anesthesia is produced is unknown, the site of action of the anesthetic may be at sensory nerve endings, neuromuscular junctions, or major nerve trunks.[9] Contrast-enhanced studies have demonstrated that the anesthetic agent does not diffuse throughout the entire arm, yet anesthesia of the entire limb is obtained. Evidence indicates that the local anesthetic does not simply diffuse from the venous system into tissue but travels via vascular channels directly inside the nerve. Regardless of where the anesthetic is infused, the fingertips are the first area to experience anesthesia, thus suggesting that the core of the nerve is in contact with the anesthetic agent initially. After release of the tourniquet, a considerable amount of the drug still remains in the injected limb for at least 1 hour.[10] This would suggest that at least a portion of the anesthetic leaves the vascular compartment and becomes fixed in tissue.

PROCEDURAL POINTS

Anesthetic Agent

Use of 0.5% plain lidocaine at a dose of 1.5 to 3 mg/kg is preferred for the upper extremity. A similar dose may be used in the leg if a *calf* tourniquet is used. For procedures in the leg, using a thigh cuff, 150 mL of 0.25% lidocaine (375 mg) has been used. The greater volume can augment drug distribution in the larger lower extremity. Bupivacaine (Marcaine, Sensorcaine) is *contraindicated* because of the potential for serious cardiovascular and neurologic complications.[11]

Some authors have suggested the use of IV ketorolac in addition to the lidocaine for superior pain control during the postprocedure period.[12,13] Mixing ketorolac with the lidocaine and injecting the combination into the operative arm is safe and effective for reducing the need for postoperative analgesics and antiemetics.[12,13] Tourniquet time is prolonged with these agents as pain under the tourniquet is the main reason for discontinuing the procedure. Opiates have not been found to be helpful when added to the lidocaine but may be given at a distant site (such as via the IV infusion in the opposite arm) for general pain control.

Peak lidocaine plasma concentrations are reached 2 to 3 minutes after deflation of the tourniquet, and side effects are minimal if the deflation is cycled after the surgical procedure. The plasma half-life of lidocaine is approximately 60 seconds,[14] but the drug demonstrates a theoretical three-compartment model similar to a direct IV infusion once the tourniquet is released.[15] Peak blood levels are related to the duration of vascular occlusion and to the concentration of the anesthetic.[14,15]

Peak plasma lidocaine levels after release of the tourniquet decrease as the time of vascular occlusion (tourniquet time) increases. If the tourniquet is inflated for at least 30 minutes and the deflation-reinflation technique is used when the procedure is finished, the plasma concentration of lidocaine should be approximately 2 to 4 µg/mL, below the 5 to 10 µg/mL level at which dose-related lidocaine reactions occur.[16] Tucker and Boas demonstrated a peak plasma lidocaine level of 10.3 µg/mL after a 10-minute period of vascular occlusion,[15] as opposed to 2.3 µg/mL if the tourniquet was inflated for 45 minutes.

More dilute solutions of lidocaine are associated with lower peak lidocaine levels. When equal doses of lidocaine are used, peak arterial plasma levels are 40% lower if the 0.5% solution is used than if the 1% solution is used.[15] For example, after 10 minutes of vascular occlusion, the peak plasma concentration of lidocaine has been demonstrated to reach 10.3 µg/mL with the 1% solution versus only 5.6 µg/mL when the drug was given under similar circumstances at a 0.5% concentration.[15]

Exsanguination

Many clinicians consider exsanguination of the extremity before injection of the anesthetic agent to be essential for success. Others do not believe that it is a critical factor. Exsanguination by simple elevation of the extremity should be done in all cases, but in certain instances one should consider avoiding the painful wrapping of the extremity with an elastic or Esmarch bandage. (Note that applying an Esmarch wrap over a fracture site is usually quite painful.) A pneumatic splint, such as the type used for prehospital immobilization, is also a reasonable alternative to painful wrapping. The process of exsanguination is believed to allow better vascular diffusion of the anesthetic.

Site of Injection

Anesthesia is usually achieved no matter where the local anesthetic is injected, but some evidence indicates that the procedure

BOX 32.1 IVRA: Step-by-Step Procedure

1. Begin an intravenous (IV) line in the uninvolved extremity (optional, but highly recommended to give fluids, sedatives, or other medications should any adverse reactions occur).
2. Draw up and dilute 1% plain lidocaine (1.5 to 3 mg/kg total lidocaine dose) for a final concentration of 0.5% lidocaine.[a]
3. Insert a small plastic IV cannula near but distal to the pathologic lesion and secure it.
4. Elevate and exsanguinate the extremity with Esmarch bandage.
5. Inflate the tourniquet (250 mm Hg), lower the extremity and remove the exsanguination device. Inflate the proximal cuff only if a double-cuff system is used.
6. Infuse the anesthetic solution.
7. Remove the infusion needle and tape the site.
8. Perform the procedure.
9. If pain is produced by the tourniquet, inflate the distal cuff first, and then deflate the proximal cuff.
10. After the procedure is complete, deflate the cuff for 5 seconds and then reinflate it for 1 to 2 minutes. Repeat this step three times. Do not deflate the cuff if total tourniquet time is less than 20 to 30 minutes.
11. Observe 45 to 60 minutes for possible reactions.

[a]*Commercial preparations with or without preservatives are acceptable.*
From Roberts JR. Intravenous regional anesthesia. JACEP. *1977;6:263.*

is more successful when the anesthetic is injected distally. Sorbie and Chacha noted the following failure rates associated with specific sites of anesthetic injection[17]: antecubital fossa, 23%; middle of the forearm or leg, 18%; and hand, wrist, or foot, 4%. In most cases a vein in the dorsum of the hand or foot is used. If local pathology precludes use of the hand, the midforearm or antecubital fossa of the elbow is an acceptable, albeit less desirable, alternative as long as the infusion catheter is well below the tourniquet to avoid systemic injection.

Although most of the literature stresses the use of this technique on the upper extremity, it may also be used successfully on the leg. It cannot, however, be used for procedures above the knee. Tourniquet pain appears to be a limiting factor when the procedure is used on the leg. One must be certain to avoid damage to the peroneal nerve by using the tourniquet in the midcalf area only.

COMPLICATIONS

Although IVRA is both safe and simple, complications do occur and are usually related to equipment failure or mistakes in technique.

Anesthetic Agent

Serious complications seldom occur if proper attention is paid to technique. True lidocaine allergy is very rare. Other reactions to lidocaine are rare and are usually systemic reactions from high blood levels.[11,16] High levels may result from miscalculation of dosages, from too rapid release of the tourniquet before the anesthetic has become fixed in tissue ("bolus effect"), or rarely, from advancement of the infusion catheter proximal to the tourniquet, thereby resulting in direct IV infusion. To minimize the potential risk of toxic systemic lidocaine release, do not deflate the tourniquet within 20 minutes of the injection. This allows the anesthetic to become fixed in the tissues minimizing the potential bolus effect into the systemic circulation.

Generally, the central nervous system effects of lidocaine are minor and result in mild reactions such as dizziness, tinnitus, lethargy, headache, or blurred vision. This should not occur in more than 2% to 3% of patients and requires no treatment.[11] Transient hypotension and bradycardia may develop but are generally self-limited.

The most common complication related to the anesthetic agent is rapid systemic vascular infusion, which occurs when a blood pressure cuff malfunctions or slowly leaks. Similar complications may occur if the cuff is deflated earlier than 20 to 30 minutes after the induction of anesthesia. Both complications are the result of a bolus effect of the anesthetic, similar to an IV injection.

Auroy and colleagues reported 23 seizures in 11,229 cases,[18] with no cardiac arrest or fatalities, and deemed IVRA safer than general anesthesia or peripheral nerve blocks. However, seizures occurring after tourniquet deflation have been reported with tourniquet time as long as 60 minutes and with the lowest effective dose at 1.5 mg/kg.[19] Seizures are generally not recurrent and are treated with oxygen and anticonvulsant drugs. Transient cardiovascular reactions, such as bradycardia and hypotension, are possible with large doses of lidocaine. A systematic review of systemic local anesthetic toxicity associated with IVRA resulted in 64 cases reported between 1964 and 2005. Cardiac arrests and deaths were reported in 13 patients and bupivacaine was used in most of these patients.[19]

Additional Complications

Other major complications reported with IVRA are nerve injuries and compartment syndromes.[19] Younger age, higher tourniquet pressures and longer tourniquet times can all increase the likelihood of a nerve complication.[20,21] Thrombophlebitis, skin discoloration, and urticaria can occur following the IV administration of anesthetics.

A particularly bothersome problem is infiltration or dislodgement of the infusion catheter during exsanguination and tissue extravasation of the anesthetic agent. In addition, some leakage of anesthetic can occur after the infusion needle has been removed. Both problems may result in poor anesthesia but may be minimized if a small, well-secured plastic infusion needle is used instead of a metal scalp vein ("butterfly") needle and if the puncture site is tightly taped after withdrawal of the catheter.

This procedure cannot be used for manipulations or operations in which the pulse must be monitored as a guide to reduction (e.g., supracondylar fractures of the humerus) because the tourniquet occludes arterial flow. Use of the Bier block in patients with sickle cell disease is not well documented. It should be used with caution until the ischemic effect of the tourniquet on the red blood cells of such patients has been clarified. In all patients, tourniquet time should not exceed 90 minutes. Ischemia for less than this amount of time is not associated with serious sequelae.

REFERENCES ARE AVAILABLE AT Elsevier eBooks+

CHAPTER 33

Systemic Analgesia and Sedation for Procedures

Craig Rowland Torres-Ness

Procedural sedation and analgesia (PSA) refers to the use of analgesic, dissociative, and sedative agents to relieve the pain and anxiety associated with diagnostic and therapeutic procedures. PSA is an integral element of emergency medicine residency and pediatric emergency medicine fellowship training and curricula, and graduates of these programs are skilled in the practice of PSA. Moreover, by virtue of their training, emergency clinicians are proficient in resuscitation, vascular access, and advanced airway management, which permits them to effectively recognize and manage the potential complications associated with PSA.[1,2]

In a study of all practitioners, the most common clinical errors associated with PSA were delayed recognition of respiratory depression and arrest, inadequate monitoring, and inadequate resuscitation,[3] mistakes that are unlikely to be made by emergency clinicians. The safety of PSA techniques by emergency clinicians has been well documented in numerous series in both children and adults.[4–8] Safe and successful application of PSA requires careful patient selection, customization of therapy to the specific needs of the patient, and careful monitoring of patients for adverse events. Emergency clinicians must ensure that all patients receive pain relief and sedation commensurate with their individual needs during any procedure.

TERMINOLOGY

The progression from minimal sedation to general anesthesia is a nonlinear continuum that does not lend itself to division into arbitrary stages. Low doses of opioids or benzodiazepines induce mild analgesia or sedation, respectively, with little danger of adverse events. If, however, clinicians continue administering additional medication beyond this initial level, progressively altered consciousness ensues with a proportionately increased risk for respiratory and airway complications. If further medications are administered, the patient will advance along this continuum until protective airway reflexes are lost and general anesthesia is ultimately reached. This continuum of sedation is not drug specific in that varying states from mild sedation to general anesthesia can be achieved with virtually all nondissociative PSA agents (e.g., opioids, benzodiazepines, barbiturates, etomidate, propofol).

In 1985 the American Academy of Pediatrics (AAP) and the National Institutes of Health issued guidelines for the management and monitoring of children receiving sedation for diagnostic and therapeutic procedures in response to the growing use of opioids and sedative-hypnotic agents in the outpatient setting and a number of sedation-related deaths.[9,10] In these documents, three levels of sedation were defined (conscious sedation, deep sedation, and general anesthesia) to create a common language for describing drug-induced alterations in consciousness (Box 33.1).[11,12] A key development in the field of PSA has been revision of the original terminology and adoption of clearer descriptions of varying types and degrees of sedation (see Box 33.1). Though historically popular, the widely misinterpreted and misused term "conscious sedation" has fallen into disfavor[13]; it has been labeled as "confusing,"[14] "imprecise,"[13] and an "oxymoron"[13,14] and has been replaced with the term "moderate sedation."[11]

Despite improvements in PSA terminology, the system is imperfect and there is still no objective way to assess the depth of sedation. Levels of responsiveness remain at best crude surrogate markers of respiratory drive and retention of protective airway reflexes. This is especially true for all levels of sedation in young children (infants and toddlers) who do not understand or are unreliable in following verbal commands. Although respiratory depression and respiratory arrest can be detected quickly with standard interactive and mechanical monitoring, there is no safe and practical way to assess the status of protective airway reflexes. Data are currently insufficient to determine whether deep sedation is associated with impairment of protective reflexes or whether such danger is encountered only when "pushing" deep sedation to the point at which it approaches or reaches general anesthesia.

PSA GUIDELINES

Before the promulgation of PSA guidelines by specialty societies and governmental agencies, clinicians simply administered sedatives in varied clinical settings and used individual judgment to determine the need for specific monitoring devices and supporting personnel. Since 1985 at least 27 sets of PSA guidelines have been published, each crafted for the unique and differing settings in which PSA is practiced.[15] Naturally, not all are in agreement.[6] The intent of each of these guidelines is to better standardize the manner in which PSA is performed to enhance patient safety. Those most pertinent to emergency clinicians are from the American College of Emergency Physicians (ACEP),[4] the AAP,[16] and the American Society of Anesthesiologists (ASA).[17]

In the early 1990s the Joint Commission on Accreditation of Healthcare Organizations, an independent, not-for-profit organization that evaluates and accredits hospitals in the United States, took a special interest in PSA, with the central theme being that the standard of sedation care provided should be comparable throughout a given hospital. Thus patients sedated in the emergency department (ED) should not receive a significantly different level of attention or monitoring than those sedated for a similar-level procedure in the operating room or in the endoscopy suite. To ensure this, the Joint Commission requires specific PSA protocols to be applied consistently throughout each institution. These hospital-wide sedation policies will vary from site to site based on the specific needs and expertise available within each institution. In 2023 the Joint Commission released new standards for pain management, sedation, and anesthesia care.[18]

At each hospital accreditation survey, the Joint Commission determines whether practitioners practice PSA consistent with their hospital-wide sedation policy and whether they provide sufficient documentation of such compliance. Clinicians must be familiar with their hospital's sedation policies and should work with their medical staff to ensure that such policies are suitably detailed, yet reasonable and realistic. Unduly restrictive policies do a disservice to patients by

BOX 33.1 PSA: Terminology and Definitions

GENERAL

- **Analgesia**[1]**:** Relief of pain without intentional production of an altered mental state such as sedation. An altered mental state may be a secondary effect of medications administered for this purpose.
- **Anxiolysis**[1]**:** A state of decreased apprehension concerning a particular situation in which there is no change in a patient's level of awareness.
- **PSA**[2]**:** A technique of administering sedatives, analgesics, dissociative agents, or any combination of such agents to induce a state that allows the patient to tolerate unpleasant procedures while maintaining cardiorespiratory function. PSA is intended to result in a depressed level of consciousness but one that allows the patient to maintain airway control independently and continuously. Specifically, the drugs, doses, and techniques used are not likely to produce loss of protective airway reflexes.

CURRENT SEDATION STATE: TERMINOLOGY

- **Minimal sedation (anxiolysis)**[1]**:** A drug-induced state during which patients respond normally to verbal commands. Although cognitive function and coordination may be impaired, ventilatory and cardiovascular function is unaffected.
- **Moderate sedation (formerly conscious sedation)**[1]**:** A drug-induced depression of consciousness during which patients respond purposefully to verbal commands, either alone or accompanied by light tactile stimulation. Reflex withdrawal from a painful stimulus is not considered a purposeful response. No interventions are required to maintain a patent airway, and spontaneous ventilation is adequate. Cardiovascular function is usually maintained.
- **Dissociative sedation**[3]**:** A trancelike cataleptic state induced by the dissociative agent ketamine and characterized by profound analgesia and amnesia with retention of protective airway reflexes, spontaneous respirations, and cardiopulmonary stability.
- **Deep sedation**[1]**:** A drug-induced depression of consciousness during which patients cannot be easily aroused but respond purposefully after repeated or painful stimulation. The ability to independently maintain ventilatory function may be impaired. Patients may require assistance in maintaining a patent airway, and spontaneous ventilation may be inadequate. Cardiovascular function is usually maintained.
- **General anesthesia**[1]**:** A drug-induced loss of consciousness during which patients cannot be aroused, even by painful stimulation. The ability to independently maintain ventilatory function is often impaired. Patients frequently need assistance in maintaining a patent airway, and positive pressure ventilation may be required because of depressed spontaneous ventilation or drug-induced depression of neuromuscular function. Cardiovascular function may be impaired.

REFERENCES

1. Joint commission on accreditation of Healthcare Organizations. *Accreditation Manual for Hosp.* 2001. JCAHO. http://www.jcaho.org.
2. American College of Emergency Physicians. Clinical Policy for Procedural Sedation and Analgesia in the Emergency Department. *Ann Emerg Med.* 2014:63–247.
3. Green SM, Krauss B. The semantics of ketamine [editorial]. *Ann Emerg Med.* 2000:36–480.

PSA, *Procedural sedation and analgesia.*

discouraging appropriate levels of analgesia and sedation. Most hospitals pattern their sedation policies after the Joint Commission standards and definitions, but there is still variation between institutions and restrictions are not uncommon.[19] It is also important to note that the unique ketamine dissociative state does not fit into the existing Joint Commission definitions of sedation and anesthesia.[12] A ready solution is to assign a distinct definition for "dissociative sedation" (see Box 33.1).

The Joint Commission requires that PSA practitioners who are permitted to administer deep sedation be qualified to rescue patients from general anesthesia.[11] Emergency clinicians typically perform all levels of sedation except general anesthesia. Moderate sedation suffices for the majority of procedures in adults and cooperative children, although it will not be adequate for extremely painful procedures (e.g., hip reduction, cardioversion). Deep sedation can facilitate such procedures, but with greater risk for cardiorespiratory depression than is the case with moderate sedation. Moderate sedation is frequently insufficient for effective anxiolysis and immobilization in younger, frightened children, and deep or dissociative sedation is an appropriate alternative.

The Centers for Medicare & Medicaid Services (CMS) has published similar requirements for hospital anesthesia services that also includes the provision of PSA throughout a given institution. Health care institutions wishing to bill Medicare must adhere to these guidelines and provide supporting documentation when requested. In 2011 CMS issued revised guidelines to help clarify various provisions of their anesthesia services requirements.[20] The new CMS guidelines emphasize that hospital policies governing the provision of anesthesia services (including PSA) must be based on nationally recognized guidelines; the source of these guidelines may include a number of specialty organizations, including ACEP.[4] CMS also notes that "The ED is a unique environment where patients present on an unscheduled basis with often very complex problems that may require several emergent or urgent interventions to proceed simultaneously to prevent further morbidity or mortality," and that, "...emergency medicine-trained physicians have very specific skill sets to manage airways and provide the ventilation necessary for patient rescue. Therefore these practitioners are uniquely qualified to provide all levels of analgesia/sedation and anesthesia (moderate to deep to general)."[20]

EVALUATION BEFORE PSA

The practice of PSA has three essential components performed in sequence: the initial presedation evaluation, sedation during the procedure, and postprocedure recovery and discharge from the ED. In all but the most emergency situations, perform a directed history and physical examination before PSA. If this evaluation suggests additional risk,

TABLE 33.1 ASA Physical Status Classification

ASA CLASS	DESCRIPTION	EXAMPLES	SUITABILITY FOR SEDATION
1	Normal healthy patient	Unremarkable past medical history	Excellent
2	Patient with mild systemic disease—no functional limitation	Mild asthma, controlled seizure disorder, anemia, controlled diabetes mellitus	Generally good
3	Patient with severe systemic disease—definite functional limitation	Moderate to severe asthma, poorly controlled seizure disorder, pneumonia, poorly controlled diabetes mellitus, moderate obesity	Intermediate to poor; consider benefits relative to risks
4	Patient with severe systemic disease that is a constant threat to life	Severe bronchopulmonary dysplasia; sepsis; advanced degrees of pulmonary, cardiac, hepatic, renal, or endocrine insufficiency	Poor; benefits rarely outweigh risks
5	Moribund patient not expected to survive without the operation	Septic shock, severe trauma	Extremely poor

ASA, American Society of Anesthesiologists.
From Krauss B, Green SM. Sedation and analgesia for procedures in children. *N Engl J Med*. 2000;342:938.

reconsider the advisability of sedation. High-risk cases may be better managed in the more controlled environment of the operating room.

Presedation assessment is a Joint Commission requirement, and most hospitals have developed specific protocols to facilitate consistent documentation of the required items. In general, however, all the appropriate parameters are already documented in the general ED record or are obvious by simply evaluating the patient's complaint. Except in emergency situations, discuss the risks, benefits, and limitations of any PSA with the patient or parent or guardian in advance and obtain verbal agreement. Formal written informed consent is not required as a standard of care (but may be an institutional requirement), although documentation, as discussed earlier, is essential.

General

Assess the type and severity of any underlying medical problems. This is usually best documented by the standard ED medical record, history, physical examination, and nursing notes. Another tool used for this purpose is the ASA physical status classification for preoperative risk stratification (Table 33.1). Verify current medications and allergies and inquire about previous adverse experiences with PSA or anesthesia.

Airway

Inspect the airway to determine whether any abnormalities (e.g., severe obesity, short neck, small mandible, large tongue, trismus) are present that might impair airway management. Consider assessments such as Mallampati scoring or the distance between the chin and hyoid bone (see Fig. 4.3).

Cardiovascular

Perform cardiac auscultation to assess for disturbances in rhythm or other abnormalities. In patients with known cardiovascular disease, evaluate their degree of reserve because most PSA agents can cause vasodilation and hypotension.

Respiratory

Perform lung auscultation to assess for active pulmonary disease, especially obstructive lung disease and upper respiratory infections that may predispose the patient to airway reactivity.

Gastrointestinal

The risk of aspiration during procedural sedation is extremely rare, with only a few reported cases of aspiration-related deaths. These incidents occurred mostly during upper gastrointestinal endoscopy and did not involve children or healthy adults. There is no evidence indicating that deviating from the ASA fasting guidelines for elective procedures increases the risk of aspiration or other adverse events[17,21–28]

In 2020 The International Committee for the Advancement of Procedural Sedation provided the first fasting and aspiration prevention recommendations specific to procedural sedation. Their recommendations are summarized in Fig. 33.1 and serve as a set of guidelines that more closely reflect the realities of the ED.[29] In summary, common sense should apply and clinical judgment should prevail, but it is standard for PSA to be performed in the ED on patients in the nonfasting state.[30]

Hepatic and Renal

The implications of delayed metabolism or excretion of PSA agents in infants younger than 6 months, in the elderly, and in patients with hepatic or renal abnormality should be considered.

PERSONNEL AND INTERACTIVE MONITORING

The most important element of PSA monitoring is close and continuous observation of the patient by an individual capable of recognizing complications of sedation (Fig. 33.2). This person must be able to continuously observe the patient's face, mouth, and chest wall motion. Equipment or sterile drapes must not interfere with such visualization. Such careful observation allows prompt detection of adverse events such

Presedation assessment: risk factors			
	Negligible risk factors	Mild risk factors	Moderate risk factors
		Patient • Severe systemic disease • Moderate obesity (BMI 30–39; 85th–95th percentile in children) • Age 12 months or less • Hiatal hernia Procedure/sedation • Upper endoscopy • Bronchoscopy • Propofol principal sedation	Patient • Severe systemic disease that is a constant threat to life • Severe obesity (BMI of 40 or higher; greater than 95th percentile in children) • Obstructive sleep apnea • Airway abnormalities (micrognathia, macroglossia and laryngomalacia) • Hyperemesis, esophageal disorders, bowel obstruction
Elective procedures			
	Negligible aspiration risk	Mild aspiration risk (any of the above)	Moderate aspiration risk (any of the above) Refer for anesthesia care
Clear liquids[1]	Unrestricted	Unrestricted	Fasting approximately 2 hrs[2]
Breast milk	Unrestricted	Fasting approximately 2 hrs[2]	Fasting approximately 4 hrs[2]
Food, formula, nonhuman milk	Fasting approximately 2 hrs[1]	Fasting approximately 4 hrs[2]	Fasting approximately 6 hrs[2]
Urgent or emergency procedures			
	No delay based on fasting time	No delay based on fasting time	No delay based on fasting time. Anesthesia care if available; if not, consider ketamine as sole agent

Fig. 33.1 Risk stratification tool regarding aspiration in procedural sedation and analgesia from the Internal Committee for the Advancement of Procedural Sedation. [1]Clear liquids are generally considered to include water, fruit juices without pulp, clear tea and black coffee. [2]Fasting intervals not absolutes and reasonable exceptions are permissible. (From Green SM, Leroy PL, Roback MG et al. International Committee for the Advancement of Procedural Sedation. An international multidisciplinary consensus statement on fasting before procedural sedation in adults and children. *Anaesthesia*. 2020;75(3):374-385.)

as respiratory depression, apnea, partial airway obstruction, emesis, and hypersalivation.

PSA personnel should understand the pharmacology of analgesic and sedative agents and their respective reversal agents. They must be proficient in maintaining airway patency and assisting ventilation if needed. PSA requires a minimum of two experienced individuals, most frequently one clinician and one nurse or respiratory therapist. The clinician typically oversees drug administration and performs the procedure, whereas the nurse or respiratory therapist continuously monitors the patient for potential complications. The nurse or respiratory therapist should also document the medications administered and the response to sedation and measure vital signs periodically. The nurse or respiratory therapist may assist in minor, interruptible tasks but must remain focused on the patient's cardiopulmonary status, and this responsibility must not be impaired. An individual with advanced life support skills should also be immediately available, which is a requisite easy to fulfill in the ED setting.

During deep sedation, the individual dedicated to patient monitoring should have experience with this depth of sedation and no other responsibilities that would interfere with the advanced level of monitoring and documentation appropriate for this degree of sedation.[31] Individual hospital-wide sedation policies may have additional requirements regarding how and when deep sedation is administered based on the patient's specific needs and the clinician's expertise.

It is not mandatory to have intravenous (IV) access in situations in which sedation is administered by the intramuscular (IM), oral, nasal, inhalational, or rectal routes, but it may be preferable based on the anticipated depth of sedation, comorbid conditions, or additional drug titration. When sedation is performed without IV access, an individual skilled in initiating such access should be immediately available.

EQUIPMENT AND MECHANICAL MONITORING

The routine use of mechanical monitoring has greatly enhanced the safety of PSA. With current technology, oxygenation (via pulse oximetry), ventilation (via capnography), and hemodynamics (via blood pressure and electrocardiogram

Procedural Sedation and Analgesia

1

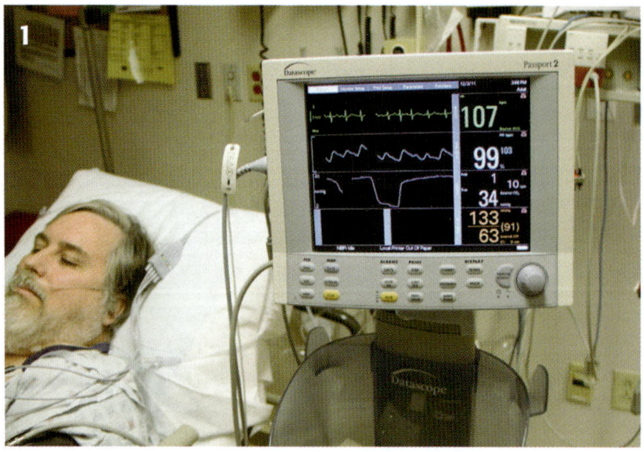

After a thorough presedation assessment, attach the patient to the monitoring system. Routine use of pulse oximetry, capnography, ECG monitoring, and blood pressure monitoring greatly enhances the safety of PSA.

2

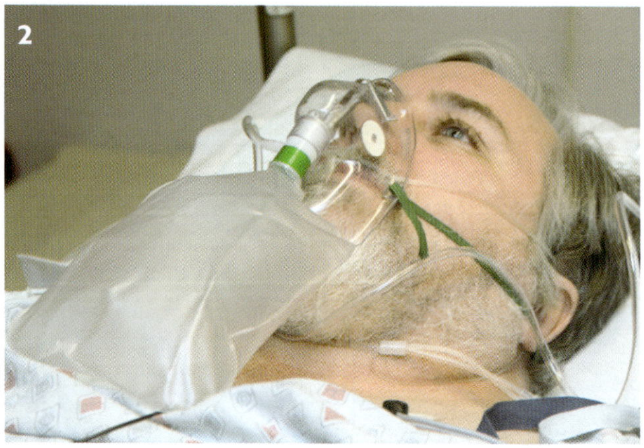

Apply supplemental oxygen, especially for patients undergoing deep sedation with agents such as propofol. In addition to pulse oximetry, observe the rise and fall of the chest, for the earliest indication of apnea. Ideally, capnography should be used in all situations in which high-flow oxygen is administered.

3

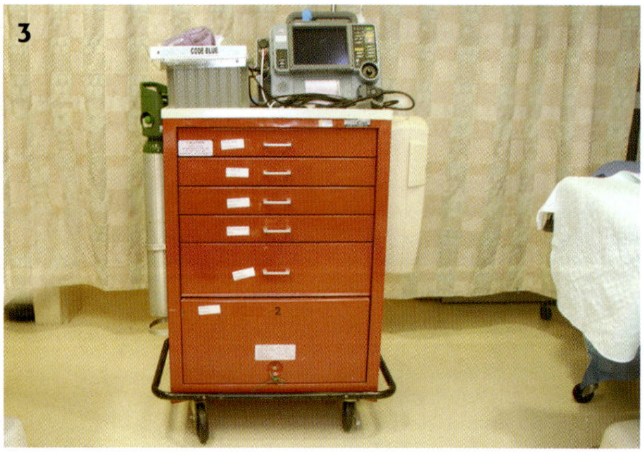

Ensure that all necessary age-appropriate resuscitation equipment is available, including oxygen, a bag-valve-mask device, suction, reversal agents, and a defibrillator (for patients with significant cardiovascular disease).

4

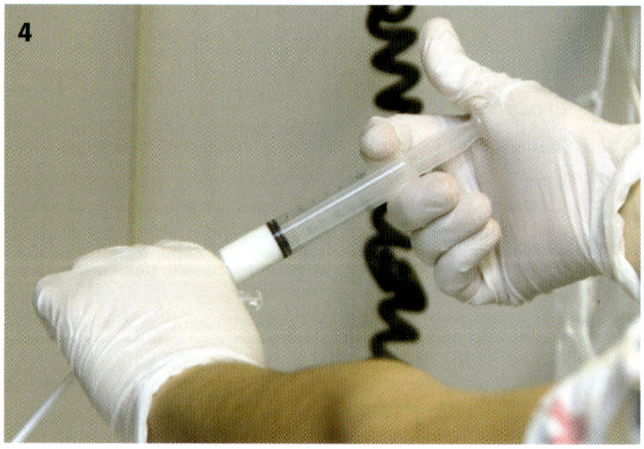

Administer the agent selected. The choice of appropriate medications is discussed in detail in the text. Here, propofol is being administered.

5

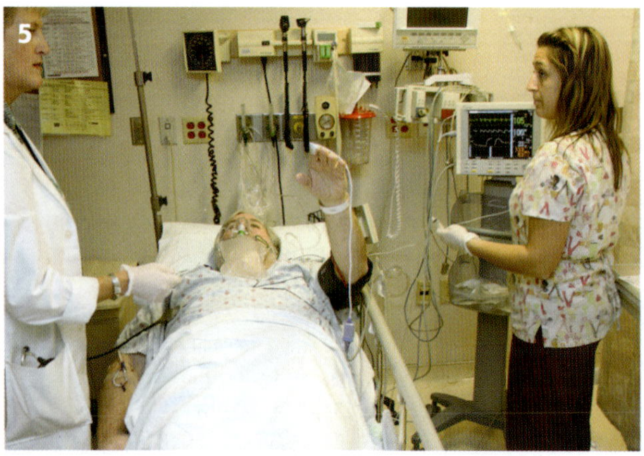

PSA requires a minimum of two experienced individuals: one to perform the procedure and one to continuously monitor the patient for potential complications. The person monitoring the patient must be focused on the patient's cardiopulmonary status.

6

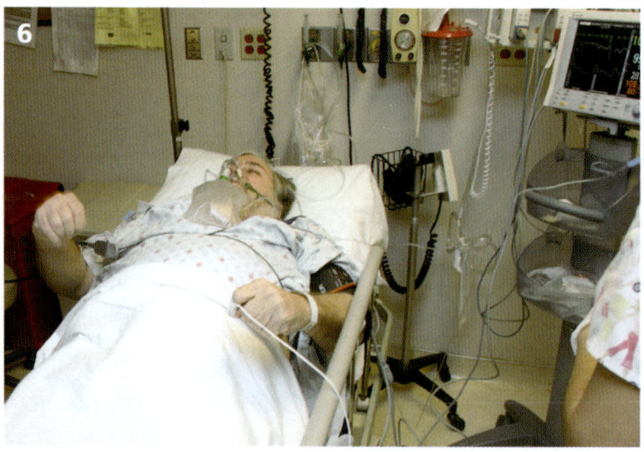

Perform the procedure. Here, the patient is being cardioverted for new-onset atrial fibrillation. After the procedure, monitor the patient until there is no further risk for cardiorespiratory depression. Before discharge, be sure that the patient is alert and oriented with stable vital signs.

Fig. 33.2 Procedural sedation and analgesia *(PSA)*.

[ECG]) can all be monitored noninvasively in nonintubated, spontaneously breathing patients.

Pulse Oximetry

Mechanical monitoring for PSA should include continuous pulse oximetry with an audible signal. Pulse oximetry measures the percentage of hemoglobin that is bound to oxygen. If the patient is breathing room air (21% oxygen), pulse oximetry will detect a decrease in alveolar ventilation rather quickly. Most patients undergoing procedural sedation in the ED are given supplemental oxygen by nasal cannula. With preoxygenation or the continued use of supplemental oxygenation during a procedure, the pulse oximetry will take significantly longer to drop despite the complete absence of ventilation. With preoxygenation it may take 4 to 5 minutes of apnea before the pulse oximetry will drop significantly. Hence, pulse oximetry is not a substitute for monitoring ventilation because of the variable lag time between the onset of hypoventilation or apnea and a change in the oxygen saturation of hemoglobin molecules.

Capnography

Capnography is a very useful tool that provides a continuous, breath-by-breath measure of the respiratory rate and CO_2 exchange. Capnography readings are not affected by the presence or absence of additional oxygen. When sedated patients begin to hypoventilate, the end-tidal CO_2 will rise. When apnea occurs, the end-tidal CO_2 drops to zero. Importantly, capnography can detect the common adverse airway and respiratory events associated with PSA.[32–44] Capnography detects the earliest airway or respiratory compromise and will show abnormally high or low end-tidal CO_2 pressure well before pulse oximetry detects falling oxyhemoglobin saturation, especially in patients receiving supplemental oxygen. Early detection of respiratory compromise is especially important in infants and toddlers, who have smaller functional residual capacity and greater oxygen consumption than older children and adults.[45–47] Capnography provides a non–impedance-based respiratory rate directly from the airway (via an oral-nasal cannula). This is more accurate than impedance-based respiratory monitoring, especially in patients with obstructive apnea or laryngospasm, in whom impedance-based monitoring will interpret chest wall movement without ventilation as a valid breath.

Multiple studies of patients undergoing PSA in a variety of clinical settings have demonstrated that capnography identifies respiratory depression earlier[33,48] and more freque ntly[39,47,49–51] than standard monitoring techniques (e.g., pulse oximetry, observation). Moreover, several additional studies have demonstrated that the use of capnography reduces the incidence of hypoxic events in both children[52] and adults.[53–56] However, there is no evidence that capnography reduces the incidence of serious adverse events such as neurologic injury (secondary to hypoxia), aspiration, or death.[57–59] As a result, capnography is not an agreed-upon standard for procedural sedation in the ED. The American College of Emergency Physician's current clinical policy on PSA gives the use of capnography a level B recommendation (recommendations for patient care that may identify a particular strategy or range of strategies that reflect moderate clinical certainty [i.e., based on evidence from one or more Class of Evidence II studies or strong consensus of Class of Evidence III studies]), stating, "Capnography may be used as an adjunct to pulse oximetry and clinical assessment to detect hypoventilation and apnea earlier than pulse oximetry and/or clinical assessment alone in patients undergoing PSA in the ED."[4]

ECG Monitoring

Although continuous ECG monitoring cannot be considered mandatory or standard of care in the absence of cardiovascular disease, such monitoring is simple, inexpensive, and readily available.

Resuscitation Equipment and Supplies

Gather all necessary age-appropriate equipment for airway management and resuscitation in the sedation area, including oxygen, a bag-valve-mask device, suction, and drug reversal agents. For subjects with significant cardiovascular disease, include a defibrillator as well.

Vital Signs

Measure vital signs periodically at individualized intervals, in most cases including measurements at baseline, after drug administration, on completion of the procedure, during early recovery, and at completion of recovery. During deep sedation it is reasonable to assess vital signs approximately every 5 minutes. Patients are at highest risk for complications 5 to 10 minutes after IV medications are administered and during the immediate postprocedure period when external stimuli are discontinued. Continuous monitoring of the ECG, blood pressure, pulse rate, and pulse oximetry via a standard monitor generally fulfills the monitoring requirements. There are no standards mandating the frequency of vital sign documentation in the medical record. Thus in the absence of institutional requirements, frequency is generally guided by the specific patient scenario, medications used, and depth of sedation, with common sense prevailing in most cases.

SUPPLEMENTAL OXYGEN

Substantial variation in practice exists with regard to the use of supplemental oxygen during PSA. The premise is a logical one: increasing systemic oxygen reserves should naturally delay, or perhaps avert, hypoxemia should an airway or respiratory adverse event occur. However, the price paid for this well-intentioned safeguard is the loss of pulse oximetry as an early warning device.[13,16,32] Hyperoxygenated patients will desaturate only after the apnea is prolonged. Indeed, the time required for preoxygenated, apneic, healthy adults, and adolescents to desaturate to 90% averages more than 6 minutes.[60,61] As a result of this, supplemental oxygen is commonly avoided when capnography is not being utilized, allowing pulse oximetry to provide warning should interactive monitoring fail to detect ventilatory compromise.[62]

Deitch and colleagues have shown in a series of randomized controlled trials that high-flow supplemental oxygen decreases the incidence of hypoxia during propofol sedation (number needed to benefit of 4),[51] whereas lesser amounts of oxygen (3 L/min) do so only marginally with propofol and not at all with lighter levels of sedation.[34,50] This benefit has been shown to be even more significant in the pediatric

TABLE 33.2 Complications After Sedation

COMPLICATION	ETIOLOGY
Delayed awakening	Prolonged drug action Hypoxemia, hypercapnia, hypovolemia
Agitation	Pain, hypoxemia, hypercapnia, full bladder Paradoxical reactions Emergence reactions
Nausea and vomiting	Sedative agents Premature oral fluids
Cardiorespiratory events	
Tachycardia	Pain, hypovolemia, impaired ventilation
Bradycardia	Vagal stimulation, opioids, hypoxia
Hypoxia	Laryngospasm, airway obstruction, oversedation

From Krauss B, Brustowicz R, eds. *Pediatric Procedural Sedation and Analgesia*. Lippincott Williams & Wilkins; 1999:145.

population.[63] As a result, clinical practice guidelines recommend the use of supplemental oxygen (with capnography if available) for adult and pediatric patients undergoing propofol or other deep sedation.[64,65] For lighter levels of sedation, supplemental oxygen has no established benefit and may impair detection of respiratory depression when using pulse oximetry without capnography.[65]

DISCHARGE CRITERIA

Monitor all patients receiving PSA until they are no longer at risk for cardiorespiratory depression (Table 33.2). Before discharge be sure that patients are alert and oriented (or have returned to an age-appropriate baseline) with stable vital signs. Many hospitals have chosen to use standardized recovery scoring systems similar to those used in their surgical post-anesthesia recovery areas (Table 33.3). Although no generally accepted minimum durations for safe discharge have been established, one large ED study found that, in children with uneventful sedation, no serious adverse effects occurred more than 25 minutes after final medication administration.[66] This suggests that in most cases, prolonged observation beyond an hour is unlikely to be necessary.

Make sure that all patients leave the hospital with a reliable adult who will observe them after discharge for postprocedural complications. Document the name of the individual in the hospital record. Give written instructions regarding appropriate diet, medications, and level of activity (Boxes 33.2 and 33.3). Even though patients may appear awake and able to comprehend instructions, they may not remember details once they leave the ED.

To be eligible for safe discharge, children are not required to walk unaided or demonstrate that they can tolerate an oral challenge because most PSA agents are emetogenic. Forcing fluids after sedation can lead to emesis before or after discharge. The AAP guidelines require only that "the patient can talk (if age appropriate)" and "the patient can sit up unaided (if age appropriate)."[17] When infants and young children are discharged after their evening bedtime, caution parents to position the child's head in the car seat carefully. Significant forward flexion might cause airway obstruction if the child falls asleep on the way home.

GENERAL PRINCIPLES

Therapeutic mistakes that result in inadequate analgesia and sedation include using the wrong agent, the wrong dose, the wrong route or frequency of administration, and poor use of adjunctive agents. With proper training and technique, adequate PSA can be provided in almost any circumstance. Understanding titration principles is critical to providing safe and effective PSA. Clinicians must have a thorough knowledge of the pharmacokinetics, dosing, administration, and potential complications of the PSA agents that they use. Time of onset from injection to the initial observed effect must be appreciated, especially when using drugs in combination, to avoid stacking of drug doses and oversedation.

The correct agent (or combination of agents) and the route and timing of administration depend on the following factors: How long will the procedure last? Will it be seconds (e.g., simple relocation of a dislocated joint, incision and drainage of a small abscess, cardioversion), minutes (e.g., complex manipulation of a fracture for reduction, breaking up loculations in a large abscess and then packing it), or prolonged (e.g., complex facial laceration repair)? How likely is it that the procedure will need to be repeated (e.g., fracture reduction)? Can topical, local, or regional anesthesia be used as an adjunct? Does the patient require sedation only for a noninvasive diagnostic imaging study?

Before drug administration, every effort should be made to minimize a patient's anxiety and distress, particularly in children. The emotional state of a patient on induction strongly correlates with the degree of distress on emergence and in the days immediately after the procedure.[67–70] Avoid being pressured by consultants to cut corners or rush PSA. Incorporating into the presedation preparation a discussion with the consultant about the sedation plan and the length of time required to safely prepare and sedate the patient can avoid the risks associated with hurried sedation.

For pediatric PSA, the clinician should appreciate the adult dose of the sedative being administered and consider this the maximum threshold. Understand that the initial dose of midazolam for PSA in a 100-kg patient on a milligram-per-kilogram basis is far less than the 0.1 mg/kg used in a child to avoid unexpected mishaps in drug dosing.

ROUTES OF ADMINISTRATION

For nondissociative agents, titrate IV medications to the patient's response for the best method of achieving rapid and safe analgesia and sedation. Wait the appropriate time for the medications to produce the intended effect before adding more doses. When using opioids, administer doses in 2- to 3-minute increments and observe for side effects such as miosis, somnolence, decreased responsiveness to verbal stimuli, impaired speech, and diminished pain on questioning

TABLE 33.3 Sample Recovery Scoring Systems

Steward Recovery Score	
Consciousness	
Awake	2
Responding to stimuli	1
Not responding	0
Airway	
Coughing on command or crying	2
Maintaining good airway	1
Airway requiring maintenance	0
Movement	
Moving limbs purposefully	2
Nonpurposeful movements	1
Not moving	0
Modified Aldrete Score	
Vital Signs	
Stable	1
Unstable	0
Respirations	
Normal	2
Shallow respirations or tachypnea	1
Apnea	0
Level of Consciousness	
Alert, oriented or returned to preprocedural level	2
Arousable, giddy, agitated	1
Unresponsive	0
Oxygen Saturation	
95%–100% or preprocedural level	2
90%–94%	1
<90%	0
Color	
Pink or preprocedural color	2
Pale or dusky	1
Cyanotic	0
Activity	
Moves on command or preprocedural level	2
Moves extremities or uncoordinated walking	1
No spontaneous movement	0
Sedation Score	**Action**
>8	Consider discharge if no score = 0
7–8	Vital signs q20min
4–6	Vital signs q10min
0–3	Vital signs q5min—consider further evaluation if prolonged

From Krauss B, Brustowicz R, eds. *Pediatric Procedural Sedation and Analgesia*. Lippincott Williams & Wilkins; 1999:157.

BOX 33.2 Sample Adult Disposition Instructions After PSA

1. Do not drive or operate heavy machinery for 12 hours.
2. Eat a light diet for the next 12 hours.
3. Take only your prescribed medications as needed, including any pain medication you were discharged with. Avoid alcohol.
4. Do not make any important decisions or sign important documents for 12 hours. You may be forgetful because of the medications that were administered.
5. If you experience any difficulty breathing or persistent nausea and vomiting, return to the emergency department.
6. You should have a responsible person with you for the rest of the day and during the night.

PSA, *Procedural sedation and analgesia.*

as appropriate initial end points. For sedative-hypnotics, use similar incremental dosing and end points such as ptosis (rather than miosis), somnolence, slurred speech, and alterations in gaze. Repeated doses may be given in a titrated fashion based on the patient's response during the procedure.

BOX 33.3 Sample Pediatric Disposition Instructions After PSA

Your child has been given medicine for sedation and/or pain control. These medicines may cause your child to be sleepy and less aware of the surroundings, thus making it easier for accidents to happen while walking or crawling. Because of these side effects, your child should be watched closely for the next few hours. We suggest the following:

1. No eating or drinking for the next 2 hours. Infants may resume half-normal feedings when they are hungry.
2. No playing for 12 hours that requires normal coordination, such as bike riding or jungle gym activities.
3. No playing without an adult to watch and supervise for the next 12 hours.
4. No baths, showers, cooking, or use of potentially dangerous electrical appliances unless supervised by an adult for the next 12 hours.

If you notice anything unusual about your child, call us for advice or return to the emergency department for reevaluation.

PSA, *Procedural sedation and analgesia.*

The oral, transmucosal (i.e., nasal, rectal), and IM routes are more convenient means of administration when IV access is not necessary, but they are much less reliable for timely dose titration to a desired response. The refinement of intranasal drug delivery has significantly increased the efficacy of this route of administration.[71,72] Before the development of metered-dose atomizers, the degree of absorption and effectiveness of intranasal drug administration were operator dependent.[73,74] Furthermore, drug formulations with concentrations appropriate for intranasal administration are now more readily available.[75]

The main advantage of these other routes is for pediatric patients in whom IV access may be problematic or for procedures that may require only minimal sedation in conjunction with the use of local anesthetics. These routes are also advantageous for simple sedation during diagnostic imaging.

With the exception of ketamine, agents administered intramuscularly have erratic absorption and a variable onset of action. Accordingly, prolonged preprocedural and postprocedural observation may be necessary. When required the IM route offers little advantage over oral or transmucosal administration.

Another PSA route is via inhalation of nitrous oxide. This gas can either be delivered by a demand-flow system using a handheld mask or be delivered to young children using a nose mask in a continuous-flow system under close clinician supervision.

Because individual needs may vary widely, the application of arbitrary ceiling doses of analgesic and sedative regimens is unwarranted. The true ceiling dose of an agent is the level that provides adequate pain relief or sedation without major cardiopulmonary side effects such as respiratory depression, apnea, bradycardia, or hypotension.

There are two absolute contraindications to PSA: severe clinical instability requiring immediate attention and refusal by a competent patient. Relative contraindications include hemodynamic or respiratory compromise, altered sensorium, or an inability to monitor for adverse events (e.g., MRI without remote monitoring). However, even in many of these circumstances, appropriate agents can be given to provide analgesia and sedation while minimizing the chance for further deterioration. Although safely sedating patients at the extremes of age is challenging and requires additional care, as well as reductions in drug dosing (because of decreased drug metabolism and excretion), age is not a contraindication to PSA.

DRUG SELECTION STRATEGIES

The majority of nonpainful or minimally painful ED procedures in older children and adults can be performed without systemic sedation and analgesia. Skilled practitioners can frequently combine a calm, reassuring bedside manner with distraction techniques, careful local or regional anesthesia, or both.[76–79] Many procedures, however, cannot be technically or humanely performed without PSA. These situations can be divided into three categories.

Insufficient Analgesia. Despite a cooperative patient, for some procedures it is impossible to achieve effective pain control with local or regional anesthesia. Examples of procedures requiring systemic PSA include fracture reductions, dislocation reductions, incision and drainage of large loculated abscesses, wounds that require scrubbing such as "road rash," cardioversion, bone marrow aspiration/biopsy, and extensive burn debridement.

Insufficient Anxiolysis. Despite effective local or regional anesthesia, some patients will be so frightened that procedures cannot be technically or humanely performed without PSA. Young children requiring repair of lacerations are frequently terrified, and older children and adults may be highly anxious in anticipation of such repairs in sensitive or personal regions (e.g., face, genitalia, perineum).

Insufficient Immobilization. Despite effective local or regional anesthesia and anxiolysis, PSA may be indicated to prevent excessive motion during procedures that require substantial immobilization (e.g., repair of complex facial lacerations, diagnostic imaging studies). Immobilization is most commonly an issue with young children and those with mental or psychiatric impairments.

General Considerations. Clinicians must therefore base customization of their selection of drugs (e.g., anxiolysis, sedation, analgesia, immobilization) on the unique needs of the patient and their individual level of experience with specific agents (Table 33.4). A risk-benefit analysis should be performed before every sedation (Box 33.4). The benefits of reducing anxiety and controlling pain should be carefully weighed against the risk for respiratory depression and airway compromise. Factors influencing the extent of pharmacologic management for pediatric patients are listed in Box 33.5. Some general drug selection strategies are discussed later and shown in Boxes 33.6–33.8.

Minor Procedures in Cooperative Adults and Older Children. Such procedures can usually be managed with topical, local, or regional anesthesia. Systemic PSA is typically unnecessary, although mild anxiolysis (e.g., nitrous oxide, oral midazolam) can make these patients more comfortable.

More Complex Procedures of Longer Duration in Cooperative Adults and Older Children. Supplementation of topical, local, or regional anesthesia with either nitrous oxide or IV midazolam and fentanyl permits customization of the depth of sedation and pain relief to the specific needs of each patient.

Procedures in Uncooperative Adults or Patients with an Intellectual Disability. Essentially all procedures in uncooperative adult-sized patients are difficult without systemic PSA. Depending on operator experience, IV midazolam, IV propofol, IV etomidate, or IM/IV ketamine or midazolam may be used in these situations. Given that the sedatives midazolam, propofol, and etomidate lack specific analgesic properties, many emergency physicians attempt to control pain with an opioid such as fentanyl before the procedure. Midazolam can be titrated intravenously to a relatively deep level of sedation, although as discussed previously, the risk for adverse effects increases with the depth of sedation. Ketamine can also provide the profound analgesia and immobilization necessary to perform painful procedures. However, in adults there is a risk for unpleasant emergence reactions (e.g., bad dreams, hallucinations). Fortunately, these can be mitigated or eliminated with the coadministration of

TABLE 33.4 Indications for PSA and Sedation Strategies[a]

CLINICAL SITUATION	INDICATION	PROCEDURAL REQUIREMENTS	SUGGESTED SEDATION STRATEGIES
Noninvasive procedures	CT Echocardiography Electroencephalography MRI Ultrasonography	Motion control Anxiolysis	Comforting alone Chloral hydrate PO (in patients <3 yr old) Methohexital PR Pentobarbital PO, IM, or IV Midazolam IV Propofol or etomidate IV
Procedure associated with low pain and high anxiety	Dental procedures Flexible fiberoptic laryngoscopy Foreign body removal, simple Intravenous cannulation Laceration repair, simple Lumbar puncture Ocular irrigation Phlebotomy Slit-lamp examination	Sedation Anxiolysis Motion control	Comforting and topical or local anesthesia Midazolam PO/IN/PR/IV Nitrous oxide
Procedures associated with a high level of pain, high anxiety, or both	Abscess incision and drainage Arthrocentesis Bone marrow aspiration and biopsy Burn debridement Cardiac catheterization Cardioversion Central line placement Endoscopy Foreign body removal, complicated Fracture or dislocation reduction Hernia reduction Interventional radiology procedures Laceration repair, complex Paracentesis Paraphimosis reduction Sexual assault examination Thoracentesis Thoracostomy tube placement	Sedation Anxiolysis Analgesia Amnesia Motion control	Propofol or etomidate IV Propofol and fentanyl IV Propofol and ketamine IV Ketamine IM/IV Midazolam and fentanyl IV

[a]There is no universally accepted or clinically correct dose, medication, or combination. Many regimens are acceptable. This table is intended as a general overview. Sedation strategies should be individualized. Although the pharmacopoeia is large, clinicians should familiarize themselves with a few agents that are flexible enough to be used for the majority of procedures. In all cases, it is assumed that practitioners are fully trained in the technique, appropriate personnel and monitoring are used as detailed in this chapter, and specific drug contraindications are absent.

CT, Computed tomography; *IM*, intramuscularly; *IN*, intranasally; *IV*, intravenously; *MRI*, magnetic resonance imaging; *PO*, orally; *PR*, per rectum; *PSA*, procedural sedation and analgesia.

From Krauss B, Green SM. Procedural sedation and analgesia in children. *Lancet*. 2006;367(9512):766-780.

midazolam.[80] Ketamine should be used with extreme caution in older adults because its sympathomimetic properties may aggravate underlying coronary artery disease or hypertension. Occasionally, procedures in extremely uncooperative adults or patients with an intellectual disability are best managed in the operating room with general anesthesia.

Minor Procedures in Uncooperative Older Children and in Young Children. Minor procedures (e.g., small lacerations, IV cannulation, venipuncture, removal of superficial foreign bodies) in uncooperative children can frequently be managed by skilled practitioners with a combination of nonpharmacologic techniques (e.g., distraction, guided imagery, hypnosis, comforting, breathing techniques) in conjunction with topical anesthesia, careful local anesthesia, and when necessary, brief forcible immobilization (by personnel or a restraining device). In other cases, supplementing nonpharmacologic techniques with topical or local anesthesia and anxiolysis with oral midazolam may be sufficient to permit successful wound repair. Although oral administration is most popular and least invasive, the nasal or rectal routes can also be used depending on operator experience and preference.

Major Procedures in Uncooperative Children. Major painful procedures (e.g., fracture reduction, incision and drainage of large loculated abscesses, or tube thoracostomy) require systemic PSA. Options include IM/IV ketamine, IV propofol, IV etomidate, or IV midazolam. Given that the sedatives midazolam, propofol, and etomidate lack specific analgesic properties, many emergency physicians attempt to control pain with an opioid such as fentanyl before the

BOX 33.4 Risk-Benefit Analysis for PSA

- Why is PSA needed in the first place? Is the procedure very painful, frightening, or requiring extreme cooperation?
- Are the risks of PSA appropriate for the procedure involved?
- If the patient is a child, do the parents or guardian consent to the use of PSA?
- How long will the procedure take? If it is a short procedure, is it worth the added risk and expense to the patient? If it is a longer procedure, is there an appropriate agent that can be titrated to allow adequate PSA throughout the entire length of the procedure?
- Are there significant side effects that limit a particular drug's usefulness?
- Are enough nurses and support personnel present to safely allow the use of PSA?
- What is the recovery period for a given agent? Are there enough treatment areas and staff in the ED to allow adequate observation during recovery?
- When did the patient last eat? Is a delay in waiting for a sufficient fasting time worth the time lost in performing the procedure?

ED, *Emergency department;* PSA, *procedural sedation and analgesia.*
From Krauss B, Brustowicz R, eds. Pediatric Procedural Sedation and Analgesia. *Lippincott Williams & Wilkins; 1999:294.*

procedure. Ketamine may be the best option in such children because dissociative sedation can consistently provide immobilization and analgesia while maintaining protective airway reflexes and upper airway muscular tone.

PHARMACOPOEIA

There is no universally correct or preferred medication or drug regimen. Many options are acceptable and successful. The best choice is an agent whose pharmacologic properties are familiar to the operator, which is used frequently by the operator, is easily titratable, and has a short duration of action or is readily reversible. All drugs should be given in adequate doses because underdosing of opioids or sedatives provides no useful purpose. Dosing recommendations for PSA drugs are provided in Table 33.5, and specialized protocols for midazolam or fentanyl, propofol, and ketamine are presented in Boxes 33.6–33.8, respectively. Individual agents are discussed in the following sections.

Sedative-Hypnotic Agents

Chloral Hydrate

Pharmacology. Chloral hydrate is a pure sedative-hypnotic agent without analgesic properties. When administered orally, the average time to peak sedation is approximately 30 minutes, with a recovery time of an additional 1 to 2 hours.[81,82] Residual motor imbalance and agitation may persist for several hours beyond this period.[83] Rectal administration is erratically absorbed and therefore not recommended.

Adult Use. Chloral hydrate is not routinely used in adults.

Pediatric Use. Because of its slow onset, inability to titrate, and prolonged duration of action, chloral hydrate is seldom used to sedate children in the ED. However, it is still used in many outpatient settings for diagnostic studies, as well as therapeutic procedures in the dental clinic.[82,84–90] Although the liquid formulation is no longer available in the United States, some hospital pharmacies compound their own formulation.[91] The drug is not recommended for use in children older than 3 years.[92]

Adverse Effects. Despite a wide margin of safety, chloral hydrate can cause airway obstruction and respiratory depression, especially at higher doses (75 to 100 mg/kg).[1,82,85,87,88] The incidence was 0.6% in one large series.[82] There is no known dosage threshold of chloral hydrate below which this potential complication can be consistently avoided,[1,87] and accordingly, standard interactive and mechanical monitoring precautions apply to chloral hydrate as they do to other PSA agents.

Because it is a halogenated hydrocarbon, overdoses of chloral hydrate can be arrhythmogenic and produce ventricular dysrhythmias. β-Blockers may be most effective in terminating ventricular arrhythmias. Despite reports of potential carcinogenicity, the AAP has judged that the evidence is currently insufficient to avoid single doses of chloral hydrate for this reason alone.[93] According to a recent review, there is significant concern about the risk of adverse events and the possibility of compounding errors related to the use of chloral hydrate.[94]

Midazolam

Pharmacology. Benzodiazepines are a group of highly lipophilic agents that possess anxiolytic, amnestic, sedative, hypnotic, muscle relaxant, and anticonvulsant properties. They lack direct analgesic properties and thus are commonly coadministered with opioids. Caution must be exercised when using benzodiazepines and opioids together because the risk for hypoxia and apnea is significantly greater than when either is used alone.[95]

Midazolam is by far the most common benzodiazepine used for PSA and is preferred over the longer-acting lorazepam and diazepam. The time to peak effect for midazolam is approximately 2 to 3 minutes when given intravenously. Unlike diazepam, midazolam and lorazepam are water soluble, thus making parenteral administration less painful and mucosal absorption faster. Midazolam is readily reversed with flumazenil, and individuals undergoing PSA with midazolam are good candidates for this antidote should reversal be required.

Adult Use. Midazolam can be used effectively for moderate and deep sedation through careful IV titration to effect, typically together with fentanyl (see Box 33.6).

Pediatric Use. Advantages of midazolam over other benzodiazepines for pediatric PSA are its short duration of action, reversibility, and availability in multiple routes of administration. Midazolam may be used for the same indications and in the same manner as in adults. Some children require larger doses than would be typical for adults on a milligram-per-kilogram basis,[96] and paradoxical responses (e.g., hyperexcitability) are not uncommon.[83,97,98] Midazolam does not reliably render a child motionless, and therefore methohexital or pentobarbital is generally preferred for neuroimaging.[89,99,100]

To avoid the need for IV access in frightened children, midazolam has been alternatively administered via the IM,[101]

BOX 33.5 Factors Influencing the Extent of Pediatric Pharmacologic Management

AGE

Selected drugs and routes of administration have age limitations and are not recommended above or below a certain age (e.g., demand-flow nitrous oxide in children <5 years, nasal and rectal routes of administration in children >6 years).

TIME OF DAY

A toddler seen at naptime or at 9 p.m. who is tired and sleepy will usually require smaller dosing and possibly a lower level of PSA than required at 9 a.m. Young children with facial lacerations at night, after their normal bedtime, may require only topical anesthesia and a quiet room for 20 to 30 minutes to achieve a painless laceration repair while the child sleeps.

FASTING STATUS

Young children can be extremely difficult and uncooperative when hungry, tired, or both. In anticipation of PSA, many children are kept without oral intake from the time that they are triaged in the ED. This can further increase hunger and irritability, especially if the child waits 1 to 2 hours to be seen by a clinician.

AVAILABILITY OF STAFFING AND EQUIPMENT

Staffing availability can affect the use and timing of sedation and is especially important in busy EDs with multiple sedations occurring concurrently and in smaller units that are set up for only one sedation at a time.

LOCATION OF THE INJURY

Injuries located in areas of cosmetic concern (especially on the face) or near sensory organs (e.g., ears, eyes, mouth, nose) will often require a high degree of agitation control and a concomitant level of PSA.

PREVIOUS MEDICATIONS

An accurate history of previous medication administration is important in situations in which a child is referred from another facility because this can affect the type and timing of PSA agents that can be given. In particular, a child may have received opioids or sedative-hypnotics before transfer and may still be sedated on arrival, thus necessitating an adjustment in the PSA regimen.

LEVEL OF ANXIETY

The level of anxiety of both the child and the accompanying adult or adults must be accurately assessed. Children manifest anxiety in many different ways, and emergency clinicians must be facile at recognizing the varying expressions of anxiety, especially in young children. A child with a facial laceration quietly sitting on the stretcher during the initial examination will not necessarily be a calm and cooperative patient during repair of the laceration (infants and toddlers). The nursing assessment at triage of the state of the child and accompanying adult or adults can be very helpful in some cases in determining the need for PSA. A child who was frightened and uncooperative in triage may be calm and compliant during a procedure. Unfortunately, the reverse is also true. When confronted with an extremely anxious child, ED personnel should ascertain what the parents have told the child about the upcoming procedure. Many parents, in the hope of lessening their child's anxiety, will tell the child that they will get a "shot" or a "needle" and that the procedure will "only hurt for a minute." This type of parental preparation, especially in young children who do not have the cognitive ability to mediate their anxiety, often results in a significant increase in the child's anxiety and a decrease in the child's ability to cooperate, especially if the child has had a previous negative experience with a procedure in the ED. It is also important to assess the parents' level of anxiety because this will determine the degree to which they can assist during the procedure. An extremely anxious parent or a parent who must take care of other siblings during the procedure will find it difficult to assist in distracting the child or otherwise helping the child cope with the procedure.

PREVIOUS EXPERIENCE

Children's previous experience in hospitals can greatly affect their response to the current situation. Direct experience is not the only way to create anxious, frightened, and uncooperative patients, though. Images from television, stories from peers, or previous witness of a sibling being forcibly restrained for repair of a laceration can leave a powerful and lasting impression. This type of influence should be especially suspected in children whose anxiety seems out of proportion to the present situation. Eliciting from the parents a history of a previous difficult experience in the ED can be a decisive factor in determining the degree of sedation required. Children who have had a recent unpleasant laceration repair and who now have a new laceration may well require PSA as opposed to simple anxiolysis (either pharmacologic or nonpharmacologic) had there been no previous trauma.

CHILD'S BEHAVIOR AT ROUTINE PRIMARY CARE VISITS

Inquiring into how a child behaves during routine primary care visits can yield important information on how the child reacts to stressful situations, how cooperative the child will be with the anticipated procedure, and whether pharmacologic management is needed. Children who cry but hold still when vaccinated may be more compliant than children who are described by their parents as being "afraid of doctors" or "wild" during visits to the primary care physician.

ED, *Emergency department;* PSA, *procedural sedation and analgesia.*

oral,[97,102–106] intranasal,[102,107–110] and rectal routes.[111] However, the inability to effectively titrate with these routes dictates that a reliable depth of sedation cannot be predictably or regularly achieved. Consequently, these non-IV routes are primarily reserved for pure anxiolysis or mild sedation (or both) for minimally painful procedures. Respiratory depression can also occur via these routes.[106]

Adverse Effects. When administered by skilled practitioners using standard precautions (see Box 33.6), the safety profile for midazolam is excellent.[6,7,112] However, when administering benzodiazepines, one must maintain continuous vigilance for respiratory depression.[1,83,95,112,113] Such respiratory depression is dose dependent and greatly enhanced in the presence of ethanol or other depressive drugs, especially opioids. These effects are exaggerated in the elderly. Deaths from undetected apnea have occurred,[95] thus underscoring the critical role of continuous interactive and mechanical monitoring.

Benzodiazepines induce minimal cardiovascular depression. Although hypotension can occur, it is rare when the

BOX 33.6 Procedure for Moderate to Deep Sedation With Intravenous Midazolam and Fentanyl

CAVEATS

- Do not consider this procedure if you lack experience with the drugs or do not have the time to perform procedural sedation and analgesia properly. Do not attempt this procedure if the pulse oximeter, suction, oxygen, or bag-mask device is not working, the intravenous line is not secured, or the room is too small or not set up for procedural sedation and analgesia.
- This is a two-person procedure, one to monitor the patient and one to perform the procedure.
- The individual response to the drugs is variable and dependent on the patient's underlying physiologic state and the presence of concomitant drugs and medications.
- The maximum drug effect occurs 2 to 3 minutes after administration. Proceed slowly and patiently and allow the medication to take full effect before giving the next dose.
- Have naloxone and flumazenil immediately available for oversedation or respiratory depression.
- If the patient seems overly sedated, begin the procedure. The pain of the procedure often stimulates respiration and lessens sedation.

CONTRAINDICATIONS—ABSOLUTE (RISKS ESSENTIALLY ALWAYS OUTWEIGH BENEFITS)

- Active hemodynamic instability
- Active respiratory distress or hypoxemia

CONTRAINDICATIONS—RELATIVE (RISKS MAY OUTWEIGH BENEFITS)

- Respiratory depression or altered level of consciousness
- Anticipated difficulty if ventilatory assistance should become necessary (e.g., facial deformity or trauma, small mandible, large tongue, trismus)

PROTOCOL

- Establish intravenous access.
- Preoxygenate the patient.
- Connect appropriate monitoring equipment to the patient. Administer supplemented oxygen if deep sedation is anticipated.
- The pulse, respiratory rate, blood pressure, and level of consciousness should all be recorded initially and periodically throughout the procedure, depending on the depth of sedation.
- Suction equipment, oxygen, a bag-valve-mask assembly, and reversal agents should be available immediately. An age-appropriate resuscitation cart with oral and nasal airways, endotracheal tubes, and a functioning laryngoscope must be nearby.
- The order of drugs is one of personal preference. The ratio of analgesia to sedation is determined by the nature of the procedure. Some procedures require primary analgesia and secondary anxiolysis or sedation (e.g., incision and drainage of an abscess, bone marrow aspiration, arthrocentesis, burn debridement, central catheter placement). In this case, administer fentanyl first. Others require primary anxiolysis or sedation with secondary analgesia (e.g., lumbar puncture, simple foreign body removal); administer midazolam first.
- Administer a local anesthetic if indicated after procedural sedation and analgesia are initiated (this often serves to help gauge the effectiveness of systemic analgesia).
- Perform the procedure. Additional doses of fentanyl or midazolam may be required if further pain or anxiety is noted based on the response and length of the procedure.
- If hypoxemia, oversedation, or slowed respirations are seen during or after the procedure, the patient should first be stimulated while oxygen is applied and the airway repositioned. If the patient's response is insufficient, assist ventilations with a bag-valve-mask device. Reversal agents should be considered if there is not a prompt response to assisted ventilation.
- Continue close observation until the patient is awake and alert, and release the patient with a friend, parent, or relative only after a sufficient discharge score has been attained.

agents are carefully titrated. One reason that midazolam is ideal for painful procedures is its significant amnesic effect. Even though patients appear to feel pain during the procedure, it is often not remembered.

Pentobarbital

Pharmacology. Pentobarbital is a barbiturate capable of profound sedation, hypnosis, amnesia, and anticonvulsant activity in a dose-dependent fashion. It has no inherent analgesic properties. When carefully titrated intravenously, sedation is evident within 5 minutes with a duration of approximately 30 to 40 minutes.[99]

Adult Use. Pentobarbital has no advantage over midazolam for adult PSA and is rarely used for this purpose.

Pediatric Use. Pentobarbital was once the IV sedative of choice in many centers for diagnostic imaging in children.[86,89,99,114,115] However, slower onset and prolonged sedation compared with other agents has reduced its use in the ED.[91,116] Pentobarbital, like midazolam, is available in multiple routes of administration (IV, IM, oral, and rectal).

Adverse Effects. Like other barbiturates, pentobarbital can lead to respiratory depression and hypotension because it is a negative inotrope.[86,89,99,100]

Ultrashort-Acting Sedative-Hypnotic Agents

Ultrashort-acting sedatives (i.e., propofol, etomidate, thiopental, methohexital) can rapidly produce potent sedation when administered intravenously, and all exhibit rapid awakening (<5 minutes) after discontinuation of the drug. This makes them particularly useful to facilitate short painful procedures in the ED.

Substantial controversy surrounded the early administration of these agents for ED PSA.[117] Proponents have cited their extremely rapid onset and recovery as enormous advantages over other sedatives. Critics have cited the level of continuous vigilance required to achieve a desired effect while simultaneously avoiding significant cardiopulmonary depression because these agents can result in rapid swings in levels of consciousness. Research that includes thousands of ED patients for propofol and hundreds for etomidate has subsequently demonstrated that the safety profiles of these agents are the same or better than those of other agents in the PSA

BOX 33.7 Procedure for Deep Sedation With Propofol

INDICATIONS

- Brief, painful procedures for which deep sedation is indicated, including fracture and dislocation reduction, incision and drainage of abscesses, cardioversion, tube thoracostomy, bone marrow aspiration or biopsy, and central line placement.

CONTRAINDICATIONS

Absolute (Risks Essentially Outweigh Benefits)

- Known or suspected allergy to propofol.

Patients at Higher Relative Risk

- Patients older than 55 years, debilitated, or with significant underlying illness (i.e., ASA physical status score of 3 or 4) are at an increased risk for propofol-induced hypotension and other complications. When the benefits of using propofol outweigh the risks, administer lower doses more slowly. Patients should ideally have their volume status optimized before receiving propofol.
- Because there is no clear consensus on the optimal fasting time before sedation, decision-making should balance the relatively low probability of aspiration with the patient's underlying risk factors, the timing and nature of recent oral intake, the urgency of the procedure, and the depth and length of sedation required.

PERSONNEL

- The minimum personnel present during deep sedation should be an emergency clinician and an ED nurse. When available, consider adding a separate emergency clinician who is solely dedicated to drug administration and patient monitoring.

PRESEDATION

- Physicians should perform a standard presedation assessment with special attention paid to the potential for airway management during deep sedation.
- Suction, airway, and resuscitation equipment should be available immediately.
- Preoxygenate the patient.
- Because propofol does not have analgesic properties, pretreatment with fentanyl (1 μg/kg) or coadministration with ketamine (0.5 mg/kg) should be considered for painful procedures.
- Assuming that capnography is in place to identify respiratory depression, high-flow oxygen is recommended because it has been shown to decrease the risk for hypoxia with propofol (number needed to benefit of 4).

PROPOFOL ADMINISTRATION: GENERAL

- Propofol induces sedation approximately 30 seconds after bolus injection, with typical resolution of clinical effects occurring within 6 minutes.
- The most common ED dosing is an initial bolus dose of 1 mg/kg followed by 0.5 mg/kg every 2 to 3 minutes as needed to achieve or maintain the desired level of sedation.
- Propofol is typically titrated to slurring of speech, lid ptosis, or both, depending on the depth of sedation and degree of relaxation needed for the procedure.

INTERACTIVE AND MECHANICAL MONITORING

- Patients should have their airway patency, oxygen saturation, electrocardiographic tracing, and level of consciousness monitored continuously.
- The addition of end-tidal CO_2 monitoring (capnography) can provide the earliest possible warning of impending airway and respiratory complications before clinical examination or pulse oximetry and is particularly important when supplemental oxygen negates pulse oximetry as a warning device.

POTENTIAL ADVERSE EFFECTS

- Respiratory depression or apnea leading to assisted ventilation (0% to 3.9%).
- Transient hypotension (2.2% to 6.5%).
- Emesis (0% to 0.5%).
- Pain with injection (2% to 20%).

RECOVERY AND DISCHARGE

- Patients receiving propofol should be monitored until they have returned to their baseline mental status.
- Qualified personnel should accompany patients who require transport before recovery.

ASA, *American Society of Anesthesiologists;* ED, *emergency department.*

pharmacopoeia.[32] Given the rapid onset and offset of propofol, consider (when available) an additional dedicated clinician (separate from the individual performing the procedure) to oversee administration of medication.[79,118]

Propofol

Pharmacology. Propofol is one of the most commonly used agents for PSA in the ED because of its efficacy and safety profile (Fig. 33.3). When administered by IV bolus, its onset of action is typically within 30 seconds. The half-life for blood-brain equilibration is approximately 1 to 3 minutes, and its clinical effects typically resolve within 5 to 7 minutes. Longer procedures can be facilitated by repeated dosing. Patients are typically awake and alert within 15 minutes after discontinuation. Propofol exhibits inherent antiemetic and perhaps euphoric properties, and patient satisfaction is typically high. In contrast to early dogma, propofol is safe for use in patients with an allergy to eggs or soy products. The only true contraindication is an allergy to propofol.[64,119]

Adult and Pediatric Use. Deep sedation can be achieved reliably in both adults and children with a single IV loading dose of propofol. Repeated bolus dosing is preferred, but an IV drip can be administered as needed to enhance or prolong sedation.[33,118–126]

Adverse Effects. Transient apnea and respiratory depression can occur with propofol but typically resolve spontaneously before intervention is necessary. Reported rates of assisted ventilation range from 0% to 4.6%.[118] Similarly, transient hypotension (via direct negative inotropy as well as arterial and venous dilation) is common but typically resolves spontaneously without treatment. Injection site pain is noted less frequently in the ED setting than in the operating room,

BOX 33.8 Procedure for Dissociative Sedation With Ketamine

DEFINITION OF DISSOCIATIVE SEDATION

- A trancelike cataleptic state induced by the dissociative agent ketamine and characterized by profound analgesia and amnesia with retention of protective airway reflexes, spontaneous respirations, and cardiopulmonary stability.

CHARACTERISTICS OF THE KETAMINE "DISSOCIATIVE STATE"

- Dissociation: After the administration of ketamine, the patient passes into a fugue state or trance. The eyes may remain open, but the patient does not respond.
- Catalepsy: Normal or slightly enhanced muscle tone is maintained. On occasion, the patient may move or be moved into a position that is self-maintaining. Occasional muscular clonus may be observed.
- Analgesia: Analgesia is typically substantial or complete.
- Amnesia: Total amnesia is typical.
- Maintenance of airway reflexes: Upper airway reflexes remain intact and may be slightly exaggerated. Intubation is unnecessary, but occasional repositioning of the head may be needed for optimal airway patency. Suctioning of hypersalivation may occasionally be necessary.
- Cardiovascular stability: Blood pressure and pulse rate are not decreased and are typically mildly increased.
- Nystagmus: Nystagmus is typical.

INDICATIONS

- Short, painful procedures, especially those requiring immobilization (e.g., facial laceration, burn debridement, fracture reduction, abscess incision and drainage, central line placement, tube thoracostomy).
- Examinations judged likely to produce excessive emotional disturbance (e.g., pediatric sexual assault examination).

CONTRAINDICATIONS: ABSOLUTE (RISKS ESSENTIALLY ALWAYS OUTWEIGH BENEFITS)

- Age younger than 3 months (higher risk for airway complications).
- Known or suspected schizophrenia, even if currently stable or controlled with medications (can exacerbate the condition).

CONTRAINDICATIONS: RELATIVE (RISKS MAY OUTWEIGH BENEFITS)

- Major procedures stimulating the posterior pharynx (e.g., endoscopy) increase the risk for laryngospasm, whereas typical minor ED oropharyngeal procedures do not.
- History of airway instability, tracheal surgery, or tracheal stenosis (presumed higher risk for airway complications).
- Active pulmonary infection or disease, including upper respiratory infection or asthma (higher risk for laryngospasm).
- Known or suspected cardiovascular disease, including angina, heart failure, or hypertension (exacerbation caused by the sympathomimetic properties of ketamine). Avoid ketamine in patients who are already hypertensive and in older adults with risk factors for coronary artery disease.
- Central nervous system masses, abnormalities, or obstructive hydrocephalus (increased intracranial pressure with ketamine).
- Glaucoma or acute globe injury (increased intraocular pressure with ketamine).
- Porphyria, thyroid disorder, or thyroid medication (enhanced sympathomimetic effect).

PERSONNEL

- Dissociative sedation requires two persons, one (a nurse) to monitor the patient and one (a physician) to perform the procedure. Both must know about ketamine's unique characteristics.

PRESEDATION

- Perform a standard presedation assessment.
- Educate accompanying family members about the unique characteristics of the dissociative state if they will be present during the procedure or recovery.
- Frame the dissociative encounter as a positive experience. Consider encouraging adults and older children to "plan" specific, pleasant dream topics in advance of sedation (believed to decrease unpleasant recovery reactions). Emphasize, especially to school-aged children and teenagers, that ketamine delivers sufficient analgesia, so there will be no pain.

KETAMINE ADMINISTRATION: GENERAL

- Ketamine is not administered until the physician is ready to begin the procedure because the onset of dissociation typically occurs rapidly.
- Ketamine is initially administered as a single IV loading dose or IM injection. There is no apparent benefit from attempts to titrate to effect.
- In settings in which IV access can be obtained with minimal upset, the IV route is preferable because recovery is faster and there is less emesis.
- The IM route is especially useful when IV access cannot be consistently obtained with minimal upset and in patients who are uncooperative or combative (e.g., the mentally disabled).
- IV access is unnecessary for children receiving IM ketamine. Because unpleasant recovery reactions are more common in adults, IV access is desirable in these patients to permit rapid treatment of these reactions should they occur.

KETAMINE ADMINISTRATION: IV ROUTE

- Administer an IV loading dose of 1.5 to 2.0 mg/kg in children or 1.0 mg/kg in adults, with this dose being administered during a 30- to 60-second period. More rapid administration produces high central nervous system levels and has been associated with respiratory depression or apnea.
- Additional incremental doses of ketamine may be administered (0.5 to 1.0 mg/kg) if initial sedation is inadequate or repeated doses are necessary to accomplish a longer procedure.

KETAMINE ADMINISTRATION: IM ROUTE

- Administer IM ketamine, 4 to 5 mg/kg in children; the IV route is preferred for adults.
- Repeat the IM ketamine dose (full or half dose) if sedation is inadequate after 5 to 10 minutes (unusual) or if additional doses are required.

Continued

BOX 33.8 Procedure for Dissociative Sedation With Ketamine—cont'd

COADMINISTERED MEDICATIONS

- Prophylactic anticholinergics are no longer recommended.
- Prophylactic benzodiazepines are no longer recommended for children; however, they should be available to treat rare, unpleasant recovery reactions should they occur. Prophylactic IV midazolam, 0.03 mg/kg, may be considered for adults (number needed to benefit, 6).
- Prophylactic ondansetron can slightly reduce the rate of vomiting (number needed to benefit, 9 or higher).

	ROUTE OF ADMINISTRATION	
	IV	**IM**
Advantages	Ease of repeated dosing, less vomiting, slightly faster recovery	No IV access necessary
Peak concentrations and clinical onset (min)	1	5
Typical duration of effective dissociation (min)	5–10	20–30
Typical time from dose to discharge (min)	50–110	60–140

PROCEDURE

- Adjunctive physical immobilization may occasionally be needed to control random motion.
- An adjunctive local anesthetic is usually unnecessary when a dissociative dose is used.
- Suction equipment, oxygen, a bag-valve-mask device, and age-appropriate equipment for advanced airway management should be immediately available. Supplemental oxygen is not mandatory but may be used when capnography is used to monitor ventilation.

INTERACTIVE MONITORING

- Close observation of the airway and respirations by an experienced health care professional is mandatory until recovery is well established.
- Drapes should be positioned so that airway and chest motion can be visualized at all times.
- Occasional repositioning of the head or suctioning of the anterior pharynx may be indicated for optimal airway patency.

MECHANICAL MONITORING

- Maintain continuous monitoring (e.g., pulse oximetry, cardiac monitoring, capnography) until recovery is well established.
- The pulse and respiratory rate should both be recorded periodically throughout the procedure. Blood pressure measurements after the initial value are generally unnecessary because ketamine stimulates catecholamine release and does not depress the cardiovascular system in healthy patients.

POTENTIAL ADVERSE EFFECTS

Percent estimates are for children; corresponding adult estimates are not yet reliable enough to report.

- Airway misalignment requiring repositioning of the head (occasional)
- Transient laryngospasm (0.3%)
- Transient apnea or respiratory depression (0.8%)
- Hypersalivation (rare)
- Emesis, usually well into recovery (8.4%)
- Recovery agitation (mild in 6.3%, clinically important in 1.4%)
- Muscular hypertonicity and random, purposeless movements (common)
- Clonus, hiccupping, or short-lived nonallergic rash on the face and neck

RECOVERY

- Maintain minimal physical contact or other sensory disturbance.
- Maintain a quiet area with dim lighting, if possible.
- Advise parents or caretakers not to stimulate the patient prematurely.

DISCHARGE CRITERIA

- Return to the pretreatment level of verbalization and awareness.
- Return to the pretreatment level of purposeful neuromuscular activity.
- A predischarge requirement of tolerating oral fluids or being able to ambulate independently not required or recommended after dissociative sedation.

DISCHARGE INSTRUCTIONS

- Nothing by mouth for approximately 2 hours
- Careful family observation and no independent ambulation for approximately 2 hours

ASA, *American Society of Anesthesiologists;* ED, *emergency department;* IM, *intramuscular;* IV, *intravenous.*
From Green SM, Roback MG, Kennedy RM et al. Clinical practice guideline for emergency department ketamine dissociative sedation: 2011 update. Ann Emerg Med. *2011;57:449-461.*

where higher doses are generally administered.[33,118–126] Propofol usually causes pain on injection in awake individuals. Injecting slowly through a large vein, not a dorsal hand vein, and administering 2 to 3 mL of 2% lidocaine slowly into the vein before propofol infusion will lessen the pain of injection.

Etomidate

Pharmacology. When administered by IV bolus, the onset of action of etomidate is typically within 30 seconds, and patients are usually awake and alert within 30 minutes after discontinuation.

Adult Use. Deep sedation can be achieved reliably with single loading doses.[127–130] Dosing can be repeated as needed to enhance or prolong sedation. Etomidate may be somewhat less effective overall than propofol and, given its additional adverse effect of myoclonus, appears to be a less desirable choice than propofol for deep sedation.[32,53]

Pediatric Use. The safety and efficacy profile of etomidate appears to be similar to that in adults.[131–133] For short-duration painful ED procedures, etomidate 0.2 mg/kg intravenously administered after fentanyl was associated with effective sedation, successful procedural completion,

TABLE 33.5 Drug Dosing Recommendations for PSA[a]

DRUG	CLINICAL EFFECTS	INDICATIONS	ADULT DOSE[b]	PEDIATRIC DOSE	ONSET (min)	DURATION (min)	COMMENTS
Sedative-Hypnotics							
Chloral hydrate (Noctec)	Sedation, motion control, anxiolysis No analgesia Not reversible	Diagnostic imaging (age < 3 yr)	Not recommended	PO: 25–100 mg/kg, after 30 min may repeat 25–50 mg/kg Maximum total dose: 2 g or 100 mg/kg (whichever is less) Single use only in neonates	PO: 15–30	PO: 60–120	Effects unreliable if age > 3 yr Avoid in patients with significant cardiac, hepatic, or renal disease Rectal absorption is erratic May produce paradoxical excitement Because drugs cannot be titrated with the PO route, monitor closely for oversedation
Etomidate (Amidate)	Sedation, motion control, anxiolysis No analgesia Not reversible	Procedures requiring sedation and/or anxiolysis	Sedation: 0.1 mg/kg IV; repeat if inadequate response	Not FDA approved in children	IV: <1	IV: 5–15	Adverse effects include respiratory depression, myoclonus, nausea, and vomiting Adrenocortical suppression occurs but is of no clinical significance
Midazolam[c] (Versed)	Sedation, motion control, anxiolysis No analgesia Reversible with flumazenil	Procedures requiring sedation and/or anxiolysis	IV: Initial dose 1 mg, then titrated to max of 5 mg IM: 5 mg or 0.07 mg/kg	IV (0.5–5 yr): Initial dose of 0.05–0.1 mg/kg, then titrated to max of 0.6 mg/kg IV (6–12 yr): Initial dose of 0.025–0.05 mg/kg, then titrated to max of 0.4 mg/kg IM: 0.1–0.15 mg/kg PO: 0.5–0.75 mg/kg IN: 0.2–0.5 mg/kg PR: 0.25–0.5 mg/kg	IV: 2–3 IM: 10–20 PO: 15–30 IN: 10–15 PR: 10–30	IV: 45–60 IM: 60–120 PO: 60–90 IN: 60 PR: 60–90	Reduce the dose when used in combination with opioids May produce paradoxical excitement Because drugs cannot be titrated with the PO/PR/IN routes, monitor closely for oversedation
Methohexital (Brevital)	Sedation, motion control, anxiolysis No analgesia Not reversible	Diagnostic imaging	Anesthesia induction IV: 1 mg/kg (less for sedation) *Caution*: limited research	PR: 25 mg/kg IV (*caution*, limited research): 0.5–1 mg/kg	PR: 10–15	PR: 60	Avoid in patients with temporal lobe epilepsy or porphyria Because drugs cannot be titrated with the PR route, monitor closely for oversedation

TABLE 33.5 Drug Dosing Recommendations for PSA[a]—cont'd

DRUG	CLINICAL EFFECTS	INDICATIONS	ADULT DOSE[b]	PEDIATRIC DOSE	ONSET (min)	DURATION (min)	COMMENTS
Pentobarbital (Nembutal)	Sedation, motion control, anxiolysis No analgesia Not reversible	Diagnostic imaging	Not recommended	IV: 1–6 mg/kg, titrated in increments of 1–2 mg/kg to desired effect IM: 2–6 mg/kg, max of 100 mg PO/PR (<4 yr): 3–6 mg/kg, max of 100 mg PO/PR (>4 yr): 1.5–3 mg/kg, max of 100 mg	IV: 3–5 IM: 10–15 PO/PR: 15–60	IV: 15–45 IM: 60–120 PO/PR: 60–240	May produce paradoxical excitement Avoid in patients with porphyria Because drugs cannot be titrated with the PO/PR routes, monitor closely for oversedation
Propofol (Diprivan)	Sedation, motion control, anxiolysis No analgesia Not reversible	Procedures requiring sedation and/or anxiolysis	Load 1 mg/kg IV; may administer additional 0.5-mg/kg doses as needed to enhance or prolong sedation	Load 1–2 mg/kg IV; may administer additional 0.5-mg/kg doses as needed to enhance or prolong sedation	IV: <1	IV: 5–15	Frequent hypotension and respiratory depression Avoid with egg or soy allergies
Thiopental (Pentothal)	Sedation, motion control, anxiolysis No analgesia Not reversible	Diagnostic imaging	Not recommended	PR: 25 mg/kg	PR: 10–15	PR: 60–120	Avoid in patients with porphyria Because drugs cannot be titrated with the PR route, monitor closely for oversedation
Analgesic[d]							
Fentanyl (Sublimaze)	Analgesia Reversible with naloxone	Procedures with moderate to severe pain	IV: 50 μg, may repeat q 3 min, titrate to effect	IV: 1 μg/kg per dose, may repeat q 3 min, titrate to effect IN: 1-2 μg/kg, max dose 100 μg	IV: 3–5 IN: 2	IV: 30–60 IN: 30–60	
Dissociative Agent							
Ketamine (Ketalar)	Analgesia, dissociation, amnesia, motion control Not reversible	Procedures with moderate to severe pain or requiring immobilization	IV: 1–1.5 mg/kg slowly over 30–60 s, may repeat one-half dose q 10 min prn	IV: 1.5 mg/kg slowly over 30–60 s, may repeat one-half dose q 10 min prn IM: 4–5 mg/kg, may repeat after 10 min (one-half dose)	IV: 1 IM: 3–5	IV: dissociation, 15; recovery, 60 IM: dissociation, 15–30; recovery, 90–150	Multiple contraindications[e]

Continued

Inhalational Agent							
Nitrous oxide (Nitronox)	Anxiolysis, analgesia, sedation, amnesia (all mild)	Procedures requiring mild analgesia or sedation (age >4 yr)	Preset mixture with a minimum of 40% O_2 self-administered by a demand-valve mask (requires a cooperative patient)	Preset mixture for a cooperative child; continuous-flow nasal mask in an uncooperative child with close monitoring	<5	<5 following discontinuation	Requires specialized apparatus and gas scavenger capability Several contraindications[f] Synergistic effect with recent opioids or sedative-hypnotics—use with caution in this setting
Reversal Agents (Antagonists)							
Naloxone (Narcan)	Opioid reversal	Opioid toxicity	IV/IM: 0.4–2 mg	IV/IM: 0.1 mg/kg per dose up to max of 2 mg/dose, may repeat q 2 min prn	IV: 2	IV: 20–40 IM: 60–90	If shorter acting than the reversed drug, serial doses may be required
Flumazenil (Romazicon)	Benzodiazepine reversal	Benzodiazepine toxicity	IV: 0.2 mg, may repeat q 1 min up to 1 mg	IV: 0.02 mg/kg per dose, may repeat q 1 min up to 1 mg	IV: 1–2	IV: 30–60	If shorter acting than the reversed drug, serial doses may be required Do not use in patients chronically taking benzodiazepines, cyclosporine, isoniazid, lithium, propoxyphene, theophylline, tricyclic antidepressants

[a]Alterations in dosing may be indicated depending on the clinical situation and the practitioner's experience with these agents. Individual dosages may vary when used in combination with other agents, especially when benzodiazepines are combined with opioids.
[b]Use lower doses in geriatric patients and those with significant cardiopulmonary disease.
[c]Midazolam is preferred over other benzodiazepines (e.g., diazepam, lorazepam) for procedural sedation and analgesia because of its shorter duration of action and multiple routes of administration.
[d]Fentanyl is preferred over other opioids (e.g., morphine, meperidine) for procedural sedation and analgesia because of its faster onset, shorter recovery, and lack of histamine release.
[e]Generally accepted contraindications to ketamine include age younger than 3 months; history of airway instability, tracheal surgery, or tracheal stenosis; procedures involving stimulation of the posterior pharynx; active pulmonary infection or disease (including active upper respiratory infection); cardiovascular disease, including angina, heart failure, or hypertension; significant head injury, central nervous system masses, or hydrocephalus; glaucoma or acute globe injury; psychosis; porphyria; and thyroid disorder or thyroid medication.
[f]Generally accepted contraindications to nitrous oxide include pregnancy (patient or personnel), preexisting nausea or vomiting, trapped gas pockets (e.g., middle ear infection, pneumothorax, bowel obstruction).
ED, Emergency department; *FDA*, US Food and Drug Administration; *IM*, intramuscularly; *IN*, intranasally; *IV*, intravenously; *PO*, orally; *PR*, per rectum; *prn*, as needed; *PSA*, procedural sedation and analgesia.
Adapted from Krauss B, Green SM. Sedation and analgesia for procedures in children. *N Engl J Med*. 2000;342:938.

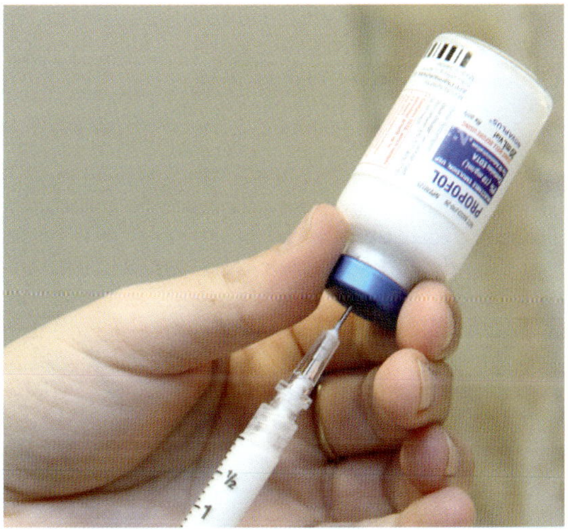

Fig. 33.3 Propofol is commonly used for painful emergency department procedures. It is safe, effective, and very short acting. It can be cautiously combined with the short-acting narcotic fentanyl or with ketamine. All the safety caveats for procedural sedation and analgesia apply. The pain of a propofol injection can be minimized by choosing a large vein not on the dorsum of the hand and slowly injecting 2 to 3 mL of 2% lidocaine into the vein before injection of propofol. Note: It is recommended to wear gloves, preferably sterile, and use sterile procedure when handling propofol to minimize risk of contaminating the bottle with bacteria.

and readily managed respiratory events in children (oxygen supplementation, stimulation, or airway repositioning).[134] Etomidate has also been compared to ketamine for orthopedic procedures in children, with equal rates of success and favorable safety profiles.[135]

Adverse Effects. The primary adverse effects of etomidate are respiratory depression, myoclonus, nausea, and vomiting.[132–136] Respiratory depression has been reported to be less common with propofol PSA than with methohexital, fentanyl/midazolam, or etomidate.[137] Myoclonus is common yet generally benign, but it may be disconcerting and can interfere with the procedure. It consists of transient jerking or twitching movements that can be mistaken for seizure activity. Transient adrenal suppression occurs with etomidate in septic patients but appears to lack clinical significance for single doses when used for ED PSA.[32,136,138]

Thiopental and Methohexital

Pharmacology. Because of their lipid solubility, barbiturates are rapidly absorbed rectally. When given by the IV route, both thiopental and methohexital produce sedation within 1 minute. Clinical recovery is rapid (≈15 minutes) as a result of rapid redistribution from the central nervous system to the periphery.

Adult Use. Thiopental is seldom used for procedural sedation in the United States, although it is used in other countries.[139] Because there is limited published experience using IV barbiturates for ED PSA,[140] propofol and etomidate are typically preferred. However, recent studies directly comparing methohexital with other agents have demonstrated similar safety and efficacy profiles.[141,142]

Pediatric Use. Rectal thiopental and methohexital can reliably produce sedation suitable for CT or MRI and obviates the need for IV access.[143–149] Respiratory depression is unusual when using typical doses (see Table 33.5) but can occur.[143,144,146–148] There is limited published experience using these IV barbiturates for ED PSA,[140] and propofol would appear to be a better choice.

Adverse Effects. Barbiturates cause potent respiratory depression; in one ED report, apnea occurred in 10% of patients.[150] Barbiturates also frequently cause hypotension at typical IV doses, so their use should be avoided whenever possible in patients with volume depletion or cardiovascular compromise.

Analgesic Agents

Fentanyl

Fentanyl is the most common opioid used for PSA because of its rapid onset, brief duration, rapid reversibility with naloxone, and lack of histamine release.[8] It is often combined with other agents such as propofol, etomidate, and midazolam to provide additional effect and pain relief. The effects of fentanyl can be reversed immediately with naloxone should excessive sedation or respiratory depression occur. The longer-duration opioids morphine and hydromorphone are preferred for nonprocedural or preprocedural pain control and are frequently given initially for acute analgesia followed by fentanyl to facilitate the needed procedure. Although longer-acting opioids can be readily used for analgesia during PSA, they will be associated with longer recovery times and a higher incidence of histamine-related effects (e.g., nausea and vomiting, hypotension, pruritus). Fentanyl lacks these effects and is therefore preferred.

Pharmacology. Fentanyl is 100 times more potent than morphine and has no intrinsic anxiolytic or amnestic properties. A single IV dose has a rapid onset (<30 seconds) with a peak at 2 to 3 minutes and brief clinical duration (20 to 40 minutes). This increase in potency and onset of action is in part related to its greater lipid solubility, which facilitates passage of the drug across the blood-brain barrier. The effects of fentanyl can be rapidly and completely reversed with opioid antagonists (e.g., naloxone, nalmefene).

Adult Use. Because of its pharmacokinetics, IV fentanyl is an ideal agent when analgesia is required for painful procedures; it can be easily and rapidly titrated.[8] Because anxiolysis and sedation do not occur at low doses (1 to 2 μg/kg), concurrent administration of a pure sedative, most commonly midazolam, is advisable, especially in children (see Box 33.6).

Pediatric Use. The combination of fentanyl and midazolam remains a popular PSA sedation regimen in children, with a strong safety and efficacy profile when both drugs are carefully titrated to effect.[7,112,151,152] Any necessary level of mild to deep sedation can be achieved with these agents.

Fentanyl can also be given intranasally, making it an ideal agent for analgesia in pediatric patients where IV access can be difficult and traumatizing. To maximize absorption, administer less than 1 mL per nostril. Fentanyl concentrations of 50 μg/mL are readily available making it easy to administer the recommended 1 to 2 μg/kg intranasal dose in most children.[153]

Adverse Effects. Like all opioids, fentanyl can cause respiratory depression.[7,8,112,151,152] When used for PSA, standard interactive and mechanical monitoring is required. Because the opioid effect is most pronounced on the central nervous system respiratory centers, apnea precedes loss of consciousness. If apnea should occur, verbal or tactile stimulation should be attempted before the administration of opioid antagonists. As discussed earlier, caution must be exercised when using benzodiazepines and other PSA agents and opioids together because the risk for hypoxia and apnea is significantly greater than when either is used alone.[6,95]

In the absence of significant ethanol intoxication, hypovolemia, or concomitant drug ingestion, hypotension is rare, even with very large doses of fentanyl (doses of 50 μg/kg are common in adult and pediatric cardiac surgery). Because of its safe hemodynamic profile, fentanyl is an ideal analgesic agent for use in critically ill or injured patients. In addition, nausea and vomiting are rare in comparison to analgesia with morphine or hydromorphone. A commonly observed reaction to fentanyl is nasal pruritus, and patients frequently attempt to scratch their nose during the procedure.[8]

A rare side effect of fentanyl with potential for respiratory compromise is chest wall rigidity. This complication has not been problematic in the ED and is related to higher doses (>5 μg/kg as a bolus dose) than those used for PSA and has not been reported in any ED series.[7,8,151,152] If it should occur, chest wall rigidity can usually be reversed with opioid antagonists, positive pressure ventilation, or both. Equipment for urgent pharmacologic paralysis should be available if reversal and positive pressure ventilation are unsuccessful.

Diamorphine

Diamorphine is a nasal opioid that is not currently available in the United States.[71,72,154] Diamorphine has an onset and duration of action similar to that of morphine; however, its higher water solubility permits potent doses to be delivered in the small (0.1 mL) volumes necessary for comfortable intranasal administration. In two studies of children and teenagers with fractures, intranasal diamorphine, 0.1 mg/kg, provided a similar level of analgesia with faster onset as IM morphine, 0.2 mg/kg. Intranasal spray administration was better tolerated than the injection, and there were no adverse events [71,72,154] Diamorphine may prove to be a useful initial analgesic for children and teenagers with acute pain, although in practice, an IV line would most likely be established to permit titration to full pain relief and PSA for any procedures needed (e.g., fracture reduction). The role of diamorphine in adults remains to be determined.

Other Short-Acting Opioids

Sufentanil, alfentanil, and remifentanil are other short-acting opioids that have a potential role in PSA. Currently, however, there is insufficient published experience to warrant their routine use. Although intranasal sufentanil, 0.75 μg/kg, appeared promising in one small pediatric trial,[155] in another, doses of 1.5 μg/kg resulted in oxygen desaturation in 8 of the 10 children studied.[108] This low toxic-to-therapeutic ratio and inability to titrate would appear to limit the utility of intranasal sufentanil by itself. However, a 2014 proof of concept trial using a lower dose of intranasal sufentanil (0.5 μg/kg) with intranasal ketamine (0.5 mg/kg) showed promise with high patient acceptance and few adverse events.[156] In the one published report of IV remifentanil with midazolam for PSA, there was an unacceptably high incidence of hypoxemia.[157] Currently, there does not appear to be a clinically important advantage with these drugs versus fentanyl.

Ketamine

Pharmacology. Ketamine produces a unique state of cortical dissociation that permits painful procedures to be performed more consistently and effectively than with other PSA agents (Video 33.1). This state of dissociative sedation is characterized by profound analgesia, sedation, amnesia, and immobilization (Fig. 33.4) and can be rapidly and reliably produced with IV or IM administration.[12] Ketamine is widely used worldwide and has demonstrated a remarkable safety profile in a variety of settings.[5,7,158–161] Clinicians administering ketamine must be especially knowledgeable about the unique actions of this drug and the numerous contraindications to its use (see Table 33.5).

Ketamine differs from other PSA agents in several important ways. First, it uniquely preserves cardiopulmonary stability. Upper airway muscular tone and protective airway reflexes are maintained. Spontaneous respiration is preserved, although when administered intravenously, ketamine

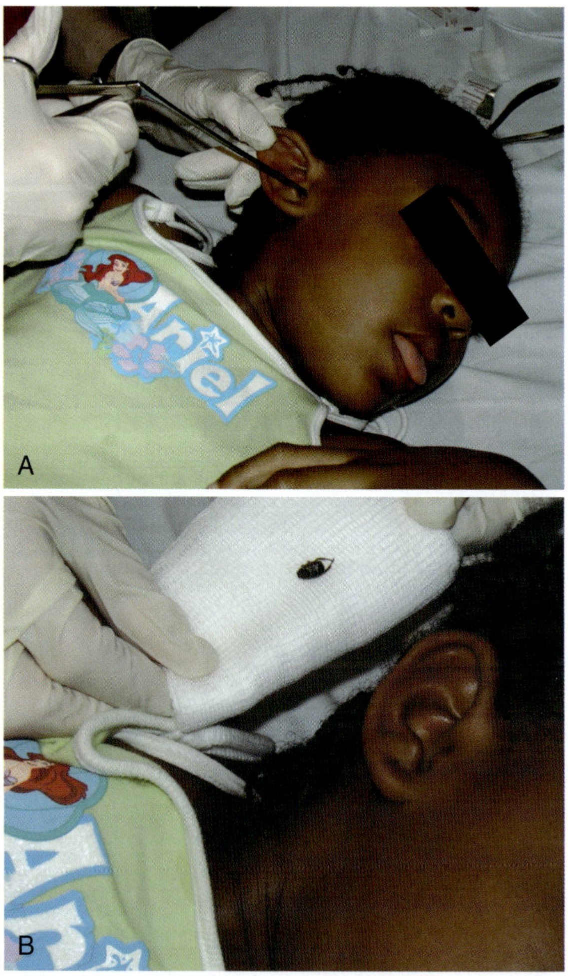

Fig. 33.4 (A) Child undergoing insect removal from the ear under ketamine sedation. No child or adult can cooperate for this painful procedure, and general anesthesia is often the other option to ketamine. The blank stare is common. (B) Insect successfully and atraumatically removed.

must be given slowly (over a period of 30 to 60 seconds) to prevent respiratory depression. Second, it differs from other agents in that it lacks the characteristic dose-response continuum to progressive titration. At lower doses ketamine produces analgesia and disorientation. However, once a dosage threshold (≈1 to 1.5 mg/kg intravenously or 3 to 4 mg/kg intramuscularly) is achieved, the characteristic dissociative state appears. This dissociation has no observable levels of depth, and thus the only value of ketamine "titration" is to maintain the presence of the state over time. Finally, the dissociative state is not consistent with formal definitions of moderate sedation, deep sedation, or general anesthesia (see Box 33.1) and must therefore be considered from a different perspective than agents that exhibit the classic sedation continuum.[12,16]

Ketamine is most effective and reliable when given intravenously or intramuscularly. Ketamine has a rapid circulation time when given intravenously, with onset of dissociation noted within 1 minute and effective procedural conditions (dissociation) lasting for approximately 10 to 15 minutes. When given intramuscularly, the same effect is achieved within 5 minutes, with effective procedural conditions (dissociation) for approximately 15 to 30 minutes. The typical duration from dosing to dischargeable recovery is 50 to 110 minutes when given intravenously and 60 to 140 minutes when given intramuscularly.[158,161]

As with benzodiazepines, ketamine undergoes substantial first-pass hepatic metabolism. As a result, oral and rectal administration results in less predictable effectiveness and substantially higher doses are required. Clinical onset and recovery are considerably longer than when given parenterally, and thus these routes are rarely used in the ED.[111,162]

Ketamine can occasionally induce excessive salivation, and to combat this, some have historically coadministered atropine or glycopyrrolate. However, there is no evidence that either of these anticholinergic agents diminishes the risk for airway or respiratory adverse events,[163–165] and their routine prophylactic use is no longer recommended.[163] Instead, they can be reserved for treatment should excessive secretions occur (Fig. 33.5).

Adult Use. The safety and efficacy of ketamine are well established in adult ED patients .[163,166–172] Such experience is corroborated by the wide and successful use of ketamine in adults throughout the developing world for both minor and major surgery, particularly in areas lacking resources for inhalational anesthesia.[158,159,170,171]

Ketamine presents potential risk to patients with coronary artery disease because it is sympathomimetic and produces mild to moderate increases in blood pressure, heart rate, and myocardial oxygen consumption. Accordingly, other sedatives are preferred in the setting of known or possible ischemic heart disease, congestive heart failure, or hypertension.[163,171] There is no accepted maximum age for ketamine; instead, emergency physicians must weigh the risks and benefits of ketamine in older adults who may have unrecognized coronary artery disease.

Hallucinatory so-called emergence reactions have been reported in up to 30% of adults receiving ketamine (though rare in children) and can be fascinating and pleasurable or, alternatively, unpleasant and nightmarish.[158] In adults, coadministered IV midazolam (0.03 mg/kg) can modestly reduce their incidence (number needed to benefit of 6),[169] although

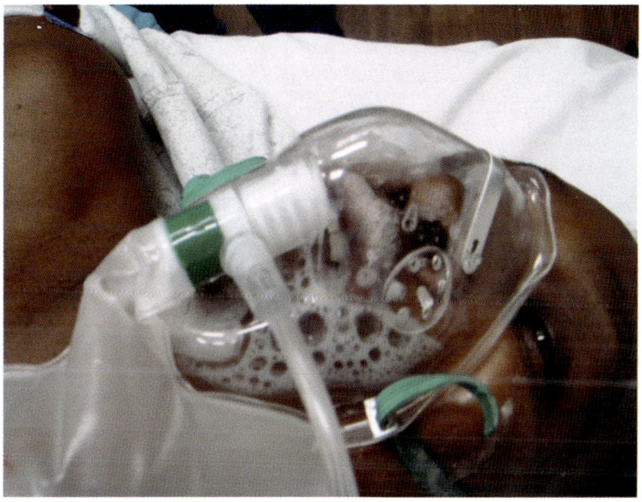

Fig. 33.5 Ketamine can occasionally induce excessive salivation, generally easily handled with minimal suctioning. Routine use of atropine or glycopyrrolate is not recommended; however, they can be administered should excessive secretions be noted.

not all such reactions are clinically important and this therapy should be considered optional.[173]

Pediatric Use. Ketamine is an ideal agent to facilitate short, painful procedures in children because of its superbly documented ED safety and efficacy.[5,7,158,161,163,164,174] The IM route is simple and effective, with venous access being unnecessary. IV administration is attractive because a lower cumulative dose can be used and recovery is faster than with the IM route. The primary caution with this route is that the initial bolus of ketamine must be administered slowly (over a 30- to 60-second period) or respiratory depression and transient apnea can occur.[161] Intranasal ketamine has become a popular alternative to opioids for analgesia[153,175] and more recently, for PSA in children.[176] A dose of 6 mg/kg in one pediatric ED study was shown to be safe and effective for PSA.[176]

Unpleasant recovery reactions are uncommon in children and teenagers and are typically mild when they do occur.[177,178] Benzodiazepine coadministration does not measurably reduce the incidence of such reactions in children (unlike adults),[163,164,174–178] and these agents should be reserved for treating preprocedural anxiety or unpleasant reactions if they occur.[163]

Adverse Effects. In a meta-analysis of ketamine administration in 8282 pediatric patients, the overall incidence of airway and respiratory adverse events was 3.9%—primarily airway malalignment but also including transient laryngospasm (0.3%) and transient apnea (0.8%). None of these patients were intubated or had adverse sequelae.[163] The frequency of such events was slightly higher when unusually high doses of ketamine were administered; otherwise, there was no clinically important association with age, doses within the typically recommended range, or other clinical factors.

Vomiting was noted in 8.4% overall in this same meta-analysis, with early adolescence representing the greatest risk and a lower incidence of emesis occurring in younger and older children.[174] It occurs more frequently with the IM route than with the IV route, and there is no evidence to support any dose relationship within the usual range of clinically administered doses.[174] When emesis occurs, it is typically late during the recovery phase when the patient is alert and can clear the airway without assistance.[163] Vomiting does occur in some patients after discharge, including some who do not vomit in the ED.[163] Although ondansetron prophylaxis (0.15 mg/kg up to a maximum of 4 mg intravenously) does reduce vomiting with ketamine, the magnitude of this effect is modest (number needed to benefit of 13), and thus it cannot be considered mandatory.[179]

In over 40 years of regular use, there have been no documented reports of clinically significant ketamine-associated aspiration in patients without established contraindications.[163] Because of its unique preservation of protective airway reflexes, ketamine may be preferred over other agents for urgent or emergency procedures when fasting is not ensured.[5,6,158,180]

Mild agitation (whimpering or crying) during recovery was noted in 7.6% of children in the large meta-analysis, with more pronounced agitation occurring in 1.4%. Such recovery reactions are not related to age, dose, or other factors to any clinically important degree, except for a higher incidence with subdissociative (<3 mg/kg intramuscularly) dosing.[174] In contrast to traditional thinking, adolescents are not at substantially higher risk.[174]

Despite the modest impact of prophylactic midazolam in reducing adult recovery agitation, in children, two controlled trials and a large meta-analysis failed to note even a trend toward a measurable benefit.[174–178] Children have far fewer recovery reactions than adults do, and their reactions are milder when they do occur. Midazolam is therefore not recommended for routine prophylaxis but is optimally reserved to treat unpleasant ketamine-associated recovery reactions when they do rarely occur.[163]

Ketamine is relatively contraindicated in patients with central nervous system masses, abnormalities, or hydrocephalus; however, there is no compelling evidence that it needs to be avoided in the setting of acute head trauma.[163,181–184] Repeated reports that ketamine can increase intracranial pressure have prompted traditional caution against use of this drug in the setting of real or potential neurologic compromise,[1,6,158,163,185–187] and there are case reports of deterioration in patients with hydrocephalus.[188,189] However, newer suggestive evidence indicates that in most patients the resulting increases in pressure are minimal, assuming normal ventilation,[181,182,188,190] and that the corresponding cerebral vasodilatory effect of ketamine may actually improve overall cerebral perfusion.[181,182,191]

Dissociative sedation may represent a risk in patients with acute globe injury or glaucoma given the inconclusive and conflicting evidence of increased intraocular pressure (IOP) with ketamine.[192–196] However, two recent studies have shown that ketamine has little to no effect on IOP in noninjured globes, but further studies are needed to assess the safety of its use in patients with ocular injury.[197,198]

Ketamine-Propofol Combination (Ketofol) for PSA in the ED

The PSA combination of ketamine and propofol, referred to by the portmanteau "ketofol," is both popular and still somewhat controversial.[199] Ketofol is safe and effective in both adults and children[200–207]; however, the dispute is whether the combination exhibits any clinically important advantage over use of either drug alone.[199] Although this question has not been definitively answered, several large recent reviews and meta-analyses suggest that the combination may have a shorter recovery time and fewer adverse effects than either agent alone.[208–211]

An important allure to ketofol proponents is how these two completely different sedatives balance each other's deficits. Propofol is a sedative but lacks the analgesia that ketamine can amply provide. Ketamine mitigates propofol-induced hypotension, and propofol mitigates ketamine-induced vomiting and recovery agitation. The drugs exhibit synergistic and perhaps smoother sedation,[201] and the combination has the theoretical benefits of minimizing the propofol dose and obviating the need for coadministered opioids.[199]

Critics note that the existing ketofol literature fails to demonstrate superior procedural conditions or less respiratory depression than occurs with each drug alone[200] and question the added complexity of administering two drugs when one is sufficient. They argue that the purported advantages related to hemodynamics and the total propofol dose are not clinically important. Ketofol uses a subdissociative dose of ketamine, and thus ketamine may just be replacing fentanyl as an analgesic rather than as a sedative.[199]

Ketofol dosing is based on weight for both adults and children. One regimen uses an initial IV loading dose of ketamine of 0.5 mg/kg, followed by a 0.5 to 1.0 mg/kg IV propofol bolus, with subsequent titration of propofol alone.[201–203,205] A second strategy mixes propofol and ketamine together 1:1 in the same syringe (both at 10-mg/mL concentrations) and then titrates in increments of 0.25 mg/kg of each drug to a usual effective dose of approximately 0.75 mg/kg.[199,204,206,207]

Careful observation for respiratory depression is required, and the precautions listed for both agents should be stringently observed.

Nitrous Oxide

Pharmacology. Inhaled nitrous oxide provides anxiolysis and mild analgesia. It is commonly dispensed at concentrations between 30% and 50%, with oxygen composing the remainder of the mixture. Nitrous oxide quickly diffuses across biologic membranes and, accordingly, has a rapid onset of action (30 to 60 seconds). Its maximum effect occurs after approximately 5 minutes, and the clinical effect wears off quickly on discontinuation. At typical PSA concentrations, there is preservation of hemodynamic status, spontaneous respirations, and protective airway reflexes.[212–215] Nitrous oxide is widely used in dentistry at higher concentrations.[216]

Nitrous oxide has an excellent safety profile; however, as a sole agent, it cannot reliably produce adequate procedural conditions.[212–215] Given its relatively weak analgesic properties, in many cases nitrous oxide needs to be supplemented with an IV opioid or local or regional anesthesia (or both).

Adult and Cooperative Child Use. The safest method of administering nitrous oxide is via a self-administered demand-valve mask (Fig. 33.6).[213–215] Patients must generate a negative pressure of 3 to 5 cm H_2O within the handheld mask or mouthpiece to activate the flow of gas. They can thus self-titrate the dose by inhaling at will through the mask. Naturally, this will be effective only when the patient is cooperative.

This technique provides a built-in fail-safe measure in that if patients become somnolent, the mask will fall from their face and gas delivery will cease.

Nitrous oxide can be used as an adjunctive anxiolytic during mildly painful procedures or during the administration of local or regional anesthesia for other procedures. It may also be administered during difficult or high-anxiety procedures such as pelvic examination or during difficult IV attempts.

A double-tank system is commonly used to deliver the nitrous oxide and oxygen mixture. The system relies on a mixing valve preset to deliver a fixed ratio and will deliver gas only when oxygen is flowing. The double-tank system contains a fail-safe device that automatically stops the flow of nitrous oxide when the oxygen supply is depleted.

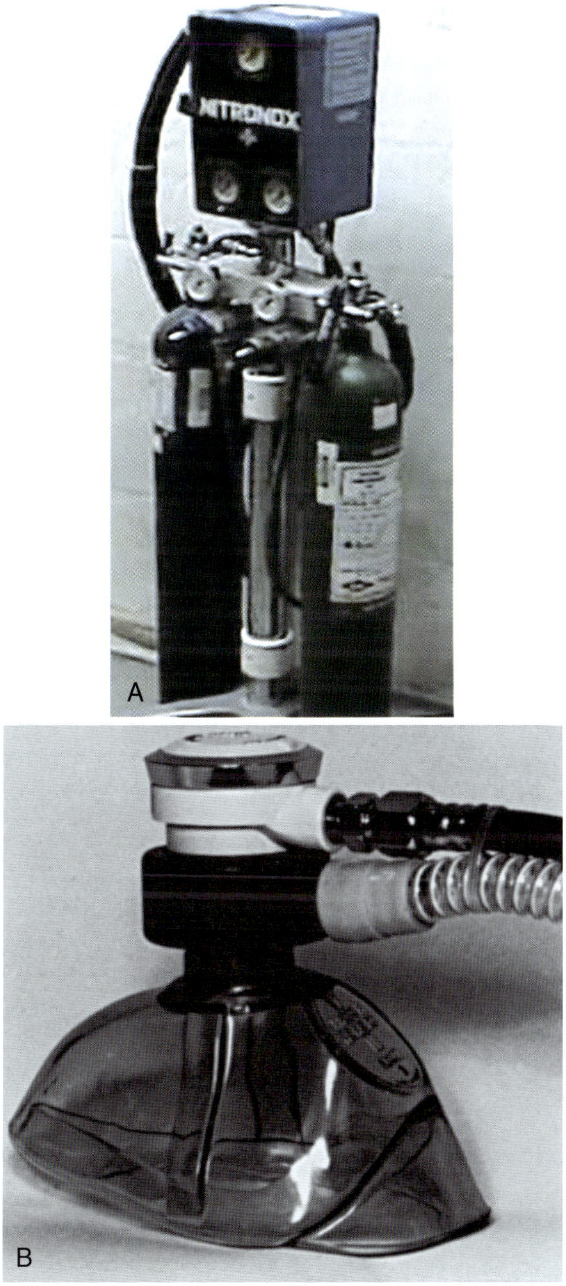

Fig. 33.6 (A) Demand-flow nitrous oxide/oxygen system. (B) Example of a free mask for a nitrous oxide system. The patient must hold the mask in contact with the face. (A, Courtesy Nitronox delivery system by Matrix Medical, division of Henry Schein.)

Uncooperative Child Use. The primary limitation of self-administration is that it is ineffective in uncooperative patients, including most frightened young children. Continuous-flow nitrous oxide via a mask strapped over the nose or over the nose and mouth has been used in this population (Fig. 33.7).[217–220] Nitrous oxide can effectively produce moderate or deep sedation when administered in this manner; however, this technique necessitates an additional clinician dedicated to continuous gas titration to avoid oversedation. In addition, it appears that the continuous-flow technique is associated with a higher rate of emesis (10%) than self-administration is (0% to 4%),[212–215,217–220] which may be a potential hazard if a mask is strapped tightly over the child's mouth.[218]

Adverse Effects and Precautions. A number of generally minor adverse effects may be seen, including nausea, dizziness, changes in voice, euphoria, and laughter.[212–215] Nitrous oxide should be avoided in patients with closed-space disease such as bowel obstruction, middle ear disease, pneumothorax, or pneumocephalus. Because of its property of high diffusibility, it has the potential to increase the size of the closed space. This should be unlikely for short-term use in typical PSA concentrations.

Make sure that a scavenging system is in place to collect exhaled nitrous oxide, and take care to ensure compliance with occupational safety regulations. Avoid exposure of pregnant ED staff members to nitrous oxide because it is a known teratogen and mutagen.

Although the potential for abuse by ED staff exists, such abuse is rare if simple steps are taken. As with other agents, maintain a strict protocol of accountability. Add a simple locking device to the cylinders of gas. In addition, lock the delivery valve or mouthpiece in the same location as controlled substances.

Antagonists

Do not routinely administer reversal agents after the administration of opioids or benzodiazepines for PSA, but rather reserve them for the rare situations of oversedation or significant respiratory depression. The downside of reversal agents is that one must wait for the antagonist to dissipate before analyzing any residual effect of the PSA agent, with the caveat that long-acting PSA agents may last longer than the administered antagonist. Serious resedation after antagonism is not usually an issue with fentanyl or midazolam, but caution is advised, especially when large doses of PSA agents and large doses of antagonists have been used. Obviously, the length

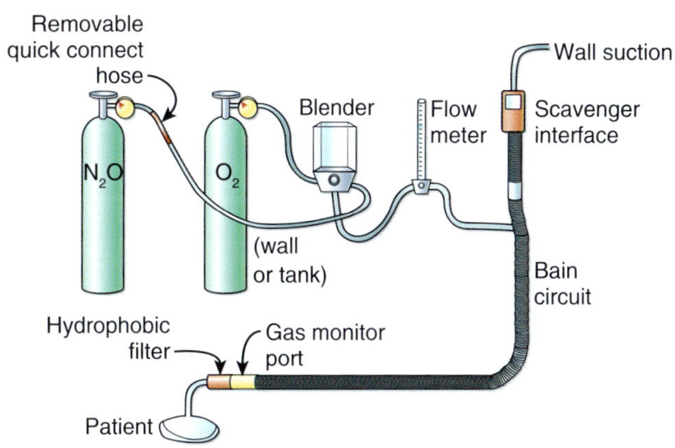

Fig. 33.7 Nitrous oxide/oxygen continuous-flow system.

of observation varies with the amount of antagonist that has been administered.

Naloxone

Naloxone is an antagonist that competitively displaces opioids from opiate receptors. It rapidly reverses the analgesic and respiratory depressant effects of opioids. It may be administered intravenously, intramuscularly, subcutaneously, intranasally and even sublingually,[200] and dosing has been standardized for infants and children.[221] Naloxone will not induce systemic opioid withdrawal symptoms in a patient without preexisting physiologic dependence. However, some patients will experience nausea with opioid reversal, and patients with persistent pain after their procedure will be quite uncomfortable. Rapid reversal may also lead to return of anxiety and stimulation of the sympathetic nervous system. If the situation permits, careful titration of small amounts of naloxone (0.1-mg aliquots intravenously) may permit partial rather than complete reversal. The only absolute contraindication to the use of naloxone is administration to a neonate born to an opioid-dependent mother because of the risk of precipitating life-threatening opioid withdrawal. The length of observation is dose related, but usually no more than 60 to 90 minutes after reversal will be sufficient if no more than 1 mg of naloxone has been administered intravenously.

Nalmefene

Nalmefene is a long-acting opioid antagonist with a duration of action significantly longer than that of naloxone.[222,223] Nalmefene may be given intravenously, intramuscularly, or subcutaneously, although intravenously is the preferred route.[223,224] Intravenously, it can be titrated in incremental doses of 0.25 μg/kg every 2 to 5 minutes until the desired effect is attained. Although either naloxone or nalmefene will reverse the analgesia of opioids, naloxone is the preferred agent. For ED PSA, short-acting opioids such as fentanyl are commonly used, and administration of a reversal agent with a duration of action as prolonged as that of nalmefene does not confer any additional benefit. Furthermore, nalmefene would interfere with postprocedure control of pain with opioids.

Flumazenil

Flumazenil is a benzodiazepine antagonist that can promptly reverse benzodiazepine-induced sedation and respiratory depression.[1,16,225,226] In the setting of PSA, flumazenil is a safe and effective method of reversing oversedation caused by benzodiazepines. It is not routinely used to reverse PSA because of the potential for resedation, and many clinicians prefer to allow patients to recover on their own. Flumazenil has not been shown to substantially decrease the time of observation in the ED required for a patient undergoing PSA. Flumazenil lowers the seizure threshold and may rarely lead to life-threatening seizures. It should be avoided in patients with known benzodiazepine dependence, seizure disorder, cyclic antidepressant overdose, and elevated intracranial pressure.[202] It should also be given cautiously to patients who are taking medications known to lower the seizure threshold (cyclosporine, tricyclic antidepressants, propoxyphene, theophylline, isoniazid, lithium).[227] These issues, however, are not usually involved in PSA in the ED. It has not been shown that simply taking therapeutic doses of these medications contraindicates the use of flumazenil, but flumazenil-induced seizures are generally associated only with drug overdose. Rapid reversal may also lead to return of anxiety and sympathetic stimulation. If the situation permits, careful titration of small amounts of flumazenil (0.1- to 0.2-mg aliquots intravenously) will reduce the risk for adverse effects and may permit partial rather than complete reversal. Observation times vary. For example, 1 hour after reversal will allow accurate assessment of residual sedation if less than 1 mg of flumazenil has been used to reverse conscious sedation with midazolam.

ACKNOWLEDGMENT

This chapter was previously superbly authored by Steven Green and Baruch Krauss and they are responsible for the majority of the content.

REFERENCES ARE AVAILABLE AT Elsevier eBooks+

SECTION VI

Soft Tissue Procedures

CHAPTER 34

Principles of Wound Management

Richard L. Lammers and Kathryn E. Redinger

Managing acute traumatic wounds is one of the most common procedures in emergency medicine. Although many aspects of traumatic wound management remain controversial, the clinician can follow some basic principles to maximize the chances of successful healing. This chapter gives the clinician a general approach to wound care and describes indications and techniques for wound management.

Wound care involves much more than the closure of divided skin. The primary goal of wound care is not technical repair of the wound, but to provide optimal conditions so that the natural reparative processes of the wound may proceed. The cornerstones of wound care are cleaning, debridement, closure (when appropriate), and protection. The primary objectives in wound care are to:

- Preserve viable tissue and remove nonviable tissue
- Restore tissue continuity and function
- Optimize conditions for the development of wound strength
- Prevent excessive or prolonged inflammation
- Avoid infection and other impediments to healing
- Minimize scar formation
- Provide appropriate anesthesia during wound management

Patients seeking care in the emergency department (ED) because of acute wounds report that their top priorities include infection prevention, return to normal function, a good cosmetic outcome, and minimal pain during repair.[1,2] This chapter reviews the current strategies for attaining these goals.

BACKGROUND: WOUND HEALING

For centuries, patients with wounds have commonly experienced inflammation, infection, and extreme scarring; in fact, these processes were considered part of normal wound healing. Emergency clinicians should have a basic understanding of the process of wound healing. Highlights of this complex phenomenon related to clinical decision-making are presented here.

Wounds extending beneath the epithelium heal by forming scar tissue. Among the various proposed overlapping phases from injury to repair, inflammation, epithelialization, fibroplasia, contraction, and scar remodeling/maturation constitute the main phases of this natural repair process.[3–6]

Inflammation is a beneficial response orchestrated by polymorphonuclear and mononuclear leukocytes concentrating at the injury site to phagocytose dead and dying tissue, foreign material, and bacteria in the wound, essentially performing a biologic debridement.[5] As white blood cells die, their intracellular contents are released into the wound. In excessive amounts, the contents form the purulence characteristic of infected wounds. Some exudate is expected even in the absence of bacterial invasion, but infection with accumulation of pus interferes with epithelialization and fibroplasia, which impairs wound healing. Wounds contaminated with significant numbers of bacteria or foreign material may undergo a prolonged or persistent inflammatory response and not heal. Granuloma formation surrounding retained sutures is an example of chronic inflammation.

While white blood cells remove debris within the wound, keratinocytes at its surface begin to migrate across the tissue defect during epithelialization. In most sutured wounds, the surface of the wound develops an epithelial covering impermeable to water within 24 to 48 hours. Surface debris, dead tissue, and eschar formation can impair this process. The epithelium thickens and grows downward into the wound along skin sutures. Although there is some "adhesiveness" at the wound edges during the first few days, this is eventually lost because of fibrinolysis.

By the fourth or fifth day, newly transformed fibroblasts in the wound begin synthesizing collagen and protein polysaccharides, thereby initiating the stage of scar formation known as *fibroplasia*. Collagen is the predominant component of scar tissue.[5] Wound strength is a balance between the lysis of old collagen and the synthesis of new collagen that "welds" the wound's edges. The amount of scar tissue that forms is influenced by physical forces (e.g., the stresses imposed by movement) acting across the wound. When the wound edges are approximated naturally or by mechanical closure within the first 24 hours, the wound can heal by "first (or primary) intention." In contrast, a wound with extensive tissue loss and not closed by sutures or other means heals by "secondary intention," a combination of processes that include contraction, collagen formation, and epithelialization (Fig. 34.1).[6] *Contraction* consists of movement of the skin edges toward the center of the defect, primarily in the direction of the underlying muscle.

Significant gains in tensile strength do not begin until approximately the fifth day after the injury. Strength increases rapidly for 6 to 17 days, more slowly for an additional 10 to 14

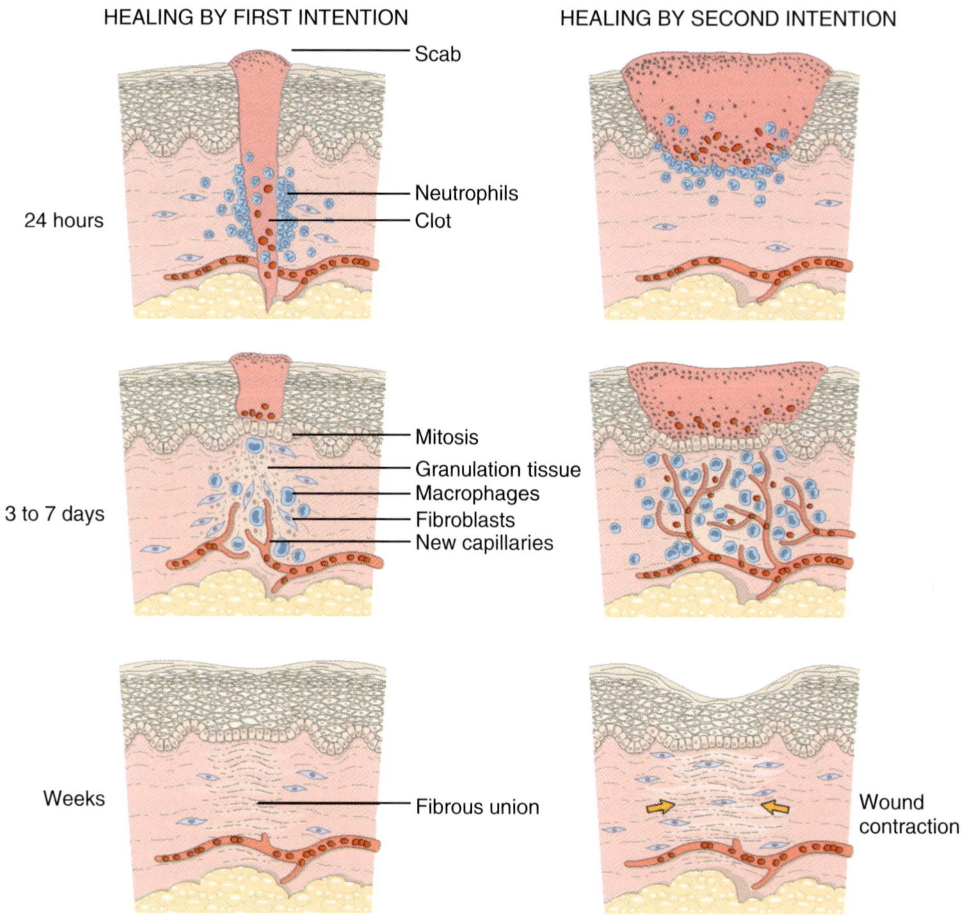

Fig. 34.1 Steps in wound healing by first or primary intention *(left)* and secondary intention *(right)*. Note the large amounts of granulation tissue and wound contraction in healing by secondary intention.

days, and imperceptibly for as long as 2 years (Fig. 34.2). The strength of scar tissue never quite reaches that of unwounded skin, approaching a maximum of 80%.[3,6] Although the process of collagen formation is essentially completed within 21 to 28 days, the scar widens for another month, and collagen continues to *remodel* and strengthen the wound for up to 1 year.[3,5] The normal desirable outcome of this complex process is a wound that is either fully reepithelialized or filled with an avascular scar.[6]

Decisions regarding the optimal time for suture removal and the need for continued support of the wound with tape are influenced by the following: (1) the tensile strength of the wound, (2) the period of scar widening, and (3) the cosmetically unacceptable effect of epithelialization along the suture track. Scars are quite red and noticeable at 3 to 8 weeks after closure. The appearance of a scar should not be judged before it is well into its remodeling phase. The cosmetic appearance of wounds 6 to 9 months after injury cannot be predicted at the time of suture removal.[7] Therefore scar revision, if necessary, should be postponed until 6 to 12 months after injury.

One of the most important factors in predicting the cosmetic result of a wound is its location. A 2006 study demonstrated that lacerations on the torso, leg, or foot received the lowest cosmetic scores from patients enrolled when asked 14 days and 3 months after wound repair. Possible contributing factors may be that the location of the wound also correlates with the propensity for wound contamination and subsequent infection. Additionally, lacerations on extremities in areas with

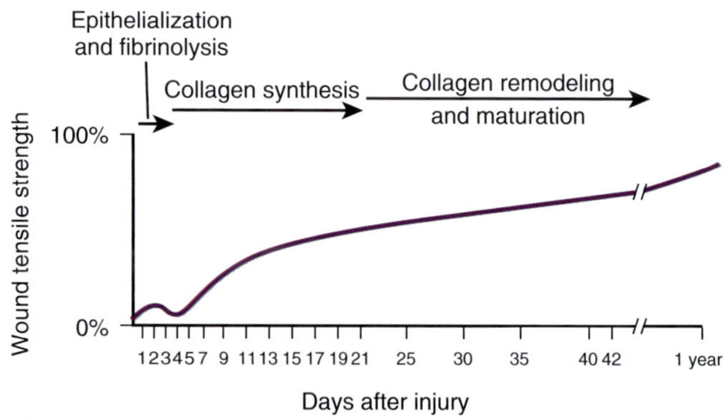

Fig. 34.2 Various phases of wound healing. Note that the tensile strength of scar tissue never reaches that of unwounded skin. The values of tensile strength displayed are approximate and demonstrate the general concept of wound healing.

greater mobility may increase tension on the healing tissue or be exposed to reinjury.[8] In general, wounds on concave surfaces heal with better cosmetic results than wounds on convex surfaces. Other factors affecting cosmesis include wound size, depth, and skin color.[9] Small, superficial wounds in lax, light-colored skin, especially areas with thin skin, result in less noticeable scars. Wounds on convex surfaces look better after primary closure than after secondary healing. Static and dynamic forces and the propensity toward keloid formation may influence the long-term cosmetic appearance of wounds more than the surgical skills of the clinician who repaired the wound.[7] Repigmentation occurs for 3 to 5 years, even in large wounds that heal by secondary intention.[9] Patients should be advised to wear sunscreen over the scar, especially during the first few years after injury, because unprotected exposure to the sun can alter the pigmentation as the wound heals and may result in noticeably darker pigmentation than the surrounding skin.[10,11]

INITIAL EVALUATION

The approach to management of a particular wound and the decision to close a wound immediately or after a period of observation is based primarily on factors that affect the risk for infection, and secondarily on cosmesis and long-term functionality. The history and physical examination should be directed toward identifying these factors. Some wounds may appear benign but conceal extensive and devastating underlying tissue damage. The following findings should alert the provider of a more complicated injury including an extremity wound caused by a roller or wringer device, a high-pressure injection gun, high-voltage electricity, heavy and prolonged compressive force, or the bite of a human or a potentially rabid animal. These findings radically alter the overall management of the patient.

History

In the initial evaluation of a wound, identify all the extrinsic and intrinsic factors that jeopardize healing and promote infection, including (1) the mechanism of injury, (2) the time of injury, (3) the environment in which the wound occurred, and (4) the patient's immune status, including reviewing the patient's past medical history for predictors of poor wound healing, such as diabetes or other chronic illness, and the patient's tetanus status.

If the reported mechanism of injury does not appear to correlate with the resulting injury, the clinician should also obtain a social history ensuring that the patient is in a safe environment and not the victim of intimate partner violence, abuse, or self-injurious behavior.[12]

Wound Age

In general, the likelihood of a wound infection increases with time from the injury to definitive wound care. Definitive wound care includes cleaning and debridement, if necessary, but it does not always mean closure of the wound. A delay in wound cleaning may allow bacteria contaminating some wounds to proliferate to infective levels, especially in heavily contaminated wounds. In highly vascular areas, such as the face and scalp, wounds can be closed without increased risk for as long as 24 hours after injury. Some wounds should never be closed, such as small, contaminated lacerations on the bottom of the foot, whereas others can be closed many hours after the injury without increasing infection rates.

There is no evidence in the medical literature defining the optimal time for initially closing acute traumatic wounds,[13,14] with no generally accepted standard. The "golden period"—the maximum time after injury that a wound may be closed safely without significant risk for infection—is not a fixed number of hours. The studies attempting to address this question have reported conflicting results.[15–21] The likely reason is that many factors interact to determine risk of infection, including amount of contamination and devitalized tissue, patient age and state of health, and wound size and location.[16] Thus closure decisions should not be based solely on time considerations in a particular patient.

Skillful cleaning and debridement may extend the safe period, allowing a clinician to convert a contaminated wound to a clean wound that can be closed during initial wound management. Delayed primary closure is a reasonable alternative when there is clinical concern for infection at the initial assessment. Primary closure of persistently contaminated wounds increases the risk of wound infection, whereas delayed primary closure decreases the risk of infection but may prolong healing time.[13]

In most instances, the clinician cannot eliminate infection risks, but adequate wound care can favorably affect the probability and severity of infection. Simply prescribing antibiotics in the hope that infection will somehow be averted is an unrealistic expectation and can lead to antibiotic-resistant microorganisms.

In summary, any time frames for closing wounds are suggestions. Clinical judgment regarding the potential for wound infection should be incorporated into the final decision-making process.

Other Historical Factors

Patient age appears to be an important factor in host resistance to infection. Individuals who are at the extremes of age, such as young children and the elderly, have the greatest risk for infection.[16,22] Infection rates are reported to be higher in patients with concurrent medical conditions such as diabetes mellitus, immunologic deficiencies, malnutrition, anemia, uremia, congestive heart failure, cirrhosis, malignancy, alcoholism, arteriosclerosis, arteritis, collagen vascular disease, chronic granulomatous disease, smoking, chronic hypoxia, renal failure, and liver failure. Morbid obesity, in addition to other conditions in which patients are taking steroids or immunosuppressive drugs, or undergoing radiation therapy, are all higher risks for infection. Shock, remote trauma, distant infection, bacteremia, retained foreign bodies, denervation, and peripheral vascular disease also increase wound infection rates and can slow the healing process.[6,16,22]

Additional information pertinent to decision-making in wound management includes the following:

- *Associated symptoms* (severe pain, paresthesia, or anesthesia)[10]
- *Current medications* (specifically, anticoagulants, steroids, and immunosuppressive drugs)
- *Allergies* (especially to local anesthetics, antiseptics, analgesics, antibiotics, and tape)
- *Tetanus immunization status*
- *Potential exposure to rabies* (in bite wounds and mucosal exposures)
- *Potential foreign bodies* (embedded in the wound, especially when the mechanism of injury is unknown, or the injury was associated with breaking glass or vegetative matter)[23]
- *Previous injuries and deformities* (especially with extremity and facial injuries)
- *Associated injuries* (underlying fracture, joint penetration, crush injury, deep penetrating injury, animal or human bite)
- *Other factors* (access to follow-up, patient understanding of wound care, compliance)

Physical Examination

All wounds should be examined for tissue destruction, degree of contamination, potential foreign bodies, and damage to underlying structures. The examiner should wear clean or sterile powder-free, latex-free gloves and avoid droplet contamination from the mouth. Examine the wound under good lighting and after the bleeding is controlled. Create a bloodless field, if necessary, with a tourniquet or sphygmomanometer (Video 34.1). Assess distal perfusion, motor and sensory function (prior to the use of anesthetics), nearby tendon function, and document findings.

Mechanism of Injury and Classification of Wounds

The magnitude and direction of the injuring force and the volume of tissue on which the force is distributed determine the type of wound that is sustained. Three types of mechanical forces—shear, tension, and compression—produce soft tissue injury. The resulting disruption or loss of tissue determines the configuration of the wound. Wounds may be classified into six categories:

1. *Abrasions.* Wounds caused by forces applied in opposite directions result in the loss of epidermis and possibly dermis (e.g., grinding of skin against a road surface).
2. *Lacerations.* Wounds caused by shear forces produce a tear in tissues. Shear forces require little energy to produce a wound (e.g., a knife cut). Consequently, little tissue damage occurs at the wound edge, the margins are sharp, and the wound appears "tidy." Tensile and compressive forces also cause separation of the tissues. The energy required to disrupt tissue by tensile or compressive forces (e.g., forehead hitting a dashboard) is considerably greater than that required for tissue disruption by shear forces because the energy is distributed over a larger volume. These lacerations often have jagged, contused, "untidy" edges, which have a higher risk for infection.[22]
3. *Crush wounds.* Wounds caused by the impact of an object against tissue, particularly over a bony surface, compress the tissue. These wounds may contain contused or partially devitalized tissue and have higher infection rates if not appropriately debrided.
4. *Puncture wounds.* Wounds with a small opening, whose depth cannot be entirely visualized, are caused by a combination of forces. They are particularly prone to infection because they are difficult to thoroughly clean and may retain foreign bodies.[4]
5. *Avulsions.* Avulsions are wounds in which a portion of tissue is completely separated from its base, which is lost, or left with a narrow base of attachment (a flap). Shear and tensile forces cause avulsions.[24] Skin tear avulsions often result from low-force friction or shearing forces that separate the layers of the skin (epidermis and dermis) from the underlying tissue. These wounds often occur in older adults with minimal impact because of vulnerable thin skin.
6. *Combination wounds.* Wounds can also have a combination of configurations. For example, a stellate laceration caused by compression of soft tissue against underlying bone can create wounds with elements of both crush injury and tissue separation. Missile wounds involve a combination of shear, tensile, and compressive forces that puncture, crush, and sometimes avulse tissue.[23]

Contaminants (Bacteria and Foreign Material)

Infection rates in studies of traumatic wounds range from 1% to 32%.[18,25] Numerous factors affect the risk for wound infection, but the primary determinants of infection are the amount of bacteria and dead tissue remaining in the wound, the patient's immune response, and local tissue perfusion.

All traumatic wounds are contaminated with bacteria. The number of bacteria remaining in the wound at the time of closure is directly related to the risk of infection. A critical number of bacteria must be present in a wound before a soft tissue infection develops. In experimental wounds, fewer bacteria are required to infect wounds caused by a compressive force ($\geq 10^4$ bacteria/g of tissue) than by a shear force ($\geq 10^6$ bacteria/g of tissue).[26]

The nature and amount of foreign material contaminating the wound often determines the type and quantity of bacteria implanted. In general, visible contamination of a wound increases the risk for infection.[22] The presence of undetected, reactive foreign bodies in sutured wounds almost guarantees an infection. Although bullet or glass fragments rarely produce wound infection, these foreign bodies may carry particles of clothing, gun wadding, or soil into the wound. Minute amounts of organic or vegetative matter, feces, or saliva carry highly infective doses of bacteria. The bacterial inoculum from human bites often contains 1 billion or more organisms per milliliter of saliva.[27] Inorganic particulate matter, such as sand or road surface grease, usually introduces a few bacteria into a wound and has little chemical reactivity. These contaminants are relatively innocuous. Soil that contains a considerable proportion of clay particles or a high organic content (such as that found in swamps, bogs, and marshes), however, has an elevated risk for infection.[28]

In industrialized countries, most wounds encountered in emergency medicine have low initial bacterial counts. If wound cleaning and removal of devitalized tissue are instituted before bacteria within the wound enter their accelerated growth phase (3 to 12 hours after the injury), bacterial counts will usually remain below the threshold needed to initiate infection.[11,29]

Devitalized Tissue

Devitalized and necrotic tissue in a traumatic wound should be identified and removed. If left in place, it will allow bacteria to proliferate, inhibit leukocyte phagocytosis, and create an anaerobic environment suitable for certain bacterial species.[23]

Wound Location

The wound's anatomic location is important in the risk for infection. Bacterial densities on the surface of the skin range from a few thousand to millions per square centimeter.[28] Distal extremity wounds are more at risk for the development of wound infections than are injuries on most other parts of the body.[16,17] Levels of endogenous bacteria on hairy parts of the scalp, the mouth, axilla, nails, foreskin, perineum, and vagina may be high enough to serve as a potential source of infection in wounds in these locations.[23] The high vascularity in areas such as the scalp, face, or perineum appears to offset the risk posed by the large numbers of endogenous microflora. In contrast, wounds in ischemic tissue are notoriously susceptible to infection.[30]

Underlying Structures

If injury to underlying structures such as nerves, vessels, tendons, joints, bones, or ducts is found, the clinician may choose to forego wound closure and consult a surgical specialist (Fig. 34.3). Procedures such as joint space irrigation reduction and debridement of compound fractures, neurorrhaphy, vascular anastomosis, and hand flexor tendon repair are best accomplished in the controlled aseptic setting of the operating room, where optimal lighting, proper instruments, and assistance are available.

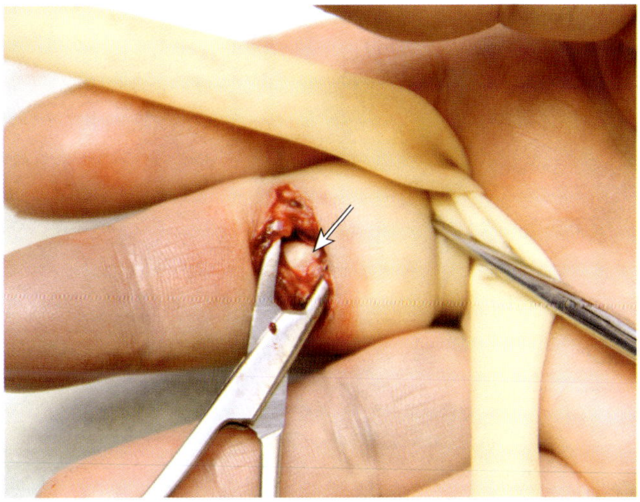

Fig. 34.3 This patient had weak, hesitant, but full flexion of the finger, thus suggesting at least a partial tendon laceration. The tendon was nearly 90% lacerated *(arrow)* and would have ruptured with any stress. Close examination of this wound, with careful blunt dissection down to the tendon itself *and the finger in the position of injury*, revealed significant trauma to the delicate flexor tendon that required consultation with a specialist. Use of a proximal tourniquet for a bloodless field and instruments to explore finger wounds is mandatory to increase sensitivity for finding injury to deep structures. This wound can be repaired within a few days by a hand specialist, but if discovered weeks later, problems are likely.

CLEANING

Clean the wound as soon as possible after evaluation. Although most wounds are initially contaminated with less than an infective dose of bacteria, given time and the appropriate wound environment, bacterial counts may quickly rise to infective levels. The goals of wound cleaning and debridement are as follows: (1) to remove bacteria and reduce their numbers below the level associated with infection; and (2) to remove particulate matter and tissue debris that would lengthen the inflammatory stage of healing or allow the growth of bacteria beyond the critical threshold.

There are two general wound-cleansing techniques: irrigation and scrubbing. Irrigation, recommended for most wounds, involves a steady flow of solution across the wound's surface. This crucial step in wound management hydrates the wound, removes deeper debris, and reduces the risk of infection. Normal saline or tap water is often used as an irrigation fluid. Many studies have demonstrated that the use of tap water as irrigation fluid provides a cost-effective and time-efficient method of low-pressure, high-volume irrigation with infection rates that are comparable to traditional techniques.[31–33] Soaking a wound in a saline or antiseptic solution before the clinician arrives is an outdated practice of no proven value and may increase bacterial count; hence, it is not recommended.[34]

Patient Preparation

Before examining, cleaning, exploring, or repairing a wound, allay the patient's fears and encourage cooperation by explaining the procedure and assuring the patient that everything possible will be done to minimize pain. In general, all wound care should be performed with the patient in a supine position because fainting is a common occurrence during wound preparation and repair (Fig. 34.4). Relatives and friends can be allowed to stay with the patient, but they should be cautioned to report any dizziness or nausea, and should remain seated throughout the procedure.

Anyone cleaning, irrigating, or suturing wounds should wear protective eyewear and gloves to reduce the possibility of exposure to pathogens. Although mucosal exposure to blood or tissue products that are contaminated by HIV is considered a relatively minimal risk for subsequent infection, universal precautions are currently recommended, and a mask should be considered. Minimal aseptic technique requires gloves during the cleaning procedure. Clean, but nonsterile technique has been shown to save time and resources without increasing wound infection rates.[35,36]

Thorough cleansing of bacteria, soil, and other contaminants from a wound cannot be accomplished without the patient's cooperation. Scrubbing most open wounds is painful, and the patient's natural response is to withdraw the injured area away from the provider. Local or regional anesthesia should precede the examination and cleansing of a wound (Video 34.2). Applying topical lidocaine preparation, such as LAT (lidocaine-adrenaline-tetracaine) gel or EMLA (eutectic mixture of local anesthetics) cream, is suitable for short lacerations (<4 cm), lacerations located on the head, and simple finger lacerations in children and adults.[37] Studies have demonstrated that applying ice to the injection site prior to local anesthetic injection might reduce the pain and discomfort caused by the injection.[38,39]

Despite adequate anesthesia, the patient may be too apprehensive to cooperate. If reassurance does not alleviate the fears of young children, consider both moderate procedural sedation and physical restraining techniques, such as swaddling the arms using a pillowcase or bed sheets.

Mechanical Scrubbing

Scrubbing the internal surface of a wound is controversial. Although scrubbing a wound with an antiseptic-soaked sponge decreases the risk of infection by removing foreign particulates, bacteria, and tissue debris,[40] an abrasive sponge may inflict more damage on the tissue.[23] Since the amount of damage caused by scrubbing correlates with the porosity of the sponge, a fine-pore sponge (e.g., 90 pores/inch) should be used to minimize tissue abrasion. Mechanical scrubbing should be reserved for wounds contaminated with significant amounts of bacteria or foreign material (Fig. 34.5A–B) or should be considered if irrigation alone is ineffective in removing visible contaminants from a wound.

Initially scrub a wide area of skin surface surrounding the wound with an antiseptic solution to remove contaminants that might be transferred into the wound by instruments, suture material, dressings, or the clinician's gloved

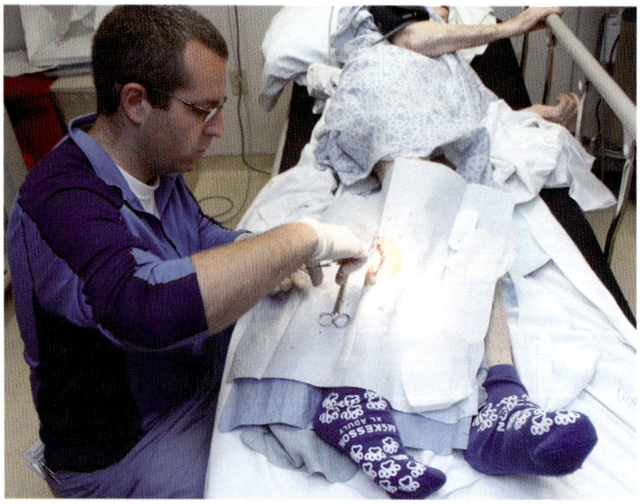

Fig. 34.4 The ideal setup for evaluation and repair of a laceration is a supine patient, a seated clinician at the correct height for the procedure, and a bloodless field with good lighting.

hand during wound management. It is important to remove all nonabsorbable particulate matter; any such material left in the dermis may be retained in the healed tissue and result in a disfiguring "tattoo" effect. Detergents have an advantage over saline by minimizing friction between the sponge and tissue, thereby limiting damage to tissue during scrubbing. Detergents also dissolve particles and thus help dislodge them from the wound's surface. Unfortunately, many of the detergents available are toxic to tissues.[10,34] Use caution when considering detergents.

Antiseptics During Cleaning

For many years, antiseptic solutions have been used for their antimicrobial properties in and around wounds (Table 34.1). Studies on the use of antiseptics in wounds demonstrate a delicate balance between killing bacteria and injuring tissue.[41,42] Intact skin can withstand strong microbicidal agents, whereas leukocytes and the exposed cells of the skin and soft tissue can be damaged by these agents.

Povidone-iodine (Betadine) as a 10% stock solution is widely available. Although the undiluted solution may be used to prepare the skin surrounding a wound, it may be harmful to some tissue; therefore it should not be placed within the interior of the wound. Diluted povidone-iodine solution in concentrations of less than 1% appears to be safe and effective for cleaning contaminated traumatic wounds,[40] but the precise concentration that provides the most benefit is unclear. Even dilute povidone-iodine may be particularly irritating when used for scrubbing contaminated wounds. In contrast, povidone-iodine surgical scrub (7.5% iodine) and hexachlorophene (pHisoHex]) both contain anionic detergents that are harmful to tissues. The effect on the actual wound infection rate is unknown. A recent randomized controlled trial of povidone-iodine as a skin disinfectant in preventing wound infections in simple traumatic nonbite lacerations did not demonstrate a reduced rate of infections. Similar to other studies, there was a significant association between the observed rate of infection and wound location.[43] Hydrogen peroxide is hemolytic, and there is little reason to use it except to clean surrounding skin encrusted with blood and coagulum, or to soak off adherent blood-saturated dressings. Peroxide should not be used on granulation tissue because oxygen bubbles lift newly formed epithelium off the wound surface.

Chlorhexidine is a biguanide with broad-spectrum bactericidal properties that inactivates gram-positive and -negative bacteria through penetration of outer and inner cell membranes. Chlorhexidine is thought to be less toxic on granulation cells, but still associated with tissue damage that can impede proper wound healing.[44] In vitro studies have demonstrated that chlorhexidine gluconate (CHG)-alcohol (Hibiclens) is toxic to both fibroblasts and keratinocytes.[41] When diluted to decrease its cytotoxic effect on these cells, it is no longer able to sufficiently kill *Staphylococcus aureus*.[42] In a recent meta-analysis seeking to compare the risk of surgical site infection (SSI) between CHG-alcohol and povidone-iodine (PVP-I) according to the CHG concentration, both 2% and 0.5% formulations demonstrated a reduction in surgical site infections when used as a skin preparation agent.[45]

Nonantiseptic, nonionic surfactants are attractive alternatives to these toxic cleansing agents. In contrast to antiseptic solutions, these preparations cause no tissue or cellular damage, leukocyte inhibition, or impairment of wound healing. The solutions cause no corneal injury, have minimal risk of conjunctival irritation, and do not cause pain on contact with the wound.[46] Poloxamer 188 (Shur-Clens, ConvaTec or Pluronic F-68, Thermo), a group of pluronic polyols, is nontoxic but has no antibacterial activity. Scrubbing experimental wounds with Shur-Clens reduced infection rates (though not statistically better than normal saline or povidone-iodine), thus proving it can cleanse a wound effectively and atraumatically.[40,41] Pluronic polyols may be a desirable choice if the wound is near mucous membranes. The use of antiseptic preparations in wounds can be considered in high-risk, contaminated wounds where the benefits outweigh the risks.

Irrigation

It is important to distinguish between skin antiseptics and irrigating solutions. In general, commercially available antiseptics should be used only to clean intact skin and not exposed wound surfaces. Most open wounds can be irrigated effectively with copious amounts of saline or tap water.[31,40] Although irrigation may not be required for low-risk, highly vascular, uncontaminated facial and scalp wounds,[47] randomized, prospective trials are needed to answer this question.

Properly performed irrigation (Video 34.3) effectively removes particulate matter, bacteria, and devitalized tissue that is loosely adherent to the edges of the wound and trapped within its depths. The effectiveness of irrigation is primarily determined by the hydraulic pressure at which the irrigation fluid is delivered.[31,48] Low-pressure irrigation is defined at 1 to 2 psi, whereas high-pressure irrigation is greater than 8 psi. Port devices spiked into plastic intravenous bags that are squeezed by hand to deliver a stream of fluid, bulb syringes, or gravity flow irrigation devices all deliver fluid at very low pressures.[48–50] Although irrigation at either low or high pressures will reduce levels of *S. aureus*, higher pressures should be more effective at ridding wounds of small particulate matter.[50] Commercial high-pressure irrigation systems commonly used in operating rooms remove significant numbers of bacteria and a substantial amount of particulate matter from the wound surface. Care must be taken to ensure that any method of irrigation is not exerting too much pressure because tissue damage can occur at pressures of 70 psi.[31] Wound irrigation is

Wound Cleansing: Mechanical Scrubbing and Irrigation

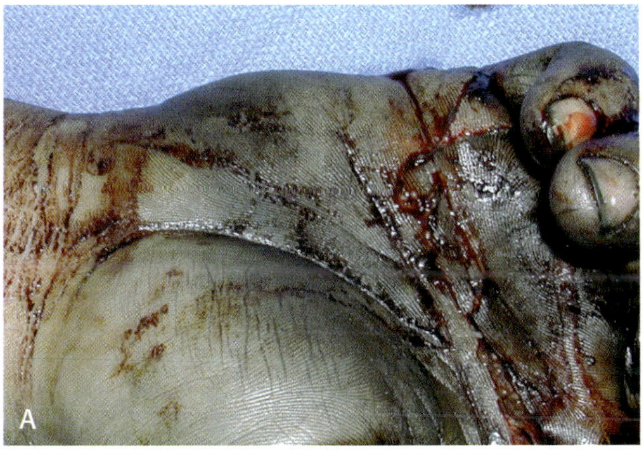

Grossly contaminated wounds such as this need to be thoroughly cleansed prior to repair, by mechanical scrubbing and/or irrigation.

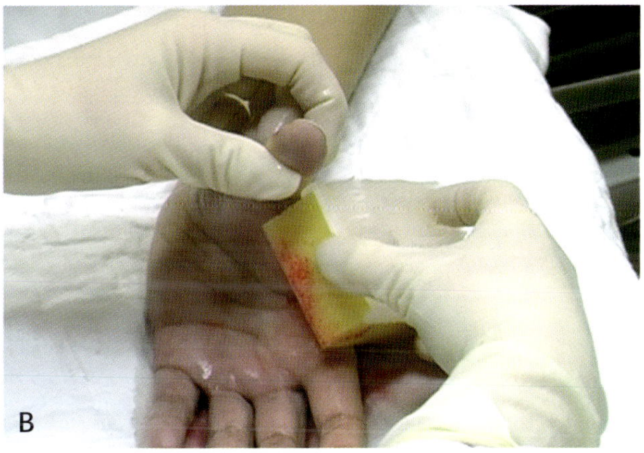

Reserve mechanical scrubbing for wounds contaminated with significant amounts of bacteria or foreign material. Use a fine-pore sponge (e.g., 90 pores/inch) to minimize tissue abrasion.

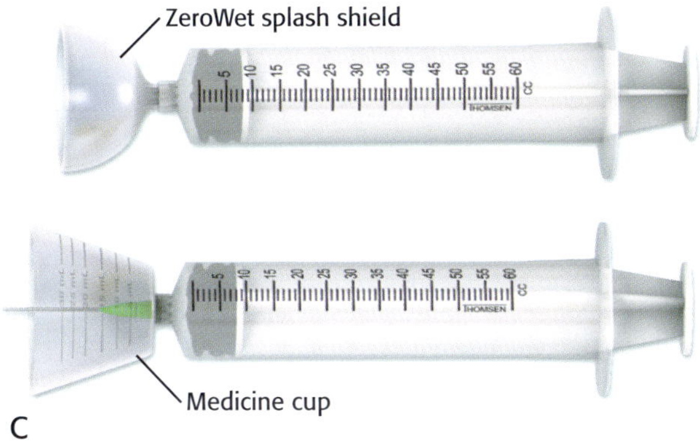

Top, ZeroWet splash shield attached to the end of a syringe. The shield is held near or against the skin and protects the user from splashes from the high-pressure laminar flow nozzle. *Bottom*, a makeshift splash protector can be made from a medicine cup.

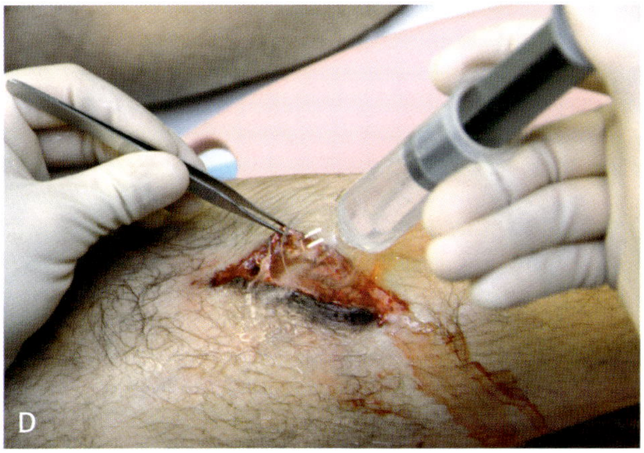

Use of the ZeroWet device. Note that the clinician is holding the laceration open with forceps to allow irrigation of the deep structures.

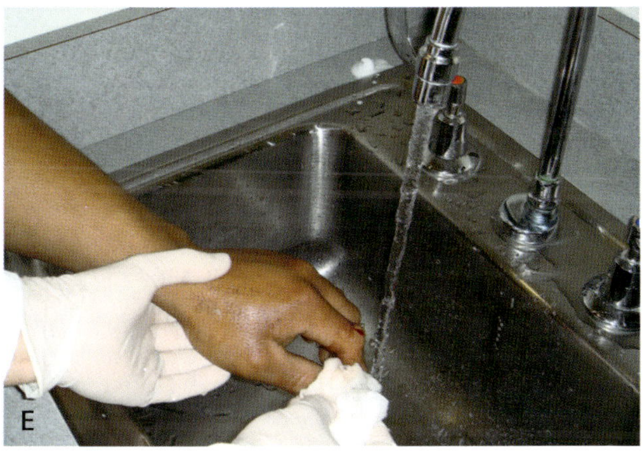

Tap water and nonsterile gloves are commonly used to copiously irrigate wounds of the extremities by taking advantage of the volume and force parameters from the faucet. Anesthetize lacerations before cleaning. Be mindful of the potential for the patient to faint.

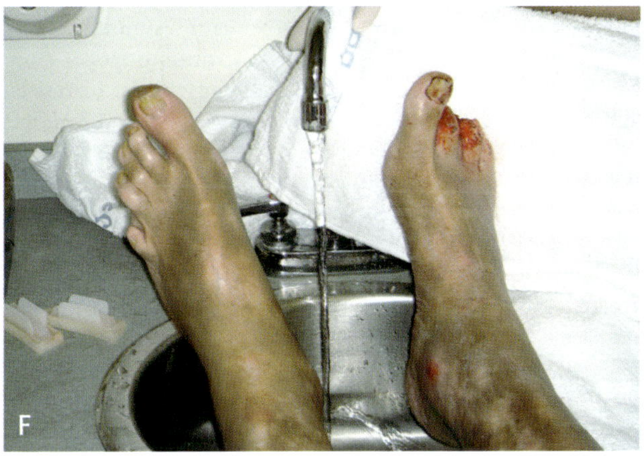

For foot wounds, the patient is placed on a stretcher and wheeled to the sink.

Fig. 34.5 Wound cleansing: mechanical scrubbing and irrigation. Wound irrigation with tap water is acceptable.

TABLE 34.1 Summary of Agents Used for Wound Care

AGENT	BIOLOGIC ACTIVITY	TISSUE TOXICITY[a]	SYSTEMIC TOXICITY[a]	POTENTIAL USES	COMMENTS
Povidone-iodine surgical scrub (Betadine 7.5%)	Virucidal; strongly bactericidal	Detergent component toxic to wound tissue	Painful in open wounds	Hand cleanser	Iodine allergy possible
Povidone-iodine solution (Betadine 10%)	Virucidal; bactericidal	Potentially toxic at full strength; 1% solution has no significant tissue toxicity	Extremely rare	Wound periphery cleanser; dilute to <1% for wound irrigation	Dilute 10:1 (saline to Betadine) if used to irrigate wounds
Chlorhexidine gluconate (Hibiclens)	Bactericidal	Toxic to tissues, including eyes	Extremely rare	Hand cleanser	Avoid in open wounds, eyes, or ears
Poloxamer 188 (Shur-Clens); Pluronic F-68	No antibacterial or antiviral activity	None known; does not inhibit wound healing	None known	Wound cleanser	Nontoxic in wounds and eyes
Hexachlorophene (pHisoHex)	Bacteriostatic against gram-positive bacteria	Potentially toxic to wound tissue	Possibly teratogenic with repeated use	Alternative hand cleanser	Systemic absorption causes neurotoxicity
Hydrogen peroxide	Very weak antibacterial agent	Toxic to tissue and red cells	Extremely rare	Wound periphery cleanser	Foaming activity removes surface debris and coagulated blood

[a]Based largely on in vitro studies and animal data.

easily achieved in the ED with a large-volume syringe, 35 or 65 mL, and an 18- or 19-gauge catheter or needle to deliver irrigation volumes of at least 250 mL. The pressure that can be delivered with a syringe varies with the force exerted on the plunger and the internal diameter of the attached needle. A simple irrigation assembly consisting of a 19-gauge plastic catheter or needle attached to a 35-mL syringe produces 25 to 40 psi when the barrel of the syringe is pushed with both hands.[48] High-pressure irrigation can also be achieved through IV tubing by placing a pressure cuff around a saline bag and inflating it to 400 mm Hg.[11] A running faucet can also generate up to 45 psi but is dependent on the distance from the faucet to the wound. Irrigating extremity lacerations by holding them under a faucet of tap water is a common and accepted practice for wound preparations. Fears of introducing new infectious material with a nonsterile irrigant are unfounded (assuming public water treatment systems are available in the community) (Fig. 34.5E–F). The advantage of using tap water from a faucet is that large volumes of irrigant can be quickly applied to an open wound at pressures required to remove debris and bacteria. The disadvantages of this technique are that irrigation pressures are difficult to control, and the patient may faint if allowed to stand at a sink.[51–53] If tap water is used to irrigate wounds, it may also be safely delivered through a syringe at the bedside.

Warmed irrigating solutions are more comfortable for patients, even after the wound is anesthetized.[54] Irrigation should continue until all visible, loose particulate matter has been removed.

A potential complication of wound irrigation is that infectious material can be splashed into the clinician's face, even when the tip of the irrigation device is held below the wound's surface. Several commercial devices are available to contain the splatter, including devices that fit on the end of a syringe (Fig. 34.5C–D) and devices that fit on the screw top of saline bottles (for this device the company reported variable pressure from 4 to 15 psi). An alternative strategy is to pierce the base of a small medicine cup with a shorter, large-bore needle. The cup can be placed upside down to cover the area to be irrigated and the syringe with the 19-gauge needle can be inserted through the base of the cup (see Fig. 34.5C). The wound should be positioned to allow continuous drainage of fluid during irrigation by any method.

Antibiotic Solutions for Irrigation

A variety of antibiotic solutions have been instilled directly into wounds or used as irrigation solutions, including ampicillin, a neomycin-bacitracin-polymyxin combination, tetracycline, penicillin, kanamycin, and cephalothin. Although there have been no reports of topical sensitization or toxic tissue levels of the antibiotic, studies have found inconsistent effectiveness in reducing infection rates.[55] The indications for using antibiotic solutions to clean wounds have not been defined, and this practice is not considered standard.

Recommendations for Cleaning the Wound

The prerequisites for any wound-cleaning technique are a calm or sedated patient, satisfactory anesthesia, and thorough cleaning of the skin surface adjacent to the wound. The primary goal of wound cleaning is to rid the wound of major contaminants and lower the infective dose of bacteria (Video 34.4). Two strategies are recommended. A contaminated or "dirty" wound can be irrigated, or both scrubbed and irrigated, with a 0.9% saline solution. As an alternative, the wound can be scrubbed with pluronic polyols and irrigated with a normal saline solution. Only pluronic polyols or saline should be used near the eyes. Perform scrubbing with a soft, fine-pore sponge, and use high-pressure techniques for irrigation. Avoid using hydrogen peroxide on open wounds. Either gentle scrubbing with pluronic polyols and normal saline high-pressure irrigation or irrigation alone is a satisfactory method for cleaning minimally contaminated wounds.[40]

Preparation for Wound Closure

Before debridement or wound closure, prepare and drape the wound. Avoid shaving body hair because preoperative wounds that were shaved demonstrated higher infection rates.[23] For wounds in hair-bearing areas, hair can be removed by clipping if it interferes with the procedure. Stubborn hairs that repeatedly invade the wound during suturing can be coated with petrolatum jelly or a water-soluble ointment to keep them out of the field. Do not shave eyebrows because critical landmarks for exact approximation of the wound edges would be lost. Although shaved eyebrows will grow back eventually, shaving also produces an undesirable cosmetic effect. Clip hair rather than shaving it.

Disinfect the skin surface adjacent to the wound (not the wound itself) with a standard 10% povidone-iodine or CHG (Hibiclens) solution. Paint the solution widely on the skin surrounding the wound but do not let it seep into the wound's interior (Fig. 34.6A).

After hand washing, the clinician and any assistants involved in the procedure must wear clean gloves, either sterile or nonsterile.[36] Sterile gloves are not required, and their use does not decrease infection rates. However, sterile gloves fit better on hands and better control instruments and sutures. Wear face masks, especially if you have an upper respiratory bacterial infection. Because droplets of saliva may leak from around the edges of a face mask, avoid talking in proximity to the wound. Use a single-fenestrated drape or multiple folded drapes around the wound site. Place a sterile glove on a patient who has a hand wound to provide a sterile field in lieu of a fenestrated drape. The area to be sutured can then be exposed by cutting a hole in the glove at the wound site, and the extremity can be placed on a sterile towel (Fig. 34.6B). This technique provides a clean field without the need to adjust the drape continually or to operate through a small opening.

Explore the entire depth and extent of every wound to locate hidden foreign bodies, particulate matter, bone fragments, or any injuries to underlying structures that may require repair (Fig. 34.6C–D). Avoid the temptation to initially explore wounds in search of a foreign body and to assess depth with a finger (Fig. 34.6E) because embedded glass, metal fragments, or sharp pieces of bone may cut the clinician and cause exposure to blood-borne pathogens. Visualize directly with good lighting in a bloodless field, explore the wound with a metal probe, and use radiographs as safer approaches to wound exploration. Despite these measures, lacerations through thick subcutaneous adipose tissue are treacherous because substantial amounts of particulate matter can be completely obscured in deep soft tissue folds. Unless a careful search is undertaken, contaminants may be inadvertently left in the depths of a sutured wound, resulting in infection. Some clinicians are reluctant to extend lacerations to clean or explore them properly; however, opening the wound to permit adequate visualization is often necessary for successful wound exploration.

Debridement

Debridement of foreign material and devitalized tissue is of undisputed importance in managing a contaminated wound. Use this technique to remove tissue embedded with foreign matter or bacteria. Devitalized tissue impairs the wound's ability to resist infection and prolongs inflammation. Debridement also creates a tidy, sharp wound edge that is easier to repair, resulting in a scar with a better cosmetic outcome.

If the wound is already clean and the edges are viable, sharp debridement may not improve the outcome. Irregular wounds have greater surface areas than linear lacerations. Because skin tension is distributed over a greater length, the scar's width is usually less with jagged wounds than if the wound is converted to an elliptical defect with tidy edges. If the edges are devitalized or contaminated, the wound edges must be debrided (Fig. 34.7A–B). To avoid a wide scar in this situation, undermine the wound and consider judicious removal of soft tissue within the wound to decrease the tension between the wound edges.

Excision

Excision is the most effective type of debridement because it converts a contaminated traumatic wound into a clean wound. If significant contamination occurs in areas with laxity of tissues, and if no important structures such as tendons or nerves lie within the wound, the entire wound may be excised (Fig. 34.7C). Complete excision of grossly contaminated wounds such as animal bites allows the primary closure of such wounds with no greater risk of infection than occurs with relatively uncontaminated lacerations.[23]

When a puncture wound is excised, make the axis of the excision parallel to a wrinkle, a skin line, or a line of dependency. Make the long axis of this lenticular excision three to four times as great as the short axis (Fig. 34.7D). Premark the skin with a surgical marking pen or make a superficial "scoring" mark (cutting only down to the epidermis) around the wound with a No. 15 scalpel blade. Place tension on the surrounding skin with a finger or a skin hook. While steadying your hand on the table or the patient, use the No. 15 blade and cut through the skin at right angles or at slightly oblique angles to the surface of the skin. If complete excision of the entire depth of the wound is not necessary, use tissue scissors to cut the edge of the wound by following the path premarked in the epidermis with the scalpel blade. If complete excision is desired, incise each wound edge past the deepest part of the wound. Excise and remove the wedge of tissue carefully without contaminating the fresh wound surface.

Plan the excision carefully because excessive removal of tissue can create a defect that is too large to close. Wounds on the trunk, the gluteal region, or the thigh are amenable to excision. In contrast, simple excision of a wound on the palm or the dorsum of the nose will make approximation of the resulting surgical wound edges difficult. In hair-bearing areas of the face, particularly through the eyebrows, angle the incision parallel to the angle of the hair follicles to avoid linear alopecia (Fig. 34.7E).

Selective Debridement

Complete excision is impossible for most wounds because of insufficient skin elasticity and area, so selective debridement must be used. Stellate wounds and wounds with an irregular,

Wound Preparation and Exploration

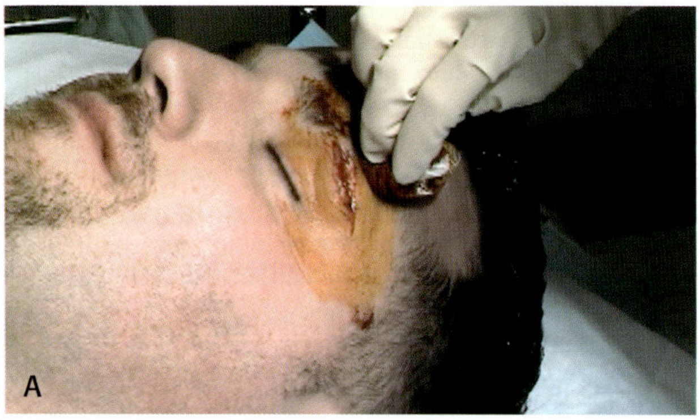

Disinfect the skin surface adjacent to the wound with 10% povidone-iodine or chlorhexidine gluconate, but do not allow it to seep into the wound.

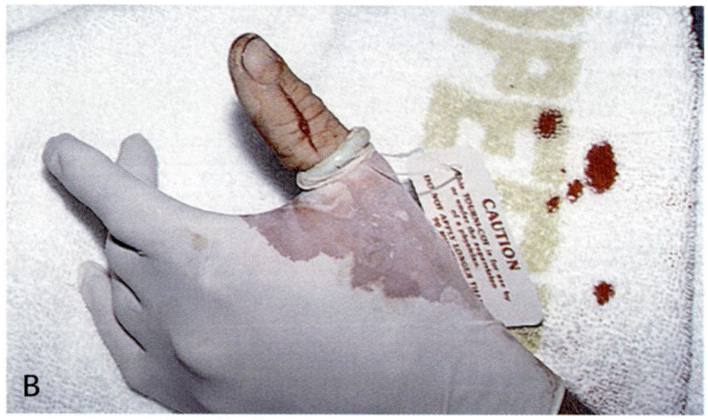

A nonsterile clean glove on the hand with the finger cut out and a finger tourniquet to provide a bloodless field make examination and suturing of a wound easier.

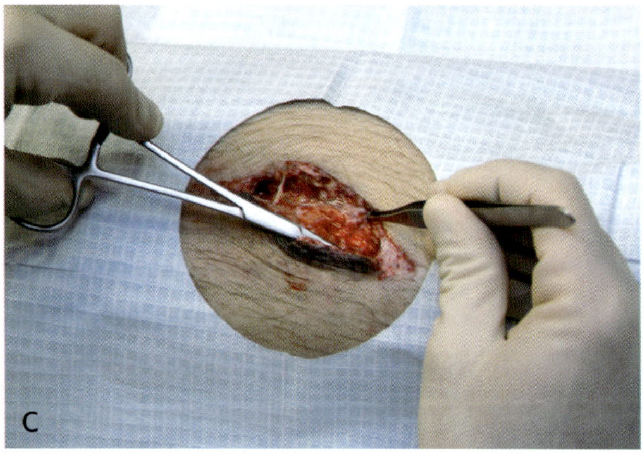

Explore the depths of the wound and examine for injured structures, foreign bodies, and the extent of injury.

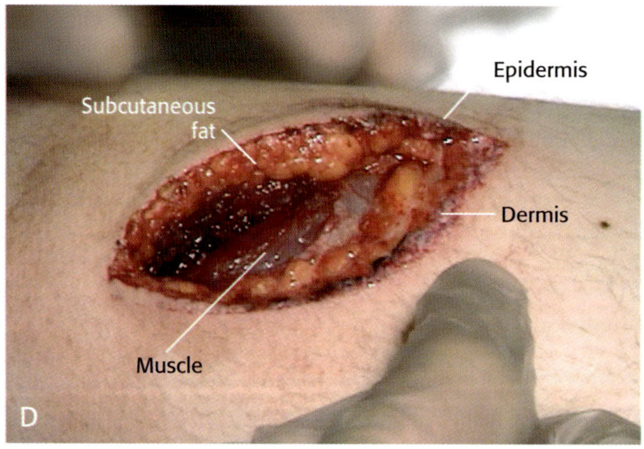

Anatomy of a deep laceration.

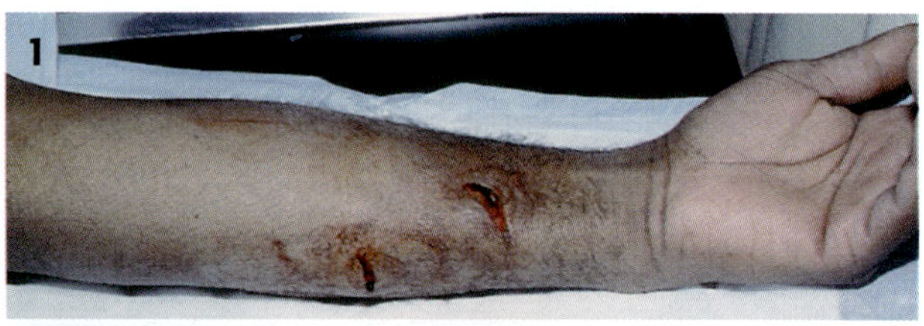

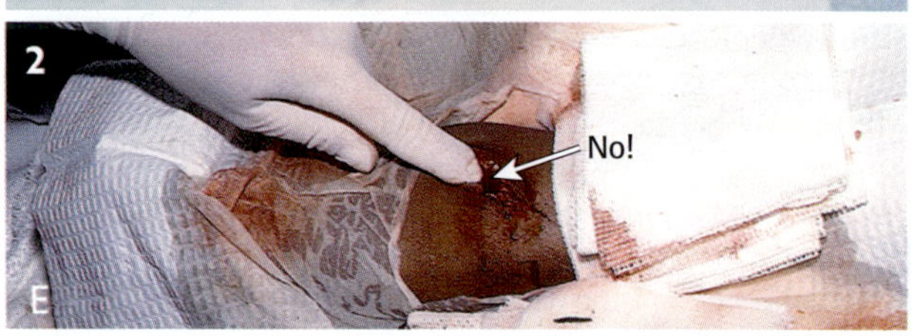

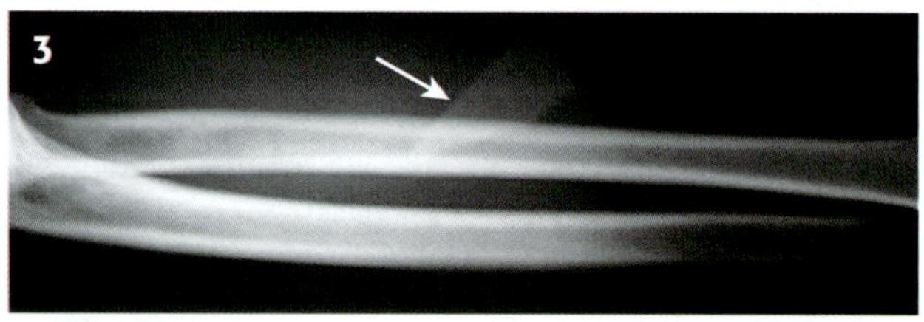

1, This patient punched out a window, a setup for retained glass. *2*, Do *not* explore this laceration with a finger. *3*, Instead, use radiographs and instruments to search for foreign bodies (the *arrow* defines a large piece of glass that could cut the examining finger). Many patients are unaware of the presence of large foreign bodies in a deep wound, although they should be questioned about the possibility or sensation of retained material.

Fig. 34.6 Wound preparation and exploration.

meandering course have greater surface area and less skin tension per unit length than linear lacerations. In some cases, excision of an entire wound would result in the loss of too much tissue (i.e., produce a gaping defect and excessive tension on the edges of the wound when closed). Avoid this problem by selective debridement and approximation of the irregular wound edges. This technique involves sharp debridement of devitalized or heavily contaminated tissue in the wound piece-by-piece and eventually matching one edge of the wound to the other. Selective debridement is time-consuming but preserves more of the surrounding viable tissue.

Identifying devitalized tissue in a wound remains a challenging problem. Tissue with a narrow pedicle or base, especially distally based narrow flaps on extremities, is unlikely to survive and should be excised. Approximately 24 hours after the wound occurs, a sharp line of demarcation often occurs and can help distinguish devitalized skin and viable skin,[23] but in most fresh wounds, usually only a subtle bluish or blanched

Wound Debridement

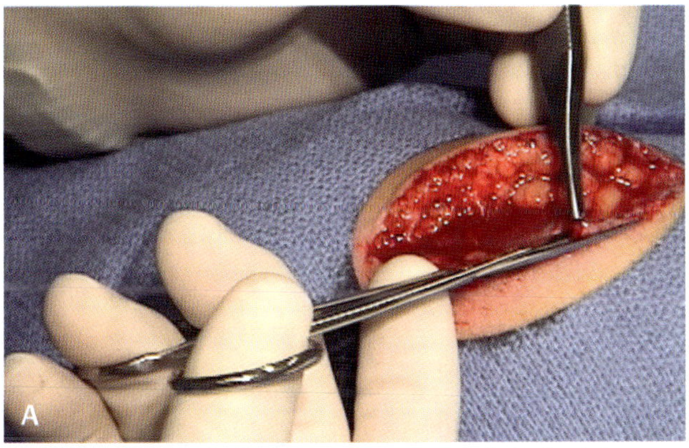
A

Sharp debridement is the best way to remove devitalized tissue and create a more cosmetic result. Here, the wound edges are trimmed with iris scissors.

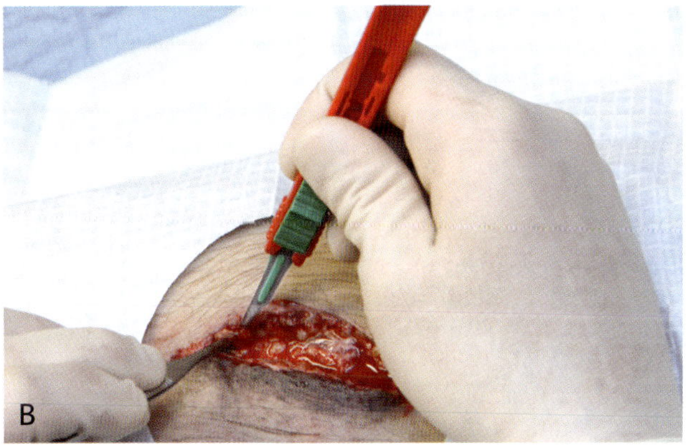
B

A scalpel can also be used. Alternatively, the skin is first sharply incised with a scalpel for a clean edge, and then the rest of the subcutaneous tissue is removed with scissors.

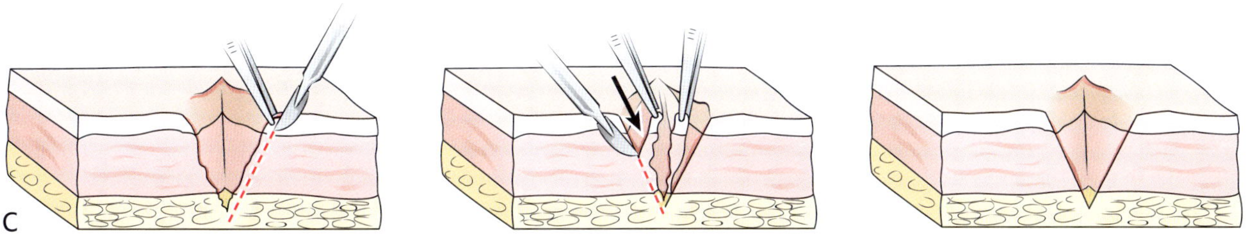
C

Excision is the most effective type of debridement because it converts a contaminated wound into a clean one. The entire wound may be excised if no important structures (such as tendons or nerves) are present. Grossly contaminated wounds may be excised and sutured primarily.

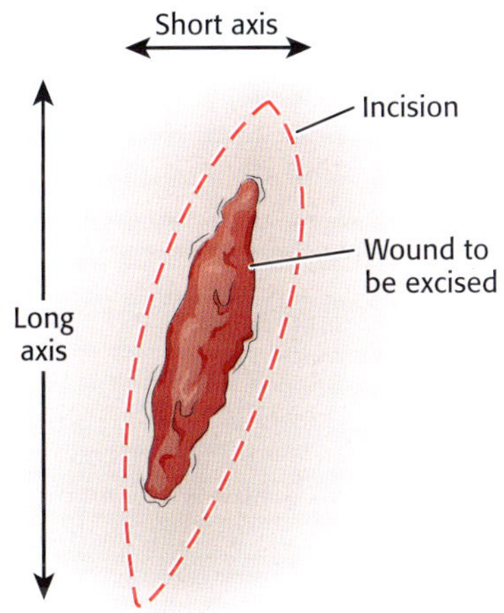

D

The long axis of an excision around a wound should be three to four times as great as the short axis.

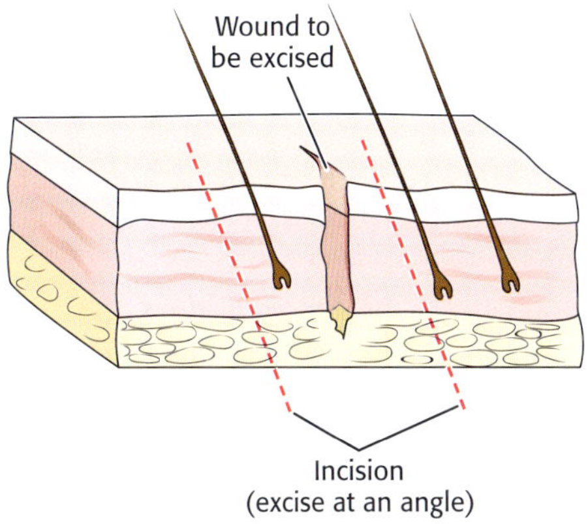

E

Excision through an eyebrow. Use an angled incision to remove tissue in the eyebrow, thus avoiding further injury to hair follicles.

Fig. 34.7 Wound debridement.

discoloration is present. Try to predict tissue viability by comparing the capillary refill of injured tissue with that of the adjacent skin. If circulation is adequate, viable tissue also becomes hyperemic soon after the release of a proximal tourniquet.

In heavily contaminated wounds, especially those with abundant adipose tissue, remove all exposed fat and all fat impregnated with particulate matter. The subcutaneous adipose tissue attached to large flaps or to avulsed viable skin should be debrided before reapproximation of the wound; removal of this fatty layer allows better perfusion of the flap or the graft. Contaminated bone fragments, nerves, and tendons are almost never removed. Every effort should be made to clean these structures and return them to their place of origin because they may be functional later. Fascia and tendons perform important functions despite potential loss of viability. If they can be cleaned adequately, these tissues should not be debrided. They may be left in wounds as free grafts and be covered by viable flaps of tissue.[23]

Instruments recommended for debridement include two fine single- or double-pronged skin hooks, a scalpel with a No.

15 blade, tissue scissors, hemostats, and small tissue forceps. Using gentle tissue pressure, stabilize the jagged wound edges with skin hooks or forceps, and use the scalpel or scissors to cut away devitalized tissue from one end of the wound to the other. After debridement or excision, irrigate the wound again to remove any remaining tissue debris.

Control of Hemorrhage

Hemostasis is essential at any stage of wound care. Persistent bleeding obscures the wound and hampers exploration and closure of the wound. If bleeding is not a problem before wound debridement, it may become a hindrance during cleaning or after the wound's edges are excised. If it is significant, hematoma formation in a sutured wound can separate the wound edges, impair healing, and cause dehiscence or infection.

Several practical methods of achieving hemostasis are available. Provide direct pressure with gloved fingers, gauze sponges, or packing material, and elevate the wound. This technique is usually effective in immediately controlling a single bleeding site or a small number of sites until the cut ends of vessels constrict and coagulation occurs. In a patient with multiple injuries and several urgent problems, control hemorrhage temporarily with a compression dressing. Apply several absorptive sponges directly over the bleeding site and secure them in place with an elastic bandage (e.g., Ace wrap) or elastic adhesive tape (Elastoplast). Then apply pressure with the elasticity of the bandage and elevate the bleeding part. Wound care can then be deferred while the clinician attends to more pressing matters.

Although simply crushing and twisting the end of a small vessel with a hemostat avoids dissection further into the wound, this method provides unreliable hemostasis. Ligation of the vessel with fine absorbable suture material is preferred. Clamp the bleeding ends of vessels with fine-point hemostats to provide immediate hemostasis. Because nerves often course with these vessels, clamp them only under direct visualization. The tip of the hemostat should project beyond the vessel to hold a loop of a ligature in place (Fig. 34.8A). With an assistant lifting the handle of the hemostat, pass a synthetic 5-0 or 6-0 *absorbable suture* around the hemostat from one hand to the other. Tie the first knot beyond the tip of the hemostat. Once the suture is securely anchored on the vessel, release the hemostat.[56] Three knots are sufficient to hold the ligature in place. Cut the ends of the suture close to the knot to minimize the amount of suture material left in the wound.

Ligate vessels with diameters greater than 2 mm. Vessels smaller than 2 mm that bleed despite direct pressure can be controlled by pinpoint, bipolar electrocautery. A dry field is required for an effective electrical current to pass through the tissues. If sponging does not dry the field, use a suction-tipped catheter. Minimize trauma by using fine-tipped electrodes to touch the vessel or the electrocautery unit's active electrode to a small hemostat or fine-tipped forceps while gripping the vessel. Keep the power of the unit to the minimum level required for thrombosis of the vessel. Self-contained, sterilizable, battery-powered coagulation units are alternatives to electrocautery. These devices cauterize vessels by the direct application of a heated wire filament. Although these units may damage more surrounding tissue than electrocautery units do, they are compact, simple, and well suited for use in the ED (Fig. 34.8B).

A cut vessel that retracts into the wall of the wound may frustrate attempts at clamping, ligation, or cauterization. First, control bleeding by downward compression on the tissue. Pass a suture through the tissue twice via a figure-of-eight or horizontal mattress stitch, and then tie it. This stitch will constrict the tissue containing the cut vessel (Fig. 34.8C).

Large superficial varicosities may bleed spontaneously or from minor trauma. They may bleed profusely, especially when the patient stands up and increases venous pressure. Use a simple figure-of-eight suture to halt the bleeding (Fig. 34.8D).

Epinephrine is an excellent vasoconstrictor. Place topical epinephrine (1:100,000) on a moistened sponge and apply it to a wound to reduce the bleeding from small vessels. When combined with local anesthetics, such as lidocaine with epinephrine, concentrations of 1:100,000 and 1:200,000 prolong the effect of the anesthetic and provide some hemostasis in highly vascular areas. Use vasoconstrictors only in situations in which widespread small-vessel and capillary hemorrhage in a wound cannot be controlled by direct pressure or cauterization. Hemostasis of a specific vessel may be achieved by directly injecting the soft tissues around the base of the bleeding vessel with a small amount of lidocaine with epinephrine solution, even though the wound has previously been anesthetized. The combination of pressure and vasoconstriction may halt the bleeding long enough for the vessel to be ligated or cauterized, or to allow the wound to be closed and a compression dressing applied.

Fibrin foam, gelatin foam, and microcrystalline collagen may be used as hemostatic agents. Their utility is limited in that vigorous bleeding will wash the agent away from the bleeding site. Their greatest value may be in packing small cavities from which there is constant oozing of blood. Another novel hemostasis technique uses 2-octyl-cyanoacrylate (Dermabond) to achieve hemostasis of skin avulsions on the fingertips, which are known to bleed aggressively. A tourniquet should first be used to minimize bleeding, and moisture should be dabbed away from the wound. Then the Dermabond can be layered on at least twice. This method is an off-label, anecdotal use of this product, and the consequence of exposing dermal skin layers directly to it have not been evaluated to date.[57]

Do not spend excessive time attempting to tie off several small bleeding vessels while the patient slowly exsanguinates (Fig. 34.9). In highly vascular areas such as the scalp, it is sometimes best to suture the laceration after exploration and irrigation of the wound despite active bleeding; the pressure exerted by the closure will usually stop the bleeding. If bleeding is too brisk to permit adequate wound evaluation and irrigation, control hemorrhage by clamping and everting the galea or dermis of each wound edge with hemostats (Fig. 34.10 A–B). Raney clamps or a large hemostat is an excellent way to stop scalp bleeding; they are used during neurosurgical procedures (Fig. 34.10C). If the edge of the entire scalp is compressed the bleeding will generally stop. In most simple wounds with persistent but minor capillary bleeding, apposition of the wound edges with sutures, followed by a compression dressing, provides adequate hemostasis.

Tourniquets

If bleeding from an extremity wound is refractory to direct pressure, electrocauterization, or ligation, or if the patient has exsanguinating hemorrhage from the wound, place a tourniquet proximal to the wound to control the bleeding temporarily. Tourniquets are also helpful in examining extremity lacerations by providing a bloodless field. However, tourniquets can cause injury in three ways:

Hemorrhage Control

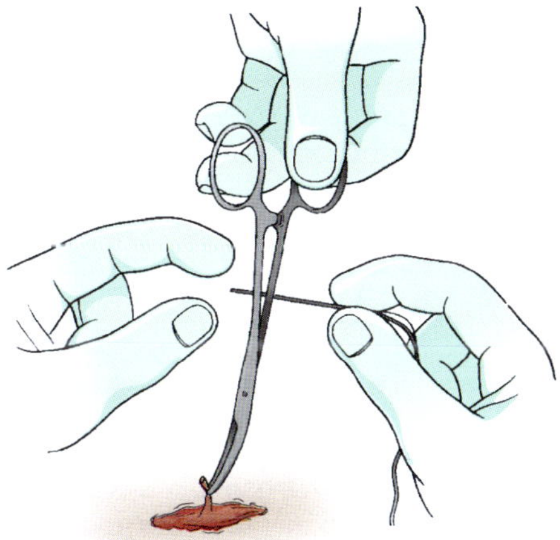

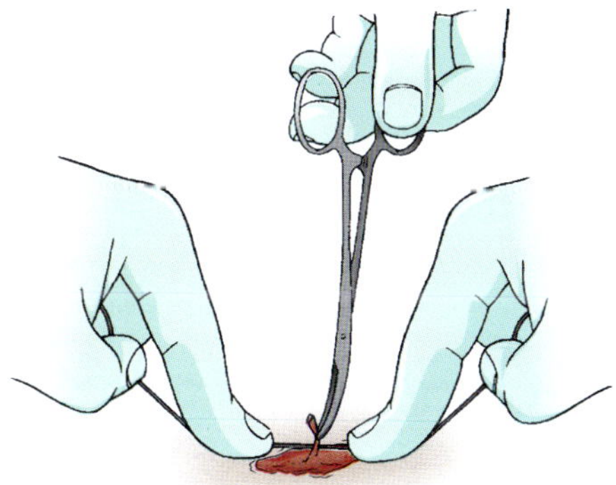

A

When tying off a bleeding vessel, the tip of the hemostat should project beyond the clamped vessel. An assistant raises the handles of the hemostat as a ligature is passed under them.

Stretch the ligature thread between the index fingertips and carry it under the projecting tips of the hemostat.

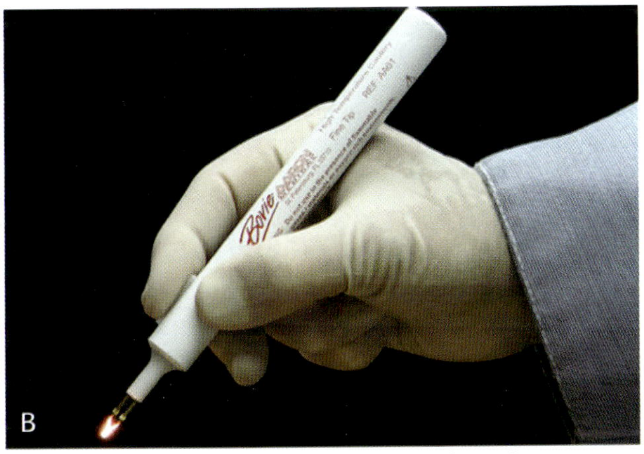

Battery-powered cautery can be used to coagulate minor subcutaneous bleeders.

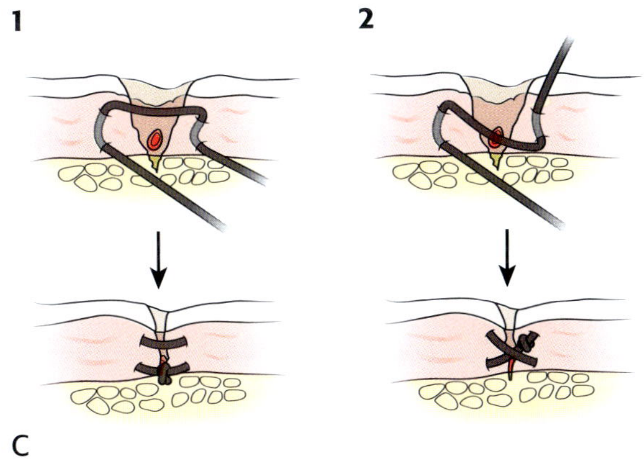

Ligation of a retracted, bleeding vessel. *1*, Horizontal mattress technique. *2*, Figure-of-eight technique.

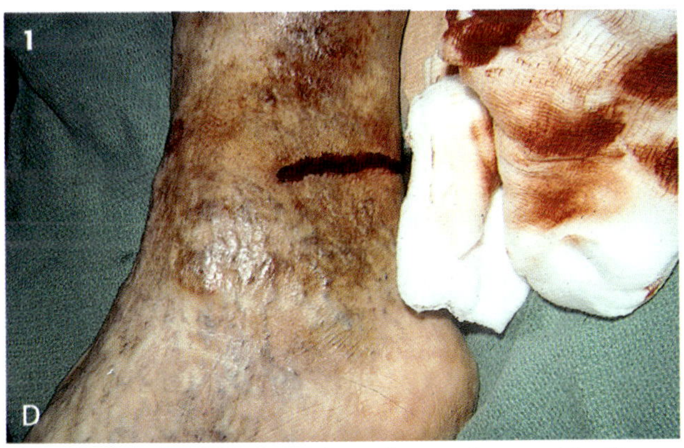

This elderly patient experienced massive spontaneous bleeding from a ruptured varicose vein. Blood loss was substantial and recurrent when she walked.

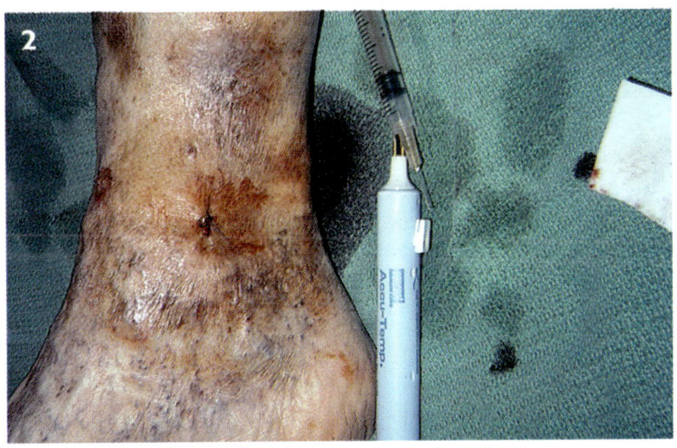

After cautery, a figure-of-eight suture was placed. Simple cautery without suturing is not always effective. A pressure dressing is applied after hemostasis is verified by walking.

Fig. 34.8 Hemorrhage control.

1. They can produce ischemia in the extremity.
2. They can compress and damage underlying blood vessels and nerves.
3. They can jeopardize the survival of marginally viable tissue.

Although problems rarely develop from tourniquets in routine wound care, potential problems can be minimized if (1) a limit is placed on the total amount of time that a tourniquet is applied and (2) excessive tourniquet pressure is avoided. It

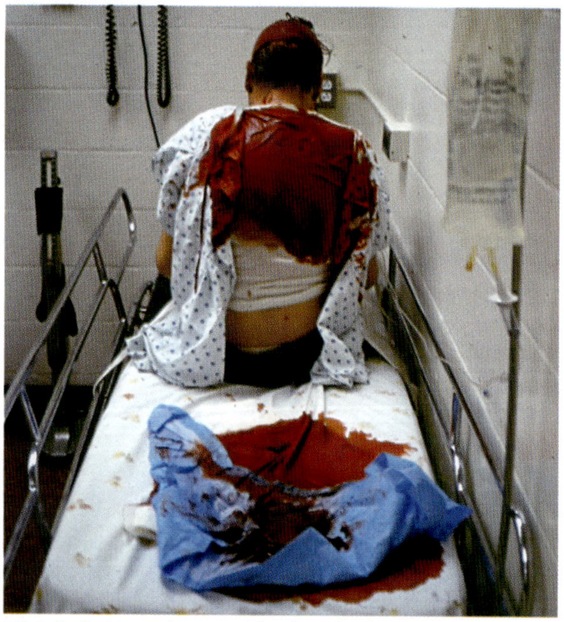

Fig. 34.9 Scalp lacerations can bleed profusely. This patient's pressure dressing fell off while he was on a stretcher in the back hall, and he experienced significant blood loss from a large scalp laceration. His intoxication prevented him from supplying his history of hemophilia.

is also imperative that all tourniquets be removed before discharging the patient. A small tourniquet may be overlooked if a bulky dressing covers it.

A single-cuff tourniquet (sphygmomanometer cuff) placed around an arm or a leg stops most distal venous or arterial bleeding without crushing any underlying structures. The length of time that a tourniquet may remain in place is limited by the development of pain underneath and distal to the tourniquet. This occurs within 15 to 30 minutes in a conscious patient, which is well within the limits of safety.[22]

Before application of the tourniquet, elevate the injured extremity and manually exsanguinate it to prevent persistent venous oozing (Fig. 34.11A). Wrap an elastic bandage (e.g., Ace wrap or Esmarch) circumferentially around the extremity, starting distally and moving in a proximal direction. Place a cuff that is 20% wider than the diameter of the limb around the arm proximal to the wound, inflate it to 250 to 300 mm Hg or 70 mm Hg higher than the patient's systolic blood pressure, and then clamp the tubing. Remove the bandage and lower the extremity. Because tourniquets impair the circulation and may produce neurapraxia, limit their use in the ED to a maximum of 2 hours.[11,23]

Tourniquets on digits have a greater potential for complications. The maximum tourniquet time that is safe for a finger is 30 to 45 minutes.[11] Also, finger tourniquets can exert excessive pressure over a small surface area at the base of the finger and injure digital nerves or cause pressure necrosis of digital vessels. For this reason, standard rubber bands should not be used as tourniquets. Instead, place a 0.5-inch Penrose drain around the finger's base and stretch it to no more than two-thirds of its circumference (Fig. 34.11B). This will provide safe and effective hemostasis. The pressure under a Penrose drain ranges between 100 and 650 mm Hg, but it can easily be controlled.[58] A few millimeters of difference in total stretch greatly affects the pressure applied by this type of tourniquet.[59] In digits, tourniquet pressures of only 150 mm Hg are needed for hemostasis.

A surgical glove placed over a patient's cleaned hand can also serve as a finger tourniquet (Fig. 34.11C). Remove the tip of the glove covering the injured digit, and then roll it proximally along the patient's finger to form a constricting band at the base. Another advantage of this technique is that contamination of the wound during closure is less likely. Rolled surgical gloves produce pressures ranging from 113 to 363 mm Hg, depending on the thickness, the amount of glove finger removed, the number of rolls, and the size of the glove in relation to the size of the patient's hand.[59] Ring-shaped exsanguinating digit tourniquets are available commercially (Tourni-Cot) (Fig. 34.11D). There is a real danger of forgetting to remove such a small tourniquet and unintentionally incorporating it into the dressing.

These techniques provide bloodless fields in which to examine, clean, and close extremity wounds. Debridement of questionably devitalized tissue in a wound is best accomplished without a tourniquet or pharmacologic vasoconstriction because bleeding from tissues is often an indication of their viability.

CLOSURE

The various techniques for wound closure are presented in Chapter 35. The remainder of this chapter addresses issues related to wound management (e.g., secondary closure, wound dressings, use of antibiotics, aftercare instructions, and suture removal).

Open Versus Closed Wound Management

Wounds that heal spontaneously (i.e., by secondary intention) undergo much more inflammation, fibroplasia, and contraction than do those whose edges are reapproximated by wound closure techniques. During wound healing, contraction covers the defect, but it may result in a deformity (contracture) or loss of function. Left to itself, the healing process may be unable to close a defect completely in areas in which the surrounding skin is immobile, such as on the scalp or in the pretibial area (Fig. 34.12). Exposed tendons, bone, nerves, or vessels may desiccate in an open wound. If the patient is careless with an otherwise adequate dressing that covers an open wound, the wound may be further contaminated. Surgical closure of wounds minimizes inflammation, fibroplasia, contracture, scar width, and contamination.

However, surgical closure of wounds can cause complications. Closure of contaminated wounds increases the probability of wound infection, with possible complications of impaired healing, dehiscence, and sepsis. For instance, raised pretibial flap lacerations in elderly patients often necrose when sutured, but survive and heal well by secondary intention if placed back into position with tape or tissue glue. Sutures in themselves are potentially detrimental to healing and can increase the risk for infection. Each suture inflicts a small intradermal incision that damages the surface epithelium, dermis, subcutaneous fat, blood vessels, small nerves, lymphatics, and epithelial appendages such as hair follicles, sweat glands, and ducts. Each suture is another piece of foreign material that can provoke inflammation. When a suture is removed, bacteria that have settled on the exposed portion of the suture are pulled into the suture track and deposited there.

Therefore the clinician must estimate the risk for infection before closure. It may be closed if the wound is judged

Hemorrhage Control of Scalp Lacerations

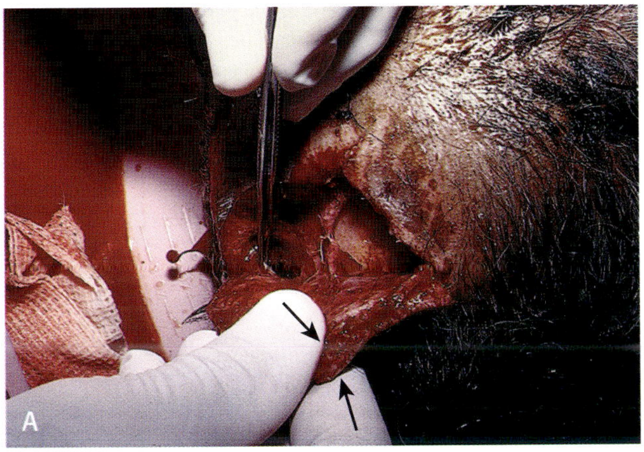

Scalp lacerations may bleed profusely, and arterial vessels may not retract if they are in tough fibrous tissue. This forceps was used to crush a small pumping artery. Placing large (3-0 nylon) sutures that incorporate all scalp layers, defined as all tissue between the thumb and index finger *(arrows)*, is preferred to attempting to cauterize or ligate small bleeders.

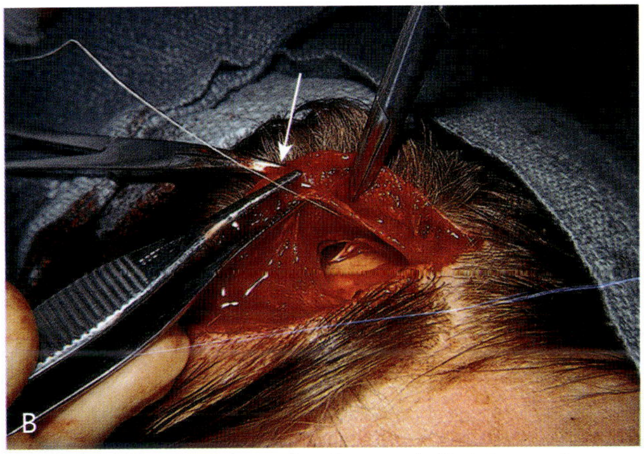

A hemostat placed on the scalp edge can similarly be used on a single bleeder.

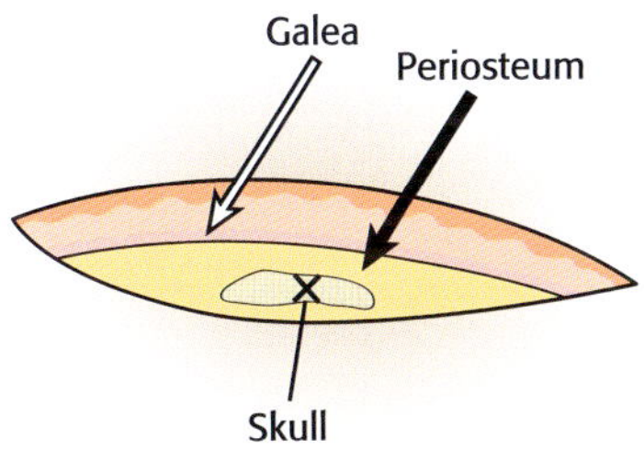

Note that the suture will incorporate all layers of the scalp. Both the galea and the periosteum are identified along with exposed skull *(x)*. The periosteum is not sutured.

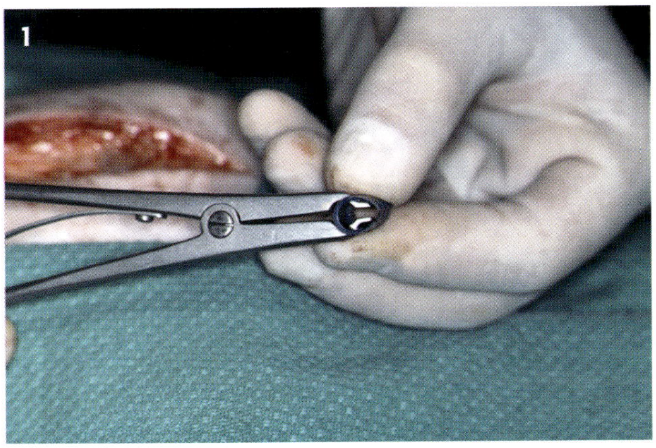

Load the Raney clip onto the applicator.

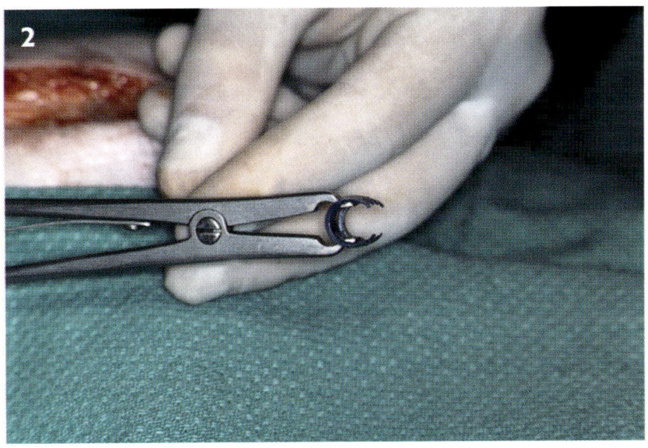

Lock the handles of the applicator to open the clip.

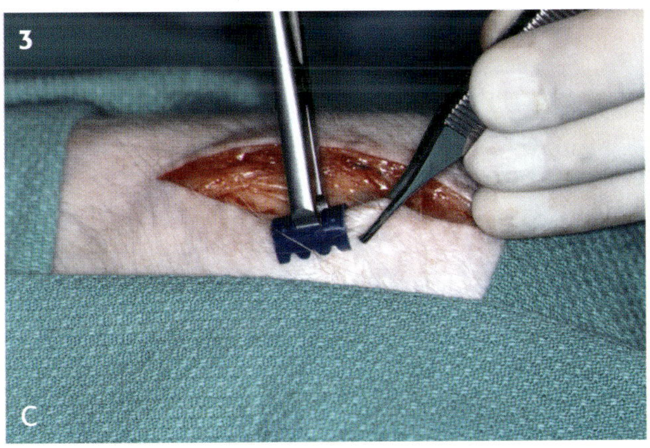

Slide the clip onto the wound edge.

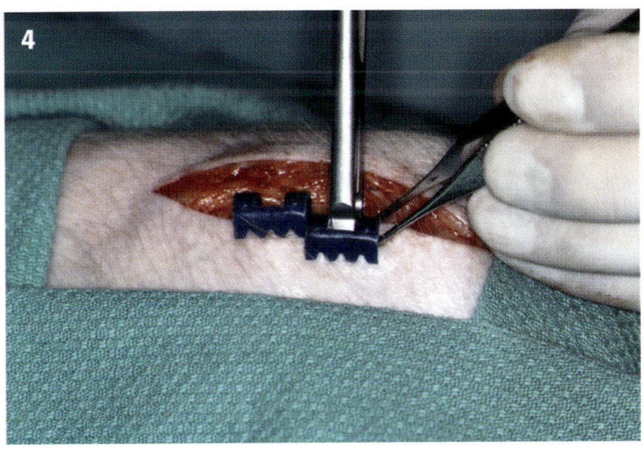

Release the clip by unlocking the applicator.

Fig. 34.10 Hemorrhage control of scalp lacerations. Note that the periosteum is often misidentified as the galea. The galea is adherent to the subcutaneous tissues, not covering the bone. (C, From Custalow CB. *Color Atlas of Emergency Department Procedures.* Saunders; 2005:136-137.)

Hemorrhage Control: Tourniquets

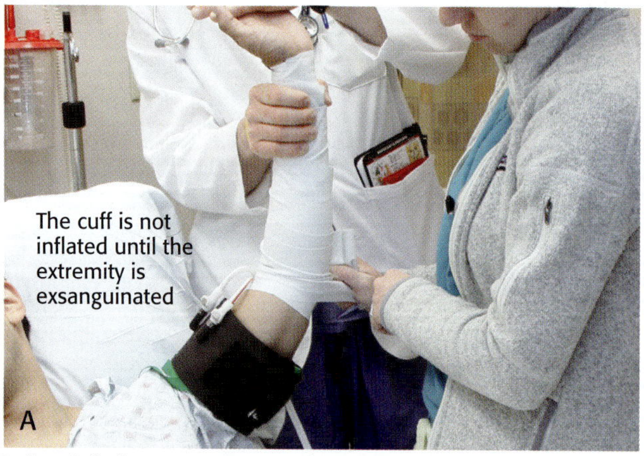

Before inflating a tourniquet such as a blood pressure cuff, wrap an elastic bandage (e.g., Ace wrap or Esmarch) around the extremity in a distal-to-proximal fashion. Inflate the cuff to 250 to 300 mm Hg or 70 mm Hg higher than systolic pressure. (The above photo is only a demonstration; gloves should obviously be worn in the case of a bleeding patient.)

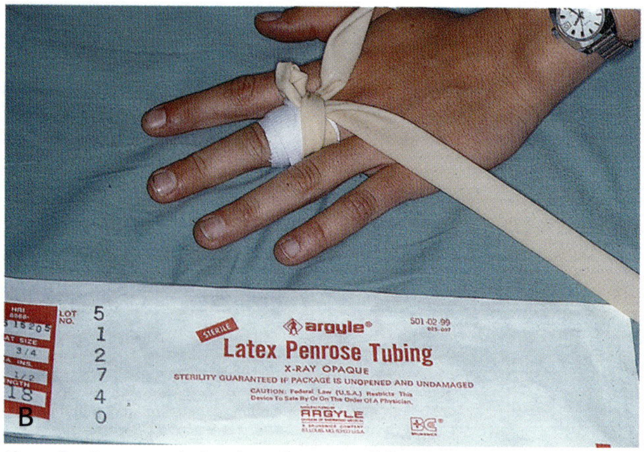

Use of a Penrose drain placed over padding for a finger tourniquet. Do not stretch the drain to more than two thirds of its circumference. This will provide safe and effective hemostasis.

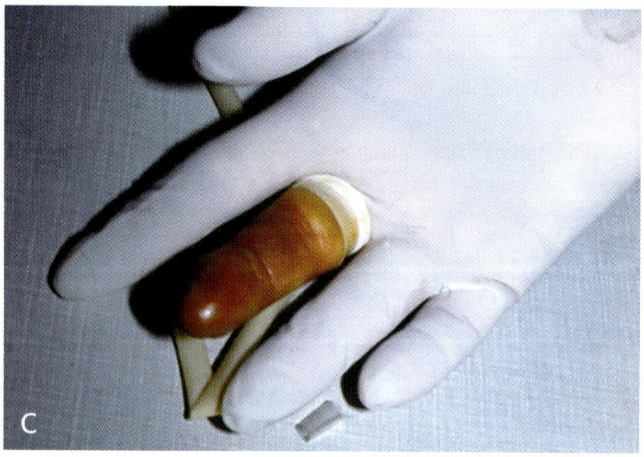

Use of a sterile glove to provide a clean field and serve as a finger tourniquet. The distal end of the glove is clipped, and the glove finger is rolled proximally over the digit. A Penrose drain is also incorporated into this tourniquet.

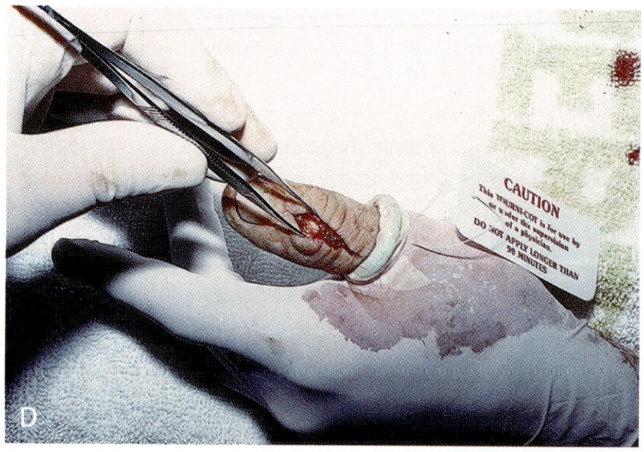

Commercial tourniquet for finger lacerations (Tournicot Mar Med Company). Various sizes are available. The accompanying warning tag has been left exposed to remind the operator of the tourniquet device. Note how the tendon injury can be seen once a bloodless field is obtained.

Fig. 34.11 Hemorrhage control: use of tourniquets.

to be clean or rendered clean by scrubbing, irrigation, and or debridement. If the wound remains contaminated despite the best of efforts, it must be left open to heal by secondary intention. If the wound's status is uncertain, delayed primary closure should be considered.

Delayed Primary or Secondary Closure

There is a common misconception that all wounds must be either sutured within a few hours or left open and relegated to slow healing and an unsightly scar. If there is a substantial risk that the closure of a particular wound might result in infection, the decision to close or to leave the wound open can be postponed. After cleaning, wounds left unsutured appear to have higher resistance to infection than closed wounds. The condition of the wound after 3 to 5 days will then determine the best strategy (Fig. 34.13).

Although cleaning and debridement should be accomplished as rapidly as possible, there is no urgency in closing a wound. Edlich and associates[23] pointed out that "the rationale for delayed primary closure is that the healing open wound will gain resistance to infection and permit an uncomplicated closure." Despite its effectiveness, delayed primary closure is a technique that is seldom used by many clinicians (Fig. 34.14). It is a highly effective means of managing wounds that have significant risk for infection. After 4 to 5 days, a well-irrigated and cleaned wound may be closed primarily with good strength and appearance. Open wound management is usually an outpatient procedure. The technique consists of careful cleaning and debridement, followed by packing of the wound with sterile, saline-moistened, fine-mesh gauze. The packed wound is covered with a thick, absorbent, sterile dressing. Depending on the specifics of the wound and the ability of the patient to perform their own wound care, the packing may be

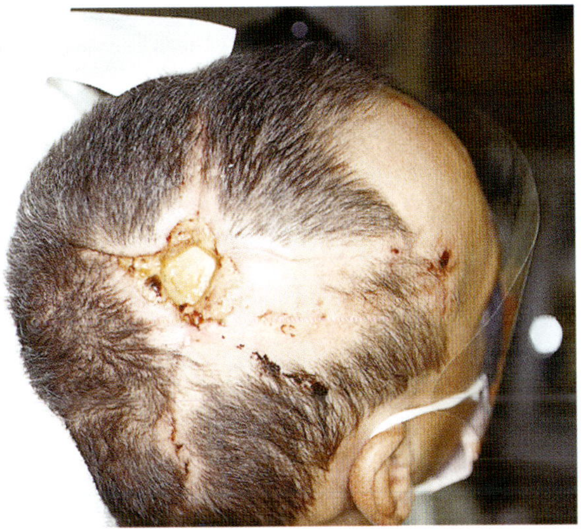

Fig. 34.12 In areas in which the skin is immobile, as in the scalp, wounds left open may not heal.

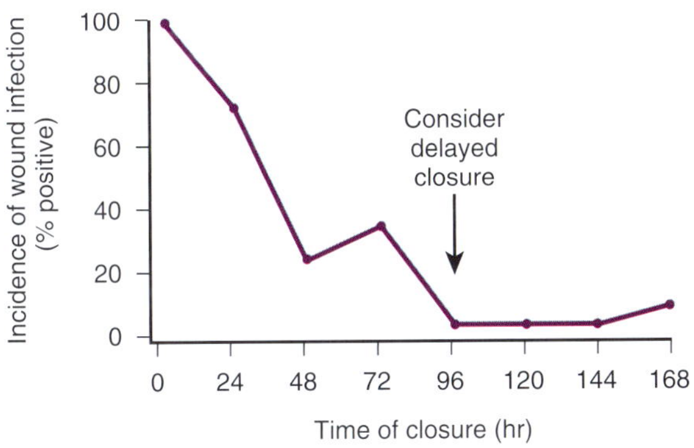

Fig. 34.13 Incidence of wound infection over time when delayed closure is performed. Delayed closure is best accomplished on the fourth or fifth day to minimize the risk for infection. (From Edlich RF, Thacker JG, Rodeheaver GT et al. *A Manual for Wound Closure.* 3M Medical Surgical Products; 1979.)

changed daily at home or in the ED, or it may be left undisturbed for several days. Sterile, saline-soaked packing is standard, and there is no need to instill wounds with antiseptics. Prophylactic antibiotics are occasionally prescribed, but their use is neither mandatory nor of proven benefit. After 48 to 72 hours, the wound is reevaluated for closure. If no evidence of infection is present, the wound margins can be approximated *(delayed primary closure)*, or the wound can be excised and then sutured *(secondary closure)* with minimal risk for infection. Because the wound is closed before the proliferative phase of healing, there is no delay in final healing, and the results are indistinguishable from those of primary healing.

Certain wounds should almost always be managed open or by delayed closure (Fig. 34.15). Such wounds include those that are already infected and those heavily contaminated by soil, organic matter, or feces. Wounds associated with extensive tissue damage, such as high-velocity missile injuries, explosion injuries involving the hand, complex crush injuries, and most bite wounds, are also included in this category. Deep or contaminated lacerations on the bottom of the foot, such as those occurring when the patient steps on an unknown object while wading in a stream or running through a field, or wounds that are deep punctures, are ideal candidates for delayed closure. Some are never sutured but left open for primary healing. Human bite wounds (extending past the dermis) should never be closed primarily, even if they appear clean, and are often opened or extended further for cleaning. Clinicians disagree about which animal bite wounds may be closed initially, and scientific evidence is lacking.[14] Most would suture cosmetically deforming injuries, including facial bites and bite wounds that can be excised completely.[60] Others would primarily suture dog bites not involving an extremity. In severe soft tissue injuries, delayed closure allows time for nonviable tissue to become demarcated from uninjured tissue. Debridement can then be accomplished with maximal preservation of tissue.

PROTECTION

Dressings

After wound repair, wipe away dried blood on the skin's surface with moistened gauze to minimize subsequent itching and cover the wound with a nonadherent dressing. Depending on the specifics of the wound and the type of repair, a dressing can consist of a simple dry gauze pad, a complex multilayer dressing, or an occlusive dressing. Some wounds, such as sutured scalp lacerations, do not routinely require any dressing. Although they are infrequently used on acute, traumatic lacerations managed in the ED, occlusive dressings have been shown to accelerate healing in a variety of wounds.[61] Various specialized (and expensive) synthetic dressings are available, including vapor-permeable adhesive films, hydrogels, hydrocolloids, alginates, synthetic foam dressings, silicone meshes, tissue adhesives, barrier films, and collagen-containing dressings.[62,63]

Function of Dressings

Dressings serve various functions. They protect the wound from contamination and trauma, absorb excess exudate from the wound, immobilize the wound and surrounding area, exert downward pressure on the wound, and improve the patient's comfort. Occlusive dressings on burns or abrasions maintain a moist environment and prevent painful exposure to air and dehydration of the wound's surface.[61,64] Sutured wounds are particularly susceptible to infection from surface contamination during the first 2 days after wound repair. Dressings protect the wound from contamination during this vulnerable period.

One of the primary functions of gauze dressing is to absorb the serosanguineous drainage that exudes from all wounds. Absorbent dressings also reduce the development of stitch abscesses. Surface sutures produce small indentations at their entrance points; tiny blood clots and debris overlie these indentations and allow bacterial growth at the site. Small "stitch abscesses" can develop; they are initially undetectable but are nevertheless destructive to epithelium. Stitch abscesses rarely infect the entire wound but can slightly increase the scar's width and produce noticeable, punctate suture marks.

The most common type of dressing is constructed in three layers: a nonadherent contact layer, an absorbent layer, and an outer wrap (Fig. 34.16A). Ideally this dressing provides nonadherence without maceration. The optimal appearance of an abrasion or an open wound under a dressing is a moist red surface with capillary and epithelial growth.

Delayed Primary Closure

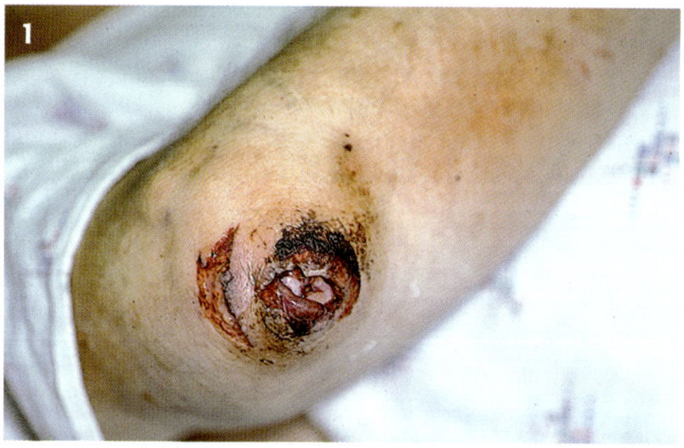

This dirty and contused extremity wound, now 18 hours old, is an ideal candidate for delayed primary closure.

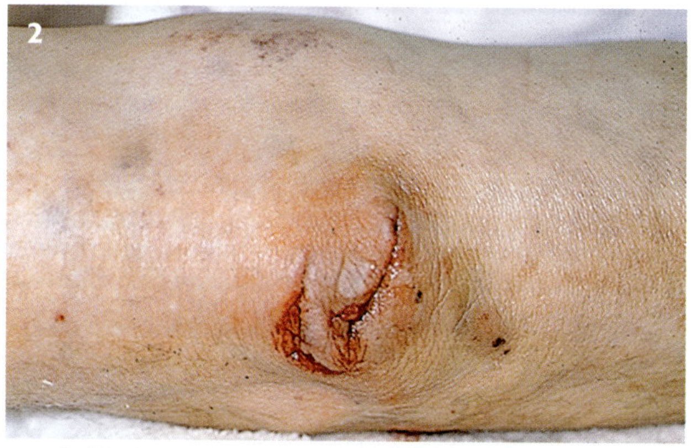

At arrival in the emergency department, the wound is anesthetized, scrubbed, irrigated, and sharply debrided.

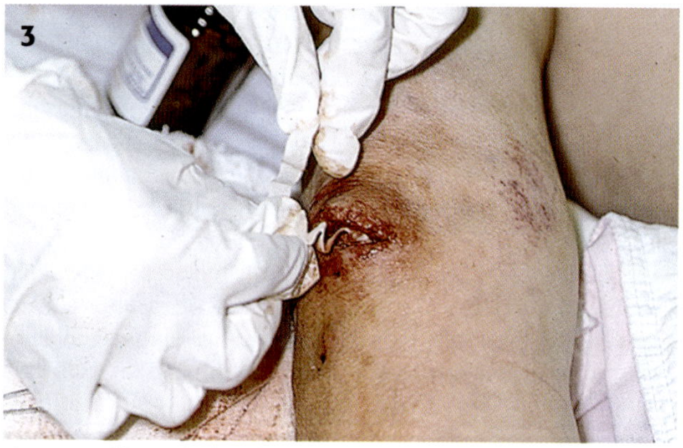

The wound is packed with sterile gauze and covered with a dry dressing. No antibiotics were prescribed and the wound was left undisturbed.

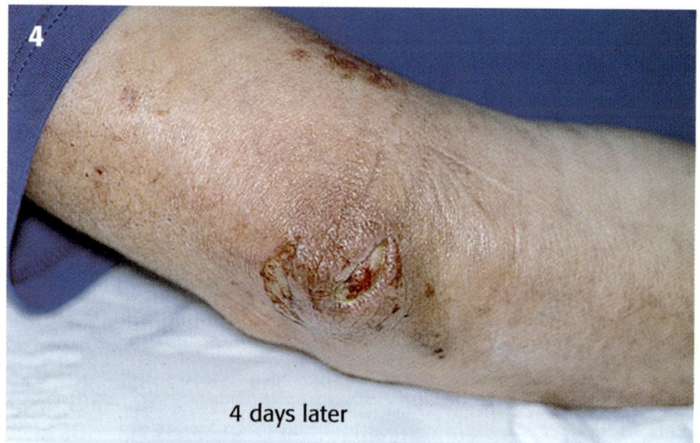

Four days later the packing is removed and the wound is minimally debrided.

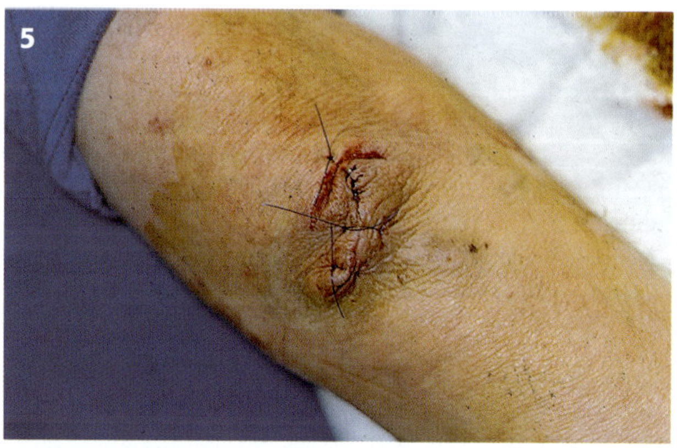

Interrupted sutures are placed as though this is a fresh, clean wound. At suture removal 10 days later, only a linear scar was evident.

Fig. 34.14 Delayed primary closure. Not all wounds must be repaired on the first visit but may be left open to slowly heal. A delayed primary closure in 3 to 4 days is often the best choice for dirty or old lacerations.

Contact Layer: Dry, Semiocclusive, and Occlusive Dressings

Wounds covered with permeable dressings, such as plain gauze, tend to dry out. Although this is acceptable for dressing sutured wounds, drying of the wound surface damages a shallow layer of exposed dermis, which impedes epidermal resurfacing of abrasions, burns, and incisions.[61,62,65] Wound desiccation results in further epidermal necrosis, crust formation, and increased inflammation. Coarse weaves of gauze, regularly available in the form of multilayered pads, absorb blood and exudate, but the dressing will adhere if the interstices of the fabric are relatively large. Capillaries, fibrin, and

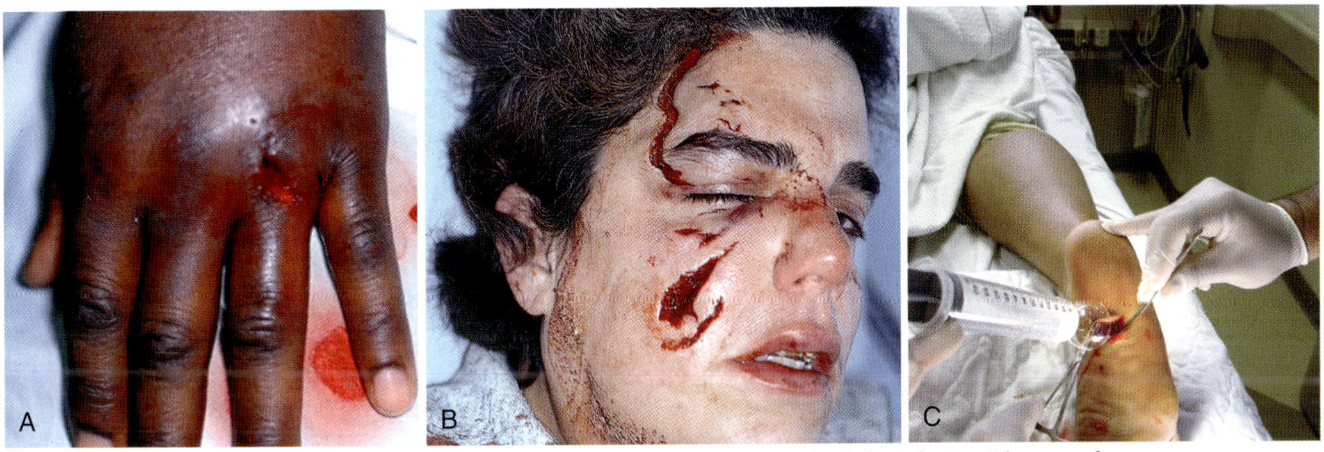

Fig. 34.15 (A) Human bites are never closed primarily because of risk for infection. They are often opened and extended to facilitate cleaning and a search for other injuries or foreign bodies (FBs) such as fragments of teeth. (B) Dog bites in a cosmetic area may be closed primarily. Large cosmetic defects are best closed in the operating room by a surgeon with adequate time to correctly prepare the wound. (C) This wound on the bottom of the foot, sustained by stepping on an unknown object while running in a stream, should not be closed but rather left open to heal primarily. Always check for FBs in these wounds. Ask an assistant to hold the wound open while you perform pressure irrigation. This was initially a much smaller puncture wound extended to search for a suspected FB and to clean and pack the wound open. Sutures were never required, and the wound healed in 7 days.

granulation tissue will penetrate and become enmeshed in the material. If the proteinaceous exudate from the wound dries by evaporation, the scab usually clings to the dressing. Some clinicians use this effect to "debride" the wound when the gauze is removed. However, it may also destroy healing tissue, particularly the new epithelium. Even though debridement of the wound with wet-to-dry dressings is quick, careful debridement with surgical instruments is more controlled and less traumatic.

Adherence to the wound can be prevented if the dressing is nonabsorbent, occlusive, or finely woven. If the wound is kept moist by covering it with an occlusive film or nonadherent covering soon after wound management, and if the film is left in place for at least 48 hours, the epidermis will migrate over the surface of the dermis faster than when a dry scab is allowed to form.[62] Protection of wounds that are healing by secondary intention with occlusive or semiocclusive dressings has several advantages[9] including more rapid healing, less pain from exposure to air, better cosmetic result, fewer dressing changes, and protection from bacteria. Occlusive dressings make good temporary coverings for wounds requiring delayed closure several days after injury.[61]

Petrolatum gauze (e.g., Adaptic, Kendall, Xeroform, Betadine) is commonly applied next to the surface of the wound to prevent the wound from sticking to the dry gauze in the absorbent layer and to protect the regenerating epithelium (Box 34.1). Always use nonadherent material to cover skin grafts. Some clinicians use fine-mesh gauze (41 to 47 warp threads/inch^2) rather than petrolatum gauze on abrasions, especially on wounds that are heavily contaminated because removal of this type of dressing debrides only the small tufts of granulation tissue that become fixed in the mesh pores and leaves a clean, even surface. Once a healthy, granulating surface is present and reepithelialization is proceeding, nonporous dressings can be used. Fine-mesh gauze is also used next to exposed tissue in wounds being considered for delayed primary closure. Though petrolatum gauze is beneficial for nonadherence of subsequent dressings to wounds, studies have shown that the petroleum may decrease the tensile strength of the knots in a suture.[66]

There are over a thousand types of occlusive dressings available today.[61] Occlusive dressings are ideal for covering abrasions[64] and burns, but they are also used on lacerations and chronic wounds. Some experts report that they should be avoided if a wound is highly exudative, infected, or at high risk for infection.

There are four main types of occlusive dressings designed for the surfaces of wounds: films, hydrocolloids, foams, and hydrogels (Table 34.2).[61] *Films* are transparent polyurethane-derived membranes that provide an occlusive effect; they include Omniderm (Omikron Scientific, Ltd.), OpSite (Smith &Nephew, Ltd.), Tegaderm (3M), and Bioclusive (Systagenix). They are best for wounds with minimal drainage and those that require frequent monitoring. *Hydrocolloids* are semiocclusive, waterproof dressings with soluble cellulose or gelatin backing, such as DuoDERM (ConvaTec) and Tegasorb (3M). They can be used in wounds with a moderate amount of exudate. *Hydrogels* are products with starch polymers and water, such as Curagel (Kendall) and Telfa (Covidien). Because they provide moisture to wounds, they are suitable for dry or painful wounds. *Foams* are moderately absorbent polyurethane or silicone products that are semiocclusive and provide a cushion effect.[61,62] *Silicon* dressings such as Mepitel (Mölnlycke Health Care) can be used to treat fragile wounds, like skin tears.[67]

One fear of using occlusive dressings is that microorganisms will proliferate in the moist environment beneath the occlusive film and increase wound infection rates. However, occlusive dressings such as DuoDERM serve more as a barrier to external pathogenic bacteria.[62] Although skin bacteria under occlusive dressings can multiply, even chronic wounds contaminated with large numbers of bacteria are routinely treated with occlusive dressings successfully.[61]

Adhesive-backed dressings (e.g., DuoDERM and OpSite) may adhere to an open wound and remove new epidermis; however, the adhesive usually only adheres to dry intact skin, which is located around the wound.[61] These film dressings

Wound Dressing

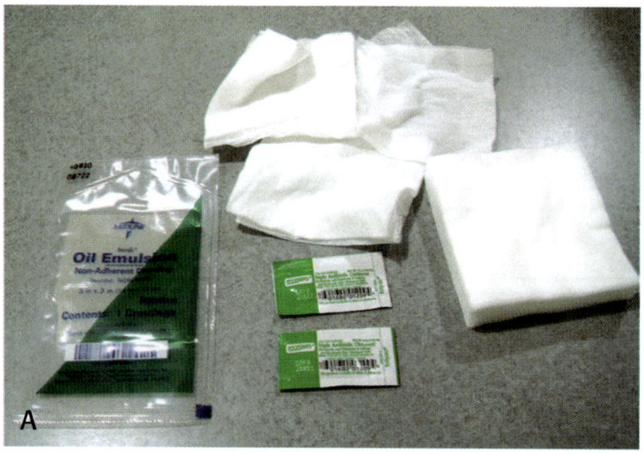

A common three-layer dressing consisting of antibiotic ointment, Adaptic, and gauze.

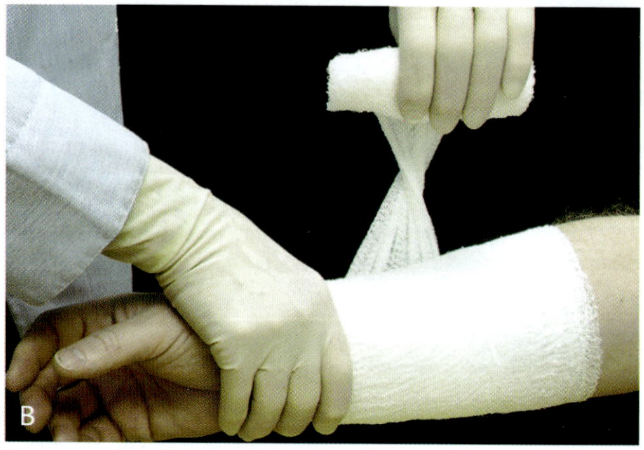

Snugness of the bandage is increased by 180-degree rotation of the bandage roll after each circular turn to create a reverse spiral.

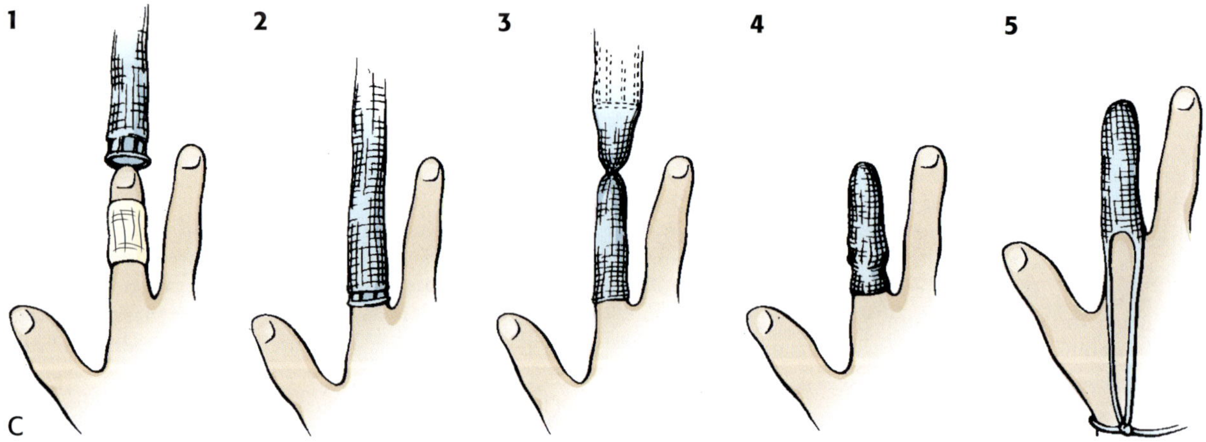

Tube gauze finger dressing applied loosely. Throbbing pain under this dressing mandates removal. *1*, The inner layer is nonadherent gauze. The middle layer is 2- × 2-inch gauze sponges wrapped circumferentially and held in place with tape. *2*, Begin with No. 2 tube gauze at the base of the finger. Hold this end with one finger while the tube gauze applicator is pulled toward the fingertip. A twisting motion firms the wrap about the digit; about 90 degrees is necessary. Excessive stretch or twisting can compromise the circulation. *3*, When the fingertip is reached, make a 360-degree twist, but avoid placing a constricting twist around the finger itself. *4*, Pass the applicator toward the base of the finger with an additional 90-degree twist. Repeat once more; thus, three layers are in place. *5*, Cut enough gauze to reach the base of the finger, and tape it there. As an alternative, pull the final layer beyond the tip while leaving it long enough to reach to and around the wrist (about three times the finger length). Split this gauze into two strands; bring them dorsally to the wrist, knot, and loosely wrap around the wrist.

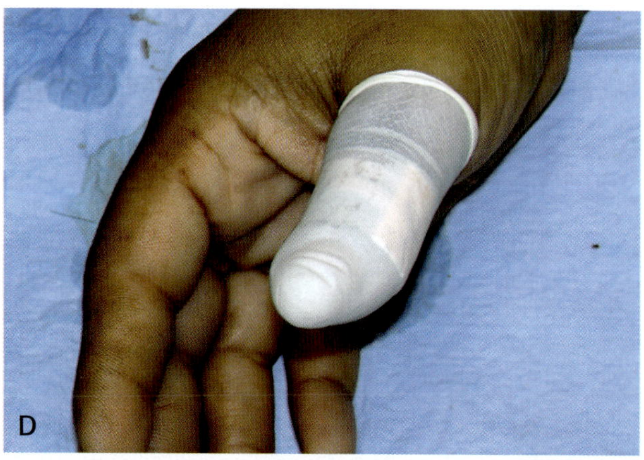

For a distal finger dressing, covering the gauze with a finger cut from a clean glove provides protection from dirt and wetness.

Fig. 34.16 Wound dressings.

have low absorptive capabilities and do not allow exudate to drain out the edges of the dressing. Exudate pooling overlying the wound will macerate skin. Between dressing changes, coat the wound with petrolatum or an antibiotic ointment before applying these products.[9] Wounds covered with certain occlusive dressings or with silver sulfadiazine (Silvadene, Marion Laboratories) appear to be blanketed with pus; this exudate represents the beneficial proliferation of macrophages and polymorphonuclear leukocytes.[68]

BOX 34.1 Advantages of Occlusive Dressings

- More rapid healing
- Less pain from exposure to air
- Better cosmetic results
- Fewer dressing changes
- Better protection from bacteria

Data from Eaglstein WH. Effect of occlusive dressings on wound healing. Clin Dermatol. *1984;2:107.*

Absorbent Layer

When dressing wounds with considerable drainage, use sufficient gauze to cover the wound and absorb all the drainage. Change the dressing whenever it becomes soiled, wet, or saturated with exudate. Once a dressing becomes moist, pathogens can pass through the mesh-like structure to the underlying wound. Consequently, a dressing that is used to absorb exudate or debride the wound must be changed more frequently

TABLE 34.2 Summary of Dressings Used for Acute Wound Care

AGENT AND TYPE	PROPERTIES	ADVANTAGES	DISADVANTAGES	CLINICAL APPLICATIONS	EXAMPLES
Gauze	Cotton or synthetic; woven; plain or petrolatum-impregnated gauze	Cost-effective	Poor absorbance; dehydrates the wound; impedes wound reepithelialization; adherence causes pain with dressing changes	Primary dressing; must be changed every 12–24 h	Curity Xeroform
Film	Transparent; self-adhesive; waterproof, but gas and water vapor permeable; flexible	Transparency allows for frequent wound inspection; adhesive does not stick to wound and thus low pain with dressing changes	Not absorbent; trapped excess exudate can cause wound maceration	Primary or secondary dressing; best for wounds with low exudate; ideal for flexible areas such as hands and joints; can be changed every 7 days	Tegaderm Transeal Bioclusive Omniderm
Foam	Polyurethane or silicone center and semiocclusive outer layer; adherent or nonadherent	Moderate absorption; cushions wounds	As wound exudate decreases, can dehydrate the wound; nonadherent foam may require a film covering	Good for wounds with high exudate; ideal over bony areas; can be changed from daily to weekly	Optifoam Mepilex
Hydrogel	Water-based gel; sheet or amorphous form	Donates moisture; reduces wound pain	Nonadherent and requires a secondary dressing	Good for dry wounds or with low exudate; changed every 1–3 days	Curagel Tegagel
Hydrocolloid	Adhesive semiocclusive waterproof	Moderate absorption; conforms to wound	Discharge can be malodorous and appears purulence-like	Changed every week	DuoDERM NuDerm
Silicon	Porous, soft silicon; nonadherent	Reduces wound pain	Expensive	Good for fragile wounds, like skin tears; changed every week	Mepitel

than one designed solely to occlude. Absorbent dressings on draining wounds can be changed daily to avoid bacterial overgrowth beneath the dressing.[61] Aspirate fluid accumulating under an occlusive dressing and change the dressing every 1 to 2 days during the first week, or until the exudate no longer accumulates.

Outer Layer

Bleeding may persist despite attempts to provide good hemostasis. Compressive dressings help prevent hematoma formation and eliminate dead space within a wound. They are particularly useful for extensively undermined wounds and facial wounds in which subcutaneous capillary bleeding and swelling can exert tension on fine skin sutures and jeopardize skin closure. Pressure dressings should be used to immobilize skin grafts. Surgical tape can serve as a pressure dressing in areas where bandages cannot be applied easily, such as fingertips.

Apply pressure dressings to all ear lacerations to prevent hematoma formation and subsequent deformation and destruction of cartilage. Envelop the ear in the dressing to distribute pressure from the outer bandage evenly across the irregular surface of the pinna. Pack moistened cotton into the concavities of the pinna until the cotton is level with the most lateral aspect of the helical rim. Cut square pieces of gauze to fit the curvature of the ear and place them behind (medial to) the pinna. Place several more gauze squares on the lateral surface of the ear. Secure the packing in place with a circumferential head bandage, but do not encompass the opposite ear because it would just as easily cause pressure necrosis of that ear if left unprotected.

Bandage traumatic wounds to compress, immobilize, secure, and protect the wound and underlying dressing. Most bandaging is performed on extremities, where dressings are difficult to secure with tape alone. Rolls of cotton (e.g., Kerlix, Kling) are well suited for this purpose. Wind the bandage around the extremity and advance it proximally with circular, overlapping turns. Take care to avoid making wrinkles in the bandage, which may create pressure points, and be careful not to make loose turns, which shorten the effective life of the dressing. When joint surfaces are crossed, anchor the cotton distally with several turns, then unroll it obliquely across the joint several times in a figure-of-eight pattern, and anchor it again proximally with two complete turns. Repeat this process until the bandage is securely in place. Fasten the ends of the bandage to the skin with strips of adhesive tape.

Bandages over the forearm and the lower extremities are particularly prone to slippage because of the constant motion of these parts and the marked changes in the diameter of the extremity over a short distance. To help prevent this problem, rotate the roll of the bandage 180 degrees after each circular turn to produce a reverse spiral and reduce the bandage's mobility (Fig. 34.16B). A simple dressing for a single digit uses tube gauze or covers it with a finger cut from a surgical glove (Fig. 34.16C–D). When bandaging digits, be cautious not to create a band-like dressing that can slip down the finger and cause constriction and ischemia.[69] This can be especially problematic in children.[70] Always include the hand and wrist in the dressing to create an anchor point and reduce circumferential bunching.

Certain chemically treated wide-mesh weaves have the properties of cling and stretch, which hold them snugly in place but expand if edema develops. An elastic cotton roll (Kerlix) allows the bandage to conform to body contours, provides some mobility to bandaged joints, and permits the wound to swell without the circumferential bandage constricting the extremity. An inelastic Kling bandage better immobilizes the part. Use rigid immobilization with plaster splints or braces to protect wounds in mobile areas, such as around large joints.

Scalp wounds do well when left uncovered; bulky occlusive dressings of the scalp are discouraged. Encourage the patient to shower daily to remove debris from a sutured scalp laceration. If a dressing is thought necessary, hold it in place with a bandage. Change the outer layer of the dressing when it becomes externally contaminated, saturated with exudate, or when inspection and wound cleaning are required.

Dressings vary in their absorbency, adhesiveness, occlusiveness, opacity, and insulating properties. Further research may identify types of dressings that are best suited for different phases of the healing wound. Currently a two- or three-layer dressing is used for most traumatic wounds. Base the choice of material for the contact layer on the characteristics of the individual wound (see Table 34.2).

Splinting and Elevation

Wounds and sutured lacerations may be immobilized to enhance healing and to provide patient comfort (Fig. 34.17). Immobilization of an injured extremity promotes healing by protecting the closure and by limiting the spread of contamination and infection along lymphatic channels. Wounds overlying joints are subjected to repeated stretching and movement, which delays healing, widens the scar, and potentially disrupts the sutures. Short-term splints are beneficial for lacerations that overlie joints and are frequently necessary for the protection of wounds involving the fingers, hands, wrists, volar aspect of the forearms, extensor surface of the elbows, posterior aspect of the legs, plantar surface of the feet, and the extremities when skin grafts have been applied. A plaster or aluminum splint may be incorporated into a bandage to reduce the mobility of the injured part.

Elevate injured extremities in all but the most trivial injuries. Elevation limits edema formation, allows more rapid healing, and reduces throbbing pain. Patients given this information are often more motivated to elevate the extremity as instructed. Use slings to elevate wounds involving the forearm or the hand. The patient can also wrap a pillow around an injured hand to promote elevation at home (Fig. 34.17A). Another technique to suggest is to lie down on a sofa with the injured extremity resting on the back of the sofa. With severe injuries, begin elevation in the ED (Fig. 34.17B).

Ointments

The safety and efficacy of topical antibiotic preparations used on wound surfaces are unproven, and no universal standard exists. Many clinicians routinely suggest using antibiotic ointments over sutured wounds, whereas others opt for a simple dry dressing. Use of a triple-antibiotic preparation containing neomycin, bacitracin, and polymyxin (Neosporin) provides a broad spectrum of protection against infection in abrasions without systemic absorption, toxicity, or the emergence of resistant strains of bacteria. There is some evidence that Neosporin ointment, Silvadene cream, and mupirocin (Bactroban), in addition to their inert bases and vehicles, either improve wound healing or slightly reduce infection rates.[71]

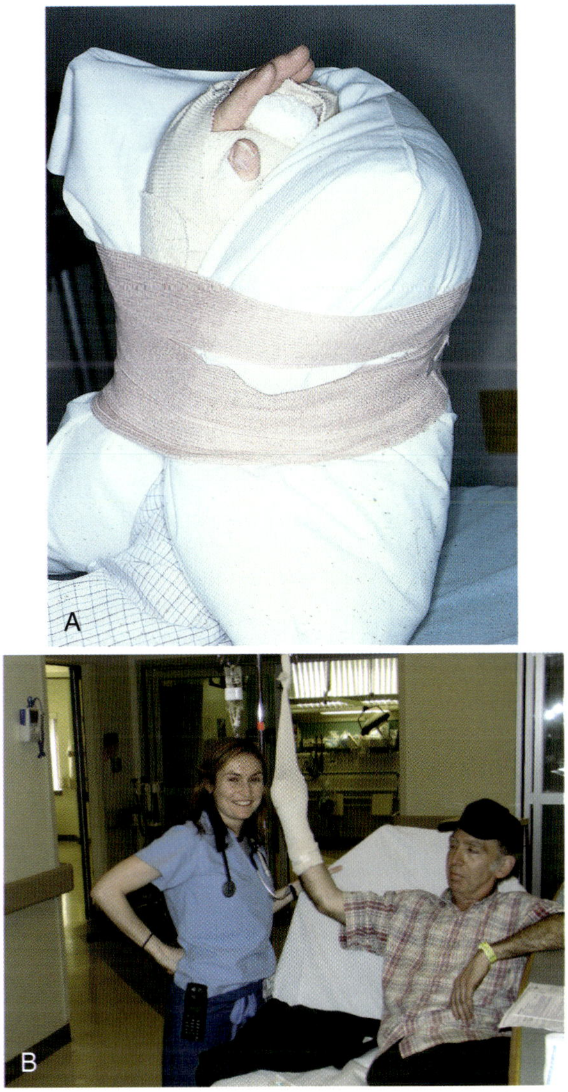

Fig. 34.17 (A) A pillow wrapped around a bandaged hand promotes elevation at home. Note that this sutured hand laceration also has a plaster splint for comfort. In general, immobilization promotes healing. (B) Elevation of a severe hand injury in the emergency department with a stockinette, splint, and intravenous pole while awaiting the surgeon.

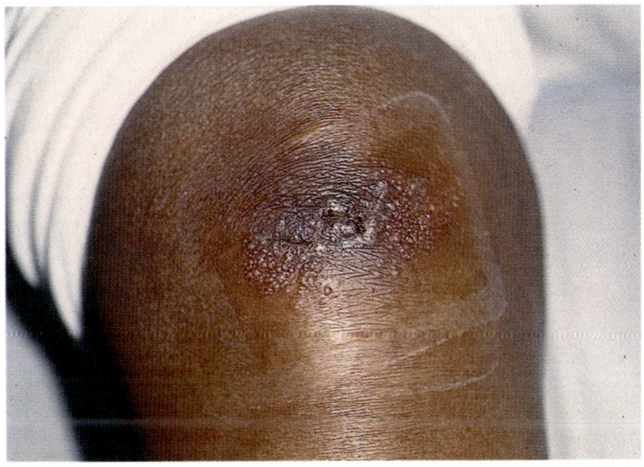

Fig. 34.18 This patient used a neomycin-containing ointment on a minor wound, and redness, swelling, pruritus, and skin changes developed. The patient thought that it was an infection, but it was contact dermatitis from the neomycin. Plain bacitracin ointment will not cause this relatively common reaction. Bacitracin and Silvadene are alternative topicals, but any topical preparation is probably of minimal value.

In comparing mupirocin and nitrofurazone ointment, mupirocin has higher antibacterial capabilities against *Streptococcus* and *Staphylococcus* species in crush wounds, but topical nitrofurazone can increase the proliferation of granulation tissue.[72] Although there is a risk for allergic sensitization or contact dermatitis with preparations containing neomycin, allergic reactions are uncommon (roughly 1%)[73] unless the ointment is used repeatedly (Fig. 34.18).

One obvious benefit of using topical antibiotics is that ointments prevent the wound surface from adhering to the dressing. Use ointments to reduce a crust that covers and separates the wound's edges. Lacerations surrounded by abraded skin are especially predisposed to coagulum formation. In such cases, instruct the patient to cleanse the wound frequently and to follow the cleansing with an application of ointment during the first few days.

Strong topical corticosteroids have detrimental effects on healing. Application of 0.1% triamcinolone acetonide in an ointment slows healing in wounds by as much as 60%, whereas hydrocortisone probably does not interfere with epithelialization.[74] Some clinicians believe that single and low doses of oral corticosteroids probably have no effect on wound healing but that repeated, large doses of steroids (≤40 mg of prednisone per day) inhibit healing, particularly if used before the injury or during the first 3 days of the healing phase.[75] There is some evidence that topical vitamin A may reverse some of the antiinflammatory and immunosuppressive effects of corticosteroids.[76]

The exact value of ointments in lacerations treatment is unknown. However, routine use of ointments after wound cleaning encourages patients to inspect the wound. Ointments without antibiotics used solely for moisture to the wound have a higher infection rate and should not be used.[77] Antibiotic ointments can be placed over abrasions or sutured lacerations. Do not use ointments on wounds closed with tissue adhesive because the ointment will dissolve the adhesive.

Wound Cultures

Tissue taken for culture at the time of wound preparation and closure in the ED serves no useful purpose and is not recommended. The results of such cultures cannot logically guide future antibiotic selection. It is not necessary to routinely culture all minimally infected wounds after closure. Cultures should be considered if there is a subsequent infection that is extensive, unusual, or otherwise concerning, if the patient is immunocompromised, or if there is suspicion of methicillin-resistant *Staphylococcus aureus* (MRSA). All wounds grossly infected at follow-up should also be assessed for a foreign body.

It is common to encounter a minor infection or inflammation of the suture tracks at the time of suture removal, as evidenced by a small drop of pus when the suture is removed. Such minor infections, so-called stitch abscesses, usually do well with warm soaks or topical antibiotic ointments and do not require wound cultures or systemic antibiotics.

Systemic Antibiotics

Most traumatic soft tissue injuries sustain a low level of bacterial contamination. Uncomplicated wound infection rates in ED patients range from 2% to 5%, *regardless of clinician intervention*. In several clinical studies of relatively uncontaminated and uncomplicated traumatic nonbite wounds (which represent the majority of wounds managed in the ED), prophylactic antibiotics administered in various routes and regimens did not reduce the incidence of infection.[78] Studies of antibiotic prophylaxis for animal bite wounds have produced variable results, and no large study providing stratification of the many prognostic factors has been conducted.[79]

As multiple studies on prophylactic antibiotic regimens for wounds treated in the ED have failed to demonstrate a benefit, there is no clear practice standard.[80] In most soft tissue wounds in which the level of bacterial contamination after cleaning and debridement is low, antibiotics are not recommended. Heavily contaminated wounds (such as wounds in contact with saliva, pus, or feces) often become infected despite antibiotic treatment. Nevertheless, antibiotics may have marginal benefit when the level of contamination is overwhelming, or if the amount of questionably viable tissue left in the wound is considerable (e.g., with crush wounds). Antibiotics may be considered for extremity bite wounds, puncture-type bite wounds in any location, intraoral lacerations that are sutured, orocutaneous lip wounds, wounds that cannot be cleaned or debrided satisfactorily, and highly contaminated wounds (e.g., those contaminated with soil, organic matter, purulence, feces, saliva, or vaginal secretions). They may also be considered for wounds involving tendons, bones, or joints; for wounds requiring extensive debridement in the operating room; for wounds in lymphedematous tissue; for distal extremity wounds when treatment is delayed for 12 to 24 hours; for patients with orthopedic prostheses; and patients at risk for the development of infective endocarditis.[11,81]

Although some consider prescribing prophylactic antibiotics for immunocompromised patients (diabetics and others), a true benefit has not consistently been demonstrated in any subset. Many resistant strains of bacteria now encountered in clinical practice (patients and in the community) have been linked to the excessive use of needless antibiotics. Other disadvantages of routine antibiotic use include unnecessary expense and potential side effects (e.g., rash, anaphylaxis, diarrhea, vomiting). It seems most prudent to avoid routine antibiotic prophylaxis and opt for meticulous wound care, close follow-up, and the selective use of antibiotics for proven infection. If antibiotics are being considered in a specific case, give them as soon as possible after wounding and continue them for only 2 to 3 days in the absence of development of an infection. If the risk for infection is high enough to warrant antibiotics, delayed primary closure may also be considered.

Many patients have difficulty determining whether their wounds are infected and mistake the normal healing process for infection; therefore follow-up is usually necessary in high-risk patients.[82,83]

The choice of antibiotic, particularly for bite wound prophylaxis, is as controversial as the indications for use.[84] Many species of bacteria cause animal bite wound infections, thus making complete coverage impossible.[81,85] Antibiotic regimens vary with the species of the biter and with evolving bacterial resistance. The duration of antibiotic prophylaxis is also in question. It is customary practice to provide antibiotics for 72 hours. (See additional comments on animal bites at the end of this chapter.)

Tetanus Immunoprophylaxis

Although tetanus is rare, it still occurs in the United States and is a preventable disease. Therefore any wound should be assessed for its potential to cause tetanus, and prophylaxis should be considered in the ED. Approximately 70% of Americans older than 6 years have protective levels of tetanus antibodies, but levels decline as age increases, with elderly females having the lowest levels of protection. New immigrants are most likely to have inadequate immunity. Hence, efforts at preventing tetanus should especially be addressed in immigrants and the elderly. The recommendations of the Centers for Disease Control and Prevention for tetanus prophylaxis are listed in Fig. 34.19 and Table 34.3.[86]

When questioning patients about their tetanus immunization status, determine if they ever completed the primary immunization series, and if not, how many doses were given. Patients who have not completed a full primary series of injections (three or four doses) may require both tetanus toxoid and passive immunization with tetanus immune globulin. Tetanus immune globulin will decrease, but not eliminate, the subsequent development of clinical tetanus. Tetanus and diphtheria immunizations are often given together (as DT or DTaP for pediatrics, and Td or Tdap for adults). The preferred active tetanus immunization in patients 7 years of age and older is Tdap or Td. For passive immunity, prepare 500 units of tetanus immune globulin. Give most of this dose intramuscularly and infiltrate the remainder around the wound.[86]

Mild local reactions consisting of erythema and induration are common (≈20%) after tetanus toxoid injections; occasionally, they are accompanied by fever and mild systemic symptoms. Reactions are approximately twice as common if diphtheria immunization is coupled with tetanus immunization. This hypersensitivity reaction, not an infection, does not represent an absolute contraindication to further immunizations. A minor febrile illness, such as an upper respiratory infection, is not a reason to delay immunization. Although serious reactions are rare, a hypersensitivity reaction consisting of tenderness, erythema, and swelling or serum sickness develops in some patients with high antibody levels. Generalized urticarial rashes and anaphylaxis are the severe reactions associated with the tetanus vaccine. Although peripheral neuropathy and Guillain-Barré syndrome have also been reported, there is inadequate evidence to accept or reject a causal relationship.[86] The only absolute contraindication to tetanus toxoid is a history of anaphylaxis or a neurologic event. In such cases, tetanus immune globulin can be given safely. Pregnancy is not a contraindication to either toxoid or immune globulin, although some suggest that the toxoid be used "with caution" during the first trimester. Given the excellent amnestic response to the toxoid, it is likely that the primary immunization series, coupled with intermittent boosters every 5 to 10 years, depending on the cleanliness of the wound, conveys immunity for most of one's life. However, a significant percentage of elderly patients do not develop protective antitoxin antibody titers after 14 days when given tetanus toxoid boosters.

Treatment decisions are based on the differentiation between clean and contaminated wounds. Even though any break in the skin can harbor *Clostridium tetani*, traditional definitions of tetanus-prone wounds include the following: injuries more than 6 hours old; wounds contaminated by

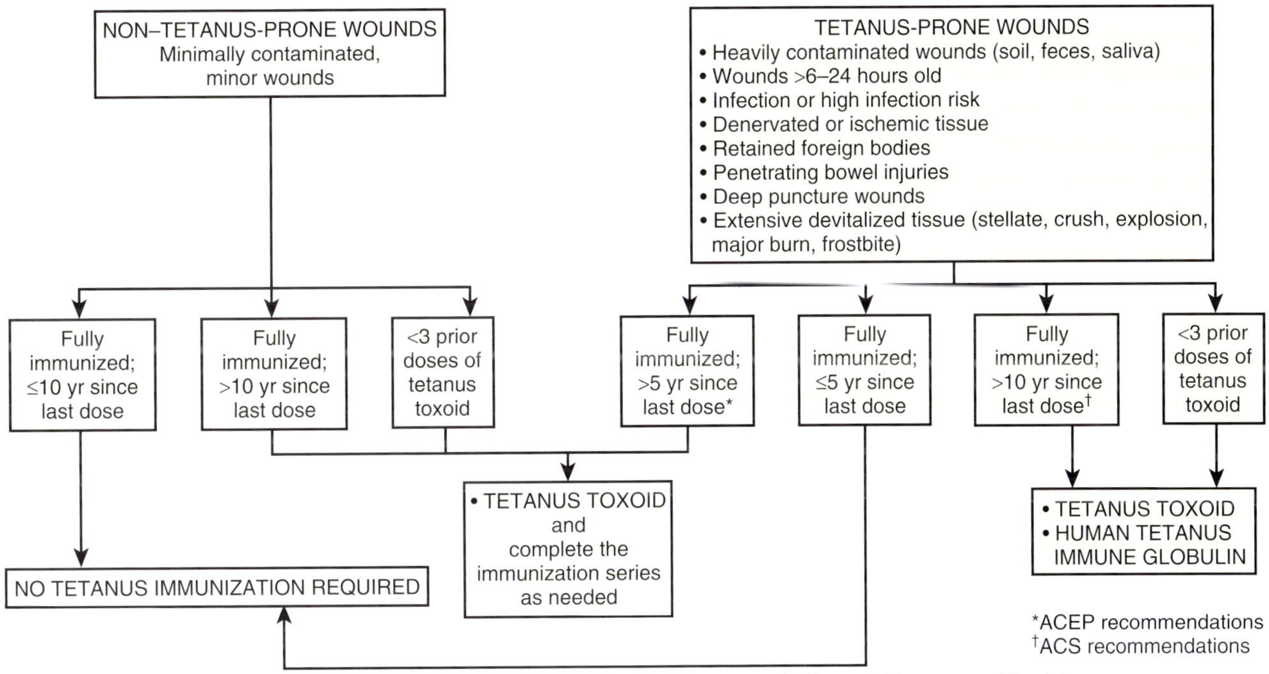

Fig. 34.19 Tetanus immunization guidelines. *ACEP*, American College of Emergency Physicians; *ACS*, American College of Surgeons.

TABLE 34.3 Summary of Tetanus Vaccine Recommendations

	Clean, Minor Wounds		All Other Wounds	
VACCINE HISTORY	TDAP OR TD	TIG	TDAP OR TD	TIG
Unknown or fewer than three doses	Yes	No	Yes	Yes
Three or more doses	No	No	No	No

Td, Tetanus and diphtheria; *Tdap*, tetanus, diphtheria, and acellular pertussis; *TIG*, tetanus immune globulin.
From Hamborsky J, Kroger A, Wolfe S. *Epidemiology and Prevention of Vaccine-Preventable Diseases*. 13th ed. Centers for Disease Control and Prevention; Public Health Foundation; 2015:341.

feces, saliva, purulent exudate, or soil; wounds with retained foreign bodies or containing devitalized or avascular tissue; established wound infections; penetrating abdominal wounds involving bowel; deep puncture wounds; and wounds caused by crush, burns, or frostbite.

Tetanus can develop despite prior immunization, and it can result from chronic skin lesions in minor or clean wounds. In 10% to 20% of cases, no previous wound can be identified. Patients' recall of past immunizations is imperfect, and immunity may be, on rare occasions, inadequate after a complete series of tetanus toxoid.[86] Tetanus boosters given more frequently than advised increase the incidence of adverse reactions to subsequent injections. However, the benefits of overtreatment seem to outweigh the risks.

PATIENT INSTRUCTIONS

Successful wound healing is partly dependent on the care given to the wound once the patient leaves the ED. Patient satisfaction depends not only on the cosmetic result but also on the expectation of that result.[8] Both are reasons why patients should receive thorough and clear instructions.

Inform the patient that no matter how skillful the repair, any wound of significance produces a scar. Most scars deepen in color and become more prominent before they mature and fade. The final appearance of the scar cannot be judged until 6 to 12 months after the repair.[7] Some wounds heal with wide, unattractive scars despite ideal management and closure. Wounds more likely to have significant scars are those that cross perpendicular to joints, wrinkle lines, or lines of minimum tension (Kraissl lines), and those that retract more than 5 mm. Wounds that are likely to scar are those that are located over convexities or in certain anatomic locations (e.g., anterior upper part of the chest, back, shoulders) where hypertrophic scars are common. A wound crossing a concave surface may result in a bowstring deformity; one crossing a convexity may leave a scar depression. To avoid these complications, a Z-plasty procedure can be performed during initial wound management, or the scar can be revised later. Tell the patient to expect suboptimal outcomes in these situations.[23]

Patients may experience dysesthesia in or around a scar, particularly about the midface. Gentle rubbing or pressing on the skin may relieve the symptoms. If wounds extend to subcutaneous levels and involve lacerated cutaneous nerves, patients may be bothered by hypoesthesia distal to the wound. The dysesthesia and anesthesia usually resolve in 6 months to 1 year.[9]

After 48 hours, the patient may remove the dressing on uncomplicated wounds and check for evidence of infection: redness, warmth, increasing pain, swelling, purulent drainage, or the "red streaks" of lymphangitis. Not all patients can identify these signs and often overlook an early infection or overcall one in the presence of normal healing. Patients with complicated or infection-prone wounds should be examined by a clinician or nurse in 2 to 3 days.[83] Inform patients that a painful wound is often a sign of infection or suture reaction, and pain should prompt inspection of the wound. If no sign of infection is present after 48 to 72 hours, the patient can care for the wound until it is time for removal of the sutures.

Because the edges of a wound are sealed by coagulum and bridged by epithelial cells within 48 hours, the wound is impermeable to bacteria after 2 days.[6,87] Instruct the patient to protect the wound and keep the dressing clean and dry for 24 to 48 hours. In this initial period change the dressing only if it becomes externally soiled or soaked by exudate from the wound. If possible, keep the injured part elevated.

After 1 to 2 days, daily gentle washing with mild soap and water to remove dried blood and exudate is beneficial, especially in areas such as the face or the scalp. Still, vigorous scrubbing of wounds should be discouraged. Patients may bathe with sutures in place but should not immerse the wound for a prolonged time. Although diluted hydrogen peroxide can remove blood from the skin's surface, it should not be used as a cleaning agent on the healing wound itself. A wound should be protected with a dressing during the first week, and the dressing should be changed daily. Sutured scalp lacerations are usually left open, and showering is encouraged.

If a splint protects an injured extremity or finger, it should be left undisturbed until the sutures are removed. Patients with intraoral lacerations can be instructed to use warm saltwater mouth rinses at least three times a day.

Patients may ask about the efficacy of various creams and lotions (e.g., vitamin E, aloe vera, cocoa butter) in limiting scar formation. Currently, there are insufficient data to evaluate topical agents' use in reducing scar formation or appearance.[88] Their use is acceptable and may prompt some patients to regularly participate in wound inspection and cleaning.

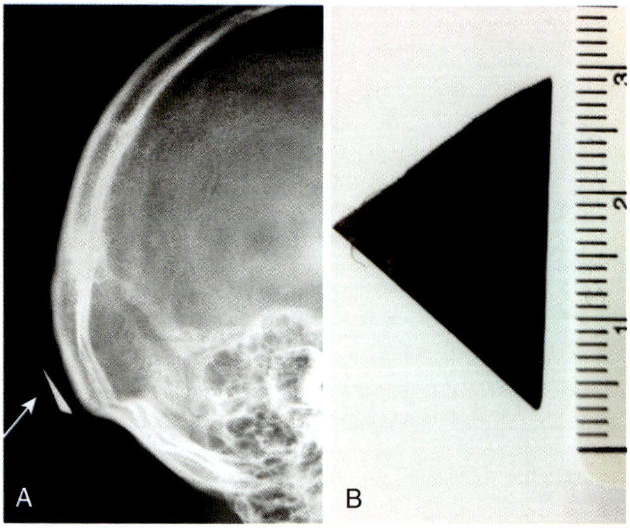

Fig. 34.20 Scalp wounds rarely become infected. This patient was seen twice with a scalp wound infection and given two courses of antibiotics with initial improvement, all before the blade of a utility knife *(arrow)* was discovered in the wound. He was intoxicated during a bar fight and resisted wound closure in the emergency department, so it was done hastily and not thoroughly explored.

SECONDARY WOUND CARE

Reexamination

Patients with simple closed wounds may be released with appropriate home care instructions and told to return for removal of the sutures at an appropriate time. It is prudent to have a wound check in 3 to 5 days for all wounds. In particular, all high-risk wounds, such as bite wounds and other infection-prone wounds, should be reexamined in 2 to 3 days for signs of infection. Inspect the wound if the patient experiences increasing discomfort, develops a fever, or believes the wound is infected. Evaluate wounds being considered for delayed primary closure in 3 to 5 days.[10]

Wounds in which extensive dissection of subcutaneous tissue has been performed may develop an intense inflammation similar in appearance to low-grade, localized cellulitis. It is rarely necessary to open these wounds. Remove one or two stitches to relieve some of the tension caused by mild swelling, if necessary. Cleanse daily with water accompanied with a mild soap and apply warm compresses, and this type of wound reaction should subside within 24 to 48 hours.

If a wound becomes infected, evaluate for a retained foreign body as the nidus of the infection (Fig. 34.20). In most sutured wounds that become infected, remove the sutures to allow drainage. If a wound exhibits a minor infection, remove a few sutures or all of them. Pack grossly infected wounds open to allow further drainage. Treat infected wounds with daily cleansing, warm compresses, and antibiotics. Leave wounds that have been opened to heal by secondary intention, which involves wound contraction, granulation tissue formation, and epithelialization.

Most wound infections can be treated in the outpatient setting with oral antibiotics and follow-up. Lymphangitis does not mandate intravenous antibiotics or hospitalization.

Suture Removal

The optimal time for suture removal varies with the wound's location, the wound's healing rate, and the amount of tension on the wound. Certain areas of the body, such as the back of the hand, heal slowly, whereas facial or scalp wounds heal rapidly. Systemic factors such as malnutrition, neoplasia, and immunosuppression affect the speed of wound healing. Therefore only general guidelines can be given for the timing of suture removal. At the time that suture removal is being considered, one or two sutures may be cut to determine whether the edges of the skin are sufficiently adherent to allow removal of all the sutures. Removing sutures too early invites wound dehiscence and widening of the scar, whereas leaving sutures in longer than necessary may result in epithelial tracks, infection, and unsightly scarring.

Percutaneous sutures stimulate an inflammatory reaction along the suture track. Infection around a suture can lead to the formation of a stitch mark. Other factors that determine the severity of stitch marks include the length of time stitches are left in place, skin tension, the relationship of the suture to the edge of the wound, the region of the body, and the patient's tendency for keloid formation. The eyelids, palms, soles' skin, and mucous membranes seldom show stitch marks. In contrast, oily skin and the skin of the back, the sternal area, the upper part of the arms, the lower extremities, the dorsum of the nose, and the forehead are likely to exhibit permanent imprints of suture material on the skin surface.

If sutures are removed within 7 days, generally no discernible needle puncture or stitch marks will persist. However, at 6 days the wound is held together by a small amount of fibrin and cells, and it has minimal strength. The tensile strength of most wounds at this time is adequate to hold the wound edges together, but only if there is no appreciable dynamic or static skin force pulling the wound apart. Minimal trauma to an unsupported wound at this point could cause dehiscence. The clinician should decide on the proper time to remove the sutures after weighing these various factors. If early suture removal is necessary (such as on the face), wound repair can be maintained with strips of surgical skin tape. The key to wound tensile strength after suture removal is an adequate deep tissue layered closure.

Some general guidelines exist for suture removal. Remove sutures on the face on the fifth day after the injury or remove alternate sutures on the third day and the remainder on the fifth day. On the extremities and the anterior aspect of the trunk, leave sutures in place for approximately 7 days to prevent wound disruption. Leave sutures on the scalp, back, feet, hands, and joints in place for 10 to 14 days, even though permanent stitch marks may result. Some clinicians recommend the removal of the sutures used to repair eyelid lacerations as early as 72 hours to avoid epithelialization along the suture track along with subsequent cyst formation.

Removing sutures is usually relatively simple. Cleanse the wound and any remaining crust overlying the wound's surface or surrounding the sutures. Wipe the skin with an alcohol swab. Cut each stitch with scissors or the tip of a No. 11 scalpel blade at a point close to the skin's surface on one side. Grasp the suture knot on the opposite side with forceps and pull it across the wound (Fig. 34.21). The amount of exposed suture dragged through the suture track is thereby minimized. It is difficult to remove sutures with very short ends. At the time of suture placement, cut the length of the suture ends so they equal the distance between sutures. This makes it easier to grasp the suture during subsequent removal while avoiding entanglement during the knotting of adjacent sutures.

Once the skin sutures are removed, the width of the scar increases gradually over the next 3 to 5 weeks unless it is supported. Support is provided by previously placed subcutaneous stitches that bring the skin's edges into apposition or by applying skin tape at the time of removal. A nonabsorbable, subcuticular suture can be left in place for 2 to 3 weeks to provide continued support for the wound. Although complications such as closed epithelial sinuses, cysts, or internal tracts can occur from prolonged use of this stitch,[89] they are unusual and can be avoided by placement of a buried subcuticular stitch with an absorbable suture.

Small stitch abscesses may occur in wounds when sutures remain in place for more than 7 to 10 days. Localized stitch abscesses resolve after removing the sutures and applying warm compresses, and without antibiotics in simple cases.

If time and effort have been invested in cosmetic closure of the face, protect the repair with skin tape after the skin sutures have been removed. Wound contraction and scar widening continue for about 40 days after the injury. Because the desired result is a scar of minimal width, the tape can be used for as long as 5 weeks after removal of the sutures. With exposure to sunlight, scars in their first 4 months redden to a greater extent than the surrounding skin. In exposed cosmetic areas and when prolonged exposure to the sun is anticipated, appropriate sun protection and avoidance strategies should be used (e.g., a hat and sunscreen). Sunscreen may have a role in protecting scars from the sun, but more studies are needed to understand its impact better.

COMPLICATIONS

There are several reasons why wounds fail to heal; some are related to decisions made at the time of wound closure, and others are consequences of later events. Some of the impediments to healing include ischemia or necrosis of tissue, hematoma formation, prolonged inflammation caused by foreign material, excessive tension on the edges of the skin, and immunocompromising systemic factors. A primary cause of delayed healing is wound infection. Wound cleaning and debridement, atraumatic and aseptic handling of tissue, and protective dressings minimize this complication. Inversion of the edges of a wound during closure produces a more noticeable scar, whereas skillful technique can convert a jagged, contaminated wound into a fine, inapparent scar. The patient's actions also affect wound healing. Delays in seeking treatment for injuries may affect the outcome of the wound. Furthermore, in the first few days after an injury, the patient must take responsibility for protecting the wound from contamination, further trauma, and swelling.

Infection is one of the most common causes of dehiscence. If the patient is careless or unlucky, reinjury can reopen a wound despite the protection of a thick dressing. If the suture size is too small, the stitch may break. A stitch too fine or tied too tightly may cut through friable

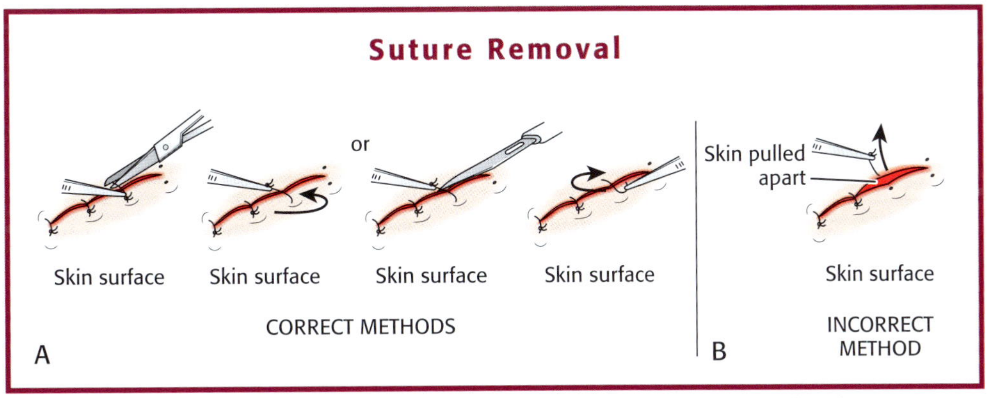

Fig. 34.21 Technique for removal of sutures. (A) Pull toward the wound line rather than (B) away from it, which causes the wound to tear apart. After suture removal, supporting the wound with surgical tape (Steri-Strips) may be advisable if tension or minor dehiscence is present.

tissue and pull out. Knots that have not been tied securely may unravel. The suture material may be extruded or absorbed too rapidly. Finally, if a stitch is removed too early (i.e., before tissues regain adequate tensile strength), the wound loses necessary support and can reopen. If the wound edges show signs of separating at the time of suture removal, alternate stitches can be left in place, and the entire length of the wound supported by strips of adhesive tape.

Several factors determine the final appearance of a scar. Infection, tissue necrosis, and keloid formation widen a scar. Wounds located in sebaceous skin or oriented 90 degrees to dynamic or static skin tension lines result in wide scars. Dynamic tension is primarily a result of nearby joint movement. Wounds located in areas of high static skin tension will gape initially and often heal with wide scars despite adequate closure, whereas wounds in areas of loose or lax skin often heal with fine, narrow scars.[23]

Miscellaneous Aspects of Wound Care

A wide variety of mechanisms creates traumatic wounds, and clinicians must sometimes adjust wound management techniques to match special circumstances.

The ED Approach to Puncture Wounds

Puncture wounds are common, yet no prospective studies identify the most effective way to manage puncture wounds in the ED. Aside from evaluating tetanus immunization status and considering the possibility of a foreign body, the clinician has few proven options to prevent infection in a puncture wound. Scrubbing the surface of the puncture, evaluating the opening for retained foreign matter, and trimming jagged skin and tissue edges may be helpful. The value or appropriateness of coring, probing, or irrigating the puncture track has not been established. Deep irrigation is usually ineffective unless the puncture site is converted into a larger laceration to make the full depth of the puncture accessible. Still, routine enlargement of a puncture track is not recommended. For through-and-through punctures, the track can often be debrided by pulling gauze through the wound (Fig. 34.22).

It is impossible to accurately predict the outcome of a puncture wound, though it may be determined at the time of the injury. Gross contamination or deep foreign bodies may not be appreciated for days. No prospective randomized trials have evaluated prophylactic antibiotic administration's role in preventing infection in puncture wounds. Hence there are no standards on the use, type, or duration of prophylactic antibiotic therapy, even in high-risk patients. Most clinicians forego routine antibiotics and opt for simple cleaning and appropriate follow-up.

Gunshot Wounds

A subset of gunshot wounds may be definitively handled in the ED with outpatient follow-up. Studies by Ordog and colleagues[90,91] documented a very low infection rate in gunshot wounds treated with standard wound care on an outpatient basis, even when the missile was left in place and minor fractures were present. Because most gunshot wounds are puncture wounds, only minimal deep wound cleaning is possible. Superficial soft tissue wounds with entrance and exit wounds in proximity may be debrided by passing sterile gauze back and forth through the wound track (Fig. 34.23). Though prescribed frequently, no data support the routine use of antibiotics following gunshot wounds.

Animal Bites

Many aspects of treating animal bites are controversial, and no universal standards exist. Most bites are caused by dogs or cats that are family pets. Numerous organisms can be cultured from an infected bite wound caused by a dog or cat, and cultures may guide antibiotic therapy in infected wounds.[85] However, cultures that are performed during the initial treatment of an animal bite are not predictive of subsequent infection or infecting organisms. The predominant pathogens in animal bites are the oral flora of the biting animal and human skin flora. Approximately 85% of bites harbor potential pathogens, and the average wound yields five types of bacterial isolates; almost 60% have mixed aerobic and anaerobic bacteria.[92] Skin flora such as staphylococci and streptococci are isolated in approximately 40% of bites. The gram-negative rod *Pasteurella canis (multocida)*, *S. aureus*, and *Streptococcus viridans* are common culprits in bite wound infections. *Pasteurella* species are isolated from 50% of dog bite wounds and 75% of cat bite wounds. Cat bites are usually puncture wounds that cannot be completely cleaned because of the sharp, pointed shape of their teeth. Compared with dog bites, cat bites may become infected quickly after the bite (within 24 hours), thus suggesting *Pasteurella* infection (Fig. 34.24). Cat bite wounds tend to penetrate deeply, with a higher risk for osteomyelitis, tenosynovitis, and septic arthritis when compared with dog bites, which are associated with crush injury and wound trauma. *Capnocytophaga canimorsus*, a fastidious gram-negative rod, can cause bacteremia and fatal sepsis after animal bites, especially in asplenic patients or those with underlying hepatic disease. Anaerobes isolated from dog and cat bite wounds include *Bacteroides*, fusobacteria, *Porphyromonas*, *Prevotella*, propionibacteria, and peptostreptococci. Puncture wounds from a dog can be problematic because they are difficult to clean unless they are through-and-through wounds (Fig. 34.25). Some clinicians have advocated primary closure of large dog bite lacerations that are centrally located on the body; however, markedly contused lacerations are good candidates for delayed primary closure (see Fig. 34.15B).

Infected animal bites should be treated with antibiotics, but the use of prophylactic antibiotics for animal bites is controversial. Depending on location, dog bites may have an infection rate of 3% to 5%, whereas cat bites may become infected 50% of the time.[81] Antibiotics for either prophylaxis or infection should have in vitro activity against *P. canis*. Prophylactic amoxicillin-clavulanate (875/125 mg twice daily) given for 3 to 5 days may reduce infection rates after cat or dog bites, especially for a puncture wound, when the patient is seen more than 8 hours after the bite, or when wound cleaning has been inadequate.[81,92] Some clinicians administer prophylactic antibiotics for all cat bites, for a dog bite that has been sutured, for hand wounds, for bite wounds close to a bone or joint, or for bites associated with deep tissue or crush injury. Although this is a reasonable and common approach, there are no data strongly supporting this practice. Alternative antibiotic combinations include clindamycin (300 mg four times daily) *plus* doxycycline (100 mg twice daily), or

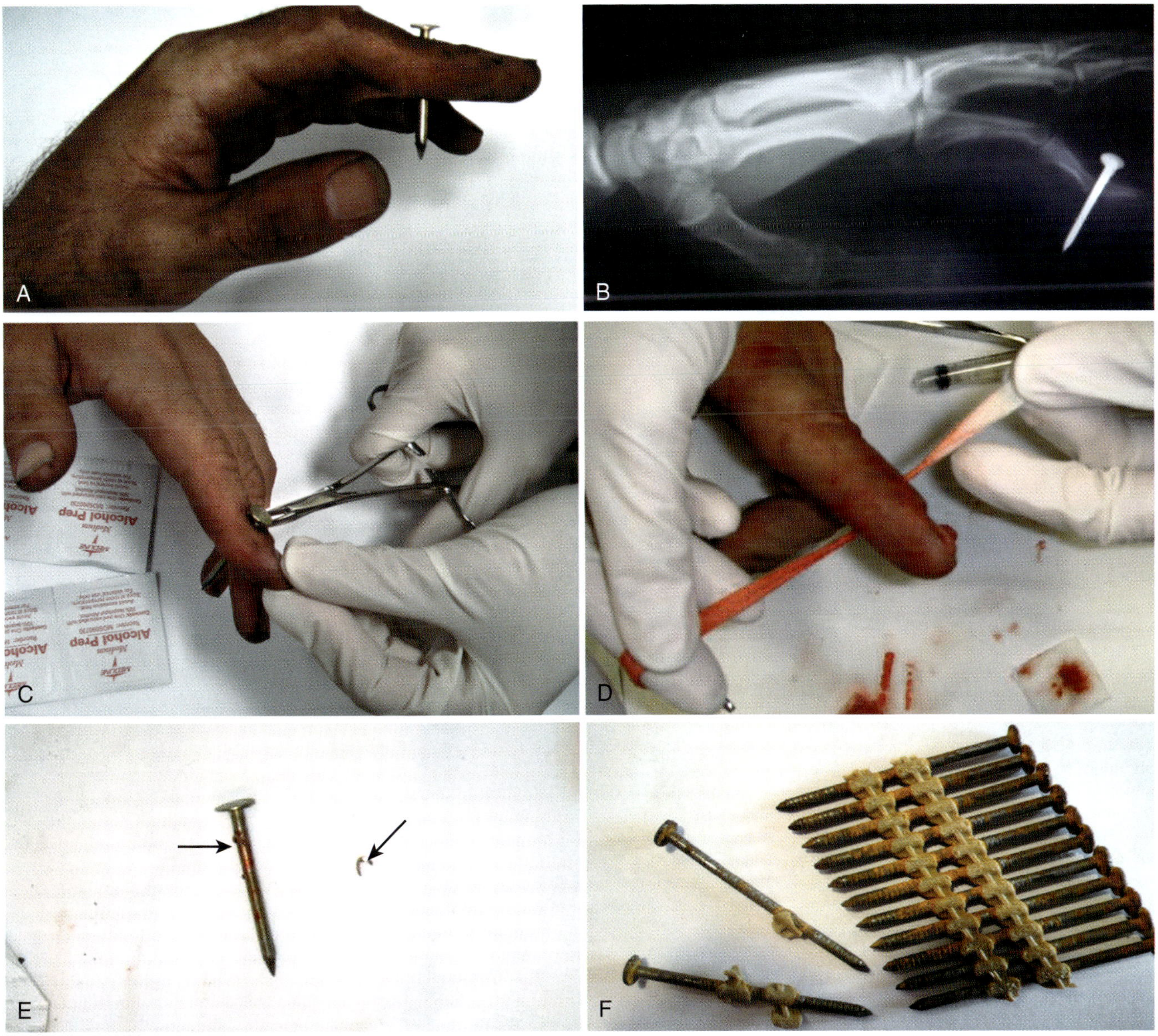

Fig. 34.22 Puncture wounds cannot be cleaned meticulously, and they may contain debris. The ultimate course of a puncture wound is likely set at the time of injury, and they often do well. If an infection is seen at follow-up, a foreign body (FB) is highly likely. (A–C) This nail gun puncture of the distal finger joint was able to be debrided by (D) passing a small hemostat through the puncture wound and pulling gauze through the wound. (E) A small piece of metal, used to attach the nails together *(arrows)*, was removed with this maneuver. (F) Note that nails from a nail gun clip are held together with a piece of metal or glue that may hamper removal or be unintentionally left in the wound. A splint and 3 days of cephalexin prophylaxis (because of the discovered foreign body) were provided, and this wound healed well.

trimethoprim-sulfamethoxazole (one double-strength tablet twice daily). Antibiotics that do not have adequate activity against *P. canis* include first-generation cephalosporins (such as cephalexin), penicillinase-resistant penicillins (such as dicloxacillin), macrolides (such as erythromycin), and clindamycin alone.

The best way to approach bite wounds is to adhere to the basic principles of wound care. Search for underlying fractures or tooth fragments with deep animal bites. When a wound results from the bite or scratch of either a wild or a domestic animal, give rabies prophylaxis if indicated (Tables 34.4 and 34.5).[93]

Human Bites

Human bite wounds are problematic for several reasons: these wounds are contaminated with human saliva; they may hide foreign material; deep structural damage may complicate the injury; and wound care may be delayed. Pathogens include aerobic bacteria (such as streptococci and *S. aureus*) and anaerobic bacteria (such as *Eikenella*, *Fusobacterium*, *Peptostreptococcus*, *Prevotella*, and *Porphyromonas* species). When cultured, most infected human bites harbor three to four pathogens, including both aerobes and anaerobes. Limited case reports suggest that viral pathogens including hepatitis, HIV, and herpes simplex virus, may be transmissible by human bites;

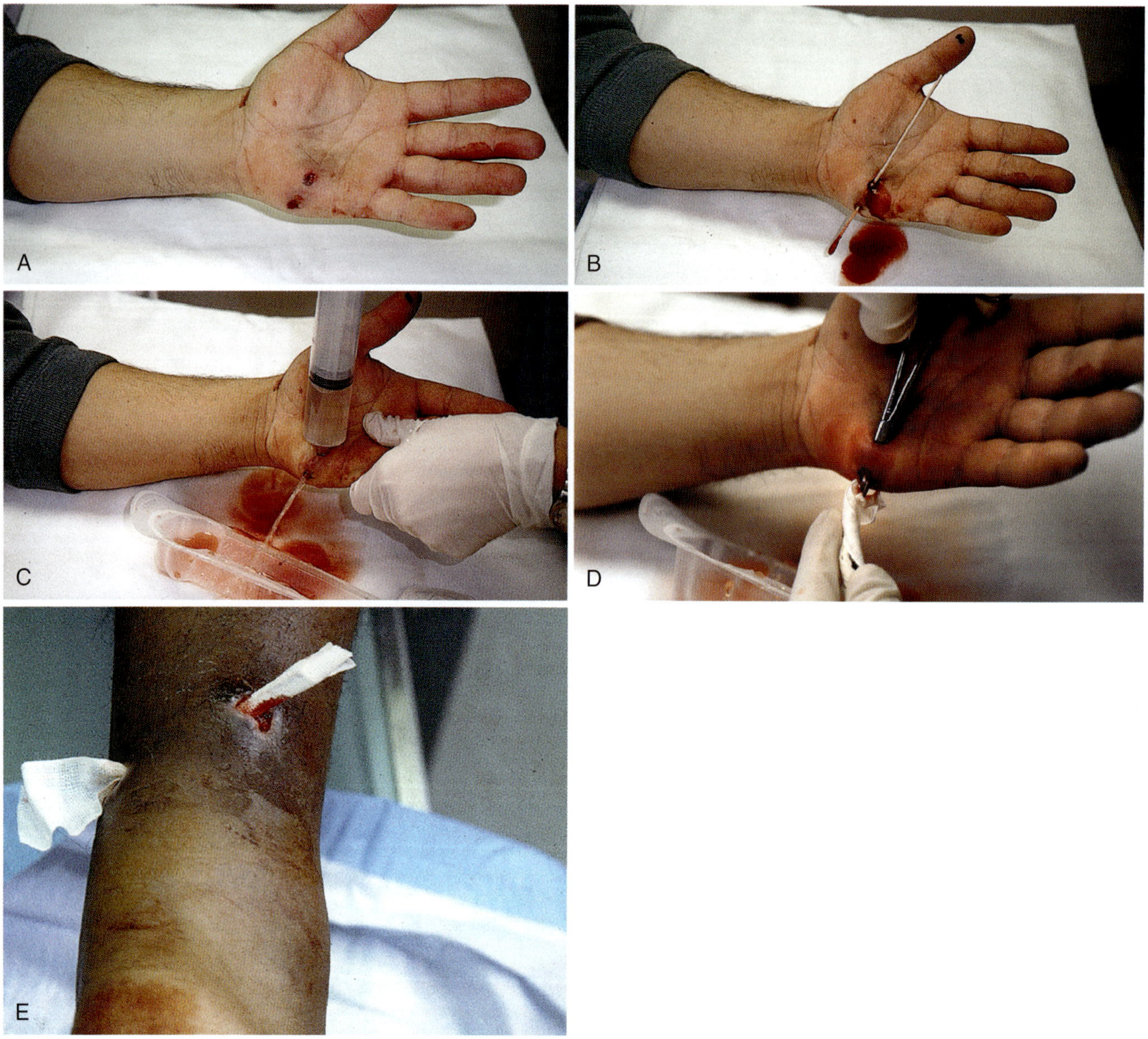

Fig. 34.23 Patients with minor gunshot wounds may be treated as outpatients, even when bullet fragments remain, and minor fractures are present. (A–B) This through-and-through injury traversed the hypothenar eminence. No bullet remained and no bones were involved. (C) Usually, it is impossible to irrigate a puncture wound, but in this case, note the saline at the exit site. (D) After the entrance wound is debrided of the powder burn, pass an instrument through the wound. Grasp the gauze packing with the instrument and pull it into the wound. Pull the gauze *back and forth to debride the wound track*. Similarly, place clean packing. (E) For a similarly cleansed gunshot wound of the leg, leave the gauze packing in the track for 48 hours. No antibiotics were given, the pack was removed at wound check in 48 hours, and the patient did well.

however, data are lacking to guide the clinician on the best approach in the ED for these potential infections. Prophylaxis is not suggested if the wound does not penetrate the dermis, is not over a joint, and does not involve the hands, feet, or cartilaginous structures.[94]

Clenched fist injuries caused by contact with another person's teeth during a fight, or "fight bites," are among the most serious human bite wounds. Lacerations typically occur over the dominant hand's third and fourth metacarpophalangeal or proximal interphalangeal joints. Even small lacerations or punctures are highly prone to infection. Joint penetration is common. Relaxation of the fist may disseminate organisms into the deep compartments and the deep tendon spaces of the hand, predisposing the patient to deep soft tissue infection, septic arthritis, and osteomyelitis. Many patients ignore these wounds until the onset of pain, swelling, or purulent discharge; as a result, these injuries are often complicated by established infection at the initial ED visit. In addition, some patients are not always forthcoming about the origin of wounds involving interpersonal violence, thereby leading to incorrect ED treatment of a seemingly minor injury (Fig. 34.26).

Irrigate bite wounds copiously with tap water or sterile saline and remove grossly visible debris. Many clinicians will extend a small laceration to allow visualization of the underlying structures and better cleaning. Look for tooth chips, tendon injury, and joint penetration. Wounds involving tendons or joint spaces are more serious and require close follow-up.

In general, leave all human bite wounds open (unsutured), even when treated soon after the injury and with seemingly benign wound conditions. Pack them with gauze until follow-up. Do not use deep sutures. On reevaluation within a few days, perform delayed primary closure if desired. Facial bite wounds are an exception; primary closure may be considered for these wounds. Consider splinting the hand in a position of function with a short-arm volar splint for a few days to minimize joint movement. Advise the patient to elevate the injured area.

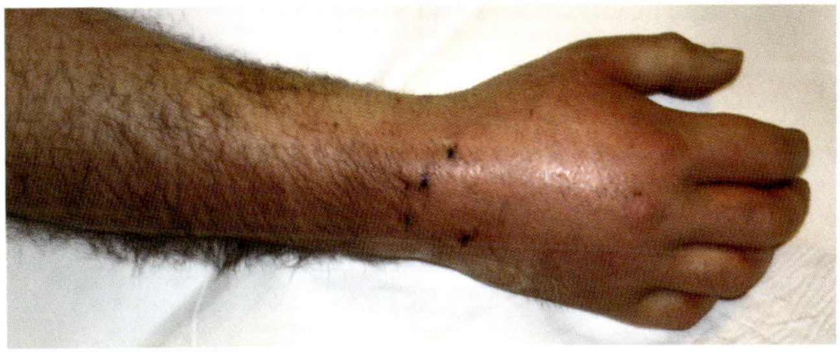

Fig. 34.24 Cat bites are puncture wounds that become infected rather quickly. See text for discussion of antibiotics.

Most clinicians administer *prophylactic* antibiotics for 3 to 5 days for human bites, although there are no studies that demonstrate the effectiveness of this practice, or to identify the best antibiotic. Most infections are polymicrobial, but use of antibiotics with activity against *S. aureus*, *Eikenella corrodens*, *Haemophilus influenzae*, and β-lactamase–producing oral anaerobic bacteria, is advised. Amoxicillin-clavulanate (875/125 mg twice daily) for 3 to 5 days is a common recommendation for monotherapy. Alternative empirical combination regimens include clindamycin (450 mg three times daily) *plus* trimethoprim-sulfamethoxazole (1 double-strength tablet twice daily), or ciprofloxacin (500 mg to 750 mg twice daily), or moxifloxacin (400 mg once daily) for 3 to 5 days.

Grossly infected wounds should be treated with intravenous antibiotics, but the need for hospitalization is based on the patient's profile and the clinician's assessment of the severity of the infection in addition to the need for close monitoring.

Serious Wound Infections

Most wound infections are easily recognized and can be treated in the outpatient setting with oral antibiotics, suture removal, evaluation for a retained foreign body, and a follow-up examination within a few days. Consider inpatient treatment for a patient with systemic complaints (fever, malaise, nausea), worsening infection at follow-up, an unreliable

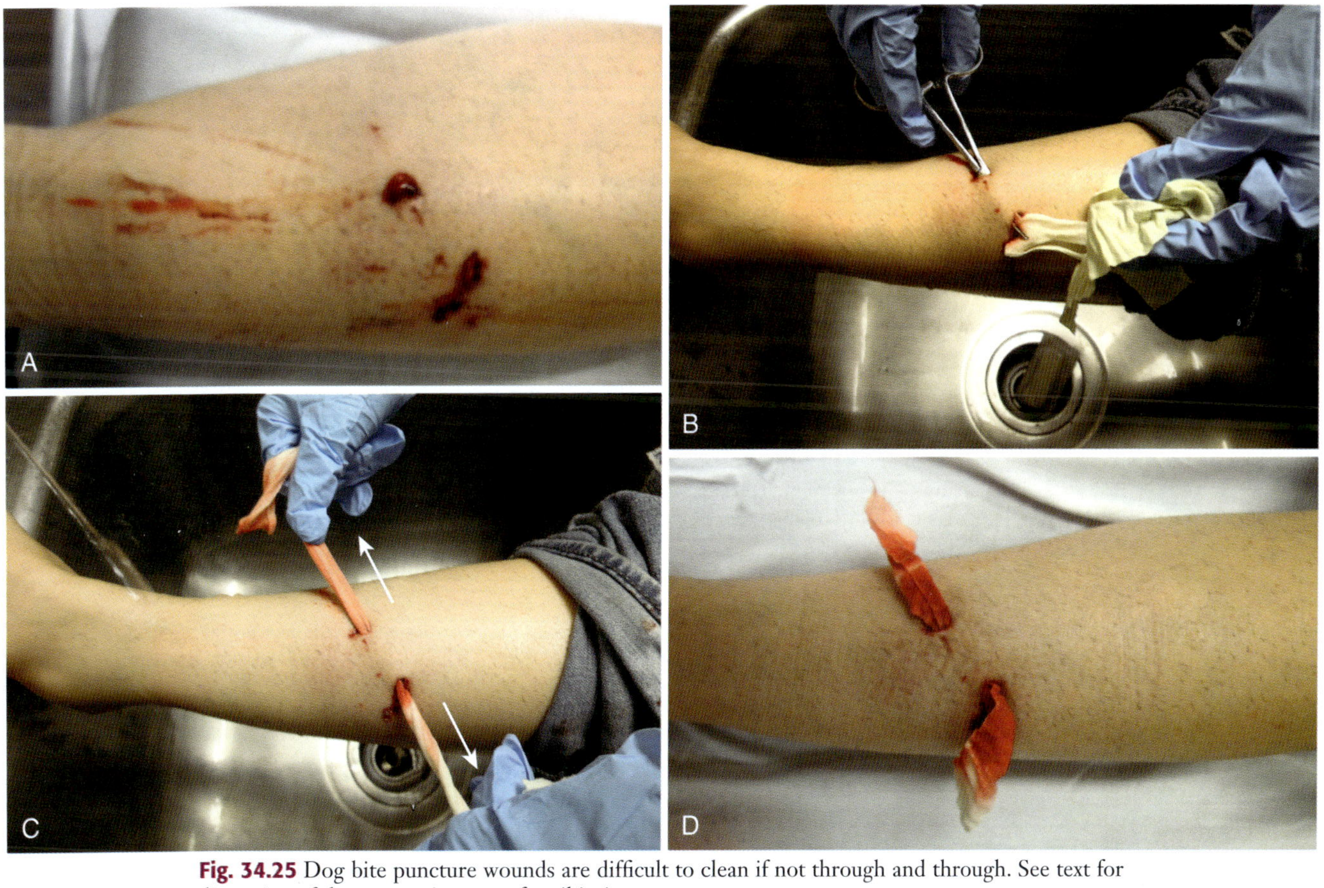

Fig. 34.25 Dog bite puncture wounds are difficult to clean if not through and through. See text for discussion of the appropriate use of antibiotics.

TABLE 34.4 Rabies Postexposure Prophylaxis Guide

ANIMAL SPECIES	CONDITION OF ANIMAL AT TIME OF ATTACK	TREATMENT OF EXPOSED PERSON[a]
Domestic		
Dog and cat	Healthy and available for 10 days of observation	None unless rabies develops in the animal[b] Local wound healing should be included in the treatment of the exposed person for each category
	Rabid or suspected rabid	RIG and HDCV
	Unknown (escaped)	Consult public health officials. If treatment is indicated, give RIG[c] and HDCV.
Wild		
Skunk, bat, fox, coyote, raccoon, bobcat, and other carnivores	Regard as rabid unless proved negative by laboratory tests[d]	RIG[c] and HDCV
Other		
Livestock, rodents, and lagomorphs (rabbits and hares)	Consider individually. Local and state public health officials should be consulted on questions about the need for rabies prophylaxis. Bites of squirrels, hamsters, guinea pigs, gerbils, chipmunks, rats, mice, other rodents, rabbits, and hares almost never call for antirabies prophylaxis.	

[a]All bites and wounds should be immediately cleansed thoroughly with soap and water. If antirabies treatment is indicated, both rabies immune globulin (RIG) and human diploid cell rabies vaccine (HDCV) should be given as soon as possible, regardless of the interval after exposure. Local reactions to vaccines are common and do not contraindicate continuing treatment. Discontinue vaccine if fluorescent antibody tests of the animal are negative.
[b]During the usual holding period of 10 days, begin treatment with RIG and HDCV at the first sign of rabies in a dog or cat that has bitten someone. The symptomatic animal should be killed immediately and tested.
[c]If RIG is not available, use antirabies serum, equine. Do not use more than the recommended dosage.
[d]The animal should be killed and tested as soon as possible. Holding for observation is not recommended. Vaccination may be discontinued if immunofluorescence tests of the animal are negative.
These recommendations are only a guide. In applying them, consider the animal species involved, the circumstances of the bite or other exposure, the vaccination status of the animal, and the presence of rabies in the region. Local or state public health officials should be consulted if questions arise about the need for rabies prophylaxis.
From Rao AK, Briggs D, Moore SM et al. Use of a modified preexposure prophylaxis vaccination schedule to prevent human rabies: recommendations of the Advisory Committee on Immunization Practices — United States, 2022. *MMWR Morb Mortal Wkly Rep*. 2022;71(18):619-627.

TABLE 34.5 Rabies Postexposure Prophylaxis Schedule, United States

VACCINATION STATUS	TREATMENT	REGIMEN[a]
Not previously vaccinated	Local wound cleansing	All postexposure treatment should begin with immediate thorough cleansing of all wounds with soap and water.
	RIG	20 IU/kg of body weight; if anatomically feasible, up to half the dose should be infiltrated around the wounds and the rest administered IM in the gluteal area on day 0. Note: RIG should not be administered in the same syringe or into the same anatomic site as the vaccine because RIG may partially suppress active production of antibody. No more than the recommended dose should be given.
	Vaccine	HDCV or PCECV, 1 mL IM (deltoid area[b]), one each on days 0, 3, 7, and 14.[d]
Previously vaccinated[c]	Local wound cleansing	All postexposure treatment should begin with immediate thorough cleansing of all wounds with soap and water.
	RIG	RIG should not be administered.
	Vaccine	HDCV or PCECV, 1 mL IM (deltoid area[b]), one each on days 0 and 3.

[a]These regimens are applicable for all age groups, including children.
[b]The deltoid area is the only acceptable site of vaccination for adults and older children. For younger children, the outer aspect of the thigh may be used. The vaccine should never be administered in the gluteal area.
[c]Any person with a history of preexposure vaccination with HDCV, PCECV, or PVRV, previous postexposure prophylaxis with HDCV, PCECV, or PVRV or prior vaccination with any other type of rabies vaccine and a documented history of antibody response to the previous vaccination.
[d]A five-dose regimen (0, 3, 7, 14, and 28) should be administered to patients with immunosuppression. An antibody titer should be checked 7–14 days after the final dose to assess their response.
HDCV, Human diploid cell rabies vaccine; *IM,* intramuscularly; *IU;* international units; *PCECV,* purified chick embryo cell vaccine; *PVRV,* purified vero cell rabies vaccine; *RIG,* rabies immune globulin. Four formulations of three inactivated rabies vaccines are currently licensed for preexposure and postexposure prophylaxis in the United States.
From Rao AK, Briggs D, Moore SM et al. Use of a modified preexposure prophylaxis vaccination schedule to prevent human rabies: Recommendations of the Advisory Committee on Immunization Practices—United States, 2022. *MMWR Morb Mortal Wkly Rep*. 2022;71(18):619-627. https://doi.org/10.15585/MMWR.MM7118A2

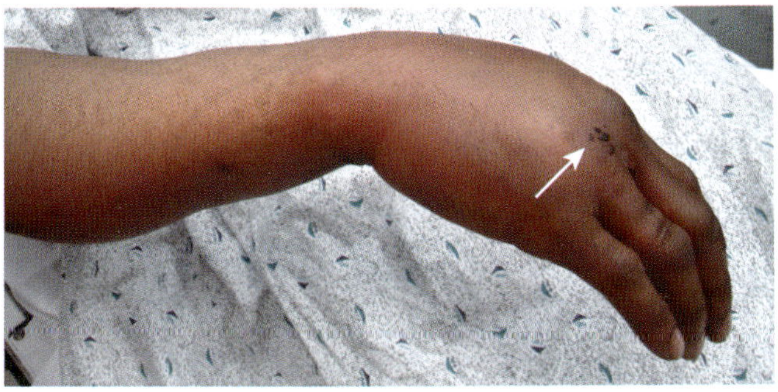

Fig. 34.26 Human bite. This patient was seen on a Monday morning with a small puncture wound on the dorsal surface of his hand *(arrow)*, and he claimed that it was an injury sustained at work. Hence, minimal wound care was given. In reality, it was a human bite from a bar fight the night before. In 3 days, a serious infection was obvious, and hospitalization was required. Note that the wrist is flexed, a patient-held position that is common and increases hand edema.

patient, or an immunocompromised patient. Some infections, such as a subgaleal infection in a scalp laceration, can be serious and will require prompt, aggressive treatment (Fig. 34.27).

Digital Nerves

Numbness in the area of digital innervation, concomitant injury to a digital artery (flash, pulsating bleeding), or an electric shock sensation when exploring a laceration should alert the clinician to a possible digital nerve injury. If there is uncertainty about nerve injury, the diagnosis can be established during a follow-up visit. However, lacerations of digital arteries that impair the distal circulation must be identified early during the initial evaluation.

Debridement of hand and finger lacerations should be minimal, and wound cleaning should be gentle yet thorough. Digital nerves that are transected distal to the metacarpophalangeal joint may be candidates for surgical repair. It is unclear at which point along the course of a digital nerve a transection can be repaired successfully, so referral to a hand specialist is essential. Frequently injuries proximal to the distal interphalangeal joint are not repaired, but many other factors will influence operative decisions. Repair of a digital nerve will often result in return of good sensory function, but it takes months, and repair can prevent painful neuromas from developing. Most hand surgeons will not repair digital nerves at the initial visit. Instead, they advise wound cleaning, skin closure, splinting, and outpatient follow-up in 24 to 36 hours, followed by delayed nerve repair.

Accidental Soft Tissue Injection with an EpiPen

An EpiPen provides self-injected subcutaneous epinephrine (0.3 mg or 0.15 mg) for emergency treatment of anaphylaxis (Fig. 34.28).

Occasionally the device is inadvertently discharged, usually into a finger, producing intense distal vasospasm (Fig. 34.29). The patient has a blanched finger and minor sensory disturbances. The natural history of untreated vasospasm is unknown; although ischemia may last for an hour or two, it may be self-limited. Digit amputation from this event has not been reported. Nonetheless, clinicians faced with an obviously ischemic finger may consider an intervention. Local heat and

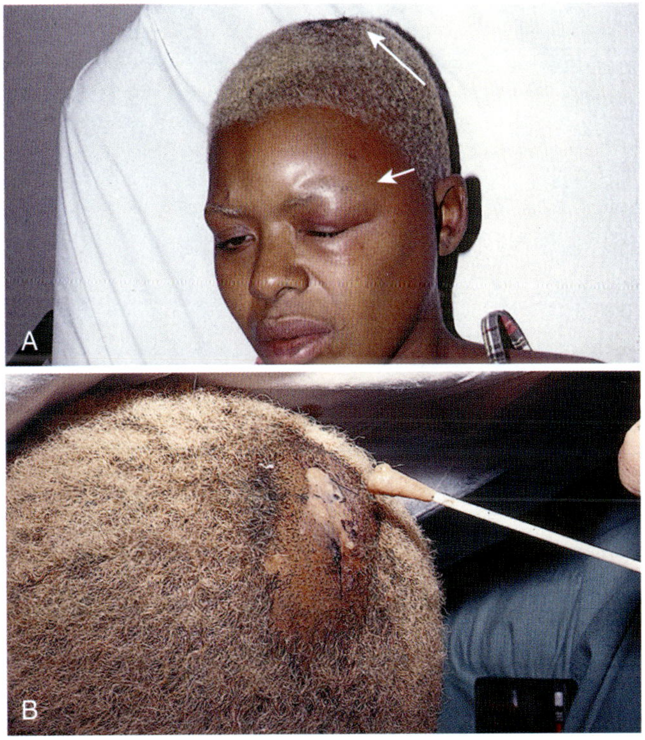

Fig. 34.27 Scalp lacerations rarely become infected because of the excellent blood supply to the area. (A) This patient had a painful swollen area under a sutured scalp laceration *(long arrow)* and impressive forehead and facial swelling *(short arrow)* from a laceration on top of the head. It was originally thought to be a hematoma. (B) Removal of sutures revealed frank pus and an extensive subgaleal abscess that required drainage and intravenous antibiotics. This infection can drain into the brain, face, neck, or mediastinum.

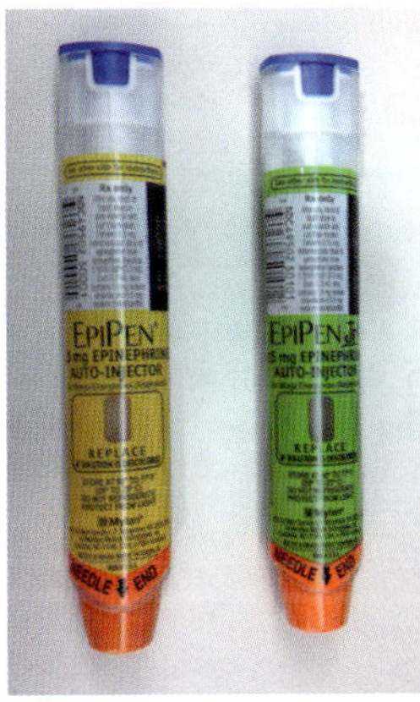

Fig. 34.28 The EpiPen and EpiPen, Jr. Each injector issues only one dose of epinephrine, and each delivers a total volume of 0.3 mL. The adult version injects 0.3 mg of epinephrine (it contains epinephrine in a 1:1000 concentration, so there is 1 mg of epinephrine in 1 mL of volume). The EpiPen, Jr. injects a similar 0.3-mL volume but uses a 1:2000 dilution of epinephrine, so only 0.15 mg of epinephrine is delivered with the injection.

nitroglycerin ointment are of no proven benefit. Placing a pulse oximeter on the fingertip can indicate the degree of resultant hypoxia, an indirect quantification of ischemia, and can also be used to assess reversal therapy.

Injecting the digit with the α-adrenergic antagonist phentolamine (Regitine) can be safely performed in the ED to

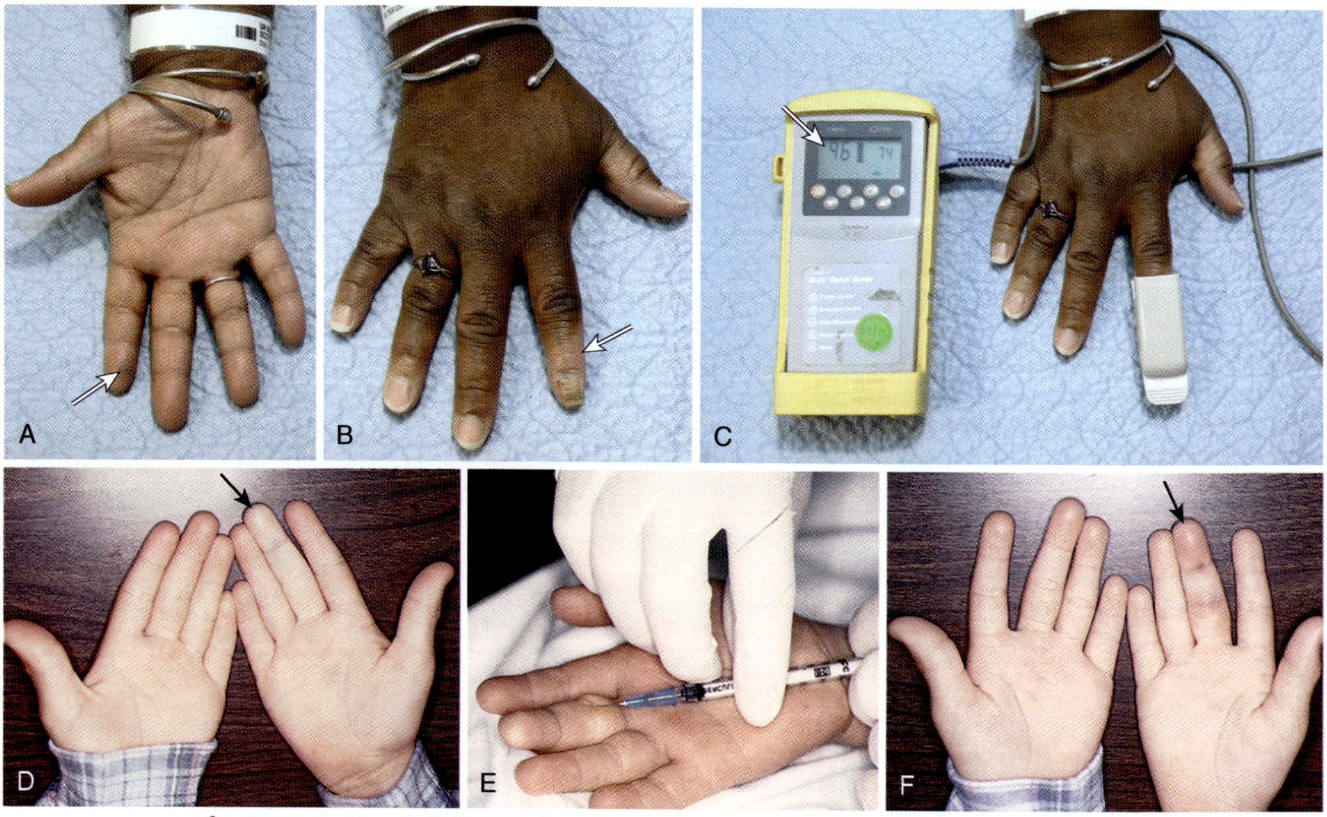

Fig. 34.29 Accidental discharge of an EpiPen into a finger will usually cause intense distal vasoconstriction. (A) This patient sustained such an injection into the volar tuft of the index finger *(arrow)* 2 hours before evaluation in the emergency department. (B) Blanching of the distal end of the finger *(arrow)* caused by the vasoconstriction. (C) A pulse oximetry probe was applied to the finger, and normal saturation (96%) *(arrow)* was found. She was simply observed for another hour, the blanching resolved, and she was discharged without intervention. (D) This patient had a similar injection on the volar surface of the middle finger. Blanching is obvious *(arrow)*. (E) Phentolamine and lidocaine were injected along the volar surface of the finger. (F) Five minutes later the finger was hyperemic *(arrow)*. No further intervention was required.

immediately and permanently reverse the ischemia (see Fig. 34.29D–F). Phentolamine is reconstituted and diluted in 2% plain lidocaine at a ratio of 1.5:1 or diluted with saline at a ratio of 1:1.[95] Inject a small aliquot of the mixture with a 25- to 27-gauge needle. Both a digital block and direct injection of the reversal agent into the site of epinephrine injection have been described. Injecting the actual site of penetration is intuitively the best option, but few case studies have been reported.[96] Within 5 to 10 minutes, the ischemia is reversed, and no further action is required.[95,97]

REFERENCES ARE AVAILABLE AT Elsevier eBooks+

CHAPTER 35

Methods of Wound Closure

Richard L. Lammers and Lovita E. Scrimshaw

WOUND TAPE

Surgical tape strips are now routinely used to close simple wounds. Tape strips can be applied by healthcare personnel in many settings, including emergency departments (EDs), operating rooms, clinics, and first aid stations. Advantages include ease of application, reduced need for local anesthesia, evenly distributed wound tension, no need for suture removal, no residual suture marks, minimal skin reaction, superiority for some grafts and flaps, and suitability for use under plaster casts. One main advantage of wound tape over standard sutures and wound staples is its greater resistance to wound infection.[1] The low rate of wound infection and low risk of dehiscence with wound tape are similar to those of tissue adhesive.[2] Wound closure strips are the most cost-effective means for the closure of low-tension lacerations and provide results comparable with a tissue adhesive.[3–6] Wound tape may provide better cosmetic results than tissue adhesive, especially in wounds <2 cm.[2,7,8]

Background and Tape Comparisons

Currently, several brands of tape with different porosity, flexibility, strength, and configuration are available. Steri-Strips (3M Corporation) are nonwoven microporous tapes with ribbed backing (Fig. 35.1 and Video 35.1) They are porous to air and water, and the ribbed backing provides extra strength. Shur-Strip (Deknatel, Inc.) is another nonwoven microporous tape. Cover-Strips (Beiersdorf) are woven tape that have a high degree of porosity. They allow not only air and water, but also wound exudates to pass through the tape. Clearon (Ethicon, Inc.) is a synthetic plastic tape whose backing contains longitudinal parallel serrations to permit gas and fluid permeability. An iodoform-impregnated Steri-Strip is intended to further retard infection without sensitization to iodine. Other tape products include Curi-Strip (Kendall), Nichi-Strip (Nichiban Co., Ltd.), Cicagraf (Smith & Nephew), Suture Strip (Genetic Laboratories), and Steri-Strip S (formerly marketed as ClozeX).[9–16] One comprehensive study of wound tapes compared Curi-Strip, Steri-Strip, Nichi-Strip, Cicagraf, Suture Strip, and Suture Strip Plus for breaking strength, elongation under stress, air porosity, and adhesiveness.[17] Curi-Strip, Cicagraf, and Steri-Strip exhibited equivalent dry breaking strength. However, when wet (a condition that can occur in the clinical setting), Cicagraf outperformed all tapes. Suture Strip Plus may stretch under tension and allow wound dehiscence. Nichi-Strip was the most porous to air, and Cicagraf was almost vapor impermeable. Nichi-Strip and Curi-Strip had the best adherence to untreated skin. When the skin was treated with tincture of benzoin, however, Steri-Strip dramatically outperformed all other products. When all study parameters were considered, Nichi-Strip, Curi-Strip, and Steri-Strip achieved the highest overall performance rankings (Video 35.2).

Indications

The primary indication for tape closure is a superficial straight laceration under little tension. If necessary, tension can be reduced by placing deep closures. Areas particularly suited for tape closure are the forehead, chin, malar eminence, thorax, and non–joint-related areas of the extremities. Tape may also be preferred for wounds in anxious children when suture placement is not essential. In young children who are likely to remove the tape, tape closure must be protected with an overlying gauze bandage.

In experimental wounds inoculated with *Staphylococcus aureus*, tape-closed wounds resisted infection better than wounds closed with nylon sutures. Tape closure works well under plaster casts when superficial suture removal would be delayed. Wound tape effectively holds flaps and grafts in place, particularly over the fingers, the flat areas of the extremities, and the trunk (Fig. 35.2). Tape closure can also be applied to wounds after early suture removal, particularly on the face, to maintain approximation of the wound edges while reducing the chance of permanent suture mark scarring. Finally, because of the minimal skin tension created by tape, it can be used on skin that has been compromised by vascular insufficiency, altered by prolonged use of steroids, and in the fragile skin of the aged. For example, wounds on the pretibial area are difficult to close, especially in the elderly because of tissue atrophy. Wound tape provides an alternative or adjunct to suture closure in this situation.[18]

Contraindications

Tape closure has limitations as well. Tape does not work well on wounds under significant tension or on irregular wounds, on concave surfaces, or in areas of marked tissue laxity. In many cases, tape does not provide satisfactory apposition of the wound edges without concurrent underlying deep closure. Naturally moist areas, such as the axilla, the palms of the hands, the soles of the feet, and the perineum, prevent tape from sticking well. Tape does not adhere well to wounds with secretions, copious exudates, or persistent bleeding. It is of little value on lax and intertriginous skin, on the scalp, and other areas with a high concentration of hair follicles. Tape strips are also at risk for premature removal by young children.

Do not place tape tightly and circumferentially around digits because it has insufficient ability to stretch or lengthen (Fig. 35.3). If placed circumferentially, the natural wound edema of an injured digit can make the tape act like a constricting band, which can lead to ischemia and possible necrosis of the digit. Use semicircular or spiral placement techniques if digits are to be taped.

Equipment

For simple tape closure, the equipment required includes forceps, scissors, and tape of the proper size (see Fig. 35.1). Most taping can be done in the ED with 0.25-inch × 3-inch strips. For wounds larger than 4 cm, however, 0.5-inch–wide strips provide greater strength. Most companies manufacture strips up to 1 inch wide and 4 inches long.

Procedure

Proper wound preparation, irrigation, debridement, and hemostasis must precede tape closure. Dry the area of tape application thoroughly to ensure proper adhesion. Do not attempt to apply tape to a wet area or over a wound that is slowly oozing blood because it will usually result in failure of the tape to stick to the skin. On fingers, tape can be applied to a wound that is kept dry by temporarily placing a tourniquet at the base of the finger (see Fig. 35.3).

The technique of applying tape is shown in Fig. 35.4. After the wound has been dried, apply a liquid adhesive such as tincture of benzoin or Mastisol (Eloquest Healthcare Inc.) to the skin adjacent to the wound to increase adhesion of the tape. All tapes come in presterilized packages. Open them directly onto the operating field. Handle tape with gloved hands. With the backing still attached, cut the tape to the desired length or long enough to allow approximately 2 cm to 3 cm of overlap on each side of the wound. After removing the end tab, gently peel

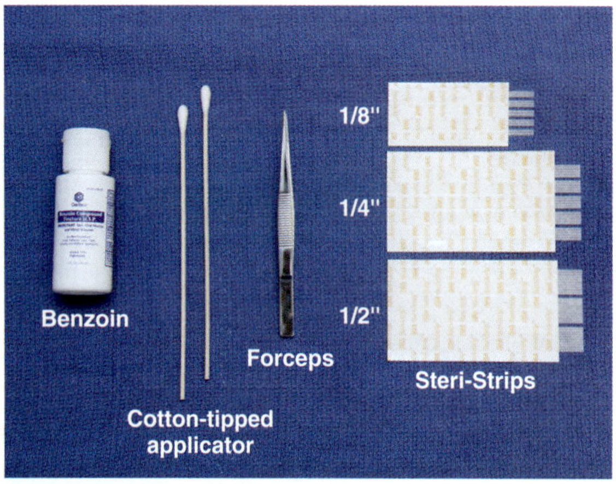

Fig. 35.1 Equipment required for the application of wound tape. Scissors will also be needed to cut the tape to the proper length. Wound tape (Steri-Strip brand depicted here) comes in a variety of widths. The use of benzoin helps Steri-Strips stay in place longer.

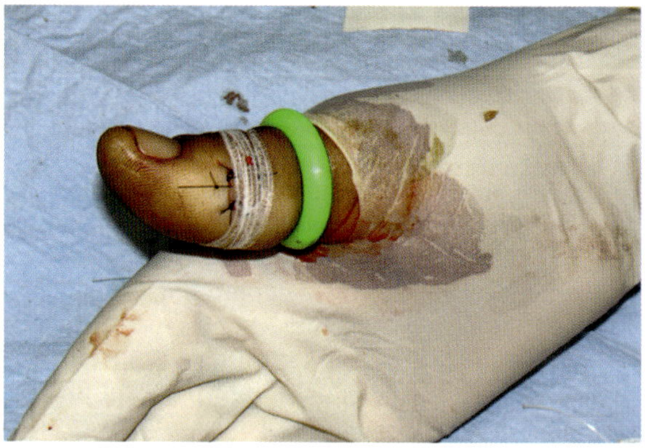

Fig. 35.3 After suturing this proximally based flap, Steri-Strips are applied under a tourniquet to compress the flap, arrest motion of the flap, and lessen buildup of fluid. Tissue movement and fluid buildup are some reasons why flaps and avulsed skin fail to heal. Tape should be placed in a semicircular or spiral pattern on digits to avoid constriction.

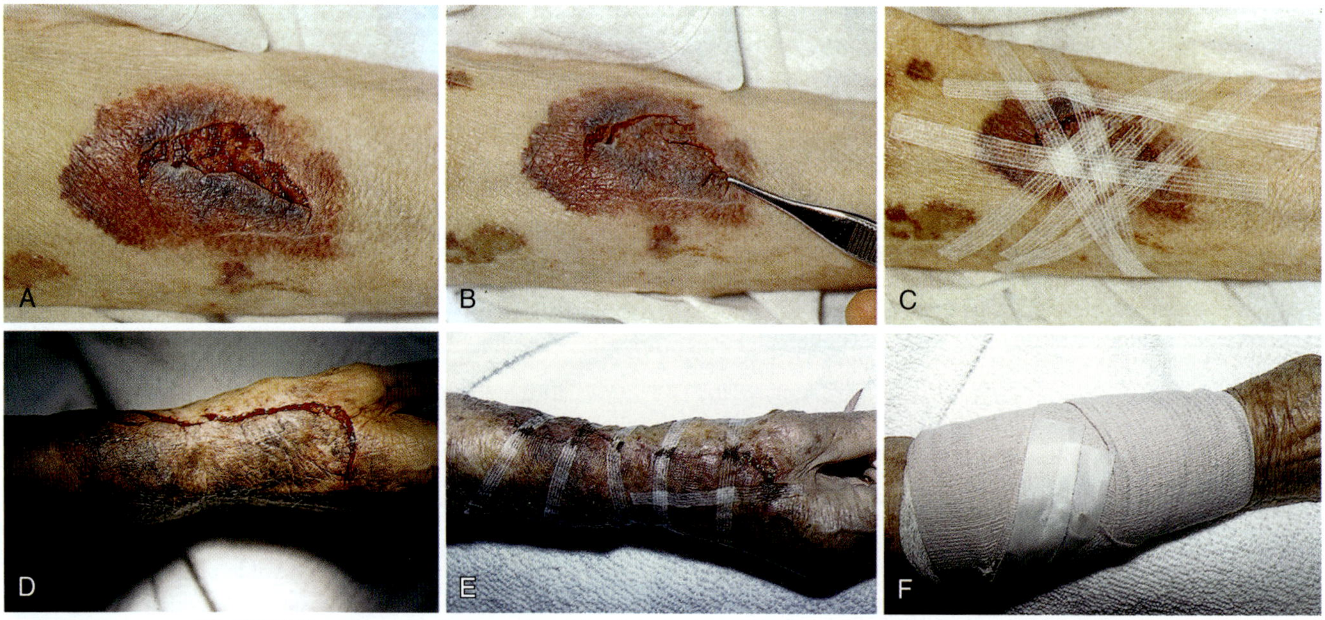

Fig. 35.2 Wound tape in the care of avulsion injuries is preferred over sutures (see Fig. 35.5). A skin avulsion in the elderly following minor trauma is an ideal wound to repair with closure tape because such injuries cannot be closed with sutures. The goal is to provide approximation of the avulsed skin and apply pressure to avoid movement of the skin flap or accumulation of fluid under the avulsion. Tissue glue can augment this procedure. (A) An elderly female who was taking steroids had extremely thin skin and sustained a skin avulsion that could not be repaired with sutures. (B) The skin edges are uncurled, stretched, and anatomically replaced. (C) The wound should heal while closure tape keeps the skin in place. Tissue glue (Dermabond) was also dabbed on various parts of the edges to allow egress of fluid. (D) Another elderly patient with a large avulsion injury on the forearm. (E) Repair with Steri-Strips and skin glue. (F) A compression dressing, such as an elastic bandage or a Dome paste (Unna boot) dressing, can be applied to minimize movement of the flap and decrease buildup of fluid under the flap.

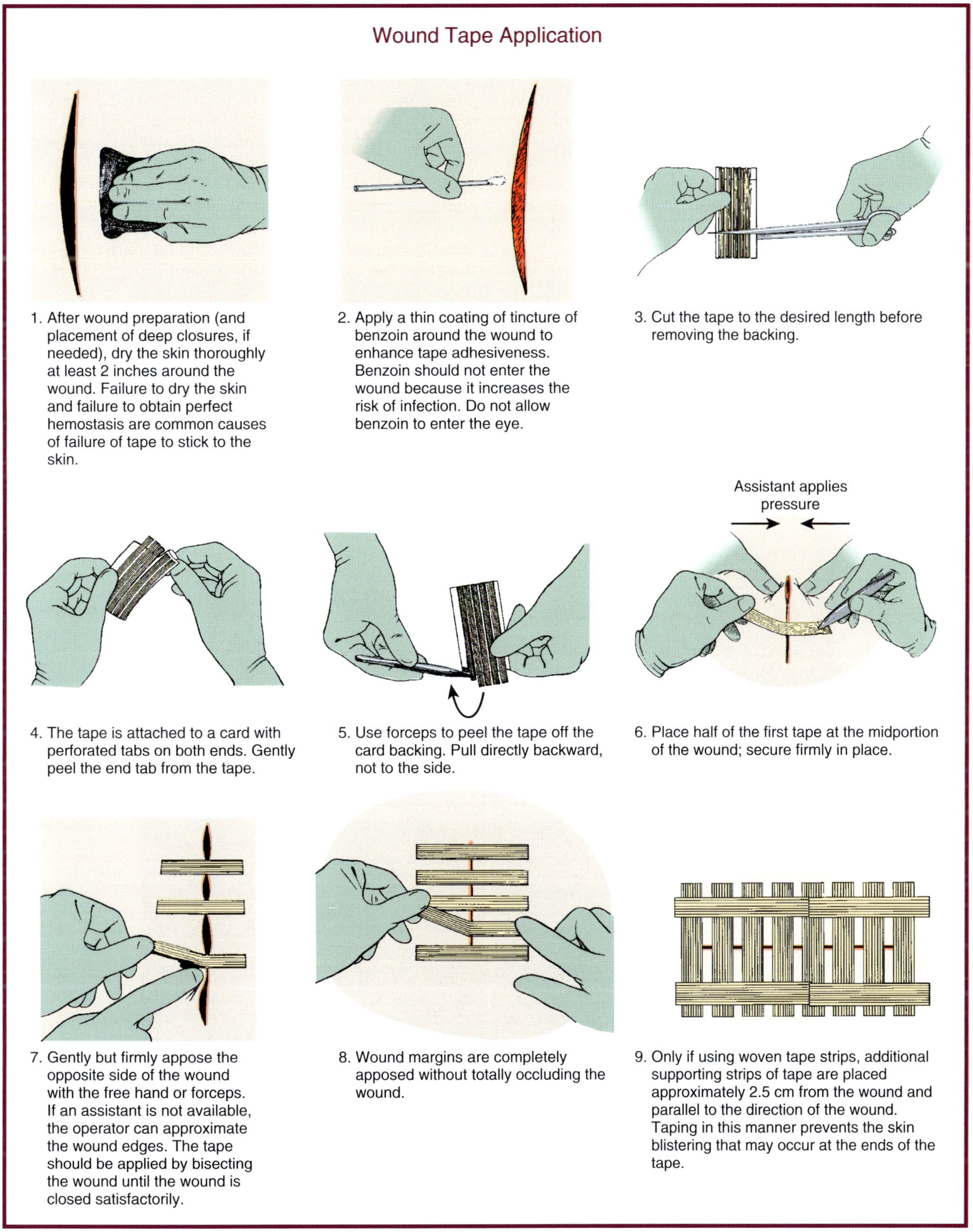

Fig. 35.4 Proper technique for the application of wound tape.

off the tape from its backing using forceps by pulling straight back. Do not pull to the side because the tape will curl and be difficult to apply to the wound. Place half of the tape securely on one side at the midportion of the wound. Gently but firmly appose the opposite wound edge to its counterpart. Apply the second half of the tape next. Hold the wound edges as close together as possible and at equal height to prevent the development of a linear, pitted scar. Apply additional tape by bisecting the remainder of the wound. Place a sufficient number of tape strips so that the wound is completely apposed without totally covering the entire length of the wound. An arrangement of tape strips parallel to each other and perpendicular to the wound provides good tape adherence over time.[15] Finally, if using a woven tape, place additional cross strips to add support and prevent blistering caused by unsupported tape ends. Cross strips are unnecessary when using nonwoven tape, such as Steri-Strip or Shur-Strip, because nonwoven tapes have sufficient ability to elongate, which also prevents blister formation.[15,16] The use of cross strips with nonwoven tape actually decreases the longevity of tape adherence.[15]

Do not cover taped wounds with occlusive dressings. Adhesive bandages (e.g., Band-Aids) and other impermeable dressings promote excessive moisture, leading to premature separation of tape strips from the wound. An adhesive bandage may also adhere to the tapes and pull them off the skin during dressing changes. If necessary, keep the tape in place for approximately 2 weeks or longer. Instruct the patient to clean the taped laceration gently with a slightly moist, soft cloth after 24 to 48 hours. However, emphasize that if excessive wetting or mechanical force is used, premature tape separation may result. Instruct patients to gently trim the curled edges of the closure tape with fine scissors to avoid premature loss of the tape.

Pretibial lacerations, particularly in the aged and in those with thin skin, may be challenging to manage. Some studies of pretibial lacerations suggest using wound tape alone.[17,18] However, wounds in this location are under great tension, and wound tape alone may be inadequate. Several studies have shown good results with a combination of tape and sutures.[19–23] The approach by Silk[19] showed improved healing time and decreased need for skin grafting (Fig. 35.5). Steri-Strips are placed parallel to and 1 cm from the wound edges, and then 2-0 silk sutures are used to approximate the wound margins. For flap-type lacerations, an immobilizing suture placed in the middle of the flap would act much like a button, lessening the tension along the wound margins. Kitcat et al. found that placing wound tape perpendicular to the wound is also beneficial for supporting closure of thin skin.[24] Bain and colleagues advocate using tissue glue rather than tissue tape to support suture placement.[25]

Complications

Complications are uncommon with tape closure. The wound infection rate in clean wounds closed with tape compares favorably with rates for other standard closures. The cosmetic result of closure with wound tape is also comparable with other closure methods.[1,4–6] Premature tape separation

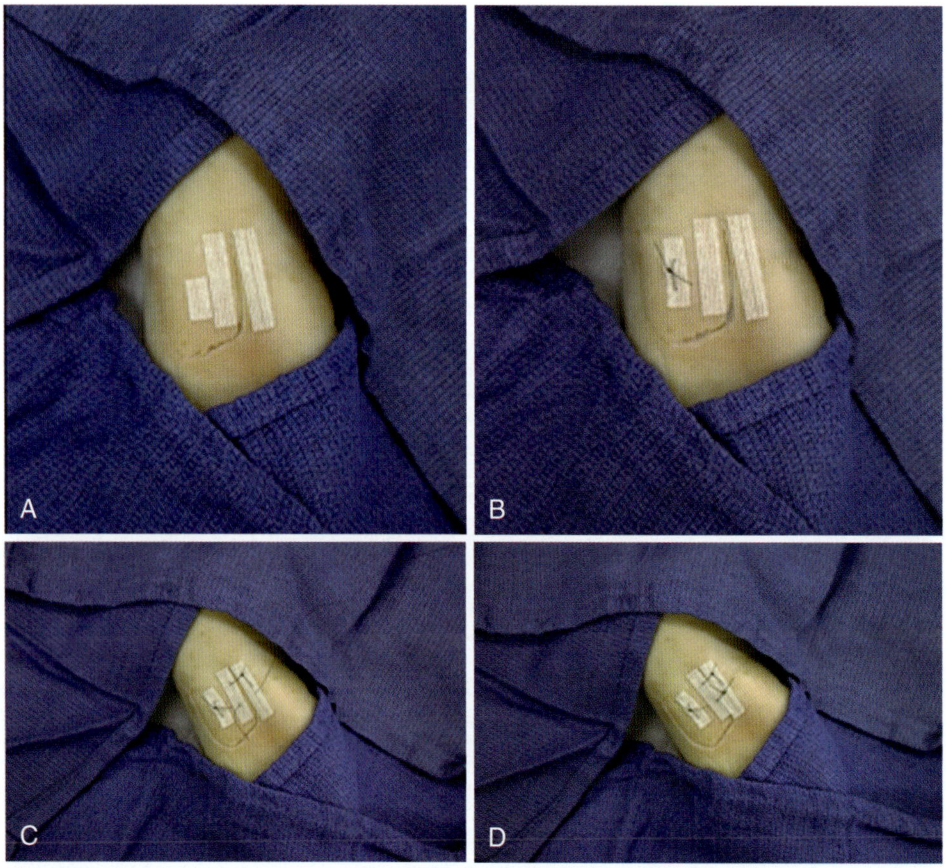

Fig. 35.5 (A) Strips of wound tape are placed parallel to the wound on both sides, approximately 1 cm from the wound margin. A strip of tape is also placed in the center of the thin flap. These strips will support the stitches and prevent them from tearing through the fragile tissue. (B) A stitch is placed through the center strip of tape, tacking the flap to the base of the wound and reducing the tension along the wound margins. (C) The needle is passed through the two strips that are parallel to the wound, and the knot is tied with minimal tension. (D) Additional strips of tape are placed around the other two sides of the flap, which is sutured in place. (Modified from Silk J. A new approach to the management of pretibial lacerations, *Injury* 32:375, 2001.)

can occur. Tape may loosen prematurely over shaved areas as hair grows back. Other complications include (1) skin blistering, which occurs if the tape is stretched too tightly across the wound, and (2) wound hematoma, which can result in inadequate hemostasis.

When a tincture of benzoin is used, it should be applied carefully to the surrounding, uninjured skin. Spillage into the wound can increase the risk of infection. Benzoin vapor can cause pain when applied near an open wound that has not been anesthetized. Benzoin can also injure the conjunctival and corneal membranes of the eye.

Summary

Modern tape products and techniques serve a valuable role in the management of minor wounds in the ED. In selected wounds, tape closure is as successful as suture closure. Closure tape should be considered for superficial wounds in cosmetically unimportant areas and for wounds on relatively flat surfaces that are too wide for simple dressings but do not require sutures.

TISSUE ADHESIVE/TISSUE TAPE COMBINATION MATERIAL

While these may not readily be available to the emergency clinician, combination materials such as Leukosan Skin Link have shown promise as a faster method of wound closure with comparable cosmetic results when compared with suturing.[26,27] Another combination product is the Zip Closure; however, its use is limited to linear wounds only.[28]

TISSUE ADHESIVE (TISSUE GLUE)

Tissue adhesive (also called *tissue glue*) provides a simple, rapid method of wound closure that is likely underused. Tissue adhesive has been approved for use in the United States since 1998. Two types of tissue adhesive are available: 2-octylcyanoacrylate (Dermabond, Ethicon, Inc.; derma+flex QS, Chemence Medical Products; SurgiSeal, Adhezion Biomedical) and *N*-butyl-2-cyanoacrylate (Indermil, Connexicon Medical Ltd.; Histoacryl, TissueSeal LLC). GluSeal (GluStitch, Inc.) and LiquiBand (Advanced Medical Solutions) both are blends of an octylcyanoacrylate and butylcyanoacrylate. Animal studies have shown octylcyanoacrylate-based adhesive to have significantly greater strength and flexibility than butylcyanoacrylate-based adhesive. Dermabond Advanced has better viscosity as well as strength and flexibility among the products in this catagory.[29,30] Dermabond, like other tissue adhesives, is packaged in sterile, single-use ampules (Fig. 35.6 and Video 35.3). These bonding agents can be used on superficial wounds, even in hair-bearing areas. Tissue adhesives polymerize on contact with water, body tissue, or blood causing strong adhesion.[31] These substances are biodegradable but remain in the wound until well after healing.[32,33] Tissue adhesive has also been shown to be useful in closure of scalp lacerations using hair apposition techniques (see later section on "Scalp Lacerations") and in both repairing nail bed lacerations and securing the nail plate to the nail bed (see later section on "Nail Bed Lacerations").

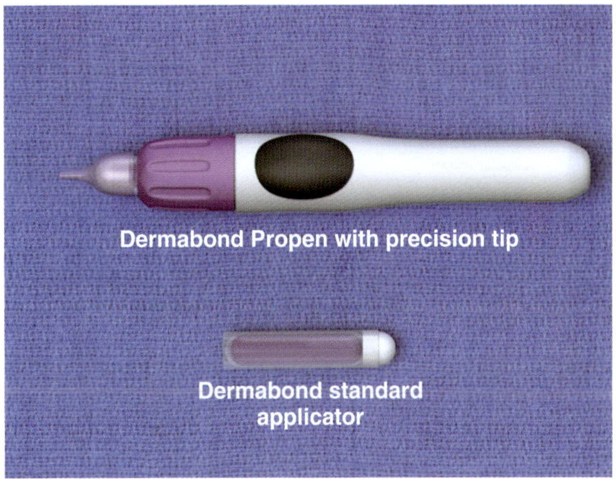

Fig. 35.6 Tissue adhesive, 2-octylcyanoacrylate, comes in a variety of commercially available dispensers.

Procedure

Tissue adhesive can be used to approximate wounds that do not require deep-layer closure and do not have significant tension on the edges of the wound (Fig. 35.7). In preparation for closure, clean and anesthetize the wound. Debride the wound if necessary. It is especially important to control bleeding from the wound.

Hold the wound edges with forceps, gauze pads, wound tape, or fingers. Squeeze the small, cylindrical plastic container to expel droplets of tissue adhesive through the cotton-tipped applicator at the end of the container. Apply the adhesive in at least three to four thin layers along the length of the wound's surface and extend it approximately 5 to 10 mm from each side of the wound. The purple color of the solution facilitates placement of the droplets. Support and hold the wound's edges together for at least 1 minute while the adhesive dries. Low-viscosity tissue adhesives may seep into the wound or trickle off rounded surfaces during application. This tendency toward migration or "runoff" can be minimized by using high-viscosity adhesives[34] (e.g., Dermabond HV Topical Skin Adhesive), positioning the wound horizontally, or applying the adhesive slowly. Contain runoff with wet gauze or by creating a barrier of petrolatum.

Wound closures with tissue adhesive can be reinforced by pulling the edges of the wound into apposition with a few strips of porous surgical tape before the adhesive is applied. Tissue adhesive can be placed on top of surgical tape, but tape should not be placed on top of dried tissue adhesive. Once the adhesive has dried completely, further protect the closure with a nonocclusive bandage.

Tissue adhesives can also be used to treat superficial skin tears that do not extend past the dermis. After the wound and skin flap are cleaned, lay the flap over the base of the wound and approximate the edges of the wound. Express any remaining blood and serum from under the flap, and ensure the entire area is dry. Apply a thin adhesive layer over the wound margins and 1 cm to 2 cm beyond the margin. After the first layer dries, apply a second layer of adhesive. To facilitate the drying of tissue adhesive, a warm overhead light may be brought near the wound.[35] A dressing is not required unless there is a reason to protect the wound from repeated injury.[36,37]

The primary advantage of tissue adhesive is the speed of closure. Wounds can be closed in as little as one-sixth the time required for repair with sutures. Application is rapid and painless. The use of tissue adhesive avoids suture marks adjacent to the wound and reduces the risk of needlestick injuries to healthcare personnel. Wounds closed with tissue adhesive

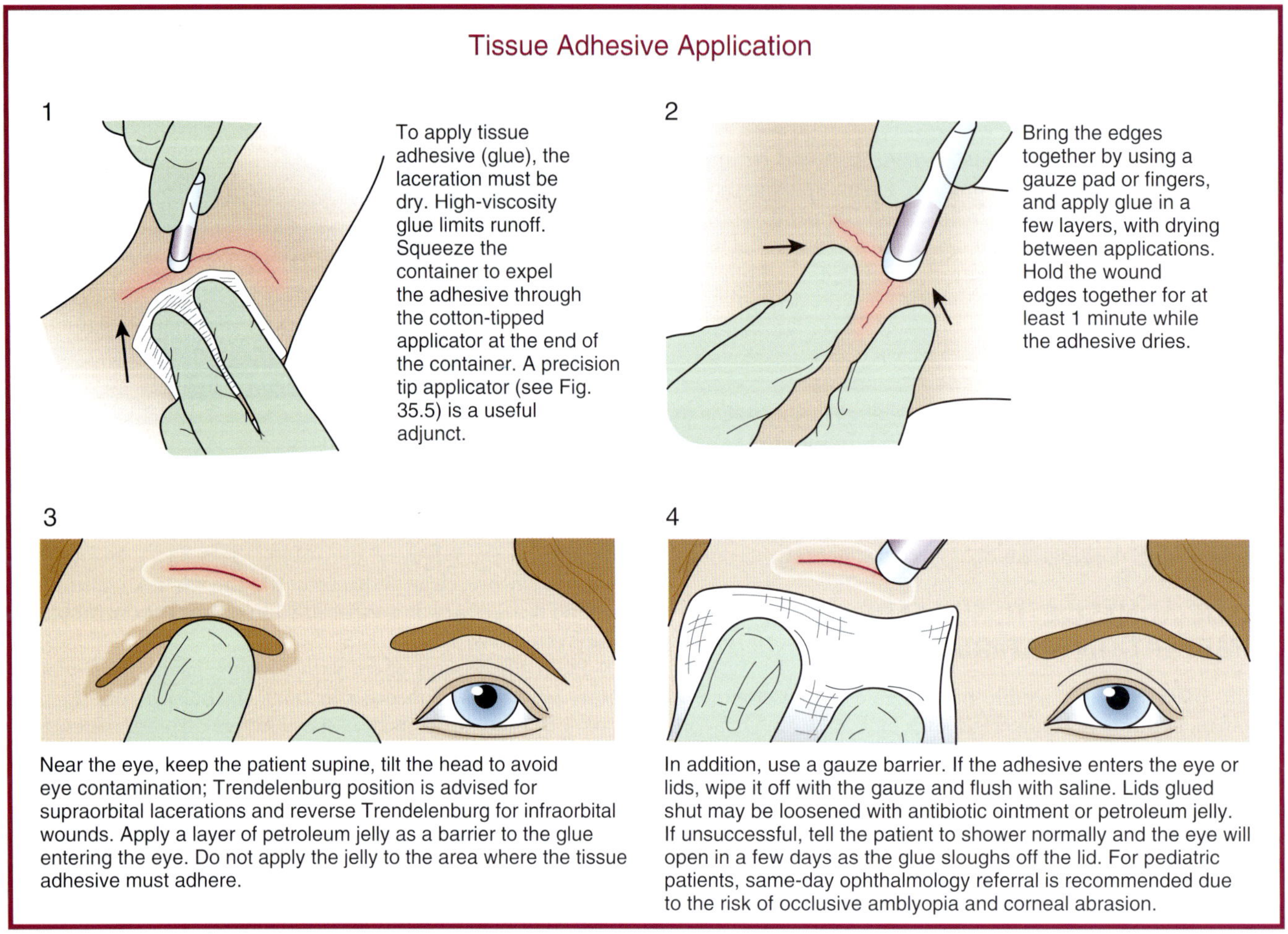

Fig. 35.7 Application of tissue adhesive. Note: glue that touches a latex glove, gauze, or a plastic instrument (but not vinyl gloves or metal instruments) will cause them to stick to the patient.

have less tensile strength in the first 4 days than do sutured wounds,[38,39] but 1 week after closure, the tensile strength and overall degree of inflammation in wounds closed with tissue adhesive are equivalent to those closed with sutures.[33,40,41] Cosmetic results are similar to those obtained with suture repair.[39,42–51] Tissue adhesive serves as its wound dressing and has an antimicrobial effect against gram-positive organisms.[52,53] The material sloughs off in 5 to 10 days, saving the patient from another visit to a clinician. Do not apply ointments or occlusive bandages onto wounds closed with tissue adhesive.

Complications

Tissue adhesive is classified as nontoxic. Some authors warn against placing it within the wound cavity.[39,40] However, several investigators have applied specially formulated octyl-2-octylcyanoacrylate (*liquid adhesive bandage*) directly to open minor lacerations, abrasions, and partial-thickness wounds. Recent studies suggest that intraoral use of tissue adhesive is safe (see section on "Lip and Intraoral Lacerations" later in this chapter). Though rare, exudates, pain, tenderness, swelling, and foreign body reactions have been reported after tissue adhesive has entered the wound.[54,55] When compared with sutures, oral wounds closed with tissue adhesive had equivalent rates of healing and complications.[56,57]

If hemostasis is inadequate or an excessive amount of adhesive is applied too quickly, the patient can experience a burning sensation or sustain a local burn from the heat of polymerization. After polymerizing, tissue adhesive can fracture with excessive or repetitive movement. Although gentle rinsing is permitted, if the adhesive is scrubbed or soaked, it will peel off in a few days before the wound is healed.[39,58]

If the clinician's gloved fingers, gauze, or plastic instruments come into contact with the tissue adhesive during the application, the glove item may adhere to the patient's skin. Tissue adhesive can be removed with antibiotic ointment or petrolatum jelly, or more rapidly with acetone.[48] Indermil (Connexicon Medical) must be stored under refrigeration.

Given their ease-of-use tissue adhesives may pose the risk of clinicians failing to adequately clean wounds beforehand.[59] Tissue adhesives should not be used to close infected wounds.

If the edges of the wound cannot be held together without considerable tension, tissue adhesive should not be used.[48] Percutaneous sutures provide a more secure immediate closure compared with tissue adhesive.[33] It should also not be used over or near joints or on wounds under significant static or dynamic skin tension. There is a slightly higher risk for wound dehiscence in closures with tissue glue than with sutures.[60,61] See Fig. 35.7 for information on managing eyelids that are accidentally glued shut.

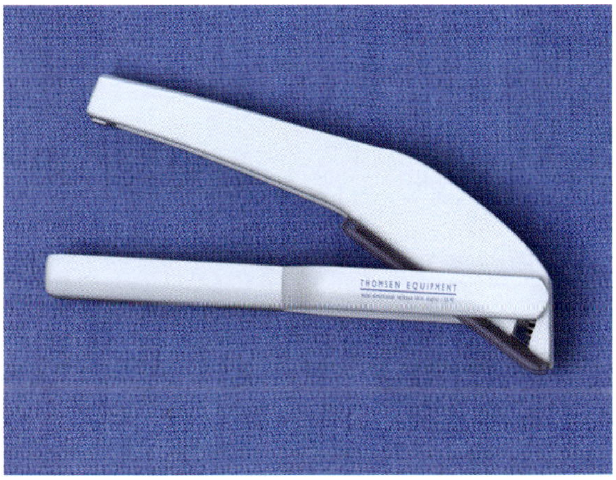

Fig. 35.8 Skin stapling device. Skin staples may be used for relatively linear lacerations with straight, sharp edges on the extremity, trunk, or scalp. Their main advantage is speed of closure. Their main disadvantage is lesser cosmesis compared with meticulous suture closure.

WOUND STAPLES

Background

Automatic stapling devices have become commonplace for closure of surgical incisions and traumatic wounds (Fig. 35.8). Clinical studies of patients with stapled surgical incisions have found no significant difference between stapling and suturing when infection rates, healing outcome, and patient acceptance are compared.[62–65] Wound stapling (Video 35.4) and nylon suture closure of skin compared favorably in wound tensile strength, complication rates, patient tolerance, closure efficiency, scar width, color, general appearance, suture or staple marks, infection rates, and cost. In animal models, staples caused less wound inflammation and offered more resistance to infection within contaminated wounds.[67–78]

The most significant advantage of wound stapling over suturing is speed of closure. The most significant downside is an inferior cosmetic outcome compared with meticulous suture closure. On average, stapling is three to four times faster than suturing traumatic wounds.[59] When clinician time and cost of instruments are considered, the difference in cost between stapling and suturing is either minimal or favors stapling.[68,69]

Indications and Contraindications

The indications for stapling are limited to relatively linear lacerations with straight, sharp edges located on an extremity, the trunk, or the scalp. Staples may be especially useful for superficial scalp lacerations in an agitated or intoxicated patient. Because of their superficial placement in the adult scalp (usually above the galea), staples are not recommended for deep scalp lacerations. Staples may not provide the same hemostasis that is possible with deep sutures. They should not be placed in scalp wounds if computed tomography head scans are to be performed because staples produce scan artifacts. Similarly, staples should not be used if the patient is expected to undergo magnetic resonance imaging because the powerful magnetic fields may avulse the staples from the surface of the skin. Staples should not be used on the face, neck, hands, or feet.

Equipment

Standard wound care should precede wound closure. In many cases, when debridement and dermal (deep) closure are unnecessary, only tissue forceps are needed to assist in everting wounds.

Many stapling devices are commercially available. The Precise stapler is the most versatile and least expensive (3M Corporation). Different units that hold between 5 and 25 staples can be purchased. The 10-staple unit will suffice for most lacerations. Other devices include the Proximate 11 (Ethicon, Inc.), Appose (Covidien), and Reflex One (ConMed).

A novel device, the Insorb (Incisive Surgical, Inc.) absorbable stapler, uses absorbable staples (made of polylactic and polyglycolic acids) placed intradermally. The device has shown both time and cost savings in repair of abdominal and breast surgical wounds comparable with intradermal sutures.[70,71] The device is not widely available in the emergency setting.

Procedure

Before stapling, it is sometimes necessary to place deep, absorbable sutures to close deep fascia and reduce tension in the superficial and dermal layers. To facilitate the stapling process, the wound's edges should be everted, preferably by a second operator (Fig. 35.9, *step 1*). The assistant precedes the operator along the wound and everts the edges of the wound with forceps or pinches the skin with the thumb and forefinger. Stapling flattened wound edges may place the staple precisely but results in inversion of the wound. Once the edges are held in eversion, the staple points are gently placed across the wound. The center of the staple device should be placed over the center of the wound to ensure the best closure and to avoid overriding or misaligned edges (which can be difficult in an uncooperative patient). When the stapler handle or trigger is squeezed, the staple is advanced automatically into the wound and bent to the proper configuration (Fig. 35.9, *steps 2 and 3*). The operator should not press too hard on the skin surface to prevent placing the staple too deeply and causing ischemia within the staple loop. When placed properly, the crossbar of the staple is elevated a few millimeters above the skin's surface (Fig. 35.9, *step 4*). A sufficient number of staples should be placed to properly apposition the edges of the wound along its entire length. (One suggested method is to place a staple in the midpoint of the length of the wound and then bisect either side of the wound with additional staples. Continue the process until the edges of the wound are well opposed.) After the wound is stapled, an antibiotic ointment may be applied. Stapled wounds may be left uncovered, or a sterile dressing may be applied. The patient can remove the dressing and gently clean the wound in 24 to 48 hours. Scalp lacerations can be cleansed by showering within a few hours.

Removal of staples requires a special instrument made available by each manufacturer of stapling devices. The lower jaw of the staple remover is placed under the crossbar, and the handle is squeezed (Fig. 35.9, *steps 5 and 6*). This action compresses the crossbar and bends the staple outward, thereby releasing the points of the staple from the skin. Many primary care physicians do not routinely stock the instrument. If referred to a primary care physician's office for removal of staples, the patient can be given a disposable staple removal device to bring with them. If well instructed, patients or their

Wound Staples

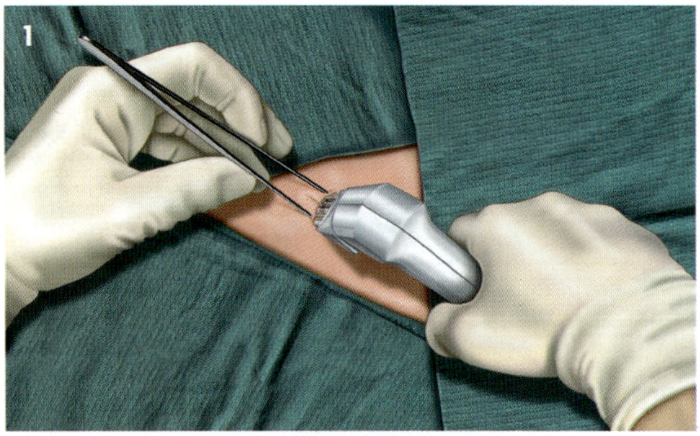

Approximate and evert the skin edges by hand or with forceps before they are secured with staples. If possible, have an assistant perform this duty. Failure to evert the wound edges is a common error that may cause an unacceptable result.

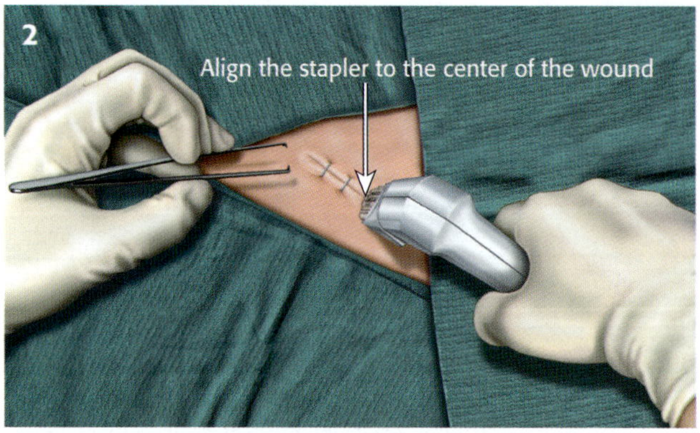

Align the center of the stapler over the center of the wound. Squeeze the stapler handle to advance one staple into the wound margins. Do not press too hard on the skin to prevent placing the staple too deeply.

3

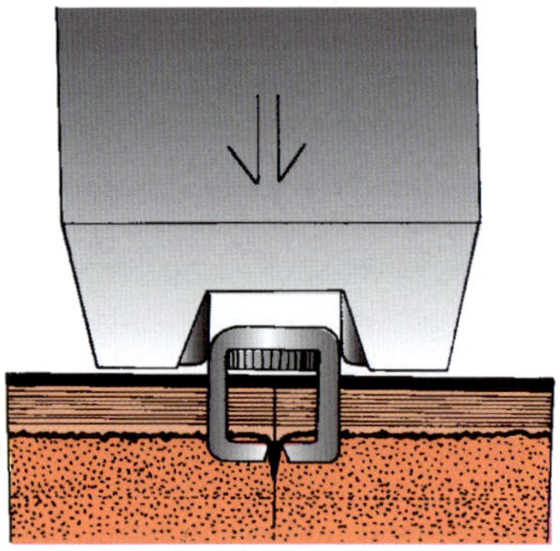

As the handle is squeezed, an anvil automatically bends the staple to the proper configuration.

4

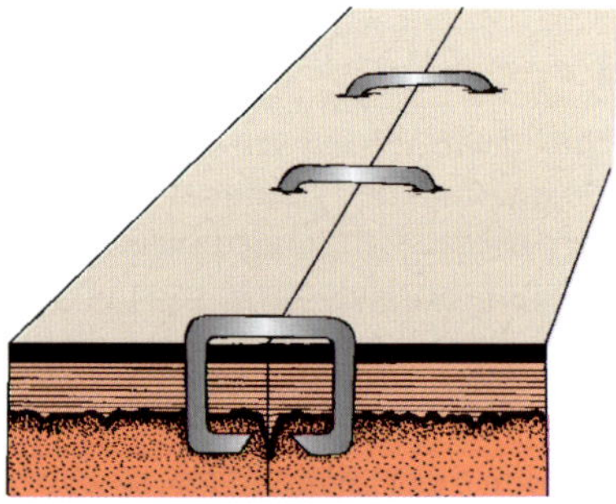

Allow a small space to remain between the skin and the crossbar of the staple. Excessive pressure created by placing the staple too deep causes wound edge ischemia, as well as pain on removal. Note that the staple bar is 2 to 3 mm above the skin line.

5

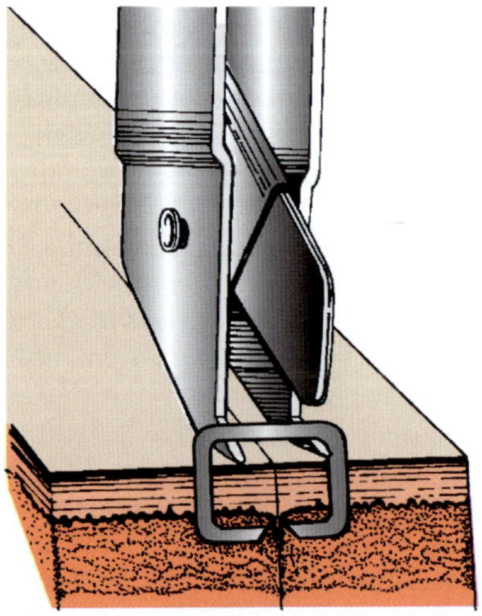

Supply the patient with a staple remover when being referred to an office for removal or for self-removal. To remove the staple, place the lower jaw of the remover under the crossbar of the staple.

6

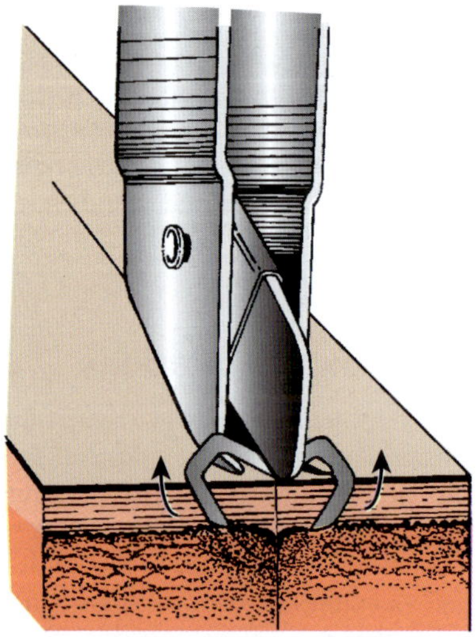

Squeeze the handle gently, and the upper jaw will compress the staple and allow it to exit the skin.

Fig. 35.9 Wound staples. Failure to align the center of the staple device directly over the center of the laceration is a common cause of inadequate staple closure. (Steps 1 and 2, from Custalow C. *Color Atlas of Emergency Department Procedures.* Elsevier; 2005; steps 3–6, from Edlich RF. *A Manual for Wound Closure.* 3M Medical-Surgical Products; 1979.)

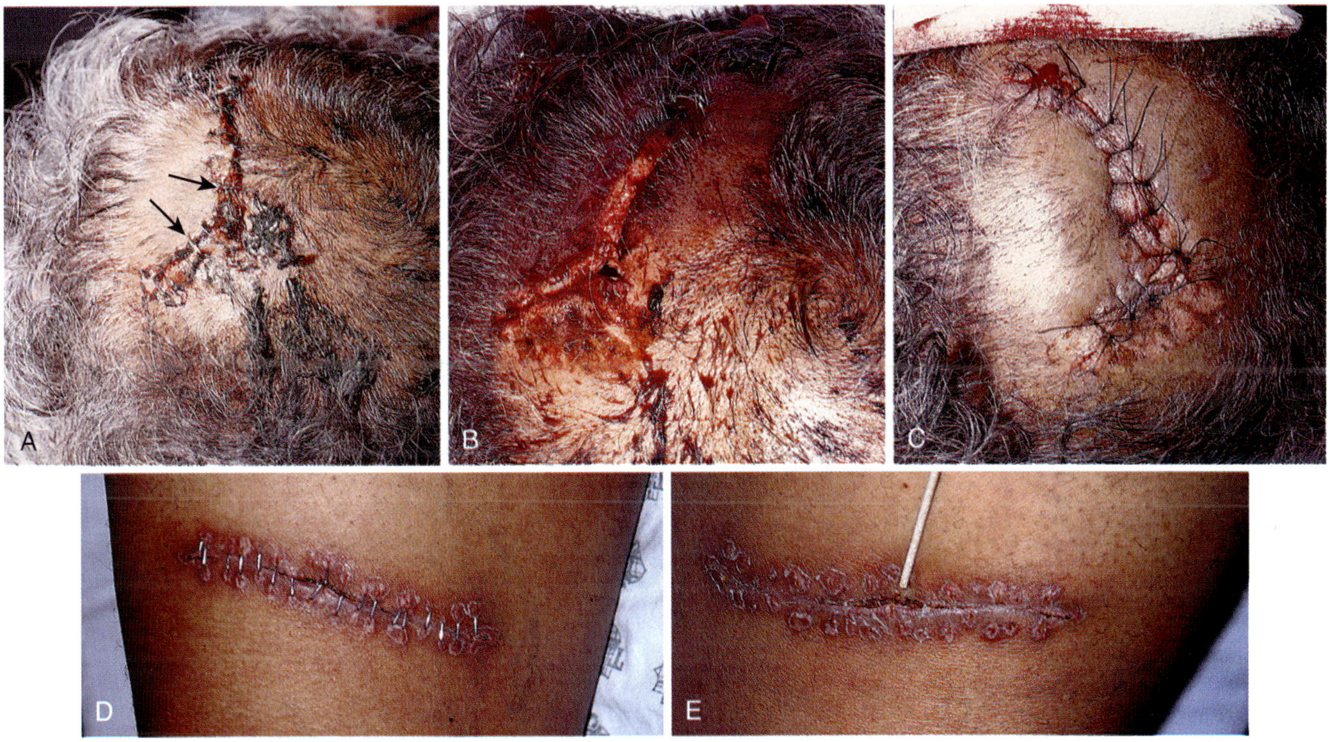

Fig. 35.10 (A) A very poor result occurred when staples (some marked with *arrows*) were used to close this deep scalp laceration. The edges of the wound were not everted, staples were not in the midline, sections of the skin overlapped significantly, poor hemostasis was obtained, and the galea could not be closed by the superficial staples. The patient did not wash his hair as instructed. (B) Three days later during inspection of the wound, the staples were removed and (C) the laceration was closed with 3-0 interrupted nylon sutures. The clinician should attempt to obtain a cosmetic closure on all scalp lacerations because as patients lose their hair, a previously hidden, unsightly scar emerges. In general, staples should not be used to close full-thickness scalp lacerations, especially wounds that are actively bleeding. (D) Sloppy stapling on an extremity with inversion rather than eversion of the edges of the wound. Some staples are totally misaligned and barely include the opposite skin edge. (E) The staples were left in too long, which caused a poor cosmetic result.

parents (for pediatric patients) can remove their staples with the removal device.[72] The interval between staple application and removal is the same as for standard suture placement and removal. Staples can cause significant scarring if left in place too long (Fig. 35.10).

Complications

Patient acceptance, comfort, rates of wound infection, and dehiscence are similar with staple-closed wounds and sutured wounds. However, removing staples can be somewhat more uncomfortable than removing sutures.

The stapler tends to invert the wound edges during the closure. This can be prevented by everting the edges of the skin before stapling (see Fig. 35.10). Eversion may be accomplished with forceps or by pinching the skin with the thumb and index finger, a procedure that requires some practice. It is important to place the middle of the staple exactly in the midline of the wound.

Staples will cause marks in the skin that are similar to sutures. However, in patients who tend to scar more easily, the scar resulting from staples may be more pronounced than that produced by sutures, especially if the staples are left in place for prolonged periods.

Wound stapling achieves results generally comparable with those of sutures for the closure of traumatic, linear lacerations in noncosmetic areas, such as the scalp, trunk, and extremities. Stapling is much faster than suturing. Wound stapling does not differ significantly from suturing in terms of cost, infection rates, wound healing, and patient acceptance, but cosmesis may suffer, especially if the staples are left in too long (see Fig. 35.10D–E).

SUTURES

In the United States, most traumatic wounds are closed by suturing.

Equipment

Instruments

In addition to the instruments used for debridement, a needle holder and suture scissors are required for suturing (Fig. 35.11). The mechanical performance of disposable needle holders distributed by different surgical instrument companies varies considerably.[73] The needle holder should match the size of the needle selected for suturing; the needle holder should be large enough to hold the needle securely as it is passed through tissue, yet not so large that the needle is crushed or bent by the instrument.

Instruments used to debride a grossly contaminated wound should be discarded and replaced with fresh instruments for

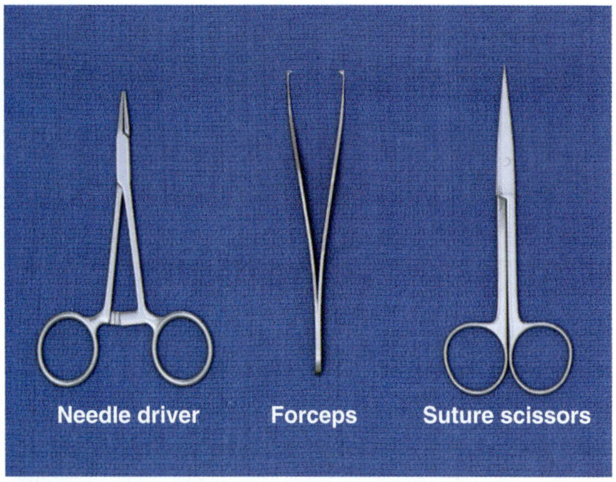

Fig. 35.11 Basic suturing equipment includes a needle driver, forceps, and suture scissors.

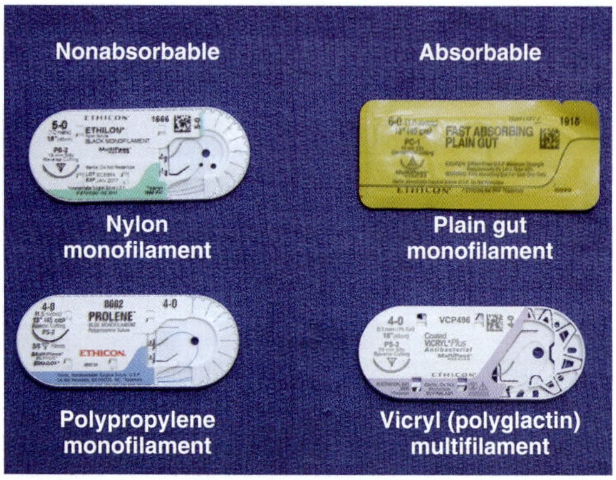

Fig. 35.12 A wide variety of both absorbable and nonabsorbable suture material is available. Other variables include suture size (e.g., 4-0, 5-0, 6-0), needle size, and type (e.g., PS-2, reverse cutting, conventional cutting). These variables are discussed in detail in the text.

closure. Instruments covered with coagulated blood can be cleansed with hydrogen peroxide, rinsed with sterile saline or water, and then used for suturing. In addition, 2.5-loupe magnification may improve inspection of wounds and facilitate the repair of facial and hand wounds.[74]

Suture Material

Various suture materials are available to satisfy clinician preferences (Fig. 35.12). There are no definitive standards on which to base the use of suture material for a particular wound or site. For most wounds that require closure of more than one layer of tissue, the clinician must choose sutures from two general categories: an absorbable suture for the deeper, subcutaneous (SQ) layer and a nonabsorbable suture for surface (percutaneous) closure. Some recent studies suggest the usage of absorbable sutures for surface closure.[75–77]

Sutures can be described in terms of four characteristics:

1. Composition (i.e., chemical and physical properties).
2. Handling characteristics and mechanical performance.
3. Absorption and reactivity.
4. Size and retention of tensile strength.

TABLE 35.1 Commonly Available Suture Material

ABSORBABLE SUTURE	NONABSORBABLE SUTURE
Monofilament	
Plain gut	Dermalon (nylon)
Chromic gut	Ethilon (nylon)
PDS (polydioxanone)	Novafil (polybutester)
Maxon (polyglyconate)	Prolene (polypropylene)
Biosyn (glycomer 631)	Steel Surgilene (polypropylene) Tevdek (Teflon coated)
Monocryl (poliglecaprone 25)	Silk
Multifilament	
Dexon (polyglycolic acid)	Ethibond (polyethylene)
Coated Vicryl (polyglactin 910)	Mersilene (braided polyester) Nurolon (nylon) Surgilon (nylon) Ti-Cron (polyester)

Composition

Sutures are made from natural fibers (cotton, silk), from sheep submucosa or beef serosa (plain gut, chromic gut), or synthetic material such as nylon (Dermalon and Surgilon, Medtronic; Ethilon and Nurolon, Ethicon Inc.), Dacron (Ethiflex and Mersilene, Ethicon Inc.), polyester (Ti-Cron, Medtronic), polyethylene (Ethibond, Ethicon Inc.), polypropylene (Prolene, Ethicon Inc.; Surgipro, Medtronic), polyglycolic acid (Dexon, Medtronic), and polyglactin (Vicryl, coated Vicryl, Vicryl Rapide, Ethicon Inc.). Stainless steel sutures are rarely, if ever useful in wound closure in the ED setting because of handling difficulty and fragmentation. Some sutures are made of a single filament (monofilament); others consist of multiple fibers braided together (Table 35.1).

Handling and Performance

Desirable handling characteristics in a suture include smooth passage through tissue, ease in knot tying, and stability of the knot once tied (Table 35.2). Smooth sutures pull through tissue easily, but knots slip more readily. Conversely, sutures with a high coefficient of friction have better knot-holding capacity but are more difficult to slide through tissue. Smooth sutures will loosen after the first throw of a knot is made, and thus, a second throw is needed to secure the first in place. Rougher, multifilament types of suture make it more difficult to tighten a knot further after the first throw is made.

Multifilament sutures have the best handling characteristics of all sutures, whereas steel sutures have the worst. In terms of performance and handling, significant improvements have been made in the newer absorbable sutures. Gut sutures have many shortcomings, including relatively low and variable strength, a tendency to fray when handled, and stiffness despite being packaged in a softening fluid. Multifilament synthetic absorbable sutures are soft and easy to tie and have few

TABLE 35.2 Characteristics of Suture Material

SUTURE MATERIAL	KNOT SECURITY	TENSILE STRENGTH	TISSUE REACTIVITY	DURATION OF SUTURE INTEGRITY (DAYS)	TIE ABILITY (HANDLING)
Absorbable					
Surgical gut	Poor	Fair	Greatest	5–7	Poor
Chromic gut	Fair	Fair	Greatest	10–14	Poor
Coated Vicryl	Good	Good	Minimal	30	Best
Dexon	Best	Good	Minimal	30	Best
PDS	Fair	Best	Least	45–60	Good
Maxon	Fair	Best	Least	45–60	Good
Biosyn	Poor	Good	Minimal	14–21	Good
Monocryl	Good	Best	Minimal	7	Good
Vicryl Rapide	Good	Good	Minimal	5	Good
Nonabsorbable					
Ethilon	Good	Good	Minimal	—	Good
Novafil	Good	Good	Minimal	—	Good
Prolene	Least	Best	Least	—	Fair
Silk	Best	Least	Greatest	—	Best

PDS, Polydioxanone.
Modified with permission from Hollander J, Singer A. Laceration management. *Ann Emerg Med*. 1999;34:351. Data from Regula C, Yag-Howard C. Suture products and techniques: what to use, where, and why. *Dermatol Surg*. 2015;41:S190-S191.

problems with knot slippage. Polyglactin 910 (coated Vicryl) sutures have an absorbable lubricant coating. The frictional drag of these coated sutures as they are pulled through tissue is less than that of uncoated multifilament materials, and resetting of knots after the initial throw is much easier. This characteristic allows retightening of a ligature without knotting or breakage and with smooth, even adjustment of suture line tension in running subcuticular stitches. Synthetic monofilament sutures have the troublesome property of "memory": a tendency of the filament to spring back to its original shape, which causes the knot to slip and unravel. Some nonabsorbable monofilament sutures are coated with polytetrafluoroethylene (Teflon) or silicone to reduce their friction. This coating improves the handling characteristics of these monofilaments but results in poorer knot security.[68]

Three square knots will secure a stitch made with silk or other braided nonabsorbable material and four knots are sufficient for synthetic, absorbable, and nonabsorbable monofilament sutures. Five knots are needed for the Teflon-coated synthetic Tevdek (Teleflex). When coated synthetic suture material is used, attention to basic principles of knot tying is even more important. An excessive number of throws in a knot weakens the suture at the knot. If the clinician uses square knots (or a surgeon's knot on the initial throw, followed by square knots) that lie down flat and are tied securely, knots will rarely unravel.

Absorption and Reactivity

Sutures that are rapidly degraded in tissue are termed absorbable; those that maintain their tensile strength for longer than 60 days are considered nonabsorbable (see Table 35.1). Plain gut may be digested by white blood cell lysozymes in 10 to 40 days; chromic gut will last 15 to 60 days. Remnants of both types of suture, however, have been seen in wounds more than 2 years after placement. Ethicon catgut is rapidly absorbed within 10 to 14 days and is associated with less inflammation than chromic catgut.[78] Polydioxanone (PDS; Ethicon) and Vicryl produce less tissue reaction and erythema than polypropylene.[79] Vicryl is absorbed from the wound site within 60 to 90 days and Dexon (Medtronic), within 120 to 210 days.[80] When placed in the oral cavity, plain gut disappears after 3 to 5 days, chromic gut after 7 to 10 days, and Dexon after 16 to 20 days.[81] When used on the skin surface, fast-absorbing catgut disappears in 9 to 13 days.[82] In contrast, SQ silk may not be completely absorbed for as long as 2 years.

Comparison of suture strength versus wound strength is a measure of the usefulness of a suture. Sutures may lose strength and function before they are completely absorbed in tissues. Sutures made of natural fibers such as silk, cotton, and gut are the weakest. Sutures made of Dacron, nylon, polyethylene, and polypropylene have greater tensile strength. Braided synthetic absorbable sutures lose nearly all their strength after approximately 21 days. In contrast, monofilament absorbable sutures (modified polyglycolic acid, Maxon, Davis & Geck; and PDS) retain 60% of their strength after 28 days.[83] Gut sutures treated with chromium salts (chromic gut) have prolonged tensile strength; however, all gut sutures retain tensile strength erratically. Polyglycolic acid suture is stronger than a plain or chromic gut suture. Polypropylene remains unchanged in tissue for longer than 2 years.[84] Catgut is stronger than the wound for no more than 7 days; chromic catgut, Dexon, and Vicryl are stronger for 10 to 21 days; and nylon, wire, and silk are stronger for 20 to 30 days.[85]

All sutures placed within tissue will damage host defenses and provoke inflammation. Even the least reactive suture impairs the ability of the wound to resist infection.[84] The magnitude of the reaction provoked by a suture is related to the quantity of suture material (diameter × total length) placed in the tissue and to the chemical composition of the suture. Among absorbable sutures, polyglycolic acid and polyglactin sutures are the least reactive, followed by chromic gut. Nonabsorbable polypropylene is less reactive than nylon or Dacron.[86,87] Significant tissue reaction is associated with catgut, silk, and cotton sutures. Absorbable polyglycolic acid sutures are less reactive than those made of nonabsorbable silk. Avoid placing highly reactive sutures in contaminated wounds.

The chemical composition of sutures is a factor in early infection. The infection rate in experimentally contaminated wounds closed with polyglycolic acid sutures is lower than when gut sutures are used.[84] However, other authors have compared plain gut and nonabsorbable nylon sutures for skin closure in children, and Vicryl Rapide and monofilament nylon in adults, and found comparable cosmetic results and infection rates.[88]

Lubricant coatings on sutures do not alter suture reactivity, absorption characteristics, breaking strength, or the risk for infection.[84] Multifilament sutures provoke more inflammation and are more likely than monofilament sutures to produce infection if left in place for prolonged periods. Monofilament sutures elicit less tissue reaction than do multifilament sutures, and multifilament materials tend to wick up fluid by capillary action and "hide" bacteria. PDS provides the advantages of a monofilament suture in an absorbable form, thus making it a good choice as a subcuticular stitch. Vicryl Plus and Monocryl (Ethicon Inc.) have been found to have less bacterial adherence when compared with Vicryl, making these two materials reasonable choices for subcuticular closure in contaminated wounds.[89] Polypropylene sutures have a low coefficient of friction, and subcuticular stitches with this material are easy to pull out.[90]

Size and Strength

The size of suture material (thread diameter) is related to the tensile strength of the suture; threads with greater diameter are stronger. The strength of the suture is proportional to the square of the diameter of the thread. Therefore a 4-0 suture of any type is larger and stronger than a 6-0 suture. The correct suture size for approximation of a layer of tissue depends on the tensile strength of that tissue. The tensile strength of the suture material should be only slightly greater than that of the tissue.

Synthetic absorbable sutures have made the older, natural suture material unnecessary for most wound closures. Polyglycolic acid (Dexon) and polyglactin 910 (coated Vicryl) have improved handling characteristics, knot security, and tensile strength. Their absorption rates are predictable and tissue reactivity is minimal. The distinct advantages of synthetic nonabsorbable sutures over silk sutures are their greater tensile strength, low coefficient of friction, and minimal tissue reactivity.[84,91] They are extensible and elongate without breaking as the edges of the wound swell in the first few days after wound closure. Stiff suture materials can lacerate the encircled tissue as the wound swells. The monofilament synthetic suture Novafil (Medtronic) has elasticity that allows a stitch to enlarge with wound edema and to return to its original length once the edema subsides. In contrast to silk sutures, synthetics can easily and painlessly be removed once the wound has healed.

The suture material most useful to emergency clinicians for wound closure is coated Vicryl for SQ layers and synthetic nonabsorbable suture (e.g., nylon or polypropylene) for skin closure.[92] Fascia can be sutured with either absorbable or nonabsorbable material. In most situations, 3-0 or 4-0 suture is used for the repair of fascia, 4-0 or 5-0 absorbable suture for SQ closure, and 4-0 or 5-0 nonabsorbable suture for skin closure. The lips, eyelids, and skin layer of facial wounds are repaired with 5-0 or 6-0 suture,[93] whereas 3-0 or 4-0 suture is used when the edges of the skin are subjected to considerable dynamic stress (e.g., wounds overlying joint surfaces) or static stress (e.g., scalp).

Studies comparing surface closure with absorbable and nonabsorbable sutures have yielded contradictory results. Some authors report that absorbable sutures have been used as an alternative to nonabsorbable sutures for simple skin closure with similar cosmetic results, rates of wound dehiscence, and infection rates in both adult and pediatric lacerations.[88,94–97] Sutures that were evaluated include fast-absorbing gut, Vicryl Rapide, and Monocryl. Absorbable suture used for skin closure obviates the need for suture removal, and thus may be particularly advantageous in children. However, in some studies, the absorbable sutures were removed in 7 to 10 days. Some authors advise usual patient follow-up for skin closed with absorbable sutures to remove any remaining suture material and to evaluate for complications.[94,95] If removal is necessary, extraction of multifilament absorbable surface sutures is more difficult and may be more painful than removal of monofilament nonabsorbable suture material.

Needles

The eyeless, or "swaged," needle is used for wound closure in most emergency centers (Fig. 35.13). Selection of the appropriate needle size and curvature is based on the dimensions of the wound and the characteristics of the tissue to be sutured. The needle should be large enough to pass through tissue to the desired depth and then to exit the tissue or skin surface far enough that the needle holder can be repositioned on the distal end of the needle at a safe distance from the tip of the needle (Fig. 35.14). Although it is tempting to use the fingers to grasp the tip of the needle to pull it through the skin, this practice risks a needlestick and blood-borne pathogen exposure. The clinician should either reposition the needle holder or use forceps to disengage the needle from the laceration.

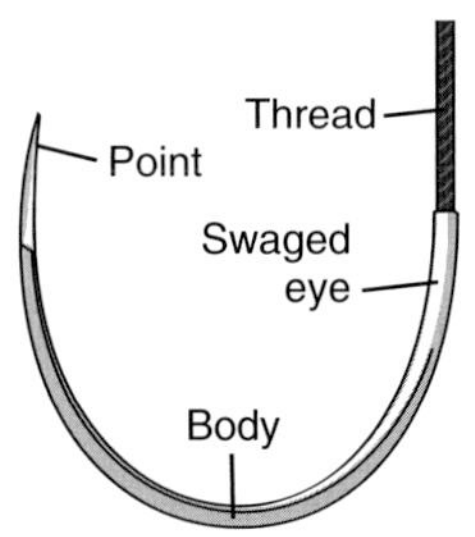

Fig. 35.13 The eyeless, or "swaged," needle. (From *Suture Use Manual: Use and Handling of Sutures and Needles.* Ethicon; 1977:29.)

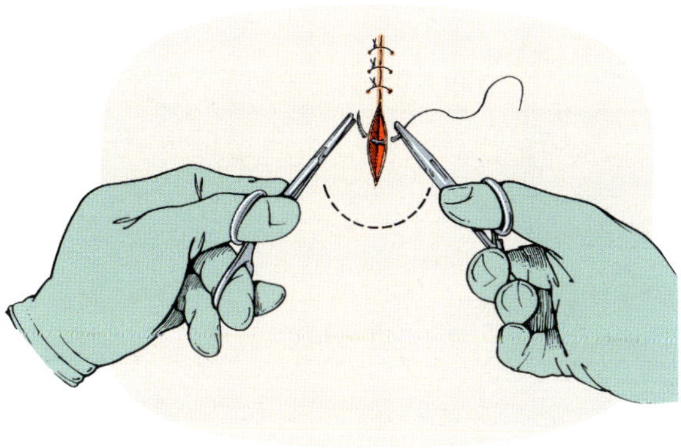

Fig. 35.14 The needle should be large enough to pass through tissue and should exit far enough to enable the needle holder to be repositioned on the end of the needle at a safe distance from the point.

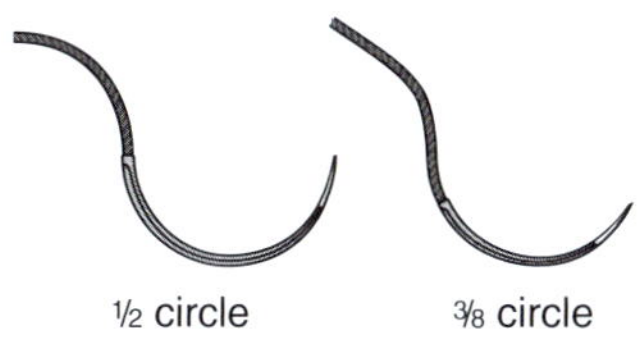

Fig. 35.15 One-half and three-eighths circle needles, used for most traumatic wound closures.

In wound repair, needles must penetrate tough, fibrous tissue (skin, SQ tissue, and fascia) yet should slice through this tissue with minimal resistance or trauma and without bending. The type of needle best suited for closure of SQ tissue is a conventional cutting needle in a three-eighths or one-half circle (Fig. 35.15). Double-curvature needles (coated Vicryl with PS-4-C cutting needles, Ethicon) may be easier to maneuver in narrow, deep wounds. For surface closure, a conventional cutting-edge needle permits more precise needle placement and requires less penetration force (Fig. 35.16).[98]

Suturing Techniques

See Figs. 35.17 and 35.18.

Skin Preparation

Before suturing, the clinician should ensure adequate exposure and illumination of the wound, and placement of the patient at the appropriate height. The clinician should assume a comfortable standing or sitting position at one end of the long axis of the wound.

The skin surrounding the wound is prepared with a povidone-iodine solution and covered with sterile drapes. A clear plastic drape (Steri-Drape, 3M Corporation) can be used to provide a sterile field and a limited view of the area surrounding the wound. Some surgeons do not drape the face but prefer to leave the facial structures and landmarks adjacent to the wound uncovered and within view. If no drapes are used on the face, the skin surrounding the wound should be widely cleansed and prepared. Wrapping the hair in a sheet or placing the patient's hair in an oversized scrub hat prevents stray hair from falling into the operating field. For a finger laceration, a sterile glove with the portion overlying the wound removed can be placed on the patient's hand to avoid using a drape.

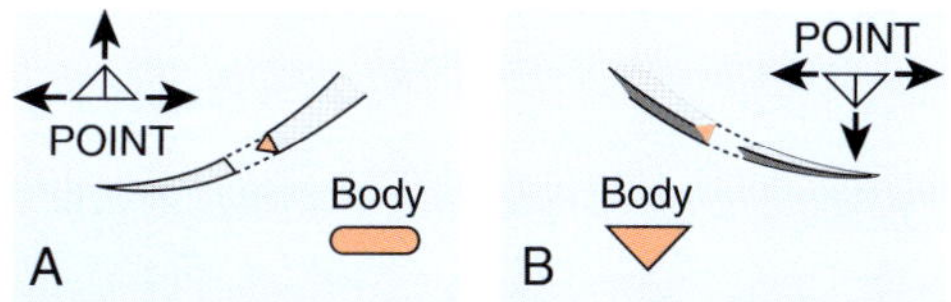

Fig. 35.16 Types of needles. (A) The conventional cutting needle has two opposing cutting edges and a third edge on the inside curvature of the needle. The conventional cutting needle changes in cross section from a triangular cutting tip to a flattened body. (B) The reverse cutting needle is used to cut through tough, difficult-to-penetrate tissue such as fascia and skin. It has two opposing cutting edges and a third cutting edge on the outer curvature of the needle. The reverse cutting needle is made with a triangular shape extending from the point to the swage area, with only the edges near the tip being sharpened. (From *Suture Use Manual: Use and Handling of Sutures and Needles*. Ethicon; 1977:31.)

Closure Principles

There is a tendency to overuse sutures for minor lacerations that will heal nicely with no intervention. Therefore before suturing, one must assess the need for the procedure (Fig. 35.19).

Three principles apply to suturing lacerations in any location: (1) minimize trauma to tissues; (2) relieve tension exerted on the edges of the wound by layered wound closure and undermining when necessary; and (3) accurately realign deep anatomic landmarks and skin edges by layered closure and precise suture placement.

Minimizing Tissue Trauma

The importance of carefully handling tissue has been emphasized since the early days of surgery. Skin and SQ tissue that has been stretched, twisted, or crushed by an instrument or strangulated by a suture that is tied too tightly may undergo necrosis; increased scarring and infection may result. When the edges of a wound must be manipulated, the SQ tissues should be lifted gently with toothed forceps or a skin hook while avoiding the surface of the skin.

When choosing suture size, the clinician should select the smallest size that will hold the tissues in place. Skin stitches should incorporate no more tissue than is needed to coapt the wound edges with little or no tension. Knots should be tied securely enough to approximate the edges of the wound without blanching or indenting the skin surface.

Relieving Tension

Many forces can produce tension on the suture line of a reapproximated wound. Static skin forces that stretch the skin over bones cause the edges of a new wound to gape, and they also continuously pull on the edges of the wound once it has been closed. Traumatic loss of tissue or wide excision of a wound may have the same effect. The best cosmetic result occurs when the long axis of a wound happens to be parallel to the direction of maximal skin tension; such alignment brings the edges of the wound together.

Muscles pulling at right angles to the axis of the wound impose dynamic stress. Swelling after an injury creates additional tension within the circle of each suture. Skin suture marks result not only from tying sutures too tightly but also from failing to eliminate any underlying forces distorting the wound. Tension can be reduced during wound closure in two ways: undermining of the wound edges and layered closure.

General Suturing Technique

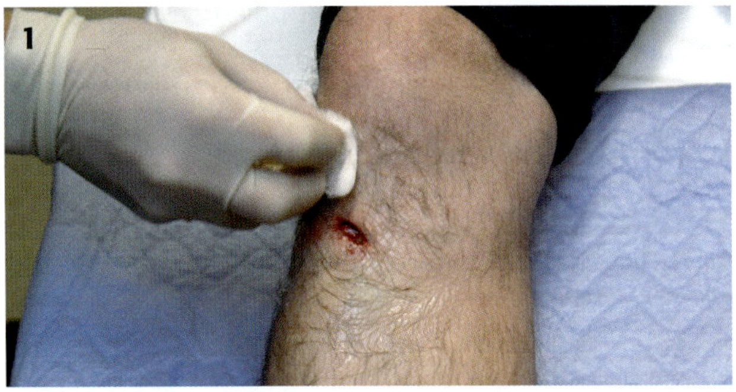

Cleanse the skin surrounding the wound with an antiseptic such as chlorhexidine or povidone-iodine. Avoid introducing antiseptic into the wound because it may be toxic to tissue.

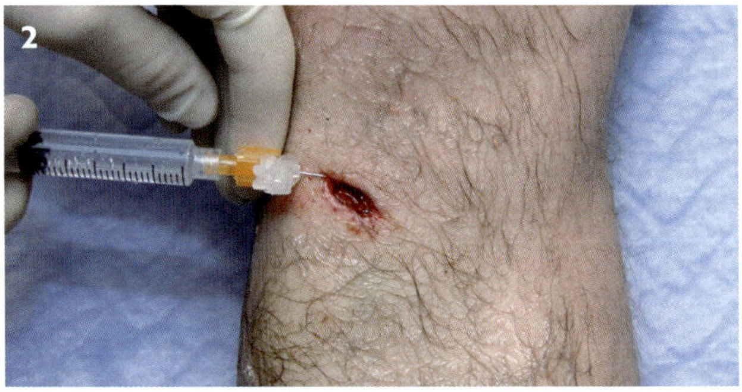

Anesthetize the wound prior to exploration and irrigation. Introduce the needle through the wound (as opposed to through the epidermis).

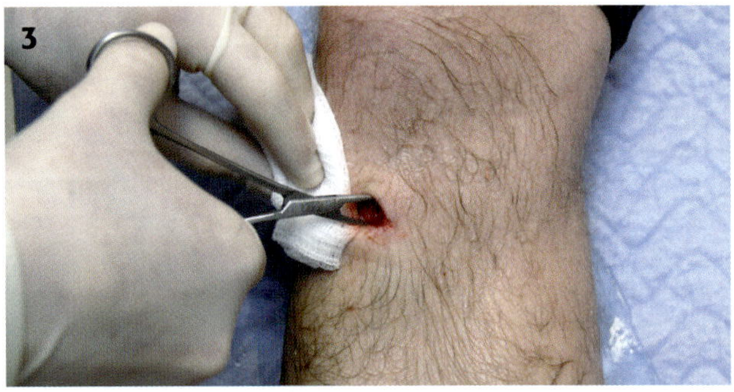

Explore the wound to exclude the presence of foreign bodies, gross contamination, or injuries to deep structures. Debride grossly contaminated or devitalized tissue.

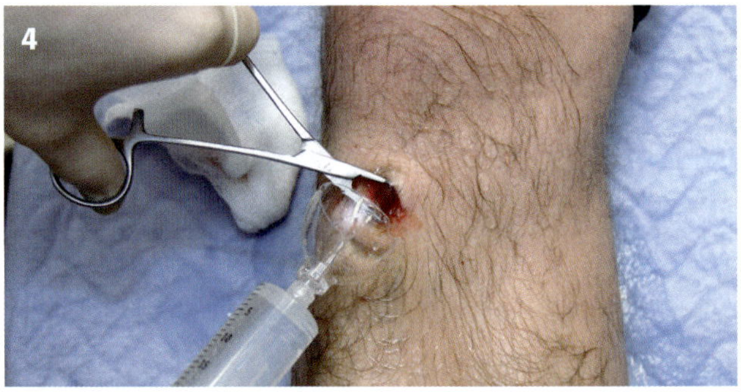

Irrigate the wound thoroughly until it is visibly clean. Use of a large syringe with a splash guard is ideal. Retract the wound edges with an instrument to facilitate thorough irrigation.

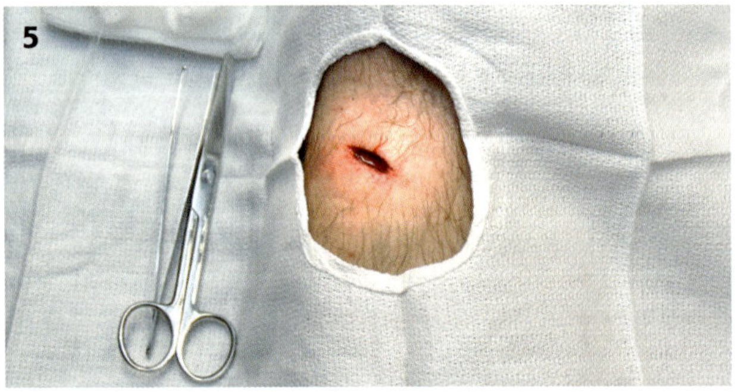

Apply a sterile drape, gather the instruments, and ensure that the field is appropriately lit.

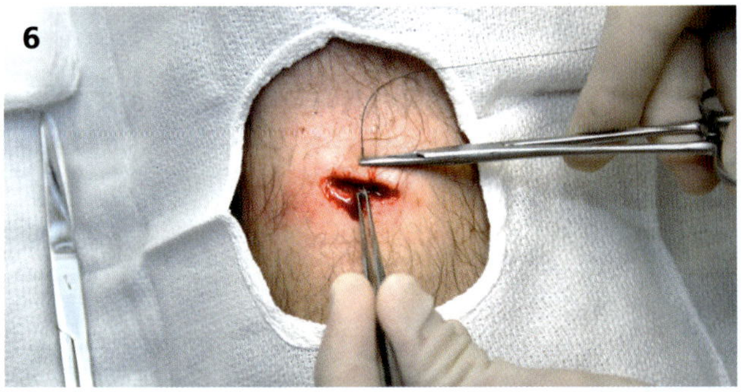

Place the first suture at the center of the wound so that it bisects the laceration into two equal segments.

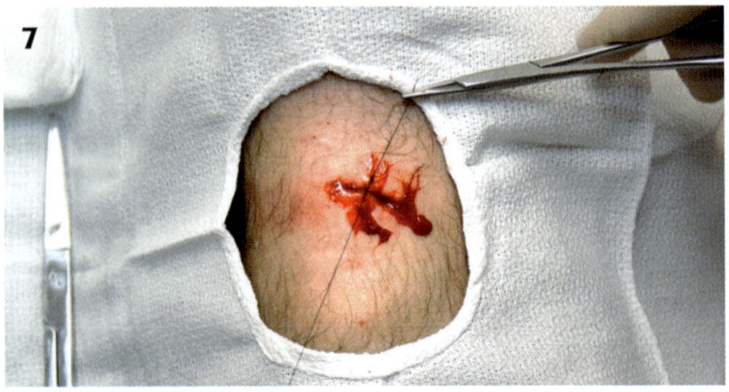

Tie the knot. The first throw should be a double throw (i.e., surgeon's knot) to prevent it from loosening. Place an additional three (single) throws and then cut the sutures while leaving 1- to 2-cm tails.

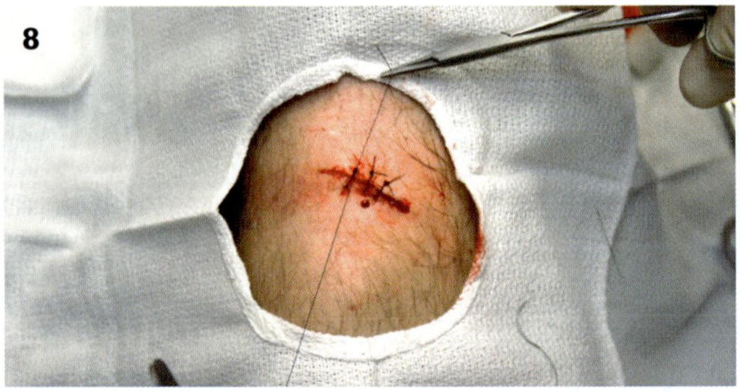

Continue to place additional sutures by further bisecting each segment of the laceration. After the last stitch has been placed, cleanse the area and apply an appropriate dressing.

Fig. 35.17 General suturing technique.

Instrument Tie

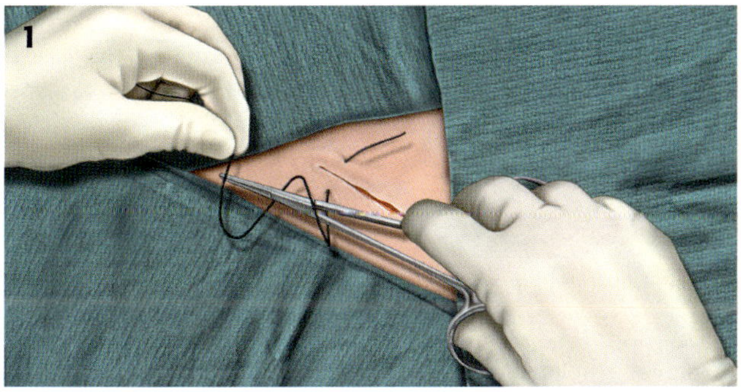

Place the needle driver parallel to the wound and wrap the suture end twice over the needle driver. This forms the surgeon's knot, which prevents the first throw from loosening.

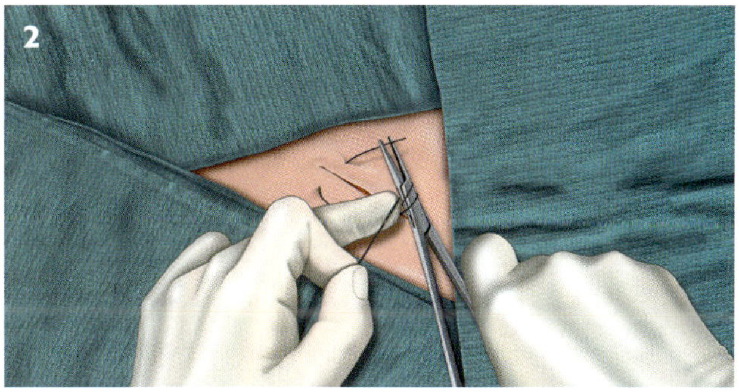

Rotate the needle driver 90 degrees and grasp the short suture end on the opposite side of the laceration.

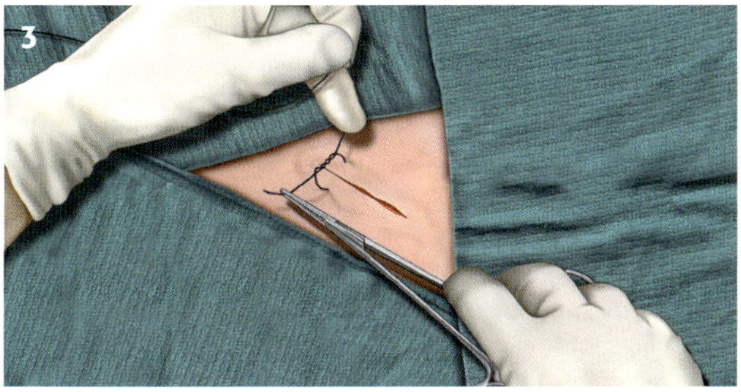

Gently pull the suture ends to the side of the laceration opposite their origin. Tighten only enough to approximate the skin edges; avoid overtightening, which may lead to tissue strangulation.

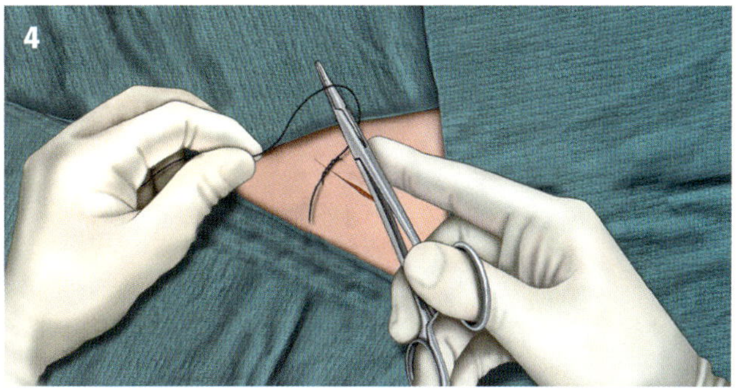

To begin the second throw, again place the needle driver parallel to the laceration. Wrap the long suture end over and around the needle driver once. (Only one wrap is used on throws 2 to 4.)

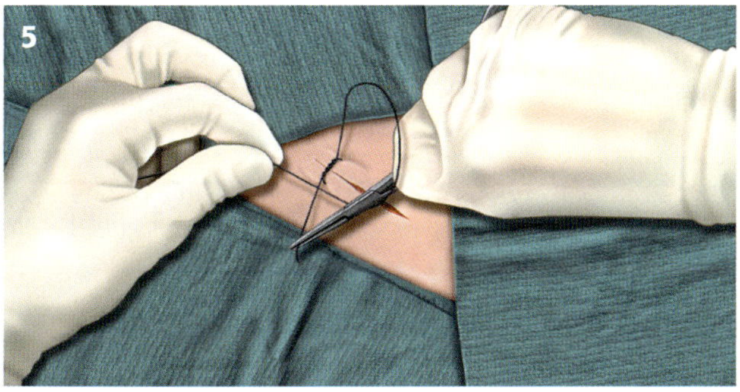

Rotate the needle driver 90 degrees and grasp the short suture end on the opposite side of the laceration.

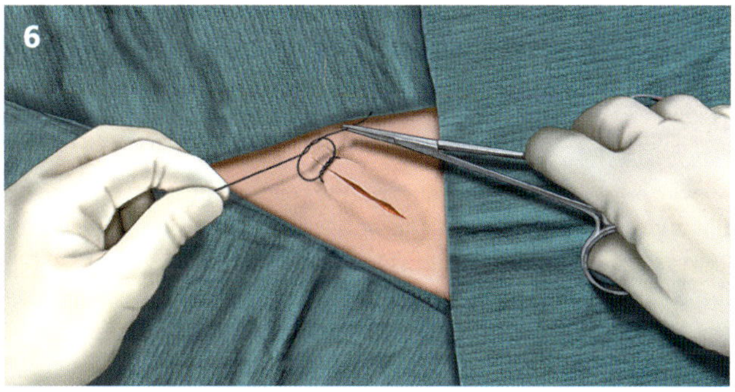

Pull the suture ends to the side of the laceration opposite their origin. On the second and subsequent throws, you can tighten the knot down snugly.

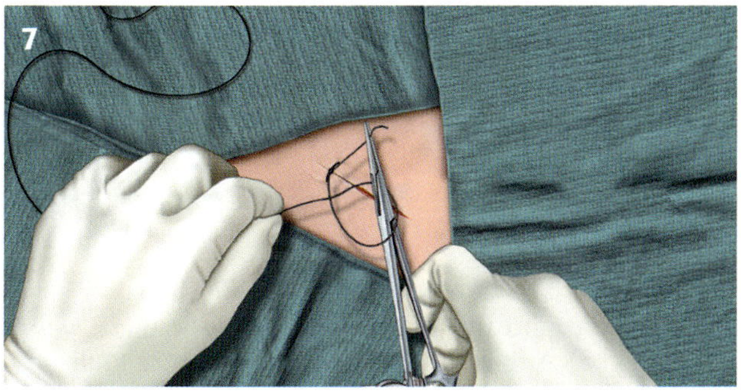

Place an additional two throws (for a total of four), as depicted in *steps 4 through 6*. Remember to place the needle driver parallel to the wound and pull the long suture end *over* the driver; this will ensure that all knots tied are square knots.

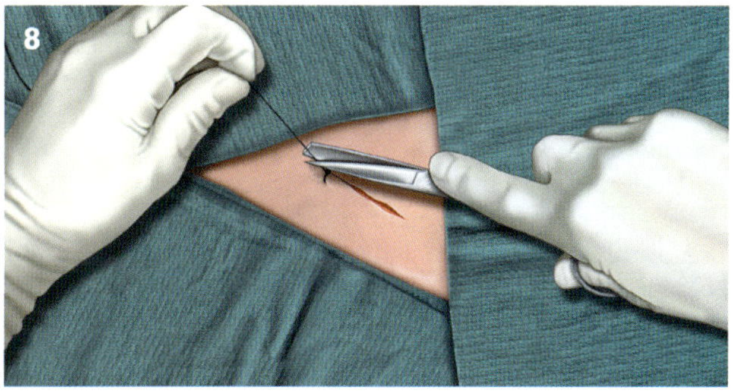

After the last throw, cut the ends of the suture while leaving 1- to 2-cm tails. Avoid cutting the ends too short, which may lead to knot unraveling or difficulty during suture removal.

Fig. 35.18 Instrument tie. (From Custalow C. *Color Atlas of Emergency Department Procedures.* Elsevier; 2005.)

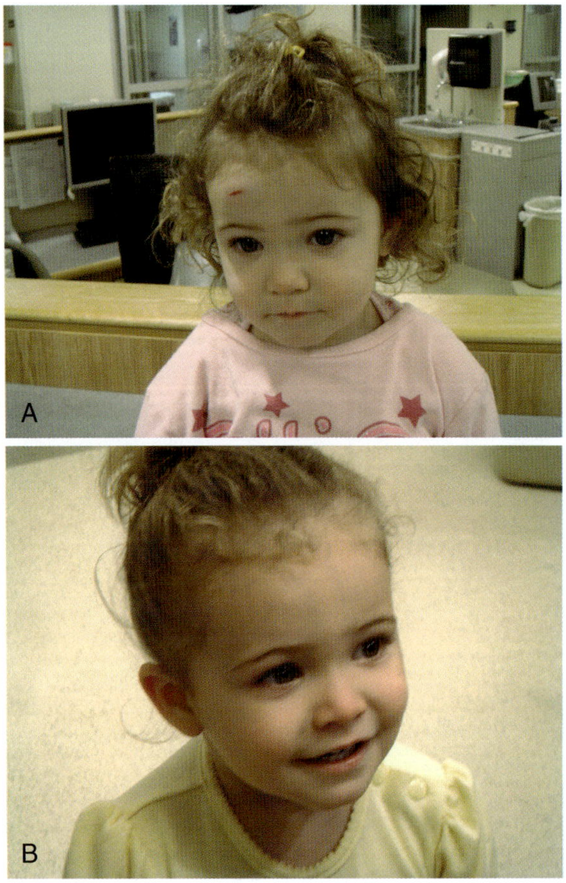

Fig. 35.19 Not all wounds require suturing. (A) This child sustained a superficial forehead laceration just through the epidermis. The swelling accentuated the defect. Treatment was simply keeping the laceration clean. (B) Four months after the injury, an excellent result was achieved. As the laceration was healing, it became red and more noticeable (as do all scars), but eventually faded.

Undermining. The force required to reapproximate the edges of a wound correlates with the subsequent width of the scar. Wounds subject to significant static tension require the undermining of at least one tissue plane on both sides of the wound to achieve a tension-free closure. To undermine a wound, the clinician frees a flap of tissue from its base at a distance from the edge of the wound approximately equal to the width of the gap that the laceration presents at its widest point (Fig. 35.20).

The depth of the incision can be modified, depending on the orientation of the laceration to skin tension lines and the laxity of skin in the area. A No. 15 scalpel blade held parallel to the surface of the skin is used to incise the adipose layer or the dermal layer of the wound. The clinician can also accomplish this technique by spreading scissors in the appropriate tissue plane. Undermining allows the edges of the skin to be lifted and brought together with gentle traction. Potential complications of this procedure include injury to cutaneous nerves and creation of a hematoma under the flap. Because undermining may harm the underlying blood supply, this technique should be reserved for relatively uncontaminated wounds when no other methods adequately relieve wound tension.[98] Undermining is not beneficial for wounds under low or moderate tension.[99]

Layered Closure. The structure of skin and soft tissue varies with the location on the body (Fig. 35.21). Most wounds

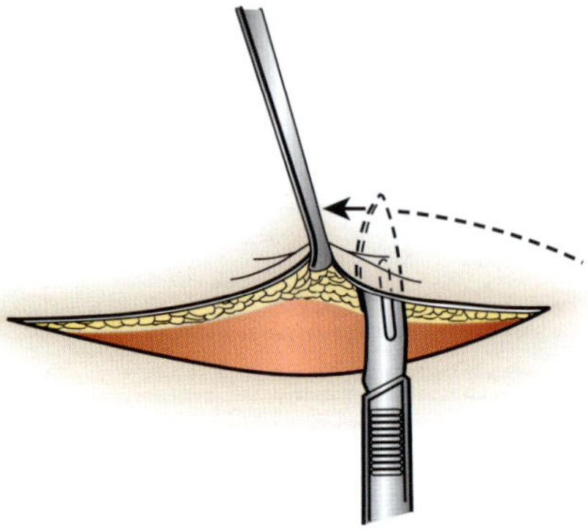

Fig. 35.20 The technique of undermining can markedly improve cosmetic results by relieving wound tension. The scalpel is used to find an appropriate site; a natural plane often exists at the junction of the epidermis and dermis.

handled in an ED require approximation of no more than three basic layers: fascia (and associated muscle), SQ tissue, and skin surface (papillary layer of the dermis and epidermis). Any "dead space" (or unapposed edges) within a wound may fill with blood or exudate and increase the risk for developing a wound infection. Closure of individual layers obliterates this dead space (Fig. 35.22).

Approximation of a lacerated muscle hastens healing and return of function to the muscle. However, the fascia, not muscle, should be sutured. Muscle tissue itself is too friable to hold a suture. Layered closure is particularly important in the management of facial wounds; this technique prevents scarring of muscle to the SQ tissue and consequent deformation of the surface of the wound with contraction of the muscle. If a deep, gaping wound is closed without approximation of underlying SQ tissue, a disfiguring depression may develop at the site of the wound. Finally, layered closure provides support to the wound and considerably reduces tension at the skin surface.

Several exceptions exist to the general rule of multilayered closure. The adipose layer of soft tissue should not be closed separately. A "fat stitch" is not necessary because little support is provided by closure of the adipose layer and additional suture material may increase the risk of infection.[100]

Scalp wounds are generally closed in a single layer. For lacerations penetrating the dermis in the fingers, hands, toes, feet, and the sebaceous skin of the nasal tip, the amount of SQ tissue is too small to warrant layered closure; in fact, SQ stitches may leave tender nodules in these sensitive locations. Layered closure is not recommended for wounds without tension, those with poor vascularity, and those with a moderate or high risk for infection. With single-layer closure, the surface stitch should be placed more deeply.[85]

Suture Placement

SQ Layer Closure

Once the wound has been assessed and appropriately managed for fascial reapproximation, the SQ layer should be addressed (Video 35.5). Although histologically the fatty and fibrous SQ tissue (hypodermis) is an extension of (and continuous with) the reticular layer of the dermis, suturing these layers is traditionally referred to as an *SQ closure*. One approach is to close the length of this layer in segments by placing the first stitch in the middle of the wound and bisecting each subsequent segment until closure of the layer has been completed. This

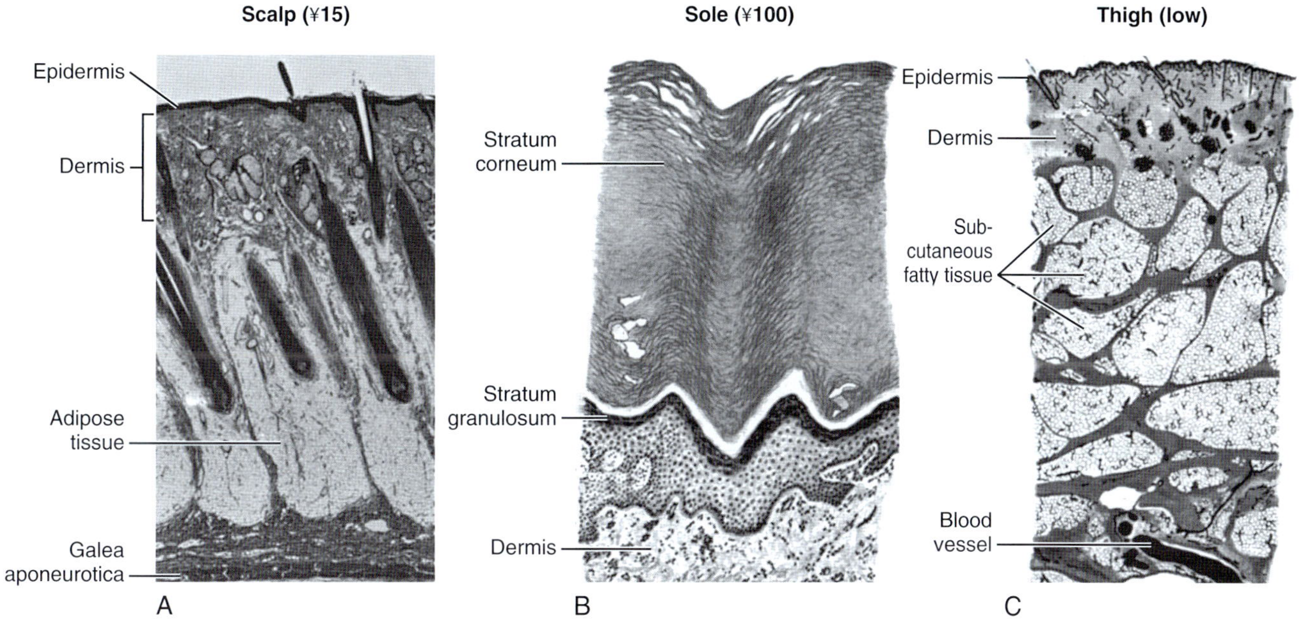

Fig. 35.21 Variation in the structure of skin. (A) Section of the skin of the scalp, ×15. (B) Section of human sole perpendicular to the free surface, ×100 (after A.A. Maximow). (C) Section through human thigh perpendicular to the surface of the skin (after A.A. Maximow). Blood vessels are injected and appear black (low magnification). (A, Courtesy H. Mizoguchi; B and C, From Bloom W, Fawcett DW. *A Textbook of Histology.* 10th ed. Saunders; 1975.)

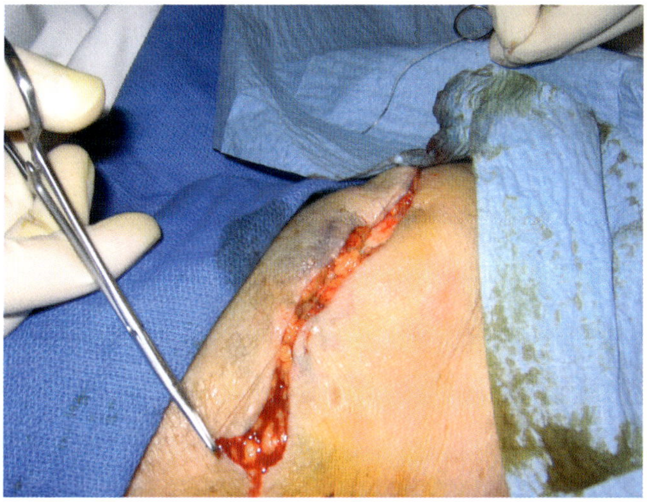

Fig. 35.22 Note how a subcutaneous suture almost closes the wound with minimal tension on the edges of the skin while obliterating any subcutaneous space. Tie and bury the knot by pulling the sutures in the long axis of the wound as shown.

technique is useful for the closure of wounds that are long or sinuous, and it is particularly effective for wounds with one elliptical and one linear side. The needle is grasped with the tip of the needle holder perpendicular to the needle. This angle provides the most stable grip on the needle. In some cases, however, SQ sutures may be easier to place if the needle is loaded at a 135-degree angle between the long axis of the needle and the needle driver (Fig. 35.23).[101]

Some clinicians can suture more rapidly if the fingers are placed on the midshaft of the needle holder rather than in the rings of the instrument (Fig. 35.24). The suture enters the SQ layer at the bottom of the wound (Fig. 35.25A) or, if the wound has been undermined, at the base of the flap (see Fig. 35.25B) and exits in the dermis. Once the suture has been placed on one side of the wound, it can be pulled across the wound to the opposite side (or the edges of the wound pushed together) to determine the matching point on the opposite side. The needle is then advanced to this point. The needle should enter

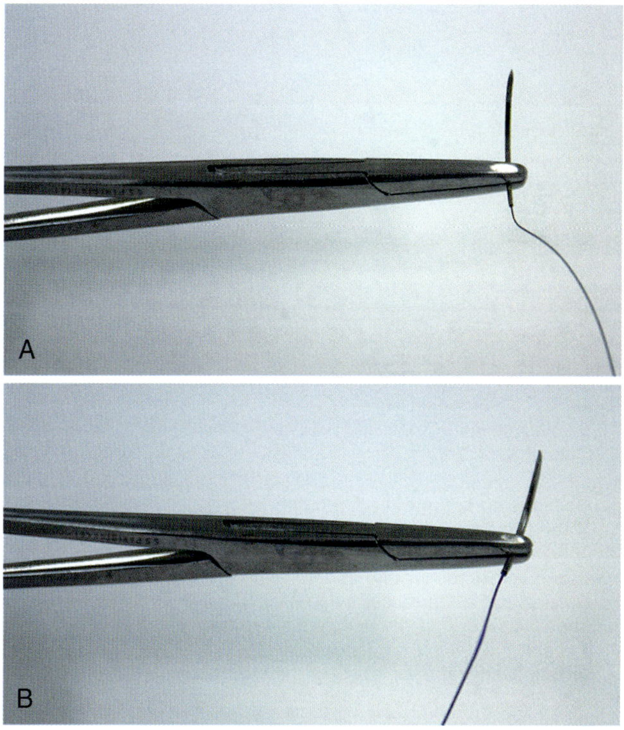

Fig. 35.23 A simple modification to the angle of the needle may make subcutaneous suturing easier. (A) In most situations, the needle should be loaded perpendicular to the needle driver. (B) If the wound is narrow, the needle can be grasped at a slightly obtuse, 135-degree angle to the needle driver. (Modified from Ahmed AM, Orengo I. Surgical Pearl: alternate method of loading needle to facilitate subcuticular suturing. *J Am Acad Dermatol.* 2007;56:S105.)

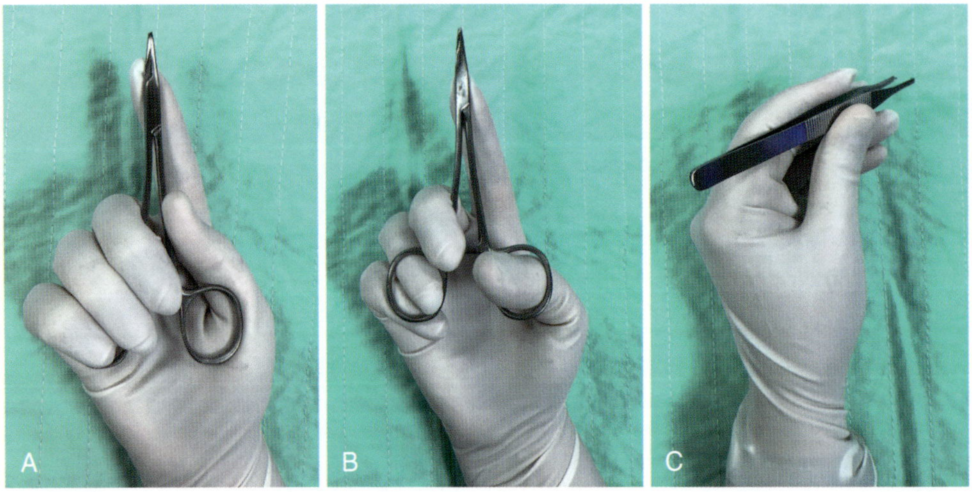

Fig. 35.24 (A) Thenar grip technique of handling the needle holder. The index finger is placed on the side of the needle holder, where it guides placement of the needle. Neither the index nor the middle finger is placed in the ringlet hole. This method allows more rapid suturing. (B) An alternative method is the thumb-ring finger grip. (C) Hold the forceps in your nondominant hand as you would hold a pencil or a dart.

Subcutaneous Sutures

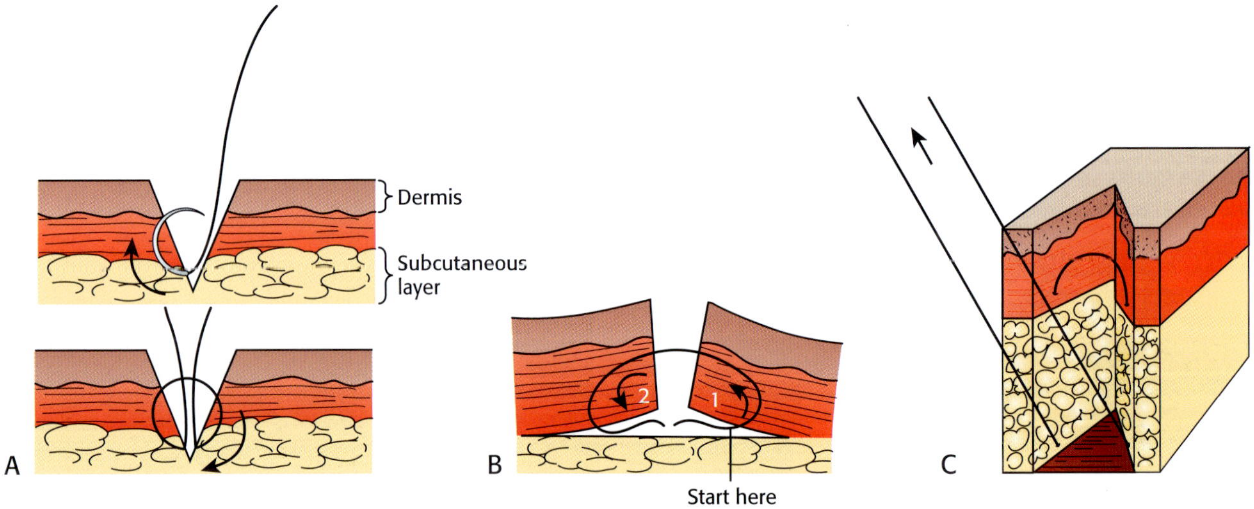

Place the suture in the subcutaneous layer at the bottom of the wound, and pass it upward so that it exits in the dermis. Pull the suture across the wound to determine the correct level of dermal entry on the opposite side. Pass the needle downward through the dermis on the opposite side so that it exits at the bottom of the wound.

If the wound has been undermined, the needle enters at the base of the flap and is passed upward through the dermis.

Pull the two tails of the suture in the same direction along the axis of the wound to appose the wound edges, and then tie the knot. Subcutaneous knots are "buried" at the bottom of the wound to prevent painful nodules beneath the epidermis and to keep the bulk of the foreign material away from the skin surface.

Fig. 35.25 Subcutaneous sutures.

the dermis at the same depth as it exited from the opposite side, pass through the tissue, and exit at the bottom of the wound (or the base of the flap). The edges of the wound can be closely apposed by pulling the two tails of the suture in the same direction along the axis of the wound (see Fig. 35.25C). When the knot in this SQ stitch is tied, it will remain inverted, or "buried," at the bottom of the wound. Burying the knot of the SQ stitch avoids a painful, palpable nodule beneath the epidermis and keeps the bulk of this foreign material away from the skin's surface. Most emergency clinicians construct knots with the instrument tie technique (see Fig. 35.18). Hand and instrument knot-tying techniques are described and illustrated in wound care texts.[102,103]

Once the knot has been secured, pull the tails of the suture taut for cutting. Hold the scissors with the index finger on the junction of the two blades. Slide the scissors' blade down the suture's tail until the knot is reached. Cut the tails with the cutting edge of the blade tilted away from the knot. This technique prevents the scissors from cutting the knot itself and leaves a 3-mm tail, which protects the knot from unraveling. Suture the entire SQ layer in this manner.

After the SQ layer has been closed, the distance between the skin edges determines the approximate width of the scar in its final form. If this width is acceptable, insert surface sutures. Despite undermining and placement of a sufficient number of SQ sutures, on occasion a large gap between the edges of the wound may persist. In such cases, use a horizontal dermal stitch to bridge this gap (see Fig. 35.31).

Surface Closure

The epidermis and the superficial layer of dermis are sutured in a single layer with nonabsorbable synthetic suture. The choice of suture size, the number of sutures used, and the depth of suture placement depend on the amount of skin tension remaining after SQ closure.

If the edges of the wound are apposed after closure of the deeper layers, small 5-0 or 6-0 sutures can be used to match the epithelium on each side. Place skin stitches closer to each other and closer to the edge in wounds with greater tension and separation, or consider using an interrupted vertical mattress suture. Layered closure is important in such wounds. If the edges of the wound remain separated, or if SQ stitches were not used, a larger-size suture placed deeply may be required.

The wound's location determines the number of sutures used in closing any wound, the amount of tension on the wound, the vascularity of the injured tissue, and the degree of accuracy required by the clinician and patient. For example, sutures on the face are often placed between 1 and 3 mm apart. However, Sklar et al. found that placing sutures in cutaneous surgical wounds of the head or neck either 2 mm or 5 mm apart did not affect wound healing or cosmesis, as long as the wound edges are nearly apposed by low skin tension or a SQ closure.[104] Similarly, Stoecker et al. found that the spacing of sutures in surgical wounds either 5 mm or 10 mm apart on the trunk or extremities have similar outcomes.[105] Unless the edges of the wound are uneven, sutures should be placed in a mirror-image fashion such that the depth and width are the same on both sides of the wound. In general, the distance between each suture should be approximately equal to the distance from the exit of the stitch to the edge of the wound.[102]

The skin surface may be closed by placing sutures in segments (Fig. 35.26). When suturing the skin, right-handed operators should pass the needle from the right side of the wound to the left. The needle should be driven through tissue by flexing the wrist and supinating the forearm; the course taken by the needle should result in a curve identical to the curvature of the needle itself (see Fig. 35.26, *steps 1 and 2*, and Fig. 35.27). The angle of exit for the needle should be the same as its angle of entrance so that an identical volume of tissue is contained within the stitch on each side of the wound (see Fig. 35.26, *steps 3 and 4*).

Once the needle exits the skin on the opposite side of the wound, regrasp it with the needle holder and advance it through the tissue; care should be taken to avoid crushing the point of the needle with the instrument. Forceps are designed for handling tissue and thus should not be used to grasp the needle tightly. Forceps can stabilize the needle by holding it within the tissue through which the needle has just passed. An assistant can keep excess thread clear of the area being sutured, or the excess can be looped around the clinician's fingers. If the point of the needle becomes dull or bent before all the attached thread has been used, the suture should be discarded.

Complications

Sutures act as foreign bodies in a wound; any stitch may damage a blood vessel or strangulate tissue. Therefore the clinician should use the smallest size and the least number of sutures to adequately close the wound.[84] However, if spaced too widely, surface stitches will leave a "crosshatch" pattern of marks.

Avoid encompassing too much tissue with a small needle. Forcefully pushing or twisting the needle to bring the point out of the tissue may bend or break the body of the needle. Using a needle of improper size will defeat the best suturing technique.

If sutures are tied too tightly around the edges of the wound or if individual stitches are under excessive tension, blood supply to the wound may be compromised, thereby increasing the chance of infection. If a stitch is too tight, suture marks may form even after 24 hours.

If the techniques described are applied to most wounds, the edges will be matched precisely in all three dimensions, with the least number of sutures required to appose the edges and relieve tension, while avoiding excessive scarring.

Eversion Techniques

If the edges of a wound invert or if one edge rolls under the opposite side, a poorly formed, deep, noticeable scar will result. Excessive eversion that exposes the dermis on both sides will also result in a larger scar than if the edges of the skin are perfectly apposed, but inversion produces a more visible scar than eversion does. Because most scars undergo some flattening with contraction, optimal results are achieved when the epidermis is slightly everted without excessive suture tension (Fig. 35.28). Wounds over mobile surfaces, such as the extensor surfaces of joints, should be everted. In time, the scar will be flattened by the dynamic forces acting in the area.

Numerous techniques can be used to avoid inversion of the wound's edges. If the clinician angles the needle obliquely away from the laceration, a surface stitch can be placed so that it is deeper than it is wide and the stitch encircles more tissue in the SQ layer than at the surface. In other words, the stitch is wider at its deepest part and narrower at the surface. If this "bottle-shaped stitch" is intended to produce some eversion of the wound edges, the stitch must include sufficient SQ tissue (see Fig. 35.26, *step 4*).

To produce eversion with a stitch, lift and turn the edge of the wound outward with a skin hook or fine-toothed forceps before inserting the needle on each side (Fig. 35.29, *plate 1*). Eversion can also be achieved simply by pressing on the skin adjacent to the wound with closed forceps (see Fig. 35.29, *plate 2*).

Vertical mattress sutures are particularly effective in everting the edges of the wound, and they can be used exclusively or alternated with simple interrupted sutures (see Fig. 35.29, *plate 3*). In wounds that have been undermined, a SQ stitch placed at the base of the flap on each side can by itself evert the wound (see Fig. 35.29, *plate 4*).

Interrupted Stitch

The simple interrupted stitch (Video 35.6) is the most frequently used technique for closure of skin. It consists of

Simple Interrupted Sutures

1

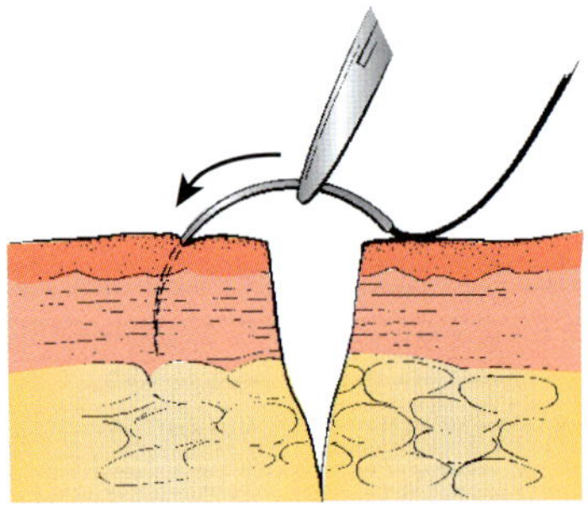

Hold the needle pointing downward by excessively pronating the wrist so that the needle tip initially moves farther from the laceration as the needle penetrates deeper into the skin. Drive the needle tip downward and away from the cut edge into the subcutaneous layer.

2

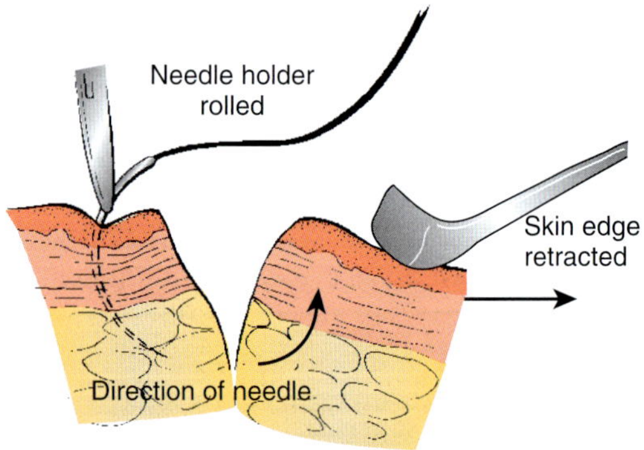

Advance the needle into the laceration. The needle tip is directed toward the opposite side at the same level by rolling the needle holder. The arc of the needle pathway is controlled by retracting the skin edge. This method incorporates more tissue within the stitch in the deeper layers of the wound than at the surface. As an alternative, if a small needle is used in thick skin or the distance across the wound is great, the needle can be removed from the first side, remounted on the needle holder, and advanced to the opposite side.

3

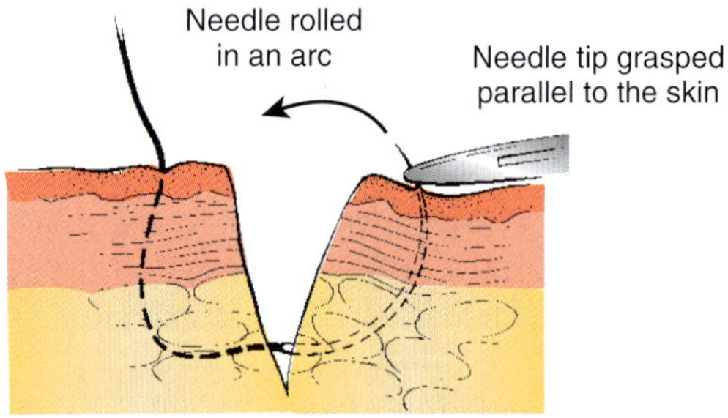

Advance the needle upward toward the surface so that it exits at the same distance from the wound edge as on the contralateral side of the wound. Grasp the needle behind the tip and roll it out in the arc of the needle.

4

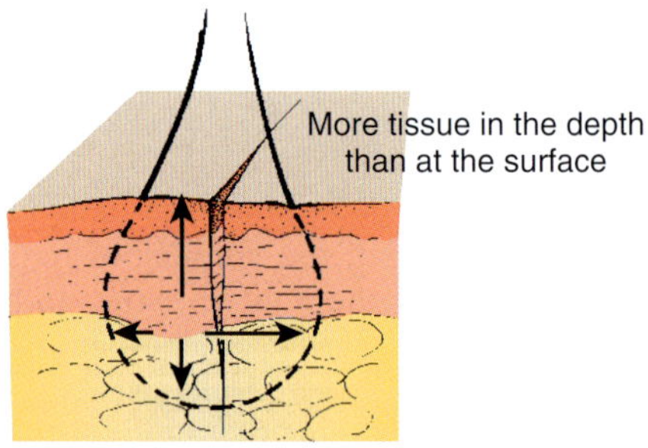

The final position, with more tissue in the depth than in the surface. The distance from each exit of the suture to the laceration is half the depth of the dermis.

5

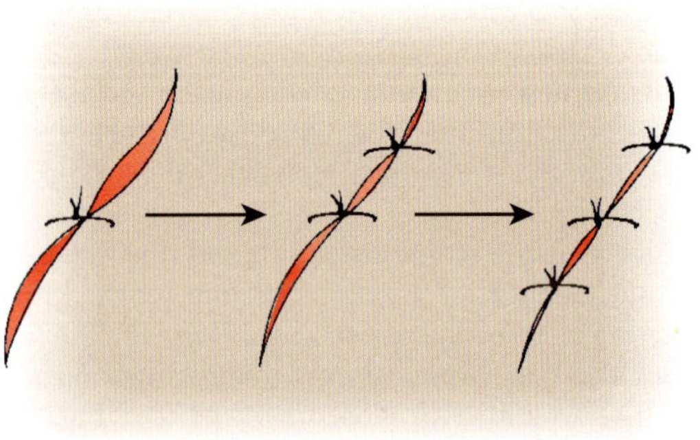

Close the surface of the wound in segments rather than from one end. Place the first suture in the center of the wound for a straight suture line.

6

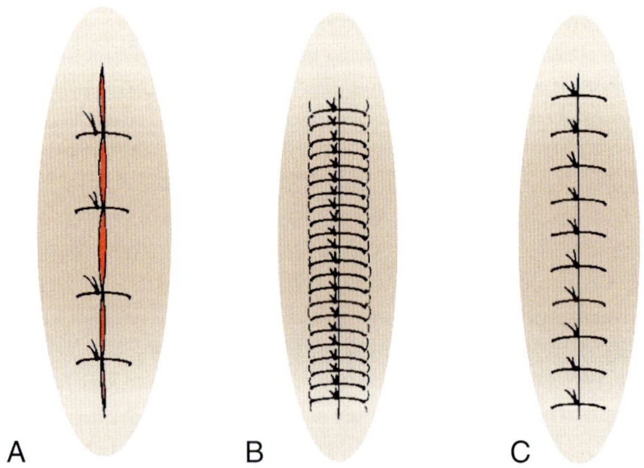

A, Too few stitches used. Note the gaping between the sutures. **B**, Too many stitches used. **C**, Correct number of stitches used for a wound under an average amount of tension.

Fig. 35.26 Simple interrupted sutures. See also Figs. 35.17 and 35.18. (Steps 1–4, from Kaplan EN, Hentz VR. *Emergency Management of Skin and Soft Tissue Wounds: An Illustrated Guide.* Little, Brown; 1984:86.)

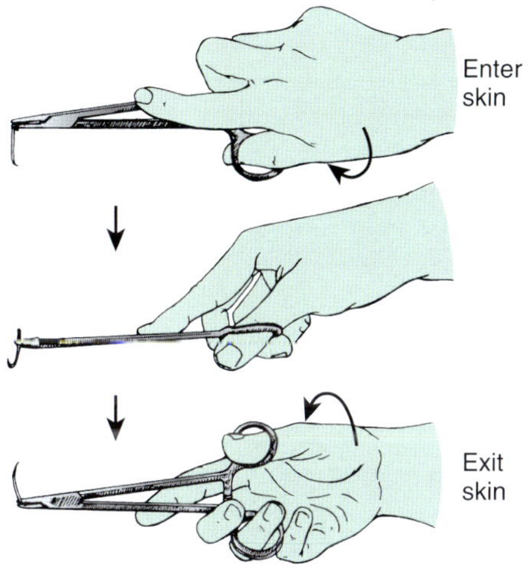

Fig. 35.27 Motion of the needle holder mimics the curve of the needle. Rotate the wrist (pronate) so that the needle enters the skin perpendicularly, not at an angle, as the wrist supinates. This helps evert the edge of the wound. (From Anderson CB. Basic surgical techniques. In: Klippel AP, Anderson CB, eds. *Manual of Outpatient and Emergency Surgical Techniques*. Little, Brown; 1979.)

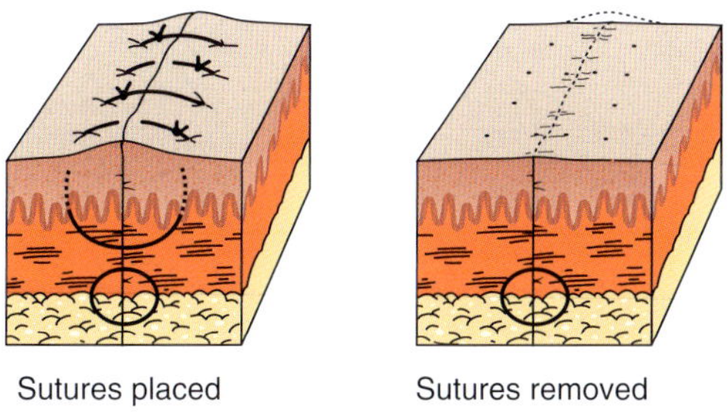

Fig. 35.28 Skin edges that are slightly everted will gradually flatten to produce a level wound surface when the sutures are removed. An inverted wound produces a shadow and is more visible. In addition, eversion allows subcutaneous tissue to heal. The black oval beneath the surface stitch represents a subcutaneous stitch. (From Grabb WC. Basic technique of plastic surgery. In: Grabb WC, Smith JW, eds. *Plastic Surgery: A Concise Guide to Clinical Practice*. Little, Brown; 1979.)

separate loops of suture tied individually. Although tying then cutting each stitch is time-consuming, the advantage of this method is that if one stitch in the closure fails, the remaining stitches continue to hold the wound together (see Fig. 35.26).

Continuous Stitch

A continuous stitch is an effective method for closing relatively clean, low-risk wounds that are under little or no tension and are on flat, immobile skin surfaces. In a continuous, or "running," stitch, the loops are the exposed portions of a helical coil tied at each end of the wound. A continuous suture line can be placed more rapidly than a series of interrupted stitches. A continuous stitch has the additional advantages of strength (with tension being evenly distributed along its entire length), fewer knots (which are the weak points of stitches), and more effective hemostasis. This stitch will accommodate mild wound swelling. The continuous technique is useful as an epithelial or surface stitch in cosmetic closures; however, if the underlying SQ layer is not stabilized in a separate closure, a continuous surface stitch tends to invert the edges of the wound.

The continuous suture technique has some disadvantages. If a loop breaks at one point, the entire suture line may unravel. Likewise, if an infection develops and the incision must be opened at one point, cutting a single loop may cause the entire wound to reopen. A simple continuous stitch has the tendency to produce suture marks if used for the closure of large wounds and if left in place for more than 5 days. However, if all tension on the wound can be removed with SQ sutures, stitch marks are seldom a problem. Additionally, this technique should not be used to close wounds overlying joints.

Among the variations of the continuous technique, the simple continuous stitch is the most useful to emergency clinicians (Fig. 35.30A). Place an interrupted stitch at one end of the wound and cut only the free tail of the suture. Next, encircle the tissue in a spiral pattern. After each passage of the needle, tighten the loop slightly, and hold the thread taut in your nondominant hand. The needle should then travel perpendicularly across the wound on each pass. Place the last loop just beyond the end of the wound and tie the suture, using the last loop as a tail to tie the knot. One can also use a locking loop with continuous suturing to prevent slippage of the loops during suturing (see Fig. 35.30B). The interlocking technique allows use of the continuous stitch along an irregular laceration.

Continuous Subcuticular Stitch

Nonabsorbable sutures used for surface closure outlast their usefulness and must be removed. On occasion, wounds require an extended period of support, longer than that provided by surface stitches. Some patients with wounds that require skin closure are unlikely or unwilling to return for removal of the sutures. Some sutured wounds are covered by plaster casts. On occasion, the patient (child or adult) is likely to be as frightened by and uncooperative with suture removal as they were for suture placement. Surface sutures are more likely to produce stitch marks in children because the wounds are under greater tension than those in adults. The continuous subcuticular (or dermal) suture technique is ideal for these situations; the wound can be closed with an absorbable subcuticular stitch, thereby obviating the need for later suture removal. In patients prone to keloid formation, the subcuticular technique can be used in lieu of surface stitches to avoid disfiguring stitch marks. However, running subcuticular stitch in facial wounds is associated with hyper- or hypoesthesia when compared with simple interrupted suture.[106] Buried, absorbable subcuticular stitches do not appear to provoke more inflammation than percutaneous running stitches with monofilament nylon. As stitch marks are not a problem, a nonabsorbable subcuticular suture can be left in place for a longer period than a surface suture can.

Although this technique is commonly used for cosmetic closures, closure of the subcuticular layer alone may not alter the scar's width. This technique does not allow perfect approximation of the vertical height of the two edges of a wound, and in cosmetic closures, it is often followed by a surface stitch. The subcuticular stitch requires a 4-0 or 5-0 suture of either absorbable material or nonabsorbable synthetic monofilament. An absorbable suture can be buried within the wound, whereas a nonabsorbable suture is used for a "pullout" stitch. The absorbable synthetic monofilament suture PDS (Ethicon) is designed for subcuticular closure. It passes through tissues as easily as nonabsorbable monofilament sutures do and is absorbed if left in the wound.

Eversion Techniques

1

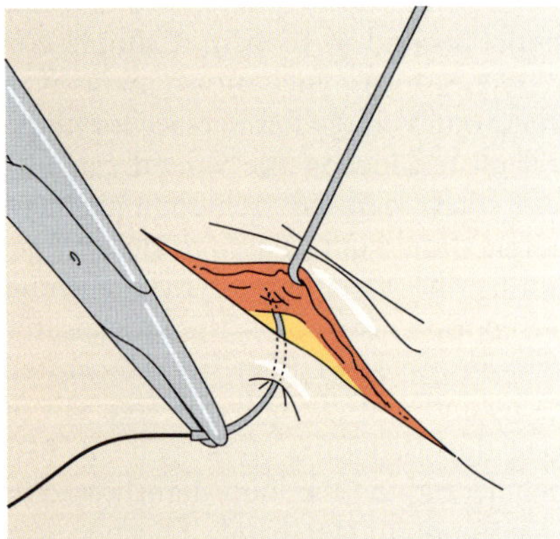

Use of forceps or a skin hook to evert the wound edge. This technique allows the operator to see the needle path, thereby ensuring that the proper depth has been reached, and promotes eversion of the skin edges.

2

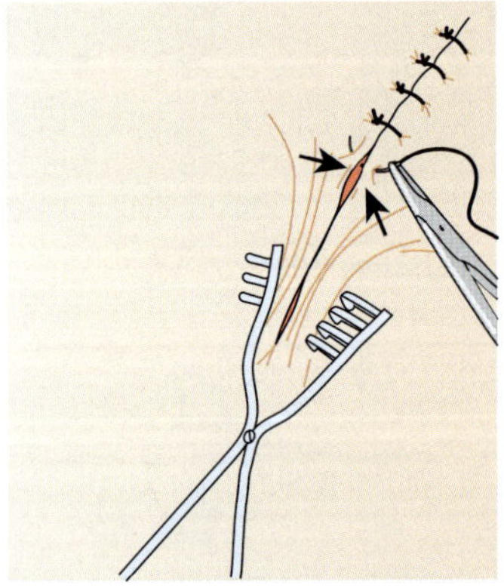

Eversion of the wound edge by forceps. Great care must be taken to avoid a needlestick.

3

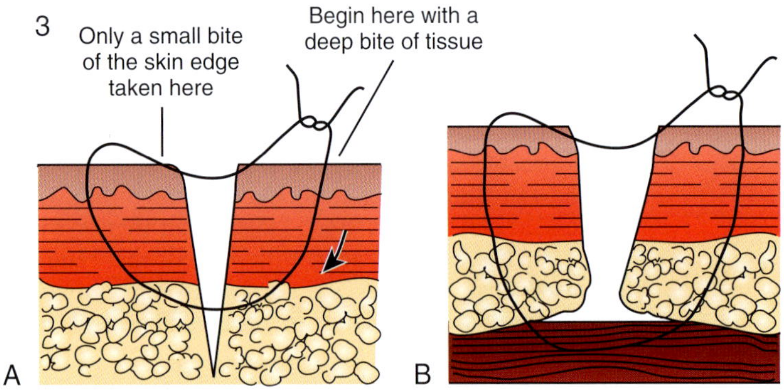

A vertical mattress suture is the best technique for producing skin edge eversion. **A**, The usual type of mattress suture for approximating and everting wound edges. **B**, "Tacking" type of vertical mattress suture extending into the deep fascia to obliterate dead space under the wound. Note that only a small bite of skin is included on the inner suture.

4

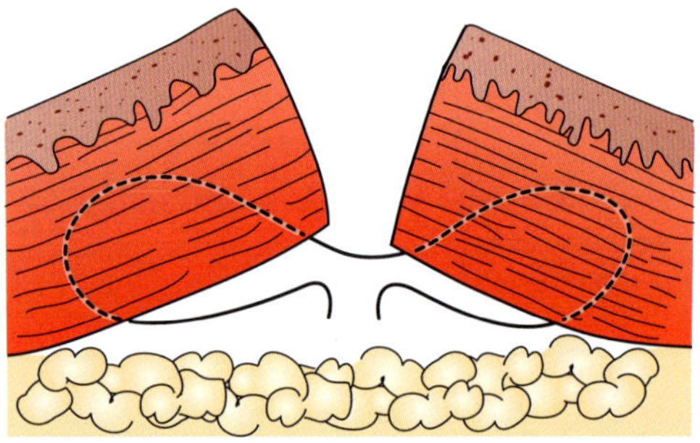

Deep dermis suturing technique. The suture enters the base of the flap, is brought up into the dermis, and exits just proximal to the wound edge along the base of the flap to be tied and cut.

Fig. 35.29 Eversion techniques. (Steps 2 and 3, from Converse JM. Introduction to plastic surgery. In: Converse JM, ed. *Reconstructive Plastic Surgery: Principles and Procedures in Correction, Reconstruction, and Transplantation.* Vol 1, 2nd ed. Saunders; 1977; step 4, from Stuzin J, Engrav LH, Buehler PK. Emergency treatment of facial lacerations. *Postgrad Med.* 1982;71:81.)

Before beginning the subcuticular stitch, approximate the SQ layer with interrupted sutures to minimize tension on the wound. Start the pullout subcuticular stitch at the skin surface approximately 1 cm to 2 cm away from one end of the wound. Insert the needle and exit the dermis at the apices of the wound (see Fig. 35.30C, *plate 1*). Take bites through tissue in a horizontal direction, with the needle penetrating the dermis 1 mm to 2 mm from the skin surface. Make the intradermal bites small, of equal size, and at the same level on each side of the wound. Place each successive bite 1 mm to 2 mm behind the exit point on the opposite side of the wound so that the entrance and exit points on either side are not directly apposed when the wound is closed. Take small bites to avoid puckering of the skin surface. Do not accidentally interlock the stitch. Some clinicians prefer to place a fine (6-0) running skin suture on the surface, in addition to the subcuticular suture, for meticulous skin approximation. Remove the skin suture in 3 to 4 days to avoid suture marks.

If a subcuticular stitch is used on lengthy lacerations, it is difficult to remove. One option is to place "reliefs," which are periodic loops, through the skin every 4 cm to 5 cm along the length of the stitch, to facilitate removal later (see Fig. 35.30C, *plate 2*). Cross the suture to the opposite side, and pass the needle from SQ tissue to the surface of the skin. Carry the suture over the surface for approximately 2 cm before reentering the skin and SQ tissue. Continue the subcuticular stitch at approximately the same point at which the next bite would have been placed had the relief not been used.

At the completion of the stitch, place the needle through the apex and exit the skin 1 cm to 2 cm away from the end of the wound. Tighten the stitch by pulling each end taut. If reliefs have been used, pull on them to take up any slack in the stitch. Secure the two ends of the stitch by taping them to the skin surface with wound closure tape, by placing a cluster of knots on each tail close to the skin surface, or by tying the two ends of the suture to each other over a dressing. The subcuticular stitch will become lax as tissue swelling subsides 48 hours after wound closure. Tighten the stitch at this time.

Subcuticular closure can be accomplished with absorbable sutures that do not penetrate the skin. Begin closure with a dermal or SQ suture placed at one end of the wound and secure it with a knot. After placement of the continuous subcuticular stitch from apex to apex, pull the suture taut, and tie a knot with a tail and a loop of suture (see Fig. 35.30C, *plate 3*). Bury the final knot by inserting the needle into deeper tissue and exit with the needle several millimeters from the edge of the wound. Pull on the end of the needle so the knot disappears into the wound. The advantage of this technique is that there are no suture marks on the skin.

Nonabsorbable subcuticular sutures can be left in place for 2 to 3 weeks, thus providing a longer period of support than surface sutures without stitch marks. If skin sutures are used in conjunction with a subcuticular stitch, remove the surface stitches in 3 to 4 days. A subcuticular closure in itself is stronger than a tape closure. If the subcuticular technique is used exclusively to approximate the skin surface, apply skin tape to correct surface unevenness and to provide more accurate apposition of the epidermis.

The primary disadvantage of the subcuticular stitch is that it is time-consuming, especially when supporting surface stitches are used. Another, faster method that avoids penetrating the skin is the interrupted subcuticular stitch (Fig. 35.31).

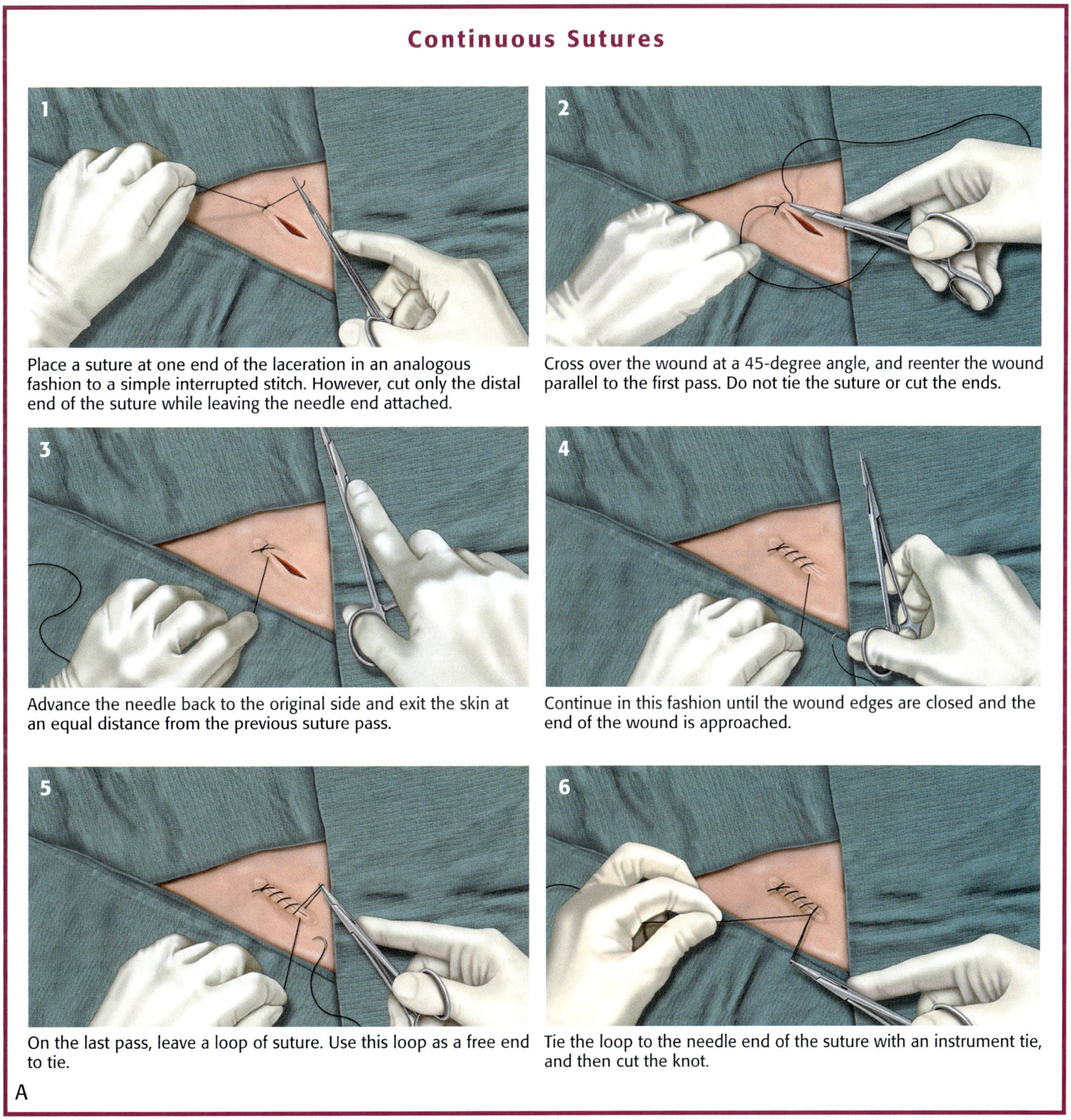

Fig. 35.30 (A) Continuous sutures.

Continued

Continuous Locked Sutures

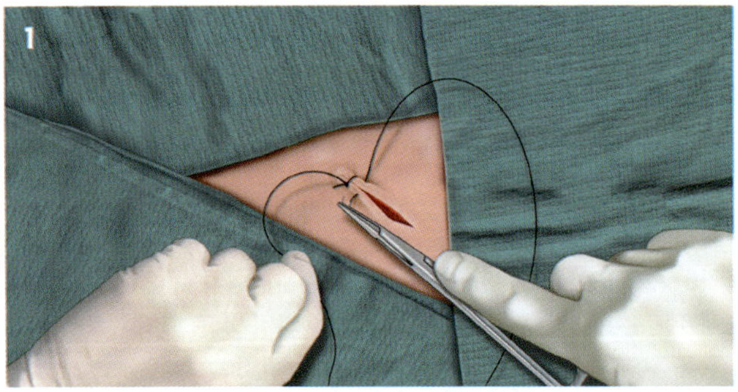

Begin the repair as you would a regular continuous stitch (Fig. 35.30A, *steps 1 and 2*). As the needle exits the near side, "lock" the suture by passing through the circle of the previous suture loop.

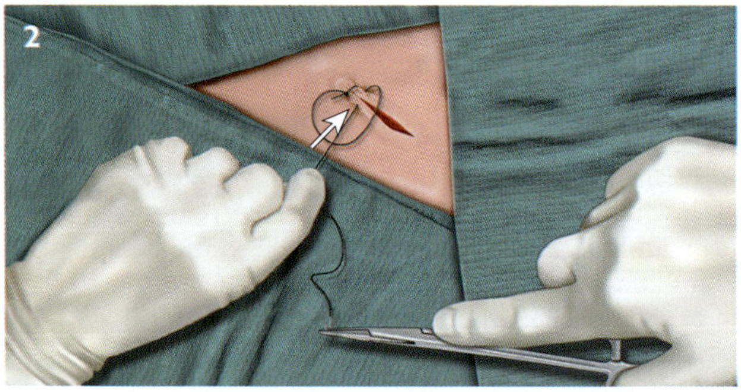

As the suture is pulled through the circle *(arrow)*, it will become locked.

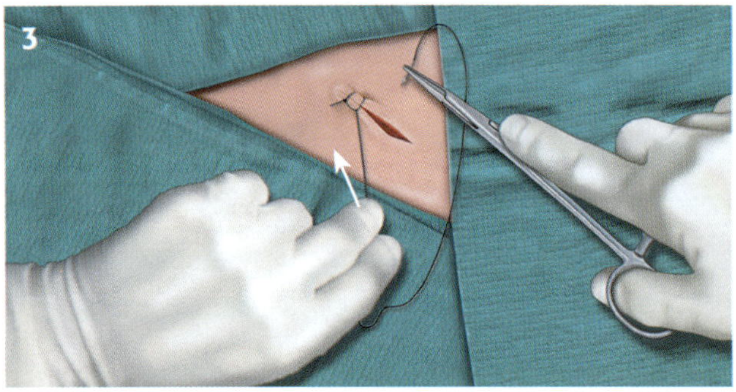

Keep tension evenly distributed across the suture as it is pulled down to the skin. The lock should be parallel to the wound edge *(arrow)*.

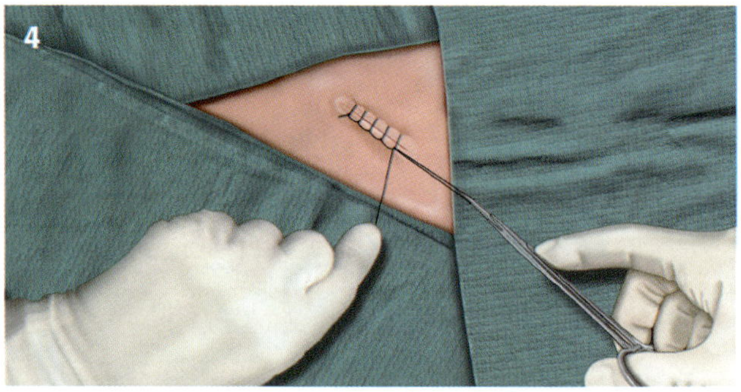

Continue in this fashion by locking each throw along the way. On the last pass, leave a loop of suture and use it to tie to the needle end of the suture.

B

Fig. 35.30, cont'd (B) Continuous locked sutures.

Wounds with strong static skin tension may benefit from a few interrupted dermal stitches placed horizontal to the skin surface instead of a continuous subcuticular stitch.

Mattress Stitch

The various types of mattress stitches of use to the emergency clinician are interrupted stitches. The *vertical mattress stitch* (Video 35.7) is an effective method of everting skin edges (Fig. 35.32A; see also Fig. 35.29, *plate 3*). A vertical mattress stitch may be used to take a deep bite of skin, thereby eliminating the need for layered closure in areas where excessive tension does not result. When the superficial loop is placed first, the tails can be pulled upward while the deep loop is placed; this technique ensures eversion of the wound in less time than needed with the traditional technique.[107]

The *horizontal mattress stitch* (Videos 35.8 and 35.9) is an SQ stitch that is oriented 90 degrees to the interrupted SQ stitch, described previously (Fig. 35.32B). The horizontal mattress stitch apposes the skin edges closely while providing some degree of eversion. A horizontal mattress suture may be ideal for areas where eversion is desirable but there is little SQ tissue.

The *half-buried horizontal mattress stitch* is particularly useful in suturing the easily damaged apex of a V-shaped flap (see Fig. 35.32B). In performing the "corner stitch", penetrate the skin at a point beyond the apex of the wound with the suture needle and exit through the dermis. Elevate the corner of the flap, and pass the suture through the dermis of the flap. Then, place the needle in the dermis at the base of the wound and return it to the surface of the skin. Place all dermal bites at the same level. Tie the suture with sufficient tension to pull the flap snugly into the corner without blanching the flap. The tip of a large flap with questionable viability may be further jeopardized by postoperative swelling, so a cotton stent can be placed underneath the knot of the corner stitch. The cotton absorbs the tension produced by swelling.

The only disadvantage of the horizontal and vertical mattress stitches is that they cause more ischemia and necrosis inside their loops than do either simple or continuous stitches. With mattress sutures, alternating the side of the wound margin on which the knot is tied has been found to reduce wound tension and may reduce the risk of edge necrosis.[108]

The *inverting horizontal mattress stitch* is a variation of the horizontal mattress stitch (Fig. 35.33). This stitch produces wound inversion and should only be used when wound inversion is desired, such as when recreating the alar crease of the nose or the rolled helical rim of the ear.[109,110] In most other wounds, inversion will create a depressed and more noticeable scar.

Figure-of-Eight Stitch

A figure-of-eight stitch is useful for wounds with friable tissue, on the eyelids where the skin is too thin for buried sutures, or in areas in which buried sutures are undesirable (Fig. 35.34,

Continuous Subcuticular Sutures

1

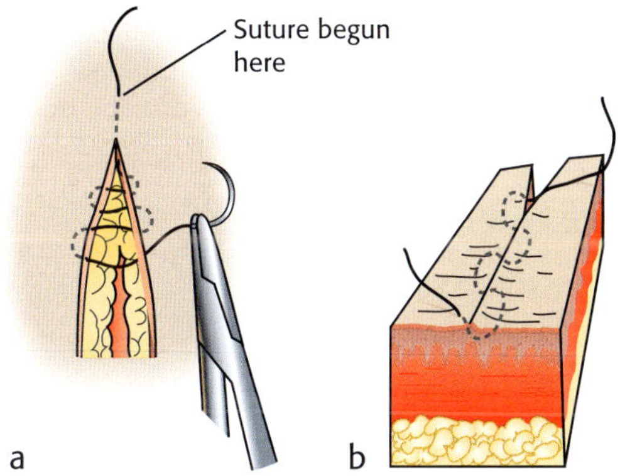

Pullout subcuticular stitch. For deep wounds, first place interrupted sutures to relieve tension on the skin edge. The suture is introduced into the skin in line with the incision, approximately 1 to 2 cm away.

2

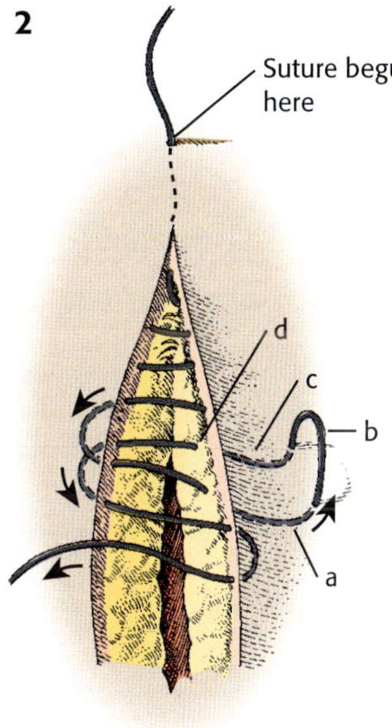

In constructing the relief to facilitate suture removal, the suture is crossed to the opposite side by going into the subcuticular area beneath the skin for approximately 2 cm before exiting *(a)*. The suture is then carried over the epidermis for approximately 2 cm *(b)* and then back under the dermis again *(c)*. Reentry is made into the wound area *(d)* at approximately the same location where the next "bite" would have been placed had the relief not been used.

3

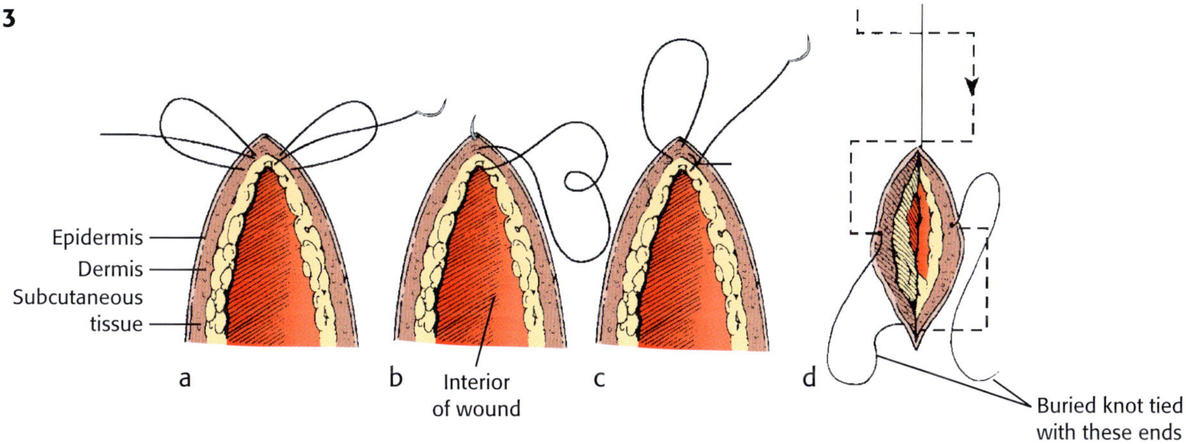

Subcuticular closure without epidermal penetration. **a**, The initial knot is secured in dermal or subcutaneous tissue. **b**, The short strand is cut, and the needle is inserted into the dermis at the apex of the wound. **c**, The needle in the dermis close to the corner of the wound and exiting the wound at the same horizontal level. **d**, After the subcuticular stitch has been completed, a knot is tied with the tail and the loop of the suture.

C

Fig. 35.30, cont'd (C) Continuous subcuticular sutures. (A–B, from Custalow C. *Color Atlas of Emergency Department Procedures*. Elsevier; 2005; C, 1–2, from Grimes DW, Garner RW. "Reliefs" in intracuticular sutures. *Surg Rounds*. 1978;1:47; 3, modified from Stillman RM. Wound closure: choosing optimal materials and methods. *ER Reports*. 1981;2:43.)

plate 1).[111] This stitch reduces the amount of tension placed on the tissue by the suture, which allows the stitch to stay in place when a simple stitch would tear through the tissue. The disadvantage of this technique is that more suture material is left in the wound (Video 35.10). A vertical variation of the figure-of-eight stitch is sometimes used to approximate close, parallel lacerations (see Fig. 35.34, *plate 2*).[112] Another technique involves a vertical mattress stitch (Fig. 35.35).

Correction of Dog-Ears

When the edges of a wound are not precisely aligned horizontally, there will be excess tissue on one or both ends. This small flap of excess skin that bunches up at the end of a sutured wound is commonly called a *dog-ear*. This effect also occurs when one side of the wound is more elliptical than the opposite side or when excision of a wound is not sufficiently elliptical because it is either too straight or too nearly circular.

If a dog-ear is present, it can be eliminated on one side of the wound in the following manner. Elevate the flap of excess skin with forceps or a skin hook. Make an incision at an oblique angle from the apex of the wound toward the side with the excess skin. Undermine the flap and lay it flat. Trim the resulting triangle of skin, and complete the closure (Fig. 35.36, *plate 1*). An alternative method consists of carrying the

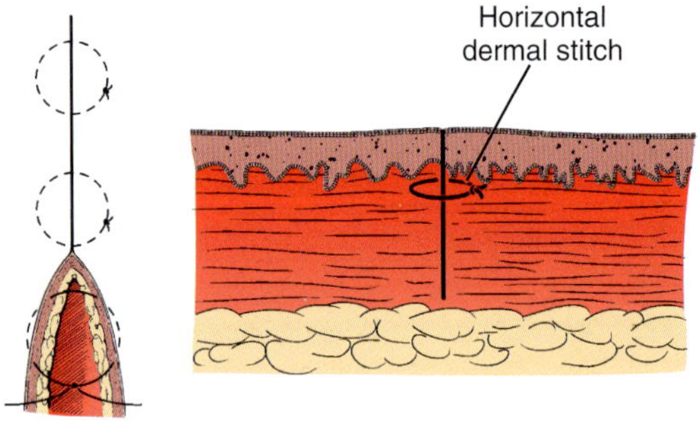

Fig. 35.31 Interrupted subcuticular stitch (also called a horizontal dermal stitch). Absorbable sutures are used. (A vertical suture also closes the deep tissue.)

incision directly from the apex in line with the wound. Pull the flap of excess tissue over the incision while using skin hooks to retract the extended apex of the wound. Excise excess tissue and suture the remainder of the wound. If dog-ears are present on both sides of one end of the wound, excise the bulge of excess tissue in an elliptical fashion and close the wound (see Fig. 35.36A). A tissue-sparing method for correction of small dog-ears, called the "snug tip" technique, may be useful in facial wounds or other areas of cosmetic importance (see Fig. 35.36B).[113]

Stellate Lacerations

Repair of a stellate laceration is challenging. Usually resulting from compression and shear forces, these injuries contain large amounts of partially devitalized tissue. The surrounding

Vertical Mattress Suture

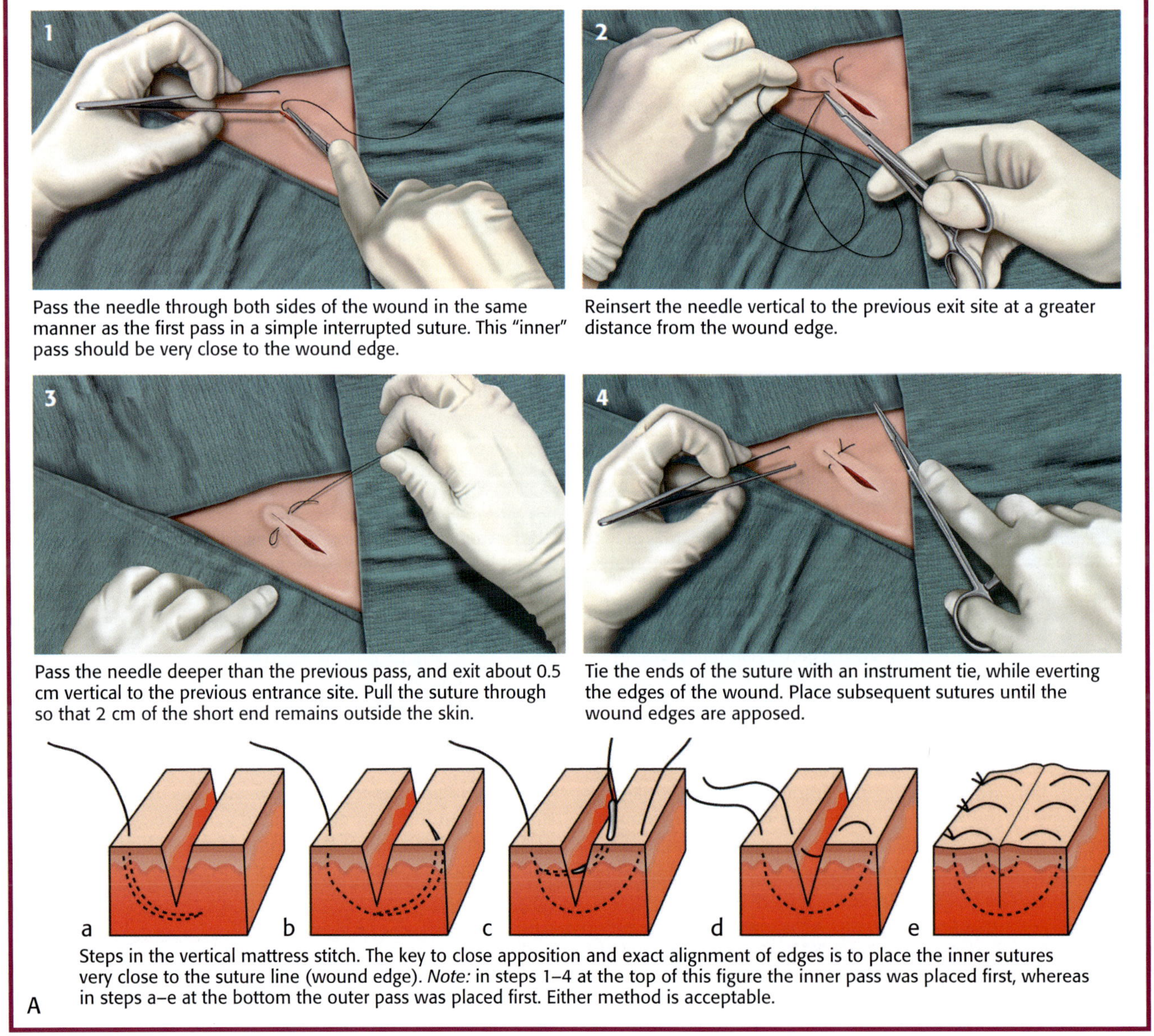

1. Pass the needle through both sides of the wound in the same manner as the first pass in a simple interrupted suture. This "inner" pass should be very close to the wound edge.
2. Reinsert the needle vertical to the previous exit site at a greater distance from the wound edge.
3. Pass the needle deeper than the previous pass, and exit about 0.5 cm vertical to the previous entrance site. Pull the suture through so that 2 cm of the short end remains outside the skin.
4. Tie the ends of the suture with an instrument tie, while everting the edges of the wound. Place subsequent sutures until the wound edges are apposed.

Steps in the vertical mattress stitch. The key to close apposition and exact alignment of edges is to place the inner sutures very close to the suture line (wound edge). *Note:* in steps 1–4 at the top of this figure the inner pass was placed first, whereas in steps a–e at the bottom the outer pass was placed first. Either method is acceptable.

Fig. 35.32 (A) Vertical mattress sutures.

Horizontal Mattress Suture

Standard Horizontal Mattress

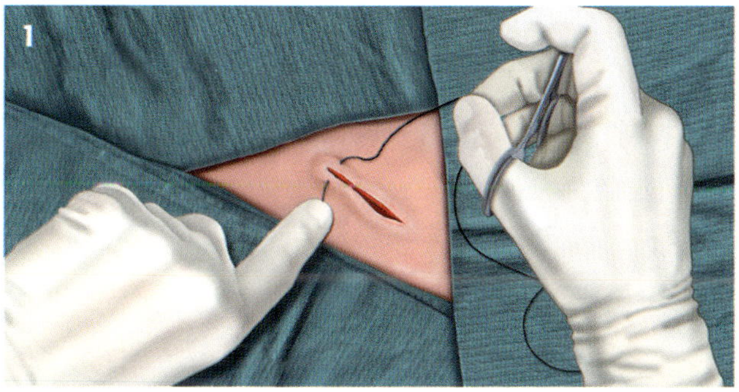

Pass the needle through both sides of the wound in the same manner as the first pass in a simple interrupted suture.

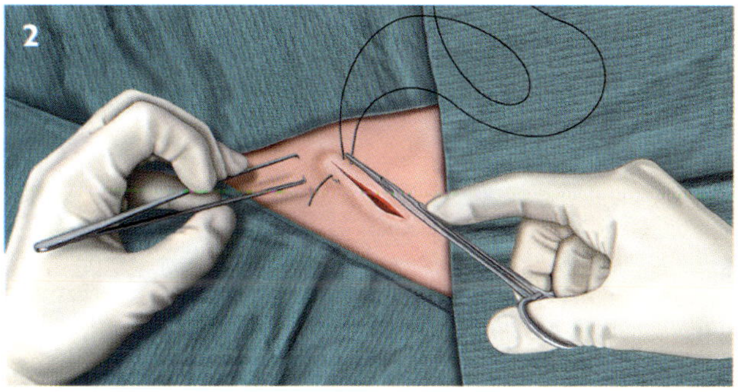

Reinsert the needle approximately 5 mm from and horizontal to the previous exit site. Exit the wound on the opposite side, parallel to the first pass and at the same distance from the wound edge.

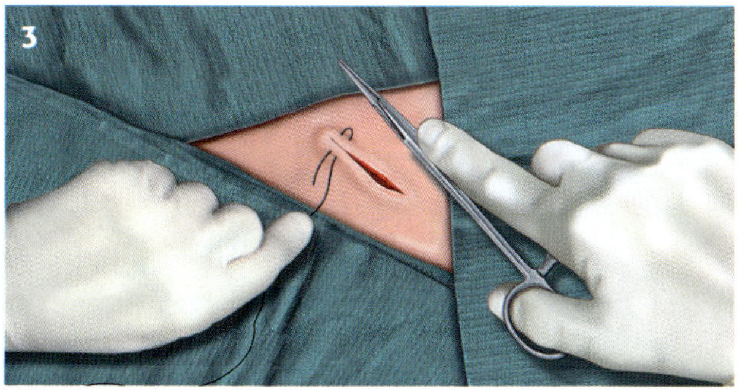

Pull the suture through so that approximately 2 cm of the short end of the suture remains outside the skin.

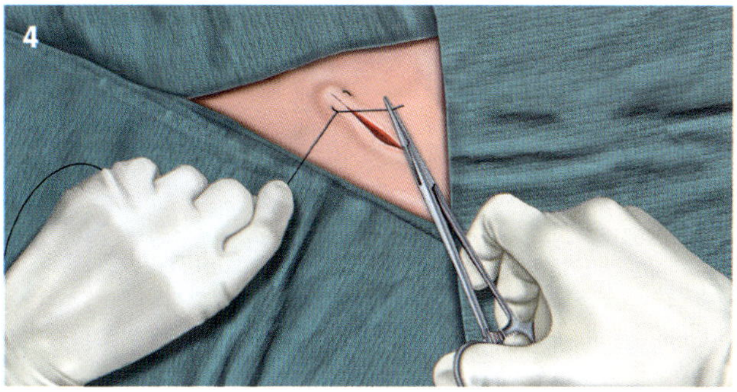

Tie the ends of the suture with an instrument tie, while everting the edges of the wound. Place subsequent sutures until the wound edges are apposed.

Half-Buried Horizontal Mattress

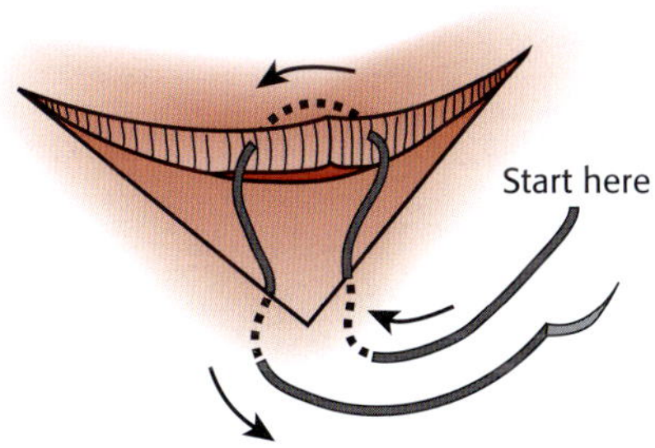

a

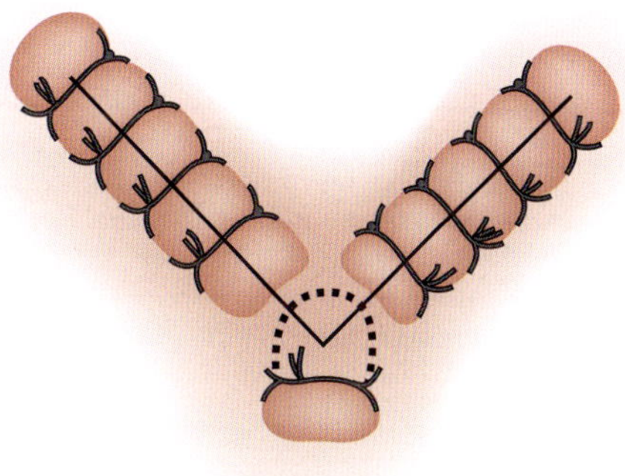

b

a and *b*, Corner stitch: Approximation of a flap with a half-buried horizontal mattress stitch, followed by interrupted sutures for the rest of the wound.

B

Fig. 35.32, cont'd (B) Horizontal mattress sutures. (From Custalow C. *Color Atlas of Emergency Department Procedures*. Elsevier; 2005.)

soft tissue is often swollen and contused. Much of this contused tissue cannot be debrided without creating a large tissue defect. Sometimes tissue is lost, yet the amount is not apparent until key sutures are placed. In repairing what often resembles a jigsaw puzzle, the clinician can remove small flaps of necrotic tissue with iris scissors; large, viable flaps can be repositioned in their beds and carefully secured with half-buried mattress stitches. If interrupted stitches are used to approximate a thin flap, take small bites in the flap and larger, deeper bites in the base of the wound. A modification of the corner stitch can be used to approximate multiple flaps to a base (Fig. 35.37, Video 35.11). Alternatively, reposition thin flaps of tissue in a stellate laceration with beveled edges and stabilize the wound with a firm dressing.

Stellate lacerations cannot always be closed immediately, especially if considerable soft tissue swelling is present. In some instances, it may be best to consider delayed closure or revision of the scar at a later date. In complicated lacerations,

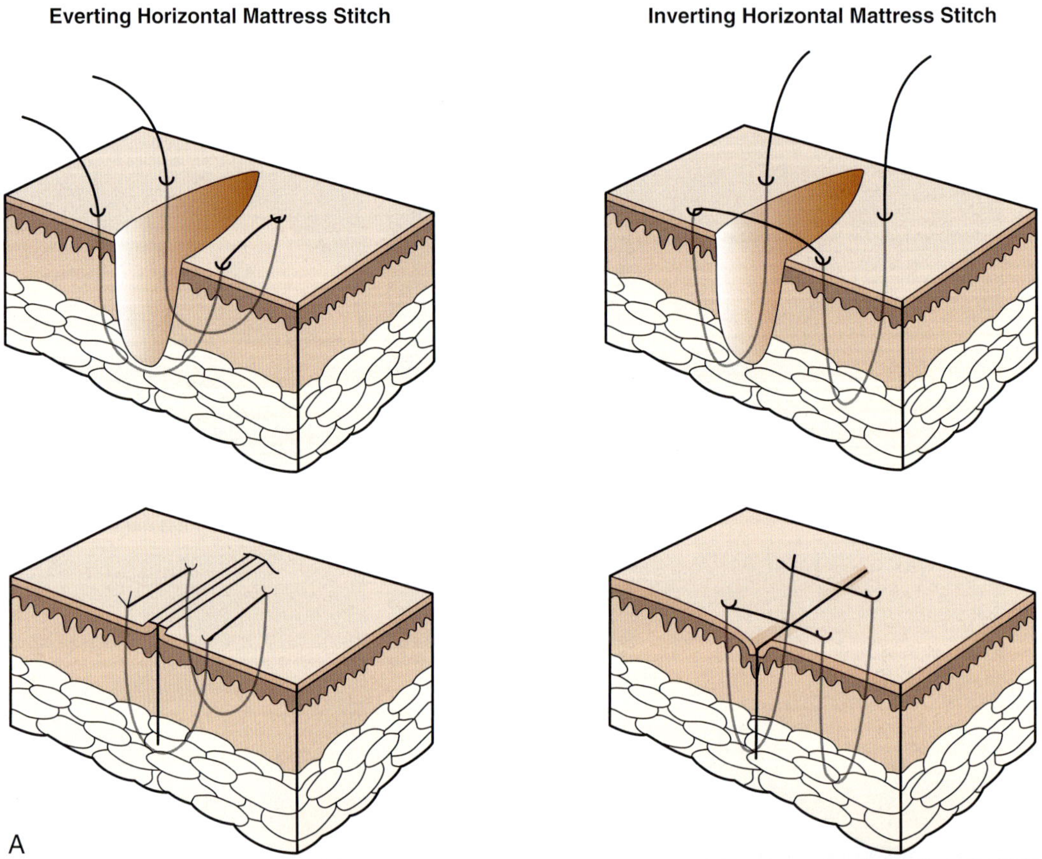

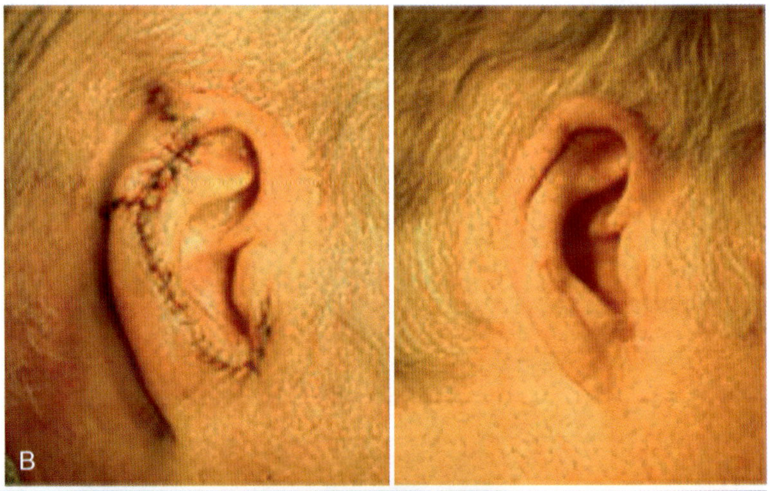

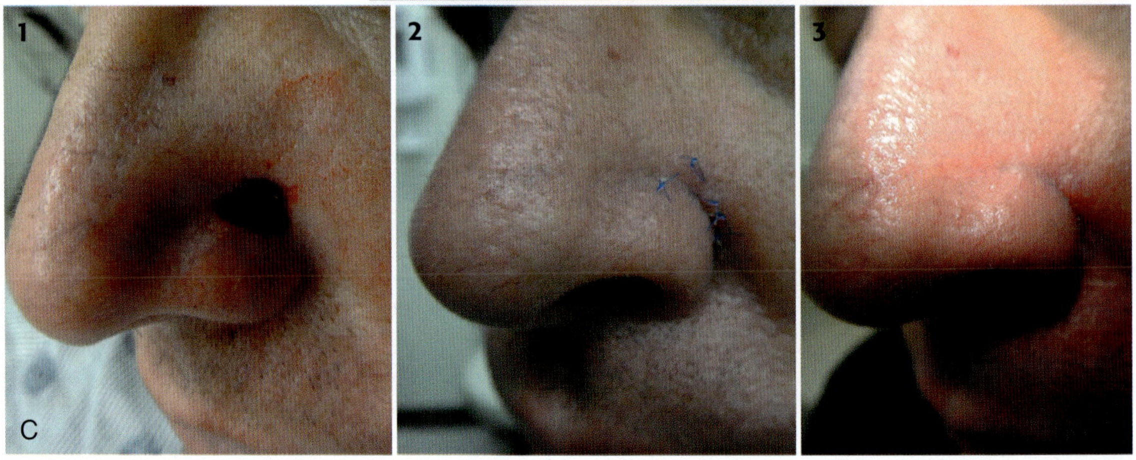

Fig. 35.33 Inverting horizontal mattress sutures. (A) Traditional everting horizontal mattress stitch and inverting horizontal mattress stitch. (B) Application of the inverting horizontal mattress suture to the helix of the ear and final cosmetic result with recreation of the helical rim. (C) *1*, Skin defect of the nasal ala. *2*, Inverting horizontal mattress suture at 1-week follow-up. *3*, Recreation of the alar crease seen 2 weeks after initial repair. (A–B, from Wentzell J, Lund J. The inverting horizontal mattress suture: applications in dermatologic surgery, *Dermatol Surg.* 2012;38:1536. C, From Malone C, Wagner R. Recreation of the alar crease using the inverted horizontal mattress suture, *J Am Acad Dermatol.* 2015;73:e112.)

Figure-of-Eight Sutures

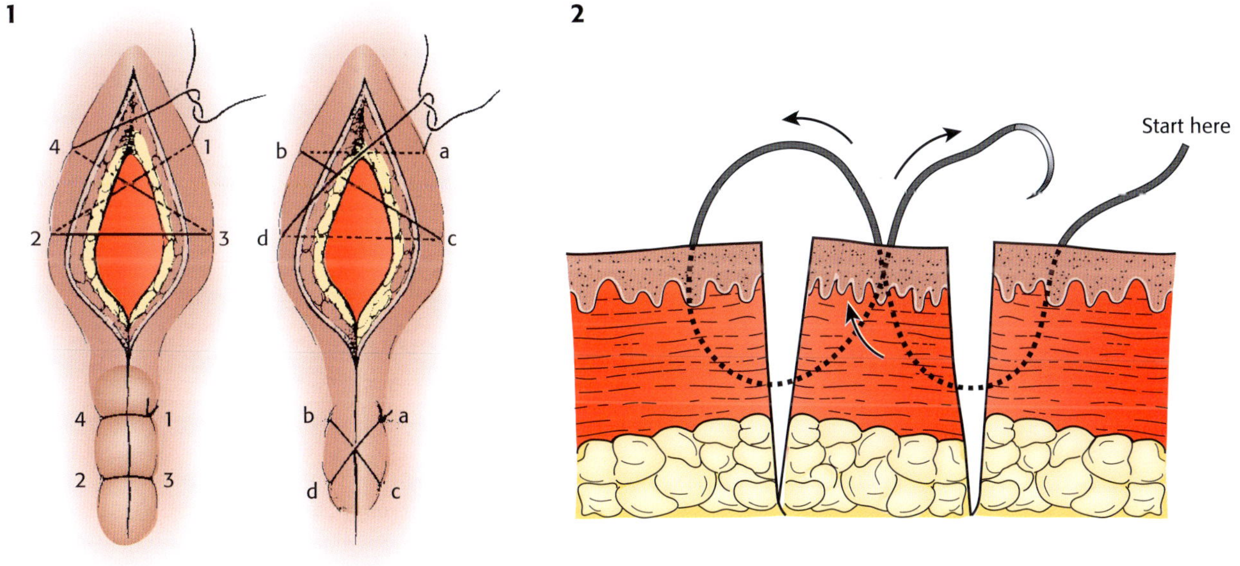

Figure-of-eight stitch, two methods. These stitches are useful in wounds with friable tissue or in areas where buried sutures are undesirable. This stitch reduces the amount of tension placed on the tissue by the suture.

Vertical figure-of-eight suture technique. It can be used to close parallel lacerations.

Fig. 35.34 Figure-of-eight sutures. (Plate 1, modified from Dushoff IM. About face. *Emerg Med.* 1974;6:11; plate 2, from Mitchell GC. Repair of parallel lacerations [letter]. *Ann Emerg Med.* 1987;16:924.)

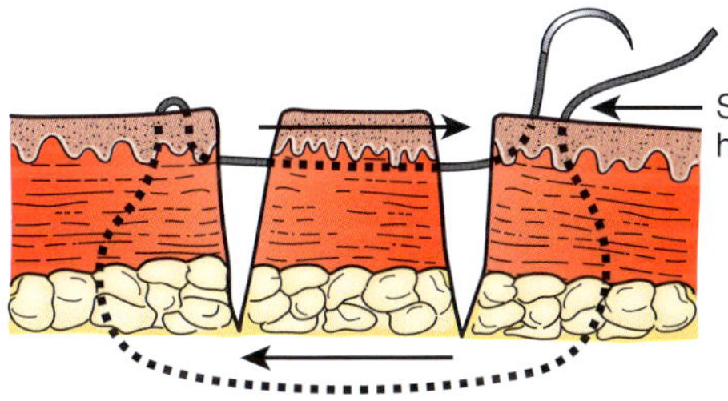

Fig. 35.35 Technique for closure of parallel lacerations in which the central tissue island has an intact base. (Modified from Samo DG. A technique for parallel lacerations, *Ann Emerg Med.* 1988;17:297.)

inexact tissue approximation may be all that is possible initially. For small stellate lacerations, it may be possible to excise the lesion totally and convert it to a linear repair.

Repair of Special Structures

See Videos 35.12–35.15.

Facial Wounds (General Features)

The ideal result in the repair of a facial laceration is an extremely narrow, flat, and inapparent scar. Facial and forehead lacerations that follow natural skin creases or lines will heal with a less noticeable scar than those that are oblique or perpendicular to the natural wrinkles of the skin (Fig. 35.38). In addition to basic wound management, a few additional techniques can be used to achieve satisfactory cosmetic results.

Although necrosis of partially devitalized wound edges contributes to wide scars, facial skin with apparently marginal circulation may survive because of excellent vascularity. SQ fat, which in other locations may be debrided thoroughly, should be preserved if possible in facial wounds to prevent eventual sinking of the scar and to preserve normal facial contours. Therefore conserve as much tissue as possible when debriding most facial wounds (Fig. 35.39). Carefully avoid underlying structures in the face. For example, the cheek contains both the seventh cranial nerve and the parotid gland. Clear drainage from a cheek laceration indicates parotid gland or Stensen's duct involvement and warrants specialist consultation.[114]

A layered closure has long been considered essential in the cosmetic repair of many facial wounds. However, Singer and associates called into question the importance of layered closure in all facial wounds.[115] These investigators found similar cosmetic outcomes and scar widths in small facial wounds less than 3 cm in length and 10 mm in width that were repaired with and without deep dermal sutures. Further confirmation of these results is needed.

If a layered closure is undertaken, approximate the dermis with an SQ stitch or with a combination of SQ and subcuticular stitches to bring the edges of the wound together or to within 1 mm to 2 mm of apposition. This may be close enough that the use of additional sutures seems almost unnecessary. If a SQ stitch is the only stitch used to close the deeper layers, pass the needle through the dermal-epidermal junction, or within 1 mm to 2 mm of the surface of the skin, without

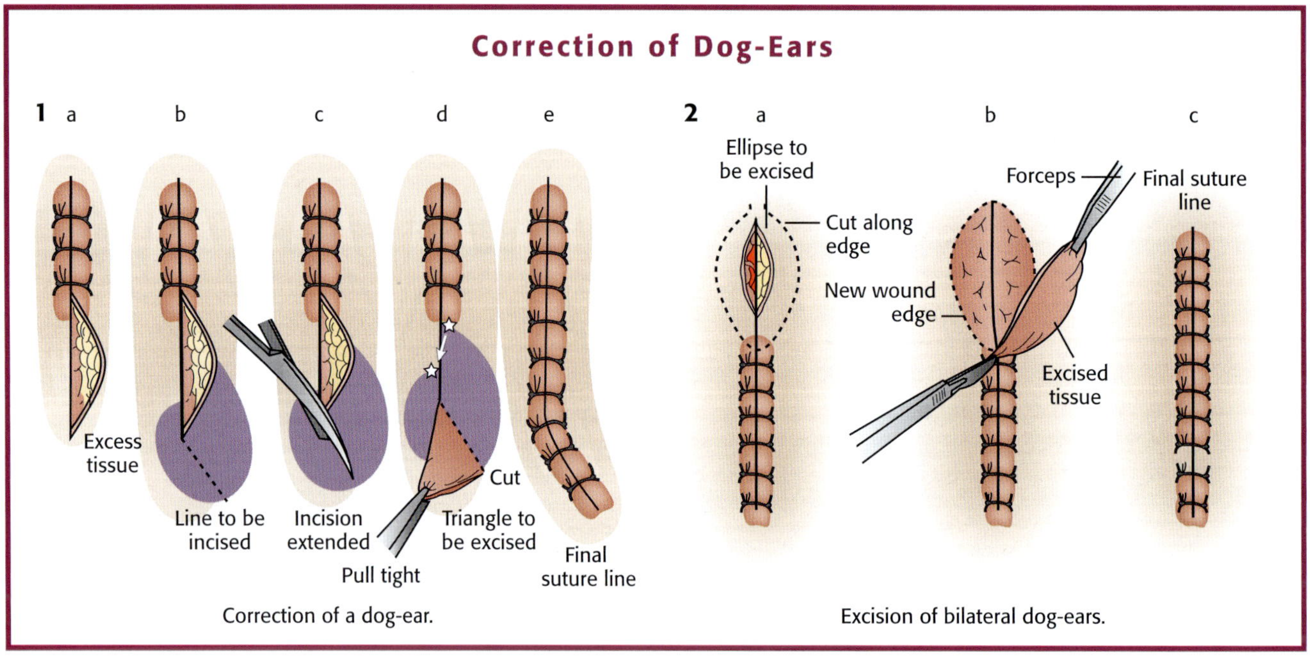

A

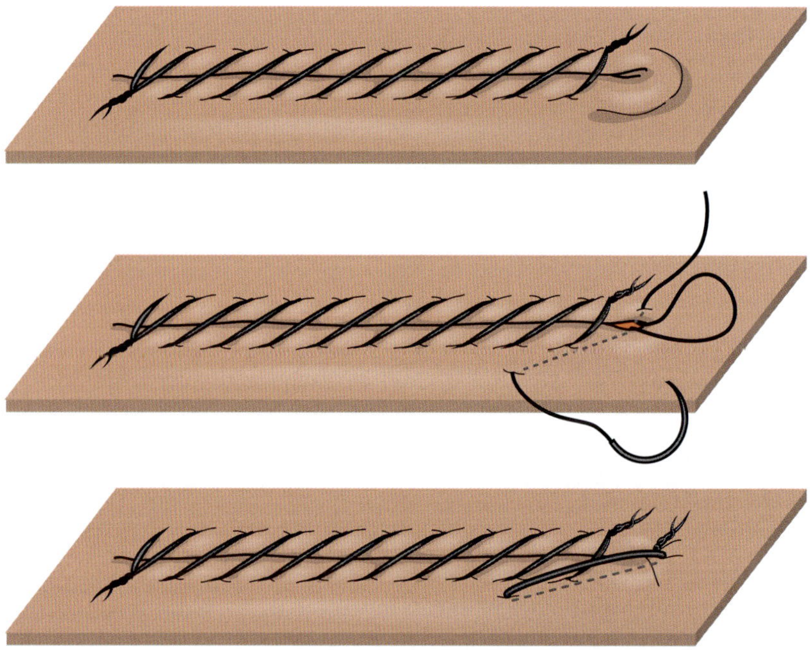

B

Fig. 35.36 Correction of a dog-ear: two methods. (A) Excision technique. The critical maneuver is shown, where the skin is pulled tight to align the starred areas and identify the triangular piece of excess tissue to be excised *(1d)*. Note that a straight laceration becomes somewhat curved with this technique. (B) Tissue-sparing technique. Insert the needle into the apex of the dog-ear, push it through the end of the wound opening, place it into the side of the wound, and then exit 3-4 mm lateral to the wound axis. (A, from Dushoff IM. A stitch in time. *Emerg Med.* 1973;5:1. B1–3, modified from Cronin M, Li Y, Cronin TA Sr, Cronin TA Jr. The snug tip stitch: a tissue-sparing technique for the correction of small dog ears. *Dermatol Surg.* 2021;47:1004-1005.)

causing a dimpling effect. Tie the stitch snugly by pulling the two ends of the suture in the same direction (see Fig. 35.25C).

In cosmetic areas, a surface stitch should not be used to relieve a wound of significant tension. A surface stitch on the face is most appropriately used to match the epidermal surfaces precisely along the length of the wound. If the edges of the wound are separated more than approximately 2 mm to 4 mm after closure of the SQ layer, use a 5-0 or 6-0 subcuticular suture to eliminate the tension produced by this separation and to provide prolonged stability. Alternatively, use a few *guide stitches* to hold sections of the wound together before definitive closure with surface stitches. Guide stitches allow the surface stitches to be placed with little tension on each individual stitch; they match irregular edges and protect the

Management of Stellate Lacerations

1

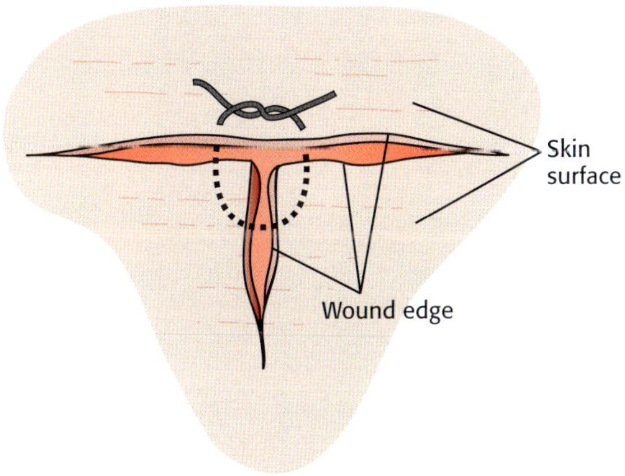

View from above a stellate laceration showing closure with half-buried mattress stitches. For some stellate lacerations it is best to cover with Steri-Strips and revise the scar later or, if small, excise the laceration and convert it to a linear repair.

2

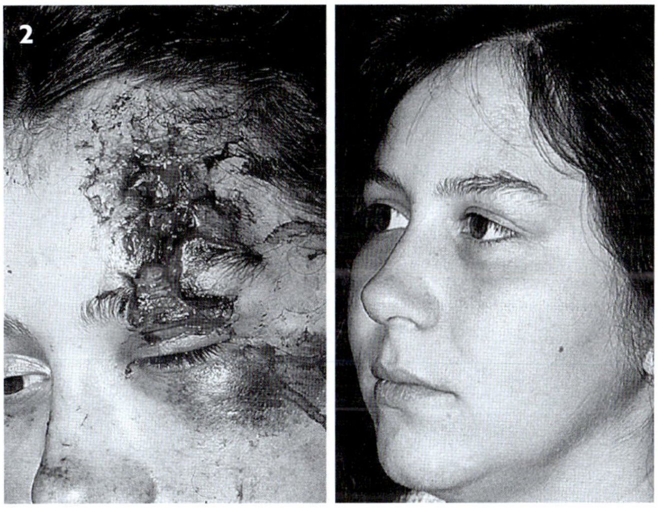

Left, significant soft tissue contusion with stellate lacerations. *Right*, the result at 1 year. No tissue was débrided; instead, meticulous attention was paid to accurate soft tissue realignment with fine suture (7-0).

Fig. 35.37 Management of stellate lacerations.

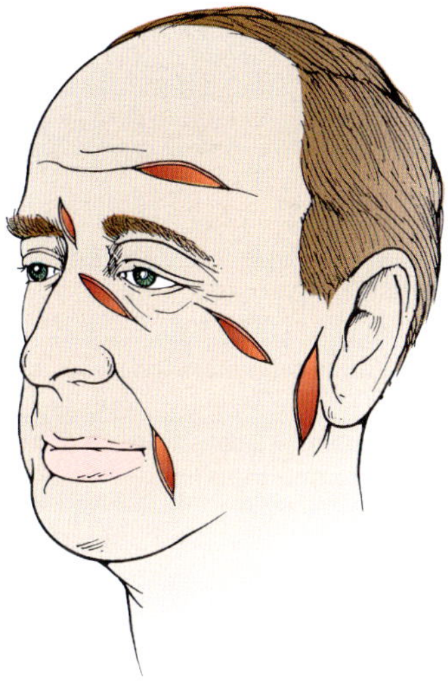

Fig. 35.38 Lacerations following natural skin lines (shown here) heal with a less noticeable scar than those that are oblique or perpendicular to natural lines (or wrinkles).

SQ stitches from disruption. Place the first guide stitch at the midpoint of the wound and subsequent guide stitches to bisect the intervening spaces. Once the definitive surface stitches have been placed, the guide stitches, if slack, can be removed. Because a needle damages tissue with each passage through the skin, use guide stitches only when necessary.

In a straight laceration, achieve better apposition during surface closure by stretching it lengthwise with finger traction or with skin hooks. When the needle is placed on one side of the wound, and that side is higher than the opposite side, take a shallow bite. Use the needle to depress the edges of the wound to the proper height, and allow the needle to "follow through" to the other side and pin the two sides together. If the first side entered is lower, elevate the needle when entering the second side to match the epithelial edges.

If the skin edges are apposed closely by the SQ stitch or a subcuticular stitch, a small, shallow *epithelial stitch* can be used in lieu of the standard, deeper, surface stitch to correct discrepancies in vertical alignment (Fig. 35.40). Achieve precise alignment of wound edges by inserting the needle as close to the edge as possible without tearing through the tissue. A 6-0 synthetic nonabsorbable suture is an excellent material for this stitch. A continuous stitch is preferable because it can be placed quickly, but interrupted stitches are acceptable. Space epithelial stitches no more than 2 mm to 3 mm apart and encompass no more than 2 mm to 4 mm of tissue. Once skin closure is complete, make final adjustments in the tension on a continuous suture line before tying the end of the stitch. If any discrepancies in level persist, use interrupted sutures or tape to flatten these few irregularities. The disadvantages of epithelial stitches are that they are time-consuming and add more suture material to the wound. Discrepancies in level can often be corrected with surgical tape.

Surgical tape is useful as a secondary support to protect the surface stitch from the stress produced by normal skin movement (Fig. 35.41). Facial wounds tend to swell and place excessive stretch on a surface stitch. Minimize this by applying a pressure dressing and cold compresses to the wound after closure. Surgical tape can serve to a limited extent as a small pressure dressing. In simple, low-tension facial wounds, wound closure with surgical tape provides results equivalent to closure with tissue adhesive.[116]

Forehead

Although the forehead is actually a part of the scalp, lacerations in this region are treated as facial wounds. Vertical lacerations across the forehead are oriented 90 degrees to skin tension lines. The resulting scars are more noticeable than

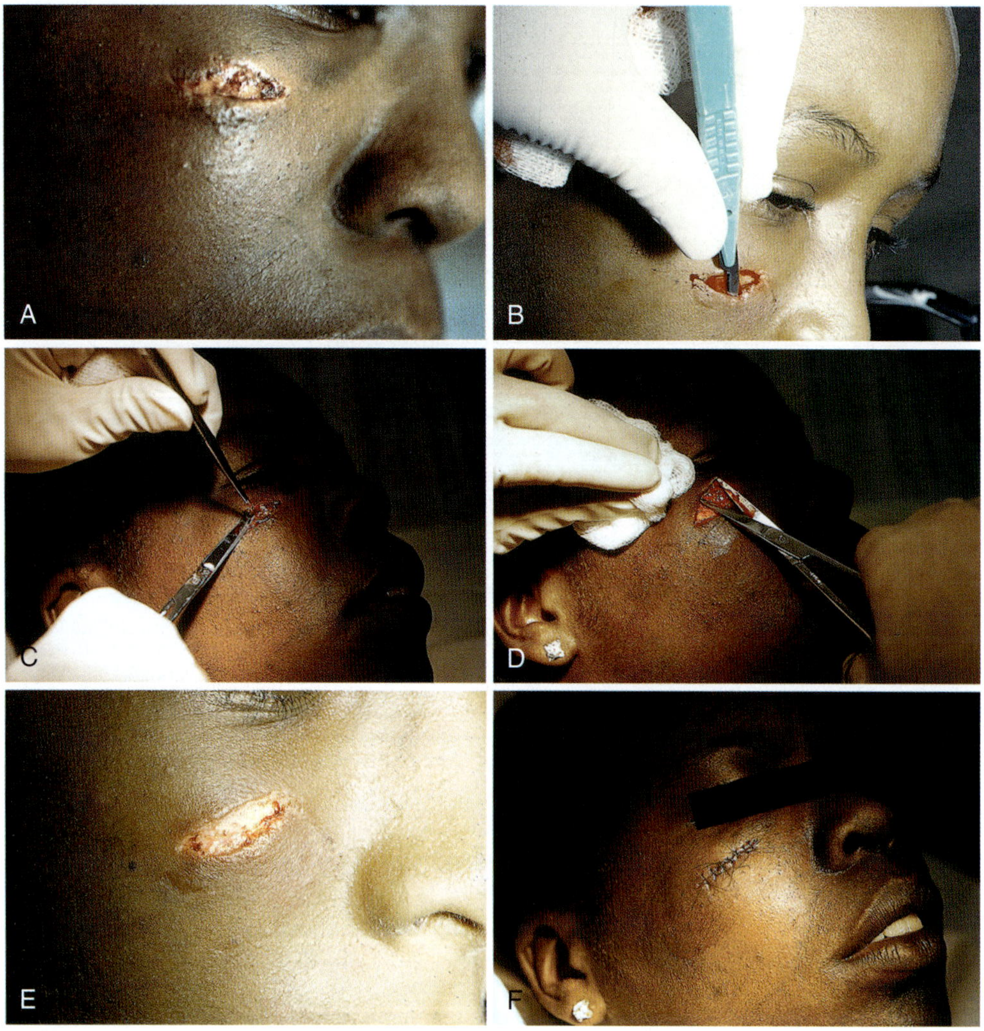

Fig. 35.39 (A) This female was punched in the face, sustained a laceration of her cheek, and went to the emergency department 35 hours later. The wound was not infected, but it had contracted and was beginning to heal by granulation. Under local anesthesia, the wound was opened, irrigated, and minimally debrided, and the skin edges were trimmed. (B) Using a No. 15 blade, a 1-mm-deep incision was made in the skin along the edges of the wound border. (C) The incised edges were then cut away with tissue scissors. (D) The wound was undermined to relieve tension on the skin. (E) The wound is clean, undermined, and ready to close. (F) The wound was closed with 6-0 interrupted sutures, which were removed in 5 days. No antibiotics were used, and only a small linear scar resulted.

those from horizontal lacerations. Midline vertical forehead lacerations may result in cosmetically acceptable scars with standard closure techniques; uncentered lacerations may benefit from S-plasty or Z-plasty techniques during the initial repair or during later revision of the scar.

Superficial lacerations may be closed with skin stitches alone, but deep forehead lacerations must be closed in layers. First, approximate significant periosteal defects before closing more superficial layers (Fig. 35.42). If skin is directly exposed to bone, adhesions might develop that in time may limit the movement of skin during facial expressions. Close the frontalis muscle fascia and adjacent fibrous tissue as a distinct layer; if left unsutured, the retracted ends of this muscle may bulge beneath the skin. If the gap in a muscle belly is later filled with scar tissue, movement of the muscle may pull on the entire scar and make it more apparent.

A U-shaped flap laceration with a superiorly oriented base poses a difficult problem. Immediate vascular congestion and later scar contraction within the flap produce the "trapdoor" effect, with the flap becoming prominently elevated (Fig. 35.43, *plates 1 and 2*). To minimize this effect, approximate the bulk of the SQ tissue of the flap to a deeper level on the base side of the wound. This way the skin surfaces of the two sides are apposed at the same level (see Fig. 35.43, *plate 3*). Apply a firm compression dressing to eliminate dead space and hematoma formation within the wound. Despite these efforts, secondary revision is sometimes necessary. Frequently, swelling of the flap resolves over a 6- to 12-month period. Because flap elevation can be quite disconcerting, forewarn the patient and family about a possible trapdoor effect.

When a forehead laceration borders the scalp and the thick scalp tissue must be sutured to thinner forehead skin, use a horizontal or vertical mattress stitch with an intradermal component (see Fig. 35.43, *plates 3E and 3F*).

Note that even a minor forehead contusion or laceration may bleed subcutaneously and, in a few days, produce blackness around the eyes (Fig. 35.44). Forewarn patients about this. So-called "raccoon eyes" were once thought to represent a fracture, and although often associated with fractures, this is usually a common, benign finding.

Windshield injuries involving the forehead can be challenging to manage (see Fig. 35.44C) because multiple superficial cuts can harbor small glass particles and the injuries do not readily lend themselves to closure with suture. Supraorbital blocks can anesthetize the forehead while the clinician meticulously looks for glass in each skin defect, often feeling pieces only with forceps or a small hemostat. Some pieces of glass are best felt with an instrument; others are appreciated as shining objects under a good light source.

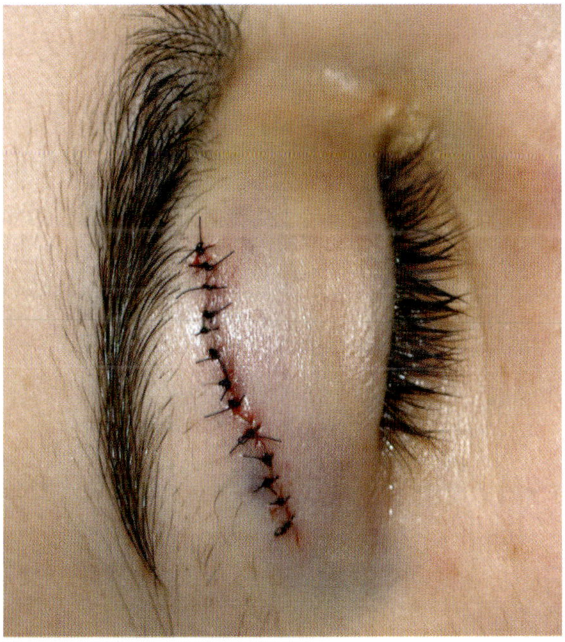

Fig. 35.40 Epithelial stitches. If the skin edges are well apposed by a subcutaneous or subcuticular stitch, epithelial stitches can be used to correct discrepancies in vertical alignment. Achieve precise alignment by inserting the needle as close to the edge as possible without tearing the tissue, no more than 2 mm to 3 mm apart and encompassing no more than 2 mm to 4 mm of tissue. This wound should be carefully evaluated for an occult globe injury.

Eyebrow and Eyelid Lacerations

Manage jagged lacerations through eyebrows with little, if any, debridement of untidy but viable edges. The hair shafts of the eyebrow grow at an oblique angle, and vertical excision may produce a linear alopecia, whereas with simple closure, the scar remains hidden within the hair.

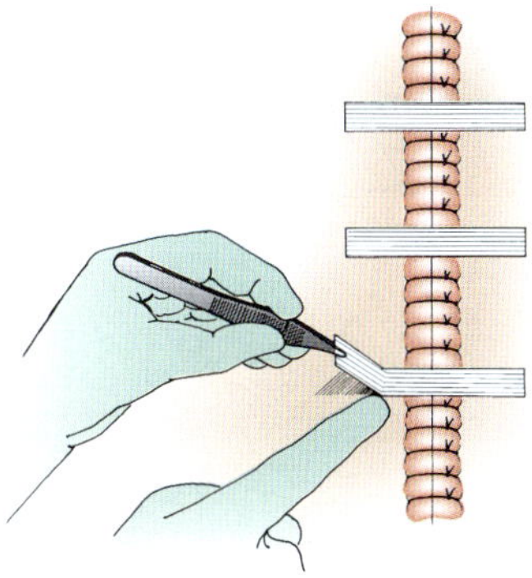

Fig. 35.41 Wound closure tape can be used to provide additional support while sutures are in place and after they are removed. This may be especially useful in cosmetic areas such as the face.

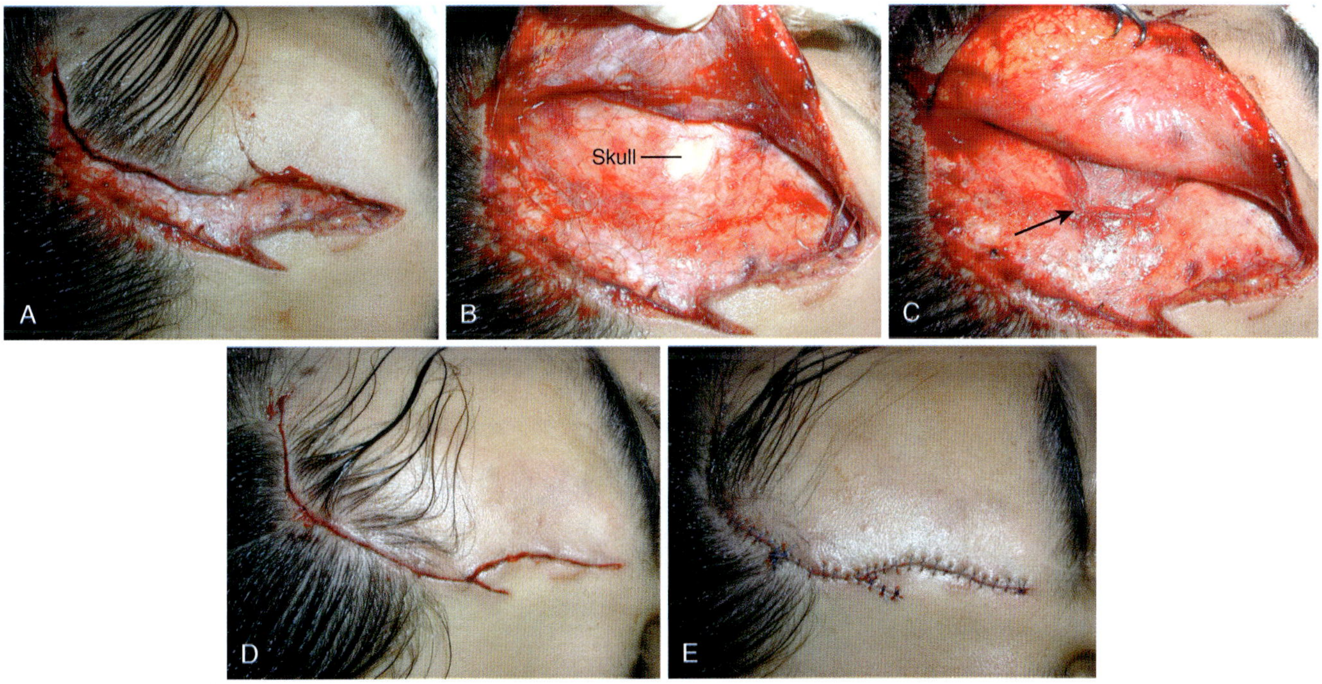

Fig. 35.42 (A) This patient sustained a full-thickness flap (partial avulsion) type of forehead laceration. (B) The surface of the skull is visible in the upper portion of the wound. Injuries such as these must be closed in layers. (C) The galea aponeurosis is repaired with absorbable suture. (D) Additional subcuticular and subcutaneous stitches were placed meticulously, which resulted in excellent apposition of the wound edges. (E) The surface is repaired with a combination of simple interrupted and continuous epithelial sutures.

Repair of "Trapdoor" Injuries

1

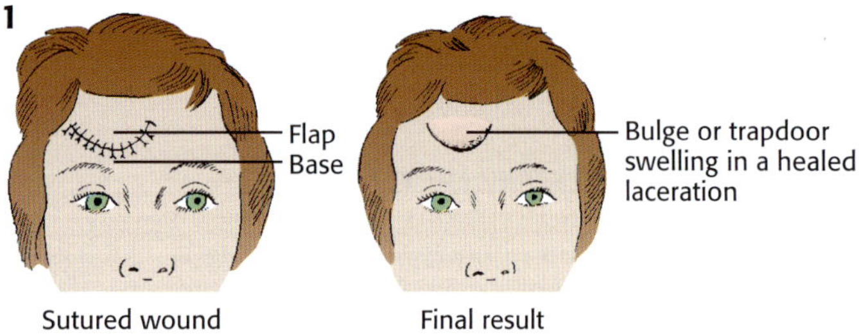

Elevation of a forehead flap. The trapdoor effect is a natural healing process of elliptical or round lacerations. Patients should be advised of this phenomenon.

2

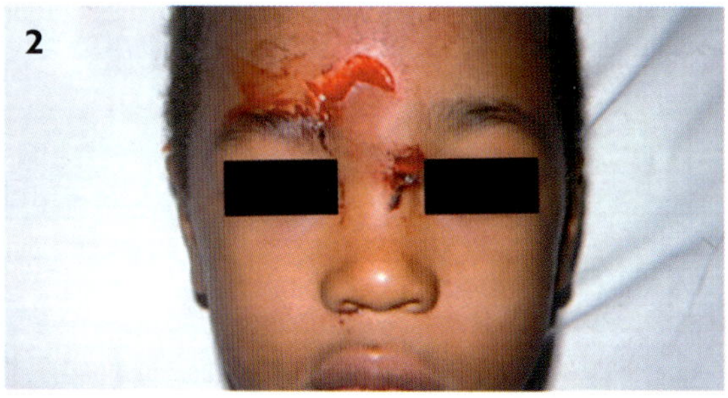

This flap-type laceration of the forehead will heal with a puffed-up center (trapdoor), even under the best of circumstances.

3

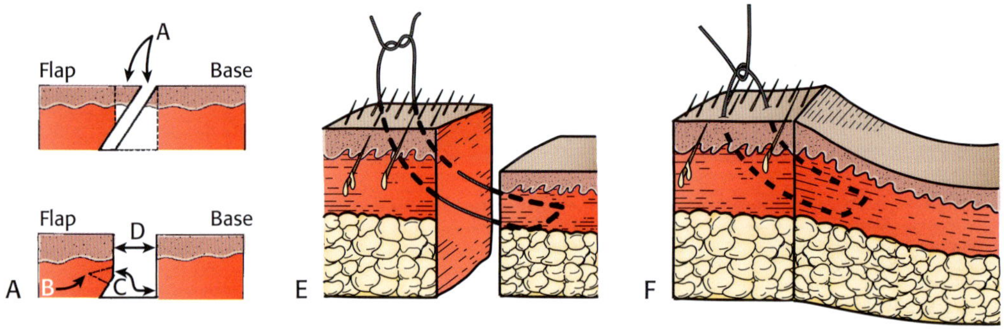

Repair of a U-shaped flap laceration with a superiorly oriented base to minimize the trapdoor effect. **A**, Excision of edges. **B**, Undermining. **C**, Approximation of subcutaneous tissue on the flap to subcutaneous tissue at a deeper level on the base. **B** and **C**, When a laceration in the thin skin of the forehead borders the thicker skin of the scalp, a horizontal mattress suture with an intradermal component can enhance healing by bringing tissues to the same plane. These figures show eversion of thinner skin to obtain adequate approximation with thicker scalp tissue. **D**-**F**, Skin closure.

Fig. 35.43 Repair of trapdoor injuries. (Plate 1, from Grabb WC, Kleinert HE. *Techniques in Surgery: Facial and Hand Injuries*. Ethicon; 1980; plate 3, from Converse JM. Introduction to plastic surgery. In: Converse JM, ed. *Reconstructive Plastic Surgery: Principles and Procedures in Correction, Reconstruction, and Transplantation*. Vol 1. 2nd ed. Saunders; 1977.)

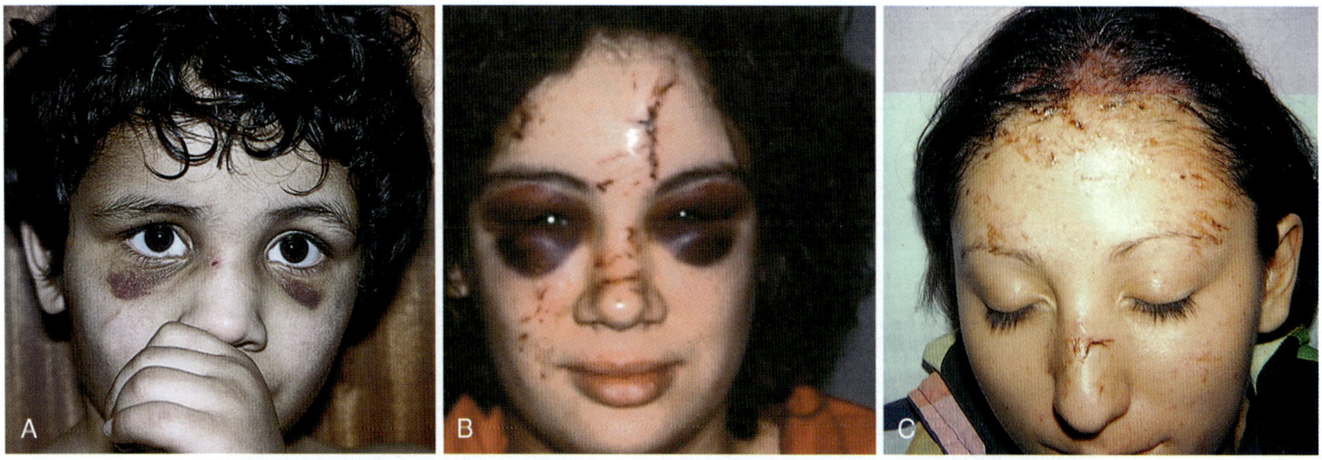

Fig. 35.44 (A) Patients should be informed that minor forehead or nasal bridge trauma can produce benign blackness around the eyes in a few days. (B) "Raccoon eyes" are most often benign; however, this phenomenon can be impressive. (C) Under bilateral supraorbital nerve blocks, multiple small lacerations from this windshield injury are explored with a metal instrument and good lighting to remove tiny pieces of glass. Most superficial cuts can be left alone and others sutured with 6-0 nylon suture.

If partial excision is unavoidable, angle the scalpel blade in a direction parallel to the axis of the hair shaft to minimize damage to the hair follicles.

Align points on each side of the lacerated eyebrow precisely. Precede SQ closure with a single percutaneous stitch on each margin of the eyebrow. Use the edges of the eyebrow as landmarks for reapproximation. Do not shave the eyebrow because these landmarks will be lost. Shaved eyebrows grow back slowly and sometimes incompletely. Shaving them often results in more deformity than caused by the injury itself. Take care not to invert hair-bearing skin into the wound.

The thin, flexible skin of the upper eyelid is relatively easy to suture. Careful examination of the globe itself should be undertaken before eyelid repair. A soft 6-0 suture (or smaller) is recommended to close simple lacerations. Traumatized eyelids are susceptible to massive swelling; compression dressings and cool compresses can be used to minimize this problem.

The emergency clinician must recognize that eyelid lacerations, especially complicated ones, require the expertise of an ophthalmologist with experience in ocular plastic surgery. Lacerations that traverse the lid margin require exact realignment to avoid entropion or ectropion. Injuries penetrating the tarsal plate frequently cause damage to the globe (Fig. 35.45A). A deep horizontal laceration through the upper lid that divides the thin levator palpebrae muscle or cuts its tendinous attachment to the tarsal plate can result in ptosis. In most cases, an ophthalmologist should repair the injury primarily. A laceration through the portion of the upper or lower lid medial to the punctum frequently damages the lacrimal duct or the medial canthal ligament. It requires specialized techniques for repair (see Fig. 35.45B). Adipose tissue seen within any periorbital laceration may be retrobulbar fat herniating through the wound, and further evaluation is required (see Fig. 35.45C). Leave the repair of lid avulsions, extensive lid lacerations with loss of tissue, and complex types of lid lacerations to ophthalmologists.

Ear Lacerations

The primary goals in the management of lacerations of the pinna are expedient coverage of exposed cartilage and prevention of wound hematoma (Fig. 35.46). Cartilage is an avascular tissue, and when ear cartilage is denuded of its protective, nutrient-providing skin, progressive erosive chondritis ensues. The first step in the repair of an ear injury is to trim away jagged or devitalized cartilage and skin. If the skin cannot be stretched to cover the defect, remove additional cartilage along the wound margin. Depending on the location, as much as 5 mm of cartilage can be removed without significant deformity. Approximate the cartilage with 4-0 or 5-0 absorbable sutures placed at folds or ridges in the pinna, representing major landmarks. Sutures tear through cartilage; therefore the anterior and posterior perichondrium are included in the stitch. Do not apply more tension than is needed to touch the edges together.

Next, in through-and-through ear lacerations, approximate the posterior skin surface with 5-0 nonabsorbable synthetic suture. Once closure of the posterior surface is completed, approximate the convoluted anterior surface of the ear with 5-0 or 6-0 nonabsorbable synthetic suture, joining landmarks point by point (see Fig. 35.46C–D). In repair of the helical fold, use the inverting horizontal mattress stitch (see prior section in this chapter on mattress suture). On the free rim, evert the skin to avoid notching later. Take care to cover all exposed cartilage. In heavily contaminated wounds of the ear (e.g., bite wounds) that already show evidence of inflammation, debride the necrotic tissue, cover the cartilage with a loose approximation of skin, and give the patient antibiotics. Once the lacerated ear has been sutured, enclose it in a compression dressing (see Chapter 64). Complex or complicated ear lacerations generally require specialist consultation and early follow-up.

Nose Lacerations

Lacerations involving the margin of the nostril are complicated and should be repaired accurately to ensure that unsightly notching does not occur (Fig. 35.47). In the medial portion of the nostril and superior columella, the lower lateral cartilages are quite close to the margin and relatively superficial. If the extent of the laceration is not recognized or repaired, wound healing may cause superior retraction of the margin of the nostril. Carefully palpate nasal wounds for underlying bone injury. If bony deformity is noted, consider consulting a plastic surgeon, because the fragments may require surgical wiring.[117] Secondary repair of complications is difficult.

In repairing superficial lacerations of the nose, reapproximation of the edges of the wound is difficult because the skin is inflexible. Even deeply placed stitches will slice through the epidermis and pull out. When the edges of the wound cannot be coapted easily before skin closure, place 6-0 absorbable sutures in the fibrofatty junction with an SQ stitch. Because it is difficult to approximate gaping wounds in this location, keep debridement to a minimum. Fortunately, the nose has a rich supply of blood and often will heal without debridement. Nasal cartilage is frequently involved in wounds of the nose, but it is seldom necessary to suture the cartilage itself.

Align the free rim of the nostril precisely to avoid unsightly notching. The inverting horizontal mattress stitch may be useful in the alar crease of the nostril to help with inversion (see prior section in this chapter on mattress suture). Many clinicians recommend early removal of stitches to avoid stitch marks, yet the oily nature of skin in this area makes it difficult to keep the wound closed with tape. A running subcuticular stitch may be preferable when repairing nasal lacerations, but simple interrupted stitches are also acceptable.[117] If the wound is gaping before closure, a subcuticular stitch can provide support for a prolonged period. If there is significant tissue injury, consultation with a facial plastic surgeon may be warranted.

Lip and Intraoral Lacerations

Lip lacerations are cosmetically deforming injuries, but if the clinician follows a few guidelines, these lacerations usually heal satisfactorily.

The contamination of all intraoral and lip wounds is considerable, and they must be thoroughly irrigated. Regional nerve blocks are preferred over local anesthetic injection because the latter method distends tissue, distorts the anatomy of the lip, and obscures the vermilion border. Loss of less than 25% of the lip permits primary closure with little deformity. The following types of wounds require initial surgical consultation or later reconstructive surgery: loss of more than 25% of the lip, extensive lacerations directly through the commissure of the mouth, and deep scars in the vermilion of the upper lip (which can later result in a redundancy of tissue).

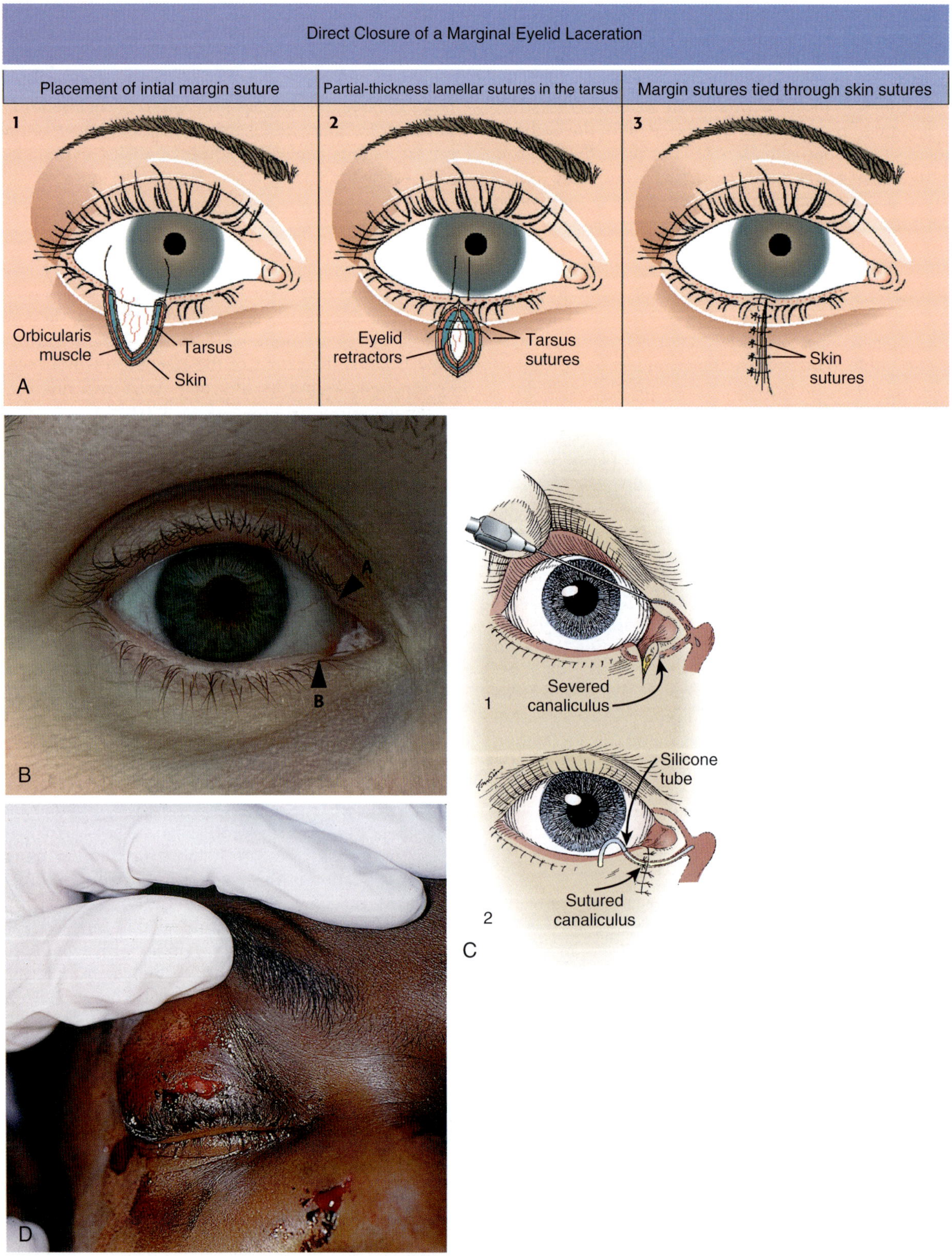

Fig. 35.45 (A) A laceration of the eyelid margin is a complicated repair usually performed by an ophthalmologist or plastic surgeon. The principles of repair are demonstrated here. *1*, The suture is placed precisely in the plane of the meibomian glands at the eyelid margin, approximately 2 mm from the edges of the wound and 2 mm deep. This placement should provide adequate eversion of the margins. *2*, Partial-thickness lamellar sutures are placed across the tarsus and tied anteriorly. *3*, The anterior skin and muscle lamella are closed with fine sutures, and these are tied over the long marginal sutures to prevent them from touching the cornea. (B) *Arrows* point to anatomic locations of puncta (*A*, upper punctum; *B*, lower punctum); the puncta may not be visible unless the lids are everted. (C) Method of identifying and repairing the canaliculus. This repair is best left to the ophthalmologist, but the emergency clinician must recognize the potential for a canaliculus injury. (D) Deep laceration of the left upper lid with herniation of orbital fat. For fat to prolapse, the orbital septum (and potentially the globe itself) must have been perforated. This is a wound requiring operating room exploration and repair.

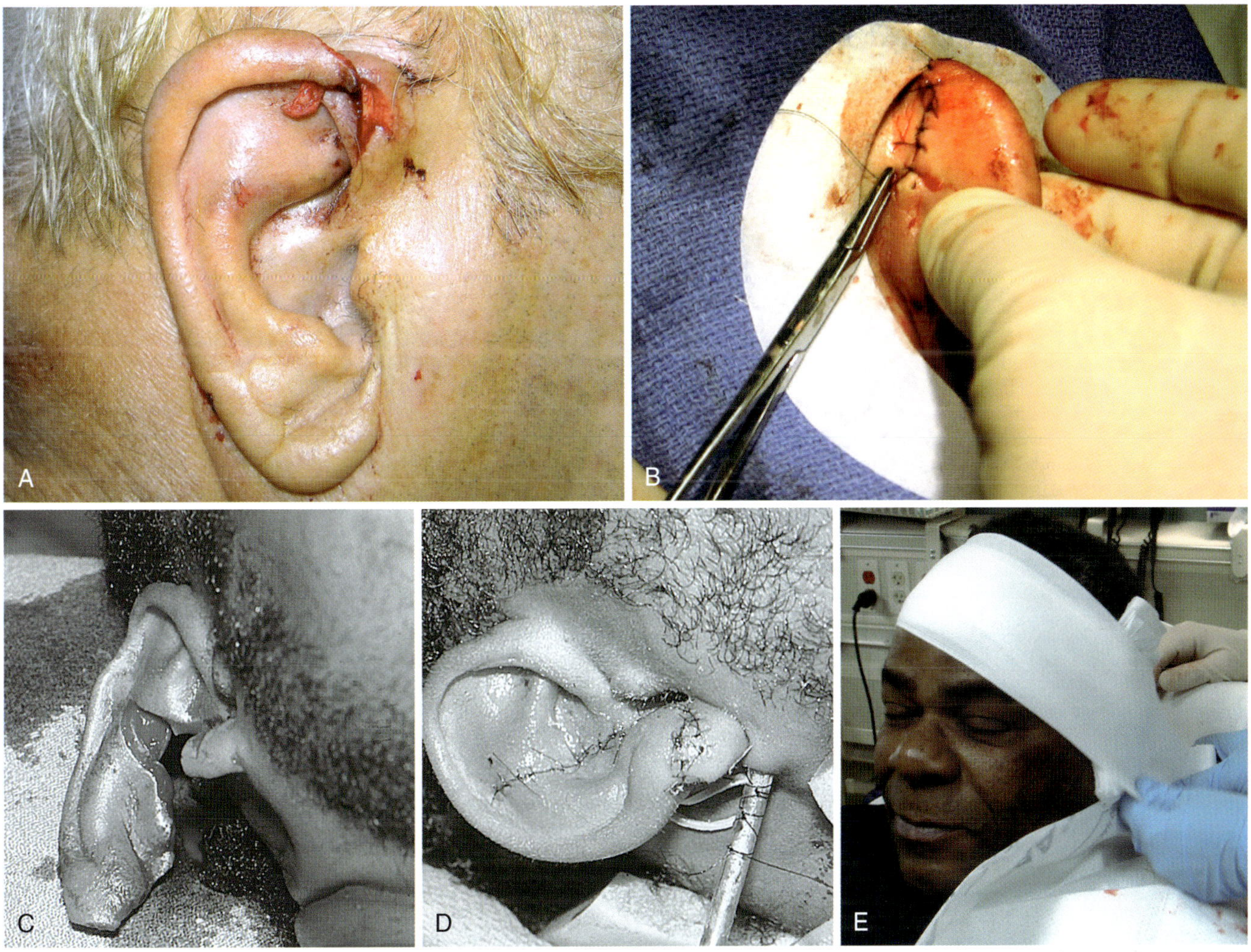

Fig. 35.46 (A) Lacerations of the ear require a special repair aimed at covering cartilage and preventing hematoma formation. With this through-and-through laceration of the margin of the pinna, the cartilage is trimmed just enough to allow the skin to be approximated to cover all exposed cartilage. Sutures are not used in the cartilage itself for this laceration, but the edges are approximated by skin sutures that incorporate the perichondrium. (B) The repair is easiest if the posterior pinna is sutured first. (C–D) Lacerations of the helical rim that traverse the two skin surfaces and the cartilage require a three-layer repair with accurate reapproximation of the auricular cartilage, as is done for the nose, to avoid notching. The cartilage is repaired by placing 5-0 or 6-0 clear absorbable suture through the perichondrium and cartilage. The skin is repaired with 6-0 or 7-0 nonabsorbable suture. (E) An ear compression dressing should be used to prevent hematoma (see Chapter 64) for discussion of anesthesia and dressing for this injury.

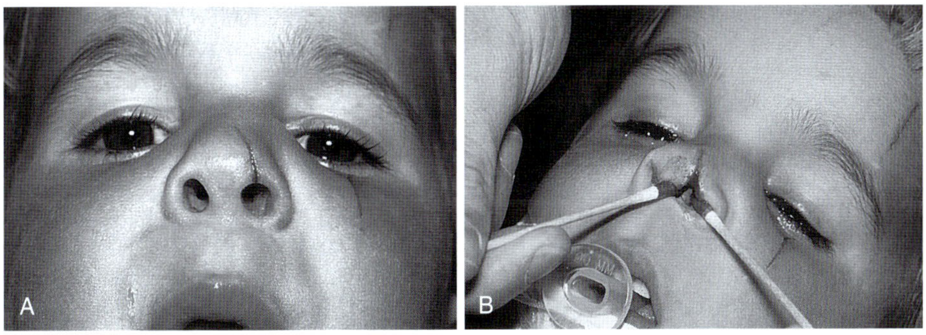

Fig. 35.47 (A) Initially benign-appearing laceration of the left nostril of a 2-year-old patient. (B) However, further investigation shows a full-thickness injury with a laceration of the lower lateral cartilage. A three-layer closure with reapproximation of the cartilage was performed.

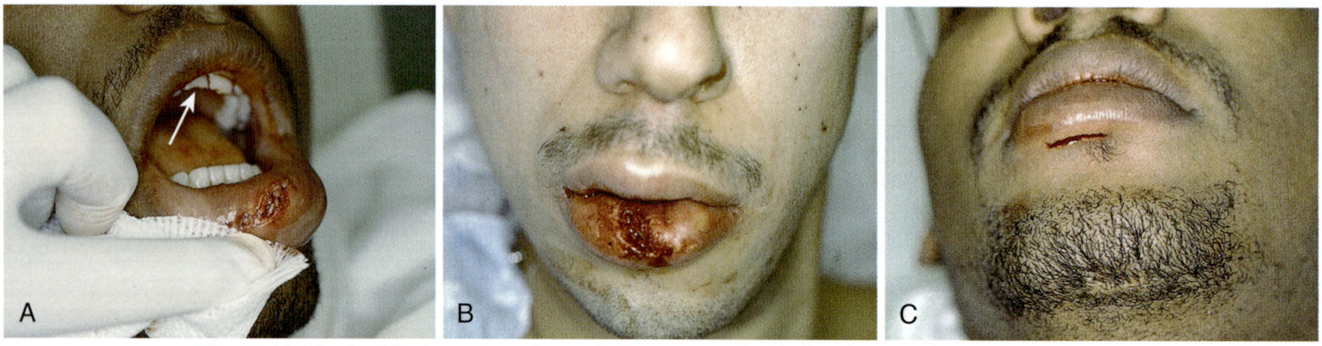

Fig. 35.48 Check all lip lacerations for tooth fragments embedded in the wound. (A) This superficial mucosal laceration produced by the teeth can be cleaned, minimally trimmed, and left open to heal. Note the broken upper teeth *(arrow)*; fragments may be embedded in the laceration. Healing produces a whitish tissue that can be mistaken for infection. (B) This extensive laceration of the mucosa requires a layered suture closure. (C) Small through-and-through lacerations made by the teeth can be irrigated and closed with skin and mucosal sutures in two layers. Small defects in the mucosa may be left open. Large through-and-through injuries and lacerations of the tongue margins require sutures to achieve anatomic healing. The muscle layer should be closed separately (with absorbable sutures) to prevent hematoma formation. In general, buried sutures are better tolerated by the patient.

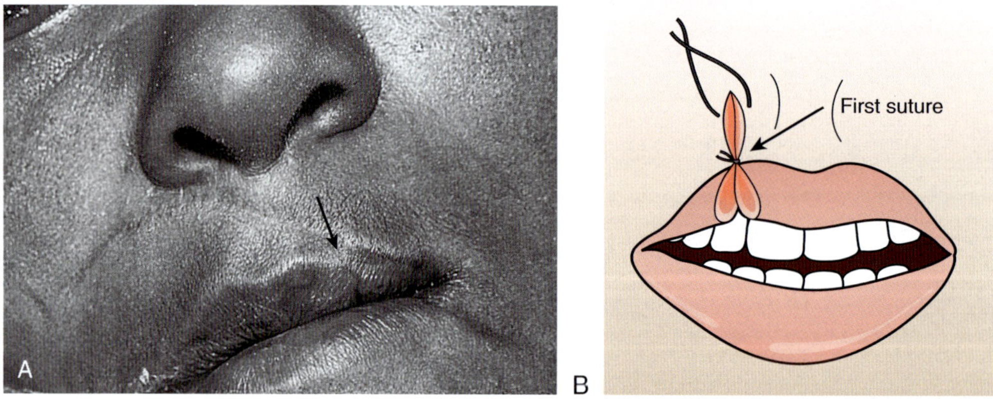

Fig. 35.49 (A) A poorly aligned vermilion border *(arrow)* distorts the lip contour. (B) To prevent this complication, place the first stitch at the vermilion-cutaneous border to obtain proper alignment.

Small puncture-type lacerations heal well only if the skin is closed and the small intraoral laceration is left open (Fig. 35.48A). Such injuries commonly occur when the victim's tooth lacerates the lip as a result of a punch to the face. Check all lip lacerations for retained tooth fragments. In general, small lacerations of the oral mucosa that do not involve muscle heal well without sutures. However, if a mucosal laceration creates a flap of tissue that falls between the occlusal surfaces of the teeth or if a laceration is extensive enough to trap food particles (e.g., ≥2 to 3 cm in length), the laceration should be closed. Small flaps may be excised. Accomplish closure with 4-0 Vicryl or Dexon in a simple interrupted suturing technique. These materials are soft and less abrasive than gut sutures, which become hard and traumatize adjacent mucosa. Vicryl Rapide promotes less inflammation than either gut or Dexon sutures.[118] Nylon sutures have sharp ends that are annoying and painful; thus, this suture material should be avoided inside the mouth. In general, when possible, close muscle and mucosal layers separately. Sutures in the oral cavity easily become untied by the constant motion of the tongue. Tie each of these sutures with at least four square knots. These sutures need not be removed; they either loosen and fall out within 1 week or are rapidly absorbed.

Recent studies demonstrate the good safety and efficacy of tissue adhesives, which are suitable for intraoral laceration repair.[119] Suthar et al. found improved wound healing of intraoral surgical wounds when closed with n-butyl-2-cyanoacrylate rather than suture.[120]

Small through-and-through lacerations can be thoroughly cleaned and closed in two layers (skin and mucosa). It is acceptable to leave the mucosal side open if the defect is small (see Fig. 35.48C). Close large through-and-through lip lacerations in three layers. With a multilayer closure, approximate the muscle layer with a 4-0 or 5-0 absorbable suture securely anchored in the fibrous tissue located anterior and posterior to the muscle.

The vermilion-cutaneous junction of the lip is a critical landmark that, if divided, must be repositioned with precision. Even a 1-mm step-off is apparent and cosmetically unacceptable. Approximate the vermilion border with a 5-0 or 6-0 nonabsorbable guide stitch before any further closure to ensure proper alignment throughout the repair (Fig. 35.49). Close the vermilion surface of the lip and the buccal mucosa with

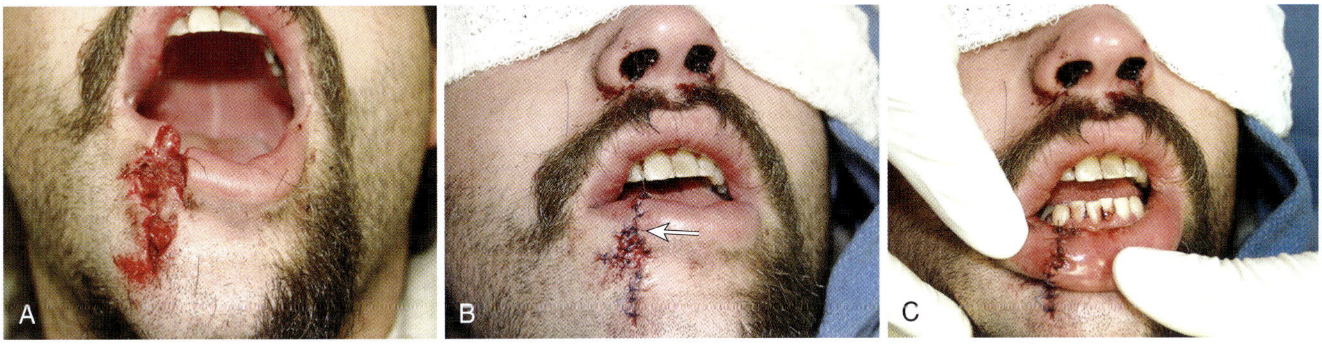

Fig. 35.50 (A) This patient sustained a large through-and-through lip laceration that will require a layered closure. A submental nerve block may be used, or a local anesthetic (lidocaine with epinephrine) can be injected if it does not distort the tissue landmarks. The muscle layer should be repaired with 4-0 or 5-0 absorbable suture. (B) The vermilion border *(arrow)* must be repositioned precisely to prevent permanent disfigurement. A 5-0 or 6-0 guide stitch should be placed at the border before any other closure. Nonabsorbable monofilament sutures are then used to close the skin. (C) Absorbable sutures are used to close the buccal mucosa.

interrupted stitches of 4-0 or 5-0 absorbable suture. Finally, close the skin with 6-0 nonabsorbable suture (Fig. 35.50).

Evaluate all lacerations that penetrate the oral mucosa for the presence of tooth fragments, especially if teeth are missing or chipped. Intensify the search if the patient returns with an infection of a sutured wound. Probe the wound with forceps to identify fragments not seen directly in the wound. In the setting of marked facial swelling, take a radiograph of the soft tissue to help identify embedded tooth fragments.

Tongue Lacerations

Some controversy exists regarding when to suture tongue lacerations. Small, simple, linear lacerations, especially those in the central portion of the tongue, heal quickly with minimal risk for infection. Many small tongue lacerations in children or from falls or seizures do not require sutures. In general, lacerations involving the edge or pass completely through the tongue, flap lacerations, and all lacerations bisecting the tongue must be sutured (Fig. 35.51). Small flaps on the edge of the tongue may be excised, but large flaps should be sutured. If dilute peroxide mouth rinses and a soft diet are used for a few days, healing can be rapid. In recent studies, tissue adhesive is a safe and beneficial option for tongue laceration rep air.[119,121,122] Persistent bleeding from minor lacerations brings most patients to the ED, and closure with deep sutures may be necessary to prevent further bleeding.

Repair of a tongue laceration in any patient is difficult, but in an uncooperative child, the procedure may prove impossible without general anesthesia. A Denhardt-Dingman side mouth gag aids in keeping the patient's mouth open. Anesthetize a localized area of the tongue topically by covering the area with 4% lidocaine-soaked gauze for 5 minutes. Determine the maximum safe dose of local anesthetic and avoid exposure to greater doses. Large lacerations require infiltration anesthesia (1% lidocaine with buffered epinephrine) or a lingual nerve block. If the tip of the tongue has been anesthetized, a towel clip or suture can be used to maintain protrusion of the tongue in an uncooperative patient. Further anesthesia and subsequent wound cleansing and closure are possible while an assistant applies gentle traction on the tongue.

Use size 4-0 absorbable sutures to close all three layers (inferior mucosa, muscle, and superior mucosa) in a single stitch; alternatively the stitch should include half the thickness of the tongue, with sutures placed on the superior and inferior surfaces, as well as on the edge of the tongue. Sutures on the tongue frequently become untied. This problem can be prevented if the stitches are buried. Avoid nylon sutures because the sharp edges are uncomfortable. Closure of the lingual muscle layer with a deep absorbable suture alone may be sufficient to control bleeding and return motor function to the lacerated tongue; mucosal healing is rapid.

Scalp Lacerations

The scalp extends from the supraorbital ridges anteriorly to the external occipital protuberances posteriorly and blends with the temporalis fascia laterally. The scalp has five anatomic layers: skin, superficial fascia, galea aponeurotica, subaponeurotic areolar connective tissue, and periosteum (Fig. 35.52). Clinically, however, the scalp may be divided into three distinct layers. The outer layer consists of the skin, superficial fascia, and galea (the aponeurosis of the frontalis and occipitalis muscles), which are firmly adherent and surgically considered as one layer. The subaponeurotic layer and the periosteum form the second and third layers. The integrity of the outer layer is maintained by inelastic, tough, fibrous septa which keep wounds from gaping open unless all three portions have been traversed. Wounds that gape open signify a laceration extending beneath the galea layer (Fig. 35.53). The galea itself is loosely adherent to the periosteum by means of the slack areolar tissue of the subaponeurotic layer. The galea is firmly attached to the underside of the SQ fascia and is rarely identified as a distinct layer in the depths of a wound. The periosteum covers the skull. The tissue-thin periosteum is often mistakenly identified as the galea, but the periosteum is flimsy and adherent to the skull and cannot be sutured.

Several unique problems are associated with wounds of the scalp. Multiple scalp wounds that are hidden by a mat of hair are easily overlooked. Stellate lacerations are common in this region, not only because the scalp is vulnerable to blunt trauma but also because its superficial fascial layer is inelastic and firmly adherent to the skin. Stellate lacerations pose additional technical problems in closure and have a greater propensity for infection. Shear-type injuries can cause extensive separation of the superficial layers from the galeal layer. Debris and other contaminants can be deposited several centimeters

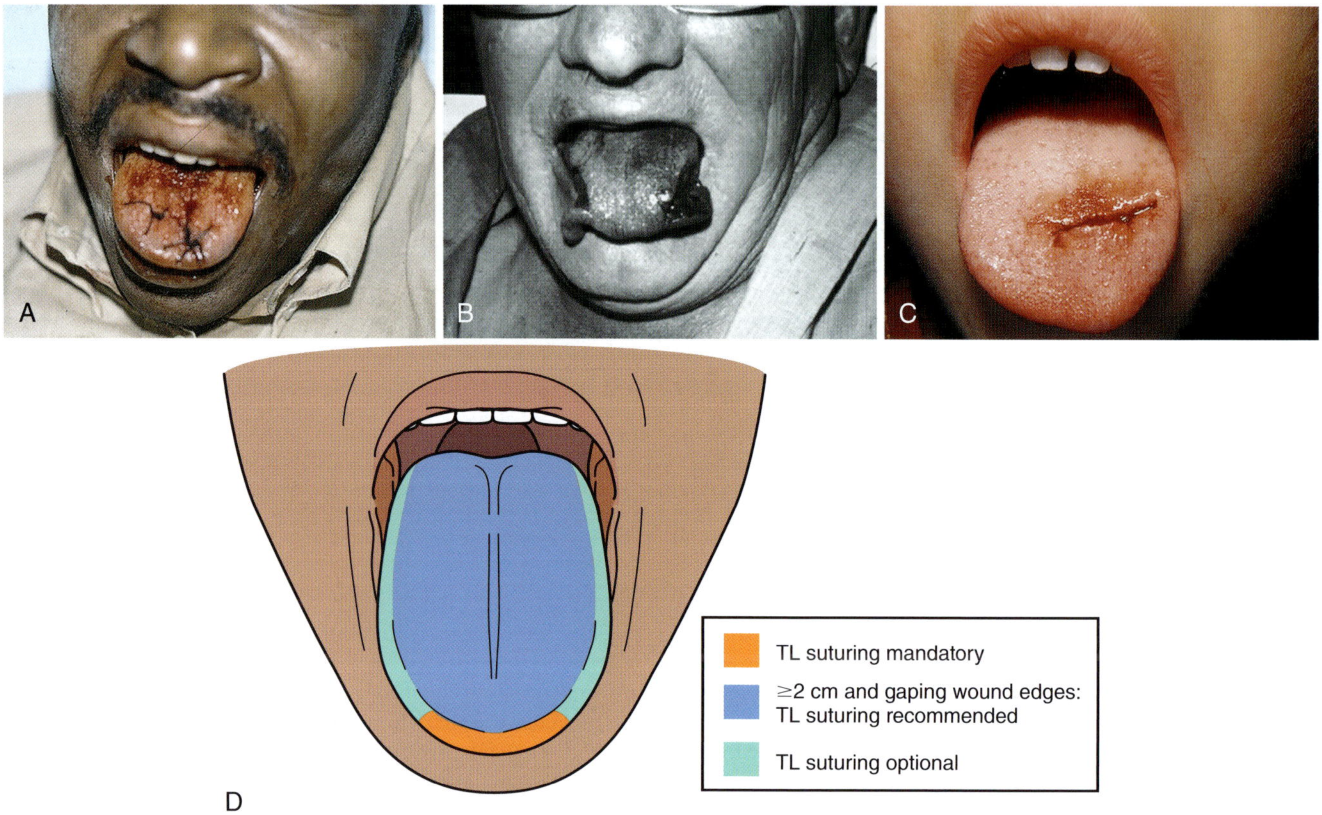

Fig. 35.51 (A) A lacerated tongue usually heals well without sutures, but they were placed in this patient because of a large rent in the middle of the tongue. Dexon, Vicryl, or silk sutures (avoid nylon) are ideal for suturing the surface of the tongue. Bleeding is usually controlled with direct pressure and local infiltration of lidocaine with epinephrine; others require deep sutures for hemostasis. Many seemingly large central tongue lacerations (such as occur during a seizure) heal well with no suturing if the margins of the tongue are intact. (B) When a forked tongue is possible or flaps are pronounced, the tongue requires anatomic repair. (C) This laceration will heal well without sutures. (D) Locations on the tongue in which suturing is recommended. *TL*, Tongue laceration. (D, from Seiler M, Massaro SL, Staubli G, Schiestl C. Tongue lacerations in children: to suture or not? *Swiss Med Wkly.* 2018;148:w14683.)

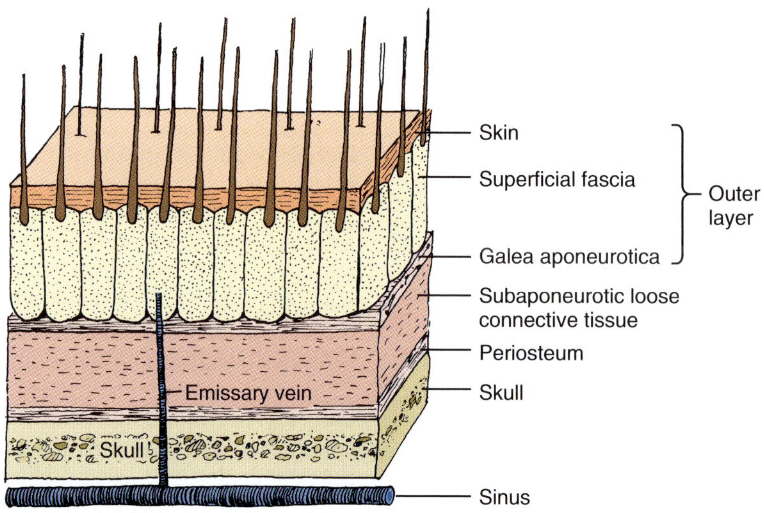

Fig. 35.52 Anatomy of the scalp. The skin, superficial fascia, and galea constitute the outer layer. Blood vessels in the fascia are the major source of bleeding in scalp lacerations.

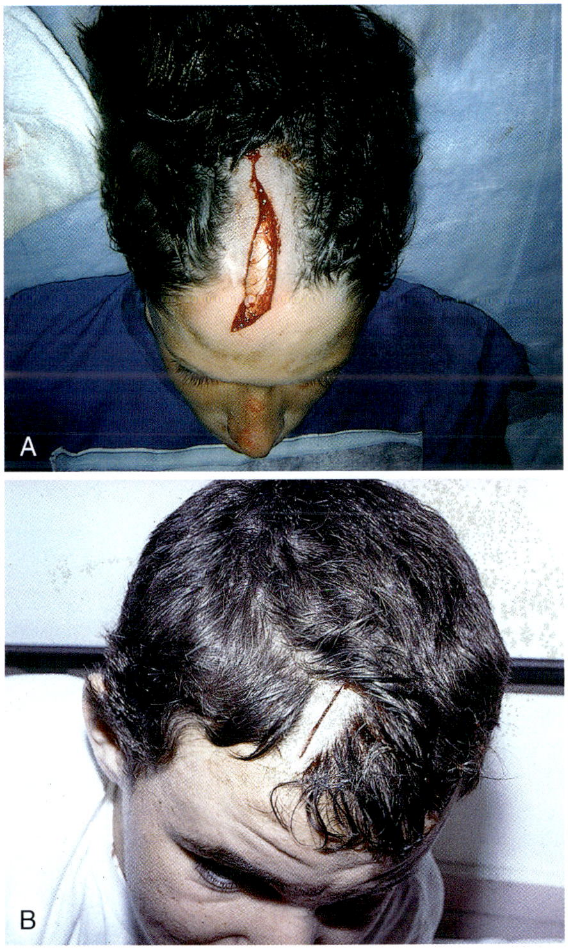

Fig. 35.53 (A) The galea has been transected in wounds that gape open like this one, and to achieve hemostasis and obtain the best closure, the galea should be sutured. (B) This nongaping wound does not include the galea and can be closed with superficial sutures.

from the visible laceration; therefore careful exploration plus cleaning of scalp wounds is important. When scalp wounds are debrided, obviously devitalized tissue should be removed, but as much tissue as possible should be conserved because closure of large defects on the scalp is difficult.

The presence of a rich vascular network in the superficial fascia results in profuse bleeding from scalp wounds. Severed scalp vessels tend to remain patent because the fibrous SQ fascia hinders the normal retraction of blood vessels that have been cut and allows persistent or massive hemorrhage with simple lacerations. The subgaleal layer of loose connective tissue contains emissary veins that drain through diploic vessels of the skull into the venous sinuses of the cranial hemispheres. In scalp wounds that penetrate this layer, these vessels may carry bacteria to the meninges and the intracranial sinuses. Thus, a scalp wound infection can result in osteomyelitis, meningitis, or a brain abscess. Closure of galeal lacerations ensures control of bleeding and protects against the spread of infection.

Profuse bleeding, especially from extensive scalp lacerations, is best controlled by suturing (see also Chapter 34). Unless the vessels are large or small, ligation of multiple scalp vessels seldom provides effective hemostasis, and considerable blood loss can occur during the attempt. Ask an assistant to maintain compression around the wound while you complete

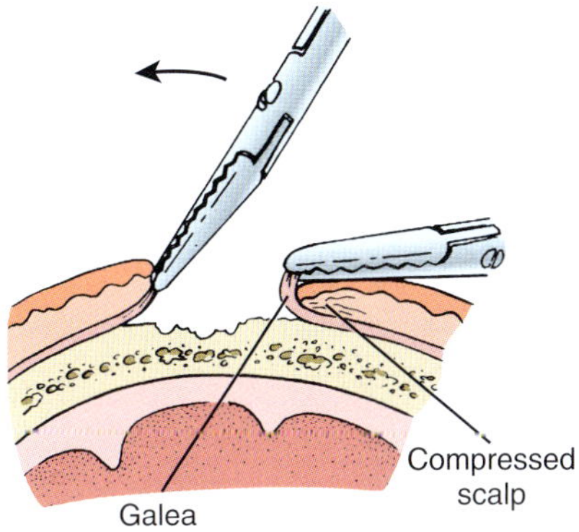

Fig. 35.54 To temporarily control bleeding from vessels in the fascia, the galea can be everted to compress the fascia.

the closure of the wound. A simple procedure that often provides hemostasis of scalp wounds is to place a wide, tight rubber band or Penrose drain around the scalp from the forehead to the occiput. Bleeding can also be temporarily controlled by grasping the galea and the dermis with a hemostat and everting the instrument over the edge of the skin (Fig. 35.54). The disadvantage of this technique is that tissue can be clamped too tightly by the hemostat, crushed and devitalized. If the SQ tissue is also everted for a prolonged period, necrosis can occur.

If an assistant is not available to apply direct pressure, use local anesthetics containing epinephrine because this is sometimes effective in controlling persistent bleeding from small vessels in a scalp wound. If bleeding from the edge of the scalp wound is vigorous and definitive repair must be postponed while the patient is resuscitated, Raney scalp clips or a hemostat can be applied quickly to the edge of the scalp wound to control the hemorrhage.

Before wound closure, visually examine the underlying skull and palpate it for skull fractures (Fig. 35.55). In wounds that can be visualized or explored, more small skull fractures are detected with the clinician's eyes and gloved finger than with radiographs. Do not mistake a tear in the galea or the periosteum for a fracture during palpation inside the wound. Direct visualization of the area should resolve the issue. Stab or puncture wounds in the scalp and forehead, such as from a nail, spike, screwdriver, knife, or ice pick, are difficult to evaluate. Without a laceration to explore, such wounds may seem benign, and the patient can initially appear relatively asymptomatic, yet the skull or brain has been penetrated. When evaluating a puncture or stab wound to the head, a computed tomography scan may provide unexpected findings of a skull fracture, linear or depressed, or an underlying brain injury or early hemorrhage. In wounds that expose bone but do not penetrate the skull, prolonged exposure may leave a nidus of dead bone in which osteomyelitis could develop. If the exposed bone is visibly necrosed, consider a consultation with neurosurgery for partial removal of the bone with rongeurs until active bleeding appears. Clip hair surrounding the scalp wound far enough from the edge of the wound so that suturing can proceed without entangling the hair or burying it in the wound. As stated in other sections, avoid shaving, and instead clip hair to avoid further injury. If hairs along the wound edges become embedded in the wound, they will stimulate excessive granulation tissue and delay healing.[123] Place Vaseline or tape on stubborn hairs that persistently fall into

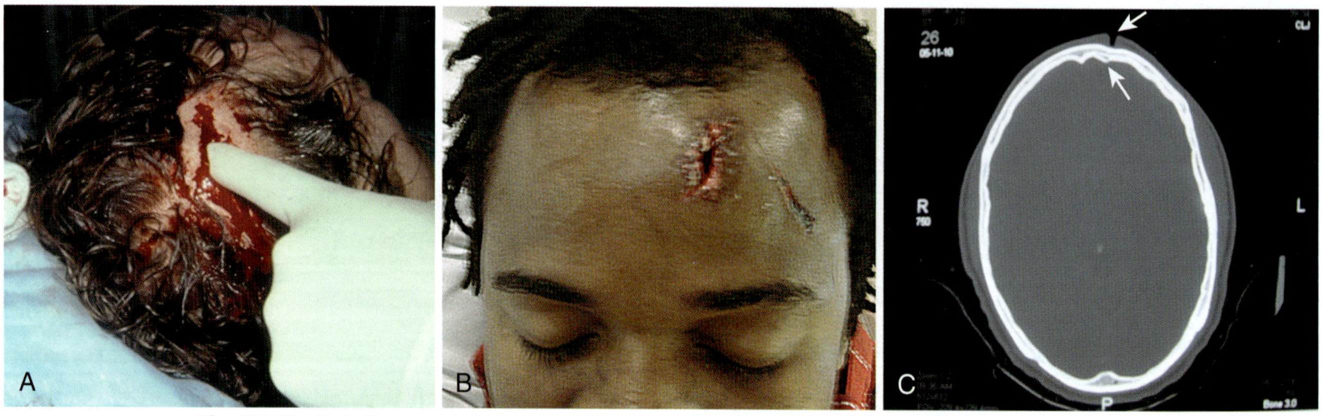

Fig. 35.55 (A) A finger and direct vision can be used to identify skull fractures. Do not mistake a rent in the soft tissues as a fracture. (B) Puncture wounds in the forehead and scalp from such objects as a knife, nail, screwdriver, or ice pick can penetrate the skull and brain, and initially the patient appears well and the wound looks benign. This patient was in a bar fight and was "stabbed" in the forehead. He had no complaints. The wound could not be fully explored but appeared to be benign. (C) Computed tomography scan demonstrating a depressed skull fracture *(arrows)*.

the wound to help hold them back. Although clipping scalp hair is not popular with some patients, failure to adequately expose an area may result in improper cleaning and closure of scalp wounds. Because of the extensive collateral blood supply of the scalp, most lacerations in this area heal without problem, even after delayed treatment. Nonetheless, wound cleaning must be sufficient to avoid the devastating complication of scalp infection.

With microvascular techniques, large skin sections avulsed from the scalp can be re-implanted. Some of the same techniques for amputated extremities are used to salvage the avulsed scalp.[124]

Unlike most wounds involving multiple layers of tissue, scalp wounds can usually be closed with a single layer of sutures that incorporate skin, SQ fascia, and the galea (Fig. 35.56). The periosteum does not need to be sutured; in fact, sutures generally do not hold in this friable, thin tissue. Separate closure of the galea introduces additional suture material into the wound and may increase the risk for infection. However, separate closure may be necessary in extremely large wounds to provide a more secure approximation of the galea than can be obtained with a large-needle, single-layer closure. In this situation, an inverted stitch (with an absorbable 3-0 or 4-0 suture) will bury the knot beneath the galea.

In superficial wounds, approximate the skin and SQ tissue with simple interrupted or vertical mattress stitches using nonabsorbable 3-0 nylon or polypropylene suture on a large needle. Avoid smaller suture material because it tends to break when firm knots are tied. Leave the ends of the tied scalp sutures at least 2 cm long to facilitate subsequent removal. The use of blue nylon rather than black may make suture removal easier. Absorbable sutures may provide similar cosmetic and functional outcomes in scalp laceration repair.[125]

Sutured scalp lacerations do not need to be bandaged. Instruct patients that they can wash their hair in 2 hours (Fig. 35.57). If bleeding persists, use an elastic bandage as a compression dressing. Place gauze sponges over the laceration to provide direct local pressure beneath the elastic bandage.

An easy method of scalp laceration repair is the hair apposition technique (HAT; Fig. 35.58A).[126–131] HAT should not be used in deep wounds as it only apposes the superficial layers of the scalp. Advantages of this technique include cosmetic results similar to suturing, increased speed of repair, no need for clipping of hair, and no need for return visit for suture or staple removal.[132] The HAT technique should not be used with lacerations greater than 10 cm in length, irregular wound margins, hair less than 3 cm in length, and continued bleeding. Wounds between 1 cm and 3 cm in length may be repaired with the modified HAT technique (Fig. 35.58B).[133] Care must be taken to place only a small drop of glue onto the twist of hair (not the scalp) to prevent tissue glue from entering the wound.[133] In the HAT technique, the hair is twisted and no actual knot is tied in the hair. The patient should be instructed to wait 2 days prior to hair washing. The patient should be informed that the glue will gradually fall off within 2 weeks. If the drop of glue fails to fall off, it may be simply removed with tweezers or comb.

Nail Bed Lacerations

Injuries to the nail and nail bed (also called the nail matrix) are common problems in emergency medicine, yet controversy exists over proper management (Fig. 35.59). As a general rule, repair nail bed lacerations unless they are well approximated. An exception is a nail bed laceration that causes a simple subungual hematoma.

Subungual Hematomas

Subungual hematomas develop from a nail bed laceration. Some nail bed lacerations are minor and of no consequence, whereas others result in a poor outcome unless the bed is repaired.[134,135] A simple subungual hematoma, in which the nail is firmly adherent and disruption of the surrounding tissue is minimal, is not an indication to remove the nail to search for nail bed lacerations, even in the presence of a tuft fracture (Fig. 35.60 and Videos 35.16, 35.17).[136] Despite the presence of a nail bed laceration, a good result can be expected as long as the tissue is held in anatomic approximation by the intact fingernail.

If a large subungual hematoma is associated with an unstable or avulsed nail, suture the nail bed. Remove the nail completely and repair the nail bed under a bloodless field (Fig. 35.61). Always use absorbable sutures in the nail bed so they

Closure of Scalp Lacerations

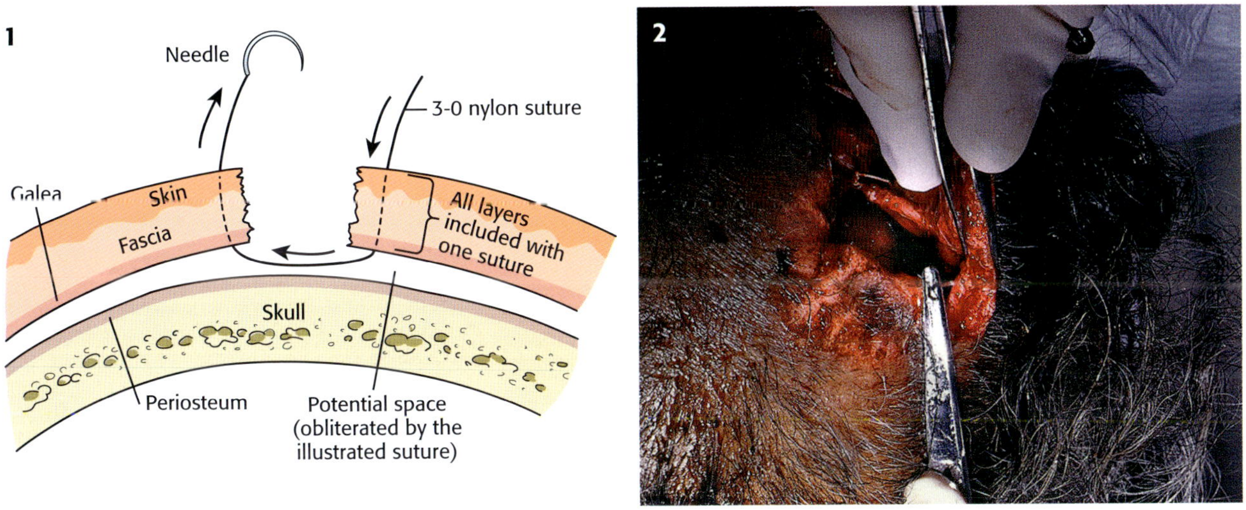

To close a scalp laceration that extends through the galea, use a long needle, forceps, and 3-0 sutures (blue polypropelene sutures make removal easier). Incorporate the skin, subcutaneous tissue, and galea in a single stitch. If this technique is used, individual buried sutures in the galea are not required, and hemostasis is ensured. At the base of this wound is the periosteum, a thin, tissue-like covering of the skull that is often mistaken for the galea. Periosteum is not sutured. The galea is actually adherent to the avulsed flap.

A good way to include all layers of the scalp in the closure is to use forceps to manipulate the tissue so that the needle can penetrate the galea as it transverses to the skin.

Fig. 35.56 Closure of scalp lacerations.

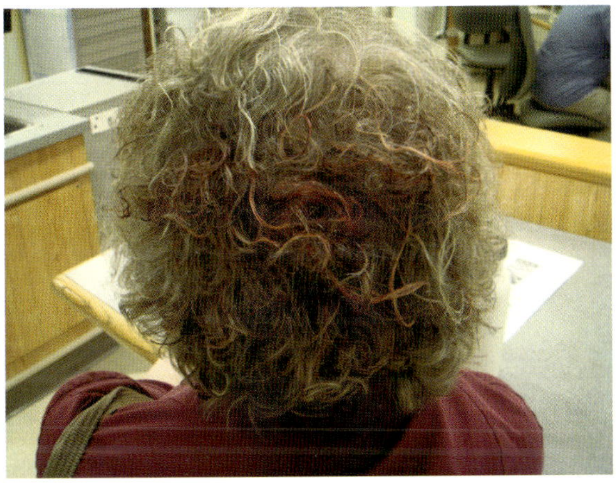

Fig. 35.57 Once the scalp is sutured, the patient is encouraged to wash the hair at home that day to remove blood and debris. Prohibiting bathing with sutures in place in any part of the body has no scientific merit.

do not have to be removed. A good outcome depends on maintaining the space under the eponychium (cuticle) as the laceration heals and the new nail grows out, which is a slow process.

Partial Nail Avulsions

If the nail is partly avulsed (especially at the base) or loose, lift the nail to assess and potentially repair the nail bed. If the nail is intact, it is best to leave it in place if the nail bed laceration can be repaired (Fig. 35.62). The method for atraumatically removing a nail is demonstrated later in Fig. 35.67.

Nail Bed Repair

When the integrity of the nail bed is significantly disrupted, a rippled nail may develop (see Fig. 35.62F). Anatomic repair of the nail bed may minimize subsequent nail deformity (Videos 35.18 and 35.19). Approximate a simple nail bed laceration with 6-0 or 7-0 absorbable suture (to obviate the need for suture removal); either Vicryl Rapide or chromic gut may be used for nail bed repair.[137,138] If available, use loupe magnification and a finger tourniquet to maintain a bloodless field (Fig. 35.63). Repair the proximal and lateral nail (onychial) folds first. Attach a sturdy needle to a 4-0 thread for suturing lacerated nails. Insert the needle perpendicularly to the nail because the needle penetrates most easily in this position. The point of the needle carves a rigid path through the nail. Unless the entire length of the needle is allowed to follow this path as it passes through the nail, the needle is likely to bend or break. Alternatively, use an electrical cautery instrument or a heated paper clip to perforate the nail and permit easy passage of the needle.

Protect the exposed nail bed by reapplying the avulsed nail (best choice) or by applying a sterile nonadherent dressing, such as Silastic sheet, sterile polypropylene foil (obtained from the sterile infusion reservoir used on IV tubing), or gauze packing for approximately 2 to 3 weeks. Reinsertion of the nail occasionally results in infection, so clean the nail carefully. After cleaning, suture the avulsed nail in place or secure it with wound closure tape or tissue glue. If only the distal portion of the nail has been avulsed, it can still be used as a temporary splint or "dressing" to protect and maintain the integrity of the underlying nail bed (see Fig. 35.63).

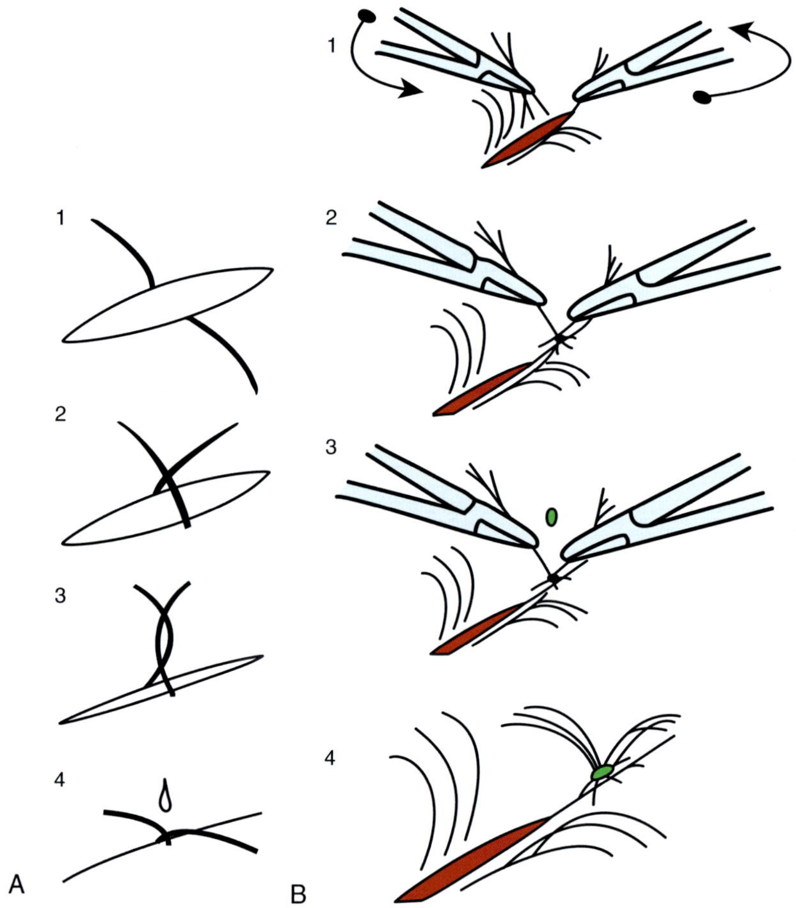

Fig. 35.58 (A) Hair apposition technique (HAT) for superficial scalp lacerations in which hair is greater than 3 cm in length. *1*, Select 4 to 5 hair strands on each side of the laceration; separately twist each group of hair strands to form bundles. *2*, Cross the bundles using artery forceps. *3*, Twist the bundles around each other once; there is no need to form an actual knot. *4*, Place one small drop of glue on the twist of hair (not on the scalp) to secure. Repeat, every 1 to 2 cm along the wound, bisecting the wound just as if using sutures. (B) Modified HAT, which is useful for hair lengths of 1 to 3 cm. *1*, On each side of the wound, a bundle of 5 to 15 hairs is grasped by a clamp and the clamps are twisted around one another. *2*, Tighten the twist of hairs to appose the wound margins. *3*, One small drop of tissue glue is placed on the twist of hairs. *4*, Repeat this every 1 cm to 1.5 cm to secure the entire laceration. (A, From Ong M, Ooi S, Saw et al. A randomized controlled trial comparing the hair apposition technique with tissue glue to standard suturing in scalp lacerations (HAT study). *Ann Emerg Med.* 2002;40:21. B, From Karaduman S, Yurukrumen A, Guryay S et al. Modified hair apposition technique as the primary closure method for scalp lacerations. *Am J Emerg Med.* 2009;27:1050.)

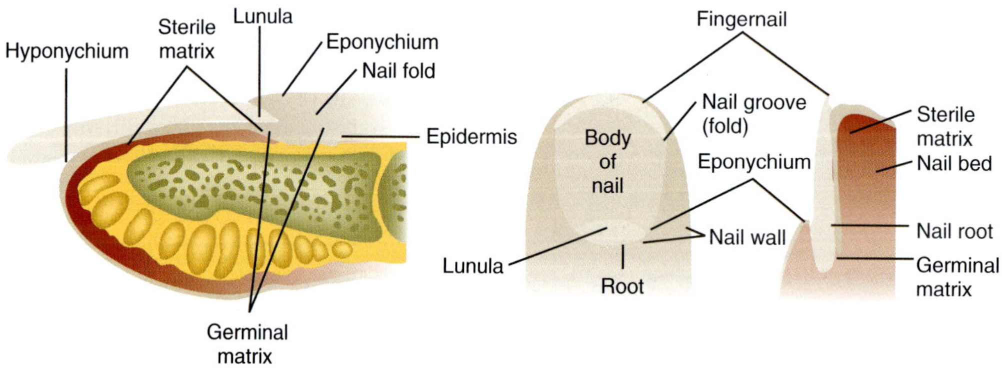

Fig. 35.59 Anatomy of the fingernail. The fingernail rests on the nail bed, also termed the matrix. The distal end of the nail covers the sterile matrix; the proximal end arises from and covers the germinal matrix. The tissue adherent to the proximal dorsal surface of the nail is the eponychium (also termed the cuticle), and the potential space between the nail and the eponychium is the nail fold.

The figure-of-eight technique can be used to secure the nail, which minimizes additional trauma to the nail bed and eponychium (Fig. 35.64).[137–140] This technique has also been used to secure sterile polypropylene foil in the event that the nail is too injured to be replaced (Fig. 35.65).[140]

Tissue adhesive is a time-saving option for repairing nail bed lacerations in both adult and pediatric patients (Fig. 35.66).[141,142] Tissue glue obviates the need for suture removal and produces similar cosmetic and functional results.[115,143] Tissue glue is applied on nail bed lacerations after meticulous alignment. The glue can also be used to secure the nail plate under the eponychial fold. A tourniquet is often necessary to maintain a bloodless field during tissue adhesive application.

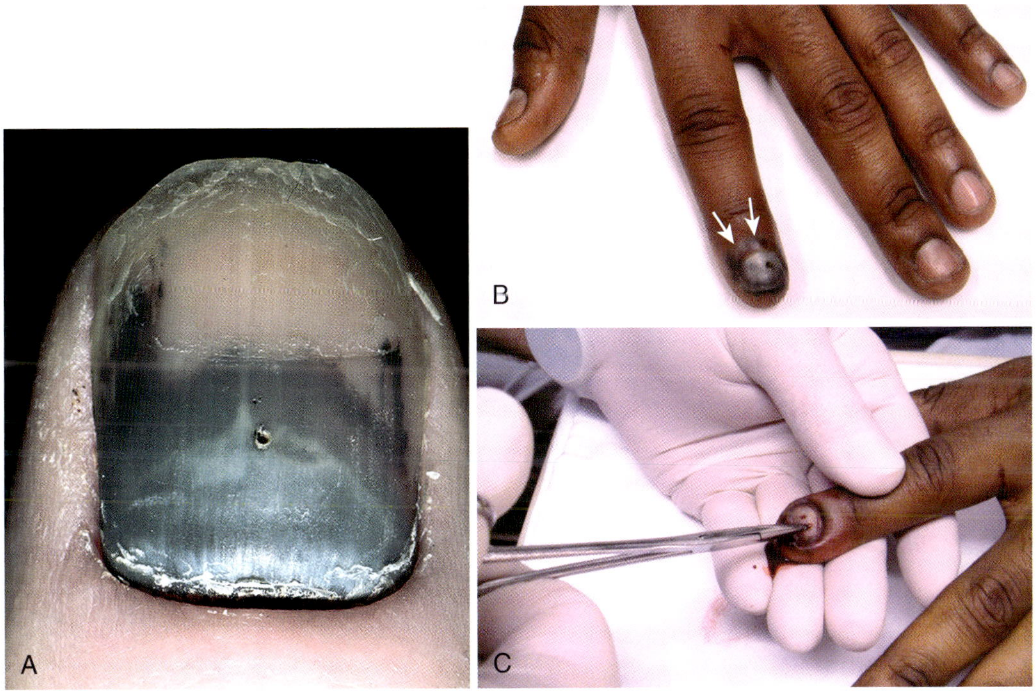

Fig. 35.60 (A) This subungual hematoma occupies most of the nail and should be drained by simple nail trephination. The injury does not require nail removal or repair of the nail bed because the nail is still firmly attached to the matrix. Even though a nail matrix laceration (the source of the bleeding) is present, the cosmetic result will be excellent. The presence of an underlying digital tuft fracture does not change management. This hole is too small and did not evacuate all the blood. (B) There are two issues with this injury. First, an inadequately sized hole was placed (too small) and did not drain the subungual hematoma. All blood should be drained in the emergency department before discharge to ensure proper treatment. Note the subtle ecchymosis under the eponychium *(arrows)*. This can occur only if the nail base was avulsed. The base of the nail is lying just under the skin. Compare it with (A) where no blood is seen in the paronychial area as the nail base remains intact. (C) After the hole is enlarged and the blood is totally drained, and without removing the nail, a hemostat is used to pull the nail forward and manipulate the base back into its proper position under the eponychium.

Complete Nail Avulsions

If the entire nail is avulsed but intact, it should be replaced after repairing the nail bed laceration for three reasons: (1) it acts as a splint or mold to maintain the normal anatomy of the nail bed, (2) it covers a sensitive area and facilitates dressing changes, and (3) it maintains the fold for new nail growth. If the proximal portion of the nail is not replaced, either of two complications may result: (1) longitudinal scar bands may form between the proximal nail fold and the germinal matrix and cause a permanent split or deformity of the nail, or (2) the space between the proximal nail fold and the germinal matrix of the nail bed may be obliterated within a few days.[144] Consequently, splints over proximal nail beds should be maintained for 2 to 3 weeks. The proximal portion of the traumatized nail often needs to be trimmed so that it will fit more easily into the nail fold. It is usually necessary to suture or glue the nail in place. A replaced nail may grow normally and act as a free graft, but it is often dislodged by a new nail. If the nail was lost or irreparably destroyed, insert a piece of nonadherent, petrolatum-impregnated gauze (such as Adaptic [Acelity] or Xeroform [DeRoyal]) between the proximal nail fold and the germinal matrix. Nails grow at a rate of 0.1 mm/day, and approximately 6 months is required for a new nail to reach to the fingertip.

Complicated Nail Bed Injuries

If the germinal matrix of the nail bed is avulsed but intact, reimplant the nail with a 5-0 or 6-0 absorbable suture using a mattress stitch. If an open fracture exists, do not allow any part of the matrix to remain trapped in the fracture line.

If the nail bed is found to be extensively lacerated, it may be prudent to refer the patient to a hand surgeon, who can raise a flap of tissue extending from the proximal nail fold, explore the wound for foreign bodies, and clean under the nail bed. A fingertip avulsion that involves the germinal matrix or an isolated nail bed avulsion should not be allowed to heal on its own (i.e., by secondary intention). If the exposed germinal matrix is left open to granulate, it will form scar tissue that could produce a distorted and sensitive digit. If part of the germinal matrix has been lost, refer the patient to a surgical consultant for a matrix graft.[145]

Recheck wounds 3 to 5 days after repair. At that time, remove and replace any nonadherent material that was inserted under the proximal nail fold, and assess the wound for infection. The use of absorbable suture for nail bed repair makes suture removal unnecessary. Sutures that were used to reattach the nail are removed in 2 weeks, and the old nail is allowed to fall off as the new nail grows. The value of antibiotics is unproven. Advise all patients with nail injuries of

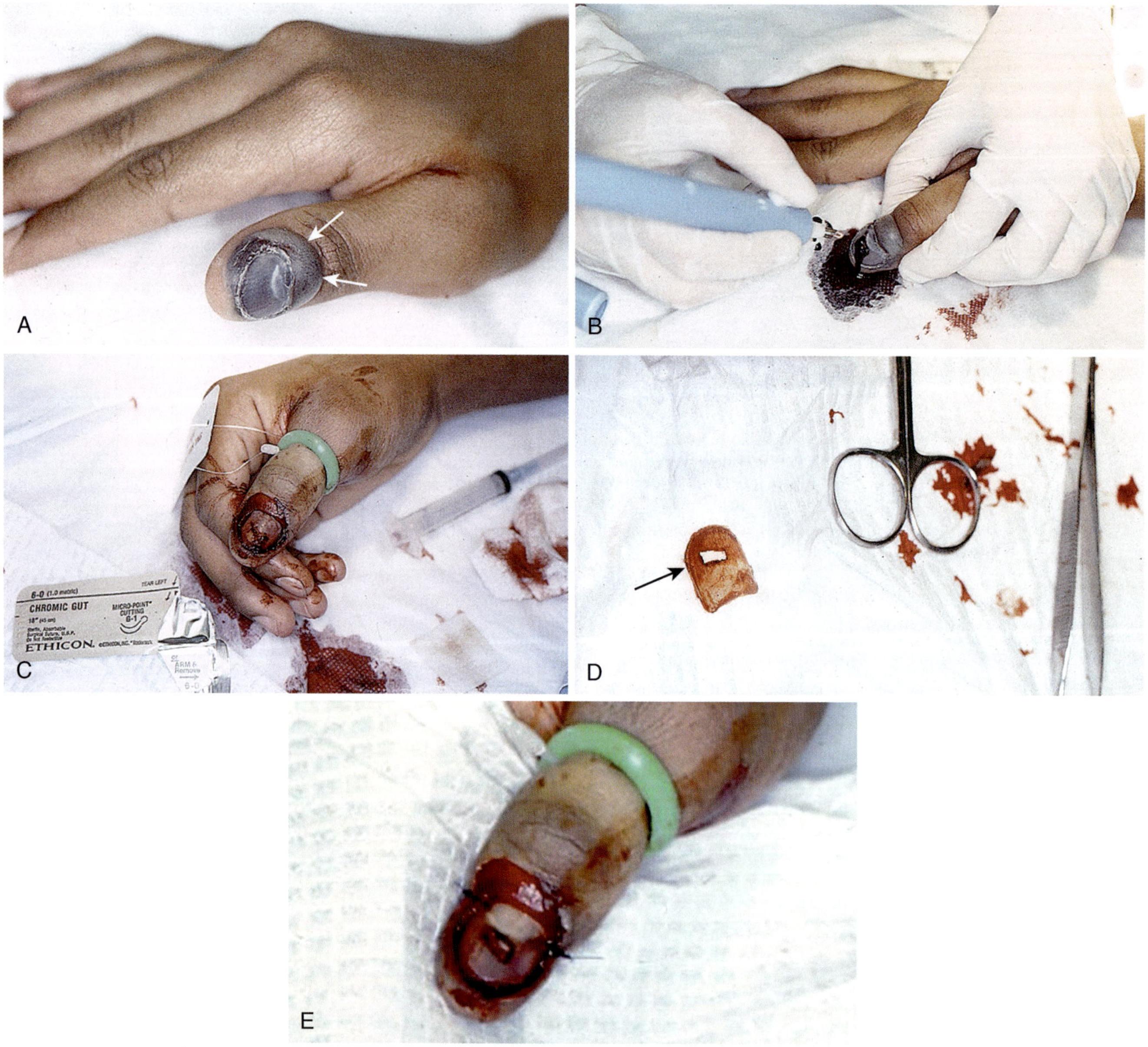

Fig. 35.61 (A) Classic "finger slammed in a door" with forced flexion and avulsion of the base of the nail. This large subungual hematoma can be misleading, but it is associated with blood under the cuticle *(arrows)* proximal to the nail, a clue that this is not a simple injury. (B) When the blood is drained, the extent of the injury is more obvious. (C) Careful removal of the nail exposes a laceration of the nail bed, which is sutured with absorbable suture. (D) A drainage hole is placed in the nail *(arrow)* because it will be used as a temporary splint for the nail bed and to keep the cuticle space open to prevent scarring. (E) The avulsed nail is placed under the eponychium to its base and sutured in place for 3 to 4 weeks while a new nail grows. This replaced nail may be removed, or it is pushed out by the new nail.

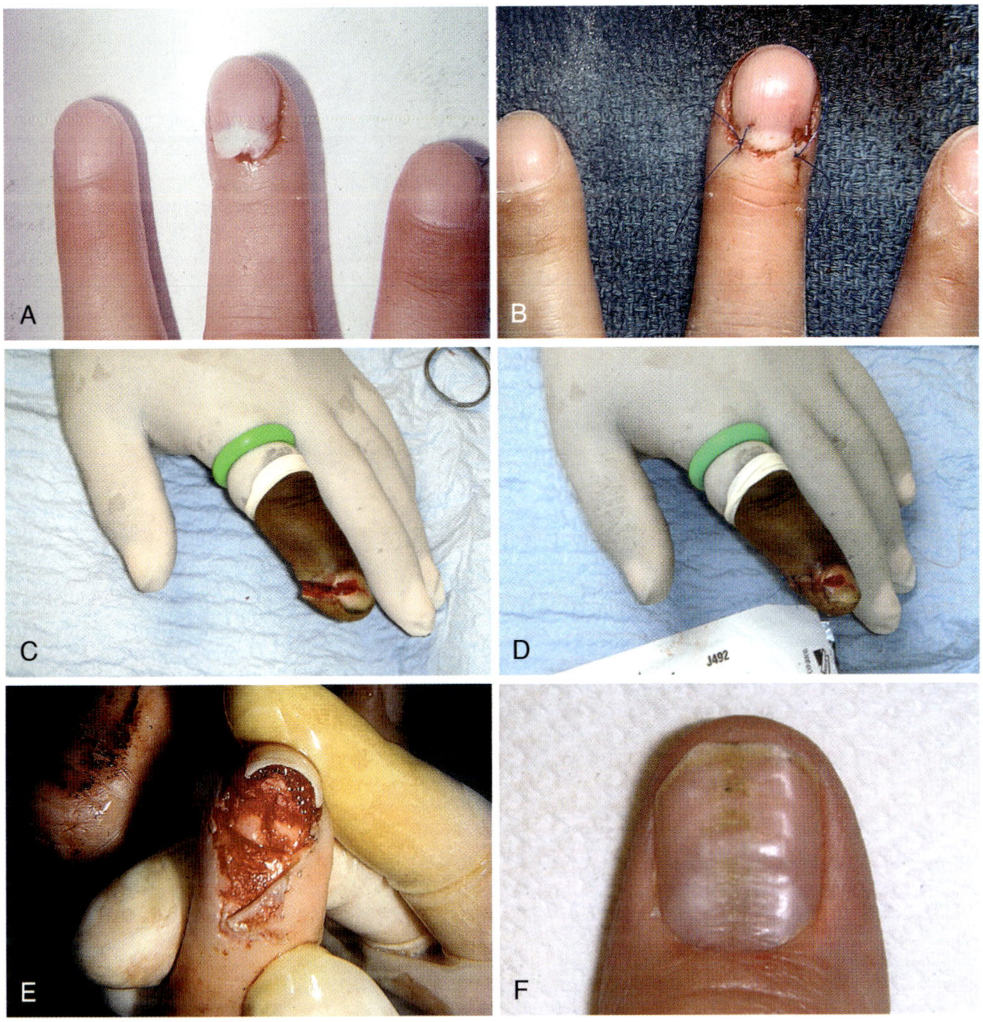

Fig. 35.62 (A) This fingernail was avulsed at the base, a common result of having a door slam on the digit. The nail is tightly adherent to the nail bed, so it is not removed but simply replaced under the eponychium to its former position. (B) Sutures are placed in the nail to keep it stable. This nail may simply start to grow on its own. (C) A saw-induced laceration of the fingertip with an open fracture, nail bed laceration, and skin laceration. (D) Only part of the nail was removed and the nail bed repaired through the window. The skin is closely approximated. Such injuries usually heal well with attention to detail, and infection is unusual despite the open fracture. Oral antibiotic therapy for 5 to 7 days is reasonable. (E) Because this avulsed nail is unstable and subungual bleeding is present, the nail can be removed and the nail bed inspected. Any large nail bed laceration should be repaired meticulously with absorbable suture (6-0). After repair of the nail bed, a drainage hole is placed in the nail, and the nail is replaced under the eponychium (cuticle) and fixed in place with sutures that incorporate the nail edge and the skin bilaterally. In 2 to 3 weeks, the new nail will begin to push out the old nail (usually growing under it while maintaining the eponychium), and the old nail is removed. The exposed nail bed will be sensitive for a while. See Fig. 35.67 for a simple technique to remove the fingernail. (F) This nail is permanently deformed with ridges. Although crush injury to the nail bed is probably responsible for this deformity, repair of the nail bed might have minimized the resultant deformity.

Nail Bed Repair

1

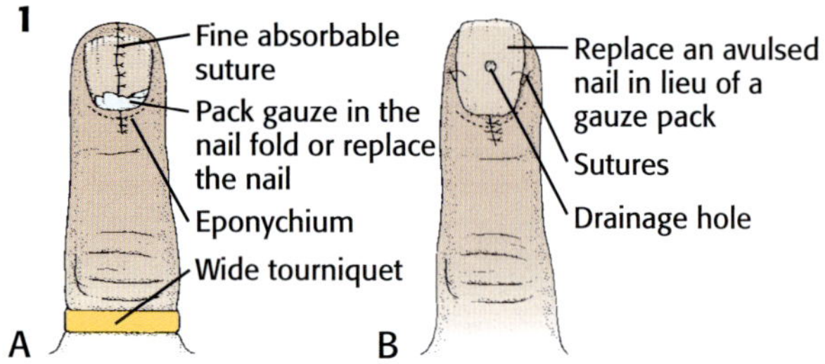

A laceration involving the nail bed, germinal matrix, and skin fold must be carefully approximated. First, the nail is completely removed. **A**, Fine, absorbable sutures are used to repair the nail bed under a bloodless field provided by a finger tourniquet. The avulsed nail (trimmed at the base) or a gauze pack is gently placed between the matrix and the eponychium for 2 to 3 weeks to prevent scar formation. **B**, If the original nail is replaced (the best option), it may be sutured or taped in place. A large hole in the nail will allow drainage. The old nail is gradually pushed out by a new one. If the nail matrix is replaced quickly and atraumatically, the nail may act as a free graft and grow normally. Note: Only absorbable sutures are used to repair the nail bed.

2

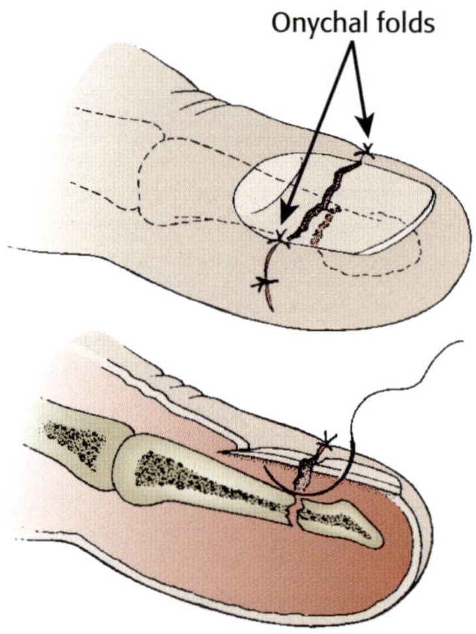

Repair of a distal finger laceration involving the nail and the onychial fold. In this case, the nail is still adherent to the nail matrix and acts as a natural splint. If the nail is loose or completely transected, it is prudent to remove the entire nail and then carefully suture the nail bed under direct vision.

3

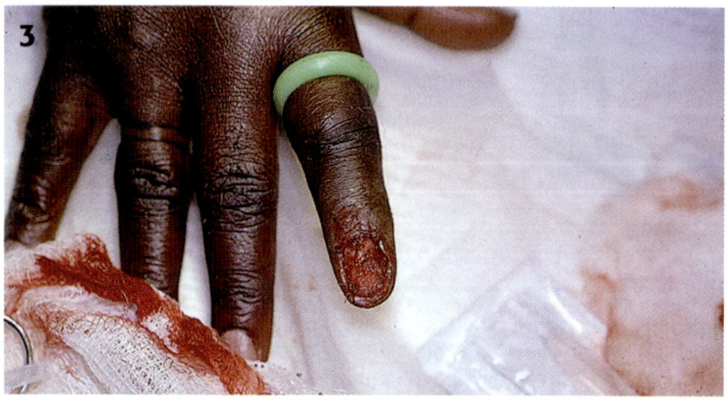

This nail was removed and the nail bed repaired with absorbable suture.

4

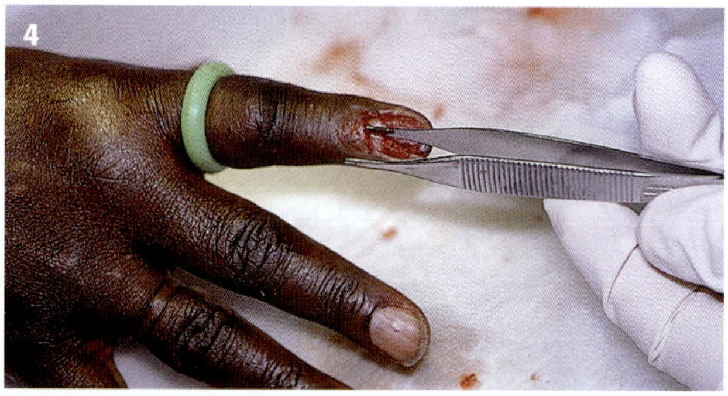

Because the nail was macerated and unable to be replaced, gauze is used to maintain the eponychial space for 2 to 3 weeks. A small piece of gauze is placed with forceps to gently pack open the space to prevent scar formation.

Fig. 35.63 Nail bed repair. (Plate 2, from Dushoff IM. Handling the hand. *Emerg Med.* 1976;8:111.)

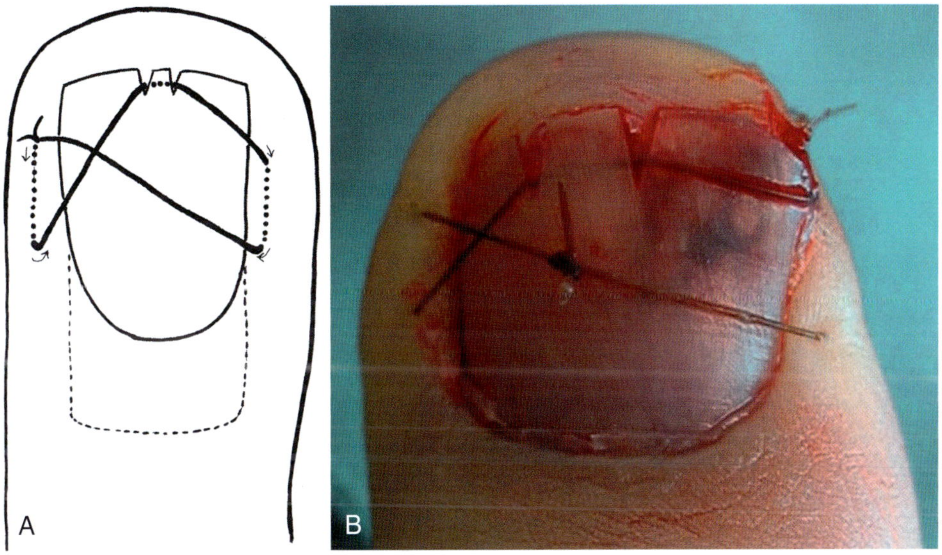

Fig. 35.64 Transverse figure-of-eight suture for securing the nail. Two small wedges are cut into the distal aspect of the nail and the nail is placed under the eponychial fold. A 4-0 (5-0 in children) absorbable or nonabsorbable suture is placed distal-to-proximal on one side of the paronychium. Suture is slid through the wedges of the distal nail, placed distal-to-proximal in the opposite paronychium, and then tied, resulting in a figure-of-eight pattern. The distal entry point is about the midpoint of the exposed nail plate and may be used even if the nail is only partially intact. The finger should be dressed with a bulky, nonadherent dressing. (From Bristol S, Verchere C. The transverse figure-of-eight suture for securing the nail. *J Hand Surg Am.* 2007;32:125.)

a possible cosmetic defect in the new nail that may occur regardless of the repair technique.

Removal of a Nail

If a partially avulsed or intact nail requires removal (Video 35.20), take care to not injure the nail bed. The nail is usually firmly attached to the bed but can be separated by advancing and opening small scissors in the plane between the nail and the bed. Once loosened, pull the nail from its base with a hemostat (Fig. 35.67).

Tuft Fractures

Once the nail bed has been lacerated, a tuft fracture is considered an open fracture. The use of antibiotics for nail bed laceration is controversial. Most injuries do well with good wound care and reasonable follow-up. Antibiotics are not used after nail trephination, even in the presence of a tuft fracture. Infection is rare, but antibiotics may be considered for significant crush or highly contaminated injuries. The approach to an open tuft fracture varies from formal operating room debridement and intravenous antibiotics to thorough ED cleaning and oral antibiotics with early follow-up. Consultation with a hand specialist is warranted. Splinting is protective. Search for a traumatic mallet finger with flexion or crush injuries (Videos 35.21 and 35.22).

Drains in Sutured Wounds

Drains are used primarily to keep wounds open for drainage of existing purulence or blood that may otherwise collect in the wound. Drains do not prevent infection. When no infection exists, using drains in soft tissue wounds "prophylactically" is rarely required in the ED setting. Drains in uninfected wounds may wick surface bacteria into the wound and impair resistance of the wound to infection. Drains placed in experimental wounds contaminated with subinfective doses of bacteria behave as foreign bodies by enhancing the rate of infection, regardless of whether the drain is placed entirely within the wound or brought out through the wound.[146]

If the wound is considered to be at high risk for infection, instead of suturing the wound with a drain in place (in anticipation of infection), it may be safer to leave the wound open and consider delayed primary closure later when the risk for infection subsides. Drains should not serve as substitutes for other methods of achieving hemostasis in traumatic wounds.

Lacerations Over Joints

Lacerations over joints may enter the joint itself or injure adjacent tendons or muscle groups. It may be difficult to determine whether the joint has been violated. A plain radiograph of a large joint such as the knee may demonstrate air within the joint, which is evidence of joint penetration (Fig. 35.68). If a wound penetrates the joint cavity, open debridement may be required, but the approach varies with the joint involved.

Fingertip Amputations

Treatment of fingertip amputations has undergone an evolution from complicated grafts and flaps to nonsurgical follow-up and primary healing (Figs. 35.69 and 35.70). If bone is not involved, a good result can be expected with attentive wound care, occasionally minimal debridement, and protective dressing changes. It may take 6 to 12 weeks for healing to occur, but acceptable length, function, and sensation can

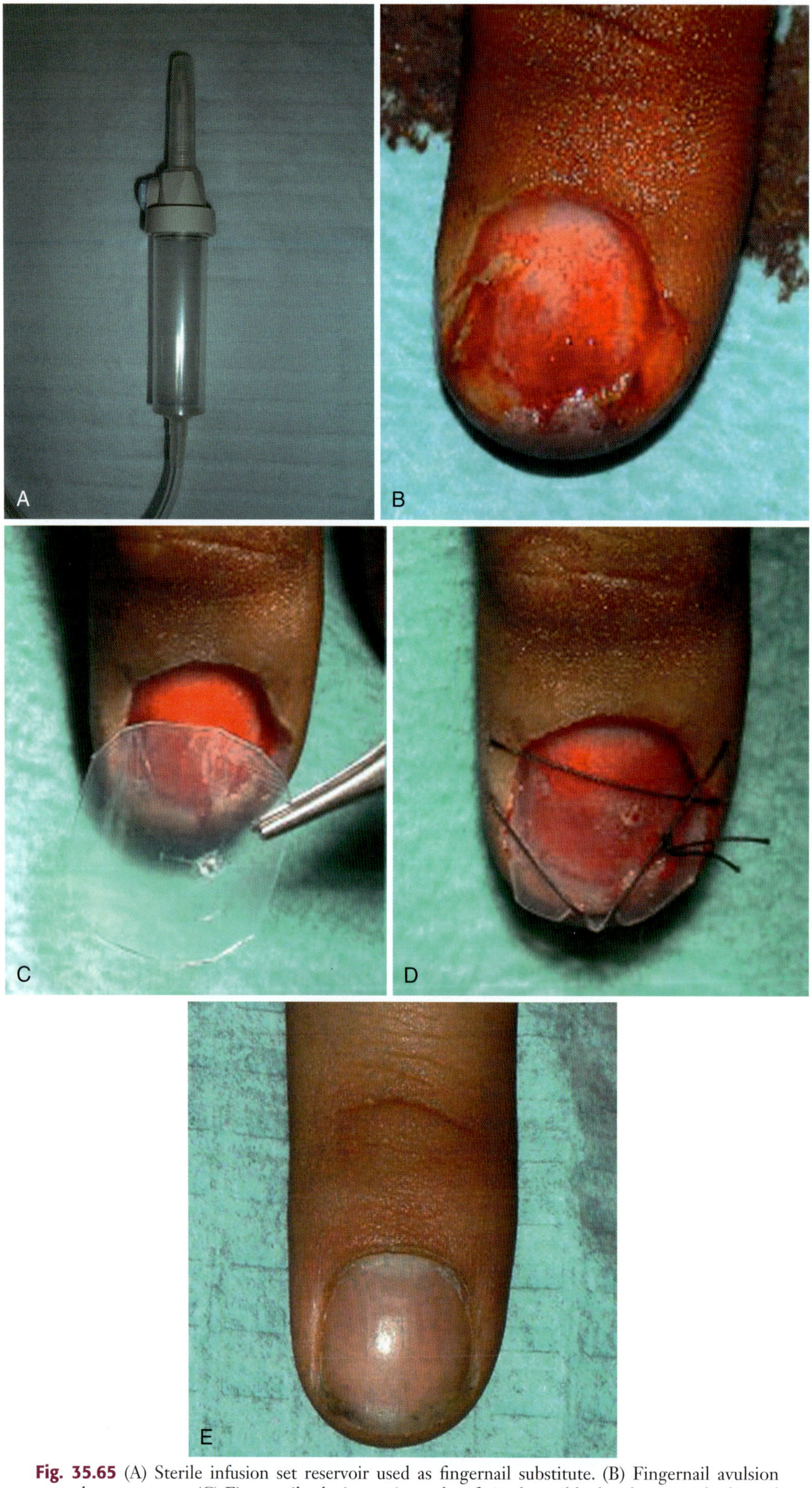

Fig. 35.65 (A) Sterile infusion set reservoir used as fingernail substitute. (B) Fingernail avulsion secondary to trauma. (C) Fingernail substitute trimmed to fit in the nail bed and to provide the nail bed protection while healing. (D) Secured fingernail substitute. (E) Clinical outcome at 1 year. (From Tos S, Artiaco S, Coppolino S et al. A simple sterile polypropylene fingernail substitute. *Chirurgie de la main.* 2009;28:144.)

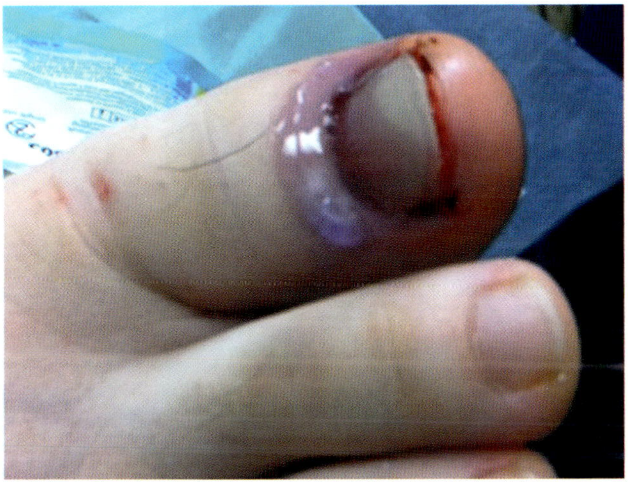

Fig. 35.66 Dermabond used for securing the nail to the nail bed. (Courtesy Michelle Lin, MD. From Rezaie S. Trick of the trade: nail bed repair with tissue adhesive glue, *Acad Life Emerg Med.* 2014.)

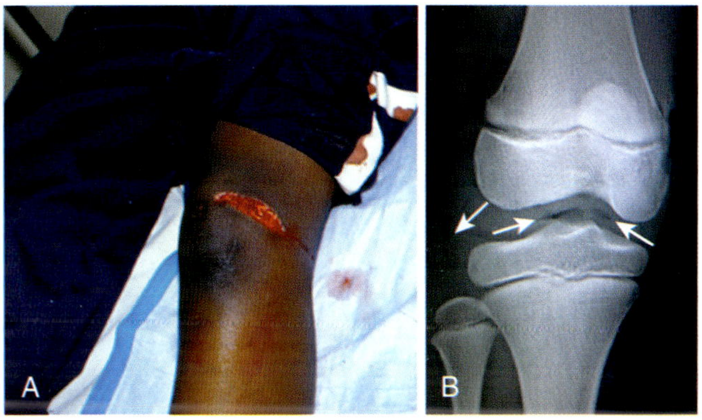

Fig. 35.68 (A) This laceration looks benign but may involve the knee joint or quadriceps tendon. A radiograph to look for air in the joint or a saline arthrogram should be performed. (B) Air in the joint space *(arrows)* on a plain radiograph proved joint space violation.

Nail Removal

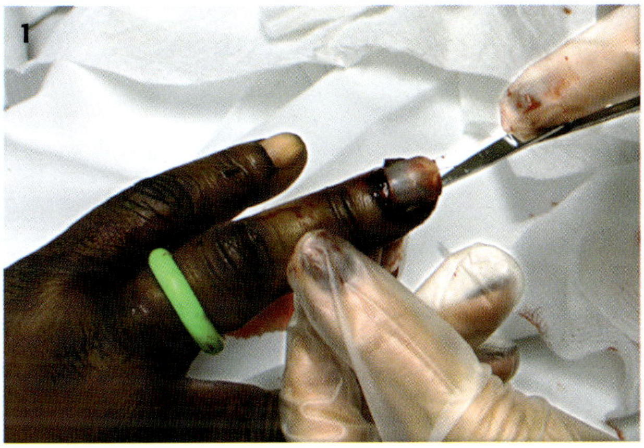

To remove a fingernail or toenail atraumatically, the blades of iris scissors are held parallel to the nail bed to avoid lacerating the matrix. A digital block is necessary. The closed blades are slowly advanced in the plane between the nail and the nail bed and then gently spread to loosen the nail. The scissors are advanced and spread in stages until the base of the nail is reached and the entire nail is loose. The nail is grasped with a hemostat and pulled from the base.

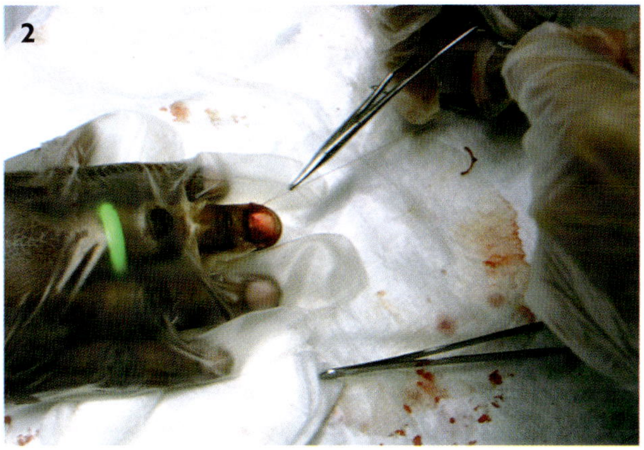

Once the nail is removed, repair any nail bed lacerations with absorbable suture.

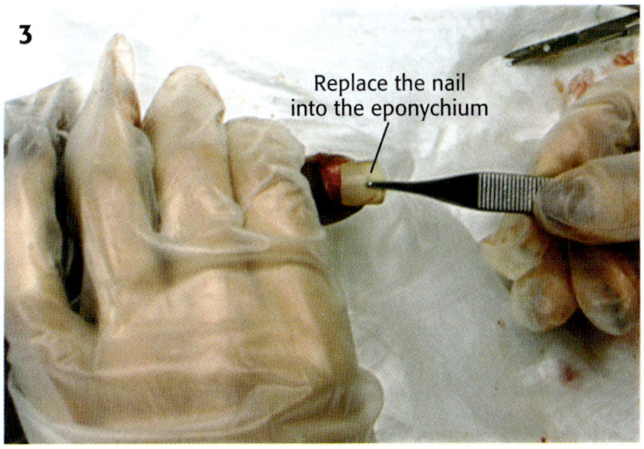

Replace the nail into the eponychial fold.

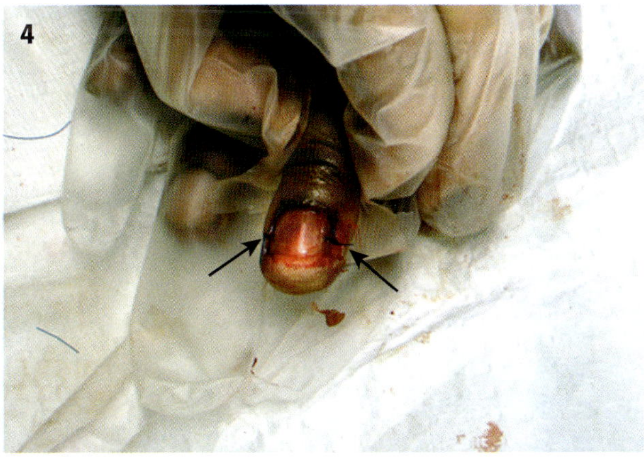

Suture the nail in place with nonabsorbable stitches.

Fig. 35.67 Nail removal.

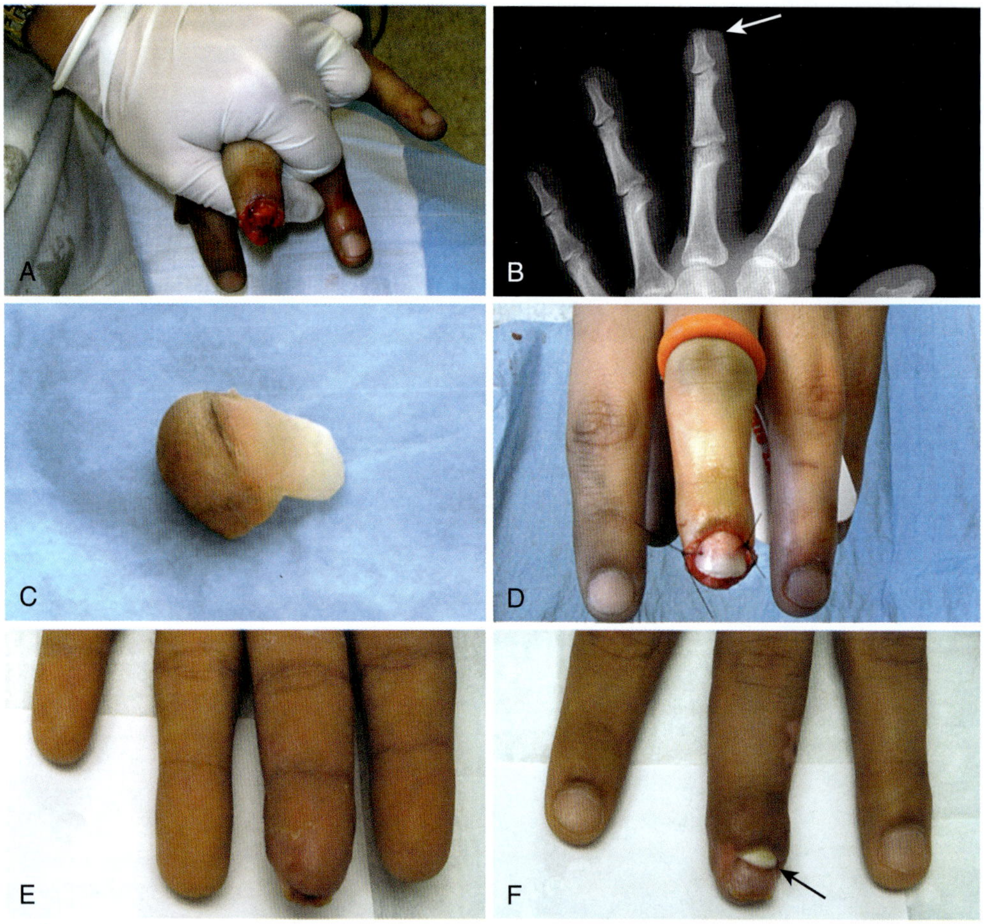

Fig. 35.69 (A–B) Guillotine amputation of the fingertip through the distal end of the nail *(arrow)*. The distal phalanx is not involved. Approaches vary widely, and referral can be made in a few days if not immediately available. (C) Although it is tempting to replace the amputated tip, many would allow this wound to heal spontaneously, albeit slowly (8 to 12 weeks), and not perform skin grafts or flaps. (D) The amputated nail is placed under the eponychium and sutured into place. A rounded but shortened tip with sensation can be expected. Periodic debridement and use of the nail as a splint resulted in a good final appearance. (E–F) In only 4 weeks, this amputation has nearly healed to the original length and contour with only dressing changes and minimal debridement. Note that a new nail is growing *(arrow)* and the replaced nail has been removed.

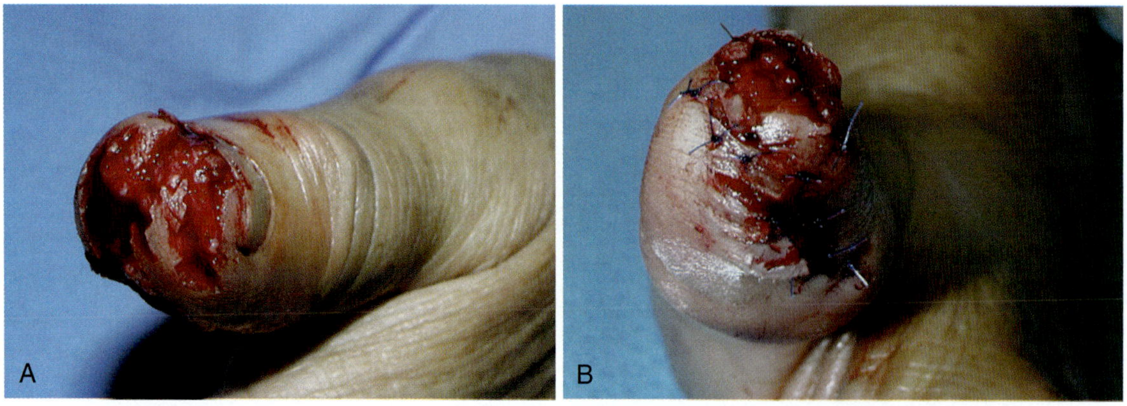

Fig. 35.70 (A–B) This macerated tip has islands of skin left and good tissue volume and will do quite well with sutures to restore the basic anatomy. Healing will take 4 to 5 weeks.

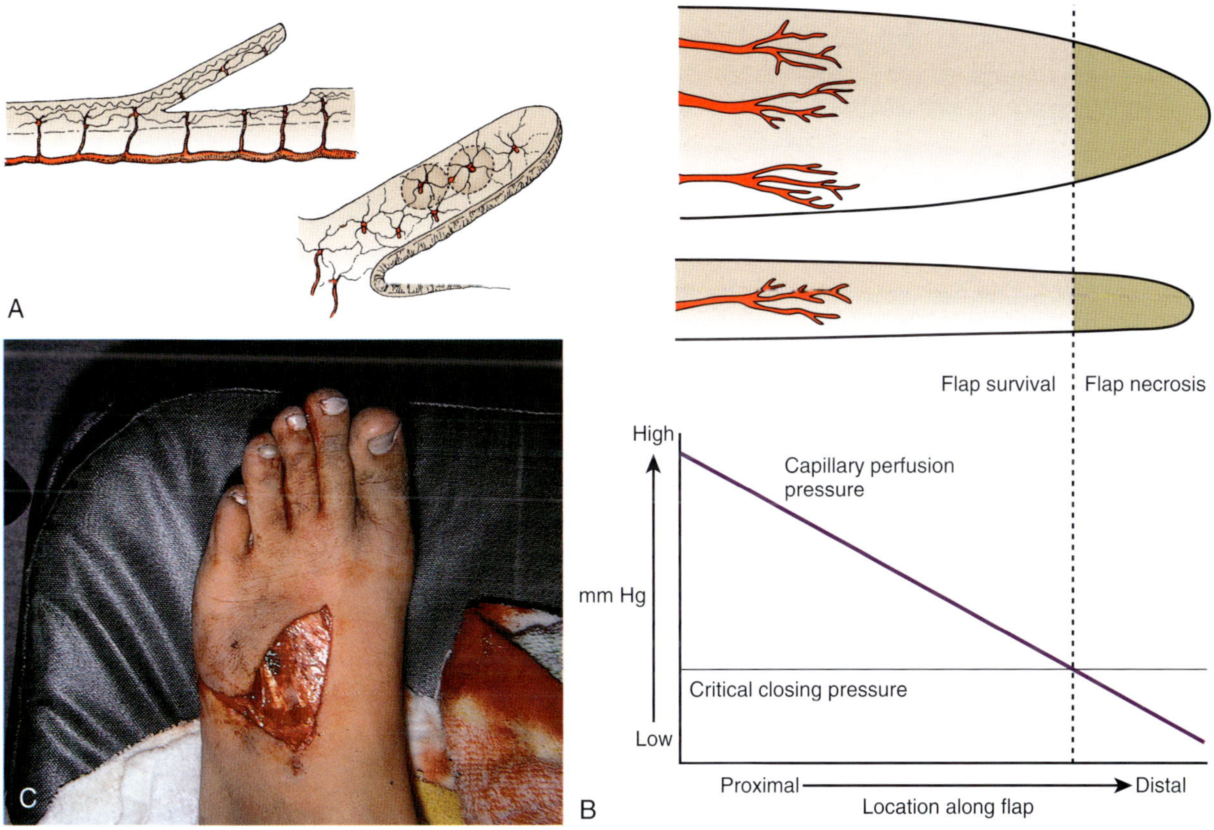

Fig. 35.71 (A) Vascular territories in skin flaps. Multiple perforating vessels exist and are interconnected at the periphery of their vascular territory. When some of these vessels are cut, the blood supply can be replaced with nearby perforating vessels, and then tissue necrosis does not occur. (B) Fallacy of the length-to-width ratio. The slope of decreasing perfusion pressure versus length does not change with the incorporation of additional vessels (flap a versus flap b) at the same perfusion pressure. Flap necrosis occurs when perfusion pressure decreases below the critical closing pressure of the capillary bed. (C) This distally based flap is at risk for necrosis because of impaired venous and lymphatic drainage rather than from loss of the arterial supply. As with all flap repairs, it should be replaced by undermining the base to relieve tension (if possible), a compression dressing to limit movement and fluid buildup under the flap, and elevation of the extremity. Even if only a portion survives, closure can be performed in the emergency department. Impaired venous drainage from a proximally based flap is less problematic.

be expected. A motivated patient and follow-up with a knowledgeable specialist are required. There are no data or standard that mandate long-term antibiotics for such injuries, but it is reasonable to provide gram-positive antibiotic coverage for 7 to 10 days.

DISTALLY AND PROXIMALLY BASED FLAP LACERATIONS

Minor flap lacerations can be managed primarily in the ED. Large flaps, such as scalping lacerations, are best handled by a consultant. Both proximally and distally based flaps are not always simple lacerations. The major problem is vascularity: venous drainage at the end of a distally based flap and the potential for ischemic necrosis in any flap configuration. The body has the ability to augment the circulation in some flaps (Fig. 35.71A). The length-to-width ratio of the flap is not the main variable in the survival of the flap (Fig. 35.71B). Perfusion pressure is the most critical factor. Intravascular perfusion pressure decreases along the length of the flap. If intravascular perfusion pressure is less than interstitial pressure at the distal end of the flap, capillaries will collapse (the *critical closing pressure*). As edema is generated by ischemia and inflammation, interstitial pressure increases which decreases chances for tissue survival.

Many proximally and distally based flaps (Fig. 35.71C) may be closed in the ED and monitored on an outpatient basis. Healing of a distally based flap is hampered by loss of venous and lymphatic drainage and by subsequent edema of the flap, which decreases capillary flow. Warn the patient about the possibility of flap necrosis and the need for revision or even skin grafting later. Partial flap survival is better than total loss of the flap, so flaps with questionable viability should not be removed. Flaps are similar to free skin grafts, and the keys to a more successful outcome include undermining part of the flap to relieve tension, limiting buildup of fluid under the flap

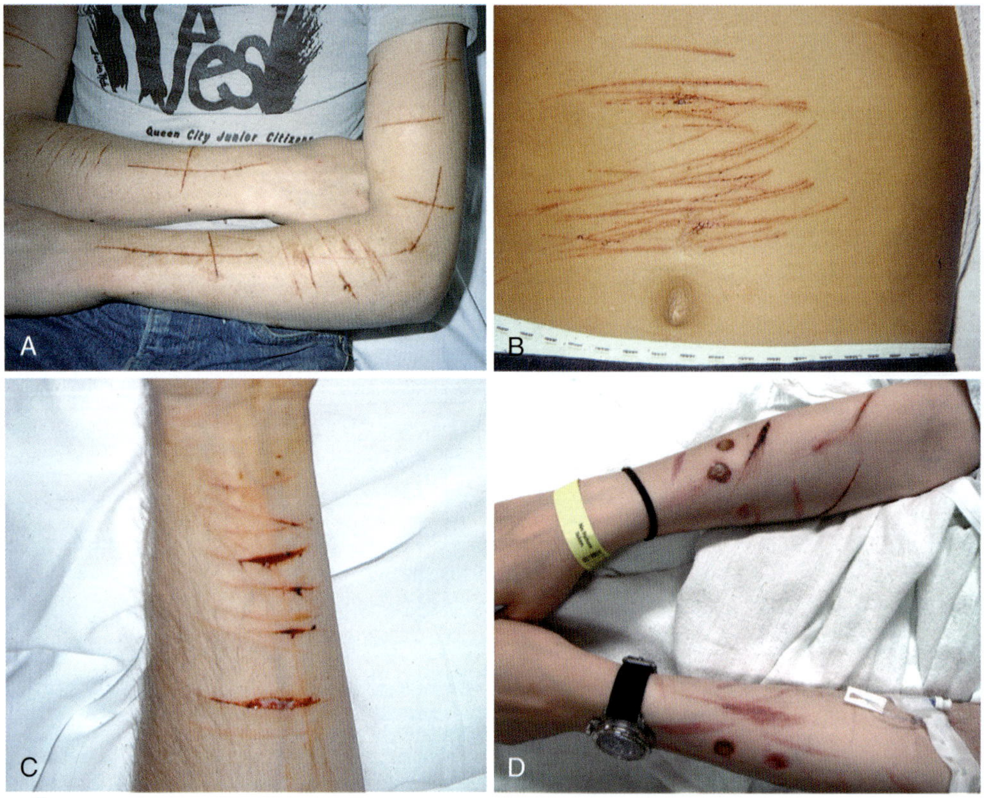

Fig. 35.72 (A–C) These patients had minor lacerations and were brought to the emergency department simply for tetanus prophylaxis or for other vague or unrelated reasons. These are characteristic of self-inflicted wounds that are representative of serious underlying psychiatric issues, and further evaluation is required. (D) These cigarette burns are also self-inflicted, though the patient initially stated that she was burned with grease while cooking.

with a compression dressing, and decreasing movement of the flap as it heals. Cautious minor defatting may be performed on the underside of the flap. Tissue adhesive instead of multiple sutures can be helpful.

Self-inflicted wounds with a vague or inaccurate history may be encountered in the ED. Characteristic self-injury patterns are depicted in Fig. 35.72. These patterns of injury should be recognized and appropriate psychiatric follow-up provided. In most cases, wounds that are repaired should be evaluated 3 to 5 days later to assess for complications.

REFERENCES ARE AVAILABLE AT Elsevier eBooks+

CHAPTER 36

Soft Tissue Foreign Body Removal

David Scordino

INTRODUCTION

Foreign bodies (FBs) are a frequent cause of visits to the emergency department (ED). FBs of the eye, rectum, ear, nose, oropharynx, esophagus, and gastrointestinal (GI) tract pose different historical and physical examination challenges, different diagnostic approaches, and strategies for removal and are discussed in separate chapters in this book. This chapter will focus on soft tissue FBs. When evaluating for a soft tissue FB a high index of suspicion must be maintained based on the history and physical findings. A thorough history and physical examination are essential to assess the risk for a FB. During assessment, FBs may not be obvious, especially when the wound may appear closed, but they should be considered whenever the history is particularly concerning. For example, a patient with an apparent "sprained foot" who was walking without shoes and experienced a sharp, sudden pain in the foot may have a needle, toothpick, or any other similar type of FB (Fig. 36.1). Certain mechanisms of injury, such as punching or kicking out a window or stepping on an unknown object while walking in a field or stream, are often associated with a retained FB. Mechanisms that make FBs less likely include lacerations from metal objects; however, if considerable force was applied during the injury and the object is not available for inspection, radiographic imaging may be warranted because bone may have been encountered and a small section might have splintered off the offending object. The history should also include whether the patient perceives or suspects an FB. Steele and associates found that the negative predictive value of patient perception was 89% but that the positive predictive value was just 31%.[1] Importantly, the patient's past medical history should be explored for allergies to local anesthetics, bleeding diatheses, diabetes mellitus, vascular disease, uremia, immunocompromised state, or other diseases that would affect wound healing or management.

Before the physical examination, be sure to have enough examination time and proper space, lighting, and equipment. Confirming that the patient is willing to undergo the procedure is important because cooperation is essential to optimize success. Attempts at removing an FB in an uncooperative patient, such as one who is intoxicated, drugged, cognitively limited, or confused, are potentially injurious to both the examiner and the patient. In most noncritical situations, if a patient is uncooperative, perform the examination again when the patient can participate. In benign cases, follow-up can occur a few days later.

During the physical examination, carefully palpate the periphery of all wounds to elicit tenderness because retained FBs often produce pain during palpation. In addition, some FBs can migrate away from the wound or perceived entry point. Some superficial FBs may be palpated through the skin, but surprisingly large FBs may be found in seemingly minor wounds without much external evidence. In some cases, the external characteristics of the wound do not yield firm evidence regarding the presence or absence of an FB. Deeper FBs may not be palpable and must be localized by other techniques.

Exploration is an important part of the bedside evaluation, whether done initially or after further imaging studies (Fig. 36.2). This requires adequate pain control, good lighting, proper equipment, a bloodless field, a cooperative patient, and appropriate positioning to visualize as much of the wound as possible (Figs. 36.3 and 36.4). A metal probe may help identify the FB by feel or sound. Glass, as an example, is difficult to identify by sight in soft tissue, but touching it with metal causes a characteristic grating sound. Probing a wound with a gloved finger to locate or identify an FB is strongly discouraged because of the risk of the FB penetrating the glove and exposing the clinician to infections such as human immunodeficiency virus (HIV) and hepatitis (Fig. 36.5).

DIAGNOSIS: AUGMENTING THE PHYSICAL EXAMINATION THROUGH IMAGING

Some emergency clinicians mistakenly believe that in the absence of adipose tissue, if the base of the wound can be clearly visualized and explored, a FB can always be ruled out. Orlinsky and Bright found the reliability of exploration to be related to the depth of the wound.[2] In their study, only 2 of 133 superficial wounds deemed adequately explored had an FB on plain films, but 10 of 130 wounds had FBs beyond the subcutaneous fat despite negative explorations. Anderson and coworkers reported that the treating physicians initially missed 37.5% of the FBs.[3] In many of these cases, a radiograph of the injured area was not taken. Avner and Baker detected glass with routine radiographs in 11 of 160 wounds (6.9%) that were inspected and believed by the clinician to be free of glass.[4,5] Clinicians evaluating for FBs should maintain a low threshold for ordering or performing imaging studies. Options for imaging include plain radiographs, ultrasound (US), computed tomography (CT), magnetic resonance imaging (MRI), and fluoroscopy. See Table 36.1 for a summary.

Plain Radiography

Plain radiographs are readily available, easily interpreted, and cost significantly less than CT, formal US, or MRI.[6] The ability of plain films to detect FBs in soft tissue depends on the object's composition (relative density), configuration, size, and orientation (Fig. 36.6). Detection of FBs on plain films can be enhanced by requesting an underpenetrated soft tissue technique and by obtaining multiple views to prevent FBs from being obscured by superimposed bone or soft tissue folds.[7] Plain films are often sufficient; however, digitized radiographs may be manipulated to enhance identification of a suspected FB. Indirect evidence of a FB may include trapped or surrounding air, a radiolucent filling defect, or secondary bony changes such as periosteal elevation, osteolytic or osteoblastic alterations, or pseudotumors of bone.[7]

Metallic objects are readily visualized on radiographs. Despite a common misconception that glass must contain lead to be visualized on a plain radiograph, almost all glass objects in soft tissue (bottles, windshield glass, lightbulbs, microscope cover slips, laboratory capillary tubes) are at

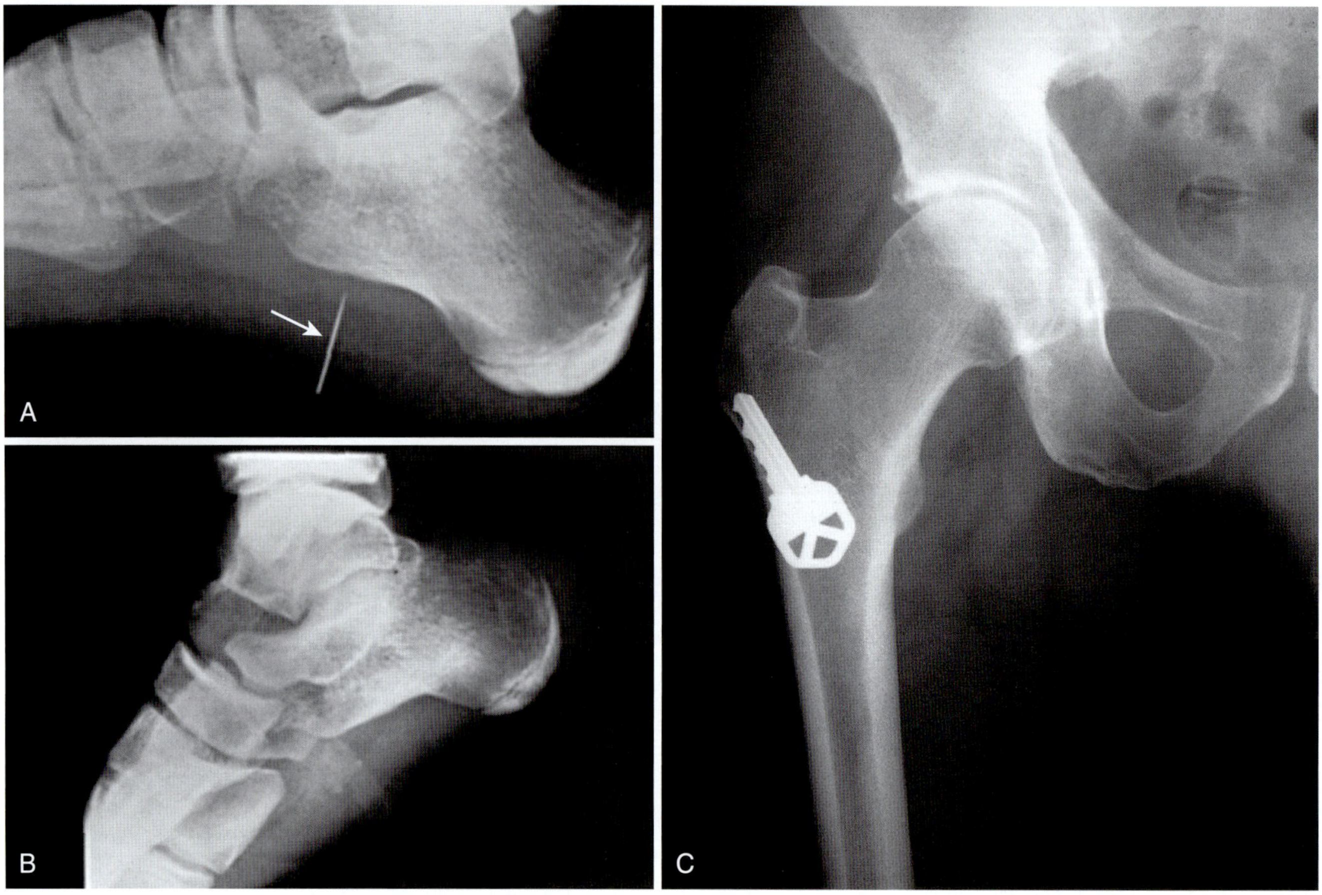

Fig. 36.1 (A) A common foreign body (FB) in the foot is a splinter, toothpick, pin, or needle that is impaled while walking barefoot on a carpet. This sewing needle *(arrow)* was obvious, but in the absence of a history of an FB, some FBs may be mistaken for a simple puncture wound, heel spur, stress fracture, contusion, or tendinitis. (B) Postoperative radiographs demonstrate complete removal. (C) This patient fell, landed on a metal pipe, and sustained a deep laceration in the thigh. A radiograph was taken to rule out a fracture, and the key was seen but thought to be an artifact (i.e., an item left on the backboard). During the examination, the key was found embedded in the wound. It had been in the patient's pants pocket and was forced into the wound by the pipe during the injury.

least somewhat radiopaque and can be detected by plain radiographs unless they are obscured by bone or are very small (<1 mm) (Fig. 36.7).[6,8,9] The absence of a glass FB on multiple projections is strong, though not absolute evidence that glass is not contained in a wound. Other nonmetallic objects readily visualized include teeth, bone, pencil graphite, asphalt, and gravel.[6,10] Aluminum, which has traditionally been deemed radiolucent, can occasionally be visualized on plain films if the object is projected away from the underlying bone. Ellis demonstrated that pure aluminum fragments as small as 0.5 × 0.5 × 1 mm could be identified in a chicken wing model simulating a human hand or foot.[11] Ellis cautioned that other aluminum FBs, such as pull tabs from cans, may not be visualized in other body parts such as the esophagus or stomach.[11]

Certain FBs such as vegetative material (thorns, wood, splinters, and cactus spines) are radiolucent and not readily visualized on plain radiographs. These materials absorb body fluids as they sit in situ and become isodense with the surrounding tissue. Because of their varying chemical composition and density, plastics may or may not be visible on plain films.[12]

Besides simply diagnosing FBs, radiographs can also be used to estimate the general location, depth, and structure of radiopaque FBs. If one strategically attaches a marker (needle or paper clip) to the skin surface at the wound entrance before taking a radiograph, the FB will be seen in relation to the entrance wound (Fig. 36.8). This also helps identify the path that leads to the FB and the relative distance from the surface to the FB.[13] Needles at two angles may also be used to aid in localization (Fig. 36.9).

Liberal use of plain film radiography makes sound clinically relevant medicolegal practice. A review of 54 wound FB claims against 32 physicians from 22 institutions found glass, a radiopaque substance, to be the most common material. However, in only 35% of the cases involving glass were plain films taken. Cases with a glass FB without a radiograph ordered were associated with unsuccessful defense (60%) and higher indemnity payments.[14]

Ultrasound

US has become the modality of choice for imaging radiolucent FBs such as wood and thorns because most soft tissue FBs are hyperechoic on US. In addition, if in place for more than 24 hours, most FBs will be surrounded by a hypoechoic area corresponding to granulation tissue, edema, or hemorrhage, which may aid in diagnosing the FB.[15] Metal will leave

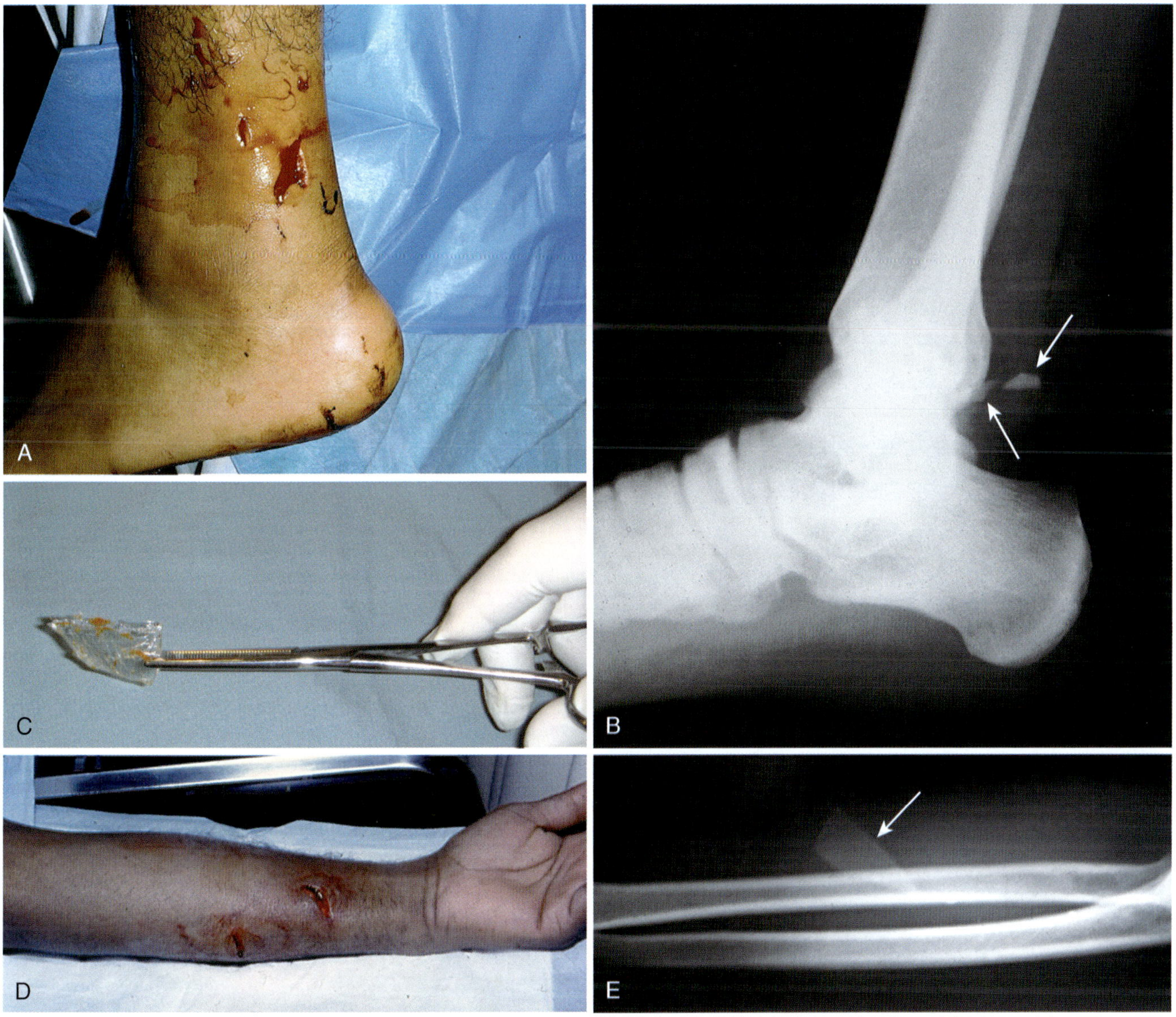

Fig. 36.2 Some wound mechanisms are classic for the presence of a foreign body (FB). Note that even small pieces of all types of glass are readily seen on a plain radiograph. (A) This intoxicated patient kicked out a window and sustained seemingly minor puncture wounds. He did not believe that glass was in the wound, there was little pain, and no FB could be palpated externally. (B) A radiograph revealed a large shard of glass *(arrows)* deeply embedded in the wound. (C) The shard of glass was removed, but only after 20 minutes of exploration. (D) Another classic scenario for a retained glass FB is putting the arm through a window. An FB was not suspected or sensed by the patient or clinician. (E) When a radiograph was taken, a large shard of glass *(arrow)* was readily detected. Despite its size, removal was difficult and time-consuming.

a linear trail of echoes deep to the FB, referred to as the *comet tail artifact*. A wooden object leaves an acoustic shadow without artifact.[16,17]

US may be performed at the bedside. To do so, use a high-frequency transducer (at least 7.5 MHz, such as a high-frequency linear vascular probe) because most FBs are small and superficial. A lower frequency may also be necessary if a deeper FB is suspected, but it may miss small FBs.[18] A spacer may be needed to adjust the "focal zone" (i.e., where the beam is the narrowest and signal intensity is the highest). US may be particularly difficult in the hand or foot, which have many echogenic structures and web spaces that may limit visualization when the FB is adjacent to bone.[15,17,19] Keep in mind that the presence of air, scars, calcification, sutures, and sesamoid bones in surrounding tissue may lead to false-positive results.[19,20]

Advantages of US include low cost, no ionizing radiation, the ability to define the object in three dimensions, and real-time bedside imaging which may be used during removal.[7] Many studies report that US is highly sensitive for detecting FBs by adequately trained personnel, either radiologists, technicians, or emergency physicians.[2] It is not easy to cite a precise sensitivity or specificity because of the wide variation in these studies with regard to FB size, material, and location; operator experience; and the models used in these studies.[20–22]

Ultrasound: Foreign Body Removal

by Christine Butts, MD

Many FBs are radiopaque and can easily be seen with traditional radiography. Such FBs include glass, metal, and some plastics. Other foreign materials, such as splinters, spines, and thinner plastics, are radiopaque and easily missed on radiographs. US is an optimal modality for both identifying retained FBs and aiding in their removal. Several studies have evaluated the sensitivity and specificity of US in identifying FBs in soft tissue. The findings have been variable, depending on the type and size of FB.[1,2]

General Considerations

A preliminary radiograph may be helpful in narrowing down the area to be evaluated with US, particularly when there is a large area where the FB may be found. Asking the patient to identify the point of maximal tenderness may also help narrow down the overall area to be examined. Once the area has been clarified, a high-frequency (10 to 12.5 MHz) transducer should be selected. Higher frequencies will convey sufficient resolution to distinguish foreign material from normal soft tissue structures.

Each type of foreign body has specific identifiable characteristics; however, certain general findings suggest the presence of foreign material. The finding of soft tissue edema, represented by anechoic (black) or hypoechoic (dark gray) areas within the normal soft tissue, is highly suggestive of recent tissue disruption (Fig. 36.US1).

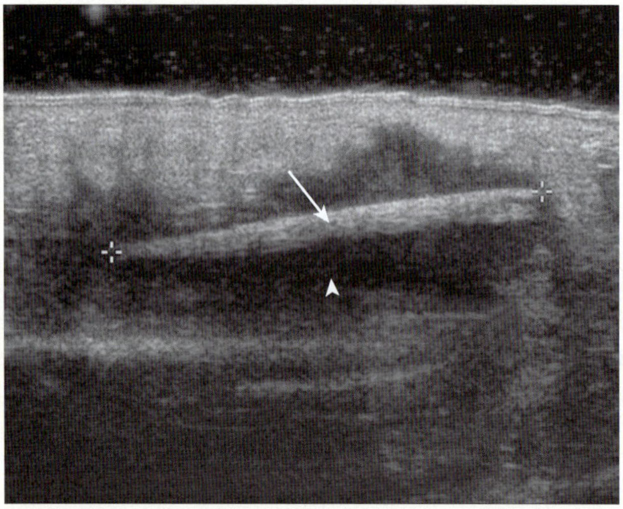

Fig. 36.US1 Wooden foreign body in the foot. The foreign body is hyperechoic *(arrow)*, whereas the surrounding hypoechoic region *(arrowhead)* is indicative of edema or pus.

The area in question should be evaluated from several different angles to find the object in its long axis. A small foreign body may easily be overlooked if only a small portion of it is seen.

Additionally, using a "stand-off" pad may be helpful, especially when dealing with superficial structures such as the hand or foot. A slim, fluid-filled structure, such as a 100-mL bag of saline or a glove filled with water, is placed over the area of interest. The transducer is then placed on top of this pad. This extra layer creates an acoustic window to allow greater resolution and eliminate some superficial artifacts that may impede the examination.

Metallic FBs are strongly echogenic and are very straightforward to locate. They will appear bright white and often give off strong reverberation artifacts (Fig. 36.US2).

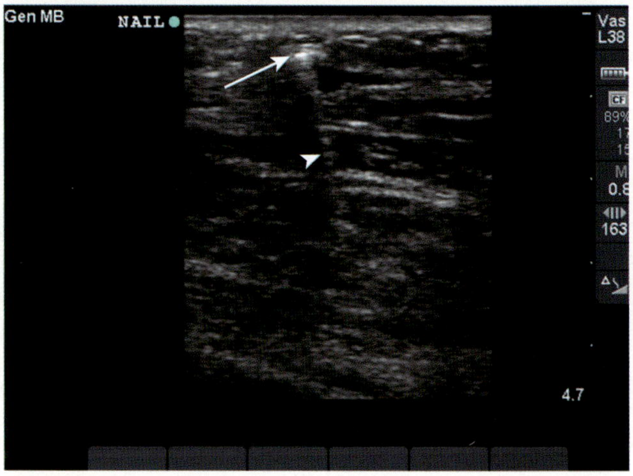

Fig. 36.US2 Metallic foreign body identified as a brightly echogenic *(white)* object *(arrow)* with a comet tail artifact seen extending deep into the soft tissue *(arrowhead)*.

Glass FBs appear very similar to metallic objects in that they are highly echogenic (white). Glass may cause a reverberation artifact, but more typically, it will cause acoustic shadowing to extend deep to the object (Fig. 36.US3).

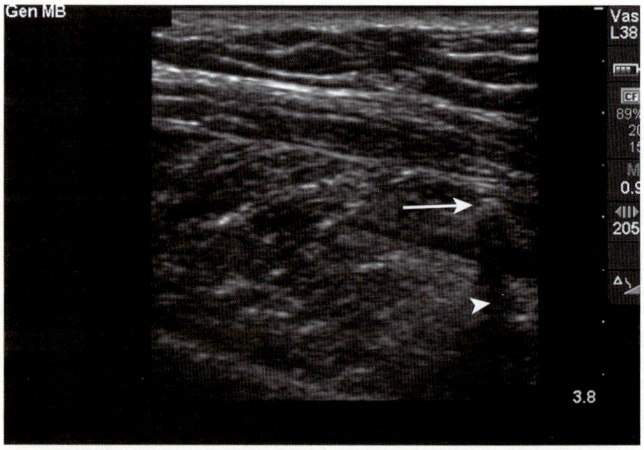

Fig. 36.US3 Glass foreign body *(arrow)* identified as a hyperechoic *(white)* object causing a strong shadow *(arrowhead)* within the otherwise normal-appearing soft tissue.

Wooden objects (such as splinters) are more challenging to locate, particularly with very small FBs. Wooden FBs do not create as strong an echogenic focus as other types of material do and may appear only slightly brighter than normal tissue (Fig. 36.US4). Very subtle shadowing may be seen extending deep to the object. The presence of surrounding edema is often key to locating the FB.

Continued

Ultrasound: Foreign Body Removal—cont'd

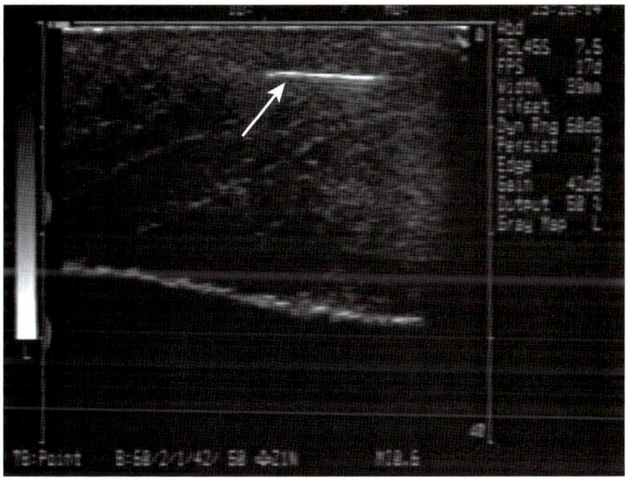

Fig. 36.US4 Sonographic appearance of a retained wooden foreign body *(arrow)*.

Removal

Once the object has been localized, it can be removed either blindly or under direct sonographic guidance.

Another technique that may be helpful, particularly with smaller objects, is to insert two 25-gauge needles under sonographic guidance. These needles should be inserted at right angles to each other so that the tips of each of them rest at the foreign body. The clinician can then cut the skin and overlying soft tissue and dissect down to the intersection of these two needles.[23–25]

From Rumack CM. Diagnostic Ultrasound. 4th ed. Elsevier; 2010.

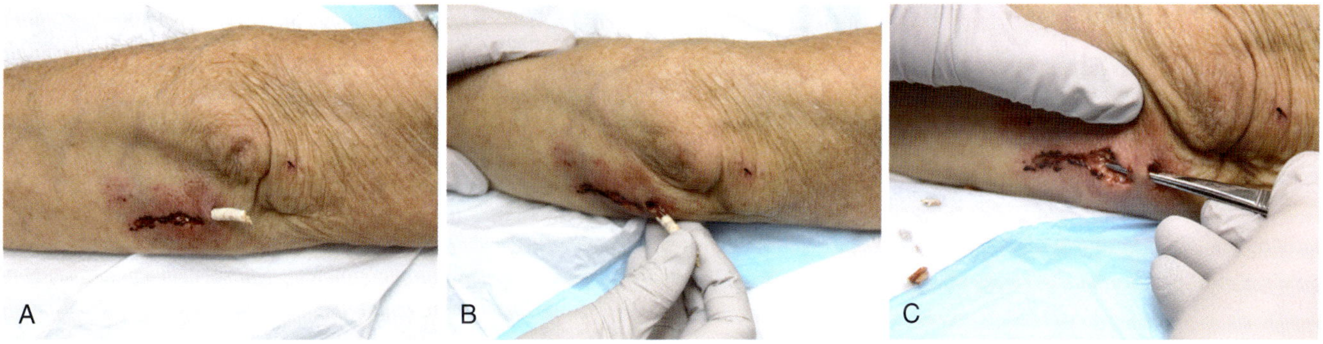

Fig. 36.3 (A) This patient has an obvious wooden foreign body (FB) on the dorsal aspect of the proximal part of the forearm. (B) Manual removal of the object was not difficult. (C) However, thorough exploration of the wound cavity via an incision over the entire length of the FB tract revealed multiple small wooden fragments. Wood fragments retained in a wound will always cause an infection. Proper exploration requires adequate analgesia, good lighting, hemostasis, and a cooperative patient. Use of a metal probe may help identify the foreign object by feel or sound (see Fig. 36.17).

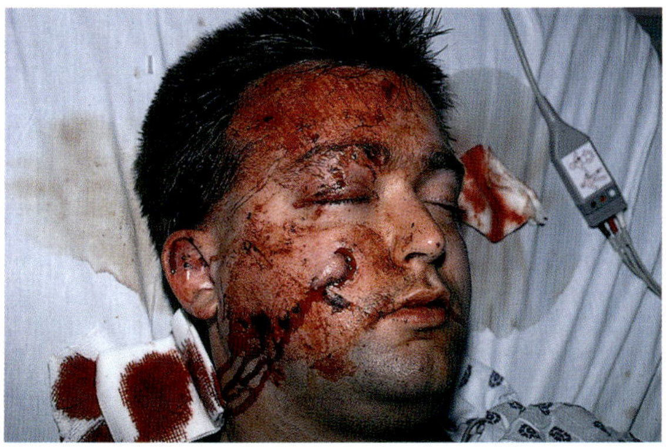

Fig. 36.4 A windshield forehead injury usually harbors multiple retained pieces of glass that are difficult to find. Probing with a needle or forceps in each wound to feel or hear contact with the fragments may help find them. A supraorbital nerve block is ideal to facilitate probing.

CT

CT depends on x-ray absorption; thus, it generally visualizes the same material detected on plain films, but subtle differences in soft tissue densities may help identify FBs not seen on radiographs.[6,10] CT produces a better three-dimensional image than plain films do and may visualize objects embedded in or behind bone. However, CT is more costly and exposes the patient to more ionizing radiation than radiography or US does, and its use should therefore be judicious.

As an example, wood is unlikely to be visible initially on CT, but after 1 week, the wood absorbs surrounding blood products. It may become higher in attenuation than muscle and fat. It may then appear on CT as a linear area of increased attenuation on a wide window setting such as a bone window.[5]

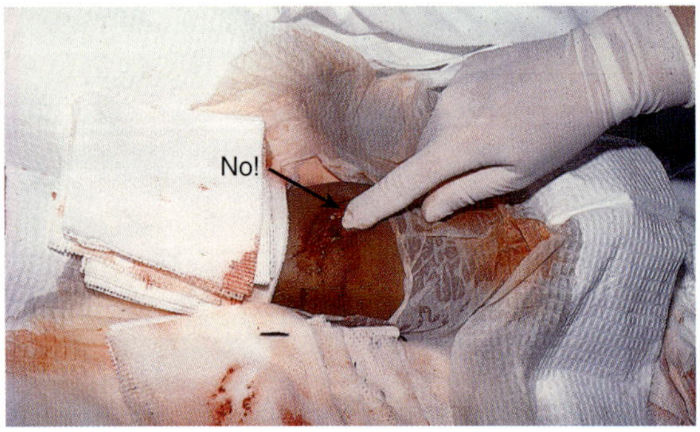

Fig. 36.5 What is wrong here? Though historically suggested as a useful technique to find foreign bodies, probing the depths of a wound with a gloved finger may result in a puncture wound in the operator. The practice is strongly discouraged because of the prevalence of hepatitis and human immunodeficiency virus infection.

MRI

Although MRI is expensive and not as readily available to emergency clinicians as plain films and CT are, it may be superior to CT in detecting small, nonmetallic, radiolucent FBs such as plastic, particularly in the orbit.[26] MRI may not visualize wood, which may appear as a linear signal with associated inflammation and look hypointense with respect to muscle on T1- and T2-weighted sequences, on which it appears as a signal void.[5] Plastic is more easily visualized with MRI than with CT. MRI cannot be used for metallic objects and gravel, which contain various ferromagnetic particles that produce signal artifacts and a theoretical risk of shifting within the magnetic field and causing structural damage.[6] This is particularly important when evaluating FBs in the eye, brain, or deep structures of the neck, face, or extremities. FBs may be difficult to differentiate from other low-signal structures on MRI, such as tendon, scar tissue, and calcium.[27]

Fluoroscopy

Like radiography, fluoroscopy can visualize objects that are radiopaque but not radiolucent such as wood and plastic.[28,29] Using correct technique and shielding, radiation scatter to imaging personnel is minute, less than 0.0001 Sv/h.[30] Fluoroscopy also offers the advantage of real-time bedside imaging.[28,30] Fluoroscopic image-intensifying equipment may follow a wound's entrance, localize the material, grasp the FB, and remove it without making a larger incision. Ariyan described a technique in which two needles are placed in the soft tissue from opposite directions and pointing toward the FB.[31] The extremity is rotated while the clinician watches the image under the image intensifier to obtain a three-dimensional effect. An incision is made perpendicular to the plane of the needles, and the object is removed. Although the technique of fluoroscopy is relatively easy to learn, the lack of instruction and availability is the major limitation to its use in the ED.[30–32]

FOREIGN BODY REMOVAL

Indications and Contraindications

One should judiciously evaluate and manage each FB scenario individually. The composition and location of an FB, the patient's medical status, as well as vocational and avocational activities, greatly affect decision-making related to FB removal, including the best time and place for removal. Reactive material, such as wood, should be removed immediately when accessible because retained wood will invariably lead to inflammation and infection. Other inert material, such as glass or plastic, may often be removed electively. Some innocuously located glass and metallic FBs may frequently be left permanently embedded in soft tissue. With deeply embedded, small, inert material (BB, bullets, etc.) that is not located near any vital structures, the time, effort, and trauma involved in removal may be excessive when compared with the possible adverse effects of the foreign material remaining in place. An ill-conceived extended search for an elusive but otherwise harmless FB often results in frustration for the clinician and discomfort, dissatisfaction, and possible injury for the patient.

If localization is certain and removal can be accomplished within a manageable period without worsening the injury, an attempt at removal is generally indicated on the initial visit (given the availability of clinicians and support staff).

When reviewing the decision regarding when and how to remove the FB, the possibility of the FB migrating to involve vital structures, though quite remote, should be discussed with the patient. Cases of reported missile embolization in the vascular system are influenced by missile caliber, impact velocity, physical wound characteristics, point of vessel entrance, body position and movement, and blood flow velocity.[33] Retained bullets usually remain in soft tissue but can rarely make their way into the vascular system. Schurr and colleagues reported a paradoxical bullet embolization from the left external iliac vein to the left iliac artery via a patent foramen ovale.[34] When clinicians first examined the patient, a bullet was noted on the chest radiograph, and an isolated chest wound was suspected. However, the bullet had apparently entered the chest, traversed the abdomen to the iliac vein, and then embolized back to the chest and arterial system.

After the initial history, examination, and preoperative and preanesthetic documentation of the patient's neurovascular status, a decision must be made regarding the time and place of removal. More difficult or time-intensive procedures should be referred and may need to be managed by a specialist in the operating room, keeping in mind that even surprisingly large or presumed superficial FBs can still often prove quite elusive.

If a FB is left in place, inform the patient why it was not removed. This should also be carefully explained and documented whenever the patient is referred for delayed removal. Regardless of whether the FB is removed, clean all wounds appropriately and update tetanus prophylaxis if indicated. In cases of retained FBs warn patients what to watch for.

Equipment and Preparation

Good space and lighting, a comfortable patient and operator position, a standard suture tray, and a scalpel are usually adequate equipment for the removal of most simple FBs (Fig. 36.10). Tissue retractors, special pickups, and loupes may be added if needed.

Local soft tissue injection or selected nerve blocks with buffered bupivacaine or lidocaine (or both) are the recommended anesthesia for removing most soft tissue FBs. If the clinician senses undue apprehension or anxiety in the patient,

TABLE 36.1 Imaging Summary

	RADIOGRAPHY	US	CT	MRI	FLUOROSCOPY
Materials visualized	Metal Glass Graphite Plastic (variable)	Wood Thorns Organic matter Metal Glass	Metal Glass Wood (late) Plastic (variable) Organic material (variable)	Glass Plastic Organic matter	Metal Glass Plastic (variable)
What type of material cannot be visualized	Wood Thorns Organic matter Plastic (variable)	Deep FBs	Wood (early) Plastic (variable) Organic material (variable)	Wood (variable) METAL!	Wood Thorns Organic matter Plastic (variable)
Pros	Cheap Available Easy to interpret	Bedside use for real-time extraction Relatively inexpensive	3D images with some improved visualization of FBs vs. plain film	Improved detection of radiolucent objects vs. CT	Useful for real-time bedside extraction
Cons	Unable to visualize all material May miss small FBs in areas adjacent to bone	Results vary based on operator experience Difficult visualization in the hands and potential for false positives	Expensive Increased exposure to ionizing radiation	Expensive Not readily available in all EDs Dangerous for metallic FBs	Unfamiliar technique to most ED clinicians Not widely available
Conclusions	Reasonable initial approach, particularly for metal and glass Obtain multiple views via a soft tissue technique	Recommended for radiolucent structures such as vegetative material (wood, thorns, etc.) Allows direct visualization Can assist with operative removal Potentially a bedside procedure depending on the clinician's skill level	Recommended approach for intracranial, intraorbital FBs Has a role for repeated visits and concerns for retained FBs Limited role during initial evaluation	Role limited on initial evaluation Has a role with repeated visits and concern for retained FBs	Use limited to individual clinicians with experience and availability

3D, Three dimensional; *CT*, computed tomography; *ED*, emergency department; *FB*, foreign body; *MRI*, magnetic resonance imaging; *US*, ultrasonography.
A reasonable initial approach for localizing nonvisualized FBs in the ED is to obtain multiple-projection plain radiographs with a soft tissue technique. This technique will visualize the majority of FBs, especially metal and glass. US should be considered for objects known to be radiolucent, such as wood or thorns. The role of CT and MRI for evaluation of FBs in the ED is limited, but they are the definitive imaging tests in confusing cases. For suspected intraorbital or intracranial FBs, CT is recommended. CT or MRI is also warranted *when a previously negative explored wound exhibits recurrent infection, poor healing, or persistent pain*. CT or MRI may be the appropriate initial test for patients with nonspecific swelling to define FBs and possible alternative diagnoses such as abscesses, masses, or other inflammatory processes.[6] Bedside US and fluoroscopy (for radiopaque FBs) may be used to guide difficult FB extractions if initial attempts at removal are unsuccessful and the proper equipment and experienced personnel are available.

use of sedation (parenteral, rectal, or oral) is advised. Sedation may be especially helpful in children. If the patient is uncooperative, postpone exploration to a more appropriate time and setting (e.g., under regional or general anesthesia in the operating room).

To successfully remove an FB in the soft tissue of an extremity, a time-limited arterial tourniquet can help provide a bloodless field. Inflate a blood pressure cuff or portable self-contained pneumatic cuff above arterial pressure on the upper part of the arm, forearm, leg, or thigh. To limit bothersome back bleeding, elevate the extremity and wrap it with an elastic bandage to exsanguinate the extremity before inflating the tourniquet. A Penrose drain or specialized tourniquet may be used at the base of a finger or toe. Alternatively, use a sterile

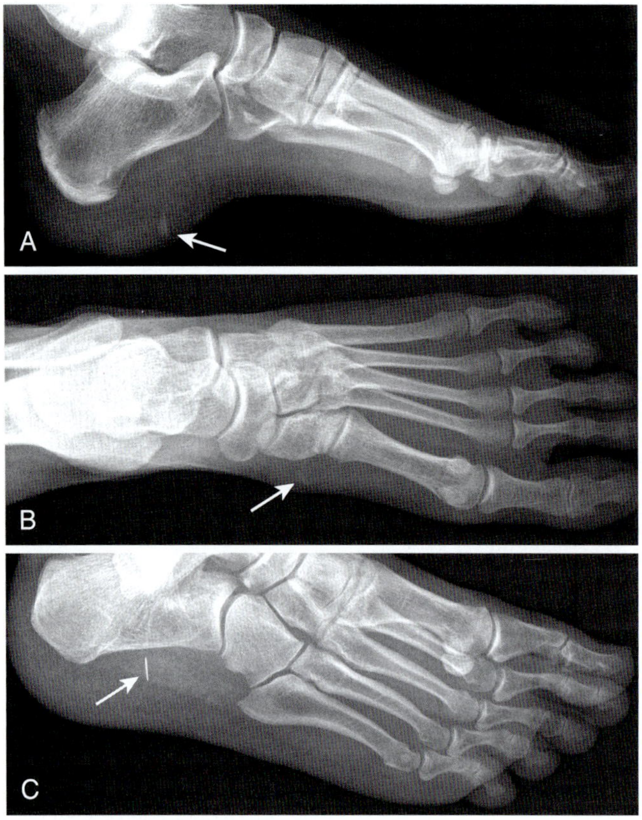

Fig. 36.6 Radiographic appearance of various foreign bodies. *Arrows* point to (A) glass (B) pencil lead (graphite, but not wood, is radiopaque), and (C) a metallic pin. Plain radiographs should be taken in multiple projections. Do not ignore subtle soft tissue irregularities. Generally absent on radiographs are aluminum, plastic, wood, thorns and other organic objects, such as fish spines, and small pieces of gravel.

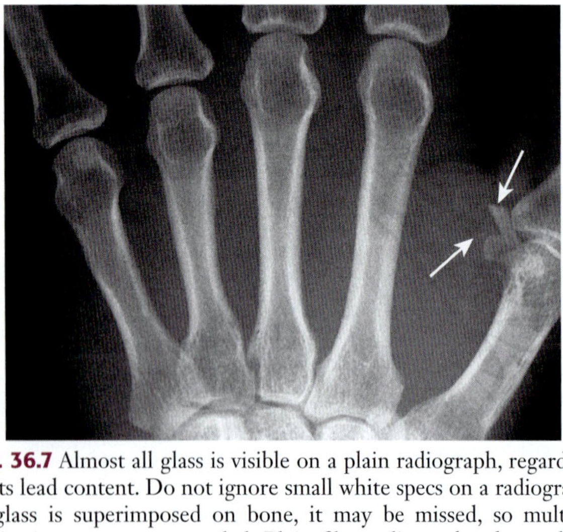

Fig. 36.7 Almost all glass is visible on a plain radiograph, regardless of its lead content. Do not ignore small white specs on a radiograph. If glass is superimposed on bone, it may be missed, so multiple projections are recommended. Plain film radiography shows sharp corners characteristic of glass. Proximity of the foreign body to the bone may be deceiving.

glove as a finger tourniquet. Cut the fingertip of the glove on the involved finger and roll the glove down to the base of the finger. Most patients can tolerate an ischemic tourniquet for 15 to 30 minutes, and it is safe to stop the circulation to an extremity for this length of time.

Procedure

The specific technique for removal of an FB is tailored to each clinical situation. In general, FBs should be removed only under direct vision. Grasping blindly into a wound with a hemostat to remove an FB should be avoided. This technique is especially dangerous in the hand, foot, neck, or face, where sensitive or vital structures may easily be damaged.

After obtaining appropriate informed consent and following sterile preparation, consider enlarging the entrance wound with an adequate skin incision creating an advantageous situation for visualization of FBs. Numerous techniques are used, depending on the clinical scenario (Fig. 36.11). Attempting to remove an FB through a puncture wound or an inadequate skin incision is a common error that is both frustrating and self-defeating. After a proper skin incision, explore the wound carefully by spreading the soft tissue with a hemostat. Frequently, the FB can be felt with an instrument before it can be seen (see Fig. 36.11, *plate 1*). After placing a tourniquet on an extremity, follow the track of the FB, although it often cannot be identified when surrounded by muscle or fat. If the FB, such as one made of fiberglass or plastic, is difficult to visualize, is located in the superficial soft tissue, or has contaminated the surrounding soft tissue, excising a small block of tissue rather than removing the FB alone may be necessary. Excise the tissue block only under direct vision and after nerves, tendons, and vessels have been identified and excluded from the excision area.

If a FB such as a thorn or needle enters the skin perpendicularly, a linear incision may pass to one side or the other of the FB, and it may be difficult to determine where the FB lies in relation to this incision (see Fig. 36.11, *plate 2*). For this reason, the search must then be extended into the walls of the incision rather than simply through the skin.[35] In such cases, excise a small ellipse of skin and undermine the skin for 0.5 cm to 1.0 cm in all directions. Next, compress the tissue from the sides in the hope that the FB will extrude and can then be grasped with a hemostat.

After FB removal, it is important to irrigate and cleanse the wounds. If a small incision has been made in a noncosmetic area (such as the bottom of the foot), leave the incision open and bandaged. The area may be periodically soaked in hot water for a few days. A return visit is necessary only if signs of infection develop. If a large incision has been made, the skin may be sutured primarily as long as no other contraindications are present. In cases where gross contamination has occurred or significant tissue injury, do not close the wound on the initial visit. Leave the wound open but packed. Suture the skin after 3 to 5 days if the wound is free of inflammation or infection (known as delayed primary closure; see Chapters 34 and 35 for details).

Special Scenarios and Techniques

Puncture Wounds in the Sole of the Foot

See Videos 36.1 and 36.2. Puncture wounds in the feet from unknown objects and under unknown circumstances present problems to the clinician. In general, puncture wounds in the feet are at risk for retained FBs and infection. It is impossible to adequately explore a puncture wound. In noncosmetic areas, therefore a puncture wound can be converted to

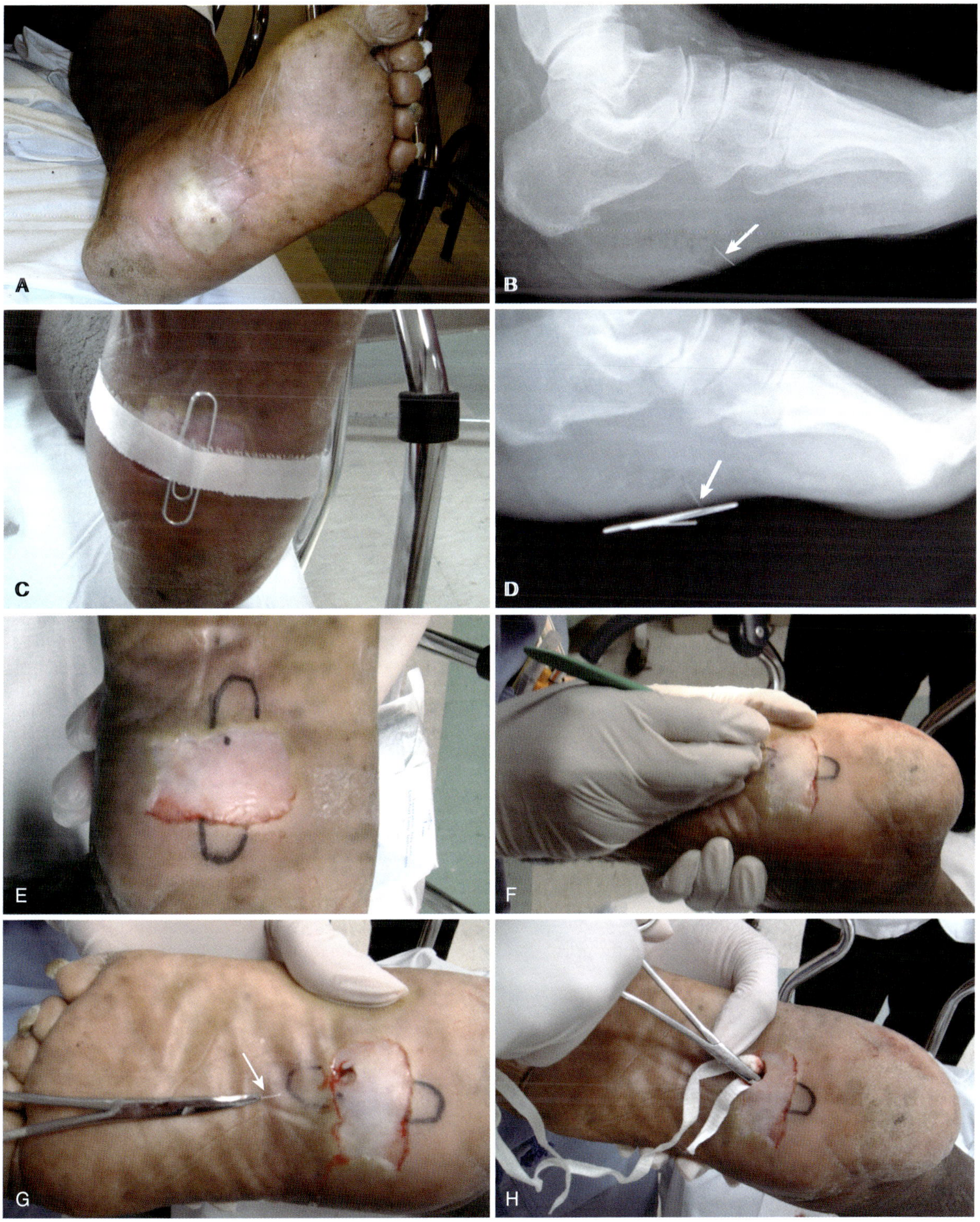

Fig. 36.8 (A) This patient had an obvious diabetic foot abscess. (B) A radiograph was taken to rule out osteomyelitis or soft tissue gas. To everyone's surprise, including the patient's, a sewing needle *(arrow)*, origin and timing unknown, was the source of the infection. (C–D) A paper clip was taped to the skin to localize the depth and position of the foreign body *(FB; arrow)* on the radiograph. An anteroposterior radiograph (not shown) also localized the FB. (E) For orientation, the outline of the paper clip was traced on the foot. A *dot* marks a possible entrance site. (F) A generous incision was made over the projected site of the FB. (G) The needle *(arrow)* was felt and extracted with a hemostat. (H) The wound was left open and packed with a cotton wick.

a laceration to adequately explore and cleanse the wound (Fig. 36.12). Under most circumstances, delayed primary closure is recommended (see Chapter 34). This topic, including stepping on a nail and puncture wounds on the sole, is discussed extensively in Chapter 52.

Subungual FBs

Wooden splinters are commonly embedded under the fingernail. Such FBs must be removed completely because of the high risk of subsequent infection. When identified, perform a digital block before manipulating the nail or nail

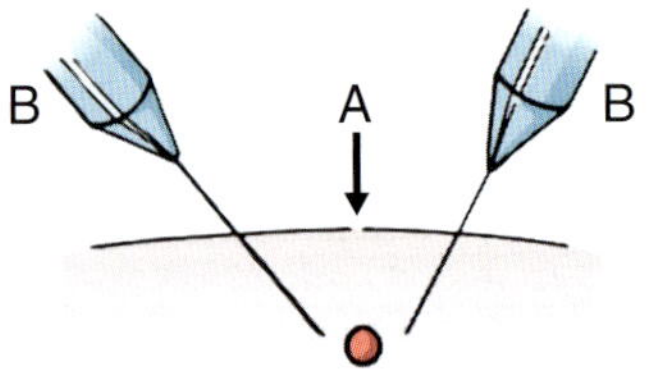

Fig. 36.9 When a small entrance wound *(A)* is noted but the foreign body (FB) is not seen, noninvasive localization is preferable to blind probing. Metal markers taped to the skin or needles inserted close to the FB under local anesthesia *(B)* and radiographed at different angles provide a guide to localization and extraction of the FB. (Reproduced from *Hospital Medicine*, January 1981, with permission of Cahners Publishing Co.)

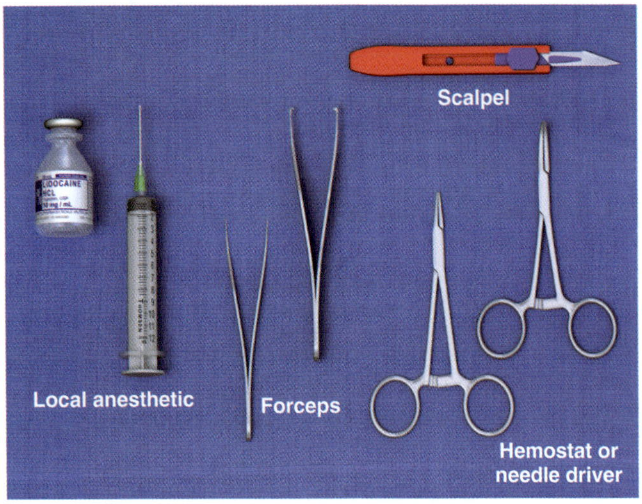

Fig. 36.10 The contents of a standard suture tray, with the addition of a scalpel, are usually adequate for the removal of most foreign bodies.

bed. Pay special attention to deeply embedded subungual FBs.[36] Some cases may require removing a small portion of the nail with double-pointed heavy scissors to expose the FB and grasp the foreign material with splinter forceps (Fig. 36.13).

One technique is to bend the tip of a sterile hypodermic needle and slide it under the nail. The needle is used to hook the FB and then remove it. Alternatively, slide a 19-gauge hypodermic needle under the nail to surround a small splinter. Bring the needle tip against the underside of the nail and secure the splinter. Remove the needle and splinter as a unit.[37] Another possible technique is to shave the overlying nail plate with a No. 15 scalpel blade via light strokes in a proximal-to-distal direction. This creates a U-shaped nail defect and exposes the sliver's entire length.[38]

Remove the entire nail if complete removal cannot be achieved with the techniques described earlier (see Chapters 34, 35 and 52). This allows all the fragments to be visualized and removed. The proximity of the distal phalanx to the subungual area is a constant concern for the development of osteomyelitis and requires follow-up.

Metallic Fragments and Bullets

See Videos 36.3–36.5. High-velocity fragments (e.g., bullets, BBs) are easy to visualize radiographically and relatively simple to remove if embedded in areas that are anatomically accessible (Fig. 36.14). Before removal, assess the area where the fragments are embedded to determine which structures are involved and which structures might be encountered during removal. Defer removal of deeply embedded metallic FBs unless symptoms of infection develop. Infection is rare because such FBs usually become encysted over time.

Surgery is rarely performed solely to remove bullets. Retained bullets rarely cause complications or infection, and aggressive attempts to find and remove bullets generally cause more harm than good. Retrieval is often quite difficult unless the fragments are very superficial. Gunshot wounds themselves need no intervention beyond simple cleaning and perhaps minor debridement of the entrance or exit wound. Gunshot wound tracks do not need debridement unless there is gross contamination or significant tissue devitalization. Entrance or exit wounds should not be closed. Antibiotics are usually unnecessary for minor uncomplicated gunshot wounds in otherwise healthy patients. Still, they may be beneficial in patients with multiple injuries, multiple comorbidities, gross wound contamination, significant tissue devitalization, large wounds, or delays in treatment.

There is a concern about lead toxicity from bullet fragments. If a bullet is bathed in synovial, pleural, peritoneal, or cerebrospinal fluid, the lead may leach out over time and can produce a significant elevation in blood lead levels. Though rare, lead fragments in contact with synovium are a reason for concern and potentially a reason for removal (see the previous discussion). In one study, Farrell and associates found that patients with retained lead FBs had statistically significant elevated blood lead levels.[39] The study did not differentiate the location of the FB and whether patients were, in fact, symptomatic from plumbism. Nevertheless, it may be prudent for the patient's primary care provider to monitor blood lead levels in patients with known lead FBs to prevent the future development of lead toxicity. The value of routine prophylactic antibiotics for metallic FBs left in soft tissue has not been proved and antibiotics are generally not used.

For superficial metallic FBs, a sterile magnet can be used to facilitate the removal of small metallic fragments.[40] Introduce the magnet into the entry site, with a small scalpel and hemostat used to extend and open the wound as needed. When the magnet comes in contact with the metal, a click is heard, and the FB is removed while it is attached to the magnet. If resistance to extraction occurs, exploration can be done with the FB attached to the magnet. Sometimes, instead of introducing the magnet directly into the wound, it can be placed on the overlying skin to guide superficial small FBs out of the wound.[41] Try not to grasp or touch the bullet because it can interfere with ballistics evidence during any subsequent legal investigation.

FBs in Fatty Tissue

FBs in fatty tissue can be removed by making an elliptical incision around the entrance wound. Grasp the incised skin loosely with an Allis forceps. Undercut the incision until the FB is contacted. Remove the FB, skin, and entrance track in one block. Remove a small portion of subcutaneous fat along with the FB to minimize infection. FBs in fat are very mobile, and probing may further displace them. FBs embedded in fat and perpendicular to the skin can also be removed, as shown in Fig. 36.11. As always, the removal of soft tissue, including adipose, should be done in as conservative a manner as possible, as any tissue removal may have implications in scar formation.

Foreign Body Removal Techniques

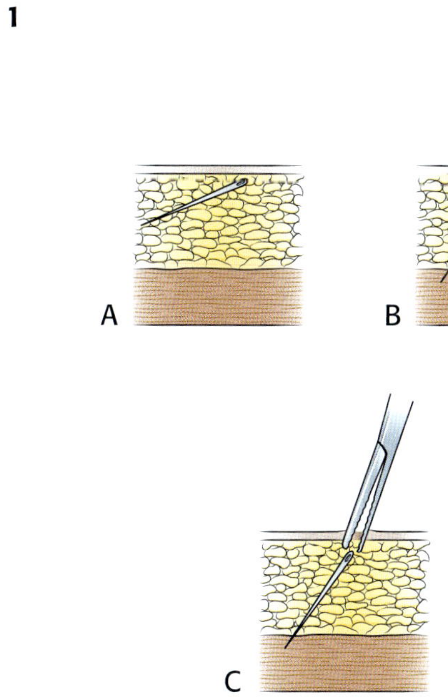

A, A sewing needle completely embedded below the surface is easily located with a radiograph. **B**, After the application of local anesthesia, a small incision over the superficial end permits removal with a hemostat. **C**, The hemostat is introduced through an adequate incision, spread to open the tissue, and used to "feel" the FB as the hemostat is advanced.

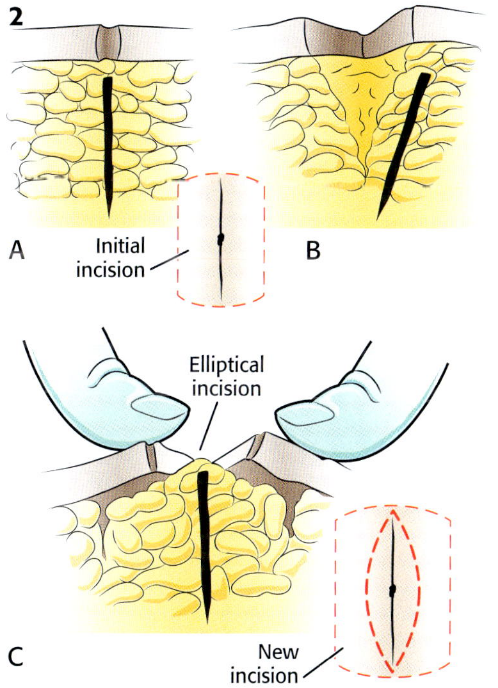

If a linear skin incision is used to locate a mobile FB that is perpendicular to the skin in subcutaneous fat (**A**), the FB may be displaced (**B**). **C**, A modified elliptical incision is made and the skin edges are undermined to displace the FB into the middle of the wound. Pressure with the thumbs may be applied to the skin to force the FB into view.

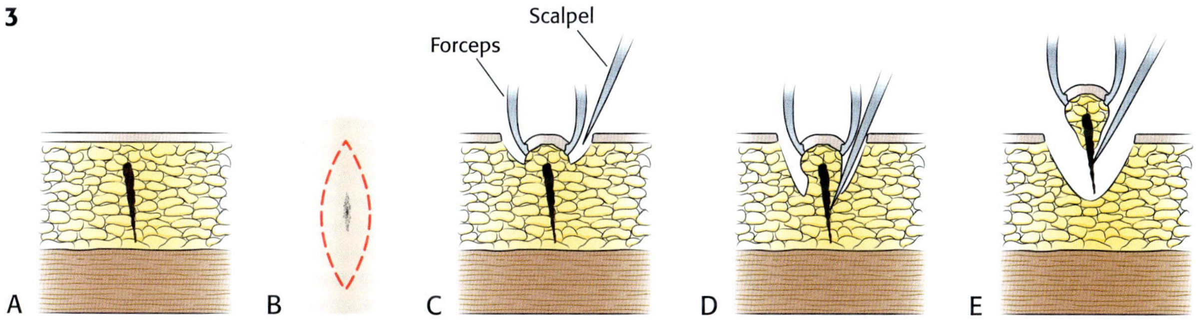

FBs in deep fat (**A**) may be approached by making a small elliptical incision around the entry point (**B**). **C**, The incision is then laterally undercut and grasped (without pulling) with forceps. **D**, The ellipse is then further undercut until contact with the FB is made. **E**, The FB may be grasped and removed along with the entry tract and the soiled local fat.

Fig. 36.11 Foreign body (FB) removal techniques. (1 and 3, From *Hospital Medicine*, January 1981, with permission of Cahners Publishing Co. 2, From Rees CE. The removal of FBs: a modified incision. *JAMA*. 1939;113:35. Copyright 1939, American Medical Association.)

Pencil Lead/Graphite

Use careful judgment in removing pencil graphite when it is lodged in the skin. Graphite invariably leaves a pigmented tattoo in the soft tissue, and it is preferable to excise the material en bloc (see Fig. 36.11) when pencil lead is found in a cosmetic area. The graphite specks cannot be irrigated or scrubbed off, tattooing results if they are not removed. Furthermore, a pencil lead FB may resemble a malignant melanoma over time. US has been shown to be useful in differentiating between pencil lead FBs and melanoma.[42]

Fishhooks

See Videos 36.6–36.8. Traditionally, four fishhook removal techniques have been described: advance and cut, string-yank, needle cover, and retrograde.[43] The preferred method depends on the type of fishhook, location, depth of penetration, and conditions under which the removal is to take place (Fig. 36.15).[44–46] Initially, note whether the fishhook is single or multiple and determine the number and location of barbs. Remove or cover any remaining exposed hooks to prevent subsequent injury. As with most injuries, document

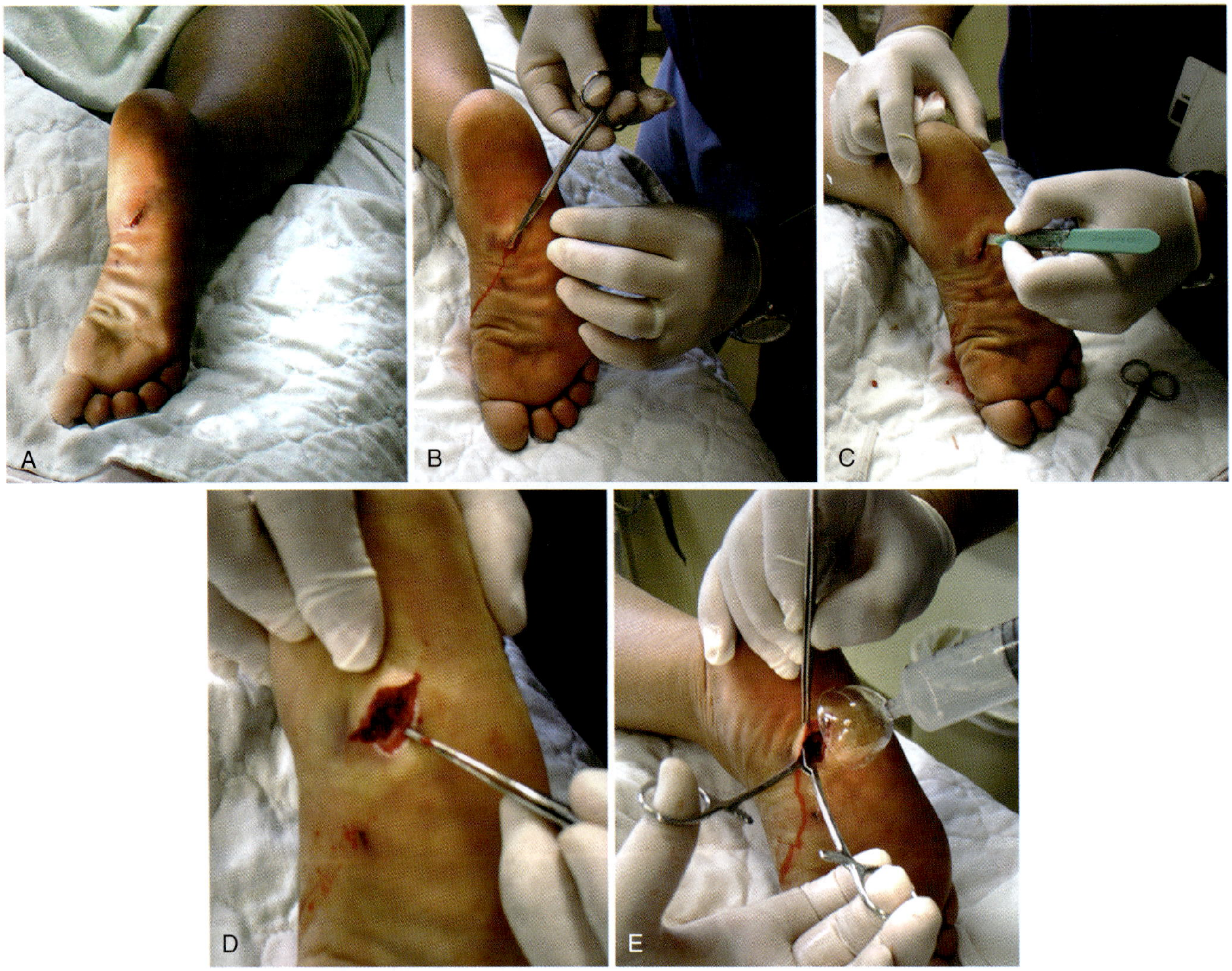

Fig. 36.12 This patient stepped on "something" while walking through a polluted urban creek, a setup for a foreign body and infection. Mandatory radiographs were negative. (A) Under proper lighting (and a calf blood pressure cuff for a tourniquet), the patient is placed prone. Local lidocaine with epinephrine is infiltrated *through the cut skin edges*, not via the intact sensitive skin. (Alternatively, a posterior tibial nerve block could be used.) (B) Inspection reveals a dirty skin flap that is cut off. (C) Because a puncture wound cannot be explored or irrigated, this wound should be lengthened with a scalpel to allow further care. (D) The depths of the wound are explored. (E) An assistant holds the wound open with a hemostat so that copious irrigation can be accomplished. This wound should be *packed open* and checked in 24 to 48 hours, *not closed primarily with sutures*. Delayed closure can be performed in 4 to 5 days if necessary, but this injury healed well without sutures. Prophylactic antibiotics are of no proven value but may be given.

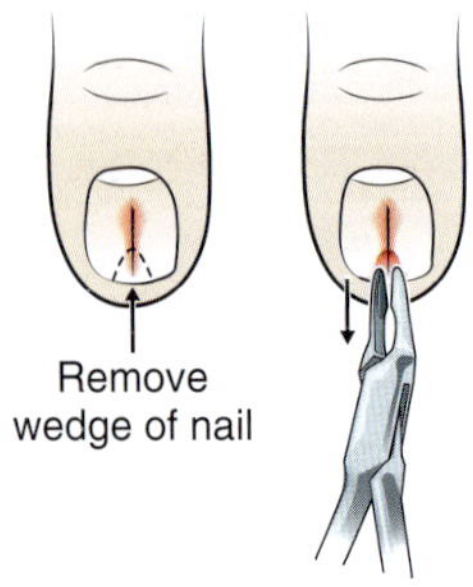

Fig. 36.13 For a foreign body (FB) deep in the nail bed, take as small a wedge of nail as will allow access to the proximal end of the splinter, and then extract the FB with splinter forceps. All wood particles should be removed. A digital nerve block is usually necessary.

the patient's vascular and neurologic status before and after removal. As with all wounds, administer tetanus prophylaxis if indicated. Prophylactic antibiotics are not generally necessary.

Advance and Cut Technique

To perform the advance and cut technique for removal, advance the fishhook and cut proximal to the barb (Fig. 36.16, *plate 1*). This method is particularly well suited for superficially embedded fishhooks. Generally, infiltrate local anesthetic (1% lidocaine) into the tissue overlying the barb. Force the barb through the surface of the anesthetized skin and clip it off. Move the rest of the hook retrogradely, along the direction of entry. Because this technique is almost always successful, it can be considered a first-line option.

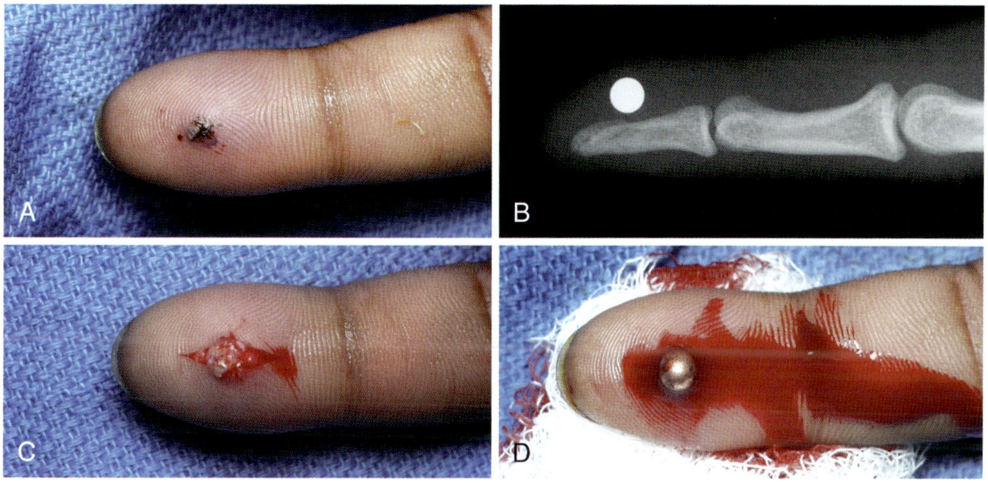

Fig. 36.14 (A–B) High-velocity fragments such as bullets or BBs are often easy to locate and visualize radiographically. Here, a BB is found embedded in the volar tuft of a finger. (C) After a digital block, a small linear incision is made with a scalpel. (D) The BB is removed without difficulty.

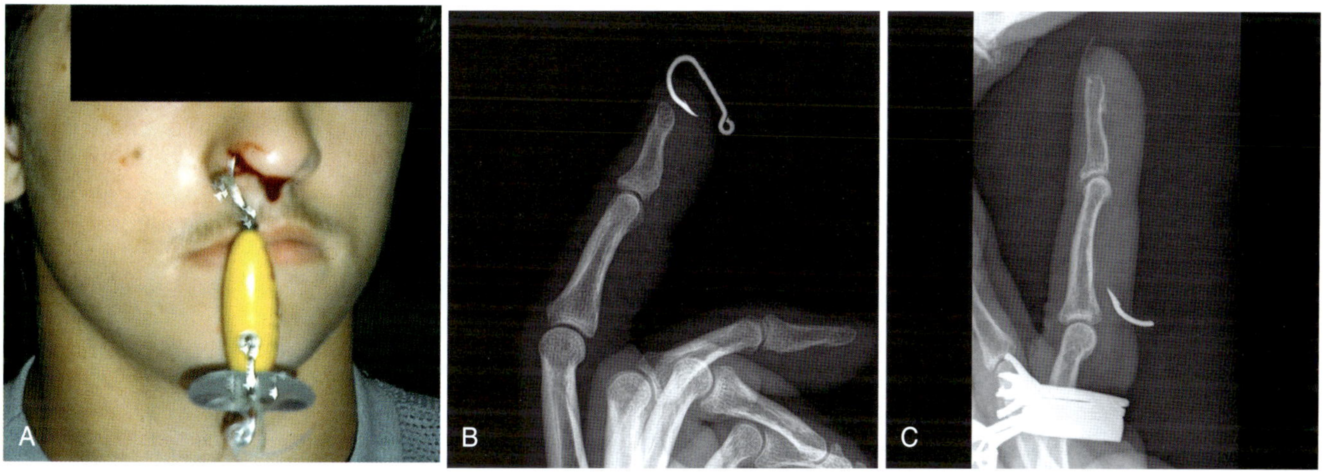

Fig. 36.15 Fishhooks. (A) Fishing lure embedded in the nasal ala. This type of injury may occur while casting the line. (B) Fishhook embedded in the distal tuft of the finger. Note that the barb is completely embedded in subcutaneous tissue, thus making removal by simply pulling the hook out impossible. (C) This patient cut off the portion of the embedded hook external to the skin before coming to the emergency department. Patients will commonly do this; however, it makes removal more difficult because there is very little hook exposed that can be manipulated during attempts at removal.

String-Yank Technique

In the field or stream, removal of a fishhook may be accomplished without local anesthesia by using the string-yank technique. This technique may be used in the emergency department (ED) as well. Some clinicians prefer to use local 1% lidocaine to facilitate removal. For the "stream" technique (see Fig. 36.16, *plate 2*), pass a looped string or fishing line around the belly of the hook at the point where it enters the skin. Wrap approximately 1 ft of string around the dominant hand to provide strong traction. Hold the shank of the hook parallel to and in approximation to the skin with the index finger of the opposite hand. Use the thumb and middle finger of the opposite hand to stabilize and depress the barb, which helps the index finger disengage the barb from the subcutaneous tissue. When the barb has been disengaged, give a sharp pull (i.e., a quick tug with a snapping motion) with the dominant hand to remove the hook. Take care to keep bystanders out of the expected path of the hook because it often flies out of the patient.

Needle Cover Technique

For this technique use an 18-gauge needle to cover the barb (see Fig. 36.16, *plate 3*). After adequate local anesthesia has been achieved, pass the needle through the entrance wound of the hook parallel to the shank of the hook to sheath the barb and allow the hook to be backed out while the barb is covered. An alternative to this procedure is to insert a No. 11 blade parallel to the shank of the hook down to the barb and use the point of the blade to free the subcutaneous tissue that is engaged on the barb. Cover the barb with the point of the No. 11 blade and back the hook out, with the blade protecting the barb.

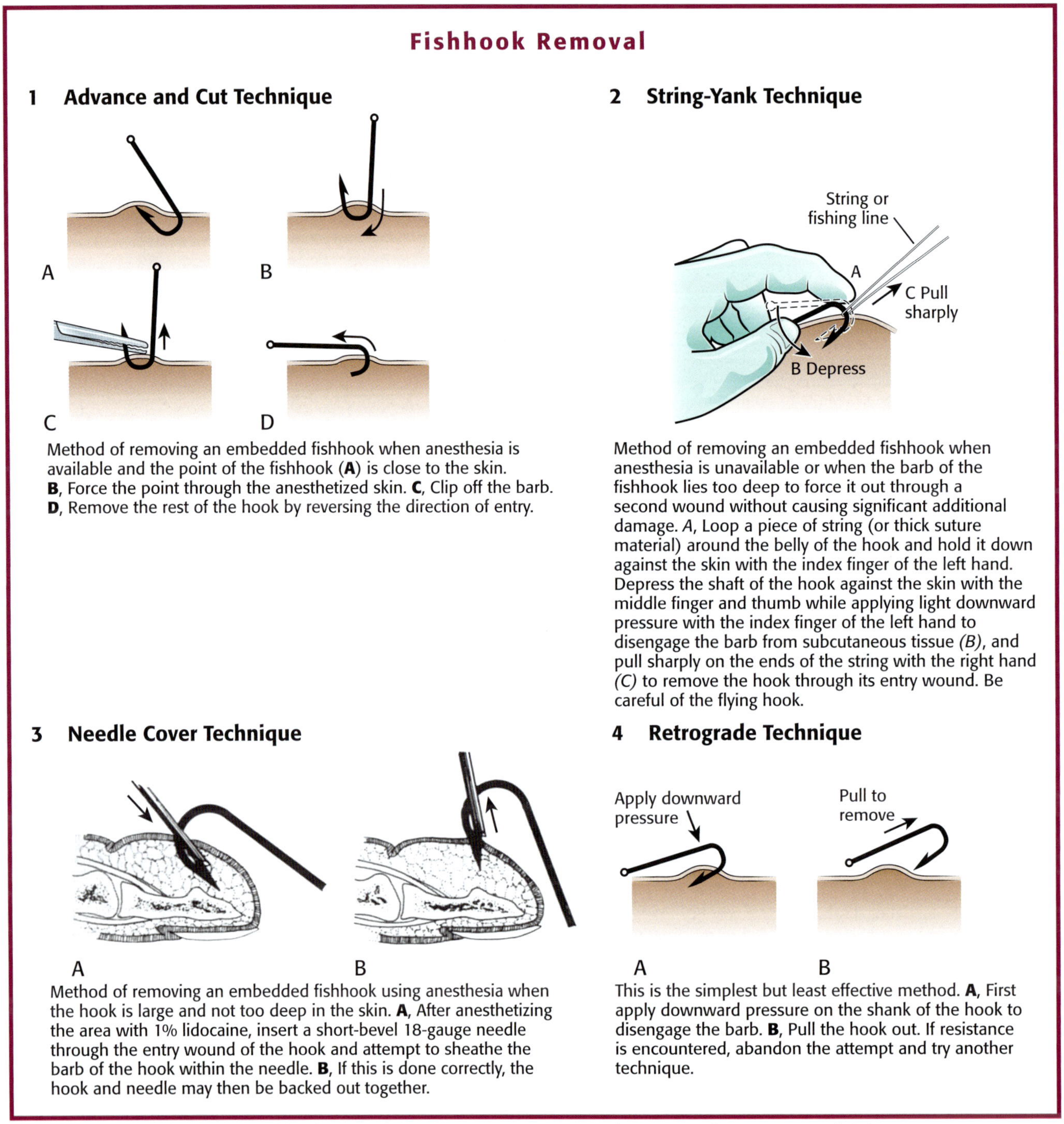

1 Advance and Cut Technique. Method of removing an embedded fishhook when anesthesia is available and the point of the fishhook (**A**) is close to the skin. **B**, Force the point through the anesthetized skin. **C**, Clip off the barb. **D**, Remove the rest of the hook by reversing the direction of entry.

2 String-Yank Technique. Method of removing an embedded fishhook when anesthesia is unavailable or when the barb of the fishhook lies too deep to force it out through a second wound without causing significant additional damage. *A*, Loop a piece of string (or thick suture material) around the belly of the hook and hold it down against the skin with the index finger of the left hand. Depress the shaft of the hook against the skin with the middle finger and thumb while applying light downward pressure with the index finger of the left hand to disengage the barb from subcutaneous tissue *(B)*, and pull sharply on the ends of the string with the right hand *(C)* to remove the hook through its entry wound. Be careful of the flying hook.

3 Needle Cover Technique. Method of removing an embedded fishhook using anesthesia when the hook is large and not too deep in the skin. **A**, After anesthetizing the area with 1% lidocaine, insert a short-bevel 18-gauge needle through the entry wound of the hook and attempt to sheathe the barb of the hook within the needle. **B**, If this is done correctly, the hook and needle may then be backed out together.

4 Retrograde Technique. This is the simplest but least effective method. **A**, First apply downward pressure on the shank of the hook to disengage the barb. **B**, Pull the hook out. If resistance is encountered, abandon the attempt and try another technique.

Fig. 36.16 Fishhook removal. (From *Hospital Medicine*, July 1980, with permission of Cahners Publishing Co.)

Retrograde Technique

This is the simplest, but least effective method. By applying downward pressure on the shank of the hook, disengage the barb to allow successful removal (see Fig. 36.16, *plate 4*). If resistance is encountered, abandon the procedure and attempt removal with another technique. If the barb is not already protruding from the skin, the retrograde technique may cause less tissue trauma.

Wooden Splinters

Removal of wooden splinters is a common FB removal procedure. By simply grasping the end of a superficial, protruding splinter, it may be adequately removed, but care should be taken not to leave small pieces of material in the wound. Some splinters cannot be visualized at the point of entry but can easily and readily be palpated beneath the skin. When a wood FB is in subcutaneous tissue, it is advisable to cut down on the long axis of the FB to remove it via a skin incision rather than pulling it out through the entrance wound (Figs. 36.17 and 36.18). Although an incision may seem extensive and creates a laceration where only a puncture wound existed, opening the track allows thorough cleaning and removal of all the small pieces of the splinter that might otherwise remain. Any remaining piece of wood can lead to infection. The deeper the splinter, the more likely that small

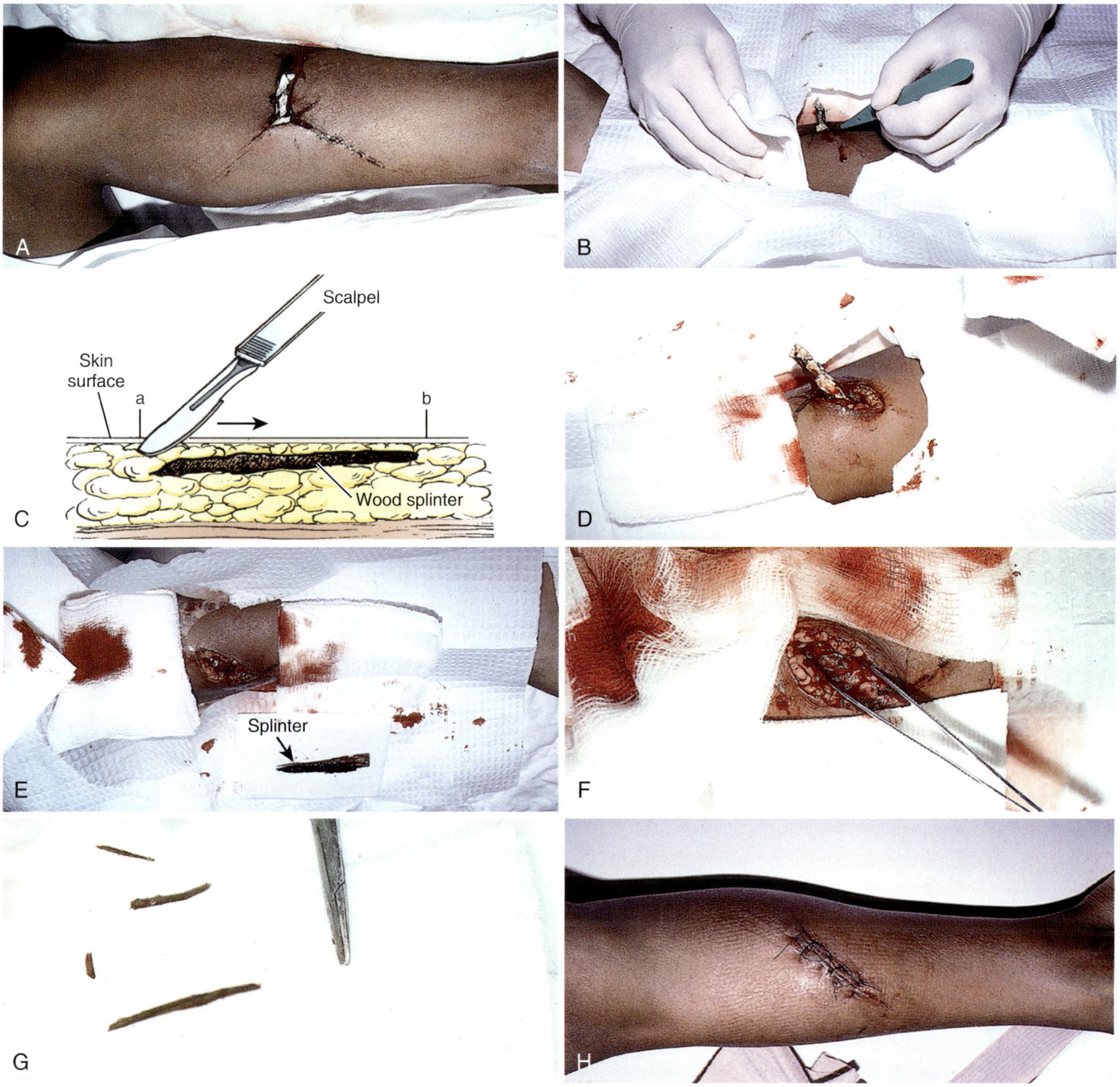

Fig. 36.17 (A) The course and depth of penetration of this large wooden splinter in the leg are uncertain, but it is axiomatic that all pieces of wood must be removed to prevent infection. (B–D) To ensure complete removal of foreign bodies, an incision is made over the entire course of the splinter. (E–G) All pieces of wood are carefully removed under direct vision. (H) The laceration is sutured primarily. Although it may be tempting to simply pull the splinter out and irrigate the puncture track, such actions often lead to retained particles and complications.

pieces of the splinter will remain in the deep part of the wound. If the incision is linear, it may be sutured. Occasionally, the fastest method of removing small wooden splinters is to completely excise the entrance track and the FB en bloc, followed by linear closure. Particular mention should be made of certain wood splinters that are pliable and reactive, such as California redwood and northwest cedar. Any wood that is easily fragmented requires meticulous care to ensure removal of all material.

Traumatic Tattooing

Ground-in foreign material or tattooing of the skin is a difficult problem because permanent disfigurement may occur (Fig. 36.19). These injuries occur most often from falls on blacktop surfaces or asphalt or falls from bicycles or motorcycles on various surfaces. Many cases may be managed with adequate local anesthesia and meticulous debridement with a sponge, scrub brush, or toothbrush. If all foreign material cannot be removed with these methods, carefully consider secondary excision of the tattooed area and primary closure with subsequent plastic surgery to repair the defect. However, it is usually impossible to completely remove traumatic tattooing in the ED. Referral for more extensive surgical treatment after local wound care is quite acceptable. Dermabrasion may be an

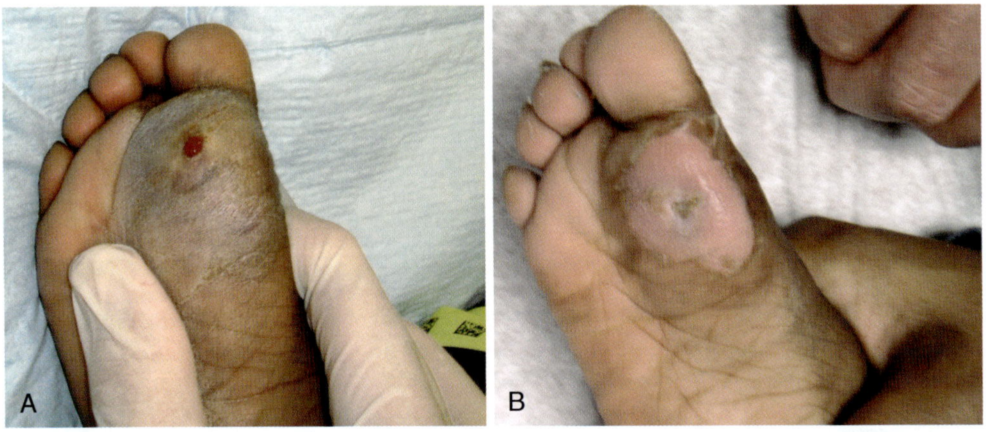

Fig. 36.18 (A) A splinter was removed from the foot of this 3-year-old 7 days earlier, and a few days after removal it began to swell. A retained foreign body (FB) was suspected. Plain radiographs were negative. A small pyogenic granuloma is seen. After ketamine sedation, a 5-mm core of tissue was removed, but no FB was found on extensive exploration. This was an abscess from the puncture. The wound was packed open and cephalexin was given. (B) It healed well (1 week later), but if it recurs, computed tomography or magnetic resonance imaging would be indicated to search for an occult FB.

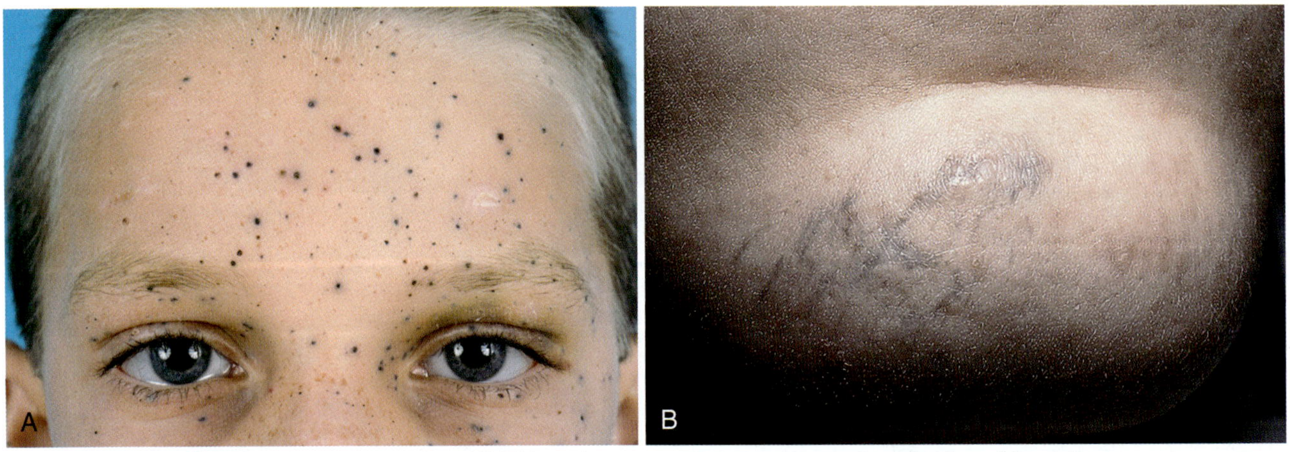

Fig. 36.19 Traumatic tattoos. (A) This patient was seen approximately 1 week after a blast injury. Traumatic tattoos are evident. The patient subsequently underwent successful laser removal of most of the pigment. (B) Traumatic tattoo of the chin. Bluish discoloration and slight erythema, predominantly caused by silica, are apparent. (A, From Flint PW, Haughey BH, Lund VJ et al. eds. *Cummings Otolaryngology: Head & Neck Surgery.* 5th ed. Elsevier; 2010. B, From Bolognia JL, Jorizzo JL, Shaffer JV, eds. *Dermatology.* 3rd ed. Elsevier; 2012.)

acceptable delayed treatment when the tattooing is superficial.[47] An alternative is to refer patients to a dermatologist for laser removal of traumatic tattoos. Certain lasers, such as an yttrium-aluminum-garnet (YAG) laser, have proved an excellent alternative.[48] The process is more specific in removing embedded material without harming the surrounding tissue. The type of material will determine the number of treatments required. Not all tattoos can be removed completely.[49]

Marine FBs

Although most marine FBs, such as shell fragments, may be treated like other FBs, a number of marine animals carry toxins and may leave FBs that require special consideration. Saltwater marine FBs may be contaminated with *Vibrio* species, which can cause serious infections including necrotizing fasciitis. These organisms are usually sensitive to tetracyclines, aminoglycosides, or third-generation cephalosporins. Even if all foreign material has been removed, stings from marine animals may initiate a prolonged local irritation that simulates cellulitis.

Coelenterates

Coelenterates, including the Portuguese man-of-war, true jellyfish, fire coral, box jellyfish, and sea anemones, inject several different toxins that are responsible for many marine envenomations by embedding venom-containing organelles, called *nematocysts*, into the victim's skin (Fig. 36.20). The tentacles of coelenterates may contain thousands of nematocysts, which allow many to be deposited by even minor skin contact. After deposition, nematocysts discharge their venom. Reactions may be local or systemic, and the pain may be severe and is often described as "shock like," "itching," "burning," or "throbbing." Substances

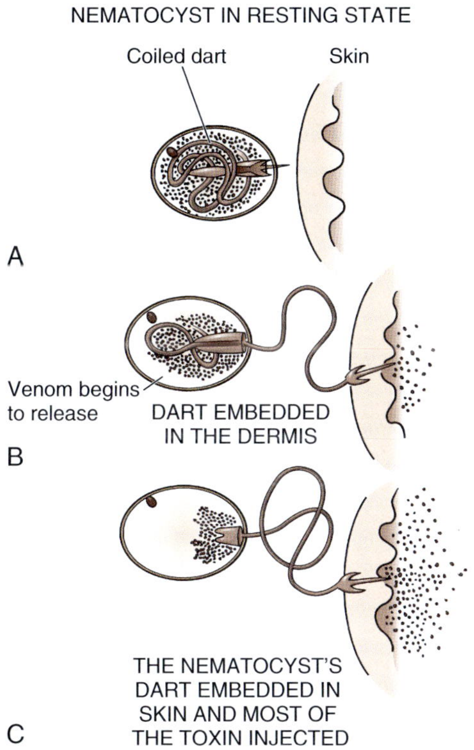

Fig. 36.20 (A) Magnified view of a venom-containing nematocyst in its resting or "cocked" state. (B) After contact with the skin, a dartlike tail is extended and penetrates the dermis, and (C) venom is injected. Further stimulation of the attached nematocyst can expel more venom (see text for the decontamination and removal technique).

such as tetramine, histamine, and 5-hydroxytryptamine are thought to be responsible for this localized reaction, whereas proteinaceous substances are implicated in the systemic response. Systemic reactions usually consist of fever, chills, and muscle spasms, but severe reactions may result in neurologic sequelae ranging from malaise and headache to paralysis and coma. Potential cardiopulmonary manifestations include dysrhythmias, hypotension, syncope, bronchospasm, laryngeal edema, and cardiorespiratory failure.[50,51]

Initial wound care should focus on decontamination and removing unfired nematocysts, decreasing pain and systemic reactions. Vinegar (5% acetic acid) is the initial decontaminating agent of choice because it will inactivate the unfired nematocysts of most (but not all) species of jellyfish, Portuguese man-of-war, and sea anemones.[50,52,53] Apply it continuously for 30 minutes or until the pain is gone.[51] *Do not apply fresh water* to the area because the osmotic shock will activate any remaining unfired nematocysts and cause them to discharge toxin and increase pain and toxicity. Other suggested, but unproven, remedies include meat tenderizer, ammonia, baking soda, urine, olive oil, sugar, and papaya latex.

After the wound has been decontaminated, remove any remaining tentacle fragments. Extract large fragments with forceps; however, individual nematocysts are very small (<1 mm in length) and are not easily visible. To remove the remaining nematocysts, scrape the skin with a hard edge, such as a credit card held perpendicular to the skin. An alternative is to apply shaving cream and shave the area gently to eliminate the remaining fragments.[51] Do not use sand to remove nematocysts because sand can increase the discharge of venom. If the pain persists, it should be assumed that organelles still remain and further cleansing is required.

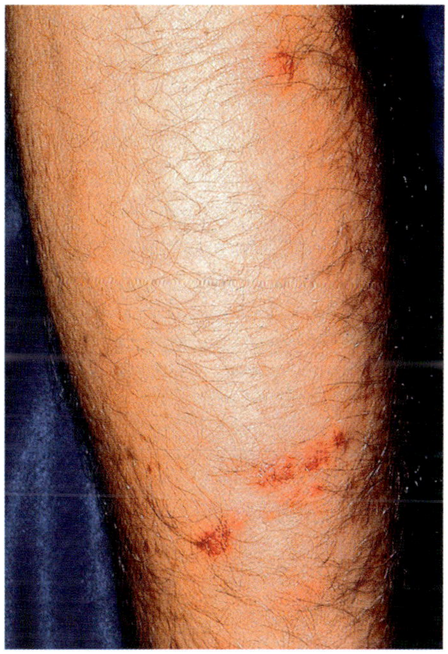

Fig. 36.21 Fire coral stings. (From James WD, Berger TG, Elston DM, eds. *Andrews' Diseases of the Skin: Clinical Dermatology.* 11th ed. Saunders; 2011.)

After decontamination, use topical anesthetics or steroids. Prophylactic antibiotics are unnecessary. Follow routine wound care. Treat allergic and systemic reactions appropriately. Applying warm or cold packs to the area has not been shown to reduce pain.[52] Antivenin is available only for box jellyfish envenomation, but its use remains incompletely understood and controversial.

In summary, a 2013 Cochrane review found inconclusive evidence defining the most effective treatment for jellyfish envenomation, but a 2016 article suggested several interventions may be effective for nemocyst inhibition. These authors wrote that topical vinegar for at least 30 seconds can help some species, while seawater, baking soda slurry, and water warmed to 42°C to 45°C can help, along with oral analgesics.[54,55] Ultimately, species-specific interventions are the most effective, but there is inadequate research to make definitive recommendations.

Coral

Coral is composed of a calcium carbonate core and thousands of small marine animals. Fire coral, a specific type of coral, is another type of coelenterate that produces toxicity with stinging nematocysts. After contact, a burning and intense pruritus may occur along with a series of skin eruptions. Within minutes of contact, pruritus, erythema, and urticaria-like lesions may appear, and blister formation may result within hours (Fig. 36.21). Eventually, the lesions will become lichenoid, but complete resolution may not occur for 15 weeks after contact. Ultimately, hyperpigmented areas will form at the point of initial contact. Immediate care with oral antihistamines and topical steroids tends to reduce, but not prevent, the symptoms.

"Coral cuts," which can be deep lacerations, occur in divers and snorkelers exploring coral reefs. With these wounds, delayed healing may occur with the secondary development of cellulitis or ulceration, perhaps due to contamination of the wound with bacteria or microparticles of coral.[50] Treatment consists of copious saline irrigation. Hydrogen peroxide may help remove small coral particles from the wound.[50] Do not close the wound; wet-to-dry dressings are advised instead.

Sponges

Sponges produce both an irritant and a contact dermatitis. The irritant dermatitis occurs due to sponge spicules embedded in the victim's skin. Remove the spicules with adhesive tape (applied to the skin and then peeled back), and then bathe the area with vinegar.[50] Contact dermatitis, believed to be caused by a toxin, produces erythema, pruritus, and vesicles similar to those with poison oak.[50] Treatment is initial immersion in vinegar followed by local steroid creams.

Sea Urchins and Starfish

Sea urchins and starfish are free-living echinoderms covered with venomous, sharp, brittle spines and venom-secreting pincers near the mouth. If sea urchins or starfish are handled or inadvertently stepped on, these spines may become embedded in the patient and a severe local reaction may result from venom in the spines. Systemic symptoms occur and include muscle weakness, paralysis of the lips, tongue, and face, hypotension, abdominal pain, and respiratory distress. Local pain responds quite well to immersion in hot water (43.3°C to 46.1°C [110°F to 115°F]) for 30 to 90 minutes. Retained spines may become infected or cause delayed (≤1 to 2 months) FB granulomas. This reaction is not adequately understood but may be due to an intense and persistent inflammatory reaction. Spines that penetrate joints may induce synovitis. Echinoderm spines may discharge a purple dye that may be mistaken for a retained spine (Fig. 36.22).[51] Spines are usually visible on radiographs and should be removed, although they are brittle and can break off in the skin. A YAG laser may be an effective alternative to remove sea urchin spines. Surgical extraction using an operative microscope may be necessary if spines are located in a joint or near a nerve.[50] Otherwise, if removal is difficult, leave the spine until it is resorbed or a local reaction occurs. If appropriate, open the wound and drain it to allow it to close by secondary intention.

Catfish

Several species of catfish in North America contain toxic venom, and a sting from the dorsal or pectoral spines can embed an FB. The spine secretes venom from an epidermal gland at its base.[56] The pain is usually ephemeral, and because no specific antitoxin exists, treatment consists of local care and analgesics. Immerse the affected part in hot water (≈43.3°C [110°F]) for at least 30 minutes if the pain is severe. This is believed to provide relief of symptoms by decreasing vascular and muscle spasm.[57] Local injection of the wound with alkalized bupivacaine provides local analgesia and may neutralize the toxin.[56] Inspect the wound and remove any remaining spines (Fig. 36.23). A radiograph may be taken to confirm the absence of FBs, but catfish spines and cartilage may be radiolucent. Bedside US may be helpful, depending on the clinician's level of experience. Thoroughly clean and irrigate the wound. Update the patient's tetanus prophylaxis if necessary. Some authors recommend empirical antibiotic therapy to cover gram-negative bacilli (e.g., *Aeromonas hydrophila*), but infection is rare, and routine antibiotic prophylaxis is not standard.[56]

Stingrays

Stingray envenomation usually occurs when a person accidentally steps on a creature resting on the bottom in shallow water and covered by sand (Fig. 36.24). This causes the stingray to lash out its whiplike caudal appendage, or tail, which contains one to four venom-containing serrated spines. Portions of the spine may become buried in the victim's skin. Each spine is covered with a sheath containing venom glands, and in addition to immediate toxin-induced pain, pieces of the

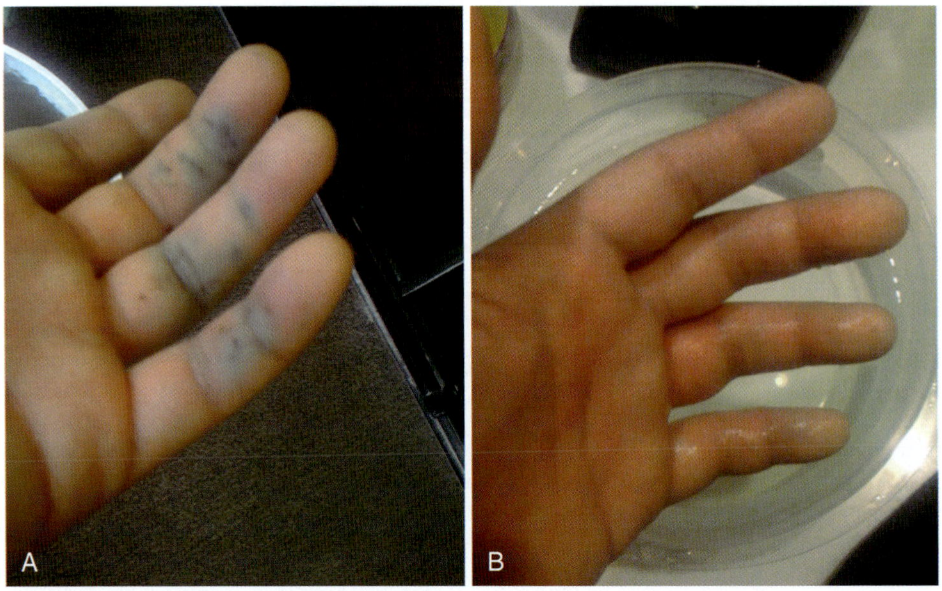

Fig. 36.22 (A) Multiple sea urchin punctures in the hand soon after injury and following a soak in hot water. (B) The same hand after 6 days without intervening therapy other than soaking. Lack of discoloration indicates absorption of dye from the sea urchin spines and probable absence of retained fragments. (From Auerbach PS, ed. *Wilderness Medicine*. 6th ed. Mosby; 2011.)

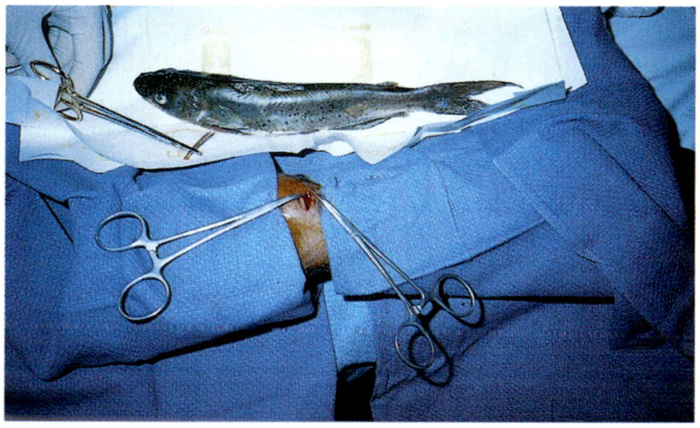

Fig. 36.23 To ensure total removal, remove the spine of a catfish by incising the puncture site as opposed to simply pulling it out.

spine or sheath may remain embedded in the wound. These fragments, though often difficult to locate, do not dissolve and must therefore be removed. Persistent pain and inflammation, even weeks to months after the attack, mandate consideration of a retained FB, but a persistent and difficult-to-treat irritative process can occur in the absence of a retained spine or sheath. Immediate local and systemic reactions develop as a result of injection of a complex toxin. Systemic reactions may be severe and can include muscle cramps, vomiting, seizures, hypotension, arrhythmias, and (rarely) death.[58]

Treatment consists of irrigation with saline followed by immersion in hot water at 42°C to 45°C for 30 to 90 minutes to inactivate the heat-labile toxin. Local digital blocks without vasoconstrictors provide effective analgesia for hand wounds. Explore and debride all wounds, removing all spine remnants and integumentary sheath.[50] Wounds should heal by secondary intention. The venom can cause significant local tissue necrosis, and surgical debridement may be required.

Tetanus and Antibiotic Therapy

Prophylactic antibiotic therapy for marine injuries is common, although there are no convincing data to support or refute this practice. Unlike other soft tissue infections, marine injuries become infected with unusual gram-negative organisms, particularly *Vibrio* species. Although few studies have evaluated the effects of specific antibiotics, it is recommended that quinolones, trimethoprim-sulfamethoxazole, tetracyclines, third-generation cephalosporins, or aminoglycosides be used in lieu of penicillin, ampicillin, erythromycin, or first-generation cephalosporins.[51] It is always difficult to differentiate chronic inflammation caused by toxins and foreign material from true infection, and surgical exploration is often required in persistent cases. Administer tetanus prophylaxis as per routine recommendations.

Cactus Spines

The size of cactus spines fluctuates considerably. The difficulty of removal is generally inversely proportional to the size of the FB.[59] Larger embedded cactus spines are managed like wood splinters and sea urchin spine FBs. More advanced imaging techniques (US, CT, or MRI) may be required for the localization of deeply embedded spines.

Deeply embedded cactus spines generally produce granulomatous reactions, but infections are rare.[60] Dermatitis from embedded cactus spines is a well-described phenomenon. Hence, try to remove deeply embedded spines after carefully weighing the benefit and potential harm related to deep

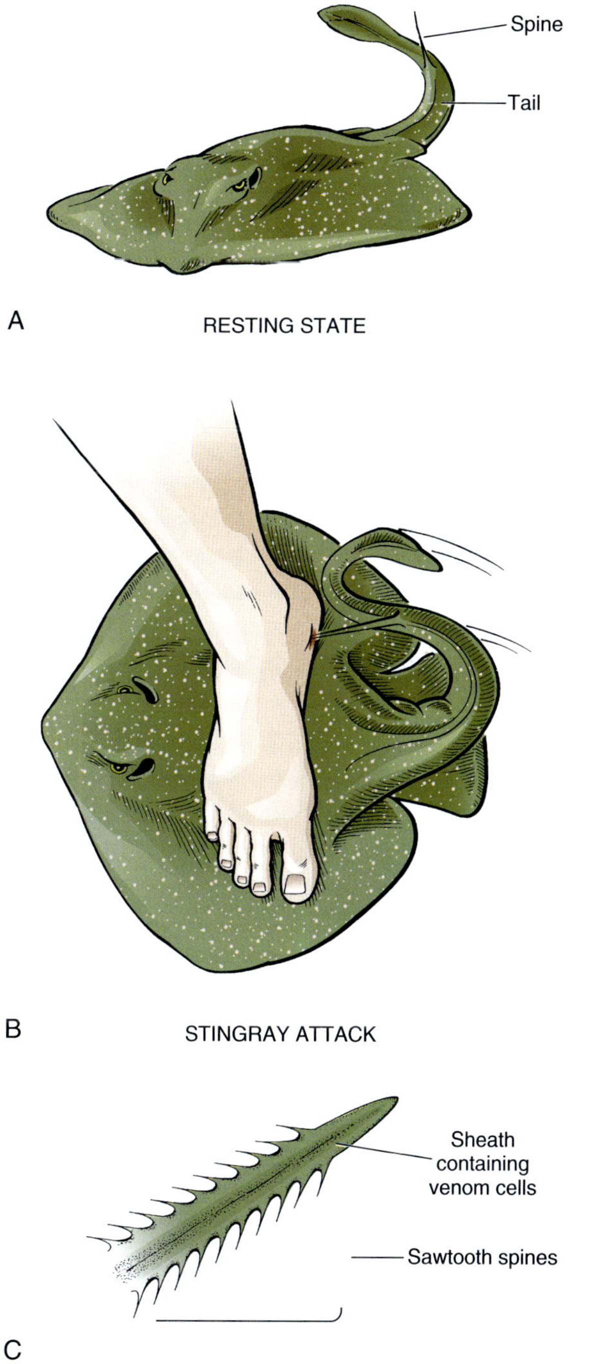

Fig. 36.24 (A) Stingray resting on the bottom of the ocean, usually covered by a layer of sand. (B) An unsuspecting victim steps on the stingray, and the whiplike tail impales the foot (even through a heavy boot) with one or more spines. (C) The spine has backward-facing barbs covered by a sheath with venom-containing cells, which causes a toxic envenomation and the potential for multiple foreign bodies.

exploration, especially in a sensitive location.[59] Using forceps, remove superficially embedded, medium to large cactus spines by direct axial traction on each spine. Smaller spines (glochids) may be difficult and tedious to remove individually. Apply an adherent facial mask gel to remove the spines en masse with the gel (Fig. 36.25). Depilatory wax melted in a microwave oven and applied warm, commercial facial gels, and household glue (e.g., Elmer's) have all been recommended.[59,61–63]

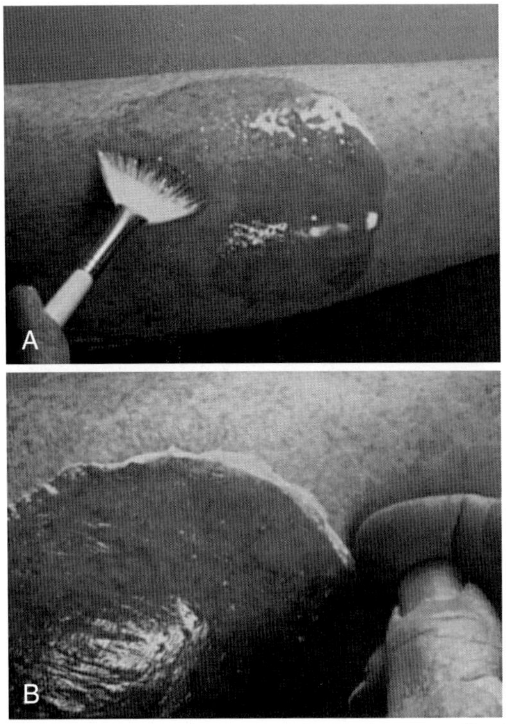

Fig. 36.25 A thousand or more glochids may become affixed to the skin by contact with a single pad of polka dot cactus. (A) To remove them, professional facial gel is spread with a fan brush, thin at the edges. (B) The gel rollup is started by picking at the edge with the fingernails. When the gel is peeled off, all the very small spines come with it. (From Lindsey D, Lindsey WE. Cactus spine injuries. *Am J Emerg Med.* 1988;6:362.)

Over-the-counter "home use" facial mask gels are not adherent enough to be effective without multiple (eight or more) applications.

Ring Removal

See Videos 36.9–36.12. Frequently, a ring must be removed to prevent laceration of tissue or vascular compromise. The type of ring, its material, composition, purpose, and sentimental value may have implications for the best technique for removal. Harder metals, medical devices, or very thick rings may be difficult to cut through or increase the risk of injury during removal. Medical devices rings may contain electrical components and thus, when cut, cannot be repaired.

Many rings can be removed by thoroughly lubricating the finger with a water-soluble lubricant (e.g., K-Y jelly). Use a circular motion with traction on the ring. A digital or metacarpal block may facilitate this procedure. However, the string-wrap method or physically cutting the ring off may be necessary. Preferably, remove all rings before the edema is extensive enough to cause pain or vascular compromise.

String-Wrap Method

Perform a proximal digital or metacarpal block to provide sufficient anesthesia and minimize tissue distention at the ring site. Before removal of the ring, wrap a wide Penrose drain circumferentially in a distal-to-proximal direction to reduce the soft tissue swelling (Fig. 36.26). Leave the wrap in place for a few minutes to reach the maximum effect. Warn nonanesthetized patients that pain may increase from both compression and unwinding; patients have been described to panic during the procedure because of these symptoms.[64]

First, pass a 20- to 25-inch piece of string, umbilical tape, or thick silk suture between the ring and the finger. Shorter lengths are discouraged because one may need to repeat the wrapping procedure midway. If marked soft tissue swelling is present, pass the tip of a hemostat under the ring to grasp the string and pull it through. Wrap the distal string clockwise around the swollen finger (proximal to distal) to include the proximal interphalangeal (PIP) joint and the entire swollen finger. Start the wrapping next to the ring. Wrap it snugly enough to compress the swollen tissue. Place successive loops of wrap next to each other to keep any swollen tissue from bulging between the strands. When the wrapping is complete, carefully unwind the proximal end of the string in the same clockwise direction to force the ring over that portion of the finger that has been compressed by the wrap. The PIP joint is the area that is most difficult to maneuver over and causes the most pain.

Occasionally, the finger must be rewrapped if it was not done carefully the first time. It is not uncommon to produce abrasions or other kinds of trauma in the skin during this procedure. If the finger with the ring is lacerated or there are underlying fractures, it is prudent to cut the ring off instead of attempting this technique.

Finger Compression Devices

Commercially available finger compression devices are available. These devices slide over the finger and provide focal compression to reduce swelling. Following manufacturer guidance is recommended but in summary, 5 minutes of compression, recheck, and then alter the angle of compression and repeat these sessions until enough swelling reduction has been achieved to remove the ring with lubrication and traction.

Certain rings are made of extremely hard material such as tungsten carbide or ceramic. In these cases, cracking the material with standard locking pliers can break the ring. Place the pliers on the ring and adjust the jaws to fit tightly, and then remove and readjust them while increasing tension with each subsequent adjustment. Continue until the material cracks and falls apart. Some rings may be lined with a metal band. Use a standard ring cutter to remove the band.

Ring Cutter

A ring cutter should be used when the swelling is excessive or other methods fail (Fig. 36.27). A ring cutter has a small hook that fits under the ring and serves as a guide for the saw-toothed wheel that cuts the metal. The cut ends of the ring are spread with large hemostats (e.g., Kelly clamps), and the ring is removed. If the tension is too great to spread the ring, another cut 180 degrees apart from the original ring cut can be performed. This will allow the ring to fall off in two pieces. A jeweler can subsequently repair cut rings.

Certain hardened metal rings, such as tungsten carbide, may not be amenable to the use of a ring cutter; however, there are ring cutters available on the market capable of cutting through titanium and tungsten (e.g., Ring Rescue, www.ringrescue.com/ring-rescue-kit). If this is not available, case studies have demonstrated that a dental-tipped drill or dental volvere can be used successfully. However, because of the nature of these instruments and the possibility of injury from them (such as lacerations from the blade, thermal burns, or ocular FBs), take precautions to limit further damage to

Ring Removal: String-wrap Method

1

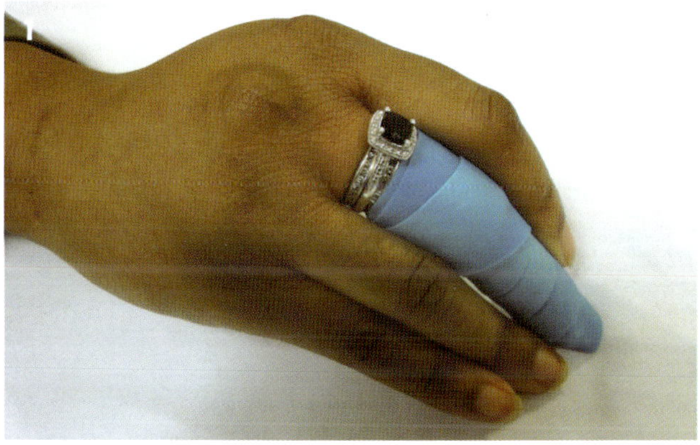

Lessen the edema by compressing the finger with a Penrose drain left tightly wrapped for 3 to 5 minutes.

2

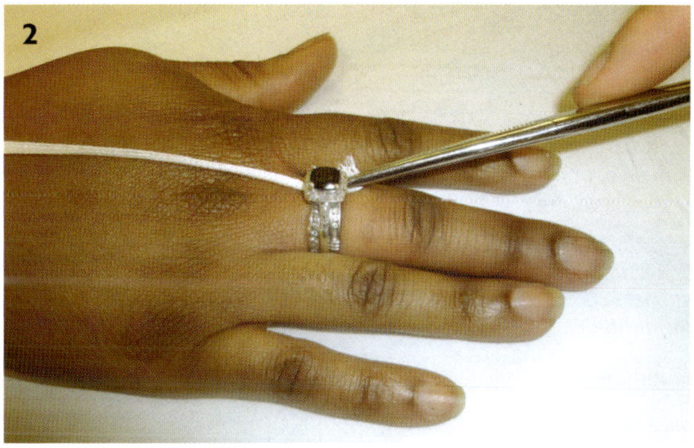

Slide a small hemostat under the ring, grab a long piece of umbilical tape, and pull it under the ring.

3

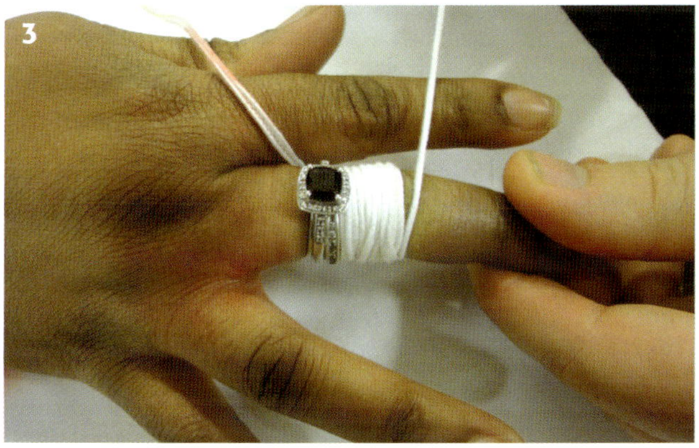

Begin to carefully wrap the tape around the finger in a proximal-to-distal fashion.

4

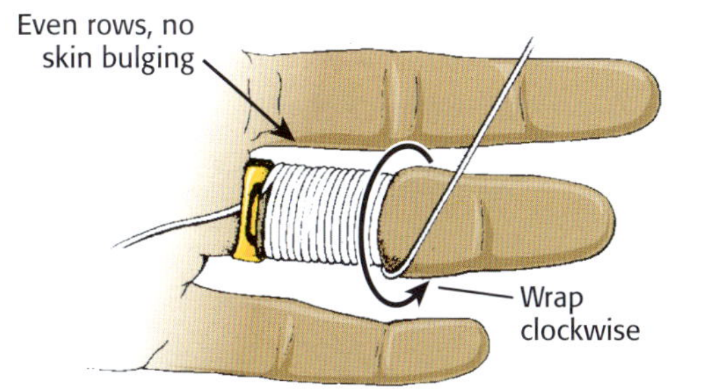

Continue winding the distal strand to compress the skin distal to the ring. Take time to place successive loops next to each other, and keep tissue from bulging between the strands.

5

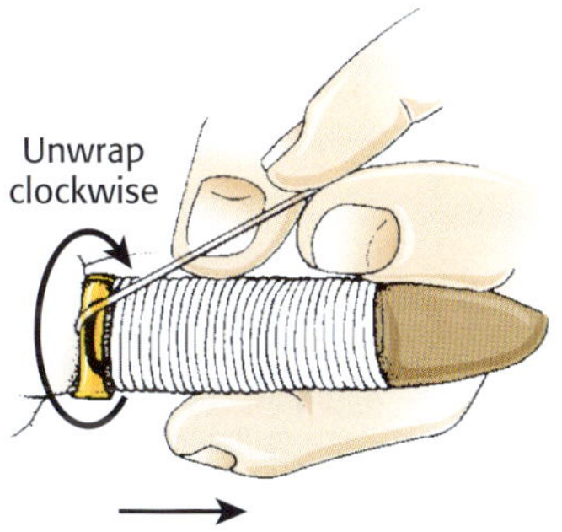

Remove the ring by unwrapping the proximal strand in the same direction that it was wrapped. The most difficult area to negotiate is the proximal interphalangeal joint. You may have to repeat the wrapping procedure to totally remove the ring.

6

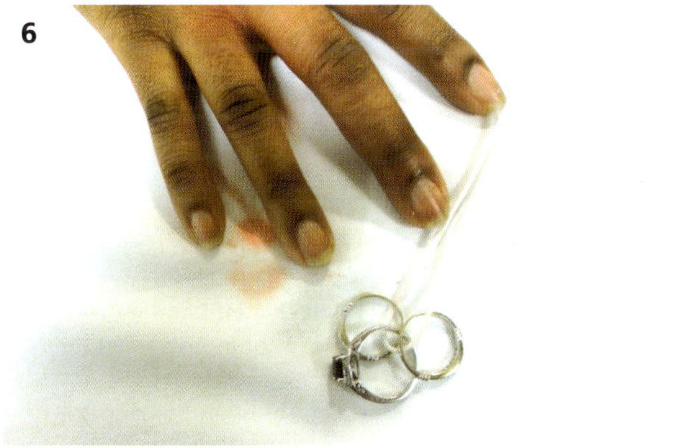

Successful removal of the rings.

Fig. 36.26 Ring removal: string-wrap method.

the finger, as well as the use of eye protection to shield the patient's and operator's eyes.

Body Piercing and Removal

See Video 36.13. The art of body piercing predates most history books. Over the past decade, an enormous increase in body piercing has occurred. Accordingly, so have the complications associated with the practice.[65] For centuries the ears were the most common place. Today, the lips, tongue, eyebrow, nose, navel, nipples, and genital areas have become body piercing sites. To date, there are limited studies on infection after piercings in areas other than the ears. Three major types

Ring Removal: Ring Cutter Method

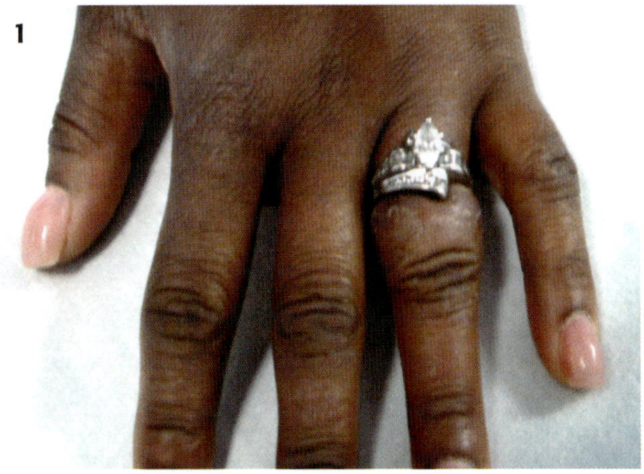

This ring is too tight to be removed by the string-wrap technique. Note that the skin is deeply indented.

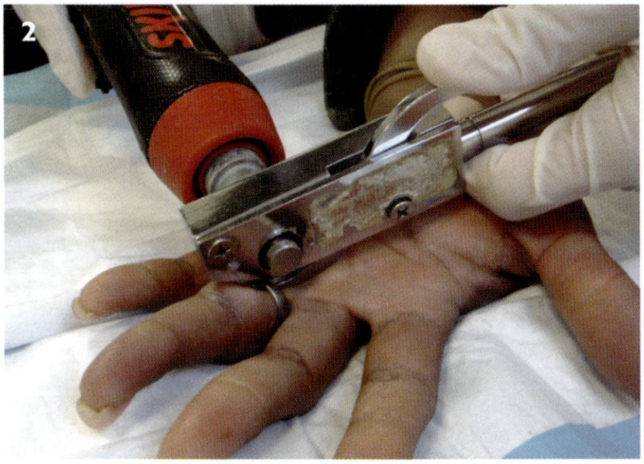

An electric ring cutter is the best option.

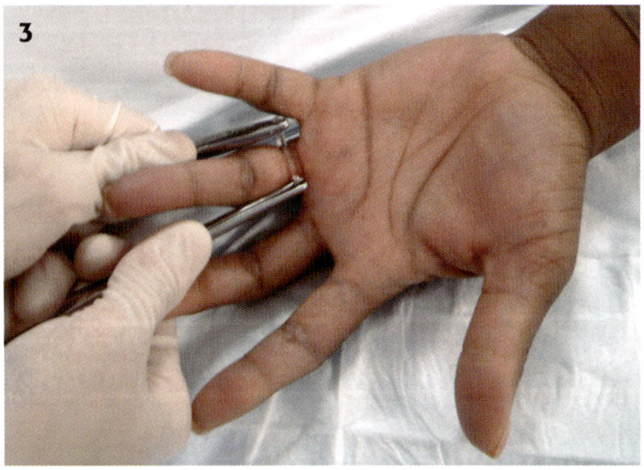

When the ring is cut through, grab the cut ends with hemostats and separate the sides. This ring can be repaired by a jeweler to a nearly new condition.

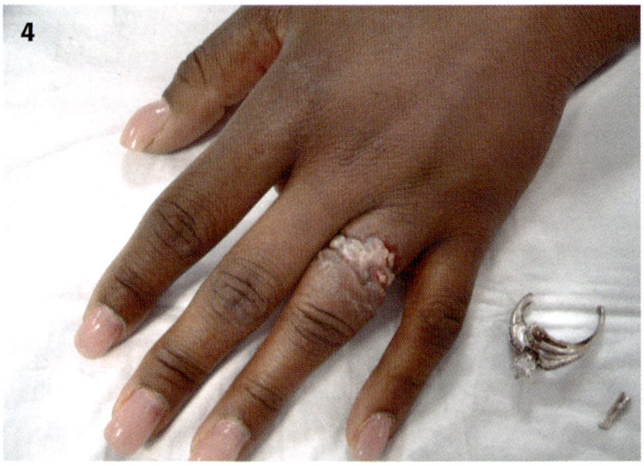

Note the macerated tissue under the ring.

Fig. 36.27 Ring removal: ring cutter method.

of jewelry are used: (1) barbell studs, which are straight bars with a ball threaded onto both ends; (2) labret studs, which are straight bars with a ball threaded on one end and a disk permanently fixed on the other end (more commonly used on the lips); and (3) a captive bead ring, which consists of a bead with small dimples on opposite sides and an incomplete ring with rounded ends to fit into the dimples (Fig. 36.28). The bead is held "captive" by tension from both sides of this incomplete ring. The bead ring is a variation of this: one bead is permanently fixed to one end, and an opening is made by removing the free end of the ring.[66]

The most common reason for removal is infection (Fig. 36.29). Other symptoms such as bleeding, edema, allergic reaction, and keloid formation may also prompt removal. Occasionally, tongue piercings must be removed to permit intubation. Hold the bar with forceps and unscrew the bead on the other end to remove barbell- and labret-type studs. To remove a captive bead ring, hold the ring on both sides of the captive bead to release tension on the bead. This will dislodge the bead from the ring, which is holding it in place. If the

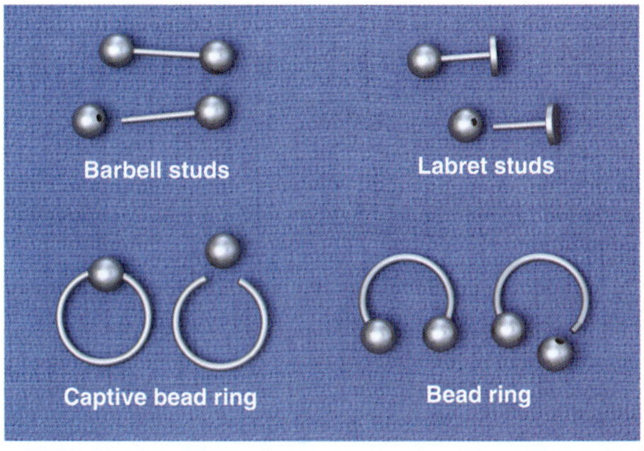

Fig. 36.28 Various types of piercing jewelry. To remove a barbell stud or labret stud, unscrew the ball that is threaded onto the bar. To remove a captive bead ring, snap the ball out of the incomplete ring (it is held in place simply by tension and is not screwed in). You may need to insert needle-nose pliers into the center of the ring and spread it to pry the ring open. To remove a bead ring, unscrew the ball from one end of the ring.

Body Piercing Removal

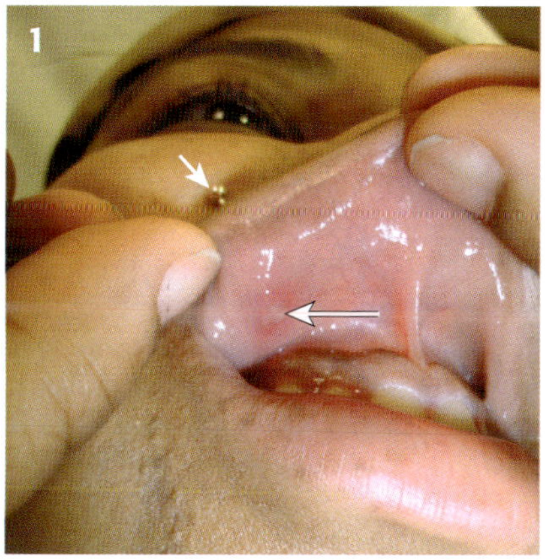

This patient has a labret stud piercing. Note that the ball is visible externally *(short arrow)*; however, the disk portion has migrated internally and the buccal mucosa has closed over it *(long arrow)*.

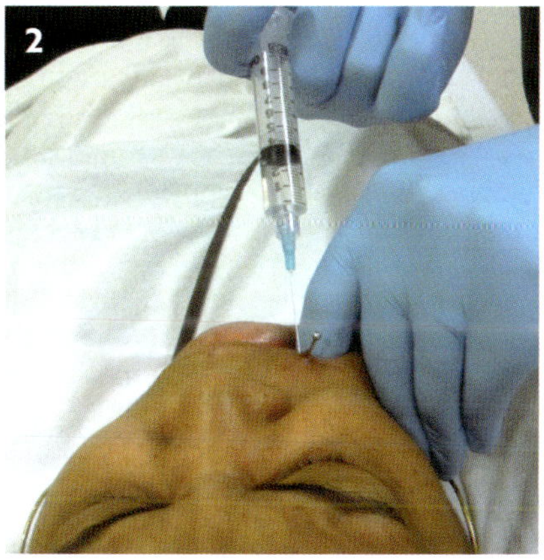

Infiltrate the region with local anesthetic. Alternatively, an infraorbital nerve block could be used (see Chapter 30).

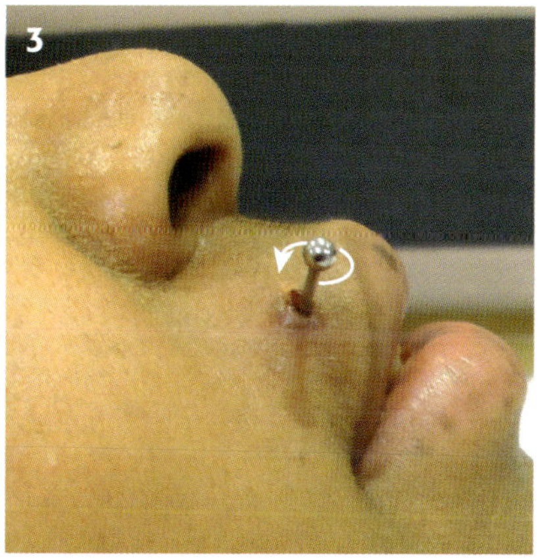

Next, unscrew the ball on the end of the bar.

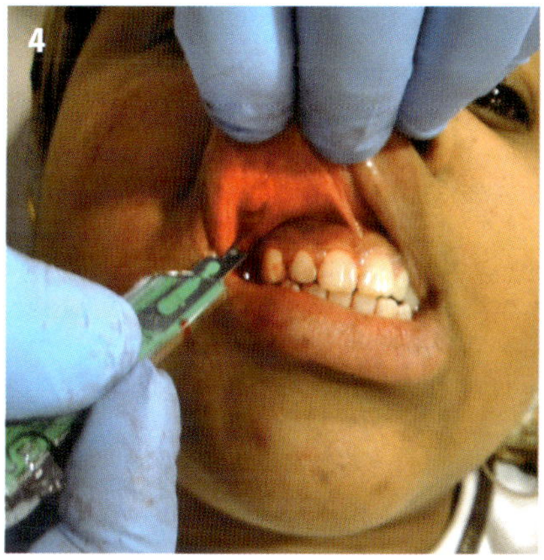

Make an incision in the buccal mucosa over the embedded disk.

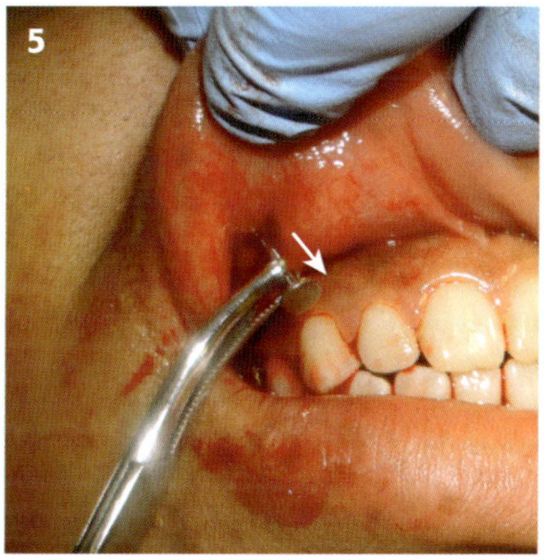

Use a hemostat to find and remove the bar from the lip.

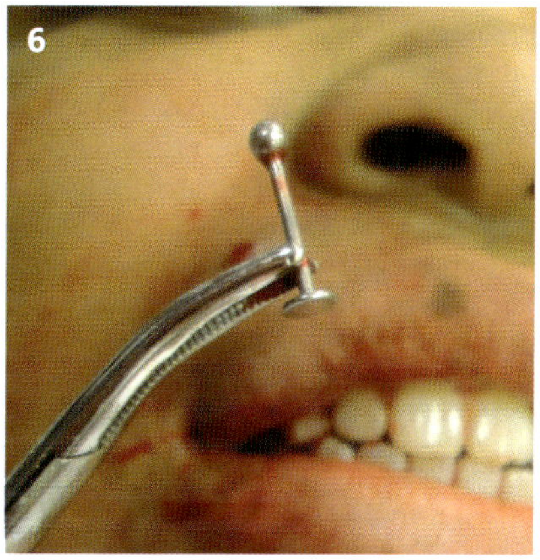

The labret stud, successfully removed and reassembled.

Fig. 36.29 Body piercing removal. This piercing became infected when the mucosal portion of the metal bar migrated into tissue. An incision was required to find and grasp the metal bar.

jewelry is near the mouth or nose, take care to prevent aspiration of the bead. The complete microbiology of infections related to body piercing has not yet been determined. However, organisms such as *Staphylococcus epidermidis* and *Staphylococcus aureus*, along with *Pseudomonas aeruginosa*, have been commonly implicated pathogens. Other infectious complications from body piercing such as septic arthritis, endocarditis, hepatitis B and C, and HIV have been reported.[67,68]

Most commonly, however, local wound infections predominate and can be managed with warm compresses, antibacterial soap, and topical antibacterial ointment once the FB is removed. The possibility of leaving the piercing in place while treating the infection has yet to be studied.

Postoperative Suture Removal

FBs in the form of nonabsorbed suture material are frequently encountered in the postoperative period. Drainage, localized pain, tenderness, and an inflammatory reaction along the suture line are characteristic of a retained FB (suture abscess). In this instance, probing the wound with a sterilized needle bent into the shape of a crochet hook is frequently successful. Hooking the suture material through the sinus tract and removing it allows the wound to heal over the tract.

Tick Removal

Tick populations over the past decade have spread and diseases once felt to be endemic in specific areas are now found in increasingly greater parts of the world. As a result, tick-borne diseases are now being seen in these newer areas and clinicians should be aware of the possibility of these infections as the ticks spread.

It is important to remove ticks early because of tick-borne disease, including the hard tick of the Ixodid family. Rocky Mountain spotted fever, Lyme disease, tularemia, and ascending paralysis are among the many infections identified as tick-borne diseases. It is important to note that the rate of disease transmission before 48 hours of attachment is exceedingly low.[69] Removal of Ixodid ticks is difficult because the mouthparts become cemented within 5 to 30 minutes of contact with the host's skin. Removal will become more difficult the longer the tick is attached. Inadequate or partial removal of the tick may cause infection or chronic granuloma formation. Removal by mechanical means is recommended.[70] Nonmechanical, traditional, and folk methods of forcing the tick to disengage (e.g., the use of petroleum jelly, fingernail polish, a hot match, or alcohol) are not advised and can cause the tick to regurgitate, thereby increasing the possibility of transmission of infection.

The use of straight or curved forceps or tweezers is the recommended method of removal. If these instruments are not available, use a gloved hand. Grasp the tick as close to the patient's skin surface as possible and gently apply steady axial traction (Fig. 36.30). Take care not to squeeze, crush, twist, or jerk the tick's body because this may expel infective agents or leave mouthparts in the skin. If mouthparts are left behind after removal of the body, they may be removed with tweezers. If one is still unable to remove the mouthparts, consider excision under local anesthesia to prevent local infection.

Many patients have great anxiety about the development of tick-borne diseases after tick removal. Prophylactic antibiotic treatment of all tick bites is a controversial area. Some studies have demonstrated that single-dose doxycycline (200 mg) may prevent the development of Lyme disease,[69] and many experts recommend using this single dose in patients with tick bites. Children younger than 8 years may be given a single dose of doxycycline (4 mg/kg). Amoxicillin prophylaxis is not effective. When a patient is in an area where the incidence of Lyme disease is high or when a partially engorged deer tick in the nymphal stage is discovered on the body, the patient is more likely to benefit from prophylaxis. Regardless of whether prophylaxis is given, instruct patients about the symptoms and signs of Lyme disease and encourage them to return or seek medical evaluation if these symptoms develop.

Zipper Entrapment

The skin of the penis may become painfully entangled in a zipper mechanism (Fig. 36.31). Unzipping the zipper frequently lacerates the skin and increases the amount of tissue caught in the mechanism. Although the clinician may anesthetize the skin and excise the entrapped tissue, a less invasive method can be considered.

Cutting the median bar between the faceplates of the zipper mechanism remains the most common method. The interlocking teeth of the zipper then fall apart when the median bar (diamond or bridge) of the zipper is cut in half (Fig. 36.32), and the skin is subsequently freed. A bone cutter or wire clippers and a moderate amount of force may be required to break the bar. Adding mineral oil followed by traction has been demonstrated to achieve some success. Patients with penile lacerations warrant urologic follow-up to assess for urethral injury.

Infiltration of Radiographic Contrast Material

The infiltration of high-osmolality intravenous contrast material has the potential to cause skin necrosis, but the use of low-osmolality dye, which is well tolerated in soft tissues, has essentially eliminated this problem (Fig. 36.33). The use of high-pressure power injectors, often when the technologist is out of the room, calls for careful inspection of the intravenous site before injection. However, because of the high-pressure rapid autoinjection of contrast material and the absence of a technician in the room, extravasation of contrast material is not a rare event and occurs even with meticulous technique. Infiltration occurs in approximately 0.5% to 1% of autoinjections. Once contrast material has infiltrated, no intervention has been demonstrated to ameliorate the local reactions, which are usually mild. Swelling, erythema, and

Tick Removal

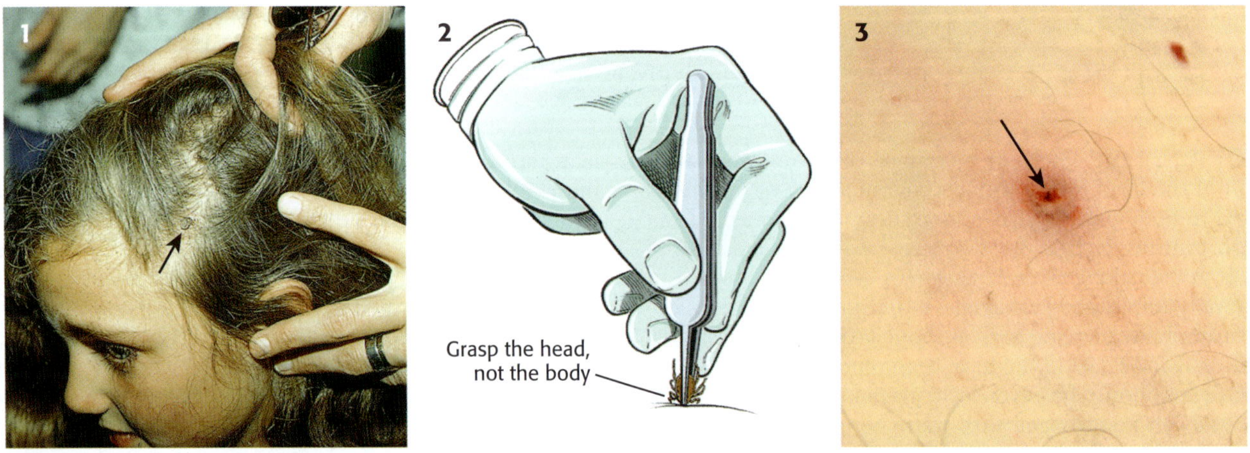

Ticks should be removed as soon as possible to minimize the transmission of tick-borne pathogens and to limit their fixation to the skin by a secreted cement compound. This engorged tick has been attached for about a day and has burrowed under the skin. Most home remedies are worthless.

A recommended approach is to grasp the tick with forceps near its head where it enters the skin (avoid the soft body) and gently pull it out. Some advise twisting the head counterclockwise, but this has not objectively been found to be more effective.

If pieces of the tick remain *(arrow)*, they should be dug out. Anesthetize the area and use a scalpel with a No. 11 blade to excise the embedded mouthparts. The erythema surrounding this tick bite is not erythema migrans (which is characteristically an oval-shaped rash, with or without central clearing), but rather local irritation from the initial removal attempt.

Fig. 36.30 Tick removal.

mild discomfort at the infiltration site may occur. It is best to resist the temptation to use excessive heat or cold. Elevation of an extremity is appropriate but of unproven value. Injection of steroids and other agents has no known benefit. Low-osmolality dye is usually totally resorbed in a few days, with no serious consequences in the vast majority of cases. Progress of the dye's egress may be followed with radiographs. Most contrast material extravasations resolve with no long-term consequences with conservative management. If large volumes of contrast material are injected (>75 to 100 mL), especially in confined areas such as the dorsum of the hand, skin necrosis from the pressure or a compartment syndrome may develop, but this is rare. The clinician should resist attempts to routinely remove even large volumes of extravasated contrast material by incision or aspiration. Although some contrast material may be removed with surgical techniques during fasciotomy, the benefit is unknown. Surgical intervention is rarely required and is based on compartment pressure measurement and clinical evaluation. Patients with small-volume and minimally symptomatic extravasations may be discharged. Large-volume extravasations warrant consultation or further observation.

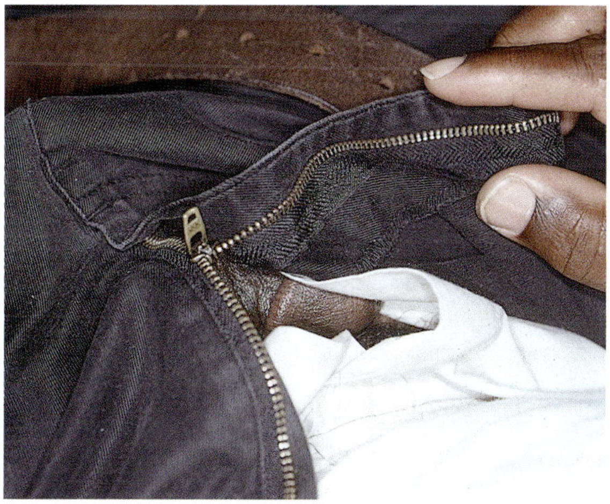

Fig. 36.31 Penile skin caught in a zipper creates a rather painful and embarrassing situation for the patient. Instead of anesthetizing and excising the skin, consider cutting the zipper as demonstrated in Fig. 36.32.

TASER Darts

The Thomas A. Swift Electric Rifle, or TASER, is a conducted electrical weapon used in many areas by police to subdue violent patients (see Chapter 70). The TASER fires two barbed electrodes on long copper wires (Fig. 36.34). The barbs attach to skin or clothing and create an arc that delivers an electrical jolt, which causes overwhelming pain and involuntary muscle contraction and incapacitates the subject. The electricity is of such high frequency that it is believed to stay near the surface and not penetrate to the depth of internal organs. The barbs are designed to not penetrate deeper than 4 mm, and police are taught to remove them by stretching the surrounding skin and tugging sharply. If this fails, cutting down on the dart after local anesthesia should facilitate removal.[71,72] Patients may need medical evaluation after ED removal of the darts for the underlying state of agitation that required the use of a TASER, complications of electrical injury, injury from the fall after incapacitation, and injury from the barb, especially if struck in the mouth, eye, neck, or groin. Most patients do well with minimal intervention and proper wound management if the patient is not unduly agitated and the TASER did not involve the critical areas of the body just mentioned.

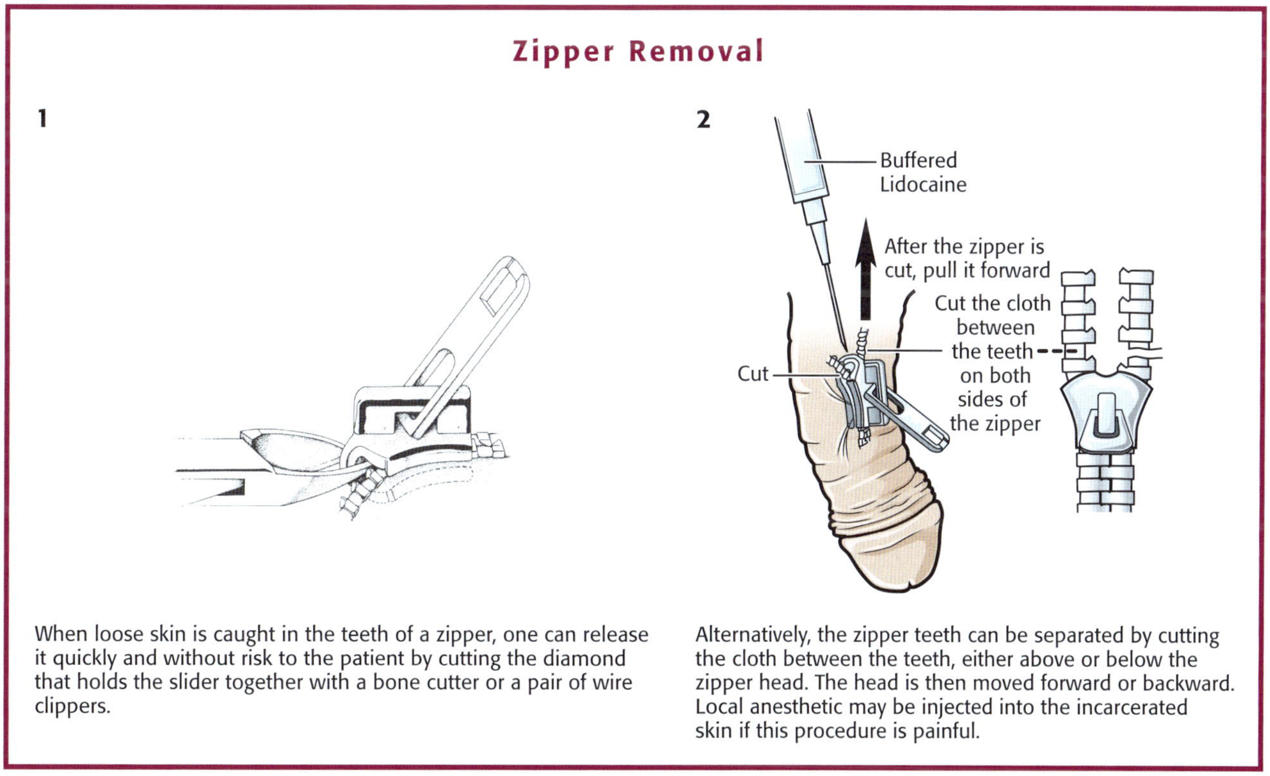

Fig. 36.32 Zipper removal. (From *Emergency Medicine*. October 15, 1982:215.)

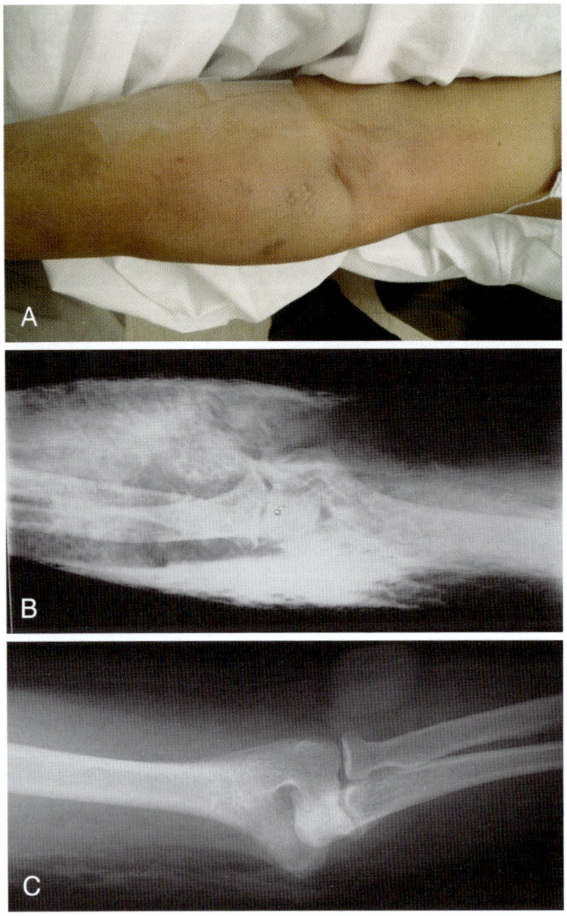

Fig. 36.33 The entire volume (100 mL) of nonionic low-osmolality contrast material (Isovue) for a computed tomography scan was pressure-injected into the antecubital soft tissue when the intravenous line infiltrated. High-volume injections are automatically administered by a programmed auto-injector; the technician is not in the room to stop it. (A) There was only mild pain but considerable soft tissue swelling, and most of the redness and blistering occurred when the technician taped an unprotected ice pack directly to the skin and nearly caused frostbite. (B) Radiographic evidence of the infiltration. (C) Within 36 hours, the dye was absorbed, without further treatment. No skin necrosis occurred, as has been seen when older ionic high-osmolality agents infiltrate. There is no known way to ameliorate the potential soft tissue injury. The antecubital fossa is the preferred site for an intravenous line for injection of contrast material, and such an extravasation on the dorsum of the hand may be more serious. Do not attempt to remove the contrast material by aspiration or surgical incisions.

Human and Animal Bite FBs

The most common FB after a human bite is a piece of tooth. These FBs can be difficult to find and may not be appreciated if the patient does not admit or disclose the bite wound. Usually, the bite puncture is small and not easily cleaned or visualized. The puncture can be widened with a formal incision to aid in cleaning and evaluation for tendon integrity, injury to the joint capsule, fracture, or an FB (Fig. 36.35). Occasionally, small pieces of teeth can become embedded in a wound, such as with dog, cat, or snake bites (Fig. 36.36). Radiographic detection is variable, and exploration is often the only alternative. Approach to wound management and antibiotic recommendations are covered in Chapter 34.

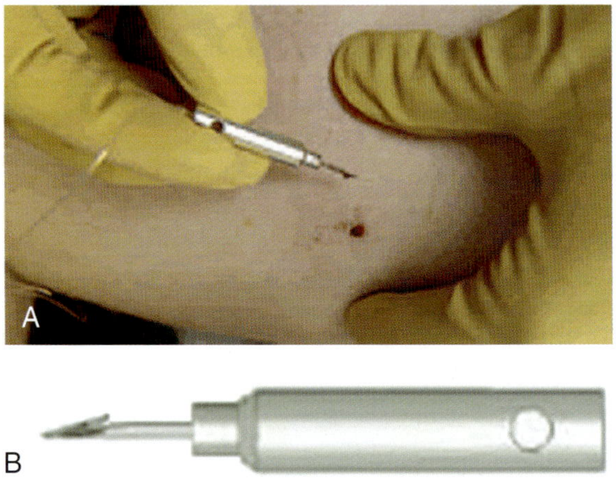

Fig. 36.34 (A–B) Barbed TASER darts can be removed by a quick pull or through a small incision made over the barb.

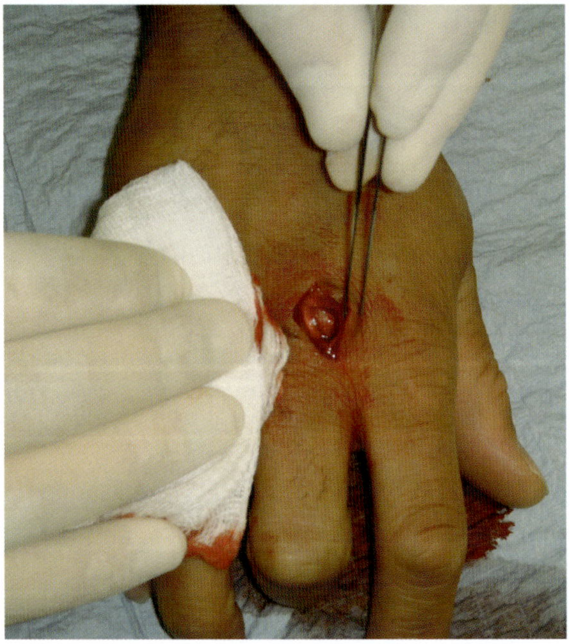

Fig. 36.35 This human bite puncture wound was enlarged with an incision to aid in cleaning and search for a foreign body, usually a piece of tooth. Even though this wound appears clean, it should not be closed with sutures.

Pyogenic Granuloma (Lobar Capillary Hemangioma)

A pyogenic granuloma is a benign acquired polypoid, friable vascular lesion of the skin (hand, neck, foot, fingers, and trunk) and mucous membranes (Fig. 36.37). They are common in children; in pregnancy, the lesion is termed *epulis gravidarum* (pregnancy tumor). The cause is unknown, but there is some association with topical retinoids and the protease inhibitor indinavir; they are not due to infection but are not granulomas. They grow rather rapidly over a few weeks, are occasionally associated with minor trauma, have a glistening dark red appearance, and may bleed. Histologically, a pyogenic granuloma is a hemangioma. Various topical therapies (silver nitrate, cryotherapy), laser, or cautery are available, but removal by sharp dissection with primary suturing is usually curative (Fig. 36.38). The recurrence rate may be as high as 40% with nonsurgical intervention.[73]

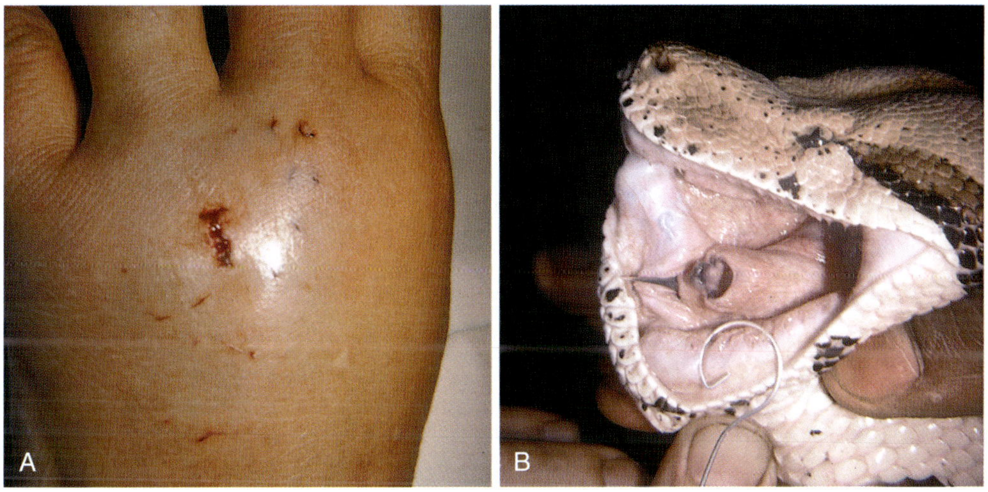

Fig. 36.36 (A–B) The bite of a boa constrictor, though not poisonous, may contain small tooth fragments. As with cat and dog bites, radiographic evaluation is variable and exploration may be required.

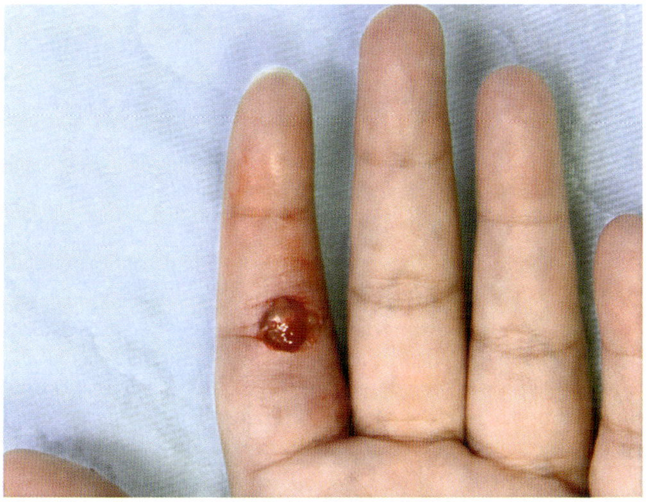

Fig. 36.37 Pyogenic granuloma. Despite their name, these lesions are neither pyogenic (i.e., infectious) nor granulomas. Rather, they are a type of hemangioma. Pyogenic granulomas can develop rapidly over a period of weeks and are common in pregnant females.

Hair-Thread Tourniquet

Hair or thread fibers adherent to infants' clothing occasionally become tightly wrapped around a child's digits or genitals (Fig. 36.39).[74] If they are left in place, amputation may eventually occur. The offending fibers may be difficult to visualize, and the child is often brought for evaluation only after signs of distal ischemia appear. Occasionally, the fiber can be grasped with toothless forceps or a small hemostat and then unwrapped. More commonly, fibers cannot be identified because they are deeply embedded in swollen tissue. Removal not requiring minor surgery includes use of a chemical depilatory, such as the over-the-counter product Nair (calcium thioglycolate), to dissolve or weaken the hair. A generous amount of depilatory cream is worked into the involved area and allowed to dissolve or weaken the hair, which is then removed mechanically. If a depilatory is not successful in 30 to 60 minutes, surgical removal is indicated.

A No. 11 blade can be used to cut the constricting bands under a regional nerve block.[75] It may be difficult to identify individual hairs that are deeply embedded in a swollen digit and even more difficult to assess the success of the intervention. Frequently, multiple hairs are involved. Because the bands may be quite deep, the incision should avoid known neurovascular tracts. Barton and coworkers recommend a dorsal, rather than a lateral, incision on the digits.[74] If the soft tissue on the distal end of the digit has been rotated after a circumferential dermal laceration from the tourniquet, the distal tissue can be realigned with the proximal tissue and two dorsolateral sutures placed or tissue adhesive glue applied to maintain the digit in alignment.

Generally, conservative wound care is sufficient once the band has been removed. Application of an antibiotic ointment may enhance healing and allow easier removal of serous drainage from the circumferential laceration. Clinical reassessment in 24 hours will indicate whether any constricting bands remain.

Wearable Medical Devices

As technology continues to evolve, wearable medical devices are becoming more prevalent. Some of these technologies involve monitoring, including physiological monitoring and blood sampling. Removing these devices should, in most cases, involve some device investigation before removal to ensure optimal safety.

Devices can be roughly categorized (Fig. 36.40). Currently, many of the devices have minimal degrees of invasiveness, but caution should be exercised whenever wearable medical devices are removed. As technology continues to evolve, these devices may increase in their complexity and have varying degrees of invasiveness.

AFTERCARE

Tetanus

Wounds with FBs should be considered contaminated wounds, and tetanus status should be updated according to the recommendations for patients with contaminated wounds.

Antibiotics

There is no consensus or standard for the use of antibiotics after removal of wound FBs. Antibiotics may be indicated for

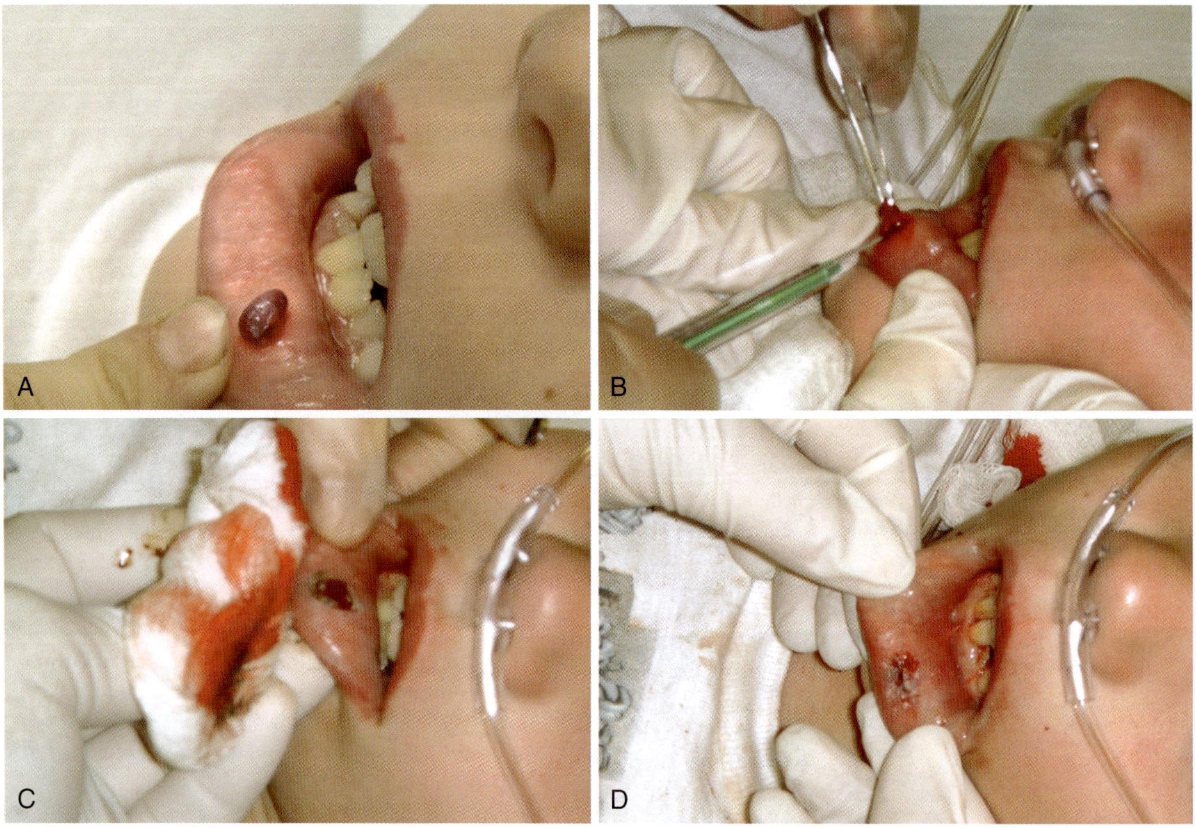

Fig. 36.38 (A–D) Pyogenic granuloma removed by sharp dissection under ketamine anesthesia and primary suturing.

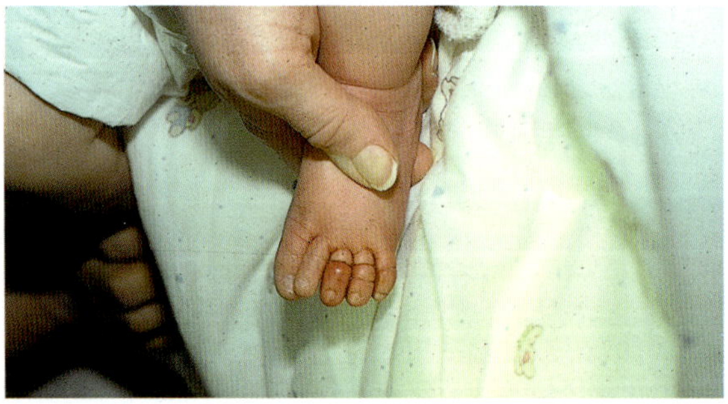

Fig. 36.39 This child has multiple hair tourniquets compromising the circulation to two toes. The hairs are deeply embedded in the skin creases and cannot be visualized. An over-the-counter depilatory (such as Nair) smeared into the fold may dissolve the hair in 30 to 45 minutes, but if unsuccessful, an incision must be performed. The best way to ensure removal of the constriction is to cut the depth of the folds with a scalpel blade (using a dorsal incision to avoid the neurovascular bundle) and attempt to extricate individual fibers. A digital nerve block may be performed for anesthesia. Return of circulation should be obvious by the change in temperature and color in the affected digit or digits before it is assumed that all the fibers have been cut.

immunocompromised patients, but there are no data to support the routine use of antibiotics in patients with wounds that have been thoroughly cleaned and from which all foreign material has been extracted. Prophylaxis may be considered if there was excessive time between injury and removal or obvious contamination or when it is difficult to adequately clean the wound. Under these circumstances, it is more prudent to opt for an open wound and delayed closure.

If prophylactic antibiotics are prescribed, a first-generation cephalosporin or penicillinase-resistant penicillin has traditionally been the first-line choice. In patients with contraindications to penicillins and cephalosporins and with the increasing incidence of community-acquired methicillin-resistant *S. aureus* in many areas, clindamycin, trimethoprim-sulfamethoxazole, or tetracycline may provide alternative coverage.[76] However, infections associated with FBs are not likely to be from methicillin-resistant *S. aureus*. Under certain circumstances, alternative antibiotics may be indicated. For infected plantar punctures through a shoe, a fluoroquinolone to cover *P. aeruginosa* is appropriate coverage, although most *Pseudomonas* infections are complex and may need extensive debridement and intravenous antibiotics. Saltwater marine FBs may be contaminated with *Vibrio* species, which are usually sensitive to tetracyclines, aminoglycosides, or third-generation cephalosporins. Freshwater FBs, on the other hand, are more likely to harbor *A. hydrophila*, which can be treated with tetracyclines.

Discharge Instructions

The patient should be informed that despite every effort there can be no absolute guarantee that all foreign material has been identified or extracted, regardless of whether some or any FB was removed during the initial exploration. Prudent clinicians should always suggest close follow-up and should leave open the possibility that an occult FB may still remain in the wound. Discharge instructions should also include the signs and symptoms of problems related to retained material. Some centers routinely add this caveat on all discharge instructions

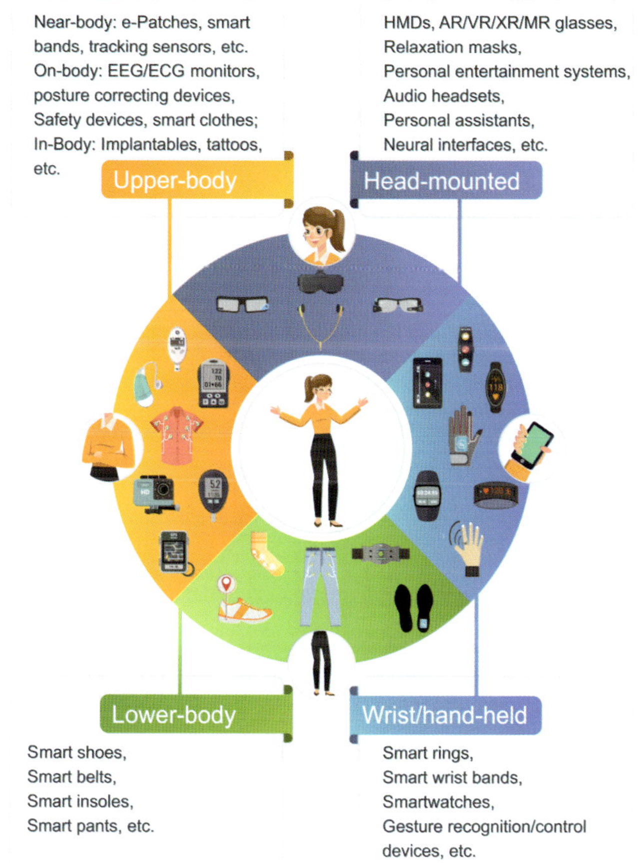

Fig. 36.40 Types of wearable medical devices. *AR*, augmented reality; *ECG*, electrocardiogram; *EEG*, electroencephalogram; *HMDs*, head-mounted displays; *MR*, mixed reality; *VR*, virtual reality; *XR*, extended reality. (From Ometov A, Shubina S, Klus L et al. A survey on wearable technology: history, state of the art and current challenges. *Comput Netw*. 2021;193:108074.)

to patients treated for lacerations or soft tissue defects. Written instructions should inform patients that additional steps may be undertaken if foreign material is subsequently suspected. Discharge instructions should indicate that close, continued, and careful follow-up is important with any evaluation for FB, FB removal, and post-FB removal assessment. Consider adding a wound check appointment in 3 to 5 days as part of the discharge instructions.

FOREIGN BODY REACTIONS

If the FB is not removed or cannot be removed, an FB reaction may occur. Some FBs produce an inflammatory reaction or infection a few days after introduction into the body. Other objects may not cause problems for weeks, months, or even years until they flare up for no apparent reason. The primary factors that affect the extent of tissue reactions are contamination and whether the material is inert or reactive with human tissue. Reactive FBs, such as wood, will eventually produce inflammation, whereas inert FBs, such as bullets, rarely do. Some inert FBs carry dirt particles, clothing, or other sources of bacterial contamination. Expeditious removal may be necessary, even if the FB itself is relatively small and unlikely to cause a reaction.

A purulent bacterial infection may develop in the presence of any FB; therefore any abscess or cellulitis that recurs or

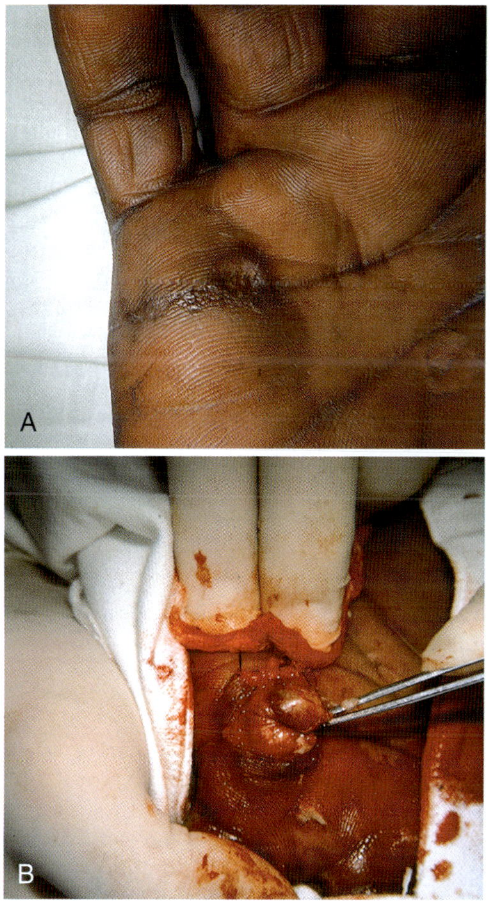

Fig. 36.41 This foreign body (FB) granuloma developed after the FB was stable for 6 months. There was no gross infection and it was dissected en masse.

wounds that do not heal as expected should always be investigated for retained FBs.[77,78] Karpman and coworkers found a 15% rate of infection (*S. aureus* and Enterobacteriaceae) in a series of 25 patients treated for cactus thorn injuries on the extremities.[60] Certain thorns (black thorns, rose thorns), redwood and northwest cedar splinters, toothpicks, hair, and stingray or sea urchin spines are noted for their ability to initiate chronic FB reactions. Sea urchin spines and other marine FBs are covered with slime, calcareous material, and other debris that commonly initiate a FB granuloma. The inflammatory reaction seen with cactus thorns may be an allergic reaction to fungus found on the cactus plant.

Many FB reactions are thought to result from an inflammatory response to organic material, or they may represent infection from bacteria introduced at the time of the wound. Clinically evident reactions may be delayed for weeks or even years after injury (Fig. 36.41). The chronic infection or inflammatory reaction may not be accompanied by the production of pus. Still, it may be quite painful or result in loss of function. FBs may also be associated with the formation or development of a chronic pseudotumor, a sinus tract, or an osteomyelitis-like lesion of bone and soft tissue.[77] In addition, organic material has been noted to induce chronic tenosynovitis, chronic monarticular synovitis, and chronic bursitis.

Rapidly traveling projectiles with considerable inherent heat (e.g., bullets) are less likely to cause infection but are more apt to cause other difficulties. Damage to surrounding areas can occur during passage through tissue. Rarely do retained lead FBs, such as bullets or shotgun pellets, leach out lead into the general circulation and produce systemic lead poisoning unless they are in contact with synovium (Fig. 36.42). If this process does occur, it may take years to develop and can result in vague or nondescript symptoms (e.g., fatigue, arthralgia, headache, or abdominal pain) many years after the initial injury. Elevated blood lead levels are more likely to occur if body fluids such as joint, pleural, peritoneal, or cerebrospinal fluid bathe the lead. Bullets retained in muscle or other soft tissue are not likely to produce any sequelae related to their lead content. However, Farrell and colleagues reported unsuspected elevated lead levels in patients with retained lead fragments who were seen in the ED with a variety of complaints.[79] Lead levels of up to 50 μg/dL were reported. Levels greater than 45 μg/dL are generally considered an indication for chelation therapy. The relationship between the retained lead and the symptoms was unclear, but this report verifies the observations of others that retained lead FBs in selected areas can significantly elevate blood lead levels and may produce symptomatic plumbism.

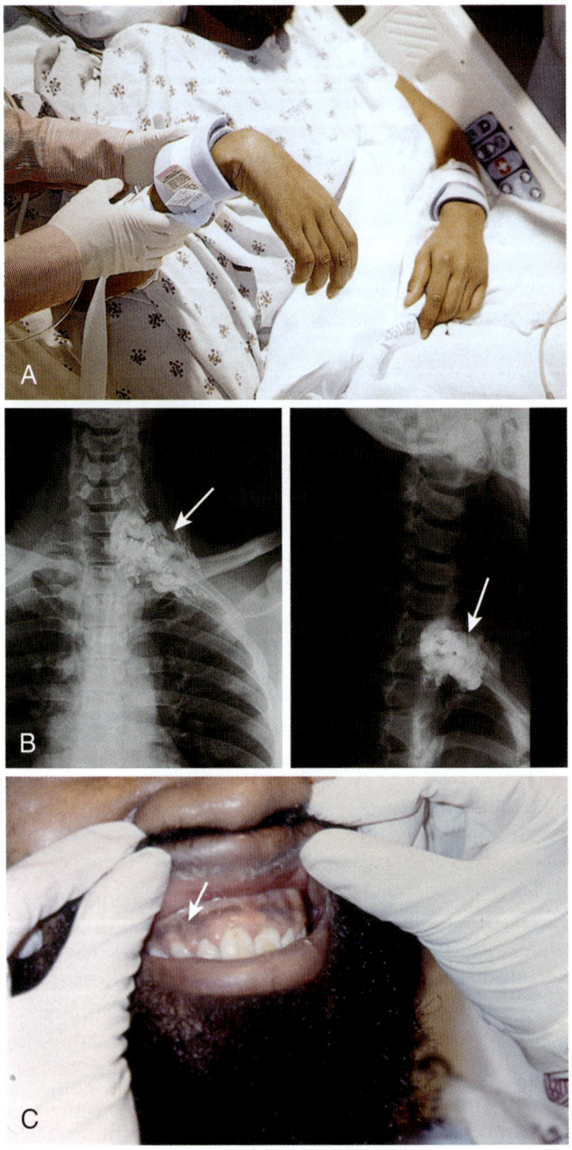

Fig. 36.42 There is no need to routinely remove retained bullets. Most lead foreign bodies are well tolerated, but if a bullet is bathed in synovial, pleural, peritoneal, or cerebrospinal fluid (CSF), the lead may leach out over time and produce a significant elevation in blood lead levels. The symptoms are often vague, and the relationship between the retained lead and the patient's clinical scenario may be difficult to sort out. (A) This patient had chronic neurologic findings, including wristdrop, and was wheelchair bound. (B) The symptoms were due to chronic lead poisoning from a 20-year-old retained bullet *(arrows)* in or near the spinal canal, possibly being bathed by CSF. (C) Note the lead lines in the gingiva, indicative of lead poisoning.

CONCLUSION

FBs are a common presenting issue within the ED. A high index of suspicion and a low threshold for imaging should be maintained for individuals with a history of traumatic injury to evaluate for retained FB. Removal of the FB depends in part of the type of object and the area of the body involved. A thorough evaluation of the wound is critical to both assessing and removing any foreign body. Adequate light, anesthesia, and possible sedation are important in achieving removal. Complicated or time-intensive removals can be referred, but those from organic material have a high propensity for infection or subsequent skin reactions and should be dealt with sooner rather than later. When discharging a patient, it is important to communicate that a foreign body could be or is present and the indications of infection which should prompt return. Tetanus should be updated when indicated. Prophylactic antibiotics should be considered on a case-by-case basis, considering the foreign body, the suspect depth of the injury, any deep tissue involvement, and the patient's comorbidities. Any patient presenting with concerning features for infection after trauma should be considered for having a retained foreign body. A wound check appointment in 3 to 5 days is an important consideration in monitoring wounds and helps to minimize the risk of complications.

ACKNOWLEDGMENT

The authors and editors thank Daniel Stone, Ted Koutouzis, and Matthew Levine for their contributions to this chapter in previous editions.

REFERENCES ARE AVAILABLE AT Elsevier eBooks+

CHAPTER 37

Incision and Drainage

Kerry A. Forrestal

INTRODUCTION

Incision and drainage (I&D) procedures are commonly performed in the emergency department (ED). According to the CDC in their National Hospital Ambulatory Medical Care Survey: 2021 Emergency Department Summary Tables, almost 1.1 million procedures were performed in that year.[1,2]

Soft tissue abscesses (Fig. 37.1) arise in many areas for a number of reasons and can be complicated by certain comorbidities. These factors will modify treatment.[3] Despite being such a commonly performed procedure, considerable variability in practices addressing abscesses remains.[4]

The emergence and predominance of methicillin-resistant *Staphylococcus aureus* (MRSA) as the cause of cutaneous abscesses during the past several decades had necessitated major revisions in long-standing guidelines for antibiotic administration. Considering this significant epidemiological change, MRSA should be considered as a probable cause in most skin and soft tissue infections.

ABSCESS ETIOLOGY AND PATHOGENESIS

Localized pyogenic infections may develop in any region of the body. Abscesses begin as localized superficial cellulitis. Some organisms cause necrosis and liquefaction. Liquifaction is mediated by enzymes from both invading organisms and defending cells, as well as the accumulation of leukocytes and cellular debris. These include bacterial hydrolytic enzymes or lysosomal hydrolytic enzymes.[5,6]

Necrosis is not a simple byproduct of infection, but a defense mechanism directed to introduce antimicrobial enzymes from dying host cells and recruit inflammatory cells into the area of infection. This is followed by loculation and subsequent walling off of these products via fibrin deposition, all of which result in the formation of pockets called abscesses.[6]

Any process or event that causes a breach in the skin's defensive epithelial barrier increases the risk for the development of an abscess. This includes primary dermatologic conditions as well as trauma. In some cases, no insult can be identified. An isolated abscess is often associated with local symptoms only, lacking fever, systemic complaints, or abnormal blood tests. Systemic signs of toxicity or fever suggest deeper tissue involvement, bacteremia, or both. As the process progresses, the area of liquefaction increases until it "points" and eventually ruptures into the area of least resistance. This may be toward the skin or the mucous membrane, into the surrounding tissues, or into a body cavity. If the abscess is particularly deep, spontaneous drainage may not occur. The lymphatic tissues may be involved causing a linear inflammation following lymphatic channels termed lymphangitis or commonly described as "streaking." In some cases, a fistulous tract can arise and lead to the formation of a chronic draining sinus. This development—or the recurrence of an abscess that was previously drained—should broaden the etiologic differential. For example, recurrent abscesses in the perineal or lower abdominal area should raise suspicion of inflammatory bowel disease as the trigger, and recurring abscesses in the axilla or groin should raise the possibility of hidradenitis suppurativa (HS). Chronic abscesses may be associated with an immunocompromised state or intravenous drug use (IVDU), and recurrent abscesses may suggest the possibility of a retained foreign body, underlying osteomyelitis, malignancy, or the presence of an atypical or drug-resistant organism (Fig. 37.2).

The cause of an abscess depends on its anatomic location and flora indigenous to that area. Different organisms cause disease based on environmental exposure (Table 37.1).

Staphylococcal strains, which are normally found on the skin, produce rapid necrosis, early suppuration, and localized infections with large amounts of creamy yellow pus, the typical manifestation of an abscess. Conversely, group A β-hemolytic streptococcal infections tend to spread through tissues and cause a more generalized infection characterized by erythema, edema, a serous exudate, and little or no necrosis, typical manifestations of cellulitis. Anaerobic bacteria, which proliferate in the oral and perineal regions, produce necrosis with profuse brownish, malodorous pus[6] and may cause both abscesses and cellulitis (Table 37.2).

Normal skin is extremely resistant to bacterial invasion, and few organisms can penetrate uninjured epidermis. In a normal healthy host with intact skin, the topical application of even very high concentrations of pathogenic bacteria does not result in infection. The requirements for infection usually include a high concentration of pathogenic organisms, structures such as hair follicles in the adnexa; occlusion of glands or other structures that prevent desquamation and normal drainage; a moist environment[7]; adequate nutrients; and trauma to the corneal layer, which allows organisms to penetrate deeper tissues. Tissue perfusion may also play a role in preventing infection. Trauma may result from abrasions, shaving, insect bites, hematoma, injection of chemical irritants, incision, or

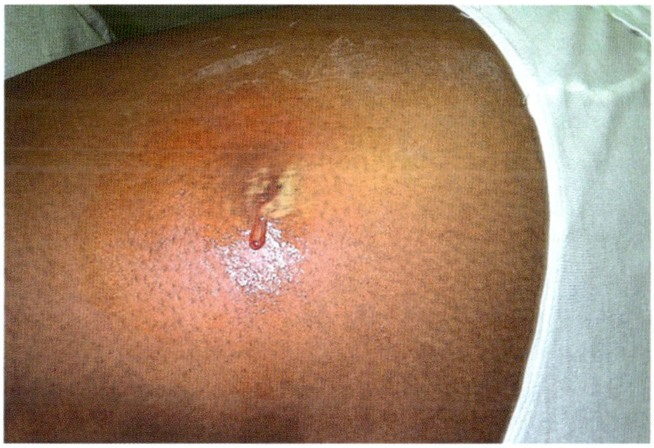

Fig. 37.1 Cutaneous soft tissue abscesses such as this are commonly encountered in the emergency department. Incision and drainage are required for definitive treatment; antibiotics alone are not sufficient. Multiple recurrent abscesses in the same area raise suspicion for a foreign body or underlying osteomyelitis. This abscess began to spontaneously drain releasing purulent contents. The abscess was caused by methicillin-resistant *Staphylococcus aureus* (MRSA). (Courtesy Public Health Image Library. https://phil.cdc.gov/details.aspx?pid=7826.)

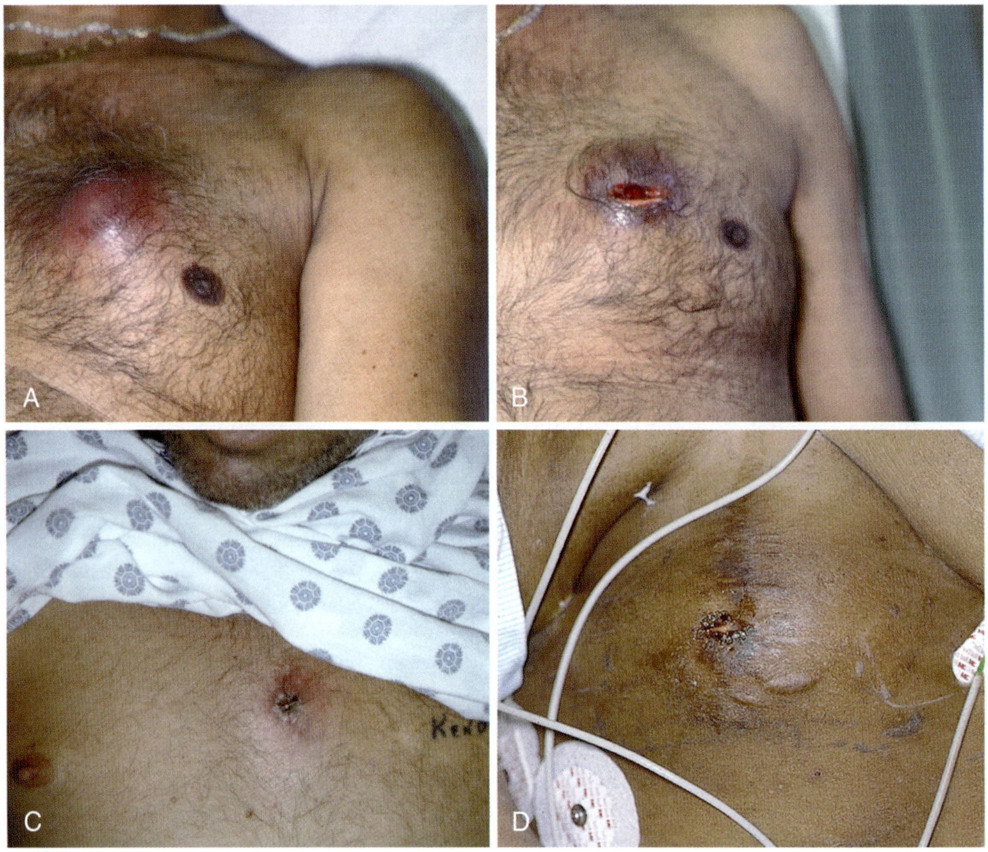

Fig. 37.2 An abscess that appears in an atypical place or recurs after successful initial treatment should raise the possibility of rare or underlying conditions. (A) This patient had a large "abscess" on the lateral chest wall that initially drained unusual gelatinous material, not frank pus. (B) At follow-up 3 days later, the abscess was much improved. The contents of the abscess had been sent for pathologic analysis because it had an unusual consistency, and a highly undifferentiated soft tissue malignancy was demonstrated. The fluid was sterile. Normally, analyzing or culturing the contents of an abscess will not yield helpful information, but in this case the unusual consistency of the collection prompted further analysis. (C) This IV drug user had an "abscess" of the chest wall drained in various emergency departments several times over a 2-month period, and it seemed to initially respond to drainage and antibiotics. He still had an area of cellulitis, minor fluctuance, and continued drainage near the center of the chest. This is an atypical place for a simple cutaneous abscess. Magnetic resonance imaging demonstrated osteomyelitis and an abscess of the sternoclavicular joint that was draining to the skin and simulating a recurrent cutaneous abscess. He required extensive surgical debridement and prolonged antibiotics. The etiologic organism was never ascertained, but *Pseudomonas* is often present. (D) This patient underwent a sternotomy for bypass surgery a few months previously. She had been treated sporadically for a minor wound infection, but then a draining fluctuant mass developed at the inferior border of the sternum. This is the external manifestation of extensive sternal osteomyelitis.

occlusive dressings that macerate the skin. The presence of a foreign body can potentiate skin infections by enabling a lower number of bacteria to establish an infection. For example, abscesses occasionally develop at suture sites in otherwise clean wounds. In addition, abscesses can develop at any site used for body piercing. Ear piercings through the pinna cartilage seem to be at particular risk for infection because of the avascularity of auricular cartilage.[8]

When favorable factors are present, the normal flora that colonizes cutaneous areas flourish and infect the skin and deeper structures. In persons performing manual labor, the arms and the hands are infected most frequently. In females, the axilla and submammary regions are frequently infected because of minor trauma from shaving, contact with undergarments, moist environment, and an abundance of bacteria in these areas. Infections may develop anywhere on the body in intravenous (IV) drug users, although the upper extremities are the most affected.[9–11] In this population, deep soft tissue abscesses can be caused by an afflicted individual's attempts to access deep venous structures when peripheral venous access sites are exhausted. In addition, areas with compromised blood supply are more prone to infection because normal host defenses, including cell-mediated immunity, are less available.[9]

Bacteriology of Cutaneous Abscesses

The microbiology and the underlying cause of skin and soft tissue abscesses are related to their location.[12] Abscesses involving the extremities are generally the result of a breach in the skin's integrity from trauma such as cuts, abrasions, or needle punctures. Abscesses involving the head, neck, and perineal region are usually associated with obstruction of the apocrine sweat glands. These types of abscesses increase

TABLE 37.1 Possible Organisms Based on Environmental Source and Potential Antibiotic Treatment

ENVIRONMENTAL SOURCE	ORGANISM(S) OF CONCERN	ANTIBIOTIC (IF NEEDED)
Mammalian bite	*Eikenella, Pasteurella*	• Penicillin • Ceftriaxone • Sulfamethoxazole-trimethoprim • Tetracyclines • Fluoroquinolones
Saltwater	*Vibrio*	• Doxycycline • Piperacillin and tazobactam • Ticarcillin and clavulanate • Ciprofloxacin
Freshwater	*Aeromonas*	• Doxycycline plus either • Ciprofloxacin or • Ceftriaxone
Meat or fish exposure	*Erysipelothrix rhusiopathiae*	• Penicillin • Cephalosporin
Hot tub	*Pseudomonas*[7]	• Ciprofloxacin • Antipseudomonal penicillins • Cephalosporins • Carbapenems • Aztreonam[5]
Fish tanks, pools	*Mycobacterium marinum*[8]	• Clarithromycin with ethambutol • Doxycycline • Trimethoprim-sulfamethoxazole • Ciprofloxacin • Azithromycin

TABLE 37.2 Infectious Agent, Clinical Reaction and Fluid Characteristics

AGENT[9]	REACTION	EXUDATE
Staphylococcus	Rapid necrosis, early suppuration, and localized infections	Large amounts of creamy yellow pus
Group A β-hemolytic *Streptococcus*	Spread through tissues and cause a more generalized infection characterized by erythema, edema, little or no necrosis	A serous exudate
Anaerobic bacteria	Produce necrosis, cellulitis, and necrosis	Profuse brownish, malodorous pus
Sterile abscesses	Inflammation	Serous, sterile exudate

in frequency after puberty because of the increased apocrine and sebaceous gland activity. Perirectal abscesses are typically the result of bacterial spread from adjacent anal glands. Vulvovaginal abscesses usually result from obstruction of a Bartholin gland, which then causes duct and gland edema and subsequent infection. Pilonidal abscesses are hypothesized to be caused by sacrococcygeal infections from ingrown hairs in the intergluteal cleft. In 2002, Brook[13] compiled the findings from more than 15 bacteriologic studies of 676 polymicrobial abscesses. *S. aureus* and group A β-hemolytic streptococci were the most prevalent aerobes in skin and soft tissue abscesses and were isolated in specimens from all body sites. Gastrointestinal and cervical flora (enteric gram-negative bacilli and *Bacteroides fragilis*) were found most often in intraabdominal, buttock, and leg lesions. Group A β-hemolytic streptococci, pigmented *Prevotella*, *Porphyromonas* species, and *Fusobacterium* species—all normal residents of the oral cavity—were most found in lesions of the mouth, head, neck, and fingers.

In two studies of the bacteriology of cutaneous abscesses in children, Holsenback et al.[14] and Fenster et al.[15] both found increased incidence of MRSA relative to previous studies and the most common site of an abscess in younger children to be the buttocks. Holsenback's study noted an MRSA incidence of 79% in their population of 318 subjects.[14] Fenster reported that bacteremia is rare in immunocompetent children, withholding antibiotics was felt to be first-line treatment, and packing did not confer any benefit.[15]

If an unexpected or atypical organism is found in an abscess culture, the clinician should consider an underlying process that is not readily apparent from the history or physical examination. For example, tuberculosis or fungal isolates are sometimes found in immunocompromised patients (e.g., those with diabetes or acquired immunodeficiency syndrome). Finding *Escherichia coli* suggests an enteric fistula or even self-inoculation of feces in some patients with a psychiatric illness such as Munchausen's syndrome. Recurrent abscesses without an obvious underlying cause could indicate clandestine drug use. What appears to be a typical recurrent abscess may be a manifestation of an underlying septic joint, osteomyelitis, or rarely, metastatic or primary cancer (see Fig. 37.2).

Frei et al. noted in their 2010 article that "Pediatric hospitalizations for methicillin-susceptible *S. aureus* and CA-MRSA skin and soft tissue infections are on the rise."[16] There is no evidence that this trend has abated.

Although most abscesses contain bacteria, 5% of abscesses are sterile, especially those associated with IVDU. Clinically, sterile abscesses cannot be differentiated from those caused by bacteria. They are caused by injected irritants that are not fully absorbed, causing local inflammation at the site of injection. Somewhat atypical abscesses develop in parenteral drug users. Injection of a cocaine-heroin mixture ("speedball") may predispose users to abscesses by inducing soft tissue ischemia.[17] The phrase "speedball" refers to any combination of a stimulant drug (cocaine or amphetamine) and a depressant (opioid or benzodiazepine). Jenkins and colleagues compared the microbiology of abscesses in IVDU patients versus patients without a history of IVDU and found that streptococcal species and anaerobes were identified more commonly than *Staphylococcus* in IVDU patients.[10]

Special Considerations

Parenteral drug users, patients with insulin-dependent diabetes, hemodialysis patients, cancer patients, transplant recipients, and individuals with acute leukemia have an increased frequency of abscess formation when compared with the general population. There are several reasons why these patients are at increased risk for abscess formation: intrinsic or acquired immune deficiency, an increased incidence of staphylococcal carriage (IV starts), potentially compromised tissue perfusion, and frequent needle punctures, which allow a mode of entry for pathogenic bacteria.[17–19]

At initial evaluation, the patient may emphasize an exacerbation of the underlying disease process or an unexplained fever, with symptoms of an abscess being a secondary complaint. In these situations, abscesses tend to have exotic or uncommon bacteriologic or fungal causes and typically respond poorly to therapy. Patients with diabetes-induced ketoacidosis (DKA) should be evaluated extensively for an infectious process[17]; an examination of the perineum should be included with the physical examination of toxic patients for Fournier's infection. Digital rectal examination for perirectal abscess as the infectious trigger of DKA has been suggested in the past; however, CT imaging is a reasonable approach if suspected. This is also true for patients who are immunocompromised.[20] Patients who use IV drugs frequently use veins in the neck and in the femoral areas, which can produce abscesses and other infectious complications at these sites.[21] Any abscess near a vein of the antecubital fossa or dorsum of the hand should alert the clinician to possible IV drug use; however, substance users may also inject directly into the skin ("skin-popping"), which can cause cutaneous abscesses distant from veins (Fig. 37.3). Skin-popping scars in the context of a new skin abscess in the same vicinity may signal occult IVDU. A foreign body may serve as a nidus for abscess formation. Patients with a history of IVDU frequently break needles in skin that multiple injections sites have toughened, so the clinician should maintain a high index of suspicion for retained needle fragments. This argues strongly against digital probing of abscess cavities in these populations. If an abscess is recurrent or if the patient is a known or suspected IV drug user, consider radiographs to search for foreign bodies, an underlying septic joint, or osteomyelitis.[21] Ultrasound is a valuable adjunct to evaluate foreign bodies that are not radiopaque either done as a point of care ultrasound by the emergency medicine physician or provider or a study done by the ultrasound technician. A 2003 study in England found that in a population of 70 IV drug users, 20% (14) had broken needles off in their skin. Some of these individuals had multiple retained needle fragments, totaling 23 needle fragments among the group. Only two-thirds of these were retrieved.[21]

MRSA: Methicillin-Resistant *Staphylococcus aureus*

First acknowledged in the 1960s as a cause of infection in patients in healthcare settings, MRSA has now become the most common identifiable cause of community-acquired skin and soft tissue infections in many metropolitan areas in the United States. Methicillin resistance in *S. aureus* is defined as an oxacillin minimum inhibitory concentration (MIC) of greater than or equal to 4 μg/mL. The spread of this organism is considered an epidemic, and it is very virulent and aggressive.[22] One study found an MRSA prevalence as high as 75% to 80% in some parts of the country.[23]

MRSA has historically been broken down between health care-associated MRSA (HA-MRSA) and community-acquired MRSA (CA-MRSA) based both on their clinical epidemiology and molecular structures. The CA-MRSA and HA-MRSA classifications, however, are no longer epidemiologically distinct as now either MRSA grouping can develop in either realm. Community-onset HA-MRSA infections have been observed with increasing frequency. This was illustrated in a study of 209 patients documented as colonized with MRSA while in the hospital, but had no infection. Of those who were discharged, 49% developed their first MRSA infection within 18 months following hospital discharge. Typically, MRSA was considered "hospital acquired" if it developed during admission or soon after discharge. Huang et al. followed patients for 18 months and nearly half developed HA-MRSA in that time frame. The authors argued for a longer period of surveillance for HA-MRSA.[24] In another series of 102 patients with CA-MRSA infections, 29% had molecular typing consistent with HA-MRSA.[25]

Despite the epidemiological blurring, there remain molecular differences with clinical impact and as no new naming convention exists, it is expedient to use the current designations to discuss those differences.

HA-MRSA, then, is defined as MRSA infection that occurs following hospitalization (hospital onset, formerly "nosocomial") or MRSA infection that occurs outside the hospital within 12 months of exposure to a health care setting (e.g., history of surgery, hospitalization, dialysis, or residence in a long-term care facility).[23] HA-MRSA is usually associated with severe, invasive diseases, including skin and soft tissue infection, bloodstream infection, and pneumonia. *S. aureus*

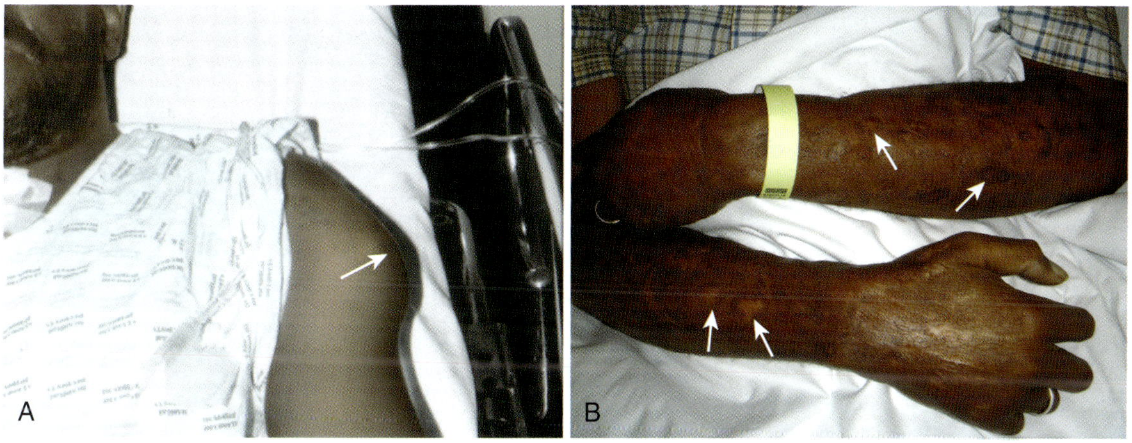

Fig. 37.3 This patient had a large abscess in the deltoid area *(arrow)* and could offer no explanation for it. This is a common scenario for a drug user who injects directly into the skin. (B) The characteristic circular skin lesion from "skin-popping" found on the arms *(arrows)* confirmed the clinical suspicion. Even though a drug screen was positive for opioids, the patient denied drug use and attributed the leg lesions to frequent trauma on the job. Drug users with abscesses are at risk for numerous infections, including brain abscess, endocarditis, and occult osteomyelitis.

continues to be a significant cause of surgical site infections.[26] HA-MRSA strains tend to be resistant to multiple drugs. MRSA is one of the few pathogens routinely implicated in nearly every type of hospital-acquired infection. This is probably partly related to the organism's capacity for "biofilm" formation on indwelling lines and tubes in hospital settings. Biofilm is the bacterially produced matrix of hydrated extracellular polymeric substances (EPS) that form their immediate environment. EPS are mainly polysaccharides, proteins, nucleic acids, and lipids; they provide the mechanical stability of biofilms and mediate their adhesion to surfaces.[27–29] This facilitates survival and multiplication of MRSA on these surfaces, necessitating prolongation of the duration of treatment with antibiotics. Another consequence of this durable microcolony is promoting the potential for the development of further genetic resistance.[30]

It follows then that CA-MRSA is defined as MRSA infection that occurs in the absence of health care exposure. It is often associated with skin and soft tissue infections in young, otherwise healthy individuals.[30] CA-MRSA was initially reported in injection drug users in the early 1980s and has since become the most frequent cause of skin and soft tissue infections seen in US EDs and ambulatory clinics. Most CA-MRSA strains are sensitive to non–β lactam antibiotics, although a multidrug-resistant isolate has been described in males who have sex with males.[31] This latter strain contains the pUSA03 plasmid and carries resistance genes for β-lactams, fluoroquinolones, tetracycline, macrolides, clindamycin, and mupirocin.

Virulent CA-MRSA causes rapid and destructive soft tissue infection. A single clone probably accounted for most MRSA isolates discovered during the 1960s; by 2004, six major MRSA clones had emerged.[23,32] In 1980 the spread of MRSA from hospitals into communities became evident. More recently, community-acquired infections have occurred more frequently, even in people without known risk factors. A small pustule can become a large abscess in 24 to 48 hours (Fig. 37.4). Such lesions are often mistaken for a spider bite or drug use because of their rapid progression and seemingly spontaneous onset in an otherwise healthy person. These observations have led to the identification of some risk factors for CA-MRSA, including skin trauma (e.g., lacerations, tattoos, IV and intradermal drug use, shaving), incarceration, shared razors or towels, and close contact with others colonized or infected with MRSA.[33] Importantly, many patients with CA-MRSA have no identifiable risk factors for acquisition of the disease.[34] CA-MRSA tends to be more virulent than HA-MRSA and is associated with more frequent serious complications such as osteomyelitis, joint infections, sepsis, and death. Fortunately, these organisms tend to be susceptible to a broader array of antibiotics.[35]

In an assessment of the prevalence of MRSA globally, Shoaib and colleagues[32] compiled data that also addresses a relatively new reservoir for MRSA that is termed "livestock-associated" or LA-MRSA, likely promoted by the use of antibiotics in the livestock industry. LA-MRSA is transmissible to humans who handle livestock, but less so from an infected person to a non-infected person. The designation "livestock" should not be construed to suggest that only livestock animals such as cows or pigs are affected. LA-MRSA has been identified in companion animals such as dogs and cats.

Additionally, the researchers discussed the rise of vancomycin-resistant *S. aureus* (VRSA) with prevalence rates ranging from 1.3% to 20%.[36]

MRSA has also emerged as a potential sexually transmitted infection. In 2007 Roberts and colleagues described their treatment of two patients who came to their urban ED with abscesses, probably transmitted by heterosexual oral-genital contact, both tested positive for MRSA.[37] A 2010 case report drew a similar conclusion. It reported orogenital transmission of MRSA to an immunocompetent 22-year-old male who tested orally positive for MRSA and group B (genital) *Streptococcus* after oral contact with a female partner in whom MRSA-positive gluteal lesions had previously been diagnosed.[38] MRSA abscesses have been described following skin-to-skin contact during a lap dance. In a retrospective chart review, Roberts and colleagues found that 18% of the 524 subcutaneous abscesses treated in their urban ED in 2006 were confined to the genital area. Almost three-fourths of the 272 outpatient wound cultures performed on that year's patient population were positive for MRSA.[37]

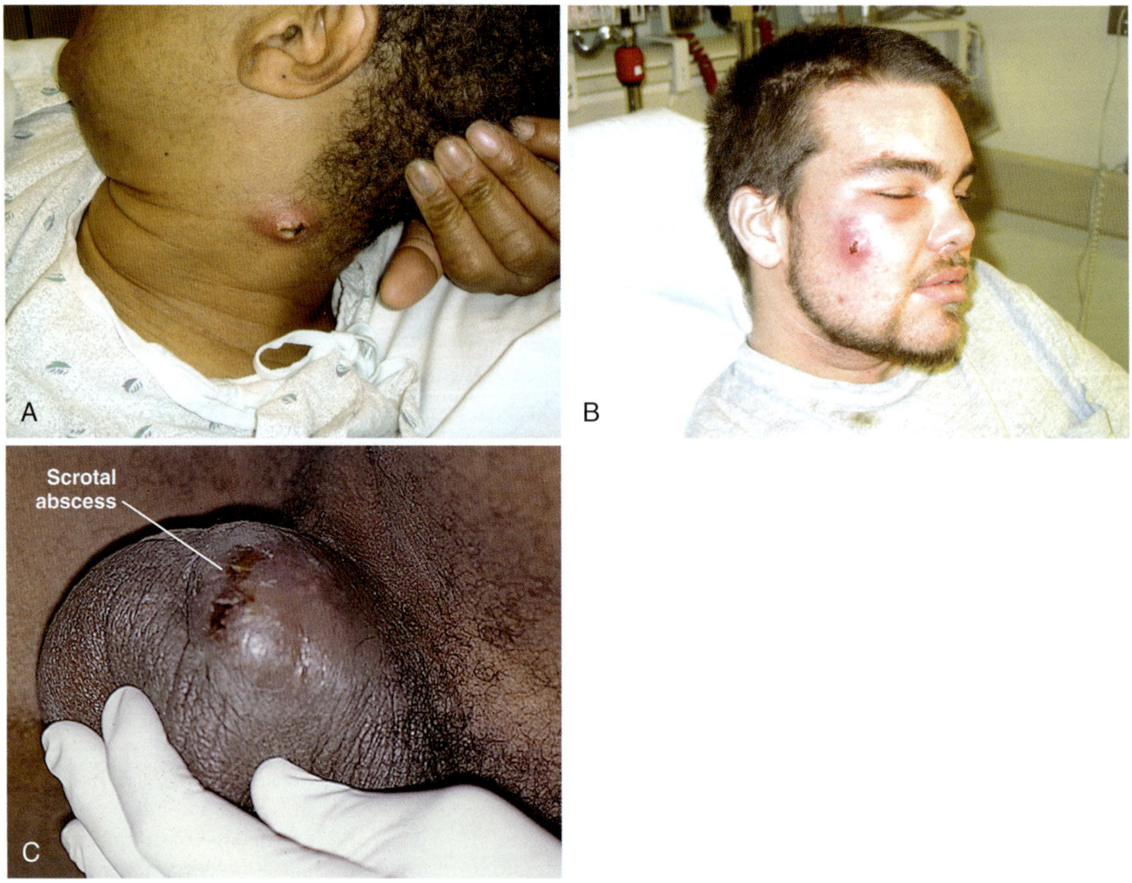

Fig. 37.4 (A–C) Examples of community-acquired methicillin-resistant *Staphylococcus aureus* (CA-MRSA) infections. These aggressive infections can spread rapidly. The patient frequently describes a small pustule that becomes an abscess in 24 to 48 hours. Patients often believe that it is a "spider bite" because of its rapid onset in an otherwise healthy person with no other reason for the lesion. A CA-MRSA abscess, though clinically aggressive, is usually treated like any other cutaneous abscess.

The economic burden of MRSA infections alone in the United States is substantial. A 2013 study by Lee et al. estimated it at 13.8 billion per year (18 billion in 2023 dollars) on society, depending on the CA-MRSA definitions and incidences. When all antibiotic resistance is considered for economic impact, according to the Centers for Disease Control and Prevention (CDC), antimicrobial resistance adds a $20 billion surplus in direct health care costs in the United States, which is exclusive of about 35 billion dollars in loss of productivity annually.[39]

The most recent updates to therapy for MRSA can be found at the NIH library including chemotherapeutics for MRSA and nano-medicinal therapies that are beyond the scope of this discussion.[40]

MANIFESTATIONS OF CUTANEOUS ABSCESSES

The diagnosis of cutaneous abscess formation is usually straightforward. The presence of a fluctuant mass in an area of induration, erythema, and tenderness is clinical evidence that an abscess exists (see Fig. 37.1). An abscess may appear initially as a definite, tender, soft tissue mass. Still, in some cases, a distinct abscess may not be readily evident. If the abscess is deep, as is true of many perirectal, pilonidal, and breast abscesses, the clinician may be misled by a firm, tender, indurated area without a definite mass. If the findings on physical examination are equivocal, needle aspiration or ultrasound examination may be performed to assist in the diagnosis.[41]

This approach may also identify a mycotic aneurysm (dilation of an arterial wall due to infection) or an inflamed lymph node simulating an abscess. A specific entity commonly mistaken for a discrete abscess is the sublingual cellulitis of Ludwig angina (see Chapter 65). Parenteral injection of illicit drugs can produce simple cutaneous abscesses that unpredictably advance to extensive necrotizing soft tissue infections.[17] The emergency clinician must maintain a high index of suspicion to avoid missing this potentially life-threatening condition. Cellulitis and abscess formation can lead to bacteremia and sepsis, especially in immunocompromised patients.[20] The pain of an abscess often brings the patient to the hospital before it spontaneously ruptures, or the patient can have a draining abscess that appears to have undergone spontaneous rupture and is self-resolving. The patient may have even punctured the abscess in attempt to drain it. In most cases, a formal I&D procedure will be necessary to effectively manage the condition, even though copious drainage may not be encountered. Although no formal drainage may be required after the spontaneous rupture of a simple cutaneous abscess, conditions such as a perirectal abscess, Bartholin gland abscess, and breast abscess are usually best managed with further appropriate drainage. Packing of wounds is no longer considered a standard of care and should be reserved for very specific instances.

IMAGING

ULTRASOUND: Soft Tissue Infection

by Christine Butts, MD

Ultrasound offers a distinct advantage when evaluating a patient with suspected soft tissue infection and may change management. A recent study from *Academic Emergency Medicine* by Tayal and colleagues evaluated the effect of soft tissue ultrasound on managing cellulitis in the ED.[45] The authors found that in patients with a low suspicion for abscess, ultrasound changed management in 56% of cases. Peritonsillar abscesses are difficult to diagnose from the physical examination alone, and some clinicians may feel hesitant to attempt blind drainage. Ultrasound of suspected peritonsillar abscesses is reliable in making the diagnosis. The overall size of the abscess, as well as its proximity to the carotid artery, can be evaluated with ultrasound, which may improve the confidence of the clinician in attempting drainage.[46,47]

General Considerations

Typically, a high-frequency (7.5 to 10 MHz) transducer should be used to evaluate the superficial soft tissues. The higher frequency will allow the clinician sufficient resolution to identify changes consistent with soft tissue infection. To identify fluid pockets, the entire area should be scanned in detail, using multiple planes. Surrounding structures in the area should also be evaluated, especially when incision and drainage is planned. An intracavitary transducer should be used when evaluating the posterior pharynx for potential peritonsillar abscess.

Normal Soft Tissue

Normal soft tissue is characterized by well-defined layers, with clear demarcation between these layers (Fig. 37.US1). The top of the screen corresponds to the most superficial soft tissue, including the epidermis and dermis. It should appear hyperechoic (light gray to white), thin, and clearly separate from the underlying layers. Subcutaneous tissue is found beneath the dermis and is of varying thickness. However, as with the most superficial layers, this layer should appear thin and well demarcated from the surrounding layers. Underneath the subcutaneous tissue, muscle will typically be seen as layers of striated tissue separated by bright layers of fascia.

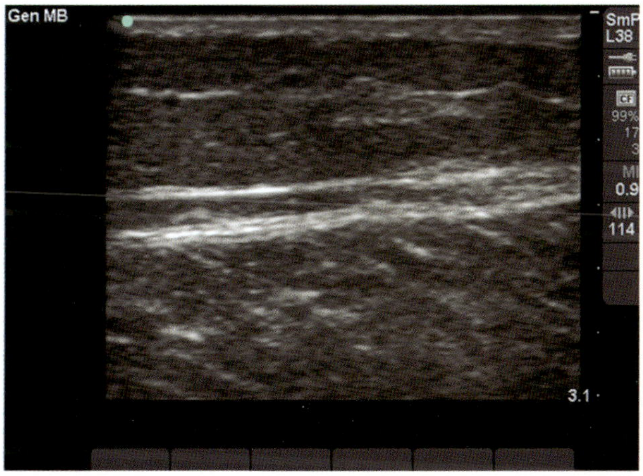

Fig. 37.US1 Ultrasound image of normal soft tissue. In this image, the tissue planes are clearly defined, with well-demarcated boundaries between the layers. This clean, organized appearance is lost with soft tissue edema and cellulitis.

Cellulitis

Cellulitis is recognized on ultrasound by thickening of the skin and subcutaneous layers (Fig. 37.US2). The tissue may also appear more hyperechoic than normal soft tissue. When a significant amount of edema is present within the tissue, bands of hypoechoic (dark gray) or anechoic (black) fluid may be seen within the area of thickened tissue. This is known as "cobble stoning" (Fig. 37.US3). Cobble stoning appears as thin bands of fluid throughout the tissue and

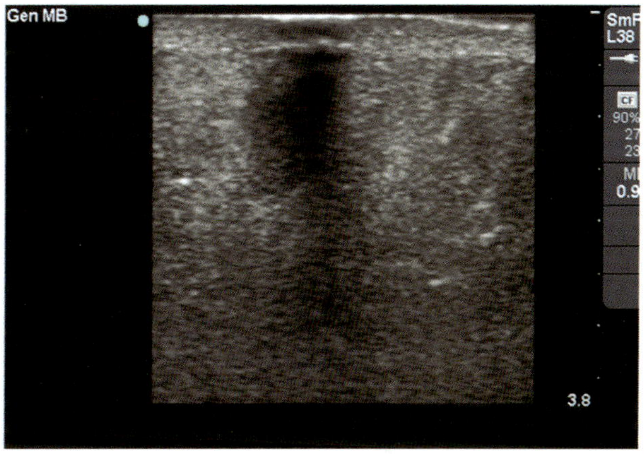

Fig. 37.US2 Ultrasound image of cellulitis. Thickening of subcutaneous tissue can be seen with loss of organized tissue planes. A small artifact is seen at the center of the image.

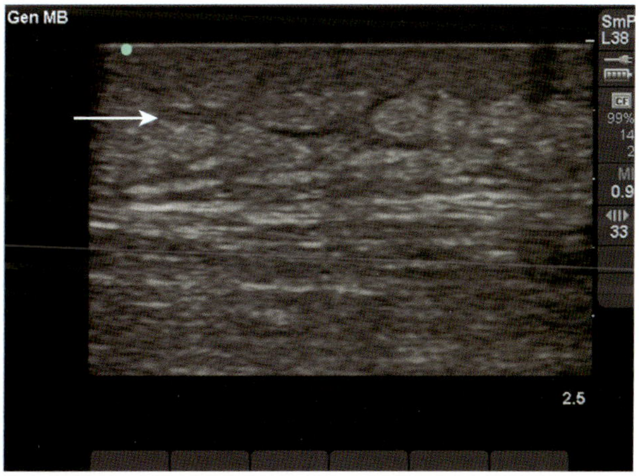

Fig. 37.US3 Ultrasound appearance of cobblestoning. Thickened subcutaneous tissue can be seen in this image with strands of hypoechoic *(dark gray)* fluid interwoven between the tissue *(arrow)*. This interweaving gives the appearance of a "cobblestoned" street and is consistent with soft tissue edema.

Continued

ULTRASOUND: Soft Tissue Infection—cont'd

can be distinguished from an abscess by the lack of a discrete fluid collection.

Abscess

An abscess is seen as a focal, discrete fluid collection within an area of cellulitis (Fig. 37.US4). The surrounding cellulitis is the key to distinguishing an abscess from other fluid collections such as cysts. The character of the fluid may be variable, depending on the content of the abscess. Complete collections of fluid will appear as anechoic (black) areas, whereas areas with more solid components will appear to have "internal echoes" within the collections (Fig. 37.US5). Once a focal fluid collection has been located, it can be evaluated in detail to determine the overall size and depth from the surface. Peritonsillar abscesses appear as rounded hypoechoic (dark gray) to anechoic (black) collections of variable size. In addition to confirming the presence of an abscess, the location and depth of the carotid artery can also be judged before an attempt at aspiration.[45–47]

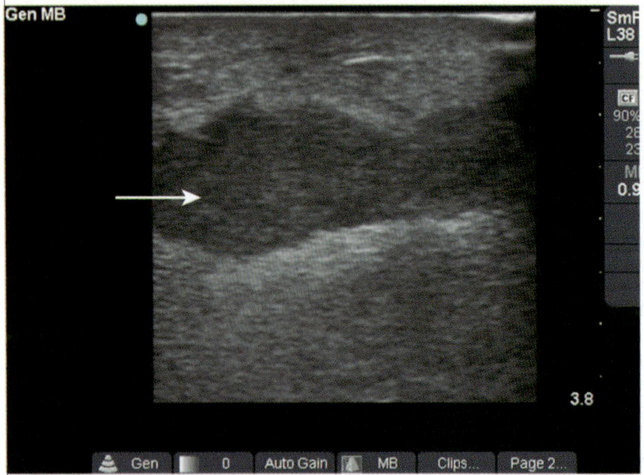

Fig. 37.US4 Ultrasound appearance of an abscess. A large, well-contained hypoechoic *(dark gray)* fluid collection *(arrow)* can be seen surrounded by thickened subcutaneous tissue.

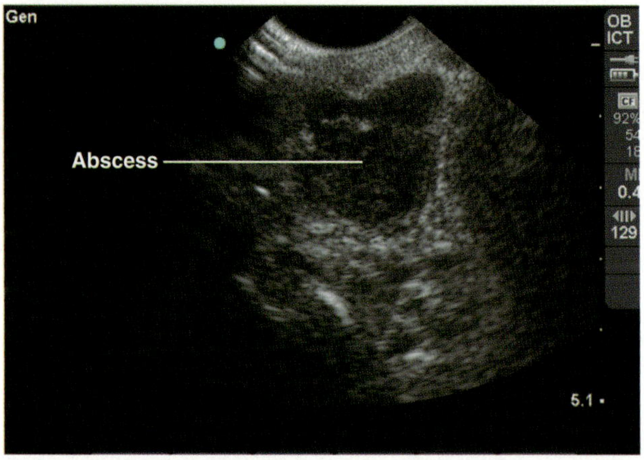

Fig. 37.US5 Ultrasound image of a peritonsillar abscess. A rounded area of mixed density (both anechoic and hypoechoic areas) is seen in the center of the image.

Ultrasound-Guided Needle Aspiration

Radiologists have been performing ultrasound-guided needle aspiration of abscesses for some time,[41] and emergency clinicians are now becoming more comfortable with the procedure. High-resolution ultrasound technology is being used to obviate "blind" procedures done in the ED (e.g., joint aspiration and central line placement). For ultrasound-guided drainage of a cutaneous abscess, use a high-resolution probe (7.5 to 10 MHz) and place an ultrasound probe cover to reduce the chance of contaminating the probe. The higher the frequency (above 7.5Mhz), the lower the depth of penetration, however, you get better quality images close to the surface (7.5MHz = 20 cm). Place the transducer over the main body of the abscess and insert the needle through the skin adjacent to the transducer. Adjust their relative relationships to keep with the depth and location of the abscess cavity. Guide the needle, seen as a bright artifact, directly into the abscess. Watch the abscess cavity collapse as pus drains out. Scan the entire area of the suspected abscess and beyond to capture unexpected extensions of the abscess. Be sure to drain all pockets.

CT Imaging

For simple cutaneous abscesses, it is unlikely that CT scanning would be of any utility. In circumstances such as a perirectal abscess of uncertain extent, peritonsillar abscesses questionably proximal to the carotid artery, or multiple abscesses in sensitive areas with underlying vascular structures such as in the axilla, CT scanning is a reasonable course of action, and when necrotizing fasciitis is also in the differential. As this will take time, it is advisable to make sure the patient's pain is managed while imaging is obtained.

LABORATORY FINDINGS

A complete blood count (CBC), blood cultures, and Gram stain are not standard or required for the treatment of straightforward cutaneous abscesses in the ED. Recommendations for culturing abscesses encountered in the ED are confusing, and clinical practice varies.

The American College of Emergency Physicians[42] and the American Academy of Family Physicians[43] do not support the practice of abscess cultures as part of standard care whereas the Infectious Diseases Society of America 2014 practice guidelines for the diagnosis and management of skin and soft tissue infections states that "Gram stain and culture of pus from carbuncles and abscesses are recommended, but treatment without these studies is reasonable in typical cases."[44]

In the circumstances of a lack of response to therapy or other complications, a culture may identify an unusual or resistant organism. Additionally, cultures in these situations will distinguish MRSA from non-resistant abscesses and could provide useful sensitivity information when managing complicated cases.

Cultures, then, should be performed for[44]:

- Recurrent, unusual, or atypical abscesses
- Poor response to initial surgical drainage
- Secondary spread of the infection occurs
- If bacteremia develops
- Development of an abscess in patients already taking antibiotics
- Immunosuppressed patients
- Those with signs of systemic illness
- Patients who have not responded adequately to initial treatment
- If there is concern for a cluster or outbreak of infection
- Patients with severe local infection

Severe local infection can be defined as an abscess larger than 5 cm in diameter, multiple lesions, or extensive surrounding cellulitis. However, the degree of surrounding cellulitis qualifying as "extensive" is ill defined.

When obtaining a specimen for culture, the most accurate and complete culture results will be obtained if one aspirates pus with a needle and syringe before I&D. The material should be cultured for aerobic and anaerobic bacteria. Most clinicians, however, still culture free-flowing purulent material obtained with a cotton swab during the procedure. For uncomplicated ED abscesses, this culture technique is standard and adequate to isolate aerobic organisms, including MRSA. A "sterile" culture from a specimen collected with a standard cotton swab after incision is frequently the result of improper anaerobic culture technique.

In selected patients, such as immunocompromised hosts or IV drug users, isolation of possible anaerobic organisms by needle aspiration with a syringe through appropriately cleaned (e.g., with chlorhexidine) skin before I&D will enhance the results of culture and can add information that may be clinically relevant to subsequent therapy. There is a general misconception that foul-smelling pus is a result of *E. coli*. This foul odor is caused by the presence of anaerobes; the pus associated with *E. coli* is odorless. The discovery of solid or suspicious material in an abscess should prompt histologic evaluation because a malignancy may mimic cutaneous abscesses (see Fig. 37.2A–B).

Most patients with an uncomplicated cutaneous abscess will have a normal CBC and will not experience fever, chills, or malaise. Therefore, without extenuating circumstances, it is not recommended to analyze blood from patients with typical cutaneous abscesses because laboratory test results do not lead to a specific therapeutic path. An abscess may produce leukocytosis, depending on the severity and duration of the purulent process; however, the presence or absence of leukocytosis has virtually no diagnostic or therapeutic implications. Bacteremia may occasionally be manifested as a peripheral abscess resulting from septic emboli, and it usually produces clinical characteristics dissimilar to those associated with simple cutaneous abscesses. A cutaneous abscess itself rarely produces bacteremia.

Gram stain is not indicated in the care of uncomplicated simple abscesses. However, patients who appear "toxic" or immunocompromised and those who require prophylactic antibiotics (see the section on "Prophylactic Antibiotics" later in this chapter) may benefit from Gram stain in addition to cultures. Gram stain results have been shown to correlate well with subsequent culture results, so in compromised hosts the test can be used to direct the choice of antibiotic therapy. Anaerobic infections should be suspected when multiple organisms are noted on Gram stain, when a foul odor is associated with the purulence, when free air is noted on soft tissue radiographs, and when no growth is reported on cultures.[13]

Finally, some argue for the routine culturing of abscesses to provide a framework for local epidemiology and resistance patterns.

Management of Very Early Abscesses

Surgical I&D is the definitive treatment of a soft tissue abscess[48]; antibiotics alone are often inadequate. Drainage of a suppurative focus generally results in marked resolution of the symptoms in most uncomplicated cases. In the initial stages, only induration and inflammation may be found in an area destined to produce an abscess. Premature incision, before localization of pus, will not be curative and may theoretically be deleterious by extending the infectious process and, theoretically, bacteremia can result from manipulation. In some cases, applying heat to an area of inflammation may ease the pain, speed resolution of the cellulitis, and facilitate the localization and accumulation of pus. Nonsurgical methods are not a substitute for surgical drainage and should not be continued for more than 24 to 36 hours before the patient is reevaluated.

PROPHYLACTIC AND THERAPEUTIC ANTIBIOTIC THERAPY

For simple abscesses in immunocompetent hosts, I&D alone is likely to be quite adequate and curative, even if the causative organism is MRSA. Routine administration of antibiotics after I&D is not universally recommended, although the topic is subject to ongoing investigations. There is, however, some degree of disagreement in the literature.

In 2007, Hankin and Everett did a literature survey noting the paucity of studies and lack of controversy on the subject. They wrote, "Our review of the literature found five studies and one abstract, spanning a 30-year period, which address the issue of clinical outcomes of abscess I&D with or without outpatient oral antibiotics." They concluded "patients treated with I&D alone exhibit resolution of their infection at the same rate as patients who are treated with I&D plus antibiotic therapy."[49]

Additionally, the Infectious Diseases Society of America (ISDA), Evidence Based Medicine (EBM) Guidelines, and Nederlands Huisartsen Genootschap (NHG) all recommend against antibiotics in the treatment of skin abscesses, with specific exceptions such as immunocompromise, artificial joints, and systemic illness.[50]

In 2017, Daum et al.[50] conducted a multicenter, prospective, double-blind trial that found "as compared with alone, clindamycin or TMP-SMX in conjunction with incision and drainage improves short-term outcomes in patients who have a simple abscess." The two antibiotics used were clindamycin and TMP-SMX, with cure rates of 83.1% for TMP-SMX and 81.7% for clindamycin, which were superior to that of the control group at 68.9%. The rate of new infections by 30 days was less for clindamycin, 6.8% than for TMP-SMX, 13.5% and both were superior to placebo at 12.4%. There is of course the caveat that adverse reactions were higher in the clindamycin group, 21.9%, than with TMP-SMX 11.1% or placebo. All adverse events resolved without sequelae.

Additionally, Talan et al. in 2016 found that cure rates when using trimethoprim-sulfamethoxazole were higher (80.5%) versus (73.6%) in the placebo group (difference, 6.9 percentage points; 95% confidence interval [CI], 2.1 to 11.7; $P = .005$). Of note, the MRSA positivity rate in their sample was 45.3%. Additionally, subsequent surgical intervention was lower in the treatment group (3.4% vs. 8.6%; difference, −5.2 percentage points; 95% CI, −8.2 to −2.2).[51]

The research is ongoing. As always, it must be remembered that the use of antibiotics is not without potential harms to both the individual patient through adverse effects and the broader community through increased antibiotic resistance.[52,53] Taken together, the decision whether to use antibiotics is multifactorial based on the patient's comorbidities, disease burden (one or multiple abscesses, size, and location), history, barriers to health (smoking, alcohol, drugs, and compliance), and local epidemiological patterns.

Even though research continues about the benefit of antibiotic therapy in conjunction with I&D of uncomplicated cutaneous abscesses in healthy, immunocompetent patients (without the specific types of valvular heart disease discussed later), there is strong consensus for antibiotic treatment of abscesses associated with the following conditions[56]:

- Severe or extensive disease (e.g., involving multiple sites of infection)
- Purulent cellulitis (e.g., drainage or exudate in the absence of a drainable abscess)
- Rapid progression in the presence of associated cellulitis
- Signs and symptoms of systemic illness
- Associated comorbid conditions
- Immunosuppression
- Extremes of age
- Abscess in an area difficult to drain (e.g., face, hand, and genitalia)
- Associated septic phlebitis
- Lesions that are unresponsive to I&D alone
- IV drug use documented or strongly suspected

It can be argued that a previous unrelated episode of treatment failure with I&D alone should be added to this list. There is no criteria for "severe" cellulitis. Purulent cellulitis is usually caused by MRSA. Nonpurulent cellulitis, defined as cellulitis with no purulent drainage or exudate and no associated abscess, is usually due to β-hemolytic streptococci.

Empirical therapy for MRSA, pending culture results, is recommended for patients who have not responded to non-MRSA treatment, for those with a previous history of or risk factors for MRSA, and for those with severe infection or systemic signs and symptoms. Empirical therapy for infection with β-hemolytic streptococci is likely to be unnecessary under these circumstances. The duration of therapy for skin and soft tissue infections has not been well defined, although no differences in outcome were observed in adult patients with uncomplicated cellulitis receiving 5 versus 10 days of therapy in a randomized, controlled trial.[54] In the Food and Drug Administration licensing trials for complicated skin and soft tissue infections, patients were typically treated for 7 to 14 days. However, in the outpatient setting of uncomplicated infections, 3 to 5 days of antibiotic therapy is reasonable but should be individualized based on the patient's clinical condition and response to treatment. Accordingly, a wound inspection or primary care follow-up early in treatment is a critical component of the care plan.

Patients with a history of IVDU who have an abscess and fever require parenteral antibiotic therapy after blood has been drawn for culture, until bacterial endocarditis can be ruled out.[40] Additionally, patients who have extensive cellulitis or are clinically septic require immediate IV antibiotics, as well as aggressive surgical drainage of any significant abscess. By administering IV ampicillin/sulbactam (2 g/1 g) every 6 hours, Talan and colleagues[55] achieved 100% eradication of pathogens from major abscesses in hospitalized IV drug users and non–drug users using this regimen.

The recommendation for immunocompromised patients for empirical coverage of CA-MRSA in outpatients with skin and soft tissue infection is TMP-SMX. Newer agents such as tedizolid and dalbavancin were also cited in the Practice Guidelines for the Diagnosis and Management of Skin and Soft Tissue Infections as appropriate for these patients. These 2014 recommendations remain the most up-to-date recommendations from the Infectious Disease Society of America as of the writing of this chapter.[44]

If coverage of both β-hemolytic streptococci and CA-MRSA is desired, options include the following: clindamycin alone or the use of TMP-SMX or a tetracycline in combination with a β-lactam (e.g., amoxicillin or cephalexin), or linezolid alone. The use of rifampin as a single agent or as adjunctive therapy for the treatment of skin and soft tissue infections is not recommended.[56] Facial abscesses should be handled cautiously and checked frequently. Any abscess above the upper lip and below the brow may drain into the cavernous sinus, so manipulation may predispose to septic thrombophlebitis of this system. Treatment with antistaphylococcal antibiotics and warm soaks after I&D has been recommended pending resolution of the process. Areas away from this zone of the face can be treated in a manner similar to that used for other cutaneous abscesses. There is a subset of patients who are "borderline" for admission and IV antibiotics.

A relatively unstudied but common and currently accepted strategy for patients with soft tissue infections (especially CA-MRSA infections) that are borderline, by clinical judgment, for hospital admission and therapeutic IV antibiotics is to administer a single dose of IV antibiotic in the ED, followed by oral antibiotics and close outpatient follow-up. When a CA-MRSA infection is likely, IV vancomycin or linezolid is a reasonable option. Oral linezolid has been shown to be as effective as the IV form.[57]

Prophylactic Antibiotics

Prophylaxis for Endocarditis After Incision and Drainage

The risk of endocarditis after I&D of a cutaneous abscess is low[58] and it is difficult to predict which patients will develop an infection and which particular therapeutic procedures will subject the patient to the highest risk for infection. However, bacteremia may occur with manipulation of infected tissue, and mortality rates are substantial for MRSA-associated endocarditis (30% to 37%).[56] Given this risk, it is reasonable that patients at the highest risk for cardiac complications related to transient bacteremia be pretreated with appropriate antibiotics within 1 hour preceding the procedure.[59,60] Guidelines issued by the American Heart Association (AHA) in 2007 recommend antibiotic prophylaxis for procedures involving the respiratory tract, infected skin, or infected musculoskeletal tissue only in patients with cardiac conditions with the highest risk for an adverse outcome from infective endocarditis.[61] They reaffirmed that position in 2021 with their AHA Scientific Statement in *Circulation*.[61] These conditions are listed in Box 37.1.

The vast majority of infectious endocarditis cases stem from gram-positive streptococci, staphylococci, and enterococci infection. Together, these three groups account for 80% to 90% of all cases, with *Staphylococcus aureus* specifically responsible for around 30% of cases in the developed world.[62] Therefore, the therapeutic regimen should include an agent active against these organisms, such as an antistaphylococcal penicillin or a cephalosporin. For patients who cannot tolerate a β-lactam or if MRSA is suspected, vancomycin or clindamycin can be substituted.

In addition to various streptococci species, other common colonizers of the oropharynx, such as the HACEK organisms (*Haemophilus*, *Actinobacillus*, *Cardiobacterium*, *Eikenella*, and *Kingella*) can less frequently be the culprit bacteria. Numerous other bacteria have been previously identified as well but comprise only about 6% of total cases. Finally, fungal endocarditis represents only about 1% of cases but can be a fatal complication of systemic *Candida* and *Aspergillus* infection in the immunocompromised population.

Two clinical situations deserve special mention. First, because of the frequent incidence of valvular damage in IV drug users, prophylactic antibiotics may be indicated before I&D of abscesses in these patients. It is prudent to inquire about previous endocarditis or auscultate for a heart murmur if IV drug use is suspected or known and administer antibiotics under these circumstances. No clear recommendations exist. Second, any patient with a documented history of endocarditis must receive prophylactic antibiotics before the I&D procedure. Cutaneous abscesses may result from active endocarditis and prophylactic antibiotics may obscure subsequent attempts to identify the causative organism. Two or even three sets of blood cultures (aerobic and anaerobic) should be considered before antibiotic therapy for those at risk for endocarditis. Patients with a diagnosis of mitral valve prolapse have traditionally been included for treatment with prophylactic antibiotics, but the indication for this is unclear and antibiotic prophylaxis for uncomplicated mitral valve prolapse is no longer part of the AHA guidelines.[61]

Prophylaxis for Bacteremia in other Conditions

Two older studies dating back to the 1980s[63,64] debated whether simple I&D was associated with bacteremia. The newer study held that bacteremia was highly unlikely and noted several issues with the design of the older study, while Bobrow called for a larger study to validate this finding. Ibrahim and Siddique's 2024 article[54] in *StatPearls* did not recommend routine antibiotics for the prevention of endocarditis in a simple cutaneous I&D. There was a notable exception in treating dental abscesses in certain populations including

- Patients with prosthetic cardiac valves
- Patients with a prior history of infective endocarditis
- Patients who have undergone cardiac transplantation and have valve regurgitation caused by a structurally abnormal valve
- Patients with congenital heart disease with:
    - Unrepaired cyanotic congenital heart disease, including palliative shunts and conduits
    - Repaired congenital heart defects, specifically those corrected with prosthetic material or devices placed during surgery or catheter intervention within the first 6 months following the procedure
    - Repaired congenital heart disease with residual defects present at the site or adjacent to the site of a prosthetic patch or device

Likewise, no studies of any size were found suggesting that bacteremia after I&D is probable. Finally, no case reports suggest that this is an issue.

Immunocompromised patients may benefit from the prophylactic administration of antibiotics in preparation for I&D of cutaneous lesions. In contrast to patients with risks for endocarditis, immunocompromised patients are at risk for septicemia secondary to brief bacteremia. IV drug users have a high incidence of diseases associated with human immunodeficiency virus (HIV),[65] and the treating clinician must anticipate various degrees of immunodeficiency among them. Because no specific standard of care exists, clinical judgment must guide the use of antibiotics in these situations. No specific guidelines have been offered for the antibiotic regimen to be used before I&D of infected cutaneous tissue in patients at risk for conditions other than endocarditis. The choice of antimicrobial agent is based on the organism anticipated to cause the bacteremia. Although the location of the abscess will give some clue to the organism involved, most abscesses contain multiple strains of bacteria. Not all bacteria are potent pathogens, so their mere presence does not predict their role in subsequent morbidity. Because *Staphylococcus* continues to be the most common cause of cutaneous abscesses, a broad-spectrum antistaphylococcal drug is indicated. Prophylaxis can consist of a single IV dose given half an hour before I&D. A first-generation cephalosporin or penicillinase-resistant penicillin is a good

BOX 37.1 Cardiac Conditions With the Highest Risk for Adverse Outcome From Endocarditis

Prosthetic cardiac valve or prosthetic material used in valve repair
Previous infective endocarditis
Congenital heart disease (CHD)[a]
Unrepaired cyanotic CHD, including palliative shunts and conduits
Completely repaired congenital heart defect with prosthetic material or a device, whether placed via surgery or catheter intervention, during the first 6 months after the procedure[b]
Repaired CHD with residual defects at the site of or adjacent to the site of a prosthetic patch or prosthetic device (which inhibits endothelialization)
Cardiac transplantation with the development of cardiac valvulopathy

[a]*Except for the conditions listed previously, antibiotic prophylaxis is no longer recommended for any other form of CHD.*
[b]*Prophylaxis is recommended because endothelialization of prosthetic material occurs within 6 months after the procedure.*
From Wilson W, Taubert KA, Gewitz M, et al. Prevention of infective endocarditis. Circulation. *2007;116:1736.*

initial choice. Vancomycin may also be considered. Others may prefer cefazolin, 1 g intravenously, for adults. This regimen covers staphylococcal and streptococcal species, many gram-negative organisms, and many anaerobes. Although it has not been studied, it is reasonable to also give antibiotics before I&D to all patients who will subsequently be administered therapeutic antibiotics. The ideal duration of therapeutic antibiotics is unknown. As a general guideline, immunocompromised patients should receive antibiotics for 5 to 7 days and immunocompetent patients for 3 to 5 days after the procedure, depending on the severity of the condition and their clinical response at follow-up.

RECURRENT INFECTIONS

The first-line approach to preventing recurrent soft tissue infections is education regarding personal hygiene and appropriate wound care. Patients should be directed to keep wounds covered with clean, dry bandages, maintain good personal hygiene with regular bathing and frequent hand washing with soap and water or an alcohol-based hand gel, especially after touching the wound or items that came in contact with the wound; and avoid reusing or sharing personal items that have contacted the infected area. Environmental hygiene measures should be considered in patients with recurrent skin and soft tissue infections in the household or community setting. Focus cleaning efforts on high-traffic surfaces (i.e., surfaces that come in frequent contact with skin daily, such as counters, doorknobs, and toilet seats) that may contact bare skin or uncovered infections. An approach to individual treatment of recurrent CA-MRSA soft tissue infections is outlined in Box 37.2.

Oral antimicrobial therapy is recommended for treating active infections only and is not routinely recommended for decolonization. In the case of multiple recurrent infections, consider consulting an infectious disease expert and referring the patient to wound care.

BOX 37.2 Strategies to Eradicate CA-MRSA Carrier States in Patients With Recurrent CA-MRSA Soft Tissue Infections

Recurrent CA-MRSA soft tissue infections have been linked to a carrier state in affected individuals, with the nose and skin areas being colonized. It may be difficult to totally or permanently eradicate colonization, and there are no proven methods to accomplish this. The following strategies have been used in an attempt to eradicate the carrier state in individuals with recurrent CA-MRSA soft tissue infections. The appropriate time to implement these procedures is not known, but it would be reasonable to institute first-line techniques if more than two to three episodes of proven CA-MRSA infection are documented.

FIRST-LINE

Apply 1 cm of mupirocin (Bactroban) ointment (an intranasal form is available) to the anterior nares three times a day for 7 days,[a] plus

Daily total body wash with (4%) chlorhexidine (Hibiclens) for 5–7 days.[b]

SECOND-LINE

Obtain specimens for culture to ascertain sensitivity to various antibiotics.

Repeat mupirocin and chlorhexidine as above.

Rifampin, 300 mg twice a day, plus trimethoprim-sulfamethoxazole DS or doxycycline (100 mg) twice a day for 1–2 weeks.[c]

[a]*May cause burning, pruritus, dry membranes, and erythema. Avoid long-term use. Do not substitute bacitracin.*

[b]*May cause skin and eye irritation. Apply for 5 minutes and then rinse thoroughly.*

[c]*Do not use rifampin alone because resistance may develop. It can cause an orange color of urine and tears and stain contact lenses. Adjust the dose for patients with renal impairment. Do not use in those with impaired hepatic function.*

For multiple recurrent infections, consider consultation with an infectious disease expert.

CA-MRSA, *Community-acquired methicillin-resistant* Staphylococcus aureus.

I&D PROCEDURE

Procedure Setting

Definitive I&D of soft tissue abscesses can be performed in either the ED or the operating room (OR) (Videos 37.1 and 37.2). Another consideration in infection control while doing this procedure given the increased use of ultrasound is contamination by MRSA of the probe itself. Frazee et al. in 2010[66] reported that MRSA was found on 14 of 20 (70%) cultures taken after skin and soft tissue infection scanning. These cultures produced heavy growth of a clinically important pathogen, including 13 *S. aureus* (5 MRSA).

The choice between ED and OR for the procedure depends on several important factors. The location of the abscess may dictate management in the OR. Large abscesses or abscesses located deep in soft tissues require a procedure involving a great degree of patient cooperation, which may only be achieved under general or regional anesthesia. Proximity to major neurovascular structures, such as in the axillae or antecubital fossa, may necessitate more extensive imaging and surgical consultation. Infections of the hand (with the exception of distal finger infections) have traditionally been managed in the OR because of the many important structures involved and the propensity for limb-threatening complications.

Lack of adequate anesthesia is the most common factor limiting I&D in the ED. The current increased use of ED procedural sedation (see Chapter 33) has changed previous OR cases to ones that can be managed well in the ED. If the clinician believes that the abscess cannot be fully incised and drained because of inadequate anesthesia, the patient should be taken to the OR for management under general anesthesia. In addition to limiting proper drainage, it is inhumane and unethical to subject a patient to extreme pain when alternatives are available.

Equipment and Anesthesia

A standard suture tray provides adequate instruments if a scalpel and packing material are added (Fig. 37.5). Although sterility is impossible during the procedure, one should avoid contamination of surrounding tissue. Some clinicians prefer to use an obligatory skin scrub with an antiseptic solution, but the value of this step is dubious. Most clinicians use nonsterile gloves while draining pus, but practices vary.

It is often difficult to achieve local anesthesia by direct infiltration because of the poor function of local anesthetic agents in the low pH of infected tissue. Furthermore, distention of

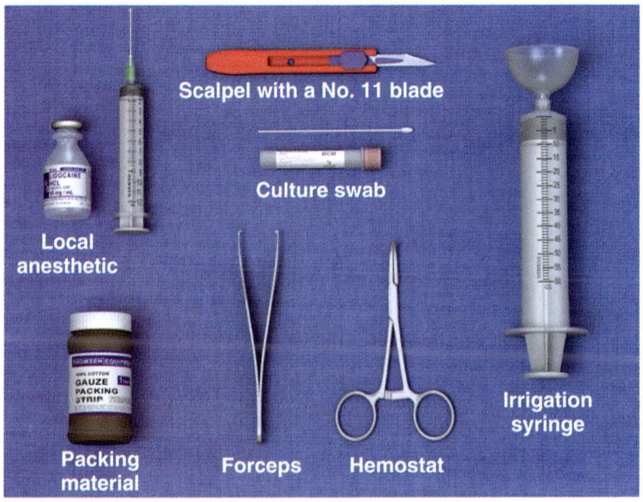

Fig. 37.5 Equipment required for incision and drainage. Most items can be found in a routine suture kit. The scalpel, culture swab, and packing material need to be gathered separately.

sensitive structures by a local injection is painful and, hence, poorly tolerated by most patients. Skin anesthesia is usually possible, but total anesthesia of the abscess cavity cannot generally be achieved. If a regional block can be performed (see Chapters 29 to 32), this type of anesthesia is preferred.

Alternatively, a field block, which is a circumferential infiltration of anesthetic around the abscess, may be used. It should be noted that infected tissue is very vascular and local anesthetics are, therefore, absorbed quickly. The skin over the dome of an abscess is often quite thin, thus making skin anesthesia difficult. If a 25-gauge needle is used carefully, one can frequently inject the dome of the abscess subcutaneously. This technique would be reminiscent of placing a Tb test intradermally. Without moving the needle tip, the anesthetic solution spreads over the dome through the subcutaneous layers into the surrounding skin and provides excellent skin anesthesia. If the needle is in the proper plane (best accomplished by holding the syringe parallel rather than perpendicular to the skin), the surrounding skin blanches symmetrically during infiltration without having to reposition the needle (Fig. 37.6, *step 2*).

In an extremely anxious or uncomfortable patient, judicious use of preoperative sedation (see Chapter 33) with IV opioids and sedatives or with nitrous oxide makes the procedure easier for both the patient and clinician. Ketamine, propofol, or a combination of these drugs is a popular option in the ED setting. Some clinicians recommend the use of topical ethyl chloride, a vapocoolant spray. If the injection of a local anesthetic or the initial skin incision is done immediately after blanching of the skin, it may provide momentary anesthesia.

Incision

To minimize visible scar formation, all incisions should conform to skin creases or natural folds (Figs. 37.7 and 37.8). Care should also taken in areas such as the groin, posterior aspect of knee, antecubital fossa, and neck so that vascular and neural structures are not damaged.

A No. 11 or 15 scalpel blade, held perpendicular to the skin, is used to nick the skin over the fluctuant area, and then a simple linear incision is carried the total length of the abscess cavity (see Fig. 37.6, *step 3*). This will afford complete drainage and facilitate the subsequent breakup of locations. Attempting to drain an abscess with an inadequate incision is counterproductive and makes packing changes, if done, more difficult.

Exceptions regarding aggressive incision are abscesses in cosmetic areas, in areas under significant skin tension (e.g., extensor surfaces), and in areas with extensive scar tissue (e.g., sites of multiple previous drainage procedures). In these special circumstances, a stab incision or simple aspiration alone may be attempted initially, to limit tissue injury and resultant scar formation. Use of this less aggressive approach requires that the patient be counseled that multiple decompressions (e.g., via needle aspiration) or delayed aggressive I&D may be required. The abscess must be reassessed in 24 to 48 hours to determine whether additional intervention is needed.

Needle Aspiration

An alternative to I&D is needle aspiration, though this is much less commonly used, given that it is less effective than I&D. In a randomized clinical control trial comparing outcomes with I&D to ultrasound-guided needle aspiration, the overall success of producing purulent drainage with needle aspiration was 26% compared with an 80% success rate in patients who underwent I&D.[67]

Wound Dissection

Following a standard incision, the operator should probe the depth of an abscess to assess its extent and ensure proper drainage by breaking open loculations (see Fig. 37.6, *step 5*). An ideal instrument for this procedure is a hemostat (or a cotton swab for small abscesses), which is placed into the abscess cavity, spread, and then manipulated throughout the cavity (Fig. 37.9). An operator's gloved finger has been suggested as an ideal way to assess the depth of the abscess cavity and to break up loculations, but this is a dangerous practice that should be avoided. Of particular concern is an abscess caused by skin-popping IV drugs as these abscesses occasionally harbor broken needle fragments (see Fig. 37.9C–D). In addition, patients who engage in this practice have a high incidence of hepatitis and HIV infection. Clinicians are often surprised at the depth or extent of abscesses discovered during probing. Sharp curettage of the abscess cavity is not usually required and may produce bacteremia. Although tissue probing is generally the most painful aspect of the procedure and total local anesthesia is difficult to attain, this portion of the intervention should not be abbreviated. If pain persists, additional local anesthetic can be administered through the cut skin edges and into deeper tissues to provide additional anesthesia (Fig. 37.10A). If the procedure is limited because of pain, use of appropriate analgesia or anesthesia is mandated.

In cases where a large volume of pus is expected or encountered, a blunt-ended suction device can extract the copious pus while also assisting in breakup of loculations (see Fig. 37.10B)

Wound Irrigation

Following the breakup of loculations, some clinicians advocate copious irrigation of the abscess cavity with normal saline to ensure debris removal from the wound cavity (see Fig. 37.6, *step 6*). Though seemingly beneficial, irrigation of the abscess cavity has not been demonstrated to augment healing or affect outcome, and hence may be eschewed.[68] Hyperemic tissue may bleed profusely, but the bleeding usually stops in a few

Incision and Drainage

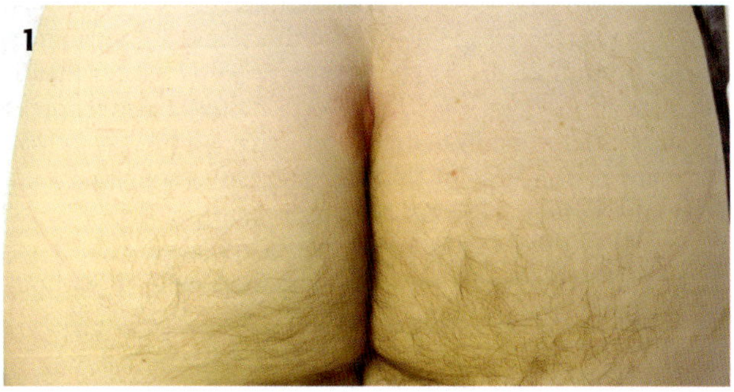

Identify and confirm the location of the abscess. This patient has a pilonidal abscess, which is found at the superior portion of the gluteal cleft.

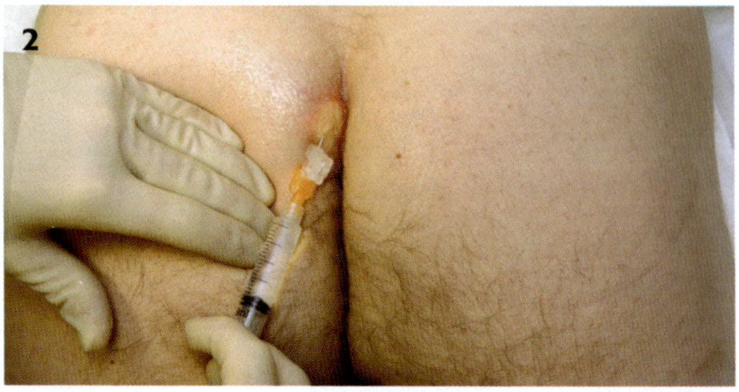

Anesthetize the region. Use a 25-gauge needle to inject the dome of the abscess. Hold the needle parallel to the skin during injection. Blanching will occur as the anesthetic spreads.

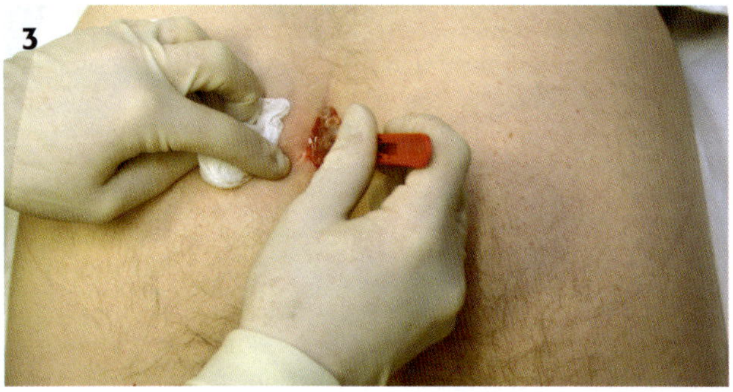

Use an 11-blade scalpel to make a linear incision over the total length of the abscess cavity. If possible, the incision should conform to skin creases or natural folds.

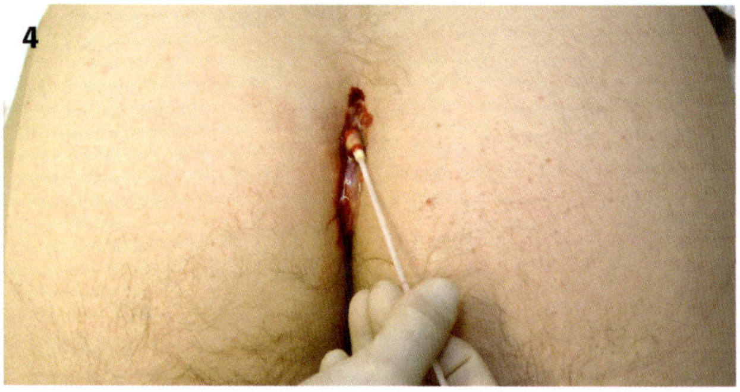

Culture the purulent drainage.

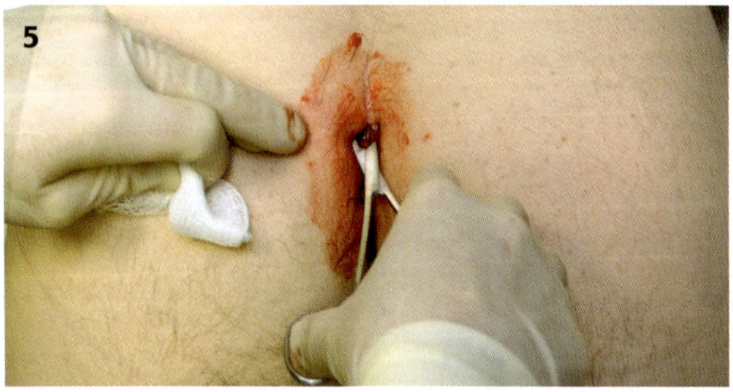

Probe the depth of the abscess and use a hemostat to break open loculations. This can be painful; inject additional anesthetic if needed through the cut skin edges and into the deeper tissues.

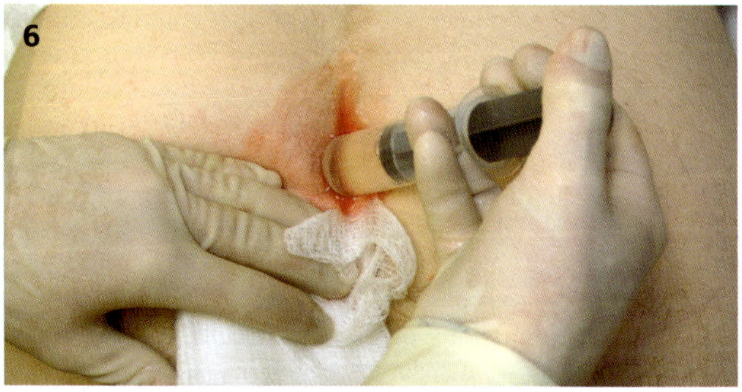

Irrigate the abscess cavity to assist with removal of residual debris.

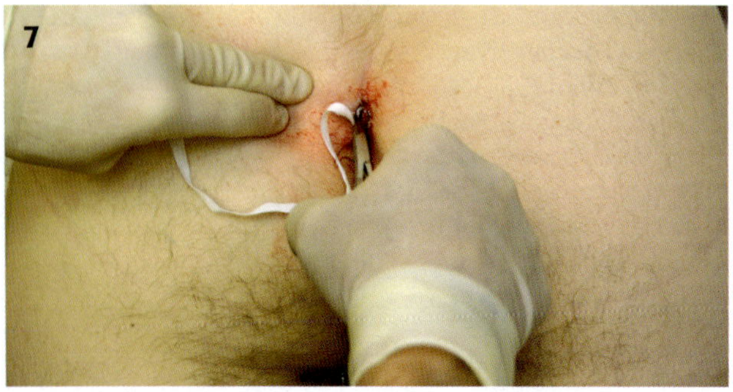

Loosely pack the abscess cavity with gauze wick. The purpose of the packing is to keep the incision open, which allows continued drainage of the cavity. Avoid overpacking the abscess.

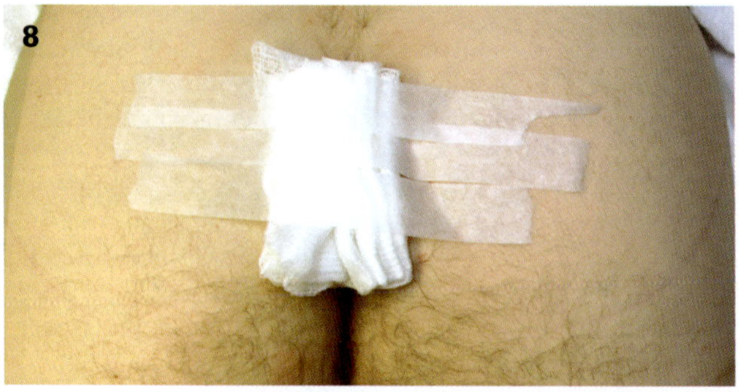

Place an absorbent gauze dressing over the packed abscess. Arrange for follow-up care, which usually entails a repeat exam in 1 to 3 days.

Fig. 37.6 Incision and drainage. Packing the cavity with gauze is a common intervention, but this procedure has not been proven to be of significant value and can cause more pain for the patient. Routine culturing and irrigation are discouraged and left to the discretion of the clinician.

minutes with direct pressure. Using lidocaine with epinephrine for numbing prior to the incision can help. Abscesses of the extremities can be drained with the use of a tourniquet to provide a bloodless field.

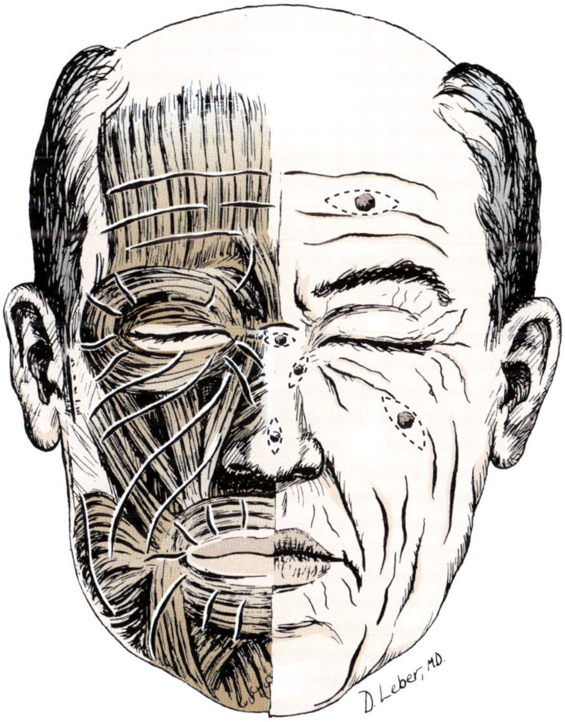

Fig. 37.7 Relationship of the elective lines of tension in the face to the underlying mimetic musculature. Only in the lower eyelid are these lines not perpendicular to the muscles. The left side of the drawing shows the use of this principle when common facial lesions are excised or a facial abscess is drained. (From Schwartz SI, Lillehei RC, eds. *Principles of Surgery*. 2nd ed. McGraw-Hill; 1974.)

Packing and Dressing

Historically, I&D has involved opening an abscess cavity, draining as much pus as possible, breaking up loculations, then packing with ribbon with or without impregnated antimicrobial, and leaving the abscess open to heal by secondary intention (Figs. 37.11and 37.12). Current literature does not support this approach.

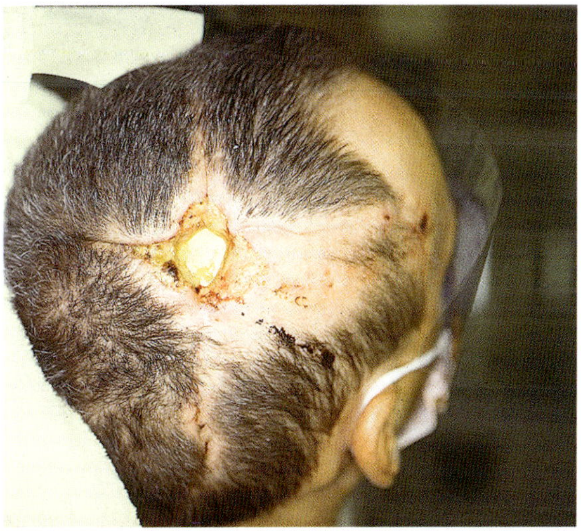

Fig. 37.8 A simple linear incision is preferred over an X-shaped or crosshatched incision. In this case, a cutaneous postsurgical scalp abscess was drained by an X incision and the tips of the flap necrosed, which left a slowly healing, full-thickness wound.

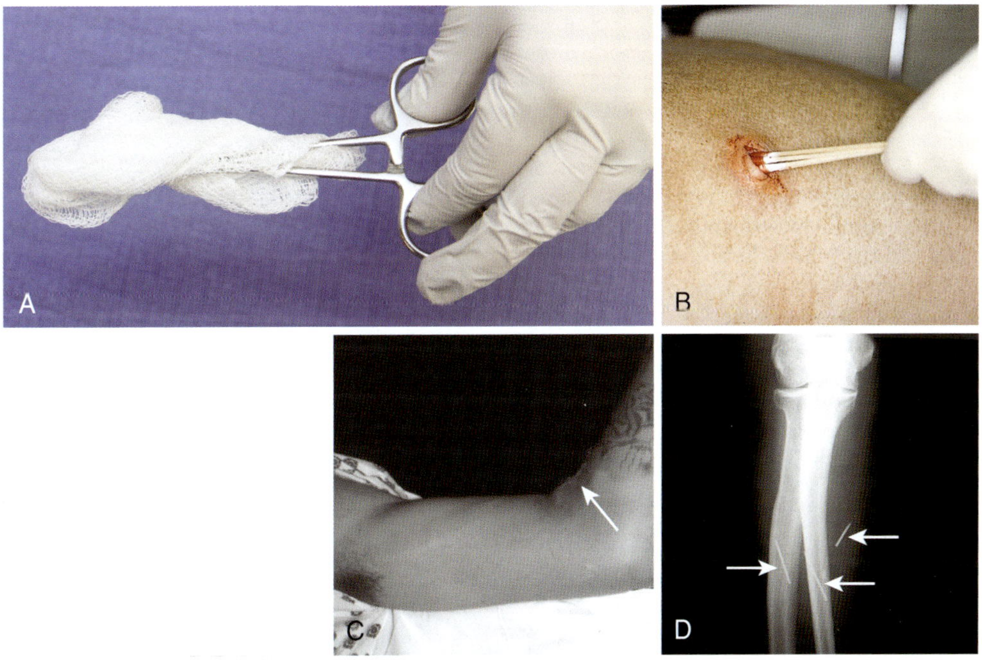

Fig. 37.9 Options for wound dissection. (A) A hemostat wrapped with gauze is an ideal instrument to break up loculations. (B) Alternatively, cotton-tipped swabs can be used. (C) This intravenous drug user had an abscess *(arrow)* in the antecubital fossa. These foreign bodies pose a risk to the clinician; finger probing of abscesses should be avoided. (D) When a radiograph was obtained, three needle fragments *(arrows)* were found embedded in the wound. The patient was positive for human immunodeficiency virus and claimed no knowledge of the presence of the needles.

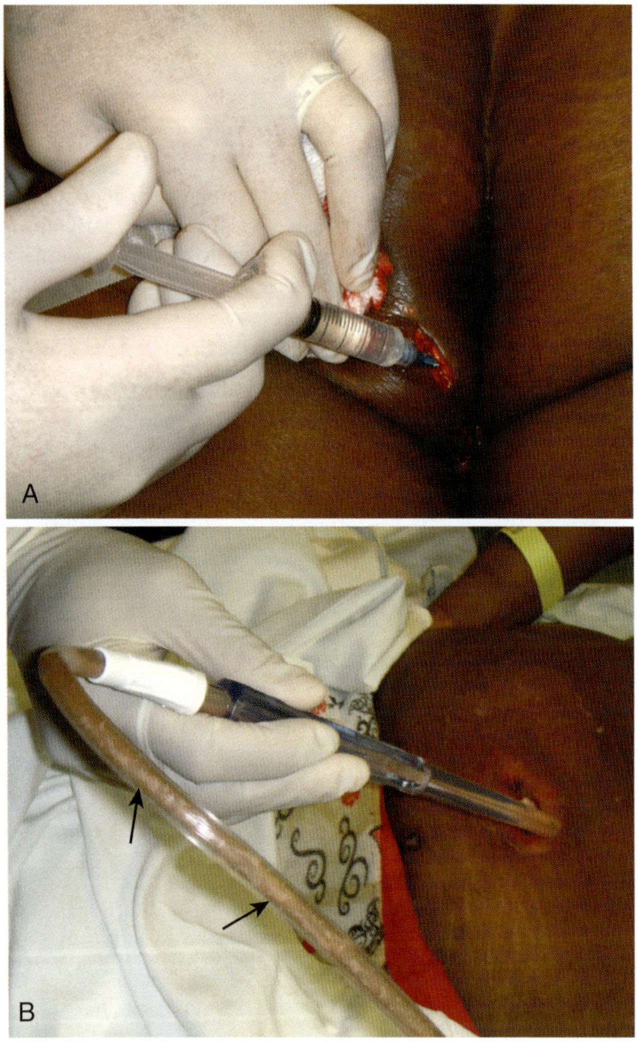

Fig. 37.10 (A) If pain persists while an abscess is being drained, pull the skin open and inject additional anesthetic into the subcutaneous tissue under direct vision. (B) This large abscess is draining copious pus. A tonsil suction device is used to both break up loculations and extract pus. Note the copious pus in the tubing *(arrows)*.

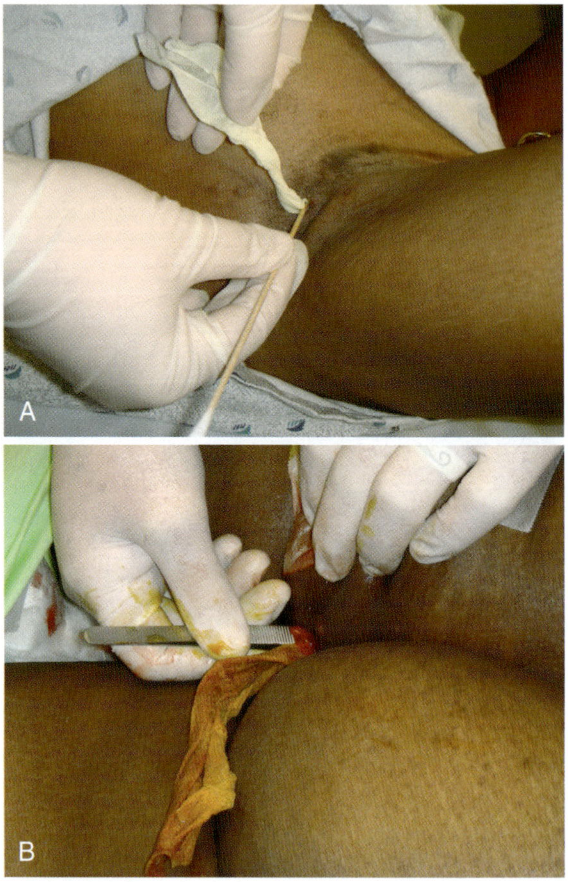

Fig. 37.11 Wound packing. (A) The traditional packing material is ¼-inch to ½-inch gauze, plain or with iodoform. (B) A 4-cm × 4-cm gauze pad soaked in povidone-iodine (Betadine) can be used to pack a large abscess, but care should be taken to avoid losing or forgetting about packing material in the base of a large abscess. Use an instrument to introduce the packing into the bottom of the abscess. Use only enough gauze to keep the incision open and avoid tight packing. Many clinicians now do not use packing at all for easily drained abscesses, as the value of packing is questionable and is not an absolute standard. Loop drainage is another alternative (see also Fig. 37.12).

In their 2023 meta-analysis Stout et al. reviewed 19 papers addressing the various techniques available to practitioners including traditional I&D, primary closure, primary closure with negative pressure (Wound vac), loop drainage (Box 37.3), and needle aspiration. They found a 75% empirical success rate of the traditional I&D procedure in the resolution of SSTI infection was accepted based on the median historic and contemporary evidence. Taking the median percentile, where available across the relative studies, the empirical efficiency of each SSTI management option can be ranked as follows[69]:

- Modified I&D with primary closure and suction therapy: 96%
- Loop drainage: 93.6%
- Traditional I&D: 75%
- Traditional I&D with primary closure: 75%
- Modified I&D with a straight catheter: 75%
- Needle aspiration: 54.5%

Loop technique was also found to be superior to traditional I&D in Gottlieb and Peska's meta-analysis in *The American Journal of Emergency Medicine* from January 2018. Their results were that the loop technique had a failure rate of 4.10% versus a failure rate of 9.43% for traditional I&D odds ratio of 2.63 (95% CI 1.04 to 6.63) in favor of higher failures in the CID group.[70]

Regarding healing times of traditional I&D versus primary closure technique, Singer et al. conducted a literature review in 2010 that showed healing times for primary closure were shorter (7.8 days [95% confidence interval {CI}, 7.3 to 8.3]), which was significantly shorter than that after secondary closure (15.0 days [95% CI, 14.3 to 15.7]; absolute difference, 7.3 days [95% CI, 6.9 to 7.6]). The rates of abscess recurrence were similar with both techniques (7.6% [95% CI, 4.6 to 10.6]) and those after secondary closure (11.1 days [95% CI, 7.5 to 14.7]; odds ratio, 0.66 [95% CI, 0.35 to 1.15]).[62]

Specific literature on healing times for other techniques is not found; however, it can be interpolated that healing times for loop procedure would fall between traditional I&D and primary closure.

In the Stout et al. study, mention is made of negative pressure appliances positively affecting outcomes. For treatment in the ED setting this would be more complicated than necessary for the majority of abscesses.

Vessel Loop Method of Incision and Drainage

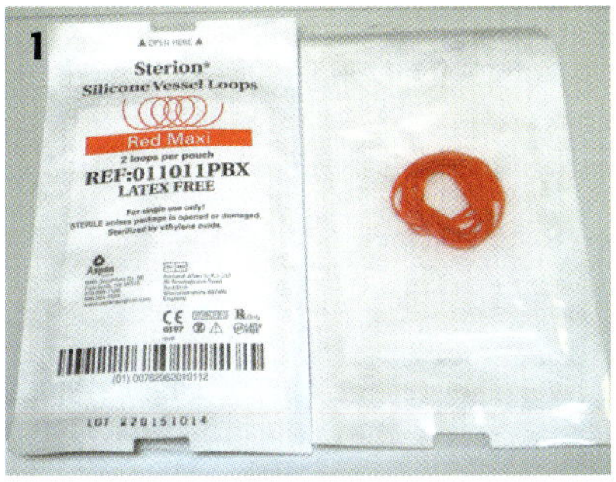

Instead of traditional gauze packing, a sterile silicone loop is used. This is commonly referred to simply as a "vessel loop" and is readily available from the operating room (this device is used by vascular surgeons).

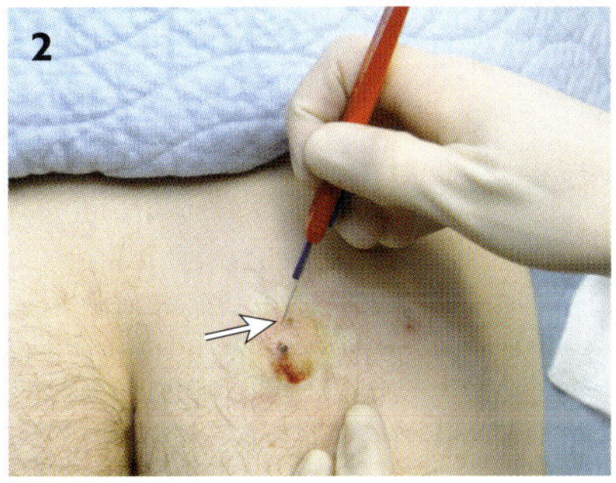

After sterile preparation and anesthetic infiltration, make a small (5–10 mm) incision at the periphery of the abscess. If possible, make the incision where the abscess is already pointing, noted by the *white arrow*.

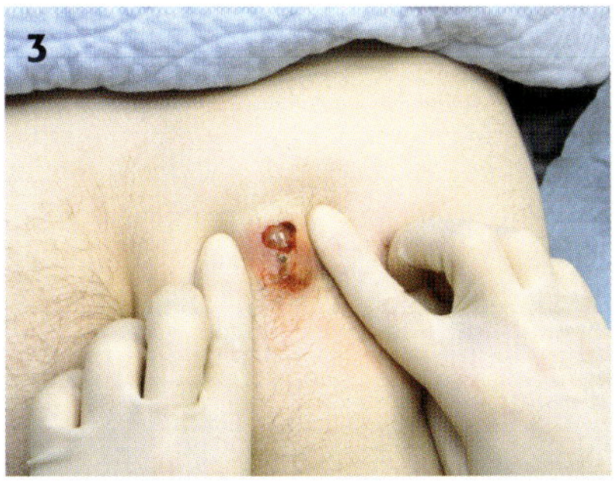

Express as much pus as possible from the incision. Obtain cultures if clinically indicated.

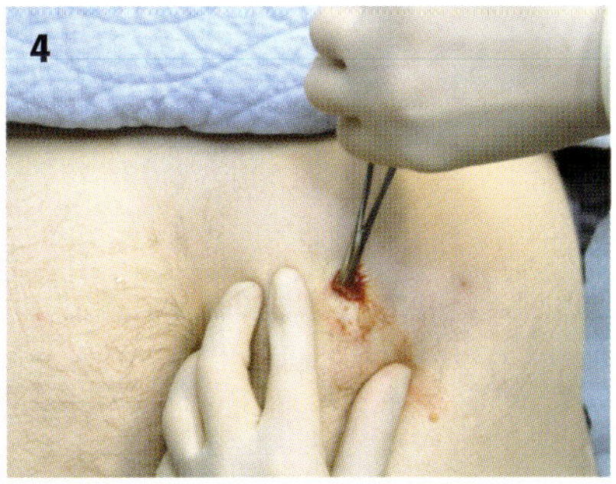

Use a hemostat to probe the abscess cavity and break up loculations.

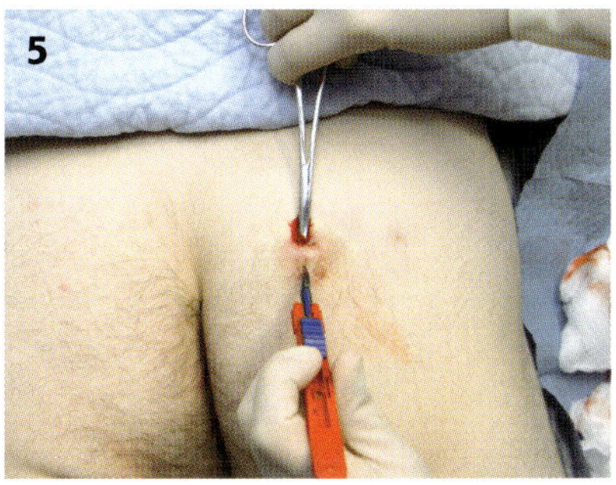

Probe with the hemostat to find the opposite edge of the abscess cavity. Position the tip of the hemostat underneath the area of the second incision, tent the skin, and make another stab incision over the hemostat tip.

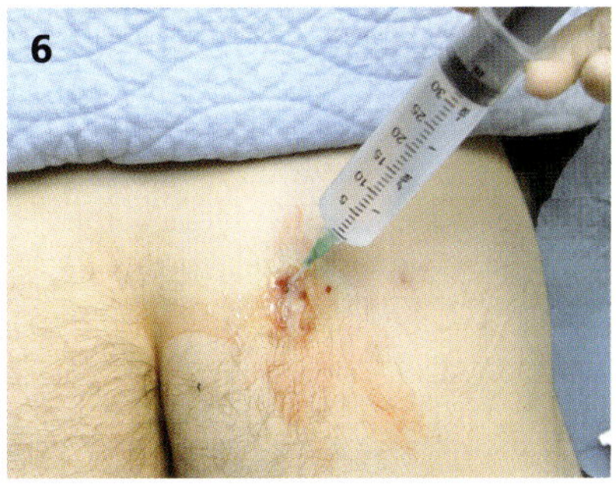

Optionally irrigate the cavity with a syringe and plastic intravenous catheter.

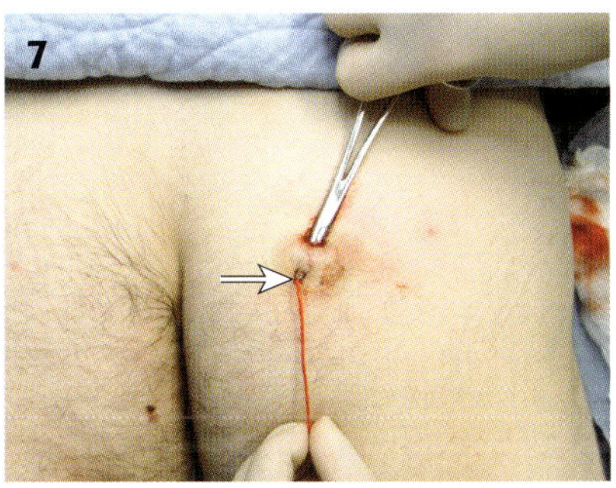

Place the hemostat through the cavity so that it exits the second incision. Grab the end of the vessel loop *(arrow)*.

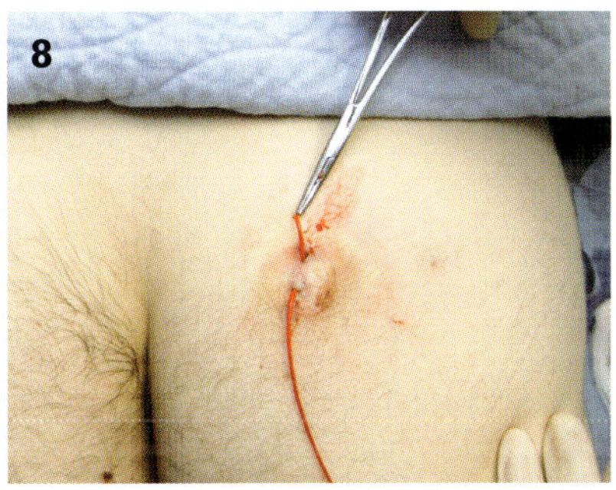

Pull the vessel loop through the abscess cavity so that it exits through the first incision.

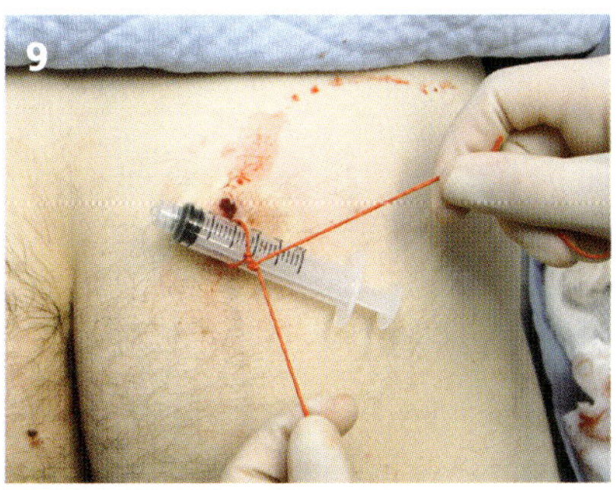

Tie the two ends of the vessel loop together. To avoid excessive skin tension, tie the loops over a syringe. Tie at least five knots, as the loop material is slippery. Tie the last two knots tightly, by stretching the loop almost to the breaking point.

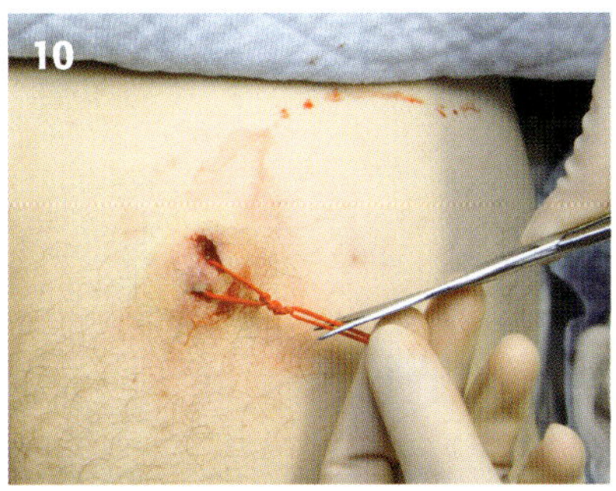

Remove the syringe, and then trim the ends of the vessel loop. Note that it is not tied tightly against the skin. Refer to the text for information on discharge instructions and loop removal.

Fig. 37.12 Vessel loop method of incision and drainage. For more details, see references 169-171.

BOX 37.3 Abscess Drainage by the Loop Drainage Technique

Historically, drainage of an abscess has involved the creation of a large skin incision to ensure adequate initial drainage of purulent material, followed by filling the abscess cavity with packing to promote continued drainage. The loop drain technique, an old technique now undergoing renewed interest, confers several advantages over the classic I&D. There are no packing changes, smaller incisions result in better cosmesis, and incisions drain as long as the loop is in place. This technique, though perhaps counterintuitive to classic teaching, provides excellent results for abscesses that previously would have been subjected to traditional incision, drainage, packing, and repacking protocols.

WHAT TYPE OF DRAIN TO USE

The original article describing this technique used a silicone vessel loop, a small Penrose drain, or a sterile rubber band. A readily available product is a vessel loop used by surgeons (Fig. 37.13, *step 1*).

TECHNIQUE

Step 1: Make a small (5–10 mm) incision with a No. 11 scalpel blade at the periphery of the abscess but still within its borders (see Fig. 37.13, *step 2*). Make the first incision where the abscess is pointing or already draining. Then probe the cavity with a hemostat and break up loculations (see Fig. 37.13, *step 4*). Pus should flow out of this puncture incision.

Step 2: With the hemostat inside the abscess cavity, find the opposite edge of the abscess cavity and position the tip of a hemostat underneath the area where you will make the second incision (see Fig. 37.13, *step 5*). Tent the skin from underneath. Make another stab with a No. 11 scalpel blade over the hemostat tip. Slide the tip of the hemostat through the new incision. At this stage, you should have two small incisions with a hemostat going into one, tunneling through the abscess cavity, and coming out of the other incision. There should be a maximum separation between the two incisions of up to 4 cm. If the abscess is larger than this, you can place more loops, depending on the shape of the abscess cavity.

Step 3: Using the hemostat that has traversed the cavity, grab the end of the loop drain and pull it back through the wound (see Fig. 37.13, *steps 7 and 8*). There should be a long end of the loop drain exiting each incision.

Step 4: Tie the two ends of the drain together without tension. Too much tension is painful and can necrose the skin between the incisions. One way to avoid excessive skin tension is to place a syringe between the skin and the drain while you are tying it (see Fig. 37.13, *step 9*). Tie the knots flush with the syringe; when the syringe is pulled away, there will be a loosely placed loop that will exert no tension on the incision sites. A finger should be able to be passed between the skin and loop. The drain is going to be slippery, so make about five knots. Tie the last two very tightly by stretching the loop almost to the breaking point. Trim the ends of the drain (see Fig. 37.13, *step 10*). An option at this point is to irrigate the abscess cavity through the stab incision. Cover the operative site with gauze as drainage will continue.

DISCHARGE INSTRUCTIONS

With the dressing removed and the loop still in place, the patient should bathe or shower twice a day for the first 3 days to promote continued drainage. Change the dressing at least twice daily or whenever saturated. Gently pull the loop back and forth once or twice a day to help keep the wound open.

WHEN TO REMOVE THE DRAIN

Remove the drain when the discharge stops and cellulitis improves. Simply cut the loop and pull it out. The loop is generally removed in approximately 5–10 days but may be removed sooner with a small abscesses or rapid healing. The patient now has only two small puncture sites that will heal over rather than a large scar that must heal by secondary intention.

From Tsoraides SS, Pearl RH, Stanfill AB, et al. Incision and loop drainage: a minimally invasive technique for subcutaneous abscess management in children. J Pediatr Surg. *2010;45:606-609.*

In sum, primary closure is non-inferior to traditional I&D and heals more quickly. Packing increases pain, delays closure, and complicates care.[70] Loop drainage has a lower failure rate than either of the previous techniques and healing times can reasonably be expected to fall between the open and closed techniques (see Video 37.3). Needle aspiration continues to have a limited role in smaller collections in specific areas, i.e., tonsil or breast given its relatively high failure rate when broadly compared with other techniques. Negative pressure devices have not seen wide deployment for abscesses treated in the ED. As always, each situation is different, and the provider will judge when to deploy which technique.

FOLLOW-UP EXAMINATION

A drained abscess should be reevaluated in 1 to 3 days. Most lesions are reevaluated 48 hours after the procedure. Patients with diabetes or patients with impaired healing capacity, mental impairment, or physical disabilities may require a home care nurse or hospital admission for more frequent wound care. Involvement of case managers to help set up care can be helpful. Wounds that are at high risk for complications, such as those about the face or hands or those with significant cellulitis, require close follow-up depending on the specific scenario. The patient should be encouraged, if possible, to play an active role in wound care. If complicated wound care is required, referral to wound care centers rather than multiple repeated ED visits should be the rule. Appropriate dressing changes should then follow until healing is completed. When all signs of infection (e.g., erythema, drainage, pain, and induration) have resolved and healthy granulation tissue is present, the patient may be discharged from medical care.

SPECIFIC ABSCESS THERAPY

Folliculitis, Furuncles, and Carbuncles

Folliculitis, furuncles, and carbuncles are common ED presentations in healthy patients with no specific predisposing risk factors, due to chronic colonization with a *staphylococcus* bacterium. Those in close contact with infected individuals are also at increased risk for similar infections. The pathogenesis

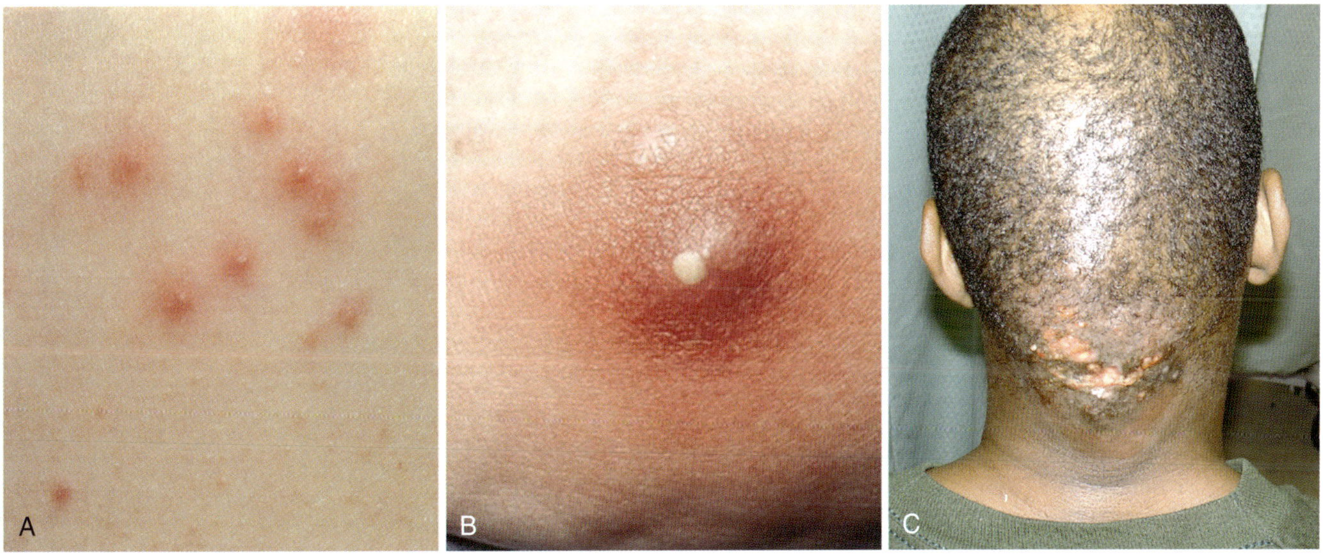

Fig. 37.13 (A) *Staphylococcus aureus* is a common cause of folliculitis, although other bacteria such as *Pseudomonas* may be responsible. Treatment consists primarily of local measures such as warm compresses and antibacterial soaps and ointments. (B) Furuncles are circumscribed abscesses of the skin and subcutaneous tissue that usually involve a hair follicle. (C) A carbuncle is a complicated abscess on the nape of the neck. It is very common in patients with diabetes. Carbuncles are usually caused by *S. aureus*, including community-acquired methicillin-resistant *S. aureus*. Because of its many crypts, loculations, and intercommunicating small abscesses, treatment by simple incision and drainage is often not readily curative. When fluctuance is appreciated, incision is indicated. One should avoid multiple small incisions because tissue circulation may be compromised. Antibiotics may augment healing of this abscess, but wide surgical excision may be required. (A, From Weston WL, Lane AT, Morelli JG, eds. *Color Textbook of Pediatric Dermatology*. 4th ed. Mosby; 2007. B, From Long SS, Pickering LK, Prober CG, et al. *Principles and Practice of Pediatric Infectious Diseases Revised Reprint*. 3rd ed. Churchill Livingstone; 2009.)

of staphylococcal disease is a complex host-bacterium interaction. *S. aureus* can invade the skin by way of a hair follicle or any size open wound. This can lead to destruction of the local tissue followed by vasodilation of the blood vessels, increasing the blood flow to the affected area (hyperemia). Subsequently, an exudative reaction occurs, with polymorphonuclear cell invasion. The process will extend, following the path of least resistance, and form an abscess. The abscess may then extend and form sinus tracts. Eventually dissemination may occur through invasion of blood vessels, leading to infection of other organ systems including osteomyelitis, meningitis, and endocarditis.[3]

Inflammation of a hair follicle caused by bacterial invasion is known as folliculitis. Folliculitis is a common inflammatory skin syndrome of the young and middle-aged but can be observed in all age groups. The underlying pathogenic mechanisms are unclear, but microbial involvement has been suggested.[71] Staphylococci, especially *S. aureus*, are mainly cultured from inflamed lesions and pustules[72,73] but fungal involvement (e.g., *Malassezia* species) has also been documented.[74] *Pseudomonas aeruginosa* is a rare cause of folliculitis. *Pseudomonas* folliculitis can develop after contact with contaminated water from swimming pools, hot tubs, and spa baths.[75]

Fungal folliculitis may be seen alone or in conjunction with *Staphylococcus* in individuals who use antibacterial antibiotics, oral corticosteroids, immunosuppressive treatments, topical steroids, have hyperhidrosis, or are obese.[76] Treatment generally consists of warm compresses to the affected area and antimicrobial soaps. If multiple sites are involved systemic antibiotics may be required. Recurrence may warrant repeat treatment along with chlorhexidine baths and bacitracin to the nares.

Furuncles, or "boils," are acute circumscribed abscesses of the skin and subcutaneous tissue that usually involve the hair follicles (Fig. 37.13). They are most frequently seen on the face, neck, buttocks, thigh, perineum, breast, and axilla. Pedicure-associated nontuberculous mycobacteria furunculosis has been reported. This is believed to be associated with the foot baths used and suboptimal cleaning methods.[77]

Carbuncles are groups of interconnected furuncles, most frequently seen at the base of the neck where the skin is thickest. The thickness of the skin leads to lateral extension. *S. aureus* is the most common organism seen. Large carbuncles can cause systemic symptoms and complications. A common risk factor for carbuncles is diabetes. Large carbuncles often require widespread surgical excision rather than simple I&D. Systemic therapy may be indicated in patients with widespread lesions, systemic symptoms, or in immunosuppressed patients.[18]

Most cases of recurrent staphylococcal skin infections are caused by autoinfection from skin lesions or nasal reservoirs. Treatment is directed at prevention, through eliminating the organisms. This can be accomplished by applying bacitracin to the nares, chlorhexidine baths, and good hygiene. If unsuccessful, systemic oral antistaphylococcal treatment is required, usually for 2 to 3 weeks. Close contacts often require treatment as well.[3,78]

S. aureus can cause suture abscesses. A suture abscess is often misdiagnosed as a wound infection, but is a local nidus of inflammation, infection, or both caused and potentiated by suture material. Such an abscess usually appears after sutures have been in place for 3 to 5 days, with single or multiple discrete areas of erythema and tenderness being noted at the site where the suture penetrates the skin. Simply removing the suture (a drop of pus may be expressed) and providing warm compresses and topical antibiotic ointment is generally all that is needed. The wide opening of the wound and systemic antibiotics are seldom required. When the suture is buried, a small incision should be followed by probing the wound with a small hook or bent needle (see Chapter 35) to snare the suture for removal.

Hidradenitis Suppurativa

HS is a chronic, relapsing, inflammatory follicular occlusive disease process that affects the apocrine sweat glands in the axilla, the inguinal region,[79] and the perineum (Fig. 37.14; Video 37.4). Its prevalence is 1% to 4% in industrialized countries; most affected individuals are young females.[80–82] The condition results from follicular inflammation and subsequent occlusion of the apocrine ducts by keratinous debris, which leads to ductal dilation, inflammation, and rupture into the subcutaneous area. The clinical manifestations vary, ranging from recurrent inflamed nodules and abscesses to draining sinus tracts and bands of severe scar formation. The associated pain, malodor, drainage, and disfigurement that accompany HS contribute to a profound psychosocial impact of the disease on many patients.[83] Depression and anxiety are associated with HS and completed suicide rates in those with HS are more than double the rates in controls.[84] Dysregulation of the immune response is thought to play a role, with some studies showing a response to immunosuppressive agents.[85,86] Occlusion of the hair follicle predisposes to secondary bacterial infection and subsequent abscess formation. In its early stages, it is indistinguishable from a simple furuncle. Progression and recurrence, however, lead to the distinctive appearance of multiple foci coupled with areas of induration and inflammation in various stages of healing. This chronic process can create draining fistulous tracts, often involving large areas that are not amenable to simple I&D procedures (see Fig. 37.14C).[87]

Genetic factors appear to be an important contributor in HS.[85,87] A hormonal impact has been suggested by observations of the rarity of HS in prepubertal children and improvement in HS during treatment with anti-androgenic agents.[87–93]

Other factors thought to be related include obesity and smoking. In a French case-control study of 302 clinically assessed patients with HS and 906 controls, 76% of the patients with HS versus 25% of the controls were current smokers. Additionally, a body mass index (BMI) of 30 or greater was present in 21% of patients with HS versus only 9% of controls, and a BMI between 25 and 29 was present in 22% of HS patients versus 17% of controls.[94] Conversely, weight loss has a positive effect on HS. The number of patients reporting HS symptoms after weight loss decreased by 35%. A weight loss of more than 15% was associated with a significant reduction of disease severity.[95] Environmental factors including antiperspirants and shaving[96] were implicated in the past, but later studies have not found any association.[97]

Bacterial cultures of specimens from HS lesions are frequently sterile or reflect organisms seen in other soft tissue abscesses. *Staphylococcus* is the most commonly isolated organism,[97] with *E. coli* and β-hemolytic streptococci being other essential pathogens. Enteric flora are often found in the perineal region. Many of these abscesses have multiple isolates, and anaerobic bacteria are frequently cultured. CA-MRSA is an increasing cause of such abscesses.

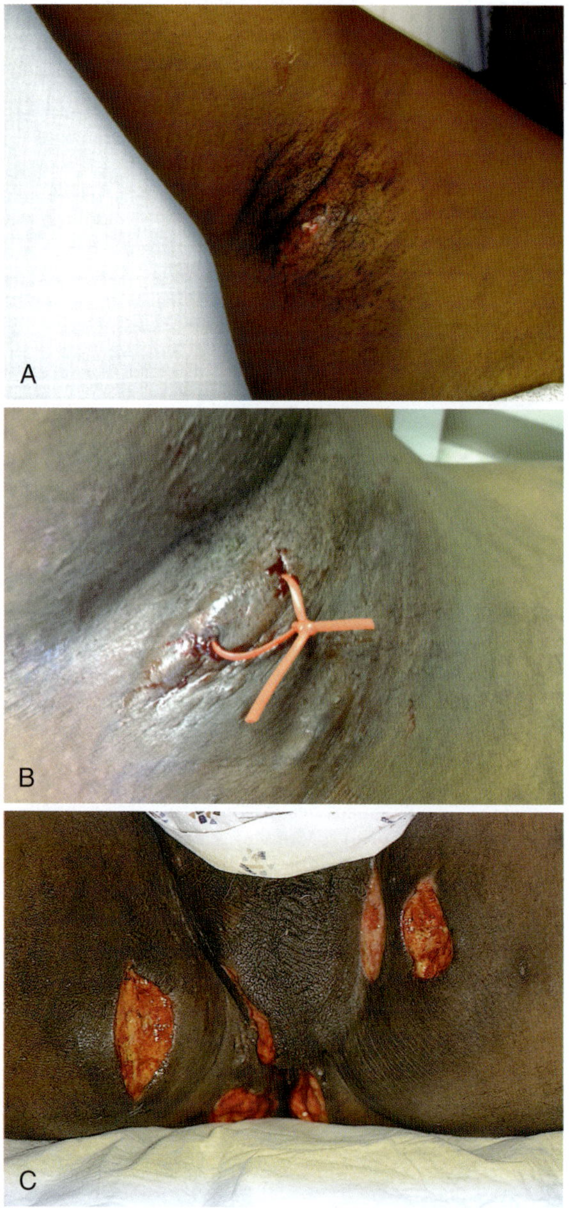

Fig. 37.14 (A) Axillary abscesses are common and recurrent. Community-acquired methicillin-resistant *Staphylococcus aureus* is an increasing cause. (B) Vessel loop drainage of an axillary abscess. (C) Hidradenitis suppurativa of the groin or axilla is a complicated series of abscesses that may not be amenable to simple incision and drainage. In this patient with involvement of the groin, extensive surgery was required to excise recurrent infection.

Clinical manifestations may be influenced by sex. Primary sites of involvement in females are the groin, upper inner thigh, axilla, chest, and buttocks or gluteal clefts.[98,99] In males, primary sites of involvement are the groin or thigh, axilla, perineal or perianal regions, and buttocks or gluteal cleft.[98–100] Both sexes regularly show involvement in non-intertriginous skin, particularly at skin compression and friction sites. Beltlines, waistbands, and brassiere straps or bands are also common locations.

Multiple disorders have been associated with HS including diabetes, obesity, dyslipidemia, hypertension, cardiovascular disease, Crohn's disease, and acne vulgaris. Long-standing, poorly controlled HS may lead to significant physical and emotional consequences such as strictures and contractures,[96] lymphatic obstruction, lymphedema of limbs and genitalia, malaise, depression, suicide, and long-term effects of chronic suppuration including anemia, hypoproteinemia, amyloidosis, infectious complications (lumbosacral epidural abscess, sacral bacterial osteomyelitis), arthritis, squamous cell carcinoma, and anemia.[101,102]

Multiple therapeutic approaches exist for the management of HS.[95] Any fluctuant area requires drainage, as described in the section on the I&D procedure. In patients with extensive cellulitis, a broad-spectrum, antistaphylococcal antibiotic should be used. Unfortunately, HS cannot be cured with localized I&D and/or antibiotics. If I&D is required for the relief of a secondary abscess, it should be made clear to the patient that this procedure does not cure the underlying disease.[99,103] The chronic nature of the disease produces multiple areas of inflammation and subcutaneous fistulous tracts that induce routine recurrences. The patient must be informed of this unfavorable prognosis and should be referred to a dermatologist or surgeon for long-term care.

Milder forms of the disease are initially treated with conservative measures. Many different approaches have been tried, with only limited degrees of success. Few controlled studies of treatment strategies have been performed. Patients are often counseled to lose weight, stop smoking, avoid skin trauma, wear light clothing, refrain from shaving, stop using scented deodorants, and improve personal hygiene. The benefits of these efforts are unknown. Topical clindamycin is often utilized as a first-line therapy for mild HS. A randomized 3-month trial supported its efficacy for mild inflammatory lesions and demonstrated the relative safety and tolerability of this regimen.[104] Oral antistaphylococcal antibiotics are most commonly used, with varying results.[104] Retrospective reviews looking at the efficacy of combination therapy (clindamycin and rifampin) have been promising, with some patients experiencing long-term remission, although diarrhea is a common side effect.[105,106] There have been reports of success with topical clindamycin,[107] hormone therapy in females, and laser therapy.[104]

Immunosuppressive therapy has been showing some promise. Previously immunosuppressive therapy with tumor necrosis factor-α inhibitors (infliximab, adalimumab, and etanercept)[107–110] had been successful in treating a few intractable cases. More recently, trials of adalimumab and secukinumab have been showing greater efficacy.[110]

In 2016 Kimball et al. published a report that adalimumab shows efficacy in treatment of HS in the Pioneer I and II trials. For the study, 307 patients were enrolled and clinical response rates at 3 months were higher in the treatment group (41%) than the control group (26%) in Pioneer 1. In Pioneer II, the differences were even greater 58.9% versus 27.6%.[110]

In February 2023, the *Lancet* published an article by Kimball et al., which demonstrated efficacy of secukinumab in HS. The SUNRISE and SUNSHINE studies were identical, multicenter, randomized, placebo-controlled, double-blind phase three trials done in 219 primary sites in 40 countries. They recruited 541 patients and found that 45% of patients in the experimental group had a sustained remission till the end of the follow-up at 52 weeks versus 34% in the placebo group when the medication was given every 2 weeks.[111] The study was funded by the manufacturer.

Advanced stages of the disease are managed by wide or local excision. Recurrence is more likely with smaller excisions than wider excisions. Delayed closure[112,113] may offer better results, but this has not been directly compared with primary closure. Wide excision may warrant skin grafting.[113]

Breast Abscess

Breast abscesses are localized collections of pus in the breast tissue (Video 37.5). They can occur in lactating and nonlactating breasts. They occur more commonly in African Americans, obese individuals, and smokers.[114,115] They are caused by normal skin bacteria that enter through a break or crack in the skin, usually the nipple (Fig. 37.15). The infection becomes established in parenchymal tissue and causes pain, swelling, and localized hyperemia. In its early stages, when cellulitis predominates, a breast abscess can be difficult to diagnose. In unclear cases, antibiotics may be curative. Cellulitis may progress to frank abscess formation. Females with a significant breast abscess can be quite ill and appear toxic.

The estimated incidence of inflammatory processes of the breast (mastitis) in lactating females ranges from 2% to 33%.[116] In lactating females, the infection is usually precipitated by milk stasis after weaning or missed feedings and usually occurs in the first 6 weeks of breastfeeding or during the weaning phase. The cause is usually bacterial invasion through a cracked or abraded nipple by *S. aureus*, including MRSA, or streptococci originating from the mouth of the nursing child.[117–119] Manifestations include redness, heat, pain, fever, and chills. Treatment consists of antistaphylococcal antibiotics, continued breast emptying with a breast pump, and application of heat. During treatment it is essential to encourage continued breast emptying to promote drainage. Nursing can be continued with either mastitis or breast abscess.[120] Breast abscesses are more common in lactating females. People who smoke and those with diabetes are at risk. These are also risk factors for recurrence. In addition, abscesses may be a complication of nipple piercing[121] or breast implants inserted under appropriate medical care,[122] as well as via illicit cosmetic procedures.[123] Most primary breast abscesses are caused by *S. aureus*, with MRSA becoming increasingly prominent.[115]

Less prominent pathogens include strains of *Streptococcus pyogenes*, *E. coli*, *Bacteroides*, *Corynebacterium* species, coagulase-negative staphylococci (e.g., *Staphylococcus lugdunensis)*, *P. aeruginosa*, *Proteus mirabilis*, and anaerobes.[121] Mixed flora are more commonly found in recurrent abscesses.[115]

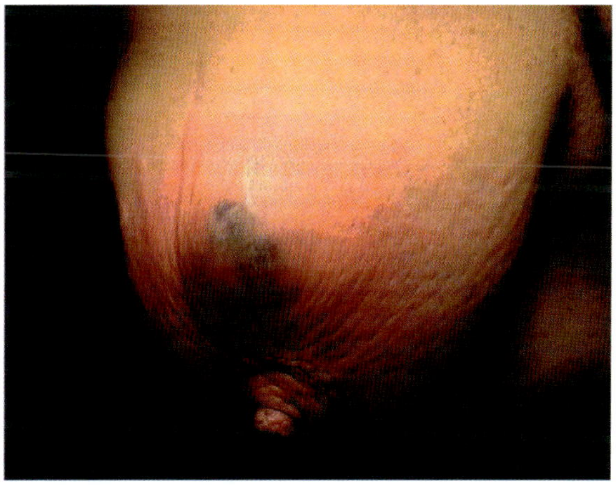

Fig. 37.15 Breast abscess. These abscesses are more common in lactating than in nonlactating females. If available, consultation with a breast surgeon is optimal and drainage may be deferred if the patient is nontoxic and the patient can be seen urgently by a specialist. Initial treatment recommendations call for ultrasound-guided needle aspiration and antibiotics, as opposed to traditional incision and drainage. Multiple aspirations may be required. (From Bland KI, Copeland EM III, eds. *The Breast*. 4th ed. Saunders; 2009.)

In the setting of nonsevere infection, in the absence of risk factors for MRSA, outpatient therapy may be initiated with dicloxacillin or cephalexin, pending culture results.[115] In the setting of β-lactam hypersensitivity, clindamycin may be used. If the community prevalence of MRSA is high, treatment with clindamycin or TMP-SMX should be considered. In the setting of severe infection, empiric inpatient therapy with vancomycin should be initiated.

Before undertaking any invasive intervention for a breast abscess, consultation with a breast specialist should be strongly considered. These patients need follow-up and may need more than one procedure to cure their infection.

Ultrasound-guided needle aspiration, as opposed to formal I&D, is becoming the standard of care for most breast abscesses.[124] Multiple aspirations may be required. When repeat aspirations are required, hospitalization may be the best way to facilitate treatment. Compared with I&D, aspiration causes less scarring, does not interfere with breastfeeding, and does not require procedural sedation.[124a] Christensen and associates[125] recommended that ultrasound-guided needle drainage replace surgery as first-line treatment of uncomplicated puerperal and nonpuerperal breast abscesses. Emerging treatment parameters favor ultrasound-guided needle aspiration for abscesses less than 3 cm in diameter and ultrasound-guided catheter drainage for abscesses 3 cm in diameter or larger.[126] Ultrasound images of breast abscesses appear as inhomogeneous, hyperechoic masses (Fig. 37.16). Repeat aspiration daily or every other day helps achieve complete resolution, with a mean of 3.5 aspirations.[126] Surgical drainage is warranted in the setting of compromise to the overlying skin and in cases in which the abscess is not responding to needle aspiration and antibiotics.[125,126]

Recurrent abscesses are a common, troublesome complication after traditional treatment with I&D and antibiotics.[127,128] Fortunately, the reported recurrence rate associated with ultrasound-guided aspiration or drainage procedures is quite low.[124–126] Patients with persistent recurrences should be managed by a surgeon for total excision of the involved area.

Although a breast abscess is rarely a harbinger of malignancy, it could be the initial manifestation of a metastatic process.[129–131] After needle aspiration or catheter drainage, send the aspirate for culture and cytologic examination, and perform a post drainage mammogram and ultrasound to evaluate for underlying or coexistent malignancy.[130] Inflammatory breast cancer would be an example of a malignancy presenting as an abscess. While aggressive, it is a very rare type of breast cancer representing perhaps 1% to 3% of the 240,000+ cases of all breast cancers every year (Fig 37.17A–C).

Pilonidal Abscess

Pilonidal sinuses are common malformations in the sacrococcygeal area (Fig. 37.18; Video 37.6). The cause of the sinus formation is unclear, and the malformation may occur during embryogenesis. Although pilonidal sinuses are present from birth, they do not usually manifest clinically until adolescence or early adulthood. Pilonidal cyst formation is thought to be secondary to blockage of a pilonidal sinus. The blockage is most commonly the result of hair in the region, and the lesion may in part be a foreign body (hair) granuloma. The result of this obstruction is repeated soft tissue infection, followed by drainage and partial resolution, with eventual recurrence of accumulation. Pilonidal abscess formation most frequently affects young adults with a 2:1 male to female ratio. The sinuses and cysts are lined with stratified squamous epithelium and, after excision, may be found to contain wads of hair and debris. When cultured, pilonidal abscesses generally yield mixed fecal flora with a preponderance of anaerobes.[132] The specific mechanism for the development of pilonidal disease is unclear, although hair and inflammation are contributing factors.[133]

As a person sits or bends, the natal cleft stretches, traumatizing hair follicles and thus creating pores. The pores collect debris and serve as a fertile environment for roots of hairs to lodge and become embedded. As the skin is drawn taut over the natal cleft with movement, negative pressure is created in the subcutaneous space drawing hair deeper into the pore, and the friction causes the hairs to form a sinus. Pilonidal disease typically develops in people with deep natal clefts. Subsequently, hairs become ingrown, bacteria invade, and an abscess develops in the sacrococcygeal region. At the current time, CA-MRSA infections are not common.

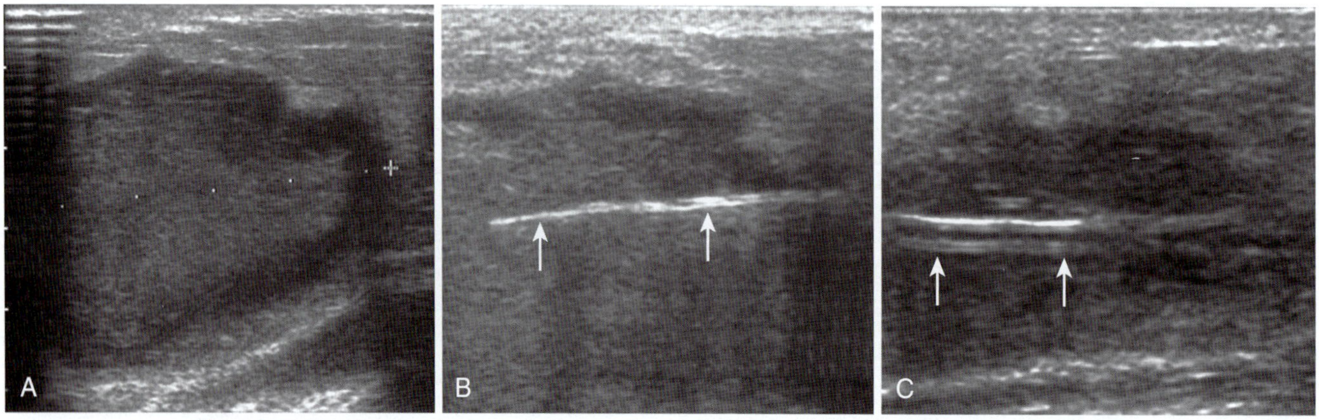

Fig. 37.16 Longitudinal images of ultrasound-guided drainage of an abscess in the lower inner quadrant of a 27-year-old woman's right breast 8 weeks after delivery. (A) Well-defined, slightly loculated, inhomogeneous hypoechoic abscess measuring 6 cm × 4 cm. *Dots* extend across the abscess, with the cursor at one margin of the abscess. (B) Pigtail catheter (7 Fr) containing a trocar *(arrows)* in the abscess cavity. (C) After removal of the trocar and aspiration of 70 mL of pus. The *parallel lines* represent the walls of the catheter *(arrows)*. (From Ulitzsch D, Nyman MKG, Carlson RA. Breast abscess in lactating women: US-guided treatment. *Radiology*.2004;232:904.)

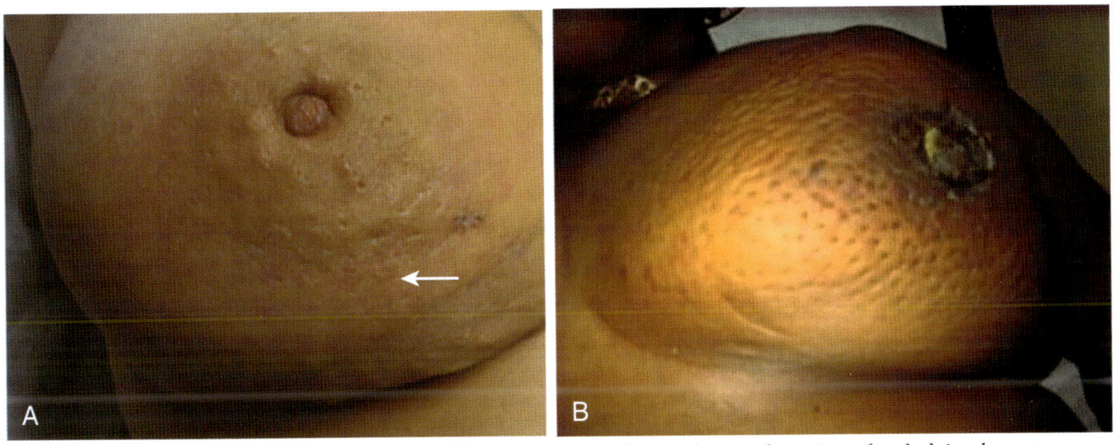

Fig. 37.17 Orange peel skin or "peau d'orange" is a skin texture change that can be a sign of underlying breast cancer

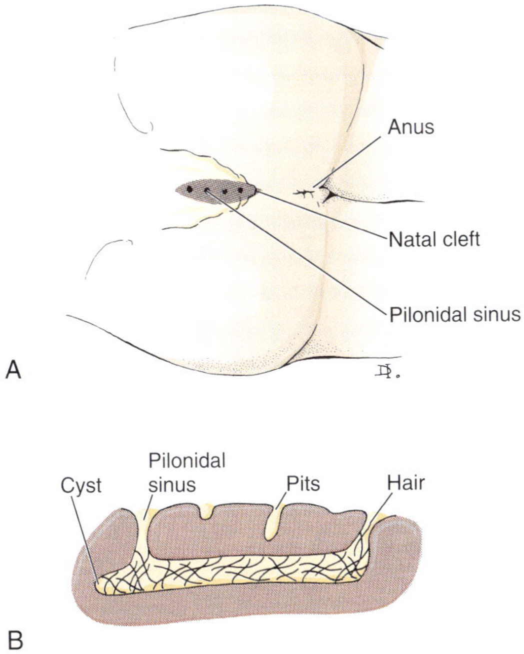

Fig. 37.18 Pilonidal sinus. (A) Sinuses occur in the midline, some 5 cm above the anus in the natal cleft. (B) Longitudinal section showing sinuses and pits. (From Hill GJ II, ed. *Outpatient Surgery*. 3rd ed. Saunders; 1988.)

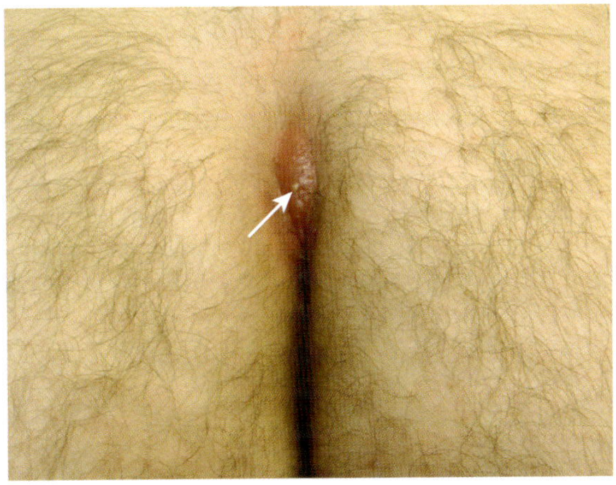

Fig. 37.19 Pilonidal abscess. An erythematous, indurated, fluctuant, and tender mass is found at the superior gluteal cleft. Small dimples or openings *(arrow)* can be seen on the surface of the abscess. Incision and drainage of pus, debris, and hair is an appropriate emergency department intervention, but these tend to recur and may require additional surgical treatment.

Patient presentation is highly variable. They may be completely asymptomatic with just a pilonidal cavity and sinus, or present with acute infection and drainage, or even chronic inflammation with drainage. There may even be multiple areas of drainage. Patients with a pilonidal abscess will seek care for back pain and local tenderness. On examination, the area is found to be indurated. Frank abscess formation may not be appreciated as sometimes the abscess is deep. One will usually see barely perceptible dimples or tiny openings at the rostral end of the gluteal crease (Fig. 37.19). A hair or slight discharge may be noticed at the opening. The discharge will usually be purulent or bloody. One may find a more caudal cyst or abscess, possibly with a palpable sinus tract connecting the two. The sinus and cyst may be draining chronically, or they may become infected as the size increases and blockage occurs.[133]

Treatment of an acutely infected cyst is the same as previously discussed for any fluctuant abscess: all hair and pus should be removed, and the lesion should be packed (see Figs. 37.6 and 37.12). The abscess cavity may be quite large and thus necessitates a lengthy incision to ensure complete drainage.[133] The incision should be made laterally, off-midline, or over the area of maximal fluctuance. A retrospective study examined 48 patients who had undergone lateral incisions and matched them with 48 patients who had undergone midline incisions. Those who had undergone midline incisions took approximately 3 weeks longer to heal than those drained with a lateral incision.[134] In general, reported median healing times after I&D vary between 12 and 63 days.[135,136] The area may be repacked at 2- to 4-day intervals as an outpatient procedure, although some prefer to discontinue packing after the first week. Antibiotic therapy is not generally required.

An I&D, however, is not the definitive procedure for pilonidal disease, as recurrence rates are up to 50% following primary intervention and as high as 10% to 30% after subsequent interventions.[137]

In a retrospective review of 73 consecutive patients with a first episode of acute pilonidal abscess treated by I&D, 42 (58%) healed primarily, with a median time to healing of 5 weeks; 9 of the 42 developed recurrence of pilonidal disease at a median follow-up of 60 months.[138] The overall cure rate following I&D was 45%. The patient should be referred to a general surgeon to remove the cyst and sinus after the inflammatory process has resolved. Small abscesses may be incised and drained as an outpatient procedure performed under local anesthesia. Still the disease process is often extensive, and general anesthesia may be required to achieve complete drainage. The extent of the cyst cavity and the volume of pus encountered on initial incision can be surprising.

Closure strategies for these potentially large wounds vary. Primary closure is associated with faster wound healing and a quicker return to work, but a delayed closure is associated with a lower likelihood of recurrence.[138]

Antibiotics are not commonly needed when treating these abscesses. They are reserved for concurrent surrounding cellulitis. However, patients with underlying immunosuppression, MRSA, concurrent systemic illness, or at high risk for endocarditis should be considered for ancillary antimicrobial prophylaxis in conjunction with surgical management.[44,48]

Perirectal Abscesses

Most anorectal infections originate in the cryptoglandular area located in the anal canal at the level of the dentate line. Abscesses within these glands can penetrate the surrounding sphincter and track in various directions, with larger abscesses occurring within the perianal, intersphincteric, ischiorectal, and supralevator spaces. A small number of anorectal abscesses have a noncryptoglandular cause such as Crohn's disease, atypical infection (e.g., tuberculosis, lymphogranuloma venereum), malignancy, or trauma.[139]

The prevalence of anal abscesses in the general population is probably much higher than seen in clinical practice as the majority of patients with symptoms referable to the anorectum do not seek medical attention. It is estimated that there are between 68,000 and 96,000 cases per year in the United States.[140] The mean age for presentation of anal abscess and fistula disease is in the third and fourth decades of life.[140] Adult males are three times as likely to develop an abscess and/or fistula compared with females.[140] The condition is seen more in the summer and spring months. Although often a concern of the patient, data do not support that there is an increased risk from hygiene, anal-receptive intercourse, diabetes, obesity, race, or altered bowel habits.[140]

Perirectal infections can range from minor irritation to fatal illness. Clandestine infections often occur in diabetics. Successful management depends on early recognition of the disease process and adequate surgical therapy. Small abscesses can initially be managed on an outpatient basis with simple I&D, described previously. Because of the morbidity and mortality associated with inadequate treatment of these conditions, patients with large and deep abscesses should be promptly admitted to the hospital for evaluation and treatment under general or spinal anesthesia (Fig. 37.20).

It is important to understand the anatomy of the anal canal and the rectum to appreciate the pathophysiology of these abscesses and their treatment (Fig. 37.21). The mucosa of the anal canal is loosely attached to the muscle wall. At the dentate line, where columnar epithelium gives way to squamous epithelium, there are vertical folds of tissue called the rectal columns of Morgagni that are connected at their lower ends by small semilunar folds called anal valves. Under these valves are invaginations termed anal crypts. Within these crypts are collections of ducts from the anal glands. These glands are believed to be responsible for the genesis of most, if not all, perirectal abscesses. These glands often pass through the internal sphincter but do not penetrate the external sphincter.

The muscular anatomy divides the perirectal area into compartments that may house an abscess, depending on the direction of spread of the foci of the infection (Fig. 37.22).[141]

The circular fibers of the intestinal coat thicken at the rectum-anus junction to become the internal anal sphincter. The muscle fibers of the levator ani fuse with those of the outer longitudinal fibers of the intestinal coat as it passes through the pelvic floor. These conjoined fibers are connected by fibrous tissue to the external sphincter system, which consists of three circular muscle groups.

Pathophysiology

As described previously, the anal glands are mucous-secreting structures that terminate in the area between the internal and external sphincters. It is believed that most perirectal

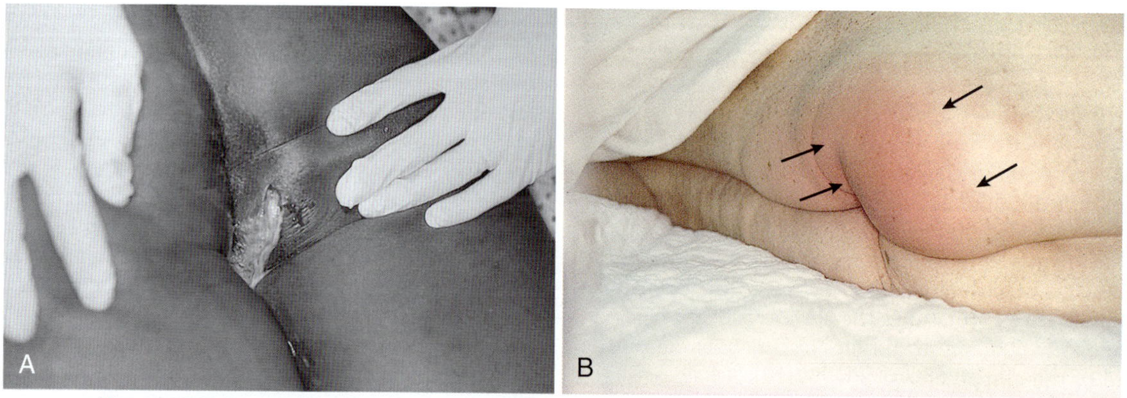

Fig. 37.20 Perirectal abscess. Most cases require general surgical consultation for drainage. (A) If a perirectal abscess spontaneously ruptures and drains, formal incision, drainage, and packing should still be performed. (B) A deep, poorly localized perirectal abscess of this size simply cannot be adequately drained in the emergency department (ED). *Arrows* outline the area of induration. This patient requires extensive drainage under general anesthesia. A CT scan may further evaluate the location of the abscess. Broad-spectrum intravenous antibiotics may be started in the ED before definitive surgical intervention. If necessary, a stab incision in the ED to initiate drainage may be attempted, especially if definitive operating room treatment is delayed.

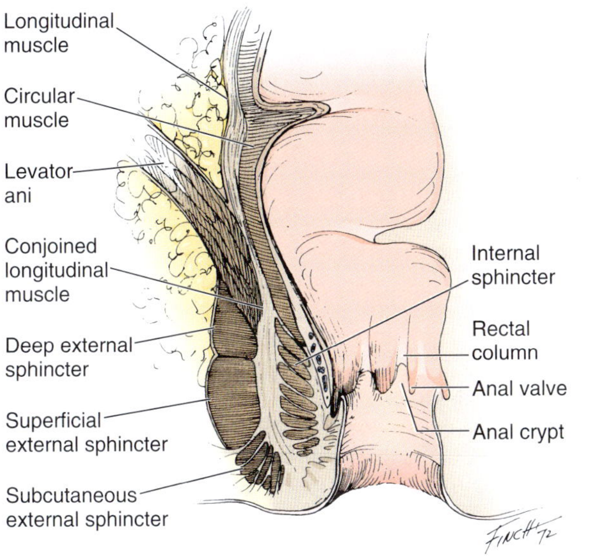

Fig. 37.21 Schematic coronal section of the anal canal and rectum. (From Schwartz SI, Lillehei RC, eds. *Principles of Surgery*. 2nd ed. McGraw-Hill; 1974.)

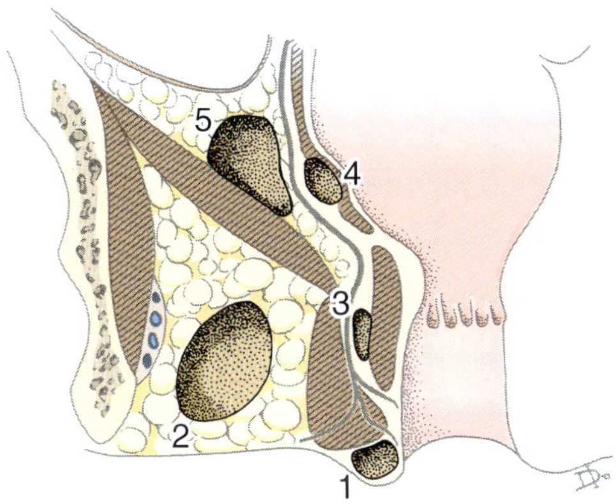

Fig. 37.22 Classification of perirectal abscesses. *1*, Perianal. *2*, Ischiorectal. *3*, Intersphincteric. *4*, High intramuscular. *5*, Pelvirectal. (From Hill GJ II, ed. *Outpatient Surgery*. 3rd ed. Saunders; 1988.)

infections begin in the intersphincteric space secondary to blockage and subsequent infection of the anal glands. Normal host defense mechanisms are overwhelmed, and this results in invasion and overgrowth by bowel flora.[142]

An ischiorectal abscess is formed if the infection spreads across the external sphincter laterally. If the infection dissects rostrally, it may continue between the internal and external sphincters and give rise to a high intramuscular abscess. The infection may also dissect through the external sphincter over the levator ani to form a pelvirectal abscess.[142]

The typical microbial composition of a perianal abscess is mixed comprising *Escherichia coli*, *B. fragilis*, *Staphylococcus aureus*, *Streptococcus* species, *Proteus vulgaris*, and *Peptostreptococcus* species. Brown et al. in their 2009 study found that the prevalence of MRSA in the patient population was 19%, and when this organism was cultured, the patient only received adequate coverage 33% of the time.[143]

When infection of an anal crypt extends by way of the perianal lymphatics and continues between the mucous membrane and the anal muscles, a perianal abscess forms at the anal orifice. A perianal abscess is the most common variety of perirectal infections. A perianal abscess lies immediately beneath the skin in the perianal region at the lowermost part of the anal canal. It is separated from the ischiorectal space by a fascial septum that extends from the external sphincter and is continuous with the subcutaneous tissues of the buttocks. The infection may be small and localized or very large, with a wall of necrotic tissue and a surrounding zone of cellulitis.[3] Perianal abscesses may be associated with a fistula-in-ano. A fistula-in-ano is an inflammatory tract with an external opening in the skin of the perianal area and an internal opening in the mucosa of the anal canal. A fistula-in-ano is usually formed after the partial resolution of a perianal abscess, and its presence is suggested by the recurrence of these abscesses with intermittent drainage. The external opening of the fissure is usually a red, elevated piece of granulation tissue that may exhibit purulent or serosanguineous drainage on compression. In many cases the tract can be palpated as a cord. Patients with anal fistulas should be referred for definitive surgical excision.[142]

Ischiorectal abscesses are fairly common. They are bounded superiorly by the levator ani, inferiorly by the fascia over the perianal space, medially by the anal sphincter muscles, and laterally by the obturator internus muscle. These abscesses may commonly be bilateral; if so, the two cavities communicate through a deep postanal space to form a "horseshoe" abscess.

Intersphincteric abscesses are less common. The internal and external sphincters bind them and may extend rostrally into the rectum, thereby separating the circular and longitudinal muscle layers. Causes of perirectal abscesses other than the cryptoglandular process have been documented but are fairly rare. Hemorrhoids, anorectal surgery, episiotomy, or local trauma may cause abscess formation by altering the local anatomy and thus destroying natural tissue barriers to infection. Perirectal abscesses may serve as a portal of entry for organisms responsible for necrotic soft tissue infections such as Fournier's gangrene.[144]

Physical and Laboratory Findings

A perianal abscess is not generally difficult to diagnose. The severe throbbing pain in the perianal region is acute and aggravated by sitting, coughing, sneezing, and straining. There is swelling, induration, tenderness, and a small area of cellulitis in proximity to the anus. Rectal examination of a patient with a perianal abscess reveals that most of the tenderness and induration are located below the level of the anal ring. Deeper abscesses may be difficult to localize and identify. Computed tomography is often the first imaging study, given its ready availability. The sensitivity of computed tomography for anorectal abscesses, however, is only 77%.[145] Therefore magnetic resonance imaging should also be considered when clinical suspicion is high.

Transperineal ultrasound for abscesses has been reported to have sensitivities ranging from 84.9% to 100% in several studies evaluated by Wright et al. in 2015.[146] As always if the initial imagining does not fit the clinical picture, a different modality should be employed given the ready availability of MRI, CT, and US.

Patients with ischiorectal abscesses have fever, chills, and malaise, but at first there is less pain than with a perianal abscess. Initially on physical examination, one will see an asymmetry of the perianal tissue; later, erythema and induration are apparent. Digital examination reveals a large, tense, tender swelling along the anal canal that extends above the anorectal ring. If both ischiorectal spaces are involved, the findings are bilateral.

Patients with intersphincteric abscesses usually have dull, aching pain in the rectum rather than in the perianal region. No external aberrations of the perianal tissues are noted, but tenderness may be present. On digital examination one frequently palpates a soft, tender, sausage-shaped mass above the anorectal ring; if the mass has already ruptured, the patient may give a history of passage of purulent material during defecation.[147]

Diagnosis of pelvirectal abscesses may be very difficult. Usually, fever, chills, and malaise are present, but because the abscess is so deeply seated, few or no signs or symptoms are present in the perianal region. The rectal or vaginal examination may reveal a tender swelling that is adherent to the rectal mucosa above the anorectal ring.

Marcus et al. found that white blood cell counts were not elevated in 23 of 91 patients who had a confirmed perirectal abscess.[148] Cultures of perirectal abscesses usually show mixed infections involving anaerobic bacteria, most commonly *B. fragilis* and gram-negative enteric bacilli. MRSA, though less common, should also be considered in endemic areas.[143]

Treatment

Small, well-defined perianal abscesses without deeper perirectal involvement are the only perirectal infections that lend themselves to outpatient therapy. All other perirectal abscesses should be drained in the OR, so surgical consultation is required. The result of I&D is almost immediate pain relief and rapid infection resolution. Indications for inpatient drainage are failure to obtain adequate anesthesia, systemic toxicity, extension of the abscess beyond a localized area, or recurrence of a perianal abscess. The presence of a fistula-in-ano may cause recurrence.[141]

Drain a perianal abscess through a cruciate incision because if a simple linear incision is used, the abscess cavity has a propensity to close prematurely without adequate drainage. With either technique, make an incision over the most fluctuant area. If a simple linear incision is used, lightly pack the abscess cavity for at least 24 hours to ensure adequate drainage. It is extremely painful to probe a perianal abscess and to break up loculations, so liberal analgesia is advised, and conscious sedation is appropriate. Advise the patient to begin sitz baths at home 24 hours after the procedure. Replace the packing at 48-hour intervals until the infection has cleared and granulation tissue has appeared. This usually occurs within 4 to 6 days. Cultures are generally not required in the treatment of an anal abscess as antibiotics are not generally needed. Cultures may be useful to distinguish between a cryptoglandular abscess (typically due to colonic flora) and an abscess of the perianal skin (typically due to staphylococcal species). Cultures may also be useful in patients who would typically be treated with antibiotics, including those with valvular heart disease, immunosuppression, extensive cellulitis, and diabetes; patients who have been on multiple courses of antibiotics; have pain out of proportion to findings, or who may have an unusual pathogen (e.g., immunocompromised patients); and patients with leukemia or lymphoma who may have unusual or resistant bacteria.[19]

Perirectal abscesses are recognized as a relatively common cause of fever in granulocytopenic patients. These abscesses have a different bacteriologic profile: *P. aeruginosa* organisms are isolated most frequently. These patients are initially seen later because pain develops later, and fever may be the first manifestation. Therefore, any patients who are granulocytopenic with vague anorectal complaints, especially those with fever, should be examined carefully for perirectal abscesses. Any abscess found should be drained immediately under appropriate anesthesia, and extensive IV antibiotic coverage should be initiated.

Infected Sebaceous Cyst

An infected sebaceous cyst is a common entity that appears as a cutaneous abscess. MRSA is increasingly causing such infections. Sebaceous cysts, caused by obstruction of sebaceous gland ducts, can occur anywhere on the body. The cyst becomes filled with a thick, cheesy, sebaceous material, and the contents frequently become infected. Sebaceous cysts can be quite large and may persist for many years before they become infected. When infected, they appear clinically as tender, fluctuant subcutaneous masses, often with overlying erythema.

The initial treatment of an infected sebaceous cyst is simple I&D (Fig. 37.23). The loop drainage technique may not be suited for this abscess. The thick sebaceous material must be expressed because it is too thick to drain spontaneously. A significant difference exists between infected sebaceous cysts and other abscesses. A sebaceous cyst has a definite pearly white capsule that must be excised to prevent recurrence. Traditionally, in the presence of significant inflammation, it is preferable to drain the infection initially and remove the shiny capsule on the first follow-up visit or at a later visit when it can be more easily identified. Alternatively, the entire cyst can be removed during the initial incision. At the time of capsule removal, the edges are grasped with clamps or hemostats, and the entire capsule is removed by sharp dissection with a scalpel or scissors. After excision of the capsule, the area is treated in the same manner as a healing abscess cavity. Simple drainage without excision of the capsule often leads to recurrence.

Paronychia

Paronychia is an infection localized around the nail root (Fig. 37.24; Videos 37.7 and 37.8). It is a common infection, probably caused by frequent trauma to the delicate skin around the fingernail and the cuticle. These types of infections have also been linked to "insults" induced by nail cosmetics (mechanical trauma, irritant reactions, and allergic reactions)[149] and to several occupations (e.g., hair cutting and meat handling).[150] When a minor infection begins, the nail itself may act like a foreign body. Usually, the infectious process is limited to the area above the nail base and underneath the eponychium (cuticle), but occasionally, it may spread to include tissue under the nail as well and form a subungual abscess. *Staphylococcus* is the most common cultured organism from these lesions; however, anaerobes and numerous gram-negative organisms may be isolated.[151] Paronychia in children is often caused by anaerobes and is believed to be the result of finger sucking and nail biting. Occasionally, a group A β-hemolytic streptococcal infection will develop in a paronychia in a child with streptococcal pharyngitis who engages in thumb sucking.[154] Paronychia involving CA-MRSA has been reported.[154,155] Paronychia has also been reported in association with antiretroviral therapy for HIV infection[154] and with use of epidermal growth factor inhibitors.[155]

A paronychia is a swelling and tenderness of the soft tissue along the base or the side of a fingernail (Fig. 37.25). Pain, often around a hangnail, usually prompts a visit to the ED. The infection begins as cellulitis and may form a frank abscess. If the nail bed is mobile, the infectious process has extended

Sebaceous Cyst Excision

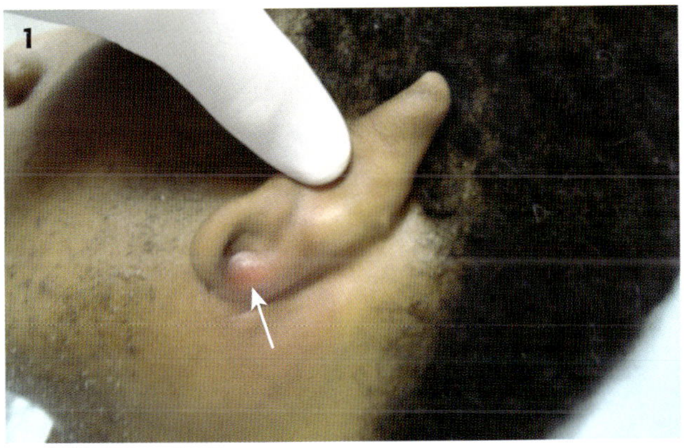

This patient has an infected sebaceous cyst on the posterior of the earlobe *(arrow)*. These lesions are typically tender, fluctuant, subcutaneous masses, often with overlying erythema.

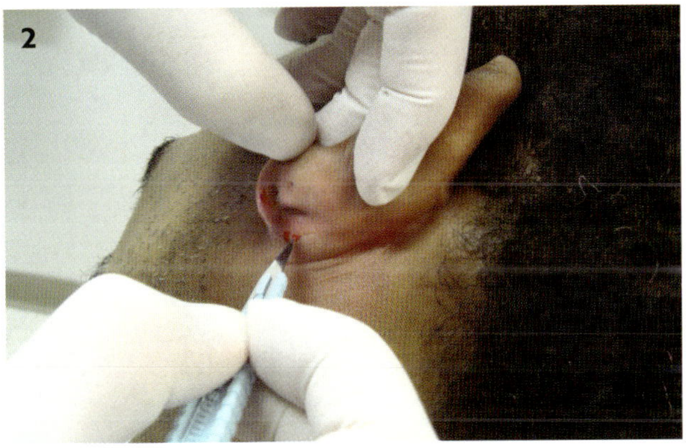

Drain the cyst as you would a typical abscess. The thick sebaceous material must be expressed manually, because it is too thick to drain spontaneously.

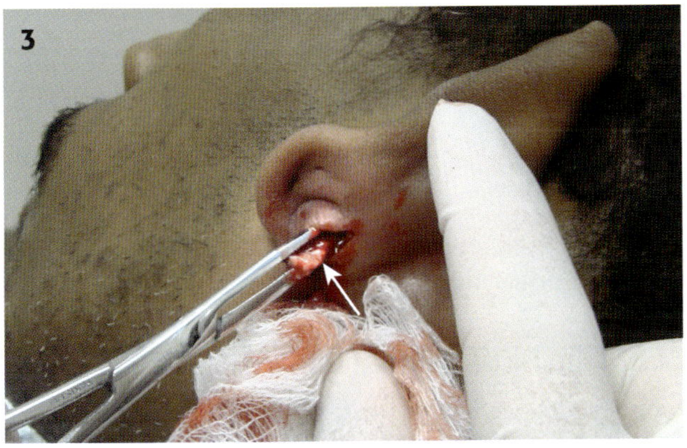

Sebaceous cysts differ from simple abscesses in that they have a distinct capsule with a pearly white appearance *(arrow)*. This capsule must be removed to prevent recurrence. This may be done initially or on a return visit once the inflammation has subsided.

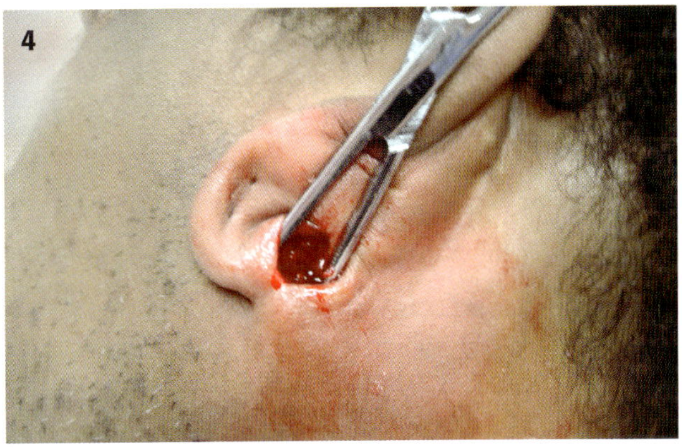

Appearance of the cavity after excision of the capsule. Treat the lesion as you would any other abscess, with wound packing and timely follow-up care.

Fig. 37.23 Excision of an infected sebaceous cyst. Loop drainage is not applicable to this abscess due to the need for capsule removal.

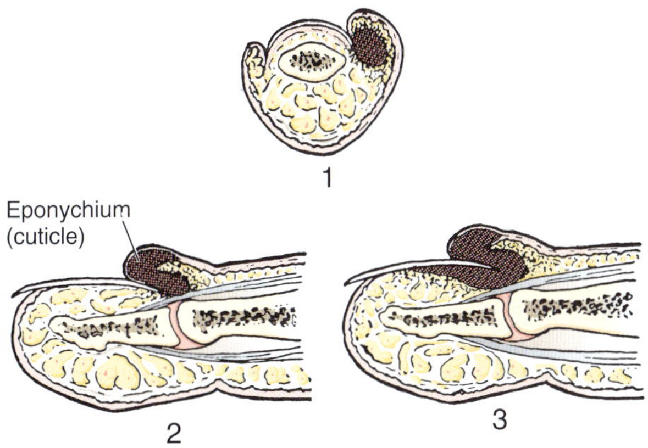

Fig. 37.24 Paronychia. *1*, Abscess at the side of the nail. *2*, The infection has extended around the base of the nail. It has raised the eponychium but has not penetrated under the nail. *3*, End stage of paronychia, with a subeponychial and subungual abscess. (From Wolcott MW, ed. *Ferguson's Surgery of the Ambulatory Patient*. 5th ed. Lippincott; 1974.)

under the nail, and a more extensive drainage procedure should be performed. Although no comparative trials of surgical management versus oral antibiotics have been performed,[156] some general guidelines for managing paronychias have become established in clinical practice. If soft tissue swelling is present without fluctuance, treatment consists of frequent warm soaks (three times a day) and a short course of oral antibiotics. Topical antibiotics with or without topical corticosteroids have also been used.[157] Incision will be of little value at the early cellulitic phase. Antibiotic treatment of localized infection is summarized in Table 37.1. If significant cellulitis is present, a broad-spectrum antistaphylococcal antibiotic (cephalosporin or semisynthetic penicillin) may be tried.

When a definite abscess has formed, drainage is usually quickly curative. Several invasive operative approaches have been suggested. Actual skin incision or removal of the nail is rarely required, and neither procedure should be the initial form of treatment. One can invariably obtain adequate drainage by lifting the eponychial fold away from the nail matrix to

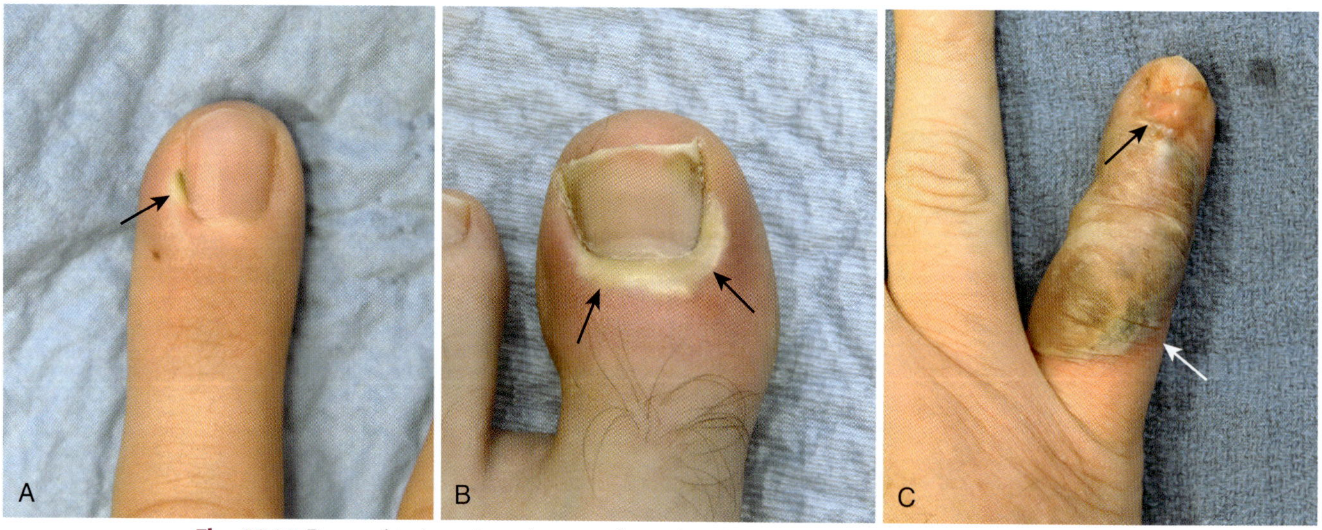

Fig. 37.25 Paronychia in various degrees of severity. (A) Paronychia of the index finger. In this early stage of abscess formation, the collection is limited to the lateral nail fold *(arrow)*. (B) More advanced paronychia of the great toe. The abscess has spread around the base of the nail and lifted the eponychium *(arrows)* but has not yet spread under the nail. There is associated cellulitis on the distal portion of the toe. (C) Even more advanced paronychia, with subungual extension *(black arrow)* and cellulitis extending up the finger and onto the dorsum of the hand *(white arrow)*. This patient required removal of the nail and intravenous antibiotics.

allow the pus to drain. This is usually curative because a paronychia is not a cutaneous abscess per se, but rather a collection of pus in the potential space between the cuticle and the proximal end of the fingernail. Drainage may be accomplished after a digital nerve block is performed. After softening the eponychium by soaking, advance a No. 11 scalpel blade, scissors, or a 21- to 23-gauge needle parallel to the nail and under the eponychium at the site of maximal swelling (Fig. 37.26). When using the needle approach, some patients may tolerate the procedure without needing digital blockade. Pus escapes rapidly, with immediate relief of pain. A tourniquet placed at the base of the finger may limit bleeding and aid the clinician in determining the exact extent of the infection during the drainage procedure.

If more than a tiny pocket of pus is present, fan the knife tip or needle or spread the scissors under the eponychium while keeping the instrument parallel to the plane of the fingernail (see Fig. 37.26, *steps 5 and 6*). When a large amount of pus is drained, slip a small piece of packing gauze under the eponychium for 24 hours to provide continual drainage. Given the prevalence of MRSA, cultures are generally indicated. Antibiotics are frequently prescribed, although they are not essential if drainage is complete or the surrounding area of cellulitis is minimal. An alternative to systemic antibiotics is to keep the operative site bathed in antibiotic ointment. After the anesthesia has worn off, start the patient on frequent soaks in warm tap water at home. In most cases, the patient may easily remove the packing. At 24 to 36 hours, soak the finger in warm water and pull the gauze out; a repeated visit to a clinician is not required if healing is progressing, but follow-up examinations should always be encouraged. Once the packing is removed, cover the area with a dry, absorbent dressing. Apply an antibiotic ointment periodically to the site for several days.

Most paronychias resolve in a few days, and one to two postoperative visits should be scheduled to evaluate healing and reinforce home care. For compliant patients with a small paronychia, home care alone may suffice after the initial drainage. Clinical infection lasting longer than a few weeks should prompt evaluation for osteomyelitis of the distal phalanx, a well-known but rare complication of even a properly drained paronychia.

Chronic Paronychia (Table 37.3)

Patients occasionally come to the ED complaining of a chronic, indolent paronychial infection. These seldom respond to ED intervention. Frank purulence is rarely present, and conservative treatments are often unsatisfactory. Recent scholarship contends that a chronic paronychia is a form of hand eczema with a trigger of an environmental allergen. In this context, topical steroids are considered the best treatment. Antifungals have a role if the compromised area is subsequently colonized with candida. Refer these patients to a dermatologist or hand surgeon because of the prolonged treatment required.[158]

Herpetic Whitlow

Herpetic whitlow is an extremely contagious infection of the distal phalanx caused by herpes simplex virus (type 1 or 2) (Fig. 37.27). Herpes infection of the hand predominantly presents in a bimodal age distribution: children younger than 10 years and young adults between 20 and 30 years of age. In children, herpetic whitlow tends to be associated with gingivostomatitis caused by herpes simplex 1, whereas adults most commonly harbor herpes simplex 2. Inoculation occurs through a discontinuity in the skin.[159] Health care providers exposed to oral secretions (e.g., dental hygienists and respiratory therapists) and patients with other herpes infections are most commonly infected.[160]

After a 2-day to 2-week incubation period, an infected individual may experience prodromal signs and symptoms such as fever, malaise, lymphadenitis, and axillary lymphadenopathy. In the affected finger the infection is characterized by tenderness, followed by throbbing or burning pain (out of proportion

TABLE 37.3 Common Hand Infections, Usual Offending Organisms, and Appropriate Therapeutic Regimens

CONDITION	MOST COMMON OFFENDING ORGANISMS	RECOMMENDED ANTIMICROBIAL AGENTS	COMMENTS
Paronychia	Usually *Staphylococcus aureus* or streptococci; *Pseudomonas*, gram-negative bacilli, and anaerobes may be present, especially in patients with exposure to oral flora	First-generation cephalosporin or antistaphylococcal penicillin; if anaerobes or *Escherichia coli* are suspected, oral clindamycin (Cleocin) or a β-lactamase inhibitor such as amoxicillin-clavulanate potassium (Augmentin)	I&D should be performed if infection is well established If infection is chronic, suspect *Candida albicans* Early infections without cellulitis may respond to conservative therapy
Felon	*S. aureus*, streptococci	First-generation cephalosporin or antistaphylococcal penicillin	I&D should be performed if infection is well established Oral antibiotic therapy is usually adequate
Herpetic whitlow	Herpes simplex virus	Supportive therapy	Antivirals may be prescribed if infection has been present for <48 h For recurrent herpetic whitlow, suppressive therapy with an antiviral agent may be helpful Consider antibiotics if secondarily infected I&D is contraindicated

I&D, Infection and drainage.
Adapted from Clark DC. Common acute hand infections. *Am Fam Physician*. 2003;68:167.

to the findings on physical examination), edema, and erythema. Vesicles containing clear, bloody, or cloudy fluid form and mark the most infectious stage of the process. Vesicles may coalesce to form a bulla. Viral vesicles typically involve the digits, but can also involve other areas of the hand. The lesions are usually quite painful but are self-limited and resolve in 2 to 3 weeks. Unlike bacterial infections, the pulp space is soft and not tense. The treatment of herpetic whitlow is conservative. Drainage of herpetic whitlow is contraindicated as it may induce a secondary bacterial infection and delay healing. Treatment is symptomatic and consists of splinting, elevation, and analgesia as needed. Oral antiviral agents effective against herpes infections (acyclovir, famciclovir, or valacyclovir) can shorten the course of the disease if given early. Infection recurs in 30% to 50% of cases, but the initial infection is usually the most severe. Acyclovir, 200 mg taken orally three to four times a day, can decrease recurrence rates.[161]

Preventing the spread of the infection must be considered. An occlusive dressing decreases the chance of viral transmission, but health care providers with herpetic whitlow should limit and perhaps even refrain from patient contact, especially until all lesions have crusted over, and viral shedding has stopped.[159] Compliance with universal precautions will decrease the likelihood of patient-to-provider transmission.

Felon

A felon is an infection of the pulp of the distal end of the finger (Fig. 37.28). The usual cause is trauma with secondary invasion by bacteria. A felon may develop in the presence of a foreign body, such as a thorn or a splinter, but often a precipitating trauma cannot be identified. Finger-stick felons are common in patients with diabetes. An important anatomic characteristic of this area is that many fibrous septa extend from the fat pad's volar skin to the phalanx's periosteum; these septa subdivide and compartmentalize the pulp area. When an infection occurs in the pulp, these structures make it a closed-space infection. The septa limit swelling, delay the pointing of the abscess, and inhibit drainage after incomplete surgical decompression. Pressure may increase in the closed space and initiate an ischemic process that compounds the infection. The infection can progress to osteomyelitis of the distal phalanx, septic arthritis, and flexor tenosynovitis. Although the septa may facilitate an infection in the pulp, they also provide a barrier that protects the joint space and tendon sheath by limiting proximal spread of the infection.

In most cases the offending organism is *S. aureus*, but mixed infections and gram-negative infection may also occur. IV drug use and felon infections in particular were risk factors for CA-MRSA.[17,153] These changing patterns, along with the often protracted course of felons and concern for osteomyelitis, make this one of the few soft tissue infections in which culture may be helpful.

A patient in whom a felon is developing will describe a gradual onset of pain and tenderness of the fingertip. In a few days, the pain becomes constant and throbbing and gradually becomes severe. In the initial stages, physical examination may be unimpressive because the fibrous septa limit swelling in the closed pulp space. As the infection progresses, swelling and redness become obvious. Occasionally, one may elicit point tenderness, but frequently, the entire pulp space is extremely tender. The patient characteristically arrives with the hand elevated over the head because the pain is so intense in the dependent position. Cessation of pain indicates necrosis and nerve degeneration.

During the early stages of cellulitis, a felon may be controlled by treatment consisting of elevation, oral antibiotics (see Box 37.2), and warm water or saline soaks. For more developed felons, proper treatment consists of early and

Paronychia Drainage

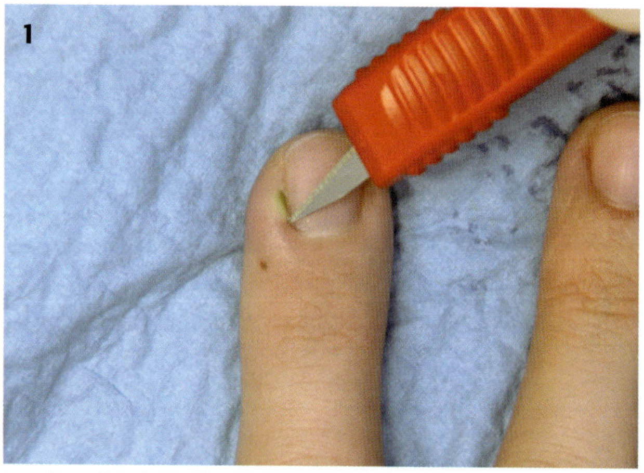

In selected patients the procedure can be completed without anesthesia. After softening the eponychium by soaking, advance a No. 11 scalpel blade under the eponychium parallel to the nail.

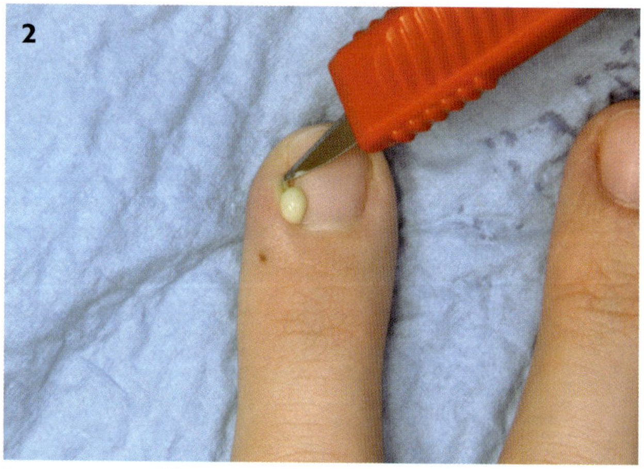

Pus escapes rapidly, with immediate relief of pain. Antibiotics are not required for minor cases. Instruct the patient to frequently soak the digit in warm water at home.

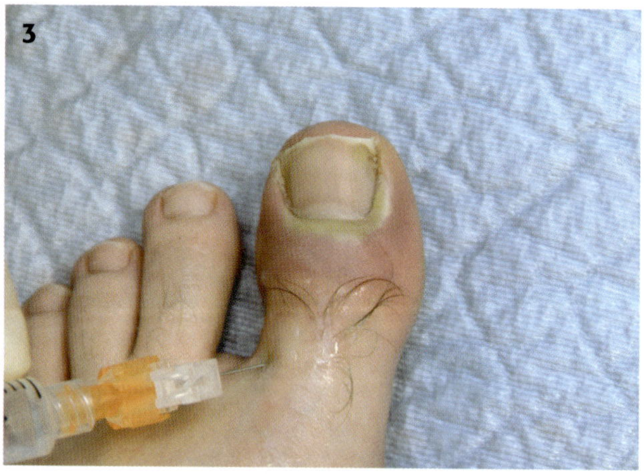

Many patients, especially those with a large paronychia, will require a digital block before the procedure. (See Chapter 31 for details on digital blocks.)

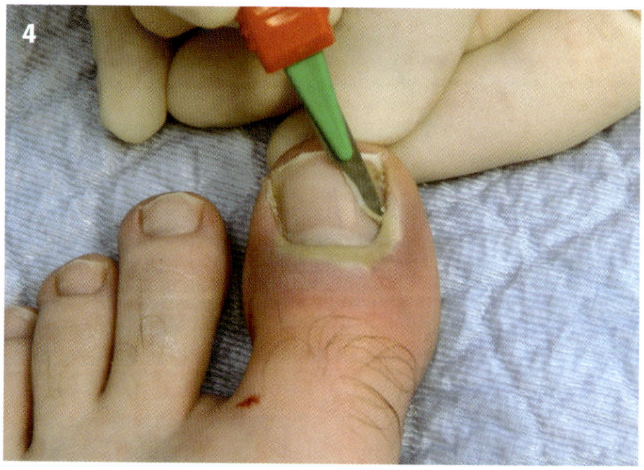

Lift the eponychial fold away from the nail. Here, the blunt side of a No. 15 blade is being used. No sharp incision is required; simply lifting the eponychium away from the nail is sufficient.

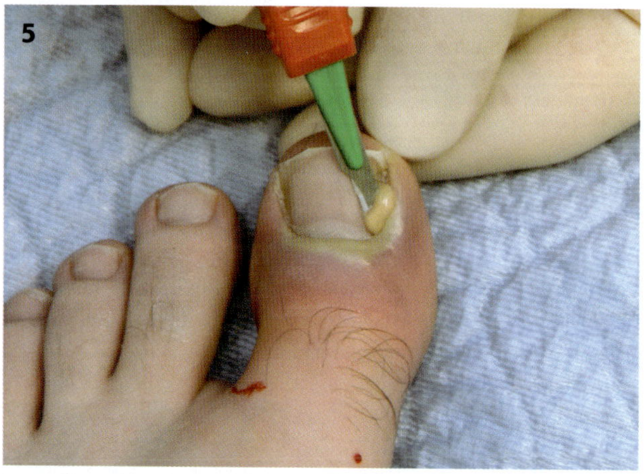

Pus will readily escape as the fold is lifted.

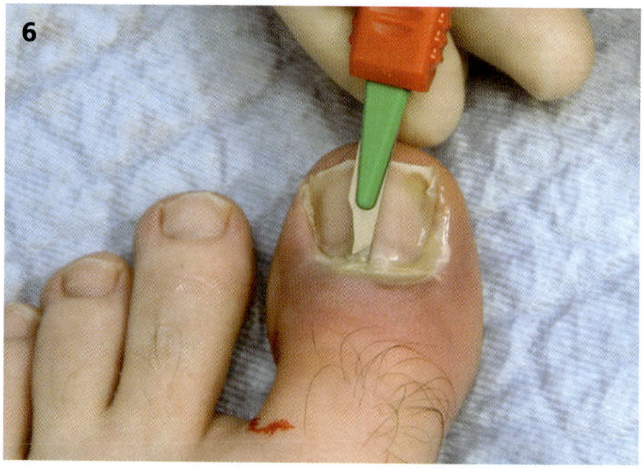

Keep the scalpel parallel to the nail and continue to lift the eponychium to release all the pus. Place a small piece of packing gauze under the eponychium for 24 hours, encourage warm soaks, and prescribe antibiotics if cellulitis is present.

Fig. 37.26 Paronychia drainage.

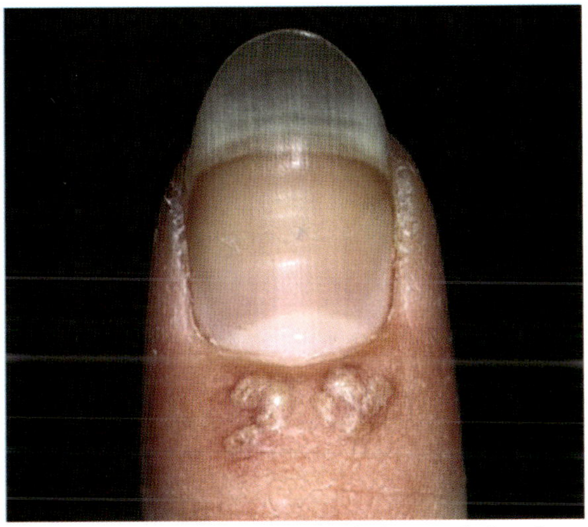

Fig. 37.27 Herpetic whitlow. Clinical findings include pain out of proportion to the results of examination, erythema, and vesicular lesions. Herpetic whitlow may be confused with paronychia. However, incision and drainage is contraindicated because it may lead to bacterial superinfection. (From Habif TP. *Clinical Dermatology.* 5 ed. Mosby; 2009.)

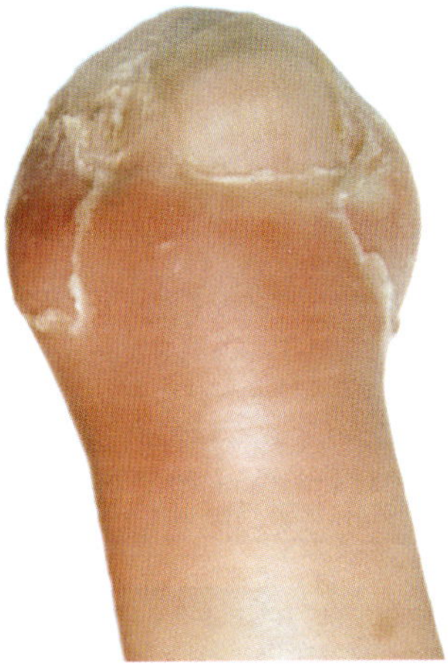

Fig. 37.28 A well-developed felon. In this advanced case the patient had little pain at initial evaluation. The distal phalanx was almost completely resorbed because of pressure, inflammation, and chronic osteomyelitis. This infection is extensive and warrants consultation with a hand specialist.

complete I&D.[161] Antibiotics alone are not curative once suppuration has occurred. Delaying surgery may result in permanent disability and deformity.

A minor felon can usually be drained on an outpatient basis after the application of a digital nerve block. A long-acting anesthetic (bupivacaine) will prolong the anesthesia. A tourniquet (1.25-cm Penrose drain) applied proximally can be used to allow an incision into a bloodless field. Surgical drainage must be performed carefully to avoid injury to nerves, vessels, and flexor tendons. Most felons can be managed with a limited procedure, but many surgical options have been advocated, none of which has been proved to be superior for all circumstances.[159] Traditional incisions ("hockey stick" or "fish mouth") have a propensity for complications such as sloughing of tissue and postoperative fat pad anesthesia or instability and are rarely used. The preferred initial treatment is a simple longitudinal incision over the area of greatest fluctuance,[161] 3 to 5 mm distal to the distal interphalangeal joint. The incision may be made laterally or along the volar surface (Fig. 37.29A), although injury to the sensory nerve or digital artery is more of a concern with the lateral incision given its proximity to these structures. Frank pus may be encountered during incision, but usually only a few drops are expressed. More often one drains a combination of necrotic tissue and interstitial fluid. A foreign body should be sought even if that history is not given. A potential drawback to an incision in the middle of the fat pad is the production of a scar in a very sensitive and commonly traumatized area. The incision must not extend to the distal interphalangeal crease because of the danger of injuring the flexor tendon. The subcutaneous tissue is bluntly dissected with a hemostat to provide adequate drainage. A gauze pack may be placed in the wound for 24 to 48 hours to ensure continued drainage. Recurrent or more severe infections may require a more aggressive approach by a hand specialist. Follow-up recommendations for patients with a diagnosis of felon should include referral to a hand surgeon.

No matter which incision is made, it must not be carried proximal to the closed pulp space because of the danger of entrance into the tendon sheath or the joint capsule. A snug dressing, splinting, elevation, and adequate opioid analgesics are prerequisites for a successful outcome. Most felons are treated empirically with antibiotics for at least 5 days. A broad-spectrum cephalosporin is a reasonable choice pending cultures (if done). Antibiotics effective against CA-MRSA should also be considered given its increasing incidence.[3]

The patient should be rechecked in 2 to 3 days. On the first postoperative visit, perform a digital block and remove the packing if present. Irrigate the incision copiously with saline and remove any additional necrotic tissue. If there is continued drainage, replace the drain for 24 to 48 hours, but it can usually be removed and a dressing reapplied. Soaking may be advised. At the first revisit, check the sensitivities of the bacterial cultures and decide to continue or change antibiotics.

Some clinicians advocate radiographic evaluation for retained foreign bodies at the initial visit, and a baseline evaluation of the bone for subsequent evaluation of osteomyelitis. Other clinicians reserve radiographs for wounds not showing significant improvement in 5 to 7 days. Evidence of osteomyelitis, however, may not be found radiographically for several weeks after the appearance of the lesion. Persistent infections necessitate more radical I&D and may require IV antibiotics. After adequate drainage, osteomyelitis may respond surprisingly well to outpatient antibiotic therapy, with almost complete regeneration of bone being achieved if the I&D procedure has been adequate.

Difficult or persistent cases require evaluation and care by a hand surgeon. Early consultation is advisable in these cases to avert catastrophic complications such as loss of function or amputation.

Subungual Hematoma

Subungual hematomas are typically caused by hitting a fingertip with a hammer, slamming a finger in a door (Fig. 37.30; Videos 37.9–37.11), or dropping a weight on a foot. Patients present with terrible throbbing pain that increases with the pressure under the nail. There is an associated blue-black discoloration under the affected nail, indicative of a hematoma. The source of the pain is pressure in a contained space, pressing against nerve fibers and not from the soft tissue injury or bony injury alone.

Felon Drainage

1

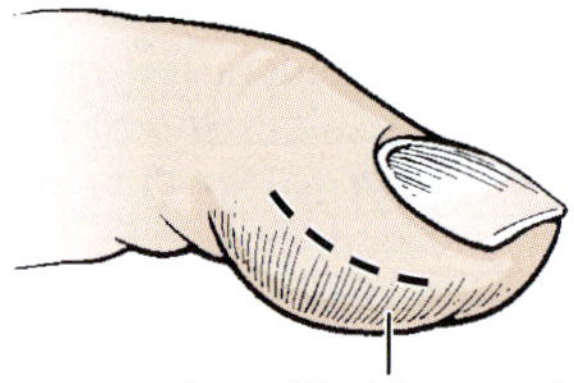

The preferred initial incision for draining a felon is made directly into the area of most fluctuance *(1)*. More aggressive incisions should be reserved for complicated cases because they have greater morbidity and require more complicated wound care. The unilateral longitudinal approach is a good first choice. Some prefer a similarly located through-and-through incision (see below).

2 3

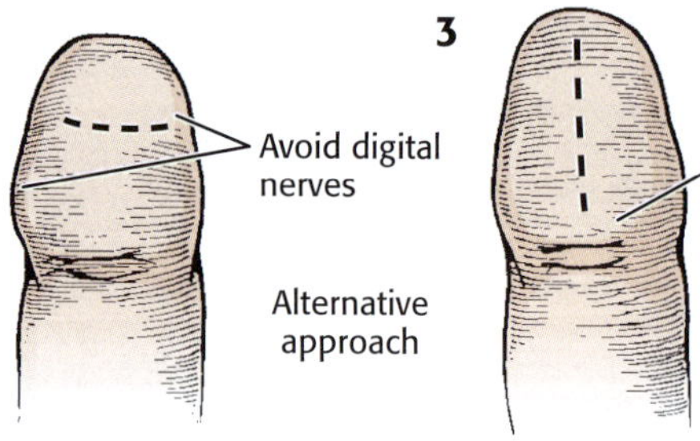

A fat pad incision is generally avoided but can be acceptable for localized infections. They may be associated with a painful scar in an area that is often traumatized. The transverse fat pad incision should avoid the digital nerves *(2)*, and the longitudinal fat pad incision should avoid the flexor tendon *(3)*.

A

1

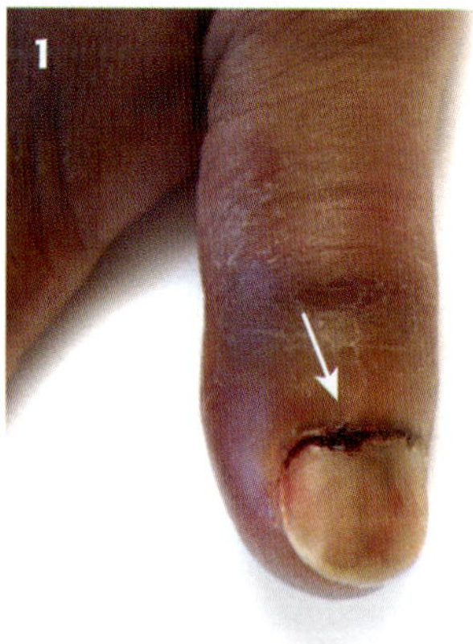

This patient has an extensive paronychia *(arrow)* but did not seek medical attention.

2

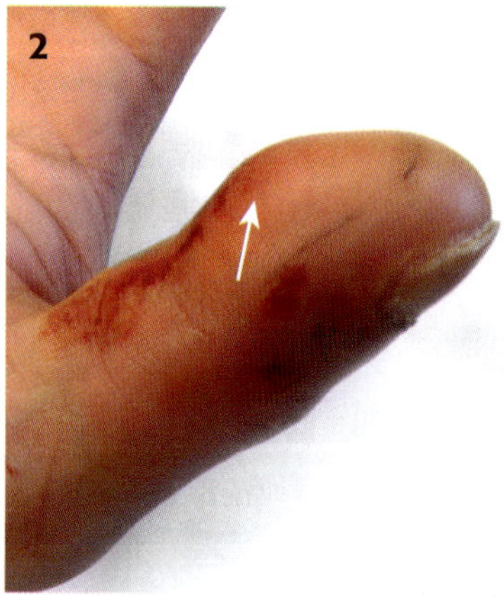

The infection has spread volarly and progressed to a felon. Drainage of both areas is required.

3

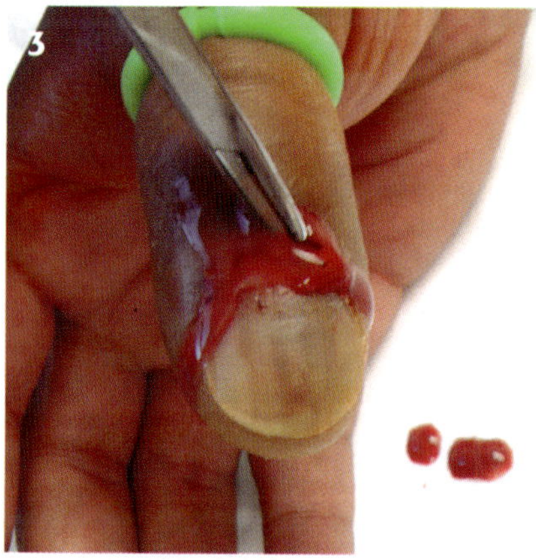

The eponychium is lifted, which resulted in immediate drainage of large quantities of pus.

4

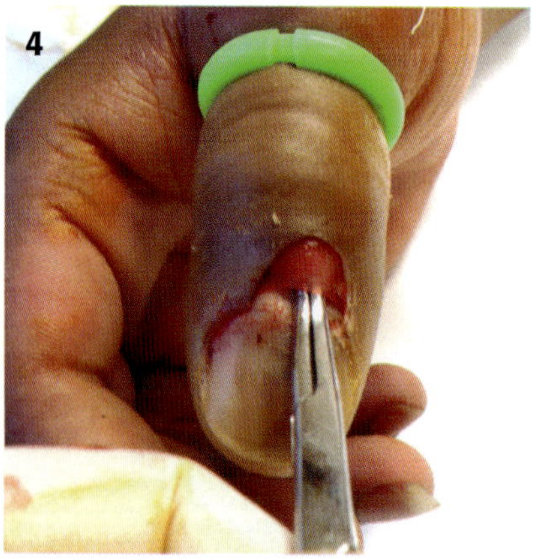

A hemostat is placed under the eponychium to facilitate complete evacuation of the pus.

5

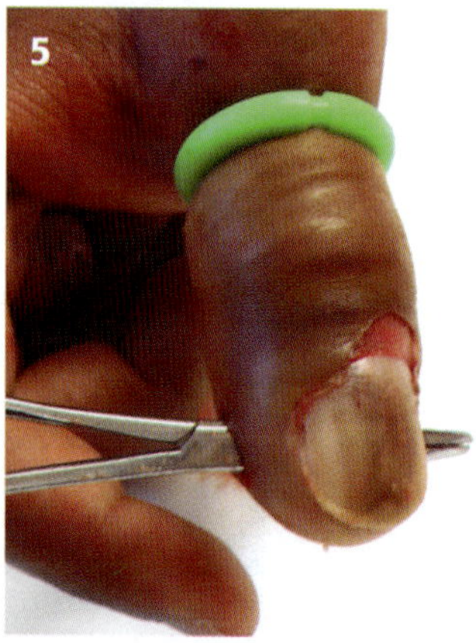

To drain the felon, a through-and-through incision is made on the volar side. A hemostat is used to break up loculations in the fat pad and then to grab gauze for a pull-through pack.

6

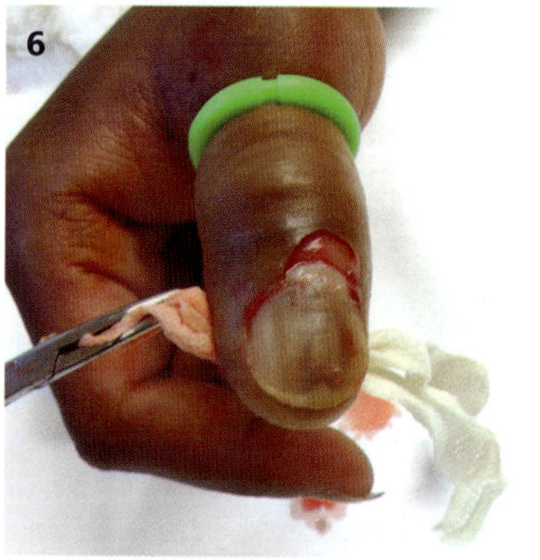

The gauze pack is pulled through the incision and left in place for 24 to 48 hours to ensure continued drainage.

B

Fig. 37.29 Felon drainage. For a felon the author prefers the through-and-through drainage procedure shown in B; an alternative is to open the abscess at the point of maximum fluctuance. Antibiotics should be used postprocedurally. Culture can aid in the selection of long-term antibiotics, but most initially cover for community-acquired methicillin-resistant *Staphylococcus aureus*.

Subungual hematomas may be simple (i.e., the nail and nail fold are intact) or accompanied by significant injuries to the nail fold and digit. The nail matrix is the tissue under the base of the nail that permits nail growth and migration. Its longitudinal fibers anchor the dermis to the periosteum of the distal phalanx.[162,163]

The matrix begins 7 to 8 mm under the proximal fold, and its distal end is the white crescent called the lunula. Scarring of the matrix, as occurs with nail trauma, can disrupt nail growth and lead to nail deformity or permanent loss of the nail. When describing the injury, the clinician should estimate the percentage of nail bed that is affected by the hematoma and discuss associated trauma to the nail margins or surrounding tissue. The examination should include tests of the extensor and flexor tendons, of circulation by capillary refill, and of the area's sensitivity.[163]

If fracture of the distal phalanx is suspected (e.g., if the fingertip is unstable or the mechanism of injury suggests a fracture), obtain anteroposterior and lateral x-ray films. Radiographs can help differentiate tendinous from bony mallet type injuries. Crush injuries are associated with three types of distal phalanx fractures: longitudinal, transverse, and comminuted. If the fracture is angulated, displaced, unstable, or intraarticular or involves a third or more of the articular surface, refer the patient to a hand surgeon.[164] Because trephination in patients with a distal phalanx fracture theoretically converts a closed fracture into an open one, there is concern about infectious and cosmetic complications. In the two studies that examined this possible association,[165] with fracture subsets totaling 26, no infections occurred. These studies suggest that the presence of an underlying fracture does not contraindicate nail trephination for fear of causing infection. No data support the routine use of prophylactic antibiotics following trephination if an underlying fracture is present.

Subungual hematomas should be trephinated if they are acute (less than 24 to 48 hours old), are not spontaneously draining, are associated with intact nail folds, or are painful. After 48 hours, most subungual hematomas have clotted and trephination is typically ineffective.

Nail removal is unnecessary, even if there is an underlying distal phalanx fracture, if the nail margins and nail are intact.[164,165] If the nail is split, avulsed or disrupted, or a nail bed laceration extends to the skin, the nail should be removed and the underlying nail bed repaired (see further discussion in Chapter 35). Simple trephination of an uncomplicated subungual hematoma, even if it involves the entire subungual area, results in a good outcome functionally and cosmetically.[164] Trephination should also be considered if the hematoma covers more than half the intact nail or if it is smaller but painful.

Prophylactic antibiotics are not necessary for patients with uncomplicated subungual hematomas that have been trephinated. An underlying tuft fracture does not mandate antibiotic prophylaxis. For more serious injuries, a slight risk for infection exists, but in most cases rigorous wound cleaning and careful soft tissue repair constitute adequate treatment.[166]

Methods of Trephination

All methods of trephination require aseptic technique. Clean the nail thoroughly and place the digit in a sterile field. Follow universal precautions because the fluid under the nail is under pressure and can spurt.[167] Ensure that adequate analgesia has been achieved. Anesthesia is not always required, but a digital block can be used to calm an anxious patient and is commonly performed.

An 18- or 21-gauge needle can be rotated between the thumb and the index finger while gentle pressure is applied so that the sharp end of the needle corkscrews through the nail.[167] When using a needle, the "give" is harder to feel, so the clinician should proceed slowly until blood is drawn. Because the hole made with a needle is small, a second hole may be required.

An alternative needle-based approach is being used by a group of Turkish dermatologists. Kaya and associates[168] use extra fine, 29-gauge insulin syringes for evacuation of hematomas. After the nail is trimmed, the needle is inserted parallel to the nail plate and advanced to the distal edge of the hematoma. This technique is especially effective for small hematomas of the second, third, and fourth toenails, which are hard to trephine.

Hot cautery is the most common form of trephination and is usually done with a paper clip which has been straightened and heated in a flame (Figs. 37.31 and 37.32). Place the hot end on the nail above the center of the hematoma and apply gentle pressure until the nail is breached and the hematoma expressed. A give is felt as the instrument passes

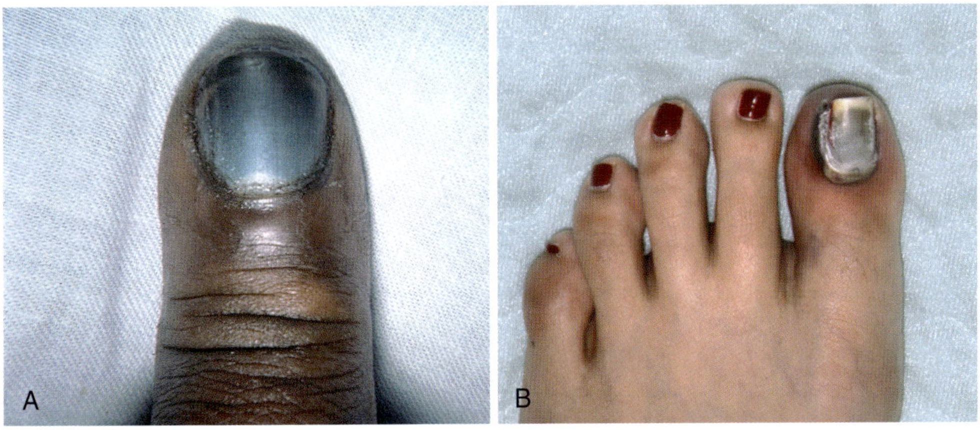

Fig. 37.30 Subungual hematoma. (A) Subungual hematoma with a totally blackened nail bed. Do not remove this intact nail, even though the nail bed is lacerated, or if there is a total hematoma and underlying minor tuft fracture. In this example, blood accumulated only under the nail, not in any paronychial areas. (B) Subungual hematoma of the great toe after dropping a heavy object on the foot (a common injury).

through the nail. Stop the pressure at this point to avoid damage to the nail bed. Blood exits rapidly, and the blackened nail regains its normal color (see Fig. 37.32, *step 3*). The blood usually remains fluid for 24 to 36 hours and can easily be expressed with slight pressure. Multiple holes may be needed for continued drainage. Do not use hot cautery trephination on artificial nails because they are flammable. Hot cautery with a paper clip is easy to perform, but hematomas treated in this way tend to reform. It has also fallen out of favor secondary to the need to use an open flame in front of the patient. In addition, most paper clips are made of aluminum, which is difficult to heat to penetrate the nail sufficiently. A portable hot-wire electrocautery unit can be used, but obtaining an adequate drainage hole is difficult without adapting the instrument (see Fig. 37.32). It can be modified to burn a larger hole by "fattening" the end of the wire loop and rotating the device slowly as the nail is penetrated or by removing a small rectangle of nail. In addition to being convenient, the cautery device is desirable because the wire stays hotter longer, thereby enhancing nail penetration.

Outcome

It is difficult to predict the fate of the fingernail after drainage of a subungual hematoma. Obviously, there must be a nail bed laceration if bleeding occurs, but with a stable nail bed, repair is unnecessary. Even if a small tuft fracture is present, most do well with simple drainage. Some patients will lose the nail, but if the nail root or nail bed is not significantly disrupted and the nail remains implanted, a normal-appearing nail is the usual final result. After a hematoma has been drained, the nail should be cleaned thoroughly, and a dry dressing applied. Patients should be advised to keep the digit dry for 2 days. Any fracture should be splinted and given appropriate follow-up at a surgical clinic.

Conditions With a Similar Appearance

One condition that may be mistaken for a simple subungual hematoma is closed avulsion of the base of a fingernail occurring in conjunction with a subungual hematoma from a nail bed laceration. A common mechanism is slamming a finger in a car door, which causes sudden flexion of the distal phalanx in conjunction with a crush injury of the nail bed. The nail is usually stable, so generally no repair of the nail bed appears to be required. However, if the subungual hematoma extends past the confines of the nail bed, such as in the paronychial space (under the skin of the cuticle), there must be a communication between the nail bed and this space. This produces a paronychial hematoma, with blood occupying the space where pus would be located in an infectious paronychia (Fig. 37.33). When this condition is present, the avulsed proximal portion of the fingernail overlies the nail fold of the cuticle but is appreciated only after the overlying skin is opened. Open reduction (replacement) of the nail must be performed. The

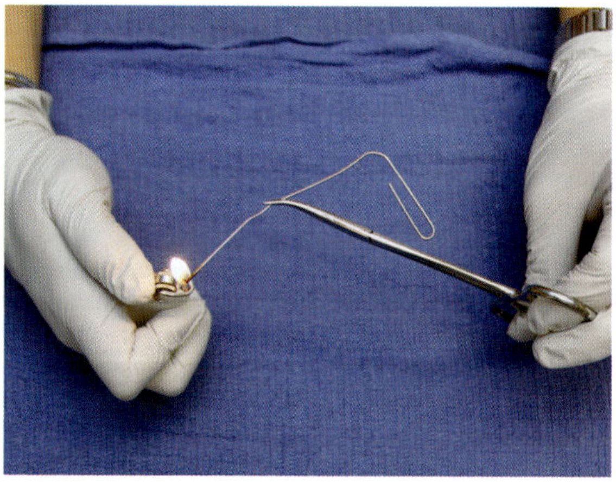

Fig. 37.31 A straightened paper clip, held with a hemostat and heated with a flame, can be used for hot cautery trephination.

Nail Trephination

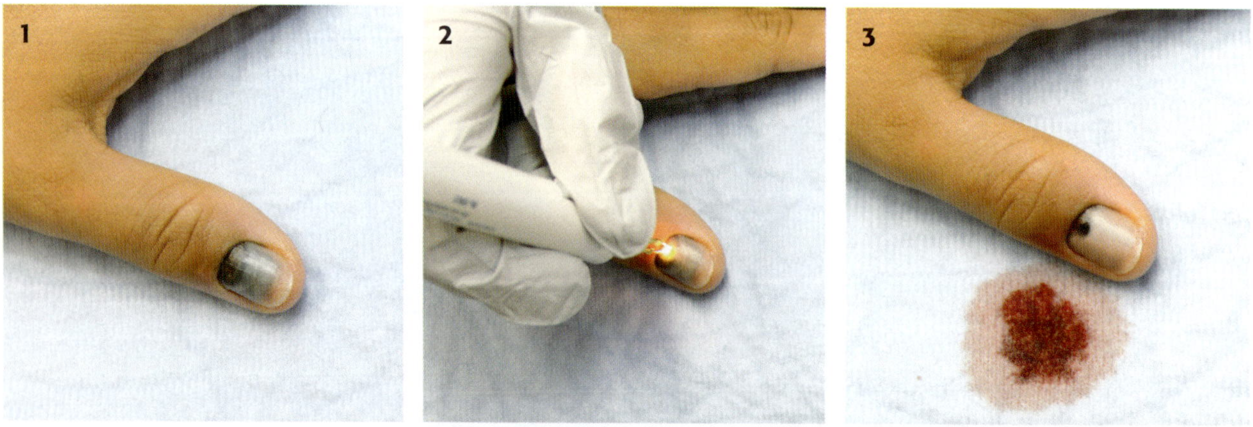

1 This patient has a painful subungal hematoma and requires trephination. Cleanse the area with antiseptic prior to trephination. Anesthesia with a digital block can optionally be used.

2 Place the hot cautery device (here, a disposable cautery pen) over the center of the hematoma and apply gentle pressure. A "give" is felt and blood is rapidly expressed as the hematoma is released. Multiple holes may be required.

3 Successful trephination is demonstrated by relief of pain and return of the normal color of the nail bed.

Fig. 37.32 Nail trephination.

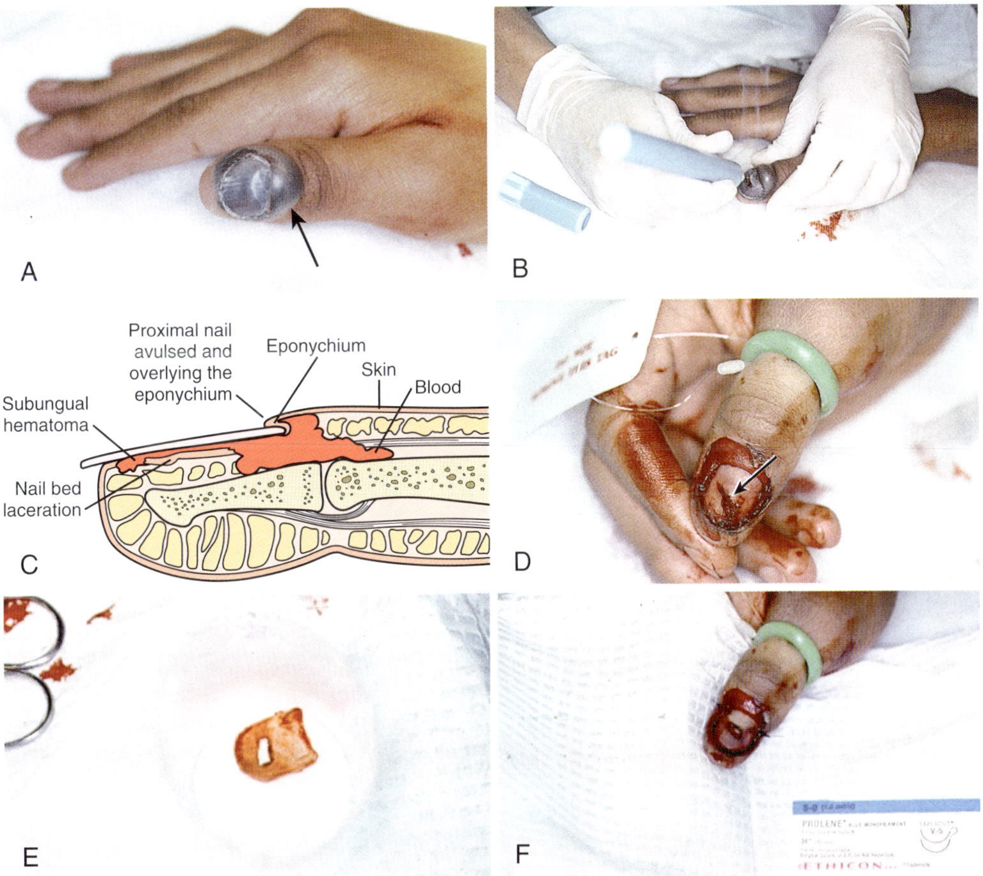

Fig. 37.33 Complicated subungual hematoma. (A) This patient slammed his finger in a car door and sustained acute flexion of the distal phalanx and a crush injury. It appears to be a simple subungual hematoma, but note the blood in the paronychial space *(arrow)*. There is communication between the nail bed laceration and the eponychium. (B) All the blood did not drain when the nail was trephinated. Blood accumulated in this area because the base of the fingernail has been avulsed from its origin and now lies between the eponychium (cuticle) and skin. This is appreciated when the skin is debrided. (C) Illustration of the affected area. (D) With the nail removed, the nail bed laceration *(arrow)* can be seen and repaired. (E) The old, trephined nail. (F) The nail can now be replaced and sutured in its original position to keep the eponychial space open, or the space can be packed with gauze for a few weeks to discourage scar formation and subsequent nail deformity. Note the drainage hole in the original nail.

replaced nail often grows normally, but a lost or deformed nail is possible. Repair of the nail bed laceration is optional at this juncture but may not be required if the nail is stable. Once the injury is anatomically aligned, splinting and soaking follow as for a simple subungual hematoma. These injuries rarely become infected, and there is no evidence that the prophylactic use of antibiotics is necessary.

Subungual hematomas/discolorations can also be a manifestation of diseases such as Kaposi's sarcoma in an AIDS patient. Additionally, consider melanoma as happened with Bob Marley, the famous Jamaican singer and songwriter, who died of the cancer. These conditions should be considered when no trauma has occurred and the findings on physical examination are not consistent with a simple subungual hematoma.

REFERENCES ARE AVAILABLE AT Elsevier eBooks+

CHAPTER 38

Burn Care Procedures

Thomas W. Kramer and Anthony S. Mazzeo

Burn injuries are common in the United States. The CDC estimates that in 2021 there were 398,000 fire or burn related injuries, along with 252,000 contact burns from hot objects or chemicals.[1] An analysis that compared claims based data and public health data estimated about 600,000 individuals suffering burn injuries in 2020.[2] According to the American Burn Association (ABA) Annual Burn Injury Report 2024 there were approximately 32,000 hospitalizations annually from 2019 to 2023, with 32,746 admissions in 2023. Children accounted for about 18% of all burn cases during that time frame; while male patients account for about 66% of all injuries. The overall mortality rate for burn patients was 3.3%, although patients with cutaneous burns alone had a mortality of only 1.9%, and those with inhalation injury had a 20.6% mortality. Overall, the case rate is about 1.0 per 10,000 individuals with the highest incidence of 1.8 per 10,000 individuals occurring in children <10 and males 50 to 60 years of age.[3]

Burns are most commonly accidental and occur outside of the workplace (75%), but accidental workplace burns account for 10% of total burns. About 625 burns annual are thought to be from abuse/assault, with an additional half that number self-inflicted. Among patients admitted with burn injuries, the most common etiologies of burns were flash/flames (42%), scalds (32%), and contact (11%). About 57% of all cases are less than 10% Total Body Surface Area (TBSA), 10% are between 10 % to 20% TBSA, and 6% of patient have greater than 20% TBSA. About 47% of all cases need surgical intervention. Burn centers also care for non-burn etiologies such as Stevens-Johnson and other cutaneous disorders, which affect these numbers.

Of those patients requiring admission for serious burns, 64% are white, 23% black or African American, and the remainder from other non-white populations; approximately 16% identify as Hispanic or Latino. Black or African American patient are overrepresented compared to being 14% of the general population, meanwhile Hispanic or Latino patients are slightly under unrepresented compared to being 20% of the general population. Racial and ethnic data also show health disparities with longer lengths of hospital stay. 32% of patients experiencing burns are covered by Medicaid (compared to 19% national covered by Medicaid), while 16% of all burn patients are uninsured (compared to 11% nationally uninsured).

Special populations include children and older adults. Of children with burn injuries, the majority are less than 5 years-of-age. Most cases were scald injuries, with typical etiologies being bathing, food/drink, and food preparation. Suspected abuse was reported in 3.9% of cases. Older adults (65 and over) are also at high risk, with burns often being more serious, requiring longer hospital length of stay, and having increased mortality at 9.8%. Additionally, inhalation injuries were more common in this age group. People experiencing homelessness were also overrepresented at 4% compared to being <1% of the total population, with 12% experience severe burns >20% TBSA.[4]

Overall, the incidence of burn injury has declined in recent decades and advances in medical care have improved the morbidity and mortality of burn patients.[2,3] Enhancements in resuscitation, surgical and anesthetic techniques, intensive care, infection control, nutrition, and metabolic support have all contributed to dramatic improvements in the survival, preservation of body function, physical appearance, and emotional outcomes of patients with this injury. The initial care provided to burn patients by emergency medical providers can improve outcomes by minimizing the conversion of superficial burns to deep burns and by improving the long-term functional and cosmetic outcomes of the affected tissues.

The classification of burns is based on three criteria[4]: depth of skin injury, percentage of TBSA involved, and source of injury (thermal, chemical, electrical, or radiation). The seriousness of a burn injury is determined by the characteristics and temperature of the burning agent, the duration of exposure, the location of the injury, the presence of associated injuries, and the age and general health of the victim (Table 38.1).

The ABA defines minor burns as uncomplicated superficial or partial-thickness burns involving less than 5% TBSA in children (<10 years old) or the elderly (>50 years old), and less than 10% TBSA in adults; additional criteria are less than 2% TBSA for full-thickness burns.[5] Moderate or major burns include injuries that involve a greater TBSA, as well as burns in areas of specialized function, such as the face, hands, feet, and perineum. More serious burns also include those caused by a high-voltage electrical injury or those with associated inhalation injuries or other major trauma.

Throughout the course of history, clinicians have experimented with burn therapies to relieve pain and promote healing. Many treatment regimens and home remedies have been successful, largely because minor burns generally do well with a modicum of intervention and commonsense wound care. Although little has changed in the care of minor ambulatory burns over the past three decades, treatment of major burns has significantly improved, including the development of sophisticated burn centers, increased knowledge of burn wound physiology, and prevention of infection.

WOUND EVALUATION

The depth of a burn wound cannot always be determined accurately on clinical grounds alone at initial evaluation and burn injury can be a dynamic process that may change over time, particularly during the 24 to 48 hours after the burning process has been arrested. It is common, for example, for a seemingly minor or superficial burn to appear deeper on the second or third return visit (Fig. 38.1). This phenomenon is not a continuation of the burning process that can be altered by clinician intervention but is considered to be a pathophysiologic event related to tissue edema, dermal ischemia, or desiccation.

Estimating Burn Depth

Currently two standard sets of nomenclature are used to describe burns. The more current classification is anatomically descriptive by thickness, whereas historically burns have been classified by degree.[5] Superficial burns (first degree) involve the epidermis only. Partial-thickness burns (second degree) extend into the dermis and are further sub-classified as superficial partial-thickness and deep partial-thickness burns. Full-thickness burns (third degree) extend into the subcutaneous (SQ) tissue with

TABLE 38.1 Characteristics of Burns, by Depth

CLASSIFICATION OF BURN	ETIOLOGY	APPEARANCE	SENSATION	TIME TO COMPLETE HEALING	SCARRING
Superficial					
Superficial epidermal layers	Sunburn, other UV exposure Short flash flame burns	Dry, red Blanches with pressure	Present May be quite painful	3–7 days	No
Partial Thickness					
Varying depth, blisters, or bullae formation					
Dermal appendages spared (e.g., sweat glands, hair follicles)					
Includes entire epidermis and some portion of the dermis					
Superficial partial thickness	Water scald Longer flash burn	Blisters, peeling skin Blanches with pressure Skin red and moist under blisters	Painful Exposure to air and temperature painful	7–21 days	Unusual if no infection and proper follow-up Pigment change may be seen Burned area may be sensitive to frostbite, windburn, and sunburn for many months Itching may be problematic for weeks after healing
Deep partial thickness	Flame Water immersion Oil, grease, hot foods (e.g., soup)	Variable color Wet or waxy dry, does not blanch Blisters easily removed, skin peeling off	Pressure only	>21 days	Severe; risk for contracture
Full Thickness					
Loss of all skin elements, thrombosis and coagulation of vessels	Flame, steam, oil grease Immersion, scald Caustic chemical, high voltage	Leathery appearance, white or charred, dry, inelastic; blanching with pressure May be present under blisters	Deep pressure only	Never heals Requires grafting	Very severe, high risk for contracture

UV, Ultraviolet.
Modified after Clayton MC, Solem LD. No ice, no butter: advice on management of burns for primary care physicians. *Postgrad Med*. 1995;97:151; and Morgan ED, Bledsoe SC, Barker J. Ambulatory management of burns. *Am Fam Physician*. 2000;62:2015.

destruction of all dermal layers. An additional fourth-degree is sometimes used to describe injuries deeper than the SQ tissue to the underlying muscle, tendon, or bone (Fig. 38.2).

In superficial burns (epidermis only) (Fig. 38.3A) the skin is reddened but is intact and not blistered. This injury ranges from mildly irritating or even pruritic to exquisitely painful. Minor edema may be noted. Common causes include ultraviolet light (as in sunburn) and brief thermal "flash" burns. Superficial burns may blister within 24 to 36 hours, and the patient should be warned about this possibility. Frequently, the epidermis may flake or peel within 5 to 10 days. Healing occurs spontaneously, usually without scarring.

Partial-thickness burns involve the epidermis and extend into the dermis to include the sweat glands and hair follicles. Superficial partial-thickness burns involve only the papillary dermis (Fig. 38.3B). These burns are pink, moist, blanching, and extremely painful. Blisters are common and the skin may slough. The burn blanches with pressure, and mild to moderate edema is common. Hair follicles often remain intact. Superficial second-degree burns are the most common burns seen in the emergency department (ED). The usual causes are scalds, contact with hot objects, or exposure to chemicals. Barring infection or repeated trauma, these burns heal spontaneously and usually without scarring in approximately 2 weeks. These areas may be sensitive to sunburn, windburn, and skin irritation for months after the original injury has healed.

Deep partial-thickness burns involve the reticular dermis and appear mottled white or pink (Fig. 38.3C). There is obvious edema and sloughing of the skin, and any blisters are usually ruptured. Blanching can be present but is less pronounced.

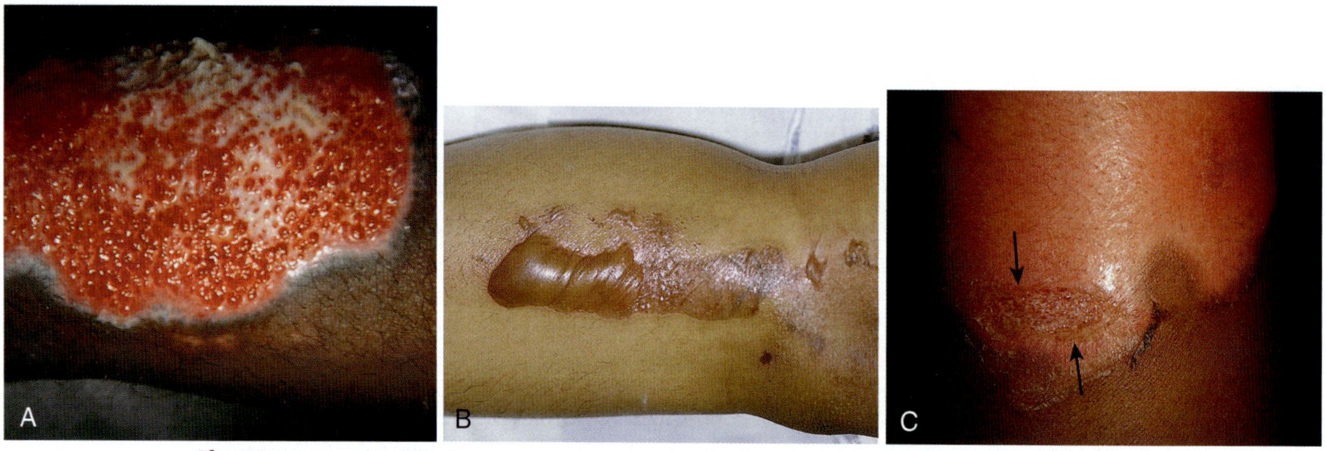

Fig. 38.1 It may be difficult to accurately assess the depth or severity of a burn on the first visit. (A) This full-thickness burn will not heal without a skin graft. (B) This blistered hot water burn is probably partial thickness, but full-thickness burns can develop under blisters. (C) At 2 weeks, a partial-thickness burn and a small area of full-thickness burn *(arrows)*.

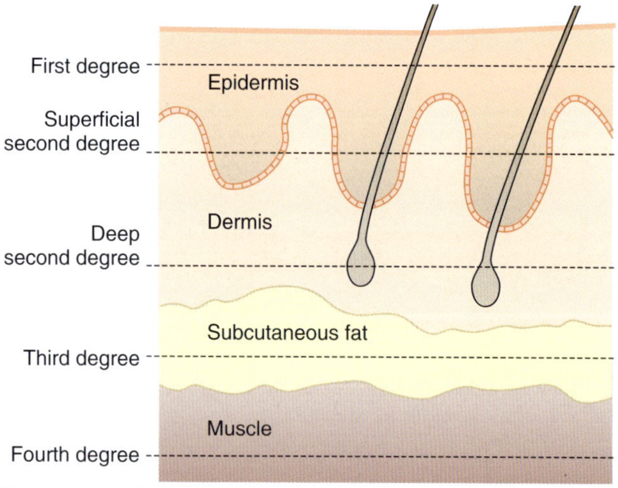

Fig. 38.2 Depths of a burn. Superficial burns are confined to the epidermis. Partial-thickness burns extend into the dermis (dermal burns). Full-thickness burns extend through the epidermis and dermis. So-called fourth-degree burns involve injury to underlying tissue structures such as muscle, tendons, and bone. (From Townsend CM, Beauchamp RD, Evers BM et al. eds. *Sabiston Textbook of Surgery*. 19th ed. Saunders; 2012.)

These burns are generally less painful initially and may have decreased sensation, but perception of pressure will be preserved. Within a few days, however, these burns can become exquisitely painful. This type of burn may be converted to a full-thickness injury by further trauma or infection.

Full-thickness burns result in destruction of the dermis and may extend into SQ tissue (Fig. 38.3D). These burns usually appear dry, leathery, and pearly white or charred in color. They are typically painless. Common causes include flame, steam, oil and grease submersion, caustic chemicals, and high-voltage electrical burns. Circumferential full-thickness burns on an extremity or the torso cause a loss of elasticity that may impair the circulation or ventilation and necessitate an escharotomy.

Deeper burns, sometimes called fourth-degree burns, extend deeply into SQ tissue, muscle, fascia, or bone (Fig. 38.3E). These burns are characteristically caused by contact with molten metal, flame, or high-voltage electricity.

The depth of burn is the most important factor in wound healing and scar formation. In general, superficial and superficial partial-thickness burns involve the papillary dermis, with its rich vascular plexus, and the epidermis, which permits spontaneous healing by reepithelialization from the dermal appendages, including hair follicles, sebaceous glands, and sweat glands. This usually occurs within 2 weeks with minimal scarring. Deep partial-thickness and full-thickness burns involve the reticular dermis and SQ fat and generally lack sufficient epithelial appendages for spontaneous healing. If healing does occur, it will occur slowly and produce unstable skin, hypertrophic scarring, and contracture. These deep burns typically need care in a specialized burn center as they are often best treated by excision and skin grafting (Table 38.2).

Although bedside evaluation of very superficial or deep wounds presents little diagnostic difficulty, clinical assessment of a mid-dermal or "indeterminate" burn is often less accurate. Even though it is useful to initially characterize the extent of the burn, it should be noted that the early appearance of a burn wound may not accurately reflect the true extent of the soft tissue injury. Reexamination and follow-up are critical because burn wounds may change during the 24 to 72 hours after the injury. Indeterminate burns may eventually heal spontaneously, or they may convert to deeper wounds requiring excision and skin grafting (see Fig. 38.1).

Estimating Burn Size

Calculating burn size is necessary to determine a treatment plan and fluid requirements, and can also aid in prognosis. Overestimating the burn size is a common error, especially in children, therefore it is important to take the time to accurately estimate the burn size. Superficial burns do not count in the calculation of total burn surface area when utilizing fluid resuscitation formulas; including these burns in the calculation of TBSA is a common error and results in an overestimate of the total burned areas.

Several formulas are available to estimate TBSA in burn patients. In 1944 Lund and Browder published the now famous Lund-Browder chart (Fig. 38.4).[6] In their landmark paper, they used direct measurements and body surface area formulas to produce a chart that clinicians can use to estimate %TBSA. Burn centers typically utilize the Lund-Browder chart for estimating burn size. The initial Lund-Browder chart was developed from human anatomic studies derived from 11 adults (3 female and 8 male) and produced a unisex chart. A

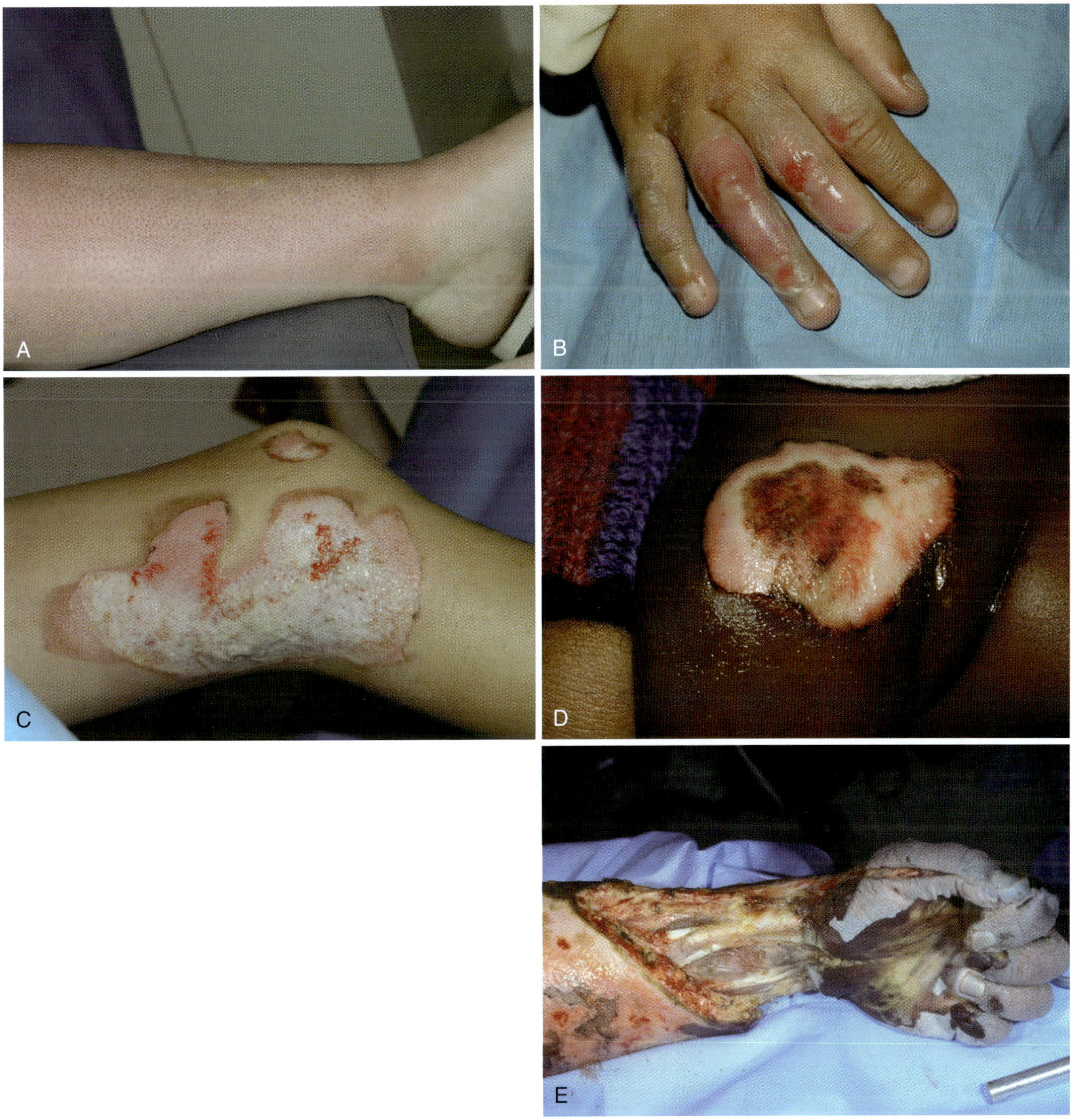

Fig. 38.3 Depth of thermal injury. (A) Patient with sunburn on the lower extremity (a superficial or first-degree burn with associated blisters on the anterior tibial surface). (B) Partial-thickness injury of the hand (superficial partial-thickness burn). (C) Partial-thickness injury extending beyond the subcutaneous layers (deep partial-thickness burn). (D) Full-thickness (third-degree) burn. (E) Full-thickness injury with extensive tissue loss (fourth-degree burn). (From Davis PJ, Cladis FP, Motoyama EK, eds. *Smith's Anesthesia for Infants and Children.* 8th ed. Mosby; 2011.)

2004 study involving 60 volunteers determined that the Lund-Browder chart significantly underestimates the size of chest burns in large-breasted females. The investigators developed a table that incorporates a correction using brassiere cup size.[7]

The simplest method for estimating TBSA in adults is the "rule of nines." This formula was developed in the late 1940s by Pulaski and Tennison, who observed that the percentage of each body segment was approximately a multiple of nine (Fig. 38.5).[8] Similar formulas for children adjust for their disproportionately large head surface area.

The size of a burn can also be estimated by using the patient's hand as representing approximately 1% TBSA. With this method, the palm and fingers are considered a rectangle of about 1% TBSA. However, two studies using planimetry have determined that the hand actually represents from 0.5% to 0.78% of a patient's TBSA.[9]

Regardless of the method used, it is important for the emergency provider to take time to quantify the %TBSA as accurately as possible. It should be reemphasized that fluid recommendations DO NOT include superficial burns in the

TABLE 38.2 American Burn Association's Grading System for Burn Severity and Disposition of Patients[a]

	Type of Burn		
	MINOR	MODERATE	MAJOR
Criteria	<10% TBSA burn in adult	10%–20% TBSA burn in adult	>20% TBSA burn in adult
	<5% TBSA burn in young or old	5%–10% TBSA burn in young or old	>10% TBSA burn in young or old
	<2% full-thickness burn	2%–5% full-thickness burn	>5% full-thickness burn
		High-voltage injury Suspected inhalation injury Circumferential burn Concomitant medical problem predisposing the patient to infection (e.g., diabetes, sickle cell disease)	High-voltage burn Known inhalation injury Any significant burn involving the face, eyes, ears, hands, feet, genitalia, or joints Significant associated injuries (e.g., fracture, other major trauma)
Disposition	Outpatient management	Hospital admission, consider referral to burn center, structured outpatient care	Referral to a burn center[b]

[a]Burn, partial-thickness or full-thickness burn, unless specified; young, patient younger than 10 years; adult, patient 10 to 50 years of age; old, patient older than 50 years.
[b]Decision to refer to a burn center is according to physician judgment on a case-by-case basis. The above list contains guidelines set by the ABA for consideration for referral.
TBSA, Total body surface area (percentage) affected by the injury.
Adapted from American Burn Association. Hospital and prehospital resources for optimal care of patients with burn injury: guidelines for development and operation of burn centers. *J Burn Care Rehabil.* 1990;11:98; with additional information from Hartford CE. Care of outpatient burns. In: Herndon DN, ed. *Total Burn Care*. Saunders; 1996:71.

%TBSA, rather they are based on %TBSA of partial and full-thickness (and fourth-degree) burns.

HISTOPATHOLOGY OF BURNS

One thermal wound theory describes three zones of injury in burns (Fig. 38.6):

1. Zone of coagulation: dead, avascular tissue that must be debrided.
2. Zone of stasis: injured tissue in which blood flow is impaired. Desiccation, infection, or mechanical trauma may lead to cell death.
3. Zone of hyperemia: minimally injured, inflamed tissue that forms the border of the wound. Hyperemia usually resolves within 7 to 10 days but may be mistaken for cellulitis.

Histologically, full-thickness burns are characterized by confluent vascular thrombosis involving arterioles, venules, and capillaries. Edema secondary to loss of microvascular integrity results not only from the effects of direct thermal injury but also from the release of vasoactive mediators such as complement and histamine. Histamine increases catalytic activity of the enzyme xanthine oxidase, with resultant production of hydrogen peroxide and hydroxyl radicals. These by-products increase the damage to dermal vascular endothelial cells and result in progressive vascular permeability.

The cellular debris and denatured proteins of the eschar provide a milieu that supports the proliferation of microorganisms. The devitalized tissue (eschar) sloughs spontaneously, usually as a result of the proteolytic effect of bacterial enzymes. The greater the degree of wound bacteriostasis, the greater the delay in sloughing.

Partial-thickness burns result in incomplete vascular thrombosis, usually limited to the upper dermis. The dermal circulation is restored gradually, generally over a period of several days, thus resulting in a significant interval of relative ischemia. The eschar in deep partial-thickness burns is thinner than in a full-thickness burn and sloughs as a result of reepithelialization rather than bacterial proteolysis.

OUTPATIENT VERSUS INPATIENT CARE

One of the first steps in burn care is to select patients for whom outpatient care is appropriate. For patients determined to require inpatient care, the decision to admit or transfer the patient will depend on the burn care capabilities of the initial treating facility.

Candidates for outpatient treatment are generally adults and children who do not meet the ABA criteria for burn center referral, however some of these patients may still require inpatient care for a variety of medical or psychosocial reasons. Burns that should be initially considered for inpatient management are large burn areas; deep burns involving the hands, face, feet, neck, or perineum; burns resulting from abuse or attempted suicide; burns occurring in association with other trauma or inhalation injuries; and chemical or electrical burns. Guidelines set forth by the ABA[1] regarding criteria for referral to a burn center include the following:

- Partial-thickness burns greater than 10% TBSA.
- Burns involving the face, hands, feet, genitalia, perineum, or major joints.
- Full-thickness burns in any age group.
- Electrical burns, including lightning injury.
- Chemical burns.
- Inhalation injury.
- Burn injury in patients with preexisting medical disorders that could complicate management, prolong recovery, or affect mortality.
- Any patient with burns and concomitant trauma in which the burn injury poses the greatest risk for morbidity or mortality after emergency or surgical stabilization of the traumatic injuries. In such cases if the trauma poses the

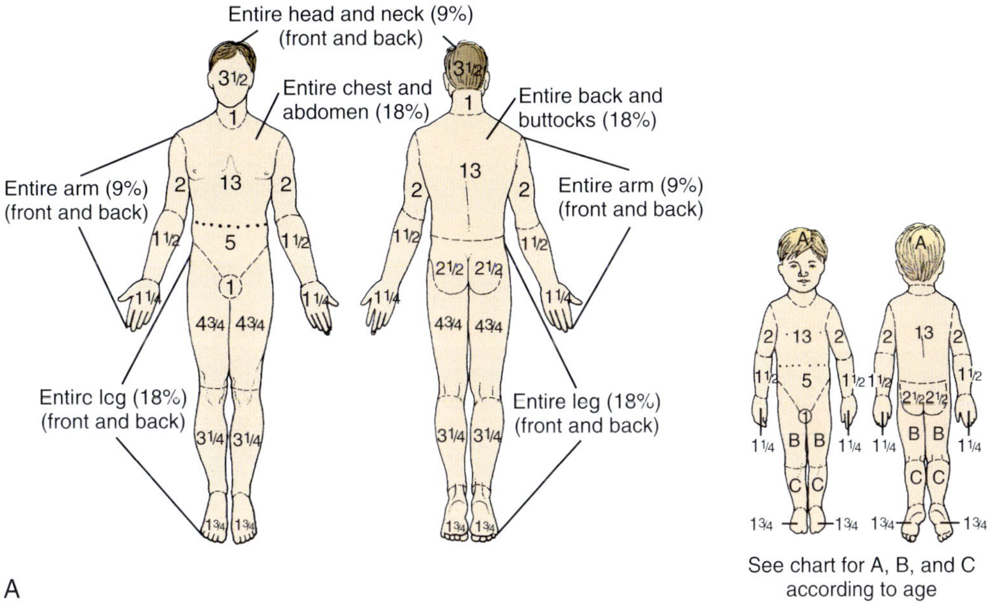

A

AGE	Birth–1 yr	1–4 yr	5–9 yr	10–14 yr	15 yr	Adult
Head	19	17	13	11	9	7
Neck	2					
Ant trunk	13					
Post trunk	13					
R buttock	2½					
L buttock	2½					
Genitalia	1					
R U arm	4					
L U arm	4					
R L arm	3					
L L arm	3					
R hand	2½	6½	8	8½	9	9½
L hand	2½	6½	8	8½	9	9½
R thigh	5½	5	5½	6	6½	7
L thigh	5½	5	5½	6	6½	7
R leg	5					
L leg	5					
R foot	3½					
L foot	3½					

B BODY AREA

Fig. 38.4 Lund-Browder charts. (A) The Lund-Browder charts are somewhat more accurate than the rule of nines in estimating the total body surface area (TBSA) burned. (B) Proportion of TBSA of individual areas according to age. When compared with adults, children have larger heads and smaller legs. Other areas are relatively equivalent throughout life. The rule of nines is not accurate in determining the percentage of TBSA burned in children.

greatest immediate risk, the patient's condition may be stabilized initially in a trauma center before transfer to a burn center. Physician judgment will be necessary in such situations and should be in concert with the regional medical control plan and triage protocols.

- Burned children in hospitals without qualified personnel or equipment for the care of children.
- Burn injury in patients who will require special social, emotional, or rehabilitative intervention.

Note, these guidelines are not absolute mandates and clinical judgment and patient characteristics may allow for deviation from these guidelines.[10] Discussion with a burn center can help determine the optimal treatment and disposition plan for the unique patient and the characteristics of the burn.

Patients who are at risk for poor outcomes with even minor burns include patients with concomitant medical problems such as diabetes mellitus, peripheral vascular disease, congestive heart failure, and end-stage renal disease; patients taking steroids or other immunosuppressive agents, patients who are very young or very old, those who are mentally impaired, have drug or alcohol dependency, those who are experiencing homelessness, those who are malnourished, and patients without a sufficient home support system. Inpatient treatment might be considered in these circumstances even for burns considered "minor" by ABA criteria, whereas very minor burns in these patients may still be treated appropriately in the outpatient setting. Other considerations for admission include pain control, the ability to return for follow-up care, the degree of incapacity, the ability to receive wound care at home, and the overall social situation; all should influence the final decision of whether admission or transfer is warranted.[11]

Additional guidelines that can assist emergency providers in determining the need for admission following an acute burn injury include:

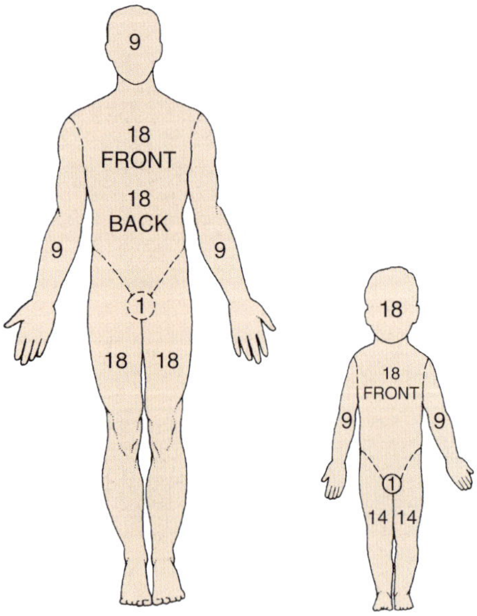

Fig. 38.5 The "rule of nines." The rule of nines is a rough estimate of the total body surface area (TBSA) burned. Note that adults and children are different. This formula frequently overestimates the extent of a burn in clinical practice. As a rough guide, the area covered by the individual's palm and fingers is approximately 1% TBSA. See Fig. 38.4 for a more accurate method of determining TBSA burned in children.

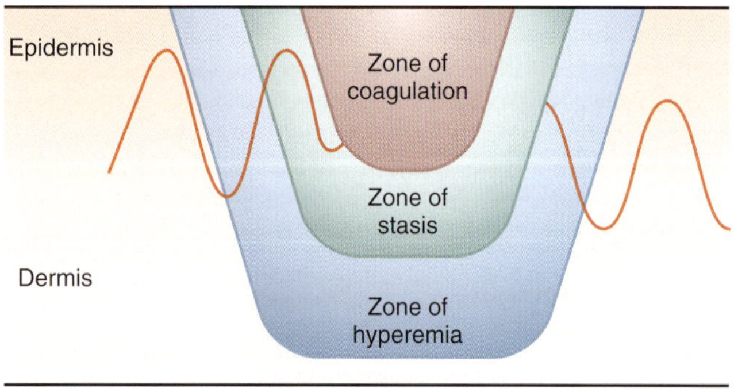

Fig. 38.6 Zones of injury after a burn. The zone of coagulation is the portion that is irreversibly injured. The zones of stasis and hyperemia are defined in response to the injury. (From Townsend CM, Beauchamp RD, Evers BM et al. eds. *Sabiston Textbook of Surgery*. 19th ed. Saunders; 2012.)

- Patients requiring intravenous (IV) access. Following a burn there is an immediate capillary leak of plasma-like fluid that can last for 18 to 24 hours. In burns involving greater than 20% TBSA, the leak occurs in both burned and nonburned tissues. If not replaced, this fluid loss can lead to hypovolemic shock and renal failure. IV fluid resuscitation is indicated for patients younger than 10 years or older than 50 years with partial and full-thickness burns greater than 10% TBSA, and for burns greater than 20% TBSA in all other age groups.
- Anticipated surgery. Deep burns are best treated by early surgical excision and skin grafting. This permits faster wound healing, provides more stable skin, and reduces contractures. Hospital admission may facilitate wound care and preparation for surgery.
- Respiratory problems. Patients with respiratory distress requiring oxygen therapy and those suspected of inhaling toxic fumes or vapors should be admitted for respiratory care and intubation with mechanical ventilation if indicated (Box 38.1). Direct bronchoscopic evaluation of the airway may assist in the evaluation and diagnosis of tracheobronchitis or pneumonitis from a smoke inhalation injury.
- Need for special nursing care. Specialized wound care, dressings, and nursing care are often required for burns involving the face, hands, feet, perineum, and genitalia and may be considered for inpatient care if outpatient care is not feasible. Patients unable to care for themselves or those lacking support to assist them may also require admission.
- Special burn injuries. Chemical injuries are often more severe than the initial examination would suggest. Unlike most thermal burns, tissue destruction may continue many hours after injury. Patients with chemical injuries should be admitted whenever the injuries are of indeterminate depth, affect a large area, are deep and require surgical excision, if there are systemic manifestations of chemical toxicity, or when the chemical responsible for the injury requires a specific antidote. Swelling from deep circumferential burns may constrict the chest or limbs and result in compartment syndrome. Such burns should be monitored frequently to determine the potential need for escharotomy or fasciotomy (Fig. 38.7). If the patient's condition prevents a reliable clinical examination, direct measurement of compartment pressures can provide an objective measurement of intracompartmental pressure and assist in the decision to perform these surgical procedures. Adult and pediatric patients with extensive burn injuries that require fluid resuscitation with large volumes of crystalloid should be monitored closely for the development of abdominal compartment syndrome.[12] Patients with mechanical burns involving large areas of skin loss or with significant frostbite injuries are often admitted for specialized wound care and parenteral pain management. Patients with electrical injuries may require admission for cardiac monitoring, specialized wound care, and/or IV fluids.

BOX 38.1 General Approach to Blisters With Minor Burns[a]

IF TREATED LESS THAN 48 HOURS AFTER THE BURN

1. Leave all intact blisters alone.
2. If blisters have ruptured, treat them as dead skin and debride them completely.

ON FOLLOW-UP OR MORE THAN 48 TO 72 HOURS AFTER THE BURN

1. Debride large (>6 cm in diameter) intact blisters and all blisters that have ruptured. Large, firm blisters on the palms and soles may be left intact longer.
2. Do not debride small or spotty blisters until they break or until 5 to 7 days after the burn.

FIVE TO 7 DAYS AFTER THE BURN

1. Debride all blisters completely.

[a]All blisters and burned skin are debrided in the presence of infection. Note: Multiple approaches to blisters are acceptable, and practice varies considerably.
Intact blisters provide significant pain relief. Be prepared for an exacerbation of pain immediately after debridement. Prophylactic analgesia is recommended.

PROCEDURE

Emergency Treatment

Home or field treatment and ED care often overlap. Initial treatment of a thermal injury begins immediately following the

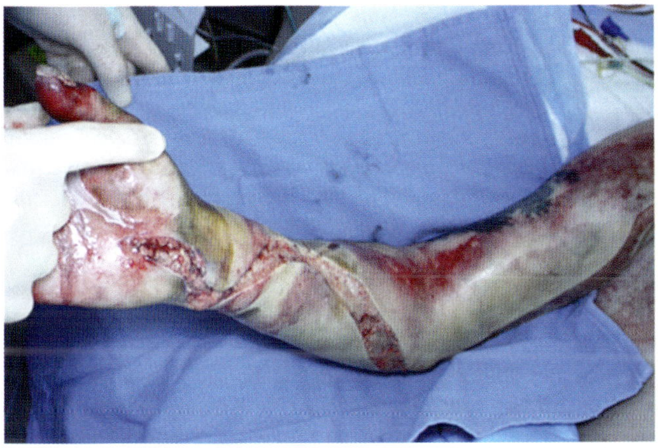

Fig. 38.7 This patient sustained circumferential full-thickness burns on the arm, and compartment syndrome developed. Escharotomy was required.

burn. Patients should be rapidly removed from the source of injury whenever possible. Flames are extinguished by smothering the fire with a blanket, jacket, or equivalent item; by dousing the fire with water; or by using a chemical fire extinguisher. Most chemical injuries are best treated by irrigating the affected area with copious amounts of water. Patients with electrical injuries are removed from contact with the electrical source as soon as it is safe to do so.

Cooling is most beneficial for small burns if started within 3 minutes of injury and can be of additional benefit for the first few hours after the burn. Doing so has been shown to reduce pain significantly and can limit tissue damage by decreasing thromboxane production. When cooling a burn wound, it is important to avoid hypothermia or freezing of tissue because this may deepen the injury. Room-temperature or cold tap water irrigation, immersion, or compresses (20°C to 25°C) will provide some pain relief without the risk of further injuring burned tissues and inducing hypothermia, which can occur with iced solutions (Fig. 38.8). Placing ice on a burn should not be done. Sterile dressings are not required for field treatment; a moist towel or nonadherent sheet may be used. Nonmentholated shaving cream makes an excellent temporary covering for out-of-hospital use if a dressing is not available. Home remedies, such as butter or Vaseline, are best avoided and can be difficult and painful to remove. Remove jewelry and gross debris in the field if possible.

Initial Care of Major Burns

Major burns require the specialized resources of a burn center. In such cases, emergency providers should initiate the resuscitation, consult the burn center for referral, and transfer the patient as soon as possible. Initial resuscitation should follow standardized trauma protocols, including a primary and secondary survey, and provide immediate interventions directed at cardiovascular support and airway management, as needed. IV catheters can be inserted initially through burned skin when unburned sites are not available. Early IV access permits the administration of necessary medications, including parenteral narcotics to relieve the pain, and resuscitative fluids.

Patients with burns exceeding 20% TBSA *should receive IV fluid resuscitation with lactated Ringer's (LR) solution* or other balanced solution. The balanced solutions are preferred because large saline infusions can produce a hyperchloremic acidosis.

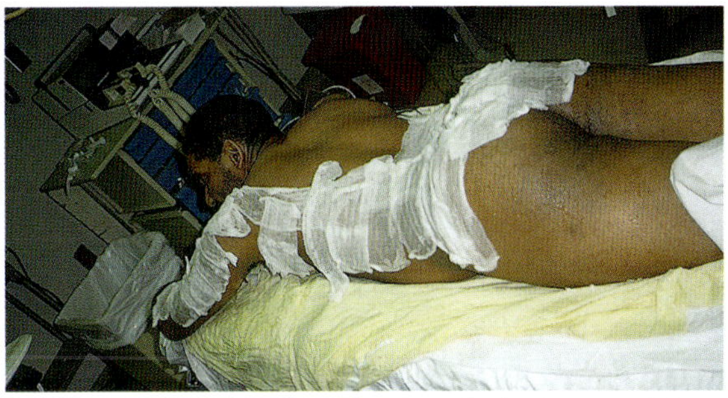

Fig. 38.8 To cool a burn that cannot easily be immersed in water, cover the area with unfolded gauze pads that have been soaked in room-temperature saline. Continue to frequently soak the gauze with cool saline or tap water drawn up in a syringe. Adding a few ice chips to the liquid is helpful, but do not cover the burn with ice. Towels are generally too bulky for this procedure. Narcotics are the best way to control pain in any burn and should be used liberally.

Bolus fluid resuscitation is not necessary as fluids are lost via capillary leak and via the raw skin, and significant fluid loss does not occur within the first hour.

For patients with visibly large burns, ABA recommendations initiating an age-based fluids rate while calculating exact fluid needs: 125 mL/h for patients 5 years old or less, 250 mL/h for patients 6 to 13 years old, and 500 mL/h in patients age 14 and above. Exact fluids needs can be calculated once a thorough assessment of TBSA can be performed.[13]

Current advanced burn life support (ABLS) fluid resuscitation guidelines advise that adults receive a total of 2 mL LR × body weight in kilograms × % partial and full-thickness burns in the first 24 hours. For pediatric patients (under age 14 and weight less than 40 kg), the ABLS advises a total of 3 mL LR × body weight in kilograms × % partial and full-thickness burns in the first 24 hours. It should be noted that 24 hours starts at the time of the burn and not the time care begins. After the total amount is calculated, fluids should be administered as a constant infusion rather than by bolus administration. Half of the calculated fluid requirement should be given in the first 8 hours and the remaining half provided over the following 16 hours (Box 38.2). These fluid quantities are guidelines and urine output monitoring should be used in adjusting the rate or volume to meet the target outputs of 0.5 mL/kg per hour for adults and 1 mL/kg per hour for children weighing under 40 kg.

Historically, the Parkland or Brooke formulas have been used to estimate fluid needs. It should be noted that the *2018 Advanced Burn Life Support Manual* specifies that research has shown that the Parkland formula's 4 mg/kg × %TBSA formula commonly results in excessive edema formation and over-resuscitation.[13] Whether this is because first-degree burns may have been erroneously included in the %TBSA is unclear.

The US Army Institute of Surgical Research has advocated a simpler formula for estimating hourly fluid requirements in burn patients. For adult patients up to 80 kg, this formula recommends 10 mL/h × %TBSA of partial and full-thickness burns; for patients heavier than 80 kg it recommends adding 100 mL/h for every additional 10 kg of body weight. This simpler formula may be more useful for prehospital providers or ED resuscitation (Box 38.3). These formulas estimate hourly fluid requirements and must be adjusted up or down to achieve a urine output of 0.5 to 1.0 mL/h. Regardless of the formula used, insertion of a Foley catheter may be necessary

BOX 38.2 ABA ABLS Initial Fluid Recommendations for Burn Patients in First 24 Hours

1. Lactated Ringer's (LR) is the fluid of choice.
2. Estimate %TBSA (count partial and full-thickness burn only).
3. Obtain actual body weight in kilograms.
4. Utilize appropriate formula as detailed below:
   - **Adults With Thermal and Chemical Burns:**
     2 mL LR × patient's body weight in kg × %TBSA (partial and full thickness only)
   - **Children 14 Years or Younger and Body Weight of Less Than 40 kg**
     3 mL LR × child's weight in kg × %TBSA (partial and full thickness only)—add normal maintenance fluid to the fluid requirements, consider including dextrose in maintenance fluids for infants and young children who may rapidly deplete glycogen stores, particularly for those 2 years and younger.[40]
   - **Adult Patients With High-Voltage Electrical Injuries**
     If there is evidence of deep tissue injury or red pigments in urine use:
     4 mL LR × patient's body weight in kg × %TBSA (partial and full thickness only)

Infuse half of the calculated 24-hour fluid needs in the first 8 hours following the burn. Infuse the second half of the 24-hour fluid needs in the next 16 hours (hours 9–24).

Increase or decrease the fluid rate based on the patient's urine output. Adjust fluids to maintain urine output at 0.5 mL/kg per hour in adults and 1 mL/kg per hour in children.

ABA, *American Burn Association;* ABLS, *advanced burn life support;* TBSA, *total body surface area.*

BOX 38.3 Simplified ED Burn Fluid Resuscitation: Rule of 10

1. Estimate burn size (%TBSA) to the nearest 10.
2. %TBSA × 10 = initial fluid rate in mL/h (for adult patients weighing 40 kg to 80 kg).
3. For every 10 kg above 80 kg, increase the rate by 100 mL/h.

ED, *Emergency department;* TBSA, *total body surface area.*
From Chung KK, Salinas J, Renz EM et al. Simple derivation of the initial fluid rate for the resuscitation of severely burned adult combat casualties: in silico validation of the rule of 10. J Trauma. *2010;69:S49-S54.*

to accurately measure hourly urine output in the setting of major burns requiring targeted fluid resuscitation.

Patients exposed to carbon monoxide should have carboxyhemoglobin levels measured and empirically receive 100% oxygen. The duration of oxygen administration will depend on the level and symptoms, but often require 6 hours or more. Once considered a traditional empirical treatment, there is no proven benefit of hyperbaric oxygen therapy for carbon monoxide poisoning. A Cochrane review from 2011 (http://www.summaries.cochrane.org/CD002042) concluded that there is insufficient evidence to support the use of hyperbaric oxygen for the treatment of patients with carbon monoxide poisoning. The Cochrane review of published trials found conflicting, potentially biased, and generally weak evidence regarding the usefulness of hyperbaric oxygen for the prevention of neurologic injury.[13a] Consultation with a local hyperbaric center is reasonable in some cases, but it is not standard that this intervention be routinely implemented. Critically ill and pregnant patients are still often offered hyperbaric treatment, but controversy over the efficacy and safety persists even for these subgroups. The ABA advocates that transfer to a burn center should not be delayed in order to implement hyperbaric oxygen therapy (Videos 38.1 and 38.2).

Cyanide is released from some fires, such as mattress fires and burning of upholstery. Patients suspected of having been exposed to significant levels of cyanide and manifesting symptoms of cyanide toxicity should receive hydroxocobalamin (Cyanokit [BTG Specialty Pharmaceuticals]). If not available, the Cyanide Antidote Kit (amyl nitrite, sodium nitrite, sodium thiosulfate) may be used despite the lack of proven benefit of this traditional cyanide therapy. Cyanide testing results may not be available in the emergency setting, and it is reasonable to empirically administer hydroxocobalamin or the sodium thiosulfate portion of the cyanide kit to burn patients in coma or to those exhibiting a significant metabolic (lactic) acidosis after smoke exposure.

In addition to the increased mortality with larger areas of TBSA involved, the mortality of patients with burns is also increased when concomitant inhalation is present. The Baux score was developed a half-century ago by Professor Serge Baux to estimate the mortality of burns. This score was updated in 2010 using data from the National Burn Registry to include the effect of inhalation injury to mortality (Box 38.4).[14]

Major burn patients have an impaired ability to regulate their core body temperature and will quickly become hypothermic if not managed appropriately. Core temperature should be measured frequently, and active and passive warming strategies should be implemented to prevent hypothermia from developing. This includes minimizing exposure by covering patients with sheets and blankets, warming IV fluids, warming the room, or applying radiant or convective warming systems. In anticipation of transfer to a burn center or while awaiting surgical consultation, removal of any wet cooling dressings and covering the wounds with dry gauze dressings can help decrease hypothermia risk.

Initial Care of Minor Burns

Prompt cooling of the burned areas is an almost instinctive response and is one of the oldest recorded burn treatments, having been recommended by Galen (129–99 CE) and Rhazes (852–923 CE). Because many patients with minor burns seek medical attention after initial self-instituted prehospital cooling, it is unlikely that the clinician can favorably affect the burned tissue with any intervention in the ED. With the exception of pain relief and removal of debris, the primary benefits of burn cooling are probably experienced only if the burn is cooled promptly, within the first 3 minutes after injury, thus making prehospital care important.

In the ED, room-temperature or cold tap water irrigation, immersion, or compresses (20°C to 25°C) are optimal for burned tissues without the problems of hypothermia that iced solutions can cause. If not done before arrival in

BOX 38.4 Baux Score and Modified Baux Score to Predict Mortality in Burn Injury

Original Baux Score: % Mortality = Age + %TBSA
Modified Baux Score: % Mortality = Age + %TBSA + 17 × (inhalation injury: yes = 1, no = 0)

APPENDIX: CALCULATION OF THE PREDICTED PROBABILITY OF DEATH FROM THE LOGISTIC REGRESSION MODEL BASED ON THE REVISED BAUX SCORE

$$\text{Revised Baux Logistic Model} = \frac{e^{-8.8163+(0.0775*\text{rBaux})}}{1+e^{-8.8163+(0.0775*\text{rBaux})}} \quad \text{(Equation 2):}$$

Which can be programmed into a hand held calculator or obtained from the following nomogram:

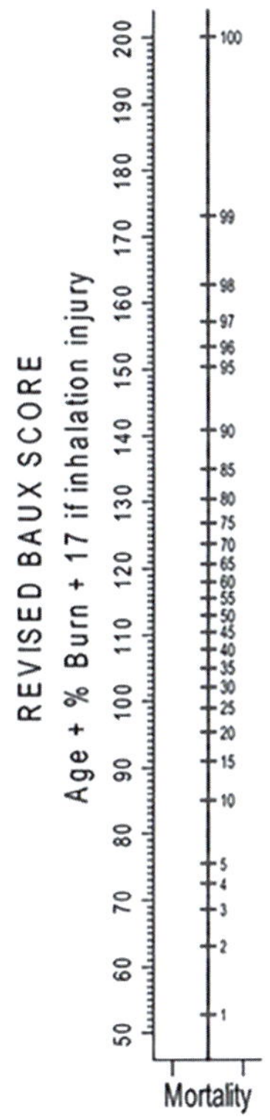

To estimate mortality, find the Revised Baux Score on the left hand axis and read mortality on the right axis. For example, a patient aged 50 with a burn area of 33% and an inhalation injury would have a revised Baux Score of 50 + 33 +17 =100, and a predicted mortality of 26%.

Plot of the observed mortality versus the group midpoint computed within 10 groups of the revised Baux score.

From Osler T, Glance LG, Hosmer DW. Simplified estimates of the probability of death after burn injuries: Extending and updating the Baux score. *J Trauma Acute Care Surgery*. 2010;68(3):690–697. doi: 10.1097/TA.0b013e3181c453b3.

the ED, immediate cold-water immersion in the ED may still have some value in limiting the extent of a burn and can provide significant pain relief. It is acceptable to add a few ice chips to the water, but packing the wound in ice should be avoided. The potential benefits of burn cooling are listed in Box 38.5.

All involved clothing and jewelry (such as rings), along with any gross debris, should be removed from the burned area. Chemical burns, particularly those involving the eyes, require prolonged tap water irrigation. The burn should otherwise be covered with a moist, sterile dressing (see Fig. 38.8). The gauze may be kept cool and moist to provide continued pain relief; the patient will often let the clinician know when additional cooling is desired. Sterile saline has no proven benefit over tap water even when the skin is broken.

BOX 38.5 Advantages of Prompt Burn Cooling

Limit extent of thermal damage
Reduction or cessation of pain
Elimination of local hyperthermia
Inhibition of postburn tissue destruction
Decreased edema
Reduced metabolism and toxin production

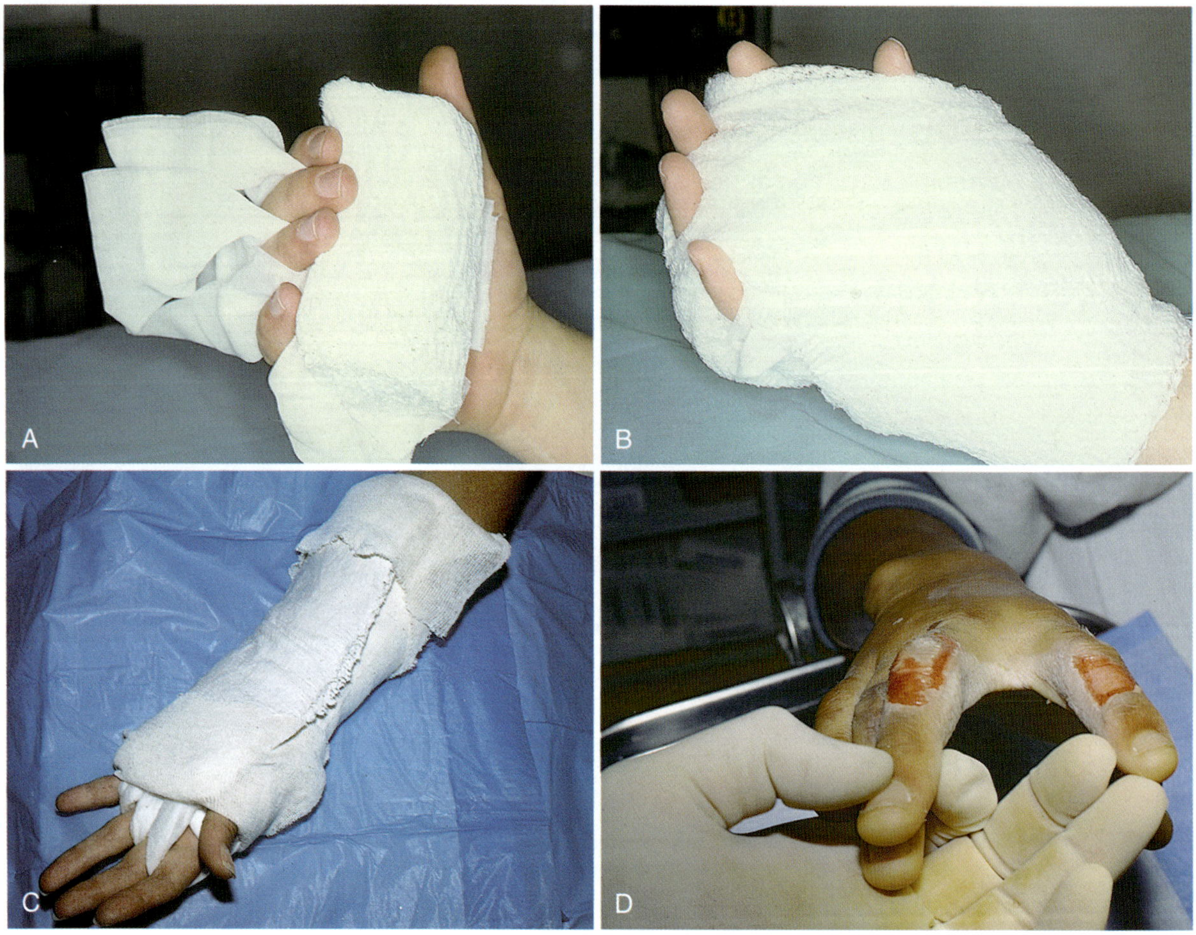

Fig. 38.9 Outpatient burn dressing of the hand. Patients with serious hand burns should be referred to a burn center and may require admission. (A) After the application of an antibiotic ointment or a dry, nonadherent dressing, separate the fingers with fluffs in the web spaces and (B) enclose the entire hand in a position of function (here with the help of a roll of Kerlix). (C) If the wrist is involved, a removable plaster splint may be applied over the dressing. (D) The result of a minor burn involving the hand when the fingers were not wrapped individually. Initially, there were only a few blisters, but this patient now has partial-thickness skin loss because of an improper burn dressing that caused maceration of normal skin between the fingers. Not only were the fingers incorrectly wrapped together in one gauze wrap, but the first wound check was also incorrectly scheduled in 6 days, too long for the first wound inspection of a hand burn.

In the ED and prehospital phase, prompt analgesics, including opiates, are the best way to control pain and should be prioritized in the early phase of burn care.

All burns are considered tetanus-prone, and tetanus toxoid should be administered if patients are unsure of their tetanus immunization status or if it has been more than 10 years since the last immunization. Nonimmunized patients should receive tetanus toxoid and immunization with subsequent boosters in accordance with current guidelines.

Outpatient Care of Minor Burns

Minor burns are generally those that will heal spontaneously and do not require surgery or specialized wound care. Unlike larger burns, these wounds are not associated with immunosuppression or hypermetabolism and are not as susceptible to infection. Treated conservatively, most minor burns will heal without significant scarring. Many complications seen with minor burns are thought to result from overtreatment rather than undertreatment. Examples include the use of dressings that can adhere to newly forming skin and the overzealous use of topical or systemic antibiotics.

The most important characteristic of a dressing is that it controls fluids within the wound. Burn dressings that keep the surface of the wound moist and avoid pooling of fluids will speed healing. The best material for this purpose is a generous amount of simple dry gauze applied over a nonadherent dressing or topical preparation. The outer layer of dressing should be porous to permit evaporation of water from the absorbent dressing material. Wound preparation and basic bandaging should include the following steps (Fig. 38.9):

1. Cleanse the burned area gently with warm water or saline, a mild cleansing agent such as soap or dilute chlorhexidine, and a clean cloth or gauze. It is not necessary to shave the hair in or around the wound. Avoid chlorhexidine in close proximity to the eyes; it is reasonable to use a baby shampoo formulation with warm water if available. There is no benefit to vigorously washing a minor wound with strong antiseptic preparations.

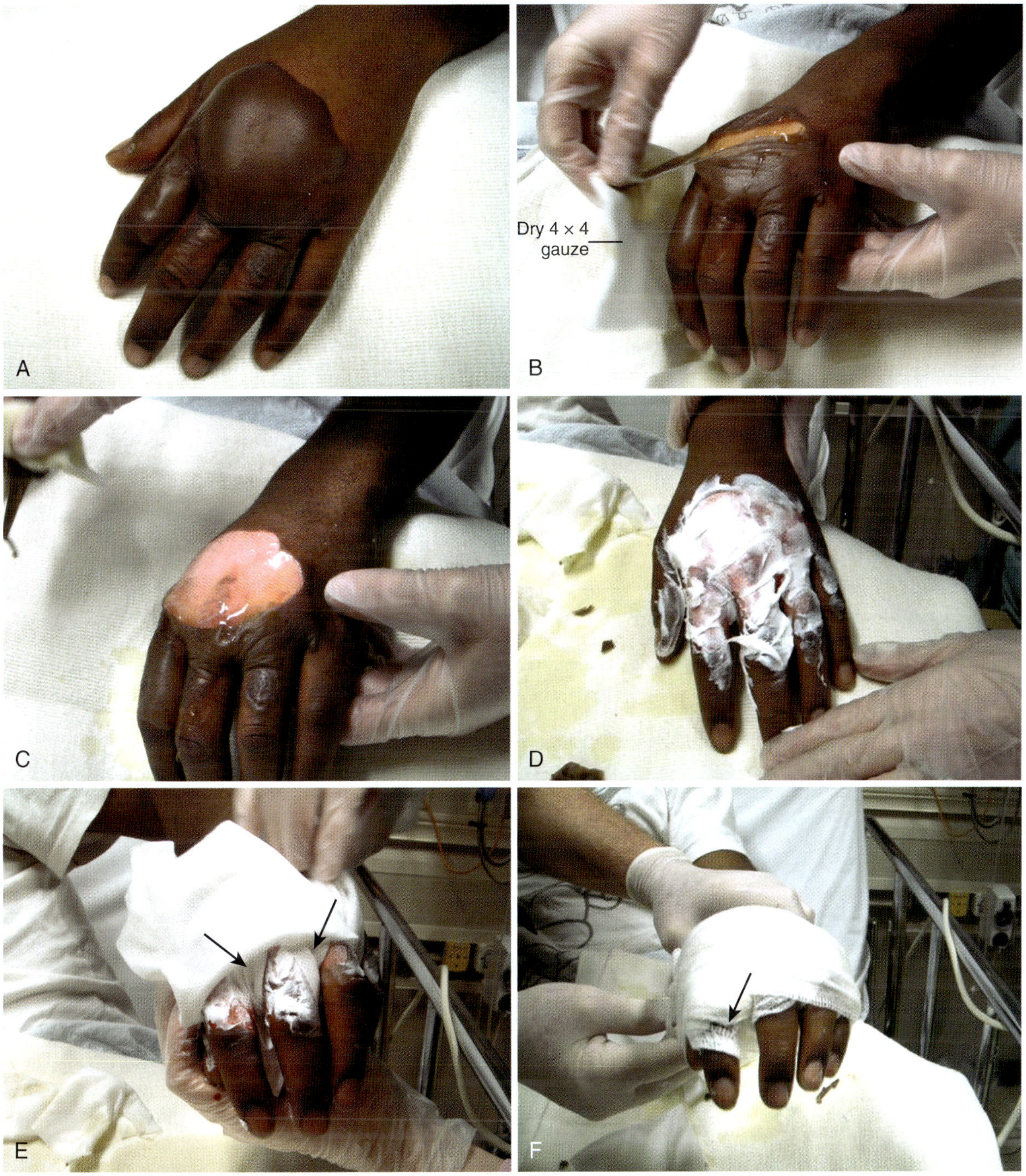

Fig. 38.10 Debridement and dressing of a blistering burn. (A) Exactly when to debride burn blisters is controversial and probably of no consequence to the final outcome (see text), although blisters often thin after the first 24 to 48 hours and are therefore easier to debride at that time. Eventually, however, all dead tissue must be removed. (B and C) The easiest and quickest way to debride blisters is to grasp the dead loose skin with dry 4- × 4-inch gauze and pull it off quickly rather than with slow meticulous instrument techniques. Provide analgesia that is appropriate for the clinical condition. (D) Apply an appropriate ointment to the denuded tissue. (Silvadene is shown here, but *it is no longer recommended.*) (E and F) The debridement itself is not especially painful, but when the underlying tissue is exposed, pain increases. Hence, dress the burn quickly after debridement.

2. Although some authors recommend leaving blisters intact, many sources advise that providers debride blisters. Sloughed skin should be debrided by peeling the devitalized skin from the wound (Fig. 38.10A–C). Blisters can be opened with scissors and forceps after thorough skin cleansing. If necessary, provide analgesia for any painful debridement. On the initial debridement, attempt to remove only grossly devitalized tissue. Additional debridement of the wound can take place, if needed, during subsequent follow-up visits when the wound has matured.
3. Consider applying a layer of antibiotic ointment directly to the wound. Historically, silver sulfadiazine cream (Silvadene [Pfizer Inc.]) was routine for superficial and

partial-thickness burns, but some evidence has shown that silver sulfadiazine is consistently associated with poorer healing and outcomes compared with many other dressing options, thought to be due to its toxic effects on keratinocytes.[15] Use of silver sulfadiazine is not longer recommended. An alternative antibiotic ointment is preferred.

4. Apply fine-mesh gauze or commercial nonadherent gauze such as Adaptic (3M) or petrolatum gauze impregnated with 3% bismuth tribromophenate (Xeroform [Cardinal Health]); or other dressing as recommended by your local burn center to the burn wound.
5. Cover and pad the wound with loose gauze fluffs. If fingers and toes are involved, pad the web spaces and the digits individually and separate them with strips of gauze (Figs. 38.9D and 38.10E–F). Wrap the entire dressing snugly (but not tightly) with an absorbent, slightly elastic gauze material (Kerlix [Cardinal Health]).
6. Instruct the patient to elevate the affected limb to prevent swelling, which may cause delayed burn conversion or wound infection.

Open Burn Care

Following cleansing of the wound with water, soap, and/or chlorhexidine and debridement of blisters and any loose skin, wounds that are not amenable to a dressing, such as those on the face, can be managed initially by the application of a bland topical antibiotic such as bacitracin; silver sulfadiazine is no longer recommended. The wound can be washed two or three times per day, followed by reapplication of the topical agent. This is the preferred method for managing burns on the face and neck.

Burn Dressings

There is a large variety of burn dressings available and the landscape is ever evolving. As noted previously the most common dressings in the emergency setting are fine-mesh gauze and nonadherent gauze. Many synthetic and biosynthetic dressings are available, but evidence comparing the outcomes achieved with each is limited. These dressing include biosynthetic dressings that are designed to allow reepithelialization before separating spontaneously from the wound; silver containing dressings designed to minimize bacterial colonization without inhibiting wound healing; silicon-coated dressings designed to be a nonadherent and reduce dressing change trauma; and hydrogel dressings designed to maintain a moist healing environment in wounds with higher levels of exudate.[15–17]

These preparations have theoretical benefits under certain circumstances, but are not proven to have superior performance over simple gauze dressings for minor outpatient burns.[18] These products are most often used by burn centers and have little applicability for minor burns in patients discharged from the ED. For patients admitted or transferred to a burn center, simple gauze dressings are appropriate. Many burn centers prefer that topical agents not be applied before transfer so that the full extent of the burn can be assessed immediately on arrival at the burn center.

Burn centers will also use biologic dressings, although they are not routinely used in the emergency care of patients who do not require burn center referral. Biologic dressings are natural tissues, including skin that consists of collagen sheets containing elastin and lipid. The benefits of biologic dressings include a reduction in surface bacterial colonization, diminished fluid and heat loss, avoidance of further wound contamination, and prevention of damage to newly developed granulation tissue. Examples of biologic dressings include cadaveric human skin and commercially available porcine xenograft or collagen sheets.

Specific Clinical Issues in Minor Burn Care

Analgesia

Pain is a critical feature of any burn injury. Relief of pain by the appropriate and judicious use of analgesics is of the utmost importance in the initial care of all burn patients. Prehospital pain control by emergency medical service is very appropriate when standard contraindications do not exist. Analgesia should be provided before extensive examination or debridement is performed. Inadequate analgesia is probably the most common ED error in the treatment of burn injuries, especially when burns occur in children.

Regional or nerve block anesthesia is an excellent alternative when possible, and if feasible, nitrous oxide analgesia may be used. Ketamine may also be a reasonable alternative. Oral opioids may be inadequate for the initial treatment of significant burns but can be used for continued outpatient analgesia. Local anesthetics may be injected in small quantities when appropriate, such as for the debridement of a deep ulcer or other small burn. Topical analgesics have no established role in burn care. A properly designed dressing will do much toward preventing further discomfort after discharge; however, home burn care and dressing changes may be quite painful. For this reason, an adequate supply of an oral analgesic should be provided, and responsibility in analgesic use should be encouraged.

Pruritus

Postburn pruritus is one of the most common and distressing complications of burn injury and is estimated to affect 87% of burns.[19] It typically develops in the subacute phase and is therefore not a common issue for the emergency provider in the acute treatment phase. Despite the limited literature on the treatment of postburn pruritus, available therapies include oral antihistamines, topical antihistamines, and topical moisturizers. The use of topical therapies should be withheld until sufficient wound healing has occurred.

Edema

Minor burns lead to immediate inflammation mediated by the release of histamine and bradykinins, which cause localized derangements in vascular permeability with resultant burn wound edema. This edema can be harmful in several ways. First, the increase in interstitial fluid increases the diffusion distance of oxygen from capillaries to cells and thereby increases hypoxia in an already ischemic wound. Second, the edema may produce untoward hemodynamic effects by a purely mechanical mechanism: compression of vessels in muscular compartments. Third, edema has been associated with the inactivation of streptococcicidal skin fatty acids, thus predisposing the patient to burn cellulitis.

Successful management of burn edema hinges on immobilization and elevation. Most patients are unfamiliar with the medical definition of elevation and are not aware or convinced of its value. Patient education in this regard is critical; however, certain burns (e.g., burns in dependent body areas) are prone to edema despite everyone's best intentions. It is for this reason that lower extremity burns in general and foot burns in particular are prone to problems. Major burns of the hand should be elevated while the patient is still in the ED. This can be accomplished by hanging the injured hand from an IV pole with a stockinette to support the bandaged hand (Fig. 38.11). Additionally, minimizing the risk for edema by avoiding over-resuscitation with IV fluids is critical to minimize risk for tissue edema.

Use of Topical Preparations and Antimicrobials

Minor burns result rarely result in significant impairment of normal host immunologic defenses, and burn wound infection is not usually a significant problem. Topical antimicrobials are of unproven value but are often used even on the most minor burns; however, some believe that these agents may impair wound healing. Most patients expect some type of topical concoction, so a discussion of their use—or nonuse—is prudent.

Topical antimicrobials were designed for the prevention and care of burn wound sepsis or wound infection, primarily in hospitalized patients with major burns, and there is no convincing evidence that their use alters the course of superficial and superficial partial-thickness burns. As noted, thorough skin cleansing and an appropriate burn dressing are key in minimizing complications in all burns. Nonetheless, topical antimicrobials are often soothing to minor burns, and their daily use prompts the patient to look at the wound, assess healing, perform prescribed dressing changes, or otherwise become personally involved in the care. Keep in mind that if a topical antimicrobial is used, its effectiveness is decreased in the presence of proteinaceous exudate, thus necessitating regular dressing changes if the antimicrobial benefit of topical therapy is to be realized. Once-daily dressing changes are most practical and are commonly prescribed, and no convincing data indicate that this regimen is inferior to more frequent dressing changes.

All deep partial-thickness and full-thickness burns should receive topical antimicrobial therapy because the eschar and burn exudate are good bacterial culture media and deep escharotic or subescharotic infections may not be easily detected until further damage is done. As stated, this intervention can await definitive therapy in a burn unit.

Criteria for choosing a specific topical agent include its in vitro and clinical efficacy, local and systemic toxicity, superinfection rate, ease and flexibility of use, cost, patient acceptance, and side effects. It is important to note that no firm scientific data convincingly support the use of any specific topical antimicrobial for minor outpatient burns.

Topical Agents

Broad-Spectrum Antibiotic Ointments. Many nonprescription topical antimicrobials are used for minor burn therapy despite a paucity of literature attesting to any benefits. Included are bacitracin zinc ointment, polymyxin B–bacitracin (Polysporin). These are all soothing, cosmetically acceptable for open treatment (such as on the face), and effective antiseptics under burn dressings. Some researchers caution against agents containing neomycin because of a potential for sensitization. Though commonly applied by patients without adverse effects, topicals that contain neomycin (Neosporin) have the potential for inducing contact dermatitis. Plain bacitracin or polymyxin B–bacitracin ointment is commonly recommended as the routine topical agents for most burns.

Silver Sulfadiazine (Silvadene). This poorly soluble compound is synthesized by reacting silver nitrate with sodium sulfadiazine. It is still a commonly used topical agent for outpatients, but evidence has shown that silver sulfadiazine typically performs worse than other wound treatment options, likely due to its toxic effects on keratinocytes. Recent studies have identified that silver sulfadiazine likely retards wounds healing, impairs epithelialization, can discolor skin, and can cause hypersensitivity reaction.[18,20] Silver sulfadiazine has broad gram-positive and gram-negative antimicrobial spectrum including β-hemolytic streptococci, *Staphylococcus aureus* and *Staphylococcus epidermidis*, *Pseudomonas* spp., *Proteus* spp., *Klebsiella* spp., Enterobacteriaceae, *Escherichia coli*, *Candida albicans*, and possibly herpesvirus hominis.

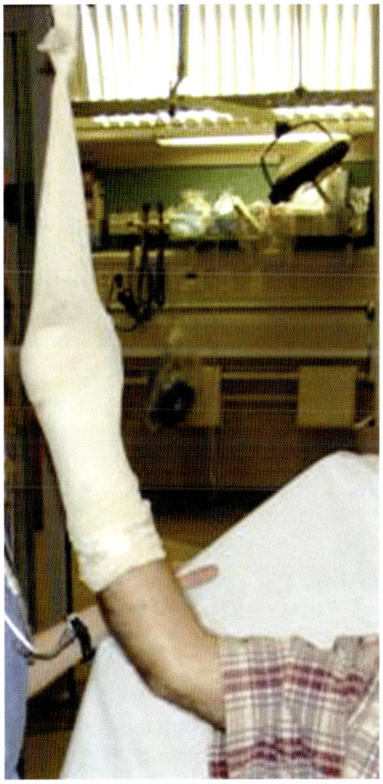

Fig. 38.11 Begin elevation of a burned hand in the emergency department. After a hand dressing is applied, suspend the arm from an intravenous pole with stockinette. A plaster or fiberglass splint may also be incorporated into the dressing.

Silver sulfadiazine is well tolerated by most patients (see Fig. 38.10D), has minimal systemic effects, and is painless on application. It must be applied daily or twice daily, and the thick white cream can be difficult, and therefore painful, to remove. There are no well-designed studies confirming improved burn healing or a reduced rate of infection with silver sulfadiazine. As noted, it may impede reepithelialization and hence many burn specialists prefer plain antibiotic ointment as the topical agent of choice because of its cost, equal efficacy, and good patient acceptance.

Silver sulfadiazine is contraindicated for term pregnancy and in newborns (i.e., because of possible induction of kernicterus). Allergy and irritation are unusual, although there is potential cross-sensitivity between silver sulfadiazine and other sulfonamides. One downside of silver sulfadiazine is that it often interacts with wound exudate to form a pseudomembrane (pseudoeschar) over partial-thickness injuries. This pseudomembrane is often difficult and painful to remove. Removing the pseudomembrane is necessary to monitor the wound state and facilitate reepitheliazation.

Aloe Vera Cream. Aloe vera cream is commercially available in a 50% or higher concentration with a preservative. It exhibits antibacterial activity against at least four common burn wound pathogens: *Pseudomonas aeruginosa*, *Enterobacter aerogenes*, *S. aureus*, and *Klebsiella pneumoniae*. Aloe vera cream is an acceptable, inexpensive option for open or dressed outpatient care of minor burns.

Honey. Honey has long been advocated as an inexpensive and effective topical treatment for minor outpatient burns. The physicochemical properties of honey (osmotic effect, pH) give this substance the antibacterial and antiinflammatory properties that support its use. Some trials have shown honey to be superior to other treatments, such as silver sulfadiazine, with regard to superficial and partial-thickness burn wound healing.[21] Honey is not widely used, but it has been promulgated as a safe, effective, and inexpensive dressing for the outpatient management of burn wounds.

Corticosteroids. High-potency topical steroid preparations have no beneficial effects on the rate of healing or limitation of scarring of thermal burns. Their use is not supported.[22]

FOLLOW-UP CARE OF MINOR BURNS

The specifics of outpatient follow-up of minor burns are controversial and often based on clinician preference and personal bias rather than on good literature. Follow-up should be individualized for each patient and should be based on the reliability of the patient, the extent of the injury, the frequency and complexity of dressing changes, and the amount of discomfort anticipated during a dressing change. Depending on the characteristics of the patient and the resources available to them, follow-up plans may include primary care physician rechecks, follow-up at a wound care center, home health visits by a wound care team, or even return to an ED or "fast-track" setting. Outpatient wound care centers often have excellent facilities to monitor outpatient burns with clinician oversight.

If a topical antibiotic agent is used, the dressing should be changed daily with removal and reapplication of the topical preparation. The wound should be rechecked by a clinician after 2 to 3 days and periodically thereafter, depending on wound size, compliance, healing, and social issues. If a dry dressing is chosen, follow-up every 3 to 5 days is usually adequate. The purpose of any burn dressing changes or home care regimen is defeated if the patient cannot afford the material or is not instructed on burn care. Many EDs supply burn dressing material on patient release. A complete pack may include antibiotic ointment or cream, gauze pads, an absorbent gauze roll, a sterile tongue blade to apply the cream, and tape (Fig. 38.12). Providing limited supplies of the items necessary for dressing changes may enhance compliance with follow-up if the patient must return for additional supplies.

Daily home care can be performed by the patient with help from a family member or visiting nurse (Box 38.6). The dressing should be removed each day and the burn area gently washed with a clean cloth or a gauze pad, tap water, and a bland soap. Sterile saline and prescription soaps are not required. The affected area may be put through a gentle range of motion during dressing changes, if indicated. After the burn is cleaned, the patient inspects it in the hope that complications can be recognized and prompt further follow-up. After complete removal of the old cream, a new layer is applied and covered with absorbent gauze.

If the undermost fine-mesh gauze of a dry dressing is dry and the coagulum is sealed to the gauze, the patient should allow the dressing to remain and simply reapply the overlying gauze dressing. If the wound is moist and macerated, the fine-mesh gauze should be removed, and the wound cleaned and redressed. When epithelialization is complete, the crust will separate, and the gauze can be removed at that time.

In the postacute phase, dryness in healing skin may be treated with mild emollients or other readily available over-the-counter skin care moisturizing lotions. Natural skin lubrication mechanisms usually return by 6 to 8 weeks. Sun exposure should be minimized during wound maturation because this may lead to hyperpigmentation. When the patient is outdoors, sun avoidance strategies should be used, or at the very least, a commercially available sunblock should be applied over healed burned areas. Exposure of the recently healed burned area to otherwise minor trauma (chemicals, heat, sun) can result in an exaggerated skin response. Pruritus is common and may be treated with oral antihistamines or a topical moisturizing cream.

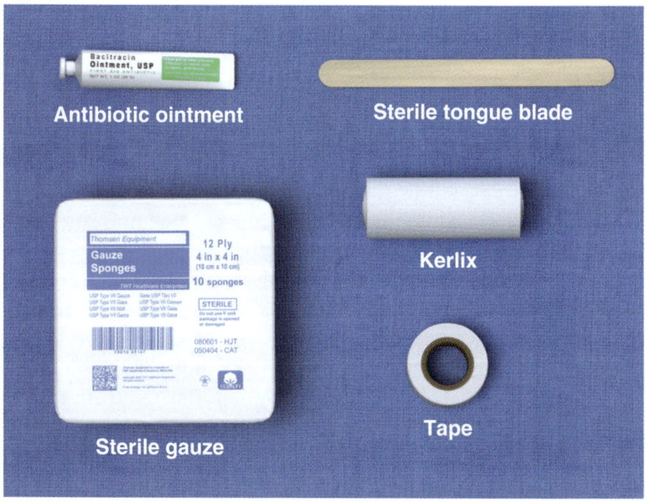

Fig. 38.12 Providing patients with burn dressing material on discharge encourages proper home care. Dispensing only limited supplies of the items may enhance compliance with follow-up visits.

BOX 38.6 How to Change a Burn Dressing at Home: Patient Instructions

1. Take pain medicine 30 minutes before dressing change if you find dressing changes to be painful.
2. If the burn is on the hand, foot, or other areas that are difficult to reach, have someone help you.
3. Have all materials available. Gloves may be worn.
4. Remove the dressing and rinse off all burn cream or ointment with tap water, under a shower, or in the bathtub. The area can be gently washed with mild soap and a clean cloth or gauze pads.
5. Look at the burn and assess the healing, blistering, and amount of swelling. Note any signs of infection.
6. Gently exercise the area through range of motion.
7. Apply the burn ointment with a sterile tongue blade.
8. Cover the cream with fluffed-up gauze.
9. Wrap the area in bulky gauze.
10. Repeat this dressing change daily.

Outpatient Wound Center Care for Burn

Many outpatient wound centers are ideally equipped to treat minor burns. If available, it is prudent to consider this option as a means of longitudinal follow-up. Many centers make available daily or periodic burn treatment consisting of dressing changes, whirlpool debridement, and range-of-motion exercises. An additional advantage is that medically trained personnel evaluate the burn daily, thereby decreasing clinician visits and enabling identification of problems before serious complications develop. Visiting home wound care services may also be appropriate for individual patient needs.

Burn Wound Healing

Burn wound healing differs from healing of other soft tissue wounds. The duration is variable but is often proportional to burn depth. Within 1 to 3 weeks and following the initial inflammatory response, neovascularization of the burn occurs and is accompanied by fibroblast migration. Collagen production begins but it is often deposited randomly, thereby leading to scar formation. Reepithelialization follows collagen deposition. The persistence of necrotic tissue and eschar in the wound will impede all aspects of healing. Proper wound debridement is associated with faster wound healing and minimizes scar formation. The extent of scar formation is often related directly to healing time.

Healing of superficial burns occurs by reepithelialization from the wound edge and from residual dermal elements containing epithelial cells. This process generally requires 10 to 14 days. After healing, the initial epithelial layer is often fragile and is easily reinjured. The application of bland, lanolin-containing creams for 4 to 8 weeks after initial healing may reduce dryness and cracking of the healing wound.

Deep burns lack residual dermal elements within the wound and heal by reepithelialization from the wound edge only. Healing is often slow and unsatisfactory, frequently taking longer than 3 weeks, and an unstable epithelium is produced that is prone to hypertrophic scarring and contractures. This is a particular problem in burns that extend across joints and limit motion. Burns that take longer than 2 to 3 weeks to heal are also prone to infection, which may be reduced by using topical antimicrobial agents. Deep wounds should be referred for surgical consultation and may require early excision, grafting, and physical therapy.

SPECIAL MINOR BURN CARE CIRCUMSTANCES

Blisters

See Video 38.3. Management of blisters in minor burns is controversial. In reality, there is little one can do wrong when it comes to a clinical approach to blisters in minor burns (Fig. 38.13). Management arguments are generally theoretical or based on local tradition; the ultimate outcome of a minor burn is rarely determined by how one treats blisters. Intact blisters do offer some pain control and a physiologic dressing that rarely becomes infected; however, most large blisters spontaneously rupture after 3 to 5 days and eventually require debridement. When the integrity of the blister is breached, the fluid becomes a potential culture medium. Clinical choices for blister management include debridement (immediate and delayed) or simply leaving the blister intact. Aspiration is generally not recommended; however, trials comparing aspiration of blisters to debridement continue to show inconsistent results, with at least one recent trial showing no significant difference in pain, infection, or cosmesis.[23] In general, ruptured blisters should be debrided.

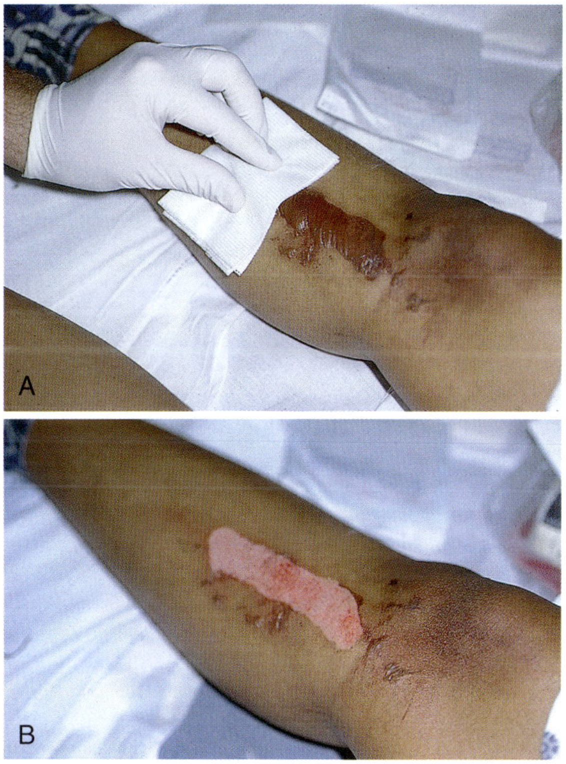

Fig. 38.13 It is difficult to do anything wrong with minor burn blisters, and many regimens are acceptable. Eventually, however, any unroofed blisters will have to be debrided. (A) An expeditious and relatively painless way to debride a burn is to use a dry gauze pad to grasp the dead skin and (B) peel it off. Meticulous instrument debridement is often time-consuming and stressful to the patient. Be aware that pain occurs when air comes in contact with the debrided skin, and prophylactic analgesia should therefore be provided. Large burns can be debrided under procedural sedation.

Some studies suggest that intact burn blisters may allow reversal of capillary stasis and less tissue necrosis. Burn exudate (as contained within intact blisters) is beneficial in stimulating epidermal cell proliferation and intact blisters may provide some pain relief, as evidenced by the sudden increase in pain immediately after debridement. Increased pain should be anticipated, and analgesia offered as appropriate when debridement is necessary. The steps listed in Fig. 38.10 act as a general approach to burn blisters.[24]

Minor Burn Infections

Prophylactic systemic antibiotics are not warranted in the routine treatment of outpatient burns. It may be difficult to separate the erythema of the injury or healing process from cellulitis, but minor burns rarely become infected. There are always bacteria on the skin; normal skin usually harbors nonvirulent pathogens such as *S. epidermidis* and diphtheroids. Therefore all burns are contaminated but not necessarily infected. Because thermal trauma results in coagulative necrosis, burn wounds contain a variable amount of necrotic tissue which, if infected, acts much as an undrained abscess and prevents access of antibiotics and host defense factors.

The microbial flora of outpatient burns varies with time after the burn. Shortly after injury, the burn becomes colonized with gram-positive bacteria such as *S. aureus* and *S. epidermidis*. After this period there is a gradual shift toward inclusion of gram-negative organisms, 80% of which originate from the patient's own gastrointestinal tract. Common organisms seen on days 1 to 3 include *S. epidermidis*, β-hemolytic streptococci, *Bacillus subtilis*, *S. aureus*, enterococci, *Mima polymorpha*, *Enterobacter* spp., *Acinetobacter* spp., and *C. albicans*. One week after the burn these organisms may be seen along with *E. coli*, *P. aeruginosa*, *Serratia marcescens*, *K. pneumoniae*, and *Proteus vulgaris*. Anaerobic colonization of burn wounds is rare unless there is excessive devitalized tissue, as may occur with a high-voltage electrical injury.

A healing burn may produce leukocytosis and a mild fever in the absence of infection, especially in children. Early (days 1 to 5) burn infections are generally caused by gram-positive cocci, especially β-hemolytic streptococci. Streptococcal cellulitis is characterized by marked spreading erythema extending outward from the wound margins. Despite the plethora of organisms and the presence of some gram-negative pathogens in superficial burn cultures, standard gram-positive cellulitis coverage is appropriate initial therapy in most cases.

Effective topical treatment at the time of initial burn care and subsequent dressing changes are meant to delay bacterial colonization, maintain the bacterial density of wounds at low levels, and produce a less diverse wound flora. Because outpatient management of burns should be attempted only when the risk for infection is minimal, the use of systemic antibiotics is unnecessary for minor burns, even in the setting of delayed treatment, diabetes, and steroid use. Unnecessary antibiotic use may select for resistant organisms.

In minor burn care, wound cultures are not required or recommended, although may be considered when overt infection develops, especially when it occurs when a topical or systemic antibiotic is being used. Sterile wound biopsy for culture is most satisfactory for the assessment of intraescharotic, subescharotic, or invasive infections and allows quantification of bacterial flora.

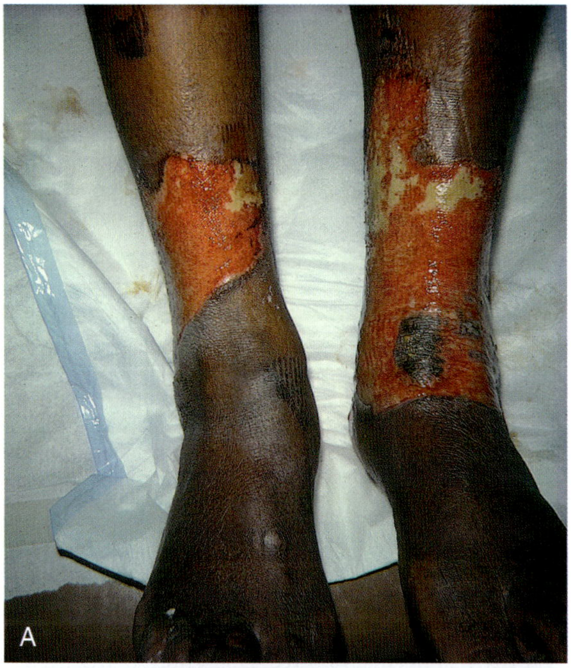

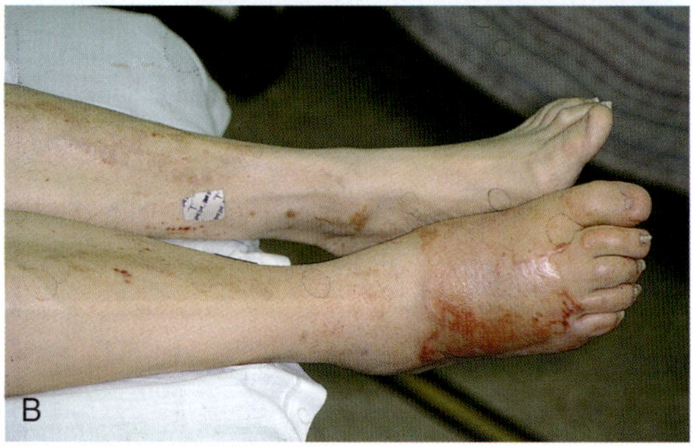

Fig. 38.14 Burns of the feet are special burns that require careful evaluation and an individualized treatment plan, even if the burn surface area is relatively small. It is difficult for many patients to provide ideal burn care at home when the feet are involved. (A) It is tempting to initially treat a seemingly minor superficial partial-thickness foot burn in an outpatient setting, but the patient's compliance and social situation must be ideal for a successful outcome. Unless home health care, a wound care center, or other similar arrangements are available to the patient, hospitalization may be most prudent until these arrangements can be solidified. (B) Example of a foot burn that is a potential disaster, in this case because of late treatment of a diabetic patient.

Foot Burns

Despite their relatively small surface area, foot burns tend to heal poorly, usually because of excessive edema; therefore they are generally considered major burns. Foot burns are the most common burn category to fail outpatient therapy, and therefore may require admission and inpatient care (Fig. 38.14). Zachary and coworkers[25] reported on a series of 104 patients with foot burns. In no patient admitted on the day of injury did burn cellulitis develop; in contrast, 27% of delayed-admission patients had cellulitis. Their study also noted a higher incidence of hypertrophic scarring with the need for skin grafting in the delayed-admission group. Overall, fewer days of hospitalization were required for the initially admitted group.

Specific problems in the care of foot burns include pain, wound drainage, difficulty changing dressings without assistance, inability of even motivated patients to comply with the requirements for elevation, and prolonged convalescence. The benefits of hospital admission include splinting, intensive local burn care, physical therapy, and bed rest with elevation to minimize edema. For these reasons, admission should be considered for all but the most minor of foot burns. Close outpatient follow-up wound checks are required for those foot burns appropriate for outpatient care.

Hand Burns

Because of its functional significance, burns involving the hand can result in significant functional loss even when the TBSA burned is small. Losing the use of one or both hands can be disabling and affect the patient's activities of daily living regardless of whether the cause of the loss is a burn dressing, the late onset of scar contractures, or loss need for amputation.

As with other burns, the depth and extent of the burn determine the severity of the injury. The entire surface of one hand represents only 2.5% TBSA, yet even small burns can cause a disproportionate loss of function. Deep partial- or full-thickness hand burns, even if quite small, often warrant referral for early excision and grafting to limit scarring and maintain function. The skin on the dorsum of the hand is thinner than that on the palm and is more susceptible to burn injury so it must remain flexible to allow finger motion. Any exposed tendon or bone, such as may be seen with an electrical burn, constitutes a true fourth-degree injury, and either flap closure or amputation may be necessary to heal the wound.

Many of the issues complicating outpatient management of foot burns are relevant to the care of hand burns. If appropriate for outpatient care, standard wound care should be performed and the fingers should be carefully separated and bandaged individually. Small, intact blisters that do not interfere with hand function should be left intact to serve as a biologic dressing. Elevation of the hand is very important in the first few days after a burn injury to minimize edema. Deep partial- or full-thickness burns on the dorsum of the hand should be splinted after bandaging to avoid the development of contractures or a boutonnière deformity.

Hospital admission or burn center referral should be considered for all significant hand burns, particularly full-thickness injuries and circumferential burns involving the digits (Fig. 38.15). If outpatient treatment is appropriate, the patient should have appropriate follow-up, comprehensive instructions, and the resources to perform daily dressing changes and range-of-motion exercises of the fingers and wrist during these dressing changes. An initial follow-up visit should occur in 48 to 72 hours. Ideally, the patient should be seen twice in the first week after injury and then may be reduced to once a week when appropriate until the burn is healed.

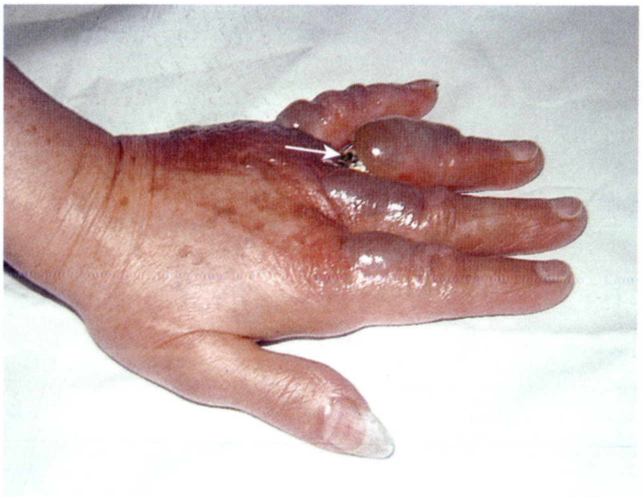

Fig. 38.15 This badly burned hand requires referral to a surgeon or burn center and should not be definitively handled in the emergency department. Note the very tight ring *(arrow)*.

Facial Burns

Facial burns commonly result from unexpected ignition flash burns (e.g., from a stove, oven, or charcoal grill) or from car radiator accidents (Fig. 38.16A–B). Facial burns from these sources usually do well, but singeing of facial hair, significant edema, and pain often result. However, facial burns from these causes may produce airway problems and might require skin grafting. Singed nasal hairs or any sign of significant heat exposure to the face should prompt an evaluation for airway injury (Fig. 38.16C).

Concurrent globe or corneal injury is quite rare because of protective blinking reflexes. If the eye is burned, it is usually in the setting of a life-threatening concomitant burn injury. Burns involving the eyelids can cause significant scarring. Fluorescein staining and slit-lamp examination should be performed to confirm or exclude the diagnosis of corneal injury (Fig. 38.17). Treatment of a corneal injury can involve irrigation, topical ophthalmic antibiotics, and consideration of eye patching versus protective soft contact lens. Referral to an ophthalmologist is prudent. Facial burns are otherwise treated in the usual fashion and with an open (no dressing) technique. Patients are instructed to wash their face two or three times a day with a mild soap and then apply a thin layer of antibiotic ointment. Car radiator burns result from the combination of a hot liquid and steam burn (see Fig. 38.16B). Antifreeze exposure to skin does not produce a caustic injury, nor is it systemically absorbed. Neck burns are treated in a similar fashion.

A flash burn from smoking cigarettes while using nasal oxygen causes a facial burn that is commonly seen in the ED (Fig. 38.16D). These burns may involve the nose and lips and may have melted plastic particles on the skin or in the nose, and can be quite painful. Although such patients generally do well, facial burns can make the continued use of nasal cannula oxygen problematic until healing takes place. Inhalation burns are rare in this circumstance, but careful evaluation of the upper airways and assessment of lung function are prudent. Many patients using oxygen may not be able to tolerate even minor physical insults and have fragile conditions that require careful evaluation, short-term observation in some cases, and close follow-up for delayed healing and infection. Hospitalization for burn care and general supportive measures may be prudent for all but minor burns in this patient population.

All patients with head or neck burns should be evaluated carefully for a concomitant inhalation injury. Such patients may have a history of being in an enclosed space and direct evidence of injury, such as oral burns, blisters, soot, or hyperemia, or have indirect evidence, such as dyspnea, wheezing, arterial hypoxemia, or an elevated carboxyhemoglobin level. The best diagnostic test for significant inhalation injury is fiberoptic bronchoscopy.

Inpatient care should be considered for all patients with significant facial burns. Outpatient pain control may be difficult in those with major facial burns, the degree of edema may be difficult to predict, and home care can be problematic. There are no universally agreed standards for admission versus outpatient treatment of facial burns.

Corneal contact burns, as from accidental contact with a curling iron, are often manifested rather dramatically as opacified, "heaped-up" corneal epithelium (see Fig. 38.17). Despite their appearance, the end result is usually excellent. Treatment is the same as for a corneal abrasion.

Oral Commissure Burns in Children

See Video 38.4. Oral commissure burns are usually seen in toddlers who have bitten an electrical cord. These injuries rarely cause issues beyond the local injury, but the damage to the commissure can impact both the child's function and cosmesis. These children should be referred urgently to an oral or plastic surgeon for continuing management and possible surgical repair, as well as for surveillance for possible delayed hemorrhage from the labial artery as the eschar sloughs at approximately one week after the injury. Parents should also be instructed on this possibility of delayed bleeding, shown how to apply direct pressure to the area and told to return to the ED if the bleeding occurs.

Abuse of Children and Older Adults

Recognition of the possibility of deliberate abuse by burning in the pediatric and geriatric populations is essential.

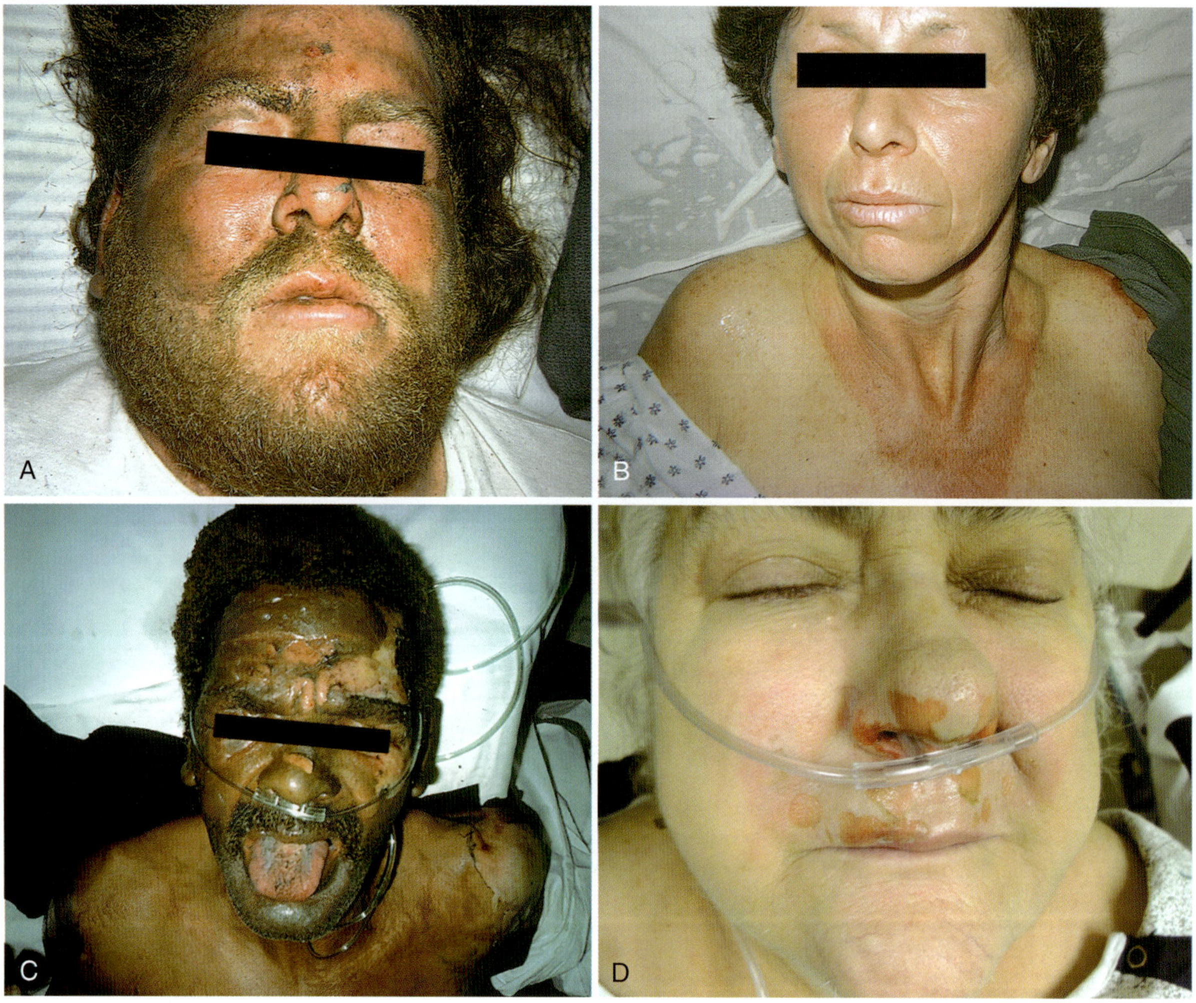

Fig. 38.16 (A) Flash burns on the face from lighting a gas stove. These burns are painful and may cause edema, but they usually do well. Note the singed facial hair. The eyes are usually protected by rapid reflex blinking, and carbon monoxide poisoning and pulmonary burns are not an issue. Most can be handled in the outpatient setting with bacitracin ointment and no dressing. Pain control may be problematic and opioids are often prescribed. (B) Facial and neck burns when a radiator cap was removed and the patient was sprayed with steam and hot antifreeze. (C) This patient has a severe facial burn with smoke inhalation, as evidenced by soot in the pharynx and singed nasal hairs. Tracheal intubation is recommended for this patient. (D) A flash burn in a patient who was smoking a cigarette while using nasal oxygen.

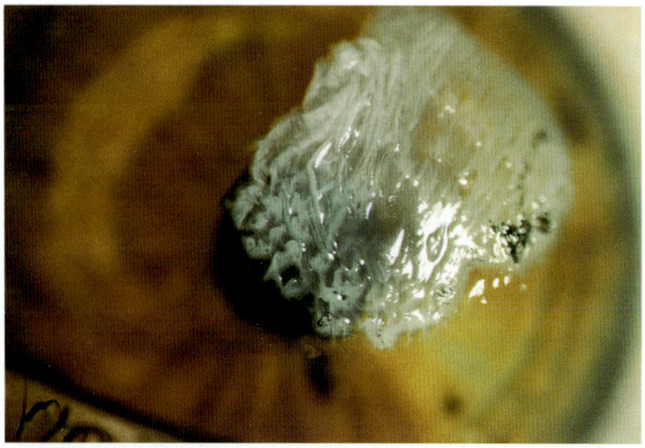

Fig. 38.17 A thermal burn of the cornea. Note the opacified, "heaped-up" appearance of the epithelium. (From Kanski JJ, ed. *Clinical Diagnosis in Ophthalmology*. Mosby; 2006.)

In addition, children younger than 2 years have a thinner dermis and a less well-developed immune system than adults do. Older patients (>65 years) likewise tolerate burns poorly. These two populations are the most prone to abuse, often by family members (Fig. 38.18). For these reasons, both these groups of patients require careful consideration for abuse and often require inpatient burn care.

Immersion burns are a common type of abuse and are characterized by circumferential, sharply demarcated burns on the hands, feet, buttocks, and perineum. Cigarette burns and burns from hot objects such as irons should be obvious. Contact burns on "nonexploring" parts of the child also warrant suspicion. A delay in seeking treatment may be a tip-off that a burn resulted from abuse. In older populations, the presence of confirmed self-inflicted burns such as cigarette burns suggests psychiatric disease (see Fig. 38.18E).

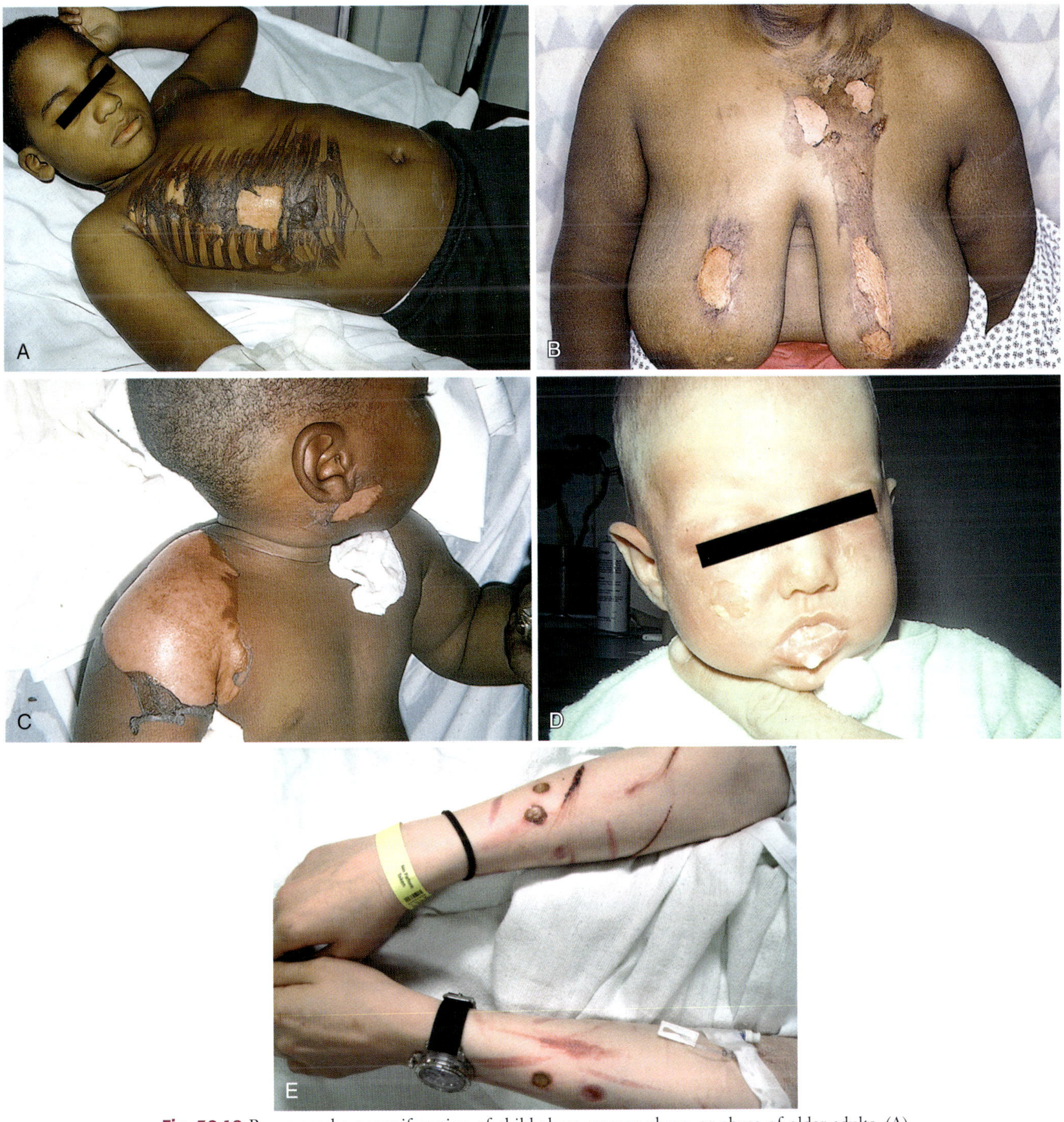

Fig. 38.18 Burns can be a manifestation of child abuse, spouse abuse, or abuse of older adults. (A) Abuse burns from contact with a hot metal grate as a result of a child allegedly falling. (B) This burn was the result of spouse abuse caused by throwing hot soup during an argument. Domestic abuse is often denied initially, but the delayed arrival at the hospital was a clue. (C) Burns of the face and neck are common when a toddler pulls hot liquid from a stove. This case was never proved to be child abuse, but burns in young children are often due to abuse, especially if they are in atypical places. Although the body surface area of this burn is relatively small, the patient's age and the burn's location, coupled with the possibility of child abuse, require that this child be hospitalized. (D) This infant received a severe blistering sunburn at the beach despite being in the shade most of the day. Reflection of sunlight from the sand and water can injure the delicate skin of an infant, who should have sunscreen applied. (E) Self-inflicted cigarette burns in a psychiatric patient.

Burns in Pregnancy

There is little information in the literature concerning the special problems of pregnant burn patients. Complications of the burn injuries in pregnant individuals include abortion and premature labor, although patients with burns covering less than 20% TBSA tend to do well.

Because the resistance of pregnant females to infection is lower than that of nonpregnant females, control of burn wound infection is paramount. Gestational age appears to have no direct bearing on prognosis. Silver sulfadiazine cream should be avoided near term because of the reported potential for kernicterus.

SPECIFIC BURNING AGENTS

Hot Tar Burns

Asphalt is a product of the residues of coal tar and is commonly used in roofing and road repair. It is kept heated to approximately 232°C (450°F). When spilled onto the skin, the tar cools relatively rapidly, but the retained heat is sufficient to produce a partial-thickness burn. Fortunately, full-thickness burns are unusual. Cooled tar is nonirritating and does not promote infection. When cooled tar is physically removed, the adherent skin is usually avulsed (Fig. 38.19). Careless removal of the tar may inflict further damage on burned tissues. Agents such as alcohol, acetone, kerosene, or gasoline have been used to remove the tar, but these are flammable and may cause additional skin damage or a toxic response secondary to absorption.

There is no great need to meticulously remove all tar at the first visit. Obviously devitalized skin can be debrided, but adherent tar should be emulsified or dissolved rather than manually removed (Fig. 38.20). Polyoxyethylene sorbitan is the water-soluble, nontoxic, emulsifying agent found in Neosporin and several other topical antibiotic creams. Note that the cream formulations, not the ointments, contain the most useful tar dissolvers. The creams contain a complex mixture of ethers, esters, and sorbitol anhydrides that possess excellent hydrophilic and lyophilic characteristics when used as nonionic, surface-active emulsifying agents. With persistence, most tar can be removed (emulsified) on the initial visit, although this may be unnecessary as previously detailed.

Another household product, De-Solv-It ([Orange-Sol Blending and Packaging, Inc.] multiuse solvent), also appears logical for topical ED use. De-Solv-It has a surface-active moiety that wets the chemical's surface and emulsifies tar and asphalt. Because De-Solv-It is itself a petroleum-based solvent, it should be applied only briefly, and the operator should wear gloves and protective eyewear during application. It should be used only for external exposure to tar or asphalt. After removal, the skin should be cleansed gently and dressed appropriately.

Many clinicians instead prefer to emulsify the majority of tar on an outpatient basis. A generous layer of polysorbate-based ointment can be applied under a bulky absorbent gauze dressing. The patient is then released home, and the residual tar is easily washed off after 24 to 36 hours (see Fig. 38.19B). Several dressing changes may be required. Once the residual tar is removed, the wound is treated as any other burn (see Fig. 38.20). Other options have been suggested, including mineral oil, petrolatum, and butter-soaked gauze.

Chemical Burns

Chemical burns generally occur in the workplace, and the offending substance is usually well known. More than 25,000 chemicals currently in use are capable of burning the skin or mucous membranes. Commonly used chemical agents capable of producing skin burns are shown in Box 38.7.

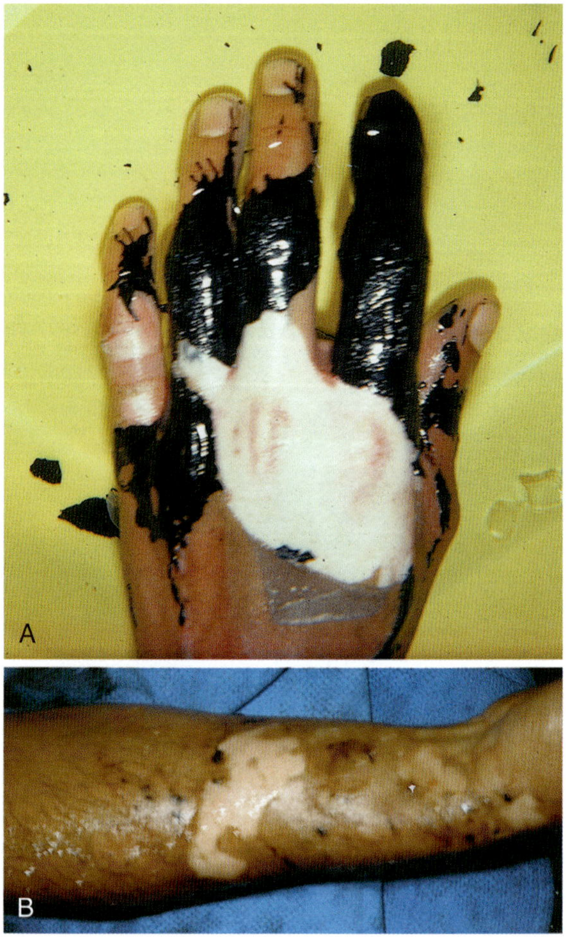

Fig. 38.19 (A) There is no compelling reason to remove all tar on the first visit. Physical removal of cooled tar usually results in avulsion of the underlying skin. Skin that is obviously loose should be debrided, but adherent tar is best liquefied with an emulsifying agent. Neomycin cream, not ointment, is a suggested emulsifier, but others are acceptable (see text). Final removal may be delayed for several days to permit loosening of the tar. Frequent dressing changes and application of an emulsifying agent can be performed by the patient to remove the tar over a period of a few days. (B) This extremity was covered with an emulsifying agent and with gauze, and the residual tar was washed off easily 36 hours later.

Injury is caused by a chemical reaction rather than a thermal burn. Reactions are classified as oxidizing, reducing, corrosive, desiccant, vesicant, or protoplasmic poisoning. The injury to skin continues until the chemical agent is physically removed or exhausts its inherent destructive capacity. The degree of injury is based on the strength, concentration, and quantity of the chemical; duration of contact; location of contact; extent of tissue penetration; and mechanism of action.

Immediate flushing with water is recommended for all chemical burns, with the exception of those caused by alkali metals. Flushing serves to cleanse the wound of unreacted surface chemical, dilute the chemical already in contact with tissue, and restore lost tissue water. Flushing should be thorough and may require at least 30 minutes (or as much as 2 hours) for maximal benefit, depending on the nature of the chemical.

Acid and Alkali Burns

Chemical burns cause progressive tissue damage until the chemical is inactivated or removed. Acids damage tissue by

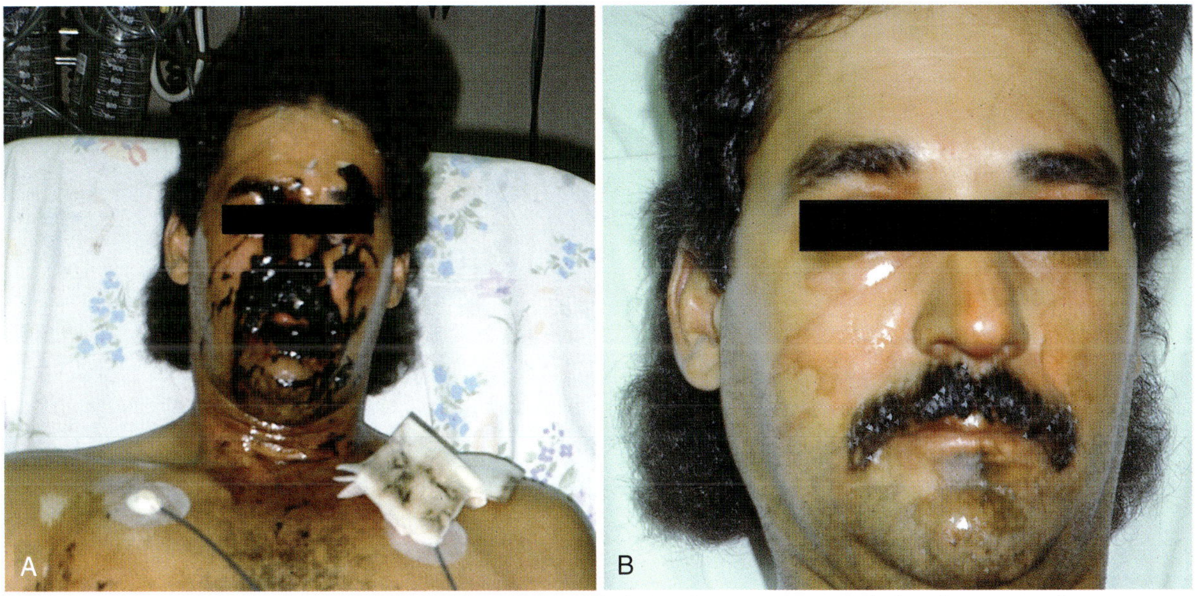

Fig. 38.20 (A) Tar stuck to the face can (B) be emulsified with various agents and a lot of patience and persistence. Fortunately, tar burns are not usually full-thickness burns.

BOX 38.7 Commonly Used Acids and Alkalis

ACIDS	ALKALIS
Picric	Sodium hydroxide
Tungstic	Ammonium hydroxide
Sulfosalicylic	Lithium hydroxide
Tannic	Barium hydroxide
Trichloroacetic	Calcium hydroxide
Cresylic	Sodium hypochlorite
Acetic	
Formic	
Sulfuric	
Hydrochloric	
Hydrofluoric	
Chromic	

coagulation necrosis, a process that limits the depth of penetration into tissue. Alkalis react with lipids in skin and result in liquefaction necrosis. This process permits penetration of the chemical into tissues until neutralized. Thus exposure to alkali is more likely to produce deep tissue wounds. Skin exposed to caustic substances should be decontaminated aggressively until neutralized and the resulting wounds considered deep until demonstrated otherwise.

Desiccant acids, such as sulfuric acid, create an exothermic reaction with tissue water and can cause both chemical and thermal injury. With extensive immersion injuries, acids may be absorbed systemically, thereby leading to systemic acidosis and coagulation abnormalities.

Chemical burns may be excruciatingly painful for long periods of time. Discomfort can be out of proportion to what one might expect from the perceived depth or extent of the burn. When caring for a chemical burn, the emergency care team should remove all potentially contaminated clothing. Any dry (anhydrous) chemical should first be brushed off the patient's skin. The involved skin should then be irrigated with large amounts of water under low pressure. Any remaining particulate matter should be carefully debrided during irrigation.

Strong alkali burns may require irrigation for 1 to 2 hours before tissue pH returns to normal. Prompt irrigation with a dilute acid (e.g., vinegar, or 2% acetic acid) may hasten neutralization and patient comfort.

Contact Burns From Wet Cement

The major constituent of Portland cement, an alkaline substance, is calcium oxide (64%), combined with oxides of silicon, aluminum, magnesium, sulfur, iron, and potassium. There is considerable variability in the calcium oxide content of different grades of cement, with concrete having less and fine-textured masonry cement having more. The addition of water exothermically converts the calcium oxide to calcium hydroxide ($Ca[OH]_2$), a strongly corrosive alkali with a pH of 11 to 13. As the cement hardens, the calcium hydroxide reacts with ambient carbon dioxide and becomes inactive.

Both the heat and the $Ca(OH)_2$ produced in this exothermic reaction can result in significant burns. Because of its low solubility and consequent low ionic strength, long exposure to $Ca(OH)_2$ is required to produce injury. This usually occurs when workers spill concrete into their boots or kneel in it for a prolonged period. The burn wound and the resultant protein denaturation of tissues produce a thick, tenacious, ulcerated eschar. Concrete burns are insidious and progressive. What may appear initially as a patchy, superficial burn might in several days become a full-thickness injury requiring excision and skin grafting. The pain associated with these burns is often severe and more intense than the appearance of the wound might suggest (Fig. 38.21). Interestingly, many workers are not warned of the dangers of prolonged contact with cement, and because the initial contact with cement is usually painless, exposure may not be realized until the damage is done.

Treatment starts with removal of any loose particulate cement or lime, usually by brushing it off, removal of contaminated clothing, and irrigation of the wound copiously with tap water (the pH of the effluent is tested and irrigation continued if the effluent is still alkaline). If available apply compresses of dilute acetic acid (vinegar) to neutralize the remaining alkali and provide relief of pain after irrigation. Apply antibiotic ointment to the eschar during the early postburn period.

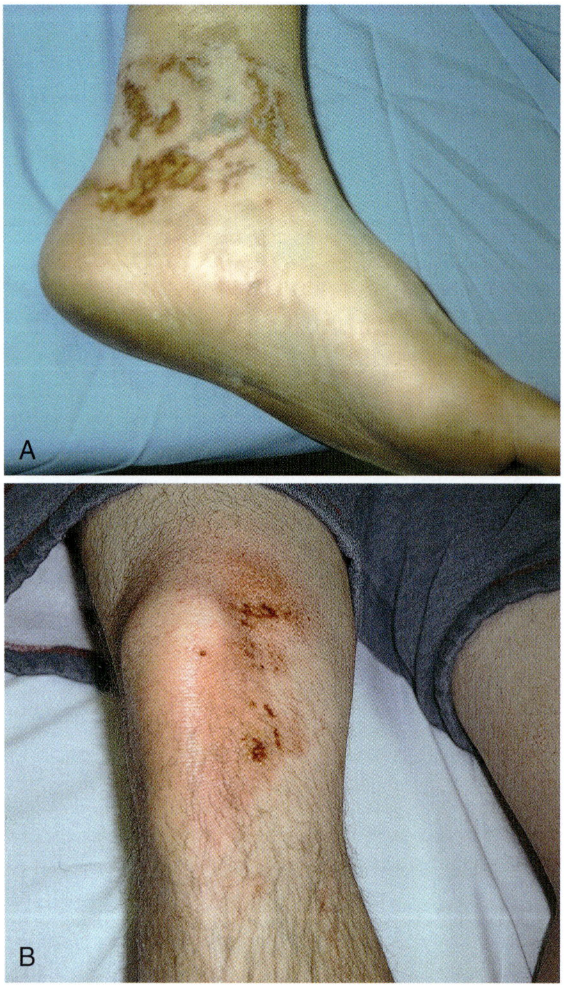

Fig. 38.21 Alkali burns from wet cement develop insidiously, are extremely painful, and are frequently full-thickness injuries. They are most common (A) on the feet when cement leaks over the top of the boots or (B) from kneeling in wet cement while working. The alkali can penetrate clothing.

The depth of burns from wet cement can be difficult to assess in the first several days. If it becomes apparent that the burns are full-thickness burns, early excision and skin grafting are recommended. Cement burns should be differentiated from cement dermatitis, which is far more common. The latter is a contact sensitivity reaction, probably from the chromates present in cement. The contact dermatitis can initially be treated as a superficial partial-thickness burn.

Air Bag Keratitis and Thermal Burns

Safety legislation has mandated increased use of air bags to protect automobile occupants in the event of collision. Burns from air bags can be thermal, friction, or chemical (Fig. 38.22). The automobile air bag is a rubberized nylon bag that inflates on spark ignition of sodium azide to yield nitrogen gas, ash, and a small amount of sodium hydroxide. Within seconds, the superheated air is vented, and this can produce a thermal burn if it contacts an extremity, the face, or the upper part of the torso.[26] If the air bag ruptures, the alkaline contents of the bag are dispersed as a fine, black powder that usually causes no problems unless the eyes are exposed. Patients with eye exposure exhibit clinical evidence of a chemical keratoconjunctivitis, including photophobia, tearing, redness, and decreased visual acuity. Tear pH is usually elevated, and there may be particulate matter in the fornices.

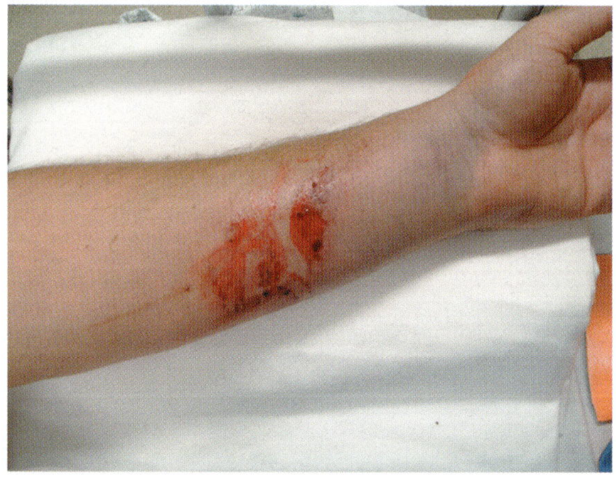

Fig. 38.22 A burn on the forearm from a first-generation air bag can be a combination of friction and chemicals. They are usually minor.

The severity of an ocular alkaline burn is related to the duration of exposure and the concentration and pH of the chemical. For this reason, prompt, copious irrigation of the eyes with frequent assessment of tear pH is essential to prevent or minimize the injury. A rising pH suggests that trapped particulate matter is releasing additional chemical. Corneal edema and conjunctival blanching are signs of serious injury and can necessitate immediate ophthalmologic consultation.

Hydrocarbon Burns

Hydrocarbons are capable of causing severe contact injury by virtue of their irritant, fat-dissolving, and dehydrating properties. Cutaneous absorption may cause even more dangerous systemic effects. Gasoline, the usual agent involved, is a complex mixture of C_4 to C_{11} alkane hydrocarbons and benzene; the hydrocarbons appear to be the major toxic agent.

The depth of injury is related to the duration of exposure and the concentration of the chemical agent. Gasoline immersion injuries resemble scald burns and are usually partial thickness. Occasionally, gasoline-injured skin exhibits a pinkish brown discoloration, possibly related to dye additives. A common source of gasoline exposure is motor vehicle collisions in which a comatose patient has been lying in a pool of gasoline.

The lungs are the usual site of systemic absorption and are often the only major route of excretion. The resultant high pulmonary concentrations may lead to pulmonary hemorrhage, atelectasis, and acute respiratory distress syndrome. To treat hydrocarbon burns, remove contaminated clothing, administer prolonged irrigation or soaking of the contaminated skin, debride significant burns caused by lead-containing gasoline (to reduce systemic lead absorption), and apply topical antibiotic ointments.

Phenol Injury

Phenol is a highly reactive aromatic acid alcohol that acts as a corrosive. Carbolic acid, an earlier term for phenol, was noted to have antiseptic properties and was used as such by Joseph Lister in performing the first antiseptic surgery. Hexylresorcinol, a phenol derivative, is in current use as a bactericidal agent. Phenols, in strong concentrations, cause considerable eschar formation, but skin absorption also occurs and can result in systemic effects such as central nervous system depression, hypotension, hemolysis, pulmonary edema, and death. Phenol penetrates deeper in a dilute solution than in a more concentrated form, and the ideal agent for removing phenolic compounds is full-strength polyethylene glycol (PG 300 or 400). Polyethylene glycol is nontoxic and nonirritating and may be used anywhere on the body, and if immediately available can be used to remove the surface chemical before water irrigation. Water irrigation for decontamination should not be delayed while awaiting polyethylene glycol.

Hydrofluoric Acid Injury

Hydrofluoric acid (HFA) is one of the strongest inorganic acids known; it has been widely used since its ability to dissolve silica was discovered in the late 17th century. Currently, HFA is used in masonry restoration, glass etching, and semiconductor manufacturing; for control of fermentation in breweries; and in the production of plastics and fluorocarbons. It is also used as a catalyst in petroleum alkylating units. It is available in industry as a liquid in varying concentrations up to 70%. It is also readily sold in home improvement and hardware stores. Significant concentrations of HFA are present in many home rust removal products, aluminum brighteners, automobile wheel cleaners, and heavy-duty cleaners in concentrations of less than 10%. Despite its ability to cause serious burns, unregulated and poorly labeled HFA products are used on a regular basis. The public and many clinicians are generally unaware of the potential problems with this acid (Fig. 38.23).

Although HFA is quite corrosive, the hydrogen ion plays a relatively insignificant role in the pathophysiology of the burn injury. The accompanying fluoride ion is a protoplasmic poison that is capable of binding cellular calcium and causing liquefaction necrosis; the ionic shifts that result, particularly shifts of potassium, are believed to be responsible for the severe pain associated with HFA burns. It is notorious for its ability to penetrate tissues and cause delayed pain and deep tissue injury. This acid can penetrate through fingernails and cause nail bed injury. With home products, the unwary user does not realize that the substance is caustic until the skin (usually the hands and fingers) is exposed for a few minutes to hours, at which time the burning begins and becomes progressively worse. At this point the damage is done and the absorbed HFA cannot be washed off. With higher-strength industrial products, symptoms are often almost immediate.

In high concentrations, the fluoride ions may penetrate to bone and produce demineralization. Exposure of skin to concentrated HFA involving as little as 2.5% TBSA can lead to systemic hypocalcemia and death from intractable cardiac arrhythmias; it has been calculated that exposure to 7 mL of anhydrous HFA (HFA gas) is capable of binding all the free calcium in a 70-kg adult. Hyperkalemia and hypomagnesemia can also develop. If the hands are exposed, the acid characteristically penetrates the fingernails and injures the nail bed and cuticle area. As with most caustics, the pain is generally out of proportion to the apparent external physical injury. HFA burns produce variable areas of blanching and erythema, but blisters or skin sloughing are rarely seen initially. Skin necrosis and cutaneous hemorrhage may be noted in a few days.

Immediate treatment should begin with copious irrigation with water. Another approach is to wash the area with a solution of iced magnesium sulfate (Epsom salts) or a 1:500 solution of a quaternary ammonium compound such as benzalkonium chloride (Zephiran) or benzethonium chloride (Hyamine 1622). Magnesium and calcium salts form an insoluble complex with fluoride ions, thus preventing further tissue diffusion. Though frequently recommended, topical preparations are often ineffective in limiting injury or controlling pain.

If there is no or only minimal visible evidence of skin injury and minimal pain, the burn may be dressed with topical calcium gluconate paste. This is not commercially available in the United States but is easily compounded in the pharmacy by mixing 3.5 g to 7 g of pulverized calcium gluconate with 5 oz of a water-soluble lubricant. This will form a thick paste with a calcium gluconate concentration of 2.5% to 5.0%. Some have suggested dimethyl sulfoxide as a vehicle to aid in skin penetration of the calcium. Plastic wrap can be used over a standard dry burn dressing to cover the calcium paste on the limbs. A vinyl or rubber glove filled with the paste can be used to cover the fingers and hands. Completely redress the wound and reapply the paste every 6 hours for the first 24 hours. As with most topical treatments of HFA burns, calcium gluconate is only minimally effective in relieving pain, and its value is probably overestimated in the literature.

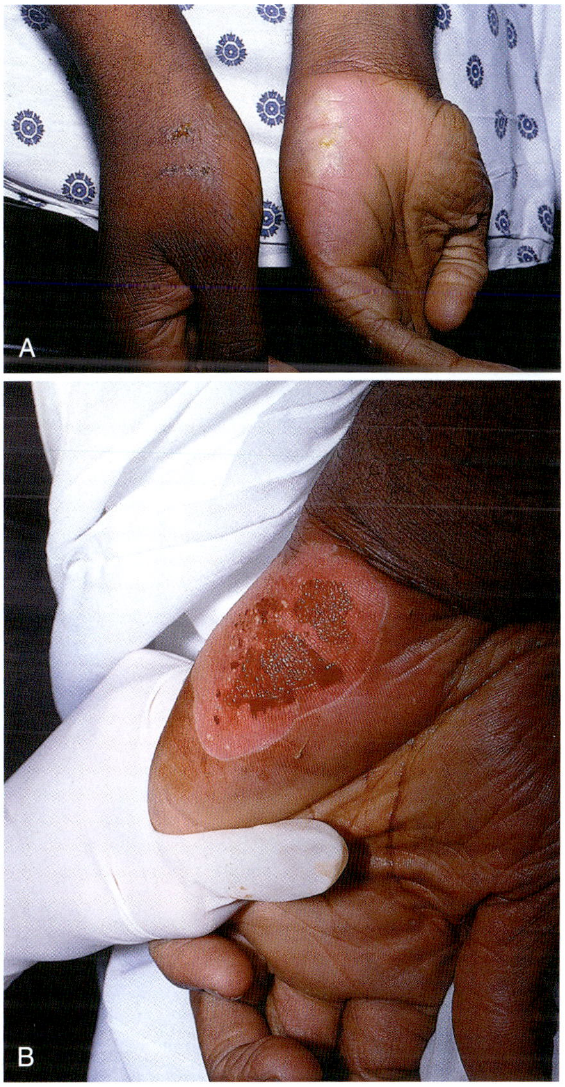

Fig. 38.23 (A) Initially, this very painful hydrofluoric acid burn of the thenar and hypothenar eminence appeared minimal. (B) Despite infiltration with calcium gluconate, a deep burn developed 3 days later.

A digital or regional nerve block with long-acting bupivacaine is an excellent way to provide prolonged pain relief if the hands are involved, but this does nothing to ameliorate the injury. In most cases, opioid analgesia is required. If bullae or vesicles have formed, they should be debrided to decrease the amount of fluoride present, and the wound should then be treated as any partial-thickness burn. Burns with HFA of less than 10% strength will heal spontaneously, usually without significant tissue loss, but pain and sensitivity of the fingertips

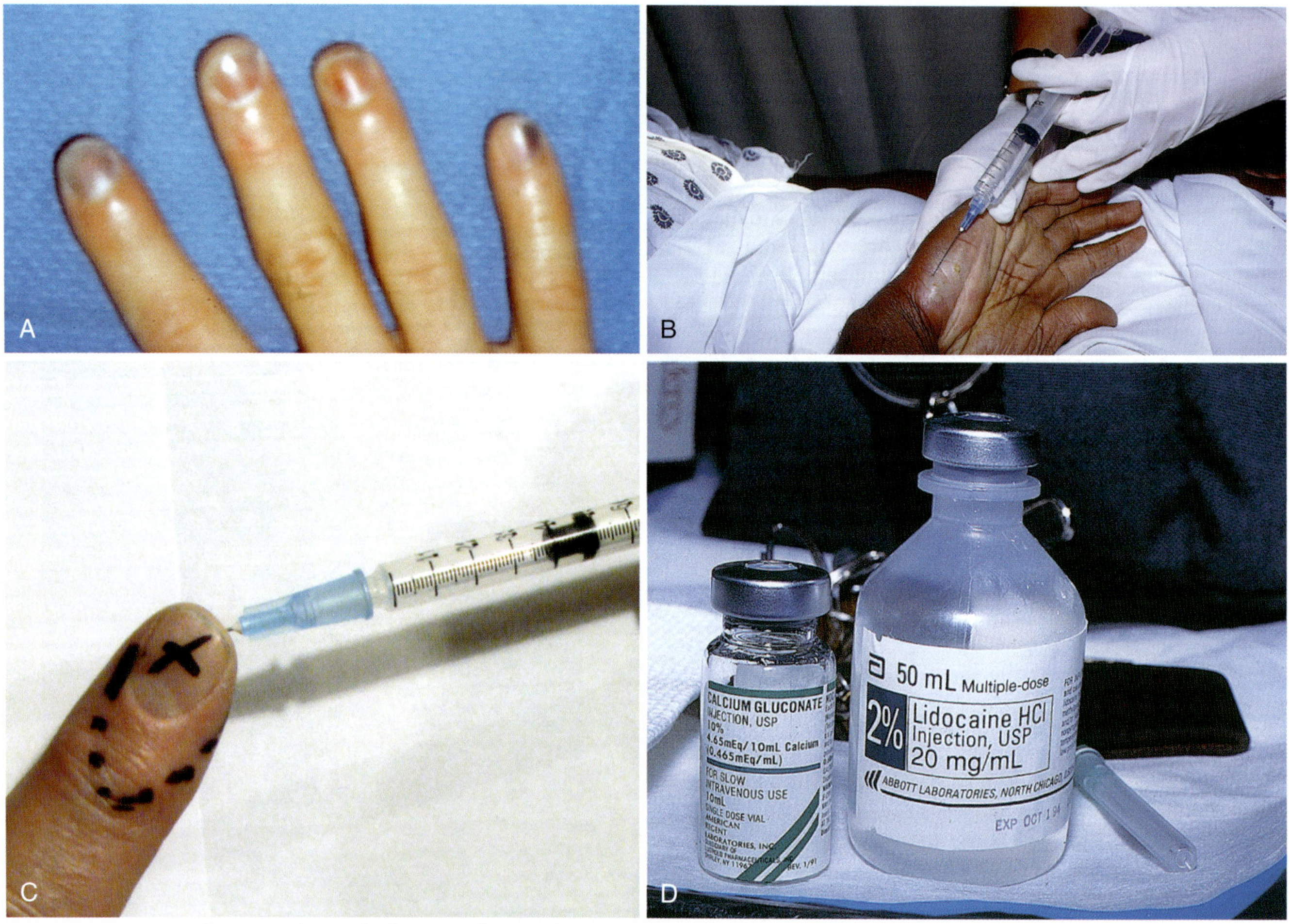

Fig. 38.24 (A) Hydrofluoric acid (HFA) burns of the fingertips are extremely painful despite minimal clinical findings; initially only hyperemia and minor ecchymosis are apparent. HFA can penetrate the intact fingernail and produce a significant injury to the nail bed. (B) The area of burn can be injected with calcium gluconate minimally diluted with plain lidocaine. Using a small-gauge needle, generously infiltrate the entire area of the burn. (C) Before performing digital block anesthesia to painlessly infiltrate the fingertips with calcium gluconate, ask the patient to outline the painful areas with a felt-tipped marker to ensure accurate placement of the antidote. In the treatment of HFA burns, topical therapy is often ineffective. Calcium gluconate may be injected subcutaneously with a 25- to 27-gauge needle into the nail bed via the fat pad under a digital nerve block. Do not remove fingernails routinely if burns are mild, such as those seen with household products containing less than a 10% concentration of the acid. Intraarterial calcium infusions are often quite successful in relieving pain and limiting necrosis. (D) Combine the calcium gluconate with a small amount of lidocaine for injection.

may persist for 7 to 10 days. In addition, the fingernails may become loose.

Initial treatment of a more concentrated exposure begins as described earlier and includes immediate debridement of necrotic tissue to remove as much fluoride ion as possible. After debridement, inject a 10% solution of calcium gluconate (note: avoid calcium chloride for tissue injections) intradermally and subcuticularly with a 30-gauge needle about the exposed area, using approximately 0.5 mL per square centimeter of burn. Pain relief should be almost immediate if this therapy is adequate, and the degree of pain is a measure of the effectiveness of treatment. Soft tissue can be injected without prior anesthesia, but if the fingertips or nail beds are involved, they may be injected after a digital nerve block has been performed (Fig. 38.24). Before anesthesia and injection of calcium, the patient can outline the affected areas with a pen to ensure accurate injection of the antidote (see Fig. 38.24C). Fingers are best injected with a 25- or 27-gauge needle (a tuberculin syringe works well). Nails frequently become loose in a few days, but they often return to normal and do not require removal, particularly when lower-concentration nonindustrial products are involved.

Although infiltration of calcium gluconate can be somewhat effective, the technique has certain limitations. Injections are painful, and the calcium gluconate solution itself causes a burning sensation. Because of the volume restrictions, not enough calcium may be delivered to bind all the free fluoride ions present. For example, 0.5 mL of 10% calcium gluconate contains 4.65 mg (0.2325 mEq) of elemental calcium, which will neutralize only 0.025 mL of 20% HFA.

Some have advocated intraarterial calcium infusions in the treatment of serious HFA burns of the extremities. Though very effective, this technique is not recommended for burns secondary to dilute HFA (i.e., concentrations <10%) because the morbidity is usually quite mild. When using this technique, 10 mL of 10% calcium gluconate is diluted in 50 mL of a 5% dextrose and water solution. The dilute solution is administered by slow infusion into an arterial catheter. It is unclear which artery best delivers the calcium to injured tissues. If only the radial three digits are involved, probably only the radial artery needs to be cannulated. Otherwise, a percutaneous catheter is inserted into the brachial artery. However, some investigators have advocated use of the radial artery in all cases, and because the arterial supply of the hand is interconnected, this may be a reasonable recommendation.[27] When arterial access has been accomplished, the solution is infused slowly over a 4-hour period. At this point the catheter is left in place and the patient is observed. If pain returns at any time over the next 4 hours, the infusion is repeated. If the patient is pain free over the 4-hour observation period, the catheter is removed, the burn is dressed, and the patient is released home. This technique may be initiated in the ED, but many clinicians are reluctant to cannulate an artery and infuse calcium in the ED, and hospitalization or referral to burn center can be considered.

Advantages of the intraarterial method are elimination of the need for painful SQ injections and avoidance of the volume limitations of the SQ route while providing substantially more calcium to neutralize the fluoride. Disadvantages of intraarterial calcium therapy include the possibility of local arterial spasm (which can be treated with vasodilators such as phentolamine or removal of the catheter), local arterial injury or thrombus, and the long duration of treatment required.

Infusing calcium into the general venous circulation is of no benefit for HFA burns. Some authors have advocated the use of regional IV calcium gluconate, similar to the method used with the Bier block for regional anesthesia.[28] Case reports have noted variable success, but this technique has neither been well studied nor rigorously compared with other options. This method would be useful only for upper extremity burns. To perform regional calcium therapy, place an IV catheter in the dorsum of the hand on the involved extremity. Partially exsanguinate the arm by elevation and wrapping with an elastic bandage. Apply a Bier block tourniquet or a heavy-duty blood pressure cuff to the arm above the burn, and inflate it to 20 to 30 mm Hg above the systolic pressure to stop blood flow to and from the arm. Because slow deflation of a regular blood pressure cuff may thwart success of the procedure, using this specialized tourniquet is recommended. Then dilute 10 mL of 10% calcium gluconate with 30 mL to 40 mL of saline, and infuse the solution into the venous catheter. Keep the solution in the arm by keeping the tourniquet on for 20 to 30 minutes. Some patients cannot tolerate arm ischemia for this period, thus limiting the effectiveness of this procedure. Theoretically the calcium diffuses out of the venous system and into the injured tissues. After 20 to 30 minutes, deflate the cuff to restore normal circulation to the extremity. It may require 10 to 20 minutes after deflation of the tourniquet before the patient experiences relief of pain. This procedure is safe, but its efficacy is variable.

HFA burns involving the eye are potentially devastating injuries that deserve special mention. Ophthalmologist referral is critical. Ocular exposure to liquid or gaseous HFA will result in severe pain, tearing, conjunctival inflammation, and corneal opacification or erosion. Complications include decreased visual acuity, globe perforation, uveitis, glaucoma, conjunctival scarring, lid deformities, and keratitis sicca. Optimal therapy for ocular HFA burns, other than initial irrigation, is unknown. Irrigation may be performed with water, isotonic saline, or magnesium chloride. We advise copious saline irrigation. Topical antibiotics and cycloplegics, along with light pressure patching, are also recommended. The use of topical steroids has been advocated by some to lessen corneal fibroblast formation, but other attempted therapies such as subconjunctival injections of calcium gluconate and ocular irrigation with quaternary ammonium compounds have been associated with additional injury.

Chromic Acid Injury

Chromium compounds are used extensively in industry, mainly in metallic electroplating. Chromic acid is commonly used in concentrated solutions containing up to 25% sulfuric acid. It causes sufficient skin damage to allow absorption of the toxic chromium ion if intensive irrigation is not undertaken immediately. Heated (60°C to 80°C) chromic acid makes the problem of chromium absorption much worse.

Dichromate salts containing hexavalent chromium are the most readily absorbed and the most toxic because they can cross cell membranes. The mortality rate from these burns is very high if the burn exceeds 10% TBSA. Chromium absorption leads to diarrhea, gastrointestinal bleeding, hemolysis, hepatic and renal damage, coma, encephalopathy, seizures, and disseminated intravascular coagulation.

To treat, immediately excise the burned tissues to lessen the total body dichromate burden. Wash wounds with a 1% sodium phosphate or sulfate solution and dress them with bandages soaked in 5% sodium thiosulfate solution. These actions reduce the hexavalent chromium ion to the less well-absorbed trivalent form.

Institute chelation therapy with ethylenediaminetetraacetic acid (EDTA) and give IV sodium thiosulfate and ascorbic acid. Hemodialysis, peritoneal dialysis, or exchange transfusion may be indicated.

Phosphorus Burns

White phosphorus is a translucent, waxy substance that ignites spontaneously on contact with air. For this reason, it is usually stored under water. It is used primarily in fireworks, insecticides, rodenticides, and military weapons.

Phosphorus causes both thermal burns from the flaming pieces and acid burns from the oxidation of phosphorus to phosphoric acid. The burns classically emit a white vapor with a characteristic garlic odor.

Treat these burns first by immersion in water. Debride any gross debris. Wash the wound with a 1% copper sulfate solution, which reacts with the residual phosphorus to form copper phosphate. Copper phosphate appears as black granules, which allow for easy debridement. After debridement, remove the residual copper with a thorough water rinse, dress the wound, and treat it as any other burn.

Elemental Alkali Metal Burns

The commonly encountered alkali metals (sodium, lithium, and potassium) are highly reactive with water and with water vapor in the air and produce their respective hydroxides with liberation of hydrogen gas. Therefore water should never be used for extinguishing or débriding the metal. A class D fire extinguisher or plain sand may be used to smother the fire, followed by the application of mineral oil or cooking oil to isolate the metal from water and allow safe debridement. Then, treat the burn as an alkali burn.

Magnesium burns in a less intense fashion but otherwise acts as other alkali metals do. These burns may be particularly injurious, however, because if all the metallic debris is not removed, the small ulcers that form will slowly enlarge and can become quite extensive.

The initial topical treatment of unusual chemical burns is outlined in Table 38.3.

Electrical Burns

Electrical burn wounds occur when energy traveling through the body across a potential difference is converted to heat, and has the ability to destroy deep tissues, including muscles, tendons, and nerves (Fig. 38.25). In addition, electrical injuries can arise from the arc produced when electricity passes through the air and from flames caused by the ignition of clothing. Electrical injuries from high-voltage or high-current sources (>1000 V and >5000 mA) are more likely to result in deep soft tissue damage, whereas low voltage or low current (<1000 V and 5 mA to 60 mA) causes less soft tissue damage but is more likely to result in cardiac arrhythmias.[29] Due to the deeper tissue injury caused by electrical burns, patients with serious electrical burns require more fluid resuscitation than those with thermal burns.

TABLE 38.3 Chemical Burn Treatment

TREATMENT	CHEMICAL SUBSTANCE	
Water lavage	Chromic acid	Tannic acid
	Potassium permanganate	Sulfosalicylic acid
	Cantharides	Trichloroacetic acid
	Lyes (hydroxide salts)	Cresylic acid
	Clorox	Acetic acid
	Dichromate salts	Formic acid
	Picric acid	—
Calcium salt injection	Oxalic acid	—
	Hydrofluoric acid	—
Oil immersion	Sodium metal	—
	White phosphorus	—
	Mustard gas	—
Avoid water lavage	Sodium metal	—
	Potassium metal	—
	Lithium metal	—
Specific Approaches		
Excision	Sodium metal	—
Weak acid lavage (vinegar)	Lyes (hydroxide salts)	—
Calcium gluconate injection	Hydrofluoric acid	—
Copper sulfate solution	White phosphorus	—

TEN and SJS

Toxic epidermal necrolysis (TEN) and Stevens-Johnson syndrome (SJS) are severe blistering diseases. They are primarily associated with taking certain medications that cause apoptosis of keratinocytes, which results in the separation of large areas of skin at the dermal-epidermal junction and produces the appearance of a scald. More than 200 medications have been associated with this condition, although infections and immunizations have also caused TEN and SJS. A major factor in improving outcomes has been high-quality intensive support and trained nursing care with expertise in wounds. Therefore these disorders are often ideally suited to treatment at burn centers.

The distinction between TEN and SJS is one of extent, with lesions occupying less than 10% TBSA qualifying as SJS (Fig. 38.26) and lesions involving greater than 30% TBSA being called TEN (Fig. 38.27); when the extent of

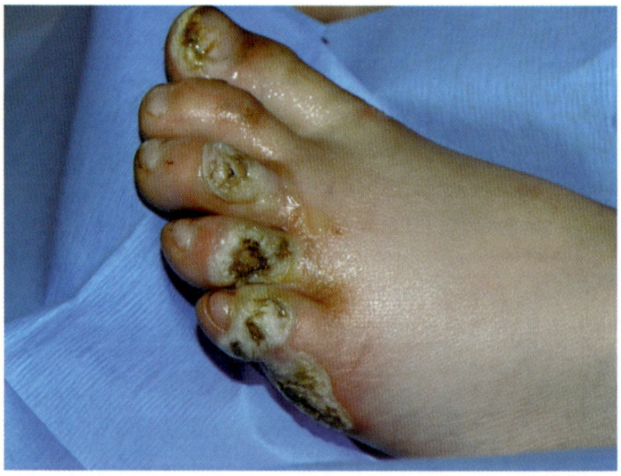

Fig. 38.25 Electrical burn. The patient experienced a contact burn across the dorsa of the toes from an exposed electrical wire. (From Davis PJ, Cladis FP, Motoyama EK, eds. *Smith's Anesthesia for Infants and Children*. 8th ed. Mosby; 2011.)

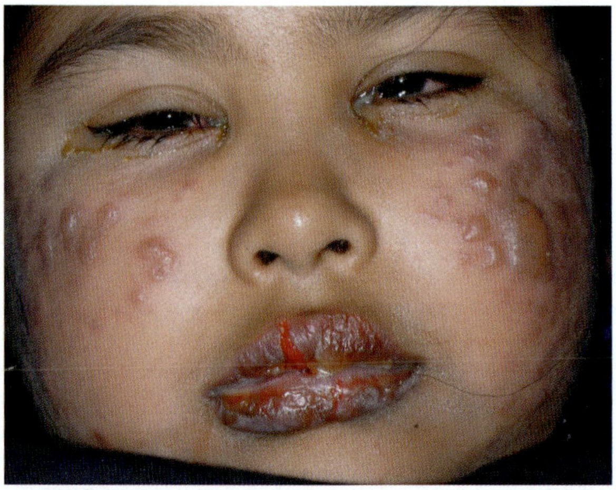

Fig. 38.26 Stevens-Johnson syndrome (SJS). Purpuric macules became bullous. Note the inflammation of the conjunctivae and lips. In SJS the lesions occupy less than 10% of total body surface area. (From Paller AS, Mancini AJ, eds. *Hurwitz Clinical Pediatric Dermatology*. 4th ed. Saunders; 2011.)

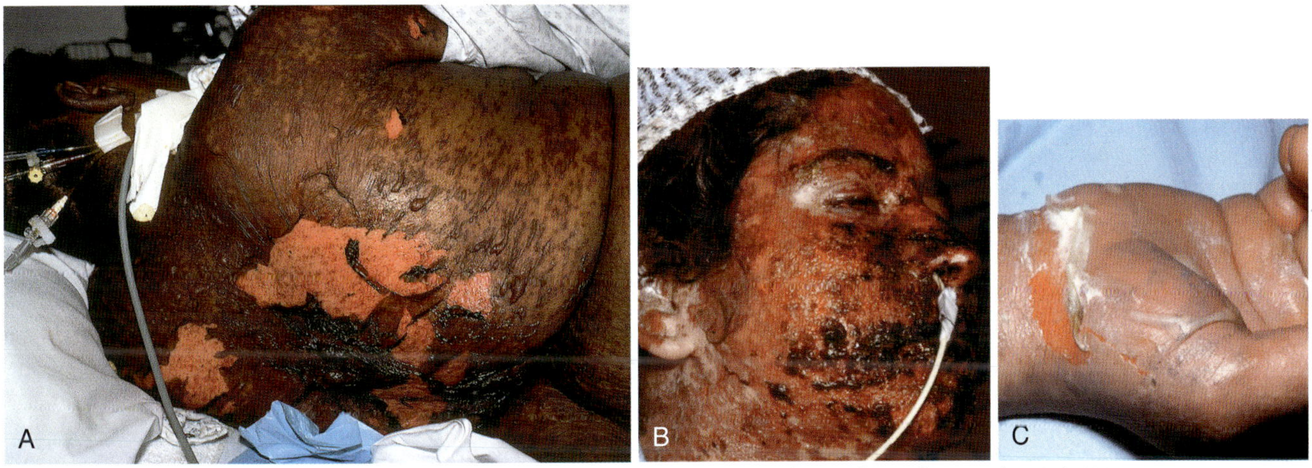

Fig. 38.27 Toxic epidermal necrolysis. (A) Detachment of large sheets of necrolytic epidermis (>30% total body surface area) led to extensive areas of denuded skin. A few intact bullae are still present. (B) Hemorrhagic crusts with mucosal involvement. (C) Epidermal detachment of the palmar skin. (From Bolognia JL, Jorizzo JL, Rapini RP, eds. *Dermatology*, 3th ed. Saunders; 2012.)

involvement lies between 10% and 30%, an intermediary term is coined, SJS-TEN overlap. These disorders are rare with an annual incidence of 0.4 to 1.2 and 1.2 to 6.0 per million persons, respectively, and are more common in females and older adults. Severely immunocompromised persons are particularly at risk. Death occurs on average in every third patient with TEN. More than 200 drugs, including antibiotics (particularly sulfonamides), nonsteroidal antiinflammatory drugs, and anticonvulsants, have been implicated.

Various theories exist to explain the precise sequence of molecular and cellular events responsible for the development of TEN. The 1- to 3-week interval between the onset of TEN and the commencement of drug therapy favors an immune etiology. Cytotoxic T cells are seen in cutaneous lesions, and it is hypothesized that necrolysis is due to their recognition of complexes between drug metabolites and major histocompatibility complex class I molecules on the surface of keratinocytes. Exfoliation is due to the death of keratinocytes via apoptosis, and data suggest that the latter is mediated by interaction of the death receptors, transmembrane proteins, Fas, and its ligand FasL. This activates the proteolytic cascade (caspases), which leads to cellular disintegration.[30]

Clinical Features

TEN and SJS are usually characterized by fever, corneal irritation, and painful swallowing (representing oral mucocutaneous involvement). These symptoms can precede the rash by 1 to 3 days. In more than 99% of patients, erythema and erosions of the buccal, ocular, and genital mucosa develop and are painful. Diagnosis may require skin biopsy as the condition might be difficult to clinically differentiate from other conditions such as staphylococcal scalded skin syndrome or other dermatologic emergencies. The epithelium of the respiratory tract is involved in 25% of cases of TEN, and gastrointestinal lesions can occur. The skin lesions first appear as erythematous, dusky red, or purpuric macules, irregular in size and shape, that tend to coalesce. Nikolsky's sign (blistering following pressure with the finger) may be evident. A gray appearance of the macule heralds necrosis of the epidermis, which soon separates from the dermis and leaves a raw painful area. Wound infections (*S. aureus* and *P. aeruginosa*) and fluid and electrolyte loss often follow. Death is mainly due to sepsis, acute respiratory distress syndrome, and multiorgan failure. Reepithelialization and healing of wounds can occur within 3 weeks but may be prolonged. There are, however, late sequelae such as scarring and pigmentary abnormalities, as well as serious ophthalmic complications (e.g., symblepharon, conjunctival synechiae, entropion), which can range from sicca syndrome to blindness.

Management

Initial management of TEN requires immediate discontinuation of all medications, including possibly causative antibiotics. Supportive care is similar to that required in the treatment of thermal burns. Depending on the body surface area involved patients may require the resources of a burn center that has dermatology consultants available. Medical attention is paid to correction of fluid and electrolyte abnormalities, renal insufficiency, nutrition, control of pain and temperature, and possible sepsis. Involvement of respiratory mucosa may warrant intubation and ventilation. The wounds are carefully debrided and a biopsy specimen is taken to confirm the diagnosis. Regular hydrotherapy and topical antimicrobials are used to decrease infection. Prophylactic empiric intravenous antimicrobials are not advised unless clinically indicated. Silver sulfadiazine and mafenide are best avoided because they may be implicated in causing the disorder.

Regular examination by an ophthalmologist is also recommended in patients with TEN. The eyelids should be cleansed daily and followed with a daily application of antibiotic ointment. Attention to oral hygiene is also important because oral lesions are common.

Several case reports, uncontrolled series, and small trials suggest the utility of specific therapies for the treatment of TEN/SJS; however, even with systematic reviews, there is no strong evidence-based standards to promote any particular therapy. Studies have included corticosteroids, cyclosporine, cyclophosphamide, etanercept, intravenous immunoglobulin (IVIG), plasmapheresis, and *N*-acetylcysteine, but these therapies are not established as standard of care. The most promising results seem to have been achieved with the use of cyclosporin, etanercept, or the combination of IVIG and systemic corticosteroids; however, data are weak and use remains controversial, with some indication that IVIG may even increase mortality. Importantly, subsequent research has not demonstrated a significant mortality advantage for patients using either high- or low-dose IVIG compared with patients treated with supportive care only, so IVIG alone is not currently established as standard of care therapy.[31–33]

Mortality of TEN approaches 30%, depending on stage of diagnosis at presentation, supportive measures, age, and comorbidities. A modified scoring system for patients with TEN has been published by Bastuji-Garin and colleagues that predicts the mortality of these patients (Table 38.4).[34] An additional scoring system called ABCD-10 also exists. In a small study of 196 patients SCORTEN was found to be superior in mortality prognostication.[35] Although rarely useful for the emergency provider, these scoring systems may aid in patient and family education, and the collaborative decision to hospitalize at a nonburn center or arrange for transfer to a burn center.

TABLE 38.4 SCORTEN Score for Predicted Mortality in TEN[a]

RISK FACTOR	0	1
Age	<40 years	≥40 years
Malignancy	No	Yes
Heart rate	<120	≥120
Serum BUN (mg/dL)	<27	>27
%BSA involved	<10%	>10%
Serum bicarbonate (mEq/L)	≤20	<20
Serum glucose (mg/dL)	<250	>250
NUMBER OF RISK FACTORS	**MORTALITY RATE**	
0–1	3.2%	
2	12.1%	
3	35.3%	
4	58.3%	
5 or more	90%	

[a]SCORTEN Scale as reported in article by Bastuji-Garin S, Fouchard N, Bertocchi M et al. SCORTEN: a severity-of-illness score for toxic epidermal necrolysis. *J Invest Dermatol.* 2000;115(2):149-153.

BSA, Body surface area; *BUN*, blood urea nitrogen; *TEN*, toxic epidermal necrolysis.

Frostbite

Frostbite is the result of exposure to low environmental temperatures (Fig. 38.28). The formation of ice crystals within extracellular fluid causes direct cellular injury and cellular dehydration through transmembrane osmotic shifts. In addition, a secondary vascular effect of cooling leads to endothelial damage and progressive dermal ischemia.

Initial management of acute frostbite should entail determination of the core temperature and a full physical examination. The frostbitten part should be rapidly rewarmed in a water bath (temperature of 40°C to 42°C) with adequate analgesia for 15 to 30 minutes while avoiding rubbing, trauma, or reexposure to cold environments. Treatment of deep injury consists of elevation of the injured part to control edema, adequate analgesia, splinting, and the application of topical antibiotics. While there is no definitive evidence, it is recommended that blisters be left intact in the initial ED treatment phase when possible. As of 2023 ABA has released guidelines conditionally recommending early (<12 hours from rewarming) thrombolytics, either intravenous or intraarterial, for severe frostbite patients to decrease the need for amputation or allow for more distal level of amputation needed.[36,37] The use of antithromboxane drugs such as aspirin or ibuprofen has been shown to be useful, as has the application of aloe vera. In 2024 the Food and Drug Administration (FDA) approved the drug iloprost for the treatment of severe frostbite. It is effective up to 3 days after the injury, so its use will likely be determined by specialists caring for the patient rather than in the ED.[38] The avoidance of refreezing is critical to reduce complications. Patients should be educated on this important precaution. Premature amputation should be avoided, but amputation may be necessary for definitive closure.

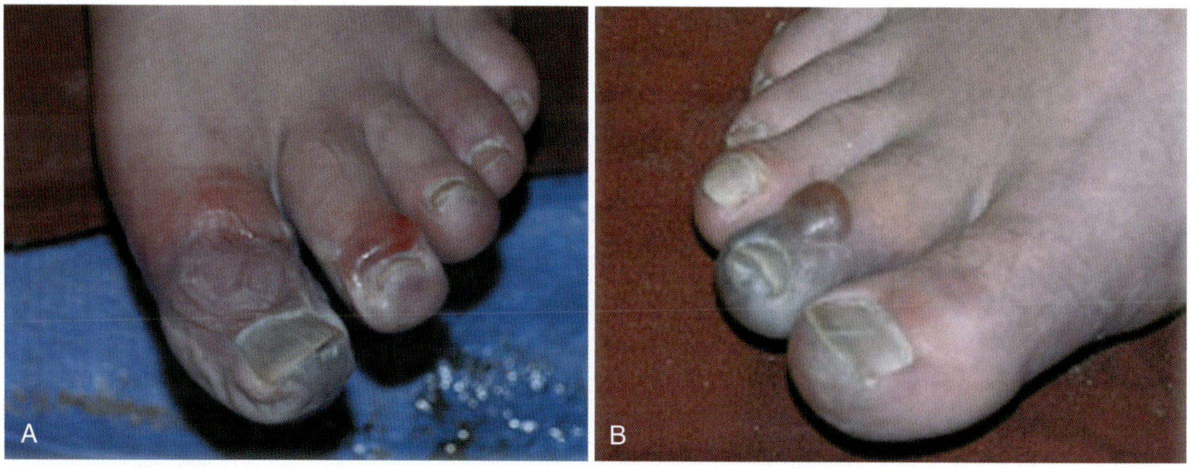

Fig. 38.28 Frostbite. Initial management includes rapid rewarming in a water bath (temperature of 40°C to 42°C) for 15 to 30 minutes. Hemorrhagic blisters should be left intact; white or clear blisters may be debrided. Avoidance of refreezing is imperative.

Long-term consequences include a predilection for future frostbite, vasospastic syndromes, and cold hypersensitivity.

Radiation Burns

Accidents involving ionizing radiation are not common, but when they occur, the clinical findings may range from erythema to charring of the superficial layers of skin. Whole-body exposure of more than 100 rad causes acute radiation syndrome within hours of exposure. This is characterized acutely by nausea, vomiting, diarrhea, fever, fatigue, and headache. The symptoms may resolve transiently during a latent period only to recur as hematopoietic, gastrointestinal, or vascular complications.[39]

EMERGENCY ESCHAROTOMY

Full-thickness burns result in an eschar that is inelastic and may become restrictive and result in compartment syndrome. Intracellular and interstitial edema can develop and progress, both because of fluid resuscitation and as a direct result of transcapillary extravasation of fluid from the thermal injury. As the soft tissues become edematous and pressure rises under the unyielding eschar, first venous and then lymphatic, capillary, and ultimately arterial flow to the underlying and distal unburned tissue may be compromised. Full-thickness and extensive partial-thickness circumferential extremity burns are most likely to impede peripheral blood flow. Circumferential chest burns may restrict chest wall movement and impair ventilation, and circumferential neck burns may result in tracheal obstruction. In such cases, immediate escharotomy may be indicated.

On occasion, because of high-volume fluid resuscitation, noncircumferential and deep partial-thickness burns require surgical decompression to prevent the complications of nerve or muscle damage. Once signs and symptoms of vascular impairment are present, the clinician must act quickly to prevent tissue hypoxia and cellular death. This pathophysiology may be manifested within a time frame that requires an emergency clinician to intervene. Clinical assessment of tight compartments may be aided by measurements such as capillary refill, Doppler signals, pulse oximetry, and direct measurement of compartment pressures. Escharotomy, when required, is usually performed within the first 2 to 6 hours of a burn injury.

It is not standard of care that emergency clinicians be skilled in emergency escharotomy, nor can it be expected that this procedure will be done in the ED. The technique is described here for circumstances when escharotomy must be performed by a non–burn specialist.

Indications

The indications for escharotomy are based on clinical examination, compartment pressure, or both. A high index of suspicion and a low threshold for intervention are essential for a successful outcome. Skin temperature and palpation of pulses are unreliable and imprecise indicators of the adequacy of circulation because of peripheral vasoconstriction and local edema. A patient with circulatory compromise significant enough to warrant escharotomy may complain of deep aching pain, progressive loss of sensation, or paresthesias, but these parameters are difficult to quantitate in a severely burned, sedated, or mechanically ventilated patient. However, motor activity and peripheral pulses may remain intact despite severe underlying muscle ischemia. Muscle compartments with pressures in excess of 30 mm Hg should be decompressed. Measurements should be taken before and after escharotomy to ensure adequate decompression.

In a patient with absent distal arterial flow but otherwise adequate blood pressure, immediate escharotomy is indicated.

Technique of Escharotomy

Because full-thickness burns are insensate to pain and involve coagulation of superficial vessels, anesthesia may not be needed. Patients with deep partial-thickness burns may still possess pain sensation, and escharotomy may be performed with local anesthesia or systemic analgesia. A properly executed escharotomy releases the eschar to the depth of SQ fat only. This results in minimal bleeding, which can be controlled with local pressure or electrocautery. These incisions, even though life or limb-saving, represent potential sources of infection for the burn patient and should be treated as part of the burn wound. The wounds should be loosely packed with sterile gauze impregnated with an appropriate topical antimicrobial. Fasciotomy, which involves a deeper incision, may be needed for thermal or electrical burns.

Limbs

Under sterile conditions, incise the lateral and medial aspects of the involved extremity with a scalpel or electrocautery 1 cm proximal to the burned area and 1 cm distal to the involved area of a constricting burn (Fig. 38.29). Carry the incision through the full thickness of skin only and this should result in

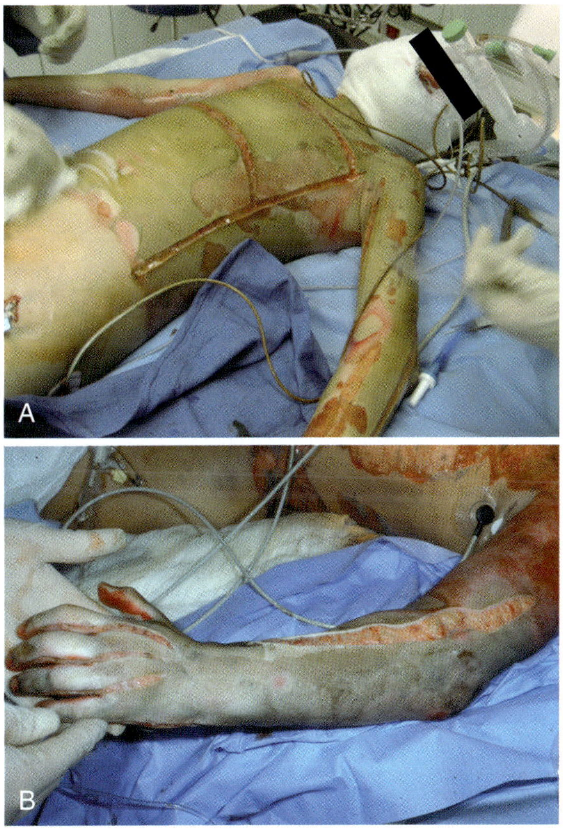

Fig. 38.29 Escharotomy. (A) Patients with deep, nearly circumferential or circumferential chest wall burns may require escharotomy to facilitate ventilation. If performed properly, escharotomy of the torso will markedly enhance compliance. (B) Properly performed escharotomy will result in immediate improvement in extremity blood flow. (From Vincent JL, Abraham E, Moore FA et al., eds. *Textbook of Critical Care*. 6th ed. Saunders; 2011.)

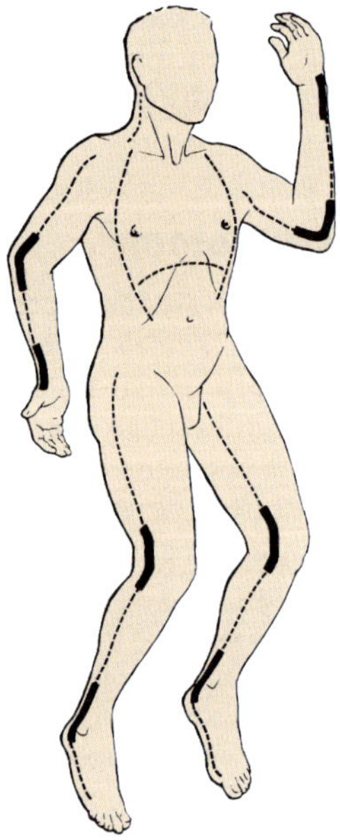

Fig. 38.30 Preferred sites for escharotomy incisions. *Dotted lines* indicate the escharotomy sites. *Bold lines* indicate areas where caution is required because vascular structures and nerves may be damaged by escharotomy incisions. (From Davis JH, Drucker WR, Foster RS et al. *Clinical Surgery*. Mosby; 1987.)

immediate separation of the constricting eschar to expose SQ fat. Because joints are areas of tight skin adherence and potential vascular impingement, incisions should cross these structures (Fig. 38.30). Take care to avoid vital structures, such as the ulnar nerve at the elbow, the radial nerve at the wrist, the superficial peroneal nerve near the fibular head, and the posterior tibial artery at the ankle. In circumferential burns of the feet, if escharotomy is indicated, extend the incision to the great toe medially and the little toe laterally. In circumferential burns of the hands in which escharotomy is indicated, extend the incisions to the thenar and hypothenar aspects of the hands (see Figs. 38.29 and 38.30). Softening of the compartment, improved distal tissue perfusion, return of sensation, Doppler flow signal strength, and oximetry values indicate adequate release.

Chest

Full-thickness circumferential chest or upper abdominal burns may impair respiration. Nearly all these patients are expected to be intubated and mechanically ventilated. Evidence of the need to release the eschar include increased airway pressure or an inability to ventilate. Escharotomy of the chest wall should extend from the clavicle to the costal margin in the anterior axillary line bilaterally, while avoiding breast tissue. This may be joined by transverse incisions to result in a chevron-shaped subcostal incision (see Fig. 38.29).

Neck

Neck escharotomy should be performed laterally and posteriorly to avoid the carotid and jugular vessels.

Penis

Penile escharotomy is performed midlaterally to avoid the dorsal vein.

Complications

Complications of escharotomy include bleeding, infection, and damage to underlying structures. Complications of inadequate decompression include muscle necrosis, nerve injury (such as footdrop), and even amputation of the limb. Systemic complications of inadequate decompression include myoglobinuria and renal failure, hyperkalemia, and metabolic acidosis.

CONCLUSION

Patients with circumferential or nearly circumferential burns should be evaluated for the risk of developing compartment syndrome and deep tissue ischemia. Emergency clinicians should not hesitate to perform an escharotomy before transfer of the patient to a burn center if there is evidence of reduced limb perfusion or impaired ventilation.

ACKNOWLEDGMENTS

The significant contributions of Courtney A. Bethel, MD, Leigh Ann Price, MD, and Kevin B. Gerold, MD, to earlier editions remain appreciated.

REFERENCES ARE AVAILABLE AT Elsevier eBooks+

CHAPTER 39

Post–Cosmetic Procedure Interventions

Jonathan Cohen, Kerry E. Gregory, and Stephanie Caterson

BACKGROUND

Derived from the Greek word *plastikos*, meaning to mold or give form, plastic surgery has been described as a surgical specialty that encompasses the entire skin envelope and its contents.[1] With its origins dating back to ancient Egypt,[2] modern-day plastic surgery has evolved from the reconstruction of disfiguring wounds sustained during World War I to the current standard of providing complex reconstruction, composite tissue transplantation, and advanced aesthetic procedures with the overall intention of restoration of form and function.

In the United States in 2020 alone, an estimated $16 billion was spent on cosmetic procedures with nearly 16 million cosmetic total procedures performed; 2,314,720 cosmetic surgical and 13,281,235 cosmetic minimally invasive procedures, respectively, performed in 2020 alone (Boxes 39.1 and 39.2).[3] Despite increasing utilization of ambulatory surgery centers and office-based surgery centers for cosmetic surgery and minimally invasive procedures, this practice is generally regarded as safe with low complication rates.[4–7] It is important to note that patient safety, favorable outcomes, and decreased emergency department (ED) visits and hospitalization rates are associated with physician training and experience, appropriate patient selection, type of procedure, and facility accreditation.[8–10]

Demand for these services continues to increase. As social norms have become more accepting of cosmetic procedures coupled with the effect of direct-to-consumer marketing via social media.[11,12] Within this expanding market, the emergence of health care providers performing cosmetic procedures outside of their scope of practice is of concern, especially as patient perception and understanding of board certification and training are often varied.[13–15] Further research is necessary to compare complication rates, ED visits, and need for hospitalization following cosmetic procedures performed by these providers outside of the "core four." As with any consumer-driven market, cost is often associated with perceived value when purchasing cosmetic services; within this equation the importance of outcomes and safety inputs are often overlooked by patients, which in turn results in higher costs and complication risks.[16]

MEDICAL TOURISM

Each year millions of Americans travel outside the United States to seek medical care.[17,18] Medical tourism is an estimated $100 billion market annually. It is predicted that this industry will experience continued growth largely in response to patient demand for low-cost cosmetic procedures, flexibility in scheduling, and the opportunity to maximize social downtime in a favorable climate.[18–20] It is important to note that quality cosmetic care performed by board-certified physicians in regulated facilities is accessible outside of the United States (Table 39.1).

Cost savings upwards of 90% when compared with US prices for these services is an undeniable motivator for medical tourism. In response to these market pressures, domestic practices near areas with accessible foreign transit have realized an increase of low-cost practices that must perform higher volumes of procedures in order to remain competitive with foreign facilities with lower operational and regulatory burdens.[21–23]

As the market expands, an increasing number of patients are returning to the United States with postprocedural complications requiring ED visits and subsequent hospital admissions. For example, one retrospective study suggests a 38% infection rate following breast augmentation surgery performed abroad compared with less than 3% in US-based breast augmentation surgery.[24–26] In the absence of a comprehensive database tracking postprocedural complications arising from medical tourism, the true scope of this problem is largely unknown. In a recent 16-patient case series by Venditto et al., the reported costs of managing these types of complications ranged from $392 to $154,700.79 individually, with a mean of $26,657.19.[27] In this patient cohort, only six patients had private health insurance. Overall, 63% of hospital charges were reimbursed in comparison with 9% of billed physician services. It is unknown if any of these patients had prearranged postoperative care scheduled in their home community other than utilization of ED services. One patient was seen twice over a 2-year period following complications of separate procedures performed in the United States and the Dominican Republic. It should be noted that the patients in this cohort had access to an academic medical center with robust specialty services, which contrasts with many patients living in rural or underserved areas.[28]

EMTALA

The Emergency Medical Treatment and Active Labor Act (EMTALA) was passed in 1986 in response to the practice of "patient dumping" in EDs and refusal of care based on the ability to pay for services. Within this legislation, hospitals receiving Medicare funding are required to perform medical screening examinations to assess patient need for emergency services, with the provision of stabilization either in-facility or via transfer to a receiving hospital.[29]

Ideally, once stabilized in the ED, care for patients experiencing postprocedure complications performed locally can be coordinated with their provider; interventions may include routine follow-up care, hospital admission, transfer, and or operative management. In contrast, complications arising from medical tourism-related procedures, performed either domestically or abroad, specialty consultation and follow-up care coordination often represent further challenges, particularly in rural areas where an estimated 25 million Americans have limited access to plastic surgery services.[30,31]

It is recommended that each emergency medical program and its specialty consultant groups review current institutional guidelines and by-laws regarding services provided by on-call consultants.[32] This recommendation is underscored by the passage of the "No Surprises Act," signed into law in 2022, which is intended to protect privately insured patients from out-of-network charges and enable uninsured/self-pay

BOX 39.1 Top Cosmetic Procedures Sought by Patients, 2021–22

1. Liposuction
2. Facelift
3. Breast augmentation
4. Tummy tuck
5. Breast lift

Responses reflect both surgeries completed and consults provided for procedures scheduled before year-end. Other procedures mentioned by respondents included rhinoplasty, gluteal fat grafting ("Brazilian butt lift"), fat transfer to face, breast implant removal (explant), and labiaplasty.

From Cosmetic Surgery Trends. www.plasticsurgery.org/documents/News/Trends/2022/trends-report-cosmetic-surgery-2022.

BOX 39.2 Top Minimally Invasive Cosmetic Procedures Sought by Patients, 2021–22

1. Botulinum toxin type A (Botox)
2. Soft tissue fillers
3. Noninvasive fat reduction
4. Nonsurgical skin tightening
5. Skin care treatments

From Cosmetic Surgery Trends. www.plasticsurgery.org/documents/News/Trends/2022/trends-report-cosmetic-surgery-2022.

TABLE 39.1 Most Common Plastic Surgery Procedures Worldwide, 2021

	Total	Share of Total
Liposuction	1,903,063	14.8%
Breast augmentation	1,685,471	13.1%
Eyelid surgery	1,446,890	11.3%
Rhinoplasty	995,149	7.7%
Abdominoplasty	991,361	7.7%
Breast lift	781,404	6.1%
Lip enhancement/perioral procedure	717,596	5.6%
Fat grafting (face)	589,494	4.6%
Buttock augmentation	523,331	4.1%
Breast reduction	507,363	4.0%

From The International Society of Aesthetic Plastic Surgery isaps.org/media/vdpdanke/isaps-global-survey-2021.

patients to receive good faith estimates of billing costs prior to receiving nonurgent medical care.

RISK OF COMPLICATIONS

Cosmetic surgery is considered "elective" and is ideally performed on healthier patients. Independent risk factors of post–cosmetic procedure complications and hospital admission are often associated with those rating as a class 3 or higher according to the American Society of Anesthesiologist (ASA) (increased age, obesity, poorly controlled diabetes, and nicotine use). A preexisting history of bleeding disorders and recent/current steroid use has also been described as risk factors.[28,29] Common complications arising from cosmetic surgical procedures are pain, postoperative nausea and vomiting, surgical site infection, wounds, incisional dehiscence, pulmonary embolism (PE), deep vein thrombosis (DVT), and bleeding. Within the ED setting, identification of critical illness and infection is the primary objective as wound care and aesthetic concerns can be managed during either hospital admission or on a less-urgent outpatient basis.

EVALUATION OF THE POST–COSMETIC PROCEDURE PATIENT

History

Accessing patient history may be rather straightforward via electronic medical record (EMR) if the presenting patient is linked to care within the same institution or system. For patients returning from domestic or foreign medical tourism, gathering a thorough procedural history may be problematic. It is recommended to obtain as much of the following information as is possible:

- Date, location, and type of procedure(s)
- Operative report, postop instructions, follow-up plan
- Number of procedures performed
- Use of anesthesia (endotracheal, monitored anesthesia care, tumescent, local)
- Past surgical/procedural history
- History of implant placement (size, manufacturer) both recent and/or distant
- Location of incisions/sutures/wound dressings/drains/donor sites (fat grafting, skin grafting)
- Medication regimen—both home medications and postoperative medications (antibiotics, antiemetics, analgesics, etc.)
- Pain scale

It is important to ascertain what procedures were performed, as it is common practice to perform multiple procedures involving multiple sites within the same surgery. Data from the American Society for Plastic Surgeons (ASPS) describe recent trends for combination procedures, with the goal of longer-lasting results and reducing the need for multiple recovery periods.[33]

Additionally, patients are generally given verbal and written instructions for care following procedures. It is common that patients will not have the instructions available at ED presentation and/or have been experiencing difficulty with understanding their postoperative instructions.[34–39]

Assessment

As with any surgical patient, one must not only assess the patient for early complications but also be mindful of the patient's comfort level, questions, and concerns. Subtle changes to the patient's vital signs, urine output, and pain level could signal an impending complication or indicate a worsening of an existing one. Elevated blood pressure due to pain can precipitate bleeding and/or hematoma formation, which can result in life-threatening anemia, compression of essential underlying structures (i.e., airway compromise in head and neck surgeries), skin flap compromise, wound dehiscence, and/or functional morbidity. It is essential to complete a full skin assessment and evaluate all incisions.

For all postoperative patients, it is imperative to consider broad differential diagnoses for presentations of postoperative nausea and vomiting, which may include inhalational anesthesia, opioids, cardiac ischemia, hypoxia, metabolic abnormalities, ileus, viscus perforation, peritonitis, urinary tract infection, pyelonephritis.[40,41]

Communication With Surgical Provider

Most surgical practices provide an "on-call" service to address patient concerns and facilitate communication with providers caring for their patients in emergency situations, as they want to be contacted with complications from their procedures and appreciate collaboration with treating providers. This often includes a discussion to coordinate patient management, particularly if the patient is unstable and is likely to require return to the operating room. To facilitate this process, the discussion should include a description of the current ED course. Details including patient's presenting complaint, applicable surgical history, vital signs, pertinent physical examination finding, surgical dressing and drain status, current/pending laboratory studies and or diagnostic imaging, and medications given should be communicated. Consultation with the patient's surgical team is a mainstay of ED care.[33]

COMMON COSMETIC PROCEDURES AND ASSOCIATED COMPLICATIONS

Injectables

Botulinum toxin type A (BoNT-A) is commonly referred to as Botox. It is derived from the bacteria *Clostridium botulinum* and is a Food and Drug Administration (FDA)–approved nonsurgical treatment for facial rejuvenation. There are also several noncosmetic therapeutic uses including treatment of chronic migraines, hyperhidrosis, and bladder dysfunction. It is the most commonly performed aesthetic procedure in the United States, representing a $4.4 billion market in 2021.[3] This service is easily accessible to patients and is performed by injectors with varied experience and clinical training.

The mechanism of cosmetic effect is via prevention of acetylcholine release from presynaptic motor neurons resulting in muscle paralysis, which provides the intended aesthetic effect of reducing the appearance of wrinkles. The procedure is generally safe, and complications are mostly self-limited.

Uncommon but more serious complications have been reported, most often with therapeutic use. These complications include cardiac arrhythmia, myocardial infarction, anaphylaxis, and death. Postprocedural deaths have not been reported in cosmetic use. Therapeutic use, larger doses, and underlying cardiovascular illness are attributed to the risk of serious adverse events.[42]

Common BoNT-A Postprocedural Complaints and Management

Asymmetry

Under correction/overcorrection

Management is largely reassurance

Headache and Flulike symptoms

Management with supportive treatment.

Ecchymosis and Pain

Preprocedural avoidance of nonsteroidal antiinflammatory drugs (NSAIDs) and aspirin.

Nonopioid analgesics

Application of ice packs to the affected area, limited to 15-minute intervals to avoid soft tissue injury.

Gentle massage (if greater than 4 hours after injection).

Eyelid Ptosis

Alpha-adrenergic ophthalmic eye drops are useful to correct mild to moderate symptoms via contraction of the superior tarsal muscle (Fig. 39.1).[43,44]

Ectropion

For comfort and prevention of possible corneal injury and exposure keratitis, consider lubricating eye drops, eyelid taping, and/or ocular moisture chambers: the latter of which can be purchased online in the form of specialty patches, goggles, and glasses.[45] Consider ophthalmology consult.

Dermal Fillers

Commonly used in the outpatient setting for soft tissue augmentation, there are several options of dermal fillers that are commercially available. The most common are hyaluronic acid–derived dermal fillers. In addition, synthetic formulations, collagen-based fillers, and autologous fat grafting (surgical procedure) are used as well. Common treatment areas include the lips, nasolabial fold, mid-face, periocular, and perioral facial elements.

Complications are typically mild and self-limiting, many of which can be attributed to injector technique. These complications include poor aesthetic result (under/over correction), localized pain, ecchymosis, edema, contour defects, pigmentation irregularities, and to a lesser extent postprocedural infection, hypersensitivity reactions, and nodule formation. The most concerning complication is iatrogenic arterial occlusion and resultant blindness. The mechanistic cause of this rare but severe complication is direct placement and retrograde flow of "filler material" into the vasculature or by localized swelling.[46] Rapid detection is essential as vision loss may be permanent.

Additionally, the use of nonapproved commercial-grade silicone has the inherent risks of disfigurement and systemic illness.[46]

Dermal Filler Complication Evaluation and Management

- Assessment of visual acuity

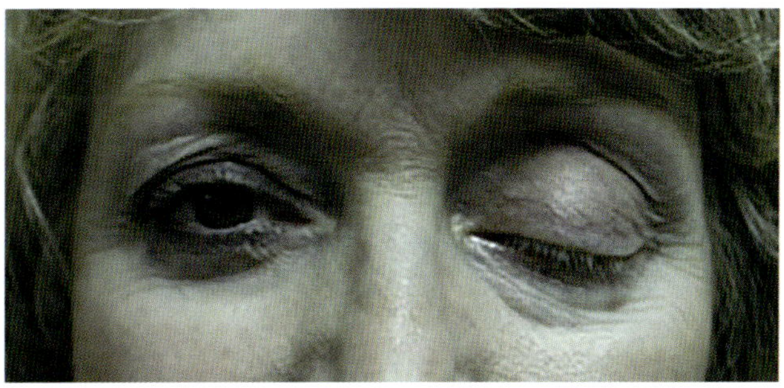

Fig. 39.1 Left upper eyelid ptosis following BoNT-A injection. Reported resolution in 10 weeks.[44]

- Ophthalmology consult, preferably retinal specialist, as indicated
- Standard therapy for central retinal artery occlusion may be employed, however remains unvalidated[47]
  - Ocular massage
  - Instillation of ophthalmic drops
  - Intravenous (IV) acetazolamide, mannitol, methylprednisolone
  - Sublingual isosorbide dinitrate
  - Hyperbaric oxygen
- Reversal with hyaluronidase injection

Breast Augmentation

Breast augmentation is one of the most common cosmetic surgical procedures performed worldwide, with an estimated 365,000 surgeries completed in the United States in 2021.[48] There are multiple methods for breast enhancement including implants, utilization of autologous free flaps, and/or fat transfer/grafting. Incisional approaches may vary based on a combination of factors (i.e., surgeon recommendation, breast characteristics, patient preference); however, the most common incisions are seen in the inframammary, periareolar, and transaxillary areas. The transumbilical breast augmentation procedure is a less commonly utilized technique.[49,50] Implant placement may be either subglandular or submuscular. Postoperative pain is often more pronounced with submuscular placement. The potential benefit of this approach is a more natural cosmetic result and optimized tissue evaluation on subsequent mammograms. Implant style, shape, and size are selected based on which best artistically compliments the overlying soft tissue. Current design options include round versus anatomically shaped, smooth versus textured implants, and saline versus silicone gel with variability in gel cohesion, projection, volume, and shape.[50]

Complications arising from breast augmentation include pain, bleeding, hematoma, seroma, infection, incisional dehiscence, and implant exposure. In addition, patients may experience asymmetry, capsular contraction, rippling, and implant migration.

BREAST AUGMENTATION COMPLICATIONS, EVALUATION, AND MANAGEMENT

Postoperative Pain

Immediate postoperative pain following submuscular implant placement with normal physical examination findings is generally caused by muscle spasm.

Treatment:

- Muscle relaxant, compression bra, and rest are mainstays of treatment.
- Utilize caution with heat or ice therapy as there is often postoperative loss of sensation. Prolonged heat or cold therapy can lead to further tissue damage.
- Utilize prescription drug monitoring program data. If providing prescription opioids during stable ED discharge, consider coprescribing naloxone.
- Surgical consultation, with patient's surgical team highly preferred.

Hematoma

Hematoma following breast surgery is often a unilateral, rapidly developing soft tissue swelling caused by bleeding, which may require surgical intervention (Fig. 39.2).[51] Incidence tends to be rare, accounting for 2.7% of postoperative complications with a median occurrence time of 14 hours (interquartile range [IQR] 5 hours to 9 days) after surgery. Of those who develop hematomas, hypertension was the suspected cause in 10% of these patients.[51] Less commonly, hematomas may present days to weeks following surgery.

Treatment:

- Laboratory studies to assess potential anemia, coagulopathy, infection
- Resuscitation with IV fluids/blood transfusion, as indicated
- Hold anticoagulant medication
- Surgical consultation, with patient's surgical team highly preferred
- Strip drains (if present), as indicated[52]

Infection

The patient with a postoperative infection may present with fever (>38°C), chills, erythema, edema, drainage from incisions, pain, and/or sepsis with hypotension and tachycardia.

Treatment:

- Assess for superficial infection versus periprosthetic infection:
- Areas of soft tissue demonstrating concern for erythema/cellulitis, incisional erythema, incisional dehiscence should be outlined with a surgical marker or pen, accompanied by date and time. The use of military time (24-hour clock) would be optimal, as ED waiting room and departmental patient boarding times routinely extend beyond a team shift (Fig. 39.3).
- Obtain routine laboratory studies, preoperative labs, blood cultures, as indicated.
- Initiate antibiotic therapy, as indicated (Fig. 39.4).
- Ultrasound evaluation for fluid collection, stranding, or inflammation around the implant.

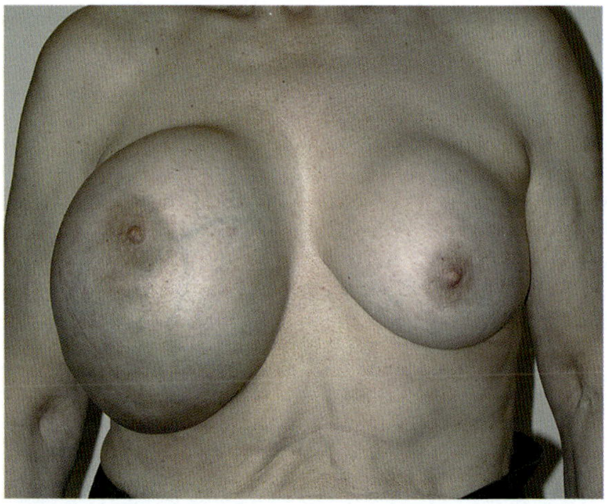

Fig. 39.2 Delayed presentation of hematoma formation following breast augmentation.

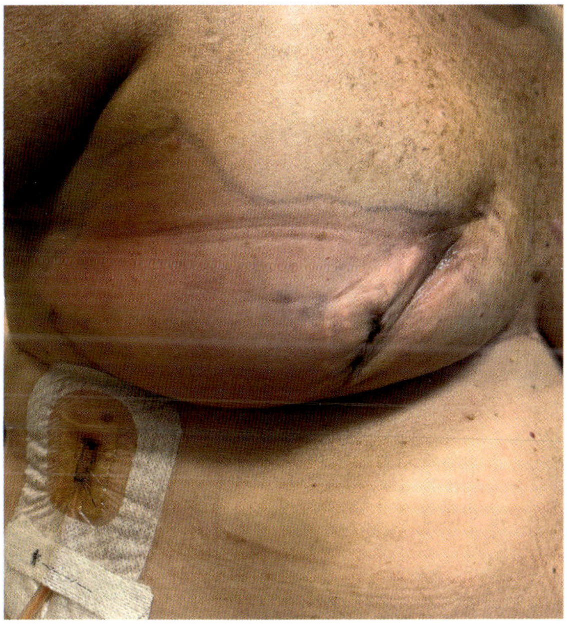

Fig. 39.3 Soft tissue erythema and cellulitis following breast implant placement for cancer reconstruction.

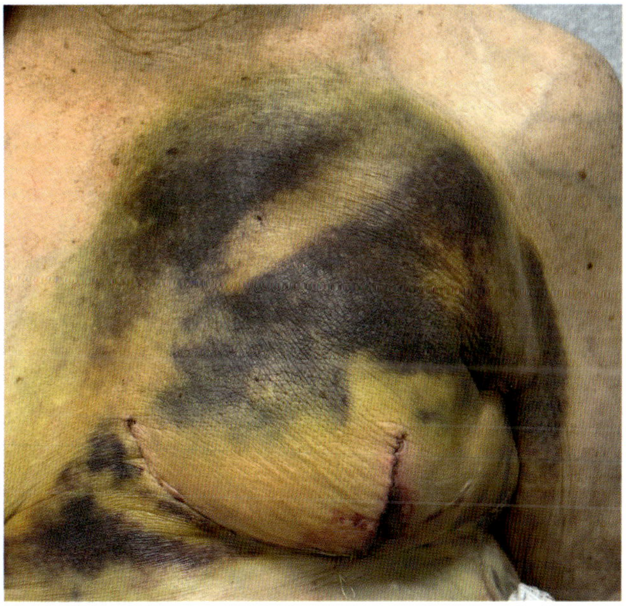

Fig. 39.5 Anterior chest ecchymosis and seroma formation status post implant-based breast reconstruction.

Treatment as suggested from the EMRA Antibiotic Guide, 20th edition	
OUTPATIENT	
Nonpurulent cellulitis	• Cephalexin 500 mg PO 4 times daily (5–10 days) • Cefuroxime 500 mg PO 2 times daily (5–10 days) • Cefadroxil 1 g once daily (5–10 days) • If severe PCN allergy: clindamycin 450 mg PO 3 times daily (5–10 days)
Purulent cellulitis	• TMP/SMX (DS) 1–2 tabs PO 2 times daily • Clindamycin 450 mg PO 3 times daily • Doxycycline 100 mg PO 2 times daily
There is no evidence to support the practice of giving one dose of IV antibiotics prior to a course of outpatient oral antibiotics.	
INPATIENT	
Nonpurulent cellulitis	• Cefazolin 1–2 g IV 3 times daily • Clindamycin 600 mg IV 3 times daily • If MRSA suspected, add vancomycin 15–20 mg/kg IV 2–3 times daily
Purulent cellulitis	• Vancomycin 15–20 mg/kg IV 2–3 times daily
Purulent cellulitis/ suspected implant infection	***Surgical evaluation with possible I and D**

Fig. 39.4 Emergency Medicine Residents' Association (EMRA) skin and soft tissue infection antibiotic guidelines. *MRSA*, methicillin-resistant *Staphylococcus aureus*; *PCN*, penicillin; *PO*, orally; *TMP/SMX*, trimethoprim-sulfamethoxazole.

- Surgical consultation for consideration of implant removal versus salvage, with patient's surgical team highly preferred.[53]

Seroma

Seroma formation is a common side effect of aesthetic surgery, breast cancer surgery, and abdominal wall hernia repair, with incidences ranging between 15% and 85% following mastectomy and 11% following abdominoplasty (Fig. 39.5).[54] Seromas are an accumulation of serous fluid within a "dead space" containing plasma and lymphatic fluid, and they generally form within a few days to a few weeks after surgery. The patient may present similarly to hematoma with unilateral swelling, discomfort, and possibly with mild redness. Treatment includes the following:

- Obtain routine laboratory studies
- Rule out or treat potential infectious process(es)
- Ultrasound evaluation. This can confirm fluid collection; sterile aspiration may be necessary if there is pain, functional deficit, or significant pressure on the incision/wound closure (risk for wound dehiscence). Caution is advised where an implant is involved as this may require ultrasound guidance to perform safely.
- Strip drains (if present), as indicated
- Document last oral intake
- Surgical consultation, with patient's surgical team highly preferred

Implant Exposure

Wound dehiscence with exposure of the breast implant is a rare complication in cosmetic breast augmentation (1.1% to 2.5% of cases).[55] The incidence of occurrence in postmastectomy breast reconstruction is estimated up to 35% and is often aggravated by the presence of an infection (Fig. 39.6).[55] Prompt surgical evaluation and treatment could salvage the reconstruction. Treatment includes the following:

- Cover exposed implant with gauze dressing.
- Obtain routine laboratory studies, preoperative labs, blood cultures. Avoid obtaining wound cultures in the ED setting given risk of contamination with skin flora. Operative deep wound cultures are preferable.
- Obtain IV access.
- Initiate antibiotic therapy and maintenance fluids.
- Strip drains (if present).

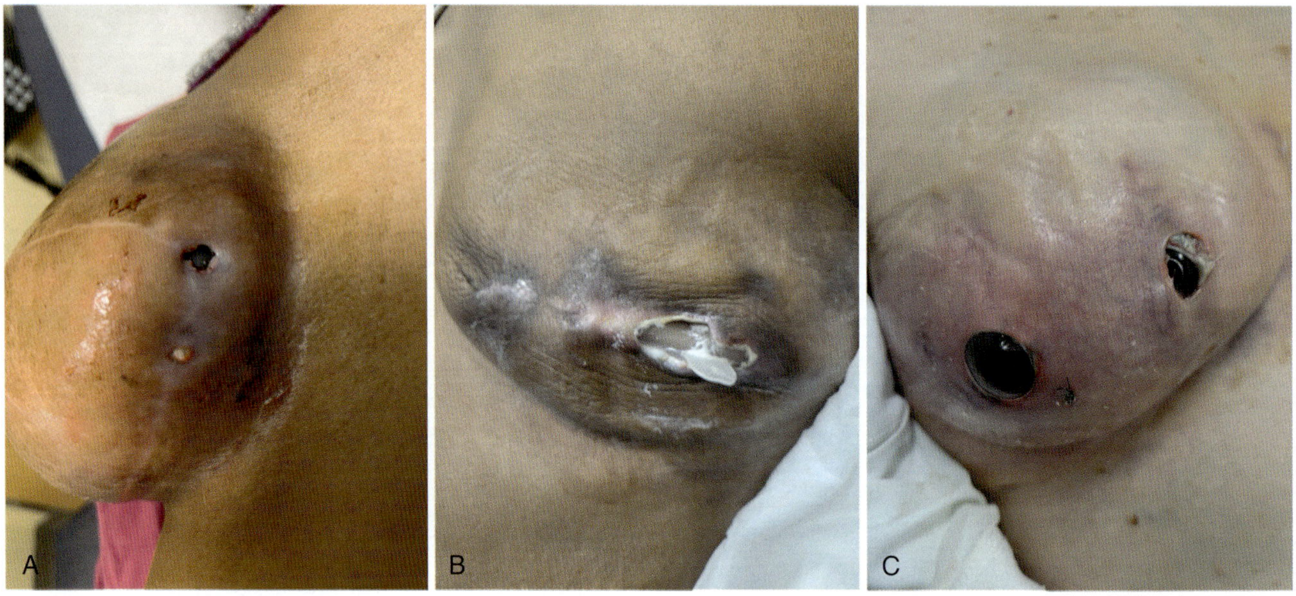

Fig. 39.6 (A) Lateral view of breast implant exposure. (B) Lateral view of breast tissue expander exposure. (C) Anterior view of right breast with multiple areas of breast implant exposure.

- Document last oral intake and initiate NPO (nothing by mouth) patient status.
- Consult with patient's surgical team (highly preferred).

Breast Implant–Associated Anaplastic Large Cell Lymphoma

Patients presenting with delayed seroma formation at least 1 year following implant placement, without evidence of infection or recent trauma should undergo evaluation for breast implant–associated anaplastic large cell lymphoma (BIA-ALCL), which is a rare T-cell non-Hodgkin lymphoma. It is thought to originate within the capsule of textured breast implants following both cosmetic and reconstructive procedures. The incidence of delayed seroma formation following implantation is estimated to be between 0.1% and 0.2%, with BIA-ALCL representing roughly 9% to 13% of these cases.[56] On average, patients present 8 to 10 years after implant placement with development of unilateral spontaneous fluid collection (60% to 90%). Other findings include capsular mass (10% to 40%) and axillary lymphadenopathy.[56,57] The patient should be referred to the plastic surgeon who placed the implants, a local plastic surgeon if that physician is unavailable, or an oncologist for full workup.

Diagnosis

- Ultrasound evaluation of breast and regional lymph nodes (looking for periprosthetic fluid).
- MRI has been shown to be superior to other modalities if ultrasound is inconclusive during initial evaluation (again looking for periprosthetic fluid and/or masses within the implant capsule).
- Ultrasound-guided, fine-needle aspiration of the periimplant fluid should be sent for cytology and flow cytometry per the American Society of Plastic Surgeons.
  - Cytology: CD30, ALK
  - Flow cytometry: T cells
- Confirmed cases require surgical resection of the implant and capsule as well as oncology consultation.
- BIA-ALCL cases are reported to PROFILE (*P*atient *R*egistry and *O*utcomes for breast *I*mplants and anaplastic large cell *L*ymphoma etiology and *E*pidemiology).

Reduction Mammoplasty

Surgical management of macromastia is commonly performed in the outpatient setting for symptomatic relief. Patients routinely endure emotional distress and social stigma in addition to chronic neck, shoulder, and back pain. The benefits of this procedure are well documented to improve the patient's physical and psychological well-being.[58] Preoperative physical examinations often reveal bra strap shoulder grooving, physical deconditioning, and recurrent rashes of the inframammary fold. Incisional approach and the use of surgical drains are largely based on surgeon preference.[59] For larger volume reductions, removal of the nipple areola complex (NAC) may be required. During this procedure, the NAC is excised and prepped for return as a skin graft into the correct anatomic position. The NAC is sutured into place and secured with a bolster dressing. These dressings remain in place until postoperative follow-up (minimum of 5 days).

Complications include nonsurgical wounds, seromas, fat necrosis, and infection. Reoperation rates for scar formation have been demonstrated as less than 7%, postoperative infection 7.3%, hematoma 2.8%, and seromas 1.2%. Larger volume reductions and patient-specific risk factors (advanced age, anticoagulant medication, obesity, poorly controlled diabetes, nicotine use, and cardiovascular disease history) have been attributed to increased risk of complication.[60]

Mastopexy

The breast lift is one of the most commonly performed aesthetic surgeries.[33] It is routinely performed in the outpatient setting for the correction of ptosis (breast tissue laxity) arising from the natural process of aging, heredity, pregnancy, breastfeeding, massive weight loss (>50 lb) and conversely an elevated body mass index (BMI).[61] Surgery involves excision and tightening of the lower breast pole to elevate the NAC above the inframammary fold. There are multiple approaches to the procedure, which may also include utilization of autologous fat grafting and breast implant placement (augmentation-mastopexy). Postoperative complications include those associated with reduction mammoplasty in addition to autologous fat grafting and implant placement, if used in combination.

Mastopexy Complication Evaluation and Management

- Consultation with operative team
- Evaluate for hemodynamic instability
- Rule out infectious process
- Symptomatic relief of postoperative pain, nausea and vomiting

Hematoma

- Operative washout for significant hematoma.
- Bedside aspiration or drainage via interventional radiology may be considered in the stable patient.
- Conservative management:
    - Continued monitoring of closed suction drains (if present)
    - Massage and warm compresses

Wound Formation

- Consider performing a culture of the wound with bordering erythema or purulence.
- Local wound care:
    - Consider moist dressings (wet-to-dry with normal saline and gauze or silver-hydrofiber).
- Extensive wounds may require operative debridement and consideration of vacuum-assisted closure dressing placement (Fig. 39.7).
- Hospital admission versus outpatient surgery follow-up.
- For medical tourism patients, consider referral to in-network plastic surgeon, general surgeon, and/or wound care center.

NAC Necrosis and Small Incisional Wounds/Dehiscence

- Local wound care (Fig. 39.8).
- Reassurance that revision procedures can restore cosmesis.
- Outpatient clinic follow-up with operative team, with patient's surgical team highly preferred.

Seroma

- Small-volume seromas can be managed with needle aspiration during clinic follow-up.
- Large-volume seromas may require drainage with ultrasound guidance.
    - In absence of pain, concern for incisional dehiscence or systemic illness, seromas can be managed nonurgently.

Abdominoplasty and Panniculectomy

The abdominoplasty procedure (tummy tuck), with or without liposuction, is commonly performed in the outpatient setting for removal of abdominal fat, correction of skin laxity and striae formation, and often includes repair of abdominal wall muscle diastasis (plication of diastasis recti). More than 11,800 abdominoplasty procedures were performed in the United States in 2019.[62] The procedure is associated with aesthetically pleasing outcomes and high patient satisfaction. In contrast, panniculectomy is a largely functional procedure for removal of the large skin apron commonly associated with bariatric surgery and large-volume weight loss. Generally, repair of abdominal wall muscle diastasis is often not performed with a panniculectomy.

Abdominoplasty may be performed via multiple surgical approaches and in most cases with placement of surgical drains as seroma formation is common following this procedure.

Contraindications for this elective procedure include unfavorable preoperative risk stratification, abdominal wall hernia, unrealistic procedural outcome expectations, and body dysmorphic disorder. In addition, relative contraindications include patient history of thromboembolic disease,

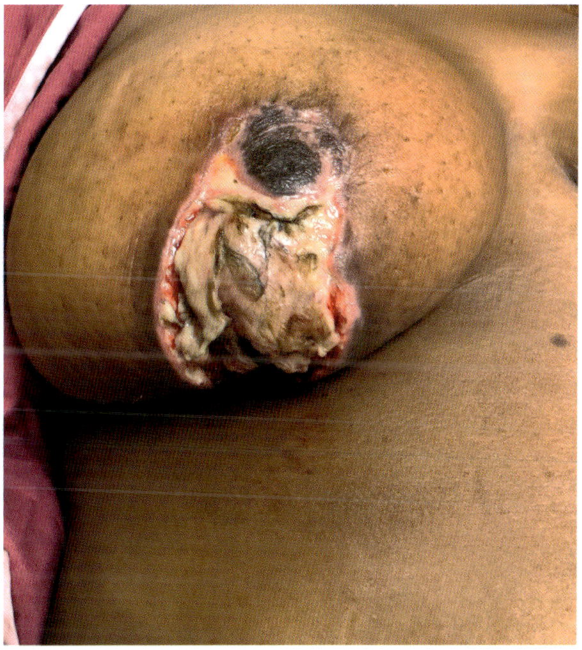

Fig. 39.7 Vertical incisional dehiscence following reduction mammoplasty requiring surgical debridement.

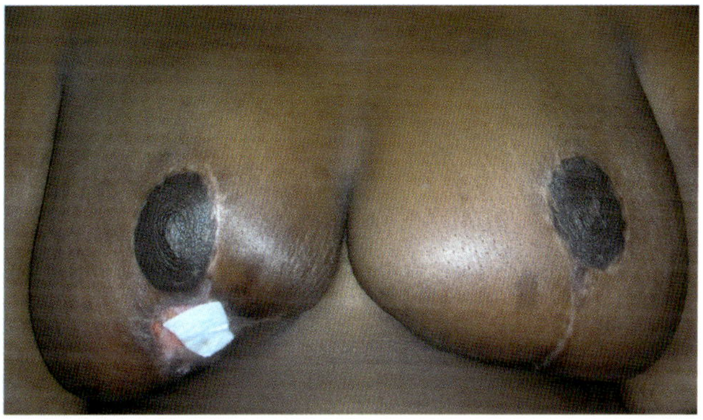

Fig. 39.8 Reduction mammoplasty with free nipple graft placement. Vertical incisional wound treated with local wound care.

cardiovascular disease, poorly controlled diabetes, morbid obesity, and nicotine use. Prior history of abdominal surgery is carefully considered (given scar formation and altered vascular supply) as well as history of keloid and hypertrophic scarring.[63] For the medical tourism patient, in addition to the known risks associated with prolonged travel following a surgical procedure, preoperative testing and surgical planning are often less rigorously employed which in turn may increase the risk of postprocedural complications and poor outcomes.[38,64]

Abdominoplasty Complications

Abdominoplasty complications include infection, PE and DVT, hemorrhage, and seroma formation in addition to less acute and more commonly experienced complications of incisional dehiscence, wounds, and fat necrosis. Complication management includes the following:

- Consult with operative team
- Treat for hemodynamic instability
- Rule out thromboembolic and infectious processes
- Evaluate for hematoma, seroma, fluid collection
- Drain management (if present)
- Provide symptomatic relief of postoperative pain, nausea and vomiting

Seroma

Roughly 11% of abdominoplasty patients develop postsurgical seroma.[65] Alteration of surgical technique has been demonstrated to reduce seroma formation, while use of abdominal binders, compressive garments, and surgical drains have been shown to be inferior. Seromas are generally self-resolving, however, in some cases require percutaneous drainage or surgical treatment.

Recommended initial management in the ED includes the following[66]:

- Surgical drains present
  - Daily output <50 mL daily—continued care and outpatient follow-up
  - Persistent daily output >50 mL—placement of seroma catheter
- No surgical drains in place
  - Small, localized seroma
    - Consider bedside aspiration (preferred under ultrasound guidance given risk of bowel perforation)
    - Abdominal binder placement
    - Outpatient follow-up
  - Large diffuse seroma
    - Placement of seroma catheter via radiology consultation
    - May require excision of seroma cavity

Wound Formation

- Incisional dehiscence commonly occurs in areas of tension (Fig. 39.9).
- Consider performing a culture of the wound with bordering erythema or purulence.
- In the absence of infection or seroma formation, local wound care is advised.
  - Silver sulfadiazine for areas of eschar formation
  - Sharp debridement of devitalized tissue
  - Moist dressings/wound packing in areas of incisional dehiscence

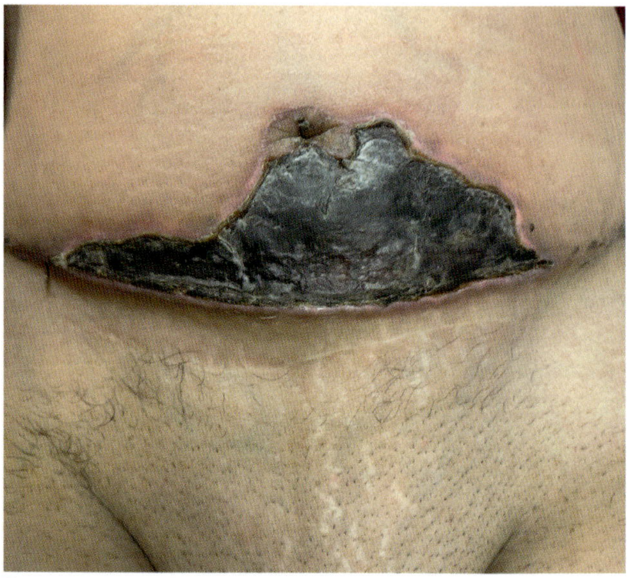

Fig. 39.9 Wound/eschar formation status post lower abdominal incision with distal well-healed surgical scar from prior surgery.

Liposuction

Liposuction is used for the removal of adipose tissue via various-sized blunt-tipped metal cannulas.[67] Small skin incisions are made as the entry points to access subcutaneous tissue. Be mindful that while this is performed through a 1-cm access incision, long metal cannulas are passed repeatedly (and relatively blindly) into the body, sometimes enhanced further by heat or ultrasound at the tip to intentionally dissolve surrounding tissues. In addition to the traditional suction-assisted liposuction, newer techniques such as power-assisted liposuction, ultrasound-assisted liposuction, and laser-assisted liposuction are used to varying degrees. To facilitate aspiration and hemostasis and, to some degree, provide postprocedural anesthesia, a wetting solution is infiltrated into the procedural area. There are several formulations ranging from "wet" to "tumescent," comprised of either normal saline (NS) or lactated Ringer's solution (LR) in differing combinations of lidocaine, epinephrine, and sodium bicarbonate. The tumescent technique incorporates a 3:1 ratio of infusion to the volume of aspirate[67] and has been demonstrated to prevent intravascular depletion (i.e., third space formation). Perioperative fluid management is critical, particularly when significant volumes are suctioned (>5 L of total aspirate).

Complications

Fatal thromboembolism is the most reported serious complication, followed by perforation of viscera, fat embolism, lidocaine toxicity, sepsis, and hemorrhage.[68] More commonly, patients may experience contour irregularities, pain, localized ecchymosis, and edema which generally resolve without issue. Liposuction complication management includes the following:

- Consult with operative team
- Treat for hemodynamic instability
- Rule out thromboembolic and infectious processes
- Evaluate for hematoma, seroma, fluid collection
- Manage drains (if present)

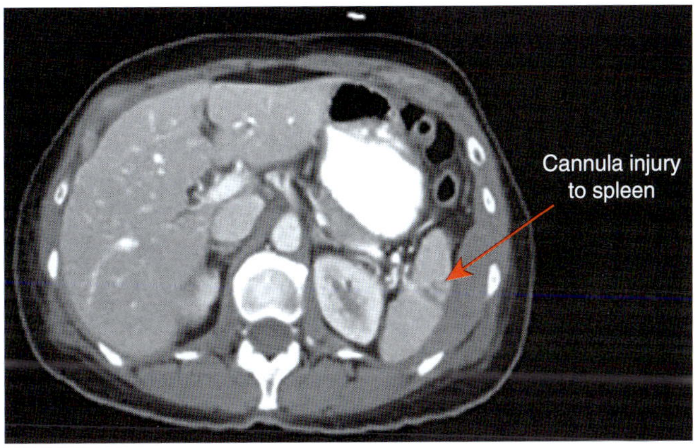

Fig. 39.10 Computed tomography image demonstrating splenic injury related to liposuction cannula.

- Provide symptomatic relief of postoperative pain, nausea and vomiting

Visceral Perforation

Perforation is the second leading cause of death after PE with a reported incidence of less than 0.1% (Fig. 39.10).[69] The literature suggests that the risks of visceral perforation are greater in patients with a rounded or distended abdominal shape, greater abdominal adiposity, presence of hernias, abdominal scars, and fibrotic adhesions following prior liposuction procedures.[69] The ileum is most frequently affected, followed by the large intestine, liver, spleen, vena cava, deep circumflex artery, pleura, and ureters.[69] Perforation injuries are often not detected during surgery.[70] Patient presentation may be subtle with "pain out of proportion to examination," with associated anorexia and absence of bowel movement or flatus.[70] Their examination may include abdominal distension/rigidity, reduced or absent bowel sounds, peritoneal signs, crepitus of surgical area, and/or change in drain color.

- Surgical consultation with the patient's surgical team is highly preferred.
- Abdominal plain film (upright) and/or abdominal CT with IV contrast may show free air.
- Strip drains (if present), as indicated.
- Obtain routine and preoperative laboratory studies.
- Obtain IV access.
- Initiate maintenance fluids.
- Document last oral intake and initiate NPO patient status.[71]

Local Anesthetic Systemic Toxicity

The recommended maximum safe dosing of lidocaine for infiltration is 4.5 mg/kg and 7 mg/kg with use of epinephrine. In contrast, Klein's research has long demonstrated the safety of higher doses with tumescent lidocaine anesthesia (TLA) during liposuction.[72] The American Academy of Dermatology guidelines outline maximum dosing of 55 mg/kg when used with epinephrine for use in TLA, given its slow rate of absorption, the vasoconstrictive effect of epinephrine, and the relative amount that is removed during the liposuction procedure.[73,74] Despite general acceptance that TLA poses low risk of local anesthetic systemic toxicity, it is important to understand the catastrophic effects of lidocaine toxicity, as it is widely used in both surgical and ED settings. Lidocaine toxicity is often experienced shortly after administration; however, during TLA, maximum serum concentrations have been reported upwards of 12 hours following use, which is both dose and patient specific.[75] Patients may present with subtle or profound CNS and cardiovascular (CVS) symptoms (Fig. 39.11).

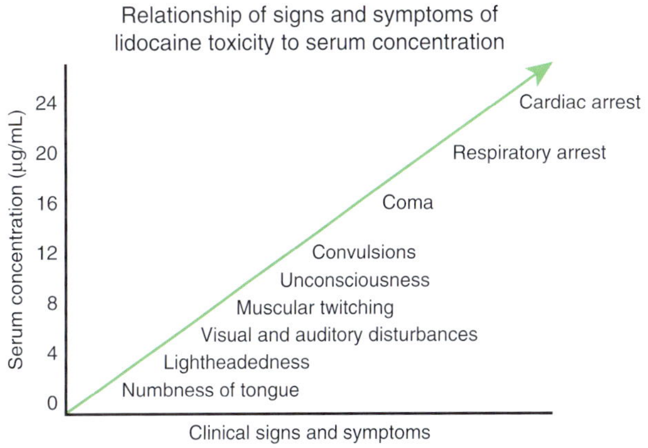

Fig. 39.11 Elevated serum concentrations of lidocaine and their relationship to adverse outcomes.

Skin Necrosis

In the absence of systemic injury, soft tissue necrosis may be managed with local wound care and routine outpatient follow-up (Fig. 39.12).

- If present, initiate treatment of associated secondary infection.
- Consider admission for predicted patient difficulty with self-managing care.
- Provide dressing supplies, wound care instructions, and precautions outlining the need for return to ED in the interim of planned clinic follow-up.

Autologous Fat Grafting

This procedure utilizes the transfer of one's own fat from one anatomic area into another. The intended result is correction of contour deformities and augmentation of an intended treatment

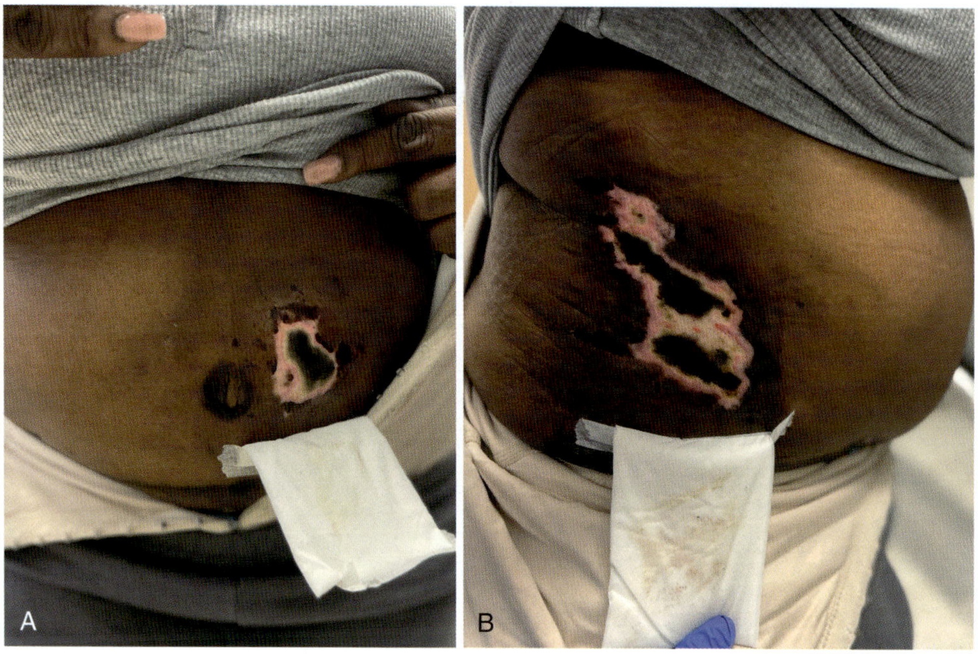

Fig. 39.12 Abdominal wounds status post large-volume liposuction procedure in medical tourism patient with history of prior abdominoplasty. Hospital admission from emergency department during initial presentation. Upon discharge, wounds managed with silver sulfadiazine, wound care dressings and outpatient follow-up, with near resolution following 6 months of local wound care. (A) Anterior abdominal wound wall view. (B) Lateral abdominal wall view.

site. This process is used commonly in facial rejuvenation (i.e., lips, cheeks), breast augmentation, and to the gluteal region.

The most common large-volume autologous fat grafting procedure, referred to as the "Brazilian butt lift" or "BBL," was first described in the 1980s. With a nearly 300% increase in BBLs being performed between 2011 and 2016, it is regarded as one of the fastest growing cosmetic procedures.[76,77] While advances in technique continue to improve patient safety and the longevity of the intended result, the BBL is regarded as the cosmetic procedure with the highest inherent risk, largely due to the development of both fatal and nonfatal fat embolism syndrome (FES).[78] In the absence of more accurate data, the procedure has an estimated mortality rate between 1 in 2350 to 1 in 6241 cases, which translates into roughly 20 times higher risk than other outpatient surgical procedures.[79–81] Within the Miami-metropolitan area alone, 25 patient deaths have been reported between 2010 and 2022, 92% of which occurred at high-volume, low-budget clinics.[82] In response to the rise of BBL-associated FES deaths, the Aesthetic Surgery and Education Research Foundation (ASERF) Task Force outlined several practice recommendations to reduce FES risks, most notably the avoidance of injecting into deep fascial planes, the use of cannula sizes smaller than 4 mm, and ensuring that injection of grafted material be pointed upwards (Fig. 39.13).[78,83]

FES is a potentially life-threatening condition characterized by circulatory obstruction via both mechanical and biochemical-mediated inflammatory processes resulting in end-organ injury. Nonfatal FES is relatively common following trauma, CPR, orthopedic surgery, and to a lesser extent with nontraumatic illness.[84–86] During the BBL procedure, injected fat may enter the circulation via transected gluteal vessels. Classically identified by the triad of respiratory, neurologic dysfunction, and development of petechiae to nondependent areas, it should be noted that hypoxia is the most commonly observed sign, followed by mental status changes, and skin manifestations (Fig. 39.14).[87]

FES diagnosis:

- The diagnosis of FES is largely based on clinical presentation, with a high index of suspicion in a patient status post recent gluteal fat grafting procedure.
- The Gurd criteria is a diagnostic tool requiring at least one of the major criteria and at least four of the minor criteria be present.[87]
  - Major criteria
    - Altered mental status
    - Hypoxia
    - Petechia (conjunctival/nondependent body surfaces)
  - Minor criteria
    - Fever
    - Tachycardia
    - Retinal emboli
    - Unexplained anemia
    - Thrombocytopenia
    - Fat macroglobulinemia
    - Decreased renal function (anuria or oliguria)
    - Elevated erythrocyte sedimentation rate (ESR)
- Routine laboratory studies, arterial blood gases, and CT scan can aid in the diagnosis.
- Management for FES is largely supportive care.[88]

Surgical Drains

As in the case of medical tourism, the patient is often left confused about how to manage their surgical drains. All too often, they turn to the ED for drain management and/or removal (Table 39.2). Closed suction drains are commonly

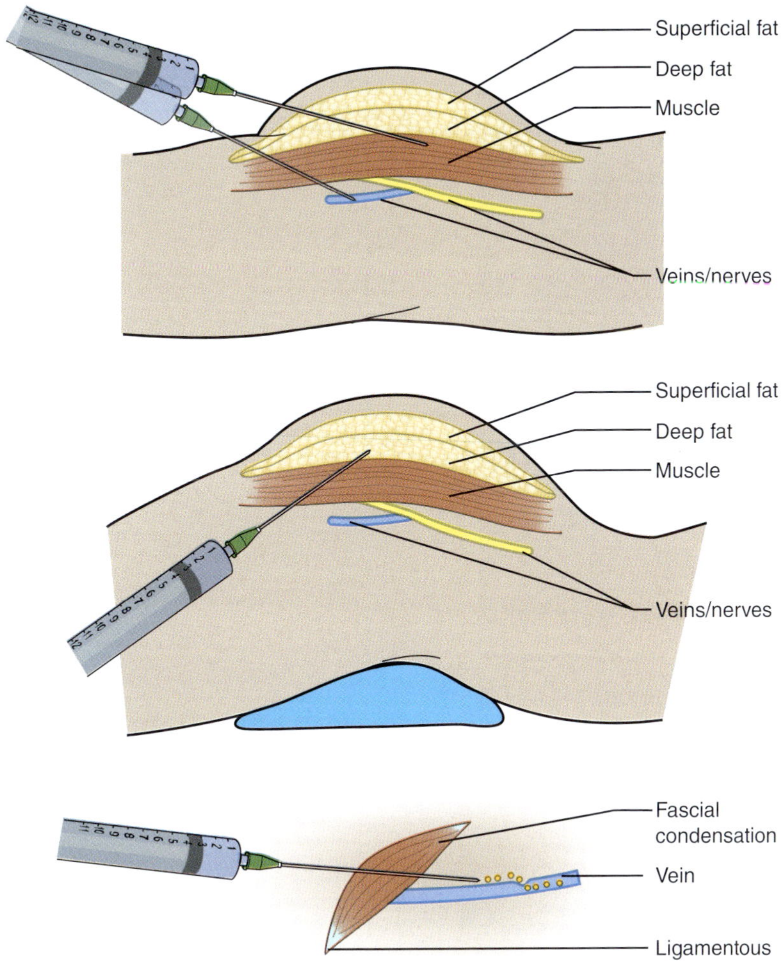

Fig. 39.13 Demonstration of suboptimal gluteal fat grafting technique and introduction of fat emboli into the circulation. (Adapted from Ghavami A, Villanueve NL. Gluteal augmentation and contouring with autologous fat transfer: part I. *Clin Plast Surg*. 2018;45(2):249-259.)

used to collect and remove fluid and assist with closure of surgical dead space (Fig. 39.15). Most surgeons utilize specific volume criteria when determining the optimal time for removal with the relative consensus being 30 mL or less in a 24-hour period.[89] However, studies demonstrate that longer drain duration increases the risk for infection in the surgical site. One retrospective cohort study found that the rate of infection escalates by 76.2% with each additional week of drain dwelling noting that a drain duration over 21 days is significantly more likely to cause infection.[89]

Stripping of Surgical Drains

Required materials include examination gloves, alcohol preparation pad, and a container for drain fluid (if present) (Video 39.1).

1. If the drain is full, release the bulb or reservoir suction (remove the cap from the drainage bulb).
2. Empty fluid into sample container or other vessel to facilitate later appropriate disposal.
3. Squeeze the bulb centrally and recap the collection bulb (to facilitate suction).
4. Place nondominant hand at the drain insertion site to hold the tube stable and avoid pulling the drain out while stripping.
5. With alcohol pad between the dominant hand thumb and index finger (to reduce friction), gently pinch the drainage tube just distal to the nondominant hand.
6. While continuing to pinch the drain, slide the dominant hand along the drainage tube toward the collection bulb (while holding the drain at the insertion site with the nondominant hand).
7. Repeat as necessary to remove fluid or clot material from the tubing.
8. Uncap and squeeze the collection bulb to expel air if necessary.
9. Squeeze the bulb centrally again, and replace the stopper cap onto the collection bulb.
10. Ensure the drain maintains suction.

Removal of Surgical Drains

Required materials include examination gloves, 4 × 4 gauze/drain sponge, tape, suture scissors/scalpel, and disposal receptacle.

1. Remove all dressings carefully.

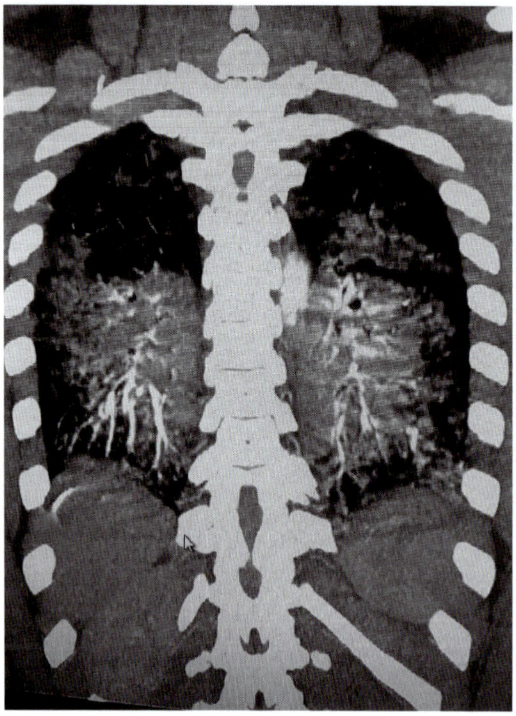

Fig. 39.14 Computed tomography scan image demonstrating embolic burden upon emergency department presentation status post "Brazilian butt lift" procedure.[88]

2. Inspect the entry point of the tubing into the body. If the drain has been sewn in, cut the suture and be sure that the entire suture has been removed from the body.
3. Release the suction from the bulb or reservoir (remove the cap from the drainage bulb).
4. Gently place a 4 × 4 gauze at the entry point of the tubing into the body using nondominant hand. Applying a small amount of counter pressure to the skin will decrease the discomfort for the patient as well as catch additional drainage that may escape during drain removal.
5. Slowly and steadily pull the drain out with the dominant hand while applying counter pressure to the entry site with the nondominant hand. If resistance is met, pause and have the patient take a deep breath and exhale. Sometimes the relaxation of the muscles is all that is needed to reduce the resistance on the drain tubing.
6. Exercise caution if the drain does not appear to budge at all—even with a gentle tug. Drains that have inadvertently been sewn into the deeper closure will require surgical intervention for removal.
7. As the drain is removed, expect some immediate serous drainage and possible fibrinous strands. The drainage should be brief, and the fibrinous material can be gently extracted from the drain site.
8. Clean the drain site with antiseptic solution and apply antibiotic ointment, gauze, and tape. Inform the patient that this area will likely drain for several days and that the dressing should be changed daily until well healed.

TABLE 39.2 Problem-Focused Drain Management

PROBLEM	SOLUTION
Drain is not holding suction	Ensure the drain stopper is securely in place and the bulb is completely compressed. On the drain tubing, the black dot is located 2 inches from the fenestrations of the drain. The surgeon intentionally places the black dot at the skin edge. If the black dot is several inches away from the drain site or the fenestrations of the drain are visible outside the skin, it is safe to remove the drain as it is not likely functioning. Do not attempt a reinsertion.
Drain is partially or fully removed	Do not attempt to replace. Place dressing over the drain insertion site. Consider imaging if there is concern for seroma/hematoma/other fluid collection.
Drain site pain or erythema	Insertion site pain is common. Often this can happen if the drain is not secure or is a bit too mobile. Secure drain with tape or clear dressing. If there is concern for cellulitis bordering the drain site, in absence of systemic illness, consider treatment for soft tissue infection.
Drain site is leaking fluid	Drain may be clogged, causing build up. Stripping repeatedly may help unclog the drain and may facilitate the passage of clot material. If not, you may reinforce the dressing around the drain until definitive management plan has been established.
Drain output diminished or absent	Examine the surgical site for swelling/erythema. Check for drain function (see above). Check drain color—clear straw-colored fluid is normal. Review the drain output trends over the last few days. If the output has consistently decreased, this is reassuring. If the drain output is less than 20 mL/day over the last couple of days and they have no local care established, it is safe to remove.
Drain bulb contains "clots" or solid material	The closer that the patient is after surgery, the more likely there will be clots, tissue, other sediment. Remind the patient to strip the drain 2 to 3 times a day until the fluid becomes clearer.

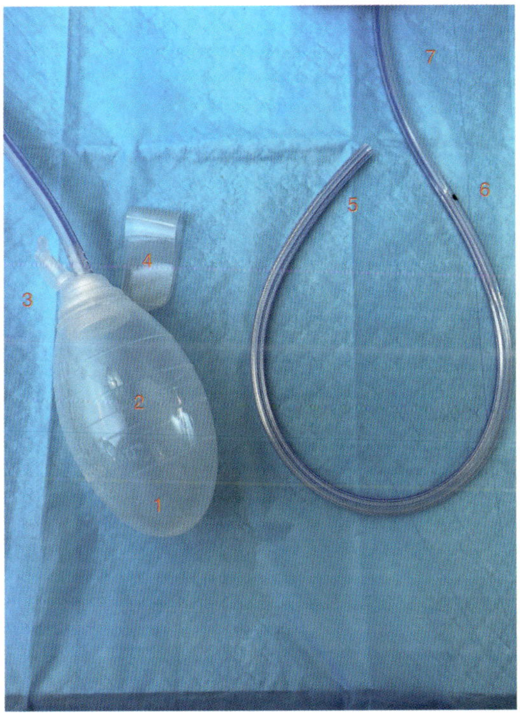

Fig. 39.15 Components of a surgical drain as numbered on the photograph. *1*, Collection bulb; *2*, volume indicator; *3*, drainage port and stopper cap; *4*, attachment tab for securing to patient clothing; *5*, fenestrated drainage tubing; *6*, black dot indicator, which demonstrates transition from solid drainage tubing to fenestrated drainage tubing; *7*, solid drainage tubing.

CONCLUSION

Although regarded as generally safe, cosmetic procedures are not without risk. While the overall complication rate for some cosmetic procedures is less than 1%, as discussed in this chapter, serious morbidities can occur and should be included in your clinical decision-making process.[90] Due to their general healthy state, cosmetic procedure patients may be able to mask major complications longer, so a sharpened sense of awareness is essential in identifying and treating emergent problems particularly given the often deceptively noninvasive nature of aesthetic surgery. As demand for these services continues to expand, increased incidence of associated complications should in turn be predicted. ED care for these patients should remain focused on treating critical illness with the understanding that issues related to cosmesis, pain, and local wound care can often be managed safely in the outpatient setting.

REFERENCES ARE AVAILABLE AT Elsevier eBooks+

SECTION VII

Gastrointestinal Procedures

CHAPTER 40

Esophageal Foreign Bodies

Michael Joseph Bono

Patients with foreign bodies (FBs) lodged in the esophagus commonly present to the emergency department (ED) for evaluation and treatment. Though most are accidental, FBs may sometimes be swallowed purposefully. Patients may have a sensation of a recently passed FB, minor irritation, life-threatening airway obstruction, or other significant complications. Because of the anatomic and physiologic features of the esophagus, FBs in this area of the gastrointestinal (GI) tract can present unique clinical challenges to the clinician.

GENERAL FEATURES

Anatomy

The esophagus is a muscular tube 20 cm to 25 cm in length extending from the hypopharynx to the stomach. The upper third of the esophagus is striated skeletal muscle, and the remainder is smooth muscle. There are three anatomic areas of narrowing where FBs are most commonly entrapped: in the upper esophageal sphincter, which consists of the cricopharyngeus muscle; in the midesophagus at the crossover of the aortic arch; and in the lower esophageal sphincter (LES) (Fig. 40.1). The LES is the narrowest point of the esophagus and the entire GI tract.

Epidemiology

There are almost 100,000 cases of FB ingestions reported annually in the United States, and they are the eighth most common cause of calls to poison control centers.[1] Patients with retained esophageal FBs generally fall into one of the following categories: pediatric patients, psychiatric patients, prisoners, and adults who either are edentulous or have underlying esophageal pathology.

Children account for 75% to 85% of esophageal FBs seen in the ED, with the peak incidence occurring between the ages of 18 and 48 months.[1–3] The incidence is similar in boys and girls. Inquisitive children frequently place objects in their mouths and unintentionally swallow them. Children most commonly ingest coins, but they also swallow buttons, marbles, beads, screws, and pins.[2–5] In contrast to adults, children who have entrapped, accidentally swallowed FBs do not normally have underlying esophageal disorders. However, this is not the case in children with esophageal meat or food impaction, and these patients will need further evaluation for underlying esophageal disease,[6–8] the most common of which is eosinophilic esophagitis (55%), or stricture (27%).[9]

Patients with an anatomic abnormality of the esophagus or a motor disturbance are more prone to FB entrapment.[10,11] Anatomic abnormalities include strictures, webs, rings, diverticula, and malignancies. Motor disturbances include achalasia, scleroderma, and esophageal spasm. Adults who have dentures or underlying esophageal anatomic or motor abnormalities may accidentally ingest food boluses, chicken bones, fish bones, glass, toothpicks, fruit pits, or pills when eating.

Prisoners and psychiatric patients ingest a wide variety of objects, some of which may be quite unusual including spoons, razor blades, pins, nails, or practically any other object.[11,12] Patients who intentionally ingest foreign objects frequently ingest more than one, with an average between 4 and 5 (Video 40.1).[12]

Complications

Impacted FBs of the esophagus must be removed or dislodged. The time frame under which this must be carried out varies widely and depends on many circumstances. In general, however, the esophagus does not tolerate FBs well or for prolonged periods because it is prone to edema, pressure necrosis, infection, and eventually perforation. FBs can travel through the esophagus in a matter of seconds or may adhere to the mucosa. Retained objects may become less symptomatic after time, and the clinician must resist the urge to allow esophageal FBs to "pass by themselves" or "dissolve." Once FBs become stuck in the mucosa, they may become less symptomatic, but they rarely pass on their own. The one exception may be children with coins or other smooth round FBs such as small marbles, especially those lodged at the LES. Approximately one-third of these objects may pass spontaneously within 24 hours, and some authorities have advocated an observational approach, although this may be more poorly accepted by parents.[5] Button batteries must be immediately removed because of the risk of rapid esophageal erosion and perforation.

The literature is replete every year with a wide array of case reports and small reports of series of complications that can arise from retained esophageal FBs (Box 40.1), including benign mucosal abrasions, lacerations, esophageal stricture, and necrosis from corrosive agents such as button batteries. Esophageal perforation[13–15] can lead to life-threatening conditions such as retropharyngeal abscess,[16]

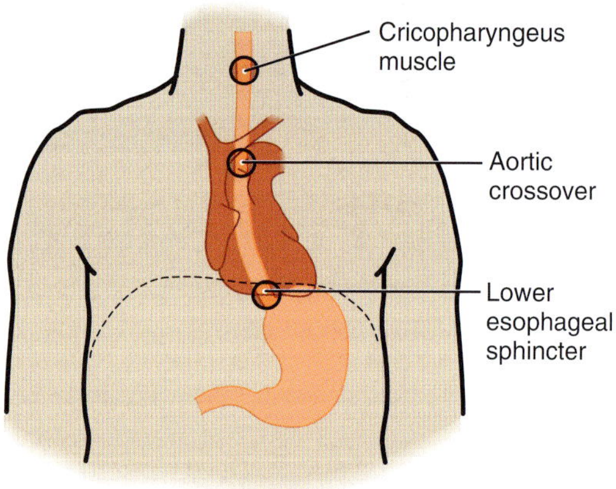

Fig. 40.1 Blunt esophageal foreign bodies are most commonly lodged at one of three anatomic areas of narrowing: the cricopharyngeus muscle, the level of the aortic crossover, and the lower esophageal sphincter.

TABLE 40.1 Level of Entrapment of Esophageal FBs

LEVEL	PEDIATRIC (%)	ADULT (%)
Cricopharyngeus muscle	74	24
Aortic crossover	14	8
Lower esophageal sphincter	12	68

FB, Foreign body.

BOX 40.1 Complications of Esophageal FBs

Airway compromise secondary to tracheal compression
Aspiration pneumonia
Esophageal necrosis
Esophageal perforation
Esophageal stricture
Failure to thrive
Mediastinitis
Mucosal abrasion
Paraesophageal abscess
Pericardial tamponade
Pericarditis
Pneumothorax
Pneumomediastinum
Retropharyngeal abscess
Tracheoesophageal fistula
Vascular injury, including aortic perforation
Vocal cord paralysis

FB, *Foreign body.*

mediastinitis, pericarditis, pericardial tamponade,[17] pneumothorax, pneumomediastinum, tracheoesophageal fistula, and vascular injuries, including injuries to the subclavian vein and aorta.[18] Complications are more common when FBs are entrapped for longer than 24 hours[13] and when they are sharp.[2,14,15]

Clinical Findings

Esophageal FB impaction is usually an acute condition, particularly in adults who have a clear history of ingestion. Children often remember an ingestion, but some will have a vague history or symptoms. As many as one-third of children with proven esophageal FBs are asymptomatic on initial evaluation[2–8]; therefore a high index of suspicion is indicated, especially in children who were seen with an object in their mouth that subsequently cannot be found. This is particularly true if transient coughing or gagging occurred, even though the actual ingestion was not witnessed. Poor feeding, irritability, fever, stridor, cough, wheezing, and aspiration can all be caused by an esophageal FB in a child, especially a young infant.[2–8]

Dysphagia is a common initial complaint with esophageal FBs. Drooling is suggestive of high-grade obstruction, and inability to handle oral secretions is a sign of a complete obstruction. Infants with a clandestine esophageal FB can exhibit wheezing or a chronic cough. They may appear to have bronchospasm and may be treated for asthma by a number of clinicians before an FB is suspected. Stridor from an FB can mimic epiglottitis.

The esophagus is well innervated proximally, and patients can typically accurately localize FBs in the oropharynx or upper third of the esophagus. However, scratches or abrasions of the esophagus can create a persistent FB sensation. Upper esophageal FBs may cause gagging or vomiting. In rare cases, an upper esophageal FB can impinge on the trachea, especially in children, and mimic infection by inducing wheezing, stridor, or frank respiratory distress. The lower two-thirds of the esophagus is not as well innervated, and FBs in this location typically cause vague symptoms of discomfort, fullness, or nonlocalizing pain. Swallowed coins that lodge in the lower part of the esophagus in children may cause no overt symptoms until feeding is attempted.

The location of retained esophageal FBs is related to age and areas of physiologic narrowing of the esophagus (Table 40.1). Children more typically have objects entrapped in the upper part of the esophagus at the level of the cricopharyngeus muscle, whereas adults more commonly have entrapment at the LES.[2–8]

Evaluation

The most useful aspect of the evaluation is often the history. The time of the ingestion, size and shape of the ingested object, and any current symptoms should be ascertained. Findings on physical examination are frequently normal in patients with esophageal FBs, unless complete obstruction is present. Patients with complete obstruction will often be drooling, spitting, and unable to handle oral secretions. Even though a patient may be asymptomatic at the initial encounter, transient coughing or gagging should raise the index of suspicion for an esophageal FB. Examination of the oropharynx, neck, respiratory system, cardiac system, and abdomen is important in the evaluation of potential complications.

After treating life-threatening conditions such as airway compromise, the goal of ED evaluation is to localize the FB to determine what, if any, interventions need to be undertaken to remove it or assist its transit into the stomach. Once an FB passes into the stomach, it has a greater than 90% likelihood of passing through the entire GI tract without complications.[19,20]

Even irregular and seemingly dangerous FBs will often transit the entire GI tract with relative ease.

RADIOLOGY OF ESOPHAGEAL FOREIGN BODIES

Background

Radiographic imaging of a patient with a suspected esophageal FB is a common practice and is particularly useful for detecting radiopaque FBs. Traditionally, an inability to quickly identify the object by physical examination encouraged the use of plain radiography in an attempt to verify and localize the retained FB. However, the limitations of plain radiography require that other diagnostic approaches also be considered.

Indications

Many patients with a suspected esophageal FB warrant radiographic evaluation with few exceptions, including those patients who have an obvious complete obstruction with an inability to manage their secretions. These patients need endoscopy to relieve the obstruction. If there is any question of aspiration, a chest radiograph may be indicated. Patients with a history of sharp, nonradiopaque FBs such as toothpicks will also need urgent endoscopy. If there has been a delay in presentation in the case of a sharp FB and there are any signs of infection such as fever or chest pain, computed tomography (CT) may be indicated to evaluate for perforation or mediastinitis. Those patients with an FB sensation that is visualized in the upper pharynx on examination and removed may forego radiographs. In nonverbal patients, including preschool children and those with cognitive disabilities, maintain a low threshold for screening radiography in cases with a suspicious history. Examples include a child seen with an object in the mouth that "disappeared" or a patient with symptomatology suggestive of an esophageal FB, such as drooling, gagging, or unexplained respiratory symptoms.

Plain Radiographs

Plain radiographs reliably verify and localize radiopaque FBs such as glass and metal of sufficient size, and are the main method of radiologic evaluation for these objects.

A complete oropharyngeal radiographic series includes the nasopharynx to the lower cervical vertebra in both lateral and anteroposterior views. Patients should be positioned upright with the neck extended and the shoulders held low. Use of a soft tissue technique enhances the discrimination of weak radiopaque FBs. Phonation of "eeeee" during radiography prevents motion artifact from swallowing, distends the hypopharynx, and enhances soft tissue landmarks. As previously mentioned, FBs are most frequently entrapped at one of three locations of physiologic narrowing in the esophagus: the cricopharyngeus muscle (Fig. 40.2), the aortic crossover (Fig. 40.3), and the LES (Fig. 40.4). Objects that become lodged in the middle portion of the esophagus most likely represent esophageal pathology, such as stricture related to tumor or eosinophilic esophagitis.[10]

Posteroanterior (PA) and lateral views of the chest are used to evaluate the remainder of the esophagus. Both projections are indicated to identify multiple objects and FBs visible in only one plane. Esophageal FBs typically lie in the vertical plane and are differentiated from airway bodies or calcifications by their location posterior to the tracheal air column on lateral radiographs. As a rule, flat objects such as coins perch in the coronal plane in the esophagus and in the sagittal orientation in the trachea. Intraesophageal air and air-fluid levels represent indirect evidence of esophageal obstruction, and may

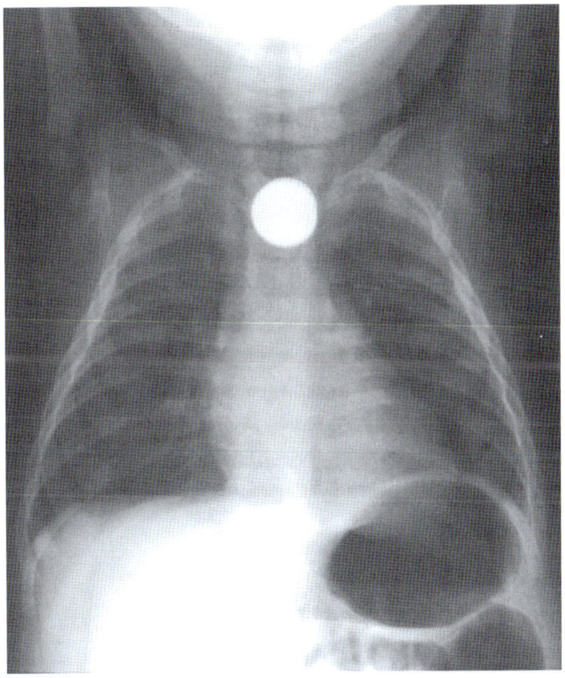

Fig. 40.2 Posteroanterior radiograph of an esophageal foreign body (coin) lodged at the level of the cricopharyngeus muscle. This is the most common area of the esophagus to harbor a coin in children. Coins remaining in the upper tract are usually removed unless there is a steady progression with observation. This coin would probably be symptomatic in an infant and cause respiratory distress, drooling, wheezing, and possibly stridor. The chance of spontaneous passage is approximately 20% to 25%.

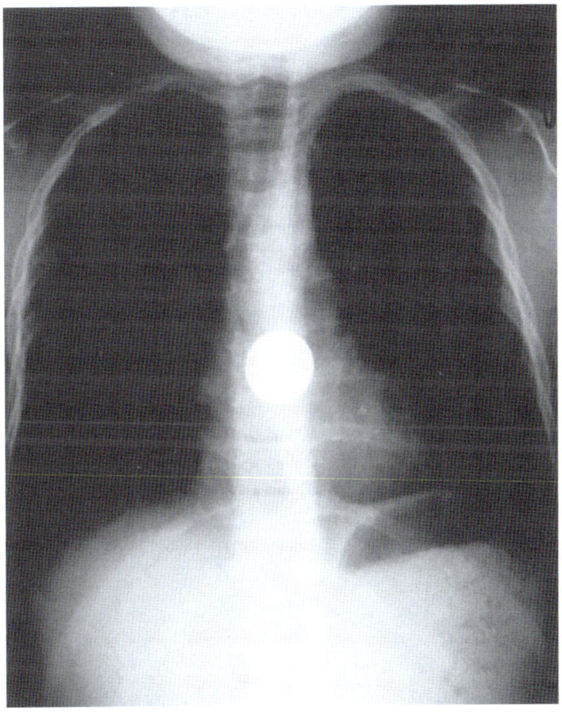

Fig. 40.3 Posteroanterior radiograph of an esophageal foreign body (coin) lodged at the level of the aortic crossover. The chance of spontaneous passage is approximately 20% to 25%.

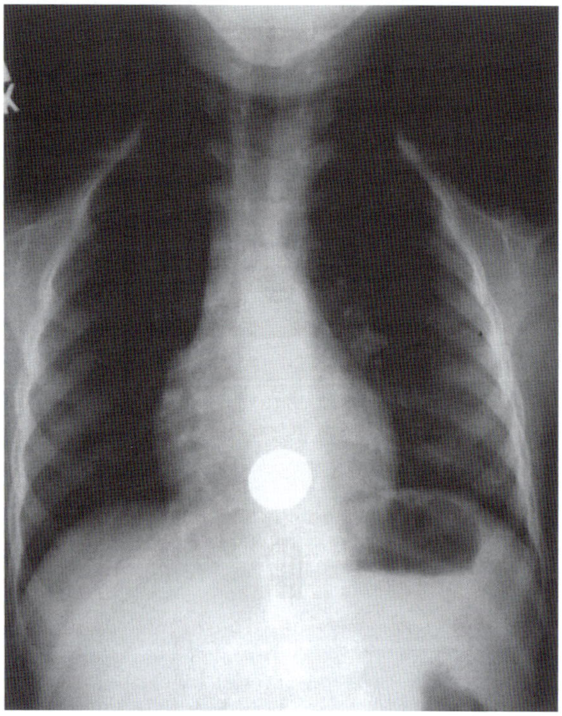

Fig. 40.4 Posteroanterior radiograph of an esophageal foreign body (coin) lodged at the level of the lower esophageal sphincter. Coins in this area are most likely to pass and be favorably manipulated by medication (see Table 40.2). The chance of spontaneous passage is approximately 25% to 60%; chances increase with prolonged observation. (From Waltzman ML, Baskin M, Wypij D et al. A randomized clinical trial of the management of esophageal coins in children. *Pediatrics* 2005;116:614; Soprano JV, Fleisher GR, Mandl KD. The spontaneous passage of esophageal coins in children. *Arch Pediatr Adolesc Med.* 1999;153:1073.)

aid in the verification of radiopaque FBs. Soft tissue swelling, extraluminal air, and aspiration pneumonitis can occasionally help identify complicated impactions radiographically.

In children, a film from the nasopharynx to the anus is frequently obtained to allow visualization of the entire nasopharynx, throat, and esophagus, in addition to the abdomen in case the FB has passed into the stomach or beyond. Radiation exposure can be minimized if adult-sized radiograph cassettes are used. Swallowed coins or other FBs may become lodged in the nasopharynx, usually after gagging or vomiting, and could be missed if this area is not included on the radiograph. In adults, if neck or chest films are negative, abdominal films are sometimes obtained for reassurance of the presence of the FB in the stomach.

Unfortunately, many ingested FBs are nonopaque, including nonbony food, plastic, wood, and aluminum. The visibility of low-opacity FBs can be improved using low-dose radiography, especially in neck films.[21,22] Some pull tabs from beer cans may be seen if oriented in the coronal plane. A metal detector has been reported to help localize radiolucent aluminum pull tabs.[23] Calcification of fish and chicken bones is often incomplete, but cooking alters the structure of bones and can make them radiolucent on plain films. The degree of bony calcification varies with the fish species and between different samples of the same species, thus preventing useful guidelines.[24,25] For these reasons, plain films generally provide little substantive evidence in the majority of cases of fish or chicken bone dysphagia. Plain radiographs detect only 25% to 55% of endoscopically proven bones, and carry a high rate of false-negative and false-positive interpretations.[22–25] Because of the lack of diagnostic value for detecting bones, many clinicians do not routinely order plain radiographs and instead initially opt for CT in cases in which radiographic evaluation is required.[22,24,26]

Plain radiography of the neck is limited by the radiographic properties of ingested materials and the complicated anatomy of the upper aerodigestive tract. The base of the tongue, palatine and lingual tonsils, vallecula, and piriform recesses are common regions for entrapment of small, sharp objects, and deserve careful interpretive attention (Fig. 40.5). Superimposition of the mandible contributes to suboptimal resolution of this region on lateral neck films. Calcified airway cartilage can masquerade as FBs and contributes to false-positive rates as high as 25%.[26] Normal ossification of airway cartilage begins in the third decade and progresses with age. The typical curvilinear contour and well-defined margins of bony FB fragments may help distinguish them from normal laryngeal calcifications. The orientation of bony FBs is variable. The C6 vertebra approximates the level of the cricopharyngeus, a common site of FB impaction. Increased prevertebral soft tissue width, air within the cervical esophagus, and soft tissue emphysema are rare indirect findings that may help identify radiolucent objects.[26]

Computed Tomography

See Video 40.2. CT of the neck and mediastinum is an easy, rapid, cost-effective, and accurate noninvasive means of detecting or excluding esophageal FBs (Fig. 40.6)[22,26] and has gained support in the setting of suspected FB entrapment.[22,26] CT further excels at localization and characterization of the impacted FB and identification of associated complications, such as perforation.[13,22,26] CT has a sensitivity and accuracy of 97% and 98%, respectively, for the diagnosis of esophageal FBs compared with a sensitivity and accuracy of 47% and 52%, respectively, for plain films.[22] CT provides improved diagnostic utility for fish bone FBs over plain radiography when obtained either with or without barium enhancement.[24,25] The sensitivity of CT can be improved with 3D reformations. These allow better visualization of the FB and any esophageal injury.[22] Use of CT in patients in whom clinical suspicion for a retained FB is high has the potential to reduce the number of unnecessary endoscopies.[26]

The use of intravenous (IV) contrast with CT is not indicated, unless there is concern for an inflammatory process (abscess, peritonitis, fistula formation), or vascular injury (aortic or caval perforation). Use of oral contrast with CT in the setting of suspected FB remains controversial.[22,27] If used, it can impair visualization on endoscopy. Use of oral contrast is generally reserved for those rare cases where either esophageal perforation is suspected (water-soluble media should be used), or a nonradiopaque FB is suspected and the radiologist wants a small amount of contrast to "outline" the potential FB.[22]

Contrast-Enhanced Esophagograms

Background

A contrast-enhanced esophagogram is a test that is almost never indicated in the ED as a routine intervention to evaluate

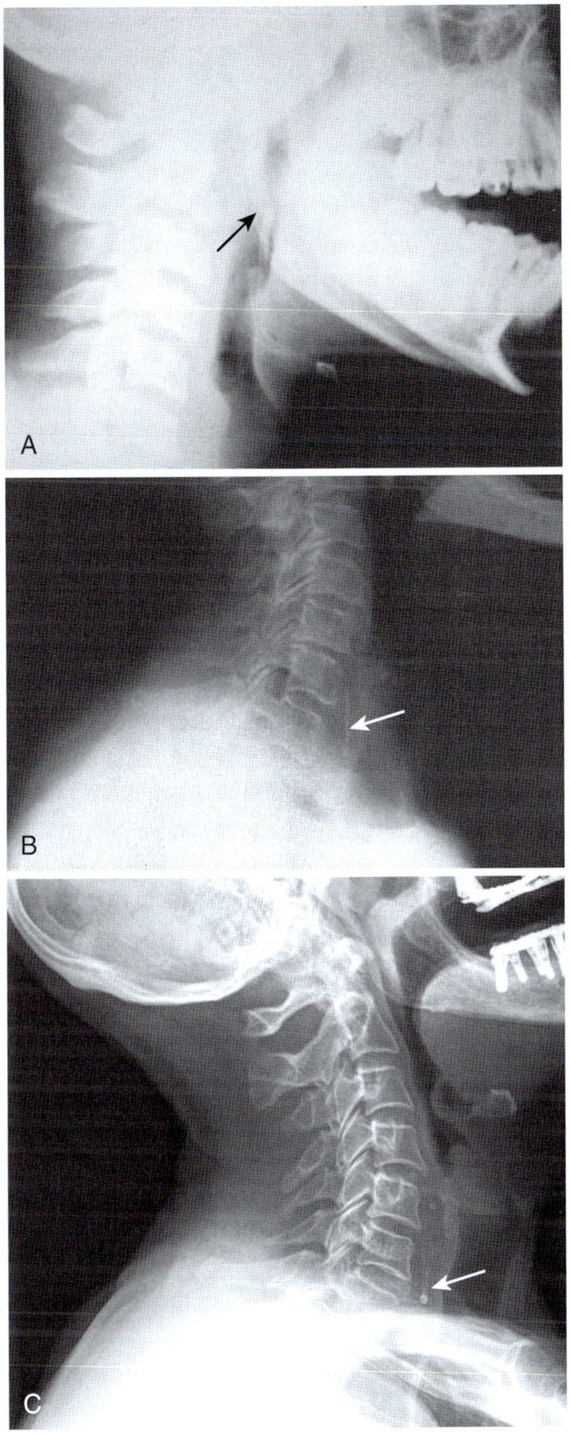

Fig. 40.5 (A) Lateral neck radiograph showing a chicken bone *(arrow)* lodged in the pharynx with associated soft tissue swelling. Plain radiographs have poor diagnostic accuracy for detecting bones in the esophagus, and they are often eschewed in favor of a computed tomography scan if radiographic evaluation is deemed necessary. (B) A chicken bone in the proximal end of the esophagus *(arrow)*, where it is more readily seen on a radiograph. (C) Another example of a chicken bone in the proximal end of the esophagus *(arrow)*.

for an esophageal FB. It has largely been replaced by CT and endoscopy for evaluation of FBs. This technique uses swallowed contrast material to help identify the presence and location of an impacted radiolucent FB, the degree of obstruction, any underlying anatomic abnormalities, and the presence of perforation. Contrast material (barium) may interfere with the detection and extraction of FBs at endoscopy, and may increase the risk for aspiration pneumonitis. Therefore routine, serial contrast-enhanced esophagograms after negative plain radiography in patients with known or suspected FBs are unnecessary for diagnostic purposes in most cases. Selective use is reasonable, but CT or endoscopy are interventions with a higher and more cost-effective yield. The American Society for Gastrointestinal Endoscopy guidelines suggest "avoiding contrast radiographic examinations" before endoscopic removal.[13]

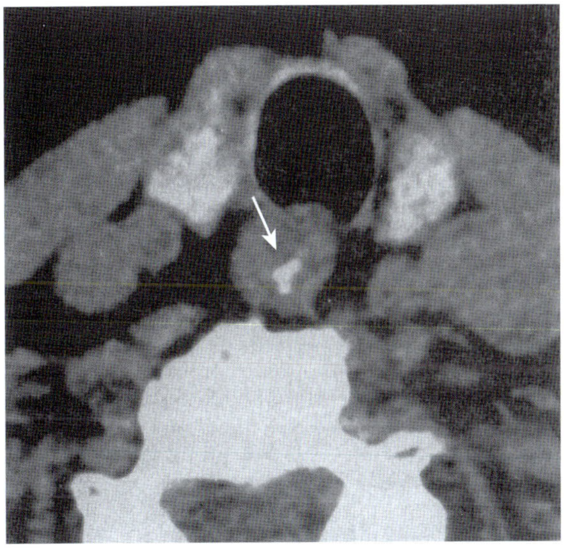

Fig. 40.6 Computed tomography scan demonstrating an esophageal foreign body.

The rare indication in the ED would be a questionable FB or perforation where the radiologist or consultant requests the procedure to "outline" a possible FB to better visualize it, or to evaluate for leakage of contrast material.

Procedure

Esophagograms couple voluntary ingestion of an enteric contrast agent (Gastrografin or barium) and plain radiography. Immediately after ingestion, erect and horizontal radiographs are performed at right-angle projections (PA and lateral, or right and left anterior oblique). In addition to anatomic abnormalities, radiolucent FBs may be identified by contrast delineation or filling defects within the contrast column (Fig. 40.7).

The initial choice of contrast agent is debated and should be individualized according to the threat of aspiration and perforation. Water-soluble Gastrografin is indicated first in most cases of suspected perforation because it causes less mediastinal inflammation if extravasation; however, it can give rise to severe chemical pneumonitis if aspirated, and is relatively contraindicated in patients with complete esophageal obstruction. Patients without evidence of complete esophageal obstruction are instructed to swallow progressively larger aliquots of contrast agent up to approximately 50 mL. If these films are normal, the procedure is repeated with half-strength and then full-strength barium to delineate small esophageal injuries. Note that water-soluble contrast material (Gastrografin) causes more pulmonary reaction than barium does when inadvertently aspirated, and should be used in small aliquots if aspiration or complete esophageal obstruction is a concern.

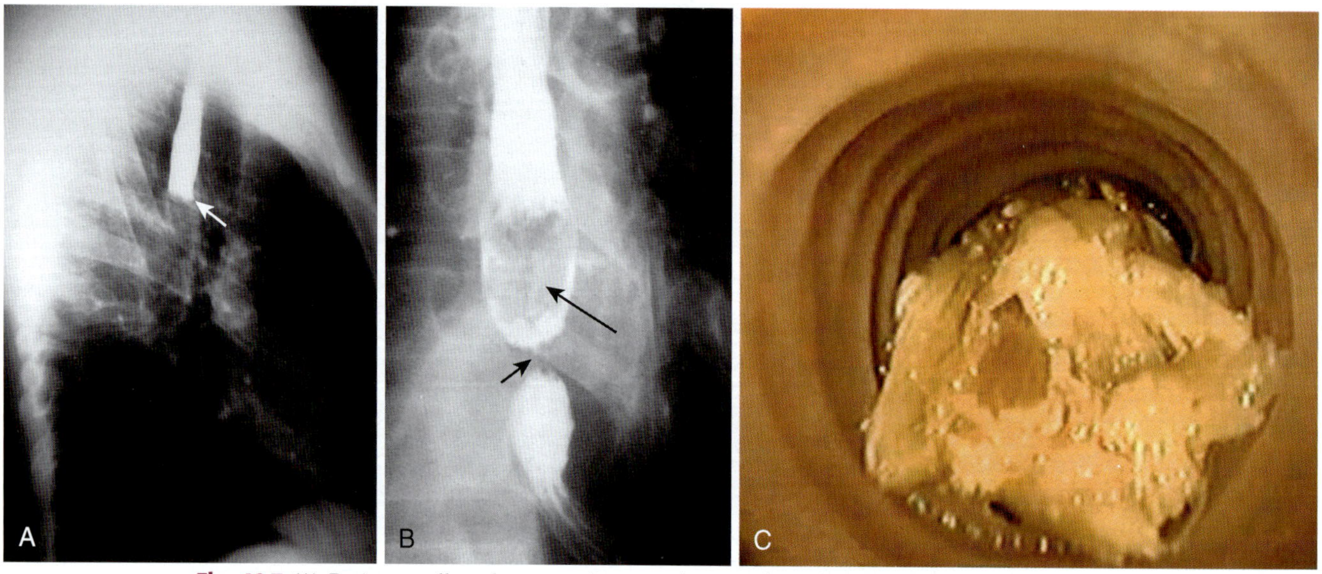

Fig. 40.7 (A) Barium swallow demonstrating complete esophageal obstruction in the proximal to midportion of the esophagus *(arrow)*. (B) Barium esophagogram demonstrating a large piece of meat *(long arrow)* lodged above an esophageal stricture *(short arrow)*. Many patients with lodged meat have underlying esophageal pathology. (C) A bolus of meat seen in the distal end of the esophagus with an endoscope. The scope provides a means for removal and esophageal evaluation simultaneously. This young person had a ringed esophagus as his pathology.

Follow-up Radiographs

Often FBs are visualized in the stomach, or procedures performed in the ED (described later) result in the FB moving into the stomach. A variety of organizations have proposed recommendations for how to manage FBs in the stomach and intestines (Table 40.2).

Conclusions

Diagnostic radiography for esophageal FBs is indicated in many cases with the exception of those with a complete obstruction where there is no concern for aspiration. Plain radiographs clearly assist the clinician in several situations: (1) screening of children, adults with dementia, and nonverbal patients with a history or symptoms suspicious for purposeful or inadvertent FB ingestion that can be assumed to be radiopaque; and (2) localization of known radiopaque FBs to clarify the necessity for and means of FB extraction. Conversely, attempts to verify radiolucent FBs, including bones, by plain radiography are often misleading. CT is more accurate and sensitive than plain films in diagnosing FBs, and in most cases, contrast is not needed.

VISUALIZATION OF ESOPHAGEAL AND PHARYNGEAL FOREIGN BODIES

Patients with an FB sensation in their oropharynx typified by a "stuck fish bone" or "chicken bone" sensation need to have some form of visualization of their oropharynx performed as part of the physical examination. The three procedures are direct pharyngoscopy, which is simply direct visualization or examination using a tongue blade with a light source that may be a pen light, wall light, or head light; indirect laryngoscopy, which involves using a handheld mirror reflecting a light to allow visualization of the epiglottis, vallecula, arytenoids, arytenoids folds, and vocal cords (a procedure that requires experience and a cooperative patient); or nasopharyngoscopy, a procedure using a flexible nasopharyngoscope. If an FB is visualized (Fig. 40.8), it should be removed with forceps and the oropharynx carefully reexamined for any injury or additional FB.

ESOPHAGOSCOPY

See Video 40.3. Esophagoscopy is the definitive diagnostic and therapeutic procedure for impacted esophageal FBs.[5,7,13] Although esophagoscopy is not a procedure performed by the emergency provider, its proper role in the ED evaluation of FBs should be understood. With esophagoscopy, the presence and location of the FB along with any underlying lesion can be documented. The clinician can then remove the object and reevaluate the esophagus after removal of the FB to rule out perforation or underlying pathology. Esophagoscopy may be necessary even if a radiologic contrast-enhanced study does not reveal complete obstruction because radiologic studies are not always conclusive.[13,20,26] Esophagoscopy may be necessary to exclude predisposing pathology or resultant perforation, even when symptoms presumed to be caused by an esophageal FB have resolved.

Esophagoscopy is the preferred method for removal of sharp or pointed objects such as bones, open safety pins, and razors. In the case of sharp objects prone to causing esophageal perforation, IV antibiotics should be administered before the procedure. Endoscopy is the preferred way to remove an impacted meat bolus and to evaluate for possible esophageal pathology at the same time. Esophagoscopy is also indicated for a FB retained for more than 24 to 48 hours, both to remove it and to examine for esophageal wall erosion or perforation. Esophagoscopy is the only appropriate removal technique for multiple or large esophageal

TABLE 40.2 Summary of Recommendations for Esophageal Foreign Bodies[10,20,38,50]

FOREIGN BODY TYPE	LOCATED IN THE ESOPHAGUS	LOCATED IN STOMACH OR BOWEL
Coin	Remove within 24 hours if still present	Stomach: radiograph weekly Remove if no progression within 3–4 weeks
Button battery	Remove emergently	Stomach: repeat radiograph in 2 days Past pylorus: repeat radiograph in 3–4 days
Magnet	Remove all magnets within endoscopic reach (proximal duodenum or stomach)	Remove all magnets within endoscopic reach (proximal duodenum or stomach) Daily radiograh to assess progression
Sharp object	Remove emergently endoscopically	Remove all objects >2.5 cm wide or 6 cm long that are within endoscopic reach (proximal duodenum or stomach) urgently Daily radiograph to assess progression
Blunt object	Remove endoscopically within 24 hours	Remove all objects >2.5 cm wide or 6 cm long that are within endoscopic reach (proximal duodenum or stomach) Weekly radiograph

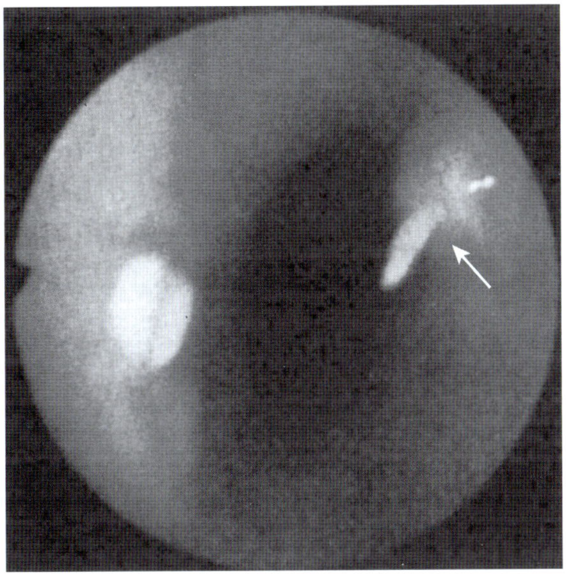

Fig. 40.8 An esophageal foreign body *(arrow)* seen on nasopharyngoscopy.

FBs. This technique is also indicated for patients with an FB proved to have passed into the stomach and must be removed, as well as for those who have persistent symptoms possibly caused by esophageal wall injury. Flexible endoscopic procedures can usually be performed without general anesthesia, even in most children.[5,7] The success rate of flexible endoscopy in patients with retained esophageal FBs exceeds 96%.[15,28]

Esophagoscopy can be significantly more expensive than other maneuvers, such as Foley catheter removal or esophageal bougienage (described later),[28,29] largely because of charges for the surgical suite, but it has a higher success rate. ED removal of esophageal FBs in children by experienced endoscopists, while the child is under procedural sedation administered by the emergency provider, has been described.[30] In selected cases this approach can shorten the interval to completion of the procedure and reduce expense.

ESOPHAGEAL PHARMACOLOGIC MANEUVERS

Background

As the LES is the narrowest portion of the entire GI tract, most FBs that reach the stomach eventually move through the GI tract without further problems. Because a large number of entrapped esophageal FBs are lodged at the LES, especially in adults, several therapeutic maneuvers have been proposed to assist transit into the stomach, including pharmacologic relaxation of the LES. In theory, agents that promote smooth muscle relaxation should improve mobility through the LES. Although some clinicians use pharmacologic adjuncts for all esophageal FBs, objects lodged at the LES will probably benefit most from such interventions. Nonspecific pain relief, anxiolysis, vomiting, and spontaneous passage over time may account for the success attributed to many pharmacologic manipulations of esophageal FBs as there is little scientific evidence that any of these agents offer any benefit over placebo.

Indications and Contraindications

The indication for pharmacologic relaxation of the LES is the presence of a smooth or blunt FB such as a coin or food bolus. Angulated, abrasive, or sharp FBs should not be treated with pharmacologic modalities but instead should be removed by esophagoscopy. Analgesics and sedatives are routinely indicated if pain is present or the patient is excessively anxious.

Glucagon

Pharmacology

Glucagon was historically a prototype for the spasmolytic agents. Glucagon theoretically relaxes esophageal smooth muscle and decreases LES resting pressure. Glucagon has no effect on the upper third of the esophagus, a common site of coin impaction in children, where striated muscle is present and some voluntary control is operative. It only minimally affects the middle third of the esophagus. Peristalsis is not affected by glucagon. Results with glucagon have been mixed, and the only randomized study, done in children, showed no better results than those achieved with placebo.[31] Nonrandomized studies in adults showed that glucagon is approximately equivalent to placebo, and a recent metanalysis which included 1185 subjects showed no benefit over placebo, with success rates of approximately 30% in each goup.[19,32,33] The North American Society for Pediatric Gastroenterology, Hepatology and Nutrition has stated that glucagon "may be considered in patients with distal esophageal impactions" or in "facilities where endoscopic care is not readily available."[27] As glucagon has little downside and emergency providers may be asked to administer it by their consultants for esophageal food impactions, it is reasonable to understand its use despite the lack of scientific evidence for efficacy.

Indications and Contraindications

Glucagon is used for smooth FBs or food impactions at the LES that are suspected because of a patient's complaint of pain or "something stuck" in the lower part of the chest or epigastrium. The clinical diagnosis is usually straightforward, especially if complete esophageal obstruction is present and the patient is unable to tolerate oral secretions. Glucagon is not effective in relieving upper and middle esophageal obstruction, and it is not widely recommended for use in children. In addition, glucagon is not usually effective in patients with fixed fibrotic strictures or rings at the gastroesophageal junction. Glucagon is contraindicated if the patient has an insulinoma, pheochromocytoma, Zollinger-Ellison syndrome, hypersensitivity to glucagon, or a sharp esophageal FB.

Administration of Glucagon

The therapeutic dose is 0.25 to 2 mg administered intravenously (Table 40.3) over a period of 1 to 2 minutes in a seated patient, although one study found that in normal subjects 1 mg of glucagon provides no significant additive benefit over 0.5 mg. The patient is given water orally within 1 minute after the injection of glucagon to stimulate normal esophageal peristalsis; this helps push the food through the relaxed LES into the stomach. Glucagon has a rapid onset and short duration of action: GI smooth muscle relaxes within 45 seconds, and its duration of action is approximately 25 minutes. If no results are seen within 10 to 20 minutes, a second administration of 0.25 to 2 mg may be tried. Success rates are higher when glucagon is combined with gas-forming agents or even carbonated beverages.[34] It is recommended that a small volume of some oral fluid be routinely given to enhance the activity of glucagon.

Complications

Glucagon is associated with a few minor side effects. If administered too rapidly, it can cause nausea and vomiting. Therefore adult patients must be alert and mobile enough to avoid aspiration. Occasionally vomiting dislodges the impacted food bolus. Theoretically, there is a risk for rupture of the obstructed esophagus during induced emesis, so slow injection is preferred to minimize this side effect.

Administration of glucagon is also associated with dizziness. Mild elevation of blood glucose levels is also common but not of clinical concern, and blood glucose levels do not need to be monitored. No fatalities have been reported. Although theoretically glucagon can stimulate release of catecholamine in patients with pheochromocytoma and can induce hypoglycemia from reflex release of insulin with an insulinoma, these endocrine tumors are rare. Nonetheless, precipitation of either profound catecholamine or insulin reactions with the use of glucagon should direct a workup for these underlying tumors.

TABLE 40.3 Recommended Pharmacologic Therapies for Esophageal FBs

CLASS AND AGENTS	SITE OF ACTION	DOSE AND ROUTE	ADVERSE EFFECTS
Spasmolytics			
Glucagon	LES	1–2 mg IV[a]	Nausea, vomiting, hyperglycemia, hypersensitivity
Nitroglycerin	Body and LES	0.4–0.8 mg SL[b]	Hypotension, tachycardia, bradycardia
Nifedipine	LES	5–10 mg SL[c]	Hypotension, tachycardia *Use with caution*
Gas-Forming Agents			
Tartaric acid	Distal and proximal	15 mL tartaric acid (18–20 g/100 mL)[d]	Vomiting, increased intraesophageal pressure
Sodium bicarbonate	Distal and proximal	15 mL sodium bicarbonate (10 g/100 mL)[d]	Vomiting
Carbonated beverage	Distal and proximal	100 mL PO	Increased intraesophageal pressure

[a]May be repeated once or used in conjunction with nitroglycerin.

[b]1 to 2 inches of nitroglycerin paste applied under an occlusive dressing may be an alternative.

[c]A capsule is punctured, chewed, held in the mouth for 3 minutes, and then swallowed. Because of *hypotension*, a 5-mg dose may be used in older adults. *Do not use if the patient has cardiovascular disease, is hypotensive, or has also recently been given nitroglycerin.*

[d]Alternatively, dissolve 2 to 3 g tartaric acid and 2 to 3 g sodium bicarbonate in 30 mL water.

FB, Foreign body; *IV*, intravenously; *LES*, lower esophageal sphincter; *PO*, per os (orally); *SL*, sublingually.

Further Evaluation and Therapy

If the patient experiences relief of symptoms after the administration of glucagon, a postprocedure radiograph or contrast-enhanced study may be obtained to confirm passage of a radiopaque object, but this is not mandatory (Fig. 40.9). Adult patients with successful FB passage into the stomach may be discharged home, but careful follow-up should be obtained to rule out coexistent esophageal pathology because a significant number of patients (65% to 80%) will have underlying esophageal disorders.[10] Pediatric patients with food boluses lodged in the esophagus also have a higher rate of underlying esophageal disease and should be referred for further evaluation; this is not the case for accidentally swallowed FBs in children.[6,8–10,12] If glucagon fails to produce relief of the symptoms or resolve the radiograph findings, its use does not preclude any other approaches from being used.

Nitroglycerin and Nifedipine Pharmacology

Both sublingual nitroglycerin and nifedipine have been used in a manner similar to glucagon to relieve LES tone and allow the passage of a distal esophageal FB, however literature is sparse and is largely limited to case reports.[35,36] Although these two agents have been used less than glucagon for the treatment of esophageal FBs, both are useful for the relief of chest pain associated with esophageal smooth muscle spasm and may be administered concurrently with glucagon. Nifedipine significantly reduces LES pressure without changing contraction amplitudes in the body of the esophagus. Thus nitroglycerin may relieve partial or complete obstruction of the middle or lower part of the esophagus secondary either to intrinsic esophageal disease or to simple FB impaction; and nifedipine, like glucagon, is most likely to succeed when the bolus is lodged at the gastroesophageal junction.

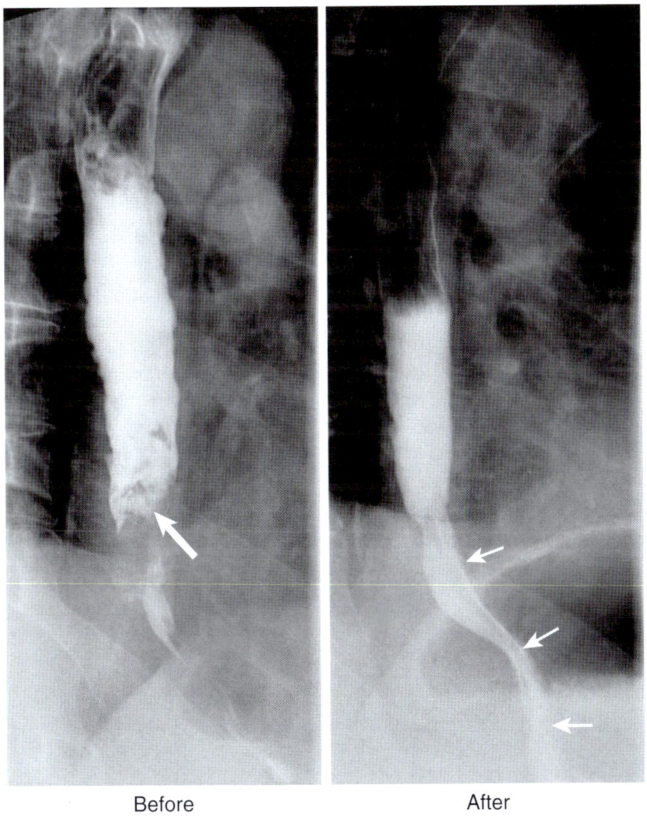

Fig. 40.9 This patient had meat impacted in the distal end of the esophagus, which is clearly visible on the "before" contrast-enhanced esophagogram *(arrow)*. He was treated successfully with simultaneous administration of glucagon and an effervescent sodium bicarbonate drink. On the "after" esophagogram, the contrast material can be seen flowing down the distal end of the esophagus and into the stomach *(arrows)*. (Note: Gastrografin contrast medium was used in this study.) This patient will require endoscopy post removal to evaluate for underlying esophageal disease.

Indications and Contraindications

Similar to clinical indications for the use of glucagon, any patient with an impacted smooth esophageal FB, especially a food bolus, may be a candidate for nitroglycerin or nifedipine (or both). In addition, similar to the mode of action of glucagon, neither of these agents is expected to relax a fixed fibrotic stricture or ring at the gastroesophageal junction.[35] Nevertheless, because both agents have a relatively benign side effect profile, if the patient has no contraindication to their use, they may be tried with or without previous documentation of the distal esophageal obstruction with a contrast-enhanced study. Contraindications to their use include a history of allergic reactions, a sharp esophageal FB, hypovolemia, and hypotension.

Use and Complications

Doses of 1 or 2 (0.4 mg) sublingual nitroglycerin tablets, 1 to 2 inches of nitroglycerin paste, or 5 to 10 mg of nifedipine have been reported.[35,36] Some patients with esophageal FBs may have some degree of dehydration because of the inability to swallow liquids or their own saliva. These patients may be prone to hypotension from the vasodilation associated with the use of either agent. Ideally, rehydration should precede therapy with these agents. *Do not* use both agents simultaneously. The smaller dose of nifedipine is suggested in older adults or those with cardiovascular disease.

Further Evaluation and Therapy

As with the use of glucagon, if nitrate therapy fails to produce relief of symptoms or resolve the radiographic findings, its use does not preclude trying another method. If a patient experiences symptomatic relief, a postprocedure radiograph may be obtained to confirm passage of a radiopaque object, but this is not mandatory. Adult patients may be discharged home, but careful follow-up should be obtained to rule out coexistent esophageal pathology because a significant number of patients will have underlying esophageal disorders.

Gas-Forming Agents

Pharmacology

The use of gas-forming agents for the treatment of distal esophageal food impaction, especially meat boluses, was first described in 1983.[37] The combination of tartaric acid solution followed immediately by a solution of sodium bicarbonate or even carbonated beverages has been reported. In theory, use of this acid-base mixture or a carbonated beverage may produce sufficient carbon dioxide to distend the esophagus, relax the LES, and push impacted food through the gastroesophageal junction into the stomach.[19,34,38]

Indications and Contraindications

Gas-forming agents are indicated for the relief of smooth distal esophageal FB impaction, with or without prior FB confirmation by a radiographic study (see Fig. 40.9). They are often given to patients with food impaction or retained coins. Although gas-forming agents are more likely to succeed with distal esophageal impactions, they have also been successful in relieving obstructions in the proximal part of the esophagus. Concurrent administration of spasmolytic agents may improve the effectiveness of gas-forming agents.

Use and Complications

A solution of 15 mL of tartaric acid (18.7 g/100 mL), followed by 15 mL of a sodium bicarbonate solution (10 g/100 mL), or 1.5 g to 3 g of tartaric acid and 2 g to 3 g of sodium bicarbonate dissolved in 15 mL of water can be used.[37] Carbonated beverages (100 mL) have also been successful in the transit of FBs into the stomach[19,34,38] and are more readily available in the ED. Many patients with esophageal FB impaction have been noted to retch after receiving gas-forming agents, which theoretically puts patients at risk for esophageal trauma, including rupture. Gas-forming agents should not be given to patients with impactions of greater than 6 hours' duration, or to patients with chest pain that might be indicative of an esophageal injury.

Further Evaluation and Therapy

As with the use of glucagon, nitroglycerin, or nifedipine, even if administration of the gas-forming agent is successful, as judged by relief of symptoms, follow-up evaluation is important to determine the underlying esophageal abnormality that potentially led to the FB impaction.

Papain

The use of papain, a proteolytic enzyme used commercially as a meat tenderizer, is NOT recommended for treatment of an esophageal food FB. The North American Society for Pediatric Gastroenterology, Hepatology and Nutrition states that it "is contraindicated."[5] Papain is not currently recommended because of the unacceptable risk for complications and the availability of safer, more effective interventions. It has been associated with esophageal injuries, pulmonary edema, and hemorrhages.[19,34] There is one published report of a retrospective series with no complications from using this agent,[39] but the preponderance of data and expert opinion would suggest against its use in the ED.

REMOVAL OF ESOPHAGEAL FOREIGN BODIES

In the United States the most prevalent method for removing FBs lodged in the esophagus is referral for removal under direct visualization via endoscopy, normally done in either an endoscopy suite or operating room under sedation. Endoscopy is costly[20,28,29] and time-consuming, and if the patient is being seen after hours, the procedure requires additional personnel to come into the hospital to care for the patient. With procedural sedation becoming more common in EDs, procedures to remove lodged esophageal FBs, when appropriate, are becoming more common. Currently three procedures are used in the ED to remove FBs lodged in the esophagus, and these are somewhat dependent on the type and location of the FB. These procedures include Magill forceps removal, Foley catheter removal, and esophageal bougienage. Each will be described separately. Another strategy, "watchful waiting," is reserved for single, smooth, asymptomatic FBs (usually coins) typically at the LES in children and will also be discussed.

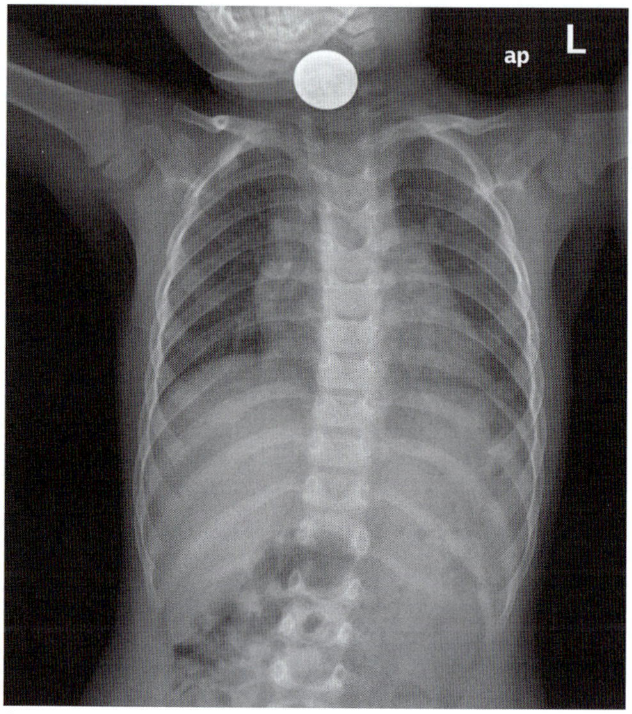

Fig. 40.10 A coin lodged at the level of the cricopharyngeus muscle in a 2-year-old child.

Magill Forceps Removal of Foreign Bodies

Background

See Video 40.4. In children, the most common accidentally ingested FB is a coin, and the most common location for the FB to be lodged is at the cricopharyngeus muscle (Fig. 40.10). When children have a single coin at the level of the cricopharyngeus muscle confirmed by radiographs, they are candidates for Magill forceps removal. The procedure requires sedation (see Chapter 33), and thus airway equipment must be available, in addition to monitoring equipment and expertise in its use. In centers that are using this procedure, success rates have ranged from 95% to 100%.[40] All centers reporting this procedure used sedation and visualization with a laryngoscope or video-assisted system. The procedure was performed rapidly, usually in less than a minute.[40] Complications were rare and typically consisted of minor bleeding or vomiting. Magill forceps removal seems to be ideally indicated for stable children with a coin at the cricopharyngeus muscle in a facility that is well equipped and staffed and experienced in managing procedural sedation and airways in children.

Procedure (Fig. 40.11)

1. Ensure that adequate procedural sedation and appropriate monitoring are both implemented. Place the patient supine on the stretcher with the head slightly extended in the "sniffing position."
2. Insert the laryngoscope or video-assisted laryngoscope. Suction may be necessary.
3. Visualize the upper part of the esophagus, where the FB is normally lodged.
4. Grasp the FB with the Magill forceps and then slowly remove it.
5. Visualize the esophagus after removal for any injuries such as erosion or bleeding.
6. Recover the patient from procedural sedation.

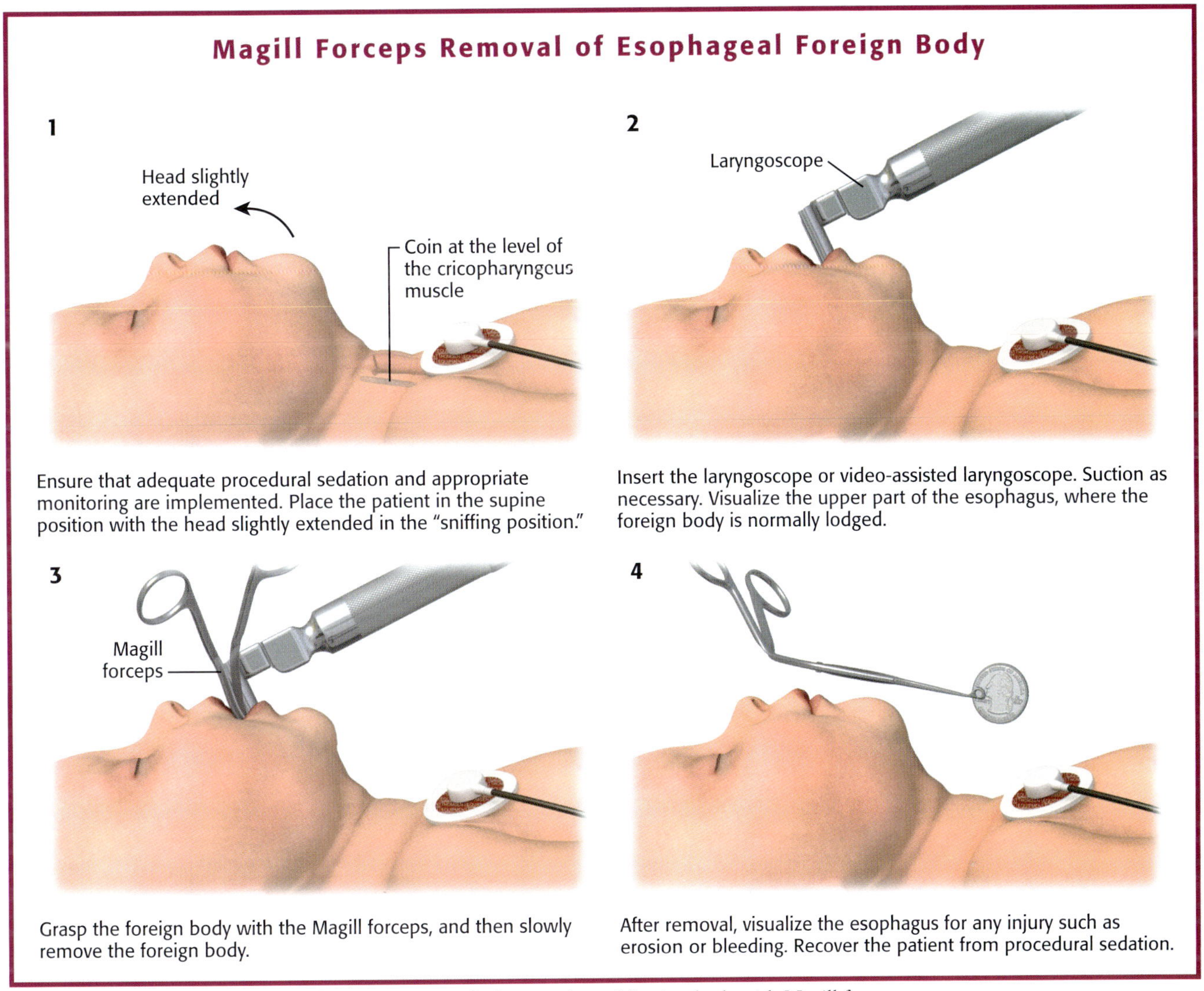

Fig. 40.11 Removal of an esophageal foreign body with Magill forceps.

Aftercare

No specific aftercare is necessary if no complications have occurred from the procedure. If there is any evidence of esophageal injury, the patient should be referred to gastroenterology immediately. Children who ingest FBs are at risk for future ingestions, with the "repeat offender" rate being as high as 18% to 20%.[9–11]

Foley Catheter Removal of Foreign Bodies

Background

Foley catheter removal of esophageal FBs was first described in the thoracic surgery literature in 1966[41] and in the emergency medicine literature in 1981.[42] The technique has essentially been unchanged since the first reports and is now used by emergency providers, radiologists, otolaryngologists, and general surgeons.[43,44] The classic patient for this technique is a small child who is brought to the hospital shortly after swallowing a coin that is documented by radiography, but the procedure may be used for a wide variety of smooth FBs in patients of all ages. Success rates for Foley catheter removal of FBs have been cited from 85% to 100%, with complication rates of 0% to 2%.[44] Many of the reported complications were caused by nasal insertion of the catheter, and complication rates are lower when the catheter is inserted orally and at centers that perform the procedure frequently. Foley catheter extraction of FBs costs significantly less than endoscopy.[45] Fluoroscopic assistance may be preferable, but it is not essential. Whether the procedure is performed in the ED or a radiology suite, equipment and personnel capable of emergency pediatric airway management should be present.

Indications

Recently ingested smooth, blunt objects that are radiographically opaque are most suitable for balloon catheter extraction. Recently ingested FBs carry little likelihood of causing pressure necrosis, perforation, or other significant injury; however, 24 to 48 hours' duration of impaction should be the upper limit for consideration of this technique.[19,46–48]

Coins are particularly amenable to Foley manipulation, but food boluses and button batteries have also been extracted successfully.[19] Radiographically opaque objects are most easily located with plain radiographs. Radiolucent objects can be manipulated, but uncertainty about location may require contrast-enhanced esophagography.

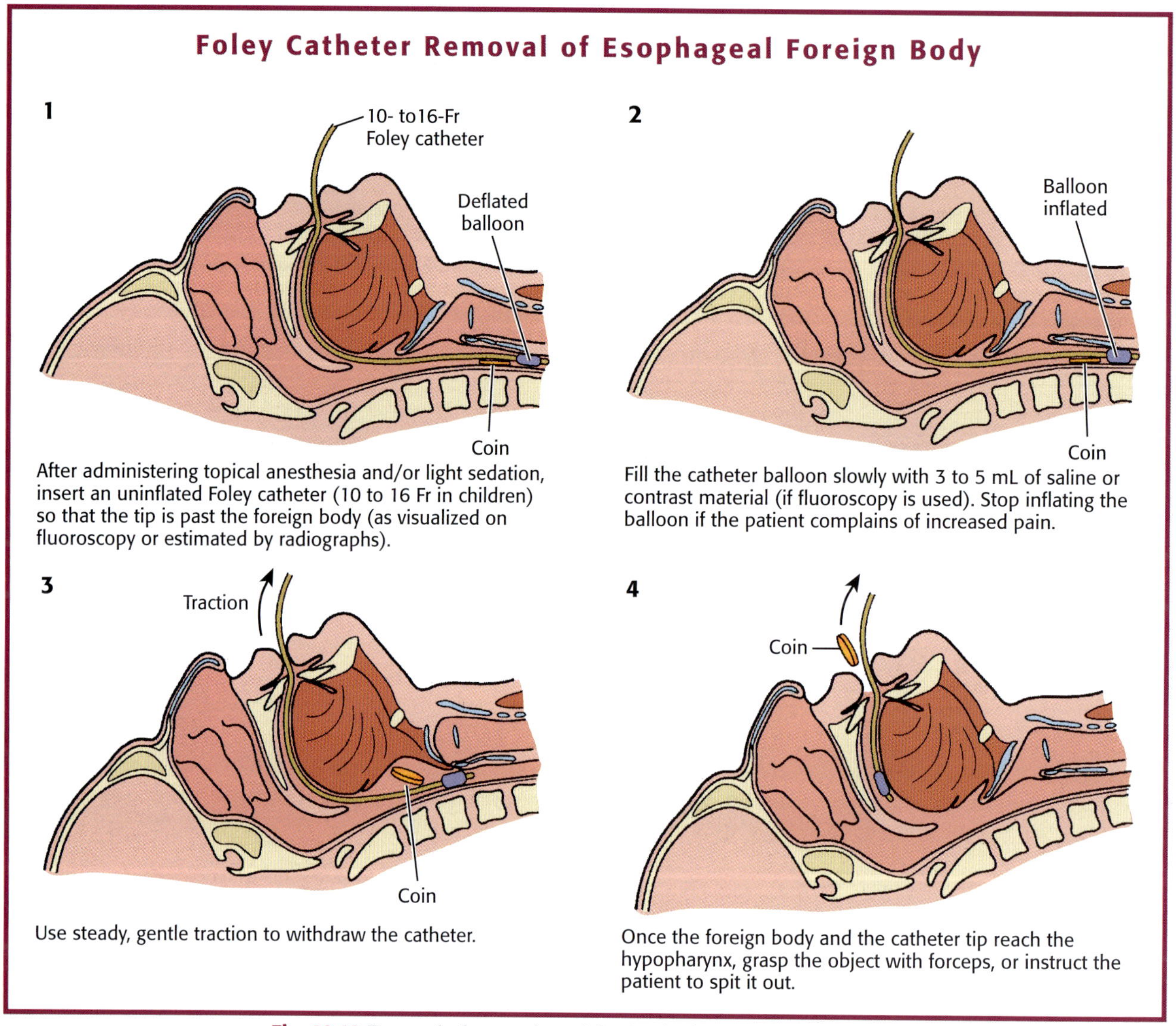

Fig. 40.12 Removal of an esophageal foreign body with a Foley catheter.

Contraindications

Contraindications to catheter removal of esophageal FBs include total esophageal obstruction, as manifested by an air-fluid level on a plain radiograph or contrast-enhanced esophagogram, or when patients are unable to handle oral secretions. The presence of a total obstruction prevents passage of the tip of the catheter distal to the FB. Clinical evidence of esophageal perforation or airway distress requires immediate intervention and precludes blind esophageal manipulation. The presence of multiple esophageal FBs also precludes use of the Foley catheter. Sharp, irregularly shaped FBs should not be removed with this technique because esophageal perforation or laceration can result, and the balloon may burst during the procedure. Finally, lack of expertise or equipment to handle an airway problem arising during the procedure is a contraindication.

Procedure (Fig. 40.12)

1. Coach the patient on the procedure. Topical oropharyngeal anesthesia may be used (although this may increase the risk for aspiration). Light sedation may be used.
2. Place the patient in the Trendelenburg, lateral decubitus, or prone position.
3. Insert an uninflated catheter (10 to 16 Fr in children) so that the tip is past the FB (as visualized on fluoroscopy or as estimated based on radiographs).
4. Fill the catheter balloon slowly with 3 to 5 mL of saline or contrast material (if fluoroscopy is used). Stop inflating the balloon if the patient complains of increased pain.
5. Use steady, gentle traction to withdraw the catheter.
6. Once the FB and the tip of the catheter reach the hypopharynx, grasp the object with forceps, or instruct the patient to spit it out.
7. Obtain another radiograph to ensure that multiple FBs were not present.
8. If the catheter slips by the FB, reinsert the catheter, inflate it with an additional 2 to 3 mL of fluid, and make one additional attempt at withdrawal.
9. If fluoroscopy is not used and no FB is retrieved, another radiograph should be obtained because 10% to 20% of the time the FB will pass distally into the stomach.

Complications

Complication rates of 0% to 2% have been reported.[44] Many complications (nosebleeds or displacement of the FB into the nose) have been related to nasal insertion of the catheter.

Complication rates are lower when the catheter is inserted orally and generally lower at centers that perform the procedure frequently. No deaths have been reported. Laryngospasm and aspiration are rare complications. Failure to either remove the object or displace it into the stomach ranges from 6% to 18%.[8,49–51] New techniques using Fogarty balloon catheters have been reported for difficult-to-remove smooth objects.[52]

Aftercare

Children who have an FB removed successfully with a Foley catheter need no further follow-up if they remain asymptomatic. If the FB was moved into the stomach, clinical follow-up should be adequate to verify movement of gastric FBs through the alimentary tract. Discharge instructions should include warnings about the potential symptoms of GI obstruction, perforation, and hemorrhage. Parents of children who swallow coins can be instructed to watch for coins in their stool. Adults with esophageal FBs that have been removed successfully should be referred for evaluation of possible esophageal pathology, as should children with food impactions. Should an FB remain lodged in the esophagus, immediate referral for endoscopy is necessary.

Esophageal Bougienage

Background

Displacement of esophageal FBs into the stomach can be done with nasogastric or orogastric tubes or via esophageal bougienage. Esophageal bougienage is a technique for dislodging impacted esophageal coins by blind mechanical advancement of the coin into the stomach, a procedure first described in 1965.[53] The technique has greater than a 95% success rate with essentially no reported complications when used for the proper indications.[49,50,54,55] Rates as high as those with endoscopy have been reported.[54,55] Furthermore, bougienage is approximately 10% of the cost of endoscopic removal.[28,55]

This technique does not allow visualization of the esophagus or retrieval of the object. There have traditionally been warnings against forceful advancement of esophageal FBs, but growing evidence verifies the efficacy and safety of blind esophageal bougienage as first-line therapy for coin ingestions in properly selected patients. Although early articles suggested that esophageal bougienage should be performed exclusively by pediatric surgeons, the technique is easily mastered and used by emergency clinicians.[28,29,55]

Indications and Contraindications

Strict patient selection is paramount for successful and uncomplicated bougienage. The criteria have changed little since initially proposed and define a group in whom a round, smooth object can be forcibly passed into the stomach with little risk.[28,29,55] Although many swallowed objects meet this description, only coins hold clear supportive evidence in the literature. Because many patients with impacted food or meat have underlying esophageal pathology, we do not suggest that it be used in the ED for this condition. Selection criteria include a single, smooth FB lodged less than 24 hours in a patient with no respiratory distress or history of esophageal disease, including previous FBs, or surgery. The FB should be likely to pass beyond the stomach without complications. The procedure should not be performed in patients who do not satisfy these criteria. It is important to ascertain the duration of esophageal impaction to avoid performing the procedure when there may be underlying esophageal injury. Plain radiographs may be used to verify coin location and the absence of multiple esophageal bodies. Preprocedure esophagograms are not required.

Procedure (Fig. 40.13)

1. Coach the patient (and parents) on the procedure. Place the patient in an upright position.
2. Achieve topical anesthesia with gargled 2% to 4% viscous lidocaine, atomized 2% lidocaine, or topical benzocaine spray.
3. Flex the patient's neck, open the mouth, and ask the patient to protrude the tongue. Use a tongue blade if necessary. In some patients a bite block may be needed; several tongue blades can be taped together for this purpose.
4. Pass a well-lubricated, appropriately sized bougie (Table 40.4) posteriorly along the roof of the mouth and caudally to the hypopharynx.
5. The patient may gag momentarily; ask the patient to swallow and gently pass the dilator past the cricopharyngeus muscle.
6. Ask the patient to phonate while passing the bougie at this point.
7. Once past the cricopharyngeus, extend the neck to enable the bougie to pass distally to the stomach with little resistance.
8. Withdraw the bougie after a single pass.
9. Terminate the procedure immediately if pain or resistance to advancement is encountered.
10. Obtain a postprocedure radiograph to ascertain passage of the coin into the stomach.

Complications

Gagging and self-limited nonbloody vomiting can occur after the procedure and may reveal the dislodged coin. Patients may experience a residual FB sensation for several hours. Pulmonary aspiration and inadvertent passage into the airway are potential complications. Likewise, traumatic pharyngeal and esophageal injury, ranging from mild self-limited bleeding to frank esophageal perforation with concomitant infection, are possible but rare.

Aftercare

Plain radiographs of the chest and abdomen can verify passage of the FB into the stomach and to check for any potential complications. Discharge asymptomatic patients with appropriate precautions, including the need to return if signs of respiratory compromise, chest or abdominal pain, dysphagia, hematemesis, persistent vomiting, or other concerns are present. Follow-up abdominal radiographs may be performed to document passage of the coin if it is not identified in feces within 1 week.

SPECIAL SITUATIONS

Childhood Coin Ingestion

Coins are the most commonly ingested objects by preschool-age children with more than 250,000 ingestions and 20 deaths in the United States in a 10 year period.[5] In most cases the ingestion is quickly realized by a caretaker, and in the majority of cases the coins pass uneventfully.[5,6,46–48,56,57] Rarely, an

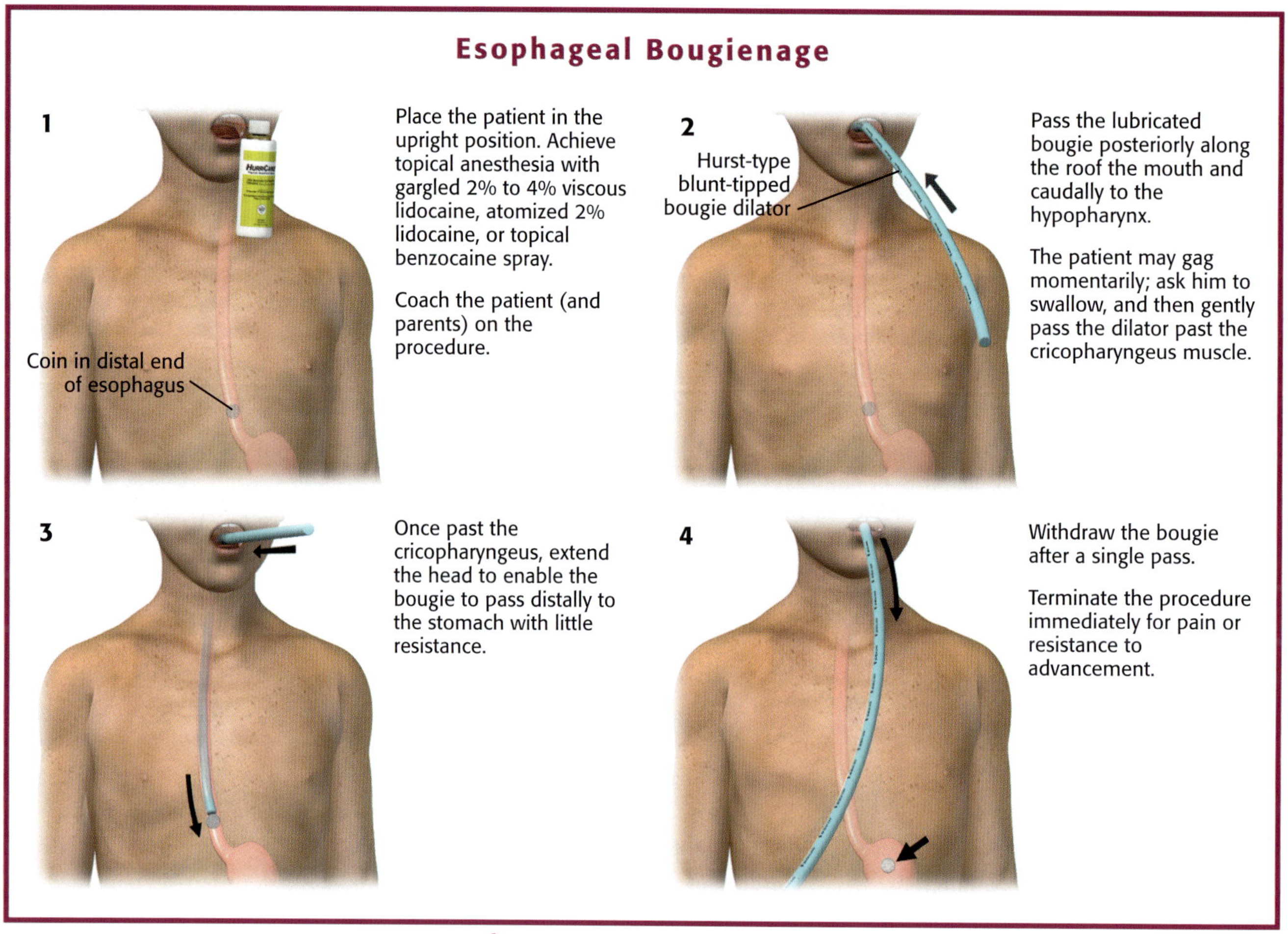

Fig. 40.13 Esophageal bougienage.

TABLE 40.4 Hurst Dilator Size by Age for Esophageal Bougienage

PATIENT AGE (YEARS)	HURST DILATOR SIZE
1–2	28 Fr
2–3	32 Fr
3–4	36 Fr
4–5	38 Fr
>5	40 Fr

esophageal coin can be clandestine for many weeks or months and produce a variety of vague respiratory or GI symptoms.[58] Many coin ingestions are not witnessed,[5,6,8,59] so maintain a high index of suspicion for children with dysphagia, drooling, or crying, who may have esophageal FBs.

Most coins pass from the esophagus to the stomach with only transient symptoms. The child may be in pain for a few minutes as the coin migrates, but on arrival at the ED, the child is often asymptomatic. Coins that remain in the esophagus are likely to, but do not always, produce continued symptoms, such as drooling, pain, dysphagia, and refusal to eat or drink. Rarely, esophageal coins can cause airway distress by external compression of the trachea and simulate an asthmatic attack. Coins below the diaphragm are usually asymptomatic, and the presence of pain or symptoms requires further evaluation. Coins in the trachea produce immediate and obvious respiratory distress.

Although up to 44% of children with esophageal coins may be asymptomatic, and up to two-thirds of coins will be in the stomach at the time of ED evaluation, it is prudent to obtain plain radiographs in all children with a suggestive history.[5,6,8,19] In most cases a single film that includes the pharynx, esophagus, and stomach will suffice to prove or exclude an ingested coin (Fig. 40.14). Another advantage of obtaining radiographs is to rule out multiple FB ingestions, which are not uncommon in children.[20,26,60,61] Only a single PA chest film is needed to prove the presence of a coin, but a lateral projection is also suggested. If the flat surface of the coin is seen (see Figs. 40.2 to 40.4), this orientation ensures an esophageal position. If the edge of the coin is seen, this orientation suggests that it has traversed the vocal cords, but a coin in the airway is often not subtle and produces obvious distress. It is advisable to also routinely obtain a lateral radiograph to determine whether multiple coins are stacked on top of each other (Fig. 40.15).

Once a coin's presence has been documented, a decision concerning removal must be made. The approach varies and there is no agreed upon standard. Overall, approximately 25% of coins will pass spontaneously, even if the coin is located proximally. Observation for 8 to 24 hours is a reasonable approach for asymptomatic children if the ingestion has

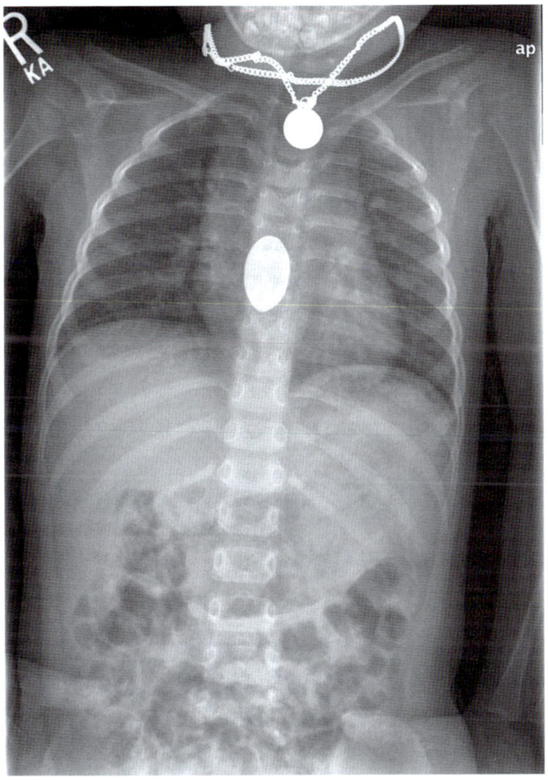

Fig. 40.14 For children who are suspected of having ingested a coin, a single radiograph that includes the pharynx, esophagus, and stomach will usually suffice to prove or exclude an ingestion. Here, the child swallowed a souvenir penny, which is seen in the region of the aortic crossover.

taken place within 24 hours. Coins in the upper and middle third of the esophagus are less likely to pass spontaneously, and some prefer to remove them as soon as the diagnosis is made.[2,62,63] Coins in the distal end of the esophagus will pass spontaneously in one-third to one-half of patients within 24 hours.[6,8,11,26,27,62,63]

The decision regarding management of these patients depends on a number of factors including clinician comfort and experience with removal techniques, local protocols and procedures developed by the medical staff of each institution, and comfort level of the caretakers with various therapeutic options. Regardless of the approach, a radiograph should be taken just before removal to ensure that spontaneous passage has not occurred.

One suggested protocol (Fig. 40.16) involves radiologically localizing the coin, and if the child is symptomatic, immediately removing the coin. If the patient is asymptomatic, the coin may be removed immediately, or the patient may be observed either as an inpatient or at home. If the child is asymptomatic, one common practice is to allow the child to drink a carbonated beverage and eat a small amount of soft food in the ED, wait approximately 1 to 2 hours, and obtain another radiograph. If sent home with an asymptomatic retained FB, the patient is allowed to eat or drink but should be rechecked in 12 to 24 hours with the knowledge that up to 50% of asymptomatic coin FBs will pass into the stomach spontaneously.[19,27]

The techniques of Magill forceps removal, esophageal bougienage, and Foley catheter removal have been described earlier. All are options for single coins present in the esophagus for less than 24 to 48 hours. Another option for coins impacted at the LES is pharmacologic relaxation of the sphincter to aid passage into the stomach, although scientific evidence for efficacy is lacking. The most common method to remove esophageal coins in use today is esophagoscopy.

Approximately two-thirds of ingested coins are in the stomach at the time of first evaluation, and such patients can be released home safely to allow almost certain spontaneous passage with a normal diet. Spontaneous passage of a coin from the stomach to the anus usually requires 3 to 7 days. There is no need for routine cathartic use. Parents should be advised to check the stool for the coin and return for repeated radiographs if the coin is not found in 1 to 2 weeks. Most coins are passed unknowingly by the patient. Any abdominal discomfort or distention warrants reevaluation in the ED. If a follow-up radiograph demonstrates a persistent coin in the intestines for more than 3 to 4 weeks, an obstructive lesion may be present, and further evaluation is warranted.

Finally, there are theoretical concerns about US pennies, which contain 97.5% zinc. Theoretically zinc can lead to mucosal ulceration from its caustic nature.[63]

Fish or Chicken Bones in the Throat

Patients who complain of a "bone" in their throat usually arrive at the ED within several hours of the onset of symptoms, and have generally tried a home remedy such as swallowing a piece of bread. These patients are typically able to pinpoint the location of their discomfort and have a FB sensation that is exacerbated by swallowing. Patients who are markedly symptomatic, vomiting, or unable to swallow require definitive treatment. Those with minor complaints may be evaluated safely over a period of a few days, often as outpatients.

In cooperative patients, careful examination of the oropharynx should be done by either direct or indirect laryngoscopy, or both. If the bone is seen, it should be removed with forceps.

If the patient feels pain in the upper part of the throat, special attention is directed to the tonsils because bones often lodge in this area (Fig. 40.17). Strands of saliva may mimic a bone, and small bones may be difficult to see. More commonly, the area of complaint is below the oropharynx. In these patients, indirect laryngoscopy or nasopharyngoscopy should be the first step, once again removing the bone if one is seen. This can also be accomplished with local oropharyngeal anesthesia by topical spray and direct visualization with a laryngoscope blade or commercial videoscope blade, and then removal of any bone with forceps.

Most patients with an oropharyngeal FB will not have an easily identified or visualized object on examination. These patients present a diagnostic dilemma for several reasons. Only 17% to 25% of patients complaining of a FB sensation after eating chicken or fish have an endoscopically proven bone present, and only 29% to 50% of endoscopically proven bones are seen on plain films.[22,24,26,64,65] The symptoms in patients with an FB sensation but no FB on endoscopy are believed to be caused by esophageal abrasions.

For these reasons, a two-tiered, but individualized approach to managing these patients is proposed.[26,64,65] The patient receives a physical examination and the bone is removed if seen. Carefully examine the tonsils, posterior pharynx, and base of the tongue, which are common places for bones to lodge. If the bone is removed and the symptoms disappear, no further intervention is required and follow-up

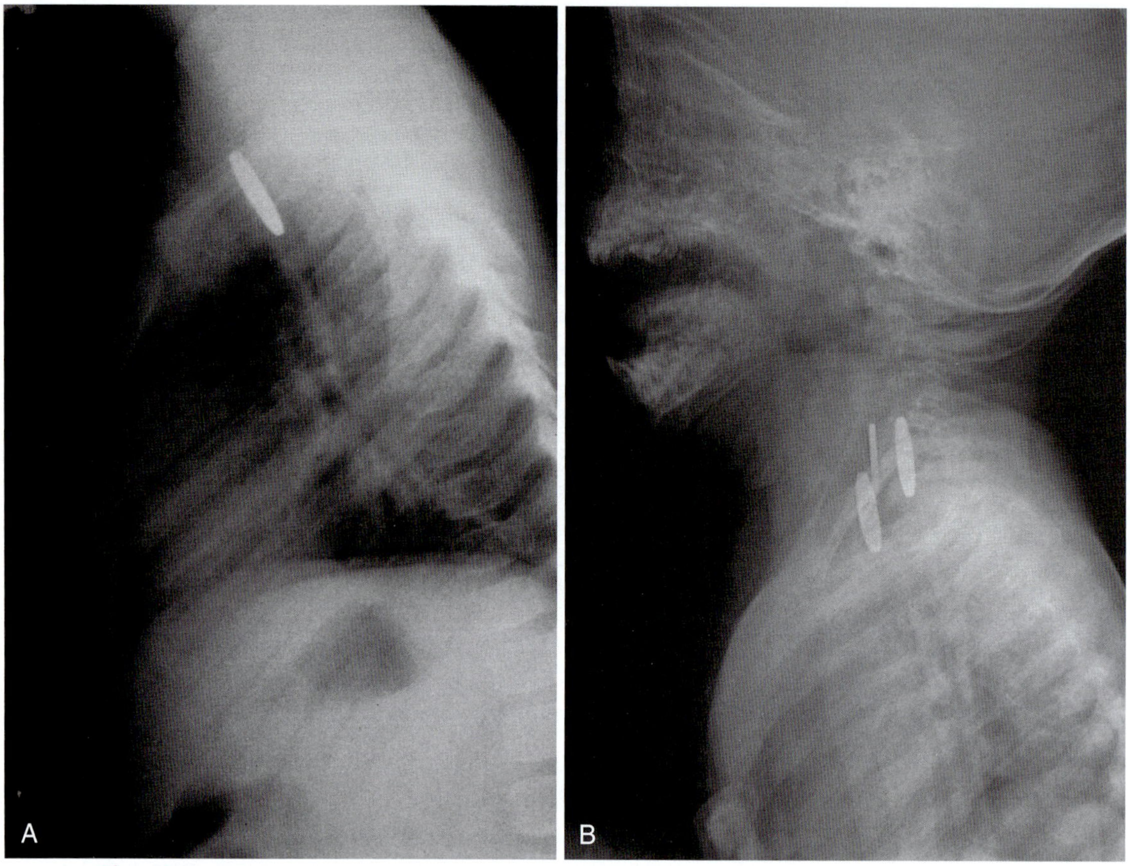

Fig. 40.15 (A) Lateral radiograph of a child showing *four stacked coins* at the same location. A posteroanterior (PA) view suggested a single coin. Multiple swallowed coins are common in children. It is important to obtain both PA and lateral films to ascertain the exact number and location of swallowed coins. (B) A single coin was seen on the PA chest film, but this lateral film suggests *three coins*. However, they do not seem to be stacked directly on top of each other. This digital radiograph was accidentally exposed three times; in fact, only one coin was swallowed and radiographed three times during minimal movement.

will be as needed. Removal of a bone usually provides immediate and complete relief of symptoms. Persistent symptoms are cause for further evaluation based on individual circumstances.

If no bone is seen on physical examination, the bone may have passed after causing local irritation that persists, or the bone is present and not visualized because of location or consistency. Minor symptoms in the upper part of the throat probably represent persistent local irritation. Minimally symptomatic patients can be discharged and reevaluated in 24 hours. Those with complaints of an FB below the visualized pharynx, or with bothersome persistent symptoms, should be evaluated with a CT scan of the neck or possibly the chest if the symptoms are distal. Positive scans are an indication for endoscopic removal of the bone. If the CT scan reveals no FB or postbone complication and the patient is stable, the patient can be discharged home with follow-up within 24 hours. Patients with oropharyngeal abrasions will usually be asymptomatic at that time. If still symptomatic on follow-up, endoscopy is advocated.

A small bone lodged in the esophagus for a few days is annoying and painful, but it is not generally an emergency. However, impacted bones can cause serious sequelae, often weeks later, and continued complaints cannot be ignored. Importantly, a lodged bone will not dissolve and rarely passes spontaneously once lodged in the mucosa. Referral and possible endoscopy are necessary if complaints persist for more than 2 to 3 days, even if the examination and CT scan are negative.

Sharp Objects in the Esophagus

See Video 40.2. Sharp objects cause the majority of complications seen in patients with esophageal FBs. Such objects include tacks, pins, open paper clips, bobby pins, toothpicks, and razor blades (Fig. 40.18). They will not usually pass spontaneously and should be removed urgently. The only appropriate removal technique is under direct visualization with endoscopy. Swallowed dentures or partial plates are a particular hazard in older adults and people with dementia or other mental challenges. Frequently there is no history of such, and patients can have a variety of complaints, such as a sore throat or persistent vomiting (Fig. 40.19). Prisoners and psychotic patients are known to clandestinely swallow multiple bizarre and sharp objects.

Attempts at radiographic localization are appropriate for metallic or radiopaque FBs. Most objects in the stomach, even those considered problematic, will travel the remainder of the GI tract if less than 6 cm in length or 2.5 cm in diameter. If larger than this, consult a gastroenterologist (see Table 40.2). If radiographs show the FB in the esophagus, endoscopic

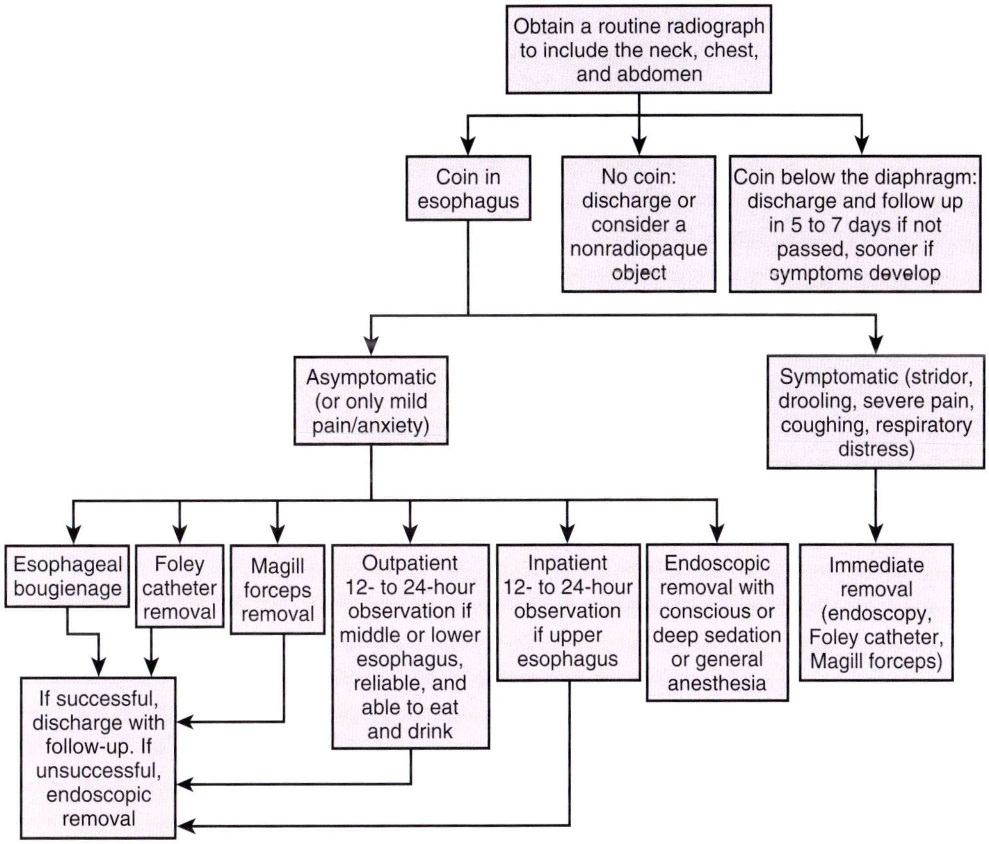

Fig. 40.16 Flow diagram outlining an approach to the management of swallowed coins.

removal is indicated, and attempts to remove such objects in the ED by other methods are not advised.

Nonradiopaque Objects in the Esophagus

Objects such as toothpicks, aluminum pull tabs from beverage cans, plastic, and food boluses may not be visualized on plain radiographs and will normally not pass spontaneously. Toothpicks cause a higher percentage of complications than any other type of esophageal FB.[66] As with fish bones, toothpicks often lodge in the tonsils or posterior pharynx and can be seen on direct vision. The imaging modality of choice is CT. Removal is mandatory and time-sensitive for sharp objects, especially toothpicks.

Impacted Food Bolus

A large bolus of food may become impacted in the esophagus, usually at the LES. This occurs most frequently in older adults, those intoxicated while eating, or those with dentures. Frequently, underlying esophageal pathology is present such as a stricture or web, even in the young (see Fig. 40.6). Children with an impacted food bolus often have underlying esophageal pathology, and it may occur following previous surgery for congenital esophageal malformations. The diagnosis is usually straightforward, and patients may be in significant distress, gagging, and unable to swallow. A barium swallow may be used to confirm the diagnosis, but this is rarely necessary and is discouraged as it impairs visualization on endoscopy, and in cases of complete obstruction, risks pulmonary aspiration. Most sources suggest avoiding contrast radiographic exams before endoscopic removal of esophageal FBs.[19,26,46,62] Proceeding directly to endoscopy appears to be the most reasonable approach. Food boluses may be amenable to pharmacologic relaxation of the LES, but the definitive intervention is endoscopy to both remove the bolus and evaluate the esophagus for pathology.

The most logical ED approach is initial aggressive relief of symptoms (judicious narcotics, sedatives, antiemetics), followed by endoscopic removal. Papain is contraindicated. Removal of impacted food is an urgent issue but need not be done immediately on arrival at the ED or in the middle of the night with inadequate resources; endoscopy can wait several hours. Frequently, pain relief and a few hours of relaxation will allow the bolus to slowly pass; if so, follow up with gastroenterology for evaluation of any esophageal pathology is advised (this is true for food boluses in patients of any age). Vomiting occasionally dislodges the impaction.

Button Battery Ingestion

Button batteries lodged in the esophagus should be considered an emergency because of the potential for serious morbidity and mortality.[19,20,26,27,67] They must be emergently removed. These batteries range in size from 7 mm to 25 mm and are radiopaque (Fig. 40.20). Batteries appear as round densities, similar to an impacted coin, but some demonstrate a "double-contour" configuration.[68] It is important to distinguish between a coin and a button battery because button batteries require immediate removal. Batteries consist of two metal plates joined by a plastic seal. Internally, they contain an electrolyte solution (usually concentrated sodium or potassium hydroxide) and a heavy metal such as mercuric oxide, silver oxide, zinc, or lithium.

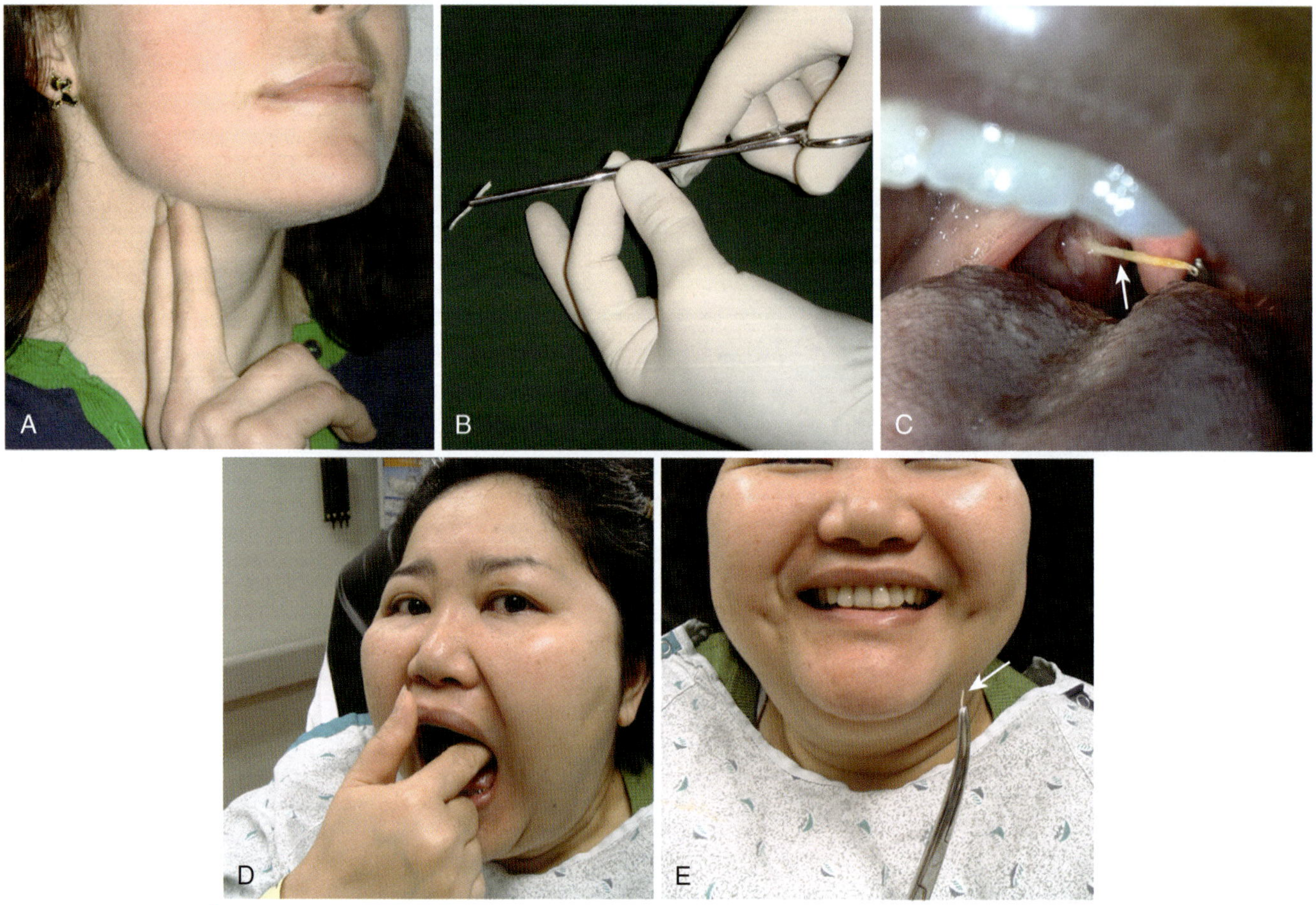

Fig. 40.17 Many fish bones become impaled in the soft tissues of the upper digestive tract. (A) This patient felt a bone catch in her throat while eating fish. As is often the case, she was able to consistently localize the foreign body to the right submandibular area, thus suggesting that it could be seen by direct visualization. (B) With only a tongue blade, local anesthetic spray, and good lighting, a fish bone was found embedded in the tonsil and was easily removed with forceps. Removal provided immediate and total relief, as is usually the case. Strands of saliva can mimic a fish bone, so be careful when probing and grasping. (C) Fishbone visualized *(arrow)* embedded in a patient's right tonsil. (D and E) This patient felt a fish bone in her left pharynx, and a small bone *(arrow)* was removed from her left tonsil, a common place to find a bone with such symptoms. (C, Courtesy Geoff deLaurier, MD, and Jerahme Posner, MD.)

If ingested, these batteries often lodge in the esophagus. Mechanisms of injury include electrolyte leakage, injury from electrical current, heavy metal toxicity, and pressure necrosis. Of particular concern is the development of corrosive esophagitis or perforation as a result of caustic injury and prolonged mucosal pressure. Though essentially harmless in the stomach and intestines, batteries lodged in the esophagus should be considered an emergency because even new batteries are subject to corrosion and leakage, which can result in mucosal necrosis within a few hours of contact with the esophagus.[19,20,26,27,69–73]

Esophageal impaction of batteries mandates immediate removal. Options include Magill forceps removal, Foley catheter removal, esophageal bougienage, or esophagoscopy. Esophagoscopy allows direct esophageal evaluation and a more controlled extraction. In addition, the "invasive" nature of batteries may lead to rapid edema, thus making the catheter technique more difficult. In some localities rapid transfer of button battery ingestions to trauma centers or referral centers has resulted in more rapid removal of the batteries.[71,72]

Once in the stomach, button batteries do not require removal. They may be monitored radiographically to demonstrate passage, with little risk for GI injury or heavy metal poisoning, even if the battery opens (see Table 40.3).[5,22,26,63]

Magnets

Swallowed small magnets from toys and household items have become a serious health hazard in children. All such swallowed magnets within endoscopic reach must be urgently removed.[5,7,26,27,74] Some children with complications from multiple magnet ingestion have underlying conditions such as developmental delay or autism, but older children can inadvertently swallow magnets when using them to imitate a pierced tongue. In 2014 there was federal legislation to restrict the sale of neodymium magnets (also called high-powered or rare earth magnets) which was overturned, then reinstated in 2022.[75,76] These

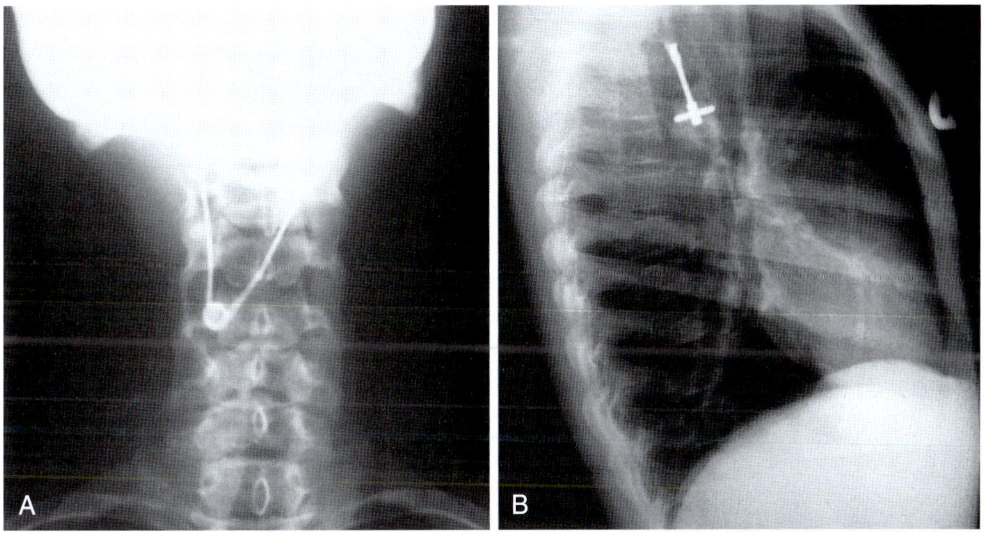

Fig. 40.18 (A) Posteroanterior radiograph of an open safety pin lodged in the upper part of the esophagus. Sharp foreign bodies (FBs) in the esophagus are best removed by endoscopic visualization. (B) This 10-year-old child was brought to the emergency department (ED) with severe chest pain. No history of an FB was given. Even when the radiograph demonstrated this metallic object in the esophagus, how it got there remained a mystery. Objects such as this are removed under anesthesia with an endoscope, and no ED intervention, except for relief of pain, is indicated.

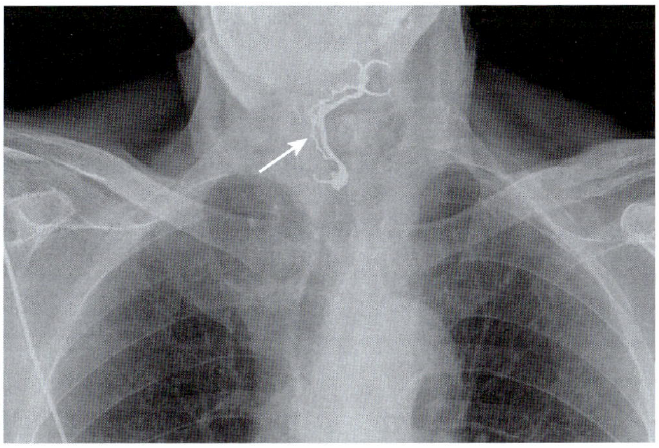

Fig. 40.19 This nursing home patient was seen in the emergency department twice for a sore throat and inability to eat. He had swallowed his partial denture *(arrow)*, but this history could not be obtained and the foreign body was discovered when a chest radiograph was taken. Endoscopic removal was indicated.

toy magnets are small round strong magnets made from rare earth elements and are much stronger than traditional magnets used to make toys, and if multiple magnets are swallowed, they will become adherent inside the bowel (Fig. 40.21). Multiple magnet ingestion is common, occurring up to 57% of the time.[77–79] Multiple magnets, especially if ingested at different times, may attract each other across layers of bowel and lead to pressure necrosis, fistula, volvulus, perforation, infection, or obstruction.[74–79] A piece of bowel may be pinched by two magnets that are swallowed simultaneously and are in different loops of bowel. Hence, suspected magnet ingestion requires urgent evaluation. Radiographs of the neck and abdomen should be obtained to prove magnet ingestion,[26,79] but radiographs cannot determine whether bowel wall is compressed between the magnets. Identification of magnets that appear to be stacked but slightly separated raises concern for bowel entrapment.

Management of swallowed magnets depends on the timing, location, type, and number of magnets. Because even single magnets have some risk, endoscopic removal is recommended if the magnets are within endoscopic reach. Magnets in the esophagus or stomach should be promptly removed via endoscopy.[5,7,26,27] Single magnets passed beyond the stomach can generally be managed conservatively initially, but serial outpatient radiographs should be obtained to confirm that the magnet is progressing through the GI tract. Theoretically, the child should be kept away from any magnetic or metallic material (such as metallic buttons or buckles in clothing) until the magnet has passed. Management of patients with multiple magnets beyond endoscopic reach depends on the symptoms and progression. Asymptomatic patients who have swallowed multiple magnets beyond endoscopic reach should be admitted and monitored closely with serial radiographs and physical examination every 4 to 6 hours.[5] Alternatively, magnets can be removed by enteroscopy or colonoscopy if accessible. Symptomatic patients or any patient with multiple magnets that do not progress on serial radiographs should undergo surgery for operative removal of the magnets.[5,26,27,79]

The Patient in Distress

See Video 40.4. Pharyngeal or upper esophageal FBs can cause respiratory distress or respiratory arrest, usually in infants and older adults. The Heimlich maneuver can be attempted in the prehospital setting or the ED when the situation is appropriate. The first intervention is to ensure an adequate airway, which can be obvious by the situation or may require laryngoscopy or other means of direct visualization. Forceps may be required to remove obstructions

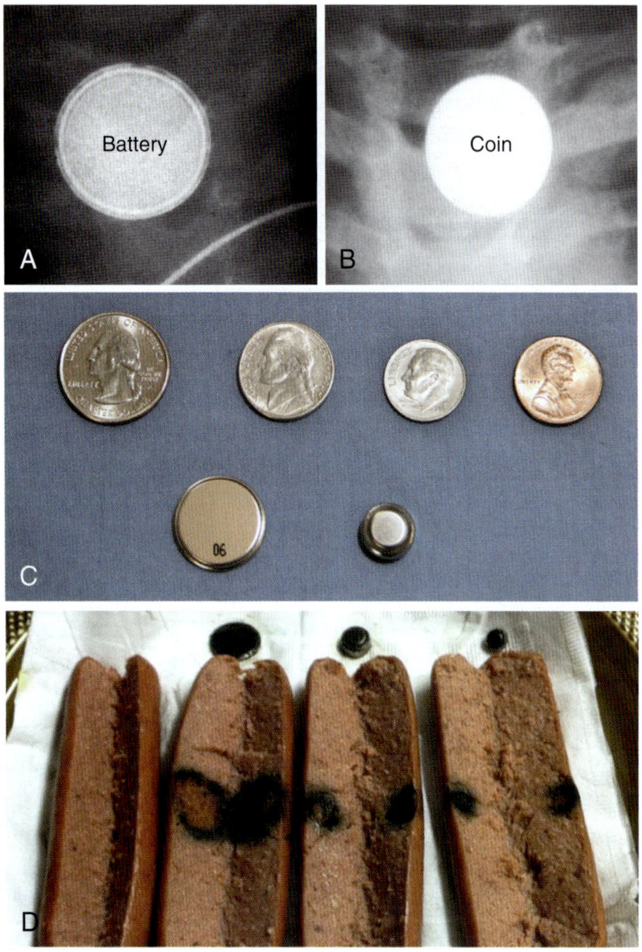

Fig. 40.20 Button batteries have a wide range of sizes and can mimic coins on radiographs. Note that the battery (A) has a double-density circular appearance at the border, whereas the coin (B) has a homogeneous density with smooth borders. (C) Button batteries range from 7 to 25 mm and are similar in size to coins. (D) An example of the potentially rapid, destructive, and caustic power of button batteries in the esophagus. In this model, intact batteries of different sizes were inserted into a hot dog. Larger batteries with greater areas of surface contact caused damage within 30 minutes, and after 3 hours *(image shown)* caustic changes were seen with each of the batteries tested. Immediate removal of all batteries from the esophagus seems prudent. (A–B, From Kost KM, Shapior RS. Button battery ingestion. A case report and review of the literature. *J Otolaryngol.* 1987;16:4. D, Courtesy Adnan Ameer, Rais Vohra, Christian Tomaszewski, and Steve Marcus.)

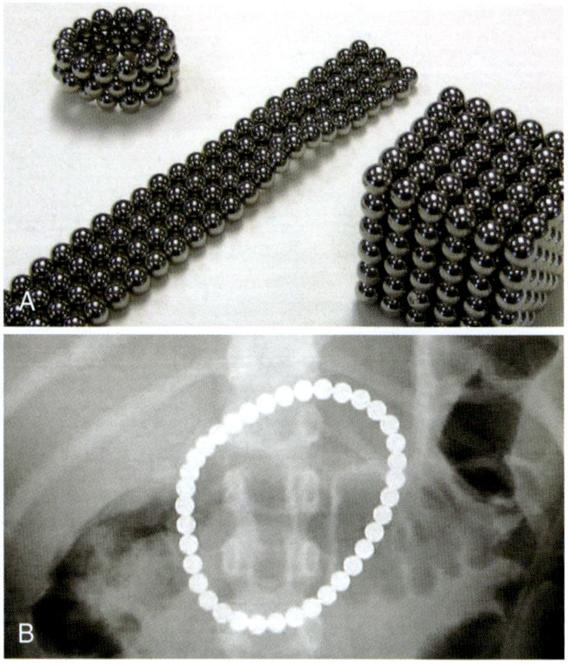

Fig. 40.21 Buckyballs are strong round toy magnets that when swallowed aggregate strongly in the bowel and may cause intestinal perforation or necrosis if the bowel wall is compressed. They should be removed if in the esophagus or stomach. Careful observation is acceptable for asymptomatic patients with multiple magnets that are not readily removed, but symptomatic patients require surgical removal if bowel pathology is suspected.

under direct vision. Because FBs may mimic multiple other pathologies, the approach to an acutely choking patient is challenging and every situation individual. Upper esophageal FBs can compress the trachea and cause stridor and respiratory compromise, which are indications for immediate removal.

ED Evaluation of FB Sensation in the Throat

FB impactions in the esophagus are usually straightforward, but patients may seek treatment in the ED because of a lump in the throat or difficulty swallowing with no apparent reason or history of FB ingestion. Such complaints require an examination and an investigation based on the clinical encounter and individual circumstances. Complete evaluation of these complaints is beyond the scope of this chapter, but initial modalities available to the clinician to evaluate these complaints include barium swallow, CT, and pharyngoscopy or laryngoscopy. The need for consultation is based on the clinical scenario.

If no cause is suspected by the history or examination, globus pharyngeus may be the causative factor. This may be associated with anxiety or a panic attack. The sensation of a painless lump in the throat is called globus pharyngeus or globus hystericus. It has many causes other than FBs. Palpate, visualize, or review the anatomic structures in the area: the chin, laryngeal cartilage, cricothyroid cartilage, tracheal rings, sternum, and cricopharyngeal muscle.

FB sensation may be caused by infection, acid reflux, esophageal spasm, esophageal strictures, pill esophagitis, benign and malignant tumors, hiatal hernia, scleroderma, and many other causes. Globus sensations may also persist after an FB has been completely removed because of mucosal injury. Neurologic causes include botulism, myasthenia gravis, cerebrovascular accident, and amyotrophic lateral sclerosis. If the patient otherwise appears well and is able to drink liquids and keep hydrated, referral to a gastroenterologist as an outpatient is standard.

REFERENCES ARE AVAILABLE AT Elsevier eBooks+

CHAPTER 41

Nasogastric and Feeding Tube Placement

Leonard E. Samuels

Nasogastric (NG) intubation is commonly used to evaluate or treat bowel obstruction, ileus, or gastric hemorrhage, preoperatively or postoperatively, or to administer food or medication into the gastrointestinal (GI) tract. Patients with long-term feeding tube complications and those requiring replacement or other manipulation of tubes are frequently seen and treated in the emergency department (ED).

PROPERTIES OF NG AND FEEDING TUBES

Polypropylene is the material most commonly used for Levin and Salem sump NG tubes (Fig. 41.1), but it is too rigid for long-term use as a feeding tube. Polypropylene tubes are less likely to kink than others but are more capable of creating a false passage during placement. Latex (rubber) tubes are moderately firm, require greater lubrication for passage, are relatively thick walled, and induce a greater foreign body reaction than tubes made of other common materials. Latex, especially in latex balloons, deteriorates more rapidly than other materials.[1]

Foley catheters are primarily latex, although silicone Foley catheters are available for patients with latex allergies. Silicone tubes are thin walled, pliable, and nonreactive; however, the walls of silicone tubes are weaker and may rupture if fluid is introduced into a kinked tube.[2] Polyurethane tubes are nonreactive and relatively durable. Rigidity varies from manufacturer to manufacturer, depending on the thickness of the tube. A stylet may aid in the passage of polyurethane and silicone tubes, but it increases rigidity and the potential for tissue dissection, especially with tubes that have a small distal end-bulb.[3] Some feeding tubes have weights, which are usually made of tungsten and are nontoxic if released into the GI tract.

NASOGASTRIC TUBE PLACEMENT

Indications and Contraindications

The simplest NG tube is the Levin tube, which has a single lumen and multiple distal "eyes." The advantage of the Levin tube is its relatively large internal diameter (ID) in proportion to its external diameter. The theoretical disadvantage is that a Levin tube should not be left hooked up to suction after the initial contents of the stomach have been drained because the suction will cause the stomach to invaginate into the eyes of the tube, blocking future tube function and potentially causing injury to the stomach lining. Levin tubes are therefore rarely used in the ED. The Salem sump tube is preferred over the Levin tube for chronic use as a drainage device because it has a separate (blue-colored) channel that vents the distal main lumen to the atmosphere (Fig. 41.2). While this vent helps prevent an excessive vacuum from forming at the tip of the tube, the narrow lumen or entrances of the vent may clog with debris, inhibiting its performance. Even intermittent suction and wall unit vacuum can exceed the venting capacity of the second lumen: vacuum should be intermittent and set less than 120 mm Hg after initial emptying of the stomach. The most used size is 16 Fr, although larger and smaller sizes are available.

The major indication for NG tube placement and suction is to aspirate the stomach contents in patients with gastric

Nasogastric Tube Placement

Indications

Decompression of stomach (e.g., obstruction or perforation)
Reduce incidence and risk of vomiting
Monitor and evaluate upper gastrointestinal bleeding
Prolonged ileus
Administration of medication or oral contrast in a patient unable to swallow
Detection of transdiaphragmatic stomach herniation

Contraindications

Midface injury, basilar skull fracture, or coagulopathy (orogastric placement may be a better option)
History of gastric bypass or lap banding
Esophageal strictures or alkali injury

Complications

Bleeding	Vomiting/retching
Intracranial placement	Perforation
Pulmonary placement	Sinusitis
Pneumothorax	Aspiration

Equipment

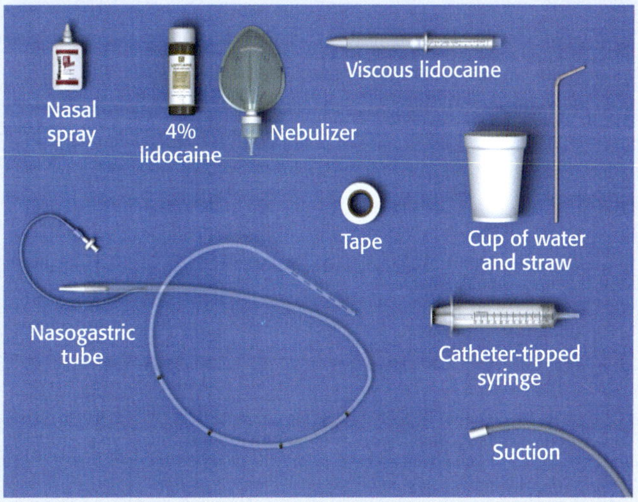

Review Box 41.1 Nasogastric tube placement: indications, contraindications, complications, and equipment.

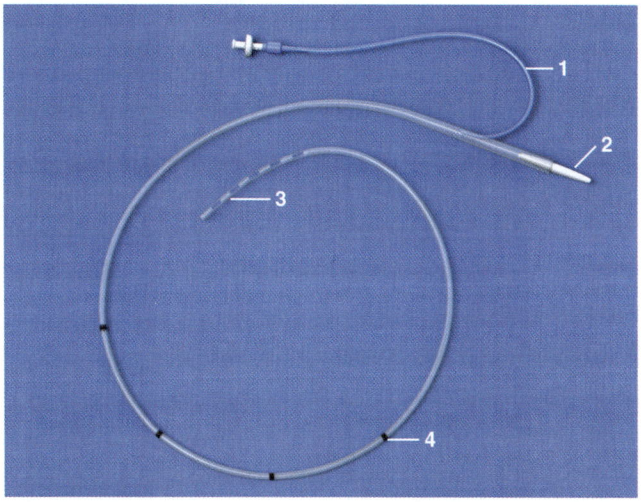

Fig. 41.1 Salem sump tube. This tube contains a second lumen that allows venting during continuous suction. *1*, Pigtail extension (blue) of the air vent lumen. *2*, Connector for attachment of the suction lumen to the vacuum line. *3*, Gastric end with suction eyes. *4*, Insertion depth markers.

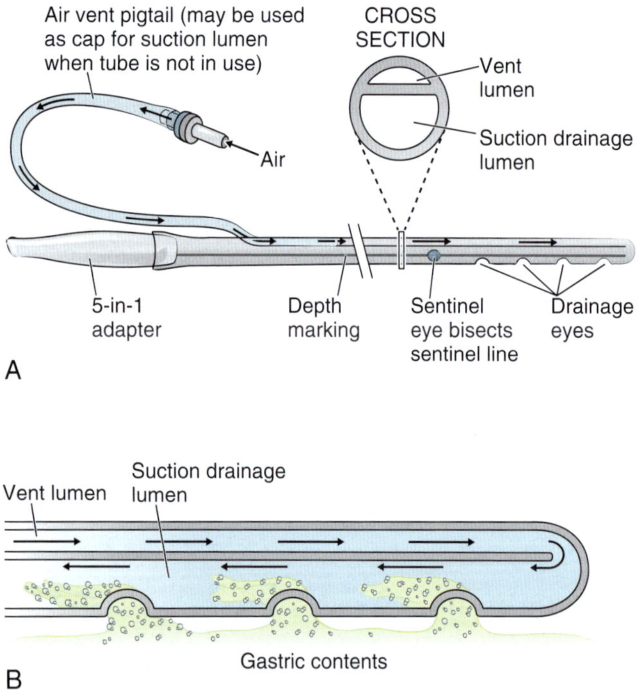

Fig. 41.2 Diagram of the Salem sump tube. (A) General design. (B) Diagram of the double-lumen principle for suction. (A–B, Courtesy Argyle Division of Sherwood Medical, St. Louis, MO.)

bleeding, gastric outlet or intestinal obstruction, gastric or bowel distention, prolonged ileus, or gastric, esophageal, or bowel perforation. Draining the dilated stomach of excessive contents lessens the chance of vomiting and possibly aspiration and provides marked relief of symptoms in patients with intestinal obstruction. The presence or anticipation of depressed mentation potentially justifies NG tube placement to protect the airway, especially if the stomach is full or vomiting is uncontrolled. Bag-valve-mask ventilation often distends the stomach with air, and a postintubation NG tube can improve ventilation, prevent vomiting, and increase patient comfort. Trauma patients may need an NG tube as part of the evaluation for GI injury or to decompress the stomach before surgery or peritoneal lavage. A radiopaque NG tube may help delineate transdiaphragmatic hernia of the stomach after trauma. A deviated NG tube is a nonspecific sign of traumatic aortic rupture. An NG tube may be used to instill air into the stomach for documentation of a suspected gastric perforation by enhancing visualization of free air under the diaphragm on an upright chest film. In patients unable to swallow, an NG tube may be passed to administer medications or oral contrast material for a computed tomography (CT) scan.

Except when frankly bloody fluid is obtained, an NG aspirate is diagnostically unhelpful in evaluating upper GI bleeding. Identification of bile in NG aspirates is unreliable and uncorrelated with the presence of bleeding.[4] Although insertion of an NG tube may prompt earlier endoscopy, the procedure has not been demonstrated to improve clinical outcomes.[5] Patients who vomit a significant amount of proven bloody material have had upper GI bleeding; they do not need an NG tube for diagnosis. Such patients are best evaluated by endoscopy. When rapid bleeding is suspected, stomach aspiration may have a role in diagnosis to confirm the presence of bleeding in patients without hematemesis. However, NG aspiration uncovers less than half the patients with upper GI hemorrhage and thus cannot be used to rule out upper GI bleeding. Even a rapidly bleeding duodenal ulcer may not produce blood in the stomach. Some contend that emptying a markedly dilated stomach of blood and stomach contents may reduce the rate of bleeding, but data are lacking. Patients with presumptive upper GI bleeding, which includes those with melena, those younger than 50 years, and those with a hematocrit lower than 30, need upper endoscopy.[6,7] Patients passing clots or blood per rectum or those with known previous lower GI bleeding are usually experiencing lower GI bleeding.[7] Suctioning up small bits of darkish material, bloody mucus, or obtaining positive Gastroccult or guaiac tests probably represent sequelae of the procedure, whereas a clear appearance and negative tests still miss most bleeding distal to the stomach. Patients with a bleeding pattern indicative of a Mallory-Weiss tear may need neither an NG tube nor endoscopy.

NG tubes can provide the earliest indication of high-volume esophageal or gastric bleeding. Although variceal rupture may potentially be caused by insertion of instruments into the esophagus, several studies suggest that passage of an NG tube is generally safe, even in patients with esophageal varices although risk increases with increased MELD-Na score and varices located in the lower third of the esophagus.[8] Use of NG tubes for the evaluation and monitoring of upper GI bleeding should be judicious rather than universal.

Most other causes of vomiting are best controlled with medication. Postoperative ileus ends sooner and patients recover faster without an NG tube after various studied abdominal surgeries.[6,9] NG tubes prolong the hospital stay, pain, and hyperamylasemia in those with mild to moderate pancreatitis.[10] Many patients are better off without an NG tube from the point of view of safety, comfort, and speed of recovery.

In an awake and alert patient with a preserved gag reflex, passage of an NG tube has not been demonstrated to result in significant pulmonary aspiration. NG tubes are contraindicated in patients with a special predisposition to injury from placement of the tube. Patients with facial fractures who have sustained an injury to the cribriform plate may

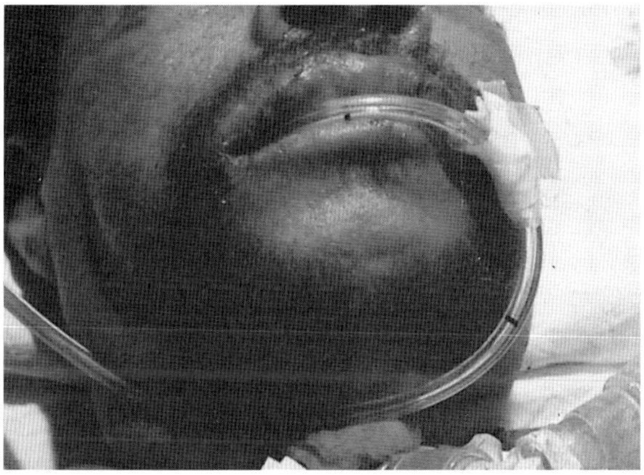

Fig. 41.3 A nasogastric (NG) tube may enter the cranium or facial soft tissues in patients with severe head or facial trauma. Those with a coagulopathy may experience significant bleeding from nasal or pharyngeal trauma during passage of an NG tube. In such cases, a standard NG tube inserted through the mouth (as shown here) may be a better alternative.

sustain intracranial penetration with a blindly placed nasal tube.[11] Severe coagulopathy is a relative contraindication to passage of an NG tube. In patients with a coagulopathy or significant facial or head trauma, passing the desired tube through the mouth may be a better alternative (Fig. 41.3). Patients who have esophageal strictures or a history of alkali ingestion may experience esophageal perforation. Gagging will decrease venous return and increase cervical and intracranial venous pressure. Comatose patients may vomit during or after NG tube placement. Indwelling NG tubes predispose patients to pulmonary aspiration because of tube-induced hypersalivation, depressed cough reflex, or mechanical or physiologic impairment of the glottis.[9] Aspiration is also quite common with nasoenteric feedings in debilitated patients, hence the use of a gastrostomy feeding tube for this condition. An NG tube should be avoided when possible in patients who have undergone gastric bypass surgery or lap banding procedures.

Extended irrigation of the stomach with water in a patient with upper GI hemorrhage can lower serum potassium levels,[12] and animal studies suggest that cold water lavage can cause rather than control bleeding.[13,14] No study has shown irrigation to be effective in the control of bleeding,[15,16] and vigorous lavage with cold water may lower the body temperature. Erythromycin has been demonstrated to be effective in clearing the stomach for endoscopy,[17,18] and its success is better substantiated than irrigation.

Equipment

Passage of standard NG or feeding tubes can be messy and may be accompanied by coughing, retching, sneezing, bleeding, and spilled water or stomach fluid. For this reason, both the patient and clinician should be gowned; cleanup may be reduced if the bib area is covered with a towel and a supply of tissues or washcloths is available. For standard NG tube placement, a piston or bulb syringe (with a catheter slip-tip) should be available. NG feeding tubes should have a compatible 50- or 60-mL syringe (some are Luer compatible, and others are slip-tip compatible). Make sure that the feeding tube is designed for duodenal passage if this is desired; such tubes are usually longer than regular feeding tubes.

Tape torn into 4-inch strips (or wider tape split in half the last 2.25 inches of the 4-inch length), or a commercial NG tube holder (e.g., suction tube attachment device, Hollister) should be handy for securing the tube after placement. Intubated patients often have a very secure endotracheal (ET) tube holder; the NG tube can sometimes be taped to the holder, and sometimes be taped to the ET tube itself. Alcohol pads may be useful to clean greasy skin, and cotton-tipped applicators with tincture of benzoin can be used on the skin in the area where taping will occur. Cloth tape is preferred.

Procedure

See Videos 41.1–41.3. Most NG tubes are placed at the bedside in an awake patient. Explain the procedure to the patient. Written informed consent is not standard. If the patient is alert, raise the head of the bed so that the patient is upright. Place a towel over the patient's chest to protect the gown and place an emesis basin on the patient's lap.[19] Position the tube (typically a 16- or 18-Fr sump) so that the insertion distance can be estimated and mark the distance with tape or by noting the markers printed on the proximal end of the tube. A simple method is to measure the tube from the xiphoid to the earlobe and then to the tip of the nose. Then add 15 cm (6 inches) to this number (Fig. 41.4, *step 5*).[20] Most NG tube placement videos use the nose-ear-xiphoid distance alone to estimate appropriate depth, but the omission of extra insertion length resulted in 96% of tubes being placed to insufficient depth in one study.[21] If placed too deeply, the tube can coil excessively in the stomach or progress into the duodenum. Check the nares for patency by direct visualization, by gentle digital nasal examination, and by having the patient sniff while first one and then the other nostril is occluded. Pass the tube down the more patent naris.

Relief of Discomfort

The pain and gagging associated with tube placement can be ameliorated by using vasoconstrictors, topical anesthetics, and antiemetics. Because patients rate NG tube placement as one of the most painful procedures performed in the ED, use these adjuncts whenever time and the clinical situation permit (Figs. 41.5 and 41.6). Spray topical vasoconstrictors, such as phenylephrine or oxymetazoline into both nares in case one side proves to be problematic (see Fig. 41.4, *step 2*). The nares, nasopharynx, and oropharynx should all be anesthetized at least 5 minutes before the procedure. Gagging is reduced if the pharynx is anesthetized as well as the nose—consider encouraging a sniff of excess topical anesthetic. Lidocaine may be nebulized and delivered by face mask with the equipment used to administer bronchodilators to asthmatics (see Fig. 41.4, *step 3*). This method has been found to be superior to lidocaine spray for reducing gagging and vomiting and increasing the chance of successful passage.[22,23] Cullen and coworkers concluded that nebulized nasal and pharyngeal lidocaine (4 mL of a 10% solution) reduces the discomfort associated with passage of an NG tube better than placebo and without any lidocaine-related toxicity.[24]

After a topical vasoconstrictor and anesthetic are administered, lubricate the tube with viscous lidocaine or lidocaine jelly.[25] Lubrication and anesthesia of the nares can be facilitated by using a syringe (without needle) filled with 5 mL of an anesthetic lubricant, such as 2% lidocaine gel (see Fig. 41.4, *step 4*). Simply putting anesthetic jelly on

Nasogastric Tube Placement

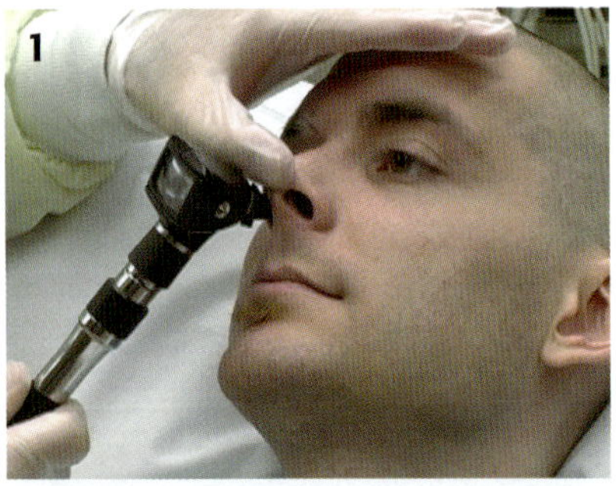

Choose the most patent naris by visual inspection and the sniff test. Alternatively, insert a gloved finger into each nostril to assess patency.

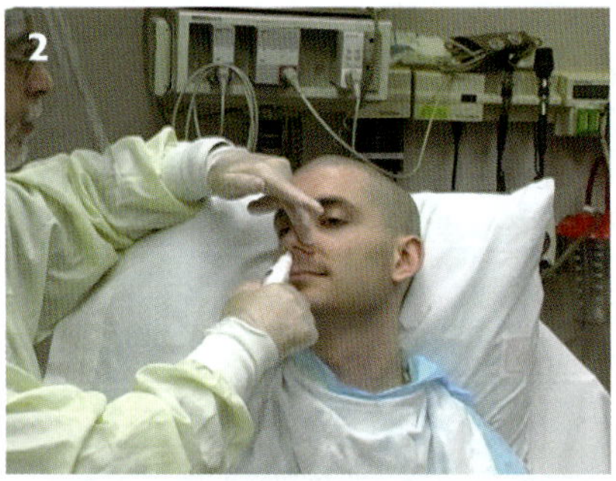

Apply a topical vasoconstrictor, such as phenylephrine or oxymetazoline.

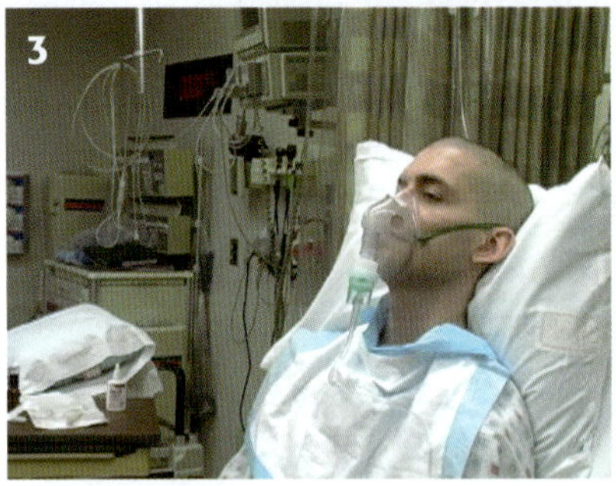

Anesthetize the naris, nasopharynx, and oropharynx at least 5 minutes before the procedure.

Nebulized lidocaine is ideal because it reduces both nasal and pharyngeal discomfort.

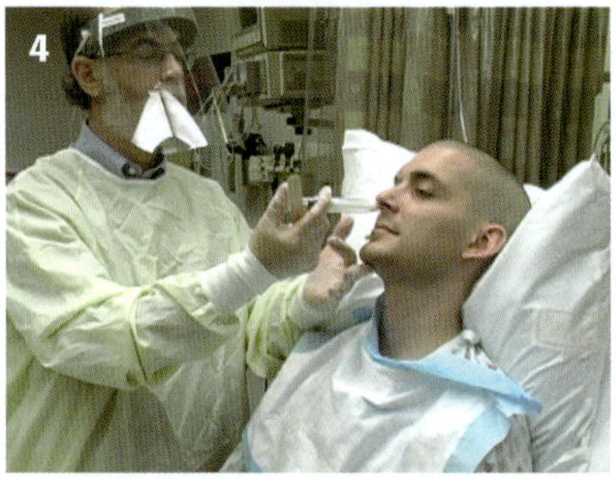

Apply 2% viscous lidocaine along the floor of the nasal cavity, and allow it to drip into the nasopharynx and be swallowed.

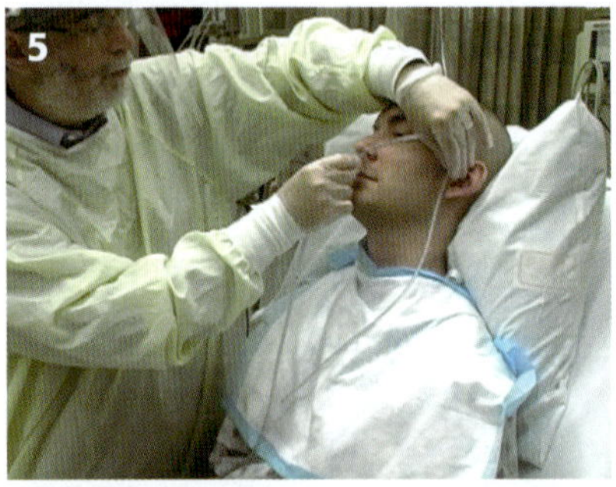

Measure the distance from the tip of the nose to the earlobe to the xiphoid process.

Add another 15 cm to this distance.

Note the total distance on the nasogastric tube markers.

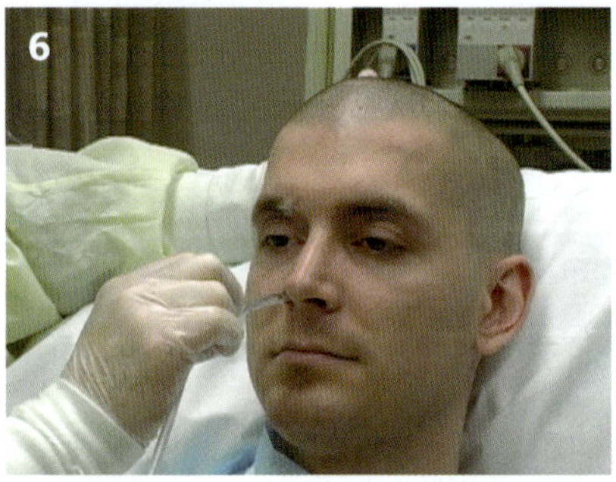

Slowly insert the nasogastric tube along the floor of the nostril under direct vision until it passes into the oropharynx.

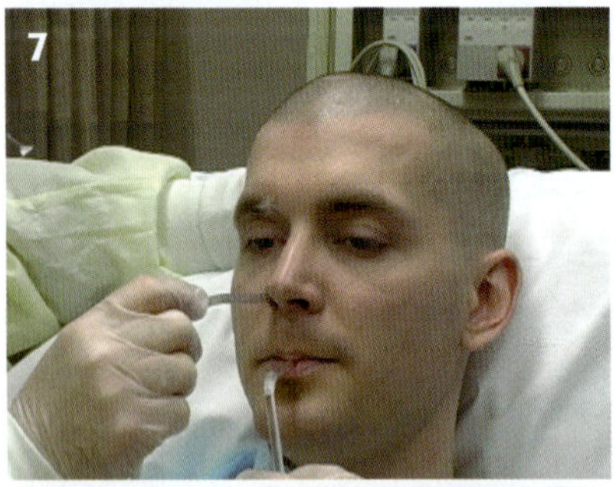

While the patient sips water from a straw, rapidly pass the tube to the predetermined depth. Coordinate tube advancement with the swallowing mechanism to promote easy passage.

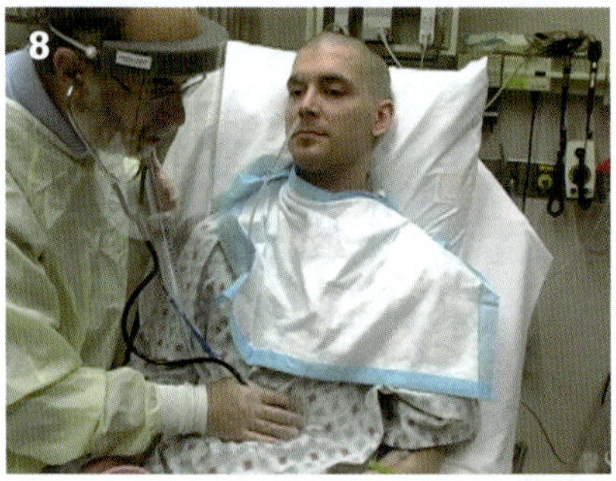

Assess tube placement with air insufflation and aspiration.

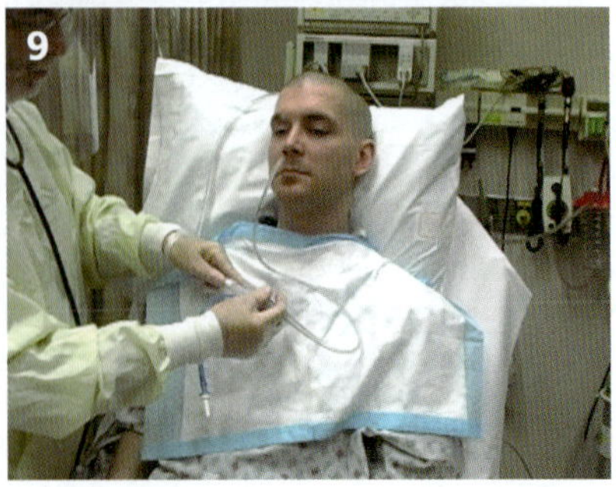

Attach the tube to intermittent wall suction.

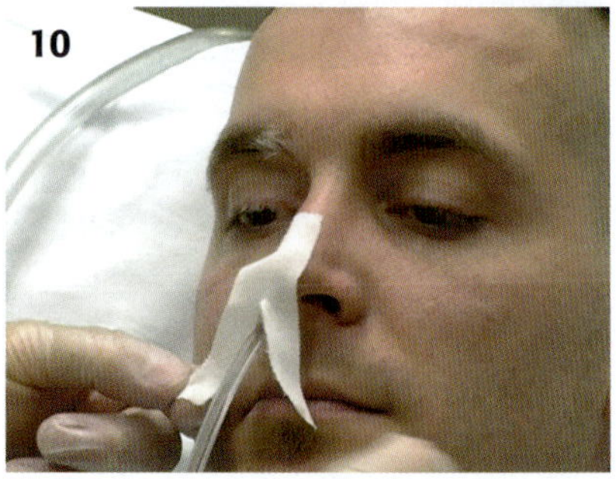

Secure the tube to the nose with tape.

Fig. 41.4 Nasogastric tube placement.

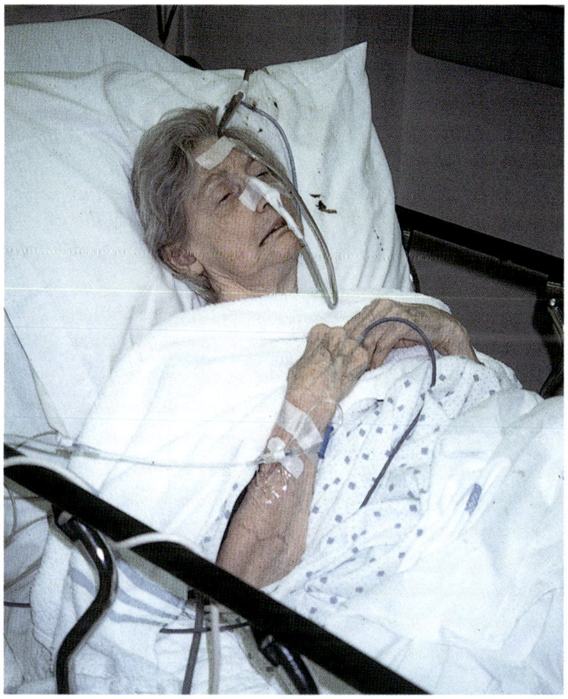

Fig. 41.5 Insertion of a nasogastric (NG) tube has been termed one of the most painful and unpleasant procedures performed in the emergency department, and it should not be used unless specifically indicated. Whenever possible, some form of topical anesthesia for both the nose and the pharynx should be used at least 5 minutes before passing an NG tube. Merely coating the tube with xylocaine ointment prior to insertion is of no anesthetic value.

the tube just before insertion will not provide adequate anesthesia. Topical anesthetics are generally quite safe, but pay attention to the total dose of anesthetic administered to avoid toxicity.[26] Note that each milliliter of a 10% lidocaine solution contains 100 mg of lidocaine and can be absorbed systemically. In rare cases, topical benzocaine has caused methemoglobinemia, even with the relatively small amounts used for endoscopy.[27]

Although no standard exists and supportive data are sparse, some clinicians administer a dopamine antagonist (e.g., metoclopramide) or serotonin antagonist (e.g., ondansetron) antinauseant 5 minutes before passage of an NG tube to potentially reduce nausea and gagging and, secondarily, to improve the pain and prolongation of the procedure that gagging engenders.

Under direct vision insert the tube gently into the naris along the floor of the nose under the inferior turbinate and NOT upward toward the nasal bridge (Fig. 41.6; also see Fig. 41.4, *step 6*). If mild resistance is felt in the posterior nasopharynx, apply gentle pressure to overcome this resistance. If significant resistance is encountered, it is better to try the other nostril because bleeding or dissection into retropharyngeal tissue may occur if force is used. Once the tube passes into the oropharynx, pause to help the patient regain composure and enhance the chance for cooperation with the rest of the procedure.

If the patient is alert and cooperative, a common option is to ask the patient to sip water from a straw and swallow while you advance the tube into and down the esophagus (see Fig. 41.4, *step* 7) as this may facilitate passage of the

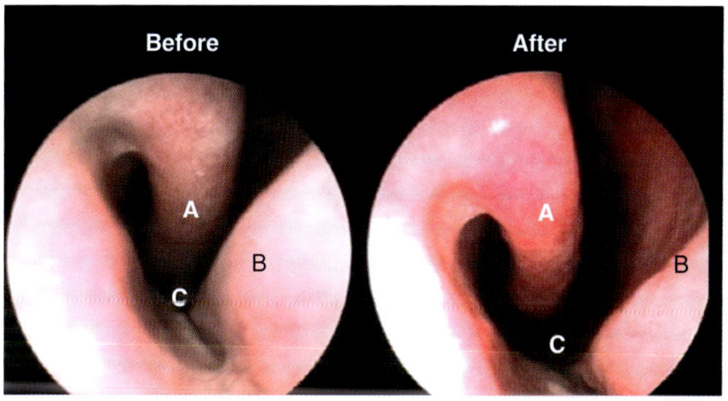

Fig. 41.6 Endoscopic view of the nasal cavity before and after the application of oxymetazoline nasal spray. The nasogastric tube is passed under the inferior turbinate, which is made more patent after the application of topical vasoconstrictors. The operator should actually look into the nose during insertion to properly guide the tube, not force it blindly. *A*, Inferior turbinate; *B*, nasal septum; *C*, pathway of the nasogastric tube. (From Thomsen T, Setnik G, eds. *Procedures Consult—Emergency Medicine Module*. Elsevier Inc.; 2008.)

tube. Once the tube is in the nasopharynx, flex the patient's neck to direct the tube into the esophagus rather than the trachea. In an intubated, anesthetized, and paralyzed patient, two stacked positive pressure breaths lasting 1 to 2 seconds each via a face mask provide similar relaxation of the upper esophageal sphincter for a brief 4- to 5-second window, and this markedly increases successful tube placement.[28] The ET tube is swung sideways to enable a sufficient seal to deliver a pressure wave with the bag valve mask.

Some gagging during the procedure is common and is not an indication to halt attempts at passage. Withdraw the tube promptly into the oropharynx if the patient has excessive choking, gagging, coughing, a change in voice, or condensation appears on the inner surface of the tube because this indicates the possibility of passage of the tube into the trachea. With the mouth open, inspect the tube in the posterior pharynx to detect coiling. If the tube is lateral to the midline, this suggests correct position in the esophagus. Once the tube is in the esophagus, advance it rapidly to the previously determined depth. Passing the tube slowly prolongs discomfort and may precipitate more gagging.[19]

Confirmation of Tube Placement

Before the NG tube is secured, confirm successful placement by nonradiographic means or by auscultation. Use more than one method when in doubt because all methods of confirmation have some possibility of error. Radiographic evaluation is the most definitive way to confirm the position of an NG tube, but it is not standard to routinely obtain radiographic confirmation. Radiographs may be more useful in the obtunded patient. Alert and cooperative patients will feel when a tube is entering the trachea or lungs and will be very symptomatic and therefore obviously alert the clinician. Patients who are struggling or have altered sensorium may not give any sign when the tube passes into the lungs, and therefore careful confirmation of placement, usually with radiography, is critical for these individuals. Ultrasound, when successful, is also highly reliable (see Ultrasound Box).[29]

ULTRASOUND: Assistance in Nasogastric Tube Placement *by Christine Butts, MD*

Ultrasound has emerged as a new modality to assist in placement verification of nasogastric tubes, both during the procedure and as a confirmatory test after the procedure.

Place the high-frequency transducer on the patient's neck transversely between the cricoid cartilage and the suprasternal notch, slightly off to the side with the orientation button to the patients' left (Fig. 41.US1). Obtaining a clear view of the esophagus sometimes involves slight angling of the probe and occasionally even benefits from some minor tracheal manipulation, usually leftward displacement. With these maneuvers, it is probably possible to visualize the esophagus over 90% of the time (Fig. 41.US2).[30]

When the nasogastric tube passes the probe image level, the esophagus acquires a bright echogenic density with posterior shadowing (Fig. 41.US3). The nasogastric tube's strong interaction with the ultrasound may obscure clear visualization of the esophageal wall. A brighter echogenic density is obtained if there is a metal guidewire in the tube, as is common in feeding tubes but not in Salem sump tubes.

If 20 cm of the tube has been passed but the esophageal appearance has not changed, the tube is likely in the trachea or coiled in the mouth and failing to pass. Sometimes the empty esophagus is not easily seen, and then it becomes even more

Continued

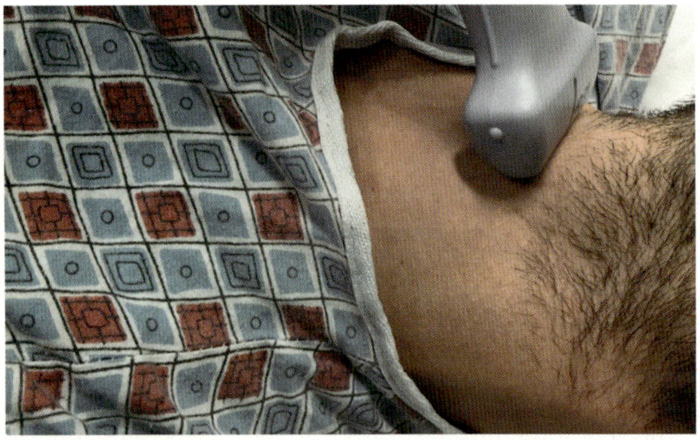

Fig. 41.US1 Proper positioning of the high-frequency transducer between the cricoid and the suprasternal notch.

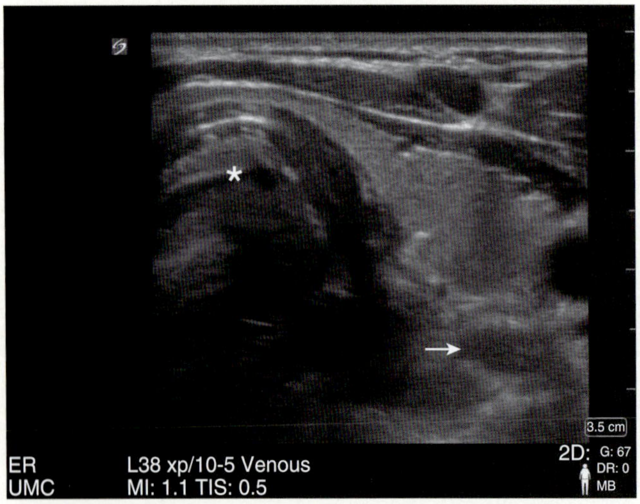

Fig. 41.US2 Angling of the probe and gentle tracheal *(asterisk)* manipulation facilitates visualization of the collapsed esophagus *(arrow)*.

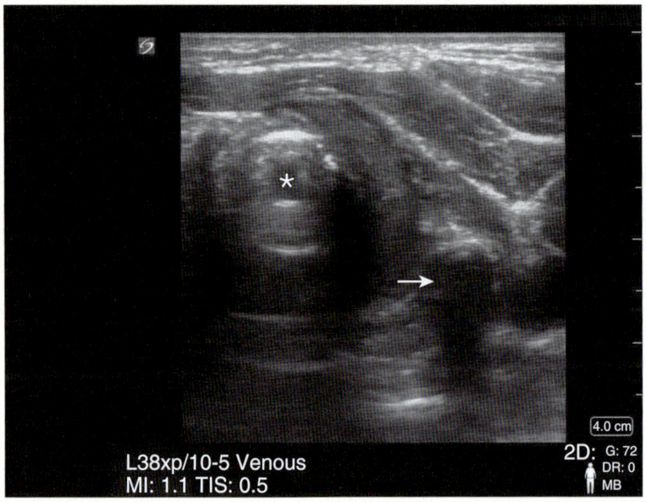

Fig. 41.US3 When the nasogastric tube passes the probe, the esophagus becomes brightly echogenic and creates posterior shadowing *(arrow)*. In this image, an endotracheal tube *(asterisk)* can be visualized in the trachea.

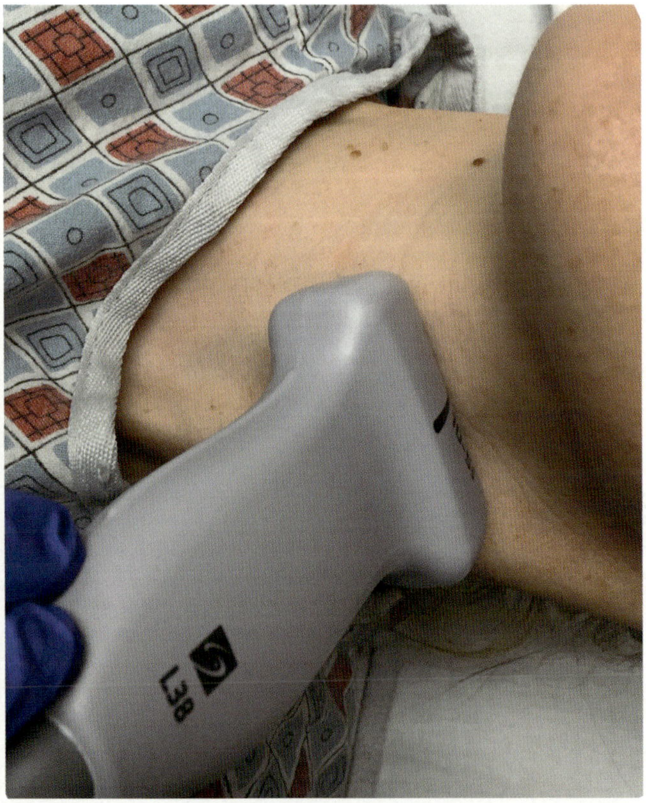

Fig. 41.US4 Lateral cross-sectional views may help confirm that the nasogastric tube is clearly outside of the trachea.

Continued

ULTRASOUND: Assistance in Nasogastric Tube Placement—cont'd

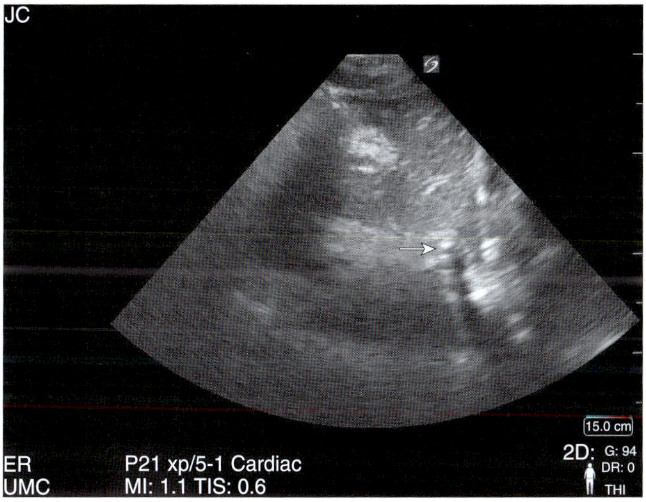

Fig. 41.US5 Visualization of the nasogastric tube in the stomach *(arrow)*. Note the prominent shadow from the tube.

important to distinguish the course of the tube and ensure that the tube is in an extratracheal soft tissue space and not in the trachea. A lateral cross-sectional view with the probe pointed across from the side (by sliding the probe around the neck from the original transverse position, as shown in Fig. 41.US4) or oblique angles of the probe may allow the nasogastric tube to be visualized as being clearly outside the trachea.

Confirmation of tube placement in the stomach is less reliable, even after successful placement. Place the low-frequency probe over the epigastric area and try to visualize the tube. Fluid can be injected through the tube, creating a visible "foggy" disturbance in the stomach. Such confirmation reliably indicates proper placement, but when absent does not imply the tube must be replaced; rather, alternative confirmatory measures should be employed prior to using the tube for instillation of materials. Visualization of the nasogastric tube in the epigastrium on still shots is possible (Fig. 41.US5). Note that still views of the nasogastric tube in the epigastric region can look similar if the tip is in the stomach, distal esophagus, or proximal duodenum.

A quick, simple, but unreliable method of confirmation is to insufflate air into the NG tube and auscultate for a rush of air over the stomach (see Fig. 41.4, *step 8*). If increased pressure is required to instill the air or if no sounds are heard, the tube may be malpositioned or kinked. Suspect an esophageal location if the patient immediately burps on insufflation. Left pulmonary tubes and tubes which have advanced past the stomach into the small bowel often sound so similar to properly placed tubes that misplacements are not detected.[3]

Aspiration of stomach contents, especially if pH-tested, is more reliable and can be performed if the tube position is in question. If the pH is less than 4, there is an approximately 95% chance that the tube is in the stomach and nonrespiratory placement is almost guaranteed.[31] Although aspirated fluid can occasionally be obtained from the lung or pleural space, the pH should be 5.5 or higher.[32] Approximately 4% of correctly placed tubes have aspirates with a pH higher than 5.5. Causes include duodenal reflux, antacids, H_2 blockers, or recent instillation of formula or medications.[32]

If awake and cooperative, ask the patient to talk. If the patient cannot speak, suspect respiratory placement. Note that with small-bore tubes, patients may still be able to speak despite tracheal placement.[33]

Once the correct tube position is tentatively confirmed, secure the tube. If the patient requires abdominal or chest radiographs for other diagnostic purposes, place the NG tube before obtaining the films if the patient's condition permits. An NG tube deviated to the right may occasionally be seen in patients with traumatic rupture of the aorta, but this is not a reliable indicator.

Securing the Tube

The NG tube is generally secured to the patient with tape attached to both the tube and nose (see Fig. 41.4, *step 10*). Excellent purpose-made tape NG holders exist. A butterfly bandage (or tape on each side of the nose) that coils around the NG tube is a typical approach. If the skin is greasy, clean before tape application. Tincture of benzoin applied with a cotton-tipped applicator may be helpful in securing the tube to the nose: make sure to let it dry completely before applying the tape. Mastisol liquid adhesive (Ferndale Laboratories, Inc.) is reportedly more effective than tincture of benzoin to help tape stick, but less commonly available. If the tape fails to stick or requires repositioning, replace both the tape and the tincture of benzoin. It is wise to also secure the tube to the patient's gown so that a tug on the tube will encounter this resistance before pulling on the tape securing the tube to the patient's nose. A rubber band tied around the tube with a slipknot (Fig. 41.7) and pinned to the gown near the patient's shoulder is effective. It is critical to ensure that the tube is secured in such a way that it does not press on the medial or lateral aspect of the nostril. Necrosis or bleeding can result if a tube is not secured correctly.

When a Salem sump is used, keep the blue pigtail above the level of the fluid in the patient's stomach or the stomach contents may leak back through the vent lumen. If a patient needs to ambulate with a sump tube in place, fit the blue pigtail into the plastic connector at the end of the suction lumen. This creates a closed loop that should not leak.

Placement Issues

If the patient is intubated, deflate the balloon of the ET tube briefly to allow passage of the NG tube. In a nonintubated unconscious patient, the NG tube is easily misplaced into the pulmonary tree. This complication may be missed during the procedure in cases in which the gag and cough reflexes are suppressed and the patient cannot talk. In addition, the absence of swallowing may prevent successful passage of the tube. A soft nasopharyngeal airway, well lubricated, is at times

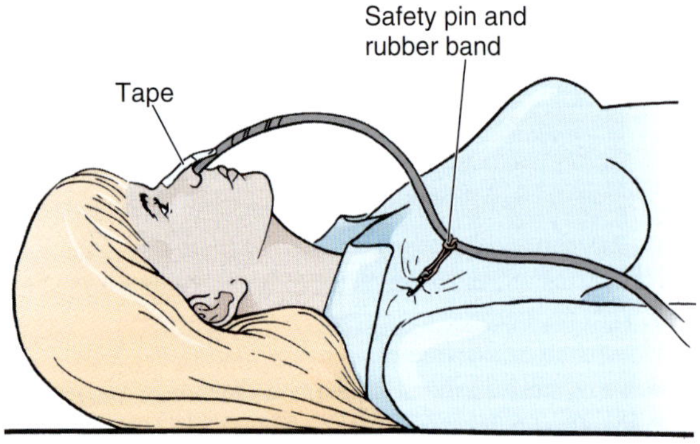

Fig. 41.7 Attach the nasogastric tube to the patient's gown with a rubber band and a safety pin so that a tug on the tube pulls the gown and not the tape holding the tube in the patient's nose.

easier to pass nasally than an NG tube, and then the lubricated NG tube can be passed through it. In addition, it affords some protection to the nasal mucosa if multiple attempts at passing the NG tube are necessary or if it is particularly important to minimize bleeding or trauma. Cooling an NG tube increases its rigidity and coiling it can increase the curvature of the tube, both of which may help pass the tube. Alternatively, the NG tube and larynx can be visualized with a laryngoscope, video laryngoscope, nasopharyngeal laryngoscope, or the GlideScope (Verathon) (see Fig. 41.9B). Under laryngeal visualization, manipulation and lifting of the jaw and neck flexion can help align the tube for passage under direct vision into the esophagus.[34] Displacing the larynx laterally, pressing on the same side as the nostril where the NG is inserted, is also reported to aid tube passage.[35]

In comatose or ventilated patients, several techniques may aid passage of the NG tube. Using Magill forceps to grip the tube or stenting the end of the tube with a gum bougie passed into the most distal tube eye can help stiffen and control the tube. The combination and sequence of techniques used will depend on the clinician's expertise, the equipment available, and the level of sedation.

If less traumatic strategies fail, an ET tube can be prepared with an ID that is slightly larger than the external diameter of the NG tube (e.g., a 7-mm-ID ET tube for nasal passage or an 8-mm tube for the oral technique). Slit it along its lesser curvature from the proximal end to a point 3 cm from its distal end. Lubricate the tube well inside and outside. Pass the slit ET tube directly through the nose into the esophagus.[36] Passage into the esophagus is facilitated by the stiffness of the larger ET tube and does not require active swallowing. Pass the NG tube to depth through the ET tube, remove the ET tube from the esophagus and nares, slit it the rest of the way and remove it. Alternatively, pass the NG tube through the nose into the pharynx and pull it out of the mouth until insertion depth is reached at the nose (or you can pass it deeper and pull it back later). Pass a slit ET tube (often 8 mm) into the esophagus through the mouth, then thread the tip of the NG tube into the ET tube and advance it into the stomach (Fig. 41.8). Remove the slit ET tube from the esophagus. When the distal part of the ET tube is visible, slit the unslit 3-cm distal part with scissors. Remove the ET tube and the NG tube will remain in place.[37] Advance any slack tubing with Magill forceps into the stomach, then pull it back nasally to the final depth required for the NG tube.

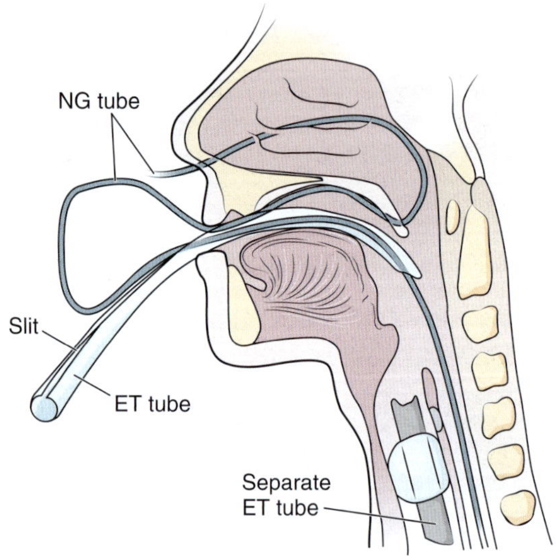

Fig. 41.8 Diagrammatic representation of separation of the nasogastric *(NG)* tube from the guiding endotracheal *(ET)* tube through the slit in the guiding ET tube. The NG tube has first been passed through the nose and is pulled out through the mouth. The tip of the tube is then threaded into the guiding ET tube to ensure passage down the esophagus. The guiding ET tube is removed from the esophagus before being separated from the NG tube. Note the previous placement of another ET tube in the trachea (partially shown) to avert passage of the guiding ET tube into the trachea. (Modified from Sprague DH, Carter SR. An alternate method for nasogastric tube insertion. *Anesthesiology.* 1980;53:436.)

In a particularly passive, intubated, sedated, unconscious, or toothless patient, guiding the NG tube with fingers into the pharynx is occasionally successful (Fig. 41.9A).[38] Displacing the larynx forward by manually gripping and lifting the thyroid cartilage can aid in inserting the tube,[39] as can simple jaw elevation.

Ultimately, if all other methods fail, place a flexible fiberoptic bronchoscope or esophagoscope into and through the esophagus under direct visualization.[39] Thread a guidewire into the stomach. Place the NG tube over the guidewire into the stomach and then remove the guidewire.[40]

Complications

Complications of standard NG tube placement are similar to the problems noted with placement of an NG feeding tube. The complications related to tube misplacement are discussed in that section. In addition, clinicians placing an NG tube in a patient with neck injuries should be cautious of potentiating cervical spine injuries with excessive motion during passage (especially in association with coughing and gagging in an awake patient). Furthermore, passage of an NG tube in an awake patient with a penetrating neck wound may exacerbate hemorrhage should coughing or gagging result. Particularly serious forms of tube misplacement are pulmonary placement (Fig. 41.10) and intracranial placement (Fig. 41.11). In confusing cases, a CT scan will clarify most misplacement issues (Figs. 41.12 and 41.13). NG tubes, when in place for prolonged periods, can cause innocuous gastric bleeding and gastric erosions.

Tension gastrothorax can develop in patients with an intrathoracic stomach. It can occupy much of the left hemithorax and thus displace the heart and lungs and cause a clinical

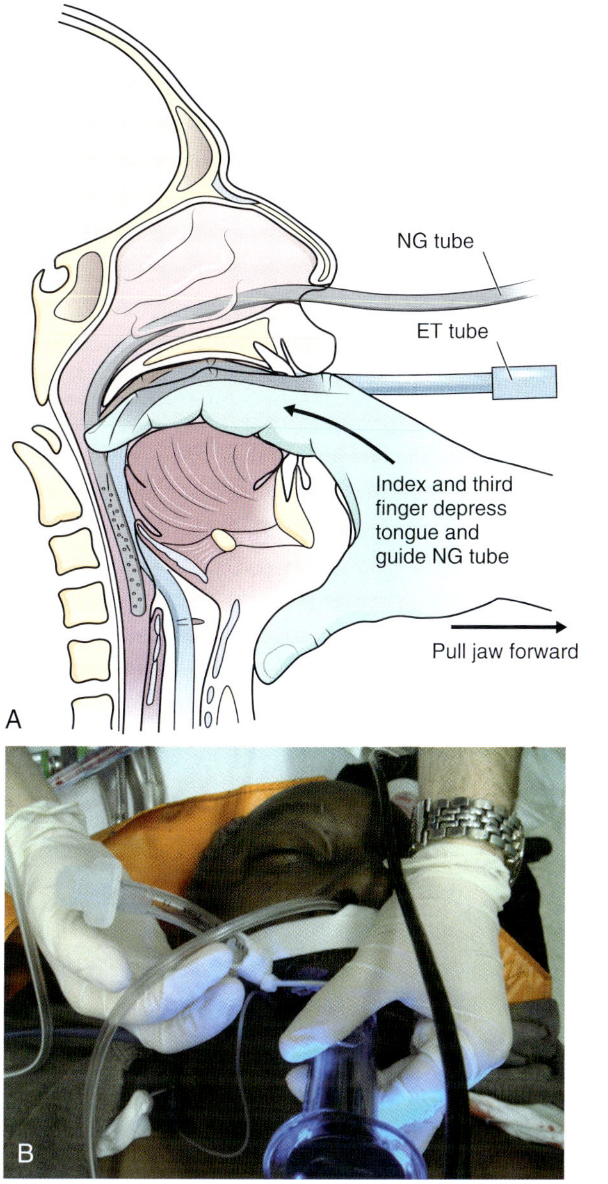

Fig. 41.9 (A) Passage of a nasogastric *(NG)* tube through the nose of an intubated patient can be difficult. An endotracheal tube *(ET)* is in the trachea via the mouth. Place the second and third fingers in the posterior pharynx. Depress the tongue with the fingers. Guide the NG tube down the esophagus by passing it through the second and third fingers. Importantly, place the thumb under the jaw and pull the jaw forward. (B) In this intubated patient, a video laryngoscope (GlideScope) can be used to manipulate the larynx and visualize the passage of the nasogastric tube.

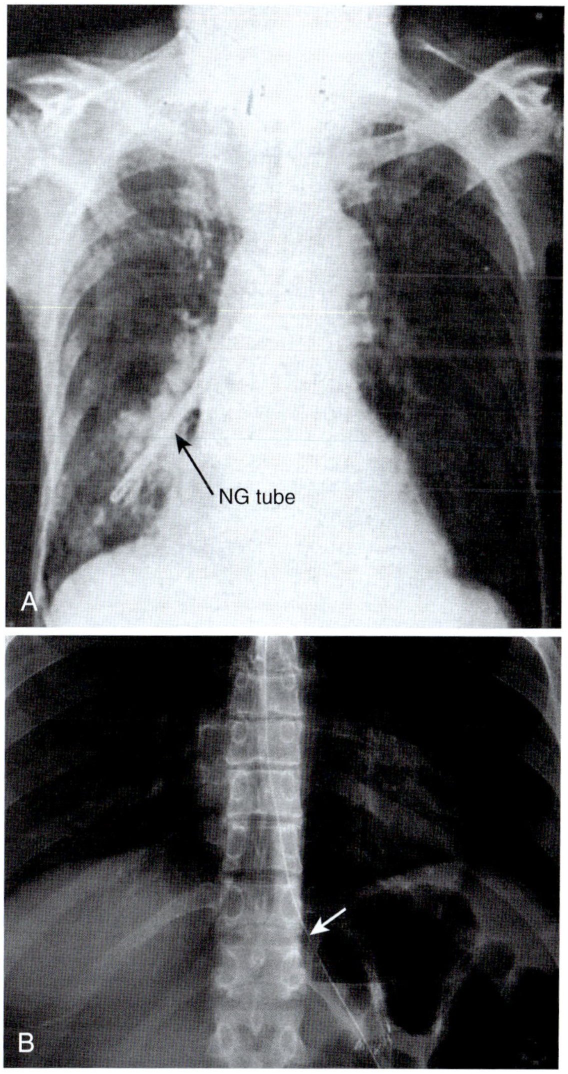

Fig. 41.10 (A) Levin tube inadvertently placed in the right main stem bronchus; an alveolar infiltrate consistent with early pneumonia is also shown. (B) Proper position of the nasogastric *(NG)* tube *(arrow)* is best verified with a radiograph. (A, From Johnson JC. Letter to the editor: back to basics for morbidity-free nasogastric intubation. *JACEP.* 1979;8:289. B, From Thomsen T, Setnik G, eds. *Procedures Consult—Emergency Medicine Module*. Elsevier; 2008.)

syndrome identical to tension pneumothorax. Even though successful passage of an NG tube will relieve tension gastrothorax, the high pressures of a tension gastrothorax may develop because torsion of the stomach in the chest prevents egress of air; such torsion may also prevent ingress of the therapeutic NG tube. The condition is rare enough that its occurrence and management are documented largely via case reports.[41–44] As of 2017 one series of three cases of traumatic gastrothorax found emergency endoscopy had a 100% treatment success rate.[45] Endoscopic relief would be followed by a nasogastric tube. An additional case report found tension gastrothorax was relieved with transthoracic puncture of the stomach with a 16-gauge catheter-over-the-needle device inserted into the second intercostal space in the midclavicular line and then removing the needle. The catheter was left in place attached to intravenous tubing with the distal end under a water seal.[46] A single 16-gauge puncture of the stomach is unlikely to leak and cause pleuritis; such punctures have long been used for placement of percutaneous endoscopic gastrostomy (PEG) tubes. Inserting a chest tube into the stomach is not advisable because gastric fluid may leak into the pleural space. Once the tension on the stomach is relieved, it may be possible to pass the NG tube to prevent the reoccurrence of the problem. The stomach, no longer tense and wedged in the chest, can twist to allow the tube to pass, after which the transthoracic catheter should be removed. Surgical correction of the condition which permitted intrathoracic herniation of the stomach is usually necessary to ensure it does not reoccur. Tension gastrothorax has also been reported in children as a complication of late onset congenital diaphragmatic hernia.[43,44] In all cases, emergency

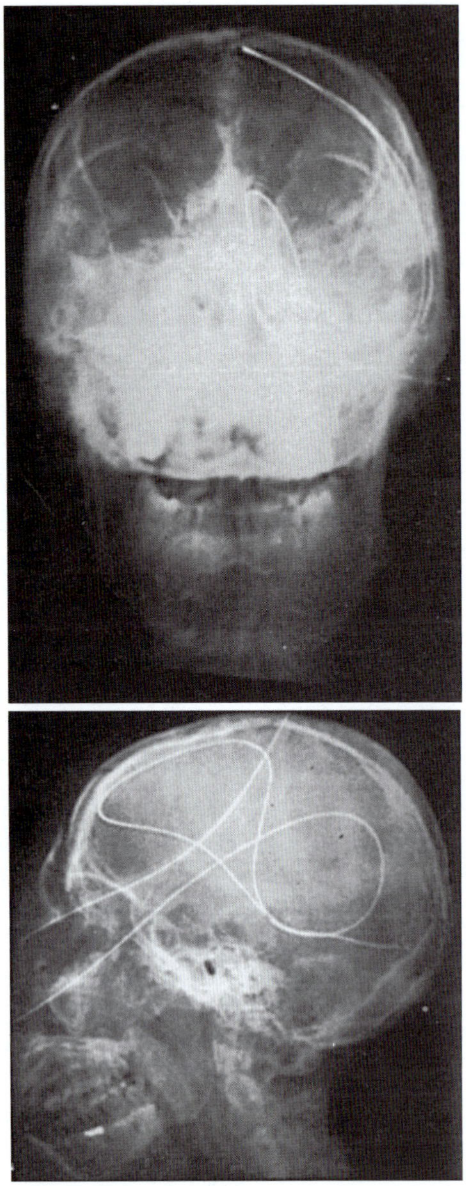

Fig. 41.11 Anteroposterior and lateral skull radiographs demonstrate intracranial insertion of a nasogastric tube in a patient with multiple skull fractures. (From Johnson JC. Letter to the editor: back to basics for morbidity-free nasogastric intubation. *JACEP.* 1979;8:289.)

surgery is needed if prompt relief by less invasive measures is not possible.

REPLACEMENT OF NASOENTERIC FEEDING TUBES

Indications and Contraindications

The most common indication for replacement of a feeding tube in the ED is unintentional removal of a preexisting feeding tube. In one prospective study, 38% of tubes were removed unintentionally. Although some of these tubes had fallen out or had been coughed out, more than half were pulled out by the patient.[47] Tube rupture, deterioration, or clogging may also necessitate replacement. Management of a clogged or nonirrigating feeding tube is discussed in the later section on clogged feeding tubes.

Feeding Tube Site

Three major classes of enteral feeding tubes are in common use and are classified according to the site of insertion and according to the location of the tip of the tube. Tubes can enter through the nares, a cervical ostomy, or an abdominal ostomy. Enteral tubes are often categorized by the location of the tip of the tube. Tubes may terminate primarily in the stomach, such as a gastrostomy (G) or PEG tube (Fig. 41.14). They may terminate in the jejunum (J tube) (Fig. 41.15) or in both the stomach and the small intestine (a PEG-J tube). To confuse the issue, some tubes enter the stomach and terminate in the stomach (G tube) or in the proximal part of the small bowel (J tube), whereas others enter the GI tract directly through the wall of the small bowel (J tube).

Most gastric tubes are PEG tubes. They are placed endoscopically with local anesthesia and without a surgical incision. J tubes that enter the small bowel directly are inserted surgically under general anesthesia, require a surgical incision, and result in a surgical scar at the insertion site. Gastric feeding results in better digestion than intestinal feeding does. Jejunal feeding reduces reflux and aspiration.[48] Normally, approximately 20% of the gastric antral contents pass into the duodenum, with 80% refluxing back into the body of the stomach for further mixing, so proximal duodenal feeding is of limited benefit in preventing aspiration.[49,50] If the feeding tube is placed in the antrum of the stomach or in the small bowel, enteral feeding solution passing into the small bowel may not be tolerated and can result in diarrhea and paradoxical decreased nutrition.[49,50]

Procedure: Nasoenteral Feeding Tubes

The clinician should explain the procedure to the patient before passage of the tube. Replacement of a nasoenteric feeding tube requires greater time and effort if the patient is uncooperative or has a physically obstructing lesion. It is generally advisable to restrain the hands of patients with dementia, those who are impaired, or other patients who are unable to cooperate with the procedure. Prepare the nares before passage of the tube using the procedure for primary NG tube placement. If a feeding tube stylet is used, lubricate and insert it into the feeding tube before introducing it into the naris. Tube stylets can be lubricated with water-soluble jelly. If using the Dobhoff, Entri-Flex (Biosearch), or another tube with preapplied lubricant, you may need to activate the lubricant with a 5-mL flush of water. Never allow the stylet to protrude beyond the end of the feeding tube because these stiff, small-diameter wires have the capacity to scratch the esophagus and allow the creation of a false passage. The stylet may lock into position on the tube at the proximal end and should be properly secured.

When the patient is uncooperative or cannot drink, introduce 5 to 15 mL of water into the mouth or into the proximal end of the feeding tube with a syringe; this may induce swallowing and facilitate passage of the tube. Although the patient may not swallow for several minutes, wait for swallowing because this may mean the difference between a coiled or pulmonary tube placement and successful passage.

Confirmation of Placement

Auscultatory confirmation of tube placement can be misleading, so confirm proper placement of the tube with a radiograph

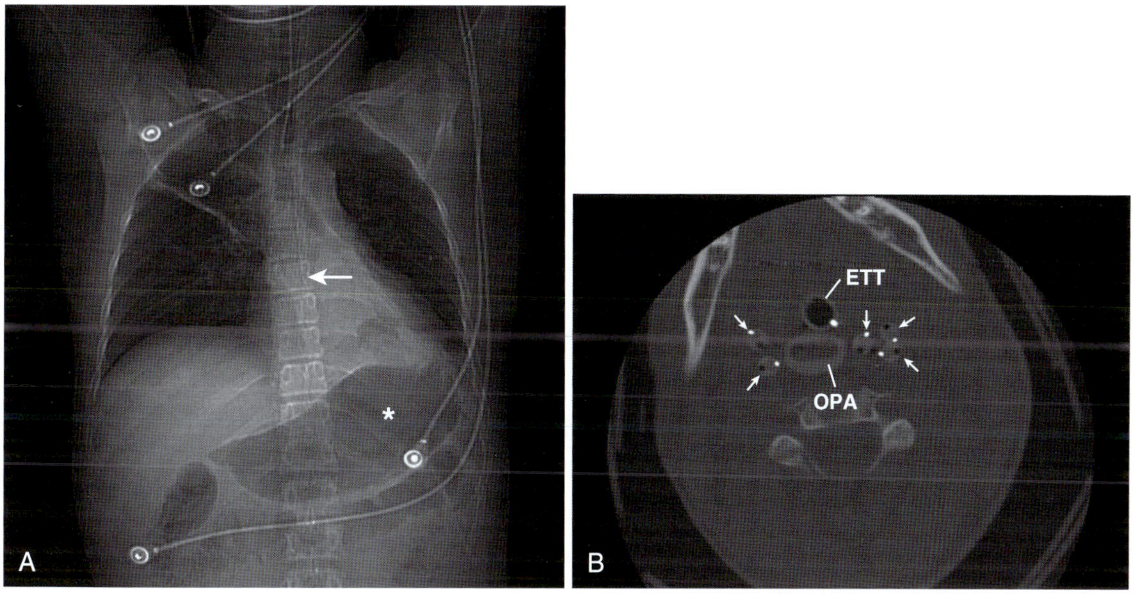

Fig. 41.12 (A) In this scout view of a thoracic computed tomography scan, the tip of the nasogastric tube descends only to the level of the T7 vertebrae *(arrow)*. The stomach is overinflated with air *(asterisk)*. (B) An axial image from the neck reveals that the nasogastric tube is coiled multiple times in the pharynx *(arrows)* and thus never reached the stomach. *ETT*, Endotracheal tube; *OPA*, oropharyngeal airway.

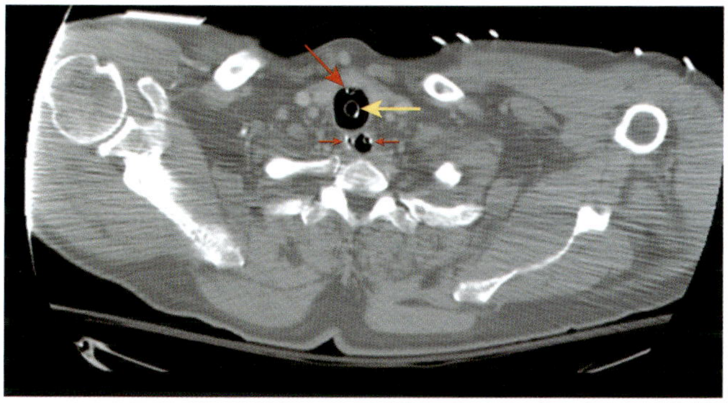

Fig. 41.13 This axial computed tomography (CT) scan at the superior thoracic level demonstrates tracheal placement of a nasogastric tube (NGT). The NGT is seen twice in the esophagus *(small red arrows)*, which suggests that it first descended and then coiled and ascended in the esophagus. It then coiled again, turned downward, and ultimately came to rest in the trachea *(large red arrow)* anterior to the endotracheal tube *(yellow arrow)*. Luckily, no oral contrast media was injected through the NGT before the CT scan.

before feeding.[3] However, radiographic confirmation of tube placement may also be misleading. In viewing the radiograph, it is particularly important to study the area around the carina. An esophageal tube shows at most a mild change in course, whereas a tracheally placed tube usually deviates significantly as it travels into the right or left main stem bronchus. The end of an NG tube may appear to be in the stomach yet may actually be in the left lung behind and below the top of the diaphragm.[51] When a stylet has been used for passage, leave it in the feeding tube for the radiograph because the tube's course is not always visible without it. The stylets of most tubes are designed to allow insufflation and aspiration while in place. Even when stomach entry is certain, the intestinal location may be misleading on a radiograph. A nasoenteric tube may lie completely to the left of midline and yet have its tip in the duodenum, or it may occupy a position overlying the right side of the abdomen yet not have entered the duodenum. A contrast-enhanced study is necessary to ascertain duodenal position when pulmonary placement has been ruled out.[52,53]

Examine the radiograph also for the presence of mediastinal air or pneumothorax, which may suggest pulmonary or esophageal puncture. An esophageal puncture should be evaluated with endoscopy and may require surgery, depending on the size of the rent.

The end-bulb of many nasoduodenal tubes will pass into the duodenum after positioning the patient in the right decubitus position for an hour. Some researchers recommend pretreatment with metoclopramide to enhance gastric emptying.[54–56] One investigator found that metoclopramide enhances duodenal passage of nasogastrically placed feeding tubes in diabetic, but not nondiabetic, patients.[52] Gastric antral motility in diabetic patients is often impaired; metoclopramide helps restore normal synchronized activity in these patients but has little effect on emptying in those with normal antral function. The usual dose of metoclopramide is 10 mg, administered intravenously. In addition, 3 mg/kg of erythromycin lactobionate given intravenously over a 1-hour period works similarly and may be effective even if metoclopramide fails.[57] Endoscopy or fluoroscopy may be necessary if positioning and metoclopramide are not successful.

Complications

Pulmonary intubation is an uncommon but well-known and potentially fatal complication of insertion of nasal feeding tubes (see Fig. 41.10A). Coughing and respiratory distress are the most common symptoms of respiratory passage of an NG tube, but there may be relatively few apparent symptoms in patients with dementia, altered mental status, or comatose patients.[58] Decreased mentation and an absent cough reflex are predisposing factors for unrecognized nasopulmonary intubation with NG

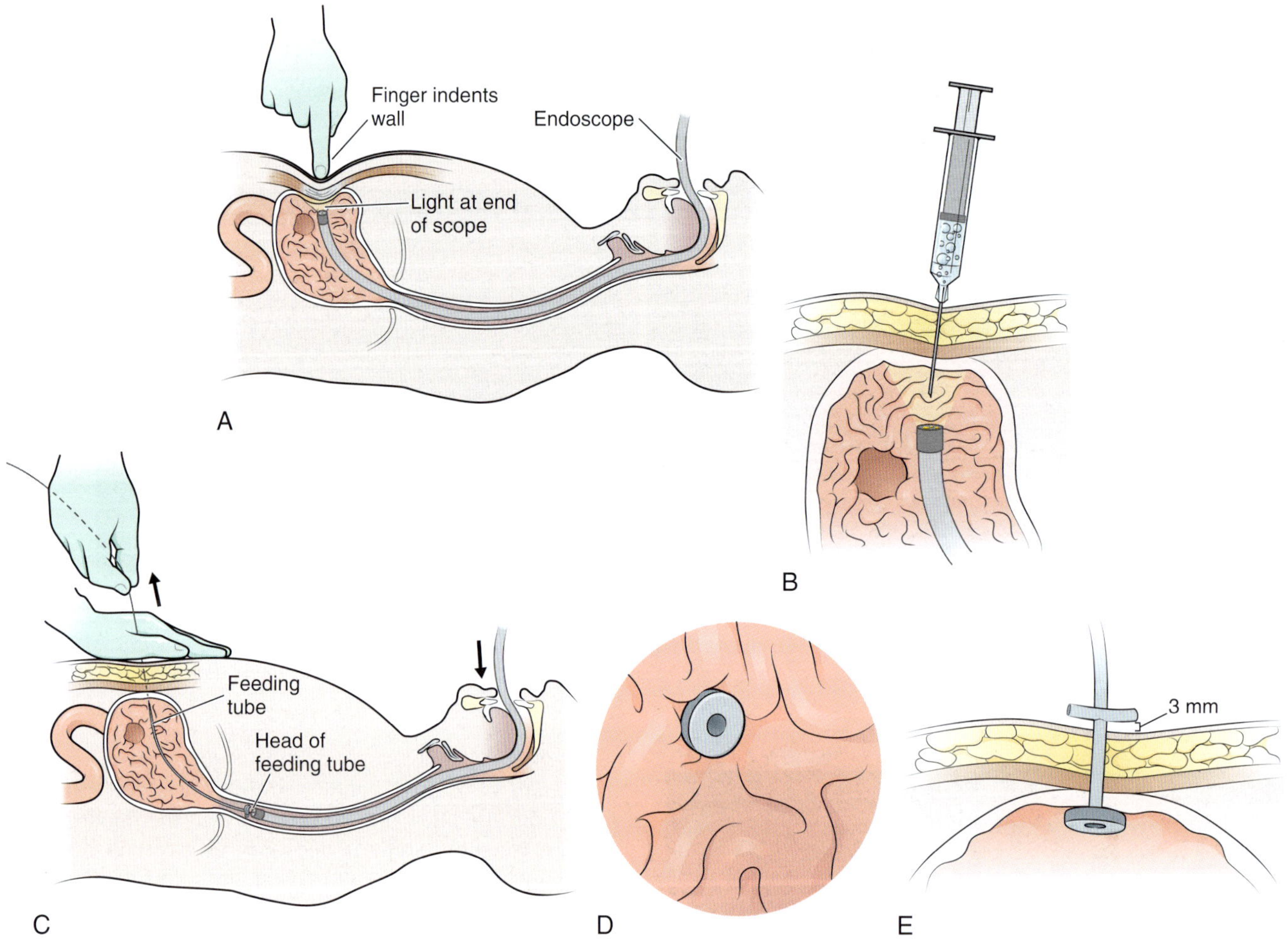

Fig. 41.14 Placement of a percutaneous endoscopic gastrostomy tube. (A) Under conscious sedation, pass a lighted endoscope into the stomach. Indent the skin with a finger to determine the optimal puncture site where the stomach and abdominal wall are closest, with no bowel between. (B) Fill a syringe with saline and advance it percutaneously to the selected entry point until the tip of the needle is seen entering from the gastric lumen through the endoscope. If air is aspirated and no needle tip is seen, the needle is in the bowel, not the stomach. (C) Push and pull the scope/snare/feeding tube combination into position (*arrows* show direction of travel). (D) Pull the head of the feeding tube into contact with the gastric mucosa. (E) Use an external bolster or crossbar to keep the tube snug against the skin and gastric wall, but not so tight that it causes ischemia of the intervening tissue.

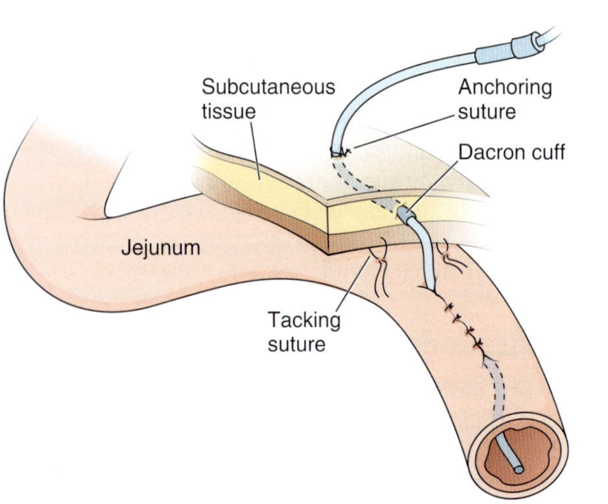

Fig. 41.15 Formation of a Witzel tunnel and final permanent placement of a jejunal catheter. (From Wiedeman JE, Smith VC. Use of the Hickman catheter for jejunal feedings in children. *Surg Gynecol Obstet.* 1986;162:69.)

tubes.[3] Misplacement is far more likely in patients with ET or tracheostomy tubes, conscious or not, perhaps because tracheal stimulation by a misplaced tube is less likely to be appreciated or communicated. A small end-bulb (e.g., 2.7 mm in diameter) can slip past a tracheal high-volume, low-pressure cuff and easily pass to the periphery of the lung.[3,58–62] Pneumothorax may result when an NG tube dissects into or is withdrawn from the pulmonary parenchyma.[63] Bloody aspirate from a tube should heighten awareness of possible tissue damage.

A clogged or nonfunctional NG tube may be difficult to remove. Fluoroscopy may allow careful insertion of a guidewire or stylet into an in situ tube to facilitate removal. Fluoroscopy may also identify the mechanical problem interfering with removal of the tube. Segments bent double are probably the most common cause. Knots, though uncommon, do occur. Do not use excessive force to remove an NG tube because serious injury to the patient may result.

Premature removal of an NG tube is the most frequent complication of the use of NG feeding tubes. For long-term use or frequent removal of an NG tube by a patient, a gastric feeding tube will probably be inserted. To help prevent removal of an NG tube by an uncooperative patient, or if it will be in long-term, secure the NG tube to a loop anchor passed in the same naris. The anchor works by aversive stimulation of the soft palate and nose, with distraction from the NG tube rather than by mechanical stabilization of the tube.

Sax and Bower recommend a technique for creating a separate NG tube anchor.[64] Cut a soft, weighted nasoenteric tube approximately 12 inches from the top. Pass a heavy (2-0) silk suture through the tube to exit the side hole. Insert the guidewire with care because it must not protrude from the inserted end. Sedate the patient if uncooperative. Insert the tube through the anesthetized naris into the nasopharynx, grasp it with Magill forceps, and pull to remove it through the mouth (Fig. 41.16A). Trim excess tubing without cutting the silk suture. Make a closed loop by tying the silk suture in front of the nose. Leave the loop long enough so that it does not apply continuous pressure to the nose or palate while at rest. Pass the nasal feeding tube through the same nostril and secure it to the loop (see Fig. 41.16B). This anchor is simpler to construct and more comfortable than anchors that pass through the opposite nostril.[64]

Complications of properly placed nasoenteric tubes include nasopharyngeal erosion, esophageal reflux, tracheoesophageal fistula, gagging, rupture of esophageal varices, and otitis media.[65] One survey of nasogastrically fed patients found that the most distressing features of having an NG tube for feeding were deprivation of tasting, drinking, and chewing of food; soreness of the nose; rhinitis; esophagitis; mouth breathing; and the sight of other patients who were eating.[66]

Checking feeding tolerance is difficult with small-gauge feeding tubes. Aspiration of tubes to check for residuals is not recommended with tubes 9 Fr in size or smaller. Aspiration is likely to clog the tubes because they collapse under pressure and relatively small particles can occlude the tube. For the same reasons, the residual is likely to be inaccurate.[67] Ultrasonic measurement of gastric residuals is not widely used but shows promise.[68–70]

Patient or Nursing Instructions

To maintain patency of the catheter, small tubes should be flushed with 20 mL to 30 mL of tap water at least two to three times daily and after the administration of medication.[53,67] Medications should be in liquid form or completely dissolved or they may clog the tube. (Methods of dealing with a clogged tube are discussed later in this chapter.) The tube should be anchored to the nose and face in such a way that it is not in contact with the skin at the nasal opening. This reduces tube discomfort and prevents necrosis of the alae, nares, and distal septum. Patients who exhibit a tendency to pull on their tubes need adequate restraints. Patients receiving tube feedings should have their head elevated to at least 30 degrees above the horizontal.[67]

PHARYNGOSTOMY AND ESOPHAGOSTOMY FEEDING TUBES

Cervical pharyngostomy and cervical esophagostomy tubes are unlikely to be replaced in the ED, but the concept of these feeding tubes is illustrated in Fig. 41.17. Complications of pharyngostomy and esophagostomy include local soft tissue irritation, accidental extubation because of excessive length of the external tube, pulmonary aspiration from vomiting, arterial erosion with exsanguination, and esophagitis or stricture of the esophagus from reflux.

GASTROENTEROSTOMY AND JEJUNOSTOMY TUBES

See Video 41.4. A nursing home patient with a nonfunctioning or displaced feeding tube represents a common ED scenario. The clinician cannot always determine the location of the original feeding tube by simply looking at a patient who arrives in the ED for replacement of the tube. Nevertheless, the emergency clinician should attempt to ensure that the terminal end of a replaced tube is in the same viscus as the original was. External inspection may or may not reveal where a feeding tube should terminate. Contrast-enhanced studies and fluoroscopy usually provide such information (Fig. 41.18).

G tubes are available in various types (Fig. 41.19). Tubes are kept in place by either a modified end (such as a mushroom tip) or an inflatable balloon. A de Pezzer (mushroom) tube, a Corflo tube (CORPAK MedSystems), or a Foley G tube is designed only for intragastric termination. Some tubes have two lumens, one terminating in the stomach for decompression and the other in the small bowel for feeding. These can be confused with tubes that have two entrances to one lumen (one for continuous feeding and the other for medications) and tubes that have a second lumen leading to an inflatable balloon. An original tube is not usually a Foley or balloon-tipped tube. An original PEG tube is pictured in Fig. 41.20. Note that on cross section, this original long tube has no balloon or port to inflate a balloon but has a mushroom end that is removed by traction.

Foley catheters are not ideal as long-term feeding tubes. They clog easily and the balloon disintegrates in stomach acid. They may be used temporarily but should be replaced with specialized feeding tubes when feasible (Fig. 41.21). A call from a nursing home indicating that a tube has been pulled out should be answered with the advice that a Foley catheter be used immediately to keep the stoma open. Always inflate the balloon with saline and use a bolster to prevent migration of the tube.

The clinician has a few options when faced with the task of replacing a feeding tube. Unfortunately, old records or nursing home personnel rarely give specific information that is helpful to the emergency clinician. If only a stoma exists, one may request that the nursing home describe or send the prior tube to the ED. If no surgical scar is seen at the stoma site, the tube is almost certainly a G tube or a G tube that terminated in the jejunum. When in doubt, pass a Foley catheter and, leaving the balloon uninflated, tape it to the skin and refer the patient to a consultant or the original referring clinician. Some type of tube must be placed to stent the stoma, or the stoma will quickly close (in a matter of hours) and the patient might require a more complicated procedure to regain access. The only real concern of placing a gastric tube into the jejunum is that the balloon will produce intestinal obstruction if it is fully inflated.

If the tube is nonfunctioning yet still in place, the clinician must make a judgment regarding the risk versus benefit of removal and replacement, versus an attempt at unclogging the tube (see the subsequent discussion on unclogging). The major concern is that a new tube may be misplaced (i.e., into the peritoneal cavity). If it appears that a skin incision

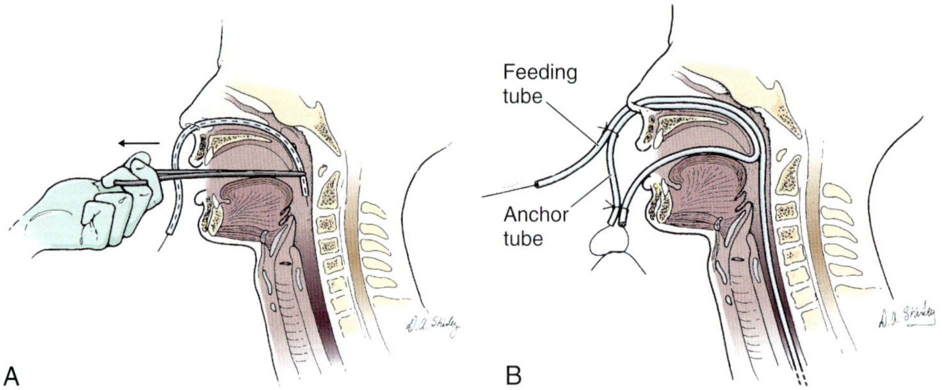

Fig. 41.16 Placement of a nasogastric (NG) tube anchor to secure a companion NG or feeding tube in an uncooperative patient who repeatedly pulls out the feeding tube. (A) Using forceps, grasp the tube in the pharynx and pull it out through the mouth (*arrow* shows direction of travel). This will serve as an anchor tube. (B) Tie the ends of the short anchor tube together to form a loop, and tie the companion NG or feeding tube to the anchor loop.

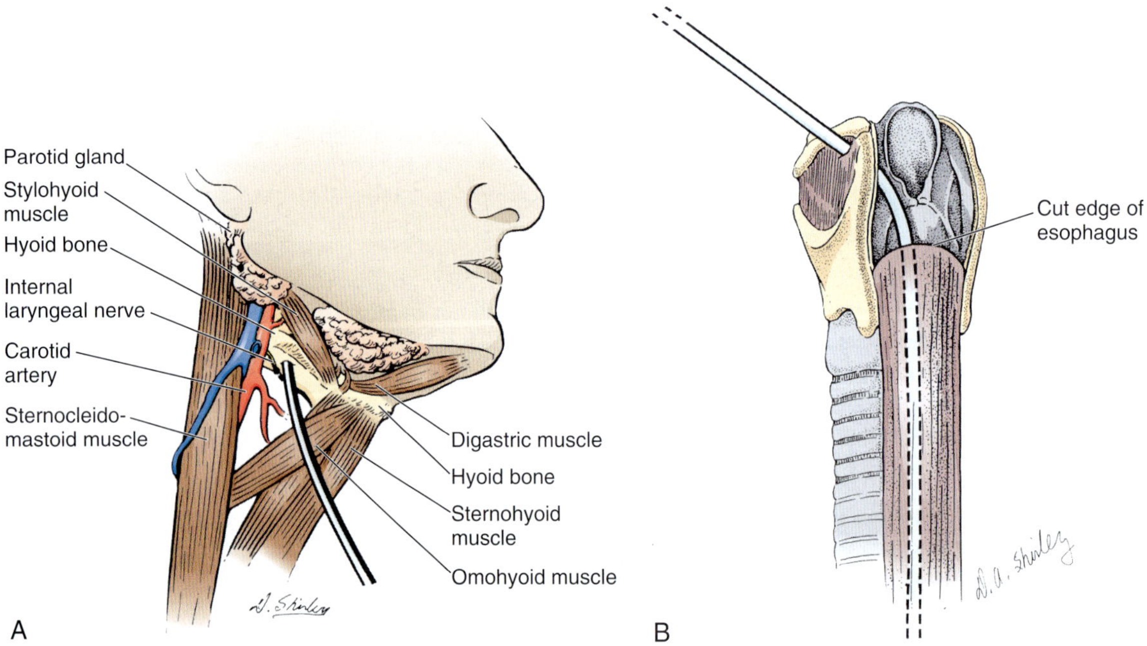

Fig. 41.17 (A) Pharyngostomy feeding tube. (B) Pathway for an esophagostomy or pharyngostomy feeding tube.

was used to place the tube, it is unlikely that the patient has an easily removable tube. If the patient has signs of a complication (e.g., infection, ileus, intestinal obstruction), surgical consultation is warranted. Note that a migrated tube, with the balloon or tube obstructing the gastric outlet, is a common cause of gastric distention, persistent vomiting, or signs of intestinal obstruction. This is easily remedied (see procedural description in section on Complications and Fig. 41.22).

Most PEG tubes do not have sutures joining the stomach with the abdominal wall, so there is potential for a replaced tube to end up in the peritoneal cavity. Adhesions, however, usually keep the stomach appropriately positioned, but only after the tract has matured. Nonoperative tube replacement techniques are safe only through an established tract between the skin and the bowel. Catheter replacement should not be attempted in the immediate postoperative period. A simple gastrostomy takes approximately a week to form a tract.[71] A stable tract may take 2 or 3 weeks longer to form if healing is compromised.

Poor nutrition is the most common element compromising wound healing in patients requiring a feeding tube. A Witzel tunnel may take up to 3 weeks after the operation to mature sufficiently for safe nonoperative tube replacement (see Fig. 41.15).

Equipment for Replacing a Dislodged Tube

Equipment for replacing a feeding tube through a matured site includes gloves, a stethoscope, a feeding tube, an external bolster, lubricant, a basin, and a syringe that fits the tube. Tincture of benzoin, tape, and absorbent dressing material may be used to dress the wound, although many are better left undressed.[72] Some feeding tubes require special plugs or connectors. Others need to be pinched with a clamp when not in use to prevent leakage. Some tubes are placed with the aid of accompanying guidewires or stents.

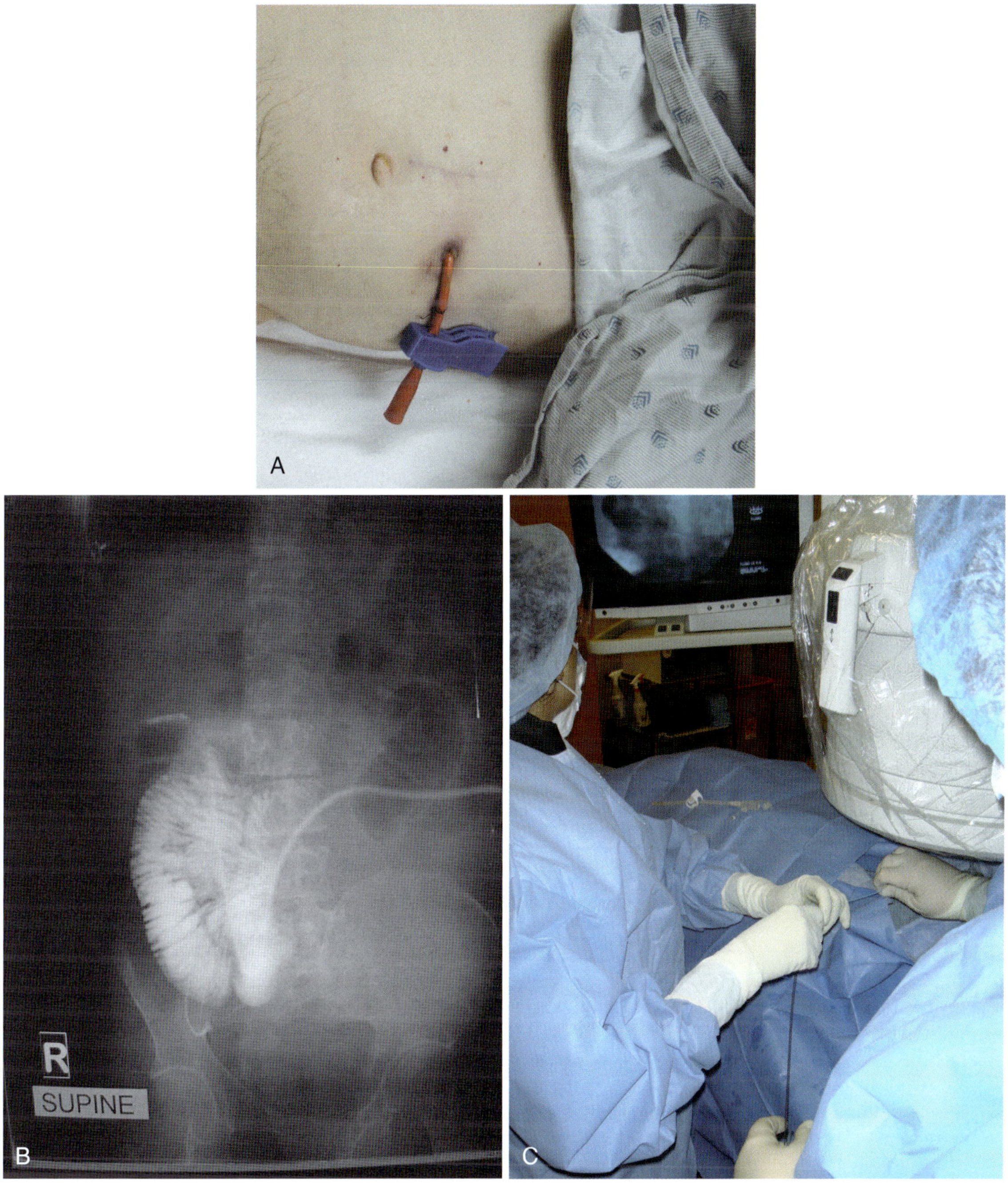

Fig. 41.18 (A) Without old records, the exact type and positioning of this nonfunctioning feeding tube are unknown. The operative scar on the abdominal wall suggests an implanted tube, not a simple gastric tube. (B) Injection of contrast material before removal of the tube demonstrates the tip of the tube ending in the small bowel, not the stomach. (C) If the tube has been removed and questions remain about the type of tube and circumstances of placement, a new tube is best placed under fluoroscopy with guidewire assistance.

The easiest tube to replace is one that has been removed in the ED or dislodged for only a few hours (Fig. 41.23). The stoma closes quite quickly, so replacement is best done as soon as possible. Gently probe the stoma site with a thin blunt object such as a cotton-tipped applicator, to determine patency and direction of the tract. In selected cases, a hemostat can gently dilate the opening to accept a replacement tube. Do all such attempts carefully to avoid creating a false tract. Use local anesthetic around the stoma if exploration causes pain. Bleeding is common. After the tube is passed, restrain the hands to avoid removal of the tube by uncooperative patients.

Removal of a Transabdominal Feeding Tube

A feeding tube may need to be removed because it is irreversibly clogged, leaking, or broken; persistently develops kinks; is too large or too small; causes a hypersensitivity reaction; is associated with an abscess; or is not the appropriate length for feeding into the desired viscus. Before a new transabdominal feeding tube is inserted, remove the old tube. Most, but not all tubes, can be removed without endoscopy. Before attempting to remove the tube in place, it is imperative to know whether it is safe to remove. Standard de Pezzer or mushroom

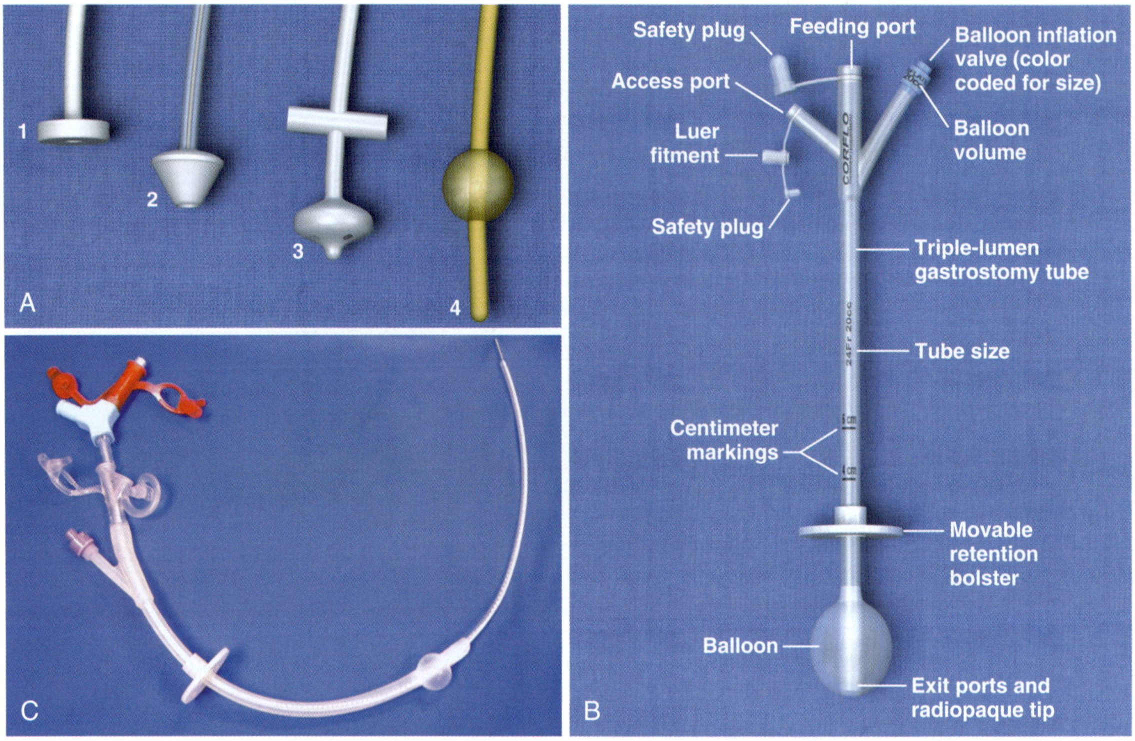

Fig. 41.19 (A) Various types of gastrostomy tubes. *1*, Silicone catheter (American Endoscopy). *2*, Polyurethane catheter with a collapsible foam flange (to collapse, the tube should be cut). *3*, Latex catheter with a movable external bolster and an internal mushroom or de Pezzer–type flange on the end (American Endoscopy). *4*, Balloon (Foley) catheter. (B) A user-friendly gastrostomy tube is supplied by VIASYS MedSystems. The CORFLO-dual GT gastrostomy tube is packaged with lubricant, a prefilled syringe for inflating the balloon, and an extension set. The color-coded inflation valve indicates tube size (12 to 24 Fr). The silicone tube uses a retention balloon and a movable bolster. Note that the retention bolster is designed to prevent inward migration of the tube and not to be an anchoring device sutured to the skin. (C) A gastric balloon jejunal feeding tube enters the stomach and delivers feedings into the jejunum.

catheters that have been modified with bolsters or rings at the time of endoscopic or surgical insertion may no longer be safe to remove with traction. Tubes are occasionally secured with sutures or rigid internal bumpers or stays. It is rare, however, to encounter a tube that cannot be removed with traction/countertraction. Modest force may be required. Use a hand for countertraction and be prepared for a pop and splattering of gastric contents (Fig. 41.24). The tube and end mushroom will narrow with traction, and the tube should come out easily. The inner crossbar, if present, may remain in the stomach when the rest of the feeding tube complex is removed by traction. The crossbar will pass in stool and is unlikely to cause obstruction in adults. In small children, obstruction is a possibility, and the crossbar should be removed by endoscopy.[72]

Recently placed feeding tubes may need to be left in until a tract has formed (1 to 3 weeks, depending on the procedure), even if the tube is nonfunctional.

A simple Foley catheter G tube is the easiest to remove. Deflate the Foley balloon and the tube should slide right out. If the Foley balloon cannot be deflated, cut the tube to allow the balloon to deflate. Do not cut the catheter so close to the abdomen that it will be impossible to maintain a grip on it for removal by traction if the balloon still does not deflate. The balloon may also be punctured to cause it to deflate. To puncture a Foley balloon, apply traction on the catheter to draw the balloon up against the ostomy (Fig. 41.25). Using the taut feeding tube as a guide, pass a small-gauge needle along the tube to puncture the balloon. It may be necessary to try again on the other side of the catheter because the balloon may be inflated asymmetrically and contact with the needle may be established on one side and not the other. Be careful not to track away from the ostomy into the patient's abdominal wall or to cause separate punctures of the stomach. Allow a minute for the balloon to deflate before making another attempt at removal by traction.

If it is not possible to pull the inner bolster or mushroom out through the ostomy, another somewhat controversial option is to cut the tube at the skin, push the remaining short stump into the stomach, and rely on later rectal passage. Although obstruction or impaction is infrequent, it can occur, and this alternative has the potential to be problematic in children or patients who have had previous impaction, potential for bowel obstruction, or stool-passing problems. Rigid or large internal mushrooms and bolsters, the very kind that cause the most difficulty with percutaneous removal, are also more likely to cause difficulty with rectal passage. In no case should a device be released into the gut with a long length of tubing attached. Remember that double-part tubes may have an additional length of tubing for duodenal or jejunal feeding that extends far past the inner bolster. Korula and Harma reported successful intestinal elimination of 63 of 64 G tubes that were cut at the skin entrance and advanced into the stomach through the stoma.[73] These cases included tubes with internal bumpers, and success occurred regardless of the nature of the patient's

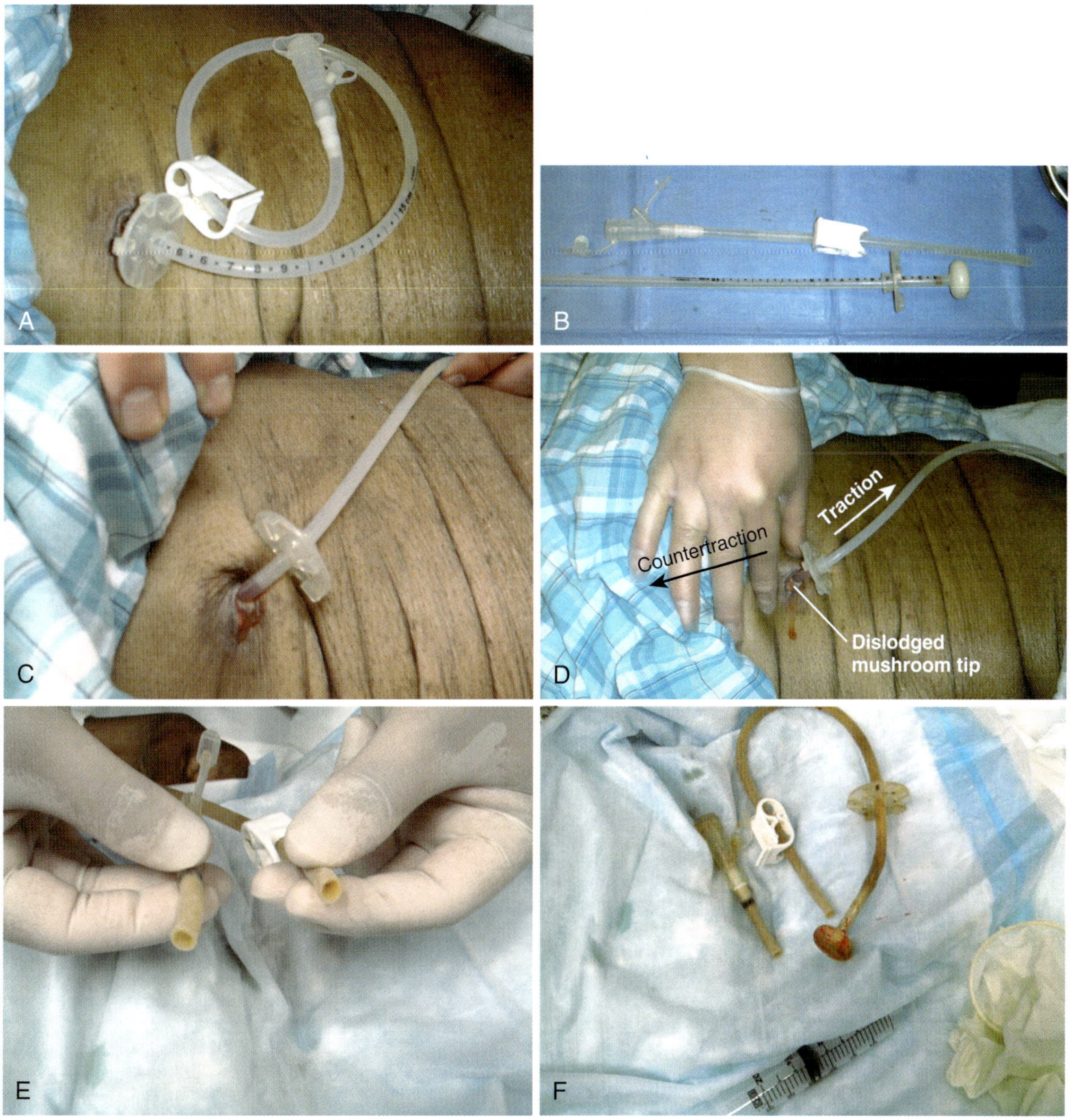

Fig. 41.20 (A) This type of tube serves as the original percutaneous endoscopic gastrostomy (PEG) device. It has a mushroom head, not a balloon. (B) When replaced, a balloon-type tube (upper tube) is used in place of the original mushroom tip tube (lower tube). (C) This original tube is leaking because the mushroom tip has been pulled out of the stomach lumen and is lodged in the soft tissue of the abdominal wall. (D) If the tube tract has matured (at least 2 weeks after placement), it may be removed by traction/countertraction. Significant force may be required; be prepared for a pop and splattering of gastric contents. (E) It is easy to determine whether there is a balloon at the end of a PEG tube that cannot be removed. Simply cut the tube, and if there is no additional port or channel to inflate the balloon, then (F) it must be the type of tube that can be removed by traction.

underlying medical disorder, age, or method of original tube placement. However, no patient had suspected obstruction or potential for obstruction (e.g., no previous radiotherapy, inflammatory bowel disease). The one lodged tube required endoscopic removal from the pylorus. In most cases, passage of the tube was documented by sequential radiographs, with a mean interval of 24 days until passage (range, 4 to 181 days).

Some clinicians and surgeons strongly condemn cutting off the tube at the skin, even when the risks posed by the procedure are very low. It is always advisable to contact the patient's private clinician before cutting the tube. In some cases, endoscopic retrieval of the tube remnant is preferred over allowing rectal passage, and the tube should not be cut until just before or during endoscopy to ensure that migration does not occur before endoscopy.

Securing a Transabdominal Feeding Tube

If an external bolster is used, no additional means of securing the tube is necessary if the patient is not prone to pulling it out. Some clinicians tape tubes to the skin rather than using a bolster or use special adhesive devices designed to control the tube and prevent ingress or egress, such as the Drain/Tube Attachment Device or Flexi-Trak (ConvaTec). Tape is particularly vulnerable to problems because the stress that the tape places on the skin as the tube pulls on the tape can

G-Tube Replacement (With Foley Catheter)

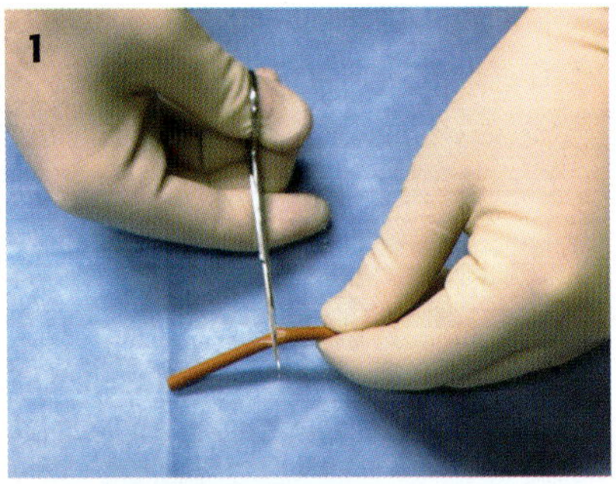

To make a bolster, cut a 3-cm segment of tubing from the proximal end of another Foley catheter. (A red rubber catheter is used in this case). A bolster will prevent migration of the tube, which can cause gastric obstruction.

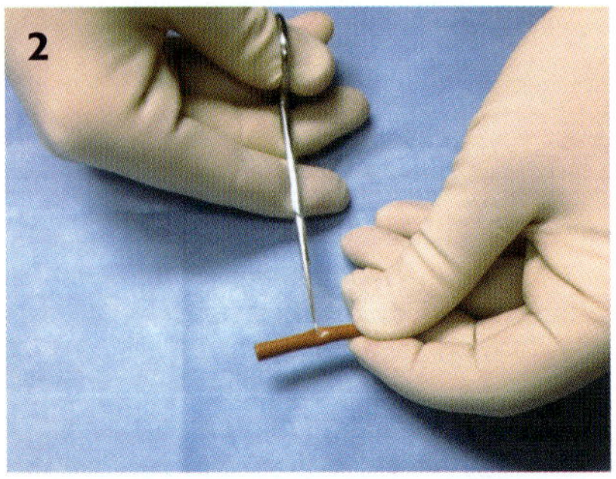

Cut a small hole (on each side) in the middle of the 3-cm segment.

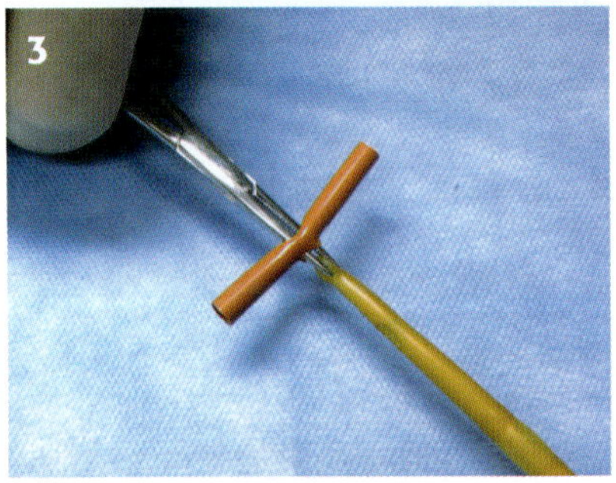

Insert a hemostat through the holes in the new bolster and grasp the feeding tube.

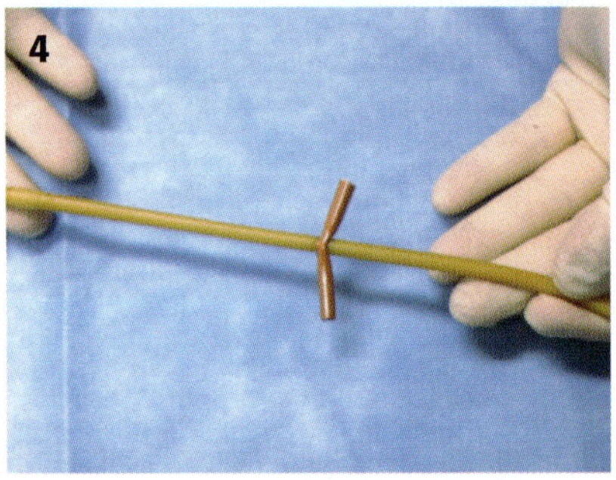

Pull the feeding tube through the bolster.

It should be placed 1 cm above the external abdominal skin.

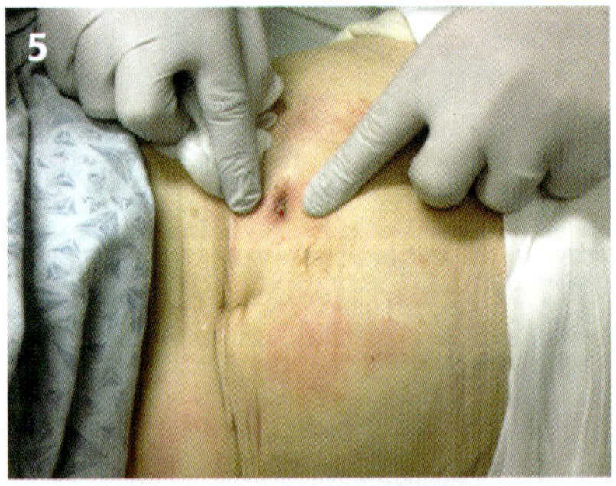

Identify and inspect the stoma.

Surrounding scars may suggest that the tube is in fact an implanted jejunal tube, not a simple G tube.

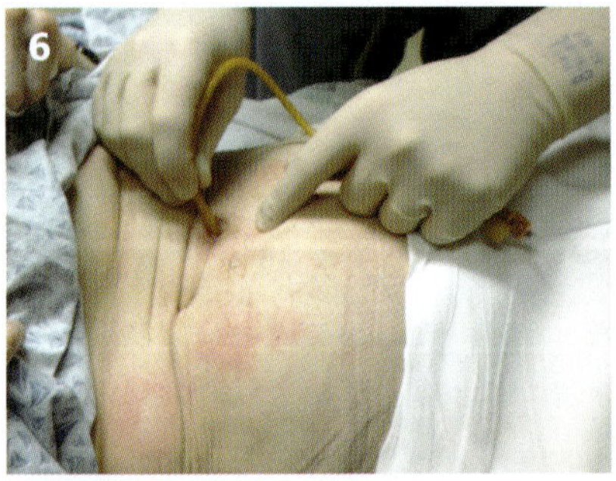

Lubricate the tube and gently pass it into the stoma.

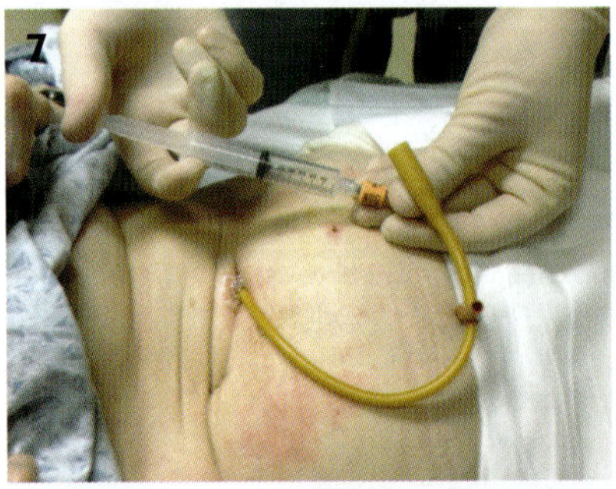

Inflate the balloon with saline once it is in proper position.

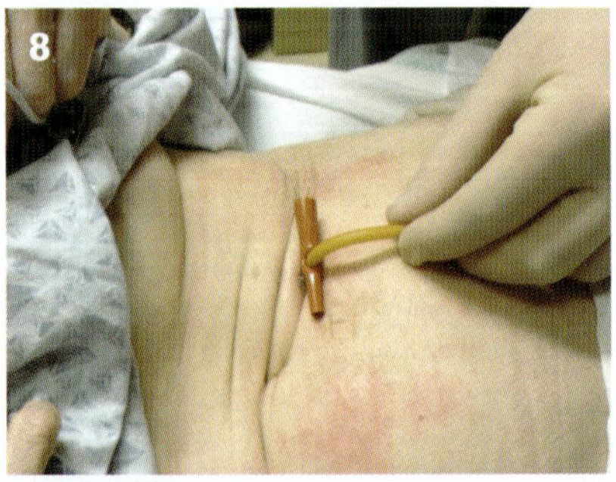

Advance the bolster so that it is 1 cm above the skin.

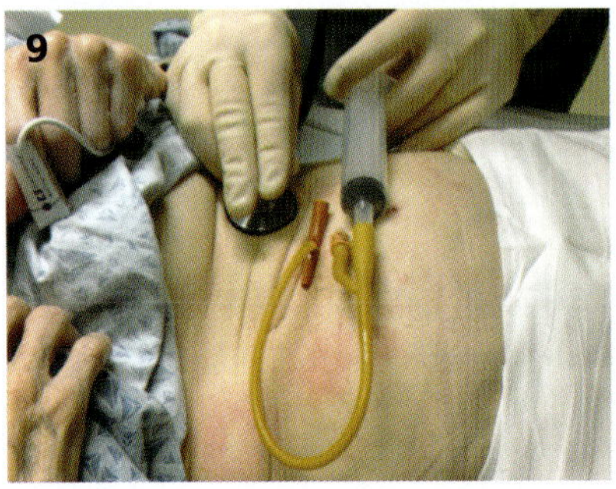

Confirm proper tube placement with auscultation and aspiration.

A contrast-enhanced radiograph may be also be obtained.

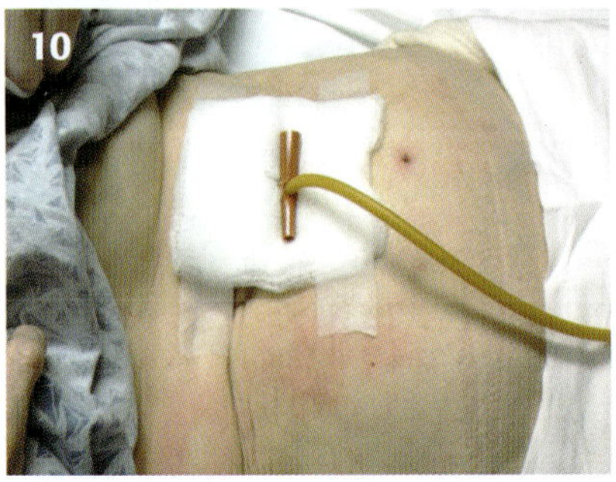

Remember that Foley catheters are not ideal feeding tubes but are useful in temporarily maintaining stoma patency.

Disintegration of the catheter latex may occur in a few months.

Fig. 41.21 G-tube replacement (with a Foley catheter). Foley catheters are not ideal feeding tubes but can be useful temporarily to maintain stoma patency.

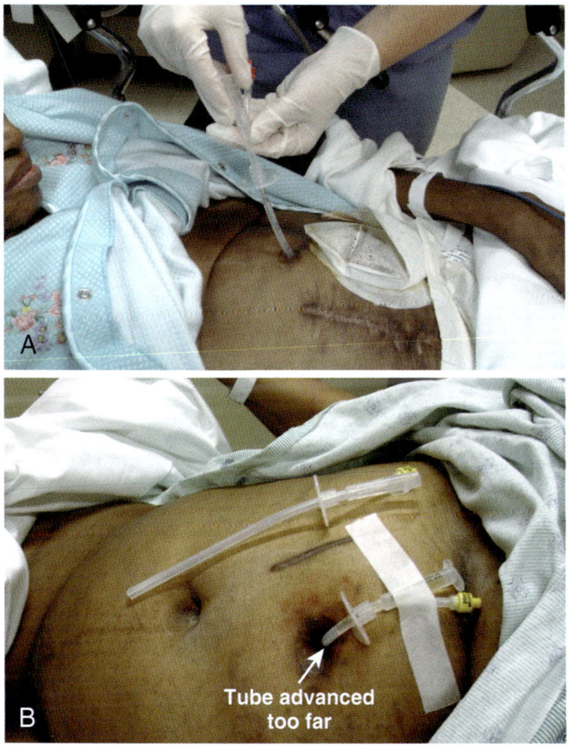

Fig. 41.22 (A) Whenever possible, use a formal feeding tube instead of a Foley catheter. (B) A common dilemma. This patient had gastric distention, and persistent vomiting after tube feedings. The tube had simply migrated distally (note the comparison of the new tube and positioning of the indwelling one) because the bolster was too far proximal. Withdrawing the tube and repositioning the bolster alleviated the problem.

lead to skin damage. Strong adhesive tape can also damage the skin on removal. Tape that is not sufficiently adhesive can let go, particularly if it gets wet. Because tape is less durable, home or nursing home caregivers who are less skilled may retape the tube (Fig. 41.26). If the tape is replaced at home, it may be placed under too much tension and cause thinning of the abdominal wall at the stoma. If too much slack is allowed, the tube may be pulled in. Strong tape can also damage the tube during tape changes if it adheres too strongly to the tube. Special adhesive devices or bolsters are preferred. All transabdominal feeding tubes not secured by suture should have some restraining tape, bolster, or device to prevent tube ingress into the abdomen.

Verification of Placement

The position of the G tube may be checked by air insufflation and aspiration of gastric fluid, as is done with nasoenteric tubes. Air should enter the stomach without resistance and should produce immediate borborygmi. Gastric fluid should return with aspiration. It may be necessary to insert a small volume of water to obtain good return. Water pooling in soft tissue may be aspirated back through a misplaced catheter. Good tube placement is indicated when more fluid returns with aspiration than was originally placed into the catheter.

There is no universally agreed standard about performing a confirmatory contrast-enhanced study for all easily replaced feeding tubes. Most clinicians verify position routinely with a contrast-enhanced radiograph whereas others are satisfied in select cases with clinical criteria alone. Radiographic verification is easily performed and interpreted in the ED. Routine use of postplacement contrast-enhanced radiography to confirm proper placement should be mandatory when the tube tract is immature (i.e., <1-month duration), when passage of the replacement catheter has been difficult, when the clinician is unable to aspirate intestinal contents, or when the patient is unable to communicate any symptoms that might occur with tube misplacement.[74] Peritoneal infusion of feeding solution can be fatal.

Correct tube placement is easy and readily verified radiographically with a small amount of contrast material passed into the tube (Fig. 41.27). Use a catheter-tipped syringe to introduce water-soluble contrast solution (e.g., diatrizoate meglumine-diatrizoate sodium [Gastrografin]) into the tube. Barium is contraindicated because of the potential for peritoneal contamination. Inject 20 mL to 30 mL of water-soluble solution to document the intraluminal tube position. Take a supine abdominal film 1 to 2 minutes after instillation of dye to optimize visualization of the gut. Because the film must be obtained quickly, it is easiest to perform the injection in the radiology suite, followed by a radiograph in only a few minutes. If the contrast material does not flow freely into the tube, the procedure should be terminated immediately, and the position of the tube questioned. With proper positioning, contrast material will outline the part of the gut containing the tube (e.g., stomach with a G tube). An irregular or rounded blotch with wispy edges or streamers suggests peritoneal leakage. In questionable cases, injection of dye can be performed under fluoroscopy.

Complications

Viscus puncture, viscus-abdominal wall separation, and creation of a false tract with subsequent misplacement of the tube are risks associated with dilation procedures. Complications of gastrostomy include wound infection around the catheter, performance of an unnecessary laparotomy for suspected leakage, gastrocolic fistula, pneumatosis cystoides intestinalis, bowel obstruction, peritonitis, and hemorrhage.[75] Jejunostomies can cause most of these complications, as well as other types of fistulas and small bowel obstruction from adhesions or volvulus around the jejunostomy site.[56,76] The most common complications of gastrostomy and gastroenterostomy are local skin erosion from leakage, wound infection, hemorrhage, and dislodgment of the tube.[67] Peritonitis and aspiration are the most critical complications of gastrostomy feedings.[67,77] Jejunostomies are less prone to stomal leakage and cause less nausea, vomiting, bloating, and aspiration than do gastrostomies.[78,80]

Dislodgment of G and J tubes is most common in the 2 weeks after creation of the ostomy.[79,81] Extrusion of the G tube is usually caused by excessive tension applied to the tube. Only gentle contact of the gastric and abdominal walls is desirable. Uncooperative patients should be restrained, and mittens are often particularly helpful. Sutures and large mushrooms or balloons do not prevent purposeful removal of the G tube by an uncooperative patient.

A small amount of drainage is to be expected at the tube entry site. Local leakage of gastric juices may macerate and irritate the skin, which can predispose the site to local infections and abscesses and encourage the development of small granulomas.[78,80] Granulomas are particularly common in children. They can be treated with silver nitrate at the time of

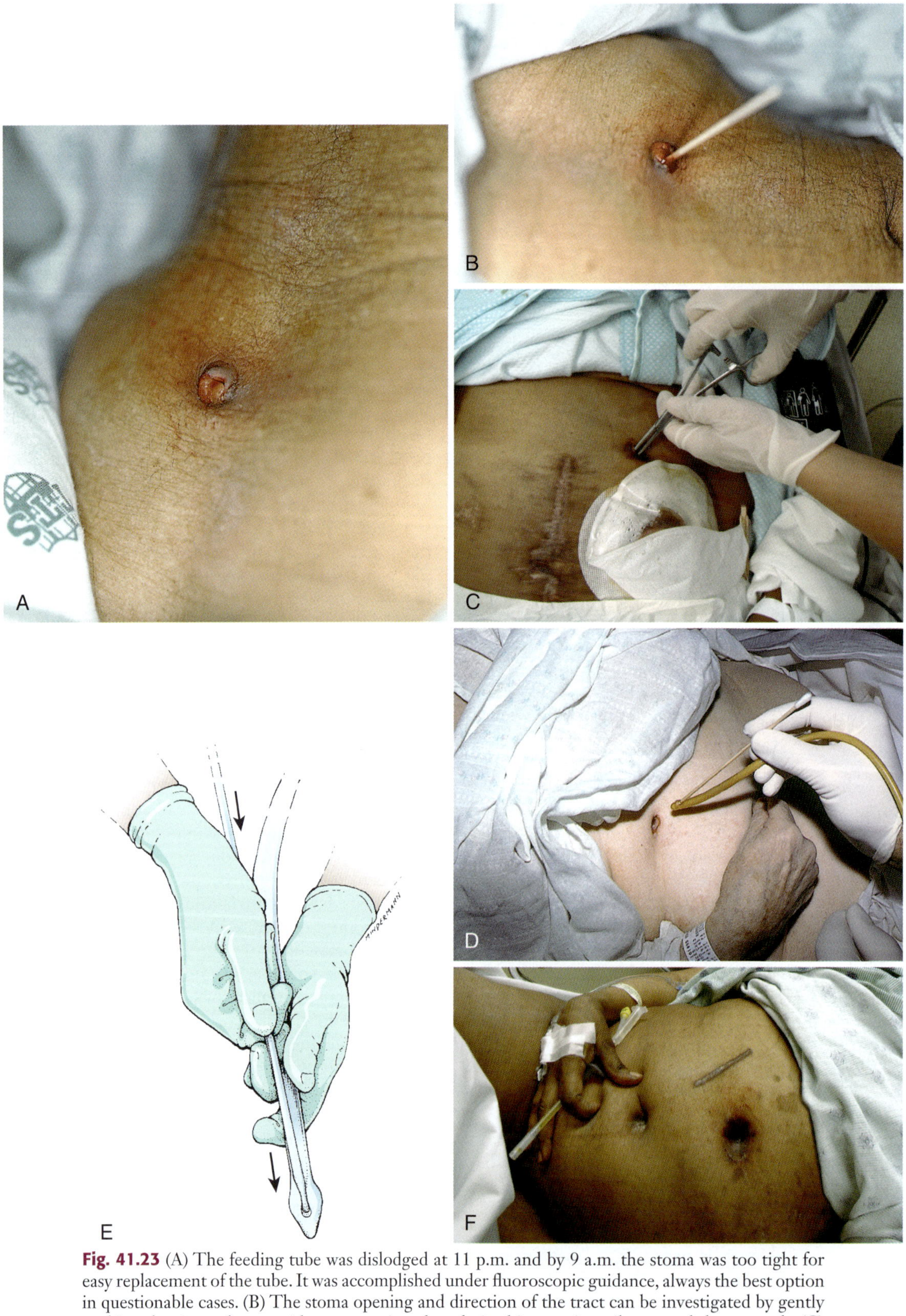

Fig. 41.23 (A) The feeding tube was dislodged at 11 p.m. and by 9 a.m. the stoma was too tight for easy replacement of the tube. It was accomplished under fluoroscopic guidance, always the best option in questionable cases. (B) The stoma opening and direction of the tract can be investigated by gently probing the site and tract with a cotton-tipped swab; in this case, it easily entered the stomach. (C) This tight stoma was carefully dilated with a hemostat under local anesthesia. A false passage can easily be created, and this area usually bleeds readily. (D) To give a Foley catheter sufficient rigidity to aid in passage, the end of a cotton-tipped swab was inserted in the side port of the distal end of the catheter, and traction was applied to the catheter. (E) If a de Pezzer catheter is used, an endotracheal tube stylet distends the flange for passage, and the tip reforms once in the stomach. (F) This patient removed her recently replaced feeding tube, with the balloon inflated, while still in the emergency department awaiting transfer. This could have been avoided if her hands were restrained.

dressing changes. Any dressing used around the entry site of an enteral nutrition tube should absorb fluid and not encourage persistent moisture.[71] An unusually large stoma may promote a leak. Although insertion of a larger tube or firmer traction on the tube might be transiently effective, these measures often result in further enlargement of the stoma. Rigid gastrostomies promote leakage by widening the stoma as they pivot. Insertion of a soft, pliant feeding tube through the widened stoma is often easy and allows later contraction of the stoma.[1] If these techniques are ineffective, temporary removal of the feeding tube may allow the stoma to shrink. Large amounts of drainage around the stoma site may occur with high residual volumes.[82] The residual should be checked, and feedings withheld until residuals are less than 100 mL. Feeding residuals should be checked every 4 hours when a patient is receiving continuous-drip feeding.[82]

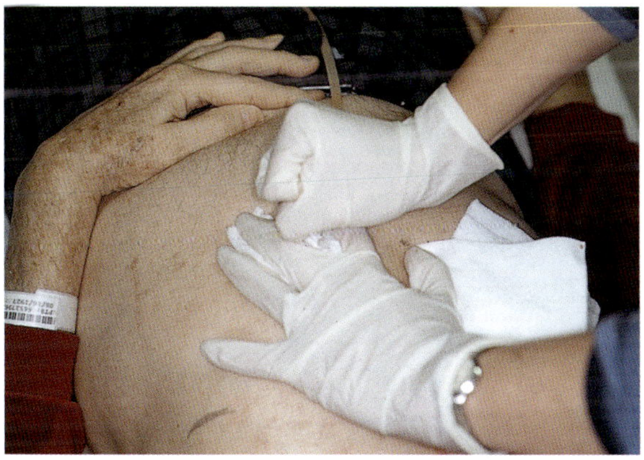

Fig. 41.24 Gentle, firm traction using the flat part of the opposite hand for countertraction will remove most percutaneous endoscopic gastrostomy tubes, even those with internal mushroom bumpers. Modest force may be required; be prepared for a sudden pop and splattering of gastric contents.

Pneumoperitoneum after percutaneous gastrostomy is neither unusual nor dangerous. Benign pneumoperitoneum may be present as long as 5 weeks after PEG.[75,82] Pneumatosis cystoides intestinalis can occur through the defect in the bowel wall created for the enterostomy tube. Though often clinically insignificant, its occurrence suggests air under pressure in the small bowel. NG suction and diet change generally permit resolution of the problem. Catheter or feeding tube removal is not usually required.[83]

Clinically significant pulmonary aspiration can occur with G-tube feeding. Methods of checking for silent pulmonary aspiration include assessing tracheal aspirates with a glucose oxidant reagent strip or placing methylene blue in the formula and monitoring tracheal aspirates for pigmentation.[65,84,85]

A Foley balloon accidentally inflated in the small bowel or esophagus can lead to perforation or obstruction.[86,87] Carefully inflate the balloon soon after it has entered the stomach to prevent perforation of the viscus.

A G tube may migrate in the stomach and obstruct the gastric outlet. This complication is manifested clinically by vomiting and high residuals of feeding solution. Volvulus and jaundice may also occur as a result of balloon migration. To

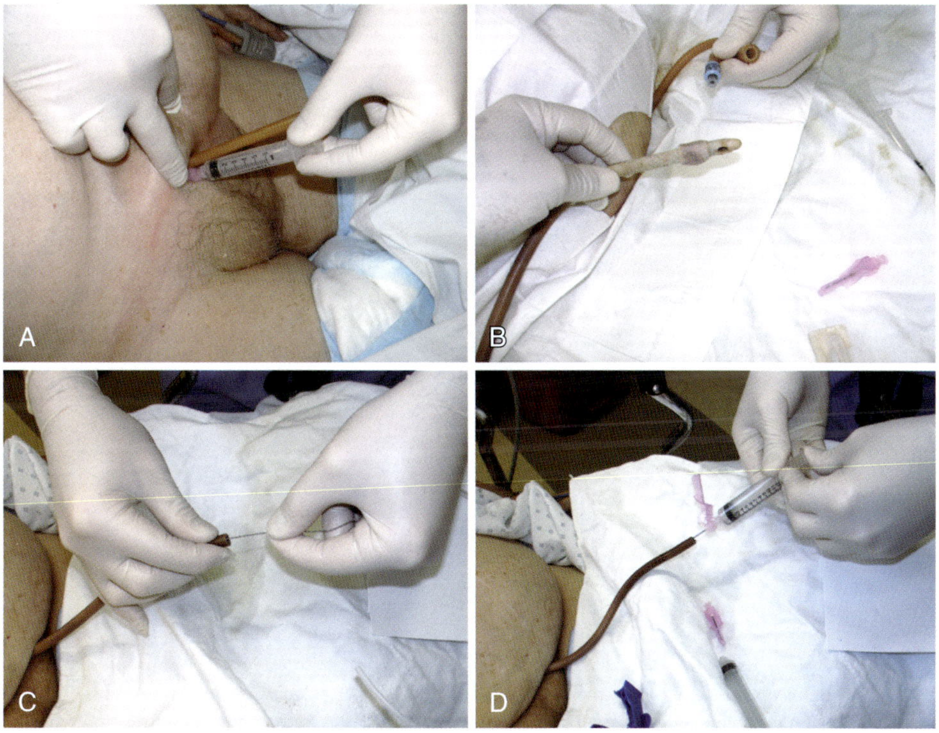

Fig. 41.25 (A) If a Foley balloon will not deflate, use traction to bring the balloon against the abdominal wall. Gently pass a small needle along the course of the catheter while puncturing the balloon as many times as necessary. Wait a few minutes for the fluid to egress. (B) Once the balloon is deflated, it can be withdrawn. Note the encrusted condition of this long-standing Foley catheter used as a percutaneous endoscopic gastrostomy tube. (C) Occasionally, the wire from a central line kit can clear the inflation lumen and allow deflation. (D) If the valve mechanism malfunctions, cut the catheter and attempt to drain the balloon by placing a needle in the inflation channel and flushing and withdrawing fluid.

correct inward migration, first deflate the balloon. Pull the tube back just deep to the desired final position. Reinflate the balloon and pull it the rest of the way back into position. The external bolster should be repositioned or one made and positioned, or inward migration will probably reoccur.[82] If the balloon is not deflated before repositioning, the bowel in which it is wedged may be drawn back with it, thereby preventing relief of the obstruction and possibly precipitating intussusception.

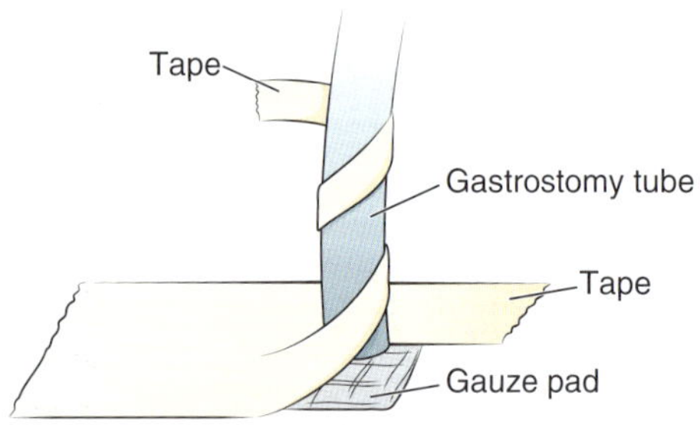

Fig. 41.26 Tape is best avoided to minimize skin maceration. If needed, this is a simple but less secure technique for securing a gastrostomy tube to the skin.

A gastrocolic fistula is usually manifested as copious diarrhea. Once it is confirmed, treatment consists of removal of the G tube. Later creation of a gastrostomy in a different location may be possible. The patient may require hospital admission for surgical correction, nutritional support and monitoring of fluid and electrolyte status.

An external bolster that is snugged down too tightly might result in a short stoma and embedding of the internal bolster in the abdominal wall. An abscess may result. Overly tight external bolsters should be loosened. The correct position is 1 cm from the external surface of the abdomen.

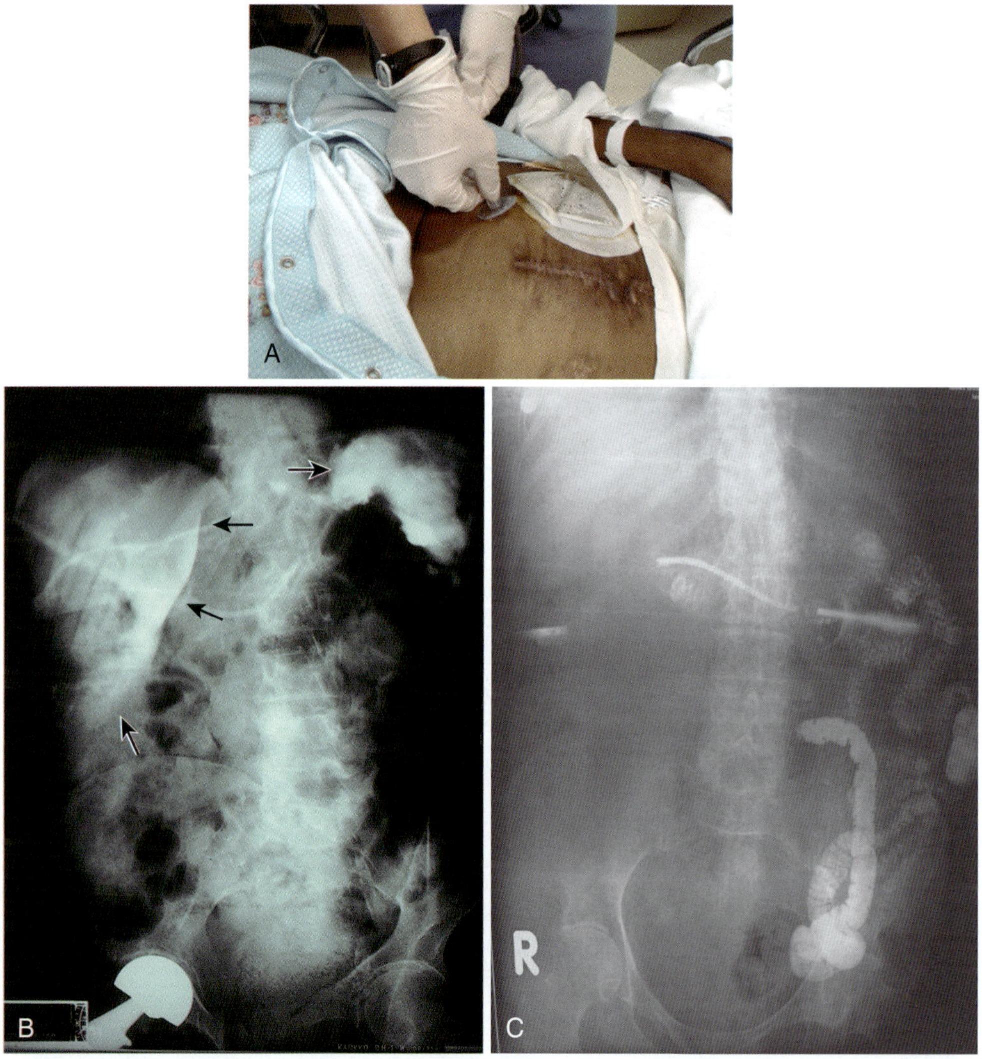

Fig. 41.27 (A) Although this feeding tube seemed to be replaced easily in an uncommunicative nursing home patient, gastric contents could not be aspirated; therefore a contrast-enhanced study was performed. (B) Note the free flow of contrast material throughout the abdomen, especially outlining the liver *(arrows)*. This film indicates placement of the feeding tube into the peritoneum. Placing food through this tube could be disastrous. It is prudent to routinely obtain a contrast-enhanced study after replacement of a percutaneous endoscopic gastrostomy tube in the emergency department. Instill 20 mL Gastrografin/10 mL saline into the tube and take a radiograph in 3 to 5 minutes. (C) Contrast-enhanced study demonstrating correct placement of a feeding tube. Note the outline of the gastric rugae and the characteristic mucosal folds of the small intestine.

CLOGGED FEEDING TUBES

Clogging, leaking, fracture, and kinking are problems common to all feeding tubes. Clearing a clogged tube may be a temporary benefit but is rarely a long-term solution. Hence, whenever feasible, replace nonfunctioning or leaking tubes with new ones. Although it may be only a temporary solution, if the tube has a complex placement or the clinician is unsure how the tube is secured internally, it is prudent to attempt to unclog the tube rather than replace it. Large G tubes are the least likely to clog. G tubes at least 28 Fr in size can tolerate food processed at home with a blender and viscous feeding solutions. Isosmotic feeding solutions are tolerated by fairly narrow tubes and cost one-sixth of what elemental feedings cost. Isosmotic feedings will clog needle catheters.[54] When tube lumens are 14 Fr or smaller, all pills and the contents of all capsules should be dissolved in water to prevent obstruction of the tube.[71]

Kinking is a frequent cause of tube blockage during the immediate period after reinsertion. Withdrawing the tube a few centimeters usually relieves the kink and obstruction. A persistently recurring kink requires removal of the tube and insertion of a fresh tube.

Accumulated feeding solution or medication precipitates are very difficult to clean or remove. Milking a pliant tube backward may remove some of the cheesy precipitates. Guidewires or stylets may clear the proximal portion of a clogged tube lumen but are unsafe to use in subcutaneous areas of the lumen because they can puncture the tube and injure the patient or create a leak in the tube. Bionix Medical Technologies supplies tube decloggers in two lengths and several diameters for clearing clogs in G and J tubes (Fig. 41.28). After selecting a declogger shorter than the feeding tube, insert it gently into the tube until the end of the screw hits the clog and then rotate it clockwise to bury the end in the clog. Next, slide the declogger up and down to break up and dislodge the clog. Insertion, rotation, and sliding might have to be repeated several times until the dislodged material can be flushed into the patient with saline or water. Gravity alone may be insufficient to allow fluid to pass through the feeding tube into the patient and is a better test of successful declogging than is passage of fluid with a syringe. Theoretically the pointed screw end of the declogger can puncture the tube, or if a declogger that is too long is put in, it may puncture the bowel or stomach directly. According to the company, no cases have been reported.

Fogarty arterial embolectomy catheters can be used to unclog J and G tubes. Insert the soft tip of the Fogarty catheter into the feeding tube and advance it while monitoring the insertion distance to avoid penetrating farther than the length of the feeding tube. Premeasure the allowable length of insertion. A No. 4 embolectomy catheter is suitable for a 10- or 12-Fr feeding tube, and a No. 5 embolectomy catheter is suitable for a 14-Fr feeding tube. When the catheter meets an obstruction, inflate the balloon. This usually opens the obstruction sufficiently for passage of the catheter. Once the Fogarty has been manipulated to a point just proximal to the internal feeding opening, withdraw it while gently inflating and deflating the balloon intermittently. Do not withdraw the catheter when the balloon is inflated because the catheter and feeding tube tend to move as a unit. Repeat this procedure several times if necessary. Once declogging is successful, inject contrast material to confirm the position and integrity of the tube.[88]

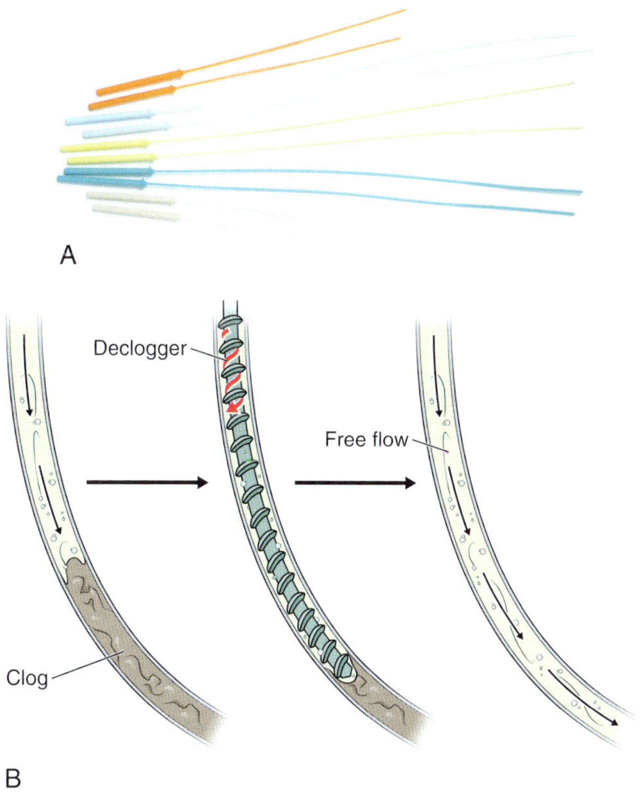

Fig. 41.28 (A–B) Bionix tube declogger. Two lengths and several diameters are available. Caution must be observed any time that the screw end of the declogger passes from view because the potential exists to extend or puncture out of the tube and into the patient. (Redrawn courtesy Bionix Medical Technologies. Bionix Enteral Feeding DeCloggers are a registered trademark of Bionix Medical Technologies. https://www.BionixMed.com.)

Irrigation with carbonated beverages and high-pressure irrigation with small-volume syringes have also been recommended as techniques for unclogging feeding tubes. Although irrigation seems like a straightforward and simple solution, these techniques are generally ineffective; furthermore, the possibility exists for dangerous tube rupture with internal leakage. Tubes unclogged by forceful irrigation or by deep luminal probing should be radiographed after injection of contrast material to check the integrity of the tube.

REFERENCES ARE AVAILABLE AT Elsevier eBooks+

CHAPTER 42

Balloon Tamponade of Gastroesophageal Varices

Meghan S. Breed

INTRODUCTION

Managing patients with acute gastrointestinal bleeding from gastroesophageal varices can be one of the most challenging scenarios in emergency medicine. These patients often have advanced liver disease and arrive to the emergency department (ED) with massive hematemesis, airway compromise, encephalopathy, hemodynamic instability, severe anemia, thrombocytopenia, and coagulopathy. Gastroesophageal varices (Fig. 42.1) are one of the most common causes of upper gastrointestinal bleeding and have the highest mortality rate.[1] Esophageal varices are present in 50% to 60% of patients with compensated cirrhosis and up to 85% in patients with decompensated cirrhosis and develop as a result of portal hypertension.[2,3] In patients with established gastric or esophageal varices, the annual incidence of acute hemorrhage ranges from 5% to 15%; however, rates of recurrent hemorrhage can be as high as 60% per year.[2–4]

Advances in resuscitation, critical care, pharmacology, and endoscopy have significantly reduced the mortality rate associated with acute variceal bleeding. Mortality rates at 6 weeks in patients with acute variceal bleeding currently range from 15% to 20%.[5–7] Despite advances in management, up to 20% of patients with acute variceal bleeding do not respond to standard therapy.[8] Rescue therapies for this group of patients are limited and include surgery, placement of a transjugular intrahepatic portosystemic shunt or a covered esophageal metal stent, and balloon tamponade.[8] This chapter details the indications and contraindications for balloon tamponade in patients with acute variceal bleeding, the techniques for placement, and the potential complications of this intervention. Although this procedure is rarely needed, physicians with knowledge of the technique can attempt to place these potentially lifesaving devices.

BACKGROUND

In 1950 Sengstaken and Blakemore developed and described the use of a double-balloon device to control variceal hemorrhage. Since that time, the Sengstaken-Blakemore tube has become the most widely known balloon tamponade device. The Sengstaken-Blakemore tube has an esophageal and a gastric balloon, along with a gastric aspiration port that allows continuous suction of stomach contents (Fig. 42.2A). In 1968 Edlich and colleagues developed the Minnesota tube and modified the Sengstaken-Blakemore tube by adding an esophageal aspiration port and increasing the capacity of the gastric balloon.[8a]

Currently, three balloon tamponade devices are commercially available: the Linton-Nachlas, the Sengstaken-Blakemore, and the Minnesota tubes (Video 42.1).[9] In contrast to the Sengstaken-Blakemore and Minnesota tubes, the Linton-Nachlas tube is a single-balloon device that consists of a gastric balloon and a gastric suction port for aspiration and lavage (Fig. 42.2B). Because placement of these tubes remains a relatively rare procedure, most hospitals stock only one type of device. Regardless of the type of device, success rates for the control of hemorrhage with balloon tamponade tubes range from 30% to 90%.[10]

Balloon Tamponade of GE Varices

Indications

Unstable patients with massive variceal bleeding in the following scenarios:

- Endoscopy is not available
- Endoscopy is unsuccessful at controlling bleeding
- Consultant physicians are unavailable and vasoactive agents have failed to stop bleeding

Contraindications

History of esophageal stricture
Recent esophageal or gastric surgery

Complications

Airway obstruction
Esophageal rupture
Aspiration pneumonitis
Pain
Ulceration of lips, mouth, tongue, or nares
Esophageal and gastric mucosal erosions
Arrhythmia
Dislodgment of previous variceal bands

Equipment

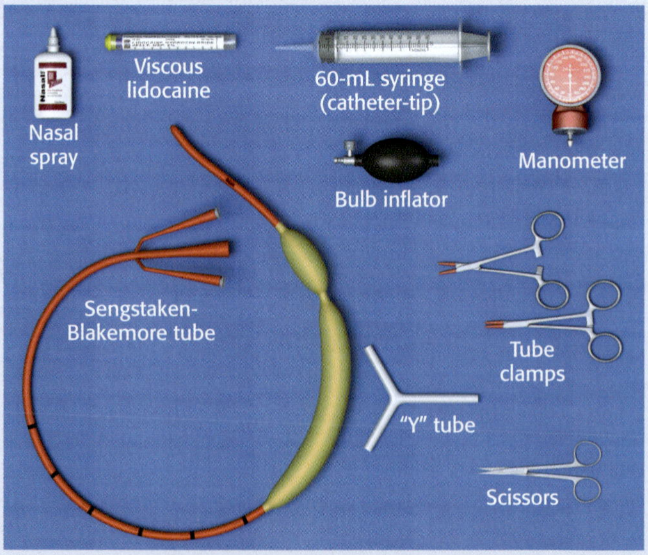

Review Box 42.1 Balloon tamponade of gastroesophageal varices: indications, contraindications, complications, and equipment.

TABLE 44.1 Clinical Indications for Laparotomy After Blunt Trauma

MANIFESTATION	PITFALL
Unstable vital signs with strongly suspected abdominal injury	Alternative sources of shock
Unequivocal peritoneal irritation	Unreliable
Pneumoperitoneum	Insensitive; may be due to a cardiopulmonary source or invasive procedures (diagnostic peritoneal lavage, laparoscopy)
Evidence of diaphragmatic injury	Nonspecific
Significant gastrointestinal bleeding	Uncommon, unknown accuracy

From Marx J, Isenhour J. Abdominal trauma. In: Marx JA, Hockberger RS, Walls RM et al, eds. *Rosen's Emergency Medicine: Concepts and Clinical Practice*. 6th ed. Mosby; 2006:509.

Furthermore, given its exquisite sensitivity, a negative peritoneal aspiration allows the clinician to proceed to alternative management steps and the patient to forego unnecessary laparotomy. Second, DPL has been used in less exigent circumstances as a means of predicting solid or hollow visceral injury requiring laparotomy. However, in this venue its sensitivity to the presence of hemorrhage may prompt unnecessary laparotomy in patients with self-limited lacerations of the liver, spleen, or mesentery.[5] CT specifically evaluates all intraperitoneal structures, as well as the retroperitoneum, a region inaccessible to DPL. Because the resolution and the speed with which it can be undertaken have vastly improved, CT has become an invaluable adjunct in the management of blunt trauma and has largely replaced DPL in stable patients. It is most useful in identifying injury to solid organs with accompanying IPH and greatly assists nonoperative management of these injuries. The ability of CT to discern hollow viscus and pancreatic pathology has continued to improve as the modality has evolved.[4] With regard to hollow viscus injury, it is when serial clinical evaluations cannot be performed that gut perforation leads to preventable mortality. This is especially true in patients with severe closed-head injury or high spinal cord injury, in whom physical assessment of the abdomen is quite compromised. It is for these express scenarios that some authorities still recommend performing a DPL. The clinician's concern for hollow viscus injury should be heightened if US or CT demonstrates minimal amounts of free intraperitoneal fluid without evidence of solid organ damage.[6]Two paradigms have brought US to the forefront. First, this modality has been adopted as the primary triage instrument, in lieu of DPL, for the detection of IPH on the basis of identifying which pouches and gutters are filled with fluid.[7] Clinical success in this role has been mixed, with reported sensitivity for IPH of 65% to 95%.[8] In addition, to be useful in this role, a competent technician and interpreter and the appropriate equipment must be present in real time. Emergency clinicians and surgeons can be trained in this technique to a level of competence sufficient for this need. In centers that rely on US, DPL can serve as a reliable study when US equipment is unavailable, performance of US is technically difficult, or the results of US are indeterminate, especially when the patient demonstrates hemodynamic compromise.

DPL is a readily available procedure that can be conducted rapidly in the safe confines of the ED. The ability to undertake CT in particular or, to a lesser extent, US in a similar manner requires careful consideration of the clinical circumstances, location of equipment, and capabilities of the personnel available (Fig. 44.1).[2,4]

Penetrating Trauma

The advent of DPL was seminal in the promotion of selective management for penetrating abdominal injury. Here its role is more prominent than for blunt trauma because of the far greater likelihood of occult injury to hollow viscera and the diaphragm after a penetrating mechanism.

Instruments and missiles may penetrate the abdominal cavity via the anterior abdominal wall, flank, back, or low chest region. The intraperitoneal space is vulnerable if penetration occurs as high as the fourth intercostal space anteriorly and the sixth or seventh space laterally and posteriorly because the diaphragm may rise to these levels in the expiratory phase of respiration. Coincident thoracic penetration occurs in up to 46% of patients with abdominal injuries.[9] The likelihood of retroperitoneal injury increases when the entry site is over the flank or back, but the prospect of intraperitoneal pathology remains considerable.[10]

Stab Wounds

Because only one-fourth to one-third of patients who sustain stab wounds to the anterior aspect of the abdomen require laparotomy, diagnostic algorithms are used to decrease the rate of unnecessary surgery.[9] An optimal approach would not sacrifice sensitivity for morbid intraperitoneal injury. A pathway using a combination of clinical mandates, local wound exploration, and DPL is well established (Fig. 44.2). These clinical mandates are reasonably accurate predictors of significant intraperitoneal injury (Table 44.2). Thus the presence of one or more suggests the need for urgent laparotomy and forgoing additional diagnostic studies.

DPL fills three roles in the evaluation of patients with abdominal stab wounds: (1) rapid determination of the presence of hemoperitoneum, (2) discovery of intraperitoneal injury requiring surgery in stable patients, and (3) establishment of diaphragmatic violation. As is the case in blunt trauma patients, DPL can be invaluable as a rapid triage tool when the source of hemodynamic instability is not known. Pericardial tamponade, intrathoracic hemorrhage, and IPH may be contributing to hemodynamic instability or wholly causal. As for blunt trauma evaluation, US is the only bedside diagnostic modality for IPH that is competitive in this role, and it carries the added advantage of scanning for intrapericardial and intrathoracic hemorrhage.[9] In determining injury after stab wounds, DPL has 90% accuracy.[11] Serial examinations, CT, and laparoscopy are alternative modalities in some centers.[12] The diaphragmatic rents created by stab wounds are generally small; thus at the outset they may not create apparent clinical or radiologic abnormalities. However, morbidity from delayed herniation of bowel, particularly after left thoracoabdominal stab wounds, has been well described.[13] Physical examination is notoriously insensitive, and DPL is

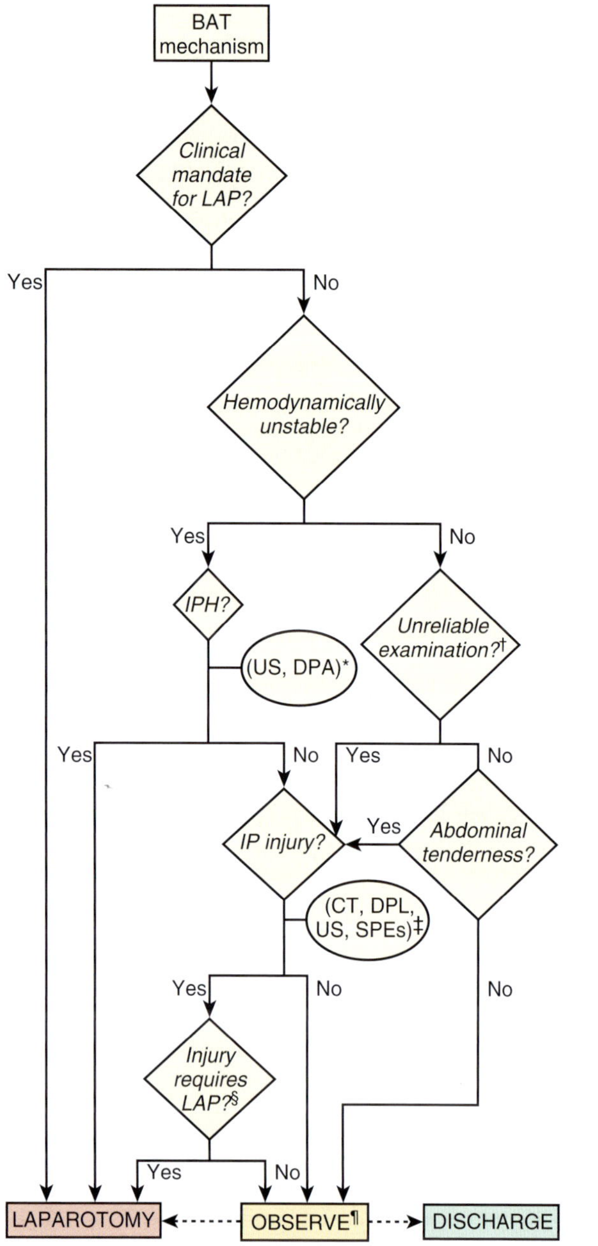

Fig. 44.1 Algorithm for blunt abdominal trauma (BAT). *Determined by unequivocal free *IP* fluid on US or positive peritoneal aspiration on DPA. †May be unreliable because of closed-head injury, intoxicants, distracting injury, or spinal cord injury. ‡One or more studies may be indicated. §The need for LAP is based on the clinical scenario, diagnostic studies, and institutional resources. The duration of observation should be 6 to 24 hours, depending on whether diagnostic tests have been performed, the results of the tests, and clinical circumstances, including the absence of factors rendering the examination unreliable. *CT,* Computed tomography; *DPA,* diagnostic peritoneal aspiration; *DPL,* diagnostic peritoneal lavage; *IP,* intraperitoneal; *IPH,* intraperitoneal hemorrhage; *LAP,* laparotomy; *SPE,* serial physical examination; *US,* ultrasound. (From Marx J, Isenhour J. Abdominal trauma. In: Marx JA, Hockberger RS, Walls RM et al., eds. *Rosen's Emergency Medicine: Concepts and Clinical Practice.* 6th ed. Mosby; 2006:508.)

currently the most sensitive means of discerning this injury in the immediate post trauma phase other than laparoscopy or laporatomy.[13] There is some evidence that coronal reconstruction of CT images provides greater sensitivity

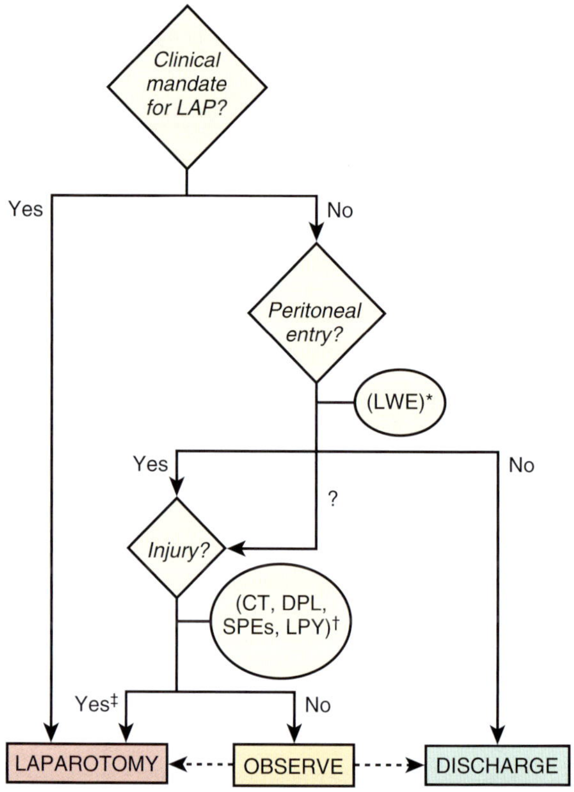

Fig. 44.2 Algorithm for anterior abdominal stab wounds. *Plain films, ultrasonography, LPY, and CT can also assess peritoneal entry. †CT, DPL, SPEs, or LPY can be used in singular or complementary fashion depending on the clinical scenario. ‡Expectant management of injuries is infrequently attempted. *CT,* Computed tomography; *DPL,* diagnostic peritoneal lavage; *LAP,* laparotomy; *LPY,* laparoscopy; *LWE,* local wound exploration; *SPE,* serial physical examination. (From Marx J, Isenhour J. Abdominal trauma. In: Marx JA, Hockberger RS, Walls RM et al., eds. *Rosen's Emergency Medicine: Concepts and Clinical Practice.* 6th ed. Mosby; 2006:503.)

for detecting small diaphragmatic tears, and as CT technology continues to evolve, it may surpass DPL for evaluation of these subtle injuries.[14] For these small wounds, magnetic resonance imaging may be diagnostic, but because of safety and accessibility concerns, it should be reserved for the nonacute phase of management. Laparoscopy has demonstrated promise in experienced hands.[13]

Gunshot Wounds

Injury to multiple organs is the rule after gunshot wounds, and mortality is significantly greater than after stab wounds.[15] The diagnostic approach is more conservative for gunshot wounds because in some studies the likelihood of intraperitoneal injury requiring operative intervention has exceeded 90% when the projectile has entered the intraperitoneal cavity (Fig. 44.3). If clinical mandates are met (see Table 44.2) or if peritoneal violation has occurred, most centers proceed to laparotomy. Nonoperative management is a reasonable option in patients who are hemodynamically stable with reliable abdominal examinations and no evidence of peritonitis or evisceration.[16] DPL is reserved for two circumstances: (1) the wound tract is neither obviously superficial nor intraperitoneal, and (2) penetration occurred in the low chest region, where diaphragmatic injury is more likely, yet the possibility of intraperitoneal injury also exists.

TABLE 44.2 Clinical Indications for Laparotomy After Penetrating Trauma

MANIFESTATION	PREMISE	PITFALL
Hemodynamic instability	Major solid visceral or vascular injury	Thorax, mediastinum
Peritoneal signs	Intraperitoneal injury	Unreliable, especially immediately after injury
Evisceration	Additional bowel, other injury	No injury in one-fourth to one-third of stab wound cases
Diaphragmatic injury	Diaphragmatic herniation	Rare clinical, radiographic findings
Gastrointestinal and vaginal hemorrhage	Proximal gut or uterine injury	Uncommon, unknown accuracy
Impalement in situ	Vascular impalement	High operative risk, pregnancy
Intraperitoneal air	Perforation of a hollow viscus	Insensitive; may be caused by intraperitoneal entry only or be due to a cardiopulmonary source

Modified from Marx JA. Diagnostic peritoneal lavage. In: Ivatury RR, Cayten CG, eds. *The Textbook of Penetrating Trauma*. Williams & Wilkins; 1996.

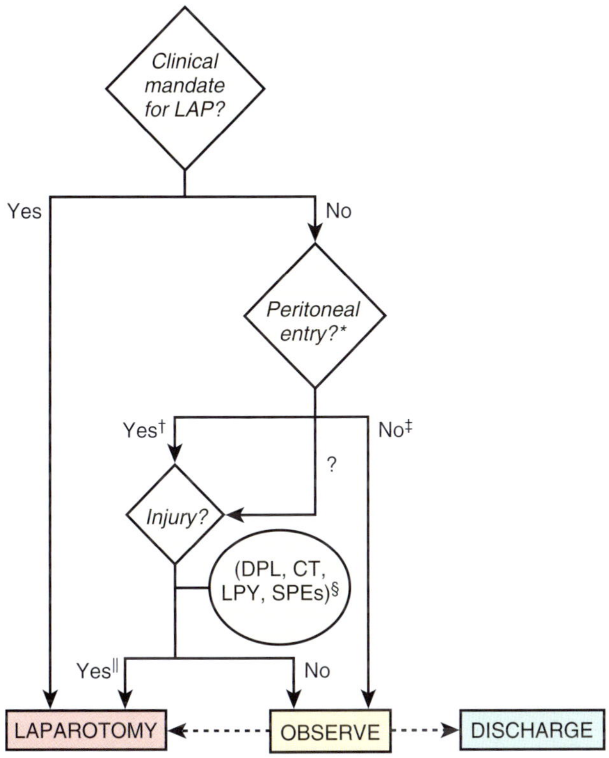

Fig. 44.3 Algorithm for abdominal gunshot wounds. *Can be assessed by the path of the missile, plain films, local wound exploration, ultrasonography, and LAP. †Most centers proceed to LAP if peritoneal entry is suspected. ‡Patients with documented superficial and low-velocity injuries can be discharged; high-velocity injuries or those of unknown depth require further tests or observation. §DPL, CT, LPY, or SPEs can be used in singular or complementary fashion depending on the clinical scenario. Expectant management of injuries caused by gunshot wounds is rarely attempted. *CT,* Computed tomography; *DPL,* diagnostic peritoneal lavage; *LAP,* laparotomy; *LPY,* laparoscopy; *SPE,* serial physical examination. (From Marx J, Isenhour J. Abdominal trauma. In: Marx JA, Hockberger RS, Walls RM et al., eds. *Rosen's Emergency Medicine: Concepts and Clinical Practice.* 6th ed. Mosby; 2006:506.)

Contraindications

DPL can be undertaken in virtually any patient irrespective of age or comorbid illness. Adjustment of the technique and site of performance allows relative contraindications to be overcome. Relative contraindications include previous abdominal surgery or infections, obesity, coagulopathy, and second- or third-trimester pregnancy. The sole absolute contraindication is when clinical mandates for urgent laparotomy already exist.

Procedure

Prior to DPL, decompress the stomach and bladder to prevent inadvertent injury. Place the patient in the supine position and administer sedatives and analgesics as appropriate. Perform DPL according to compliance with standards for body fluid precautions. Observe sterile technique throughout the procedure. Before making the skin incisions described later, prepare the site with standard skin antiseptics and drape appropriately. Prophylactic antibiotics are not indicated for routine DPL because local and systemic infections are rare.

Infiltrate the area for incision and dissection with a local anesthetic such as 1% lidocaine *with* epinephrine (Fig. 44.4, *step 1*). Delay the incision for more than 30 seconds after infiltration of local anesthetic to permit local vasospasm, which minimizes bleeding of the wound during the procedure.

Placement of the Catheter

There are two basic methods for DPL: open and closed. The two open techniques are *semi-open* and *fully open*, and both typically require an assistant. DPL is clearly within the diagnostic armamentarium of the emergency clinician and surgeon. Either may undertake it in keeping with clinical policies established at the particular trauma center.

Semi-open Technique

Make a skin incision 4 cm to 6 cm in length with a No. 11 scalpel blade. Using Army-Navy retractors, proceed with blunt dissection to expose the rectus fascia (see Fig. 44.4, *steps 2 and 3*). With the infraumbilical incision in the midline, continue

Diagnostic Peritoneal Lavage: Semi-open Technique

1

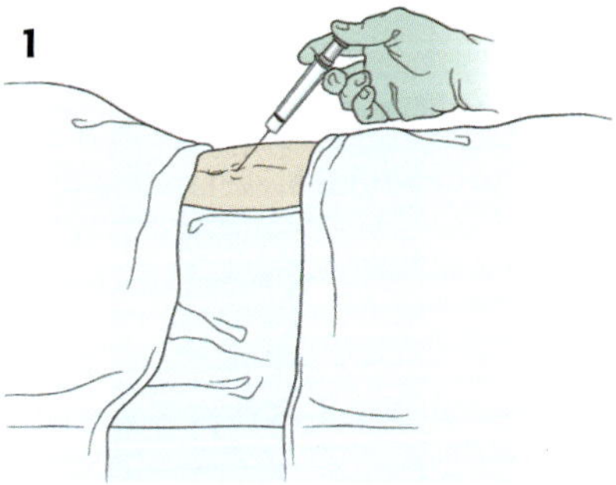

Anesthetize the skin with lidocaine with epinephrine.

2

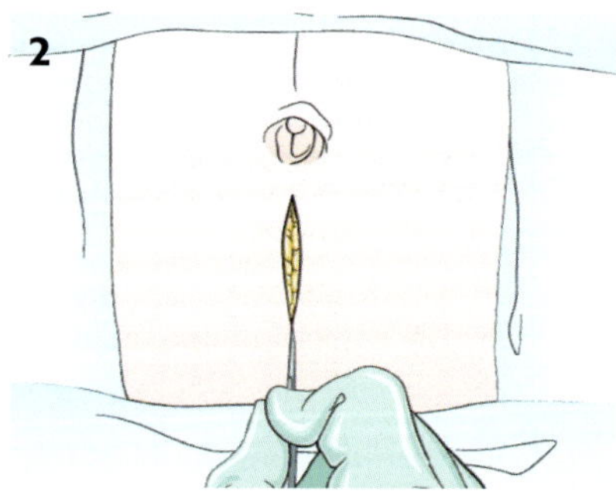

Make a 4- to 6-cm infra-umbilical midline skin incision with a No. 11 scalpel.

3

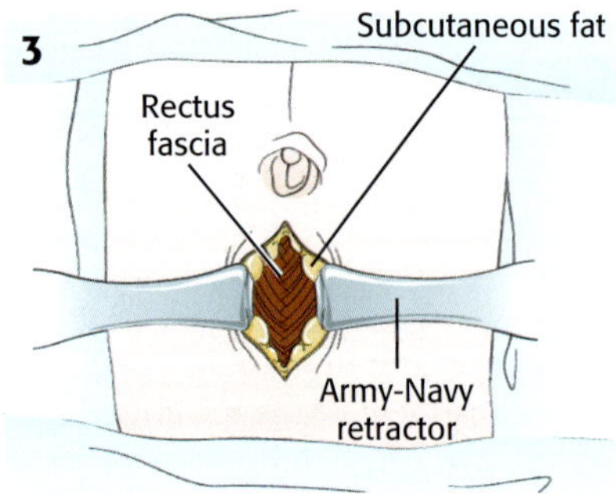

Using Army-Navy retractors, bluntly dissect to the linea alba.

4

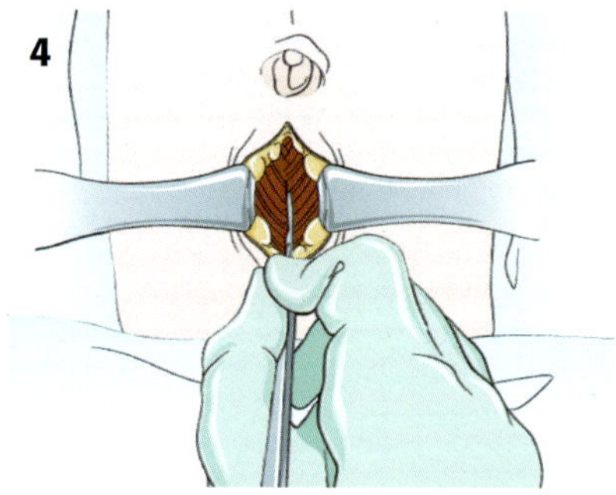

Make a small 2- to 3-mm opening in the linea alba with a No. 15 scalpel blade.

5

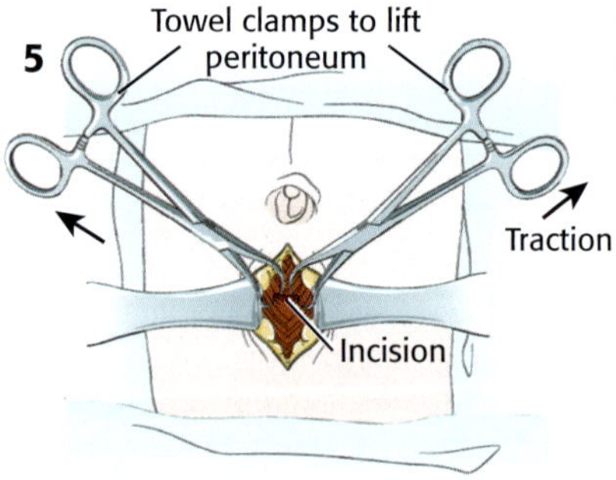

Place towel clips through this opening to grasp and lift each side of the rectus.

6

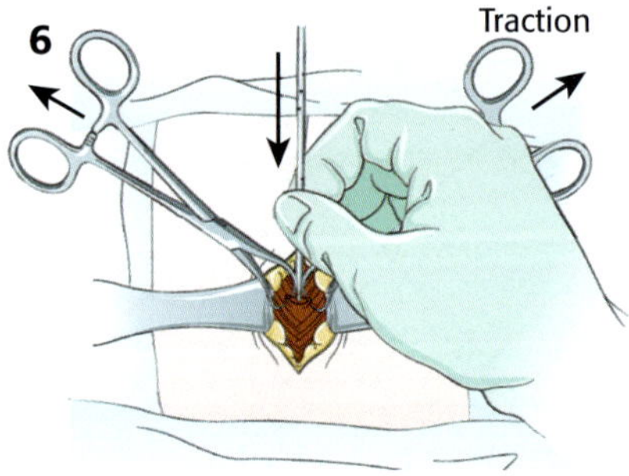

Advance the catheter and trocar 45 to 60 degrees caudally into the peritoneum.

7

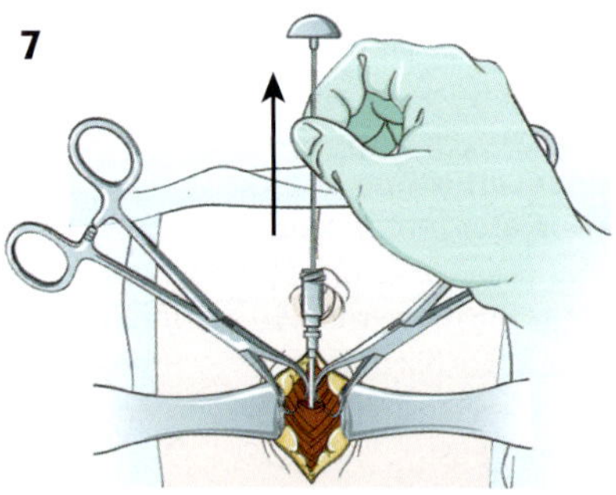

Retract the trocar within the catheter, and advance the catheter toward the pelvis.

8

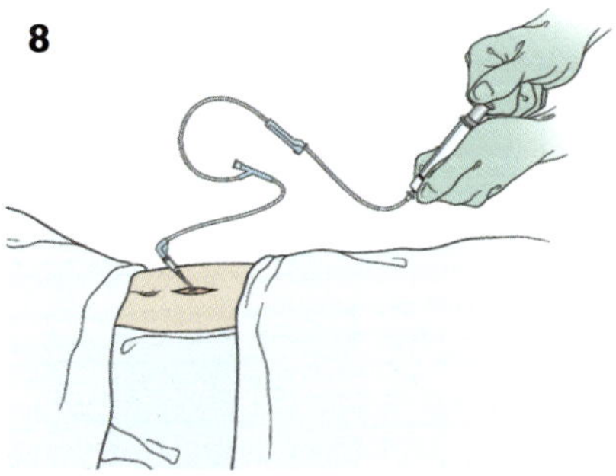

Withdraw the trochar and aspirate for blood using a 10-cc syringe.

9

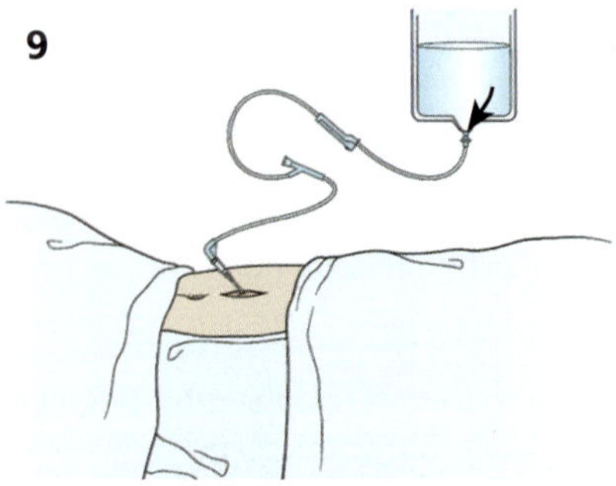

If lavage is necessary, infuse 1 L of warm normal saline and recover fluids under gravity.

Fig. 44.4 Semi-open technique of diagnostic peritoneal lavage. Note that the stomach and bladder have been decompressed under most circumstances.

blunt dissection until the linea alba is seen. Its crossing bands of crural fibers may be apparent. Make a small 2- to 3-mm opening in the linea alba with a No. 15 scalpel blade (see Fig. 44.4, *step 4*). You may notice a tough, gritty sensation when cutting the linea alba with the scalpel. Place towel clips through this opening to grasp each side of the rectus fascia (see Fig. 44.4, *step 5*). Ask an assistant to lift the two towel clips and carefully advance the catheter and trocar in a 45- to 60-degree caudad orientation. Proceed through the peritoneum into the peritoneal cavity (see Fig. 44.4, *steps 6 and 7*).

One method to decrease the likelihood of penetrating any underlying viscera is to hold the fingers low on the catheter/trocar instrument such that on entering the abdominal peritoneum, the fingers prevent deep penetration. Excessive pressure during penetration with the trocar is a common error. Apply steady one-finger pressure to the handle sufficient to "pop" through the peritoneum. After controlled peritoneal penetration of 0.5 cm to 1.0 cm in the midline, retract the trocar 1.0 cm to 2.0 cm within the catheter, and advance the catheter carefully toward the pelvis. Some operators advance the catheter toward the right or left side of the pelvis. Use a slight twisting motion during advancement to minimize visceral or omental injury.

The fully open technique extends the semi-open technique by one step. Lengthen the opening in the linea alba to open the peritoneum, and use direct visualization to advance the catheter into the peritoneal cavity. The trocar is unnecessary with the open technique.

A single technician can accomplish the two open techniques, but it is useful to have an assistant help with retraction and handling of the instruments. The fully open method is the more technically demanding and time-consuming. Reserve this method for clinical circumstances in which neither the closed nor the semi-open technique is deemed safe, or they have been attempted and failed. Examples of such circumstances include pelvic fracture, pregnancy, previous abdominal surgery, adhesions, infections, and obesity.

Closed Technique

For the closed technique, introduce the catheter into the peritoneal space in a blind percutaneous fashion. Use the simple Seldinger (guidewire) method, in which a small-gauge guide needle is inserted into the peritoneal cavity in the midline just inferior to the umbilicus (Fig. 44.5, *step 2*). Pass a flexible wire through the needle (see Fig. 44.5, *step 3*), and remove the needle but not the wire. Make a small stab with a No. 11 scalpel blade at the entry site of the wire to allow easier passage of the catheter through the abdominal wall (see Fig. 44.5, *step 4*), and then advance a soft catheter over the wire and into the peritoneal cavity. Rotate the catheter while pushing it over the guidewire to facilitate entry into the peritoneal cavity if the catheter does not advance easily. Place the catheter into the right or left pelvic gutter.

Always control the guidewire to avert intraabdominal migration of the wire. Withdraw the wire and aspirate for blood with a 10-mL syringe. Follow this with peritoneal lavage when necessary. Proponents of the guidewire technique promote its ease and rapidity. Those who prefer the semi-open method argue that the time until peritoneal aspiration, the more critical interval, is minimally different and that this method may have fewer complications and thus be more accurate than the guidewire technique. Note that for both the semi-open and closed approaches, the time until aspiration is performed should be no more than 2 to 5 minutes.

Site

The optimum location for DPL is at the infraumbilical ring at the inferior border of the umbilicus (Table 44.3). Here, between the rectus abdominis muscles there is adherence of the peritoneum and relative lack of vascularity and preperitoneal fat. Closed DPL should be conducted here. In the event of second- or third-trimester pregnancy, a suprauterine approach is used. If midline scarring is present, a fully open technique at the lateral border of the rectus abdominis in the left lower quadrant may be necessary. The left side is preferred to avoid later confusion about whether an appendectomy has been performed. In the presence of a pelvic fracture, use a fully open supraumbilical approach. This decreases the likelihood of passing the catheter through a retroperitoneal hematoma that has dissected from the fracture anteriorly and across the abdominal wall. In patients with penetrating trauma, do not perform DPL through the stab or missile entry site. This approach can contaminate the intraperitoneal cavity, potentially exacerbate the abdominal wall bleeding, and lead to a false-positive result.

Aspiration and Lavage

Once the catheter has been placed successfully into the peritoneal cavity, attach the right-angle adapter, extension tubing, and a non–Luer-Lok syringe and attempt aspiration (see Fig. 44.4, *step 8*). If 10 mL of blood is aspirated, the test is positive and the procedure is terminated. With penetrating trauma, acquisition of lesser amounts may be meaningful because of the tendency for the diaphragm and bowel to hemorrhage minimally when injured. However, no rules have been established in this regard.

If little to no blood is aspirated, lavage the peritoneal cavity with either normal saline or lactated Ringer's solution (see Fig. 44.4, *step 9*). Apply a blood pressure cuff or blood infusion pump around the plastic intravenous (IV) bag to speed the influx (i.e., decrease lavage time) if necessary. Large-bore infusion tubing (e.g., urologic irrigation tubing sets, such as the Abbott No. 6543 cystoscopy/irrigation set [Allegiance]) also shortens fluid influx time. Infuse 1 L of fluid in adults or 15 mL/kg in children. When possible, roll or shift the patient from side to side after the infusion to increase mixing. Place the IV bag or bottle on the floor (or below abdominal level), and allow the fluid to return by gravity.

If the fluid does not return, there may be several reasons. Some IV tubing contains a one-way valve. If tubing with a valve was used in error, replace it with valveless tubing and reattach it to the IV bag. Another reason for poor return is inadequate suction. To correct this problem, insert a needle into the second opening at the bottom of the IV bag or into the head of the IV bottle for aspiration of 10 mL of air. Alternatively, the catheter may be adherent to the peritoneum. If so, try to relieve some of the pressure in the IV bottle by gently wiggling and twisting the catheter or applying abdominal pressure to aid in the return of flow.

Return of 700 mL or more in an adult is generally accepted as adequate for interpretation of the findings. However, as little as 10% to 20% of the infusate may give a representative sample for both gross and microscopic determination. Send 10 mL of fluid from the return to the laboratory for cell count analysis, and send another 10 mL for enzyme analysis (see the

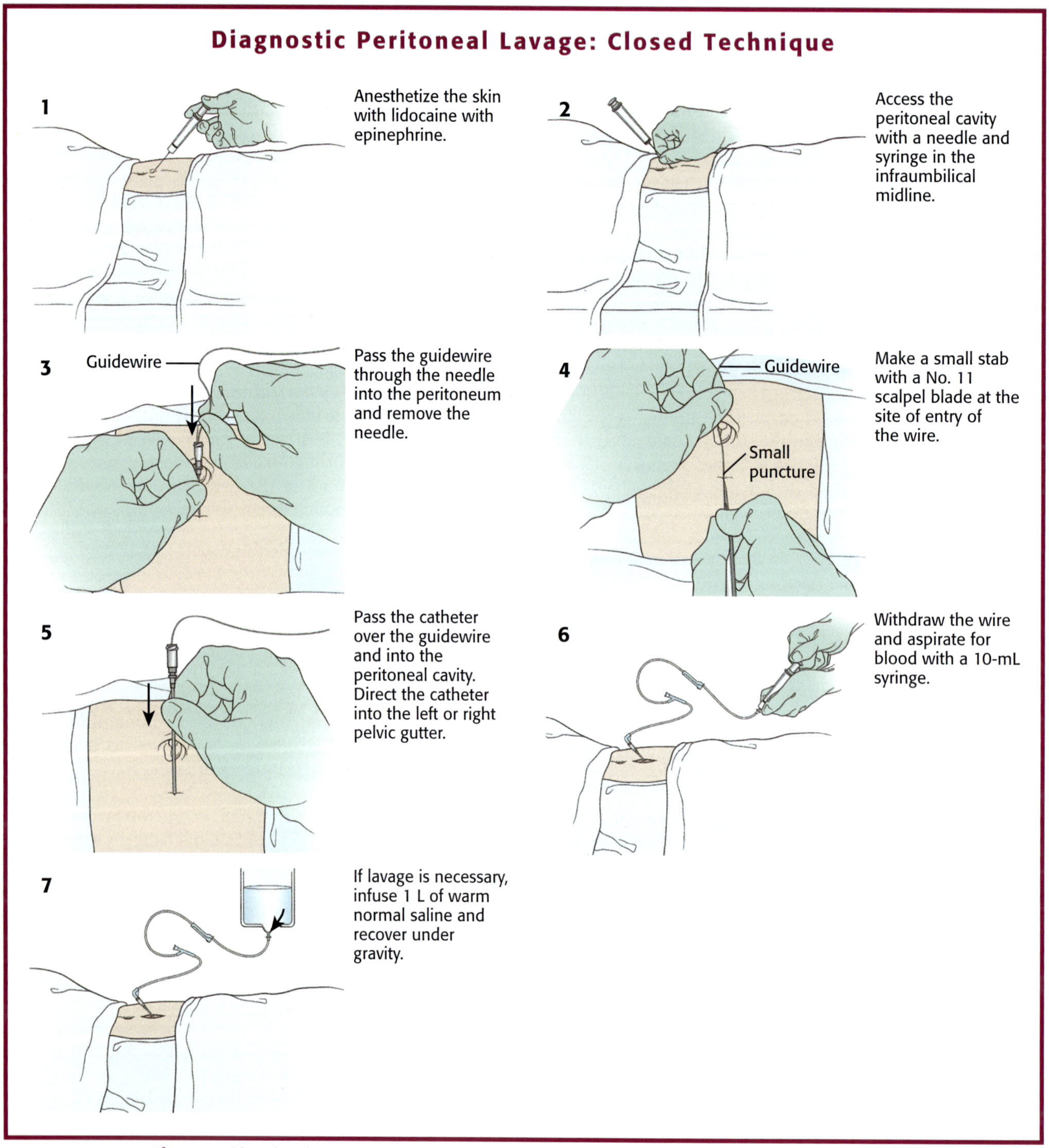

Fig. 44.5 Closed technique of diagnostic peritoneal lavage. Note that the stomach and bladder are decompressed under most circumstances.

section on "Interpretation" later in this chapter). Some operators prefer to leave the catheter in place until the returned fluid is analyzed so that lavage may be repeated if the initial results are borderline or an occult bowel perforation is suspected.

Complications

Local and Systemic

Local wound complications, including infection, hematoma, and dehiscence, are rare (Table 44.4).

Intraperitoneal

The trocar, wire, and rarely, the catheter can inflict iatrogenic intraperitoneal injury. Virtually any structure in the peritoneal cavity can be breached, including the small and large bowel, the bladder, and major vessels. Typically, if the needle is the culprit and even if the trocar is responsible, injury to these structures is minimal and self-limited, and observation of the patient is sufficient.

Technical Failure

Inability to recover peritoneal aspirate or lavage fluid can result in a false-negative interpretation. This can occur in

TABLE 44.3 Preferred Site for DPL

CLINICAL CIRCUMSTANCE	SITE	METHOD
Standard adult	Infraumbilical midline	C or SO
Standard pediatric	Infraumbilical midline	C or SO
Second- and third-trimester pregnancy	Suprauterine	FO
Midline scarring	Left lower quadrant	FO
Pelvic fracture	Supraumbilical	FO
Penetrating trauma	Infraumbilical midline[a]	C or SO

[a]The stab wound or gunshot wound site should be avoided.
C, Closed; *DPL, diagnostic* peritoneal lavage; *FO,* fully open; *SO,* semi-open.

several circumstances. It follows unwitting placement of the catheter into the preperitoneal space, which is less likely to occur with either open technique. Compartmentalization of fluid by adhesions or obstructing omentum can impede the egress of fluid. When a fully open supraumbilical or supra-uterine technique is used, the catheter may be too short to access the depths of the intraperitoneal cavity. Finally, the large diaphragmatic tears typical of blunt pathophysiology allow flow of lavage fluid from the intraperitoneal to the thoracic cavity.

False-positive findings can occur in two ways. First, iatrogenic misadventure may be responsible. Second, in penetrating trauma, particularly stab wounds, bleeding from the abdominal wall injury site into the peritoneal cavity can lead to positive findings when no injury to intraperitoneal structures has occurred.

Interpretation

Gross Blood

Recovery of 10 mL or more of blood via aspiration is considered a positive finding. Aspirates with lesser volume are generally discarded and are not factored into analysis of the lavage fluid. Grossly bloody aspirates are typically indicative of solid visceral or vascular injury, with a positive predictive value of greater than 90%.[17] Aspiration of blood is responsible for approximately 80% of true-positive DPL findings with blunt trauma and for 50% with stab wounds.[11]

A positive aspiration in a blunt trauma patient who is hemodynamically stable or has been resuscitated to apparent stability need not mandate urgent surgery. Unnecessary laparotomy will occur if there has been minimal and self-limited damage to the liver, spleen, bowel serosa, or mesentery. In this situation, CT and clinical indicators should be used in concert with the findings on DPL.

RBC Count

The recommended red blood cell (RBC) threshold varies according to the mechanism and, in the case of stab wounds, the external site of injury (Table 44.5). The optimum criterion will deliver excellent sensitivity, a high positive predictive value, and a minimal incidence of unnecessary laparotomy. Negative laparotomy incurs a prolongation of hospitalization and increases the cost of care, in addition to creating the potential for procedural complications. RBC counts greater than $10^5/mm^3$ ($10^5/\mu L$) are generally considered positive with a blunt mechanism or after stab wounds in the anterior part of the abdomen, flank, or back. Counts of $20,000/mm^3$ to $100,000/mm^3$ should be considered indeterminate.[11] For stab wounds in the low chest region, where the diaphragm is at increased risk for injury, the RBC criterion should be lowered to $5000/mm^3$ to maximize sensitivity for isolated injury to this structure,[11] although others have advocated to use $100,000\ mm^3$ to safely reduce the number of nontherapeutic procedures in the operating room.[18] With gunshot wounds involving the abdomen or low chest region, the RBC criterion of $5000/mm^3$ is applied. This is intended to increase the sensitivity of the test because intraperitoneal entry by a missile carries a greater likelihood of intraperitoneal injury. An

TABLE 44.4 Complications of DPL

CATEGORY	COMMENTS
Local and Systemic	
Hematoma incision site	Local wound care
Dehiscence incision site	Local wound care
Local wound infection	As indicated
Systemic infection	As indicated
Intraperitoneal Injury	
Bowel	Observe, usually self-limited
Bladder	Observe, usually self-limited
Vascular	Observe, usually self-limited
Technical Failure	
Inability to Recover Fluid[a]	
Preperitoneal catheter placement	Repeat DPL
Compartmentalization of fluid	US, CT
Obstructed catheter	Gentle catheter manipulation
Diaphragm injury	Reverse Trendelenburg; consider US, CT
"Short" catheter (supraumbilical or suprauterine approach)	Trendelenburg
Intraperitoneal Hemorrhage[b]	
Iatrogenic injury	As indicated by clinical markers
Stab wound, abdominal wall bleeding	As indicated by clinical markers
Pelvic fracture (RBC count)	Complementary CT

[a]May lead to false-negative DPL results.
[b]May lead to false-positive DPL results.
CT, Computed tomography; *DPL,* diagnostic peritoneal lavage; *RBC,* red blood cell; *US,* ultrasound.

TABLE 44.5 Diagnostic Peritoneal Lavage

	POSITIVE	INDETERMINATE
Blunt trauma (RBC/mm^3)	100,000[a]	20,000–100,000
Stab wound (RBC/mm^3)		
Anterior abdomen	100,000	20,000–100,000
Flank	100,000	20,000–100,000
Back	100,000	20,000–100,000
Low chest	5000–10,000	1000–5000
Gunshot wound (RBC/mm^3)	5000–10,000	1000–5000
LAM (IU/L)	>20	10–19
LAP (IU/L)	≥3	NA
WBCs (per mm^3)	>500	250–500

[a]In a hemodynamically stable patient with a pelvic fracture and a positive or equivocal red blood cell count, computed tomography should be obtained to corroborate or refute intraperitoneal injury.
LAM, Lavage amylase; *LAP*, lavage alkaline phosphatase; *NA*, not applicable; *RBC*, red blood cell; *WBCs*, white blood cells.
From Marx JA. Diagnostic peritoneal lavage. In: Ivatury RR, Cayten CG, eds. *The Textbook of Penetrating Trauma*. Williams & Wilkins; 1996.

uncomplicated DPL should not result in more than several hundred to several thousand RBCs in the peritoneal lavage fluid.

The incidence of false-positive RBC interpretation in the setting of pelvic fracture is considerable. However, aspiration of free blood in patients with critical pelvic fractures predicts active IPH in more than 80% of cases. A positive RBC count should generally prompt corroboration or refutation of intraperitoneal injury by CT. In this fashion, needed pelvic angiography and embolization will not be delayed unnecessarily should active intraperitoneal bleeding not be found (Fig. 44.6).

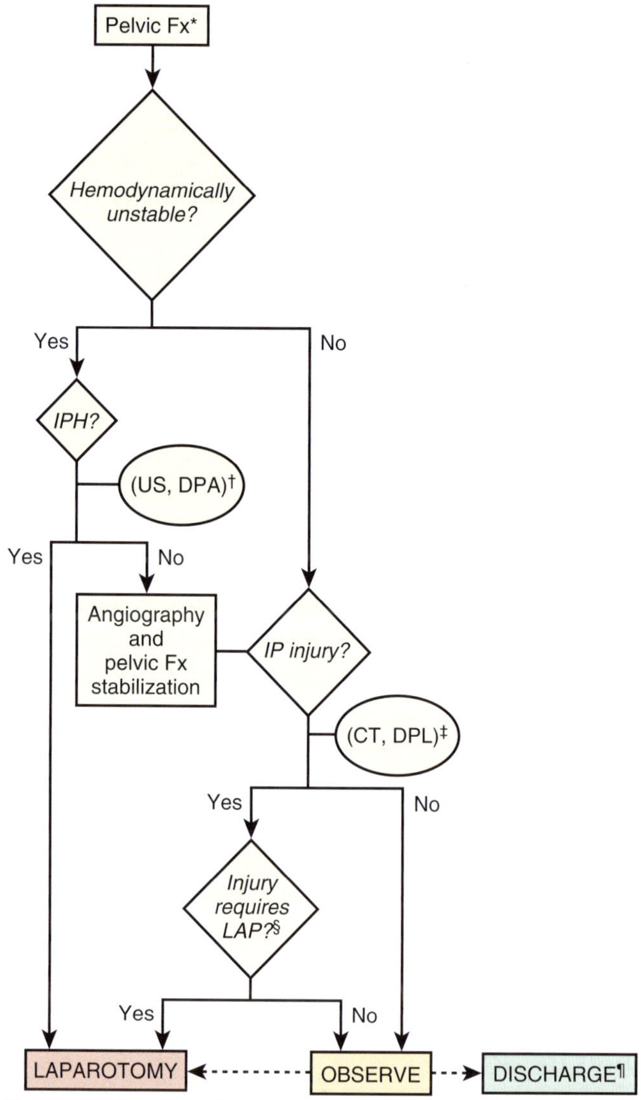

Fig. 44.6 Algorithm for the management of pelvic fractures and blunt abdominal trauma. *Certain pelvic fractures are more likely to cause pelvic vascular disruption and subsequent retroperitoneal hemorrhage. †Determined by unequivocal free intraperitoneal fluid on US or positive peritoneal aspiration on DPA. ‡One or more studies may be indicated. SPEs are generally considered unreliable because of the presence of a pelvic fracture. §The need for LAP is based on the clinical scenario, diagnostic studies, and institutional resources. ¶D/C from the perspective of need for further consideration for LAP. *CT*, Computed tomography; *D/C*, discharge; *DPA*, diagnostic peritoneal aspiration; *DPL*, diagnostic peritoneal lavage; *Fx*, fracture; *IP*, intraperitoneal; *IPH*, intraperitoneal hemorrhage; *LAP*, laparotomy; *US*, ultrasonogram. (From Marx J, Isenhour J. Abdominal trauma. In: Marx JA, Hockberger RS, Walls RM et al., eds. *Rosen's Emergency Medicine: Concepts and Clinical Practice*. 6th ed. Mosby; 2006:510.)

WBC Count

An inflammatory peritoneal response to a multitude of stimuli can occur, including stool, blood, and enzymes. The white blood cell (WBC) count in lavage effluent was at one point touted to predict small bowel injury but has since been proved unreliable. It is insensitive in the immediate postinjury period because 3 to 5 hours is necessary before the test becomes positive (see Table 44.5). Moreover, a positive finding is likely to be falsely so. Therefore the WBC level in and of itself should not determine the need for laparotomy.

Enzymes

Alkaline phosphatase is contained intramurally in the small bowel, as well as in hepatobiliary secretions released into the proximal part of the intestine. Amylase is contained in the latter only. Perforation of the small bowel allows access of these two markers to the peritoneal cavity, where they can be recovered by peritoneal lavage. Although levels of the two markers usually rise in tandem, lavage amylase has been shown to be a more accurate marker than lavage alkaline phosphatase (see Table 44.5). In contradistinction to the WBC count, these tests will be positive in the immediate postinjury period. However, they may not be economical if used on a mandatory rather than a selective basis. Neither is helpful in discerning the presence of pancreatic pathology.

Miscellaneous

Routine bile staining, Gram staining, and microscopy to identify vegetable fibers are rarely productive and are of untested accuracy. Deck and Porter reported that finding urine in the lavage fluid, as evidenced by a straw color, and creatinine in the peritoneal fluid should suggest an intraperitoneal bladder or collecting system injury.[19]

Conclusion

In the current era of readily available advanced imaging techniques such as CT and US, DPL maintains a diminished, but potentially important role in the evaluation of injured patients. It can identify life-threatening IPH in unstable patients when US is unavailable, indeterminate, or negative for free fluid. In addition, DPL can identify hollow viscus injury when CT is nondiagnostic in patients in whom serial clinical evaluations are impractical or unreliable, as in those with severe traumatic brain and spinal cord injuries. Finally, DPL remains more accurate than CT in identifying occult diaphragmatic injuries and is useful in high-risk patients without other indications for surgical abdominal exploration. It should be used in commonsense fashion. The noted laboratory parameters are guidelines and should not be embraced to the exclusion of pertinent clinical features. Optimal strategies depend largely on the capability of an institution's resources and personnel in each clinical scenario.

BOX 44.1 Pathophysiologic Classification of Ascites

I. Elevated hydrostatic pressure
   A. Cirrhosis
   B. Congestive heart failure
   C. Constrictive pericarditis
   D. Inferior vena cava obstruction
   E. Hepatic vein obstruction (Budd-Chiari syndrome)
II. Decreased osmotic pressure
   A. Nephrotic syndrome
   B. Protein-losing enteropathy
   C. Malnutrition
   D. Cirrhosis or hepatic insufficiency
III. Fluid production exceeding resorptive capacity
   A. Infections
      1. Bacterial
      2. Tuberculosis
      3. Parasitic
   B. Neoplasms

From Runyon BA. Diseases of the peritoneum. In: Wyngaarden JB, Smith LH, eds. Cecil Textbook of Medicine. *18th ed. Saunders; 1998:790-793.*

PARACENTESIS

Therapeutic abdominal paracentesis, the removal of intraperitoneal fluid, is one of the oldest medical procedures and dates to approximately 20 BCE. Paracentesis was first described in the modern medical literature by Saloman at the beginning of the 20th century, and it became a valued decompressive therapy.[20] With the advent of diuretics in the early 1950s, paracentesis fell out of favor as a treatment option. Controlled clinical trials in the late 1980s up to the present have restored its reputation by demonstrating the safety and efficacy of large-volume paracentesis (LVP) in adults and children.[21,22] Because this mode is invasive and consumes clinician hours, it is generally reserved for the treatment of patients with chronic ascites who have tense ascites or whose condition is refractory to diuretic therapy. However, paracentesis remains an important diagnostic agent for patients with new-onset ascites or to determine the presence of worrisome conditions, notably infection, in those with preexistent ascites.[23]

Clinical Features

Determination of Ascites

See Videos 44.1 and 44.2. Small amounts of ascites may be asymptomatic. Larger collections typically cause a sense of abdominal fullness, anorexia, early satiety, and perhaps nausea and abdominal pain. Substantial accumulations create symptoms of respiratory distress by restricting lung capacity.

Patients who lack obvious clinical markers may benefit from the performance of US, which can discern the presence of as little as 100 mL of fluid and determine fluid complexity (e.g., simple vs. complex fluid with septations or layering).[24] Endoscopically guided US may detect as little as 10 mL. It is more sensitive than CT in this respect and can assist in the identification of malignancy.[25] In addition, it is a useful adjunct for determining the location of fluid that may be compartmentalized by preexistent infection or surgical adhesions.

Differential Diagnosis

Causes of ascites can be categorized in several ways. On a structural basis, the causes are divided into diseases of the peritoneum and diseases not involving the peritoneum. The former group includes infection, neoplasm, collagen vascular disease, and idiopathic causes. The latter includes cirrhosis, congestive heart failure, nephrotic syndrome, protein-losing enteropathy, malnutrition, myxedema, pancreatic disease, ovarian disease, chylous effusion, Budd-Chiari syndrome, and hepatic venous occlusive disease. Pathophysiologic categories are listed in Box 44.1. In the United States, parenchymal liver pathology is overwhelmingly the most likely cause. Within this group, alcoholic liver disease, specifically cirrhosis, is responsible for approximately 85% of cases (Table 44.6).[26] Finally, ascites can be classified on the basis of a serum-ascites albumin gradient, that is, the difference between albumin values obtained simultaneously from serum and ascites samples (Box 44.2).

Indications and Contraindications

Therapeutic paracentesis is often undertaken in the ED setting to relieve the cardiorespiratory and gastrointestinal manifestations of tense ascites. LVP, or removal of more than 5 L, ameliorates the shortness of breath and early satiety that these patients experience. It may also be associated with collateral advantages, such as a reduction in hepatic venous pressure gradients, intravariceal pressure, and variceal wall tension. These parameters are considered important predictors of variceal bleeding, and the improvement after LVP may decrease the risk for bleeding.

Abdominal Paracentesis

Indications

New onset ascites
Suspected spontaneous bacterial peritonitis
To relieve the cardiorespiratory and gastrointestinal manifestations of tense ascites

Contraindications

Uncorrected coagulopathy AND clinically evident fibrinolysis or disseminated intravascular coagulation
Bowel dilation or obstruction
Pregnancy (technique should be altered as noted below)
Abdominal hematoma, engorged veins, or superficial infection at puncture site

Complications

Systemic
Hyponatremia
Renal dysfunction
Hepatic encephalopathy
Hemodynamic compromise
Significant bleeding
Death

Local
Persistent ascitic fluid leak at the wound site
Abdominal wall hematoma
Localized infection

Intraperitoneal
Perforation of vessels and viscera
Generalized peritonitis
Abdominal wall abscess

Equipment

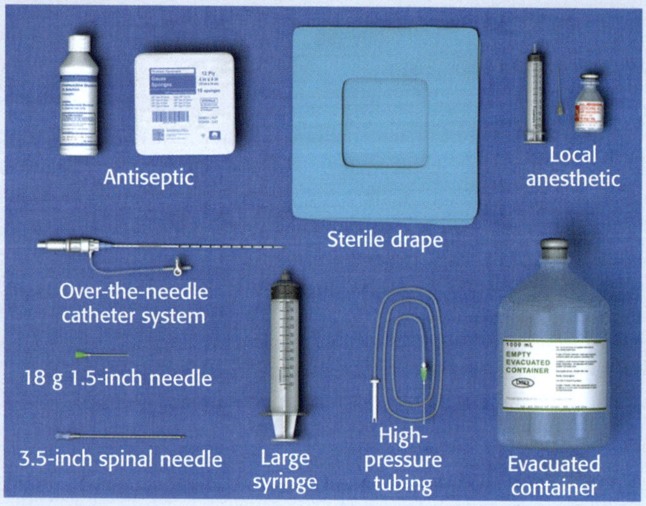

Review Box 44.2 Abdominal paracentesis: indications, contraindications, complications, and equipment.

TABLE 44.6 Causes of Ascites[a]

CAUSE	PATIENTS (%)
Parenchymal liver disease	80
Mixed	5
Malignancy	10
Heart failure	5
Tuberculosis	2
Pancreatic	1
Nephrogenous ("dialysis ascites")	<1
Chlamydia	<1
Nephrotic	<1
Surgical peritonitis in the absence of liver disease	<1

[a]Based on a series of 1500 paracenteses (unpublished) performed in a predominantly inpatient hepatology/general internal medicine setting.
From Runyon BA. Ascites and spontaneous bacterial peritonitis. In: Sleisenger MH, Fordtran JS, eds. *Gastrointestinal Disease: Pathophysiology/Diagnosis/Management*. 5th ed. Saunders; 1993:1977.

BOX 44.2 **Classification of Ascites by the Serum-Ascites Albumin Concentration Gradient**

HIGH GRADIENT (≥1.1 g/dL)
Cirrhosis
Alcoholic hepatitis
Cardiac ascites
Massive liver metastases
Fulminant hepatic failure
Budd-Chiari syndrome
Portal vein thrombosis
Venous occlusive disease
Fatty liver of pregnancy
Myxedema
Mixed ascites

LOW GRADIENT (<1.1 g/dL)
Peritoneal carcinomatosis
Tuberculous peritonitis
Pancreatic ascites
Biliary ascites
Nephrotic syndrome
Serositis in connective tissue diseases

From Runyon BA. Ascites. In: Schiff L, Schiff ER, eds. Diseases of the Liver. *7th ed. Lippincott-Raven; 1993:997.*

Diagnostic paracentesis, sometimes relegated to inpatient services, is indicated in any patient whose ascites is of new onset or in those with signs of clinical deterioration, including fever, abdominal pain or tenderness, altered mental status, or renal injury.[27–32] Diagnostic paracentesis can also be useful in the management of patients with acquired immunodeficiency syndrome (AIDS), in whom the etiology of ascites will be non–AIDS related in many cases. There are few relative contraindications to abdominal paracentesis. Certain systemic and anatomic risks should be considered, however.

Systemic

The majority of patients with liver dysfunction and cirrhosis will demonstrate abnormal coagulation panel testing and thrombocytopenia. However, the risk of bleeding and other adverse events from paracentesis is low. Therefore for patients undergoing repeated therapeutic paracentesis, in the absence of previous problems or obvious clotting issues, routinely obtaining a platelet count and international normalized ratio (INR) before the procedure is not necessary. In an investigation of 628 patients undergoing outpatient LVP, the procedure was safely performed when the INR was as high as 8.7 (mean value, 1.7) and the platelet count as low as 19,000/mm^3 (mean value, 50,000/mm^3).[33] Other studies have found bleeding rates less than 0.2% in all patients undergoing paracentesis, and studies including patients with platelet counts <50,000/mm^3 or significantly elevated INR found bleeding occurred in <1% of patients undergoing paracentesis.[34,35] These data countermand older and more conservative recommendations to administer platelets to patients with levels of less than 50,000/mm^3 or to give fresh frozen plasma to those with a prothrombin time (PT) exceeding 20 seconds (1.5 times the therapeutic level). These blood products should be reserved for clinically evident fibrinolysis and disseminated intravascular coagulation.

Anatomic

Structural impediments to the safe introduction of a paracentesis needle can include the bladder, bowel, and pregnant uterus. The bladder is normally tucked into the recess of the pelvis. However, bladders that are neuropathologically distended as a result of pharmacologic agents or medical conditions should preferably be emptied by voiding or by catheterization to avoid puncture. The intestines typically float in ascitic fluid and will move safely away from a slowly advancing paracentesis needle. Therefore US guidance may be indicated in cases of suspected adhesions or bowel obstruction. Even if penetrated by an 18- to 22-gauge needle, leakage of intestinal contents will not occur unless intraluminal pressure is significantly elevated. In second- and third-term pregnancy, an open supraumbilical or US-assisted approach is preferred. The abdomen should be inspected carefully for evidence of abdominal hematoma, engorged veins, or superficial infection, and these sites should be strictly avoided. US can also be used to visualize blood vessels within the soft tissue prior to paracentesis to optimize needle placement.

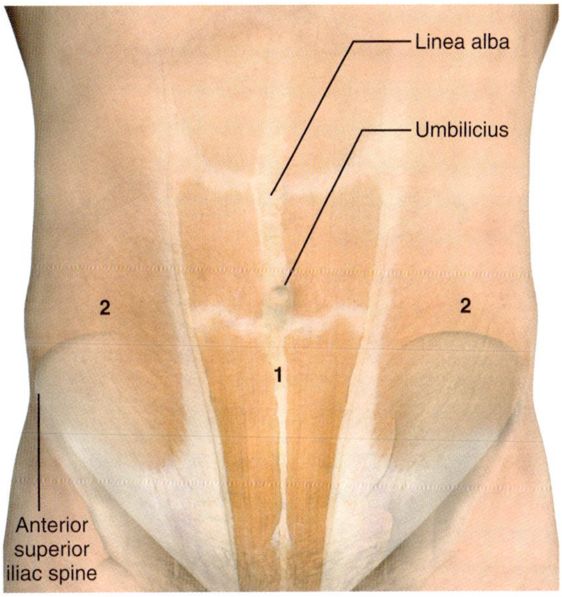

Fig. 44.7 The best site for drainage of recurrent ascites is based on success in previous similar procedures on the patient or ultrasound evaluation. The following are the preferred sites for paracentesis. *1*, The primary site is infraumbilical in the midline through the linea alba. *2*, The preferred alternative (lateral rectus) site is in either lower quadrant, approximately 4 to 5 cm cephalad and medial to the anterior superior iliac spine.

Technique

Preliminary Actions

Paracentesis should be performed after the patient has voided. It is not standard to decompress the stomach with a nasogastric tube or the bladder with a catheter before paracentesis. Place the patient in the supine position. Some clinicians prefer the supine lateral decubitus position, which will allow the fluid to collect on the dependent side. Perform paracentesis according to compliance with standards for body fluid precautions. Observe sterile technique throughout the procedure to prevent the iatrogenic introduction of bacteria into the abdominal wall tract or peritoneal cavity. Before making the skin incisions described later, prepare the site with standard skin antiseptics and drape appropriately.

Site of Entry

The best site of entrance for repeated paracentesis is determined by the patient's previous experience, so this question should be asked of the patient. Theoretically, most sites on the abdominal wall can be used, but in absence of previous experience with the individual patient, two sites are preferred. One site is approximately 2 cm below the umbilicus in the midline (Fig. 44.7), where the fasciae of the rectus abdominis muscle join to form the fibrous, thin, avascular linea alba. Large collateral veins may occasionally be present and should be avoided (Fig. 44.8), as should suspected areas of skin infection. Another preferred site is either the right or left lower quadrant, approximately 4 cm to 5 cm cephalad and medial to the anterior superior iliac spine (see Fig. 44.7).

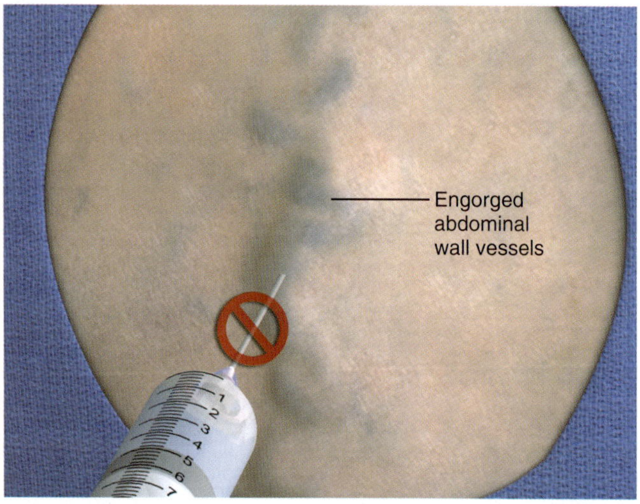

Fig. 44.8 Avoid sites on the abdominal wall with engorged veins.

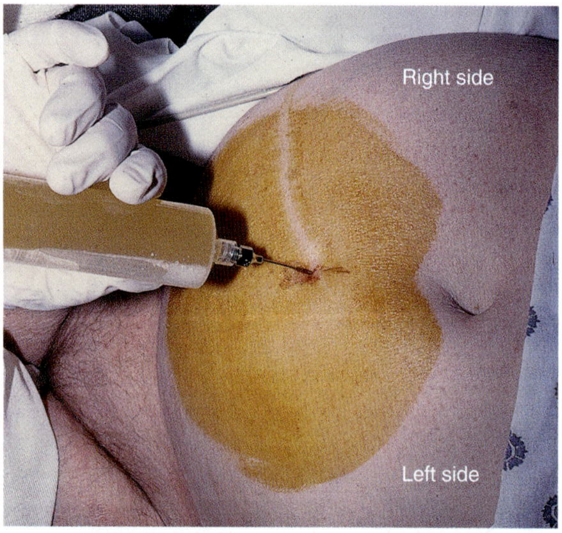

Fig. 44.9 An alternative to the sitting or supine position for diagnostic or therapeutic needle paracentesis is to place the patient in the lateral decubitus position. In this example the midline is aspirated, although lateral rectus sites may also be used. Some prefer the lateral decubitus position routinely because the bowel tends to float upward and out of the path of the needle. Note the cloudy fluid seen with spontaneous bacterial peritonitis. The patient had vague abdominal pain only, a subtle manifestation of a serious problem.

One study evaluating abdominal wall thickness and fluid depth determined the left lower quadrant was superior compared to the infraumbilical midline site.[36] The right or left lower quadrant should also be used if the patient has midline scarring or if previous experience has been positive. The entry site must be lateral to the rectus sheath to avoid the inferior epigastric artery. Patients with a large quantity of ascites can readily undergo the procedure in the supine position with the head of the bed slightly elevated. Those with lesser amounts of fluid may benefit from a lateral decubitus position with introduction of the needle into the midline or dependent lower quadrant (Fig. 44.9). Some clinicians

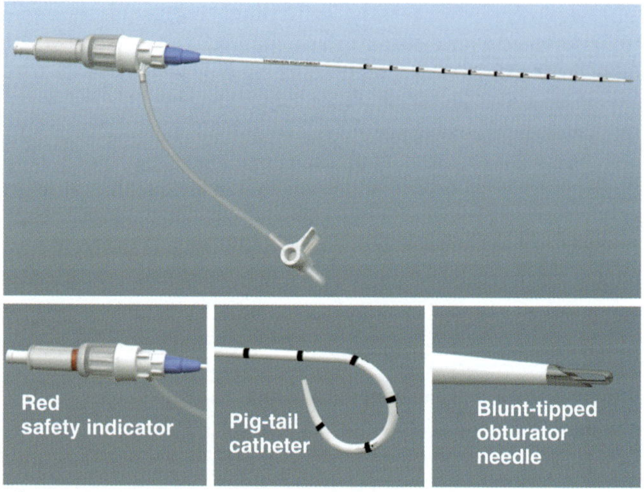

Fig. 44.10 Paracentesis can be performed with a prepackaged kit. The Safe-T-Centesis system depicted here includes safety features such as a blunt-tipped obturator needle, a color-changing indicator, and a pigtail catheter. The blunt-tipped obturator retracts with pressure to expose the sharp needle tip. This causes the color in the device to change from white to red. Once the abdominal cavity is entered and there is no longer pressure on the tip, the spring-loaded obturator covers the sharp tip of the needle to prevent damage to the underlying organs. This will cause the color to revert to white.

prefer to use the lateral decubitus position routinely because the bowel tends to float upward and away from the path of the needle. Hence, the site of needle entrance is in the midline or on the side closest to the bed. Rarely, patients may need to be placed in a facedown, hands-on-knees position. In patients with multiple abdominal scars or suspicion of compartmentalized abdominal fluid for any reason, US guidance is prudent.

Procedure

See Videos 44.3, 44.4. A prepackaged kit, such as the Safe-T-Centesis system (CareFusion), is a convenient way to perform the procedure (Fig. 44.10). Following sterile preparation of the skin, inject local anesthetic at the paracentesis site (Fig. 44.11, *step 4*). Use a standard 3.8-cm (1.5-inch) metal needle in most cases. If necessary, use a longer 8.9-cm (3.5-inch) spinal needle in obese patients. Plastic sheath cannulas tend to kink and run the risk of being sheared off into the peritoneal cavity, but a steel needle can be left in the abdomen during a therapeutic tap for intervals of an hour or longer without injury. The 15-gauge, 3.25-inch Caldwell needle/cannula is an alternative for LVP that has been shown to perform similar to a steel needle in terms of procedural complications and the volume of fluid removed. Use a smaller-gauge (20- to 22-gauge) needle for diagnostic taps because such needles lessen the likelihood of leakage of ascitic fluid through the wound site after the procedure. However, for therapeutic LVP, use an 18-gauge needle because it permits expeditious outflow.[21]

Insert the needle directly perpendicular to the skin at the preferred site (see Fig. 44.11, *step 5*). Alternatively, use

Abdominal Paracentesis

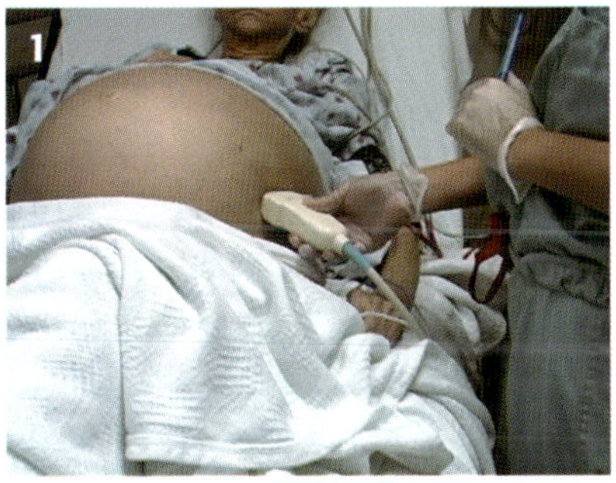

Localize the fluid collection by percussion or by ultrasound. Mark the entry site.

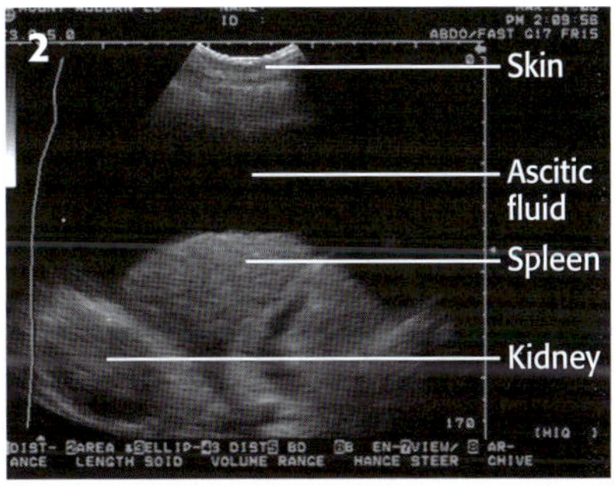

With ultrasound, identify free pockets of ascitic fluid, as well as organs such as the liver, spleen, kidney, or bowel.

See details of ultrasound techniques at the end of this chapter.

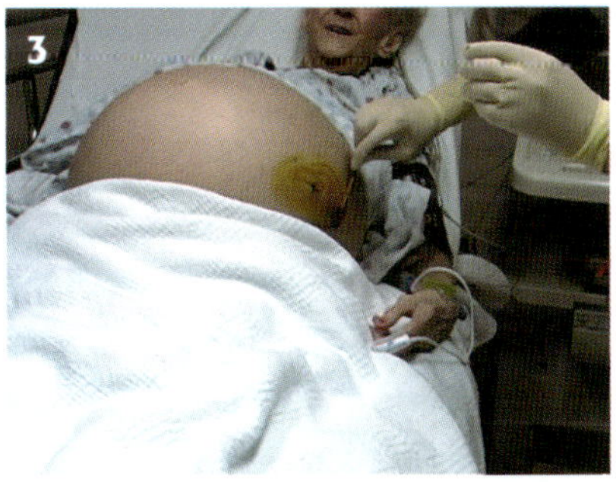

Cleanse the overlying skin with antiseptic and apply a sterile drape.

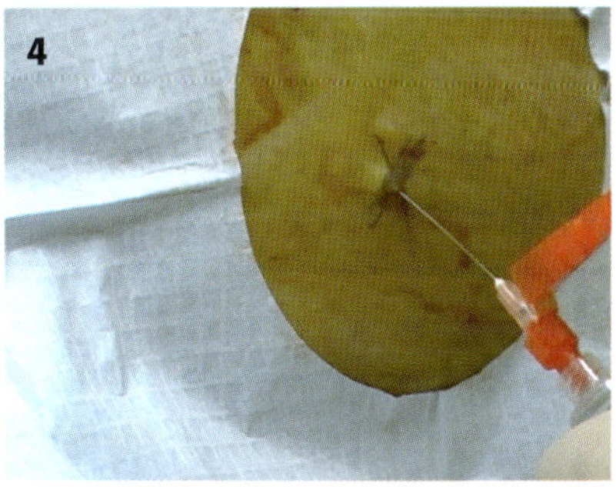

Anesthetize the skin and the proposed tract of the paracentesis needle with local anesthetic.

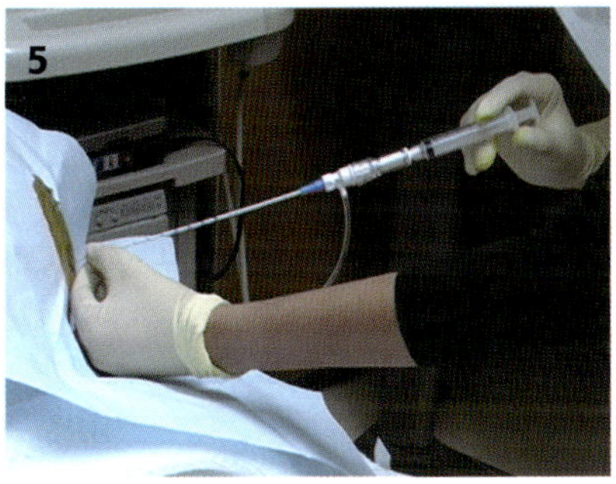

Insert the needle perpendicular to the skin and slowly advance.

See text and Fig. 44.12 for details on the Z-track method of paracentesis.

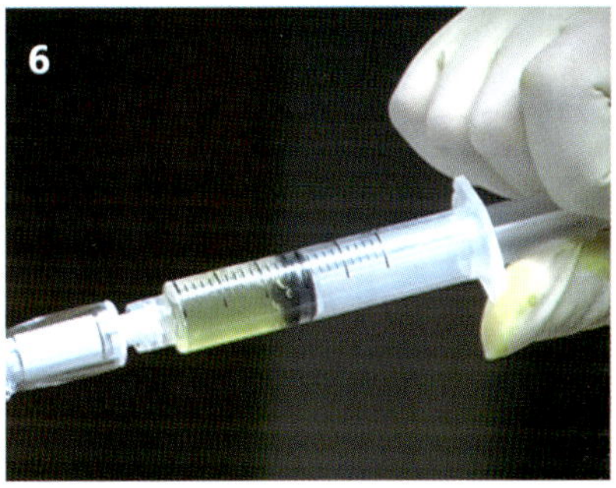

Advance the needle in 5-mm increments until fluid is returned in the syringe. Advance the catheter over the needle and into the peritoneal cavity (if a catheter-over-the-needle system is being used).

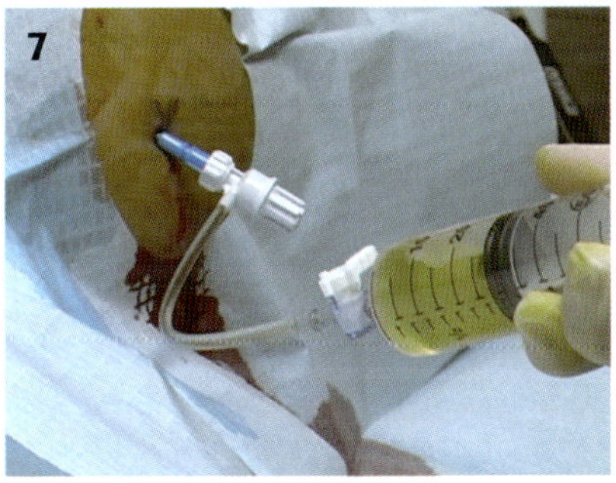

Aspirate peritoneal fluid into a 20- to 60-mL syringe for a diagnostic sample.

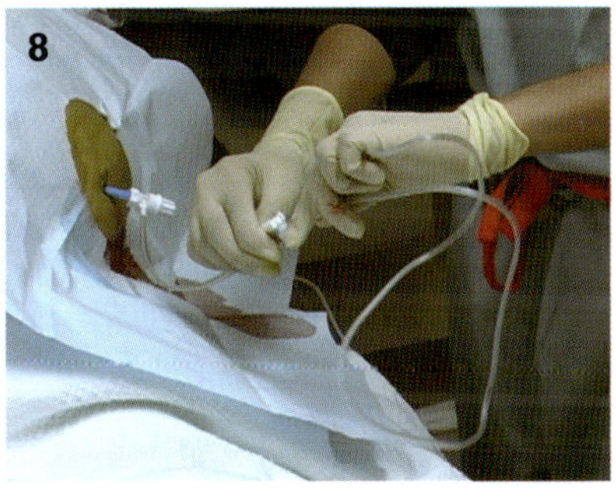

If large-volume (therapeutic) paracentesis is desired, attach the high-pressure tubing to the catheter hub.

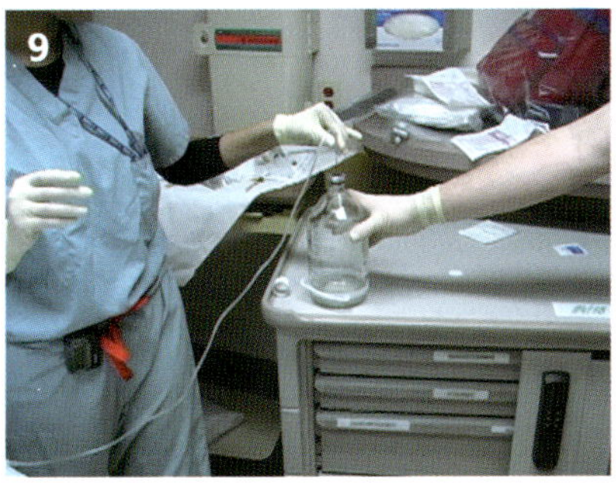

Insert the high-pressure tubing needle into the evacuated container to withdraw the fluid.

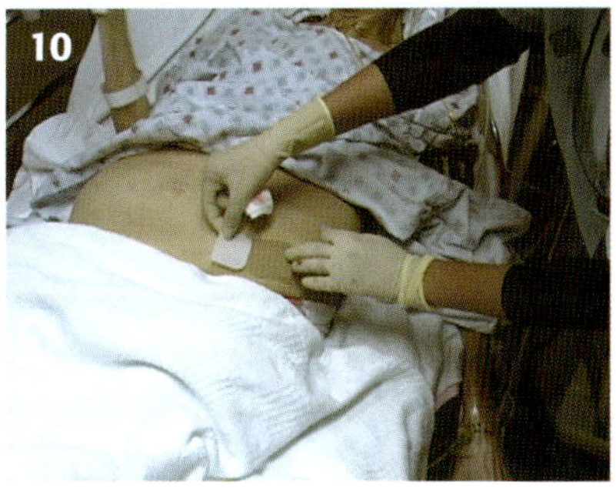

After fluid collection is completed, remove the catheter and apply an adhesive bandage (or a pressure dressing if there is persistent fluid leakage).

Fig. 44.11 Abdominal paracentesis.

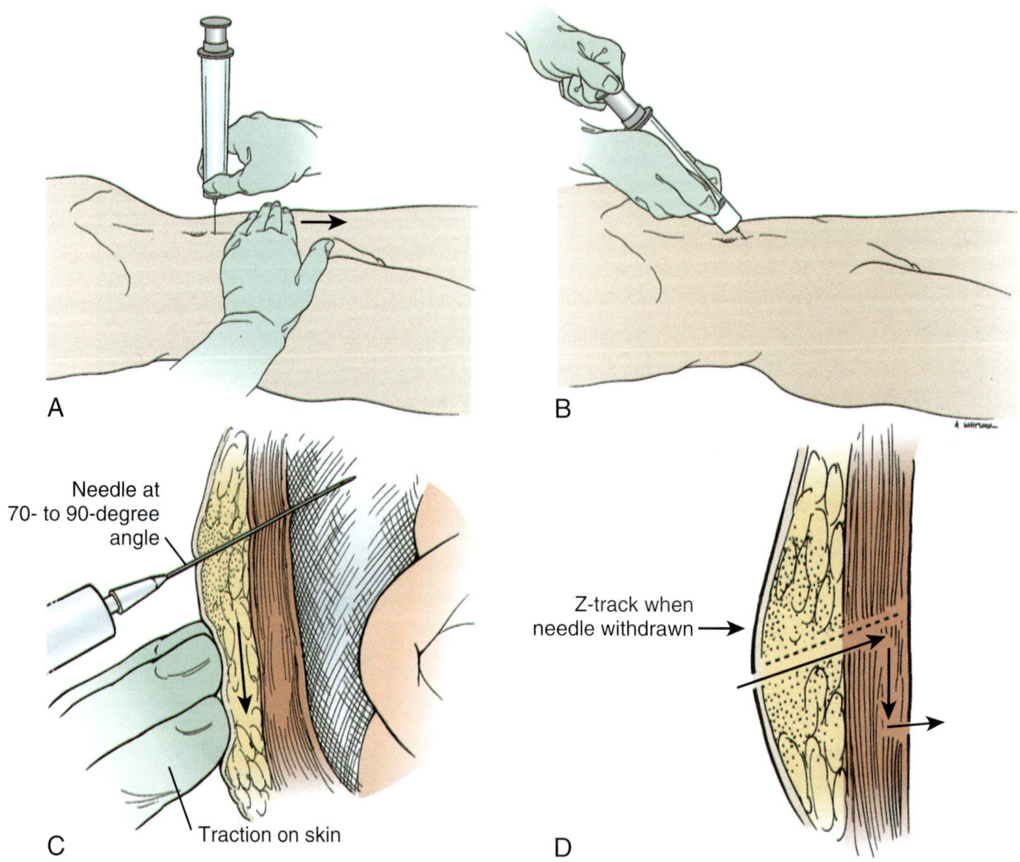

Fig. 44.12 (A) Z-track method of needle paracentesis. Pull the skin approximately 2 cm caudad in relation to the deep abdominal wall with the non–needle-bearing hand while slowly inserting the paracentesis needle perpendicular to the skin. (B) After penetrating the peritoneum and obtaining return of fluid, release the skin. Note that the needle is now angled caudally. (C–D) Use of the Z-tract method helps seal the tract and prevent persistent fluid leaks.

the Z-track method. For this method, pull the skin approximately 2 cm caudad to the deep abdominal wall with the non–needle-bearing hand while slowly inserting the paracentesis needle (Fig. 44.12). Release the skin when the needle has penetrated the peritoneum and fluid flows. This technique also holds the draining needle in place without suture or tape. A gauze pad can be used to pull on the skin, which will improve abdominal wall traction. Remove the needle after the procedure, and the skin will slide to its original position, helping seal the tract. In any case, insert the needle slowly in 5-mm increments to detect undesired entry of a vessel and to help prevent unnecessary puncture of the small bowel. Avoid continuous suction because it may attract bowel or omentum to the end of the paracentesis needle with resultant occlusion. Once fluid is flowing, stabilize the needle to ensure a steady flow. If flow ceases, gently rotate the needle and advance it inward in 1- to 2-mm increments. When fluid removal is complete, remove the needle and place an adhesive bandage over the puncture site. If there is persistent leakage of fluid, a pressure bandage may be required. Cyanoacrylate adhesive can also be utilized for persistent leakage. First place the patient so the site is in a nondependent position and apply pressure to the site with gauze for 10 minutes. Then withdraw the gauze and apply the adhesive over the puncture site. Dry air applied to the adhesive using nasal cannula can improve drying of the adhesive.

Ultrasound Guidance

See Video 44.5. US-guided paracentesis may be performed by a radiologist or an experienced emergency clinician ultrasonographer (see Ultrasound Box). This technique clearly delineates the pocket of ascitic fluid and allows visualization of loculated collections and avoidance of bowel adherent to the anterior abdominal peritoneum or blood vessels in the abdominal wall. The ultrasonographer scans the abdomen and marks the skin at the point overlying the optimal puncture site (see Fig. 44.11, *step 2*). Once the entry site is marked, keep the patient immobile and perform the procedure (as detailed previously) as soon as practical to avoid shifting of the fluid, which may decrease the utility of US guidance.

Volume of Fluid Removed

Many patients with chronic ascites are well versed on the procedure and have experienced it many times. Some undergo paracentesis on a regular basis in the outpatient

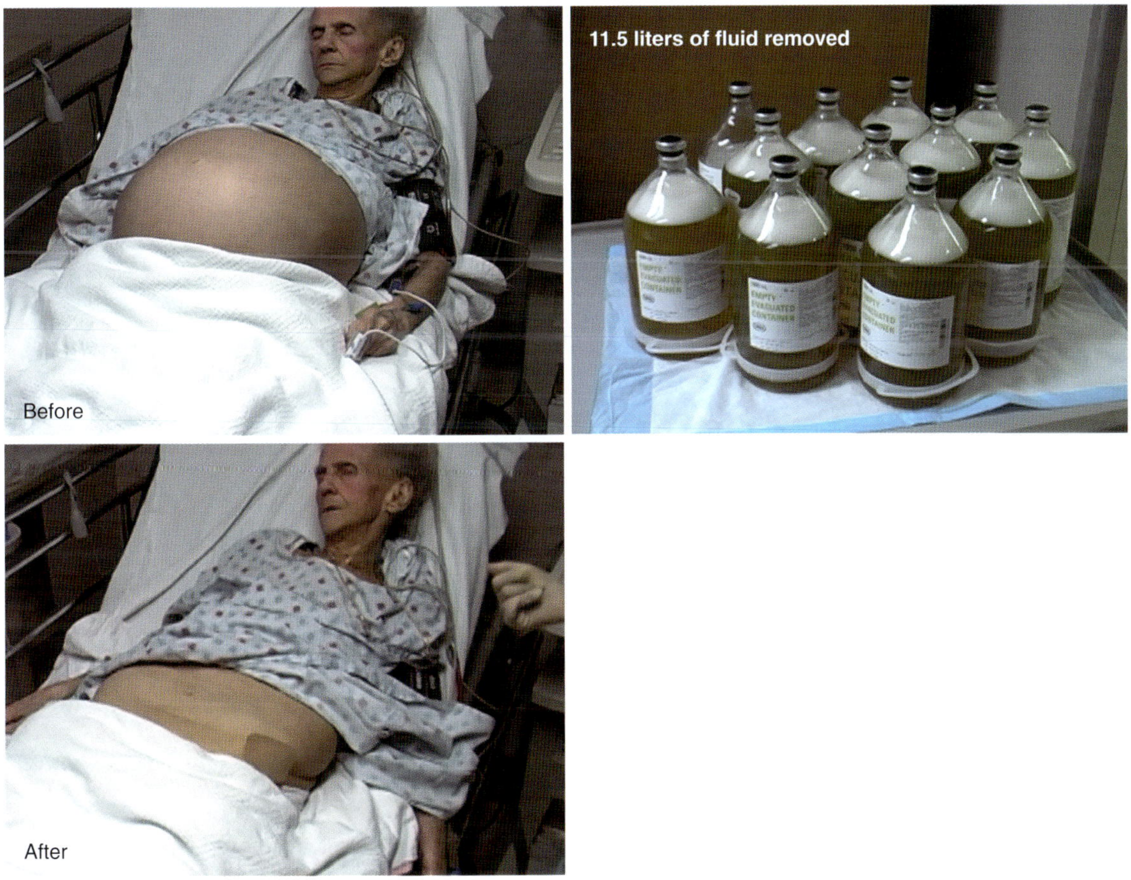

Fig. 44.13 Large-volume paracentesis in a patient with a history of recurrent ascites. See text for guidelines on the volume to remove and potential complications of removing large volumes. Note the use of blood pressure monitoring.

setting. Therefore the best guide to the volume of fluid to be removed for recurrent ascites is based on the patient's previous experience, and this question should be asked. Removal of 5 or 6 L is routine and well tolerated, and for therapeutic purposes, at least this volume should be removed. Patients seen in the ED may be less compliant with outpatient regimens and seek care only when in extremis. Hence, their ascites is likely to be much more voluminous than in those treated regularly. In general, the paracentesis volume consists of as much fluid as can be removed without excessive manipulation of the patient. Volumes greater than 5 L are termed LVP. Up to 10 to 12 L may be removed safely in most patients with chronic ascites (Fig. 44.13). For first-time paracentesis and for diagnostic purposes (ruling out bacterial peritonitis, screening for cancer), 200 to 500 mL is usually sufficient, but more can be drained if it flows easily.

Removal of large amounts of ascitic fluid during paracentesis can be accomplished with the assistance of continuous wall suction. This technique should be used for patients with large amount of ascites (chronic liver failure patients) and who regularly have large volumes removed during paracentesis. Materials required include continuous wall suction, three-way stopcock, tubing elbow, syringes (3 mL, 5 mL, and 10 mL), suction tubing, three or more suction canisters, and usual paracentesis supplies (Fig. 44.14A). The patient is prepped for paracentesis. Standard tubing is attached to the wall suction, with the other end connected to the first suction canister. Tubing is then utilized to attach the first and second canister. Each canister must have one port with self-sealing filter, which is needed to close the system (Fig. 44.14B). Seal and cap all ports. This process can be repeated creating a suction train (Fig. 44.14C). Once the suction canisters are connected, take the final suction tubing end and place into a syringe, with plunger removed. After the paracentesis catheter has been placed and flow obtained, attach the suction syringe to the catheter or first to a 3-way stopcock (Fig. 44.14D). Turn the paracentesis catheter to the open position and turn on wall suction. Fluid should begin to drain into the first canister, and once full, fluid will continue into the other canisters in order. If flow stops, a stopcock can be helpful to flush the catheter with sterile saline or the patient's ascitic fluid. The final setup is shown in Fig. 44.14E.[37]

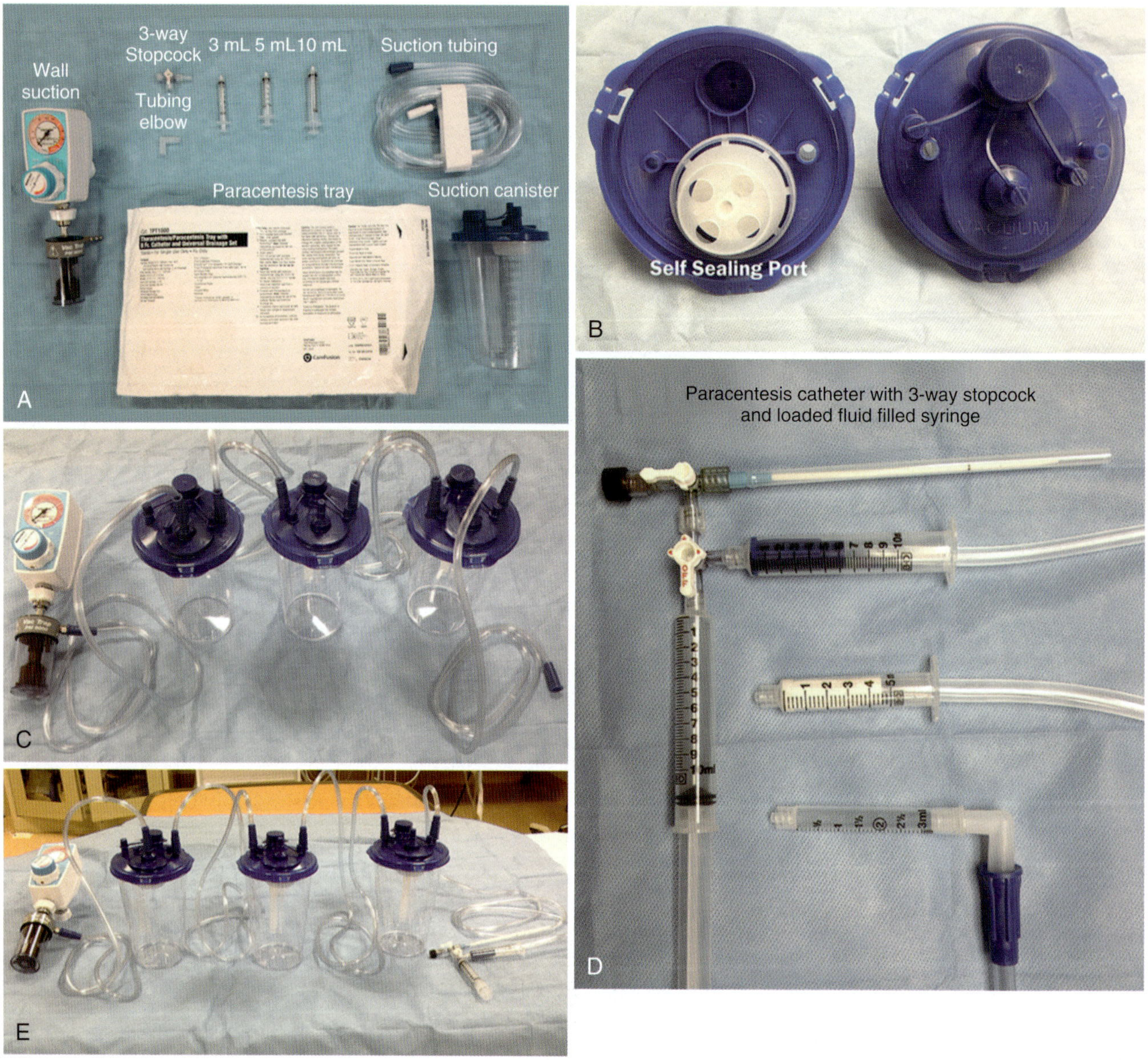

Fig. 44.14 Using continuous wall suction for large-volume paracentesis. (A) Equipment required for continuous wall suction paracentesis. (B) Self-sealing port of suction canisters. (C) Creation of suction "train." (D) Paracentesis catheter setup. (E) Final setup for continuous wall suction paracentesis. (From Jeong J, McNamee J, Rosenberg M. How to use continuous wall suction for paracentesis. *ACEP Now*. 2014. http://www.acepnow.com/article/use-continuous-wall-suction-paracentesis/.)

ULTRASOUND: Abdominal Paracentesis

by Christine Butts, MD

Although paracentesis has traditionally been performed "blindly," use of ultrasound allows the physician to confirm the presence of ascites. In addition, it allows the clinician to evaluate the most optimal location to attempt the procedure, which can be less straightforward in patients with smaller fluid collections or in whom physical examination alone is insufficient to make the diagnosis.

Equipment

Use a low-frequency transducer (2 to 5 mHz) to obtain a sufficient depth of penetration to visualize the area of interest. It is frequently helpful to set the initial depth to 20 to 25 cm to ensure that the entire abdomen is visualized.

Image Interpretation

The location of ascites is variable and depends on the amount of fluid present, as well as the position of the patient. The dependent areas of the abdomen, those evaluated with the focused abdominal sonography for trauma (FAST) examination, are ideal initial areas of evaluation. Evaluate the right upper quadrant by placing the transducer in either the transverse or the longitudinal orientation in

Continued

ULTRASOUND: Abdominal Paracentesis—cont'd

the eighth to eleventh intercostal space at the anterior axillary line (Fig. 44.US1). The transducer will probably need to be adjusted slightly to allow an optimal view of this area, either by moving up or down a rib space or by adjusting the angle of the transducer. Ascitic fluid will appear anechoic (black) and may be seen in Morison's pouch (in the hepatorenal space), near the inferior aspect of the liver, or at the superior aspect of the liver (Fig. 44.US2). Once this area has been evaluated in detail, evaluate the left upper quadrant in much the same fashion. Because the spleen is typically slightly more superior and posterior than the liver, place the transducer in the 8th to 11th intercostal space in the posterior axillary line (Fig. 44.US3). Again, make slight adjustments as needed to fully evaluate the area in question. Ascitic fluid will appear as anechoic (black) areas in the splenorenal space, as well as the potential space between the diaphragm and the spleen (Fig. 44.US4). Once these areas have been evaluated, look at the pelvis and lower part of the abdomen by placing the transducer just superior to the pubic symphysis (Fig. 44.US5). First identify the bladder to avoid any confusion. The bladder is typically seen as a well-demarcated area that is rectangular in shape in the transverse orientation and slightly triangular in shape in the longitudinal orientation (Fig. 44.US6). In contrast, free fluid will appear to have irregular borders and may seem to "seep" into the crevices of the lower part of the abdomen and pelvis. Additionally, bowel may be seen to float freely within free fluid (Fig. 44.US7). If free fluid is not appreciated in this area, evaluate the right and left aspects of the lower part of the abdomen as well. To do this, place the transducer in either the transverse or longitudinal orientation over the right and left lower quadrants, or near the areas where the traditional "blind" approach to paracentesis would be performed.

Procedure and Technique

Once free fluid has been seen, identify the area with the largest collection of fluid. Use ultrasound to identify the areas that contain the least number of loops of bowel. If the fluid collection appears to be large, use ultrasound to "mark the spot" and then put it aside. Proceed with the procedure in the typical sterile fashion in the area that has been identified and marked (Fig. 44.US8).

In cases in which the fluid collection is smaller, cover the transducer with a sterile cover to guide direct placement of the catheter.

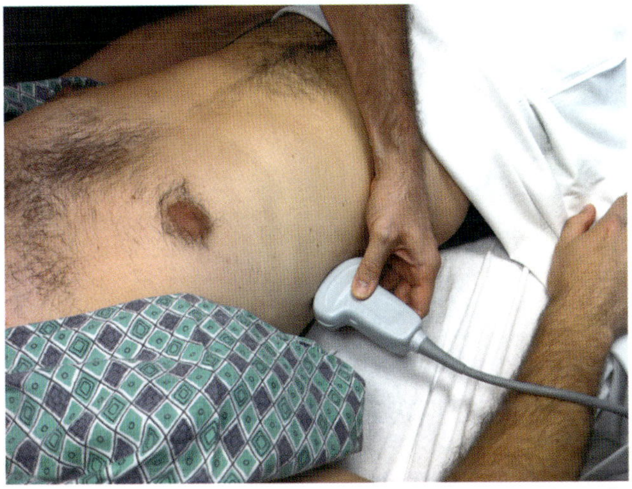

Fig. 44.US1 Placement of the ultrasound transducer in the right upper quadrant to evaluate for the presence of free fluid.

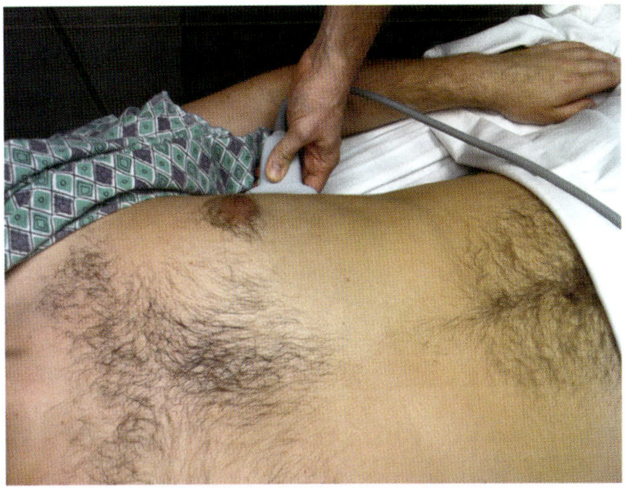

Fig. 44.US3 Placement of the ultrasound transducer in the left upper quadrant to evaluate for the presence of free fluid.

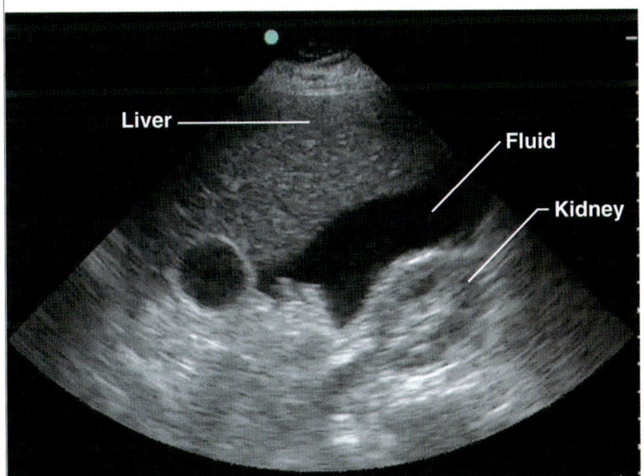

Fig. 44.US2 Free fluid in the right upper quadrant. The liver can be seen as the hypoechoic *(dark gray)* object *on the left* of the image, with anechoic *(black)* fluid seen between the liver and kidney (*on the right* of the image).

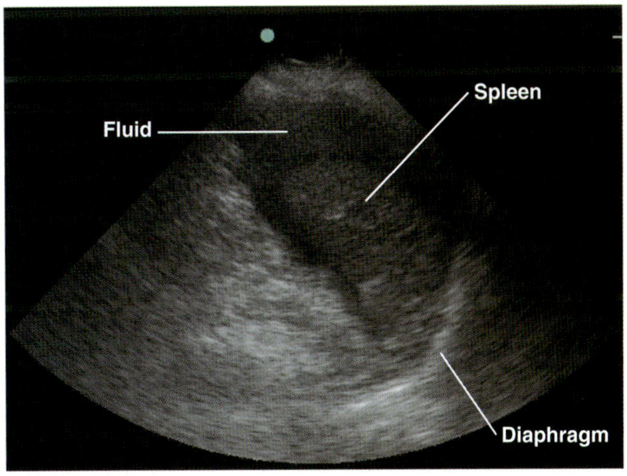

Fig. 44.US4 Free fluid in the left upper quadrant. Anechoic *(black)* free fluid can be seen surrounding the spleen at the right of the image. The diaphragm is seen as the bright white arcing structure on the far right of the image.

ULTRASOUND: Abdominal Paracentesis—cont'd

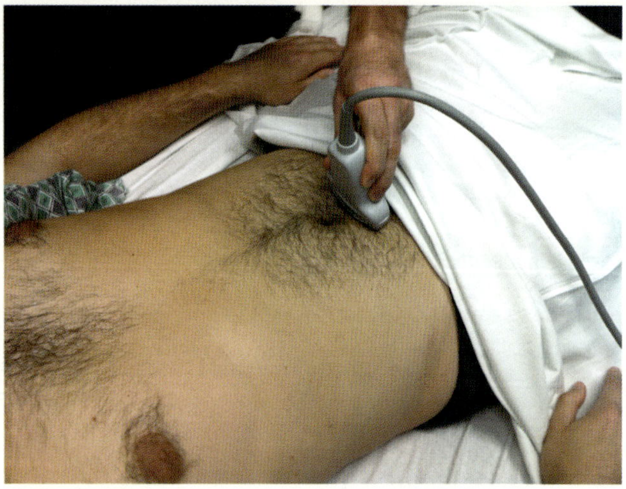

Fig. 44.US5 Placement of the ultrasound transducer to evaluate the pelvis for free fluid.

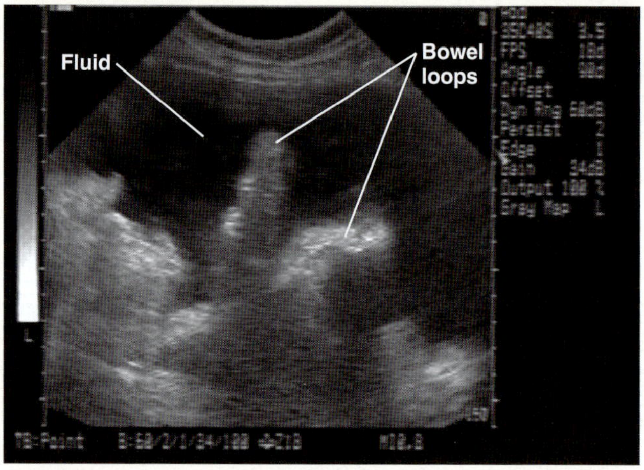

Fig. 44.US7 Large area of free fluid seen with ultrasound. Bowel loops are seen to "float" within the fluid.

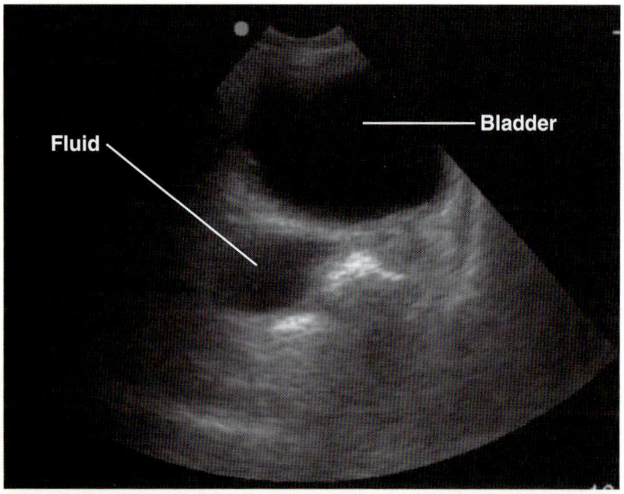

Fig. 44.US6 In this ultrasound image of the pelvis, the bladder can be seen as the rectangular object filled with anechoic *(black)* urine. An area of free fluid can be seen posterior to the bladder.

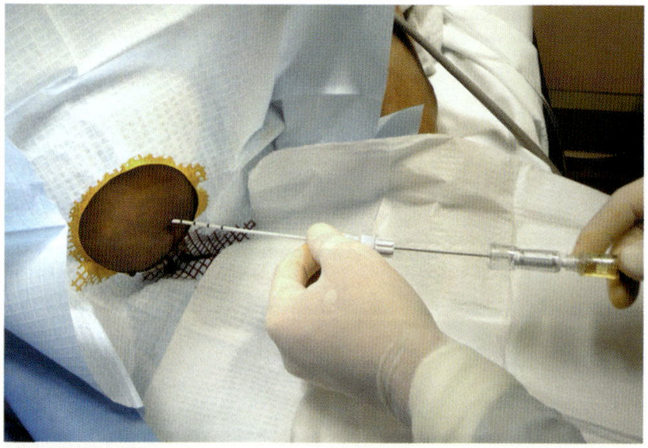

Fig. 44.US8 Place the paracentesis needle at the site that ultrasound had previously identified as being free of bowel loops and containing a large amount of fluid.

Complications

Complications of paracentesis can be divided into systemic, local, and intraperitoneal categories.

Systemic

Retrospective studies have suggested a risk for deterioration in hospitalized patients following LVP. However, the risk attributable to paracentesis is unclear given the difficulty in adjusting for the underlying severity of illness and comorbid conditions in these patients. The risk in ambulatory ED patients has not been investigated but is clearly less because paracentesis is often an outpatient procedure. Most systemic complications of paracentesis are merely temporally related or seen in seriously ill patients with end-stage liver failure who have a plethora of comorbidities.

Oft-cited but poorly documented concerns include hemodynamic compromise and other physiologic conditions caused by the overzealous removal of large volumes of ascitic fluid (greater than 5 L). This has been termed postparacentesis circulatory dysfunction (PCD), which may occur in 15% to 20% of patients undergoing LVP. It may not occur for several hours or days after paracentesis and is characterized primarily by hypovolemia (often asymptomatic), hyponatremia, and impaired renal function. The actual clinical significance of the associated disorders is unclear. Hypotension, for example, is common after paracentesis and is often not clinically significant.

Because upward of 6 L has been reportedly removed in less than 15 minutes without complication, certain authorities decry this issue as folklore. Others believe that rapid total paracentesis is accompanied by marked cardiovascular and humoral changes, some of which are explained by mechanical factors directly or indirectly related to relief of abdominal pressure.[38] Other changes, including systemic vasodilation and humoral deactivation, are of a nonmechanical nature. Hepatic encephalopathy, hyponatremia, hepatorenal syndrome, and rapid reaccumulation of ascitic fluid have also been ascribed to LVP. PCD of varying degrees is a real syndrome, and it may occur more often than suspected because many patients are discharged after the procedure. The consequences of LVP in ED patients have not been well studied, and the implications are somewhat obscure in this subset of patients. Because many patients require therapeutic paracentesis on a regular basis, ask the patient about previous experience and the usual volume of fluid removed to help guide treatment.

Because fluid and electrolyte shifts tend to be minimal after the removal of large amounts of fluid, colloid infusion is considered optional by some for patients with paracentesis of more than 5 L and is *not recommended* for paracentesis of lesser volume.[23] Others support the routine administration of albumin if more than 5 L is removed. When colloid is indicated, albumin has been the de facto choice. Being a blood product, albumin has been associated with rare complications, including anaphylaxis. The recommended infusion is 6 to 8 g of IV albumin per liter of ascitic fluid removed, or 50 g. However, colloid dextran 70 is favored by some authorities because of cost and concern for infection.

The necessity of routine plasma expansion after LVP remains controversial. No study has shown a direct survival advantage of one expander over another or in comparison to no expander. Postparacentesis plasma volume expansion does not prevent asymptomatic laboratory abnormalities. The mere fact that controversy still exists suggests that no clear indications can be promulgated to the emergency physician. The authors suggest *not* using IV albumin after taps of less than 5 L. We suggest that it may be used (6 to 8 g of albumin per liter of fluid removed, or 50 g) when more than 6 to 8 L is removed. If the patient is hypervolemic 25% albumin can be given, whereas 5% albumin is a good option if dehydration is suspected. If used, albumin is generally given immediately after the procedure, although administering it immediately before the procedure is also reasonable.

Local

Local complications include persistent leakage of ascitic fluid at the wound site, abdominal wall hematoma, and localized infection. Persistent fluid leaks may occur in up to 5% of patients and most commonly occur due to the Z-track not being performed correctly. This can be corrected with a single suture at the site of puncture.[39] Just as in cases of persistent leakage at the DPL site, cyanoacrylate glue can be utilized to stop leakage. The patient is positioned so the site is nondependent and then pressure applied to the site with gauze for 10 minutes. The gauze is then withdrawn and adhesive applied over the puncture site. To assist with drying, supplemental air can be applied to the site using nasal cannula or tubing connected to wall air or oxygen supply. An abdominal wall hematoma requiring transfusion is very uncommon, but careful observation in such cases is prudent.

Intraperitoneal

Intraperitoneal complications include perforation of vessels and viscera. In experienced hands these complications are uncommon, and in most circumstances, they are self-sealing and clinically inconsequential. However, generalized peritonitis and abdominal wall abscess have been reported after paracentesis in rare cases. The most common cause of postparacentesis IPH is bleeding as a result of a coagulopathy rather than large-vessel injury per se.[40]

Interpretation

Ascitic fluid should undergo gross inspection, but this should not be used to exclude the diagnosis of spontaneous bacterial peritonitis (SBP).[41] Routine laboratory testing includes a differential cell count, albumin assay, and cultures (Box 44.3). The prevalence of occult infection of ascitic fluid in asymptomatic outpatients undergoing therapeutic LVP for resistant ascites is low. As a result, in the absence of concerning symptoms or cloudy fluid, routine laboratory tests and culture of fluid during outpatient or ED paracentesis are not warranted.

Inspection

Ascitic fluid is typically translucent and yellow. A dark greenish brown hue may reflect biliary perforation. Cloudy fluid generally indicates particulate matter, including neutrophils; fluid with WBC counts greater than 5000/µL (i.e., >5000/mm^3) are cloudy, and those greater than 50,000/µL are purulent. Of note, fluid inspection by the clinician has a sensitivity of less than 75% for diagnosis of SBP.[41] An opaque, milky appearance may indicate elevated triglyceride levels. A blood-tinged appearance requires at least 10,000 RBCs/µL. This may reflect an iatrogenic complication, malignancy, hemorrhagic pancreatitis, or tuberculous peritonitis, although the last diagnosis creates hemorrhagic-appearing fluid very rarely.

Cell Count

Several milliliters of ascitic fluid are sufficient to obtain a differential cell count. Cirrhotic ascites should contain

BOX 44.3 Ascitic Fluid Laboratory Data to Be Obtained on Patients With Ascites

ROUTINE	UNUSUAL
Cell count	Tuberculosis smear and culture
Albumin	Cytology
Culture in blood culture bottles	Triglyceride
	Bilirubin
OPTIONAL	**UNHELPFUL**
Total protein	pH
Glucose	Lactate
Lactate dehydrogenase	Cholesterol
Amylase	Fibronectin
Gram stain	

From Runyon BA. Ascites. In: Schiff L, Schiff ER, eds. Diseases of the Liver. *7th ed. Lippincott-Raven; 1993:997.*

less than 250 WBCs/μL (Table 44.7). However, because cells may exit through the peritoneal cavity more slowly than fluid does, the WBC count can rise in the ascitic fluid during the procedure. Thus an upper limit for uncomplicated cirrhotic ascites is reported as 500 cells/μL. Lymphocytes should predominate, and clinical signs or symptoms of peritoneal infection should be absent. In cases in which SBP is a clinical consideration, the WBC criterion is 250/μL with greater than 50% polymorphonuclear leukocytes.[27]

Albumin

A serum-ascites albumin gradient can be obtained by simultaneously measuring albumin in ascites and serum and calculating the gradient. A serum-ascites albumin gradient greater than 1.1 g/dL indicates portal hypertension with greater than 95% accuracy (see Box 44.2).[42]

Culture and Gram Stain

The most valuable method for determining the presence of infection is culture. The sensitivity of this test is markedly increased by direct inoculation of blood culture bottles at the bedside as opposed to simply delivering the ascitic fluid to the laboratory. A different needle than the one used to perform the paracentesis should be used to inoculate the blood culture bottle. Gram staining of peritoneal fluid is rarely helpful in the evaluation of ascites and has poor sensitivity.[28] Approximately 10 bacteria/μL of fluid is required for a positive Gram stain. Thus the Gram stain is notoriously insensitive in patients with SBP, in whom the medium concentration of bacteria is 10^{-3} organisms/μL of fluid. Gram stain can be expected to be helpful only in cases of free gut perforation.

Miscellaneous

Optional tests include measurement of total protein, glucose, lactate dehydrogenase, and amylase. These tests will be beneficial in selected circumstances and need not be obtained on a routine basis. Immunosuppressed patients, including those with HIV/AIDS, should undergo microbiologic testing for opportunistic infections, including tuberculosis. Cytologic analysis is recommended in patients with suspicious

TABLE 44.7 Ascitic Fluid Characteristics in Various Disease States

				Cell Count		
CONDITION	GROSS APPEARANCE	SPECIFIC GRAVITY	PROTEIN (g/dL)	RBCs (>10,000/μL)	WBCs/μL (WBCs/mm³)	OTHER TESTS
Cirrhosis	Straw colored or bile stained	<1.016 (95%)[a]	<25 (95%)	1%	<250 (90%),[a] predominantly mesothelial	
Neoplasm	Straw colored, hemorrhagic, mucinous, or chylous	Variable, >1.016 (45%)	>25 (75%)	20%	>1000 (50%); variable cell types	Cytology, cell block, peritoneal biopsy
Tuberculous peritonitis	Clear, turbid, hemorrhagic, or chylous	Variable, >1.016 (50%)	>25 (50%)	7%	>1000 (70%); usually >70% lymphocytes	Peritoneal biopsy, stain and culture for acid-fast bacilli
Pyogenic peritonitis	Turbid or purulent	If purulent, >1.016	If purulent, >2.5	Unusual	>250; mainly polymorphonuclear leukocytes	Positive Gram stain, culture
Congestive heart failure	Straw colored	Variable, <1.016 (60%)	Variable, 15–53	10%	<1000 (90%); usually mesothelial, mononuclear	
Nephrosis	Straw colored or chylous	<1.016	<25 (100%)	Unusual	<250; mesothelial, mononuclear	If chylous, ether extraction, Sudan staining
Pancreatic ascites (pancreatitis, pseudocyst)	Turbid, hemorrhagic, or chylous	Variable, often >1.016	Variable, often >25	Variable, may be blood stained	Variable	Increased amylase in ascitic fluid and serum

[a]Because the conditions of examining fluid and selecting patients were not identical in each series, the percentages (in parentheses) should be taken as an indication of the order of magnitude rather than as the precise incidence of any abnormal finding.
RBC, Red blood cell; *WBC*, white blood cell.
From Glickman RM, Isselbacher KJ. Abdominal swelling and ascites. In: Isselbacher KJ, Braunwald E, Wilson JD et al., eds. *Harrison's Principles of Internal Medicine*. 13th ed. McGraw-Hill; 1994:234.

constitutional symptoms and signs.[43] Triglyceride and bilirubin studies are indicated if the gross appearance of the fluid is suggestive of increased levels. Other testing of ascitic fluid includes lactoferrin (iron-binding protein associated with SBP), calprotectin (a protein derived from neutrophils), bilirubin, and lactate. These tests have demonstrated promise, but they are not available in all centers.[44–48]

Leukocyte esterase reagent strips can be used for diagnosis of SBP. There are several types available, with sensitivity ranging between 80.6% and 96.4% and specificity ranging between 67.2% and 97.4%.[49] Testing with reagent strips may be most helpful in settings where ascitic cell count is not readily available.

Medical Therapy and Disposition

Total paracentesis may be performed safely in the ED, even in cirrhotic patients with large volumes of ascitic fluid (>5 L). However, the immediate relief provided by the procedure is temporary, and medical therapy is indicated to prevent or slow the reaccumulation of fluid. Measures include reduction of dietary sodium intake (<2000 mg/day) and the use of diuretics (spironolactone and furosemide) to promote natriuresis. It is prudent to observe patients undergoing LVP in the ED for 2 to 4 hours for hemodynamic compromise. In the absence of other indications for hospital admission, these patients may then be managed in the outpatient setting with close follow-up to ensure adequacy of their medical regimen. Overall, the clinician should base the decision to admit or discharge on the initial scenario, individual patient characteristics, and response to paracentesis.

Spontaneous Bacterial Peritonitis

SBP is an ascitic fluid infection, occurring almost always in patients with cirrhosis and ascites. It may be associated with fever or hypothermia, abdominal pain, altered mental status, abdominal tenderness, diarrhea, paralytic ileus, hypotension. It can be clinically quite subtle in some patients. Patients suspected of SBP, and after paracentesis, should be treated with empiric antibiotic therapy to improve patient morbidity and mortality. The majority of cases are due to *Escherichia coli* and *Klebsiella*. Treatment includes antibiotics. Unfortunately, studies comparing antibiotics in patients with SBP are limited. Cefotaxime 2 g intravenously every 8 hours provides optimal blood and ascitic fluid levels. Other options include cephalosporins and fluoroquinolones, such as ceftriaxone 2 g IV.[50] Recent data suggest more broad-spectrum antibiotic coverage (e.g., carbapenem) may result in reduced mortality and faster disease resolution in SBP, and thus those with critical illness, end-organ injury, recurrent SBP, or recent hospitalization may benefit from broad-spectrum antibiotics.[51,52] Broader coverage is warranted as well for patients with secondary bacterial peritonitis or polymicrobial infections.

Renal failure develops in 30% to 50% of patients with SBP, which is a significant cause of mortality.[53–55] This risk of death may be decreased with albumin infused at 1.5 g/kg body weight within 6 hours of diagnosis, followed by 1 g/kg 48 hours later, and albumin should be provided with creatinine greater than 1 mg/dL (88 mmol/L), blood urea nitrogen greater than 30 mg/dL (10.7 mmol/L), or total bilirubin greater than 4 mg/dL.[56] Albumin infusion is associated with decrease in incidence of renal impairment and mortality.[57,58]

Chronic Ambulatory Peritoneal Dialysis

Patients undergoing chronic ambulatory peritoneal dialysis are at an increased risk for peritonitis because of the presence of a chronic indwelling peritoneal catheter. Culture yield is maximized by obtaining a sample of greater than 10 mL of the peritoneal effluent under sterile conditions after a dwell time of at least 2 to 4 hours.[59] Peritonitis is defined by cloudy fluid with more than 100 WBCs/mm^3 and greater than 50% polymorphonuclear cells.[59] Although Gram stain is often negative in patients with bacterial peritonitis, it may reveal the presence of yeast and prompt timely initiation of antifungal therapy. Intraperitoneal antibiotics are superior to IV dosing, and removal of the catheter may be required for refractory or recurrent infections. Initial empirical intraperitoneal therapy usually includes a first-generation cephalosporin along with an aminoglycoside, ceftazidime, cefepime, or carbapenem.[59] Vancomycin should be considered in patients with a previous history of methicillin-resistant *Staphylococcus aureus* colonization or infection, in those who are seriously ill, or in areas with an increased local rate of methicillin resistance. The optimal treatment strategy should be discussed with the consulting nephrologist.

ACKNOWLEDGMENT

This chapter is dedicated to the memory of John A. Marx, MD, editor, author, educator, researcher, leader, humanitarian, and friend.

REFERENCES ARE AVAILABLE AT Elsevier eBooks+

CHAPTER 45

Abdominal and Groin Hernia Reduction

Aaryn K. Hammond, David E. Manthey, and Michael T. Fitch

INTRODUCTION

A *hernia* is a protrusion of any viscus from its normal cavity through an abnormal opening. Abdominal wall hernias are characterized by protrusion of intraabdominal contents (usually bowel or omentum) through an abnormal defect in the abdominal wall musculature. Hernias can develop along a congenital tract that fails to close (e.g., indirect inguinal or umbilical hernias), or along an area of weakness in the muscular and fascial layers (e.g., direct inguinal, ventral, or incisional hernias). Weakness of the musculature may be the result of aging and an accompanying loss of tissue elasticity, increased intraabdominal pressure, failure of proper healing after surgery or injury, or trauma involving the abdominal wall. It is estimated that hernias develop in 5% of males and 2% of females,[1,2] and that 75% of them occur in the groin.[3] A recent meta-analysis found a pooled prevalence of inguinal hernias of 7.7% with a predominance in males (9.61%) versus females (1.31%).[4] Groin hernias have a lifetime prevalence of 27% in males and 3% in females.[5] In children and young adults, the majority of hernias are indirect inguinal hernias of congenital origin,[6] whereas most direct hernias are acquired and become more common as a patient ages.[7] In patients who undergo abdominal surgery, incisional hernias can occur in up to 20% of cases.

Classification and Clinical Approach

When a patient is seen in the emergency department (ED) with a palpable mass that is suspected to be an abdominal hernia, the emergency clinician should consider three issues: (1) Is the palpable mass truly a hernia? (2) Is the hernia easily reducible or is it incarcerated? (3) Is the vascular supply to the bowel strangulated?

A *reducible hernia* is one whose contents can be manually returned through the fascial defect back into the abdominal cavity without surgical intervention. Patients with large reducible hernias may be asymptomatic for years and be able to self-reduce them easily but may present for evaluation when such hernias become strangulated or incarcerated. An *incarcerated hernia* is one whose contents are not reducible without surgical intervention. These hernias often have associated swelling of the hernia sac contents, making self-reduction more difficult for most patients. A *strangulated hernia* is an incarcerated hernia where the blood supply to the herniated structures is compromised, and this can result in tissue ischemia and necrosis if adequate blood flow is not restored in a timely fashion. Hernias with a small neck are more likely to become incarcerated or strangulated.

A patient with an easily reducible hernia can be discharged safely for outpatient follow-up and elective repair. While some seemingly incarcerated hernias can be reduced by careful clinician manipulation in the ED, most acutely incarcerated hernias and those with suspected strangulation represent surgical emergencies.

This chapter addresses abdominal and groin hernias, both of which are amenable to diagnosis and potential manual reduction in the ED.

HERNIA REDUCTION

Indications and Contraindications

The primary indication for attempting a hernia reduction is the identification of a hernia in the absence of strangulation. If initial attempts at manual reduction prove to be difficult, limit repetitive attempts that may increase the swelling of the herniated contents and limit the success of nonoperative reduction by a surgical consultant. Reduction of a strangulated hernia in the ED is contraindicated and operative management will be required. Surgical consultation in the ED is indicated for bowel obstruction associated with a hernia, undescended testicles or ovaries within the hernia contents, or traumatic hernias (Fig. 45.1).

Radiologic Imaging

When findings on physical examination are equivocal and the emergency clinician suspects an occult hernia, several options are available for diagnostic imaging.[8] Computed tomography (CT) scanning is the diagnostic modality used most often to confirm the presence of hernias and associated complications such as bowel obstruction or perforation (Figs. 45.2 and 45.3).[9] Magnetic resonance imaging has a high positive predictive value for patients with clinically uncertain herniations,[10,11] but its utility in the urgent setting is limited. Ultrasound examination has been shown to have good sensitivity and specificity for the diagnosis of groin hernias[12–14] and may decrease the rate of emergency surgery by improving the ability to reduce hernias.[15] Ultrasound may also have good specificity and a high positive predictive value for diagnosing postoperative incisional hernias.[8] However, ultrasound results can be operator-dependent and a difficult modality to interpret in some clinical circumstances.

Anatomy

A primary *ventral hernia* of the abdominal wall may be umbilical, epigastric, or spigelian, depending on its location (Fig. 45.4). A spigelian hernia (lateral ventral hernia) is located in the abdominal wall just lateral to the rectus abdominis muscle.[16] An *incisional hernia* is found along or near a previous surgical scar. An *inguinal hernia* is found within the inguinal triangle, which is formed by the inguinal ligament on the inferior side, the inferior epigastric artery on the superior lateral side, and the lateral edge of the rectus abdominis muscle on the medial side. Direct and indirect inguinal hernias occur superior to the inguinal ligament, whereas a femoral hernia is located inferior to the inguinal ligament (Figs. 45.5–45.7).

History and Physical Examination

A patient with a symptomatic hernia may seek treatment in the ED because of swelling or pain in the region of the

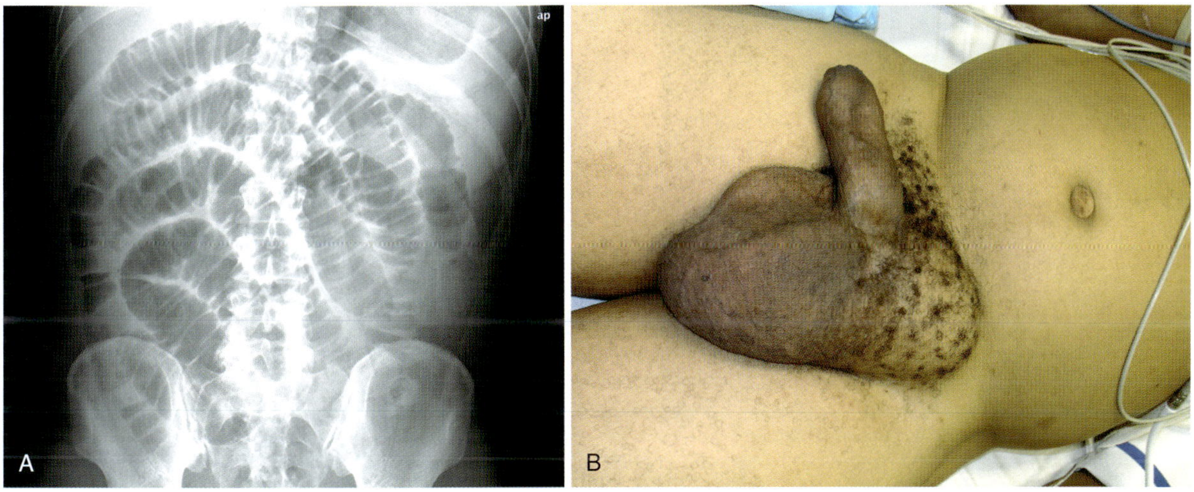

Fig. 45.1 Small bowel obstruction on plain film (A) caused by an indirect inguinal hernia (B).

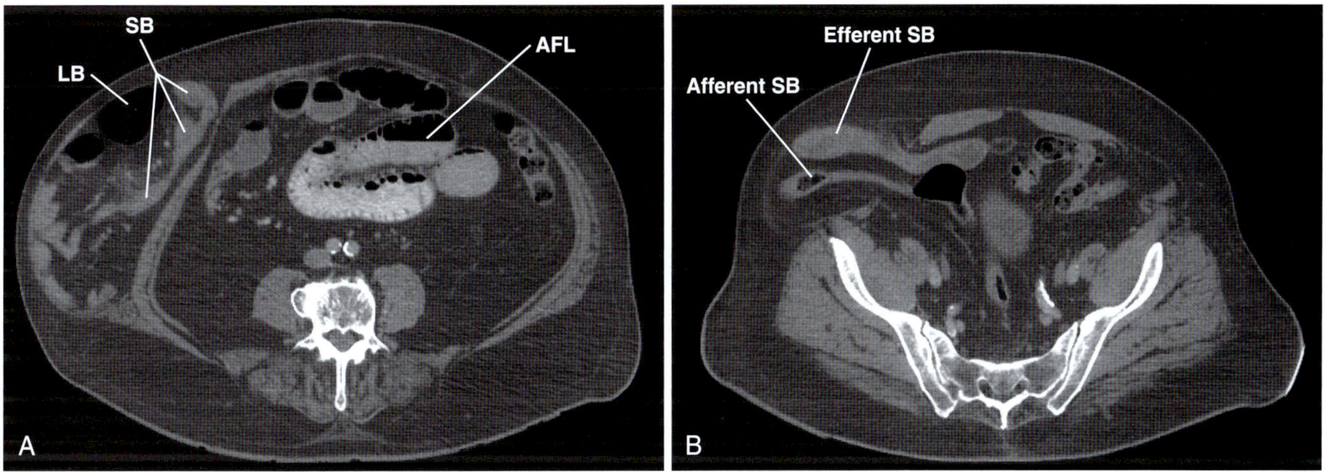

Fig. 45.2 Incarcerated spigelian hernia identified on abdominal computed tomography (CT). (A) Dilated loops of small bowel with air-fluid levels *(AFL)* are noted in the abdomen. Loops of both small bowel *(SB)* and large bowel *(LB)* are seen outside the peritoneal cavity in a lateral position, which is diagnostic of a spigelian hernia. (B) A CT slice lower in the abdomen shows the site of the hernia. The efferent loop of SB is of normal caliber; however, the afferent loop is decompressed, thus suggesting a transition point within the hernia. Operative repair was required.

hernia or abdomen. Ask whether the patient has a history of heavy lifting or straining. Inquire about signs of infection and systemic illness, such as fever, chills, and malaise. Seek symptoms associated with sustained increases in intraabdominal pressure such as chronic cough, chronic constipation, or straining to urinate. Determine whether the patient has signs or symptoms of bowel obstruction, including nausea and vomiting. Document a record of previous surgeries and hernia repairs, including any presence of synthetic mesh.

Physical examination of suspected groin hernias includes an examination of the groin and testicles, keeping in mind that the differential diagnosis of a groin mass includes entities other than a hernia (Box 45.1).

To evaluate for a hernia, palpate the inguinal canal in males by inverting the scrotal skin and passing a finger into the external ring. Ask the patient to cough or perform a Valsalva maneuver, which increases intraabdominal pressure and facilitates detection of a hernia. Examining the patient in both standing and supine positions can be helpful. Palpation of the external ring is more difficult in females because it is narrower. An indirect inguinal hernia is manifested as a swelling in the area of the inguinal ligament or as scrotal swelling in male patients. It is often painless and may be noted as an incidental finding. On examination, an indirect hernia can be differentiated from a direct hernia in several distinct ways: (1) an indirect hernia begins lateral to the inferior epigastric arteries; (2) the contents of an indirect hernia will strike the top of the finger instead of the volar pad during examination, as the hernia protrudes down the canal instead of directly across a fascial defect; (3) applying pressure over the internal ring after hernia reduction will block recurrence of the hernia during Valsalva, without impacting the bulge of a

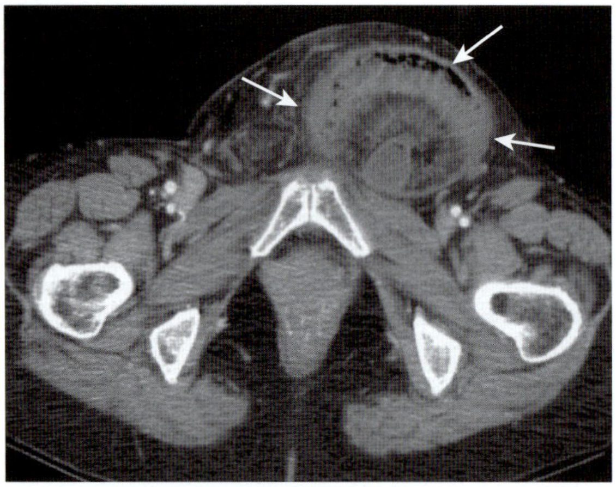

Fig. 45.3 Strangulated hernia in a 56-year-old male. An axial, contrast-enhanced, computed tomography image of the abdomen shows a strangulated left inguinal hernia with a C-shaped configuration *(arrows)*. Note the bowel wall thickening, severe fat stranding, mesenteric engorgement, and extraluminal fluid confined to the hernia sac, findings that suggest strangulation. (From Aguirre DA, Santosa AC, Casola G et al. Abdominal wall hernias: imaging features, complications, and diagnostic pitfalls at multidetector row CT. *Radiographics* 2005;25:1501-1520.)

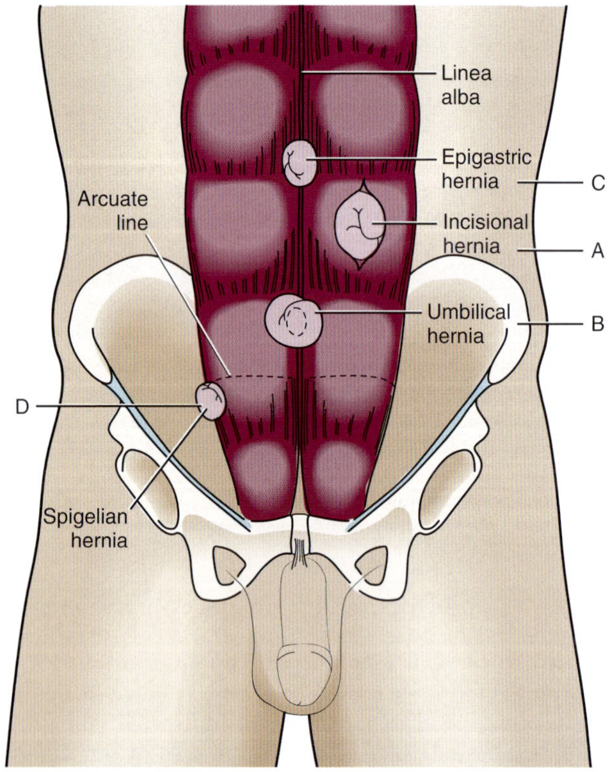

Fig. 45.4 Ventral hernias. *A*, Incisional hernia; *B*, umbilical hernia; *C*, epigastric hernia; and *D*, Spigelian hernia.

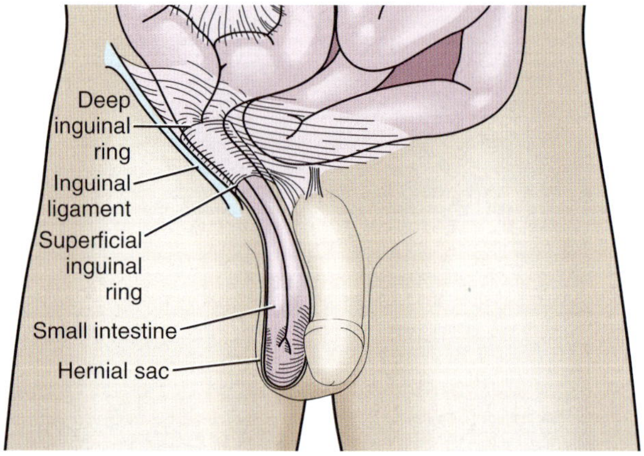

Fig. 45.5 Indirect inguinal hernia.

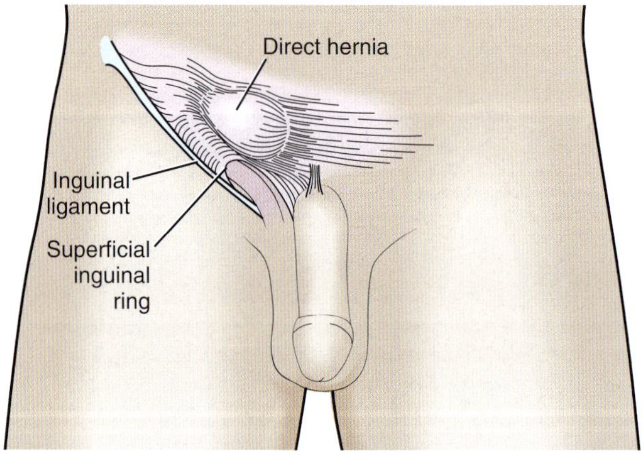

Fig. 45.6 Direct inguinal hernia.

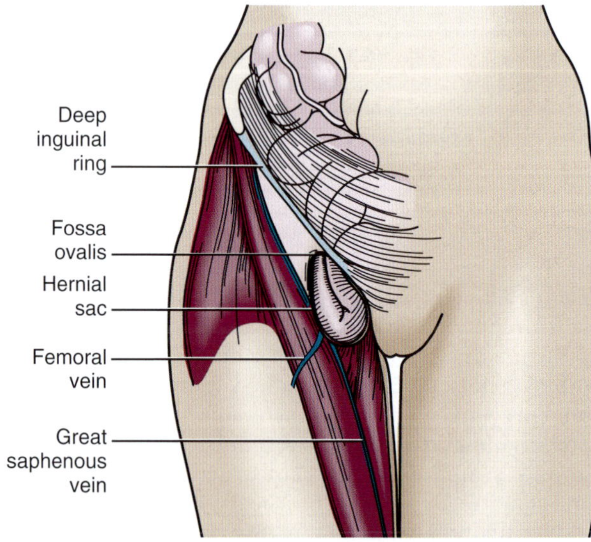

Fig. 45.7 Femoral hernia.

direct hernia during straining; and (4) a hernia that fills the scrotum is most likely an indirect hernia.

An asymptomatic hernia may be identified as a mass found incidentally on physical examination of the abdomen or groin. If a hernia is easily reducible, no specific intervention is required in the ED, but instructions should be given for appropriate outpatient surgical follow-up for potential elective repair. This is particularly important for inguinal hernias because elective repair is associated with much less morbidity than emergency repair for strangulation.[17–19]

A child with a groin hernia may have a reducible inguinal or scrotal mass that occurs with straining or crying. Consider the possibility of an incarcerated or strangulated hernia in

BOX 45.1 Differential Diagnosis of Groin Masses

Hernia
Testicular torsion
Retracted or undescended testicle
Hydrocele
Spermatocele
Venous varix
Pseudoaneurysm
Lymphadenopathy
Lymphogranuloma venereum
Epididymitis
Hidradenitis suppurativa
Groin abscess
Hematoma
Lipoma
Epidermal inclusion cyst
Tumor
Tracking of intraperitoneal blood

young children with nonspecific complaints such as vomiting, poor eating, lethargy, or irritability.

Diagnosis of Incarcerated Versus Strangulated Hernias

When the patient or emergency care provider cannot manually reduce the contents of the hernia back into the abdominal cavity, the hernia is described as *incarcerated*. Although hernias are a leading cause of bowel obstruction, patients with incarcerated hernias do not necessarily have associated bowel obstruction. Incarceration is more common with femoral hernias, small indirect inguinal hernias, and ventral or incisional hernias. Incarceration can be caused by the presence of a small fascial defect, by constriction of the defect by surrounding musculature, adhesions, or by swelling of the hernia contents. Incarceration increases the risk for strangulation and necessary bowel resection and on average, the risk doubles per 24-hour delay in intervention.[20]

A strangulated hernia is one in which the vascular supply to the herniated bowel is compromised, leading to ischemia. Strangulated hernias will often also be incarcerated, but this is not a universal finding. Ischemic injury of the bowel is suggested by a red, purple, or bluish discoloration of the skin over the hernia, significant abdominal tenderness with peritoneal signs, and radiographic findings of extraluminal air or poor perfusion of herniated bowel on a CT scan with IV contrast.[21] Ultrasound may also be utilized to detect blood flow to the bowel in the hernia sac by using color Doppler.[22] Patients with strangulated hernias may exhibit bowel obstruction, peritonitis, viscus perforation, intraabdominal abscess, or septic shock. Associated symptoms may include nausea, vomiting, fever, or abdominal distention.

PROCEDURE

See Video 45.1. The first step in successful hernia reduction is to position the patient properly to reduce intraabdominal pressure. Place the patient in a position so that gravity can facilitate hernia sac reduction back into the peritoneal cavity. Ensure patient comfort to decrease voluntary or involuntary muscle contraction and guarding, as this can increase intraabdominal pressure and make reduction more difficult. For ventral abdominal hernias, place the patient in the supine position. The Trendelenburg position (supine with the head 20 degrees downward) may facilitate reduction of inguinal hernias. Many hernias can reduce spontaneously if the patient is left comfortably in this position for 10 to 20 minutes.

A cool compress or ice pack may help to reduce swelling and facilitate reduction of a hernia that is predicted to be difficult to reduce. Before attempting reduction, use analgesics to treat the patient's pain and make the patient more comfortable. If needed, consider sedation to facilitate patient relaxation and minimize pain associated with the procedure. Options for procedural sedation include etomidate, propofol, midazolam, or ketamine. Fentanyl is usually the most common agent used for adjunctive analgesia. If the patient requires sedation to facilitate a successful manual reduction, it may be helpful to have a surgeon available while reduction is attempted and the patient is under sedation in the ED.

Before beginning the reduction, first palpate to identify the components of the hernia that will be manipulated during the procedure and the size of the opening through which the hernia is protruding. If the neck is small, the hernia will be more difficult to reduce, and a higher incidence of incarceration and strangulation may result.

When attempting to reduce the hernia, take care to not allow the contents of the hernia sac to override the edge of the hernia orifice because this can cause "ballooning" of the contents of the hernia sack around the hernia neck. Attempt to find the edge of the hernia defect and position your hand or fingers along that edge to help reduce ballooning and stabilize the edge of the fascial defect.

When available, bedside ultrasound may facilitate specifically locating the fascial defect and the hernia sac to be reduced. A high-frequency linear probe can be used to identify the extent of the fascial defect, thus allowing the clinician to guide the hernia sac back in the plane of maximal opening in the fascial defect under direct visualization. This real-time imaging allows guidance of the proximal end of the hernia contents through the defect and limits the "ballooning" that may occur without the benefit of visualization (Fig. 45.8).[23]

When first beginning an attempt at manual hernia reduction, approach slowly with soft, ongoing dialogue, and warm hands. This method encourages patient relaxation and minimizes muscular contractions resulting from pain, cold, or other physical discomfort. Begin the reduction procedure by gently guiding the proximal contents of the hernia sac back through the neck of the hernia first. In other words, reduce the hernia in the opposite order from which the contents protruded. Guiding the distal end of the contents of the hernia through the fascial defect first is not recommended and may cause the proximal contents to be displaced around the opening (ballooning) and prevent successful reduction. In order to accomplish this, it may be beneficial to pull the distal part of the hernia sac away from the body to prevent bunching of the intestines and allow the contents of the hernia to align with re-entry into the abdominal cavity. While using the other hand, pull the hernia sac and apply gentle, steady pressure on the tissue at the neck of the hernia to gradually reduce the hernia (Figs. 45.9 and 45.10). A key tip is that air in the bowel may impede your ability to reduce the hernia, so if an air bubble can be palpated, gentle steady pressure on this area may expel the air from the herniated portion of the bowel. This technique will prevent the air from becoming trapped in the herniated segment and facilitate reduction.[24]

When reducing inguinal hernias in children, place the patient supine in an approximate 20-degree Trendelenburg position, which may allow spontaneous reduction. Another positioning option is to place the patient in the "unilateral frog-leg" position (Fig. 45.11).[25] Stabilize the patient by grasping the anterior superior iliac spines to prevent lateral movement of the pelvis. Abduct the ipsilateral leg, externally rotate and flex the hip, and flex the knee to obtain the classic frog-leg position. The purpose of this position is to allow the greatest reapproximation of both the internal and external rings. After achieving this position, use the fingers of one hand to prevent the hernia contents from overriding the external ring, while using the other hand to provide steady but gentle pressure on the contents of the hernia sac. Repeated or forceful attempts are not recommended.

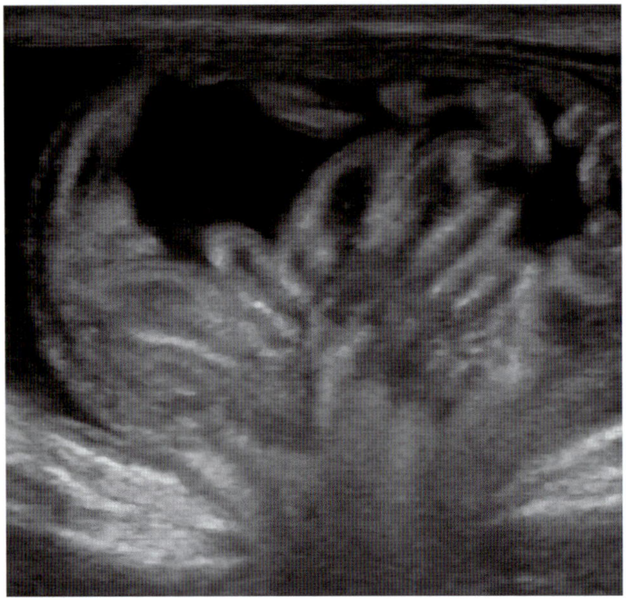

Fig. 45.8 Ultrasound of hernia. Note bowel through hernia into abdominal wall.

INTERPRETATION

In general, successful reduction can be identified by the absence of a mass, palpation of the hernia ring, and relief of pain. Continued significant pain suggests the possibility that strangulated bowel has been reduced back into the peritoneal cavity. Inability to palpate the hernia ring after reduction suggests that the hernia is in the preperitoneal position, is not completely reduced, or is not palpable because of body habitus.

COMPLICATIONS

While most bedside hernia reductions in the ED are uncomplicated, there are complications that rarely occur during the manual reduction of hernias. Underlying bowel can be injured from attempts at reduction that are too forceful. Repetitive and overaggressive attempts that are unsuccessful may aggravate the swelling and create conditions where the hernia cannot be reduced at the bedside. This complication can be avoided with appropriate patient preparation, positioning, sedation, and reduction techniques. Reduction of ischemic bowel in the setting of an undiagnosed strangulated hernia is a potential complication that may occur when the clinician inadvertently reduces ischemic bowel back into the peritoneal cavity.

In less than 1% of hernias, the strangulated or incarcerated hernia may inadvertently be reduced en masse to a

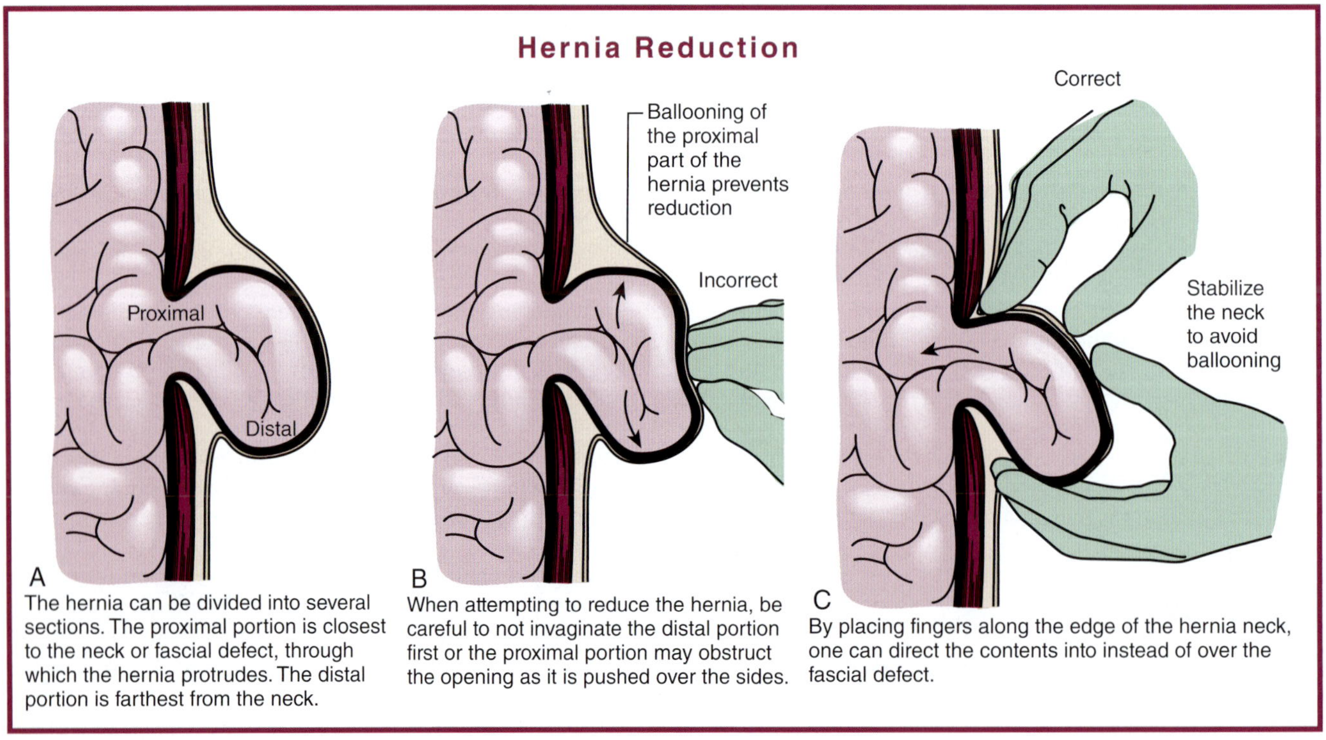

Fig. 45.9 Hernia reduction. See text for details.

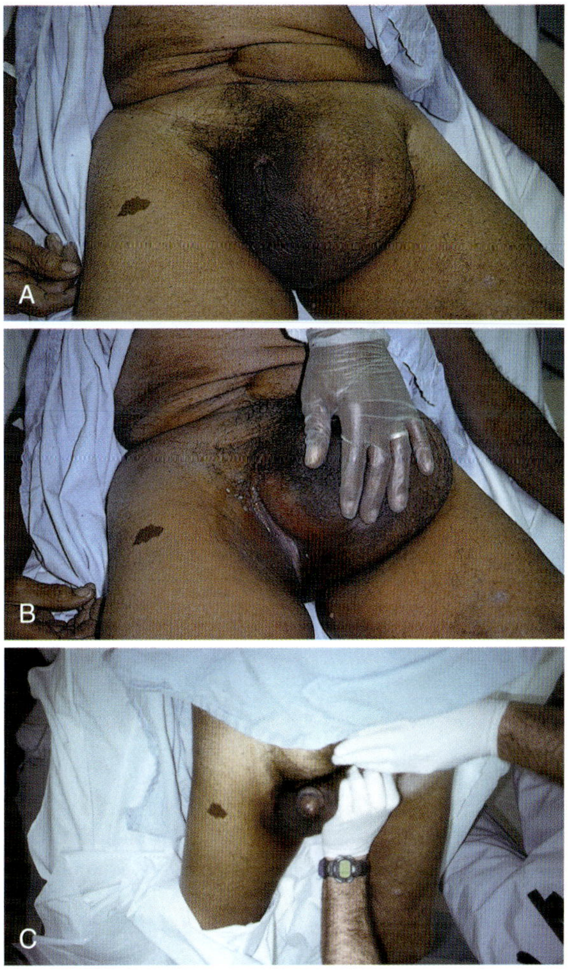

Fig. 45.10 (A) This very large hernia is challenging to reduce. (B) Merely pushing on the distal end of the mass, as shown here, will not be successful. (C) Instead, try to first reduce the contents that are more proximal by stabilizing the neck and replacing the portion of bowel closest to the fascial defect.

Hernia Reduction: Frog-Leg Technique

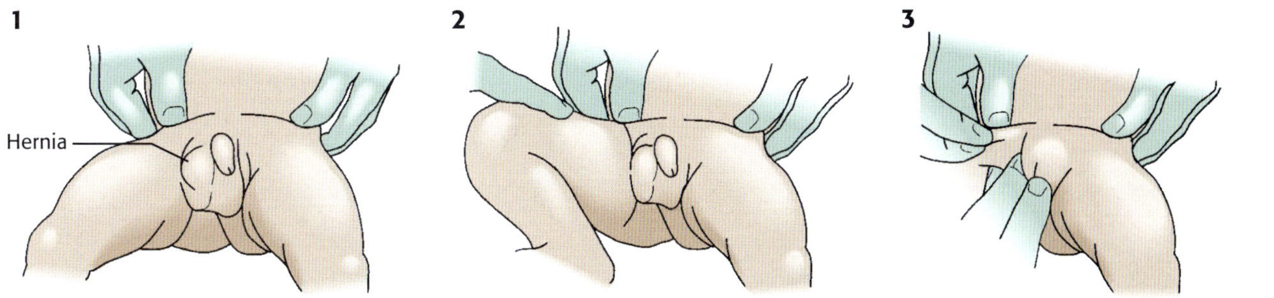

1. Stabilize the patient by grasping the anterior superior iliac spines.
2. Abduct the ipsilateral leg, and externally rotate and flex the hip to obtain the classic frog-leg position.
3. Use the fingers of one hand to prevent the hernia contents from overriding the external ring while using the other hand to provide steady but gentle pressure on the contents of the hernia sac.

Fig. 45.11 Frog-leg technique of hernia reduction.

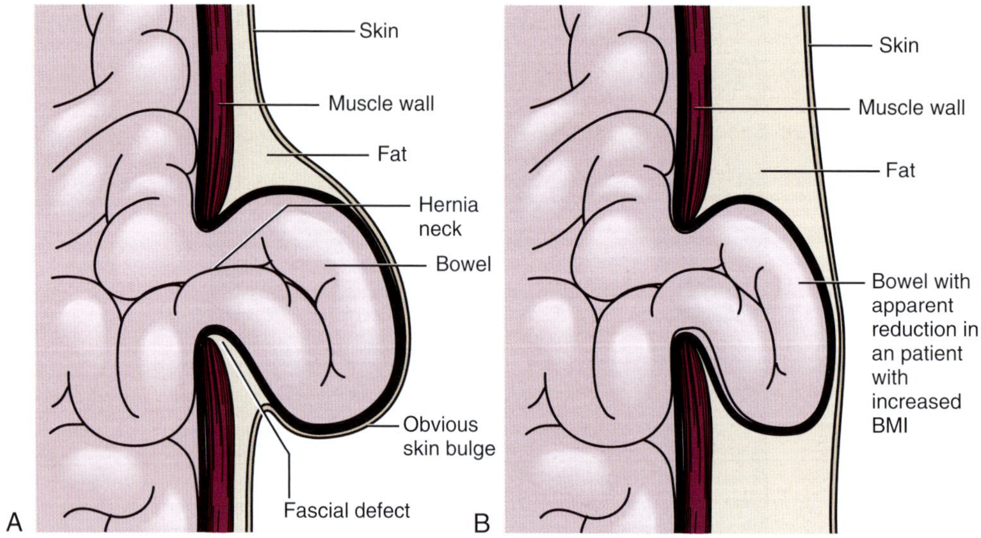

Fig. 45.12 En masse reduction. (A) When a hernia forms, it projects from the fascia into subcutaneous fat. The object of reduction is to place the hernia back into the peritoneal cavity. (B) If the hernia sac is partially reduced into the subcutaneous fat of a patient with increased body mass index *(BMI)*, it may appear reduced and not be palpable because of the patient's body habitus. However, the hernia is still susceptible to incarceration or ischemia because it has not been returned to the peritoneal cavity.

preperitoneal location (Fig. 45.12), thus making the contents no longer palpable.[26–28] In this case, the hernia has not been reduced fully into the peritoneal cavity, and the incarceration and ischemia therefore have not been relieved. Because the clinician believes that the hernia has been appropriately reduced, this can result in a delay in the diagnosis of ischemic bowel. Fortunately, this occurs in less than 1% of hernias.[29]

Persistent pain after reduction of a hernia, especially more than at the orifice of the fascial defect, should alert the physician to the possibility of either preperitoneal reduction or reduction of ischemic bowel.

REFERENCES ARE AVAILABLE AT Elsevier eBooks+

CHAPTER 46

Anorectal Procedures

Wendy C. Coates

Patients with anorectal disorders frequently seek care in the emergency department (ED). The condition may be isolated or the anorectal complaint may be an outward manifestation of a serious underlying illness. A thorough history and physical examination must precede any procedure. Because of the nature of these conditions, extreme sensitivity and professionalism are essential. In addition, it is advisable to consider using a chaperone during this examination or any procedures involving the anorectal area.

Patients may be anxious about anorectal examination or associated procedures, including the digital rectal examination (DRE). The results of DRE may lead to performing diagnostic or therapeutic procedures such as anoscopy, excision of thrombosed external hemorrhoids, drainage of anorectal abscesses or pilonidal cysts, reduction of rectal prolapse, or removal of rectal foreign bodies (FBs). For these procedures, analgesia, sedation, or both may be useful adjuncts.

ANATOMY

The rectum and anus compose the most distal portion of the gastrointestinal tract. The rectum begins at the level of the third sacral vertebra and extends distally 12 to 15 cm. Blood supply to the anorectum is derived from the superior, middle, and inferior hemorrhoidal arteries. Venous drainage from the rectum and anus returns to both the portal and systemic systems (Fig. 46.1). The dentate (pectinate) line marks the transition from the rectum to the anus and contains submucosal glands in anal crypts. Occlusion with subsequent infection of these glands causes anorectal abscesses. Sensory innervation to the rectum is primarily visceral, whereas the anus is innervated by cutaneous fibers. Therefore patients are often unaware of rectal pathology because the pain associated with it may be vague or absent. By contrast, anal lesions are usually very painful and well localized.[1]

DIGITAL RECTAL EXAM

Indications and Contraindications

The physical examination should be performed in a private location and the patient should be completely draped and relaxed. Generally, a calm atmosphere and caring examiner preclude the need for analgesic or anxiolytic agents, although they may be needed to facilitate a thorough examination. In some extremely painful conditions, such as thrombosed or gangrenous hemorrhoids, DRE may be postponed until the patient is anesthetized. If a sharp-edged FB (e.g., metal blade or broken glass) is suspected, performing a DRE may cause injury to the clinician, as well as the patient. In these cases, radiologic evaluation with subsequent operative management may be indicated.

Procedure

Consider using a chaperone for this procedure. Place the patient in the lateral decubitus position and wear protective gloves. Begin the examination with a preliminary visual inspection of the perianal area for important information regarding patient hygiene, trauma, obvious abnormalities, or sexually transmitted infections. Next, ask the patient to perform a Valsalva maneuver and look for prolapsing rectal mucosa or hemorrhoids. When the patient relaxes, prolapsed structures may retreat or remain external to the anus. By placing a gloved finger firmly against the anal sphincter, it will relax and allow entry of the examiner's gloved, lubricated finger (Fig. 46.2A). Once inserted into the anus, make a 360-degree sweep to identify any irregularities in the anorectum and prostate. After withdrawing the finger, examine stool remaining on the glove for the presence of visible or occult blood (Fig. 46.2B–C).[2] Testing for blood in stool is discussed in detail in Chapter 68.

Complications

Although it is not a firm contraindication in patients whose absolute neutrophil count is dangerously low, many would defer routine DRE, especially avoiding vigorous prostate manipulation, to minimize the likelihood of bacteremia.

ANOSCOPY

See Video 46.1.

Indications and Contraindications

When evaluating a patient for anal pathology, some practitioners use anoscopy as an adjunct to DRE. Internal hemorrhoids, tears in the distal rectal mucosa, FBs, and distal anorectal masses may be visualized. An imperforate anus is the only absolute contraindication to anoscopy; however, severe rectal pain, a common complaint in the ED, may preclude awake anoscopic examination in anxious patients or those with thrombosed hemorrhoids or other painful conditions. Internal visual inspection in these patients is better performed with sedation. If a definitive study such as sigmoidoscopy or colonoscopy is being planned by the treating physician, anoscopy can be deferred in the acute care setting.

Equipment and Setup

The anoscope is a plastic or a stainless steel tube with a removable obturator (Fig. 46.3). It may have an integrated light source or require an external light or headlamp. An appropriate examination table, topical anesthetic, lubricant, gauze, and forceps may also be required.

Positioning

Ideally, place the patient in a prone position on a proctoscopic examination table. The lateral decubitus position with the knees and hips flexed may also be adequate and is sometimes tolerated better. In the lateral decubitus position, place the patient on the left side if the examiner is right-handed (Fig. 46.4, *step 1*). In some cases, the knee-chest position facilitates the procedure but the patient should remain covered and

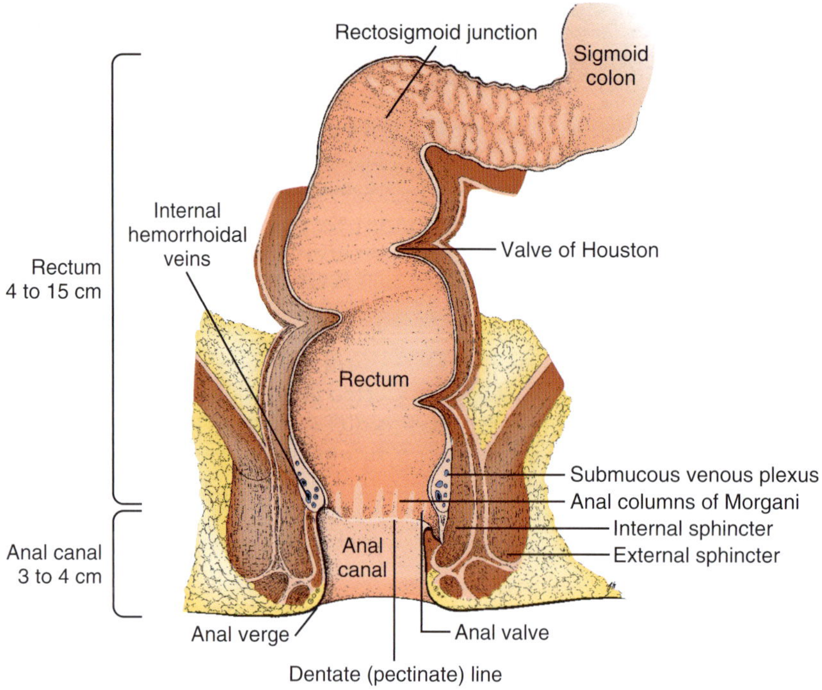

Fig. 46.1 Anatomy of the terminal gastrointestinal tract. (Redrawn from Abrahams PH, Webb PJ. *Clinical Anatomy of Practical Procedures*. Pitman; 1975.)

Digital Rectal Examination

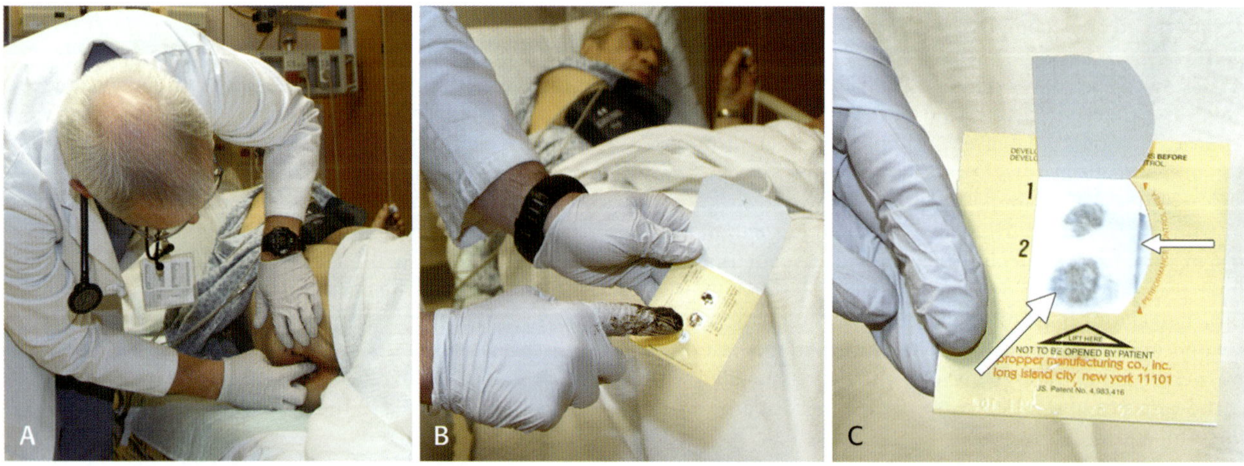

Fig. 46.2 Digital rectal examination. (A) Insert a gloved, lubricated finger into the anus and perform a 360-degree sweep to check for any irregularities in the anorectum and prostate. (B) Examine the stool for visible and occult blood. This patient had melena, which is dark and tarry in consistency and indicative of upper gastrointestinal hemorrhage. (C) This sample is positive for blood. The *large arrow* points to the blue coloration on the test area of the card, whereas the *small arrow* points to the control. The control should turn blue. See also a discussion of testing stool for blood in Chapter 68.

should only be placed in the position immediately before the procedure.

Procedure

Consider using a chaperone for this procedure. Although most patients do not require intravenous sedation and analgesia, administer these agents as needed to keep the patient relaxed and comfortable. Before anoscopy, perform a routine DRE to identify sources of bleeding or pain and to locate any palpable masses. Next, lubricate the anoscope. After DRE and with the obturator inserted completely into the anoscope, carefully introduce the scope into the anus. Use gentle, constant pressure to overcome resistance from involuntary contraction of the external anal sphincter. Gently advance the anoscope while asking the patient to bear down slightly. Pass the

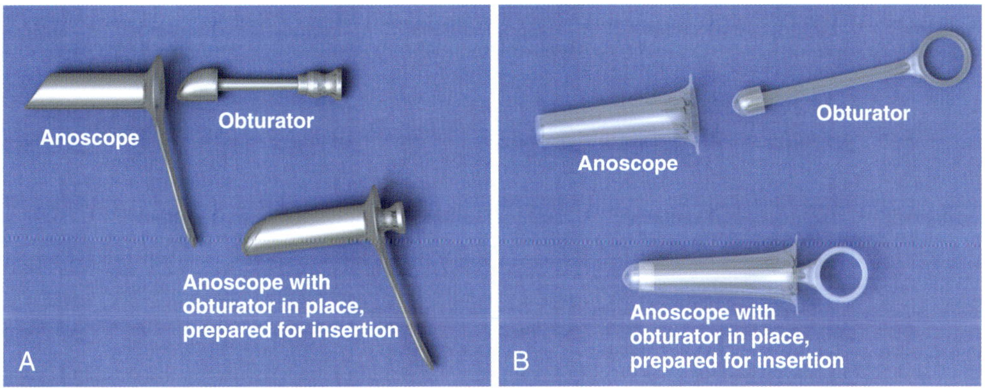

Fig. 46.3 (A) Reusable stainless steel and (B) disposable plastic anoscopes are available. Regardless of the type of anoscope used, the obturator must be fully inserted and held in place with the thumb during advancement of the device into the anorectum.

anoscope gently into the anorectum (see Fig. 45.6, *step 2*). The examiner should keep a thumb pressing on the obturator to prevent it from being dislodged. If the obturator falls back during insertion, remove the anoscope completely and replace the obturator to avoid pinching the anal mucosa. Advance the anoscope until the outer flange impinges on the anal verge.

When the anoscope is fully inserted, remove the obturator (see Fig. 46.4, *step 3*). Unless the anoscope has an internal light, use an external light source such as a penlight, otoscope, headlamp, or pelvic examination light. While gradually withdrawing the anoscope, visualize all areas of the anal canal (see Fig. 46.4, *step 4*). Swab away blood or debris to aid in visualization, and culture any abnormal discharge that is found. Note whether there is rectal bleeding or an FB beyond the reach of the anoscope. Withdraw the anoscope slowly and inspect the entire circumference of mucosa for hemorrhoids, anal fissures, ulcerations, abscesses, or tears. Near the last stage of withdrawal, be aware of reflex spasm of the anal sphincter, which may cause the anoscope to be expelled quickly. Use firm counterpressure to prevent such rapid expulsion.[3]

Complications

Although complications are rare, patients often complain of increased pain after the examination. Local mucosal irritation with subsequent bleeding is the most common complication. To prevent transmission of infectious diseases, dispose of or sterilize instruments after each use.

MANAGEMENT OF HEMORRHOIDS

Hemorrhoids are a common affliction and have been described and treated for more than 4000 years. The refined, low-fiber diet of Western nations makes hemorrhoids extremely common in North America, where 1 in 25 to 30 individuals is afflicted. One million patients annually seek medical attention with this chief complaint.[4]

Hemorrhoids are normal vascular structures in the submucosal layer of the anal canal, arising from a channel of arteriovenous connective tissues that drains into the superior and inferior hemorrhoidal veins. Hemorrhoidal tissue is composed of vascular, mucosal, and muscular tissue (Fig. 46.5). There are two types of hemorrhoids: internal and external. *Internal hemorrhoids* originate proximal to the dentate line, are covered with mucosa, and lack sensory innervation. If they are visible outside the anal verge, they can be identified by noting that their covering differs in appearance from the surrounding perianal skin. Internal hemorrhoids may prolapse and bleed, which usually produces bright red blood on toilet paper or in the toilet bowel. This bleeding is from presinusoidal arterioles and is mostly associated with brown stool and bleeding only with a bowel movement. Atypical bleeding requires further investigation. Internal hemorrhoids are rarely felt by digital palpation unless they are very large or thrombosed. Internal hemorrhoids are usually painless unless gangrenous, strangulated, extruded, or thrombosed, and then they may be extremely painful. Anal pain in the absence of such pathology suggests a problem other than simple internal hemorrhoids.[4]

Internal hemorrhoids can be further classified as first through fourth degree. First-degree hemorrhoids do not prolapse but may be identified on anoscopic examination. Second-degree hemorrhoids prolapse on straining but reduce spontaneously. Third-degree hemorrhoids prolapse on straining and can be reduced manually, whereas fourth-degree hemorrhoids prolapse and are irreducible. Fourth-degree hemorrhoids are prone to thrombosis, strangulation, and eventually gangrene (see Fig. 46.5C).

External hemorrhoids originate distal to the dentate line and are covered with squamous epithelium. This makes them easily recognizable because their covering matches the surrounding skin (anoderm). A thrombosed external hemorrhoid appears as a bluish mass covered by epidermis. Acute thrombosis occurs suddenly and is generally very painful because external hemorrhoids are innervated by the inferior rectal nerve. Many patients feel a tender mass and are unable to sit comfortably. Significant bleeding is uncommon but may occur with spontaneous rupture. Increased pressure from straining, or trauma from constipation or diarrhea, may exacerbate external hemorrhoids. Distention and trauma predispose the hemorrhoidal venous plexus to stasis with ensuing clot formation and edema.[2,4,5]

Conservative Treatment

ED management of minor *internal hemorrhoids* is conservative. Prolapsing internal hemorrhoids will not benefit long-term from conservative intervention and should receive surgical consultation. A useful mnemonic for managing hemorrhoids is WASH: water (increase fluid intake, warm water contacting the hemorrhoid via bath or directed shower),

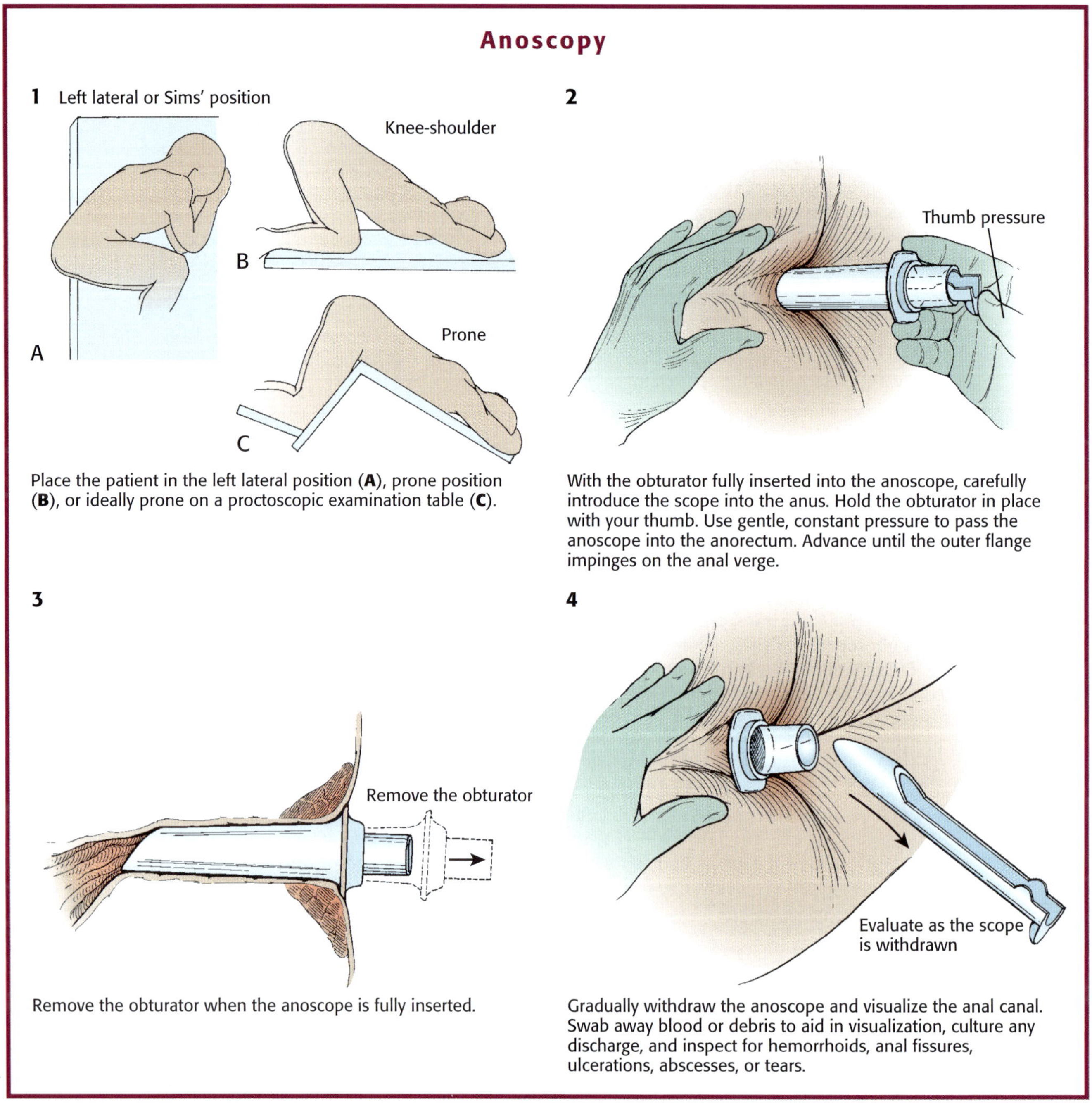

Fig. 46.4 Anoscopy. Remember to keep your thumb on the obturator during passage of the instrument until it is fully inserted). (Step 1, From Hill GJ II. *Outpatient Surgery*. 3rd ed. Saunders; 1988.)

analgesics, stool softeners, and a high-fiber diet.[2] Psyllium (e.g., Metamucil, Procter & Gamble) is often prescribed as a dietary supplement to increase fiber. Hemorrhoids that fail to respond to medical management may be treated on an outpatient basis with rubber band ligation, sclerosis, and thermotherapy consisting of an infrared beam, electric current, Co_2 laser, or ultrasonic energy. Patients who must push hemorrhoids back in after a bowel movement have symptomatic third-degree internal hemorrhoids and would benefit from elective surgical referral. This condition can easily be demonstrated by having the patient strain before DRE. *Nonreducible prolapsed internal hemorrhoids* should receive prompt surgical consultation and, frequently, admission to the hospital.[4]

Without treatment, thrombosed *external hemorrhoids* and those that have spontaneously ruptured will generally resolve over a period of 1 to 3 weeks. Residual skin tags may persist. During the interim, however, they are quite painful and may bleed. Small ruptured or nonruptured hemorrhoids that are seen acutely with minimal discomfort may be managed conservatively with warm water baths or a directed stream of water, and topical corticosteroids (e.g., Anusol HC), or Preparation H. Topical agents that contain corticosteroids or local anesthetics may promote skin breakdown if used for more than a couple of days. Because the pain is most severe within the first 48 hours, patients evaluated within this time window benefit from excision (not incision and drainage) of the contents of the thrombosed external hemorrhoid and its

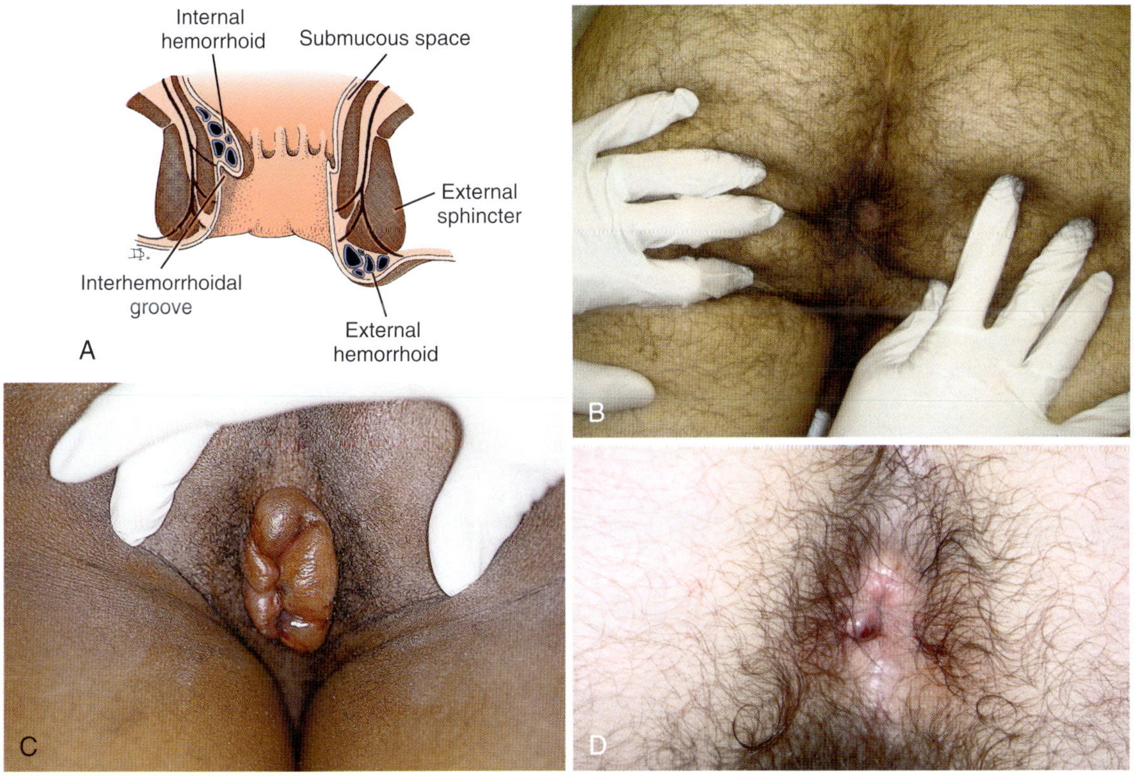

Fig. 46.5 (A) Anatomic location of internal and external hemorrhoids. (B) Thrombosed external hemorrhoid. (C) Thrombosed prolapsed internal hemorrhoids. These hemorrhoids cannot be permanently reduced and are quite painful; occasionally, partial relief can be obtained by manual reduction if they are not gangrenous. They should not be incised in the emergency department; formal hemorrhoidectomy is required if conservative measures are not successful. They are often mistaken for a partial "rectal prolapse." Sitz baths and stool softeners are frequently futile in such severe cases. (D) This small external hemorrhoid ruptured and produced minor but persistent bleeding and pain. Conservative treatment consisting of topical corticosteroids or Preparation H and frequent sitz baths will be curative in 5 to 7 days. (A, From Hill GJ II. *Outpatient Surgery*. 2nd ed. Saunders; 1980.)

overlying skin. Patients seen after this time are usually best managed with conservative treatment because the thrombosis begins the reabsorption process and the clot may have liquefied (see Fig. 46.5D).[2,5]

Surgical Excision of Thrombosed External Hemorrhoids

Indications and Contraindications

Indications for surgical excision of acutely (<48 hours) thrombosed external hemorrhoids in the ED include relief of symptoms and prevention of the formation of permanent perianal skin tags. These appendages remain as loose skin after the body reabsorbs the thrombosis and serve as a nidus for poor perianal hygiene and local irritation. Surgical consultation should be obtained in the ED for multiple painful external hemorrhoids and for profuse bleeding that is hemodynamically significant. Bleeding disorders, serious systemic illness, and hemodynamic instability are all relative contraindications to excision in the ED.

Procedure

See Video 46.2. Consider using a chaperone for this procedure. Place the patient in the prone or lateral decubitus position. Tape the buttocks apart to aid in visualization (Fig. 46.6, *step 1*). An assistant is often needed. Administer parenteral analgesics and sedatives as an adjunct to local anesthesia if necessary. Infiltrate with a local anesthetic (such as 0.5% bupivacaine or buffered 1% lidocaine with epinephrine at 1:100,000) just under the skin and over the dome of the hemorrhoid (Fig. 46.7; also see Fig. 46.6, *step 2*). The overlying skin should blanch, which indicates that anesthesia has been introduced at the appropriate depth. Inject additional anesthetic through the anesthetized tissue into the base of the hemorrhoid, if needed, rather than through the intact skin (see Fig. 46.7C).

Grasp the skin overlying the thrombosis with forceps. Make an elliptical incision around the clot and direct it radially from the anal orifice (Fig. 46.8; also see Fig. 46.6, *step 3*). Elevate the edges of the skin with forceps and excise from the edges to expose the underlying thrombosis. Remove the clot with forceps or by applying digital pressure (see Fig. 46.6, *steps 4* and *5*). Frequently, multiple individual clots will be present. If any skin ulceration is noted over the hemorrhoid, include it in the excised portion. Pack the wound loosely with standard gauze to prevent the skin edges from reapproximating prematurely.

For the trip home, place a gauze pad between the buttocks and tape the buttocks together to hold the gauze in place (see Fig. 46.6, *step 6*). Advise the patient to avoid prolonged standing or straining for the next few days. Minor bleeding may occur. Hygiene with a directed stream of warm water or sitz baths can be started a few hours after the procedure.

Excision of Thrombosed External Hemorrhoids

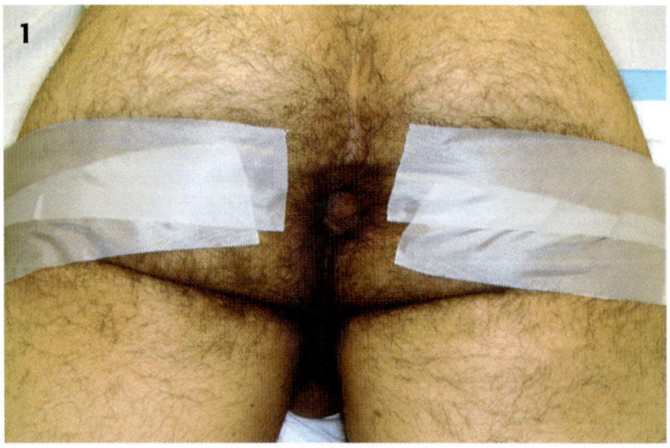

Place the patient in the prone or lateral decubitus position. Tape the buttocks apart to aid in visualization.

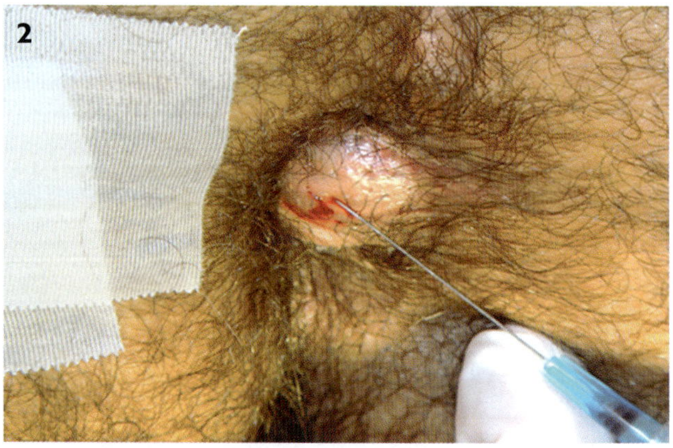

Infiltrate with a local anesthetic just under the skin and over the dome of the hemorrhoid (see Fig. 45.7).

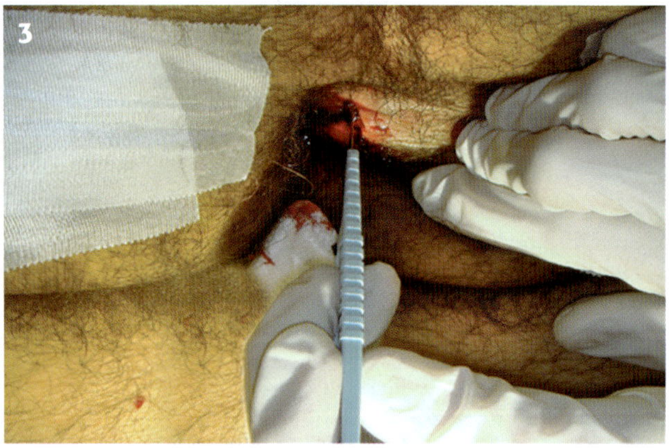

Make an elliptical incision around the clot and direct it radially from the anal orifice (see Fig. 45.8).

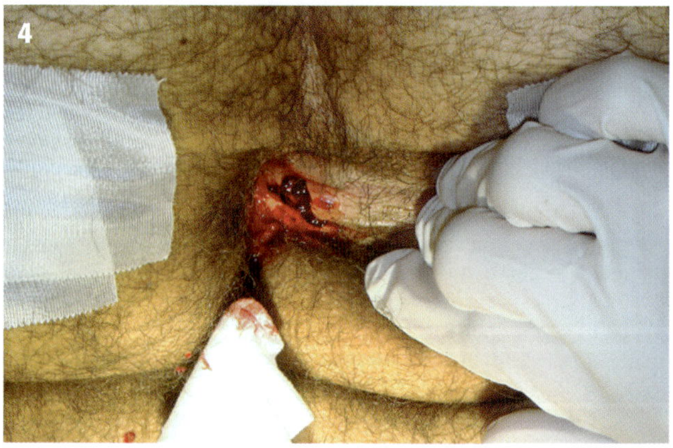

Remove the clot with digital pressure. Often, multiple individual clots will be present.

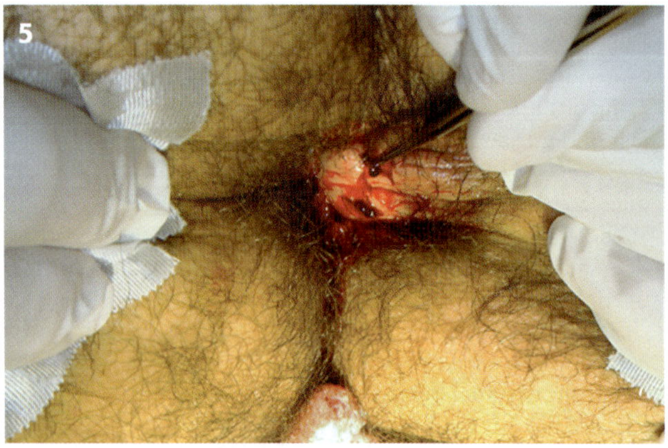

Use forceps to remove residual clots.

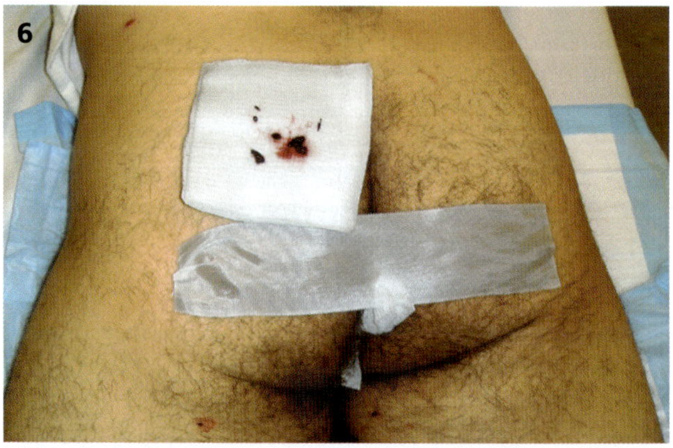

Pack the wound loosely with standard cotton gauze. Place a gauze pad between the buttocks and tape the buttocks together to hold the gauze in place.

Fig. 46.6 Excision of thrombosed external hemorrhoids.

The gauze may fall out or can be removed at the first sitz bath. After the packing has been removed, the patient may apply a soothing cream to the area for a couple of days (such as Preparation H, Anusol HC), or an astringent (such as witch hazel pads). Instruct the patient to avoid using toilet paper after a bowel movement for a few days but to wash the area with mild soap and water in the shower. Most patients are relatively asymptomatic in 48 hours and do not need a routine wound check unless the pain or bleeding persists. Once the clot has been removed, recurrent thrombosis is unlikely, but these patients are predisposed to future episodes. Long-term therapy should be directed toward avoiding constipation by increasing dietary fiber and fluid intake. Antibiotics are not routinely indicated.[2,5]

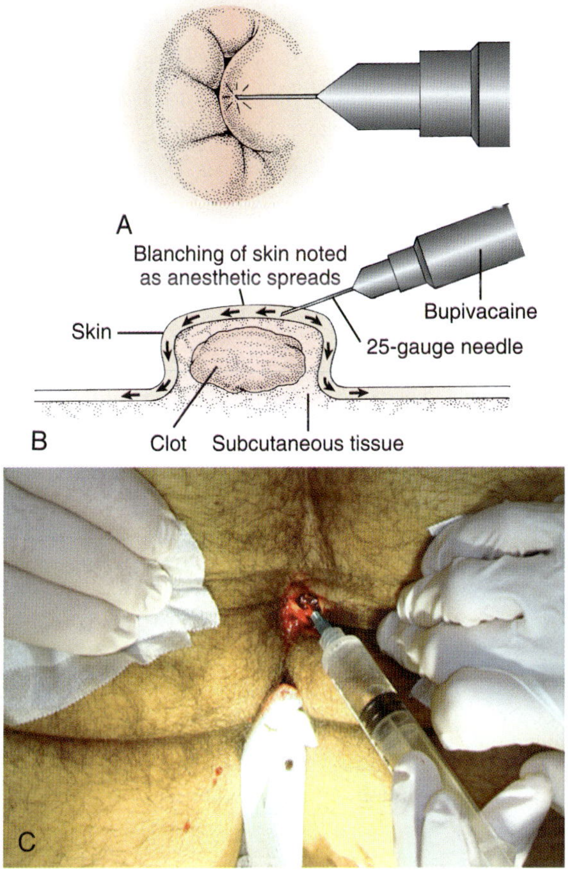

Fig. 46.7 (A) For surgical treatment of a thrombosed external hemorrhoid in the emergency department, anesthesia can usually be obtained with a *single injection* of buffered long-acting bupivacaine with epinephrine. In elective cases, apply a eutectic mixture of local anesthetics (EMLA) cream for 1 hour before the procedure. Parenteral sedation is optional. Using a 25-gauge needle, inject an anesthetic solution into the middle of the swollen hemorrhoid just below the surface of the skin. (B) Do not move the tip of the needle. With slow injection, the anesthetic will spread over the surface of the dome and into the surrounding tissue. Avoid deep field blocks at the base of the hemorrhoid because they are unnecessary and very painful. (C) If pain persists, inject additional anesthetic into deeper tissues *through the cut edges, not through the intact skin*.

If an invasive procedure would not be well tolerated by the patient, alternative nonoperative treatments include topical nitrates or topical nifedipine. Applied to the thrombosed hemorrhoid, these creams relax the anal sphincter, relieve pain, and promote healing. Systemic absorption is minimal, and the application is usually well tolerated.[4]

Complications

Although complications are rare, bleeding and infection do occur. The bleeding usually stops with direct pressure. When simple incision plus drainage is performed instead of an elliptical excision, or when the ellipse of skin is not removed completely, the edges of the skin can close prematurely and result in infection and a permanent perianal skin tag. Premature closure can also result in incomplete evacuation of the clot.

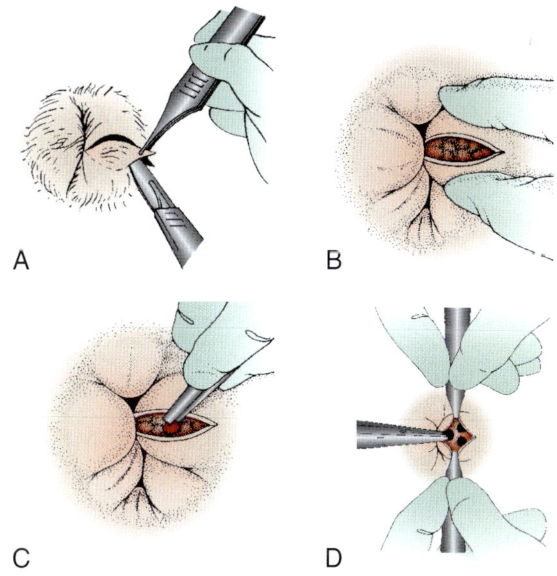

Fig. 46.8 Schematic technique as described in Fig. 46.6. (A) For the unroofing technique, make an elliptical incision to remove a piece of the overlying skin. To prevent skin tags, do not use a simple linear incision. (B) Blood clots may extrude spontaneously, but (C) remove the remaining ones with forceps or express them with the fingers. (D) Frequently, multiple clots are present, and they should all be removed. Ask an assistant to provide exposure with forceps if necessary.

MANAGEMENT OF ANORECTAL ABSCESS AND PILONIDAL CYST AND ABSCESS

These topics are covered in detail in Chapter 37.

MANAGEMENT OF RECTAL FBS

Causes of rectal FBs include autoeroticism (most common), iatrogenic or self-administered placement (thermometer, enema tip), assault, accidental ingestion, and concealment (body packing). The myriad objects that have been removed include vibrators, sex toy phalluses, aerosol cans, lightbulbs, glass bottles, billiard balls, fruits, vegetables, and small animals (Fig. 46.9). Many of these objects can be removed successfully in the ED. By following some simple guidelines, outpatient treatment can be practical and cost-effective.

Diagnosis of a rectal FB is usually made from the history. The physical examination should therefore concentrate on excluding anorectal or intestinal perforation and determining which objects will be accessible in the ED. DRE will identify objects that are low lying or palpable. Such objects are most likely to be removed successfully in the outpatient setting. Plain radiographs can supplement the examination by delineating the shape, position, and number of objects. If an FB with a sharp edge is suspected from the history or radiograph, omit the DRE to prevent injury to the provider and intestinal perforation.[6,7]

Indications and Contraindications

Although some objects may pass spontaneously, delayed removal may lead to obstipation, pain, infection, and perforation. For these reasons, FB removal is indicated according to the algorithm included in this chapter (Fig. 46.10). Rectal FB removal can lead to rectal perforation. Although many FBs

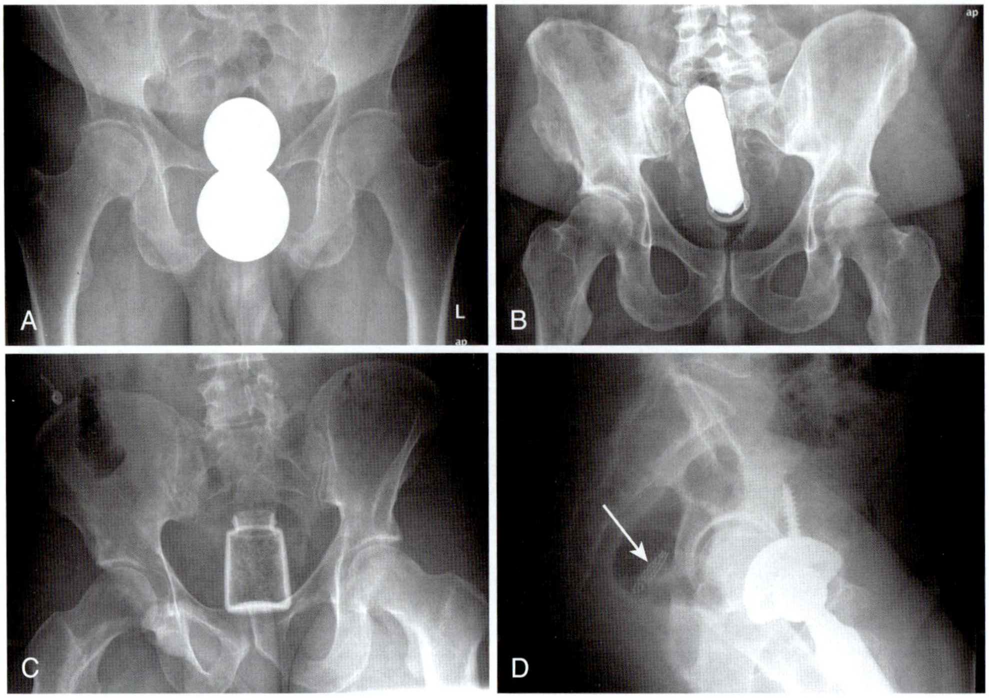

Fig. 46.9 Rectal foreign bodies. (A) Two large tungsten spheres, one on top of the other, gave a snowman-like appearance on the radiograph. They were removed manually in the emergency department (ED) with the aid of a Foley catheter and large-volume balloon. (B) A vibrator that migrated into the sigmoid colon. It required removal in the operating room under general anesthesia. (C) A small glass jar that the patient had tried to remove multiple times over a period of hours at home. On arrival at the ED, he had signs of peritonitis and was taken to the operating room, where perforation of the distal colon was discovered. Diverting colostomy was required. (D) A toothbrush that was removed manually in the ED.

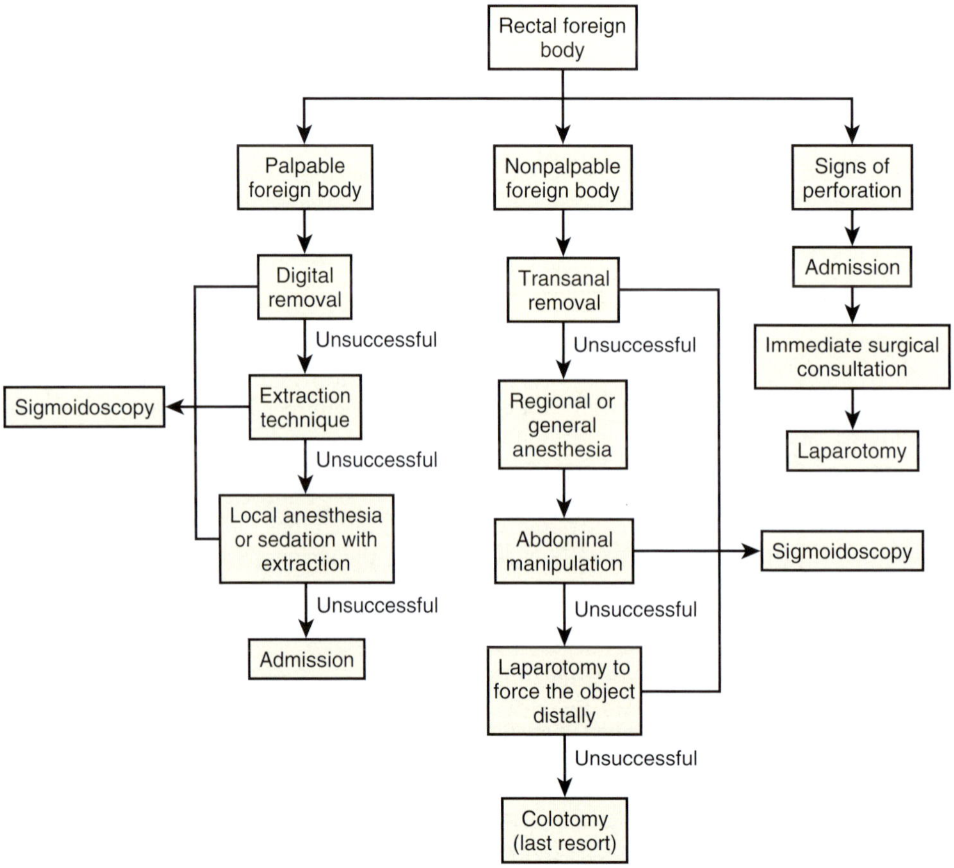

Fig. 46.10 Emergency approach to the removal of rectal foreign bodies. Foreign bodies that are fragile or associated with rectal spasm are generally managed with regional or general anesthesia. The use of supplemental analgesic, anxiolytic, and local anesthetic medications is recommended.

can be removed safely in the ED, complicated or prolonged attempts may be better performed under general anesthesia.

Removal of FBs in the ED is contraindicated in patients who have severe abdominal pain or signs of perforation, a nonpalpable FB, or sharp objects or broken glass in the rectum. Other situations precluding ED removal include a rectal FB that is unusually difficult to remove (a set time limit has elapsed, or the patient cannot tolerate removal), or when there is insufficient experience or equipment to perform the procedure. Patients who arrive at the ED under these conditions require surgical consultation.[6,7]

Equipment

The specific equipment required will often depend on the nature of the FB (Fig. 46.11). In general, the clinician will need a speculum with a light source and an instrument to grasp the FB. The speculum can be an anoscope, a rigid sigmoidoscope, a vaginal speculum, or surgical retractors. Instruments useful for grasping the FB include ring forceps, tenaculum forceps, and obstetric forceps. In some instances, a Foley catheter or endotracheal tube will be helpful. A suction dart, vacuum extractor, and plaster of Paris have also been used to aid in FB retrieval. Individual situations may lead to creative use of standard medical equipment, but one must ensure the safety of the patient and health care personnel before using a device to remove a rectal FB.

Procedure

Consider using a chaperone for this procedure. The technique for removal depends on the size, location, orientation, and composition of the FB. Place the patient either prone in the knee-chest position or in a lateral decubitus position. Alternatively, if the patient is in the lithotomy position, pressure can be placed on the abdomen to help maneuver the FB toward the distal end of the rectum. Parenteral analgesia is often required to relieve the pain from anal stretching and manipulation. Intravenous sedation is almost always required to calm the patient and facilitate relaxation of the anal sphincter. A perianal block allows greater dilation of the sphincter. Local infiltration with 0.5% bupivacaine or 1% lidocaine with epinephrine at 1:100,000 may be administered circumferentially around the anus in the submucosal tissue.

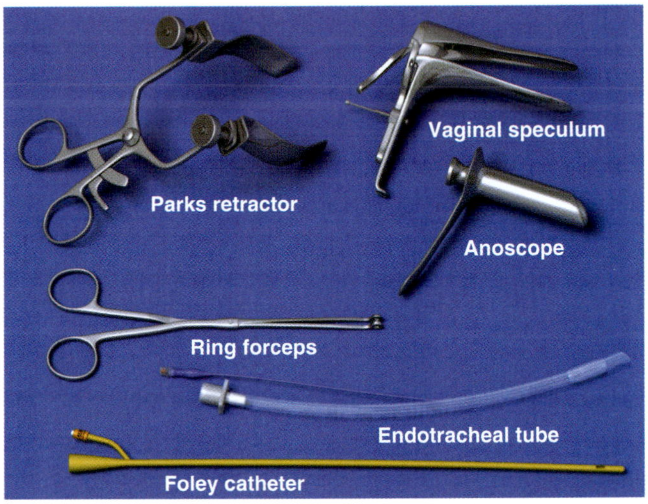

Fig. 46.11 A variety of equipment may be required to remove a rectal foreign body, and the choice of specific equipment will depend on the clinical scenario. Individual situations may lead to creative use of standard medical equipment, but one must ensure safety before using a device to remove a rectal foreign body.

After analgesia and sedation of the patient, perform a DRE to gauge the position and orientation of the FB. Suprapubic pressure from above, the examiner's finger from below, and the patient performing a Valsalva maneuver may successfully deliver the object without instrumentation. If the FB is lodged against the sacrum posteriorly, redirect it by cradling its posterior aspect between two fingers and directing it slightly proximally and anteriorly while the patient gently bears down.

If DRE reveals that the object has an accessible edge or lip, use an instrument to extract it under direct visualization (Fig. 46.12). First, insert an anoscope, rigid sigmoidoscope, vaginal speculum, or retractor into the anus as described above. If an intact object is visualized clearly, use a blunt instrument to secure it. Apply gentle traction to remove the object, the instrument, and the anoscope or speculum as a single unit. Grasp the object under direct visualization to avoid pinching or tearing the mucosa.

Rigid sigmoidoscopes offer a unique advantage in that air can be insufflated into the rectum around the FB. This technique can be particularly helpful when retrieving glass objects. Glass rectal FBs often create a vacuum in the segment of bowel just proximal to where they lie. This makes removal with simple traction almost impossible. The vacuum can be released by distending the rectal wall around the object with air. If a sigmoidoscope cannot be used to retrieve a glass object, pass one or two Foley catheters or an endotracheal tube beyond the FB and inflate the balloon or cuff. Air can be insufflated through these devices to relieve the vacuum proximal to the object. Then remove the object with the inflated balloons and gentle traction. Specific equipment is often not available to remove all FBs, and the clinician must improvise depending on the circumstances. Something as simple as two large spoons or an endotracheal tube may be used in lieu of complicated forceps and clamps.

Besides creating a vacuum, glass objects are especially difficult to remove because they can break and cause a tear or perforation in the rectal wall. If forceps are used to retrieve a glass object, coat the grasping edge with rubber or plastic or pad it with gauze. Plaster of Paris has been used to remove a hollow glass object if the object has an open end facing distally. Insert a hollow tube (e.g., an endotracheal tube, or small chest tube) into the open end. Fill the FB with plaster by injecting it through the hollow tube with a large irrigation syringe. Once the plaster cools and hardens within the tube, it can be used as a handle to remove the object with gentle traction. Be careful not to leak plaster onto the mucosa. In addition, heat is released as the plaster hardens and may cause the glass to crack or shatter. After removal, perform sigmoidoscopy to evaluate for edema and possible perforation of the mucosa. Alternatively, if a Foley catheter can be inserted into the opening of the FB, then the balloon on the catheter can be inflated and used to pull the object from the rectum. Again, relieving any proximal vacuum can be helpful. Patients with normal findings on postextraction examination and no evidence of perforation may be released home safely after a period of observation.[2,6,7]

FBs that are positioned proximal to the rectum warrant surgical consultation. Management options include observation to enable passage to the rectum or surgical removal.

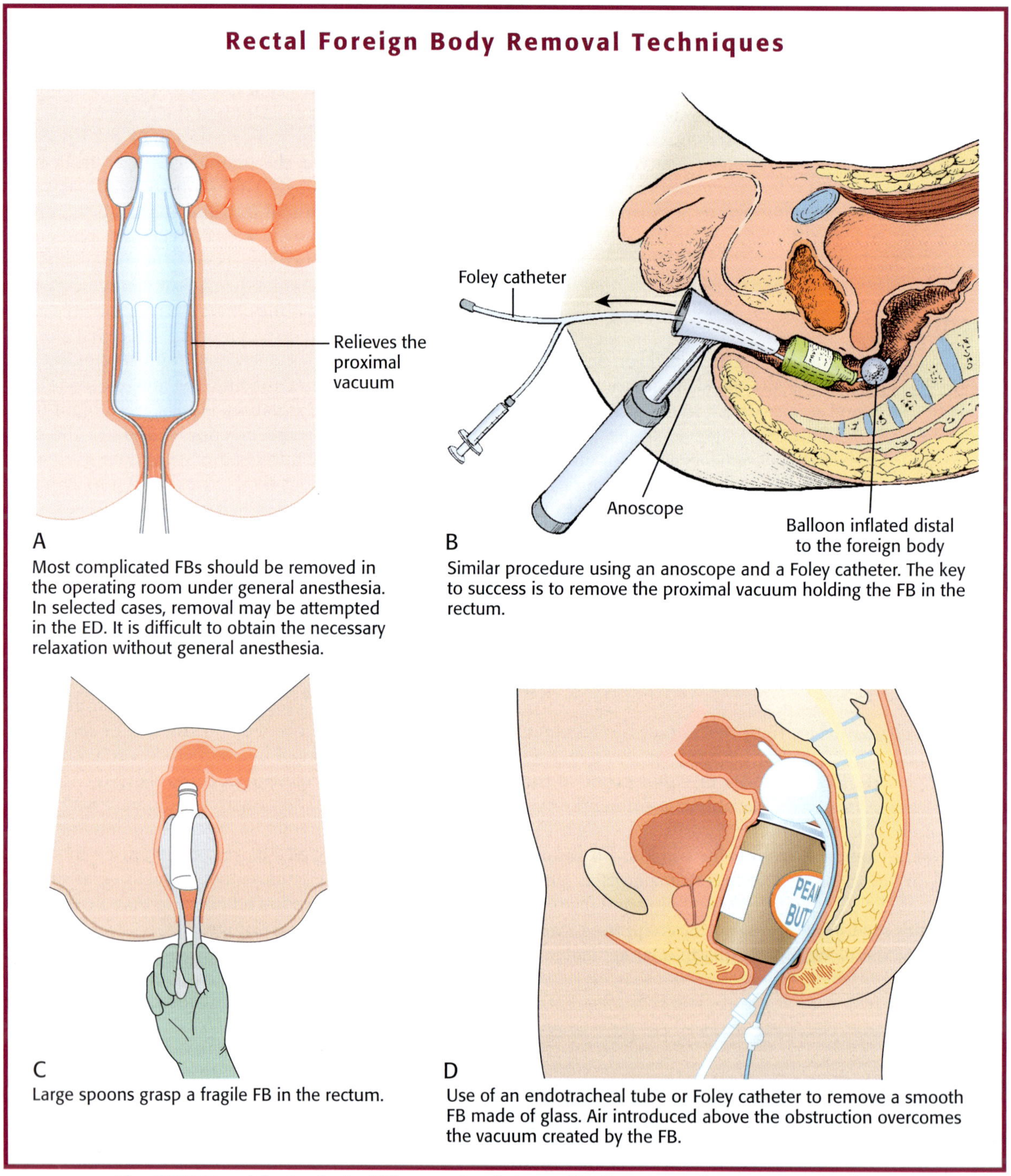

A Most complicated FBs should be removed in the operating room under general anesthesia. In selected cases, removal may be attempted in the ED. It is difficult to obtain the necessary relaxation without general anesthesia.

B Similar procedure using an anoscope and a Foley catheter. The key to success is to remove the proximal vacuum holding the FB in the rectum.

C Large spoons grasp a fragile FB in the rectum.

D Use of an endotracheal tube or Foley catheter to remove a smooth FB made of glass. Air introduced above the obstruction overcomes the vacuum created by the FB.

Fig. 46.12 Rectal foreign body *(FB)* removal techniques. *ED*, Emergency department. Difficult-to-remove FBs require operating room techniques.

Enemas or cathartics should not be used because they may increase the impaction of a rectal FB or cause it to move higher into the colon.

Complications

The most common complication is an inability to remove the rectal FB, which should prompt surgical consultation. The most serious complication of rectal FB retrieval is perforation or a deep mucosal tear, which may necessitate surgery. Cracking or shattering of glass may also require surgical exploration and retrieval. Mild mucosal edema and rectal bleeding are common sequelae of prolonged rectal FB presence and retrieval. These complications may not require any specific treatment. However, the presence of postprocedural abdominal pain, fever, sustained or profuse rectal bleeding, or discharge warrants surgical consultation.

MANAGEMENT OF RECTAL PROLAPSE

Rectal prolapse is protrusion of some or all the layers of the rectal wall through the anal orifice. Prolapse is not usually an emergency, and manual reduction is often easily accomplished in the ED. The most common complaint is protrusion

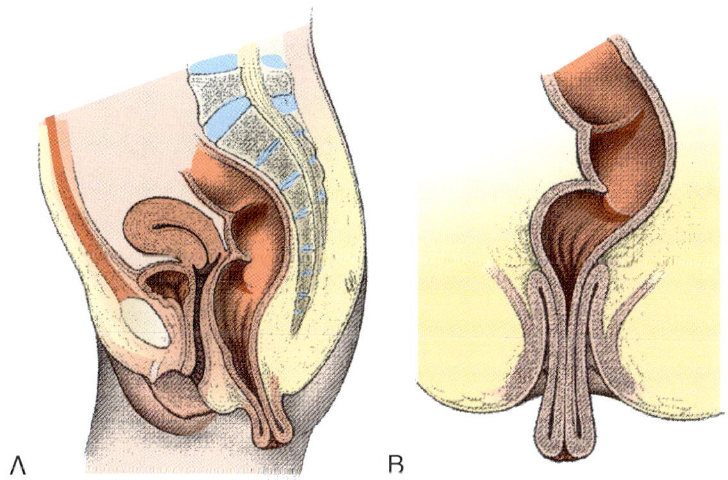

Fig. 46.13 (A) Type I procidentia (rectal prolapse). (B) Intussusception of the sigmoid colon beyond the anus. (From Kratzer GL, Demarest RJ. *Office Management of Colon and Rectal Disease*. Saunders; 1985.)

of a rectal "mass" or tissue. Patients may complain of pain on defecation, itching, incomplete evacuation, incontinence, or bloody mucosal discharge and mistake the condition for "hemorrhoids." Rectal prolapse is diagnosed by visual inspection of the anus. DRE may diagnose occult prolapse that is situated inside the anal canal. The differential diagnosis includes hemorrhoids, polyps, cystocele, and carcinoma.

There are three types of prolapse. (1) Complete prolapse, or procidentia, involves all layers of the rectum protruding through the anal orifice (Figs. 46.13 and 46.14). (2) Incomplete, or occult, prolapse describes internal prolapse that does not reach the orifice. This type is difficult to diagnose in the ED and requires no emergency intervention. (3) Mucosal prolapse is limited to protrusion of mucosa through the anal opening.

Complete and partial prolapse can be distinguished from each other by digital palpation. A thick muscular layer of tissue between the examiner's thumb and forefinger suggests complete prolapse. With partial or mucosal prolapse, radial rectal folds may be seen protruding through the rectum. This type of prolapse rarely extends more than 3 to 4 cm from the anus. Complete prolapse can extend 10 to 15 cm outside the anal verge.

Rectal prolapse is most common in children and older adults. Prolapse in children is typically incomplete, or mucosal. It usually affects children younger than 3 years and is often associated with cystic fibrosis, parasitic infection, chronic diarrhea, malnutrition, or as a sequela of chronic neurologic disease.[8] Prolapse is usually self-limited; outpatient management (after manual reduction) includes correcting constipation, avoiding straining, and referring for testing to exclude cystic fibrosis. Rectal prolapse in adults occurs most often in older females and may be recurrent. The cause is poorly understood, but it is associated with chronic constipation, chronic neurologic conditions, or pudendal neuropathies that weaken the anal sphincter.[9]

Indications for Reduction

Rectal prolapse may be reduced in the ED as a palliative measure. If unsuccessful, surgical referral is appropriate. Definitive surgery may be attempted, but occasional prolapses in debilitated patients are usually treated conservatively. Patients should be referred for outpatient proctoscopy to search for a polyp or malignancy that may have acted as a lead point. If the prolapse is incarcerated, surgical consultation should be obtained.

Procedure

Reduce a mucosal prolapse by applying gentle, constant pressure on the mass for a few minutes. In children, intravenous sedation may be necessary to allow reduction. Children are often more relaxed if they are allowed to remain on the parent's lap during the procedure. After reduction, send the child home with a pressure dressing and stool softeners. Counsel the parents on the use of dietary fiber and increased fluid intake to prevent constipation and straining. Refer the child for outpatient follow-up.[8]

For reduction of a complete prolapse, place the patient in the prone or lateral decubitus position (see Fig. 46.14, *step 1*). Parenteral sedation should be provided if the patient is anxious or has difficulty relaxing the sphincteric muscles. Tape the buttocks apart or have an assistant aid in reduction (see Fig. 46.14, *step 2*). Apply constant, gentle circumferential pressure to the prolapsed area, beginning with the portion closest to the lumen (the most distal segment). Place the thumbs on either side of the lumen while grasping the exterior walls with the fingers. Apply pressure with the thumbs while rolling the walls inward to force the prolapse back through the anus (see Fig. 46.14, *step 3*). Care should be taken to avoid poking at the tissue with the fingertips. If substantial tissue edema has developed, application of gauze soaked in sugar water may promote shrinkage and subsequent manual reduction.[9]

Complications

Complications after successful reduction are uncommon but may include bleeding and ulceration. Failure to reduce a prolapse requires surgical consultation. Apply saline-moistened gauze over the rectal tissue while awaiting consultation. A persistently prolapsed rectum can result in ulceration, strangulation, and perforation of the bowel wall.

Rectal Prolapse Reduction

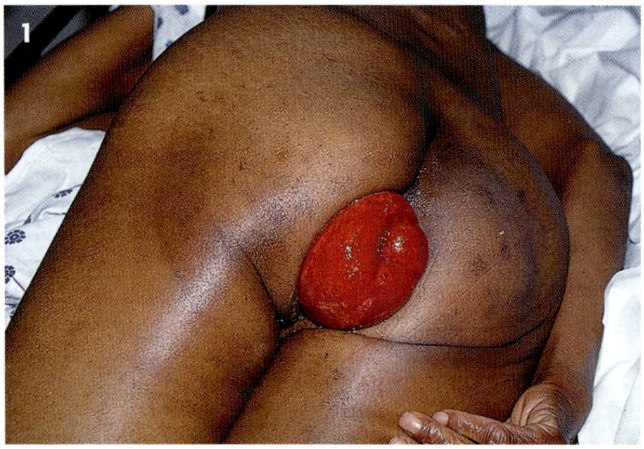

Complete (recurrent) rectal prolapse in a nursing home patient. To reduce the prolapse, place the patient in the prone or lateral decubitus position. Parenteral sedation may be required.

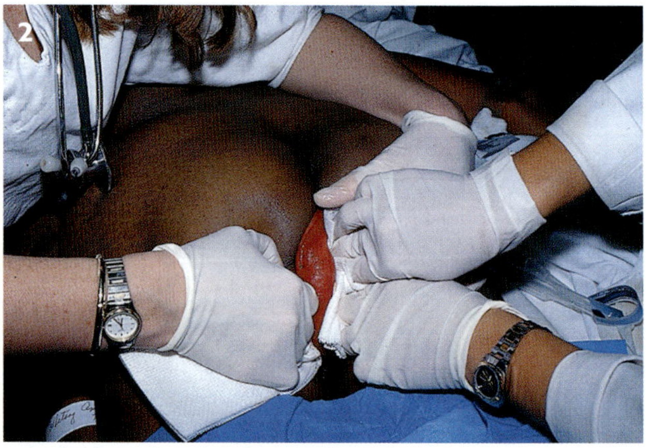

Tape the buttocks apart (or enlist the help of an assistant to spread the buttocks) to aid in reduction.

3

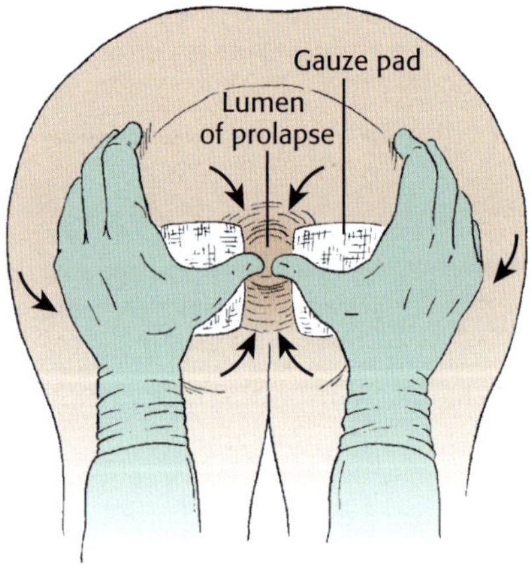

Apply constant, gentle circumferential pressure to the prolapsed area, beginning with the portion closest to the lumen (the most distal segment). Apply pressure with the thumbs while rolling the walls inward to force the prolapse back through the anus.

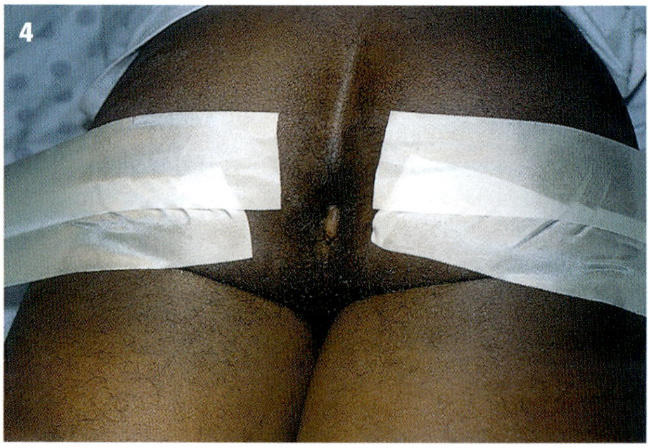

Successful reduction of the rectal prolapse.

Fig. 46.14 Reduction of rectal prolapse.

Moreover, the possibility of loss of anal sphincter tone and incontinence increases with delays in reduction of rectal prolapse.

ANAL FISSURE

An anal fissure is a small laceration or ulcer at the anal verge.[10] Anal fissures are the most common cause of sudden, searing anorectal pain. Though appearing trivial on examination, fissures can be extremely painful, even hours after a bowel movement, because of persistent spasm (Fig. 46.15). The condition is quite difficult to eradicate, is debilitating, and can last for months. It is occasionally associated with bright red rectal bleeding. An anal fissure is most commonly found in young adults, males, and females equally. In children, it can be a sign of child abuse. Anal fissures are usually associated with constipation, a hard or strained stool, or chronic diarrhea, but the exact cause is unknown. The diagnosis is relatively easy to make, and the fissure is readily seen by spreading the buttocks. The vast majority of anal fissures occur in the posterior midline, 10% to 15% occur in the anterior midline, and less than 1% occur in lateral positions. Fissures occurring in atypical locations should prompt consideration of other diseases or trauma. Multiple or recurrent fissures are associated with Crohn's disease, tuberculosis, syphilis, human immunodeficiency virus infection, and malignancy. Conservative therapy with the WASH regimen (see the section "Management of Hemorrhoids") may promote gradual healing in 4 to 6 weeks.

Most patients with acute anal fissures and almost half of patients with chronic fissures will experience healing with medical therapy. Therapy is aimed at breaking the cycle of pain, spasm, and ischemia, factors thought to be responsible for the development of the fissure. Therapies include relaxation of the internal sphincter, institution and maintenance of atraumatic passage of stool, and relief of pain. Simple measures include bulk agents, stool softeners, and probably most helpful, warm sitz baths following bowel movements to relax the sphincter. Based on the theory that anal fissures are caused by ischemia through a spasmodic internal sphincter,

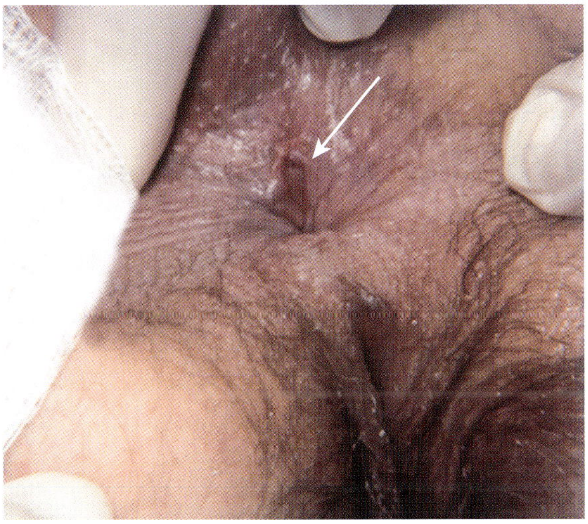

Fig. 46.15 A posterior midline anal fissure *(arrow)* is the most common type. Although some topical preparations may be helpful (see text), these lesions are painful and difficult to heal. In a child, an anal fissure may arouse suspicion of child abuse. (Courtesy the Mayo Foundation.)

pharmacological agents, including glyceryl trinitrate (GTN), diltiazem, and botulinum toxin, may be useful as alternatives to surgical sphincterotomy for chronic fissures. GTN ointment applied two to four times per day to the anus results in various healing rates, but a major side effect is dose-related headaches. Nitroglycerin 0.2% ointment applied twice daily may heal chronic ulcers via a reduction in resting anal pressure and an increase in anodermal blood flow. Diltiazem ointment (2%) appears to have efficacy similar to that of GTN but may cause fewer side effects. Diltiazem may be associated with the development of pruritus. Both diltiazem and GTN are first-line therapies. Botulinum toxin causes temporary muscle paralysis by preventing the release of acetylcholine from presynaptic nerve terminals, thereby decreasing pressure in the internal sphincter. Surgical treatment is generally reserved for fissures that have failed medical therapy and is usually curative.

REFERENCES ARE AVAILABLE AT Elsevier eBooks+

SECTION VIII

Musculoskeletal Procedures

CHAPTER 47

Prehospital Immobilization

Alison N.A. Abele and Stephen Sanko

SPINAL MOTION RESTRICTION

Background

The first widely accepted recommendations for "spinal immobilization" following blunt trauma came from the American Academy of Orthopaedic Surgeons in 1971.[1] These guidelines called for strict spinal immobilization—the use of adjuncts (i.e., cervical collar and long board) to minimize movement of the spinal column—in patients with symptoms or physical findings suggestive of spinal injuries.[1,2] Since then, recommendations for spinal immobilization have evolved considerably.

During the 1980s and 1990s indications for spinal immobilization were based primarily on the mechanism of injury, regardless of the presence or absence of symptoms or physical findings suggestive of a spinal injury.[2–5] This resulted in routine and often unnecessary prehospital spinal immobilization for all but the most trivial injuries.[6]

In 1998 Hauswald and colleagues[7] published the results of a 5-year retrospective review comparing patients from Malaysia, where cervical spine immobilization was nonexistent, to patients from New Mexico, where cervical spine immobilization based on the mechanism of injury was standard practice. The authors concluded that out-of-hospital immobilization has little or no effect on neurologic outcome in patients with blunt spinal injuries.[7] This study, and others demonstrating increased complications[8–13] and significant spinal movement, despite the use of cervical collars (c-collars) and long spine boards,[14,15] prompted the development and evaluation of prehospital clinical decision rules to selectively immobilize patients after blunt trauma.[16–19]

A 4-year prospective study in two Michigan counties found that the use of a selective immobilization protocol resulted in spine immobilization for most patients with spinal injury without causing harm to patients in which spine immobilization was withheld.[18] A larger study in Maine demonstrated that selective immobilization based on a statewide protocol resulted in only one nonimmobilized unstable cervical spine fracture in more than 32,000 patient encounters.[19]

Data demonstrating the safe application of selective spinal immobilization protocols by prehospital providers, a lack of scientific evidence demonstrating improved outcomes with the use of long spine boards, and a keen awareness of the complications associated with spinal immobilization resulted in a set of recommendations from the National Association of EMS Physicians and the American College of Surgeons Committee on Trauma[20] and the American College of Emergency Physicians[21] in 2014. These recommendations include the selective use of long spine boards following blunt trauma and elimination of their use following penetrating trauma in patients with no evidence of spinal injury.[20] In 2018 these organizations published a joint position statement updating their 2014 recommendations (Box 47.1).[22]

The effects of spinal immobilization on mortality, neurologic injury, spinal stability, and adverse effects in trauma patients remain uncertain. Due to the low incidence of actual spinal cord injury (SCI) and associated neurologic sequelae, prospective trials are difficult to safely design and perform. Nevertheless, available data suggests that we should reduce or eliminate routine prehospital spinal immobilization in favor of using validated clinical rules to determine which patients may have sustained a spinal column injury and applying spinal motion restriction strategies only to these patients. Indeed, the term spinal motion restriction has been increasingly used to describe prehospital procedures to simply maintain the spine in anatomic alignment and minimizing gross movement irrespective of adjuncts or devices. However, these new approaches will take time to promulgate through the EMS community. There is a lack of high-quality evidence on the acceptability and appropriate implementation of such tools. Until then, emergency physicians must be knowledgeable about prehospital spinal immobilization. Therefore the remainder of this section provides a detailed review of immobilization devices and techniques.

EPIDEMIOLOGY

According to the National Spinal Cord Injury Statistical Center, an estimated 17,800 new, survivable SCIs occur in the Unites States annually,[23] and 294,000 people were living with SCIs in the United States in 2020.[23] Since 2010 the most common cause of SCI is motor vehicle collision, which accounts for almost 40% of cases, followed closely by falls (32%) and acts of violence (14%), primarily gunshot wounds.[23] Sports such as American football, rugby, swimming and diving, gymnastics, ice hockey, track and field (specifically pole vaulting), cheerleading, and baseball all place participants at increased risk for spinal injuries.[23] The cost of care in both the immediate and extended care setting can be exorbitant, especially

BOX 47.1 Spinal Motion Restriction in the Trauma Patient: Consensus[a]

POINTS OF CONSENSUS

1. Unstable spinal column injuries can progress to severe neurological injuries in the presence of excessive movement of the injured spine.
2. While current techniques limit or reduce undesired motion of the spine, they do not provide true spinal immobilization. For this reason, the term "spinal motion restriction (SMR)" has gained favor over "spinal immobilization," although both terms refer to the same concept. The goal of both SMR and spinal immobilization in the trauma patient is to minimize unwanted movement of the potentially injured spine.
3. While backboards have historically been used to attempt spinal immobilization, SMR may also be achieved by use of a scoop stretcher, vacuum splint, ambulance cot, or other similar device to which a patient is safely secured.
4. Indications for SMR following blunt trauma include:
   i. Acutely altered level of consciousness (e.g., GCS < 15, evidence of intoxication)
   ii. Midline neck or back pain and/or tenderness
   iii. Focal neurologic signs and/or symptoms (e.g., numbness or motor weakness)
   iv. Anatomic deformity of the spine
   v. Distracting circumstances or injury (e.g., long-bone fracture, degloving, or crush injuries, large burns, emotional distress, communication barrier, etc.) or any similar injury that impairs the patient's ability to contribute to a reliable examination
5. SMR, when indicated, should apply to the entire spine due to the risk of noncontiguous injuries. An appropriately sized cervical collar is a critical component of SMR and should be used to limit movement of the cervical spine whenever SMR is employed. The remainder of the spine should be stabilized by keeping the head, neck, and torso in alignment. This can be accomplished by placing the patient on a long backboard, a scoop stretcher, a vacuum mattress, or an ambulance cot. If elevation of the head is required, the device used to stabilize the spine should be elevated at the head while maintaining alignment of the neck and torso. SMR cannot be properly performed with a patient in a sitting position.
6. All patient transfers create potential for unwanted displacement of an unstable spine injury. Particular attention should be focused on patient transfers from one surface to another including, for example, ground to ambulance cot. A long spine board, a scoop stretcher, or a vacuum mattress is recommended to assist with patient transfers in order to minimize flexion, extension, or rotation of the possibly injured spine.
7. Once a patient is safely positioned on an ambulance cot, transfer or extrication devices may be removed if an adequate number of trained personnel are present to minimize unnecessary movement during the removal process. The risks of patient manipulation must be weighed against the benefits of device removal. If transport time is expected to be short, it may be better to transport a patient on the device and remove it on arrival at the hospital. If the decision is made to remove the extrication device in the field, SMR should be maintained by assuring that the patient remains securely positioned on the ambulance cot with a cervical collar in place.
8. Hospitals should be prepared and equipped to carefully and quickly remove patients from a long backboard, scoop stretcher, or vacuum mattress as soon as possible after arrival at the hospital. Safe transfer may require the use of a slider board or similar device in order to maintain SMR during patient movement. Procedures should be in place to assure that a sufficient number of properly trained individuals are available to assist with patient transfers in order to minimize the risk of inadvertent displacement of a potentially unstable spinal injury.
9. There is no role for SMR in penetrating trauma.
10. SMR in children
    i. Age alone should not be a factor in decision-making for prehospital spinal care, both for the young child and the child who can reliably provide a history.
    ii. Young children pose communication barriers, but this should not mandate SMR purely based on age.
    iii. Based on the best available pediatric evidence from studies that have been conducted through the Pediatric Emergency Care Applied Research Network (PECARN), a cervical collar should be applied if the patient has any of the following:
       a. Complaint of neck pain;
       b. Torticollis;
       c. Neurologic deficit;
       d. Altered mental status including GCS < 15, intoxication, and other signs (agitation, apnea, hypopnea, somnolence, etc.)
       e. Involvement in a high-risk motor vehicle collision, high impact diving injury, or has substantial torso injury.
    iv. There is no evidence supporting a high risk/incidence for noncontiguous multilevel spinal injury in children. The rate of contiguous multilevel injury in children is extremely low at 1%. The rate of noncontiguous multilevel injury in children is thought to be equally as low.
    v. Minimize the time on backboards with consideration for use of a vacuum mattress or padding as adjuncts to minimize the risk of pain and pressure ulcers if this time is to be prolonged.
    vi. Because of the variation in the head size to body ratio in young children relative to adults, additional padding under the shoulders is often necessary to avoid excessive cervical spine flexion with SMR.

[a]*A joint position statement of the American College of Surgeons Committee on Trauma (ACS-COT), American College of Emergency Physicians (ACEP), and the National Association of EMS Physicians (NAEMSP).*
From Fischer PE, Perina DG, Delbridge TR et al. Spinal motion restriction in the trauma patient—a joint position statement. Prehosp Emerg Care. *2018;22(6):659-661.*

among the young. The average lifetime cost of medical care for patients with SCI varies depending on the level of injury and age at time of injury, and ranges from $1.2 million to more than $5.1 million, with annual costs from $45,000 to $1.1 million.[23]

PATHOPHYSIOLOGY

The direction and strength of the injurious force may help predict the type of injury sustained. The basic forces that can be exerted on the spine are flexion, extension, rotation, lateral bending, distraction (stretching), and compression (axial loading).[24,25] Of course, complex mechanisms may exert multiple forces. For example, high-speed rollover motor vehicle collisions could easily exert all the aforementioned forces.

Injuries to the upper cervical spine (C1 and C2) (Fig. 47.1) occur more often in older, osteoporotic patients than in younger patients. The spectrum of injuries in the cervicocranium includes occipital condyle fractures, occipitoatlantal dislocations, dislocations and subluxations of the atlantoaxial joint, fractures of the ring of the atlas, odontoid fractures, fractures of the arch of the axis, and fractures of the lateral mass of the axis (Fig. 47.2). Involvement of the spinal cord at this high level can cause devastating neurologic injury, and it is reasonable to believe that many of these injuries are not reported because they result in death.[26,27] Subaxial cervical spinal injuries involving C3–C7 have broad clinical implications. Approximately two-thirds of cervical injuries causing quadriplegia occur within the lower cervical spine, with fractures occurring most often in C6 and C7 and dislocations most commonly occurring between C5–C6 and C6–C7.[28]

The orientation of the facets in the thoracic spine allows significantly less flexion and extension than in the cervical or lumbar spine. In addition, the free space between the thoracic spinal cord and the borders of the spinal canal is relatively small, and the blood supply is less robust. These factors increase the susceptibility of the spinal cord to injuries at this level. At the thoracolumbar junction, there is an acute transition in stability because of the loss of rib restraint, which increases the risk for flexion-extension and rotational injuries. Disk size and shape also change, thus making this section of the spine particularly susceptible to injury. Approximately half of all vertebral body fractures and 40% of all SCIs occur between T11 and L2.[29]

The lumbar spine is protected only by the abdominal and paraspinous musculature, making it subject to distracting and shearing forces, such as those seen with lap belt injuries. There is also a higher prevalence of compression and burst fractures in the lumbar spine. These fractures commonly occur when axial loading forces straighten the natural lordosis at the moment of impact.[29]

The sacrum forms both the terminal portion of the spine and the central portion of the pelvis, which gives it added stability and makes isolated sacral fractures uncommon. Such fractures are usually caused by direct trauma or falls from a height or occur as a result of sacral insufficiency secondary to osteopenia, chronic steroid use, or previous pelvic irradiation. More often, sacral fractures occur because of high-energy mechanisms and are associated with major pelvic disruption.[30]

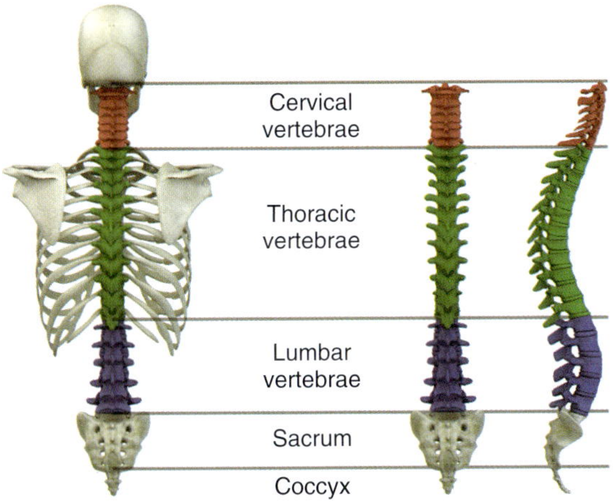

Fig. 47.1 The human spinal column.

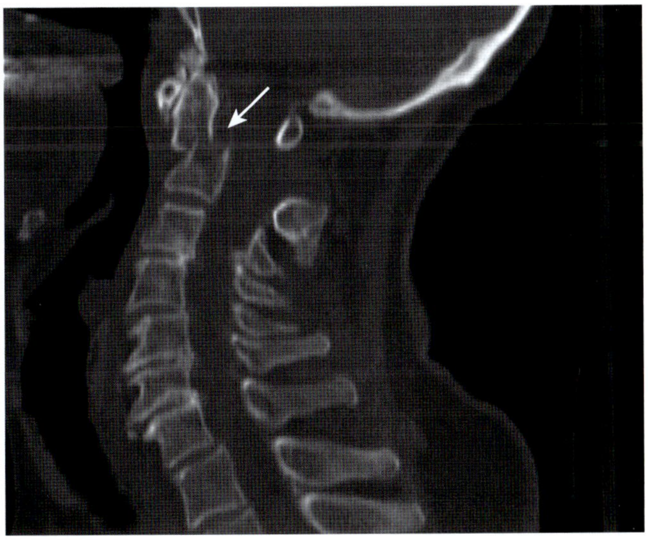

Fig. 47.2 Type III odontoid (C2) fracture *(arrow)*. A common scenario for this type of injury is an older female who falls from a standing height.

INDICATIONS

Spinal motion restriction should be considered for victims of blunt trauma who sustain an injury with a mechanism that has the potential for causing spinal injury and who have at least one of the following criteria: altered mental status, intoxication, a distracting painful injury (e.g., long-bone fracture), anatomic spinal deformity, a focal neurologic deficit or symptom (e.g., motor weakness, numbness), and/or midline spinal pain or tenderness (see Box 47.1).[22]

Extremes of age and the presence of communication barriers (e.g., language, hearing impairment) may affect the ability to accurately assess the patient's perception and communication of pain and should lower one's threshold for spinal precautions.[2,5] It is also important to remember that serious cervical cord injuries can occur in the absence of demonstrable fractures. SCI is common in older patients with cervical spondylosis, in whom an arthritic osteophyte may sever a portion of the cord as permanently as a fracture or dislocation. In such cases, there may be little subjective pain, and the mechanism of injury may appear seemingly minor.[31]

Although data are sparse, patients who have had a seizure in the field are at low risk for spinal injury.[32] Nevertheless, immobilization of postictal patients due to a presumed risk for spinal injury and inability to adequately assess the patient is commonplace. Unfortunately, attempts at immobilization often prompt further patient confusion and agitation, and struggling may exacerbate injuries that do exist (Fig. 47.3). In these situations, when there is concern for a spinal injury based on the mechanism of injury, physical findings (e.g., focal neurologic deficit, facial injuries), or patient complaints, administer sedation rather than, or in addition to, spinal motion restriction. Sedation in such patients should be accompanied by appropriate vital sign monitoring.

When spinal motion restriction is indicated, it is imperative that restrictions are upheld during any and all patient

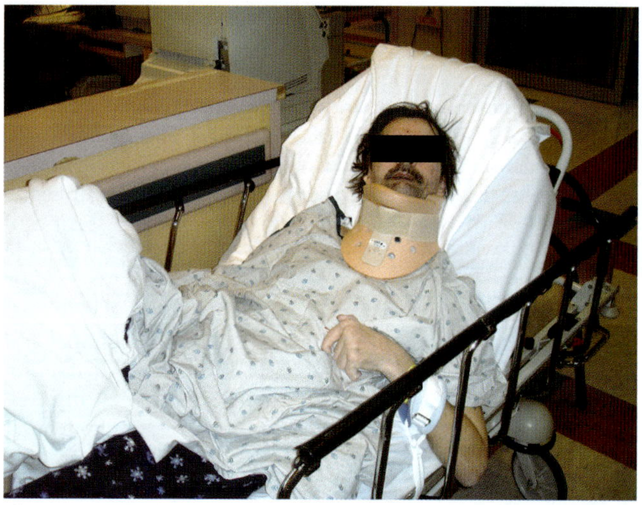

Fig. 47.3 This patient was initially postictal and combative and did not allow prehospital cervical spine immobilization. Although this is a dilemma for all involved, it is best to avoid forcing such immobilization. Sedation may be an alternative if injury is strongly suspected and immobilization is deemed clinically necessary. After recovering from his postictal state with a clear mental status and no neck pain (and National Emergency X-radiology Utilization Study rules negative), an unneeded collar was subsequently unnecessarily applied in the emergency department, to the annoyance of the patient, who then became very agitated and tried to leave. Note that the patient is shown physically restrained and is sitting upright.

transfers. For example, providers must be careful to uphold spinal precautions when transferring a patient from an ambulance gurney to hospital bed, when removing a backboard, and when logrolling a patient to assess more closely for injury, in order to prevent further harm.

In summary, there is no good evidence that cervical immobilization restricts harmful movement, and the use of c-collars may cause harm. There is evidence that c-collars reduce venous return and hence may cause an increase in intracranial pressure (ICP). Taking a patient out of a comfortable position and placing them in a collar that extends the neck does not make them safer. However, patients with altered mental status, intoxication, or focal neurologic deficits should prompt spinal motion restriction.

CONTRAINDICATIONS

Spinal immobilization with a c-collar or a backboard following blunt trauma is not necessary in patients with a normal mental status (Glasgow Coma Scale [GCS] 15), no spinal tenderness or anatomic abnormality, no neurologic findings or complaints, no distracting injuries, and no intoxication (see Box 47.1).[22]

In general, spinal immobilization with a c-collar and a backboard is contraindicated (or may require modification) when its use could harm the patient, when it is logistically impossible, or when the scene is unsafe (Box 47.2). Good clinical judgment, not blind application of protocols, is essential. For example, if application of a c-collar will cause or mask airway compromise secondary to swelling, an expanding hematoma, or other process, it should not be used. Obviously, if a patient requires a surgical airway, the EMS provider will need immediate, unencumbered access to the anterior aspect of the neck. Sometimes preexisting airways (e.g., tracheotomy tube) and associated equipment prohibit proper application of a c-collar. These situations can often be managed with an improvised cervical immobilizer, such as a collar fashioned from a towel roll or prolonged manual stabilization without traction.

BOX 47.2 Contraindications to Prehospital Spine Immobilization

May be potentially harmful (e.g., prevents identification of airway compromise)
Need for a surgical airway
Presence of a preexisting airway (e.g., tracheostomy tube)
Obesity
Impaled objects
Chronic respiratory diseases (e.g., congestive heart failure) or acute respiratory distress from any cause (e.g., ascites)
Altered mental status or agitation (e.g., intoxicated patients)
Cervical dislocation or anatomic limitation because of preexisting conditions (e.g., ankylosing spondylitis)
Logistically impractical (e.g., mass-casualty incident, hazmat incident)
Unsafe scene:

- Exposure to hazardous material, fire, or smoke
- Building explosion or collapse
- Deep or fast moving water that poses a risk for drowning
- Risk for injury from assault (e.g., gunshot, stabbing, blunt trauma)
- Any other circumstance that the emergency medical service provider deems an immediate danger to the life or health of the patient, provider, or both

[a]*Situations listed in this table can often be managed with modified spinal precautions (see text for details).*

Other conditions that may prevent spinal immobilization or require modification of standard techniques and equipment (e.g., towel roll and manual in-line stabilization) include obesity, impaled objects, underlying respiratory problems or acute respiratory distress, altered mental status (e.g., combative patients due to intoxication or psychiatric illness), and cervical dislocation with fixed angulation or anatomic limitations from preexisting conditions such as ankylosing spondylitis and kyphosis.[33]

There are also scenarios when spinal motion restriction is logistically difficult or impossible. In a mass-casualty incident or wilderness accident, maintaining spinal motion restriction may be impractical or impossible (Fig. 47.4). Moreover, spinal motion restriction may need to be delayed or modified when the scene poses a significant threat to the patient or providers (see Box 47.2).[25] In these situations, the prehospital provider may opt for rapid extrication of the patient from the scene without immobilization of the spine (Fig. 47.5).

In general, victims of penetrating trauma to the head, neck, or torso, such as gunshot wounds, with no evidence of spinal injury should not be immobilized.[22] No study has demonstrated worsening neurologic outcomes related to a lack of prehospital spinal immobilization, whereas delays to definitive care for life-threatening hemorrhage or airway obstruction can lead to increased morbidity and mortality in these patients (Fig. 47.6).[34–37] In hemodynamically stable patients with focal neurologic deficits following a penetrating injury, it may be reasonable to restrict spinal motion; however, it is

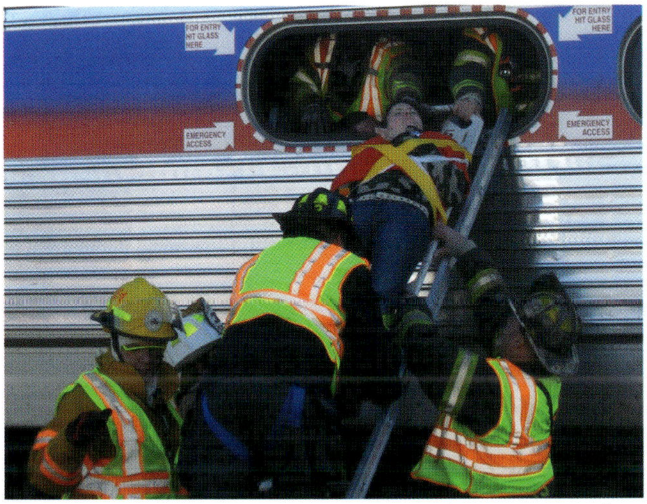

Fig. 47.4 During a mass-casualty incident such as a train accident, spinal motion restriction of multiple victims with a low probability of spinal injury may not be practical and may delay other more pressing interventions if resources are limited.

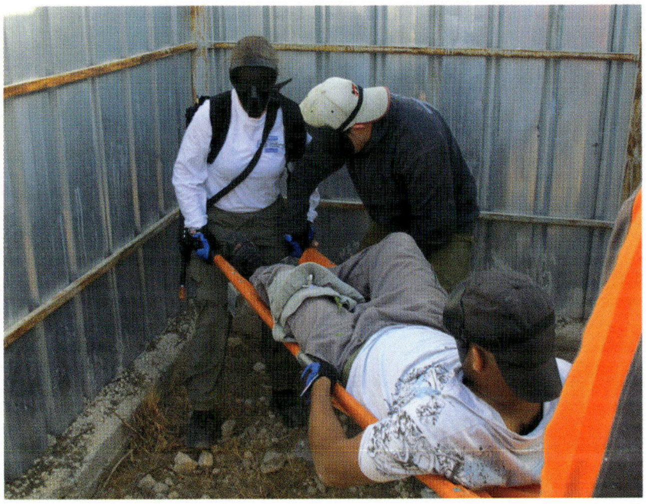

Fig. 47.5 Spinal motion restriction may need to be delayed, modified, or omitted when the scene poses a significant threat to the patient or providers, such as evacuating a wounded soldier during a sniper attack. Rescue from a toxic or poisonous environment, such as hydrogen sulfide or carbon monoxide, is a similar situation.

prudent to err on the side of expediting care at the expense of immobilization.

EQUIPMENT

C-Collars

See Video 47.1. Traditionally, c-collars have used a four-point support structure at the bottom of the collar: at the two trapezius muscles posteriorly and at the two clavicles anteriorly. Most modern collars are modified rigid head-cervical-thoracic devices that use the sternum as a fifth support structure. Current collar designs support the head with winglike flaps on the collar's upper posterior edges. Anteriorly, the collar supports the mandible. The collar's flaring design generally prevents compression of the thyroid cartilage and cervical vessels, even when applied firmly. Some collars come as single units that conform to the neck once a chin support has been assembled, whereas others come in two parts, with a front and a back that are secured with Velcro (Fig. 47.7). Some manufacturers have developed collars that have adjustable heights to account for different neck lengths. Soft collars, though comfortable, have no role in spinal immobilization because they provide minimal support and do not reduce cervical motion to any significant degree.[38]

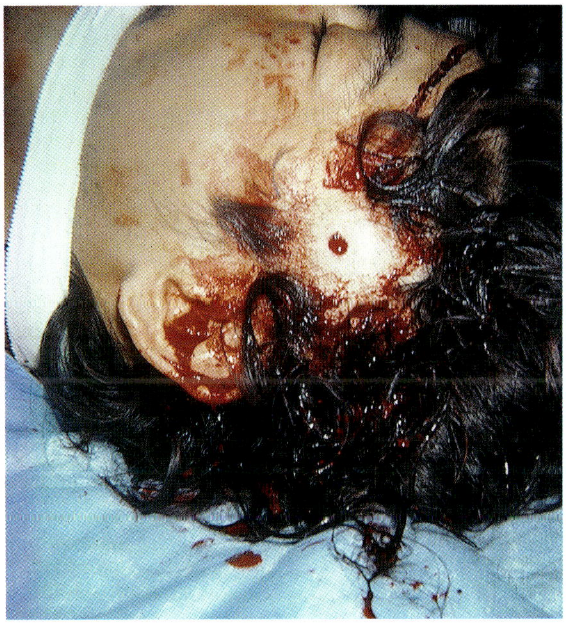

Fig. 47.6 A gunshot wound to the head is not an indication for routine cervical spine immobilization. No study has demonstrated worsening neurologic outcomes related to a lack of prehospital spinal immobilization. Immobilizing the cervical spine in these patients may lead to missed injury under the collar, airway compromise, increased intracranial pressure, and delay in resuscitation.

Investigators have attempted to evaluate c-collars in an objective fashion. The accepted "gold standard" for comparison is the halo brace, which restricts motion to 4% flexion-extension, 1% rotation, and 4% lateral bending.[39] Unfortunately, even the best c-collars (when used independently) restrict flexion and extension by only 70% to 75% and overall neck movement by 50% or less.[39] A number of studies have evaluated neck motion in volunteers immobilized supine on a backboard with various collars in place.[38,40–43] Although these studies demonstrated small differences among some of the collars, overall they merely confirm the fact that c-collars do not completely prevent motion of the cervical spine. Interestingly, some cadaver studies have shown the potential for c-collars to actually increase motion and force in the unstable cervical spine.[44] Despite these limitations, c-collars remain a widely used component of most spinal motion restriction strategies.

Cervical Extrication Splints

A large variety of short spine boards and intermediate-stage extrication devices are available for prehospital use (Fig. 47.8). Generally, these devices are manufactured from rigid lightweight material. They have a narrow board design that permits easy application in automobiles or confined spaces and are constructed with multiple openings along the edges to allow for a variety of strapping options. Ideally, these devices

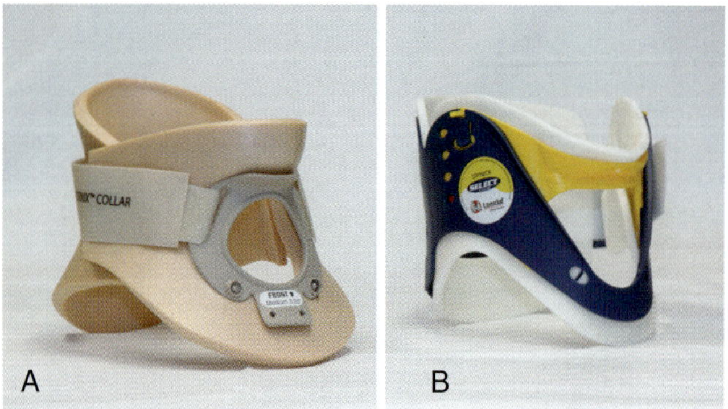

Fig. 47.7 Cervical collars. (A) Philadelphia collar. This two-piece, high-type collar comes in four sizes. The collar supports the head in a dish-shaped contour that is formed when the front and rear halves are joined by Velcro fasteners. When properly sized for a patient, this collar provides excellent support. When applied too tightly, it tends to force the mandible backward and can cause compression of the thyroid in some patients. (B) Stifneck collar. This collar is made of high-density polyethylene (a hard material) and padded with semiflexible foam margins. Note the low-reaching anterior panel, which contacts the sternum for additional support.

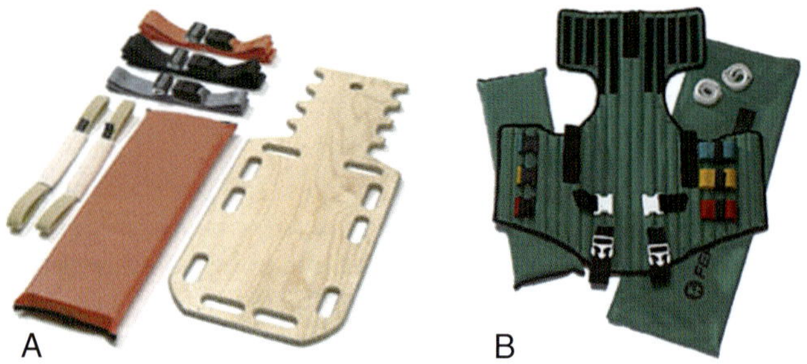

Fig. 47.8 Cervical extrication splints. (A) Rigid short boards. (B) Kendrick Extrication Device. (Courtesy Ferno-Washington, Inc.)

should also be translucent so that radiographs can be readily obtained in the emergency department (ED), and they should allow repeated use and easy cleanup.

Application of a cervical extrication splint should not produce unnecessary movement or change the position of the head, neck, shoulders, or torso. In conjunction with a good c-collar, a properly applied cervical extrication splint should effectively limit flexion, extension, lateral motion, and rotational motion of the head, neck, and torso.

One commonly used device that meets all these criteria is the Kendrick Extrication Device (KED) (see Fig. 47.8B). This device consists of two layers of nylon mesh impregnated with plastic and sewn over plywood slats to provide rigidity. It has a nylon loop behind the patient's head that is continuous with the pelvic support straps for additional strength. Part of its anterior thoracic panels can be folded backward to fit obese, pregnant, or pediatric patients.[45] When properly applied, the KED is a snug-fitting, highly adaptable immobilizer that can be used in even the most adverse circumstances.

When patients require immobilization or extrication (or both) in more difficult or treacherous environments, many EMS providers prefer the LSP half-back (Allied Healthcare Products, Inc.), which resembles a KED, but is more rugged and durable. In addition to providing spinal motion restriction, it also acts as a harness and can be used for hauling patients over flat surfaces and for vertical lifts (Fig. 47.9).[46]

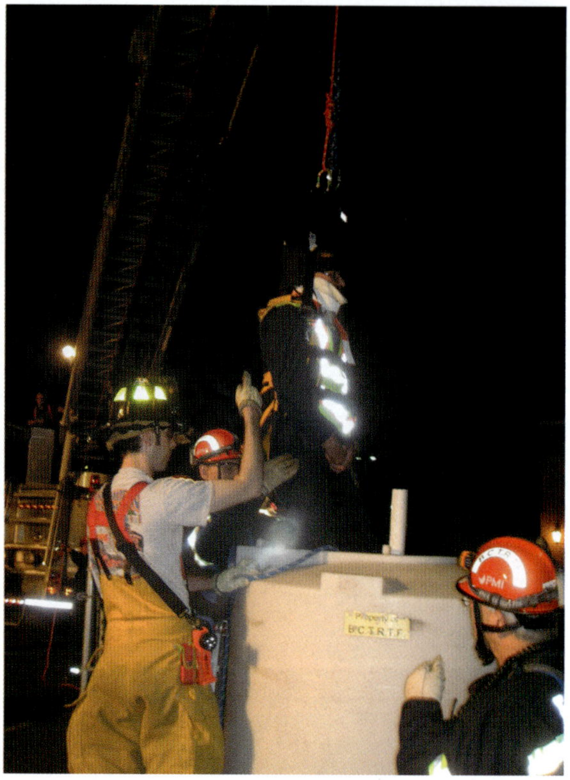

Fig. 47.9 The LSP half-back. This cervical extrication splint resembles a Kendrick Extrication Device but is more rugged and durable. In addition to providing spinal immobilization, it also acts as a harness that can be used for hauling patients over flat surfaces and for vertical lifts.

Mosesso and colleagues[47] compared six prehospital cervical immobilization devices and concluded that the devices were similar in their ability to limit motion of the cervical spine.

Full-Body Spinal Restriction

Long Spine Boards (Backboards)

See Video 47.2. Backboards are made of wood or plastic composites and can be either rectangular or tapered in shape (Fig. 47.10A). Most rescuers prefer the tapered type because it takes up less horizontal room when angled into a narrow opening or doorway. In addition, the slight narrowing of these boards on either end enhances the effectiveness of strapping.

Most backboards (have strategically placed openings along the edges that can be used to secure head-stabilizing devices, strap the patient to the board, or lift the patient). Many also feature runners, usually approximately 2.5 cm thick, on their undersides that serve both as stiffeners and as spacers. They raise the board slightly off the ground so that rescuers can get their fingers under the board during lifting. The runners, however, may make it more difficult to slide a patient onto the board.

Advantages of backboards over full-body splints include their ease of storage, low cost, and extreme versatility. The backboard can be used to slide a victim out of an automobile or to protect a victim during removal of a windshield.

Board splints, as a class, are the least comfortable of all immobilizers. Studies have demonstrated that spinal immobilization on a hard backboard causes head, back, and jaw pain.[8,13] Pain in these areas may become severe if patients are

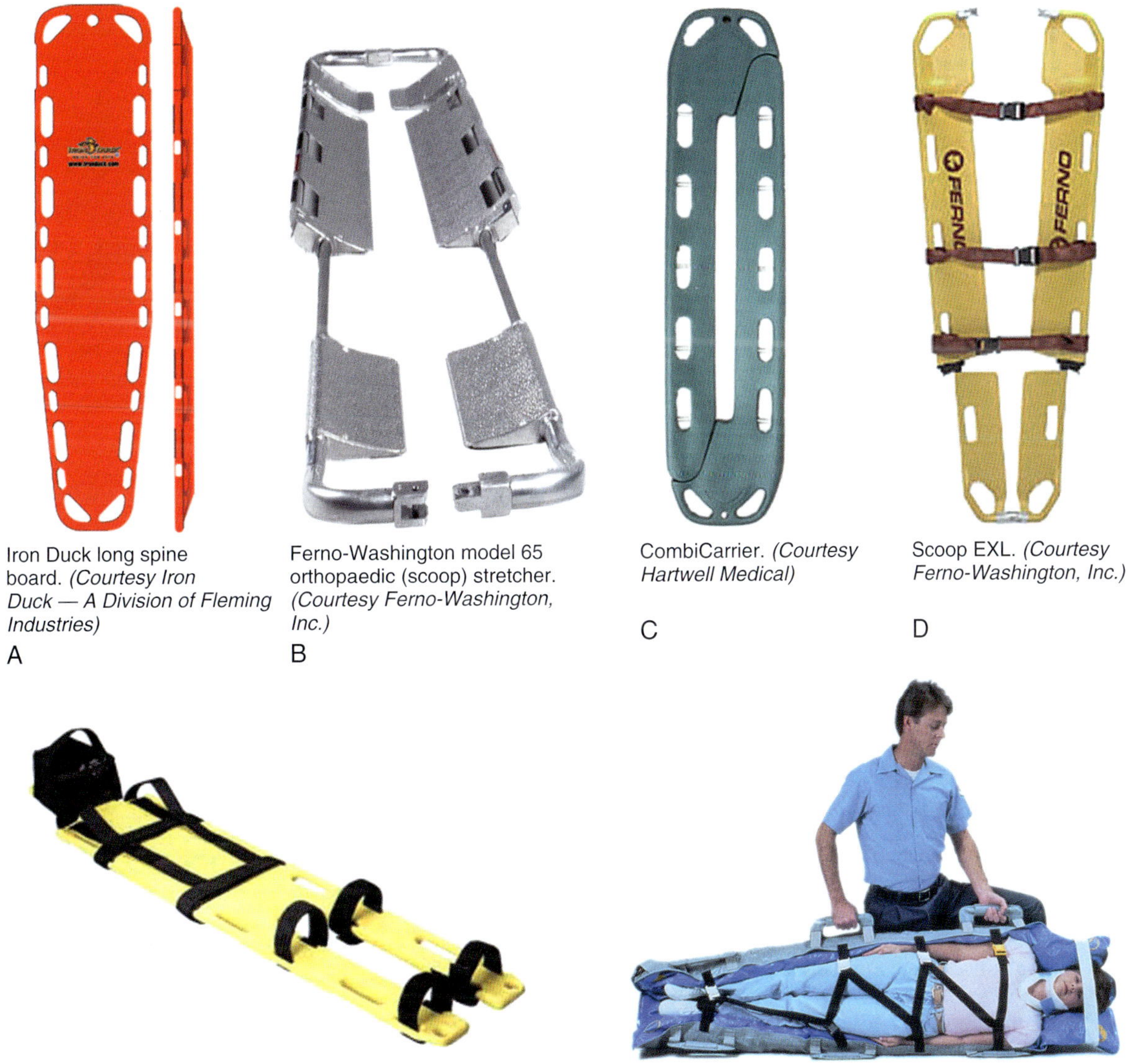

Iron Duck long spine board. *(Courtesy Iron Duck — A Division of Fleming Industries)*
A

Ferno-Washington model 65 orthopaedic (scoop) stretcher. *(Courtesy Ferno-Washington, Inc.)*
B

CombiCarrier. *(Courtesy Hartwell Medical)*
C

Scoop EXL. *(Courtesy Ferno-Washington, Inc.)*
D

Miller body splint. *(Courtesy Life Support Products, Inc.)*
E

EVAC-U-SPLINT mattress. *(Courtesy Hartwell Medical)*
F

Fig. 47.10 Full-body spine boards (backboards).

left immobilized on these boards for extended periods.[9–11] In addition, the pain caused by application of a backboard may be difficult to separate from other sources of pain in a trauma patient and might lead to costly radiographs and unnecessary radiation exposure to the patient.[2,48] Discomfort may be minimized by using padding at points of contact between a bony prominence and the board. This concept was reaffirmed by Hauswald and colleagues,[49] who found that increasing the amount of padding on a backboard decreases the amount of ischemic pain caused by immobilization. In some cases, tissue ischemia can lead to frank pressure ulcers, particularly in the older or nutritional-deficient populations.[50] Other concerning, well-described risks of long spine board immobilization include respiratory compromise,[51] aspiration in the event of vomiting, delay to care for management of emergent injuries, and restraint-related "combativeness."

Scoop Stretchers

In many cases, a litter that separates longitudinally into two halves, commonly called a scoop stretcher, is an ideal field immobilizer (see Fig. 47.10B). In fact, one study found that using the scoop stretcher caused less spinal motion than did a traditional long backboard and logroll technique.[52]

The scoop stretcher is designed to split into two or four pieces. It is comfortable, rigid, and adaptable to patients of various lengths and provides unobstructed radiographic transparency of the entire spine. If necessary, it can be applied almost instantly or removed without disturbing the position of the victim. The scoop stretcher also provides good lateral stability because of the trough-like shape of its top surface, and it is stable enough to be used for carrying. When cervical motion restriction is desired, a c-collar can be used with the scoop stretcher. In keeping with current recommendations regarding rigid long boards (see Box 47.1), the scoop should be removed once the patient is transferred to the ambulance cot and the practice of placing a long spine board under the scoop or transferring a patient to a spine board for transport should be abandoned. If the patient must be transported to the hospital on a scoop stretcher, removal is achieved by unfastening the latches at the top and the bottom of the device (see the section on "Procedure" later in this chapter).

One limitation of the scoop stretcher is the potential for trapping clothes, skin, or other objects between interlocking parts. It also interferes slightly with the ischial section of a half-ring traction splint but works well with Sager-type devices. The Ferno-Washington model 65 scoop is the most widely used stretcher of this type. Other devices such as the CombiCarrier (Hartwell Medical) and the Scoop EXL (Ferno-Washington, Inc.) offer lightweight polymer construction and additional spinal support (see Fig. 47.10C and D).

Full-Body Splints

A variety of full-body splints are available and may be used by some prehospital providers. One popular device is the Miller body splint, which consists of a polyethylene shell injected with closed-cell foam that is radiographically translucent and provides buoyancy in water (see Fig. 47.10E). This full-body splint has a removable head harness and a thoracic harness, as well as pelvic and lower extremity belts. The space between the lower extremities facilitates wrapping with bandage material in the event of fractures. In addition, it is shaped so that it can easily fit into a basket-type rescue stretcher. Similar spine immobilization systems are available for pediatric patients (e.g., Pedi-Pac, Ferno-Washington, Inc.).

Another full-body splint designed to reduce the pain associated with many of the immobilization devices described previously is the vacuum mattress splint (e.g., EVAC-U-SPLINT, Hartwell Medical, and Immobile-Vac, MDI) (see Fig. 47.10F). It consists of a vinyl-coated polyester envelope filled with thousands of 1.1-mm-diameter polyester foam spheres. A manual or electric vacuum pump is used to evacuate the interior to a pressure of approximately 0.25 atm. The reduction in internal pressure causes the mattress to conform to the contours of the patient's body. Vacuum splints have been shown to produce lower sacral interface pressure and lower mean pain scores than traditional hard backboards[11,53] and may provide better immobilization in patients with known SCI.[54,55] It should also be pointed out, however, that vacuum splints are larger and more cumbersome than backboards, thus making ambulance storage more difficult.

Lateral Neck Stabilizers

Lightweight objects such as blocks (10 × 10 × 15 cm) made of medium-density foam rubber are commonly used to provide additional lateral stabilization of the head and neck. Foam blocks are inexpensive and disposable and do not slip on the backboard. Disposable cardboard devices that have the same advantages as foam blocks are also available (Fig. 47.11A).

Another commercial device is the Universal Head Immobilizer (Ferno-Washington, Inc.). It is a lateral neck stabilizer designed to quickly and easily fasten the patient's head to a scoop stretcher or spine board (see Fig. 47.11B). The Universal Head Immobilizer is made of a Herculite nylon and a polyethylene foam platform that fastens to the stretcher with Velcro straps. The lateral pillows are then attached to the nylon platform by means of large Velcro interfaces.

It should be noted that, although sandbags are effective devices for lateral immobilization, they may cause significant movement of the neck if the board is suddenly tilted (e.g., to decrease the risk for aspiration in a vomiting patient). Therefore their use is no longer recommended. Additionally, tightly securing the head to any device without similarly securing the body has the potential to increase forces on the cervical spine during transportation and transfer. Because any manner of strapping is unlikely to completely prevent movement of the torso, the head should always be able to shift axially as a unit with the body.

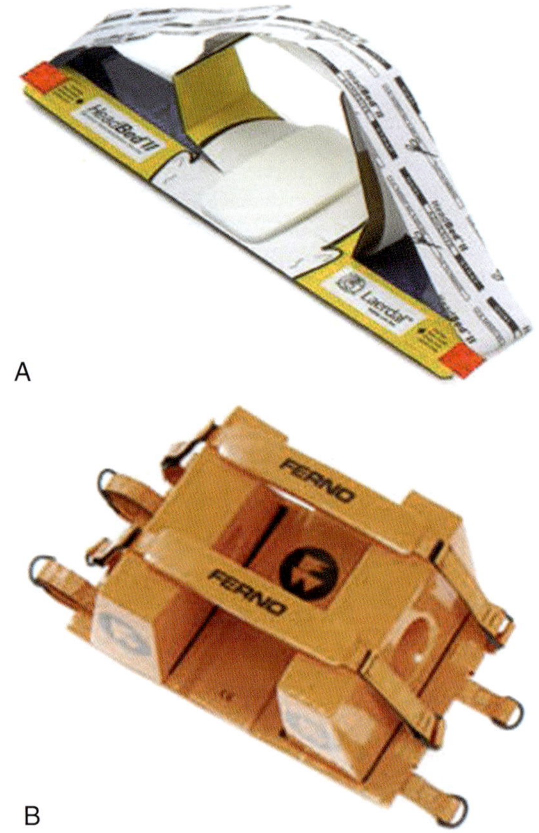

Fig. 47.11 Lateral neck stabilizers. (A) The HeadBed, a cervical immobilization device made of a water-resistant corrugated board. (B) Universal Head Immobilizer. (A, Courtesy Laerdal Medical Corporation. B, Courtesy Ferno-Washington, Inc.)

Foam Padding

Padding increases comfort and can help prevent further injury. It can also help support an injured extremity or impaled object or allow an obese or kyphotic patient to lie supine on a long backboard or stretcher (Fig. 47.12).[40] Pregnant females may benefit from padding under the right hip to help shift the gravid uterus off the inferior vena cava and increase venous return.[56] Padding applied under the neck and shoulders prevents hyperflexion in children with large occiputs (Fig. 47.13) or in individuals wearing certain types of helmets (e.g., bicycle, motorcycle, rock climbing) that cannot be removed in the field.

PROCEDURE

Cervical Spinal Motion Restriction

The priority in cervical spinal motion restriction is maintaining the head and spine in the neutral position. If patients can cooperate, instruct them to keep their head and neck in the neutral position and remain still. Next, place both hands on the sides of the patient's head to manually stabilize the cervical spine and minimize flexion, rotation, or bending. Be sure to

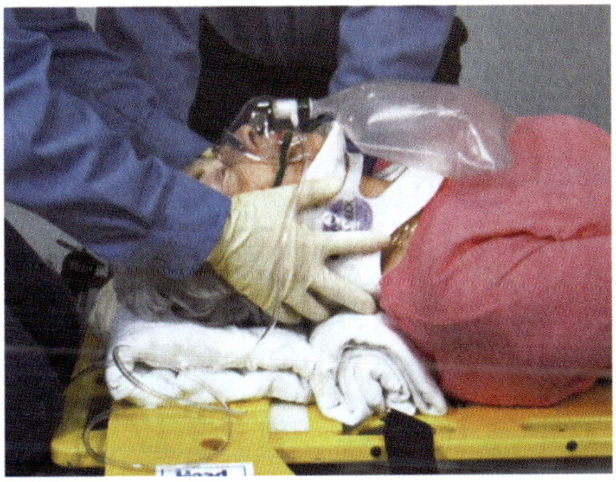

Fig. 47.12 Padding increases comfort and theoretically may prevent further injury. It can also help support an injured extremity or impaled object or allow an obese or kyphotic patient to lie supine on a long backboard.

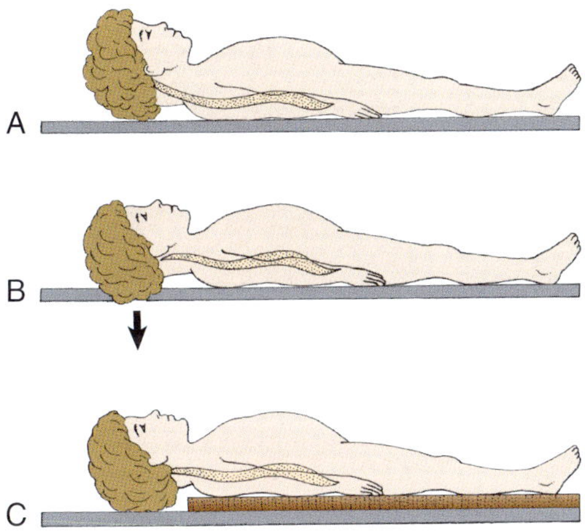

Fig. 47.13 (A) Young child immobilized on a standard backboard. Note how the large head forces the neck into flexion. Backboards can be modified by an occiput cutout (B) or a double mattress pad (C) to raise the chest, the actual clinical consequences of which are unknown. (Adapted from Herzenberg JE, Hensinger RN, Dedrick DK et al. Emergency transport and positioning of young children who have an injury of the cervical spine. *J Bone Joint Surg Am.* 1989;71:15.)

avoid cervical traction as it can theoretically increase the risk for SCI. The preferred mechanism of manual in-line stabilization is to position yourself at the patient's head, placing both hands on either side of the patient's neck, thumbs on the jaw and fingers extending down toward the shoulder area. Once the cervical spine has been manually stabilized, examine the neck for swelling, ecchymosis, deformity, bony tenderness, or penetrating wounds. Application of a c-collar follows and is generally a straightforward procedure (Fig. 47.14). The rescuer's intentions should be thoroughly explained to the patient throughout the procedure.

Once the collar is in place, caution conscious patients against movement of the head. Investigate any persistent complaints of pain or dyspnea by removal and possible replacement of the collar while manual stabilization is maintained. The size of the collar should be determined from the manufacturer's suggested guidelines. For example, the Stifneck collar (Laerdal Medical Corporation) is available in various sizes and uses the distance from the top of the shoulder to the chin to determine the appropriate size. Use the tallest collar that does not cause hyperextension. For extremely short necks, a special c-collar such as the No-Neck (Laerdal Medical Corporation) is recommended. In cases in which a c-collar of the proper size is not available, construct an improvised device from available materials (Fig. 47.15).

It should also be remembered that application of a c-collar should not be attempted until the patient's head has been brought into a neutral position and manual in-line stabilization has been applied.[39] If the patient experiences cervical muscle spasm, increased pain, neurologic complaints (e.g. paresthesias, weakness), or airway compromise, immediately halt any further movement of the head and neck. In these situations, immobilize the head and neck in the position they are found or in the position of comfort by using an alternative technique (e.g., blanket, towel roll, manual in-line stabilization).

Thoracolumbar Spinal Motion Restriction

Studies have shown that healthy individuals are able to self-extricate from a vehicle with less spinal motion than when extricated by emergency medical technicians.[57,58] Consequently, ambulatory patients or those who are able to self-extricate without undue pain should have a c-collar applied and be allowed to move themselves to an EMS cot. Backboards should be removed as soon as possible after use, and patients should not be placed unnecessarily on rigid boards during interfacility transfer (see Box 47.1).

Sitting Position

To immobilize patients who require extrication and are found in a sitting position, providers can use a short backboard or commercially available cervical extrication device (e.g., KED) or perform rapid extrication using manual in-line stabilization, a c-collar, and a long spine board. At least two rescuers should be present to apply an extrication splint to a sitting patient. Open the device butterfly style and gently slide it behind the victim via a rocking motion (Fig. 47.16, *step 1*). If necessary, carefully rock the patient forward a few degrees to facilitate placement of the splint. Once behind the victim, free the splint's pelvic support straps from their retainers and allow them to dangle at the patient's sides. Next, bring the lateral thoracic panels around the chest just beneath the patient's shoulders. Grasp these panels and slide the splint upward until the top edges of the panels firmly engage the patient's axillae. Now use the thoracic straps to secure the splint, beginning with the middle strap, then the bottom strap, and finally the top strap (see Fig. 47.16, *step 2*). The straps should be snug, but not so tight that they interfere with respiration.

Fasten the pelvic support straps next. They can be slipped one at a time beneath the patient's lower extremities and brought directly beneath the pelvis with a back-and-forth motion. If the pelvic straps are not applied properly, considerable slippage may occur when the patient is lifted. Connect the free end of each pelvic strap to buckles located at the patient's hip on the outside of the splint. Once a strap is ready to be buckled, it can be either attached to the buckle on its own side or moved across the patient's lap and engaged with the opposite buckle. Many prehospital care providers prefer the latter method because it allows the patient's knees to remain together without discomfort. It is also a good idea to pad the

Cervical Collar Application

A Posterior-First Method

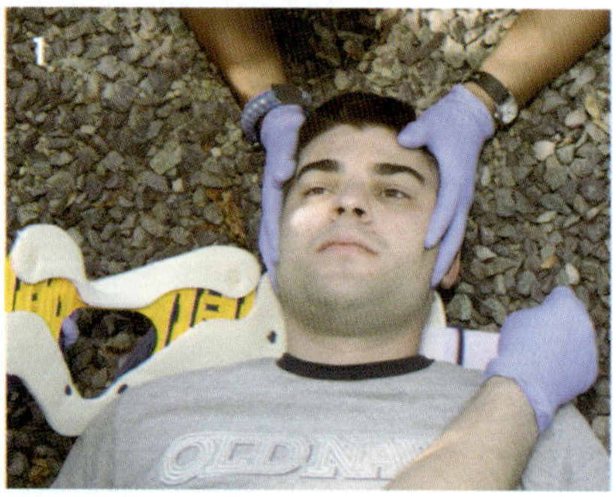

While one provider applies in-line stabilization (*not* traction!), slide the posterior portion of the collar behind the patient's neck. Maintain in-line stabilization in the neutral position until the patient is fully immobilized.

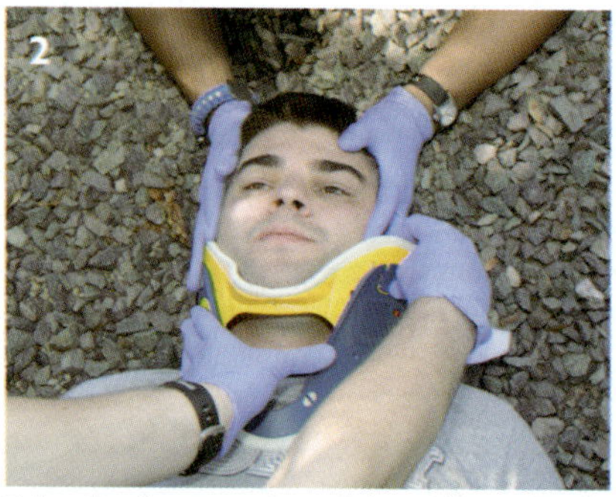

Bring the front portion of the collar around, under the patient's chin. Ensure that the chin is well supported by the chin piece. Difficulty positioning the chin piece may indicate the need for a shorter collar.

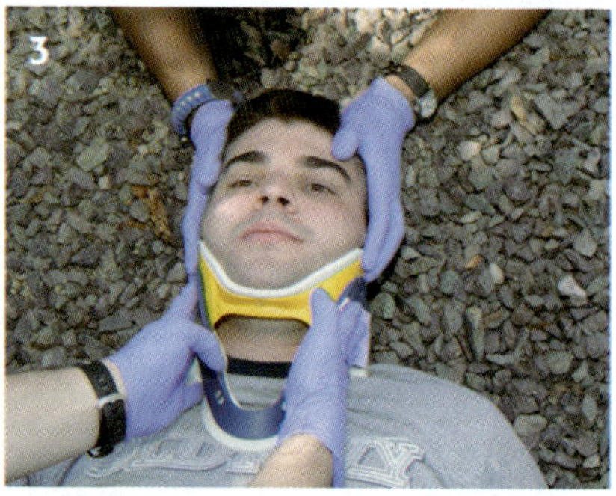

Attach the loop Velcro from the posterior portion of the collar to the hook Velcro on the anterior portion. Recheck the position of the patient's head for proper alignment. Tighten the collar as needed until proper support is obtained.

B Anterior-First Method

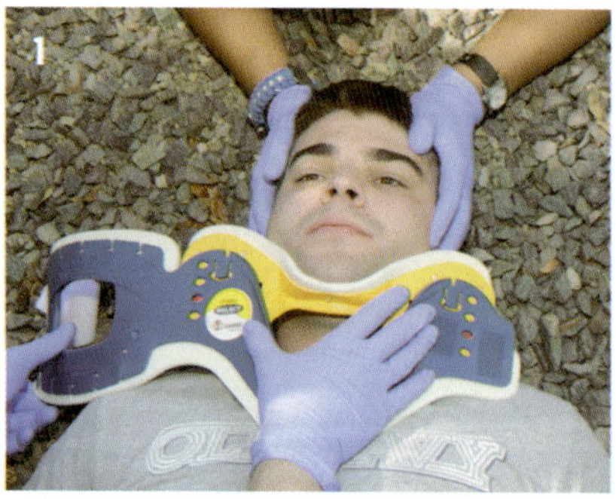

While in-line stabilization is provided, position the chin piece under the patient's chin.

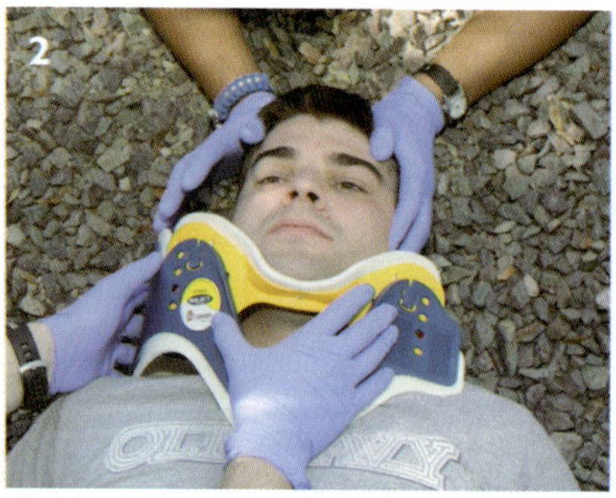

Slide the posterior portion of the collar behind the patient's neck.

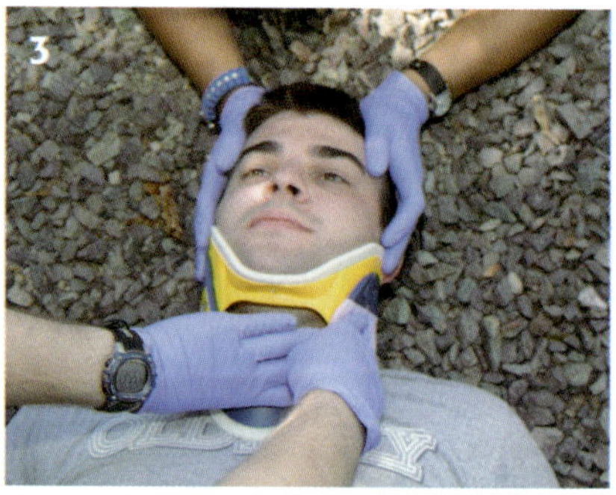

Secure the collar and assess proper placement as described above.

Fig. 47.14 Cervical collar application.

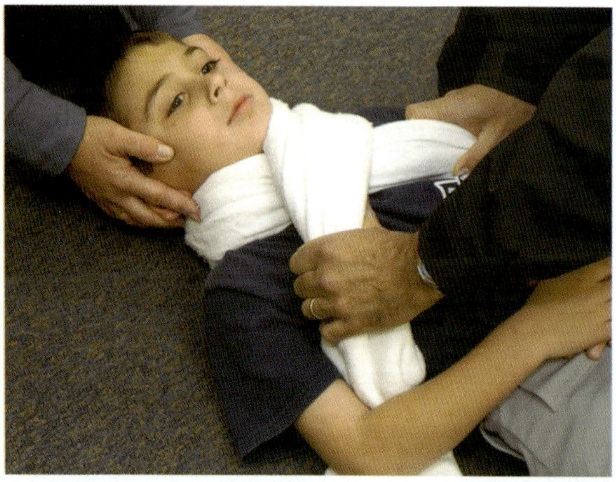

Fig. 47.15 Horse collar. Most extrication collars are available in three to five factory sizes. If a collar is not sized properly to fit a particular patient, it performs no function. Patients with extremely long necks or especially short ones can be immobilized by means of a horse collar fashioned from a blanket or towel. The blanket (or towel) is rolled to the thickness desired and slid under the patient's neck while a bystander applies manual stabilization; the ends of the blanket (or towel) are then brought across the anterior aspect of the patient's chest. (Courtesy AtlantiCare Regional Medical Center, Emergency Medical Services.)

groin area when placing the pelvic support straps because these straps may cause the patient considerable discomfort.

This procedure may need to be modified for certain injuries and preexisting conditions. For example, patients with pelvic fractures may not tolerate placement of the pelvic support and bottom straps, and the gravid abdomen of a pregnant patient may prevent placement of the middle strap.

Next, secure the head to the device (see Fig. 47.16, *step 3*). When using the KED, wrap the head panels snugly around the head and neck while another rescuer applies the diagonal head straps. It may be necessary to place padding behind the head to maintain a neutral position. Use the forehead as a point of engagement for one strap and the c-collar for the other.

As a final step, tighten all buckles until the entire splint is firmly in place. The patient can now be moved. If the patient is to be lifted from a vehicle, bring the ambulance cot (with a spine board if needed to facilitate extrication) as close to the patient as possible (see Fig. 47.16, *step 4*). While one rescuer supports the patient's knees, the other rescuer uses the handholds on the splint to lift the patient. The patient should be rotated and laid in a supine position onto a backboard or cot as needed. Loosen the pelvic straps to allow the legs to be

Kendrick Extrication Device (KED)

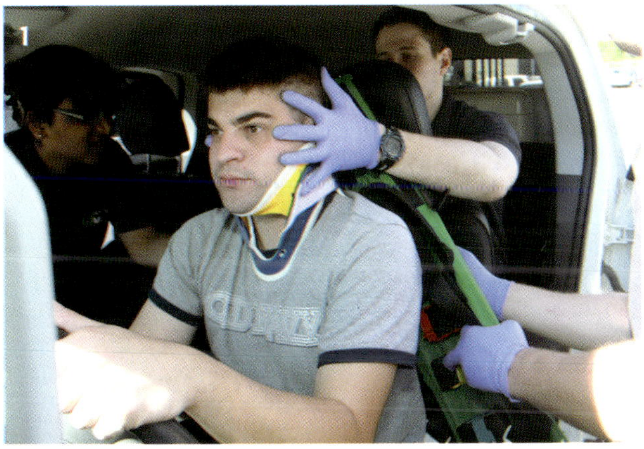

Apply a cervical collar and maintain in-line stabilization throughout the procedure. Gently slide the KED behind the patient; it may be necessary to rock the patient forward a few degrees to facilitate placement of the device.

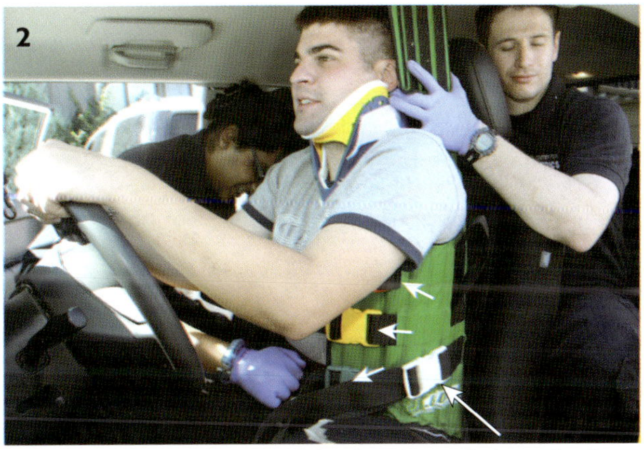

Bring the lateral panels around the chest beneath the patient's shoulders. First secure the thoracic straps *(short arrows)*, and then fasten the pelvic support straps *(long arrow)*. See text for details.

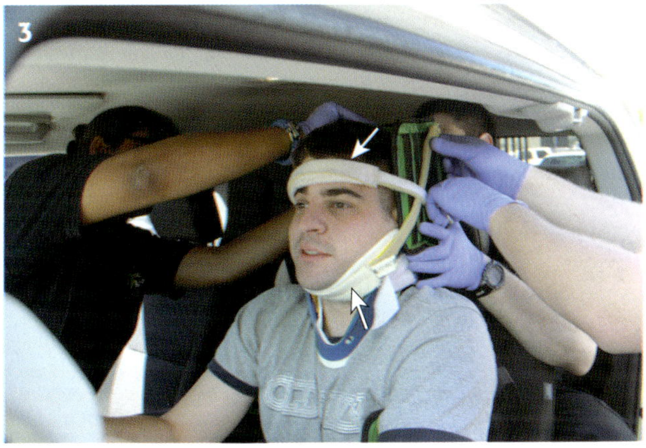

Next, secure the patient's head to the device. Wrap the head panels snugly around the head and neck while another rescuer applies the diagonal head straps *(arrows)*.

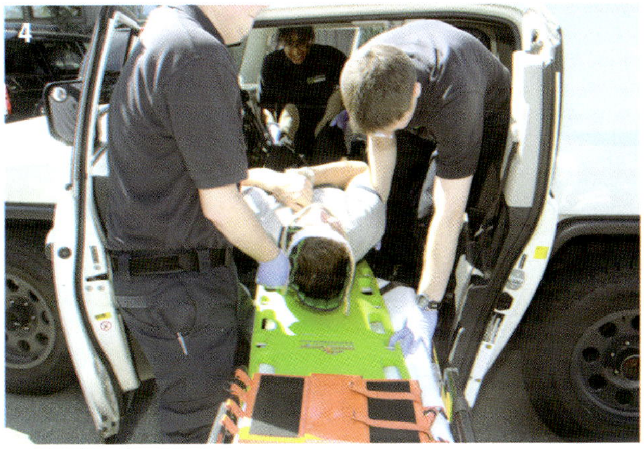

Bring the ambulance stretcher (with a backboard on it) as close to the patient as possible. Rotate the patient out of the vehicle and onto the backboard. Loosen the pelvic straps, and secure the patient to the board.

Fig. 47.16 Kendrick Extrication Device. Use of other short boards follows the same principles as depicted here.

lowered onto the backboard. The legs can then be extended and secured or left in the flexed position with a pillow placed under the knees for support.

If needed, apply a lateral immobilizer to help prevent movement of the head and neck and secure the body with straps. Once the patient is on the stretcher, the thoracic straps may need to be readjusted. The device should be removed as soon as possible, with care to avoid unnecessary movement of the spine until significant injuries are ruled out.

Recumbent Position

A patient who is found in a recumbent position should be placed in a supine position, if not already in one. If repositioning is necessary, examine the back during the process. Physical examination, spinal immobilization, airway management, and transport are easier to accomplish with the patient in the supine position.

Patients who are found supine do not require the use of a cervical extrication splint. They should, however, receive initial manual in-line cervical stabilization and a c-collar. The patient can then be secured to a full-body spinal immobilizer, such as a scoop stretcher, backboard, or full-body splint if indicated (see Box 47.1).

Scoop Stretcher

A patient who is in a supine position can be moved by means of a scoop stretcher. In a conscious patient, rescuers should explain that they are about to apply a scoop-type stretcher beneath the patient's body. Prior to beginning, apply a c-collar and maintain manual in-line cervical stabilization until the patient is completely secured to the stretcher.

Place the scoop on the ground next to the patient and open the latches that regulate its length. Adjust the length to fit the full length of the patient's body and reengage (lock) the latches. Next, release the latches at each end and separate the stretcher into two halves. Place each half next to the patient. One rescuer then gently pushes half the stretcher under one side of the patient. In some cases, it may be necessary to have another rescuer rock the patient to allow proper positioning. Repeat the procedure with the opposite half of the scoop until both halves are aligned beneath the patient. Engage the latch at the head of the device first. Then bring the lower ends together and engage the foot latch to complete the integrity of the stretcher. Strap the patient's torso into place and immobilize the head with a suitable lateral neck stabilizer. The patient can then be lifted onto another device for transport, such as a stokes basket or ambulance litter. After placement on another device (e.g., ambulance cot), the scoop stretcher can be removed without disturbing the patient's position.

Full-Body Spine Boards (Backboards)

There are several ways of placing a patient onto a spine board. The precise technique used will depend on the space available and the position of the patient within that space. Apply a c-collar or maintain manual cervical in-line stabilization throughout the procedure and avoid spinal compression or traction. For lengthwise extrication, as from an automobile seat, the patient can be slid, either feet first or head first, onto the backboard. It is important that the patient be moved as a unit during this process. Place one end of the backboard on the seat or doorsill of the automobile. One rescuer stabilizes the opposite end of the board, while at least two other rescuers lift and slide the patient's body onto the board. Once the patient is secured to the board, slide the board out of the vehicle and onto a waiting stretcher. The patient should be removed from the longboard as soon as possible using the *logroll maneuver* or a lift-and-slide technique described hereafter.

If the patient is in the recumbent position, logroll or slide the patient onto the board. The logroll maneuver requires the presence of at least three rescuers. Position one rescuer at the patient's head to apply manual in-line cervical stabilization (Fig. 47.17, *step 1*). It is this person's responsibility to oversee and direct body movement throughout the procedure. Next, position the backboard alongside the patient's body (see Fig. 47.17, *step 2*). To minimize thoracolumbar movement, extend the patient's arms at the sides with the palms resting on the lateral aspect of the thighs.[59] To keep the patient from reaching for a rescuer or object during transfer, some rescuers prefer to have patients cross their arms across the thorax. Place the backboard against the injured (more painful) side of the body so that the patient can be rolled onto the uninjured (less painful) side. Position the other rescuers on the side that the patient will be rolled toward, with one rescuer at the mid chest and the other at the legs. The rescuer at the chest should reach across the victim and take hold of the shoulder and hips while the other rescuer grasps the hips and lower part of the legs. When everyone is ready, the rescuer at the head gives the command to roll the patient onto the side (see Fig. 47.17, *step 3*). If possible, examine the patient's back at this point. Slide the backboard under the patient, and when everyone is ready, the rescuer at the head gives the command to roll the patient back onto the board (see Fig. 47.17, *step 4*). Before applying straps, it is often necessary to center the patient on the board.

To center the patient on the long spine board, support the cervical spine, shoulders, and hips and slide the patient first caudally, then cephalad, in a zigzag pattern to avoid applying uneven lateral or rotational force onto the spine. Alternatively, during lateral extraction, slide a recumbent patient sideways onto the spine board. This improvised technique also requires the presence of three or four rescuers, one of whom can maintain control of the patient's head and neck.

The lift-and-slide technique, sometimes referred to as a six-person lift or bridge lift, is a technique that may reduce the amount of motion at an unstable vertebral segment when compared with the logroll. Del Rossi and coworkers demonstrated this in cadaver studies,[60] but the difference has never been shown to be clinically relevant and the logroll remains nearly ubiquitous. One disadvantage of this technique is the inability to visually assess the spine during the lift.

To perform the lift-and-slide, rescuers line up opposite each other on both sides of the patient, ideally with at least two rescuers per side. An additional rescuer is located at the patient's head to provide in-line stabilization and coordinate the lift. When all are ready, they place hands underneath the patient in an alternating fashion and lift the patient directly upward a few inches. At this point, another rescuer inserts the carrying device (e.g., backboard, stokes basket, vacuum mattress) and the patient is lowered and secured. For heavier patients, additional rescuers may be needed. Rescuers may place their head on the shoulder of the person across from them to form an arch and reduce the strain on the lower back. In some cases, such as in environments with limited space, standing over the patient and lifting straight upward may be required.

When necessary, various techniques can be used to secure a patient to the backboard. In addition to the standard thoracic, pelvic, and lower extremity straps, use of an abdominal strap may reduce lateral motion without compromising respiration.[61] Proper strap placement and firm contact between the straps and the patient are also important in limiting lateral motion (see Fig. 47.17, *step 5*).[62] Commercial products such as Spider- Straps are also available or webbing may be used in a zigzag alternating fashion.

After the body has been strapped to the board, the head can be secured. If necessary, padding should be placed under the occiput to maintain the head in the neutral position. Apply a lateral neck stabilizer (e.g., foam blocks, HeadBed device [Laerdal Medical Corp.]) and secure the head in place with tape or straps (see Fig. 47.17, *step 6*). Most taping techniques involve the use of one piece across the forehead and one piece across the c-collar. Remember, taping across the neck may make airway management difficult. Placing straps across the head and neck may cause hyperextension or axial stretching of the neck. For this reason, omitting the lower strap is recommended. The head should only be secured as tightly as necessary to minimize motion; it should be able to easily slide axially if the torso shifts during transportation. Thus if the body is not secured to the board, the head should similarly not be fastened to the board.

Standing Position

Traditionally, standing patients were placed on a backboard by positioning the board behind the patient, stabilizing the head, and lowering the patient and the backboard backward until the patient was lying on it. However, there is no evidence that this protects the spine from further injury. Current recommendations are to apply a c-collar and allow ambulatory patients to walk to the stretcher and assist them into supine position on the mattress.[22] Nevertheless, there may still be a role for using a backboard or other rigid device placed behind the patient when a stretcher is not available (as in a wilderness or technical rescue environment) and the patient is unable to comfortably lower themselves to a ground-level extrication device, such as a longboard or scoop stretcher. In this case, the device should be placed behind the patient while at

Full-Body Spine Board (Backboard): Logroll Maneuver

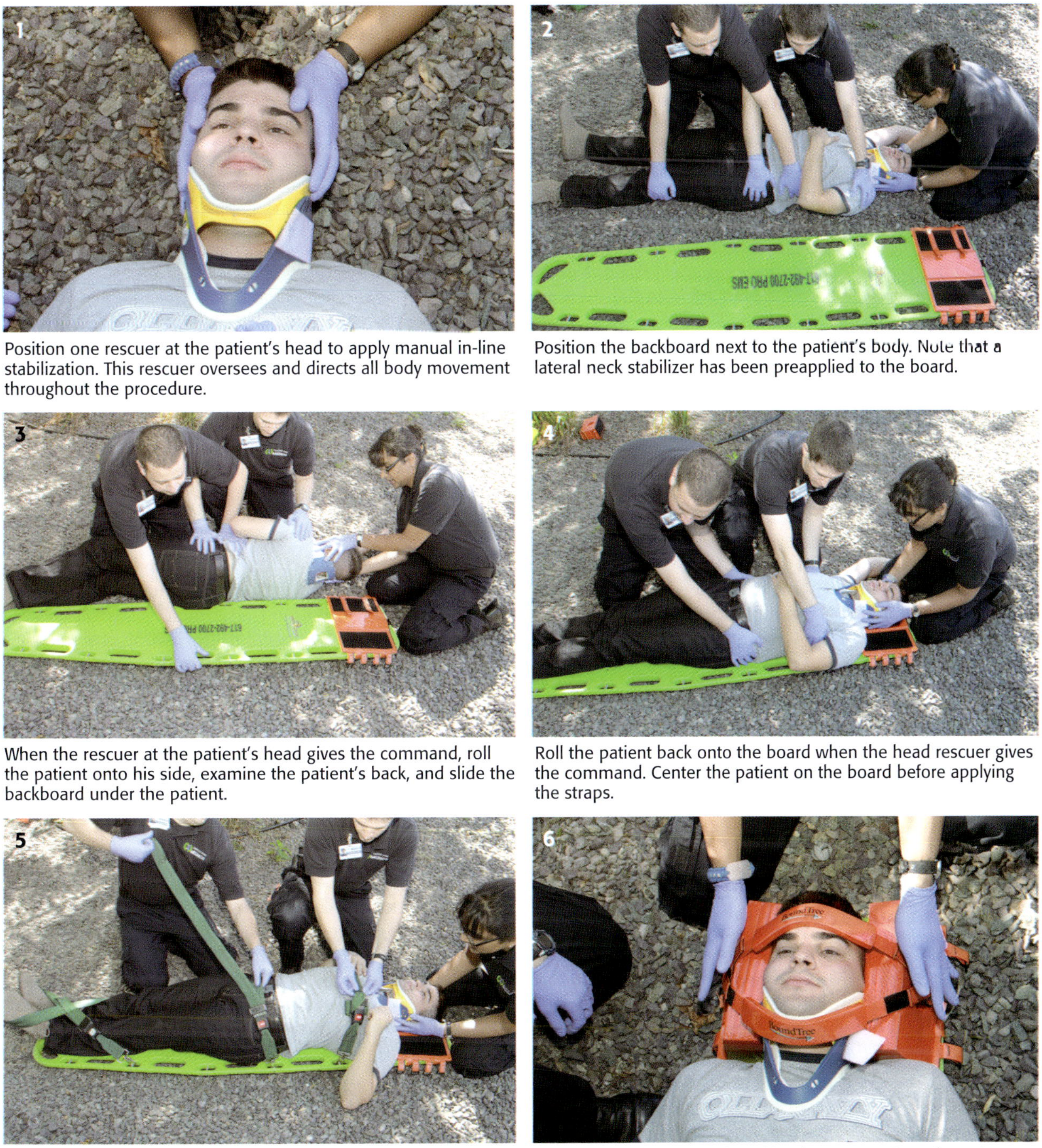

1. Position one rescuer at the patient's head to apply manual in-line stabilization. This rescuer oversees and directs all body movement throughout the procedure.

2. Position the backboard next to the patient's body. Note that a lateral neck stabilizer has been preapplied to the board.

3. When the rescuer at the patient's head gives the command, roll the patient onto his side, examine the patient's back, and slide the backboard under the patient.

4. Roll the patient back onto the board when the head rescuer gives the command. Center the patient on the board before applying the straps.

5. Strap the patient to the board. Proper strap placement (chest, pelvis, and legs) and firm contact between the straps and the patient are important in limiting lateral motion.

6. Apply a lateral neck stabilizer, like the Ferno Universal Head Immobilizer shown above. Secure it in place using the supplied straps or tape.

Fig. 47.17 Full-body spine board (backboard): the logroll maneuver.

least one rescuer on each side (more may be needed for large patients) grasps the handles underneath the patient's arms and slowly tips the patient and board backward until the board is completely on the ground. There is no need to provide manual head stabilization during this maneuver, but the patient should be reminded to keep his head still.

PEDIATRIC PATIENTS

Little information is available on the proper selection and application of spinal immobilization devices for children. Most of the data available were derived from studies of adults and might not be fully applicable to children, especially those under 8 years of age. Half the total growth in head circumference is achieved by the age of 18 months, giving children a disproportionately large head in comparison to the rest of the body. Before 8 years of age, these anatomic and developmental differences result in a higher incidence of upper cervical spine injuries (C1–C2). Because injuries in this area are frequently unstable, proper cervical immobilization in the neutral position is critically important.

Age alone should not be the primary factor in deciding when to employ spinal motion restriction. Current data suggest that spinal motion restriction should be considered for children and adolescents involved in trauma who complain of neck pain, exhibit torticollis or a neurologic deficit, are altered (including GCS < 15, signs of intoxication, agitation, somnolence), or are involved in a high mechanism accident.[22]

In the neutral position, the pediatric cervical spine is normally lordotic or extended.[63] However, because the occiput is large, positioning the child's body on a standard backboard may force the neck into flexion or a relative kyphosis. The clinical significance of this is currently unclear, but theoretically it may be hazardous for young children. Therefore the standard backboard should be modified to adapt to the child's larger head size. As a rough guide, the external auditory meatus should be on the same level as the midpoint of the shoulder. Suggested modifications include a cutout in the backboard that accommodates the occiput or a pad under the back at the level of the chest (see Fig. 47.13). If not modified, the standard backboard in conjunction with the disproportionately large head of a child may force the neck into hyperflexion and potentially aggravate an underlying cervical spine injury. Nypaver and Treloar[64] showed that all children required elevation of the back (mean height, 25.4 ± 6.7 mm) for correct neutral position on a spine board. Children younger than 4 years required greater elevation than did those 4 years or older. It must be pointed out, however, that there have been no published reports of an SCI resulting from the use of standard immobilization techniques and equipment in children.[64]

COMPLICATIONS

Cervical Immobilization

Improper application of a c-collar can occur if the wrong size is used, or too little care is exercised during placement. The best means of preventing either error is strong clinician involvement in training and continuing education of EMS crews together with vigorous feedback regarding correct and incorrect application. In addition, adherence to the manufacturer's collar-specific recommendations for size and application should be emphasized.

A collar that is too small for a patient may be either too tight for the girth of the neck or too short to provide adequate immobilization. Too large a collar commonly results in hyperextension and possibly neck distraction, which can exacerbate a preexisting spinal injury. Underlying spinal abnormalities from conditions such as ankylosing spondylitis, rheumatoid arthritis, or kyphosis can also contribute to exacerbation of injuries with c-collar application.[33]

Given the higher head size to body ratio in young children, it may be necessary to provide additional padding under the shoulders to minimize excessive cervical spine flexion.

Improper or prolonged application of an extrication collar may impede venous return and raise ICP.[65] Although the clinical significance of increased ICP produced by cervical immobilization is still unknown, two studies have confirmed that application of a rigid c-collar causes a statistically significant and sustained rise in ICP.[66,67] Kolb and colleagues[66] reported a 24.8-cm H_2O increase in cerebrospinal fluid pressure in 20 adult patients undergoing lumbar puncture. Hunt and associates[67] reported a 4.6-mm Hg mean rise in ICP in 30 patients with severe traumatic brain injury. The largest rise in ICP was noted in patients with a baseline ICP higher than 15 mm Hg. The authors of these studies concluded that the elevation in ICP produced by cervical immobilization might have deleterious effects in patients with acute or sustained intracranial hypertension.[66,67]

Long-term use of the Philadelphia extrication collar (Philadelphia Cervical Collar Co.) as part of the treatment plan for an underlying cervical spine injury has been associated with pressure ulcers.[68] Because some collars (e.g., Philadelphia and Stifneck [Laerdal Medical Corporation]) have been shown to exert higher capillary closing pressure at contact points, it is suggested that only collars with favorable skin pressure patterns and superior patient comfort (e.g., Nec-Loc, Jerome Medical) be used for long-term application.

One final complication should be mentioned. A patient who, for whatever reason, actively resists placement of a c-collar or other splint should not be forced to wear it (see Fig. 47.3). Postictal and intoxicated patients may present such a dilemma. Immobilization of a combative patient cannot be accomplished without considerable muscular exertion, not only by rescuers, but also by the patient. If fractures do exist, it is possible that struggling and using muscles attached to these fractured fragments may cause further injury. If the patient permits manual stabilization, this should be used as an alternative. Sedation should be used judiciously to enhance compliance, and administration of sedatives should be accompanied by appropriate vital sign monitoring.

THORACOLUMBAR IMMOBILIZATION

In general, complications are more likely to occur from failure to immobilize spinal injuries rather than from the process of immobilization itself. When complications do arise, they may be related to improper choice or use of equipment or prolonged immobilization.

Patients are generally strapped in place on a spine board to prevent sliding during transport. If too few straps are used or if the straps are loosely applied, motion during transport can occur. Even when applied correctly, spinal immobilization on a hard board may be extremely uncomfortable for patients and may induce pressure-related tissue damage. In one study, 100% of healthy volunteers reported significant pain after only 30 minutes on a long spine board.[8] Occipital headaches, as well as mandibular, lumbar, and sacral pain, developed in these individuals. Other studies have demonstrated elevated tissue interface pressure in patients on spine boards without air mattress padding.[9,69,70] These studies underscore the need to use adequate padding when patients require immobilization on a longboard, as well as removal from the board as soon as possible.

Excessive strapping can interfere with respiratory function in both children[71] and adults.[51,72,73] In healthy children 6 to 15 years old, forced vital capacity (FVC) has been shown to decrease from 4% to 59% during spinal immobilization.[71] Totten and Sugarman[51] evaluated the effect of two spinal immobilization methods (wooden backboard and vacuum mattress) on eight respiratory function measurements in healthy volunteers. In comparing baselines for each method, six of the eight measures (FVC, FVC%, forced expiratory volume in 1 second [FEV1], FEV1%, peak expiratory flow [PEF], and forced expiratory flow [FEF25-75%]) were reduced by an average of 15%. Although this may not be a problem in healthy volunteers, the effects on patients with chest trauma or preexisting respiratory disease may be significant.[52]

Patients immobilized on a backboard are also at risk for aspiration if they vomit. If vomiting does occur, logroll the patient and board as a unit and suction the airway as needed. Although this procedure may be associated with some spinal movement, airway protection takes priority.

CONCLUSION

Although spinal immobilization has not been shown to decrease the likelihood of spinal injury and is associated with a variety of complications, prehospital spinal immobilization remains commonplace. Nevertheless, recent evidence supports a widespread shift to selective spinal motion restriction by prehospital providers. Until these new recommendations become universal, emergency medicine practitioners should know when spinal motion restriction is indicated, recognize properly and improperly applied devices, minimize unnecessary immobilization time, and work with prehospital providers to ensure appropriate indications and proper use.

EXTREMITY IMMOBILIZATION

Upper Extremity

Background

The earliest evidence of upper extremity splinting comes from the Egyptians circa 300 BCE. In 1903 archaeologists from the Hearst expedition discovered two specimens whose open fractures had been treated with wooden splints and bandages. Their bones showed no signs of healing, so the individuals probably died soon after their injuries; however, numerous other ancient Egyptian specimens have demonstrated evidence of well-healed forearm fractures.[74]

The purpose of splinting is to prevent motion of broken or dislocated bone ends. Carefully applied splints decrease pain while minimizing further damage to muscles, nerves, and blood vessels. Splinting also reduces the risk of converting a closed injury to an open one.[75] Nevertheless, injuries to adjacent structures may still occur, so circulation, motor function, and sensation distal to the injury must be carefully assessed both before and after splint placement and monitored closely during transport.

Over the last three decades, prehospital splinting materials, equipment, and techniques have evolved considerably. Today's prehospital providers can choose from a wide assortment of ready-to-use splints made from a variety of sturdy lightweight materials.

INDICATIONS AND CONTRAINDICATIONS

Indications for splinting an extremity are usually clear. Pain after trauma, with or without deformity, should arouse suspicion of underlying bone or joint injury. Other signs include swelling, discoloration, deformity, crepitus, and loss of neurovascular function. However, absence of these findings does not rule out an underlying fracture or dislocation. Thus in most cases where a musculoskeletal injury is suspected, a splint should be applied and maintained.

There are no absolute contraindications to splinting suspected extremity fractures or dislocations. However, in the setting of multisystem trauma with life-threatening injuries, rapid transport may be more important than extremity splinting. Averting loss of life takes precedence over loss of limb.

Equipment

Various types of splints are currently available for immobilizing upper extremity injuries. Emergency care providers should be well trained and familiar with their equipment. The type of splint used is less important than the expertise of the provider. Upper extremity splints can be divided into two basic types: rigid and soft.[76] Table 47.1 provides splint recommendations for a variety of upper extremity injuries.

Rigid Splints

Rigid and semirigid splints are the mainstays of EMS fracture care (Fig. 47.18A–C). These splints are made of many different materials, including cardboard, plastic, aluminum, wire, and wood. They are fastened to the injured extremity with tape, gauze, cravats, or Velcro straps. Rigid splints are generally nonflexible (some commercially available splints may have some flexibility in their design) and, when applied properly, immobilize the limb in a rigid fashion to maintain stability. Although most commercial rigid splints are prepadded, many will still benefit from additional soft padding to cushion the splint and increase comfort. This is particularly true over bony prominences. When applying rigid splints, leave the fingertips exposed so that the distal circulation can be continuously monitored.

Cardboard splints are excellent for long-bone fractures in the upper part of the arm. They can be formed into many

TABLE 47.1 Management of Specific Upper Extremity Orthopedic Injuries

SITE	SUGGESTED IMMOBILIZATION TECHNIQUES
Clavicle	Sling and swath
Shoulder	Sling and swath as it lies
Humerus	Cardboard or vacuum splint with a sling and swath
Elbow	Cardboard or vacuum splint as it lies, realign if circulation deficit exists
Forearm	Cardboard, malleable metal, air, or vacuum splint with a sling and swath
Wrist	Pillow, cardboard, malleable metal, or vacuum splint applied in the position found
Hand	Pillow, cardboard, or malleable metal splint in the position of function
Finger	Tongue depressor or small malleable metal splint

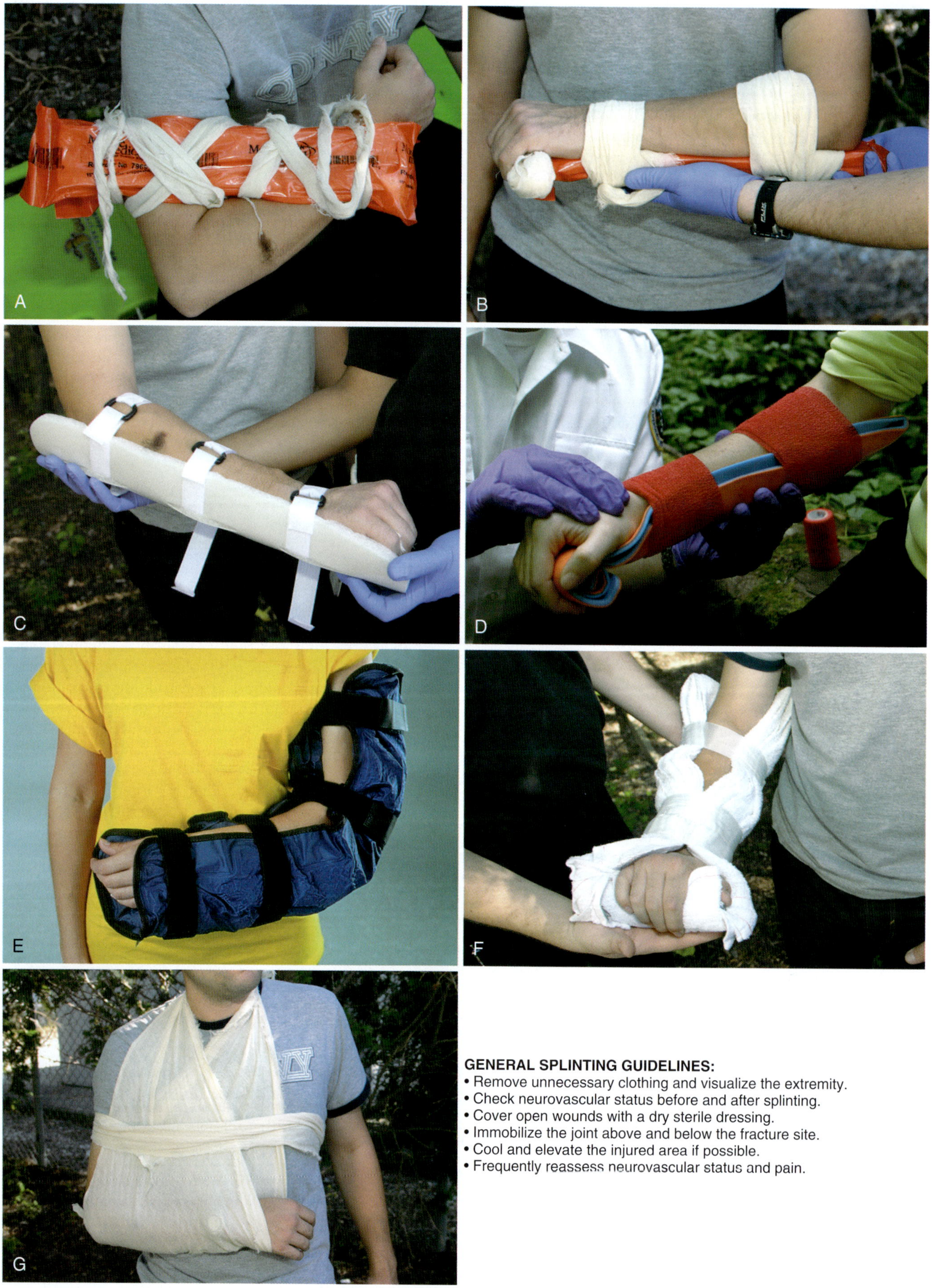

Fig. 47.18 Upper extremity splints. (A–C) Padded rigid splints. (D) SAM Splint. (E) EVAC-U-SPLINT vacuum splint. (F) Soft towel splint (a pillow can be used in a similar manner). (G) Sling and swath. (D, Courtesy SAM Medical Products. E, Courtesy Hartwell Medical.)

shapes and are easy to apply, inexpensive, lightweight, radiolucent, and compatible with magnetic resonance imaging. Splints made from wax-impregnated cardboard are also water resistant. Plastic, aluminum, wire, and wood splints, though less malleable, are also appropriate choices. An inexpensive aluminum splint that is popular with emergency care providers and is found in many wilderness medical kits is the SAM Splint (Sam Medical Products) (see Fig. 47.18D). The SAM Splint is built from a thin core of soft aluminum alloy sandwiched between two layers of closed-cell foam. The SAM Splint is extremely pliable. Bent into any of three simple curves, it is extremely strong and provides support for any fractured or injured extremity. In addition, it is water resistant, lightweight, radiolucent, reusable, and not affected by extreme temperatures or altitudes. These characteristics make it an ideal tool for emergency care providers and outdoor enthusiasts.

Vacuum splints (see Fig. 47.18E) are a special type of rigid splint in which the air is evacuated from a closed bag containing tiny foam beads. Flexibility of the splint before removal of the air allows molding of the splint to conform to the patient's position. Removal of the air compresses the contents into a solid mass and results in a rigid splint that encases the extremity, immobilizing it in the position it was found. As a result, vacuum splints in general are more comfortable than other rigid splints. Vacuum splints are radiolucent and do not apply external pressure, thus ensuring maximum circulation to the injured extremity.

Soft Splints

Soft splints include air splints, pillows, slings, and swaths. Depending on the type of injury being treated, immobilization with pillows, slings, or swaths alone may be inadequate because they allow significant motion. Therefore when treating fractures and dislocations, these splints are most effective when used in conjunction with some form of a rigid device. However, even when used alone, pillows, slings, or swaths provide cushioning and some limitation of motion that may be adequate for less severe injuries such as sprains and contusions.

Air splints are soft splints that become rigid when inflated. Besides providing immobilization, they help compress the underlying soft tissue, reducing local hemorrhage. These devices are sensitive to differences in atmospheric pressure and temperature. Therefore their inflation must be closely monitored to ensure that the underlying tissue is not subjected to pressure-induced ischemia and the development of a compartment syndrome. One study suggested a maximum splint pressure of 15 mm Hg to reduce the risk for ischemia.[77] During long ambulance transport times, deflate the splint for 5 minutes every 1.5 hours.

Disadvantages of most air splints include an inability to continuously monitor pulses and susceptibility to puncture. Air splints are designed to conform to a specific shape when inflated and should not be used on angulated fractures. In addition to being radiolucent, some types can be inflated with a refrigerant to provide concurrent cooling.

Pillow splints (see Fig. 47.18F) can be fashioned from any soft bulky material and are excellent choices for hand or wrist injuries. These splints are extremely comfortable and are easily applied.

Slings and swaths are generally used in combination with a rigid or a soft splint. When used alone they can effectively immobilize injuries to the shoulder, clavicle, and humerus (see Fig. 47.18G).

Procedure

Utilize the following guidelines to properly apply a splint to an injured extremity. First, communicate with patients to ensure that they understand what is being done, and when possible, administer an appropriate analgesic to minimize discomfort prior to splint placement. Remove any unnecessary clothing to adequately visualize the injured extremity. Stabilize the fracture site manually to limit unnecessary movement and prevent further injury. Check the patient's neurovascular status (i.e., pulse, motor function, and sensation) before and after the application of a splint. For a severely angulated extremity with neurovascular compromise, reduce the deformity with gentle longitudinal traction (not exceeding 10 lbs. of pressure) before splinting. Make only one attempt at fracture reduction. If resistance or pain is encountered, splint the extremity in the position found. Cover open wounds with a dry sterile dressing before applying the splint. When possible, immobilize the joint above and below a suspected fracture site. Once the splint has been applied, cool and elevate the injured area to help reduce swelling and pain. Assess distal neurovascular status frequently. Any deterioration requires immediate evaluation of the splint to determine whether excessive pressure is being applied. In addition, continue to assess and treat pain.

Rigid Splints

To apply a rigid splint, have an assistant provide support and gentle traction above and below the injury. Apply the splint on the side of the extremity away from any open wounds. The splint should be large enough to immobilize the joint above and below a suspected fracture or the bone above and below a dislocation and should be well padded to reduce the risk for pressure necrosis. Secure the splint to the extremity with gauze, tape, cravats, or Velcro straps (see Fig. 47.18A and C).

Apply vacuum splints in much the same manner as other rigid splints. While an assistant stabilizes the injured site and applies traction, wrap the splint around the extremity and secure it in place with the attached straps. Evacuate the air from the splint with a hand pump until the splint becomes rigid.

Soft Splints

The application procedure for an air splint depends on whether the splint is equipped with a zipper. If the splint does not have a zipper, first place the splint over the rescuer's arm until the bottom edge lies above the wrist. Use this hand to grasp the hand of the patient's injured extremity and use the free hand to provide support and gentle traction above the injury (Fig. 47.19A). An assistant then slides the splint onto the patient's arm (see Fig. 47.19B). Smooth out any wrinkles and inflate the splint until finger pressure makes a slight indentation (see Fig. 47.19C). Open a zippered air splint and place it around the injured area. Close the zipper and inflate the splint as described previously. With air splints that completely enclose the hand, continuously assess the distal circulation by checking fingertip color, temperature, and capillary refill.

Apply pillow splints by encasing the injury in the pillow and securing it with tape, cravats, or gauze (see Fig. 47.18F). If possible, keep the nail beds exposed to allow frequent neurovascular checks.

Air Splint Application

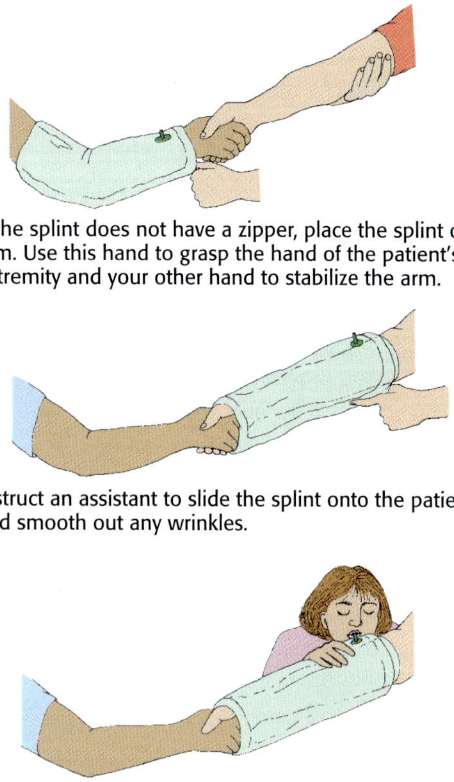

A

If the splint does not have a zipper, place the splint over your arm. Use this hand to grasp the hand of the patient's injured extremity and your other hand to stabilize the arm.

B

Instruct an assistant to slide the splint onto the patient's arm, and smooth out any wrinkles.

C

Inflate the splint until finger pressure makes a slight dent. Continuously assess the distal circulation while the splint is inflated.

Fig. 47.19 Air splint application.

To apply a sling, have an assistant support the injured arm in a flexed position across the patient's chest (Fig. 47.20). Place the long edge of the triangular bandage lengthwise along the patient's side opposite the injury with its tip over the uninjured shoulder. Bring the other tip over the injured shoulder to enclose the arm in the sling. Adjust the sling so that the arm rests comfortably with the hand higher than the elbow. Tie the ends of the sling together at the side of the neck and pad the knot for comfort. Finally, wrap the point of the sling at the elbow around the front of the forearm and pin. With the sling properly applied, rest the patient's arm comfortably against the chest with the fingertips exposed.

To apply a swath, place a cravat of sufficient length under the uninjured arm and over the injured arm at the level of the mid humerus. Tie the ends circumferentially around the thorax so that the injured extremity is secured snugly to the chest (see Fig. 47.18G). In adults, two cravats may have to be tied together in an end-to-end fashion to produce a swath of sufficient length.

COMPLICATIONS

Potential complications of upper extremity splinting include pressure necrosis, conversion of a closed injury to an open one, and loss of neurovascular function. With the use of air splints there is the additional risk of pressure-induced tissue ischemia and compartment syndrome.[77]

CONCLUSION

Injuries to the upper extremities, though not life-threatening, may be limb-threatening and can have significant immediate or long-term effects. Maintain a high index of suspicion for underlying neurovascular injury; check neurovascular status before and after applying a splint and frequently during transport. Administration of appropriate analgesia will minimize patient discomfort.

LOWER EXTREMITY

Background

Injuries to the lower extremities, including sprains, fractures, and dislocations, are also commonly encountered by prehospital care providers. Inability to ambulate and bystander inability to safely lift a patient often prompts use of 9-1-1 for ED access. As with upper extremity injuries, application of a splint is an essential part of the prehospital management of lower extremity injuries (Fig. 47.21). Many of the principles, techniques, products, and complications discussed for upper extremity splinting also apply to injuries to the lower extremity; the SAM Splint (see Fig. 47.18D) and pillow splint (see Fig. 47.18F) are just two examples. Table 47.2 provides recommendations for immobilizing a variety of lower extremity injuries. One fundamental difference between splinting upper and lower extremity injuries is the use of a traction splint in the management of femoral fractures. The remainder of this section focuses on the use of traction splints.

The use of traction and countertraction for alignment and reduction of fractures dates from the time of Hippocrates.[78] In the late 1800s Sir Hugh Owen Thomas developed the first full-ring traction splint for the definitive management of fractured femurs.[74,78] However, because the Thomas full-ring splint was difficult to apply on the battlefield, it was later modified by his nephew, Sir Robert Jones, and other surgeons to a half-ring design, which made it easier to apply in a combat setting. During World War I, the modified splint was credited with reducing the mortality rate associated with fractured femurs from 80% to 15%.[79] Since then, several additional modifications that carry the name of their inventors (e.g., Glenn Hare, Joseph Sager, Allen Klippel) have furthered the development of lower extremity traction splints. Today, traction splints are a nearly universal piece of equipment found on most ambulances, and their application is an integral part of the prehospital care provider's skill set. The main purpose of the traction splint is to immobilize a fractured femur.[79,80]

In the setting of a fractured femur, muscle spasm and overlap of fragments may cause the thigh to lose its cylindrical shape and adopt a more spherical appearance (Fig. 47.22).[80] The resultant decreased tissue pressure and increased volume may allow 1 to 2 L of blood to accumulate at the fracture site.

Traction splints are designed to align fracture segments and restore the cylindrical shape of the thigh (Fig. 47.23). This in turn increases tissue pressure, decreases the potential space for blood loss, and inhibits further hemorrhage. In addition, traction splints help reduce pain, prevent further damage to neurovascular structures, and reduce the incidence of fat embolism.[79,80]

Sling Application

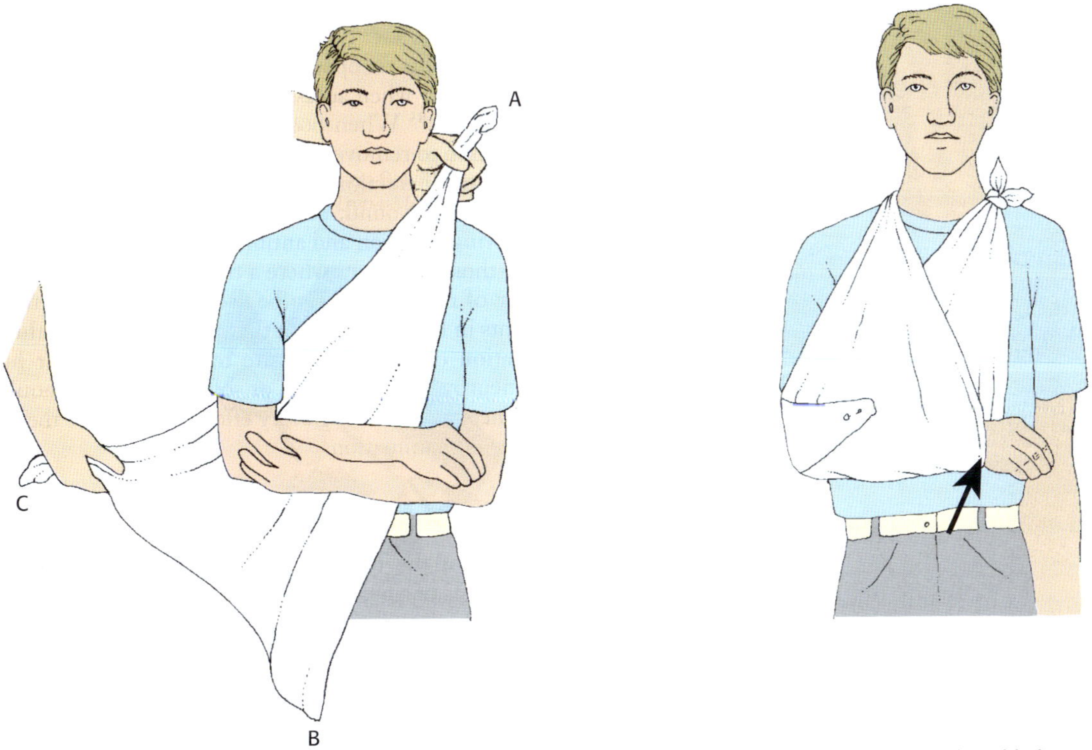

First, place tip *A* over the uninjured shoulder. Next, bring tip *B* over the injured shoulder to enclose the arm. Then, draw tip *C* around the front and secure with a pin.

The completed sling. A swath may be added to provide further immobilization (see Fig. 46.18*G*).

Fig. 47.20 Sling application. Note that the wrist is supported by the sling *(arrow)* as the tendency is to flex the wrist with any upper extremity injury.

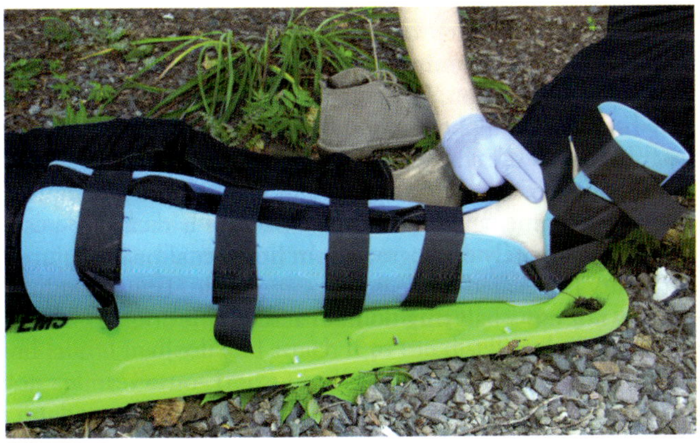

Fig. 47.21 Prefabricated padded leg splint. Similar to the arm splints described earlier, many prefabricated leg splints are commercially available. Their application and use mirror the general principles of splinting described in Fig. 46.18.

TABLE 47.2 Management of Specific Lower Extremity Orthopedic Injuries

SITE	SUGGESTED IMMOBILIZATION TECHNIQUES
Hip	Secure the injured leg to the uninjured leg, ideally padded between, and/or with a long external splint secured proximally and distally Full-body immobilization (backboard, Reeves flexible stretcher, scoop stretcher, vacuum mattress, etc.), with the limb padded and secured
Midshaft femur	Traction splint, contralateral leg stabilization, or rigid splint
Knee	Cardboard or vacuum splint in the position found
Tibia/fibula	Cardboard, air, or vacuum splint
Ankle	Pillow, cardboard, or air splint
Foot	Pillow or air splint
Toe	Tape to the adjacent toe

INDICATIONS

Application of a lower extremity traction splint is indicated whenever an isolated midshaft femur fracture is suspected.[76,81,82] Clinical signs of a fractured femur include thigh pain associated with limb shortening, angulation, crepitus, swelling, or ecchymosis.

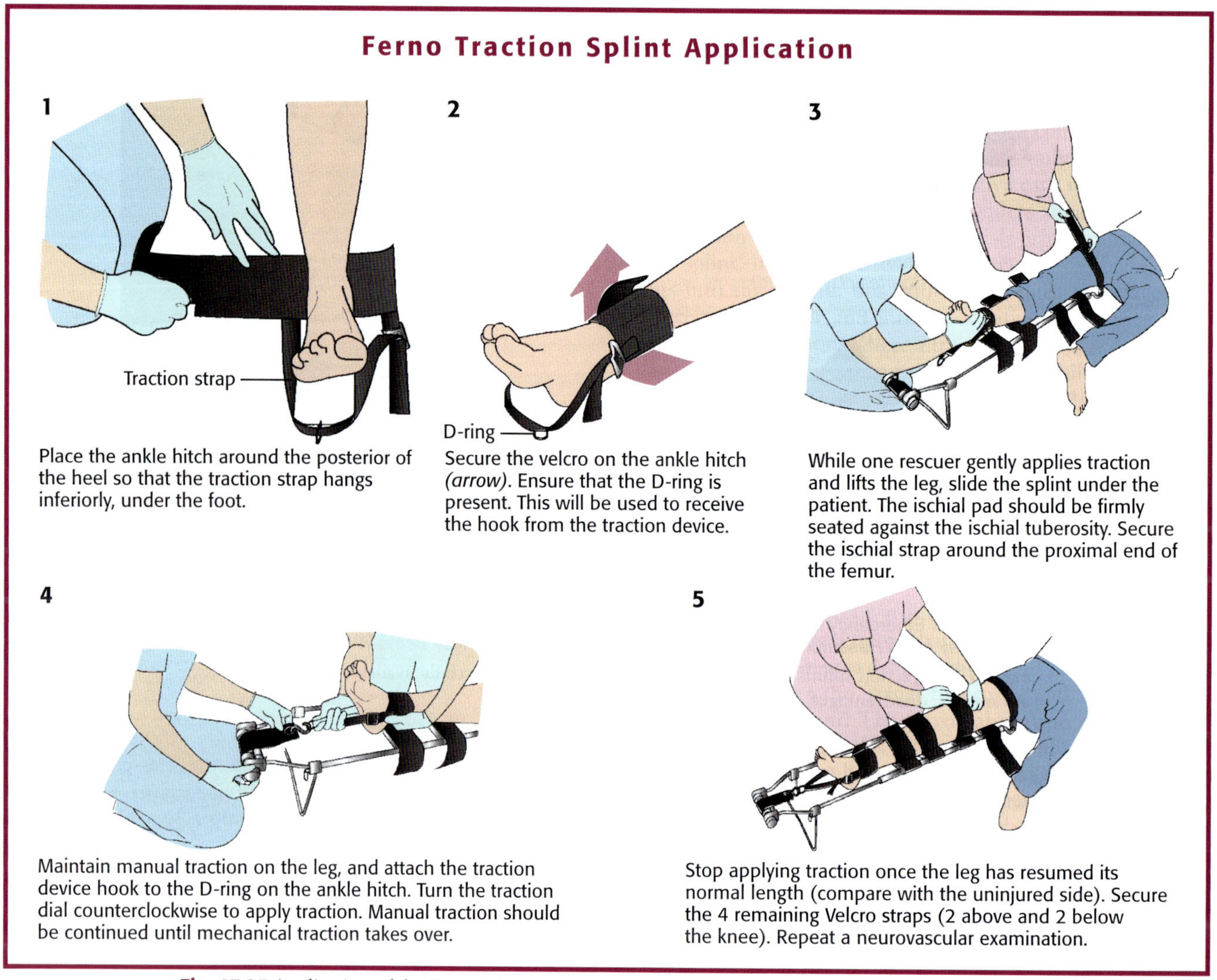

Fig. 47.25 Application of the Ferno Traction Splint. Note that the splint should be adjusted so that it is 12 inches longer than the uninjured leg before application. (From Ferno-Washington, Inc.)

CONCLUSION

When properly applied, traction splints reduce the pain, hemorrhage, and potential injury to adjacent structures that are associated with femoral fractures. Close attention to the manufacturer's application instructions and frequent patient reassessment will help reduce complications.

PELVIC IMMOBILIZATION

Background

Pelvic fractures cause significant morbidity and mortality, especially in older individuals. The decreased bone density in older individuals contributes to the likelihood of sustaining pelvic fractures from low- to moderate-energy mechanisms, such as falls from a standing height. The findings on physical examination may be subtle, such as slight asymmetry of the lower extremities, so a high index of suspicion is important. In younger individuals, pelvic injuries are usually caused by high-energy mechanisms, most commonly motor vehicle collisions.[87] Major pelvic trauma can lead to severe, uncontrollable hemorrhage, hypovolemic shock, and multisystem organ failure (Fig. 47.27).[88]

In the prehospital setting, early stabilization of fracture segments to control hemorrhage, gentle handling, and immediate transport to a trauma center are the cornerstones of treatment.[89] However, even the most experienced prehospital provider may find it difficult to identify pelvic injuries in the field. Hence, prehospital providers should not hesitate to stabilize the pelvis if a fracture is suspected.

INDICATIONS AND CONTRAINDICATIONS

Apply a pelvic circumferential compression device to any patient with significant pelvic pain, tenderness, or evidence of pelvic instability after trauma, especially if the patient is hypotensive.[90] There are no definite contraindications to pelvic stabilization in patients with presumed pelvic fractures.

PROCEDURE

Stabilization of the pelvis consists primarily of compressing the bony ring. This can be accomplished using a variety of devices, including a simple sheet, commercially available pelvic circumferential compression devices (also known as *pelvic binders*) such as the SAM Sling (SAM Medical

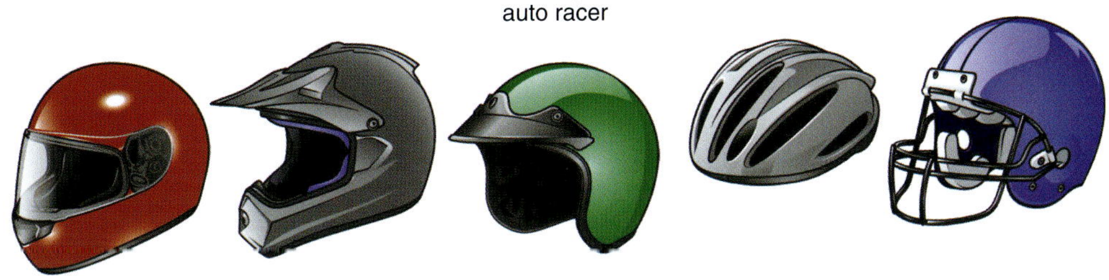

Fig. 47.31 Types of helmets.

Trainers' Association (NATA), The Sports Institute at UW Medicine, National Collegiate Athlete Association (NCAA) and the Harborview Injury Prevention and Research Center (HIPRC), published updated consensus recommendations that emphasized the need for preevent planning, having experienced personnel, and transport using a spinal board (minimizing the total duration of board use) to a regionalized trauma center (see Box 47.3).[113,114] The potential for helmets to interfere with plain films of the spine was demonstrated in two studies,[115,116] though nonmetallic helmets were less likely to interfere with computed tomography.[117] Thus removal prior to imaging may be indicated depending on the imaging mode available or desired.

Motorcycle and motorsport helmets should be removed in the prehospital setting.[76] Motorcycle helmets with a full-face guard make it very difficult to assess and manage the airway and to evaluate injuries to the head and neck. The helmet's large size and design may cause significant neck flexion if left in place. While decreasing the likelihood of injury, the increasing use of head and neck restraint devices (e.g., the HANS device [Fig. 47.32A] and the SHRFlex device [Fig. 47.32B]) in professional motorsports has further complicated cervical spine management and helmet removal.

CONTRAINDICATIONS

The only absolute contraindications to helmet removal are neck pain or paresthesias associated with the procedure or an inability to remove the helmet because of an impaled object (e.g., deer antler through a motorcycle helmet).[118,119] Relative contraindications to helmet removal include unfamiliarity with the technique, lack of sufficient assistance, and situations in which provider judgment is that helmet and equipment removal may worsen spinal alignment during transport.[120]

PROCEDURE

Sport Helmet Removal

When a face mask is present, if not immediately removing the helmet, remove the mask at the earliest opportunity, before transportation and despite the absence of any respiratory complaints.[105,106,121] A variety of tools (e.g. FM Extractor [Collins Surgical], Trainer's Angel [Trainer's Angel], anvil pruner, polyvinyl chloride pipe cutter, or power screwdriver) and techniques are used for face mask removal.[110] All emergency care providers should have tools for face mask removal readily available and be familiar with their use. The choice of equipment is less important than the skill and experience

BOX 47.3 Spinal Motion Restriction in the Trauma Patient: Recommendations[a]

KEY RECOMMENDATIONS

1. Athletic programs should have an emergency action plan (EAP) developed in conjunction with local emergency medical services agencies specific to prehospital spine injury care. Best practices are for an athlete with a suspected spinal injury to be transported to a designated Level 1 or 2 trauma center as quickly and safely as possible.
2. Sports medicine teams should conduct a preevent medical time out before each athletic event (practices and competitions). Participating in these "time outs" should include medical personnel from both teams, EMS personnel and game officials.
3. When feasible, those with the highest level of training and experience in removal techniques should participate in equipment removal. Athletic trainers are recognized as the medical professional with the most training and experience in athletic equipment removal.
4. Removal of the helmet and shoulder pads can occur in the emergency room or on the field. There are potential advantages to on-field removal prior to transport to the hospital, such as improved airway management, access to the chest for CPR, and expedited care of the athlete. The decision to remove equipment before transport should be based on a variety of factors, such as the medical status of the injured athlete, type of equipment worn, number of onsite rescuers and training and experience of on-the-field and emergency room rescuers in equipment removal.
5. If a spine board is used in the care of an athlete with a suspected cervical spine injury, nonathlete data recommend that time on the board be minimized; however, the board is left in place for transport to the hospital.
6. If feasible, spine-injured athletes should be transported to a medical facility that can deliver immediate and definitive care in the event the athlete has a significant cervical spine injury. This includes an emergency department with certified emergency medicine physicians, personnel trained in equipment removal, advanced imaging services, spine surgeon consultation in house or readily available, 24/7 operating access, and critical care monitoring and rehabilitation services.

[a]*A joint position statement of the American College of Surgeons Committee on Trauma (ACS-COT), American College of Emergency Physicians (ACEP), and the National Association of EMS Physicians (NAEMSP).*

Modified from Courson R, Ellis J, Herring SA et al. Best practices and current care concepts in prehospital care of the spine-injured athlete in American Tackle Football March 2-3, 2019; Atlanta, GA. J Athl Train. *2020;55(6):545-562; and Mills BM, Conrick KM, Anderson S et al. Consensus Recommendations on the prehospital care of the injured athlete with a suspected catastrophic cervical spine injury.* Clin J Sport Med. *2020;30(4):296-304.*

CPR, *Cardiopulmonary resuscitation.*

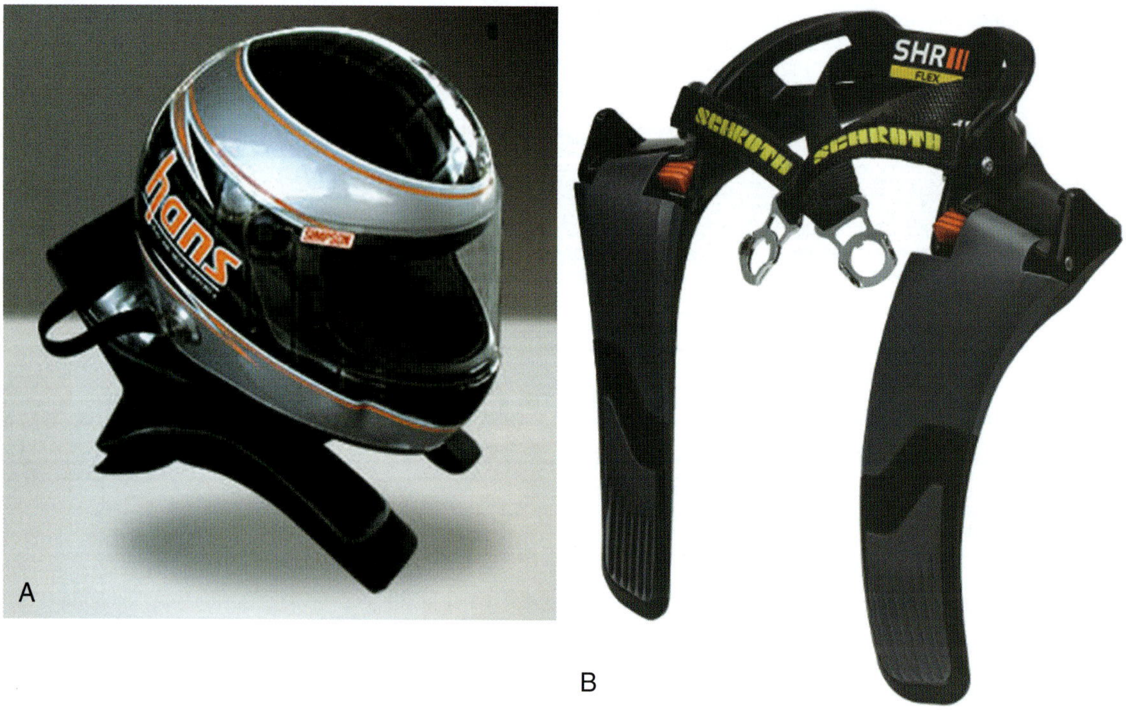

Fig. 47.32 (A) HANS device. (B) SHR Flex device. (A, Courtesy HANS Performance Products. B, Courtesy SCH Roth Racing, https://www.schrothracing.com.)

of the personnel using it.[122] To remove the face mask of a football helmet, cut the four plastic loop straps that secure the face mask to the helmet. Remove hockey and lacrosse face masks by unscrewing the external screws holding them in place. Maintain in-line stabilization to keep the head and neck in the neutral position during the entire procedure. With practice, the face mask of any helmet can be quickly and safely removed with minimal movement of the cervical spine.[112]

The NATA protocol for helmet and shoulder pad removal discussed in this chapter has been shown to effectively limit motion of the cervical spine when removal of equipment is necessary.[123] Proper removal of a helmet and shoulder pads requires at least two (and preferably three or four) individuals, one of whom maintains manual in-line stabilization of the cervical spine throughout the procedure.[108]

One rescuer manually stabilizes the head and neck in the neutral position by placing their hands on each side of the helmet with the thumbs pointing up (Fig. 47.33, *step 1*). A second rescuer then removes the chin strap by cutting or unsnapping it (see Fig. 47.33, *step 2*). Next, this rescuer removes the left or right cheek and jaw pads from the helmet by first slipping the flat blade of a screwdriver or bandage scissors between the pad snaps and the helmet's inner surface and twisting slightly. Once separated from the helmet, remove the pads by sliding them out firmly and slowly. Remove the opposite side in the same manner. Note that some helmet models (e.g., Riddell Revolution [Riddell]) are padded with a number of air-filled bladders that must be deflated (rather than removed) before removal of the helmet (Fig. 47.34).[124] In this case, the second rescuer deflates the air inflation system by releasing the air at the external ports with the inflation needle that comes with the helmet. Alternatively, an 18-gauge needle or air pump needle may be tried. If an inflation needle is not available (or an 18-gauge needle or air pump needle does not work), directly puncture the bladders with an 18-gauge needle.

The second rescuer then takes over in-line immobilization of the head by using one hand to grasp the patient's mandible between the thumb and the first two fingers while placing the other hand under the occiput (see Fig. 47.33, *step 3*). The first rescuer then places a thumb inside each ear hole of the helmet and curls their fingers along the bottom edge of the helmet (see Fig. 47.33, *step 4*). Remove the helmet by rotating it off the head in a gentle fashion without pulling laterally.[121] Remove shoulder pads by cutting the straps underneath the arms and the anterior straps holding the pads together (see Fig. 47.33, *step 5*). If a cervical orthosis (e.g., neck roll, cowboy collar, or butterfly restrictor) is present, disconnect it from the helmet and shoulder pads before removal.

When possible, remove the shoulder pads and helmet simultaneously to prevent the head from falling into extension. If the shoulder pads cannot be removed simultaneously, manually stabilize the head in the neutral position during the procedure. The hands of the second rescuer can be moved superiorly as the helmet is being removed so that the thumb and first fingers grasp the maxilla at each side of the nose in the maxillary notch (see Fig. 47.33, *step 6*).

After removal of the helmet, place a c-collar while maintaining in-line stabilization. Remember that if the helmet cannot be removed and access to the chest area is required, remove the anterior half of the shoulder pads and leave the posterior portion to maintain cervical position with the helmet in place.

During patient transfer, current guidelines recommend using the log-roll-pull technique when turning prone injured athletes, as opposed to log-roll-push. For supine patients, the

Football Helmet and Shoulder Pad Removal

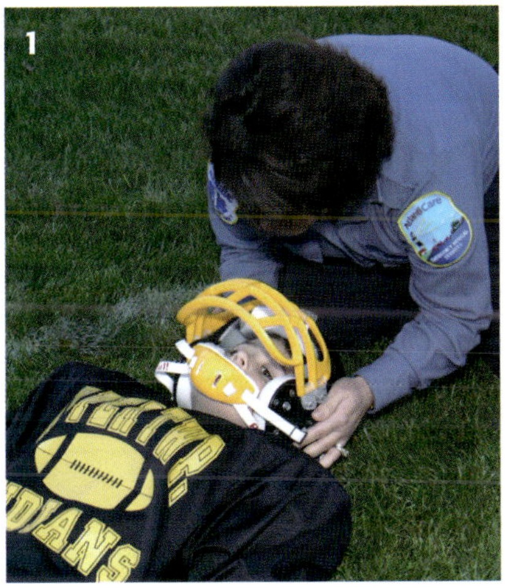

One rescuer manually stabilizes the patient's head and neck in the neutral position by placing his or her hands on each side of the helmet, with the thumbs pointing up.

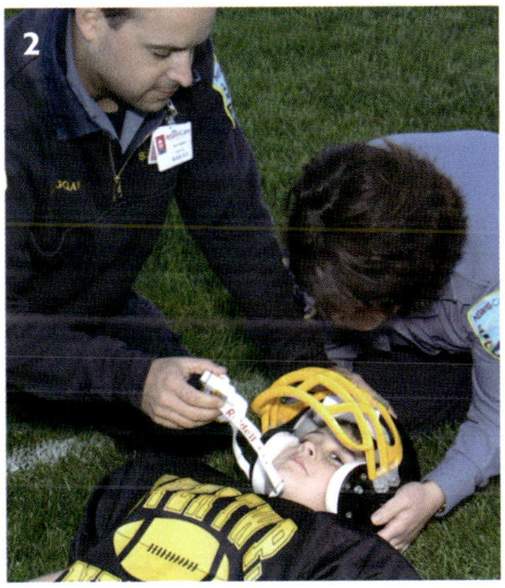

A second rescuer then removes the chin strap by cutting or unsnapping it.

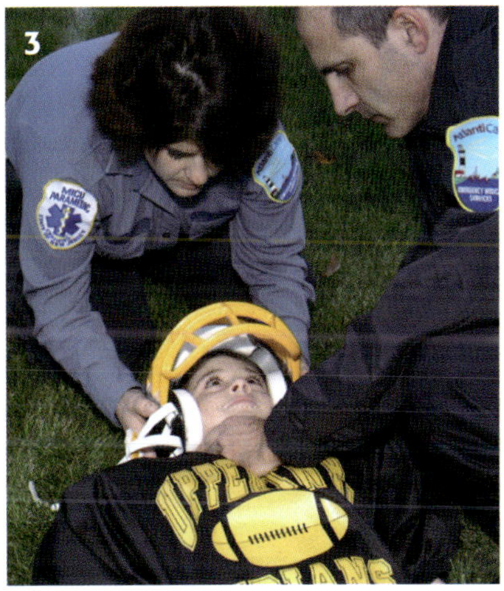

The second rescuer then takes over in-line immobilization of the head by using one hand to grasp the patient's mandible between the thumb and the first two fingers while placing the other hand under the occiput.

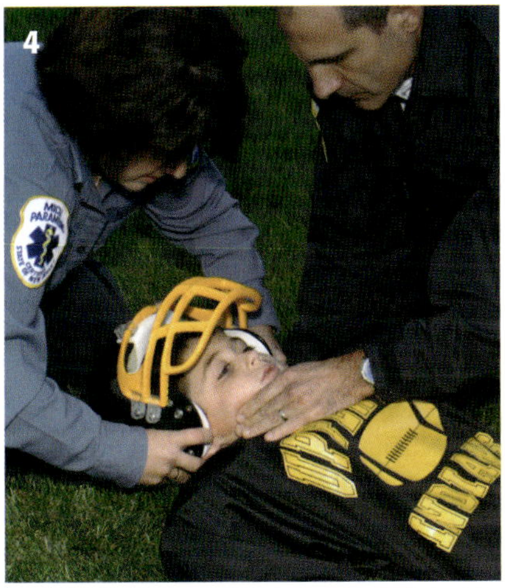

The first rescuer then places a thumb inside each ear hole of the helmet and curls his or her fingers along the bottom edge of the helmet. Without pulling laterally, the helmet is removed by gently rotating it off the head.

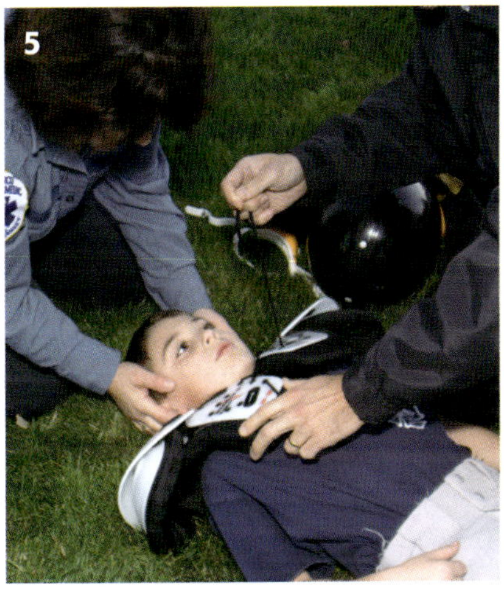

The shoulder pads are removed by cutting the straps underneath the arms and the anterior straps holding the pads together.

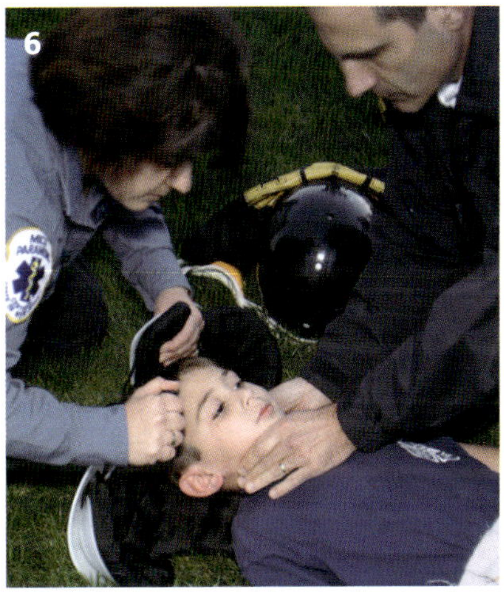

The hands of the second rescuer stabilize the head as the shoulder pads are removed. When possible, the helmet (with the face mask removed) and shoulder pads should remain in place until the initial clinical and radiographic evaluation is completed in the ED.

Fig. 47.33 Football helmet and shoulder pad removal. Proper removal of a helmet and shoulder pads requires at least two rescuers. Note that this figure does not demonstrate removal of the face mask and cheek/jaw pads, which is recommended before helmet removal. See text for details.) *ED*, Emergency department. (Courtesy AtlantiCare Regional Medical Center, Emergency Medical Services.)

eight-person lift-and-slide technique results in less spinal movement during transfer.

Motorcycle Helmet Removal

For the reasons described earlier, motorcycle helmets should be removed in the prehospital setting. The removal method endorsed by the American College of Surgeons in 1997 is the method most often used today (Fig. 47.35).[125] Providers should be aware that significant cervical motion can occur during removal of a motorcycle helmet if the shoulders are not properly elevated; a folded sheet or jacket placed behind the patient's shoulders may help limit any cervical motion associated with the procedure.[126]

If attempts to remove the helmet result in pain or paresthesias, the advanced trauma life support guidelines recommend removing the helmet via a technique described by Aprahamian and coworkers.[127] This technique uses a cast

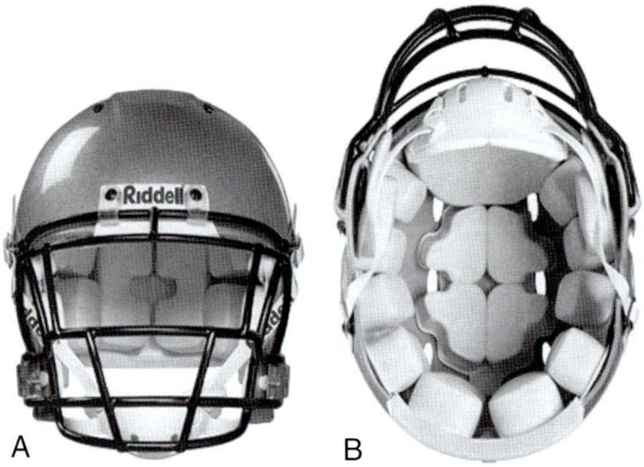

Fig. 47.34 Riddell Revolution football helmet. These helmets are padded with a number of air-filled bladders that must be deflated (rather than removed) before removal of the helmet. (A) Frontal view. (B) Inside view. See text for details. (Courtesy Riddell.)

Motorcycle Helmet Removal

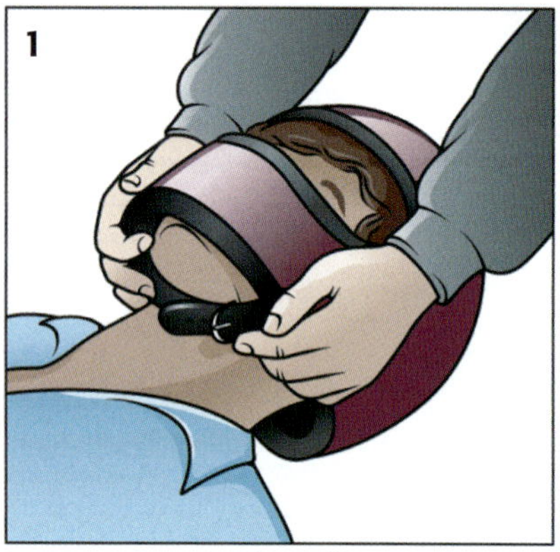

One rescuer maintains in-line immobilization by placing his or her hands on each side, of the helmet with the fingers on the victim's mandible. This position prevents slippage if the strap is loose.

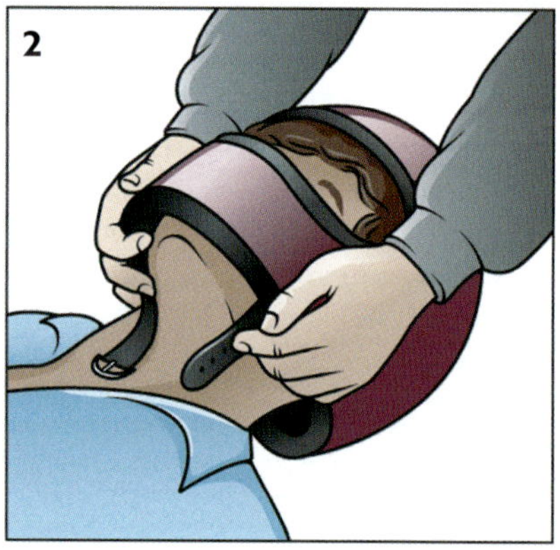

A second rescuer cuts or loosens the strap at the D-ring.

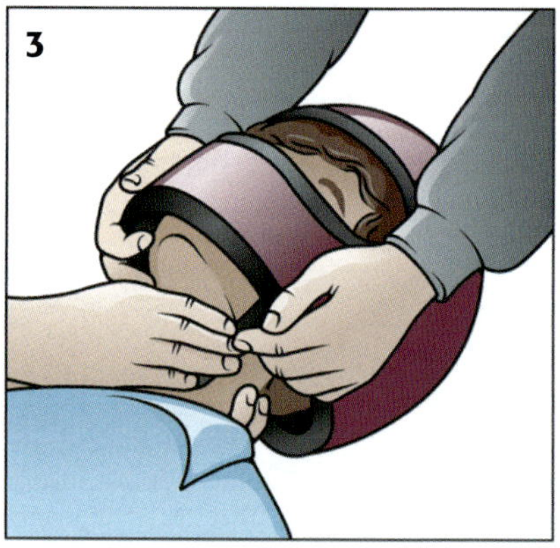

The second rescuer places one hand on the mandible at the angle, the thumb on one side and the long and index fingers on the other. With the other hand the rescuer applies pressure from the occipital region. This maneuver transfers the in-line immobilization responsibility to the second rescuer.

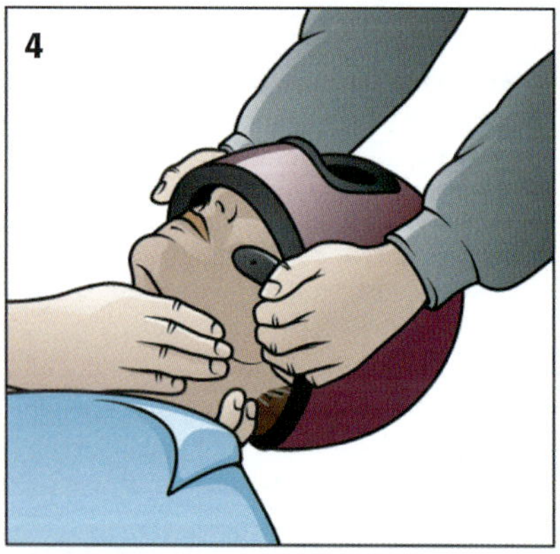

The rescuer at the top moves the helmet. Three factors should be kept in mind:

- The helmet is egg-shaped and therefore must be expanded laterally to clear the ears.
- If the helmet provides full facial coverage, glasses must be removed first.
- If the helmet provides full facial coverage, the nose may impede removal. To clear the nose, the helmet must be tilted backward and raised over it.

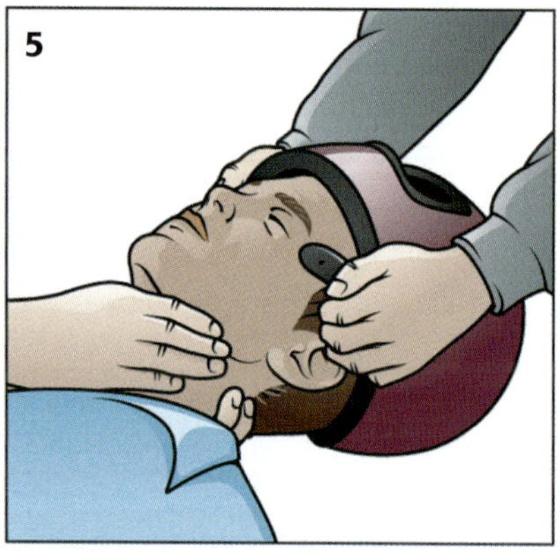

Throughout the removal process the second rescuer maintains in-line immobilization from below to prevent unnecessary neck motion.

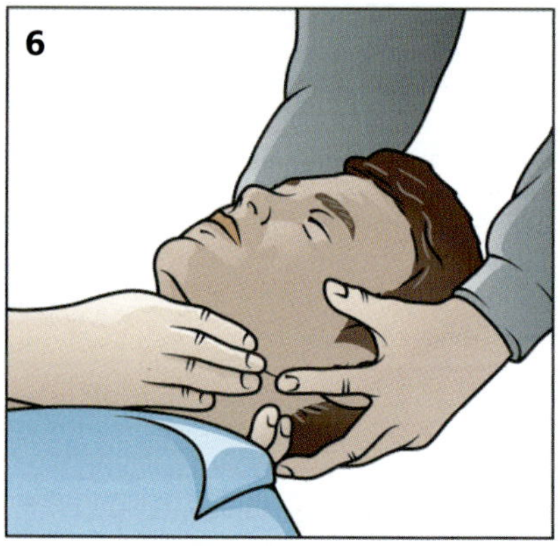

After the helmet has been removed, the rescuer at the top replaces his or her hands on either side of the victim's head with the palms over the ears.

Fig. 47.35 Motorcycle helmet removal. (From Norman E. McSwain, Jr., MD, FACS, and Richard L. Garrnelli, MD, FACS—American College of Surgeons Committee on Trauma, April 1997.)

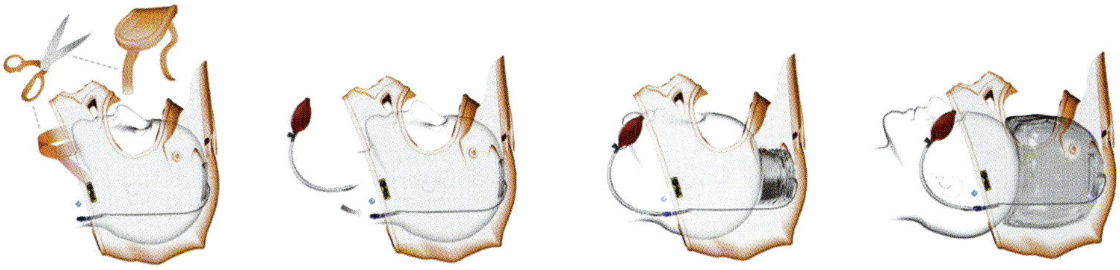

Fig. 47.36 Eject Helmet Removal System. This device uses a small air bladder that is neatly folded in an accordion fashion and placed underneath the helmet liner. A small tube runs under the padding and fastens to the bottom of the rim of the helmet to provide easy access. The device may be prefitted into the rider's helmet or inserted at the time of removal by using an insertion tool that allows the airbag to be slid up inside the top of a helmet. (Courtesy Shock Doctor, http://www.ejectsafety.com.)

saw to bivalve the helmet in the coronal plane. Following division of the outer rigid shell, incise the inner foam material and remove it while maintaining the head and neck in neutral alignment. Although this approach does provide an alternative method of removing the helmet, the intense vibrations produced during use of the cast cutter may exacerbate an underlying spinal injury. In addition, this technique may be slow and difficult with modern, well-fitting, high-quality helmets.[128]

The preferred method of helmet removal in organized motorsports is the Eject Helmet Removal System (formerly the Hats Off System), which consists of an inflatable air bladder that can be placed into the helmet before use or introduced into the crown of the helmet with a specially designed insertion tool. When inflated with a hand pump or CO_2 cartridge, it purportedly loosens the helmet to allow easy removal (Fig. 47.36).[128] Despite little scientific data supporting its use, the IndyCar Racing League, American Speed Association, and American Motorcycle Association have made the Eject Helmet Removal System mandatory at all of their events. In addition, the Championship Auto Racing Teams and National Association for Stock Car Auto Racing strongly recommend its use.

COMPLICATIONS

It is theorized that underlying cervical spine injuries may be exacerbated by failure to adhere to proper helmet removal techniques, though clinical data is lacking.[110] In a cadaveric model, Donaldson and colleagues[129] demonstrated that even when using proper technique, there is a significant amount of motion during removal of helmets and shoulder pads. Larger studies are needed to determine whether there is a real and significant risk in the clinical setting.

CONCLUSION

Prehospital care providers must take caution when evaluating and treating an athlete with a suspected head and neck injury. In general, removal of athletic helmets and shoulder pads at the scene should be considered when appropriate and when adequately trained personnel are available, though it is reasonable to transport without removal when equipment is maintaining the spine in neutral alignment, and when there are no other emergency conditions that require their removal. Face masks, however, should be removed early in the management of these patients. Motorcycle and motorsport helmets, as well as sports and other helmets worn without shoulder pads, should be removed routinely to provide access to the patient's airway and allow proper spinal motion restriction. When indicated, prehospital helmet removal can be accomplished in a safe and effective manner by well-trained prehospital care providers.

The primary concern of removing helmets and protective padding is causing additional injury to the patient. It may also prolong on-scene time and delay transport to the hospital.

REFERENCES ARE AVAILABLE AT Elsevier eBooks+

CHAPTER 48

Management of Amputations

Emily Rose

Rapid and appropriate emergency care of a patient with an amputated body part is crucial to the potential salvage and preservation of function. This chapter discusses the emergency management priorities of patients with amputation injuries, the acute care of amputated parts before they are replanted, and the management of distal digit amputations and dermal "slice" wounds.

Amputation may be partial or complete. Injuries with any interconnecting tissue between the distal and proximal portions, even if it is only a small piece of bridging skin, are considered incomplete (or partial) amputations. The peak incidence of traumatic amputations occurs between the ages of 15 and 40 years and approximately 80% of injuries occur in males. Motor vehicle collisions are the leading mechanism of injury, followed by industrial and agricultural accidents. Crush injuries occur most commonly, and sharp guillotine amputations are least common. Partial amputations occur as often as total amputations. Seventy percent of amputations overall occur in the upper extremity and distal amputations are more common than proximal.

Successful revascularization of amputated parts may ensure viability, but neurologic, osseous, and tendinous healing is critical for ultimate function. If there is incomplete neurologic recovery, limited range of motion, and intolerance to cold, the replanted part may have little functional value for the patient. Rehabilitation from replantation surgery may be prolonged, (often >1 year) and repeat surgical procedures are often required. The decision to replant or revise the stump is multifactorial and includes the type of injury (location and mechanism), associated injuries, underlying health of patient, occupation, patient preference, among many other factors.[1]

BACKGROUND

Replantation attempts (with rare success) have been described for hundreds of years but the ability to consistently replant amputated parts is now possible with advances in microvascular surgical techniques. Upper limb and hand replants were first described in 1962. The first successful microvascular anastomosis of a digital vessel was described in 1965, and now replantation success rates range from 50% to >90%.[2–7] Survival of the replanted tissue was the criterion for success for the original pioneers in replant surgery, but with further technological and surgical refinements, today's surgeons emphasize functional recovery and aesthetics as well as viability. Replantation of a part that is painful or useless or that interferes with function is a disservice to the patient and is less desirable than early restoration of function without replantation. With advancements in technology, there are also alternatives to replantation such as targeted reinnervation, advanced prostheses, transplantation of composite tissue, or the potential for upper extremity transplantation to restore upper extremity function. The operative plan must be tailored to each individual patient with consideration of the patient's needs, underlying health, ability to undergo and comply with rehabilitation, support network, and likely functional outcome.

INDICATIONS

The mechanism of injury is the most important determinant of implant survival. Replantation is more likely to occur with sharp/penetrating injury, distal level of amputation, lack of multilevel involvement, and when the injury is isolated to the extremity.[2] Preservation of the amputated part is indicated whenever there is a potential for replantation. Revascularization and reanastomosis of partially and completely amputated parts should be provided when there is hope of preservation or restoration of function. Aesthetic considerations, patient avocations, and in some cases the patient's religious or social customs may also influence the decision to proceed with surgery.[8–10] Ultimately, the microsurgical team and patient must reach the decision together after an explanation of the risks and potential results.

Replantation is more commonly performed for upper extremity amputation because a lower extremity prosthesis often provides a good functional outcome and can often be superior to outcomes with replantation. Upper extremity prostheses are less able to achieve fine motor activity and a "bad hand" may be more functional than a "good amputation" in the upper extremity. Additionally, there is less muscle (which is less vulnerable to crush injury and allows a longer ischemia time) and increased collateral circulation in the upper extremity, which improves replantation success. Review Box 48.1 summarizes the general indications for replantation. Single-digit amputations that are both proximal to the distal interphalangeal (DIP) joint and distal to the flexor digitorum superficialis may be replanted successfully with good functional recovery (Fig. 48.1). The decision to replant single-digit amputations often depends on the digit involved. Revision amputation only of the little finger may be preferred for recovery speed.[11] The thumb accounts for 40% to 50% of hand function with its utility in pinch and grip. Even if a replanted thumb has a limited range of motion, it is more functional than any other available reconstructive procedure or prosthetic device.[12] Hand function requires orchestration of multiple finger interactions to pinch, grasp, and perform fine motor manipulation. Measures of hand function include sensation, range of motion, and grip strength. In multiple-digit amputations, the interaction of involved fingers is included in the calculation in surgical planning.[11,13–17] Multifinger replantations are more cost effective and may result in better functional outcomes.[14] The underlying health of the patient is often more predictive of good outcomes than chronologic age and there are no fixed age limits for replantation. However, children consistently have better outcomes due to their superior neuroplasticity, regenerative capacity, and adaptability to rehabilitation.[18,19] The decision to replant is made on a case-by-case basis by the microsurgical team, who must weigh all the factors involved. In general, patients can expect to achieve 50% of original sensation and motor function of the replanted part, with younger patients and more distal amputations having the best outcomes.[6,7,20]

Management of Amputations

Indications

Young stable patient
Thumb
Multiple digits injured
Sharp wounds with little associated damage
Upper extremity (children)

Contraindications

Absolute

- Associated life threats
- Severe crush injuries
- Inability to withstand prolonged surgery

Relative[a]

- Single digit, unless thumb
- Avulsion injury
- Prolonged warm ischemia (>12 hr)
- Gross contamination
- Prior injury or surgery to part
- Emotionally unstable patient
- Lower extremity

Complications

Infection
Poor function

Equipment

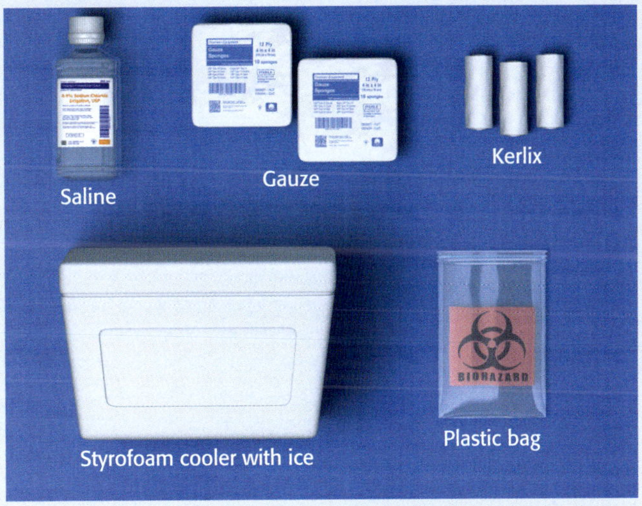

Review Box 48.1 Management of amputations: indications for reimplantation, contraindications, complications, and equipment. [a]If the patient is a child or if there are multiple losses, salvage reimplantations are attempted and the relative contraindications are ignored.

CONTRAINDICATIONS

Contraindications to replantation include life-threatening injury or significant comorbidity that prohibits a lengthy operation.[18] Relative contraindications include severely crushed or mangled parts or profuse contamination. Contraindications to replantation are listed in Review Box 48.1 and are discussed in the following sections. The amputated part should be treated carefully because portions may be used as a graft even if the entire part cannot be replanted. For example, an amputated fingertip not suitable for replantation may be an ideal donor source for a skin graft on the stump. In addition, even when replantation is contraindicated, tissue (e.g., skin, bone, tendon) from the amputated part may be useful in restoring function to other damaged parts. Do not discard amputated tissue until all possible uses of the severed parts are considered.

GENERAL CONSIDERATIONS

Mechanism of Injury

The potential for successful replantation in terms of survival, as well as useful function, is often related to the mechanism of injury. Guillotine-type injuries are the least common but have the best prognosis because of the limited area of destruction. Crush injuries are the most common but produce more tissue injury and therefore often have a poorer prognosis. Avulsion injuries have the worst prognosis because a significant amount of vascular, nerve, tendon, and soft tissue injury is involved.

Ischemia Time

Irreversible ischemic injury occurs in muscle tissue after 2 to 4 hours of warm ischemia and 6 to 8 hours of cold ischemia. Digits have less muscle tissue and are therefore less susceptible to ischemic damage (increasing warm ischemia time to 6 to 12 hours and cold ischemia time to 12 to 24 hours).[21] However, ischemic time alone does not preclude replantation attempt as successful replantation after prolonged ischemia time has been reported (hand reimplantation after 54 hours of cold ischemia; digit replantation after 33 hours of warm and 94 hours of cold ischemia).[22,23] Techniques such as interosseous muscle stripping to prevent necrosis may improve replantation success in scenarios of prolonged ischemia time.

PATIENT ASSESSMENT AND MANAGEMENT

The initial care and treatment of a patient with a traumatic amputation begins with a primary survey and stabilization of the airway, breathing, and circulation. Traumatic limb amputations often do not occur in isolation and management of a patient's injuries must be prioritized such that life-threatening injuries take precedence over limb-threatening conditions (Fig. 48.2).[24] Early hemorrhage control is essential. Bleeding should be controlled initially with direct pressure. If direct pressure is unsuccessful, the judicious use of tourniquets is endorsed as a temporary adjunct to control extremity hemorrhage.[25,26] To minimize potential complications, note the time of tourniquet application and limit tourniquet use to the time

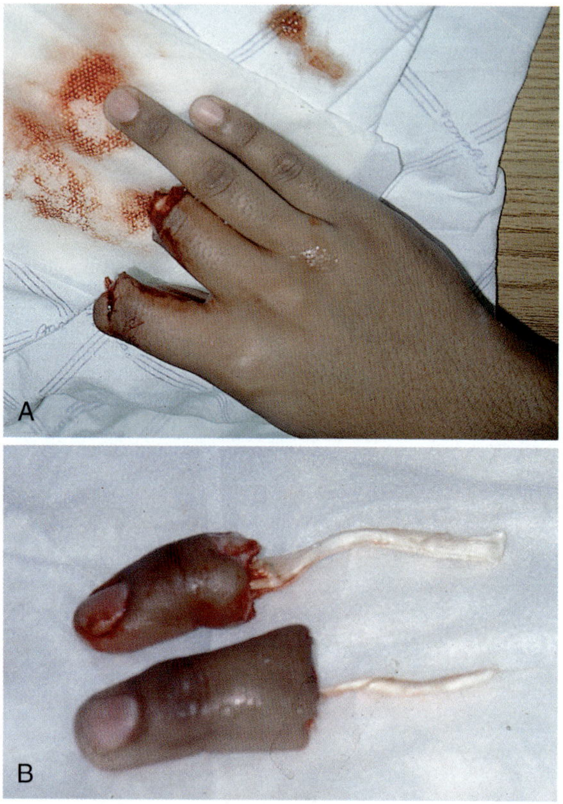

Fig. 48.1 (A–B) Single-digit amputations are not usually replanted unless the thumb is involved. This sharp amputation with little associated damage in a 20-year-old may qualify, but it is best to discuss this with the hand surgery team before giving unrealistic expectations to the patient, who may anticipate a normal result by simply "sewing it back on." Avulsion of the tendons proximal to the amputation greatly complicates this case.

necessary to control the hemorrhage. Multiple amputations are an independent risk factor for death.[18]

After the initial assessment and stabilization of the patient, initiate care of the stump and amputated part (Box 48.1). A thorough neurovascular examination should be performed and documented. Evaluate the extremities for pulses and the presence of a bruit. In partial amputations, note the hard and soft signs of vascular injury (Table 48.1). In patients with soft signs, measure the ankle-brachial index or arterial pressure index (systolic pressure of the injured extremity/systolic pressure of the uninjured extremity). A ratio of less than or equal to 0.9 raises concern for a vascular injury. Reduce and immobilize associated dislocations and fractures and evaluate the patient for associated conditions such as rhabdomyolysis and compartment syndrome.

Obtain a history regarding the exact mechanism, time, and duration of the injury, dominant hand, general medical status (notably diabetes, vascular disease, and smoking), allergies, medications, illness, previous injury to the affected part, care of the stump and amputated part before arrival in the emergency department (ED), occupation, avocations, tetanus history, and the patient's expectations. Child abuse should always be considered in fingertip injuries.[27]

Initiate tetanus prophylaxis (if indicated) and broad-spectrum systemic antibiotic therapy (with amputations involving more than a single digit, e.g., cephalosporins).[28,29] Intravenous opioids are recommended for pain; titrate the dose to the clinical condition. Digital or regional nerve blocks are effective adjuncts for pain relief but limit ongoing neurologic evaluation (see Chapters 31 and 32). Obtain preoperative labs and imaging, including radiographs of the amputated part and proximal stump that include at least one joint proximal to the injury site (Fig. 48.3). Contact the regional replantation resource center as soon as possible to arrange transportation and provide adequate time for mobilization of the replantation team.

Patients who have sustained an amputation often experience denial, shock, disbelief, and feelings of hopelessness about their injury; some even become suicidal.[30] Treat patients with supportive and realistic reassurance and avoid promises of outcome. It is important that the emergency clinician (or other nonreplantation specialist) not speculate on the specifics of the ultimate prognosis.

CARE OF THE STUMP AND AMPUTATED PART

See Video 48.1. The goals of initial care of the stump and amputated part include control of hemorrhage and prevention of further injury or contamination.

Stump

Examination of the stump may be brief and should primarily be an assessment of the degree of damage to surrounding tissue (Fig. 48.4). Remove all jewelry from the stump and irrigate with normal saline to remove gross contamination; any manual debridement and dissection should be performed by the replantation team. Do not use local antiseptics, especially hydrogen peroxide or alcohol, because they may damage viable tissue. Do not clamp arterial bleeders. Similarly, surrounding tissue should not be manipulated, clamped, tagged, or further traumatized in any way. Cover the stump wound with a saline-moistened sterile dressing to prevent further contamination and to limit damage from desiccation. Splint the stump for protection and to prevent further injury from concomitant fractures or compromised blood flow from a change in position. Splinting and elevation may also reduce swelling and help control bleeding.

Amputated Part

Remove all jewelry and irrigate the amputated part with normal saline to remove gross contamination, similar to care of the stump described previously (Fig. 48.5). The amputated part should be wrapped in saline-moistened gauze and placed in a dry and closed waterproof plastic bag (see Fig. 48.5, *step 5*). Do not place the amputated part directly in ice or cold saline. The bag containing the specimen wrapped in saline-moistened gauze should be immersed in ice water or refrigerated at 4°C. The amputated part itself should NOT come into direct contact with ice or saline or reach freezing temperatures. Do not discard any tissue as any amputated fragment could be potentially used for skin, bone, or nerve grafting.[18] Label the tissue containers with the patient's name, the amputated part contained within, the time of the original injury, and the time that cooling began.

Treatment is similar for partial amputations with vascular compromise. Irrigate the wound with normal saline. Place a saline-moistened sponge on the open tissue and wrap the

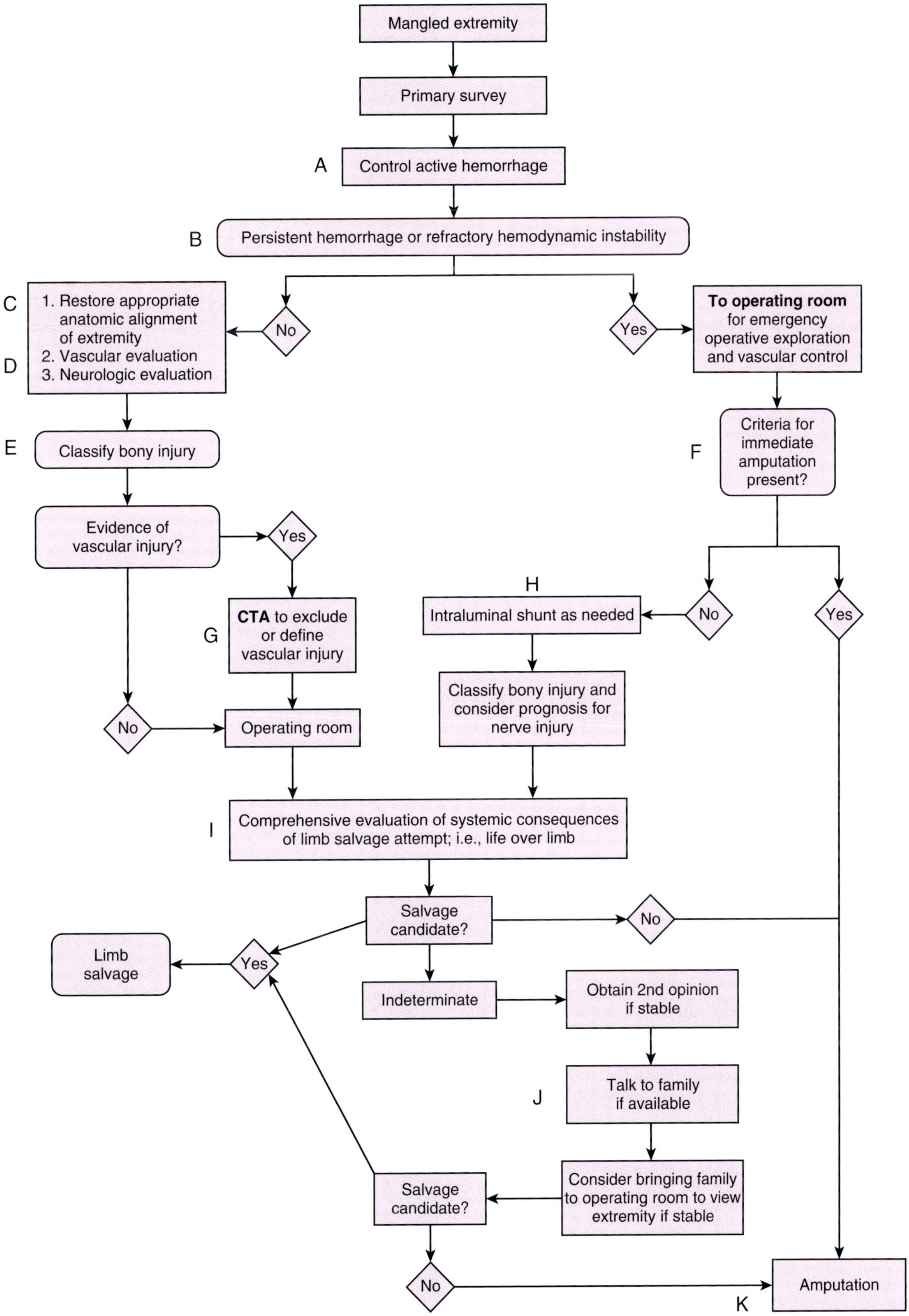

Fig. 48.2 Management algorithm for patients with mangled extremities. *CTA*, Computed tomography angiography. (From Scalea TM, DuBose J, Moore EE et al. Western Trauma Association critical decisions in trauma: management of the mangled extremity. *J Trauma Acute Care Surg*. 2012;72(1):86-93.)

BOX 48.1 Axioms for Care of Amputations

DO:

Splint and elevate
Apply a pressure dressing
Protect from further trauma or injury
Protect from further contamination
Provide analgesia
Give tetanus prophylaxis and antibiotic therapy
Obtain radiographs

DO NOT:

Apply dry ice or freeze tissue
Place tags on tissue
Place sutures in tissue
Sever skin bridges
Initiate perfusion of the amputated part
Place tissue in formalin or water

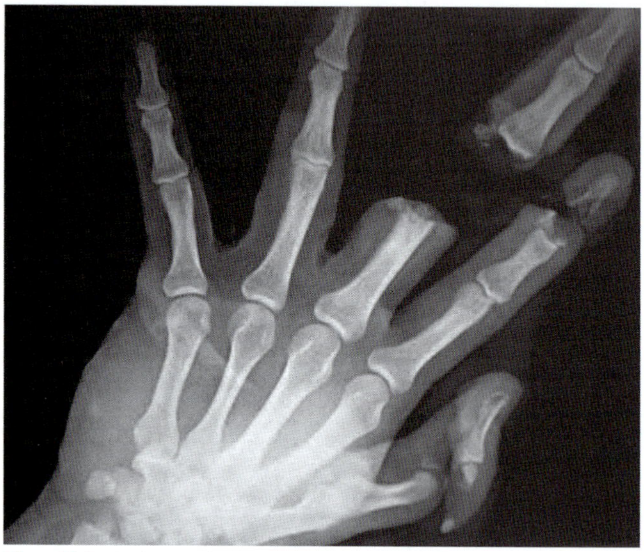

Fig. 48.3 Radiograph of hand with amputated fingers in view. (Courtesy Jonathan Gottlieb, MD.)

TABLE 48.1 Clinical Signs of Vascular Injury

HARD SIGNS OF VASCULAR INJURY	SOFT SIGNS OF VASCULAR INJURY
Absent distal pulses Active pulsatile bleeding Large expanding hematoma Bruit or thrill	Distal nerve deficit Diminished pulses Nonexpanding hematoma History of pulsatile or significant hemorrhage at time of injury

injury in a sterile dressing in which a splint has been incorporated to protect from further injury. Place ice packs or commercial cold packs over the dressing to cool the devascularized area (see Fig. 48.5, *step 8*).

SPECIAL CONSIDERATIONS

Lower Extremity Amputations

Lower limbs are not commonly replanted because replantation is fraught with potential complications and lower limb prostheses, especially those used below the knee, are well tolerated and functional.[31] Prostheses provide a secure stance and permit locomotion. Lower extremity replantation generally requires skeletal shortening, and distal nerve regeneration is often imperfect, with both deficits producing dysfunction.[32] A patient with a replanted lower extremity, with significant shortening and without sensation, typically has superior functional outcome with a prosthesis. Children are an exception and replantation may be attempted in a child with a lower limb amputation due to their potentially superior replantation functional outcomes.

Hand Function

Fine motor hand function involves pinch and grasp functions. If the index finger is amputated, the middle finger can often adequately perform the pinching function formerly provided by the index finger. Power in grasping and

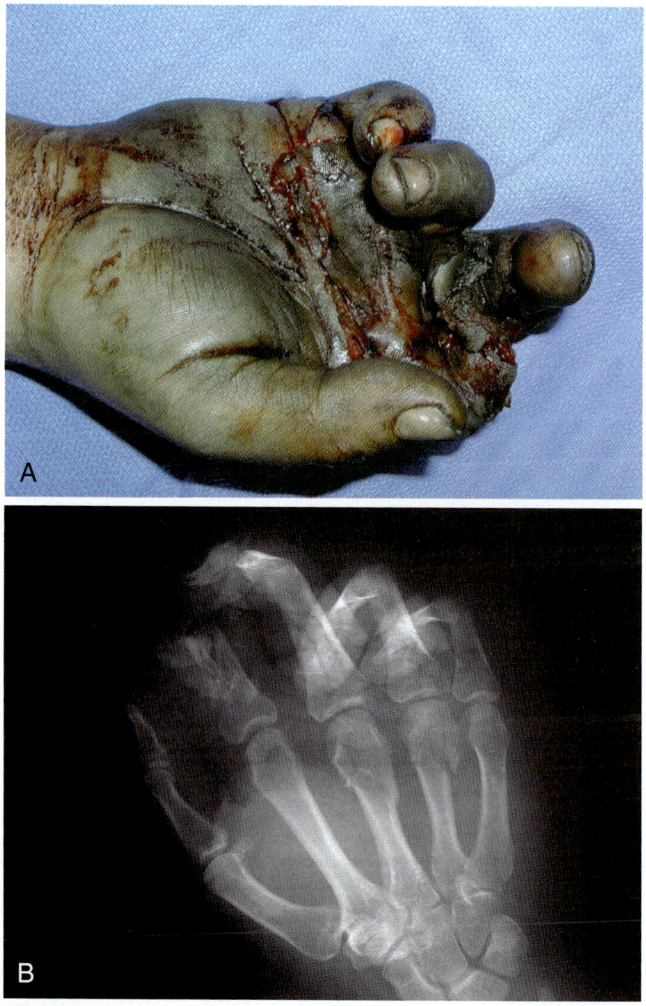

Fig. 48.4 (A) Blast injury resulting in amputation. Remove gross contamination by irrigating with normal saline. Avoid using antiseptics because they may damage viable tissue. Assess the degree of contamination, the level of the injury, and any concomitant injury. (B) Obtain radiographs of the amputated part (if available) and the proximal stump to include at least one joint proximal to the injury site. (Courtesy Stephen Pap, MD.)

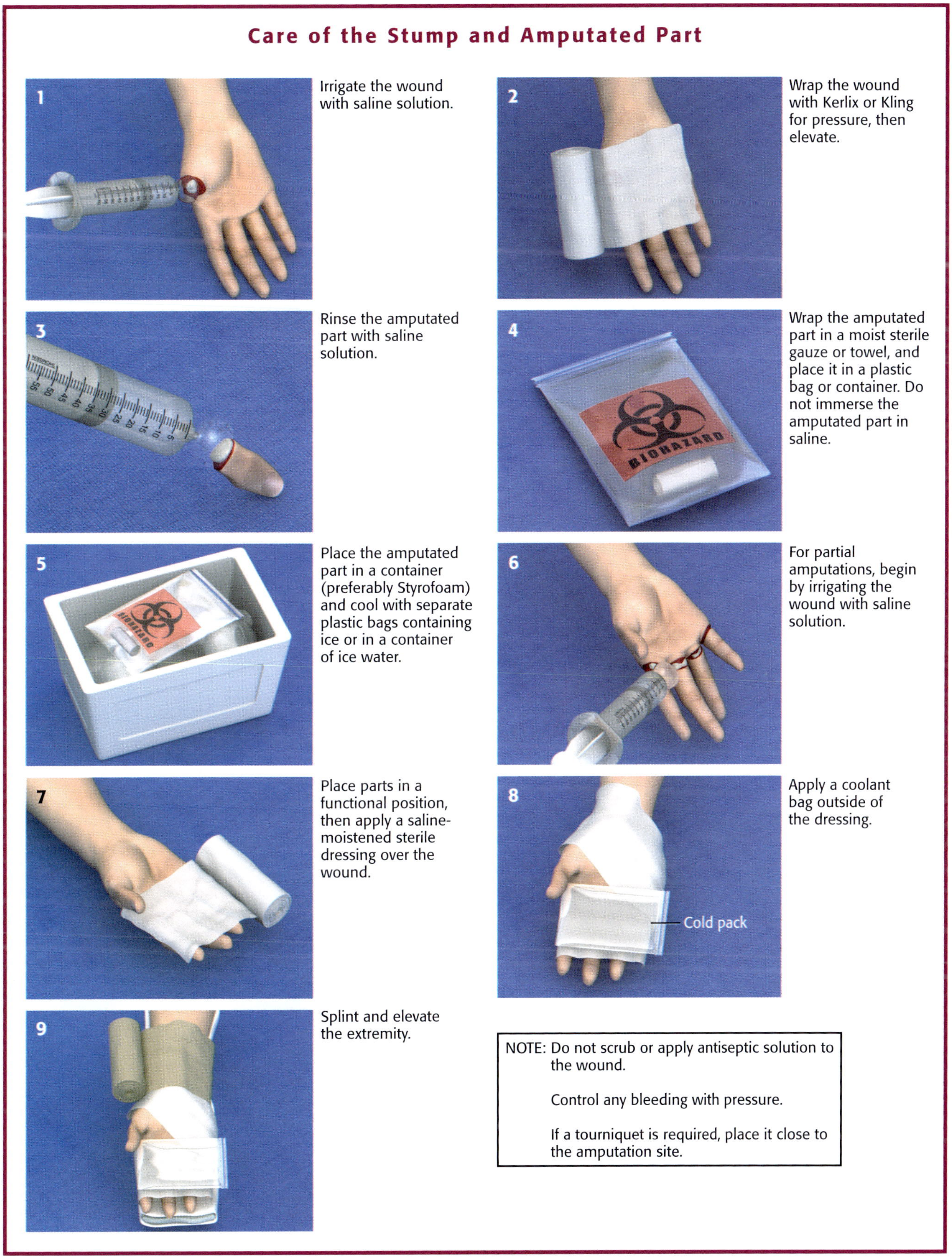

Fig. 48.5 Care of the stump and amputated part. Do not place the amputated part directly in ice or saline.

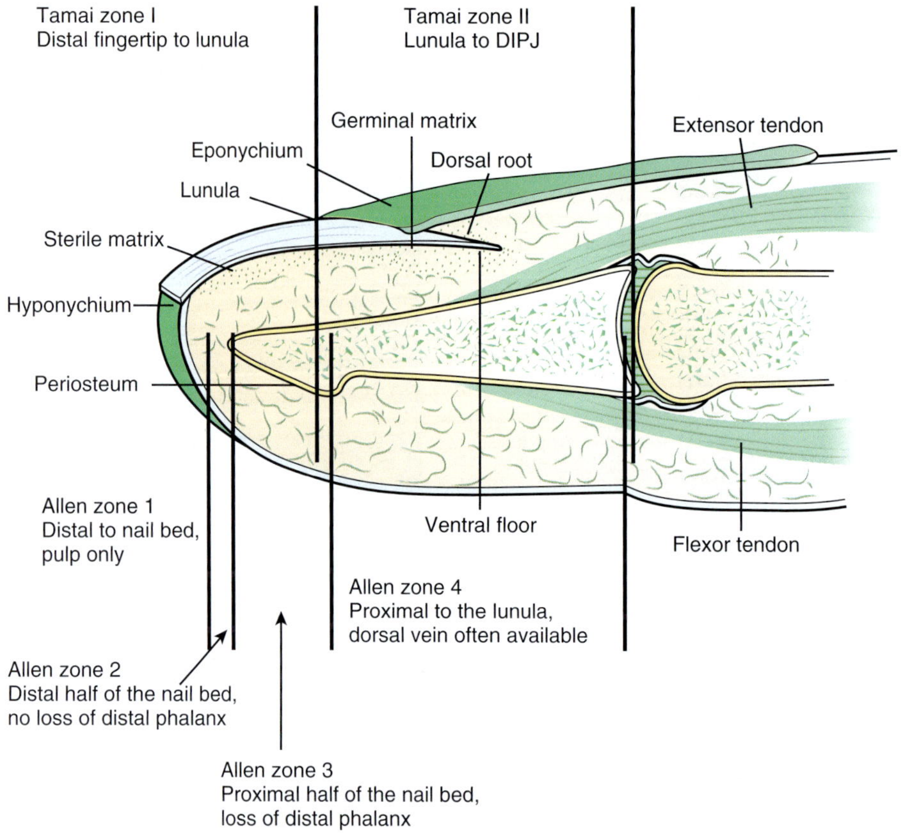

Fig. 48.6 Tamai and Allen classifications of distal fingertip amputations. *DIPJ*, Distal interphalangeal joint. (From Lee DH, Mignemi ME, Crosby SN. Fingertip injuries: an update on management. *J Am Acad Orthop Surg*. 2013;21(12):756-766.)

gripping is primarily a function of the fourth and fifth digits. An effective grip that provides the ability to hold a variety of objects is a central function of the ring and middle fingers. In addition to its function in pinching, the thumb is the major opposing force for successful grip and grasp. The thumb is the most important digit for adequate hand function, and its loss can result in 40% to 50% disability. Such disability requires aggressive attempts to replant amputated thumbs. If this is not possible or is unsuccessful, secondary alternatives are pollicization (creation of a thumb by using another digit) or toe transfers.[33]

Fingertip Amputations and Dermal Slice Wounds

There are several classification systems for distal fingertip amputations. The Tamai classification is most commonly used, though the Allen classification is the most clinically useful for hand surgeons (Fig. 48.6).

Treatment of distal fingertip injuries remains somewhat controversial, but good results are often achieved with conservative management. Factors that impact decisions on management include the involved finger, the amount of soft tissue loss, the integrity of the nail bed, and the patient's age, occupation, and management preference. The basic goals of treatment are to provide tissue coverage, an acceptable cosmetic result, and early functional recovery. Primary closure or healing by secondary intention is preferred when there is adequate soft tissue coverage and no exposed bone (Fig. 48.7). If there is no exposed bone, but significant pulp loss, treatment options include primary closure, healing by secondary intention, completion amputation, full-thickness skin grafting, or split-thickness skin grafting.[34]

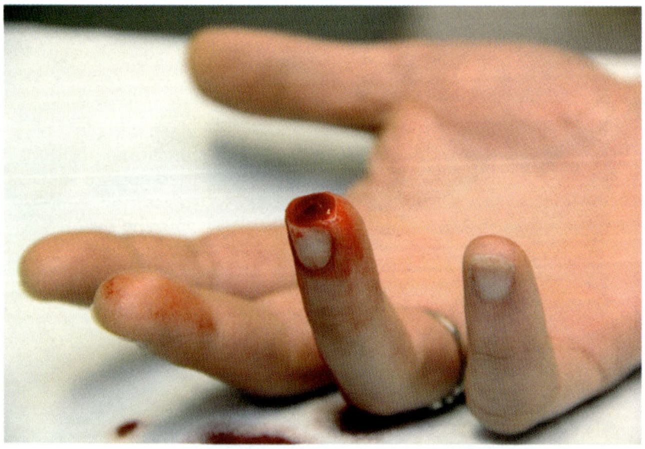

Fig. 48.7 This very minimal amputation of the fat pad with a mandolin slicer does not involve bone or the nail bed and is a common injury. It will heal very well with conservative therapy. No skin grafting is required. It will require a few weeks to heal, with periodic cleaning and debridement. Note: The ring should be removed as soon as possible.

In general, uncomplicated fingertip wounds less than 1 cm in size heal well with conservative treatment (Video 48.2). In children under 2 years of age, fingertip wounds up to 2 cm may be managed conservatively, as children in this age group have superior regenerative capacity.[34] Management is more

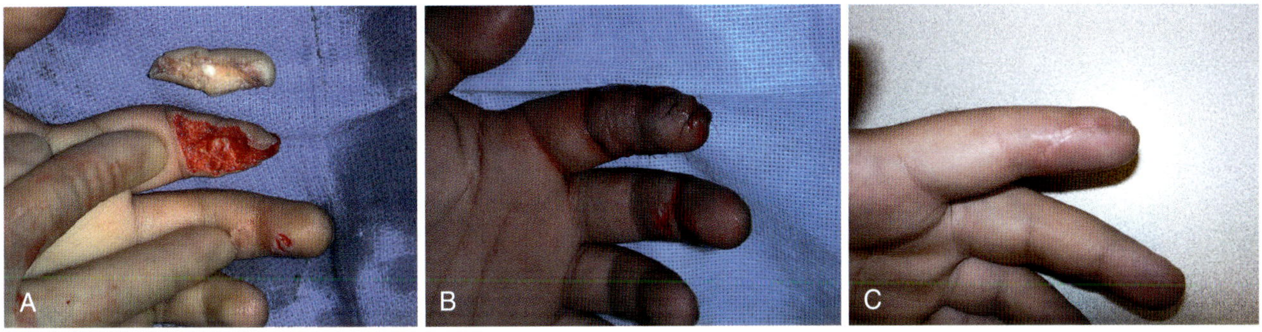

Fig. 48.8 This patient with significant volar tissue loss required microsurgical replantation. (A) Tamai level 2 volar oblique pulp amputation. (B) After completion of microsurgical replantation. (C) Four-month follow-up. (From Peterson SL, Peterson EL, Wheatley MJ. Management of fingertip amputations. *J Hand Surg Am.* 2014;39(10):2093-2101.)

challenging when there is significant loss of skin and soft tissue from the finger pad.

Volar skin is unique in its combination of toughness and sensitivity. Wounds with a significant loss of volar tissue frequently require additional treatment (Fig. 48.8). If there is significant soft tissue loss on the volar aspect of the distal finger, completion amputation and closure by a hand specialist provides the quickest recovery. In these cases, ablation of the nail bed and digital nerve transection are generally required to prevent hook nail deformity and painful neuroma formation, respectively.[34] Alternatives to completion amputation include partial-thickness skin grafts, full-thickness skin grafts, Atasoy-Kleinert V-Y flap, Kutler lateral V-Y flap, Moberg flap, or other local and distal flap coverage techniques. Semiocclusive dressings and digital caps are also being utilized with excellent outcomes.[20,34–39] A composite graft is another reconstructive option in children, where the amputated part is sutured back to the stump without formal microvascular repair. The tip may potentially necrose but serves as a biological dressing. In adults, composite graft may be attempted after the amputated portion is defatted but outcomes are inferior to those in children.[40] Although traditionally some type of grafting or advancement techniques have been used for distal guillotine amputations, conservative management is now more common, even if some portion of bone is exposed (Fig. 48.9).

For more significant distal amputations, replanting the amputated tip preserves the nail (which enhances fingertip sensation and two-point discrimination), digit length, and joint motion, and often results in better overall functional outcomes. Moreover, survival rates of finger replantation are high (approaching 90%).[41–43] Even in cases of amputations distal to the insertion of the flexor digitorum superficialis, replants are often attempted because digit function with preserved proximal interphalangeal joint motion is enhanced by the additional length, even if the DIP joint is stiff or fused.[42,44] Additionally, active range of motion is increased if this insertion site is preserved (82 degrees compared with 25 degrees with a more proximal amputation).[12] Though young children (especially <2 years of age) potentially regenerate the distal tip, functional outcomes are also excellent after replantation.[45]

As discussed previously, incomplete transections and small distal amputations without significant soft tissue loss may heal well with conservative therapy initiated by the emergency clinician. It may require a number of weeks to totally heal, but nonoperative treatment in appropriate patients provides excellent functional and cosmetic results, minimizes recovery time, and has few complications. Debride necrotic and grossly contaminated tissue and irrigate the wound thoroughly with normal saline. If bone is left exposed without soft tissue coverage, the patient will probably need an operative procedure. Alternatively, the bone may be rongeured (shortened) to allow soft tissue coverage and primary healing with better functional recovery. The nail bed tissues should be preserved, if possible, because the presence of a nail improves hand sensation and affects the cosmetic appearance. After cleansing and careful debridement, apply an occlusive dressing directly over the wound and then bandage and splint the finger for protection. Provide tetanus prophylaxis if needed. Amputations that involve the distal phalanx are frequently treated as contaminated open fractures. However, there is no evidence that antibiotics prevent infection or are superior to careful wound care, and prophylactic or empiric antibiotics are generally not recommended.[28] Wound contraction and healing usually result in acceptable cosmetic and functional recovery in 2 to 3 weeks. Arrange appropriate follow-up to ensure adequate healing and recovery.

Partial Fingertip Amputations

The emergency clinician can also manage partial fingertip amputations distal to the DIP joint without emergent consultation. These wounds are treated in a manner similar to complete amputations. However, when the amputation has a substantial amount of undamaged tissue connecting the fingertip, use sutures or bandaging and protective splinting to carefully align and stabilize the injured fingertip. Partially amputated fingertips, especially in children, may occasionally survive and regain vascularization and sensation. The patient must be warned that the distal tip may potentially become necrotic and progress to a complete amputation. Injury to the nail bed requires special attention to ensure proper alignment. If the nail bed tissues are not aligned properly, permanently disfigured nails may result. Complete or partial nail removal may be required for the placement of sutures.

Manage dermal slice wounds (see Fig. 48.7) by gently cleansing the wound and applying antibiotic ointment and a nonadherent dressing, followed by a pressure dressing. The patient should return in 48 to 72 hours for the wound to be inspected and the dressing changed. At that time, instruct the patient on the use of nonadherent dressings that should be changed daily until functional epithelialization of the wound takes place (generally 10 to 14 days). A protective finger splint or guard also minimizes the risk for further injury and pain from trauma to the sensitive wound

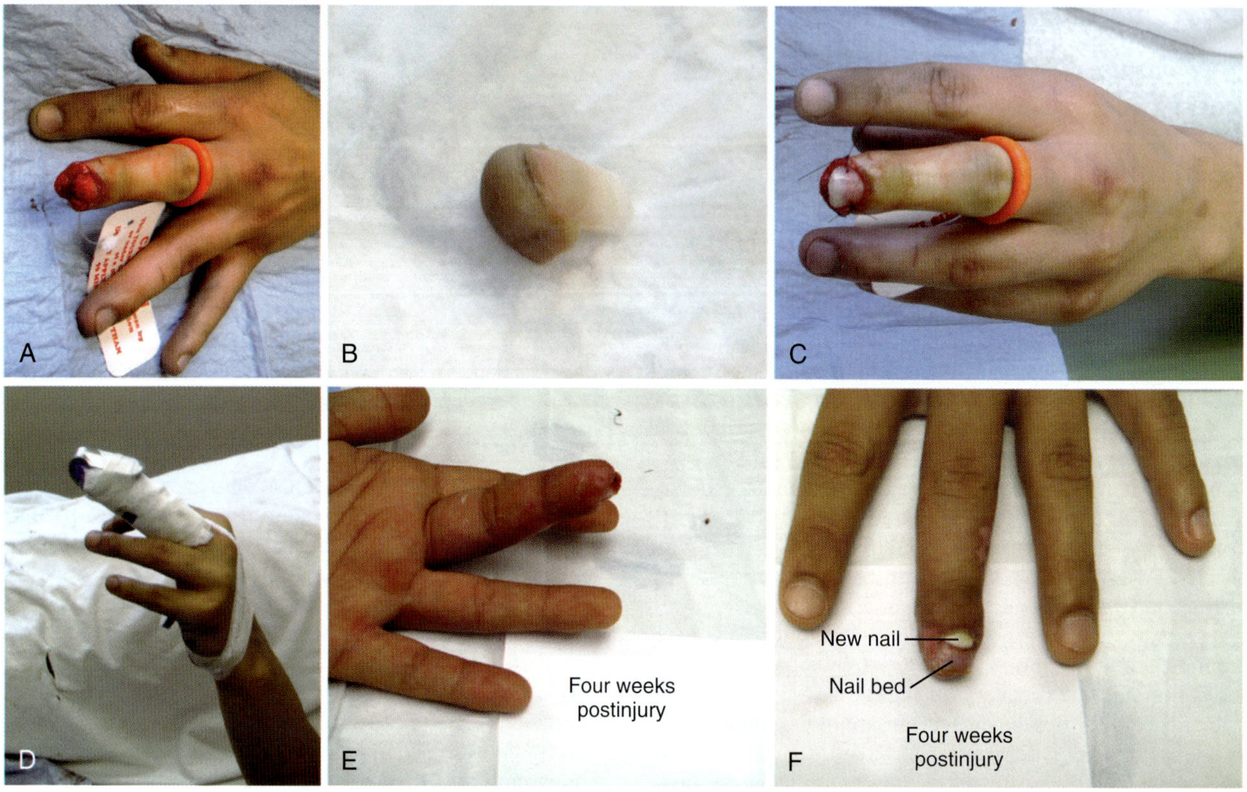

Fig. 48.9 (A) This young patient with no medical problems had his fingertip cut off by a metal press, a guillotine-type amputation that has traditionally been treated with various surgical techniques. A conservative approach is now advocated, especially in children. Note that the nail bed is now exposed because of avulsion of the nail. The distal phalanx was not injured but could be felt in the stump. (B) The avulsed tip had skin and the avulsed nail was attached. (C) After the tip was cleaned by gentle scrubbing and minor debridement of macerated tissue, the nail was dissected from the tip and sutured back under the eponychium. The amputated tip was discarded. (D) A protective splint and pressure dressing were applied. Cephalexin was given for 7 days. The patient was seen weekly for dressing changes and minor debridement. (E) At 4 weeks the finger had healed well with good sensation and an almost normal appearance. (F) The old nail was removed to reveal the growth of a new nail. At 8 weeks there was no deformity or problem, except minor shortening of the tip.

area. Protection also allows earlier return to functional use and employment. Wounds larger than 10 mm^2 and those with deep loss of digit pulp tissue may be candidates for skin grafting.

Penis, Ear, and Nose Amputations

Replantation of the penis, ear, and nose generally results in better function and cosmesis than a prosthesis or reconstructive surgery. The amputated parts and wounds should be handled in the same manner as digital amputations.

Penile amputations are uncommon; most cases are self-inflicted trauma in patients who are psychologically disturbed though punitive domestic disputes also occur. Successful replantation with microsurgical techniques is recommended. Better outcomes occur with a total ischemia time <15 hours.[46] Preservation or reconstruction of the urethra to maintain a competent urinary stream is critical for success.[46–48] The amputated penis should be managed as any other amputation with moist gauze in a waterproof bag on ice. Ears and noses are frequently partially amputated and occasionally totally amputated. Whenever possible, these body parts should be replanted unless they are severely traumatized and there is gross contamination. These wounds frequently heal well and have a high tissue survival rate and a low incidence of total necrosis. Microsurgical repair leads to improved outcomes for replantation of the ear and nose.[49–52]

COMPLICATIONS

Appropriate and expedited ED care facilitates the best possible outcome after an injury. Avoid improper management of the parts or stump and subsequent additional injury to the tissue from overzealous hemostasis or cleansing. Furthermore, avoid desiccation, maceration, or freezing of tissue from improper storage. Expedite the preoperative workup of the patient and immediately notify the replantation team, as these can be crucial factors in the patient's care.

Despite optimal initial care, replantation itself may be associated with acute or long-term complications. Multiple operations may be required, with prolonged immobilization and rigorous rehabilitation. Early surgical complications include wound infection and arterial and venous insufficiency. Late complications include cold intolerance, paresthesias, tendon adhesions, bone malunion/nonunion, neuroma formation, and contractures. Despite advanced microsurgical techniques, patients typically recover only 50% of their original function and sensation of the replanted parts, which can have negative psychosocial and economic consequences.[53]

FIELD AMPUTATIONS

Emergency physicians may be called on to perform field amputation of an extremity as a lifesaving intervention. The typical scenario is a victim who is trapped or unable to be extricated from the scene because an extremity is caught or held immobile due to debris or other heavy objects, or is lodged in a narrow space. The procedure is not detailed in this text but is contained in the video library (Videos 48.3–48.5).

ACKNOWLEDGMENT

The contributions by Dean Moore II, MD, to the previous edition are appreciated.

REFERENCES ARE AVAILABLE AT Elsevier eBooks+

CHAPTER 49

Tendon Injuries in the Hand, Wrist, Knee, and Foot

David K. Barnes and Peter E. Sokolove

EXTENSOR TENDONS OF THE HAND AND WRIST

Extensor tendons of the hand and wrist are quite superficial, covered only by skin and a thin layer of fascia, and are thus highly susceptible to injury by commonly experienced trauma. Such injuries may result from lacerations, bites, or burns, but they may also be caused by blunt injury or with seemingly superficial lacerations. The emergency physician must understand the anatomy, principles of treatment, repair technique, and postrepair care of these injuries to ensure the best possible patient outcome. For extensor tendon injuries requiring primary repair, the techniques described herein demand finesse and precision. Not all emergency physicians possess the necessary experience and comfort to perform a primary tendon repair. We recommend that most hand and wrist tendon disruptions be repaired by a hand surgeon. There may be circumstances where this is not possible because of patient or systems factors, in which case the outlined principles of tendon repair will serve as a guide based on the best available evidence from the literature. We also recommend that physicians who elect to perform primary extensor tendon repair in the emergency department (ED) discuss their plan with a consulting hand surgeon when possible to ensure all recommended treatment principles are adhered to and that close follow-up is assured. Flexor tendon lacerations should only be repaired by a hand surgeon.

Functional Anatomy

There are 12 extrinsic extensor muscles of the wrist and digits, all of which are innervated by the radial nerve. The muscles that give rise to these tendons originate in the forearm and elbow (Fig. 49.1). The extrinsic extensor tendons reach the hand and digits by passing through a fibro-osseous tendon sheath (retinaculum) located at the dorsal surface of the wrist. This synovium-lined sheath provides smooth gliding for the tendons and prevents bowstringing when the wrist is extended.[1] The dorsal retinaculum contains six compartments or subdivisions (Fig. 49.2). These compartments are numbered from the radial to the ulnar aspect of the wrist.

The first compartment contains two tendons, the abductor pollicis longus (APL) and the extensor pollicis brevis (EPB). The APL tendon is the most radial of the extensor tendons and inserts on the base of the thumb metacarpal. It is easily palpated just distal to the radial tubercle and adjacent to the radial artery when the thumb is abducted. The APL tendon permits thumb abduction and extension and some radial wrist deviation. The EPB travels with the APL through the first compartment but inserts on the base of the proximal phalanx of the thumb. The EPB tendon can be palpated over the dorsum of the thumb at the metacarpal when the thumb is extended against resistance. Both tendons can be tested by having the patient spread the fingers apart against resistance.

The second compartment also contains two tendons: the extensor carpi radialis brevis (ECRB) and the extensor carpi radialis longus (ECRL). These two tendons arise from the lateral epicondyle of the elbow. The ECRL inserts on the base of the index finger metacarpal, while the ECRB inserts on the base of the middle (long) finger metacarpal. Both tendons are powerful wrist extensors, and the ECRL also allows some radial wrist deviation. Wrist extension plays an especially important role in the mechanics of hand function because hand-grip strength is maximal only when the wrist is extended.

The third compartment contains only the extensor pollicis longus (EPL), which crosses over the ECRB and ECRL and travels along the dorsum of the thumb to insert on the distal phalanx. The EPL forms the dorsal boundary of the anatomic snuffbox; the volar boundary is formed by the EPB. The EPL can be visualized when the thumb is extended, and its strength can be tested by having the patient extend the interphalangeal (IP) joint against resistance. APL, an intrinsic extensor of the thumb, can provide some degree of extension at the IP joint. Therefore if an EPL injury is suspected, it is important to compare extension at the IP joint with that of the unaffected thumb.

The fourth and fifth compartments contain the six tendons that extend the index, middle, ring, and little (small) fingers. Each finger has its own extensor digitorum communis (EDC) tendon. The index and little fingers have an additional independent extensor tendon: extensor indicis proprius (EIP) for the index finger, and extensor digiti minimi (EDM) for the little finger. The fourth compartment contains the EIP and EDC tendons, and the fifth compartment contains only the EDM tendon. These six tendons can be seen over the dorsum of the hand where they are poorly protected and prone to injury. The tendinous, ligamentous, and fascial connections between these tendons, known as the *juncturae tendinum*, create redundant interconnections. Consequently, a patient may be able to extend a digit, albeit weakly, even when there is a complete laceration of its EDC tendon. To avoid missing a tendon injury on the dorsum of the hand, it is important to test for tendon strength against resistance and not just for active extension.

The course of the extensor tendons along the fingers is more complex, but a basic understanding of this anatomy is essential for the evaluation and treatment of extensor tendon injuries (Fig. 49.3). The EIP tendon joins its respective EDC tendon at the level of the metacarpophalangeal (MCP) joint in the index finger. Similarly, the EDM tendon parallels the course of the EDC tendon. The four EDC tendons eventually insert at the base of the proximal, middle, and distal phalanges. The most proximal insertion of the EDC tendon is at the level of the base of the proximal phalanx, and it inserts in two ways. First, there is a loose dorsal insertion just distal to the MCP joint. In addition, the EDC tendon inserts into the volar plate via the sagittal band. The sagittal band is a circumferential ligament at the level of the metacarpal head that keeps the EDC tendon centered over the metacarpal head and provides a stable connection with the volar plate located on the palmar aspect of the joint. After its primary insertion at the level of the MCP joint, the EDC tendon extends dorsally along the length of the digit trifurcating over the proximal phalanx

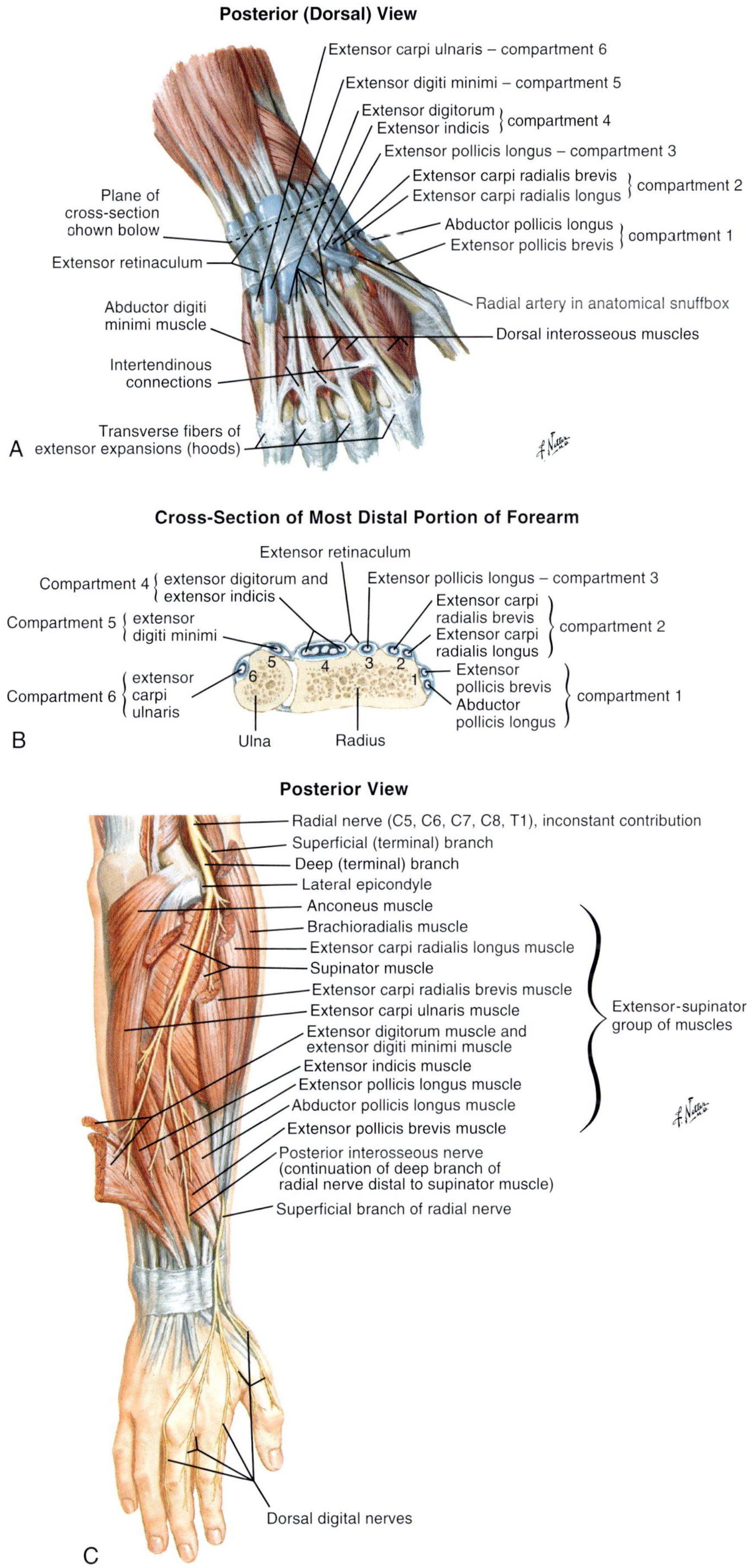

Fig. 49.1 Extensor muscles and tendons of the right wrist and hand. (A) Posterior (dorsal) view. (B) Cross-section of the most distal portion of the forearm. (C) Radial nerve in the forearm: posterior view. (Netter illustrations from www.netterimages.com. Elsevier Inc. All rights reserved.)

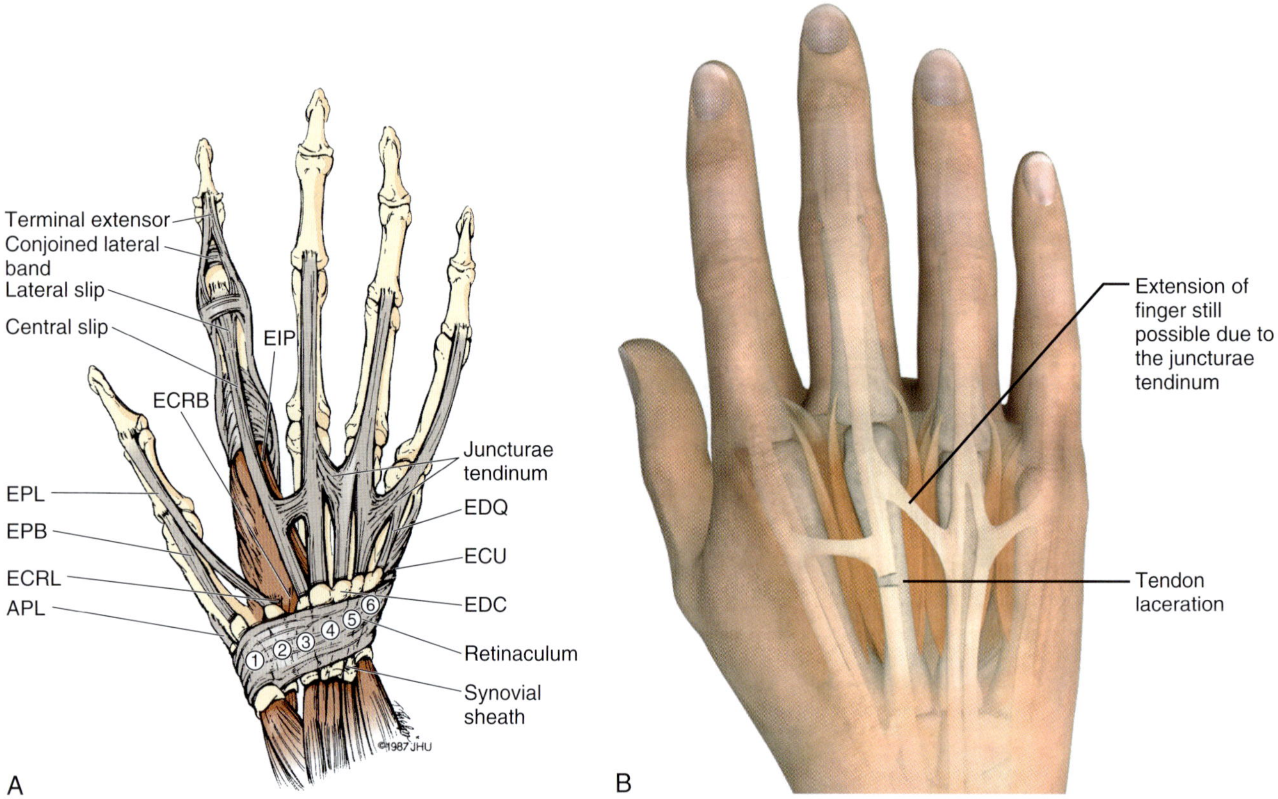

Fig. 49.2 (A) The extensor mechanism at the wrist and dorsum of the right hand. The six extensor compartments at the wrist contain *(1)* the abductor pollicis longus *(APL)* and extensor pollicis brevis *(EPB)*, *(2)* the extensor carpi radialis longus *(ECRL)* and extensor carpi radialis brevis *(ECRB)*, *(3)* the extensor pollicis longus *(EPL)*, *(4)* the extensor digitorum communis *(EDC)* II to V and the extensor indicis proprius *(EIP)*, *(5)* the extensor digiti quinti *(EDQ)*, and *(6)* the extensor carpi ulnaris *(ECU)*. An important anatomic detail is the presence of a synovial sheath around each tendon unit within each fibro-osseous canal. Note that the EDQ is also called the extensor digiti minimi by some authors. (B) Note that the juncturae tendinum allows some weak extension of the finger when the proximal extensor is completely lacerated. (A, Adapted from Thomas JS, Peimer CA. Extensor tendon injuries: acute repair and late reconstruction. In: Chapman MW, ed. *Operative Orthopaedics*. 3rd ed. JB Lippincott; 2001:1487.)

(Fig. 49.4). Its major central slip then inserts on the base of the middle phalanx (Fig. 49.5). The two lateral branches of the EDC tendon join with the lateral bands from the interossei muscles and lumbricals to form the conjoined lateral bands. The two conjoined lateral bands then fuse over the middle phalanx to form the terminal extensor mechanism (TEM) that inserts on the dorsal base of the distal phalanx (Fig. 49.6). The triangular ligament is a connection between the two conjoined lateral bands that assists in keeping these structures on the dorsal aspect of the digit.

The sixth dorsal compartment of the wrist contains only the extensor carpi ulnaris (ECU) tendon, which originates from the lateral epicondyle of the elbow and inserts on the base of the little finger metacarpal. The ECU functions to extend and ulnar deviate the wrist. It can be palpated just distal to the tip of the ulna, and its strength can be tested by forced ulnar deviation of the wrist.

General Approach to Extensor Tendon Injuries

The key to detecting extensor tendon injuries in the ED is to perform a careful and thorough history and physical examination. These injuries are easy to miss with a cursory examination. Closed injuries and some lacerations may appear innocuous at first but can result in tendon injuries that may lead to severe deformities or dysfunction if undetected (Figs. 49.7–49.9). Closed injuries can also be associated with fractures. A hand radiograph is recommended for closed hand injuries when a fracture is suspected, or for open hand injuries in which a fracture or foreign body is suspected. Open injuries that result from glass should be radiographed. Plain radiographs have a sensitivity of up to 98% for detecting radiopaque foreign bodies (e.g., gravel, glass, metal).[2]

Injuries to extensor tendons from lacerations are quite common, especially on the dorsum of the hand where the tendons are located superficially. All dorsal wrist, hand, and digit lacerations should be assumed to have an underlying tendon laceration until proved otherwise. Digital extension, albeit weak, can still occur with partial tendon lacerations of up to 90%, so visualization of the tendon and careful strength testing are required to definitively rule out a partial injury. In some cases, the specific diagnosis cannot be made on the first examination (this will be discussed later). Digit extension via the juncturae tendinum is still possible even with complete laceration of an EDC tendon on the dorsum of the hand.

After assessing the strength and neurovascular status of the injured hand, it is imperative to visually inspect the wound

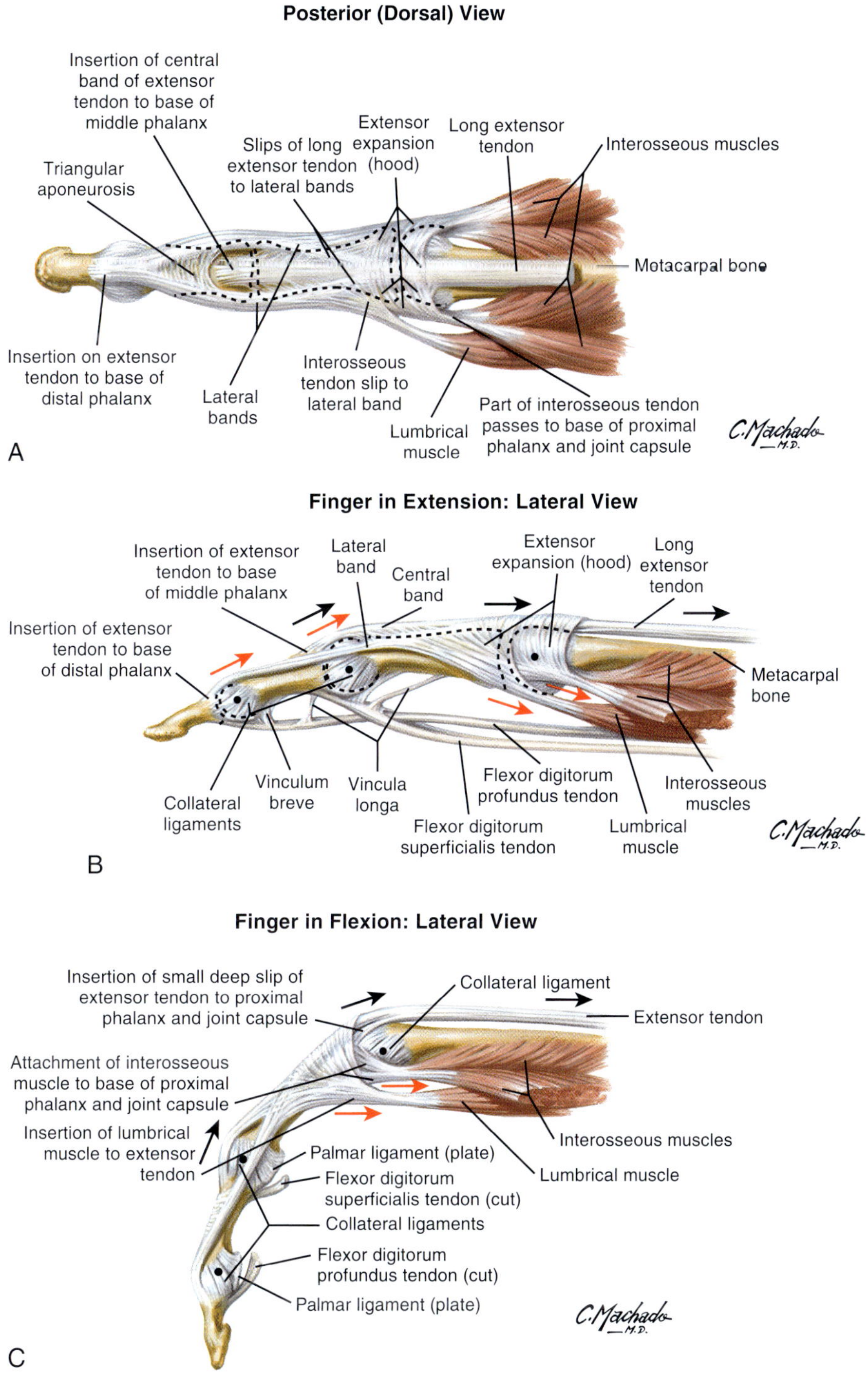

Fig. 49.3 Flexor and extensor tendons in the fingers. (A) Posterior (dorsal) view. (B) Finger in extension: lateral view. (C) Finger in flexion: lateral view. Note the directions of force when the extensor tendon is activated *(arrows)*. (Netter illustrations from www.netterimages.com. Elsevier Inc. All rights reserved.)

thoroughly. Inspection should include an assessment of the degree of wound contamination, a search for foreign bodies, and inspection for occult tendon lacerations (if not already identified). It may be necessary to extend a skin laceration to aid in the visualization of a possible tendon injury, though this should be done carefully and only to the extent necessary to visualize a tendon laceration. Because an extensor tendon is a mobile structure, it is imperative to visualize it in its entirety through its full range of motion if it is exposed. It is especially important to examine the tendon in the position that it occupied at the time of injury because the tendon injury frequently does not lie directly under the external skin wound (see Fig. 49.8).

Ultrasound is commonly used in the diagnosis of suspected tendon lacerations in the hand because it is noninvasive and provides point-of-care analysis.[3] Ultrasound has the added advantage of facilitating dynamic evaluation of tendons through their range of motion.[4] In a study of 34 patients with

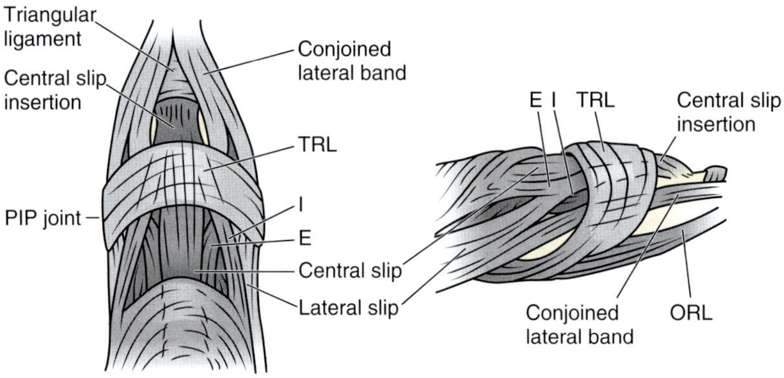

Fig. 49.4 Zone of convergence of the digital extensor mechanism, which begins at approximately the midportion of the proximal phalanx and ends at the level of the insertion of the central slip into the dorsal base of the middle phalanx. Proximal to the zone of convergence, the extrinsic and intrinsic components of the extensor mechanism are separate: the central slip is extrinsic, whereas the lateral slips are intrinsic. Within the zone of convergence there is complete reciprocal crossover of fibers from the central slip and lateral slips. The products of the completed convergence are the central slip insertion and the conjoined lateral bands, both of which have dual muscular activity. *E*, Extrinsic contribution to the conjoined lateral bands; *I*, intrinsic contribution to the insertion of the central slip; *ORL*, oblique retinacular ligament; *PIP*, proximal interphalangeal; *TRL*, transverse retinacular ligament. (From Thomas JS, Peimer CA. Extensor tendon injuries: acute repair and late reconstruction. In: Chapman MW, ed. *Operative Orthopaedics*. 3rd ed. JB Lippincott; 2001:1500.)

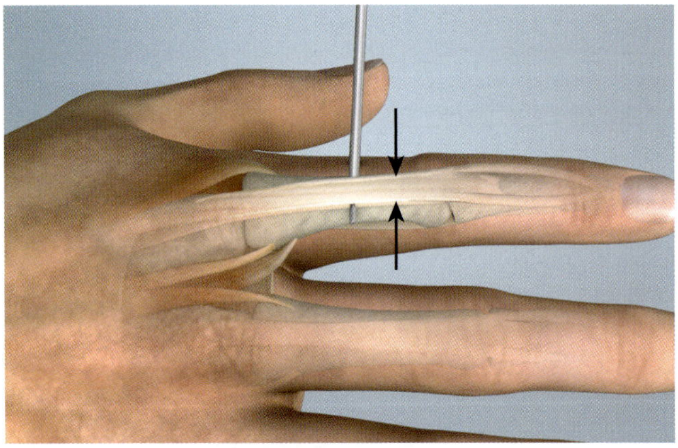

Fig. 49.5 The extensor mechanism on the dorsum of a finger. *Arrows* point to the radial and ulnar lateral band portions of the extensor mechanism, and the probe is lifting the entire structure up off the phalanx.

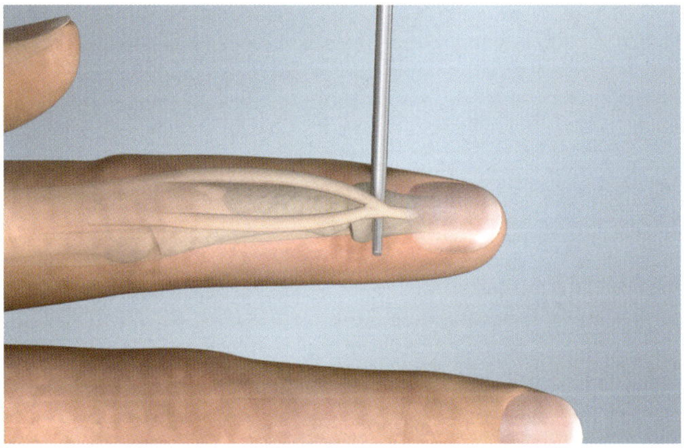

Fig. 49.6 Terminal extensor mechanism.

upper extremity tendon injuries treated by emergency physicians, ultrasound was faster and more accurate than exploration, magnetic resonance imaging (MRI), and specialty consultation.[5] Accuracy of sonography for detection of hand and digit tendon injuries greatly depends on operator experience. The process for interrogating tendons using ultrasound is discussed in detail below.

Definitive examination of any wound must occur under the best possible conditions. A bright light source, a bloodless field, adequate anesthesia, and a relaxed and cooperative patient are essential. It may be impossible to assess some patients completely during the ED visit. The examination may be limited by the patient's pain, swelling, anxiety, or altered sensorium. Therefore it would not be considered standard to diagnose the presence or the full extent of all extensor tendon injuries immediately. In some situations, the final diagnosis will be delayed until the proper circumstances permit the required conditions. Whenever logistically possible, emergency physicians should consult a specialist when an extensor tendon injury is suspected by mechanism, location of the wound, or tendon dysfunction. Under most circumstances, however, immediate on-site consultation with a hand or orthopedic surgeon is not necessary because the scenario would similarly limit any clinician's diagnostic acumen.

If the examining clinician suspects, but is unable to locate, a tendon laceration, or if a patient is unable to cooperate with the examination and the circumstances prohibit ideal initial care, patients should be referred for close follow-up for a repeat examination. In this circumstance, provide any necessary wound care, close the skin, and apply a splint to stabilize the injury. A delay of a few days for definitive diagnosis, surgical repair, or both, does not result in any significant alteration in the outcome. Delayed primary repair, without the need for tendon grafting or tendon transfer, is a well-accepted technique. In fact, many hand surgeons are reluctant to immediately repair even a complete extensor tendon laceration in a contused, potentially contaminated wound. The exact time frame under which such delayed repair results in an outcome

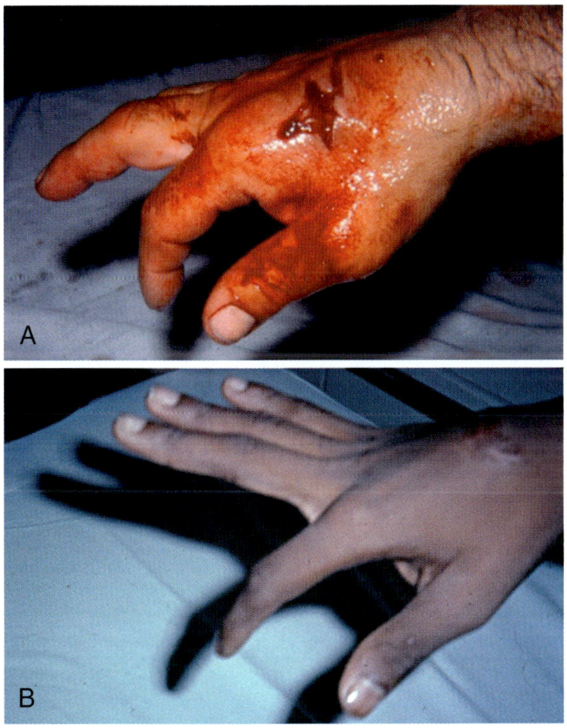

Fig. 49.7 Because of their superficial location, it is difficult to avoid at least partial injury to the extensor tendons with even superficial lacerations of the dorsum of the wrist, hand, or fingers. (A) This complete extensor tendon laceration is obvious because the index finger cannot be extended. (B) This partial tendon laceration was not appreciated on initial examination, which seemingly demonstrated full tendon function. The entire tendon could not be visualized because of an uncooperative patient. The unappreciated partial laceration progressed to a complete rupture by the time of suture removal. Expeditious delayed primary repair resulted in a good outcome.

similar to that of immediate repair has not been well defined and is best determined by the consulting surgeon. Emergency physicians should clearly document the inability to rule out a tendon injury in the ED and the mandate for follow-up within a specified time frame on the medical record and discharge instructions.[6]

Use of Antibiotics

There are no data to support or refute the use of prophylactic or empiric antibiotics for clean wounds without contamination as a routine adjunct after tendon injury. In general, prophylactic antibiotics have not been demonstrated to reduce infection rates after soft tissue injury in the setting of proper wound cleaning, nor have they been proven to reduce infection rates in the absence of gross contamination, retained foreign material, extensive contusion, or a delay in cleaning. Many physicians prescribe prophylactic antibiotics with gram-positive (e.g., antistaphylococcal) coverage if a tendon has been injured or sutured, but no universally accepted standard of care exists and an individualized approach is therefore advocated.[7] Prophylaxis is generally used for 3 to 5 days after injury absent extenuating circumstances such as immunocompromise, diabetes, a human bite, an unusual source of contamination, or peripheral vascular disease. If the sterility of a wound is in doubt, do not attempt tendon repair.

Preparation for Repair

Before attempting repair of an open extensor tendon injury in the ED, preparation and proper equipment are essential. Place the patient on a gurney that ideally has an arm board attached. Bright overhead lighting is necessary for effective wound exploration so that the presence of tendon injuries and foreign bodies can be adequately assessed. Instruments should ideally include a needle driver, two skin hooks and retractors, sharp (i.e., iris) and blunt-nosed scissors, several small hemostats, and one pair of small single-toothed (i.e., Adson) forceps.

The choice of suture material depends on the location of the tendon injury. For repair of complete tendon injuries on the dorsum of the hand, non-absorbable, synthetic braided suture is preferred.[8] Polyester suture, such as Ethibond (Ethicon) or Mersilene (Ethicon), is commonly recommended. Nylon suture is acceptable but less ideal because colored nylon may be visible under the skin. Do not use chromic or plain gut because these may react unfavorably with surrounding skin and may dissolve before the tendon heals. Silk is not desirable because of its reactivity. Most extensor tendons on the dorsum of the hand will accommodate 4-0 suture, but 5-0 suture material may be needed for smaller tendons. Small, "plastic repair" tapered needles are preferred, if available, to avoid tearing the tendon. Partial tendon injuries in the digits are best repaired with fine, synthetic absorbable suture such as polyglactin (Vicryl, Ethicon). Complex lacerations that involve tissue loss and fraying of the tendon margins (e.g., table saw injuries) represent a particularly challenging situation that may make an otherwise straightforward tendon repair more difficult. In these cases, Lalonde and Kozin recommend closing the lacerated skin and tendon together (i.e., dermatotenodesis). Take large, composite bites of skin and tendon together, 5 mm to 10 mm on either side of the wound, with 3-0 or 4-0 nylon suture tied outside the skin. Tighten the suture until the digit is in full extension.[9]

Before wound exploration or tendon repair, it is important to achieve adequate anesthesia. Many hand surgeons prefer the WALANT (wide awake, local anesthetic, no tourniquet) technique for anesthesia in which 1% lidocaine with 1:100,000 epinephrine buffered with 8.4% sodium bicarbonate is slowly infiltrated proximal to the region of interest. Adopters of this technique note fewer postoperative tendon ruptures, lower rates of tenolysis for adhesions, the ability to educate patients intraoperatively how to avoid rupturing repairs, and improved surgical technique and repair integrity because of the ability to identify and close repair gaps.[10] A standard field block or regional nerve block can also be used to anesthetize the dorsum of the hand, whereas local anesthesia or a digital nerve block can be used to anesthetize the fingers. It is important that the digits be fully anesthetized or, in the case of more proximal wounds on the hand, that the area around the wound be liberally anesthetized because many lacerations must be extended to afford access to the surgical field. It is a common error to avoid extending a laceration and to attempt examination, cleaning, or repair through a small initial skin laceration.

The choice of anesthetic composition has been the subject of long-standing controversy. Traditional teaching warned that epinephrine-containing anesthetic causes digital ischemia. However, surgeons have used epinephrine-containing anesthetics in the hand and fingers without complications for many years, and there is ample evidence supporting the safety profile and benefits of using epinephrine for digital anesthesia,

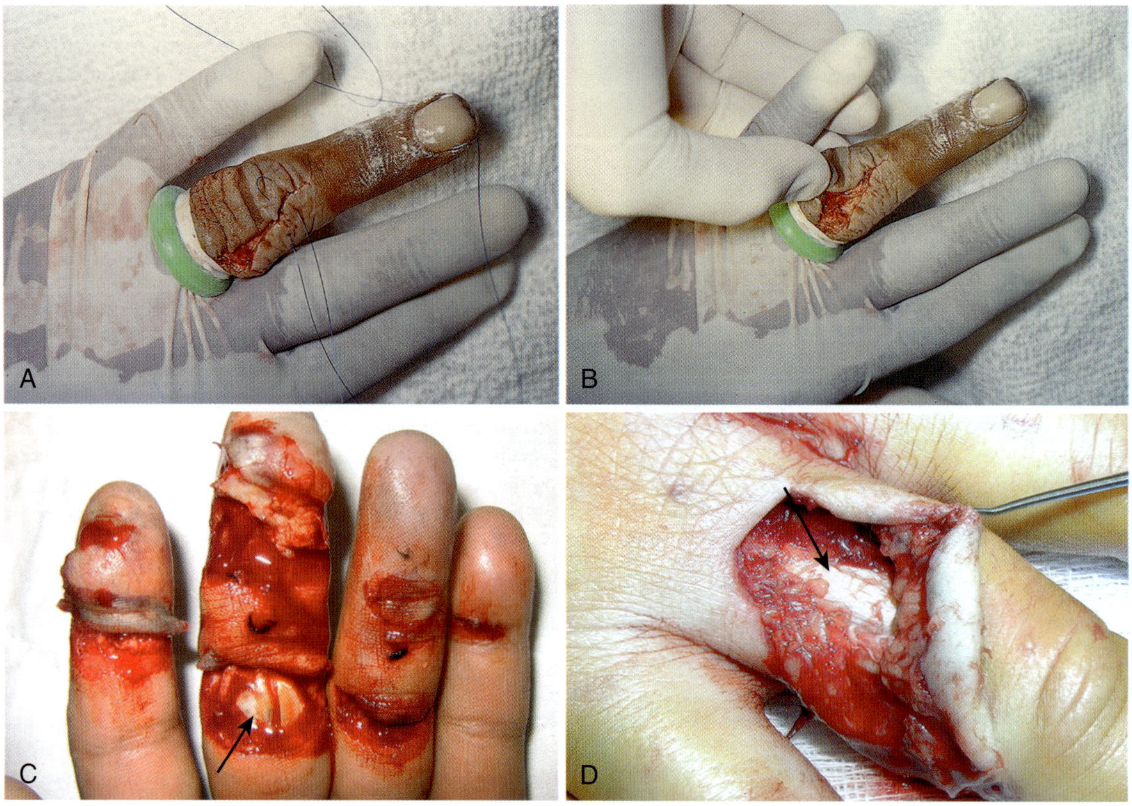

Fig. 49.8 To examine for a tendon injury, use a bloodless field. Note the sterile glove on the patient to maintain a clean field. It is almost impossible to cut the dorsum of the hand or fingers and avoid at least a partial tendon injury. (A) The location and depth of this laceration suggest an extensor tendon injury. On examination, the patient had full extension. (B) No tendon injury is visualized when the laceration was examined with the fingers in extension. When the laceration was extended and probed with the finger flexed, a 60% laceration of the extensor tendon could be viewed in the depths of the wound. (C–D) Note the typical shiny white appearance of the fully exposed tendons *(arrows)*.

especially with the advent of phentolamine rescue. In fact, the WALANT technique derives much of its benefit from the addition of epinephrine, which has the benefit of prolonging the anesthetic effect and promoting a bloodless field during wound exploration and repair.[10,11]

A bloodless field is important for adequate examination and repair of lacerated tendons. It is very difficult to find the proximal end of a retracted tendon in a bloody field. If hemostasis remains a problem after administration of epinephrine-containing local anesthetic, a tourniquet may be placed on the involved limb (see Fig. 49.8). If a tourniquet is used, wrap the patient's arm in several layers of cast padding as a comfort measure and elevate the arm for at least 1 minute to allow blood to drain by gravity prior to inflating the tourniquet. Alternatively, wrap the injured extremity from distal to proximal using an elastic bandage to exsanguinate the extremity prior to tourniquet application. Place a blood pressure cuff on the middle to upper part of the arm, wrap several more layers of cast padding around the cuff, then inflate to the limb occlusion pressure (LOP), the pressure at which the distal arterial blood flow, assessed by Doppler, is occluded. A safety margin to ensure a bloodless field is then added. If LOP is <130 mm Hg, the safety margin is 40 mm Hg; for LOP 131 to 190 mm Hg, the margin is 60 mm Hg; and if LOP is >190 mm Hg, the margin is 80 mm Hg. A margin of 50 mm Hg has been recommended for pediatric patients.[12] Once inflated, clamp the tubes of the tourniquet tightly with a hemostat. The use of cast padding during inflation helps avoid premature opening of the cuff. Use of a hemostat to clamp the blood pressure cuff tubes helps avoid cuff deflation. A blood pressure cuff tourniquet is generally well tolerated by patients for approximately 15 to 20 minutes. When longer periods are needed, a tourniquet should be let down for 5 minutes for every 30 minutes of application time.[12] If tendon repair cannot be accomplished in a single application cycle, it is likely that the injury is too complex for repair in the ED. When necessary, use parenteral analgesia or anxiolysis to help the patient tolerate a longer tourniquet time. For finger injuries, a rubber ring tourniquet at the base of the finger usually provides excellent hemostasis. Tourniquet use is relatively contraindicated in limbs with severe infection, patients with poor cardiac reserve, and severely traumatized limbs. Likewise, avoid tourniquets when possible in patients with peripheral neuropathy, deep vein thrombosis (DVT) in the affected limb, Reynaud's disease, and peripheral vascular disease.

Atraumatic surgical technique will help to minimize adhesions and scar tissue formation. Tendons should be handled delicately, avoiding crushing force or excessive punctures with forceps and needles. Forceps should be used only on the exposed, cut end of the tendon whenever possible.[13]

Patterns of Injury and Management

Treatment of extensor tendon injury depends primarily on whether the injury is open or closed, as well as the anatomic

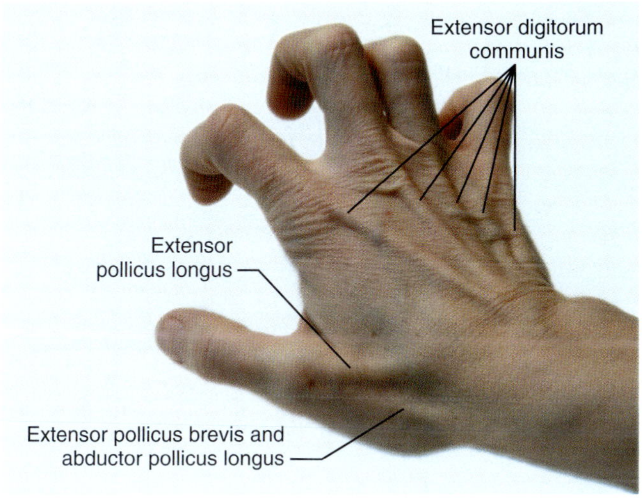

Fig. 49.9 Given the superficial location of extensor tendons, suspect a tendon injury even with seemingly superficial lacerations of the dorsum of the hand and fingers. Full function is possible with a significant tendon laceration, and delayed total rupture can occur days to weeks later if the injury is not repaired or splinted. Most partial extensor tendon lacerations do well with 3 to 4 weeks of splinting and no surgical repair. When in doubt, clean the laceration, suture the skin, splint, and refer for subsequent examination in a few days.

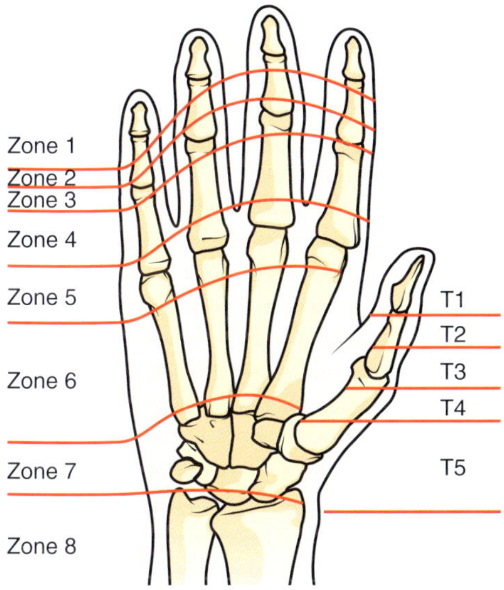

Fig. 49.10 Dorsum of the left hand. The injury classification system recommended by Verdan[14] includes eight anatomically based zones. (Adapted from Blair WF, Steyers CM. Extensor tendon injuries. *Orthop Clin North Am.* 1992;23:142.)

location of the injury. The most widely accepted classification system is that developed by Verdan,[14] which divides the hand and wrist into eight anatomical zones (Fig. 49.10). It is quite useful for emergency physicians to become familiar with this classification because in many instances the zone of injury can help determine whether tendon repair should even be attempted in the ED. For tendon injuries beyond the capability the emergency physician to repair, initial care in the ED should consist of sterile skin preparation, copious wound irrigation and inspection for foreign bodies, skin closure, splint application, and urgent referral to a hand specialist for further care. A plaster, metallic, or fiberglass splint in which a metal foam finger splint is incorporated is an ideal way to totally immobilize a finger (Fig. 49.11).

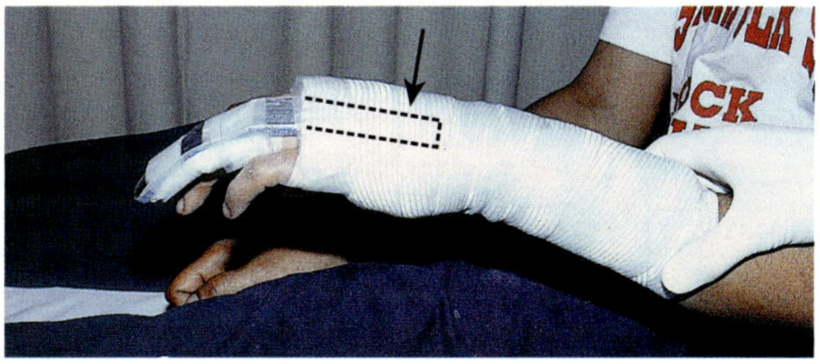

Fig. 49.11 An effective way to fully immobilize a finger with a tendon laceration is to incorporate an aluminum foam splint into the middle layers *(arrow)* of a standard dorsal plaster/fiberglass short-arm dorsal splint.

Zone 7 and 8 Injuries

Zones 7 and 8 consist of the area over the wrist and the dorsal aspect of the distal forearm, respectively.[1] Extensor tendon lacerations in these regions can be quite complex and therefore should not be repaired by emergency physicians. Because of the proximity to extensor tendons in the distal part of the forearm, lacerations such as stab wounds may appear innocuous but can result in multiple tendon lacerations. At the wrist level, the extensor tendons are covered by a retinaculum that is lined with synovium. Although this tissue allows smooth gliding of tendons during normal activity, the presence of synovium increases the risk for adhesions after tendon repair. In addition, lacerated tendons in the wrist and distal part of the forearm may retract away from the site of initial injury. This may make tendon retrieval and repair quite difficult and necessitate incision of the retinaculum and exploration of one or more compartments.

As a result of the potential complexity of these injuries, all tendon lacerations in zones 7 and 8 require surgical exploration and repair. ED management of these patients includes local wound care with primary repair of the skin, placement of a volar splint in 35 degrees of extension at the wrist and 10 to 15 degrees of flexion at the MCP joints, and prompt referral to a hand surgeon for definitive repair.

Zone 6 Injuries

Zone 6 consists of the area over the dorsum of the hand. [1,8,15] Extensor tendon injuries in this region are frequently caused by lacerations from broken glass or other sharp objects. Common pitfalls in ED management of these injuries usually relate to failed recognition that the tendon has been injured. It is important to remember that these tendons are located superficially, partial tendon lacerations may occur, and weak extension of a digit is possible with a complete tendon laceration because of transfer of extensor function through the juncturae tendinum. Lacerations of the EIP or EDM tendons are evidenced by an inability to extend independently the index or little finger, respectively. In most cases, missing zone 6 injuries can be avoided if a careful physical examination is performed, including thorough wound exploration with adequate local anesthesia and good lighting. When in doubt, splint and refer for a delayed secondary exam.

Of all extensor tendon injuries, those in zone 6 are generally the most appropriate for repair by emergency physicians. Because of the juncturae tendinum, extensor tendons in zone 6 are less likely to retract than those in zones 7 or 8; however, a severed tendon may retract when the injury is more proximal. The distal end of a severed tendon is usually easy to find by passively extending the patient's affected digit to bring the end into view. Retrieval of the proximal portion

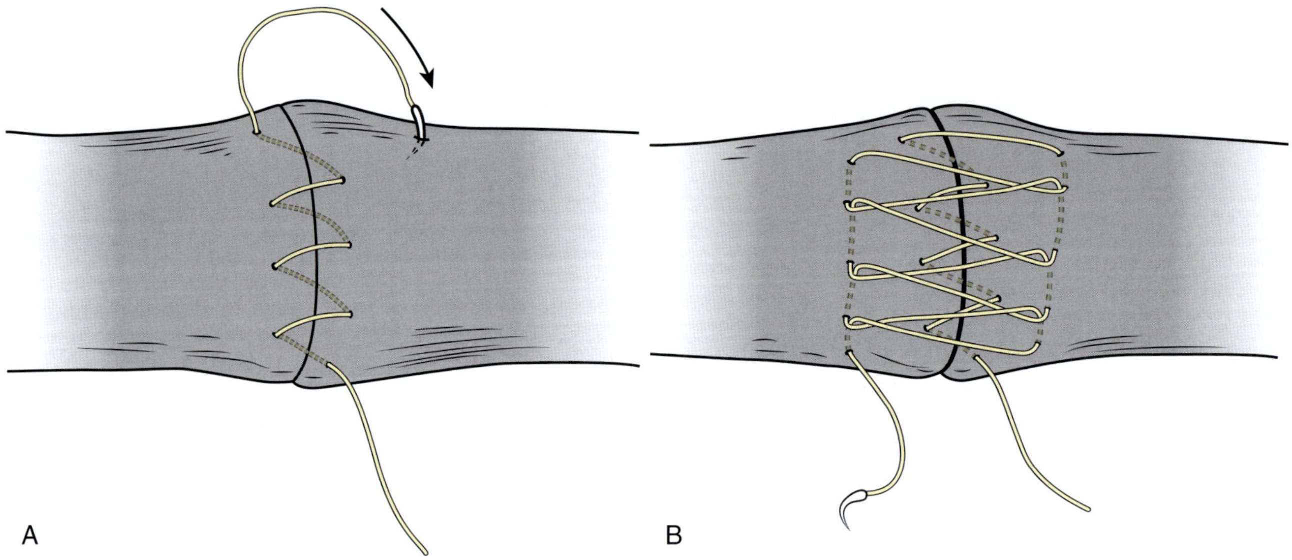

Fig. 49.12 The running interlocking horizontal mattress suture (RIHM). (A) Begin the repair with a simple running suture directed away from the clinician. (B) Complete the repair by placing a running mattress suture back toward the clinician, interlocking each returning throw underneath the previously crossed suture to lock each throw. (From Lee SK, Dubey A, Kim BH, et al. A biomechanical study of extensor tendon repairs: introduction to the running interlocking horizontal mattress extensor tendon repair technique. *J Hand Surg Am.* 2010;35(1):19-23.)

of a severed tendon is sometimes required but should be done with care to avoid damaging the ends of the tendon and surrounding tissue. It is often necessary to use a scalpel to extend the skin wound proximally in a direction parallel to the course of the injured tendon to obtain adequate exposure. One should then begin to search for the tendon by lifting up this overlying skin with forceps and inspecting the proximal portion of the wound. Sometimes the blood-stained end of a tendon tunnel can be seen; this may contain the proximal end of the tendon. By gently placing a small hemostat or toothed forceps up this tunnel, the tendon stump can often be pulled into view.

Once both ends of the injured tendon have been located, the technique used for repair will depend on the size and shape of the tendon. Whereas larger, round tendons can accommodate sutures that pass through the core of the tendon, smaller or flat tendons are difficult to repair with this technique. Most tendons in zone 6 can be repaired using one of several published techniques that maximize the strength of repair and minimize the risk of adhesions and catching. A detailed description of all available tendon repair techniques is beyond the scope of this text, but emergency physicians should be familiar with some of the more common approaches such as the modified Kessler, modified Bunnell, modified (or augmented) Becker (aka Massachusetts General Hospital), and Krackow-Thomas techniques.[6,16,17]

Both the modified Bunnell and modified Kessler techniques involve first placing a single suture into one face of the cut tendon, usually 3-0 or 4-0 nonabsorbable material. Place the suture in the tendon core by inserting the suture needle into the exposed face, then weave the suture through the lateral tendon margins. Next place the same suture through the core of the opposite half of the cut tendon. Tie the suture ends in a square knot in between the cut ends of the tendon to bring the two halves together. To improve the tensile strength of the repair, various other suture techniques have been described.[8] One option is to increase the number of suture strands that cross the repair site (e.g., four strands rather than two). A cadaver study comparing various four-strand tendon repair techniques concluded that the Massachusetts General Hospital technique was more resistant to gap formation than either the Krackow-Thomas or the four-strand modified Bunnell techniques.[18] However, this cadaver model could not assess tendon shortening or subsequent range of motion.[19] Another way to improve tensile strength is to place a peripheral suture in addition to the core suture. Place a running cross-stitch suture of synthetic, absorbable material (e.g., 5-0 polyglycolic acid, polyglactin, or polydioxanone) circumferentially around the repair site or just on the dorsal surface of the tendon across the laceration site. Alternatively, place sutures laterally along both sides of the tendon starting at approximately 1 cm of either side of the repair site.

The running interlocking horizontal mattress (RIHM) technique is recommended by some authors for primary extensor tendon repair (Fig. 49.12) This method has been shown to be as strong as the modified Becker technique and was associated with a better overall result compared with other repair methods.[20] Using 4-0 nonabsorbable suture, the RIHM begins with a simple running suture directed away from the operator. Then, using the same suture, a running mattress is directed toward the examiner, interlocking each returning throw underneath the previously crossed suture to secure each pass. Tie the suture at the near end on the outside of the tendon to complete the repair. In a cadaver model of zone 6 injuries, the RIHM repair was significantly stiffer, resulted in significantly less shortening, required less tendon exposure, and took less time to perform than both the augmented Becker and modified Bunnell techniques. There was no significant difference in failure rates. This technique has the added benefit of being able to withstand the forces of early active motion during the postoperative period. It also preserved more tendon length and decreased flexion loss, potentially improving grip strength after repair.[21,22] Smaller tendons may be repaired with a figure-of-eight or horizontal mattress suture (Fig. 49.13). Use small, tapered needles to avoid tearing the tendon.

No studies demonstrate clear superiority for any particular suture technique, and not all hand surgeons agree on the repair approach, even for the same or similar injuries. The ultimate choice of repair technique will depend largely on the operator's familiarity with extensor tendon repair as well as the size of the tendon. Regardless of the chosen suture technique, it is important to test the degree of flexion passively at the MCP joint after a zone 6 tendon repair to be certain that the tendon has not been excessively shortened.

After repair of a lacerated EDC tendon in zone 6, apply a volar splint so that the wrist and injured MCP joint are held in 15 to 20 degrees of extension. If there is an isolated EIP or EDM tendon injury, only the index or little finger must be included in the splint, but a short period of immobilization of uninjured joints is acceptable. Close outpatient follow-up is important as postrepair protocols can be complex and may require coordination with a hand surgeon and physical therapist.[23] Early active motion protocols, initiated as soon as 2 days after tendon repair, result in better total active motion, stronger grip strength, and improved overall outcomes compared to static splinting.[24]

The approach to partial extensor tendon lacerations is not well defined, and no definitive standard of care exists. Given the lack of literature on the subject, a reasonable approach may be to extrapolate from data on flexor tendon injuries. It has been demonstrated that many partial flexor tendon lacerations do well without repair,[25] but hand surgeons still disagree on the need for repair of these injuries. In a survey of hand surgeons, 30% of respondents repaired all partial flexor tendon lacerations and 45% repaired only lacerations with greater than 50% involvement of the cross-sectional area.[26] Except at the wrist level, extensor tendons are not covered with synovium and are less likely than flexor tendons to form adhesions after repair. Many surgeons therefore recommend repair of most partial extensor tendon lacerations. Although the ideal approach to these injuries is not known, it is reasonable to consider repair of partial extensor tendon lacerations to be optional if less than 50% of the cross-sectional area is involved. However, if not repaired, such injuries must be splinted for 3 to 4 weeks to ensure that a partial laceration is not converted into a complete injury. Skin closure, splinting, and referral for follow-up is a standard approach to unrepaired partial extensor tendon lacerations.

Zone 5 Injuries

Zone 5 consists of the area over the MCP joint.[27,28] Open injuries in this region should be considered secondary to a human tooth bite until proved otherwise (Fig. 49.14), especially if the injury occurs over the first or second MCP joint because this is frequently the location of a clenched-fist ("fight-bite") injury. ED evaluation must begin with a careful history and physical examination as patients may be reluctant to admit to punching someone in the mouth. The wound should be inspected through its full range of motion because the positions of the EDC tendons change with hand and finger position. It is generally recommended that radiographs be obtained for all these injuries to evaluate for metacarpal head fractures, air in the joint space, or the presence of a foreign body such as a tooth fragment (Fig. 49.15).

If, after a thorough evaluation, it is determined that a human bite in this region has resulted in a superficial skin

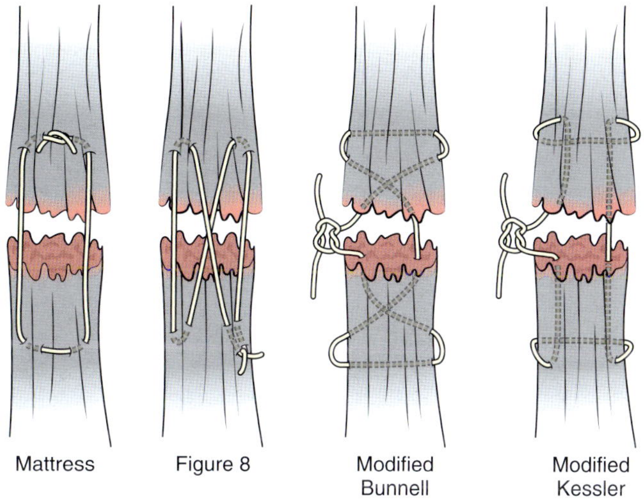

Fig. 49.13 Suture techniques used for extensor tendon repair.

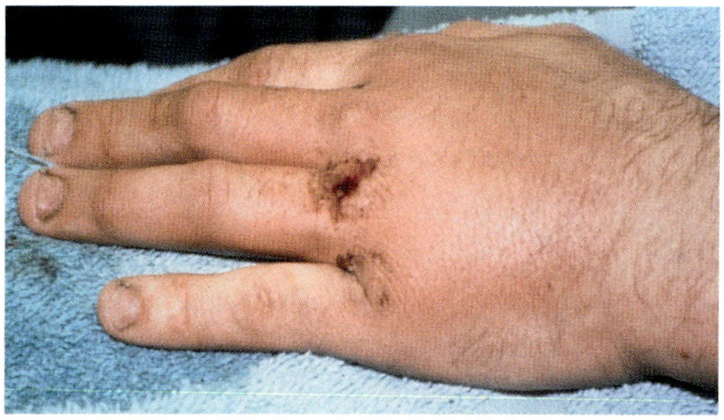

Fig. 49.14 Regardless of this patient's history, this wound is infected and highly suggestive of a human bite injury, which was vehemently denied by this patient. Human bites cause extensor tendon injuries, fractures, and joint capsule injuries and can harbor foreign bodies.

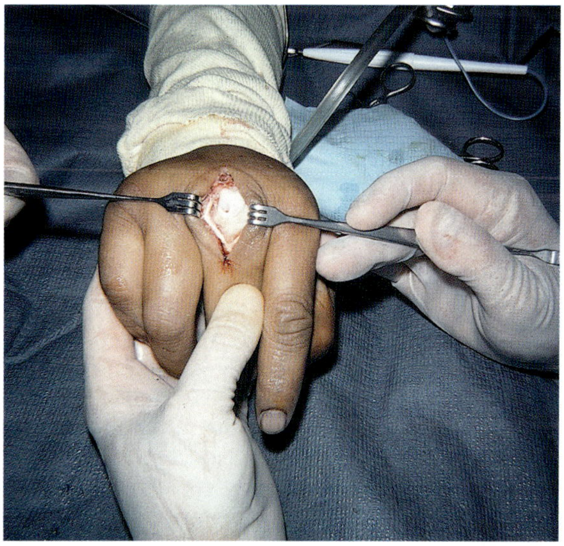

Fig. 49.15 This patient stated that he sliced his hand on a piece of metal at work (expecting a workers' compensation claim) but was unable to explain the chipped bone and piece of tooth that was found in the wound on exploration. Note that this puncture-type wound had to be significantly extended to adequately visualize the extent of the injury.

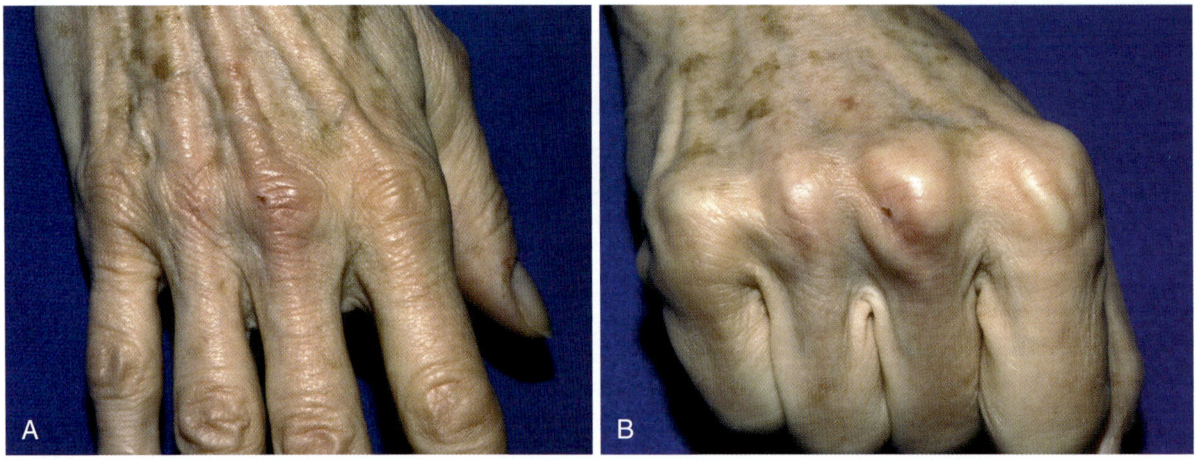

Fig. 49.16 Traumatic ulnar dislocation of the extensor digitorum tendon at the metacarpophalangeal (MCP) joint of the long finger. (A) No swelling or tenderness. The tendon is centralized. Tendon instability is not evident with the MCP joint extended. (B) Ulnar displacement of the extensor tendon increases with MCP joint flexion. (From Skirven TM. *Rehabilitation of the Hand and Upper Extremity*. 6th ed. Mosby; 2011.)

laceration only without injury to the underlying tendon or joint, outpatient management is appropriate. The wound should be copiously irrigated and left open, a volar splint applied with the wrist in 45 degrees of extension, the MCP joints in neutral position (0 degrees of flexion), and the hand dressed with a bulky dressing. The use of prophylactic antibiotics for these "low-risk" human bites on the hand is controversial, and clinical trials have yielded mixed results.[29,30] Despite the lack of compelling clinical evidence for either approach, many authors recommend at least 3 to 5 days of prophylactic antibiotics for these patients. Regardless of whether antibiotics are prescribed, patients should be seen within 36 hours for a repeat examination to evaluate for wound infection.

If a human bite results in tendon damage, either partial or complete laceration, it is reasonable to admit the patient for intravenous antibiotics even if infection is not identified. However, no specific standard of care exists. Outpatient therapy is acceptable in a reliable patient who has no evidence of infection and access to close follow-up. Delayed closure with evaluation and repair of the tendon should be undertaken by a hand surgeon after a course of antibiotic therapy.[8] Primary closure by emergency physicians of even seemingly clean and well-irrigated human bites in this region is not advised because of the increased risk for wound infection and the potential for septic destruction in cases of traumatic MCP joint arthrotomy. If an open joint is noted on physical examination, a more aggressive approach is warranted. Such patients are generally admitted for intravenous antibiotics after copious irrigation.[8] For all open zone 5 injuries, we recommend consultation with a hand surgeon to discuss the management plan and to coordinate follow-up for discharged patients. If a patient sustains a zone 5 tendon injury, and it can be determined that it was caused by a relatively clean, sharp object rather than a human bite, primary wound closure is appropriate followed by splinting as described earlier. Careful repair of lacerations involving both the EDC tendon and the sagittal band is necessary to prevent subluxation of the EDC tendon away from the center of the metacarpal head; therefore hand surgeon follow-up is recommended given the complexities of the injury and possible sequelae.

Closed extensor tendon injuries in zone 5 usually result from the acute or recurrent application of compressive force to the MCP joint capsule. Closed injuries in this region are sometimes referred to as a *boxer's knuckle*. Repetitive closed injury to the MCP joint region can produce small tears in the EDC tendon, the sagittal band, or the joint capsule. These patients tend to have chronic and recurrent pain and swelling in the MCP joint region but usually have normal radiographic findings. Acute trauma may result in the same injuries or cause more severe damage to the extensor hood. Such patients may have complete disruption of the extensor mechanism including damage to the central tendon and the sagittal band. The MCP joint is swollen, has decreased mobility, and may exhibit an extension lag. Traumatic subluxation of an EDC tendon may occur and usually involves the middle finger with ulnar subluxation (Fig. 49.16). Radial subluxation is less common, probably because of the juncturae tendinum on the ulnar side that can compensate for injuries to the sagittal band.[31] Subluxation becomes more prominent with flexion at the MCP joint. Controversy exists regarding the initial management of closed injuries in this region. Whereas some authors prefer surgical repair,[28] others use an initial trial of extension splinting.[8,27,31] Splint the affected MCP joint in extension and refer to a hand surgeon for definitive management. Operative repair is usually reserved for more delayed manifestations or patients who do not respond to splint therapy.[32]

Zone 4 Injuries

Zone 4 consists of the area over the dorsal aspect of the proximal phalanx between the MCP and proximal interphalangeal (PIP) joints.[27] The extensor tendon in this region is broad and flat and is therefore relatively easy to repair. Because the extensor tendon conforms to the roundness of the proximal phalanx, tendon injuries in this area generally result from a laceration and are almost always incomplete. As a result, extension at the PIP joint may not be impaired. It is therefore imperative that all these wounds be explored carefully while remembering that the extensor tendon lies immediately beneath the thin overlying skin. Tendons tend to not retract in this area so the injury is usually visualized on close inspection.

Hand surgeons generally repair central slip lacerations or any laceration that results in an extension deficit at the PIP joint.[32] The decision to repair a partial tendon laceration in zone 4, and whether it should be repaired by the emergency physician, is best discussed with the consulting hand surgeon. In general, because of the duality of the extensor system in this region, lacerations of a single lateral slip can either be repaired with 5-0 nonabsorbable suture or left unrepaired and splinted. Placement of running sutures or simple interrupted sutures with buried knots is appropriate for this area. As placement of core sutures is technically difficult or impossible here due to the physical properties of the tendon, other techniques such as the RIHM are recommended.[21] Patients without an extension deficit can be managed with soft tissue injury management alone with the injured PIP joint splinted in extension for 3 to 4 weeks.[32]

Splinting after tendon repair depends on the presence of tension at the repair site. Minor lacerations in zone 4 that do not result in tension on the repair site can be treated with a finger guard for 7 to 10 days and early range of motion. Larger lacerations, or those that result in tension at the repair site, should be treated with a splint that extends from the forearm to the digit. Apply the splint so that the wrist is in 30 degrees of extension, the MCP joint is at 30 degrees of flexion, and the PIP joint is in neutral position. Group the fingers so that either the index and middle fingers, or the middle, ring, and little fingers are immobilized together ensuring adequate padding between the fingers to avoid pressure necrosis of the skin.

It is important to recognize that complex partial tendon lacerations in zone 4 may result in damage to the gliding layer located between the tendon and the bone. If the patient is still able to actively extend the digit at the PIP joint, these complex partial tendon lacerations may be managed by debriding the frayed tendon ends and splinting the digit in extension rather than attempting to suture the damaged tendon. However, we recommend splinting these injuries and referring patients to a hand surgeon who can perform delayed debridement. The splint should be worn for 10 days, followed by active range of motion.

Zone 3 Injuries

Zone 3, the area over the PIP joint, is a common site of both closed and open injuries.[1,28] An open injury usually results from lacerations with a sharp object. It is important that these wounds be carefully explored in the ED to rule out penetration of the joint capsule (i.e., arthrotomy). Patients with wounds that are suspected of penetrating the joint are generally taken to the operating room for surgical exploration, irrigation, and treatment with intravenous antibiotics, but protocols vary.

Zone 3 tendon lacerations can result in long-term deformity if not carefully repaired. Partial lacerations of the central slip or lateral bands are managed variably, and it is advisable to discuss these injuries with the consulting hand surgeon. Lacerations in this area may sometimes result in a complete central slip injury. This may manifest as an acute boutonnière ("buttonhole") deformity in which the PIP joint rests in 60 degrees of flexion. The signs may be subtle and may be noticeable only by weakened extension at the PIP joint or incomplete extension by only a few degrees.

A boutonnière deformity develops when the central slip is ruptured by an open or closed mechanism that leads to unopposed action of the flexor digitorum superficialis tendon. This results in flexion at the PIP joint, protrusion of the head of the proximal phalanx between the two lateral bands, and disruption of the triangular ligament. When this occurs, the lateral bands are displaced volar to the axis of motion of the PIP joint and the lateral bands paradoxically become flexors of the PIP joint (Fig. 49.17). In addition, the extensor hood mechanism is pulled more proximally which results in increased tension on the TEM and hyperextension at the distal interphalangeal (DIP) joint. Thus a boutonnière deformity consists of flexion of the PIP joint with hyperextension of the DIP joint.

Open central slip injuries are usually managed operatively, and complex injuries may require direct attachment of the tendon to bone or tendon reconstruction. If the consulting hand surgeon chooses not to repair the tendon injury immediately, close the skin and apply a splint in the same fashion as described for zone 4 injuries. Thermoplastic splints allow immobilization of the hand without involvement of the wrist but may not be available in the ED setting. Refer these patients to a hand surgeon for prompt outpatient follow-up.

Patients with closed injuries in zone 3 are commonly encountered in the ED. They may complain of a direct blow to the dorsal PIP joint or a "jammed" finger. This injury occurs when an object such as a ball delivers a sudden axial loading force causing forced flexion of the PIP joint while it is extended. These patients commonly complain of a painful, swollen PIP joint, which often makes the examination difficult. Some of these injuries may represent PIP joint dislocations which were either manually or spontaneously reduced before the patient arrived to the ED. The tendon injury that is important to recognize in this setting is an occult, isolated central slip rupture. Patients may have decreased extension at the PIP joint, but extension is generally normal because the lateral bands are the primary extenders of this joint. With forced extension against resistance, patients usually have pain and may have decreased strength. To eliminate pain as the cause of the decreased mobility, it may be helpful to test PIP extension against resistance after performing a digital block. With acute central slip rupture, PIP joint extension may be particularly weak when the MCP and wrist joints are held in maximal flexion. In this position, a 15-degree or greater loss of active extension is highly suggestive of a central slip injury.[28]

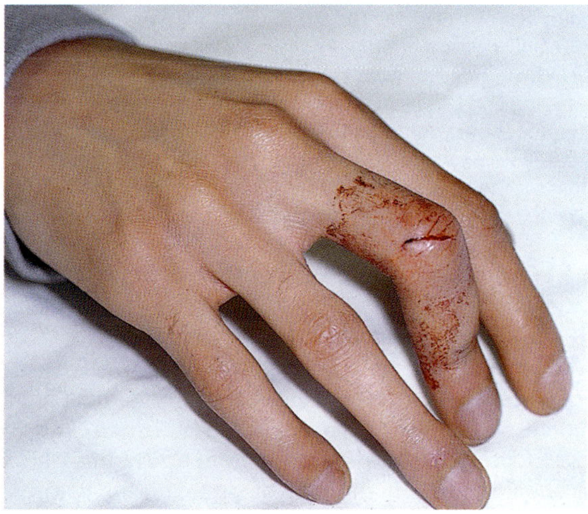

Fig. 49.17 Boutonnière deformity. This can be an open or a closed injury. Note the flexion of the proximal interphalangeal joint and extension of the distal interphalangeal joint from a laceration of the central slip mechanism.

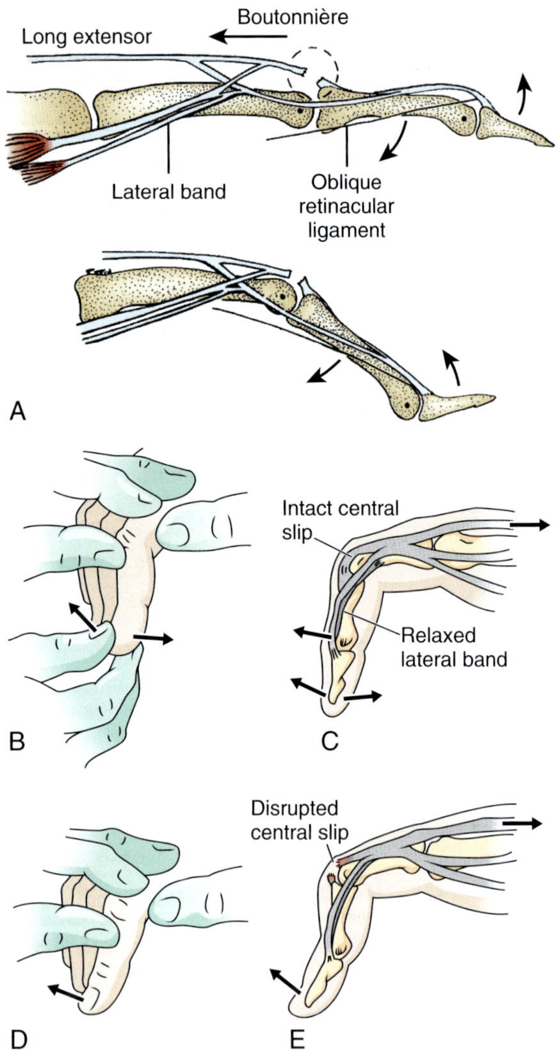

Fig. 49.18 (A) Diagram of a boutonnière deformity. (B–E) The Elson test for early diagnosis of an acute rupture of the central slip of the extensor digitorum communis tendon. Such rupture results in a boutonnière deformity in which the distal interphalangeal joint is hyperextended, as shown. (B) With the patient's finger flexed (over a straight edge) at the proximal interphalangeal (PIP) joint, palpate the dorsal surface of the middle phalanx. (C) If the central slip is intact, PIP joint flexion causes the slip to tighten distally, thereby relaxing the lateral bands and leaving the distal phalanx flail *(arrows)*. Thus when the patient is asked to extend the digit, the examiner feels pressure that is being exerted by an intact central slip. (D–E) If the central slip is disrupted, however, the examiner feels no pressure on the dorsum of the middle phalanx as the patient tries to extend the digit. It is possible for the patient to extend the injured finger successfully only by hyperextending (by action of the lateral bands) *(arrows)*.

The Elson test may also help identify this injury (Fig. 49.18 and Video 49.1).[33]

A boutonnière deformity does not usually develop in patients with closed zone 3 injuries until 10 to 21 days after injury unless the central slip and triangular ligament are both disrupted and the lateral bands subluxate toward the volar plate. To prevent the deformity from occurring, the provider should have a high index of suspicion for its presence and treat these patients conservatively. It is advisable that all patients with a swollen, tender PIP joint and pain with flexion or extension be splinted and referred for close follow-up.[34] Apply a dorsal splint overlying the PIP joint while keeping it in full extension. Initial splinting is usually performed for 3 to 6 weeks, followed by nighttime splitting for an additional 6 weeks. Use an aluminum foam-backed splint or a Bunnell ("safety pin") splint, although the latter may not be available in the ED.[32] The MCP, DIP, and wrist joints should be left free to have full, active range of motion (Fig. 49.19). If a central slip attachment fracture is present, orthopedic consultation is recommended because these patients may require surgical internal fixation.[35]

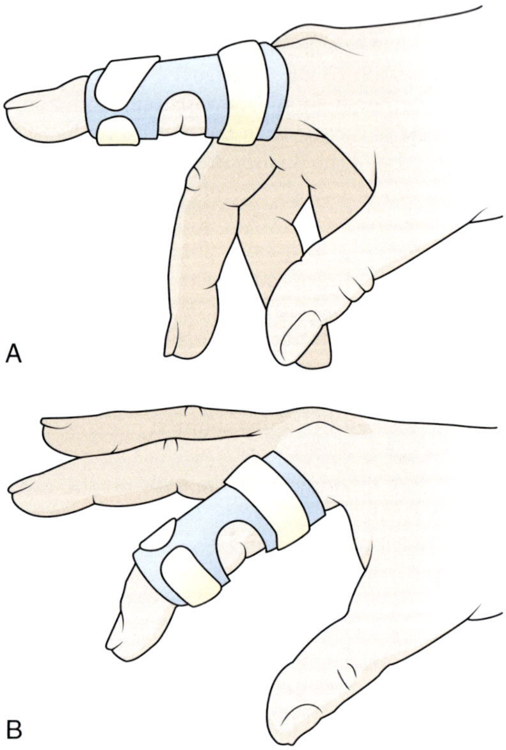

Fig. 49.19 (A) Boutonnière splint. (B) This splint allows active flexion at the metacarpophalangeal and distal interphalangeal joints.

Zone 1 and 2 Injuries

Zones 1 and 2 consist of the area over the DIP joint and the middle phalanx, respectively.[1,8,28] In zone 2, the conjoined lateral bands come together to form the TEM and are held together, in part, by the triangular ligament. The TEM inserts on the base of the distal phalanx and allows extension at the DIP joint. Complete disruption of the TEM results in an inability to extend at the DIP joint. Because of the unopposed action of the flexor digitorum profundus (FDP) tendon, the DIP joint rests in the flexed position. Injuries in zones 1 and 2 may be either open or closed. The most common closed tendon injury of the hand is known as a *mallet deformity* of the finger (Fig. 49.20A). When evaluating DIP motion, it is important to isolate the function of the extensor tendon by holding the PIP joint in full extension (see Fig. 49.20B–C). Normally, full active extension is possible.

Open tendon lacerations in zone 1 or 2 that result in a partial or complete mallet deformity warrant discussion with a hand surgeon (Fig. 49.21). Operative management consists of repair of the lacerated tendon and postrepair immobilization. Some surgeons will use only an external splint; others prefer placement of a Kirschner wire (K-wire) through the distal phalanx into the middle phalanx to help stabilize the joint. One technique for tendon repair is dermatotenodesis,

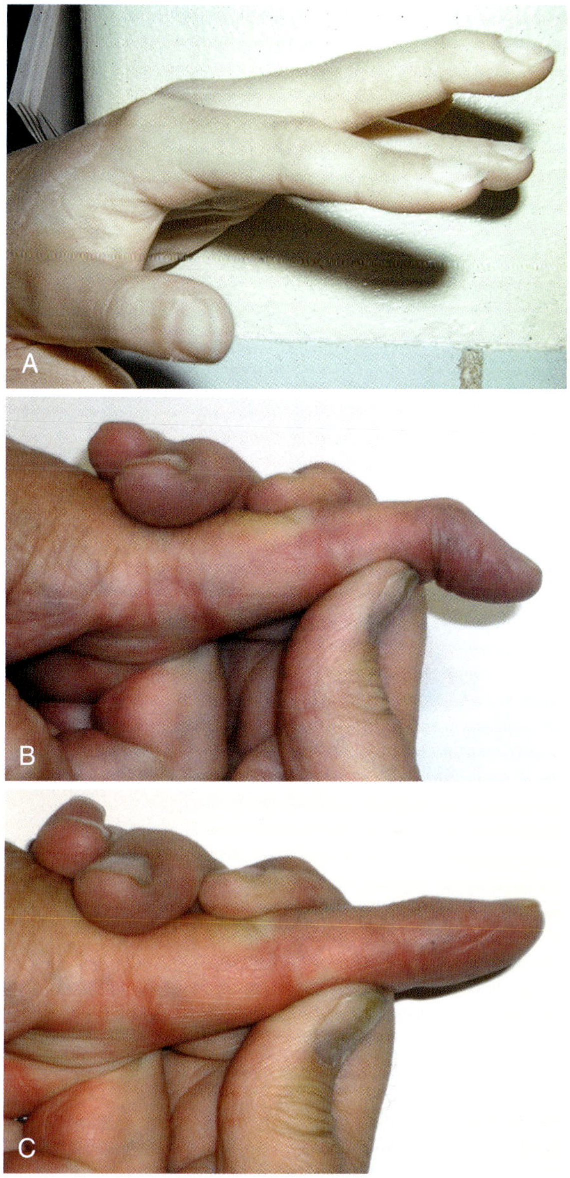

Fig. 49.20 (A) Mallet finger deformity. (B–C) When evaluating distal interphalangeal (DIP) motion for a mallet finger, isolate the function of the extensor tendon by holding the proximal interphalangeal (PIP) joint in full extension. This minimizes the contribution of the central slip to DIP extension. With the PIP joint stabilized, test active extension at the DIP joint. (B) A patient with a mallet finger will be unable to extend the distal phalanx actively, but the joint can usually be extended passively. (C) Normal extension with the PIP joint stabilized rules out a mallet finger. See Fig. 51.18 for splinting techniques for a mallet finger. (A, From Leddy JP, Dennis TR. Tendon injuries. In: Strickland JW, Rettic AC, eds. *Hand Injuries in Athletes*. Saunders; 1992:180.)

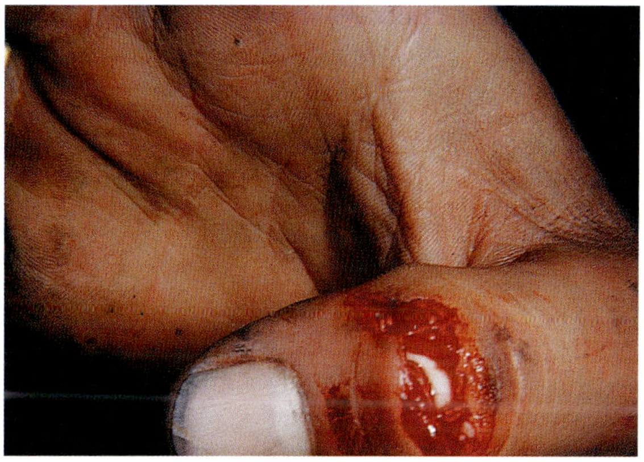

Fig. 49.21 An open mallet finger can be repaired surgically.

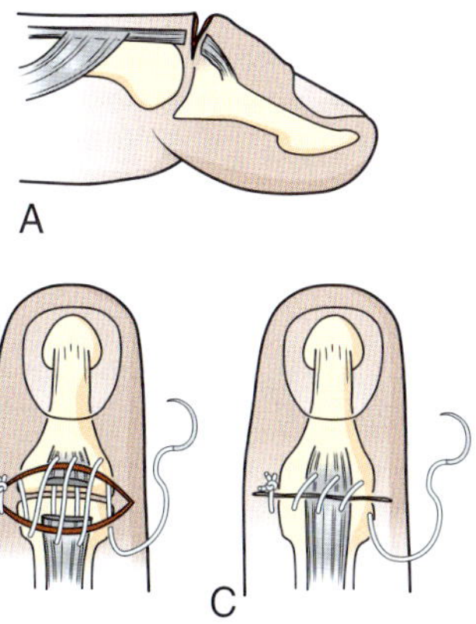

Fig. 49.22 Dermatotenodesis technique for zone 1 extensor tendon repair. (A) Fresh lacerations of the extensor mechanism over the distal joint with a mallet finger deformity are repaired with a running-type suture, which simultaneously approximates the skin and tendon (B–C). A small dressing is applied along with a splint to maintain the joint in full extension. The sutures are removed at 10 to 12 days, but the splint is continued for a total of 6 weeks. (A–C, Adapted from Baratz ME, Schmidt CC, Sugar AM, et al. Extensor tendon injuries. In: Green DP, ed. *Operative Hand Surgery*. 5th ed. Churchill Livingstone; 2005:190.)

which involves placement of a single, running roll-type suture through the tendon and overlying skin (Fig. 49.22).[1] The DIP joint is then splinted in full extension for at least 6 weeks.

Occult partial tendon lacerations are important to recognize to prevent the development of a mallet deformity. If there is a partial tendon laceration in zone 1 or 2 that does not result in any extension deficit, the approach to repair is variable and it is advisable to discuss the repair with a consulting hand surgeon. In general, partial tendon lacerations involving less than 50% of the tendon area that do not result in an extension deficit may be splinted in extension for 1 to 2 weeks without repair of the tendon itself followed by active range-of-motion therapy.[32] Partial tendon lacerations involving more than 50% that do not result in an extension deficit may be repaired by a hand surgeon or by an emergency physician who is experienced in the repair of these injuries. In either case, it is advisable to discuss with the consultant hand surgeon whether the tendon will be repaired in the ED or the operating room.

If a zone 1 or 2 partial tendon laceration is repaired in the ED, it can be approximated with a figure-of-eight, running, or cross-stitch suture pattern using 5-0 nonabsorbable suture material.[32] In general, given the diminutive size of the extensor tendon in this region, placement of core sutures is not possible. It is important that the tendon ends be approximated but not pulled too tightly; otherwise, joint stiffness and limitation of flexion will occur. After repair of a partial tendon laceration, splint the DIP joint in extension for 6 weeks with the PIP and MCP joints remaining free.[32] Patients should be warned after tendon repair that there is likely to be some residual loss of flexion at the DIP joint, even in the best case.

Closed injuries in zones 1 and 2 may result in a partial or complete mallet deformity, depending on the injury. These injuries are usually caused by an axial loading force with forced flexion of the DIP joint while it is being held in extension. A common ED presentation involving this injury is a patient who complains of pain and swelling at the DIP joint after a ball strikes the fingertip.

Closed tendon injuries in this region can generally be classified into three categories. The first type of injury consists of a closed rupture of the TEM. The second type of injury is an avulsion fracture of the dorsal lip of the distal phalanx. Known as a "bony mallet," this fracture is intraarticular, but there is no volar displacement of the remaining portion of the distal phalanx. Avoid attempting to reduce displaced fractures before splinting because any reduction is unlikely to be maintained without surgical repair; mallet fingers with associated fractures are best splinted and referred. Treat both type 1 and type 2 injuries by splinting in full extension for 6 weeks. Either a dorsal or volar splint should hold the DIP joint in slight hyperextension (5 to 10 degrees) while allowing free range of motion of the PIP joint (Fig. 49.23). With a properly fitted splint, no flexion of the DIP joint should occur. The splint can be constructed from aluminum, foam-backed splint material, or from a prefabricated stack splint (Stax, North Coast Medical, Inc.). A Cochrane review of mallet finger injury treatments found inadequate data to establish the most effective type of splint, but the stack splint does offer ease of application and improved patient comfort.[36] Be careful to avoid excessive pressure from the splint on the DIP joint area because skin necrosis may occur. Strictly maintain the DIP joint in full extension for 6 to 8 weeks, including during sleep and splint changes. Adherence to this instruction is important because patients often test its function on their own thus tearing the healing tendon fibers. The most common reason for treatment failure is patient noncompliance with prolonged splinting. Patients should support the distal fingertip in full extension whenever the splint is removed. Should DIP joint extension be lost at any point during the initial treatment period, reset the immobilization period for an additional 6 weeks.

The third type of closed injury is an intraarticular avulsion fracture of the dorsal lip of the distal phalanx with volar displacement of the remaining portion of the distal phalanx (Fig. 49.24). Such injuries are best referred for definitive treatment consisting of either surgery or more complex splinting. Normally, the DIP collateral ligaments hold the distal phalanx in place; however, if there is a large enough fracture fragment (usually >50% of the articular surface), the remaining distal phalanx fragment displaces in the volar direction secondary to unopposed action of the FDP tendon. When volar displacement of the distal phalanx occurs, this injury may require more aggressive treatment to achieve an optimal outcome.[28] Unfortunately, there are no adequate randomized controlled trials comparing operative versus conservative treatment of these injuries.[36] Operative repair usually involves open reduction and internal fixation of the fracture with placement of a K-wire for additional stabilization. It is important to remember that it is the presence of volar subluxation, not the size of the avulsion fracture, which is most often considered when determining the need for operative management.

Any injuries, whether open or closed, that result in complete disruption of the TEM may result in a swan neck deformity (Figs. 49.25 and 49.26). This deformity consists of flexion at the DIP joint (a mallet finger) and hyperextension at the PIP joint. It results from increased extension force on the middle phalanx caused by dorsal and proximal displacement of

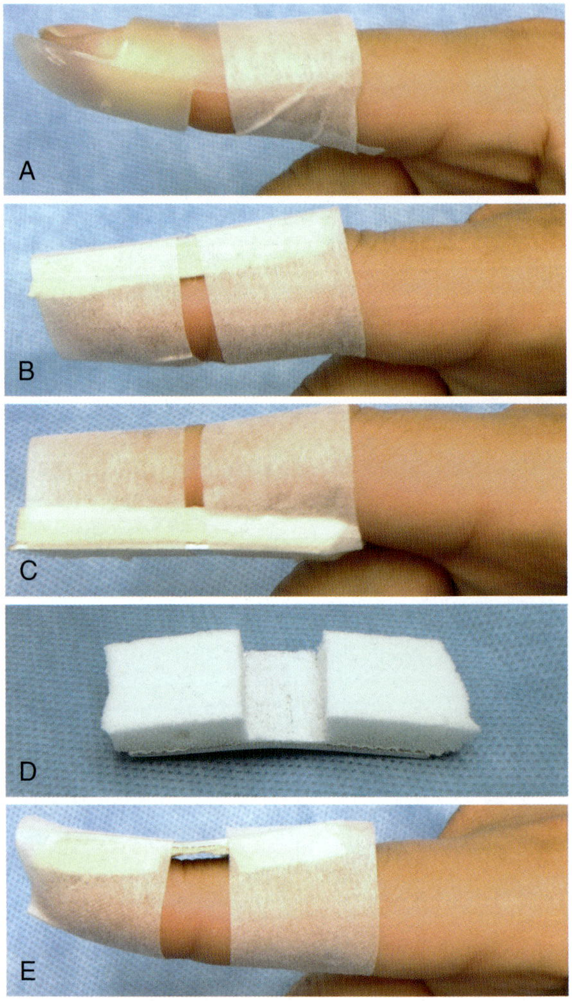

Fig. 49.23 Mallet finger splints. Be careful to avoid direct sustained pressure from the splint on the skin in the area of the distal interphalangeal (DIP) joint. Excessive pressure or hyperextension can cause skin necrosis. The splint should allow easy motion of the proximal interphalangeal joint with no flexion of the DIP joint. Immobilize the DIP joint in full extension or slight hyperextension (5 to 10 degrees). Splints are maintained continually for 6 to 8 weeks, including during sleep, with strict avoidance of any flexion during hand washing or splint changes. (A) Commercially available and an ideal and preferred volar plastic splint (Stack mallet finger splint). (B) Dorsal aluminum foam splint. (C) Volar aluminum foam splint. (D–E) Kleinert mallet finger splint. The Kleinert splint provides modest hyperextension and avoids pressure on the skin by removing the middle third of the foam padding, thereby eliminating all direct pressure on the injury site. All give good results.

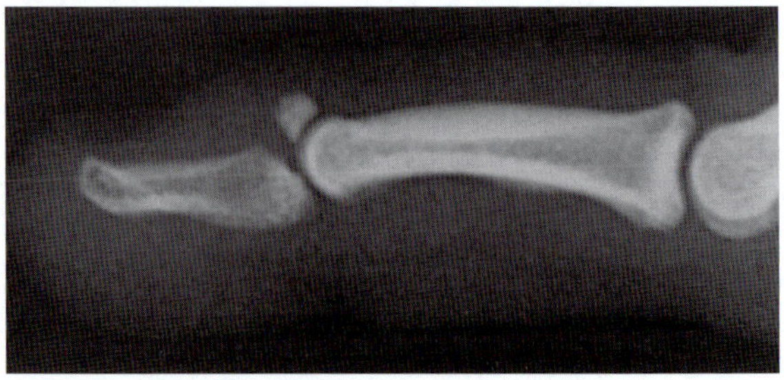

Fig. 49.24 A mallet fracture with volar subluxation of the distal phalanx. Avoid attempts to reduce any displaced fractures before splinting because any reduction is unlikely to be maintained without surgery; mallet fingers with associated fractures are best referred.

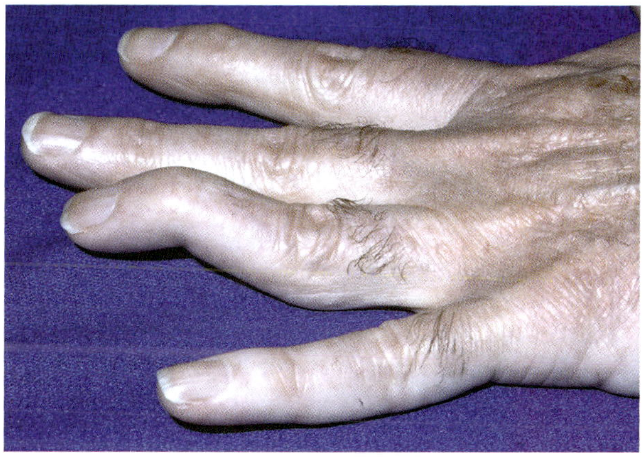

Fig. 49.25 Swan neck deformity. (From Skirven TM. *Rehabilitation of the Hand and Upper Extremity*. 6th ed. Mosby; 2011.)

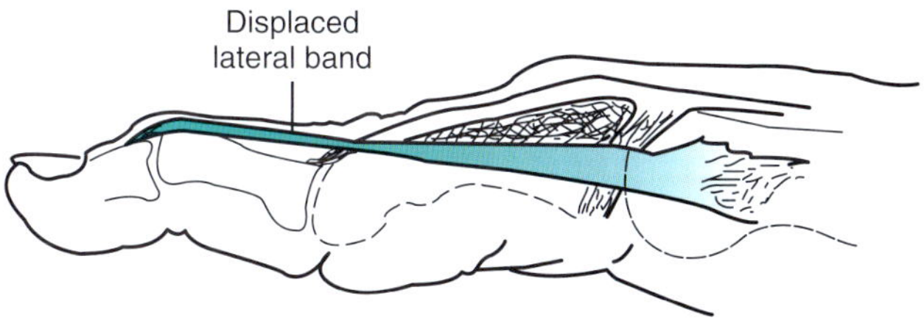

Fig. 49.26 Diagram of the swan neck deformity. Lateral bands have displaced dorsal to the axis of the proximal interphalangeal joint, where they extend the joint and allow the distal interphalangeal joint to flex. (From Rizio L, Belsky MR. Finger deformities in rheumatoid arthritis. *Hand Clin*. 1996;12:531.)

the lateral bands. This complication can be avoided if disruption of the TEM is diagnosed and addressed appropriately in the ED.

Complications

All extensor tendon repairs are subject to the usual complications of wound infection and skin breakdown secondary to prolonged splinting. Tendon rupture is a known complication after tendon repair and may result from inadequate suture technique, noncompliance with immobilization, or premature motion against resistance. When extensor tendons are repaired, the ideal suture technique should assure a high tensile strength, low rupture rate, and no tendon shortening to achieve optimal physiologic movement of the digit.[37] Sutures should be tied with square knots. All extensor tendon repairs require some period of complete immobilization during tendon healing; the necessity for patient compliance and follow-up must therefore be stressed.

Extensor tendon injuries in zone 7 tend to have the worst prognosis. Because of the presence of a synovial lining, postrepair adhesions may develop. Adhesions may lead to decreased excursion of the extensor tendons with resultant decreased mobility at the wrist. There may also be limitation of finger flexion when the wrist is flexed, as well as limitation of finger extension when the wrist is extended. Because of the lack of synovium, the low risk for adhesions, greater tendon excursion, the relatively simple anatomy, and the usual lack of associated injuries, zone 6 tendon injuries tend to have fewer complications than other areas of the hand. The tendons in zone 6, however, do tend to shorten if the ends are approximated too tightly. Shortening by as little as 1 mm may result in restriction of PIP and MCP joint flexion. This must be balanced with the need to avoid gaps in tendon closure which can lead to loss of extension and repair rupture.[38] Worse outcomes may occur with complex zone 6 tendon injuries when additional soft tissue or bony injuries are present.[39] Zone 5 injuries are particularly prone to infection because injuries in this region commonly occur from a human bite. Moreover, if the extensor hood covering the MCP joint is not repaired carefully, subluxation of the EDC tendon may occur.[15] Tendon shortening and joint stiffness may result if complex partial tendon lacerations in zone 4 are managed too aggressively. As discussed previously, these injuries are often best managed by splinting alone. A common complication of zone 3 extensor tendon injury is the development of a boutonnière deformity, which usually results from failure to diagnose or adequately immobilize a central slip injury. Similarly, undiagnosed or improperly treated extensor tendon injuries in zones 1 and 2 may lead to either a swan neck or a chronic mallet deformity of the digit. DIP joint splinting itself may result in skin ulceration or tape allergy, often occurring in the second week of treatment. Skin breakdown may ensue if the DIP joint is splinted in hyperextension because of decreased skin perfusion.

Postrepair Care and Rehabilitation

Proper care after diagnosis and repair of an extensor tendon injury is extremely important for optimal patient outcome. Even the best initial tendon repair can have a poor result if subsequently treated improperly. Rehabilitation of tendon injuries has evolved to include dynamic splinting and active range-of-motion exercises to achieve maximal motion of the affected digit. The specific details of the various rehabilitation protocols are beyond the scope of this text and best determined by the hand surgeon and physical therapist who will manage the patient in follow-up after the ED visit. The following are therefore only general guidelines, and individualized plans for splinting and immobilization should be discussed with a consulting hand surgeon.

Zone 1 and 2 injuries are usually treated with static splinting, as described previously. After 6 to 8 weeks, active range-of-motion exercises should begin. Night splinting is recommended for an additional 2 to 6 weeks after initial immobilization.[1,6,28] It is advisable to provide extra splints so that the patient can change the splint frequently to avoid pressure injury. During splint changes, it is important that the DIP joint be held in full extension, either by using the other hand, or by placing the finger against a table. If an extension lag develops at any time, continuous splinting must be repeated. Closed injuries of the central slip (zone 3) are often treated with a boutonnière splint for 4 to 6 weeks, followed by 2 to 6 weeks of gradual flexion exercises and night splinting. During the initial period of immobilization, the patient should be instructed to passively flex the DIP joint every hour to maintain gliding and proper position of the lateral bands.

Lacerations in zones 3 and 4 have traditionally been treated with static splinting from the forearm to the digits. An alternative approach is to splint only the DIP and PIP joints in extension and begin a "short-arc-motion" protocol within 1 to 2 days of repair.[40] This consists of active motion at the PIP joint progressing from 0 to 30 degrees in the first 2 weeks, then to 0 to 50 degrees in the third and fourth weeks. When compared with static splinting, this protocol may lead to better

PIP and DIP joint flexion without resulting in tendon rupture or a boutonnière deformity. Dynamic extension splints are also proving to be useful for rehabilitation of zone 3 and 4 tendon injuries.[40]

Early motion after extensor tendon repair has been found to be most useful in zones 5 through 7. A dynamic extension splint in which the wrist is extended 45 degrees and all finger joints rest in the neutral position is commonly used. A volar block allows 30 to 40 degrees of MCP joint flexion, whereas a dynamic traction mechanism passively extends the digits. Dynamic splinting is started 1 to 3 days after repair. Active motion is added at 3 to 4 weeks, and resistance is added at 7 weeks. A randomized controlled trial of zone 5 and 6 extensor tendon repairs found total active motion with dynamic splinting was superior to static splinting at 4 to 8 weeks, but not at 6 months. However, grip strength in the affected hand was improved at 6 months with dynamic splinting.[41] A short-arc-motion protocol with controlled active motion at the MCP joint has also been shown to be safe and effective when started 24 to 48 hours after repair.[17] One comparative trial reported that dynamic extension splinting and controlled active mobilization worked equally well for zone 5 and 6 tendon injuries.[42] All early range-of-motion protocols are most beneficial when managed closely by a skilled hand therapist. Patient age, associated injuries, suture type, and repair technique all affect the choice of rehabilitation protocol.[15] Most importantly, patients must be reliable and motivated to take advantage of early range-of-motion techniques. It is best to refer patients to a hand surgeon or hand therapist as soon as possible after repair so that rehabilitation can begin in a timely manner.

EXTENSOR TENDON INJURIES OF THE FOOT

The extensor tendons of the foot are less commonly injured than the extensor tendons of the hand and wrist. The most important extensors of the foot and ankle that may be injured and encountered in the ED are the tibialis anterior, extensor hallucis longus (EHL), and extensor digitorum longus (EDL) tendons.

The tibialis anterior muscle originates on the shaft of the tibia and interosseous membrane and inserts on the medial cuneiform and the base of the first metatarsal. The tibialis anterior extends the foot at the ankle joint (dorsiflexion) and inverts the foot at the subtalar and transverse tarsal joints. Rupture of the tibialis anterior tendon may be seen in both those older than 65 years and young patients who have been injured during athletic activity. Injury to this tendon commonly results from forceful attempted dorsiflexion of the ankle while it is held fixed in the plantar-flexed position. Patients generally have decreased strength of foot dorsiflexion because the toe extensors are used to accomplish this motion. Rupture or laceration of the tibialis anterior tendon should be promptly referred to an orthopedic surgeon or podiatrist for consideration of formal operative repair. Surgical repair is generally preferred while nonoperative management is reserved for those patients with contraindications to surgery or those who are inactive.[43]

The EDL and EHL tendons both originate from the shaft of the fibula and interosseous membrane. The EHL tendon inserts on the base of the distal phalanx of the great toe, whereas the EDL tendon divides into four branches that insert on toes 2 through 5 (Fig. 49.27). Both the EHL and the EDL tendons primarily result in toe extension and ankle dorsiflexion. The extensor digitorum brevis (EDB) and extensor hallucis brevis (EHB) muscles originate from the upper part of the calcaneus. The EHB tendon joins the lateral aspect of the EHL tendon before inserting on the great toe. The EDB muscle gives rise to three tendons that join the lateral side of the EDL tendons going to toes 2 through 4 (see Fig. 49.27).

Injury to the EHL and EDL tendons may result from a sharp object lacerating the dorsum of the foot. Patients may have weakness of, or an inability to extend, the involved toe or toes. The examiner may be unable to palpate the injured tendon. The decision to repair EHL or EDL tendon lacerations is controversial. Many authors favor repair because failure to repair EDL tendons may result in a claw deformity of the adjacent toes.[44] Lacerations of the EHL and EDL tendons at the level of the ankle are usually repaired, whereas lacerations on the dorsum of the foot and the toe are variably managed. Repair is favored if the patient has significant pain or any flexion deformity of the involved toe. Repair is also favored when both ends of the tendon are easily visualized in the wound and the patient is willing to undergo prolonged immobilization after repair.[45]

Because management of extensor tendon injuries of the foot is controversial, it is advisable to discuss the care of these patients with a consultant. Extensor tendon repair of the foot is not usually performed by emergency physicians, and we recommend that these injuries be stabilized and referred to an orthopedic surgeon or podiatrist for definitive treatment. Superficial cutaneous nerves are easily injured on the dorsum of the foot during wound exploration, which can lead to the formation of a chronic, painful neuroma. If the injury is repaired in the ED, the technique for repair is similar to that used for dorsal hand extensor tendon injuries (zone 6). A posterior splint that includes the toes should be applied after tendon repair. Splint the ankle at 90 degrees with the toes in the neutral position and recommend non–weight-bearing status until specialty follow-up.

FLEXOR TENDON INJURIES OF THE HAND AND WRIST

Flexor tendon injuries are more difficult to diagnose and more challenging to treat than extensor tendon injuries. Emergency physicians should not repair flexor tendons. Unique anatomic and biomechanical factors, the physiology of flexor tendons and tendon healing, and follow-up rehabilitation and physical therapy are dynamic, complex, and formidable. A satisfactory outcome is more difficult to achieve with an injured flexor tendon than with a similar degree of injury to an extensor tendon. Unlike extensor tendons, flexor tendons are influenced by complex pulley mechanisms, which are ligamentous structures that prevent tendons from bowstringing. Flexor tendons glide through delicate tendon sheathes, so even a minor defect in tendon integrity is physiologically magnified (Fig. 49.28). In addition, flexor tendon injuries are often associated with nerve and vascular injuries.

The main clinical mandate for the emergency physician is to consider or diagnose flexor tendon injuries, provide initial proper wound care, and expedite appropriate consultation and follow-up. Unlike the more superficial extensor tendons, flexor tendons are buried deep within the hand and forearm, and it is frequently not possible to visualize the tendon in the recesses of a wound. Puncture wounds of the palm can injure flexor

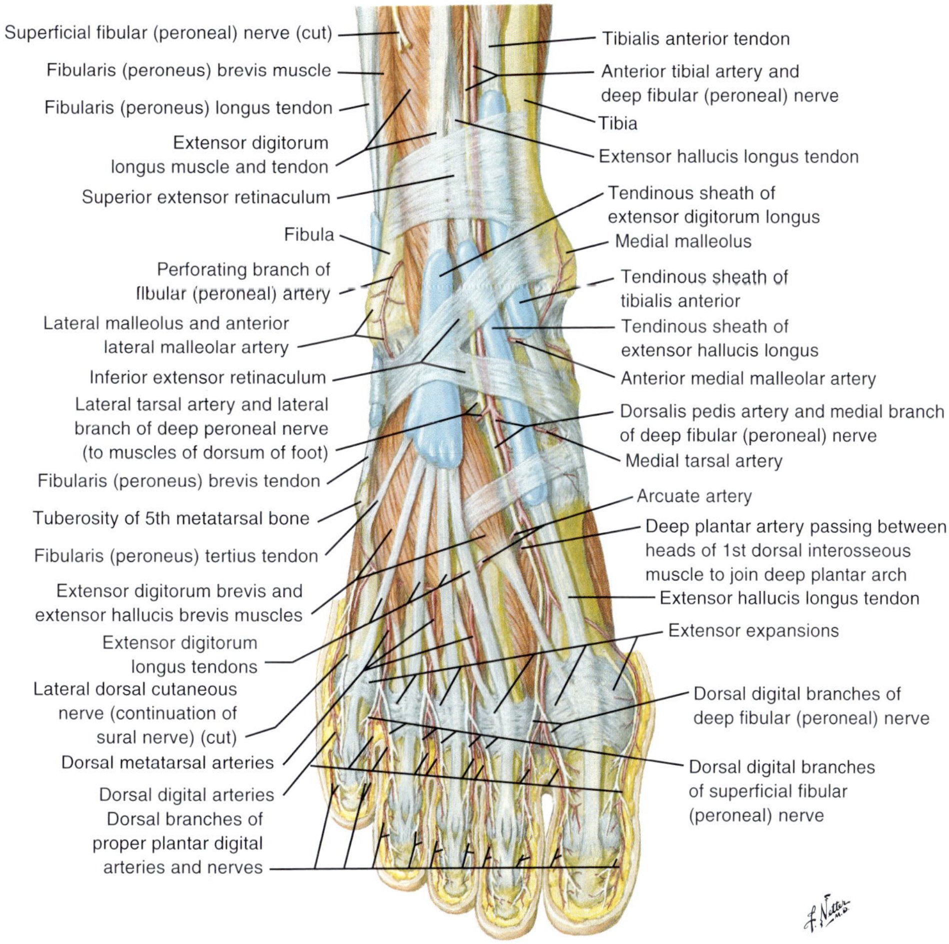

Fig. 49.27 Muscles of the dorsum of the foot: superficial dissection. (Netter illustrations from www.netterimages.com. Elsevier, Inc. All rights reserved.)

tendons, and deep puncture wounds prohibit visualization of injured structures (Fig. 49.29). Therefore a partial flexor tendon injury may be clinically silent until rupture occurs days or weeks later. Delayed repair of undiagnosed flexor tendons may be complicated by tendon retraction or scar formation, which may necessitate tendon transfer and grafting.

We recommend consultation with a hand surgeon for all clinically apparent flexor tendon disruptions. However, it may not be possible at the initial visit to diagnose flexor tendon injuries, nor the full extent of such injuries. Although there is no mandate for such immediate on-site examination when tendon integrity is uncertain, the same limitations to the examination would similarly confront a specialist. Individual scenarios and local protocols will guide the timing and degree of consultation from the ED.

Notwithstanding the previous discussion, complete flexor tendon injuries are usually apparent on physical examination, either by the resting posture of the injured hand or by testing individual tendons (Videos 49.2 and 49.3). In contrast, partial flexor tendon lacerations are commonly clinically unappreciated because functional deficits may not be evident. Clinical clues to a potential flexor tendon injury are weakness of flexor tendon function (difficult to evaluate in an acutely injured extremity), pain at the site of injury when performing active range of motion against resistance, and an abnormal resting position of the hand or finger (Fig. 49.30A–B), which can be determined by careful examination but can be particularly difficult in a child or uncooperative patient (Fig. 49.30C–D). It is rarely productive and potentially harmful to attempt extensive exploration of the deep recesses of the hand or forearm in the ED merely to visualize a suspected flexor tendon injury. Ultimately, accurate diagnosis may not be possible without surgical exploration.

While the technique and timing of repair is still a matter of debate, there is consensus that completely transected flexor tendons be repaired surgically, and many hand surgeons repair flexor tendon lacerations on the same day of the injury or at most a few days later. End-to-end surgical repair of lacerated tendons within 24 hours of injury is known as primary repair. The outcome of flexor tendon surgery depends on multiple intrinsic and extrinsic factors, but even delayed primary repair—within 3 to 4 weeks, or in some cases even 5 weeks—can result in similar outcomes.[46] Nevertheless, early repair within 1 week of injury is preferred.[47] If tendon repair is delayed until after the ED visit, the wound should be cleaned, the skin closed, and the patient referred for subsequent definitive repair.

Partial flexor tendon lacerations can lead to delayed rupture or entrapment from adhesions. Optimal management of these injuries is still debated. The conservative approach is supported by experimental evidence suggesting surgical repair of partially lacerated tendons results in weaker tendons than if the tendons are not surgically repaired.[48] Wray and colleagues suggested forgoing suturing in favor of splinting, followed by

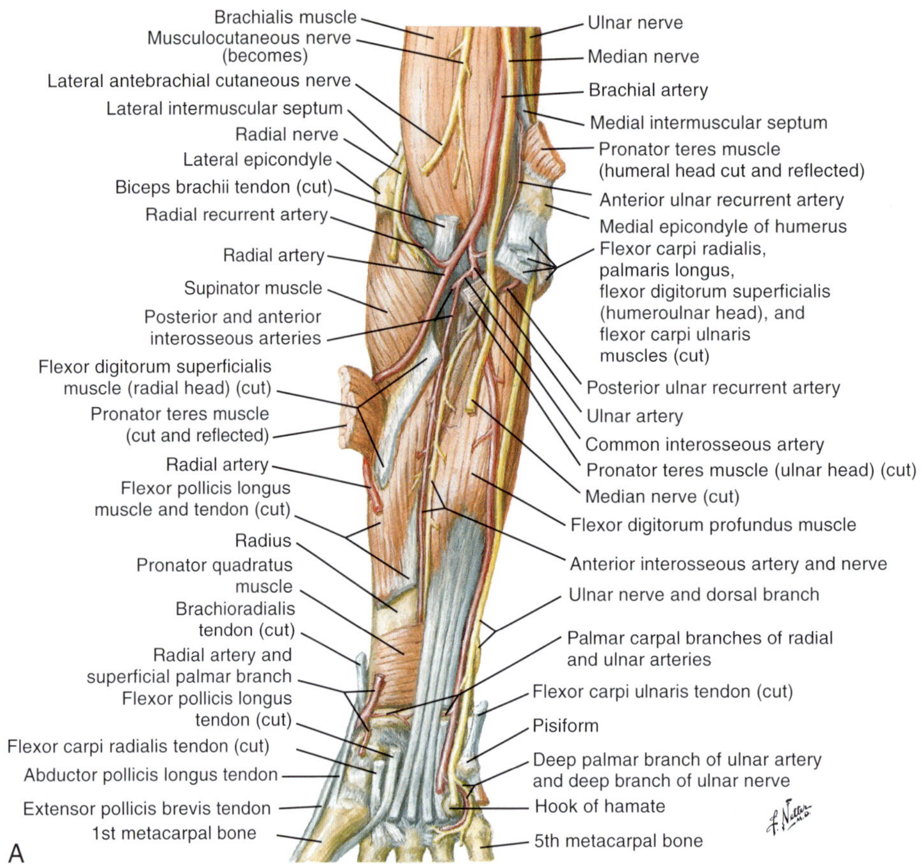

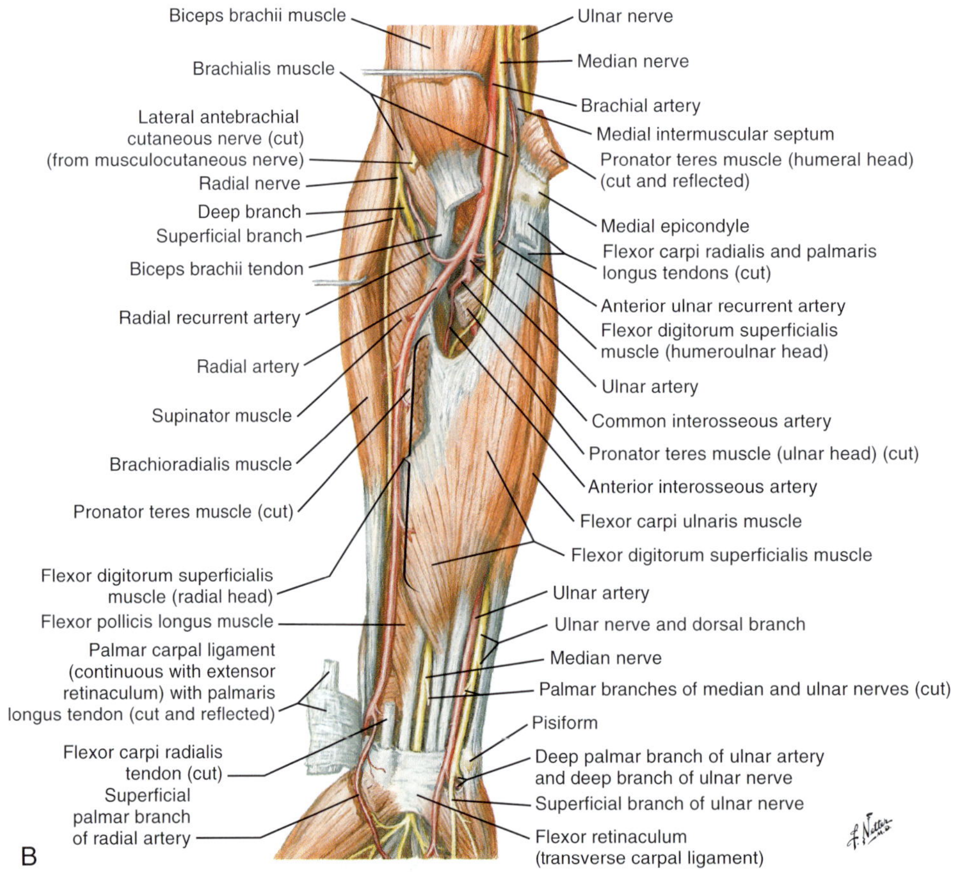

Fig. 49.28 (A) Muscles of the forearm (deep layer): anterior view. (B) Muscles of the forearm (intermediate layer): anterior view.

Continued

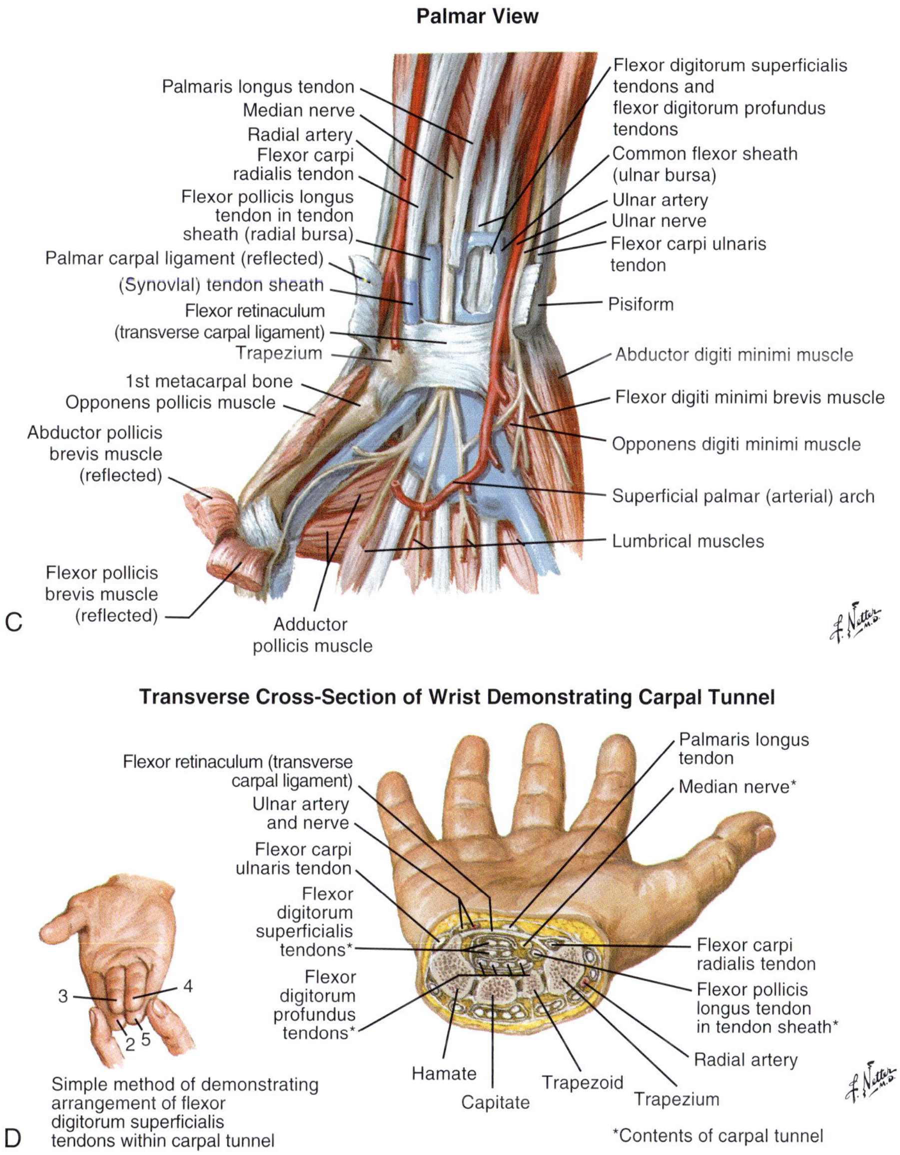

Fig. 49.28 cont'd (C) Flexor tendons, arteries, and nerves at the wrist: palmar view. (D) Transverse cross-section of the wrist demonstrating the carpal tunnel. (Netter illustrations from www.netterimages.com. Elsevier, Inc. All rights reserved.)

early mobilization of tendons with lacerations involving 25% to 95% of the cross-sectional area.[49] More recently, many authors recommend repair for lacerations involving greater than 50% of the cross-sectional area of the tendon. Lacerations involving less than 50% of the cross-sectional area may be repaired or simply debrided to prevent adhesions.[50] If a partial tendon laceration is not diagnosed at the initial visit and rupture is noted at the time of removal of the skin sutures or inspection of the wound, urgent referral to a hand surgeon would be expected to provide a similar result had the injury been diagnosed at the time of the initial ED visit. Open partial flexor tendon lacerations, if appreciated, should be treated with careful wound cleaning, skin closure, splinting, and referral for reevaluation, preferably within 1 week. All decisions concerning the type and timing of repair should be made in concert with a consultant, while keeping in mind that some decisions regarding surgical repair of partial injuries may not be made for weeks or months.

Following evaluation of a known or suspected flexor tendon injury, suture the skin and splint the hand to protect the tendon and minimize retraction. Techniques vary, and the initial splinting positions likely do not significantly impact the outcome. As a guideline, splinting the wrist in 30 degrees of flexion, the MCP joints in 70 degrees of flexion, and the IP joints in 10% to 15% of flexion is recommended.[51] No data exist to support or refute the value of prophylactic antibiotics for any soft tissue injury that has been properly cleaned. Antibiotics are recommended if the degree of contamination is significant, cleaning has been delayed, there are unusual sources of injury, or the patient is immunocompromised. Patients with evidence of infection should be considered for admission for wound debridement and intravenous antibiotics. Discharged patients should be provided with specific written instructions with a definite follow-up time frame outlined. Assistance with patient referral and follow-up will probably improve the outcome, but flexor tendon injuries often

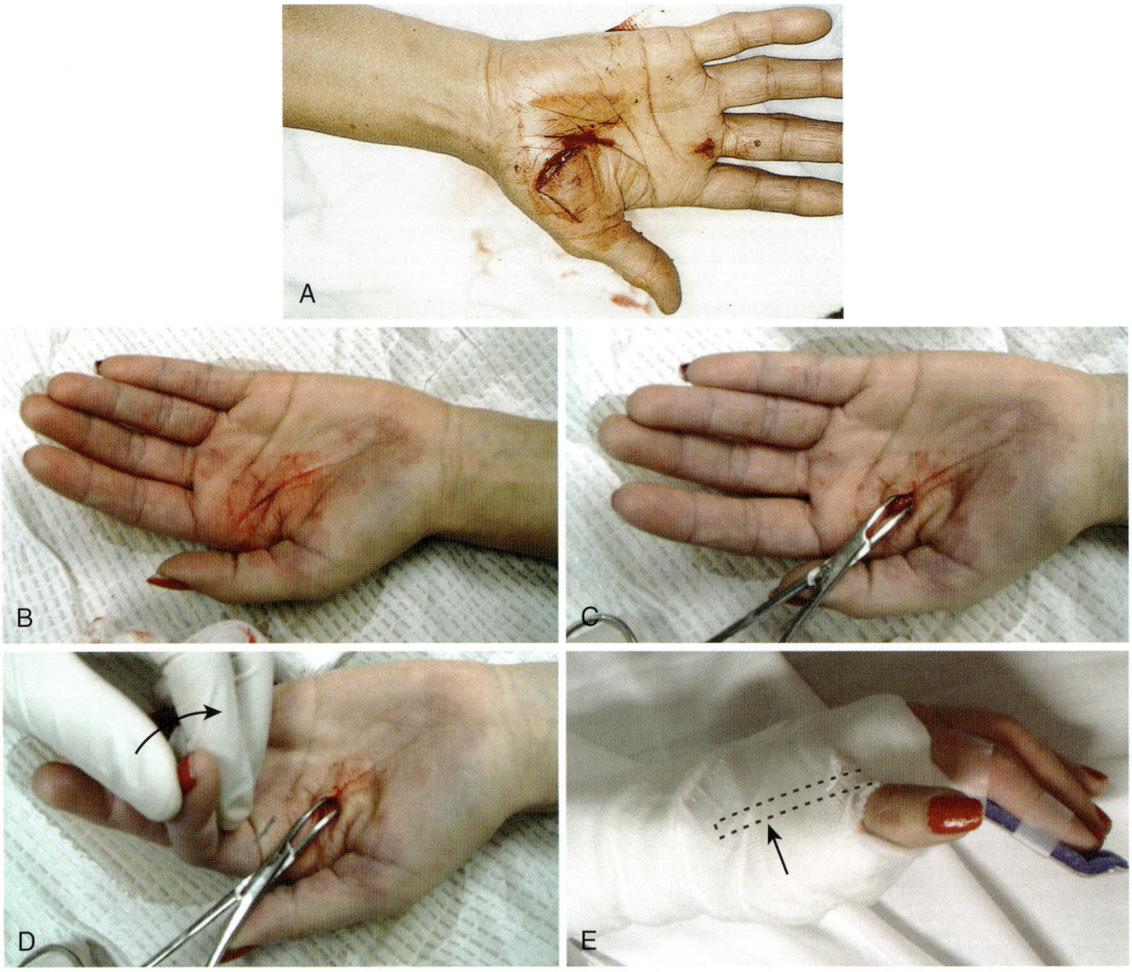

Fig. 49.29 Deep puncture wounds of the palm may injure the flexor tendons. (A) The depth of this wound precludes extensive exploration to visualize the tendon. Partial tendon lacerations may still initially allow full function. Clues to a partial flexor tendon laceration include weakness of flexion or pain with attempts at flexion against resistance, but many partial lacerations are clinically silent. Despite full function, this wound's location and depth suggest the possibility of at least a partial tendon injury. The prudent course would include meticulous wound care, splinting, skin closure, and contact with a hand specialist to arrange reexamination in a few days, while cautioning the patient that a flexor tendon injury may be present and delayed repair for up to 1 to 3 weeks yields results comparable to immediate repair. Immediate repair is often eschewed because of swelling and wound contamination. Further care may be required. (B) This palm laceration from the sharp top of a metal can seemed superficial. Function was normal. (C) When examined with the fingers in extension, the tendon was readily visualized, a surprise to the clinician given the benign and superficial appearance of the laceration. The visualized tendon was intact. (D) However, when the fingers were flexed *(arrow)*, the position of the hand when the injury occurred, a 20% to 30% laceration of the tendon was demonstrated. (E) This injury will do well with 3 weeks of splinting and no tendon repair. Follow-up with a hand surgeon in a few days is prudent. Note the outrigger aluminum splint incorporated into a short-arm plaster splint (*arrow*; see Fig. 51.11).

produce lifelong disability despite ideal care in the ED. As many as 10% require a second surgery for complications such as re-rupture or adhesions.[7,52,53]

ACHILLES TENDON RUPTURE

An Achilles tendon rupture can lead to significant morbidity. Although definitive care of such injuries is not performed in the ED, it is important to make the correct diagnosis and institute proper and prompt referral. Often initially considered a minor ankle sprain or tendonitis by both the patient and examiner, this injury is easy to miss and is not always diagnosed on the first visit.[54]

While largely an academic marker, the best predictor of acute Achilles tendon rupture is decreased tendon fibril size.[55] Clinically, rupture has been associated with steroid use, degenerative conditions, and older age, but Achilles tendon rupture can also occur in healthy athletic patients with no history of heel pain and often with seemingly minor trauma. In a 2022 systematic review, historical risk factors, including body mass index greater than 25, steroid use, living in urban areas, and high cholesterol were found to have limited supporting evidence for rupture risk. Male sex, Black race, and higher age were found to confer limited but measurable risk.[55] Fluoroquinolone antibiotics, which can cause dysplasia of collagen fibers, have been implicated in Achilles tendon rupture,

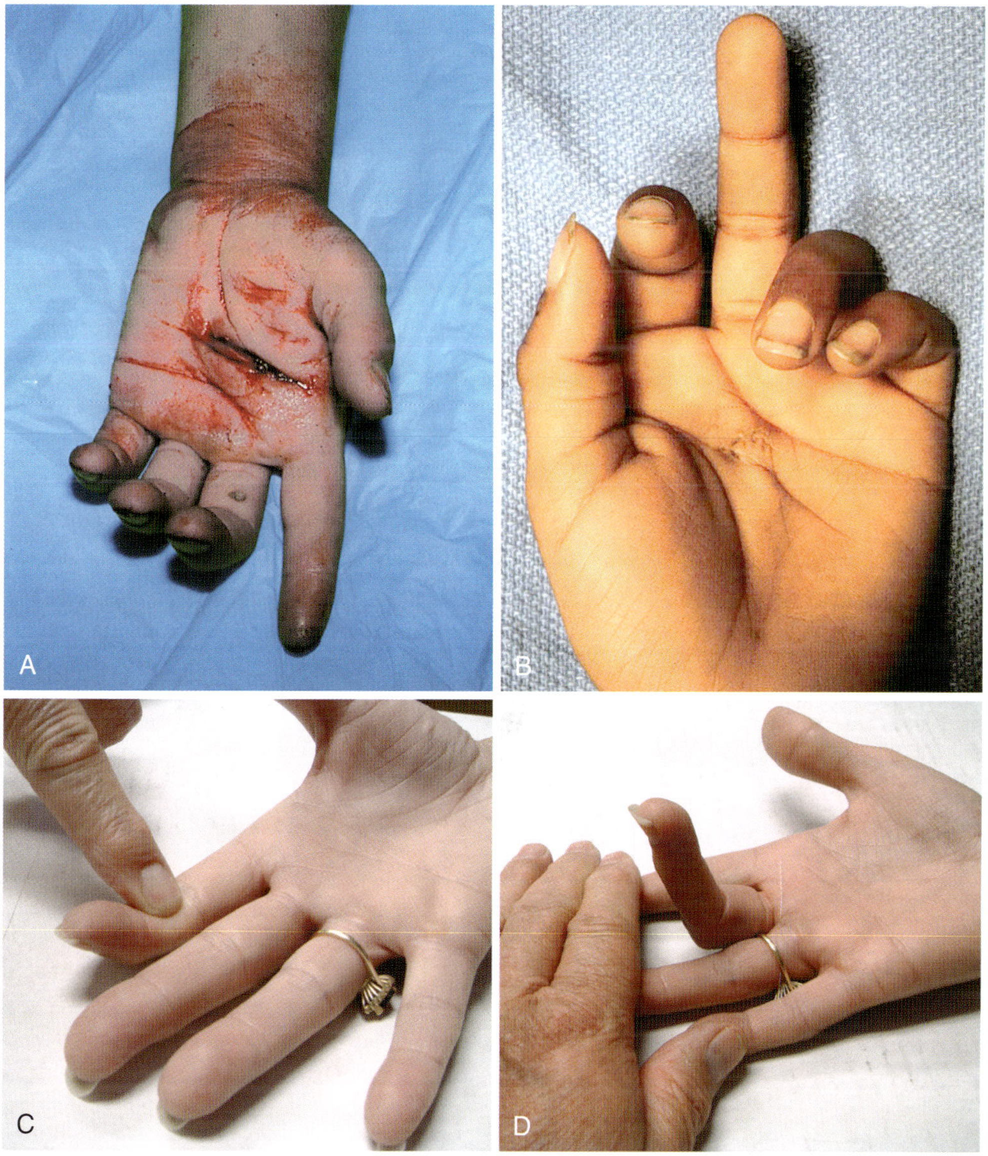

Fig. 49.30 (A) Note the obvious abnormal resting posture of the hand. This boy's palm laceration involved the flexor tendons to his index finger. With his hand at rest, his index finger lies in extension, in contrast to his other fingers, which are partially flexed. (B) Loss of the digital cascade in the middle finger illustrated here should be indicative of a flexor tendon laceration without further examination. The small glass laceration in the palm accounts for the profundus laceration, apparent only at follow-up. Children are difficult to fully examine in the emergency department. Splinting and follow-up in a few days are prudent based on the injury mechanism and location. (C) The flexor digitorum profundus tendon is examined by immobilizing the digit in question and asking the patient to flex the distal interphalangeal joint against resistance. D, The flexor digitorum superficialis tendon is examined by immobilizing the digits not being tested and asking the patient to flex the proximal interphalangeal joint against resistance. Pain and weakness associated with flexion against resistance may suggest a partial tendon laceration, but this is often a very subtle or inaccurate evaluation that must be repeated when the pain and swelling have subsided. (A, Courtesy Robert Hickey, MD, Children's Hospital of Pittsburgh.)

especially in older adults.[56] This led the Food and Drug Administration to issue a "black box" warning on the use of all fluoroquinolones for this condition in 2008.[57]

The common mechanism of rupture is sudden overload of the tendon by forceful plantar flexion of the foot, as in recreational sports involving jumping (basketball), pushing a heavy object, or stepping up, and should be suspected whenever the patient reports the sharp onset of heel pain and inability to fully load the tendon.[54] The injury is usually a complete as opposed to a partial tear, and rupture commonly occurs in the region 2 to 6 cm proximal to the tendon's insertion on the calcaneus.[56] Occasionally, the patient may appreciate an audible snap or pop. Pain may not be perceived in the tendon itself; instead, heel or diffuse ankle pain may be experienced. Because multiple structures plantar flex the foot, the initial result is weakness of ankle plantar flexion, but importantly, complete loss of motion of the foot may not occur. Characteristic ecchymosis may be evident 48 to 72 hours after injury.

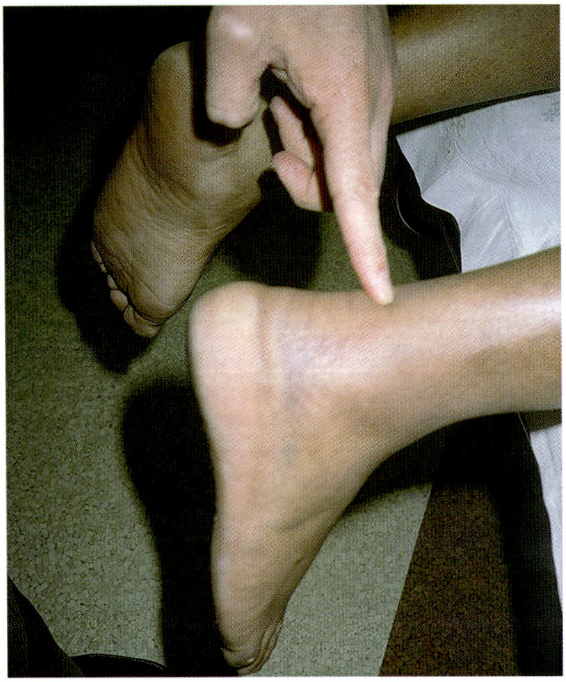

Fig. 49.31 This patient complained of a sprained ankle of 3 days' duration after jumping in a basketball game. There was moderate weakness of plantar flexion, but not complete loss. A defect in the Achilles tendon may be appreciated in some cases of Achilles tendon rupture, but not in this case. Note the characteristic bruising.

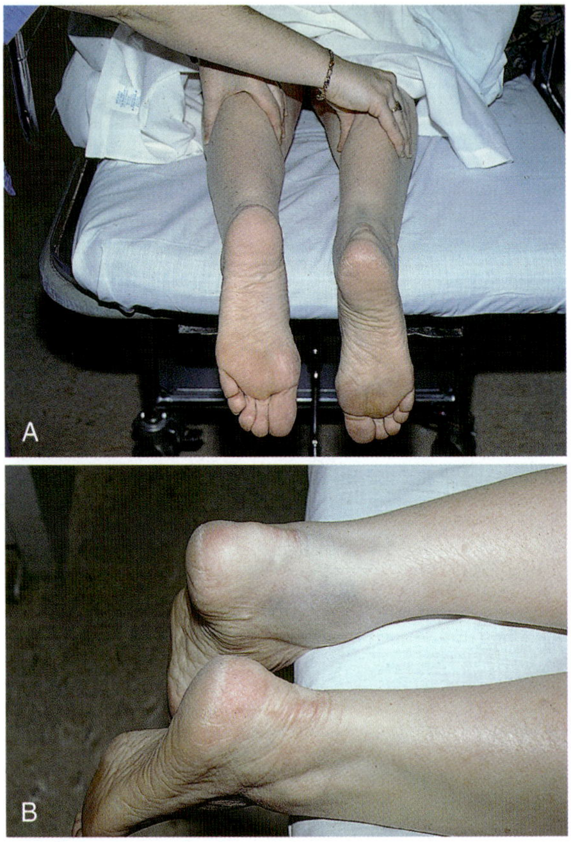

Fig. 49.32 (A) To perform the calf squeeze test (Thompson test), place the patient prone on the stretcher with the feet overhanging the edge. (B) Squeeze the calf and look for forceful passive plantar flexion of the foot. In this case the left foot (note the swelling and ecchymosis) did not move, thus confirming a complete Achilles tendon rupture.

The diagnosis may be suggested by a palpable defect in the tendon, but this can be subtle or absent (Fig. 49.31). The calf squeeze test (Thompson's test) (Video 49.4) is a physical finding that is 96% sensitive and 93% specific for Achilles tendon rupture.[58] To perform this test, have the patient lie prone with the feet overhanging the edge of the examination table. Squeeze the calf and observe for strong passive plantar flexion of the foot. If the foot does not move, a complete Achilles tendon tear is suspected (Fig. 49.32). When the diagnosis is unclear, or when the possibility of other injuries exists, emergency imaging should be performed.

With isolated Achilles tendon rupture, standard radiographs will be normal. MRI is diagnostic but not usually indicated in the ED. Point-of-care ultrasound can diagnose both complete and partial tendon ruptures.[59]

Although not specific to Achilles tendon rupture, the American College of Emergency Physicians (ACEP) identified the use of ultrasound for tendon rupture as a core emergency medicine application.[60] Healthy tendons have a bright, fibrillar appearance on ultrasound. Their echogenicity changes based on the incident angle of sound waves striking the tendon fibers, a unique property known as anisotropy. When sound waves strike perpendicular to tendon fibers, an intact tendon appears bright (hyperechoic). Echogenicity normally decreases as the sound angle moves obliquely to the tendon surface. Ruptured tendons appear hypoechoic or even anechoic, and may be surrounded by edema and hematoma which also appear hypoechoic.[61] Sonography is appealing because of its relatively low cost, portability, safety profile, the ability to compare the contralateral side easily, and the ability to perform static and dynamic evaluations. The sensitivity and specificity of ultrasound for Achilles tendon rupture, as reported in the radiology literature, are 96% to 100% and 83% to 100%, respectively.[62,63] A 2021 systematic review and meta-analysis of 808 patients found the sensitivity and specificity for ultrasound in detecting complete Achilles tendon rupture was 95% and 99%, respectively, with similar results for partial tears. The authors concluded that a negative ultrasound effectively ruled out a complete or even partial Achilles tear.[64] Although no studies have directly evaluated the diagnostic accuracy of ultrasound performed by emergency physicians for Achilles tendon ruptures, bedside ultrasound performed by emergency physicians for tendon injuries in other body areas had a sensitivity, specificity, and accuracy of 100%, 95%, and 97%, respectively.[5]

A *sonographic Thompson's test*, also known as the Realtime Achilles Ultrasound Thompson (RAUT) test, combines the benefits of physical exam and sonography. It is performed by directly visualizing the Achilles tendon with the high-frequency linear ultrasound probe while the calf muscle of the prone patient is gently squeezed. The tendon is assessed, proximally to distally, for synchronous movement, using dynamic sonography during passive dorsiflexion and plantar flexion of the ankle with the probe over the area of interest. Complete tears are recognized by retraction of the proximal tendon end, and echogenic adipose tissue (Kager's fat) may be seen to herniate between the torn ends of the tendon (Fig. 49.33). There will be continuous tendon movement at the rupture site in the case of a partial rupture because some intact fibers remain.[65] Foot and ankle surgeons not trained in ultrasound identified Achilles tendon ruptures with 86% sensitivity and

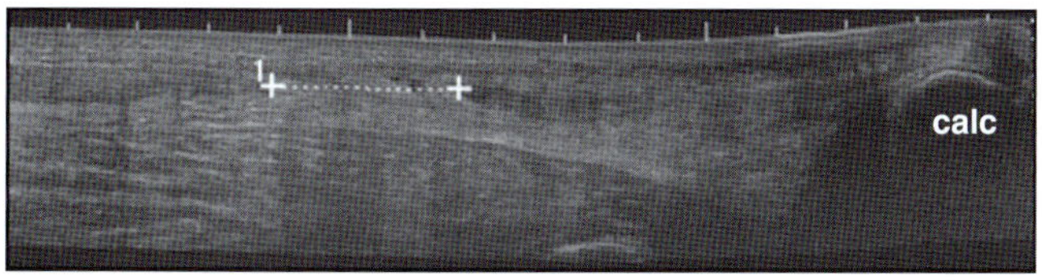

Fig. 49.33 Longitudinal ultrasound of a complete Achilles tendon rupture. There is a 2.6-cm separation between the proximal *(left)* and distal *(right)* torn tendon ends (indicated by the *dotted line* between plus marks). The calcaneus is located far to the right. Herniated echogenic fat can be seen between the injured tendon edges. (From Fessell DP, Jacobson JA. Ultrasound of the hindfoot and midfoot. *Radiol Clin North Am.* 2008;46:1027.)

92% specificity using RAUT.[66] For emergency physicians with formal ultrasound training and experience, performance may be better.

Treatment protocols vary, ranging from conservative splinting to surgical repair. A minimally invasive surgical approach with an early rehabilitation protocol is commonly recommended. This allows for earlier return to normal activities, increased patient satisfaction, and may improve functional outcomes.[67] However, in older patients without high functional demand, nonoperative treatment offers lower risk of surgical complications and may be preferable. Partial Achilles tendon ruptures are usually treated conservatively using 2-cm heel lift for 12 weeks followed by gradual reduction in heel lift and progressive tendon loading for 7 to 12 weeks.[54] Splint the foot in mild plantar flexion (gravity equinus) to protect the tendon until follow-up. Emergency physicians should be wary of the risk of DVT associated with prolonged immobilization of the lower extremity and should consider DVT prophylaxis (e.g., aspirin) on a case-by-case basis.[55,56]

KNEE EXTENSOR TENDON RUPTURE

The extensor mechanism of the knee is composed of the four strong quadriceps muscles, the femoral quadriceps tendon, the patella, the patellofemoral and patellotibial ligaments, the medial and lateral retinacula, the patellar tendon, and the tibial tubercle.[45] Both the quadriceps and patellar tendons are subject to rupture. These injuries occur predominantly in males and are associated with significant morbidity regardless of treatment. Quadriceps tendon rupture is more common in older adults and in those with systemic degenerative diseases such as diabetes mellitus, renal failure, lupus, gout, and rheumatoid arthritis. Local factors such as tendinopathy and corticosteroid injection also predispose to rupture. It may also be seen in younger patients with mechanisms such as taking a basketball jump shot. Performance-enhancing steroid use is likewise a risk factor in these patients. Patellar tendon rupture is also a serious injury but occurs more commonly in healthy patients, younger than 40 years, participating in sporting events.[68,69] High-energy trauma in patients without predisposing factors, as well as direct trauma to the anterior knee, may lead to patellar or quadriceps tendon rupture and is frequently associated with fractures and ligamentous injuries.[69]

As with Achilles tendon rupture, rupture of the knee extensor mechanism is not always initially suspected or diagnosed; it is missed on initial evaluation in nearly 40% of cases.[70] The mechanism of quadriceps tendon rupture is commonly a low-energy deceleration injury with the knee partially flexed, coupled with a strong quadriceps muscle contraction when the foot is fixed. The precipitating event may be seemingly minor, such as missing a step or jumping from a low height. A common history is an older patient who is descending steps or walking off a curb, misses a step, and attempts to keep from falling. The patient may recall a popping or tearing sensation, and the pain may be deceptively mild. The rupture may be partial but is more often complete. Quadriceps tendon rupture usually occurs transversely, just proximal to the patellar insertion, with or without an avulsion fracture of the superior pole of the patella. A suprapatellar gap may be palpated. The mechanism of patellar tendon rupture is usually an excessive load on the flexed knee during athletic activities. The patient complains of pain and inability to extend the knee or ambulate. Patellar tendon rupture generally occurs at the inferior pole of the patella. Athletic patients may continue to play with a partial tear, but a complete rupture does not allow ambulation. Bilateral complete rupture has been described, but the condition is generally unilateral.

With either type of rupture, a large hemarthrosis is often present and may prompt the incorrect diagnosis of a ligamentous injury such as an anterior cruciate ligament rupture. A palpable defect superior or inferior to the patella may be appreciated, but diffuse swelling can mask this finding (Fig. 49.34). Lack of the expected palpable defect can be misleading in the presence of a large hemarthrosis.

With complete rupture, a supine patient is unable to actively extend the knee or lift a straightened leg off the stretcher, and the knee flexes when posterior support is removed from the raised leg. Weak extension, especially in the sitting position, may be possible if portions of the medial and lateral retinaculae are intact, even with a complete rupture of the central rectus femoris. With complete rupture, the patient cannot walk as the knee gives way immediately. As one would intuit, a knee immobilizer allows the patient to apparently walk normally. Partial tears may allow the patient to walk with a peculiar forward-leaning gait that helps support the knee in extension.

Plain radiographs may demonstrate a patellar avulsion fracture. With complete quadriceps tendon ruptures, a low-riding patella (*patella baja*) may be present as the patella falls inferiorly. Conversely, a high-riding patella (*patella alta*) is often seen with patellar tendon ruptures as the quadriceps tendon and patella retract superiorly. With an intact patellar tendon, the Insall-Salvati ratio—the ratio of the patellar tendon length, measured from the base of the patella to its insertion on the tibia, to the diagonal length of the patella—measures 0.8 to 1.2. A ratio greater than 1.2 strongly suggests patellar tendon rupture.[71] MRI is definitive but is neither commonly available nor necessary during the initial visit. As with Achilles tendon rupture, sonography is a useful diagnostic imaging tool to assess for ruptures of the quadriceps and patellar tendons.[59,61] The use of dynamic ultrasound, similar to the RAUT described above, will demonstrate the separated tendon ends moving away from each other with intervening echogenic or echolucent fluid.[61,72]

Complete tears require surgical repair. There is no consensus regarding the timing of repair, although delays correlate with tendon retraction and atrophy. Therefore most authors recommend early repair, usually as soon as possible after the diagnosis.[68,69,73,74] A 2021 systematic review of 48 studies including 1135 cases of patellar or quadriceps tendon ruptures demonstrated successful outcomes after surgical repair with high rates of return to play (for athletes) or work.

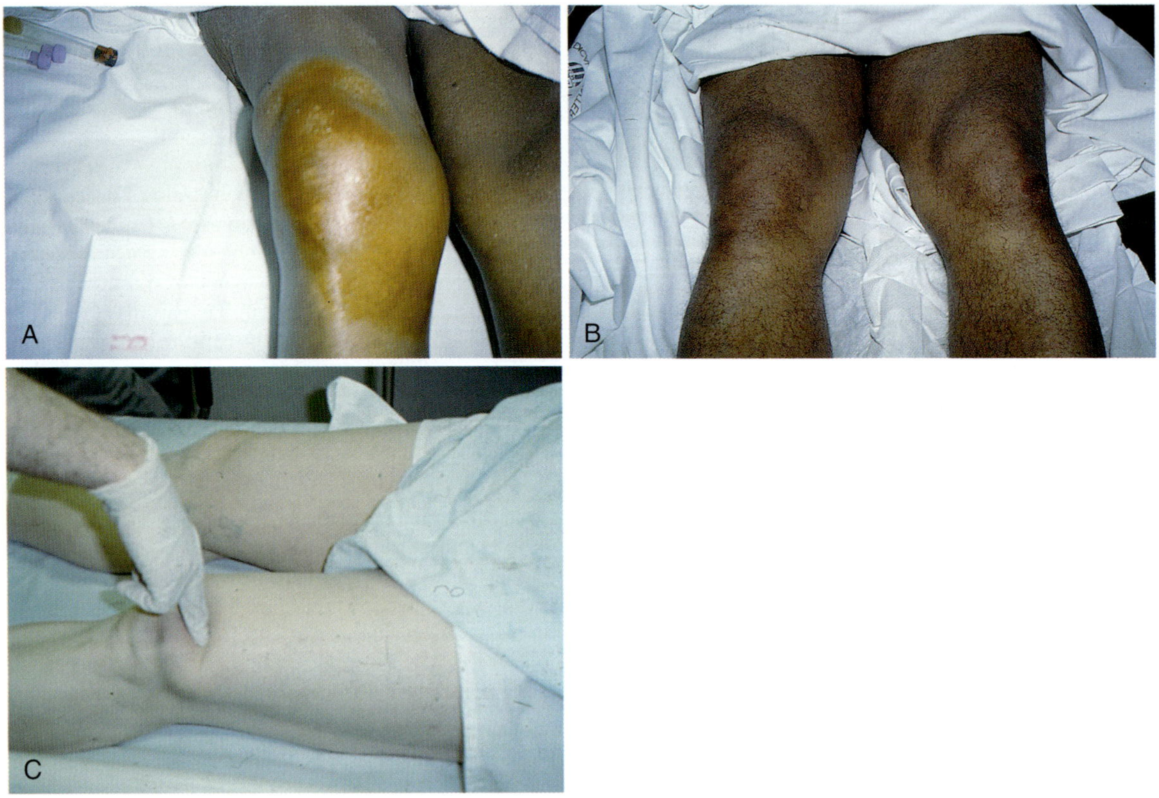

Fig. 49.34 (A) This older male lost his footing going down the stairs and missed only a single step. He felt a pop and was unable to walk. Arthrocentesis yielded a grossly bloody effluent. An obvious suprapatellar soft tissue defect and an inability to perform a straight-leg raise while supine made the diagnosis of a complete quadriceps tendon rupture obvious. (B) This male landed on both feet while jumping off a low curb and then collapsed. Pain was minimal and malingering was suspected. Diffuse soft tissue swelling, bilateral knee effusions, normal radiographic findings, and the ability to walk with bilateral knee immobilizers delayed the diagnosis of bilateral quadriceps tendon rupture until follow-up. (C) A step-off above the knee readily identified a complete quadriceps tendon rupture. The patient was unable to lift the leg off the stretcher, an activity that made the soft tissue defect obvious.

Unfortunately, the level of play varies substantially, and many athletes do not return to the same *level* of preinjury play.[75] Although definitive treatment is not undertaken in the ED, early diagnosis may improve the long-term outcome. Partial tears of either tendon may be treated surgically, or nonoperatively if there is no functional impairment. Open patellar tendon ruptures should be assumed to represent an open joint (arthrotomy) and are treated similarly to other open injuries associated with tendon disruption, including imaging to evaluate for fracture and foreign body, antibiotic prophylaxis, local wound care, and specialty consultation.

Acute injuries diagnosed in the ED should be treated with the knee fully extended in a knee immobilizer with protected weight-bearing using crutches. Patients should be referred for urgent outpatient follow-up with an orthopedic surgeon. Admission is sometimes warranted to expedite treatment.[48] In any case, the postoperative period of recovery is prolonged and difficult, especially for older adults.

REFERENCES ARE AVAILABLE AT Elsevier eBooks+

CHAPTER 50

Management of Common Dislocations

Robin Naples and Danielle Levine

Joint dislocations are frequently encountered in patients seen in the emergency department (ED). They can range from a simple finger joint dislocation to limb- or life-threatening consequences of high-energy trauma. Keys to clinical assessment and radiographic evaluation of these injuries are discussed along with methods of reduction. The emphasis of the chapter is on simple dislocations that should be diagnosed and initially managed in the ED. Fracture-dislocations that commonly require operative intervention and emergency orthopedic consultation are not discussed.

PREPARATION OF THE PATIENT

Although many authors claim that their reduction method is well tolerated without premedication, they have not usually measured the discomfort of their patients quantitatively.[1–4] There are no rigid, generally accepted guidelines for the use of pharmacologic adjuncts in the management of dislocations. Each patient and each dislocation is unique, and the treating clinician must use judgment regarding whether premedication is required, which agent or agents to use, and what dose to give. In general, the authors suggest the routine judicious use of analgesia with or without sedation for most reductions performed in the ED. A calm, cooperative patient may tolerate attempts at gentle reduction of a major joint such as the shoulder, but even the most stoic of patients may be quite uncomfortable with the manipulations necessary for reduction of a dislocated finger. A radial head dislocation in a child is usually easily treated without analgesia; however, reduction of a hip dislocation is unlikely to be successful without a significant amount of sedation and analgesia. Attempting any reduction technique in an extremely anxious patient without premedication will generally frustrate the operator and further upset the patient, and thus may hinder a successful outcome. When multiple attempts are required and significant force must be exerted because of muscle spasm or an uncooperative patient, there is an additional chance of producing complications during the reduction.

Verbal techniques for alleviating anxiety and discomfort are not to be discounted because they can be of great assistance during joint reduction. In field settings, simple hypnosis techniques have been used successfully for major joint dislocations.[5] In the ED, verbal reassurance and distracting conversation are useful adjuncts. Additionally, the use of handheld tablets and even virtual reality have been shown to aide a variety of painful procedures in the pediatric population and may be a useful adjunct.[6,7]

In most circumstances, analgesia, or sedation of some sort, or both, will be required; the intravenous (IV) route of drug administration is usually the method of choice because it allows rapid relief of patient discomfort and facilitates repetitive dosing for titration to the desired effect (see Chapter 33). Alternatives to procedural sedation and analgesia include intraarticular injection of local anesthetics, hematoma blocks, peripheral nerve blocks, and regional anesthesia (see Chapters 29, 31, and 33).

GENERAL PRINCIPLES

Clinical assessment of a patient with a dislocation must include a search for fractures or other serious injuries, especially if the mechanism involved high energy. This is most important for hip, knee, and posterior sternoclavicular dislocations. For all dislocations, perform a detailed neurovascular examination of the extremity before focusing attention on the injured joint.

Although many dislocations are clinically obvious, some may escape detection for some time as other injuries or issues dominate the clinical picture. A knee dislocation may be unmistakable in a 170-lb male who displays a deformity of the knee, but in a 400-lb patient, the knee may look deceivingly normal. The history and mechanism of injury can be quite helpful in certain circumstances. For example, a painful shoulder joint in a seizure patient should prompt assessment for a posterior shoulder dislocation, whereas a history of the knee striking the dashboard is a clue to a potential hip dislocation.

Some dislocations can be difficult to identify on plain radiographs. One should keep a high index of suspicion for dislocation when indicated. Carpal dislocations in the wrist may be subtle but are clinically suggested by severe pain and swelling. Similarly, superior dislocation of the patella may be mistaken for high riding patella typical of patellar tendon rupture. Unlike anterior shoulder dislocations, which are often easily detected on plain films, posterior shoulder dislocations may be missed on initial radiographs.

Some dislocations will have been reduced before clinician assessment. A careful history will uncover these injuries, prompt the necessary assessment of the ligamentous integrity and the possibility of an associated vascular injury, and guide proper immobilization and follow-up care. A dislocated and then spontaneously reduced knee is a severe injury that often escapes detection by even a seasoned clinician's initial evaluation. Other dislocations that are commonly first seen in a reduced state include finger dislocations, patellar dislocations, and radial head subluxations.

Although the chance that a gentle attempt at reduction will cause a fracture or neurovascular injury is extremely low, careful evaluation before and after reduction, as well as documentation of the patient's neurovascular status, is important. Frequently, the initial pain of the dislocation is distracting, and paresthesias or a weak pulse may not be readily apparent until the joint has been reduced. When the integrity of the pulse is in question, *blood pressure* at the wrist or foot may be compared with that in the uninjured extremity, or a *pulse oximeter* may be applied to the distal end of the fingers.

Prereduction radiographs are generally recommended. Reasons include difficulty distinguishing a fracture-dislocation by clinical examination and the potential for medicolegal problems if the fracture is not identified before attempts at reduction. More importantly, certain associated fractures predict a poor outcome with closed reduction and make orthopedic consultation a consideration before such attempts. Exception to this rule include suspected radial head subluxation in young children and clinical circumstances in which radiographs are not readily available (e.g., in the wilderness). Clinical conditions (i.e., vascular compromise or threatened skin penetration) may dictate the need for immediate reduction without radiographs; however, the few minutes required for initial radiographic evaluation rarely increases vascular or neurologic complications and provides very useful information to the consultant.

Postreduction films are recommended in virtually all patients who have had a dislocation reduced in the ED. Patients who have received sedatives and opioids may not remember the actual successful reduction or the immediate postreduction period. Reinjury after release from the ED without radiographic corroboration of a successful reduction can raise questions about the adequacy of the initial procedure. Occasionally, a fracture is detected on postreduction radiographs that was not obvious on the initial films, or a previously noted minor fracture may be found to reside in an intraarticular location.[8] Point-of-care ultrasound (POCUS) is safe and efficacious for diagnosing dislocations and confirming successful reduction, and will be discussed later in this chapter. As practitioners gain confidence and experience with ultrasound in this capacity, the need for both pre- and postreduction radiographs may be supplanted by the performance of ultrasound.

In general, dislocations of all types are less common in children than in adults because of the relative weakness of the epiphyseal growth plate with respect to the ligamentous support of the joint. Therefore, in children the epiphysis will tend to fracture before dislocation occurs, except in the case of radial head dislocation (nursemaid's elbow). Reduction techniques for pediatric dislocations are generally like those used for adults.

The proper terminology for dislocations describes the relationship of the distal (or displaced) segment relative to the proximal bone or the normal anatomic structure. The terms *anterior* and *posterior* are used for most dislocations. Therefore, if the head of the humerus lies anterior to the glenoid fossa, the injury is an anterior shoulder dislocation. Similarly, if the olecranon lies behind the distal end of the humerus, the injury is a posterior elbow dislocation. In the hand, wrist, and foot, one uses the terms *dorsal* and *volar*. *Palmar* and *plantar* are sometimes used in place of volar to describe the position of the dislocated part. Dislocations can be *open* or *closed* and may have associated fractures, which require a separate description.

It is generally accepted that the sooner a dislocation is reduced, the better. This alleviates the patient's discomfort, relieves neurovascular compression, and corrects distortion of the surrounding soft tissues.[9] In some studies, the success rate of reduction is higher when attempted closer to the time of injury.[10] However, there is no reason to forego an attempt at closed reduction of an "old injury" in the vast majority of dislocations. Although chronic dislocations persisting several days, weeks, or longer are often difficult to reduce in a closed manner, such cases are infrequent and should not deter the physician from attempting closed reduction.

A certain percentage of all types of dislocations are not amenable to closed reduction. Inability to complete a closed reduction is generally the result of interposition of soft tissue structures or fracture fragments and not necessarily due to improper technique. If sedation and analgesia are adequate to permit relaxation of the patient's muscle tone, reduction should be relatively straightforward. When reduction under adequate sedation and analgesia is unsuccessful after several attempts, further attempts at closed reduction are inappropriate. Generally, orthopedic consultation should be obtained after two or three failed attempts.

Once an attempt at reduction is completed, recheck the neurovascular status that was documented before the reduction was performed. For the elbow, hand, and forefoot joints, perform passive range of motion to assess the stability of the reduction and to ensure a smooth gliding joint that is free of intraarticular obstruction. For the shoulder, one must be cautious after reduction as full passive range of motion may cause repeated dislocation. Testing the ability to place the palm of the ipsilateral hand on the contralateral shoulder can safely assess successful range of motion and confirmation of reduction.

In addition to close monitoring of the medicated patient, proper aftercare involves adequate immobilization of the injured joint for comfort and to prevent repeated dislocation. Recommendations for follow-up care depend on the injury and its severity.

TIMING OF REDUCTION

Questions often arise concerning the necessity of immediate versus delayed reduction, with the clinician fearing disastrous neurovascular consequences if a dislocation is not manipulated immediately on arrival at the ED. There is rarely an instance in which prereduction radiographs, even portable films, cannot be obtained before treatment. Even if the pulse is weak or the fingers are numb, a few minutes' delay is usually acceptable to gain important radiographic information on the type of dislocation and the presence of an associated fracture and to provide documentation for follow-up clinicians. Important clinical information may be difficult to obtain, or the specific initial injury may be impossible to reconstruct once the joint has been reduced (Fig. 50.1). Of equal importance, a dislocation with concomitant neurovascular injury should be reduced with the least amount of trauma possible, which often requires a few minutes for induction of analgesia and sedation, a time during which radiographs can be obtained. If a vascular or neurologic abnormality is documented before reduction, the joint should be reduced by the timeliest and least traumatic procedure available. Each case should be handled individually by taking the specific injury, available resources, and the clinician's experience into account. Although multiple unsuccessful or forceful attempts at reduction in the ED should be avoided with all dislocations, this is especially important in patients with vascular or neurologic compromise. Occasionally, the more prudent course is reduction under general anesthesia, but this decision must take into consideration the availability of consultation and other resources.

The remainder of this chapter covers dislocations of the various joints apart from carpal (wrist) dislocations, which are complex and require orthopedic consultation, and temporomandibular joint dislocations, which are discussed in Chapter 64.

SHOULDER DISLOCATIONS

The human shoulder joint is remarkable for its degrees of motion. The glenohumeral joint has the greatest range of motion of any joint in the body, largely because of the loose joint capsule and the shallow nature of the glenoid fossa.[10] However, these anatomic features that allow for great mobility contribute to its instability, making it the most frequently encountered large joint dislocation. Posterior dislocation is uncommon, mainly because of the anatomic support of the scapula and the thick muscular support in this area. Anterior support is less pronounced, with the inferior glenohumeral ligament serving as the primary restraint to anterior

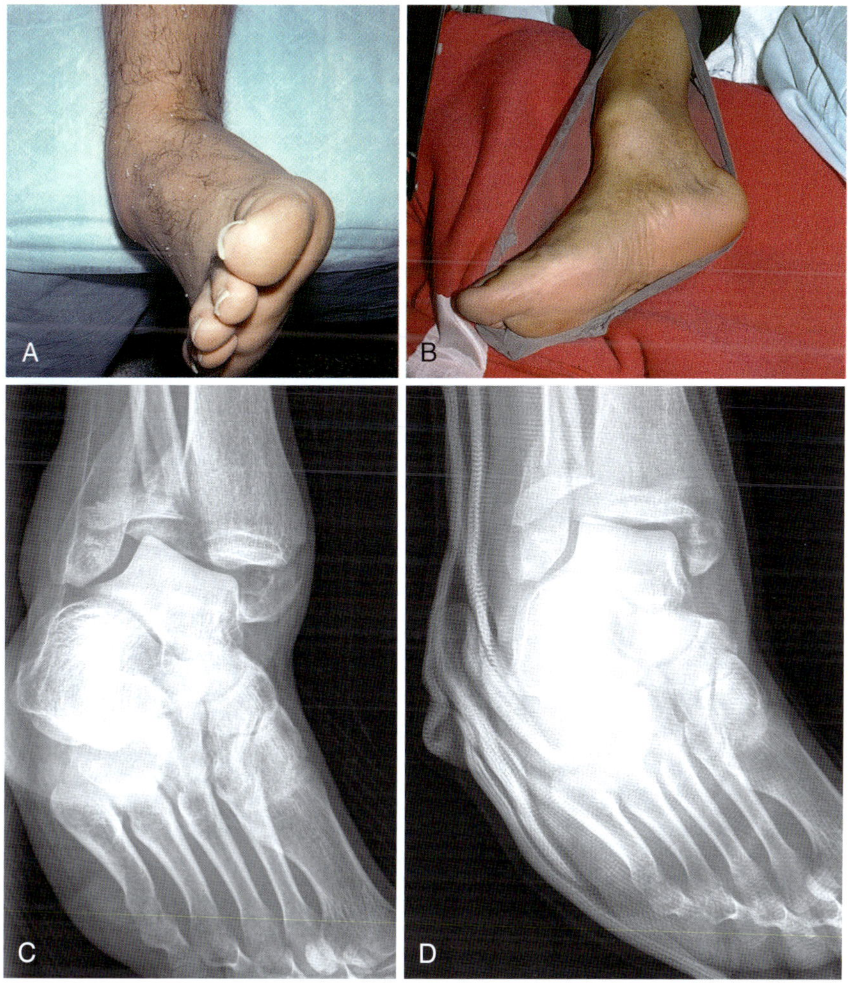

Fig. 50.1 (A–B) Because the distal pulse is weak and the toes are numb, it may be tempting—and is commonly advocated and acceptable—to immediately reduce these obvious dislocations while the patient is still on the ambulance stretcher. Because proper analgesia or sedation (or both) is required, it is often prudent, although not mandatory, to take a few minutes to also obtain at least a portable radiograph. (C) Note the very significant fracture-dislocation on the prereduction radiograph. (D) Once the reduction is accomplished, there is a remarkable difference that suggests a less impressive injury. *The specific initial injury will be impossible to reconstruct from the postreduction physical examination alone.* The few minutes required to properly prepare the patient for reduction and to document the initial injury will not result in a more serious adverse outcome than has been prognosticated by the initial injury. However, when the patient has sustained multiple trauma and extremity films are a low priority, early reduction without radiographs may be warranted.

dislocation.[11] The depth of the glenoid fossa is somewhat increased by the fibrocartilaginous glenoid labrum, which forms the rim of this structure.

Most shoulder dislocations are anterior (i.e., the humeral head becomes situated in front of the glenoid fossa). Posterior dislocations are the next most common, but they only account for 2% to 5% of shoulder dislocations.[12] Less common variations include inferior (luxatio erecta), superior, and intrathoracic dislocations.

Anterior Shoulder Dislocations

As stated earlier, shoulder dislocations are the most common major joint dislocation encountered and reduced in the ED, with anterior dislocations comprising the vast majority. The usual mechanism of injury is indirect and consists of a combination of abduction, extension, and external rotation.[10,11] Only rarely is the mechanism a direct blow to the posterior aspect of the shoulder. Occasionally, especially with recurrent dislocations, the mechanism is surprisingly minor and can be puzzling to the clinician. An anterior dislocation can be induced by mere external rotation of the shoulder while rolling over in bed or reaching behind oneself for the seat belt. When the first dislocation occurs at a younger age, the recurrence rate is higher. If the first dislocation occurs before 20 years of age, there is an 80% to 92% rate of recurrence. If the first dislocation takes place after 40 years of age, the rate of recurrence is 10% to 15%.[10]. Rotator cuff injuries, however, occur more frequently in older patients with anterior shoulder dislocations.[13]

The four types of anterior dislocations are classified according to where the humeral head comes to rest. Subcoracoid dislocations account for more than 75% of anterior dislocations. The other anterior shoulder dislocations include subglenoid dislocation and the uncommon subclavicular and intrathoracic dislocations (Fig. 50.2).[10]

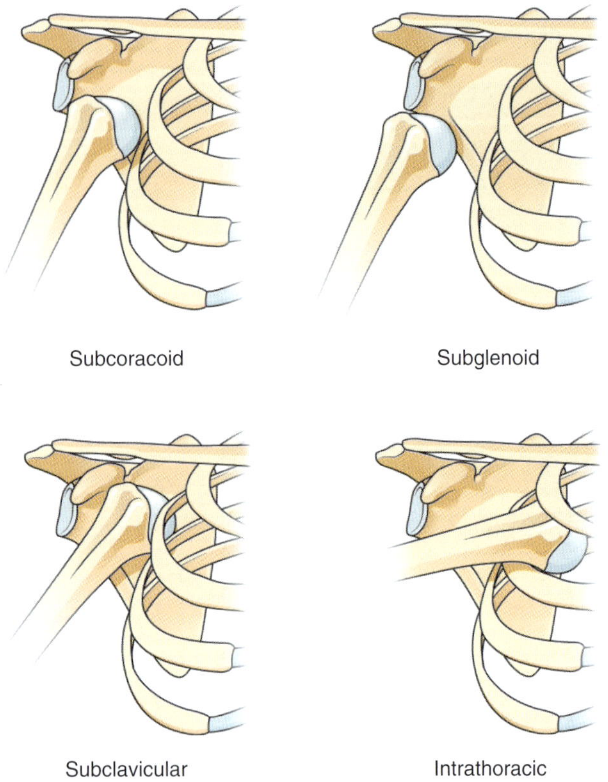

Fig. 50.2 Types of anterior shoulder dislocations.

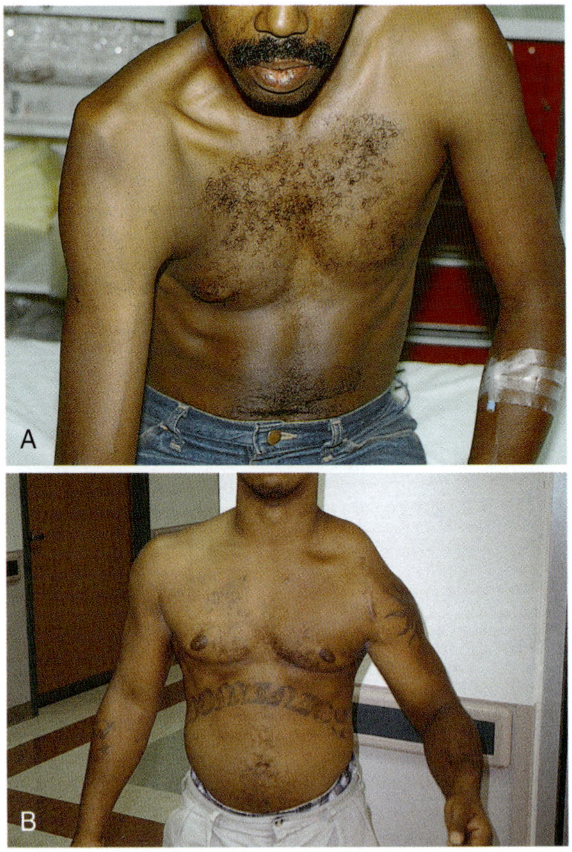

Fig. 50.3 (A) Typical manifestation of an anterior right shoulder dislocation. The shoulder is very painful, and thus the patient resists movement. The outer round contour of the shoulder is obviously flattened, and the displaced humeral head may be appreciated in the subcoracoid area. Frequently, the patient abducts the arm slightly, bends the torso toward the injured side, and supports the flexed elbow on the injured side with the other hand. (B) Obvious left shoulder dislocation. This chronic dislocation occurred frequently with minimal trauma, and the patient was able to dislocate it at will, feign a new injury, and obtain narcotics from multiple emergency departments.

Clinical Assessment

The presence of an anterior shoulder dislocation is usually obvious (Fig. 50.3). A posterior dislocation is more subtle in terms of both clinical and radiographic findings. It can be misdiagnosed as a severe contusion (Table 50.1). A patient with an anterior shoulder dislocation supports the injured extremity and leans toward the injured side while holding the arm in abduction and slight external rotation. The patient cannot adduct or internally rotate the shoulder. Visual inspection reveals loss of the rounded appearance of the shoulder because of absence of the humeral head beneath the deltoid region. The acromion is prominent and an abrupt drop-off below the acromion can be seen or palpated. An anterior fullness in the subclavicular region is visible in thinner individuals and is easily palpable in most others. Comparison with the uninjured side is a useful aid for both visual examination and palpation. Any attempt at internal rotation is quite painful and resisted by the patient. An inability to place the palm from the injured extremity on the uninjured shoulder is consistent with an anterior shoulder dislocation; after reduction, this maneuver should be possible.

Careful assessment of the neurovascular status of the affected extremity is essential. Injury to the axillary artery is rare. It occurs more commonly in older adults[13] and can be quickly assessed by a decreased or absent radial pulse or by the appearance of an expanding hematoma. It is important to evaluate the status of the axillary nerve because this is the most common nerve injury resulting from anterior dislocations.[14] Assess the sensory component of the axillary nerve by testing for sensation over the lateral aspect of the upper part of the arm in the "regimental badge" area over the deltoid muscle. Testing the motor component of the axillary nerve is a difficult undertaking in a patient with a dislocated shoulder, as it requires activation of the deltoid muscle. Less commonly, the brachial plexus may be injured by a stretch injury and produce variable nerve deficits. Perform a complete assessment of all the major nerves to the arm because other nerve injuries may occur, such as injuries to the ulnar and radial nerves.[14] A neurologic deficit does not preclude closed reduction, but in patients with a nerve injury, avoid multiple forceful attempts at reduction.

Brachial plexus injuries require an especially atraumatic reduction. If generous sedation and analgesia do not permit easy reduction in the ED, reduction of a dislocation with a nerve injury may be more prudently performed in the operating room with the patient under general anesthesia. Nerve injuries in this setting generally have a good prognosis, but the patient should be informed of the findings and the need for follow-up. The symptoms may require many months to resolve.

Vascular injuries, such as axillary artery disruption, are rare but usually obvious because of dysesthesias and coolness of the involved arm. An expanding axillary hematoma, pulse deficit, peripheral cyanosis, and pallor can be seen. Collateral circulation may produce a faint pulse in the extremity, so comparison with blood pressure on the uninjured side may be helpful. Specific lesions include complete disruption, linear tears, and thrombosis. Axillary artery injuries can occur at all ages, but they are more common in adults over 65 years of age.. The artery is particularly at risk with anterior dislocations, and dislocation with spontaneous reduction can produce the injury. Arteriography with surgical repair of the artery is required,

TABLE 50.1 Comparison of Anterior and Posterior Shoulder Dislocations: Classified According to Displacement of the Humeral Head

TYPE OF DISLOCATION	FEATURES	OTHER CLINICAL CLUES	RADIOGRAPHS
Anterior			
99% subcoracoid and subglenoid Humeral head anterior to the glenoid	Arm held in *abduction* and *slight external rotation* (abduction more prominent with subglenoid dislocation) The patient cannot adduct or *internally* rotate the shoulder	Seen from the front, the shoulder appears "squared off" Distal acromion prominent on a side view	*On AP view*: obvious dislocation *On lateral or Y view*: humeral head appears anterior to the glenoid fossa
Posterior			
95% subacromial 5% subglenoid and subspinous Humeral head posterior to the glenoid	Arm held in the sling position with adduction and internal rotation Attempts at *abduction* and *external rotation* cause extreme pain	Coracoid process prominent, glenoid fossa empty anteriorly, and humeral head bulging posteriorly	*On AP view*: vacant glenoid sign, 6-mm sign, light bulb sign *On lateral or Y view*: humeral head appears posterior to the glenoid fossa

AP, Anteroposterior.

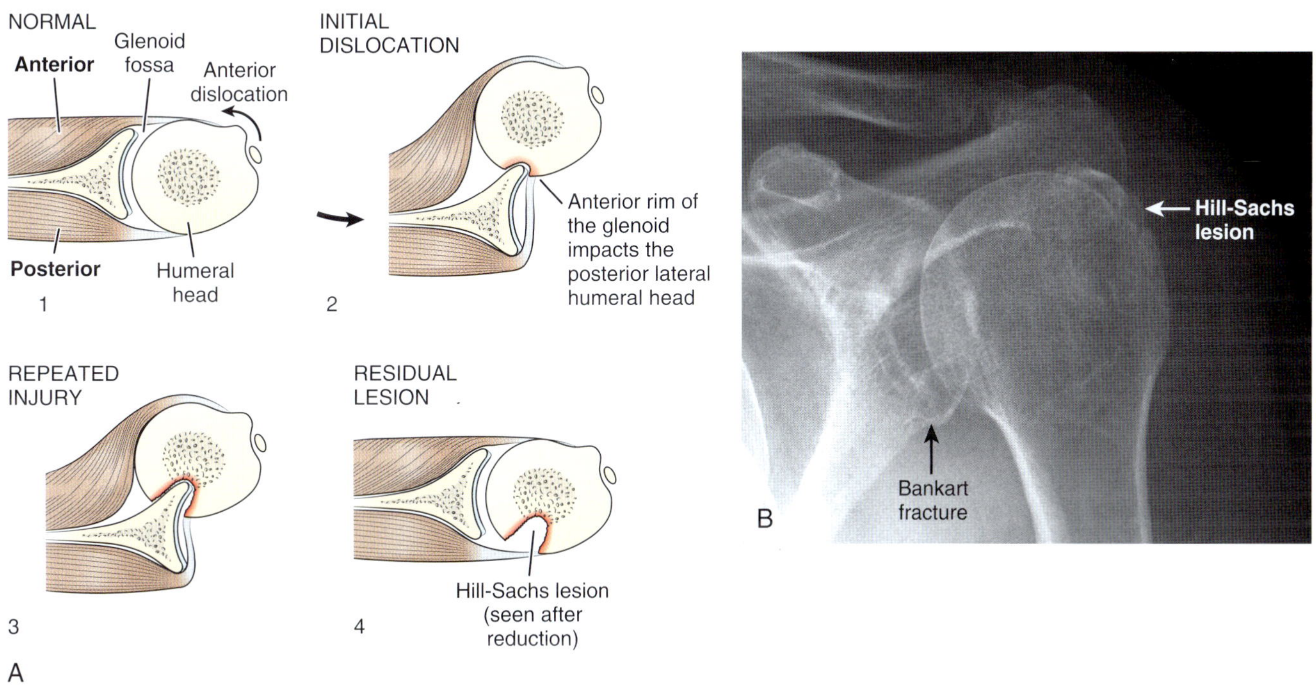

Fig. 50.4 (A) *1*, Normal. With repeated anterior shoulder dislocations, a Hill-Sachs lesion may form. *2*, During dislocation, the humeral head is damaged by the sharp anterior rim of the glenoid. *3*, With repeated dislocation, a lesion called the "hatchet sign" develops. *4*, On the reduction film the lesion is apparent. (B) Radiograph demonstrating a Hill-Sachs lesion and a Bankart fracture: a fracture of the inferior glenoid rim from impaction of the dislocated humeral head.

occasionally with fasciotomy of the forearm if the ischemia is long-standing.[15]

In many shoulder dislocations, some portion of the rotator cuff will be injured. Rotator cuff tears are easier to evaluate after reduction when the pain and swelling have subsided.

Radiologic Examination

Associated fractures are detected in 15% to 35% of anterior shoulder dislocations, with fractures of the greater tuberosity being the most common.[10] The presence of a fracture of the greater tuberosity does not change the initial management of anterior shoulder dislocations, and these fractures usually heal well after closed reduction in routine fashion.[10] The Hill-Sachs deformity, a sign of repeated dislocations, produces a groove in the posterolateral aspect of the humeral head and may be seen on prereduction or postreduction films (Fig. 50.4). The Hill-Sachs deformity is caused by impaction of the humeral head against the glenoid rim after dislocation. It rarely has any clinical significance but may result in a loose body within the joint.[13] Impaction of the humeral head against the glenoid during dislocation may also cause disruption of the anteroinferior portion of the cartilaginous labrum of the glenoid or the inferior aspect of the bony glenoid, an injury known as a *Bankart lesion*. It has been implicated as one source of recurrent dislocations but does not affect immediate ED management.[13]

Fractures of the humeral neck are frequently displaced with attempts at closed reduction, which can lead to avascular necrosis (AVN) of the humeral head.[16] The fact that humeral neck fractures are a known complication of shoulder relocation[10] supports the value of prereduction radiographs of anterior shoulder dislocations. However, some argue that clinically obvious recurrent dislocations and first-time anterior dislocations without a blunt traumatic mechanism (information usually offered by the patient) can be reduced without prior radiographs because fracture is quite unlikely in these situations.[17]

One retrospective case-control study found that the presence of any of three risk factors (age >40 years, first episode of dislocation, traumatic mechanism of injury defined as a fall greater than one flight of stairs, a fight or assault, or a motor vehicle collision) predicted clinically important fractures with a sensitivity of 97.7%.[18] However, in a prospective study by Atef and colleagues, associated injuries were found in 60% of patients with anterior shoulder dislocation, a much higher frequency than previously thought; rotator cuff tears were most commonly noted, but the injuries ranged from axillary nerve injury to greater tuberosity fracture.[19]

Anterior dislocations are not subtle on routine anteroposterior (AP) radiographs, and this view detects the most important fracture to identify, that of the humeral neck (Fig. 50.5). An adequate AP view, when combined with the typical clinical examination, allows successful detection of most anterior

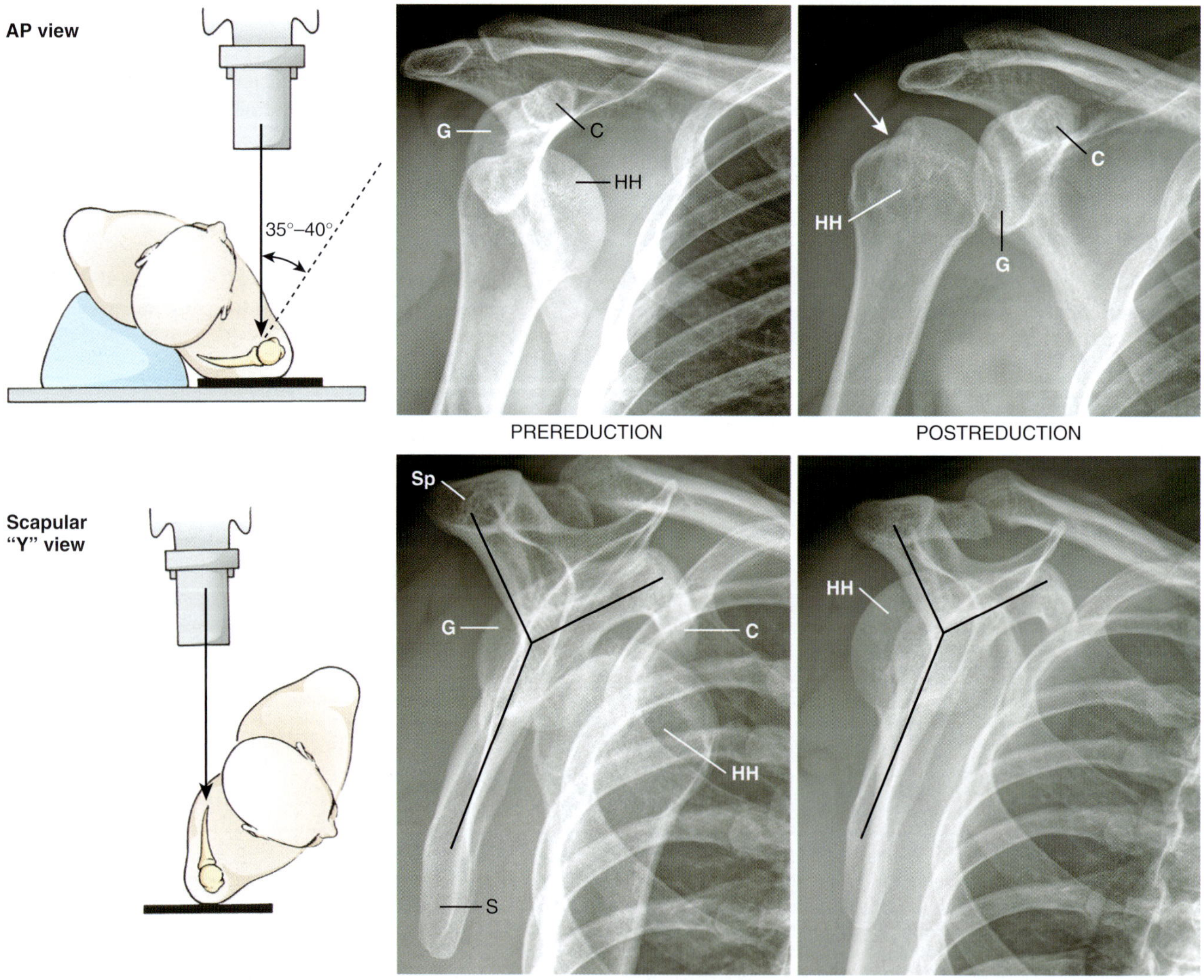

Fig. 50.5 Anteroposterior *(AP)* and scapular Y views of an anterior subcoracoid dislocation. The AP views *(top row)* are fairly easy to interpret. On the prereduction film, the humeral head is clearly dislocated from the glenoid fossa and is seen underneath the coracoid process. The correct anatomic relationship of the humeral head and glenoid is demonstrated on the postreduction film. Note the presence of a Hill-Sachs lesion *(arrow)* on the superior aspect of the humeral head. The scapular Y view *(bottom row)* is more difficult to understand. The limbs of the Y are composed of the scapular spine, the coracoid process, and the scapular body *(gray lines)*. The glenoid fossa is found at the convergence of these limbs in the center of the scapula. On the prereduction view, the humeral head is found *anterior*, or *medial*, to the glenoid and under the coracoid, thus confirming the presence of an anterior dislocation. In a posterior dislocation, the humeral head is *posterior*, or *lateral*, to the glenoid (see Fig. 50.6). On the postreduction view, the humeral head is correctly positioned in the middle of the Y, over the glenoid. *C*, Coracoid process; *G*, glenoid fossa; *HH*, humeral head; *S*, scapular body; *Sp*, scapular spine. (Diagrams from Heppenstall RB. *Fracture Treatment and Healing*. Saunders; 1980:374.)

shoulder dislocations. A true AP view of the shoulder is taken at a right angle to the scapula and requires rotation of the patient to 30 to 45 degrees.

The typical lateral views obtained include a scapular Y view (see Fig. 50.5), a transthoracic view, and an axillary view. These views rarely add to the AP film in patients with an obvious anterior dislocation, but they are of value in posterior dislocations (Fig. 50.6). The usefulness of additional views for anterior shoulder dislocations is primarily to detect fractures, and the previously mentioned lateral views (especially the transthoracic view) are quite limited in this respect. The apical oblique view has been found to be more valuable than the oblique scapular projection for acute shoulder trauma.[20] This view is obtained by angling the beam 45 degrees caudad with the patient in a 45-degree oblique position (Fig. 50.7).

Postreduction radiographs are obtained to document the success of the reduction. Occasionally, they will reveal a fracture not detected on prereduction radiographs.

POCUS by emergency physicians has been found to be highly sensitive and specific for the diagnosis of shoulder dislocations and reductions. Overall, POCUS demonstrated 100% sensitivity and 100% specificity, with 96.8% sensitivity and 99.7 specificity for diagnosis of associated fractures.[21] POCUS can be easily performed during the initial examination of the patient, thus reducing the time to diagnosis compared with plain radiography.[22] One multicenter study reported that POCUS reduced the time to diagnosis by 50 minutes.[23] Furthermore, in cases requiring procedural sedation, POCUS can rapidly confirm proper reduction while the patient remains sedated. No differences in accuracy between transducer types have been reported. Ultrasound is an operator-dependent

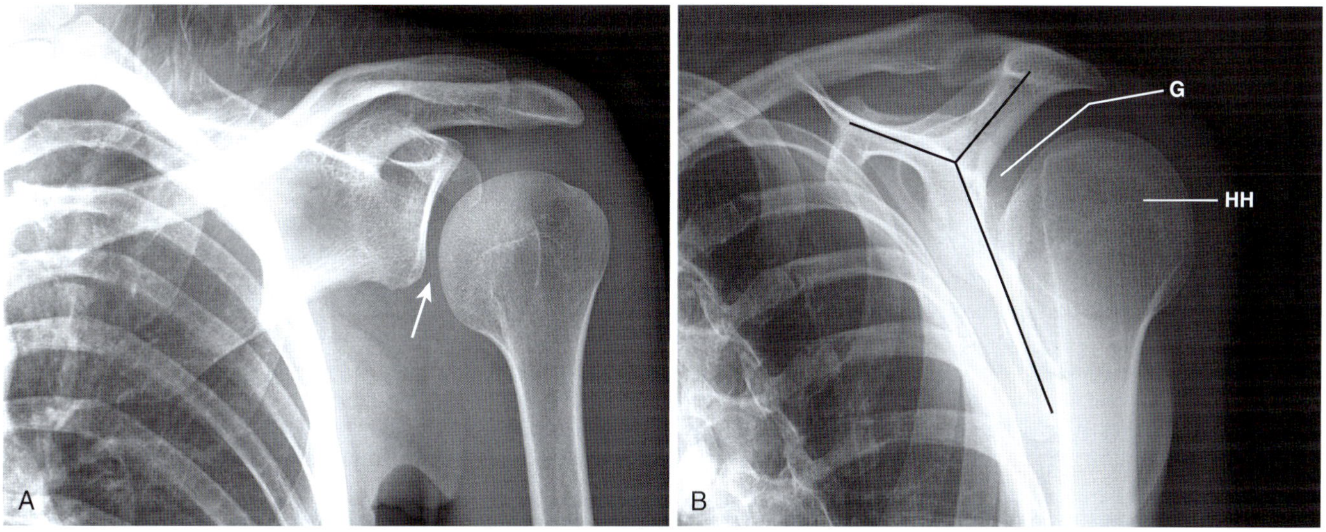

Fig. 50.6 Posterior shoulder dislocation. (A) Anteroposterior (AP) view of a patient with a posterior dislocation. A *posterior dislocation* may be difficult to appreciate on an AP view because it is *not inferiorly displaced and may appear to be in the glenoid fossa*. Note the space between the glenoid fossa and the humeral head *(arrow)*. It does not look normal. (B) The scapular Y view reveals that a posterior dislocation is present. Note that the humeral head lies *posterior, or lateral, to the glenoid fossa* rather than being centered over it. *G*, Glenoid; *HH*, humeral head.

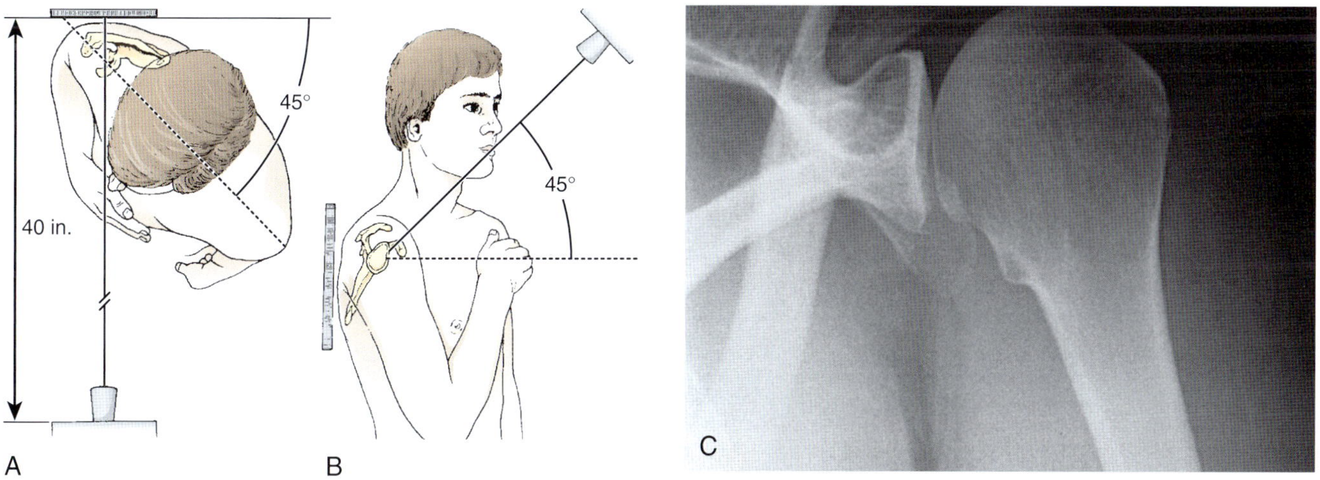

Fig. 50.7 (A–B) Positioning for an apical oblique view. The affected shoulder is placed at a 45-degree oblique position and the central ray is angled 45 degrees caudad. The affected arm is adducted. (C) Normal apical oblique view. (From Heppenstall RB. *Fracture Treatment and Healing*. Saunders; 1980:392.)

skill; thus adequate training and reinforcement of skills are necessary for routine use.

Reduction Techniques

See Video 50.1. Hippocrates (450 BCE) is generally credited with the first detailed description of reduction techniques, and it is believed that a drawing in the tomb of Upuy (1200 BCE) is the earliest depiction of such a method.[10] The Hippocratic technique involves placement of the operator's foot in the axilla to allow countertraction. This technique is problematic and not recommended by some authors.[2,10] Likewise, the Kocher method, which involves forceful leverage of the humerus, is associated with an increased rate of complications and is generally discouraged in favor of other techniques.[10,11]

This section discusses several methods of reduction that are well studied, proven to be safe, and easy to master. Regardless of the reduction technique used, gradual, gentle application of the technique is essential. Although all the techniques discussed are generally acceptable and many authors state that their techniques are quite painless,[1–4] few studies have quantified the actual pain reported by patients.[24] As noted previously, intraarticular lidocaine may offer significant relief of pain during reduction of anterior shoulder dislocations (Fig. 50.8 and Videos 50.2–50.4) A 2022 meta-analysis showed that intraarticular lidocaine had similar success rates as procedural sedation and led to decreased length of stay and complication rates, thus making it a useful alternative to procedural sedation and analgesia.[25] Ultrasound may be used to assist intraarticular lidocaine injection in both adults and pediatric patients.[26,27] When using intraarticular lidocaine, any blood present should be aspirated from the glenohumeral joint before injecting the anesthetic. Note that 10 to 20 mL of 1% lidocaine has been used with the intraarticular technique and that it may take as long as 15 to 20 minutes for adequate analgesia.

The use of regional nerve blocks (suprascapular and scalene) under ultrasound guidance have also been used to provide analgesia for closed reduction of anterior shoulder dislocations. Nerve blocks are a viable option for patients over 65 years of age or patients with significant cardiopulmonary comorbidities for whom procedural sedation may present elevated risks.[28] Studies have demonstrated similar analgesia and reduction success rates when compared to procedural sedation, but with significantly less one-on-one practitioner time and a lower ED length of stay[25,29,30] (see Chapter 31). Furthermore, the use of an ultrasound-guided axillary nerve block as an adjunct to a suprascapular nerve block for reduction of anterior shoulder dislocation has been reported.[31]

It is important to note that neither local nor regional anesthesia produces muscle relaxation, but they may obviate the need for IV access and prolonged observation. Operator judgment is an important part of the decision as to whether reduction should be attempted without premedication. Advantages of such an approach include avoidance of potential complications from drug therapy, reduced staff requirements, and theoretically, more rapid patient disposition. Certainly, a patient who is markedly intoxicated may require little if any supplemental sedative therapy. However, all patients who are reluctant or too anxious to cooperate with an attempt at reduction without medication and those with a high degree of muscle spasm should receive premedication. Generally, only one attempt is made; if unsuccessful, further attempts at reduction are made after the IV administration of sedatives (Video 50.5) When in doubt, it is best to use pharmacologic adjuncts (see Chapter 33). In addition, positioning the patient for any given reduction method should be optimized for the specific technique (Video 50.6). Several factors will help in deciding which reduction technique is best in each clinical situation. Do not use forceful techniques such as traction-countertraction in patients who are not sedated. The clinician's comfort level with a given technique is always a factor as the greatest success rates will probably result from techniques with which the clinician is most familiar. The time and resources available to the clinician must also be considered because methods such as the Stimson maneuver require more time and the availability of weights and straps. In addition, certain reduction techniques can be performed without assistance, whereas others require an additional person to apply countertraction or to help with manipulation of the scapula or humeral head. Ideally, the emergency clinician should become familiar with multiple different techniques for reducing anterior shoulder dislocations because no single method has a 100% success rate nor is any technique ideal in every situation.

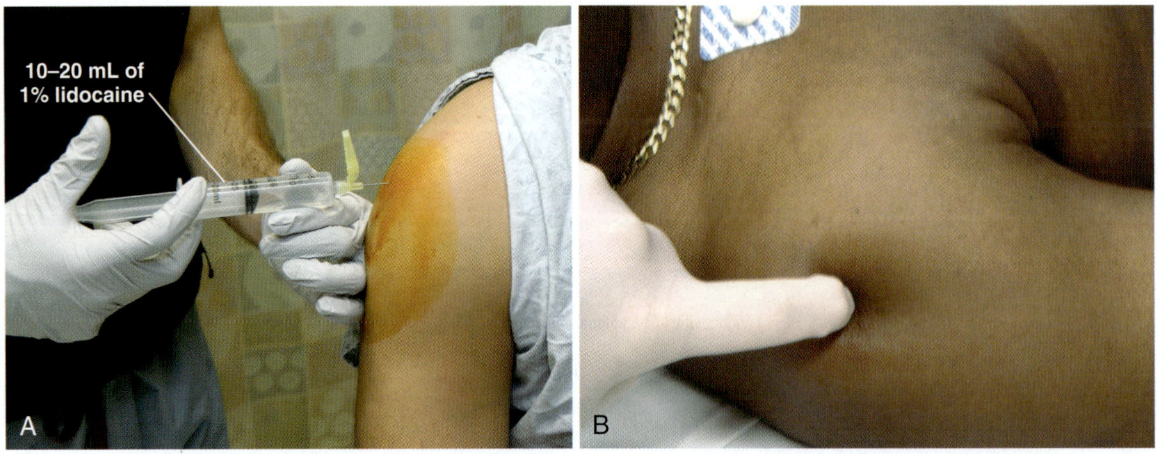

Fig. 50.8 (A) Intraarticular injection for the reduction of an acute anterior shoulder dislocation can be very effective. After aspirating blood from the joint, 10 mL to 20 mL of 1% plain lidocaine is injected slowly through the lateral sulcus. Allow 15 to 20 minutes for the lidocaine to take effect. (B) The empty glenoid fossa is easily identified when considering an injection of lidocaine into the joint to facilitate reduction of a dislocated shoulder.

Stimson Maneuver

The Stimson maneuver is a classic technique that offers the advantage of not requiring an assistant (Fig. 50.9A and Video 50.7). Place the patient prone on an elevated stretcher and suspend approximately 2.5 to 5.0 kg (5 to 10 lb) of weight from the wrist.[10,11] The weights can be strapped to the wrist, or a commercially available Velcro wrist splint can be placed and the weights hung from the strap with a hook.[32] The slow, steady traction produced with this method often permits reduction, but 20 to 30 minutes may be required. If needed, facilitate reduction by externally rotating the extended arm.

Variations of this method include the recommendation for flexion of the elbow to further relax the biceps tendon and the application of manual traction instead of weights.[33,34] Rollinson[35] allowed the arm to hang under its own weight after a supraclavicular block and reported a 91% success rate with usually no more than a gentle pull on the arm after 20 minutes in this position. Each variation of the Stimson method can be used in combination with the scapular manipulation technique described later. Indeed, a success rate of 96% has been reported with the combined prone position, hanging weights, IV analgesia and sedation, and scapular manipulation.[32]

Disadvantages of the Stimson method include the time required to achieve reduction and possible dangers to the patient associated with the positioning required for this technique. There is a potential danger of patients slipping off the elevated bed. A "seat belt" strap or bedsheet may be placed around the patient and stretcher to avoid movement of the patient off the stretcher. Airway access to a patient in the prone position may be more difficult in the setting of an overly intoxicated patient or one who becomes overly sedated. Logistically, the Stimson method may be difficult. One must have a bed that elevates to a suitable height for length of the patient's arm and a convenient method to hang the weights.

Scapular Manipulation Technique

This method is popular because of its ease of performance, reported safety, and acceptability to patients (see Fig. 50.9B and Video 50.8). To date, no complications from the scapular manipulation technique have been reported in the literature.[24,32,36] Shoulder reduction via this method focuses on repositioning the glenoid fossa rather than the humeral head, and less force is required than with many other methods. Its success rate is high, generally greater than 90% in experienced hands.[32,36,37] Some studies report higher success rates in patients who have had repeated dislocations and lower rates in patients with an associated greater tuberosity fracture.[37] The initial maneuver for scapular manipulation is traction on the arm as it is held in 90 degrees of forward flexion. This may be performed with the patient prone and the arm hanging down, as described for the Stimson method, with or without flexion of the elbow to 90 degrees. Alternatively, this traction may be applied by placing an outstretched arm over the seated patient's midclavicular region while pulling the injured extremity with the other arm. Regardless of the means of arm traction, slight external rotation of the humerus may facilitate reduction by releasing the superior glenohumeral ligament and presenting a favorable profile of the humeral head to the glenoid fossa.[38]

The prone patient position is recommended for those not familiar with the technique because it facilitates identification of the scapula for manipulation (medial rotation of the tip). Nonetheless, the technique can be performed with the patient supine given that the patient's shoulder is flexed to 90 degrees and the scapula is exposed during gentle upward traction on the humerus. Although seated scapular manipulation offers the advantage of not requiring the patient to go through the awkward and potentially uncomfortable assumption of the prone position, it is a technically more difficult variation of scapular manipulation, especially if sedation is going to be necessary. When using the prone position, place the injured shoulder over the edge of the bed to allow the arm to hang perpendicular for the application of traction (see Fig. 50.9A).[36]

After the application of traction, manipulate the scapula to complete the reduction. Anderson and associates[36] recommended manipulation of the scapula after the patient's arm is relaxed; however, success is possible with no delay in performing this second step.[24] Manipulate the scapula by stabilizing the superior aspect of the scapula with one hand and pushing the inferior tip of the scapula medially toward the spine. Place the thumb of the hand stabilizing the superior aspect of the scapula along the lateral border of the scapula to assist the pressure applied by the thumb of the other hand. A small degree of dorsal displacement of the scapular tip is recommended as it is being pushed as far as possible in the medial direction.[36]

When the patient is properly positioned with the affected arm hanging perpendicularly, the lateral border of the scapula may be difficult to find in larger patients. This border is generally located quite laterally with the patient in this position, and it must be properly located before any attempt at reduction. The reduction itself is occasionally so subtle that it may be missed by both the patient and operator. A minor shift of the arm may be the only clue that reduction has been successful. Careful palpation of the subclavicular area to locate the position of the humeral head before repositioning the patient may be used to determine the success of the reduction.

Best-of-Both Technique

A variation of the seated scapular manipulation technique is the "best-of-both" (BOB) maneuver (see Fig. 50.9C).[39] To perform the BOB maneuver, position the patient seated sideways on the stretcher with the unaffected shoulder and hip against the fully elevated head of the stretcher. Stand on the foot end of the gurney at the patient's affected side and use one hand to apply downward force on the proximal end of the patient's bent forearm. Use the other hand to grasp the patient's hand and gently rotate the arm internally or externally as needed. Once downward force is being applied, ask an assistant to perform the scapular manipulation maneuver described earlier.[39]

External Rotation Method

The external rotation method offers the advantage of requiring only one person and no special equipment (see Fig. 50.9D and Videos 50.9 and 50.10). The technique needs no strength or endurance on the part of the operator and is well tolerated by patients.[2] The actual pain experienced by patients with this technique has not been quantified, but Plummer and Clinton[2] stated that it can be performed with "little, if any sedation." In this technique, the basic maneuver is slow, gentle external rotation of the fully adducted arm. In 1957, Parvin described a self-reduction external rotation technique in which the patient sits on a swivel-type chair and grasps a fixed post positioned waist high and slowly turns the body to enact external

Anterior Shoulder Dislocation Reduction

A. Stimson Maneuver

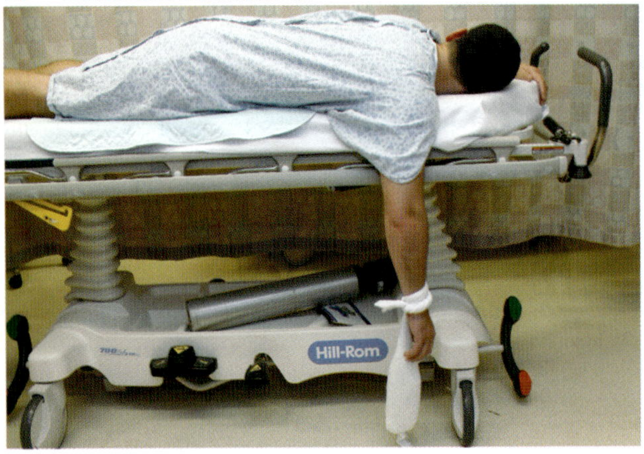

Place the patient prone on the edge of the stretcher. Be careful that a sedated or intoxicated patient does not fall off the table. Belts or sheets can be used to secure the patient to the stretcher, 5-kg weights are attached to the arm, and the patient maintains this position for 20 to 30 minutes, if necessary.

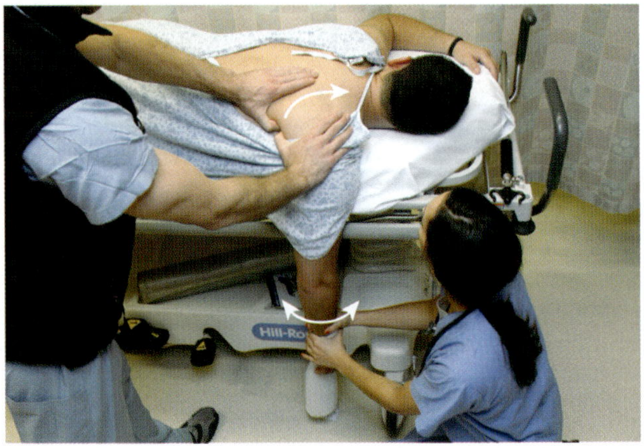

The addition of scapular manipulation and/or gentle external and internal rotation of the shoulder with manual traction may aid in reduction.

B. Scapular Manipulation

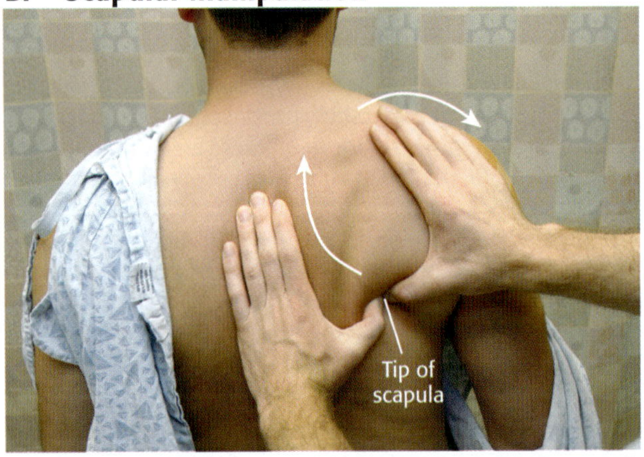

Rotate the inferior tip of the scapula medially and dorsally toward the spine with the tips of your thumbs.

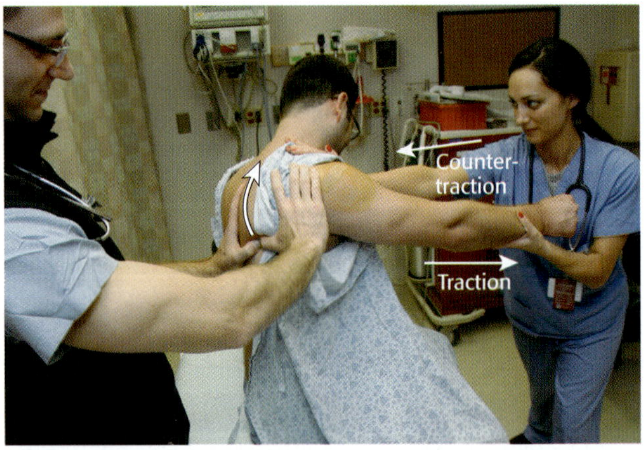

The procedure can take place with the patient prone (as in the Stimson technique) or with the patient seated. For the latter, have an assistant apply traction on the arm while applying countertraction on the ipsilateral clavicle.

C. Best-of-Both Technique

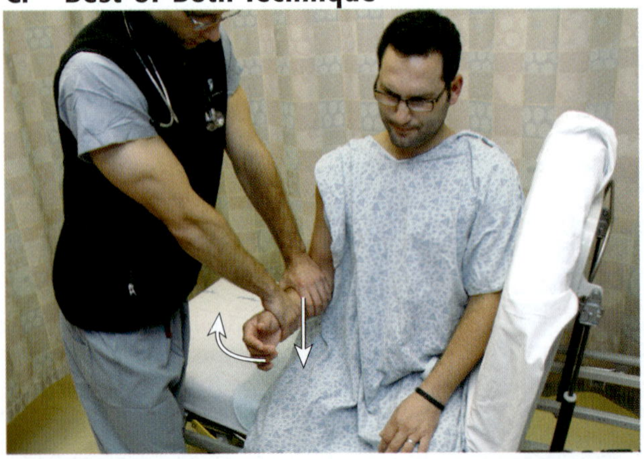

Position the patient seated sideways with the unaffected shoulder and hip against the upright head of the stretcher. Apply downward force on the patient's flexed forearm, and gently rotate the arm internally or externally as needed.

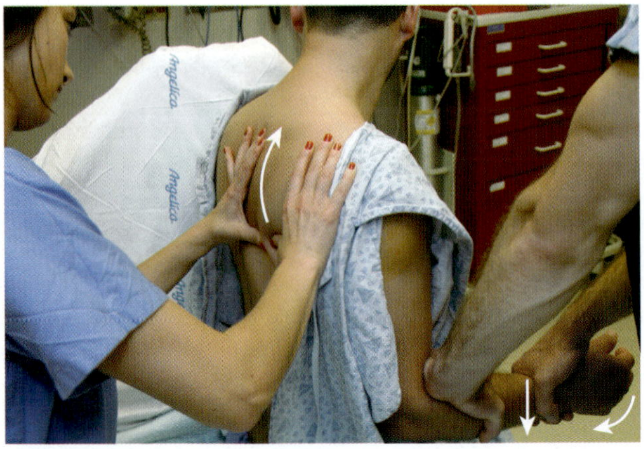

Once downward force is applied, instruct an assistant to perform scapular manipulation as described previously.

Fig. 50.9 Anterior shoulder dislocation reduction methods. *ED*, Emergency department.

Anterior Shoulder Dislocation Reduction

D. External Rotation

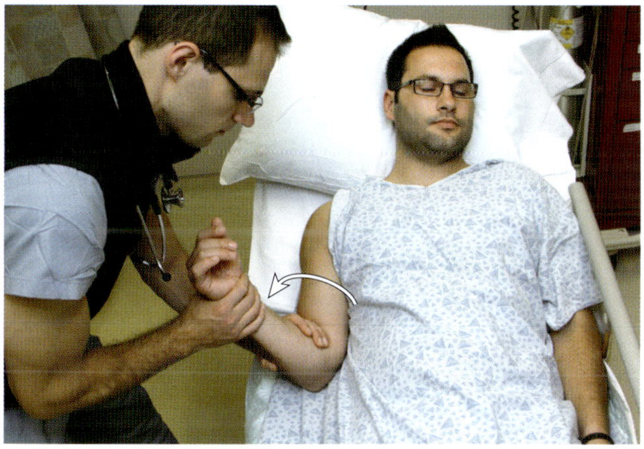

Fully adduct the arm and flex the elbow to 90 degrees. Hold the patient's wrist and guide the arm into slow and gently external rotation. Halt momentarily if the patient experiences pain. Continue the rotation until the forearm is laying on the bed. No traction is applied.

E. Milch Technique

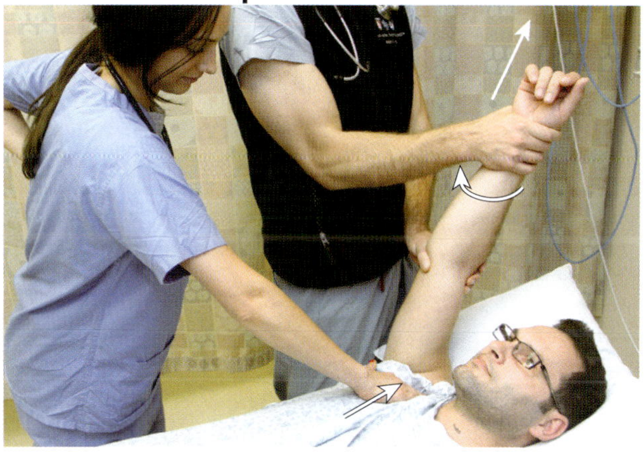

First abduct the arm to an overhead position by grasping the patient's arm at the elbow or wrist. Once fully abducted, apply gentle longitudinal traction with slight external rotation. If reduction does not occur quickly, push the humeral head upward into the glenoid fossa.

F. Traction-Countertraction Method

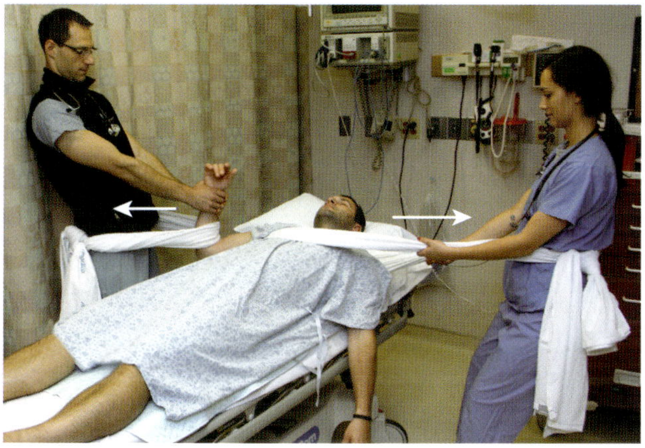

Wrap one sheet around the affected axilla and the assistant's waist. The assistant leans back to apply countertraction. Wrap another sheet around the patient's flexed arm and your waist. Lean back to apply traction.

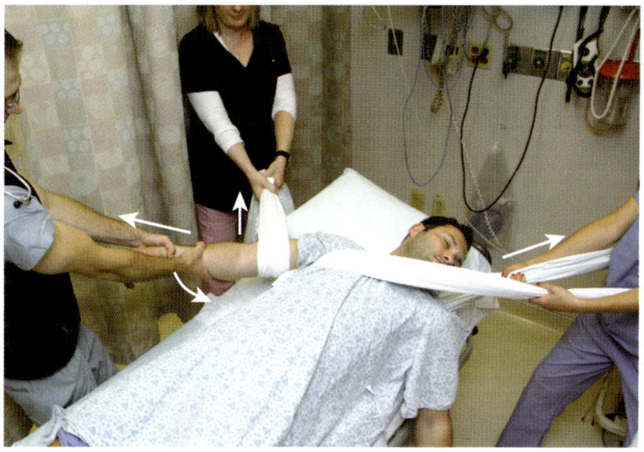

Reduction can be facilitated by gently adducting the arm (after traction is applied) while a second assistant provides gentle lateral traction on the humerus.

G. Spaso Technique

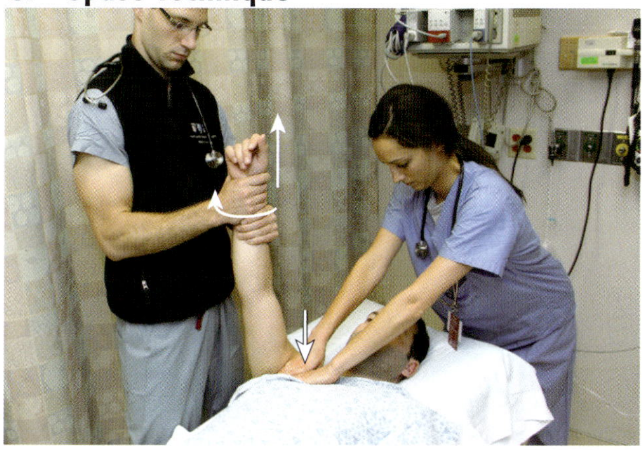

With the patient supine, gently lift the arm toward the ceiling while applying gentle vertical traction. Instruct an assistant to apply countertraction. Apply gentle external rotation during the procedure.

H. Vertical Traction Reduction Technique

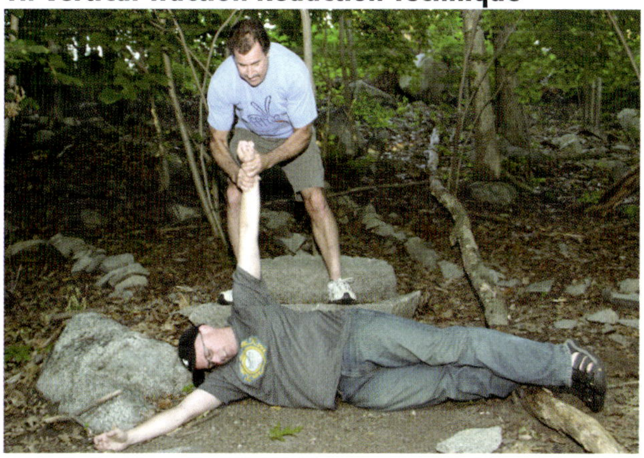

While the patient lies on the unaffected side, lift him a short distance off the ground by grasping the abducted arm of the injured side. This is a field technique and should not be used in the ED.

Fig. 50.9 (cont'd)

rotation.[40] Parvin reported that the reduction usually takes place at 70 to 110 degrees of external rotation.[40]

Since Parvin's initial study, this method has been described with the patient supine and the affected arm adducted tightly to the patient's side.[1,41] Flex the elbow to 90 degrees and hold it in the adducted position with the operator's hand closest to the patient. Use the other hand to hold the patient's wrist and guide the arm into slow and gentle external rotation. The procedure may require several minutes because each time the patient experiences pain, the procedure is halted momentarily. Although the report of Mirick and coworkers[1] mentioned using the forearm as "a lever," a later description clearly recommends allowing the forearm to "fall" under its own weight.[2] No additional force should be applied to the forearm, and no traction is exerted on the arm.

The end point of the reduction may be difficult to identify because reduction is frequently very subtle. It is therefore recommended that external rotation be continued until the forearm is near the coronal plane (lying on the bed, perpendicular to the body), a process that usually takes 5 to 10 minutes.[2] If the patient's dislocation persists after full external rotation, apply steady gentle traction at the elbow. Reduction may occasionally be noted when the arm is rotated back internally. The success rate of this technique when performed by emergency clinicians has been reported as over 80%.[41]

Milch Technique

Proponents of the Milch method praise its gentle nature, high success rate, lack of complications, and tolerance by patients (see Fig. 50.9E).[4] It can be described as "reaching up to pull an apple from a tree." The basic steps of this technique are abduction, external rotation, and gentle traction of the affected arm. Finally, if needed, the humeral head can be pushed into the glenoid fossa with the thumb or fingers.

In describing this technique, Milch[42] wrote that the fully abducted arm was in a natural position in which there was little tension on the muscles of the shoulder girdle. He postulated that this was related to our ancestral "arboreal brachiation" (swinging from trees). The primary step in this technique is to abduct the affected arm to an overhead position. Russell and colleagues[38] had their patients raise their arm and put their hand behind their head as a first step. Although this seems odd, patients can usually do this quite readily with little assistance and be quite comfortable in this position. Alternatively, abduct the arm by grasping the patient's elbow or the wrist. Lacey and Crawford[43] found that the prone position, with the patient's shoulder close to the end of the bed, facilitated this step.

Once the arm is fully abducted, apply gentle longitudinal traction with slight external rotation. If reduction does not occur quickly, push the humeral head upward into the glenoid fossa with the thumb or fingers of the other hand. Studies have reported success rates of 90% or greater.[4,38] In a comparison study of external rotation and the Milch technique for reduction of anterior shoulder dislocations without sedation, success rates were equivalent but external rotation was noted to be easier and less painful for the patient.[41]

Traction-Countertraction

This traction-countertraction method is commonly used in the ED, largely because of tradition, clinician comfort, and a high success rate (see Fig. 50.9F). Clinician familiarity is an advantage of this technique, but it requires more than one operator, some degree of force, and occasionally, endurance. This technique is usually quite uncomfortable for the patient, and premedication is recommended before any attempt. In a 2014 comparison study of traction-countertraction versus modified scapular manipulation, modified scapular manipulation was better tolerated by patients and had a better success rate on first attempt; traction-countertraction was more successful on second attempt.[44]

With the patient supine, wrap a sheet or strap around the upper part of the patient's chest and under the axilla of the affected shoulder. Ask an assistant to hold the sheet, preferably by wrapping it around the assistant's waist to take advantage of body weight rather than arm strength to apply the countertraction. Traction may then be applied onto the extended arm by the clinician, but this generally results in operator fatigue, especially if the operator relies on biceps strength to provide continuous traction. Instead, flex the elbow of the affected side to 90 degrees and wrap a sheet or strap around the proximal part of the forearm and then around the operator's waist. Elevate the bed to the point at which the sheet can sit at the level of the operator's ischial tuberosities. This allows the operator to comfortably lean back and use body weight to supply the force of traction, thereby reducing the possibility of operator fatigue. The portion of the sheet that is positioned on the patient's forearm tends to ride up; flexion of the elbow beyond 90 degrees will minimize this problem. Alternatively, the operator merely leans backward with the arms fully extended, again using the continuous weight of the body rather than the strength of the biceps to provide constant traction.

Once traction has been applied, the operator must be patient because the procedure may take quite a few minutes to be successful. The premedication is probably inadequate if the patient resists the procedure or is notably uncomfortable during attempts at reduction. Do not hesitate to order supplementary medications. Gentle, limited external rotation is sometimes useful to complete the reduction.[10] Applying traction to an arm that is slightly abducted from the patient's body is often successful, but some operators prefer to slowly bring the arm medial to the patient's midline while maintaining traction or to have an assistant apply a gentle lateral force to the midhumerus to direct the humeral head laterally. Successful reduction is usually presaged by slight lengthening of the arm as relaxation occurs, and a noticeable "clunk" may occur at the point of reduction. A brief wave of fasciculations in the deltoid may also be seen at the time of reduction.

Spaso Technique

The Spaso technique was first reported by Spaso Miljesic as a simple, single-operator technique requiring minimal force (see Fig. 50.9G and Video 50.11).[45] A 2015 study comparing the Spaso technique to external rotation found both to be equally efficacious; however, the Spaso technique was faster, more efficient, and more easily performed.[46] Place the patient in the supine position and grasp the affected arm around the wrist or distal end of the forearm. Gently lift the affected arm vertically toward the ceiling and apply gentle vertical traction. While maintaining traction continuously, externally rotate the arm. Reduction may be subtle but is generally signaled by hearing or feeling a "clunk." Completion of this technique may require several minutes of gentle traction to allow the muscles of the patient's shoulder to relax.

Fast, Reliable, and Safe (FARES) Method

This method was first described in 2009 (Fig. 50.10 A–D and Video 50.12).[47] Proponents tout high success rates, favorable reduction times, and low levels of pain during reduction, even when performed without analgesia.[48,49] With the patient lying supine, use both hands to grasp the patient's wrist on the affected side. Keep the patient's elbow extended with the forearm in neutral rotation. Slowly abduct the patient's arm. While keeping gentle longitudinal traction on the arm, apply brief (2 to 3 seconds) and short-range (5 cm above and below the horizontal level) vertical oscillating movements. When the arm is abducted past 90 degrees, gently externally rotate the arm while maintaining longitudinal traction, abduction, and vertical oscillating movements. Reduction is usually achieved by 120 degrees of abduction. Once reduction is complete, gently internally rotate the arm to rest the forearm across the chest wall.

Boss-Holzach-Matter (Davos) Technique

This method requires clear instructions from the clinician and compliance from the patient (Fig. 50.11 and Video 50.13). The patient flexes the ipsilateral knee as much as possible, then passes both hands in front of the flexed knee. The wrists are then tied together with an elastic band or ace wrap. The elbows are kept close to the thigh to keep the shoulders relaxed. The clinician then sits on the patient's foot (if performed in the wilderness, a rock or log can be used) and instructs the patient to lean the head back and let the shoulders roll forward. By extending the neck, the patient exerts a constant traction on the injured shoulder and allows the dislocation to be reduced without any additional maneuvers on the physician's part.[50] In a 2016 study, 86% of patients achieved reduction on first attempt, 21% of whom required no analgesia.[51]

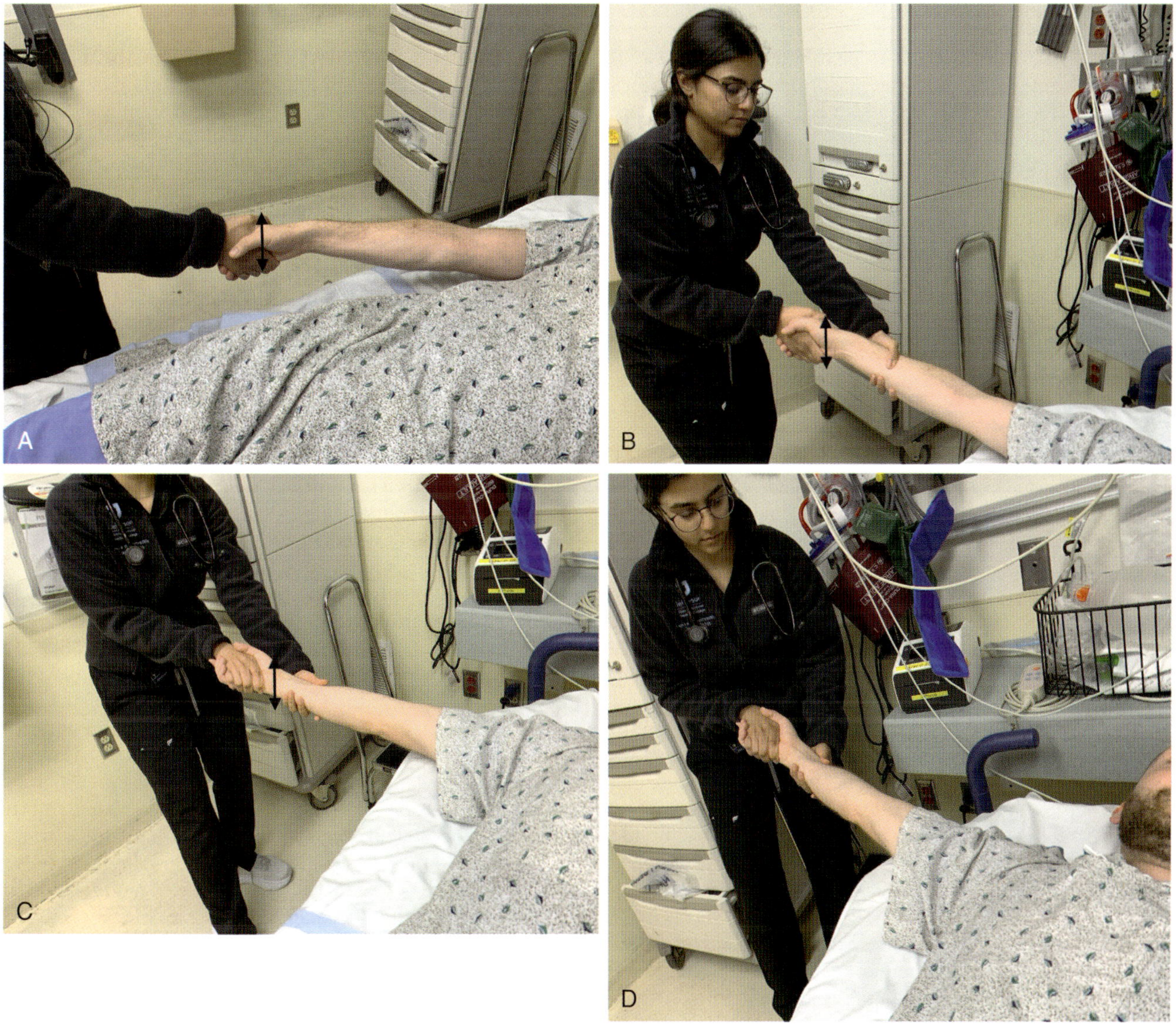

Fig. 50.10 (A) Grasp the patient's wrist on the affected side. Keep the patient's elbow extended with the forearm in neutral rotation. Apply brief (2 to 3 seconds) and short-range (5 cm above and below the horizontal level) vertical oscillating movements. (B) Slowly abduct the patient's arm, while keeping gentle longitudinal traction on the arm. Continue vertical oscillating movements (C) When the arm is abducted past 90 degrees, gently externally rotate the arm while maintaining longitudinal traction, abduction, and vertical oscillating movements. (D) Reduction is usually achieved by 120 degrees of abduction.

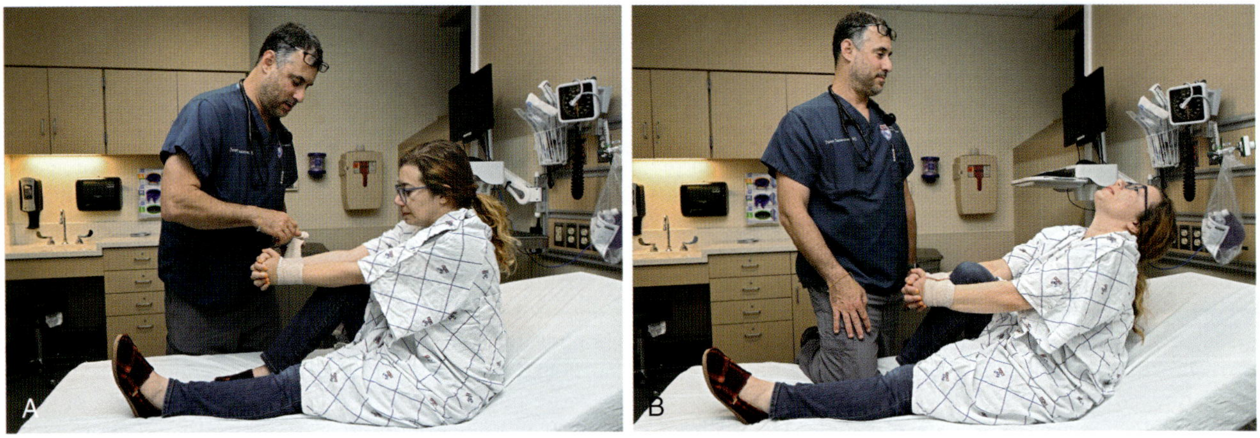

Fig. 50.11 (A) Flex the ipsilateral knee as much as possible. Bind the wrists together and place them in front of the flexed knee. (B) Apply weight to the patient's foot. Instruct the patient to extend their neck and lean back, while letting their shoulders roll forward with arms extended.

Other Methods

Poulsen[52] reported a method termed the vertical traction reduction technique that may be performed in field settings (see Fig. 50.9H and Videos 50.14 and Video 50.15). In this technique the patient lies on the unaffected side and is lifted a short distance off the ground by grasping the abducted arm on the injured side. The patient's body weight acts to affect the reduction. Poulsen's success rate was 74% in a series of 23 patients, all of whom were premedicated. However, the author[52] also postulated that this technique could place undue stress on the brachial plexus or axillary vessels. Use of this technique should be avoided if other options are available.

The modified chair technique[53] is performed while the patient sits sideways in a chair. The patient allows their arm to be abducted over the chair's backrest, which is often set up with a pillow or folded sheet placed over it for comfort. The operator uses both hands to hold the patient's forearm at the proximal and distal ends. The operator then applies external rotation until reduction is achieved, with an audible or palpable clunk. In a study of 141 patients who underwent this technique, 96.5% had reduction on the first attempt without use of any anesthesia.[53]

Prakash's method[54] can be done without anesthesia.[55] Reduction is attempted in a sitting position, though the patient can stand if that is more comfortable. The clinician holds the dislocated arm at the elbow and wrist. Next, the shoulder is externally rotated in the position of deformity to bring the arm into the coronal plane, without any adduction or abduction. The shoulder should be maintained in maximal external rotation for 2 to 3 minutes. Next, the arm is gradually adducted while external rotation is maintained. Finally, the arm is internally rotated so that the hand touches the opposite shoulder. Reduction can be achieved without any audible clunks.

A 2020 study examined the effectiveness of three different methods for self-assisted reduction taught via smartphone video link.[56] Patients who presented to the ED with anterior shoulder dislocation were randomized to the Stimson, Milch, or Boss-Holzach-Matter technique. Each patient was given a link to watch a short instructional video on a smartphone and instructed to attempt self-reduction. Success rates for the Milch and Boss-Holzach-Matter (55% and 53%, respectively) were higher than that of the Stimson method (16%).[56] This has implications for care as the use of telemedicine expands.

Postreduction Care

After an attempt at reduction, the neurovascular status of the affected extremity should be rechecked, and the results documented in the patient's medical record. Indirect evidence that the reduction has been successful includes an immediate decrease in pain, restoration of the round shoulder contour, and increased passive mobility of the shoulder. No harm is done by putting the joint through a limited range of motion. If the patient can tolerate placement of the palm from the injured arm on the opposite shoulder, it is quite likely that the shoulder reduction was successful (Fig. 50.12A). For patients with possible axillary nerve injury, close to 90% will recover with expectant management. Nevertheless, it is prudent to refer these patients for early orthopedic follow-up.[57]

Postreduction radiographs are recommended to make a careful search for new fractures. Although most greater tuberosity fractures do not alter patient management, patients with greater tuberosity fractures displaced more than 1 cm after closed reduction almost always have an associated rotator cuff tear[58] and should receive prompt orthopedic consultation because they may require operative repair.

Traditional postreduction treatment focuses on the importance of preventing the shoulder from dislocating again after the patient is discharged. This is best accomplished by immobilizing the joint with a commercially available shoulder immobilizer or a sling and swath to limit external rotation and abduction (see Chapter 51). Orthopedic follow-up is recommended for all anterior shoulder dislocations because the incidence of rotator cuff injury is as high as 64%, which may complicate restoration of normal function.[59] As a general rule, the older the patient, the shorter the recommended time of immobilization.[10] Those older than 60 years should have early follow-up (e.g., 5 to 7 days) to allow early mobilization and avoid persistent shoulder joint stiffness or adhesive capsulitis. Younger patients are usually immobilized for approximately 3 weeks and can be instructed to follow up within 1 or 2 weeks of the event. As mentioned earlier, young age confers risk of recurrent dislocation, but it is not clear if prolonged immobilization decreases recurrence rates. A 2015 meta-analysis found that immobilization for more than 1 week did not reduce recurrence rates.[60]

Since the early 2000s, the wisdom of immobilization in internal rotation has been questioned. Several studies have shown that placing the arm in internal rotation actually

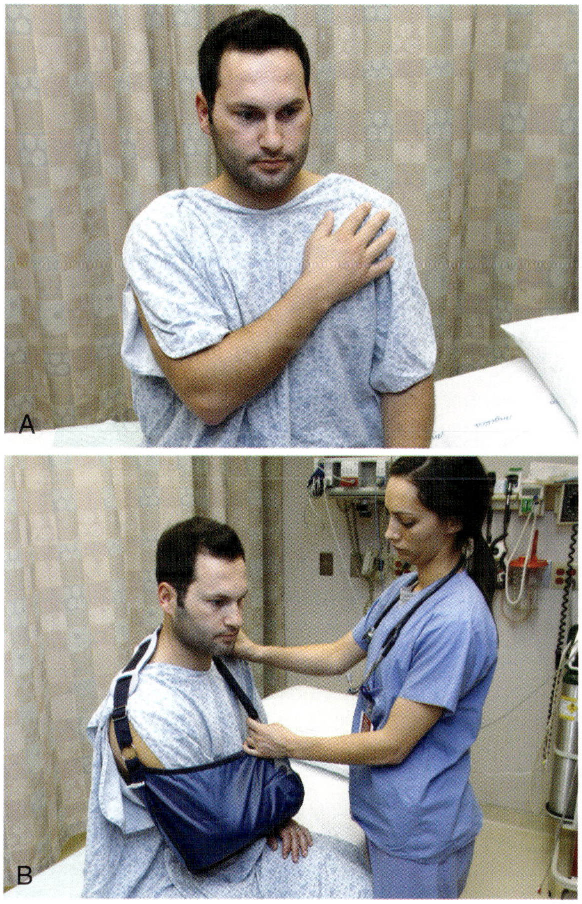

Fig. 50.12 (A) If a patient with a shoulder injury can place the palm of the injured arm on top of the contralateral shoulder, it is unlikely that a shoulder dislocation is present. Alternatively, completion of this maneuver after an attempt at reduction provides strong evidence that the reduction was successful, even if the patient is still sedated. (B) The best way to immobilize any reduced shoulder dislocation is uncertain and unlikely to be of consequence for a few days (see text). A typical shoulder immobilizer or a simple sling is appropriate pending orthopedic referral and follow-up.

increases labral detachment from the glenoid rim, whereas some degree of external rotation maximizes contact between the detached labrum and the glenoid rim.[61–63] In one study, cadavers were used to measure the force of contact between the labrum and the glenoid rim in different arm positions. The authors of this study found that maximum contact force was actually generated in 45 degrees of external rotation, whereas no contact force was generated with the arm in internal rotation.[63] Unfortunately, the question of which position (e.g., internal versus external rotation) is superior for postreduction immobilization remains unanswered. Clinical studies thus far have shown conflicting results.[64–67] A 2020 meta-analysis found that early external immobilization resulted in a lower rate of recurrence compared with internal immobilization.[68] However, external immobilization certainly presents quality of life concerns, as patients may have significantly diminished comfort and functionality with their upper extremity immobilized in such a position for an extended period of time. One may consider all of these factors when selecting an immobilization method. It is not unreasonable to immobilize the extremity in a manner consistent with the recommendations of the orthopedic surgeons at one's institution until further evidence is presented. When in doubt, a simple sling or the traditional shoulder immobilizer will certainly suffice pending 5- to 7-day follow-up (see Fig. 50.12B).

Discharge the patient with oral analgesics to minimize discomfort and instruct them to return if the clinical condition worsens. Periodically, one may encounter a return visit from a successfully treated patient who is in severe pain from hemarthrosis. In one series of patients older than 60 years, Trimmings[69] reported excellent pain relief by aspirating the hemarthrosis 24 to 48 hours after shoulder reduction. This can be accomplished by using the technique of arthrocentesis described in Chapter 54. In addition, intraarticular instillation of 10 mL to 20 mL of 1% lidocaine (or a longer-acting local anesthetic) may be helpful for further pain relief.

Posterior Shoulder Dislocations

Posterior shoulder dislocations account for approximately 2% to 5% of all shoulder dislocations (Video 50.16).[12] Because they are so uncommon, posterior dislocations have the potential to be missed. In fact, delays in diagnosis for weeks to months have been reported.[70,71] This may lead to increased rates of dislocation arthropathy and chronic pain.[14] The mechanism of injury is almost always indirect and consists of a combination of internal rotation, adduction, and flexion.[10] Classic precipitating events include seizure, electrical shock, and falls. Some patients may not be seen until at a point well past the original event.[70] In addition, patients with seizures may not complain of pain or a limited range of motion in the immediate postictal period because of their altered mental status.

Clinical Assessment

Though clinically less obvious than anterior dislocations, posterior shoulder dislocations do occur in a typical, recognizable manner. Mistakes may be made if the clinician is overly reliant on AP radiographs, which are potentially misleading[70] and may result in misdiagnosing the injury as a soft tissue contusion or acromioclavicular (AC) strain. The principal sign of a posterior dislocation is an arm that is somewhat fixed in adduction and internal rotation (Fig. 50.13). Abduction and external rotation are limited, and attempts to perform these movements generally elicit pain.[10,71] Inspection and palpation reveal loss of the normal anterior contour of the shoulder, as well as a prominent coracoid and acromion. The shoulder is flattened anteriorly and rounded posteriorly, and the humeral head may be palpable.[10,71]

Comparison with the opposite shoulder should be undertaken with caution because this injury may occasionally occur bilaterally. Perform a neurovascular assessment in the standard manner, but such complications are unusual with posterior dislocations.

Radiologic Examination

The key point regarding radiographs for posterior shoulder dislocations is the subtle nature of this dislocation on a single AP film (Figs. 50.14A and 50.15A) and the diagnostic importance of the scapular Y view (see Fig. 50.14B) or the axillary view (see Fig. 50.15B). Diagnosis of posterior shoulder dislocation is quite easy with the axillary view, whereas the routine AP and lateral views are difficult to interpret in approximately half the cases.[70] The axillary view is generally available in the radiology department and can be obtained with as little as 20 to 30 degrees of abduction and the plate placed on the shoulder.[70] In addition to easy visualization of the posteriorly situated humeral head, the axillary view often reveals an impression fracture of the humeral head (see Fig. 50.15B). The scapular Y view is produced by superimposing the head of the humerus over the coracoid, acromion, and body of the scapula, which form a Y shape. In the event of a posterior shoulder dislocation, the head of the humerus will lie posterior to the glenoid (away from the chest wall) (see Figs. 50.6B and 50.14B).

Even though axillary and scapular Y views are diagnostic, clues to posterior dislocation do exist on AP films. The internally rotated humeral head appears symmetric on an AP film and is in the shape of a light bulb, as opposed to the normal club-shaped appearance created by the greater tuberosity (Fig. 50.16). With posterior dislocation, the space between the articular surface of the humeral head and the anterior glenoid rim is widened, and there is a decrease in the half-moon–shaped overlap of the head and the fossa.[71] There may also be a compression fracture on the medial aspect of the humeral head, as indicated by a dense line. This is known as the trough sign.[72] A fracture of the lesser tuberosity should always prompt a search for the presence of a posterior shoulder dislocation.

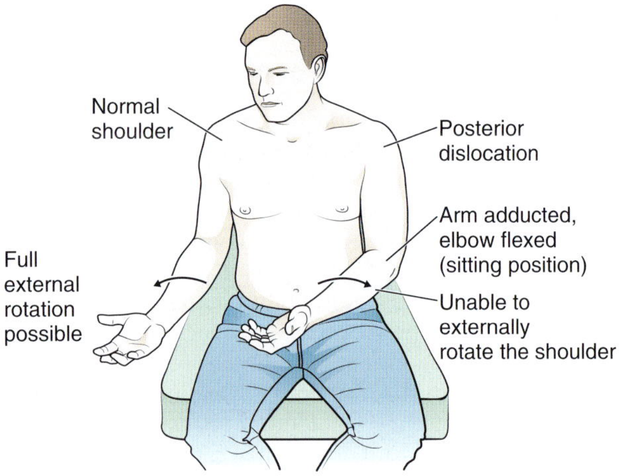

Fig. 50.13 A posterior dislocation may be difficult to appreciate on radiographs. A clue to a posterior shoulder dislocation is the arm locked in adduction and internal rotation and the patient's inability to rotate the shoulder externally with the elbow flexed at 90 degrees.

As mentioned earlier in this section, ultrasound is a useful tool for the diagnosis of shoulder dislocations, including posterior shoulder dislocations and may be used as an adjunct to the physical exam when dislocation is clinically suspected but not radiographically apparent.[21,73]

Reduction Technique

Reduce an acute posterior dislocation by applying traction on the internally rotated and adducted arm combined with anteriorly directed pressure on the posterior aspect of the humeral head (Fig. 50.17A).[10,70] Generous premedication is usually indicated, and countertraction may be applied with a sheet looped in the affected axilla, similar to the procedure described for anterior dislocations. Lateral traction on the upper part of the humerus is recommended if the humeral head is locked on the posterior glenoid. Hawkins and colleagues suggested that posterior dislocations with an impression defect of the humeral head greater than 20% of the articular surface require open reduction.[70] Posterior dislocations that have been diagnosed late are difficult to reduce in a closed manner, but an attempt with adequate premedication is generally indicated.

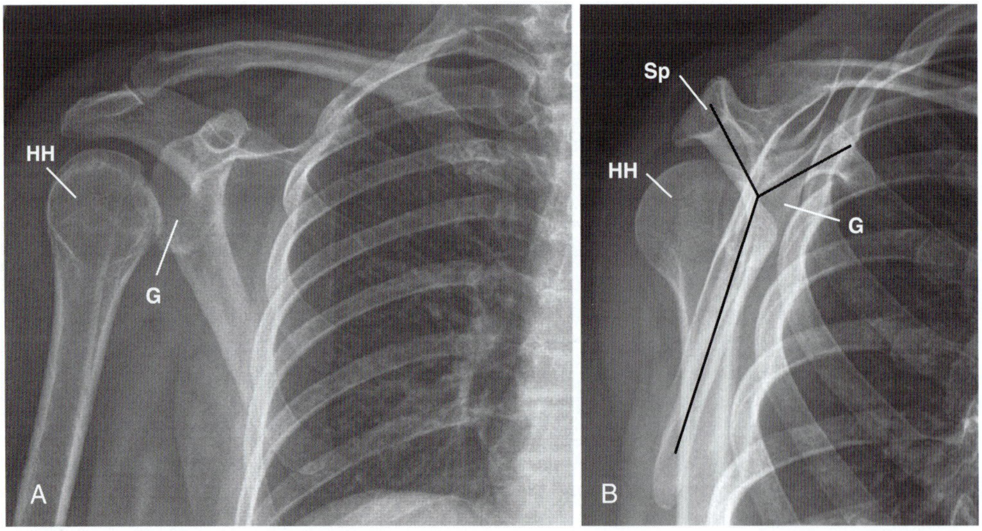

Fig. 50.14 Posterior shoulder dislocation seen on a scapular Y view (see also Figs. 50.5 and 50.6). (A) The anteroposterior view does not definitively show the dislocation. Because the dislocation is directly posterior, there is no superior or inferior displacement of the humeral head. On superficial observation, the head of the humerus appears to maintain a normal relationship with the glenoid fossa and the acromion process. However, definite abnormalities exist on this film. The space between the humeral head and the glenoid fossa is abnormal, and because of the extreme internal rotation of the humerus, the head and neck are seen end on and resemble a light bulb. (B) On the scapular Y view it becomes obvious that the humeral head is posteriorly dislocated. It projects posteriorly under the scapular spine rather than in its normal location, centered over the glenoid fossa. *G*, Glenoid fossa; *HH*, humeral head; *Sp*, scapular spine.

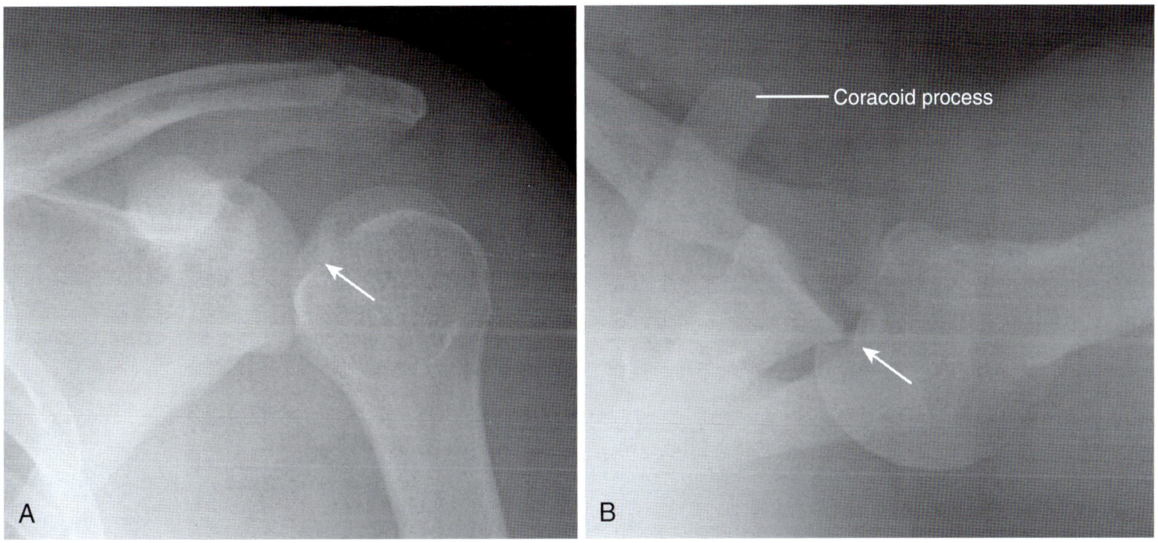

Fig. 50.15 Posterior shoulder dislocation, seen on axillary view. (A) The dislocation is not immediately evident on the anteroposterior view. The humeral head appears as a light bulb, which indicates internal rotation and is a subtle sign that a posterior dislocation might be present *(arrow)*. (B) On the axillary view the humeral head is seen to lie posteriorly and is impacted on the rim of the glenoid *(arrow)*. When viewing axillary films, use the coracoid process to orient yourself to anterior and posterior (the coracoid is an anterior structure). (From Andrews JR, Wilk PE, Reinold MM. *The Athlete's Shoulder.* 2nd ed. Churchill Livingstone; 2008.)

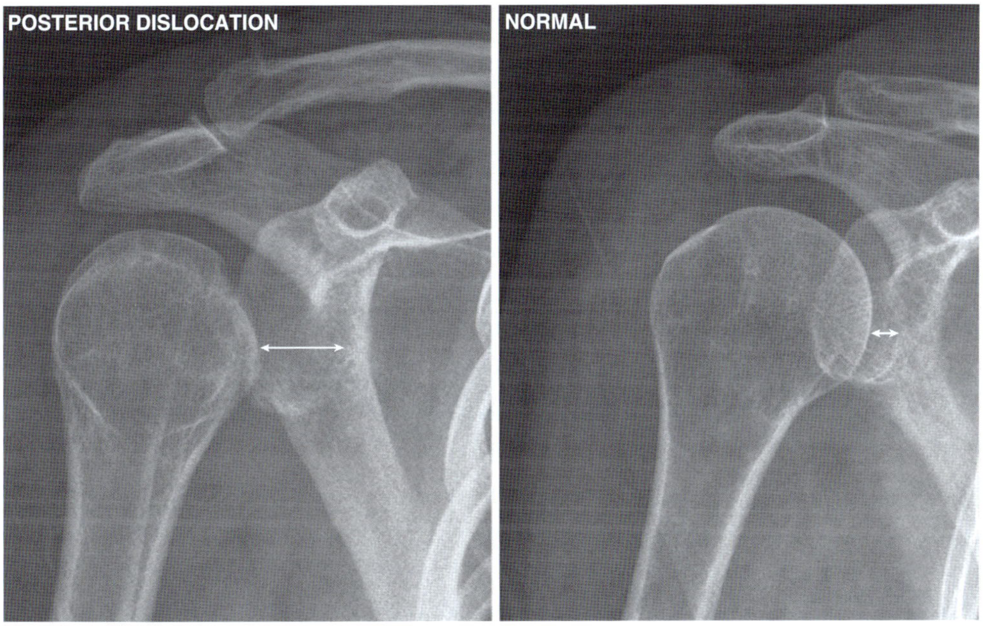

Fig. 50.16 Anteroposterior views comparing posterior dislocation and a normal shoulder joint. Posterior shoulder dislocation causes internal rotation of the humeral head, which makes the head appear as a light bulb rather than its normal club-shaped appearance. In addition, note that the space between the articular surface of the humeral head and the anterior glenoid rim is widened *(arrows)*, and there is a decrease in the overlap between the head and the fossa.

Postreduction Care

As with anterior dislocations, neurovascular examination and radiographs should be repeated after attempts at reduction. Successful reduction is suggested by a patient's ability to place the palm of the injured arm on the opposite shoulder. Given the rarity of these injuries, orthopedic consultation is often sought early in the care of these patients. An analysis and review of the literature of posterior dislocations suggests the majority (65%) of posterior shoulder dislocations will have an associated injury (fracture, reverse Hill-Sachs injury, or rotation cuff tear), underscoring the importance of orthopedic consultation.[12]

Unusual Shoulder Dislocations

Luxatio Erecta

Inferior dislocations of the shoulder, known as *luxatio erecta*, are quite rare but also quite obvious (Videos 50.17 and 50.18).

Posterior and Inferior Shoulder Dislocation Reduction

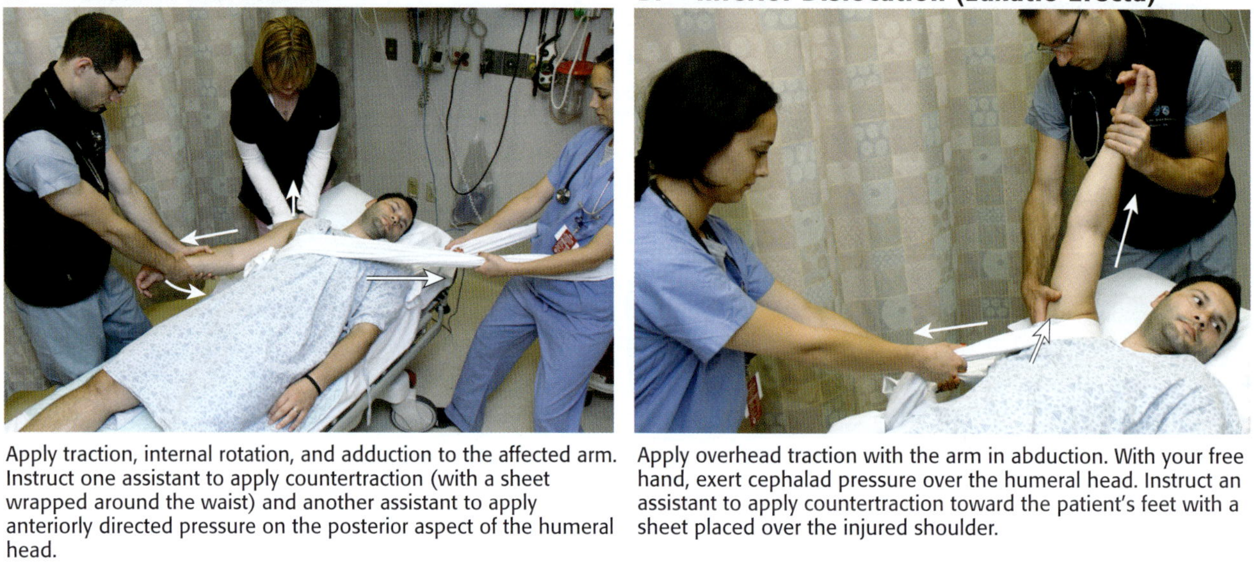

Fig. 50.17 Posterior and inferior shoulder dislocation reduction methods.

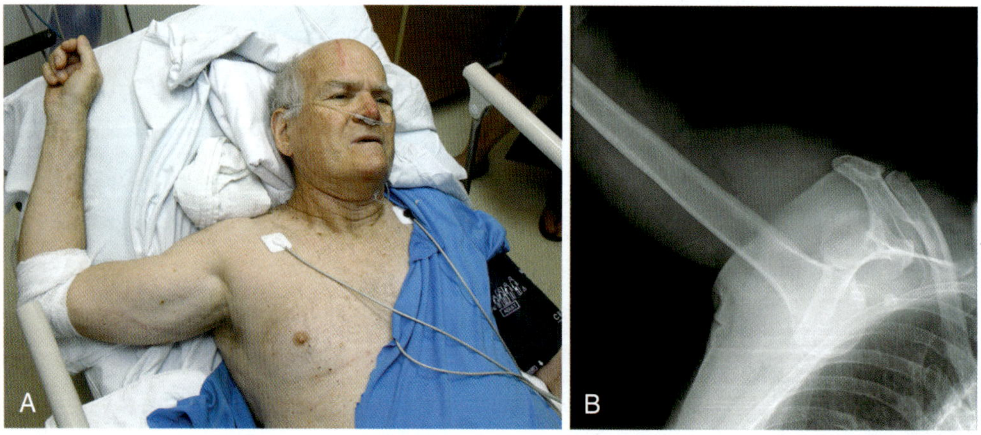

Fig. 50.18 Luxatio erecta. (A) This is a rare inferior shoulder dislocation, and patients may hold their arm in marked abduction with the elbow flexed and the forearm resting on their head. (B) Radiographic appearance of luxatio erecta.

The patient has the arm locked in marked abduction with the flexed forearm lying on or behind the head (Fig. 50.18).[74] Occasionally, the humerus may have less abduction, thus potentially obscuring the diagnosis.[75] The humeral head can be palpated along the lateral chest wall. With this injury, the inferior capsule is almost always torn. Associated injuries include fractures of the greater tuberosity, acromion, clavicle, coracoid process, and glenoid rim. Neurovascular compression may be present, but this is usually reversed once reduction is accomplished.[10] Long-term complications include adhesive capsulitis and recurrent dislocations.

To reduce an inferior shoulder dislocation, apply overhead traction (generally with the arm in full abduction) in the longitudinal direction of the arm, and exert cephalad pressure over the humeral head much as with the Milch technique (see Fig. 50.17B).[10,75] If needed, apply countertraction toward the patient's feet by using a sheet placed over the injured shoulder. After reduction, bring the abducted arm into adduction against the body and supinate the forearm.[76]

Alternatively, use the "two-step" maneuver described by Nho and associates,[77] in which the luxatio erecta is first converted to an anterior dislocation. To perform this maneuver, place one hand on the medial condyle of the elbow and the other hand around the shaft of the humerus. Push anteriorly on the shaft of the humerus while stabilizing the medial condyle of the elbow and rotate the humeral head from an inferior to an anterior position. The authors then describe using the external rotation method to reduce what is now a typical anterior dislocation.[77]

Scapular dislocation or "locked scapula" is a rare condition characterized by obvious protrusion of the lateral border of the scapula and significant swelling of the medial border because of tearing of the musculature.[78] To reduce the scapula, apply traction on the abducted arm and apply medial pressure on the scapula.[78]

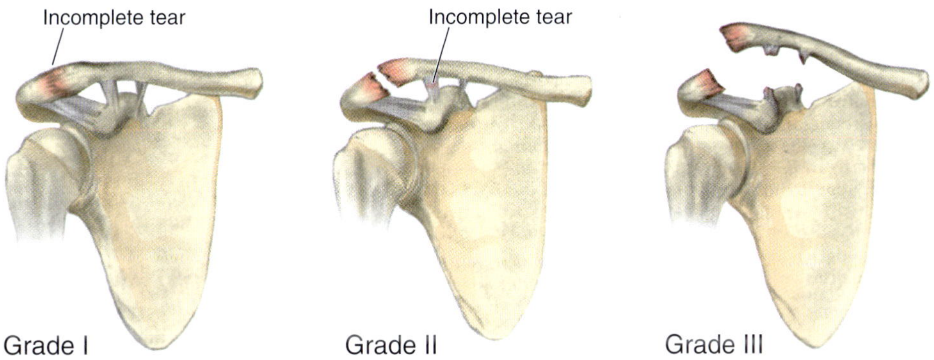

Fig. 50.19 Grade I to III acromioclavicular separation. (See text for description.) (From Heppenstall RB. Fractures and dislocations of the distal clavicle. *Orthop Clin North Am.* 1975;6:480.)

AC JOINT SUBLUXATION AND DISLOCATION

The AC joint is a true diarthrodial joint that consists of a synovial cavity surrounded by a relatively lax capsule and the weak AC ligament. This structure allows the gliding motion necessary for shoulder movement. The major stability of the AC joint comes from two ligaments. The AC ligament is primarily responsible for joint stability in the AP direction. The coracoclavicular ligament, which has posterior (conoid) and anterior (trapezoid) components, anchors the distal end of the clavicle to the coracoid process of the scapula and therefore supports the joint in a superior-inferior direction. In general, AC injuries arise from a direct force such as a fall on the point of the shoulder with the arm adducted.[79] AC joint injuries are categorized according to the Rockwood classification (types I to VI) (Fig. 50.19).[79]

First Degree (Type I)

This injury consists of a minor tear in the AC ligament. The coracoclavicular ligament is intact. The clinical findings are limited to tenderness around the AC joint. Radiographs show little, if any change in position of the clavicle in relation to the acromion.[58] Management of this condition consists of a sling for comfort, ice, and mild analgesics. Generally, the symptoms subside with 7 to 10 days of rest.[79] Orthopedic referral is not usually necessary unless return to normal function is delayed beyond 2 weeks.

Second Degree (Type II)

In addition to a complete tear of the AC ligament, the coracoclavicular ligament is stretched or incompletely torn.[58] The patient generally supports the injured arm and has slight swelling and definite tenderness over the AC joint. Radiographs demonstrate a definite change in the relationship of the distal end of the clavicle to the acromion. However, in type II injuries the inferior edge of the clavicle should not be separated from the acromion by more than half its diameter,[58] and the coracoclavicular distance is the same as that on the uninjured side.[10]This injury can be treated in closed fashion with a sling.[79] Orthopedic referral is recommended, and some still recommend a sling-strap device that elevates the arm and depresses the clavicle for these injuries.[58]

Third Degree (Type III)

In this injury, the distal end of the clavicle is essentially free floating because both the AC and coracoclavicular ligaments are completely disrupted.[58] The arm is supported by an uncomfortable-appearing patient, and the distal end of the clavicle is usually seen to be riding high above the acromion. The diagnosis is generally obvious, and radiographs are used mainly to rule out an associated fracture. Radiographic criteria for this degree of injury include the inferior border of the clavicle raised above the acromion or a discrepancy in the coracoclavicular distance between the normal and affected sides (Fig. 50.20).[79] These injuries require orthopedic referral, and a fair bit of controversy exists regarding their subsequent management.[79] Larsen and coworkers[80] conducted a prospective, randomized trial of conservative versus operative management of significant AC separations and concluded that conservative management was generally better, with possible exceptions made for patients with significant cosmetic deformity and for those who frequently keep their arm at 90 degrees of abduction. Even though optimal therapy is still unclear, a logical approach includes ED treatment with a sling and early orthopedic referral.

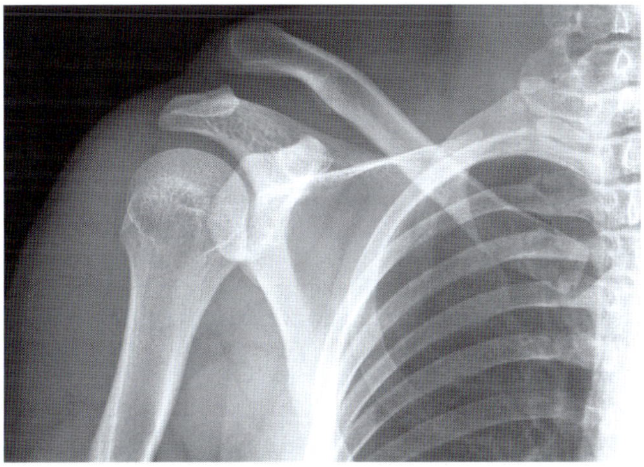

Fig. 50.20 Third-degree acromioclavicular (AC) separation. In a third-degree AC separation, the clavicle is seen riding high above the acromion. This is due to disruption of both the AC and coracoclavicular ligaments.

Fourth, Fifth, and Sixth Degrees (Types IV to VI)

In type IV injury, the distal end of the clavicle is free floating and posteriorly displaced into or through the trapezius muscle. Type V injury is characterized by inferior displacement

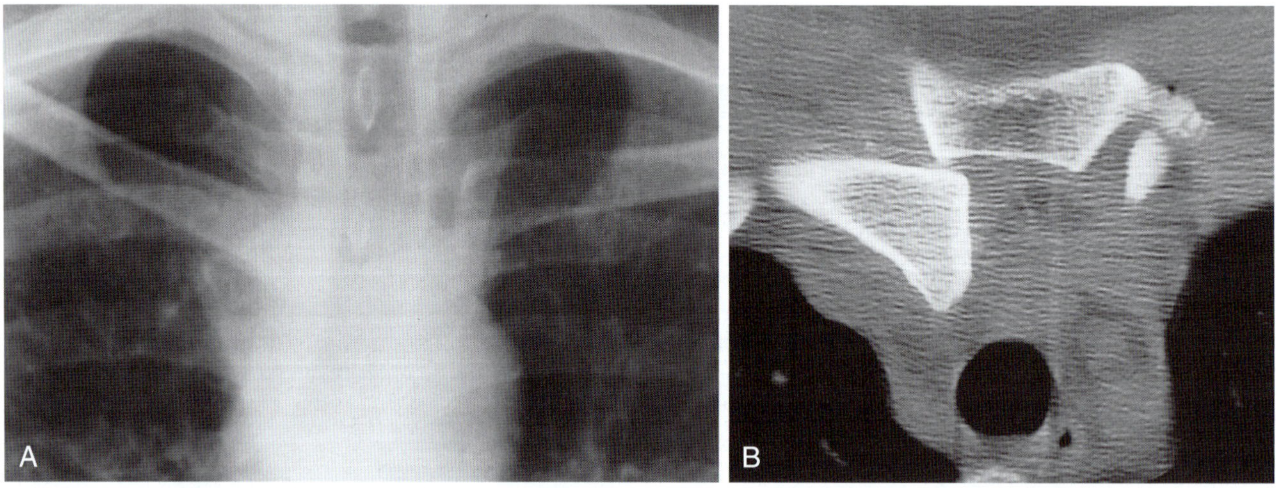

Fig. 50.21 Sternoclavicular joint: posterior dislocation. (A) Frontal chest radiograph showing asymmetry in the position of the medial margins of the clavicle, with the right clavicle (on the injured side) being located inferior to the left clavicle. (B) An axial computed tomography scan confirms posterior dislocation of the right sternoclavicular joint. (From Resnick D Kransdorf MJ, eds. *Bone and Joint Imaging*. 3rd ed. Saunders; 2005.)

of the scapula with a marked increase (two to three times normal) in the coracoclavicular interspace.[79] Type IV and V dislocations generally require surgery, and orthopedic referral is necessary. Type VI injury involves dislocation of the distal end of the clavicle inferiorly. Because this is usually the result of major trauma, other fractures are often present and should be sought.[79]

Radiographic Examination

The diagnosis of AC dislocation is usually made clinically by noting pain and local tenderness at the AC joint in the absence of other findings. Radiographs are generally indicated to rule out associated fractures and to aid in assessing the degree of injury. A single radiograph of the injured shoulder often suffices, but some clinicians prefer to obtain views of the opposite shoulder for comparison, though their efficacy has never been proven. While it has traditionally been recommended that "weighted" films (attaching 10- to 15-lb weights to each wrist) be obtained, these do not enhance interpretation of plain films and only add to the patient's discomfort. Thus they are not recommended for routine use.[81]

STERNOCLAVICULAR DISLOCATIONS

Even though the sternoclavicular joint is the least stable joint in the body, sternoclavicular dislocations are rare.[82] The primary supports of this joint are the sternoclavicular and costoclavicular ligaments. Anterior dislocations are much more common and usually the result of an indirect mechanism involving a blow thrusting the shoulder forward,[58] or they may be atraumatic, caused by ligamentous laxity in teens and young adults.[82] Posterior dislocations also usually result from a blow to the shoulder but can also be caused by a direct superior sternal or medial clavicular blow.[82] Injuries resulting from motor vehicle accidents account for the vast majority of sternoclavicular dislocations, followed by athletic injuries.[57] Posterior sternoclavicular dislocation (also known as retrosternal dislocation because the medial end of the clavicle dislocates both posteriorly and medially) is potentially life-threatening because injury to the great vessels or compression of the airway might occur.[82] Patients may complain of dyspnea, choking, or hoarseness with tracheal compression; dysphagia with esophageal compression; ipsilateral upper extremity pain and swelling with subclavian vessel occlusion; or paresthesias if the brachial plexus is compromised.[83] Any suggestion of these complications should prompt immediate surgical consultation.

The clinical manifestation of these injuries is usually straightforward and consists of pain, swelling, tenderness, and deformity of the joint. Patients may complain of pain that is worse with arm movement and when they are supine. Plain radiographs of this joint are difficult to interpret and generally include an apical lordotic-type view with the radiographic tube angled 45 degrees cephalad. Confirmation of the diagnosis is best made with a thoracic computed tomography (CT) scan, which may also identify high rib fractures, pulmonary contusion, or pneumothorax (Fig. 50.21).[82] CT angiography should be obtained to identify associated vascular injury when indicated. Children may have epiphyseal disruption with retrosternal displacement of the medial aspect of the clavicle.[84]

To reduce both types of sternoclavicular dislocation, place a rolled blanket or a sandbag between the scapula and spine to separate the medial aspect of the clavicle from the manubrium. Apply traction on the 90-degree abducted, 10-degree extended arm in line with the clavicle and then push (anterior dislocation) or lift (posterior dislocation) the clavicle back into position.[82] Posterior dislocations may be difficult to reduce and to maintain via closed reduction. Therefore some authors recommend reduction in an operating suite unless complications necessitate immediate reduction.[82] Given the rarity of this injury and the potential for major underlying complications, early consultation is recommended for suspected posterior sternoclavicular dislocations. Once reduced, a clavicle strap may be used to immobilize both anterior and posterior dislocations for up to 6 weeks.[83]

ELBOW DISLOCATIONS

The elbow is second only to the shoulder as a site of major joint dislocations in adults; it is the most dislocated joint in

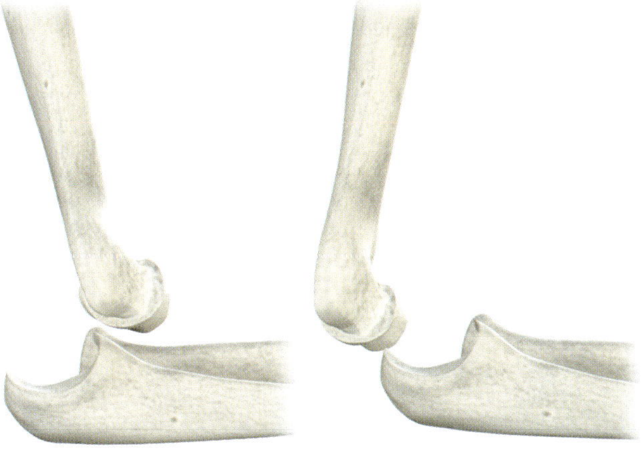

Fig. 50.22 Classification of elbow dislocations.

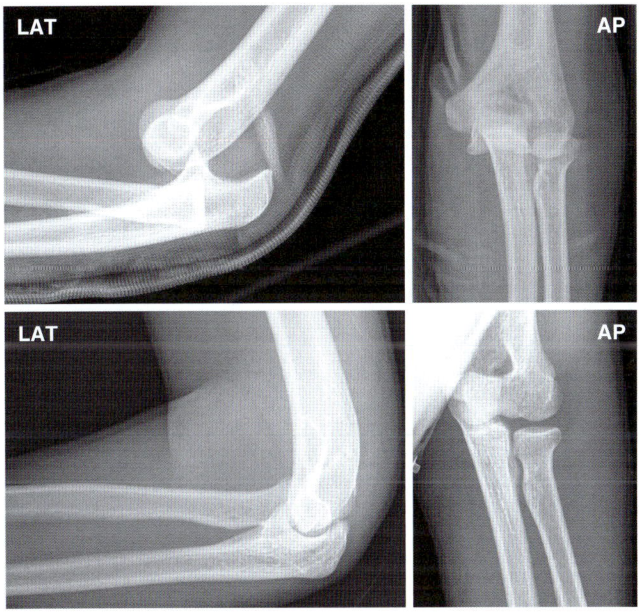

Fig. 50.23 Posterior elbow dislocation. *Top row*, prereduction films; *bottom row*, postreduction films. *AP*, Anteroposterior; *LAT*, lateral.

children (Videos 50.19 and 50.20). Anatomically, the principal articulation of the humerus and ulna is a stable hinge joint with the intercondylar groove of the distal end of the humerus nestled in the olecranon fossa. Because of the stability of the elbow, any dislocation is expected to be accompanied by considerable soft tissue damage. Associated fractures of the radial head and coronoid process of the ulna are common. Elbow dislocations are usually simply divided into posterior and anterior dislocations (Fig. 50.22). However, there are actually several additional types of elbow dislocations, including lateral, divergent, and isolated dislocations of the radius.[85] In the rare divergent dislocations, the radius and ulna are dislocated in opposite directions, either anterior and posterior or medial and lateral.[85]

Studies have shown that many patients report long-term problems including residual pain and joint stiffness after elbow dislocation.[86] However, the most serious complication of elbow dislocation is injury to the brachial artery. This injury is possible with any type of elbow dislocation and is a frequent occurrence with open dislocations.[85] Vascular compromise can be delayed in onset and result from either unsuspected arterial injury or progressive soft tissue swelling. The circulatory status of the arm must be carefully monitored even after successful reduction.[85] In most cases, orthopedic consultation should be sought before disposition. Patients with any variety of elbow dislocation who have significant or immediate soft tissue swelling or hematoma formation or those who have questionable vascular integrity or neurologic findings are often admitted to the hospital or ED observation unit.

Injury to the median and ulnar nerves may be the result of stretch, severance, or entrapment. It is difficult to clinically distinguish these causes; therefore management of nerve injuries is frequently expectant.[85] It is imperative to conduct a careful neurologic examination before and after reduction because any increase in findings may indicate entrapment and the need for surgical intervention.[85] Myositis ossificans is also a potential complication of elbow dislocations secondary to hemarthrosis, which underscores the advisability of orthopedic consultation early in the course of care.

Posterior Dislocations

Posterior dislocations make up the vast majority of elbow dislocations (Videos 50.21–50.23).[58] The usual mechanism is a fall on an outstretched hand with the elbow in extension. Findings on clinical examination are usually diagnostic unless severe soft tissue swelling is present. The patient has a shortened forearm that is held in flexion, and the olecranon is prominent posteriorly. The normally tight triangular relationship of the olecranon and the epicondyles of the distal end of the humerus is disturbed in a posterior dislocation. A defect may also be palpated above the prominence of the olecranon.

Radiologic Examination

Two radiographic views, an AP and a true lateral, should be obtained (Fig. 50.23). The diagnosis is obvious with proper radiographs. A careful search for fractures of the distal end of the humerus, radial head, and coronoid process must be undertaken because they commonly occur in this injury.[85] In children younger than 14 years, the fracture is usually a separation of the medial epicondyle because the epiphyseal plate gives way before the medial collateral ligament of the elbow. Postreduction radiographs are also necessary to confirm reduction and disclose any associated fractures.[87]

Reduction Techniques and Postreduction Care

As with shoulder reductions, some authors claim that their method of elbow reduction is virtually painless,[40,88] but this has not been objectively documented. In general, patients with posterior elbow dislocations are quite uncomfortable, and it is beneficial to administer IV analgesics early in the course of care, preferably before positioning for radiographs. In addition to or in lieu of parenteral sedation and analgesia, the elbow joint may be injected with a local anesthetic (e.g., 3 to 5 mL of 2% plain lidocaine) before attempting reduction. Before injection, aspirate the joint to remove any blood.

Recommended Initial Approach

A prone technique is advantageous because patients tolerate this position quite well. Hang the flexed elbow over the edge of the bed and position an assistant with their back toward the patient such that the patient's humerus can be encircled with both hands and pressure applied with the thumbs on the

Posterior Elbow Dislocation Reduction

A. Initial Recommended Approach

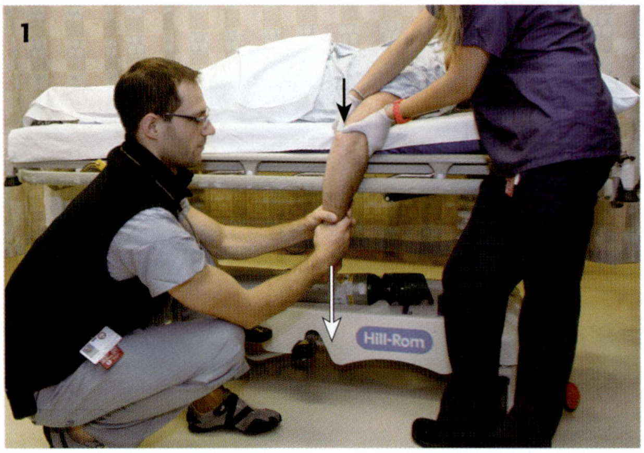

1, Position the patient prone and hang the flexed elbow over the bed. Instruct an assistant to grasp the humerus with both hands and apply pressure on the olecranon with the thumbs *(black arrow)*. Apply longitudinal traction on the humerus *(white arrow)*.

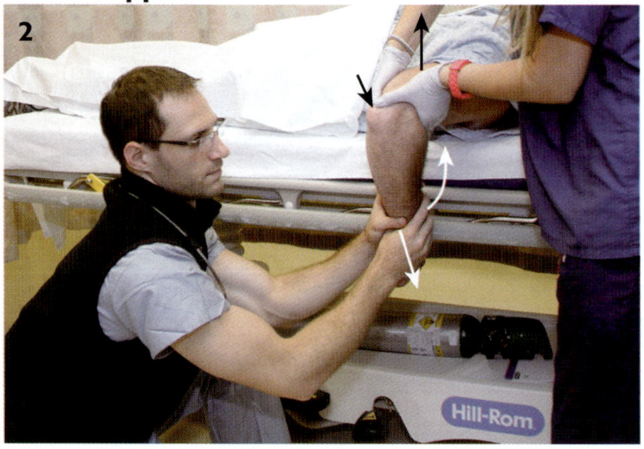

2, If reduction is not accomplished, try to further flex the elbow while applying traction *(white arrows)*, or instruct the assistant to lift the humerus while pushing down on the olecranon *(black arrows)*. Reduction is generally noted by a definitive "clunk."

B. Traction-Countertraction

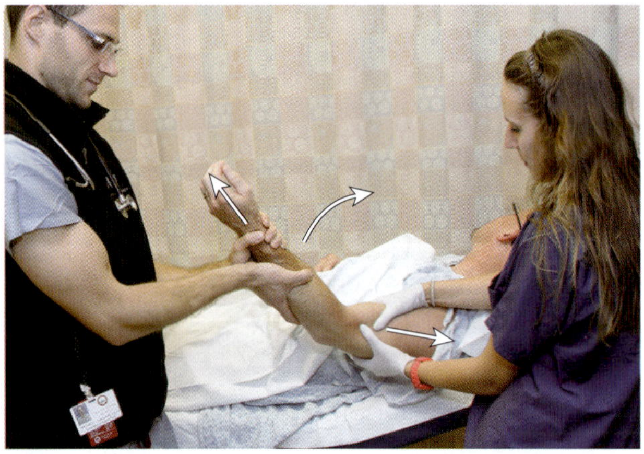

With the patient supine, instruct an assistant to stabilize the humerus. Grasp the wrist and apply in-line traction. Slightly flex the elbow, and hold the wrist supinated as traction is applied.

C. Chair/Back of Bed Method

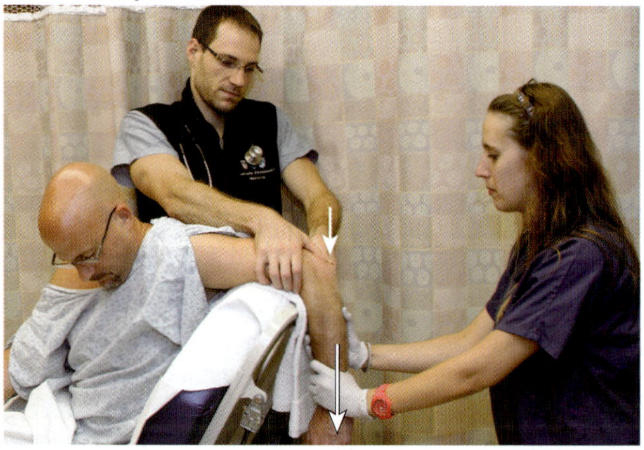

Hang the patient's arm over the padded back of a chair or over the edge of the bed. Apply pressure to the posterior aspect of the olecranon to achieve reduction. Traction may be applied to the forearm.

Fig. 50.24 Posterior elbow dislocation reduction methods.

posterior aspect of the olecranon (Fig. 50.24A). This pressure on the olecranon is intended to lift it up and away from the humerus. Apply longitudinal traction on the arm with the elbow in slight flexion. If reduction is not accomplished, an attempt may be made to further flex the elbow, or the assistant can be instructed to lift the humerus. Reduction is generally noted by a definite "clunk."

Traditional Traction Method

Place the patient in the supine position and have an assistant stabilize the humerus with both hands (see Fig. 50.24B).[89] Grasp the wrist and apply slow and steady in-line traction. Slightly flex the elbow to keep the triceps mechanism loose, and hold the wrist supinated while applying traction. Reduction is usually signified by a "clunk" that is heard or felt. If this method is not successful after a reasonable period of traction (10 minutes), gently flex the forearm to effect reduction. Alternatively, apply downward pressure on the proximal volar surface of the forearm to free up the coronoid process.

Alternatives

Several authors have described variations of a prone method of reduction that are reportedly well tolerated by patients.[40,88,89] In the method described by Minford and Beattie,[88] position the patient with the arm hanging over the padded back of a chair or over the edge of the bed (see Fig. 50.24C). Apply pressure to the prominent posterior aspect of the olecranon to achieve reduction. Alternatively, apply traction with the elbow flexed over the edge of a chair. Pull down on the hand while using the thumb to guide the olecranon into place. Parvin[40] positioned the patient as for the Stimson method of shoulder relocation, prone on a stretcher with the arm hanging down, and applied gentle downward traction on the wrist.

Anterior Elbow Dislocation Reduction

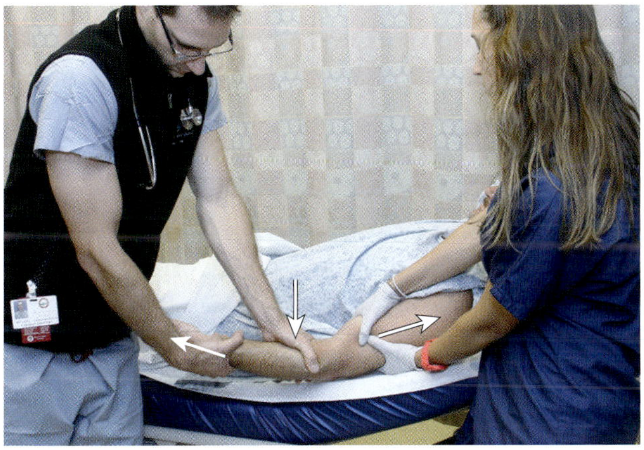

Apply in-line traction and backward pressure on the proximal end of the forearm while an assistant provides countertraction on the humerus. A clunk usually indicates that reduction is achieved.

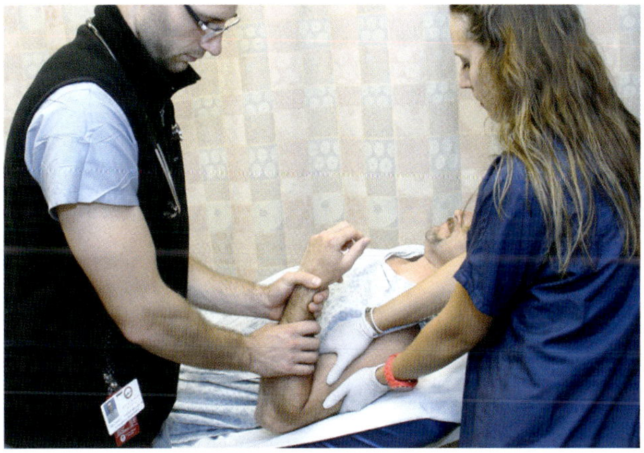

Flex the arm beyond 90 degrees to ensure that the joint has been reduced. Splint the elbow in at least 90 degrees of flexion with a posterior long-arm splint.

Fig. 50.25 Anterior elbow dislocation reduction method.

Postreduction Care

Once reduction is achieved, put the elbow through a gentle range of motion to ensure that the reduction is stable and there is no mechanical block to movement.[85] An inability to move the elbow through a smooth range of motion after reduction is often caused by an entrapped medial epicondyle fracture fragment, which requires operative intervention.[85] Immobilize the elbow in at least 90 degrees of flexion with the forearm in slight pronation by using a long arm posterior splint (see Chapter 51). After immobilizing the joint, recheck the neurovascular status of the extremity and obtain postreduction radiographs.

After reduction, any signs of delayed vascular compromise are first addressed by loosening the splint and decreasing the degree of flexion. This may restore adequate blood flow.[85] If not, immediate surgical consultation is necessary for emergency arteriography, exploration of the brachial artery, or both.[87] Brachial arterial injury may not be immediately apparent because of the presence of collateral circulation. The risk for vascular compromise is a reason to consider in-hospital observation. Alternatively, observe the patient in the ED or ED observation unit for 2 to 3 hours after reduction to evaluate for delayed neurovascular compromise before discharge.

The optimal duration of immobilization is unknown. However, a 2017 randomized multicenter trial found early range of motion to be safe and associated with faster recovery time and return to work when compared to plaster immobilization for 3 weeks.[90]

Anterior Dislocations

Anterior dislocations of the elbow are quite rare; they usually result from a direct posterior blow to the olecranon with the elbow flexed.[85] On physical examination, the arm is elongated and extended with anterior tenting of the proximal end of the forearm and prominence of the distal end of the humerus posteriorly.[85] These injuries are the result of a great deal of force; they are frequently open and accompanied by significant neurovascular injury. An avulsion of the triceps mechanism may also occur.[85]

To reduce anterior dislocations of the elbow, apply in-line traction and backward pressure on the proximal end of the forearm (Fig. 50.25). An assistant provides countertraction by grasping the humerus with both hands. Given the infrequent nature of anterior dislocations and the high probability of a severe associated injury, the emergency clinician should consider early orthopedic consultation.

RADIAL HEAD SUBLUXATION (NURSEMAID'S ELBOW)

Radial head subluxation is a common pediatric orthopedic issue that generally occurs between the ages of 1 and 3 years. The mean age is just older than 2 years, but this entity has been reported in infants younger than 6 months[91,92] and in older children up to the preteen years.[93] There is a slight predilection for this injury to occur in girls and in the left arm.[92,94] The classic mechanism of injury is longitudinal traction on the arm with the wrist in pronation, as occurs when the child is lifted up by the wrist (Fig. 50.26A).[92] There is no support for the common assumption that the relatively small head of the radius in relation to the neck of the radius predisposes the young to this injury.[95] The pathologic lesion is generally a tear in the attachment of the annular ligament to the periosteum of the radial neck, with the detached portion becoming trapped between the head of the radius and the capitellum (see Fig. 50.26B).[95]

Clinical Assessment

The history offered by the caretaker may not be that of the classic pulling-type mechanism. Schunk,[92] in a series of 83 patients, reported that only 51% described such a mechanism whereas 22% reported a fall. In patients younger than 6 months, the mechanism in the majority of cases is simply rolling over in bed.[91] Therefore isolated radial head subluxation in children younger than 6 months does not automatically

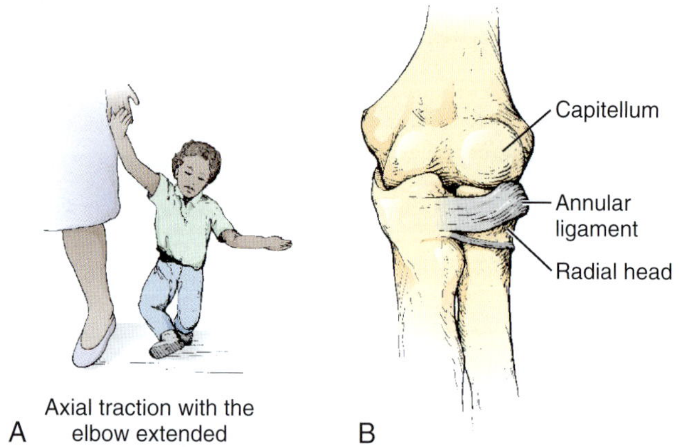

Fig. 50.26 Radial head subluxation (nursemaid's elbow). (A) The classic mechanism for this injury is longitudinal traction on the arm with the wrist in pronation. (B) The pathologic lesion is usually a torn piece of the annular ligament becoming trapped between the radial head and the capitellum of the humerus. (From Fleisher GR, Ludwig S, eds. *Textbook of Pediatric Emergency Medicine*. Williams & Wilkins; 1988:1322.)

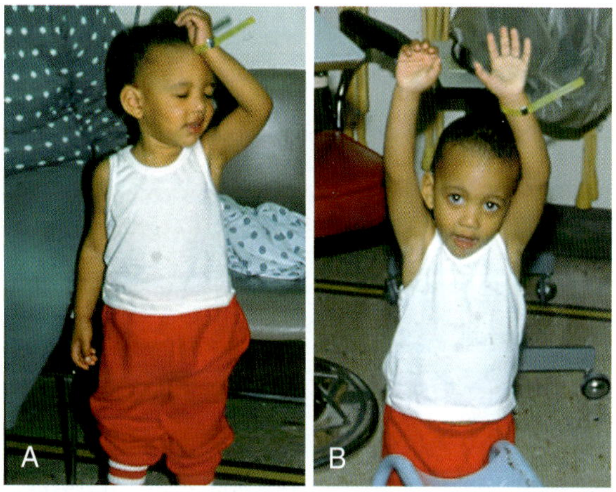

Fig. 50.27 Typical findings in a child with subluxation of the right radial head (nursemaid's elbow). It may be difficult to determine exactly where the pathology exists, and the wrist is often thought to be the area of injury. This child will not use the injured right arm but has minimal discomfort as long as the elbow is not manipulated. (A) The affected arm hangs down at the side, slightly flexed and pronated. (B) Once the subluxation is reduced, full activity is generally regained in a matter of minutes.

necessitate a child abuse investigation. The typical patient with radial head subluxation is in no distress and holds the involved arm slightly flexed and the wrist pronated at the side (Fig. 50.27). This has been termed the *nursemaid's position*.[96] The exact area of pain is often difficult to locate. The child will refuse to use the arm, and this may be the chief complaint.[93] An older child will usually point to the dorsal aspect of the distal end of the forearm when asked where it hurts, which may mislead the clinician to suspect a distal radial buckle fracture.

Although tenderness about the elbow has been reported occasionally, there is often little tenderness or swelling in the elbow region.[92,93] In a cooperative child, the arm and shoulder are carefully palpated to discern any tenderness. Areas of focus on palpation should include the clavicle and distal end of the radius because these are common sites for pediatric fractures. When patient anxiety interferes with reliable assessment of tenderness in a child whose arm is in the classic nursemaid's position, the examiner can stand at a distance and have the parent or caretaker palpate the extremity to ascertain tenderness. This may also be done with a cooperative patient to reassure a doubtful parent regarding the absence of a fracture. If no tenderness is noted on palpation, it is appropriate to attempt reduction without prior radiographs.[97]

Although resistance to or pain with supination is a frequent finding in patients with radial head subluxation,[92] one need not test for this finding until the time of reduction.

Radiographic Examination

Radiographs are not generally needed with the classic findings of a child with an arm in the nursemaid's position that is not tender (or minimally tender in the radial head area) on palpation and an appropriate history.[97] In these cases, findings on radiographs are generally normal, and if obtained, the positioning of the child's arm by the x-ray technician often effects reduction.[92] Nevertheless, Frumkin[95] described three cases of nursemaid's elbow in which a line drawn through the longitudinal axis of the radius did not normally bisect the capitellum on prereduction radiographs but did so after reduction. Radiographs are sometimes recommended if the child is not moving the arm normally 15 minutes after reduction.[96] However, this time frame may be too short because reuse can be delayed for more than 30 minutes, particularly in children initially seen some time after the injury. Quan and Marcuse[93] recommended an approach in which no radiographs are obtained on the first visit, including in children released from the ED before regaining full use of the arm. At the time of a 24-hour follow-up visit, radiographs are obtained only if repeat attempts at manipulation are not successful.

Even though this condition does not generally require radiographs, they can be valuable if external signs of trauma are present (e.g., swelling, abrasions, ecchymoses) or if the child does not use the arm normally within 24 hours after the subluxation is thought to be reduced. Other less common conditions that can have similar findings are fractures, joint infections, tumors, and osteomyelitis.

POCUS is an additional tool that may be used to help exclude an alternate etiology of elbow pain or confirm the presence of a suspected radial head subluxation. Ultrasound may be used to exclude a posterior fat pad, a finding associated with supracondylar fracture, in patients with suspected radial head subluxation.[98] All patients with normal elbow ultrasound had successful reduction of the radial head subluxation with return to full function.[98] Ultrasound may also be diagnostic in radial head subluxation. The "hook sign," caused by the hyperechoic J-shaped supinator muscle above the radial head, has been shown to be 100% sensitive for the diagnosis of radial head subluxation.[99,100] As with other conditions, ultrasound can be a useful radiation-sparing adjunct to the physical examination and may additionally assist in reassuring an anxious caregiver of the diagnosis prior to reduction attempts.

Reduction Techniques

Supination Method

Reduction of nursemaid's elbow (Fig. 50.28 and Videos 50.24–50.27) is generally performed without premedication. If the subluxation has been present for hours, oral or nasal midazolam can be a useful adjunct to overcome the child's anxiety related to manipulation (see Chapter 33). It is important to

Nursemaid's Elbow Reduction

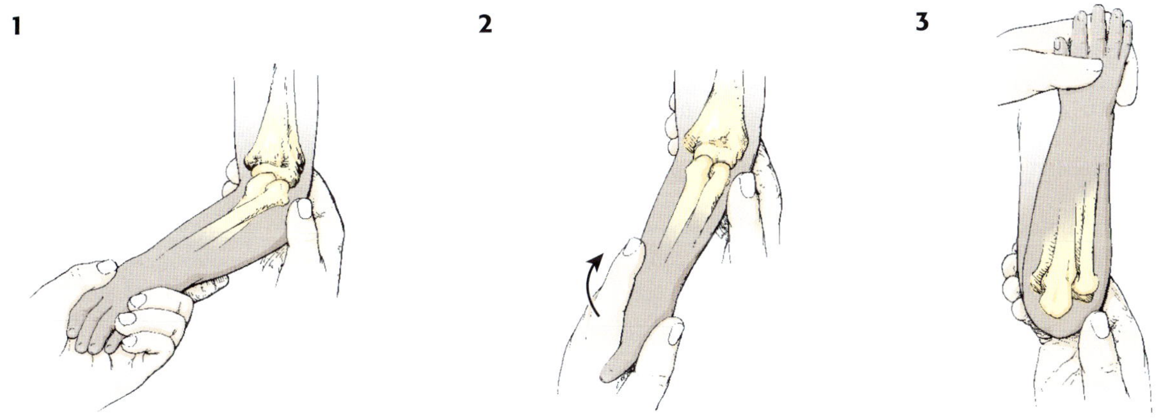

1. Grasp the elbow with one hand and place your thumb over the region of the radial head.
2. Grasp the wrist with your other hand and supinate the extended forearm in a steady and deliberate manner. Apply slight traction to the arm.
3. Once supinated, flex the arm. An audible or palpable click signifies successful reduction but is not always noted.

Fig. 50.28 Nursemaid's elbow (radial head subluxation) reduction. (From Fleisher GR, Ludwig S, eds. *Textbook of Pediatric Emergency Medicine*. Williams & Wilkins; 1988:1322.)

explain to the caretaker that the reduction will probably cause the child discomfort and precipitate crying, but that this is transient and a clue to the diagnosis. Position the child seated on the lap of an assistant (often a parent) who stabilizes the arm by holding the humerus adducted to the side. Grasp the elbow with one hand and place the thumb over the region of the radial head. Although it has been stated that the thumb can apply pressure on the radial head, this positioning is mainly useful for palpation of the reduction "click." Grasp the child's wrist with the other hand and supinate the extended forearm in a steady, deliberate manner. Slight traction before supination is generally recommended, but it is unclear whether this increases the likelihood of successful reduction. Once supinated, flex or extend the arm; however, flexion is the most common maneuver and may be somewhat more successful than extension.[92] An audible or palpable click signifies successful reduction but is not always noted. Once the reduction has been performed, the child usually cries for a few minutes. Generally, the operator should leave the room and then return in 10 to 15 minutes to repeat the examination. Full use of the arm should be evident (see Fig. 50.27B).

Pronation Method

This technique is performed with the child positioned as for the supination method. However, the forearm is not supinated. Instead, the forearm is rapidly hyperpronated and flexed.

Multiple studies have found a variable combination of improved success and less pain with this method.[101–103] Similarly, a 2017 meta-analysis concluded hyperpronation to be more successful and less painful than the supination method.[104]

After Attempted Reduction

If a click is detected, the child will generally regain use of the affected arm quickly (almost always by 30 minutes).[93] Therefore, if a definite click is detected, it is reasonable to observe the child for up to 30 minutes before further intervention. If there is still no use at 30 minutes, the operator may try to determine whether supination is still painful, which would suggest the need to repeat the attempt. In children in whom a click is not detected, the majority will not use the arm by 30 minutes.[93] Therefore a repeated attempt at reduction is recommended after 10 to 15 minutes of nonuse in children who did not have a click during the primary reduction. Two or more attempts are required to produce the click in up to 30% of patients.[93]

If the child has not regained use of the arm after a few attempts and a reasonable period of time, some authors recommend that radiographs be obtained.[96] Radiographs may also help relieve parental anxiety. Alternatively, instructions may be given for 24-hour follow-up if normal function is not restored, with consideration of radiographs at the time of follow-up.[93] In two series of patients with nursemaid's elbow, 6 of 10 patients released without normal arm use had spontaneous restoration of function, whereas the other 4 required remanipulation (which successfully restored function).[92,93] Delayed use of radiographs may decrease overall radiation exposure in a child with a radial head subluxation.

The use of a posterior splint to protect the elbow of a child who refuses to use the affected arm after a presumed reduction is of uncertain value. However, some form of immobilization (e.g., splint, sling, or both) may be valuable in a child with significant residual discomfort after a prolonged period of subluxation or in whom recurrent subluxations have taken place.

On occasion, a successful reduction painfully resubluxates with movement; in this case, immobilization and referral may be necessary.[95] If reduction has been achieved clinically and maintained in the ED, analgesics or a follow-up visit is unnecessary. Because other pathology can rarely mimic this condition (e.g., occult fracture, osteomyelitis, joint infection, tumor), full, unrestricted, and painless use of the arm must be evident by 24 hours. If not, further workup is warranted.

The emergency clinician should consider parental education regarding prevention of radial head subluxation. Parents or caregivers should be instructed to lift toddlers who are at an age most at risk for these injuries from beneath their axilla, as opposed to forcibly lifting or pulling them by the wrist or hand.

HAND INJURIES

The hand is extremely susceptible to dislocation injuries because of its frequent use and exposed nature. Proper motion and function of the hand are intimately related to normal anatomic alignment.[105] The emergency clinician must therefore be skilled in the diagnosis and management of dislocations involving the hand. An improperly managed hand injury can result in significant long-term or permanent disability.

Anatomically, the joints of the digits are quite similar and consist of a hinged joint with a tongue-in-groove type of arrangement.[105] The soft tissue support includes two collateral ligaments attached to a volar plate (Fig. 50.29). The volar plate is composed of dense fibrous connective tissue that is thickened at its distal attachment and thinner at its proximal attachment to allow folding with joint flexion.[105,106] Dorsal dislocation of a digit requires failure of the volar plate, whereas lateral dislocation disrupts a collateral ligament and induces at least a partial tear in the volar plate.

Radiographic examination of all hand injuries is relatively straightforward and includes at least two views (AP and lateral) of the injured area (Fig. 50.30). The most important radiographic error in evaluating joint injuries in the hand is failing to get a true lateral view of the injured joint.[106] This may lead to missing a fracture or a loose body in the joint.

Anesthesia is generally required for proper management of dislocations involving the hand. It is most often accomplished with a finger or wrist block (see Chapter 31), although a more proximal regional or Bier block may be used on occasion (see Chapter 32). Getting a secure grip on the digits may be difficult and could complicate the reduction. Wearing rubber gloves or wrapping gauze around the fingers may be useful.

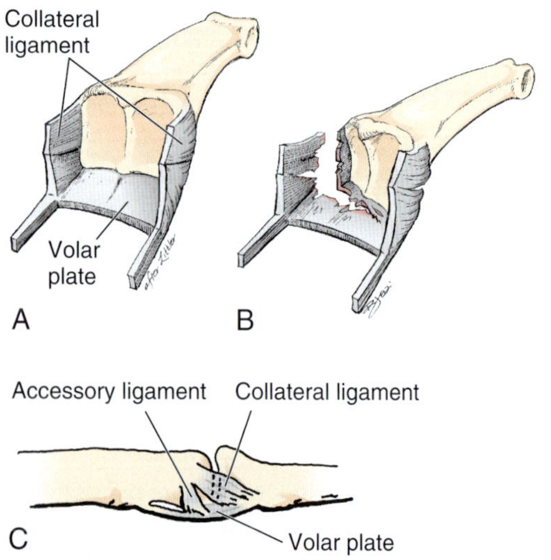

Fig. 50.29 (A–B) The collateral ligament-volar plate relationship. The metacarpophalangeal and interphalangeal joints derive their strength from a combination of the two collateral ligaments and the volar plate. Dislocations of these joints require tearing of at least two parts of this three-part structure. (C) Lateral view demonstrating the collateral ligament-volar plate relationship. (A–B, From Carter P, ed. *Common Hand Injuries and Infections*. Saunders; 1983:114. C, Redrawn from Eaton RG. *Joint Injuries of the Hand*. Charles C. Thomas; 1972.)

Thumb Dislocations

The opposable thumb is an essential structure for countless activities (Video 50.28). Despite its strong ligamentous and capsular support, the exposed positioning of the thumb makes it a frequent site of dislocations and subluxations. The metacarpophalangeal (MCP) joint in the thumb is similar to the MCP joints in the fingers but has a stronger volar plate and collateral ligaments.[106]

Interphalangeal Joint Dislocation of the Thumb

The single interphalangeal (IP) joint of the thumb has strong cutaneous-periosteal attachments, and dislocations of this type are therefore frequently open.[106] Dislocations at the IP joint are generally dorsal and can be reduced in a manner similar to that for IP dislocations of the finger (Fig. 50.31A–B). First, recreate the mechanism of injury by applying longitudinal traction and hyperextension to distract the phalanges. Next, flex

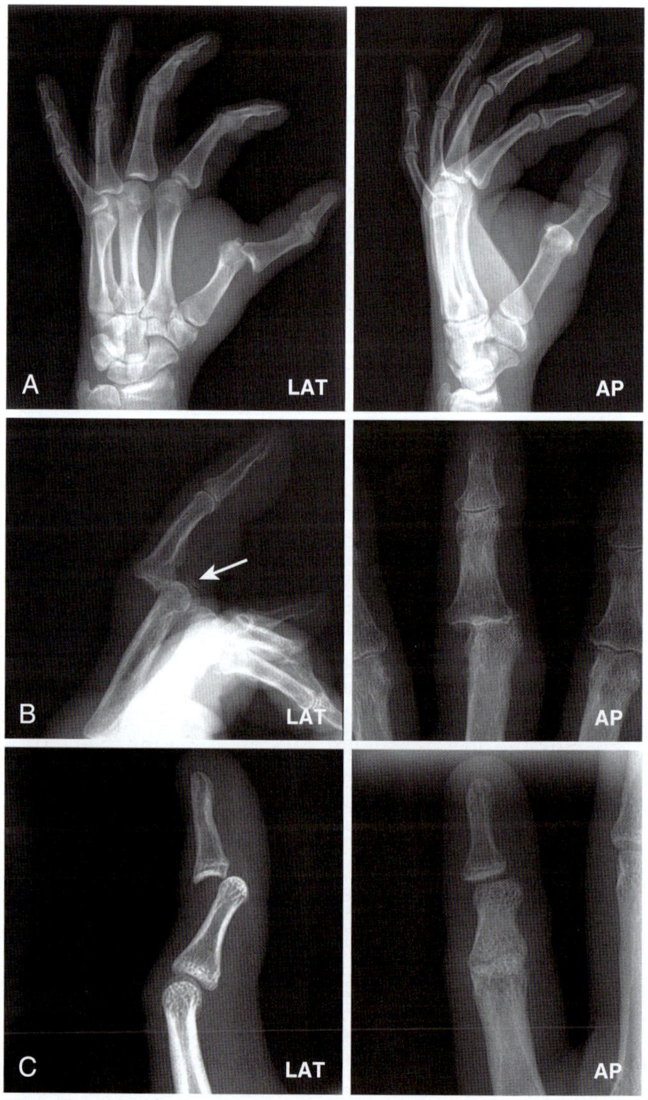

Fig. 50.30 Phalangeal dislocations. (A) Dorsal dislocation of the metacarpophalangeal joint of the thumb. (B) Dorsal dislocation of the proximal interphalangeal joint of the middle finger. Note the presence of a small volar plate fracture *(arrow)*. (C) Dorsal dislocation of the distal interphalangeal joint of the little finger. Dorsal dislocations are much more common than volar ones. *AP*, Anteroposterior; *LAT*, lateral.

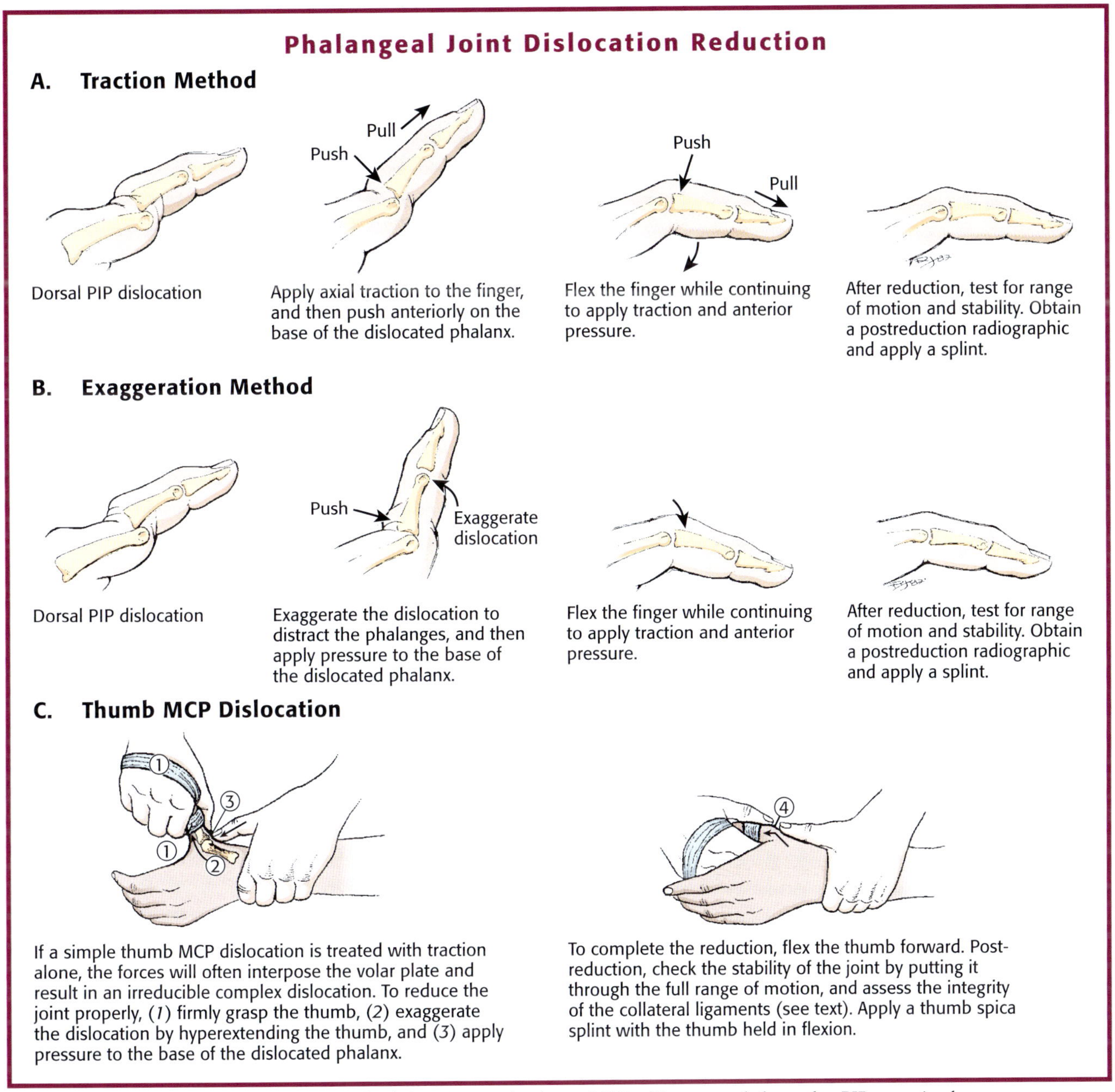

Fig. 50.31 Phalangeal dislocation reduction. *MCP,* Metacarpophalangeal; *PIP,* proximal interphalangeal.

the IP joint with continued traction and apply direct pressure on the base of the distal phalanx to complete the reduction.[106]

After reduction, test the range of motion and stability of the joint and obtain postreduction radiographs. If adequate reduction has been achieved, splint the thumb in slight flexion for 3 weeks.[106] Orthopedic or hand specialist referral is advisable.

Metacarpophalangeal Joint Injury of the Thumb

Dorsal Dislocation

The MCP joint of the thumb can be dislocated dorsally by a hyperextension injury. The proximal phalanx will come to rest in a position dorsal to the first metacarpal (Fig. 50.32; also see Fig. 50.30A). There are two basic types of MCP dislocation (this applies to the fingers also): simple and complex. In a complex MCP dislocation, the volar plate becomes entrapped dorsal to the metacarpal head (Fig. 50.33), with the flexor tendons and lumbricals acting to completely entrap the metacarpal head.[106] The simple type is amenable to closed reduction, whereas the complex type requires operative reduction because of the interposed soft tissue.[105,106] It is important to note that a simple MCP dislocation can be converted into a complex one during reduction.[105]

Clinical features that suggest a complex MCP dislocation include a proximal phalanx that is less acutely angulated than with a simple dislocation (i.e., <60 degrees).[106] Dimpling may also be noted over the thenar eminence as a result of pressure from the entrapped metacarpal head.[105] On radiographs of simple dislocations, the joint surfaces are in close contact, whereas they are separated in complex dislocations. The presence of a sesamoid bone in the joint space is diagnostic of a complex MCP dislocation (Fig. 50.34).[105]

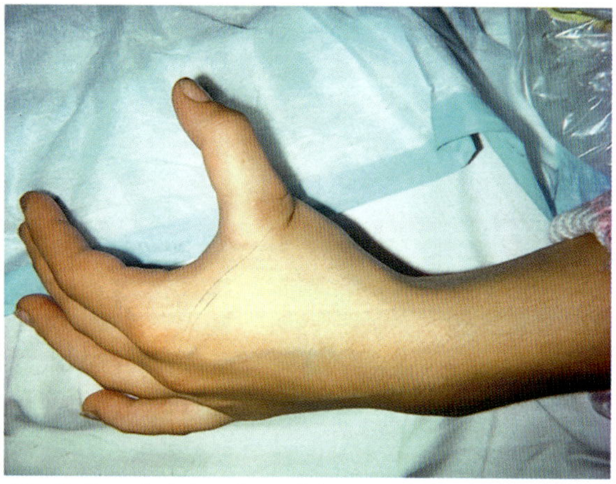

Fig. 50.32 Dorsal dislocation of the metacarpophalangeal joint of the thumb.

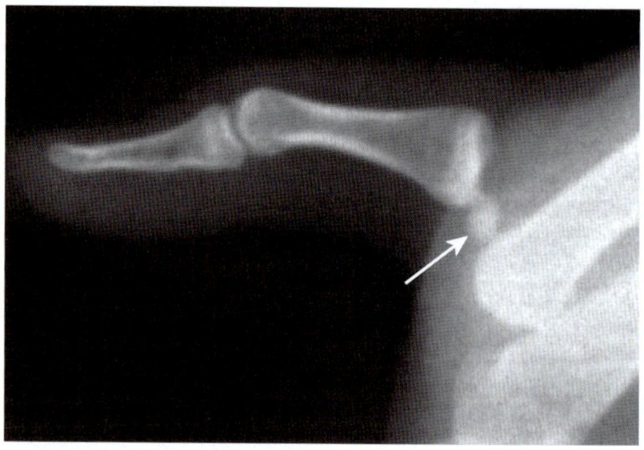

Fig. 50.34 Irreducible metacarpophalangeal joint dislocation of the thumb. Note the sesamoid bone *(arrow)*, which indicates interposition of the volar plate between the two ends of the bone and may prevent closed reduction. (From Carter P, ed. *Common Hand Injuries and Infections*. Saunders; 1983:115.)

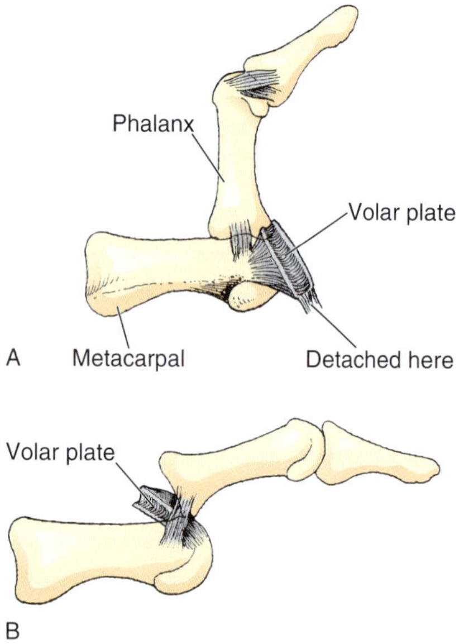

Fig. 50.33 (A) In a simple dorsal metacarpophalangeal joint dislocation (note the right angle between the phalanx and the metacarpal), the volar plate remains in front of the metacarpal head, although it is detached from its weaker metacarpal insertion. (B) In a complex dislocation (note the more parallel alignment between the phalanx and the metacarpal), the volar plate becomes entrapped in the joint, and this makes reduction by closed methods impossible. (From DePalma AF. *Management of Fractures and Dislocations: An Atlas*. Saunders; 1970:1177.)

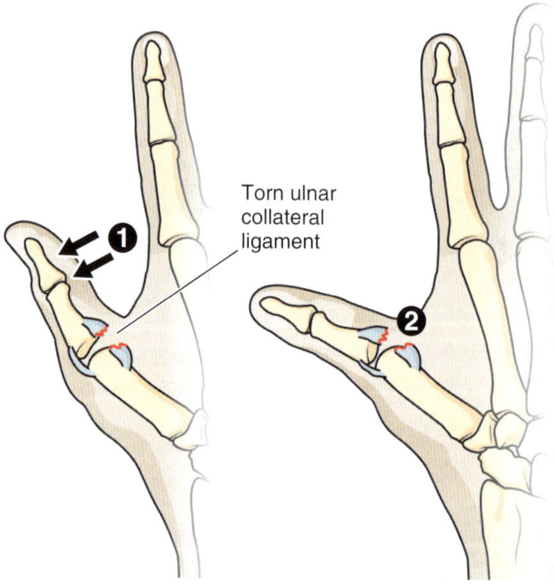

Fig. 50.35 Rupture of the ulnar collateral ligament (gamekeeper's thumb). *1*, This injury is caused by forcible abduction. If unrecognized and untreated, progressive metacarpophalangeal (MCP) subluxation may occur *(2)*, which interferes with grasping and causes significant permanent disability. Suspect this injury when there is a complaint of pain in this region. Look for tenderness on the medial side of the MCP joint. (Modified from McRae R. *Practical Fracture Treatment*. Churchill Livingstone; 1981:162.)

To reduce a simple MCP dislocation, hyperextend the joint as far as possible with the wrist in flexion to relax the tendons (see Fig. 50.31C). Once maximal hyperextension is achieved, push the base of the proximal phalanx distally while bringing the joint back into flexion.[105] Applying simple traction alone as an initial maneuver risks trapping the volar plate and creating a complex dislocation.[105] After reduction, test the stability of the joint by putting it through a full range of motion. Assess the integrity of the collateral ligaments with the MCP joint in flexion (see later). Simple MCP dislocation injuries generally require casting for 3 weeks with the joint in moderate flexion.[106]

Volar Dislocation

Volar dislocations are rare and generally associated with collateral ligament ruptures. They are commonly irreducible because of interposition of one or both extensor tendons and the dorsal capsule.[105] Orthopedic consultation is required.

Ulnar Collateral Ligament Rupture

Also known as *gamekeeper's* or *skier's thumb*, this injury results from a laterally directed force at the thumb MCP joint causing rupture of the ulnar collateral ligament (Fig. 50.35). The usual mechanisms include falling with a ski pole in the hand or having the thumb alone draped over the steering wheel in an auto crash. These injuries are most often initially seen in the reduced state with just a complaint of pain in the area. Early recognition of this injury is essential to prevent further disability because this ligament is important for the grasping function of the thumb. A strain or partial tear probably cannot be diagnosed in the ED. It is therefore prudent to immobilize

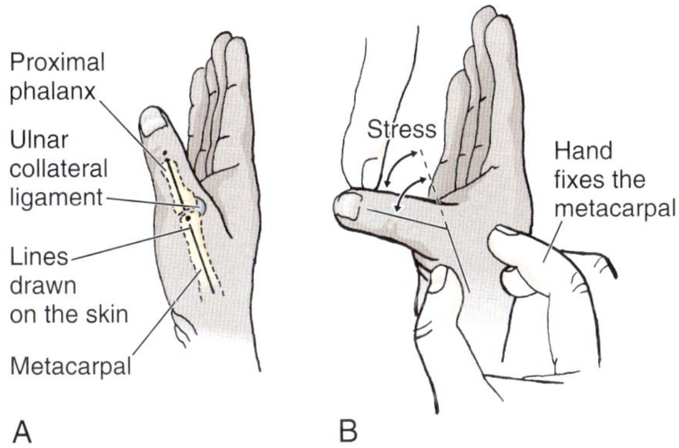

Fig. 50.36 Stress testing of the ulnar collateral ligament of the thumb. This is done both clinically and with an anteroposterior radiograph. (A) A line is drawn on the skin with a pen. The line is along the long axis of the metacarpal and the proximal phalanx. (B) Deviation of the straight line during stress indicates instability. The metacarpal is fixed with the operator's other hand. Note that with acute injuries of the thumb, a simple sprain may be diagnosed when an ulnar collateral ligament injury is partial or severe and stress tests are negative because of swelling and spasm. Therefore it is prudent to splint all significantly sprained thumbs and reexamine them in a few days if the symptoms persist.

all significantly "sprained thumbs" in a thumb spica splint for a few days and reexamine those with significant injuries. A complete or severe ligamentous tear is generally diagnosed by stress testing of the MCP joint (Fig. 50.36). Radiographs occasionally demonstrate an avulsion-type fracture. The exact positioning of the thumb for stress testing is debatable, but the metacarpal should be stabilized with the thumb and index finger of one hand while applying stress with the other hand. Louis and associates[107] recommended stressing the joint in full flexion because virtually no lateral movement of the MCP joint should be noted in this position. Instability in full flexion of greater than 35 degrees is indicative of a complete rupture. Hossfeld and Uehara[106] suggested testing the MCP joint in 20 to 30 degrees of flexion to lessen the stabilizing effects of the volar plate; the results should be compared with stability on the other side.

Cast partial injuries to the ulnar collateral ligament for 3 weeks; complete rupture usually requires operative repair.[107] An associated nondisplaced fracture may be treated in closed fashion, whereas a displaced fracture is an indication for operative repair.[107]

Carpometacarpal Dislocations of the Thumb

Carpometacarpal (CMC) dislocations of the thumb are uncommon (Fig. 50.37); when present, they often occur with an associated fracture. Because closed reduction is generally unstable, operative stabilization by percutaneous placement of Kirschner wires (K-wires) is usually required.[106]

Finger Dislocations

The basic anatomic structure of the fingers is like that of the thumb, with the exception that the fingers have more lateral support from the MCP joints, making collateral ligament injury here much less common than in the thumb (Videos 50.29–50.31). The treatment principles are also similar. It is advisable to order radiographs for a specific finger (not just "hand" films). Complete views of the finger will include an AP view, a true lateral view, and an oblique view. A true lateral

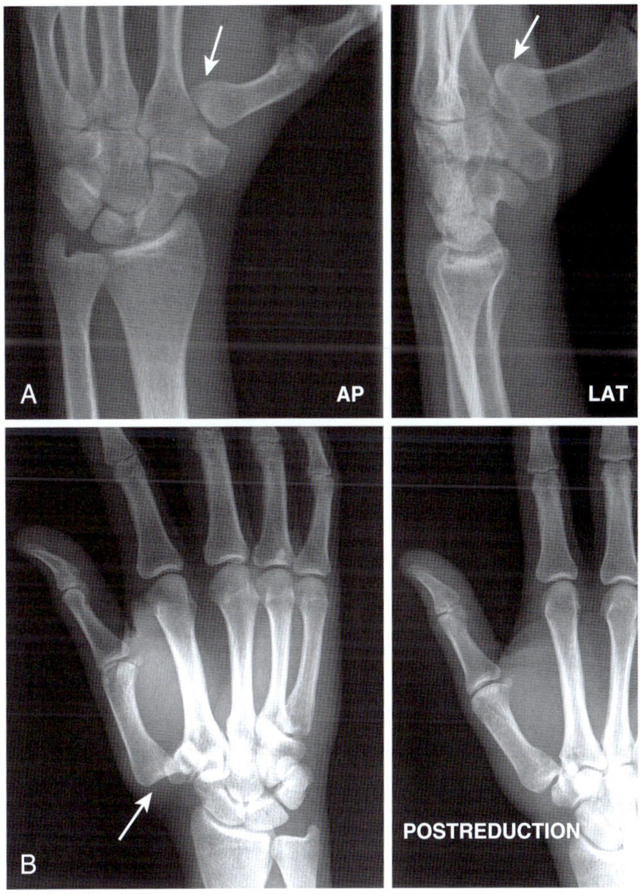

Fig. 50.37 Carpometacarpal (CMC) dislocation of the thumb (*arrows* in A and B). (A) Anteroposterior (*AP*) and lateral (*LAT*) radiographs of a CMC dislocation of the thumb, which is an uncommon injury. The patient sustained this injury when an air bag deployed during a motor vehicle collision. These dislocations are not generally amenable to closed reduction and usually require Kirschner wires. (B) Pre- and postreduction films of a CMC dislocation.

view is extremely important for detection of subtle dislocations or small avulsion fractures on the volar surfaces (Fig. 50.38).

Proximal Interphalangeal Joint Dislocations

The proximal interphalangeal (PIP) joint is extremely important, and any loss of motion in this joint may severely restrict normal function.[105] This joint is also prone to stiffness, so careful treatment of injuries in this area is essential. Injuries to the PIP joint are generally slow to heal and often result in an increase in joint size as a result of scar tissue formation.[105] Because of this propensity for a less-than-perfect outcome, it is advisable to refer PIP injuries after emergency care.

Proper examination of the PIP joint (Fig. 50.39) includes the application of ulnar and radial stress to test the integrity of the collateral ligaments and hyperextension to determine the integrity of the volar plate. Inability to actively extend the flexed PIP joint against resistance suggests a central slip rupture, which may progress to a boutonnière deformity (see Chapter 49).[105] Such an examination should be carried out *after* any successful joint reduction. This examination should also be conducted on a painful PIP joint that is radiographically normal to detect soft tissue injury in a spontaneously or field-reduced dislocation. This is extremely important in athletes because coaches often reduce these injuries.[105]

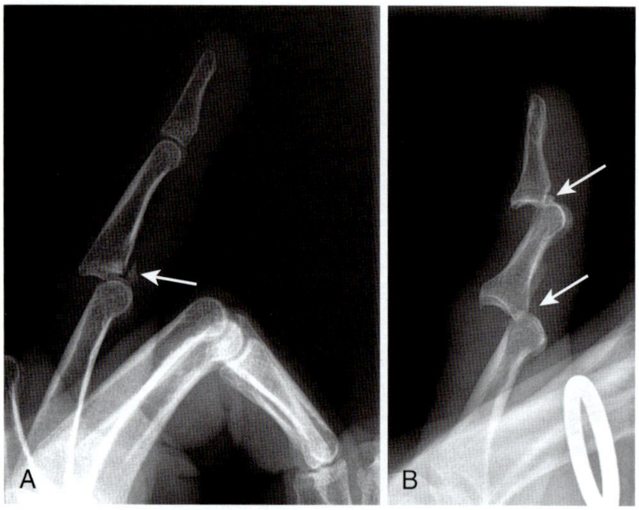

Fig. 50.38 Fracture-dislocations of the proximal (PIP) and distal interphalangeal (DIP) joints. True lateral radiographs are required to maximize sensitivity for small avulsion fractures. (A) A volar avulsion fracture *(arrow)* is readily seen on this dorsal DIP dislocation. (B) The fractures are more difficult to appreciate on this unfortunate patient who sustained dislocations of both the DIP and PIP joints in a fall *(arrows)*.

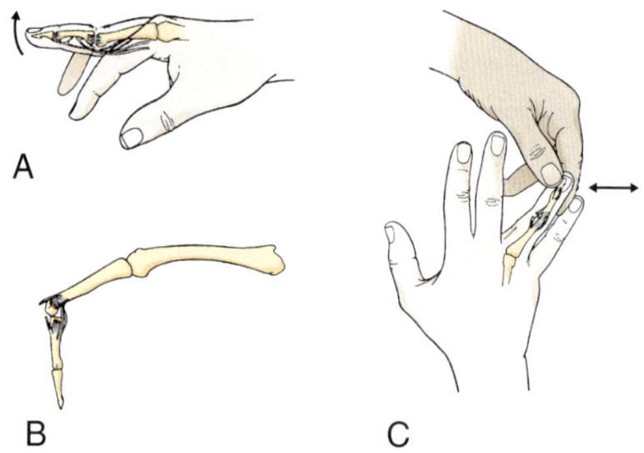

Fig. 50.39 Postreduction stress applied to a dislocated proximal interphalangeal (PIP) joint. (A) If the volar plate has been completely disrupted, the PIP joint will hyperextend with both passive and active motion. (B) Inability to actively extend the PIP joint indicates rupture of the central slip of the extensor tendon. (C) Passive lateral stress is applied to check the integrity of the collateral ligaments. (A–C, From DePalma AF. *Management of Fractures and Dislocations: An Atlas*. Saunders; 1970:1203-1204.)

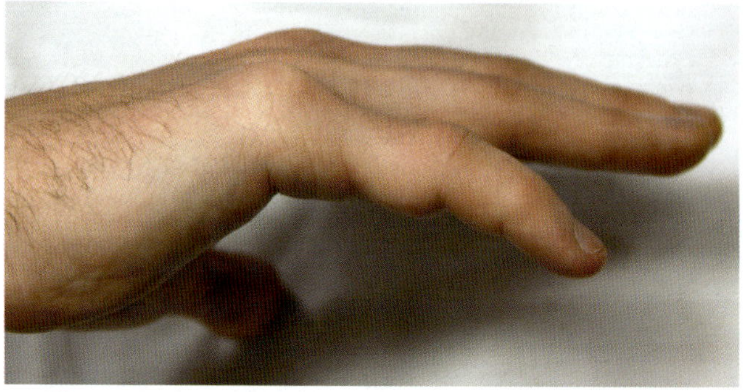

Fig. 50.40 Dorsal proximal interphalangeal joint dislocation.

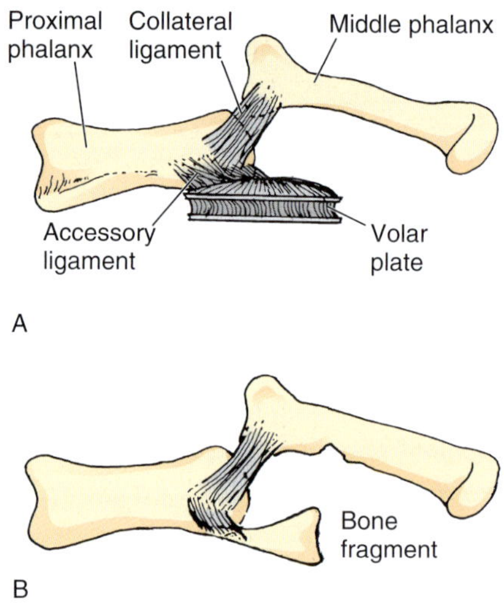

Fig. 50.41 A dorsal proximal interphalangeal joint dislocation (A) may involve rupture of the volar plate itself or (B) may involve avulsion of varying amounts of bone from the middle phalanx. If a large fragment of bone is avulsed from the base of the phalanx, the dislocation is unstable after reduction. The collateral ligaments will tear in varying degrees and should be assessed with stress testing after reduction.

Dorsal PIP Dislocations

Dorsal PIP dislocations are among the most common types encountered in the ED (Fig. 50.40; also see Fig. 50.30B). The mechanism is usually a blow to the end of the finger, such as from a thrown ball, that creates an axial load and hyperextends the finger.[106] The middle phalanx comes to rest dorsal to the proximal phalanx (Fig. 50.41). An associated disruption of the volar plate is generally present.[105,106] The deformity is obvious on clinical examination, and radiographs clearly demonstrate the injury. An associated fracture of the volar lip may be detected. If this fracture affects greater than 33% of the joint surface, closed reduction will be unstable because the collateral ligament is attached to the bony fragment. In these cases, operative repair will be necessary.[106]

A dorsal PIP dislocation can be reduced after a digital block. The usual method (see Figs. 50.31A–B) is to exaggerate the injury by slight traction and hyperextension, thereby distracting the middle phalanx. Apply pressure to the base of the middle phalanx as the finger is brought into flexion. These injuries usually reduce easily, and failure of routine attempts should raise suspicion of interposed soft tissue and the need for orthopedic consultation.

After reduction is completed, place the joint through a range of motion to ensure stability of the reduction. If stable, splint the joint in 20 to 30 degrees of flexion for 3 weeks.[105,106] Alternatively, buddy taping to an adjacent finger for 3 to 6 weeks allows early active motion and prevents hyperextension, which should be avoided.[106] Because PIP injuries can be slow to heal and are complicated by stiffness, it is advisable to refer these patients for orthopedic follow-up.

Volar PIP Dislocations

Volar PIP dislocations are uncommon injuries and virtually always accompanied by injury to the central slip of the extensor tendons. If the dislocation is reduced before the ED visit and there is no indication that the dislocation was volar, this injury may be incorrectly treated by splinting in mild flexion as though it were the more common dorsal dislocation. However, with disruption of the central slip of the extensor tendons, immobilization in flexion will lead to the development of a boutonnière deformity.[105,108] Even when this injury is

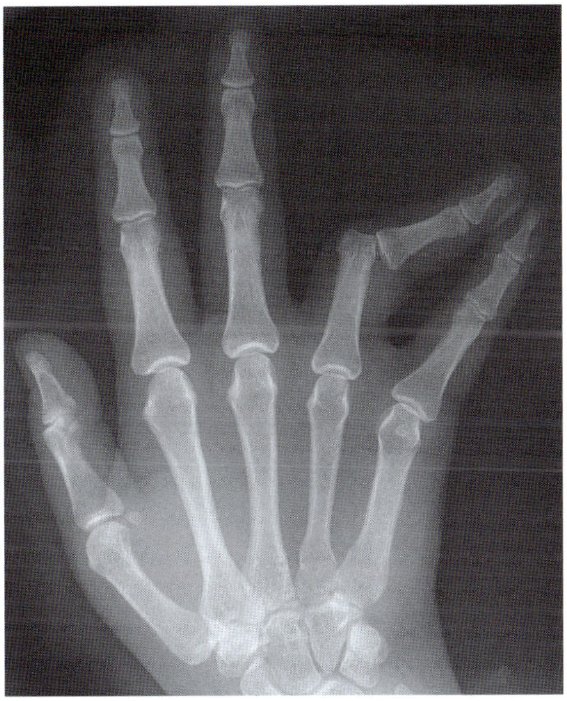

Fig. 50.42 Lateral proximal interphalangeal dislocation. These injuries are fairly common and will have dramatic and obvious clinical findings. The dislocation is often reduced in the field, before emergency department evaluation.

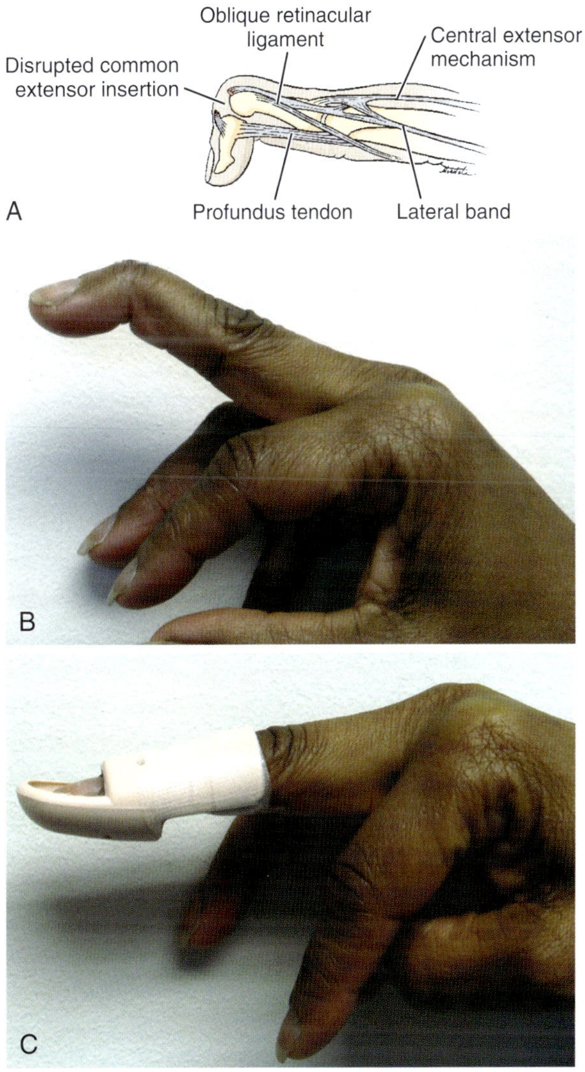

Fig. 50.43 (A) A mallet finger injury is not a dislocation; it is a rupture of the extensor tendon to the distal phalanx. It can occur with or without (demonstrated here) an avulsion fracture after seemingly minor trauma. (B) This mallet deformity was caused by a baseball striking the fingertip end on and producing acute flexion of the joint. (C) A stack splint, *with the proximal interphalangeal joint left free to allow relaxation of the distal interphalangeal joint*, is kept in place for 6 to 8 weeks. Caution the patient to avoid flexing the joint to "test it out" during splint changes. Wire fixation may be required.

recognized and treated properly, some impairment of mobility may occur. It is generally best to seek early orthopedic consultation for these injuries because some require operative repair. If the emergency clinician accomplishes a closed reduction, postreduction films must demonstrate normal congruity of the joint surfaces, and a central slip attachment fracture must be excluded.[108] If so, splinting of only the PIP joint in full extension should be undertaken for 3 weeks and early orthopedic follow-up ensured.[105]

Lateral PIP Dislocations

Lateral PIP dislocations are common and often reduced in the field. The patient will frequently describe dramatically how the finger was pointing in an unnatural manner (Fig. 50.42). The injury can be detected by applying ulnar and radial stress to the PIP joint. If still dislocated, re-create the injury and then apply longitudinal traction to reduce the dislocation. Treat partial tears of the collateral ligaments by buddy taping the finger for 3 to 6 weeks.[105] Management of complete tears is controversial, with some advocating operative therapy for all such injuries and others using varying durations of immobilization or buddy taping.[105] Referral is suggested for all but the mildest of PIP collateral ligament injuries.

Distal Interphalangeal Dislocations

As in the thumb, the distal phalanx is attached firmly to skin and subcutaneous tissue by osteocutaneous fibers. For this reason, dislocations of the distal interphalangeal (DIP) joint are frequently open.[105] A DIP dislocation is usually dorsal, and the mechanism is a blow to the end of the finger. Despite the dislocation, the DIP joint may retain some range of motion, so it is important to not overlook these injuries.[109] Lateral radiographs are diagnostic.

Management of a dorsal DIP dislocation involves reduction in a fashion like that described for other IP joint injuries (see Fig. 50.31). Hyperextend the finger and apply traction to distract the joint, and then apply pressure on the base of the distal phalanx during flexion. Following reduction, check the joint for stability and place the finger in a dorsal splint for 10 to 12 days.[105]

An injury to the DIP joint that may be confused with a dislocation is the mallet finger (Fig. 50.43). This injury is often caused by forced flexion of an extended finger (e.g., struck by a baseball). The patient is unable to extend the fingertip, but the joint appears normal on passive extension by the examiner. The injury is a rupture of the extensor tendon, with or without avulsion of a small piece of bone. Unless the injury is properly splinted or surgically immobilized, permanent deformity will occur (see Chapter 49).

MCP Dislocations

The pathology and management of finger MCP dislocations are identical to those of the thumb, as discussed earlier. The same classification of simple and complex applies; the complex type requires operative repair. Dimpling on the palmar surface suggests the presence of a complex dislocation. It is important to remember that application of traction alone for a simple MCP dislocation may convert it to a complex dislocation. For dorsal dislocations, flex the wrist to relax the tendons and hyperextend the joint as far as possible. Then apply pressure on the base of the proximal phalanx to effect reduction. After reduction of a simple dorsal MCP dislocation, buddy taping is generally sufficient to secure the reduction.[105] Volar dislocations are rare and require orthopedic consultation.

CMC Dislocations

CMC dislocations are rare injuries that are frequently misdiagnosed. The usual site of injury is the fifth CMC joint, which is dorsally dislocated.[106] The injury is generally the result of a high-energy mechanism, such as a motor vehicle crash or a fall. The diagnosis can be quite difficult to make because the appearance may be subtle even on a lateral radiograph. Associated fractures and other injuries are frequently present, and percutaneous fixation is usually required.[106]

Carpal Dislocation/Dissociation

Dislocation and dissociation of the carpal bones are significant injuries that require identification in the ED and expeditious immobilization and reduction to ensure the best ultimate outcome. Nonetheless, these injuries often produce significant long-term disability, such as chronic pain and weakness, premature arthritis, and AVN. Specific intervention to establish anatomic alignment is usually undertaken on diagnosis or within a few days of the injury, so identification in the ED, initial splinting, and proper referral are paramount. Definitive treatment is beyond the scope of this chapter and is performed by a consultant, often a hand surgeon.

The most common carpal injuries are scapholunate dissociation and lunate and perilunate dislocation, although a number of variations exist.[105] These injuries are often sustained by a fall on an outstretched hand. Carpal dislocations and dissociations produce pain, weakness, decreased range of motion, and often significant soft tissue swelling, with many symptoms seemingly out of proportion to the radiographic findings. Specific radiographic diagnosis is frequently difficult, and it is not uncommon for definitive diagnosis to be missed on initial ED evaluation. CT or magnetic resonance imaging may be required to delineate the specifics of the injury. Marked swelling on the dorsal surface of the hand or wrist, in the absence of a definitive fracture on plain radiographs, is a common scenario, and such findings should prompt consideration of carpal dislocation or dissociation (Fig. 50.44).[105] If a diagnosis is not forthcoming, splinting and reevaluation of a markedly swollen and painful hand or wrist in 2 to 3 days is prudent.

Scapholunate dissociation is a serious, frequently missed injury that is characterized by a widened space (>3 mm) between the scaphoid and lunate bones on a plain radiograph. This is best visualized on a posteroanterior view with the hand closed in a fist and the wrist in ulnar deviation (Fig. 50.45). It is indicative of disruption of ligaments stabilizing the two carpal bones. Even though the symptoms and swelling may be impressive, the radiographic findings are subtle and often overlooked, with initial and subsequent complaints being attributed to a severe bruise or sprain. When identified, the hand and wrist are immobilized in the ED by a splint in neutral position or in 10 to 15 degrees of wrist dorsiflexion. Referral should also be initiated.

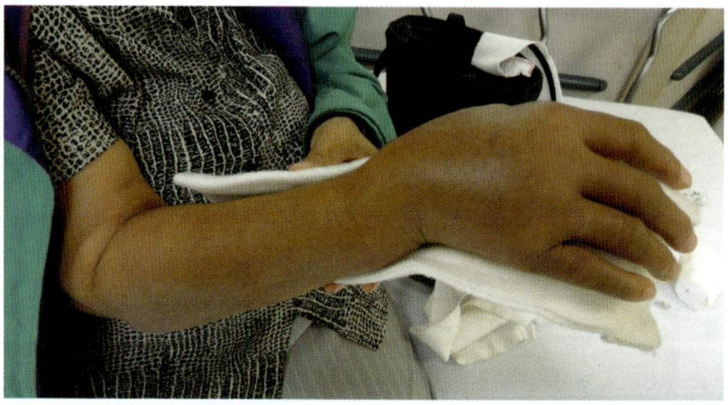

Fig. 50.44 With this much soft tissue swelling 2 days after a fall on an outstretched hand, something more than a sprain or bruise is likely. If no fracture is seen on radiographs, consider carpal bone fracture or dissociation as the culprit. Scaphoid fracture, scapholunate disassociation, or lunate or perilunate dislocation should be considered. Computed tomography or magnetic resonance imaging may be required to define the exact pathology. Note that patients with such injuries hold the wrist in flexion, worsening the edema by compression of dorsal hand veins.

Lunate dislocation and perilunate dislocation (Figs. 50.46 and 50.47) can also occur from trauma and produce pain, swelling, and disability. Plain radiographs will usually delineate the pathology. Identification, splinting in a neutral position or in 10 to 15 degrees of wrist dorsiflexion, and referral are the mainstays of ED treatment.

HIP DISLOCATIONS

The hip is generally a stable ball-and-socket joint (Videos 50.32–50.35). The head of the femur is deeply situated in the acetabulum, and ligamentous and muscular support is very strong. Therefore hip dislocations are usually the result of significant force, and a careful search for other limb- or life-threatening injuries must be undertaken. The common mechanism of native hip dislocation during motor vehicle accidents involves the flexed knee striking the dashboard when the hip is in flexion causing a posterior dislocation.[110]

Associated fractures are quite common with hip dislocations. In fact, up to 70% of hip dislocations are accompanied by an associated fracture.[111] If a fracture complicates the dislocation, orthopedic consultation is generally indicated. However, the emergency clinician should be able to reduce simple hip dislocations, which are dislocations without an associated fracture or with a very minor fracture.[112,113]

Hip dislocations may occasionally be missed in the setting of severe trauma because other injuries garner more attention. Common complications of hip dislocation include sciatic nerve injuries and AVN of the femoral head. Sciatic nerve injuries are seen in approximately10% of posterior hip dislocations.[114] AVN of the femoral head is one of the more disabling complications associated with hip dislocation. Although it is generally stated that early reduction will reduce the frequency of this complication, patients with native hip dislocation often have other significant traumatic injuries that require stabilization and intervention.[115] Providers should provide expeditious evaluation and diagnosis of patients with suspected native hip

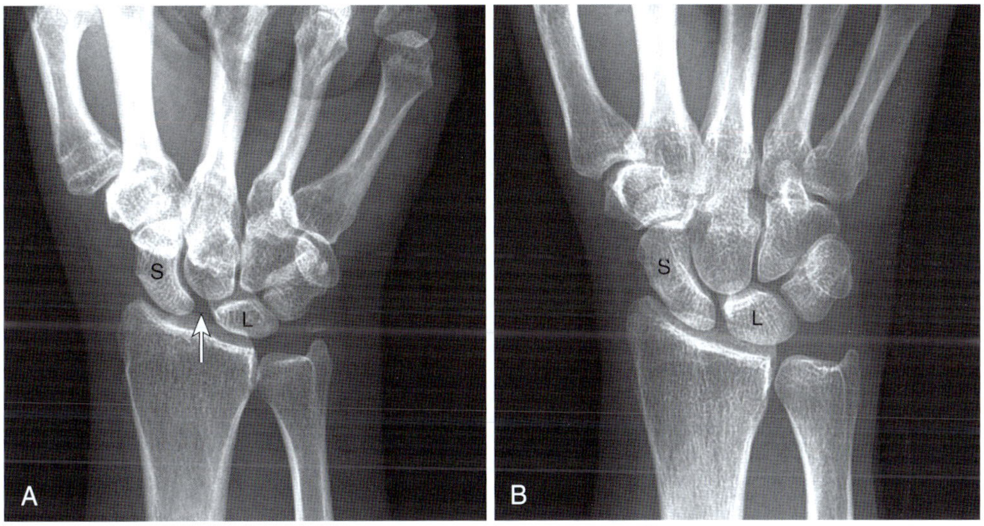

Fig. 50.45 Scapholunate disassociation is easy to miss on a plain film. (A) A posteroanterior view of the wrist demonstrates a widened space between the scaphoid *(S)* and the lunate *(L)* *(arrow)* because of ligamentous disruption from an impaction injury. Orthopedic consultation is required for this injury. (B) A normal wrist shows that the typical distance between the scaphoid and lunate should be approximately the same as that between the scaphoid and the radius.

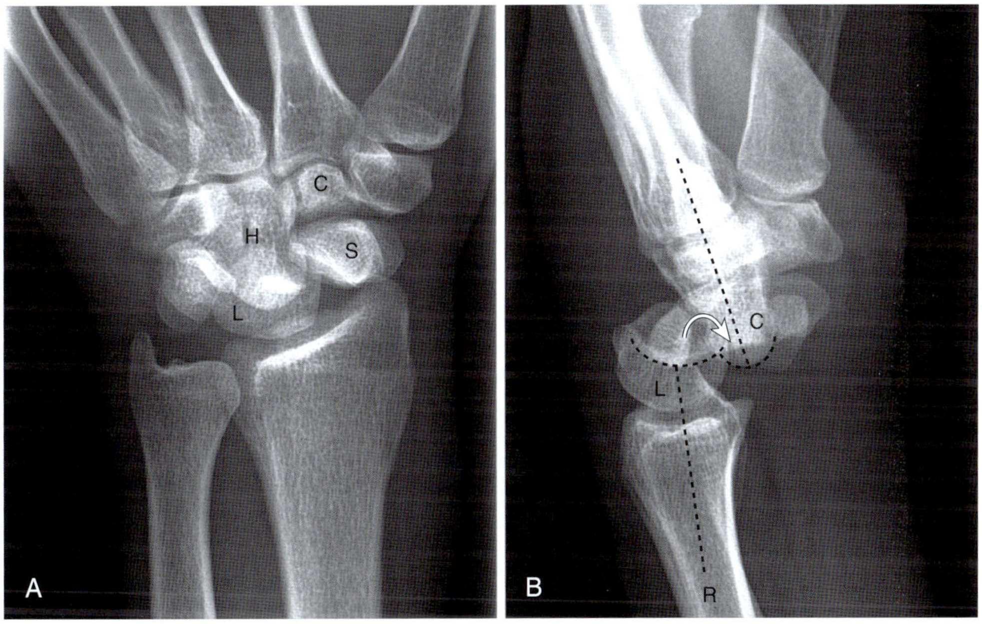

Fig. 50.46 Perilunate dislocation. (A) A posteroanterior view of the wrist does not show the normal two crescentic rows of carpal bones but rather shows significant overlap of the hamate *(H)* and the lunate *(L)*, as well as the capitate *(C)* with the scaphoid *(S)*. (B) A lateral view shows that the lunate remains in alignment with the end of the radius *(R)*, but the remainder of the carpal bones have been dislocated.

dislocation with a goal to perform reduction within 6 hours of time of injury to decrease incidence of AVN.[116,117] If evidence of nerve injury exists, the dislocation should be treated as an emergency and reduced as early as possible.

Radiographic Examination

Dislocation of the hip is generally obvious on the standard AP pelvic film that is often taken during trauma resuscitation (Fig. 50.48). A lateral or oblique view of the hip may help clarify the type of dislocation and allow detection of associated fractures.

Analgesia and Anesthesia

Dislocation of a prosthetic hip can usually be managed with moderate amounts of IV premedication in the ED. Premedication recommendations for other acute traumatic dislocations run the gamut from general anesthesia for all reductions[112,115] to IV sedation only. Similar to the growing body of evidence of ED-administered nerve blocks for upper extremity dislocations (shoulder, elbow), there have been reports describing the use of fascia iliaca compartment blocks and femoral nerve blocks to successfully reduce a dislocation of a total hip arthroplasty.[118,119] Most clinicians would agree that some type

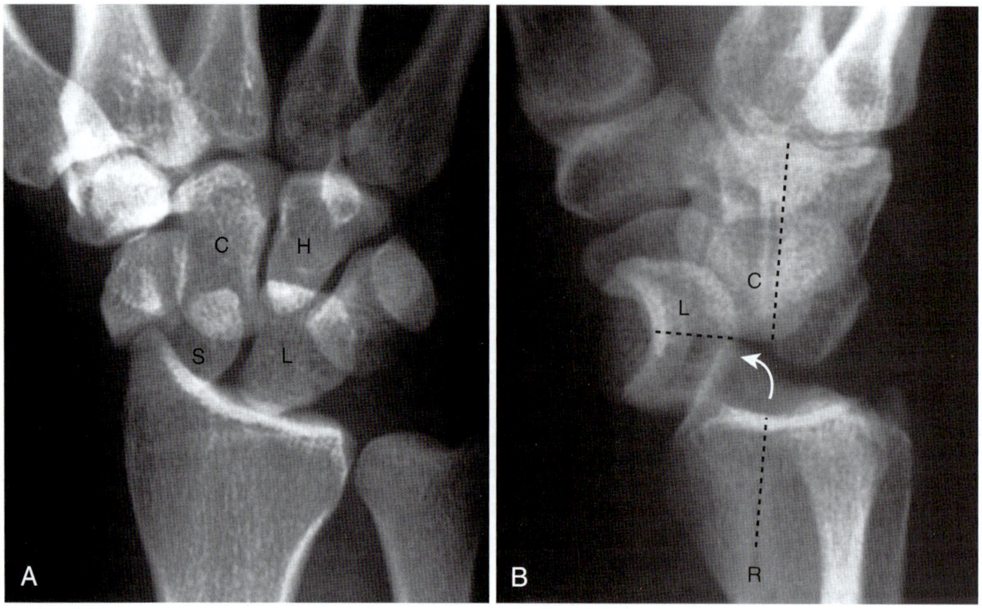

Fig. 50.47 Lunate dislocation. (A) On a posteroanterior view of the wrist, significant overlap is seen of the capitate *(C)* and scaphoid *(S)*, as well as the hamate *(H)* and lunate *(L)*. Furthermore, clear overlap appears between the scaphoid and the radial styloid. All these findings suggest dislocation. (B) On the lateral view, the carpal bones remain in alignment with the distal end of the radius *(R)*, but the lunate has rotated and dislocated in the palmar direction *(arrow)*. (From Mettler FA, ed. *Essentials of Radiology*. 2nd ed. Saunders; 2005.)

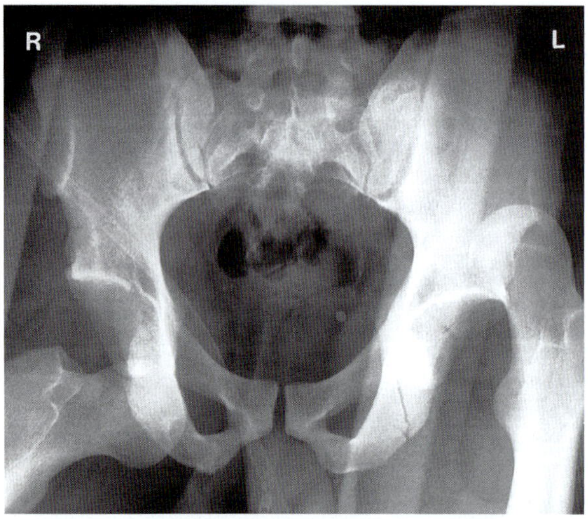

Fig. 50.48 This patient was in a motor vehicle accident and has both an anterior and a posterior dislocation of the hips. Posterior dislocation occurs 90% of the time and is seen here on the *left*, with the femoral head displaced superior and lateral to the acetabulum. On the *right* is an anterior dislocation with the femoral head displaced inferiorly and medially. This patient also has a fracture of the pelvis and possibly the left acetabulum and will require a computed tomography scan to unravel the extent of all injuries. (From Mettler FA, ed. *Essentials of Radiology*. 2nd ed. Saunders; 2005.)

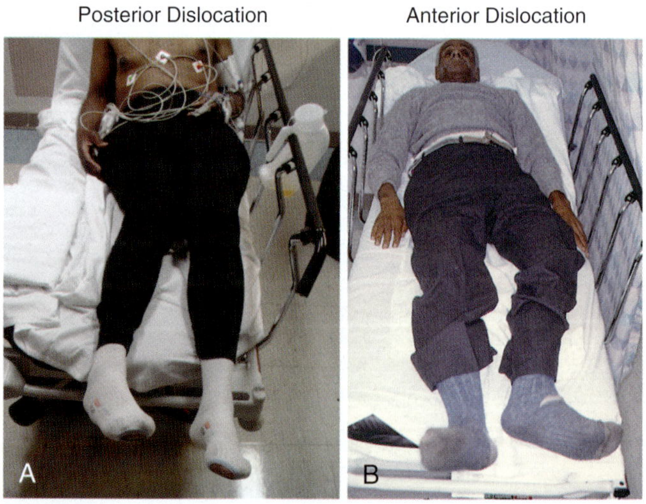

Fig. 50.49 (A) Posterior hip dislocation in a patient with a hip prosthesis. The right leg is adducted, flexed at the knee, shortened, and internally rotated. (B) The much less common anterior dislocation. The left leg is shortened, abducted, flexed at the knee, and externally rotated, similar to the appearance of a hip fracture.

of IV premedication is necessary, and patients often require deep sedation if the procedure is to be successful in the ED.[120] Nevertheless, if reasonable attempts fail in the ED, one should not hesitate to opt for spinal or general anesthesia.

Posterior Hip Dislocation

Posterior dislocation is the most common type of hip dislocation. Posterior dislocations generally occur secondary to a blow to the flexed knee with the hip in varying degrees of flexion (e.g., a knee striking the dashboard in a head-on motor vehicle collision). The greater the amount of flexion and adduction of the hip at the time of the injury, the less the chance of an associated fracture.[115] The femoral head is forced out of the acetabulum and rests behind it. The sciatic nerve is located just behind the hip joint and may be injured with a posterior hip dislocation. The clinical picture includes a shortened, internally rotated, and adducted leg (Fig. 50.49A).

Reduction Techniques

Several basic methods of hip reduction have been reported. Some techniques involve placing the patient in the prone

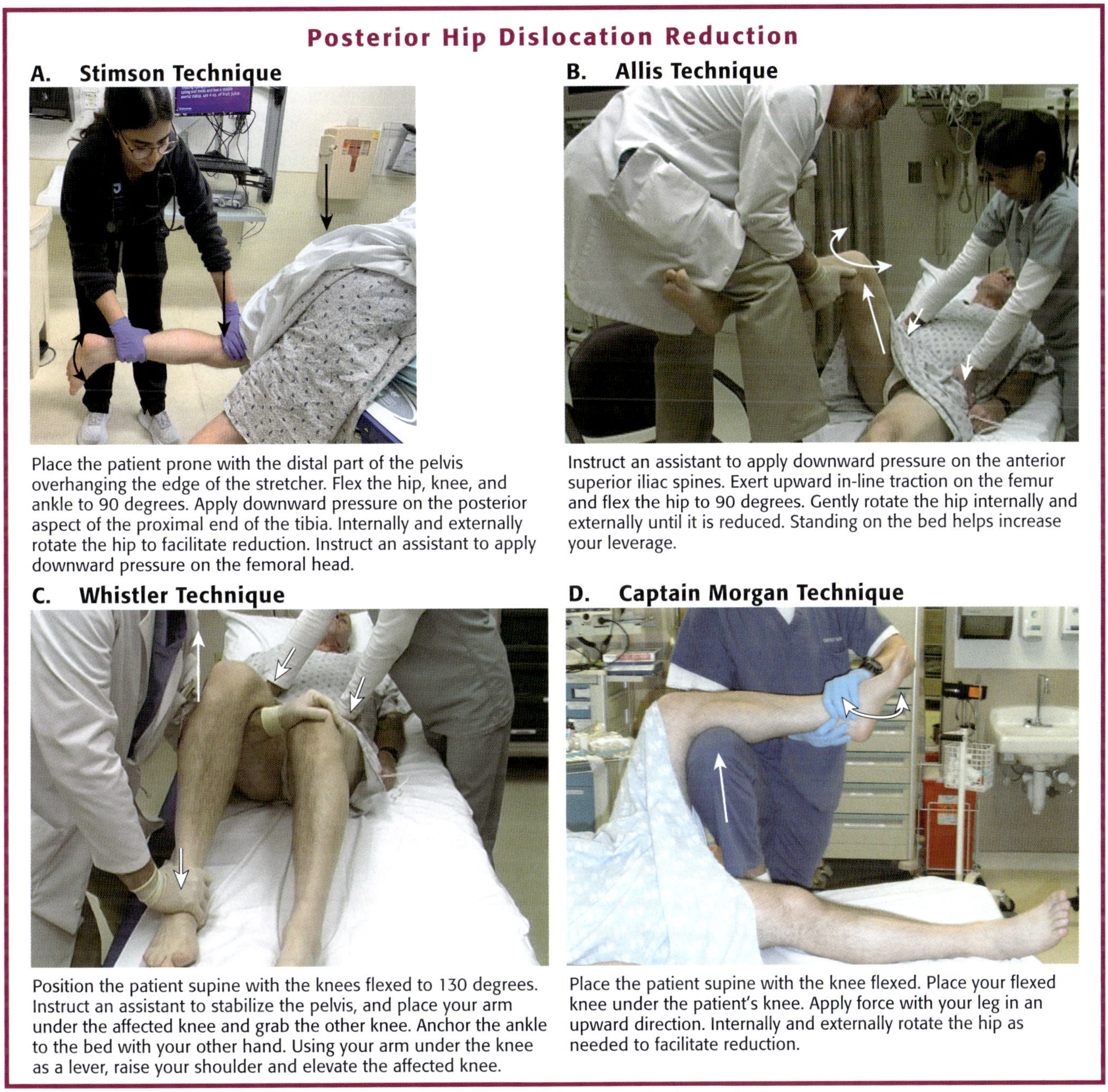
Posterior Hip Dislocation Reduction
A. Stimson Technique
Place the patient prone with the distal part of the pelvis overhanging the edge of the stretcher. Flex the hip, knee, and ankle to 90 degrees. Apply downward pressure on the posterior aspect of the proximal end of the tibia. Internally and externally rotate the hip to facilitate reduction. Instruct an assistant to apply downward pressure on the femoral head.
B. Allis Technique
Instruct an assistant to apply downward pressure on the anterior superior iliac spines. Exert upward in-line traction on the femur and flex the hip to 90 degrees. Gently rotate the hip internally and externally until it is reduced. Standing on the bed helps increase your leverage.
C. Whistler Technique
Position the patient supine with the knees flexed to 130 degrees. Instruct an assistant to stabilize the pelvis, and place your arm under the affected knee and grab the other knee. Anchor the ankle to the bed with your other hand. Using your arm under the knee as a lever, raise your shoulder and elevate the affected knee.
D. Captain Morgan Technique
Place the patient supine with the knee flexed. Place your flexed knee under the patient's knee. Apply force with your leg in an upward direction. Internally and externally rotate the hip as needed to facilitate reduction.

Fig. 50.50 Posterior hip dislocation reduction methods.

position (e.g., the Stimson technique), whereas others require that the patient be supine with downward stabilization of the pelvis performed by an assistant. The supine position may be preferable in multiply injured patients because of the difficulty involved in closely monitoring a critically ill patient in the prone position.

Stimson Technique

In the prone or gravity method described by Stimson, the patient is positioned so that the distal portion of the pelvis overhangs the edge of the stretcher (Fig. 50.50A). Flex the hip, knee, and ankle to 90 degrees and apply downward pressure on the posterior aspect of the proximal end of the tibia.[121] Gently rotate the hip internally and externally to facilitate reduction. If needed, an assistant may apply direct downward pressure on the femoral head. The modified Stimson technique is an alternative and more comfortable way to provide downward pressure on the tibia. The operator grasps the patient's ankle, places a knee on the patient's calf, and uses body weight to apply pressure.[122] This method is believed to be the least traumatic; however, associated thoracoabdominal injuries or a need for deep sedation, which may pose an airway risk, may make the prone position risky for the patient.[115]

Allis Technique

For the Allis technique, place the patient supine and have an assistant stabilize the pelvis by applying downward pressure at the anterior superior iliac spines (see Fig. 50.50B). Exert upward traction in line with the deformity and flex the hip to 90 degrees. Gently rotate the hip internally and externally until it is reduced.[115] Some prefer to stand on the patient's stretcher so that body weight can be used for leverage. Howard[123] suggested modifying this technique by applying lateral

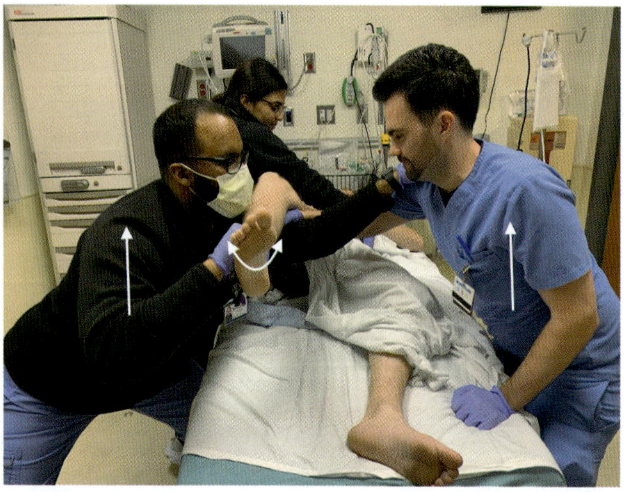

Fig. 50.51 Stand on the ipsilateral side to the injury with an assistant standing on the contralateral side. Flex the affected hip and knee to 90 degrees. Place one arm under the flexed knee while the other hand grips the lower leg at the ankle in facilitate reduction through internal and external rotation. Link arms with an assistant under the patient's leg, resting your hand on each other's shoulder. A second assistant can provide stabilization at the pelvis. Slowly stand up to provide traction to the affected leg.

traction on the flexed upper part of the femur to disengage the head of the femur from the outer lip of the acetabulum.

Whistler Technique

Another method known as the Whistler technique was described by Walden and Hamer (see Fig. 50.50C and Video 50.36).[124] Place the patient in the supine position with both knees flexed to 130 degrees. While an assistant stabilizes the pelvis, stand beside the affected limb. Place an arm under the affected knee and grab the unaffected knee. With the other hand, anchor the ankle of the affected leg firmly against the stretcher. Using the arm placed under the knee as a lever, raise your shoulder to elevate the affected knee. This allows the femoral head to move anteriorly around the acetabular rim and relocate.[124] Although experience with this technique is limited, it appears to be a promising, gentle reduction method.

Captain Morgan Technique

Another gentle method for reducing posterior hip dislocations is like the Whistler technique but uses the clinician's knee as opposed to the arm (see Fig. 50.50D and Video 50.37). To perform the Captain Morgan technique,[125] place the patient supine with the affected knee flexed. Stand on the affected side and place your flexed knee underneath the patient's flexed knee. Apply force with your leg in an upward direction. Internal or external rotation can be added as needed. One case series described an extremely high success rate with this method of reduction, with only one failed attempt secondary to bony fragments in the joint space, which required open reduction.[125]

East Baltimore Lift

The East Baltimore Lift method positions the patient in the supine position for the reduction (Fig. 50.51).[126] The provider stands on the ipsilateral side to the injury with an assistant standing on the contralateral side. The affected limb is flexed so the hip and knee are at 90 degrees. The provider places one arm under the flexed knee while the other hand grips the lower leg at the ankle. The assistant passes their arm under the leg linking arms, allowing their hands to rest on each other's shoulders. A second assistant provides stabilization at the pelvis. The height of the bed should be adjusted so that the provider and assistant are squatting slightly at 45 degrees. The provider and assistant slowly stand up while providing traction to the affected leg. With one hand on the ankle, the provider can also provide internal and external rotation to facilitate reduction.[126] This technique has the advantage of utilizing two providers to exert upward force rising from a slight squatting position requiring less physical demand of the physicians. However, this advantage can also be seen as the maneuver's downfall, as it requires several personnel (three for the reduction and an additional person supervising the sedation).

PGI technique

The Postgraduate Institute of Medical Education and Research has developed a method for reduction that in limited study has shown great efficacy (Fig. 50.52A–D).[127] It only requires one provider, and does not require force or dangerous positioning of either the provider or the patient. With the patient in the supine position, the provider uses their dominant hand to flex the knee of the affected leg to 120 degrees. While maintaining flexion of the knee, the affected hip is gradually abducted by the provider's nondominant hand. At 45 degrees of abduction, gentle external rotation is performed to reduce the femoral head.[127]

Once reduction is achieved, the legs are immobilized in slight abduction by placing an abduction pillow or another object between the knees. Radiographs should be repeated to confirm reduction, and the patient should be admitted to the hospital.

Dislocations of Hip Prostheses

Dislocation of a hip prosthesis is a separate issue (Fig. 50.53 and Video 50.38). Unlike primary dislocations, which require significant trauma, a prosthetic hip may dislocate with minimal force, such as rolling over in bed or trying to get out of a chair. Most dislocations occur in the first 3 to 4 months after surgery, but recurrent dislocation may take place much later.[128] The majority of dislocations are posterior. The emergency physician should consider consultation with the orthopedic surgeon who placed the prosthesis.

The three major causes of prosthetic hip dislocations include (1) assumption of a position that exceeds the stability of the prosthesis, (2) soft tissue imbalances, and (3) component malposition.[110]

Emergency clinicians have been shown to be highly successful in reducing prosthetic hip dislocations.[129–131] Reduction techniques are similar to those described earlier; however, the urgency is not as paramount because problems with bone necrosis do not exist. Although complications are occasionally unavoidable, the clinician must be aware that forceful reduction of a dislocated hip prosthesis may dislodge the acetabular cup, fracture underlying osteoporotic bone, or loosen the prosthesis. Unlike other hip dislocations, patients with prosthetic hip dislocations will often not require hospital admission and may be discharged after discussion with the consulting orthopedic surgeon. The most common way to reduce such dislocations is shown in Fig. 50.54.

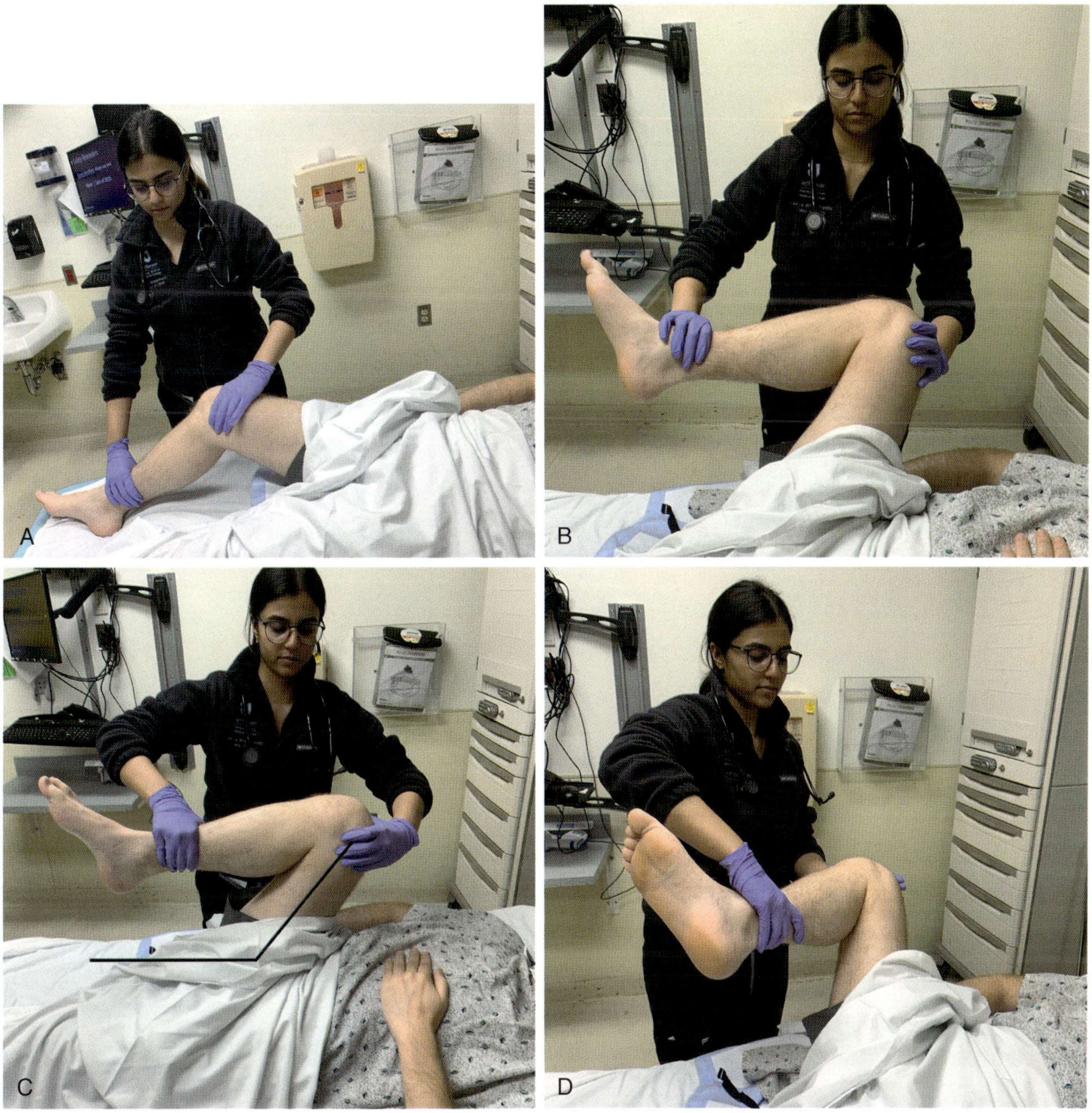

Fig. 50.52 (A) Place your dominant hand on the knee of the affected leg and your other hand in the supramalleolar region. (B) Flex the knee of the affected leg to 120 degrees. (C) Use your nondominant hand to gradually abduct the leg. (D) At 45 degrees of abduction, gently externally rotate the leg to reduce the femoral head.

Anterior Hip Dislocation

Anterior hip dislocations are less common than posterior dislocations and account for 10% to 15% of all hip dislocations.[110,115] There are three general types of anterior hip dislocations that are defined by the place where the femoral head comes to rest (Fig. 50.55): iliac or subspinous, pubic, and inferior or obturator dislocation. Anterior hip dislocations generally result from forced abductions of the thigh, which may occur with motorcycle accidents, falls, or motor vehicle collisions.[115] The clinical picture varies with the type of dislocation. With the obturator (inferior) type, the leg is abducted and externally rotated with varying degrees of flexion. In the other types, the hip is usually extended and externally rotated.[115]

Reduction Techniques

The Stimson gravity method may work for anterior hip dislocation, although it is not recommended for the pubic type (Fig. 50.56).[115] Alternatively, the Allis maneuver can be applied in the modified Walker fashion. Place the patient in a supine position and have an assistant stabilize the pelvis while applying lateral countertraction on the thigh. Flex the hip slightly and apply traction along the long axis of the femur. Gently adduct and internally rotate the leg to affect reduction.[115]

For the reverse Bigelow technique, place the hip in partial flexion and abduction. Apply traction in the line of the deformity, then adduct, sharply internally rotate, and extend the hip. Caution should be exercised when using this technique because the sharp internal rotation may result in fracture

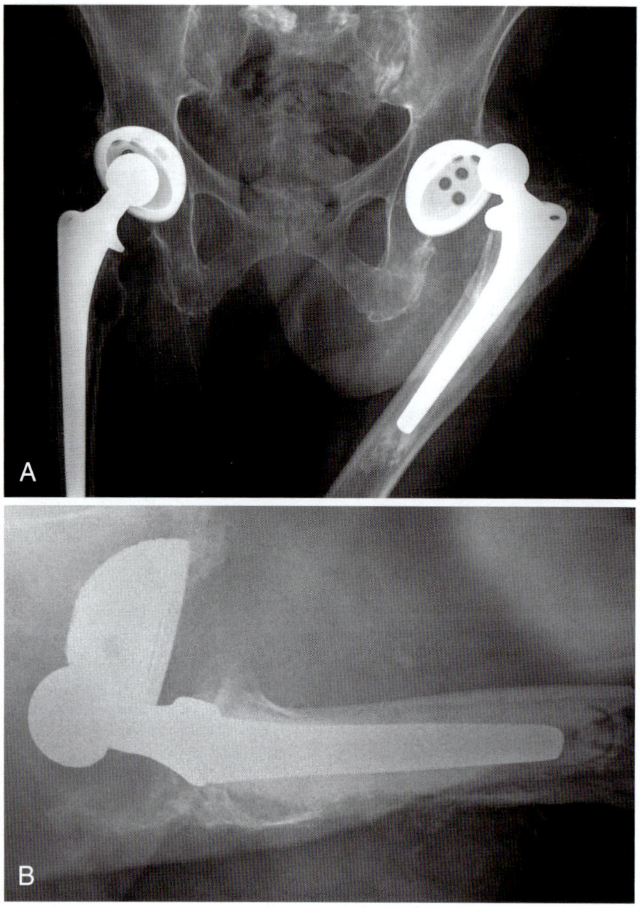

Fig. 50.53 Prosthetic hip dislocation. (A) This patient has bilateral hip replacements. This posteroanterior radiograph shows left-sided dislocation, with the femoral component displaced in a superior direction. (B) A cross-table lateral view demonstrates that this is a posterior dislocation (posterior is at the *bottom* of the image, anterior at the *top*). The majority of prosthetic dislocations are posterior.

of the femoral neck in patients with osteoporotic bone.[110] As with posterior dislocations, admission to the hospital is required for patients with these injuries.

KNEE (FEMUR, TIBIA) DISLOCATIONS

Although the knee is a simple hinge joint, dislocations are quite rare because of its strong ligamentous support. The major ligaments include the anterior and posterior cruciate and the collateral ligaments. The usual mechanism of a knee dislocation involves a great deal of force, such as a motor vehicle crash or a sporting injury.[132] However, knee dislocation has been reported with greater frequency after minor mechanisms, such as stepping off a curb or into a hole, usually in association with a twisting action.[133,134] Patients with increased body mass index may be more likely to dislocate a knee with surprisingly minor trauma, coined low-velocity or ultra-low velocity injuries, such as when stepping into a hole causes a twisting motion (Fig. 50.57). These patients are more commonly females and are at increased risk of vascular injury when compared to high-energy mechanism multi-ligament disruptions.[133–136] As with other joint dislocations, knee dislocations are described with respect to the position of the distal bone in relation to the proximal one (i.e., tibia in relation to the femur).[137] The more common types are shown in Fig. 50.58.

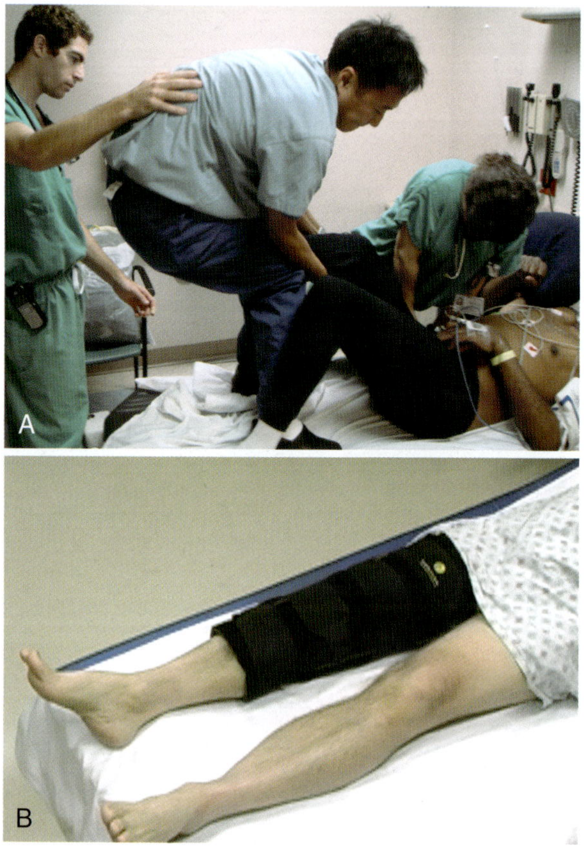

Fig. 50.54 (A) A common method of reducing a posterior hip dislocation is to stand on the bed as shown. Apply traction with external rotation to move the femoral head away from the metallic cup. Assistants protect the operator and provide countertraction. (B) After reduction, a knee immobilizer prevents dislocation again as hip motion is hampered.

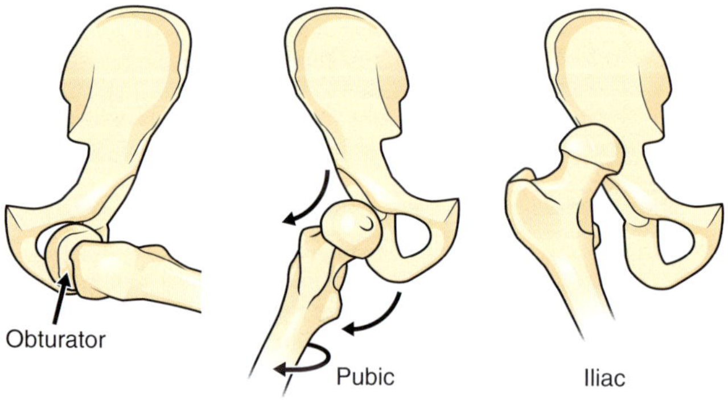

Fig. 50.55 Anterior dislocations of the hip: obturator, pubic, and iliac. (From Simon R, Koenigsknecht S. *Orthopedics in Emergency Medicine.* Appleton-Century-Crofts; 1982:367.)

There are five general types of knee dislocation, including anterior (Fig. 50.59), posterior, lateral, and the less common medial and rotatory.[132] Rotatory dislocations may be anteromedial, anterolateral, posterolateral, or posteromedial.[132]

Clinical Assessment

Knee dislocations are usually clinically obvious; however, in up to 50% of cases the dislocation may have spontaneously reduced before evaluation in the ED and be manifested only

Anterior Hip Dislocation Reduction

Modified Allis Technique

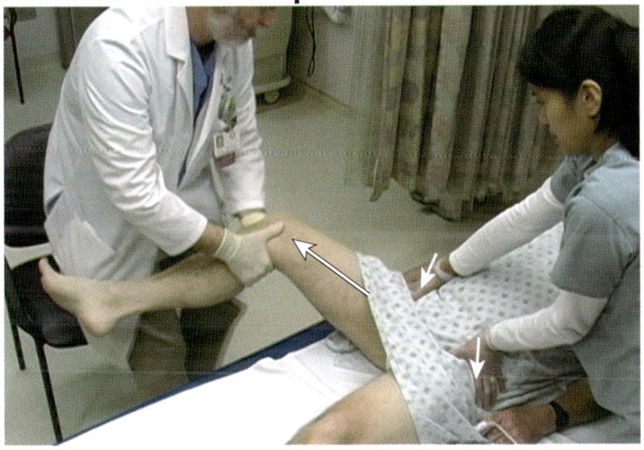

Place the patient supine and instruct an assistant to stabilize the pelvis. Flex the hip slightly and apply traction along the long axis of the femur.

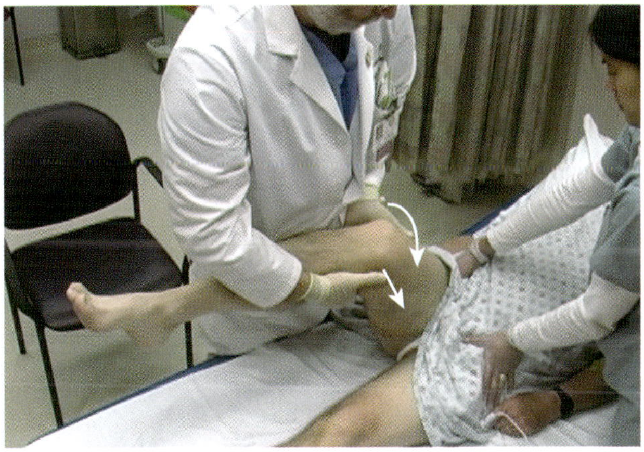

Gently adduct and internally rotate the leg to reduce the dislocation.

Fig. 50.56 Anterior hip dislocation reduction.

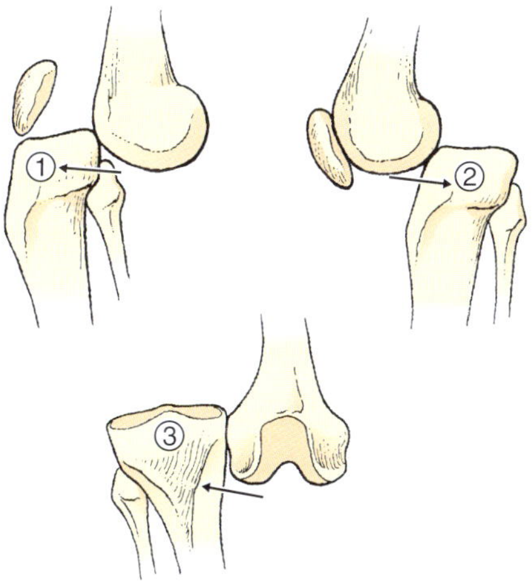

Fig. 50.57 The three most common types of knee dislocations: anterior (*1*), posterior (*2*), and lateral (*3*). (From DePalma AF. *Management of Fractures and Dislocations: An Atlas*. Saunders; 1970:1621.)

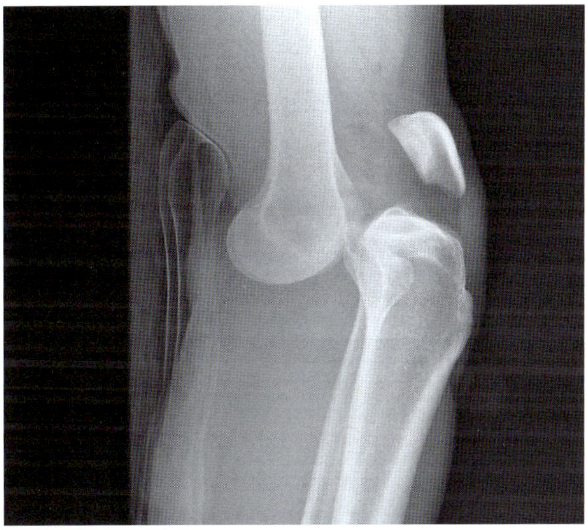

Fig. 50.58 Anterior knee dislocation seen on a lateral radiograph. The patient sustained this injury when he was struck by a vehicle.

as severe knee pain with hemarthrosis (Video 50.39).[132,138] When a spontaneously reduced knee dislocation is associated with other major trauma, the diagnosis can be missed. Patients with increased body mass index may have a seemingly normal appearance of their knee, but an obvious deformity will be visible on the initial radiographs (see Fig. 50.57). A grossly unstable knee that does not appear to be dislocated is probably a reduced dislocation and carries the same risk for vascular and other complications as a dislocated knee.[139] A severely unstable knee can be defined as one that has greater than 30 degrees of recurvatum (hyperextension) on lifting the leg off the stretcher by the heel or one that exhibits gross instability after reduction. Because pain and muscle spasm may limit the physical examination for stability, a knee hemarthrosis, usually a large one with signs of posterior or calf hemorrhage, is a potential tip-off to a reduced dislocation.

An impressive effusion may not be present with a knee dislocation because the joint capsule is often disrupted and extravasation occurs into the surrounding tissue, usually posteriorly.[137] The most important part of the clinical assessment is the vascular status of the extremity (see the section "Vascular Injury"). Nerve injury is less common, but peroneal nerve injury is a recognized complication, particularly with a posterolateral dislocation.[137] Peroneal nerve injury should be suspected if the patient is unable to dorsiflex the ankle (footdrop) or has decreased sensation on the dorsum of the foot. Posterolateral dislocations may be irreducible because the medial femoral condyle buttonholes through the joint capsule.[137] A clue to this injury is the presence of a dimple sign at the medial joint line.

Vascular Injury

The most feared complication of a knee dislocation is severance or internal injury of the popliteal artery (Fig. 50.60). Injury to the popliteal artery may complicate both anterior

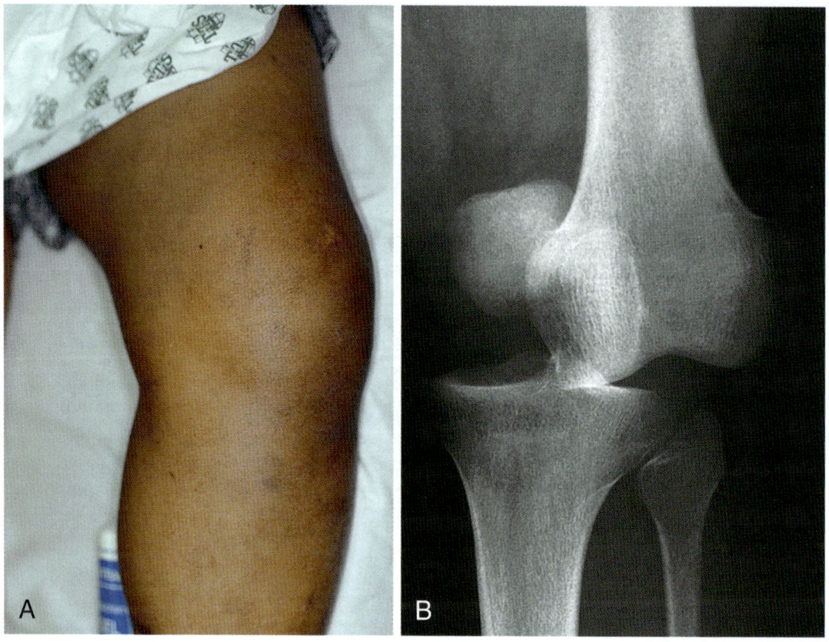

Fig. 50.59 (A) In a patient with increased body mass index, a dislocated knee may not be obvious on initial inspection. This patient stated that she stepped into a hole and twisted her knee (a classic mechanism for dislocation), which caused the clinician to suspect only ligamentous injury or a sprain with a hemarthrosis. (B) A radiograph demonstrated the seriousness of this seemingly benign injury. If spontaneous reduction occurs before evaluation in the emergency department, this diagnosis may not even be considered. Arterial injury (especially popliteal artery) is a serious complication of a knee dislocation. An arteriogram is the gold standard for evaluation of arterial injuries, which can initially be subtle or delayed (see Fig. 50.60).

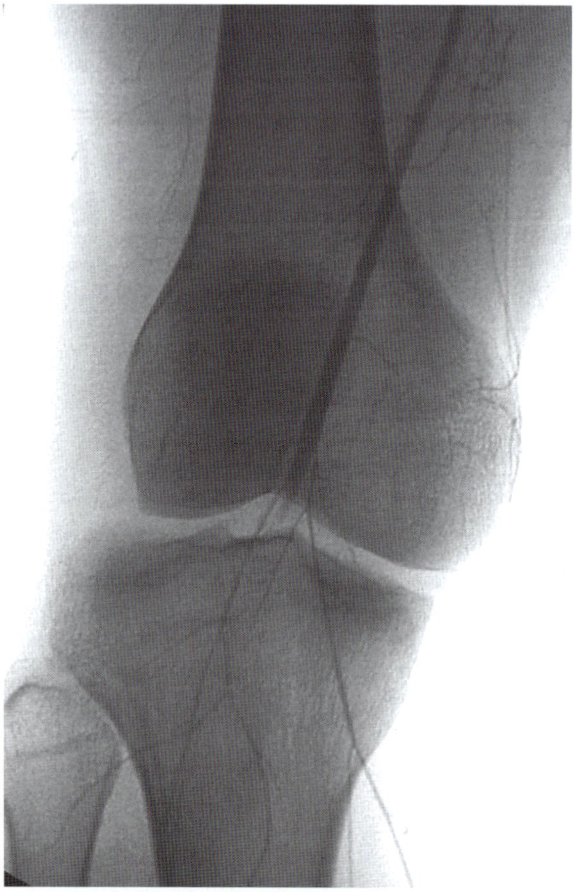

Fig. 50.60 Complete occlusion of the popliteal artery after posterior knee dislocation. This injury can be subtle or delayed. (From Valji K, ed. *Vascular and Interventional Radiology*. 2nd ed. Saunders; 2006.)

and posterior knee dislocations and occurs because the artery is relatively fixed both proximally and distally.[137,140] If popliteal artery injury occurs, it is often due to transection with posterior dislocations or intimal tearing due to traction forces during anterior dislocations.[138] In addition, Varnell and associates[141] noted that vascular injury was as common in a severely unstable knee (e.g., field reduced) as in an acutely dislocated knee. The reported incidence of popliteal artery injury in a dislocated knee has a wide range, from 3.3% to 18%.[140,142–144] The seriousness of this complication is largely due to the fact that the collateral circulation about the knee is poor, and the end result of injury to the popliteal artery (or vein) may be amputation, particularly if recognition is delayed.[142,143] It should also be noted that nerve injuries are more common in patients with a vascular injury.[142,143]

It has previously been stated that popliteal artery disruption may be present despite a normal pulse. While such a statement has been refuted over the years, simple palpation of the artery may not be sensitive enough to detect a decreased pulse. An ankle-brachial arterial pressure index (ABI) should be performed to compare blood pressure in the ankle with that in the arm. In addition, consider digit pulse oximetry to compare the uninjured leg with the injured one. Most recently, a review by Weinberg et al.[145] found that a palpable dorsalis pedis and posterior tibial pulses along with an ABI of 0.9 or greater is 100% sensitive in ruling out vascular injury. Surgical exploration is still recommended for patients with hard signs of vascular injury and arterial imaging for those with pulse discrepancy or an ABI less than 0.9.[137] However, it is noted that the hard physical signs of arterial injury might be delayed for 24 to 48 hours. Thus although focused clinician examination may be quite accurate in most cases, any dislocated knee should prompt serious concern about the vascular integrity of the leg given the sometimes

Knee Dislocation Reduction

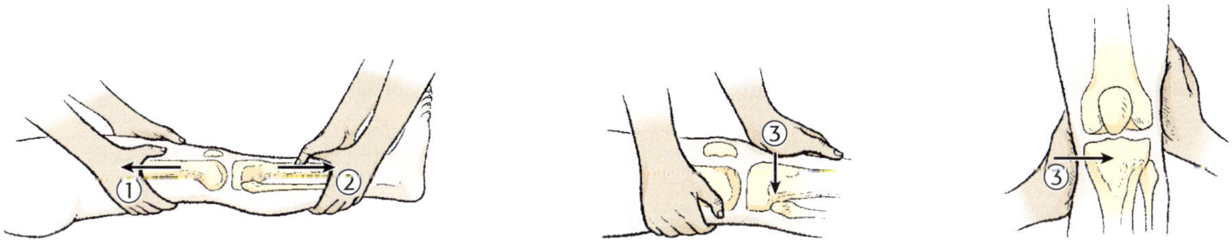

Apply (*1*) countertraction and (*2*) traction on the extremity. Often this maneuver alone will reduce the joint because of the severe ligamentous disruption associated with the dislocation.

Additional maneuvers may be required, depending on the type of dislocation. Apply posteriorly directed pressure on the tibia for anterior dislocations.

For a medial dislocation, apply a lateral force to the medial side of the tibia. Adjust the reducing force according to the type of dislocation present.

Fig. 50.61 Knee dislocation reduction.

subtle or delayed manifestation of vascular injuries. For this reason, serial clinical vascular examinations should occur every 2 to 4 hours for a 48-hour period.[137]

Knee dislocations are usually clinically obvious or easily visible on plain radiographs. Therefore it is occult knee dislocations (i.e., dislocated and spontaneously reduced) that are problematic for the emergency clinician to diagnose. Internal derangement with a knee hemarthrosis (often of the size noted with a torn anterior cruciate ligament) is a common first sign that the knee had previously been dislocated and spontaneously reduced. For this reason, all knee injuries with significant swelling, hemarthrosis, or a dislocating mechanism of injury should be evaluated with the specific intent of ruling out vascular injury.

If vascular compromise is detected on clinical assessment, it is appropriate to reduce the knee dislocation without obtaining radiographs, although a few minutes to obtain portable radiographs and to administer IV medication would be unlikely to make a difference in the outcome. Use of Doppler ultrasound for pulse checks and ABI should also be considered with these injuries (see Chapter 1). Early consultation should be sought for knee dislocations because of the high incidence of complications and the frequent need for operative intervention. The decision to pursue arterial imaging in a patient with a dislocated knee is best made in consultation with an orthopedic surgeon.

Reduction Technique

The need for IV sedation and analgesia depends on the clinical situation, but it should be considered routine whenever possible (see Chapter 33; Fig. 50.61 and Video 50.40). The basic initial approach for all types of knee dislocation is to apply traction to the extremity. This alone is often all that is required for reduction because of severe disruption of the ligamentous support of the knee. For anterior dislocations, lift the distal end of the femur to effect reduction. For posterior dislocations, lift the proximal end of the tibia to complete the reduction.[146] For medial, lateral, and rotatory dislocations, a similar approach is acceptable, with pressure exerted in the medial or lateral direction as needed.

After reduction, splint the extremity in 15 degrees of flexion. A posterolateral dislocation may be irreducible in the ED, and operative intervention should be considered if reduction is not easily accomplished.[146]

Postreduction Care

Appropriate aftercare for knee dislocations requires serial reassessment of the neurovascular status of the extremity, postreduction films, and admission to the hospital. Use a knee immobilizer to provide stabilization and comfort. These injuries cause severe ligamentous and other derangements in the knee and generally require operative stabilization with a long period of recovery and physical therapy.

DISLOCATIONS OF THE FIBULAR HEAD

The fibula can be dislocated at its proximal articulation in the knee joint. This is most commonly an anterior dislocation.[146] The fibular head is normally nestled in a stable manner behind the lateral tibial condyle with two supporting tibiofibular ligaments.[147] The tibiofibular joint has a separate synovial cavity, and therefore a typical knee joint effusion will not be seen with this dislocation. When the knee is flexed, the stability of this joint is decreased because of relaxation of the fibular collateral ligament. The typical mechanism of injury is a fall on a flexed, adducted leg, often combined with ankle inversion.[146] This mechanism is seen in sports and parachute landings. Posterior dislocations can result from a twisting mechanism or a direct blow to the area while the knee is flexed.[137]

Anterolateral dislocation is the most common type. It is accompanied by obvious prominence of the fibular head anteriorly; no associated neurovascular problems are noted. The less common posterior dislocation may be accompanied by peroneal nerve injury.[137] Patients have varying degrees of disability, and some may walk on the leg with only mild discomfort.[147] On radiographic examination the three cardinal signs of anterior dislocation are lateral displacement of the fibula on an AP film, a widened proximal interosseous space, and anterior displacement of the fibular head on a lateral view (Fig. 50.62). If high clinical suspicion exists for fibular head dislocation and radiographs are nondiagnostic, CT is the next study of choice.[147,148]

Reduction Technique

To reduce an anterior fibular head dislocation, place the patient supine and flex the affected knee to 90 degrees to relax the biceps femoris tendon. Dorsiflex and externally

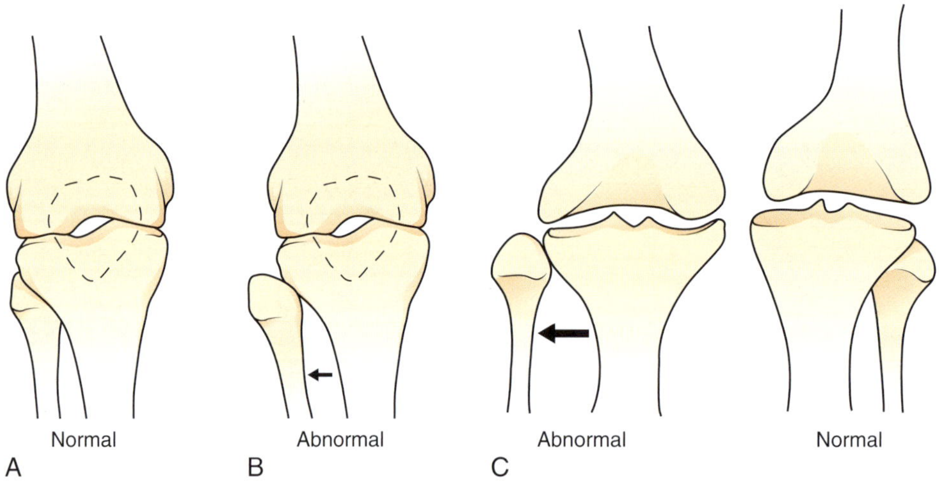

Fig. 50.62 Anterolateral fibular head dislocation compared with a normal knee. The interosseous distance is widened and the proximal end of the fibula is displaced laterally. (A) Normal anteroposterior projection of the knee. (B) Lateral displacement of the proximal end of the fibula. (C) Use of bilateral comparison views to highlight the fibular displacement.

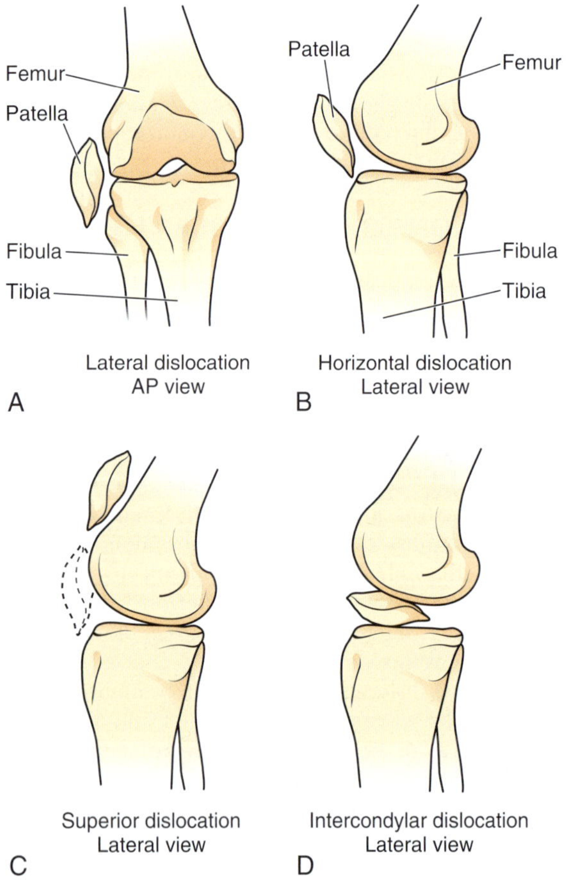

Fig. 50.63 (A–D) Various types of patellar dislocation. Lateral dislocation is the most common. *AP,* Anteroposterior.

rotate the foot and apply direct pressure to the fibular head; reduction is usually signified by a snap.[146,147] The method for reduction of a posterior dislocation is the same except that direct pressure is applied in a forward direction. Patients should not bear weight for 2 weeks and should receive orthopedic referral. Immobilization is probably unnecessary.[146]

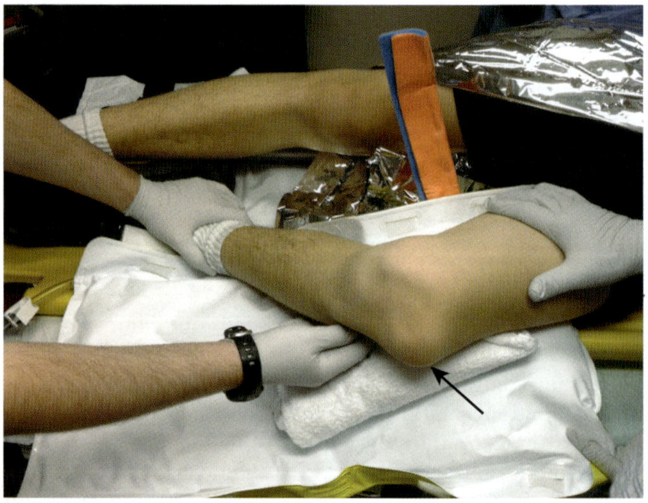

Fig. 50.64 Lateral patellar dislocations are usually clinically obvious. The knee is held in flexion, and the patella *(arrow)* can be seen and palpated along the lateral aspect of the knee.

PATELLAR DISLOCATION

Patellar dislocations are common, especially in adolescents. The usual mechanism is a powerful quadriceps contraction combined with a strong valgus and external rotation component.[149] This may be seen in activities such as dancing or making a "cut" in sports play. The patella may also dislocate with a direct blow to the flexed knee.[146] Factors predisposing to patellar dislocation include chronic patellofemoral abnormalities such as genu valgum and femoral anteversion.[149] Patellar dislocation is described by the relationship of the patella to the knee joint. Lateral dislocations are the most common by far.[149] Other types include superior, medial, and intercondylar (Fig. 50.63).

Clinical Assessment

Lateral dislocation of the patella is generally clinically obvious (Fig. 50.64). The knee is held in some degree of flexion and the patella can easily be seen and palpated on the lateral side

Lateral Patellar Dislocation Reduction

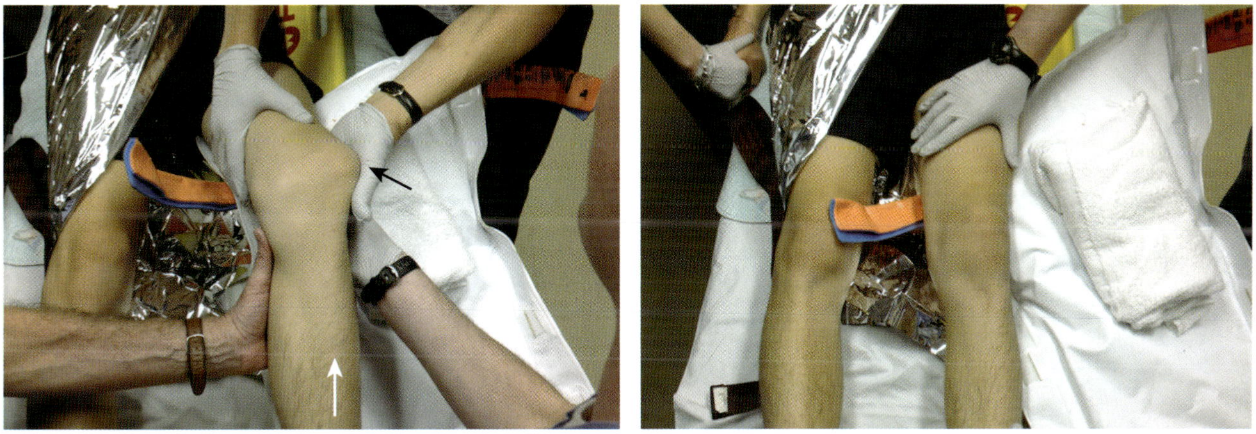

Gently extend the knee *(white arrow)* and apply medial pressure on the patella *(black arrow)* while lifting up the most lateral edge of the patella over the femoral condyle.

Reduction is usually quite simple and the knee will regain a normal appearance. Immobilize the leg in extension with a splint or knee immobilizer. Arrange for orthopedic follow-up.

Fig. 50.65 Lateral patellar dislocation reduction.

of the knee. Tenting of the patella is often detectable unless significant soft tissue swelling is present.

The patella may be spontaneously reduced in the field with simple leg straightening. The patient will report that the leg "went out" and may describe seeing the lateral deformity caused by the displaced patella. Clinical clues to a spontaneously reduced patella include the presence of a knee effusion and tenderness along the medial edge of the patella. Fairbank's test or the patellar "apprehension" sign is elicited when the patella is pushed laterally and the patient grabs for the knee, a response indicative of the sensation of repeated injury.[146]

Radiographs

Prereduction films are difficult to obtain because the patient's knee is usually in flexion. Some recommend prereduction films when possible in all patients[146]; however, it is easy to reduce these injuries before radiographs are obtained. The diagnosis is usually obvious, and there are no reports in the literature of complications from gentle reduction. Osteochondral fractures are detectable in approximately half the patients with patellar dislocations, but many of these fractures are visible only on arthroscopy.[149] Postreduction radiographs are recommended, as are prereduction studies, when the diagnosis is uncertain. The clinical diagnosis of patellar dislocation in an older patient should be made with caution because these are primarily injuries involving the young.

Reduction Technique and Postreduction Care

Reduction of a lateral patellar dislocation is usually quite simple (Videos 50.41–50.43). Premedication is often not required if the patient can be verbally reassured. If the patient is anxious or in great discomfort, premedication with parenteral analgesia or regional nerve block[150] should be considered (see Chapters 31 and 33). The two basic maneuvers for patellar relocation are extension of the knee and gentle medial pressure applied to the patella while lifting the most lateral edge of the patella over the femoral condyle (Fig. 50.65).[146]

Immobilize the leg in extension with a splint or commercially available knee immobilizer (see Chapter 51). Orthopedic follow-up is necessary because of the need for physical therapy and the high rate of persistent instability.[146] However, hospitalization is not required for routine lateral dislocations of the patella. Recurrent dislocations and those associated with an osteochondral fracture might require operative repair.

Patellar dislocations in other locations are often irreducible, and orthopedic consultation should be sought. Intracondylar, superior, and vertical axis (dorsal fin) dislocations are extremely rare and require operative reduction. The rare horizontal dislocation may relocate with closed reduction, but surgical reduction is often necessary.

ANKLE DISLOCATIONS

The ankle joint is a modified saddle joint in which the talus is nestled in the mortise formed by the distal ends of the tibia and fibula.[151] The ligamentous support of the ankle is quite strong, and pure dislocations are uncommon. Usually, there are associated fractures of the ankle joint (Fig. 50.66). Ankle dislocations are described by the relationship of the talus to the tibia. Posterior dislocations of the ankle are more common than anterior dislocations, and they usually result from a fall on a plantar-flexed foot. Patients with posterior dislocations often have an associated fracture of one or more of the malleoli[151] occasionally seen only after reduction. The clinical picture usually consists of significant deformity and disability.

Anterior dislocations generally result from forced dorsiflexion, or a blow directed posteriorly onto the distal end of the tibia while the foot is fixed. The talus is prominent anteriorly, and the dorsalis pedis pulse may be lost secondary to pressure from the talus. Superior dislocations are uncommon and result in diastasis of the tibiofibular joint. These injuries are usually the result of a significant axial force, such as a fall from a significant height. Therefore clinicians should search

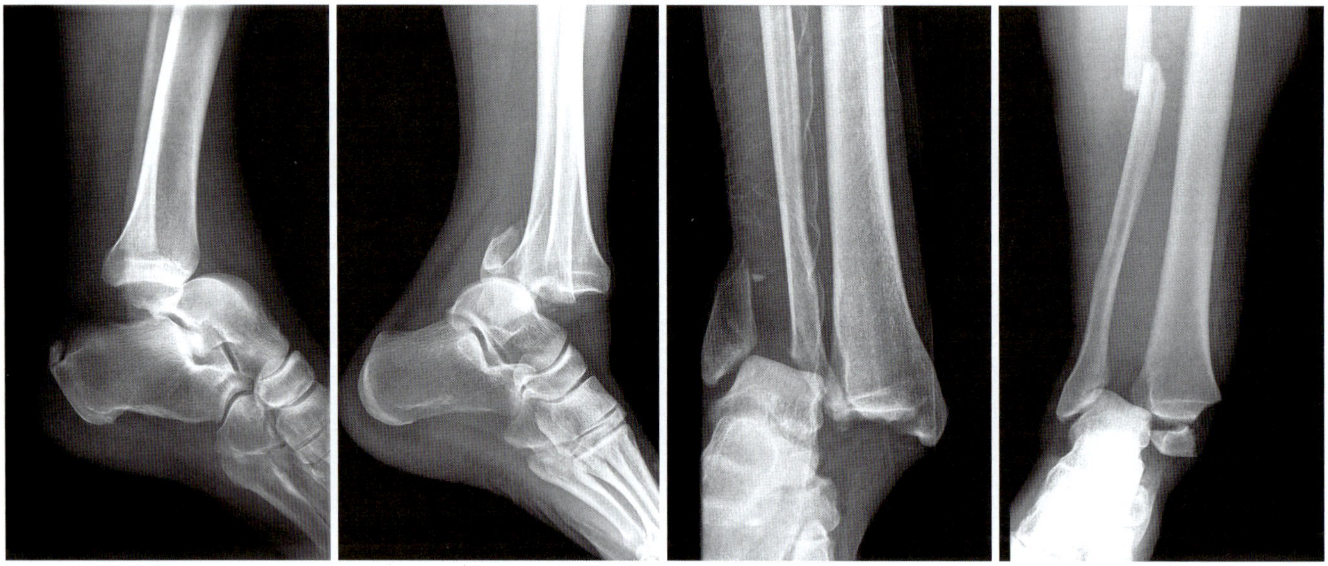

Fig. 50.66 Types of ankle dislocation. Note that there are usually associated fractures of the tibia, fibula, or both.

for concomitant calcaneal or low spine fractures. Lateral dislocations of the ankle are always associated with fractures of the malleoli or distal end of the fibula.

Radiographic Examination

Because of the high rate of associated fractures and the clinical difficulty in assessing for the presence or the exact nature of a dislocation, it is recommended that prereduction radiographs be obtained for all suspected ankle dislocations (see Figs. 50.1 and 50.66). It is acceptable to reduce the dislocation without a radiograph if severe vascular compromise is present but, for most cases, the few minutes taken to obtain bedside radiographs and administer IV medications rarely affect the outcome. It may be impossible to accurately determine the exact type of dislocation unless prereduction films are obtained. AP and lateral views usually suffice for emergency management; other views can be ordered if necessary after the joint is relocated.

Reduction Techniques

Unless a strong contraindication is present, it is advisable to administer IV sedation and analgesia to patients with an ankle dislocation early in their care, preferably before conducting any manipulations or radiologic studies (Fig. 50.67 and Videos 50.44–50.46). Reduction is always painful in an awake patient, and sufficient premedication must be administered. For posterior dislocations, place the patient supine, and flex the *knee slightly* to relax the Achilles tendon. An assistant can do this, or the patient can be positioned such that the knee hangs over the end of the bed. Grasp the foot with both hands; place one hand on the heel and the other on the forefoot. Apply traction on the slightly plantar-flexed foot. Have a second assistant apply downward pressure on the distal end of the tibia and move the heel anteriorly to affect reduction.[151]

For anterior dislocations, the initial steps and positioning are the same as those for posterior dislocation. However, instead of plantar flexion, dorsiflex the foot to free the talus. The second assistant applies upward pressure on the distal end of the tibia while the operator applies traction and pushes the foot in a posterior direction.[151]

Lateral dislocations are really fracture-dislocations, and orthopedic consultation is generally required as part of the ED course. The emergency clinician will often need to reduce these injuries because of the extreme lateral deformity and occasional compromise of the dorsalis pedis artery by stretch. Open dislocations (in the absence of vascular compromise) may be better handled by operating room washout before attempting reduction. If a lateral fracture-dislocation is to be reduced in the ED, the approach is quite like that for posterior ankle dislocations. However, instead of pressure in the AP direction, the foot is moved medially after the application of traction.[151]

Postreduction Care

After reduction, splint the ankle at 90 degrees with a long leg posterior splint. Application of a stirrup splint in addition to the posterior splint will provide additional stability (see Chapter 51). The necessity of admission to the hospital must be determined in consultation with an orthopedic surgeon. Many patients with these injuries have associated fractures that require surgical intervention.

DISLOCATIONS OF THE FOOT

The importance of the foot is recognized by anyone who has had to spend time ambulating with an injury in this area. For purposes of this discussion, dislocation injuries of the foot can be divided into those of the hindfoot and those of the forefoot.

Hindfoot Injuries

Injuries to this area are uncommon and usually result from high-energy transfer. The major dislocations are subtalar and talar dislocations and midtarsal fracture-dislocations (Lisfranc injury). Although radiographic findings are often subtle and

Ankle Dislocation Reduction

A. Posterior Dislocations

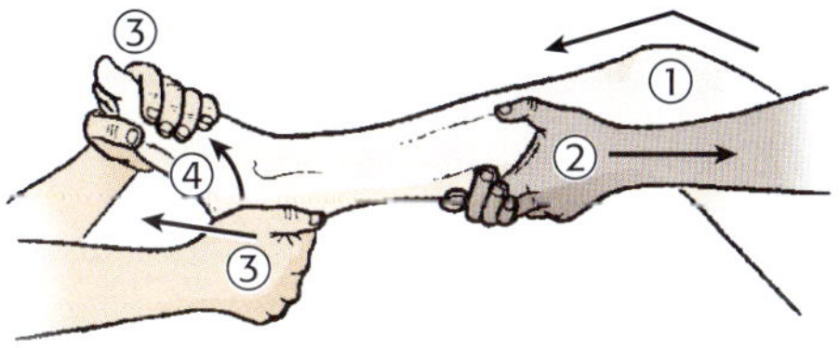

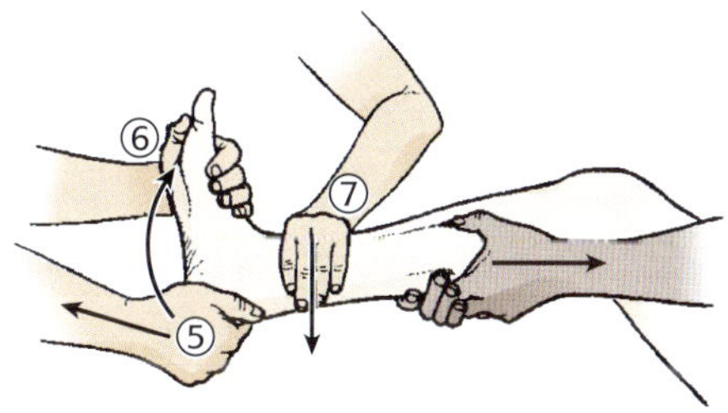

(*1*) Slightly flex the knee. (*2*) Instruct an assistant to provide countertraction on the leg. (*3*) Grasp the heel with one hand and the dorsal metatarsals with the other. (*4*) Slightly plantarflex the foot and apply straight downward counterpressure on the foot.

(*5*) Pull the foot forward with longitudinal traction on the heel. (*6*) Dorsiflex the foot. (*7*) Instruct a second assistant to provide counterpressure on the front of the lower part of the leg.

B. Anterior Dislocations

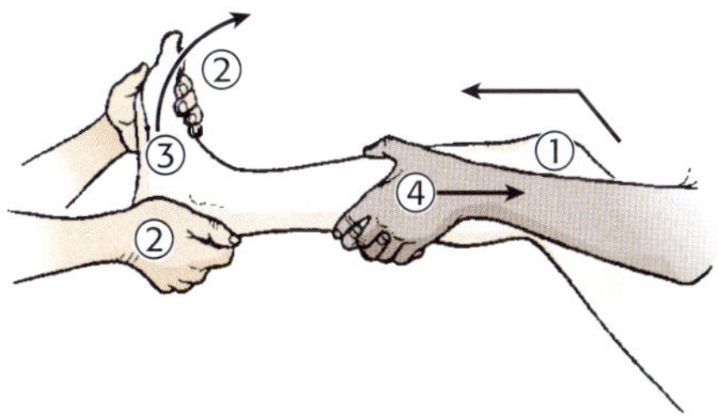

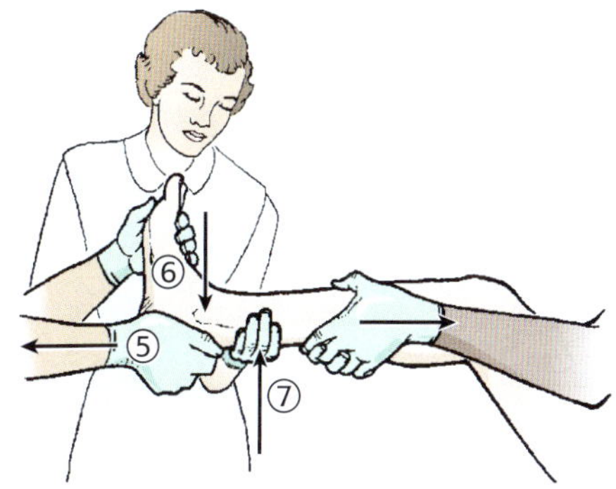

(*1*) Flex the knee. (*2*) Grasp the forefoot with one hand and the heel with the other. (*3*) Dorsiflex the foot to disengage the talus. (*4*) Instruct an assistant to provide countertraction on the leg.

(*5*) Apply straight longitudinal traction. (*6*) Push the foot directly backward. (*7*) Instruct a second assistant to apply countertraction on the back of the lower part of the leg.

Fig. 50.67 Ankle dislocation reduction.

easily overlooked, a Lisfranc injury is complex and always a fracture-dislocation because of the rigid nature of the region (Figs. 50.68 and 50.69). These injuries require orthopedic management and are not discussed here.

Subtalar Dislocation

This uncommon injury generally occurs secondary to sports, falls from heights, or motor vehicle crashes. The calcaneus, navicular, and forefoot are displaced from the talus (Fig. 50.70).[152] The medial subtalar dislocation type is a result of hindfoot inversion, often involving a low-energy mechanism such as a sprain leading to the moniker *basketball foot* for this injury.[152] This injury is usually seen in young adult males. Medial dislocations constitute the majority (85%) of these injuries, with lateral dislocations, caused by severe eversion with axial loading, making up the rest.[152]

The diagnosis is usually obvious because the talus is prominent and often tents the skin of the proximal part of the foot. The medial type has been termed an *acquired clubfoot*; the lateral type as an *acquired flatfoot*.

It is usually possible to reduce these injuries with IV premedication. Position the patient in a supine fashion and flex the hip and knee much as for reduction of a posterior ankle dislocation. Place one hand on the forefoot and grasp the heel with the other hand. Apply firm longitudinal traction to effect reduction. Dangling the leg over the end of the bed allows the operator to use body weight to assist in traction. Once traction is applied, the deformity is initially increased (inversion and plantarflexion for medial; eversion and dorsiflexion for lateral) and then reversed to effect reduction.[152]

Dislocation of the Talus

In this extremely rare injury, the talus is essentially extruded from its normal position and comes to lie anteriorly. This injury is generally open,[153] is not amenable to closed reduction, and virtually always progresses to AVN.[153] Talectomy and arthrodesis are often required,[153] and orthopedic referral should be undertaken on an emergency basis if vascular compromise of the foot is present.

Forefoot Dislocations

Much of what is pertinent to the diagnosis and management of forefoot dislocations has already been discussed in the management of dislocations of the finger and hand MCP joints. Anatomically, the joints are quite similar.

Metatarsophalangeal Dislocations

These uncommon injuries are generally the result of hyperextension resulting in dorsal dislocation of the great toe metatarsophalangeal (MTP) joint (Fig. 50.71A).[154] Among the

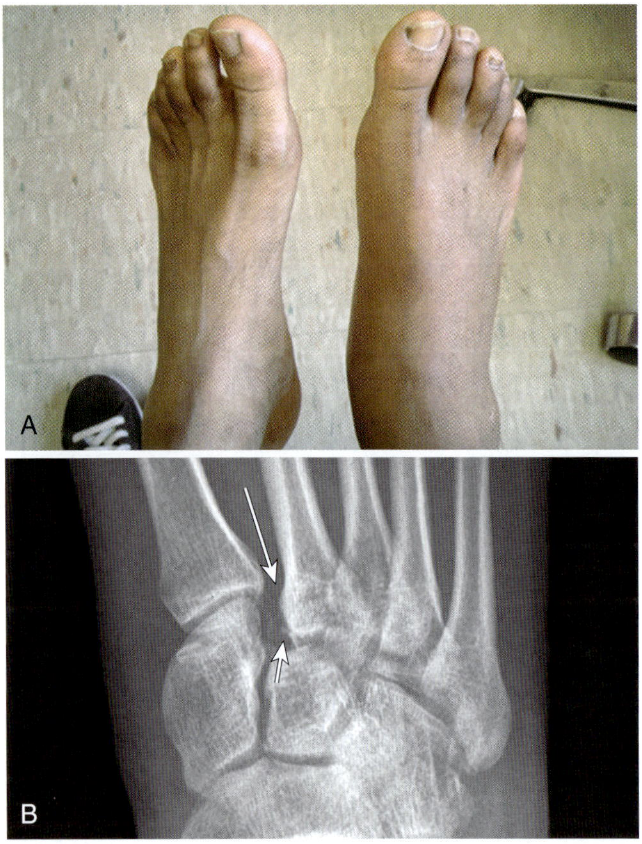

Fig. 50.68 (A) A Lisfranc fracture-dislocation is a serious and debilitating injury that is easily missed. This patient complained of extremely severe pain in the foot and was unable to walk after falling down the steps while intoxicated, so the mechanism was unclear. Drug seeking was suspected; however; *note the significant soft tissue swelling* of the right foot suggestive of internal injury. (B) This radiograph was initially read as a minor avulsion fracture around the base of the second metatarsal, but a closer review shows widening of the space between the first and second metatarsals and *lateral displacement of the rest of the metatarsals (arrows)*. This injury often requires operative repair, and permanent disability is common in the best of circumstances.

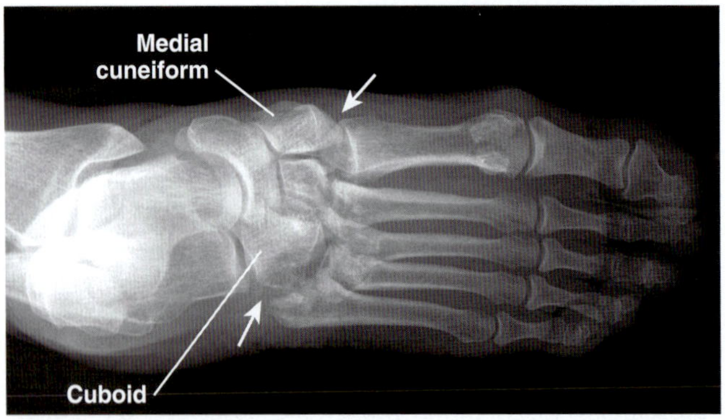

Fig. 50.69 Lisfranc fracture-dislocation. Note that the first through fifth metatarsals are shifted laterally with respect to the tarsal bones. This is termed a homolateral dislocation. Poor alignment between the first metatarsal and medial cuneiform and between the fifth metatarsal and cuboid is a clue that this substantial injury is present *(arrows)*. Also note the irregularities at the bases of the second through fifth metatarsals, which may represent fractures in this region. Computed tomography or magnetic resonance imaging may be needed to fully assess this subtle, yet complex injury.

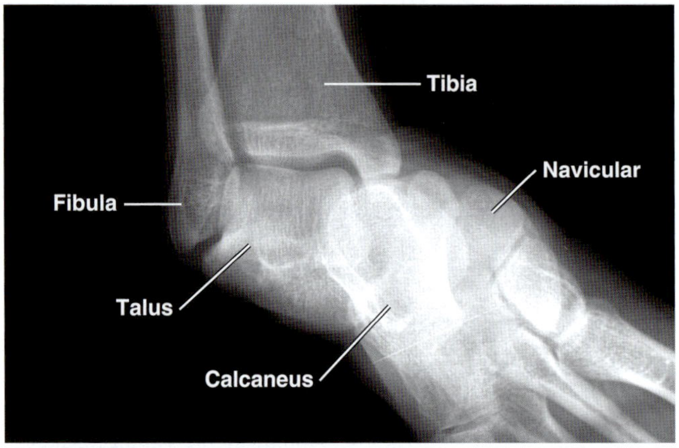

Fig. 50.70 Medial subtalar dislocation. Note that the tibia, talus, and fibula retain a normal anatomic relationship but that the calcaneus, navicular, and forefoot are displaced medially.

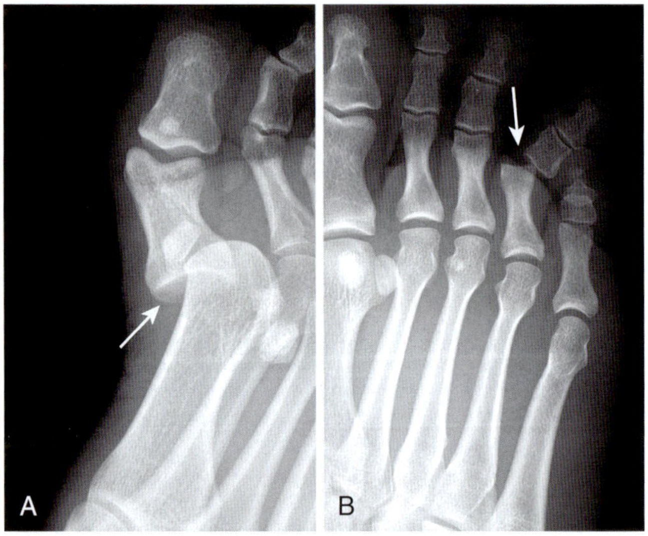

Fig. 50.71 Toe dislocations. (A) Dorsal dislocation of the first metatarsophalangeal joint *(arrow)*. (B) Lateral dislocation of the fourth proximal interphalangeal joint *(arrow)*. Reduction of toe dislocations follows the same technique as described for finger dislocations (see Fig. 50.31).

lesser toe MTP joints, lateral or medial displacement of the digit on the metatarsal head is more common and usually the result of jamming the toe on a piece of furniture.[155] As with MCP dislocations, they can be simple or complex. Complex dislocations of the first toe can be suspected by the presence of sesamoid bones in the joint space on prereduction radiographs.[155] Complex MTP dislocations are often irreducible.

For simple MTP dislocations, reduction is accomplished by increasing the deformity through hyperextension and then applying traction while exerting thumb pressure over the base of the dislocated proximal phalanx. Plantar flexion of the foot may be used to relax the flexor tendons.[154] Operative intervention is required after reduction if crepitus is present on motion, the joint is unstable, or an intraarticular loose body is noted on postreduction radiographs.[154]

Interphalangeal Dislocations

In the foot, IP dislocations result from an axial load on the toe, such as from kicking a wall (see Fig. 50.71B). These dislocations are generally dorsal and can be reduced as in the hand. Specifically, the toe should be dorsiflexed to exaggerate the deformity and then undergo traction followed by plantar flexion. Dislocations of the first toe IP joint are usually buddy-taped to the second toe for 2 to 3 weeks, whereas those of lesser toes can be taped for 10 to 14 days.[154] Reduction of dorsal dislocations may be difficult because of entrapment of the plantar plate inside the joint. As in the hand, complex dislocations or those that do not respond to closed reduction may occur. Such dislocations require open reduction and internal fixation.[154]

CONCLUSION

The following points are important regarding the assessment and management of dislocations:

1. A search for other more serious injuries should be undertaken when there is a high-energy mechanism of injury.
2. Neurovascular assessment should be performed early in the evaluation and appropriately documented.
3. Radiographs and IV premedication are generally indicated before attempts at reduction.
4. Reduction attempts should involve gentle, gradual application of force and patience on the operator's part.
5. After completing reduction, the operator should recheck the patient's neurovascular status, request postreduction radiographs (except with radial head subluxations), and in certain circumstances, assess the stability and range of motion of the joint.
6. A definite percentage of dislocations are irreducible, and the need for multiple attempts should halt prolonged and forceful attempts in the ED and prompt orthopedic consultation.
7. Dislocations accompanied by neurologic injury should be reduced by the most expeditious and least traumatic method.

REFERENCES ARE AVAILABLE AT Elsevier eBooks+

CHAPTER 51

Splinting Techniques

Carl R. Chudnofsky and Arielle C. Paul

Splints are used frequently in the emergency department (ED) for temporary immobilization of fractures and dislocations and for definitive treatment of soft tissue injuries.[1,2] Patients with a variety of nontraumatic musculoskeletal disorders (e.g., gout, inflammatory joint diseases, infections, burns) also benefit from short-term immobilization. Immobilization is the mainstay of fracture therapy, but though intuitively beneficial, it is difficult to find firm scientific data that support the use of splinting for soft tissue injuries.[3,4] Although the general principle of immobilizing sprains and contusions is strongly supported by custom and personal preference, its exact influence on healing, number of complications, and ultimate return to normal activity is not known. In most studies of ankle sprains, for example, the function and pain of the injured joint are similar at 6 weeks' follow-up, regardless of whether treatment consisted of ad lib walking, a simple elastic bandage, a posterior splint, or a formal cast.[5,6] However, the results of a recent umbrella review of 24 systematic reviews of acute ankle sprain management strongly favor functional treatment over immobilization.[7]

Patients are routinely seen in the ED with injuries that are amenable to splinting to relieve pain and augment healing. Although a strict standard of care cannot be promulgated, the use of short-term splinting in the ED for acutely painful conditions remains a common practice. Emergency clinicians have virtually abandoned the use of circumferential casts in favor of premade commercial immobilizing devices or splints constructed of plaster of Paris or fiberglass. The impetus for this change is primarily related to the complications occasionally associated with circumferential casts, liability issues, and ease of application brought about by new technology. In most instances, properly applied splints provide short-term immobilization equal to that of casts while allowing continued swelling and thus reducing the risk for ischemic injury. Other obvious advantages of splints are that patients can take them off when immobilization is no longer needed or can remove them temporarily to bathe, exercise the injured part, or perform wound care. Most splinting techniques are handed down from house staff or experienced clinicians, but the procedure is often suboptimal and haphazard.[8] This chapter presents guidelines for adequate immobilization of injuries commonly encountered by emergency clinicians. Details of the construction and application of commonly used custom-made plaster splints are provided.

INDICATIONS AND CONTRAINDICATIONS

Theoretically, immobilization facilitates the healing process by decreasing pain and protecting the extremity from further injury. Other benefits of splinting are specific to the particular injury or problem being treated (Fig. 51.1). For example, in the treatment of fractures, splinting helps maintain bony alignment. Splinting deep lacerations that cross joints reduces tension on the wound and helps prevent wound dehiscence. Immobilizing tendon lacerations may facilitate the healing process by relieving stress on the repaired tendon. The discomfort of inflammatory disorders such as tenosynovitis or acute gout is greatly reduced by immobilization. Deep space infections of the hands or feet, as well as cellulitis over any joint, should similarly be immobilized for comfort. Limiting early motion may also reduce edema and theoretically improve the immune system's ability to combat infection. Hence, selected puncture wounds and mammalian or human bites of the hands and feet may be immobilized until the risk for infection has passed. Splinting large abrasions that cross joint surfaces prevents movement of the injured extremity and reduces the pain produced when the injured skin is stretched. Finally, patients with complex trauma should have fractures and reduced dislocations adequately splinted while other diagnostic and therapeutic procedures (e.g., fluid resuscitation, airway control, computed tomography [CT] scans, tube thoracostomy) are completed. Immobilization decreases blood loss, minimizes the potential for further neurovascular injury, reduces the need for opioid analgesia, and may decrease the risk for fat emboli from long-bone fractures.

EQUIPMENT (REVIEW BOX 51.1)

Support Materials

Plaster of Paris

Plaster of Paris is the most widely used material for ED splinting.[9] Its name originated from the fact that it was first prepared from the gypsum of Paris, France. When gypsum is heated to approximately 128°C, most of the water of crystallization is driven off and a fine white powder is left behind—plaster of Paris. When water is added to the plaster, the reaction is reversed, and the plaster recrystallizes or "sets" by incorporating water molecules into the crystalline lattice of the calcium sulfate dehydrate molecules.

Today, plaster is impregnated into strips or rolls of a crinoline-type material. The crinoline allows easy application, helps keep the plaster molded to the proper form during the setting process, and adds support to the finished splint. Plaster rolls and sheets are available in a variety of setting times and widths (2-, 3-, 4-, or 6-inch widths). The distinct advantage of plaster over commercially available premade splints is that plaster can more easily be molded and tailored to the individual's anatomy, thereby negating the "one-size-fits-all" approach. In addition, plaster rolls and strips are generally less expensive than premade splints.

Prefabricated Splint Rolls

The use of plaster splints in the form of prefabricated splint rolls (e.g., OCL, BSN Medical) is very popular among emergency clinicians. These splint rolls have 10 to 20 sheets of plaster enclosed between a thick layer of protective foam padding on one side and a thin layer of cloth on the other. Like custom-constructed splints, they are secured to the extremity with an elastic bandage. The major advantage of prefabricated splint rolls is that significant time is saved because the splint and padding come ready to apply. In addition, prefabricated splint rolls are ideal for intermittent splinting and can be removed and reapplied by the patient as needed. However, prefabricated plaster splint rolls are more expensive than simple plaster rolls, and they lack some of

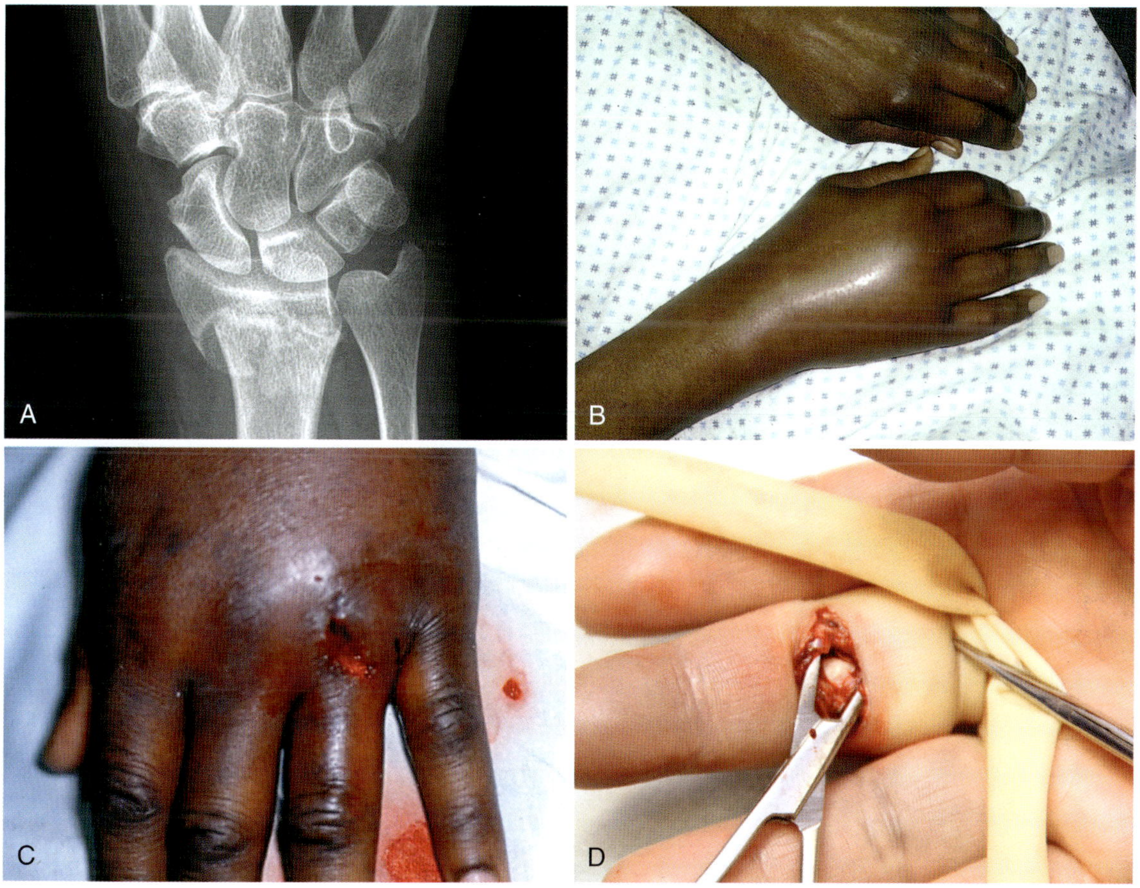

Fig. 51.1 Indications for splinting. Splinting is traditionally thought of as a treatment of fractures, such as the comminuted distal radius fracture depicted in (A). However, splinting is also beneficial in a wide variety of other conditions, such as (B) acute gout, (C) human and mammalian bites of the hand, and (D) tendon injuries. Other indications include inflammatory disorders such as tenosynovitis, deep lacerations that cross joints, and deep space infections of the hands and feet.

the versatility and custom-fit qualities of self-made plaster splints.

Prefabricated splint rolls composed of layers of fiberglass between polypropylene padding (e.g., Ortho-Glass, BSN Medical; 3M Scotchcast One-Step, 3M) are now commonplace in many EDs. Fiberglass splint rolls offer the same time-saving aspect as prefabricated plaster splint rolls but require only 3 minutes to set, thus making application faster. In addition, splints made of prefabricated fiberglass rolls cure more rapidly (20 minutes), have no messy residue (i.e., they can be hydrated in a conventional sink without a special trap), can be washed and reapplied, and are stronger and lighter than splints constructed of prefabricated plaster rolls. Another advantage is the polypropylene padding, which wicks moisture away from the skin better than polyester, nylon, or cotton padding does.[10] Prefabricated fiberglass splint rolls are more expensive than both simple plaster rolls and prefabricated plaster splint rolls and, like prefabricated plaster splints, lack some of the versatility and custom-fit qualities of self-made plaster splints.

Woodcast Composite Splinting Material

A new synthetic material that has had a limited presence in the United States but looks promising in European studies is Woodcast (Onbone Oy).[11–13] Woodcast is made from spruce tree chips and biodegradable plastic, making it nontoxic and environmentally friendly. The material comes in slabs ranging from 1 to 4 mm thick from which the provider can cut out the desired shape for a specific splint. Woodcast splits are applied in the same manner as conventional splints (Fig. 51.2) and have comparable stiffness.[11] Like splints made from plaster of Paris and fiberglass, increasing the thickness of the split increases its ultimate strength. The composite material is easily molded to the contour of an extremity or digit by heating for 15 minutes to a temperature of 65°C using one of the Woodcast heating devices (Fig. 51.3). The material takes approximately 15 minutes to set, providing sufficient time for applying and molding the splint. If needed, setting time can be reduced to 5 to 10 minutes with application of ice packs. Woodcast splints can be rewarmed and remolded after application and gloves are not required when handling the material. Compared to conventional splinting materials, Woodcast splints cause fewer skin reactions and are associated with similar rates of healing and patient satisfaction.[12,13]

Protective and Miscellaneous Equipment

Stockinette

A single layer of stockinette is commonly used over the skin and under cotton (Webril, Medtronic) padding, circumferential casts, and splints. It protects the skin and, when folded back over the ends of the plaster, creates a smooth, professional-looking, padded rim. Stockinette is available in 2-, 3-, 4-, 8-, 10-, and 12-inch widths.

Splinting Techniques

Indications

Immobilization of a variety of clinical conditions:
- Fractures and dislocations
- Deep lacerations that cross joints
- Tendon lacerations
- Inflammatory disorders (e.g., gout, tenosynovitis)
- Deep space infections of the hands or feet
- Cellulitis overlying a joint
- Selected puncture or bite wounds

Contraindications

No absolute contraindications

Complications

- Ischemia
- Heat injury
- Pressure sores
- Infection
- Dermatitis
- Pruritus
- Joint stiffness
- Cast pain
- Compartment syndrome

Equipment

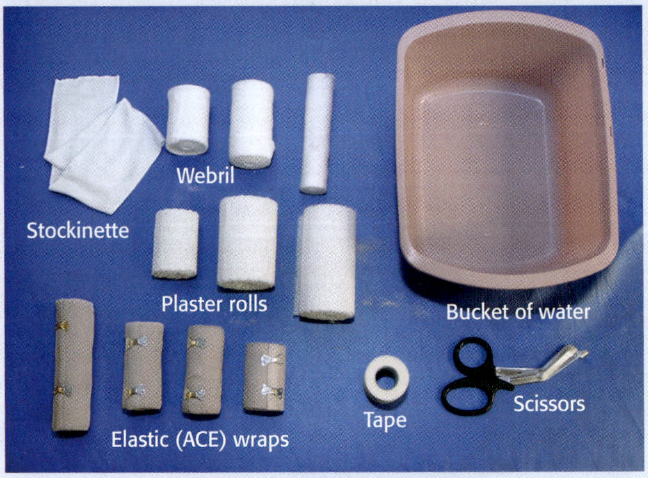

Equipment for plaster splints

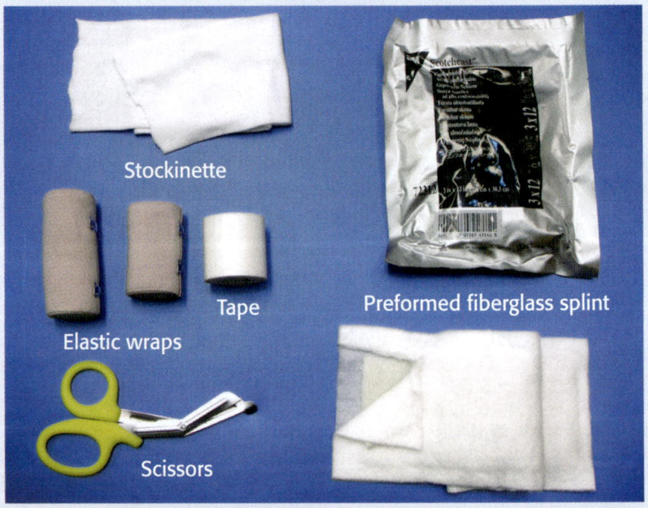

Equipment for preformed fiberglass splints

Review Box 51.1 Splinting techniques: indications, contraindications, complications, and equipment.

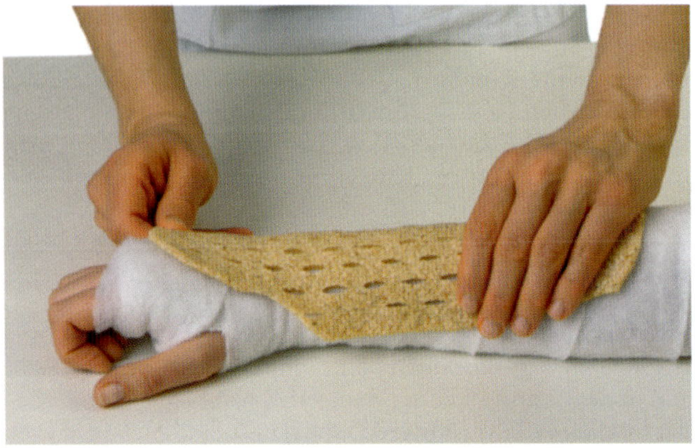
Fig. 51.2 Woodcast splint. After heating, Woodcast splints are applied in the same manner as conventional splints. (Courtesy Onbone Oy.)

Padding

Padding under the splint protects the skin and bony prominences and accommodates swelling of the injured extremity. Most commercially available splints contain adequate padding in the premade product, but in some instances, additional padding is prudent. In general, the older thin cotton padding known as sheet wadding has been replaced by newer material such as Webril (Curity), Specialist (Johnson & Johnson) cast padding, and others (e.g., Delta cast padding). Webril is soft cotton with a much coarser weave than sheet wadding; consequently, it has greater tensile strength, adheres better, and can be applied more evenly. Specialist padding uses micropleated cotton fibers that relax when moistened. This results in uniform, felt-like padding that conforms to the surface being wrapped. Felt (0.5-inch thick) may also be used to pad bony prominences.

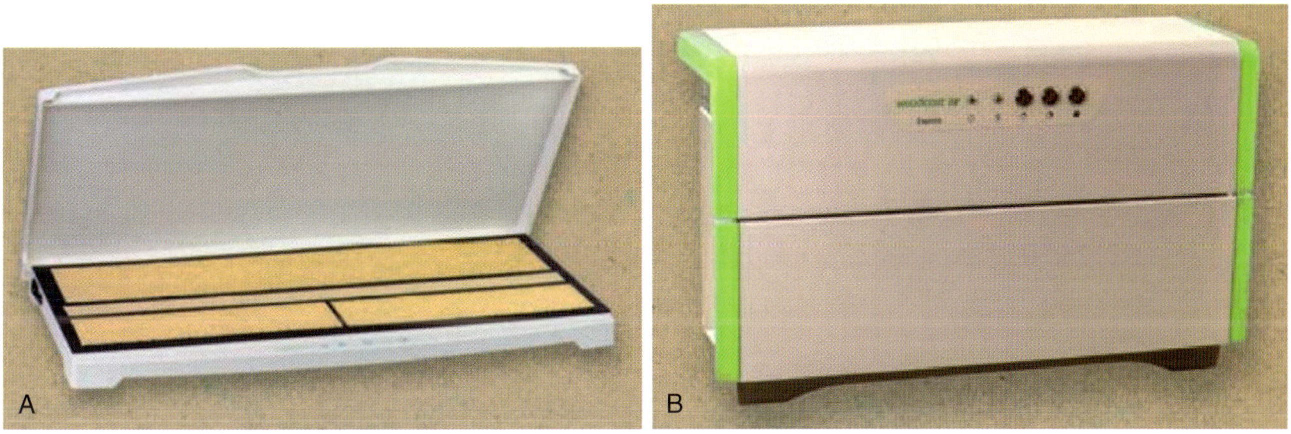

Fig. 51.3 Woodcast heating devices. (A) Woodcast standard heating device is designed for heating all flat Woodcast materials. (B) Woodcast express heating device can be used to heat flat material to create a new splint and to reheat a split that has already been applied to improve its fit. The express device heats the material much faster than the standard device. (Courtesy Onbone Oy.)

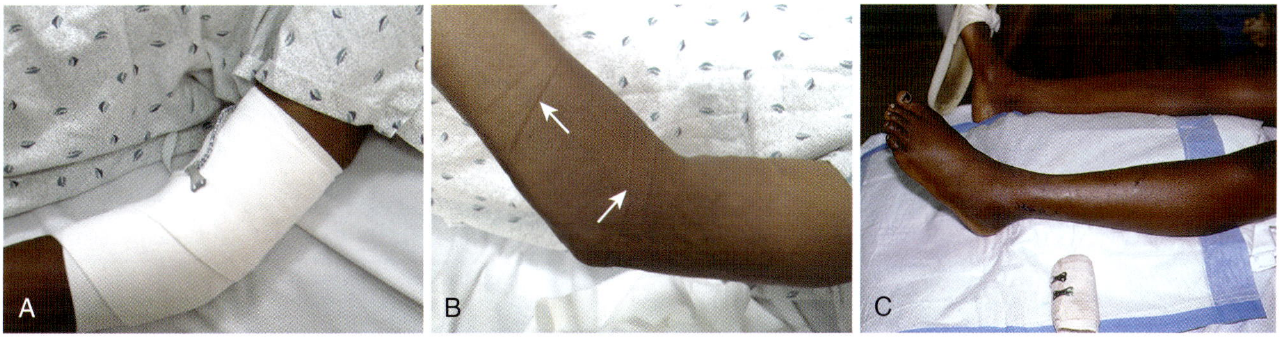

Fig. 51.4 Elastic bandages. (A) An elastic bandage is a popular home treatment of many painful conditions, such as sprains and contusions. An actual medical benefit is unproven. (B) Wrapping an extremity too tightly may cause additional injury or distal swelling. This patient complained of a swollen hand after an elbow injury. Note the grooves in the skin *(arrows)* indicating that the wrap was the culprit that caused the hand swelling. (C) A markedly swollen foot after application of a useless elastic bandage on the lower part of the leg.

Elastic Bandages

Elastic bandages are used to secure the splint in place. Elastic bandages are available in 2-, 3-, 4-, and 6-inch widths. Some bandages use metal clips, whereas others use a Velcro-type mechanism to secure the bandage in place. Metal clips should be taped in place to avoid inadvertent removal.

Patients often use or request an elastic bandage for many soft tissue injuries. Although applying an elastic bandage to an injured part is popular, it is of minimal benefit alone. The downside is that the bandage may be wrapped too tightly and cause additional injury or distal swelling (Fig. 51.4).

Adhesive Tape

Use adhesive tape to prevent slippage of the elastic bandages, to line the cut edges of a bivalved cast, and to buddy-tape digits. Coban tape can be used in a similar manner and has the advantage of adhering only to itself.

Utility Knife, Scalpel, and Plaster or Trauma Scissors

Use a utility knife, a No. 10 scalpel blade, or plaster or trauma scissors to cut and shape dry plaster.

Bucket

Use a large bucket (preferably stainless steel) for wetting plaster. Do not prepare the plaster in the sink unless it is equipped with a special drain designed to accept plaster residue without clogging. A bucket is not required for the minimal amount of water used to soften premade fiberglass splints. They can be activated by placing them directly under the faucet.

Protective Gear

Use gowns or sheets to prevent soilage of both the patient's and the clinician's clothing. Use gloves (vinyl or latex) and safety glasses to prevent skin or eye damage from plaster dust, wet plaster, or uncured fiberglass polymer. Wearing gloves also decreases clean-up time for the clinician.

GENERAL PROCEDURE OF CUSTOM SPLINT APPLICATION

See Videos 51.1 and 51.2. This following text refers to the application of custom-made plaster splints unless otherwise stated (Figs. 51.5 and 51.6). If periodic wound care is required, apply a more easily removable splint (e.g., OCL, BSN Medical; Ortho-Glass; Velcro-type splint, described later) in lieu of the standard splint (Fig. 51.7). Address the issue of removability before the splint is applied. In addition, use of Webril (Curity) cast padding is described, but other suitable cast padding may be substituted. Caveats for proper ED splinting are listed in Box 51.1.

Plaster Splint Application: Standard Method

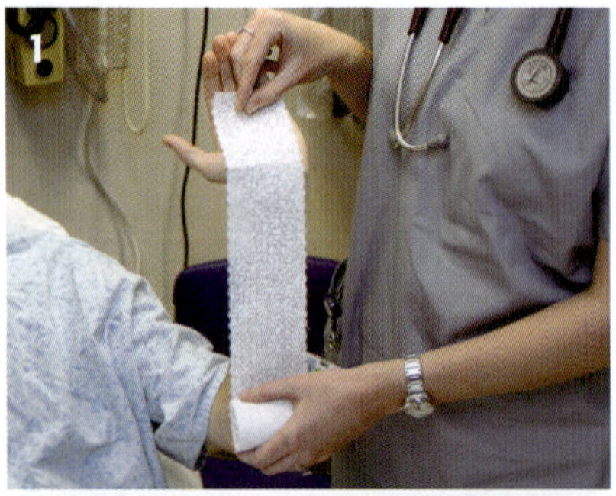

Measure the length of plaster to be used against the area to be splinted. Roll out the appropriate layers of plaster (roughly 8 layers for upper extremities, 12–15 for the lower).

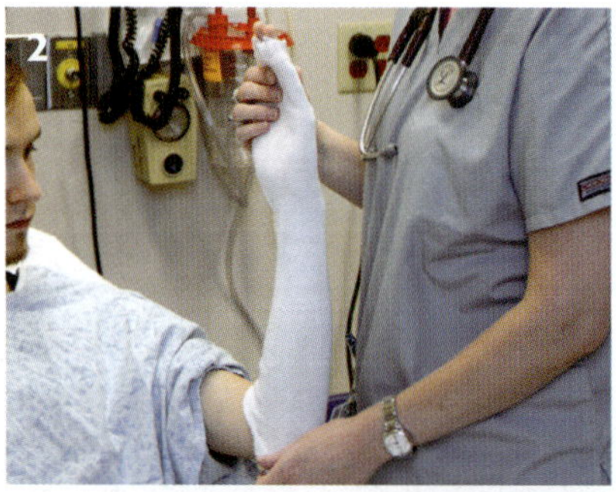

Place a single layer of stockinette over the extremity. The stockinette should extend 10–15 cm beyond both ends of the area to be splinted. Generally, use a 3-inch stockinette for the arm, and a 4-inch for the leg.

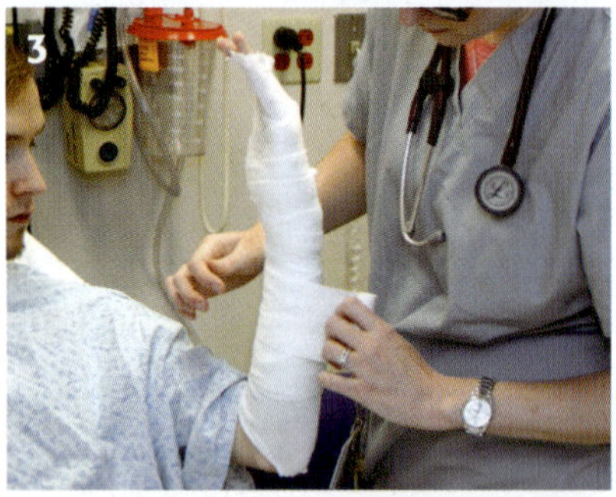

Wrap 2 to 3 layers of Webril around the entire area to be splinted, overlapping each pass by 25% to 50%. Avoid wrinkling, which may cause pressure sores. See text for precautions regarding potential ischemic injury.

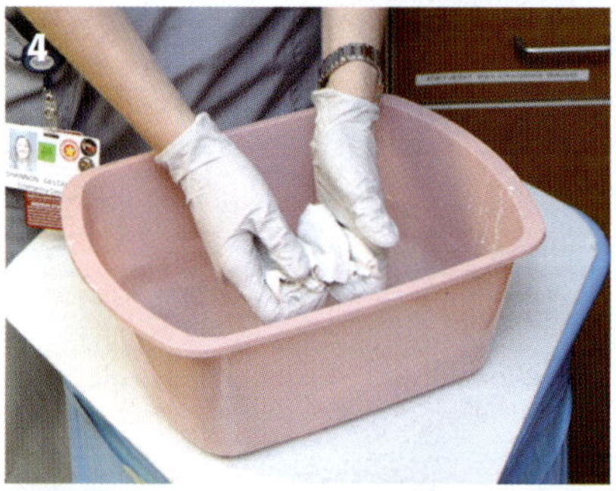

Submerge the plaster strips in a bucket of water until the bubbling stops. Do not use water hotter than 24°C (75°F). Using warmer water may cause thermal injury, because the plaster releases heat when activated.

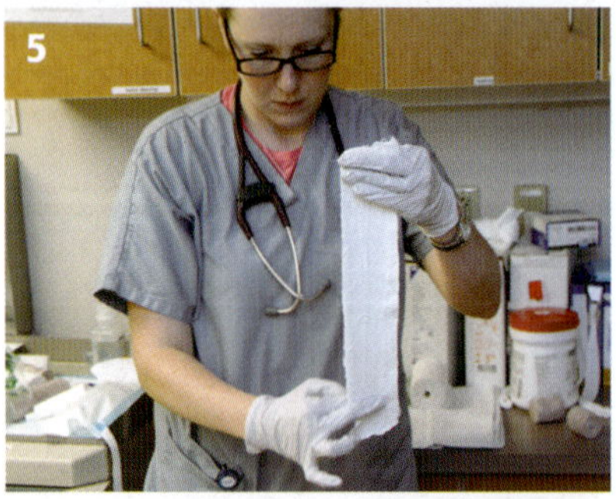

Smooth the plaster between your fingers and remove all excess water. Lay the plaster out on a table and smooth further to remove all wrinkles and ensure uniform lamination of all layers.

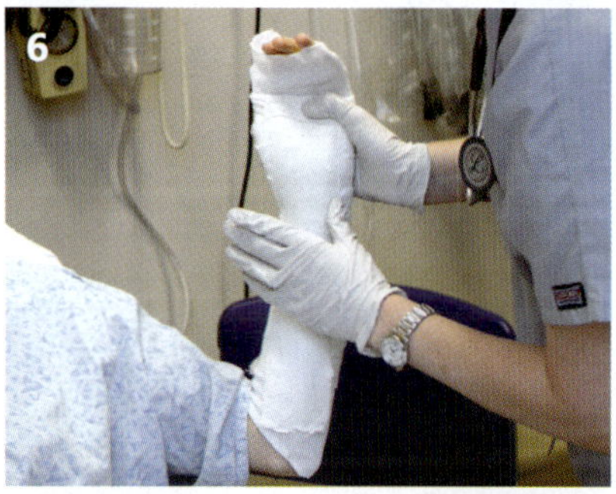

Apply the plaster over the Webril and smooth it over the extremity. Avoid using your fingertips, which may leave indentations in the plaster. A layer of Webril may be placed over the plaster to prevent it from sticking to the elastic wrap.

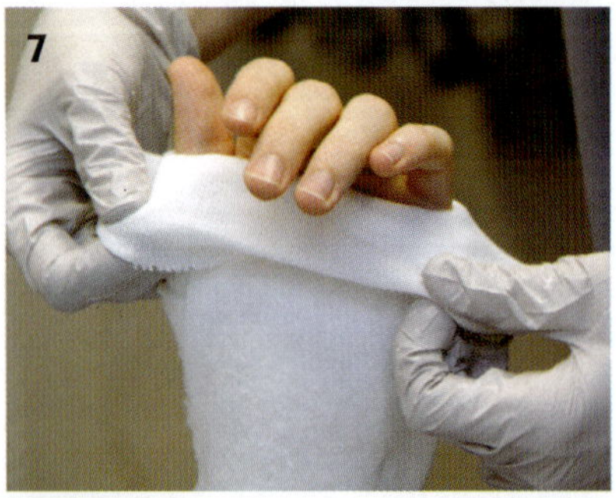

Fold the stockinette over the edge of the plaster and Webril. This helps to hold the splint in place, and provides a smooth padded edge.

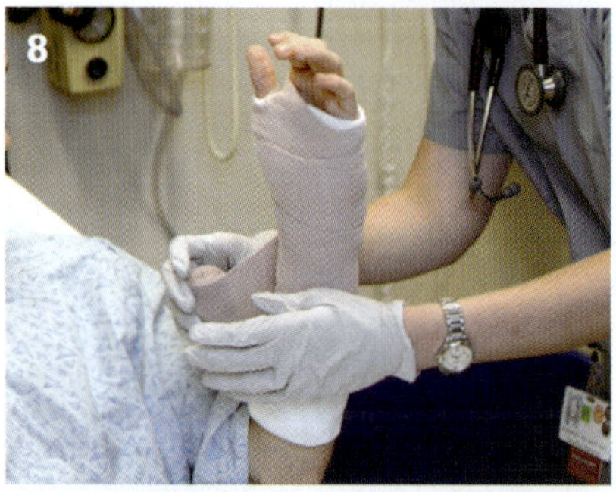

Secure the splint to the extremity with an elastic wrap by proceeding in a distal-to-proximal fashion. Do not wrap the elastic bandage too tightly.

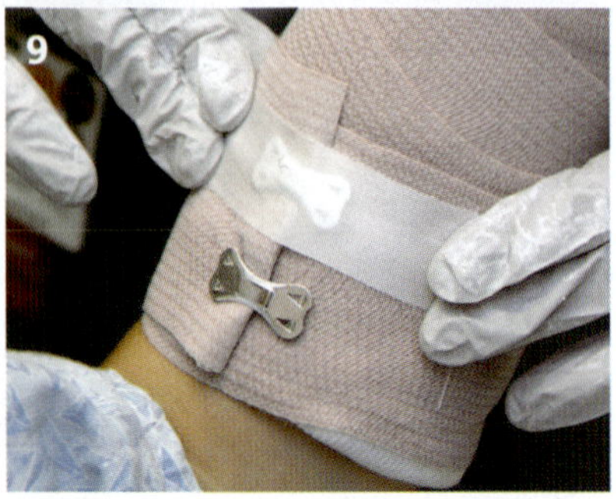

If metal clips are used to secure the elastic wrap, cover them with tape to prevent them from falling off. Alternatively, the wrap can simply be secured with tape.

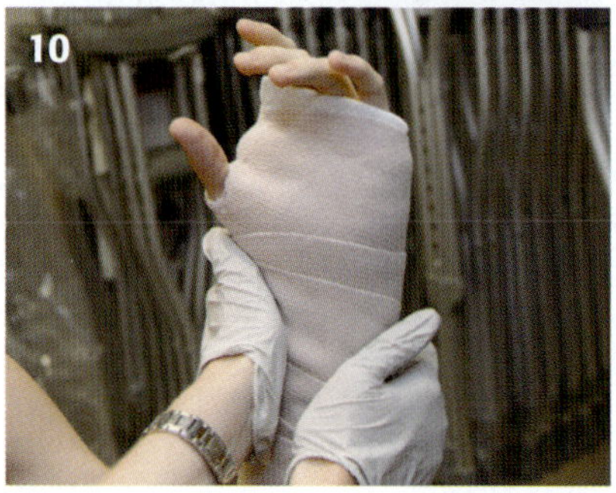

Place the extremity in the desired position, and use the palms of your hands to mold the splint to the contour of the extremity. Again, avoid using your fingertips, which may leave indentations that result in pressure sores.

Fig. 51.5 Plaster splint application: standard method (volar wrist splint depicted here).

Plaster Splint Application: Alternative Method

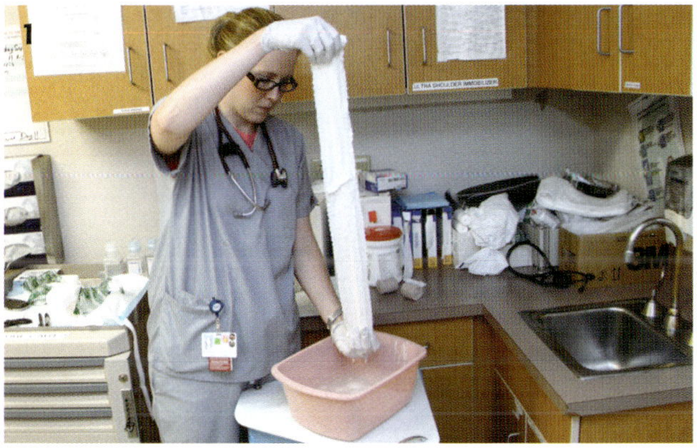

Measure the splint and apply stockinette as depicted in steps 1 and 2 of Fig. 50.3. Additionally, premeasure 5 to 6 layers of Webril of the same length as the plaster. Soak and prepare the plaster.

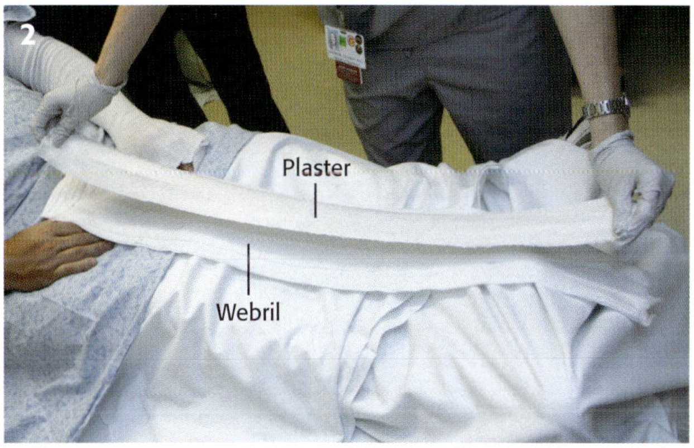

Lay out 3 to 4 layers of Webril, which will serve as padding for the splint. Place the plaster (which has already been smoothed) on top of these layers of Webril.

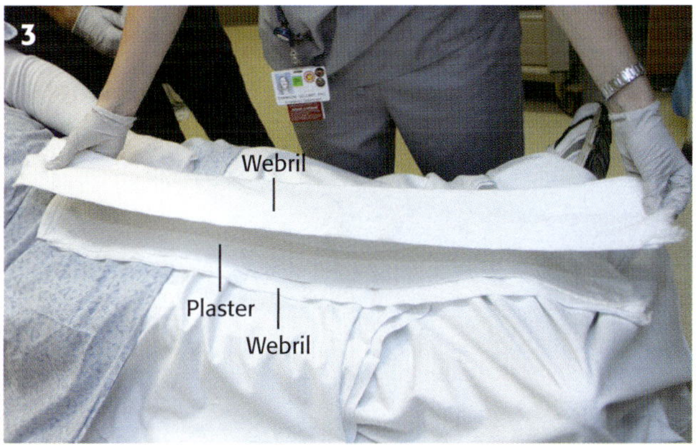

Place an additional layer of Webril on top of the plaster, which will prevent it from sticking to the elastic wrap. Essentially, you are sandwiching the plaster between layers of Webril.

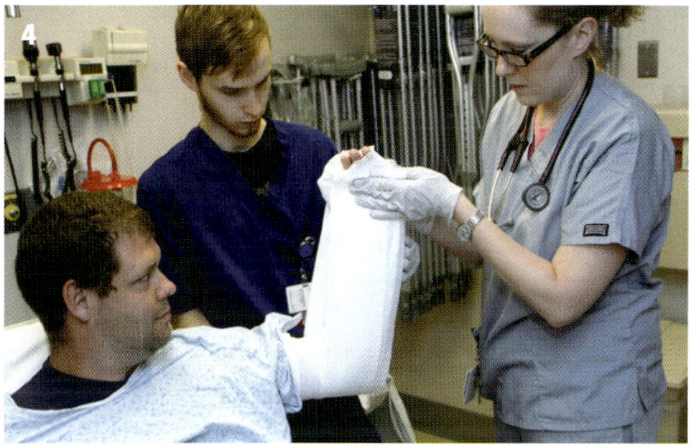

Apply the splint to the extremity. Enlist the help of an assistant to hold the splint in place.

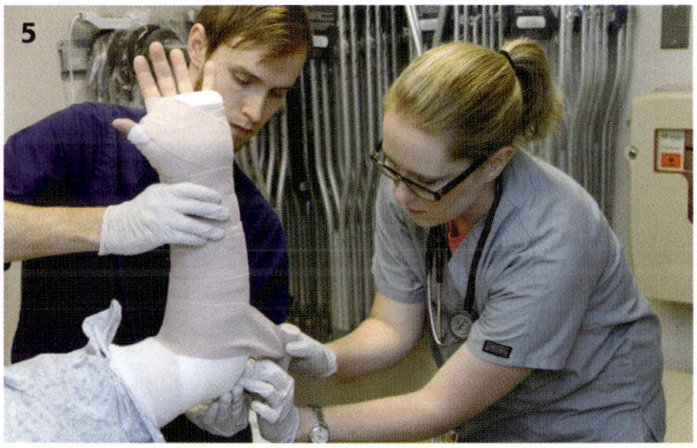

Secure the splint to the extremity with elastic bandages by wrapping in a distal-to-proximal fashion. Remember to fold the stockinette over the edges of the plaster and Webril.

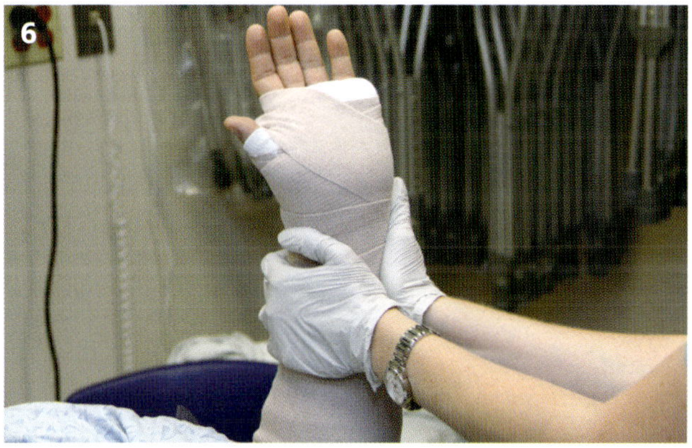

Position the extremity as desired, and then gently mold the splint using the palms of your hands.

Fig. 51.6 Plaster splint application: alternative method (sugar-tong splint depicted here). This technique may be used if significant swelling is anticipated as Webril (the same diameter as the plaster) is placed directly over the wet plaster rather than wrapped circumferentially around the extremity.

Patient Preparation

If the clinical situation permits, cover the patient with a sheet or gown to protect clothing and the surrounding area from water and plaster. Nursing staff and housekeeping also appreciate this courtesy. Properly drape hallway patients if areas of the body are exposed. Carefully inspect and examine the involved extremity before splinting, and clearly document the presence of all skin lesions and soft tissue injuries. Clean, repair, and dress all wounds in the usual manner. When open

Prefabricated Fiberglass Splint Application

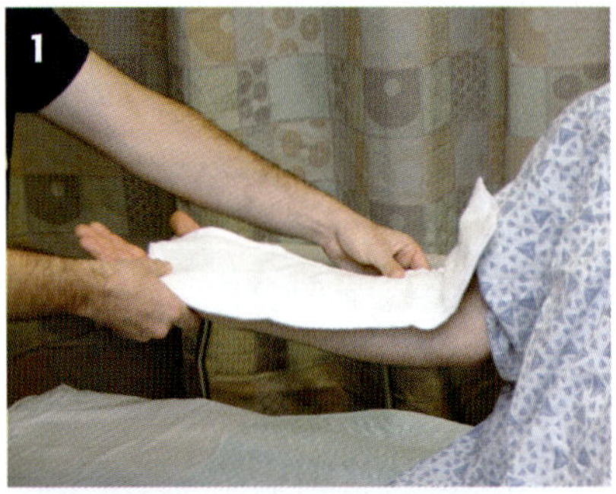

Measure the length of splint to be used against the area to be splinted. These splints are available in a variety of lengths and widths.

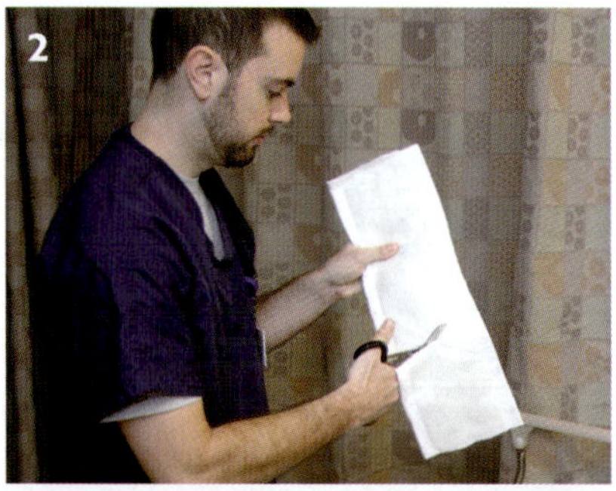

Cut the splint to length using a pair of trauma shears. Round the corners of the cuts to avoid sharp edges of fiberglass.

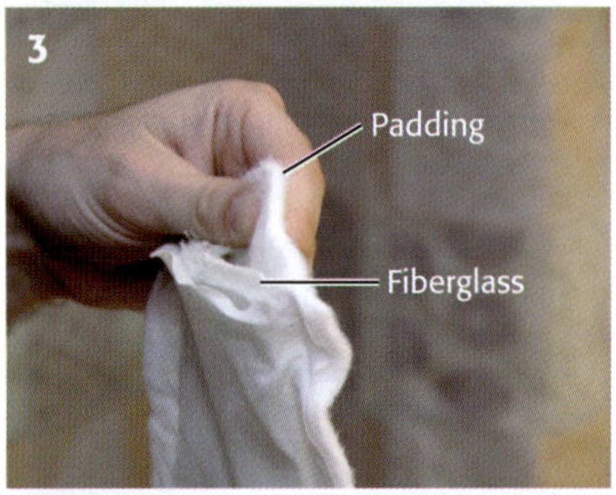

Stretch the cotton padding several inches beyond the edge of the fiberglass on both ends of the splint to assure that there will be no fiberglass in contact with the skin.

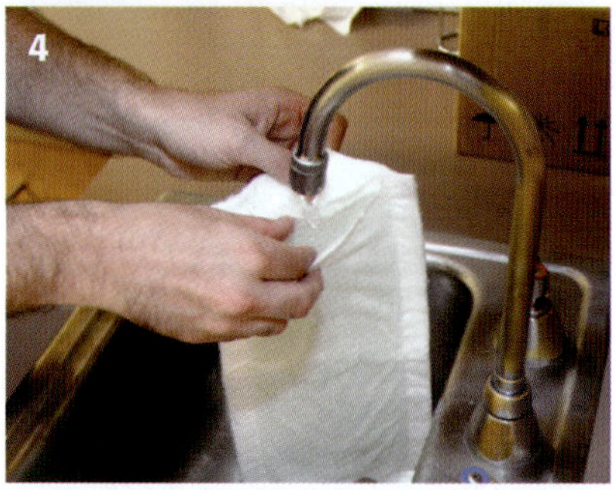

Prefabricated fiberglass splints require minimal wetting. Simply open one end of the pouch and run tap water over the fiberglass. When water exits the bottom, it is ready to apply. Excess water may be wrung out.

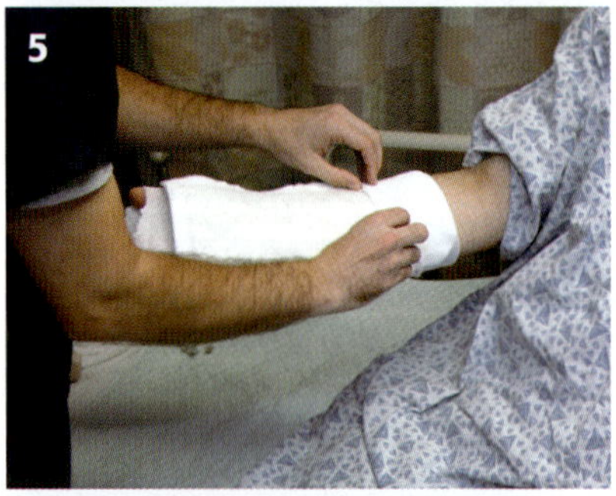

Apply the splint to the extremity. If stockinette is used (optional though recommended), fold the edges of the stockinette over the splint. This provides comfort and also holds the splint in place during application.

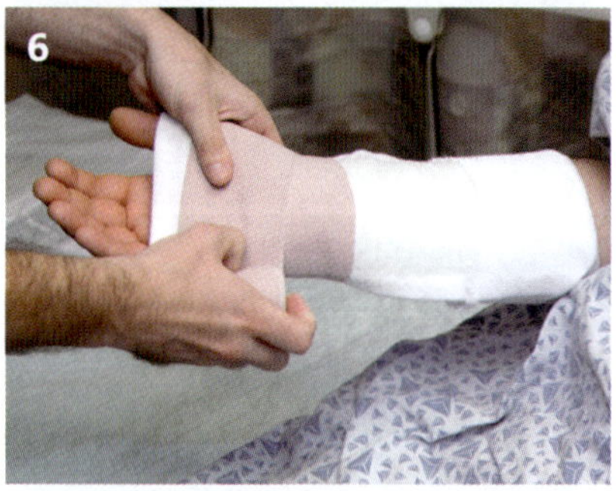

Secure the splint to the extremity using elastic bandages wrapped in a distal-to-proximal fashion.

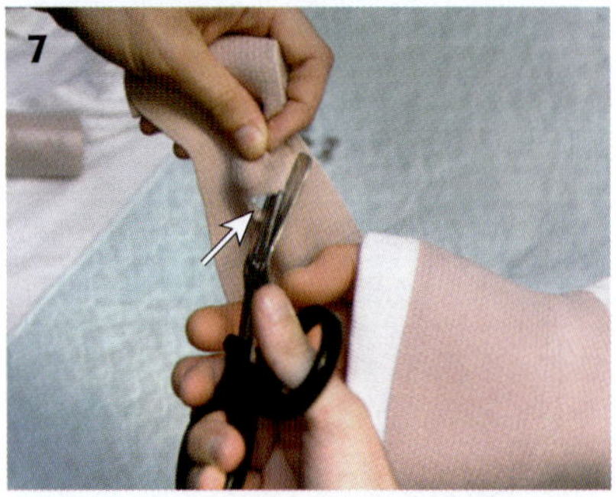

For splints that involve the hand, cut a hole in the center of the elastic bandage, in the loop that is in the region of the thumb.

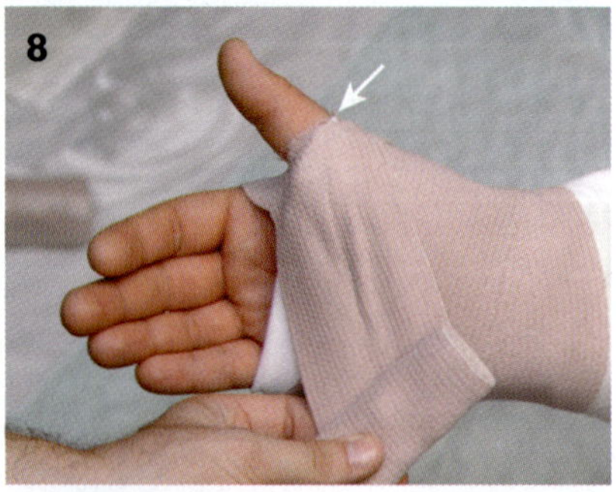

Bring the thumb through the hole. This provides a perfect fit, reduces bunching of the elastic in the web space, and allows for more thumb mobility.

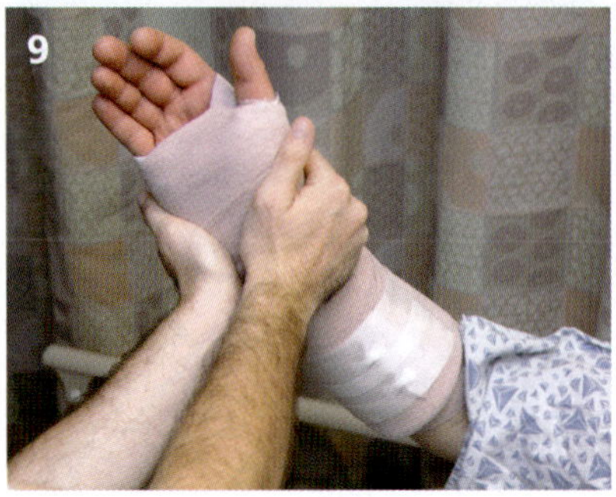

Place the extremity in the desired position, and mold the splint with your palms to the contours of the body. Avoid using fingertips, which may leave indentations in the fiberglass.

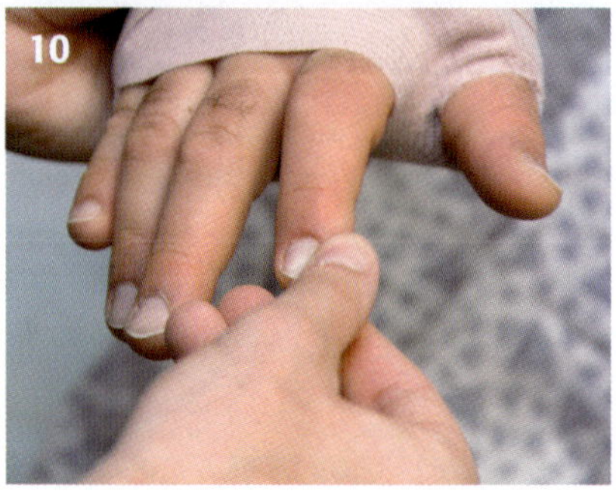

After splint application, observe for vascular compromise or increased patient discomfort. If either occur, loosen the elastic wrap. Never discharge a patient with increasing pain after splint application.

Fig. 51.7 Prefabricated fiberglass splint application (volar wrist splint depicted here).

BOX 51.1 Caveats for Proper ED Splinting

- Always use cool, clean water.
- Do not oversaturate the plaster splint. Minimal water is required for fiberglass splints.
- Make the splint *smooth* when placing it on the patient to avoid bumps and pressure points.
- Smooth and mold the splint without squeezing. Use the palms of the hands, not the fingers, to mold the splint to fit the contour of the body part.
- Place the padded side against the skin. Extra cotton padding is optimal.
- Simply roll elastic bandages over the extremity without undue tension.
- Protect or pad the edges.
- Leave the fingertips exposed to check for circulation and sensation.
- Keep the patient still until the splint has dried and hardened.
- The postsplint check includes function, arterial pulse, capillary refill, temperature of the skin, and sensation (FACTS).
- Emphasize and demonstrate splint elevation to the patient.
- Tape over the metal clips used to fasten the elastic bandage to keep them in place and avoid ingestion by a child.

ED, *Emergency department.*

BOX 51.2 Areas of the Upper and Lower Extremity That Require Additional Padding

UPPER EXTREMITY

Olecranon
Radial styloid
Ulnar styloid

LOWER EXTREMITY

Upper portion of the inner aspect of the thigh
Patella
Fibular head
Achilles tendon
Medial and lateral malleoli

fractures or joints are to be immobilized, cover the soft tissue defect with saline-moistened sterile gauze.

Padding

When the splint involves the digits, place padding between the fingers and toes to prevent maceration of the skin. This can be done with pieces of Webril or gauze cut to the appropriate length.

Following placement of padding between the fingers and toes in self-made splints, use a stockinette over the skin as the first protective layer (see Fig. 51.5, *step 2*). Extend the stockinette at least 10 cm to 15 cm beyond the area to be splinted at both ends of the extremity. Later, after the plaster has been applied, fold the stockinette back over the ends of the splint to create smooth, padded rims and to help hold the splint in place when applying elastic bandages (see Fig. 51.5, *step 7*). To avoid pressure damage, do not pull the stockinette too tightly over bony prominences such as the heel. In addition, prevent wrinkling over flexion creases by slitting and overlapping the stockinette at bony prominences. One may also use two separate pieces of stockinette (one at each end of the splint) to produce the smooth padded rims. As a general rule, use 3-inch-wide stockinette for the upper extremity and 4-inch-wide stockinette for the lower extremity.

After the stockinette has been properly positioned, wrap Webril around the entire area that will be exposed to plaster. Apply at least two or three layers of Webril, with each turn overlapping the previous turn by 25% to 50% of its width (see Fig. 51.5, *step 3*). Make sure that the Webril extends 2.5 cm to 5.0 cm beyond the ends of the splint so that it, too, can be folded back over the splint to help create smooth, well-padded edges. Place extra padding over areas of bony prominence, such as the radial condyle or the malleoli (Box 51.2). Although this can be done with Webril, Mother's Cotton adds an additional measure of protection without the worry of wrinkling or ischemic injury. If significant swelling is anticipated, use three or four layers of Webril. Be careful to avoid wrinkling because this can result in significant skin pressure when a tight splint is worn for a long period. Prevent wrinkles by proportionately stretching or even tearing the side of the Webril that must wrap around the larger portion of an extremity. Joints that must be immobilized in a 90-degree position, such as the ankle, make continuous Webril wrapping difficult. To avoid wrinkles around the ankle, place the joint in the proper position before padding. Wrap the Webril around the malleolar and midtarsal regions first, and then cover the bare calcaneal region with overlapping vertical and horizontal Webril strips until the entire heel region is evenly padded. Use the same approach in similar areas such as the elbow. Choose a width of Webril appropriate for the extremity to be splinted. In general, use the 2-inch width for the hands and feet, the 3- or 4-inch width for the upper extremity, and the 4- or 6-inch width for the lower extremity.

A final caveat when using Webril is to be aware of the potential for ischemic injury. This rare complication is most likely to occur in an extremity that continues to have significant swelling after the patient is released from the ED. Ischemia may result because the concentrically placed Webril can become a constricting band. If this situation is anticipated, it can easily be prevented. Cut through the Webril along the side of the extremity that is opposite the plaster splint. Then, secure the splint to the extremity in the usual manner. Alternatively, place two or three layers of Webril (the same diameter as the plaster) directly over the wet plaster (see Fig. 51.6). Position the Webril-lined splint over the area to be immobilized and secure it in place with an elastic bandage.

Plaster Preparation

The choice of plaster setting time depends on the nature of the injury and the expertise of the clinician. Use extra-fast setting plaster when rapid hardening is desired to help maintain alignment of an acutely reduced fracture. However, for the majority of ED splints, plaster with slower setting times (e.g., Specialist Plaster Bandage Fast Setting, BSN Medical) is recommended.[14] Plaster that sets more slowly is easier for some

TABLE 51.1 Setting Times of Fast- and Extra-Fast Drying Plaster

PLASTER	SETTING TIME (min)
Fast drying	5–8
Extra-fast drying	2–4

BOX 51.3 Effect of Water Temperature and Different Additives on the Setting Time of Plaster

Accelerates Setting Time	Slows Setting Time
Reusing the dip water	Cool dip water
Higher dip water temperature	Glue
Salicylic acid	Gum
Zinc	Borax
Magnesium	
Copper	
Iron	
Aluminum	
Salt	
Alum	

clinicians to use because it affords more leeway in applying and molding the splint. Furthermore, plaster with a longer setting time produces less heat, thus reducing both patient discomfort and the risk for serious burns.[15] Table 51.1 lists the setting times for commonly used plaster. These setting times can be adjusted by adding different substances to the plaster during the production process (Box 51.3). Given plaster with equal setting times, the most important variable affecting the rate of crystallization is water temperature. Warm water hardens a splint faster than cold water does and should not be used when extra time is needed for splint application.

The ideal length and width of plaster depend on the body part to be splinted and the degree of immobilization required. The best way to estimate length is to lay the dry splint next to the area to be splinted. It is best to use a generous length because wet plaster shrinks slightly from its dry length. In addition, if the wet splint is too long, the ends can be folded back easily. Plaster width varies according to the type of splint being made and the body part that is injured, but generally, it should be slightly greater than the diameter of the limb to be splinted. Specific recommendations regarding splint length and width are discussed in the sections describing individual splints.

The thickness of a splint depends on the size of the patient, the extremity that is injured, and the desired strength of the final product. An ankle splint may crack quickly and become useless if only eight layers are used, but this thickness may be ideal for a wrist splint. In general, it is best to use the minimum number of layers necessary to achieve adequate strength. Thicker splints are heavier and more uncomfortable. It is also important to note that plaster thickness is a major determinant of the amount of heat given off during the setting process. More than 12 sheets of plaster create an increased risk for significant burns, especially when using extra-fast drying plaster, when using dipping water with a temperature higher

BOX 51.4 Variables That Increase Heat Production During Crystallization

MAJOR

Increased splint thickness
Setting time
High dip water temperature
Wrapping the extremity for support while drying

MINOR

High humidity
High ambient temperature
Reusing the dip water

[a]*Faster setting times produce more heat.*
[b]*Dip water temperature has been a minor determinant of heat production in some studies. Use room-temperature not hot water to make a splint.*

than 24°C, or when a pillow is placed under or around the extremity for support during the setting process (Box 51.4). For an average-sized adult, splint the upper extremities with 8 sheets of plaster and the lower extremities with 12 to 15 sheets. Such layering usually provides the strength necessary for adequate immobilization while reducing the patient's discomfort and the risk for significant burns. In a 136-kg (300-lb) patient, however, up to 20 layers may be required to make a durable ankle splint.

Keep the dipping water clean and fresh. Reusing water that has been used previously for wetting plaster increases the amount of heat given off during crystallization and causes the plaster to set more quickly. As a rule of thumb, keep the temperature of the water at approximately 24°C. This temperature allows a workable setting time and has not been associated with increased risk for significant burns. As the temperature of the dipping water approaches 40°C, the potential for serious burns increases, even with splint thicknesses consisting of fewer than 12 plies. It is interesting to note that water temperature has been shown to be only a minor consideration in heat production in some studies (see Box 51.4).

Splint Application

Completely submerge the dry splint in the water bucket until the bubbling stops (see Fig. 51.5). Remove the splint and gently squeeze out excess water until the plaster has a wet and sloppy consistency. Place the splint on a hard table or countertop (a protective covering is recommended to prevent water or plaster damage) and smooth out the splint (with gloved hands) to remove any wrinkles and ensure uniform lamination of all layers. Lamination helps increase the final strength of the splint. Position the splint over the Webril and gently smooth it over the extremity. Plaster is usually somewhat adherent to Webril, but an assistant may be required to hold the splint in place during positioning. Once the splint has been properly positioned over the extremity, fold back the underlying stockinette and Webril to help hold it in place. Secure the splint with an appropriately sized elastic bandage by wrapping it in a distal-to-proximal direction. Finally, place the extremity in the desired position and mold the wet plaster to the contour of the extremity with only the palms of the hand. Finger indentations may cause ridges, which can produce pressure points.

Molding the wet splint to conform to the body's anatomy is probably the most important, yet the most frequently overlooked step to ensure adequate immobilization. The act of molding may cause some pain, so be sure to forewarn the patient. Mold with the palm or flat side of the fingers to avoid putting ridges or indentations in the underlying plaster. Complete all manipulation of the wet plaster before it reaches a thick, creamy consistency. Any movement after this time, which is known as the critical period, results in an imperfect crystalline network of calcium sulfate molecules and greatly weakens the ultimate strength of the splint. While the plaster is setting, do not wrap a pillow or blanket around the extremity for support because this leads to inadequate ventilation around the splint and greatly increases the amount of heat produced (see Box 51.4).

If an elastic bandage is applied directly over wet plaster, it may be incorporated into the drying plaster, thus making subsequent removal of the bandage difficult. To make it easier for patients to remove and reapply the splint, wrap a single layer of Webril or roll gauze around the wet plaster loosely before applying the elastic bandage. This prevents the wet plaster from becoming stuck to the elastic bandage. Use only one layer of Webril over the plaster because multiple layers are associated with high drying temperatures.

Before the patient is released from the ED, check the extremity for adequate immobilization and evaluate the patient for any evidence of vascular compromise or significant discomfort. If either occurs, loosen the elastic bandage. If the discomfort persists, place additional padding over the painful areas. If this measure, too, is unsuccessful, make a new splint while paying special attention to proper molding so that the wet plaster does not become indented. By resting tender tissue, splinting usually relieves the discomfort quickly, and patients generally say that they feel better soon after the splint has been applied. In general, a splint should decrease the patient's pain, not increase it; hence, do not readily release a patient who complains of increased pain after a splint has been placed. Such complaints may be due to manipulation during splinting, but increased pain should be further addressed or explained.

After a properly fitting, comfortable splint has been applied, place two strips of tape along each side of the splint to prevent the elastic bandage from slipping. It is also prudent to place tape over any metal fasteners used to secure the elastic bandages because these objects can fall off and be swallowed or aspirated by infants and small children. Use enough tape to include the entire circumference of the area under the fasteners, not just small pieces of tape that may not adhere to the moist splint. Finally, provide a sling for patients with upper extremity injuries and, if required, crutches (and instructions for their proper use) for those with lower extremity injuries.

Patient Instructions

Give patients both verbal and written instructions on splint care and precautions. Stress the importance of elevation in helping to decrease pain and swelling. Demonstrate this as well because most patients do not understand the medical definition of elevation. At night, wrap and secure a pillow around the injured extremity to help the patient keep it satisfactorily elevated. If the injury is less than 24 hours old, encourage the application of ice bags or cold packs. It is useless to apply cold packs over plaster, but it can be beneficial to apply them over Webril or an elastic bandage directly over an injury. It may be necessary to remove the splint to ice the injury. In theory, cold therapy stiffens collagen and thus reduces the tendency for ligaments and tendons to deform. Cold therapy also decreases muscle spasm and excitability, reduces blood flow (thereby limiting hemorrhage and edema), raises the pain threshold, and decreases inflammation. Because the thermal conductivity of subcutaneous tissue is poor, apply cold packs for at least 30 minutes at a time. This guideline is in contrast to the popular recommendation of "ice 20 minutes on, 20 minutes off," which often does nothing more than cool the skin. Do not use cold packs for more than the first 24 to 48 hours because cold can interfere with long-term healing. Instruct the patient to not stress the splint for at least 24 hours because plaster does not approach optimal strength until evaporation has reduced the water content of the plaster to approximately 21% of its initial hydrated level. This process of removing excess water by evaporation is called *curing*, and it generally takes several days to be completed. However, by 24 hours the water content of the plaster has usually been reduced enough to produce a strong, resilient splint. In addition, because the chemical process involved in the formation of plaster is reversible, the patient should avoid getting the splint wet. If the injury permits, the splint can be removed for showering and then reapplied. Alternatively, one or more plastic bags may be placed over a splint before showering.

Splints may crack, break, or disintegrate with wear, and a useless splint should be removed or replaced. Give patients general guidelines for length of immobilization and appropriate follow-up care. Avoid long-term immobilization, particularly in the older patients, because this can produce permanent disability. It is extremely important for the patient to continue to check for signs of vascular compromise. If the patient experiences a significant increase in pain, numbness or tingling of the digits, pallor of the distal end of the extremity, decreased capillary refill, or weakness, instruct the patient to return to the ED or to see their primary clinician without delay. As with casting, increased pain after splinting is a warning sign that should prompt a return visit, not telephone advice. Avoid giving excessive doses of opioids during the first 2 to 3 days after splinting to allow pain to prompt a follow-up visit.

UPPER EXTREMITY SPLINTS

Long Arm Splints

Long Arm Posterior Splint

Indications. Use a long arm posterior splint (Figs. 51.8 and 51.9) to immobilize injuries to the elbow and proximal end of the forearm. It completely eliminates flexion and extension of the elbow but does not entirely prevent pronation and supination of the forearm. Therefore it is not recommended for immobilization of complex or unstable distal forearm fractures unless used in conjunction with a long arm anterior splint (see later in this section). Alternatively, a double "sugar-tong" splint can be applied (see later in this section).

Construction. Construct a long arm posterior splint with 8 to 10 layers of 4- or 6-inch-wide plaster. Start the splint on the posterior aspect of the proximal end of the arm. Extend it down the arm to the elbow and then along the ulnar aspect of

Long Arm Posterior Splint

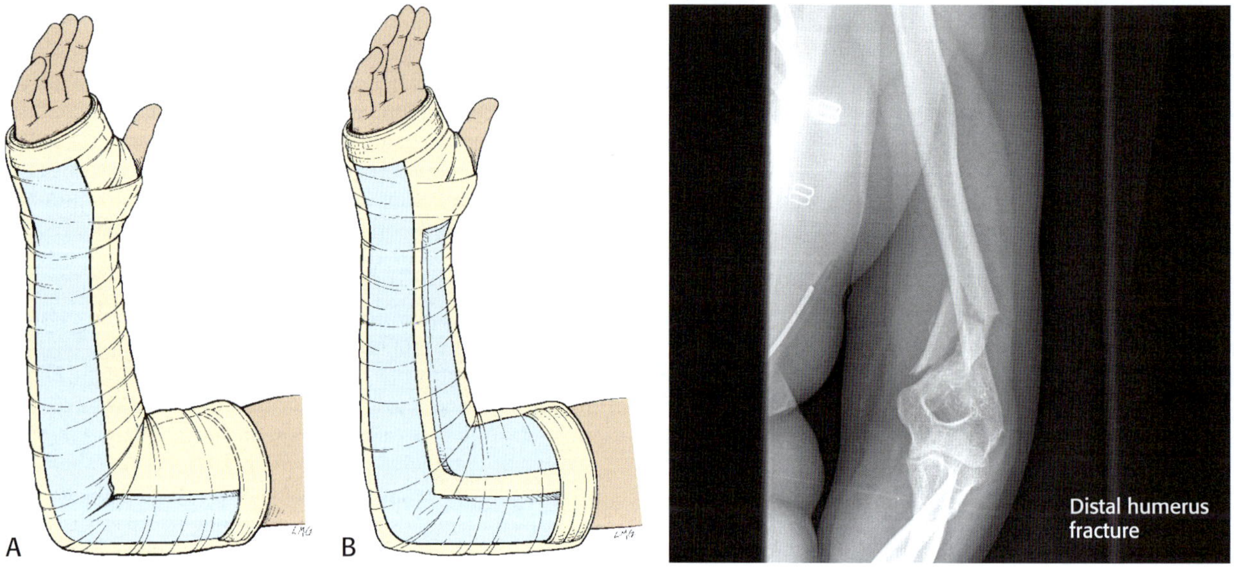

Application

A, Extend the splint from the posterior aspect of the humerus to the elbow and then along the ulnar aspect of the forearm to the distal metacarpals. Flex the elbow to 90 degrees, maintain the forearm in the neutral (thumb-up) position, and place the wrist in a neutral or slightly extended (10 to 20 degrees) position.

B, An anterior splint that mirrors the posterior splint may be used to increase stability and prevent supination and pronation. An anterior splint is never used alone.

Indications

Injuries of the elbow and distal end of the forearm, including:
- Distal humerus fractures (shown above)
- Supracondylar fractures
- Olecranon fractures
- Elbow dislocations

Fig. 51.8 Long arm posterior splint.

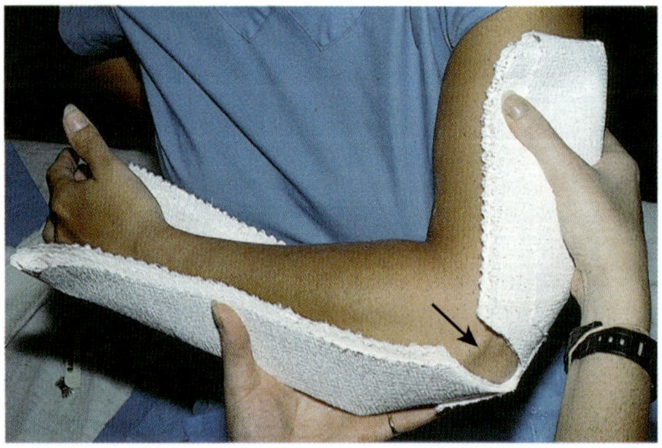

Fig. 51.9 When preparing a splint (such as a long arm splint) that involves a right angle, cut out a notch *(arrow)* to allow a smooth bend. Note that padding needs to be applied before splinting.

the forearm and hand to the level of the metacarpophalangeal (MCP) joints.

Application. Apply a stockinette and Webril as described previously. Cut a hole in the stockinette to expose the thumb, and place extra padding over the olecranon to prevent pressure injury. Position the arm with the elbow flexed to 90 degrees, the forearm neutral (thumb upward), and the wrist neutral or slightly extended (10 to 20 degrees). Ask an assistant to hold the wet splint in place, particularly when applying both a posterior and an anterior splint. Once the splint has been properly positioned, fold the ends of the stockinette and Webril back and secure the splint in place with 2-, 3-, or 4-inch elastic bandages. Finally, fold the sides of the splint up to create a gutter configuration and carefully mold the plaster around the extremity with the palms of the hand. The fingers and thumb should remain free to prevent stiffness from unnecessary immobilization.

Long Arm Anterior Splint

Indications. A long arm anterior splint is never used alone but, rather, as an adjunct to a long arm posterior splint to improve immobilization by increasing stability and preventing pronation and supination of the forearm (see Fig. 51.8B).

Construction. Construct a long arm anterior splint in the same manner as described for a long arm posterior splint. It mirrors the posterior splint by running down the anterior aspect of the arm to the antecubital fossa, where it continues along the radial aspect of the forearm to the distal end of the radius.

Application. Use stockinette, Webril, and positioning similar to the way described for the application of a long arm posterior splint. When using both an anterior and a posterior long arm splint, have an assistant available to hold the wet splint in place. Place the anterior splint first and then position the posterior splint. Once both splints have been properly positioned, fold the ends of the stockinette and Webril back and secure the

Double Sugar-Tong Splint

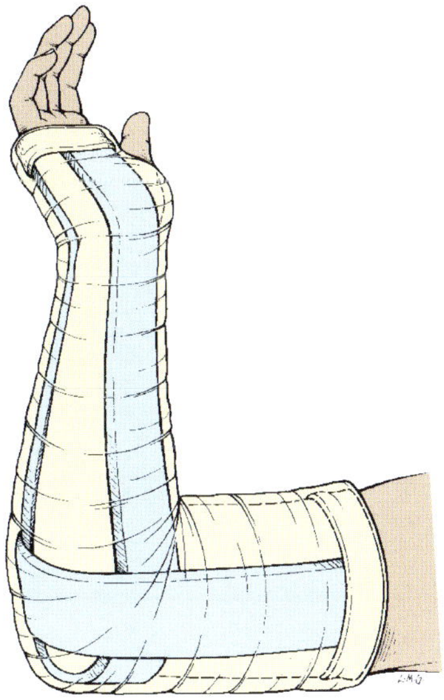

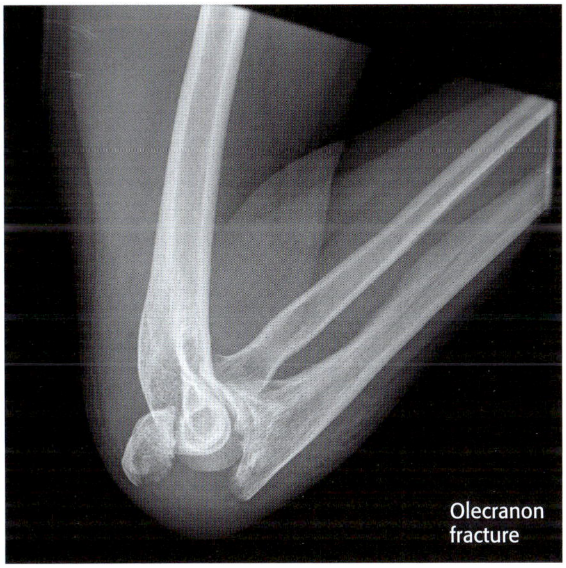

Application

Apply the forearm portion of the double sugar-tong splint first. Begin the splint at the metacarpal heads on the dorsum of the hand, and then extend it along the dorsal surface of the forearm and around the elbow. Continue along the volar surface of the forearm and stop at the level of the metacarpophalangeal joints.

Begin the arm portion on the medial aspect of the proximal part of the arm, and then run it down over the forearm splint and around the elbow. Continue up the lateral aspect of the arm (once again going over the forearm splint) until it reaches the starting point.

Keep the elbow flexed at 90 degrees, the forearm in the neutral (thumb-up) position, and the wrist in a neutral or slightly extended (10 to 20 degrees) position. Allow the fingers and thumb to remain free to avoid stiffness.

Indications

Injuries of the elbow and distal part of the forearm, including:
- Distal humerus fractures
- Supracondylar fractures
- Olecranon fractures (shown above)
- Elbow dislocations

Indications are similar to those for the long arm splint. Since the double sugar-tong splint prevents supination and pronation, it may be preferable for some fractures of the distal humerus and of the forearm and elbow.

Fig. 51.10 Double sugar-tong splint.

splint in place with 2-, 3-, or 4-inch elastic bandages. Finally, fold up the sides of the splint to create a gutter configuration and carefully mold the plaster around the extremity with the palms of the hands. Keep the patient's fingers and thumb free to prevent stiffness from unnecessary immobilization.

Double Sugar-Tong Splint

Indications. Use a double sugar-tong splint (Fig. 51.10) like a long arm posterior splint to immobilize injuries to the elbow and forearm. However, because it prevents pronation and supination of the forearm, it is preferable for some distal forearm and elbow fractures.

Construction. The splint consists of two separate pieces of plaster, a forearm splint and an arm splint. Construct each piece with eight layers of 3- or 4-inch plaster. The forearm portion of the splint runs from the metacarpal heads on the dorsum of the hand along the dorsal surface of the forearm around the elbow. It continues along the volar surface of the forearm to the palm of the hand and stops at the level of the MCP joints. The arm portion of the splint begins on the anterior aspect of the proximal end of the humerus. It runs down the arm over the forearm splint and around the elbow. It then continues up the posterior aspect of the arm, once again going over the forearm splint, until it reaches the starting point.

Application. Use a stockinette, Webril, and positioning similar to the way described for the application of a long arm posterior splint. Secure the two splints in place with 2-, 3-, or 4-inch elastic bandages starting with the forearm splint at the hand. Once the forearm splint is secured in place, wrap the arm portion of the splint beginning at its proximal end. Keep the patient's fingers and thumb free to prevent stiffness.

Forearm and Hand Splints

See Video 51.3.

Volar Splint

Indications. Use a volar splint (Fig. 51.11) to immobilize a variety of soft tissue injuries to the hand and wrist. It is also used for temporary immobilization of triquetral fractures, lunate and perilunate dislocations, and second through fifth metacarpal head fractures. For these more serious injuries, some clinicians prefer to add a dorsal splint to create a more

Volar Splint

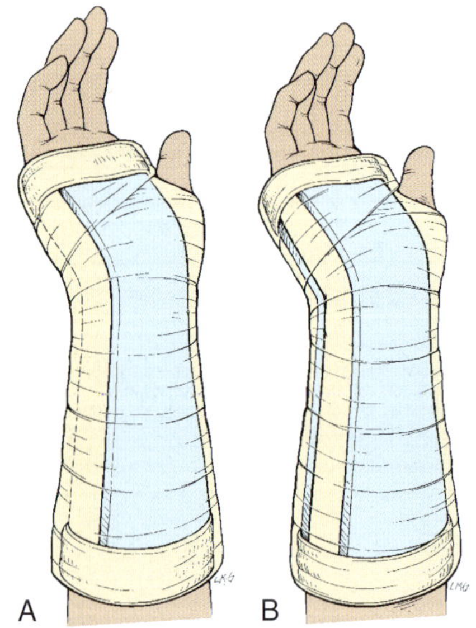

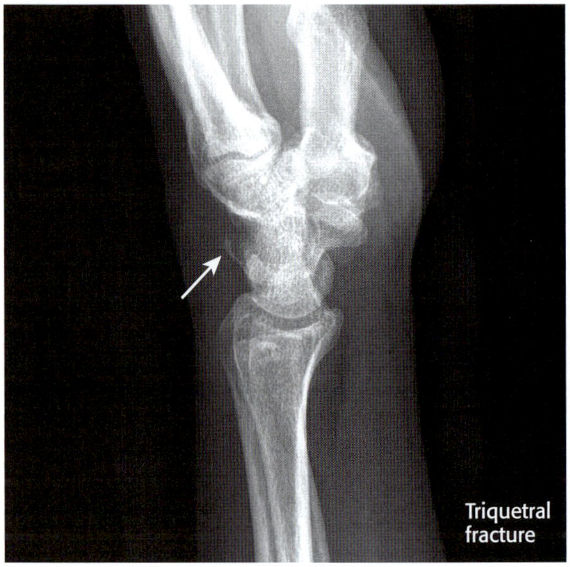

Application

A, Begin the splint in the palm at the metacarpal heads and extend it along the volar surface of the forearm to a point just proximal to the elbow. If any of the fingers are injured, extend the splint to incorporate the involved digits. Place the forearm in the neutral (thumb-up) position with the wrist slightly extended (10 to 20 degrees). Wrist flexion should be avoided.

B, For more serious injuries, add an additional dorsal slab to create a bivalve splint.

Indications

Soft tissue injuries of the hand and wrist
Orthopedic injuries of the hand and wrist, including:
- Triquetral fractures (shown above)
- Lunate and perilunate dislocations
- Second through fifth metacarpal head fractures
- Minimally displaced distal radius and ulna fractures

The volar splint does not eliminate supination and pronation of the forearm and therefore is not ideal for more complicated distal radius and ulna fractures.

Fig. 51.11 Volar splint. This splint does not eliminate pronation or supination of the forearm.

stable bivalve effect (see Fig. 51.11B). Because a volar splint does not completely eliminate pronation and supination of the forearm, it may not be ideal for distal radial and ulnar fractures, although many clinicians use this splint for nondisplaced or minimally displaced distal ulnar and radial fractures.

Construction. Construct the splint with 8 to 10 layers of 3- or 4-inch-wide plaster. The splint begins in the palm at the metacarpal heads and extends along the volar surface of the forearm to just proximal to the elbow. If there is an injury to any of the fingers, extend the splint to incorporate the involved digit or digits.

Application. Apply a stockinette and Webril as described previously. Cut a hole in the stockinette to expose the thumb. If the splint is going to incorporate one or more digits, insert a piece of Webril or gauze between the digits to prevent skin maceration. Place the forearm in the neutral position (thumb upward) with the wrist extended slightly (10 to 20 degrees). Avoid wrist flexion. After properly positioning the wet plaster, fold back the ends of the stockinette and Webril and use a 3- or 4-inch elastic bandage to secure the splint in place. Fold the sides of the splint up around the forearm to create a gutter effect and carefully mold the plaster to conform to the contours of the palm and wrist. Some clinicians prefer to extend the splint to the fingertips and then fold the wet plaster back toward the palm, which allows the fingers to "grasp" the rounded distal end when at rest. With either method, keep the thumb and fingers free to move unless they are injured and are being intentionally immobilized by the splint.

Sugar-Tong Splint

See Video 51.4.

Indications. Use a sugar-tong splint (Fig. 51.12) for fractures of the distal end of the radius and ulna. The advantage of this splint over a volar splint is prevention of pronation and supination of the forearm. In addition, it immobilizes the elbow, which is desirable for the first few days after a distal forearm fracture.

Construction and Application. Construct and apply this splint in the same manner as the forearm portion of the double sugar-tong splint described earlier.

Thumb Spica Splint

See Video 51.5.

Indications. Use a thumb spica splint (Fig. 51.13) to immobilize injuries and fractures of the scaphoid, lunate, thumb, and first metacarpal. It is also used for the treatment of de Quervain tenosynovitis. Traditionally, a thumb spica splint or cast was thought to be a requirement for properly immobilizing scaphoid fractures; however, there is no totally agreed standard. Clay and coworkers[16] stated that the optimal method of casting scaphoid fractures has not been definitively

Forearm Sugar-Tong Splint

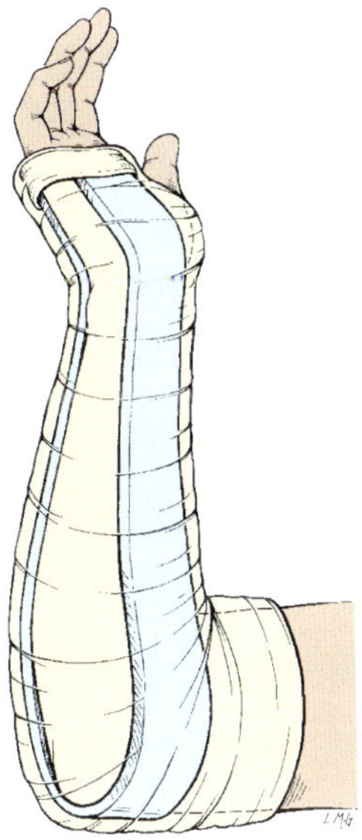

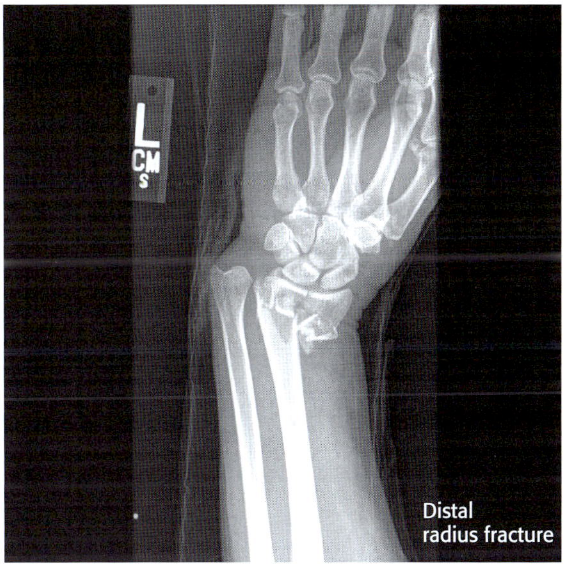

Application

Begin the splint at the metacarpal heads on the dorsum of the hand, extend it along the dorsal surface of the forearm, and then around the elbow. Continue along the volar surface of the forearm and stop at the level of the metacarpophalangeal joints.

Keep the elbow flexed at a 90-degree angle, the forearm in the neutral (thumb-up) position, and the wrist in a neutral position or slightly extended (10 to 20 degrees).

Indications

Distal radius and ulna fractures (shown above)
Distal forearm fractures

The forearm sugar-tong splint, unlike the volar wrist splint, prevents supination and pronation of the forearm. Additionally, it immobilizes the elbow, which is desirable for the first few days after a distal forearm fracture.

Fig. 51.12 Forearm sugar-tong splint. This splint will eliminate pronation and supination of the forearm.

established. They were unable to prove a difference in patient comfort, recovery of function, or incidence of nonunion between a Colles cast and a traditional scaphoid cast that included the thumb.

The incidence of nonunion of scaphoid fractures is approximately 10%, regardless of the type of immobilization in the ED, but it is greatest with unstable proximal pole fractures. Because some scaphoid fractures heal poorly under the best of circumstances, it seems prudent to provide thumb immobilization in the initial splinting. Failure to do so, such as when a "sprained wrist" is suspected, should not be construed as being beneath the accepted standard of care. Most volar splints will at least partly immobilize the base of the thumb, so the discussion may be moot.

Construction. Construct the splint with eight layers of 3-inch-wide plaster. Extend the splint from just distal to the interphalangeal joint of the thumb to the midforearm level.

Application. Place the forearm in the neutral position with the wrist extended 25 degrees and the thumb in the wineglass position (Fig. 51.14). Apply a stockinette and Webril from the base of the palm to the midforearm level. It is difficult to place a stockinette around the thumb. Instead, cut a hole in the stockinette to expose the thumb, and then pad the exposed thumb with small vertical strips of Webril or wrap it with 2-inch Webril. Place the dry plaster over the radial aspect of the forearm from just beyond the thumb interphalangeal joint to the midforearm level. Once in position, mark the location of the first MCP joint and make a small (1 cm to 2 cm) perpendicular cut 1 cm distal to the mark on each edge of the plaster (see Fig. 51.13, *inset*). This allows the splint to be molded around the thumb without creating a buckle in the plaster. If the plaster distal to the cut notches is too wide to mold around the thumb without overlapping, trim the edges to the desired width. Wet the plaster and secure it in place with a 2- or 3-inch elastic bandage. It is important to carefully mold the wet plaster around the thumb and palm and to maintain the thumb in the wineglass position while the plaster is drying.

Ulnar Collateral Ligament Injury (Gamekeeper's or Skier's Thumb)

Forced abduction with hyperextension of the thumb is the usual mechanism for injury to the ulnar collateral ligament. This is a rather disabling injury that requires early recognition because improper treatment can result in chronic pain, pinch weakness, and loss of stability of the thumb. Characterized by MCP joint pain, tenderness of the ulnar side, and laxity of this joint with valgus stressing, this is not a simple sprain. Although immobilization with a thumb spica splint or figure-of-eight thumb splint may suffice as definitive treatment (Fig. 51.15), surgery is often recommended for more advanced injuries. Splinting in the ED with referral to a consultant is prudent for all significant thumb soft tissue injuries consistent with an ulnar collateral ligament injury.

Ulnar Gutter Splint

See Video 51.6.

Thumb Spica Splint

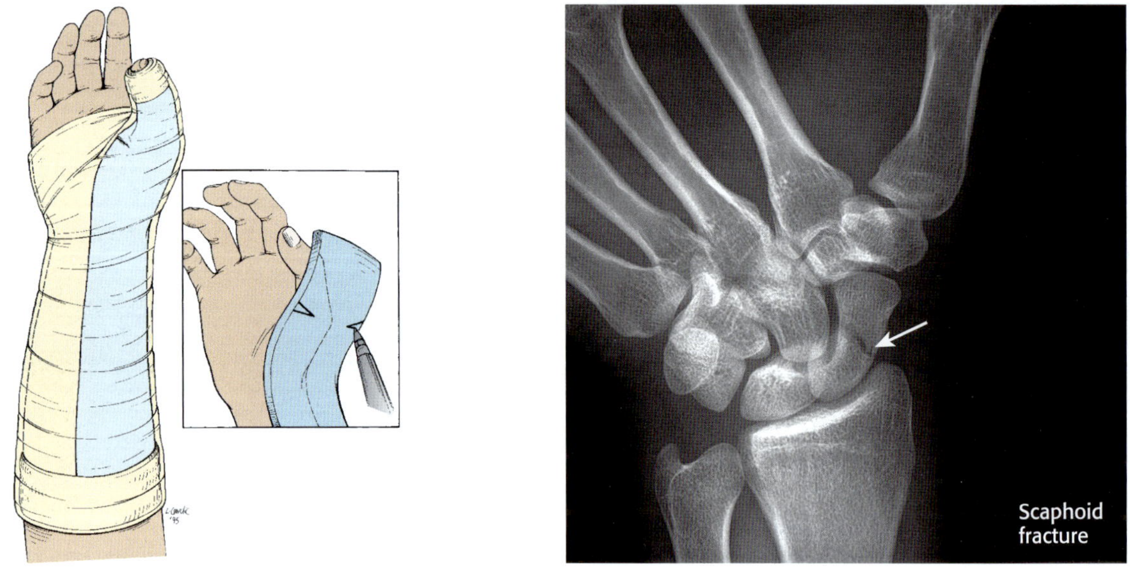

Application

Extend the splint from just distal to the interphalangeal joint of the thumb to the midforearm level.

Place the forearm in the neutral position with the wrist extended 25 degrees and the thumb in the wineglass position (see Fig. 51.12).

Inset: Make a small (1- to 2-cm) perpendicular cut 1 cm distal to the first metacarpophalangeal joint on each edge of the plaster to allow molding of the splint around the thumb without creating a buckle in the plaster.

Indications

Scaphoid fractures (shown above)
Lunate, thumb, and first metacarpal fractures
de Quervain tenosynovitis

Fig. 51.13 Thumb spica splint.

Indications. Use an ulnar gutter splint (Fig. 51.16) to immobilize fractures and serious soft tissue injuries of the little and ring fingers and fractures of the neck, shaft, and base of the fourth and fifth metacarpals.

Construction. Make the splint with six to eight layers of 3- or 4-inch plaster. It incorporates both the little and the ring fingers. It runs along the ulnar aspect of the forearm from just beyond the distal interphalangeal joint of the little finger to the midforearm level.

Application. Apply a stockinette and Webril as usual. Place additional Webril or gauze between the little and ring fingers to prevent maceration of the skin. Position the forearm in the neutral position with the wrist in slight extension (10 to 20 degrees), the MCP joints in 50 degrees of flexion, and the proximal and distal interphalangeal joints in slight flexion (10 to 15 degrees). When immobilizing a metacarpal neck fracture (i.e., boxer's fracture), flex the MCP joint to 90 degrees. Once in proper position, fold the sides of the splint up to form a gutter. Finally, fold the ends of the stockinette and Webril back to help hold the splint in place while it is secured to the extremity with a 2- or 3-inch elastic bandage.

Radial Gutter Splint

Indications. Use a radial gutter splint (Fig. 51.17) to immobilize fractures and serious soft tissue injuries of the index and long fingers and fractures of the neck, shaft, and base of the second and third metacarpals.

Construction. Make the splint with six to eight layers of 3- or 4-inch plaster. It runs along the radial aspect of the forearm from just beyond the distal interphalangeal joint of the index finger to the midforearm level.

Application. Apply a stockinette (with a hole cut to expose the thumb) and Webril as described previously. Insert an additional piece of Webril or gauze between the index and long fingers to prevent maceration of the skin. Place the hand and fingers in the *position of function* or in the *intrinsic position* (see Fig. 51.14). Neither position has been proved to be superior for the first few weeks of splinting, which makes them both acceptable for initial immobilization in the ED. In the position of function, the forearm is in the neutral position with the wrist in slight extension (10 to 20 degrees), the MCP joints in 50 to 60 degrees of flexion, and the proximal and distal interphalangeal joints in slight flexion (5 to 10 degrees) (see Fig. 51.14A). When immobilizing a metacarpal neck fracture, the intrinsic position is often used, with the MCP joint flexed to 90 degrees and the fingers extended (see Fig. 51.14B).

Place the dry plaster over the extremity and mark the location of the thumb. Cut a hole in the dry plaster to expose the thumb. Dip the plaster and position the wet splint over the extremity. Fold back the ends of the stockinette and Webril to

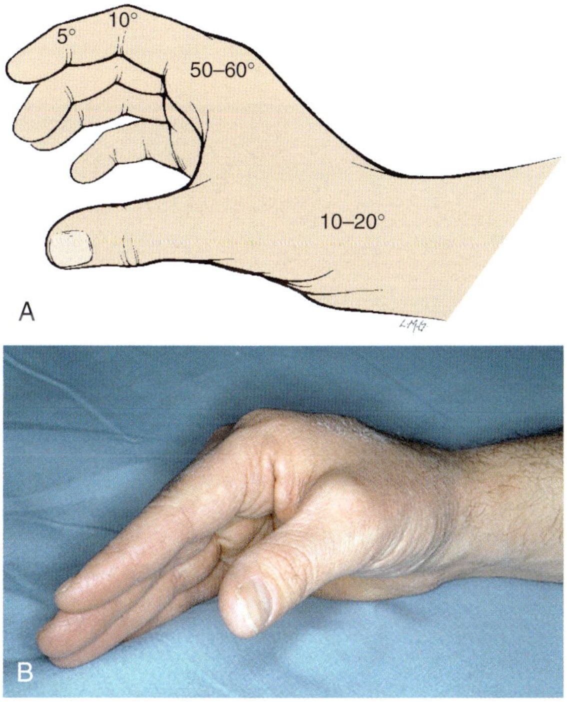

Fig. 51.14 (A) The wineglass position, also termed the position of function, is a safe splint position for the hand and fingers for short-term splinting (7 to 14 days). The wrist should allow alignment of the thumb with the forearm, the metacarpophalangeal (MCP) joint should be moderately flexed, and the interphalangeal joints should be only slightly flexed. The thumb should be abducted away from the palm. (B) For longer splinting, the fingers should be extended to prevent flexion contractures. This is referred to as the intrinsic position. The MCP joint is flexed at 90 degrees. Either position is acceptable for initial short-term splinting in the emergency department.

Figure-of-Eight Thumb Splint

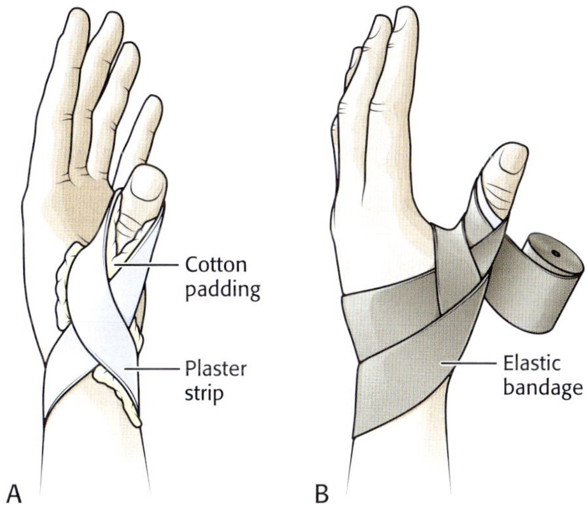

Indications

Skier's/gamekeeper's thumb (ulnar collateral ligament injury)

Application

A, Cut a length of Webril and plaster approximately 14 to 16 inches long. Center the splint on the web space, cross over the dorsal aspect of the thumb in a figure-of-eight fashion, and overlap the cut edges around the styloid process of the ulna.
B, Wrap with a small elastic bandage while overlapping in a figure-of-eight formation. Mold and position the splint after placement.

Fig. 51.15 Figure-of-eight thumb splint.

help hold the splint in place and secure it to the extremity with a 2- or 3-inch elastic bandage.

Finger Splints

See Videos 51.7–51.9. Use finger splints for sprains, fractures, tendon repairs, or infections. Minor finger sprains can often be managed with dynamic splinting (e.g., buddy taping) (Fig. 51.18A) or a commercially available foam splint with aluminum backing (one-surface splint) (Fig. 51.18B), but fractures, tendon repairs, and some soft tissue injuries benefit from formal splinting (e.g., thumb spica and ulnar and radial gutter splints). Specific conditions, such as mallet finger, require a specialized splint (plaster or Stack splint) (Fig. 51.18C). When complete immobilization of a finger is required (e.g., unstable phalangeal fractures), an "outrigger" finger splint that incorporates the wrist may be used (Fig. 51.18D). Both the position of function and the intrinsic position are acceptable for initial splinting.

Pitfalls of Hand Dressings and Splints

The two most common problems with hand dressings and splints are putting them on too tightly and leaving them on too long (Table 51.2). One must be especially careful to avoid wrapping elastic bandages too snugly. Before discharge from the ED, instruct patients to loosen an elastic bandage if it feels too tight, and be sure that they have access to emergency follow-up care. It is often advisable to start patients on a regimen of early protected motion. This means that the patient removes the splint for a specified period, performs a prescribed exercise, and then replaces the splint. A splint is not an all-or-none device, and the patient is generally weaned from it slowly before it is discarded entirely. A stiff hand is a nonfunctional one, and stiffness is often a consequence of prolonged immobilization. It is important for patients to be made aware of their responsibility for the injured hand.

Sling, Swathe and Sling, and Shoulder Immobilizer

Sling

Use a sling to maintain elevation and provide immobilization of the hand, forearm, and elbow (Fig. 51.19). It is most often used in conjunction with a plaster splint or cast. A number of commercial slings are available to choose from. Many of them are fairly economical and simple to use, whereas others are more expensive and do not allow the versatility of a simple, inexpensive triangular muslin bandage. When applying a sling, make it long enough to adequately support the wrist and hand. A sling that is too short will allow the wrist and hand to hang down (ulnar deviate) and can result in ulnar nerve injury.

Swathe and Sling

Use of a swathe and sling is the treatment of choice for most proximal humeral fractures and shoulder injuries, such as reduced dislocations. The sling supports the weight of the arm, and the swathe immobilizes the arm against the chest wall to minimize shoulder motion.

Ulnar Gutter Splint

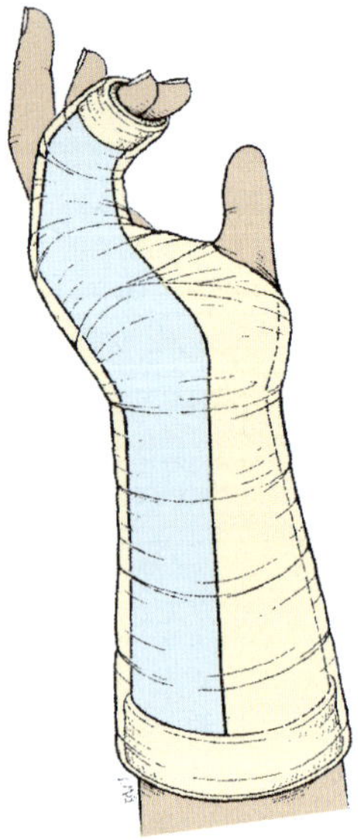

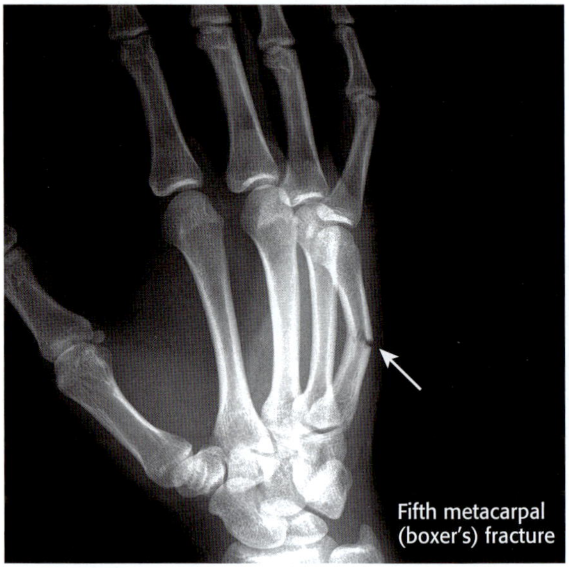

Application

The ulnar gutter splint incorporates both the little and the ring fingers. Therefore place Webril or gauze between the digits to prevent maceration of the skin. Run the splint along the ulnar aspect of the forearm from just beyond the distal interphalangeal joint of the little finger to the midforearm level.

Maintain the forearm in the neutral position with the wrist in slight extension (10 to 20 degrees), the metacarpophalangeal (MCP) joint in 50° of flexion, and the proximal and distal interphalangeal joints in slight flexion (10 to 15 degrees). When immobilizing a metacarpal neck fracture, flex the MCP joint to 90 degrees.

Indications

Injuries of the ulnar side of the hand, including:
- Fourth and fifth metacarpal fractures (shown above)
- Serious injuries of the ring and little fingers

Fig. 51.16 Ulnar gutter splint.

Shoulder Immobilizer

In most EDs, the swathe and sling have been replaced by commercially available shoulder immobilizers. Its advantage is that it may be removed for showering and range-of-motion exercises and is easily reapplied by the patient (a desirable option in the care of a shoulder dislocation). If the shoulder immobilizer is used for more than a few days, pad the axilla to absorb moisture and decrease skin chafing.

A Velpeau bandage is a sling and swathe device that positions the forearm diagonally rather than horizontally across the chest with the hand elevated to the level of the shoulder. It offers no particular advantage over a standard sling and swathe, is difficult to apply, cannot be removed easily, and is not well tolerated with prolonged immobilization.

Figure-of-Eight Clavicle Strap

In the past, clavicle fractures were often treated with an uncomfortable and complex figure-of-eight bandage. Despite its early popularity, this device never proved to be superior to a simple sling (in terms of cosmesis, functional outcome, or pain relief).[17,18] Moreover, use of a figure-of-eight clavicle strap may actually promote nonunion or increase the deformity at the fracture site. When compared with a simple sling, a figure-of-eight clavicle strap is very uncomfortable, prohibits bathing, often causes chafing and discomfort in the axilla, and may predispose to axillary vein thrombosis.[4] Thus most emergency clinicians have abandoned the figure-of-eight dressing in favor of a simple sling, which is sufficient to treat most clavicular fractures.

LOWER EXTREMITY SPLINTS

Knee Splints

Knee Immobilizer

Indications. A knee immobilizer (Fig. 51.20) is commonly used for mild to moderate ligamentous and soft tissue injuries involving the knee. It is removable and extremely easy to apply, which makes it popular among patients and clinicians alike. In most EDs, it has replaced the bulkier plaster splint. Its use should be restricted to injuries that do not require immediate surgical intervention, traction, or casting. For these injuries, in which temporary but more complete immobilization is needed, use a plaster knee splint because it provides better stabilization and costs much less than a knee immobilizer. The exact scientific benefit of a knee immobilizer is poorly studied and difficult to document. However, it clearly helps relieve pain and, at least theoretically, hastens healing.

Radial Gutter Splint

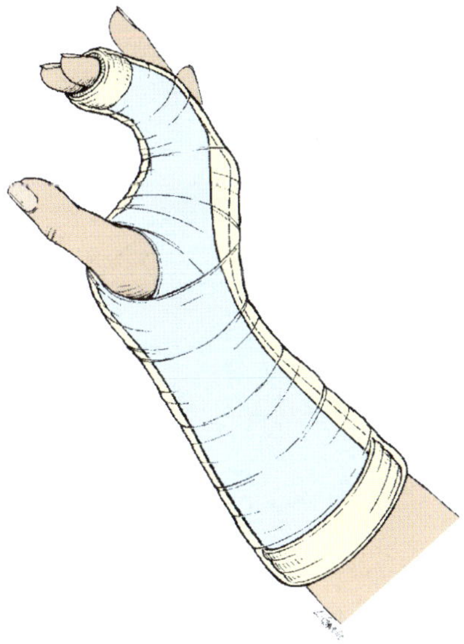

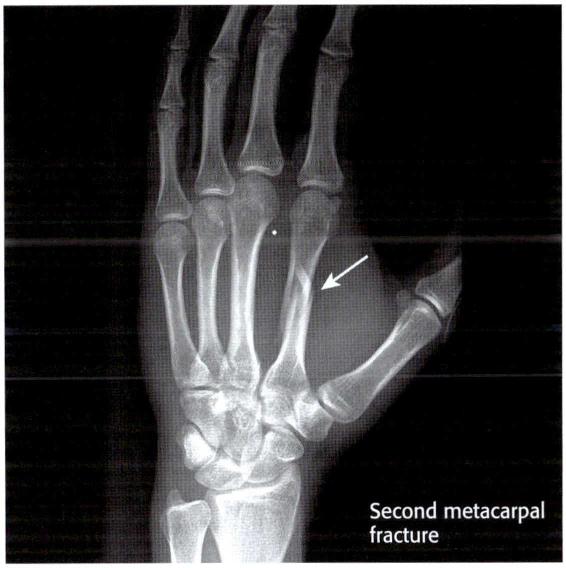

Application

The radial gutter splint incorporates both the index and the long fingers. Therefore, Webril or gauze should be placed between the digits to prevent maceration of the skin. Run the splint along the radial aspect of the forearm from just beyond the distal interphalangeal joint of the index finger to the midforearm.

Maintain the forearm in the neutral position with the wrist in slight extension (10 to 20 degrees), the MCP joint in 50 degrees of flexion, and the proximal and distal interphalangeal joints in slight flexion (10 to 15 degrees). When immobilizing a metacarpal neck fracture, flex the MCP joint to 90 degrees.

Indications

Injuries on the radial side of the hand, including:
- Second and third metacarpal fractures (shown above)
- Serious injuries to the index and middle fingers

Fig. 51.17 Radial gutter splint.

Application. Knee immobilizers are available in small, medium, large, and extra-large sizes. To choose the appropriate size, place the knee immobilizer next to the injured leg so that the tapered end lies distal to the patient's knee; if present, the cutout patellar area on the anterior aspect of the splint lies adjacent to the knee joint. In this position, the splint should extend distally to within a few inches of the malleoli and proximally to just below the buttocks crease. To apply the knee immobilizer, slide the open splint under the injured leg, wrap it around the extremity, and secure it in place with the Velcro straps. A knee immobilizer can be applied directly over clothing, thus obviating the need to remove or cut the patient's pants.

Posterior Knee Splint

Indications. In many EDs, the knee immobilizer has virtually replaced the plaster knee splint for mild to moderate injuries to the knee. However, a plaster knee splint can be particularly useful in patients whose extremities are too large for a knee immobilizer, in the treatment of angulated fractures, or for temporarily immobilizing injuries that require immediate operative intervention or orthopedic referral. The posterior (gutter) knee splint (Fig. 51.21A) is the type most commonly applied, but as alternatives, two parallel splints can be placed along each side of the leg and foreleg to create a bivalve effect (see Fig. 51.21B), or a long leg U-splint can be applied (see later). A bilateral knee splint is slightly more difficult to apply than a posterior knee splint, but it may provide better immobilization of the lateral and medial collateral ligaments and can be used for injuries to these structures.

Construction. Construct a posterior knee splint with 12 to 15 layers of 6-inch plaster. It should run from just below the buttocks crease to approximately 5 to 8 cm above the malleoli. The sides of the splint are folded upward to form a gutter configuration.

Application. Apply a stockinette in the usual manner and wrap the leg with 4- or 6-inch Webril. Have an assistant elevate the leg and hold the splint in place while securing it to the extremity with 4- or 6-inch elastic bandages. If no aide is available, place the patient in the prone position and have him use his toes to elevate the lower part of the leg off the bed to allow sufficient room to wrap the Webril and elastic bandages around the injured extremity. Lay the splint along the posterior surface of the extremity, and secure it in place with 4- or 6-inch elastic bandages.

Jones Compression Dressing

Indications. A Jones compression dressing is commonly used for short-term immobilization of soft tissue injuries of the knee. It immobilizes and compresses the knee, thereby

Finger Splinting Techniques

A. Buddy Taping

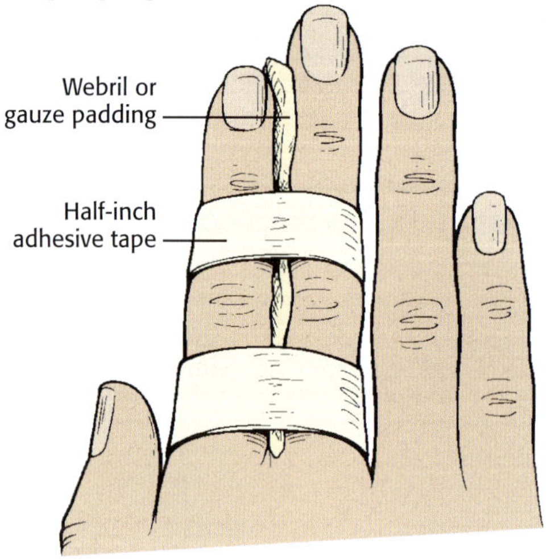

Taping between the digital joints (toes or fingers) allows the normal adjacent finger to protect the collateral ligament of its injured neighbor. Place Webril between the digits to prevent maceration of the skin.

B. Dorsal Aluminum Foam Splint

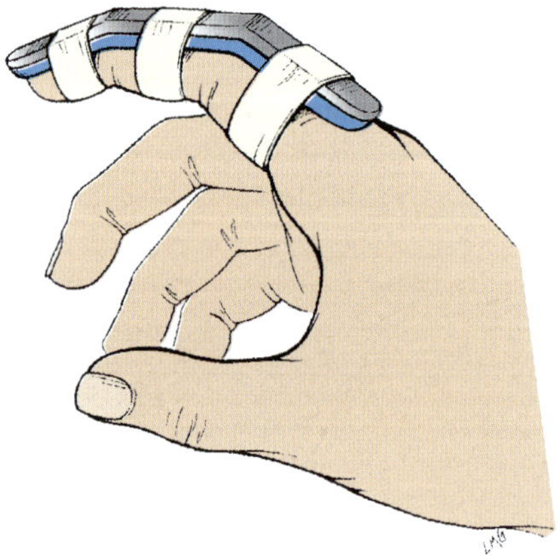

The bone is subcutaneous dorsally, and splints here afford better immobilization of the digit. The dorsal splint also allows preservation and use of tactile sense, which encourages function and better splint acceptance on the part of the patient.

C. Mallet Finger Splints

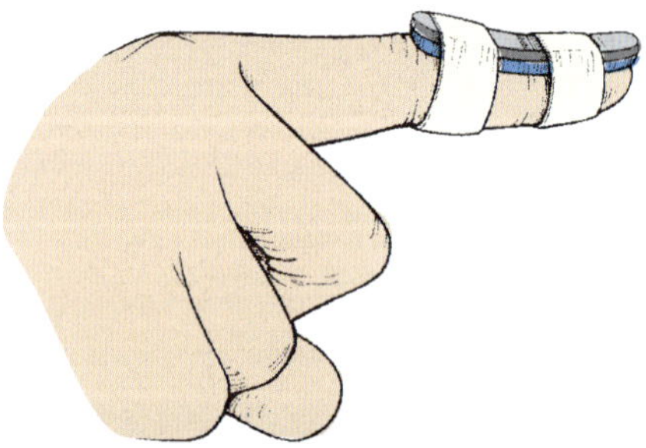

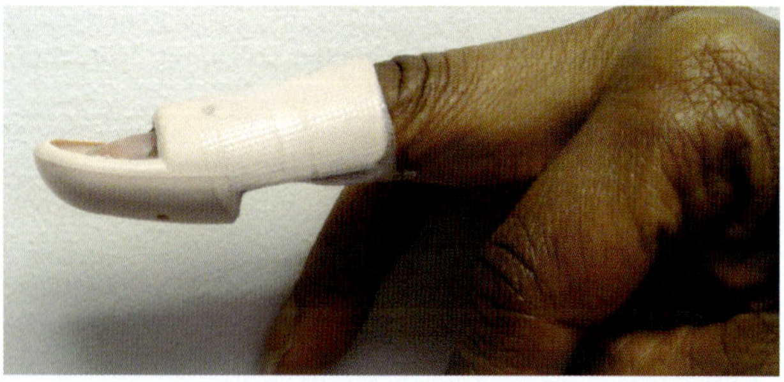

Top: The dorsal splint immobilizes only the distal interphalangeal joint, which allows use of the finger. Hyperextension of this joint predisposes to skin sloughing and should be avoided. The patient should be advised to not flex the joint during splint changes.

Bottom: A Stack splint is designed especially to treat a mallet finger. Long-term immobilization (8 weeks) or surgical fixation is required for this injury.

D. "Outrigger" Finger Splint

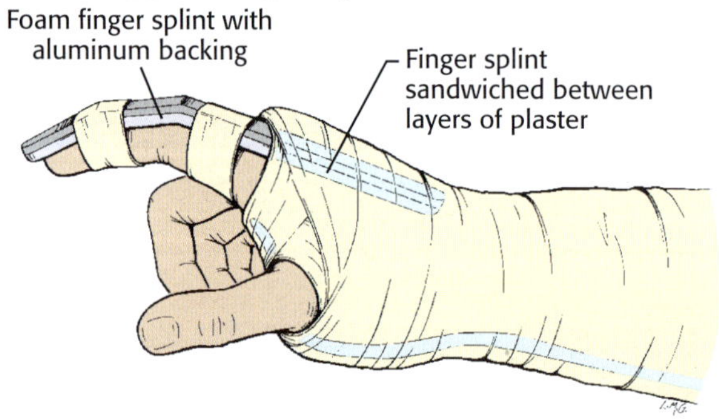

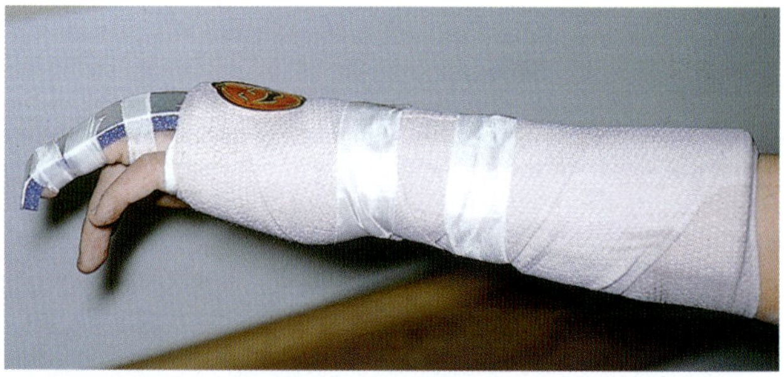

A padded aluminum splint is incorporated into the middle of a plaster splint to form an outrigger configuration. The plaster splint is applied to the dorsum of the hand and wrist with an elastic bandage; the finger is then taped to the aluminum splint. This provides complete immobilization of the finger.

Fig. 51.18 Finger splinting techniques.

TABLE 51.2 Useful Estimates of Splint Times for Various Hand Problems

INJURY	SPLINT TYPE	IMMOBILIZATION TIME[a]
Mallet finger	FIN	8 weeks
Boutonnière deformity	FIN	6 weeks
Distal phalanx—soft tissue	FIN	1–2 weeks
Extensor tendon	DHWF	3 weeks
Sprain-strain[b]		
Interphalangeal joint	FIN	1–2 weeks
Wrist	DHWF	1–2 weeks
Hand burn	DHWF	5–7 weeks
Infection		
Digit	DHWF	5–7 days
Hand	DHWF	5–7 days
Severe hand contusion	DHWF	5–7 days
Fracture		
Distal phalanx	FIN	2–3 weeks
Middle phalanx	FIN	2–3 weeks
Proximal phalanx	DHWF	2–3 weeks
Metacarpal	DHWF	2–3 weeks
Carpal tunnel	DHWF	Night only
de Quervain's disease	DHWF	2–3 weeks
Trigger finger	FIN	Night only

[a]These are average times only. Every patient is treated as an individual when a splint is used. Clinical judgment is critical.
[b]Diagnosis of a sprain should be made only after a thorough effort has been made to rule out a fracture or dislocation. This is particularly true in the wrist.
DHWF, Digit-hand-wrist-forearm; *FIN*, finger.

reducing both pain and swelling. However, because it does allow slight flexion and extension of the knee, it should not be used for injuries that require strict immobilization. In addition, it is difficult to maintain the splint for more than a few days.

Construction. A Jones dressing is fashioned from 6-inch Webril and elastic bandages.

Application. To apply a Jones dressing, place the patient supine on the stretcher. If available, ask an assistant to elevate the patient's leg to facilitate wrapping. If no help is available, place a pillow under the patient's heel to lift the extremity off the stretcher. Wrap Webril around the extremity from the groin to a few inches above the malleoli. Use two or three layers of Webril and overlap the previous turn by 25% to 50%. Complete the dressing by wrapping 6-inch elastic bandages (two are usually required) around the Webril. If more support is required, repeat the process with another two or three layers of Webril held in place by additional elastic bandages.

Ankle Splints

Posterior Splint

See Video 51.10.

Indications. A posterior ankle splint (Fig. 51.22) is one of the most common splints applied in the ED. As noted in the introductory section, the entire concept of splinting an acutely sprained ankle has been questioned, with no firm evidence to support better outcomes with splinting or casting versus functional management (early mobilization with an external support). Nonetheless, an acutely sprained ankle is painful, and if nothing else, splinting for a few days helps alleviate the pain.

Use a posterior splint primarily to immobilize severe ankle sprains, fractures of the distal ends of the fibula and tibia, and reduce ankle dislocations. It can also be used for fractures of the tarsal and metatarsal bones or for other foot conditions that require immobilization. With particularly severe or unstable injuries, an additional anterior splint may be used to provide extra immobilization resembling that of a formal cast (Fig. 51.23). For severe lateral or bilateral ligamentous injuries, add a U-splint or stirrup splint (see later) to the posterior splint for increased immobilization. With minor soft tissue injuries, patients may have partial weight bearing on ankle splints after 24 hours. If the patient will be bearing weight, wearing a cast shoe over the splint makes it easier to walk and increases the longevity of the splint. Generally, though, walking on the splint is prohibited if immobilization for more than 2 or 3 days is desired.

Construction. Make the posterior splint with 4- or 6-inch-wide plaster strips. It should extend from the plantar surface of the great toe or metatarsal heads along the posterior surface of the foreleg to the level of the fibular head. If it hurts to move the toes, incorporate them into the splint (after padding is placed between the digits). It is a common mistake to apply a posterior splint that does not extend far enough to support the ball of the foot. Use 15 to 20 layers if partial weight bearing is allowed because this splint frequently breaks or cracks when walked on.[19]

Application. The easiest way to apply a posterior splint is to place the patient in the prone position with the knee and ankle flexed at a 90-degree angle. Failure to place the ankle in a 90-degree angle results in a plantar-flexed splint. A supine patient may help maintain the ankle in a 90-degree angle by pulling up on the foot with a wide stockinette stirrup. Flexing the knee to a 90-degree angle relaxes the gastrocnemius muscle and facilitates ankle motion. With the knee and ankle in the proper position, apply a stockinette and pad the foot and leg with Webril as described earlier. Use extra padding over bony prominences, particularly the malleoli. To prevent skin maceration, place pieces of Webril or gauze between the toes if they are to be included in the splint. Lay the wet plaster over the plantar surface of the foot and secure it in place by folding back the ends of the stockinette and Webril and wrapping with one or two 4-inch-wide elastic bandages. Carefully mold the wet plaster around the malleoli and instep to ensure maximum comfort and immobilization. Leave the toes partially exposed for later examination of color and capillary refill.

Shoulder Slings

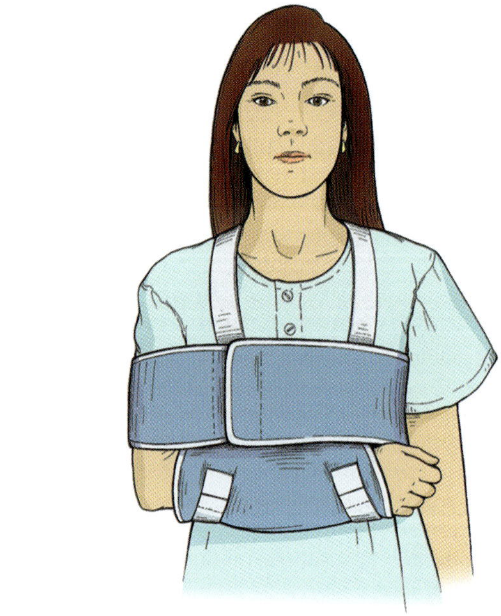

The shoulder immobilizer is used for most proximal humerus fractures and shoulder injuries. It may be removed for showering and range-of-motion exercises and is easily reapplied by the patient.

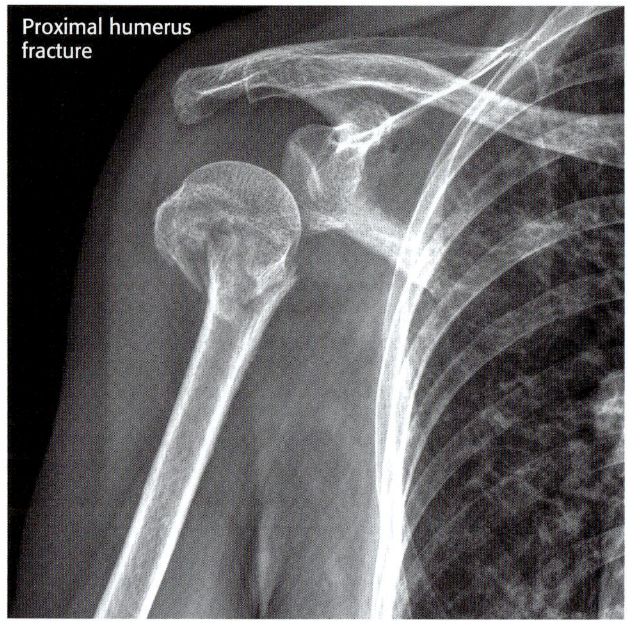

Proximal humerus fractures are common injuries in the elderly, especially after a fall. A shoulder sling is the immobilization device of choice.

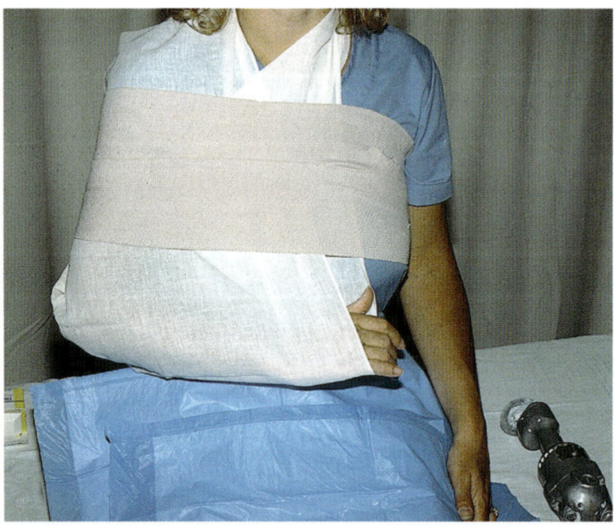

An elastic bandage and sling provide similar shoulder immobilization. Note that the wrist is supported by the slings.

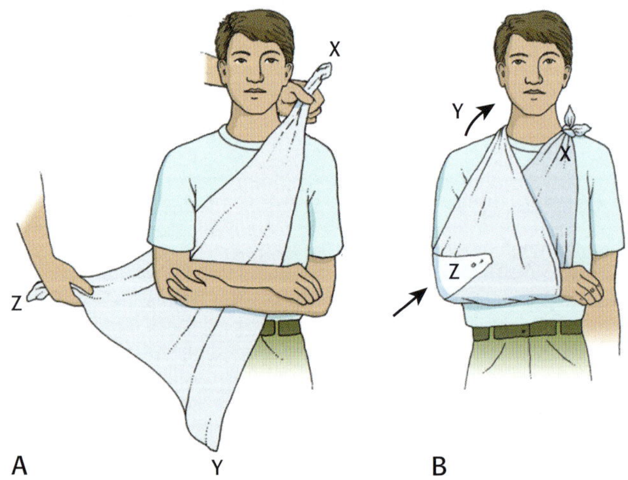

A, Stepwise application of a triangular muslin sling. (1) Place tip *X* over the uninjured shoulder. (2) Bring tip *Y* over the injured shoulder to enclose the arm. (3) Draw tip *Z* around the front and pin. **B,** Completed triangular muslin sling. (*Note*: When applying a sling it is important to have adequate support of the wrist and hand. A sling that is too short will allow the wrist and hand to hang down [ulnar deviate] and can result in hand edema and ulnar nerve injury.)

Fig. 51.19 Shoulder slings.

Anterior-Posterior Splint

Indications. An anterior splint is never used by itself, but it can augment a posterior splint to create a bivalve effect (see Fig. 51.23). Use it for serious fractures and soft tissue injuries of the ankle.

Construction. Cut a piece of plaster several centimeters shorter than the one used for the posterior splint, but as this splint does not bear weight, only 8 to 10 layers are required.

Application. Position the patient and apply padding as described for a posterior splint. After the wet posterior splint has been applied, place the anterior splint over the anterior aspect of the ankle and foreleg parallel to the posterior splint. Hold the two in place with elastic bandages as described earlier for a posterior splint alone. An assistant is needed to apply an anterior-posterior splint because it is extremely difficult to hold both splints in place while wrapping the elastic bandages.

Knee Immobilizer

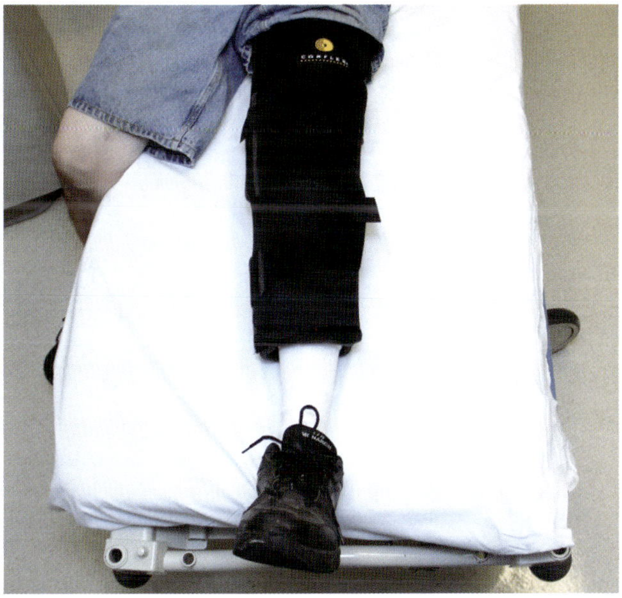

Application

Choose the appropriate-size knee immobilizer for the patient. The tapered end should be distal to the knee. The splints simply wrap around the leg (and can be applied over clothing) and are secured with Velcro straps.

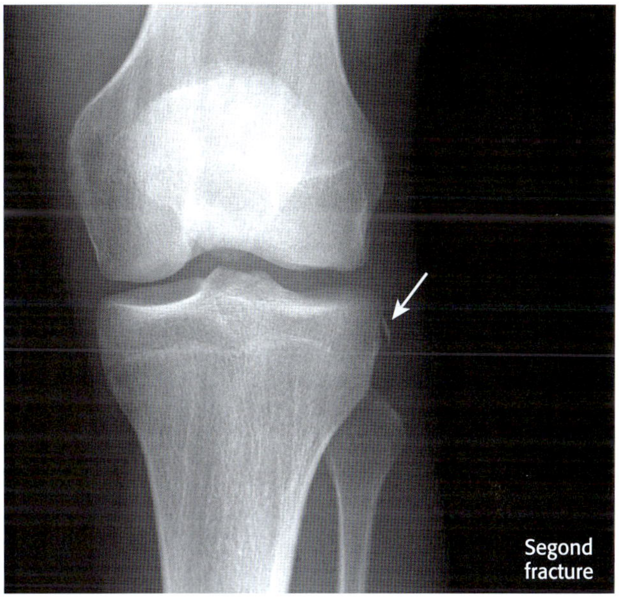

Indications

Ligamentous and soft tissue injuries of the knee.

Above, a *Segond fracture* is demonstrated. Note the small bony avulsion fracture on the lateral aspect of the tibial plateau. Although at first glance this appears to be a rather innocuous injury, a Segond fracture is highly associated with tears of the anterior cruciate ligament. This patient should be treated with a knee immobilizer until orthopedic follow-up can be arranged.

Fig. 51.20 Knee immobilizer.

Once secured, carefully mold both splints over the instep and ankle joint.

U-Splint (Stirrup Splint)

See Video 51.11.

Indications. Use a U-splint or stirrup splint (Fig. 51.24) primarily for injuries to the ankle. It functions like a posterior splint, and either one provides satisfactory ankle immobilization. In one study that compared these splints in normal volunteers, the U-splint allowed less plantar flexion and broke less often with plantar flexion than did the posterior splint.[19] In addition, because it actually covers the malleoli, a U-splint may protect the medial and lateral ligaments from further injury better than a posterior splint can.

Construction. Construct a U-splint of 4- or 6-inch-wide plaster strips. The splint passes under the plantar surface of the foot from the calcaneus to the metatarsal heads and extends up the medial and lateral sides of the foreleg to just below the level of the fibular head.

Application. Position the patient and pad the extremity as described for a posterior splint. Lay the wet plaster across the plantar surface of the foot between the calcaneus and the metatarsal heads with the sides extending up the lateral and medial aspects of the foreleg. Secure it in place with 4-inch elastic bandages. Wrap the elastic bandage around the extremity starting at the metatarsal heads and continuing around the ankle in a figure-of-eight configuration. Once the ankle has been wrapped, use another 4- or 6-inch elastic bandage to secure the remainder of the splint in place. Carefully mold the splint around the malleoli. The plaster may overlap on the anterior aspect of the ankle; this overlap does not interfere with the splint's ability to accommodate further swelling. Note that if a U-splint is combined with a posterior splint, apply the posterior splint first.

Walking Boots

Indications. Use a walking boot (e.g., CAM Walker Boot) for the treatment of moderate to severe soft tissue injuries of the ankle, including second- and third-degree sprains (Fig. 51.25A).[20] In addition, many orthopedic surgeons use it for isolated, nondisplaced lateral malleolar fractures.[21] A walking boot provides a degree of immobilization similar to that of a U-splint but is easier to remove for bathing and dressing, and the Velcro straps allow adjustment for edema.

Refer patients in a walking boot for follow-up with an appropriate specialist. Advise them of the importance of partial or non–weight bearing as indicated by the type and degree of injury. When cleared by the follow-up physician, a walking boot allows easy transition to full weight bearing. Studies have shown that rapid mobilization after ankle

Posterior Knee Splint

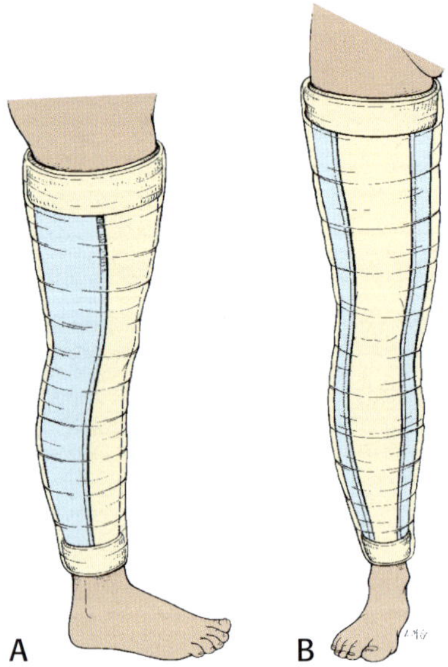

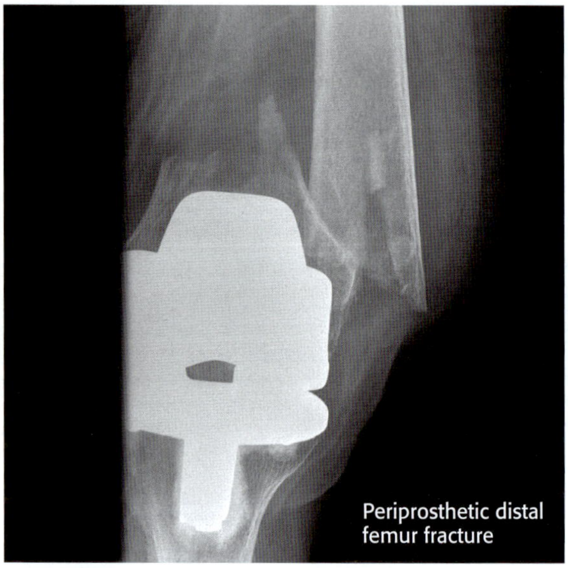

Application

A, Extend the posterior knee splint from just below the buttocks crease to approximately 2 to 3 cm above the malleoli.

B, Alternatively, place two parallel splints along each side of the leg and foreleg to create a bivalve effect. Although this variation is more difficult to apply, it may provide better immobilization of the lateral and medial collateral ligaments.

Indications

Angulated fractures around the knee (shown above)
Temporary immobilization of injuries prior to operative repair
Knee injuries in patients with extremities too large for a knee immobilizer

The knee immobilizer has largely replaced the posterior knee splint in modern emergency department practice.

Fig. 51.21 Posterior knee splint.

injuries improves functional outcome and reduces disability time.[7]

Application. Walking boots come in a variety of sizes from extra small to extra large, depending on the manufacturer. The boot should fit comfortably with the patient's calcaneus snugly in the heel of the boot and the patient's toes close to but not extending over the front edge of the boot. Once the appropriate size has been determined, place the patient's bare foot and ankle into the boot, and adjust the Velcro straps for a secure, but comfortable fit.

Semirigid Orthosis

Indications. In patients with lateral ankle sprains associated with a stable joint, a functional brace with early mobilization is frequently more comfortable and results in earlier return to normal function than complete immobilization in a plaster splint or cast (see Fig. 51.25B).[7] Consequently, functional bracing with early mobilization has become the treatment of choice in most EDs. However, it should be pointed out that there is no documented difference in long-term outcome between the two methods of treatment.

Application. Most functional ankle braces resemble a U-splint with air bladders (Aircast, Inc.) or foam padding (DeRoyal, Inc.) for cushioning the malleoli. The braces are secured about the ankle with Velcro straps. The device can be worn within the patient's shoe over a sock and helps eliminate ankle instability.

Hard Shoe (Cast or Reese Shoe)

Indications. Use a hard shoe to help reduce pain on ambulation in patients with fractures or soft tissue injuries of the foot. This device can also be used over a splint or cast to allow partial weight bearing. A hard shoe is commonly used for fractured toes that have been buddy taped.

Application. If a cast shoe is going to be used for a patient with a fractured toe, first buddy-tape the injured digit to the adjacent toe (Fig. 51.26). After this is done, the patient can slip the hard shoe on like a sandal. Fasten the shoe with ties or Velcro straps.

Ankle Wraps and Bandages

There are no data supporting the routine use of ankle wraps for simple sprains, but some pain relief may be afforded by a proper wrap. Some type of temporary immobilization is commonly used in the ED and usually requested and expected by patients. For minor ankle injuries, a simple elastic (Ace) bandage can be applied in a figure-of-eight configuration. Apply the wrap to give only lateral support with minimal compression. It should not be tight enough to impair venous drainage, a common problem when patients apply their own elastic wraps (see Fig. 51.4).

An Unna boot placed over Webril is an alternative to a simple elastic bandage (see Fig. 51.25C). The Unna boot is constructed from a semisolid paste roll that hardens as it dries. Apply an Unna boot in a figure-of-eight configuration, similar to a simple elastic bandage. Once in place, wrap the ankle with

Posterior Ankle Splint

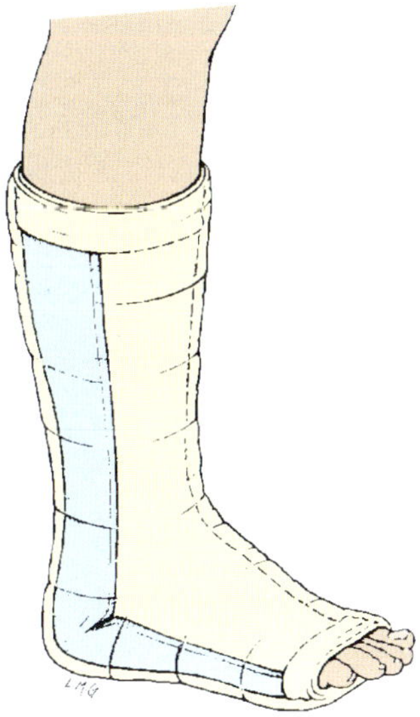

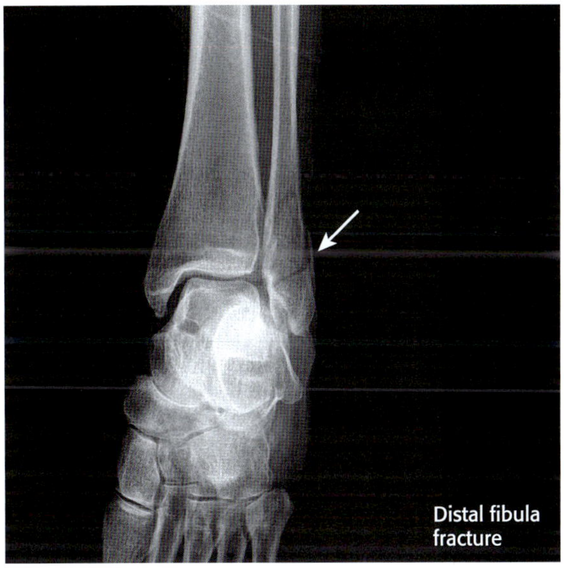

Application

Extend the splint from the plantar surface of the great toe (or metatarsal heads) along the posterior surface of the foreleg to the level of the fibular head. The ankle should be at a 90-degree angle.

Indications

Fractures of the distal ends of the fibula and tibia (shown above)
Severe ankle sprains
Reduced ankle dislocations

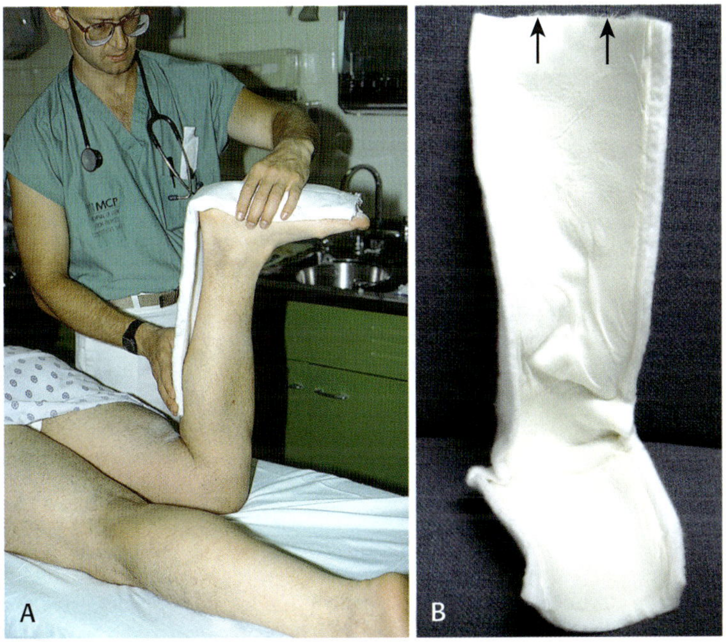

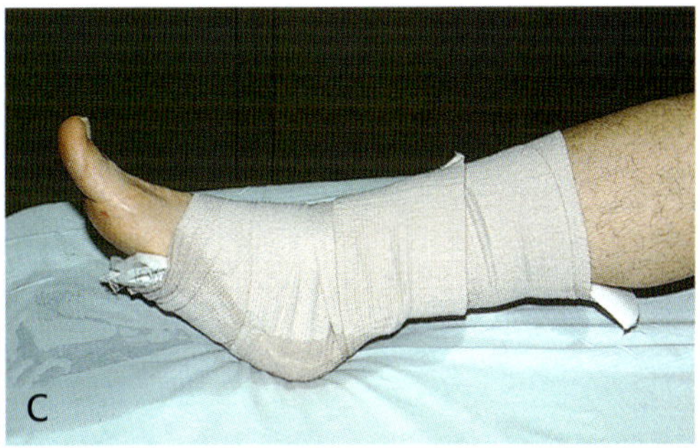

A, Apply the splint with the patient prone and the knee bent to 90 degrees, thereby relaxing the calf muscles. Position the ankle at 90 degrees so that the foot is flat for partial weight bearing. **B,** This is an unacceptable fiberglass splint. Note the very sharp frayed fiberglass edges *(arrows)* and the multiple internal ridges and folds that will produce soft tissue trauma when worn. **C,** Three things are wrong with this posterior ankle splint: (1) It does not extend distally enough to support the entire foot. (2) The ankle is not maintained at a 90-degree angle. (3) The edges and ankle area are not molded or protected. Overall, the splint is sloppy and ineffective.

Fig. 51.22 Posterior ankle splint. Note unacceptable splints in parts B and C.

roller gauze or an elastic bandage. The entire dressing can be cut off by the patient at home.

Soft Cast

Indications. A soft cast is basically a modified Jones compression dressing for the ankle. Use it for minor ligamentous and soft tissue injuries of the foot and ankle that do not require prolonged or complete immobilization. A soft cast can help reduce the pain and swelling often associated with mild ankle sprains, and it gives support for early weight bearing.

Construction. Make the soft cast of 3- or 4-inch Webril and elastic bandages.

Application. Place the patient in a supine position with the foot and ankle extending off the end of the stretcher. Alternatively, ask an assistant to elevate the leg or place pillows under the knee and foreleg. Wrap the ankle and foot with five to seven layers of Webril starting at the metatarsal heads and continuing around the ankle in a figure-of-eight configuration. Extend the Webril 5 cm to 7 cm above the malleoli

Anterior-Posterior Ankle Splint

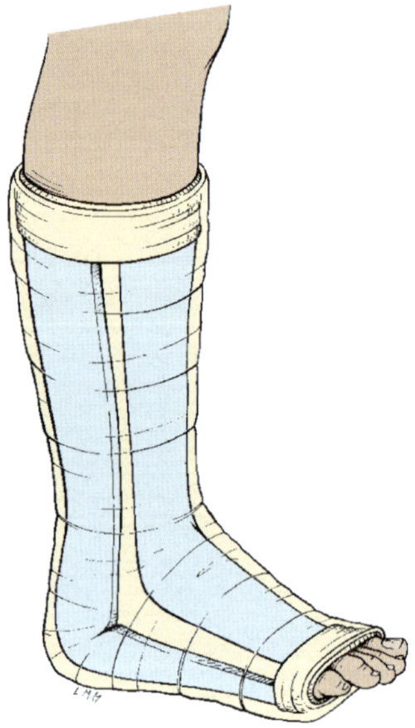

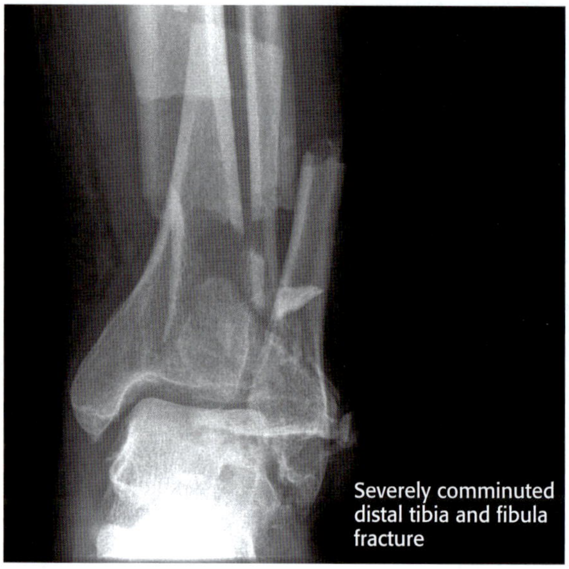

Application

Apply the posterior splint as described in Fig. 51.20.

For the anterior portion, begin on the dorsal surface of the foot at the level of the metatarsophalangeal joints. Extend the splint along the anterior portion of the foreleg, to the same height as the posterior splint. Maintain the ankle at a 90-degree angle.

Indications

Serious fractures and soft tissue injuries of the ankle.

The anterior portion of the splint is never used by itself; it is always used to augment the immobilization provided by the posterior ankle splint.

Fig. 51.23 Anterior-posterior ankle splint.

and overlap each turn by 25% to 50% of its width. After the Webril is in place, wrap an elastic bandage around the foot and ankle in a similar fashion. Additional layers of Webril and elastic bandages are seldom required. A cast shoe can be used with this dressing.

COMPLICATIONS OF SPLINTS

Ischemia

A compartment syndrome (see Chapter 55) leading to ischemic injury and ultimately to a Volkmann ischemic contracture is the most worrisome complication of cylindrical casts. Although the risk for ischemia is drastically reduced with splinting, Webril or elastic bandages can cause significant constriction. To reduce the likelihood of constriction occurring, do not pull the elastic bandage excessively tight. If the patient has a high-risk injury, cut the Webril lengthwise before the plaster is applied. Stress the importance of elevation, no weight bearing, and application of cold packs, and carefully review the signs and symptoms of vascular compromise with every patient. All patients whose injuries have the potential for significant swelling or loss of vascular integrity should receive follow-up care in the first 24 to 48 hours. *Never ignore complaints of increasing pain under a splint.* Patients with splint-related discomfort must be reevaluated clinically and should not be treated with a telephone prescription for opioid analgesics (Fig. 51.27).

Heat Injury

Fiberglass splints produce minimal heat when drying, but plaster generates considerable heat as it hardens. Many clinicians are unaware of the potential for drying plaster to produce second-degree burns.[15] Thermal injury can occur with both cylindrical casts and plaster splints. Some clinicians have reported a higher incidence of burns with the use of plaster splints, although the reasons for this are unclear.[22,23] Box 51.4 lists factors that can increase the amount of heat produced during plaster recrystallization. Their effects are additive, and this fact should be taken into account when applying a splint. For example, if 15 sheets of plaster are needed for strength in a particular splint, one should not increase the heat production further by using extra-fast drying plaster or reusing warm dip water. To avoid plaster burns, use only 8 to 12 sheets of plaster when possible, use fresh dip water with a temperature near 24°C, and never wrap the extremity in a sheet or pillow during the setting process. Peak temperatures usually occur between 5 and 15 minutes after plaster wetting.

The patient should be warned that the hardening process produces warmth. The heat of drying may produce pain in patients with hemophilia-related hemarthroses. Splinting these patients may require that the plaster splint be placed only long enough to verify proper fit; the splint is then reapplied after setting (and cooling) of the plaster. If any patient complains of significant burning while the plaster is drying, *do not ignore this complaint*! Immediately remove the splint, and promptly cool the area with cold packs or cool water. Patients

U-Splint (or Stirrup/Sugar-Tong Splint)

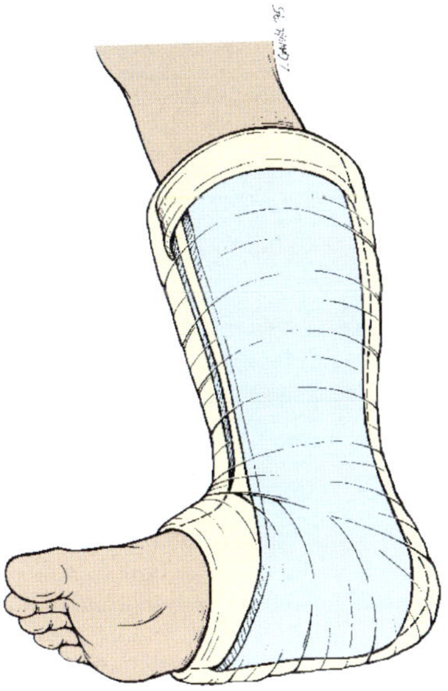

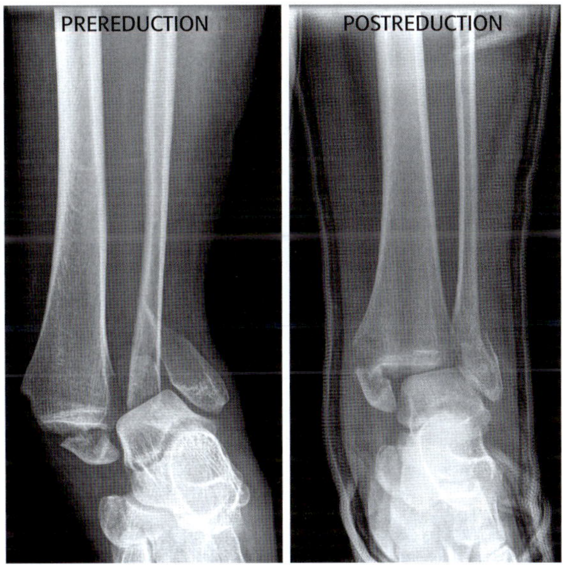

Application

Apply the splint under the plantar surface of the foot and extend it up the medial and lateral sides of the foreleg to just below the level of the fibular head. Keep the ankle at a 90-degree angle.

For immobilization of the knee, extend the sides of the splint proximally to the groin to create a long leg splint.

Indications

Injuries of the ankle, including:
- Fractures of the distal tibia and fibula
- Postreduction stabilization of ankle dislocations (above)

The U-splint can be combined with the posterior ankle splint to provide both anterior-posterior and medial-lateral stability.

Fig. 51.24 U-splint (also referred to as a stirrup or sugar-tong splint).

with vascular insufficiency or sensory deficits (e.g., diabetic neuropathy, stroke) are at high risk for plaster burns and require close observation during the drying process.

Pressure Sores

Pressure sores are an uncommon complication of short-term splinting (Fig. 51.28).[24] They can result from stockinette wrinkles, irregular wadding of Webril, incorrectly padded or unpadded bony prominences, irregular splint ends, plaster ridges, or indentations produced from using the fingers rather than the palms to smooth and mold the wet plaster. Attention to detail during padding and splinting reduces the incidence of pressure sores. However, whenever a patient complains of a persistent pain or burning sensation under any part of a splint, remove the splint and inspect the symptomatic area closely. The padding incorporated in premade plaster and fiberglass splints is generally all that is needed for safe short-term splinting. However, the life of a splint applied in the ED may be longer than intended by the clinician; therefore it is prudent to err on the side of additional padding when placing splints on patients who may overuse the splint, such as those who will not use crutches, or for those who may not have ready access to follow-up.

Infection

Bacterial and fungal infections can occur under a splint.[25] Infection is more common in the presence of an open wound but may occur with intact skin or in a skin lesion produced by prolonged splinting. The moist, warm, and dark environment created by the splint is an excellent nidus for infection. Toxic shock syndrome has been rarely reported from a staphylococcal skin infection that clandestinely developed under a splint or cast. In addition, it has been shown that bacteria can multiply in slowly drying plaster. To avoid infection, clean and debride all wounds before splint application, and use clean, fresh tap water for plaster wetting. If necessary, apply a removable splint that allows periodic wound inspection or local wound care.

Dermatitis

Occasionally, a rash develops under a plaster cast or splint.[26–30] Allergy to plaster is exceedingly rare, but there are several reports of contact dermatitis when formaldehyde and melamine resins are added to the plaster.[28,29] The rash is usually pruritic with weeping papular or vesicular lesions. Because these resins are unnecessary for ED splints, their use should be avoided whenever possible. Dermatitis has also been reported with the use of fiberglass splinting material.[31]

Pruritus

Itching under a cast can be problematic. Patients, especially children, use various objects such as pencils, coat hangers, or forks to get to the itch. This can cause skin maceration and possible infection, or a foreign body can be left under the cast (Fig. 51.29).

Joint Stiffness

Some degree of joint stiffness is an invariable consequence of immobilization (Fig. 51.30). It can range in severity from mild

Splints for Ankle Sprains

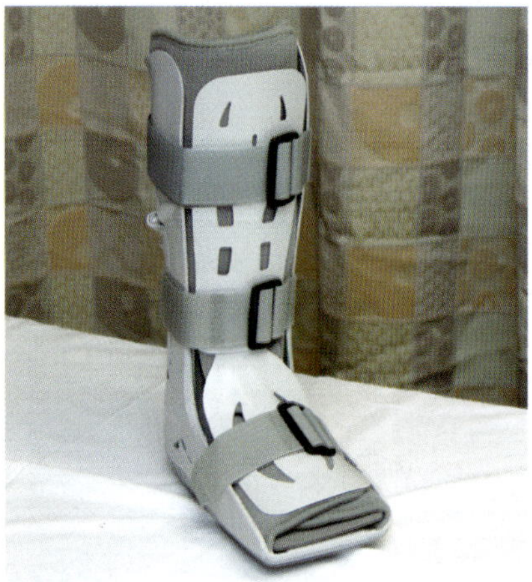

A walking boot can be used for the treatment of moderate to severe soft tissue injuries of the ankle, including second- and third-degree sprains and isolated, nondisplaced lateral malleolar fractures. A walking boot provides a similar degree of immobilization as a U-splint but is easier to remove for bathing and dressing, and the Velcro straps allow adjustment for edema.

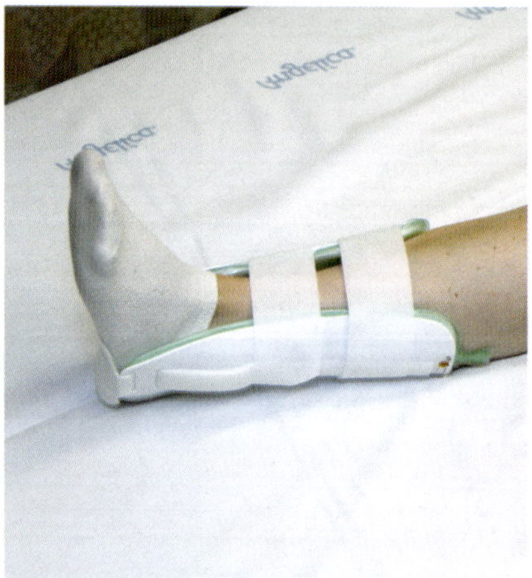

Prefabricated semirigid orthoses such as the Aircast (pictured above) are often used for patients with minor ankle sprains. The Aircast can be worn inside the patient's shoe to provide early mobility along with increased ankle stability.

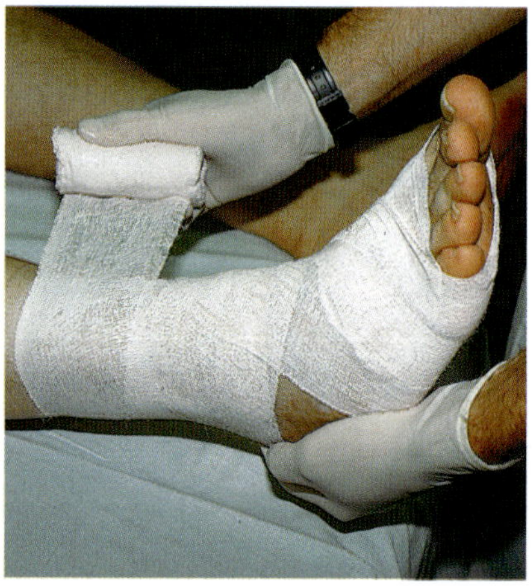

The Unna boot or an Ace wrap provides effective immobilization of an ankle soft tissue injury. The Unna boot is applied from a semisolid paste roll. The wrap is then covered with gauze or an elastic bandage. The entire dressing can be cut off by the patient at home. For similar short-term immobilization without plaster, a modified Jones dressing can be used. Copious Webril is wrapped around the ankle and foot and covered with an elastic bandage. A cast shoe can be used with this dressing.

Fig. 51.25 Splints for ankle sprains.

Hard Shoe Splint

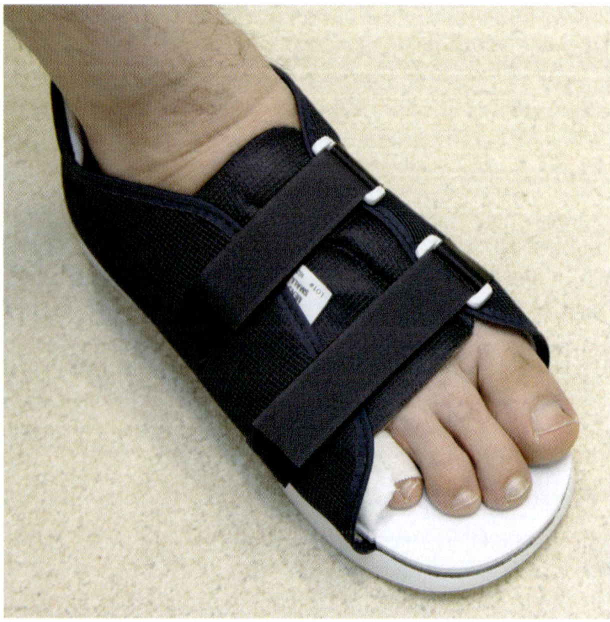

Indications

Reduction of ambulatory pain in patients with fractures or soft tissue injuries of the foot
Used over a splint to allow partial weight bearing

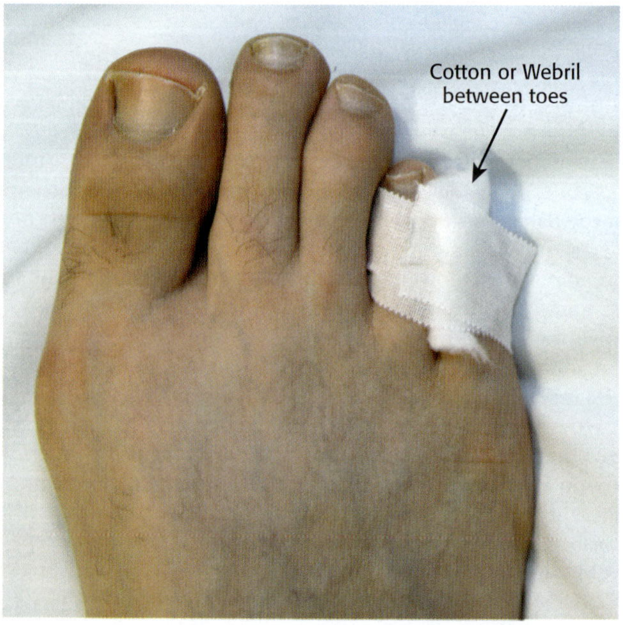

If the shoe is going to be used for a fractured toe, first buddy-tape the toe to the adjacent digit. Remember to place a piece of cotton or Webril between the toes to prevent skin maceration.

Fig. 51.26 Hard shoe splint.

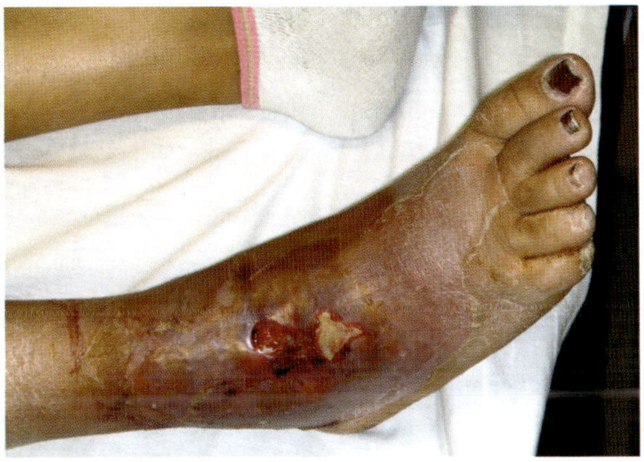

Fig. 51.27 If a patient complains of a cast being too tight, it probably is. The cast must be removed to inspect the area for infection or other problems. Complaints of pain under this cast were incorrectly met with a phone call to suggest elevation and a call-in prescription for narcotics.

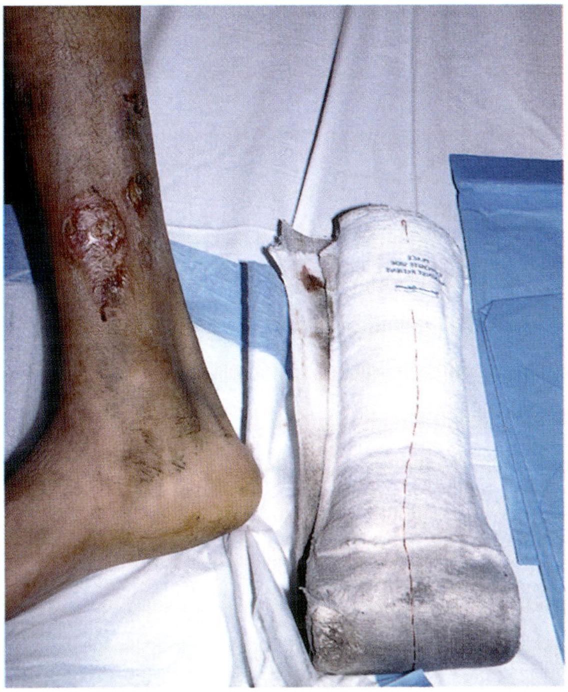

Fig. 51.28 The problem with this splint is that it was intended to be used for only a few days, but the patient wore it and walked on it for 3 weeks. Note the resultant full-thickness skin loss. No padding was used under the premade splint. Skin grafting was eventually required.

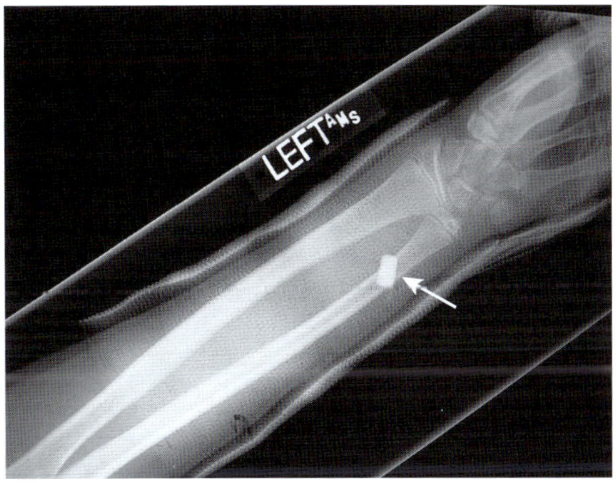

Fig. 51.29 This 9-year-old tried to scratch an itch under his splint with a pencil and the eraser fell off *(arrow)*. This resulted in skin irritation and infection, requiring removal of the splint.

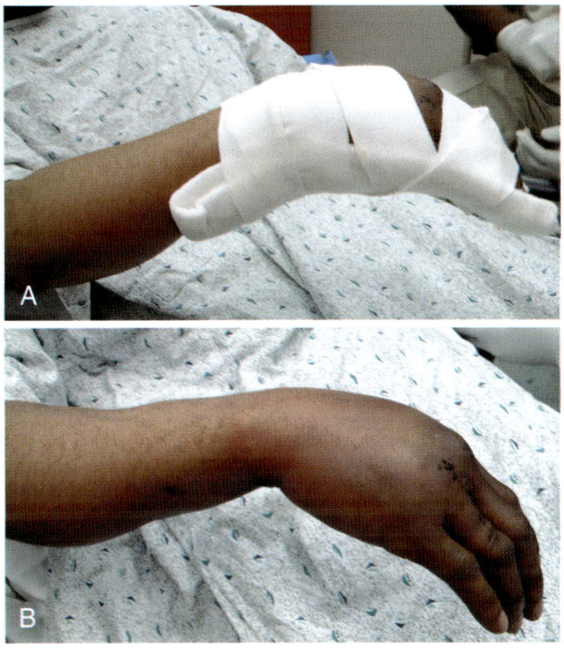

Fig. 51.30 (A) Never splint an injured wrist in flexion even though the patient prefers this position. (B) When immobilizing an infected human bite, this splint was not held in position until hardened, and the patient reflexively flexed the wrist.

to incapacitating and can result in transient, prolonged, or in some cases, permanent loss of function. Stiffness appears to be worse with prolonged periods of immobilization, in older patients, and in patients with preexisting joint diseases such as rheumatoid arthritis or osteoarthritis. Thus splints should be left on for only the time necessary for adequate healing. Table 51.3 lists several injuries that commonly require splinting, along with some suggestions for length of immobilization. Fractures, dislocations, or other conditions that require prolonged immobilization (>7 days) should have orthopedic follow-up. Tell patients that a splint is only a short-term device and that prolonged immobilization can be detrimental. For minor injuries, suggest that patients use their own judgment about when to remove the splint, but a definite end point should be set.

Cast Pain

See Video 51.12. Cast-related pain is a common complaint that brings patients to the ED. Because of the potential for ischemia with circumferential casts, fully investigate all complaints, and rule out vascular compromise. If a patient states that a cast is too tight, it probably is (see Fig. 51.27). Do not prescribe narcotics for cast pain until a properly fitting (i.e., one that is not too tight) cast has been ensured.

Perform a detailed history and physical examination on all patients complaining of cast pain. The nature and onset of the pain are of particular importance. A dull, nonspecific pain

TABLE 51.3 Suggested Length of Immobilization for Conditions That Frequently Require Splinting

TYPE OF CONDITION	IMMOBILIZATION (DAYS)
Contusions	1–3
Abrasions	1–3
Soft tissue lacerations	5–7
Tendon lacerations	Variable[a]
Tendinitis	5–7
Puncture wounds and bites	3–4
Deep space infections and cellulitis	3–5
Mild sprains	5–7
Fractures and severe sprains	Variable[b]

[a]Considerable controversy surrounds the length of immobilization for tendon lacerations, and duration is therefore best left to the consultant surgeon.
[b]Usually requires prolonged immobilization, which is best determined by an orthopedic surgeon.

that has worsened gradually since the time of injury may be the only clue to an early compartment syndrome (see Chapter 55). A sudden onset of throbbing pain associated with swelling and redness suggests a possible deep venous thrombosis. In both these cases, rapid intervention is the key to decreasing morbidity and mortality. During the physical examination, pay particular attention to areas of tenderness and the effect of active and passive movement on the severity of the pain.

With a compartment syndrome, tenderness over the involved compartment is a common finding, and stretching or contracting ischemic muscle elicits significant pain. Evaluate for the presence and quality of distal pulses, the amount of edema fluid present, distal sensation, capillary refill, and color and temperature of the digits. The five Ps (pain, pallor, paresthesias, paralysis, and pulselessness) are pathognomonic for ischemia. Unfortunately, they seldom occur simultaneously, and their presence together is usually a late finding that carries a poor prognosis. Hence, the emergency clinician must maintain a high index of suspicion for possible ischemia and remove the cast if any possibility of vascular compromise exists. Almost any cast can be bivalved, with Webril and stockinette also cut, and the bivalved cast reapplied after inspection without significant loss of short-term immobilization.

Cast Removal

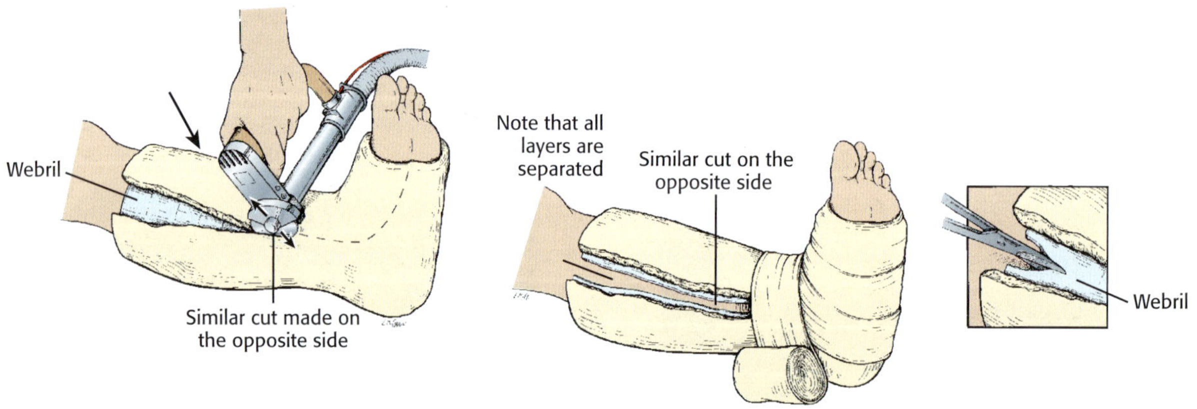

The cast saw vibrates; it does not rotate. It will not cut the patient. Note that the underlying Webril padding is cut to relieve pressure but is not removed.

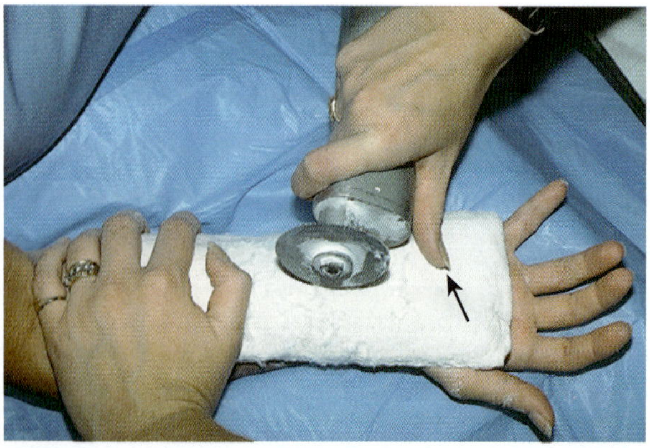

The blade is controlled by placing the thumb *(arrow)* on the splint and lowering the saw blade to the plaster. The blade is raised and lowered for each cut; it is not drawn across the plaster like a knife.

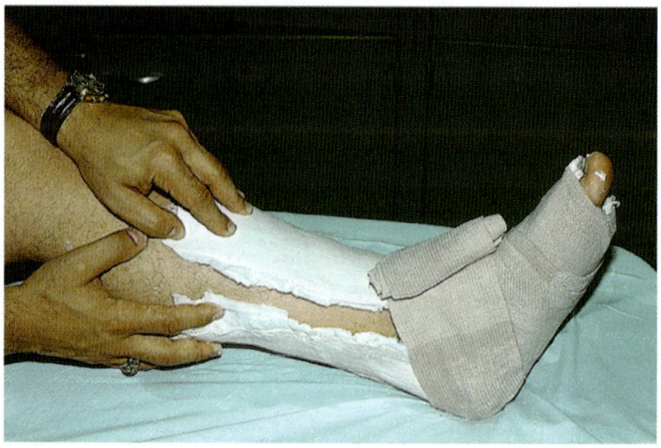

This cast was too tight, and it was therefore bivalved from calf to forefoot with a cast saw. After separation of the edges of the cut cast, the anterior and posterior components were secured in place with an elastic bandage. A bivalved cast provides temporary immobilization equal to that of an intact cast. Extra padding can be used to protect the skin from the cut edges.

Fig. 51.31 Cast removal.

To loosen a cast, use an oscillating cast saw to cut along the medial and lateral aspects of the cast (Fig. 51.31). This is called *bivalving the cast*, and it allows the halves to be spread and reapplied in a less constricting manner while still maintaining proper immobilization. To use an oscillating power saw, proceed in a series of downward cutting movements facilitated by wrist supination, and remove the blade between cuts to prevent it from getting hot enough to burn the skin. This is particularly important if synthetic material has been used in the cast. Additionally, do not allow the blade to slide along the skin, and never use the saw on unpadded plaster. In an apprehensive patient, demonstrate that the cast saw blade only vibrates (it does not turn) and that it does not cut the skin.

After the medial and lateral sides of the cast are completely cut through, separate the two halves with a cast spreader, and cut the padding lengthwise with scissors. Note that the padding may also contribute to the pressure, so once the plaster is bivalved, compression from padding must also be relieved. This may be sufficient to relieve early ischemia if the problem is simple postinjury swelling, but both the padding and the cast can be totally removed to inspect the injured area if necessary. If ischemia cannot be ruled out, measure compartment pressures (see Chapter 55) and obtain an orthopedic consultation.

If vascular integrity is established and no other problems are found, replace the bivalved cast. First, pad the extremity in the usual manner with fresh Webril. Line the cut ends of the bivalved cast with white adhesive tape, and replace the cast around the extremity. Finally, secure the cast in place with elastic bandages.

If plaster sores are causing the patient discomfort, consult the clinician who placed the cast. In some cases, additional padding is all that is needed, but in others, a window should be cut out over the problem area. Because pressure sores can lead to significant tissue necrosis, refer the patient for follow-up care within 24 hours.

If the patient's problem is plaster (or, more likely, resin) dermatitis, administer topical or oral steroids and antihistamines. Provide therapy in concert with an orthopedic surgeon because the patient may require admission for other forms of immobilization until the cast can be replaced. In mild cases, changing the cast or splint and using antihistamines for symptomatic relief may suffice. All patients should receive close follow-up, and if the condition does not improve, the cast must be removed.

CONCLUSION

Splinting is an important means of temporary fracture immobilization and provides protection and comfort for a variety of soft tissue injuries. The clinician should be aware of potential complications that can occur with improper splint application, including ischemia, thermal injury, and pressure sores. Use proper technique to minimize the risk for these adverse outcomes. When ischemia is suspected, the emergency clinician should also be facile in the release of circumferential cast and splint material.

REFERENCES ARE AVAILABLE AT Elsevier eBooks+

CHAPTER 52

Podiatric Procedures

Douglas L. McGee

COMMON NONTRAUMATIC CONDITIONS OF THE FOOT

Many painful conditions of the foot are chronic and do not usually require definitive treatment in the emergency department (ED); however, patients are often seen with common conditions that require evaluation and proper referral. To accomplish this, the clinician must be cognizant of basic podiatric conditions, including painful lesions over bony prominences, heel pain, foot infections, and pain on the plantar surface of the foot.

Footpad Use

Footpads redistribute pressure over an inflamed, tender area of the foot. The particular type of footpad and its placement depend on the condition being treated (Fig. 52.1). Commercially available aperture footpads are recommended for the temporary relief of warts, corns, hyperkeratoses, and bunions. Human papilloma virus introduced into the plantar surface of the foot may produce a painful hyperkeratotic lesion, commonly referred to as a *plantar wart*, on the sole of the foot. A simple callus may be painful and result in the formation of a "hard corn" when formed over the bony prominence of a digit. Once recognized, and after other conditions are ruled out, definitive care of these lesions is rarely indicated in the ED.

When tenderness is elicited over more than one metatarsal head, the diagnosis is metatarsalgia. Pain that is progressively worse while walking but relieved by rest, often beneath the second or third metatarsal head, is typical in this case. A pad placed under the first metatarsal head to raise the second and third metatarsals may provide some relief.

A bunion develops when unbalanced forces applied to the first metatarsal cause lateral displacement of the distal end of the hallux. Bunions typically form in females wearing heeled shoes with narrow toe boxes. The patient may complain of numbness over the distal, medial aspect of the first toe as a result of compression of the terminal branch of the medial dorsal cutaneous nerve. The mechanical forces that precipitate bunion formation may also cause other painful conditions, including intermetatarsal neuromas, hammertoes, ingrown toenails, corns, and calluses. Bursitis may develop over the medial bony prominence of the first metatarsophalangeal (MTP) joint. Self-adherent bunion pads placed over the first MTP joint may provide temporary relief (Fig. 52.2). In the ED, treating patients with these common disorders includes analgesics and footpads, followed by referral for definitive care. Patients should also be instructed to avoid wearing offending shoes. In males and postmenopausal females, gout should be considered when evaluating pain over the first MTP joint, particularly in the presence of other signs of inflammation (e.g., redness, swelling, warmth).

Heel Pain Syndromes

Bony spurs on the plantar surface of the calcaneus, retrocalcaneal bursitis, calcaneal apophysitis, and other conditions may cause heel pain. Rest, nonsteroidal antiinflammatory drugs (NSAIDs), modification of physical activities or shoe wear, footpads, and orthoses are the optimal treatments for these conditions. Some clinicians also inject anesthetics or steroids for these conditions, but these treatments tend to be done by foot specialists who can follow the patient.

Heel spur pain can be quite bothersome and chronic or recurrent. This condition is not easily remedied in the ED, and after other conditions are ruled out, such as an unexpected foreign body (FB), minimal intervention with podiatric referral is often the best course of action. Patients typically have pain over the medial border of the plantar aspect of the calcaneus. The pain gradually worsens over a period of months. A bony prominence that begins as periostitis extends from the medial aspect of the calcaneal tuberosity into the central plantar fascia and may be seen on radiographs. Radiographs of the calcaneus that do not demonstrate a bony spur suggest

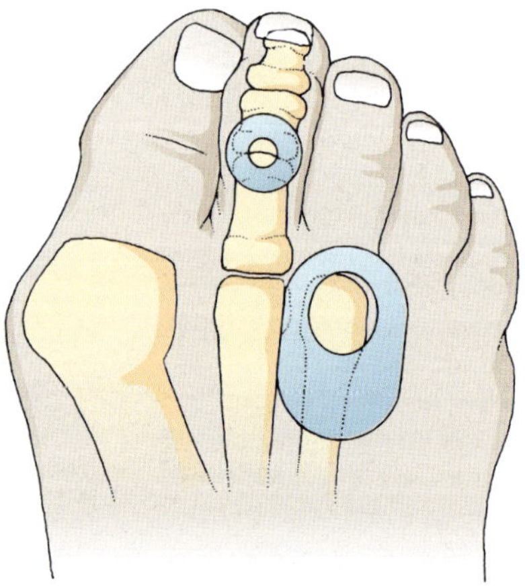

Fig. 52.1 Use of aperture pads to redistribute pressure from painful areas to surrounding structures. The center hole is placed over the lesion and the surrounding pad absorbs the friction. (Courtesy Kenneth R. Walker, DPM.)

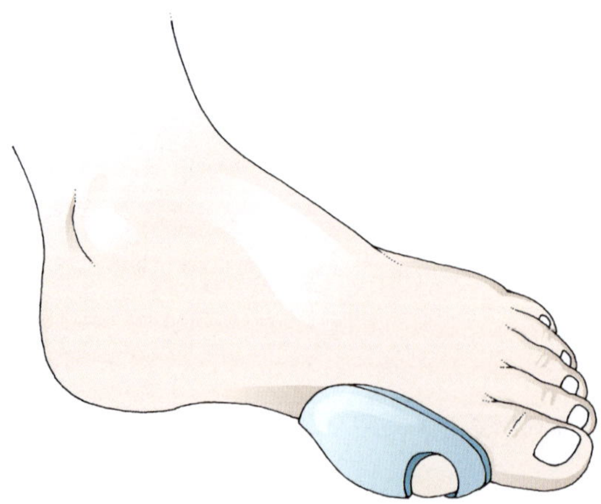

Fig. 52.2 Use of an adhesive bunion pad. The hole in the pad is placed over the bunion and the surrounding pad absorbs friction. (Courtesy Kenneth R. Walker, DPM.)

plantar fasciitis (see the later section "Painful Conditions of the Plantar Surface of the Foot"), even though many patients with plantar fasciitis have plantar calcaneal and Achilles spurs. Plantar calcaneal heel spurs are found in nearly 15% of the population, only 30% of whom have heel pain. Although many persons with heel spurs are asymptomatic, 75% of patients with heel pain have heel spurs. However, radiographs have little value in evaluating nontraumatic heel pain because they rarely demonstrate radiographic abnormalities that prompt additional treatment.

Shoe supports with a heel pad or cup, or a doughnut-shaped orthotic often help reduce the discomfort by redistributing weight. Few randomized controlled trials have evaluated steroid therapy; those that have do not provide substantial evidence supporting its long-term efficacy.[1] Treatment for the painful site is 10 mg to 20 mg of methylprednisolone injected into the medial aspect of the foot while avoiding the sensitive plantar surface. Some evidence suggests that injecting 25 mg of prednisolone acetate into the medial aspect of the heel provides partial pain relief at 1 month in comparison to lidocaine only, but no advantage can be detected at 3 months.[2] A short-leg walking cast may be effective in some patients with recalcitrant heel pain. There is little evidence to suggest that specific interventions aimed at reducing heel pain are superior to conservative, supportive treatment alone.

Retrocalcaneal Bursitis, Achilles Tendinopathy, and Calcaneal Apophysitis

Although retrocalcaneal bursitis and Achilles tendinopathy (formerly referred to as Achilles tendinitis) are anatomically distinct, the clinical findings are similar. Pain at the insertion of the Achilles tendon is worsened with prolonged standing or walking and is aggravated by passive or active range of motion in both conditions. Directed palpation can distinguish one entity from the other, but both are treated similarly. Tenderness of the Achilles tendon suggests tendinopathy, whereas tenderness between the tendon and the calcaneus suggests retrocalcaneal bursitis. Importantly, Achilles tendinopathy may develop spontaneously after the use of quinolone antibiotics, occasionally with rupture. The condition may occur during quinolone use or a few weeks after therapy; immediate discontinuation of the drug is recommended. Rest, elevation, ice, oral NSAIDs, heel pads, and an open-backed shoe provide relief in the majority of patients. Ten percent topical diclofenac applied to Achilles tendinopathy did not provide relief compared to placebo at 4 weeks.[3] A corticosteroid injection may provide some relief, but this treatment is best given by foot specialists who can follow the patient. Achilles tendinopathy treated with exercise and methylprednisolone acetate 40 mg injected periodically resulted in less morning or exercise pain compared with exercise and placebo injection.[4] Repeated steroid injection is associated with Achilles tendon rupture. Injection of platelet-rich plasma (PRP) as treatment for Achilles tendinopathy has gained some support among sports medicine physicians, but recently published studies have failed to demonstrate short- or long-term improvement in pain or function when PRP injection is compared with placebo.[5,6] Osteochondrosis of the posterior calcaneal apophysis, often referred to as *Sever disease*, may cause pain that is worsened by activity in children between 7 and 10 years of age. It is thought to represent an overuse syndrome in an athletically active child with tenderness in the posterior heel region.[7] Treat this self-limited condition with rest, ice, and heel pads. Radiographs are not indicated unless other diagnoses are suspected. Activity is resumed when the pain abates.

Painful Conditions of the Plantar Surface of the Foot

Plantar Fasciitis

Repeated microtrauma to the plantar aponeurosis causes pain on the plantar surface of the foot (Fig. 52.3A). Plantar fasciitis is typically unilateral and found in females who wear high-heeled shoes. The pain is maximally severe in the morning or after prolonged sitting and improves after walking, often referred to as *first-step pain*. Some patients with plantar fasciitis may also have a calcaneal heel spur, but the presence or absence of this radiographic finding is clinically irrelevant. Pain is elicited with palpation (Fig. 52.3B), toe walking, or passive stretching of the plantar aponeurosis. Frequently, this annoying condition resolves spontaneously, but resolution is slow, often taking as long as 6 to 18 months. Conservative therapy, including rest, stretching, elevation, ice, and NSAIDs, results in a satisfactory outcome after 6 to 8 weeks in nearly all patients. Pain improves over time in most patients, with or without NSAIDs, although the addition of NSAIDs appears to increase pain relief when compared with conservative treatments alone. The emergency clinician can do little to treat this chronic, distressing condition. Stretching exercises each morning and evening can be suggested (Fig. 52.3D). Night splinting to keep the foot dorsiflexed and custom orthoses made from the patient's foot impression can be very helpful but usually require referral to podiatry for proper fitting (Fig. 52.3C). Corticosteroid injection is used by some clinicians; however, its benefit remains unproved. A single injection may be warranted as supplemental therapy in resistant cases. Repeated injections of corticosteroids should be avoided and have been associated with rupture of the plantar fascia and fat pad atrophy. Some authors suggest the injection of autologous PRP when plantar fasciitis is chronic. The benefits of PRP remain unproved.[8] In a 2010 study, 50 units of botulinum toxin type A injected into the plantar fascia decreased pain in comparison to placebo but did not cure the disease.[9]

Forefoot Neuroma

A forefoot neuroma, also known as *Morton's neuroma*, is a painful condition of the plantar surface of the foot. It most commonly affects females who wear high-heeled shoes. The neuroma forms after chronic irritation to the digital sensory nerve between the metatarsals. A neuroma frequently occurs in the third interspace but may be found in the second (Fig. 52.4A). Patients report the sensation of a lump or cord in the interspace and describe paresthesia or numbness in the third or fourth toes. Direct compression plus release of the forefoot causes pain and often a "click" (*Mulder's sign*) (Fig. 52.4B). Rest, elevation, ice, and NSAIDs may result in some improvement, but surgical excision is often required.[10] Few data support the use of corticosteroid injections. In one study, less than 50% of patients with a foot neuroma had any benefit from injected corticosteroids.[10] Another study demonstrated complete or partial relief in 80% of patients injected with corticosteroids.[11] Although this study demonstrated a trend toward improved outcome when injected corticosteroids were compared with footwear modifications, corticosteroid injection therapy alone was not statistically better than footwear modification at 1 year.[11]

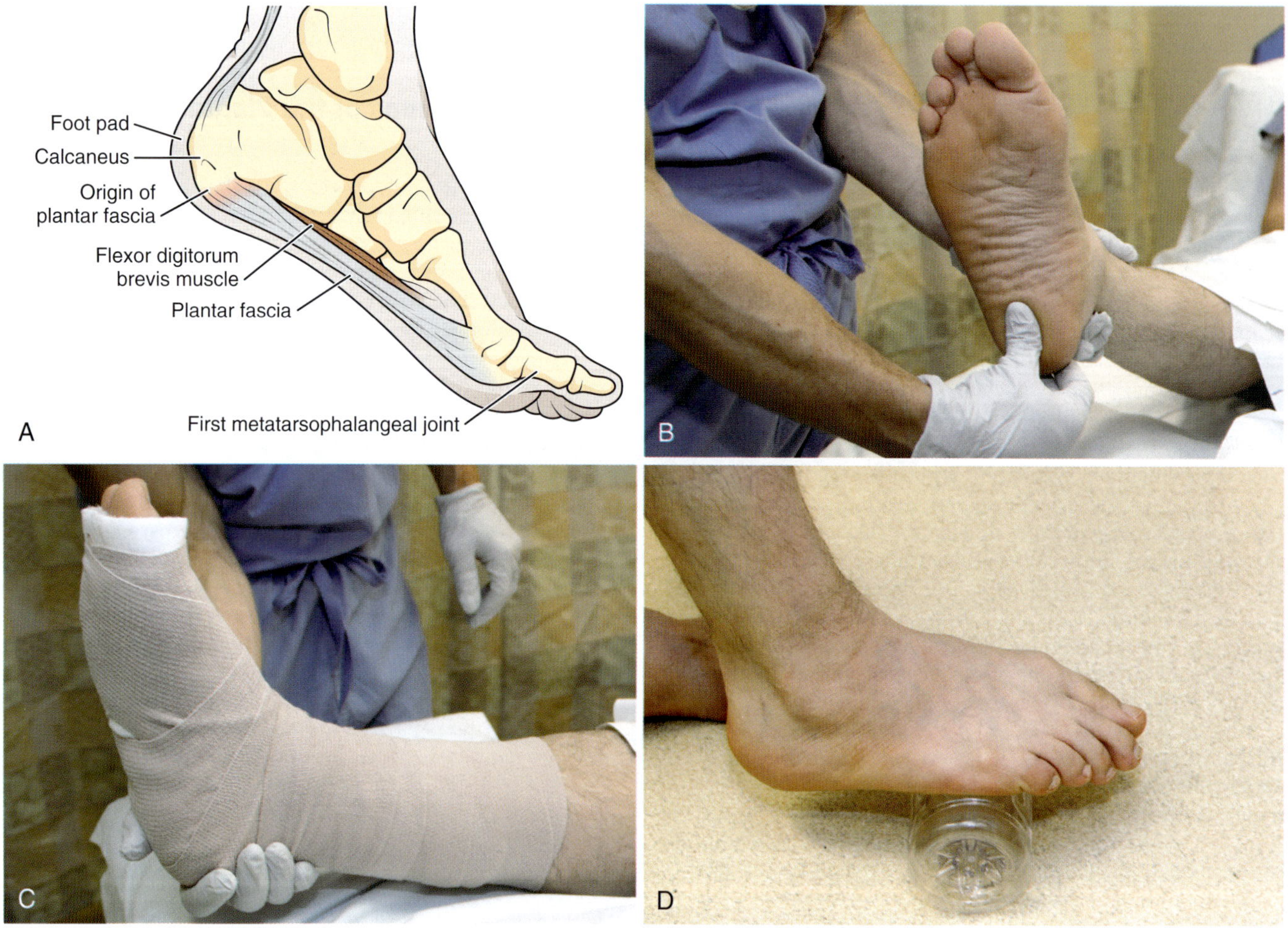

Fig. 52.3 Plantar fasciitis. (A) The plantar fascia spans the plantar aspect of the foot. The origin is the medial tubercle of the calcaneus, which is the most common site of pain. A heel spur may be seen on radiographs, but inflammation of the plantar fascia, not the spur, is the source of the pain. (B) Palpation of the tubercle of the calcaneus reproduces the pain of plantar fasciitis. (C) A posterior lower leg splint may be created for patients in the emergency department, and it is intended to be worn at night to keep the foot in a position of dorsiflexion. Referral to podiatry for custom-fit orthoses may also be beneficial. (D) Rolling the arch of the foot back and forth over a frozen water bottle will stretch the fascia and, over time, may lessen the pain of plantar fasciitis. A tennis ball can also be used.

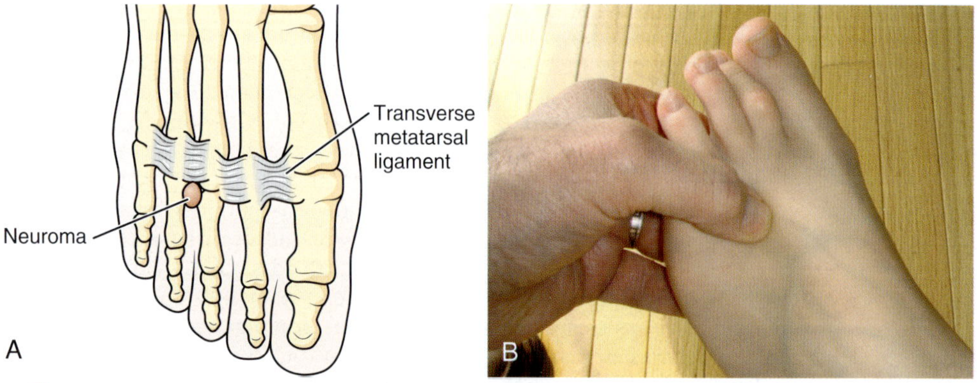

Fig. 52.4 Morton's neuroma. (A) Site of Morton's neuroma arising from a digital nerve. (B) Palpation of the distal metatarsal area may reveal pain from Morton's neuroma. Squeezing and releasing this area (not shown) can elicit pain and a clicking sensation, termed Mulder's sign.

Ganglion Cyst of the Foot

A ganglion cyst is histologically similar to the synovial sheath and contains synovial fluid. The diagnosis is easy to make when the cyst is located over a tendon on the dorsum of the foot (Fig. 52.5), but may be difficult when located among the compact structures of the plantar forefoot. A ganglion cyst usually causes edema along the involved tendon sheath. The mass should roll under the examiner's finger; a painless,

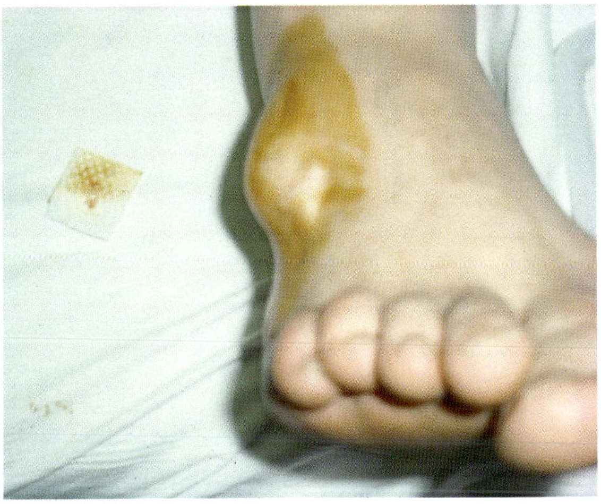

Fig. 52.5 Ganglion cysts. A small amount of gel substance was aspirated with a needle, but a cyst of this size is best totally excised surgically.

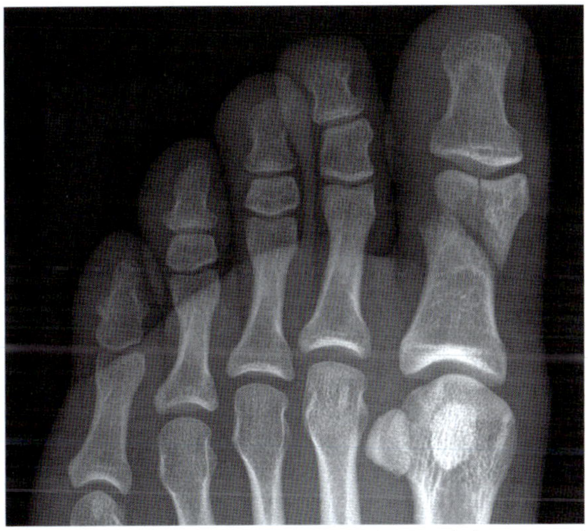

Fig. 52.6 Proper treatment of oblique displaced fractures of the proximal phalanx of the great toe includes reduction, a non–weight-bearing splint that extends beyond the great toe, and referral to a foot and ankle surgeon because surgical intervention may be required.

immovable mass suggests a soft tissue neoplasm. Painful ganglion cysts are treated by aspiration, with or without injection of a corticosteroid. After local or regional anesthesia (see Chapters 29 and 31), insert a 20-gauge needle into the cyst and withdraw yellow, thick, synovial fluid. Manually express any remaining synovial fluid after the needle is withdrawn. Corticosteroid injection is often advocated for ganglion cysts, but recurrence is common after aspiration and corticosteroid injection, as high as 57% in one study.[12] Many studies have shown that recurrence, chronic pain, neuritis, stiffness, and infection are common, even after surgical excision.[13]

TRAUMATIC CONDITIONS OF THE FOOT

Trauma to the feet and toes is common and covers a broad spectrum of injury. Lacerations, fractures, compartment syndromes, and nail bed injuries are described in other chapters of this text. Three specific injuries—toe fractures, sesamoid-bone fractures, and puncture wounds to the plantar surface of the foot—are discussed in detail here.

Toe Fractures and Fractures of the Sesamoid Bones

Emergency clinicians often treat toe fractures and can intervene to relieve the pain and encourage healing. As with any other fracture, attention to the possibility of disrupted joint cartilage, hypermobility of the fracture segments, and malposition or malunion of the fracture fragments is necessary. Fracture displacement greater than 2 mm is uncommon; reduction is rarely needed for most toe fractures. However, aggressive reduction is indicated for fractures of the proximal phalanx of the great toe because it represents the main propulsive segment of the forefoot (Fig. 52.6). A plaster cast alone without anatomic reduction is insufficient treatment. Displacement suggests axial rotation or abnormal biomechanical interaction between the hallux and its own interphalangeal or MTP joint. Stubbed great toes are common in bare-footed children. When radiographs suggest a Salter-Harris type I/II fracture, and there is a nailbed laceration, flexion deformity of the fracture site, or bleeding at the nail fold suggesting nail plate subluxation, an open fracture that may involve the physis should be considered. Oral or intravenous antibiotics, irrigation and reduction are recommended. Referral to a podiatrist or orthopedic surgeon for urgent follow-up is necessary when reduction is unsuccessful.[14]

In the acute setting, a non–weight-bearing ankle splint that extends beyond the great toe provides protection until the patient with a complicated fracture of the great toe obtains follow-up with a foot and ankle surgeon. Open fractures require careful cleaning, usually antibiotic therapy, and close follow-up. Fractures of the lesser toes generally result from jamming the toe into a nightstand or bedpost when barefoot. Radiographs of the lesser phalanges confirm the suspected fracture and may occasionally reveal an unsuspected interphalangeal or MTP dislocation. However, radiographs are not typically required, and the injured digit is easily reduced.

Closed, lesser phalangeal fractures are treated with immobilization for 6 weeks. After the fracture is reduced, the injured toe is splinted against an adjacent noninjured toe. Place a soft corn pad or other suitable material between the toes to prevent skin maceration, and hold the toes together with adhesive tape or a self-adherent wrap such as Coban (Fig. 52.7). The procedure should be demonstrated to the patient or family and supplies dispensed or prescribed so that the splint can be changed every 2 to 3 days at home. The patient will be required to wear a less restrictive, stiff-soled shoe (Fig. 52.8). A postoperative shoe (or similar footwear) may be a comfortable alternative for the first several days. Nondisplaced and stable lesser phalangeal fractures do not need orthopedic referral in most cases[15] (Video 52.1).

Jumping from a height can result in a fracture of the first MTP joint sesamoid bone (Fig. 52.9A). The great toe sesamoid bones lie in grooves on the bottom of the metatarsal head. Each bone lies within the tendon of its respective flexor hallucis brevis muscle belly. Localized pain on the plantar aspect of the first metatarsal head accompanies a sesamoid-bone fracture. Bipartite sesamoids (tibial more frequently than fibular) are common. Comparison radiographs clarify whether the radiographic abnormality represents a fracture.

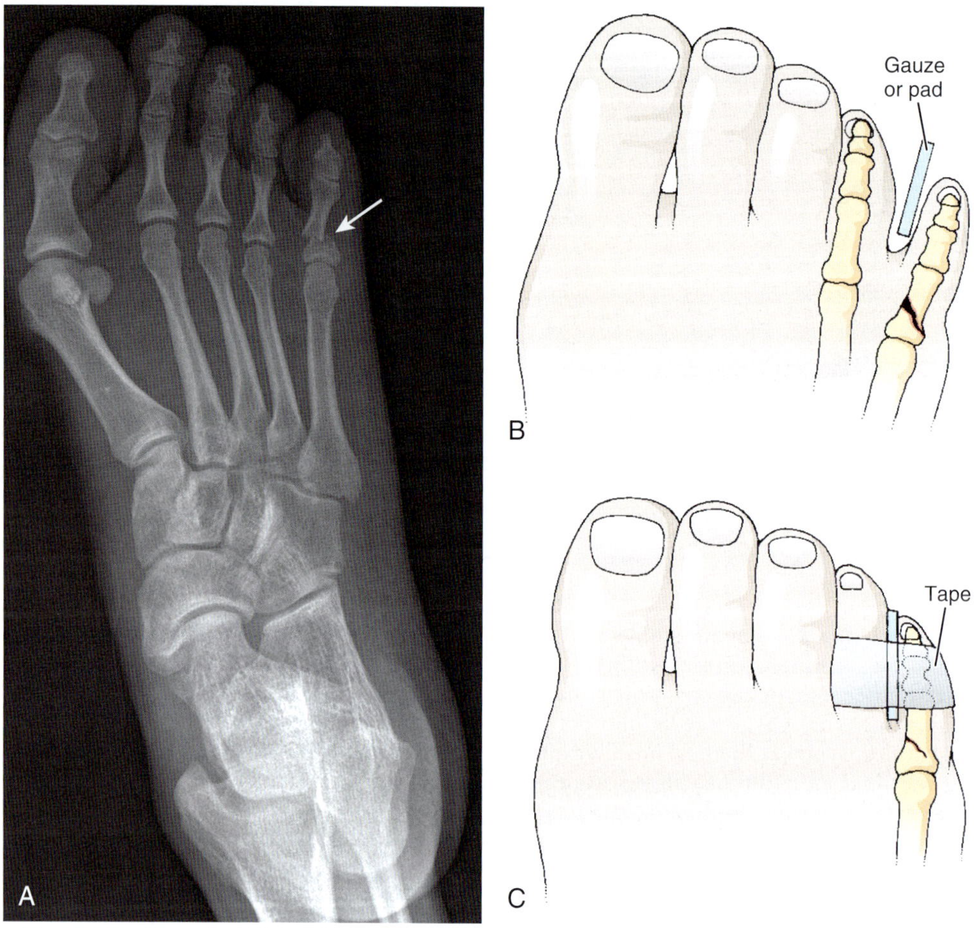

Fig. 52.7 Buddy taping. (A) Displaced fractures of the lesser toes *(arrow)* are often a result of jamming the foot into a bedpost or nightstand when barefoot and are easily reduced with in-line traction. (B) A pad is placed between the injured toe and an adjacent toe. (C) The toes are secured together with tape or a self-adherent wrap. After reduction of the misalignment by in-line traction, generally the only treatment required is a postoperative shoe and taping in place for 4 to 6 weeks. (B–C, Courtesy Kenneth R. Walker, DPM.)

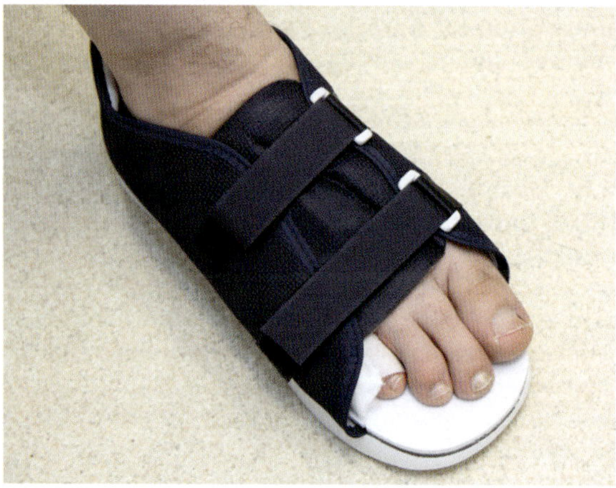

Fig. 52.8 A stiff-soled postoperative shoe prevents flexion of the foot and will provide comfort for patients with toe and sesamoid fractures.

For a tibial sesamoid injury, an aperture bunion-type pad, reinforced medially with 0.5- to 0.75-cm-thick felt, protects the sesamoid and transfers weight bearing to the surrounding structures (see Fig. 52.9B). A hard-soled shoe and NSAIDs are also helpful. Subsequent radiographs rarely show bony consolidation, but the fracture interface appears smoother.

Stress Fractures

A metatarsal stress fracture, commonly of the distal second and third metatarsals, can develop in runners, military recruits, or those with repetitive trauma to the foot (Fig. 52.10). Other risk factors are listed in Box 52.1.[16] There is pain when walking but minimal to no external findings. A bone scan or magnetic resonance imaging (MRI) may detect the subtle fracture that often eludes a plain radiograph. Occasionally, an occult FB of the foot is the culprit and can mimic a stress fracture. Females are more prone to stress fractures than males. Treatment is usually rest and alleviation of the precipitant causes.

Plantar Puncture Wounds

Plantar puncture wounds present a diagnostic and therapeutic challenge for the clinician. Considerable controversy exists regarding the proper initial management of puncture wounds in the plantar surface of the foot, and no universally accepted standard of care exists. Treatment recommendations range from simple cleaning of the wound to aggressive debridement. A reasonable approach is close inspection for retained foreign material and an initially conservative approach, but an aggressive approach is recommended if the patient returns, has an infection, or if the pain persists for more than a few days.

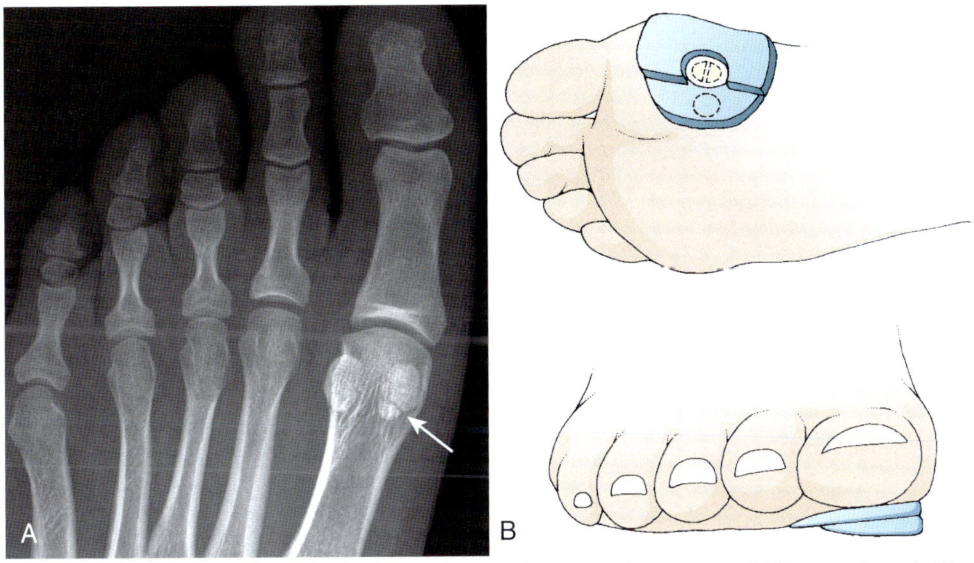

Fig. 52.9 Sesamoid fracture. (A) Jumping from a height can result in a sesamoid fracture *(arrow)*. (B) Bunion shields can be used to redistribute pressure away from fractured sesamoid bones. The hole in the pad is placed over the fracture and the surrounding pad absorbs the pressure.

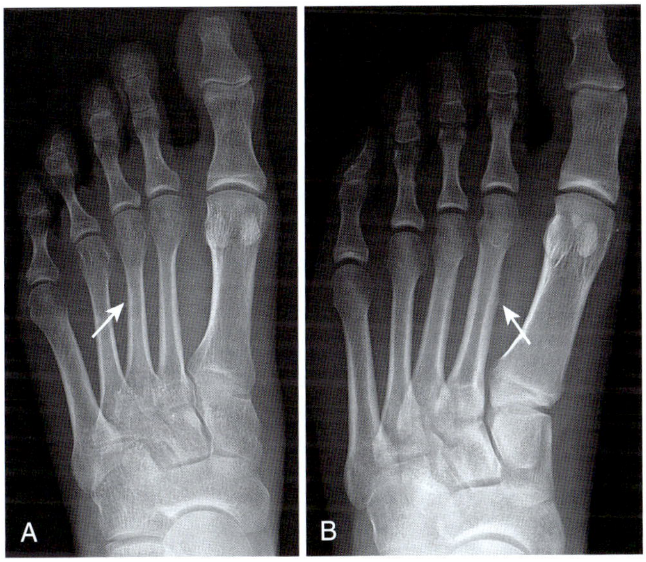

Fig. 52.10 Metatarsal stress fractures. Repetitive foot trauma can lead to metatarsal stress fractures, most commonly the second and third metatarsals *(arrows)*. These are usually subtle fractures that can be difficult to identify on conventional radiographs. (A) Slight cortical disruptions or (B) periosteal reactions indicative of healing may be seen, but often a bone scan or magnetic resonance imaging is needed to confirm the diagnosis. Treatment consists of rest and removing the precipitant causes.

BOX 52.1 Risk Factors for Stress Fractures

- Sports involving running and jumping, especially on angled, hard, or irregular surfaces
- Rapid increase in a physical training program
- Poor physical condition
- Female sex
- Hormonal or menstrual disturbances
- Osteoporosis or decreased bone density
- Nutritional deficiencies (including extreme dieting)
- Obesity and overweight
- Inappropriate footwear
- Poor flexibility

Adapted from Sanderlin BW, Raspa RF. Common stress fractures. Am Fam Physician. *2003;68:1527.*

Although nails produce many such wounds, various other objects may cause them, including other metal objects, wood, and glass. Patient response to the injury depends on the penetrating material, location and circumstances of the wound, depth of penetration, footwear, time from injury until initial evaluation, and underlying health. As superficial puncture wounds generally do well, depth of penetration may be a primary determinant of outcome.[17] Because reflexes are not fast enough to pull back when stepping on a sharp object, the clinician should assume that the entire length of a protruding nail has entered the foot (minus the thickness of the footwear). Stepping on an unknown object in a field or while walking in a stream requires a more cautious approach than a simple puncture from a known object, such as a protruding nail.

The vast majority of patients who step on a nail experience nothing more than transient pain and never seek medical attention. Because most minor puncture wounds are not seen in the ED, the true risk for infection, including osteomyelitis, is unknown. Consequently, reported infection rates vastly overstate the actual incidence. Probably no more than 2% to 8% of puncture wounds become infected, and in only a small percentage of these wounds is surgical debridement needed or does osteomyelitis develop.[18] A prospective series suggested that only the presence of symptoms (e.g., redness, tenderness, increased swelling) at 48 hours is associated with risk for infection or a potential retained FB.[19] Retained foreign material (e.g., a piece of sock or a portion of a tennis shoe sole) in the wound is an important factor in persistent infection. Because no single test detects all possible FBs, tailor the evaluation of a suspected FB to the suspected object.

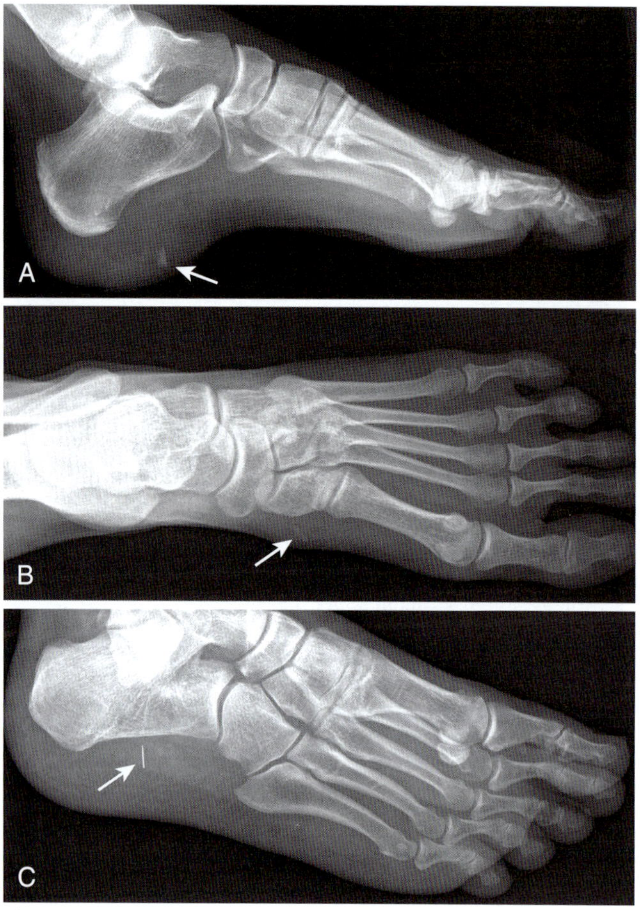

Fig. 52.11 Radiographic appearance of foreign bodies in the foot *(arrows)*. Conventional radiographs will demonstrate a variety of foreign bodies. Shown here are (A) glass, (B) pencil graphite, and (C) a metallic pin. Some objects, such as rubber or pieces of sock, will not be visible.

Evaluation

The approach to the patient depends on several factors, including the time from injury to evaluation, suspicion of an FB, and the presence of infection. The extent to which an FB is pursued depends on the history and findings on physical examination. When the patient clearly states that a needle, pin, or nail was removed intact, radiographs or local wound exploration for a retained metallic FB is not needed. Stepping on an identified intact nail does not always require a radiograph, but if there is any debate regarding a retained metallic object, plain radiographs readily demonstrate their presence. Plain radiographs also demonstrate other radiopaque objects such as glass, gravel, bone, and teeth (Fig. 52.11). Rubber or pieces of a sock will not be visible on a radiograph. If the patient steps on an unknown object, a radiograph is usually indicated unless the entire depth of the wound can be ascertained and inspected. Ultrasonography is noninvasive and does not use radiation, thus making it potentially useful for radiolucent FBs, but soft tissue, air, or calcifications may suggest a retained FB when none is present. Bedside ultrasound has been used to localize radiolucent FBs for removal. Computed tomography (CT) can demonstrate radiopaque and radiolucent objects, but its expense and greater radiation exposure than with plain films make it unsuitable as an initial screening tool. CT scanning can be useful when other screening tools fail to demonstrate a suspected FB, when infection is present, or when joint penetration is suspected. Fluoroscopy may be used to help localize metallic or radiopaque FBs during exploration and removal. It may be particularly useful for long metallic objects such as needles and pins. MRI provides no additional benefit and cannot be used when metallic objects are retained. Diabetic patients with unexplained foot pain or infection warrant investigation for a retained FB; diabetic neuropathy may mask the initial puncture injury.

Treatment

As a rule, the plantar surface of the foot should be examined under good lighting and in a bloodless field. This is best accomplished with the patient in a prone position, not in a chair (Fig. 52.12). Plantar puncture wounds explored for persistent infection often have foreign material in them. Because persistent infection does not develop in most patients, initial deep exploration in the absence of evidence or a strong suspicion of retained material cannot be advocated.[17] Routine initial deep wound exploration, including coring of the wound, is not supported by scientific research and is not recommended for simple, noninfected puncture wounds.[17] However, selected wounds may benefit from exploration to facilitate a search for FBs and to promote irrigation, cleansing, and drainage. When the wound is large and retained organic material is suspected, local wound exploration is warranted. Patients wearing rubber-soled shoes during plantar puncture wounds may retain a portion of the shoe in the wound. Exploration of the wound is most productive after local anesthesia or a regional anesthetic block and excision of the epidermal flap. An incision may be required to facilitate removal of the FB when known to be present, but it has not been proved that extensive removal of surrounding tissue increases successful removal of retained material.[17]

Some clinicians favor a coring technique when an FB is found or suspected. Although this may be too aggressive for many wounds, it may be the best way to remove particulate matter as a block (Fig. 52.13). To accomplish coring, advance a No. 11 blade completely through the dermis into the subcutaneous fat and excise a 2- to 3-mm core. Use a hemostat to grab the cutout core or to open the tract to better visualize the wound. Alternatively, use a 2- to 3-mm punch biopsy instrument to core out the tract. The tract can be packed with gauze for a few days or left open. There is no evidence that coring a plantar puncture wound produces better outcomes than conservative or expectant treatment, and it should be reserved for selected cases. Occasionally, blunt probes may facilitate exploration of the wound. It is generally impossible and probably counterproductive to attempt to probe or visualize the entire length of the puncture tract. Patients initially seen within 24 hours and without signs of infection generally require only simple topical wound care. Although irrigation of all exposed dermal tissue is recommended, high-pressure irrigation of deep tissues with distention of soft tissues is unlikely to be helpful and is not recommended. Schwab and Powers described a case series of uncomplicated puncture wounds in healthy individuals who underwent conservative treatment with cleansing and crutches.[19] Radiographs were obtained at the discretion of the treating clinician and antibiotics were not given. At the 6-month follow-up, 88% of all patients healed without complication. In the remaining 12% complications developed, including wound infection from retained FBs. No

Foreign Body Removal

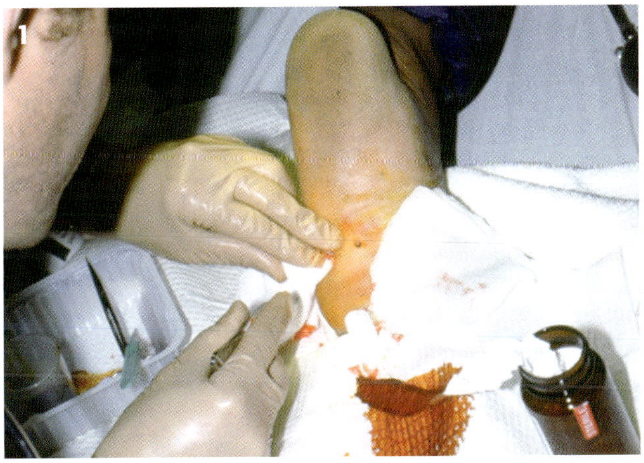

The best way to examine a puncture wound of the foot is to place the patient prone on a stretcher, have good lighting, and obtain a bloodless field (a blood pressure cuff was used here). First, remove the flap of skin at the puncture site. A local anesthetic injection (lidocaine 1%) is usually required but can be quite painful.

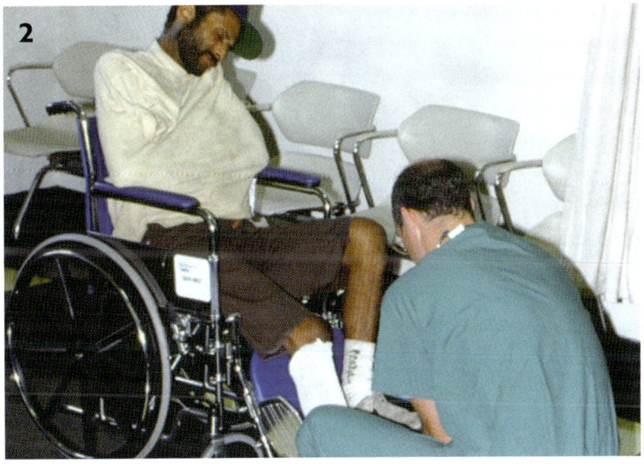

It is difficult to adequately try to examine the bottom of the foot with the patient in a hallway chair.

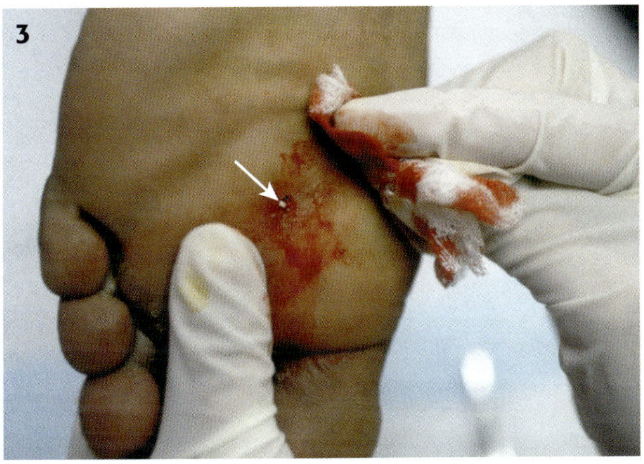

This piece of rubber *(arrow)* was introduced into a puncture when a nail went through a sneaker. It was not seen until the skin flap was removed and carefully examined.

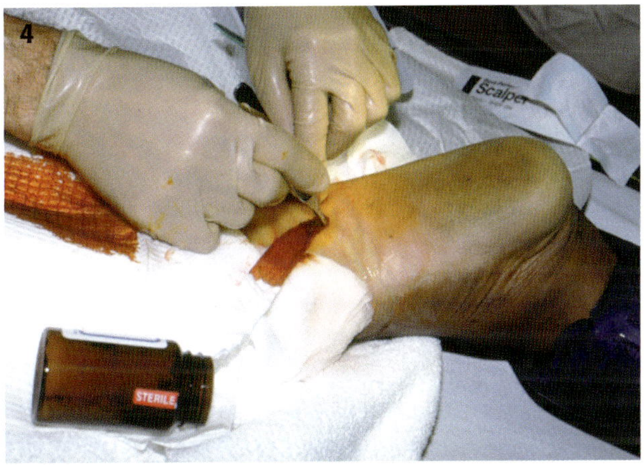

After removing the foreign body, the wound can be left open or packed, as depicted here. Packing gauze can be dry or wet with saline or iodine solution.

Fig. 52.12 Removal of a foreign body from the plantar surface of the foot.

findings on initial evaluation predicted a subsequent infection. Initial antibiotic therapy remains controversial, but there is no evidence to suggest that prophylactic antibiotics reduce the already low rate of infection. In fact, some cases of *Pseudomonas* osteomyelitis develop despite initial treatment with anti-*Pseudomonas* antibiotics. The author does not suggest routine prophylactic antibiotics for uncomplicated puncture wounds, and such treatment may theoretically select out resistant organisms.

Symptomatic patients who delay presentation after injury (≥48 hours) may have an increased probability for a retained FB when inflammation or infection develops. Local wound exploration is warranted unless the patient does not have an infection or a clearly superficial cellulitis is expected to respond to simple oral antibiotics. Recurrent infection, deep soft tissue tenderness, and increasing soft tissue swelling suggest a retained FB or deep space infection, such as osteomyelitis. Such patients require prompt specialty referral or additional diagnostic studies in the ED.

Patients with obvious signs of infection within a few days of a puncture wound usually have simple cellulitis (with or without an FB) with a gram-positive organism (Fig. 52.14). In a patient with persistent pain or swelling days to weeks after a puncture wound, the presence or absence of a deep soft tissue infection or low-grade osteomyelitis cannot be ruled in or ruled out by physical examination, plain radiographs, or laboratory tests (such as a sedimentation rate, complete blood count, or wound cultures). A high index of suspicion, coupled with additional investigation, is the prudent approach to patients with minimal findings on physical examination, normal laboratory test results, and continued pain or swelling after a seemingly simple puncture wound in the bottom of the foot. This usually entails CT, bone scan, or MRI. A study of 80 children with plantar puncture wounds and signs of infection at presentation found simple cellulitis in 59, retained FBs in 11, and osteomyelitis or septic arthritis in 10 children. Because a significant number of children in this study had retained FBs or bony infections, a cautious approach is warranted.[20]

Foreign Body Removal: Coring Technique

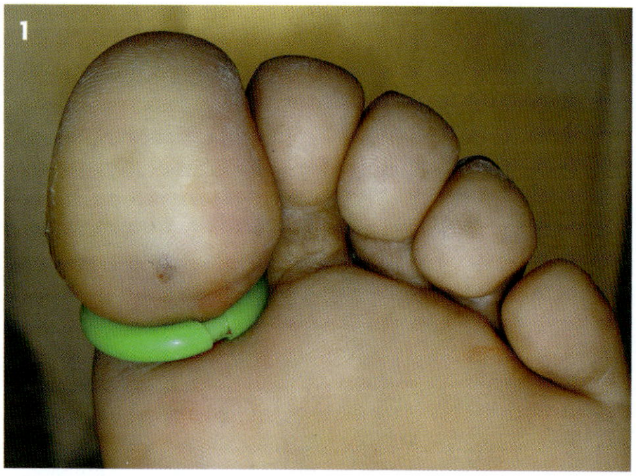

A foreign body is difficult to appreciate in this puncture wound of the big toe.

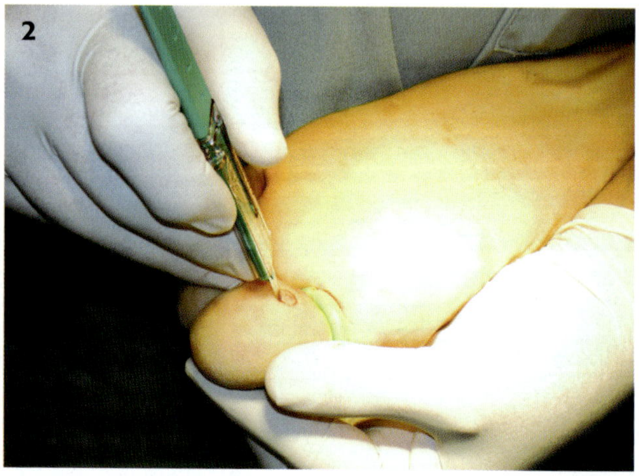

To core out a puncture, use a No. 11 blade and advance it to the hilt.

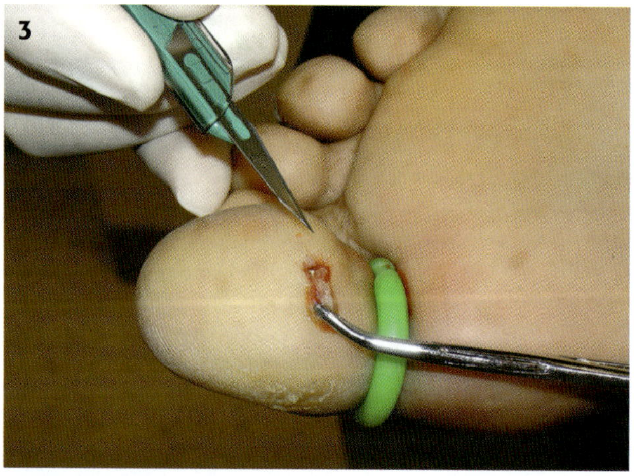

When the cored-out section was removed with a hemostat, a piece of rubber was found deep in the wound.

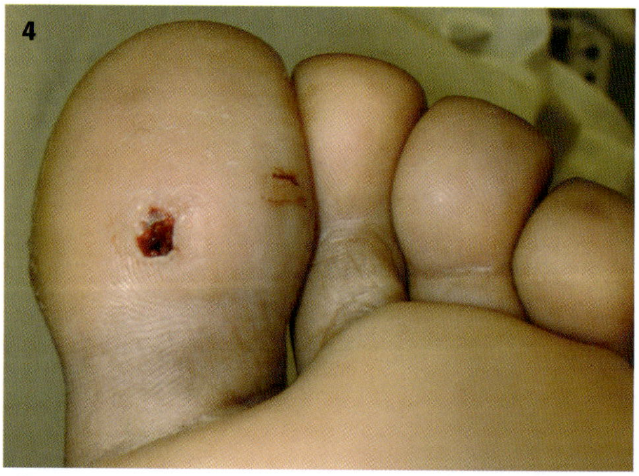

After coring out a puncture tract, the wound can be left open (as shown here) or packed (as shown in Fig 52.12).

Fig. 52.13 Foreign body removal: coring technique.

Plantar puncture wounds complicated by *Pseudomonas* osteomyelitis and osteochondritis are clinically clandestine and particularly devastating. They have been described for nearly 40 years. Some investigators have cultured *Pseudomonas* from the soles of tennis shoes, thus suggesting that puncture wounds made through athletic footwear may be inoculated with *Pseudomonas* (Fig. 52.15).[21] No evidence suggests that prescribing prophylactic anti-*Pseudomonas* antibiotics on initial evaluation of an uncomplicated wound will prevent infection in patients with subsequent deep space or bone infections.[21] Some argue that prophylactic antibiotics, at the time of puncture, may select out resistant organisms.[21] Surgical debridement and prolonged intravenous antibiotics are often required for established infections.

INGROWN TOENAIL

An ingrown toenail is characterized by progressive curving or excessive widening of the lateral margin of the toenail and impingement of the nail into the periungual soft tissue (Fig. 52.16). The toenail normally grows distally in an unimpeded manner, thereby allowing the nail to pass beyond the lateral nail fold. Nail deformity, tight-fitting shoes, and rotational deformity of the toes increase the friction between the nail and the nail fold. Toenails that have been trimmed in a curve increase the likelihood that the lateral nail margin will impinge on the lateral nail fold (Fig. 52.17). The resulting soft tissue injury may lead to hyperkeratosis, edema, and erythema of the nail fold or frank infection (Fig. 52.18). Although an ingrown toenail can be found on any toe, the majority occur on the great toe.

Evaluation

The patient has pain, edema, and erythema of the lateral nail fold. Pressure over the nail margins increases the pain. Because intense pain often precipitates an early visit to the ED, most inflammatory or infectious responses are confined locally. Recurrent ingrown toenails or those in patients with circulatory dysfunction, neuropathy, or diabetes may have underlying osteomyelitis. Cleansing the toe gently facilitates visualization of the periungual debris.

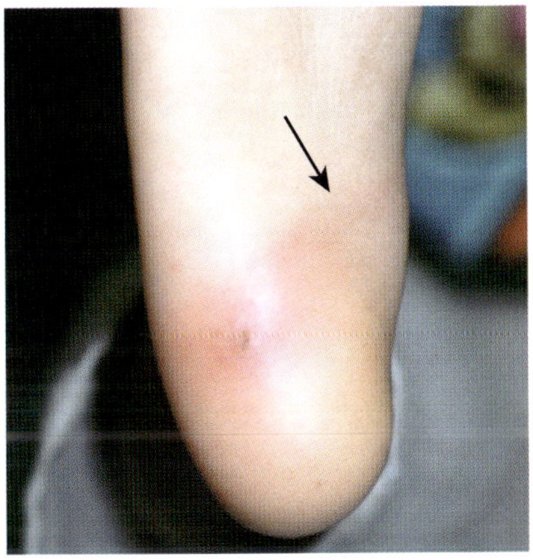

Fig. 52.14 This 5-day-old inflamed and infected puncture wound tract probably harbors a foreign body. Minor lymphangitis *(arrow)* spread up the ankle, but there were no systemic complaints, adenopathy, or leukocytosis. Excision of a core of the tract found scant pus and a threads from the patient's sock embedded in the wound. The wound was left open and did well with oral antibiotics and warm soaks.

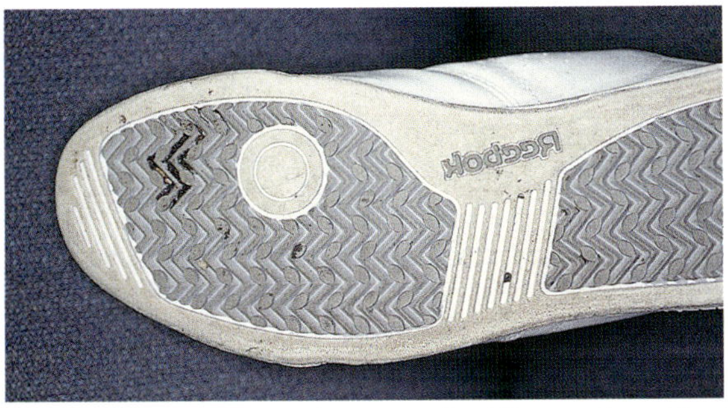

Fig. 52.15 A patient stepped on a nail while wearing this shoe. An initial evaluation in the emergency department 3 weeks earlier found no foreign body or infection. One week earlier the patient began taking antibiotics but did not improve. Findings on physical examination were quite benign, but the continued aching pain and minimal swelling suggested a deep infection. The complete blood count, sedimentation rate, and plain film were negative. Magnetic resonance imaging demonstrated osteomyelitis. *Pseudomonas* are often the offending organism in this scenario and often requires surgical debridement. Prophylactic antibiotics at the time of the puncture have not been shown to prevent this infection. The subsequent course is likely set at the time of injury and the key is to suspect this infection if pain is still present after the first week.

When the free edge of the lateral part of the nail can easily be visualized as separate from the lateral nail fold, consider other painful conditions of the toe such as trauma, gout, paronychia, and cellulitis.

Treatment

Because the toe is exquisitely tender, additional treatment will usually require digital block anesthesia. The decision to treat and what course of action to take in the ED depend on the patient's degree of discomfort. Two general courses of action are often suggested: removal of the offending nail spicule or removal of the spicule and some portion of the nail. Any degree of nail removal is usually followed by ablation of the nail bed. Nail-splinting techniques may also be effective and are less invasive than nail removal techniques.

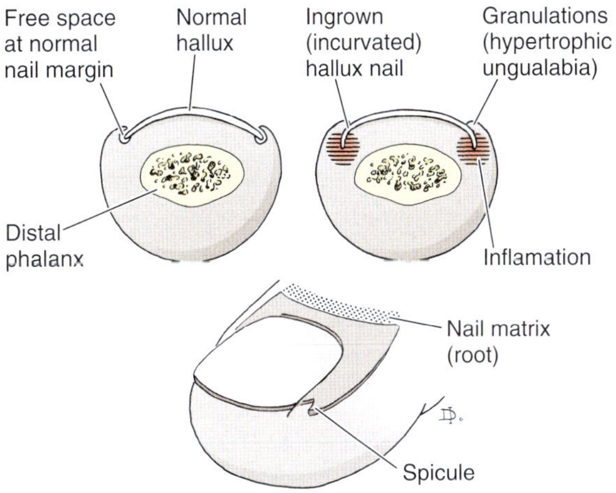

Fig. 52.16 Pathology of an ingrown toenail. The normal free space at the nail margin is obliterated by inflammation and granulation tissue, which is caused by improper nail trimming, trauma to the matrix, and faulty footwear. (From Hill GL II, ed. *Outpatient Surgery*. 3rd ed. Saunders; 1988.)

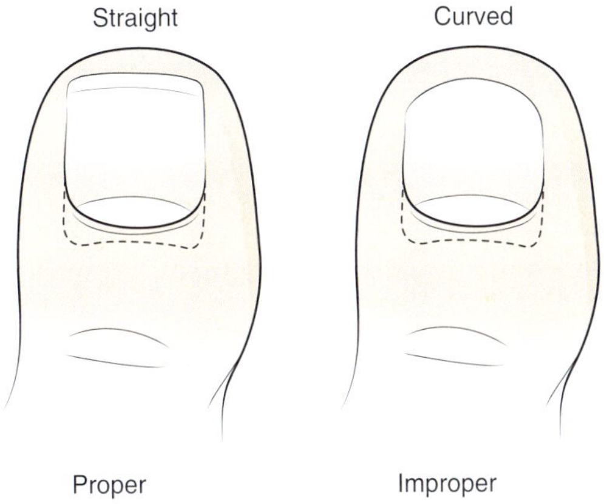

Fig. 52.17 The proper way to trim a toenail that is prone to becoming ingrown is to cut the end of the nail straight across, not at an angle. This is counterintuitive to a patient who wants the nail to conform to the contour of the toe.

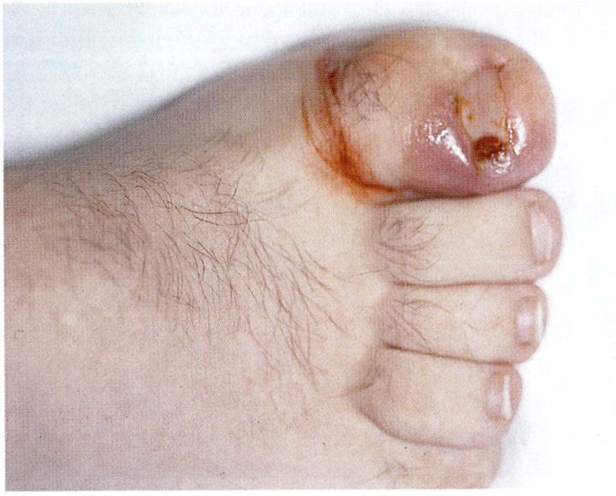

Fig. 52.18 An ingrown toenail of this degree requires removal of a portion of the nail and debridement of inflamed tissue. Antibiotics effective against gram-positive organisms are often prescribed after surgical intervention.

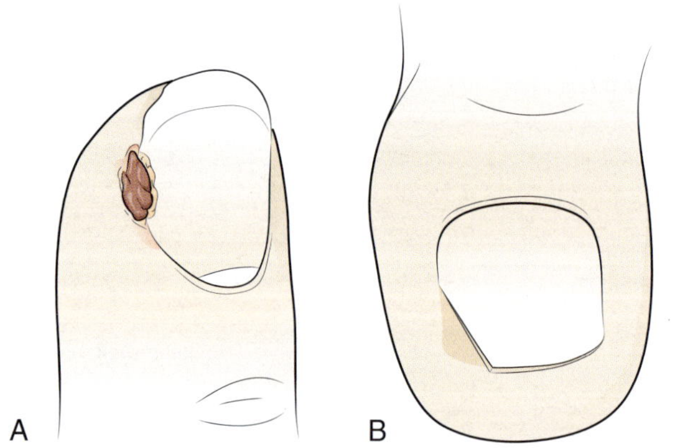

Fig. 52.19 (A) This minor ingrown toenail can be treated by removal of a portion of the distal end of the nail. (B) An oblique wedge of nail is trimmed from the lateral margin of the nail to free it from the hyperkeratotic area. (Courtesy Kenneth R. Walker, DPM.)

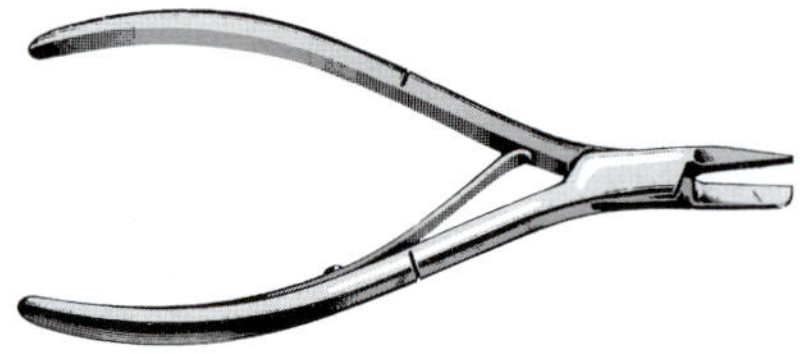

Fig. 52.20 English nail anvil used to divide the nail. (Courtesy Gill Podiatry Supply Company.)

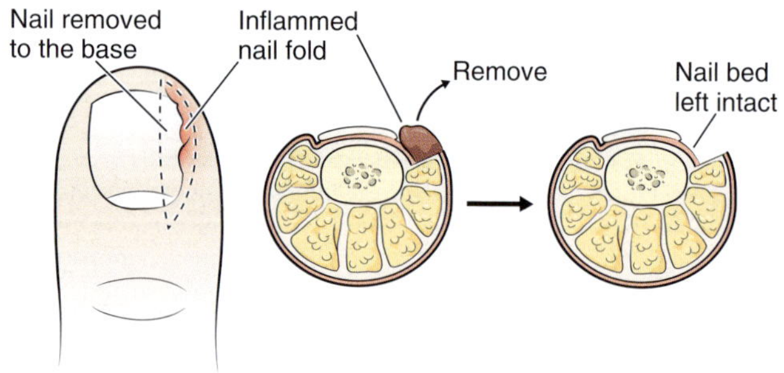

Fig. 52.21 Resection of the entire length of a toenail plus removal of inflamed tissue is usually a curative intervention for a complex ingrown toenail. The nail bed is left intact.

Removal of the Nail Spicule and Debridement of Hyperkeratosis for Minor Ingrown Toenails

When the amount of inflammation and pain and the degree of nail deformity are both minimal, such as involvement of only the distal toenail area, simple removal of the impacted nail spicule is indicated and usually curative. If the condition is advanced, complete removal of a portion of the nail may be required. All procedures are best done with a tourniquet to produce a bloodless field. After a digital block and thorough cleansing, remove an oblique segment of the nail approximately one-third to one-half the way to the proximal nail fold (Fig. 52.19). The ideal instrument is an English anvil nail splitter, which is designed to cut the nail while minimizing trauma to the underlying nail matrix (Fig. 52.20). Sharp, pointed scissors may be substituted if care is taken to minimize injury to the nail bed by maintaining upward pressure while cutting the nail. Some clinicians use a disposable electric cautery device to cut the nail after softening it by soaking in warm soapy water.

After cutting the nail spicule free from the bulk of the nail, grasp the free edge of the nail with forceps or hemostats and remove it to expose the irritated area. The nail fold typically contains impacted debris that must be removed after the nail fold has been gently retracted away from the nail. Remove debris until the epidermis or dermis is uncovered while taking care to avoid aggressive debridement that causes bleeding. A silver nitrate stick applied to the debrided area may be used to control bleeding. Dress the area with antibiotic ointment and a nonadherent dressing. Soaking the toe in warm water two or three times a day, with home redressing, is explained. Harsh chemicals are avoided in the soaking regimen. The wound should be reinspected for signs of infection at 48 to 72 hours. If the problem is resolved, no further therapy is necessary. If the problem is persistent or recurrent, referral for definitive podiatric care is reasonable. Instruct patients to wear less constricting shoes and to trim the nail straight across. Like most FB reactions, removal of the nail spicule resolves the inflammation and infection. Antibiotics given without removal of the nail spicule will not ensure a satisfactory result or add benefit after removal of the spicule. Topical antibiotics (avoid those containing neomycin) are reasonable, but systemic antibiotics are not required. Diabetic patients and those with peripheral vascular disease require closer follow-up. When the ingrown toenail is caused by a nail deformity, a podiatrist or primary clinician can perform definitive removal during follow-up evaluation.

Toenail Removal for Complex or Extensive Ingrown Toenails

See Videos 52.2–52.4. When irritation, infection, or both are more widespread or include the entire toe, removal of a portion of the nail and debridement of the inflamed tissue may be required (Figs. 52.21 and 52.22). Toenail removal may be total or partial. Total nail removal is rarely needed but may be done when both lateral nail folds are infected, particularly if the condition has been present for more than a month. Consider partial removal of the toenail when ingrown toenails are associated with chronic inflammation, infection, or severe pain. Partial nail removal accomplishes two things: removal of the offending portion of nail and destruction of the underlying nail matrix to prevent regrowth of the nail. Phenol, the most commonly applied chemical, causes neurolysis of the nerve endings and necrosis of the nail matrix in a procedure called *matricectomy*. Several studies have demonstrated that 10% sodium hydroxide solution is as effective as phenol and may be associated with less postprocedural pain and faster recovery. As most EDs do not stock phenol or sodium hydroxide solution, nail bed ablation is usually not pursued on the initial visit.

After a digital block, exsanguinate the toe by squeezing or wrapping, and apply a tourniquet at the base of the toe. Stabilize the toe with the nondominant hand. Separate the lateral third of the nail from the nail bed by advancing and separating scissors held parallel to the nail bed (Fig. 52.23). Split the nail lengthwise toward the cuticle. An English anvil nail splitter is desirable to begin the procedure, but sharp scissors or a No. 11 blade also work. Take care to perform a controlled division along the longitudinal lines of the nail for several millimeters past the proximal nail fold (cuticle). Grasp the end of the cut toenail with a hemostat or forceps. Remove the free piece of nail by twisting it toward the remaining nail. This will pull the nail root out from under the cuticle. Inspect the remnant

Ingrown Toenail Removal

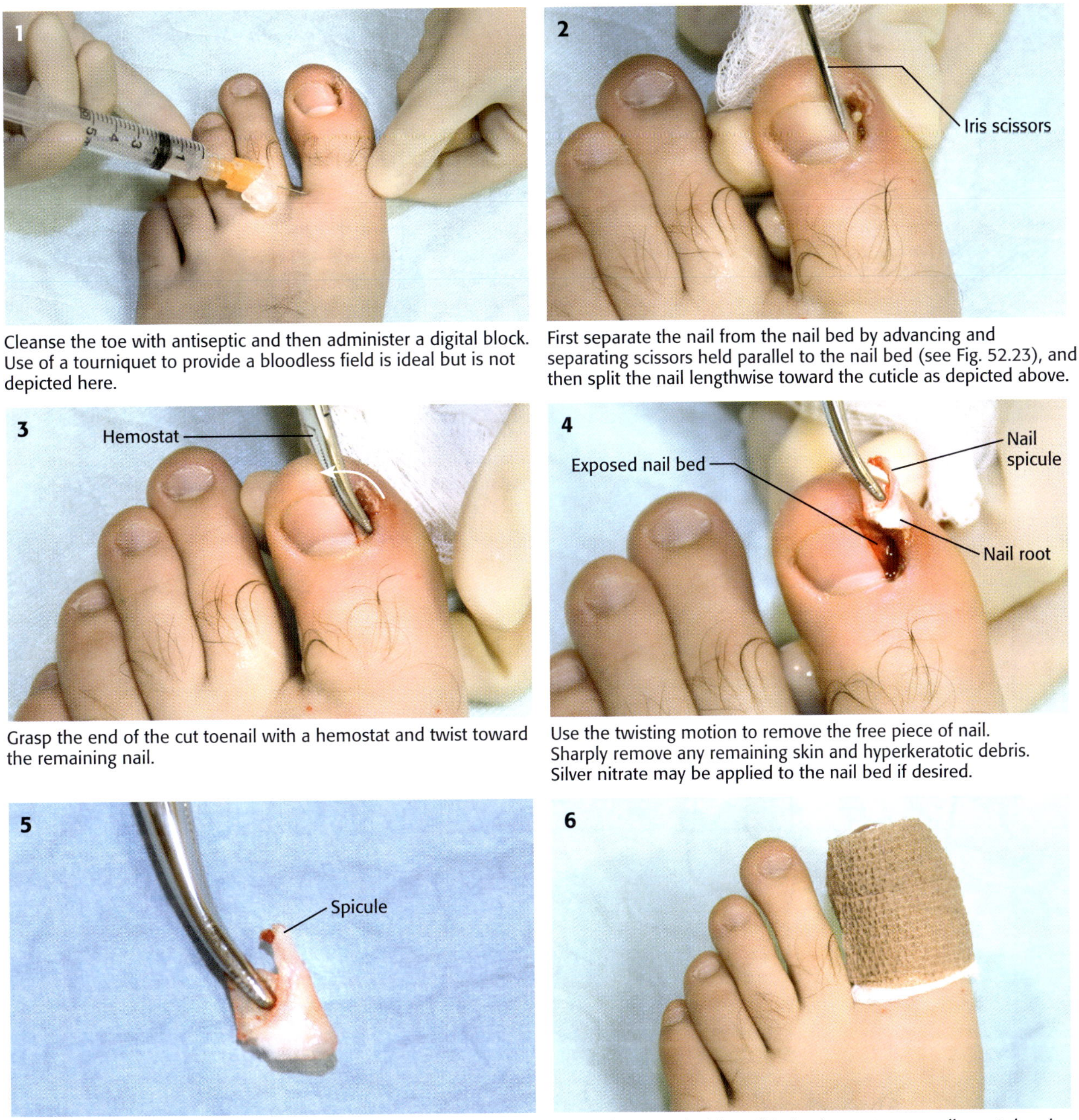

1. Cleanse the toe with antiseptic and then administer a digital block. Use of a tourniquet to provide a bloodless field is ideal but is not depicted here.

2. First separate the nail from the nail bed by advancing and separating scissors held parallel to the nail bed (see Fig. 52.23), and then split the nail lengthwise toward the cuticle as depicted above.

3. Grasp the end of the cut toenail with a hemostat and twist toward the remaining nail.

4. Use the twisting motion to remove the free piece of nail. Sharply remove any remaining skin and hyperkeratotic debris. Silver nitrate may be applied to the nail bed if desired.

5. Inspect the remnant to make sure that the entire piece of nail has been removed as desired. Note the prominent spicule present on this ingrown toenail.

6. Cover the wound with antibiotic ointment, a nonadherent dressing, and a dry sterile wrap.

Fig. 52.22 Removal of an ingrown toenail. Antibiotics effective against gram-positive organisms are prescribed for significant associated infection but are likely not required for this localized process.

to be certain that the entire piece of nail has been removed as desired. Sharply remove any remaining or swollen/heaped-up skin and all hyperkeratotic debris. After removal of the nail, most clinicians apply a silver nitrate stick to the nail bed and to granulation tissue for 2 to 3 minutes. When finished, the nail bed is open and the heaped-up tissue is now flat.

As an option and if phenol or other ablating solutions are available, the following is suggested to permanently ablate the nail bed so that a new nail will not grow (Fig. 52.24). Apply a 10% sodium hydroxide solution to the nail bed with a cotton-tipped applicator for 1 to 2 minutes to provide effective ablation of the nail matrix. Alternatively, apply a 1% solution of aqueous phenol to the nail matrix beneath the involved area of the lateral nail groove and proximal nail fold with cotton-tipped applicators. A 1% phenol solution can be prepared by diluting a 70% to 90% aqueous phenol

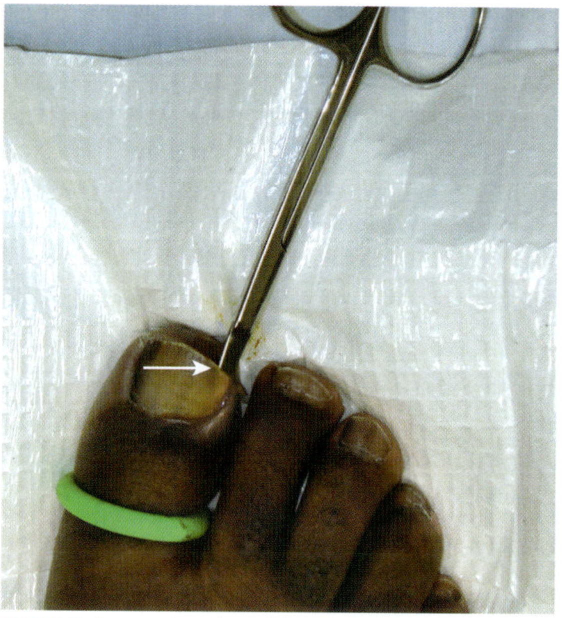

Fig. 52.23 Before cutting the nail lengthwise, separate the nail from the nail bed by advancing and spreading iris scissors held parallel to the nail bed. The *arrow* identifies the technique described in the figure regarding placing the phenol-soaked applicator under the eponychium. Note the use of a tourniquet to provide a bloodless field.

solution in an 80:1 ratio (e.g., 8 mL distilled water to 0.1 mL phenol). Remove some of the cotton if the applicator is too bulky to concentrate the solution beneath the proximal nail fold and lateral nail groove. Apply thoroughly moistened (but not saturated) applicators for three 30-second applications. Avoid forcing phenol under the remaining nail by rolling the applicator so that it rolls over the matrix and over the nail surface rather than against the split edge of the nail. Although it is necessary to cover the lateral aspect of the nail bed and lateral nail fold, do not allow excess phenol to contact the exposed nail bed or surrounding healthy tissue. After the third application, the cauterized tissue appears brown-tinged or gray. Alternatively, a 1% phenol solution can be applied for 5 minutes. Thoroughly irrigate the cauterized nail bed with water and rub the area with a gloved finger to remove all traces of phenol. Snip away any remaining debris or dead skin with scissors.

Apply antibiotic ointment (not containing neomycin) and a nonadherent dressing to the wound, followed by a dry sterile wrap. Do not forget to remove the tourniquet after the dressing has been applied. Instruct the patient to wash the wound twice daily followed by dry dressing changes. Systemic antibiotics do not hasten wound healing and are not necessary in most cases. Soaking the open wound in warm water twice a day is soothing and allows the patient to view

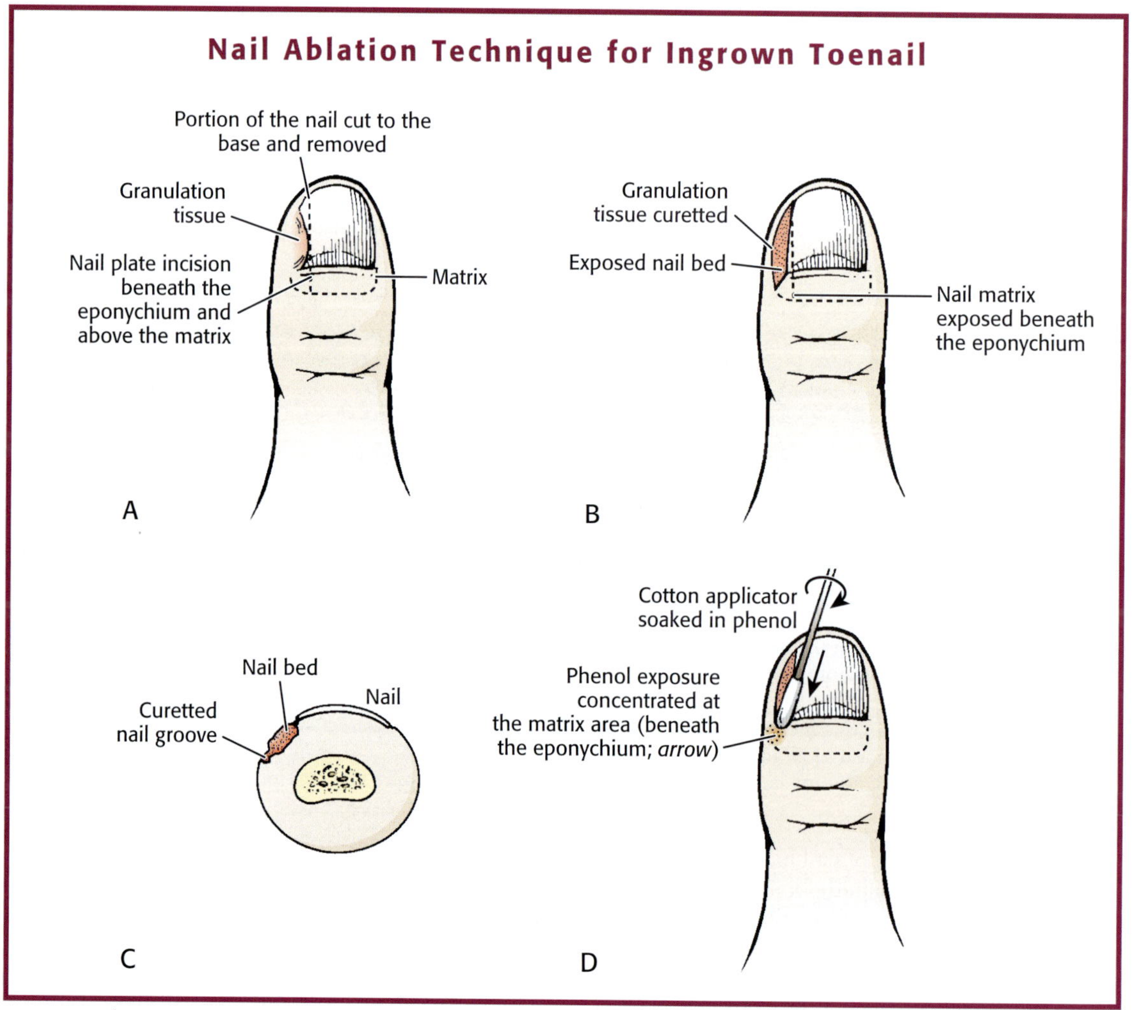

Fig. 52.24 Nail ablation technique for the treatment of an ingrown toenail. The lateral portion of the nail is cut and removed (A) to expose the nail bed. Granulation tissue is curetted (B and C), and the nail matrix is cauterized with hydrogen peroxide or phenol (D) (see text).

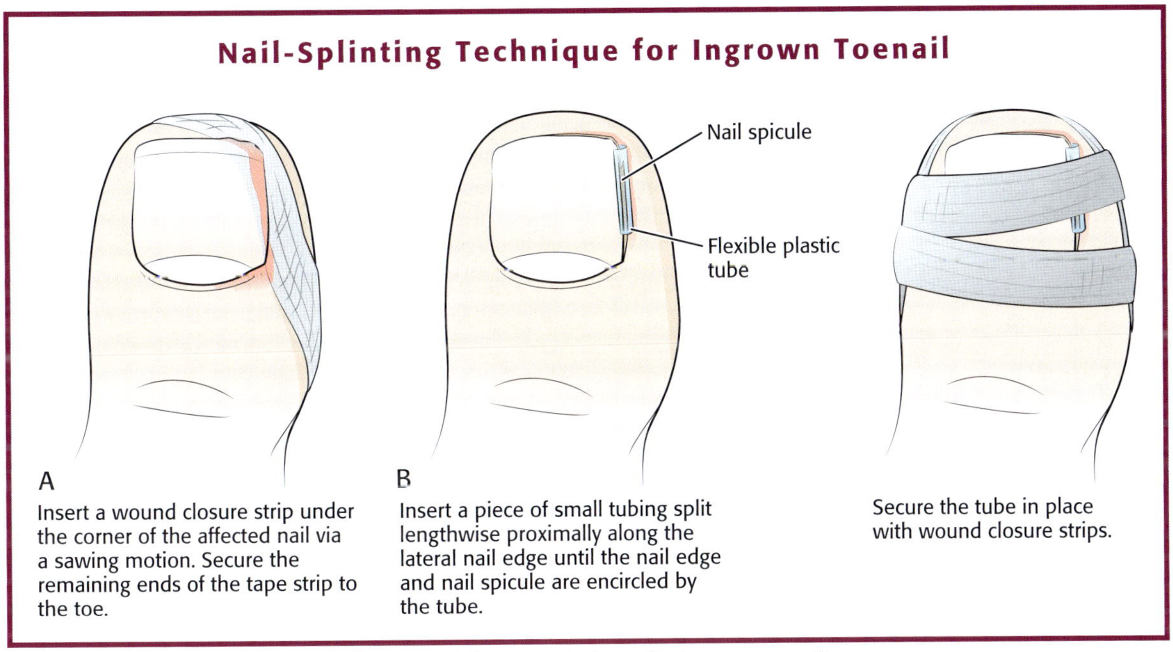

Fig. 52.25 Splinting techniques for ingrown toenails.

the healing process. The wound will heal in 2 to 4 weeks and may be accompanied by serous drainage for 2 weeks. The patient should be informed of this possibility. Complications include nail regrowth, infection, growth of an inclusion cyst, or delayed healing. If the condition returns, podiatric referral is recommended for more extensive ablation of the nail bed.

Nail-Splinting Technique

Splinting of the nail spicule at the lateral edge of the affected nail may allow the toenail to grow out without affecting the inflamed soft tissue. This technique provides time for the periungual tissue to heal while the nail continues to grow until it can be trimmed straight across. No portion of the nail is removed when the nail is initially splinted. When the degree of inflammation is minimal, elevation of the nail spicule is easily accomplished with forceps or a hemostat. A cotton pledget inserted under the lateral edge to maintain elevation is often sufficient in minor cases. Alternatively, a wound closure strip can be used to elevate the corner of the offending nail. After cleansing the edge of the nail and providing drainage if an abscess is present, insert a wound closure strip obliquely under the corner of the nail with a to-and-fro sawing motion until the corner is sufficiently elevated. Secure the tape closure around the toe (Fig. 52.25A). Instruct the patient to soak the toe in warm water daily, remove the tape closure, and reinsert a new tape strip. This procedure is repeated until the corner of the nail or the nail spicule has grown out and cleared the periungual soft tissue, at which time it can be cut straight across. When the degree of inflammation is moderate, nail splinting is accomplished by using the flexible tube procedure. Obtain a surgical drain (2 mm to 3 mm in diameter) used to perform percutaneous drainage procedures, or the small tubing in venipuncture kits. Split a 1-cm piece of the drainage tube lengthwise. Perform a digital block and elevate the lateral edge of the nail with forceps or a hemostat. Insert the split drainage tube along the lateral edge of the nail so that it completely encircles the nail spicule and push it proximately until as much of the lateral nail and nail spicule as possible are covered (see Fig. 52.25B). Some authors suggest that the tube be secured with 2-0 suture passed through the nail, but securing the tube with wound closure strips is more easily accomplished (see Fig. 52.25B). Instruct the patient to wash the affected area daily and replace loosened tape strips when needed. When the inflammation and granulation tissue have subsided and the nail spicule has grown sufficiently to not impinge on the periungual soft tissue, the tube splint is removed by the patient and the nail is cut straight across.

REFERENCES ARE AVAILABLE AT Elsevier eBooks+

CHAPTER 53

Treatment of Bursitis, Tendinitis, and Trigger Points

Neeraj Gupta and Daniel Simpson

INTRODUCTION

Bursitis and tendinitis are terms frequently used to describe a variety of common and often ill-defined regional musculoskeletal conditions characterized chiefly by inflammation, pain, and resultant disability at the involved site. They are either periarticular or contained within specific soft tissue structures. Myofascial pain syndromes are characterized by sensory, motor, and autonomic symptoms that are often associated with a trigger point, a hyperirritable point in skeletal muscle that reproduces the patient's symptoms. These musculoskeletal conditions largely rely on a clinical diagnosis in that they often cannot be confirmed by objective data such as radiographs or laboratory studies. Use of injection therapy with local anesthetics and corticosteroids for bursitis and tendinitis can relieve pain, reduce inflammation, and improve mobility. Injection therapy may provide definitive treatment of a condition or serve as an adjunct to facilitate rehabilitation therapy. Several invasive and noninvasive techniques can be used for the treatment of trigger points and myofascial pain syndromes. Successful treatment of any of these musculoskeletal conditions depends highly on an accurate diagnosis and the use of appropriate techniques.

GENERAL ANATOMIC CONSIDERATIONS

Bursae and Tendon Sheaths

Bursae are small fluid-filled sacs, subcutaneous and deep, which provide a cushion for bone and the surrounding soft tissue. They develop in relation to friction and facilitate the gliding motion of tendons and muscles. Bursae can be categorized as being deep, superficial, and adventitious. Adventitial bursae may form in response to abnormal shearing stress at sites subjected to chronic pressure, such as a bunion over the metatarsal head of the great toe. Tendon sheaths are similar in composition to bursae but differ in overall shape. Tendon sheaths are long and tubular, whereas bursae are usually round and flat.

Inflammation of bursae, as in bursitis, can be seen microscopically as a thickening of the normal thin surface of synovial cells lining the bursal wall.[1] This thickening coupled with increased production of synovial fluid leads to localized pain, swelling, erythema, and reduced movement. Aside from simple overuse, bursitis may be caused by local trauma, infection, and crystal deposition as in gout and pseudogout. Underlying systemic and autoimmune disorders, such as lupus, rheumatoid arthritis, ankylosing spondylitis, psoriatic arthropathy, and scleroderma, can also lead to bursitis. Cases of subdeltoid and subacromial bursitis have been reported after vaccinations. In septic bursitis, the inflammatory cascade is activated by bacteria. This occurs most often in superficial bursae, the most common organisms being *Staphylococcus aureus* and streptococci.[2] Bursitis can be acute, recurrent, or chronic.

Because of the adjacent location of bursae and tendons, an inflammatory process in one may also involve the other.[1,3] *Tendinitis* and *tenosynovitis* are used to describe similar inflammatory reactions in tendons and tendon sheaths, respectively. Tendinopathy is a broad term commonly used to describe the pain, swelling, or impaired performance that can affect tendons which may not be related to specific inflammation. Tendinopathy can produce destructive changes in the tendon that can be seen on ultrasound. Some forms of tendinitis may be caused by factors other than overuse, inflammation, trauma, and degenerative disease. Gonococcemia, for example, is one cause of tenosynovitis that should be considered in the appropriate setting. Another rare cause is hemodialysis. In 2008 the US Food and Drug Administration (FDA) added a black box warning to fluoroquinolone antibiotics, highlighting the potential for tendinopathy and tendon rupture. Clinicians should avoid tendon sheath injections in patients who are taking this class of drugs.

Common sites of tendinitis and bursitis in the body are depicted in Fig. 53.1.

Trigger Points

Myofascial pain related to trigger points is probably omnipresent, but it is vague and ill-defined in the literature, the specific syndromes are unknown to many clinicians, and the disorders are difficult to clarify in many patients. Hence, myofascial pain originating from trigger points is often attributed to a plethora of other conditions. Consequently, the true incidence is unknown. Examples of misdiagnosis can include fibromyalgia, overuse syndromes, statin-induced myopathy, and malingering.

Trigger points are 1- to 4-mm focal areas of hyperirritability usually found within a taut band of skeletal muscle or in the muscle fascia that are painful on compression and associated with a characteristic pattern of referred pain, motor dysfunction, and autonomic phenomena (Box 53.1).[4] Trigger points can also be identified by the "jump sign" or *local twitch response*, a brisk contraction of muscle fibers elicited by snapping palpation or rapid insertion of a needle into the trigger point itself.[4,5]

Trigger points probably develop in response to muscle fiber injury. The injury may be an acute traumatic event or more subtle repetitive microtrauma. Inflammatory mediators including bradykinin, norepinephrine, serotonin, substance P and vasoactive mediators, and pronociceptive neurotransmitters have all been identified in the center of trigger points.

Trigger points can occur in any muscle or muscle group; they are generally unilateral, but bilateral trigger points have been reported. As the stress associated with myofascial pain commonly affects both single muscles and whole muscle groups, trigger points tend to cluster. In the upper part of the trunk, a common trigger point cluster involves the muscles of the neck and shoulder area, including the trapezius, levator scapulae, and infraspinatus muscles (Fig. 53.2). In the lower part of the trunk, the quadratus lumborum, gluteus medius, and tensor fasciae latae are commonly affected. Trigger points often affect other muscles innervated by the same spinal segments, and subsequent treatment is usually directed at all muscles innervated by both the anterior and posterior branches of

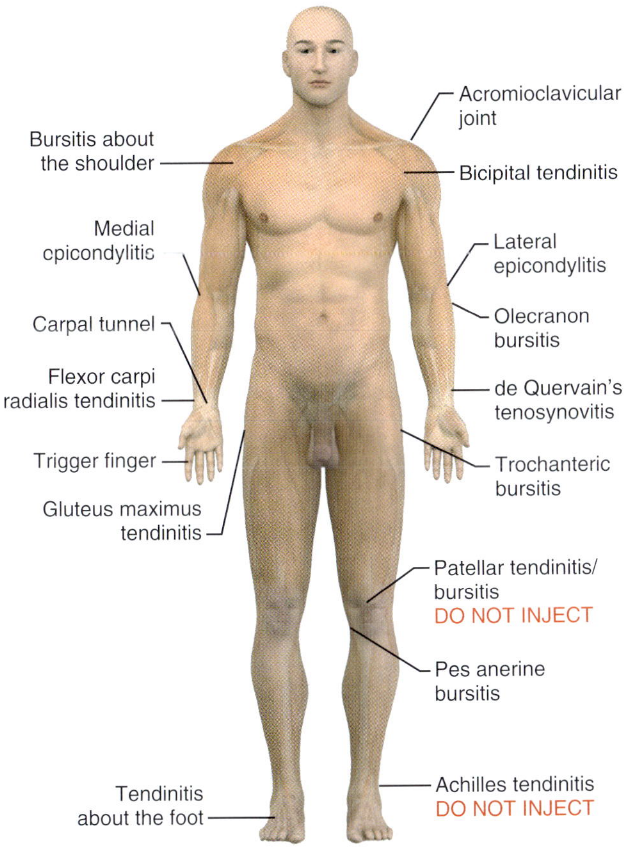

Fig. 53.1 Common sites of tendinitis and bursitis. (Redrawn from Walker LG, Meals RM. Tendinitis: a practical approach to diagnosis and management. *J Musculoskel Med.* 1989;6:24.)

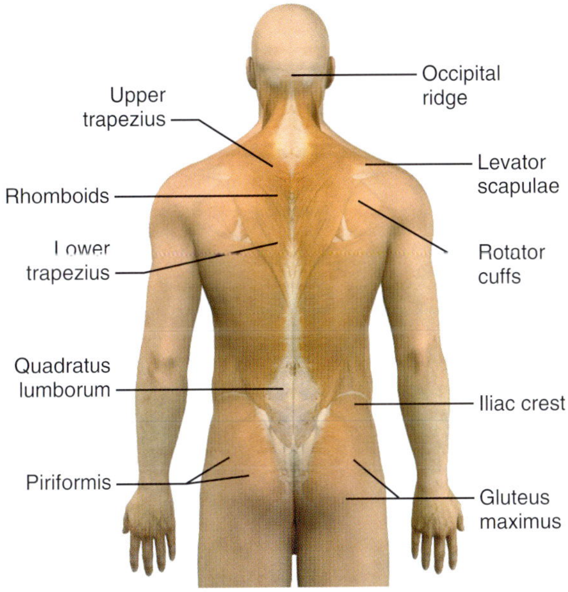

Fig. 53.2 Common trigger point clusters on the back. In the upper part of the trunk, a common trigger point cluster involves the muscles of the neck and shoulder area including the trapezius, levator scapulae, and infraspinatus muscles. The quadratus lumborum, gluteus medius, and tensor fasciae latae are commonly affected lower trunk muscles.

BOX 53.1 Clinical Characteristics of Myofascial Pain Syndromes

- Characteristic distribution pattern of the pain
- Restricted range of motion with increased sensitivity to stretching
- Weakened muscle because of pain with no muscular atrophy
- Compression causing pain similar to the patient's chief complaint
- A palpable taut band of muscle correlating with the patient's trigger point
- Local twitch response elicited by snapping palpation or rapid insertion of a needle
- Reproduction of the referred pain with mechanical stimulation of the trigger point
- Associated autonomic phenomena

the same spinal nerve. Table 53.1 lists common trigger points and their associated myofascial pain syndromes.

RATIONALE FOR INJECTION THERAPY

Bursitis and Tendinopathies

Management of the pain resulting from bursitis and tendinitis may be greatly enhanced by the proper selection and administration of local injections, especially if the patient does not respond to other treatments. Successful application of local injection and intrasynovial (bursa and tendon sheath) therapy requires an understanding of the diagnosis, accurate localization of the pathologic condition, and appropriate injection techniques. Lidocaine and corticosteroid preparations may be injected separately or together as adjuncts for pain control. In many cases, a single injection may be all that is required to ameliorate a painful condition. However, injection therapy is best viewed as an adjunct in the management of painful tendinitis and bursitis syndromes. It should not be viewed as a single quick fix, but a method to facilitate other modalities.

The precise mechanisms for the lasting analgesia and beneficial therapeutic effects of local injection therapy have not been clarified. Few clinical trials have adequately measured the efficacy of corticosteroid therapy. Although steroids are known to reduce inflammation, it is unclear whether the antiinflammatory effect is responsible for the increased range of motion and relief of pain that the patient usually experiences. Histologic studies of chronic tenosynovitis lesions demonstrate degeneration, but not inflammation.[1] It is therefore possible that the pain experienced with tendinitis and bursitis occurs as a result of mechanisms other than inflammation, such as mechanoreceptor stimulation by shearing, traction, or activation of nociceptive receptors by substance P and chondroitin sulfate. A study looking at the combination of aspiration with steroid injection versus compression bandaging and nonsteroidal antiinflammatory drugs (NSAIDs) found no differences in bursitis resolution at week 4 but did show an earlier time to resolution in the former group.[5,6]

Injection therapy is a therapy utilized by orthopedic surgeons, rheumatologists, and family practitioners. Rarely is it definitive care, hence, follow-up and additional evaluations and interventions should be considered. In short, injection therapy should be considered an adjunct to a variety of treatment modalities including pain control, physical therapy, occupational therapy, relative rest, immobilization, and exercise.

TABLE 53.1 Myofascial Pain Syndromes

MUSCLE[a]	TRIGGER POINT LOCATION	AREA OF PAIN	COMMENTS
Levator scapulae	Superior medial aspect of the scapula along the flat muscle belly; insertion sites on the transverse processes of C1–C4	Posterior cervical region, posterior aspect of the scalp, periauricular area	May cause or contribute to headache syndromes in some patients
Splenius capitis and semispinalis capitis	May occur in any part of these muscles	Over the muscles themselves, head, face	Having the patient point to the area of maximal pain may help localize the trigger point or points; may also cause dizziness
Trapezius	Angle of the neck, occipital insertion sites	Trapezius muscle itself, occiput	Inject neck trigger points carefully to avoid iatrogenic pneumothorax
Sternocleidomastoid	Sternal and clavicular origins, occipital insertion site, upper two-thirds of the muscle belly	Sternocleidomastoid muscle itself, periauricular area, frontal area, face	May also cause dizziness, ipsilateral ptosis, lacrimation, and conjunctival injection
Infraspinatus	Anywhere in the infraspinatus muscle	Arm, posterior and lateral aspects of the shoulder	May cause sympathetic hyperactivity; subject to early degeneration
Rectus abdominis	Most common in the upper 3 segments, less often in the lower muscle segments	Anterior abdominal wall (upper segment), back (lower segments)	Often flare after abdominal surgery
Pectoralis major and minor	Most common at the insertion site on the anterior medial aspect of the shoulder and in the inferior muscle belly, but may be found anywhere in the muscle	Over the trigger point, upper most part of the muscle, ipsilateral arm	Because trigger points may be found anywhere in the muscle, it is important to search the entire muscle
Intercostals	Intercostal spaces	Chest (increased during inspiration)	Often flare after chest surgery or trauma; inject carefully to avoid iatrogenic pneumothorax
Tensor fasciae latae	Muscle belly	Lateral thigh pain to the knee	Tensor fasciae latae trigger points are generally easy to locate
Anterior tibialis	Upper third of muscle	Anterior aspect of the foreleg and ankle, dorsal surface of the ankle	
Gastrocnemius and soleus	Medial and lateral muscle margins, along the midline of the muscle	Posterior of the knee, Achilles tendon near the heel	Often flare with vascular insufficiency of the lower extremities
Quadratus lumborum	Along the 12th rib, around the iliac crest, lateral border of the muscle	Area of the 12th rib (especially during deep inspiration), anterior abdominal wall	May accentuate postoperative pain or pain associated with abdominal wall scars
Gluteus medius	Along the iliac shelf; in severe cases, the entire gluteal ridge may be involved (including the gluteus minimus and maximus from the sacroiliac joint to the anterior superior iliac spine)	Most often cause hip, leg, and lower back pain; may cause remote pain in the cervical region and head	Often associated with sympathetic hyperactivity; common in late-stage pregnancy and in patients with unequal leg lengths

[a]See also Fig. 53.30 for diagrams of trigger points for specific muscles.

Additional pain control can be achieved with such options as NSAIDs, acupuncture, ultrasound, ice, heat, and electrical nerve stimulation. Besides pain relief, early participation in rehabilitative activities and exercises can be an important aspect of patient recovery. Patients receiving only analgesics may have worse outcomes than those who also incorporate exercise as part of their treatment.[3,4] Any factors that provoke the initial injury should also be identified because failure to eliminate these provoking factors can contribute to the injury developing into a chronic condition.[5]

Although opinions in the literature differ, repeated corticosteroid injections in the same site should be avoided unless at least a partial clinical response has occurred. In addition, an injection should not be repeated in the same site more than once every 3 months. Some limit corticosteroid injections at any given site to two or three injections before alternative therapy is pursued. Despite little data on the outcome of repeated injections, these recommendations are generally accepted and may limit the risk for adverse effects.[7–10]

Though considered safe and effective for short-term therapy, there are sparse scientific data defining a true benefit of corticosteroid injections for musculotendinous conditions. Inflammation is not always the cause of tendinopathy. Although true inflammatory tendinitis may respond quite well to corticosteroid injections, conditions such as posttraumatic shoulder impingement and rotator cuff tears may not benefit from local injection any more than from treatment consisting of rest, time, physical therapy, and NSAIDs. Despite appearing to initially be effective for conditions such as olecranon bursitis, lateral epicondylitis, and de Quervain's tenosynovitis, long-term relief of other conditions is often superior with other modalities. In addition, oral corticosteroids can be as effective as local injection and can be an alternative for emergency clinicians reluctant to perform an injection.

Trigger Points

Injection therapy is the most widely accepted and scientifically supported as an effective treatment modality for treatment of trigger point pain.[10] However, because it may place patients at risk for becoming dependent on injection for pain relief, some authors reserve injection therapy for patients who have not responded to other measures (Box 53.2).[11]

Various substances have been used for trigger point injections, including local anesthetics, botulinum toxin, sterile water, and sterile saline.[10,11] Dry needling, a technique that involves multiple advances of a needle into the muscle at the region of the trigger point, provides as much pain relief as an injection of lidocaine. In support of these findings, it has been proposed that the needle (not the injected substance) reduces trigger point pain by mechanically disrupting dysfunctional activity at the motor end plate.[12,13] Nevertheless, the addition of a local anesthetic is recommended to reduce the degree of postinjection soreness.

The use of steroids for trigger point injection is controversial and without a clear rationale because there is little evidence to support an inflammatory pathophysiology for trigger point pain. Hence, the use of steroids for trigger point injection is not recommended.

BOX 53.2 Modalities for Treating Trigger Point Pain[a]

NONINVASIVE TECHNIQUES

Oral medications (NSAIDs, muscle relaxants, neuroleptics, opiates)
Spray and stretch
Massage therapy
Ischemic compression

INVASIVE TECHNIQUES

Injection
Dry needling

[a]*Physical therapy, transcutaneous electrical stimulation, and ultrasound are adjuncts to both invasive and noninvasive techniques.*

INDICATIONS AND CONTRAINDICATIONS

Bursae and Tendon Sheaths

The indications for steroid injection are twofold: therapy and diagnosis. Injection therapy offers not only relief of pain, particularly when a local anesthetic is used concurrently, but also a medium to deliver therapeutic agents. In addition to relieving pain, injection therapy may aid in diagnosis. When injecting a bursa, for example, bursal fluid is sometimes collected for laboratory analysis. In addition, relief of pain helps differentiate a localized site of injury from referred or visceral pain.

Absolute contraindications to local injection therapy are limited and include specific infections such as bacteremia, infectious arthritis, periarticular cellulitis or ulceration, and adjacent osteomyelitis (Box 53.3). The procedure is also contraindicated in patients with underlying bleeding disorders. A history of hypersensitivity, either to the corticosteroid or to the vehicle by which it is delivered, is also an absolute contraindication. Finally, corticosteroid injections should not be performed in a patient who has a documented osteochondral fracture. Relative contraindications depend on both the clinician's experience and the indication for the injection. Violation of the integrity of the skin or chronic foci of infection, either locally or in the vicinity of the site of involvement, is a relative contraindication. The procedure is also relatively contraindicated in patients taking anticoagulants, in patients with poorly controlled diabetes, and in those with internal joint derangements or hemarthrosis. Patients with a preexisting tendon injury may be subject to tendon rupture if the

BOX 53.3 Contraindications to Local Injection Therapy

ABSOLUTE

Infection (bacteremia, infectious arthritis, periarticular cellulitis or ulceration, adjacent osteomyelitis)
Uncontrolled bleeding disorder
Hypersensitivity/allergy to corticosteroid or vehicle
Osteochondral fracture

RELATIVE

Anticoagulant therapy
Joint instability
Poorly controlled diabetes (steroids raise blood glucose levels)
Hemarthrosis
Decubitus ulcers
Joint prosthesis
Adjacent abraded skin
Chronic foci of infection
Internal joint derangement
Partial tendon rupture

corticosteroid injection relieves the pain and full activity is then resumed. Therefore partial tendon rupture is a relative contraindication.

Trigger Points

Consider trigger point injection once a myofascial pain syndrome has been identified (see Box 53.1 and Table 53.1). As mentioned previously, some authors reserve injection for patients who do not respond to noninvasive modalities (see Box 53.2). There are few contraindications to trigger point injection. Overlying infection is an absolute contraindication. Relative contraindications include proximity to sensitive structures, bleeding disorders, anticoagulation, or an uncooperative patient. Dry needling is as effective as injection therapy, so in those with allergy to local anesthetics, the clinician may perform dry needling to avoid the problem.

Hazards and Complications

All injection therapies can be expected to cause local effects such as pain at the site, bruising, and hematoma formation. These can be ameliorated with proper technique. Local anesthetics may be mixed with a corticosteroid preparation to increase volume, decrease postinjection pain, and assess the accuracy of bursae and tendon sheath injections. However, some clinicians prefer to inject local anesthetics alone before injecting the corticosteroid. Subcutaneous bleeding may occur at the site of injection and patients should be warned that this may occur. Advise patients to apply ice packs or cold compresses to the involved area for the first 24 hours. Clinicians must be aware of the local anatomy and aspirate after injecting every 1 to 2 mL of solution to help prevent inadvertent vascular injection. Penetration into or striking a nerve may cause sharp pain or paresthesia, and the patient should be warned of this possibility in advance.

Anesthetic Injections

Injection of a local anesthetic causes discomfort secondary to tissue irritation related to its acidity and from tissue distension caused by infiltration. Mixing the anesthetic solution with sodium bicarbonate 8.4% (9 mL of anesthetic to 1 mL of sodium bicarbonate) can reduce this pain by creating a more physiologic pH. Warming and slowly injecting the anesthetic may also be helpful.[14] Other minor reactions occasionally seen after injection of amide preparations include light-headedness or dizziness, pallor, weakness, sweating, nausea, fainting (rare), and tachycardia. These symptoms usually disappear within a few minutes after the injection and rarely require any treatment except reassurance. Frequently, it is difficult to determine whether the symptoms are the result of sensitivity to the drug or a fright (vasovagal) reaction to needles and injections. When the anatomic location of the injection permits, place the patient in a supine, prone, or reclining position during the injection to minimize the effect of a potential vasovagal reaction.

The major hazards with injection of local anesthetics are hypersensitivity reactions and accidental intravenous or intraarterial injection (see Chapter 29). Serious or fatal hypersensitivity to procaine and other regional anesthetic agents is encountered very rarely. This possibility is usually suggested by a previous history of reactions to these compounds. Ester solutions (e.g., procaine, tetracaine) that produce the metabolite para-aminobenzoic acid (PABA) account for the majority of these reactions. Amide solutions (e.g., lidocaine, bupivacaine) are rarely involved, and usually the preservative methylparaben, which is structurally similar to PABA, is responsible. When a definite history of sensitivity is present, the use of any agent from that class of anesthetic agents is absolutely contraindicated.

Corticosteroid Injections

Intrabursal corticosteroid injections have been found to be safe procedures with few complications (Box 53.4).[14,15] A maximum of 40 mg of a corticosteroid should be used. Although there is evidence of allergic reactions from corticosteroids given orally and parentally, the possibility of an allergic reaction caused by corticosteroid injection is highly unlikely, and such cases occur infrequently. Nevertheless, the clinician should be aware that anaphylaxis after injection of methylprednisolone acetate has been reported. In addition, an unusual rash after an intraarticular methylprednisolone injection, which appears to be consistent with a delayed type of hypersensitivity, has also been documented. Introducing infection is one of the most serious potential complications, but infections occurring as an aftermath of intrasynovial injections are extremely rare. Although the problem of infection is usually minimized with meticulous attention to aseptic technique, the patient should be cautioned to watch for the development of any significant pain, redness, or swelling after local injections. Routine prophylactic antibiotic administration after corticosteroid injections is not recommended.[15]

Local undesirable reactions are usually minor and reversible. After steroid injection, approximately 2% of patients may experience an acute synovitis otherwise known as *postinjection flare*.[16] Characterized by an increase in pain and joint swelling,

BOX 53.4 Potential Side Effects of Corticosteroid and Local Anesthetic

INJECTION THERAPY

Systemic Side Effects

Cushing syndrome
Facial flushing
Nausea
Impaired diabetic control
Menstrual irregularity/uterine bleeding
Hypothalamic-pituitary axis suppression
Fall in the erythrocyte sedimentation rate and C-reactive protein level
Anaphylaxis
Dysphoria
Pancreatitis
Cataracts

Local Side Effects

Postinjection flare of pain
Skin depigmentation, fat atrophy
Bleeding, bruising
Steroid "chalk" calcification
Steroid arthropathy
Nerve injury
Tendon rupture and atrophy
Joint and soft tissue infection

symptoms usually begin a few hours after steroid injection and can last as long as 3 days. These reactions can be stressful to the patient who has expected relief, rather than exacerbation, from an injection. Although quite symptomatic they should not be misinterpreted as faulty technique or an infection secondary to the injection. Histologically, steroid crystals have been seen within polymorphonuclear leukocytes, making it a true synovitis. This reaction may be difficult to differentiate from an infection, and infection must be ruled out if the symptoms last longer than 48 hours or are associated with fever, warmth, or other suspicious signs. Postinjection flare appears to be more likely to develop with the more soluble (shorter-acting) steroid solutions and may be related to the carrier in which the steroid is manufactured. When it does occur, the reaction is usually mild and can be controlled adequately with the application of ice or cold compresses and analgesics as needed.

Rarely, *afterpains* may occur and last for several hours after an injection. Although the cause is obscure, this phenomenon may result from the trauma of needle insertion, penetration of inflamed tissue, or pressure on adjacent nerves from local swelling or bleeding. Afterpains can usually be relieved by the application of moist or dry heat and analgesics until the pain abates, but it is best prevented by mixing a long-acting anesthetic, such as bupivacaine, with the steroid preparation.

Another relatively minor complication is localized subcutaneous or cutaneous atrophy at the site of the injection. This problem is chiefly of cosmetic concern and is recognized as a small depression in the skin frequently associated with depigmentation, transparency, and the occasional formation of telangiectases. These changes in the skin occur when injections are made near the surface and some of the injected steroid leaks back along the needle track. The skin depression usually recedes and the skin returns to normal when the crystals of the steroid have been completely absorbed. These changes are usually evident 6 weeks to 3 months after the initial injection and generally resolve within 6 months, although they can be permanent. In the *two-syringe technique*, the anesthetic is injected first, the needle is advanced into the bursa/peritendon area, and the syringe is then exchanged for another to inject the steroid. This technique helps prevent injection site atrophy by avoiding any leakage of the steroid suspension close to the skin's surface. Use of a small amount of lidocaine or normal saline to flush the suspension from the needle before removing it can also help avoid this problem. The *Z-track technique* is a method of creating an indirect route from the skin puncture to the ultimate site of the steroid injection. To perform this technique, the needle is inserted 0.5 cm to 1.0 cm from the actual target site. When the needle is halfway through the fat tissue, redirect it to the target site and inject both the anesthetic and the corticosteroid. Injection site atrophy is more likely to occur with preparations that are less soluble and thus longer acting.[17,18]

Minor skin depigmentation, especially in dark-skinned individuals, occurs in patients undergoing local corticosteroid injections.[18] It usually occurs within a few months after the initial injection and resolves several months later. This complication can be limited by applying pressure to the site during withdrawal of the needle. Hydrocortisone would be the preferable agent for superficial injections to minimize depigmentation.

One of the most serious complications after local steroid injection is tendon rupture. In general, the risk is very low (<1%) and appears to be related to the dose used. Some believe that injecting steroids directly into the tendon leads to a decrease in the tendon's tensile strength.[19] By using one size of needle and syringe, the operator is more likely to appreciate the increase in resistance when injecting directly into the tendon. Limiting the frequency of injections to no more than once every 3 months in the same site can help avoid this problem as well. Tendon rupture is more likely to occur in major stress-bearing tendons in athletes, such as the Achilles tendon and the patellar tendons.

There have been reports of accidental nerve injury after corticosteroid injection, particularly of the ulnar nerve (for treating medial epicondylitis) and the median nerve (for treating carpal tunnel syndrome [CTS]). Finally, within minutes to hours after injection, approximately some patients may experience facial and neck flushing. This reaction may last a few days, but it is usually a benign and self-limited reaction. Facial flushing seems to be more common with triamcinolone preparations.

Systemic absorption of local corticosteroid injections does occur, although at a slower rate than with oral steroids. As a result patients are at low risk for systemic complications, but they do occur. Specifically, intrasynovial injections of steroids have been shown to suppress the hypothalamic-pituitary-adrenal axis for 2 to 7 days.[20] This complication is more likely to occur in patients who receive repeated injections in a short period or multiple injections in different sites at one time. Corticosteroids can also exacerbate hyperglycemia in diabetics. Abnormal uterine bleeding has also been reported.

Other potential complications of corticosteroid and local anesthetic injections are outlined in Box 53.4.

CORTICOSTEROID PREPARATIONS

Commonly used corticosteroid repository preparations for the injection of bursae and tendon sheaths are described in Table 53.2. Local anesthetics such as lidocaine or bupivacaine can be mixed with the corticosteroid preparation in the same syringe. All corticosteroid suspensions, with the exception of cortisone and prednisone, can produce a significant and rapid antiinflammatory effect (in the synovial spaces). Corticosteroids should not be used for trigger point injections.

Corticosteroid preparations are categorized by their solubility and relative potency. Solutions that are more soluble have a shorter duration of action, primarily because they are absorbed and dispersed more rapidly. The addition of tertiary butyl acetate to the solution causes decreased solubility and therefore a longer duration of action. For example, triamcinolone hexacetonide, the least soluble preparation has the longest duration of action. Because the long duration of action increases its potential for subcutaneous atrophy, some authors use this preparation only for intraarticular injections.

There is little consensus in the literature regarding which corticosteroid to use and what dosage is most appropriate for a given site. Some clinicians advocate mixing both shorter- and longer-acting corticosteroids in the same syringe with little consideration for the location or type of condition. In general, use a short- or intermediate-acting agent for an acute or subacute condition such as bursitis or tendinitis is likely safest with reservation of longer-acting agents such as triamcinolone for chronic and prolonged conditions, including arthritis. Triamcinolone acetonide and methylprednisolone acetate are reasonable first choices for most ED procedures.

TABLE 53.2 Injectable Corticosteroids

INTRASYNOVIAL PREPARATIONS	POTENCY[a]	RANGE OF USUAL DOSAGE (mg)	SOLUBILITY
Short Acting			
Hydrocortisone acetate	1	12.5–75	High
Cortisone	0.8	15–25	High
Intermediate Acting			
Prednisone	3.5	2.5–5	Medium
Prednisolone acetate	4	5–30	NA
Methylprednisolone acetate[b]	5	5–40	Medium
Long Acting[c]			
Triamcinolone acetonide[c]	5	5–40	Low
Triamcinolone diacetate	5	4–40	Low
Triamcinolone hexacetonide	5	4–25	Low
Betamethasone acetate and disodium phosphate	25	1.5–6	Low
Dexamethasone acetate	25	0.8–6	Low

[a]Hydrocortisone equivalents (per milligram).
[b]Preferred for emergency department use.
[c]Best used for intraarticular injection.
N/A, Not applicable.

DOSAGE AND ADMINISTRATION

Bursae and Tendon Sheaths

The dose of any corticosteroid suspension used for intrasynovial injection may be selected arbitrarily. Factors that influence the dosage and expected response include the size of the affected area, the presence or absence of synovial fluid or edema, the severity and extent of any synovitis, and the steroid preparation selected (Table 53.3; also see Table 53.2). Dosages may need to be reduced in older adults.[15]

A useful guideline for estimating dosage is as follows: for relatively large spaces such as the subacromial, olecranon, and trochanteric bursae, use a maximum of 40 mg of methylprednisolone acetate or its equivalent. For medium- or intermediate-sized bursae and ganglia at the wrists, knees, and heels, use 10 to 20 mg. For tendon sheaths, such as flexor tenosynovitis of the digits and the abductor tendon of the thumb (de Quervain's disease), use 5 to 15 mg. Sometimes it may be necessary to give larger doses for an optimal response. Intrabursal treatment of the elbow (olecranon) or the knee (prepatellar) bursae, which contain a considerable amount of fluid, may require 30-mg to 40-mg doses.

Unlike intraarticular injections for synovitis in patients with chronic joint disease, repeated infiltration for soft tissue conditions such as bursitis and tendinitis is not generally recommended or required. However, if only a partial response occurs or if recurrence develops, a single injection can be repeated as long as there is 12-week delay between injections.[15]

Trigger Points

In contrast to injection of bursae and tendon sheaths, use small volumes of local anesthetic, botulinum toxin, sterile water, or sterile saline, or dry needling for trigger point injection.[10] In most cases 1 mL to 2 mL of the chosen agent is sufficient.

Preparation of the Site

Preparation of the site before injection requires meticulous adherence to aseptic technique. Anatomic landmarks may be outlined with a skin pencil. It is important that the injection site and needle tip remain sterile with use of the no-touch technique, although sterile drapes are not generally considered necessary. For operator protection, universal precautions should be followed.

TECHNIQUES

General Considerations

Before beginning the injection inform the patient of the specific indication or indications for treatment. Describe the procedure, including the risks and complications, and obtain informed consent. Subsequently, document the details of the procedure in the medical record. A written consent form is not standard, and its use is best based on institutional or departmental policy.

The material required for local injection procedures includes antiseptic solution, needles, syringes, a hemostat, culture and laboratory tubes, bandages, and sterile gauze (Fig. 53.3). Special trays may be stocked for this purpose. The usual sizes of needles for injection sites and corticosteroid doses are listed in Table 53.3.

Bursae and Tendon Sheaths

Local skin anesthesia is an option before injection but not universally practiced. For bursae and tendon sheaths, local anesthetics can be injected alone or with corticosteroids mixed together in the same syringe. Use the Z-track technique to limit the risk for a fistulous track in the soft tissue. Because the steroid may theoretically precipitate or layer in the barrel of the syringe during the injection, agitate the syringe immediately before using it to optimize its distribution. In addition to minimizing the pain associated with the injection, mixing an anesthetic with the corticosteroid also produces a larger volume for delivery.

The duration of action of lidocaine is approximately 1 hour, whereas bupivacaine may last 6 to 8 hours. Caution the patient that the local anesthetic effect may wear off within a couple of hours and that the beneficial effects of the corticosteroid may be delayed.

TABLE 53.3 A Guide for Needle Size and Dosage for Injection of Common Regional Disorders

DISORDER OR INJECTION SITE	NEEDLE SIZE	USUAL DOSAGE OF METHYLPREDNISOLONE ACETATE (mg)[a]
Bicipital tendinitis	1.5–2 inches, 22–25 gauge	20–40
Calcific tendinitis Subacromial bursitis	1.5–2 inches, 22–25 gauge	20–60
Radiohumeral bursitis Epicondylitis	1.5 inches, 22–25 gauge	20–40
Olecranon bursitis	1–1.5 inches, 20 gauge[b]	15–30
Ganglia on the wrist	1 inch, 22–25 gauge	10–15
de Quervain's disease	7/8 inch, 22–25 gauge	10–20
Carpal tunnel syndrome	1–1.5 inches, 22–25 gauge	20–40
Digital flexor tenosynovitis	7/8 inch, 22–25 gauge	5–10
Trochanteric bursitis	1.5–2 inches, 22–25 gauge	20–40
Prepatellar bursitis	1–1.5 inches, 22–25 gauge	15–20
Anserine bursitis	1–1.5 inches, 22–25 gauge	20–40
Bunion bursitis	1 inch, 22–25 gauge	5–10
Calcaneal bursitis	1 inch, 22–25 gauge	10–20
Superficial trigger point	1.5 inch, 22 gauge	N/A
Deep trigger point	2.0–2.5 inch, 21 gauge	N/A

[a]Empirical dose. A larger or smaller dose may be used, depending on the clinical scenario.
[b]Allows bursa aspiration and steroid injection without removing the needle.
N/A, Not applicable.

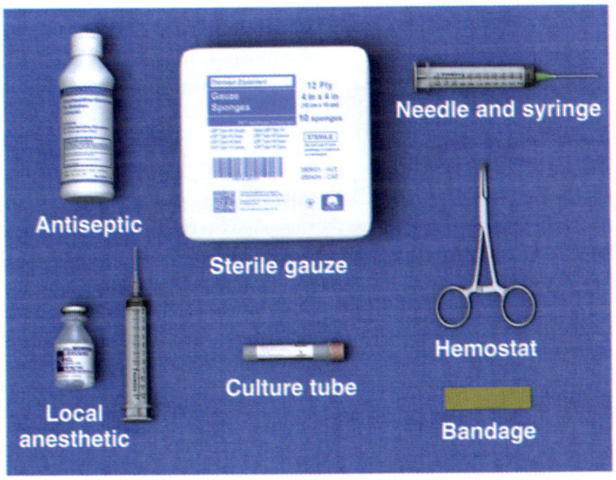

Fig. 53.3 Typical equipment required for injection therapy. Needle sizes and choice of corticosteroid and anesthetic can vary. Typical corticosteroid doses are listed in Table 53.3.

The optimum technique for joint and soft tissue injections has not been firmly established. However, one important aspect of a successful technique is accurate positioning of the needle. Aspiration of fluid confirms that the needle has correctly entered the sac. Conversely, direct injection into a painful soft tissue lesion may require some trial and error to localize the correct site. Sometimes it is advisable to reaspirate and reinject several times within the barrel of the syringe, a procedure called *barbotage*, to obtain heterogeneous mixing and maximal dispersion of the steroid throughout the synovial cavity. Although it is desirable to inject the solution directly into the bursa, direct injection into the tendon itself is best avoided. If the injection requires the application of significant pressure, the needle may be in the tendon and should be withdrawn or advanced a few millimeters. Although an accurate injection is desirable, using a generous volume of anesthetic (3 to 6 mL) to dilute and hence disperse the steroid can compensate for less-than-perfect injections. Asking the patient to use one finger to localize the area of maximum pain and tenderness is the best way to ensure the most accurate positioning of the needle. In general, if the patient cannot localize a specific area of tenderness, the diagnosis should be reconsidered or the expectations of success lowered. Diffuse pain, such as throughout the entire shoulder or knee, is probably not tendinitis or bursitis and is not likely to be relieved with a local injection.

Trigger Points

Successful treatment of a myofascial pain syndrome requires accurate diagnosis (see Box 53.1 and Table 53.1) and precise identification of the trigger point (a taut band of muscle fibers). There are three generally accepted methods for identification of trigger points: flat palpation, pincer palpation, and deep palpation.[10]

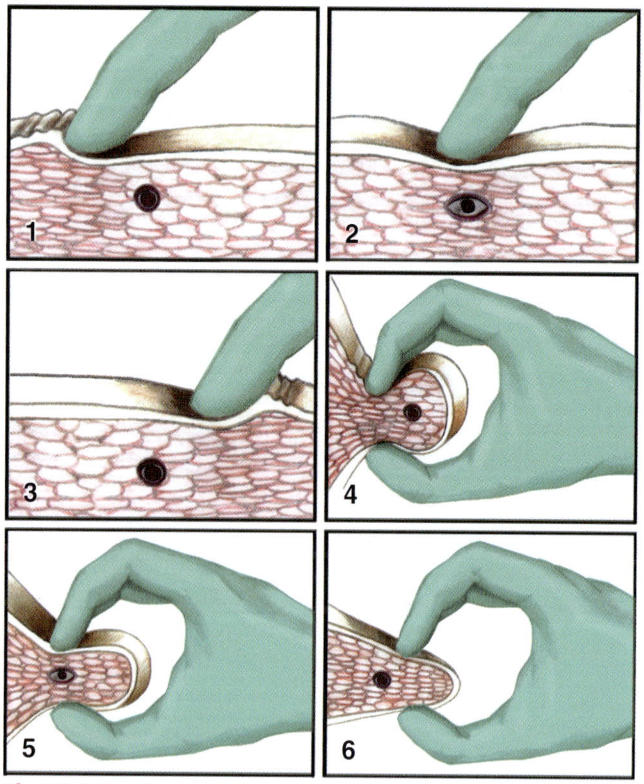

Fig. 53.4 Identification of trigger points. *1*, Push the skin to one side to begin palpation. *2*, Slide the fingertip across the muscle fibers to feel the cordlike texture of the taut band rolling beneath it. *3*, Push the skin to the other side at completion of the movement (this same movement performed vigorously is snapping palpation). *4*, Surround the muscle fibers with the thumb and fingers in a pincer grip. *5*, Feel the hardness of the taut band while rolling it between the digits. *6*, Sharply define the palpable edge of the taut band as it escapes from between the fingertips, often with a local twitch response. (Modified from Sola AE. Myofascial trigger point therapy. *Res Staff Phys.* 1981;27(8):44.)

To perform flat palpation, slide a fingertip across the muscle fibers of the affected muscle group, and at the same time, use the opposite hand to retract the skin to either side until the taut band is identified (Fig. 53.4, *1–3*). Snap the band like a violin string to precisely identify the trigger point. Pincer palpation involves firmly grasping and rolling the muscle fibers between the thumb and forefinger until the taut band is found (see Fig. 53.4, *4–6*). Use deep palpation when the taut band is obscured by superficial tissue. Place a fingertip over the muscle attachment of the area suspected of housing the trigger point and apply pressure in different directions. Reproduction of the patient's symptoms identifies the trigger point. It may be helpful to mark the trigger point with a skin marker for easy identification before treatment.

Once the trigger point has been found, therapy can be divided into invasive and noninvasive techniques (see Box 53.2). Noninvasive techniques used in the ED include spray and stretch, massage therapy, and ischemic compression therapy. Physical therapy, transcutaneous electrical stimulation, and ultrasound treatments are adjuncts that may be arranged by the patient's primary care physician. Invasive techniques involve injecting the trigger point with a local anesthetic, botulinum toxin, or dry needling.

Noninvasive Techniques

Spray and Stretch

The technique of spray and stretch was once advocated by some as the single most effective treatment of trigger point pain. Place the patient in a comfortable position; ensure that the target muscle is well supported and under minimal tension, and that one end of the trigger point is securely anchored. Anesthetize the skin overlying the trigger point with vapocoolant spray (ethyl chloride, dichlorodifluoromethane, or trichloromonofluoromethane) over the entire length of the muscle. Apply the spray at a 30-degree angle to the skin. After the first pass of spray, apply immediate pressure on the other end of the muscle to create a passive stretch. Perform multiple slow spray passes over the entire width of the muscle while maintaining passive stretch until the muscle achieves a full range of motion. Do not perform more than three repetitions before rewarming the area with moist warm heat, and do not allow each spray to last more than 6 seconds. Educate patients to not overstretch muscles after each therapy session.[21–23]

Massage Therapy

Various massage techniques including massage of the trigger point itself have been described as alternative therapies. Massage with ice, or "ice stroking," involves stroking the skin with ice and can be combined with traditional massage.[21]

Ultrasound

Ultrasound has recently been studied as a potential noninvasive method of treating myofascial pain by using sound waves to provide heat energy to muscles. Limited data suggest perhaps a modest benefit in terms of increases in pain pressure threshold.

Ischemic Compression Therapy

The principle behind ischemic compression therapy is to use pressure to induce ischemia for ablation of the trigger point. To perform this technique, apply and maintain pressure on the trigger point with increasing resistance until tension in the muscle is relieved. This is performed with braced thumbs, long, or index fingers. The patient might perceive mild discomfort but not profound pain. Repeat the process for three to four times for each trigger point encountered. Stretching should follow ischemic compression therapy to maximize benefit.

Invasive Techniques

Injection Therapy

Almost any trigger point is suitable for injection therapy. Patients who do not respond to noninvasive treatments should be strongly considered for injection. Historically, various substances have been used, including local anesthetics, botulinum toxin, sterile water, and sterile saline. Despite the different compositions, durations of action, and mechanisms of action of these substances, a common finding is that the duration of pain relief following the procedure outlasts the duration of action of the injected substance.[20] As noted earlier, the authors of a 2001 systematic review concluded that based on current medical evidence, the nature of the injected substance makes no difference on the outcome and that wet needling is not therapeutically superior to dry needling. Nevertheless, the addition of a local anesthetic has been shown to reduce the degree of postinjection soreness and is recommended by most authors.

The technique most often recommended for trigger point injection has been referred to as the *universal technique*. Position the patient in a recumbent position to assist in relaxation of the affected muscles, overall comfort, and prevention of syncope. Re-identify the previously marked trigger point of interest, and scrub the overlying skin with a topical antiseptic solution. For superficial trigger points, use a 22-gauge, 1.5-inch needle. Deeper muscles may require a 21-gauge, 2- or 2.5-inch needle (see Table 53.3). Grasp the skin overlying the trigger point between the thumb and index or middle finger of the nondominant hand. Insert the needle approximately 1 to 1.5 cm from the trigger point and advance it into the trigger point at a 30-degree angle. Aspirate to confirm that a blood vessel has not been entered, and inject a small amount (0.2 mL) of the agent. Withdraw the needle to the skin, redirect it to another area of the trigger point, and inject again. Use a fast-in, fast-out approach to elicit a local twitch response, which has been shown to increase the effectiveness of the trigger point injection and allows the entire trigger point area to be treated. Severe cramping or paresthesia suggest inadvertent nerve entry and mandates withdrawal and redirection of the needle. For best results, it is critical to elicit a local twitch response with every injection and continue the needling and injection process until the local twitch response is extinguished. Following the procedure, the muscle group that was injected should undergo a full active stretch to try to obtain full length.

Specific Regions and Clinical Entities

Bursitis and Tendinitis

Shoulder Region

See Video 53.1. Shoulder pain is a common complaint in both the emergency and primary care settings. The pain can be associated with significant disability and may result from pathology that is intraarticular or extraarticular including bicipital tendinitis, calcific (calcareous) tendinitis, and subacromial bursitis (Fig. 53.5). Because injections in this area are easy and safe to perform, these areas are frequently injected, especially in patients who have not responded to more conservative therapy such as ice, rest, and oral antiinflammatory medications. Injections may also offer a diagnostic advantage when evaluating a patient with subacromial pain or a rotator cuff syndrome in differentiating shoulder weakness caused by impingement, in which shoulder strength improves after injection, and a true rotator cuff tear, in which there is generally no change in strength following injection. A potential long-term complication of untreated persistent inflammation is the development of a *frozen shoulder* (adhesive capsulitis).[24]

Bicipital Tendinitis (Tenosynovitis) (Fig. 53.6). The biceps tendon is a common extraarticular cause of shoulder pain and injuries to the tendon can range from minor inflammation to complete rupture. Bicipital tendinitis and tenosynovitis represent nonspecific low-grade inflammation of the biceps tendon and/or its sheath that is common in those who repeatedly flex the elbow against resistance, such as weight lifters and swimmers.[4] Older patients are more likely to develop degenerative tendinosis and rupture, whereas isolated tendinitis is more common in younger patients.

The bicipital tendon courses through the joint and along the bicipital (intertubercular) groove (see Fig. 53.5), which can be appreciated when the elbow is held at 90 degrees of flexion

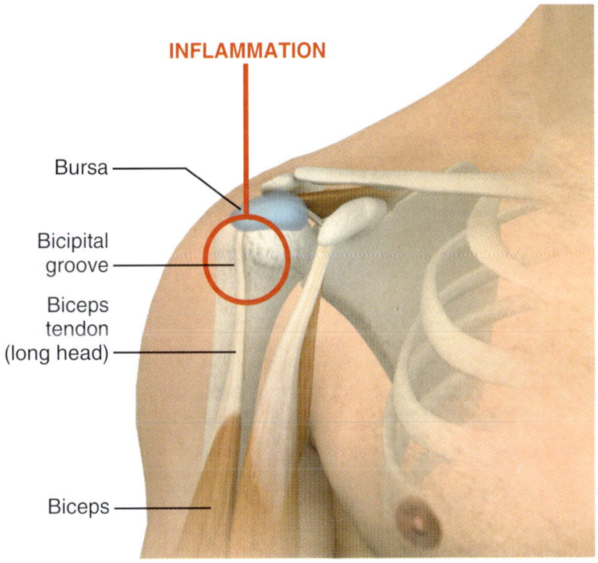

Fig. 53.5 Bicipital tendinitis and subacromial bursitis. Pain in the shoulder may be caused by biceps tendinitis or subacromial bursitis, but this is difficult to clinically differentiate from other shoulder conditions. Sudden pain and a distinct soft tissue bulge in this area can indicate rupture of the long head of the biceps.

and the arm is internally and externally rotated.[25] Patients typically complain of pain over the biceps muscle extending into the anterior shoulder. They may have restricted or normal range of motion and normal strength; however, they usually complain of tenderness on palpation over the bicipital groove. Efforts to elevate the shoulder, reach the hip pocket, or pull a back zipper all aggravate the symptoms. Tenderness over the bicipital groove does not confirm the diagnosis; however, because the supraspinatus tendon is in close proximity to the insertion of the bicipital tendon.[26] Other diagnostic clues include the Lippman test, in which rolling the bicipital tendon produces localized tenderness; the Yergason test, which elicits pain along the bicipital groove when the patient attempts supination of the forearm against resistance while holding the elbow flexed at a 90-degree angle against the side of the body; and the Speed test, in which pain is reproduced when the patient resists forward elevation of the humerus against an extended elbow (see Fig. 53.6).[25] Although helpful, these tests are only moderately specific for bicipital tendinitis. Radiographic testing is generally not warranted if the clinical diagnosis is supported; however, plain film, ultrasonography, and MRI can be helpful in diagnosing alternative or concomitant pathology such as rotator cuff syndromes which can mimic or occur in conjunction with bicipital tendonitis.[27]

Approach. Place the patient in a seated position with both hands resting comfortably in their lap. Locate the point of maximal tenderness along the bicipital tendon. Make entry with a 22- or 25-gauge, 3.9- to 5.0-cm needle through an optional lidocaine skin wheal. Avoid an intratendinous injection, which may cause weakening of the tendon and predispose the patient to tendon rupture. Advance the needle along the side of the tendon at a 30-degree angle and aim at one border of the bicipital groove to perform a *peritendinous infiltration* (see Fig. 53.6). Administer one-third of the injection at this point. Withdraw the needle slightly but keep it subcutaneous and redirect it upward approximately 2.5 cm for injection of another third of the drug. Withdraw it again

Bicipital Tendinitis

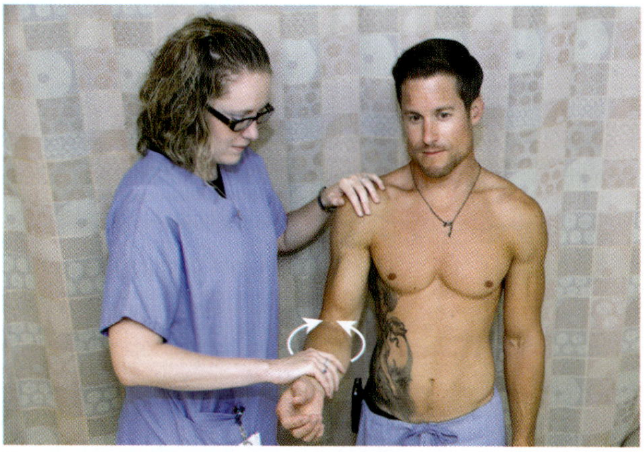

Yergason's test. Yergason's test helps determine the stability of the long head of the biceps tendon in the bicipital groove. This test, which involves resisted supination of the forearm with the elbow flexed to 90 degrees, may accurately reproduce symptoms of bicipital tendinitis.

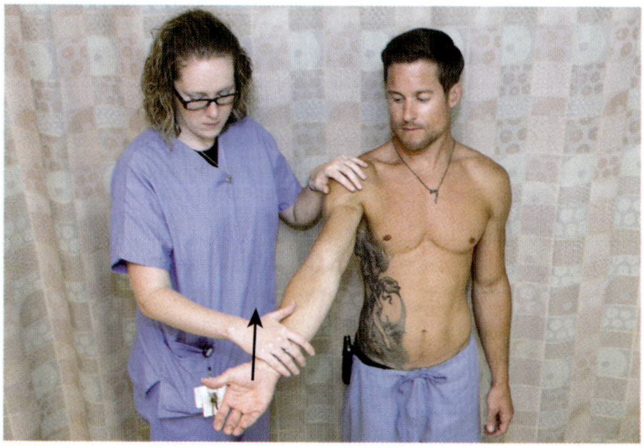

Speed's test. While the elbow is maintained in extension and the forearm in supination, perform forward flexion of the shoulder against resistance. Patients with bicipital tendinitis may have pain or tenderness in the bicipital groove with this maneuver.

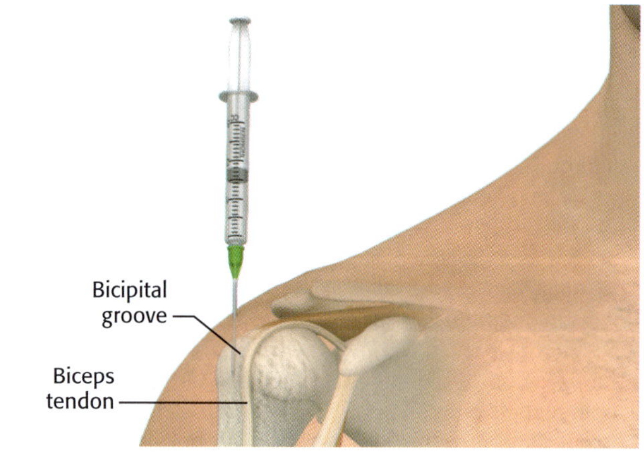

Insert the needle along the side of the biceps tendon (long head) at a 30 degree angle, aimed at one border of the bicipital groove.

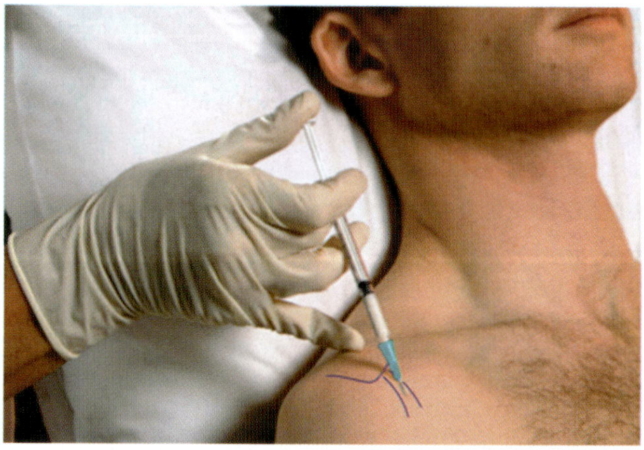

Make a peritendinous infiltration by injecting around the biceps tendon in a fan-wise distribution. Avoid intratendinous injection. Use a 10- to 20-mg equivalent of Kenalog 40 (triamcinolone acetonide).

Fig. 53.6 Bicipital tendinitis.

and redirect it downward so that it touches the bicipital border gently. Deposit the remainder of the drug at this point. With any of these injections, resistance to injection suggests intratendinous needle placement, which should be avoided. If the two-syringe technique is used, instill 1 to 1.5 mL of an intermediate-acting corticosteroid suspension, such as prednisolone tebutate, at the point of maximum tenderness. Inject the anesthetic (2 to 4 mL of 1% lidocaine, or 0.25% bupivacaine) along the upper and lower borders of the tendon. Ultrasound may aid in locating and injecting the tendon sheath.[14,28]

Calcific (Calcareous) Tendinitis, Supraspinatus Tendinitis, and Subacromial Bursitis. These inflammatory syndromes are clinically similar making their symptoms and signs difficult to differentiate. The musculotendinous rotator cuff is composed of the supraspinatus, infraspinatus, teres minor, and subscapularis muscles, which insert as the conjoined tendon into the greater tuberosity of the humerus. The subacromial bursa lies just superior and lateral to the supraspinatus tendon (Fig. 53.7). Both the tendon and the bursa are in the space between the acromion process and the head of the humerus and are particularly prone to impingement in this "critical zone." Impingement can occur when the shoulder moves forward and compresses the cuff and bursa under the anterior third of the coracoacromial arch. Injections into either the bursa or the tendon sheath area are commonly performed to relieve inflammation and overuse injuries.

In *calcific* tendinitis of the shoulder, a calcific deposit (hydroxyapatite) is located within the substance of one or more of the rotator cuff tendons (commonly the supraspinatus).[29] These calcium crystals can occasionally rupture into the adjacent subacromial bursa and cause acute pain and tenderness in the deltoid area (Fig. 53.8). The bursae in relation to the greater tuberosity and the subdeltoid (subacromial) bursa are the most common sites of calcific deposits.

During the acute or hyperacute stage, the patient holds the arm in a protective fashion against the chest wall. The pain may be incapacitating, and all ranges of motion are disturbed, with internal rotation especially limited. Tenderness is often diffuse over the perihumeral region. The patient may also complain of pain at night when lying on the affected side and with abduction of the arm. Supraspinatus tendon impingement is most apparent when the humerus is abducted and internally rotated. The Hawkins test elicits pain with forcible internal rotation while the patient's arm is passively flexed forward at 90 degrees, and the Neer test elicits pain with full forward flexion between 70 and 120 degrees (Fig. 53.9). Both tests are sensitive but not specific for supraspinatus tendon impingement. Constitutional symptoms are rare and should prompt consideration of alternative pathology, such as gout, rheumatoid arthritis, infection, or polymyalgia rheumatica. However, swelling may sometimes be apparent with the hyperacute form, and a fever and elevated sedimentation rate may even develop in some patients. When shoulder radiographs demonstrate a calcific deposit, the shadow appears "hazy" with lightening of the periphery caused by the pressure of inflammatory edema (see Fig. 53.8). Night pain may be intolerable and often requires additional analgesics for pain control.

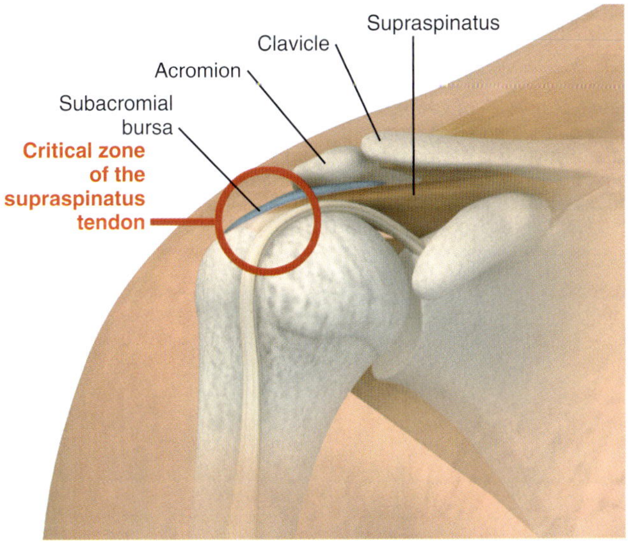

Fig. 53.7 The "critical zone." Note the close relationship of the supraspinatus tendon and subacromial bursa to the humeral head and acromion, which make an exact clinical diagnosis very difficult.

Anterior Approach. In calcific tendinitis, or supraspinatus tendinitis without calcification, use the anterior (subcoracoid) approach. With the extremity resting on the patient's lap, externally rotate the arm approximately 15 degrees. The point of insertion is over the depression that is palpable inferior and lateral to the coracoid process and medial to the head of the humerus (see Fig. 53.9).

Posterolateral Approach. With the patient sitting and the lower part of the extremity resting on the lap, make a lidocaine skin wheal at the depression approximately 1 cm inferior to the posterolateral tip of the acromion, located between the head of the humerus and the acromion. Direct a 3.9- to 5.0-cm, 22- or 25-gauge needle toward the center of the head of the humerus and upward at an angle of approximately 10 degrees. Because the bursa does not extend posteriorly beyond the middle of the acromion, it is important that the needle be positioned sufficiently anterior and inferior to the acromion (see Fig. 53.9). After the site has been penetrated 2 to 3 cm, aspirate for any fluid or calcific material. Remove the syringe but leave the needle in position. Attach another syringe containing 20 to 40 mg of methylprednisolone suspension or an

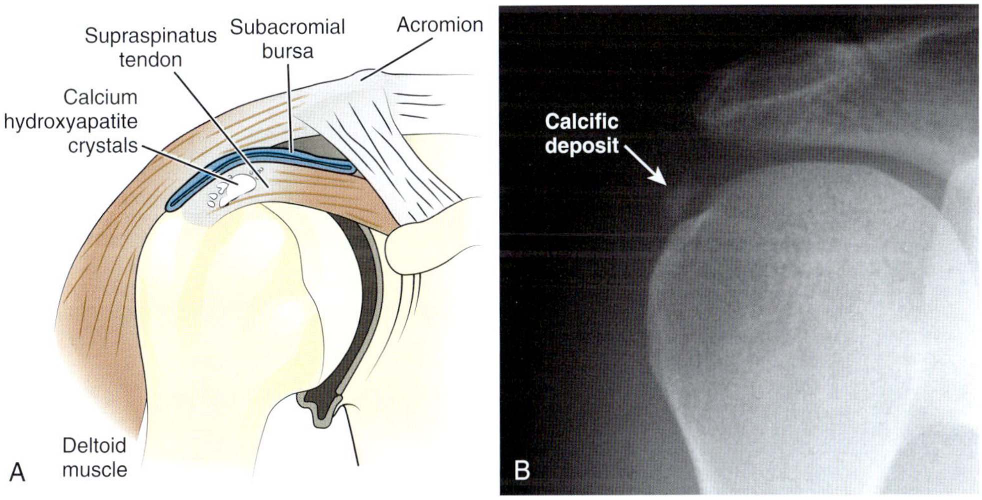

Fig. 53.8 Calcific tendinitis. (A) In calcific tendinitis of the shoulder, calcium hydroxyapatite crystals are deposited in the tendons of the rotator cuff and occasionally rupture into the adjacent bursa. (B) Abnormal calcific deposits in calcific tendinitis of the shoulder are usually demonstrated roentgenographically in the suprahumeral region or adjacent to the greater tuberosity. When the bursal calcifications appear to be dense (as on this x-ray film), they are frequently asymptomatic, whereas lightening at the margins of the calcium deposit is compatible with the presence of inflammatory edema in the rotator cuff, which produces pain and tenderness in the shoulder region. The location of the calcific deposit on the radiograph may be a useful guide for the point of entry for aspiration and injection. Direct the needle to the calcific deposit, aspirate, and deposit a portion of the steroid medication there. The calcium may subsequently disappear. Not infrequently, it does so spontaneously.

Calcific Tendinitis, Supraspinatus Tendinitis, and Subacromial Bursitis

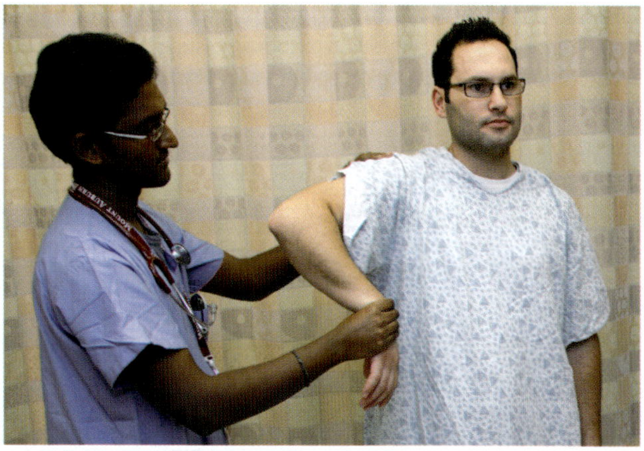

Hawkin's test. With the patient's arm and elbow flexed to 90 degrees, the examiner rotates the forearm internally (i.e., thumb pointed down so that the palm of the hand is directed as far posteriorly as possible). Pain is reproduced if there is impingement of the coracoacromial ligament.

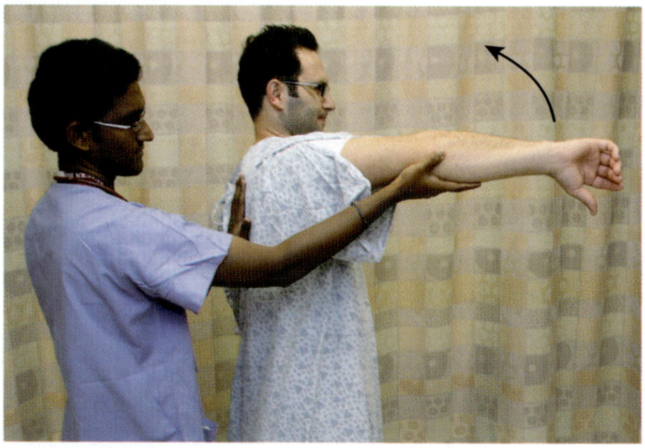

Neer's test. With one hand placed on the patient's scapula, the forearm is slowly flexed forward. The arm should be internally rotated such that the thumb is pointing downward. This test causes pain as the greater tuberosity of the humerus impinges on the acromion. Pain may be reproduced between 70 degrees and 120 degrees of forward flexion.

Anterior Approach

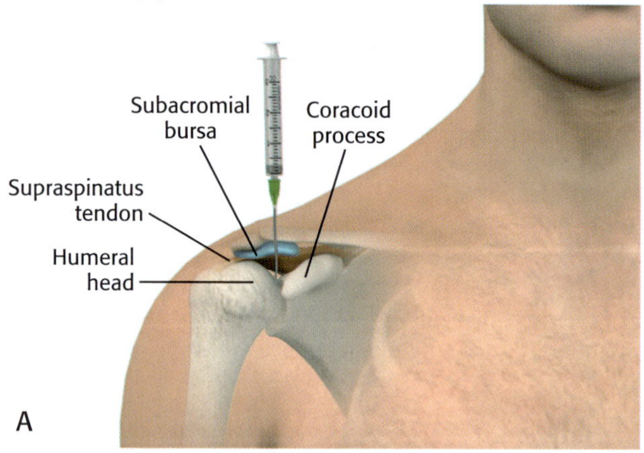

Externally rotate the arm to 15 degrees. Insert the needle over the depression that is palpable inferior and lateral to the coracoid process and medial to the head of the humerus.

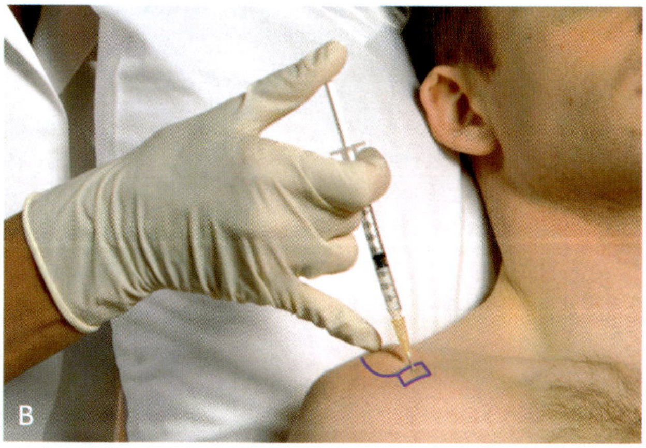

The bursa lies mainly under the acromion, but this is variable. Supraspinatus tendinopathy often occurs with subacromial bursitis.

Posterolateral Approach

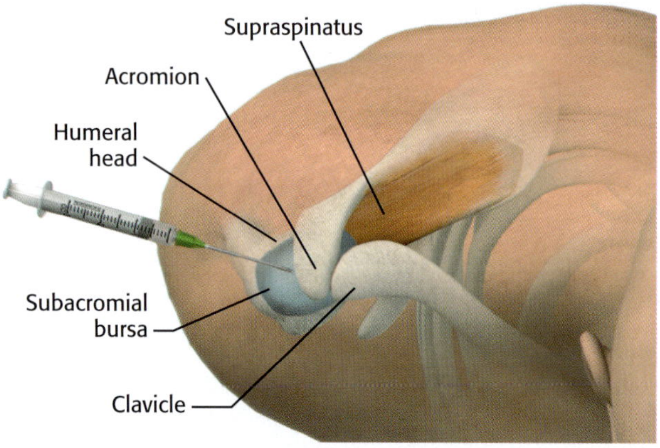

Insert the needle in the depression just inferior to the posterolateral tip of the acromion and superior to the head of the humerus.

Lateral Approach

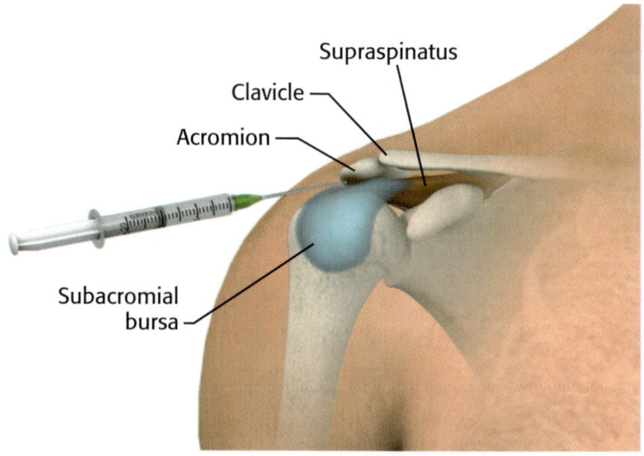

For the lateral approach, insert the needle over the superior aspect of the humeral head and under the lateral margin of the acromion.

Fig. 53.9 Calcific tendinitis, supraspinatus tendinitis, and subacromial bursitis. Subacromial bursitis pain is quite common and responds well to injection. Recurrent pain can be due to a rotator cuff tear, which requires evaluation with magnetic resonance imaging. Pain is felt in the deltoid area and can radiate down the arm. The bursa lies mainly under the acromion, but this is variable. Supraspinatus tendinopathy often occurs together with subacromial bursitis.

equivalent intermediate-acting steroid and inject the medication. Little resistance should be encountered when injecting the steroid. If resistance is appreciated, reposition the needle because it may be in the tendon substance of the rotator cuff. Follow this injection with 4 to 6 mL of 1% lidocaine (or a similar volume of 0.25% bupivacaine). Alternatively, combine the local anesthetic and steroid in the same syringe. Be generous with the volume of local anesthetic injected to ensure adequate dispersion of the steroid. A single treatment relieves most acute disorders, however, can be repeated if needed. An injection into the peritendinous space is like that described previously except that the needle is advanced deeper than with a subacromial bursal injection.

If calcific tendinitis is suspected, some recommend attempting to aspirate the calcium deposits. After the bursa has been anesthetized, use an 18-gauge needle to penetrate the calcium, which often creates a gritty sensation.[24,29] This can be performed under ultrasound guidance for a more directed approach. Barbotage can facilitate cleavage of the calcium deposits and obtain greater dissemination of the injection. Use this method as described previously by aspirating and reinjecting the steroid or anesthetic-steroid combination repeatedly. Needling followed by aspiration and lavage of the subacromial space has also been proven to be effective.

Sometimes a painful reaction develops after the analgesic has worn off. Development of bursitis is also a possibility. Warn the patient about this possibility and give appropriate analgesia. A sling may provide additional relief. Short-term use of opioids is also appropriate. Although some authors claim that patients who do not also undergo physical therapy after corticosteroid injection have satisfactory results, some evidence supports the importance of close patient follow-up, range-of-motion exercises, and physical therapy for total recovery.

Acromioclavicular Joint Inflammation. Pain arising in the acromioclavicular (AC) joint can be the result an acute injury, such as falling on an outstretched hand or from repetitive strain injuries and degeneration. With this injury, all ranges of motion of the shoulder cause pain, and the joint is tender but rarely swollen. Tenderness over the AC joint is sensitive but not specific for AC joint pathology. Be aware that an obvious deformity or mechanism of injury may suggest AC separation or dislocation. Radiographic imaging should be obtained as clinically indicated. With AC joint inflammation, crepitus is not uncommon. Adduction of the arm across the body with forward elevation to 90 degrees (the cross-arm test) may exacerbate the pain because the AC joint is compressed with this motion. Many patients obtain relatively short-term pain relief from injection therapy, some clinicians believe that AC joint injection should be performed only in patients with persistent pain despite a trial of rest, oral antiinflammatory medications, and modification of activity.[30,31]

Approach. Make an entry through an optional cutaneous lidocaine wheal over the interosseous groove at the point of greatest tenderness (Fig. 53.10). This is usually at the AC joint, which is palpated as a small V-shaped depression posteriorly at the most lateral aspect of the clavicle. In this area, the joint line is relatively superficial. Advance a 2.2- to 2.5-cm, 22- or 25-gauge needle approximately 5 mm and inject 1 mL to 2 mL of lidocaine and 5 mg to 10 mg of a prednisolone suspension. It is not necessary to advance the needle beyond the proximal margin of the joint surface.

Elbow Region

The elbow is subject to characteristic extraarticular disorders, including radiohumeral bursitis, lateral, and medial epicondylitis (*tennis elbow* and *golfer's elbow*, respectively), and olecranon bursitis *(barfly's elbow).*

Radiohumeral Bursitis, Lateral Epicondylitis, and Medial Epicondylitis. Radiohumeral bursitis occurs at the juncture of the radial head and the lateral epicondyle of the elbow. This condition is commonly found in combination with lateral epicondylitis, which is thought to result from repetitive microtrauma at the insertion of the *extensor carpi radialis brevis* (ECRB) *and other wrist extensors.* The symptoms of the two adjacent problems are indistinguishable, but tenderness overlies the radiohumeral groove with bursitis, whereas tenderness occurs chiefly at the lateral epicondyle with tennis elbow (Fig. 53.11). Although the term *epicondylitis* suggests an inflammatory cause of the pain, evidence indicates that the injury in lateral epicondylitis results from a degenerative process causing a tendinopathy.[32] Regardless of the exact pathophysiology, there is often a history of repetitive motion of the wrist such as while playing tennis, gardening, or using tools. A clinical sign supporting the diagnosis of tennis elbow is provocation of pain when the patient attempts extension of the middle finger against resistance with the wrist and elbow held in extension. Alternatively, pain is reproduced at the elbow when the patient is asked to extend the wrist against resistance.

Medial epicondylitis (golfer's elbow) is a similar condition, although it occurs on the side opposite that of lateral epicondylitis and is much less common (Fig. 53.12). This condition involves the origin of the *pronator teres* and *flexor carpi radialis* muscles. On physical examination, the patient usually complains of pain when the wrist is *flexed* against resistance or when the forearm is pronated. Palpation of the medial epicondyle also elicits tenderness.

There is evidence supporting the short-term efficacy of corticosteroid injection for both lateral and medial epicondylitis; however, newer biologic therapies such as platelet-rich plasma injections and extracorporeal shock wave therapy have led to decrease in corticoid steroid injection.[32–35] Successful injection of lateral epicondylitis produces a predictable short-term (usually less than 6 weeks) improvement in pain that is superior to that with nonsteroidal drug therapy and physical therapy.[35] However, after 6 weeks, physical therapy reduces symptoms more than corticosteroid injection does. Nevertheless, some clinicians still feel corticosteroid injection should be a first-line treatment for lateral epicondylitis. A similar effect was noted with medial epicondylitis regarding short-term pain improvement and physical therapy.[36,37]

Approach. See Video 53.2. For lateral epicondylitis, pronate the patient's forearm and flex the elbow to 90 degrees (Fig. 53.13). Palpate the radial head as a bony protrusion just distal to the epicondyle (confirm identification of the radial head by rotating the patient's forearm). The entry site is at the point of maximal tenderness, which is usually found at a location slightly distal to the lateral epicondyle. Using a 3.9-cm, 22-gauge needle, deposit 20 mg to 30 mg of methylprednisolone or equivalent intermediate-acting steroid mixed with anesthetic through a lidocaine skin wheal. Alternatively,

Acromioclavicular Joint

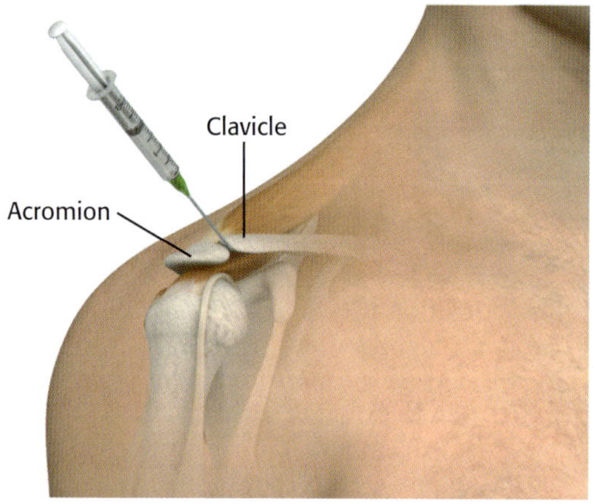

Insert the needle in the interosseous groove at the point of greatest tenderness. This is usually at the AC joint, which is a small V-shaped depression at the most lateral aspect of the clavicle.

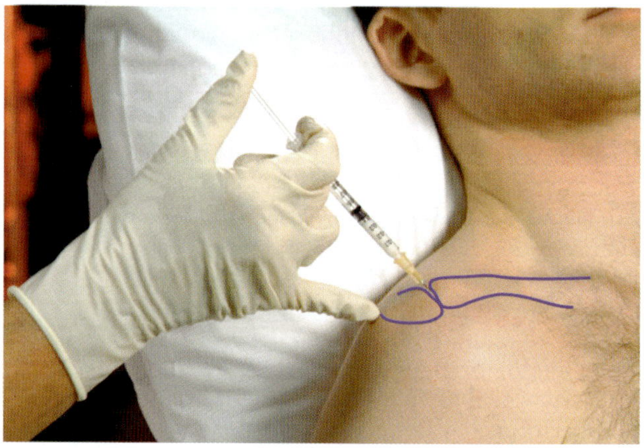

The joint is relatively superficial, and the needle will need to be advanced only about 5 mm. It is not necessary to advance the needle beyond the proximal margin of the joint surface.

Fig. 53.10 Acromioclavicular *(AC)* joint inflammation.

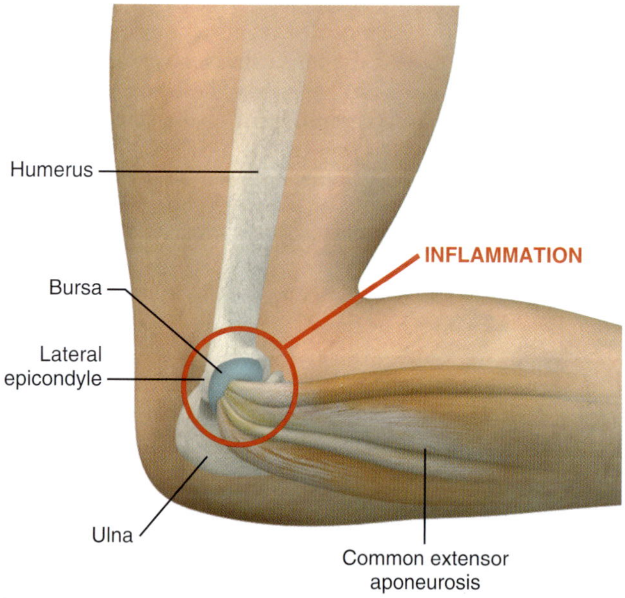

Fig. 53.11 Lateral epicondylitis. Commonly known as *tennis elbow*, this condition is common and quite painful and the result of microscopic rupture and incomplete tendinous repair of the extensor carpi radialis brevis origin on the lateral epicondyle of the humerus. Pain usually occurs over the lateral humeral epicondyle during work or recreation. Although this condition often responds well to an injection, recurrences are common. Physical therapy is indicated for recurring pain.

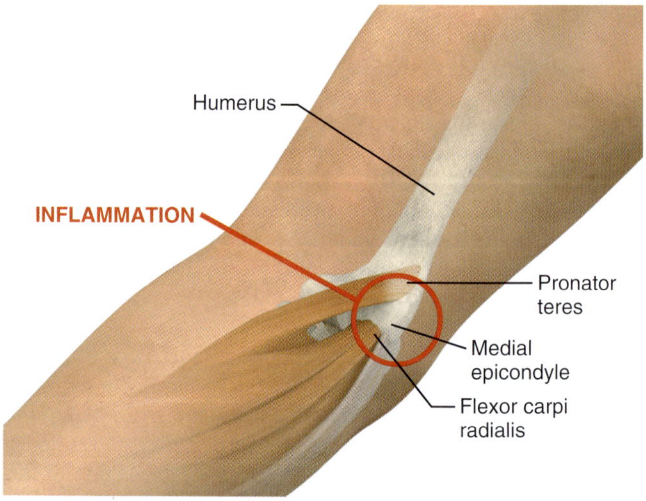

Fig. 53.12 Medial epicondylitis. Also known as *golfer's elbow*, medial epicondylitis is a flexor tendinitis with pain in the medial aspect of the elbow that is elicited by flexing the wrist. This condition is much less common than the lateral variety.

follow the steroid with 1 mL to 3 mL of local anesthetic. Inject the solution in a fanlike pattern while avoiding direct tendon injection. For radiohumeral bursitis, instill part of the repository preparation into the radiohumeral bursa and part at the lateral epicondyle (see Fig. 53.11). With medial epicondylitis (golfer's elbow) use a similar technique, but take care to avoid the ulnar nerve, which lies in the ulnar groove behind the medial epicondyle (Fig. 53.14). Damage to this nerve during steroid injection has been reported.[37]

Olecranon Bursitis (Aseptic). Olecranon bursitis is an inflammation of the olecranon bursa of the elbow, located between the skin and the olecranon process (Fig. 53.15). Swelling of the bursa is easy to detect given its superficial location and can be differentiated from an elbow joint effusion by preserved elbow extension and flexion. The most common cause of olecranon bursitis is minor trauma,[38,39] or activities that involve chronic leaning or repetitive elbow motion. As a result of the latter, olecranon bursitis is also known as *barfly elbow* or *student's elbow*. It may also be seen after an AstroTurf rug burn of the elbow during sporting activities. Other patients at risk for olecranon bursitis include gardeners, auto mechanics, carpet layers, gymnasts, and wrestlers.[39] More significant trauma, such as a direct blow to the elbow, can also cause olecranon bursitis. In this case, hemorrhage into the bursa results in acute hemorrhagic bursitis. Less

Lateral Epicondylitis

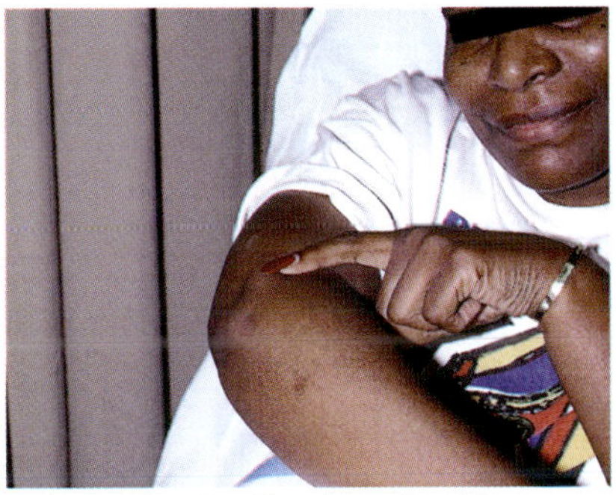

Patients often localize the pain with one finger.

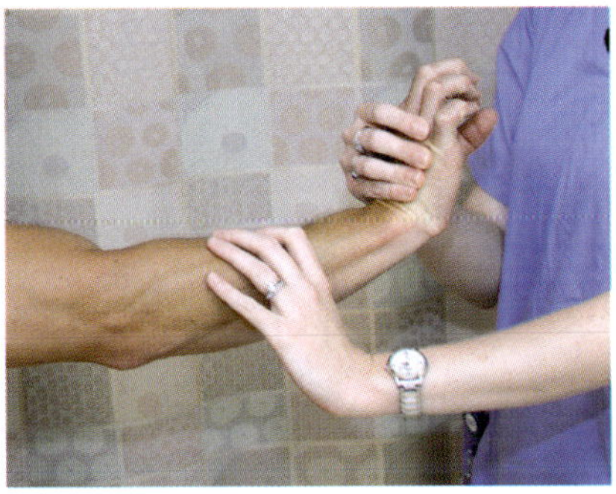

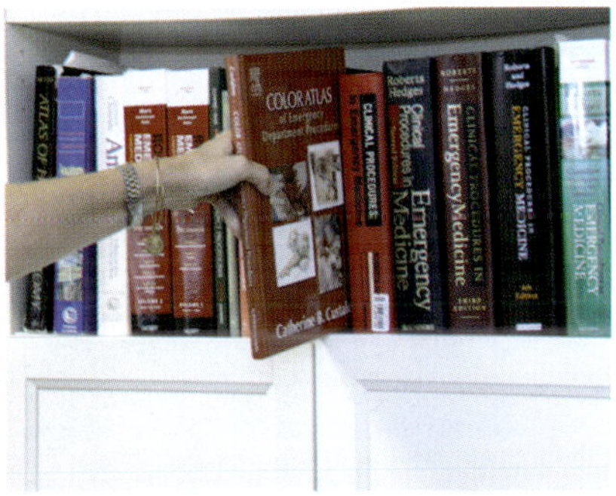

Because this is an extensor tendinitis, extending the wrist against resistance or taking a book off a shelf elicits pain with lateral epicondylitis.

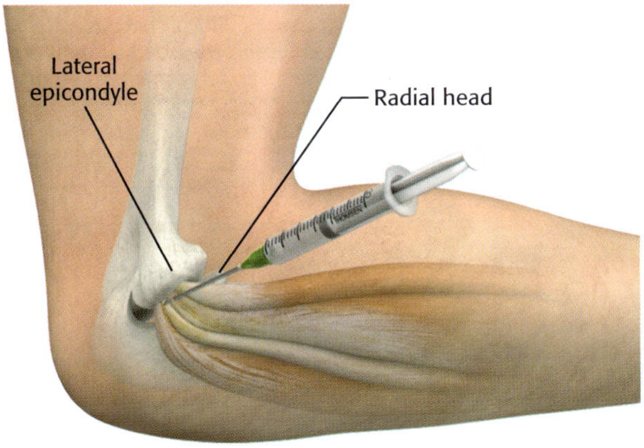

Insert the needle at the point of maximum tenderness, which is usually at a point slightly distal to the lateral epicondyle.

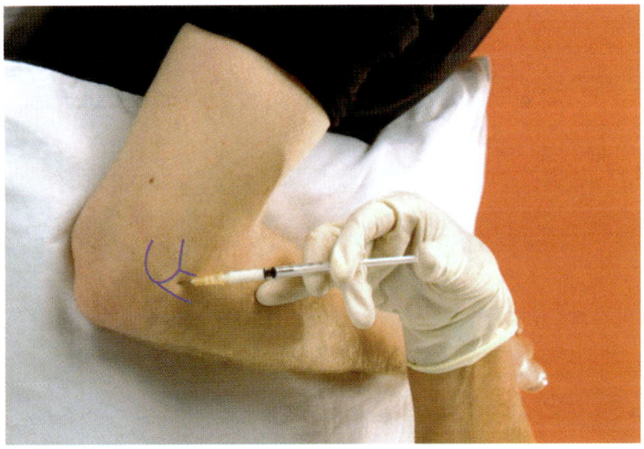

Infiltrate the injection in a fanlike distribution while avoiding direct injection of the tendon.

Fig. 53.13 Lateral epicondylitis.

Medial Epicondylitis

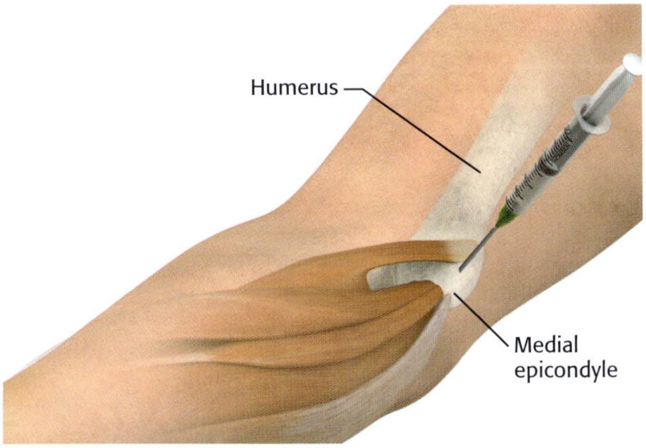

Enter the skin at the point of maximum tenderness, over the medial epicondyle.

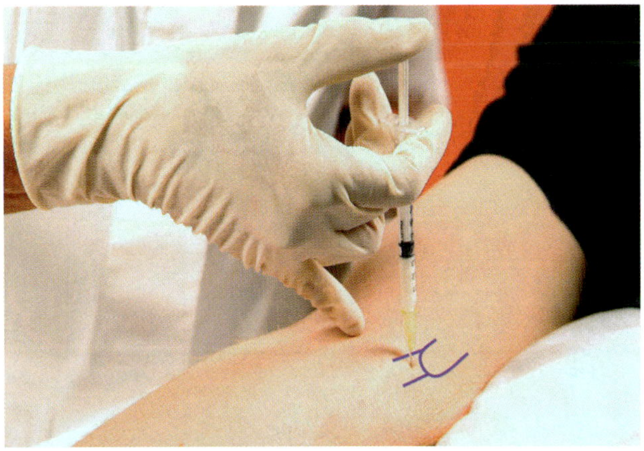

During injection, avoid the ulnar nerve, which lies in the ulnar groove behind the medial epicondyle.

Fig. 53.14 Medial epicondylitis.

Olecranon Bursitis

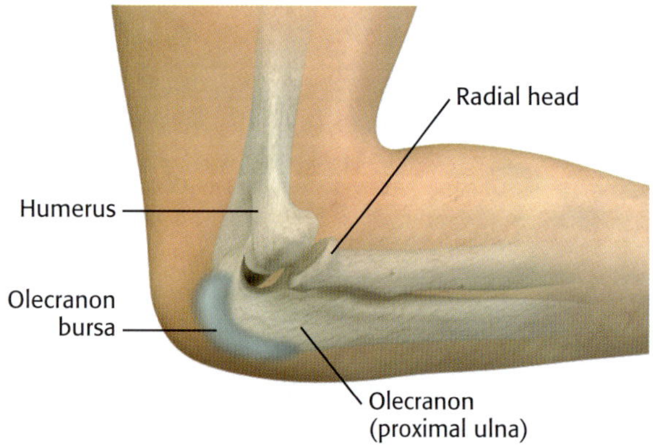

The olecranon bursa is found on the posterior aspect of the elbow and is directly superficial to the olecranon process of the ulna. Trauma is the leading cause of olecranon bursitis, but it may also be related to rheumatoid arthritis, lupus, uremia, and gout. Most cases are sterile, although septic bursitis is a clinical possibility and should be considered.

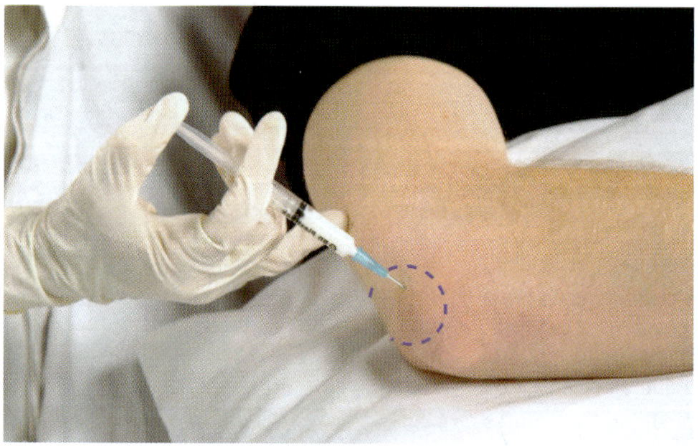

Aspiration and injection are not usually difficult because the bursa is often quite distended with fluid. Insert the needle into the most dependent aspect of the bursal sac. Minimize the risk for persistent drainage and skin contamination by inserting the needle through the skin 2 to 3 cm away from the bursa.

Aspiration and Injection of Olecranon Bursitis

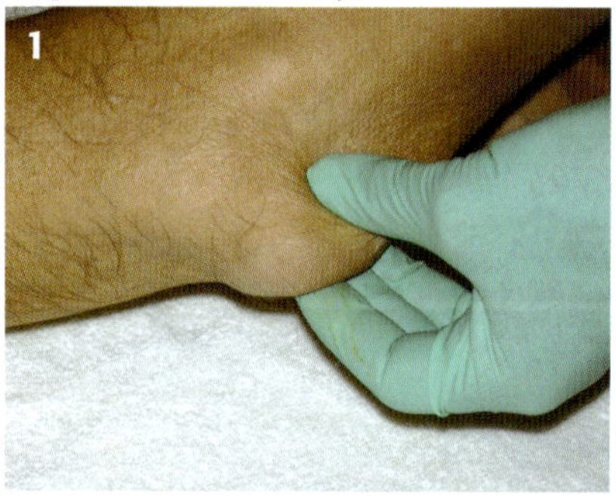

Painless swelling over the posterior aspect of the elbow is characteristic of nonseptic olecranon bursitis. The mass is soft, movable, and fluctuant.

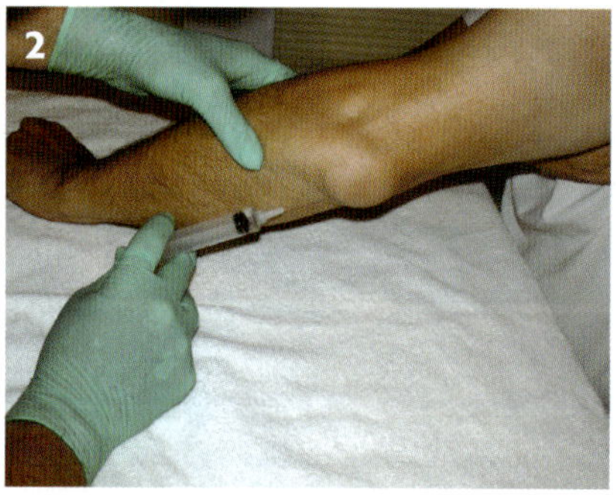

Using sterile preparation, advance a 20-gauge needle on a 10-mL syringe parallel to the forearm.

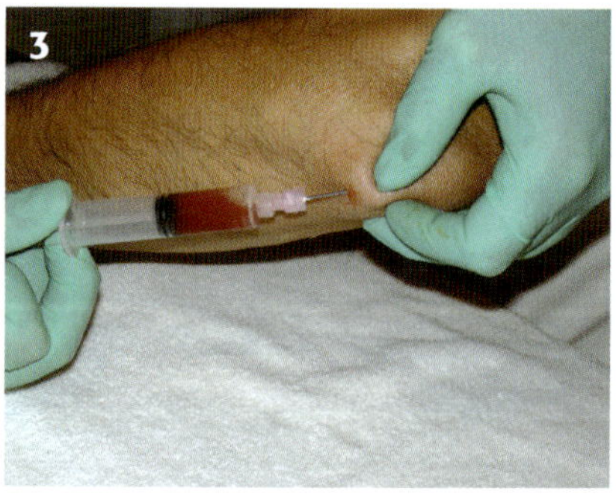

Aspirate the bursal fluid completely. Compress the bursa during aspiration. Typically, slightly blood-tinged serous fluid is obtained.

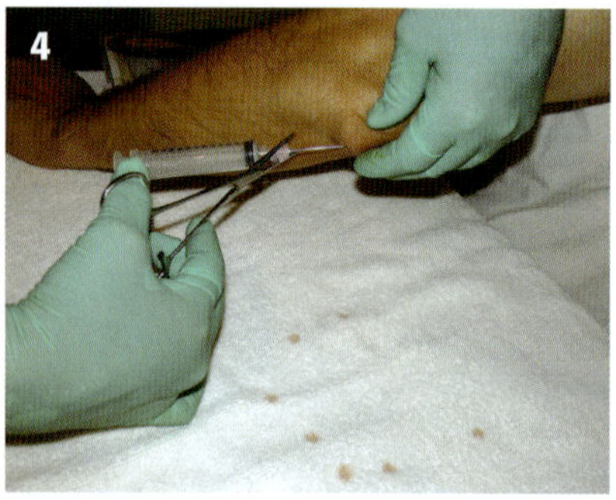

Change the aspirating syringe while the needle remains in the bursal sac.

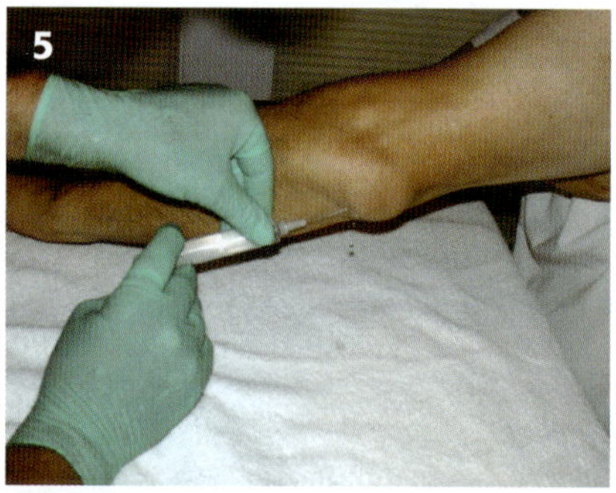

Inject a long-acting steroid preparation (such as 40 mg of methylprednisolone). Use an elastic bandage to compress the site for 12 hours.

Fig. 53.15 Olecranon bursitis.

common causes of olecranon bursitis include hemodialysis and systemic diseases such as rheumatoid arthritis, lupus, uremia, and gout.

Although most cases of olecranon bursitis are sterile, the olecranon bursa is the most frequent site of septic bursitis.[39] Therefore it is important to accurately differentiate between the two entities. Steroid injections are absolutely contraindicated in cases of confirmed or suspected septic bursitis. Frequently the diagnosis will be suggested by the history and physical examination, but it may be necessary to aspirate and analyze the fluid if septic bursitis is suspected.

In aseptic olecranon bursitis, findings on radiographs are usually normal, but soft tissue swelling may be evident. Bony spurs or amorphous calcific deposits may also be seen, especially in older patients. Occasionally with rheumatoid arthritis and gout, nodules, or tophi, may be palpated within the bursal sac. The bursa and surrounding structures are not typically tender, and there is full and painless range of motion of the involved elbow. Signs of infection such as warmth and erythema of the overlying skin are usually absent. It should be noted, however, that pain, warmth, tenderness, and erythema might be present in both septic and aseptic olecranon bursitis. If there is any suspicion of septic olecranon bursitis, aspiration should be performed, and corticosteroid injection deferred until an infectious cause has been ruled out.[40]

Aseptic olecranon bursitis may be cosmetically bothersome to the patient but does not usually cause discomfort and may resolve spontaneously. In cases of bursal swelling that is neither tender nor tense, treatment is symptomatic and includes NSAIDs, compression, and avoidance of further injury.[40] In cases of acute hemorrhagic bursitis, aspiration of the bursa followed by application of a compression dressing and ice will decrease the incidence of chronic bursitis.[40] In patients with aseptic olecranon bursitis who have large, tense, and inflamed bursae, aspiration followed by steroid injection (after infection has been excluded) has been shown to hasten the resolution of symptoms. Smith and colleagues[41] demonstrated the superiority of intrabursal methylprednisolone acetate over oral naproxen or placebo at 6 months and noted faster resolution and less reaccumulation of fluid with the steroid injection. The addition of a course of an oral NSAID after steroid injection did not affect the outcome.[41] Following aspiration and steroid injection, application of a compression dressing and a brief period of relative immobilization may be helpful.[40] Complications with development of septic bursitis, skin atrophy, and sinus tracts have been reported. Repetitive steroid injections for aseptic olecranon bursitis have been associated with triceps rupture and should be avoided.

Olecranon Bursitis (Septic). Because of its superficial location, the olecranon bursa is a common location for septic bursitis along with the pre- and infrapatellar bursa.[42] Infection of the other bursa is much less common. The infection is most likely caused by direct percutaneous inoculation of common skin organisms into the bursa as a result of trauma or contiguous spread from an overlying cellulitis.[42] Septic bursitis secondary to hematogenous spread is rare due to poor blood flow to bursal sacs. Most cases of septic bursitis are caused by *Staphylococcus aureus* (80%), followed by streptococcal organisms. Other less common organisms include coagulase-negative staphylococci, enterococci, and gram-negative organisms such as *Escherichia coli* and *Pseudomonas aeruginosa*. Isolated cases of bursitis caused by fungi (*Aspergillus terreus*, *Candida lusitaniae*), *Brucella*, and *Mycobacterium tuberculosis* have also been reported. Such unusual organisms should be considered in cases of septic bursitis that are subacute or chronic, and those discovered in an immunocompromised host.[42]

The most common cause of olecranon septic bursitis is trauma. It has been estimated that as many as 70% of cases of septic bursitis are related to trauma, either chronic and caused by repetitive injury, or acute and often associated with occupational or recreational activities. Other risk factors for the development of septic bursitis include chronic illnesses (e.g., diabetes mellitus, alcoholism), and previous inflammation of the bursa, which occurs with gout, rheumatoid arthritis, and uremia. The risk of developing septic bursitis in up to 10% of cases following corticosteroid injection was previously mentioned.[42]

At times the diagnosis of septic bursitis can be challenging. Acute gouty olecranon bursitis may have a very similar clinical picture and often can only be accurately differentiated from septic arthritis by fluid analysis (Fig. 53.16). Other conditions that may mimic bacterial septic olecranon bursitis include acute rheumatoid bursitis, aseptic bursitis secondary to oxalosis induced by dialysis, or infectious bursitis caused by unusual organisms such as *Mycobacterium*, *Serratia marcescens*, or fungi. Approximately one-third of all cases of olecranon bursitis are septic.[42]

In some cases, the diagnosis of septic bursitis is obvious (see Fig. 53.16A). The onset of pain and swelling may be quite rapid (over a period of 8 to 24 hours), as opposed to the more gradual onset of aseptic bursitis. The bursa is erythematous, tense, swollen, warm, and very painful. Flexion of the elbow is limited by pain; however, some joint mobility may be present because the bursa does not usually extend into the joint. The patient may report a history of trauma to the area, which may be evident on physical examination. A retrospective 2021 study showed that approximately one-third of patients had a fever of 38.5°C or greater.[42]

Aspiration of infected bursal fluid with culture of bacteria from the aspirate confirms the diagnosis of septic bursitis. Fluid is usually easily obtained from the tense bursa and may be cloudy or grossly purulent. The white blood cell count of the fluid in septic bursitis is usually 5000 to 100,000 cells/mm^3 or greater, and the proportion of polymorphonuclear cells usually exceeds 90%. Neither fever nor systemic leukocytosis is considered sensitive or specific for the disease. However, in immunocompromised patients (e.g., those with diabetes mellitus, or alcoholism), the white blood cell count in the bursal fluid tends to be higher.[43] Because of some overlap in the leukocyte count of bursal fluid in septic versus aseptic bursitis, it is important to remember that a low bursal white blood cell count does not exclude a septic cause. Moreover, the sensitivity of Gram stain may be 50% or less.[44] In a study of 200 patients with olecranon bursitis, cell count and Gram stain were not always helpful in the acute evaluation and treatment of new cases of septic bursitis. Therefore if clinical suspicion for septic olecranon bursitis is high, even in the presence of a normal or equivocal fluid cell count or Gram stain, steroid injection should be delayed and empirical antibiotic therapy started until the results of culture are available. Treatment of septic bursitis includes the use of antibiotics directed against penicillinase-producing *Staphylococcus*, splinting and warm soaks. Administer antibiotics for at least 2 weeks.[45,46] Consider additional antibiotic coverage against methicillin-resistant *S. aureus* based on the patient's risk factors and epidemiology. Outpatient therapy with oral antibiotics is generally acceptable, although this approach has been challenged for immunocompromised patients.[45] More recent literature, including a 2021 retrospective study, recommend against bursal aspiration or drainage and encourage empiric antibiotic treatment with results showing high rates of resolution without recurrence or need for subsequent aspiration or bursectomy. Recurrent infection or infection refractory to treatment may require surgical management.[45,46] This decision is generally guided by the clinical appearance of the bursa, in addition to associated comorbid conditions, compliance, and other factors regarding patient care. Response to antibiotic therapy

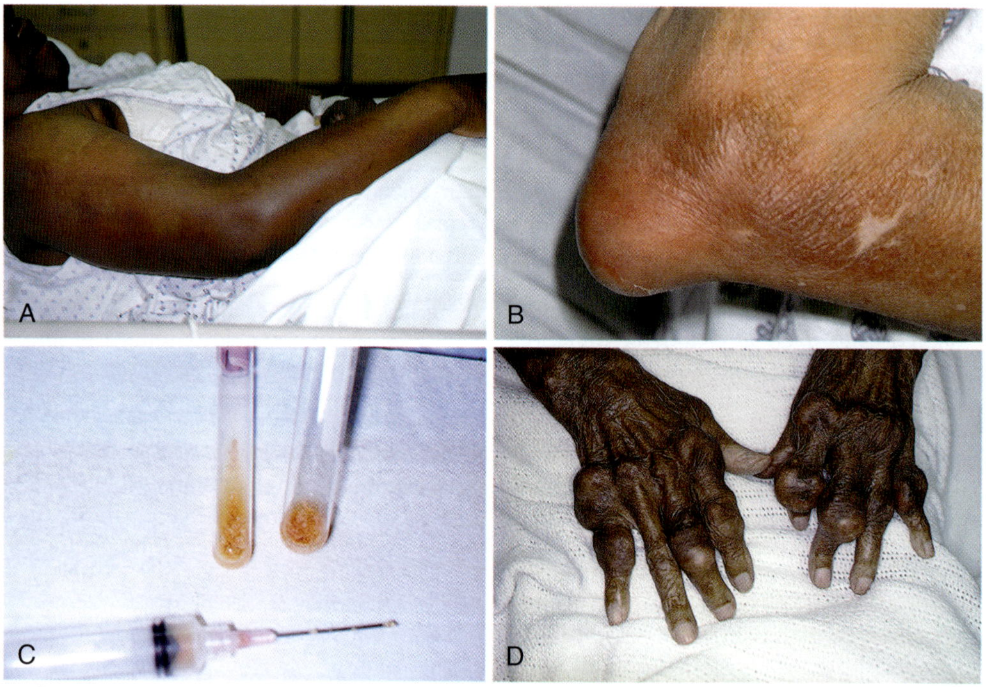

Fig. 53.16 (A) Fully developed septic bursitis is usually distinguished from nonseptic bursitis by clinical parameters. In the septic variety, there is diffuse swelling (as opposed to a discrete mass), and the area is red, warm, and quite tender. In addition, bursal fluid leukocytosis is present. (B) Acute gout can cause painful olecranon bursitis resembling septic bursitis. (C) Aspiration can yield urate paste. (D) Tophi in a patient with advanced gout.

might be slow. Thus it is important to initiate antimicrobial treatment as soon as clinical suspicion of septic bursitis exists. Additional treatment with oral NSAIDs may help reduce the pain. Standard gout medications will generally resolve acute gouty bursitis.

Approach. See Video 53.3. Insert a 2.5- to 3.9-cm, 20-gauge needle through a lidocaine skin wheal at a dependent aspect of the bursal sac (see Fig. 53.15, *steps 1–5*). To minimize the risk for persistent drainage after aspiration and for contamination of the overlying skin, penetrate the skin 2 to 3 cm from the bursa utilizing the Z-track technique. If infected or inspissated fluid is anticipated, use a 16- to 18-gauge needle to aspirate the viscous contents. Aspirate as much fluid as possible. With aseptic bursitis, the aspirated fluid may be yellow and clear, but it is often mildly serosanguinous in appearance. The leukocyte count of the aspirated fluid of aseptic bursitis should be less than 1000/mm^3. Counts of approximately 2000 to 10,000/mm^3 are associated with a higher incidence of infection or acute gout. After aspiration and injection, wrap the elbow in an elastic compression bandage for 5 to 7 days. If administering corticosteroid, inject 15 to 30 mg of methylprednisolone and 1.5 mL of lidocaine. If septic olecranon bursitis is suspected, do not perform corticosteroid injections.

Wrist and Hand Region

Ganglion Cysts of the Wrist or Hand. These cystic swellings occur frequently on the hands, especially on the dorsal aspect of the wrist (Fig. 53.17). They are easily discovered on physical examination and are usually firm, round, and have a rubbery consistency. When physical examination alone is not diagnostic, transillumination or ultrasound can help differentiate cysts from solid tumors. Ganglion cysts are common and make up approximately 60% of all soft tissue tumors affecting the wrist and hand. They usually develop spontaneously in adults between 20 and 50 years of age, with a female-to-male ratio of 3:1. Ganglion cysts may also be seen on the foot and ankle, generally on the extensor surface.

The etiology of ganglia remains obscure; there is usually no history of trauma. The word *ganglion* is derived from the Greek word meaning "cystic tumor." The mesothelium- or synovium-lined cystic structures are attached to or may arise from tendon sheaths or near the joint capsule and do not extend into the joint itself. Attachment is often by a pedicle. The wall of a ganglion is smooth, fibrous, and of variable thickness. The cyst is filled with a clear, gelatinous, sticky, or mucoid fluid of great density. The viscous fluid in the cyst may sometimes represent almost pure hyaluronic acid.

The types of ganglia vary with their location. The most common ganglia are located on the dorsal surface of the wrist and arise from the scapholunate joint. These constitute approximately 70% of ganglia. Volar wrist ganglia, which arise over the distal aspect of the radius, constitute another 20% to 25% of ganglia and are often adherent to the radial artery.[47] Flexor tendon sheath ganglia make up the remaining 10% to 15% and are found on the hand and wrist.

Close to 60% of ganglia spontaneously regress and do not require treatment.[48,49] However, they can sometimes cause pain, loss of function, or weakness (from soft tissue or nerve compression or bone erosion), prompting intervention. In addition, some patients request treatment because of cosmetic concerns. Treatment options include aspiration and surgical excision. Simple aspiration is usually an effective approach, but up to three aspirations may be required for complete resolution. It should be noted, however, that ganglia often recur after aspiration or surgery. In fact, up to half of all ganglion

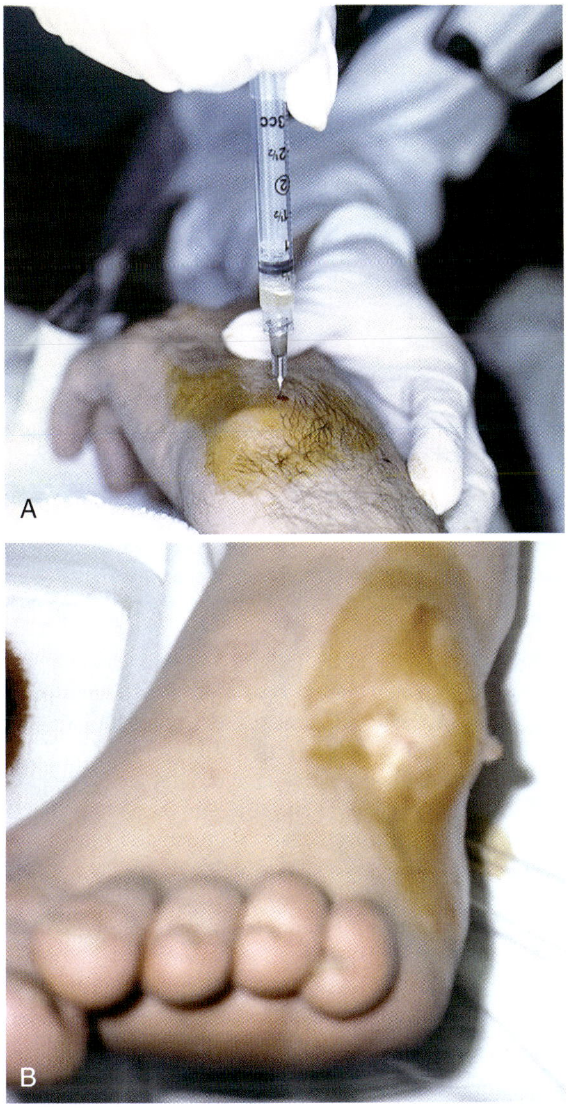

Fig. 53.17 Typical dorsal ganglion cyst of (A) the wrist and (B) dorsum of the foot.

cysts that undergo aspiration will recur within 1 year and most of those within the first 3 months. Following aspiration there is no apparent benefit to the instillation of steroids or hyaluronidase, despite previously reported literature.[50] Because aspiration is associated with considerable cost savings and shorter recovery times than surgery, and because there is no difference in recurrence rates, aspiration appears to be the initial treatment of choice.[50] In the event that nonsurgical treatment fails, surgical excision may be indicated. The old treatment of attempting to rupture the ganglion with a heavy book is not advised because of the potential for local injury. Aspiration of volar wrist ganglia should also be undertaken with caution because the radial artery often adheres to the cyst and may be at risk for injury.[51]

Approach. Following the instillation of 1% lidocaine for local anesthesia, insert a 2.5-cm, relatively large-bore needle (17 to 18 gauge) into the center of the ganglion and aspirate the contents (see Fig. 53.17A). Usually, 1 mL to 2 mL of mucinous fluid can be aspirated. Milk the contents of the cyst toward the aspiration needle to maximize the volume removed, taking care not to stick yourself with the needle. After the cyst is localized by aspiration, if desired (although there is no high-quality supporting evidence for this practice) use another smaller needle to administer 10 mg to 15 mg of methylprednisolone or a combination of methylprednisolone and hyaluronidase.[52,53] Ultrasound guidance can be utilized but does not offer benefit in terms of success or recurrence.[52,53] Following aspiration, a splint is not usually recommended as this limits range of motion prolonging recovery, and activity need not be restricted. There is no proven role for routine NSAIDs or oral steroid therapy.

de Quervain's Disease and Intersection Syndrome. de Quervain's disease, a relatively common disorder, is a stenosing tenosynovitis of the extensor pollicis brevis (EPB) and abductor pollicis longus (APL) tendons of the thumb (Fig. 53.18). Though commonly referred to as a *tenosynovitis,* which denotes inflammation of the synovial sheaths, this condition is more accurately described as a tenovaginitis, which refers to thickening of the fibrous sheath of the first extensor compartment. Histologically the thickening is caused by the accumulation of mucopolysaccharide within the tendon sheath.

It is commonly thought that the disorder occurs more often after repetitive use of the wrists, especially with a wringing motion. Hence, the syndrome has been referred to *washerwoman's sprain.* The etiology of this condition remains in question; however, the leading etiologies include the inflammatory and chronic myxoid degeneration theories. Thus it may be possible that repetitive activities exacerbate the pain associated with a condition for which the underlying cause is still under investigation. Females during pregnancy or within 12 months of childbirth are also frequently affected.

Tenderness, enlargement, and occasionally palpable crepitation are elicited just distal to the radial styloid process, where both tendons come together in an osseofibrous tunnel. Patients usually have radial wrist pain that is exacerbated with certain thumb and wrist movements. The condition may be confused with first carpometacarpal arthrosis (osteoarthritis of the thumb) and intersection syndrome. Radiographs will have normal findings in de Quervain's disease but are appropriate to obtain to rule out other pathologic abnormalities. Ultrasound may demonstrate thickening and edema of the synovial sheath but has not yet been routinely used to make or confirm the diagnosis. Rarely, gonococcal tenosynovitis might simulate this inflammatory condition (Fig. 53.19).

A useful clinical maneuver that indicates de Quervain's disease is the Finkelstein test (Fig. 53.20). With the patient's thumb grasped in their palm, apply ulnar deviation at the wrist. Severe pain at the site of the affected tendon sheaths indicates a positive test. When performing the Finkelstein test, also palpate the tender area for crepitus. If axial traction or compression (the carpometacarpal grind test) and rotation of the thumb produce pain, the condition is most likely caused by degenerative changes in the carpometacarpal joint of the thumb rather than de Quervain's disease. It should be noted that gonococcal tenosynovitis of the wrist may mimic de Quervain's disease, and one should inquire about other symptoms (e.g., sore throat, penile or vaginal discharge, or fever) and carefully look for the characteristic rash of this sexually transmitted disease (see Fig. 53.19).

Patients with mild symptoms may be managed with splinting and NSAIDs, but more severe cases typically require local corticosteroid injection.[54] In one study comparing steroid injection with immobilization and oral NSAID therapy

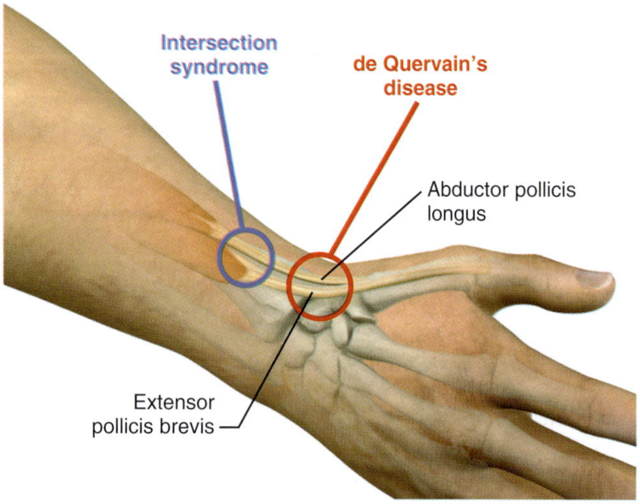

Fig. 53.18 de Quervain's disease and intersection syndrome. de Quervain's tenosynovitis occurs in the first dorsal compartment of the wrist secondary to tenosynovitis of the abductor pollicis longus and extensor pollicis brevis tendons. Symptoms, which include pain over the radial styloid, are generally caused by overuse. Intersection syndrome, often confused with de Quervain's disease, produces symptoms 4 cm to 8 cm more proximally.

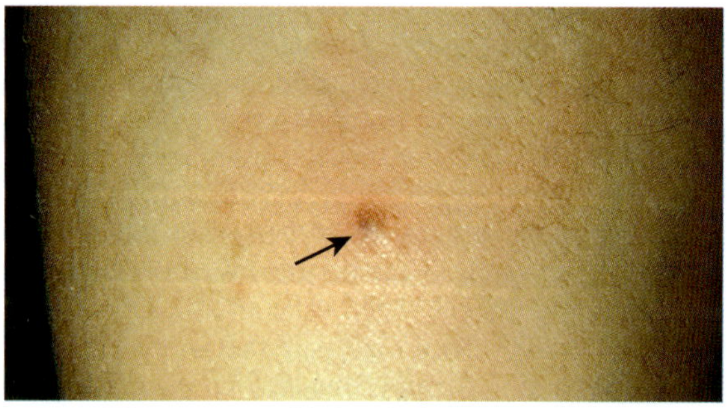

Fig. 53.19 This 25-year-old female had signs and symptoms of tenosynovitis of the wrist that was initially thought to be de Quervain's disease. A single hemorrhagic papule *(arrow)* demonstrating a septic embolus was found on the forearm and is a subtle but classic lesion of gonococcal bacteremia. One aspect of this sexually transmitted disease is tenosynovitis. Cervical cultures were positive for *Neisseria gonorrhoeae* despite the absence of vaginal symptoms.

alone, the latter was effective only in a small group of patients with minimal symptoms.[55] In another retrospective study, 84% of 58 patients were effectively managed either with a single injection (60%) or with repeat injections (24%), with only 12% requiring surgical treatment. These data support a meta-analysis of 495 subjects treated for de Quervain's tenosynovitis in which an 83% cure rate was found with injection alone versus 61% for injection and splinting, 14% for splinting alone, and 0% for rest or NSAIDs.[55] The strikingly favorable response to local injection therapy suggests that surgery to release the tendon sheaths is seldom needed. Interestingly, some evidence suggests that failure of steroid injections may be the result of an anatomic variant in which the EPB is located in a separate synovial compartment.[56] Clinical suspicion for this anatomic variant should be raised when previous steroid injections have failed and patients have pain with firm resistance to thumb metacarpophalangeal (MCP) joint extension (the EPB entrapment test).[57] Consider selective injection into the EPB tenosynovium in these patients.

Using radiographic dye to verify correct corticosteroid placement, researchers have found that when the corticosteroid and anesthetic injection did not successfully reach either the EPB or the APL compartment, the patient did not experience relief of pain. Conversely, when the medication was injected accurately, most patients reported an improvement in symptoms. If available, ultrasound may help guide the injection. A systematic review from 2023 comparing ultrasound-guided injections with standard blind technique demonstrated higher success rates with the use of ultrasound.[56]

Intersection syndrome is a condition that may easily be confused with de Quervain's disease. Because the treatment approach and the clinical course of intersection syndrome differ from that of de Quervain's tenosynovitis, it is important that the clinician also be familiar with this entity. First described in 1841 by Velpea, intersection syndrome describes a clinical entity approximately 4 cm to 8 cm proximal to the location of de Quervain's disease (see Fig. 53.18).[57,58] Intersection syndrome is thought to result from inflammation of the second dorsal compartment of the wrist, which houses the extensor carpi radialis longus (ECRL) and ECRB tendons. Other possible causes include inflammation of a bursa that develops between the APL and the ECRB tendons, and inflammation of the ECRL and ECRB tenosynovium where they cross the muscle bellies of the APL and EPB.[58,59]

Intersection syndrome is characterized by pain, tenderness, edema, and occasional crepitus 4 cm to 8 cm proximal to the radial styloid and may be mistaken for de Quervain's disease. This condition is seen in athletes who play sports that require forceful repetitive wrist flexion and extension, such as rowing, weightlifting, gymnastics, and tennis. Treatment includes rest, NSAIDs, and immobilization with a thumb spica splint in 15 degrees of wrist extension. After a 2- to 3-week trial of splinting, corticosteroid injection therapy is recommended for patients with persistent symptoms. Most patients with intersection syndrome respond well to nonoperative treatment, and surgery is generally reserved for refractory cases.[60]

Approach. See Videos 53.4 and 53.5. For injection of de Quervain's tenosynovitis, position the patient's hand so that the ulnar side of the wrist is on the table and the radial side is facing upward (see Fig. 53.20). Introduce a 2.2-cm, 25-gauge needle at the most tender point (approximately 1 cm distal to the radial styloid) through a lidocaine skin wheal and inject 10 mg to 20 mg of prednisolone or an equivalent intermediate-acting steroid suspension mixed with 4 mL to 5 mL of 1% lidocaine adjacent and parallel to the tendon sheath (peritendinous infiltration). The injection should be under the edge of the first dorsal compartment retinaculum within the first extensor compartment. If firm resistance is met or if needle movement is noted when the patient abducts and extends the thumb, the needle may be in the tendon and should be redirected to prevent intratendinous injection. Because many superficial vessels are present in this area, aspirate before injecting to verify that the needle is not in a blood vessel. Be generous with the injection volume because a common reason for failure is the inability to get medication into both tendon sheaths. Frequently, edema is visible at the radial aspect of the first metacarpal base and at the thumb MCP joint dorsally after successful injection. A lightweight thumb or wrist splint for support and protection may be used at night for several

De Quervain's Disease And Intersection Syndrome

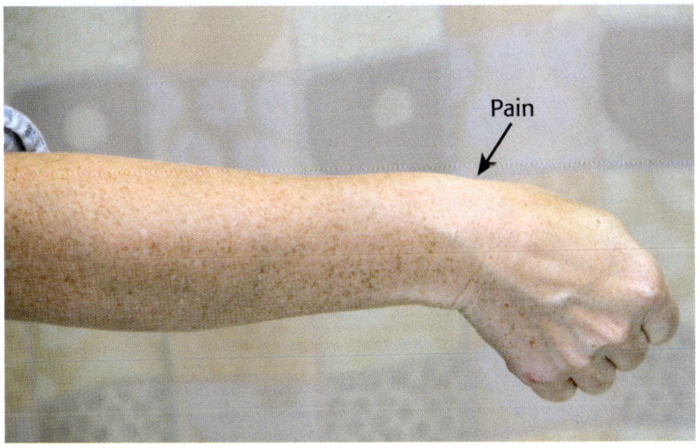

Finkelstein's test. The Finkelstein test is positive when pain is reproduced by ulnar deviation of the wrist while the patient grasps the thumb with the fingers.

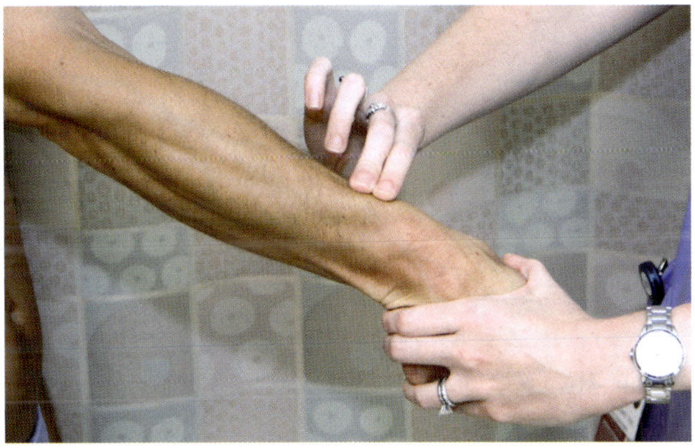

Occasionally, crepitus may be palpated over the involved area. To elicit this sign, the examiner's fingers are placed over the painful area and the patient's wrist is placed in ulnar deviation, which produces the characteristic sensation.

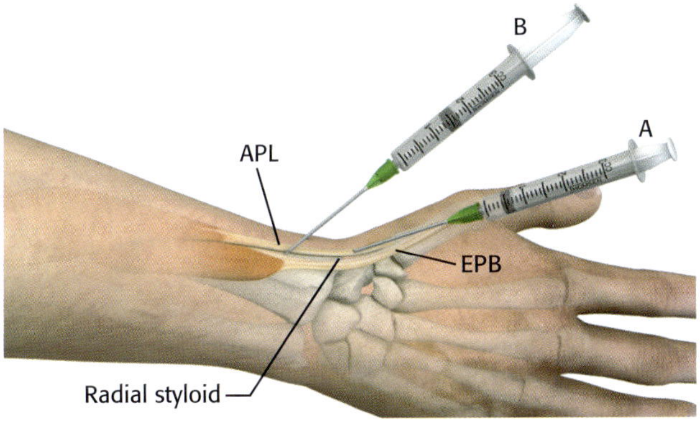

A, For de Quervain's disease, insert the needle through the most tender point, usually about 1 cm distal to the radial styloid. *B*, For intersection syndrome, the target site is again the site of maximal tenderness, which is usually 4 to 8 cm proximal to the radial styloid. (*APL*, Abductor pollicus longus; *EPB*, extensor pollicus brevis.)

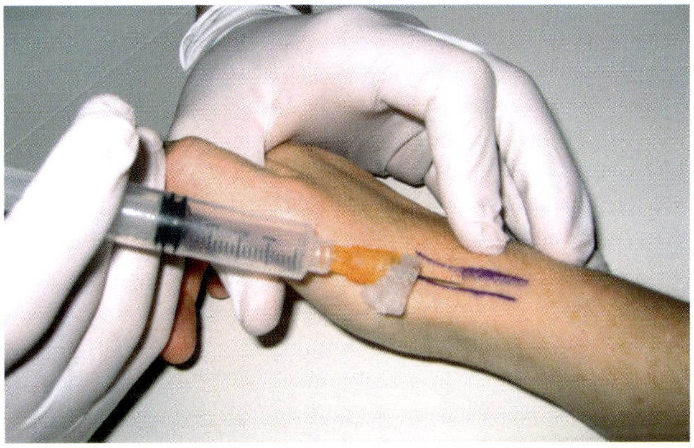

Injection for de Quervain's tenosynovitis usually produces a good result.

Fig. 53.20 de Quervain's disease and intersection syndrome.

weeks after the injection, but routine splinting after injection is not required.[55] Oral NSAIDs may be prescribed for analgesia but will probably not be a cure by themselves. There is no proven role for oral corticosteroids.

Injection for intersection syndrome is similar to that for de Quervain's disease except that the target site is at the point of maximal tenderness, which is usually 4 cm to 8 cm proximal to the radial styloid (see Fig. 53.20).

Carpal Tunnel Syndrome. CTS is the most common nerve entrapment neuropathy of the wrist.[61] Caused by median nerve compression in the fibro-osseous tunnel of the wrist, CTS is characterized by pain at the wrist that is associated with pain and paresthesia along the median nerve territory. This includes the medial aspect of the thumb, palmar side of the index and middle fingers, and radial half of the ring finger. Typically, the patient wakes during the night with burning or aching pain, numbness, and tingling. Occasionally the discomfort is extremely severe and causes the patient to seek emergency care. Clinical signs that support this diagnosis include a positive Tinel sign, which is elicited by reproducing the tingling and paresthesia by tapping (with a reflex hammer) over the median nerve at the volar crease of the wrist (Fig. 53.21). In addition, one can perform the Phalen test, described as holding the dorsal sides of the flexed wrists at a 90-degree angle against each other for several minutes to provoke symptoms in the median nerve distribution (Fig. 53.21).[61] The Phalen test is more sensitive than Tinel sign and is more specific for CTS. Severe muscle atrophy of the thenar eminence may develop in advanced or neglected cases. In many patients the disturbance is idiopathic, without a recognizable underlying cause. However, people who participate in repetitive activities of the wrist, such as typing, driving, assembly line work, and racquet sports are at risk for the development of CTS. Other conditions associated with CTS include rheumatoid arthritis (sometimes as the initial manifestation), pregnancy, hypothyroidism, diabetes, and acromegaly. CTS is a clinical diagnosis, but nerve conduction studies can help support the diagnosis. Radiography is not indicated.

Initial therapy for CTS consists of modification of activity and splinting; the latter is particularly helpful at night. Of the medications sometimes used to treat CTS, diuretics, NSAIDs,

Carpal Tunnel Syndrome

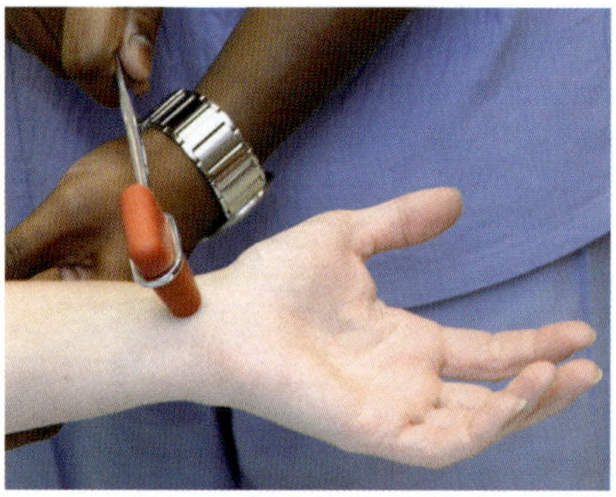

Tinel test. Tap over the median nerve at the volar wrist crease with a reflex hammer; reproduction of tingling and paresthesias supports the diagnosis.

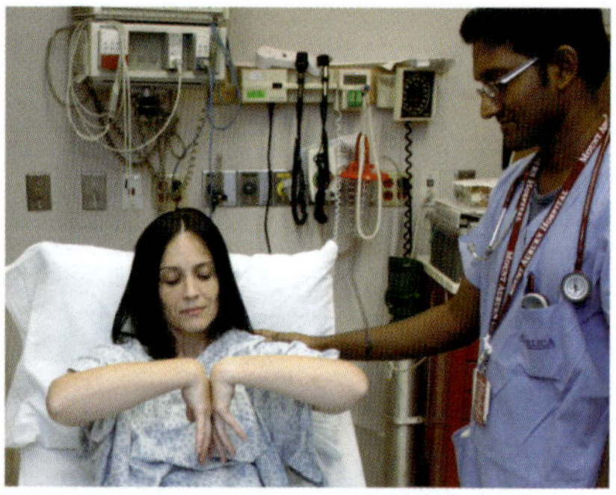

Phalen test. Instruct the patient to hold the wrists together in a flexed position for several minutes; observe for symptoms in a median nerve distribution.

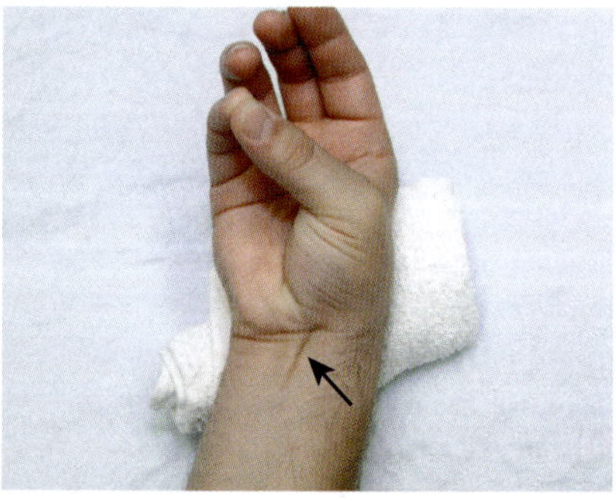

Prior to needle insertion, identify the palmaris longus tendon (*arrow*) by instructing the patient to oppose the thumb and pinky finger while flexing the wrist.

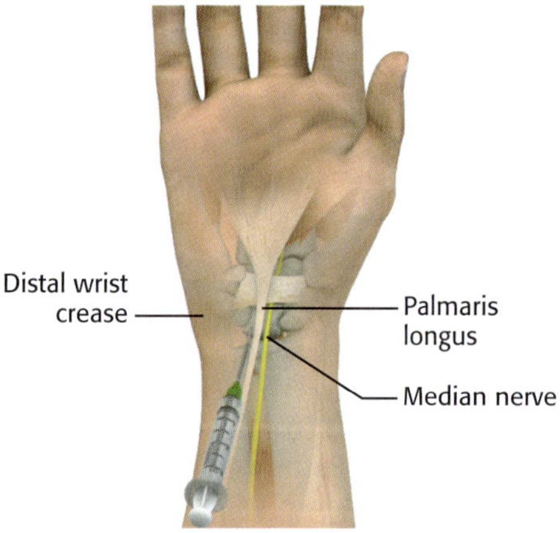

Insert the needle on the ulnar side of the palmaris longus tendon about 1 cm proximal to the distal wrist crease.

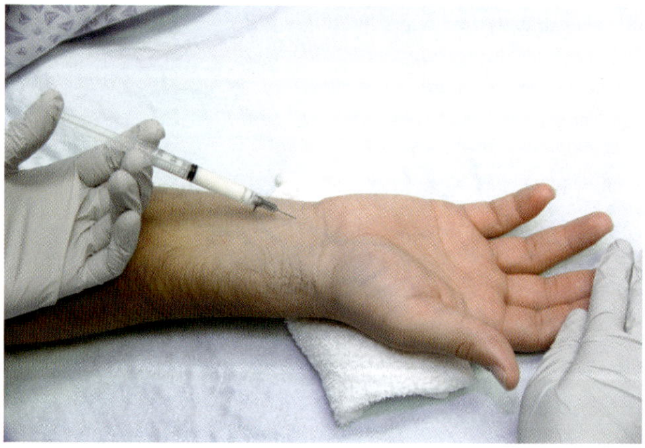

Hold the needle at a 45-degree angle, aimed toward the tip of the middle finger. Advance the needle about 1 to 2 cm. If the patient experiences paresthesias, reposition the needle tip because direct nerve injection should be avoided.

Fig. 53.21 Carpal tunnel syndrome. Recurrent pain may require surgery.

and pyridoxine have been shown to offer little to no relief.[62] In contrast, the benefits, at least in the short term (e.g., 4 to 6 weeks), of local steroid injections for CTS have been well proven. A Cochrane review of randomized trials by Marshall and colleagues, local steroid injection provided greater clinical improvement 1 month after injection than did placebo and up to 3 months after injection than oral steroid treatment. However, symptoms after local corticosteroid injection were no different from the symptoms after either NSAIDs or splinting at 8 weeks.[63] The benefits of initial steroid injection versus surgical intervention for CTS are controversial because there is little scientifically valid information from which to draw any conclusions. In one small study, Hui and associates found that surgery resulted in a better symptomatic outcome (but not grip strength) than did local steroid injection over a 20-week period.[64] It appears that local steroid injection for CTS offers improvement in symptoms, but this improvement may not be permanent or long term. Current recommendations include a trial of conservative treatment (including possible steroid injection) for patients who have mild to moderate symptoms and lack thenar wasting.[64] Surgery is indicated for patients with persistent symptoms after conservative treatment and for those with severe weakness of the thumb abductors.[64–66]

Approach. Insert the needle through a lidocaine skin wheal just ulnar to the palmaris longus tendon and approximately 1 cm proximal to the distal crease at the wrist. The palmaris longus tendon can be appreciated by having the patient pinch all the fingertips together while holding the wrist in a neutral position (see Fig. 53.21). Injecting medial (ulnar) to the palmaris longus is preferred because it avoids accidental injection of the median nerve and superficial veins. Direct a 2.5- to 3.9-cm, 25-gauge needle at a 45-degree angle to the skin surface toward the tip of the middle finger. Advance the needle 1 to 2 cm and inject 20 to 40 mg of methylprednisolone (or another intermediate-acting steroid equivalent) with or without lidocaine along the track and into the tissue space. If the patient complains of paresthesia, or the needle meets resistance during injection, redirect the needle to avoid injecting directly into a nerve or tendon, respectively. Up to 2 weeks may be required for the paresthesia to abate significantly, although it usually takes only a few days for improvement of nocturnal pain. A lightweight wrist splint may hasten recovery. Repeated injections may be given, but if a response is not elicited or permanent after two or three injections, decompressive surgery should be considered.

Digital Flexor Tenosynovitis ("Trigger Finger")

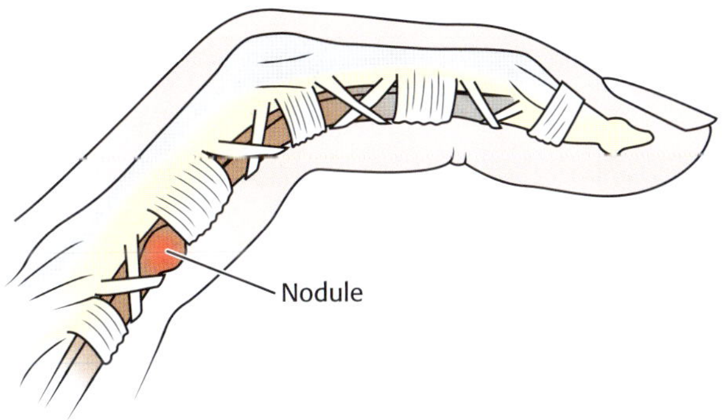

Trigger finger (stenosing tenosynovitis) can affect any digit, including the thumb, but it is most common in the ring and middle fingers. Palpation of the flexor tendon sheath over the metacarpophalangeal joint often reproduces the symptoms. Injection is often very effective, but the nodule may persist.

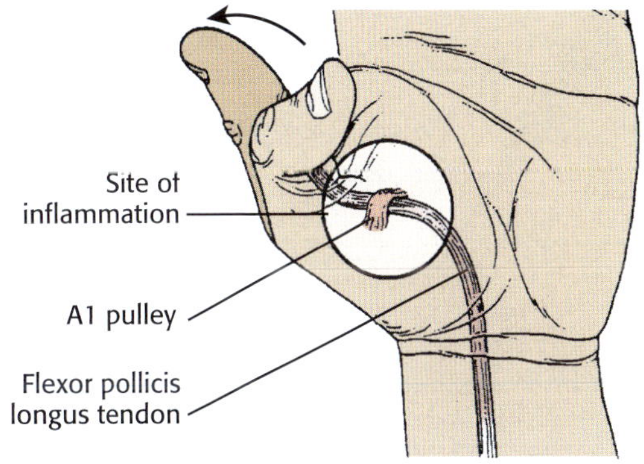

In advanced cases, inflammation at the proximal (A1) pulley of the flexor tendon sheath overlying the metacarpophalangeal joint may hold the digit in either a flexed or an extended position. Generally, the tendon becomes thickened either proximal or distal to the pulley, which causes a snapping or a locking phenomenon with finger flexion or extension.

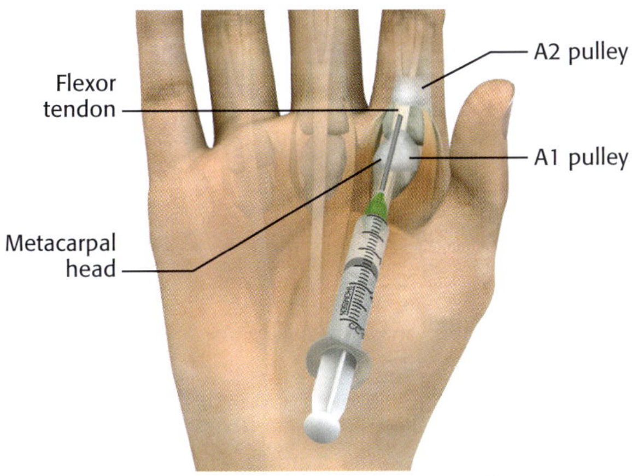

Locate the tendon point at the base of the finger flexion crease, which is located between the A1 and A2 pulleys.

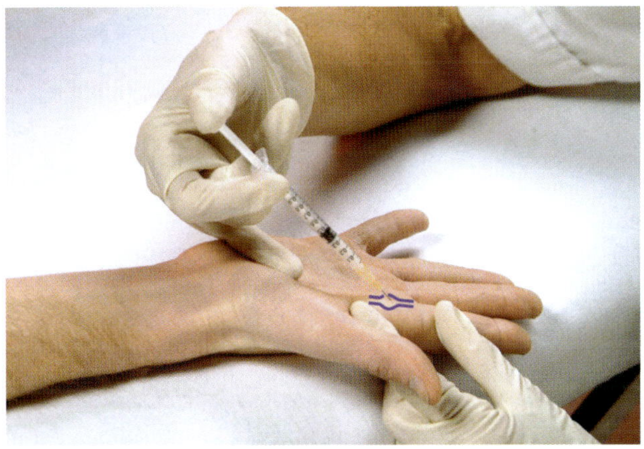

Angle the needle 30 degrees into the involved tendon sheath, parallel to the tendon fibers.

Fig. 53.22 Digital flexor tenosynovitis ("trigger finger"). (*Top right image*, From Walker LG, Meals RA. Tendinitis: a practical approach to diagnosis and management. *J Musculoskel Med.* 1989;6:41.)

Trigger Finger (Stenosing Flexor Tenosynovitis). See Video 53.6. A *trigger* or *snapping* finger is one of the most common problems of the hand, affecting roughly 2% of the general population. It is characterized by a stenosed tendon sheath at the level of the first annular pulley (A1), which is located on the palmar surface over the base of the metacarpal head (Fig. 53.22).[67,68] In this condition, the A1 pulley becomes inflamed, and a nodule develops on the tendon as it gets "pinched" under the constricted sheath. Locking occurs when the involved digit is in flexion and is especially troublesome when the patient awakens in the morning. This can occur in any finger but is seen most frequently in the ring and middle fingers.

Besides thickening and stenosing of the tendon sheath, a trigger finger may also be characterized by flexor tendon synovitis. The tendon sheaths are long and tubular, and the walls are lined with a thin layer of synovial cells. Symptoms develop when the tendon becomes trapped and is unable to glide within the tendon sheath. A nodule or fibrinous deposit may form at a site in the tendon sheath, usually over or just distal to the metacarpal head of the trigger finger. When the digit is flexed, the nodule moves with the tendon proximally, and on extension it gets "stuck" on the pulley thereby leading to intermittent catching of the tendon.[67] The nodule may be palpable on physical examination, but this is not necessary for diagnosis. CTS commonly coexists with a trigger finger and may be caused by tenosynovitis. Common causes of tenosynovitis include trauma, diabetes mellitus, and rheumatoid arthritis, although it may also be a primary and idiopathic disorder.

Conservative treatment including local rest or splinting, application of moist heat, and NSAID therapy is a common initial approach aimed at alleviating pain and allowing for smoother movements of the finger. Splinting involves immobilization of the MCP joint with slight flexion for up to 6 weeks and has been shown to be an effective option for those who want to avoid corticosteroid injections.[69] However, if these measures fail to control the symptoms, or if the symptoms are severe, corticosteroid injection is indicated. A 2009 Cochrane review found that corticosteroid injection with lidocaine was more effective than lidocaine alone at 4 months.[70] A 2013 retrospective review found that corticosteroid injection was nearly 80% effective in treating and preventing recurrence of trigger finger. Steroid injections are

Carpal/Metacarpal Inflammation

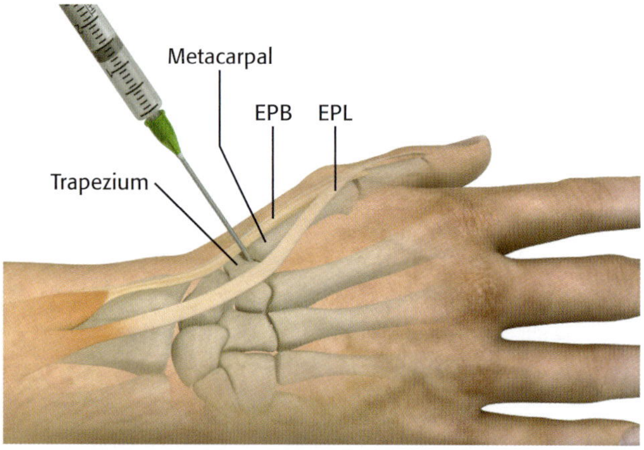

Painful and limited motion of the thumb is often caused by inflammation at the trapezium-metacarpal joint. Inject at the apex of the snuffbox while avoiding the radial artery. (*EPB*, Extensor pollicis brevis; *EPL*, extensor pollicis longus. The anatomic snuffbox is outlined by these two tendons.)

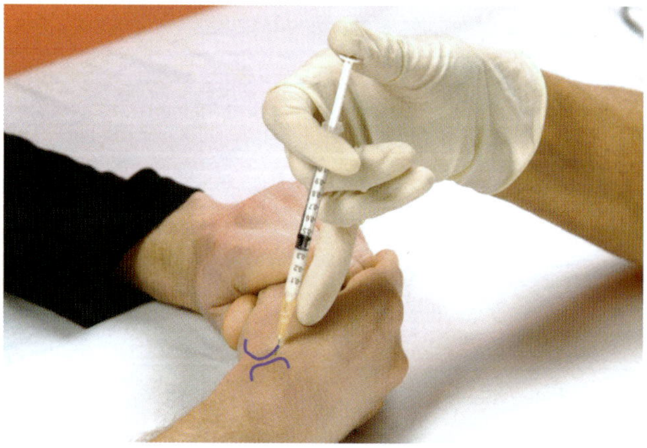

Injection therapy is usually quite successful for this very painful condition, which is common in older females.

Fig. 53.23 Carpal/metacarpal inflammation.

more successful when performed in patients with a palpable nodule or symptoms for less than 6 months. Younger age, insulin-dependent diabetes, involvement of multiple digits, and a history of other tendinopathies are associated with treatment failure.[71] There is also evidence to suggest that the efficacy of steroid injections for trigger fingers diminishes with each subsequent injection at the same site. As a general guideline, if treatment fails after three injections (separated by several weeks or months), consider surgery for treatment of the condition. In addition, patients with insulin-dependent diabetes mellitus require surgical release for trigger finger more often than do patients with non–insulin-dependent diabeties.[71] Division of the first annular pulley, digital nerve injury, scarring, and recurrence are well-known complications of surgical release.

Approach. Preparation of the site before injection requires meticulous adherence to aseptic technique. Rest the patient's hand on a table with the palm facing upward. The injection point is at the base of the finger's flexion crease between the A1 and the A2 tendon pulleys. Using a 2.2-cm, 25-gauge needle, enter the skin at a 30-degree angle and insert the needle into the tendon sheath parallel to the tendon fibers. Inject 0.25 to 0.35 mL of an intermediate-acting corticosteroid suspension mixed with 1.5 to 3 mL of anesthetic (see Fig. 53.22). If resistance is felt on insertion of the needle, an intratendinous location is suggested. Withdraw the needle slightly before injection. Similar injections can be administered in the base of the thumb metacarpal for a snapping thumb. Injection into the tendon sheath is the goal. If relapses are frequent or the clinical response is not satisfactory, surgical release is indicated.

Carpal/Metacarpal Inflammation. Overuse and aging can lead to pain at the base of the thumb and fingers. This is especially common in older females and can be quite painful. The first metacarpal articulates with the trapezium, a common site for this condition. Injection therapy is usually quite successful (Fig. 53.23).

Hip Region

Greater Trochanteric Pain Syndrome (Formerly Trochanteric Bursitis). Greater trochanteric pain syndrome (GTPS) is one of the most common causes of lateral hip pain. Formerly referred to as *trochanteric bursitis*, imaging and histopathological studies have shown that the actual bursa is rarely involved. GTPS can be confused with other conditions at or near the hip such as sacrolumbar disease, hip or femur pathology, and metastatic disease. The hallmark, though, is the demonstration of discrete tenderness on deep palpation at or adjacent to the greater trochanter.[72]

GTPS is primarily caused by tendinopathy of the gluteus medius or minimus or the bursae associated with this region (Fig. 53.24). The pain may be acute but is more often subacute or chronic; frequently, patients have already tried NSAIDs without success and have been assigned several incorrect diagnoses. Risk factors include female sex, obesity, and those with underlying lower gait disturbances and scoliosis. The chief locus of the pathologic condition is in the abductor mechanism of the hip. Pain occurs near the greater trochanter and may radiate down the lateral or posterolateral aspect of the thigh and, rarely, into the knee. The pain is described as *deep*, *dull*, and *aching* and often interferes with sleep. Lying on the affected hip, stepping from curbs, and descending steps frequently provoke the pain.

On examination, with the patient lying on the unaffected side, tenderness may be elicited over and adjacent to the greater trochanter. In contrast to true hip joint involvement, the Patrick FABERE sign (*f*lexion, *ab*duction, *e*xternal *r*otation, and *e*xtension) may be negative, and complete passive range of motion is relatively painless. Active abduction when the patient lies on the opposite side typically intensifies the discomfort, and sharp external rotation may accentuate the symptoms. Internal rotation does not usually affect the level of pain. Hip radiographs may demonstrate a calcific deposit adjacent to the trochanter; however, the incidence of this finding is low.[72]

GTPS is a self-limited condition that can improve with conservative measures such as rest, ice, oral acetaminophen and NSAIDs, weight reduction, and correction of length discrepancy. In patients with persistent pain, corticosteroid injection for GTPS can be an effective therapy. Short-term benefit has been proven in multiple studies with greatest benefit being seen around 6 weeks; however, at 12-month follow-up, other conservative measures have been proven just as beneficial.[73,74] Failure of corticosteroid therapy should prompt the clinician to seek alternative diagnoses, such as true hip joint disease, which can easily be confused with GTPS. In addition, although rare, there have been case reports of septic trochanteric bursitis caused by tuberculosis.[75]

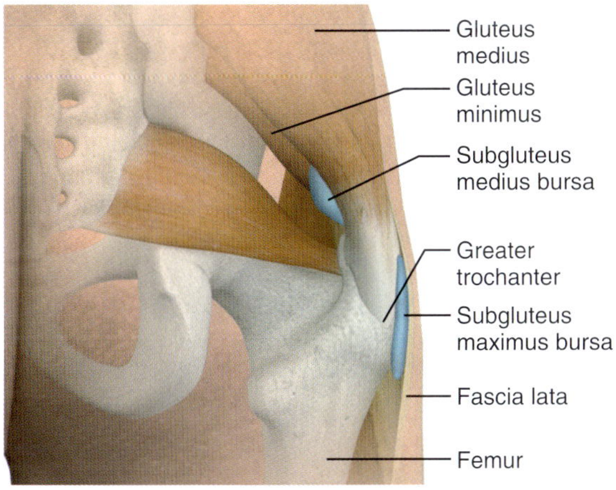

Fig. 53.24 Greater trochanteric pain syndrome. The principal bursa lies between the gluteus maximus and the greater trochanter, although other bursae may also be involved.

Approach. Place the patient in a supine or lateral recumbent position and identify the site of maximum tenderness for needle entry. Advance a 3.9- to 5.0-cm, 20- or 21-gauge needle perpendicular to the skin until the tip of the needle reaches the trochanter (Fig. 53.25). Withdraw the needle slightly and widely infiltrate the site with 3 mL to 10 mL of lidocaine and 20 mg to 40 mg of methylprednisolone or an equivalent steroid.

Ischiogluteal Bursitis. Ischiogluteal bursitis, colloquially known as Weaver's bottom, is a painful disorder characterized by pain over the center of the buttocks with radiation down the back of the leg, not to be confused with sciatica. This condition is rarely diagnosed initially and is often mistaken for lumbosacral strain, a herniated disk, or a spinal cord tumor. The ischial or ischiogluteal bursa is adjacent to the ischial tuberosity and overlies the sciatic and posterior femoral cutaneous nerves. Patients are usually asymptomatic when standing; however, when going to a seated position, the gluteus maximus muscle slides away from the bursa allowing for direct contact between the bursa and subcutaneous tissue. The condition is often associated with a sedentary lifestyle, which is where it gets its nickname. Sitting on hard surfaces, bending forward, and standing on tiptoes may all provoke the pain. Maximal tenderness is present over the ischial tuberosity. At times a

Greater Trochanteric Pain Syndrome

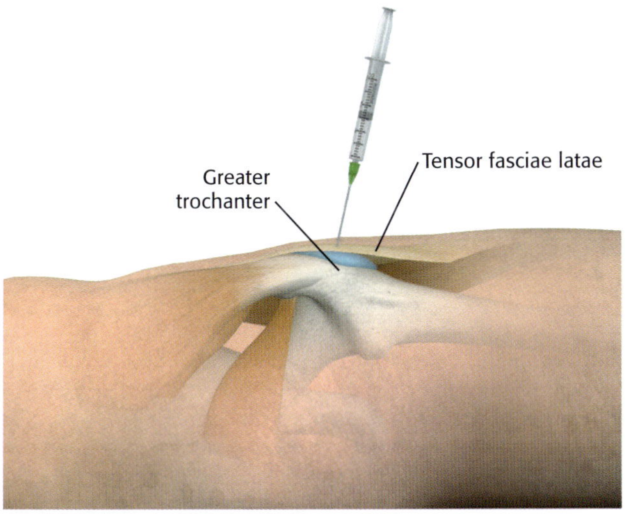

Place the patient in the lateral recumbent or supine position. Insert the needle at the area of maximum tenderness, and advance perpendicular to the skin until the needle tip reaches the greater trochanter.

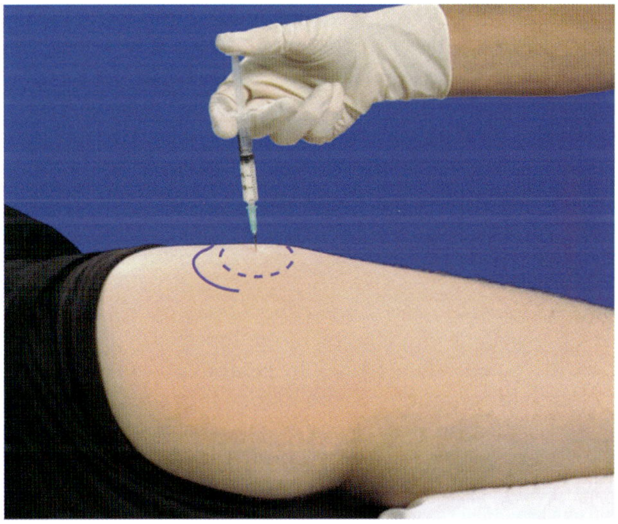

After the trochanter is reached, withdraw the needle slightly, and infiltrate the site widely with 3 to 10 mL of lidocaine and 20 to 40 mg of methylprednisolone (or the equivalent).

Fig. 53.25 Greater trochanteric pain syndrome.

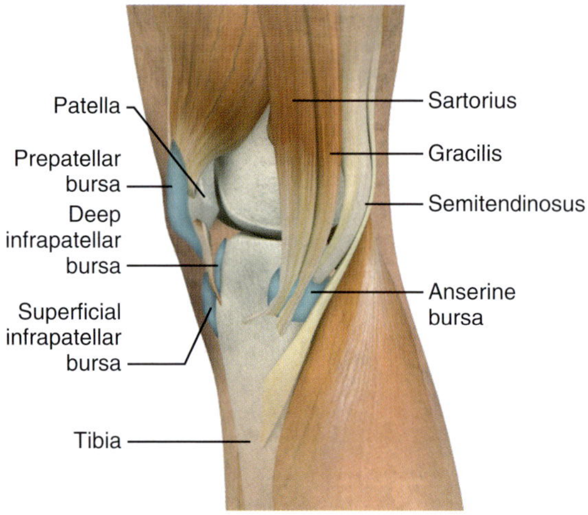

Fig. 53.26 Bursae of the knee (medial view). The prepatellar bursa lies superior to the patella, and the pes anserine bursa lies deep to the insertion of the sartorius, gracilis, and semitendinosus tendons. Prepatellar bursitis is common in carpet layers, and pes anserine bursitis is seen in dancers and runners. Infrapatellar bursitis is common in long-distance runners and can be mistaken for patellar tendinitis. Pain is felt below the patella at the midpoint of the patellar tendon and is elicited by knee extension. Note that there are two infrapatellar bursae. Osgood-Schlatter disease is similar in adolescents, a condition that should not be injected.

soft tissue mass may also be felt in this area. When it is recognized, a skillful intrabursal injection, coupled with rest, usually relieves the extreme pain.[76]

Approach. Place the patient in either a prone position or on the unaffected side with the leg flexed at 90 degrees, locating the ischial tuberosity, and insert a 5.0-cm, 20- to 22-gauge needle through a lidocaine skin wheal. Advance the needle cautiously to avoid the sciatic nerve, which lies at a depth of approximately 6.5 to 7.5 cm. If paresthesias occur (indicating contact with a nerve), withdraw and redirect the needle. Inject 5 mL to 10 mL of lidocaine and 20 mg to 40 mg of methylprednisolone into the bursa. Because of the close proximity of the bursa to the sciatic nerve, some experts advise against the use of injection therapy in this area, especially as the addition of steroids can cause soft tissue atrophy making sitting uncomfortable. Ultrasound guidance can help localize the ischial bursa.[76]

Knee Region

Prepatellar Bursitis. *Housemaid's knee* or *nun's knee* is characterized by swelling with effusion of the superficial bursa anterior to the patella (Fig. 53.26). In contrast to intraarticular pathology, passive motion of the knee is fully preserved, and the pain is generally mild, except during extreme knee flexion or direct pressure. Although the disorder is usually caused by pressure from repetitive kneeling on a firm surface, it can also develop after direct trauma, and occasionally it is a manifestation of rheumatoid arthritis or gout.[77] Although uncommon, the prepatellar bursa is one of the most frequent sites of septic bursitis. In fact approximately one-third of all cases are septic in nature.[78] Moreover, patients with septic prepatellar bursitis may not have the classic signs of infection such as erythema, warmth, or fever, making it difficult to differentiate from aseptic bursitis. The bursal aspirate should therefore always be sent for laboratory analysis.

Acute bursitis is more likely to be septic with the most common bacteria being skin flora; however, gout and direct trauma are also known causes. Chronic bursitis is more likely to be secondary to trauma and less likely infection. Symptoms of septic bursitis include localized redness, swelling, and tenderness over the patella. Fever may be present in 30% of patients. Examination may reveal subtle evidence of trauma including abrasions or puncture wounds. Patients with aseptic bursitis may experience the same swelling; however, warmth and tenderness are mild or absent in most patients.

Approach. Place the patient supine with the affected leg extended (Fig. 53.27). The bursa is located superficially, between the skin and the patella, and can often be "milked" during the procedure to facilitate aspiration. Use a 2.5-cm, 20- to 21-gauge needle to enter the bursa and aspirate as much fluid as possible. Aspiration often yields a surprisingly scant amount of clear, serous fluid because the prepatellar bursa is multilocular rather than the usual single cavity. Once aspiration is complete, instill 1 to 2 mL of lidocaine with 15 to 20 mg of a prednisolone (or an equivalent steroid) suspension. In some cases, the procedure may need to be repeated more than once (in 6- to 8-week intervals) to obtain a lasting result. Following the procedure, instruct the patient to discontinue the provocative activity and avoid direct pressure to the knees. A compressive dressing should be worn for a few days.

Suprapatellar Bursitis. Suprapatellar bursitis is usually associated with synovitis of the knee. Patients will typically complain of anterior knee and distal thigh pain. On occasion the bursa is largely separated from the synovial cavity with only a very minor communication, and the swelling and effusion are chiefly confined to the suprapatellar area. This may be traumatic in origin or a manifestation of an inflammatory arthropathy.

Approach. The procedure for aspiration and injection of the suprapatellar area is similar to that for the knee.

Pes Anserinus Pain Syndrome (Formerly Anserine Bursitis). Historically referred to as *anserine bursitis*, Pes anserinus pain syndrome (PAPS) is used to characterize pain along the medial aspect of the leg from the upper tibia to the knee. Imaging studies in PAPS patients seldom demonstrate an associated anserine bursitis,[79–81] hence the change in terminology. In the past, the syndrome was associated with horseback riding (and the disease was referred to as *Cavalryman's disease*); however, it now mainly occurs in heavy females with disproportionately large thighs in association with osteoarthritis of the knee, although it may also be seen in athletes involved in running, baseball, and racquet sports. In rare cases, there may be true bursitis of the anserine bursa, which is relatively large at 7 cm and located on the anteromedial side of the knee, inferior to the joint line at the site of insertion of the conjoined tendons of the sartorius, semitendinosus, and gracilis muscles, and superficial to the medial collateral ligament. The entity is characterized by a relatively abrupt onset of knee pain along with localized tenderness and a sense of fullness in the vicinity of the anserine bursa approximately 4 cm to 5 cm below the anteromedial aspect of the tibial plateau. Pain is exacerbated by flexion of the knee. Corticosteroid injection for PAPS has been shown in clinical trials to be an effective treatment.[82]

Prepatellar Bursitis Aspiration

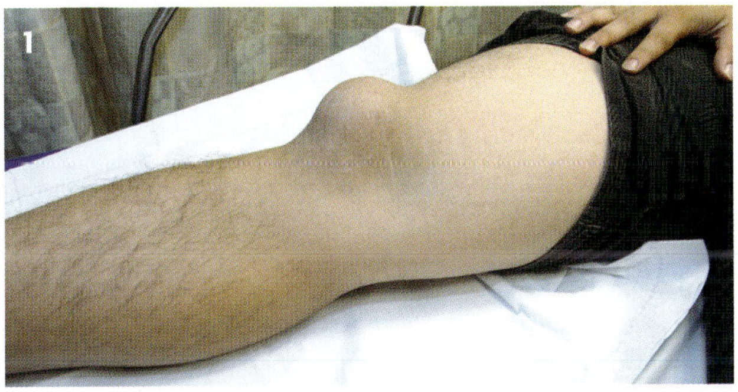

This patient has had anterior knee swelling for 6 weeks after falling directly onto his knee. This collection is confined to the prepatellar space, and passive range of motion of the knee is preserved.

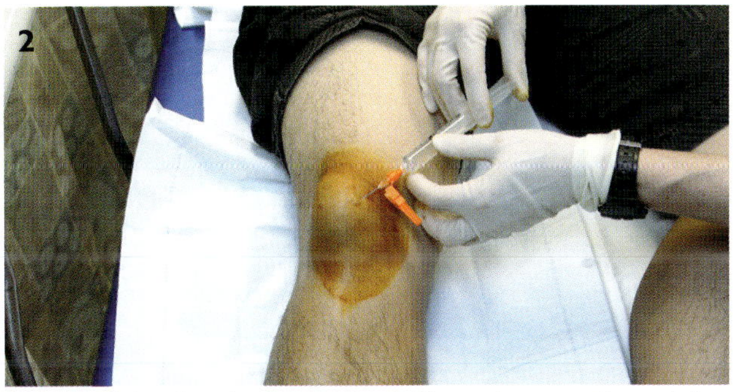

After careful antiseptic preparation, infiltrate the entry site and the anticipated trajectory of the needle with lidocaine.

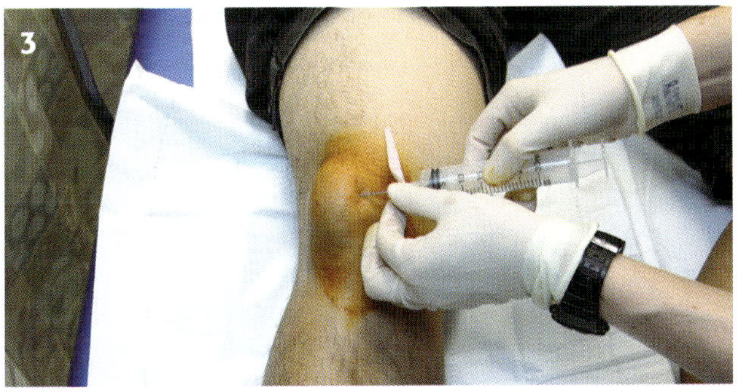

Keep the knee extended during the procedure. Insert the needle into the fluctuant area in the space between the skin and the patella; either a medial or a lateral approach may be used.

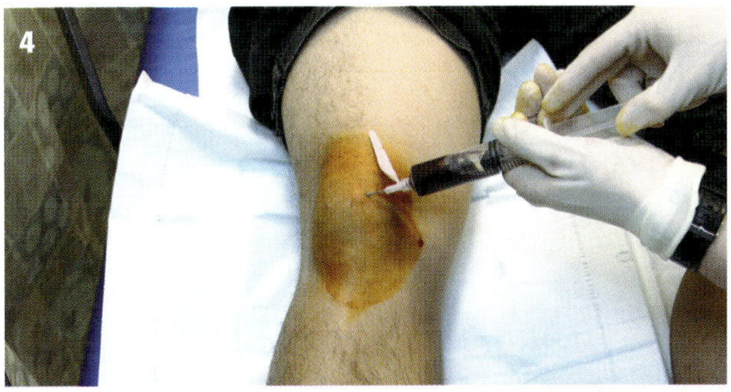

Once in the bursa, aspirate the fluid. Occasionally, a substantial volume of fluid may be obtained, so use a large syringe.

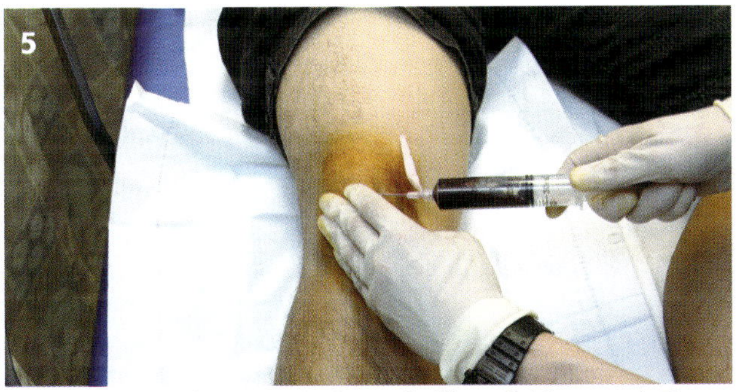

"Milk" the bursa during aspiration to facilitate fluid removal. The needle may be repositioned if needed because the prepatellar bursa is a multiloculated structure (as opposed to a single cavity).

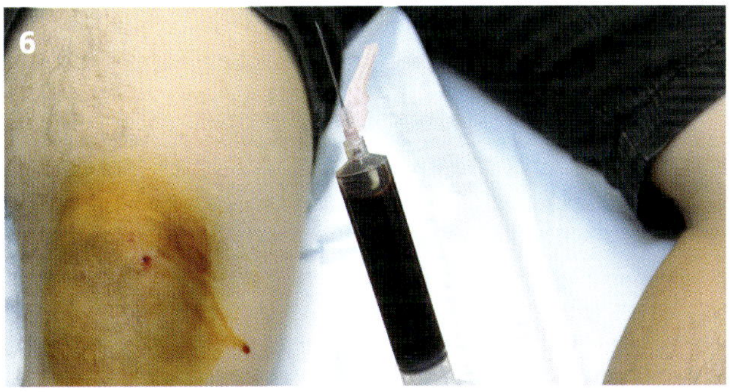

Note that this patient's aspirate was grossly hemorrhagic, consistent with his history of knee trauma.

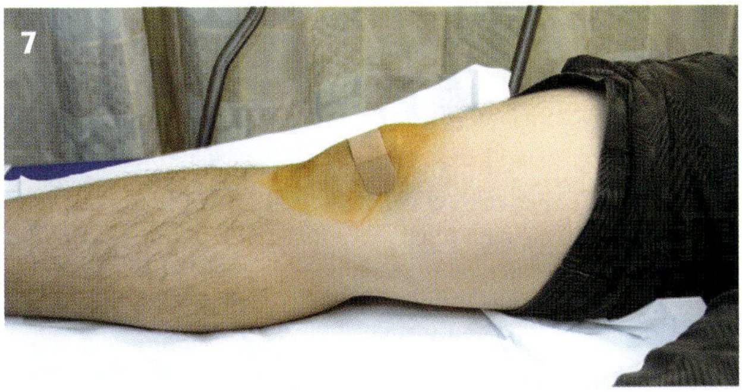

Remove as much fluid as possible. This patient's knee regained a normal appearance after the procedure.

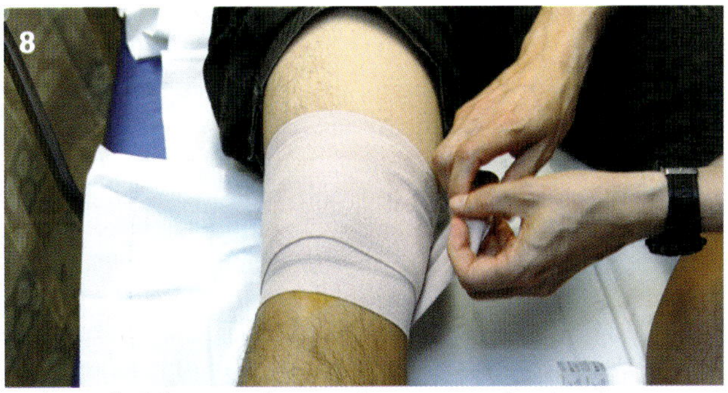

At the end of the procedure, apply a compressive dressing to reduce recurrence.

Fig. 53.27 Prepatellar bursitis aspiration.

Pes Anserine Pain Syndrome

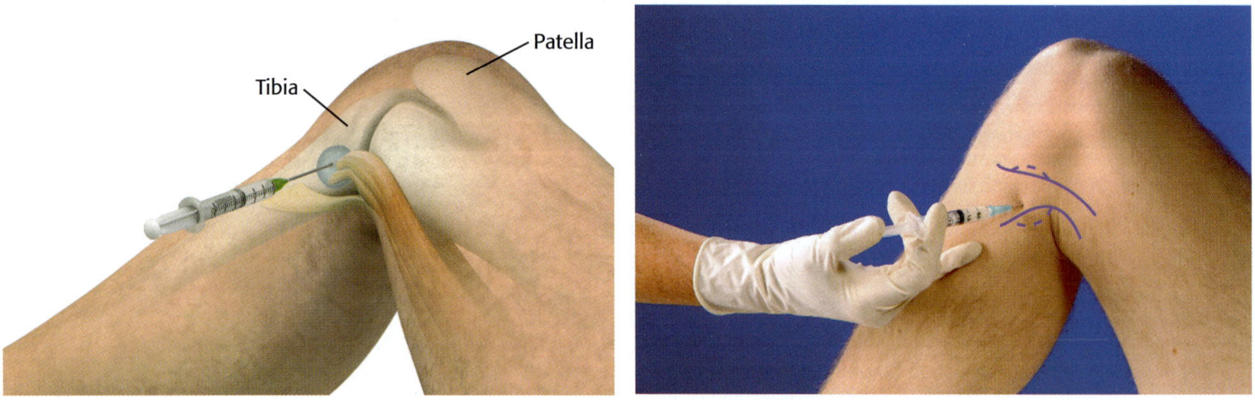

Insert the needle at the point of maximum tenderness. This will be inferior to the patella and medial to the tibial tuberosity.

Advance the needle until the tibia is reached, and then slightly withdraw the needle and inject the steroid. Avoid direct injection into the nearby tendons.

Fig. 53.28 Pes anserine pain syndrome.

Approach. See Video 53.7. Position the patient with the knee flexed 90 degrees. Using an anterior or medial approach with a 2.5- to 3.9-cm, 22-gauge needle, identify the point of greatest tenderness and gently advance the needle until the tibia is reached. Withdraw the needle 2 to 3 mm and inject 2 to 4 mL of lidocaine along with or followed by approximately 20 to 40 mg of a corticosteroid suspension (Fig. 53.28). Prompt symptomatic relief is frequently obtained, but the duration of benefit is variable and probably correlates with the patient's weight-bearing activities. It is important to avoid direct injection of the corticosteroid suspension into the nearby tendons.

Medial Collateral Ligament Bursa. This bursa is located anterior to the tibia and posterior to the medial collateral ligament. Injury to this bursa often occurs when the patient undergoes a twisting motion with concurrent external rotation of the tibia. Tenderness may be appreciated along the anteroinferior aspect of the medial collateral ligament, and the pain is exacerbated with extension of the knee. This condition may sometimes be confused with a medial meniscus tear, and magnetic resonance imaging might be necessary to differentiate the two conditions. Treatment is usually successful with conservative measures, including relative rest, compression, and NSAIDs.[83]

Popliteal Cyst. Baker cysts are herniated fluid-filled sacs of the articular synovial membrane that extend into the popliteal fossa, sometimes through the natural communication between the bursa in the posterior of the knee and the joint itself. These cysts may also be caused by swelling of the medial gastrocnemius or semimembranosus bursae alone. Baker cysts are common with prevalence in the general population of 4.7% and up to 40% in those with knee pain. They may occur secondary to trauma and are seen in patients with rheumatoid arthritis, gout, and osteoarthritis. Patients will often complain of *popliteal fossa* tenderness and swelling that may extend into the calf. Activities that involve active flexion of the knee, such as walking or jumping, exacerbate the symptoms.

The clinical manifestation of Baker cysts can mimic that of deep venous thrombosis (DVT). For this reason, symptomatic Baker cysts are also known as *pseudothrombophlebitis syndrome,* and it is important to take great care in differentiating the two.[84] In most studies, 2% to 6% of patients suspected of having DVT actually have a popliteal cyst as the cause of their knee or calf pain. Ultrasound is an important tool in this diagnosis. Many cases of Baker cyst resolve spontaneously over a few weeks. However, treatment may require surgery to correct any articular injury or to remove the cyst.

Kiel and Fredericksen reported safe and effective treatment of symptomatic popliteal cysts with ultrasound-guided aspiration of fluid through a spinal needle, fenestration of the cyst walls and septations, and injection of 1 mL triamcinolone and 2 mL 0.5% bupivacaine into the decompressed remnant.[85] Another approach involves arthrocentesis followed by injection of glucocorticoids directly into the knee joint. In a study of 30 patients with knee osteoarthritis complicated with a symptomatic Baker cyst, a single intraarticular injection of 40 mg triamcinolone acetonide resulted in an improvement in knee pain, swelling, and range of motion, in addition to a reduction in Baker cyst size. Steroid injections should be done with care because of the risk for neurovascular injury. Ultrasound may aid in treatment as well.[85]

Ankle, Foot, and Heel Region

Ankle Tendinitis. This is a relatively uncommon condition that may result from unusual repetitive activity, or rarely from acute trauma. The disorder is differentiated from ankle joint involvement by the lack of pain or restricted motion during passive flexion and extension of the ankle. Active flexion and extension of the toes produces pain and there is tenderness along the involved tendons (i.e., peroneal, tibialis anterior, flexors, extensors). Initial treatment consists of rest, NSAIDs, and immobilization, sometimes for several weeks. Some patients may eventually need operative intervention for prolonged symptoms.[86] Local steroid injections have been used successfully in patients who do not respond to conservative measures; however, the risk for tendon rupture is well documented. As a result, tendon sheath injections should be reserved for patients with persistent symptoms despite an adequate trial of conservative therapy and should be done in consultation with a foot and ankle specialist.

Heel Pain

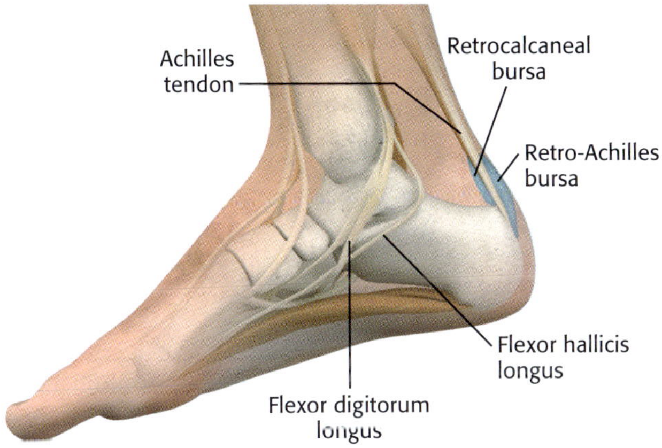

Heel pain. Talalgia may involve the tendons, bursae, or fasciae around the heel. Do not inject Achilles tendinitis since tendon rupture may occur. Fluoroquinolones can cause significant Achilles tendinopathy (see Box 52.1).

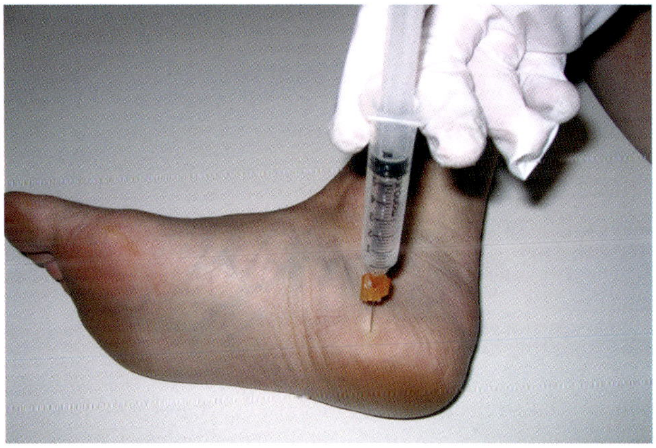

Injection of calcaneal bursitis with a heel spur. A lateral injection is preferred (see Chapter 51).

Fig. 53.29 Heel pain.

Approach. Enter the tendon sheath tangentially with a 2.5- to 3.9-cm, 22- or 25-gauge needle and inject approximately 2 to 4 mL of a mixture of corticosteroid (20 to 40 mg of methylprednisolone) and lidocaine.

Bunion Bursitis. Hallux valgus deformity of the big toe is more commonly referred to as a *bunion*. This common medical condition is found in up to 23% of all adults, especially patients over 65 and in females.[87] On rare occasions inflammation develops in the medial bursa of the first metatarsophalangeal joint of the great toe. Initial treatment is conservative and includes shoe modification, stretching, and ice; however, on occasion tense swelling occurs and decompression is required. In these cases, aspiration with culture of the fluid should be performed.

Approach. If no infection is present, the bursa is injected with 5 to 10 mg of methylprednisolone via a 2.5-cm, 20-gauge needle. Special shoes or an orthopedic correction will be needed if the swelling recurs. Often surgical intervention of the underlying deformity will be required for those who do not respond to conservative treatment.

Heel Pain. *Talalgia* may be caused by many different conditions including Achilles tendinitis, retrocalcaneal bursitis, and plantar fasciitis (Fig. 53.29). Additional discussion may be found in Chapter 52. The bursae of clinical significance around the heel include the retroachilles bursa (located in the space between the skin and the Achilles tendon), the retrocalcaneal bursa (located between the Achilles tendon and the calcaneus), and the subcalcaneal bursa. Achilles tendinitis or bursitis may be traumatic in origin but is more apt to be part of a systemic disease such as rheumatoid or gouty arthritis. Although a normal Achilles tendon is thick and strong, when affected by an inflammatory arthropathy, it is predisposed to degeneration, and because the Achilles tendon is not invested by a full synovial sheath, it is more vulnerable to intratendon instillation. Because of the potential hazard of tendon rupture after local steroid injection, avoid infiltration of steroids into this area. Rather, treat Achilles tendinitis with rest, splinting, and oral NSAIDs.

Retrocalcaneal bursitis is often seen in association with Haglund deformity, a bony ridge on the posterosuperior aspect of the calcaneus. The bursa lies anterior to the Achilles tendon and posterior to the calcaneus. Local swelling and tenderness at the posterior aspect of the heel, proximal (and sometimes lateral) to the insertion of the Achilles tendon, characterize this bursitis. Treatment is focused on minimizing pressure on the bony ridge, which includes the use of open-heeled shoes (clogs), bare feet, sandals, or a heel lift. Conservative measures such as ice, oral NSAIDs, and rest are other common treatment modalities. Corticosteroid injections are not recommended because of the risk for Achilles tendon rupture.[88,89]

The condition in this region that is most amenable to injection therapy is plantar fasciitis, which is also the most common cause of heel pain in adults.[90] The plantar fascia is located deep to the fat layer of the foot and extends from the calcaneus to the base of the digits. It is responsible for support of the medial longitudinal arch of the foot. Signs of this condition include pain on the plantar medial aspect of the heel, which is often worse in the morning after long periods of rest, and with passive dorsiflexion of the toes.[90,91] The pain may be relieved with activity. Although patients may have a heel spur, many symptomatic patients do not, and the presence of a heel spur should not be considered pathognomonic for the condition. Although still debated, the pathology is generally thought to originate from microtears in the fascia, often because of overuse. Obesity may also increase the risk for plantar fasciitis because of the excessive load on the fascia.

Most cases of plantar fasciitis eventually resolve with nonsurgical management.[92] Treatment begins with elimination of any precipitating activity, relative rest, strength and stretching exercises, arch supports, and night splints. If these conservative measures are not effective, injection of the painful heel will usually provide short-term improvement. A 2003 Cochrane review found that steroid injections for plantar fasciitis resulted in significant improvement at 1 month, but not at 3 or 6 months when compared with control groups.[93] This was seen in a 2017 Cochrane review as well.[94] Ultrasound guidance may improve the accuracy and success rates for injection, but data thus far are conflicting. It should also be remembered that there is a risk for rupture of the plantar fascia and fat pad atrophy with corticosteroid injections.[95] While the rates of this appear relatively low (<10%) in the available data, caution should be exercised when injecting steroids into a painful heel. In addition, because this condition tends to be chronic or recurring, referral to an appropriate specialist is recommended.

Approach. See Videos 53.8 and 53.9. Insert a 2.5-cm, 22- to 24-gauge needle at the spot of maximal tenderness on the medial aspect of the heel (see Fig. 53.29). Enter the plantar surface at 90 degrees by sliding into the space at the midpoint of the calcaneus. The tip of the needle should lie in the aponeurosis of the attachment to the os calcis. Inject 1 mL of lidocaine and 10 to 20 mg of methylprednisolone. Injection through the more superficial aspect of the base of the foot should be avoided because it may result in dispersion of medications into the fat pad and produce fat pad atrophy.

Trigger Points

The technique for trigger point injection (universal technique) is the same regardless of location and is described in detail earlier in the chapter (see "Invasive Techniques" section).

Myofascial Headache Syndromes

Trigger points commonly contribute to the muscle component of many headache syndromes, so it is important to carefully examine the muscles of the entire head, neck, shoulder, and back region for hypersensitive areas when evaluating patients with headaches. Trigger points are often found in the sternocleidomastoid, levator scapulae, and trapezius muscles, and less frequently in the scalp and facial muscles. The posterior strap muscles, including the splenius and semispinalis muscles, are also commonly involved. Trigger points along the muscles of mastication can lead to unilateral headaches, and also ear, tooth, and temporomandibular joint pain.[96] Trigger points in the thoracic paraspinal muscles are frequently associated with both migraine and tension headaches, whereas trigger points in the quadratus lumborum and gluteus medius have been associated with unilateral headaches.

Torticollis. Myofascial causes of torticollis usually involve the trapezius, sternocleidomastoid, and levator scapulae muscles, either alone or in a synergistic manner. The splenius and semispinalis muscles may also be involved. Carefully inject trigger points in the trapezius muscle to avoid puncture of a high-rising apical pleura.

Levator Scapulae Muscle Syndrome. Painful sensitive foci may occur at the origin of the levator scapulae muscle on the superior medial aspect of the scapula, along the flat muscle belly, or at the insertion of the transverse processes of the first four cervical vertebrae (Fig. 53.30A). Pain is usually referred to the posterior cervical region, the posterior aspect of the scalp, and the periauricular area.

Splenius Capitis and Semispinalis Capitis Muscle Syndrome. Pain resulting from the trigger points in the splenius capitis and semispinalis capitis muscles may be located over the muscles themselves or be perceived in the head and face and give rise to headaches and dizziness (Fig. 53.30B). Trigger points in the splenius capitis and semispinalis capitis muscles may be difficult to pinpoint, so having the patient point to the area of maximal tenderness is extremely helpful.

Trapezius Muscle Syndrome. The trapezius muscle is a frequent source of muscle pain and headache, especially at the angle of the neck or at the occipital insertion where trigger points are most commonly located (Fig. 53.30C). When injecting trigger points at the angle of the neck be careful to not puncture the apical pleura (Video 53.10).

Sternocleidomastoid Muscle Syndrome. The sternocleidomastoid muscle is also a frequent source of neck pain and headache. Trigger points are most often found at its sternal and clavicular origins and occipital insertions, in addition to the upper two-thirds of the muscle belly (see Fig. 53.30C). Dizziness, ipsilateral ptosis, lacrimation, and conjunctival injection may accompany trigger points located in the sternocleidomastoid muscle.[97] Pain may involve the muscle itself or be referred to as the periauricular, facial, or frontal areas.

Cervical Myofascial Pain Syndrome. This syndrome represents a chronic cause of neck pain, sometimes mistaken for radiculopathy. Trigger points can be present in the head, neck, or shoulder area causing referred pain through the cervical area. A nonfocal neurologic exam and sometimes imaging is paramount to exclude more serious causes.

Myofascial Shoulder Disorders

Myofascial shoulder pain is frequently misdiagnosed as bursitis. It is important to remember that a painful shoulder may be caused by trigger points, which are most often located in the posterior scapular muscles. Other common sites include the supraspinatus, infraspinatus, and pectoralis major muscles. The teres, deltoid, and triceps muscles are rarely involved. Occasionally, trigger points located in the splenius, semispinalis, and gluteal muscles contribute to shoulder pain syndromes and should be treated if found.

Scapula Muscles. When injecting trigger points in the lateral scapular and periscapular muscles, place the patient prone with a pillow under the chest to round the shoulders and facilitate injection. Note the anatomy and boundaries of the shoulder before injection and warn the patient to not move the shoulder. Stabilize the scapula with the nondominant thumb and fingers to prevent movement of the lower portion of the scapula, which could result in inadvertent puncture of the pleura.

Myofascial pain is also commonly associated with several muscle beds at the medial border of the scapula including the rhomboids, the serratus anterior, the subscapular muscles, and the levator scapulae. To inject trigger points in these medially situated muscles, have the patient place the ipsilateral hand behind the back. This will cause winging of the scapula and a safer approach. Direct the needle tangentially for easy access to the serratus anterior and subscapularis muscles. As with the lower portion of the scapula, care should be taken to inject the levator scapulae at an oblique angle that is nearly parallel to the thorax to help reduce the chance of accidentally inducing pneumothorax.

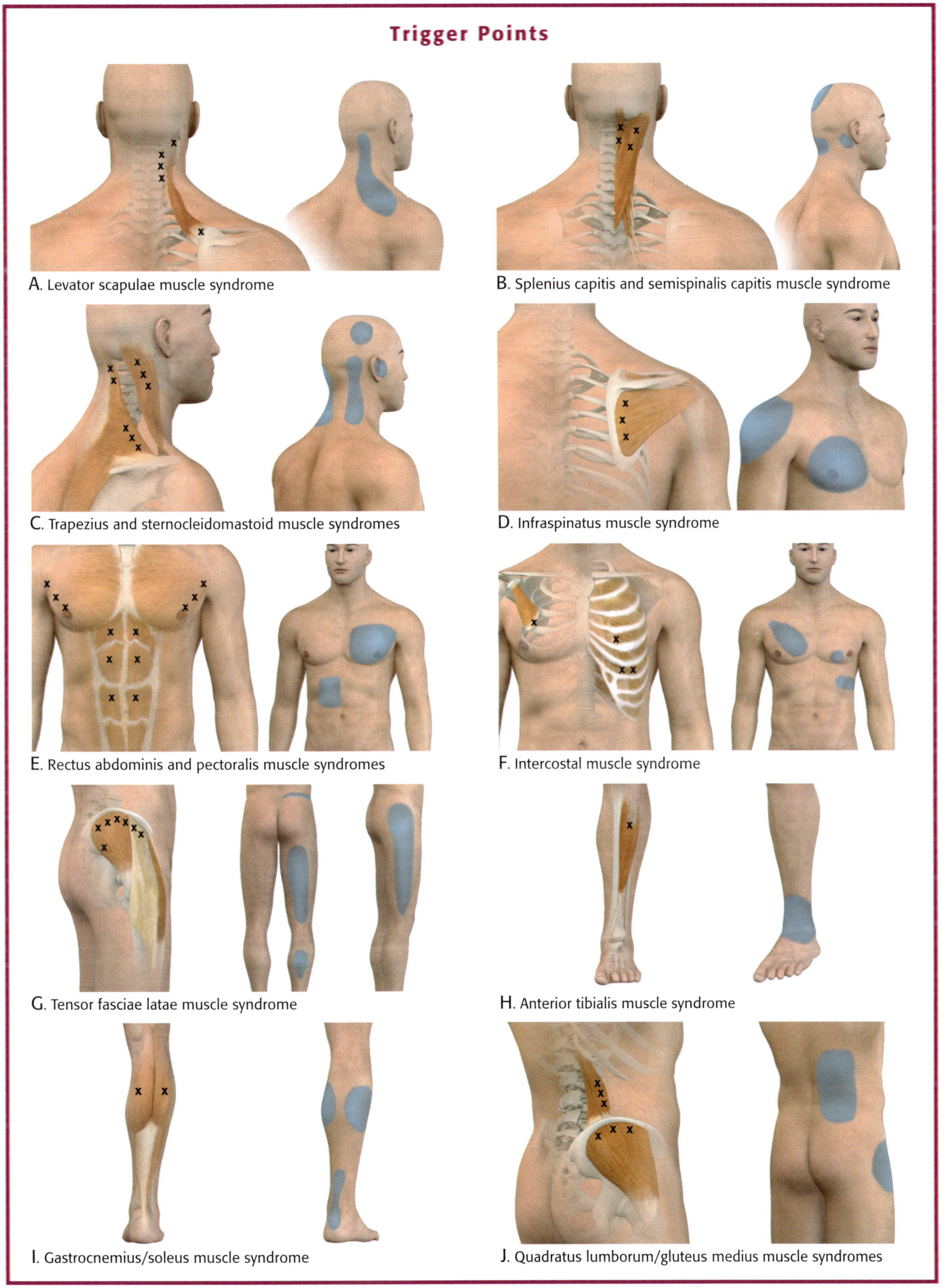

Fig. 53.30 Trigger points. See text for descriptions of the various syndromes.

Infraspinatus Muscle Syndrome. Because of its multiple functions, this muscle is subject to earlier degeneration than other muscles of the rotator cuff and is more susceptible to trigger points (Fig. 53.30D). Trigger points in the infraspinatus muscle invariably cause sympathetic hyperactivity and often contribute to dystrophy-like syndromes of the upper extremity. To identify trigger points in the infraspinatus muscle, it is important to palpate along the entire length of the muscle bundles, and across the grain of the muscle (see Fig. 53.4).

Somatic Visceral Reflex Phenomenon

Skeletal muscle trigger points may contribute to visceral pain by either induction or continuation of the spinal reflex arc.[98,99] Visceral sympathetic afferent nerves converge on the same dorsal horn neuron as somatic nociceptive afferent nerves do. Reflex sympathetic efferent nerve activity may result in spasm of the visceral sphincters and cutaneous nociceptors (leading in part to referred cutaneous pain). The rectus abdominis muscle is particularly prone to trigger point development in conjunction with visceral pain. For example, right upper quadrant trigger points are associated with gallbladder disease, left upper quadrant trigger points with esophageal and ulcer disease, right lower quadrant trigger points with dysmenorrhea, and left lower quadrant trigger points with intestinal disorders.

Treatment of abdominal wall trigger points can provide significant relief of somatic and visceral pain in appropriate patients. Consider injecting these trigger points when palpating the trigger point or placing the affected muscle under tension (e.g., performing a sit-up) produces the characteristic visceral discomfort. It should also be noted that abdominal wall trigger points are often accompanied by trigger points in the corresponding posterior paraspinal muscle segment. For example, esophageal spasm is frequently associated with trigger points on the left posterior aspect of the thorax at spinal nerve levels T3 through T6. To provide more effective pain control, treat these trigger points also.

Rectus Abdominis Muscle Syndrome. These muscles are frequent sites of anterior abdominal wall pain. They often flare up after abdominal surgery and may be a major cause of postoperative pain in some patients. Abdominal wall trigger points are commonly found in the upper three segments of the rectus muscle and can be located more easily by placing the patient in a supine position with the head and neck flexed so that the rectus muscles are under tension (Fig. 53.30E). Pain and tenderness are usually localized directly over the trigger point. Trigger points in the lower rectus segments may be a cause of low back pain. Lower segment trigger points may be associated with trigger points in the corresponding posterior lumbar spinal segments (i.e., L4, L5, S1).

Pectoralis Major/Pectoralis Minor Muscle Syndrome. The pectoralis major muscle is a frequent site of myofascial pain, particularly at its insertion on the anterior medial portion of the shoulder (Fig. 53.30E). The inferior belly of the muscle is also a common area for trigger points, so be sure to carefully search the entire muscle to avoid missing a treatable area. Pain is usually located at the trigger point, but patients with trigger points in the clavicular portion of the muscle may have referred pain in the uppermost part of the muscle, whereas others may experience referred pain in the arm.

Intercostal Muscle Syndrome. In patients with musculoskeletal chest pain, palpate the intercostal muscles for areas of tenderness. Pain emanating from the exterior intercostal muscles is usually localized near the site of the trigger point and is emphasized during inspiration (Fig. 53.30F). Intercostal muscle trigger points often flare after chest surgery or trauma. Exercise extreme care when injecting an intercostal muscle trigger point to avoid entry into the pleural space.

Knee Region

Tensor Fasciae Latae Muscle Syndrome. Because the tensor fasciae latae muscle is easy to examine, trigger points located here are easy to identify (Fig. 53.30G). Patients usually complain of pain along the lateral aspect of the thigh as far down as the knee.

Ankle, Foot, and Heel Region

Anterior Tibialis Muscle Syndrome. Trigger points located in the anterior tibialis muscle usually cause pain along the anterior aspect of the ankle, but the entire ankle may be involved in severe cases. Trigger points are most commonly found in the upper third of the muscle and typically cause pain in the anterior portion of the leg and dorsal portion of the ankle (Fig. 53.30H).

Gastrocnemius/Soleus Muscle Syndrome. Myofascial pain related to trigger points in the gastrocnemius and soleus muscles is usually located behind the knee and along the Achilles tendon near the heel (Fig. 53.30I). These trigger points are generally found along the lateral and medial margins of the muscle group or along the midline (or in both areas) and often flare in patients experiencing vascular insufficiency of the lower extremities.

Myofascial Back Pain

Patients with myofascial back pain syndromes can have presenting symptoms of chronic aching muscle pain, spasms, stiffness, and sometimes weakness. Direct palpation of the back muscles may reveal the presence of trigger points as the true cause, especially in unilateral back pain. The most common trigger points are found in the levator scapulae, quadratus lumborum, and gluteus medius muscles. Syndromes involving the quadratus lumborum and gluteus medius should be considered in all patients presenting with low back pain.

The lumbosacral muscles are also commonly involved in low back pain. Trigger points may occur secondary to nerve root or vertebral spondylolysis and cause neuropathic pain. In these cases, patients may experience only minimal or temporary relief from trigger point injections. Hence, if the patient is no better after a reasonable trial of trigger point injections, referral should be made for further diagnostics and treatment.

Quadratus Lumborum Muscle Syndrome. The quadratus lumborum is considered a hip hiker and lateral flexor of the spine. It also assists respiratory function by anchoring the 12th rib for the pull of the diaphragm. Trigger points may be found along the 12th rib, around the iliac crest, and along the lateral border of the muscle (Fig. 53.30J) and are often associated with distress on deep inspiration and 12th rib pain. Pain can be local or referred to the anterior abdominal wall. In addition, these trigger points may accentuate postoperative pain or painful abdominal scars over the lower quadrant.

Gluteus Pain Syndromes. The gluteal region is composed of several muscles that allow for extension, rotation, and abduction of the hip joint. Trigger points located in the gluteus medius may be the most critical trigger points in the lower extremities (see Fig. 53.30J). They are commonly found along the iliac shelf, and with extensive involvement along the entire gluteal ridge, including the gluteus minimus and maximus muscles from the sacroiliac joint to the anterior superior iliac spine. Trigger points in the gluteus medius may cause hip pain that mimics GTPS (common during the latter stages of pregnancy), whereas trigger points in the gluteus minimus can cause pain radiating down the lateral and posterior aspect of the leg imitating sciatica.

Similar to the infraspinatus muscle syndrome, trigger points in the gluteus medius muscle are frequently associated with sympathetic hyperactivity. In addition, when these trigger points flare, they often recruit trigger points in the quadratus lumborum, tensor fasciae latae, and other gluteal muscles, where they induce diffuse low back pain, or in the cervical muscles causing neck pain and headaches. Though less common, isolated gluteus medius pain may also occur and usually projects along the iliac crest into the posterior of the hip, thigh, and calf.

Acknowledgments

The editors and author wish acknowledge the contributions of Jason Becker and Joshua Markowitz to this chapter in previous editions.

REFERENCES ARE AVAILABLE AT Elsevier eBooks+

CHAPTER 54

Arthrocentesis

Ryan Bateman and Lea Rowson

BACKGROUND

Arthrocentesis, the puncture and aspiration of synovial fluid from an extremity joint, is a core emergency department (ED) procedure.[1] It is both a diagnostic and therapeutic tool necessary for an accurate assessment of an acutely painful, hot, and swollen joint.

INDICATIONS AND CONTRAINDICATIONS

In the acute care setting the primary indication for arthrocentesis is the collection of synovial fluid for analysis to exclude the possibility of a bacterial joint infection. Other indications for this procedure are listed in Review Box 54.1. There are few absolute contraindications to performance of an arthrocentesis with the exception of a clearly evident soft tissue infection overlying the entry site of the puncture needle.[2] Inflammatory changes secondary to an infected joint may cause warmth, erythema, and edema of the surrounding soft tissue, which may mimic a soft tissue infection. Known bacteremia is a theoretical relative contraindication to arthrocentesis because of the fear that bacteria can be introduced into the joint space during the procedure. However, hematogenous spread is the most likely etiology of septic joint in the first place.[2] This complication should be weighed against the necessary information gained by fluid analysis.

Bleeding diatheses are a relative contraindication to arthrocentesis. Multiple studies have confirmed the safety of arthrocentesis in patients on anticoagulation. A retrospective review of over 1000 patients who underwent arthrocentesis or joint injections while on direct oral anticoagulants found no evidence of increased bleeding risk.[3] Additional studies examining the safety of arthrocentesis in anticoagulated patients, including chronic warfarin therapy, have yielded similar results.[4,5] In addition, arthrocentesis to relieve a tense hemarthrosis in bleeding disorders such as hemophilia is an accepted practice after infusion of the appropriate clotting factors. As such, therapeutic anticoagulants are not an absolute contraindication to performance of arthrocentesis. Prosthetic joints are at a higher risk for infection but if infection is suspected in a joint, arthrocentesis should be performed, preferably after consultation with an orthopedic surgeon, who may prefer to do the procedure.

Articular Versus Periarticular Disease

Periarticular conditions such as trauma, tendinitis, bursitis, contusion, cellulitis, or phlebitis may mimic articular disease and suggest the need for arthrocentesis. Evaluation of acute joint pain requires the clinician to determine whether the patient's constellation of signs and symptoms derives from the joint itself or from another musculoskeletal or periarticular structure. No specific test or physical finding has high specificity for distinguishing articular from periarticular disease; however, some physical findings may prove helpful. Pain from a periarticular process is often localized, and tenderness can be elicited only with certain specific movements or at specific points around the joint. In periarticular inflammation, one can often passively range the joint with minimal discomfort, yet pain is significant when the patient attempts active motion. *Crepitus* may be elicited with tendinitis, or the pain may be traced along the course of a specific tendon. Periarticular

Arthrocentesis

Indications

Diagnosis of septic or crystal-induced arthritis
Diagnosis of traumatic bony or ligamentous injury
Instillation of medications for acute or chronic arthritis
Relief of the pain of acute hemarthrosis
Determination of communication between the laceration and joint space

Contraindications

Absolute:
Overlying cellulitis
Relative:
Bleeding diathesis

Complications

Introduction of infection
Bleeding
Allergy to local anesthetic
Pain

Equipment

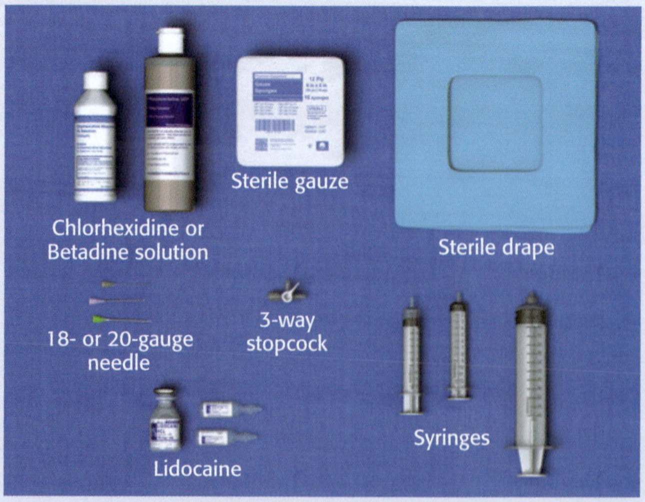

Review Box 54.1 Arthrocentesis: indications, contraindications, complications, and equipment.

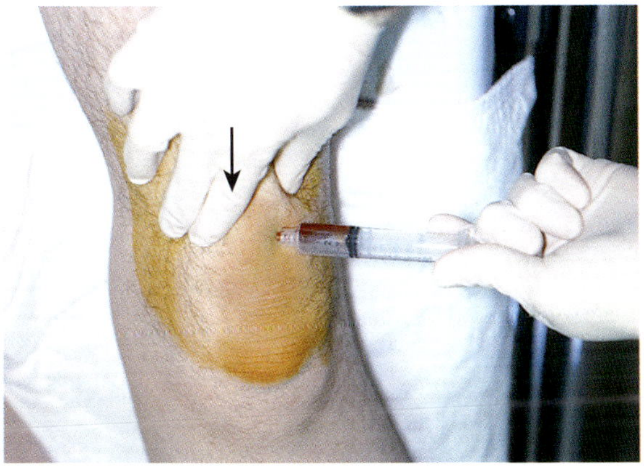

Fig. 54.1 Periarticular problems may mimic an intraarticular process. This patient developed anterior soft tissue swelling and fluctuance after trauma to the knee, representing a hematoma of the prepatellar bursa, not a hemarthrosis. Pressure applied to the edge of the swelling aids in the aspiration of blood from the bursa *(arrow)*.

pain may also be localized to one side of the joint, whereas an interarticular infection will be tender across the entire area of the joint. The entire articular capsule will be inflamed and distended and fluid can often be palpated within the joint. The knee is a good example of this process. In the knee, the effusion into the joint occurs posterior to the patella, whereas bursal swelling occurs anterior to it (Fig. 54.1). When considerable articular effusion of the knee is present, the capsule of the joint is distended, and an inverted U-shaped swelling of the joint develops. This characteristic shape occurs because the dense patellar ligament prevents distention of the capsule along its inferior border. In addition, with the knee extended a large effusion causes the patella to "float" or lift away from the femoral condyles. Complete extension and flexion are often not possible because of the joint tension produced by the effusion, which causes significant pain.[6]

The pain arising from a pathologic condition involving a joint may be diffuse or clearly localized to the joint, or it may radiate. Hip pain, for example, frequently radiates into the groin or down the front of the thigh into the knee. Shoulder joint pain commonly radiates into the elbow or the neck. Therefore complete examination of contiguous structures is essential for adequate diagnosis.

Septic Arthritis

Acute monoarticular arthritis has many causes, but septic arthritis is the most significant and if not identified can produce severe morbidity and even mortality. A missed diagnosis will lead to severe and rapid joint destruction with a mortality up to 13% in native joints.[7] Multiple risk factors for septic arthritis have been identified and include rheumatoid arthritis, advanced age, overlying skin infection, joint prosthesis, recent joint surgery, injection drug use, diabetes, and immunosuppression.[2] While many components of a patient's medical history may raise suspicion for septic arthritis, synovial fluid is needed to confirm the diagnosis. While a positive Gram stain supports the diagnosis, a negative Gram stain has a poor sensitivity and does not rule out the diagnosis.[8] Additionally, while cultures remain the most definitive study for confirmation of septic arthritis, negative cultures cannot be relied on to exclude the diagnosis either. It has also been shown that the presence of crystals in synovial fluid does not exclude the diagnosis of septic arthritis. A retrospective study of over 1000 patients who underwent arthrocentesis found 5% of patients with crystal arthritis had concomitant septic arthritis.[9]

Infection of a joint occurs by one of several mechanisms: hematogenous spread (bacteremia, infective endocarditis) from a contiguous source of infection, direct implantation, postoperative contamination, or trauma.[2,10] The noninfectious differential diagnosis includes crystal-induced arthritis, fracture, hemarthrosis, foreign body, osteoarthritis, ischemic necrosis, and monoarticular rheumatoid arthritis. In addition, osteomyelitis may mimic septic arthritis because of the proximity of the infected metaphysis to the joint space.[2] In many instances, an acutely inflamed joint from gout or other arthritides simply cannot be distinguished from infection clinically. Nonetheless, early diagnosis is essential to prevent complications such as impairment of growth, articular destruction with ankylosis, osteomyelitis, and soft tissue extension.[10]

Because an acutely swollen joint may be indicative of several disease entities, a thorough history and physical examination may help identify the etiology of the problem. Ultimately, though, arthrocentesis may be required to definitely exclude a bacterial infection (Fig. 54.2). In cases where arthrocentesis is not possible, laboratory findings may be useful in making a diagnosis, as can response to therapy. For example, the response to empirical antibiotics in gonococcal arthritis is often the only criterion used for diagnosis as the organism is difficult to culture from joint fluid.[11] Blood cultures may be positive because joint infections are often due to hematogenous spread. Patients with malignancy (especially leukemia) or those who are immunosuppressed are at particular risk for a septic cause. Infectious arthritis should be considered primarily in these patients, as well as in those with preexisting joint diseases such as rheumatoid arthritis.[9] In general, a swollen joint is not usually injected with corticosteroids until the possibility of infection has been eliminated.[12]

Staphylococcus (including methicillin resistant), *Streptococcus*, and *Pseudomonas* are the most frequently identified etiologic agents.[2] *Neisseria gonorrhoeae*, although less common, should be considered in adolescents and young adults where it has been shown to have increased prevalence.[13] Patients older than 40 years and those with other medical illnesses are more likely to have *Staphylococcus* joint infections. In children, *Staphylococcus*, *Streptococcus*, and *Escherichia coli* predominate. *Haemophilus influenzae* was a common cause of pediatric septic arthritis in the past, but widespread use of the conjugate vaccine has reduced *H. influenzae* infection rates to nearly zero.[8,14] In neonates, staphylococci, Enterobacteriaceae, group B streptococci, and *N. gonorrhoeae* are the most likely organisms. Staphylococcal or pseudomonal infections commonly develop in injection drug abusers. *Salmonella* arthritis is more prevalent in patients with sickle cell disease than in the general population; however, more common organisms still predominate. Prosthetic joints or postoperative infections have high rates of *Staphylococcus aureus*, *Streptococcus epidermidis*, Enterobacteriaceae, and *Pseudomonas* infection.[7]

Septic arthritis from methicillin-resistant *S. aureus* (MRSA) appears to be increasing in frequency. Recent studies have identified MRSA as the causative organism in 17% to 50% of confirmed cases of septic arthritis.[7,15] It appears to be more prevalent in young patients as well as intravenous drug users. MRSA-infected joints tend to progress rapidly causing significant joint and bone destruction and can be fatal. Therefore

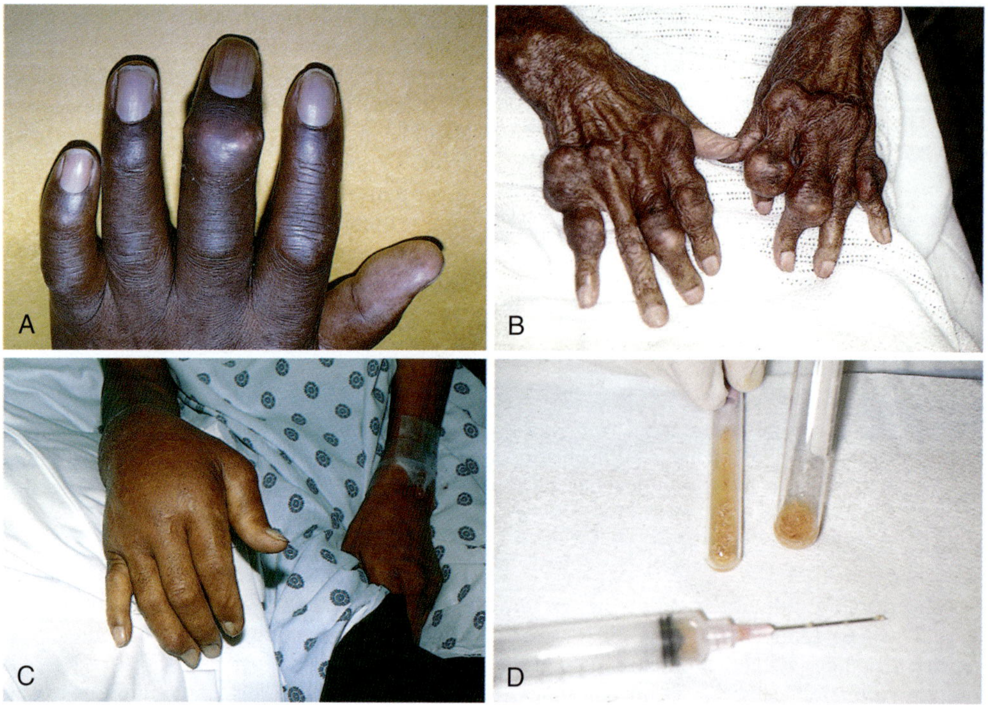

Fig. 54.2 (A–B) Tophaceous gout. These nodules are painless and full of uric acid crystals. (C) The acutely swollen and painful wrist joint in this patient is most likely due to acute gouty arthritis, which can produce fever and leukocytosis. In some cases, joint fluid analysis is the only way to differentiate gout from a septic joint. (D) Aspiration of a tophus yields a precipitated, waxy, soft uric acid conglomeration.

empiric MRSA therapy should be initiated in the ED when septic arthritis is suspected.

N. gonorrhoeae is another cause of septic arthritis and deserves special mention. Disseminated gonococcal infection occurs in 0.5% to 3% of cases of mucosal infection.[16] Gonococcal septic arthritis is more common in females, especially during pregnancy or after menstruation, because females with sexually transmitted gonorrhea infections are more likely to be asymptomatic initially. The time needed for local infection to disseminate can vary from several days to weeks. Patients will often experience systemic symptoms, including fevers, chills, and malaise, as well as migratory polyarthralgia. Gonococcal tenosynovitis without joint involvement occurs in two-thirds of patients. Dermatitis is also present in two-thirds of patients (Fig. 54.3). The most common rash consists of scattered painless, nonpruritic, 0.5- to 0.75-cm macules or papules with necrotic or pustular centers, distributed on the extremities and trunk. Eventually, the infection settles into one or two large joints to yield purulent arthritis.[13,16] Overt urethritis and vaginitis may be absent or overlooked because of concentration solely on the obvious joint pathology. Hence, it is important to realize that disseminated gonococcal infections can be associated with surprisingly minimal or even absent signs and symptoms of a genital infection source. Some joints may become inoculated through hematogenous spread from anal and oral sites of infection. Even though *N. gonorrhoeae*–infected joint fluid is usually "septic" in character, the yield of positive synovial fluid cultures has ranged from 25% to 50%. Blood cultures appear to be less helpful as they are positive in only 20% to 30% of cases.[17] Because blood and joint fluid culture has a low yield, it would be prudent to culture all possible sites of gonococcal infection, including anal and pharyngeal sites. The organism can often be identified in asymptomatic genitourinary sites, with cultures from the primary mucosal site being positive in up to 80% of infected patients.[16,17]

A positive Gram stain is immediately diagnostic of septic arthritis. However, Gram stains are positive in only 71% of gram-positive infections, 40% to 50% of gram-negative infections, and 25% of gonococcal infections. An elevated synovial white blood cell (WBC) count and a reduction in synovial fluid glucose may give supportive data. However, the synovial fluid WBC count in gonococcal arthritis is often between 10,000 and 20,000 cells/mm.[17] Although mild leukocytosis and an elevated erythrocyte sedimentation rate may occur, normal laboratory values do not exclude infection.

Hemarthrosis

Isolated nontraumatic hemarthrosis may occasionally be seen by the emergency clinician. An inflammatory reaction is likely to follow intracapsular bleeding, and the proliferative reaction and the hyperplastic synovium formed might predispose patients to recurrent hemorrhage in that joint, especially those with bleeding diatheses. The knee is the most affected joint, followed by the ankle, elbow, shoulder, and hip.[18] Hemarthrosis may also be a complication of sickle cell anemia, pseudogout, amyloidosis, pigmented villonodular synovitis, synovial hemangioma, rheumatoid arthritis, and infection.[19]

The most common cause of intraarticular hemorrhage in the setting of no or minor trauma is a hereditary clotting factor deficiency such as hemophilia. Similarly, hemarthrosis is the most common manifestation of hemophilia and severe hemophilia accounts for hemarthrosis in 75% to 90% of patients.[18] Approximately 50% of persons living with hemophilia will develop hemarthrosis at some time during their life.[20] Hemarthrosis is an infrequent complication of oral

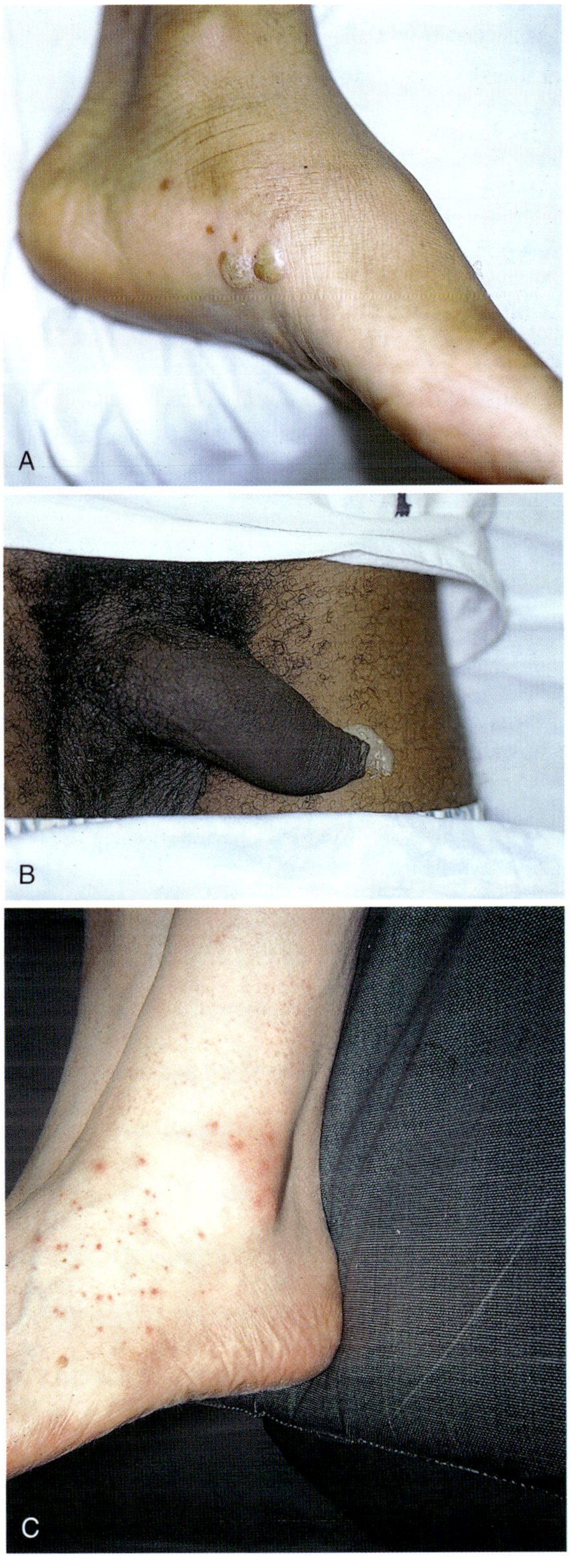

Fig. 54.3 (A) Often mistaken for insect or spider bites, these multiple embolic skin lesions (ranging from single or multiple petechiae to pustules) may be seen in patients with acutely swollen joints infected with *Neisseria gonorrhoeae*. Skin lesions are usually found on the extremities, especially the feet and hands, and may be present before a large-joint effusion accumulates or with gonococcal tenosynovitis. (B) A genital manifestation of urethritis (penile discharge) or vaginitis may be seen but can be rather clinically silent. (C) Maculopapular rash associated with *N. gonorrhoeae*.

anticoagulant therapy, which was previously thought to have significant risk.[3–5] In a retrospective study of 445 patients comparing corticosteroid injections on patients on direct acting oral anticoagulants (DOACs) versus those who were not, no adverse events of significant intraarticular or extraarticular bleeding were observed.[5] Cessation of anticoagulant therapy in these patients must be weighed against the risk for adverse clot formation (e.g., acute cerebrovascular accident).

Hemarthrosis after trauma is a frequent occurrence. It is most common in the knee and often denotes significant internal damage. Based on a cohort study of 1145 consecutive patients who developed a traumatic hemarthrosis of the knee, approximately 50% had an anterior cruciate ligament (ACL) injury. In those 16 years of age or younger, lateral patellar dislocation was the most frequent structural injury associated with traumatic hemarthrosis of the knee.[20] Likewise, intraarticular fractures can cause significant hemarthrosis and debilitating pain.

In patients with recurrent hemarthrosis, regardless of etiology, there is risk of long-term effects of joint destruction and ongoing chronic pain. In a 2019 study on rat models, 54 rats were subjected to hemarthrosis and 41 showed varying degrees of intraarticular and subcutaneous bleeding.[21] Hyperplasia and immune cell infiltration of the synovial tissue was revealed 24 to 48 hours post hemarthrosis. In addition, proteoglycan loss was apparent, most localized to the lateral tibial plateau and there was excessive bone remodeling of the cortical bone covering the femoral growth plates.[21] Similarly, there is significant correlation between the incidence of synovial thickening, bone and cartilage damage, and bleeding incidence and increasing age.[22]

Management of acute hemarthrosis depends on the cause. Although rare, hemarthrosis associated with oral anticoagulant therapy may only improve after the oral anticoagulant is reversed or discontinued. This is achieved via replacement of clotting factors with prothrombin complex concentrate, fresh frozen plasma (FFP) or administration of reversal agents.[19,20] Management of hemarthrosis in the setting of bleeding diatheses (such as hemophilia) deserves special recognition. Coagulation factor should be administered to those with suspected hemarthrosis within the first 2 hours of identification. For large joints or significant trauma, factor levels should be raised to 80% to 100%. Bleeding into smaller, peripheral joints can be managed by raising factors levels to 40% to 50%.[20]

Distension of the joint by effusion or hemorrhage causes considerable pain and disability. If the fluid is not removed, it is partially absorbed, but part of it may undergo organization and result in the formation of adhesions or bands within the joint, again leading to continued pain and bone remodeling. This is one argument for drainage of the joint. Some believe that in an otherwise healthy joint that is subjected to a single traumatic event, even a relatively large hemarthrosis will be spontaneously reabsorbed without significant sequelae and therefore presents no pressing need for drainage. Unfortunately, no literature exists to guide the best approach; hence, there is no universal standard of care regarding the need or lack of draining blood from a traumatic joint.[23,24]

Nonetheless, a large, tense, traumatic effusion is quite painful, and its presence precludes proper evaluation of an injured joint. Therapeutic arthrocentesis to drain a symptomatic traumatic effusion is a common and well-accepted practice.[6,20,23,24]

TABLE 54.1 Intrasynovial Corticosteroid Preparations[a]

PREPARATION	LARGE-JOINT DOSE (mg)	SMALL-JOINT DOSE (mg)[b]
Triamcinolone hexacetonide	20	2–6
Triamcinolone acetonide	20	2–6
Methylprednisolone acetate	40	3.5–10.5
Triamcinolone diacetate	20	2–6
Dexamethasone acetate	5	0.5–1.5

[a]Listed in approximate descending order of duration of action.
[b]The dose will depend on joint size, capsular distensibility, and degree of inflammation.
From Gray RG, Gottlieb NL. Corticosteroid injections in RA: appraisal of a neglected therapy. *J Musculoskelet Med*. 1990;7:53.

Following therapeutic arthrocentesis for hemarthrosis, it may be desirable to inject 2 mL to 15 mL, depending on joint size, of a local anesthetic into the joint to facilitate examination or provide temporary relief of the symptoms.[25,26]

Intraarticular Corticosteroid Injections

In 1951 Hollander and coworkers first demonstrated that intraarticular corticosteroid injections are useful for relief of symptoms in patients with severe rheumatoid arthritis. The use of steroids has proved to be a dependable method for providing rapid relief of pain and swelling of inflamed joints, although it is strictly local, usually temporary, and rarely curative.[25–28] It is easily performed in the emergency setting. Acute gout responds well to joint injection, and this may be preferable in patients who cannot tolerate indomethacin or colchicine.

Corticosteroid injections are most helpful when only a small number of joints are actively inflamed. The most frequently used corticosteroids for intraarticular injection are shown in Table 54.1. Diminution of joint pain, swelling, effusion, and warmth is usually evident within 6 to 12 hours after injection.

Though very rare, the most serious complication of this practice is intraarticular infection.[12] Therefore steroids should not be injected into a joint if infection is suspected. Repeated injections into one joint pose a risk for necrosis of juxtaarticular bone with subsequent joint destruction, instability, and suppression of the hypothalamic-pituitary axis from systemic absorption. Other complications include local soft tissue atrophy and calcification, tendon rupture, intraarticular bleeding, and transient nerve palsy.[27] Transient elevations in blood glucose, as well as erythema, warmth, and diaphoresis of the face and torso, may also occur after intraarticular steroid injections. Acute pain, redness, and swelling 12 to 24 hours after steroid injection can mimic infection, but with this timing it is most likely an inflammatory reaction (steroid flare) to crystal-containing steroid preparation (often methylprednisolone). Deposition of steroid crystals on the synovium can give rise to a transient, self-limited flare-up of synovitis.[9]

It is always important to determine whether local corticosteroid therapy has been used previously, not only to consider the array of clinical conditions associated with steroid use but also because crystalline corticosteroid material can hinder proper interpretation of crystals found in synovial fluid.[9]

Other Intraarticular Injections

In addition to steroids local anesthetics such as lidocaine and bupivacaine, opioids including morphine and fentanyl and other agents such as ketamine and dexmedetomidine have all been instilled into a joint to relieve pain. In postoperative cases these adjuncts have reduced analgesic use.[28a,28b,28c]

Equipment

The materials needed for arthrocentesis include skin preparation solutions (e.g., chlorhexidine), sterile gloves and drapes, local anesthetic, syringes for injecting local anesthetic and aspirating joint fluid, a three-way stopcock for draining large amounts of fluid, lavender, red, and green-topped blood tubes, and various sizes of needles and intravenous catheters (see Review Box 54.1).

Depending on the size of the effusion to be drained, a Luer-Lok syringe between 10 mL to 60 mL can be used. If a large effusion is suspected, a three-way stopcock should be placed between the needle and the syringe. This allows a broader surface to be grasp when switching syringes and also allows a separate port for injection of medications. Though still common practice in many institutions, recent evidence suggests that synovial fluid protein and glucose levels are poor differentiators of noninflammatory and inflammatory effusions and are no longer recommended (see section on "Synovial Fluid Interpretation" later).[28d] Immediately examine fresh synovial fluid in its unadulterated form for crystals. Calcium oxalate and lithium heparin anticoagulants have been reported to introduce artifactual crystals into the fluid. Joint fluid to be analyzed for crystals should be collected in a green-topped tube containing sodium heparin. Some laboratories will request the fluid simply be placed into a sterile specimen cup and hand delivered to the lab allowing their technicians to distribute it to the appropriate containers. If culturing for *N. gonorrhoeae*, the fluid should be immediately placed on proper medium and stored in a low-oxygen environment in the ED.[11]

GENERAL ARTHROCENTESIS TECHNIQUE

Joint fluid may be obtained even when there is little clinical evidence of an effusion. Although one may aspirate successfully at the point where the joint bulges maximally, certain landmarks are important. The most crucial part of arthrocentesis is defining the joint anatomy by palpating the bony landmarks as a guide. First, select a puncture site and an approach to the joint. Avoid tendons, major vessels, and major nerve branches. In most instances, the approach is via the extensor surfaces of joints because most major vessels and nerves are found beneath the flexor surfaces. In addition, the synovial pouch is usually more superficial on the extensor side of a joint. Ultrasound may be particularly helpful in locating small effusions.

Use aseptic technique, including the use of sterile gloves and instruments, to avoid infection. Do not attempt arthrocentesis if there is a definite or suspected infection overlying the joint. Allow antiseptic preparation solutions to dry for several minutes before performing the procedure. If an iodine solution was utilized, wipe the area clean with an alcohol sponge to prevent transference of iodine into the joint space, which can lead to an inflammatory process. Although the utility of draping is unproved and it may obscure the site, a sterile perforated drape may be placed over the joint.

ULTRASOUND: Arthrocentesis

by Christine Butts, MD

Ultrasound offers a significant advantage when evaluating a patient with joint pain. In patients with obesity or significant pain, limited physical examination makes the diagnosis of a joint effusion difficult. The success rate of blind arthrocentesis varies from 61% to 78% depending on the joint being assessed.[29–32] However, evaluation of an effusion within the joint space utilizing ultrasound guidance has an 80% sensitivity and 90% specificity.[30] Ultrasound has shown utility in identifying a joint effusion in patients with nondiagnostic radiographs and ultimately leading to the diagnosis of septic arthritis.[31]

Other advantages of ultrasound include lack of ionizing radiation, visualization of vascular structures, differentiation of joint fluid from synovitis, identification of extraarticular fluid collections, and ability to accommodate many patient positions and approaches.[29] Attempting blind aspiration in these patients may cause significant pain for the patient and frustration for the clinician. Ultrasound allows the physician to thoroughly evaluate the joint space for the presence of effusion and to plan the best approach for aspiration. Ultrasound is able to detect effusions with as little as 4 mL of aspirate within the joint space, which would otherwise be unable to be detected by blind physical examination alone.[31] The initial evaluation of the major joints is discussed hereafter, followed by a general approach to aspiration.

Knee

Although effusions of the knee are frequently diagnosed on physical examination alone and aspirated blindly, ultrasound allows the clinician to distinguish effusion from other conditions that may cause generalized swelling (such as bursitis).

A high-frequency transducer (7.5 MHz to 12 MHz) should be used to allow the greatest resolution. Begin with the indicator pointing toward the patient's head (in longitudinal orientation) over the anterior aspect of the knee and attempt to locate the patella (Fig. 54.US1). The patella can be seen as a brightly echogenic (white) object with posterior shadowing (Fig. 54.US2). Locating the patella is key to distinguishing prepatellar bursitis, which will appear as a dark, fluid-filled collection superficial to the patella, and a joint effusion, which will appear as a dark, fluid-filled collection deep to the patella. Once the patella has been identified, move the transducer medially or laterally to "look under" the patella into the joint space (Fig. 54.US3). Fluid will appear as a dark gray or black collection between the articular surface of the femur and fibula or tibia (Fig. 54.US4). Once this area has been evaluated, move the transducer superiorly to evaluate the suprapatellar bursa, which lies superior to the patella and deep to the quadriceps tendon. The suprapatellar bursa communicates with the joint space and frequently houses a large amount of fluid (Fig. 54.US5). Placing

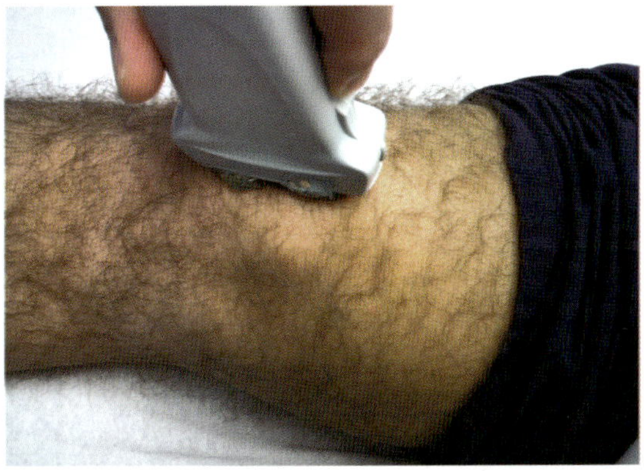

Fig. 54.US1 Placement of the ultrasound transducer in a longitudinal orientation over the patella. Such placement enables localization of the patella and serves to orient the sonographer.

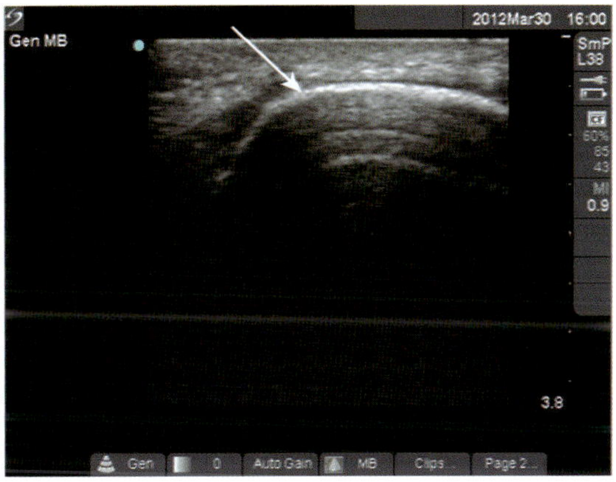

Fig. 54.US2 Ultrasound image of a normal patella. The patella is seen as a brightly echogenic *(white)* arcing line just beneath the surface *(arrow)*. Prepatellar fluid collections, such as bursitis, will be seen superficial to this area.

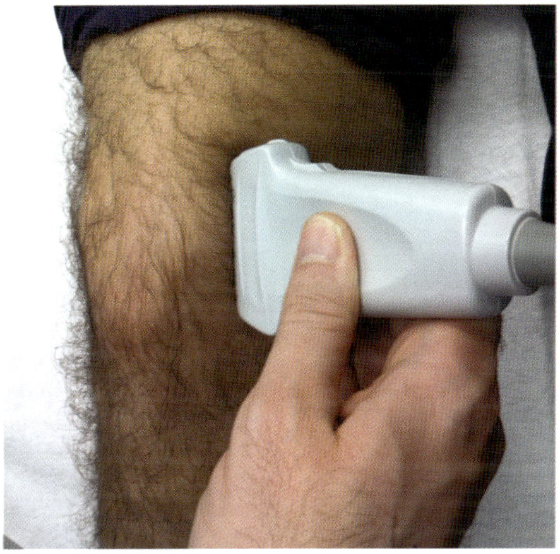

Fig. 54.US3 Placement of the ultrasound transducer to "look under" the patella into the joint space.

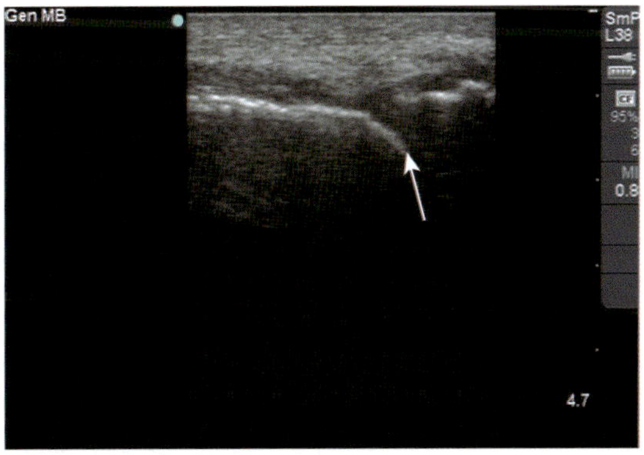

Fig. 54.US4 Ultrasound image of the junction of the femur (at the left of the image) and the tibia (at the right of the image) *(arrow)*. When an effusion is suspected, the suprapatellar recess should be evaluated in addition to this space because fluid frequently collects in the potential space superior to this junction.

ULTRASOUND: Arthrocentesis—cont'd

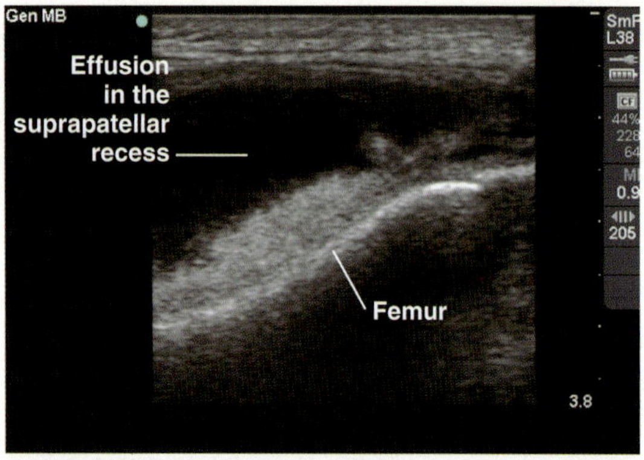

Fig. 54.US5 Ultrasound image of a joint effusion within the suprapatellar recess of the knee joint. The recess is distended with anechoic *(black)* fluid and the femur can be seen as the hyperechoic *(white)* line at the bottom of the image.

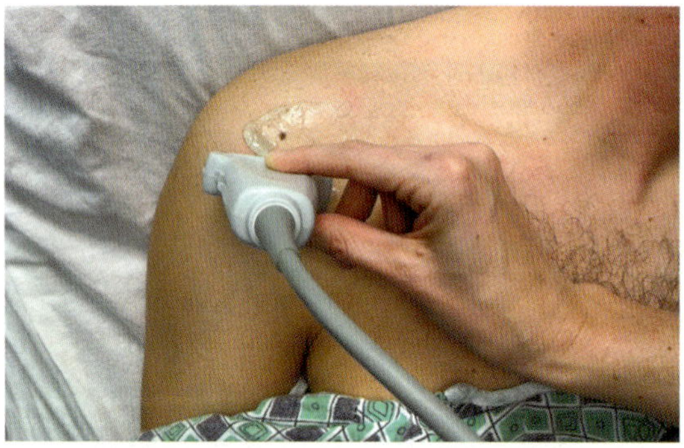

Fig. 54.US6 Placement of the ultrasound transducer over the anterior aspect of the shoulder to evaluate the biceps tendon. To obtain the best view, the patient's arm should be flexed at the elbow, supinated, and slightly abducted.

a hand on this bursa can milk fluid into the joint itself distending the joint space and making placement of the aspiration needle easier.

Shoulder

Either an anterior or posterior approach can be used to evaluate the shoulder. In the anterior approach, place the patient first in a seated position with the elbow adducted and the palm facing up. Then, place the high-frequency transducer in a transverse orientation over the approximate location of the biceps tendon (Fig. 54.US6). The biceps tendon is an extracapsular extension of the joint and will be seen to distend with fluid when a joint effusion is present. A normal tendon can be seen to lie within the biceps groove of the humerus (Fig. 54.US7). When surrounded by fluid, the tendon will be seen to "float" within an anechoic (black) area (Fig. 54.US8).

To evaluate the joint from the posterior approach, place the patient in a seated position with the affected hand on the opposite shoulder to open the joint space. Then, place the transducer at the approximate location of the articulation of the humeral head with the glenoid (Fig. 54.US9). In a normal joint, the humerus can be seen to articulate with the glenoid without any intervening fluid (Fig. 54.US10). When an effusion is present, a dark gray or black collection can be seen medial to the glenoid (Fig. 54.US11). Aspiration can be performed via an out-of-

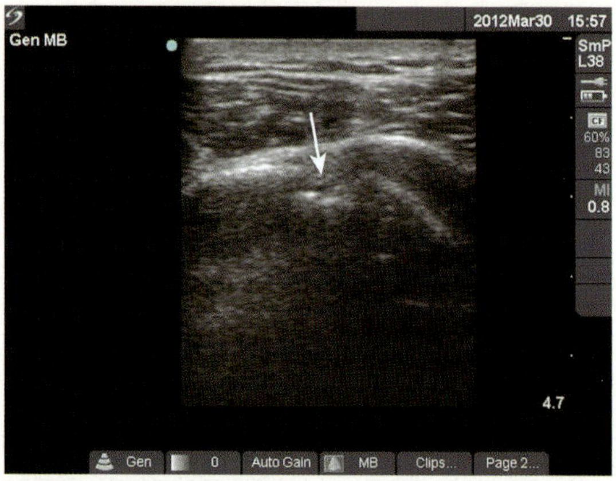

Fig. 54.US7 Ultrasound image of a normal-appearing biceps tendon. The tendon will appear as a hyperechoic *(white)* bundle within the groove of the humerus as indicated by the *arrow*.

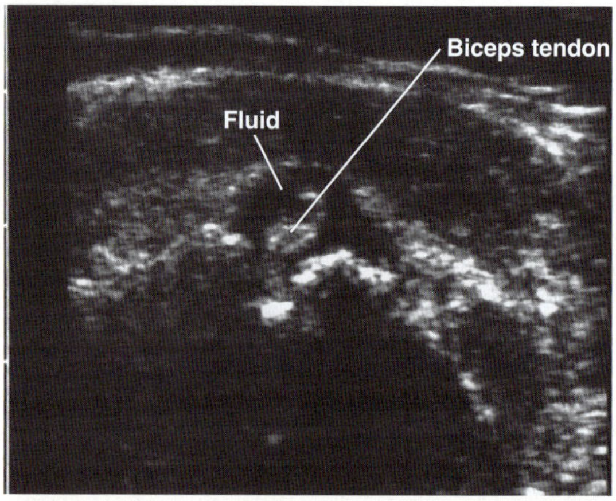

Fig. 54.US8 The biceps tendon is surrounded by anechoic *(black)* fluid. (Courtesy Verena Valley, MD.)

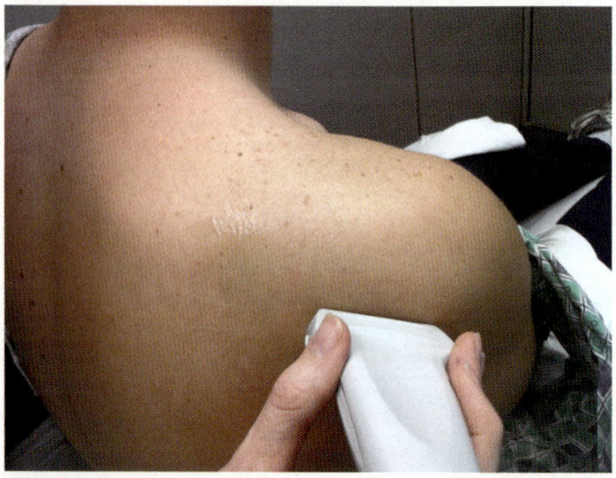

Fig. 54.US9 Placement of the ultrasound transducer over the posterior aspect of the shoulder to evaluate the glenohumeral joint. This joint line can typically be palpated to approximate the best initial position.

place approach by inserting a needle at a steep angle at the center of the side of the linear ultrasound probe.

Continued

ULTRASOUND: Arthrocentesis—cont'd

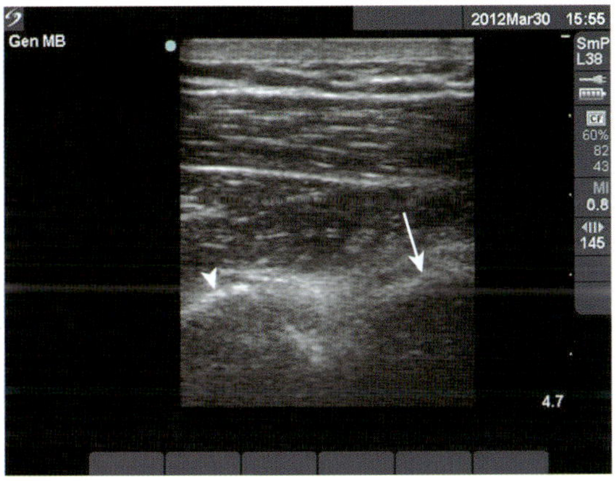

Fig. 54.US10 Ultrasound of a normal-appearing shoulder joint. Deep to the overlying musculature, the glenoid can be seen at the left of the image *(arrowhead)*. The humeral head is seen to the right of the glenoid *(arrow)*.

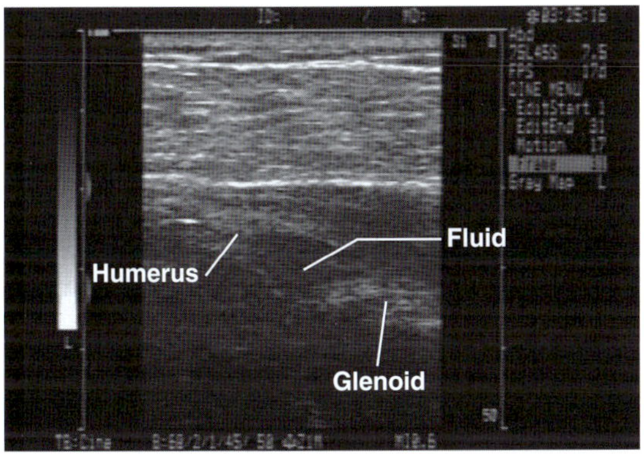

Fig. 54.US11 Shoulder effusion as viewed from a posterior approach. Free fluid will appear as an anechoic collection medial to the glenoid rim. (Courtesy Verena Valley, MD.)

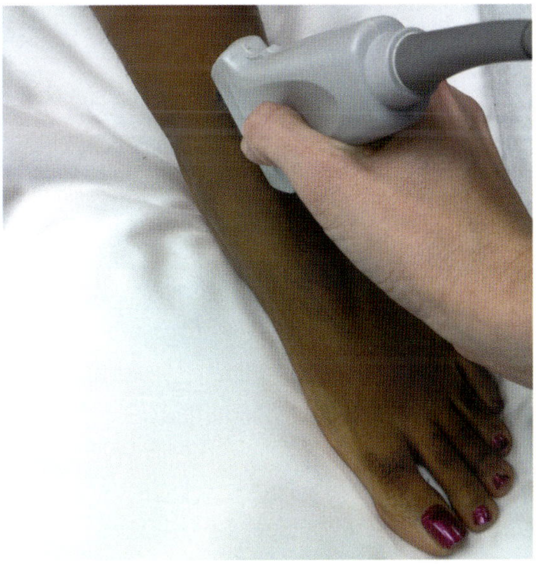

Fig. 54.US12 Placement of the ultrasound transducer over the anterior aspect of the ankle to evaluate for an ankle effusion.

Ankle

The ankle joint is best evaluated in the longitudinal axis with the transducer placed over the space between the posterior edge of the tibia and the talus (Fig. 54.US12). Slightly plantar-flexing the foot will enable the transducer to "fit" in this space. In a normal joint, the distal edge of the tibia can be seen to articulate with the talus without any intervening fluid (Fig. 54.US13). When an effusion is present, it is seen as a triangular, dark gray or black pocket between the tibia and talus (Fig. 54.US14). Ultrasound can also be used to identify the location of the dorsalis pedis artery before aspiration.

Elbow

The elbow is easily evaluated from the posterior approach. With this approach, place the transducer over the olecranon fossa with the elbow flexed to 90 degrees and the lower part of the arm supported (Fig. 54.US15) or resting on a table. In a normal elbow the olecranon fossa can be seen as a slight "divot" between the olecranon of the ulna (below the triceps tendon) and the humerus (Fig. 54.US16). When an effusion is present, dark gray or black fluid can be seen to distend this space (Fig. 54.US17).

Hip

The hip joint is unique in that physical examination may suggest the presence of an effusion, but direct confirmation is difficult with traditional examination techniques. Ultrasound will easily confirm the presence of

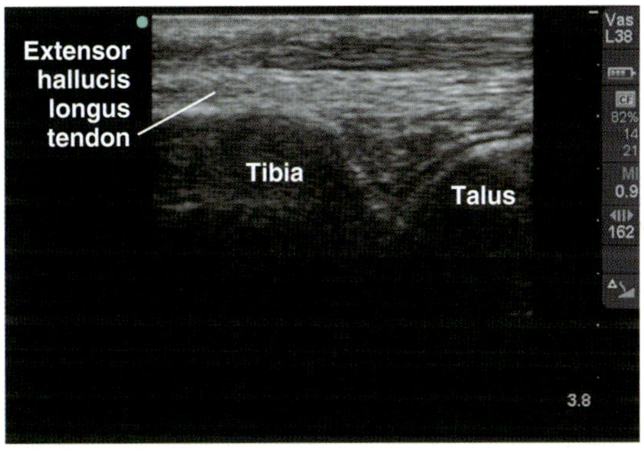

Fig. 54.US13 Ultrasound image of a normal ankle joint. At the left of the image is the tibia, with the talus seen at the right. The intervening area is free of fluid and the extensor hallucis longus can be seen superficial to this area.

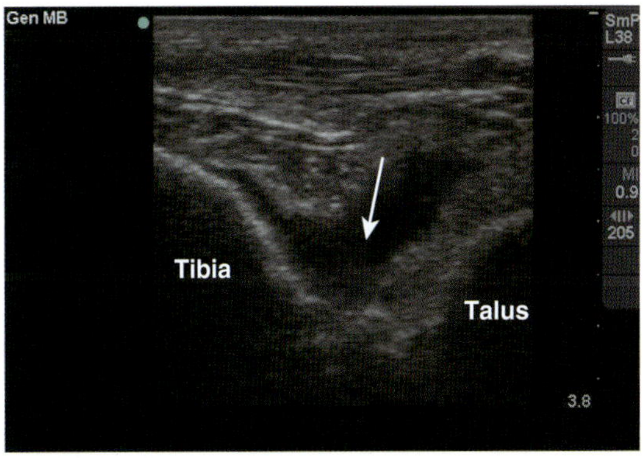

Fig. 54.US14 Ultrasound image of an ankle effusion. As with the normal image, the tibia and talus can be seen on either side of the image. However, in the intervening area, an anechoic *(black)* fluid collection can be seen *(white arrow)*.

ULTRASOUND: Arthrocentesis—cont'd

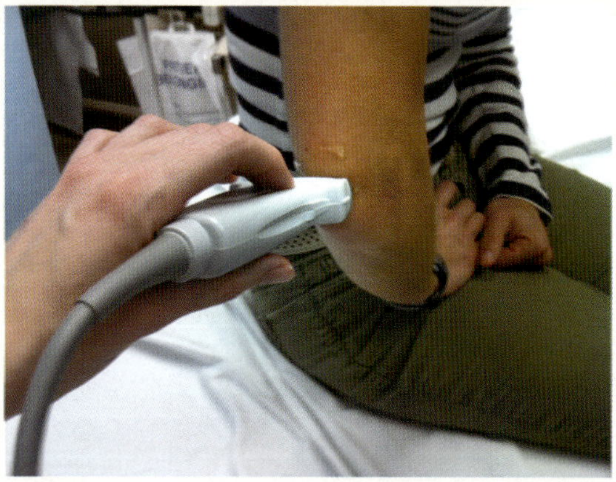

Fig. 54.US15 Placement of the transducer in the transverse plane over the area of the olecranon fossa. For best resolution, a high-frequency transducer should be used.

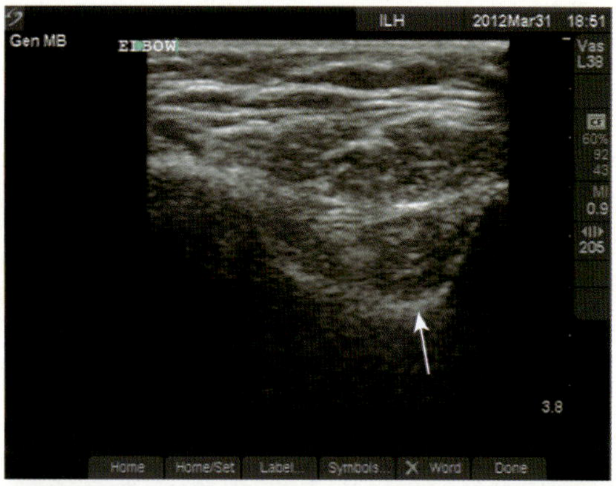

Fig. 54.US16 Ultrasound image of a normal elbow joint. The olecranon fossa can be identified as the echogenic *(white)* crescent at the bottom of the image *(arrow)*. The area just above the fossa should be evaluated for the presence of fluid indicative of an effusion.

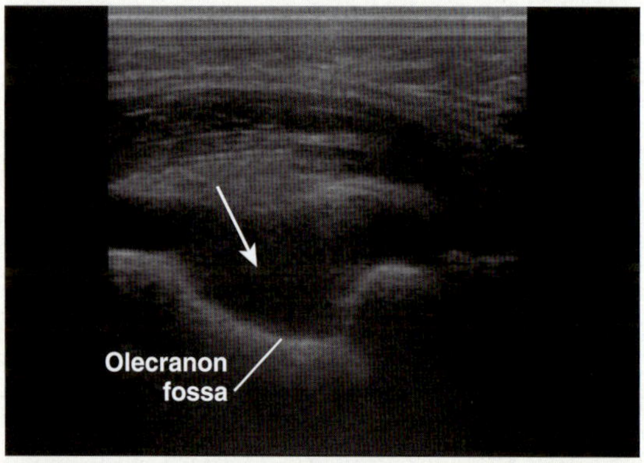

Fig. 54.US17 Elbow joint distended by anechoic fluid *(arrow)* superficial to the olecranon fossa. (From Allan PL, Baxter GM, Weston MJ, eds. *Clinical Ultrasound.* 3rd ed. Elsevier; 2011.)

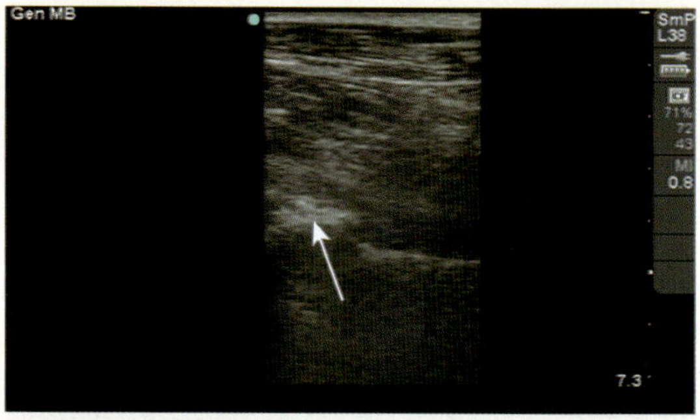

Fig. 54.US18 Normal ultrasound of the hip. The femoral head can be seen as the hyperechoic *(white)* line highlighted by the *arrow*. The area immediately superficial to the femur is devoid of any significant fluid collection.

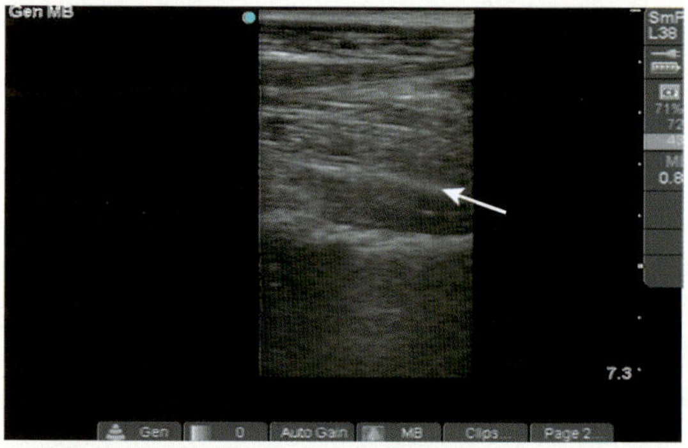

Fig. 54.US19 Ultrasound image of the hip with demonstration of the joint capsule. The joint capsule can be seen as the hyperechoic *(white)* arcing structure marked by the *arrow*.

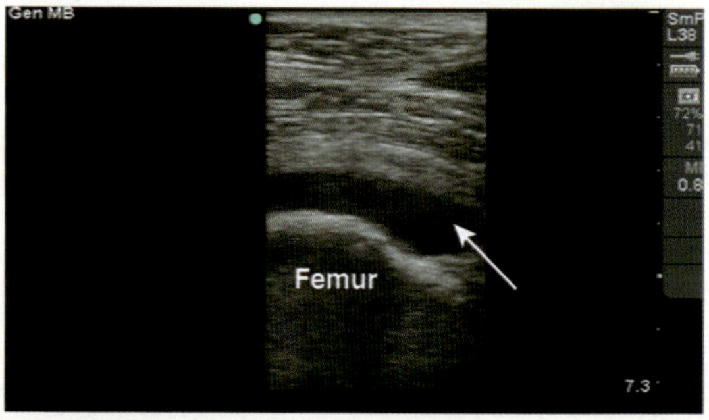

Fig. 54.US20 Ultrasound image of a hip effusion. As in a normal hip, the femur can be seen at the bottom of the image. Immediately superficial to the femur, an anechoic *(black)* fluid collection is highlighted by the *arrow*

an effusion. To evaluate the hip joint, select a low-frequency transducer (3 to 5 mHz) initially because of the depth of the joint. In very thin patients, the distance from the skin to the joint may be small enough to allow the use of a high-frequency transducer. Align the transducer in a slightly oblique axis (mimicking the orientation of the femoral neck) along the inguinal area. This view will include visualization of the femoral neurovascular bundle. Next, rotate the linear probe to aim toward the umbilicus. Look for the femoral neck and head. They will appear as brightly echogenic outlines in the expected shape of the bones (Fig. 54.US18). Once the femur has been identified, look for the joint capsule. It will appear as an arcing, hyperechoic line superficial to the bones (Fig. 54.US19). In a normal hip there will be very little tissue between these two structures. There may be a small amount of anechoic or hypoechoic fluid present in this space in a normal hip, and correlation with the unaffected side will aid in evaluation. In the presence of a significant effusion, a large anechoic or hypoechoic fluid collection will be seen between the femoral neck and the capsule (Fig. 54.US20).

Continued

ULTRASOUND: Arthrocentesis—cont'd

Aspiration

Once the joint in question has been evaluated, the optimal site for aspiration can be planned. In contrast to the traditional, blind aspiration technique, the use of ultrasound may suggest an alternative approach. Ultrasound will enable the clinician to map the best approach to the effusion. Once this approach has been clarified, one of two techniques can be applied. The site can be marked and the aspiration can then proceed blindly under sterile conditions. In other cases it may be preferable to perform the tap under direct ultrasound guidance. In these circumstances the needle is inserted either from the transverse or from the long-axis approach and guided directly into the joint space.

With appropriate local anesthesia, arthrocentesis should be a relatively painless procedure; without anesthesia, it may be quite painful and distressing to the patient. The synovial membrane itself has pain fibers associated with blood vessels, and the articular capsule and periosteum are richly supplied with nerve fibers, so both are very sensitive. The articular cartilage has no intrinsic pain fibers. It is important to have the patient relax during the procedure. Tense muscles narrow the joint space and make the procedure more difficult, often necessitating repeated attempts or resulting in inadequate drainage. Distraction of the joint may enhance the target area, especially in areas such as the wrist and finger joints. Traction not only increases the chance of entering the joint but also lessens the chance of scoring the articular cartilage with the needle.

To best accomplish anesthesia, infiltrate the skin down to the area of the joint capsule along the entire route of needle penetration. Use a local anesthetic agent such as 1% or 2% lidocaine (Xylocaine) via a 25- to 27-gauge needle. For extremely painful joints, a regional nerve block can be considered.

Use the landmarks described in "Specific Arthrocentesis Techniques" later in this chapter. Take care not to bounce the needle off bony structures as a means of finding the joint space because this may cause unnecessary pain. However, in contrast to earlier beliefs, striking bone with the arthrocentesis needle is unlikely to damage articular cartilage.[2] Attach an 18- to 22-gauge needle or intravenous catheter and needle set of suitable length to an appropriately sized syringe with or without a stopcock. Insert the needle at the desired anatomic point through the skin and subcutaneous tissue into the joint space. Use the largest needle that is practical to avoid obstructing the lumen with debris or clot. Large joints, such as the knee, can accommodate large effusions, so a 30- to 60-mL syringe is suggested because it may be difficult to change a syringe when the needle is within the joint cavity (Fig. 54.4). A three-way stopcock placed between the needle and the syringe is an option for draining large effusions (Fig. 54.5). If the syringe must be changed during the procedure, grasp the hub of the needle with a hemostat and hold it tightly while the syringe is removed. Use of a stopcock eliminates the need for any hemostat as the stopcock provides a large enough surface to be grasp directly with the fingers and held to allow removal of the syringe. Either a needle or a catheter-over-the-needle (intravenous catheter) may be used for the aspiration. If a needle is used, it should be inserted as deep as possible into the joint at the beginning of the procedure, even after aspiration of fluid is felt. This will compensate for displacement of the needle as joint space collapses when the fluid is withdrawn. If a catheter is used, the needle and catheter are introduced together and once fluid is aspirated the catheter is slid off the needle. Do not withdraw the needle from the catheter until the catheter is fully seated in the joint. Removal of the needle too early can leave the catheter outside the joint. Manipulation of the joint or catheter can now occur with little threat of tissue injury.

Aspiration of synovial fluid and easy injection and return of fluid indicate intraarticular placement of the needle tip. As a rule, try to remove as much fluid or blood as possible. If the fluid stops flowing, it indicates that the joint has been drained completely, the tip of the needle has become dislodged, or debris or clot is obstructing the needle. In this case, slightly advance or retract the tip of the needle, rotate the bevel, or lessen the force of aspiration. Never reintroduce a needle through a plastic catheter that has been left in the joint. Occasionally, reinjecting a small amount of fluid into the joint space confirms placement of the needle and may clear the needle. If fluid flows freely back into the joint and is easily reaspirated, one has probably removed all the fluid. If resistance is met, the needle has probably been jarred from the joint space and is lodged in soft tissue. In some instances, minor changes in position produced by flexion or extension of the joint may allow the fluid to flow more freely. Scraping or shearing the articular cartilage with the needle should be avoided. One should enter the joint in a straight line and avoid unnecessary side-to-side motion of the needle.

Send synovial fluid for studies as indicated by the clinical situation. Studies usually obtained include cell count with differential, crystal analysis, Gram staining, and bacterial culture and sensitivity analysis. Synovial protein, glucose, and lactate dehydrogenase determinations have been shown to be unreliable in distinguishing noninflammatory from inflammatory and infectious causes and are no longer recommended.[2,29–33] Less frequently obtained studies include rheumatoid factor analysis, lupus erythematosus cell preparation, viscosity analysis, mucin clot, fibrin clot, fungal and acid-fast stains, Lyme titer, fungal and tuberculous culture, and synovial fluid complement analysis. If the arthrocentesis is performed for the relief of hemarthrosis, the fluid need not be sent for analysis. One should be selective in ordering tests. If the volume of fluid collected is low, culture, Gram stain, and examination of the "wet preparation" under regular and polarizing microscopy have the highest priority. Prompt examination of specimens should be performed to avoid misdiagnosing borderline inflammatory fluids, missing crystals that dissolve with time, or misinterpreting the findings because of new artifactual crystals that appear over a prolonged time.

Complications

Significant complications are rare with arthrocentesis but include the following:

1. Infection. Skin bacteria may be introduced into the joint space during needle puncture. Nevertheless, infection

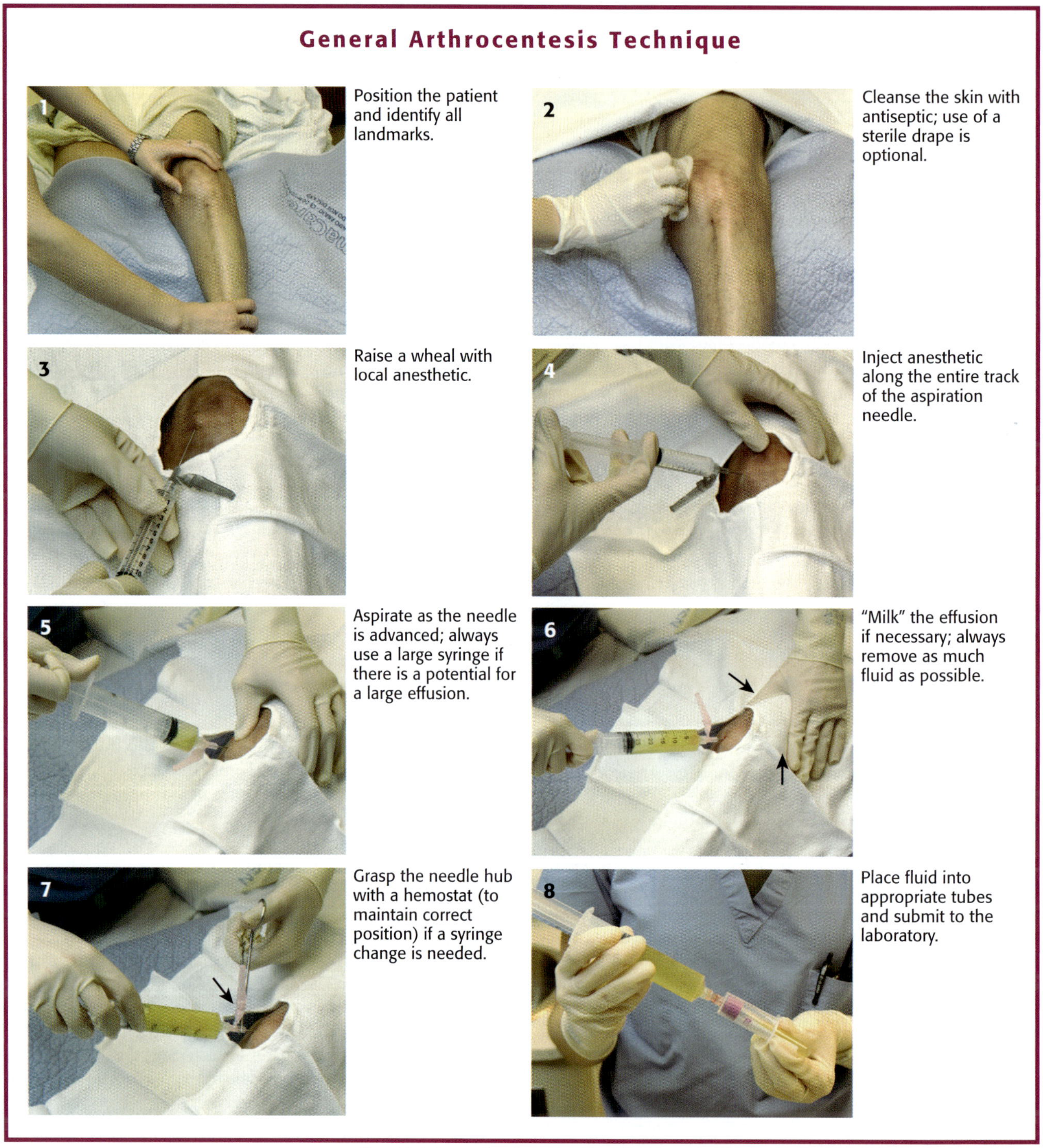

Fig. 54.4 General arthrocentesis technique.

occurs rarely because the bacteria are either quickly cleared or not viable. One can further limit this complication by maintaining rigorous sterile technique and avoiding insertion of the needle through obviously (or possibly) infected skin or subcutaneous tissue. Various studies report the incidence of infection after routine arthrocentesis to be in the range of 1 in 10,000.[10] However, in immunocompromised patients, particularly those with rheumatoid arthritis, the incidence is higher (1 in 2000 to 10,000 aspirations).[35,36] Joint aspiration in the presence of bacteremia was discussed previously. Acute pain, redness, and swelling 12 to 24 hours after steroid injection can mimic infection but is most likely an inflammatory reaction (steroid flare) to the steroid preparation (often methylprednisolone).

2. Bleeding. Bleeding with subsequent hemarthrosis is rarely a complication, except in patients with a bleeding diathesis. In those with a bleeding diathesis such as hemophilia, arthrocentesis should be delayed until clotting competence has been enhanced by infusing specific clotting factors. In general, spontaneous bleeding into a hemophiliac patient's joint is an indication for replacement of clotting factors.[19,22] Occasionally, a small quantity of blood may be aspirated along with synovial fluid. This happens most often when the joint is nearly emptied. A small amount of

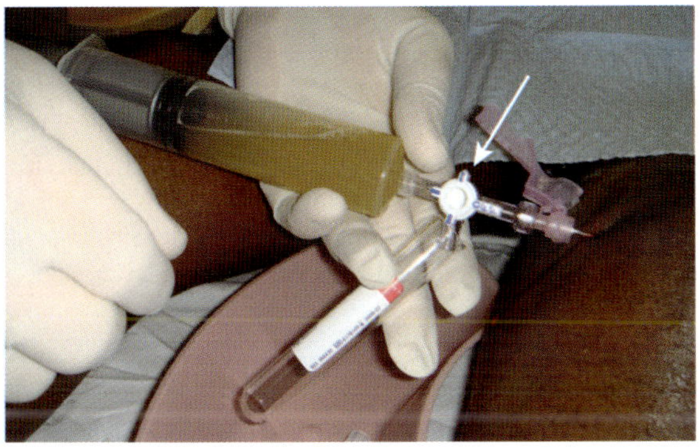

Fig. 54.5 Use of a stopcock will negate the need to change the syringe during arthrocentesis. Turn the stopcock *(arrow)* to collect and then expel fluid, or inject lidocaine or steroid without moving the needle.

blood-tinged fluid is generally the result of nicking a small synovial blood vessel and is usually inconsequential.

3. Arthrocentesis and joint injections in patients on anticoagulation have been shown to be safe. Studies have demonstrated no increase in bleeding risk in patients on DOACs, warfarin, or other anticoagulants.[3,5]
4. Allergic reaction. Hypersensitivity to the local anesthetic can usually be prevented by thorough history taking. Facial and torso flushing associated with corticosteroid injection may represent an idiosyncratic reaction to preservatives in the steroid preparation.[2] Fainting during the procedure is not uncommon and most often the result of vasovagal influences. To help prevent this, perform the procedure with the patient lying down whenever possible.
5. Corticosteroid-induced complications. See earlier section on "Intraarticular Corticosteroid Injections."

SPECIFIC ARTHROCENTESIS TECHNIQUES

Arthrocentesis has traditionally been performed as landmark technique and for most joints can still be performed successfully with this approach. This is especially true if a joint effusion is confirmed with an ultrasound evaluation prior to the procedure itself. For some joints such as the hip it is easier to do the needle advancement under direct ultrasound visualization. Arthrocentesis under real-time ultrasound direction can also be used if an attempt is unsuccessful utilizing the landmark technique. Ultrasound-directed aspirations are best performed by visualizing the joint and effusion and advancing the needle along the longitudinal axis of the probe. For small joints, application of traction is often very helpful in obtaining fluid. While applying continuous suction to the aspirating syringe, walk the needle over palpated bone until the joint is entered or fluid is obtained. However, it may be quite difficult to obtain fluid from small joints in the hand and foot. If only one drop of fluid is obtained from small joints, it is best to send it for culture.

First Carpometacarpal Joint (Fig. 54.6)

Landmarks. The radial aspect of the proximal end of the first metacarpal is the arthrocentesis landmark for this joint. Locate the abductor pollicis longus (APL) tendon by active extension of the tendon.

Position. Oppose the thumb against the little finger so that the proximal end of the first metacarpal is palpable. Apply

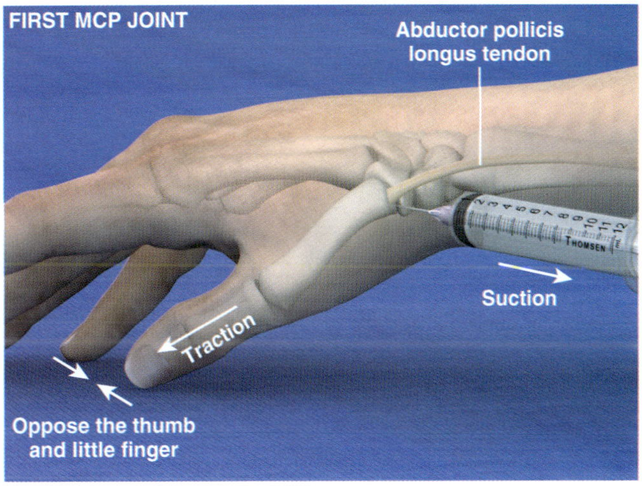

Fig. 54.6 Landmarks for arthrocentesis of the first carpometacarpal joint. All small joints pose a difficult aspiration. When aspirating small joints, apply continuous suction to the syringe, and walk the tip of the needle along the bones until the joint is entered or fluid is obtained. Apply longitudinal traction to facilitate entry into a small joint. *MCP,* Metacarpophalangeal.

traction to the thumb to widen the joint space between the first metacarpal and the greater multangular (trapezium) bone.

Needle Insertion. Insert a 22- to 23-gauge needle at a point proximal to the prominence at the base of the first metacarpal on the palmar side of the APL tendon.

Comments. Degenerative joint disease commonly affects this joint, making arthrocentesis difficult. The anatomic "snuffbox" (located more proximally and on the dorsal side of the APL tendon) should be avoided because it contains the radial artery and superficial radial nerve. A more dorsal approach may also be used.

Interphalangeal and Metacarpophalangeal Joints (Fig. 54.7)

Landmarks. The landmarks are located on the dorsal surface. For the metacarpophalangeal joints, palpate for the prominence at the proximal end of the proximal phalanx. For the interphalangeal joints, palpate for the prominence at the proximal end of the middle or distal phalanx. The extensor tendon runs down the midline.

Position. Flex the fingers to approximately 15 to 20 degrees and apply traction.

Needle Insertion. Insert a 22- to 25-gauge needle into the joint space dorsally, just medial or lateral to the central slip of the extensor tendon.

Comments. Synovitis causes these joints to bulge dorsally. Normally, it is unusual to obtain fluid in the absence of a significant pathologic condition.

Radiocarpal Joint (Wrist)

See Fig. 54.8 and Videos 54.1–54.5.

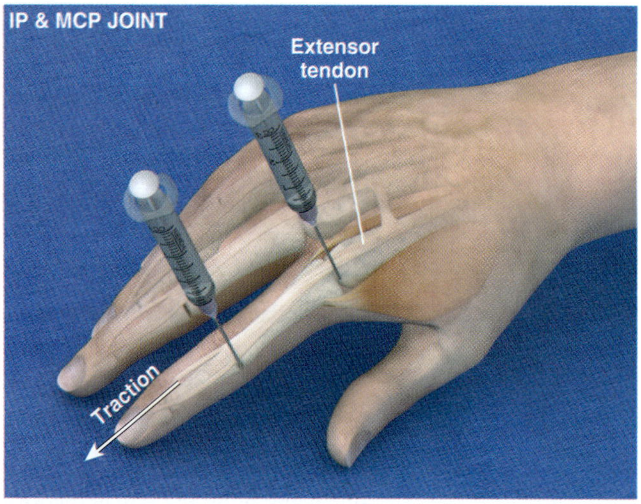

Fig. 54.7 Landmarks for arthrocentesis of the interphalangeal *(IP)* and metacarpophalangeal *(MCP)* joints.

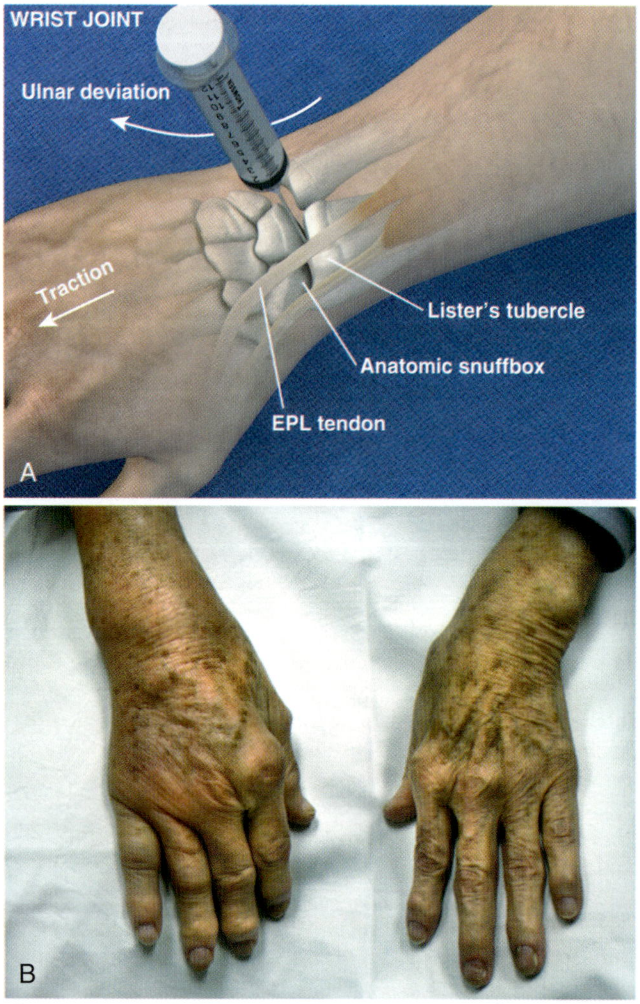

Fig. 54.8 (A) Landmarks for arthrocentesis of the radiocarpal (wrist) joint. This is a difficult joint to aspirate. (B) Acute joint effusion of the right wrist. *EPL*, Extensor pollicis longus.

Landmarks. The dorsal radial tubercle (Lister's tubercle) is an elevation found in the center of the dorsal aspect of the distal end of the radius. The extensor pollicis longus tendon runs in a groove on the radial side of the tubercle. The tendon can be palpated by active extension of the wrist and thumb.

Position. Position the wrist in approximately 20 to 30 degrees of flexion with accompanying ulnar deviation. Apply traction to the hand.

Needle Insertion. Insert a 22-gauge needle dorsally, just distal to the dorsal tubercle on the ulnar side of the extensor pollicis longus tendon. Avoid the anatomic snuffbox, located more radially, to prevent injury to the radial artery or superficial radial nerve.

Radiohumeral Joint (Elbow)

See Fig. 54.9; Videos 54.6 and 54.7.

Landmarks. The lateral epicondyle of the humerus and the head of the radius are the arthrocentesis landmarks for the radiohumeral joint. With the elbow extended, palpate the depression between the radial head and the lateral epicondyle of the humerus.

Position. With the palpating finger still touching the radial head, flex the elbow to 90 degrees. Pronate the forearm, and place the palm flat on a table.

Needle Insertion. Insert a 20-gauge needle from the lateral aspect, just distal to the lateral epicondyle and directed medially.

Comments. Elevation of the anterior fat pad or the presence of a posterior fat pad on a lateral soft tissue elbow radiograph signifies blood, pus, or fluid in the elbow joint (see Fig. 54.9B). Effusions in the elbow joint may bulge and be readily palpated (see Fig. 54.9C). Frequently, the effusion appears inferior to the lateral epicondyle. The bulge can then be aspirated from a posterior approach on the lateral side Fig. 54.9D. A medial approach is not recommended because the ulnar nerve and superior ulnar collateral artery may be damaged. Gout and septic arthritis commonly affect this joint. The most common cause of elbow hemarthrosis after trauma with no obvious fracture is a nondisplaced radial head fracture. A small hemarthrosis need not be aspirated, but removal of blood from a tense elbow joint will significantly hasten recovery and facilitate range of motion in patients with a radial head fracture.

Glenohumeral Joint (Shoulder), Anterior Approach (Fig. 54.10)

Landmarks. Anteriorly palpate the coracoid process medially and the proximal end of the humerus laterally.

Position. The patient should sit upright with the arm at the side and hand in the lap.

Needle Insertion. Insert a 20-gauge needle at a point inferior and lateral to the coracoid process and direct it posteriorly toward the glenoid rim.

Comments. Arthrocentesis of this joint is moderately difficult. Other approaches have been suggested but are less well accepted.

Knee Joint, Anteromedial Approach

See Fig. 54.11 and Videos 54.8–54.10.

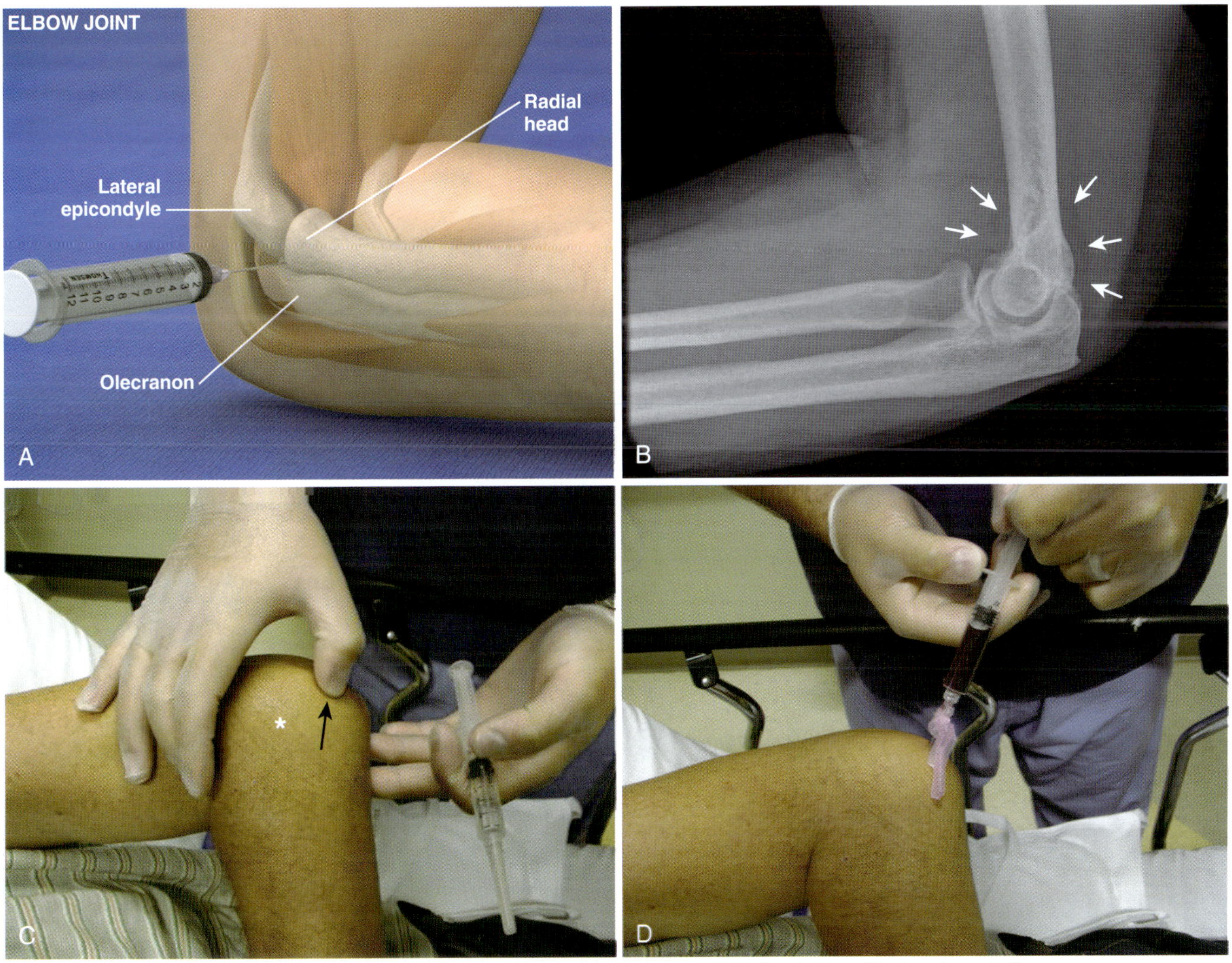

Fig. 54.9 (A) Landmarks for arthrocentesis of the radiohumeral (elbow) joint. (B) On a lateral elbow radiograph, displacement of the anterior fat pad *(arrows)* or the presence of a posterior fat pad *(arrows)* indicates blood, pus, or fluid in the joint. (C) An effusion in the elbow joint can usually be readily palpated. A palpating finger is placed over the lateral epicondyle *(asterisk)* and slid posteriorly and inferiorly toward the olecranon *(arrow)*. Usually, a depression is felt as the finger leaves the epicondyle, but a bulge is appreciated if a joint effusion is present. (D) Removal of only a few milliliters of blood will reduce pain and hasten recovery of range of motion. The most common pathology after trauma with a radiograph negative for fracture but positive for hemarthrosis is a nondisplaced radial head fracture.

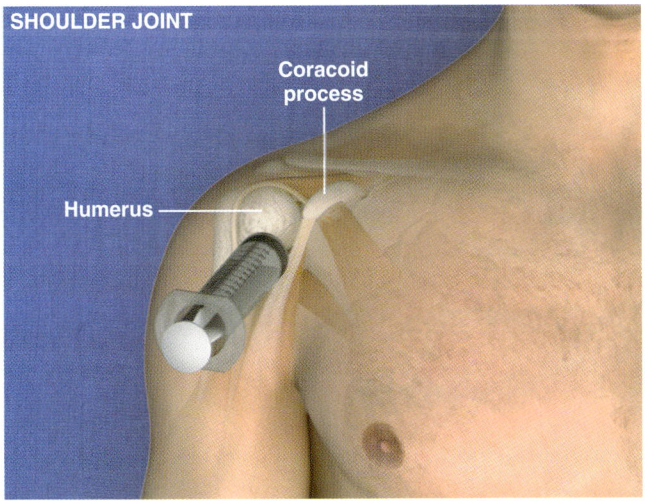

Fig. 54.10 Landmarks for arthrocentesis of the glenohumeral (shoulder) joint.

Landmarks. The medial surface of the patella at the middle or superior portion of the patella is the landmark for the knee joint.

Position. It is usually recommended that the knee be extended as far as possible. Alternatively, some practitioners prefer to flex the knee 15 to 20 degrees by placing a towel under the popliteal region to open the joint space up. Relaxation of the quadriceps muscle greatly facilitates needle placement. Keep the foot perpendicular to the floor.

Needle Insertion. Insert an 18-gauge needle or catheter and needle set at the midpoint or superior portion of the patella approximately 1 cm medial to the anteromedial patellar edge. On some patients palpation of the lateral aspect of the knee will reveal a more prominent protuberance of the joint space. In these patients the arthrocentesis needle should be directed from this location. Direct the needle between the posterior surface of the patella and the intercondylar femoral notch. The patella may be grasped with the hand and elevated to aid

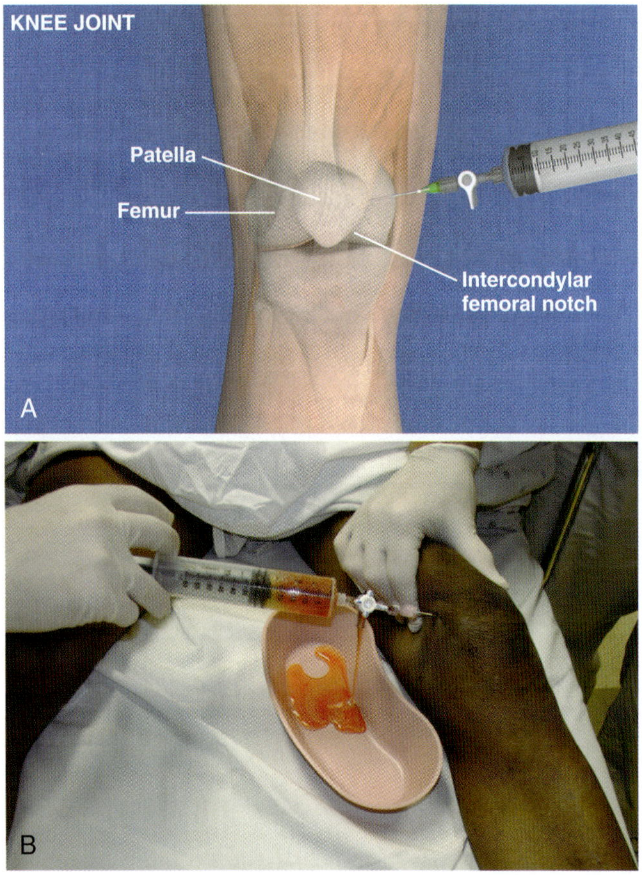

Fig. 54.11 (A) Landmarks for arthrocentesis of the knee joint. (B) Note the use of a stopcock on the syringe to allow complete drainage without repositioning the needle. Note that the syringe is held parallel to the table. Compression of the suprapatellar region by the operator or an assistant will facilitate complete aspiration. For the knee, a 60-mL syringe and an 18-gauge needle should be used to drain large effusions. Note that the red streaks of blood denote a traumatic tap rather than hemarthrosis. The blood streaks started after clear fluid had been withdrawn.

entry of the needle into the joint. Keeping the needle/syringe parallel to the bed limits internal injury.

Comments. If the patient is tense, contraction of the quadriceps will greatly hinder entering the joint. However, the knee is probably the easiest joint to enter, and removal of a tense hemarthrosis will relieve pain and facilitate examination for ligamentous injury. If fluid stops flowing, squeeze the soft tissue area of the suprapatellar region to "milk" the suprapatellar pouch of fluid. Alternatively, wrap the patient's thigh with a 6-inch elastic bandage from the groin to the suprapatellar area before beginning the procedure. The knee can easily accommodate 50 mL to 70 mL of fluid, so use a large syringe. Hold or secure the hub of the needle with a hemostat to remove the syringe without changing the position of the intraarticular needle. Alternatively, a stopcock on the needle will allow complete removal of fluid without changing the position of the needle (see Fig. 54.11B). The knee is a common site for septic arthritis (especially gonococcal) and various inflammatory or degenerative diseases.

Tibiotalar Joint (Ankle)

See Fig. 54.12; Videos 54.11 and 54.12.

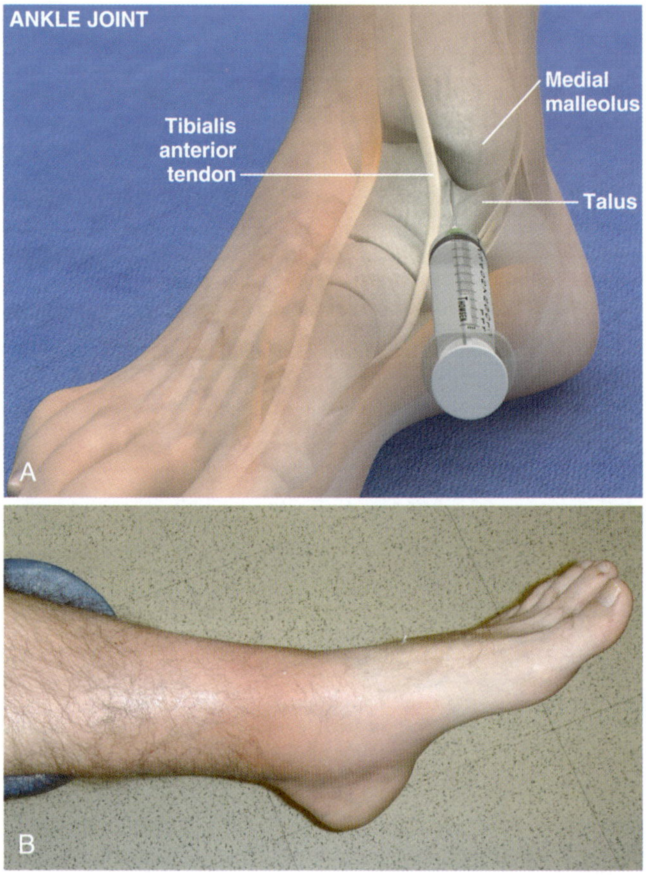

Fig. 54.12 (A) Landmarks for arthrocentesis of the tibiotalar joint. This is a difficult joint to aspirate. (B) Acute gout of the ankle is common but can mimic an infected joint, an uncommon condition. Arthrocentesis was unsuccessful, but a previous history of gout and the clinical features allowed empirical treatment of gout.

Landmarks. The medial malleolar sulcus is bordered medially by the medial malleolus and laterally by the anterior tibial tendon. The tendon can easily be identified with active dorsiflexion of the foot.

Position. With the patient lying supine, plantar-flex the foot.

Needle Insertion. Insert a 20- to 22-gauge needle at a point just medial to the anterior tibial tendon and directed into the hollow at the anterior edge of the medial malleolus. The needle must be inserted 2 cm to 3 cm to penetrate the joint space.

Comments. If the joint bulges medially, one may use an approach that is more medial than anterior and enter at a point just anterior to the medial malleolus. The needle may have to be advanced 2 cm to 4 cm with this approach.

Metatarsophalangeal and Interphalangeal Joints

See Fig. 54.13 and Videos 54.13–54.15.

Landmarks. For the first digit, landmarks are the distal metatarsal head and the proximal base of the first phalanx. For the other toes, the landmarks are the prominences at the proximal interphalangeal and distal interphalangeal joints. The extensor

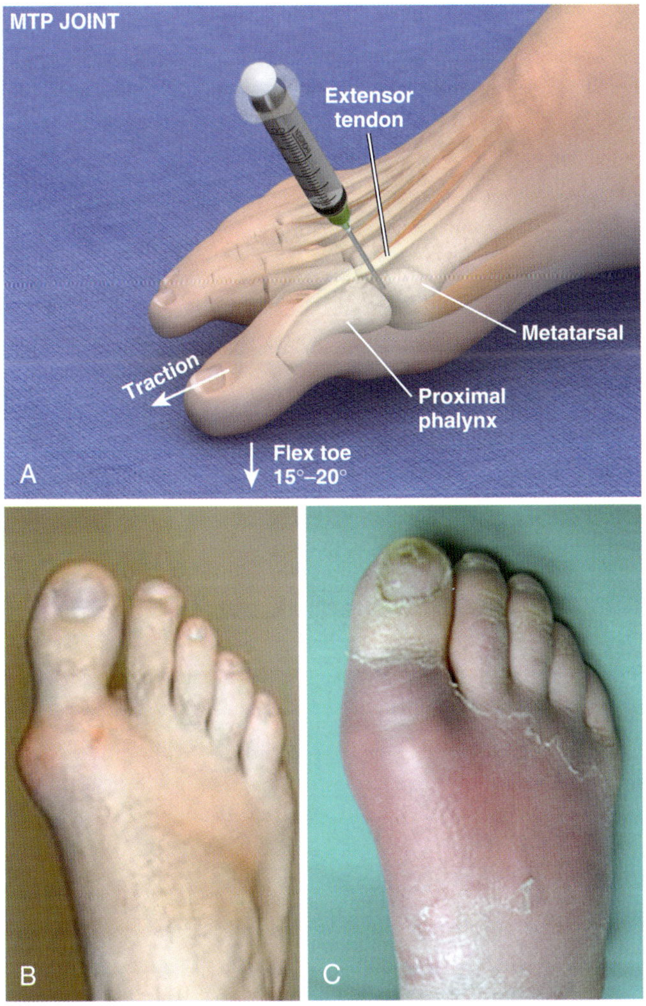

Fig. 54.13 (A) Landmarks for arthrocentesis of the first metatarsophalangeal *(MTP)* joint. This is a difficult joint to aspirate. (B) Acute gout can be mistaken for cellulitis, but this is classic podagra. Aspiration of small joints may be difficult. One can treat gout empirically with close follow-up to be certain that infection or coinfection is not present. (C) The red, warm, swollen, and painful condition of the dorsum of the foot is a common finding with gout but may suggest cellulitis. Clinical acumen may diagnose gout (e.g., woke up with sudden acute pain, diuretic use, previous gout, elevated uric acid level), but arthrocentesis is often helpful, especially if this is the first manifestation of gout.

tendon of the great toe can be located by active extension of the toe.

Position. With the patient supine, flex the toes 15 to 20 degrees. Then apply traction.

Needle Insertion. Insert a 22-gauge needle on the dorsal surface at a point just medial or lateral to the central slip of the extensor tendon.

SYNOVIAL FLUID INTERPRETATION

Synovial fluid examination is essential for the diagnosis of septic arthritis, gout, and pseudogout.[38–40] Inflammatory joint disease of previously unknown etiology can often be diagnosed precisely by synovial fluid analysis. Joint fluid is a dialysate of plasma that contains protein and hyaluronic acid. Normal fluid is clear enough to read newsprint through and will not clot. It is straw colored, flows freely, and has the consistency of machine oil. Normal fluid produces a good mucin clot and yields a positive "string sign" (see the next section). The uric acid level of joint fluid approaches that of serum, and the glucose concentration is normally at least 80% of that in serum. The clarity of the fluid reflects the leukocyte count. High leukocyte counts result in opacity, the degree of which generally correlates with the degree of elevated synovial fluid leukocytes. However, the degree of opacity cannot be used to reliably determine the synovial fluid leukocyte count and should not be used as a surrogate for laboratory cell count measurements.

String Sign

See Video 54.16. Viscosity correlates with the concentration of hyaluronate in synovial fluid. Any inflammation degrades hyaluronate, which characteristically results in low-viscosity synovial fluid. The string sign is a simple test for assessing viscosity. The practitioner measures the length of the "string" formed by a falling drop of synovial fluid extruded from a syringe or stretched between the thumb and the index finger of a gloved hand. Normal joint fluid produces a string 5 cm to 10 cm long. (Fig. 54.14) If viscosity is reduced, as with inflammatory conditions, synovial fluid forms a shorter string or falls in drops.

Cell Count

A leukocytosis consisting predominantly of neutrophils is usually seen with inflammatory arthritides; a WBC count greater than 50,000/mm^3 (i.e., >50,000/μL) is highly suggestive of a septic joint. Shmerling and colleagues[38] found a WBC count of greater than 2000/mm^3 to be 84% sensitive and 84% specific for all inflammatory arthritides. Of their septic arthritis patients, 37% had a synovial WBC count lower than 50,000/mm^3. However, 89% of their patients with a synovial WBC count greater than 50,000/mm^3 had a septic joint.[38]

Glucose and Protein

Current literature suggests that synovial protein and glucose are highly inaccurate markers of inflammation.[28d] In one study of 100 consecutive patients undergoing diagnostic arthrocentesis, the sensitivity of synovial protein and glucose was found to be 0.52 and 0.20, respectively.[36]

Serology

Though available, most serologic tests are not likely to be useful in the emergency setting. Polymerase chain reaction (PCR) is an effective means of identifying septic arthritis, even in the setting of a negative fluid culture or when antibiotics have been administered previously. PCR can also help isolate slowly growing microorganisms. Gas-liquid chromatography, a rapid and sensitive method for detection of short-chain fatty acids, may complement the currently available methods used to diagnose septic arthritis.

Counterimmunoelectrophoresis and latex agglutination are also useful and available in some centers on an emergency basis. Other immunologic markers such as complement, rheumatoid factor, and antinuclear antibodies have

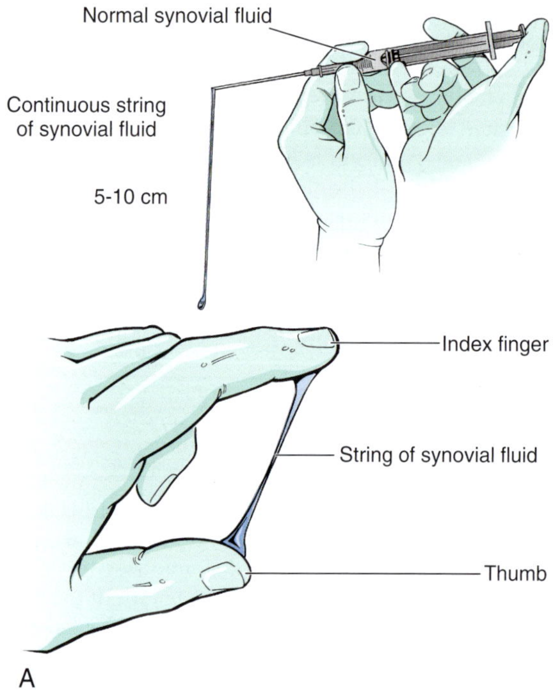

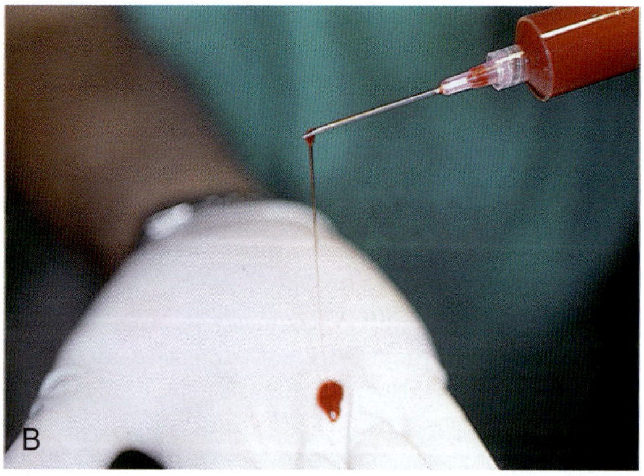

Fig. 54.14 (A) Ability of normal synovial fluid to form a long tenacious string. Inflammatory fluid will not produce this finding. (B) Bloody joint fluid from recent trauma forms a normal string sign.

little diagnostic value in the acute setting but may be useful to the clinician providing follow-up care when compared with serum levels.

Fluid Processing

Proper collection of joint fluid is essential for examination and testing. Tests for viscosity, serology, and chemistries are done on fluid collected in a red-topped (clot) tube, whereas cytology samples are collected in tubes with an anticoagulant (purple top). One should always transfer the fluid for crystal examination into a tube with liquid heparin (green top) because undissolved heparin crystals from powdered anticoagulant tubes can be seen on microscopy. Early transfer of synovial fluid to this green-topped tube is essential to prevent clotting. Culture requirements for transport and processing should be accessed before the procedure to ensure appropriate processing or plating of specimens. Some institutions now prefer that synovial fluid be hand delivered to the lab in a simple sterile container and separated into the appropriate vessels in the lab itself.

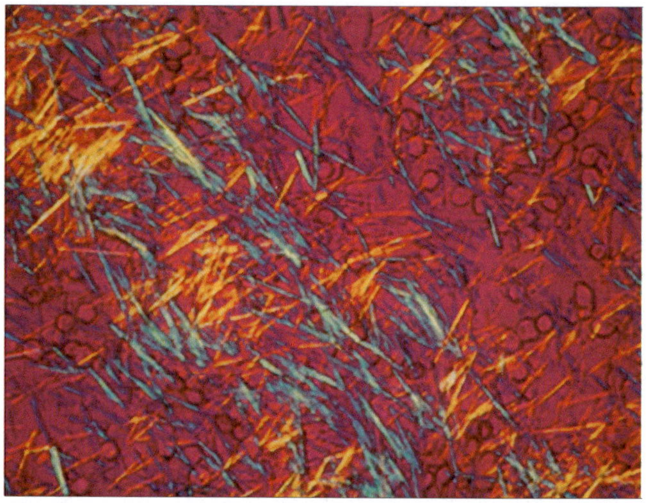

Fig. 54.15 Monosodium urate crystals under a polarizing light microscope. The crystals are positively birefringent and usually needle shaped. (From Hochberg MC, Silman AJ, Smolen JS, eds. *Rheumatology*. 5th ed. Elsevier; 2011.)

Polarizing Microscope

No synovial fluid analysis is complete until the fluid has been examined for crystals under a polarizing light microscope. The polarizing microscope used for crystal identification differs from the ordinary light microscope in that it contains two identical polarizing prisms or filters. One filter, called the *polarizer*, is positioned below the condenser. The other filter is called the *analyzer* and is inserted at some point above the objective. Examination for crystals is performed by most hospital laboratories.

The polarizer allows passage of light in only one specific orientation. The analyzer acts as a crossed filter by removing all light in the light path unless the material being examined rotates the beam from the polarizer into the plane of the analyzer. The compensator functions by imparting color of a certain wavelength (red at approximately 550 nm). Birefringent materials change the wavelength to blue or yellow, depending on the direction (negative or positive) of refringence.

Microscopic Analysis

When examining crystals under polarized microscopy, the technician orients crystals on a stage according to two axes, referred to as x and z. If the long axis of the crystals is blue when parallel to the z-axis and yellow when perpendicular to it, it is calcium pyrophosphate and termed *positively birefringent*. If the long axis of the crystal is yellow when parallel to the z-axis and blue when perpendicular to it, it is monosodium urate and termed *negatively birefringent*. Urate crystals are 2 to 10 μm and usually needle shaped (Fig. 54.15). Calcium pyrophosphate crystals range from 10 μm down to tiny crystals that have to be examined with the oil objective; they appear as rods, rhomboids, plates, or needle-like forms and are weakly birefringent (Figs. 54.16 and 54.17). Cholesterol crystals are sometimes seen and are large, very bright square or rectangular plates with broken corners.[40]

Items found in synovial fluid that can be confused with sodium urate or calcium pyrophosphate crystals include collagen fibrils, cartilage fragments, cholesterol crystals, metallic fragments from prosthetic arthroplasty, and corticosteroid esters.[40] One may also identify fat globules (see Fig. 54.17).

Note that rare cases of uric acid spherulites in gouty synovia have been reported.[9] The spherulites are birefringent and do not take up fat stains.

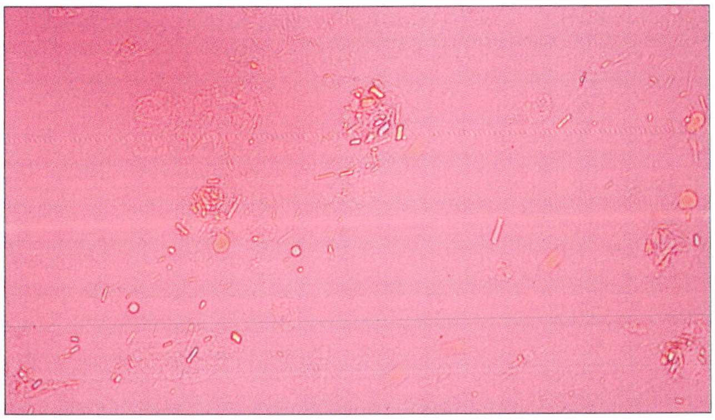

Fig. 54.16 Calcium pyrophosphate dihydrate crystals under a polarizing light microscope. These crystals are negatively birefringent and rhomboid shaped. (From Hochberg MC, Silman AJ, Smolen JS, eds. *Rheumatology*. 5th ed. Elsevier; 2011.)

Table 54.2 summarizes synovial fluid features for the joint diseases commonly encountered and studies commonly performed in the ED.

JOINT ARTHROGRAPHY

Background

See Video 54.17. Wounds near joints raise concern regarding joint penetration. Treatment and interventions may be altered significantly if a joint space has been traumatically violated. Plain radiographs may demonstrate air in the joint, which clinches the diagnosis, but in questionable cases the diagnostic approach includes injection arthrograms. Historically, these were performed by injecting methylene blue into the joint in question and assessing leakage from the wound. However, the dye can interfere with arthroscopic evaluation and produce an inflammatory reaction, so saline arthrography (SA) is now preferred. SA, or a "saline load test," was first described in 1975 but became more popular in the 1990s.[33,34]

In recent years, CT imaging has gained traction in investigating violation of the joint capsule. The presence of

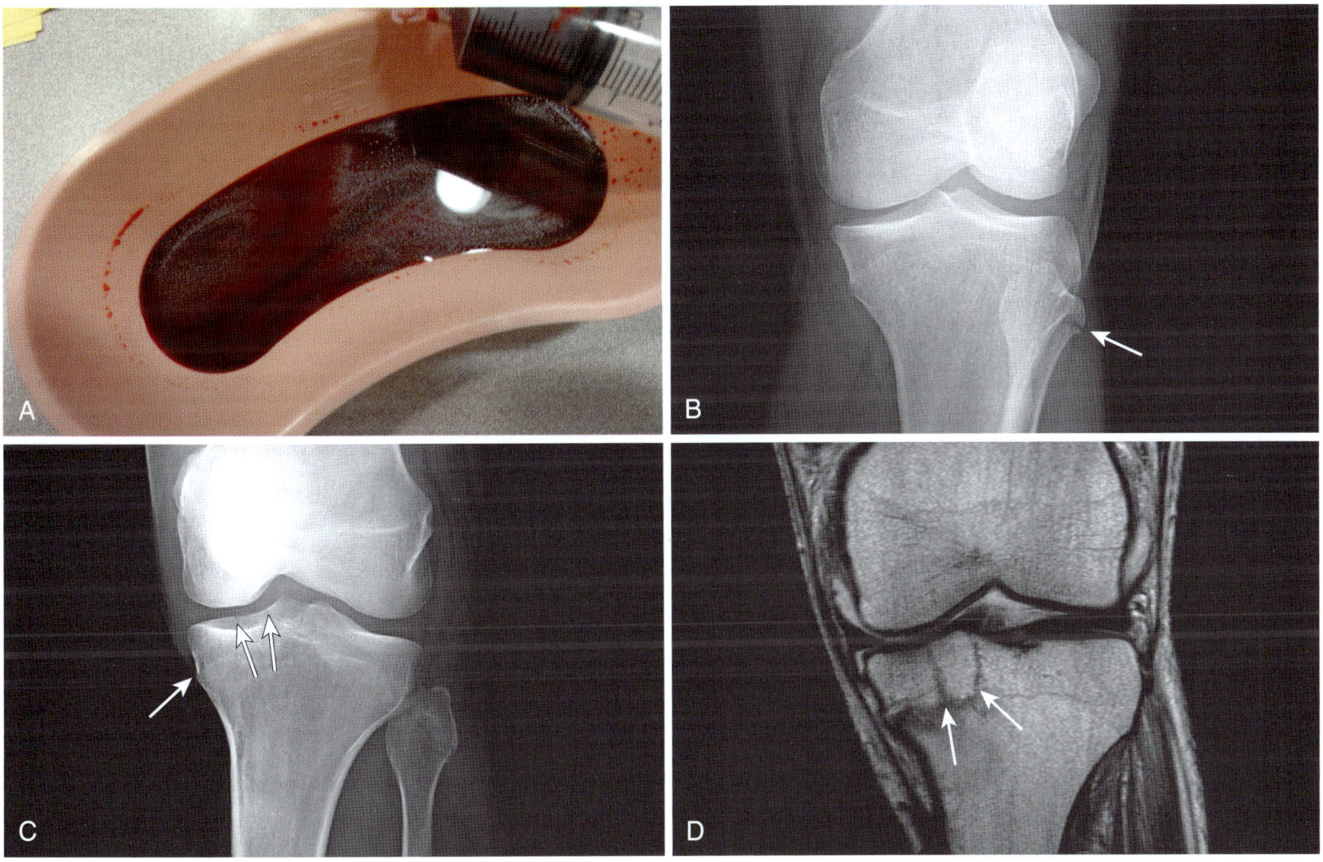

Fig. 54.17 (A) Blood aspirated from a traumatized joint is placed in an emesis basin and put under a bright light to search for lipohemarthrosis, which is clinical evidence of an intraarticular fracture. Note the characteristic greasy sheen of floating fat. Do not throw away this blood before assessing for lipohemarthrosis. (B) A fibular head fracture *(arrow)* was initially thought to be responsible for a large knee hemarthrosis, but anatomically it is extraarticular. A tibial plateau fracture is not appreciated on this radiograph. Such injuries are often occult. (C) On this view one might appreciate the radiolucent lines suggestive of a lateral tibial plateau fracture *(arrows)*, but such subtle findings are easily missed, as was the case with this patient. Therapeutic arthrocentesis was performed to alleviate pain, and an obvious lipohemarthrosis was noted. (D) Magnetic resonance imaging demonstrates an obvious lateral tibial plateau fracture *(arrows)*, which was searched for only after lipohemarthrosis was noted. Computed tomography could also be used.

TABLE 54.2 Characteristics of Synovial Fluid

	APPEARANCE	VISCOSITY	CELLS PER mm³	PMN (%)	CRYSTALS
Normal	Transparent	High	<180	<10	Negative
Osteoarthritis	Transparent	High	200–2000	<10	Occasional calcium pyrophosphate and hydroxyapatite crystals
Rheumatoid arthritis	Translucent	Low	2000–50,000	Variable	Negative
Psoriatic arthritis	Translucent	Low	2000–50,000	Variable	Negative
Reactive arthritis	Translucent	Low	2000–50,000	Variable	Negative
Spondyloarthropathy	Translucent	Low	2000–50,000	Variable	Negative
Gout	Translucent to cloudy	Low	200 to >50,000	>90	Needle-shaped, positive birefringent monosodium urate monohydrate crystals
Pseudogout	Translucent to cloudy	Low	200–50,000	>90	Rhomboid, negative birefringent calcium pyrophosphate crystals
Bacterial arthritis	Cloudy	Variable	2000 to >50,000	>90	Negative
PVNS	Hemorrhagic or brown	Low			Negative
Hemarthrosis	Hemorrhagic	Low			Negative

PMN, Polymorphic nuclear cell; *PVNS*, pigmented villonodular synovitis.

intraarticular air on CT suggests that a nearby wound has violated the joint space and thus warrants orthopedic evaluation. Multiple studies have found CT imaging has both high specificity and sensitivity and offers an alternative approach when concerned that nearby wounds may penetrate a joint space.[33,34]

Indications and Contraindications

SA should be performed in patients with penetrating injuries near a joint in which violation of the joint itself is unclear based on examination and imaging (Fig. 54.18). Smaller joints such as those in the hand are inspected visually. However, for larger joints, SA is the preferred test.

Contraindications to performing SA are essentially the same as for performing arthrocentesis. When indicated, underlying fracture of the joint should first be ruled out. An obvious open fracture would preclude the need to perform SA.

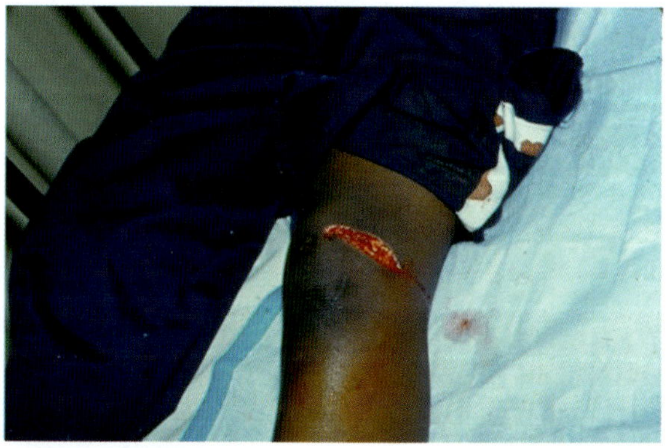

Fig. 54.18 This periarticular laceration raises the question of knee joint penetration. A plain radiograph may demonstrate air in the joint space, but a saline arthrogram may also be used. Methylene blue alone is not generally required and it can cause an inflammatory reaction and obscure arthroscopy. A small amount of methylene blue may be added to color the saline.

Equipment and Procedure

Aseptic technique is essential, but the equipment and procedure are essentially the same as for performing arthrocentesis, with minor differences. First, a source of sterile saline is required (e.g., a small bag of intravenous fluid). Second, larger joints require more saline infusion, and this is most easily performed if a stopcock is used to allow refill of the syringe (Fig. 54.19).

Because saline is not as viscous as joint fluid, a 20-gauge needle is sufficient. Once the joint space has been reliably entered, a variable amount of saline to "load" that joint is slowly injected. The amount of saline injected varies with the size of the joint. In general, inject a sufficient volume to visibly distend the joint or create resistance to injection, which may cause the patient discomfort. The sensitivity of the test in detecting small traumatic joint injuries is proportional to the volume injected. Specifically, for knee injuries, injecting 50 mL of saline was 46% sensitive and injecting 100 mL, 75% sensitive; to achieve 95% sensitivity required an average of 194 mL of saline. The following is the recommended volume of injection per joint:

- Knee: 100 to 200 mL
- Elbow: 20 to 30 mL
- Ankle: 20 to 30 mL
- Wrist: 5 mL
- Shoulder: 40 to 60 mL

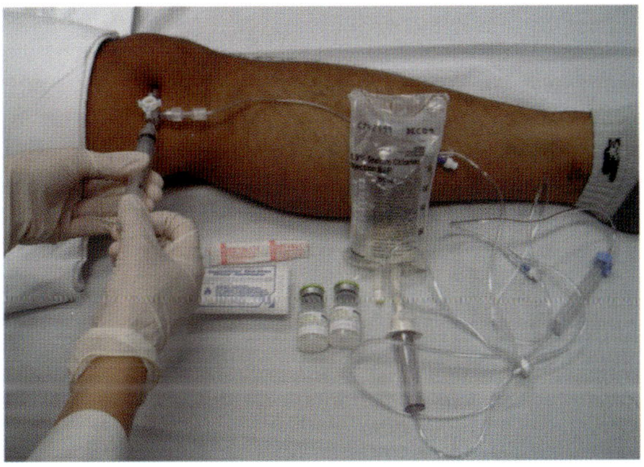

Fig. 54.19 Saline arthrography. Using a stopcock and an 18-gauge needle, enter the joint in a manner identical to that for arthrocentesis. Note that a bag of intravenous saline (or additional vials of saline) introduced into the syringe may be required to provide enough saline to distend the joint properly. Unless the joint is markedly distended, a false-negative test may result. When completed, drain the injected saline via the original needle. A positive test is egress of saline into the original wound or slow loss of saline from the joint. A small amount of methylene blue may be added to the saline.

Once the injection is complete, do not remove the needle but close the stopcock to avoid backflow. Examine the joint for evidence of leakage of fluid from the wound. This is performed in a static position but, if negative, also with some gentle passive movement of the joint. Visible leakage of fluid into the laceration confirms the diagnosis of joint space violation. A negative test is defined as absence of evidence of leakage after an appropriate amount of saline has been injected. A slow loss of fluid may indicate a small insult to the joint, and saline can be left in the joint for a few minutes to observe for this. After completion, the fluid should be evacuated for patient comfort. This is generally performed by leaving the original needle in place with a closed stopcock attached, which is then used to aspirate the saline in the joint.

Complications

Complications associated with performing SA are essentially the same as those for performing arthrocentesis. In addition, some temporary patient discomfort because of joint distention should be assumed.

CONCLUSION

Small traumatic joint penetration can be difficult to diagnose clinically. SA can help confirm the diagnosis. To be a sensitive test, it must be performed with an adequate amount of saline infusion to truly "load" the joint. If the test is positive, orthopedic consultation is indicated.

REFERENCES ARE AVAILABLE AT Elsevier eBooks+

CHAPTER 55

Compartment Syndrome Evaluation

Ross Allen Simcoe

INTRODUCTION

Open fractures, dislocations, and exposed joints are true orthopedic emergencies that must be managed aggressively to prevent morbidity and mortality. Even when managed appropriately, these injuries may be further complicated by compartment syndrome, a condition of increased pressure within a limited space that results in compromised tissue perfusion, leading to tissue ischemia, and ultimately dysfunction of the neural and muscular structures contained within that space.[1] Compartment syndrome is most often associated with significant trauma, particularly long-bone fractures (e.g., tibia, radius, ulna). However, it may also occur following less severe trauma that does not cause fractures, such as crush injuries, severe thermal burns, penetrating trauma, injury to vascular structures in the extremities and, in some cases, even minor injuries. Patients on anticoagulants, those with a bleeding diathesis, and those who continue to use an injured limb are at increased risk. Nontraumatic causes of compartment syndrome occur less often and include ischemia-reperfusion injury, excessive muscular exertion, thrombosis, bleeding disorders and coagulopathies, vascular disease, nephrotic syndrome, certain animal envenomations and bites, extravasation of intravenous (IV) fluids, injection of recreational drugs, and prolonged external pressure (e.g., from a tight circumferential bandage or cast, or from lying on an extremity for a prolonged period secondary to drug or alcohol intoxication).

Numerous drugs and toxins have been reported to cause rhabdomyolysis, possibly because of a direct effect or secondary to agitation and exertion, with the *theoretical potential* for the development of compartment syndrome (Fig. 55.1). This list is exhaustive but includes heroin, various hydrocarbons, cocaine, amphetamines, antidepressants, antipsychotics, salicylates, propoxyphene, nonsteroidal antiinflammatory drugs, succinylcholine, human immunodeficiency virus (HIV) medications, antimetabolite and cancer drugs, antimalarials, diphenhydramine, baclofen, ecstasy, ethanol, anticoagulants and thrombolytics, strychnine, statins, and phenothiazines.[2]

Causes of compartment syndrome are categorized into those that decrease compartment volume capacity, those that increase the contents of a compartment, and those that create externally applied pressure (Box 55.1).[1]

Subtleties in the early signs and symptoms of compartment syndrome or other clinical priorities render some cases simply impossible to recognize and treat early enough to thwart the ultimate disability. In fact, approximately 10% of cases of acute compartment syndrome secondary to fractures and 20% of non–fracture-associated cases will have muscle necrosis requiring debridement at the time of surgery.[3] These statistics indicate that even with diligent clinical care, it is often difficult to identify all cases before injury to muscles occurs. This is particularly true in uncooperative, unconscious, or

Compartment Syndrome Evaluation Using Stryker Device

Indications

Suspected compartment syndrome with clinical findings that are equivocal or difficult to interpret:

- Unresponsive patients
- Uncooperative patients
- Children
- Patients with multiple or distracting injuries
- Patients with peripheral nerve deficits attributable to other causes (fracture-associated nerve injury, diabetic peripheral neuropathy)

Contraindications

Absolute

None

Relative

Coagulation disorders

Overlying infection, cellulitis, or burns

Complications

Pain from needle insertion, fluid injection, or bleeding

Inaccurate readings due to poor technique, improper needle position, injected fluid or anesthetic, or external compression

Injury to underlying tissue, nerves, or blood vessels

Local or systemic infection

Equipment

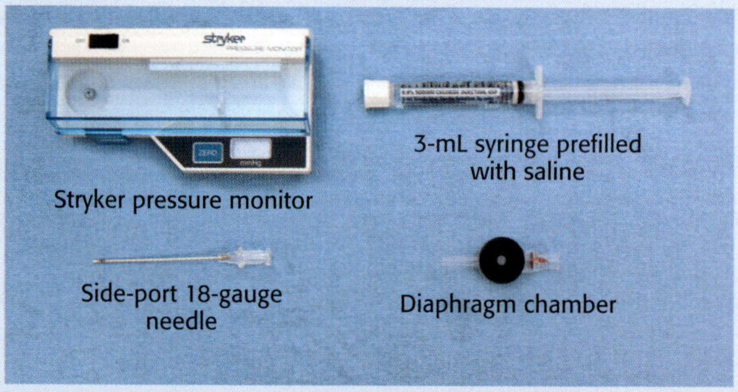

Review Box 55.1 Compartment syndrome evaluation using Stryker Device.

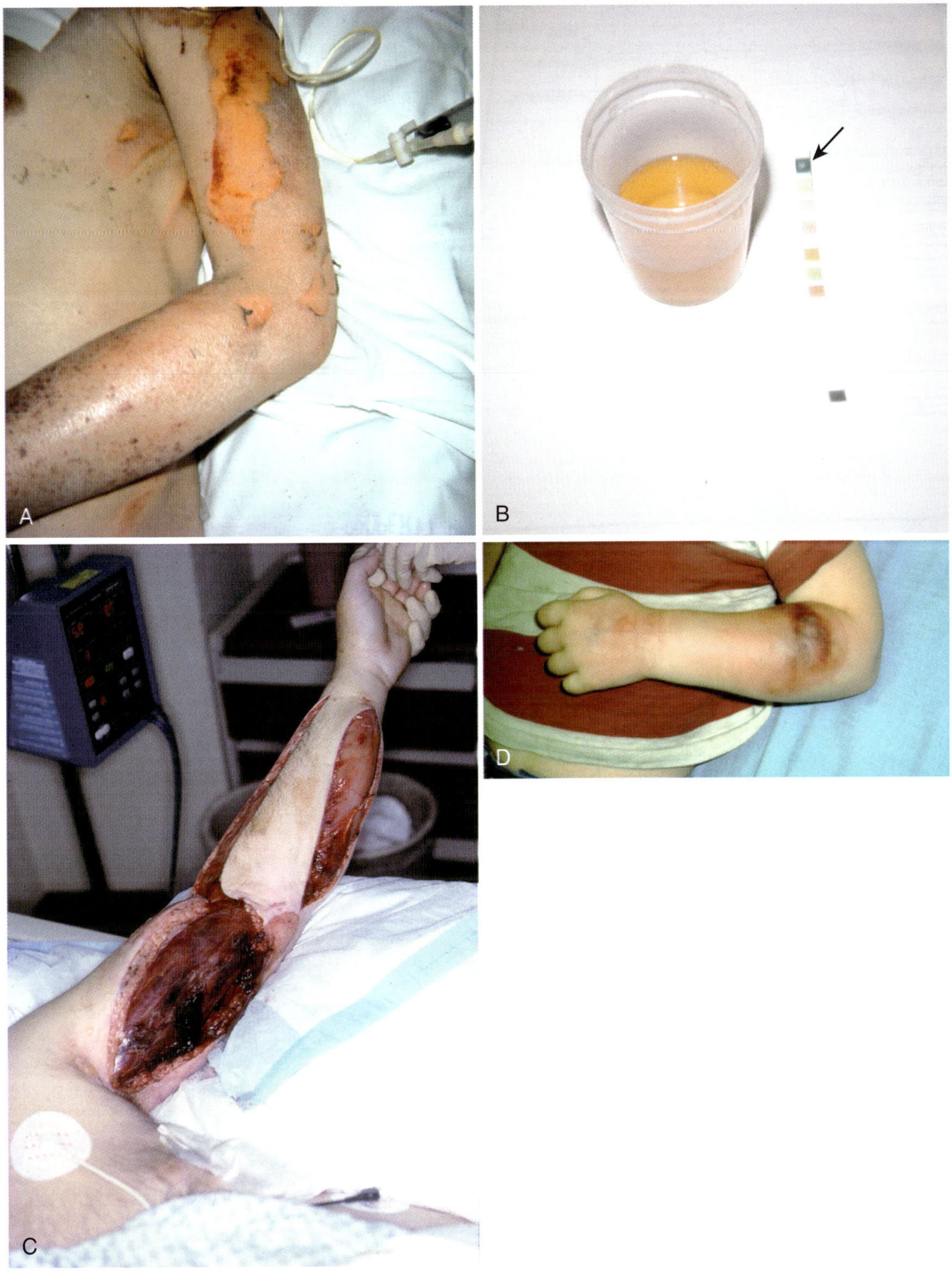

Fig. 55.1 The diagnosis of compartment syndrome is not always straightforward. (A) This patient was initially seen while in a coma from a heroin overdose and had been lying on his arm for a number of hours. He was hypotensive, in renal failure, comatose, and on a ventilator. The entire arm was swollen and rhabdomyolysis was correctly suspected. (B) Clear urine, a strongly positive dipstick for blood *(arrow)*, and no red blood cells by microscopy equate to myoglobinuria. Because of the coma, he was unable to voice any complaint of pain. (C) When he awakened 20 hours later, the pain was severe, and compartment pressures indicated the need for fasciotomy. Heroin can cause rhabdomyolysis, and hypotension/reperfusion and certainly prolonged pressure on the muscles may have exacerbated the condition. (D) The classic wringer washer injury predisposes to compartment syndrome, but industrial rollers are now usually the culprit.

BOX 55.1 Causes of Compartment Syndrome

DECREASED COMPARTMENTAL VOLUME

Closure of fascial defects
Application of excessive traction to fractured limbs
Compressive devices (casts, splints, circumferential dressings)

INCREASED COMPARTMENTAL CONTENTS

Bleeding
Major vascular injury
Coagulation disorders
- Bleeding disorder
- Anticoagulation therapy
- Thrombolytic therapy
- After placement of an arterial line

INCREASED CAPILLARY FILTRATION

Reperfusion after ischemia
- Arterial bypass grafting
- Embolectomy
- Ergotamine ingestion
- Cardiac catheterization
- Lying on the limb

Trauma
- Fracture
- Contusion

Intensive use of muscles
- Exercise or severe exertion
- Seizures
- Eclampsia
- Tetany

Burns
- Thermal
- Electric

Intraarterial drug injection
Cold
Orthopedic surgery
- Tibial osteotomy
- Hauser's procedure
- Reduction and internal fixation of fractures

Snakebite

INCREASED CAPILLARY PRESSURE

Intensive use of muscles
Venous obstruction
- Phlegmasia cerulea dolens
- Ill-fitting leg brace
- Venous ligation

Diminished serum osmolarity, nephrotic syndrome

OTHER CAUSES OF INCREASED COMPARTMENTAL CONTENTS

Infiltrated infusion
Pressure transfusion
Leaky dialysis cannula
Muscle hypertrophy
Popliteal cyst
Carbon monoxide poisoning

EXTERNALLY APPLIED PRESSURE

Tight casts, dressings, or air splints
Lying on the limb
Pneumatic antishock garment
Congenital bands

Modified from Matsen FA. Compartmental Syndromes. *Grune & Stratton; 1980.*

critically injured patients who are unable to report symptoms. Unfortunately, the vagaries of the clinical scenario that result in failure to recognize the early signs and symptoms of compartment syndrome may have severe and irreversible limb- or life-threatening consequences.

Although compartment syndrome is essentially a clinical diagnosis, objective measurement of compartment tissue pressure may assist in confirming the diagnosis and determining if operative management is required. This chapter discusses the indications, complications, and interpretation of compartment pressure monitoring, as well as the equipment and techniques required to measure and monitor compartment pressure. This chapter will not cover the metabolic abnormalities that can accompany compartment syndrome or their treatment (Review Box 55.1).

BACKGROUND

Though recognized as a clinical syndrome in the mid-19th century, the pathophysiology of ischemia in extremities was not fully described until more than a century later. Postischemic myoneural dysfunction and its associated contractures were first described in the 1870s by the German surgeon Richard von Volkmann, who recognized the effects of increased pressure causing vascular compromise of the limb.[4]

Over the past 40 years or so, various needles and equipment have been developed to measure compartment pressure (Fig. 55.2).[5–11] The *wick catheter*, originally developed to measure subcutaneous and brain tissue pressure, was modified during the mid-1970s to provide continuous compartment pressure measurements. This catheter is rarely used today because of the fear of catheter breakdown leading to errors in measurement and retained foreign bodies. The *slit catheter* was introduced in 1980.[10,11] As its name implies, this catheter has slits at its distal end that prevent clogging. The proximal end of the catheter is connected to a transducer and infusion system, which permits continuous pressure monitoring. Both the wick and slit catheters have been shown to offer similar accuracy and reproducibility as long as patency of the catheter is ensured.[11–13]

The C2Dx STIC Intracompartmental Compartment Pressure Monitoring System (Schoolcraft), formerly made by Stryker, is the most commonly used commercially available device to measure compartment pressure in the emergency department (ED) (see Review Box 55.1). This device uses a fluid-filled pressure measurement catheter, a pressure monitor, and a fluid infusion mechanism that maintains catheter patency and ensures accurate measurement. In contrast to earlier devices in which relatively large volumes of fluid were injected into the compartment to measure pressure, the

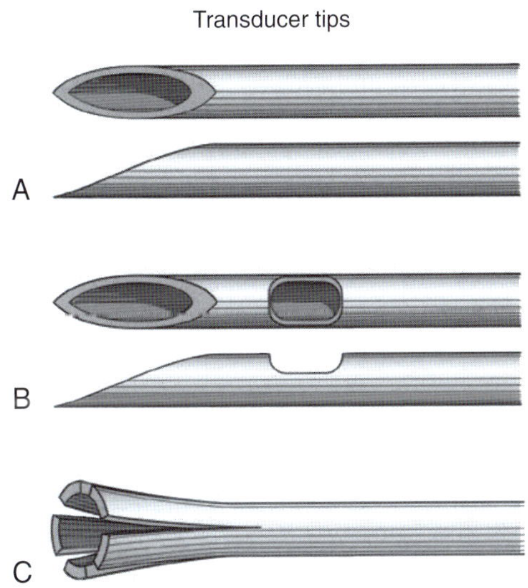

Fig. 55.2 (A) An 18-gauge straight needle. (B) An 18-gauge side-port needle. (C) A slit catheter. (From Boody AR, Wongworawat MD. Accuracy in the measurement of compartment pressures: a comparison of three commonly used devices. *J Bone Joint Surg Am.* 2005;87:2415.)

C2Dx system uses a minimal amount of saline (<0.3 mL). This helps ensure accurate measurements (Videos 55.1–55.3) while reducing the chance of further increases in compartment pressure. The C2Dx system also has the ability to record a single measurement or provide continuous compartment pressure recordings when required. Many clinicians may not have access to the C2Dx system. In these cases, Compass Compartment Pressure Monitoring Kits made by Centurion can be used instead and are easier to set up. Lastly, if neither device is available a standard arterial line pressure monitor can be used and connected to the intracompartmental catheter or needle to monitor pressures (Video 55.4). Arterial line pressure monitoring systems have widespread availability and have shown excellent measured pressures and actual pressures.[13,14]

Noninfusion systems offer a distinct advantage over conventional fluid-filled systems in that they do not produce hydrostatic pressure artifacts or require the injection of fluid for long-term or continuous measurements. Fiberoptic systems have been evaluated in the past and more recently a novel microelectromechanical sensor that is deployed within the compartment and tethered to an external monitor has shown promise in a limited case series.[15,16] For patients who have been placed in a cast, there is research being conducted on skin-cast surface pressure monitors that can monitor pressures noninvasively and without removing the cast.[17] Others have attempted to predict the onset of compartment syndrome by measuring compartment pH as a marker of compromised circulation and decreased tissue perfusion.[18] A rise in lactic acid from ischemic tissue lowers the pH of the compartment and has promise as an early predictor of compartment syndrome.

In recent years, noninvasive, less painful methods of measuring compartment pressure have been studied in patients with both acute and chronic exertional compartment syndromes. Investigations using magnetic resonance imaging (MRI), single-photon emission computed tomography (SPECT), myotonometry, electromyography, ultrasound, near-infrared spectroscopy, microwave tomography, and magnetic resonance spectroscopy have provided encouraging results in the evaluation of compartment syndrome.[19–37] In addition, externally applied devices that measure muscle tissue "hardness" are under investigation as an economic alternative to these modalities, although support for their use has been mixed.[38–40] There has been a significant amount of work in attempting to find alternative methods to diagnose acute compartment syndrome with both noninvasive and invasive technologies. Despite promising results from some studies, there has been no compelling evidence to replace needle-driven modalities, and intracompartmental pressure monitoring remains the gold standard.[11]

The remainder of this chapter describes the most commonly used devices and techniques for measuring compartment pressures in the acute setting. Each method provides rapid measurements with reasonable accuracy. The method chosen will depend on the availability of the supplies and equipment necessary for a particular procedure and the experience of the operator.

PATHOPHYSIOLOGY

Several theories have been proposed to account for the tissue ischemia associated with compartment syndrome. They include the "arteriovenous (AV) gradient" theory, which suggests that reduced AV pressure-perfusion gradients prevent adequate blood supply[42]; the "critical closure" theory, in which blood flow is arrested well before the AV perfusion gradient declines to zero[43,44]; and the "venous occlusion" theory,[45] which states that externally applied pressure, thrombotic events, and reperfusion contribute to the increased compartment pressure and, ultimately, tissue ischemia. Although the exact mechanism has not been agreed on, inherent in each of these theories is a decrease in blood flow to levels below those required to meet the metabolic demands of the tissue. Hence, the final common pathway is cellular hypoxia and muscle necrosis.

Adequate blood flow to tissues is a function of AV gradients across capillary beds. Once blood flow falls below a critical level, delivery of oxygen to these structures is impaired and aerobic cellular metabolism is no longer possible. Anaerobic metabolism then ensues until energy stores become depleted. Muscles then become ischemic, and a reduction in venous and lymphatic drainage creates increased pressure within this confined space. It is important to note that ischemia and necrosis of the musculature can occur despite an arterial pressure high enough to produce pulses, therefore merely assessing distal pulses is insufficient.[46]

A drop in blood pressure, an increase in compartment pressure, or a combination of the two can reduce AV gradients and lead to insufficient blood flow. Hypotension can occur in a variety of settings, including hypovolemia, acute blood loss, cardiac disease states (e.g., ischemia), and sepsis. An increase in the contents of a compartment, a decrease in its volume capacity, and external constriction of a compartment can all lead to increases in compartment pressure. Thus the relationship between intracompartmental pressure and the circulatory status of the extremity is an important factor in the development of compartment syndrome.[47]

At rest, normal adult compartment pressures are typically below 10 mm Hg. However, deviations of 2 to 6 mm Hg have been reported.[1,8–10,12] Data suggest that normal compartment pressures in the lower extremity at rest are higher in children.[48] The *perfusion pressure* of a compartment is defined as the difference between diastolic blood pressure and intracompartmental pressure.[49] A model using legs of volunteers has shown that a progression of neuromuscular deficits occurs when the perfusion pressure drops below 35 to 40 mm Hg.[50] Below this level, tissue perfusion is interrupted. Studies of neuromuscular tissue ischemia have demonstrated that inflammatory necrosis can occur at intracompartmental pressures between 40 and 60 mm Hg.[51,52]

Whitesides and colleagues demonstrated that when tissue pressure within a closed compartment rises to within 10 to 30 mm Hg of the patient's diastolic blood pressure, inadequate perfusion ensues and results in relative ischemia of the involved limb.[6] Heppenstall and associates further clarified this relationship by demonstrating that the difference (ΔP) between mean arterial pressure (MAP) and the measured compartment pressure is directly related to blood flow to the tissue.[53] They noted that as compartment pressure approaches MAP, ΔP decreases. Once ΔP falls below 30 mm Hg, tissue ischemia becomes more likely. In normal musculature, a ΔP of less than 30 mm Hg results in loss of normal aerobic cellular metabolism.[53] In traumatized muscle, a ΔP of less than 40 mm Hg is associated with abnormal cellular function, thus highlighting the importance of maintaining adequate systemic blood pressure in the setting of neuromuscular injury.[53]

For years, conventional wisdom maintained that immediate reperfusion of traumatized tissue would provide improved motor and neurologic function after injury. Research suggests that muscle tissue may remain viable even after prolonged periods of ischemia and that a substantial proportion of the injury is generated during reperfusion.[54,55] Tissue acidosis, intracellular and extracellular edema, free radical–mediated injury, loss of adenine nucleotide precursors, and interruption of mitochondrial oxidative phosphorylation by increased intracellular calcium have been implicated in the development of reperfusion-associated compartment syndrome.[54–59] Even in the absence of local trauma, ischemia followed by reperfusion has been shown to increase compartment pressure in canine models of hypovolemic shock.[60]

Evidence also suggests that elevated compartment pressure itself (in addition to causing ischemia) plays a role in the cellular deterioration seen with compartment syndrome.[61] In a study by Heppenstall and associates,[61] muscle ischemia caused by placement of a tourniquet was compared with an experimentally derived high-pressure compartment syndrome. The authors found no difference in the degree to which phosphocreatine levels fell between groups. However, levels of adenosine triphosphate (ATP) diminished rapidly in the compartment syndrome group in comparison to the tourniquet group. Moreover, phosphocreatine levels, ATP, and tissue pH normalized within 15 minutes of releasing the tourniquet. In the group with compartment syndrome, these levels remained low even after fasciotomy. These results suggest that elevated tissue pressure plays a synergistic role with ischemia in cellular deterioration.

CLINICAL FEATURES

Any compartment limited by fascial planes is potentially at risk for compartment syndrome. However, because of their propensity for injury and the presence of several low-volume compartments, the lower extremities are most commonly affected. In the leg, the anterior compartment is involved most often,[62] whereas the posterior compartment is most often associated with a delayed diagnosis. The hands, feet, forearms, upper part of the arms, thighs, thorax, abdomen, gluteal musculature, and back are other locations where compartment syndrome is known to occur.[1]

Risk factors for the development of compartment syndrome include recent trauma to an extremity (including acupuncture, venipuncture, IV infusions, or IV drug use), vascular injury, bleeding within a compartment, a restrictive cast or splint, a crush or compression injury, a prolonged lithotomy position, prolonged external pressure on an extremity, placement of a tourniquet during an operative procedure, and circumferential burns.[63–67]

Long-bone fractures account for approximately 75% of traumatic compartment syndromes, and the absence of a fracture in a traumatized extremity is a factor in delayed diagnosis. The tibia is most often involved, followed by bones of the forearm. Supracondylar fractures in children are at risk for compartment syndrome. Comminuted fractures increase the risk. Closed fractures are of greatest concern, but open fractures do not necessarily decompress elevated compartment pressures. Treatment of fractures, by both open and closed reduction, can increase compartment pressures. Compartment pressures may peak *immediately after reduction*. In addition, some evidence suggests that compartment syndrome may occur in the setting of chronic exertion and muscle overuse.[5,68,69] Although the exact etiology remains elusive, studies have demonstrated elevated lactate and water levels in the tibialis anterior muscle after exercise with a reduction in these levels after fasciotomy.[70,71] Increases in muscle mass (related to a rise in blood volume during exertion) and hypertrophy of muscle and fascia with chronic use and exertion have also been reported.[72–76]

The signs and symptoms of acute compartment syndrome generally appear in a stepwise fashion, with rapid progression over a few hours. This underscores the need for serial examinations, particularly in those with equivocal or subtle findings. The classic findings associated with arterial insufficiency, the "five P's" (pain, pallor, pulselessness, paresthesias, paralysis), are often described as signs of acute compartment syndrome, but these are seldom all seen together and do not need to be present to suspect the diagnosis. When this constellation of signs and symptoms are present, it is generally late in the course of the disease when tissue death and permanent dysfunction are likely.

Early signs of compartment syndrome include a burning sensation over the involved compartment, nonspecific sensory deficits, or poorly localized deep muscular pain. Common features include pain that seems out of proportion to the apparent injury and clinical examination and pain that intensifies when the musculature is passively stretched. Pallor, a pulse deficit with respect to the opposite limb, paresthesias, paresis, or paralysis are variably seen and lack diagnostic sensitivity. Neurologic complaints such as weakness and paresthesias can be confusing because peripheral nerve injury may also result from the inciting trauma. In addition, these findings are not discernable in young children[77,78] and patients with altered mental status. When present, sensory deficits typically precede motor deficits and manifest distal to the involved compartment. Paralysis is always a late finding.

The period between the injury and the onset of symptoms can be as short as 2 hours and as long as 6 days.[79] The peak interval appears to be 15 to 30 hours. Frequently, the first symptom described by patients is pain greater than expected

TABLE 55.1 Compartment Syndromes and Associated Physical Signs

COMPARTMENT	SENSORY LOSS	MUSCLES WEAKENED	PAINFUL PASSIVE MOTION	LOCATION OF TENSENESS
Foot	Digital nerves	Foot intrinsics	Toe flexion, extension	Dorsal or plantar surface of the foot
Lumbar	—	Erector spinae	Lumbar flexion	Paraspinous
Forearm				
Dorsal	—	Digital extensors	Digital flexion	Dorsal surface of the forearm
Volar	Ulnar, median nerves	Digital flexors	Digital extension	Volar surface of the forearm
Hand				
Intraosseous	—	Intraosseous	Abduction/adduction (metacarpophalangeal joints)	Dorsum of the hand between the metacarpals
Leg				
Anterior	Deep peroneal nerve	Toe extensors Tibialis anterior	Toe flexion	Anterior aspect of the leg
Superficial posterior	—	Soleus and gastrocnemius	Foot dorsiflexion	Calf
Deep posterior	Posterior tibial nerve	Toe flexors Tibialis posterior	Toe extension	Distal medial part of the leg between the Achilles tendon and tibia
Gluteal	(Rarely sciatic)	Gluteals, piriformis, or tensor fasciae latae	Hip flexion	Buttock
Upper Part of Arm				
Flexor	Ulnar and median nerves	Biceps and distal flexors	Elbow extension	Anterior aspect of the upper part of the arm
Extensor	Radial nerves	Triceps and forearm extensors	Elbow flexion	Posterior aspect of the upper part of the arm

given the clinical scenario. Although pain out of proportion to the visible injury may raise the question of drug-seeking behavior, a focused evaluation for the possibility of limb-threatening disorders must precede this diagnosis of exclusion.

Physical examination may reveal a tense compartment with a firm, "woody" feel, muscles that are weak, and hypoesthesia in the distribution of the involved nerves. Sensory deficits, including loss of two-point discrimination and decreased vibratory sensation, may be present.[80–82] The presence or absence of a palpable arterial pulse is not an accurate indicator of relative tissue pressure or the risk for compartment syndrome. Pulses may be present in a severely compromised extremity.[83] Table 55.1 lists the signs and symptoms of compartment syndrome specific to each compartment.

DIAGNOSIS

Even experienced clinicians may find it difficult to diagnose a compartment syndrome, and no specific standard of care exists with regard to a time interval from injury to definitive treatment. In an unconscious patient or in those with other life-threatening conditions that mandate other priorities, the clinical scenario simply does not allow a diagnosis to be made in a timely fashion. In cases without trauma or in patients who are unable to voice pain or cooperate with an examination, compartment syndrome is often not considered and the diagnosis is delayed. Regional nerve blocks or epidural anesthesia may also obscure the signs and symptoms of increased compartment pressure and cause further delays in diagnosis.

The difficulty in diagnosing acute compartment syndrome was highlighted in a report by Vaillancourt and coworkers.[84] In a retrospective review of 76 patients who underwent fasciotomy at major university trauma centers or teaching hospitals, the interval from initial patient assessment to diagnosis of compartment syndrome was up to 8 hours. A delay in diagnosis was most common in nontraumatic cases. The interval from the precipitating event to definitive surgery was up to 35 hours, thus reflecting the difficulty in recognizing the presence of a compartment syndrome and instituting definitive therapy in clinical practice. Such statistics describe actual care, which may be less than ideal when compared with theoretical benchmarks.

Notwithstanding the difficulties just described, the diagnosis of compartment syndrome is primarily a clinical one that may be supplemented by direct measurement of compartment pressure. In a study evaluating the utility of clinical findings in making the diagnosis of compartment syndrome, Ulmer noted that the sensitivity and positive predictive value

TABLE 55.2 Clinical Findings in Patients With Compartment Syndrome, Arterial Occlusion, and Neuropraxia

	COMPARTMENTAL SYNDROME	ARTERIAL OCCLUSION	NEUROPRAXIA
Pressure increased in the compartment	+	–	–
Pain with stretch	+	+	–
Paresthesia or anesthesia	+	+	+
Paresis or paralysis	+	+	+
Pulses intact	+	–	+

From Mubarak S, Carroll N. Volkmann's contracture in children: etiology and prevention. *J Bone Joint Surg Br*. 1979;61:290.

of clinical findings are low, whereas the specificity and negative predictive value of these findings are high.[85] Nonetheless, the study found that although the sensitivity of an individual clinical finding may be low, the probability of compartment syndrome rises considerably when more than one clinical hallmark is present.[85] Other studies have suggested that the absence of clinical evidence is more useful in excluding compartment syndrome than its presence is in confirming the diagnosis.[86–88] All things considered, compartment syndrome remains largely a clinical diagnosis, and a high index of suspicion is paramount. The decision to perform fasciotomy must be made with great care. Delaying or failing to perform fasciotomy can result in devastating and irreversible complications. Fasciotomy itself is not a benign procedure and exposes the patient to significant risk of morbidity from wound infections, repeat surgeries, and prolonged hospitalizations.[89]

The differential diagnosis of compartment syndrome is extensive and includes primary vascular, nerve, and muscle injuries that produce similar findings. Acute arterial occlusion, cellulitis, osteomyelitis, neuropraxia, reflex sympathetic dystrophy, synovitis, tenosynovitis, stress fractures, envenomations, necrotizing fasciitis, deep vein thrombosis, and thrombophlebitis are additional diseases that should be considered. Differentiating compartment syndrome from these and other orthopedic disorders requires a detailed history and thorough physical examination, often supplemented by measurement of compartment pressures (Table 55.2).

ANCILLARY STUDIES

In general, laboratory and radiographic studies are not helpful in confirming the diagnosis of compartment syndrome. However, they might be useful in identifying other diagnoses, associated conditions, and complications. Box 55.2 lists useful studies for patients in whom compartment syndrome is suspected. A 2013 retrospective study of 97 hospitalized patients by Valdez and colleagues attempted to determine if a threshold serum creatinine kinase (CK) level was associated with the development of compartment syndrome.[90] They found that a CK level greater than 4000 U/L was associated with compartment syndrome and when serial measurements were obtained, the combination of a maximum CK greater than 4000 U/L, a maximal chloride level greater than 104 mg/dL, and a minimal blood urea nitrogen (BUN) level less than 10 mg/dL had a 100% association with compartment syndrome. A later study applied the Valdez model to 930 ED patients and found the same laboratory threshold values for CK, chloride, and BUN had a specificity of 99.2%, but a sensitivity of only 2.9%.[91]

BOX 55.2 Ancillary Studies That May Be Helpful in Identifying Other Diagnoses, Associated Conditions, and Complications in Patients Suspected of Having Compartment Syndrome

LABORATORY STUDIES

- Complete metabolic profile (including electrolytes and renal function testing)
- Complete blood count with differential
- Serum and urine myoglobin
- Creatine phosphokinase
- Urinalysis to evaluate for concurrent rhabdomyolysis
- Coagulation studies

IMAGING STUDIES

- Radiography of the affected limb to evaluate for a fracture or foreign body
- Ultrasonography to rule out deep vein thrombosis or Doppler ultrasonography to evaluate blood flow to the extremity

INVASIVE COMPARTMENT PRESSURE MONITORING

Indications and Contraindications

The earliest objective manifestation of acute compartment syndrome is an elevation in the tissue pressure of one or more compartments. However, signs and symptoms do not generally develop until tissue pressure has reached a critical level (see earlier section "Pathophysiology"). In some patients the diagnosis of compartment syndrome is clinically obvious, and one can proceed directly to fasciotomy. When the clinical findings are equivocal or difficult to interpret, measurement of tissue pressure may help guide treatment. However, it must be remembered that the interpretation of such measurements always requires clinical judgment.

There are several groups of patients in whom clinical findings are difficult to obtain or interpret and who would benefit from measurement of compartment pressure. These groups include unresponsive patients, uncooperative patients, children, patients with multiple or distracting injuries, those with peripheral nerve deficits attributable to other causes (e.g., fracture-associated nerve injury, diabetic peripheral neuropathy), and those whose clinical findings are equivocal.

There are no absolute contraindications to measurement or continuous monitoring of compartment pressure. Caution should be taken when performing these procedures on patients with platelet dysfunction or other coagulation disorders. If possible, avoid inserting needles through overlying areas of infection, cellulitis, or burns.

Patient Preparation and Positioning

Explain the procedure to the patient or surrogate. Written informed consent is not a universal standard but may be an institutional requirement. Positioning the patient and extremity for measurement of the compartment pressure depends on the extremity and the compartment being studied, coexisting injuries, and the clinical status of the patient. In general, patients should be in the supine position.[92–94] The exceptions to supine positioning are discussed in subsequent sections related to the specific compartment of interest.

For most patients, measurement of compartment pressure is a painful procedure that requires adequate local anesthesia (see Chapter 29), systemic analgesia, or procedural sedation (see Chapter 33). Some patients may require more than one method of pain control. Anesthetize the skin with a small amount of local anesthetic while avoiding the underlying muscle and fascia. Inadvertent injection into the underlying structures may falsely elevate compartment pressure. Patient movement (as a result of inadequate analgesia or improper positioning) may also falsely elevate compartment pressure, particularly if the patient requires limb restraint. To minimize the discomfort of multiple attempts at localizing the correct compartment, some have advocated the use of ultrasound guidance to improve the accuracy of needle insertion.[95] However, there is currently no consensus regarding the use of ultrasound guidance in this setting.[96,97] In general, place the extremity being studied at the level of the heart and in a position that permits insertion of the needle perpendicular to the compartment being measured. This may require that an assistant hold the extremity above the stretcher. Remove any obstruction to needle entry and all objects that may constrict or exert pressure on the compartment.

Perform compartment pressure measurements with sterile technique, including standard skin preparation and draping at the planned insertion site (see Chapter 34). Avoid placing the needle through areas of overlying burn or infection. If a circumferential cast is present, bivalve the cast or, if necessary, create a window overlying the desired area with a cast saw.

Equipment

Needles commonly used for measurement of compartment pressure include a simple 18-gauge needle, an 18-gauge spinal needle (for deep compartments), and a side-port needle (C2Dx, Schoolcraft). The side-port needle may be more accurate than simple 18-gauge needles.[47] Nevertheless, simple 18-gauge needles are more readily available and more commonly used. The wick catheter and slit catheter described previously generally require specialized, cumbersome equipment not often available in most EDs and are therefore not described.

In an effort to reduce the pain associated with insertion of larger-gauge needles, Mars and colleagues evaluated the accuracy and reliability of measuring compartment pressures with smaller-gauge needles.[98] The authors compared compartment pressures measured with 18- to 25-gauge needles and found that smaller-gauged needles provided results similar to or better than the more traditional 18-gauge needles did. Furthermore, the addition of a side port did not improve accuracy.[98] Unfortunately, no additional studies have been done to corroborate these findings. As a result, most clinicians continue to use 18-gauge needles.

Pressure Measurement Systems

C2Dx Intracompartmental Pressure Measurement

See Fig. 55.3 and Videos 55.1–55.4.

Equipment

- C2Dx Quick Pressure Monitor System
- C2Dx handheld pressure monitoring unit (included)
- One side-port 18-gauge needle (included)
- One diaphragm chamber (included)
- One syringe prefilled with 3 mL of saline (included)

Setup and Procedure

1. Position the patient. Prepare and anesthetize the needle insertion site according to the guidelines described earlier.
2. Open the Quick Pressure Monitor Set and remove the contents while maintaining sterile conditions.
3. Place the needle firmly on the tapered chamber stem.
4. Remove the cap on the prefilled syringe and screw the syringe onto the remaining chamber stem. Take care to avoid contaminating the fluid pathway.
5. Open the monitor cover and inspect the device for damage or contamination. Place the chamber into the device well (black surface down) and push gently until it seats.
6. Snap the cover closed, but DO NOT FORCE IT. The latch must have "snapped" in place.
7. Hold the needle at approximately 45 degrees from the horizontal plane and slowly force fluid through the disposable system to purge it of air. *Caution:* DO NOT allow saline to roll down the needle into the transducer well.
8. Turn on the unit; it should read between 0 and 9 mm Hg.
9. Hold the device at the intended angle of insertion and press the "ZERO" button to calibrate it. After a few seconds, the display should read "00." Failure to calibrate the device while in the intended angle of insertion may result in inaccurate readings. *Note:* The display must read "00" before continuing. If it does not, follow the troubleshooting instructions provided by the manufacturer before proceeding.
10. Now insert the needle into the compartment being measured (see section "Needle Placement Techniques for Specific Compartments"). Slowly inject no more than 0.3 mL of saline into the compartment to equilibrate with the interstitial fluid.
11. Wait for the display to reach equilibrium and record the resulting pressure.
12. *For additional measurements*, turn the unit off and repeat steps 8 through 11. Recalibrate the unit to zero before each measurement.
13. For continuous monitoring with an indwelling slit catheter, refer to the instructions accompanying the system.

Arterial Line Monitoring System

Equipment

- One 18-gauge simple or spinal needle, use side-port needle if available

Compartment Pressure Evaluation: Stryker Method

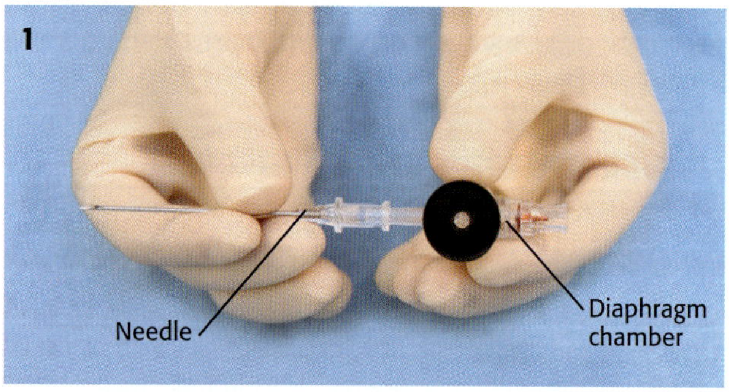

Place the 18-gauge needle with a side port on the tapered stem of the diaphragm chamber.

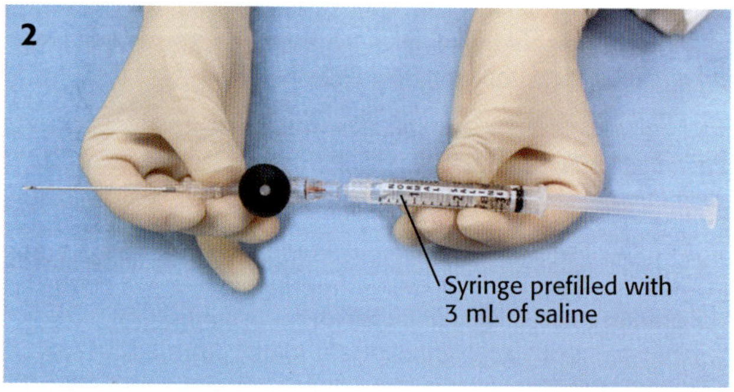

Screw syringe prefilled with 3 mL of saline onto the back of the diaphragm chamber.

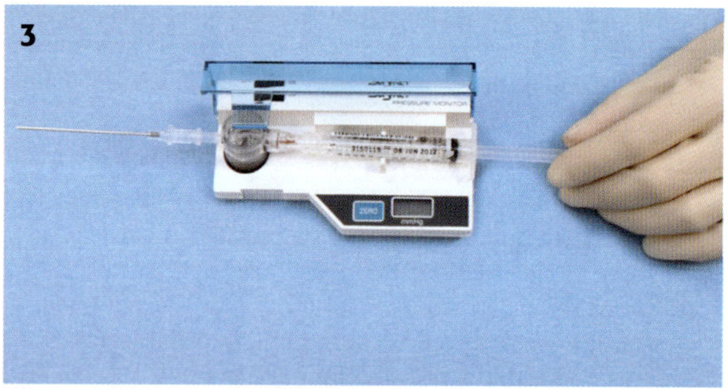

Place the diaphragm chamber assembly into the pressure monitor, black side down. Gently push the chamber until it is well seated in the device.

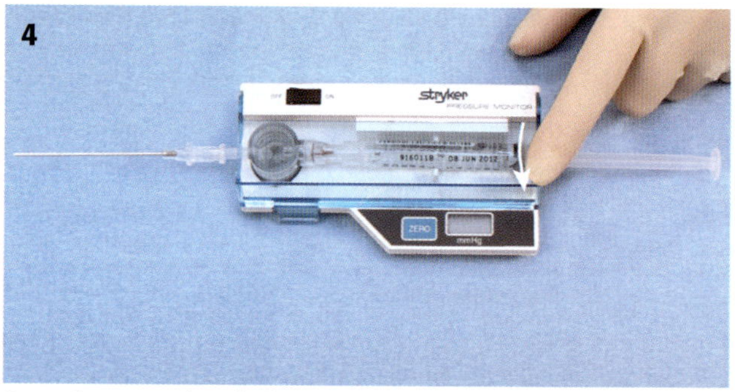

Snap the cover closed; *do not force it!* Listen for the latch to snap into place.

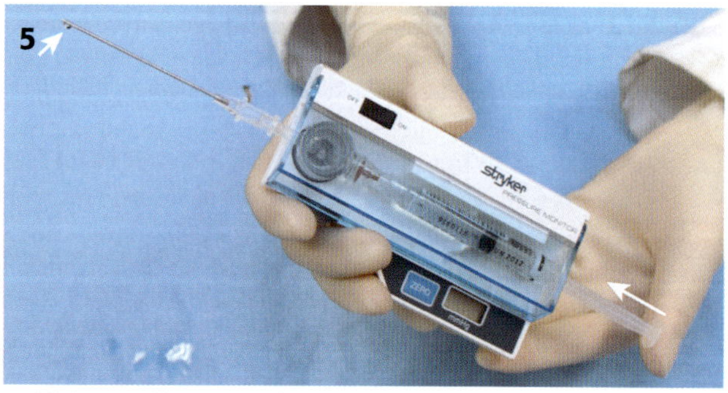

Hold the needle at a 45-degree angle up from horizontal and depress the plunger to force fluid through system and purge it of air.

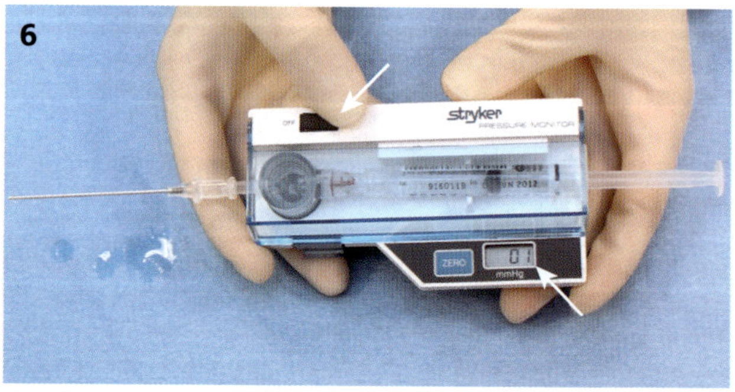

Turn the pressure monitor on. It should read between 0 and 9 mm Hg.

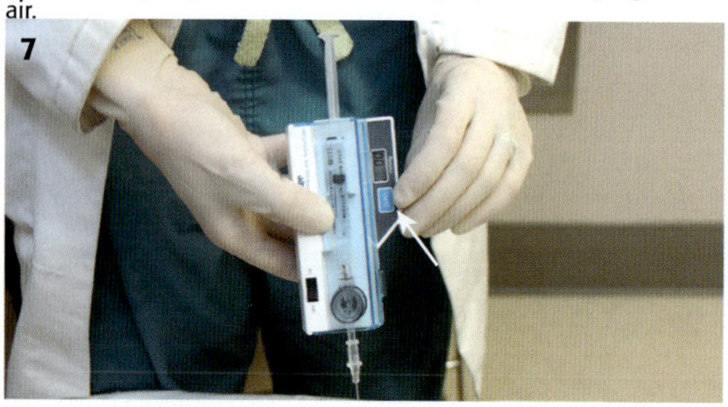

Hold the pressure monitor at the intended angle of insertion and press the "ZERO" button to calibrate the unit. The device display should read "00."

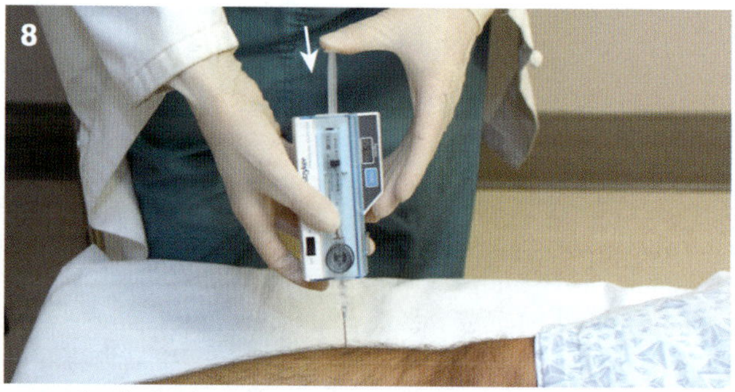

Insert the device into the compartment being measured (after skin cleansing and administration of anesthetic). Slowly inject no more than 0.3 mL into the compartment and wait for the device to record and display the pressure.

Fig. 55.3 Measuring compartment pressure with the Stryker 295-2 pressure monitor.

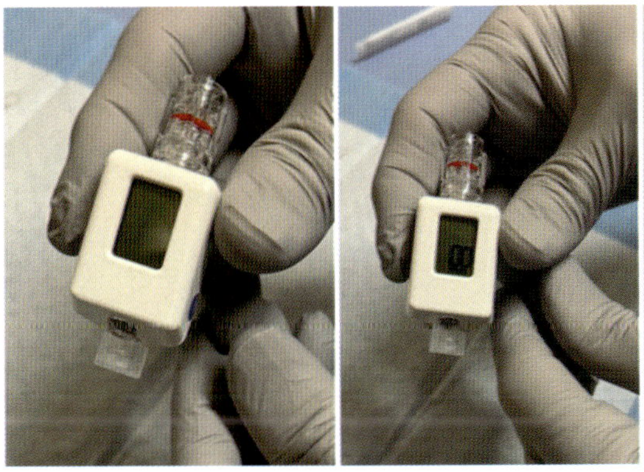

Remove the transducer from the sterile package and activate it by depression the colored button on the side of the device.

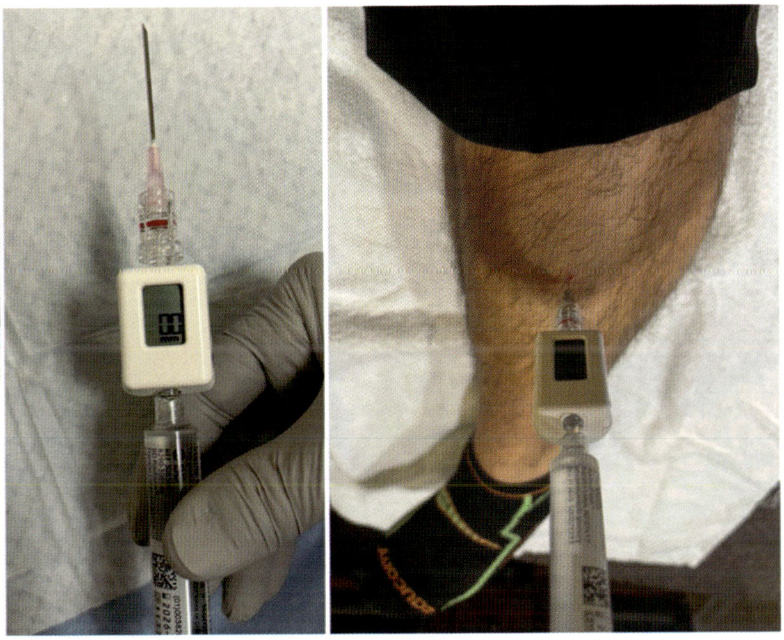

Remove the cover cap and attach a sterile saline filled syringe while at the same time attatch an 18 gage needle to the other end of the device. Flush the device with 0.5–1 mL of saline.

Insert the needle into the compartment to be measured and flush with 0.3 mL of saline. Allow the pressure to equilibrate, then read the compartment pressure.

Fig. 55.4 Measuring compartment pressure with the Centurion Compass Universal Hg transducer.

- Pressure bag
- One syringe sterile normal saline
- High-pressure tubing
- Pressure transducer with cable
- Pressure monitor
- Transducer stand that allows for adjustment of height
- Three-way stopcocks

Setup and Procedure

1. Position the patient. Prepare and anesthetize the needle insertion site according to the guidelines described earlier.
2. Set up the arterial tubing and transducer as you normally would (see Chapter 20).
3. Attach the stop cock to the distal end of the tubing. Attach the needle to the distal end of the stop cock.
4. Flush the system with saline and zero the monitor.
5. Insert the needle into the muscle of the compartment being measured (see section "Needle Placement Techniques for Specific Compartments").
6. Make sure the stop cock is open to the needle and flush the needle with 0.3 mL of saline from the syringe of sterile saline.
7. Turn the stop cock back so it is open to the monitor and read the pressure.

Compass Compartment Pressure Monitor

See Fig. 55.4 and Video 55.5.

Equipment

- One 18-gauge simple or spinal needle, use side-port needle if available
- One syringe sterile normal saline
- Compass compartment pressure monitor

Setup and Procedure

1. Position the patient. Prepare and anesthetize the needle insertion site according to the guidelines described earlier.
2. Remove the rear cap on the device and attach the needle to the distal end.
3. Attach a sterile flush to the proximal end of the device and prime the device by flushing with a small amount of saline.
4. Hold the device at the angle of insertion and push the button on the side. The monitor should read "00."
5. Insert the needle into the compartment being measured (see section "Needle Placement Techniques for Specific Compartments"). Slowly inject no more than 0.3 mL of saline into the compartment to make sure the tip of the needle is not blocked.
6. After the saline is injected allow several seconds for the reading to stabilize and read the compartment pressure.

NEEDLE PLACEMENT TECHNIQUES FOR SPECIFIC COMPARTMENTS

General Principles

Accurate pressure measurements depend on careful needle insertion and confirmation of correct placement. Proper needle insertion requires (1) reliable placement in the compartment being measured, (2) avoidance of important neurovascular structures, (3) simplicity and reproducibility, and (4) minimal patient discomfort.[99] Most compartments are superficial and easily accessible. Only the deep posterior compartment in the leg and the gluteal compartment may require a spinal needle to reach the required depth. Most approaches require that the needle enters the tissue perpendicular to the skin.

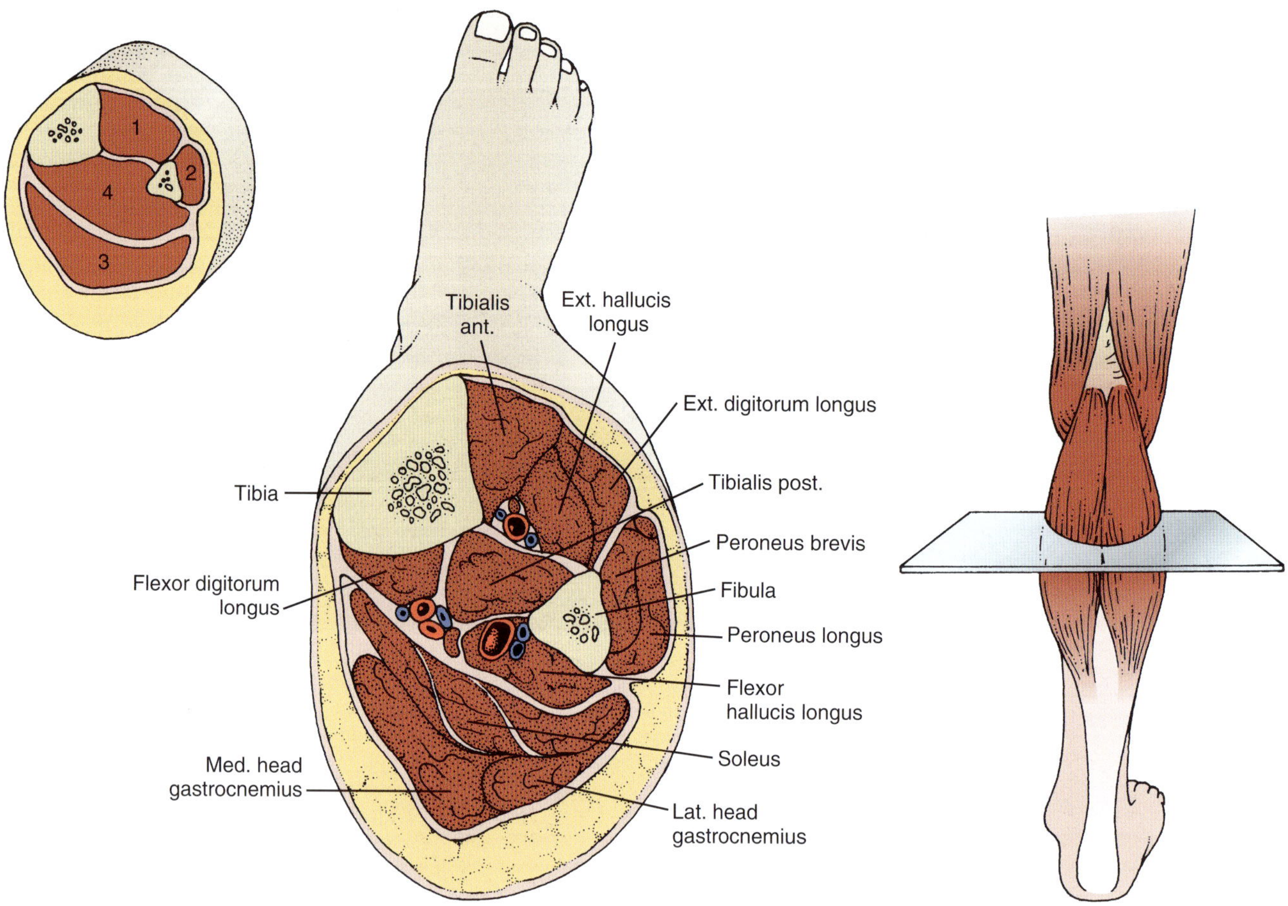

Fig. 55.5 Fascial compartments of the lower part of the leg with enclosed muscle groups *(upper left)*: *1*, anterior; *2*, lateral; *3*, superficial posterior; and *4*, deep posterior compartments.

Lower Extremity

Because of its high vulnerability to injury and limited fascial compliance, the lower part of the leg is predisposed to compartment syndrome. The foreleg traditionally has four compartments: anterior, lateral, deep posterior, and superficial posterior (Fig. 55.5).[1] The anterior compartment is the most frequent site of compartment syndrome.[50] In some patients, the tibialis posterior muscle may occupy its own compartment, separate from the rest of the deep posterior compartment.[100–102] Keep this possibility in mind when measuring compartment pressure in this area.

The easiest cross-sectional level for placement of the needle in any foreleg compartment is approximately 3 cm on either side of a transverse line drawn at the junction of the proximal and middle thirds of the lower part of the leg (see Fig. 55.5). When measuring compartment pressure in the foreleg, place the patient in the supine position with the leg at the level of the heart. An exception occurs when measuring the superficial posterior compartment. In this case, place the patient in the prone position. Prepare and anesthetize the needle insertion site as described previously in this chapter.

Anterior Compartment (Fig. 55.6A)

With the patient supine, palpate the anterior border of the tibia at the junction of the proximal and middle thirds of the lower part of the leg. Insert the needle perpendicular to the skin 1 cm *lateral* to the anterior border of the tibia to a depth of approximately 1 to 3 cm. A several-fold rise in pressure during (1) external compression of the anterior compartment just proximal or distal to the needle insertion site, (2) plantar flexion of the foot, or (3) dorsiflexion of the foot confirms proper needle depth.

Deep Posterior Compartment (Fig. 55.6B)

With the patient supine, have an assistant elevate the leg slightly off the stretcher (if the clinical situation permits). Palpate the medial border of the tibia at the junction of the proximal and middle thirds of the lower part of the leg while simultaneously palpating the posterior border of the fibula on the lateral aspect of the leg at the same level. Insert the needle perpendicular to the skin just posterior to the medial border of the tibia and direct it toward the palpated posterior border of the fibula to a depth of 2 to 4 cm (the final depth depends on the amount of subcutaneous adipose tissue). Confirm proper needle depth by observing a rise in pressure during (1) toe extension or (2) ankle eversion.

Lateral Compartment (Fig. 55.6C)

With the patient supine and the leg at heart level, have an assistant elevate the leg slightly off the stretcher (if the clinical situation permits). Palpate the posterior border of the fibula at the junction of the proximal and middle thirds of the lower part of the leg. Insert the needle into the skin just anterior to the posterior border of the fibula and direct it toward the

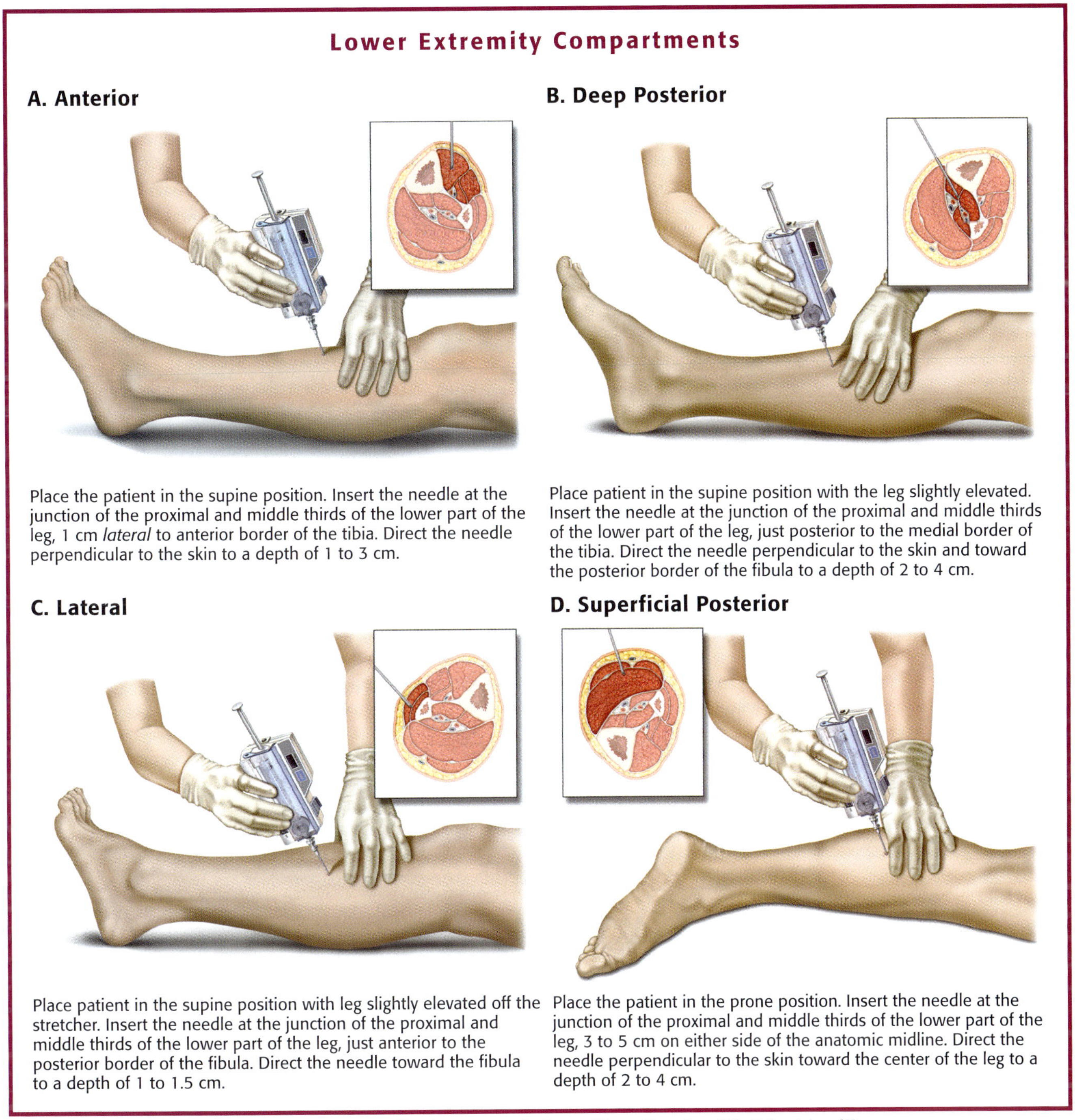

Fig. 55.6 Lower extremity needle placement techniques. (From Custalow CB. *Color Atlas of Emergency Department Procedures*. Saunders; 2005.)

fibula to a depth of 1 to 1.5 cm. If the needle contacts bone, withdraw it approximately 0.5 cm. Confirm proper needle depth by observing a rise in pressure during (1) external compression of the lateral compartment just inferior or superior to the needle's entrance or (2) inversion of the foot and ankle.

Superficial Posterior Compartment (Fig. 55.6D)

With the patient in the prone position and the leg at heart level, identify an imaginary transverse line (or draw one with a marking pen) between the proximal and middle thirds of the lower part of the leg. Insert the needle perpendicular to the skin at this level, 3 cm to 5 cm on either side of a vertical line drawn down the middle of the calf. Direct the needle toward the center of the leg to a depth of 2 to 4 cm. Confirm proper needle depth by observing a rise in pressure during (1) digital external compression of the posterior compartment just inferior or superior to the needle insertion point or (2) dorsiflexion of the foot.

Forearm

Traditionally, the forearm has been considered a two-compartment limb.[1] However, some authors place the extensor carpi radialis brevis, the extensor carpi radialis longus, and the brachioradialis muscles in a third compartment called the "mobile wad."[103–105] The forearm compartments (particularly

Upper Extremity Compartments

A. Volar

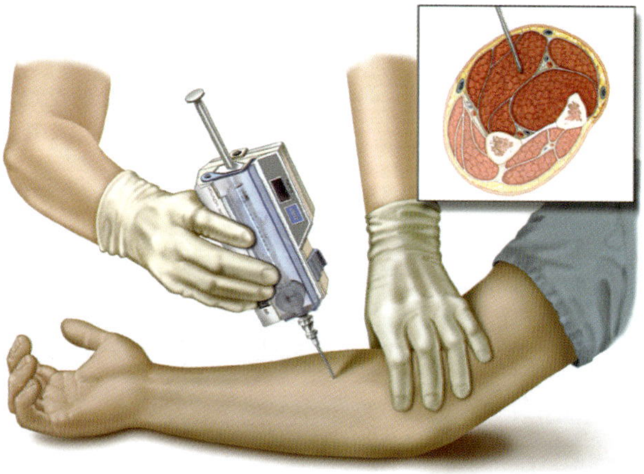

Hold the forearm in supination. Insert the needle at the junction of the proximal and middle thirds of the forearm, just medial to the palmaris longus tendon. Direct the needle perpendicular to the skin, toward the posterior border of the ulna, to a depth of 1 to 2 cm.

B. Dorsal

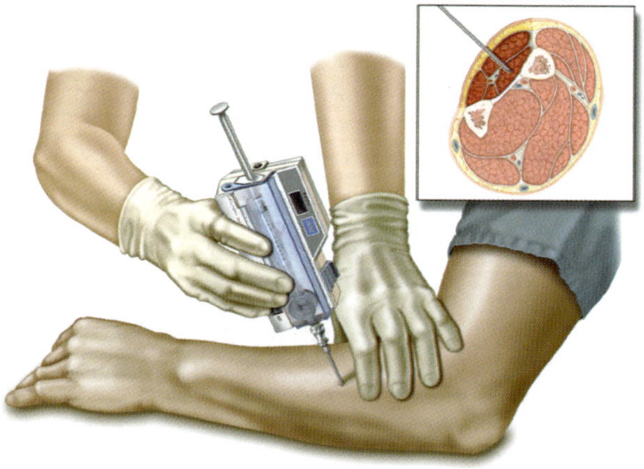

Hold the forearm in pronation with the elbow flexed and the dorsum of the forearm facing up. Insert the needle at the junction of the proximal and middle thirds of the forearm, 1 to 2 cm lateral to the posterior aspect of the ulna. Direct the needle perpendicular to the skin to a depth of 1 to 2 cm.

C. Mobile Wad

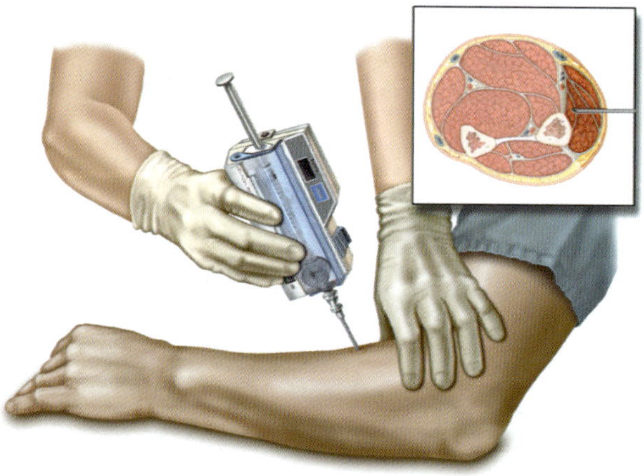

Hold the forearm in supination. Insert the needle at the junction of the proximal and middle thirds of the forearm, at the most lateral (radial) portion of the forearm. Direct the needle perpendicular to the skin to a depth of 1 to 1.5 cm.

Fig. 55.7 Upper extremity needle placement techniques. (From Custalow CB. *Color Atlas of Emergency Department Procedures*. Saunders; 2005.)

the volar compartment) are predisposed to compartment syndrome because of their use during vigorous exercise, accessibility for drug use, IV infiltration of fluid or medication, and vulnerability to injury and burns.[1,106–109]

The junction of the proximal and middle thirds of the forearm is the cross-sectional level for insertion of the needle.[103] When measuring forearm compartment pressure, place the patient in the supine position with the arm at the level of the heart. Prepare and anesthetize the needle insertion site as previously described.

Volar Compartment (Fig. 55.7A)

Hold the forearm in supination. Identify the palmaris longus tendon by having the patient oppose the thumb and small finger with the wrist flexed against resistance. Follow the tendon to the junction of the proximal and middle thirds of the forearm. Palpate the posterior border of the ulna and insert the needle perpendicular to the skin just medial (ulnar) to the palmaris longus tendon. Direct the needle toward the palpated posterior border of the ulna to a depth of 1 to 2 cm. Confirm proper needle depth by observing a rise in pressure during (1) external compression of the volar compartment just proximal or distal to the needle insertion point or (2) extension of the fingers or wrist.

Dorsal Compartment (Fig. 55.7B)

Hold the forearm in pronation with the elbow flexed and the dorsum of the forearm facing upward. Palpate the posterior

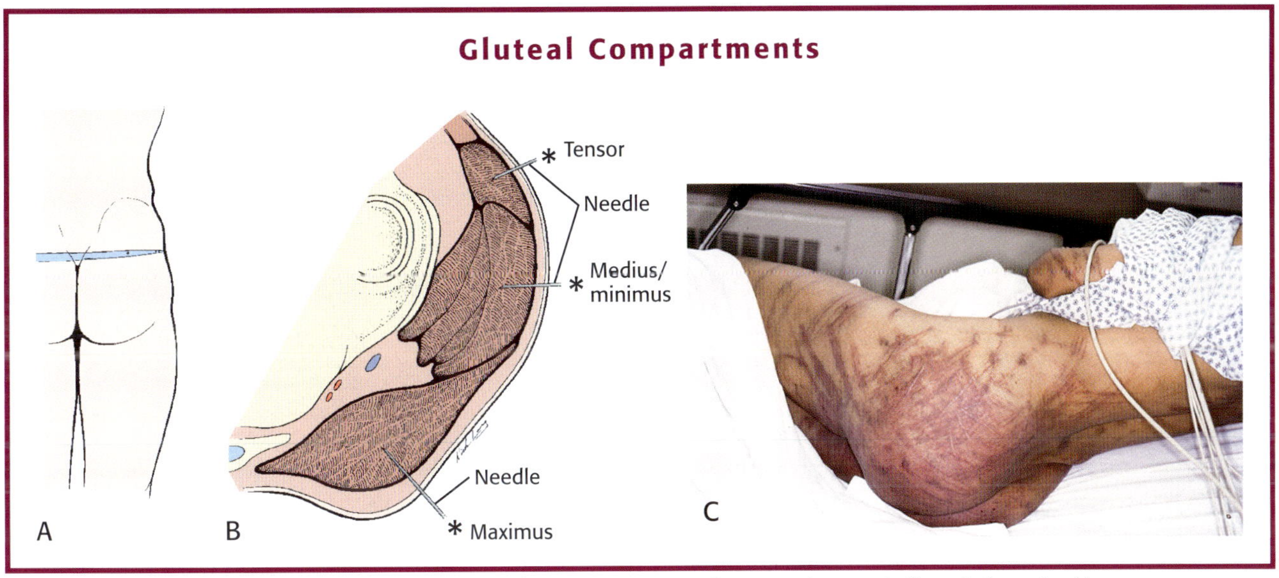

Fig. 55.8 Gluteal compartment syndrome. (A) Suggested entry points are indicated along the *blue line*. The needle should be inserted to a depth of 4 cm to 8 cm, depending on which compartment is being measured. (B) Needle tips *(asterisks)* are shown entering the muscle compartments. (C) This patient sustained extensive soft tissue trauma to the buttocks as a result of repeated blows from a stick (domestic abuse) and was at risk for rhabdomyolysis and gluteal compartment syndrome. (A–B, modified with permission from Owen CA, Moody PR, Mubarak SJ et al. Gluteal compartment syndromes. *Clin Orthop.* 1978;132:57.)

aspect of the ulna at the junction of the proximal and middle thirds of the forearm. Insert the needle perpendicular to the skin 1 to 2 cm lateral (radial) to the posterior aspect of the ulna to a depth of 1 to 2 cm. Confirm proper needle placement by observing a rise in pressure during (1) digital external compression of the dorsal compartment just proximal or distal to the needle insertion point or (2) flexion of the wrist or fingers.

Mobile Wad (Fig. 55.7C)

Hold the forearm in supination. Identify the most lateral (radial) portion of the forearm at the junction of its proximal and middle thirds. Insert the needle into the muscle tissue lateral to the radius and perpendicular to the skin to a depth of 1 to 1.5 cm. Confirm proper needle placement by observing a rise in pressure during (1) digital external compression of the mobile wad just proximal or distal to the needle entry point or (2) deviation of the wrist.

Gluteal Musculature

A two-layer fascia encases the muscle bellies of the tensor fasciae latae anteriorly and the gluteus maximus posteriorly. This fascia divides the musculature into three distinct compartments: maximus, tensor, and medius/minimus (Fig. 55.8A–B). The sciatic nerve is deep to the fascia but lies between the pelvis–external rotator complex and the gluteus maximus, which makes it vulnerable to injury when compartment syndrome occurs here. Gluteal compartment syndrome is very rare and unknown to many clinicians. Most reported cases of gluteal compartment syndrome result from prolonged immobilization and local compression in association with drug or alcohol intoxication.[110–114] Prolonged pressure from a toilet seat or significant soft tissue contusions (whipping, paddling) may predispose to this condition. Patients typically have gluteal tenderness that is often attributed to contusion or hematoma. This, combined with the rarity of a compartment syndrome in this area, frequently results in a delayed or missed diagnosis. Rhabdomyolysis should be considered in patients with gluteal compartment syndrome given the large muscle mass involved.

Gluteal Compartments

To measure gluteal compartment pressure, place the patient in the prone position with the gluteal structures at the level of the heart. Prepare and anesthetize the needle insertion site as described previously. Cutaneous landmarks for the three compartments are not consistent from patient to patient. Therefore in cases of suspected gluteal compartment syndrome, insertion of the needle at the point of maximal tenderness is considered sufficient to provide adequate pressure measurements.[110] Insert an 18-gauge spinal needle perpendicular to the skin and direct it toward the point of maximal tenderness to a depth of 4 cm to 8 cm (see Fig. 55.8B). Confirm proper needle placement by observing a rise in pressure during external compression of the gluteal musculature.

Foot

Crush injuries account for the majority of reported cases of compartment syndrome in the foot,[115–117] but it may also be seen after vascular injuries, fractures, and other high-energy injuries. Although compartment syndrome of the foot is rare, it is being reported with increasing frequency as clinicians become more aware of this entity. Despite a lack of universal agreement on the number or exact location of the anatomic compartments in the foot,[118–122] it is generally accepted that there are at least nine compartments separated into four groups: the central/calcaneal, intrinsic/interosseous, medial, and lateral (Fig. 55.9A). For measurement of pressure in any of the foot compartments, place the patient in the supine position with the foot at the level of the heart and prepare and

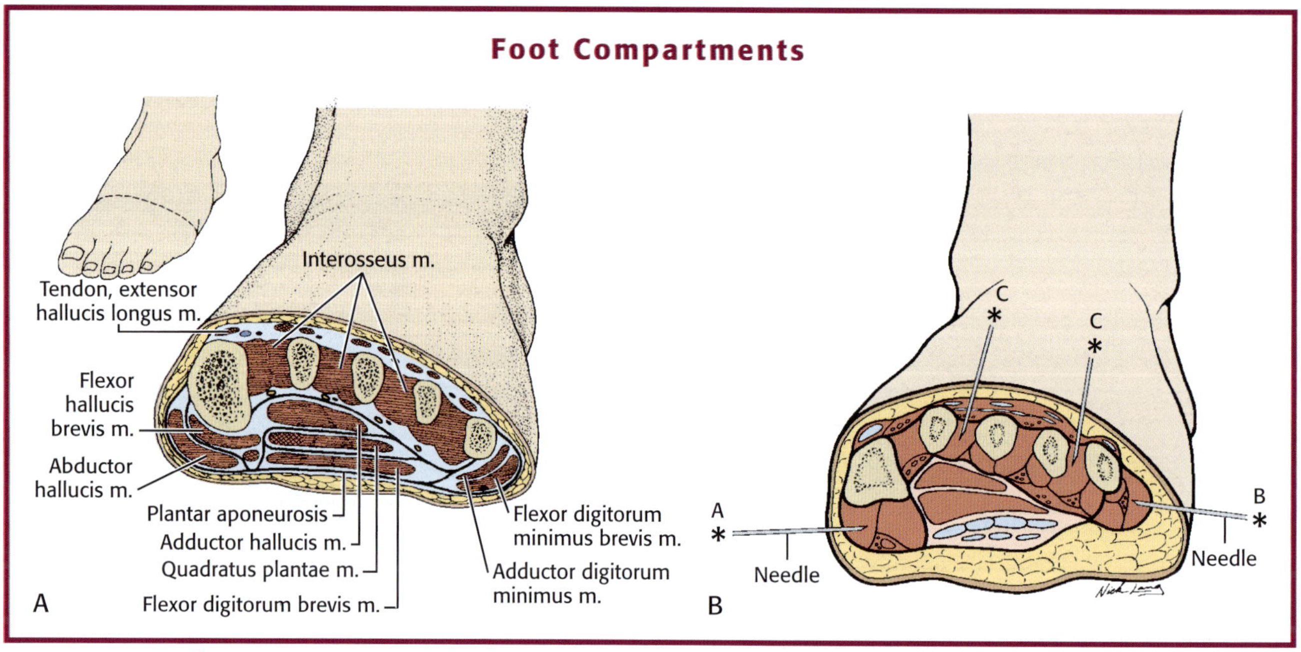

Fig. 55.9 (A) Compartments of the foot. (B) Suggested needle pathways *(asterisks)* to measure intracompartmental pressure: *A*, medial; *B*, lateral; *C*, interosseous. The central compartment is surrounded by these compartments. *m*, Muscle. (A, From Mubarak SJ, Hargens AR. *Compartment Syndromes and Volkmann's contracture.* Saunders; 1981. B, Modified from Myerson M. Acute compartment syndromes of the foot. *Bull Hosp J Dis.* 1987;47:251.)

anesthetize the needle insertion site as described previously. Note that pedal edema has been shown to increase resting tissue pressure in the foot.[123,124]

MEDIAL COMPARTMENT (FIG. 55.9B)

The medial compartment contains the abductor hallucis and flexor hallucis brevis muscles. The compartment is bounded medially and inferiorly by an extension of the plantar aponeurosis, laterally by an intramuscular septum, and dorsally by the first metatarsal. To measure pressure in this compartment, insert the needle perpendicular to the skin at the medial aspect of the foot just inferior to the base of the first metatarsal into the abductor hallucis muscle, which is approximately 1 cm to 1.5 cm deep.[125] Confirm proper needle depth by observing a rise in pressure during external compression of the medial compartment of the foot.

Central (Calcaneal) Compartment (See Fig. 55.9B)

The central compartment contains the flexor digitorum brevis, the quadratus plantae, the lumbricals, and the abductor hallucis muscles. Its boundaries are the plantar aponeurosis inferiorly, the osteofascial tarsometatarsal structures dorsally, and the intermuscular septa medially and laterally. To measure pressure in this compartment, insert the needle perpendicular to the skin at the medial aspect of the foot just inferior to the base of the first metatarsal. Advance the needle through the abductor hallucis muscle to a depth of 3 cm.[125] Confirm proper needle depth by observing a rise in pressure during external compression of the central compartment of the foot.

Lateral Compartment (See Fig. 55.9B)

The lateral compartment contains the abductor, flexor, and opponens muscles of the fifth toe. The boundaries are the fifth metatarsal dorsally, the plantar aponeurosis inferiorly and laterally, and an intermuscular septum medially.[125] To measure pressure in this compartment, insert the needle parallel to the plantar aspect of the foot just inferior to the base of the fifth metatarsal. Advance the needle to a depth of 1 to 1.5 cm. Confirm proper needle depth by observing a rise in pressure during external compression of the lateral compartment of the foot.

Intrinsic (Interosseous) Compartment (See Fig. 55.9B)

The intrinsic compartment contains the seven interossei muscles and is bounded by the metatarsals and the interosseous fascia. Pressure in this compartment is measured in two areas, the second and fourth web spaces. Avoid the first web space to prevent inadvertent puncture or disruption of the dorsalis pedis artery or the deep peroneal nerve.[125] Insert the needle perpendicular to the skin at the dorsum of the second and fourth web spaces at the base of the metatarsals, and advance the needle to a depth of 1 cm.[125] Confirm proper needle depth by observing a rise in pressure during external compression of the intrinsic compartment adjacent to the needle insertion site.

INTERPRETATION OF COMPARTMENT PRESSURE MEASUREMENTS

Compartment pressures must be interpreted within the context of the clinical picture. Inaccurate measurements are far worse than no measurement at all, and clinical evaluation is more telling than pressure measurements alone. To be most accurate, compartment pressures should be measured in the area of highest pressure and greatest tissue damage.[83,126] Inaccurate measurements may result from placement of the needle into tendon or fascia, plugged needles, defective or poorly calibrated devices, injection of fluid into the compartment, and movement during the procedure. Whitesides and colleagues found a 1 mm Hg increase in compartment pressure for every 1 mL of saline infused into the anterior compartment of the lower extremity.[6] It is difficult to assess the relevance of this finding, but recognition of the potential for its occurrence is important.

Reports of normal human compartment pressure vary in the literature. In comparing several techniques, Shakespeare and associates found an average normal pressure of 8.5 mm Hg with slightly higher resting pressure in individuals who were physically fit.[12] Willy and coworkers found a mean of 15 mm Hg (±8 mm Hg) when using an electronic transducer-tipped probe in healthy volunteers.[15] Although the generally accepted range of normal is between 0 and 10 mm Hg, others have noted pressures in normal subjects ranging from 0 to as high as 18 mm Hg.[1,8,82,127] Even though compartment pressure measurements have not been studied extensively in pediatric populations, one study reported higher resting compartment pressure in children than in adults.[48]

When properly performed, each method described in this chapter has acceptable accuracy in the clinical setting. Studies have found standard deviations of between 2 and 6 mm Hg with all the techniques described earlier.[1,8–10,12] The arterial line system used with a simple (straight) or side-port needle provides a higher degree of accuracy for simple, episodic readings. The C2Dx Intracompartmental Pressure Monitoring System provides consistent, accurate readings for both episodic and continuous pressure monitoring. The development of miniature transducer-tipped devices is ongoing.[122] Noninvasive modalities, including MRI, SPECT, myotonometry, electromyography, near-infrared spectroscopy, and ultrasound, continue to be investigated as painless alternatives to needle-driven compartment pressure measurements, and although the early results are promising, they are not currently in widespread use.[19–36]

Mubarak and coworkers[9,128] and Hargens and colleagues[129] suggested that an absolute compartment pressure of 30 mm Hg is the "critical pressure" requiring fasciotomy. Others have supported these recommendations.[126,130] However, it is important to note that a compartment pressure of 30 mm Hg does not necessarily precipitate compartment syndrome in the absence of other factors and must be interpreted within the context of the clinical scenario. Although compartment syndrome may develop in some patients at this pressure, in others it will not, as tolerance to increasing pressure appears to be variable.[1,8,12,82]

Despite a body of literature addressing measurement of compartment pressure, there continues to be no consensus regarding a specific compartment pressure threshold at which fasciotomy should be performed. Obviously, no measured compartment pressure, by itself, is an indication for fasciotomy, but it may guide consultation and further observation. A single pressure reading can be misleading, and trends in pressure provide more information to the clinician. Some argue that an absolute compartment pressure of 30 mm Hg or greater should be the threshold for fasciotomy.[9,129,130] Matsen found that no patients with a pressure lower than 45 mm Hg had symptoms of compartment syndrome,[1] whereas all patients with a pressure higher than 60 mm Hg had symptoms. Whitesides and colleagues found that fasciotomy was required when intracompartmental pressure approaches 20 mm Hg below diastolic pressure,[6] whereas McQueen and associates recommended using a perfusion pressure (diastolic pressure minus compartment pressure) of less than 30 mm Hg as a criterion for fasciotomy.[131] Heppenstall and coworkers concluded that use of either the Whitesides or McQueen criteria would produce similar results and recommended using a ΔP (MAP minus the measured compartment pressure) of 30 mm Hg or less in nontraumatized muscle and a ΔP of 40 mm Hg or less in traumatized muscle as a guide for fasciotomy.[53,61] McQueen and associates argue for continuous compartment pressure monitoring. In their review of almost 1000 trauma patients, they estimated sensitivity of intracompartmental pressure monitoring for suspected acute compartment syndrome was 94%, with an estimated specificity of 98%, an estimated positive predictive value of 93%, and an estimated negative predictive value of 99%.[132]

In summary, absolute compartment pressures of 30 mm Hg or higher garner concern for consultation or intervention for compartment syndrome. Based on pathophysiology, it appears quite reasonable to consider the difference between diastolic blood pressure and the measured compartment pressure (perfusion pressure) as a guide for diagnosing compartment syndrome and a strong consideration for fasciotomy. A compartment pressure within 30 mm Hg of the patient's diastolic blood pressure, essentially a perfusion pressure of less than 30 mm Hg, is generally considered the threshold for consideration of fasciotomy.[52,126,133]

Factors other than compartment pressure alone are important in the development of compartment syndrome and the need for fasciotomy. In patients with chronic systemic hypertension, higher compartment pressure may be necessary before nerve injury or muscle ischemia occurs. Situations in which MAP is low (e.g., hypovolemia, peripheral vascular disease) might interfere with the patient's ability to tolerate even mildly elevated compartment pressure. Finally, the duration of increased compartment pressure is also an important factor in the development and severity of compartment syndrome.

COMPLICATIONS

All invasive monitoring systems are associated with some degree of pain during insertion of the needle or catheter. Adequate analgesia and, when necessary, procedural sedation are often necessary to gain the patient's cooperation and prevent movement during pressure measurements. When using local anesthetics, avoid injections into the compartment because this can increase pain and result in inaccurate (higher) readings.

Failure to properly use pressure measurement devices may result in inaccurate results and a delay in the diagnosis of compartment syndrome. As with any invasive procedure, care must be taken to minimize bleeding and additional damage to underlying tissue, nerves, or blood vessels. The risk for both local and systemic infection is similar for all the measurement procedures described in this chapter. Strict adherence to aseptic technique and universal precautions is mandatory. This includes sterilization of catheters and the use of sterile solutions in addition to sterile gloves and supplies whenever possible.

ACKNOWLEDGMENTS

The author recognizes the original contributions of Chaiya Laoteppitaks, MD, to a previous edition of this text.

REFERENCES ARE AVAILABLE AT Elsevier eBooks+

SECTION IX

Genitourinary, Obstetric, and Gynecologic Procedures

CHAPTER 56

Urologic Procedures

Jonathan M. Watson and Jonathan E. Davis

INTRODUCTION

This chapter addresses urologic conditions that are either initially or eventually associated with an emergency procedure or may need to be performed by emergency providers in the absence of a urologic surgeon.

Testicular torsion is a scrotal emergency that can be challenging to diagnose under the best clinical circumstances. Although surgical exploration is the only definitive diagnostic and therapeutic procedure, many urologists prefer an initial diagnostic imaging study prior to surgical exploration, provided imaging can be obtained expediently while simultaneously preparing for operative intervention. This chapter addresses bedside maneuvers for testicular torsion, including manual testicular detorsion.

Emergency penile conditions include paraphimosis and priapism. This chapter addresses bedside paraphimosis reduction techniques, as well as penile aspiration-irrigation-injection for relief of ischemic priapism. In addition, relief of phimosis complicated by the inability to void by means of a dorsal slit of the penile foreskin will be detailed for completeness.

Access to and the subsequent evaluation of the bladder and urine are clinically important to all emergency providers. Various approaches to urine sampling and bladder drainage, including the techniques and complications of male and female urethral catheterization in various clinical situations and emergency suprapubic bladder access, are discussed.

Finally, a discussion of radiographic imaging of the genitourinary (GU) system is provided, with an emphasis on assessing lower urinary tract injury. Although the timing of GU radiologic examinations within the workup of the critically ill, multitrauma patient must be individualized, general guidelines for successful imaging are provided.

TESTICULAR TORSION

Introduction

Although acute scrotal pain comprises less than 1% of all emergency department (ED) visits, this presentation may provoke great anxiety for the patient or caretaker, given its highly sensitive nature. One of the most challenging aspects of scrotal complaints is that a variety of clinical conditions may present in a similar fashion: a male patient complaining of an acute, painful, swollen, and tender hemiscrotum. Although the differential is extensive, testicular torsion is the principal fertility threat that needs to be ruled out. Definitive management of testicular torsion involves surgical exploration and orchiopexy. Manual detorsion, with or without spermatic cord anesthesia can be attempted while simultaneously preparing for operative intervention.

Procedure Overview

Indications: suspected or confirmed testicular torsion.
Contraindications: alternative cause of acute scrotal pain.
Complications: worsening ischemia, increased pain.
Equipment:

- For spermatic cord anesthesia: 1% lidocaine (10 mL for an adult, or age-/weight-appropriate local anesthetic dosing for child), 27-gauge (or similar) needle for anesthetic infiltration.
- For manual detorsion: bedside sonography may be helpful in assessing for pre- and postprocedure intratesticular blood flow.

Key Procedure Sequence

1. Initiate urologic consultation and simultaneous preparation for surgical intervention.
2. Administer spermatic cord anesthesia (optional).
3. Consider systemic analgesia or light sedation.
4. Keep the patient comfortable in a reclining or supine position.
5. Stand beside the stretcher (right side if right-hand dominant, or vice versa).
6. Rotate the testicle from medial to lateral (two-thirds of torsion occurs lateral to medial).
7. Rotate 180 degrees initially; it may ultimately require two to three rotations to alleviate pain.
8. If mechanically difficult or there is increased pain, detorse in the opposite direction.
9. The end point is relief of pain or return of intratesticular blood flow on sonogram.
10. Consult urology for definitive surgical scrotal exploration.

Description

Background

An acute scrotum is defined as an acute, painful swelling of the scrotum or its contents, accompanied by local signs or general symptoms.[1] Although the list of diagnostic possibilities for a patient with an undifferentiated acute scrotum is extensive, early identification and skillful management of testicular torsion is critical as it may threaten testicular viability and future fertility if not managed expediently. Acute epididymitis is commonly the cause of acute scrotal pain in adolescents and adults. Testicular (or epididymal) appendage torsion is another frequent cause of acute scrotal pain in prepubertal boys.

Differentiating testicular torsion from alternative conditions takes precedence over a definitive diagnosis. The presence of an intact cremasteric reflex and testicular sonography are frequently utilized, yet imperfect, diagnostic tools in assessing for testicular torsion.

Anatomy and Physiology

A congenital anomaly of fixation of the testis, termed the *bell-clapper deformity*, is associated with the development of testicular torsion.[2] This occurs when the intrascrotal portion of the spermatic cord lacks firm posterior adhesion to the scrotal wall and remains surrounded by the tunica vaginalis (Fig. 56.1A). As a result of the abnormal attachment, the testis may be suspended horizontally.[3] These anatomic features predispose the affected testis to rotation.

Pathophysiology

Testicular salvage rates decrease with time from the onset of ischemia. A meta-analysis of 1140 patients in 22 series demonstrated a greater than 90% salvage rate with surgery within 6 hours of pain onset.[4] Testicular atrophy may lead to subfertility. Furthermore, testicular loss may lead to contralateral testicular dysfunction through local vasoconstriction, autoimmune pathways, or other mechanisms.[4]

The testis may torse, detorse, and retorse, so clinicians should be cautious about assigning a definitive time of onset and deferring urologic consultation based on an erroneous assumption that the testis is not salvageable. The gold standard for determining testicular viability is intraoperative visualization of the affected testis. Although all clinicians recognize the need for expedient surgery in the setting of known torsion, not all experts will agree on surgical exploration without some adjunctive testing.

When utilized in the appropriate clinical setting, ultrasound remains the most useful diagnostic modality in the evaluation of GU complaints (Fig. 56.2). A patient with compelling historical and examination findings of testicular torsion does not require any preoperative diagnostic tests. Color flow Doppler ultrasonography (CDUS) may be helpful in all other cases. The classic sonographic finding suggestive of testicular torsion is diminished intratesticular blood flow. In addition, examination of the spermatic cord with high-resolution gray-scale ultrasonography may reveal "coiling" or "kinking" of the cord at the site of torsion.[5–7] Sonography is used not only to exclude testicular torsion, but also to search for alternative causes of acute scrotal pain. In epididymitis, perfusion may be normal (or increased) due to the effects of inflammatory mediators on local vascular beds, although this is a nonspecific finding.[8,9] An infarcted appendage may be visualized on ultrasound as well.[10] It has been suggested that emergency physicians may be able to accurately assess for intratesticular blood flow in patients presenting with acute scrotal pain using bedside sonography, and ultrasound-guided manual detorsion by emergency physicians has been successfully performed.[11,12]

CDUS has long been regarded as the diagnostic modality of choice in assessing for testicular torsion. However, false-negative ultrasound results have been reported.[13–15] Many of these studies are case reports or case series, limited by small numbers and retrospective design. Doppler ultrasound may reveal seemingly adequate intratesticular blood flow in partial torsion, which can be misleading to the practitioner.

Radionuclide scintigraphy and CDUS show similar sensitivity, as well as false-negative rates, for the diagnosis of testicular torsion.[16] Given the widespread availability and expertise with ultrasound technology, however, combined with the risks of isotope radiation exposure, radionuclide procedures have fallen out of favor. The use of magnetic resonance imaging has been explored, though significant limitations include availability and time required for imaging.[17,18]

Once the diagnosis of testicular torsion is suspected, immediately place a call to notify a urologist of the suspected diagnosis, the possible need for surgical exploration, and whether testicular detorsion will be attempted while awaiting patient transport to the operating room. Time is of the essence. Do not wait for confirmation of the diagnosis to call urology.

Indications

Testicular torsion may be relieved by manual detorsion. A study of 162 cases of testicular torsion revealed that anticipated lateral to medial rotation occurred in 67% of cases, with medial to lateral rotation in the remaining 33%. This challenges the standard dogma of medial to lateral rotation, or "opening the book," as the standard method for detorsion, which may fail in one-third of cases. There may be a cranial-caudal component to torsion as well. The end point of manual detorsion is relief of pain, or the return of intratesticular blood flow as seen on ultrasound imaging.[19] Although manual detorsion may allow for reperfusion of the testis, a lesser degree of residual torsion may remain. Given that infarction can occur with as little as 180 degrees of torsion, surgical exploration after what is thought to be a successful manual detorsion may be prudent. The bottom line is that specialty consultation and plans for the possibility of surgical exploration should occur regardless of outcome of the detorsion procedure. Detorsion, however, may convert an emergent procedure to an urgent one.

Contraindications

Presence of an alternative cause of acute scrotal pain is a relative contraindication to the detorsion procedure. However, precise diagnosis may be challenging prior to definitive surgical exploration. A nonanomalous, appropriately fixated testicle should not be adversely affected by an initial trial (e.g., 180 degrees) of manual detorsion if circumstances are highly suspect for spermatic cord torsion.

Procedure: Manual Detorsion and Spermatic Cord Anesthesia

Manual detorsion is performed in the following manner. Advise the patient that the procedure will be uncomfortable and painful and offer systemic analgesia or light sedation when appropriate. The rationale for not using spermatic cord anesthesia with attempted detorsion is that the anesthesia takes away an important subjective end point: relief of the patient's pain after manipulation of the testis. Some authors, however, do advocate for spermatic cord anesthesia prior to initiating manual detorsion.

Manual Testicular Detorsion

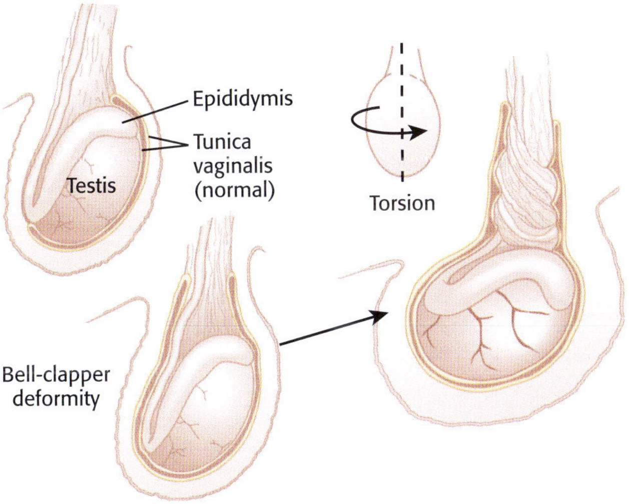

A. Anatomy of testicular torsion. Testicular torsion occurs when the testis twists within the tunica vaginalis. Patients with the bell-clapper deformity (i.e., incomplete fusion of the tunica along the epididymis, which results in incomplete attachment of the testicle to the scrotum) are at higher risk.

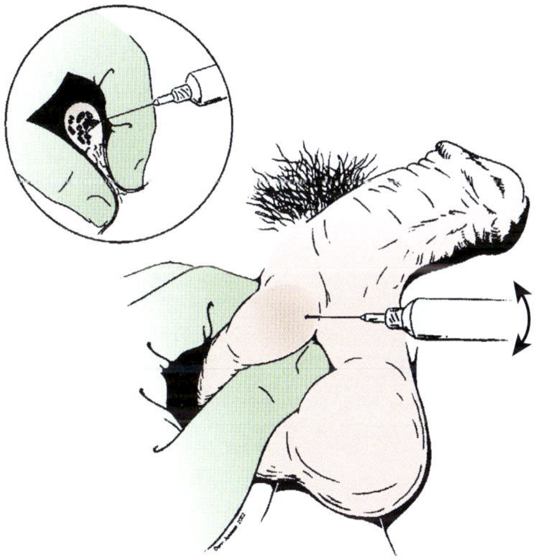

B. Spermatic cord block. Grasp the spermatic cord between your thumb and index finger. Use a 30-gauge needle to infiltrate the entire cross section of the spermatic cord and its surrounding rim with anesthetic. This will cause visual ballooning of the grasped segment of the cord. Gently massage this bulge to disperse the anesthetic. Usually about 10 mL is required. Ultrasound guidance may be used to aid in identifying structures and preventing complications

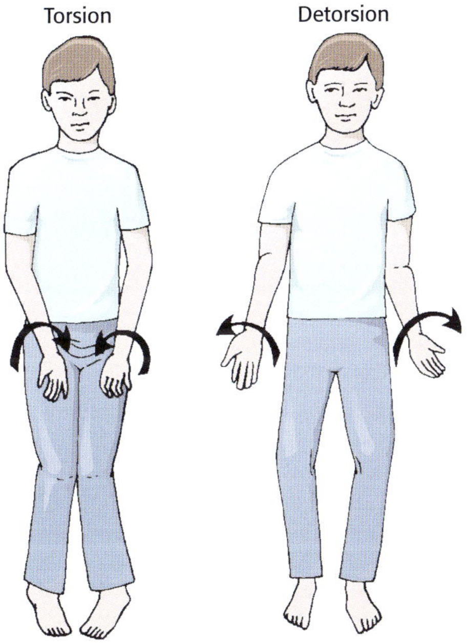

C. Testicular torsion more commonly occurs in a medial direction. Initially attempt detorsion by rotating the testis outward toward the thigh. This is most successful if attempted within the first few hours of torsion, before the onset of significant scrotal swelling. Intravenous narcotics can be administered or a cord block performed before attempting detorsion.

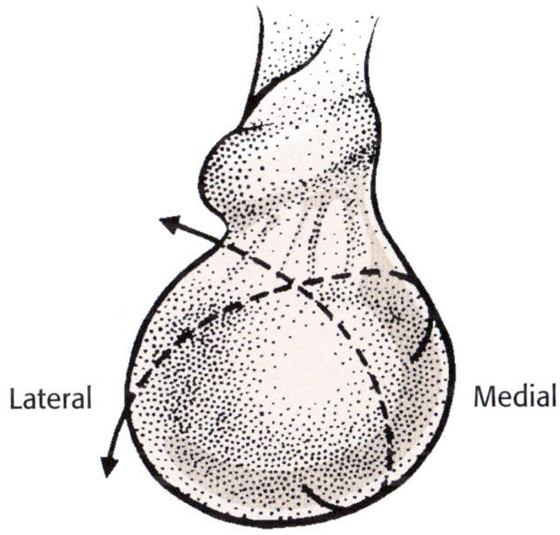

D. Detorsion maneuver. Detorsion of the testicle may require testicular rotation through two planes. To release the cremasteric muscle, rotate the testis in a caudal-to-cranial direction simultaneously with medial-to-lateral rotation. The right testis is shown.

Fig. 56.1 (A) Anatomy of testicular torsion. (B) Achieve anesthesia of the spermatic cord by injecting lidocaine at the superficial inguinal ring. (C) Manual detorsion of the testis using the "open book" technique, rotating outward toward the thigh to restore perfusion and preserve viability. (A, From Snyder HM III. Urologic emergencies. In: Fleisher GR, Ludwig S, eds. *Textbook of Pediatric Emergency Medicine*. 4th ed. Lippincott Williams & Wilkins; 2000:1585-1593. B, From Issa MM, Hsiao K, Bassel YS et al. Spermatic cord anesthesia block for scrotal procedures in outpatient clinic setting. *J Urol.* 2004;172:2358-2361. D, From Freeman S, Chapman J. Urologic procedures. *Emerg Med Clin North Am.* 1986;4:543.)

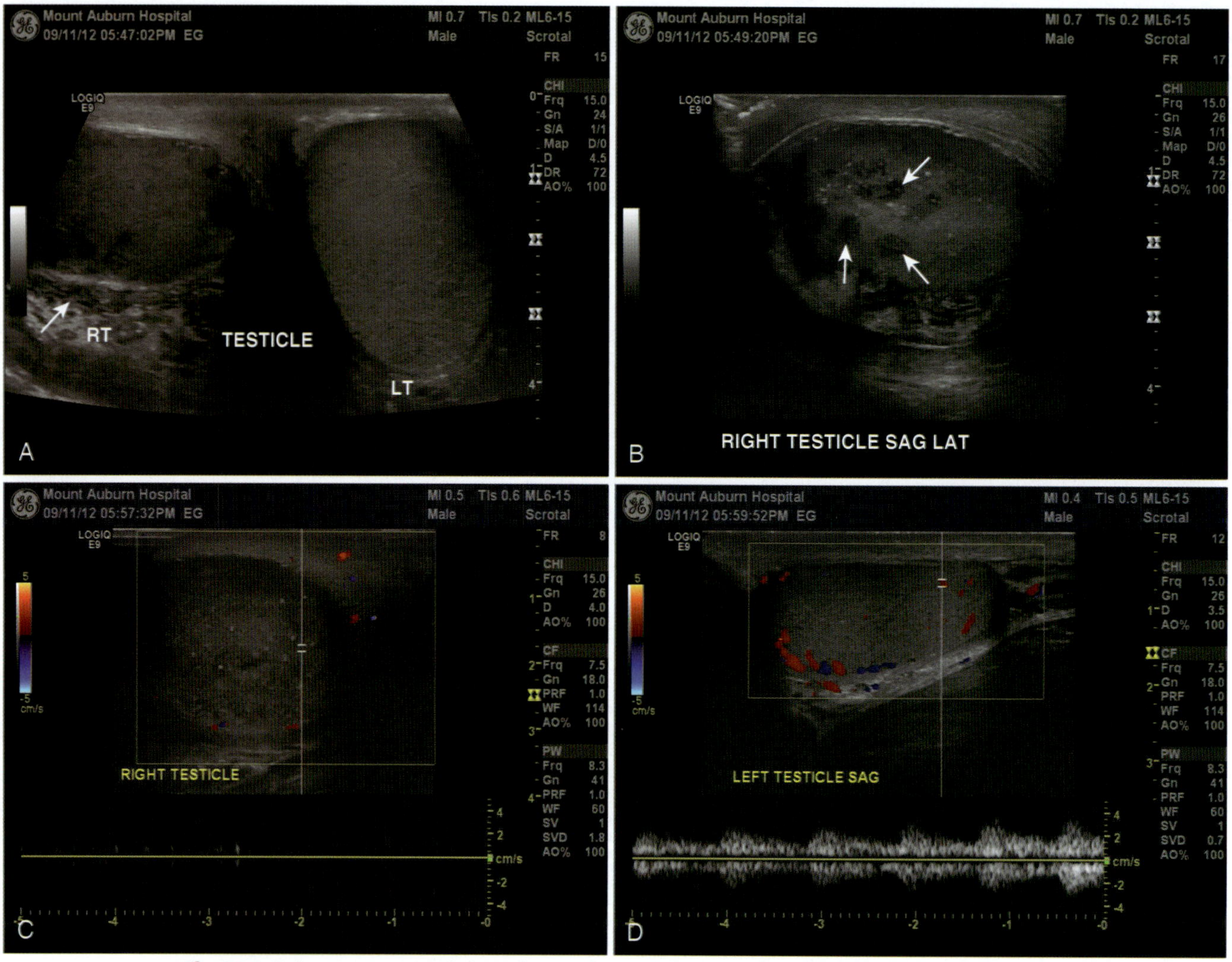

Fig. 56.2 Ischemic necrosis of the right testicle secondary to testicular torsion. This patient was evaluated in the emergency department 9 days after the onset of intermittent testicular pain. (A) Transverse view of the scrotum showing the right testicle to be in a horizontal lie. Also note the cobblestoning of surrounding tissue *(arrow)*, indicative of localized edema. (B) Sagittal view of the right testicle revealing diffuse, round, complex hypoechoic foci *(arrows)*, indicative of ischemic necrosis. (C–D) Color flow Doppler imaging revealing no flow in the right testicle and normal flow in the left. Right orchiectomy was required. *LAT,* Lateral; *LT,* left; *RT,* right; *SAG,* sagittal.

Spermatic Cord Anesthesia

See Video 56.1. Local anesthesia of the spermatic cord using 1% plain lidocaine is usually done at the external inguinal ring and ultrasound guidance may be used as an adjunct to avoid intravascular injection, hematoma formation, and perforation of the deferent duct (see Fig. 56.1B).[20] First prepare the skin with an antiseptic solution. The cord can usually be grasped between the thumb and the index finger, and 10 mL of 1% plain lidocaine (for an adult) can be directly injected in and around the cord. If the cord is swollen, as is often the case in testicular torsion, or if the testicle is lying high in the hemiscrotum as a result of spermatic cord torsion (so as to preclude grasping), the cord may be palpated at the pubic tubercle as it passes over the pubis and the lidocaine injected at this landmark.

Manual Detorsion

See Videos 56.2, 56.3. The goal of manual detorsion is to reestablish (or increase) blood flow to a previously ischemic testis. This should be done in conjunction with preparation of the operating suite in highly suspect cases.

Before initiating detorsion, ensure that the patient is as comfortable as possible in a reclining or supine position. Lithotomy position gives the examiner greatest access to the appropriate anatomy and prevents the patient from retreating during the procedure. If light analgesia and/or sedation are selected, implement them at this time.

Manual detorsion begins with the clinician standing comfortably at the side of the bed or stretcher, preferably on the patient's right side if the clinician is right-handed, or vice versa. Detorsion is begun just as one would open a book (i.e., an initial 180-degree detorsion of the patient's right testis is done in a counterclockwise fashion) (see Fig. 56.1C). The patient's left testis is detorsed 180 degrees in a clockwise fashion. Pain relief is an objective end point. If one rotation relieves some but not all the pain, continue with another rotation. The degree of torsion may range from 180 to 1080 degrees with medians of 360 to 540 degrees. As such, patients may require two or three rotations to alleviate pain. If the initial detorsion is mechanically difficult (which it will be if one is detorsing in the wrong direction) or makes the pain worse, attempt to detorse the testis in the opposite direction and observe the result. Approximately one-third of testicular torsions occur in the lateral, or unexpected, direction. Additionally, detorsion may also require testicular rotation through the caudal-cranial plane (see Fig. 56.1D). The objective success of any testicular manipulation can be substantiated by an increase in Doppler signal or the patient's relief of pain.

With successful detorsion, the testicle returns to its normal anatomic position. Resolution of induration and swelling of the spermatic cord, testis, and epididymis will depend on the degree and duration of ischemia. Thus the more severe the torsion and the longer it has been present, the longer it will take for the edema and induration to resolve. With significant ischemia, the entire epididymis can become enlarged like a link sausage (uncommon in epididymitis except in severe cases or those that are initially misdiagnosed or seen late in their clinical course), and the testis becomes quite firm, simulating a testicular tumor. In some authors' experience, these reversible changes usually resolve over 3 to 4 hours.

Aftercare

Provide systemic analgesics as needed for discomfort. Importantly, even though manual detorsion can save an ischemic testicle, it should not be substituted for definitive scrotal exploration.

Complications

In a portion of cases, the testis will torse in the opposite direction (medial to lateral) or have multiple twists. This may become apparent as the clinician assesses the results of the detorsion procedure by palpation, relief of edema, and return or increase of the Doppler signal.

Conclusions

Spermatic cord torsion may be relieved by manual detorsion. In two-thirds of cases, this is accomplished by medial to lateral rotation of the affected testicle. In the remaining one-third of cases, lateral to medial rotation is necessary to untwist the spermatic cord. In all cases, manual detorsion, even when successful, only serves as a temporizing bridge to definitive surgical management.

PRIAPISM

Introduction

Priapism is defined as prolonged erection of the penis, generally lasting over 4 hours, in the absence of sexual desire or stimulation (Fig. 56.3). This medical condition was named after Priapus, an ancient Greek god of fertility and horticulture who was endowed with oversized genitalia.

Priapism can be divided into two main categories. Ischemic priapism, also known as *low-flow priapism*, is the most commonly seen variant and is due to painful venous engorgement of the corpora cavernosa and requires emergency treatment. Nonischemic (high-flow) priapism is comparatively rare and is often painless. It is caused by increased arterial inflow to the penis as a result of traumatic arteriocavernosal fistulae and does not necessitate urgent intervention.

Ischemic priapism can be thought of as a compartment syndrome of the penis.[21] The corpora cavernosa becomes engorged with stagnant, oxygen-depleted venous blood due to either an intraluminal obstruction of venous blood flow or an inability of the penile muscle tissue to adequately contract and augment venous outflow.[22]

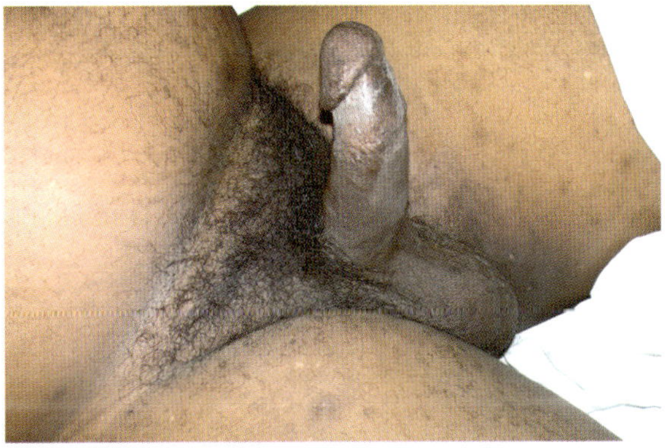

Fig. 56.3 Typical appearance of priapism. It has many causes, is typically painful, can be recurrent, and can potentially lead to impotence. Many cases can be effectively treated in the emergency department setting.

Procedure Overview

Indications: failure of an initial trial of subcutaneous or oral terbutaline (optional).

Contraindications: high-flow (nonischemic) priapism, stuttering priapism.

Complications: hematoma formation, infection, systemic absorption, and subsequent effects of α-adrenergic agents; permanent impotence may result from priapism regardless of promptness of therapeutic interventions.

Equipment: see later.

Key Procedure Sequence

1. Administer parenteral opioid analgesic or light sedation.
2. Give a trial of 0.25 mg to 0.5 mg subcutaneous terbutaline (repeat in 15 minutes), or 5 mg terbutaline by mouth (optional).
3. Give an intracorporal injection of α-adrenergic agents and, if necessary, repeat every 20 minutes for a total of three doses (minimally invasive approach).
4. If unsuccessful, aspirate 20 to 30 mL of corporal blood.
5. If detumescence is not achieved, irrigate with saline or a dilute α-adrenergic agonist solution (aspirate-irrigate-aspirate cycle, as needed).
6. A visible change from venous (dark red) to arterial (bright red) blood is a marker of success.
7. For persistent erections, consult urology for possible shunt placement (cavernosum-spongiosum shunt).
8. If the procedure is successful, loosely wrap the penis in an elastic bandage.
9. A 3-day course of an oral α-adrenergic agent is reasonable at the time of discharge.
10. Arrange for urgent urology follow-up and provide strict return precautions.

Description

Background

Priapism is manifested by a persistent, usually painful, penile erection, unrelated to sexual stimulation and not relieved by ejaculation.

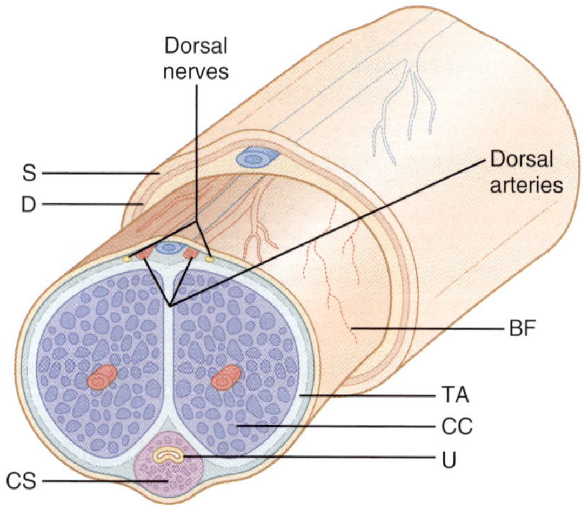

Fig. 56.4 Anatomy of the penile shaft. The corpora cavernosa communicate with each other, and thus unilateral injection or aspiration will typically suffice in the treatment of acute priapism. *BF,* Buck's fascia; *CC,* corpora cavernosa; *CS,* corpus spongiosum; *D,* dartos; *S,* skin; *TA,* tunica albuginea; *U,* urethra. (From Bostwick DG, Cheng L, eds. *Urologic Surgical Pathology.* 2nd ed. Mosby; 2008.)

Over one-third of patients with severe priapism may experience permanent erectile dysfunction despite treatment, with obvious functional and emotional sequelae.[22]

Anatomy and Physiology

Priapism is characterized clinically by a soft glans penis and spongy urethra in the presence of two erect penile bodies (corpora cavernosa) (Fig. 56.4). Two important concepts are worthy of mention. First, there is communication of blood flow between the corpora cavernosa; therefore, in most cases the operator needs to access only one of the corpora. Secondly, introduction of vasoactive or other agents into the corpora is akin to an intravenous injection; thus, systemic effects may be precipitated, particularly after partial or full detumescence is achieved.

Pathophysiology

The pathophysiology of priapism is complex. The pharmacologic basis for treatment is based on manipulating blood flow via the α- and β-adrenergic receptors. Priapism is believed to result from increased arterial inflow of blood into the corpora cavernosa secondary to dilation of the cavernosal arteries. Relaxation of the cavernosal tissue occurs and secondary compression of the emissary veins leads to engorgement of both corpora cavernosa during an erection. When the cavernosal pressure approaches the arterial pressure, blood flow is markedly reduced. Ischemic or low-flow priapism results after several hours of continuous painful erection, leading to intracavernosal acidosis and sludging of blood, with subsequent thrombosis of the cavernosal arteries, fibrosis of the corporal tissue, and potentially irreversible impotence.

High-flow priapism is less common than low-flow priapism and usually results from traumatic creation of arteriocavernosal fistulae. It is not associated with intracavernosal ischemia or acidosis and is therefore painless and may be treated electively rather than emergently.

Historically, priapism was primarily encountered as a complication of a number of medical (e.g., hematologic, neoplastic, and drug-related) conditions (Table 56.1). Today, many cases are iatrogenic, resulting from the current practice of using vasoactive substances (e.g., papaverine and phentolamine) and other newer erectile dysfunction medications to induce penile erections in males with erectile dysfunction. Sickle cell disease continues to be a leading cause of priapism.[23] Sickle cell patients may experience such a high rate of recurrence that home self-injection of vasoactive drugs into the penis

TABLE 56.1 Selected Causes of Ischemic Priapism

CATEGORY	EXAMPLES
Medications	
Impotence agents	Intracavernosal therapies (prostaglandin E1, papaverine, phentolamine)
	Oral agents (sildenafil)
Anticoagulants	Heparin, warfarin
Antihypertensives	Hydralazine, prazosin, doxazosin
Antidepressants	Trazodone, fluoxetine, sertraline, citalopram
Antipsychotics	Phenothiazines, atypical antipsychotics
Hormones	Gonadotropin-releasing hormones, testosterone
Illicit substances	Cocaine, marijuana, alcohol
Miscellaneous	Hydroxyzine, metoclopramide, omeprazole, total parenteral nutrition, general anesthetics
Hematologic/Oncologic Disorders	
Sickle cell disease	
Hematologic malignancies	Leukemia, myeloma
Other malignancies	Prostate, bladder, metastatic cancer
Central Nervous System	
Brain	Cerebrovascular accident
Brain stem	Medulla injury
Spinal cord	Spinal stenosis, spinal cord injury, lumbar disk herniation
Others	
Genitourinary trauma	Straddle injury
Infections	Malaria, rabies
Toxins	Black widow, scorpion, carbon monoxide
Metabolic	Amyloidosis, gout, hypertriglyceridemia
Idiopathic	

has been advocated. Cocaine use is one etiology that may be underreported.

Vasoactive drugs promote engorgement of the corpora cavernosa and reduction in venous outflow, which may result in low-flow or ischemic priapism.[24] Several phosphodiesterase inhibitors and prostaglandin E1 are approved by the US Food and Drug Administration (FDA) for the treatment of erectile dysfunction. These medications act by increasing penile blood flow and enhancing smooth muscle relaxation. The incidence of priapism with these medications is low, particularly with the phosphodiesterase inhibitors.[25] Penile rigidity due to a nondeflating penile prosthesis (pseudopriapism) or malignant replacement of the corpora in patients with advanced bladder or prostate cancer may be confused with true priapism.

Indications

The emergency clinician should attempt to identify reversible causes for low-flow priapism and, often in conjunction with a urologic surgeon, initiate specific corrective therapy as soon as possible. Low-flow priapism in children and young adults may be due to sickle cell disease and such cases may respond to noninvasive standard antisickling measures. The role of transfusion therapy in patients with priapism due to sickle cell disease is uncertain.[26]

Regardless of the etiology, this distressing condition is first treated with adequate analgesia, often consisting of parenteral opioids, with or without benzodiazepines.

A urologic surgeon typically manages acute priapism. However, emergency treatment for ischemic priapism will frequently need to be initiated while awaiting specialty input. The classic teaching is that the initial treatment, oral (or subcutaneous) terbutaline, is the same regardless of the inciting etiology, although the utility and efficacy of terbutaline continue to be debated.[27] Terbutaline, a β2-adrenergic agonist, is thought to increase venous outflow from the engorged corpora by way of relaxation of venous sinusoidal smooth muscle. Terbutaline is of unproved benefit; however, given its limited propensity for adverse effects, a trial is reasonable in select circumstances while awaiting specialty input.[28]

If terbutaline fails to work rapidly, the next steps generally include penile blood aspiration, saline irrigation of the corpora cavernosum, and intracorporal instillation of an α-adrenergic receptor agonist such as dilute phenylephrine or epinephrine.

Contraindications

A subtype of ischemic priapism is known as stuttering priapism. This entity is typically observed in patients with sickle cell disease. Patients experience recurrent episodes of priapism that often last less than 3 hours and are less prone to requiring emergency treatment unless symptoms become markedly prolonged.[29] High-flow (nonischemic) priapism is treated surgically (elective repair).

Procedure

A suggested algorithm for the initial treatment of acute nonischemic priapism in the emergency setting is presented in Box 56.1. Options for treatment include:

- Minimally invasive technique (direct intracorporal injection of α-adrenergic agent, without aspiration or irrigation).
- Aspiration of corporal blood
  - may be performed with or without saline irrigation,
  - following aspiration, may be followed by injection of α-adrenergic agent,
  - alternatively, corpora can be irrigated with a dilute α-adrenergic agent–containing solution.

BOX 56.1 Suggested Algorithm for the Initial Treatment of Acute Priapism in the Emergency Department

Proceed with treatment of acute priapism in the following order until detumescence is achieved:

1. Parenteral narcotic analgesia or sedation.
2. Terbutaline, 0.25 to 0.5 mg subcutaneously (may be repeated in 15 minutes), or terbutaline, 5 mg orally (one dose only).
3. Intracorporal injection of adrenergic agents. May repeat every 20 minutes for a total of three doses.
4. If unsuccessful, perform corporal aspiration of 30 to 60 mL of blood, followed by observation. If detumescence is not achieved, irrigate (inject and remove 10- to 20-mL aliquots) with a diluted α-agonist solution (e.g., phenylephrine, 10 mg in 500 mL of normal saline, or 1 mg epinephrine in 1 L of normal saline). Multiple irrigations may be required. The initial aspiration removes venous blood (dark red) and return of arterial blood (bright red) may serve as a marker of success.
5. For persistent erections, engage urology for possible corpus cavernosum-spongiosum shunt placement.
6. If treatment is successful in the emergency department, discharge is possible. A 3-day course of an oral α-adrenergic agent such as pseudoephedrine to promote continued vasoconstriction is recommended. The value of this intervention is unproven, however.

Minimally Invasive Technique: Simple Injection

See Videos 56.4 and 56.5. Relief of priapism by simple injection of vasoactive solutions into the corpus cavernosum has been reported.[30] Intercavernous injection therapy for the management of priapism is simple to perform, less traumatic, and less invasive than aspiration and irrigation. This minimally invasive procedure may be attempted as an initial approach. This same procedure may be used as a self-injection technique for home treatment of recurrent priapism. With this technique, a 25- to 27-gauge needle is used to inject vasoactive substances into the corpus at the proximal end (base) of the penis (2 cm to 4 cm distal to the shaft origin), with the goal of pharmacologically reversing priapism (Fig. 56.5A). Often this can be accomplished without anesthesia. One option is to draw up 0.5 mg (0.5 mL) of phenylephrine and add 0.5 mL of saline diluent for a final volume of 1 mL (Table 56.2). Puncture the corpus with the needle at the 10 o'clock or 2 o'clock position at the base of the penis (with 12 o'clock being the dorsal vein of the penis), aspirate blood to confirm position, and inject the solution. If detumescence is not achieved in 20 to 30 minutes, give a repeat dose, up to a total of three injections. Alternatively, 0.1 mg of epinephrine (0.1 mL of 1:1000) diluted with 0.9 mL of saline may be used (1 mL total volume). Regardless of medication utilized, only one side needs to be injected, though two or three injections might be necessary. Wait at least 20 minutes after each injection before additional interventions. Note that this is essentially an intravenous injection and thus systemic effects may occur. As such, proceed with caution in patients with cardiovascular disease. Success has also been noted by injecting the corpus cavernosum with 1 mL of the

Management of Acute Priapism

A. Minimally Invasive Method

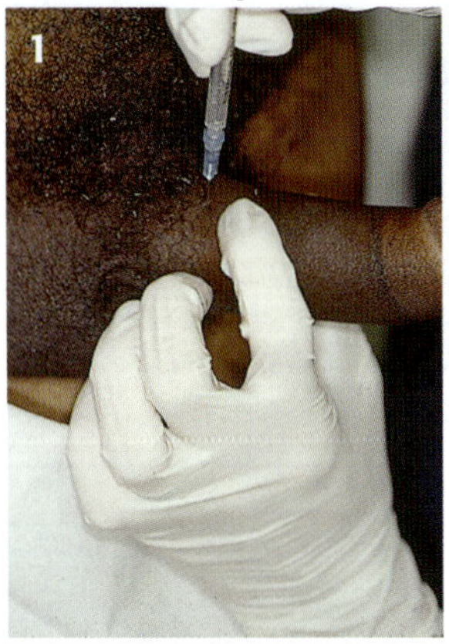

10 o'clock approach

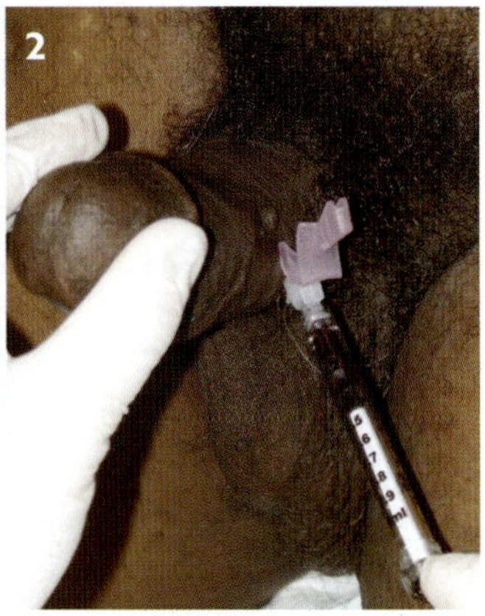

2 o'clock approach

- Anesthesia is not required. Use a small-gauge needle to inject a small aliquot of an adrenergic agent into the corpus at 10 or 2 o'clock at the proximal end of the penile shaft. (Only one side need be injected.)
- Aspirate blood *(2)* to confirm placement prior to injection.
- Consider a repeated injection after 20 minutes if unsuccessful, but be wary of the systemic effects of adrenergic agents (especially if repeated doses or injections are given during partial detumescence).
  Maximum: 3 doses, at least 20 minutes apart

Adrenergic Agents
- 0.2 to 0.5 mg of phenylephrine per dose (refer to text for instructions on dilution)
- 0.1 mg of epinephrine (0.1 mL of a 1:1000 solution) mixed with 0.9 mL of saline

(Use a 1-mL tuberculin syringe to draw up these small volumes.)

B. Aspiration and Irrigation Method

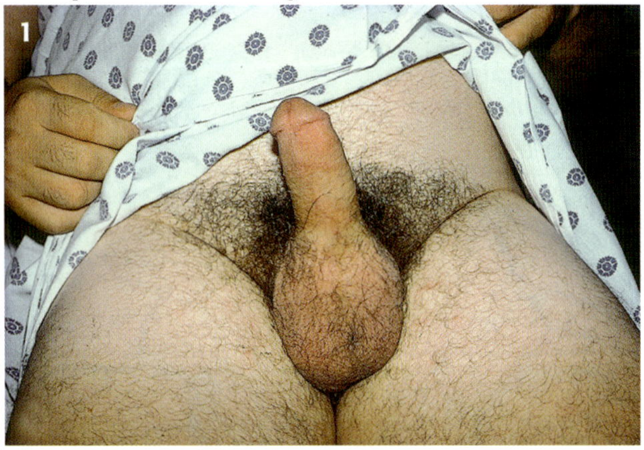

This patient experienced 18 hours of priapism after penile self-injection of papaverine as therapy for impotence.

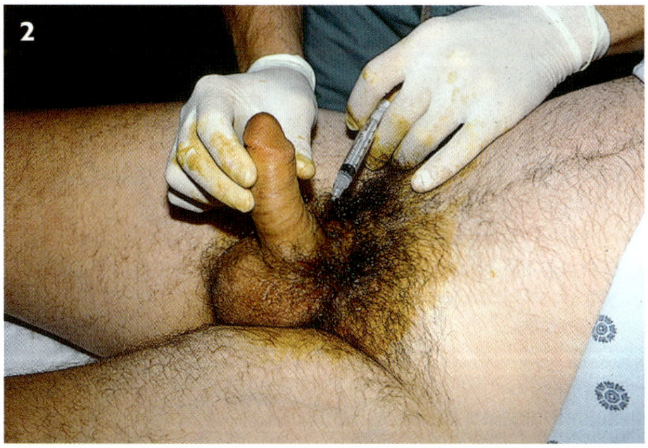

For corpus irrigation the irrigation needle can be placed through a simple skin wheal, or peform a penile dorsal nerve block by injecting 1% plain lidocaine at the base of the dorsal aspect of the penis. The dorsal nerves are relatively superficial and deep injections are not required.

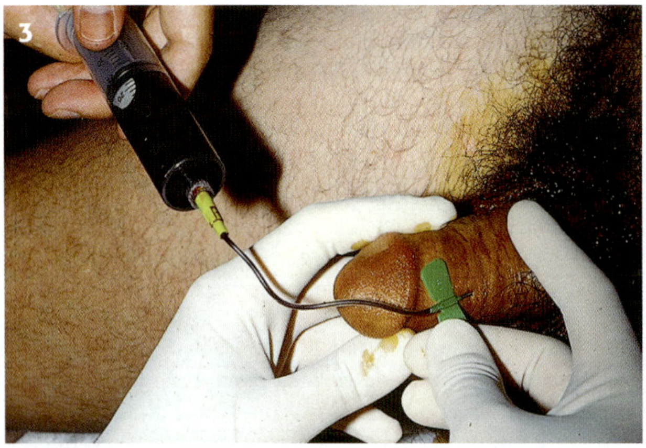

Insert no smaller than a 19-gauge butterfly needle into the corpus via the proximal penile shaft at either the 2 o'clock or the 10 o'clock position and aspirate. Only one side need be punctured. Slow steady suction will be most successful, whereas excessive suction may halt the aspiration. Do not puncture the corpus via the glans (see text). After initial aspiration, irrigate (slowly inject and withdraw) 10- to 20-mL aliquots of vasoactive solution until detumescence persists.

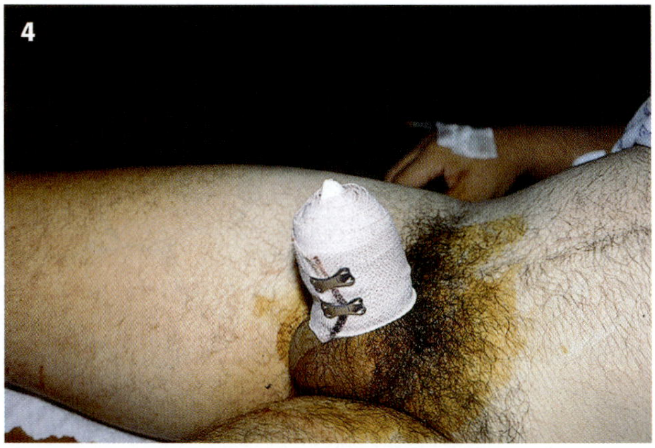

After detumescence with the first aspiration or with aspiration-irrigation-aspiration of a vasoactive medication (see text), wrap the penis with an elastic bandage to discourage reengorgement and to compress the puncture site. Note: Acceptable procedures include aspiration alone followed by instillation of a small aliquot of epinephrine (0.1 mg) and combined multiple aspirations and irrigations with a vasoactive solution. The end point is the appearance of bright red arterial blood and/or persistent detumescence.

Fig. 56.5 Management of acute priapism. The minimally invasive technique (A) consists of directly injecting the corpus with a small aliquot of an adrenergic agent. This is often successful and can be used at home by a motivated patient with recurrent priapism (such as sickle cell disease). It may require 15 to 20 minutes to be effective and, at times, repeat injections.

TABLE 56.2 Adrenergic Agents Used for Intracavernous Injections

AGENT	DOSE	VOLUME
Phenylephrine[a]	0.2–0.5 mg	Dilute with saline; final volume, 1 mL[a]
Epinephrine (1:1000)	0.1 mg (0.1 mL)	Dilute with 0.9 mL saline; final volume, 1 mL
Lidocaine (2%) with epinephrine (1.100,000) (local anesthetic solution)	40 mg lidocaine 0.02 mg epinephrine (2 mL)	1 mL injected into each side of the corpus cavernosum; final volume, 2 mL[b]

[a]Single side injected with the entire amount. See text for preparation of the phenylephrine injection solution.
[b]Total amount divided into two doses. Inject each side with half the total volume (1 mL) or inject the total volume (2 mL) into one side.
From Roberts JR, Price C, Mazzeo T. Intracavernous epinephrine: a minimally invasive treatment for priapism in the emergency department. *J Emerg Med.* 2009;36(3):285-289.

local anesthetic lidocaine (2%) with epinephrine (1:100,000) into each side, or 2 mL into one side.[30]

Aspiration/Irrigation Technique

See Videos 56.6–56.8. Box 56.2 lists the equipment needed for aspiration and irrigation of the corpus cavernosum. This procedure entails drainage of blood from the erect penis, irrigation with saline if necessary (e.g., inadequate return of blood with lack of detumescence), and finally the instillation of a vasoactive medication. Alternatively, irrigation with aliquots of a dilute vasoactive solution may be effective (aspirate-infuse-aspirate cycle as needed).

Place the patient in the supine position. Parenteral analgesia and sedation are suggested. Local anesthesia at the puncture site is recommended. An injection of 1% plain lidocaine placed at the base of the penis for a dorsal penile nerve block or placement of a circumferential penile block can be performed, but is usually not necessary (see Fig. 56.5B). Prepare and drape the penis in sterile fashion. Grasp the shaft of the penis with your nondominant thumb and index finger. Palpate the engorged corpus cavernosum laterally (2 and 10 o'clock positions) and insert a 21- to 19-gauge butterfly needle into the corpus cavernosum. Alternatively, a 20-gauge intravenous catheter may be used, but the butterfly needle is preferred. A dialysis access butterfly needle may also be used (Fig. 56.6).

If palpation fails to demonstrate the corpus, blindly inserting the needle at either 10 o'clock or 2 o'clock will usually gain access to this large vascular structure. Because there is communication of blood flow between both sides, the operator needs access to only one of the corpora. Either side may be punctured. The site of needle placement is typically anywhere from the base to the proximal shaft, 2 cm to 4 cm distal from the shaft origin. The glans should not be used as a puncture site.

The needle is advanced at a 45-degree angle, using constant suction. Blood is usually readily aspirated; once blood is obtained do not advance the needle further. Next, stabilize the needle. Avoid deep penetration to minimize the risk of injury to the cavernosal artery during this procedure.

Aspirate an initial 20 to 30 mL of corporal blood while milking the corpus with the nondominant hand. Do not apply excessive suction because this often halts the aspiration. A common error is to use too much suction with a 60-mL syringe. Using a 10-mL syringe, and changing it if it fills with blood, is preferable. Use of a butterfly reduces the danger of dislodging the needle when changing syringes.

Continue aspiration until the original egress of dark blood ceases and bright red arterial blood returns, or when complete detumescence is obtained and persists. Because multiple anastomoses exist between the two corpora cavernosa, bilateral aspiration is not required. If there is inadequate return of blood with a lack of detumescence, consider irrigating with 20 to 30 mL of saline.

BOX 56.2 Equipment Needed for Aspiration of the Corpus Cavernosum for Low-Flow Priapism

27-gauge needle (for penile block)
1-mL syringe (for local anesthetic)
1% lidocaine without epinephrine (for penile block)
Sterile drapes
Gauze sponges
Chlorhexidine preparation solution
19-gauge butterfly needles (for aspiration)
Two 10- to 30-mL syringes (for aspiration)
Sterile basin for aspirated blood
Blood gas syringe with cap
Irrigation fluid (one of the following vasoactive agents[a] is diluted with 500 mL of normal saline and 20 to 30 mL is administered in small aliquots; 5000 units of heparin added to the solution is optional):
  Phenylephrine, 10 mg/500 mL of saline
  Norepinephrine, 1 mg/500 mL of saline
  Epinephrine, 0.5 mg/500 mL of saline

[a]*Systemic absorption of vasoactive agents may occur and result in adverse cardiovascular effects.*

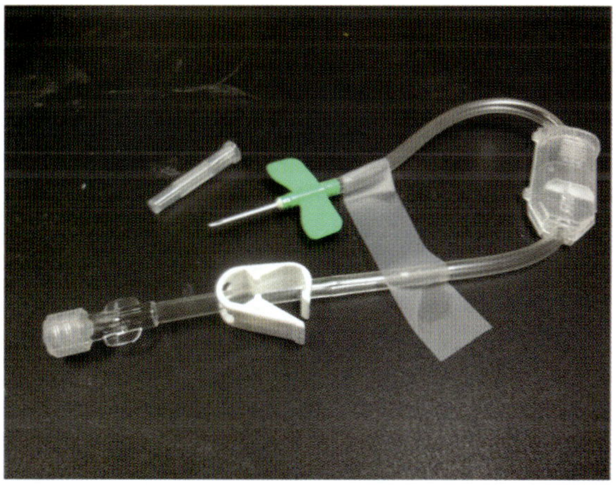

Fig. 56.6 An 18-gauge dialysis or butterfly catheter can be used for irrigation of the corpora if simple aspiration or injections of medication are unsuccessful. Utilizing needles smaller than 19-gauge caliber is often counterproductive.

If detumescence is achieved after initial aspiration with or without saline irrigation, no further treatment may be required. If this is successful, some clinicians advise instilling an aliquot of a vasoactive substance. Phenylephrine is recommended as the agent of choice as it may minimize the risk of cardiovascular side effects more commonly seen with other sympathomimetic agents.[27] Inject 0.1 to 0.5 mg of phenylephrine (in 1 mL of normal saline). It is important to note that the recommended concentration for instillation is similar to that recommended for the minimally invasive technique detailed earlier. Lower concentrations in smaller volumes should be used for patients with cardiovascular risk factors or for children. If irrigation is performed with a dilute vasoactive substance as delineated hereafter, additional medication instillation is not suggested.

If detumescence is not achieved following aspiration (with or without saline irrigation), irrigation with a dilute vasoactive substance is another option. A number of dilute irrigation solutions have been suggested, but none have been proven to be superior. Some suggest 20 to 30 mL of a phenylephrine/normal saline solution (10 mg of phenylephrine in 500 mL of normal saline) as the exchange aliquots for 20 to 30 mL of aspirated corporal blood. Some clinicians add 2500 to 5000 units of heparin to the solution, but the use of heparin is of unproven value. Alternatively, 1 mg of epinephrine can be added to 1 L of saline, with irrigation performed using 20- to 30-mL aliquots. It is important to note that corporal irrigation is performed with a significantly less concentrated solution (phenylephrine, 20 μg/mL) as compared with that used for the minimally invasive technique or vasoactive instillation of 1 mL aliquots following detumescence detailed earlier (phenylephrine, 500 μg/mL).

The corpus cavernosum has ready access to the systemic circulation and injecting a drug into it is essentially the same as an intravenous injection. When detumescence occurs, the unmetabolized drug enters the systemic circulation; therefore, vasoactive drug dosages should be monitored carefully.

Aftercare

Observe the patient in the ED for recurrence. Although the ideal observation period is unknown, 2 hours has been suggested.[30] Fig. 56.5B, *step 4* demonstrates the entire penis loosely wrapped with elastic bandage (ACE, 3M) to prevent hematoma formation at the injection site(s). Strict return precautions should be provided for priapism recurrence, and urgent urology follow-up should be ensured. A short course of an oral α-adrenergic agent, such as pseudoephedrine for 3 days, is often recommended, though the value of this intervention is of questionable value and unproven benefit.[30]

Complications

Although hematoma formation or infection can occur with properly performed aspiration, these complications are infrequent. Injected or instilled vasoactive agents can be absorbed systemically, with the potential for toxic effects. Therefore the intracavernosal use of vasoactive agents is relatively contraindicated in patients with conditions sensitive to these agents (e.g., severe hypertension, dysrhythmias, monoamine oxidase inhibitor use, etc.). Blood pressure and cardiac rhythm should be monitored throughout the procedure if the patient is at risk. Failure to aspirate blood is a potential complication, usually because of a misplaced needle, applying excessive suction, or if blood has clotted. Because impotence is a well-recognized complication of priapism regardless of the cause or the promptness of therapeutic intervention, the patient should be advised regarding this potential long-term consequence.

Conclusions

Because prolonged priapism increases the risk of subsequent erectile dysfunction, an aggressive management strategy is advised. After 4 hours of persistent priapism, there is heightened release of inflammatory cytokines in the acidotic and hypoxic corpora cavernosa. Inflammation may include smooth muscle changes including cell death and fibrosis, which may cause permanent erectile dysfunction.[31] Recurrence is not uncommon, and some patients require multiple procedures on a recurring basis. Surgical shunting procedures by the urology team might be required if these additional measures are met without success.

PARAPHIMOSIS

Introduction

Paraphimosis is the inability to completely reduce the penile foreskin distally, back to its natural position overlying the glans penis. This condition occurs exclusively in uncircumcised males and is a urologic emergency.

Paraphimosis may occur at any age, but most often occurs in the extremes of life (Fig. 56.7). The condition can be quite subtle and may be either unrecognized or misdiagnosed as an allergic reaction, penile trauma, infection, or edema resulting from systemic volume overload (e.g., congestive heart failure, nephrotic syndrome) (Fig. 56.8).

Iatrogenic paraphimosis may occur following urinary catheterization or medical examination if the foreskin is not returned to its native location overlying the glans. Poor hygiene or balanoposthitis is also associated with the development of paraphimosis. Inflammation can result in contracture of the distal foreskin. Later when the foreskin is retracted proximally over the compressible glans, the contracted foreskin forms a constrictive band and gets caught in the retracted position.

Procedure Overview

Indications: emergency reduction of paraphimotic foreskin.

Contraindications: none.

Complications: skin tears or lacerations; failure of the reduction procedure necessitates surgical intervention (dorsal slit or definitive circumcision).

Equipment: for simple manual reduction, all that is needed is a topical anesthetic lubricant. Adjunctive equipment for alternative reduction techniques and maneuvers as described in this chapter are optional.

Key Procedure Sequence

1. Apply a topical anesthetic lubricant to the distal penis (foreskin and glans).
2. Administer a systemic analgesic (optional).
3. Compress the foreskin and glans with a snugly grasped hand.
4. Use the thumbs to invert the glans penis proximally through the phimotic ring.

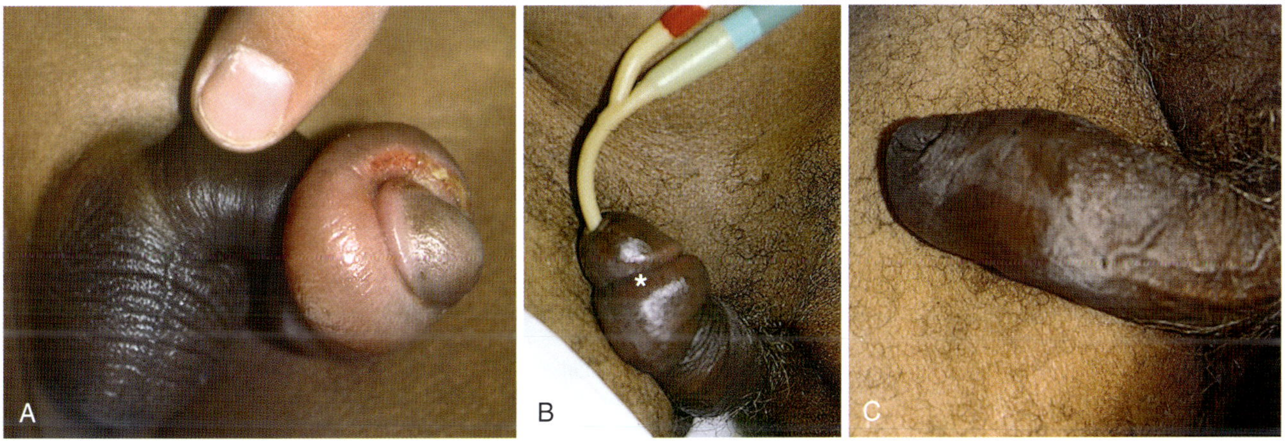

Fig. 56.7 Paraphimosis often occurs in the extremes of life. (A) Uncircumcised boy with paraphimosis. This may be mistaken for infection or localized trauma, especially if it is unclear whether circumcision has been performed, thus it may be prudent to seek this history. (B) Paraphimosis, pictured here, may be mistaken for penile trauma, angioedema, or infection. Note that the swollen tissue is proximal to the coronal sulcus *(asterisk)*. The cause of paraphimosis in this case was failure to replace the foreskin after a catheter change in an uncircumcised older patient. Before reduction, the catheter is typically removed. When the edema is minimal, the catheter may be left in place during reduction. (C) Appearance of the penis after catheter removal and foreskin reduction.

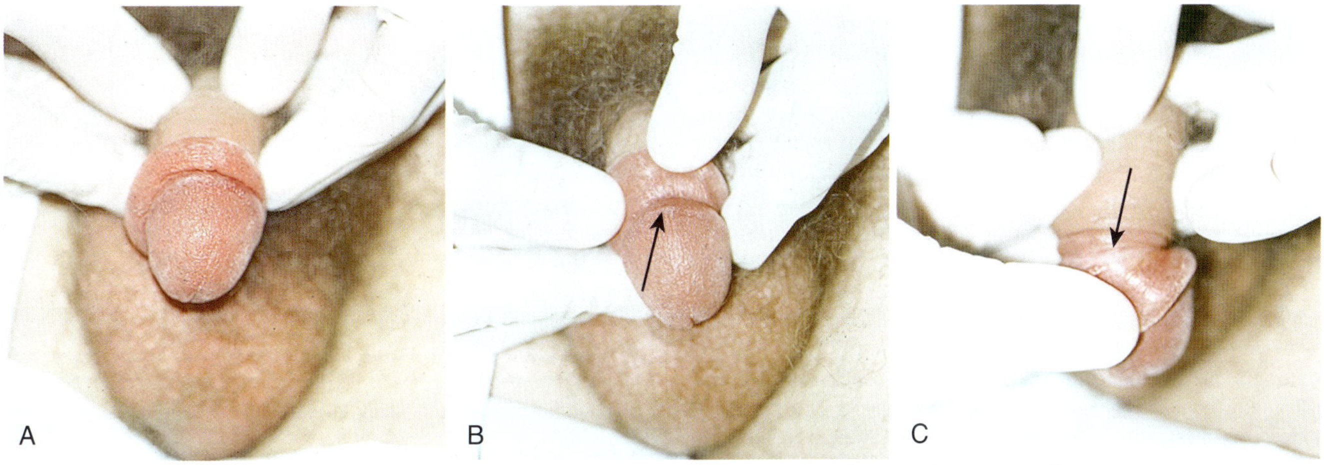

Fig. 56.8 (A) This edematous foreskin may have numerous causes, from benign edema to paraphimosis, and at first glance the inciting etiology might not be obvious. This patient has paraphimosis that is appreciated by careful inspection to identify (B) the normal coronal sulcus and (C) a phimotic foreskin band proximal to the glans.

5. Use the index and long fingers to reduce the phimotic ring distally.
6. If unsuccessful, try alternate maneuvers to reduce edema before reattempting manual reduction.
7. Consider an optional trial of glans adjuncts: administer an ice pack or a compressive bandage to reduce glans edema.
8. Consider an optional trial of foreskin adjuncts: administer micropuncture wounds, use sugar, or use hyaluronidase to reduce foreskin edema.
9. If unsuccessful, reduction of the paraphimosis surgically by dorsal slit or definitive circumcision may be necessary.
10. Arrange urgent urology follow-up following reduction.

Description

Background

Paraphimosis is a urologic emergency that must be treated promptly to prevent glans necrosis. Paraphimosis can be managed in the ED without the need for emergency specialty consultation, though if feasible, urology involvement may be necessary for postprocedure management. There are many reported methods of successful paraphimosis reduction The most commonly employed initial maneuver involves manual compression of the distal penis to decrease edema, followed by reduction of the glans penis back through the proximal constricting band of foreskin (phimotic ring).[32]

Anatomy and Physiology

The penis consists of the paired corpora cavernosa, or erectile bodies, which lie dorsal to the corpus spongiosum (see Fig. 56.4). The corpus spongiosum surrounds the penile urethra. The corpora cavernosa and the corpus spongiosum are wrapped by a thin connective tissue layer, the tunica albuginea. The glans is the distal portion (head) of the penis. The foreskin, or prepuce, in uncircumcised males lies over the glans and can be retracted proximally to expose the glans. The coronal sulcus distinguishes the glans penis from the penile shaft (see Figs. 56.7B and 56.8B).

Pathophysiology

Patients will typically present with a red, painful, and swollen glans penis associated with an edematous, proximally retracted foreskin that forms a circumferential constricting band. The penile shaft proximal to the constricting band is typically soft. Compression from the entrapped, constricting foreskin inhibits venous drainage of the glans and results in a cycle of progressive glans edema. The typical anatomy and identification of the foreskin may be obfuscated by edema, and the condition can appear asymmetric or otherwise unusual (Fig. 56.9, *step 1*). Glans edema may become so severe that arterial flow is compromised, which can result in necrosis and gangrene of the glans penis.

Indications

Emergency reduction is indicated whenever a paraphimosis exists.

Contraindications

There are no contraindications.

Procedure

Manual Reduction Technique

See Video 56.9. The current standard for reducing paraphimosis is manual reduction. This can be accomplished by using a nonirritating topical anesthetic lubricant applied to the inner surface of the foreskin (not to the shaft of the penis) and the glans to reduce friction and decrease the discomfort of the procedure. A penile block may be performed, if necessary (see Fig. 56.9, *steps 2 and 3*). If there is significant discomfort or patient apprehension, systemic analgesia or procedural sedation may be useful adjuncts. For young children, general anesthesia may be necessary.[33]

Compress the foreskin and glans with a snugly grasped hand for several minutes to reduce as much edema fluid as possible (see Fig. 56.9, *steps 4–6*). Use the thumb to push the glans through the constricting foreskin that has been encircled by the operator's entire palm (see Fig. 56.9, *step 7*). Alternatively, place the index and long fingers of both hands in apposition just proximal to the phimotic ring. Align both thumbs near the urethral meatus. Apply constant force with the thumbs to try and invert the glans penis proximally while using the index and long fingers to reduce the phimotic ring distally over the glans penis and into its normal anatomic position (see Fig. 56.9, *step 8*). Successful reduction results in the appearance of an uncircumcised penis with a phimotic foreskin (see Fig. 56.9, *steps 9 and 10*). The key to success in both these maneuvers is the application of slow, steady pressure.

Adjunctive Techniques to Assist in Manual Reduction

Several alternative methods for reducing the edema have been described in the literature. These methods can be used before attempting manual reduction, or if simple manual reduction fails.

Babcock clamps (noncrushing tissue clamps) can be used to reduce the paraphimotic foreskin (Fig. 56.10A). Apply six to eight Babcock clamps spaced evenly around the foreskin, straddling the phimotic ring (one edge just proximal and the other edge just distal to the phimotic ring). Grasp all clamps and apply simultaneous distal traction to pull the phimotic ring over the glans. After reduction, remove the clamps. It is important to inspect the foreskin for injuries.

Other techniques focus on reduction of glans or foreskin edema (or both), followed by reduction of the paraphimosis. Diminished glans edema facilitates foreskin reduction to its natural position. One maneuver is to apply an ice pack. In the "iced glove" method, use cold compression to reduce foreskin swelling and induce vasoconstriction in the glans penis (Fig. 56.10B). Half fill a large glove with crushed ice and water and tie the cuff end of the glove securely. Invaginate the thumb of the glove and then draw it over the lubricated paraphimotic penis. Hold the thumb of the glove securely in place over the glans for 5 to 10 minutes. The combination of cooling and compression may decrease edema sufficiently to permit manual reduction of the foreskin. Wrapping the penis in a compressive bandage is another alternative. A 2-inch compressive bandage can be wound snugly around the penis from the glans to the base and removed after 5 to 7 minutes.

Alternatively, techniques focusing on reduction of foreskin edema have been advocated (Box 56.3). The Dundee technique involves creating multiple micropunctures of the edematous foreskin and then expressing edema fluid. Hyaluronidase has been reported to result in rapid reduction of prepuce edema that facilitates manual reduction of the foreskin. This enzyme, when injected into the swollen retracted foreskin, causes hydrolysis of hyaluronic acid that, in turn, increases tissue permeability so the edema in the foreskin is diffused out into the surrounding penile tissue. There have even been advocates of a noninvasive way to reduce the foreskin edema via the application of granulated sugar or a dextrose solution to the penis. Sugar forms an osmotic gradient that draws out edema fluid, but this may take several hours. Publications on these alternative procedures are generally observational in design with very small numbers. To date, there have not been any large studies of comparative effectiveness; as such it is difficult to recommend any one method as superior.[34]

If the previous methods are unsuccessful, it may be necessary to incise the constricting phimotic tissue to permit reduction of the foreskin over the glans by dorsal slit procedure.[32] In adults, this can generally be carried out under penile-block anesthesia, though procedural sedation or general anesthesia may be necessary for young children.

Aftercare

Observe the patient to ensure adequate local hemostasis, ability to void spontaneously, and recovery from analgesia or sedation, if utilized. Replacing the foreskin to its native position following examination, catheter placement, sexual activity, or any other manipulation is essential to preventing recurrent episodes. Patients should be referred to a urologist for evaluation of possible surgical options, including circumcision.

Complications

Penile shaft laceration or simple tearing of edematous and taut penile skin may occur during manual or surgical paraphimotic reduction. Simple suturing is all that is required for most injuries. If reduction of a paraphimosis cannot be achieved by other means, surgical interventions should be considered.

Conclusions

Emergency manual or surgical reduction of the edematous foreskin is mandatory to restore proper circulation, relieve discomfort, and permit resolution of potentially serious sequelae: skin ulceration and gangrene. It should be performed as rapidly as achievable. Once the foreskin is successfully reduced, urgent referral for dorsal slit or definitive circumcision is prudent.

Paraphimosis Reduction

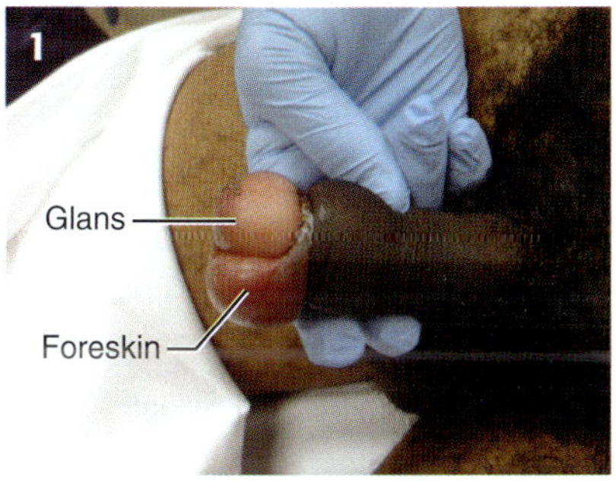

This patient had asymmetric paraphimosis. Note that the glans is edematous, as is the foreskin. A circumferential constricting band is found proximal to the glans and foreskin.

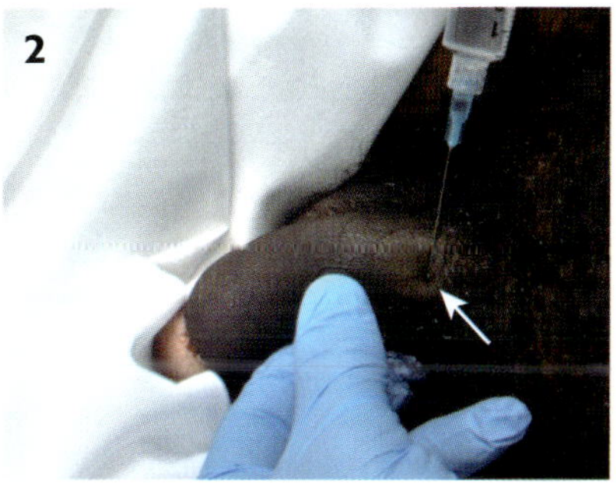

Perform a penile block in cases that will require significant manipulation. First, block the dorsal penile nerves by depositing anesthetic at the 2 and 10 o'clock positions on the dorsal aspect of the shaft of the penis.

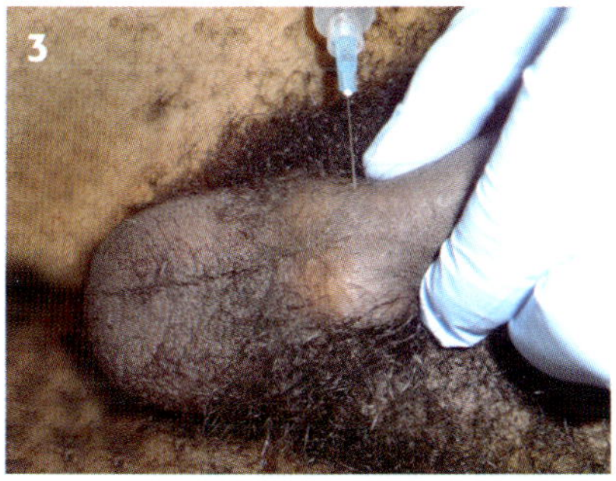

Complete a ring block of the penis by depositing anesthetic circumferentially around the proximal part of the shaft.

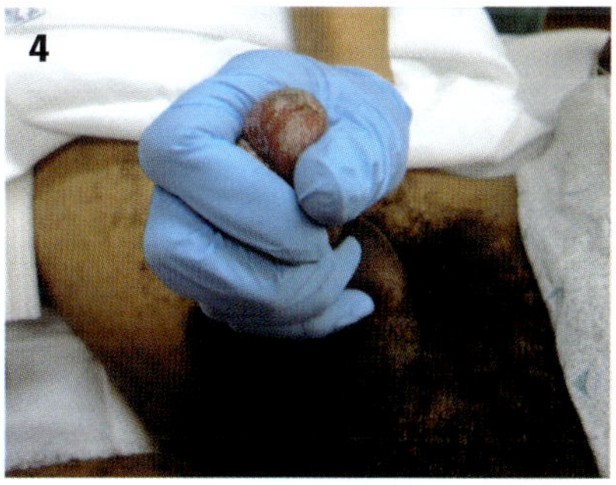

Compress the foreskin and glans by grasping it with the palm of your hand and applying pressure for several minutes.

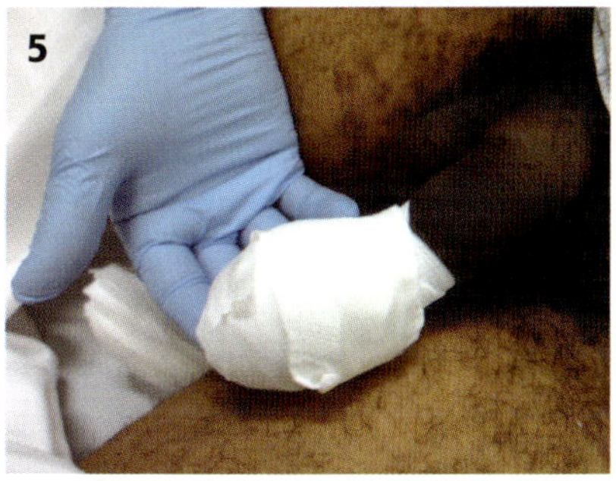

Alternatively, wrap an elastic bandage around the distal end of the penis for several minutes. This step is often omitted, which makes the procedure unnecessarily difficult.

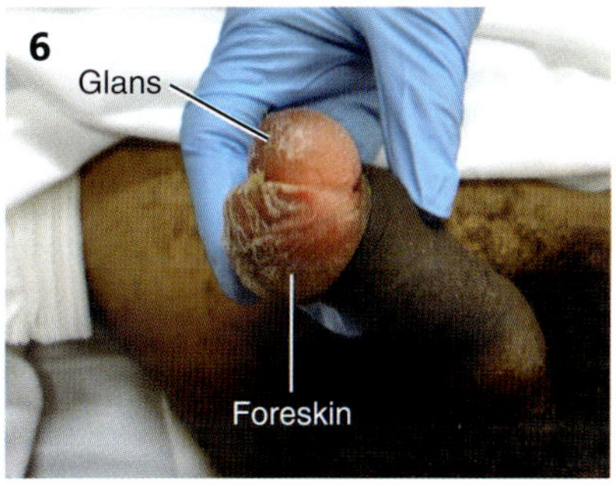

Note that manual compression substantially reduced the amount of swelling (compare with *step 1*; the foreskin and glans were taut prior to compression).

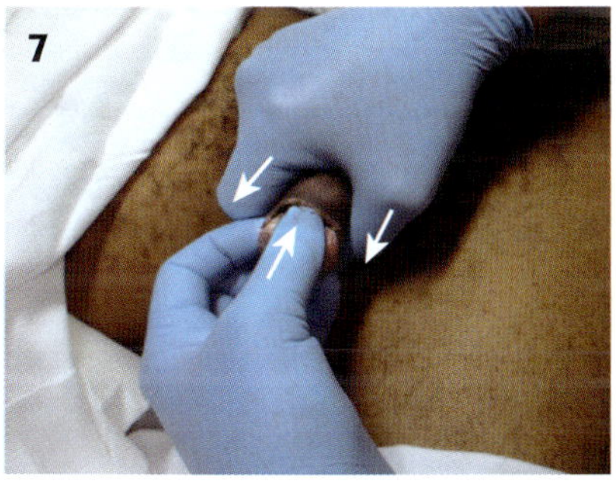

Grasp the shaft of the penis with one hand and apply force onto the urethral meatus with the thumb of your other hand. Push the glans forward while sliding the foreskin distally.

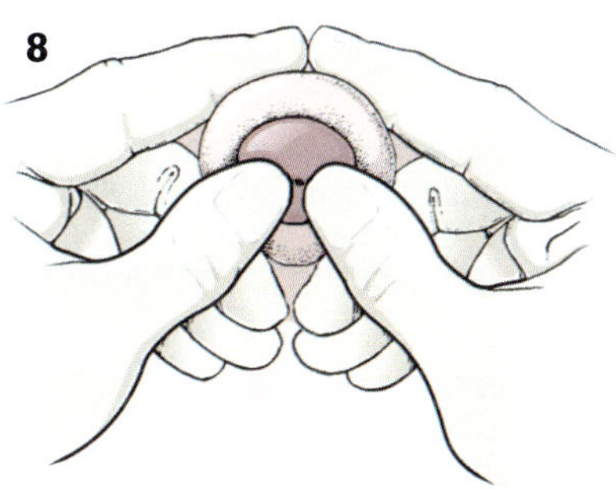

Alternatively, grasp the penis with the fingers of both hands just proximal to the phimotic ring, and use your thumbs to apply constant pressure on the glans.

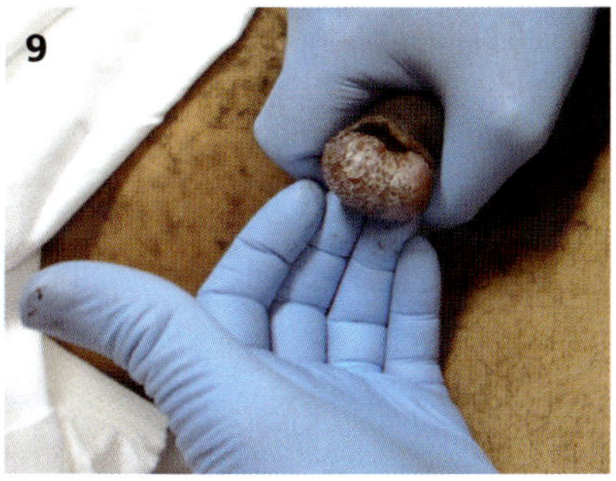

The key to success is the application of slow, steady pressure. Note that the glans has retracted into its normal position and only the edematous foreskin is visible.

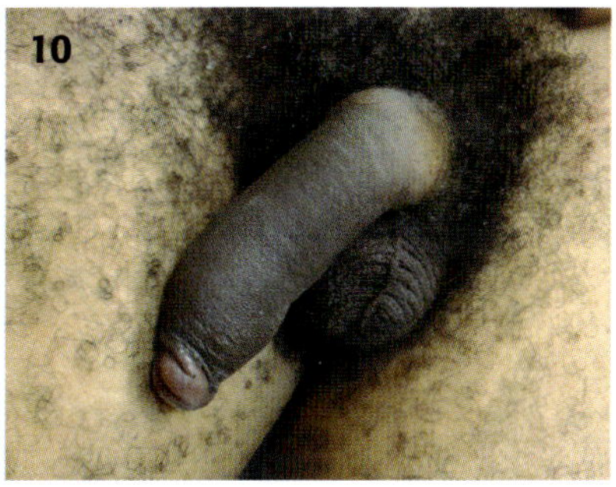

Successful reduction results in the appearance of an uncircumcised penis with a phimotic foreskin.

Fig. 56.9 Paraphimosis reduction. (Step 8, From Neuwirth H, Frasier B, Cochran ST. Genitourinary imaging and procedures by the emergency clinician. *Emerg Med Clin North Am.* 1989;7:1.)

Paraphimosis Reduction: Alternative Techniques

A. Babcock Clamps

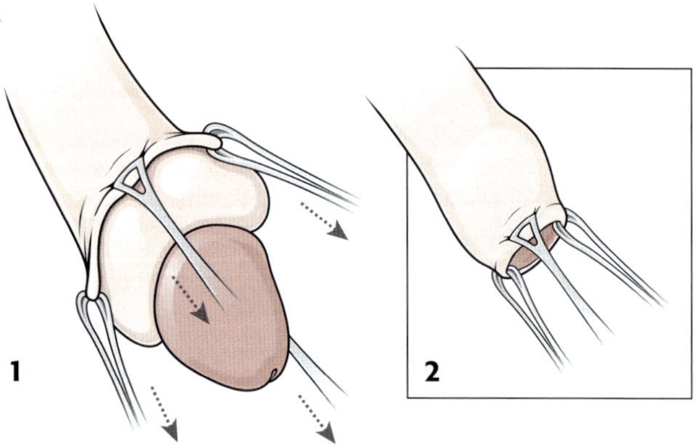

Babcock clamps will not crush tissue. *1,* Place six to eight clamps so that they are evenly spaced on the distal edge of the foreskin and straddling the phimotic ring. *2,* Grasp all clamps and apply simultaneous distal traction to pull the phimotic ring over the glans.

B. Iced-Glove Method

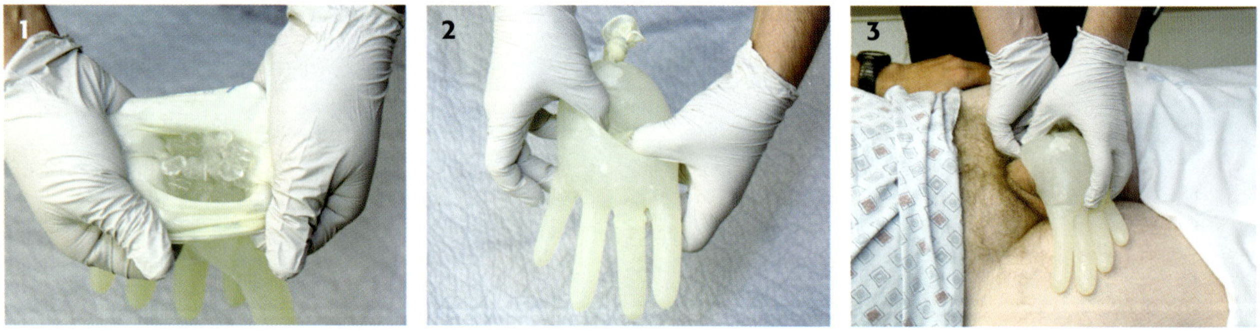

1. Fill a large glove halfway with crushed ice and water.
2. Securely tie the cuff end and invaginate the thumb of the glove.
3. Draw the invagination over the lubricated paraphimotic penis and hold it in place for 5 to 10 minutes. The combination of cooling and compression decreases edema and facilitates foreskin reduction.

Fig. 56.10 Paraphimosis reduction: alternative techniques.

BOX 56.3 Adjunctive Methods to Reduce Foreskin Edema

Dundee micropuncture technique: Make approximately 20 puncture holes in the edematous foreskin tissue with a 26-gauge (or similar) needle and express the fluid.[1]

Hyaluronidase technique: Inject 1 mL of hyaluronidase (150 U/mL) by tuberculin syringe into one or two sites in the edematous foreskin to reduce edema fluid immediately.[2]

Sugar technique: Granulated sugar has been studied, but another alternative for patients in the emergency department is to soak gauze in 50 mL of 50% dextrose solution and leave it wrapped around the paraphimotic foreskin for about 1 hour.[3]

Iced glove technique: see Fig. 56.10B.

1. *Ganti SU, Sayegh N, Addonizio JC. Simple method for the reduction of paraphimosis. Urology 1985;25:77.*
2. *Reynard J, Barua J. Reduction of paraphimosis the simple way – the Dundee technique. BJU Int. 1999;83(7):859-860.*
3. *DeVries C, Miller A. Reduction of paraphimosis with hyaluronidase. Urology 1996;48(3):464-465.*

PHIMOSIS

Introduction

Phimosis is constriction of the foreskin (prepuce) that limits its retraction proximally over the glans (Fig. 56.11). Uncircumcised infants and young children often have a physiologic phimosis due to adhesions between the prepuce and glans. This is in contrast to a pathologic phimosis, where failure to retract results from distal scarring of the prepuce. Circumcision (removal of the foreskin) rates vary widely. Circumcision renders phimosis and paraphimosis anatomically impossible.

Phimosis does not ordinarily require any treatment. However, a patient with phimosis may present acutely to the ED if unable to void spontaneously as a result of distal urethral obstruction. It may render urethral catheterization more challenging or prevent it altogether. In such situations, the phimotic opening may need to be dilated. An alternative strategy is to crush a portion of the foreskin followed by an incision (dorsal slit), using local anesthesia with or without parenteral analgesia or sedation to allow access to the urethral meatus. This procedure can be readily performed in the acute care setting when necessary.

Procedure Overview

Indications:
- Phimosis and the inability to void or the inability to perform urethral catheterization
- As definitive treatment following successful foreskin reduction in a patient with paraphimosis in selected patients
- Phimotic ring incision and foreskin reduction in a patient with an otherwise irreducible paraphimosis

Contraindications: none.

Complications: injury to the urethral meatus or glans penis, bleeding at site of tissue injury (when tissue is crushed and then cut).

Equipment: see later.

Key Procedure Sequence

1. Clean and drape the penis with sterile towels.
2. Inject local anesthesia: lidocaine without epinephrine.
3. Use toothed forceps to test for adequate local anesthesia.
4. If anesthesia is inadequate, consider dorsal nerve block or "ring block" at the base of the penis.
5. Advance both jaws of a straight hemostat proximally between the inner layer of the foreskin and glans.
6. Use the hemostat to separate preputial adhesions.
7. Remove the hemostat, reinsert one jaw, and use the hemostat to crush interposed foreskin tissue.
8. Cut the resultant crushed foreskin tissue longitudinally with straight scissors.
9. Use absorbable sutures to reapproximate leaves of foreskin resulting from the cut (if necessary).
10. With success, the prepuce is easily retracted for exposure of the glans penis and urethral meatus.

Description

Background

Phimosis is constriction of the foreskin that limits proximal retraction of the foreskin over the glans. Phimosis does not ordinarily require any treatment. However, phimosis may present acutely to the ED when a patient is unable to void spontaneously as a result of distal urethral obstruction.

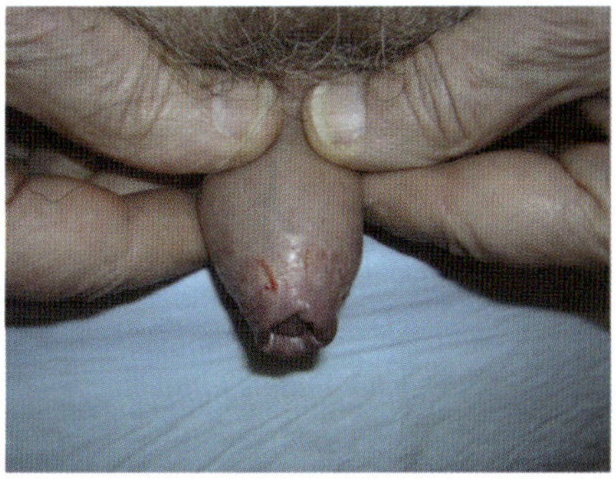

Fig. 56.11 Phimosis is constriction of the foreskin that inhibits retraction proximally over the glans. Ordinarily, treatment is not required; however, dilation of the phimotic opening may be necessary if the patient is unable to void or if urethral catheterization must be performed. (From Studdiford JS, Altshuler M, Salzman B et al., eds. *Images from the Wards: Diagnosis and Treatment.* Saunders; 2009.)

Anatomy and Physiology

A physiologic phimosis in young uncircumcised boys consists of a pliant, unscarred preputial orifice on physical examination. The foreskin gradually becomes retractile over time as a result of intermittent erections and keratinization of the inner epithelium. By 3 years of age, the foreskin can easily be retracted in 90% of patients, with nearly all becoming retractile by late adolescence.[35]

Pathophysiology

A pathologic phimosis exists when the failure to retract results from distal scarring of the prepuce. This is typically a subacute condition that may present acutely to the ED when a patient is unable to void spontaneously as a result of distal urethral obstruction. Pathologic phimosis is caused by local trauma, infection, chemical irritation, complications of circumcision (insufficient tissue removal), or poor hygiene.

Patients with acute phimosis complain of penile pain over hours to days. On examination, the physician will discover a tender foreskin that is not readily retracted. Although the prepuce may be gently manipulated to allow a better examination, forced retraction should be avoided. Forceful retraction contributes to future adhesion and stricture formation.

Indications

Dorsal slit of the foreskin is performed in any emergency situation to gain access to the urethral meatus for urethral catheterization. In the setting of paraphimosis, a dorsal slit may be used as a definitive treatment following simple foreskin reduction, or for phimotic ring incision and subsequent reduction in a patient with an otherwise irreducible paraphimosis. Elective circumcision rather than dorsal slit of the foreskin is the definitive procedure of choice in nonemergency situations.

Contraindications

None.

Procedure

Box 56.4 lists the equipment needed to perform dorsal slit of the foreskin. With the patient in the supine position, clean and drape the penis with sterile towels. Clipping the pubic hair is unnecessary. Infiltrate lidocaine without epinephrine into the dorsal midline of the foreskin just beneath the superficial fascia throughout the course of the proposed incision, starting proximally at the level of the coronal sulcus and proceeding distally to the tip of the foreskin (Fig. 56.12, *step 1*). Consider

BOX 56.4 Equipment Necessary for the Dorsal Slit Procedure

1% lidocaine without epinephrine
5-mL syringe
27-gauge needle
1 straight hemostat (Crile hemostatic forceps preferred, if available)
1 straight scissors
1 needle holder
1 absorbable suture (4-0 to 5-0 for children, 3-0 to 4-0 for adults)

Dorsal Slit (Phimosis Treatment)

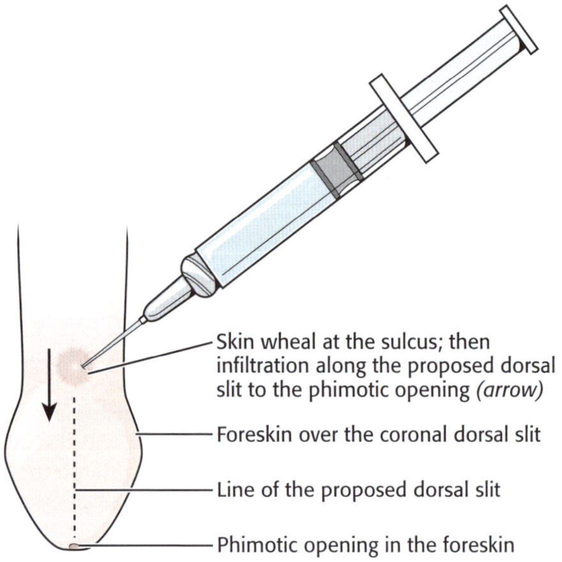

1. Infiltrate plain lidocaine without epinephrine into the dorsal midline of the foreskin just beneath the superficial fascia throughout the course of the planned incision. Begin at the coronal sulcus and proceed distally to the tip of the foreskin. Alternatively, consider a dorsal nerve block or ring block of the penis (see Fig. 56.13).

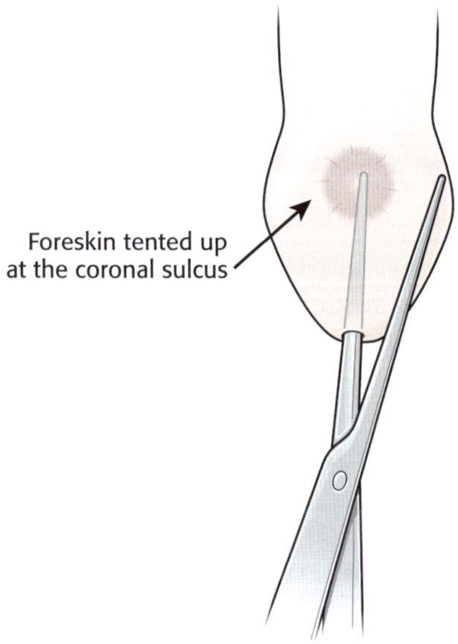

2. Insert both jaws of the hemostat proximally to the level of the coronal sulcus and carefully separate any adhesions. Remove the hemostat, then reinsert only one jaw, and advance again to the coronal sulcus. Close the instrument and crush the foreskin. Leave the hemostat in place for 3 to 5 minutes. Remove the hemostat then use straight scissors to cut along the crushed tissue.

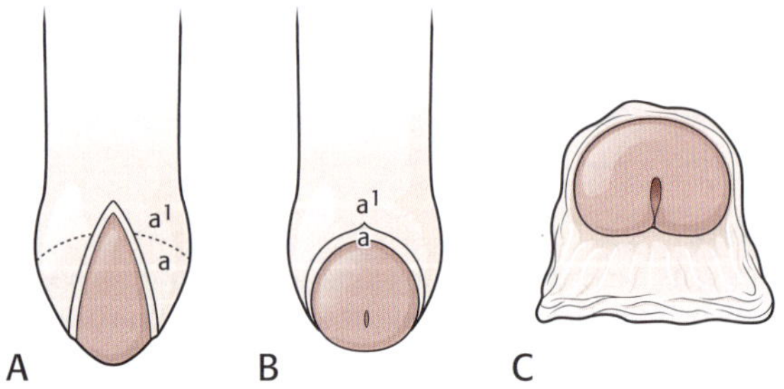

3. *A,* Use straight scissors to cut along the crushed tissue. The exposed glans is shaded. (*a*[1], outer layer of the foreskin; *a*, inner layer of the foreskin). *B,* Retract the cut edges of the foreskin drawn back around the glans penis. If hemostasis is required, first suture *a*[1] to *a* and then sew the remainder of the cut edges together. *C,* The ventral transposed foreskin will assume a beagle-ear deformity after the dorsal slit procedure has been completed.

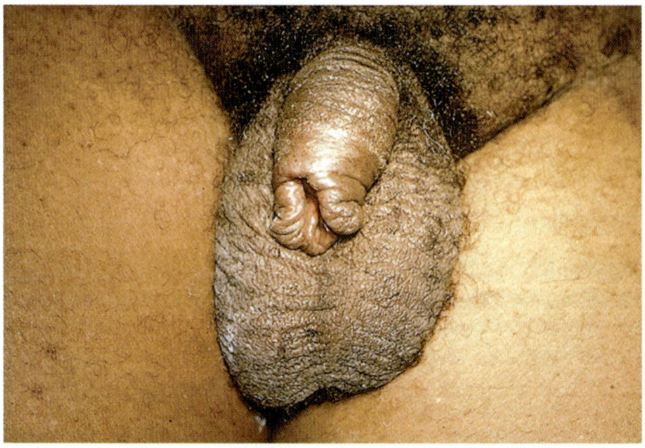

4. Postoperative appearance of the dorsal slit showing the beagle ear. A formal, complete circumcision can be performed after the inflammation has resolved, if desired.

Fig. 56.12 Dorsal slit treatment of phimosis.

mixing equal volumes of lidocaine with bupivacaine. After several minutes, grasp the foreskin with toothed forceps to test for adequate local anesthesia. The operator must be certain that the inner surface of the foreskin is also anesthetized. If this area is not numb, use a dorsal nerve block or ring block at the base of the penis (Fig. 56.13). Systemic analgesia or procedural sedation may be useful adjuncts as well.

After achieving adequate local anesthesia or procedural sedation if needed, take a straight hemostat and carefully advance both jaws of the hemostat proximally to the area of the coronal sulcus between the inner layer of the foreskin and the smooth glans penis, carefully separating any existing preputial adhesions (see Fig. 56.12, *step 2*). Take care that the meatus and urethra are visualized or palpated at all times to avoid inadvertent injury during this maneuver. Once release of adhesions is complete, open the hemostat, and place one jaw of the hemostat in the recently developed plane between the glans penis and the superior overlying inner layer of foreskin. Advance the hemostat to the level of the coronal sulcus and then close it, effectively crushing the interposed anesthetized

Regional Anesthesia of the Penis

A. Dorsal Nerve Block

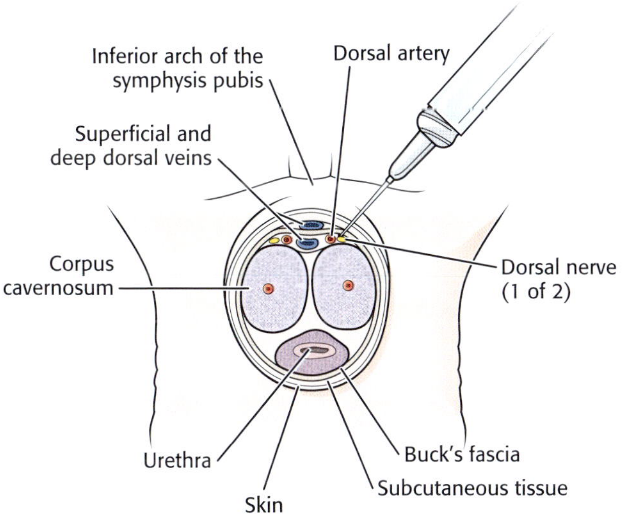

1. The penis has two dorsal penile arteries and two nerves running together and one dorsal penile vein in the midline. A dorsal nerve block at the base of the penis will provide anesthesia of only the dorsum of the penis.

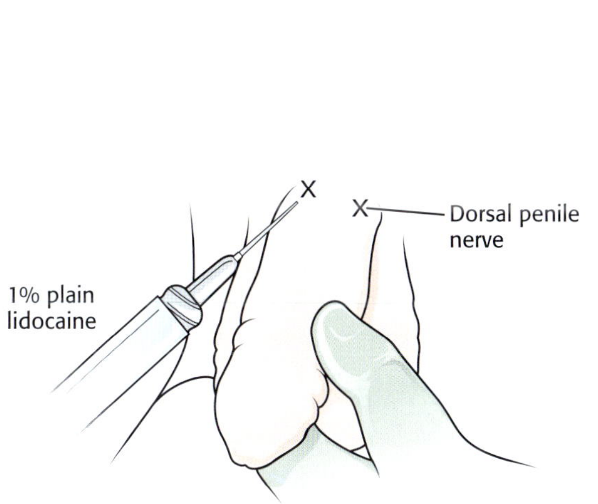

2. To perform the dorsal block, inject at the base of the penis lateral to the midline at approximately the 10 and 2 o'clock positions.

B. Ring Block

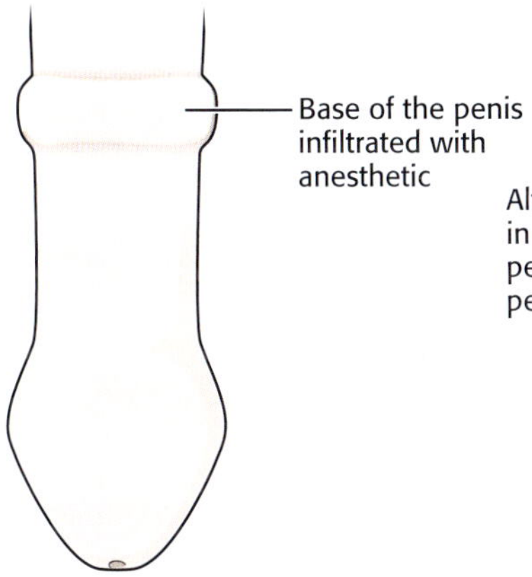

Alternatively, infiltrate subcutaneous lidocaine (without epinephrine) in a circumferential fashion for a (ring) field block at the base of the penis. This technique provides anesthesia to the entire distal end of the penis.

Fig. 56.13 Regional anesthesia of the penis utilizing a dorsal nerve block (A) or ring block approach (B). Consider the use of supplemental intravenous analgesia or procedural sedation, or both, based on the clinical scenario. (A1, From Soliman MG, Tremblay NA. Nerve block of the penis for postoperative pain relief in children. *Anesth Analg*. 1978;57:495.)

foreskin. Leave the closed hemostat in place for 3 to 5 minutes, then remove it and cut the resultant serrated crushed foreskin longitudinally with straight scissors throughout the extent of the crushed tissue.

Normally, the incised, anatomically approximated skin edges bleed and ooze. Not infrequently, these skin edges of the foreskin separate into two layers, the outer foreskin and the inner foreskin (see Fig. 56.12, *step 3*). Absorbable chromic or Vicryl (4-0 to 5-0 for children, 3-0 to 4-0 for adults) running hemostatic sutures may be placed, each beginning proximally at the apex of the dorsal slit and carried distally, reapproximating the two leaves of foreskin. Standard antibiotic ointment may be used to lubricate the suture material and facilitate passage of the suture through the delicate foreskin tissue.

After successful dorsal slit of the foreskin, the prepuce is easily retracted for cleansing of the glans penis or exposure of the urethral meatus. Postprocedural conscientious foreskin reduction to its normal anatomic position must be ensured after any distal penile manipulation to avoid paraphimosis.

If reduction of a paraphimosis cannot be achieved with other means, then surgical interventions should be considered. Fig. 56.14 describes the dorsal slit procedure for paraphimosis reduction, which involves carefully sterilizing the field, anesthetizing the penis on the dorsal aspect, followed by a linear incision.

Aftercare

Ideally, a definitive elective circumcision is recommended after a dorsal slit. Some patients complain about the appearance of

Dorsal Slit (Paraphimosis Treatment)

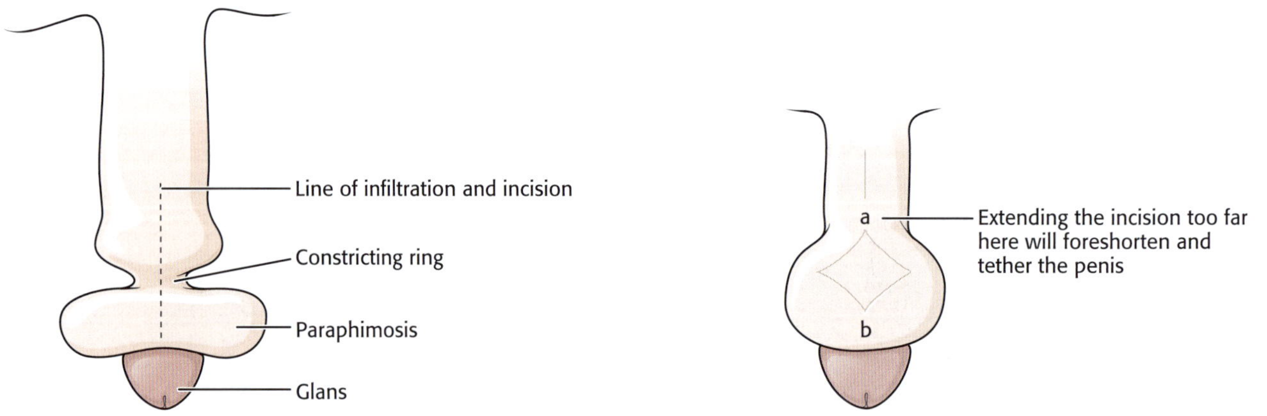

1. Infiltrate local anesthetic from the constricting band of the paraphimosis proximally along the dorsal aspect of the penis. Make an incision along this line.

2. A diamond-shaped defect will result from the linear incision of the foreskin. Approximate the two apices of the dorsal slit (*a* and *b*) after the foreskin is reduced.

Fig. 56.14 Dorsal slit treatment of paraphimosis. This procedure may be necessary if manual reduction of paraphimosis (see Fig. 56.9) is unsuccessful.

their incised foreskin ("beagle ears") and the relative inconvenience during urination, whereas others are pleased they no longer have their phimosis and decline further treatment (see Fig. 56.12, *step 4*).

Complications

Injury to the urethral meatus, urethra, and the glans penis may occur if the hemostat or straight scissors are blindly and unknowingly introduced into the urethra. Bleeding may occur if the hemostat has not adequately crushed the foreskin or if the scissor incision is made lateral to the serrated crushed tissue. The latter two problems may be readily resolved with the previously described running hemostatic suture.

Conclusions

Dorsal slit of the foreskin is performed in any emergency situation either to gain access to the urethral meatus for urethral catheterization or as definitive treatment after simple foreskin reduction, or phimotic ring incision and foreskin reduction in a patient with an otherwise irreducible paraphimosis. This minor operative procedure can be readily performed in the acute care setting when necessary.

URETHRAL CATHETERIZATION

Introduction

Urethral catheterization seems a simple task: insertion of one tube into a larger tube. Nonetheless, many difficulties might arise. Patients often remember catheterization as either painful or uneventful depending on the operator's expertise, confidence, and gentleness.

The merits of various approaches to urine specimen collection depend on the patient's age and clinical setting.

Urethral catheterization is definitive and routinely used to collect urine for analysis and culture in infants and young children who are not yet toilet trained. For older children who can follow directions, midstream urine collection is a reasonable alternative approach to specimen collection.

In adult males without anatomic lesions, first-voided midstream specimens can define the presence or absence of culture-proven bacteriuria. This certainly represents a simple, noninvasive, and user-friendly approach to urine collection in the busy ED setting.

In adult females, properly collected clean-catch midstream specimens have been found to be as bacteriologically reliable as catheterized specimens. Whether it is necessary to be a midstream specimen is a matter of some debate.[36] A few caveats are worth mentioning. Ideally, patients must sit backward on the toilet when collecting the specimen (i.e., patient facing the wall behind the toilet, which theoretically promotes labial spreading). Many studies, however, excluded patients with vaginitis, urologic abnormalities, pregnancy, or vaginal bleeding—diagnoses representing the clinical circumstances for which urine is commonly examined in young females being evaluated in the ED. In this at-risk population, catheterized urine specimens are optimal. This, however, needs to be balanced with the reality that catheterization may be coupled with unnecessary patient discomfort and resource utilization, as well as the risk of introducing bacteria into the bladder.[37]

Procedure Overview

Indications: bladder access for urinary drainage or evaluation of bladder urine.

Contraindications: when other less invasive procedures will be equally effective and informative; relatively contraindicated in certain pelvic or GU trauma until urethral integrity is assured.

Complications: mechanical (false passage or iatrogenic paraphimosis following foreskin retraction for urethral access), infection, bleeding, undesired catheter retention, complications of long-term catheter use.

Urethral Catheterization

Indications
Acute urinary retention
Obstructive uropathy
Urine output monitoring in any critically ill or injured patient
Collection of a sterile urine specimen for diagnostic purposes
Intermittent bladder catheterization in patients with neurogenic bladder dysfunction
Urologic study of the lower urinary tract

Contraindications
Situations in which a less invasive procedure is sufficient
Trauma patient with suspected urethral injury

Complications
Urethral trauma and hemorrhage
Paraphimosis (if the foreskin is not reduced after the procedure)
Infection
Undesirable catheter retention (nondeflating balloon)

Equipment

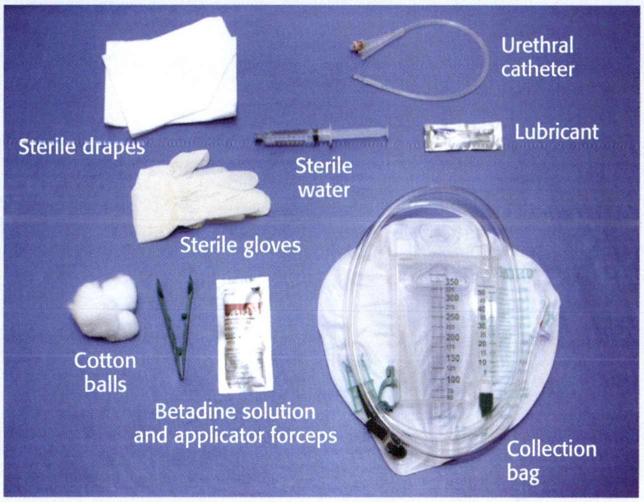

Review Box 56.1 Urethral catheterizations: indications, contraindications, complications, and equipment.

Equipment: the equipment listed in Review Box 56.1 is included in most standard catheterization trays and should be available before attempting urethral catheterization.

Key Procedure Sequence

1. Identify the urethral meatus; expose it with the nondominant hand.
2. Cleanse the meatus and surrounding tissues with antiseptic solution.
3. With the dominant hand, cleanse the area in a circular motion, from the meatus outward.
4. Lubricate the catheter (sterile) and pass it through the meatus toward the bladder.
5. For males: consider instilling 5 mL of 2% viscous lidocaine (or similar) into the urethra prior to passing the catheter.
6. For females: discard any catheter that has inadvertently entered the vagina.
7. Pass the catheter fully into the bladder, confirm its placement by the flow of urine. For males, continue to insert the catheter fully.
8. Inflate the balloon with 10 mL of air or water.
9. If resistance or obvious discomfort is felt, deflate the balloon and attempt repositioning.
10. After successful passage and balloon inflation, gently withdraw the catheter until resistance is met.
11. Connect the catheter to a drainage bag. Always reduce the penile foreskin, if present, to avoid inadvertent iatrogenic paraphimosis.

Description

Background

Patients are often apprehensive about catheterization. If the clinician shows concern regarding positioning and exposure, the patient will be reassured. Although adequate exposure may be obtained in the frog-leg position, the use of an examination table with stirrups (lithotomy position) is ideal, especially for female catheterization.

Anticipation and preparation of all anticipated materials necessary for successful urethral catheterization beforehand remain prudent. Most catheterizations are performed using a standard catheterization tray. Often these trays contain more equipment than is truly needed. This necessitates opening the tray and establishing a sterile field at the bedside, selecting those items that will be needed, and discarding the rest of the equipment. Once the penis or labia has been touched in preparation for the procedure, the touching hand (usually nondominant) is contaminated and ideally should not be handling any of the sterile equipment. When a standard catheterization tray is not used or is not available, go through the anticipated procedure mentally and secure all the appropriate equipment before actually initiating the procedure.

Anatomy and Physiology

Female Catheterization

The female urethra is a short (~4 cm) straight tube, usually of wide caliber, lying on top of the vagina. It must be approached between the double labia, and the urethral meatus is occasionally hidden and not obvious. This is in contrast to most males, except those with hypospadias. If the female patient adducts her legs, successful catheterization will be very difficult if not impossible.

The female urethral meatus is oval but may appear as an anteroposterior slit with rather prominent margins situated directly superior to the opening of the vagina and approximately 2.5 cm inferior to the glans clitoris (Fig. 56.15). It is the first of three orifices encountered when examining the female genitalia cephalad to caudad in the lithotomy position. The urethral meatus might be especially difficult to find in the young infant and the older, postmenopausal female.

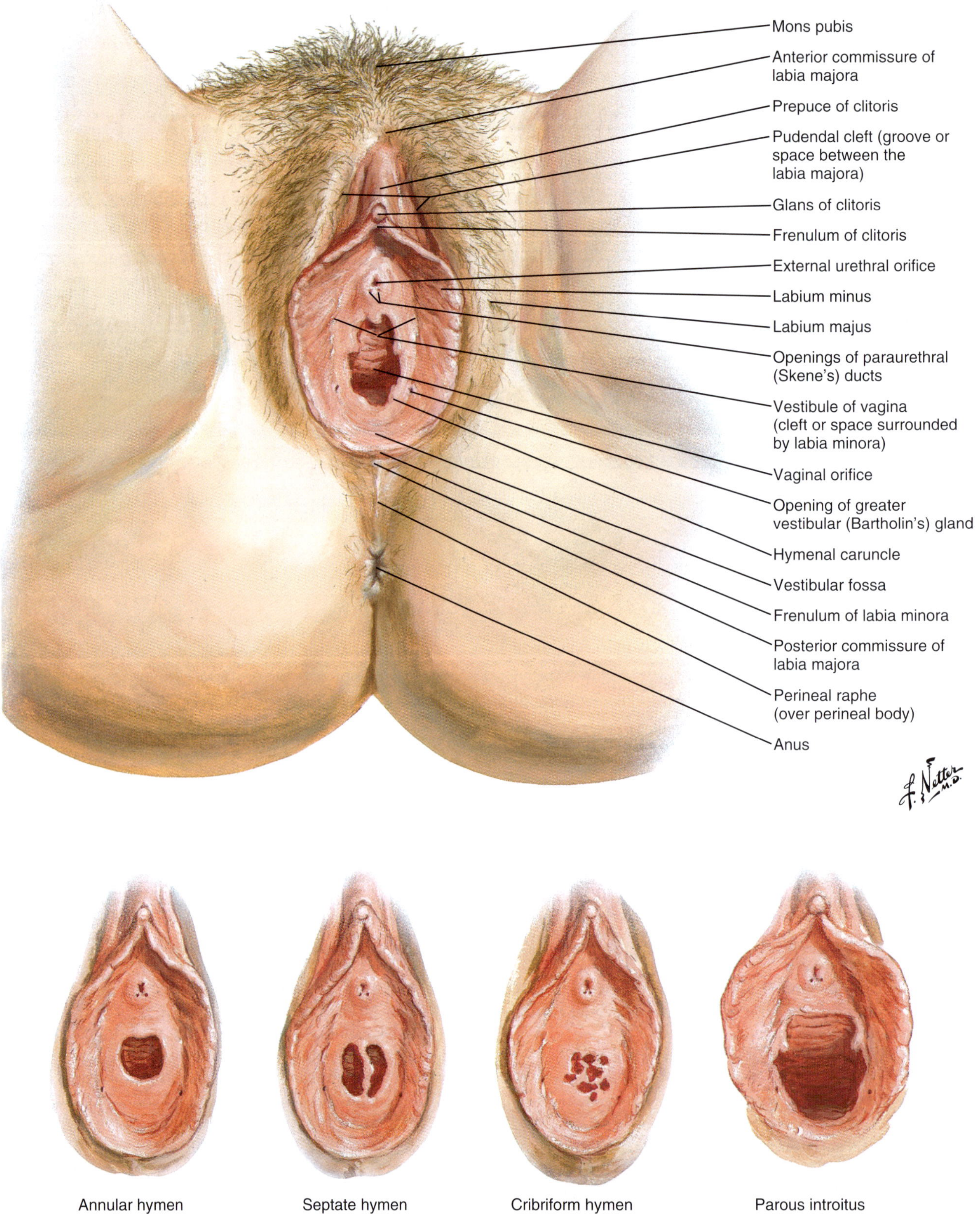

Fig. 56.15 External female genitalia. The urethral meatus is directly superior to the vaginal introitus and approximately 2.5 cm inferior to the clitoris. (Netter illustration from https://www.netterimages.com. Elsevier, Inc. All rights reserved.)

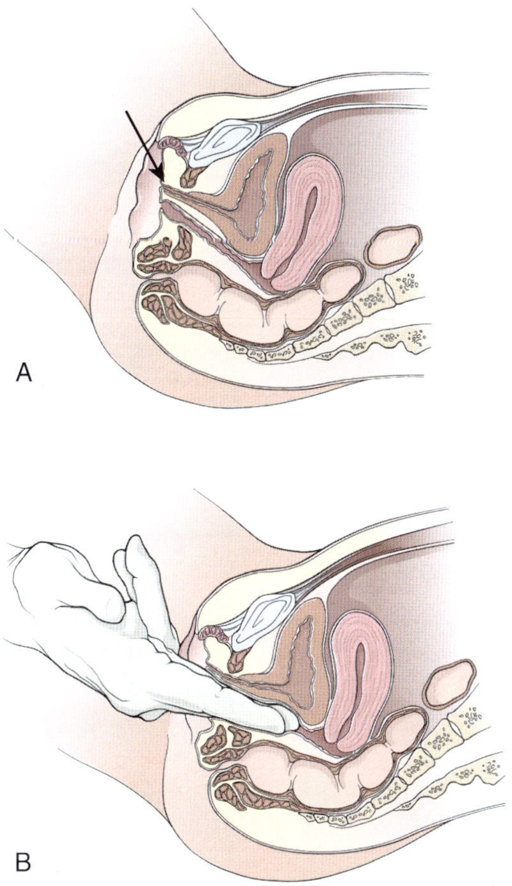

Fig. 56.16 Female urethra. (A) Normal sagittal anatomy of the female urethra *(arrow)*. (B) In a patient with a cystocele/urethrocele or prolapsed bladder, the normal anatomy may have to be recreated for passage of a catheter. Insert two fingers into the vagina and lift upward while passing the catheter.

Anticipation of this and knowledge of the anatomic variances will help to modify any patient discomfort associated with needless catheter-tip probing, which is an unsettling experience for both the patient and the proceduralist.

Occasionally, the urethral meatus recedes superiorly into the vagina and is not immediately visible because of either prior surgical procedures or atrophic postmenopausal changes. Anticipation of such challenges will allow the examiner to gently advance a nondominant index finger into the vagina in the superior midline. The urethral meatus can usually be palpated then visualized as a soft mound surrounded by a firmer ring of supporting periurethral tissue. Rarely, the meatus will have receded so far superiorly and intravaginally that it cannot be visualized at all, and catheterization must be carried out by palpation alone. From the meatus (if the patient assumes a supine position), the urethra proceeds straight back to slightly downward as it advances into the bladder just behind the symphysis pubis (Fig. 56.16A).

In females with a urethrocele or cystourethrocele, in whom the urethra or the bladder falls into the vagina, the "normal" urethral course might be significantly more posterior. The normal anatomic relationships in these situations may be recreated by spreading the index and long fingers and placing them along the superior vaginal wall and gently applying upward support (Fig. 56.16B). This reconstitutes the normal anatomic relationships and permits straight, rapid urethral catheterization. Because the female urethra is comparatively short, only half the total length of the catheter has to be inserted before it is safe to inflate the balloon.

Male Catheterization

Because the urethral meatus is usually evident in most males, it might seem a simple matter to insert a urethral catheter, yet catheterization can be quite difficult. The normal male urethra is approximately 20 cm long from the external urethral meatus to the bladder neck (Fig. 56.17). The posterior prostatic urethra is approximately 3.5 cm long, and the contiguous external sphincter or urogenital diaphragm that encompasses the membranous urethra is 4 cm from the bladder neck. In males, any catheter must be fully inserted to the balloon-inflating side-arm channel before it is safe to inflate the balloon. At the first egress of urine from the catheter, the balloon is just passing through the membranous urethra. The catheter balloon still has approximately 3 cm to 4 cm to go before clearing the bladder neck. Inflation of the Foley balloon at any point before full insertion of the catheter has the potential to result in iatrogenic urethral injury.

The male urethra is relatively fixed at the level of the urogenital diaphragm and symphysis pubis; traction downward on the penis kinks and promotes urethral folding at the level of the penile suspensory ligament (Fig. 56.18A), which creates a level of spurious obstruction. For this reason, the penis should always be held taut and upright during any urethral instrumentation, including catheterization (Fig. 56.18B). The catheter then needs to make only a single curve rather than a complex S-curve as it traverses into the bladder.

Pathophysiology

See Table 56.3: Approach to Difficulties in Male Catheterization.

Indications

Urinary catheterization and instrumentation are rarely a primary cause of urinary infection in otherwise healthy patients who urinate normally and carry small amounts of postvoid residual urine. As with any procedure, catheterization needs to be limited to those clinical situations in which the benefits outweigh the risks. The following are generally considered to be indications for urethral catheterization:

- Acute urinary retention.
- Urethral or prostatic obstruction leading to compromised renal function.
- Urine output monitoring in a critically ill or injured patient.
- Collection of a sterile urine specimen for diagnostic purposes.
- Intermittent bladder catheterization in patients with neurogenic bladder dysfunction.
- Urologic study of the lower urinary tract.

Contraindications

Urethral catheterization should be avoided when other less invasive procedures will be equally effective and informative. A traditional relative contraindication to urethral catheterization is the trauma patient with suspected urethral injury as evidenced by blood at the urethral meatus, an abnormal-feeling or high-riding prostate on rectal examination, penile, scrotal, perineal hematoma, or radiographic evidence of urethral or

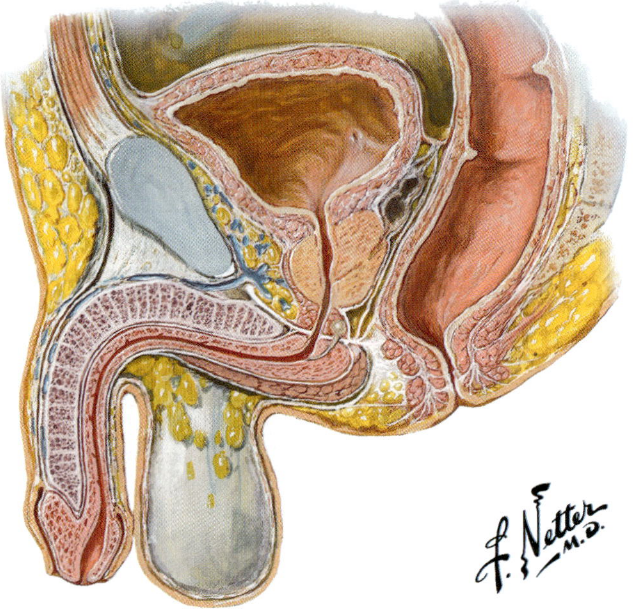

Fig. 56.17 Male urethra. The male urethra is approximately 20 cm long from the meatus to the neck of the bladder. The prostatic urethra and membranous urethra can be up to 7 cm combined. Thus it is essential to advance the urethral catheter to the maximum extent before balloon inflation to avoid urethral injury. (Netter illustration from https://www.netterimages.com. Elsevier, Inc. All rights reserved.)

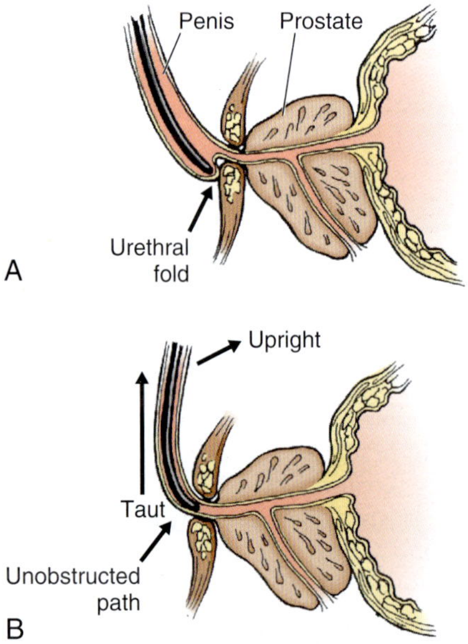

Fig. 56.18 (A) The urethra may fold and kink if the penis is not held taut and upright during passage of a catheter. Kinking may halt the advancement of a catheter in the absence of other anatomic blockage. (B) The taut and upright position allows an unobstructed path for the catheter.

bladder trauma. In the setting of a severely fractured pelvis or diastasis of the pubic symphysis, urethrogram should precede attempts at catheterization when possible. Some authors, and many clinical protocols allow for gentle attempts at catheter passage even in the presence of the previously discussed traditional contraindications.[38,39]

Procedure

Equipment

The equipment listed in Review Box 56.1 is included in most standard catheterization trays and should be at hand before attempting urethral catheterization. Check the list of contents before opening the tray as some trays do not include certain items. For most routine adult in-and-out catheterizations, a 14-Fr red rubber catheter or Foley balloon catheter is adequate (Fig. 56.19). In neonates or infants, a small feeding tube taped in place produces the least amount of urethral trauma. In older boys, a red rubber catheter or Foley balloon catheter may be used. Table 56.4 lists age-appropriate sized catheters or feeding tubes for children.[40]

A 14- to 18-Fr Coudé catheter should be considered after unsuccessful passage of a straight Foley balloon catheter or in any male patient with known enlargement of the median prostatic lobe (Fig. 56.20). If a Coudé catheter is not available, a larger 18- to 22-Fr Foley balloon catheter can be attempted. In a male patient with a urethral stricture in whom attempts at catheterization with a straight Foley or Coudé catheter have failed, retrograde cystoscopy, passage of a guidewire, or passage of filiforms and followers under the direction of a urologist is the next step. If immediate bladder access is required in any emergency, suprapubic placement of a Foley balloon catheter using the Seldinger technique can be performed (as described in the later section on "Suprapubic Cystostomy").

General Procedure (Figs. 56.21 and 56.22)

Urethral catheterization must be done using sterile technique. Both male and female patients have unique urethral meatal considerations. In the uncircumcised or partially circumcised male, control of the penile foreskin is paramount to ensuring success. Before establishing a sterile field, retract the available foreskin to its fullest extent proximal to the glans penis (Fig. 56.23A). Unfold a standard 4 × 4 gauze pad, then refold it in its longest dimension and carefully wrap it around the retracted foreskin at the level of the coronal sulcus (Fig. 56.23B). This will prevent the tendency for lubricant-associated normal anatomic foreskin reduction during catheterization and provide a continuously dry and sterile field. Encircle the folded 4 × 4 gauze pad surrounding the foreskin between the nondominant index finger and thumb, creating a ring near the distal end of the penis, and do not release until the procedure is completed. After catheterization, remove the 4 × 4 gauze pad and reduce the penile foreskin to its normal anatomic position to prevent the development of an iatrogenic paraphimosis.

After exposing the urethral meatus in the female and the glans penis and urethral meatus in the male, use an antiseptic solution soaked into cotton balls or oversized cotton-tipped applicators to cleanse the exposed meatus and surrounding tissues. This is best done by hand but can also be done using the plastic forceps in the catheterization tray. Begin the cleansing in a circular motion at the urethral meatus and proceed outward, intentionally moving any debris toward the periphery and thus creating a sterile field.

Lubricate an appropriately sized catheter (14- to 16-Fr is commonly used in adults) with viscous rather than inspissated lubricating jelly. Injection of the male urethra with 5 mL of 2% viscous lidocaine or a syringe filled with anesthetic lubricant can be helpful for topical anesthesia and urethral distention. Regardless, advise the patient of mild urethral discomfort and the potential urge to void. Gently pass the catheter by

TABLE 56.3 Approach to Difficulties in Male Catheterization

CONDITION	ISSUE	WORK-AROUND STRATEGY
Phimosis	Inability to identify the urethral meatus because of a tight phimotic opening	Dilate the phimotic opening sufficiently to identify the urethral meatus and pass the catheter Dorsal slit of the foreskin to expose the glans and urethral meatus in extreme cases
Foreskin edema	Edema may obscure the glans penis and urethral meatus	Attempt to identify the cause of the edema; exclude paraphimosis or foreign body strangulation Manually compress the swollen foreskin by hand or with cold packs If unsuccessful, snugly wrap the distal penis in a compressive dressing for 10 min
Meatal stenosis	The urethral meatus may be either congenitally or secondarily narrowed by scarring	Trial of a smaller-caliber catheter If a larger-caliber catheter is necessary, meatal dilation or meatotomy might be necessary under the direction of a urologist
Urethral stricture	May develop as a result of trauma, infection (especially STDs), lower urinary tract instrumentation, or long-term indwelling catheter drainage	Trial with a Coudé catheter However, manual force should not be used to negotiate or to dilate urethral strictures because it may lead to false passages, bleeding, and future increased scarring Consideration of urethral dilation with the use of filiforms and followers under the direction of a urologist
External urethral sphincter spasm	Voluntary or involuntary contraction of the urogenital diaphragm (external sphincter) produces spurious urethral resistance at approximately 16 cm from the meatus	Encourage the patient to lay supine and take slow, deep breaths while consciously trying to relax the perineum and rectum Plantar flexion of the toes and ankles may also aid in relaxation of the pelvic floor Gentle but steady pressure exerted on the catheter along with the aforementioned steps may aid in passage The external sphincter is composed of striated muscle and fatigues within a few minutes If continued resistance, assume an anatomic abnormality and consider RUG prior to further instrumentation
High bladder neck	Enlarged intravesical portion of the prostate with a secondary high-riding bladder neck Typically resistance encountered after the catheter has been passed 16–20 cm into the urethra	Slow instillation or injection of 20–30 mL of sterile lubricating jelly If unsuccessful, consider a trial with a Coudé catheter; may be enhanced by digital compression of the prostate during digital rectal examination
Pelvic trauma, straddle injury	Partial or complete urethral injury might occur Injudicious catheterization has the potential for conversion of a partial injury (may heal with little or no scarring) to a complete urethral injury (often requires surgical repair and usually results in some degree of postoperative morbidity) Blood at the urethral meatus, a high-riding or abnormal-feeling prostate on rectal examination, and penile, scrotal, or perineal ecchymoses might be indicative of potential urethral or bladder injury though have poor sensitivity[a]	Consider precatheterization RUG in suspected cases Maintain a low threshold for urologic consultation Suprapubic catheter placement may be necessary in certain cases

[a]Blandy JP. Acute retention of urine. *Br J Hosp Med*. 1978;19:109-111.
RUG, Retrograde urethrography; *STDs*, sexually transmitted diseases.

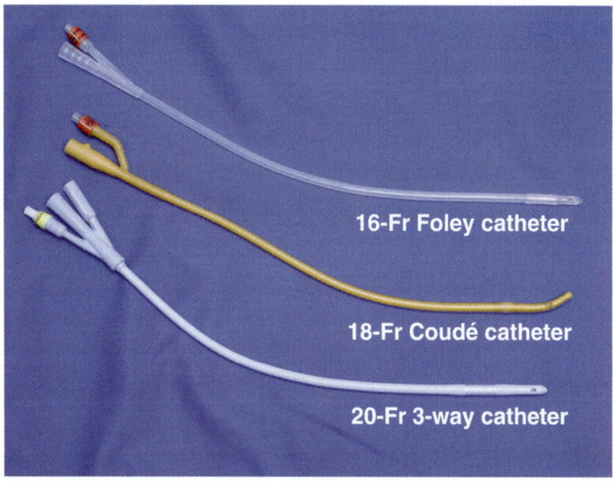

Fig. 56.19 Urethral catheters. A wide variety of types and sizes of catheters are available. For most adult catheterizations, a 14- or 16-Fr Foley catheter is sufficient. For male patients with prostatic enlargement, a 14- to 18-Fr Coudé catheter may be used (see Fig. 56.20). For patients with gross hematuria, a large (20 Fr and up) three-way catheter is ideal because it allows continuous bladder irrigation and its large diameter allows the passage of blood clots.

TABLE 56.4 Pediatric Urethral Catheter Size

AGE GROUP	PEDIATRIC CATHETER SIZE[a]
Infants (y)	5- to 8-Fr feeding tube
1–3	8-Fr feeding tube
4–6	10-Fr feeding tube
7–12	10- to 12-Fr red rubber catheter (Robinson)
>12	14-Fr red rubber catheter (Robinson)

[a]Sizes are approximate; 6-Fr is the smallest balloon catheter and is quite flimsy, and therefore 8 Fr is recommended; 12-Fr is the smallest Coudé catheter.

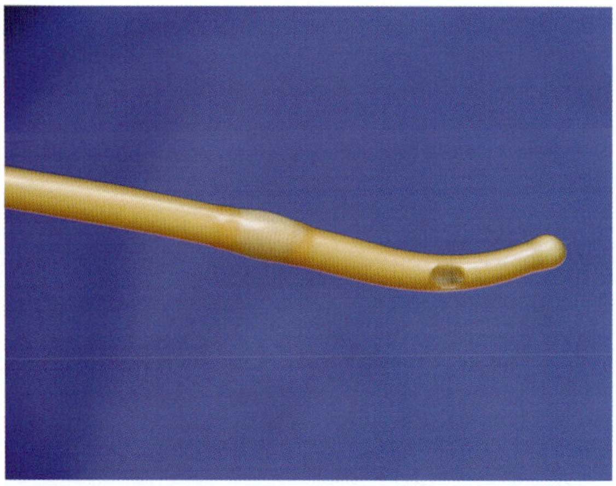

Fig. 56.20 Coudé catheter. A Coudé catheter is used for men with prostatic enlargement. It features a semirigid curved tip that helps the catheter traverse the median lobe of the enlarged prostate gland. When inserting the Coudé, the curved tip should be pointing toward the dorsal aspect of the penis.

hand, or with the aid of a hemostat or plastic forceps, into the urethra and upward into the bladder. During slow, gentle passage of the catheter, be aware of the anatomic considerations discussed previously. Any catheter that contacts a nonsterile surface or inadvertently enters the vagina should be discarded due to increased risk of subsequent infection.

After passing the catheter fully in all male patients, slowly inflate the balloon with 10 mL of air or water. Sterile water or saline is not required. Most 5-mL balloons will easily accommodate 30 mL to 50 mL of air or water without bursting. Obvious resistance or patient discomfort on balloon inflation should signal potential erroneous urethral positioning and necessitates reevaluation. If this occurs, immediately deflate the Foley balloon and reposition or slightly withdraw the catheter, then pass it fully again before balloon reinflation. If this is unsuccessful a second time, remove the catheter. At this point, retrograde urethrography (RUG) is recommended to evaluate the urethra for a potential obstructive problem or false passage (see later section on RUG). It may be difficult or impossible to pass a Foley catheter in a male with a markedly edematous penis (Fig. 56.24). If this cannot be accomplished, a suprapubic catheter may be required.

After successful catheter passage and Foley balloon inflation, slowly withdraw the catheter until the approximation of the balloon with the bladder neck precludes further withdrawal. Then connect the catheter to either a sterile leg bag or a closed-system bedside drainage bag. If the patient will be discharged with an indwelling Foley catheter, it can be initially connected to a leg bag, which is then comfortably fastened to the lower thigh and upper calf. The patient and family should be instructed regarding proper care of the catheter and drainage device. In most other cases, the catheter may be secured to either the thigh or the lower abdomen (preferred with males) with adhesive tape or simply placed under the knee and left to drain dependently into the bedside drainage bag.

Bladder Irrigation

After prostate surgery (transurethral resection) or in other clinical scenarios, blood clots may form in the bladder and cause acute urinary retention. Blood loss can be significant. This condition is usually relieved by the use of a large three-way irrigation catheter. A 22- to 26-Fr Foley three-way catheter is preferred. Infuse saline irrigation fluid continuously into the bladder, while allowing the egress of fluid and blood clots. Continue the procedure until the bladder remains decompressed or bleeding stops (see Fig. 56.21, *steps 8–10*). Gravity alone usually provides adequate ingress-egress of fluid, though gentle syringe irrigation with 60-mL aliquots of saline may be used. Irrigation can be brisk, 1 to 2 L/h or more, as long as the volume of drained saline is equal to the volume infused. Infuse saline (supplied in 2- or 4-L bags) by gravity. As stated previously, syringe irrigation of a Foley catheter with 60-mL aliquots is an acceptable alternative. The goal is to obtain clear urine.

Difficult Urethral Catheterization

Difficult urethral catheterization (DUC) is a common urologic problem. In females, this is due primarily to vaginal atrophy with retraction of the meatus into the vagina. This can typically be overcome by placing the patient in the lithotomy position, using a speculum, or guiding the catheter blindly through palpation with the provider's index and middle fingers. However, DUC in males may present greater challenges. Common causes

Male Urethral Catheterization and Bladder Irrigation

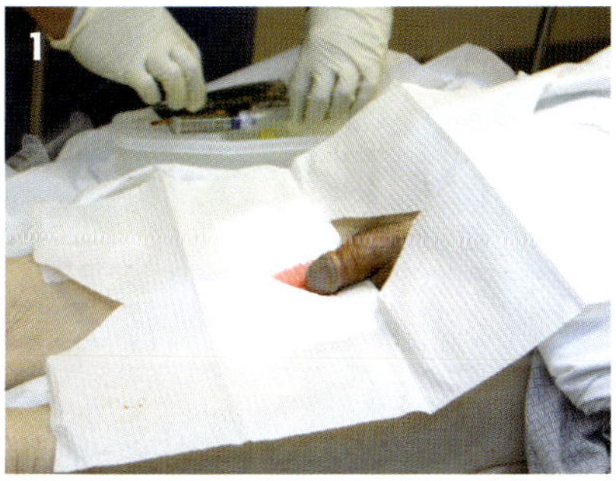

Prepare your equipment and place a sterile fenestrated drape around the penis. If the patient is uncircumcised, retract the foreskin prior to the procedure (see Fig. 56.23).

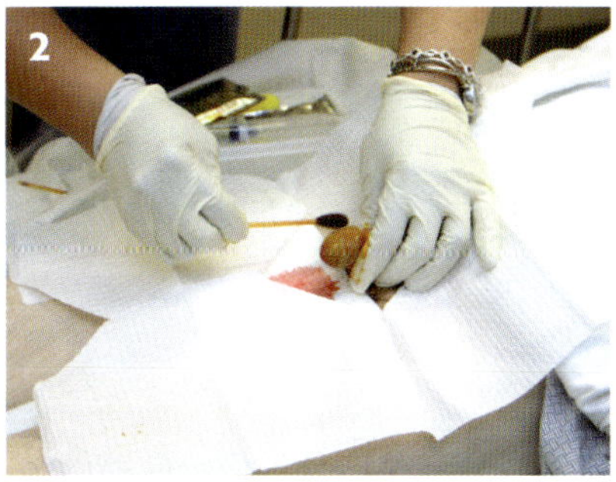

Use your nondominant hand to hold the penis, and cleanse the meatus and surrounding tissue with antiseptic. Your nondominant hand is now contaminated and should not let go of the penis or handle sterile equipment until the insertion has been completed.

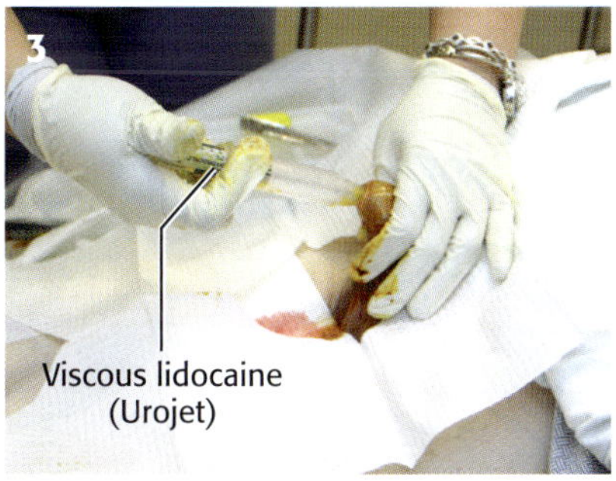

Inject the urethra with 5 to 10 mL of 2% viscous lidocaine to distend the urethra and provide topical anesthesia. A commercially available Urojet syringe (depicted here) is ideal. If possible, wait 5 to 10 minutes for maximum anesthetic effect.

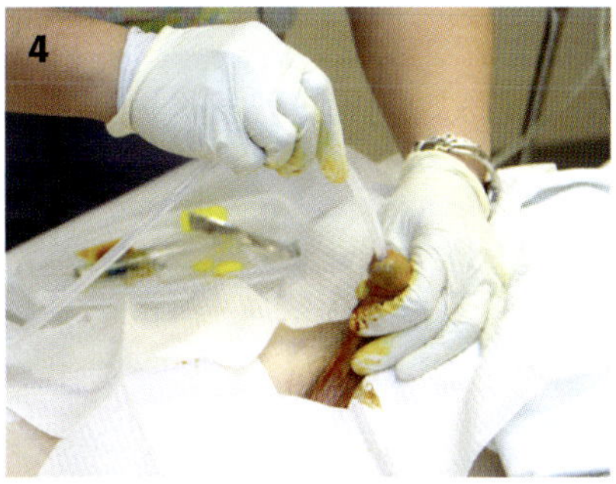

Hold the penis taut and upright with your nondominant hand while you pass the catheter into the urethra (see Fig. 56.18).

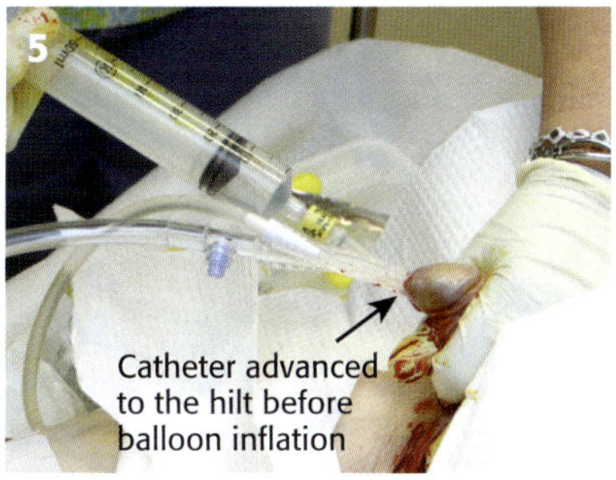

Advance the catheter to the hilt before inflating the balloon with the recommended amount of air or water. If there is obvious resistance or patient discomfort, immediately deflate and reevaluate the position of the catheter.

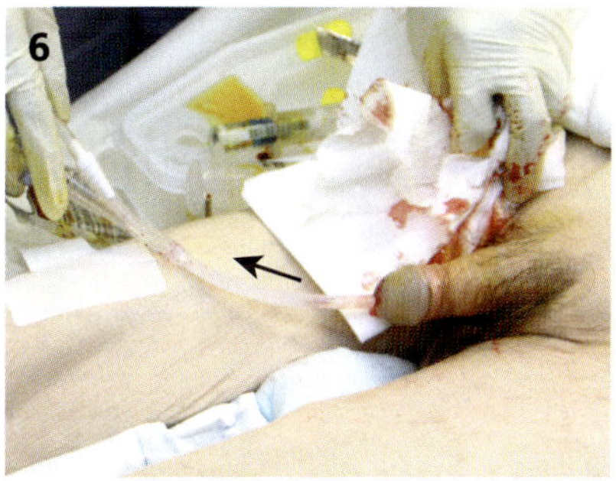

After balloon inflation, slowly withdraw the catheter until the balloon is against the bladder neck and precluding further withdrawal. Connect to a drainage system if one is not preattached.

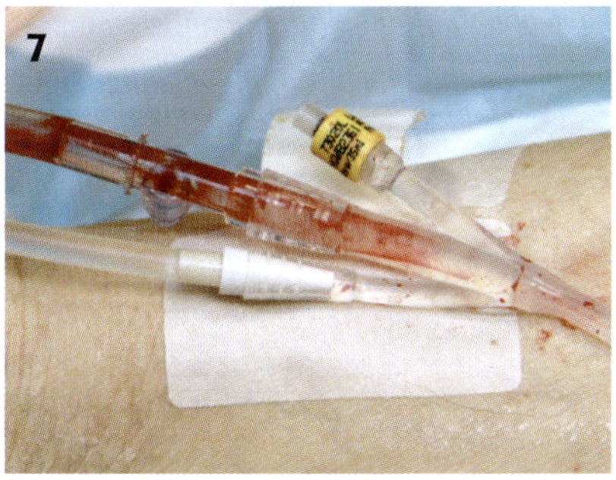

Affix the catheter to the thigh with tape or a catheter-specific attachment device. Note that a three-way catheter was placed in this patient with gross hematuria.

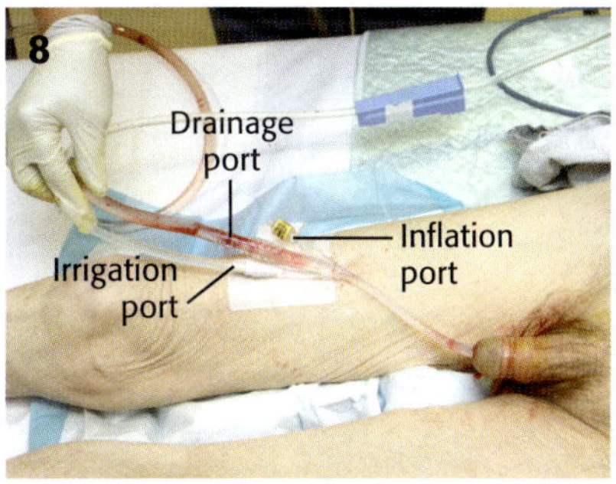

To irrigate the bladder, attach the irrigation port to a 2- to 4-L bag of saline irrigation fluid. (Hand irrigation with a 60-mL catheter-tipped syringe is an alternative.) Attach the drainage port to a large-volume collection bag.

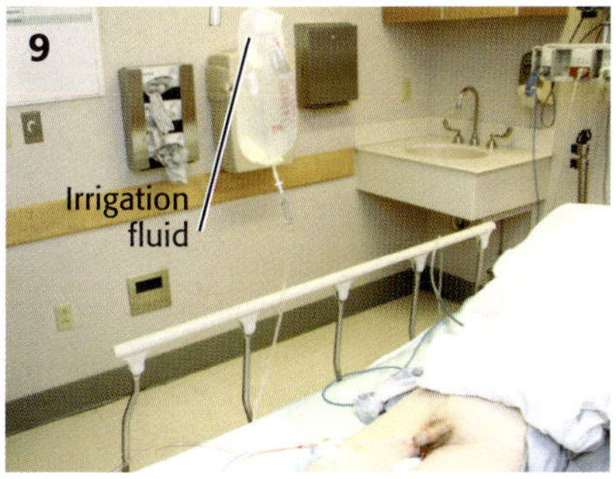

Continuously infuse the irrigant into the bladder. Rates of 1 to 2 L/hr are acceptable, provided that the amount of irrigant drained equals the amount infused.

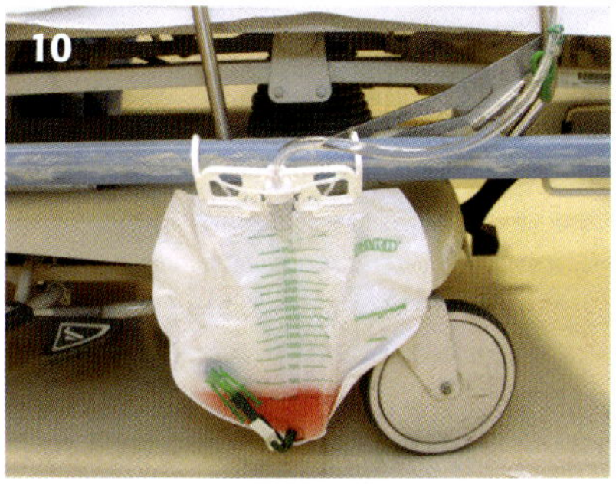

Monitor output carefully during the procedure. The goal of irrigation is to obtain clear urinary effluent.

Fig. 56.21 Male urethral catheterization and bladder irrigation.

Female Urethral Catheterization

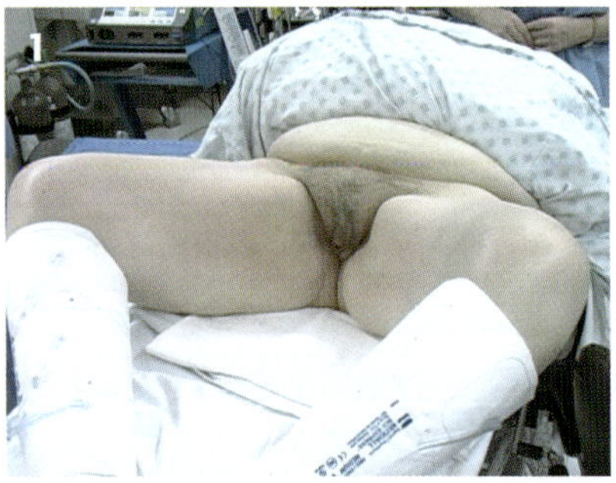

1. Place the patient in the frog-leg position: the hips externally rotated and slightly flexed and the knees bent.

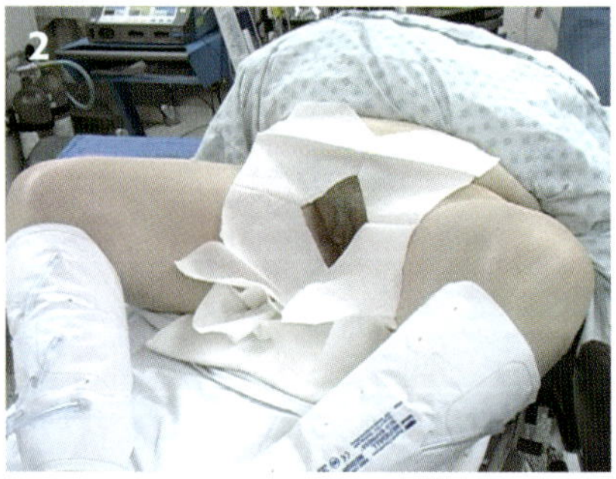

2. Place a sterile fenestrated drape over the area. Strict attention to sterile technique is required.

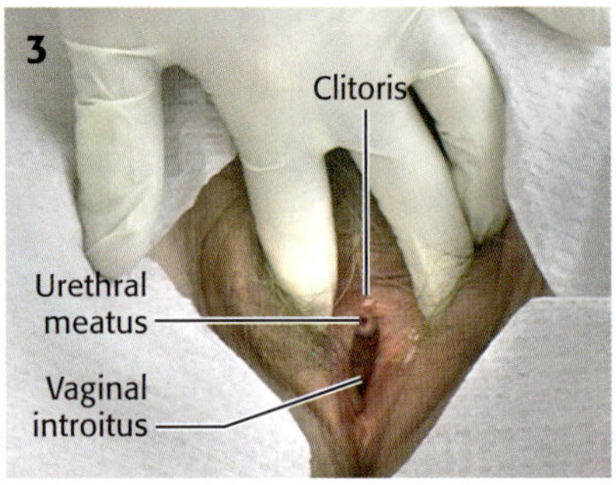

3. Use your nondominant hand to spread the labia and identify the urethral meatus. This hand is now considered contaminated and should not release the labia or handle sterile equipment throughout the procedure.

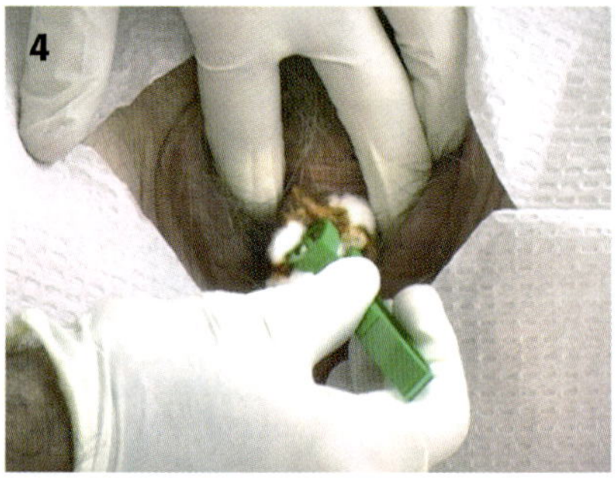

4. Cleanse the urethral meatus with antiseptic in progressively increasing concentric circles.

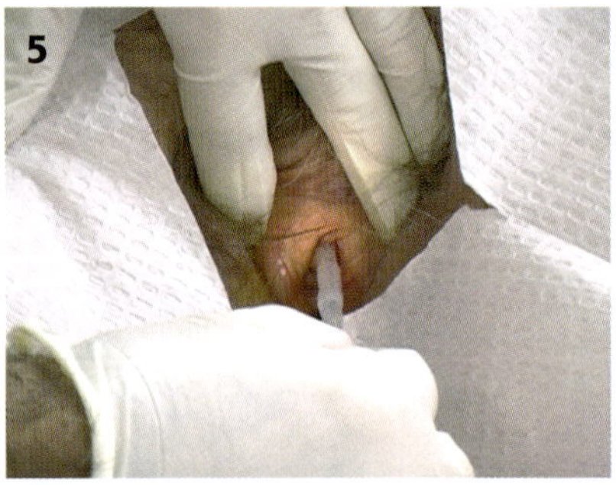

5. Insert the catheter into the meatus under direct vision. If the catheter accidentally enters the vagina, it should be discarded and a new one used (to prevent iatrogenic infection).

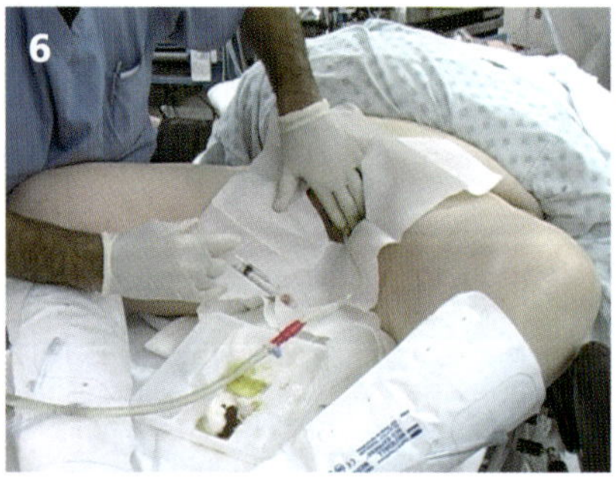

6. Once the catheter is in the bladder and urine returns in the tubing, advance the catheter several centimeters farther and inflate the balloon with the recommended amount of water or air.

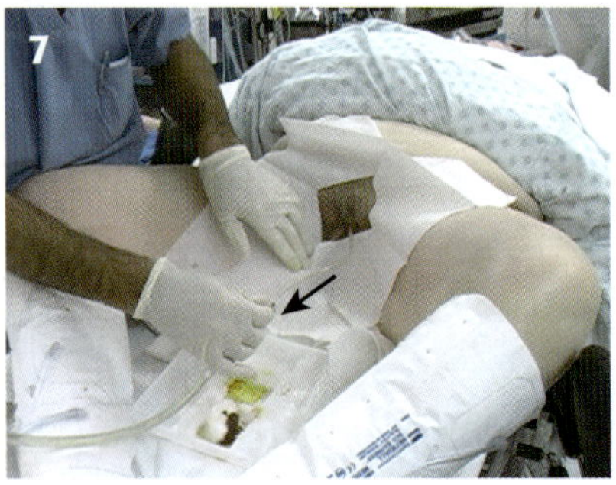

7. Gently retract the catheter until the balloon encounters the bladder neck and resistance is felt.

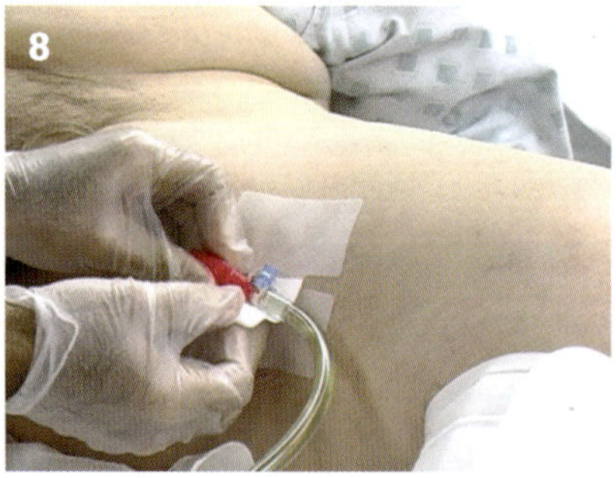

8. Attach the catheter to a collection device (if not already preconnected), and affix the catheter to the patient's thigh with tape or a connection device.

Fig. 56.22 Female urethral catheterization.

in males include urethral strictures, bladder neck contracture, false passage, and prostate disease. Trial of a Coudé catheter is generally the first-line approach to DUC (see Fig. 56.20). Alternatives utilized by urologists include flexible cystoscopy, passage of a guidewire, or filiforms and followers.[41] Suprapubic cystostomy should generally be considered an option of last resort. Various causes and approaches to DUC in the emergency care setting are presented in Table 56.3.

Aftercare

Systemic antimicrobial prophylaxis should not be used routinely in patients with short- or long-term catheterization to reduce catheter-associated bacteriuria or urinary tract infection owing to concern about selection of antimicrobial resistance.[42]

Complications

Although urethral catheterization performed by skilled personnel in appropriate circumstances has an acceptable complication rate, untoward sequelae of catheterization are not unusual.

Mechanical

False passages might be established in any area of the urethra when force is exerted on the catheter. In an uncircumcised

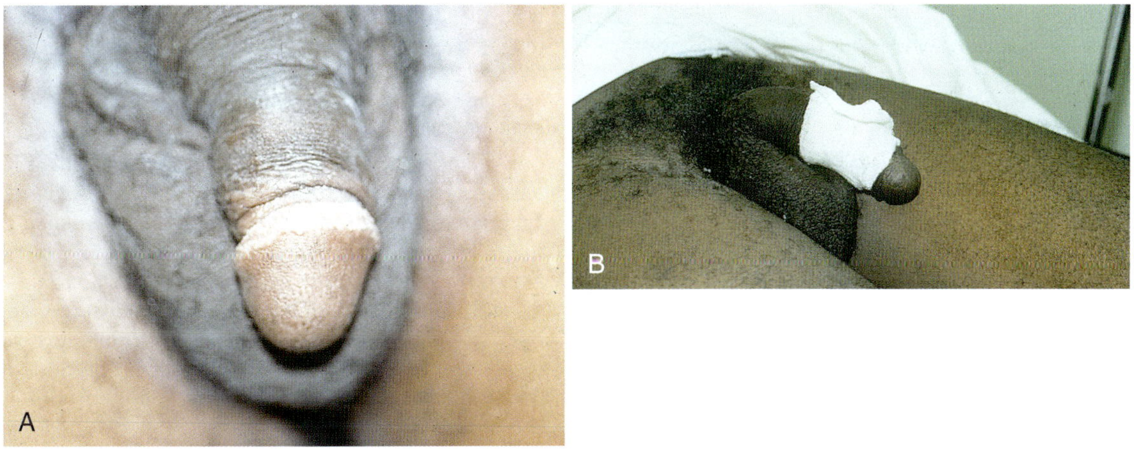

Fig. 56.23 (A) In this uncircumcised male, the foreskin has been fully retracted for placement of a catheter. (B) A gauze pad allows a firm grasp on the foreskin to prevent movement during catheterization. Reduce the foreskin to its original position once the catheter is in place.

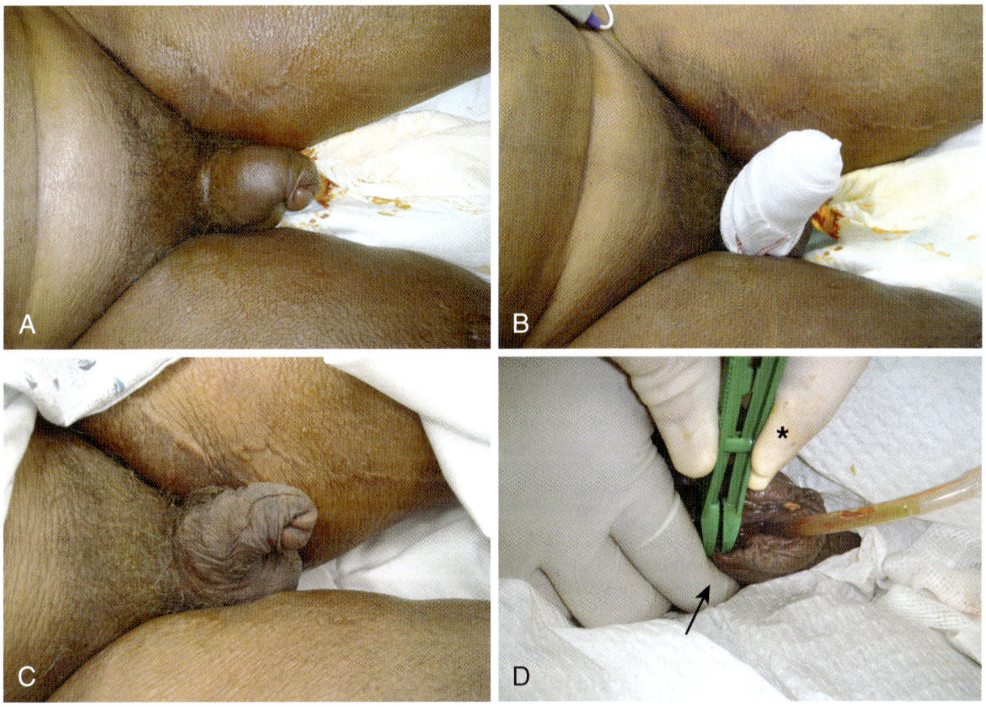

Fig. 56.24 (A) The urethral meatus cannot be found in the markedly edematous penis in this patient with massive anasarca. (B) Wrap the penis in an elastic bandage for 8 to 10 minutes. (C) Much of the edema is reduced with compression alone. (D) An assistant stabilizes the penile shaft with the thumb and index finger *(arrow)* while the operator *(asterisk)* spreads the redundant tissue with forceps to visualize the meatus deep within the swollen tissue and advances the catheter.

patient, inattention to reducing the retracted foreskin to its normal anatomic position after urethral catheterization or instrumentation could potentially lead to painful paraphimosis and associated complications.

Bleeding

Hematuria is common immediately, even after an atraumatic catheterization. Careful monitoring of symptom trajectory is prudent, as most often, postprocedure hematuria resolves rapidly and spontaneously.

Infection

The incidence of bacteriuria associated with indwelling catheterization is 3% to 8% per day, and the duration of catheterization is the most important risk factor for the development of catheter-associated bacteriuria.[42] The rate might be considerably higher in hospitalized, older, debilitated, or postpartum patients. Urinary catheterization is a leading cause of nosocomial infection.[42] Given widespread patient safety, as well as value-based reimbursement initiatives, additional scrutiny is prudent regarding the necessity of initial catheter placement, as is expeditious catheter removal as soon as feasible.

Long-Term Catheter Use

By 1 month, nearly all patients with an indwelling catheter will be bacteriuric.[42] Other less frequent complications of long-term indwelling urethral catheterization include bladder stones, recurring bladder spasm, periurethral abscesses, urethral stricture formation, bladder perforation, and urethral erosion.

Undesirable Catheter Retention

Catheters may be retained because of balloons that do not deflate (see the next section) or, rarely, because of a knot that has spontaneously developed in the catheter.

Removal of a Nondeflating Catheter. Occasionally an indwelling catheter balloon fails to deflate, leading to undesired retention of the Foley catheter in the bladder. This problem has challenged and frustrated many clinicians and has produced a number of ingenious solutions. Unfortunately, pretesting Foley catheter balloons by trial inflation and deflation before insertion does not eliminate the potential for a nondeflating Foley catheter balloon.

A common cause of the nondeflating catheter balloon is the malfunction of the flap-type valve in the balloon lumen of the catheter, which normally allows fluid to fill the balloon of the catheter but prevents passive egress (Fig. 56.25, *step 1*). The ideal solution is one that resolves the problem, deflating the balloon, without creating another problem: that is, unnecessary bladder irritation or balloon fragmentation. Of the methods recommended to decompress nondeflating catheter balloons, the only technique that approaches the ideal directly attacks this flap-valve deformity.

The inflate-deflate channel normally prevents the passive egress of inflating fluid or air. Occasionally, cutting off the inflation port will deflate the balloon, but usually, the problematic area is further along the catheter, closer to the bladder. Once the port has been removed, insert a needle attached to a syringe into the inflation channel to suck out balloon fluid (see Fig. 56.25, *step 4*). Cutting the catheter closer to the bladder may fortuitously cut off the offending area, but be careful not to cut off an excessive length of exposed catheter.

The inflation channel may have a valve defect or be filled with debris (see Fig. 56.25, *step 2*). If cutting the balloon port and using a needle attached to a syringe is unsuccessful, it is best to insert a thin, rigid wire into the balloon-port lumen in an attempt to deflate the valve-flap defect sufficiently and promote the escape of fluid from the balloon (see Fig. 56.25, *step 3*). Occasionally, the balloon itself may be punctured by this wire. The wire stylets from a central venous or angiographic catheter, guidewires from ureteral catheters, and very small, well-lubricated ureteral catheters themselves have all been reported to be successful. When a ureteral catheter guidewire was used in one series, 34 of 39 balloons were deflated without fragmentation.[43]

Once a malfunctioning balloon has been deflated, inspect the balloon itself for missing fragments. If a piece of the balloon is missing, arrange for subsequent cystoscopy to look for and remove the fragments.

Alternative methods of nondeflating catheter removal are presented in Table 56.5.

A variation on the nondeflating balloon is "cuffing," essentially an asymmetrical deflation in which the balloon does not deflate flush with the catheter. The irregularity becomes more pronounced as the catheter is withdrawn into the urethra, preventing easy withdrawal. This occurs more often when balloon fluid is quickly aspirated and less often with more gradual fluid withdrawal. Inflate the balloon again and try slow deflation if this occurs. Reinflating the balloon to a smooth surface with 0.5 mL to 1 mL of saline during withdrawal may also obviate this.

Traumatic Foley Catheter Removal

Occasionally, uncooperative or demented patients will pull out their Foley catheter with the balloon still inflated (Fig. 56.26). One would intuit that urethral injury is possible; however, there remain limited data on the incidence or type of injury from this maneuver or optimal pathways to address this situation. Usually, there is blood at the meatus, and it may be difficult to know whether the patient can spontaneously urinate. If the patient can spontaneously urinate, it would seem reasonable to gently pass another Foley catheter to avoid urethral obstruction by tears or clots and allow healing of urethral trauma with a new catheter in place. Most of the time, however, the clinician has minimal data yet is faced with the decision on how to approach this conundrum. Fortunately, this incident does not typically result in significant urethral injury. It is assumed that a new catheter will be required, either to continue the original catheter indication or to provide a stent while any urethral injury heals. In the absence of available urologic consultation, gentle attempts at passage of another Foley catheter are reasonable, without a routine retrograde urethrogram (described later in this chapter). If the catheter does not pass easily, stop and consider performing a retrograde urethrogram to assess the nature and extent of the pathology. Most of the time, simply replacing the catheter will be the most prudent approach. Prophylactic antibiotics are reasonable under these circumstances. Complete eversion and prolapse of the bladder have been rarely associated with this misadventure.[44]

Conclusions

Access to and the subsequent evaluation of bladder urine are at times clinically important to emergency practitioners. The merits of various approaches to urine specimen collection depend on the patient's age and clinical setting. Urethral catheterization generally provides a relatively safe and effective means of bladder access.

SUPRAPUBIC ASPIRATION

Introduction

Suprapubic aspiration of the bladder, first reported as a method of collecting urine for bacteriologic study in 1956,[45] offers the clinician a relatively simple means of obtaining uncontaminated bladder urine. It is utilized primarily in young children, although there are limited indications for this procedure in adults as well.

With proper technique, suprapubic aspiration consistently provides an uncontaminated urine specimen capable of distinguishing true bacteriuria from contamination. The perception and demonstration of increased discomfort and procedural failure rate, however, have led to a precipitous decline in its use, particularly outside of the neonatal intensive care unit setting.[46,47]

Despite the lack of experience by most currently practicing clinicians, the procedure may still be necessary in girls with labial adhesions and boys with phimosis. The introduction of ultrasound technology has led to a significant improvement in success rates, and likely in the comfort of the clinician performing the procedure.[48,49]

Removal of a Nondeflating Catheter

1

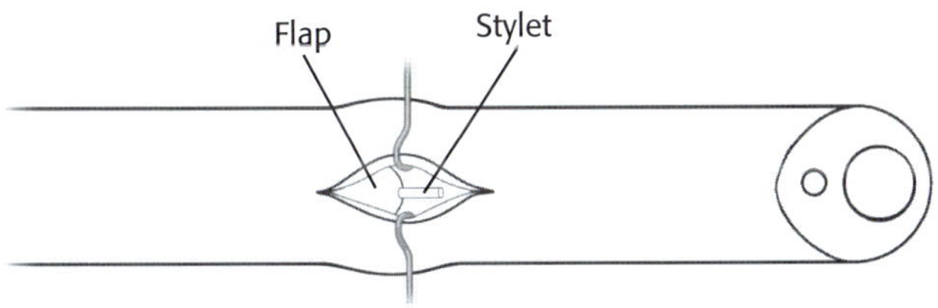

A flaplike defect in the inflating channel of a balloon catheter may prevent balloon deflation. A wire stylet (from a central venous catheter kit) can be passed down the inflating channel to raise the flap and deflate the balloon.

2

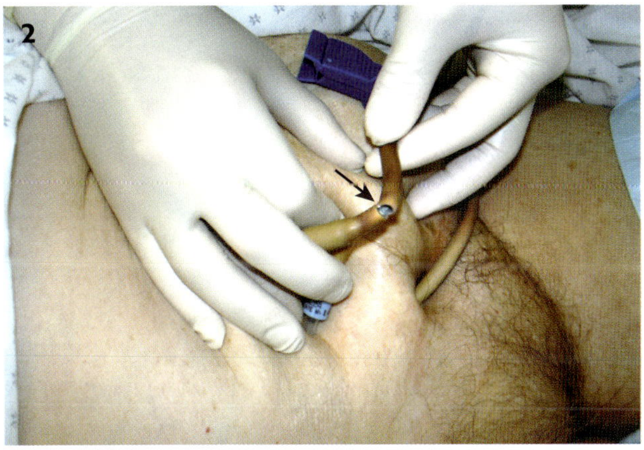

Note that the entire inflation channel is filled with debris *(arrow)*, thus preventing egress of fluid from the retaining balloon.

3

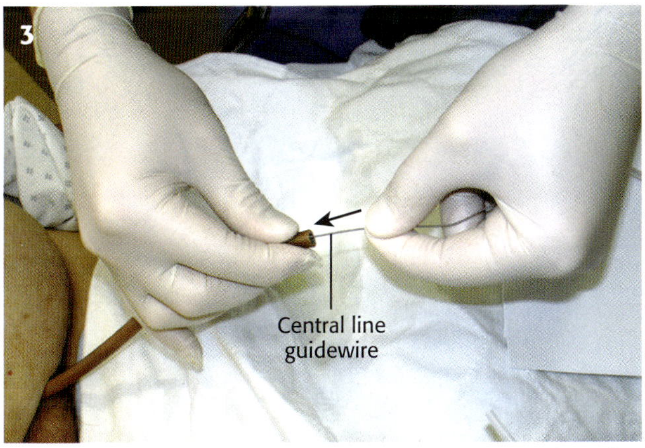

Cut the catheter, remove the inflation port, and advance the stiff end of a guidewire through the inflation channel. The wire may puncture the balloon or clear the channel so that fluid escapes.

4

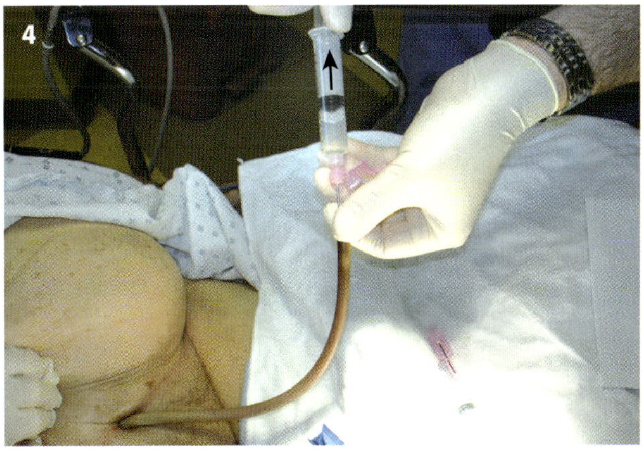

Once the channel has been cleared, insert a 20-gauge needle gently into the inflation channel to aspirate the balloon fluid.

5

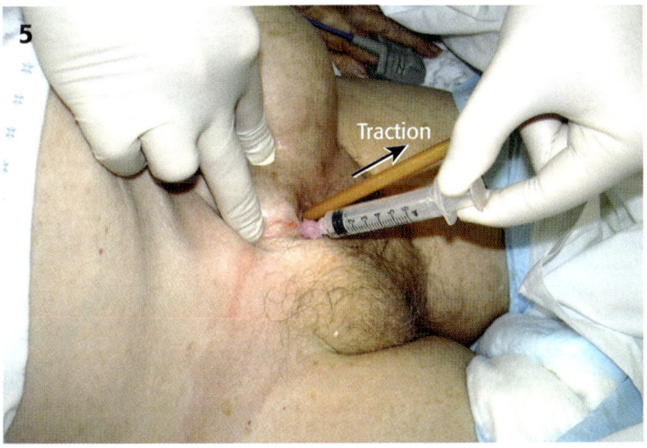

In the case of a nondeflating suprapubic balloon, you can try to insert a 25-gauge spinal needle parallel to the catheter to puncture the balloon. Maintain traction on the catheter to stabilize the balloon during the procedure.

6

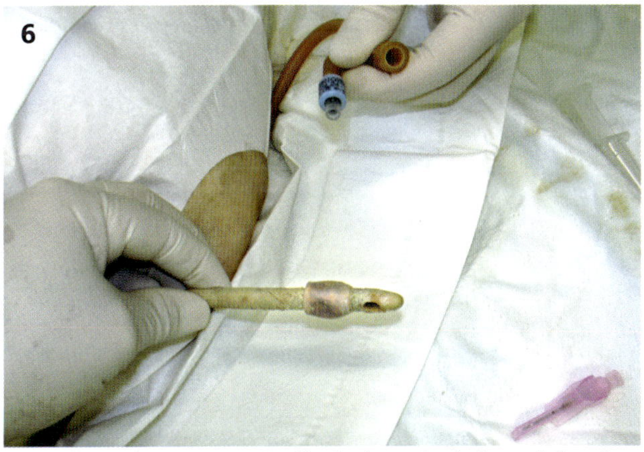

This balloon demonstrates "cuffing" where the balloon deflated asymmetrically and got caught up during withdrawal.

Fig. 56.25 Removal of a nondeflating catheter. (Step 1, From Eichenberg HA, Amin M, Clark J. Nondeflating Foley catheters. *Int Urol Nephrol.* 1976;8:171)

TABLE 56.5 Alternative Methods of Removing Nondeflating Catheters

METHOD	COMMENTS
Needle puncture of the balloon (see Fig. 56.25, *step 5*)	Overinflate the balloon (50–100 mL of saline) Draw the balloon against the bladder neck Use local anesthesia for the suprapubic approach Use a 25- to 27-gauge spinal needle to puncture the balloon Ultrasound guidance may be helpful
Hyperinflation of the balloon	High rate of balloon fragmentation: 100 of 100 in one report[a] Postprocedure cystoscopic inspection of the bladder is essential Consider adding 50–100 mL of saline into the bladder to cushion the effects of subsequent balloon rupture if no urinary retention is present Inject up to 200 mL of air into a 5-mL balloon to induce rupture
Injection of an erosive substance into the balloon port (e.g., mineral oil)	This technique has fallen out of favor High rate of balloon fragmentation: 97 of 100 in one report[a] Associated with chemical cystitis

[a]Steidle CP, Mulcahy JJ. Erosion of penile prostheses: a complication of urethral catheterization. *J Urol.* 1989;142:737-739.

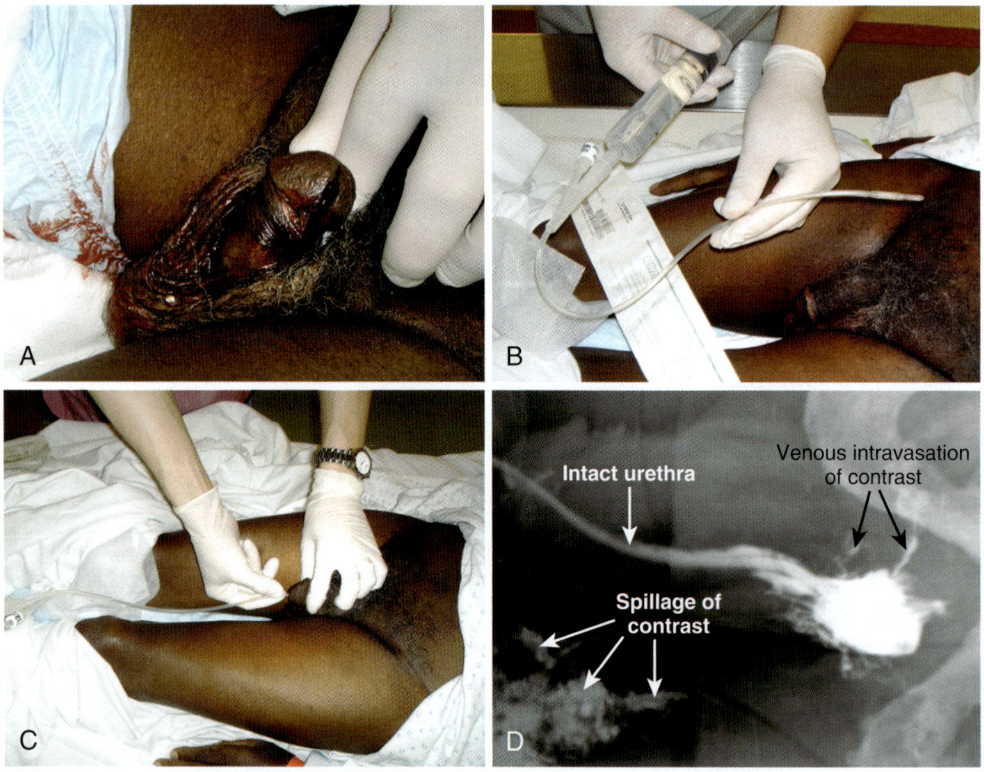

Fig. 56.26 Traumatic Foley catheter removal. (A) This patient pulled out his Foley catheter with the balloon inflated. Blood appeared at the meatus. His mental status prevented assessment of his ability to void spontaneously. Given the large volume of the previously inflated balloon and detection of gross blood, it was decided to perform retrograde urethrography, although it is not unreasonable to simply try to gently pass a new catheter depending on the overall clinical picture. (B) Place a balloon-tipped catheter into the meatus and inflate with 1 to 2 mL of air or water. (C) Squeeze the glans while an assistant slowly injects contrast material. (D) Overzealous injection resulted in venous uptake of the dye and spillage on the patient's leg. The urethra is intact. A new catheter was easily passed.

Procedure Overview

Indications: provides the clinician with a urine sample that is reliable for bacteriologic interpretation.

Contraindications: infection at proposed puncture site.

Complications: infection or hematoma at puncture site; simple penetration of the bowel with a needle is considered an innocuous event and requires no specific treatment.

Equipment: skin cleansing agent, local anesthetic, needle (usually 22-gauge) and syringe for puncture and aspiration procedure.

Key Procedure Sequence

1. Place the patient supine on the examination table.
2. Place the legs in the frog-leg position.

3. Locate the full bladder (ultrasound guidance is often helpful).
4. Prep and drape the skin.
5. Place a wheal of local anesthetic at the aspiration site.
6. Advance the needle (usually 22-gauge, 3.75- to 8.75-cm length) in the midline through the skin and subcutaneous tissues toward the bladder.
7. Actively aspirate the syringe while simultaneously advancing.
8. If the bladder is entered, urine appears in the syringe.
9. If there is no urine, withdraw the needle to a subcutaneous position and redirect it at a different angle.
10. Following adequate urine collection, withdraw the syringe and needle.

Description

Background

Utilized primarily in young children as an alternate means of urine specimen collection.

Anatomy and Physiology

See Fig. 56.27.

Pathophysiology

Results in urine specimen collection capable of distinguishing true bacteriuria from contamination.

Indications

In the neonate or the young child, suprapubic aspiration or urethral catheterization can provide the clinician with a sample that is reliable for bacteriologic interpretation. Although disconcerting to some parents, suprapubic aspiration is not a dangerous procedure, and the sensitivity of urinalysis for bacteriuria approaches 100%. For many young children, however, urine can generally be more readily collected by urethral catheterization.

For adult patients, the indications for suprapubic aspiration are more limited because these patients can usually cooperate with the clinician. Males with condom catheters or phimosis, however, may require suprapubic aspiration to minimize urethral contamination. Aspirated cultures, rather than catheterized specimens, may help assess for infection versus contamination in patients with asymptomatic bacteriuria on routine urine collection. In infections caused by organisms that in other circumstances are often discounted as contaminants (e.g., *Staphylococcus epidermidis* or *Candida albicans*), suprapubic aspiration or a catheterized specimen may be necessary to confirm the presence of such pathogens.

In patients in whom the possibility of infravesical infection is a concern (e.g., patients with chronic infections of the urethra or the periurethral glands), suprapubic aspiration may help distinguish a bladder source from a urethral source.

Contraindications

Skin or soft tissue infection in the area of the proposed anterior abdominal wall puncture site.

Procedure

Place the child supine with the legs in a frog-leg position and gently restrain as necessary (Fig. 56.27*A*, *step 1*). First locate the bladder. A full, palpable, or percussible bladder may be readily apparent, though this can be difficult to discern depending on body habitus. If there is any question about the location or the amount of bladder urine, a quick ultrasound examination is informative. The point of entry in the skin should be 1 cm to 2 cm above the superior edge of the symphysis pubis. Pass the syringe and needle perpendicular to the abdominal wall toward the bladder, usually at a 10- to 20-degree angle from the true vertical, somewhat cephalad in children (see Fig. 56.27*A*, *step 2*) and somewhat caudad in adults (see Fig. 56.27*B*). Note that the bladder of a newborn is an abdominal organ and that it will be missed if the needle is inserted too close to the pubis or angled toward the feet.

After draping the prepared skin and choosing the point of entry, raise a skin wheal of local anesthesia to reduce discomfort. After anesthetizing the skin, advance a longer, midcaliber needle (usually 22-gauge, 3.75 to 8.75 cm in length) in the midline through the skin and quickly into the bladder. Advance the needle attached to a syringe and aspirate during advancement. As soon as the bladder is entered, urine will appear in the syringe. A short needle is adequate for virtually all pediatric patients. After collecting urine, withdraw the syringe and needle. Microscopic hematuria always follows the procedure but gross hematuria is uncommon.

If urine is not obtained, do not remove the needle; rather, withdraw it to a subcutaneous position and redirect it at a different angle. Often a child may spontaneously start to void after any type of invasive stimulus (e.g., bladder irritation by a probing needle, venipuncture, or lumbar puncture). Hence, prepare to collect a spontaneously voided specimen, should that option arise. Anticipate this before beginning blood or spinal fluid collection during the bacteremic workup of the febrile neonate.

In most patients, an acceptable urine sample can be obtained with the first needle pass. If the needle points too caudad, in an effort to avoid entering the peritoneum, it is possible to enter the retropubic space, skimming the bladder muscle and never penetrating the bladder mucosa.

Aftercare

Following withdrawal of the needle, place a simple bandage over the puncture site.

Complications

Bacteremia does not typically result from suprapubic aspiration. Bowel penetration has occurred in children with distended abdomens from gastrointestinal disturbances. The combination of gaseous bowel distention and relative hypovolemia might displace and flatten the relatively empty bladder against the pelvic floor. Even when the large bowel has been penetrated, most patients typically recover uneventfully. As a general rule, simple penetration of the bowel with a needle is considered an innocuous event and requires no specific treatment.

Conclusions

Although it can be performed in a patient of any age, suprapubic aspiration is utilized for urine collection in young children only when alternative collection methods are not feasible. It consistently provides a urine specimen that is capable of distinguishing true bacteriuria from contamination. However, in many cases, alternative methods of urine collection are preferred over this procedure.

Suprapubic Aspiration

A. Pediatric

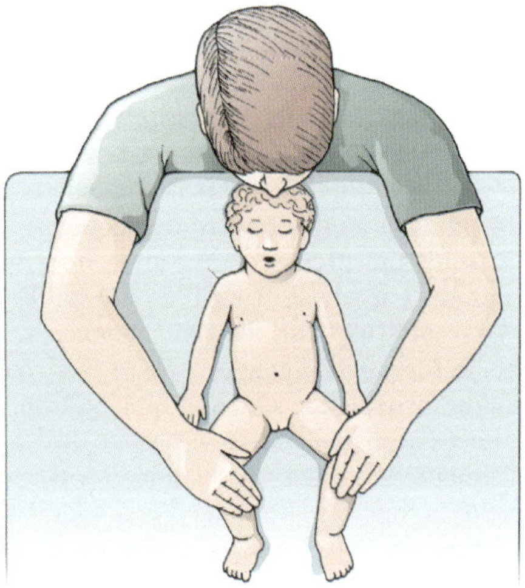

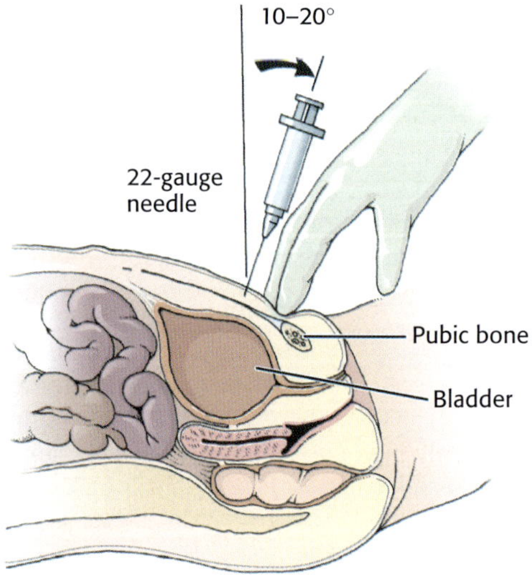

1. Restrain the infant and place her in a frog-leg position. Prepare and drape the skin, and raise a skin wheal with local anesthetic to reduce discomfort. Despite the safety of this procedure, it may be disconcerting for worried parents, and they may wish to leave the room during the aspiration.

2. Puncture the abdominal wall with a 22-gauge needle in the midline approximately 1 to 2 cm cephalad to the superior border of the pubic bone. Keep the syringe perpendicular to the plane of the abdominal wall (usually 10 to 20 degrees from the true vertical). The bladder is an abdominal organ in infants, and placing the needle too close to the pubic bone or angling toward the feet might cause the needle to miss the bladder. Localizing the bladder with bedside ultrasound facilitates this procedure.

B. Adult

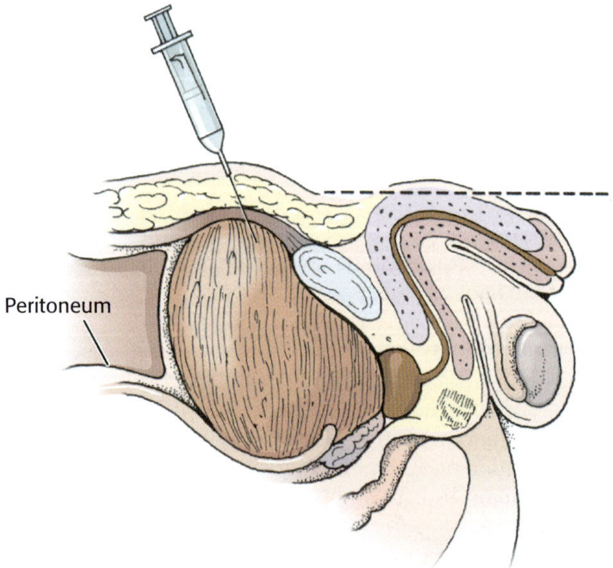

In adults, the peritoneum is pushed cephalad by the filled bladder during suprapubic aspiration. Direct the needle slightly caudad.

Fig. 56.27 Suprapubic aspiration.

SUPRAPUBIC CYSTOSTOMY

Introduction

In general, any patient requiring a urethral catheter in whom a catheter cannot be safely passed is a candidate for a suprapubic cystostomy tube.

Among the most user-friendly devices for suprapubic bladder access is the Cook peel-away sheath unit (Cook Medical). It employs the Seldinger (guidewire) technique to gain bladder access and allows suprapubic placement of a Foley balloon catheter for definitive bladder drainage. This device is readily suitable for ED use when compared with other suprapubic bladder access approaches, such as trocar-type devices.

When emergency bladder drainage is required and a transurethral Foley catheter cannot be placed, any device suitable for central venous access can be inserted suprapubically using the Seldinger technique (Fig. 56.28).

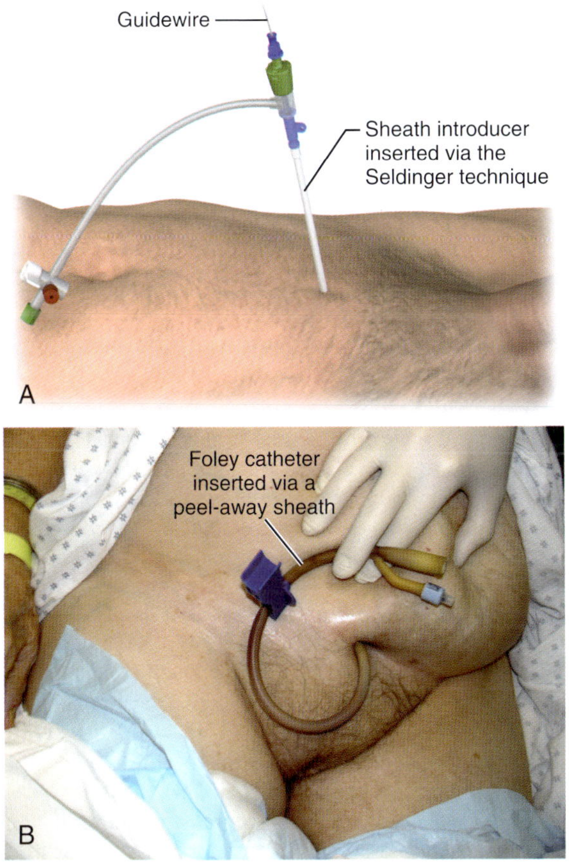

Fig. 56.28 Suprapubic cystostomy. (A) Any catheter that can be used as a central venous catheter can be inserted suprapubically via the Seldinger technique. (B) The more traditional and more permanent suprapubic cystostomy with a Foley catheter inserted through a Cook peel-away sheath introducer.

Procedure Overview

Indications: need for emergency bladder access and drainage.

Contraindications: bladder not readily definable or excessively low bladder volume; relative contraindications include history of previous lower abdominal surgery, intraperitoneal surgery, irradiation, bleeding diathesis, or concurrent antithrombotic use.

Complications: a wide variety of complications have been reported, including bowel or other organ injuries, which serve as reminders that suprapubic cystostomy is not innocuous.

Equipment: O'Brien Suprapubic Peel-Away Access Set (Cook Medical) and Foley catheter.

Key Procedure Sequence

1. Prep and drape the skin for a sterile procedure.
2. Inject local anesthesia ~2 cm to 3 cm above the pubic symphysis.
3. Locate the bladder by palpation (or ultrasound). While aspirating, advance a 22-gauge spinal needle with an attached syringe until urine returns.
4. Keep the needle in place, remove the syringe, and thread the guidewire through the needle into the bladder.
5. Once the guidewire is threaded into the bladder, remove the needle.
6. Make a stab incision at the guidewire/skin interface.
7. Pass a peel-away sheath and indwelling fascial dilator device over the wire.
8. Remove the guidewire and fascial dilator, leaving only the sheath in place.
9. Pass a Foley balloon catheter through the sheath and inflate the catheter.
10. Withdraw the peel-away sheath, leaving only the suprapubic catheter in place.

Description

Background

In situations where emergency bladder access is necessary, the Seldinger (guidewire) technique allows for suprapubic placement of a Foley balloon catheter for definitive bladder drainage.

Anatomy and Physiology

See Fig. 56.29.

Pathophysiology

In emergency situations, the majority of patients requiring suprapubic cystostomy are trauma patients with urethral disruption, or males with severe urethral stricture or complex prostatic disease.

Indications

If time allows, it is prudent to discuss the case with a urologist to explore alternative methods of bladder access and urine drainage prior to initiation of a suprapubic cystostomy. Even in the case of major trauma, many affected patients will require laparotomy for associated injuries, thus the suprapubic catheter can be placed intraoperatively.

Contraindications

Because placement of a suprapubic tube involves some risk, proper patient selection is important. Exercise caution when performing the procedure in a patient whose bladder is not readily definable. Although no absolute reported minimum bladder volume has been established, there must be enough urine in the bladder to allow the needle to fully penetrate the bladder dome without immediately exiting through the base. There must also be enough urine in the bladder to displace the bowel away from the anterosuperior surface of the bladder and the entrance of the needle. Ultrasound can be helpful in defining bladder anatomy.

Individuals who have a history of previous lower abdominal surgery, intraperitoneal surgery, or irradiation may have developed adhesions or adherence of the bowel to the anterior bladder wall. They are potentially at greater risk for bowel injury during percutaneous suprapubic cystostomy tube placement than those without previous abdominal surgery. Blind suprapubic cystostomy tube placement should be avoided in these patients. The absence of any of these risk factors does not entirely exclude the risks of bowel or intraperitoneal injury, though it reduces them significantly.

Patients with bleeding diatheses are at greater risk for postinsertion bleeding, either into the bladder, into the retropubic space, or at the site of skin entry.

Procedure

See Videos 56.10, 56.11. The following comments pertain to the placement of the Cook peel-away sheath. With modifications, the same principles apply for any type of suprapubic catheter placement.

If necessary, shave the lower abdomen and apply antiseptic topically. Fill a 10-mL syringe with 1% lidocaine, and attach it to a 22-gauge, 7.75-cm or similar spinal needle. Raise a skin wheal in the proposed site (~2–3 cm above the pubic symphysis) and infiltrate the subcutaneous tissue and rectus abdominis muscle fascia at a 10- to 20-degree angle toward the pelvis.

Locate the bladder by advancing the needle in the prescribed direction while aspirating the syringe. Urine is easily aspirated when the bladder is entered (Fig. 56.29, *step 1*).

Once the bladder has been located, remove the syringe from the needle and advance a guidewire through the needle into the bladder (see Fig. 56.29, *step 2*). Withdraw the needle, leaving only the guidewire traversing the anterior abdominal wall and positioned inside the bladder. Use a No. 11 or similar scalpel blade to make a stab incision directly posterior to the wire through the skin, subcutaneous tissue, and superficial anterior abdominal wall fascia. Then pass the peel-away sheath and indwelling fascial dilator together over the wire into the bladder (see Fig. 56.29, *step 3*). Remove the guidewire and fascial dilator, leaving only the peel-away sheath inside the bladder (see Fig. 56.29, *step 4*). Then pass a Foley balloon catheter through the indwelling intravesical sheath into the bladder (see Fig. 56.29, *step 5*). Aspirate urine to confirm proper placement. Inflate the Foley balloon with a minimum of 10 mL of air, water, or saline (see Fig. 56.29, *step 6*). A 5-mL balloon will accommodate 10 mL readily and make accidental catheter distraction less likely. Withdraw the peel-away sheath from the bladder and anterior abdominal wall and literally peel it away from the catheter, leaving only the indwelling suprapubic Foley catheter (see Fig. 56.29, *step 7*). Withdraw the catheter slowly until the inflated balloon approximates the cystostomy site (see Fig. 56.29, *step 8*).

Aftercare

Connect the catheter to a drainage bag, then dress the wound with 4 × 4 gauze pads to complete the procedure. The major difficulty with cystostomy tubes of all designs is securing them to the patient's skin. Those with retention balloons, such as the standard Foley urethral catheter, are the most secure and need only tape to attach them to the anterior abdominal wall.

Complications

A wide variety of complications have been reported, which serve as reminders that suprapubic cystostomy is not innocuous. Occasionally, the suprapubic tube or catheter cannot be positioned or maintained successfully without complications (Box 56.5).

The most serious complications involve perforation of the peritoneum or the intraperitoneal contents. Although finding the bladder using a small-gauge "scout" needle may help reduce bowel injury, even in the most apparently successful of bladder punctures, a complication may still result.

Occasionally, the clinician proceeds with suprapubic cystostomy when the bladder is not palpable and has not been located with a syringe and needle. Injury of adjacent organs is much more frequent in these circumstances. Allowing the bladder to refill over time can be an important consideration, especially if initial attempts to locate the bladder were unsuccessful. Ultrasound guidance is helpful for determining bladder size and location.

Conclusions

Suprapubic cystostomy can be readily performed when emergency bladder access is needed. This procedure, however, may be associated with significant risks to the patient. As such, when time affords, discussion with a urologist is prudent to explore alternative methods of bladder access and urine drainage.

LOWER GENITOURINARY TRACT IMAGING

Introduction

Although the signs of GU trauma in general can be quite subtle, lower urinary tract injury can often be rapidly identified and evaluated radiographically in the ED. Radiologic imaging of the upper urinary tract is generally a less urgent matter and can usually be done in the radiology suite or, when important for emergency operative decision-making, as a single-phase intravenous pyelogram (IVP) in the operating room.

The timing of any radiologic evaluation can be challenging in the emergency setting, especially when faced with a critically ill, multiply injured patient. The trauma team of clinicians involved in each resuscitation must determine the priority and extent of such an evaluation on a case-by-case basis.

In patients with urologic trauma, the lower urinary tract should be studied before the upper urinary tract (e.g., study the urethra before the bladder, study the bladder before the kidneys). As such, specific diagnostic studies should be conducted in a retrograde fashion (Fig. 56.30).

RUG and retrograde cystography are the diagnostic procedures of choice to evaluate potential injury to the lower urinary tract. These studies must be carried out in the proper sequence and in a retrograde fashion to avoid missing potential injuries. Retrograde refers to the technique of instilling contrast retrograde through the urethra or by gravity filling of the bladder. It must be distinguished from antegrade filling, in which intravenous contrast for IVP or abdominal computed tomography (CT) is excreted from the kidneys and allowed to fill the bladder passively over time.

Procedure Overview

Indications: RUG is indicated whenever uncertainty exists about the integrity of the urethra; retrograde cystography is indicated any time a bladder injury is suspected.

Contraindications: uncertainty about urethral integrity is a contraindication to blind urethral catheterization; ensuring urethral integrity with a RUG prior to Foley catheter placement is necessary for retrograde cystography; prior history of reaction to radiographic contrast material is a precaution.

Complications: tissue irritation from contrast extravasation; progression of urethral injury from overly forceful injection of contrast material.

Equipment: equipment and personnel for plain radiographs (or fluoroscopy), small Foley catheter (or Toomey syringe), contrast material for injection.

Key Procedure Sequence

Retrograde Urethrogram

1. Assemble the items and personnel needed for plain imaging (or fluoroscopy).
2. In case of pelvic fracture, keep the patient supine.

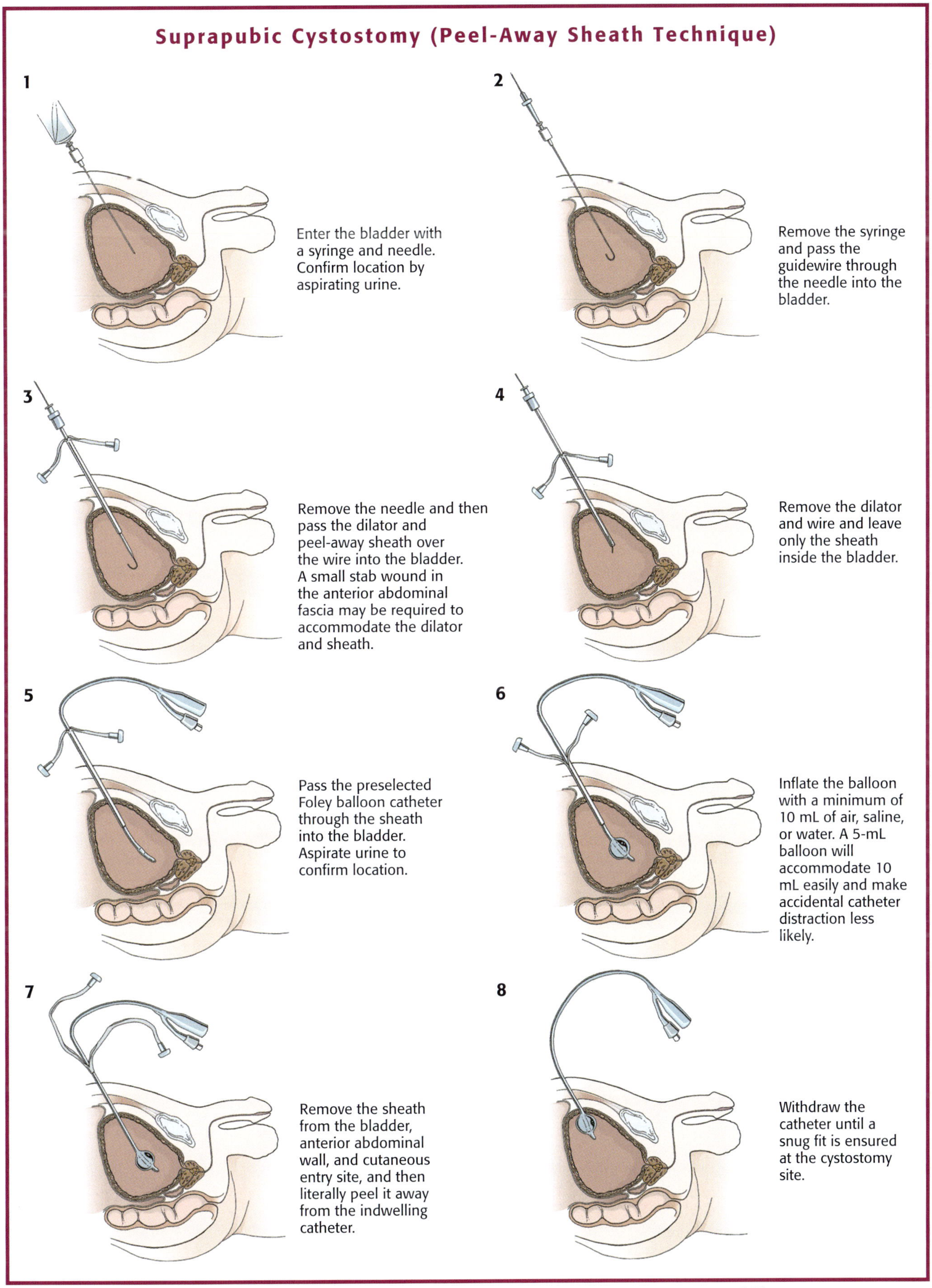

Fig. 56.29 Suprapubic cystostomy using a peel-away sheath. If this equipment is not available, an analogous procedure using any catheter suitable for central venous catheterization may be performed.

BOX 56.5 Complications of Suprapubic Cystostomy

Bowel perforation
Through-and-through bladder penetration with associated rectal, vaginal, or uterine injury
Intraperitoneal extravasation (without a previous history of surgery)
Extraperitoneal extravasation
Ureteral catheterization
Obstruction of the tubing (blood, mucus, or kinking)
Tubing dislodgement
Infection
Hematuria

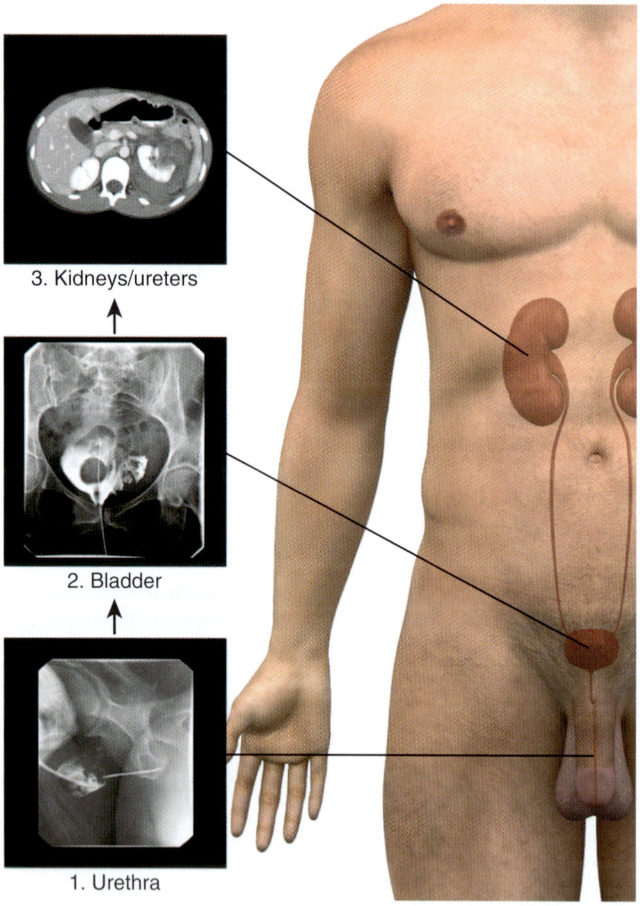

Fig. 56.30 Diagnostic approach to genitourinary (GU) tract trauma. The GU tract is studied in a retrograde fashion, proceeding from the urethra (retrograde urethrography) to the bladder (conventional or computed tomographic [CT] cystography) to the kidneys and ureters (CT urography with delayed/excretory images). These studies must be carried out in the proper sequence and in a retrograde fashion to avoid missing potential injuries.

3. In other cases, orient the hips in a slightly oblique position in relation to the stretcher.
4. Gently extend and stretch the penis along the medial thigh to maximize urethral unfolding.
5. Obtain a plain radiograph (kidneys, ureters, and bladder [KUB]) or fluoroscopy for a reference image prior to injecting the contrast.
6. Retract the foreskin, if present, and secure the glans with a folded 4 × 4 gauze pad.
7. Hold the penis securely in the nondominant hand.
8. Insert a non–Luer-Lok syringe or a small Foley catheter snugly into the meatus.
9. Before injecting contrast, stretch the penis perpendicularly across the patient's thigh.
10. Gently inject 10 to 15 mL of contrast; avoid an overly forceful injection.
11. Immediately following the contrast injection, obtain a radiograph (urethrogram).

Retrograde Cystogram

1. Assemble items and personnel needed for plain imaging (or fluoroscopy).
2. In the case of a pelvic fracture, keep the patient supine.
3. In other cases, orient the hips in a slightly oblique position in relation to the stretcher.
4. Perform a RUG to ensure urethral integrity prior to placement of the catheter needed for the cystogram.
5. Remove the central plunger from a 60-mL catheter-tip syringe and attach the tip to a Foley catheter.
6. Hold the syringe above the level of the bladder and pour contrast material into the syringe.
7. Allow the bladder to fill by gravity instillation and fill to capacity (~400 mL in an adult).
8. Clamp the catheter, obtain both anteroposterior (AP) and oblique images (or AP and lateral if oblique not feasible).
9. Obtain an AP postevacuation film after bladder drainage.
10. If bladder injury is detected, keep the catheter in place and consult urology.

Description

Background

In the resuscitation of any trauma patient, placement of a Foley catheter is a standard method of monitoring urinary output. Blood at the urethral meatus, however, may indicate a partial or complete urethral disruption and dictates the need for an RUG to delineate urethral integrity. This study can be done by the resuscitating clinician in the ED or on the operating room table by the trauma surgeon or urologist if the patient requires immediate surgical intervention for life-threatening injuries. RUG is quick, technically easy study to perform, and should be part of every emergency clinician's armamentarium. Similarly, retrograde cystography allows for the evaluation of bladder integrity.

Anatomy and Physiology

The anatomy of the male urethra is demonstrated in Fig. 56.17. The male urethra varies from 17.5 to 20 cm in length for adults and consists of anterior and posterior portions, each of which is subdivided into two parts. The membranous and prostatic segments are posterior, and the pendulous and bulbous urethral segments are anterior. The female urethra is approximately 4 cm long and extends from the bladder neck at the urethrovesical junction to the vaginal vestibule, where it forms the external meatus between the labia minora (see Figs. 56.15 and 56.16).

Pathophysiology

The male posterior urethra, which includes the membranous and prostatic urethra, is injured more frequently than the

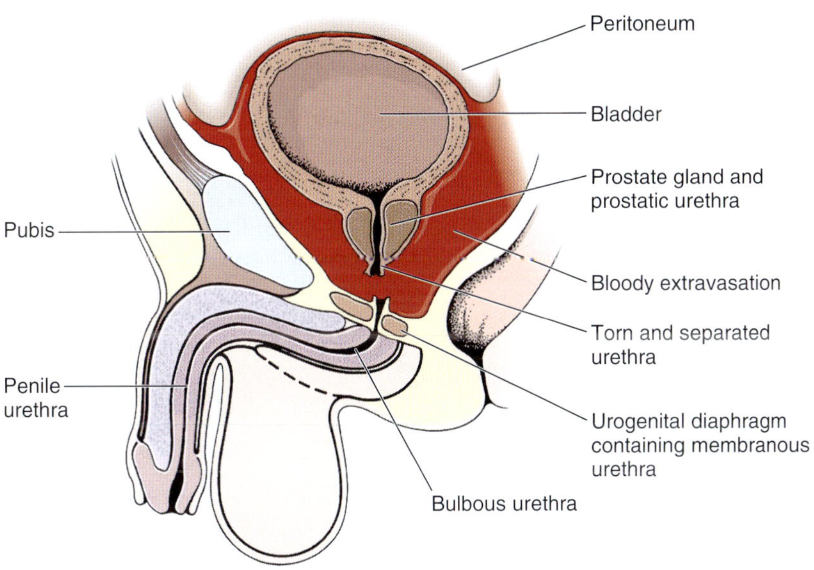

Fig. 56.31 Posterior urethral injury. A common posterior urethral injury is disruption of the membranous urethra. In this case, a distended bladder and attached prostate gland are sheared from the fixed membranous urethra. Note the development of a perivesical hematoma and the presence of a high-riding prostate gland. This scenario will prohibit the passage of a catheter.

anterior urethra. The urogenital diaphragm encloses and fixes the membranous urethra; the prostate and prostatic urethra are firmly attached to the posterior surface of the symphysis pubis by the puboprostatic ligaments. Blunt trauma and pelvic fractures, especially in the presence of a full bladder, may result in shearing forces that partially or completely avulse portions of the firmly attached posterior urethra. Usually, the bladder and prostate gland are sheared from the membranous urethra, resulting in a complete urethral disruption (Fig. 56.31). The female urethra, in contrast, is short and relatively mobile and generally escapes injury in blunt trauma. Occasionally, a significant pelvic fracture will result in a laceration or avulsion of the female urethra at the bladder neck. Direct injuries to the female urethra may also occur secondary to penetrating trauma to the vagina or perineum. These injuries often are disclosed by blood at the introitus or an abnormal vaginal examination in the female pelvic fracture patient.

Contusions or lacerations of the male anterior urethra occur when the bulbous urethra is compressed against the inferior surface of the symphysis pubis. This happens most commonly as a result of straddle injuries in males but may result from any blunt perineal trauma. Penetrating injuries or urethral instrumentation may also cause injuries to the penile urethra. Anterior urethral injuries may result in extravasation of blood or urine into the penis, scrotum, or perineum or along the anterior abdominal wall, depending on whether Buck's fascia has been violated (Fig. 56.32). This is in contrast to posterior urethral injuries, in which blood and urine extravasate into the pelvis.

Indications

RUG is indicated whenever uncertainty exists about the integrity of the urethra. The RUG is an anatomic rather than a physiologic examination, and remains critical in the identification of a possible urethral injury prior to urinary catheter insertion to preclude a potentially devastating complication.[50]

The traditional physical indications to perform a RUG in the trauma setting include blood at the urethral meatus, a nonpalpable or high-riding prostate, or evidence of urethral trauma. The value of these findings to the emergency clinician, particularly a "high-riding prostate," has been called into question, given their low sensitivity.[51,52]

Perform a retrograde cystogram any time a bladder injury is suspected. It assumes that the urethra is normal before passing the Foley catheter required for retrograde cystography.

Contraindications

Uncertainty about urethral integrity is a contraindication to blind urethral catheterization. As such, urethral integrity must be ensured prior to Foley catheter placement, which is essential for retrograde cystography. History of a prior reaction to radiographic contrast material is a relative contraindication to contrast use, depending on the route of administration selected. Intravenous administration for antegrade imaging carries a higher risk of serious adverse events as compared with retrograde injection or instillation of iodinated contrast materials necessary for lower GU tract imaging.

Procedure

Several different iodinated contrast agents are suitable for retrograde studies (urethography, cystography). Common agents, dosages, and methods of administration are listed in Table 56.6.

RUG and retrograde cystography should ideally be performed under fluoroscopy to provide real-time imaging, though plain films are an acceptable and frequently utilized alternative.

Retrograde Urethrogram

A patient with an associated pelvic fracture should remain supine throughout the entire radiographic examination. In cases of suspected urethral injury not associated with pelvic fracture, it is acceptable to obtain oblique films during the study that may complement the examination findings (e.g. supine 45-degree oblique position).

First, take a plain film (KUB) or fluoroscopic image for reference before injecting any contrast material.[53] Retract and secure the penile foreskin, if applicable, with a folded 4 × 4

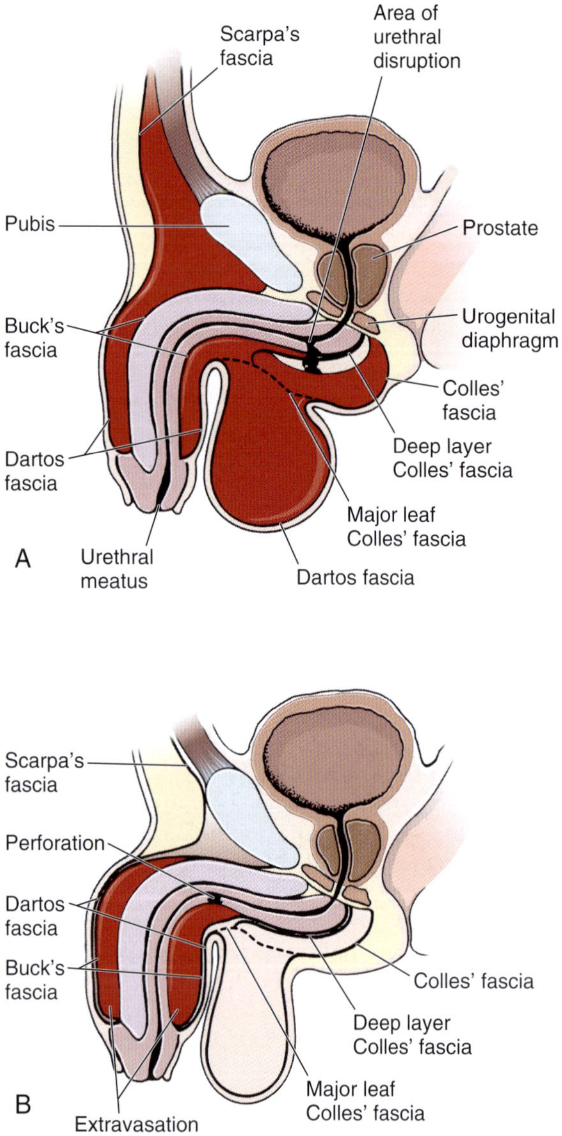

Fig. 56.32 Anterior urethral injury. (A) Disruption of the anterior urethra (bulbous urethra) occurs with straddle-type injuries in a male. Extravasation of urine and blood may occur in the perineum or scrotum or along the anterior abdominal wall. Note that in this diagram Buck's fascia has been penetrated. (B) Anterior urethral injury in which Buck's fascia remains intact. In this situation, extravasation is confirmed and results in a swollen and ecchymotic penis. Such an injury usually results from instrumentation of the anterior urethra.

gauze sponge. Second, hold the distal end of the penis in the nondominant hand to allow a snug fit of the contrast-filled syringe or catheter inside the urethral meatus. Stretch the penis laterally over the proximal thigh with moderate traction to prevent urethral folding (i.e., the double image of the proximal penile and bulbous urethra superimposed on one another) to ensure a high-quality RUG (Fig. 56.33, *step 3*).

After sterilizing the glans and urethra meatus, prepare to inject the dye. A small Foley catheter may be used (see Fig. 56.33, *step 1*). Seat the balloon portion of the catheter in the fossa navicularis of the penile urethra, and delicately inflate it with 1.0 to 1.5 mL of saline solution to ensure a snug fit. Lubrication is not recommended because it may prevent the balloon from remaining in place. Alternatively, apply steady manual pressure of the balloon against the external urethral meatus (distal to the fossa navicularis). Another option is to gently advance a catheter-tipped Toomey irrigating syringe or a regular 60-mL syringe with an attached Christmas-tree adapter or a non–Luer-Lok syringe inside the urethral meatus until a snug fit is ensured (see Fig. 56.33, *step 2*). Gently squeeze the meatus over the injecting device to prevent leaking.

Inject contrast through the catheter or syringe. If not done carefully, this technique often results in the spillage and deposition of contrast outside the urethra and onto the patient and the examination table, yielding a spurious radiographic result. As such, slowly inject anywhere from 10 mL to 60 mL of contrast material (typically less than 10 to 20 mL is all that is needed) under constant pressure into the urethra. Not uncommonly, a spasm of the external urethral sphincter will be encountered, preventing filling of the posterior urethra. Use slow, gentle pressure to overcome this resistance.[54] Overly forceful injection of contrast material may cause intravasation of contrast material into the venous plexus of the urethra, simulating an injury (see Fig. 56.33, *step 4*). Finally, during the injection of the last 10 mL of contrast, take a film (the urethrogram) (see Fig. 56.33, *step 3*). Alternatively, view the urethrogram in real time utilizing fluoroscopy.

The extravasation of contrast material from a urethral disruption usually appears as a flamelike density outside the urethral contour (see Fig. 56.33, *steps 5–7*). If any contrast material is seen within the bladder in conjunction with urethral extravasation, a partial rather than a complete urethral disruption is more likely. In a complete urethral disruption, urethral extravasation will be present without evidence of contrast within the bladder. The examiner needs to be certain that the lack of bladder contrast is not secondary to voluntary contraction

TABLE 56.6 Common Agents, Dosages, and Administration Information for Contrast-Enhanced Retrograde Urologic Imaging

AGENTS[a]	USE	PROCEDURE
Diatrizoate (Cystografin) or Dilute iohexol (Omnipaque)	Use a stock concentration of solution[b] or Use a one-half stock concentration of solution or Dilute the stock solution with saline in a ratio of 1 part contrast to 10 parts saline (resulting in a <10% solution)	*Urethrography:* 10–15 mL of dilute solution injected slowly through the urethral meatus for adults (children: 0.2 mL/kg) *Cystography:* after a plain film and with the Foley catheter in place, fill the bladder of adults with 400 mL of dilute contrast material introduced under gravity (children: 5 mL/kg)

[a]Kawashima A, Sandler CM, Wasserman NF et al. Imaging of urethral disease: a pictorial review. *Radiographics* 2004;24:S195-S216.
[b]A higher concentration may allow improved image quality; however, extravasation of contrast material into periurethral or perivesical tissues may cause a considerable inflammatory reaction at higher concentrations. Iohexol should be diluted per package insert instructions.
Data from American College of Radiology (ACR) Committee on Drugs and Contrast Media. *ACR Manual on Contrast Media*. Reston: American College of Radiology; 2023.

Retrograde Urethrography

1

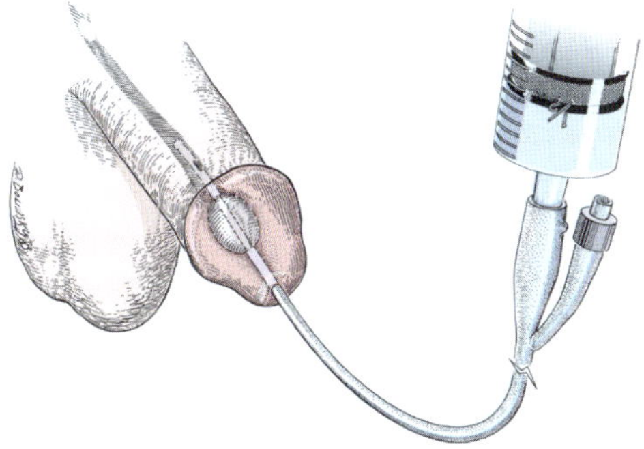

Insert the balloon portion of a Foley catheter (8 Fr) into the urethra, and slowly inflate the balloon with 2 mL of air or water to create a snug fit. Then slowly inject 10 to 60 mL of a 10% solution of contrast material through the catheter lumen. Usually only 10 to 20 mL is required.

2

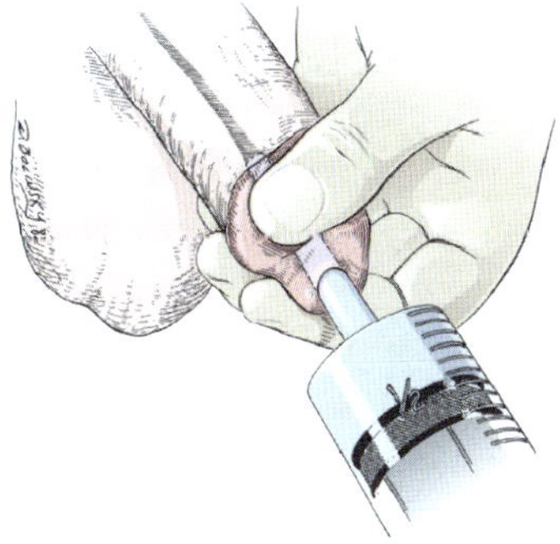

Alternatively, use a plain-tipped (non–Luer-Lok) syringe or a catheter-tipped (Toomey) syringe in the urethra. Squeeze the glans around the syringe to prevent spillage of the contrast material. Inject slowly.

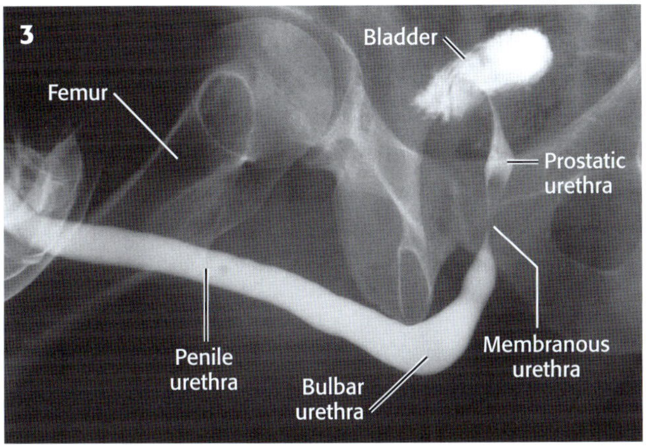

Normal retrograde urethrogram. Note that penis is pulled taut over the proximal part of the thigh to prevent urethral folding. After injection of contrast material, the entire urethra can be visualized and inspected for injury.

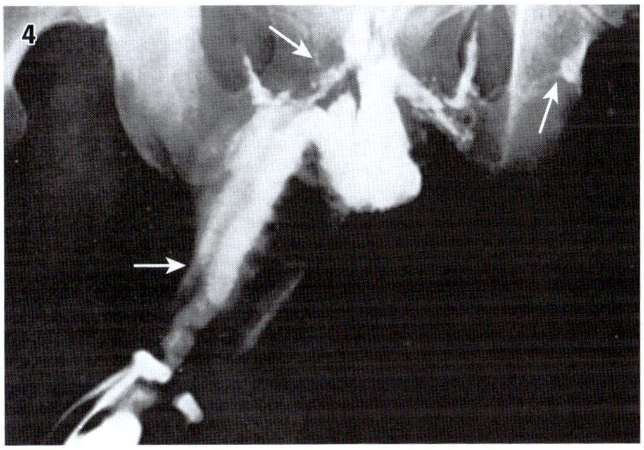

Inject the contrast material slowly. Injecting too fast causes venous intravasation *(arrows)*. This may mimic urethral extravasation but it clears immediately, as opposed to actual extravasation, which remains indefinitely. If unsure, take another film in 10 minutes. The presence of intravasation is benign but can confuse the clinician.

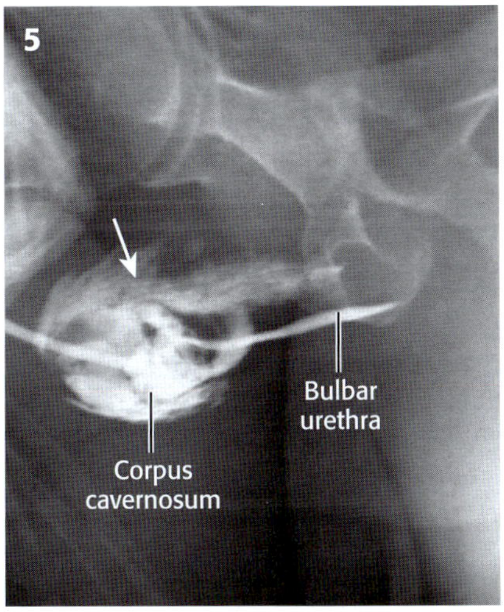

Penile urethral disruption. Extravasation of contrast material *(arrow)* is seen in the corpus cavernosum.

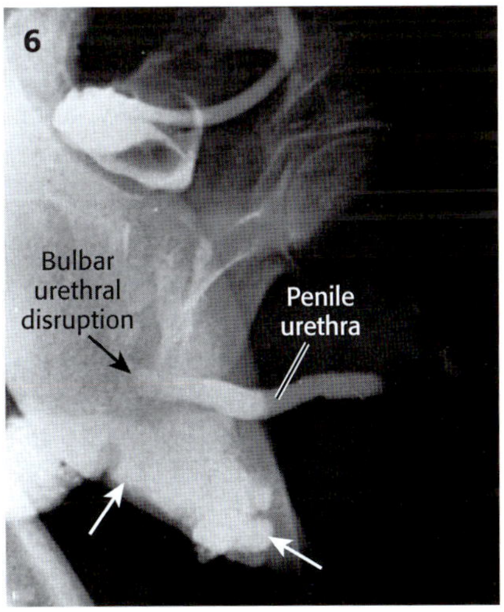

Bulbar urethral disruption. Extravasation of contrast material *(white arrows)* is seen in the scrotum.

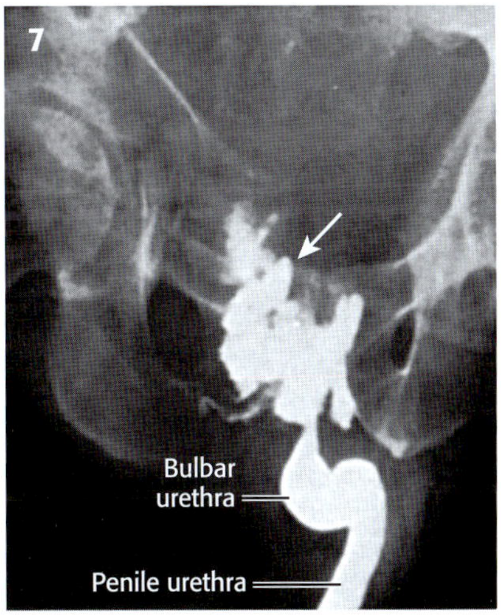

Supramembranous urethral disruption. Extravasation of contrast material *(arrow)* is noted superiorly.

Fig. 56.33 Retrograde urethrography. (Step 4, From Richter MW, Lytton B, Myerson D et al. Radiology of genitourinary trauma. *Radiol Clin North Am.* 1973;11:626; step 7, from Morehouse DD, MacKinnon KJ. Posterior urethral injury: etiology, diagnosis, initial management. *Urol Clin North Am.* 1977;4:74.)

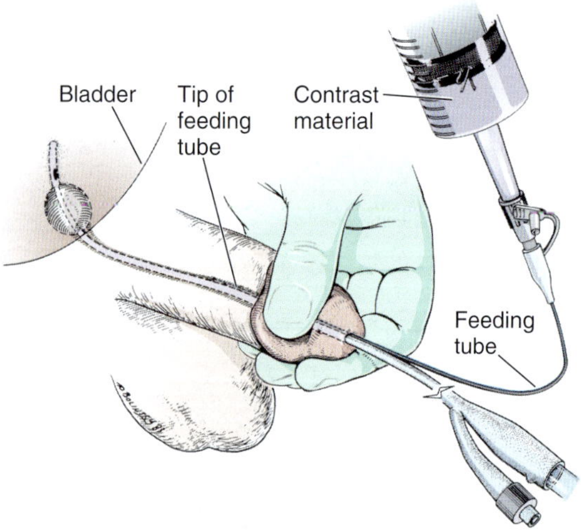

Fig. 56.34 Evaluation of a urethral injury with a Foley catheter in place. A lubricated pediatric feeding tube has been advanced into the urethra beside the indwelling Foley catheter.

of the external sphincter. Occasionally, intravasated contrast material is seen in the periurethral penile venous plexus (see Fig. 56.33, *step 4*). It is of no clinical significance and should not be mistaken for urethral extravasation. As expected, penile venous intravasation (venous plexus opacification) will clear spontaneously on any postvoid films, unlike urethral extravasation, which remains in place.

If a Foley catheter has been successfully placed into the bladder and a partial urethral injury is suspected later, such an injury can be readily demonstrated without removing the catheter. Place the lubricated end of a pediatric feeding tube into the proximal penile urethra alongside the existing Foley catheter (Fig. 56.34). Obtain a seal by compressing the glans penis with the nondominant thumb and index finger and gently inject contrast material with the dominant hand. In this method, extravasation can be demonstrated if a disruption is present. It should be noted, however, that successful placement of the Foley catheter obviates the need for further treatment of a partial urethral tear in the emergency setting because an indwelling catheter alone is often appropriate initial management for this type of injury. The finding of an associated urethral injury must be conveyed to a urologist as it will dictate the duration of definitive Foley catheter drainage.

Retrograde Cystogram

Demonstrate that the urethra is normal before passing the Foley catheter required for retrograde cystography.

Obtain a preliminary KUB or fluoroscopic image to serve as the reference film for the entire examination. Next, fill the bladder under direct operator supervision by gravity instillation of contrast material. After removing the central plunger from a 60-mL catheter-tip syringe, attach the catheter-tipped end of the syringe to the Foley catheter and hold it above the level of the patient's bladder. Pour the contrast material into the syringe and allow it to fill the bladder by gravity instillation to one of three end points: (1) 100 mL with evidence of gross extravasation on fluoroscopy or on plain film (if the examiner elects to check at this point); (2) 400 mL in an adult or any child aged 11 years or older. In children younger than 11 years, bladder capacity, and therefore appropriate contrast volumes, are estimated based on the formula ([age in years + 2] × [30]); or (3) the point of initiating a bladder contraction (see later), then add an additional 50 mL by hand injection under gentle but steady pressure.

Obtain AP and complementary oblique projections if feasible (Fig. 56.35*A1*). In the presence of a pelvic fracture, obtain all films with the patient in the supine position for the same reasons that were elucidated for RUG. A lateral film may be informative when oblique films are not possible (see Fig. 56.35*A2*). Routinely obtain an AP postevacuation film after bladder drainage to disclose posterior perforation, especially in cases of penetrating trauma (see Fig. 56.35*A3*). A dilute solution of contrast material (see Table 56.6) may be used, rather than full-strength contrast. Some authors recommend a dilute solution of contrast material (≤10%) because extravasation into the periurethral or perivesical tissues may cause considerable inflammatory reaction at higher concentrations. The dilute solutions do not appear to compromise the quality of the study, though this should remain a consideration. Retrograde cystography done by any technique other than hand-poured gravity instillation is subject to inadequate bladder filling or connector tubing-catheter disconnection. Either condition may result in spurious radiographic examination results, which have the potential to adversely impact or delay important patient management decisions.

It must be stressed that in the absence of initial gross extravasation, the bladder must be filled to 400 mL in an adult, or to an appropriate age-based capacity in a child, and the catheter clamped with a Kelly clamp. Volumes less than 400 mL have been associated with false-negative findings, especially in penetrating bladder injuries. At times, the patient may have difficulty cooperating with bladder filling because of a head injury or associated pain; and in the case of severe injury, the patient may have involuntary bladder contractions, causing contrast material to back up into the syringe. If this occurs, refill the bladder to the point of initiating a bladder contraction, clamp the Foley catheter, remove the initial syringe and replace it with a 60-mL contrast-filled syringe, unclamp the catheter, hand-inject the additional 50 mL under gentle pressure, and reclamp the catheter. The goal is to overdistend the bladder. Once the filled-bladder films have been obtained and reviewed, unclamp the Foley catheter and allow the contrast material to drain into a bedside drainage bag. Then obtain the AP postevacuation film to visualize any posterior extravasation that may have been hidden by the distended bladder during the AP filled-bladder film (see Fig. 56.35B2–B3). Once again, take care to ensure that contrast material is not spilled onto the patient or the examination table during the procedure.

Extravasation from an injured bladder may be intraperitoneal, extraperitoneal, or both. Extraperitoneal extravasation is usually seen as flamelike areas of contrast material confined to the pelvis and projecting laterally to the bladder (see Fig. 56.35B1 and B4). If the contrast material extravasates intraperitoneally, it tends to fill the paracolic gutters and outline intraperitoneal structures, particularly the bowel, spleen, or liver (see Fig. 56.35B5). It is important to distinguish extraperitoneal from intraperitoneal injury because the treatment options differ significantly: surgical repair is required for intraperitoneal injuries and for those extraperitoneal injuries that extend into or primarily involve the bladder neck, especially in females. Most other extraperitoneal injuries can be managed confidently by Foley catheter drainage alone.

Retrograde Cystography

A. Normal Examination

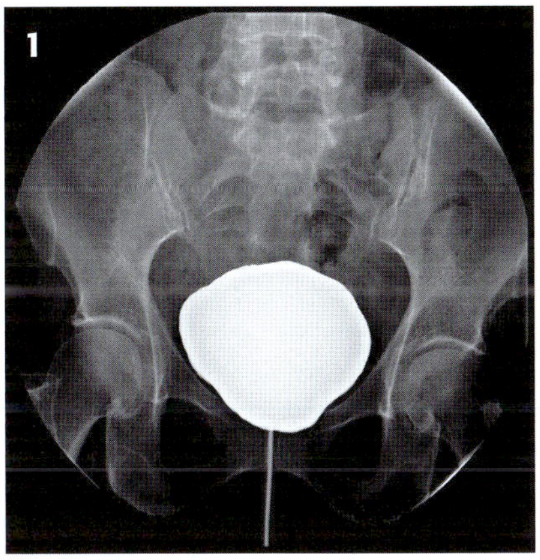

AP view. Fill the bladder with at least 400 mL (see text for details). The normal bladder has a smooth outer contour and no extravasation of contrast material is seen.

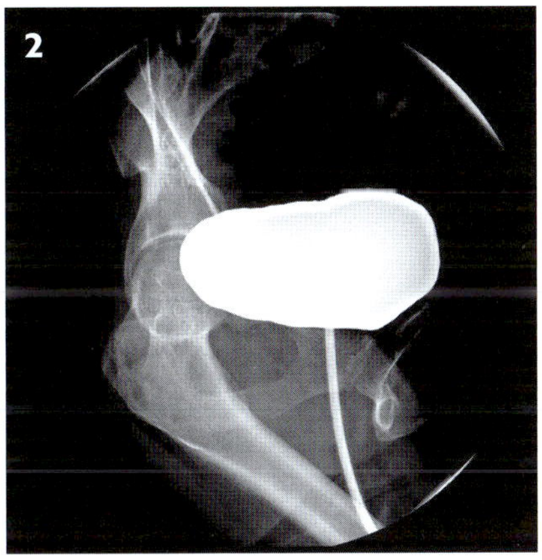

Lateral view. Obtain a lateral or oblique view to assess for posterior extravasation because the opacified bladder would prevent visualization of this injury on the AP view.

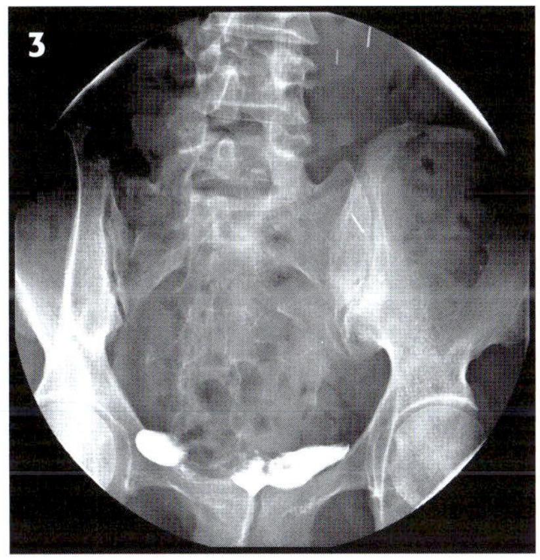

Postvoid film. Always perform a postvoid film to assess for subtle posterior perforation, especially in the case of penetrating trauma.

B. Abnormal Examinations

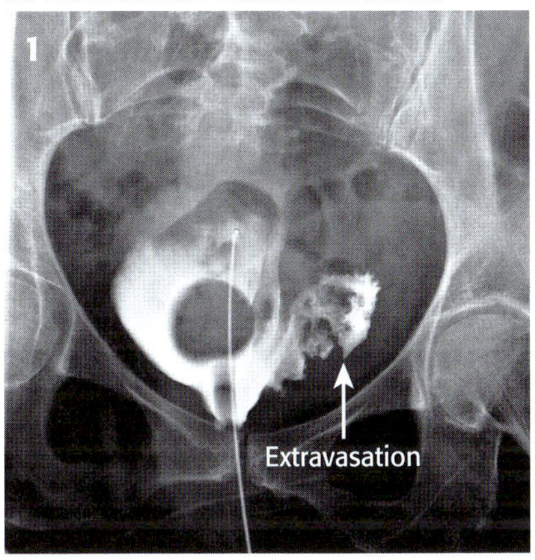

Extraperitoneal bladder perforation. Contrast material is seen adjacent to the bladder neck. The bladder itself is displaced rightward by an adjacent hematoma.

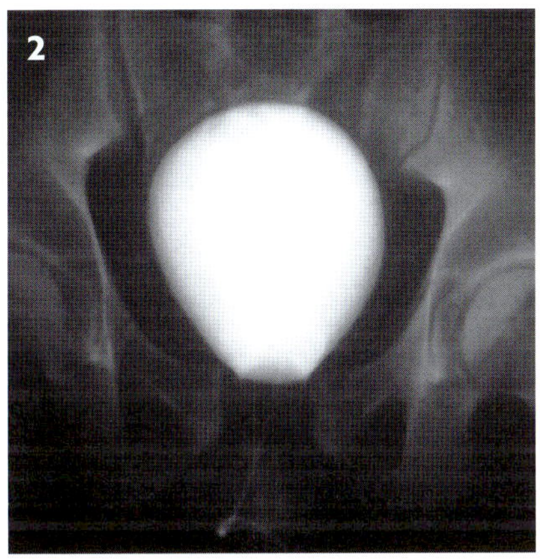

Posterior injury. On this AP film, the bladder appears normal, and no extravasation of contrast material is noted. However, postvoid films are required to rule out posterior injury.

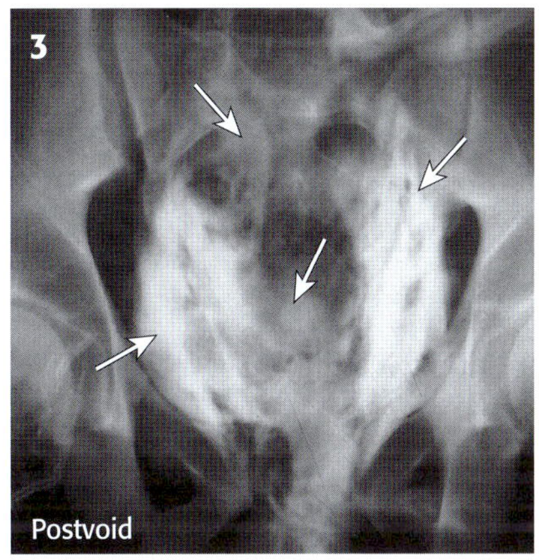

The postvoid film demonstrates substantial posterior extravasation of contrast material. This injury would have been missed if only the AP study were performed.

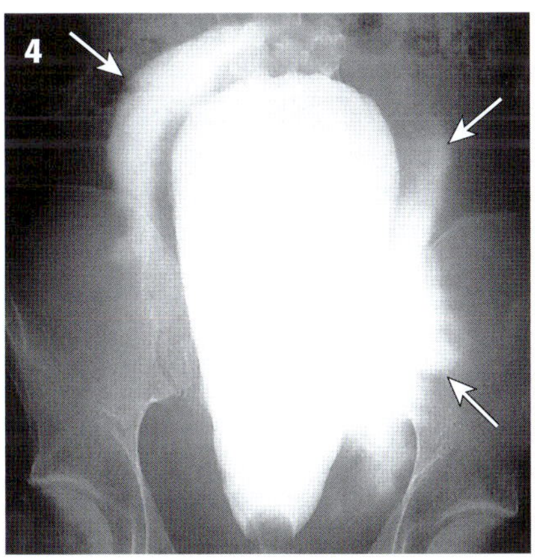

Extraperitoneal bladder rupture. Extravasated contrast material is seen surrounding the bladder *(arrows)* but no loops of bowel are outlined. This injury can typically be treated conservatively with a Foley catheter.

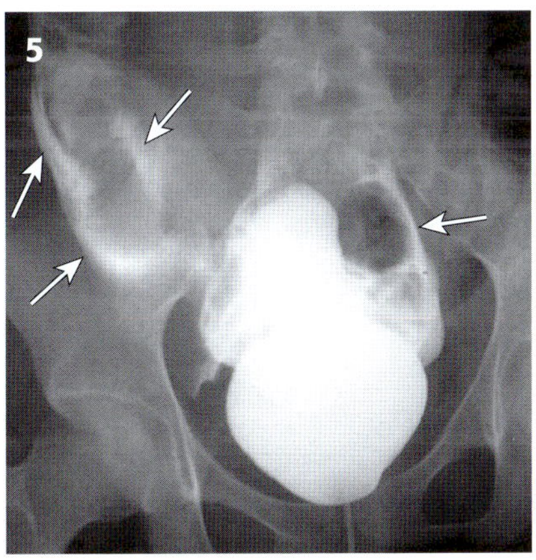

Intraperitoneal bladder rupture. Note the contrast material outlining the paravesical space, tracking up the right paracolic gutter and outlying loops of bowel *(arrows)*. This typically requires operative repair.

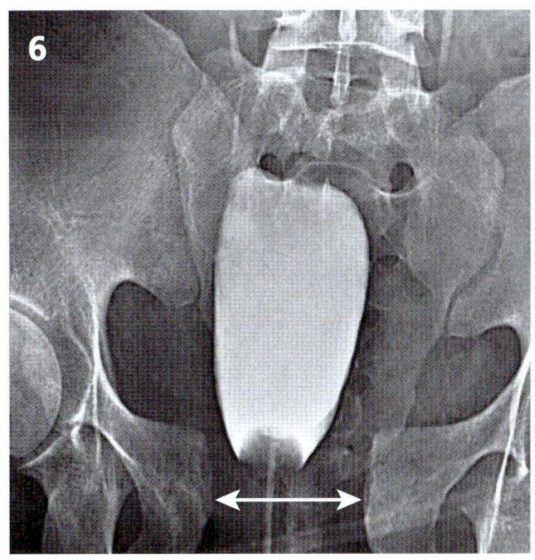

Pelvic hematoma. Note the "open-book" pelvic fracture *(arrows)*. No extravasation of contrast material is seen, however, the pear-shaped bladder indicates the presence of a pelvic hematoma.

Fig. 56.35 Retrograde cystography. *AP,* Anteroposterior.

Retrograde Computed Tomographic Cystography

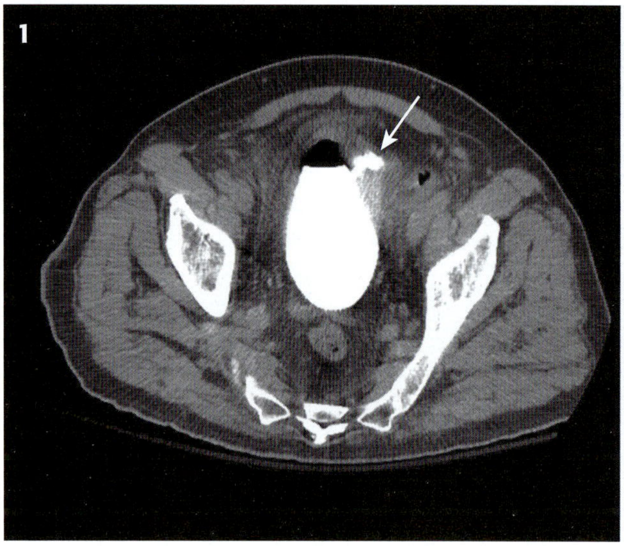

Extraperitoneal bladder perforation. Retrograde cystography may be performed in conjuction with abdominal CT scanning. Fill the bladder in the same fashion as for conventional cystography (obtaining delayed images with IV contrast material collected in the bladder is not sufficient). Above, extravasation of contrast material is noted adjacent to the left side of the bladder *(arrow)*.

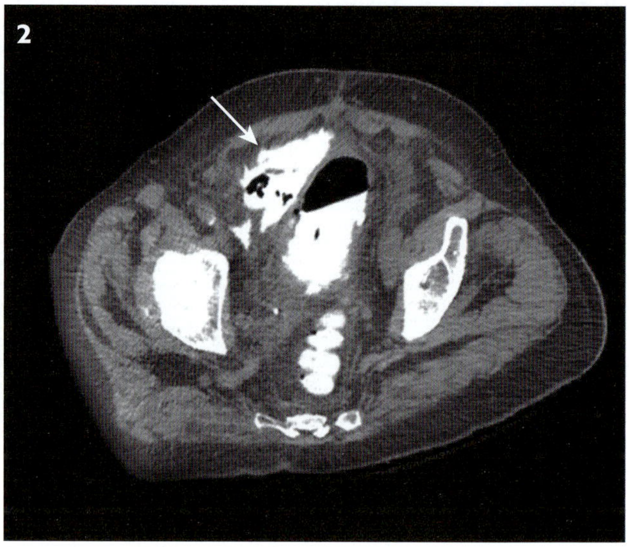

Intraperitoneal bladder perforation. This patient complained of abdominal pain after routine cystoscopy. Standard IV and oral contrast-enhanced CT imaging of the pelvis revealed nonspecific inflammatory changes in the right pelvis. CT cystography was required to diagnose the bladder perforation, as evidenced by extravasation of contrast material into the peritoneal cavity *(arrow)*.

Fig. 56.36 Retrograde computed tomographic cystography. *CT,* Computed tomography; *IV,* intravenous.

Retrograde cystography may be done in conjunction with contrast-enhanced abdominal CT scanning (Fig. 56.36). The bladder should be filled just as if a conventional retrograde cystogram were being obtained. Clamp the catheter and seek evidence for contrast ascites on the CT scan. When this is encountered, bladder injury with extravasation should be further evaluated with selective images of the pelvis.

Aftercare

Foley catheter placement following demonstration of urethral integrity with a RUG. Consult urology to aid in decision-making in any case of urethral or bladder injury.

Complications

Contrast extravasation into periurethral or perivesical tissues in the case of urethral or bladder injury, respectively, may cause considerable inflammatory reaction, particularly contrast materials of higher concentrations.

Conclusions

RUG and retrograde cystography are the diagnostic procedures of choice to evaluate potential injury to the lower urinary tract. These studies must be carried out in the proper sequence and in a retrograde fashion to avoid missing potential injuries.

UPPER GENITOURINARY TRACT IMAGING

Once injuries to the lower GU tract have been excluded with RUG and retrograde cystography, the upper tract (kidneys and ureters) should be evaluated. For adult blunt trauma patients with gross hematuria or hypotension (systolic pressure lower than 90 mm Hg), upper tract imaging is typically indicated.[55] One study found that 12.5% of such patients had major renal injury compared with only 0.2% of adults with microscopic hematuruia and a normal blood pressure.[56] In the presence of a major mechanism of injury or other extenuating circumstances, inclusion criteria for upper tract imaging may be broadened. It should be noted that these criteria are not intended for use in pediatric populations, and opinions regarding diagnostic strategies in children remain varied.

Contrast-enhanced CT is the gold standard for evaluating patients with suspected renal trauma.[56] Parenchymal injuries, vascular injuries, and urinary extravasation can all be readily identified on CT (Fig. 56.37, *plates 1 and 2*). Traumatic renal injuries are graded on a 5-point scale (Box 56.6). For patients with a mandate for emergency laparotomy, upper tract imaging can be performed in the operating room with an excretory urogram (see Fig. 56.37, *plate 3*).

Ureteral injuries can also be identified on contrast-enhanced CT imaging; however, it is essential to obtain delayed images (i.e., approximately 10 minutes after the initial intravenous contrast bolus) (see Fig. 56.37, *plates 4–6*). This delay allows the contrast material to become concentrated in the kidneys and excreted through the ureters. Ureteral injury can then be identified by extravasation of contrast material into adjacent tissues.

Upper Genitourinary Tract Imaging

1

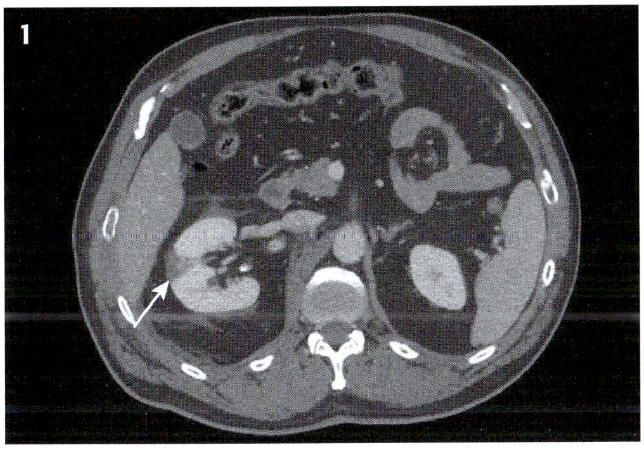

Grade 3 renal laceration. This contrast-enhanced CT scan reveals a renal laceration >1 cm in depth without urinary extravasation *(arrow)* and hence a grade 3 injury.

2

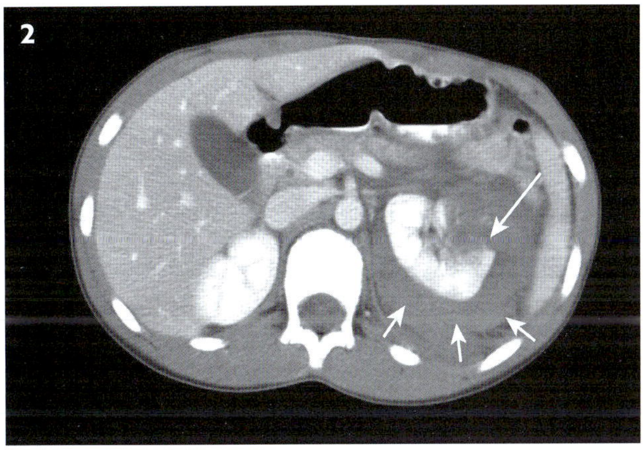

Grade 4 renal injury. This laceration extends through the renal parenchyma and into the collecting system. Extravasation of contrast material is seen *(long arrow)*, thus making this a grade 4 injury. Note the large perinephric hematoma *(short arrows)*.

3

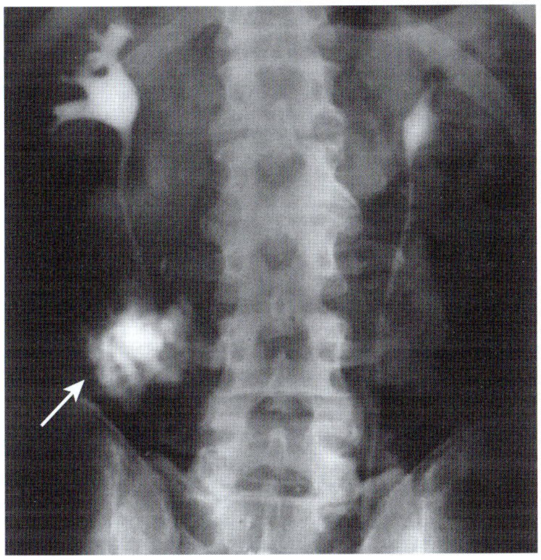

Urethral transection. This intraoperative excretory urogram reveals extravasation *(arrow)* in the upper part of the right ureter consequent to a stab wound. No contrast material is seen in the ureter below the site of injury, a finding indicative of complete transection.

4

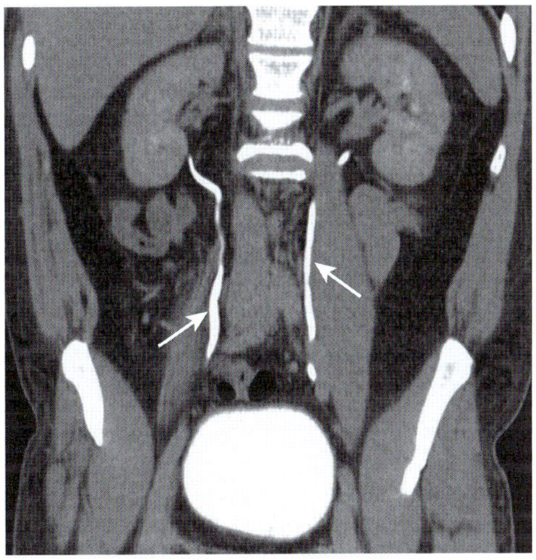

Normal CT urogram. A coronal projection of a CT urogram in the excretory phase demonstrates opacification of the proximal and middle section of the ureters *(arrows)* without evidence of extravasation of contrast material.

5

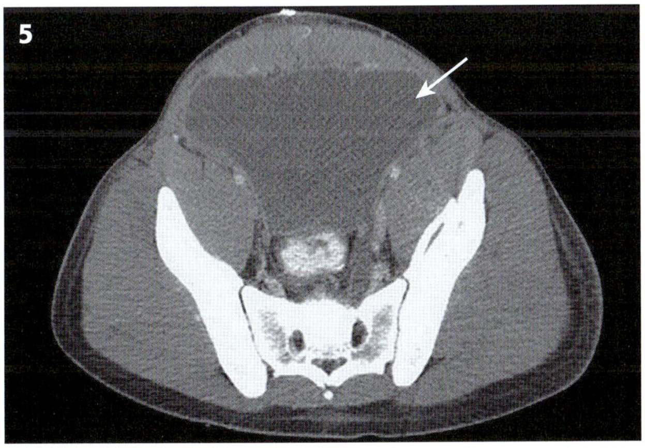

Distal ureter injury. This patient suffered a gunshot wound to his abdomen. After emergency laparotomy and bowel resection, abdominal pain worsened. The initial arterial phase CT demonstrated a large fluid collection in the inferior recesses of the peritoneum *(arrow)*.

6

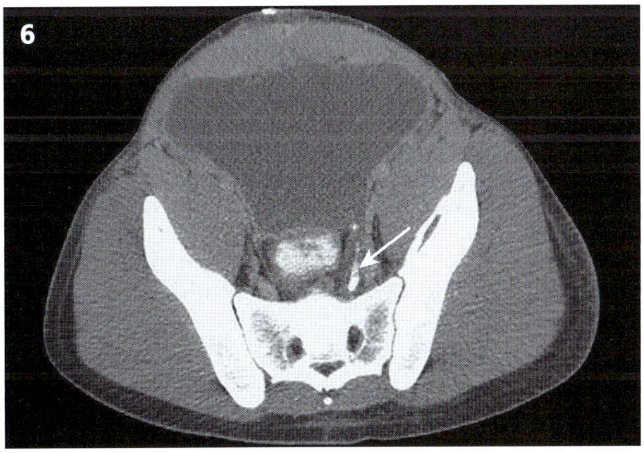

Delayed images revealed extravasation of contrast material from the distal end of the ureter *(arrow)* into the fluid collection. This part of the ureter was not explored during the initial operation.

Fig. 56.37 Upper genitourinary tract imaging. *CT,* Computed tomography. (Step 3, From Wein AJ, Kavoussi LR, Novick AC et al., eds. *Campbell-Walsh Urology*. 10th ed. 2011, Saunders. Step 4, from Haaga JR, Dogra VS, Forsting M et al., eds. *CT and MRI of the Whole Body*. 5th ed. Mosby; 2008. Steps 5 and 6, from Jankowski JT, Spirnak JP. Current recommendations for imaging in the management of urologic traumas. *Urol Clin North Am*. 2006;33:365-376.)

BOX 56.6 American Association for the Surgery of Trauma Classification System for Renal Injuries

GRADE 1 INJURIES

Hematuria with normal imaging
Contusions
Subcapsular, nonexpanding hematoma without parenchymal laceration

GRADE 2 INJURIES

Nonexpanding perinephric hematomas confined to the retroperitoneum
Renal cortical lacerations <1 cm in depth without urinary extravasation

GRADE 3 INJURIES

Renal cortical lacerations >1 cm in depth without urinary extravasation

GRADE 4 INJURIES

Parenchymal laceration extending through the renal cortex/medulla and into the collecting system
Main renal artery or vein injury with contained hemorrhage
Segmental infarction without associated laceration

GRADE 5 INJURIES

Shattered or devascularized kidney
Complete avulsion or thrombosis of the main renal artery or vein
Avulsion of the ureteropelvic junction

From Moore EE, Shackford SR, Pachter HL et al. Organ injury scaling: spleen, liver, and kidney. J Trauma. *1989;29:1664-1666.*

ACKNOWLEDGMENTS

The authors and editors wish to acknowledge the contributions made to previous editions by Michael A. Silverman, MD, Robert E. Schneider, MD, Ivan Zbaraschuk, MD, Richard E. Berger, MD, Jerris R. Hedges, MD, Martin Schiff, Jr., MD, Morton G. Glickman, MD, and Geoffrey E. Herter, MD. In addition, the authors wish to acknowledge Dr. Robert E. Schneider, who is board certified in both emergency medicine and urology, for his mentorship.

REFERENCES ARE AVAILABLE AT Elsevier eBooks+

CHAPTER 57

Emergency Childbirth

Michele Callahan

BACKGROUND

Of the more than 3.5 million births in the United States in 2023, the vast majority were delivered in a hospital setting and a clinician was present for most of these births. In institutions where on-site and timely obstetric services are available, the primary duty of the emergency physician (EP) may be only to determine that labor is active and delivery imminent. However, in the case of unavailable obstetrics, precipitous delivery, or delayed arrival of the obstetrician, the EP may be required to solely manage a patient in active labor, often with little warning.

Emergency delivery of an infant continues to be one of the most challenging and stress-inducing procedures facing EPs. Fortunately, the majority of deliveries that occur in the emergency department (ED) will proceed without any significant issues, and the majority of neonates will not require any special medical assistance. Approximately 10% of infants require some intervention after birth beyond warming, drying, and stimulation, and less than 1% will require significant resuscitative measures such as positive pressure ventilation (PPV) and chest compressions.[1,2]

Clinicians caring for females in labor need to assess the mother and fetus, prepare for delivery, and anticipate potential difficulties or complications during and after the birthing process and may be called upon to evaluate and resuscitate the newborn. This requires having readily available supplies for managing a vaginal delivery, as well as what might be needed for any potential neonatal and/or maternal resuscitation.

GENERAL APPROACH TO THE PATIENT IN LABOR

EMTALA

When a female is initially seen with contractions, the general condition of both the fetus and mother should be assessed quickly. Under the federal Emergency Medical Treatment and Labor Act (EMTALA), hospitals with an ED must conduct an appropriate screening examination to rule out true labor.[3] If the patient is having contractions where there is not enough time to safely transfer her to another hospital before delivery, or if transferring her could pose a threat to her health or the health of her unborn child, she is not considered stable for transfer. In addition, under EMTALA, a female in labor is considered unstable for interhospital transfer unless done so at the direction of the patient or a physician who certifies that the benefits outweigh the risks of transfer. In this case, the clinician should conduct a brief obstetric history, including the onset and frequency of contractions, the presence or absence of bleeding, possible loss of amniotic fluid, previous prenatal care, and due date. In the absence of active vaginal bleeding, a sterile vaginal examination and palpation of the maternal abdomen should be done to determine the stage of labor as well as the position, presentation, and lie of the fetus. Fetal well-being should be monitored by evaluating the fetal heart rate, particularly immediately after a uterine contraction. In an ED setting, fetal assessment is increasingly done via bedside ultrasonography, which can assess fetal movement and heart rate. The traditional approaches of using external Doppler or auscultation are also acceptable. The normal baseline fetal heart rate is 110 to 160 beats/min.

Pregnant patients presenting to an ED in possible labor are often sent expeditiously to a Labor and Delivery department for further assessment and care. If the patient needs to remain in the ED (there is no Labor and Delivery department available, the patient is unstable or delivery is imminent), the patient should be placed on a gurney and both the patient and fetus evaluated.

Signs of Impending Delivery

Signs of impending delivery include the presence of contractions, bloody show (expulsion of the mucous plug), rupture of membranes (often felt as a "gush of fluid"), and back pain. If the patient has the urge to defecate, push, or bear down, or visualization of the perineum shows crowning of the baby's head, delivery is imminent. All necessary equipment should be gathered and all staff (including labor and delivery and neonatal personnel) prepared for delivery and delivery in the ED.

History

Patients in labor should be asked about pertinent medical history. In particular, the following information should be obtained:

- Last menstrual period and estimated due date, if known
- Presence or absence of prenatal care
- Gravidity and parity and any prior pregnancy complications
- Number of babies (singleton, twins, etc.)
- Complications of pregnancy (preeclampsia, gestational diabetes, anemia, persistent breech presentation, etc.)
- Basic maternal medical and surgical history, allergies, and medications
- Social history, particularly during pregnancy
- When contractions began, how far apart are the contractions, how long do they last
- Any leakage of fluid
- Any vaginal bleeding
- Sensation of fetal movement, or when it was last felt

Examination

Examination of the pregnant patient in possible labor includes determination of the estimated gestation age on examination as well as a measurement of the fetal heart rate.

A rapid means of determining gestational age is measurement of fundal height, the distance from the pubic symphysis to the top of the uterine fundus. At 20 weeks of gestational age, the fundus reaches the height of the umbilicus. Estimation of fundal height may be hampered by obesity or inaccurate due to conditions like multiple gestations, growth restriction, fetal macrosomia, and polyhydramnios. In addition, as labor progresses and the fetal head drops into the pelvis, this measurement may underestimate gestational age.

Ultrasound can be used to not only determine gestational age but also to evaluate the fetal heart rate. It is considered generally safe and should be the imaging test of choice in pregnant patients. The machine should be set in "OB" mode and the scanning time minimized to decrease fetal exposure to as low as reasonably achievable (ALARA) principles.

Ultrasound is the recommended method to determine gestational age up to 13 weeks and 6/7 days' gestation by the American College of Obstetricians and Gynecologists.[4] In the first trimester, crown rump length (CRL) is the preferred measurement, but becomes less accurate as the pregnancy enters the second trimester. Other measurements useful at this stage of pregnancy are femur length, biparietal diameter, head circumference, and abdominal circumference (Fig. 57.1.)

Fetal heart rate determination should be done using a curvilinear ultrasound probe. Heart rate measurement should be done in the M-mode, not using pulse wave Doppler mode (Figs. 57.2 and 57.3). A normal fetal heart rate is 110 to 160 beats per minute; fetal bradycardia is a fetal heart rate of <100 to 120 beats/min.

External tocodynamometry, a technique to determine both labor and fetal heart responses to that labor, is a technique commonly used in labor and delivery suites. It requires specific training and is not usually available in the ED unless someone trained in its use accompanies the machine.

The minimum equipment necessary for a vaginal delivery is listed below. Ideally, this equipment should be kept in a kit close to the pediatric code cart or near the equipment needed for neonatal resuscitation.

- Sterile gloves
- Sterile 4 × 4 gauze
- Sterile towels
- Scissors
- Umbilical cord clamps
- Needle driver
- Suture and laceration repair supplies
- Lubricant gel
- Chlorhexidine or betadine

LABOR AND DELIVERY

Anatomy and Physiology

Labor is the process by which the fetus is expelled from the uterus. It begins with a sequence of regular and effective uterine contractions that result in effacement and dilation of the cervix. False labor pains known as Braxton Hicks contractions feel like a tightening or cramping of the abdomen, but do not cause cervical changes. Identification of true labor versus false labor is best determined in a dedicated obstetric unit, often with external uterine monitoring.

Labor can also be divided into *phases*. The *latent phase* of labor is the period between its onset and when labor becomes active, which generally requires 80% effacement and cervical dilation of greater than 4 cm.[5,6] *Active labor* is normally divided into three progressive stages. *The first stage* begins with cervical effacement and dilation and ends when the cervix is completely dilated. In multiparous females, this stage of labor typically lasts approximately 5 to 8 hours, as opposed to 7 to 13 hours in nulliparous females, but with much individual variation.[5,6] The *second stage* of labor begins when dilation of the cervix is complete and ends with delivery of the infant. The duration of this stage is also variable, with a median of 50 to 60 minutes in nulliparas and 15 to 20 minutes in multiparas.[5,6] The *third stage* of labor begins after delivery of the infant and ends with delivery of the placenta. The *fourth stage* of labor refers to the 1 hour immediately after delivery, the period in which postpartum hemorrhage (PPH) is most likely to occur.[3] It is recommended that maternal blood pressure and pulse be recorded immediately after delivery and every 15 minutes for the first hour to rapidly detect any ongoing hemorrhage.[5]

A precipitous delivery is defined as the delivery of an infant within 3 hours of the onset of contractions and constitutes about 3% of deliveries in the United States.[7,8] In comparison, an average labor often lasts between 6 and 18 hours from onset of contractions to delivery. Subsequent pregnancies (in multiparous females) are often associated with shorter durations of labor at around 6 to 8 hours. Risk factors for precipitous delivery include smaller fetal size, prior precipitous delivery, and hypertension.[9]

Identification of Labor

It is not uncommon for patients to have contractions late in pregnancy, although not all are true or effective labor contractions. Brief Braxton Hicks contractions of the uterus, usually confined to discomfort in the lower abdominal region and groin, are typically irregular in timing and strength. These pains do not cause any change in the cervix or result in descent of the fetus. Although these pains usually stop spontaneously, they can rapidly convert to true labor contractions; if they occur, a period of observation may be necessary.

True labor is characterized by a regular sequence of uterine contractions with progressively increasing intensity and decreasing intervals between contractions. The interval between contractions gradually diminishes from 10 minutes at the onset of labor to as short as 1 minute or less in the second stage of labor. This should be accompanied by effacement and dilation of the cervix, along with descent of the fetal presenting part into the pelvis. The term "fetal station" describes how far into the pelvis the fetal head has descended. The fetal head at the level of the maternal ischial spines is considered zero station. When the head is above this level, measurements range from −1 to −5; below this level they range from +1 to +5 as the head descends into the pelvis.

The onset of true labor may be difficult to identify given that patients are far more likely to be at home than in a hospital when labor begins.

Show or *bloody show* is a sign of approaching labor. The normal mucous plug sealing the cervix discharges as the cervix dilates. Show consists of a small amount of blood-tinged mucus discharged from the vagina and indicates that labor is already in progress or will probably occur during the next several hours to a few days. The mucous color can be pink or brown tinged because of minor bleeding. However, if more than a small amount of blood escapes with the mucous plug, an abnormal cause such as placental abruption or placenta previa should be considered. Digital vaginal examination under these circumstances is generally contraindicated.

Spontaneous rupture of membranes can occur during the course of active labor, typically evident by a sudden gush or continuous leakage of a variable amount of clear or slightly turbid vaginal fluid. Rupture of membranes before the onset of labor at any stage of gestation is referred to as *premature rupture of membranes* (PROM); if it occurs before 37 weeks of

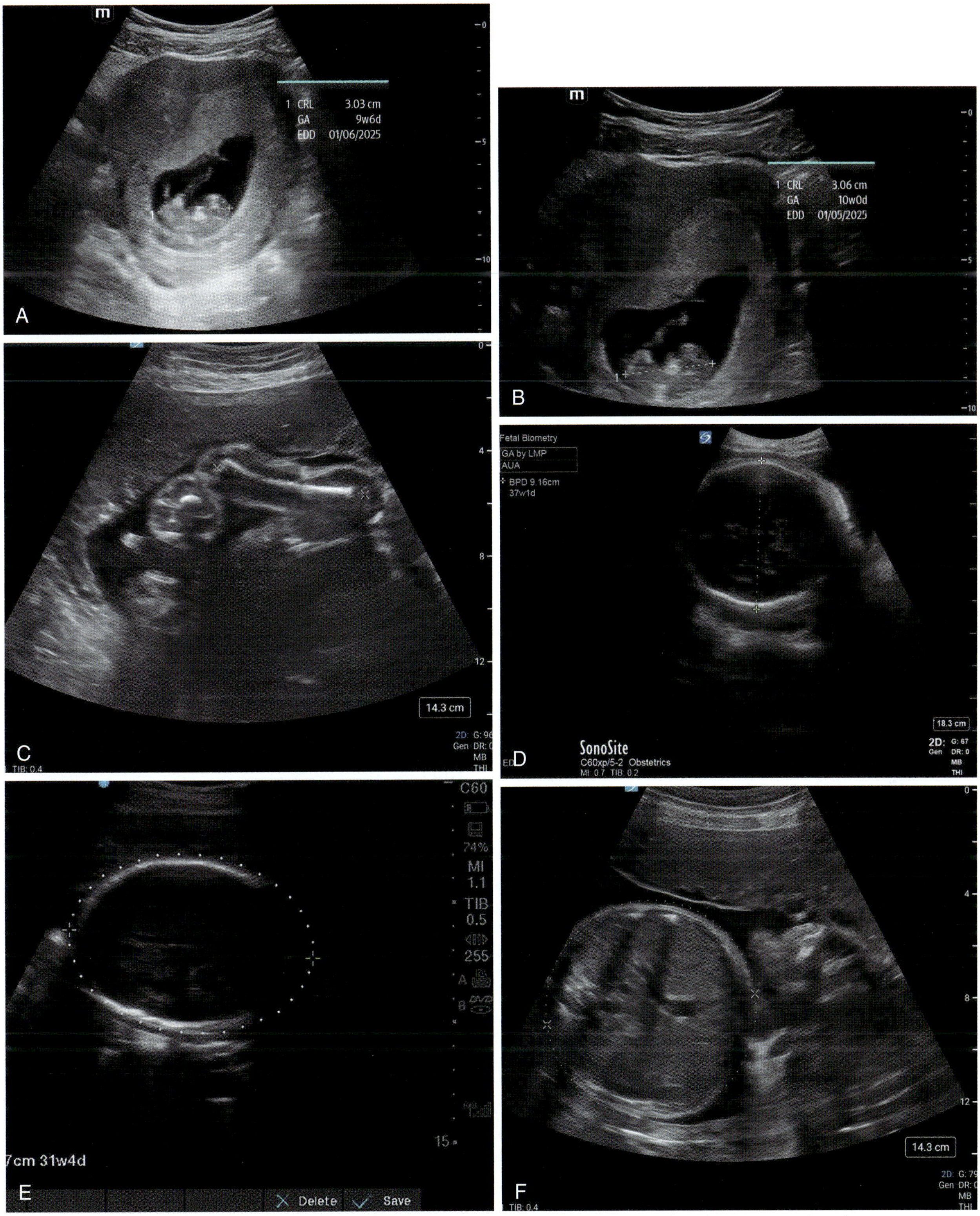

Fig. 57.1 Ultrasound for estimating gestational age. (A–B) Crown-rump length. (C) Femur length. (D) Biparietal diameter. (E) Head circumference. (F) Abdominal circumference. (A–B, Courtesy Matthew VandeHai, MD, Mitch Butterbaugh, MD, and Christine Butts, MD. C, Courtesy Matthew VandeHei, MD, Grace Carey, MD, and Christine Butts, MD. D, Courtesy Christine Butts, MD. E, Courtesy Cassandra Hardy. MD, and Jess Schmidt, MD. F, Courtesy Matthew VendeHei, MD.)

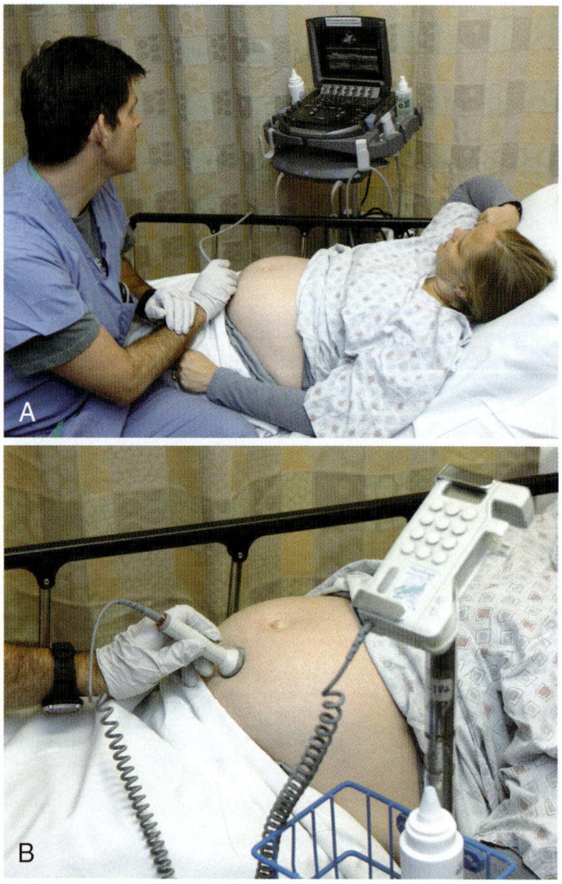

Fig. 57.2 Assessment of fetal heart rate. (A) Fetal assessment is often done via bedside ultrasonography in the emergency department. (B) Traditional methods, such as external Doppler, are also acceptable. The normal baseline fetal heart rate is 110 to 160 beats/min.

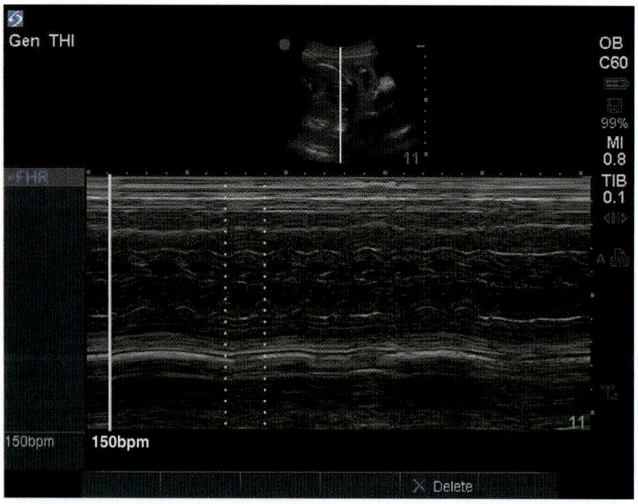

Fig. 57.3 Fetal heart rate determination using M-mode ultrasound. (Courtesy Christine Butts, MD.)

pregnancy, it is called preterm premature rupture of membranes (PPROM).

Term PROM complicates approximately 2% to 3% of pregnancies.[10] In most cases it is followed by the onset of labor and delivery within hours. The most significant maternal risk associated with term PROM is intrauterine infection (chorioamnionitis and endometritis). Fetal risks associated

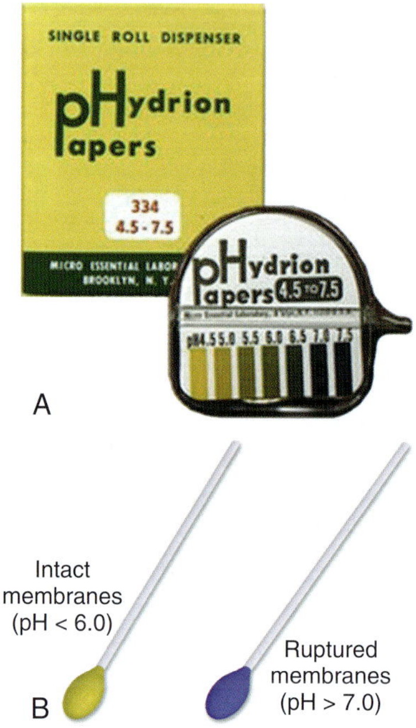

Fig. 57.4 Amniotic fluid has an *alkaline pH*, whereas normal vaginal secretions are acidic. Both (A) Nitrazine or pH paper and (B) an indicator swab will turn yellow when placed in a sample in the absence of amniotic fluid and dark blue in the presence of amniotic fluid within a few seconds.

with PROM include umbilical cord compression and ascending infection.[10] The ideal management of PROM should be deferred to the consulting obstetrician.

In cases of PPROM, birth within 1 week generally occurs regardless of management or the clinical findings. The most significant maternal risk related to PPROM is intrauterine infection, but umbilical cord compression, hemorrhage, and other complications can occur.[11] The most significant risks to the fetus are complications related to prematurity. Preterm delivery occurs in approximately 10% to 12% of all births in the United States and is the leading cause of perinatal morbidity and mortality.[10] Patients with PPROM should be admitted for monitoring.

Accurate diagnosis of PROM is helpful in further management. Suspected PROM should be confirmed by an examination that minimizes the risk of introducing infection. Avoid digital cervical examination unless the patient is in active labor or delivery is imminent. A sterile speculum examination can be performed to look for amniotic fluid leaking from the cervical os or pooling in the posterior fornix, as well as to inspect for fetal or umbilical cord prolapse and assess cervical effacement and dilation.[5,10]

Amniotic fluid may be differentiated from vaginal fluid by testing the pH of the fluid with Nitrazine paper or similar swab devices (Fig. 57.4). The pH of vaginal fluid is generally 3.8 to 4.5, whereas amniotic fluid has a pH of 7.1 to 7.3.[10] The yellow testing paper turns blue-green to deep blue in the presence of amniotic fluid. With vaginal secretions, the Nitrazine paper remains yellow. False-positive results may occur with blood, semen, bacterial vaginosis, or alkaline urine. If rupture of membranes is documented in the ED, notify the patient's obstetrician and plan for hospital admission or possible transfer. While testing for 'ferning' (arborization) was once used to determine the presence of amniotic fluid, this test is now only rarely performed in the emergency setting.

The biomarker fetal fibronectin (fFN), a glycoprotein produced by amniocytes and cytotrophoblast found in cervicovaginal secretions, may also be used as a screening tool for preterm labor as an adjunct to maternal/fetal monitoring and pelvic examination.[12,13] fFN has an excellent negative predictive value (99%) in determining the likelihood of delivery within 1 week. The test is done with a vaginal swab but must be done before any digital exam. The test is not reliable if the patient has had sexual intercourse within 24 hours, associated bleeding, or has used a gel.[12,13]

Fetal Lie, Presentation, and Position

Lie refers to the relationship of the long axis of the fetus to the long axis of the uterus. It is either longitudinal, transverse, or oblique (Fig. 57.5). Oblique lies are unstable and will convert to a longitudinal or transverse lie during labor. Longitudinal lies occur in more than 99% of pregnancies at term.[5] Transverse lies generally cannot be safely delivered vaginally.[6]

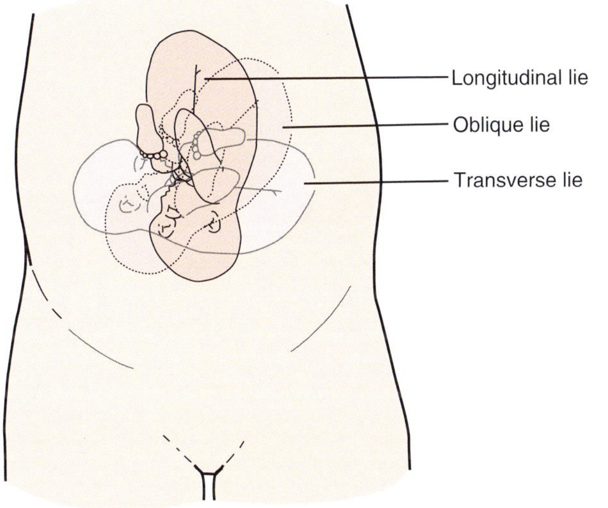

Fig. 57.5 Examples of different fetal lie. (From Gabbe SG, Niebyl JR, Simpson JL, eds. *Obstetrics: Normal and Problem Pregnancies*. Elsevier; 2007.)

The presentation, or presenting part, refers to the portion of the body of the fetus nearest to or foremost in the birth canal and is most commonly the occiput or vertex of the head. The presenting part can be felt through the cervix on sterile vaginal examination. In longitudinal lies, the presenting part is the fetal head, the buttocks (breech), or the feet (footling breech). With a transverse lie, the presenting part is the shoulder. The presentation can be cephalic, breech, shoulder, or compound (a fetal extremity with another presenting part).

Cephalic presentations are classified by the bony leading landmark of the fetal skull. Ordinarily, the head is sharply flexed so that the occipital fontanelle is the presenting part. This is referred to as a *vertex* or *occiput presentation*. Less commonly, the neck is fully extended and the face is foremost in the birth canal; this is termed *face presentation*. A partially flexed or partially extended neck position results in *sinciput* and *brow presentations*, respectively. Sinciput and brow presentations associated with preterm infants almost always convert to either an occiput or face presentation as labor progresses.

Breech presentations are classified as frank, complete, or incomplete (Fig. 57.6). A fetus presenting with the buttocks and hips flexed and the legs extended is termed a *frank breech*. Presentation of the buttocks with flexion of the fetal hips and knees results in *a complete breech* presentation. When one or both feet or knees are lowermost in the canal, an *incomplete* or *footling breech* results.

At or near term, 97% of fetuses will be vertex and 3% will be breech.[5] The incidence of breech delivery is approximately 25% at 28 weeks, 17% at 30 weeks, and 11% at 32 weeks.[5]

Position refers to the relationship of the presenting part to the maternal pelvis and may be either left or right. The occiput is the reference point in cephalic presentations, whereas the sacrum is the determining part in breech presentations. The vertex occiput anterior position is the most common and is considered normal. The other position is occiput posterior.

Labor Movements: Vertex Presentation

Full dilation of the cervix signifies the second stage of labor and heralds the delivery of the infant. Typically, the patient begins to bear down, which coincides with descent of the presenting part. Uterine contractions may last 1.5 minutes and recur after a resting phase of less than 1 minute. Delivery of a vertex-presenting infant usually occurs spontaneously. The

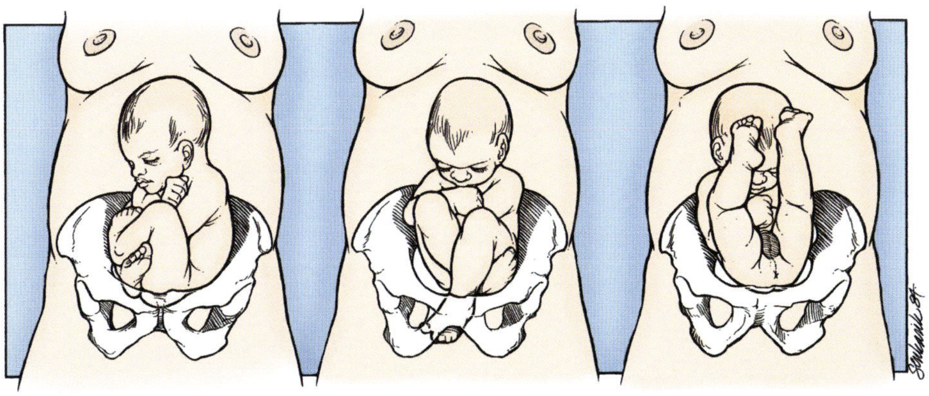

Fig. 57.6 A fetus in a complete breech presentation is flexed at the hips and at the knees. An incomplete breech shows incomplete deflexion of one or both knees or hips. With a frank breech presentation, the fetus is flexed at the hips and extended at the knees.

role of the clinician or attendant is principally to provide control of the birth process by preventing forceful, sudden expulsion or extraction of the infant with resultant fetal or maternal injury.

The mechanism of labor in vertex presentations consists of engagement of the presenting part, flexion, descent, internal rotation, extension, external rotation or restitution, and expulsion (Fig. 57.7).[5] These are often referred to as *cardinal* movements of labor. The mechanism of labor is determined by the pelvic dimensions and configuration, the size of the fetus, and the strength of the uterine contractions. Essentially, the fetus will follow the path of least resistance by adaptation of the smallest achievable diameter of the presenting part to the most favorable dimensions and contours of the birth canal.

The sequence of movements in vertex presentations is as follows:

1. *Engagement* refers to the mechanism by which the greatest transverse diameter of the head, the biparietal diameter in occiput presentations, passes through the pelvic inlet. A fetus is engaged when the presenting part is at 0 station. In a primiparous patient, it usually occurs in the last 2 weeks of pregnancy; in a multiparous patient, it can occur at the onset of labor.
2. *Flexion* of the head is necessary to minimize the presenting cross-sectional diameter of the head during passage through the smallest diameter of the bony pelvis. In most cases, flexion is necessary for both engagement and descent and occurs passively.
3. *Descent* is the downward passage of the fetal presenting part. It is gradually progressive but is not necessarily continuous. Descent is affected by uterine and abdominal contractions, as well as by straightening and extension of the fetal body.
4. *Internal rotation* occurs with descent and is necessary for the head or presenting part to traverse the ischial spines. This movement essentially turns the head such that the occiput gradually moves from its original, more transverse position anteriorly toward the symphysis pubis or, less commonly, posteriorly toward the hollow of the sacrum. This is known as occiput anterior or occiput posterior, respectively.
5. *Extension* occurs as the flexed head reaches the anteriorly directed vaginal introitus. The occiput reaches the inferior aspect of the pubic symphysis. The head is born by further extension as it rotates around the pubic symphysis and the occiput, bregma, forehead, nose, mouth, and finally, the chin pass successively over the anterior margin of the perineum. Immediately after its birth, the head drops downward such that the chin lies over the maternal anal region.
6. *External rotation* or restitution is return of the head to the correct anatomic position with respect to the fetal torso. It

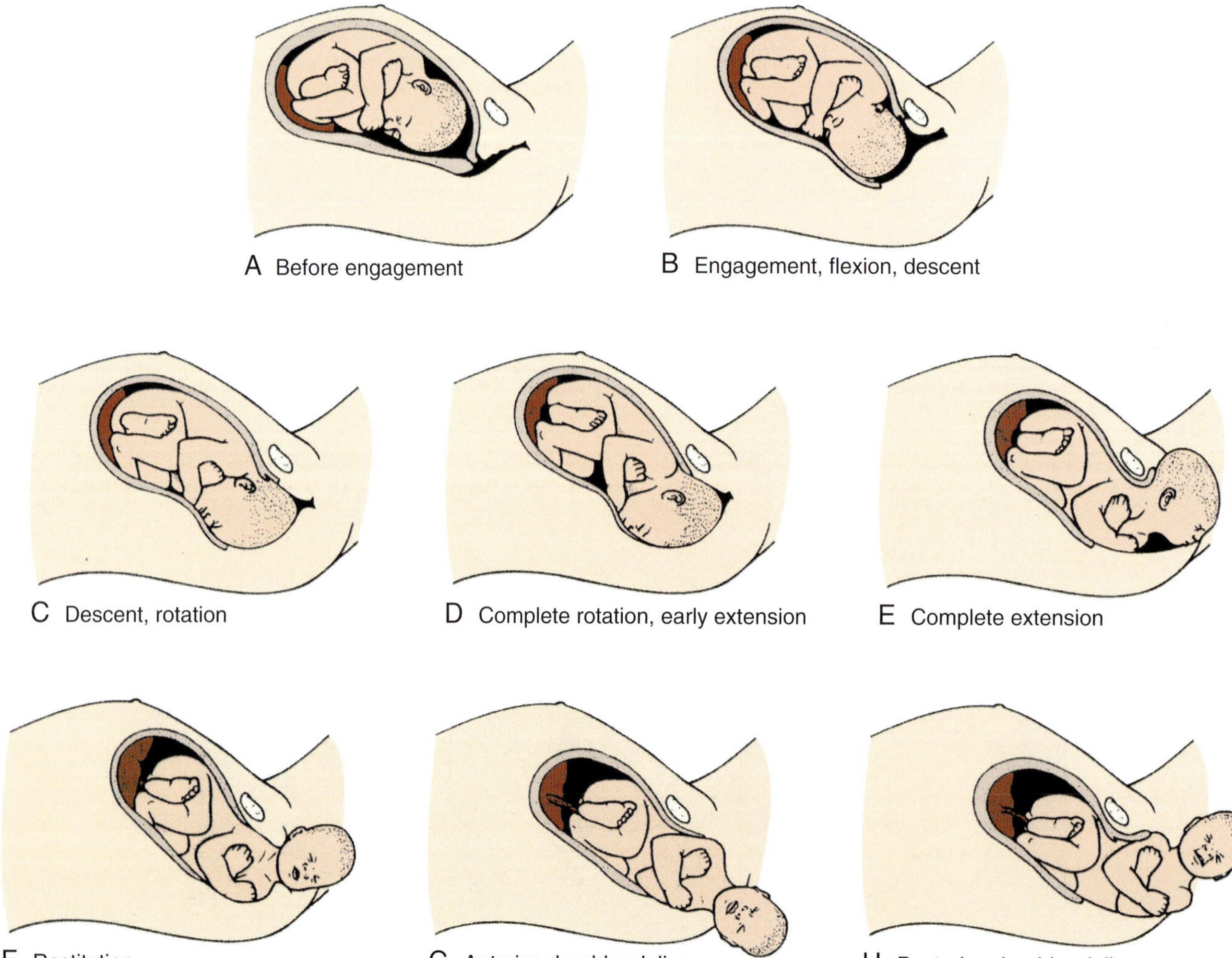

Fig. 57.7 Cardinal movements of labor. (From Gabbe SG, Niebyl JR, Simpson JL, eds. *Obstetrics: Normal and Problem Pregnancies*. 5th ed. Elsevier; 2007.)

follows delivery of the head as it rotates to the transverse position that it occupied at engagement. This is also a passive movement.

7. *Expulsion* of the remainder of the fetal body then occurs. The shoulders descend in a path similar to that traced by the head (i.e., rotating anteroposteriorly for delivery). First, the anterior shoulder is delivered beneath the symphysis pubis followed by the posterior shoulder across the perineum.

Labor Movements: Breech Presentation

The mechanism of labor for breech presentations varies (see Fig. 57.6). The widest diameter that is engaged is the bitrochanteric diameter. Usually, the hips engage in one of the oblique diameters of the pelvic inlet. As descent occurs, the anterior hip generally descends more rapidly than the posterior hip. Internal rotation occurs as the bitrochanteric diameter assumes the anteroposterior (AP) position. Lateral flexion takes place as the anterior hip catches beneath the symphysis pubis, which allows the posterior hip to be born first. The infant's body then rotates to allow engagement of the shoulders in an oblique orientation. Gradual descent occurs, with the anterior shoulder rotating to bring the shoulders into the AP diameter of the outlet. The anterior shoulder follows lateral flexion to appear beneath the symphysis, with the posterior shoulder being delivered first as the body is supported. The head tends to engage in the same diameter as the shoulders. Subsequent flexion, descent, and rotation of the head occur to bring the posterior portion of the neck under the symphysis pubis. The head is then born in flexion.

Breech delivery is associated with a greater incidence of prematurity, prolapsed cord, and increased perinatal morbidity and mortality.[5,14–16] The emergency clinician should be cognizant of the imminent vaginal delivery of a breech infant in any presentation: frank, complete, or footling. However, a breech presentation is always problematic for any clinician, even under the best of circumstances. It is not expected that the EP will always be able to successfully deliver a breech presentation.

Types of Breech Deliveries

There are three types of vaginal breech deliveries. *Spontaneous breech* is a breech delivery in which the infant is delivered spontaneously without any manipulation or traction other than supporting the infant. This form of delivery is rare with term infants, and there is little associated traumatic morbidity. *Partial breech extraction* occurs when the infant is delivered spontaneously as far as the umbilicus and the remainder of the body is extracted. *Total breech extraction* occurs when the entire body of the infant is extracted by the clinician.

Similar to cephalic presentations, the role of the clinician is to assist the patient in the birthing process and allow maternal expulsive efforts to effect delivery of the infant. Premature or aggressive assistance or traction can significantly increase the risk for fetal or maternal morbidity and this should be kept in mind when caring for a patient with a breech delivery.

To perform any vaginal breech delivery, the birth canal must be sufficiently large to allow passage of the fetus without trauma and the cervix must be completely effaced and dilated. If these conditions do not exist, cesarean section is indicated. To ensure full cervical dilation in a footling or complete breech, it is important that the feet, legs, and buttocks advance through the introitus to the level of the fetal umbilicus *before* the clinician intervenes and further delivery is attempted. The mere appearance of the feet through the vulva is not in itself an indication to proceed with delivery; this may be a footling presentation through a cervix that is not completely dilated. In this case there may be time to transfer the patient to the labor and delivery suite, preferably in the knee-chest position to minimize the risk for cord compression. Similarly, if the breech is frank, cervical dilation and outcome are improved if the infant is allowed to deliver to the level of the umbilicus. Before this, as with complete and footling presentations, there may be time to safely transfer the patient to the labor and delivery area. Tocolytics such as subcutaneous terbutaline may be considered to inhibit labor until such patients can be safely transferred.

Vaginal Examination and Preparation for Delivery

Cleanse the perineum with an antiseptic and use a sterile lubricant to decrease potential contamination. A sterile digital vaginal (not speculum) examination is performed to identify the fetal presentation and position and assess the progress of labor, except in cases of suspected bleeding. During the digital examination, take care to avoid the anal region and potential fecal contamination. Assess cervical effacement and dilation, as well as fetal station, presentation, and position. Do not withdraw the finger from the vagina until the examination is complete. The number of vaginal examinations during labor correlates with infectious morbidity, especially in cases of early membrane rupture.

Cervical effacement refers to the process of cervical thinning that occurs before and during the first stage of labor as the cervical canal shortens from a length of approximately 2 cm to a circular opening with almost no length remaining (Fig. 57.8). Effacement is expressed as a percentage from 0% (uneffaced and thick) to 100% (completely effaced). Assess the degree of cervical effacement by palpation and determine the palpated length of the cervical canal in comparison to that of an uneffaced, or normal, cervical canal.

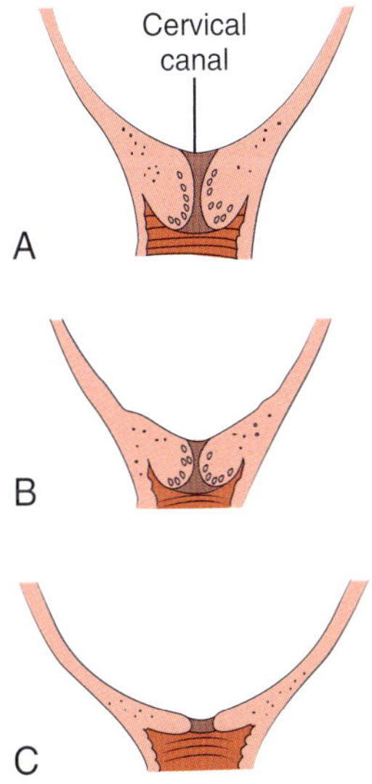

Fig. 57.8 Effacement of the cervix. (A) None. (B) Partial. (C) Complete. (From Romney S, Gray MK, Little AB et al., eds. *Gynecology and Obstetrics: The Health Care of Women*. McGraw-Hill; 1975.)

Determine *cervical dilation* by estimating the average diameter of the internal cervical os. Sweep the examining finger from the cervical margin on one side across the cervical os to the opposite margin. Express the diameter in centimeters. Ten centimeters constitutes full cervical dilation. A diameter of less than 6 cm can be measured directly. A cervix that accommodates one index finger is 1 cm, and one that accommodates two fingers is dilated approximately 3 cm. For a diameter greater than 6 cm, it is frequently easier to determine the width of the remaining cervical rim and subtract twice that measurement from 10 cm. For example, if a 1-cm rim is felt, dilation is 8 cm.

Station refers to the level of the presenting fetal part in the birth canal relative to the ischial spines, which lie halfway between the pelvic inlet and the pelvic outlet (Fig. 57.9). Zero station is used to denote that the presenting part is at the level of the ischial spines. When the presenting part lies above the spines, the distance, estimated in centimeters ranging from 1 to 5, is stated in negative figures (−5, −4, −3, −2, −1). Below the ischial spines, the presenting fetal part passes +1, +2, +3, +4, and +5 stations to delivery. This measurement is made by simple palpation. The ischial spines can be palpated at roughly the 8 and 4 o'clock positions on the vaginal examination.

Three maneuvers are used to determine fetal presentation and position. First, introduce two fingers into the vagina and advance them to the presenting part to differentiate face, vertex, and breech presentations. In vertex presentations, move your fingers up behind the symphysis pubis and then sweep them posteriorly over the fetal head toward the maternal sacrum to identify the course of the sagittal suture. Define the positions of the two fontanelles, which are

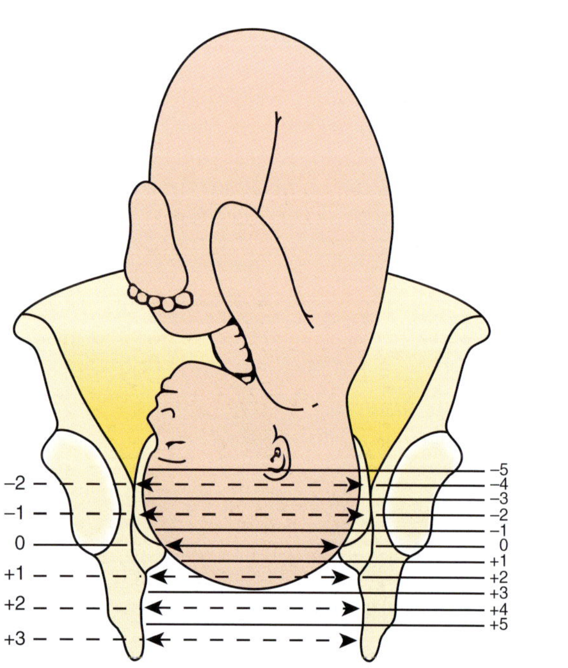

Fig. 57.9 Relationship of the leading edge of the presenting part of the fetus to the plane of the maternal ischial spines determines the station. Old and new classification are included. (From Gabbe SG, Niebyl JR, Simpson JL, eds. *Obstetrics: Normal and Problem Pregnancies.* 5th ed. Elsevier; 2007.)

located at opposite ends of the sagittal sutures, by palpation. The anterior fontanel is diamond shaped; the posterior fontanel is triangular. In breech presentations, the fetal sacrum is the point of reference, whereas in face presentations the fetal chin is used.

FETAL WELL-BEING

Assessing Fetal Heart Rate

Make the initial determination of fetal well-being by assessing the fetal heart rate with a fetoscope, bedside ultrasound, or a fetal Doppler device. Place the device firmly on the maternal abdominal wall overlying the fetal thorax and reposition it until fetal heart tones are heard. When a Doppler device is used, apply a conducting gel to the abdominal wall to interface with the Doppler receiver. To avoid confusion of the maternal and fetal heart sounds, palpate the maternal pulse as the fetal heart rate is auscultated.

The normal baseline fetal heart rate is 110 to 160 beats/min and varies considerably from a baseline measured for a minimum of 2 minutes in a 10-minute segment of time.[17,18] Rates above or below this range may indicate fetal distress. Accelerations in the fetal heart rate lasting longer than 10 seconds and less than 2 minutes commonly occur during labor and are probably a physiologic response to fetal movement.[5,17,18] Persistent fetal tachycardia occurs most frequently in response to maternal fever or amnionitis but may also indicate fetal compromise.[5,17]

As with brief accelerations in the fetal heart rate, a gradual decrease in the fetal heart rate in association with a uterine contraction with an onset to nadir of 30 seconds or more (with the nadir coinciding with the peak of contraction) is termed an *early deceleration*. Such decelerations are physiologic and probably the result of vagal nerve stimulation secondary to compression of the fetal head. Decelerations that occur independent of uterine contractions, are abrupt, or last between 15 seconds and 2 minutes, are known as *variable decelerations*. Variable decelerations are relatively common, can be classified according to their severity, and may be temporarily corrected by maternal repositioning. *Late decelerations* are those that are delayed in timing with respect to a contraction, with the nadir of the deceleration occurring after the peak of the contraction. Late decelerations can be an ominous sign and may represent cord compression or uteroplacental insufficiency and may necessitate emergency delivery.[17,18]

Changes in the fetal heart rate that indicate fetal distress are usually evident immediately after a uterine contraction, and therefore the fetal heart rate is optimally assessed at this time. Formal monitoring of labor should ideally be performed in an obstetrics unit (Fig. 57.10).[5,17]

Management of Fetal Distress

Definitive evaluation of fetal distress should be performed in the obstetric unit by the delivery team. There is no role for sophisticated fetal monitoring in the ED. In the absence of a dedicated obstetric unit, transfer to another hospital is the only option, albeit a less than ideal one. An EP working in an ED without adequate obstetric backup can do little to affect a positive outcome in high-risk situations. Eclampsia, bleeding, and abnormal fetal presentation may be identified, but the EP needs to focus attention on maternal well-being

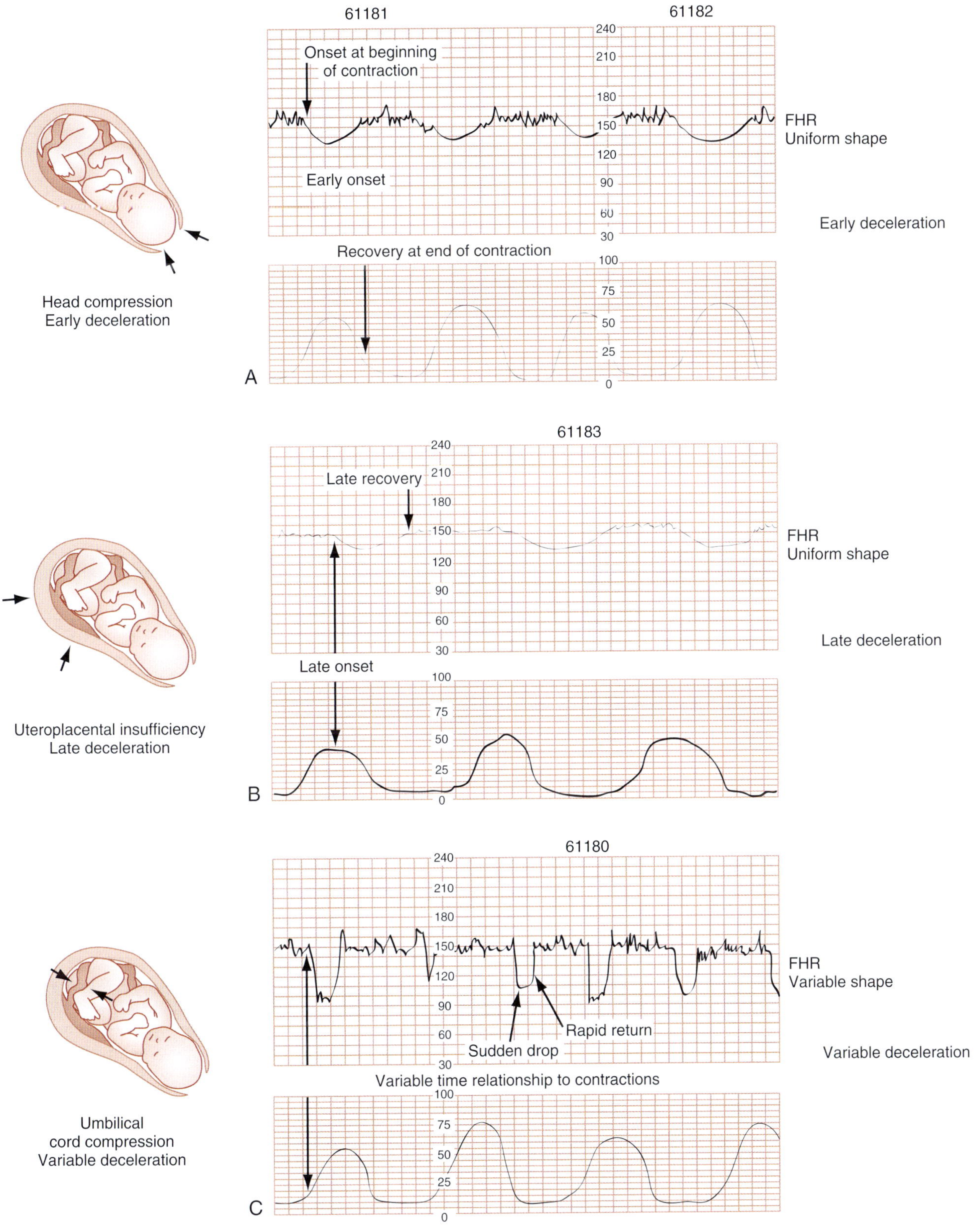

Fig. 57.10 Deceleration patterns of the fetal heart rate *(FHR)*. (A) Early deceleration caused by head compression. (B) Late deceleration caused by uteroplacental insufficiency. (C) Variable deceleration caused by cord compression. Note: fetal monitoring is not done in the emergency department; this figure is supplied for completeness. (Modified from Lowdermilk DL, Perry SE, Bobak IM, eds. *Maternity and Women's Health Care*. 6th ed. Mosby; 1997.)

while expediting transfer, referral, or both. The EP has limited options for managing fetal distress.

If fetal distress is suspected based on the resting fetal heart rate or changes after contractions, change the maternal position, typically into the left lateral decubitus position, and reevaluate. Administer supplemental oxygen to the patient to optimize fetal oxygenation.

In the absence of bleeding, perform a vaginal examination to rule out the possibility of umbilical cord prolapse.[17] *Cord prolapse* usually occurs at the same time as rupture of the membranes and is diagnosed by palpation of the umbilical cord on vaginal examination or by visualization of the cord protruding through the introitus. Cord prolapse is associated with several risk factors such as malpresentation, grand multiparity, and prematurity, as well as iatrogenic causes.[19]

PRETERM LABOR AND TOCOLYTIC THERAPY

Tocolytics are drugs used to suppress uterine contractions for patients in preterm labor and are rarely indicated or instituted in the ED. However, under extremely limited circumstances and preferably under obstetric guidance, this intervention may be initiated in the ED. The goal of delaying delivery is to enable administration of antenatal corticosteroids for lung maturation and magnesium sulfate ($MgSO_4$) for fetal neuroprotection, as well as to permit maternal transport (if indicated) to a tertiary facility.[20–24]

Before instituting pharmacologic tocolytic therapy for either preterm labor or fetal distress, initiate basic maneuvers to improve maternal and fetal status. Because uterine hypoxia may induce uterine contractions, administer supplemental oxygen and infuse 500 mL of crystalloid intravenously. Place the patient in the left lateral decubitus position to improve uterine perfusion.[25] Because uterine, cervical, or urinary tract infections account for 20% to 40% of cases of preterm labor, search for a specific cause and treat infections appropriately.[25,26] If the contractions persist and cervical changes are documented despite these basic interventions, consider pharmacologic therapy.[25] Although tocolytic agents are commonly used and have been shown to prolong pregnancy by 2 to 7 days, data suggest that tocolysis does not improve neonatal outcomes.[5,23,25] In addition, none of the commonly used tocolytic medications are approved for use by the U.S. Food and Drug Administration (FDA) for this indication. General contraindications to tocolytic therapy include severe preeclampsia, placental abruption, intrauterine infection, advanced cervical dilation, and evidence of fetal compromise or placental insufficiency.[25]

There are no clear first-line tocolytic agents to manage preterm labor (Table 57.1). Clinical circumstances and preferences should dictate treatment. Agents such as calcium channel blockers (CCBs) and the prostaglandin inhibitor indomethacin have shown varying efficacy in clinical trials.[5,17] The most commonly used tocolytic agents in the United States are the CCB nifedipine, $MgSO_4$, and the β_2-receptor agonist terbutaline.

β_2-Receptor Agonists

The most commonly used β_2-adrenergic tocolytic agent is terbutaline. The β-mimetic agents react with adrenergic receptors to reduce intracellular ionized calcium levels and prevent the activation of myometrial contractile proteins.[5] Although terbutaline stimulates β_2-receptors primarily, it has some β_1-activity, and this is responsible for its cardiovascular side effects.

TABLE 57.1 Tocolytics for the Emergency Management or Cessation of Preterm Labor

DRUG	DOSE	END POINT
Indomethacin	50–100 mg PO or 50 mg PR	May repeat 25–50 mg PO every 6 h for a maximum of 48 h
Terbutaline	0.25 mg SC	May repeat every 20–60 min Cessation of uterine contractions Intolerable maternal side effects
Magnesium sulfate	4–6 g IV over 20 min followed by an infusion at 1–3 g/h IV	Cessation of uterine contractions Signs of magnesium toxicity (e.g., respiratory depression, hypotension, somnolence)
Nifedipine[a]	10 mg PO	May repeat every 15–20 min Cessation of uterine contractions Harmful maternal side effects (e.g., hypotension) Maximum dose, 40 mg

[a]Variable doses have been used.
IV, Intravenously; *PO*, orally; *PR*, per rectum; *SC*, subcutaneously.

Terbutaline is commonly used for the treatment of preterm labor.[5,26,27] Administer terbutaline subcutaneously in a 0.25-mg dose and repeat it every 20 to 60 minutes until contractions cease or intolerable maternal side effects occur.[25,28] In 2011 the FDA required the addition of a *Boxed Warning and Contraindication* ("black box warning") against the use of injectable terbutaline for the prevention or prolonged treatment of preterm labor beyond 48 to 72 hours because of adverse effects, including maternal death.[29] Use terbutaline with caution in patients with cardiovascular disease, hypertension, hyperthyroidism, diabetes, and seizures and in those taking other sympathomimetic amines.[25] The general clinical side effects of arrhythmias, myocardial ischemia, and pulmonary edema are related to its inherent activity as a β-mimetic drug. Treatment of the majority of side effects is supportive; severe cardiovascular effects may be treated with β-blocking agents.[28]

$MgSO_4$

$MgSO_4$ is not approved in the United States for use as a tocolytic agent and has been shown to be ineffective at delaying birth or preventing preterm birth, has no apparent advantages as a tocolytic agent, and it may be associated with an increased risk of fetal, neonatal, or infant mortality.[30] Even though the use of $MgSO_4$ as a tocolytic has fallen out of favor, benefits have been shown for antenatal use for its fetal neuroprotective effects.[31,32] The mechanism of action is not fully understood; magnesium probably decreases myometrial contractility through its role as a calcium antagonist.[5] Its fetoprotective effects probably result from noncompetitive antagonism of the *N*-methyl-D-aspartate receptor or through antiapoptosis and prevention of neuronal cell loss.[33]

$MgSO_4$ is generally administered at a loading dose of 4 g intravenously over a period of 20 to 30 minutes, followed by a maintenance intravenous infusion beginning at 1 g/h.[25,34] Infusion of $MgSO_4$ often produces sweating, warmth, and flushing. Rapid parenteral administration may cause transient nausea, vomiting, headache, or palpitations.[25] The major side effect of magnesium therapy is impairment of the muscles of respiration with subsequent respiratory arrest, an effect not usually seen until the serum magnesium level exceeds 10 mEq/L. At levels of 12 mEq/L or greater, respiratory arrest may occur.

The first sign of magnesium toxicity, a decrease in the patellar reflex, typically occurs as serum magnesium levels exceed 4 mEq/L, with loss of the reflex as levels increase further. The dosing and ongoing maintenance of magnesium therapy should be guided by the clinical status of the patient rather than by laboratory values. Monitor the patellar reflex throughout therapy. Because magnesium is almost totally excreted by the kidney, it is contraindicated in the presence of renal failure. Monitor urinary output and renal function throughout therapy. If respiratory depression develops, inject 10 mL of a 10% solution of calcium gluconate or calcium chloride over a 3-minute period as an antidote. For severe respiratory depression or arrest, prompt endotracheal intubation may be lifesaving.[5]

Calcium Channel Blockers

Calcium antagonists inhibit the influx of calcium ions through the muscle cell membrane and reduce uterine vascular resistance. The decrease in intracellular calcium also results in decreased myometrial activity. CCBs, mainly nifedipine, have demonstrated benefits in postponement of birth compared with β-mimetics with respect to prolongation of pregnancy, serious neonatal morbidity, and maternal adverse effects. CCBs may have some benefits over oxytocin receptor antagonists and magnesium sulfate, although oxytocin receptor antagonists had fewer maternal adverse effects. No difference has been noted in perinatal mortality.[35]

Although dosing regimens vary, nifedipine is frequently given as an initial loading dose of 30 mg orally and then 10 to 20 mg every 4 to 6 hours.[25,28] The CCB–induced decreased vascular resistance can lead to maternal hypotension and thus decreased uteroplacental perfusion.

Cyclo-Oxygenase Inhibitors

Cyclo-oxygenase (COX) inhibitors inhibit uterine contractions, are easily administered, and appear to have few maternal side effects, although adverse effects have been reported in the fetus and newborn.[36] Indomethacin is administered as an initial oral or rectal dose of 50 to 100 mg followed by 25- to 50-mg doses every 6 hours for a total of 48 hours.[25] Ketorolac can be used as an alternative with a 60-mg intramuscular loading dose, followed by 30 mg intramuscularly every 6 hours for 48 hours.[25] Side effects include oligohydramnios and premature closure of the ductus arteriosus.

Steroids

Patients in preterm labor between 24 0/7 and 33 6/7 weeks' gestation are candidates for antenatal steroid administration if it is believed delivery will occur within the next 7 days. This may reduce the incidence of neonatal morbidity and mortality, including things such as respiratory distress syndrome, intraventricular hemorrhage, and necrotizing enterocolitis.[25] Appropriate patients should receive betamethasone, 12 mg intramuscularly every 24 hours for a total of two doses, or dexamethasone, 6 mg intramuscularly every 12 hours for a total of four doses. Dexamethasone may have benefits compared with betamethasone such as fewer intraventricular hemorrhages and decreased lengths of stay in the neonatal intensive care unit (NICU). The intramuscular route may be more advantageous than the oral route.[37]

THIRD-TRIMESTER EMERGENCIES

Bleeding during the third trimester should always be considered an emergency because shock may occur within minutes. Prepare for the two most typical causes of bleeding in late gestation, placenta previa and placental abruption (Fig. 57.11).

Placenta previa refers to implantation of the placenta in the lower uterine segment with varying degrees of encroachment on the cervical os: in complete previa, the placenta completely overlays the cervical os, and in marginal previa, it lies within 2 cm of the os. Placenta previa is classically characterized by vaginal bleeding with little or no abdominal or pelvic pain. It may occur spontaneously or with minimal trauma, including after sexual intercourse. It is important to note that patients with placenta previa may present with a self-limited sentinel bleed and severe bleeding may occur subsequently. In all cases of third-trimester vaginal bleeding, this must be a consideration and the patient seen by an obstetrician in the emergency setting.

Abruptio placentae (placental abruption) refers to separation of the placenta from its site of implantation in the uterus before delivery of the fetus. It occurs in 0.6% to 1.2% of all pregnancies, with nearly half occurring at or near term.[38] Causes include maternal hypertension, cigarette smoking, substance abuse (alcohol, cocaine), older maternal age, and trauma. Although the clinical signs and symptoms with placental abruption can vary considerably, abruptio placentae is typically associated with varying degrees of abdominal pain and uterine irritability or contractions. Vaginal bleeding may or not be present; when it is not, it is called concealed abruption.[5,38]

Stabilization of a patient with third-trimester bleeding should be initiated with large-bore intravenous access. Blood should be drawn for a complete blood count (CBC) with platelets and a type and crossmatch. If abruption is suspected, clotting studies, including a fibrinogen level and a toxicology screen for cocaine, may be indicated because of the association of abruption with disseminated intravascular coagulation and cocaine abuse, respectively. Until the diagnosis of placenta previa is excluded, digital vaginal examination is *contraindicated*

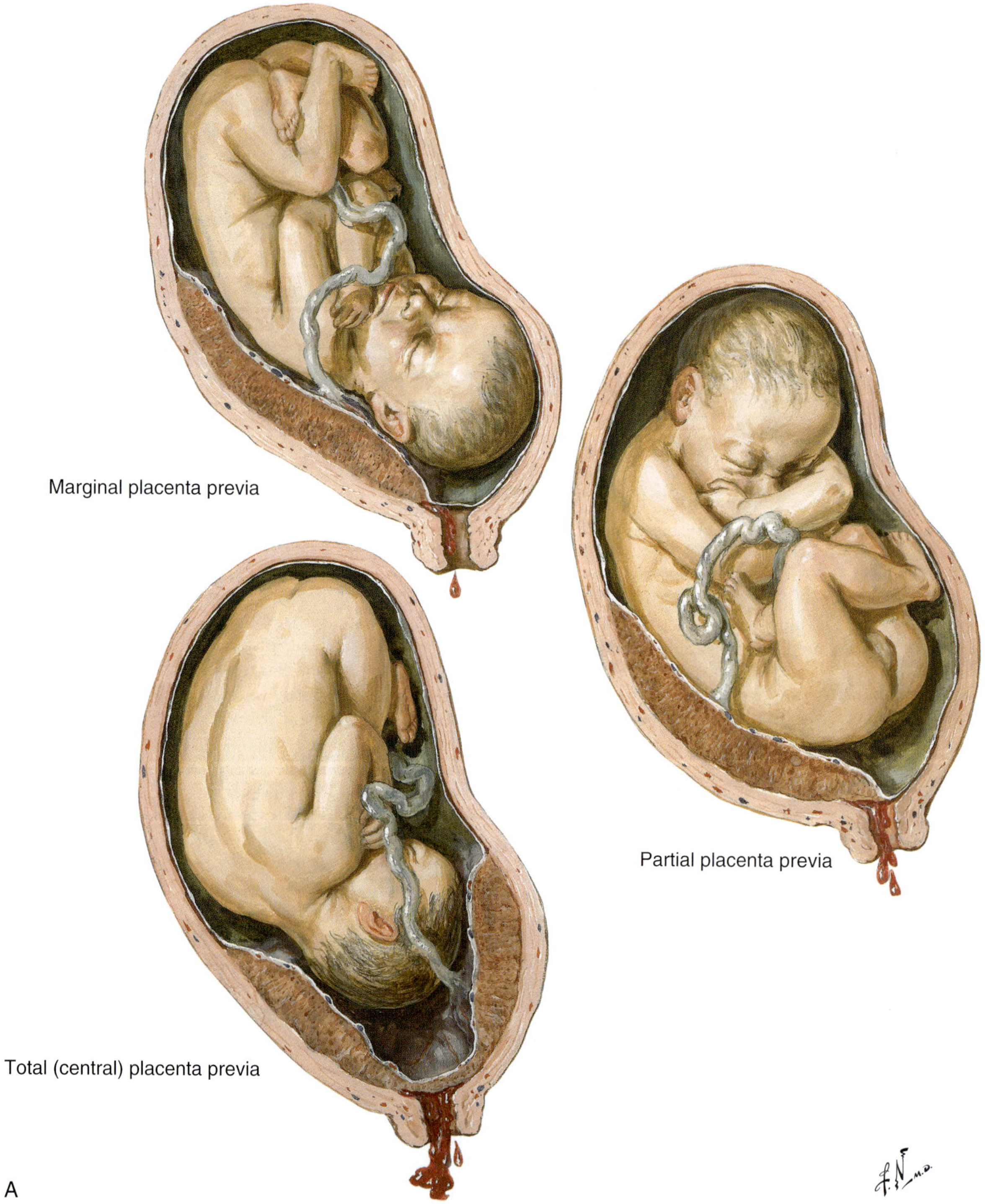

Fig. 57.11 (A) Abnormalities of placental implantation.

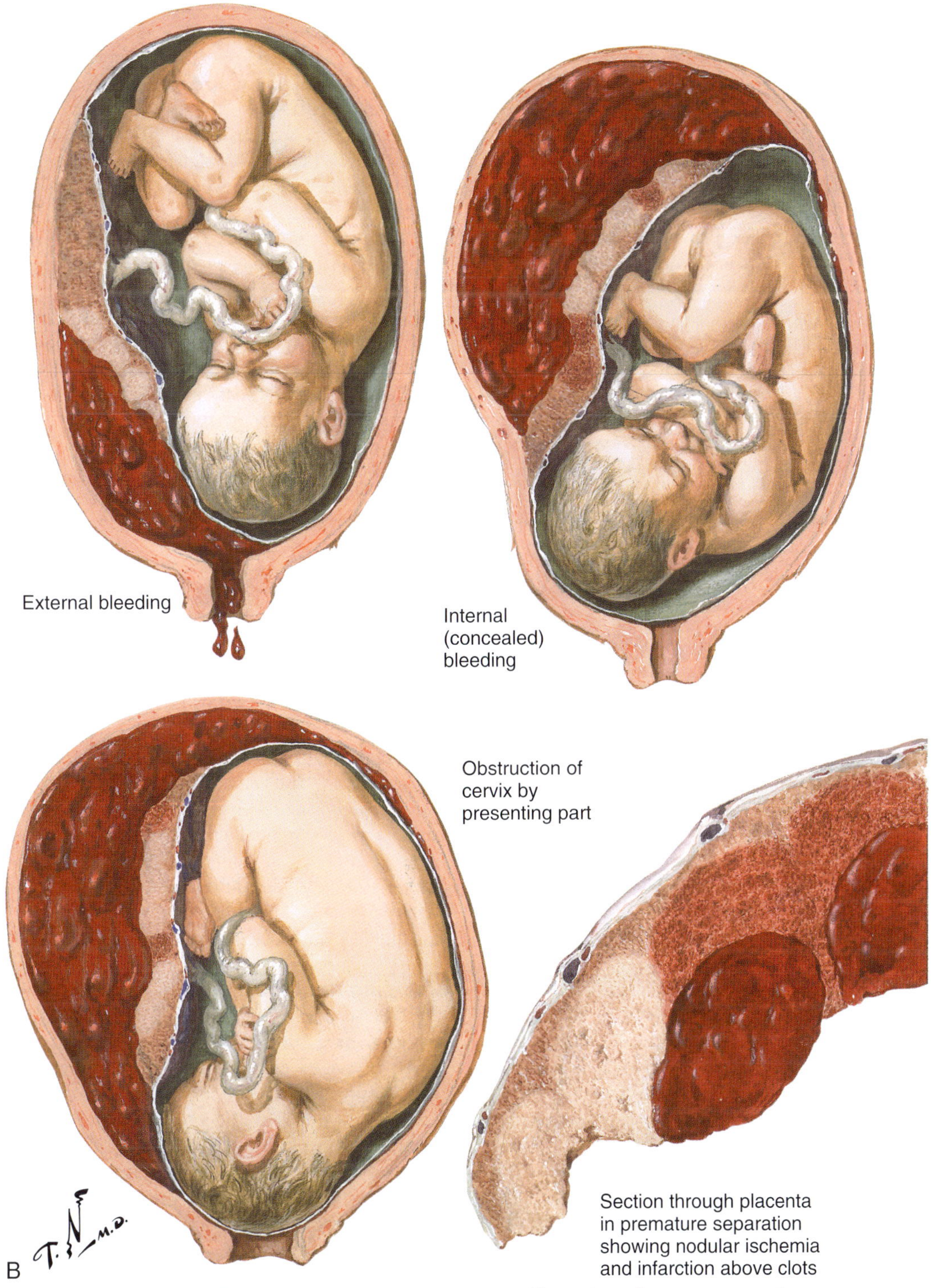

Fig. 57.11, cont'd (B) Placental abruption. (Netter illustrations from www.netterimages.com. Elsevier Inc. All rights reserved.)

because of the possibility of tearing or dislodging a placenta previa, which may result in profuse, potentially fatal hemorrhage. The patient should be placed on a cardiotocographic machine to monitor the status of the fetus.

The simplest and most precise method of placental localization is by transabdominal ultrasound. This modality is highly accurate in locating placenta previa; however, ultrasonography has limited sensitivity in detecting abruptio placentae, with a reported negative predictive value of between 63% and 88%.[5] Therefore negative findings on ultrasound should not be used to exclude placental abruption.

Patients with placental abruption may go into disseminated intravascular coagulation, and clinicians caring for these patients should be prepared to evaluate for and manage this condition.

Immediately transfer the patient to the care of an obstetrician for further evaluation.

PROCEDURE

Technique for Uncomplicated Delivery

Although complete sterility is not always possible, especially during emergency conditions, when time permits, use sterile technique and equipment. Wear sterile gloves, a gown, mask, and eye protection. Clean the perineum and vulva as for a vaginal examination and drape with sterile towels so that only the immediate area about the vulva is exposed. Be careful to avoid fecal contamination of the infant or perineum.

Ideally, place the patient on a delivery table in the dorsal lithotomy position to increase the diameter of the pelvic outlet (Fig. 57.12, *step 1*). Alternatively, position the patient on a stretcher with her hips and knees partially flexed, her thighs abducted, and the soles of her feet placed firmly on the stretcher. Additional personnel may assist in keeping the patient in this position. If the foot of the bed cannot be removed, enhance the delivery position by placing the underside of a bedpan under the patient's buttocks to provide additional space between the bed and the perineum.

Spontaneous Vertex Delivery

Spontaneous delivery of a vertex-presenting infant is divided into three phases: delivery of the head, delivery of the shoulders, and delivery of the body and legs.

Delivery of the Head

Anticipate delivery when the presenting part reaches the pelvic floor. With each contraction, the perineum bulges further and the vulvovaginal opening becomes more and more dilated by the fetal head. Just before delivery, *crowning* occurs, which is when the head is visible at the vaginal introitus and the widest portion, or the biparietal diameter of the head, distends the vulva.

Gentle, gradual, controlled delivery is desirable. Avoid explosive delivery of the head. Once the fetal head distends the vaginal introitus to 5 cm or more during a contraction, place the palm of one hand over the occipital area and provide gentle pressure to control delivery of the head (see Fig. 57.12, *step 2*). With the other hand preferably draped with a sterile towel to prevent contamination from the anus, exert upward pressure on the chin of the fetus through the perineum just in front of the coccyx in a modified Ritgen maneuver (Fig. 57.13). This maneuver extends the neck at the proper time such that the smallest diameter of the head passes through the introitus and over the perineum to protect the maternal perineal musculature. It is not uncommon for the vagina and perineum to tear with expulsive maternal effort during delivery of the head. If maternal expulsive efforts are insufficient to allow delivery of the head, an episiotomy may be considered at this time.

Gently support the head during subsequent delivery of the forehead, face, chin, and neck. With delivery of the neck, pass a finger around the infant's neck to determine whether it is encircled by one or more coils of the umbilical cord. If a loop of cord is felt, loosen it carefully and gently slip it over the infant's head (Fig. 57.14). If this cannot be done easily, clamp the cord doubly, cut the cord between the clamps, and promptly deliver the infant.

Delivery of the Shoulders

Just before external rotation the head usually falls posteriorly, almost bringing it into contact with the mother's anus. If maternal defecation occurs, avoid fecal contamination of the fetus. As rotation takes place, the head assumes a transverse position and the transverse diameter of the thorax rotates into the AP diameter of the pelvis. In most cases the shoulders are born spontaneously. Aid delivery by grasping the sides of the head and exerting *gentle* downward (posterior) traction until the anterior shoulder appears beneath the symphysis pubis (see Fig.12, *step 3*). Gently lift the head upward to aid in delivery of the posterior shoulder (see Fig. 57.12, *step 4*). The remainder of the body usually follows without difficulty.

If delivery of the body is delayed after the shoulders have been freed, assist by providing *moderate* traction on the exposed fetal body. To avoid injury to the brachial plexus, do not hook the fingers in the axilla during delivery. Always exert traction in the direction of the long axis of the infant. If traction is applied obliquely, bending of the neck and excessive stretching of the brachial plexus may occur.

Clearing the Airway

Once the head has been delivered, quickly wipe the infant's face and mouth. Routine suctioning is not indicated for vigorous newborns. Although it may be counterintuitive, current recommendations no longer advise routine oropharyngeal and nasopharyngeal suctioning of vigorous infants with meconium staining by amniotic fluid as studies have shown that this practice offers no benefit. A vigorous infant is one who has strong respiratory effort, good muscle tone, and a heart rate greater than 100 beats/min.[39] Routine intubation for tracheal suction of infants with meconium staining is also no longer recommended.[39] Per 2023 American Heart Association (AHA) guidelines, infant resuscitation should be initiated with air (21% oxygen at sea level), particularly for preterm infants less than 35 weeks, then titrated as necessary.[39]

Clamping the Cord

The infant should be positioned at or slightly below the level of the vaginal introitus before and during clamping of the cord.[39] Delayed clamping of the umbilical cord, no earlier than 1 minute after birth, in infants who do not require resuscitation can improve the short- and long-term hematologic and iron status of infants with a gestational age of 34 weeks or greater who do not require resuscitation.[39–41] Cut the umbilical cord with scissors between two Kelly clamps placed 4 to 5 cm from the infant's abdomen (see Fig. 57.12, *step 6*). Later, apply an umbilical cord clamp 2 to 3 cm from the infant's abdomen. Collect blood samples from the placental end of the cord for infant serology, including Rh determination.

After cutting the umbilical cord, evaluate the infant and, if necessary, initiate resuscitation as described in the later section on "The Newborn." Rapidly assess the infant by determining the following:

- Was the baby born after a full-term gestation?
- Does the baby have good muscle tone?
- Is the baby breathing or crying spontaneously?

If the answer to these questions is "yes," the baby will probably not need resuscitation[39] and the infant can be placed on the mother's chest for skin-to-skin contact, which promotes

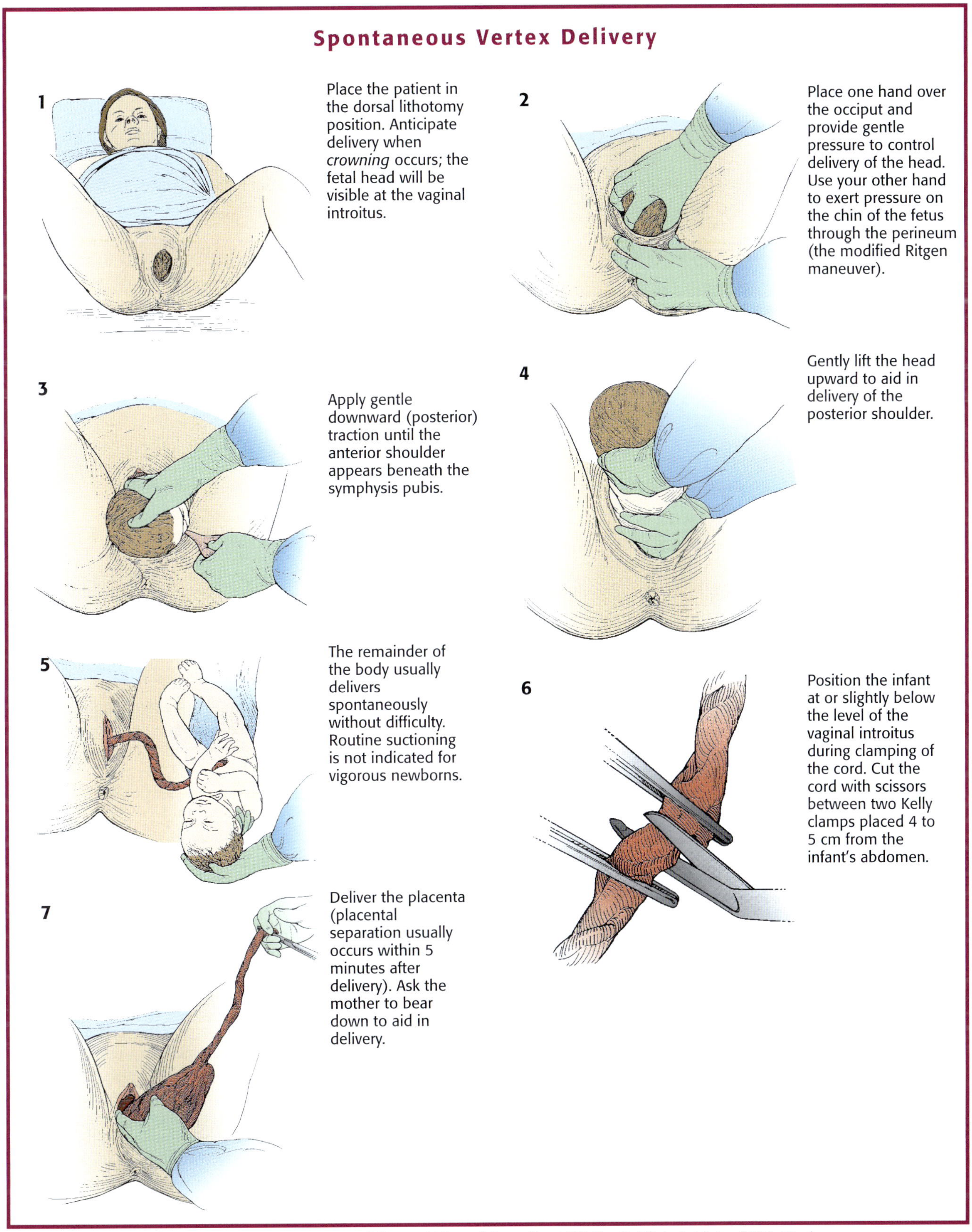

Fig. 57.12 Spontaneous vertex delivery. (Adapted from Ferri FF. *Ferri's Clinical Advisor 2013*. Mosby; 2013.)

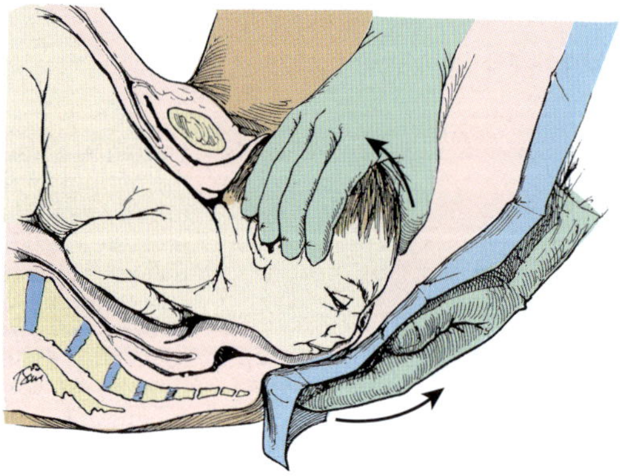

Fig. 57.13 For controlled and gentle delivery of the head, use the modified Ritgen maneuver. (From Seils A, Noujaim S, Davis K et al., eds. *Williams Obstetrics.* 22nd ed. McGraw-Hill Medical; 2005.)

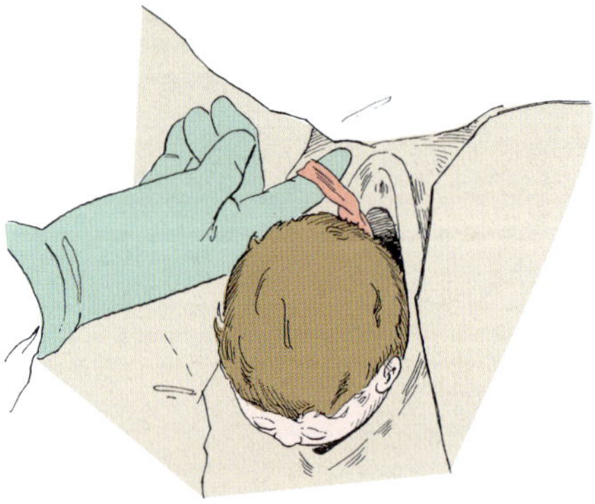

Fig. 57.14 As the head is delivered, use a finger to determine whether the umbilical cord is encircling the neck. If a loop of cord is felt, loosen it carefully and gently slip it over the infant's head.

uterine contraction and decreased bleeding as well as encouraging bonding between the mother and neonate and possibly facilitating successful breastfeeding.

Delivery of the Placenta

Placental separation usually occurs within approximately 5 minutes after delivery of the infant, although it may take longer. It can be recognized by the following signs:

- The uterus becomes globular and firmer as it contracts.
- There is a sudden gush of blood as the placenta separates from the uterine wall.
- The umbilical cord lengthens and protrudes further out of the vagina.

Ask the mother to bear down; the increased intraabdominal pressure produced by this maneuver may be enough to effect complete expulsion of the placenta (see Fig. 57.12, *step* 7). If maternal force alone is insufficient, aid in the delivery of the placenta. After ensuring that the uterus is firmly contracted and placental separation has occurred, use one hand to exert gentle pressure through the abdominal wall to lift the uterine fundus cephalad while keeping the umbilical cord slightly taut with the other hand (Fig. 57.15). Repeat this maneuver until the placenta reaches the introitus. At this time, stop uterine pressure and gently lift the placenta upward and out of the vagina. Never force expulsion of the placenta before placental separation has occurred, and never use forceful traction to pull the placenta out of the uterus. Such maneuvers may result in separation of the cord from the placenta or uterine inversion

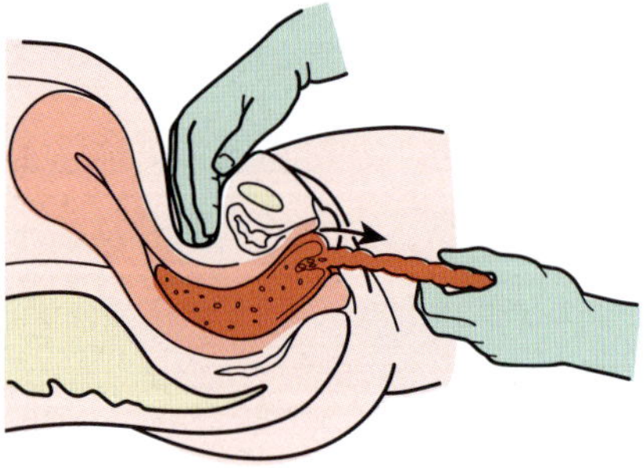

Fig. 57.15 Delivery of the placenta and fetal membranes by exerting controlled traction on the cord and suprapubic pressure with the abdominal hand to prevent uterine inversion. Care should be taken to avoid avulsion of the cord. Active management with uterotonic agents such as oxytocin administered at delivery hastens delivery of the placenta and may reduce the incidence of postpartum hemorrhage and total blood loss. (From Gabbe SG, Niebyl JR, Simpson JL, eds. *Obstetrics: Normal and Problem Pregnancies.* 5th ed. Elsevier; 2007.)

with potentially catastrophic hemodynamic consequences. Examine the placenta for completeness and save it for later evaluation by the obstetrician.[5]

Examine the vulva, vagina, and cervix for traumatic lacerations. Cervical lacerations most typically occur at the 9 or 3 o'clock position; vaginal lacerations typically occur at the point of the ischial spines. The most common areas for lacerations are the vagina, hymen, and perineum. Based on the availability of resources and the clinical setting, definitive repair of uncomplicated or minor obstetric lacerations may be performed in the ED by the EP, but this is often done by a consultant obstetrician.

After delivery of the placenta, the primary mechanism by which hemostasis is achieved at the placental site is through myometrial contraction. Agents such as oxytocin, methylergonovine, and ergonovine may be used to stimulate myometrial contraction. To prevent uterine atony and subsequent bleeding, oxytocin is often administered after delivery of the placenta.

Oxytocin is the most commonly used oxytocic drug and is usually given by continuous intravenous infusion. Twenty units of oxytocin are added to 1 L of normal saline and the solution is administered at a rate of 10 mL/min for several minutes until the uterus remains firmly contracted and bleeding is controlled. At this point, reduce the infusion rate to 1 to 2 mL/min.[3] Alternatively, ergot derivatives such as methylergonovine maleate, 0.2 mg, or ergonovine maleate, 0.2 mg, may be given intramuscularly.[5] Because of their vasoconstrictive properties, ergot preparations are relatively contraindicated in patients with hypertension, including pregnancy-associated hypertension or preeclampsia.[5] The synthetic prostaglandin misoprostol can also be given as an 800- to 1000-μg rectal dose. In the United States, oxytocic agents are not generally administered before delivery of the placenta because of concerns that the resultant uterine contraction may entrap the placenta or trap an undiagnosed twin within the uterus.[5] Even when oxytocics are administered, the hour after delivery of the placenta is the time during which PPH secondary to uterine atony is most likely to occur. For this reason, palpate the uterus frequently to ensure that it is well contracted. A normally contracted uterus will feel firm with its upper margin just below the maternal umbilicus. If the uterus is flaccid or bleeding, gently massage it through the abdominal wall.

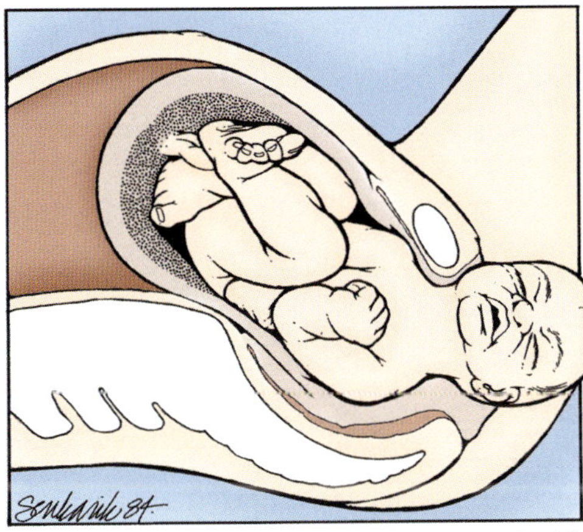

Fig. 57.16 Shoulder dystocia. When delivery of the fetal head is not followed by delivery of the shoulders, the anterior shoulder has often become caught behind the symphysis.

Occasionally, the placenta may fail to separate completely, resulting in a retained placenta or placental fragments with persistent uterine bleeding. Support the patient with intravenous fluids and blood transfusions as indicated until definitive therapy is available. Constant firm uterine massage can lessen hemorrhage and may be lifesaving.

COMPLICATIONS

Complex Deliveries

Shoulder Dystocia

Shoulder dystocia refers to impaction of the fetal shoulders in the pelvic outlet after delivery of the head and occurs in 0.6% to 1.4% of deliveries (Fig. 57.16).[42] Shoulder dystocia is associated with several risk factors, including fetal macrosomia, maternal diabetes, obesity, post-term pregnancy and multiparity, and is an obstetric emergency.

Impaction of the fetal shoulders and thorax in the maternal pelvis prohibits adequate respiration, and compression of the umbilical cord frequently compromises the fetal circulation. For these reasons, shoulder dystocia is a serious and potentially fatal complication of delivery.[43] Fetal complications include brachial plexus injury, clavicular and humeral fractures, and rarely, death.[43] Risks to the mother include genital injuries, higher-degree perineal lacerations, and a higher risk of PPH.

Management

The techniques used to treat shoulder dystocia frequently require an assistant, and delivery can result in fetal injury or hypoxia, as well as increased rates of PPH.[44] As soon as shoulder dystocia is determined to be present, the mother should be instructed to stop pushing so the dystocia does not worsen. Call for emergency assistance from a pediatrician, an obstetrician, and an anesthesiologist. Complications such as a fetal fracture or nerve injury are not unusual with shoulder dystocia during any delivery technique.

Although a variety of techniques have been described to free the anterior shoulder from its impacted position beneath the symphysis pubis, the initial technique of choice is the McRoberts maneuver because of its ease and potential for success (Fig. 57.17A).[45] In one study, approximately 40% of shoulder dystocias were relieved with the McRoberts maneuver alone.[46] To perform the McRoberts maneuver, place the mother in the extreme lithotomy position with her hips completely flexed so that her knees rest alongside her chest. This causes a flattening of the lumbar lordosis, rotates the maternal pelvis cephalad, and frequently frees the impacted anterior fetal shoulder.[5,43,45] If the McRoberts maneuver fails to effect delivery, ask an assistant to apply moderate suprapubic, *not fundal*, pressure to the maternal abdomen while providing gentle downward traction on the fetal head; this maneuver may increase success rates to up to 90% (Fig. 57.17B).[43]

If these initial maneuvers fail to achieve delivery, several other techniques exist, the choice of which will depend on clinician preference and experience. In the first maneuver, place two fingers in the vagina and exert pressure on the fetal scapula to rotate the *posterior* shoulder 180 degrees in a clockwise or counterclockwise fashion, depending on the orientation of the torso *(reverse Wood's screw)*, to free the entrapped anterior shoulder (Fig. 57.17C). Other maneuvers include the Rubin maneuver, in which rotation is achieved by applying pressure on the posterior aspect of the anterior shoulder, or the Wood's screw maneuver, in which pressure is placed on the anterior aspect of the posterior shoulder. This may cause release of the impacted anterior shoulder and result in progression of delivery.[43,47] Alternatively, attempt to deliver the posterior arm (Fig. 57.17D). In this maneuver, insert the hand along the hollow of the maternal sacrum to the level of the fetus' posterior elbow. Exert pressure at the antecubital fossa, flex the posterior forearm of the fetus, and grasp the hand or forearm. Next, carefully sweep the posterior arm of the fetus across its chest to effect delivery of the posterior arm and shoulder. Rotate the shoulder girdle into one of the oblique diameters of the pelvis and subsequently deliver the anterior shoulder.[5,45] No particular maneuver has a higher correlation to neonatal morbidity and mortality, but the use of multiple maneuvers does increase the chance for neonatal complications.[45,48] Preliminary data suggest delivery of the posterior arm should be considered immediately following the McRoberts maneuver/subrapubic pressure.[45]

The Gaskin maneuver calls for turning the patient face-down into an all-fours position on hands and knees. This positioning results in a wider anterior-posterior pelvic diameter and can facilitate the rotation of the baby. It may not be feasible in those with limited mobility.

If all these strategies fail, it may be necessary to perform a controlled destructive procedure, such as fracture of the fetal clavicle, or the cephalic replacement maneuver (Zavanelli), in which the baby's head is pushed back into the birth canal with subsequent cesarean delivery.[5] The Zavanelli maneuver should be a last resort. An episiotomy is not useful during the management of shoulder dystocia.[49] These procedures are rarely if ever performed in the ED and are usually done by obstetricians in labor and delivery suites.

Breech Delivery

Technique

In general, a "hands off" approach to a breech delivery is preferred. The only maneuver that may be useful is gently rotating the baby so it is in a sacrum-anterior position during descent. As the breech progressively distends the perineum, the posterior hip will be delivered, usually from the 6 o'clock position (Fig. 57.18, *step 1*). The anterior hip will then be delivered, followed by external rotation to the sacrum-anterior position.

Management Of Shoulder Dystocia

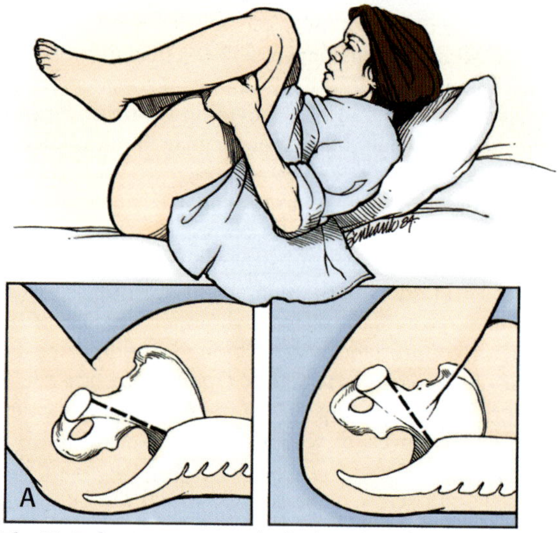

The McRoberts maneuver is the least invasive maneuver to disimpact the shoulders in shoulder dystocia. Position the patient in the extreme lithotomy position with the hips completely flexed (knee-chest position); this may free the anterior fetal shoulder.

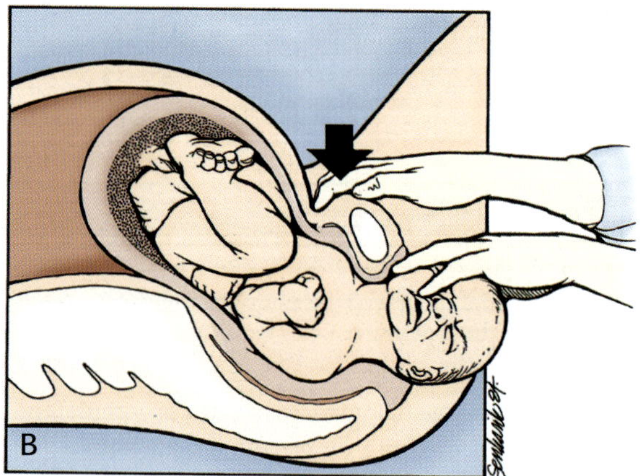

Moderate suprapubic pressure will often disimpact the anterior shoulder. Desperate traction on the fetal head is not likely to facilitate delivery and might lead to trauma. Delivery of an infant with shoulder dystocia often results in fracture of the clavicle or humerus to accomplish delivery.

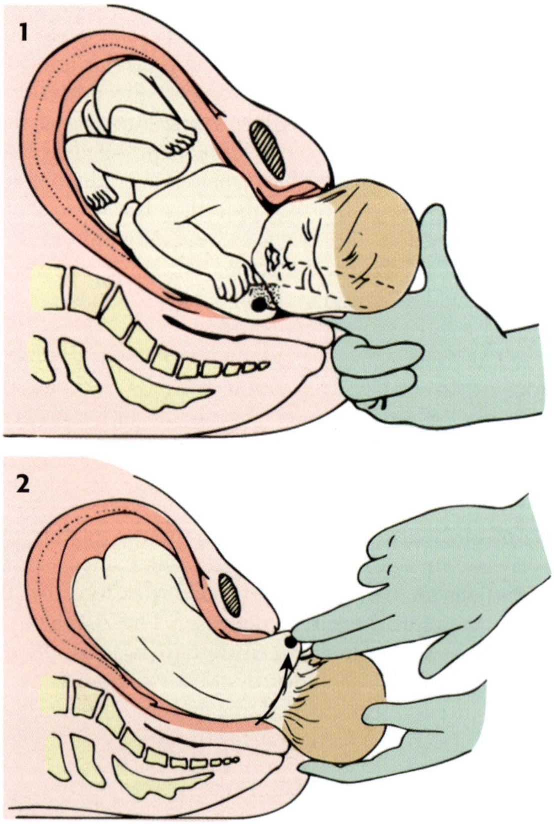

C

Rubin or reverse Wood's screw maneuver. *1*, Rotate the posterior shoulder. *2*, Deliver the rotated shoulder.

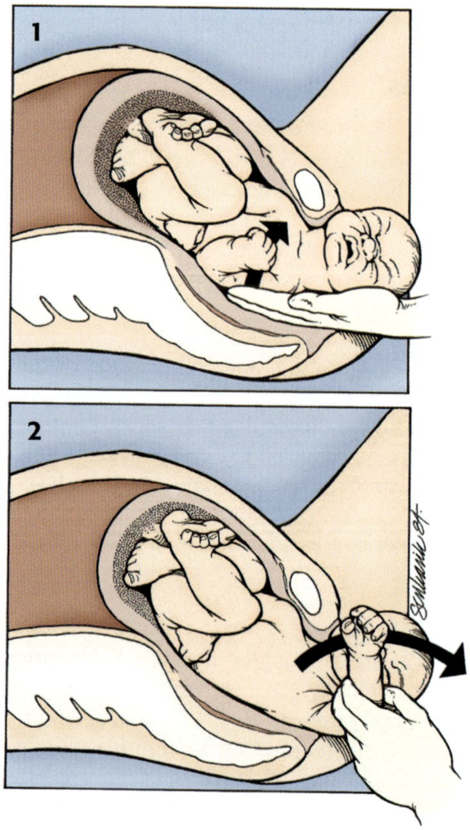

D

Posterior shoulder delivery. Insert a hand and sweep the posterior arm across the chest and over the perineum. Take care to distribute the pressure evenly across the humerus to avoid unnecessary fracture.

Fig. 57.17 Management of shoulder dystocia. (A, B, and D, From Gabbe SG, Niebyl JR, Simpson JL, eds. *Obstetrics: Normal and Problem Pregnancies.* 5th ed. Elsevier; 2007.)

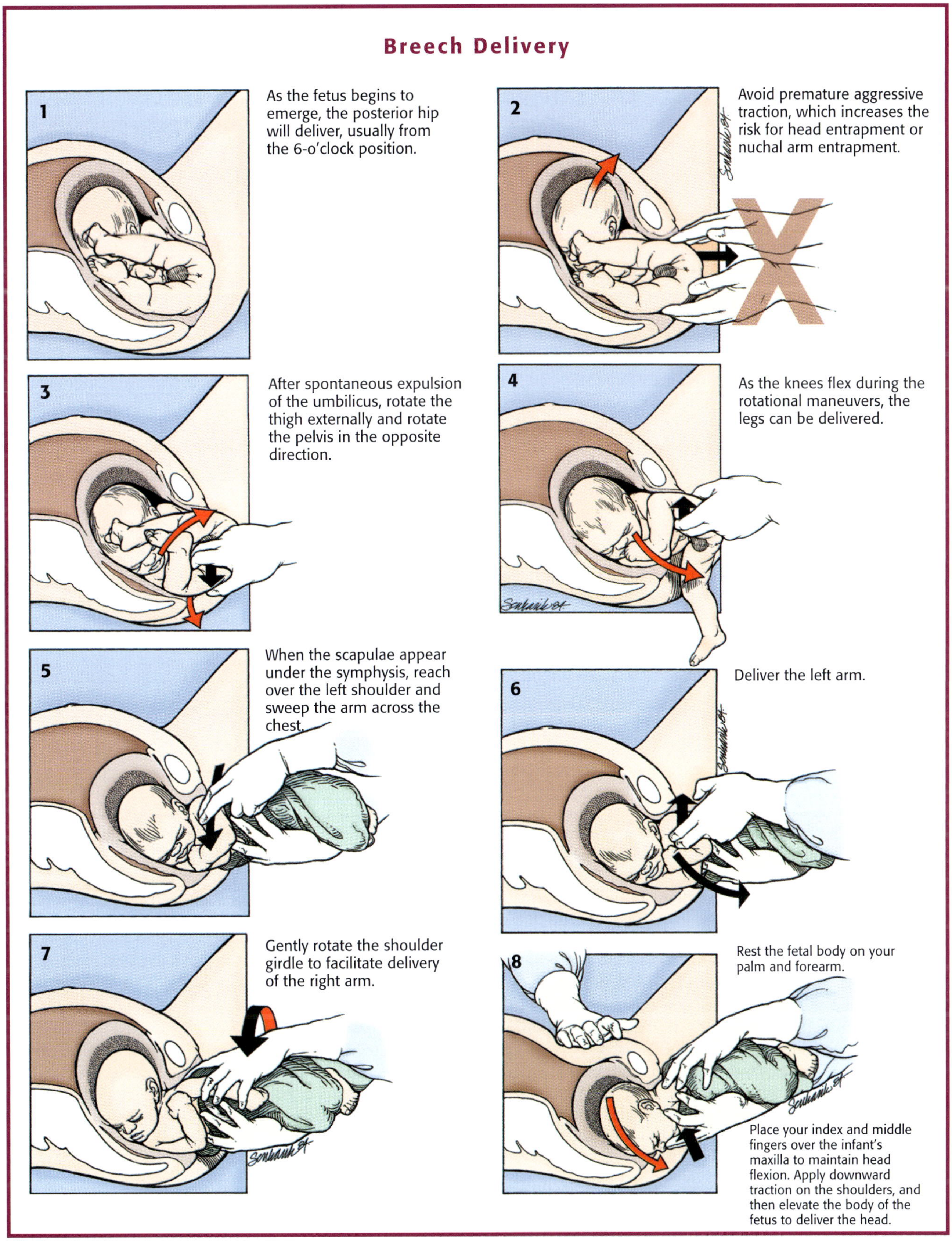

Fig. 57.18 Breech delivery.

Ideally, two attendants should be available for a breech delivery.

Delivery of the Presenting Part and Body. Many breech infants deliver spontaneously with maternal expulsion efforts alone. Avoid fetal traction and apply fetal manipulation only after spontaneous delivery to the level of the umbilicus. Continued descent of the fetus will allow delivery of the legs, which may be aided by splinting the medial part of the thighs of the fetus with the fingers positioned parallel to the femur and exerting pressure laterally to sweep the legs away from the midline (see Fig. 57.18, *steps 2–4*). If assistance is needed to deliver the legs, the Pinard maneuver may be used. This maneuver involves pressure applied to the popliteal space of the infant with resultant flexion of the knees and external rotation of the thigh. After delivery of the legs, grasp the fetal bony pelvis with both hands, with the fingers resting on the anterior superior iliac crests and the thumbs on the sacrum. Because the fetal body is slippery and difficult to hold, wrap it in a towel to assist delivery. Use the maternal expulsive efforts in conjunction with gentle downward traction. Rotate the fetal pelvis to bring the fetal sacrum into the transverse position to effect delivery of the scapulae. Two methods of shoulder delivery are commonly used (see Fig. 57.18, *steps 5–7*). In the first, with the scapulae visible, rotate the trunk so that the anterior arm and shoulder appear at the vulva and can easily be released and delivered. Next, rotate the body of the fetus in the reverse direction to deliver the other shoulder and arm beneath the symphysis pubis. In the second method, if trunk rotation is unsuccessful, deliver the posterior shoulder. Grasp the feet in one hand and draw them upward over the mother's groin. Exert leverage on the posterior shoulder, which will slide out over the perineal margin, usually followed by the arm and hand. Deliver the anterior shoulder, arm, and hand beneath the symphysis pubis by downward traction on the fetal body.

Occasionally, spontaneous delivery of the arm and hand does not follow delivery of the shoulder. If this occurs, provide upward traction on the fetal body after delivery of the posterior shoulder. Pass two fingers along the fetal humerus until the fetal elbow is reached. Using the fingers to splint the fetal arm, sweep it downward and deliver it. Deliver the anterior arm by depression of the fetal body alone. In some cases it may be necessary to sweep the anterior arm down over the thorax by using two fingers as a splint.

Delivery of the Head. After the shoulders appear, the head usually occupies one of the oblique diameters of the pelvis, with the chin directed posteriorly. Extract the head by using the Mauriceau-Smellie-Veit maneuver as follows. With the fetal body resting on the clinician's palm and forearm, place the index and middle fingers of one hand over the infant's maxilla, not the mandible, to maintain flexion of the fetal head (see Fig. 57.18, *step 8*). Hook two fingers of the other hand over the fetal neck and, while grasping the shoulders, apply downward traction until the suboccipital region appears under the symphysis pubis. Elevate the body of the fetus toward the mother's abdomen, and the fetal mouth, nose, brow, and eventually the occiput will emerge over the perineum. Avoid excessive elevation of the fetal torso to prevent hyperextension of the neck. If available, have an assistant apply suprapubic pressure to help deliver the head. If delivery of the head is not affected by the Mauriceau-Smellie-Veit maneuver, forceps delivery may be necessary but is beyond the scope of this text and most ED practitioners. Once the breech baby is delivered, further management proceeds as for a normal vertex delivery.

Rarely, *breech extraction* of an infant becomes necessary and is indicated only if there is a definite diagnosis of fetal distress unresponsive to routine maneuvers, if obstetric services are unavailable, and if cesarean section cannot be performed promptly. To perform the extraction, introduce the hand into the vagina and grasp both feet of the fetus, with the index finger placed between the fetal ankles. Apply gentle traction until the feet are pulled through the vulva. Continue gentle downward traction while grasping successively higher portions of both legs and thighs. When the breech appears at the vulva, apply gentle traction until the hips are delivered. As the buttocks emerge, rotate the fetal back anteriorly. Place the thumbs over the sacrum and the fingers over the hips and deliver the remainder of the breech as described earlier. At times, delivery of a frank breech may be necessary. Facilitated by an episiotomy, allow the breech to deliver spontaneously as far as possible. Place a finger on each side of the fetal groin and exert moderate traction. Once the knees appear outside the birth canal, flex the legs slowly to assist in delivery, and proceed with delivery as described earlier.

Nuchal Cord

Nuchal cord occurs when the umbilical cord wraps around the fetal neck 360 degrees and it occurs in approximately 10% to 30% of fetuses. Nuchal cords can be single or multiple loops and can be loosely or tightly wrapped around the neck. Risk factors include polyhydramnios and abnormally long umbilical cords, but they can occur without identifiable risk factors.

Tight nuchal cords can cause compression of the umbilical vein and obstruction of blood flow. A strangulation syndrome can be seen in infants with tightly wound nuchal cords. They show signs such as facial duskiness, petechial lesions, and subconjunctival hemorrhages. Infants may also have hypovolemia, hypotension, and hypoxia.

As the fetal head delivers, the clinician should check for the presence or absence of a nuchal cord by feeling the infant's neck. If present, the cord can usually be slipped over the head and the delivery can proceed. If it cannot be slipped over the head but is loose, it may be able to be slipped caudally over the infant's shoulders and the baby delivered "through" the looped cord. If the cord is wrapped tightly or wrapped multiple times, it may require that the cord be clamped in two places 4 cm apart and cut between the clamps. The delivery can then proceed.

Cord Prolapse

This obstetrical emergency occurs when the umbilical cord exits the cervix before or at the same time as the fetal presenting part. This results in cord compression and subsequent hypoxia and fetal bradycardia. An abnormal fetal heart rate may be the first indicator of a cord prolapse, and visualization of the cord at the cervix or vaginal introitus confirms the diagnosis.

Management of cord prolapse is directed at sustaining fetal life until delivery is accomplished. In labor and delivery settings, patients often go straight to cesarean section. In other settings, like the ED, the goal is to lift the presenting part off the prolapsed cord. If immediate obstetric services are not available, four temporizing measures can be undertaken. (1) Place the patient in the knee-chest or deep Trendelenburg position and keep the patient in this position until delivery.[50–52]

(2) Minimize compression of the umbilical cord by inserting a sterile gloved hand and exerting manual pressure in the vagina to lift and maintain the presenting part away from the prolapsed cord. (3) After manual elevation of the presenting part, instill 500 to 700 mL of saline into the bladder to raise the presenting part and maintain cord decompression. Once the bladder is filled, remove the vaginal hand.[51,52] (4) Tocolytic therapy can be administered to decrease uterine contractions and improve fetoplacental perfusion in cases of fetal bradycardia or pathological decelerations.[51,52] Unfortunately, outcomes of true obstetric emergencies managed solely in the ED are often bleak and essentially out of the hands of the EP.

Touching or manipulating the cord should be avoided as it can trigger vasospasm.

Episiotomy

Routine use of episiotomy is no longer recommended.[53,54] Selected indications include breech delivery, shoulder dystocia, occiput-posterior presentations, and imminent perineal tear, but generally is not indicated and when done in these circumstances is an independent risk factor for third- or fourth- degree perineal tears.[53] Episiotomy may be necessary to expedite delivery in situations of fetal distress. Two types of episiotomy are used: median (midline) and mediolateral (Fig. 57.19). The median approach is the easiest type to perform and repair, and results in the least amount of blood loss, heals more rapidly with minimal discomfort, and is generally more common in the United States. A major complication of median episiotomy is potential inadvertent extension of the incision into the anal sphincter or rectum, which results in third- and fourth-degree lacerations, respectively.[5] A mediolateral episiotomy seldom results in extension into the anal sphincter, but blood loss is greater, repair is more difficult, and healing may be more painful.

Technique

With vertex presentations, perform the episiotomy during the second stage of labor, when the fetal head begins to distend the perineum and becomes visible to a diameter of 3 to 4 cm during a contraction.[5] Anesthesia for episiotomy in the ED is usually limited to local infiltration of the perineum with 1% or 2% lidocaine.

Make the incision with Mayo scissors through the skin and subcutaneous tissue, the vaginal mucosa, the urogenital septum, and the superior fascia of the pelvic diaphragm (see Fig. 57.19). Make the incision up to half the length of the perineum and extend it 2 to 3 cm upward into the vaginal mucosa. If the incision is in the midline, extend the incision through the lowermost fibers of the puborectalis portion of the levator ani muscles. As the head crowns, place the index and middle fingers inside the vaginal introitus to expose the mucosa, posterior fourchette, and perineal body. Use tissue scissors to incise the median raphe of the perineum halfway to the anal sphincter. For a mediolateral episiotomy, direct the incision downward and outward in the direction of the lateral margin of the anal sphincter either to the right or to the left.

Repair the episiotomy after delivery of the infant and placenta. Repairs are usually performed by the obstetric consultant in the delivery suite but can be done by an EP experienced in the procedure (see Fig. 57.19). The goals of episiotomy repair are to restore both anatomy and hemostasis with a minimal amount of suture material. Perform the closure after delivery of the placenta and following inspection and repair of the cervix and upper vaginal canal if indicated. The principles of repair are the same regardless of the type of episiotomy.

Because there is minimal tension on the closed wound, use 2-0 or 3-0 absorbable suture, such as chromic catgut or polyglycolic acid, on a large atraumatic needle. The first step is to close the vaginal mucosa with a continuous suture from just above the apex of the incision to the mucocutaneous junction to reapproximate the margins of the hymenal ring (see Fig. 57.19, *step 1*). Ligate large actively bleeding vessels during closure with separate absorbable sutures. Next, reapproxi mate the perineal musculature with three or four interrupted sutures (see Fig. 57.19, *step 2*). Close the superficial layers by one of two methods. In the first method, use a continuous suture to close the superficial mucosa from the mucocutaneous junction outward and then continue it upward as a subcuticular skin closure, with the suture returning to and ending at the mucocutaneous junction (see Fig. 57.19, *steps 3 and 4*). Alternatively, place several interrupted sutures through the skin and subcutaneous fascia and tie them loosely. This last method of skin closure avoids burying two layers of suture in the more superficial layers of the perineum.[5] The most common complication of episiotomy is hematoma formation, which requires evacuation and drainage. Infection is an infrequent complication that usually responds to sitz baths, good hygiene, and antibiotic therapy.

Immediate Postpartum Hemorrhage

PPH is the leading cause of maternal mortality globally. It is primarily seen in developing countries, but the incidence is increasing in the United States.[55,56] PPH is generally defined as blood loss of more than 500 mL following vaginal delivery and more than 1000 mL following cesarean delivery, with signs of hypovolemia. The average blood loss with a vaginal delivery is estimated to be approximately 500 mL but clinicians consistently underestimate actual blood loss.[55,57] PPH is divided into early hemorrhage, which occurs within 24 hours of delivery, and late hemorrhage, which occurs after 24 hours and up to 6 weeks after delivery.

PPH may be sudden and massive but is frequently characterized by persistent moderate bleeding until serious hypovolemia develops. Observe carefully for blood loss, including evaluation of uterine size and consistency, during the early postpartum period. The most common cause of early PPH is uterine atony, which is involved in up to 80% of cases.[56] Less common causes include lacerations of the lower genital tract, retained placenta or placental fragments, coagulation disorders, uterine rupture, uterine inversion, and placental site bleeding.[6]

General Management

The priority of management of PPH is to control the bleeding before coagulation abnormalities or problems with organ perfusion occur. Management is similar to management of any acute blood loss, focusing on the basics of airway, breathing, and circulation, and replacing intravascular volume with crystalloid and blood products, and using massive transfusion protocols as needed, and to correct the underlying cause of the hemorrhage.

Large-bore intravenous lines are often already in place, but, if not, at least two should be established rapidly. Infusion may start with crystalloid but should be transitioned to blood

Episiotomy And Repair

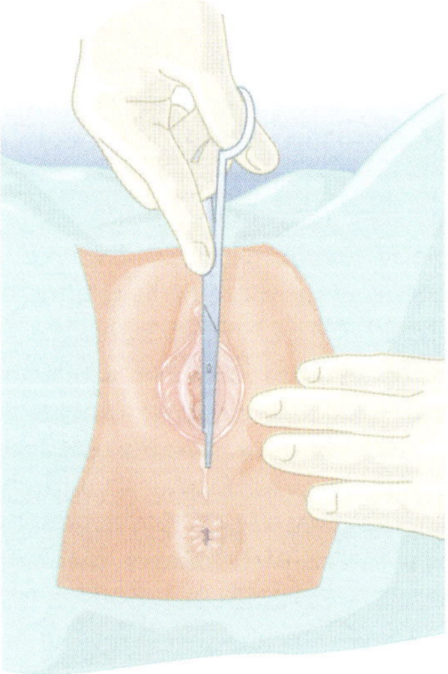

Midline Episiotomy

Make the incision through the lowermost fibers of the puborectalis portion of the levator ani muscles. Incise the median raphe of the perineum halfway to the anal sphincter.

A major complication of midline episiotomy is incision of the anal sphincter or rectum, which leads to third- and fourth-degree lacerations.

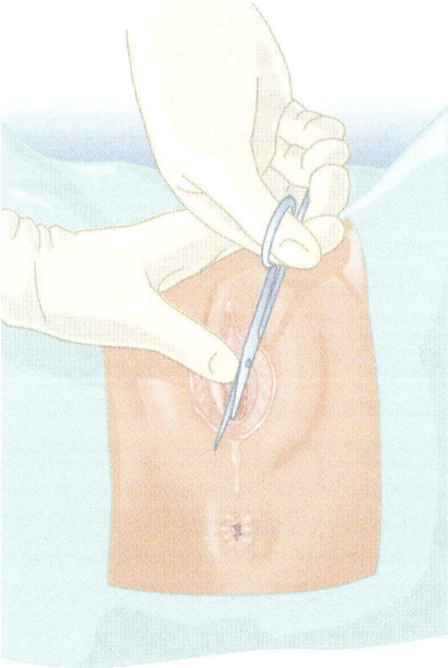

Mediolateral Episiotomy

Make the incision through the lowermost fibers of the puborectalis portion of the levator ani muscles. Direct the incision downward and outward in the direction of the lateral margin of the anal sphincter.

The mediolateral approach rarely extends into the anal sphincter but may be associated with greater blood loss and more difficult repair.

Episiotomy Repair

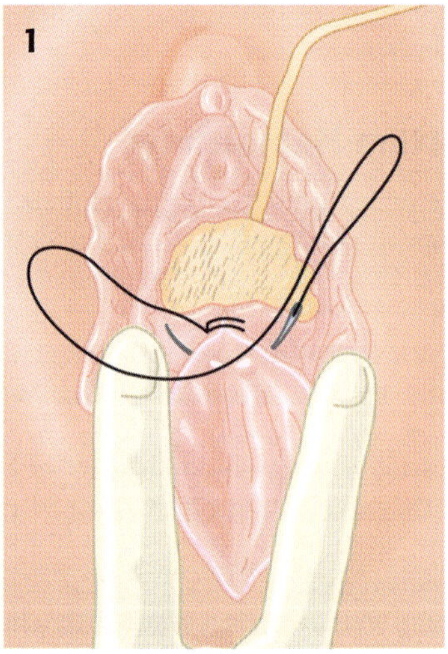

Place a taped sponge in the upper part of the vagina. Expose the full extent of the episiotomy with the left hand. Place the first suture 1 cm cephalad to the most superior margin of the episiotomy or laceration to ensure hemostasis of the repair. Use continuous locked absorbable suture to close the vaginal epithelium from the apex of the laceration to the hymenal ring.

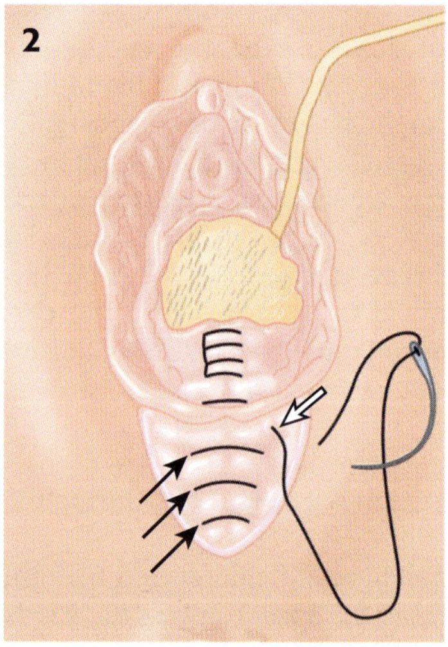

Use simple interrupted (absorbable) suture to close the deep perineal fascia and underlying levator ani muscles *(black arrows)*.

Bring the vaginal epithelial suture below the skin into the subcutaneous tissue *(white arrow)*.

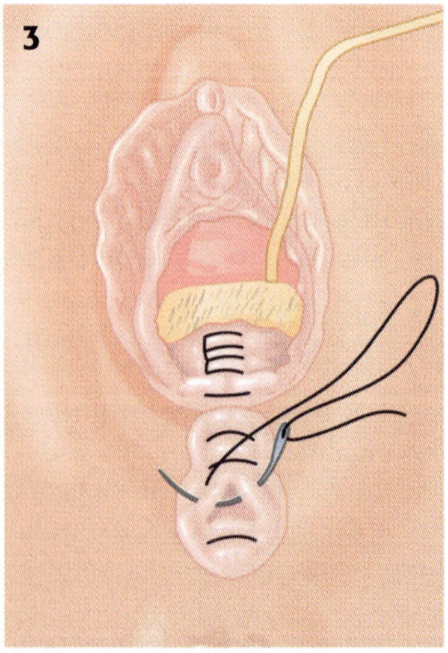

Use the vaginal epithelial suture to close the superficial fascia down to the edge of the episiotomy.

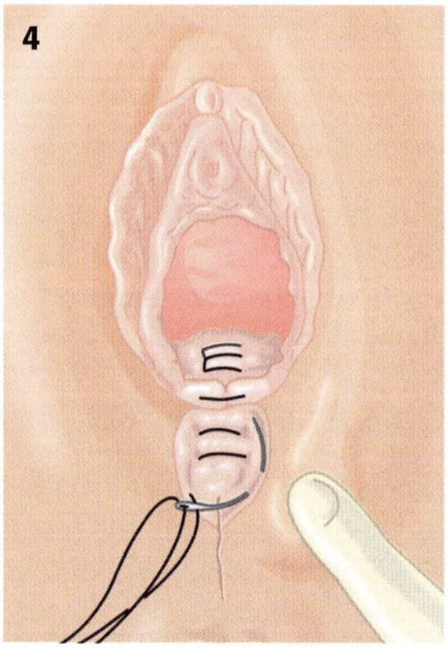

Use the same suture again as a subcuticular stitch coming back to the hymenal ring, where it is tied off.

Remove the vaginal sponge.

Fig. 57.19 Episiotomy and repair. Routine episiotomy is no longer advised, but the procedure is often performed. Simple repairs may be done in the emergency department (ED), but this is often performed by the obstetrician or in the delivery room after an ED birth. (From Hacker NF, Gambone JC, Hobel CK, eds. *Hacker & Moore's Essentials of Obstetrics and Gynecology.* 5th ed. Elsevier; 2009.)

products as soon as possible. Blood should be sent for a CBC, coagulation studies (prothrombin time [PT]/partial thromboplastin time [PTT], international normalized ratio [INR], fibrinogen), and a type and screen with an Rh, if not already done. Immediate consultation with obstetrics is necessary and, if bleeding continues, interventional radiology may also need to be consulted.

Management of Uterine Atony

The diagnosis of uterine atony, the most common cause of bleeding, is made when uterine palpation reveals a soft "boggy" uterus. The diagnosis may be suspected based on abdominal examination with confirmation made on bimanual examination as atony may be localized to the lower uterine segment. Uterine atony is initially managed with firm manual massage of the uterine fundus through the abdominal wall in conjunction with the administration of oxytocic agents (Table 57.2).

If bleeding persists, bimanual uterine compression is indicated. Use one hand to compress and massage the uterus through the abdominal wall while using the fist of the other hand to gently massage the anterior aspect of the uterus through the vagina (Fig. 57.20). Avoid vigorous downward massage, which can result in acute uterine inversion or can injure the blood vessels in the broad ligament.

Oxytocics

Oxytocin is the usual first-line drug for PPH secondary to uterine atony.[58] Oxytocin is given as an intravenous infusion. While recommendations in the literature vary, a typical initial dose is 20 to 40 units in 1 L of crystalloid infused at a rate of 200 to 500 mL/h. Titrate to sustain uterine contractions and control uterine hemorrhage. Slowing of hemorrhage should be observed within minutes of administration. If an intravenous line is not available, administer 10 units of intramuscular or intrauterine oxytocin. Do not administer oxytocin as an intravenous bolus because this can cause severe hypotension.[59]

If bleeding and poor uterine tone persist despite oxytocin therapy, emergent consultation with obstetrics is necessary, as the other drugs used are unfamiliar to most emergency clinicians.

Tranexamic Acid

Tranexamic acid (TXA) administration should be considered in patients with PPH, particularly it initial therapies such as uterine massage fail to control bleeding. TXA is an anti-fibrinolytic agent that prevents clot breakdown. The WOMAN Trial was an international, randomized, controlled trial to assess the effects of TXA administration on rates of death or surgical intervention in patients with PPH.[60] The study reported that early administration of TXA within 3 hours of birth reduces death due to bleeding from PPH by approximately one-third, with no evidence of adverse effects.[60] While the generalizability of these data to the United States is unclear, the American College of Obstetrics and Gynecology recommends considering administering TXA in patients with PPH who have not responded to initial medical therapy. TXA is given as a 1 gm IV bolus over 10 minutes; it can be repeated once within a 24-hour period if bleeding persists. Of note, some states in the United States have protocols for prehospital use of TXA.[58,61]

Management of Genital Tract Lacerations

If vaginal bleeding persists despite a firmly contracted uterus, the cervical, vaginal, perineal, and rectovaginal regions should be examined for a source of bleeding, as these are the areas where lacerations are most likely to occur. Control bleeding by direct pressure or by gentle application of ring forceps to bleeding cervical lacerations. Use absorbable suture to control bleeding from accessible lacerations. Adequate visualization of the upper part of the vagina and cervix can be difficult, and repair of lacerations may require general anesthesia and obstetric intervention regardless of the location. Genital tract hematomas may also be a significant cause of hemorrhage but are not generally recognized until several hours after delivery.

Consider retained placental fragments and coagulopathy as a cause of the bleeding. Retained placental fragments may be removed by gentle manual extraction. Use one hand to follow the path of the umbilical cord and find the maternal placental plane and use the other hand to steady the uterine fundus through the maternal abdomen. The plane should feel velvety and irregular and should be gently dissected with side-to-side

TABLE 57.2 Drugs for the Management of Immediate Postpartum Hemorrhage

DRUG	DOSE	COMMENTS
Oxytocin[a]	20–40 U in 1 L of crystalloid initially infused at 200–500 mL/h and then titrate to sustain uterine contractions and control hemorrhage	Do not administer as an IV bolus. First-line therapy. If IV access is unavailable, may use 10 units IM.
Methylergonovine maleate or ergonovine maleate	0.2 mg IM	Avoid in patients with hypertensive disease, including preeclampsia
Carboprost tromethamine	0.25 mg IM Repeat every 15 min until uterine hemorrhage is controlled or a maximum dose of 2 mg	Concurrent use of antiemetics and antidiarrheals recommended to control side effects
Misoprostol	800–1000 µg PR	Single dose; can give PO; may cause tachycardia

[a]Note the increased concentration of oxytocin when used for the treatment of postpartum hemorrhage versus that given to stimulate uterine contractions after uncomplicated delivery.

IM, Intramuscularly; *IV*, intravenous; *PO*, orally; *PR*, per rectum.

motion of the fingers until the placenta separates. This procedure is painful and associated with increased risk of infection, so analgesia and antibiotics should be administered.

If bleeding continues despite these measures, consider uterine tamponade with sterile gauze packing, insertion of an intrauterine balloon tamponade catheter (Bakri balloon [Cook Urological Inc.] or BT-cath balloon tamponade catheter [Utah Medical Products, Inc.]), or placing a Foley catheter into the atonic uterine cavity until surgical intervention or arterial embolization can be performed.[62] In severe and persistent cases, the patient may need to have an emergency hysterectomy to control the bleeding.

Uterine Inversion

Rarely, PPH is due to uterine inversion, with an estimated incidence of one in several thousand deliveries.[63] Consider uterine inversion especially when there is severe pelvic pain, absence of a palpable fundus, brisk excessive PPH, and maternal hemodynamic instability. Shock develops in up to 40% of patients.[64] The diagnosis is made by visualization or palpation of the uterine fundus in the vaginal vault or protruding through the introitus. On abdominal examination, no mass representing the uterus may be palpated, or when palpated, the uterus may have a cuplike dimpling of the fundus.[64,65]

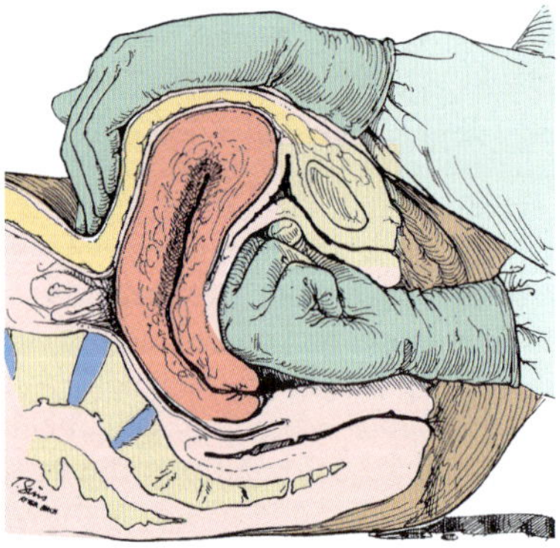

Fig. 57.20 Use uterine massage to control postpartum bleeding. Insert one hand into the vagina to compress the anterior uterine wall while massaging the posterior aspect of the uterus through the abdominal wall with the other hand.

Treat with crystalloid intravenous fluids to maintain cardiovascular stability. Reposition the uterus immediately (Fig. 57.21). Conscious sedation and general anesthesia may be necessary. Use tocolytic agents such as terbutaline or $MgSO_4$ for uterine relaxation and repositioning, and stop all oxytocic drugs.[5,64,65]

To reposition the uterus, insert one hand into the vagina with the tips of the fingers at the uterocervical junction and hold the uterine fundus firmly in the palm of the hand. Gently apply pressure to the uterine fundus in the direction of the umbilicus. Do not initially exert pressure centrally on the fundus because this will cause the uterus to become compressed and force more "layers" of the uterus to lie within the relatively tight cervical ring.[64] General anesthesia and laparotomy may be necessary for uterine positioning.

Late or Secondary Postpartum Hemorrhage

Bleeding that occurs more than 24 hours and up to 12 weeks postpartum is called late, or secondary, PPH. Causes include retained products of conception, endomyometritis, uterine vascular abnormalities (e.g., arteriovenous malformations), uterine subinvolution, and coagulopathies such as von Willebrand's disease. Management focuses on the usual resuscitation of a bleeding patient and specific treatments depend on the etiology. Emergency consultation is usually required.

Uterine Rupture

Uterine rupture is associated with significant maternal morbidity and mortality and is defined as spontaneous tearing of the uterus, sometimes resulting in expulsion of the fetus into the peritoneal space. Risk factors include previous cesarean section, multiparity, malpresentation, myomectomy, and the use of oxytocin.

Patients usually present in shock or with rapid deterioration into shock or cardiac arrest. Treatment is aggressive resuscitation with emergent consultation with obstetrics, who need to take the patient to the operating room emergently.

PERIMORTEM CESAREAN SECTION

Cardiopulmonary arrest, from either a medical cause or a traumatic event, is rare during pregnancy: the exact incidence

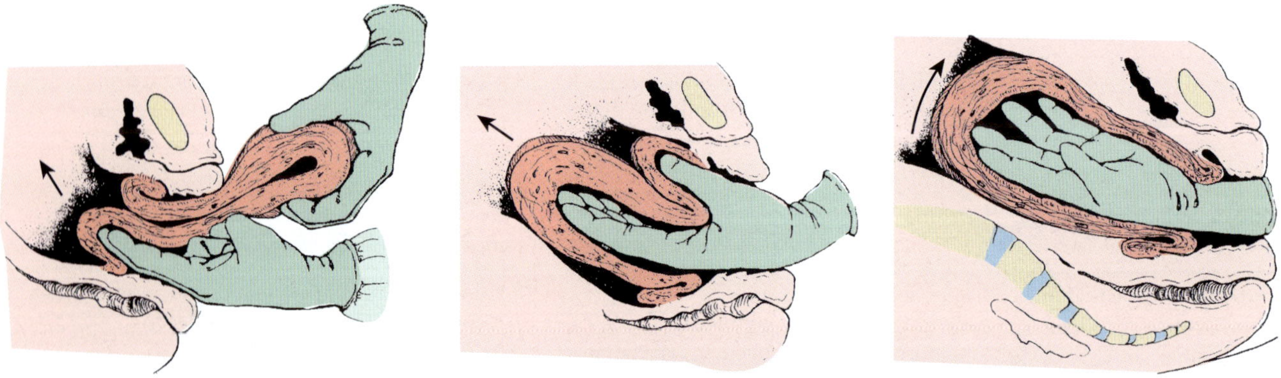

Fig. 57.21 Manual replacement of an inverted uterus. Uterine inversion should be suspected with the sudden onset of brisk vaginal bleeding in association with an absent palpable fundus abdominally and maternal hemodynamic instability. It may occur before or after placental detachment. The diagnosis is made clinically with bimanual examination, during which the uterine fundus is palpated in the lower uterine segment or within the vagina. Use sonography to confirm the diagnosis if the findings on clinical examination are unclear.

is unknown. Perimortem cesarean section (PCS) or resuscitative hysterotomy is a surgical procedure with the potential to save a viable fetus and improve maternal circulation in cases of maternal cardiopulmonary arrest.

The time from when maternal circulation ceases to extraction of the neonate is the critical factor in determining maternal and fetal outcome: initiation of the procedure within 4 minutes and delivery of the fetus within 5 minutes of maternal cardiac arrest is optimal for best outcomes. Delivery of the fetus increases maternal venous return and cardiac output by 25% to 30% and may lead to survival benefit for the mother.[66,67] PCS should be considered in any patient who experiences a cardiac arrest after 24 weeks' gestation (uterine size exceeding the level of the umbilicus) and initiated within 4 minutes of onset of maternal cardiac arrest and the absence of spontaneous circulation.[67,68]

Evidence suggests the early initiation of PCS in cases of cardiac arrest may increase the restoration of hemodynamic status and likelihood of return of spontaneous circulation in the mother.[69,70]

Indications

Although the lower limit of fetal viability varies among institutions, performance of PCS before approximately 24 weeks is not generally indicated. If the duration of gestation is not known from the history, estimate fetal maturity quickly by calculating gestational age on the basis of the date of the patient's last normal menstrual period or by measuring the height of the uterine fundus. Between 18- and 30-weeks of gestation, the age of the fetus in weeks will correspond to the distance in centimeters from the uterine fundus to the symphysis pubis (e.g., at 28 weeks' gestation the fundus lies approximately 28 cm above the symphysis pubis or halfway between the umbilicus and the costal margin).

Survival of the infant is directly related to the time elapsed from maternal cardiac arrest to delivery, prompt performance of cardiopulmonary resuscitation (CPR) on the mother, the maturity of the fetus, prearrest health status of the mother, and in certain circumstances, the availability of neonatal intensive care facilities.[71–73] In accordance with advanced cardiac life support guidelines, initiate CPR immediately on recognition of maternal arrest and continue it until the infant has been delivered. The anatomic and physiologic changes of pregnancy will inhibit the effectiveness of CPR on the mother. Aortocaval occlusion by the gravid uterus may occur after 20 weeks' gestation. It can reduce venous return and compromise maternal cardiac output, especially in the supine position. CPR should be performed in the left lateral, head-down position or with an assistant manually displacing uterus away from the inferior vena cava.[73] In addition, the decreased functional residual capacity of the lungs may impede ventilation efforts. Under these conditions, CPR generates only 30% to 40% of normal cardiac output, which severely compromises placental perfusion. The potential for infant survival decreases and the chance of neurologic damage increases as the time from maternal cardiac arrest to PCS rises. Neonatal outcome is best when PCS is performed within 4 minutes and poor if done after 20 minutes. Every attempt should be made to begin PCS within 4 minutes of cardiopulmonary arrest and complete the procedure within 5 minutes of arrest.[73,74] Fetal prognosis is generally better in the later stages of pregnancy and after the sudden death of a previously healthy mother rather than death secondary to chronic illness.[71,74] CPR should continue during and after the procedure. PCS itself may represent the most important variable for successful maternal resuscitation.[71,75] The decision to perform this procedure may be one of the most challenging that an EP will encounter. In the absence of immediate obstetric backup, it is reasonable to proceed with PCS within 4 minutes if initial maternal resuscitation efforts are unsuccessful. Prolonged attempts to resuscitate the mother are unlikely to benefit either the mother or the fetus.

Technique

See Videos 57.1 and 57.2. The most experienced person present should perform the PCS, preferably an obstetrician. Under ideal circumstances a neonatologist should also be in attendance. Do not delay the procedure to allow time for the arrival of consultants. Time should not be wasted searching for fetal heart tones or attempting to evaluate fetal viability with ultrasonography.

Extract the infant rapidly while avoiding fetal and maternal injury in the ED (Fig. 57.22). Hence, do not waste time preparing a sterile operating field or transporting the patient to an operating suite outside the ED. Use a large (e.g., No. 10) scalpel blade and make a midline vertical incision through the abdominal wall extending from the symphysis pubis to the umbilicus. Carry the incision through all abdominal layers into the peritoneal cavity. In most gravid females, the hyperpigmented "linea nigra" is apparent, and when present, use this as a guide for the incision. If available, place retractors in the abdominal wound and draw them laterally to expose the anterior surface of the uterus. Reflect the bladder inferiorly. If full, aspirate the bladder to evacuate it and permit better access to the uterus. While avoiding injury to fetal parts, make a small (≈5 cm) vertical incision through the uterus until amniotic fluid is obtained or the uterine cavity is clearly entered. Insert the index and long fingers into the incision and use them to lift the uterine wall away from the fetus. Use bandage scissors to extend the incision vertically to the fundus until a wide exposure is obtained. Gently deliver the infant, clamp and cut the cord, and evaluate and resuscitate the newborn as clinically indicated. Because the incision is relatively high in the uterus, the infant's head may not be readily accessible to the clinician. In this case, grasp the infant's feet and deliver the infant through maneuvers similar to those used for a breech delivery.

THE NEWBORN

Approximately 10% of newborns require some degree of assistance to begin breathing at birth (e.g., some sort of stimulation to breathe), but less than 1% require extensive resuscitation.[39] Evaluation of the newborn begins before delivery with assessment of maternal well-being and identification of risk factors for fetal distress: multiple pregnancies of less than 35 weeks, maternal infection or hypertension, oligohydramnios, preterm delivery at less than 36 weeks, breech presentation, meconium-stained amniotic fluid, non-reassuring fetal heart rate, emergency cesarean section, shoulder dystocia, and opiate use in normal labor.[76]

Neonatal resuscitation supplies should be available and are preferably stored near supplies used for emergency delivery or pediatric resuscitation.

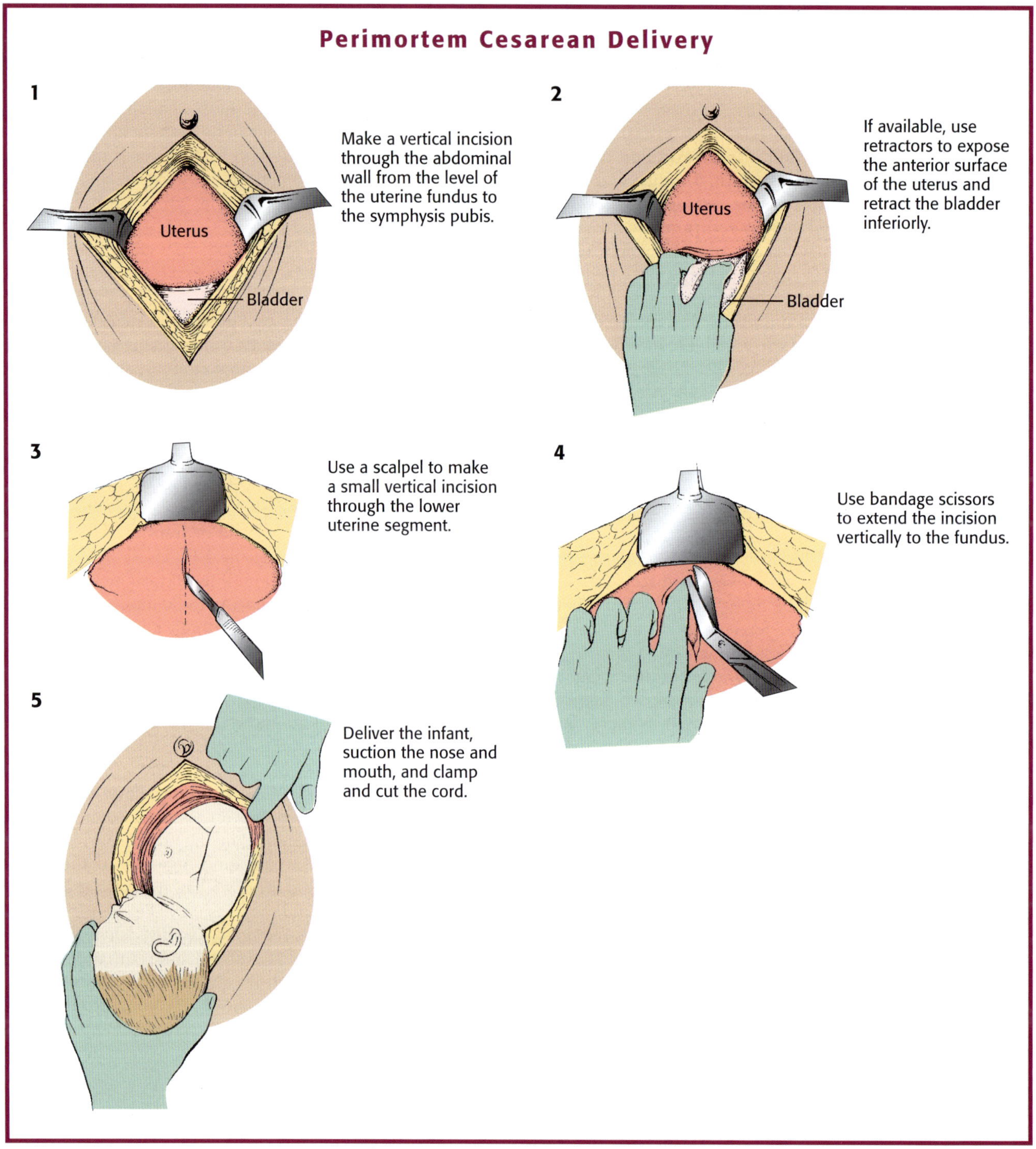

Fig. 57.22 Perimortem cesarean delivery.

Newborn resuscitation is outlined in an algorithm (Fig. 57.23) and can be divided into four categories of action: (1) initial assessment and stabilization; (2) ventilation, including bag-valve-mask (BVM) or bag-tube ventilation; (3) chest compressions; and (4) administration of medications or fluids. Although most newborns require no resuscitation or only basic steps such as warming, drying, and stimulation, others will require further intervention. The most crucial action of neonatal resuscitation is establishment of adequate ventilation.[39]

Evaluation

A rapid evaluation of the newborn can be used to identify whether additional resuscitation/supportive measures are necessary. The following questions need to be addressed:

- Is the infant full term?
- Does the infant have good tone?
- Is the infant crying vigorously?

If the answer to all three questions is yes, it is unlikely the infant will require any supportive measures beyond maintaining warmth and avoiding hypothermia. If any answer is yes,

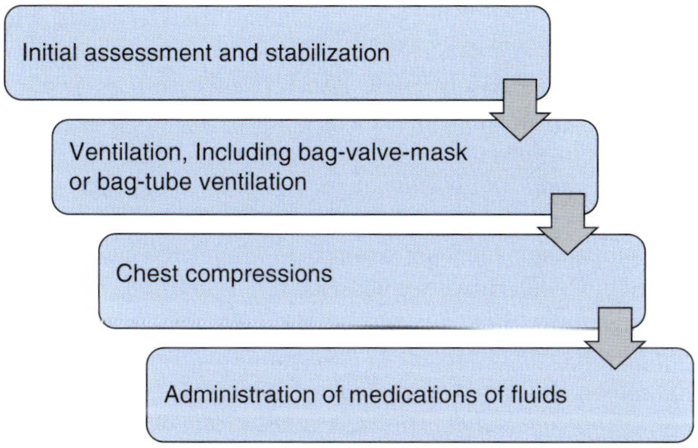

Fig. 57.23 Neonatal resuscitation algorithm. (From Sakharkar S, Tiwari D, Kabra NS. Neonatal resuscitation program algorithm with timeline- a concise flow chart for delivery room resuscitation. *Resusc Plus.* 2023;15:100445.)

TABLE 57.3 APGAR Scoring System

SIGN	0	1	2
Heart rate (beats/min)	Absent	Slow (<100)	>100
Respiratory effort	Absent	Slow, irregular	Good, crying
Muscle tone	Flaccid	Some flexion of extremities	Active motion
Reflex irritability	No response	Grimace	Vigorous cry
Color	Blue, pale	Body pink, extremities blue	Completely pink

APGAR, Appearance, pulse, grimace, activity, and respirations.

the infant should be placed on the infant warmer and should undergo additional evaluation while warming, drying and stimulating the infant.

Traditionally, the APGAR scoring system, applied at 1 and 5 minutes after birth, has been the standard of newborn evaluation (Table 57.3). APGAR is a mnemonic for the components of the score: appearance, pulse, grimace, activity, and respirations. In general, the higher the score, the better the condition of the infant. Waiting for the traditional 1-minute APGAR score to indicate the need for resuscitation has been replaced by the concept of "the golden minute." Begin basic resuscitation maneuvers, reevaluation, and PPV, if required, by the first 60 seconds after birth. Use the heart rate and respiratory effort to guide resuscitation efforts because skin color does not reliably predict oxygenation status in the newborn period.[39]

Respiration

Normally, the newborn begins to breathe and cry almost immediately after birth. After initial respiratory efforts, the newborn should be able to establish regular respirations sufficient to improve color and should be able to maintain a heart rate higher than 100 beats/min. Generally, drying and stimulation (rubbing the back or flicking the soles of the feet)

TABLE 57.4 Targeted Preductal SpO_2 After Birth

1 min	60%–65%
2 min	65%–70%
3 min	70%–75%
4 min	75%–80%
5 min	80%–85%
10 min	85%–95%

Note that oxygen administration to the newborn *is not recommended* after a routine delivery, even when there is early cyanosis. Excessive oxygenation may be toxic. For term and preterm infants requiring ventilation, the current recommendation is to begin with room air and avoid the use of supplemental oxygen. It is important to note that even in healthy newborns, oxygen saturation does not normally reach extrauterine levels until 10 minutes after birth.
SpO_2, Peripheral oxygen saturation.
From Aziz K, Lee HC, Escobedo MB et al. Part 5: Neonatal resuscitation: 2020 American Heart Association guidelines for cardiopulmonary resuscitation and emergency cardiovascular care. *Circulation*. 2020;143(16)(Supp l2):S524-S550.

are enough to induce effective respirations in the newborn.[39] Gasping and apnea after 30 seconds of stimulation are signs indicating the need for assisted ventilation and continuous pulse oximetry monitoring.[39]

It is important to note that even in healthy newborns, oxygen saturation does not reach extrauterine levels until 10 minutes after birth. Studies have demonstrated potential harmful effects from both excessive and insufficient supplemental oxygen versus room air during neonatal resuscitation. For term and preterm infants requiring ventilation, the current recommendation is to begin with room air and avoid the use of supplemental oxygen.[39] The application of supplemental oxygen should be guided by normal newborn oxygen saturation ranges (Table 57.4). Establishing adequate ventilation and oxygenation will restore vital signs in the vast majority of newborns.[39]

Heart Rate

The heart rate may be determined by auscultation or palpation of the pulse at the base of the umbilical cord. If available, a three-lead electrocardiogram (ECG) may be a more accurate and rapid measurement of neonatal heart rate during resuscitation.[39] The heart rate should consistently be greater than 100 beats/min in an uncompromised newborn. If after 30 seconds the heart rate is less than 100 beats/min, initiate PPV. If the heart rate is less than 60 beats/min despite adequate ventilation and oxygenation for 30 seconds, commence chest compressions. Because chest compressions may diminish the effectiveness of ventilation, do not initiate them until lung inflation and ventilation have been established.[39]

Color

An uncompromised newborn will be able to maintain a pink color of the mucous membranes without supplemental oxygenation. Central cyanosis is determined by examining the face, trunk, and mucous membranes, but it is not a reliable method of determining oxygen saturation in the immediate neonatal period. Acrocyanosis is usually a normal finding in the newborn and not a reliable indicator of hypoxemia. It may, however, indicate other conditions such as cold stress.[39,40]

Stabilization Technique

Following delivery of the infant and cutting the umbilical cord, place the newborn on the side in the sniffing position with the neck in a neutral or slightly extended position.[39,40] Place a rolled blanket or towel under the back and shoulders of the supine infant to elevate the torso 2 to 2.5 cm because this may help maintain head position.[40] Prevent heat loss in the newborn because cold stress can increase oxygen consumption and impede effective resuscitation.[40] Avoid hyperthermia, however, because it is associated with perinatal respiratory depression.[39,40] Place the infant under a radiant warmer, rapidly dry the skin, and wrap the infant in warmed blankets to reduce heat loss.[39,40] Alternatively, use the mother's body as a heat source for the newborn. If initial evaluation indicates that the infant is stable, dry and place the infant skin to skin on the mother's chest or abdomen, and cover both with blankets.[39,40]

Vigorous newborns should not be routinely suctioned after delivery, even those delivered through meconium-stained fluid.[39,40] Reserve suctioning (including suctioning with a bulb syringe) immediately after birth for babies who exhibit obvious obstruction to spontaneous breathing or require PPV. Endotracheal intubation and suctioning is no longer recommended for nonvigorous babies born through meconium-stained amniotic fluid.[39] If airway obstruction necessitates suctioning, first clear secretions from the mouth and nose with a bulb syringe or suction catheter (8- or 10-Fr). Aggressive pharyngeal suctioning can cause laryngeal spasm and vagal bradycardia, so limit the depth and duration of suctioning and do not exceed a negative pressure of 100 mm Hg.[39]

For newborns who do not quickly respond to conservative measures, PPV using room air is indicated within 1 minute of birth. Most newborns who require PPV can be adequately ventilated with a bag and mask. Perform assisted ventilations at a rate of 40 to 60 breaths/min (30 breaths/min if mechanical compressions are being performed). As of the 2015 AHA guidelines, higher inflation pressures and longer inflation times for the first several breaths are not recommended due to insufficient data.[39,40] Visible chest expansion is a more reliable indicator of appropriate inflation pressure than a specific manometer reading.[39,40] Heart rate measurement can be used to assess adequacy of ventilation after 60 seconds of visible chest rise with PPV. Because BVM ventilation can produce gastric distention and impede respiration, insert an orogastric tube (8-Fr) in infants undergoing prolonged PPV.

Endotracheal intubation may be indicated when BVM ventilation is ineffective, when the airway is obstructed, when chest compressions are performed, or when prolonged PPV is required.[39,40] Alternatively, a neonatal laryngeal mask airway may provide effective airway management, especially in the case of ineffective BVM ventilation or failed endotracheal intubation.[39]

Monitor the heart rate during neonatal evaluation and stabilization by either direct auscultation over the chest, palpation of the pulse at the base of the umbilical cord, or a three-lead ECG. A readily discernible heartbeat of 100 beats/min or greater is acceptable. If the heart rate is less than 60 beats/min despite adequate ventilation and oxygenation for 30 seconds, institute chest compressions while continuing to ventilate.[39,40] Deliver chest compressions on the lower third of the sternum and not over the xiphoid to avoid damage to the liver.[39] There are two techniques for performing chest compressions in the newborn. In the preferred method, position two thumbs side by side over the lower third of the sternum just below the nipple line. If the infant is large or the resuscitator's hands are too small to encircle the chest, use two-finger compressions with the ring and middle fingers.[39,40] Compress to a depth that is approximately one-third of the AP diameter of the newborn's chest so that a palpable pulse is generated.[39] Coordinate compressions and ventilations to avoid simultaneous delivery, which may compromise the efficacy of ventilation. Use a compression-to-ventilation ratio of 3:1 with 90 compressions and 30 breaths to achieve approximately 120 events/min.[39,40] If the heart rate remains less than 60 beats/min despite these interventions,[39] establish an umbilical vein (see Chapter 19 and Video 19.2), intravenous or intraosseous line and give epinephrine, 0.01 to 0.03 mg/kg of 1:10,000 concentration, repeated every 3 to 5 minutes, as needed. If is of note that intraosseous access may not be as effective in a preterm infant.[40] The medications most commonly used during neonatal resuscitation are listed in Table 57.5.[39,40]

TABLE 57.5 Medications Commonly Used in Neonatal Resuscitation

DRUG	DOSE	INDICATIONS	COMMENTS
Epinephrine[a]	0.01–0.03 mg/kg (0.1–0.3 mL/kg of a 1:10,000 solution)	Bradycardia, asystole	May be repeated every 3–5 min as indicated High-dose epinephrine in newborns is contraindicated
Volume expanders (normal saline or Ringer's solution)	10 mL/kg IV over 5–10 min	Suspected hypovolemia, shock, or blood loss	May be repeated after determination of clinical response

[a]The intravenous route is now strongly preferred, but one can consider administering epinephrine via an endotracheal tube in doses of 0.05 to 0.1 mg/kg while obtaining intravenous access.

CPR, Cardiopulmonary resuscitation.

From Aziz K, Lee HC, Escobedo MB et al. Part 5: Neonatal resuscitation: 2020 American Heart Association guidelines for cardiopulmonary resuscitation and emergency cardiovascular care. *Circulation*. 2020;143(16)(Supp l2):S524-S550.

If hypovolemia is a concern, a normal saline bolus of 10 mL/kg may be given. If hypovolemia is felt to be due to hemorrhage, emergency blood may be administered at a dose of 10 to 15 mL/kg.

It is important to note that neonatal hypoglycemia can present with lethargy, poor feeding, hypotonia, apnea, hypothermia, seizures, and irritability. Hypoglycemia in neonates is defined as a glucose of <30 mg/dL in the first 24 hours of life. It can be treated with an IV bolus of 10% dextrose in water (D10W), at a dose of 2 to 3 mL/kg. If hypoglycemia persists, a maintenance infusion of D10W at 4 to 6 mg/kg/min may be administered with frequent glucose checks.

ACKNOWLEDGMENTS

The author gratefully acknowledges the work of Samreen Vora and Valerie A. Dobiesz, who contributed this chapter to the last edition, and all the authors of previous versions of this chapter.

REFERENCES ARE AVAILABLE AT Elsevier eBooks+

CHAPTER 58

Gynecologic Procedures

G. Richard Braen, John Kiel, Morgan Sweere, Eric Tizzard, and Bryan Salvato

FEMALE PELVIC EXAMINATION

In an emergency department (ED), there are several reasons to perform a pelvic examination: lower abdominal pain, vaginal discharge, vaginal bleeding, suspected sexually transmitted infection (STI), retained foreign body, and possible Bartholin abscess (BA) of the vulva. Emergency physicians do not routinely screen for cervical cancer. The evaluation of sexual assault victims is discussed in Chapter 59.

Before performing a pelvic examination, the examiner must have a basic understanding of female pelvic anatomy (Fig. 58.1). The vulva comprises the labia majora, labia minora, clitoris, hymen, and vulvar vestibule. The labia majora extend from the mons veneris anteriorly to the perineal body and are filled with fatty tissue that varies in thickness with age—proportionately thicker in children and thinner as a female passes through menopause. The labia minora are generally entirely covered by the labia majora and are more delicate, pink, and hairless. Anteriorly, the labia minora form a hood for the clitoris and posteriorly join with the labia majora to form the fourchette. The urethral meatus is just posterior to the clitoris. The hymen separates the external genitalia from the vagina and may be obscured by the labia. There are two Bartholin glands which lie below the fascia, one on each side of the lower, posterior third of the vagina. These glands secrete lubrication through ducts located at the lower pole of the labia minora. Normal Bartholin glands are rarely palpable. Healthy vaginal mucosa is reddish pink, but during pregnancy may become dusky, almost cyanotic appearing. The cervix most commonly faces posteriorly (80%) but may face anteriorly (20%). The nonparous cervical diameter is 2 cm to 3 cm with a length of 2 cm to 4 cm. The cervix is normally pink. The cervical os changes with vaginal delivery from being smooth and circular to being fissured, oval, and slightly irregular.

Preparation for a Pelvic Examination

Before beginning an internal pelvic examination assemble the appropriate equipment. This equipment includes: a stretcher with stirrups or knee holders, various sizes of vaginal speculums, gloves, surgical lubricant, appropriate lighting, swabs, ring forceps or a Kelly clamp for the removal of foreign bodies or products of conception, transport medium for testing for sexually transmitted and vaginal infections, pH paper, slides, coverslips, "eye dropper" bottles of 10% potassium hydroxide (KOH), and normal saline for testing vaginal discharge (Fig. 58.2). Speculums may be plastic and disposable or may be metal (warmed to body temperature before insertion) but must be sized to the patient; a pediatric speculum for females with a narrow introitus (older females and young adolescents), a Smith-Pederson speculum for virginal females, a standard speculum for most, and a Graves speculum for obese females and multiparous females. Note that if stirrups or leg supports are not available, the patient can have a padded bedpan under her buttocks with the bottoms of her feet together and her knees separated. When examination in a lithotomy position is not possible, such as in older patients and those with mobility issues and joint disease, an examination may be performed with the patient in a knee-chest position, with the knees flexed and hips rotated externally.

A pelvic examination should be done with the patient in a lithotomy position. The patient should be gowned and have an empty bladder. The patient should be informed of the examination beforehand, and verbal and/or written consent should be obtained. Chaperones are necessary during the examination to protect both the patient and the examiner. The examiner should glove and prioritize privacy during the examination, reassuring the patient, and explain each phase of the pelvic examination. The patient should remain covered until the examination is performed and should be recovered as soon as possible after the examination is completed.

Performance of the Pelvic Examination

The vulva is examined visually for any lesions, and then by palpation. Females with a BA have acute, painful swelling of the posterior vulva that usually has developed over 2 to 3 days, and can progress to a point when it becomes difficult for them to sit or walk. The abscess appears erythematous, swollen, and forms a tender, spherical (3 to 4 cm in diameter) mass just lateral to the posterior fourchette. A Bartholin cyst is usually not tender and there is no associated erythema or swelling, differentiating it from an abscess. The treatment of a BA is similar to other abscesses in that incision and drainage is often required.

After examination of the vulva, separate the labia majora to expose the introitus and look for lesions, discharge, or blood. Next, insert a speculum with good lighting. If cervical cancer screening is anticipated, lubricate the speculum with water only. Otherwise, use surgical lubricant. Spread the labia, insert the speculum to its full length, and open the speculum. If the cervix is not seen, withdraw the speculum and palpate the location of the cervix with one finger, remove the finger, and follow with a second redirected speculum insertion. Inspect the cervix for blood, discharge and any lesions, particularly at the squamocolumnar junction (where the red columnar tissue of the endocervix changes to the reddish-pink squamous epithelium of the vagina). If there is a white lesion at the squamocolumnar junction that does not wipe off with a swab, consider dysplasia, carcinoma in situ, or condyloma accuminata. Collect samples for STI and vaginitis prior to withdrawal of the speculum (see later section "Vaginal Discharge and Suspected STI Sampling"). Additionally, remove any foreign body or material found (see later section "Vaginal Foreign Body Removal"). Withdraw the speculum slowly while inspecting the walls of the vagina. Close the speculum just prior to exiting the introitus.

A bimanual examination of a female with a small vagina can be accomplished with one gloved, lubricated index finger. Two fingers can be used when the introitus is larger. Gently place your opposite hand on the patient's abdomen. After palpating the labia majora, separate them, and inspect the introitus. Insert the fingers to locate the cervix. When using two fingers, place one on each side of the cervix. Pain with "side-to-side" cervical motion may indicate pelvic inflammatory disease

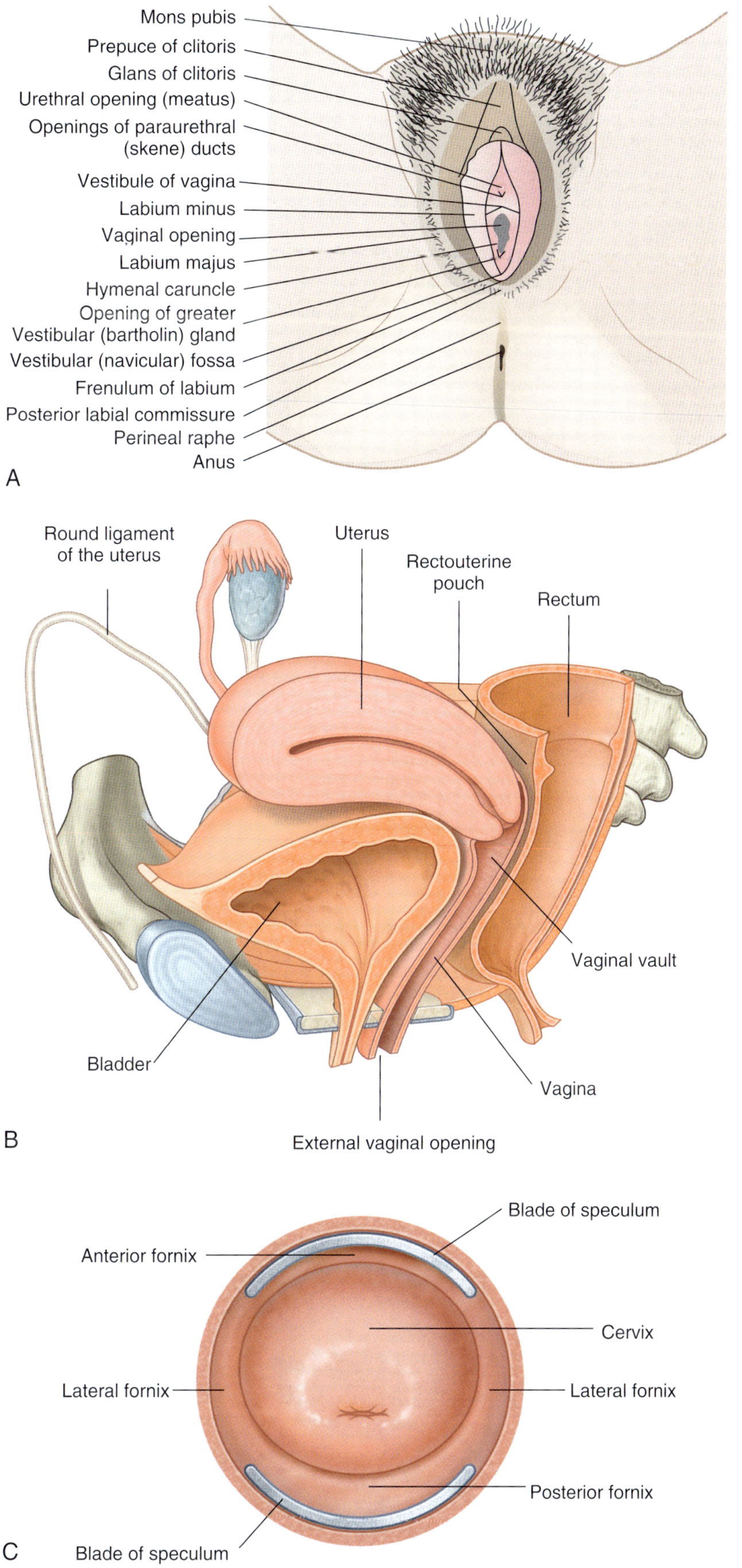

Fig. 58.1 Anatomy of the female external genitalia, vagina, and rectouterine pouch (pouch of Douglas). (A) Female external genitalia. (B) Cross-sectional view of female genitalia demonstrating the rectouterine pouch (pouch of Douglas). (C) Anatomy of cervix and posterior fornix as seen through speculum. (Modified from Drake RL. *Gray's Anatomy for Students.* 2nd ed. Elsevier; 2010.)

(PID). Using the hand on the abdomen and the intravaginal fingers, evaluate the size and shape of the uterus. An asymmetric uterus may be an indication of a fibroid tumor. After moving both fingers to one side of the cervix, palpate the adnexa of that side between the intravaginal fingers and the abdominal hand. Gently palpate the pelvic adnexa since firm palpation of normal organs may cause pain and can be misleading to the examiner. If an adnexal mass is found, estimate a 3D size in centimeters along with the degree of firmness, the degree of fixation to adjoining organs, and the degree of tenderness. Masses that can be detected with the bimanual examination include pedunculated fibroids, paraovarian cysts, tuboovarian abscesses (TOAs), and ectopic pregnancies.

Following the bimanual examination, examiners may consider a rectal examination, looking for firmness or nodules between the uterus and rectum suggestive of tumors or uterosacral ligamentous endometriosis. Rectal material should be guaiac tested for blood, which may be falsely positive for gastrointestinal bleeding if blood is present in the vagina.

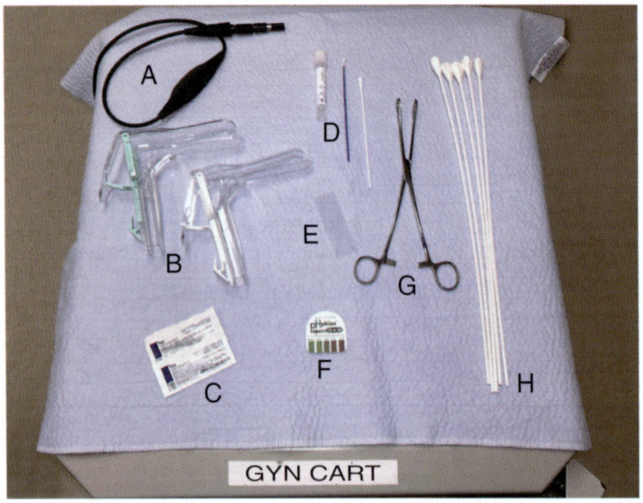

Fig. 58.2 Equipment for routine gynecologic examination. *A*, Light source; *B*, speculum; *C*, water-soluble lubricant; *D*, transport media for chlamydia and gonorrhea testing; *E*, glass slide and cover slip; *F*, pH paper; *G*, ring forceps; *H*, swabs.

Bartholin Abscess

As stated previously, the BA is an acute painful swelling located in the posterior part of the vaginal introitus (Fig. 58.3). The inflammatory swelling can be small or quite large and painful. BA occurs in about 2% of females, usually in the reproductive years.[1] The pathogenesis of the abscess is unclear but is thought to be the result of a blocked or partially obstructed Bartholin duct leading to accumulation of material with subsequent infection.

As with any abscess, the evaluation must include consideration of the patient's comorbidities and willingness to consent for the procedure. The most commonly isolated organism in a BA is *E. coli*, but *N. gonorrheae* and *C. trachomatis* are also known to cause them.

A BA can be treated in the ED in most cases, but close follow-up with gynecology is needed. These abscesses can recur, and the gynecologist may elect to do a marsupialization of the area, which reduces the recurrence rate. If the abscess is very large, if the diagnosis is uncertain, or if there are other masses, significant cellulitis, or significantly distorted tissue, involvement of the gynecologist is warranted. In addition, if the patient has significant comorbidities, unstable vital signs, a bleeding dyscrasia, or is immunocompromised, the patient should be seen by a consulting gynecologist to manage the abscess.

Incision and Drainage

Incision and drainage of a BA can be painful and anxiety-provoking for many patients (Fig. 58.4).

It is an invasive procedure that requires a written, witnessed, and signed consent form from the patient, parent, or guardian and should be witnessed with a notation made in the medical record documenting that the procedure was described, complications were discussed, and any alternatives such as antibiotics or warm compresses were offered when appropriate.

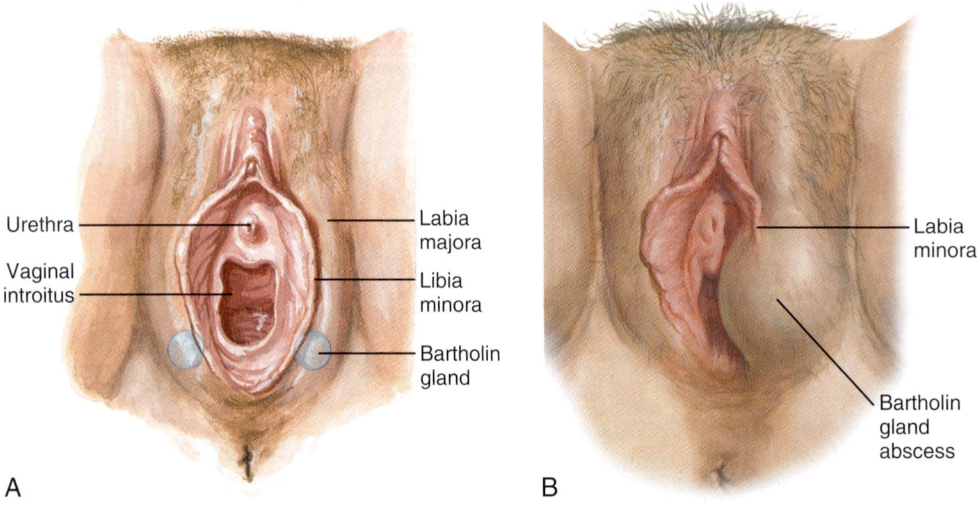

Fig. 58.3 Bartholin gland and abscess. (A) Anatomy of the female external genitalia. Note the location of Bartholin glands at 5 and 7 o'clock. (B) Bartholin gland duct cysts and abscesses are recognized by the presence of a fluctuant mass of variable size within the posterior vestibule, with the labia minora transecting the cyst. (Netter illustration from www.netterimages.com. Elsevier Inc. All rights reserved.)

Bartholin Abscess Drainage (Word Catheter)

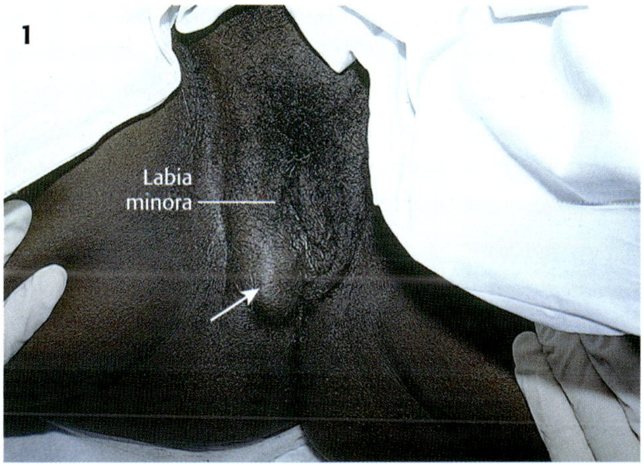

Place the patient in the dorsal lithotomy position and identify the abscess, which will be located at either the 5- or 7-o'clock position, with the labia minora transecting the abscess.

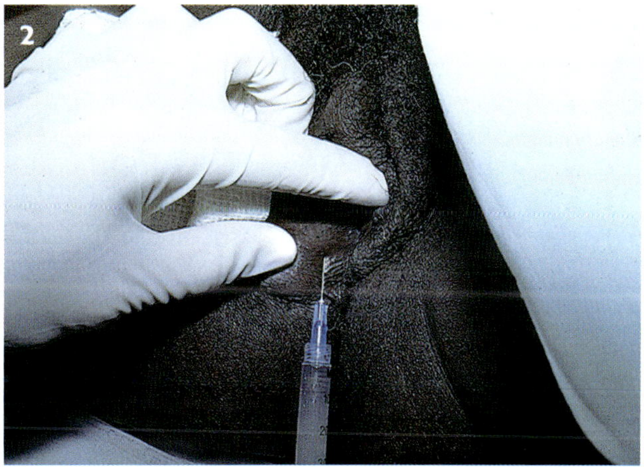

Cleanse the area with antiseptic solution. While stabilizing the abscess with your thumb and index finger, inject local anesthetic through the mucosal surface (not through the skin).

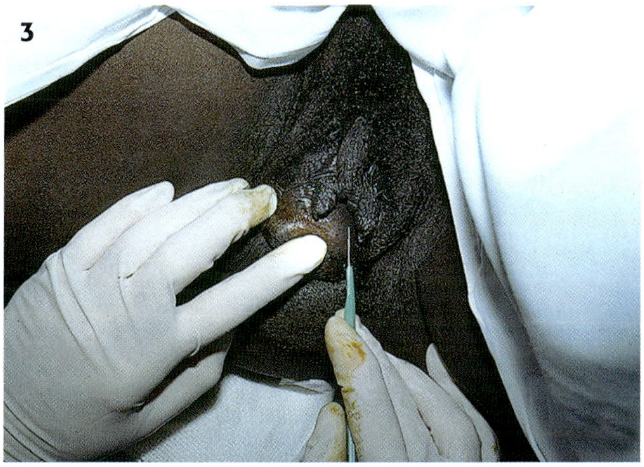

Use a No. 11 scalpel blade to make an incision in the mucosal surface of the abscess. Make the incision large enough to accomodate the catheter, but small enough to prevent extrusion of the inflated balloon.

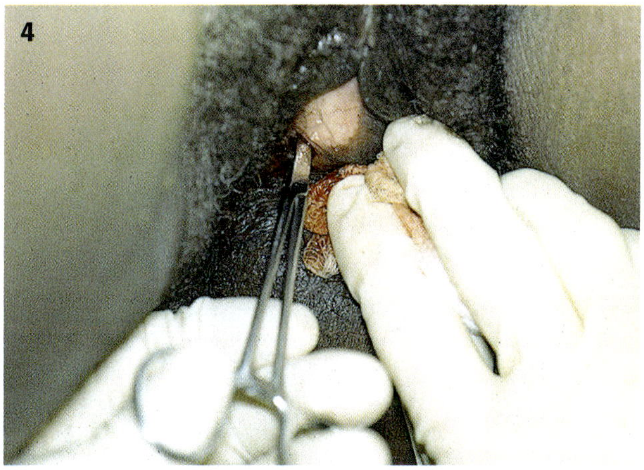

Alternatively, a hemostat can be used to puncture the abscess cavity. Stabilize the abscess with your thumb and index finger and skewer the abscess onto the hemostat.

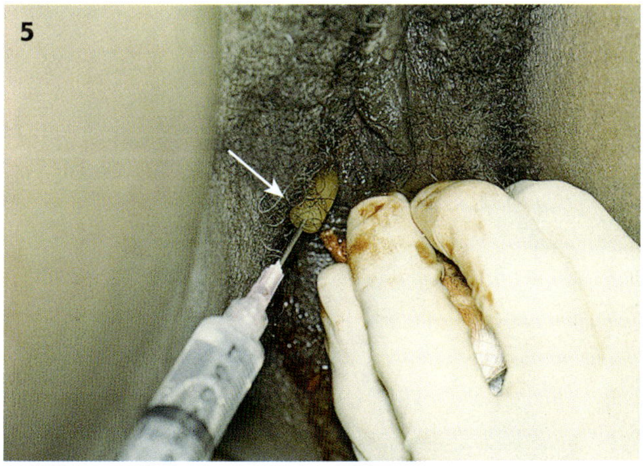

Once the abscess has been entered (heralded by a palpable pop or the free flow of pus), insert the Word catheter to the hilt and inflate with 3 to 4 mL of saline. Use a 25-gauge needle to fill the balloon.

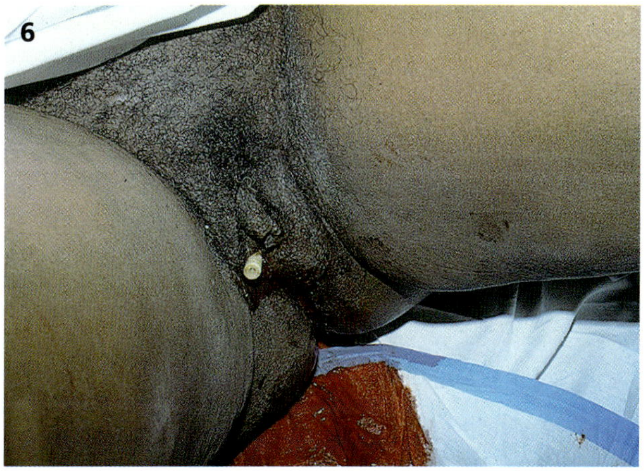

The catheter is left in place for 2 to 4 weeks to form a fistula. Antibiotics are of no proven value once drainage is performed, but practice varies.

Fig. 58.4 Drainage of a Bartholin abscess (Word catheter method). Note that the mucosal surface, not the skin, is the site of abscess drainage.

Once written consent is obtained, place the patient in the lithotomy position. Place the patient's feet in stirrups. Generously premedicate with nonopioid or opioid analgesia; consider sedatives when appropriate. Administration of nitrous oxide analgesia is also an accepted practice. Procedural sedation with propofol, etomidate, ketamine, or benzodiazepines can be considered, especially for those patients who are extremely uncomfortable.

1. Use universal precautions with gown, gloves, and mask. The contents of the abscess may be under pressure and can spray when incised.
2. Clean the affected area using sterile technique.
3. Apply topical analgesia to the mucosal surface of the introitus where the swelling is most evident. Note that the abscess incision is made on the mucosal side near the introitus, not on the skin surface. Applying viscous lidocaine to this area for 10 minutes can help reduce discomfort.
4. Administer a local anesthetic using a 25- or 27-gauge needle and 2% lidocaine. Note that the abscess contents may be under pressure and may leak or even suddenly burst during this step.
5. Approach the abscess from the vaginal introitus and, using an 11-blade scalpel, make a 5-mm incision *through the mucosal surface, not the skin,* to evacuate the contents of the abscess. If the abscess is larger, the incision can be lengthened to the diameter of the abscess, but in most cases 5 mm is sufficient (Fig. 58.5).
6. After irrigating and cleaning the area, the wound can be packed or left open. Iodoform strips can be used to pack the wound. Do not pack the wound too tightly and leave just enough material to fill the base of the wound with a small tail (0.5 cm to 1 cm) extending from the cavity. Alternatively, a vessel loop can be considered.
7. A common alternative to packing is inserting a small balloon catheter into the wound rather. The Word catheter (Cook Medical Inc.) is often recommended (Fig. 58.6). Insert the Word catheter cautiously and fill it with 3 mL of saline. Be careful not to fill it too much because the resulting pressure in the abscess cavity can be uncomfortable. This should be sufficient to hold the catheter in place. On rare occasions, it is necessary to suture the catheter in place. The Word catheter is usually left in place for 2 to 4 weeks. If it is more comfortable for the patient, gently push the external portion of the catheter into the vagina so it does not hang outside. Counsel the patient that the Word catheter is usually left in place for up to 4 weeks, but close gynecology follow-up and monitoring are needed throughout that time (Video 58.1).
8. An alternative to Word catheter placement is a marsupialization procedure. This procedure is rarely performed in the emergency setting and is usually done by gynecologists. This should not be attempted if there is overlying

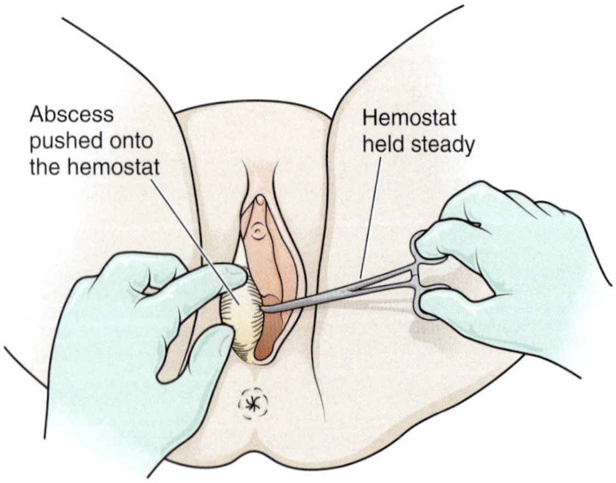

Fig. 58.5 It is technically easier to enter the Bartholin gland abscess cavity if the hemostat is held steady and the mucosal surface of the abscess, held with the thumb and index finger, is skewered onto the hemostat. Attempting to puncture a deep immobilized abscess by stabbing with the hemostat may be more difficult. Expect a palpable pop or drainage of frank pus when entering the abscess. Note that the mucosal surface, not the skin, is the site of abscess drainage.

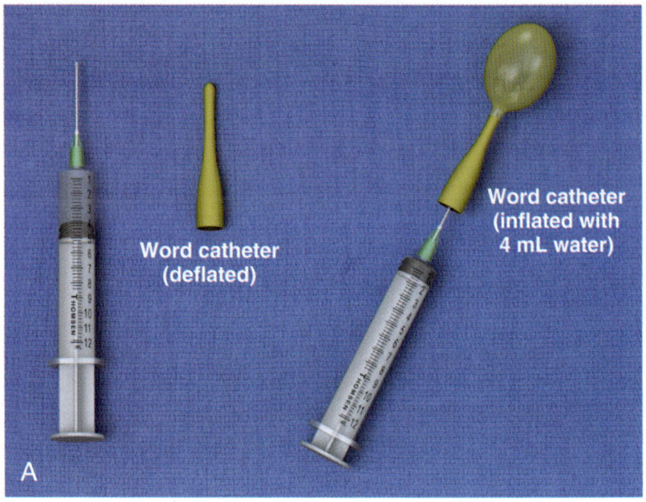

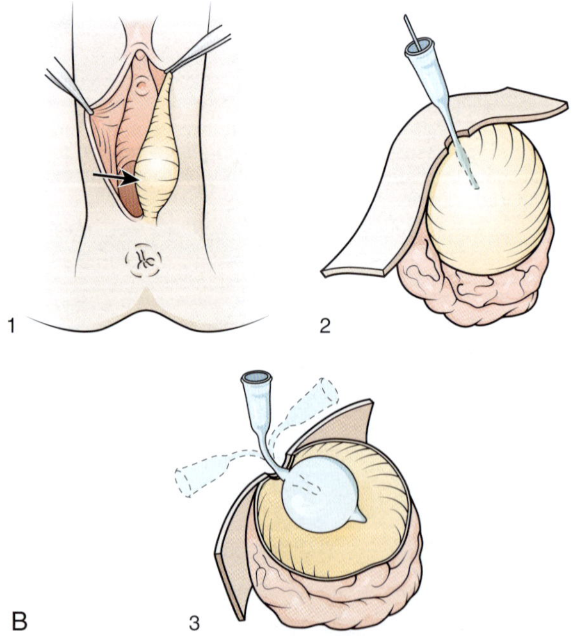

Fig. 58.6 Word catheter. (A) Inflatable bulb-tipped catheter. *Left,* uninflated; *right,* inflated with 4-mL water. (B) Use of the Word catheter for outpatient drainage of a Bartholin gland abscess. This is a fistulization procedure rather than standard incision and drainage. *1,* A stab incision is made on the mucosal surface. *2,* The catheter is inserted into the cyst cavity. *3,* The catheter is filled with 3 mL to 4 mL of water. The Word catheter is left in place for 2 to 4 weeks. (B, From Word B. Office treatment of cyst and abscess of Bartholin gland. *JAMA.* 1964;190:777.)

or surrounding cellulitis. After making the initial incision, irrigate with saline solution. Hemostats may be used to break up loculations within the abscess. Evert the wall of the cyst and use absorbable interrupted sutures to approximate it to the edge of the vestibular mucosa.

9. Close follow-up with gynecology is recommended for a repeat examination and evaluation within the next 3 days.
10. Antibiotics are controversial in treating BAs with a paucity of evidence to guide decision-making. After initial incision and drainage, antibiotic therapy is recommended for patients with systemic symptoms, surrounding cellulitis, high likelihood of being methicillin-resistant *Staphylococcus aureus* (MRSA) positive, recurrent abscesses, or if the patient is immunocompromised in any way. If these conditions are present, the patient may need observation and gynecology consultation before performing the procedure. Antibiotic coverage should provide adequate coverage for MRSA and enteric gram-negative aerobes, such as trimethoprim-sulfamethoxazole, amoxicillin-clavulanate, doxycycline, or clindamycin. Patients requiring antibiotic therapy should be treated for 7 to 10 days.
11. If the patient is well enough to be discharged, prescribe analgesics, including nonsteroidal antiinflammatory medications. Advise patients that they can resume most of their normal activities pending repeat follow-up evaluation by gynecology. However, patients should be instructed to maintain pelvic rest (nothing in the vagina) until they are examined by gynecology. Daily sitz baths can also be recommended to the patient.

COMMON CAUSES OF VAGINAL BLEEDING IN ADULT FEMALES

Causes of vaginal bleeding in adult females include menstruation, oral contraceptive use, anovulatory cycles, spontaneous abortion, ectopic pregnancy, intrauterine contraceptive devices, persistent corpus luteum, gynecologic malignancy, vaginal or cervical injury, vaginal foreign bodies, gestational trophoblastic diseases, placenta abruptio, placenta previa, vasa previa, and uterine rupture. A good history along with beta human chorionic gonadotropin (β-hCG) testing and ultrasound (US) help differentiate among some of these, but pelvic examination should be considered for most of these potential conditions, except, most notably, placenta previa where it can cause catastrophic hemorrhage. In general, avoid a pelvic examination in late third trimester bleeding.

Early Pregnancy Bleeding

One-fifth of pregnant females have vaginal bleeding during the first half of pregnancy and 2% of females have an ectopic pregnancy, with the potential of hemorrhagic shock and maternal death. Evaluation of ectopic pregnancy is discussed in the later section "Culdocentesis."

One of the most common reasons to perform a speculum examination in early pregnancy bleeding is to evaluate for a possible miscarriage, looking for cervical dilation or the presence of products of conception. Some emergency physicians palpate the os intravaginally to determine the status of cervical dilation and feel that speculum examination adds little to either the diagnosis or the plan of treatment. The exception for this is during early pregnancy bleeding associated with shock when the removal of obstructing products of conception can be a resuscitative measure. Ultrasonography and β-hCG levels typically provide the necessary information needed to manage a patient with early pregnancy bleeding, and some practitioners feel that performing a vaginal examination does not enhance diagnostic accuracy and may cause unnecessary discomfort to the patient.[2,3]

Pelvic and Lower Abdominal Pain

Pelvic examination, particularly bimanual examination, is often performed for pelvic and lower abdominal pain. The pain can be caused by problems in the urinary tract, intestinal tract, and reproductive tract (in both pregnant and nonpregnant patients). Common urinary tract conditions include ureteral colic, cystitis, and pyelonephritis. Intestinal tract conditions include but are not limited to appendicitis, diverticulitis, inflammatory bowel disease, bowel obstruction or ischemia, and a perforated viscus. Reproductive tract conditions include ectopic pregnancy, threatened abortion, endometritis, endometriosis, corpus luteal cyst, salpingitis (PID and TOA), ovarian cyst, ovarian torsion, round ligament pain, uterine fibroids, and uterine perforation. Later in pregnancy two conditions of importance are placenta previa (which is most often painless) and placenta abruption. Conditions that may cause pain in the nonpregnant patient include salpingitis (PID), TOA, ovarian cyst, ovarian torsion, endometriosis, round ligament pain, uterine perforation, or uterine fibroids. Painless third trimester bleeding may be caused by placenta previa, in which a separated placenta is near or at the cervical os. Because manipulation of the uterus may further dislodge the placenta, defer rectal examination, speculum examination, and manual examination of the vagina to an obstetric professional in cases of suspected placenta previa. PID and TOA are often associated with vaginal discharge and fever. Endometriosis is associated with dyspareunia and dysmenorrhea.

Vaginal Foreign Body Removal

Retained vaginal foreign bodies can cause pain or bleeding and may lead to a foul-smelling vagal discharge and/or vaginitis. Common vaginal foreign bodies in adults include retained tampons, broken parts of condoms, pessaries, contraceptive diaphragms, drug smuggling devices, and sexual stimulation devices. Females with psychiatric illness sometimes insert vaginal foreign bodies (vaginal polyembolokoilamania). The removal of these foreign bodies, once located, may be accomplished using a speculum and ring forceps, or a Kelly clamp. Imbedded foreign bodies may require removal in an operating room. Once the foreign body is removed, the vaginal walls should be inspected for lacerations and infection. Bleeding vaginal lacerations can be tamponaded with surgical dressing prior to repair. Deep lacerations may require operative repair by a gynecologist.

It is not uncommon for a tampon to be lodged in a horizontal position in the upper vagina, commonly following intercourse. There is frequently a foul odor. The tampon can be removed by trapping it between two of the examiner's gloved fingers. Withdraw the tampon while inverting the examining glove with the tampon inside, placing the encased tampon in the palm of the opposite glove and then inverting the second glove over the first, followed by disposal in a biohazard container.

Vaginal Discharge and Suspected STI Sampling

History and physical examination are essential components for diagnosing infectious pathology of the external genitalia, vagina, cervix, or reproductive tract, the majority of physical examination findings and historical features alone have weak likelihood ratios and limited value in diagnosing vaginal infections. These findings and features should be used in combination to estimate the probability of disease and the utility of treatment.[6] Given the often nonspecific symptoms, laboratory evaluation is mandatory to target appropriate therapy. Diagnostic options include Gram stain, culture, nucleic acid amplification tests (NAATs), and antigen-detecting immunochromatography. The usefulness of microscopic examination of discharge as a diagnostic tool may be limited by contamination and a lack of operator skill.[7] Culturing is done to assess the effectiveness of antibiotics on targeted bacteria, particularly when there has been treatment failure. According to the Centers for Disease Control and Prevention, "the performance of NAATs with respect to overall sensitivity, specificity, and ease of specimen transport is better than that of any of the other tests available for the diagnosis of chlamydial and gonococcal infections."[4]

Bacterial Vaginosis and Candidiasis

The vaginal discharge of bacterial vaginosis (BV) is homogeneous, thin, and white and when obtained from a speculum examination, can aid in diagnosis. pH paper applied to the vaginal fluid can suggest BV when the pH is over.[4,5] This pH is elevated because of a lack of the normal acid-producing lactobacillus predominance in the vagina. Vaginal fluid generally has a pH below 4.5 and is usually in the 3.8 to 4.2 range. Conversely, mucus from the cervix generally has a pH that is in the 7.0 range and care must be taken not to sample cervical mucus when testing vaginal fluid for vaginitis. Make a wet mount of a very small smear of vaginal fluid. Apply the fluid with a cotton swab to a glass slide. Mix it with a drop of 10% KOH and cover it with a coverslip. The fluid may have a fishy, amine smell (the "whiff" test) suggesting BV. When examined microscopically (40 to 100 × power), the slide may reveal clue cells (vaginal epithelial cells studded with adherent coccobacilli that look somewhat like sugar cookies covered with poppy seeds).[5]

The combination of clue cell on microscopy, a positive whiff test (caused by the release of volatile amines), a vaginal pH greater than 4.5, with a homogenous vaginal discharge will help to confirm the diagnosis of BV.

The vaginal discharge of moniliasis (candidiasis) is "cheesy" and is associated with severe itching and burning of the perineum. A mixture of vaginal fluid with KOH should lyse many bacteria allowing the examiner to identify budding yeast cells, thereby helping with the diagnosis of monilial vaginitis (candidiasis).

Trichomoniasis

A wet mount of a tiny drop of vaginal fluid and a drop of normal saline, covered with a coverslip and examined microscopically, can aid in the diagnosis of trichomoniasis but such examination has poor sensitivity (51% to 65%).[6] Trichomonads are about the size of white blood cells but are characterized by a rapid, flagella-caused movement.

NAATs are highly sensitive and detect three to five times more *T. vaginalis* infections than wet-mount microscopy,[5] so these are the preferred tests for diagnosing trichomoniasis. There is also an antigen-detection test using immunochromatographic capillary flow dipstick technology (OSOM Trichomonas Rapid Test [Sekisui Diagnostics]) that can be performed at the point of care. The OSOM Trichomonas test is rapidly available and has a sensitivity of 82% to 95% with a specificity of 97% to 100%.[7]

Cervicitis and PID

For females with a purulent cervical discharge, the diagnosis of cervicitis or PID should be considered. The cervix should be visualized during the speculum examination, assessing for mucopurulent discharge from the os. Appropriate transport culture medium and NAAT swabs should be available and a cervical swab should be obtained, placed in the medium, and sent to a bacteriologic laboratory. It should be noted that PID is a clinical diagnosis made when the patient has cervical motion tenderness or adnexal tenderness, alone or in combination. Lab testing is not required to make the diagnosis and the patient should be treated based on clinical examination.

Chlamydia and Gonorrhea

NAATs are the diagnostic tests of choice, when available, for both chlamydia and gonorrhea.[4] The difference between urine, cervical, and vaginal specimen tests is not statistically significant.[8] The sensitivity of a Gram stain of endocervical discharge for the diagnosis of chlamydia or gonorrhea is low compared to culture or NAATs and is not recommended.

CULDOCENTESIS

Culdocentesis is a procedure in which peritoneal fluid is aspirated from the retrouterine pouch by the insertion of a hollow needle through the posterior fornix of the vagina. Historically, this technique was used to diagnose ruptured ectopic pregnancies and ruptured ovarian cysts, and, rarely, to obtain cultures for diagnosis and treatment of PID. Widespread utilization of transvaginal US and β-hCG have largely replaced the use of culdocentesis. Nevertheless, culdocentesis has clinical utility to diagnose ruptured ectopic pregnancy in a patient for whom sonography is not readily available.[9]

Anatomy for Performing a Culdocentesis

Before attempting culdocentesis, the clinician must be familiar with the anatomy of the vagina and the rectouterine pouch (pouch of Douglas) (see Fig. 58.1). In adult females, the vagina is approximately 9 cm long. From its inferior to its superior aspect, the posterior wall of the vagina is related to the anal canal by way of the perineal body, the rectum, and the peritoneum of the rectouterine pouch.[10] The uterus lies at nearly a right angle to the vagina. The rectouterine pouch and the posterior wall of the vagina are adjacent only at the upper quarter (≈2 cm) of the posterior vaginal wall. The vaginal wall in this area is less than 5 mm thick.

The blood supply to the upper part of the vagina comes from the uterine and vaginal arteries, which are branches of the internal iliac artery. This area is drained by a vaginal venous plexus that communicates with the uterine plexuses. The vagina has its greatest sensation near the introitus and little sensation in the area adjacent to the rectouterine pouch.

The rectouterine pouch is formed by reflections of the peritoneum, and it is the most dependent intraperitoneal space in both the upright and the supine positions. Blood, pus, and other free fluids in the peritoneal cavity pool in the pouch because of its dependent location. This pouch separates the upper portion of the rectum from the uterus and the upper part of the vagina. The pouch often contains small intestine and, normally, a small amount of peritoneal fluid.

Indications

Culdocentesis is indicated in any adult female in whom aspiration of fluid from the rectouterine pouch will help confirm the clinical diagnosis. If US examination is not readily available in the ED or if the patient is too hemodynamically unstable to be transported to an off-site location for US, culdocentesis may be the fastest and most accurate diagnostic technique available to the emergency clinician.[11] Analysis of peritoneal fluid is also an acceptable method of differentiating inflammatory from hemorrhagic pelvic pathologic conditions. Conditions in which culdocentesis may be of diagnostic value include a ruptured viscus (particularly an ectopic pregnancy or a corpus luteum cyst), PID and other intraabdominal infections (particularly appendicitis with rupture or diverticulitis with perforation), intraabdominal injuries to the liver or spleen, and ruptured aortic aneurysms.[12]

Ectopic Pregnancy

Ectopic pregnancy can be one of the most difficult gynecologic lesions to diagnose.[13] The incidence of ectopic pregnancy is estimated to be 0.64% to 2.0%, although surveillance data are imprecise and limited for a variety of reasons.[14] Ectopic pregnancy is the most common obstetric cause of maternal death in the first trimester.[13] In a series of 300 consecutive cases of ectopic pregnancy, 50% of patients received medical evaluation at least twice before the correct diagnosis was made.

The clinical picture of ectopic pregnancy may include vascular collapse, pelvic pain, isolated rectal or back pain, amenorrhea, abnormal menses, vaginal bleeding, shoulder pain, syncope, cervical or adnexal tenderness, adnexal mass, anemia, and leukocytosis. It is important to note that blood in the peritoneal cavity does not consistently correlate with peritoneal irritation, blood pressure, or pulse rate.[15] In fact, bradycardia in the presence of significant intraperitoneal bleeding from a ruptured ectopic pregnancy is not unusual (Tables 58.1 and 58.2).

Although the risk factors for ectopic pregnancy include a history of salpingitis, use of an intrauterine contraceptive device, or tubal ligation, almost half of patients with ectopic pregnancy have no identifiable risk factor. In fact, no combination of signs, symptoms, or historical data is diagnostic of an ectopic pregnancy. To confuse the diagnosis further, a normal menstrual history is reported in approximately 50% of patients with an ectopic pregnancy. On very rare occasions, a urine pregnancy test may occasionally be negative.[16] Though rarely seen, the combination of a uterine decidual cast (Fig. 58.7) and a positive pregnancy test is virtually pathognomonic of an ectopic pregnancy. A uterine cast is decidua that has been hormonally stimulated by the ectopic pregnancy but is passed vaginally when the tissue can no longer be supported. The

TABLE 58.1 Correlation Between the Results of Culdocentesis Performed on 77 Patients With Ectopic Gestation and Various Clinical Parameters

	Classic Triad									
	BLEEDING	PAIN	ADNEXAL MASS	PERITONEAL SIGNS	PULSE ≥100 beats/min	BLOOD PRESSURE < 90/40 mm Hg	MEAN HEMATOCRIT (%)	HEMOPERITONEUM ≥100 mL	RUPTURED TUBE	TOTAL
Positive	37	54	10	26	19	9	35	52	30	54
Negative	8	8	3	1	1	0	39	0	0	8
Inadequate	13	15	6	5	4	1	38	13	7	15
Total patients	58	77	19	32	24	10	65	37	77	

There is a lack of correlation between positive culdocentesis and peritoneal signs and changes in vital signs. Patients are grouped by the result of culdocentesis (i.e., positive, negative, or inadequate). Note that only 10 patients were hypotensive and only 24 experienced tachycardia.
From Cartwright PS, Vaughn B, Tuttle D. Culdocentesis and ectopic pregnancy. *J Reprod Med*. 1984;29:88.

TABLE 58.2 Correlation Between Tubal Status and Hypotension, Tachycardia, Hematocrit, Signs of Peritoneal Irritation, and Hemoperitoneum in 77 Patients With Ectopic Gestation

CULDOCENTESIS	CULDOCENTESIS POSITIVE	PERITONEAL SIGNS	BLOOD PRESSURE <90/40 mm Hg	PULSE ≥100 beats/min	HEMOPERITONEUM ≥100 mL	AVERAGE HEMATOCRIT (%)
Ruptured (*n* = 37)	30	25	8	19	37	33.6
Intact (*n* = 40)	24	7	2	5	28	37.3
Total patients	54	32	10	24	65	

Culdocentesis is frequently positive in the absence of rupture. Patients are grouped by the presence (i.e., "ruptured") or absence (i.e., "intact") of hemoperitoneum. Note that only about half the patients with "ruptured" status had tachycardia.
From Cartwright PS, Vaughn B, Tuttle D. Culdocentesis and ectopic pregnancy. *J Reprod Med*. 1984;29:88.

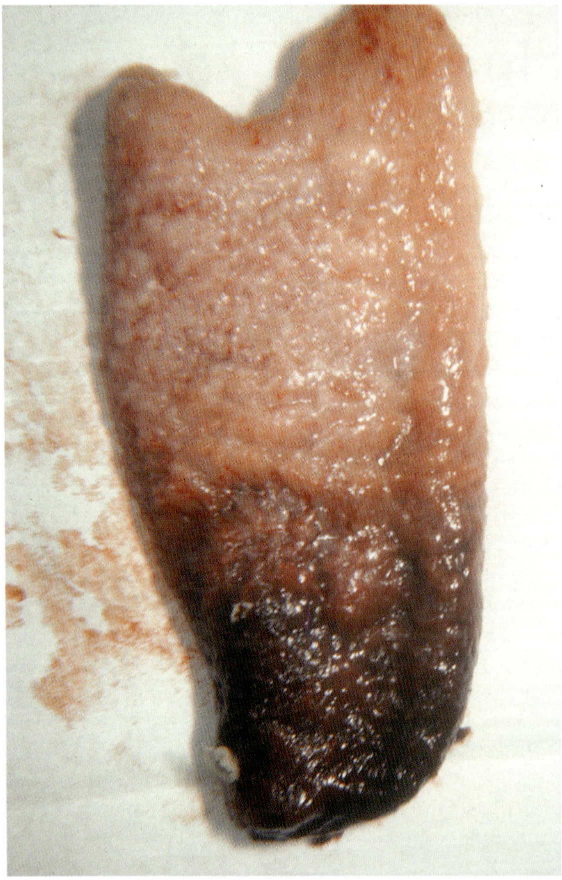

Fig. 58.7 This decidual cast, a perfect outline of the uterine cavity, was initially thought to be a product of conception when found in the vaginal vault of a pregnant female treated for abdominal pain and vaginal bleeding. The initial diagnosis was a spontaneous abortion, but this cast is *virtually diagnostic of an ectopic pregnancy*. Hypotension developed later, and the patient was found to have a ruptured tubal pregnancy.

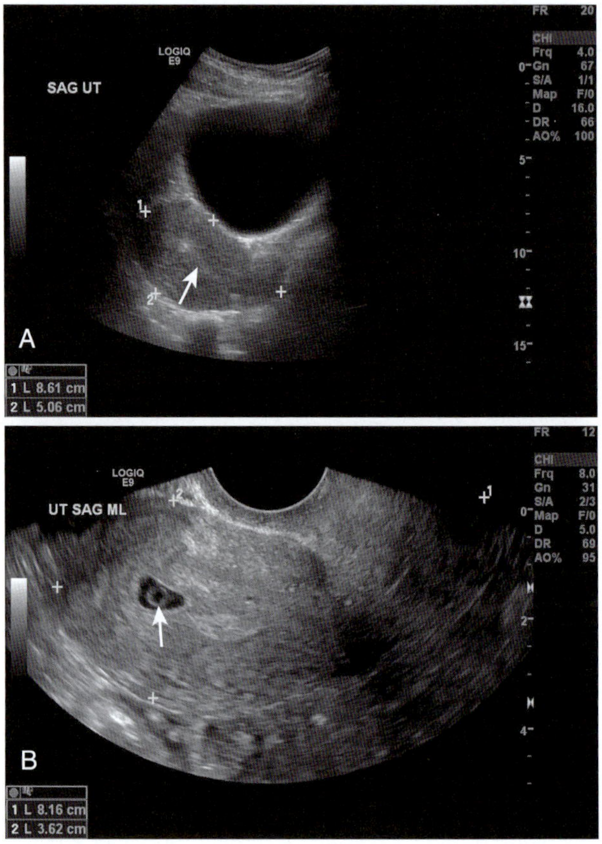

Fig. 58.8 (A) Pelvic ultrasound showing an empty uterus. The endometrial stripe *(arrow)* is clearly visible, and there is no evidence of a gestational sac. A beta human chorionic gonadotropin (β-hCG) level below the discriminatory zone (see text) could represent an early viable intrauterine pregnancy, a nonviable intrauterine pregnancy, completed abortion, or an ectopic pregnancy. If β-hCG exceeds the discriminatory zone, the chance of an ectopic pregnancy exceeds 85%. (B) Pelvic ultrasound showing the presence of a yolk sac *(arrow)* within a gestational sac in the uterus. This patient was 5 weeks pregnant by dates.

cast is an outline of the uterine cavity, but it can be mistaken for products of conception if not inspected carefully. Therefore all tissue passed vaginally should be carefully inspected before being sent to the laboratory for analysis for products of conception. An ectopic pregnancy can occasionally occur in conjunction with an intrauterine pregnancy and is called a heterotopic pregnancy. This is most commonly seen in females pregnant after medically assisted interventions such as in vitro fertilization or ovarian stimulation. Patients who have undergone a therapeutic abortion may actually have had an unrecognized ectopic pregnancy, hence the need for pathologic evaluation of any tissue obtained by uterine evacuation procedures.

The greater sensitivity of the serum and urine β-hCG assay, coupled with the increased availability of emergency medicine physicians trained to perform pelvic US, has greatly increased the chance of early diagnosis of unruptured and ruptured ectopic pregnancy.[17] Urinary β-hCG tests are sensitive at 20 mIU/mL or greater and are positive 98% of the time in the first few weeks of pregnancy.

Quantification of the serum test adds additional information as it is sensitive to 5 mIU/mL. Therefore a negative *urine* β-hCG test rules out pregnancy in greater than 98% of cases, and pregnancy in any site can be ruled out in virtually all patients with a negative *serum* β-hCG test.[18] A single quantitative β-hCG level is a poor predictor of the size of the pregnancy or the risk for ectopic pregnancy, but serial testing is quite helpful. The quantitative serum β-hCG level should be expected to double approximately every 2 days in the first trimester in a normal pregnancy.

To increase the accuracy of diagnosis, it is helpful to combine quantitative β-hCG testing with US examination (Fig. 58.8). The quantitative range in which the ultrasonographer should detect an intrauterine pregnancy varies, but an intrauterine pregnancy should be detected if the serum β-hCG level is in the range of 1200 to 1500 mIU/mL when using a *transvaginal probe* and greater than 6000 mIU/mL when using a *transabdominal probe* A completely empty uterus on ultrasound in patients with these β-hCG cutoffs is diagnostic of an ectopic pregnancy and gynecologic consultation is necessary in these patients.

Endovaginal US scanning consistently identifies a 4-week gestational sac if the β-hCG level is 2000 mIU/mL or greater. A fetal pole and cardiac activity are detectable with endovaginal US scanning at approximately 6 and 7 weeks, respectively.[19] Note that a heartbeat can occasionally be detected in an ectopic pregnancy or an extrauterine pregnancy and may be mistakenly deemed intrauterine. It is important to note that the absence of an intrauterine pregnancy by US when the β-hCG level is below the discriminatory zone (defined as the hCG level at which a normal intrauterine pregnancy can be detected by US), is *nondiagnostic* and could represent an early viable normal pregnancy, a nonviable intrauterine pregnancy, a completed abortion, or an ectopic pregnancy. These cases are called "pregnancy of unknown location." If the patient is highly symptomatic or her vital signs are abnormal, gynecologic consultation is recommended. If not, these patients require close follow-up with serial β-hCG levels and repeat US in 24 to 48 hours. When no intrauterine pregnancy is detected by US and the serum β-hCG level *exceeds the discriminatory zone*, the chance of an ectopic pregnancy ranges from 86% to 100%.[20]

Culdocentesis may play an important role in some patients in the diagnosis of ectopic pregnancy. Historically, the test has an accuracy rate of 85% to 95%; however, this may be contemporaneously limited by the infrequent use of the procedure in modern practice.[11,21,22] Romero and coworkers[23] reported that an ectopic pregnancy was found in 99% of patients with a positive pregnancy test and positive results on culdocentesis. More recent studies,[31,32] however, may suggest a lower accuracy rate, in the range of 37% to 44%. Although culdocentesis is most often positive in the presence of a frankly ruptured ectopic pregnancy, it may be diagnostic even in a nonruptured case when bleeding has been slow or intermittent. Note that many ectopic pregnancies leak varying amounts of blood for days or weeks before rupture. Hemoperitoneum has been found in 45% to 60% of cases of *unruptured* ectopic pregnancy, as proved at surgery.[14,23]

Hence, culdocentesis may be helpful in a stable patient whose US examination does not demonstrate an intrauterine pregnancy despite a quantitative serum β-hCG level in the appropriate range. Although some clinicians opt for outpatient monitoring of serial β-hCG levels in this setting, patients in whom the clinician has high suspicion for an ectopic pregnancy (e.g., a patient who has or has had significant discomfort) or in whom close follow-up cannot be ensured may be candidates for culdocentesis.[11] Even though a negative finding on culdocentesis does not rule out an early ectopic pregnancy, patients with a nondiagnostic US and a negative culdocentesis generally represent those at lower risk for "rupture" of an ectopic pregnancy during outpatient serum β-hCG monitoring. Patients with a nondiagnostic US examination and a serum β-hCG level below the threshold at which an intrauterine pregnancy should be visible on the US examination may need further evaluation. These patients, especially those with significant pain, an unexplained low hematocrit, or postural changes in vital signs (or near syncope), might be candidates for culdocentesis.

Blunt Abdominal Trauma

Historically, diagnostic peritoneal lavage (DPL) and computed tomography (CT) have been used to identify hemoperitoneum in blunt trauma patients. The use of culdocentesis has also been advocated to aid in this diagnosis.[12,24] In the ED, two factors have largely obviated the need to perform invasive procedures for diagnosis of hemoperitoneum: (1) the increasing availability of high-resolution CT and (2) emergency clinicians trained to perform the bedside US-focused assessment with sonography for trauma (FAST) examination. However, because small amounts of blood tend to collect in the rectouterine pouch, aspiration of clear peritoneal fluid is of great potential value in excluding a diagnosis of hemoperitoneum. This is especially helpful in situations in which US is unavailable or the patient is too unstable to leave the ED for a CT scan. In fact, culdocentesis may be more advantageous than DPL in some instances because there is less risk for urinary bladder perforation or bowel injury. In addition, previous abdominal surgery is not a relative contraindication to culdocentesis, as it is with DPL.[25]

Ovarian Hyperstimulation Syndrome

Ovarian hyperstimulation syndrome (OHSS) is a rare, potentially lethal complication of in vitro fertilization (IVF) associated with the use of hCG for ovulation induction. Characterized by fluid shifts out of the vasculature (third-spacing) due to increased vascular permeability, this iatrogenic condition can range in severity from mild cases—abdominal discomfort, mild nausea and vomiting, diarrhea—to severe multisystem organ dysfunction, with intractable nausea/vomiting, hydrothorax, acute respiratory distress syndrome, anuria, venous thromboembolism, and even death. The massive fluid shifts associated with OHSS often lead to fluid accumulation in the rectouterine pouch (pouch of Douglas).[32] Treatment of OHSS includes bedrest, oral rehydration with balanced electrolyte solutions, and removal of ascites in attempt to prevent organ failure.[33] Culdocentesis can be utilized for removal of this fluid, particularly if the clinician is unable to visualize a significant fluid collection in the typical locations for a paracentesis. Typical volumes of fluid removed are approximately 2 L[32–34] due to concerns for hemodynamic instability associated with larger volumes causing additional fluid shift and improvement in organ perfusion seen with removal of 2 L.

Contraindications

Contraindications to culdocentesis are relatively few and include an uncooperative patient, a pelvic mass detected on bimanual pelvic examination, a nonmobile retroverted uterus, and coagulopathies. Pelvic masses may include TOAs, appendiceal abscesses, ovarian masses, and pelvic kidneys. It has been suggested that the only major risk with the procedure is rupture of an unsuspected TOA into the peritoneal cavity. This can be avoided by careful bimanual pelvic examination to exclude patients with large masses in the cul-de-sac.[26] Although no data are available to guide the age at which culdocentesis may be performed safely, the procedure is generally limited to patients beyond puberty. This limitation is suggested on the basis of anatomy and with the consideration that the procedure is difficult to perform through a small prepubertal vagina.

Equipment

The equipment required for culdocentesis is depicted in Review Box 58.1. Either an 18-gauge spinal needle or a 19-gauge butterfly needle held by ring forceps is acceptable. It may be helpful to anesthetize the posterior vaginal wall at the site of the puncture with 1% to 2% lidocaine with epinephrine administered through a 27- or 25-gauge needle. Some physicians use a topical anesthetic (eutectic mixture of local anesthetics [EMLA], benzocaine), viscous lidocaine, or a cocaine-soaked cotton ball to anesthetize the mucosa before infiltration with a local anesthetic. Although puncture of the posterior vaginal wall at the upper fourth of the vagina is generally no more painful than a venipuncture, there is some

Culdocentesis

Indications

Diagnosis of acute pelvic conditions when ultrasound is not available or clinically feasible, including:
- Ruptured viscus (ectopic pregnancy or corpus luteum cyst)
- Pelvic inflammatory disease
- Other intraabdominal infections
- Splenic or liver injuries
- Ruptured aortic aneurysm

Contraindications

Uncooperative patient
Pelvic mass detected on bimanual examination
Nonmobile retroverted uterus
Coagulopathies

Complications

Rupture of unsuspected tuboovarian abscess
Bowel perforation
Pelvic kidney perforation
Bleeding

Equipment

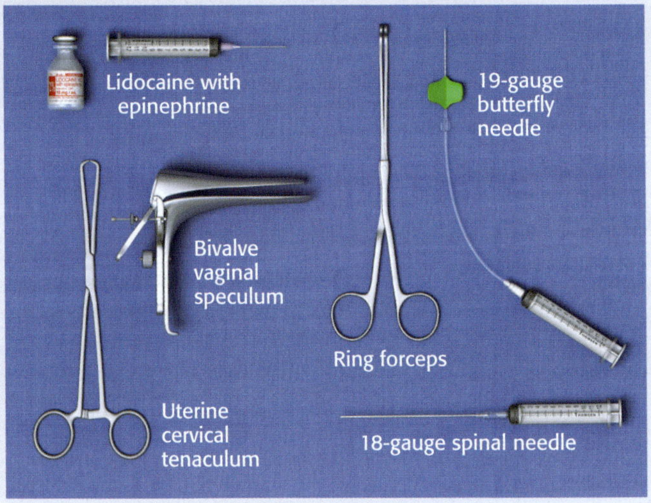

Review Box 58.1 Culdocentesis: indications, contraindications, complications, and equipment. Not shown is optional prepuncture topical anesthetic, such as a topical anesthetic-soaked cotton ball.

advantage to using a local anesthetic if multiple attempts at culdocentesis are required, as is sometimes the case. In addition, the epinephrine may produce vasoconstriction and reduce bleeding associated with the needle puncture. Culdocentesis is often stressful to the patient, and all attempts should be made to render the procedure as painless as possible. Parenteral analgesia and/or sedation should be administered when the patient is uncomfortable or anxious.

Technique

Preparation

Culdocentesis is an invasive procedure that requires a written, witnessed, and signed consent form from the patient, parent, or guardian when the patient's condition permits. If verbal consent is obtained, this action should be witnessed, and a notation made in the medical record documenting that the procedure was described, complications were discussed, and any alternatives (e.g., CT, sonography, or immediate laparoscopy) were offered when appropriate.

Once written or verbal consent is obtained, place the patient in a lithotomy position with the head of the table slightly elevated (reverse Trendelenburg position) so that intraperitoneal fluid gravitates toward the rectouterine pouch. Place the patient's feet in stirrups. Premedicate with intravenous opioids or sedatives if appropriate. Administration of nitrous oxide analgesia is also an accepted practice. Procedural sedation with propofol, etomidate, or benzodiazepines can be considered. Although the pain associated with the passage of the culdocentesis needle is generally minor, judicious use of analgesia and sedation makes the procedure easier for both the clinician and patient.

If radiographs are indicated, take them before culdocentesis to avoid confusion with procedure-induced pneumoperitoneum.

Exposure

Perform a bimanual pelvic examination before culdocentesis to rule out a fixed pelvic mass and to assess the position of the uterus. It is possible to palpate an adnexal mass if the mass exceeds 3 cm in diameter. Insert a bivalve vaginal speculum and open it widely by adjusting both the height and the angle thumbscrews (Fig. 58.9, *step 1*). Grasp the posterior lip of the cervix with the toothed uterine cervical tenaculum and elevate the cervix. Warn the patient in advance that she may feel a sharp pain when the cervix is grasped with the tenaculum. Inform the patient also that bleeding from the tenaculum puncture site or culdocentesis site, or both, may produce postprocedural spotting.

Use the tenaculum to elevate a retroverted uterus from the pouch, to expose the puncture site, and to stabilize the posterior wall during puncture with the needle. Some clinicians prefer to use longitudinal traction on the cervix to produce the same result. The vaginal wall adjacent to the rectouterine pouch will be tightened somewhat between the inferior blade of the bivalve speculum and the elevated posterior lip of the cervix. Such tightening of the vaginal wall exposes the puncture site and keeps it from moving away from the needle when the wall is punctured.

After the tenaculum is applied and the posterior lip of the cervix is elevated or traction is applied, swab the vaginal wall in the area of the rectouterine pouch with an antiseptic, followed by a small amount of sterile water. Administer a local anesthetic (1% lidocaine with epinephrine) at this point. Anesthetic may be injected through a separate 27- or 25-gauge needle or with the spinal needle that will be used for the culdocentesis. Use a cotton ball soaked in 4% cocaine or 20% benzocaine solution or apply viscous lidocaine to the area for topical anesthesia of the posterior vaginal wall approximately 15 minutes before infiltration with a local anesthetic. This combination will make the needle puncture nearly painless.

Culdocentesis

1

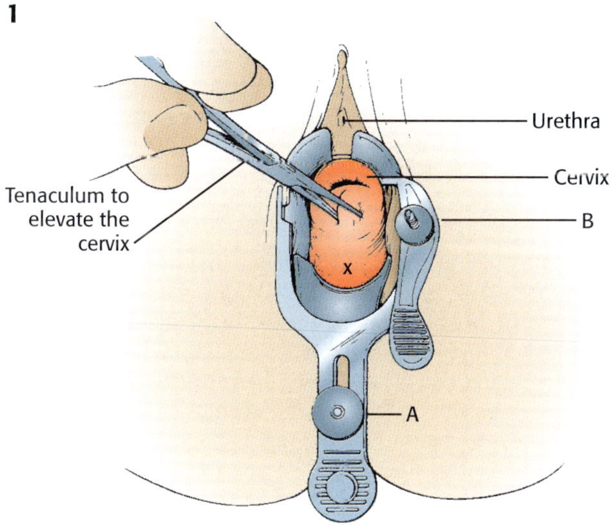

Place the patient in the lithotomy position with the head of the bed slightly elevated so that intraperitoneal fluid gravitates toward the rectouterine pouch. Premedicate with sedatives or intravenous opiates as clinically indicated. Perform a bimanual pelvic examination to exclude the presence of a pelvic mass.

Insert a bivalve pelvic speculum and open it widely by using both the height *(A)* and angle *(B)* thumbscrews. Grasp the posterior lip of the cervix with a tenaculum and elevate the cervix.

Swab the vaginal wall in the area of the rectouterine pouch with antiseptic followed by a small amount of sterile water.

Administer a local anesthetic with a separate 25- or 27-gauge needle or with the needle that will be used for culdocentesis. The site of needle entry is 1 cm posterior to the point at which the vaginal wall joins the cervix *(x)*. (*Optional:* before injecting the local anesthetic, place a cocaine [4%]- or benzocaine [20%]-soaked cotton ball on the area to be punctured for 15 minutes.)

2

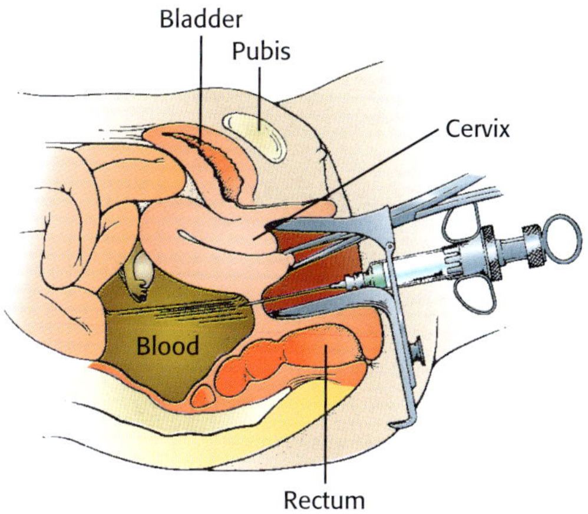

3

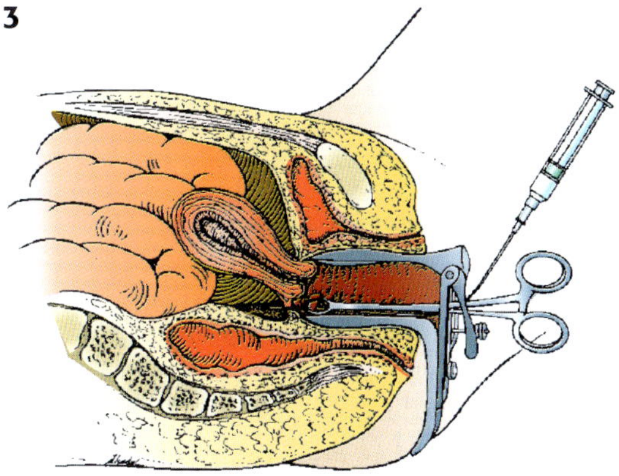

Fill the syringe with 2 to 3 mL of saline prior to puncture. Advance the spinal needle parallel to the lower blade of the speculum. Gently depress the plunger during advancement of the needle. Free flow of fluid will confirm proper needle placement in the rectouterine pouch. Pass the needle 2 to 2.5 cm. Apply gentle suction while slowly withdrawing the syringe.

Alternatively, use a 19-gauge butterfly needle held with ring forceps. This technique offers a built-in guide to needle depth and allows good control of the needle during puncture. Use the help of an assistant to aspirate while you control needle position and withdrawal.

Fig. 58.9 Culdocentesis. (1 and 2, From Vander Salm TJ, Cutler BS, Wheeler HB. *Atlas of Bedside Procedures.* Little, Brown; 1979. 3, From Webb MJ. Culdocentesis. *JACEP.* 1978;7:452.)

Attach the needle to a 20-mL syringe. A smaller syringe might not be long enough to allow adequate control of the needle, and the clinician's hand may block the view of the puncture site if a smaller syringe is used.

Aspiration

Following local anesthesia, advance the syringe and the spinal needle parallel to the lower blade of the speculum (see Fig. 58.9, *step 2*). Fill the syringe with 2 mL to 3 mL of saline (nonbacteriostatic) before puncture. After needle puncture, the free flow of fluid from the syringe will expel tissue that may have clogged the needle and confirm that the needle tip is in the proper position and not lodged in the uterine wall or the intestinal wall. Use saline rather than air because if air is used, it may be difficult to interpret the presence of free peritoneal air on subsequent radiographs. To avoid the need to change the syringe during the procedure, use 1% lidocaine for both anesthesia and confirmation of proper needle placement; however, the bacteriostatic property of this agent precludes its use if the procedure is performed to obtain fluid for culture.

Penetrate the vaginal wall in the midline 1 cm to 1.5 cm posterior (inferior) to the point at which the vaginal wall joins the cervix (see Fig. 58.9, *step 2*).[27] Pass the needle a total of 2 cm to 2.5 cm.[27,28] Apply gentle suction with the syringe while slowly withdrawing the needle. Avoid aspirating any blood that has accumulated in the vagina from previous needle punctures or from cervical bleeding because this may give the false impression of a positive tap. Bleeding from the puncture site in the vaginal wall can be minimized by adding epinephrine to the local anesthetic.

Blood or fluid may be obtained immediately but may also be obtained when the needle is withdrawn from the peritoneal

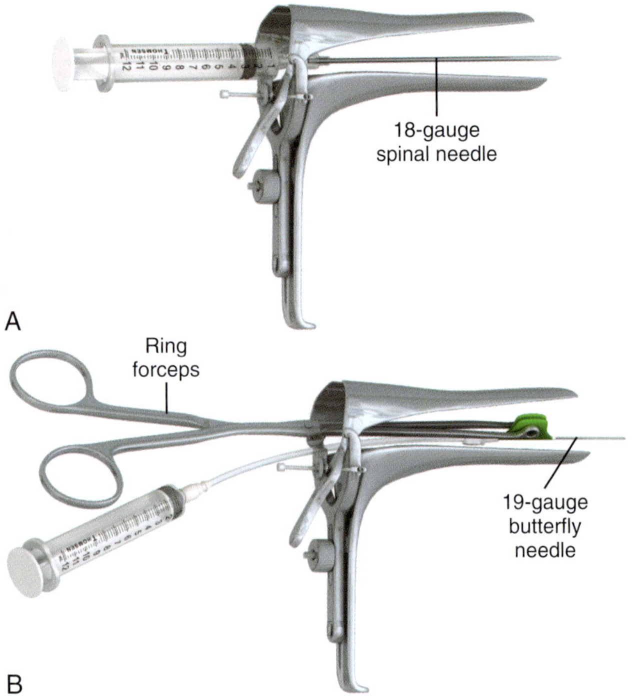

Fig. 58.10 Variations in culdocentesis technique. (A) An 18-gauge spinal needle attached to a syringe. The operator applies continuous suction during withdrawal of the needle. (B) A 19-gauge butterfly needle attached to a syringe and held with ring forceps. An assistant is required to aspirate the syringe while the operator controls the needle with the forceps.

cavity; therefore it is important to aspirate continuously while *gradually* withdrawing the needle. If no fluid is aspirated, reintroduce the needle and direct it only slightly to the left or right of the midline. Directing the needle too far laterally may result in puncture of the mesenteric or pelvic vessels. If no fluid is obtained on the first attempt, repeat the procedure.

Some physicians prefer the use of a 19-gauge butterfly needle held with ring forceps (see Fig. 58.9, *step 3*, and Fig. 58.10).[27] This technique offers a built-in guide to needle depth and allows good control of the needle during puncture. An assistant must aspirate the tubing while the physician controls positioning and withdrawal of the needle.

Aspirated fluid may be old nonclotting blood, bright red blood, pus, exudate, or a straw-colored serous liquid. Any fluid that is not blood should be submitted for Gram stain, aerobic and anaerobic culture, and cell count. Blood should be observed for clotting. Blood should also be sent to determine the hematocrit.

Interpretation of Results

Interpretation of the results of culdocentesis depends primarily on whether any fluid was obtained. In the absence of a pathologic condition, 2 to 3 mL of clear yellowish peritoneal fluid can be aspirated. The procedure has no diagnostic value when there is no return of fluid of any type (a so-called dry tap). Because a dry tap is nondiagnostic, it should not be equated with normal peritoneal fluid. In addition, when less than 2 mL of clotting blood is obtained, this is also considered to be a nondiagnostic tap because the source of this small amount of blood may be the puncture site on the vaginal wall. Such blood will usually clot. More than 2 mL of *nonclotting blood* is certainly suggestive of hemoperitoneum. However, some researchers interpret as little as 0.3 mL of *nonclotting* blood as a positive tap.[15] There is no particular significance of larger amounts of blood because absolute volume may be related to the needle's position or the bleeding rate. Brenner and colleagues[14] reported no blood from culdocentesis in 5% of patients with proven ectopic pregnancies even when rupture had occurred. In the series of 61 patients with surgically proven ectopic pregnancy reported by Cartwright and associates,[15] culdocentesis performed within 4 hours of surgery was positive in 70%, negative in 10%, and inadequate in 20%. "Positive" in their series was defined as obtaining at least 0.3 mL of nonclotting blood with a hematocrit of greater than 3%. "Negative" was defined as obtaining 0.3 mL of fluid with a hematocrit of less than 3%. An "inadequate" tap was one in which no fluid was obtained. In the 252 patients reported by Vermesh and coworkers[29] who had surgically proven ectopic pregnancies and underwent culdocentesis, 83% had a positive tap. They defined a positive tap as nonclotting blood with a hematocrit of greater than 15%.

When culdocentesis is used to diagnose a ruptured ectopic pregnancy, a "negative tap" is one that yields pus or clear, straw-colored peritoneal or cystic fluid. A large amount of clear fluid (>10 mL) indicates a probable ruptured ovarian cyst, aspiration of an intact corpus luteal cyst, ascites, or possibly carcinoma. The significance of this fluid and the interpretation of the results are outlined in Table 58.3 and Box 58.1. Elliot and colleagues[30] cautioned that obtaining greater than 10 mL of clear fluid should not automatically rule out an ectopic pregnancy because the latter may coexist with other pathologic conditions.

A "positive tap" is one in which nonclotting blood is obtained, although the presence of nonclotted blood does not confirm a tubal pregnancy. Intraperitoneal blood from any source (ectopic pregnancy, ovarian cyst, ruptured spleen) may remain unclotted after aspiration for days in the syringe as a result of the defibrination activity of the peritoneum. Return of serosanguineous fluid also suggests a ruptured ovarian cyst. The hematocrit of blood from active intraperitoneal bleeding is greater than 10%. In one series, the hematocrit of blood from a ruptured ectopic pregnancy was 15% or greater in 97% of cases.[14]

It should be emphasized that a positive finding on culdocentesis in the presence of a positive pregnancy test does not always prove an ectopic pregnancy.[29] A ruptured corpus luteum cyst in the presence of an intrauterine pregnancy test is probably the most common cause of a false-positive scenario. Whenever possible, US can help corroborate the findings on culdocentesis.

Complications

Culdocentesis is one of the safest procedures performed in the emergency setting, and there are probably fewer complications with this technique than with peripheral venous cannulation. Complications have been reported, however, the most serious being rupture of an unsuspected TOA.[27] Other complications include perforation of the bowel, perforation of a pelvic kidney, and bleeding from the puncture site in patients with clotting disorders. Because the most common complications result from puncture of a pelvic mass, careful bimanual examination of the patient should help prevent this problem. Puncture of the bowel and the uterine wall occurs relatively

TABLE 58.3 Interpretation of Culdocentesis Fluid

ASPIRATED FLUID	CONDITION AND SUGGESTED DIFFERENTIAL DIAGNOSIS
Clear, serous, straw colored (usually only a few milliliters)	Normal peritoneal fluid
Large amount of clear fluid	Ruptured or large ovarian cyst (fluid may be serosanguineous); pregnancy may be coexistent Ascites Carcinoma
Exudate with polymorphonuclear leukocytes	Pelvic inflammatory disease Gonococcal salpingitis Chronic salpingitis
Purulent fluid	Bacterial infection Tuboovarian abscess with rupture Appendicitis with rupture Diverticulitis with perforation
Bright red blood[a]	Ruptured viscus or vascular injury Recently bleeding ectopic pregnancy[a] (ruptured or unruptured) Bleeding corpus luteum Intraabdominal injury (e.g., liver, spleen, other organs) Ruptured aortic aneurysm
Old, brown, nonclotting blood	Ruptured viscus Ectopic pregnancy with intraperitoneal bleeding over a few days or weeks Old (days) intraabdominal injury (e.g., delayed splenic rupture)

[a]The hematocrit of blood from a ruptured ectopic pregnancy is usually ≥15% (97.5% of cases), but some authors use >3% as positive.

frequently but does not generally result in serious morbidity. Obviously, penetration of a gravid uterus has greater potential for harm. Occasionally, one will aspirate air or fecal matter, thereby confirming inadvertent puncture of the rectum.

Complications of Self-Managed Abortions

Self-managed abortions can lead to complications that vary from minor to severe. These events occur when an individual attempts to terminate their own pregnancy without the support of the health care environment. The complications also vary depending on the method used as well as the gestational age at the time of the abortion. The most common complications include incomplete abortion, hemorrhage, infection, and the need for surgical intervention.

Incomplete abortion is one of the more frequent complications. They can occur with medication-induced abortions, usually involving misoprostol alone or in combination with mifepristone. Studies have shown that incomplete abortion rates can be as high as 6.7% for medical abortions compared to 1.6% for surgical abortions.[35] Incomplete abortions often necessitate further medical or surgical intervention to complete the abortion.[35]

Hemorrhage is another significant complication, with medical abortions showing a higher incidence compared with surgical abortions (15.6% vs. 2.1%),[35] which can sometimes require blood transfusions or other emergency interventions.

Infection, although less common, remains a serious risk. The incidence of infection is similar between medical and surgical abortions, around 1.7%. However, in settings where abortion is illegal or access to health care is limited, the risk of severe infections such as septic shock and pelvic peritonitis increases significantly.[36]

Other complications include undiagnosed ectopic pregnancies, which can be life-threatening if not properly managed. Complications are often related to underestimated gestational age, which can increase the risk of adverse outcomes.

Heavy bleeding is a common risk, which can be dangerous if not managed properly. It might necessitate blood transfusions, emergency interventions like vaginal packing, or surgical interventions to stop the hemorrhage.

BOX 58.1 Interpretation of Culdocentesis

POSITIVE

- >0.5 mL nonclotting, bloody fluid (hematocrit >12%)
- Indicates hemoperitoneum
- When β-hCG is also positive, ectopic pregnancy is found in greater than 95%
- Nonspecific—can occur in intrauterine pregnancies and nonpregnant females (e.g., ruptured cyst, retrograde bleeding)
- Does not necessarily indicate tubal rupture
- 50% to 62% of ectopic pregnancies with peritoneal blood may be unruptured

NEGATIVE

- Serous fluid
- Excludes hemoperitoneum and tubal rupture
- Falsely negative in 10% to 15% of ectopic pregnancies (generally unruptured)

NONDIAGNOSTIC

- Dry tap or clotting blood
- Excludes neither ectopic pregnancy nor hemoperitoneum
- 15% of procedures are nondiagnostic
- 16% of ectopic pregnancies have nondiagnostic study results

β-hCG, β subunit of human chorionic gonadotropin.
From Brennan DF. Ectopic pregnancy: II. Diagnostic procedures and imaging. Acad Emerg Med. *1995;2:1090.*

Other Considerations

- *Delayed or inadequate medical care:* Individuals may delay seeking help due to fear of legal repercussions or stigma. This delay can worsen complications, making them harder to treat.
- *Toxicity from inappropriate medication use:* Incorrect dosing or use of nonrecommended substances can lead to toxicity and adverse drug reactions, posing significant health risks.
- *Psychologic impact:* In addition to physical complications, self-managed abortions can also have psychological impacts, including anxiety, stress, and emotional trauma, especially if complications arise.

Recommendations for Reducing Risks

- Education and access:
  - Providing comprehensive education about safe methods and potential risks associated with self-managed abortions.
  - Ensuring access to safe and legal abortion services to minimize the need for self-management.
- Emergency care:
  - Establishing clear pathways for individuals to seek emergency care without fear of legal consequences.

CONCLUSION

While self-managed abortions may offer autonomy, they carry significant risks that can be mitigated through proper education, access to safe medical care, and supportive health policies. Ensuring that individuals have access to safe and legal abortion services is crucial in reducing the incidence of complications from self-managed abortions.

REFERENCES ARE AVAILABLE AT Elsevier eBooks+

CHAPTER 59

The Sexual Assault Forensic Examination

Emily Haley, Rebecca C.R. Plante, and Amelia Y. Pousson

The majority of sexually assaulted individuals do not share the experience with anyone, suffering in silence. An estimated one-third of all sexual assaults are reported to law enforcement. Only 21% seek medical care.[1] After contact with law enforcement, patients are often taken to the emergency department (ED) for evaluation, examination, and treatment. Sexual assault patients may also present to the ED de novo, without prior law enforcement contact. Sexual assault accounts for 4.4% of ED visits due to violence.[2] It has been estimated that ED visits for sexual assault have increased by more than 1533% between 2006 and 2019.[1]

Often hospitals and jurisdictions affiliate with designated sexual assault examination teams to provide specialized evaluation and treatment of patients. These sexual assault response teams (SARTs)/forensic medical units (FMUs) include sexual assault nurse examiners (SANE) or forensic nurse examiners (FNEs) and provide clear advantages. However, patients may be brought to an ED that does not routinely provide specialized care for sexual assault. This chapter is designed to aid clinicians in such a general care location. Clinicians who treat sexual assault patients have a professional, ethical, and moral responsibility to provide the best medical and psychological care possible. At the same time, they must collect and preserve the proper medicolegal evidence that is unique to the evaluation of sexual assault cases.

Some sexual assault victims agree to police interviews and investigations, and others do not. Federal legislation guarantees all victims the right to a forensic examination and treatment of sexual assault regardless of their cooperation with a legal investigation or their desire to pursue prosecution initially.[3] Some states require medical personnel treating sexual assault patients to report the assault to local law enforcement, whereas others forbid such reporting without patient consent.[4,5] Clinicians must know their own state laws regarding such reports.[5]

Prepared emergency personnel can help attenuate the psychological and physical impact of sexual assault. Through proper care of the patient and careful acquisition of evidence, emergency medicine staff can provide medical treatment as well as obtain necessary forensic evidence.

DEFINITIONS

Sexual assault refers to any sexual contact between one person and another without appropriate legal consent.[6,7] Physical force may be used to overcome the victim's lack of consent, but this is not mandatory to prove assault. Coercion into sexual contact by intimidation, threats, or fear also defines sexual assault. State laws differ slightly on the definition of exact acts that constitute sexual contact and on which populations are unable to give legal consent.[4] In general, persons under the influence of drugs or alcohol, minors, and those who are mentally incapacitated are considered unable to give consent for sexual contact.

Sexual violence may also occur in the setting of intimate partner violence (IPV), defined by the Centers for Disease Control and Prevention (CDC) as abuse or aggression that occurs in a romantic relationship.[8] Sexual violence in IPV includes forcing or attempting to force a partner to take part in a sexual act, sexual touching, or nonphysical sexual events when a partner does not or cannot provide consent.[8]

Human sex trafficking is defined by US Federal law as the recruitment, harboring, transportation, provision, obtaining, soliciting, or patronizing of a person for a commercial sex act using force, fraud, or coercion or in which the person induced to perform sexual acts is younger than 18 years. These individuals often require ED evaluation and medical care for routine or urgent medical care as well as for care related to their experience of sexual violence.[9,10] EDs are key linchpins in the care of these patients, playing "a crucial role in serving the medical, psychiatric, and social needs of human trafficking survivors, as we are often their only access to medical care and resources."[10] In a survey of 100 survivors of domestic sex trafficking, 63% reported going to an ED while being trafficked.[11] Providers must recognize at-risk patients and provide appropriate care and assistance to victims and suspected victims of human trafficking and recognize multiple forms of human trafficking.

SEXUAL ASSAULT RESPONSE TEAMS AND FORENSIC MEDICAL UNITS

Before the 1990s, sexual assault examinations were mostly the responsibility of emergency clinicians. However, since the early 1990s, nurses or nurse clinicians have been performing an increasing number of sexual assault examinations. Called SANEs or FNEs, these nurses are the core members of SARTs/FMUs. Other members of SARTs/FMUs include law enforcement, victim advocates, prosecutors, and forensic laboratory personnel.

Most examinations still take place in the ED but may be done in a space near the ED or an affiliated clinic. Nurse examiners have formed the International Association of Forensic Nurses. This group has drafted standards of practice for sexual assault examiners' education and the examinations themselves. Advantages include the following:

- The practitioner performing the examination is specifically dedicated to treating the patient with a history of sexual assault, not task-switching between multiple patients in a busy ED.[12]
- The clinician has usually completed more extensive training on sexual assault examination, and evidence collection; they, accordingly, may perform a more comprehensive examination with better evidence collection.[13,14]
- Designated SANEs/FNEs may have more trauma-informed behavior deriving from a deeper understanding of and consideration for the emotional needs of the victim covered in their additional subspecialty training.[15]

EVALUATION AND TREATMENT FOR FORENSIC MEDICAL EXAMINATION

Triage and Transfer Considerations

Victims of sexual assault should be considered a priority and triaged appropriately. An initial prompt medical assessment should be performed to determine acute injuries, the need for trauma care, and assess the safety needs of patients before collecting evidence.[16] Acute medical needs take priority over evidence collection. Patients should be advised not to eat or drink, change clothes, wash, urinate, or defecate or smoke until evaluated by the examiner. If voiding occurs, preservation of a first-stream urine sample without cleansing is valuable and should be transferred as a specimen along with the patient. Samples should be appropriately labeled including initials and date and sealed; this facilitates maintenance of chain of evidence. If patients are being transferred to another facility to access SART resources, patients should be cleared medically and stable for transfer. In some regions, the SANE or FNE may travel to the location of the victim; thus the transferring team should be aware of local laws and procedures.

Triage is also a time when questions addressing the patient's safety at home and identifying suspected victims of human trafficking and IPV may be asked. The answers to these questions should be reviewed by the treating clinician. The National Human Trafficking Hotline is available for assistance and to report suspected trafficking at 888-373-7888. For additional training and awareness on human trafficking, the Department of Homeland Security offers courses through the Blue Campaign. Courses can be accessed on their website: dhs.gov/blue-campaign.[17]

Most often local jurisdictions or hospitals provide clinicians with detailed forms and instructions for the examination and documentation of sexual assault. This chapter is meant to supplement such instructions and forms. Clinicians should be familiar with local documents before performing a sexual assault examination. Careful step-by-step planning and the use of written protocols ensure the best care for victims, aid in the prosecution of guilty assailants, and the exoneration of wrongly accused subjects.

ED personnel must secure patient privacy and designate a separate area for the care of sexually assaulted patients. If medically and logistically possible, interviews should be conducted in a private room separate from the examination room. Law enforcement or other governmental agencies may provide examination kits to collect forensic evidence from victims. These kits may be available in the ED, and if available, staff should be familiar with them. If such kits are not provided by local sources, hospital staff may need to assemble their kits from material found in most EDs. Prepared kits, widely commercially available, can save a tremendous amount of nursing and clinician time. A checklist of local requirements for sexual assault examination should be included in the kits and serve as a reminder for all the necessary medicolegal procedures to be completed.

Guidelines for the evaluation of special populations, including adult male sexual assault patients, pediatric patients, gender-nonconforming patients, and accused assailants, are provided in separate sections of this chapter. The same examiners designated to perform adult female examinations may easily perform male victim and assailant examinations; however, the examination of a pediatric sexual assault patient often requires considerable additional expertise and training. When possible, medical staff with specialized training in the examination of pediatric sexual assault patients should perform these examinations. If this is not possible, the section on Child Sexual Assault Examinations should provide emergency medical personnel with a basic framework to perform an initial examination.

Consent

Consent for the evaluation and treatment of a sexual assault patient is mandatory. The patient has undergone an experience in which their right to grant or deny consent was taken from them, and obtaining consent for medical treatment and gathering evidence has important psychological and legal implications. A patient with capacity, or their designee, can decline medicolegal examination and even medical treatment. Before beginning evaluation and treatment, obtain witnessed, written, informed consent in language understandable to the patient for medical evaluation and treatment and consent for evidence collection and release to law enforcement.[16] If no local forensic examination forms are available, use the standard ED "consent to treat" forms, but ensure that the patient is well informed and gives verbal consent to each step of the examination. Although a few states mandate that medical personnel report sexual assault to law enforcement, patients may choose to not discuss the event with police.[5,16] If the patient cannot give consent for a forensic examination because of a reversible process (e.g., intoxication, an acute psychological reaction), clinicians should wait until the patient is capacitated and able to provide consent. When patients cannot give consent because of minor status or a developmental disability, the person authorized to give medical consent for the patient may give consent for the examination unless that person is a suspect in the assault. State laws differ in the age of consent for adolescents and in examiners' requirements to attempt contact of the legal guardian (unless the guardian is a suspected perpetrator).[19] Emergency personnel must be familiar with local laws concerning these requirements. In the rare case that a patient cannot give consent as a result of a potentially irreversible medical condition, such as severe head trauma and coma, seek the advice of institutional legal counsel before proceeding with a forensic examination. In some cases, the next of kin/medical power of attorney may provide the needed consent, whereas in other cases, it may be necessary to obtain a court order to proceed.

History

The history of the event should be victim-centered and include only the elements necessary to complete the required forms, to perform a focused physical examination, and to collect evidence. Questions beyond this, such as the details leading up to the assault, should be left to police investigators. Overly detailed discussion of the assault can retraumatize the patient. Limiting the history shortens the ED evaluation and helps prevent discrepancies between the ED history and the official police investigation report, which could weaken the victim's case in court. Document the pertinent medical history, including the last menstrual period; current contraception; substance use with medical relevance to chief complaint; recent perineal, anal, or genital injuries/surgeries; and preexisting medical conditions or injuries.

The history of the event required usually includes the time, date, and place of the alleged assault and a description of the use of force, threats of force, and the type of assault. Elements of force may include the type of violence used (e.g., grabbing, hitting, kicking, strangling, weapon use), threats of violence, the use of restraints, the number of assailants, assailants, any suspected substance-facilitated assault, and any loss of consciousness experienced by the patient. Sexually assaultive acts may include manual or oral fondling (of breasts, genitalia, or both); vaginal, oral or anal penetration or attempted penetration (with fingers, penis, or other objects); and/or ejaculation on or in the body. The use or non-use of a condom or lubricants should be noted. The use of physical force or violence is partly a police matter. Still, from a medical standpoint, it is desirable to correlate positive findings on the physical examination (e.g., abrasions, ecchymosis, and scratches) with a description of any force, restraint, or violence.

Include the patient's postassault activity, which is commonly requested on the necessary documentation, including douching, bathing, urinating, defecating, gargling, and brushing teeth. These activities can alter the recovery of seminal specimens and other sexual assault evidence. However, hygiene activities should not deter the clinician from collecting evidence because perpetrator DNA has been recovered from the patient's skin even after multiple showers. In addition, obtain a good history from the patient about potential injuries and body trauma that may have occurred before the assault as well as recent consensual sexual activity, seeking to document preexisting or unintentional genital trauma that might alter the expected normal genital appearance.

A patient's sex assigned at birth should be asked, as well as their current gender identity. Patients should be asked about history of previous gynecologic or urologic surgery, including gender-affirming surgery. One way to inquire about this in patient-centric manner for transgender patients is to ask: "Have you had any gender-affirming procedures?".[20] The type of procedure and timing should be elicited on history and documented in the chart. Patients with prior gender-affirming surgical procedures may also need completion of an anatomical inventory in the electronic medical record.[20–22]

Elements of the victim's history should help in deciding which potential samples to collect. The risk of negative genital swab results after sexual intercourse increases by approximately 3% per hour, however sperm may be recovered from the cervix even days after intercourse.[23,24] Cervical samples are now recommended in all cases that will involve speculum examination because of greater forensic yield. Additionally, the posterior fornix should be swabbed for sperm recovery as it might have superior yield as compared to the external genitalia; combining these sample sites yields the best results.[24] Obtain a gynecologic and urologic history in preparation for documentation of injuries and treatment plans. The history should also include the use of any method of birth control (with information regarding any missed birth control pills), last normal menstrual period, last voluntary intercourse, gravidity and parity, and recent sexually transmitted infections (STIs). As with all assaulted patients, the medical history should include current medications, tetanus immunization status, and allergies.

Patients should be directly asked about the act of strangulation using easy-to-understand terminology. Strangulation is defined as asphyxia caused by external pressure or blunt force to the neck, resulting in restriction and partial or complete closure of air passages and blood vessels.[25,26] Strangulation combined with sexual assault increases the risk of the victim experiencing future lethal violence and may be a tool used in IPV to control the victim.[25] A cross-sectional study found that 58% of nonfatal strangulation (NFS) sexual assault cases involved an intimate partner.[27] Prior NFS increased the odds of attempted homicide by six-fold and completed homicide by seven-fold.[28] NFS is categorized as a distinct criminal felony in 48 states, and forensic medical documentation can support the victim, law enforcement officers, and prosecutor in holding the perpetrator legally responsible.[29] Symptoms of strangulation may include dysphonia, dysphagia, dyspnea, hyperventilation, vision loss or impairment, agitation, impulsivity, difficulty concentrating, hearing changes, and memory loss.[26,30]

While taking the history, observe the patient's ability to understand and respond appropriately to questions. Victims of sexual assault may not possess the capacity to consent to intercourse because of a developmental disability, young age, or intoxication with drugs or alcohol. Consider reported and suspected presence of substances when the history suggests impaired consciousness and pursue indicated testing accordingly. Patients who lack consenting capacity because of a developmental disability may have sufficient prior documentation of the condition. In the instance in which an examiner suspects a previously undocumented developmental disability, a formal examination of the patient's mental capacity can be performed at a later time.

Physical Examination

Physical examination of a sexual assault patient differs from most other ED examinations in that examiners are not only caring for a patient's physical and mental well-being but also investigating a crime scene and collecting specific evidence. As always, patiently explain every step of the examination process to the patient. Remind the patient to communicate any discomfort or questions during the examination and to ask for a break from the examination if needed. In addition, remind the patient of their right to decline any portion of the examination and the ability to stop at any point. Each patient should have the opportunity to have a family member, friend, victim advocate, or any combination of such individuals in the room during all parts of the examination, if they so desire.

Collection of Clothing

If not already collected by law enforcement, collect the clothes that the victim wore during the assault for potential evidence. Ask the patient to disrobe by dropping their clothes onto a large piece of paper or a disposable underpad that is protected from the floor by a sheet. Using gloved hands, place each item of clothing in a separate paper bag. Label all collected material meticulously and describe it in the chart. Labels should include date, time, contents, and name of person who collected clothing. Bundle the paper or underpad and any material that might have fallen during the patient's disrobing and place it in a separate paper bag. Minute amounts of blood, semen, and/or saliva can produce a DNA profile. When properly dried and free of moisture, DNA can persist in swabs and on clothing for years at room temperature. Therefore ensure that clothing has air-dried before packaging (note that heat-drying may destroy evidence). The DNA profile obtained by the laboratory can be uploaded into the Federal Bureau of Investigation (FBI)'s CODIS (Combined DNA Index System) database and identify an unknown assailant. Be sensitive when taking clothing, considering evidentiary value and the patient's future release from the ED. When a victim's clothing must be collected, ensure that suitable clothing will be available for the patient to wear home after release from the ED.

General Body Examination

After the patient disrobes and is placed in a gown, examine their body for signs of trauma and foreign material. Uncover only one part of the body at a time to examine and then carefully recover it. This allows the patient to retain some modesty during the examination. Important nongenital focus areas for evaluation are the neck (particularly if there is concern for NFS injury), back, thighs, breasts, wrists, and ankles (particularly if restraints were used). Even in the absence of visible erythema, abrasion or ecchymosis, note all tender areas during the examination. Evidence from the physical surroundings of the assault can occasionally be found in the hair or on the skin. Retain such material as evidence. Document areas of trauma and evaluate further (e.g., with radiographs) as indicated by the type and extent of injury.

According to a study of 1163 sexually assaulted females from Australia, 71% had some form of general body injury, classified as mild in severity in 52%, moderate in 17%, and severe in 2% of victims.[31] Document these injuries because they correlate significantly with successful prosecution of perpetrators.[32] Bodily evidence of general injury may range from minor abrasions and areas of tenderness to obvious deformities from major blunt force or penetrating trauma. If the victim has not bathed, bodily evidence in the form of dried semen stains may be visible on the hair or the skin of the victim. In a darkened room, dried semen (and, unfortunately, many other substances) on skin may fluoresce under examination with shortwave light, such as that produced by a Woods lamp or an alternate light source, but may also be noticed equally well by its reflective appearance under regular room lighting.[33–35] Use moistened swabs to collect potential dried secretions; then air-dry them thoroughly and preserve as evidence. Visible dried secretions may be semen or saliva stains. If the history indicates oral contact or ejaculation in specific areas, these areas should be sampled using moistened swabs even if no dried secretions are visible. Fragments of the assailant's skin, blood, facial hair, or other foreign material from the assault site may be trapped beneath a victim's fingernails. Obtain fingernail scrapings by cleaning under a victim's nails with a toothpick or small swab or by cutting the nails closely over a clean piece of paper. Fingernail samples should be collected in such a way as to maximize the detection of foreign DNA and minimize the amount of the patient's cells present, using only light pressure to avoid any injury or bleeding to the patient. Fold the toothpick and debris into the paper, place it in an envelope, and package it with the other specimens. Collect tampons from menstruating individuals (including cisgender females and transgender males), air-dry them, and place them in a separate paper collection bag.

Imaging

Photographs can be a valuable addition to the documentation of bodily injury. Medical institutions may direct the use of facility-issued smart phones for documentation of injuries in the chart or employ professional-quality photographic teams. The use of reflective UV imaging may be employed to detect more detail, including strangulation signs and bite marks. Other institutions must rely on law enforcement for photographic documentation.[36] The Sexual Assault Forensic Examination (SAFE) protocol recommends that examiners should take these photographs due to the sensitive nature of the photography involved and because "patients are often more comfortable and less traumatized when [SANEs/FNEs] photographs"; institutions may require separate patient consent for photographs taken by hospital personnel.[37] Optimally, institutions should have a prearranged plan to handle media according to a written "chain of custody." The photographs should be labeled immediately and may be added to the legal evidence.[16] In some jurisdictions, photographs of physical injuries will be taken and retained by an accompanying law officer. These photographs may serve as evidence or may simply refresh the examiner's memory at the time of the trial.

Alternative light source (ALS) photography is an important tool used by forensic specialists and is recommended by the Department of Justice. While not readily available to most emergency medicine providers, it is becoming more widely used due to its ability to detect subdermal bruising and ability to detect both biologic and nonbiologic evidence such as lubricants and creams used to facilitate sexual assault.[33,36,38] All substances that fluoresce or absorb should be documented, photographed, and swabbed. Positive ALS findings are not necessarily indicative of injury, but positive ALS findings that are present after cleaning or are supported by physical examination such as tenderness to palpation are more suggestive of injury.[36,38] Providers should be aware that it may be more difficult to detect absorption on victims with darker skin tones and that this can create an unjust disparity in evidence collection.[39–41] Prior work has indicated that "dark skin color, rather than race, was a strong predictor for decreased (identified) injury prevalence" and concluded that assault forensic examiners may not be as able to readily detect injuries in individuals with dark skin tones.[39]

Oral Evaluation

If directed by the history, inspect the oral cavity closely for signs of trauma and collect evidence if indicated. Mouth injuries from forced oral sexual contact may include lacerations of the labial or lingual frenulum, mucosal lacerations, or abrasions). Injury to the lips is often produced by the patient's teeth as their lips are forced inward during forced oral penetration. Potential injuries to the posterior pharyngeal wall and soft palate include contusions, submucosal hemorrhage, and lacerations (Fig. 59.1B). Document these injuries at the initial examination because mucosal injuries heal quickly and may not be present hours or days later. Collect potential evidence with swabs rubbed between the teeth and the buccal mucosa on both the upper and lower gingival surfaces bilaterally. Spermatozoa have been identified in oral smears for hours after the attack despite brushing the teeth, using mouthwash, or drinking various fluids and may provide valuable evidence up to 12 hours after examination.[42,43] Collect any foreign material (e.g., hair) to include as potential evidence. During the oral inspection, local law enforcement may request that examiners collect buccal cell swabs to provide the crime laboratory with a sample for victim DNA reference.

Neck Examination

Strangulation may result in no physical findings or apparent injury and is often missed or under-evaluated. Approximately half of NFS victims will have some form of visible injury, often in the form of faint erythema or bruising, petechiae

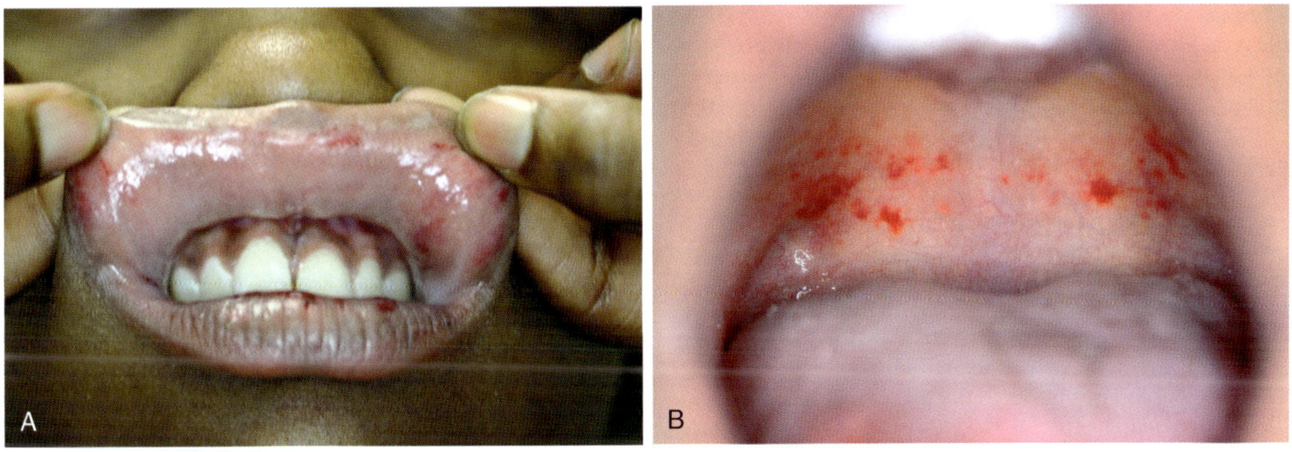

Fig. 59.1 Oral injuries incurred as a result of sexual assault. (A) Mucosal labial injury after forced oral copulation. (B) Petechial hemorrhage seen on the soft palate after a similar assault.

or patterned marks from either hands/fingerails or ligature, depending on if the strangulation was manual or with a ligature.[44] While tracheal or hyoid fractures are rare, up to half of NFS victims may have voice changes.[30,45] More serious injuries, including fractures, should be suspected if there is crepitus or dysphonia/dysphagia accompanied by rapid airway obstruction.[30,44,45]

Neurologic deficits, including changes in vision, ptosis, unilateral weakness, or a facial droop, may occur due to injury to the injury to the vascular structures including the vertebral or carotid arteries. Document all subjective and objectively observed findings on neurological examination and evaluate further (e.g., with diagnostic imaging of cerebral vasculature and/or brain) as indicated by the type and extent of injury.[26,30,45] If the event resulted in a period of hypoxia, the victim may have altered mentation including encephalopathy.[7,30,45]

Genital Examination and Evidence Recovery

Once the patient is in the lithotomy position, inspect the thighs and perineum for signs of trauma and for foreign material such as seminal stains. Use an ultraviolet light again to look at suspicious dried secretions. Many jurisdictions recommend routine collection of swabs from the external genital area because of the high likelihood of evidence being present after drainage from the vaginal vault and the inconsistent fluorescence of seminal fluid with a Wood's lamp.[7,16,37]

Pubic Hair Samples

If local crime laboratories request pubic hair samples, proceed with the following protocol. Before the internal pelvic examination, comb the patient's pubic hair for foreign material (particularly pubic hair belonging to the assailant). Place clean paper below the victim's buttocks with the patient in the lithotomy position and comb the pubic hair onto the paper. Fold these hairs and the comb into the paper and place them directly in an appropriate storage container such as a large paper envelope to be given to law enforcement. Foreign pubic hairs can often provide enough cellular DNA material from the root to enable the crime laboratory to perform DNA analysis. In addition, specialized laboratories possess the capability of performing mitochondrial DNA analysis from the hair shaft in many cases.

Significant hair transfer occurs in less than 5% of assaults.[46] For the small minority of cases in which crime laboratories desire to compare foreign suspect hairs with the victim's hair, a sample pulled from the patient may be requested. Although pulling the patient's hair from the roots may provide the best sample, this collection method is painful, considered insensitive, and not recommended by these authors during the initial evaluation. Additionally, many agencies perform DNA testing on any hair recovered initially, rendering microscopic comparison with victim hairs superfluous.[7,16] In the very rare case when it is requested, a patient can provide the hairs at a later time.

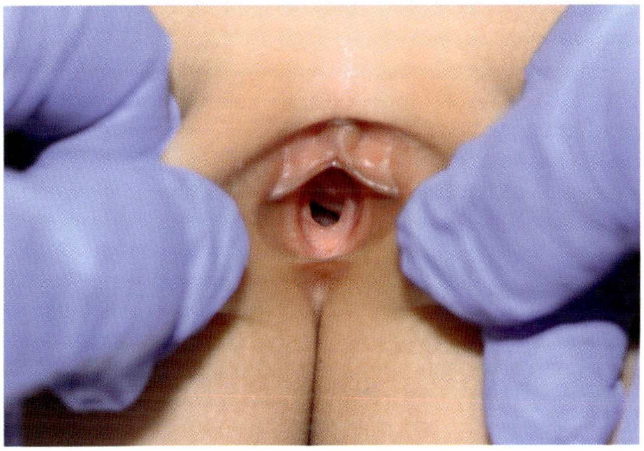

Fig. 59.2 The normal hymen in a prepubertal female as seen with inferior labial traction.

Genital examination of a sexual assault patient differs considerably from most ED pelvic examinations. First, carefully explain what you are doing to the patient. For patients with a vulva (including cisgender females, transgender females who have had vulvoplasty/vaginoplasty, and some transgender males), perform a careful visual evaluation of the vulva and vaginal introitus for signs of trauma. Use of the following techniques of separation and traction will help to move the tissues that are most likely to undergo injury into view. In performing separation, use both hands to gently separate the labia laterally in each direction and inspect the posterior fourchette and vaginal introitus. Similarly, in performing traction, use both hands to hold each labium majus and apply gentle inferior labial traction (i.e., toward the examiner); this gives a much-improved view of the hymen, especially in prepubertal females (Fig. 59.2). If these maneuvers are not performed, traumatic genital injuries may be missed.

Familiarity with typical cisgender female (Fig. 59.3) and male (Fig. 59.4) genital anatomy, including all terms, is important for accurate descriptions. Intersex adults will often be familiar with, and can inform the examiner of, any differences in their own anatomy from typical norms. When caring for transgender patients who have had gender-affirming "bottom" surgery, familiarity with the postoperative appearance of patients who have undergone phalloplasty, metoidioplasty, vaginoplasty, or vulvoplasty is also appropriate; the same terms are used for the relevant elements of anatomy constructed via gender-affirming surgery as for natal structures.[47–49] Although some novice examiners anticipate a detailed focus on detecting injuries to the hymen, the majority of sexual assault–related vaginal injuries occur to the posterior fourchette and/or fossa navicularis (Fig. 59.5).[50,51] In fact, hymenal injuries are extremely rare in sexually active adult females and are more commonly observed in sexually inexperienced adolescents (Fig. 59.6).[52–54] While injuries to the vaginal walls and cervix are more uncommon, these may be discovered during the speculum examination and should be sought in cases of sexual assault where there was penetration with an object.[55]

Reported rates of genital injury in forensically examined patients range from 6% to 20% without colposcopy to 53% to 87% with colposcopy.[50,52,56] Most importantly, examiners must be cognizant of the fact that even completely normal findings on genital examination remain consistent with forced sexual assault.[56–58] Limitations in variation of quality of the examination, use of colposcopy and tissue staining dye are a challenge in determining the true epidemiology of sexual assault without injury on genital examination but multiple studies show that injuries and normal findings can occur with both consensual and nonconsensual contact.[58,59] A study of more than 1000 sexual assault patients found that almost half of all victims with forensic evidence positive for sperm had no genital injury.[53] Another study found that genital injury was detectable in only 24% of females reporting assault with completed vaginal penetration.[60]

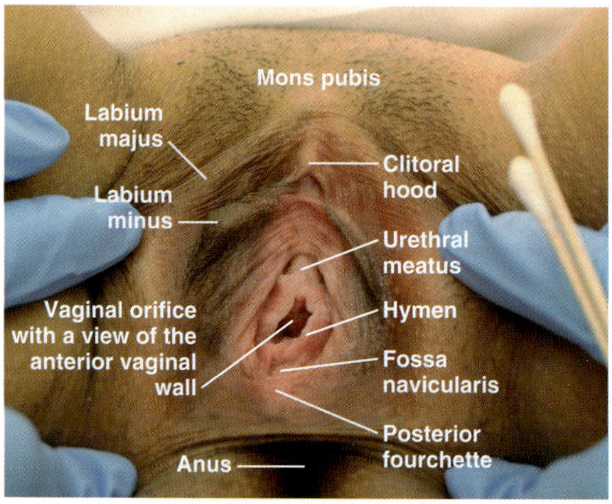

Fig. 59.3 Normal female anatomy.

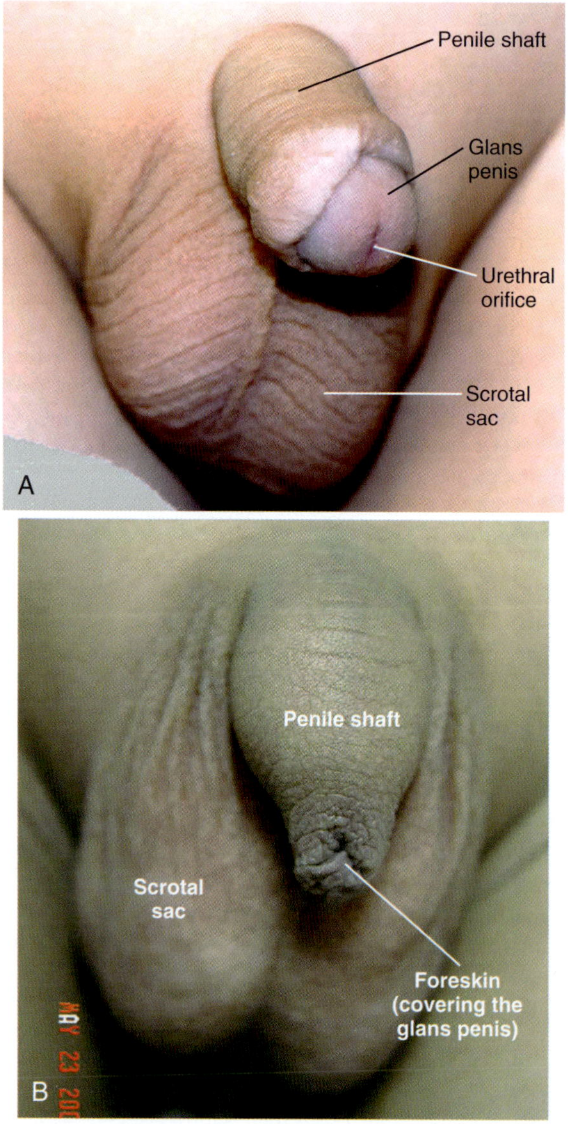

Fig. 59.4 Normal male anatomy. (A) Circumcised. (B) Uncircumcised.

Colposcopy

Teixeira first described the use of colposcopy for documentation of sexual assault in 1981.[61] Although it is not readily available, nor a standard of care in most EDs, the use of colposcopy has revolutionized the documentation of injury.[50,54] The colposcope provides magnification, a bright light source, and usually permanent documentation of injuries in the form of still images or video (mainly in digital format but occasionally traditional film). In one small study, the colposcope increased the rate of detection of genital injury from 6% to 53%.[54] Colposcopes with photo or video attachments provide excellent photographic documentation for the court and allow review by expert practitioners for court testimony without subjecting the victim to reexamination. Experienced sexual assault examiner programs are increasingly using high-quality digital single-lens reflex cameras mounted on a tripod to obtain excellent images that are indistinguishable from those obtained with colposcopy. ED practitioners may have access to such equipment. Colposcopically visible injuries have also been described in adolescent females after the first consensual intercourse; hence, genital injury does not always translate to nonconsensual vaginal penetration.[58] Conversely, totally normal findings on genital examination by colposcopy are often found after sexual assault. Even in sexually inexperienced adolescents, forced penetration can occur without leaving discernible genital injury.[58] Although previous sexual experience by the victim decreases the likelihood of finding genital injury, experts cannot fully explain the reasons why some rape

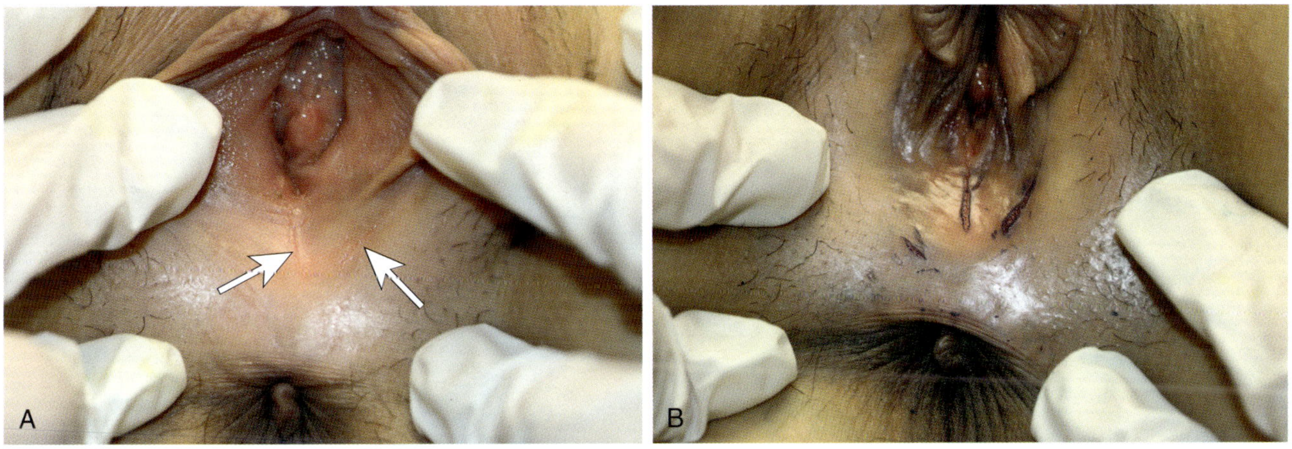

Fig. 59.5 The majority of sexual assault–related vaginal injuries occur to the posterior fourchette. (A) Superficial epithelial injuries *(arrows)* to this region may be difficult to appreciate. (B) Application of toluidine blue dye highlights the injury.

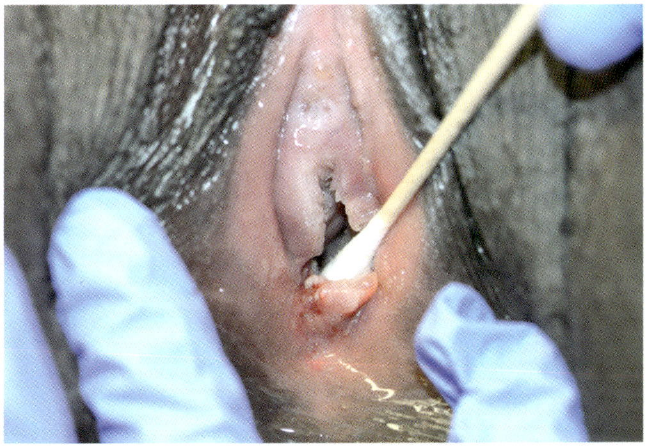

Fig. 59.6 Hymenal injury at the 6-o'clock position, usually found in adolescent girls. Such injuries are uncommon in adults.

victims sustain measurable genital injury whereas others do not.[57,59]

Swab Collection

Protocols for collection of evidence vary by legal jurisdiction. The following discussion draws from the model protocol suggested by the US Department of Justice, State of California, and the *American College of Emergency Physicians Manual*.[7,16]

Obtain standard specimens during inspection of the external genitalia, rectum, vagina, and cervix. Lubricate the speculum as usual for cisgender females. Special considerations for transgender patients include: use of the smallest speculum possible for transgender males given hypo-estrogenic state/atrophy of vulvovaginal structures and the use of an anoscope for the pelvic examination rather than a speculum for patients who have undergone surgery with vaginoplasty.[62] Lubricant use is no longer considered a potential threat to evidence recovery and should be used for patient comfort per examiner protocol. Generally, the specimens collected will be determined by the patient's history and local protocol. Several swabs from the vaginal pool and the external genitalia should be obtained and then applied over clean slides for a dry mount. In addition, collect cervical swabs. The crime laboratory may recover sperm from cervical specimens up to 12 days or more after coitus.[23,42,43,56] Label all slides and then allow them to air-dry. Package swabs and slides in paper envelopes for the local crime laboratory. Some EDs maintain specific equipment (i.e., a dry box) to aid in the drying of specimens; in others, the swabs and slides must be left out until completely dried. Obtain samples from the perineal area, flake off or swab dried secretions using a moist swab followed by a dried swab. Place flaked dried secretions in a provided container. Air-dry swabs and slides and place in an envelope, labeled and sealed accordingly.[7,16]

Due to the extreme sensitivity of new DNA tests, exercise caution to prevent contamination of samples. Wear gloves at all times during specimen collection and packaging. Consider masking and take care not to inadvertently sneeze, spit, or cough on or near samples.

Testing for STIs

The majority of SART programs in the United States do not routinely perform STI testing on adults and adolescents.[13] Among sexually active adults, identification of an STI at the time of a forensic examination likely represents infection acquired before the assault, and is unlikely to be helpful to, and may in some cases be prejudicial in, the individual's pursuit of legal action against their assailant.[63] It is important to remember that STIs remain common: the CDC estimates 1 in 5 US residents have an STI, with an incidence of 26 million new infections per year, where youth aged 15 to 24 account for nearly half of all new infections.[64–66] Given this, there is a potential medical benefit to the sexually active adolescent or adult patient in their clinician identifying and treating an extant sexually transmitted infection that should be considered on an individualized basis and with shared decision-making with the patient. Clinicians might want to consider obtaining samples for culture or nucleic acid amplification tests (NAATs) from child victims in whom the presence of an STI would be indicative of previous sexual contact.[67]

In cases where STI testing is desired or felt to be indicated, it should include NAAT for *Chlamydia trachomatis* and *Neisseria gonorrhoeae* at the site of penetration or attempted penetration. People with the potential for trichomoniasis (including cisgender females, transgender females who have had vulvoplasty/vaginoplasty, and transgender males with vaginas)

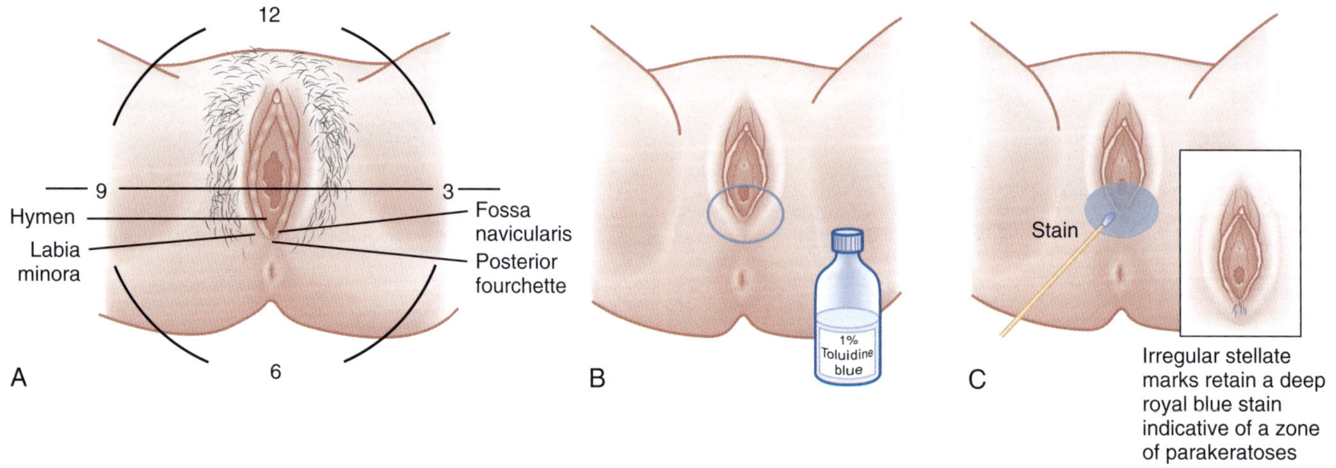

Fig. 59.7 (A) During a sexual assault, injuries are often multiple and typically occur between the 3-, 6-, and 9-o'clock positions. (B–C) Traumatic skin injuries can be highlighted by applying toluidine blue to the perineum and vaginal area and then wiping it off to show the lesions. (A, From Marx J. *Rosen's Emergency Medicine: Concepts and Clinical Practice*. 6th ed. Elsevier; 2006.)

should be offered NAAT testing for *Trichomonas vaginalis* via urine or vaginal specimen. Males who have sex with males (MSM) reporting receptive oral or anal sex within the prior twelve months should be offered screening for *C. trachomatis* and *N. gonorrhoeae* regardless of the type of sexual contact that occurred during the assault. All interested patients should be offered the opportunity to have serum samples obtained for HIV, hepatitis B virus (HBV), hepatitis C virus (HCV), and syphilis testing.

Toluidine Blue Staining and Photography

Toluidine blue dye is a nuclear stain, also used for cancer detection and mast cell staining, which highlights areas of injury. It adheres to areas denuded by abrasions and lacerations where the epidermal layer of nonnucleated cells has been removed (Figs. 59.7 and 59.8).[68] The underlying nucleated cells take up the dye. The dye can significantly enhance the examiner's ability to visualize and photographically document more subtle genital and mucosal injuries (see Fig. 59.8; also Fig. 59.5B).[40] Genital lacerations may provide corroborating evidence of specific details of a case of nonconsensual intercourse (although lesions may be seen up to 50% of the time after consensual intercourse).[41,69,70] To outline injuries, apply a 1% aqueous solution of toluidine blue dye to the perineum and wipe the excess dye off with a cotton ball moistened with lubricating jelly. After the excess dye is removed, any areas that retain the stain signify an epidermal disruption. Separate any folds of the area and carefully examine them to avoid missing injuries. Ideally, the dye should be applied before speculum examination to eliminate the possibility of iatrogenic injury. The procedure is described in Fig. 59.7 and Box 59.1. As noted, injuries detected with the aid of toluidine blue dye are not specific for sexual assault because such injuries have also been found after consensual intercourse, especially in adolescents.[40,41,69–72] Considerations for photography are similar to colposcopy.

Collect external genital samples before the application of toluidine blue to avoid washing away potential DNA evidence. The use of toluidine blue dye itself does not interfere with DNA evidence from vaginal specimens, and it has proved safe for mucosal application.[73,74]

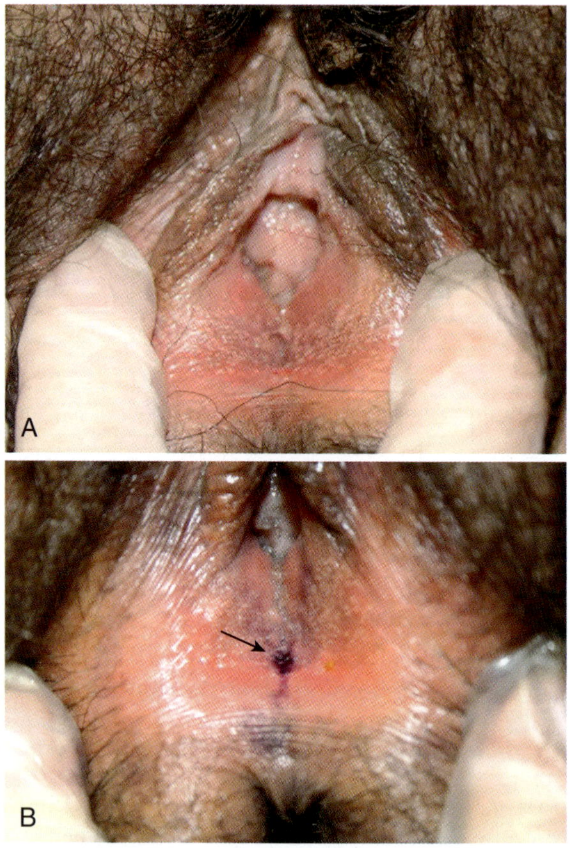

Fig. 59.8 Posterior fourchette injury (A) before and (B) after application of toluidine blue dye. Toluidine dye highlights an injury that would likely go unnoticed without dye application.

Anal Evaluation

The anal examination follows the genital examination in most cases (Fig. 59.9). Documentation of anal penetration holds significant value because it is a separate offense in addition to other forms of penetration, and therefore may increase criminal penalties. First, gently separate the anal folds to look for lacerations and abrasions, and collect two external anal swabs. If desired, apply toluidine blue as outlined in the genital section. Clean the dye off thoroughly. If anoscopy is not indicated

BOX 59.1 Toluidine Blue[a] Staining of the Perineum to Detect Microabrasion[b]

1. Collect all external genital specimens as indicated by examination before application of the dye.[c]
2. Before speculum examination or anoscopy, apply 1% toluidine blue to the entire vulva (labia majora, labia minora, posterior fourchette, perineal body, and perianal area). The anus may also be stained. Do not use dye in the vaginal vault or mucous membranes.
3. Allow it to dry for approximately 1 minute.
4. Remove excess dye with water-soluble lubricant by gently blotting the area until the excess dye is removed.
5. DO NOT rub the area.
6. Photograph the area if indicated.
7. The dye will fade in 1 to 2 days.

[a]*Pre-filled swabs consisting of a soft foam applicator tip and reservoir of 1% toluidine blue dye are widely commercially available.*
[b]*See Fig. 59.7.*
[c]*This does not interfere with DNA or semen testing.*
Modified from the technique described by the National Forensic Nursing Institute based on work by McCauley J, Gorman RL, Guzinski G. Toluidine Blue in the Detection of Perineal Lacerations in Pediatric and Adolescent Sexual Abuse Victims. Pediatrics. 1986;78(6):1039–1043 and Lauber AA, Souma ML. Use of Toluidine Blue for Documentation of Traumatic Intercourse. Obstet Gynecol. 1982;60(5):644–648.

or planned, collect the internal rectal sample as follows: separate the anal folds as much as possible by applying gentle lateral or vertical traction, clean the external anal skin with water and gauze, and then insert swabs approximately 2 cm into the anus. Gently move them in a circular motion and then remove them. Use the swabs to make slides, air-dry them, and then include them in the evidence sent to the crime laboratory. Anoscopy is indicated to document potential internal mucosal injuries in victims who report anal penetration or who describe loss of consciousness during the assault. Perform this procedure in the same manner as diagnostic anoscopy to evaluate other anal or rectal emergencies in the ED. Collecting the internal rectal specimens at the end of the anoscope is best to prevent contamination from any external sample being dragged internally. In one retrospective observational study of male patients, the use of anoscopy and colposcopy provided superior documentation of injuries over colposcopy alone.[75] The location of anoscopically detected injuries may be recorded geographically on an imaginary clock face as with vaginal injuries.

Blood Tests

Some crime laboratories request blood samples for DNA reference, toxicology analysis, or both. Include these samples with the material sent to law enforcement. When collecting blood for toxicology testing, record the exact date and time of collection on the specimen so that the criminalist may estimate the dose and timing of substances used by perpetrators to facilitate the assault. Comprehensive metabolic panels are routinely sent for patients who might elect to initiate postexposure prophylactic (PEP) medications.

Urine Tests

Perform bedside urine or laboratory serum β-human chorionic gonadotripin (β-hCG) testing in all patients of childbearing age with anatomic pregnancy potential to exclude pre-existing pregnancy prior to administering pregnancy and STI prophylaxis. Collect the patient's first available voided urine: as previously noted, preservation of a first-stream urine sample without cleansing is valuable and should be maintained or transferred as a specimen along with the patient. Local crime laboratories may require this sample to optimize recovery of potential evidence. Samples should be appropriately labeled including initials and date and sealed; this facilitates maintenance of chain of evidence.

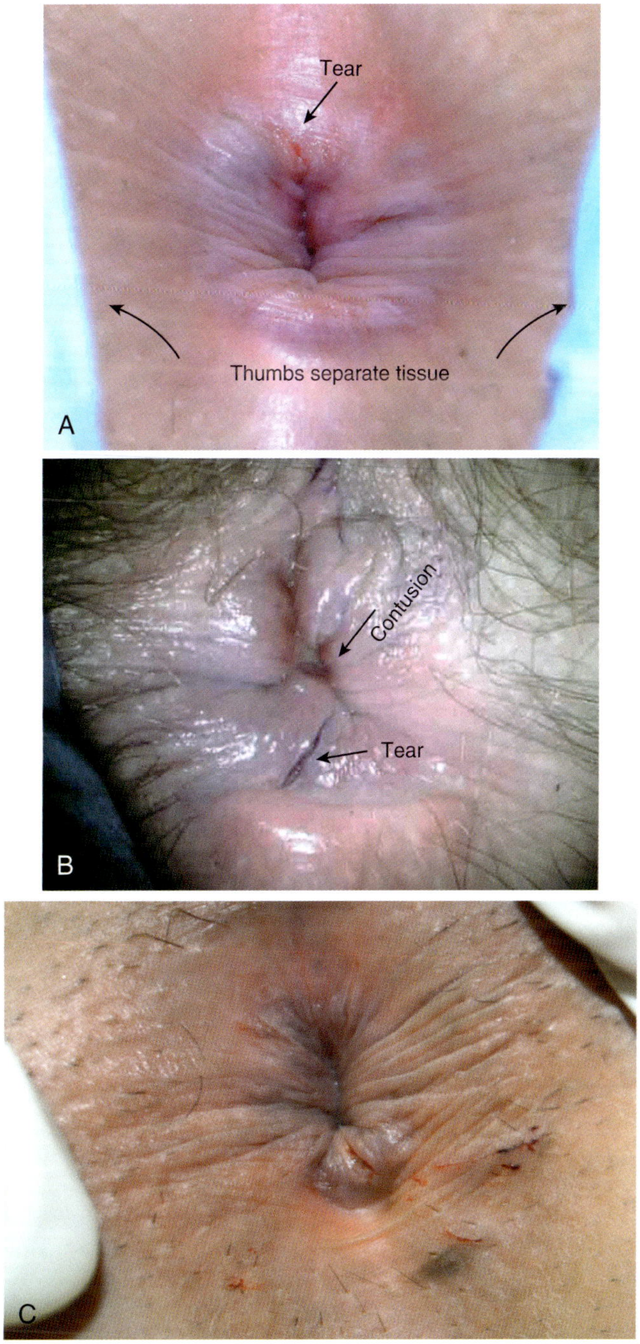

Fig. 59.9 Anal injury is best seen with separation of perianal tissues. (A) Anal tear in a 13-year-old boy after forced penile-anal penetration. (B) Anal contusion and tear *(arrows)* in an adult male after forced penile-anal penetration. (C) Multiple superficial tears to the anus and perianal region.

Spermatozoa, Semen, and DNA Testing

Motile and immotile sperm may be found microscopically in wet mounts of vaginal aspirates and in vaginal, oral, and rectal swabs.[42,43] If formally trained, examiners evaluating the slide microscopically immediately after the physical examination may find sperm in vaginal wet mount specimens, and early discovery of sperm may at times be helpful to law enforcement investigations. However, most ED examiners lack formal training in this process and crime laboratories possess much higher sensitivity for detection of sperm, thus making a negative initial wet mount unhelpful. For these reasons, most examiners do not routinely perform the wet mount examination. After consensual intercourse with a normal ejaculate, laboratory testing of vaginal secretions detects sperm in 50% of specimens 4 days after coitus.[76] However, despite penile penetration during sexual assault, crime laboratories may fail to detect sperm with reasons for failure including, but not limited to inadequate specimen collection, degradation of the ejaculate, azoospermia, failure of the perpetrator to ejaculate, vasectomy in the perpetrator, washing by the victim, or use of a condom. Collection of relevant clothing may prove most important for DNA recovery as laboratories have recovered spermatozoa DNA from laundered clothing as long as 8 months after deposit.[77]

A crime laboratory analyst initially looks for semen in a given sample by searching microscopically for sperm on a concentrated specimen and by testing for other components found in semen. The presence of spermatozoa is the only confirmatory test for semen. As DNA testing technology rapidly changes, the ability of crime laboratories to perform a specific forensic test will vary by location and over time.

Reference Samples

Crime laboratories may request reference samples from various locations on the patient's body to use in comparison testing with potential evidence from the perpetrator. These reference samples may include two buccal swabs collecting mucosal epithelial cells, a blood sample in a designated tube or filter paper card, or even two nasal swabs, especially useful in pediatric cases. The need for such samples will be determined by local protocol.

PHARMACOLOGICAL TREATMENT

STI Prophylaxis

The approach to prophylaxis for potential infections transmitted by sexual assault varies by region, disease prevalence, and local practice and can be influenced by the emotional state of the victim as well as personal and religious viewpoints (Box 59.2).

It is advisable to address the issues of STI, pregnancy, psychological distress, and follow-up in the treatment of a patient with a history of recent sexual assault. Because infection rates before the assault are not known, the risk of contracting an STI as a consequence of a sexual assault has been difficult to determine, and estimates vary widely (Table 59.1).[63,67,78–81] Jenny and colleagues found the postassault incidence of STIs to be 2% for chlamydia and 4% for gonorrhea.[79] The reported rates of 12% for trichomonas and 19% for bacterial vaginosis seem high and may reflect a preexposure infection because male transmission of these infections, especially bacterial vaginosis, is uncommon.[80,81] There are a lack of specific data on risk for the development of herpes, hepatitis B, or HIV infection from sexual assault although transmission has been noted for all of these.[80,82]

Because some patients may have relatively low compliance with attending follow-up visits, most examiners offer, at the least, treatment of gonorrhea, chlamydia, and trichomonas at the time of the initial examination. Though most often termed "prophylaxis," technically this antibiotic administration is considered "treatment," albeit given so early that the disease is subclinical. The CDC recommends empiric treatment for *C. trachomatis*, *N. gonorrhoeae*, and *T. vaginalis* in cisgender females and transgender males with vaginas and empiric

BOX 59.2 Recommended Empirical Emergency Department Testing and Pharmacologic Treatment After Sexual Assault[a]

- No routine STI cultures of adult victims. Testing of pediatric victims may be indicated as a positive test in a child is indicative of abuse. Shared decision-making can guide individualized decisions regarding testing versus empiric prophylaxis in adolescent and adult patients.
- Treat empirically for GC,[b] *Chlamydia*, *Trichomonas* (optional), and bacterial vaginosis (optional).
- Administer a tetanus booster vaccine if indicated.
- If not immunized for hepatitis B or unsure of the victim's vaccination status, give the first dose of vaccine empirically and follow with subsequent vaccination at 1 to 2 and 4 to 6 months, or age-appropriate schedule. If previously vaccinated, the patient may receive a single booster dose. In addition to vaccination, consider HBIG in nonimmune patients after high-risk exposure to a known hepatitis B–positive perpetrator, followed by a full vaccination schedule.
- Patients aged 9–26 years previously unvaccinated or incompletely vaccinated against HPV should receive HPV vaccine on examination with additional doses at 1–2 months and 6 months follow-up. Some previously unvaccinated patients aged 27–45 years may benefit from vaccine series.
- If the suspect is known or suspected to be HIV positive, treat with medications recommended by local ID experts or provided in occupational exposure kits or consider either of the following: tenofovir disoproxil fumarate 300 mg with emtricitabine 200 mg (Truvada) once daily plus raltegravir (Isentress) 400 mg twice daily or dolutegravir (Tivicay) 50 mg for 28 days.
- If the suspect is not known to be HIV positive, there is no consensus on recommendations for treatment, and clinicians must consider each patient individually.[c] This is an area of uncertainty. HIV prophylaxis may be given after a discussion of the risks and benefits with the patient.
- Obtain a pregnancy test and administer pregnancy prevention if not already pregnant and physically able to conceive.

[a]*Treatment regimens are subject to change based on sensitivities and local patterns.*
[b]*Treatment of GC will treat incubating syphilis. Prophylaxis for herpes is not recommended.*
[c]*There are no published data on the effectiveness of HIV postexposure prophylaxis after sexual assault.*
GC, *Gonococci;* HBIG, *hepatitis B immune globulin;* HIV, *human immunodeficiency virus;* HPV, *human papillomavirus;* ID, *infectious disease;* STI, *sexually transmitted infection.*

TABLE 59.1 Risk for Sexually Transmitted Diseases After Sexual Assault

DISEASE	RISK (%)
Gonorrhea	6–18
Chlamydia	4–17
Syphilis	0.5–3
HIV	<1

Assistance with postexposure prophylaxis–related decisions can be obtained by calling the National Clinician's Post Exposure Prophylaxis Hotline (PEP Line) (telephone: 888–448–4911).
From Marx J, ed. Rosen's Emergency Medicine: Concepts and Clinical Practice. 6th ed. Elsevier; 2006.

treatment for *C. trachomatis* and *N. gonorrhoeae* for cisgender males and transgender females with penises.[63,66,81] While inadequate data exist to guide empiric treatment decisions for transgender males with vaginectomy or transgender females with penectomy, shared decision-making around offering treatment remains appropriate. Patients should be instructed to avoid sexual intercourse until completion of their treatment and an additional week thereafter.[63]

With the increasing prevalence of antibiotic-resistant *N. gonorrhoeae*, ceftriaxone in a single intramuscular 500-mg dose (for patients <150 kg) and 1000-mg (for those patients ≥150 kg) is the CDC's most current recommended treatment of choice in targeting gonorrhea after sexual assault.[63] No single-dose regimen for gonorrhea is effective against coexisting *C. trachomatis* infection; patients should therefore receive a 7-day course of doxycycline, 100 mg orally twice daily.[63,81] A single dose of azithromycin is no longer recommended unless significant concern for medication noncompliance or in the case of pregnancy.[63] For people at risk of trichomoniasis, clinicians should administer empiric treatment for *T. vaginalis* with a 7-day course of metronidazole 500 mg orally twice daily. Although effective and recommended by the CDC, these medications may cause significant nausea, vomiting, and diarrhea, which can interfere with the efficacy of pregnancy prophylaxis. One option to circumvent metronidazole-induced emesis interfering with efficacy of concomitantly administered medications is to delay administration by several hours. Box 59.3 provides several options for STI prophylaxis.

Prevention of Hepatitis B

Most sexual assaults involve perpetrators whose hepatitis B status is unknown. In these cases, the CDC recommends hepatitis B vaccination at the time of examination, followed by two more vaccines at the age-appropriate vaccine dose and schedule for previously unvaccinated patients.[83] Previously vaccinated patients may receive a single booster dose only. Give the vaccine to victims as soon as possible after the assault. The CDC recommends giving it within 24 hours, but this may not be possible in all cases. When a perpetrator is known to be hepatitis B antigen–positive and the victim is known to be hepatitis B antigen–negative and has not been adequately vaccinated, the CDC recommends the administration of hepatitis B immune globulin (HBIG) in addition to vaccination.[83] If the patient is first seen by medical providers 14 days or more after the sexual exposure, HBIG is not recommended. Hepatitis B vaccine should be administered simultaneously with HBIG at a separate injection site, and the vaccine series should be completed at subsequent visits. Complete CDC recommendations for treatment of hepatitis B and other STIs in sexual assault victims can be found at the linked citations.[63,83]

BOX 59.3 **CDC-Recommended Regimens for Prevention of Gonorrhea, Chlamydia, and Trichomonas After Sexual Assault[a]**

Ceftriaxone, 500 mg intramuscularly in a single dose (for prevention of *Neisseria gonorrhoeae* infection) for patients <150 kg; 1g intramuscularly in a single dose for patients >150 kg

Plus

Metronidazole, 500 mg orally twice a day for 7 days (for females or trans males for prevention of *Trichomonas* infection and bacterial vaginosis)

Plus

Doxycycline, 100 mg orally twice a day for 7 days (for prevention of *Chlamydia* infection)

Or

Azithromycin, 1 g orally in a single dose (for prevention of Chlamydia infection only if doxycycline contraindicated---as in pregnancy or if significant concern exists for medication non-adherence)

[a]*Because of widespread resistance, fluoroquinolones are no longer recommended. Prophylaxis for hepatitis B (vaccination without hepatitis B immune globulin) is also suggested.*
CDC, *Centers for Disease Control and Prevention.*

Prevention of Hepatitis C

HCV is poorly transmitted through sexual contact, though it is possible. It is more common when there is coinfection with HIV. Unfortunately, there is no known effective postexposure prophylaxis for HCV, though treatment is available for acute infection and is more effective the earlier it is initiated. Thus patients should receive follow-up testing per guidelines.

Prevention of Human Papillomavirus

The human papillomavirus (HPV) can be transmitted during sexual assault and can lead to malignancy. In recent years, the HPV vaccine has become increasingly commonly administered and has been proven safe and highly effective. It is recommended for administration postassault for previously unvaccinated or incompletely vaccinated female and male patients who are aged 9 to 26 years.[63,81] Some adults aged 27 to 45 years may benefit from the vaccine if they are previously unvaccinated or incompletely vaccinated; this decision should be made on a case-by-case basis by the treating provider.[63] The vaccine should be given at time of initial examination with additional doses at 1 to 2 months and 6 months after initiation.

Prevention of HIV Infection

In a non–assault-related scenario, the risk for transmission of HIV from one episode of unprotected consensual receptive vaginal intercourse with an infected individual is approximately 1 in 1000. The incidence with unprotected receptive anal intercourse is significantly higher at 8 to 32 per 1000.[66,82,84] However, sexual assault victims who are forcibly penetrated often sustain tissue injury because of the violent nature of the act, which may increase the rate of transmission of the virus.[82] 40% of sexual assault victims fear contracting HIV after assault and should, at a minimum, receive counseling and the option of taking anti-HIV medication (Fig. 59.10).[85–87] Unfortunately, immediate testing of the perpetrator may not be feasible. It is estimated that a 28-day course of PEP reduces risk of HIV transmission by 80%.[85,88] The PEP recommendation specifies a 28-day medication course for patients with a history of sexual assault, who arrive for care less than 72 hours after the event and when that exposure represents a substantial risk for transmission (i.e., mucosal contact with genital secretions).[85,88] A combination of tenofovir disoproxil fumarate 300 mg with emtricitabine 200 mg (Truvada, Descovy) once daily plus raltegravir 400 mg twice daily (Isentress, Merk) or dolutegravir 50 mg (Tivicay, Viiv Healthcare), is the current preferred regimen.[85] As with occupational exposure, antiretroviral medications should be initiated as soon as possible after exposure. HIV seroconversion due to failures of PEP following sexual exposure have been reported.[89] For sexual assault exposure with a perpetrator of unknown HIV status, the CDC states PEP as well as the potential referral for consideration of preexposure prophylaxis (PrEP) for high-risk individuals must be addressed by practitioners on an individual case-by-case basis.[90,91] The CDC recommendations provide a useful framework to approach individual decisions in prescribing HIV PEP (https://www.cdc.gov/mmwr/volumes/74/rr/rr7401a1.htm).[91a]

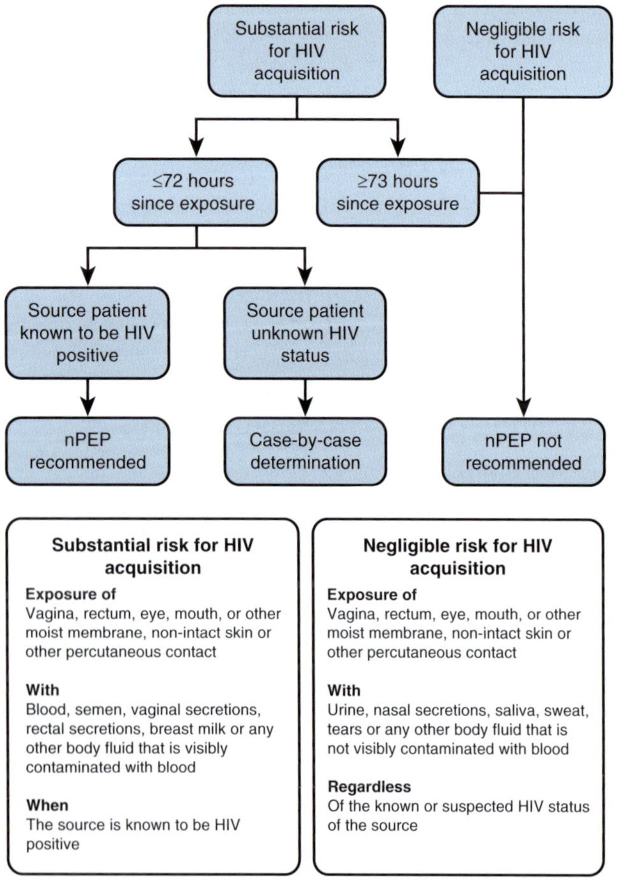

Fig. 59.10 Centers for Disease Control and Prevention algorithm for evaluation and treatment of possible nonoccupational HIV exposures. *HIV,* Human immunodeficiency virus; *nPEP,* nonoccupational postexposure prophylaxis. (From https://www.cdc.gov/hivnexus/hcp/pep/index.html.)

Pregnancy Prophylaxis

Pregnancy occurs in up to 4.7% of sexual assault victims.[92] An estimated 22,000 annual rape-related pregnancies could be avoided if all victims received pregnancy prophylaxis.[93] As an initial step, perform a urine pregnancy test before administering postcoital contraception (PcC). Modern urine pregnancy tests possess a β-hCG detection threshold approaching 20 mIU/mL to 25 mIU/mL and will usually be positive 1 to 2 weeks after conception, often before a menstrual period is missed.

Offer pregnancy prevention with available oral PcC to all patients with a history of sexual assault if local guidelines allow. Several methods can be used to prevent pregnancy after forced, nonconsenting intercourse (Table 59.2). The drug of choice for PcC is levonorgestrel, an agent that prevents ovulation but has no effect on implantation should pregnancy occur in a patient who has already ovulated, nor does the drug cause abortion. This drug is available without a prescription in the United States in commercial kits called Plan B One-Step (Teva Women's Health, Inc.), Next Choice One-Dose (Watson Pharma, Inc.), Take Action (Teva Pharmaceuticals), My Way (GAVIS Pharmaceuticals), or other generics. In 2013, the US Food and Drug Administration (FDA) extended the approved sale of Plan B without a prescription to all females of childbearing status from a more restrictive policy that limited its sale to individuals 17 years or older.[94] Plan B One-Step is a single 1.5-mg pill to be taken once as PcC. In 2010, the FDA approved an additional option for pharmacologic emergency contraception, ulipristal acetate (Ella, Afaxys, Inc.). This selective progesterone receptor modulator has been demonstrated to be as effective as levonorgestrel for prevention of pregnancy 72 hours after intercourse and more effective for

TABLE 59.2 Emergency Contraception[a,b]

BRAND	MANUFACTURER	PILLS[c]
Progestin-Only Emergency Contraception Oral Therapy: Recommended Primarily for Patients <75 kg		
Plan B One-Step	WCC	1 pill (levonorgestrel, 1.5 mg) immediately
Or		
Progesterone Receptor Agonist/Antagonist: Preferred for Patients ≥75 kg		
Ulipristal (Ella)	Watson Pharma, Inc.	One 30-mg pill immediately

[a]For the most up-to-date recommendations view https://www.cdc.gov/contraception/hcp/usspr/emergency-contraception.html.
[b]Some regimens cause nausea and an antiemetic may be used. If vomiting occurs, repeat the dose of antiemetic.
[c]Alternatively, the older Yuzpe method may be used with any combination oral contraceptive containing levonorgestrel, ethinyloestradiol 0.03 mg/0.3 mg dosed as two pills immediately and two pills after 12 hours.

longer postcoital use. Ulipristal requires a prescription and is approved for use up to 120 hours after intercourse.[95] Despite taking PcC, patients who meet criteria for obesity may be two to four times more likely to become pregnant than those who do not meet obesity criteria, though this failure is somewhat less with ulipristal; patients with the potential to experience pregnancy weighing >75 kg should be offered Ella/ulipristal acetate over Plan B/levonorgestrel.[96,97] All available evidence demonstrates no untoward effects on the fetus if pregnancy occurs despite oral PcC.[98,99] Insertion of a copper intrauterine device is another form of PcC and remains the most effective emergency contraception available, preventing more than 99% of pregnancies, but is generally outside the purview of the emergency physician.[98,99]

Religious preferences and some state legal changes due to the 2022 Supreme Court ruling Dobbs v. Jackson may deter or prohibit some hospital EDs from providing PcC. Practitioners should be aware of local legal and hospital guidelines. The website and number listed at the end of this paragraph provide practitioners information to give referral for easy access to PcC for patients who lack funds to pay for the medication. In addition, given the ever-increasing availability of new methods and drugs for PcC, examiners may want to obtain up-to-date information from either https://www.cdc.gov/contraception/hcp/usspr/emergency-contraception.html or https://www.americansocietyforec.org/ec-for-sadv.

Psychological Support and Aftercare

Sexual assault and IPV may precipitate a psychological crisis for the patient, and psychological care should begin as soon as possible, ideally initiated when the patient first arrives in the ED.[16,100,101] Reassure the victim that they will be in control of the examination, that they may ask questions at any point, and that they should notify the examiner if anything hurts or if they need a break. Ensure that the patient has a complete understanding that in the ED they have full control over their body and the examination is the first step toward psychological support and healing. Unfortunately, if this is not made a priority, full recovery may be impaired. Posttraumatic stress disorder (PTSD), manifested as numbed responsiveness to the external world, disturbances in sleep, feelings of guilt, memory impairment, avoidance of activities, and other symptoms, often develops in sexual assault victims. Attention to the initial psychological care of an assault victim in the ED is fundamental and can reduce distress during forensic examination.[100]

Many areas have a local sexual assault crisis agency that can dispatch an advocate that will accompany patients with a history of sexual assault during the interview and examination. This same agency may help to provide the follow-up psychological support that must be offered to all victims. It is critical that all examiners maintain current contact information with these agencies and use their services. The importance of this contact is emphasized in some areas by the fact that state law dictates that medical personnel contact a local sexual assault crisis agency when a victim arrives for examination.[102] In the absence of immediate local crisis services, a hospital social worker may fill this role.

Postexamination Follow-up

Medical and psychological follow-up of sexual assault victims is essential. Many protocols recommend a 2-week follow-up to reexamine any injuries and to repeat testing for STIs and pregnancy. Because of the measurable failure rate of PcC, repeated pregnancy testing is critical for a victim who does not experience an expected menses. Further follow-up evaluations may be performed at 4 or 6 weeks and 3 and 6 months to repeat serologic tests for HIV, hepatitis B, hepatitis C, and syphilis.

SPECIFIC POPULATIONS

LGBTQI+ Sexual Assault Victims

Sexual and gender minorities face unique epidemiologic risks of sexual assault. Sexual and gender minority (SGM) is an umbrella term that encompasses lesbian, gay, bisexual, and queer populations as well as transgender and intersex individuals, often abbreviated LGBTQI+.[103,104] This term is also inclusive of those whose gender identity, expression, or reproductive development varies from societal, cultural, or physiologic norms. The term transgender is used in this text to refer to individuals whose gender differs from their sex assigned at birth, while cisgender refers to individuals whose gender is the same as their assigned birth sex.

Sexual assault is more common for transgender people, with 66% of transgender adults experiencing sexual assault over the life-course (with other reported rates varying by year and geographic location of survey from 53% to 68%), compared with approximately 23% of cisgender females and 9% of cisgender males.[1,2,105–107] Sexual minority individuals are two to more than five times more likely to experience sexual assault than heterosexual individuals.[108,109] Sexual violence has been found to be even higher in some sub-populations including SGM individuals of color, transgender youth, individuals experiencing housing insecurity, and those involved in sex work. Interactions with health care providers, SANEs/FNEs, or law enforcement may be complicated by prior experiences of sexual violence as 15% of transgender individuals report being sexually assaulted while in police custody or jail, which more than doubles (to 32%) for African-American transgender people.[105,106,110] Recognition of this epidemiology allows healthcare providers caring for SGM victims of sexual assault to recognize that past experiences have bearing on present and future experiences and ensure that the forensic examination occurs in a safe environment where patients who have experienced past trauma are not retraumatized.

Best practices for this population include universal trauma-informed care, appropriate disclosure and privacy practices as they relate to potentially sensitive issues of sexual history taking, sexuality, and gender, ascertainment and use of patient pronouns and chosen names, anatomic surveys and documentation in the electronic medical record, and identification of relevant samples with sex assigned at birth to avoid confusion if DNA sample sex is incongruent with patient gender.[20–22,47,49] Specific considerations relating to the examination of patients with prior experience of gender-affirming surgery such as phalloplasty, metoidioplasty, vaginoplasty or vulvoplasty are addressed in the text. Other notable considerations include the use of lubrication to address hypoestrogenic state causing vaginal atrophy and dryness similar to what is seen in postmenopausal cisgender females and in transgender males needing vulvovaginal examination.[47] Consideration should be given to the use of blind swabs for any patient who, due to gender dysphoria, prior traumatization or anatomic issues, cannot tolerate a speculum examination.

Male Sexual Assault Victims

It is estimated that 1 in every 4 males has experienced some form of contact sexual violence and 1 in every 38 males has been the victim of attempted or completed sexual assault.[111] Sexual assaults of boys and adult males are less commonly reported than female sexual assault and believed to be not just underreported but also underrecognized and undertreated.[112,113] Male patients with a history of sexual assault deserve the same unhurried, nonjudgmental, compassionate care that female victims do, particularly in light of the fact that male victims may be less likely to get the psychological support they require. As with all patients who have been sexually assaulted, the forensic examination is guided by the history of events related by the patient. Male examinations include all the same forensic evidence collection as for female victims with the exception of vaginal and cervical specimens (other than in transgender males with vaginas where vaginal specimens may remain indicated). Penile samples from the shaft, glans, corona, and scrotum using similar techniques to those described in the general body examination section may be obtained if there is penile-oral, penile-vaginal, or penile-anal contact with the perpetrator in settings of coerced penetration (sometimes termed "made-to-penetrate"/MTP).[63,67,111]

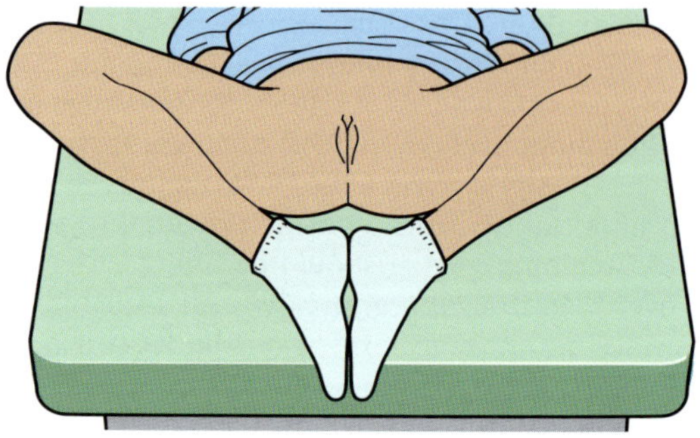

Fig. 59.11 "Frog leg" position to examine children.

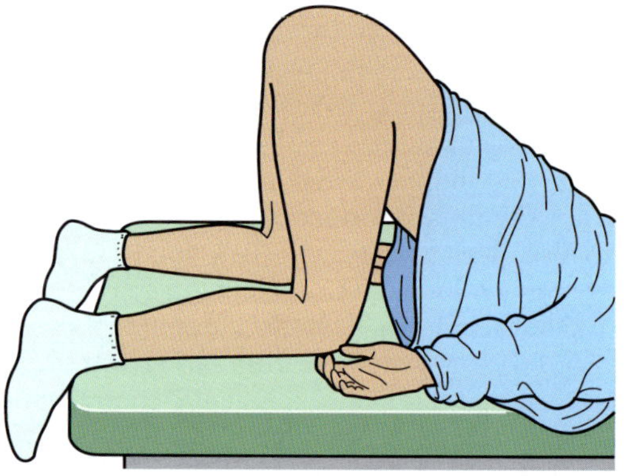

Fig. 59.12 Child in knee-chest position to facilitate examination.

Pediatric Sexual Assault Victims

In general, the care and treatment of a pediatric sexual assault patient requires expert knowledge and experience; if feasible, transfer to a pediatric center with SART/FMU access is preferred. In some cases, specialist teams may travel to the location of the patient.

ED practitioners may be the first professionals to examine a child victim. The presence of obvious genital injury and trauma should be an adequate prompt to initiate the forensic process. However, in less obvious cases, the subtle variations in developmental changes and congenital anomalies may leave many clinicians ill-equipped to render an opinion concerning findings indicative of sexual assault. The history in these cases can be challenging to obtain given the age of the patient, their developmental stage, and psychological state. Emergency providers must remain vigilant for any clues, no matter how insignificant they may appear initially. Adams and associates demonstrated that the majority of children reporting sexual abuse have normal or nonspecific genital findings.[58,114] Despite expert physical examination, the vast majority of sexually abused children cannot be physically differentiated from nonabused children.[115] Discovery of one of the rare examination markers of injury should be confirmed by experts, and a discussion of these findings, though beyond the scope of this chapter, is covered extensively in other resources.[116] The history provided by the child or caretaker should therefore remain the primary indicator that inappropriate genital contact has occurred. Any concerning elements of the history warrant an investigation of the possibility of sexual abuse.

Ask a parent (unless they are a suspect) to assist in calming, reassurance, and positioning of the child for examination. Whereas the basic lithotomy position may be used for an older, more mature child or an adolescent patient, use of alternative positioning of a pediatric female patient is essential for inspection. The frog leg position (the feet together and the knees spread widely apart) with the use of labial or gluteal (or both) separation and traction is often beneficial in children (Fig. 59.11). For a very young child with small genital orifices, the aid of a magnification source may be extremely helpful. Take care to gently separate the labia to avoid superficial examiner-induced injuries. In addition, to get a better look at the hymenal perimeter in prepubertal girls and the anus in girls and boys, ask them to turn over into the knee-chest position (Figs. 59.11 and 59.12). Inspect the genitalia carefully in an unhurried, child-friendly manner. Genital findings that are deemed definitive of sexual abuse or penetration or are nonspecific are included in Box 59.4.[67,117] Many normal hymenal differences exist from one child to the next, and the definitive diagnosis of "abnormal" is often difficult even for experts. When any doubt exists in the ED, completely describe the findings and refer the child for later examination by experts.

When disclosure or genital injuries confirm possible penetration of the child, collect specimens for potential evidence. On all conscious prepubertal children, collect the specimens without inserting a pediatric speculum. If there is no bleeding or significant trauma, procedural sedation is rarely indicated. With very young children, the practitioner may have only one opportunity to collect vaginal specimens without causing agitation and prohibiting further examination. Forcing specimen collection under physical restraint is considered a second assault on the child. External anal and vulvar swabs are usually collected quite easily. Lack of estrogen in prepubertal children may increase hymenal sensitivity making vaginal samples difficult to obtain. Therefore many local protocols do not require collection of internal samples. For extraordinary circumstances, internal samples should remain the very last evidence collected. Make every effort possible to avoid swab contact with hymenal tissue during collection. For the rare

BOX 59.4 Acute Findings on Examination Diagnostic of Sexual Contact in Children[a]

ACUTE TRAUMA TO EXTERNAL GENITAL/ANAL TISSUES, WHICH COULD BE ACCIDENTAL OR INFLICTED

- Acute laceration(s) or bruising of labia, penis, scrotum, perianal tissues, or perineum
- Acute laceration of the posterior fourchette or vestibule, not involving the hymen
- Residual (healing) injuries to external genital/anal tissues (These rare findings are difficult to diagnose unless an acute injury was previously documented at the same location.)
- Perianal scar
- Scar of posterior fourchette or fossa

INJURIES INDICATIVE OF ACUTE OR HEALED TRAUMA TO THE GENITAL/ANAL TISSUES

- Bruising, petechiae, or abrasions on the hymen
- Acute laceration of the hymen, of any depth; partial or complete
- Vaginal laceration
- Perianal laceration with exposure of tissues below the dermis
- Healed hymenal transection/complete hymen cleft (A defect in the hymen between 4 o'clock and 8 o'clock that extends to the base of the hymen, with no hymenal tissue discernible at that location.)
- A defect in the posterior (inferior) half of the hymen, wider than a transection, with an absence of hymenal tissue extending to the base of the hymen

INFECTIONS TRANSMITTED BY SEXUAL CONTACT, UNLESS THERE IS EVIDENCE OF PERINATAL TRANSMISSION OR CLEARLY, REASONABLY, AND INDEPENDENTLY DOCUMENTED BUT RARE NONSEXUAL TRANSMISSION

- Genital, rectal, or pharyngeal *Neisseria gonorrhea* infection
- Syphilis
- Genital or rectal *Chlamydia trachomatis* infection
- *Trichomonas vaginalis* infection
- HIV, if transmission by blood transfusion has been ruled out

DIAGNOSTIC OF SEXUAL CONTACT

- Pregnancy
- Semen identified in forensic specimens taken directly from a child's body

[a]*These findings support a disclosure of sexual abuse and are highly suggestive of abuse even in the absence of a disclosure, unless a timely and plausible description of accidental injury is provided by the child and/or caretaker. Physical findings should be confirmed using additional examination positions and/or techniques. Diagnoses of sexually transmitted infections must be confirmed by additional testing to avoid assigning significance to possible false positive screening test results. Photographs or video recordings of these findings should be evaluated and confirmed by an expert in sexual abuse evaluation to ensure accurate interpretation.*

From Adams JA, Kellogg ND, Farst KJ et al. Updated guidelines for the medical assessment and care of children who may have been sexually abused. J Pediatr Adolesc Gynecol. *2015;2:81-87.*

cases involving severe vaginal trauma or suspected internal genital injury (active bleeding) that will possibly require surgical repair, conduct the examination under deep procedural sedation or refer for examination by a consulting gynecologist under general anesthesia. Clinicians should consult local child abuse centers and state agencies for protocols regarding immediate STI specimen collection, referral, and follow-up services.

Inebriated Sexual Assault Victims and Drug-Facilitated Sexual Assault

Alcohol and other drugs play an important role in many sexual assaults.[118–122] Often the victim's last memory is of using drugs or alcohol and then passing out. A common scenario is for the victim to have one glass of wine (or another usual drink), suddenly feel nauseated, and then wake up hours later in a different location and lacking intervening memory. Some remember short segments of activity that may indicate some type of sexual acts. Victims may lack any memory at all but desire to be "checked" for intercourse. A comprehensive medical-forensic examination should be conducted on these individuals. Without a history from the victim, examiners should collect samples from every potential oral or genital contact, including the neck, breasts, vulva, and from all orifices (oral, vaginal, and/or anal).

Extreme sensitivity must be used when discussing positive genital findings with a victim who has no memory of any sexual activity. Many times, the imagined sexual acts can create just as severe a traumatic response as an actual remembered sexual assault. For the unconscious victim, there is no memory of events to fill in the blanks, only their imagination of what may have happened.

Drug-facilitated sexual assaults can be difficult to diagnose due to limitations in testing and are often underestimated.[118–120] Aside from ethanol, there is no dominant category-specific agent associated with drug-facilitated sexual assault (DFSA).[122] While popular media has raised public awareness of drugs used to facilitate sexual assault under the term *date-rape drugs*, numerous CNS depressant, over-the-counter, prescription, and illicit substances have been associated with this crime including, but not limited to, benzodiazepines (e.g., Valium, Xanax, Rohypnol), opioids (e.g., oxycodone, Vicodin, Oxycontin), muscle relaxants (e.g., Soma, Flexeril), antihistamines (e.g., Benadryl), hallucinogens (e.g., ecstasy, marijuana, ketamine), and central CNS depressants (e.g., GHB/γ-hydroxybutyrate).[122,123] In previous decades, laboratory testing implicated flunitrazepam and GHB in a minority of cases, estimated as 3% to 5% of total cases of DFSA.[124] In many cases it is unclear whether a drug was taken voluntarily, or whether it was surreptitiously given to the assaulted victim. Obtain samples of both blood and urine, if possible, for toxicology (including ethanol), with exact times of collection documented. To optimize potential recovery, at least 100 mL urine should be collected if <120 hours have elapsed since the incident. Most drugs will be undetectable in the blood more than 24 hours after ingestion but if collection is possible in that time span, at least 12 mL of blood should be obtained in a gray-top tube (containing sodium fluoride/potassium oxalate). Samples for DFSA investigation should be stored refrigerated.[125]

As a full accounting of all substances used in DFSA is outside the scope of this chapter, the authors recommend the use of dedicated up-to-date reference lists such as the ones formulated and maintained by the Society of Forensic Toxicologists Drug-Facilitated Crimes Committee.[125] A routine hospital urine drug screen is inadequate to evaluate a sexual assault victim for DFSA and forensic laboratories may offer an evaluation for multiple drugs in an expanded spectrum toxicology panel.[122,125] However, testing may not be adequately sensitive to test for all substances used during DFSA. A positive drug test does not prove DFSA, and it may be impossible to distinguish voluntary ingestion from clandestine administration. Opportunistic DFSA of victims with preassault voluntary ingestion of alcohol or other substances is likely more common than clandestine DFSA by assailants.[126,127]

LEGAL ISSUES

Chain of Custody

Samples and other evidence need to be carefully and formally transferred to the police, a crime laboratory, or a forensic pathologist. Label each sample with the patient's name, hospital number, date, time of collection, area from which the specimen was collected, and collector's name. Package these specimens according to local crime laboratory specifications and transfer them to the next appropriate official (police officer, pathologist, or other individual) along with a written confirmation of chain of custody, including a list of the specimens, the signature of each person who collected them, and the signature of each person who received them. If this documentation is inadequate or the documentation chain is broken, important evidence may be deemed inadmissible in court.[7,37]

Suspect Examinations

As forensic evidence collection in the form of DNA retrieval continues to evolve, EDs may see more requests from local law enforcement for collection of evidence from suspects. EDs should be familiar with local and state protocols, especially regarding consent. Some jurisdictions permit examination of suspects without consent, given the imminent degradation of potential biological evidence. Other jurisdictions require that suspects give consent or, at the very least, that police obtain a search warrant from the court. The sooner that a suspect is apprehended and brought in for a medical-forensic examination, the better the quality of forensic biological evidence.

Law enforcement should be in attendance during the examination of any suspect to ensure the safety of the examiner, the witness, and the cooperation of the suspect. Be sure that the suspect and victim do not encounter one another in the hospital setting during the examination period. Examine the victim and suspect in separate locations within the ED or clinical setting. It is beneficial to conduct the examination and history of the victim before the suspect's examination, to search for physical findings on the suspect that were indicated by the victim's history. For example, if during the victim's history they relate that they scratched the suspect's left shoulder in defense, the examiner should examine, document, and preferably photograph the presence (or absence) of an injury on the suspect's left shoulder.

The physical and evidentiary examination of the suspect is similar to that of the victim. The primary differences lie in history taking, reference samples, and more "blind" samples. During the examination of a suspect, law enforcement officers, rather than the suspect, provide the history of the event. Collect reference samples of blood and buccal swabs if possible. Previously recommended, head and pubic hair reference samples are no longer required in most areas and practitioners should refer to local protocols for guidance on this. Apply special attention not only to nail scrapings but also to swabbing all the fingers for possible vaginal epithelial cells from digital penetration. Female DNA persists in the male fingernail scrapings for up to 6 hours or more.[128] The shaft and corona of the glans penis should be swabbed along with separate swabs of the scrotum for vaginal secretions. Criminalists often recover a female victim's DNA from the scrotal swab even if the perpetrator wore a condom. With an unwashed penis, swabs almost uniformly show evidence of female cells up to 24 hours after coitus.[129]

Examining suspects requires the same amount of professional sensitivity and respect that any patient receives within the ED. It is not within the realm of the clinician's expertise to determine whether the suspect is guilty or innocent.

Testimony

When the local government decides to proceed with a sex crime case against an alleged perpetrator, the district attorney will commonly contact the examiner to give legal testimony. A concise and complete well-documented chart may negate the need for a clinician to appear in court. The examiner should work with the district attorney to prepare testimony when the case is being prosecuted. As is the case for all ED patients, chart notes should be written objectively and carefully in the expectation that the ED evaluation and evidence collection may be presented in court. The examining clinician is most often considered a percipient witness and not necessarily an expert in the area of sexual assault. The law requires that one testify only to one's best recollection and to what is indicated in the chart. Factual information in answer to questions should be given only if one knows the facts; assumptions should be avoided. One should not be afraid to acknowledge the limits of one's knowledge or expertise. Statements such as "there were marks on the body consistent with bite marks" are preferable to statements such as "there were bite marks." The court decides if a person was sexually assaulted, and the clinician is there to give information about the patient's findings and statements, what was found, and what was done for treatment.

ACKNOWLEDGMENT

The editors and authors wish to acknowledge the contributions of Carolyn Joy Sachs, Malinda Wheeler, and G. Richard Braen to this chapter in previous editions; Beverly Kerr, Supervising Criminalist at Los Angeles County Sheriff's Department; Mary Hong, Sr. Forensic Scientist-DNA Supervisor at Orange County Crime Laboratory; and Patricia A. Huck, Criminalist II of the LAPD Crime Laboratory for their technical forensic advice. The authors of this edition also wish to thank Jennifer DiNoto, MSN, RN, CEN, FNE-A/P at Greater Baltimore Medical Center, Glen Burnie, MD.

REFERENCES ARE AVAILABLE AT Elsevier eBooks+

SECTION X

Neurologic Procedures

CHAPTER 60

Management of Increased Intracranial Pressure and Intracranial Shunts

Alessandra Conforto and Jonathan G. Wagner

Headache and head injury are common chief complaints seen in the emergency department (ED). If either is accompanied by vomiting, decreased level of consciousness, focal neurologic findings, or abnormal vital signs, the possibility of increased intracranial pressure (ICP) should be considered. Acutely increased ICP is a neurologic emergency that must be managed rapidly to prevent further brain injury and death. In some cases, the accompanying clinical symptoms may be vague or subtle and make diagnosis difficult. Familiarity with the pathophysiology of increased ICP facilitates its diagnosis and management.

PATHOPHYSIOLOGY OF ICP

Alexander Monro, an anatomist in the 18th century, described the intracranial contents as containing a fixed volume. The fixed-volume theory was supported by George Kellie a few years later and became known as the Monro-Kellie doctrine. This doctrine has since guided our understanding of intracranial dynamics and the principles of autoregulation. In brief, the doctrine states that ICP is a function of the volume and compliance of each element within the intracranial compartment. Therefore an increase in the volume of one component will displace other structures, and eventually increase ICP.

The components of the calvaria are the brain parenchyma, cerebrospinal fluid (CSF), the venous blood supply, and the arterial blood supply (Fig. 60.1). CSF and the venous blood supply have the greatest ability to change their volume to compensate for increases in pressure. These dynamic changes in the relative proportion of the cranial content may not affect the patient if ICP elevation is not excessive. However, if a pathologic process overwhelms the compensatory mechanisms, the result will be a nearly exponential increase in ICP (Fig. 60.2).

Normal supine ICP ranges from 5 to 15 mm Hg. Transient increases in ICP as high as 80 to 100 mm Hg occur with coughing, sneezing, or straining. Other factors that can transiently increase ICP are movement, pain, and fever. A space-occupying lesion such as a tumor, hematoma, abscess, or foreign body can also raise ICP. Fig. 60.3 demonstrates that the area and cause of the increased ICP will determine where shifts occur to result in brain herniation.

Brain

Brain volume can be increased by edema, idiopathic intracranial hypertension (IIH), tumor, or bleeding. There are three types of edema that typically affect the brain parenchyma: vasogenic, cytotoxic, and interstitial. Vasogenic edema results from increased permeability of the capillaries, which leads to passage of excess fluid into the extracellular space. Cytotoxic edema is due to accumulation of intracellular fluid in brain tissue (neurons and glia) secondary to dysfunction of the adenosine triphosphatase pump. Interstitial edema occurs when fluid accumulates because of blockage of CSF absorption.

IIH, formerly known as pseudotumor cerebri or benign intracranial hypertension, is a chronic condition characterized by increased CSF pressure not caused by a tumor, edema, hydrocephalus, or change in CSF composition. It occurs most frequently in females with an increased body mass index. Symptoms may include headache, nausea, and blurry vision. The headache is typically worse on waking or with exertion. In general, patients with IIH have normal findings on neurologic examination except for the frequent presence of papilledema. The precise pathophysiology behind IIH remains unclear, with several proposed etiologies, including: cerebral venous outflow abnormalities (e.g., venous stenosis); increased CSF outflow resistance at either the level of the arachnoid granulations or CSF lymphatic drainage sites; obesity-related increased abdominal and intracranial venous pressure and obesity-related chronic inflammation; altered sodium and water retention mechanisms; abnormalities of vitamin A metabolism; and sex hormone dysfunction.[1–3] Severe and untreated cases of IIH can lead to permanent vision loss. There is some crossover with the more serious and life-threatening diagnosis of cerebral venous thrombosis (CVT), and therefore magnetic resonance (MR) (ideally with venography) or computed tomography (CT) venography of the cerebral venous system is recommended in patients with presumed IIH to rule out CVT.[4,5] Other commonly associated conditions are listed in Box 60.1.

Brain tumors encompass neoplasms that originate in the brain itself *(primary brain tumors)* or involve the brain as a metastatic site *(secondary brain tumors)*. Primary brain tumors include tumors of the brain parenchyma, meninges, cranial nerves, and other intracranial structures (the pituitary and

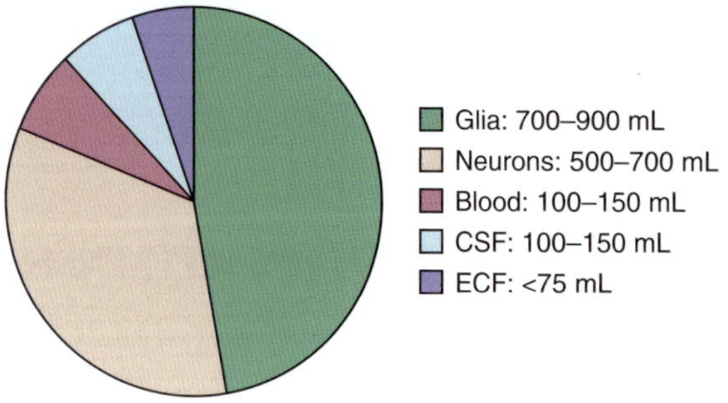

Fig. 60.1 Intracranial contents and their volumes in healthy adults. *CSF,* Cerebrospinal fluid; *ECF,* extracellular fluid.

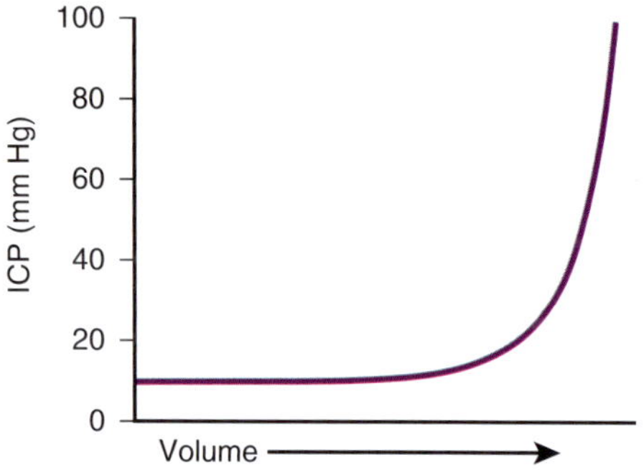

Fig. 60.2 The intracranial volume-pressure relationship demonstrates the limits of compensatory mechanisms. Small changes in intracranial volume markedly increase intracranial pressure. *ICP,* Intracranial pressure.

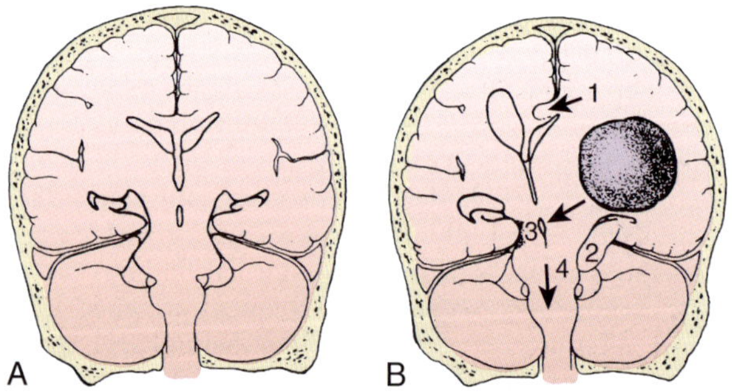

Fig. 60.3 Intracranial shifts as a result of supratentorial lesions. (A) Relationships of the various supratentorial compartments as seen in a coronal section. (B) Herniation of the cingulate gyrus under the falx *(1);* herniation of the temporal lobe into the tentorial notch *(2);* compression of the opposite cerebral peduncle against the unyielding tentorium, which produces Kernohan's notch *(3);* and downward displacement of the brain stem through the tentorial notch *(4).* (From Plum F, Posner JB. *The Diagnosis of Stupor and Coma.* 2nd ed. Davis; 1972.)

pineal glands) (Fig. 60.4). Primary central nervous system lymphoma refers to high-grade B-cell non-Hodgkin lymphoma confined to the central nervous system. Secondary brain tumors, the most common type, originate elsewhere in the body and metastasize to the intracranial compartment.

Bleeding in the brain can occur spontaneously, such as in the case of hemorrhagic stroke or spontaneous subarachnoid hemorrhage, or can be a result of trauma. In addition to the mass effect of the blood itself, the associated edema contributes to further increases in ICP. Diffuse axonal injury (DAI) may occur in isolation or in conjunction with intracerebral bleeding. With DAI, it is believed that the axons sustain significant injury and edema via shearing effect.[6]

BOX 60.1 Clinical Conditions and Factors Associated With Idiopathic or Benign Intracranial Hypertension (Pseudotumor Cerebri)

Hematologic disorders
- Iron deficiency anemia
- Pernicious anemia
- Polycythemia vera
- Thrombocytopenia

Lupus
Cushing disease
Hypoparathyroidism
Hypothyroidism
Endocrine conditions and disorders
- Addison disease
- Menstrual irregularities, menstrual cycle
- Pregnancy

Medical/surgical conditions with impaired cerebral venous drainage
- Otitis media, mastoiditis
- Idiopathic dural sinus thrombosis
- Radical neck surgery
- Chronic pulmonary disease with venous hypertension
- Heart failure with venous hypertension
- Congenital heart disease
- Renal failure
- High-flow arteriovenous malformation
- Chronic obstructive pulmonary disease
- Sleep apnea
- Growth hormone
- Cimetidine

Common drugs
- Systemic steroid withdrawal
- Topical steroid withdrawal (infants)
- Oral contraceptives
- Tetracycline/minocycline
- Nitrofurantoin
- Sulfamethoxazole
- Vitamin A excess
- Glucocorticoids
- Nalidixic acid
- Levothyroxine
- Lithium
- Isotretinoin
- Nonsteroidal antiinflammatory drugs
- Tamoxifen
- Cyclosporine

Dietary considerations
- Hypovitaminosis A
- Obesity
- Malnutrition

Cerebrospinal Fluid

CSF is produced by the choroid plexus at a daily rate of 400 mL to 600 mL (~20 mL/h) with complete turnover of total volume occurring four to five times per day in young adults

(Fig. 60.5).[7] It flows from the ventricles into the cisternae of the subarachnoid space and is drained by the arachnoid villi of the dural sinuses to maintain a constant volume of 100 mL to 150 mL. *Obstructive hydrocephalus* occurs when flow is blocked at any point in the ventricular system by clotted blood, tumor, colloid cyst, edema, or primary stenosis. *Communicating hydrocephalus* is due to impedance of flow beyond the ventricular system at the level of the basal cisternae or lack of absorption by the arachnoid villi. Communicating hydrocephalus can occur with both infection and subarachnoid hemorrhage (Fig. 60.6).

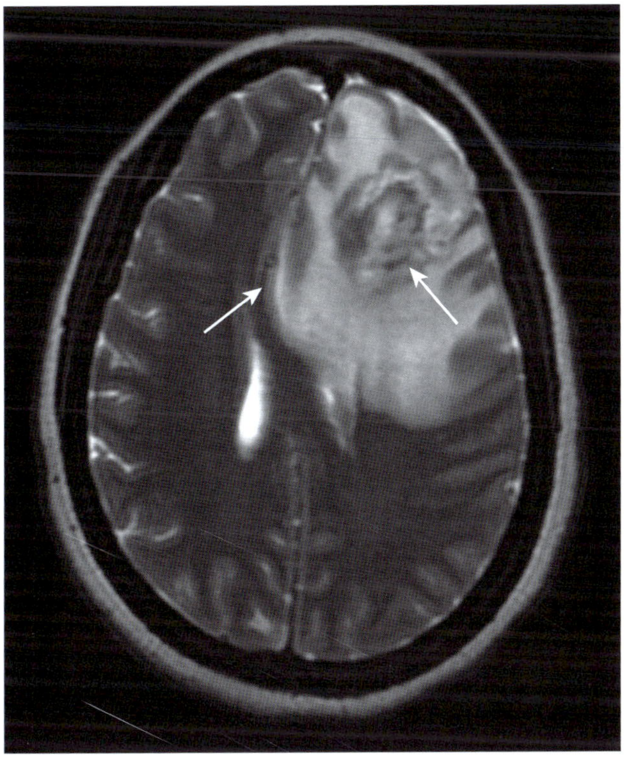

Fig. 60.4 T2-magnetic resonance image of a patient with a left frontal mass *(right arrow)* and surrounding parenchymal edema, consistent with glioblastoma. The lesion has exerted a mass effect on the brain causing 7 mm of midline shift *(left arrow)* and subsequent subfalcine herniation.

Blood

Up to a certain range, cerebral blood flow (CBF) is maintained by an autoregulatory mechanism despite fluctuations in cerebral perfusion pressure (CPP) (Fig. 60.7). Constant CBF can typically be maintained at any CPP between 60 mm Hg and 160 mm Hg. Once CPP is out of the autoregulatory zone, CBF is linearly related to CPP. CPP lower than 60 mm Hg can lead to ischemia, whereas CPP higher than 160 mm Hg can result in hypertensive encephalopathy.

SIGNS AND SYMPTOMS

Findings on neurologic examination can be normal in a patient with a mild increase in ICP because of the brain's compensatory mechanisms. Patients with a complaint of headache

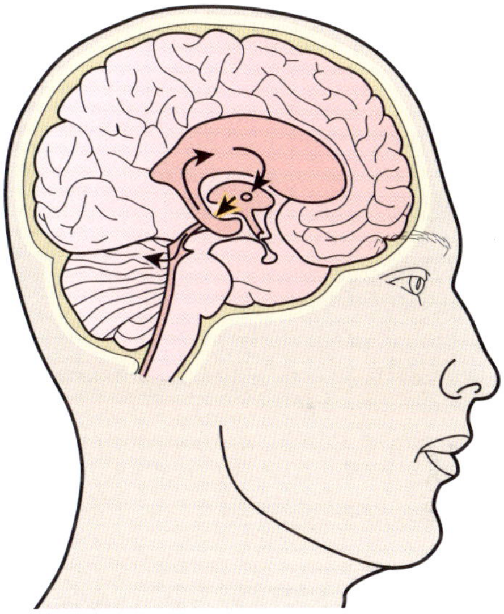

Fig. 60.5 Cerebrospinal fluid production and flow. (From Rengachary SS, Wilkins RH, eds. *Principles of Neurosurgery*. Mosby; 1994.)

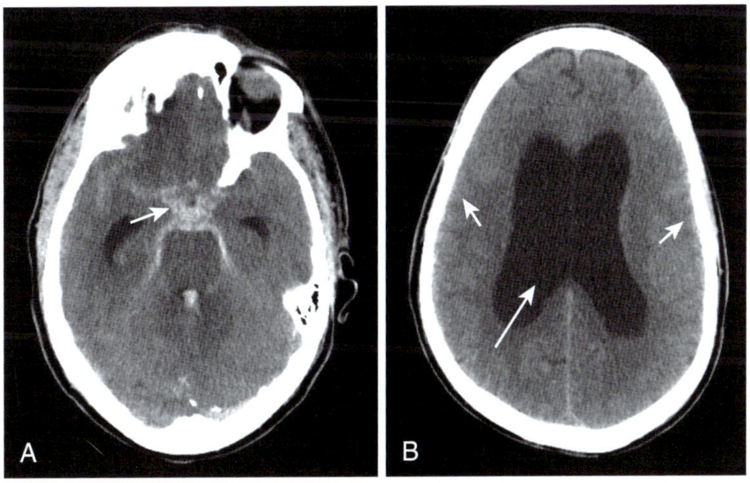

Fig. 60.6 Subarachnoid hemorrhage. (A) Hyperdense blood from subarachnoid hemorrhage can be seen collecting in the basal cistern *(arrow)*. (B) Image from the same patient, more superior in the cranium. Note the ventricular enlargement *(long arrow)* and effacement of the peripheral sulci *(short arrows)*. These findings are indicative of hydrocephalus, and external ventricular drainage by a neurosurgeon should be considered.

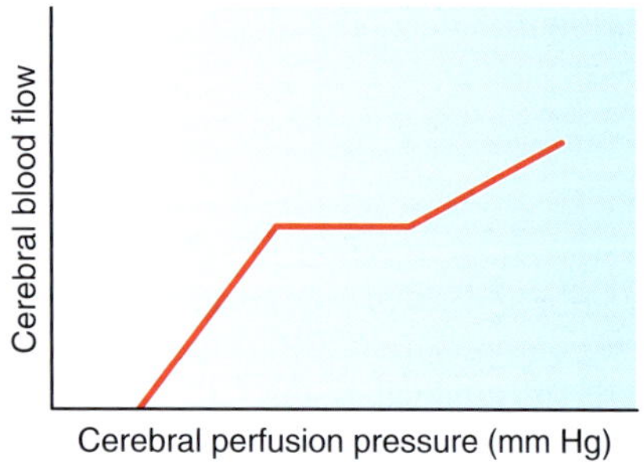

Fig. 60.7 Cerebral autoregulation. *CPP,* Cerebral perfusion pressure; *ICP,* intracranial pressure.

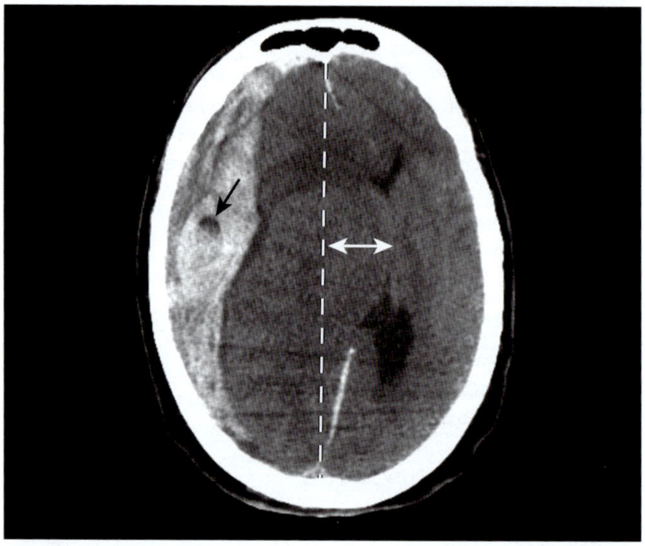

Fig. 60.8 Acute subdural hematoma. The large hyperdense *(white)* collection on the right side of the brain is an acute subdural hematoma. The finding of hypodense areas *(black arrow)* within the subdural is referred to as the "swirl" sign, which suggests active bleeding. Also seen is approximately 3 cm of midline shift *(white arrow),* which indicates subfalcine herniation. Immediate reduction of intracranial pressure and surgical intervention are required.

or head injury may not initially manifest the more dramatic and worrisome symptoms of increased ICP such as vomiting, syncope, altered mentation, or Cushing reflex (bradycardia, increased blood pressure, and irregular respirations). ICP correlates poorly with clinical symptomatology. One of the earliest clinical signs is decreased venous pulsation on funduscopic examination, but this may be difficult to appreciate in an acutely ill patient in a busy ED. Moreover, the initial findings on head CT may not reveal the true extent of injury, especially in early stroke or when DAI has occurred. However, as compensatory mechanisms fail, CT findings, as well as clinical symptoms, will become more evident.

Signs and symptoms of severely increased ICP include a decreasing level of consciousness, papilledema, cranial nerve palsies, and lateralizing neurologic deficits. When any one of these signs is noted, particularly when CT confirms the presence of a mass effect, such as hydrocephalus or a midline shift, emergent intervention is necessary (Fig. 60.8). Specifically, medical management should be initiated immediately in the ED while awaiting neurosurgical consultation for possible invasive measures to reduce ICP.

MEDICAL TREATMENT OF INCREASED ICP

Oxygenation

Management of the airway and breathing is paramount in patients with brain injury. If the patient is hypoxic, supplemental oxygen is critical in preventing further ischemia. Patients with clinical signs of cerebral herniation and those at risk of aspiration or impending respiratory decompensation should undergo rapid-sequence intubation (RSI) to protect their airway and better control blood levels of oxygen and carbon dioxide (partial pressure of oxygen [Po_2] and partial pressure of carbon dioxide [Pco_2]). Apneic patients should receive bag-valve-mask ventilation while preparing for intubation and apneic oxygenation via a high-flow nasal cannula (rate of 15 L/min or higher) during airway securement to avoid transient hypoxia and worsening brain ischemia.

Sedation and Paralytics

A rapid neurologic examination that assesses the patient's pupillary reflexes, motor response to voice and painful stimuli, and the ability to interact with their surroundings should be performed before sedation and RSI. To blunt the hemodynamic response to intubation, fentanyl, at an intravenous (IV) dose of 2 to 5 μg/kg, can be given over 30 to 60 seconds while preoxygenating the patient.[8] Fentanyl is an excellent drug for control of pain, which if untreated, can lead to increased ICP. Fentanyl can also be given during the pretreatment phase of RSI (3 minutes before administration of the paralytic agent) if time allows. Caution should be exercised, however, to avoid precipitous drops in blood pressure, which can threaten CBF and exacerbate brain injury. Therefore fentanyl should be avoided in hypotensive patients and hypovolemic patients. Caution should also be exercised in brain-injured patients with concomitant trauma, who may have exaggerated episodes of hypotension with opioids and sedatives. Pretreatment lidocaine, which was traditionally believed to decrease the sympathomimetic response to intubation, is no longer recommended as multiple studies have shown conflicting and insufficient evidence to support its use.[8,9] A defasciculating dose (typically one-tenth the intubating dose) of a nondepolarizing neuromuscular blocking agent given prior to intubation has also fallen out of favor as no sufficient evidence has supported this practice.[8,10]

In patients who are normotensive or hypotensive, etomidate (0.3 mg/kg IV) is the induction agent of choice due to its minimal effect on systemic blood pressure and its lowering of ICP.[11,12] Ketamine, at a dose of 1 to 2 mg/kg IV, can also be used as it does not appear to increase ICP, as previously believed, and should be considered in severely hypotensive patients due to its ability to increase blood pressure and its analgesic effects that minimize the adverse sympathetic stimulation of laryngoscopy.[13] In hypertensive patients, thiopental (50 to 100 mg IV or 3 to 5 mg/kg IV) or propofol (1 mg/kg IV) can be used for induction.[11,12,14]

Succinylcholine (1.5 mg/kg in adults and up to 2.5 mg/kg in pediatric patients) is the ideal paralytic agent in patients with increased ICP due to its rapid onset, short duration of action, and consistent and reliable effects.[15] Longer-acting nondepolarizing agents (e.g., rocuronium or vecuronium) are appropriate when contraindications to succinylcholine exist (see Chapter 5). Ideally, paralytics should be short-acting to facilitate close monitoring of the patient's neurologic status.

Propofol has gained acceptance as the sedative of choice in patients with increased ICP because of its short duration of action and depression of cerebral metabolism and oxygen consumption. This is hypothesized to have a neuroprotective effect; however, there is no evidence that it improves mortality or 6-month outcomes.[16] When compared to midazolam, propofol has been shown to produce a better quality of sedation and increased seizure threshold.[17] This agent should be used with caution as higher doses of propofol can cause significant hypotension and extended periods of its use can be associated with significant morbidity.[14]

Oxygenation and Hyperventilation

As the airway is secured, adequate supplemental oxygen should be provided, with titration down rapidly from the initial fraction of inspired oxygen of 1.0 used for RSI to ensure oxygen saturation greater than 90%.[6]

In general, hyperventilation should be avoided in patients with brain injury, particularly in the first 24 hours as low Pco_2 levels cause cerebral vasoconstriction, resulting in decreased CBF in the critical hours following injury.[6,16] Hyperventilation is also associated with poor survival and neurologic outcomes.[16,18] For the majority of brain-injured patients, the target is thus eucapnia with a Pco_2 of 35 to 40 mm Hg.[16] Nevertheless, if a patient displays evolving signs of brain herniation (e.g., anisocoria, hemiparesis, asymmetric posturing, Cushing reflex, or rapid deterioration in GCS score), transient hyperventilation may be necessary to arrest the process. Current recommendations target a Pco_2 of 30 to 35 mm Hg in these scenarios as a temporizing measure (15 to 30 min) until surgical or other interventions to lower ICP can occur.[16]

Head Position

If not in shock, routinely elevate the patient's head to decrease ICP, risk of aspiration, and in those who are intubated, rates of ventilator-associated pneumonia. This position allows drainage of cerebral veins. Feldman,[19] Ng,[20] and their colleagues demonstrated that elevation of the head to 30 degrees significantly reduces ICP in most patients without impairing CBF, CPP, or cerebral metabolism. In hypotensive patients, head of bed elevation should be maintained, and the hypotension should be corrected with vasopressor therapy. If head elevation is to be used, MAP must be maintained above 90 mm Hg to facilitate a CPP of approximately 60 mm Hg.[21] It is also important to avoid neck rotation and flexion or any other intervention that could result in compression of the jugular vein. If the jugular veins are compressed, venous outflow from the head can be further compromised, increasing ICP. Therefore the head and neck should be kept in a neutral position.

Fluid and Blood Pressure Management

The goal in fluid management is to maintain euvolemia; head-injured patients with hypotension have double the mortality of normotensive patients. Patients with increased ICP may be hypovolemic from profuse vomiting, decreased fluid intake, or hemorrhage. Distributive shock may also be present and occurs as a result of loss of vasomotor sympathetic tone, especially in patients with concomitant cervical spine injury. Only isotonic or hypertonic fluids should be used (normal or hypertonic saline), as hypotonic fluids may lead to worsening brain edema. Vasopressors may also be necessary to maintain a recommended SBP > 100 mm Hg for patients 50 to 69 years old or ≥110 mm Hg for patients 15 to 49 or >70 years old to decrease mortality and improve outcomes.[16]

Hyperosmolar Therapy

Mannitol effectively and rapidly reduces ICP. Mannitol can be given at doses of 0.25 to 1 g/kg (with the highest dose used in emergency situations) infused every 2 to 4 or more hours.[22] Current recommendations favor bolus therapy over continuous infusion. Mannitol can cause a precipitous drop in blood pressure (and hence CPP) in patients who are hypovolemic. Thus mannitol is contraindicated in those with preexisting hypotension (typically defined as systolic blood pressure lower than 90 mm Hg).[16] The effect of mannitol on ICP is transient; repeated doses lose their ability to decrease ICP over time. It may also cause renal damage as serum osmolarity increases. Like hyperventilation, mannitol should be viewed as a bridge to definitive neurosurgical intervention and its use reserved for patients with signs of impending herniation.

Mannitol has two properties: it initially acts as a volume expander and then serves as an osmotic agent. On administration of mannitol, intravascular volume expands and blood viscosity decreases, resulting in augmentation of CBF. Once volume expansion has occurred, osmotic movement of fluid from the brain parenchyma to the intravascular compartment begins and results in a decrease in ICP. The osmotic effect usually occurs within 15 minutes. The half-life of mannitol ranges from 90 minutes to 6 hours.[23] Its effect is most pronounced in patients with CPP lower than 70 mm Hg.[23]

Hypertonic saline is a good alternative to mannitol in patients who are found to be hypotensive. Hypertonic saline is an ideal resuscitation fluid for patients with concomitant head injury and hemorrhagic shock as it effectively expands intravascular volume while causing osmotic diuresis of the brain. Hypertonic saline is typically used as a 3% solution in 150-mL boluses, as a 7.5% solution in 75-mL boluses, or as a 23.4% solution in 30-mL boluses. There is no consensus on the preferred concentration or volume of administration.[22–24] Hypertonic saline can be re-dosed if needed and its onset of action occurs rapidly.

Although the use of mannitol and hypertonic saline have both been endorsed by the Brain Trauma Foundation and a large consortium of pediatric societies in the past, no clear evidence favors the use of one or the other in normotensive or hypertensive patients.[22,23,25] Meta-analyses comparing mannitol and hypertonic saline head-to-head in patients with elevated ICP, from a variety of causes (traumatic brain injury, stroke, tumors), found that hypertonic saline appears to have greater efficacy in managing elevated ICP, but clinical outcomes have not been systematically compared.[26,27] However, in patients with hypotension, hypertonic saline is clearly preferred. A serum osmolarity of 320 mmol/L has previously been stated to be the upper limit of safety with both mannitol and hypertonic saline; however, this has been safely exceeded in practice without deleterious effects.[22,28]

Seizure Prophylaxis

Controlling seizure activity is paramount in the early stages of traumatic brain injury to avoid hypoxia and aspiration, as well as elevation of ICP and possible herniation. In the absence of a seizure, it is currently controversial whether prophylactic anticonvulsant medication should be routinely administered after spontaneous intracranial hemorrhage. If a seizure occurs, anticonvulsant therapy is warranted. Following traumatic brain injury, there is low-quality evidence supporting the use of prophylactic phenytoin during the first 7 days following injury to prevent early posttraumatic seizures, with the recognition that this has no effect on the occurrence of late seizures or mortality.[29] Rapidly acting benzodiazepines such as lorazepam and diazepam are first-line therapy for actively seizing patients, followed by anticonvulsant agents such as pentobarbital or phenytoin. Fosphenytoin can be given more rapidly (up to 150 mg/min IV by infusion) than phenytoin, which can be administered no faster than 50 mg/min IV. Phenytoin can induce hypotension and lower CPP, even at rates below 50 mg/min. A randomized control study comparing levetiracetam and phenytoin for seizure prophylaxis in cases of severe head injury and stroke showed equivalent efficacy.[30] A subsequent meta-analysis study suggests that levetiracetam has a better safety profile compared to phenytoin.[31] Although beneficial effects of prophylactic anticonvulsants on outcomes have not been established, the risks associated with administration of anticonvulsants are small in comparison to the potentially devastating secondary injury that results from uncontrolled seizure activity.

Patients who are paralyzed, either chemically or by their neurologic disease, are difficult to monitor for seizure activity without the use of electroencephalography (EEG). These patients may manifest seizures by subtle rhythmic movements of the extremities, tonic gaze deviation, an elevation in heart rate or blood pressure, or spikes on an ICP monitor (if one is placed by the neurosurgeon). Whenever possible, avoid using paralytic agents (other than during intubation) so that seizure activity can be monitored. If seizures are not controlled despite upward titration of benzodiazepines, phenytoin, or other agents, endotracheal intubation and induction of a barbiturate or propofol coma may be necessary. Pentobarbital has been used to treat uncontrolled elevations in ICP when other medical and surgical treatments have failed. It decreases CBF, metabolism, oxygen consumption, and cerebral edema. It also scavenges free radicals.[32] Pentobarbital is given at a loading dose of 10 mg/kg over a 30-minute period followed by infusion at 1 to 3 mg/kg per hour with an EEG monitor available for burst suppression. Intensive monitoring of the patient's hemodynamic status is necessary because of pentobarbital's hypotensive effect.

Steroids

Steroids have been shown to be beneficial in patients with edema associated with brain tumors. Steroids decrease CSF production, stabilize membranes, and restore normal membrane permeability.[33–35] Dexamethasone is usually administered at 10 to 20 mg IV as a loading dose, followed by 4 to 10 mg every 6 hours. No studies support the use of steroids in head-injured patients; in fact, steroid use in this population has been found to increase mortality.[36,37] In addition, glucocorticoids are not believed to be useful in the management of intracranial hemorrhage or cerebral infarction, but do have some utility in central nervous system infections that are associated with elevated ICP (i.e., brain abscess and bacterial meningitis).

Glucose Control

Head-injured patients tend to be hyperglycemic in response to stress. Patients treated with steroids for tumor-related edema may also develop hyperglycemia. Optimization of blood glucose levels is important in the management of these patients to avoid cellular edema in brain tissue. Hypoglycemic states can exacerbate brain injury and therefore should be scrupulously avoided. However, the long-term value of tight glycemic control in the management of acute brain injury with increased ICP is unclear.

Temperature Control

Fever increases brain metabolism, resulting in increased CBF, and can elevate ICP by increasing the volume of blood within the fixed space of the cranial vault. Studies have shown that in patients with ICH or TBI, elevated temperatures are associated with worse outcomes.[38,39]

Based on this data and the relationship between increased metabolic demand and increased CBF, elevated temperatures (greater than 37.0°C) should be aggressively treated with antipyretics and cooling measures in patients with increased ICP (with specific avoidance of shivering as it too can increase cerebral metabolism).

Conversely, lower body temperatures have been associated with a decrease in CBF, ICP, and metabolism. The previous method of keeping core temperatures lower than 30°C has been abandoned due to increased incidence of cardiac arrhythmias, severe coagulopathy, and the difficulty of maintaining such profound hypothermia. Although one study has shown a benefit in survival and decreased ICP with mild hypothermia (32 to 34°C),[40] in the setting of traumatic brain injury and stroke it is not currently recommended and should only be considered if all other treatment modalities have been ineffective in lowering ICP.[41]

Skull Trephination

Skull trephination, also known as trepanning, trepanation, or burr hole placement, is a technique that has been traced back to the Neolithic age.[42] Though rarely performed by nonsurgeons, it can be a lifesaving procedure for severely head-injured patients. In a patient with an acute epidural hematoma and deteriorating findings on neurologic examination (such as decreasing level of consciousness, anisocoria, or hemiparesis), skull trephination has been shown to improve both short- and long-term neurologic outcomes.[43,44] Trephination is also an appropriate treatment for acute subdural hematoma, but this requires incision through the dura mater and is less realistic for nonneurosurgeons (Figs. 60.9 and 60.10). Trephination may be lifesaving if performed before transport in selected patients from remote-practice environments without neurosurgical capability. This heroic procedure is not standard, nor is it an expected skill for most emergency clinicians; nonetheless, it may be attempted when the situation is dire.

Trephination in the ED should be performed only in the temporal regions. Trephination in the parietal and occipital regions is associated with a much higher risk for hemorrhage and air embolism due to their proximity to the dural venous sinuses. These approaches should generally be performed only after the results of CT are available for guidance.[43]

In practice environments without access to CT, it is not unreasonable to attempt this procedure before transport of the patient when all other measures to lower ICP have failed and signs of evolving brain herniation are present. The blind approach for temporal trephination is depicted in Fig. 60.11 and involves locating an area 2 cm anterior and 2 cm superior to the tragus on the side of the suspected hematoma.[43] In the majority of cases, the appropriate side for trephination is ipsilateral to pupillary dilation and contralateral to motor paresis.

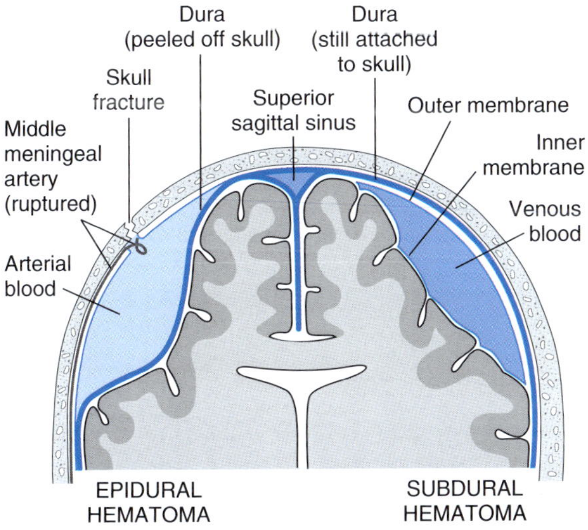

Fig. 60.9 Epidural hematoma *(left)*: rupture of a meningeal artery (usually associated with a skull fracture) leads to accumulation of arterial blood between the dura and skull. Subdural hematoma *(right)*: damage to bridging veins between the brain and superior sagittal sinus leads to accumulation of blood between the dura and the arachnoid. (From Mitchell R, Kumar V, Fausto N, et al. *Pocket Companion to Robbins & Cotran Pathological Basis of Disease*. 8th ed. Saunders; 2011.)

The temporal area (between the ear and the orbit) should be shaved and prepared with chlorhexidine or povidone-iodine using sterile technique. Local anesthetic can be used to infiltrate the area of the planned incision; however, this is not necessary in an unconscious patient and adds unnecessary time to the procedure (Review Box 60-1).

Once the proper location is identified, either with a blind approach or by using the results of CT, make a 4-cm vertical incision through the skin and temporalis fascia. Divide the temporalis muscle. Once the periosteum is identified, incise it. Expose the skull by elevating the periosteum (using a periosteal elevator if available). Insert a trephine or hand drill into the area underneath the periosteum.[43] While holding the drill perpendicular to the skull, apply continuous gentle downward pressure and rotate the drill in an alternating clockwise-counterclockwise motion. As progress is made with the hand drill, gradually reduce pressure to avoid inadvertent "plunging" into the brain parenchyma. The operator will know when penetration through both the outer and inner tables of the skull has been accomplished when resistance against the drill is no longer appreciated. After skull penetration has been accomplished, remove the round piece of bone that has been cored out (with the diameter of the drill) and place it in saline.

In many cases, epidural blood and clots under pressure will extrude from the site upon complete penetration of the skull. However, insertion of a suction catheter into the trephinated space may be necessary for full evacuation of clotted material. If easily identified, the bleeding artery (usually the middle meningeal artery) may be clamped.[43] After successful trephination, the patient's status should immediately be reassessed

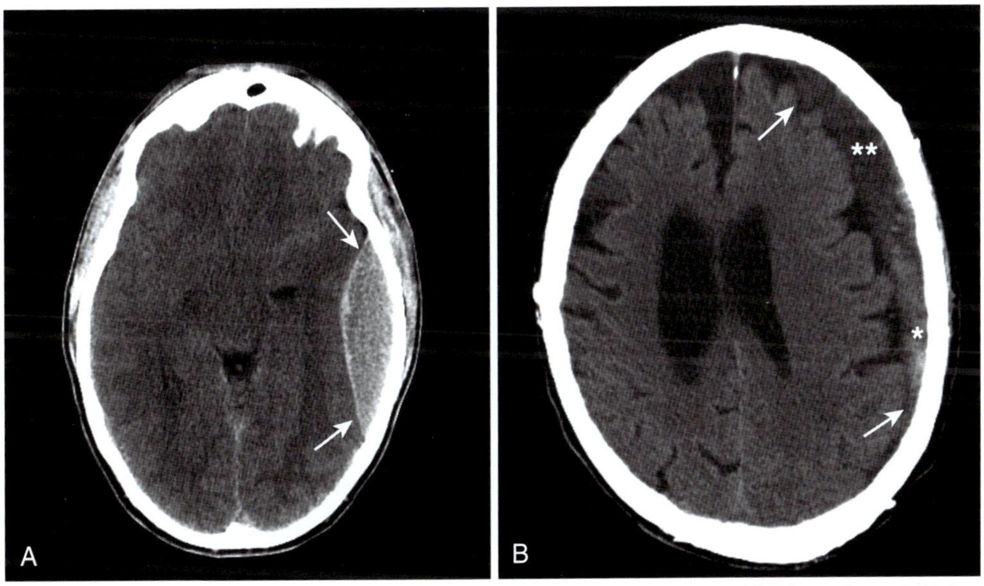

Fig. 60.10 Epidural and subdural hematomas. (A) Acute epidural hematoma. The hyperdense *(white)* appearance of this lesion indicates that it is acute. The inner margins of epidurals *(arrows)* have a convex appearance, which results in a lens-shaped hematoma. Note that the hematoma does not cross the suture lines (temporal-sphenoid anteriorly, temporal-parietal posteriorly). (B) Acute-on-chronic subdural hematoma. The heterogeneous density of this lesion (hypodense anteriorly *[double asterisk]*, hyperdense posteriorly *[asterisk]*) suggests an acute-on-chronic hemorrhage. The inner margins of subdurals *(arrows)* are concave, which results in a crescent-shaped hematoma. Subdural hematomas may cross suture lines (note that this hematoma extends from the frontal to the parietal regions). Both these examples demonstrate effacement of the lateral ventricles and midline shift, which are indicators of increased intracranial pressure.

Emergency Skull Trephination

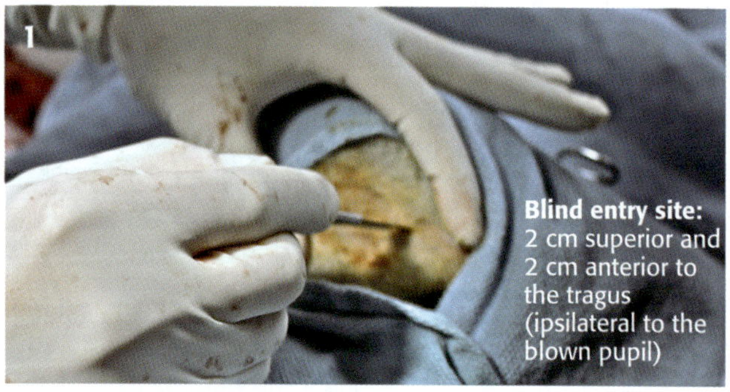

Shave, prepare, and drape the entry site. Use CT to guide the location of the burr hole placement. If CT is not available, choose a site 2 cm anterior and 2 cm superior to the tragus.

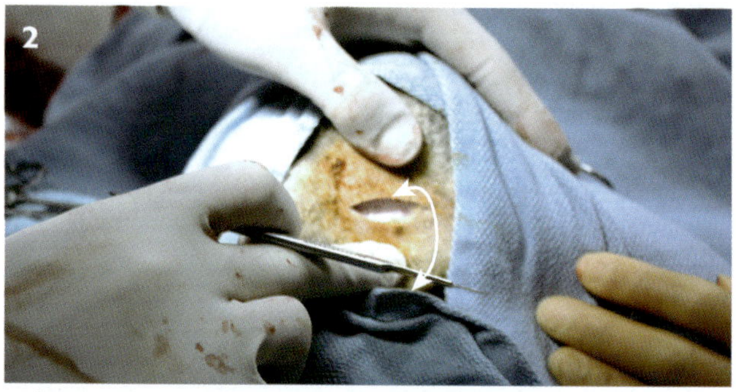

Make a 4-cm vertical incision extending down to the periosteum. Optionally apply Raney clips to the skin edges to control bleeding.

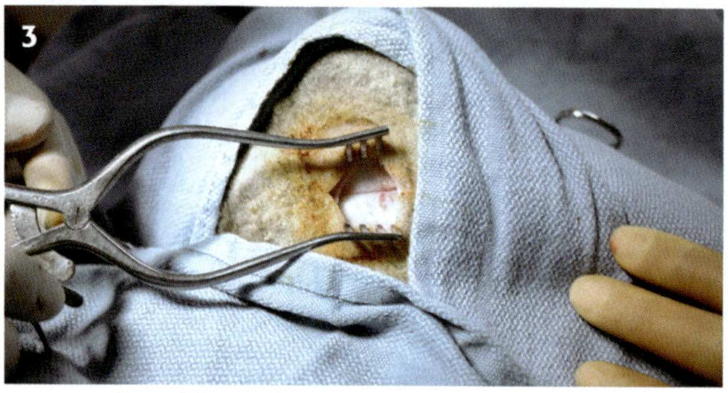

Insert a self-retaining scalp retractor to provide exposure. The exposed area should be about 2.5 cm in diameter.

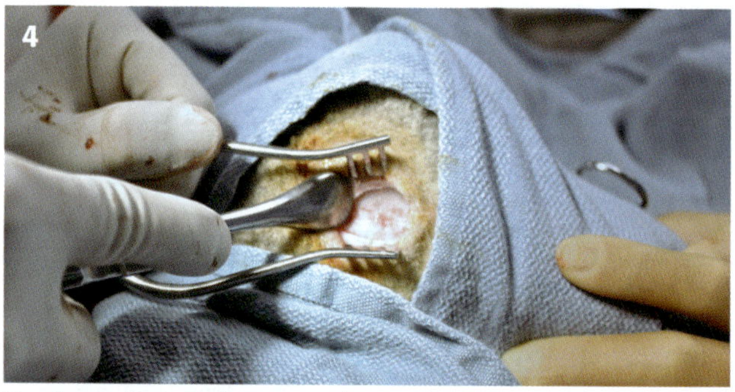

Use the periosteal elevator to elevate the periosteum off the skull.

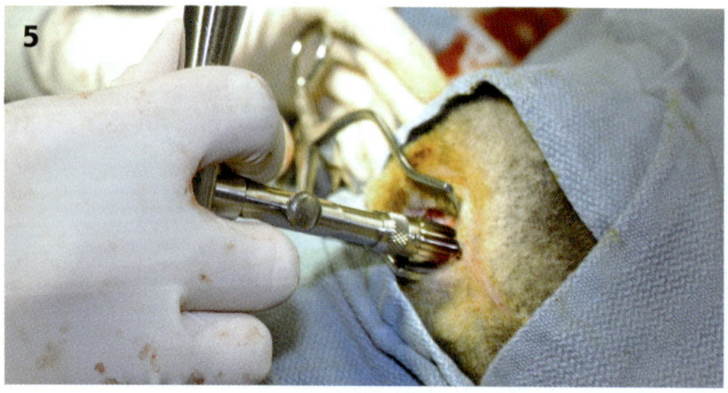

Adjust the centering point of the trephine so that it protrudes 1/8 inch. With the trephine at a 90-degree angle to the skull, apply gentle pressure with a clockwise-counterclockwise rotating motion.

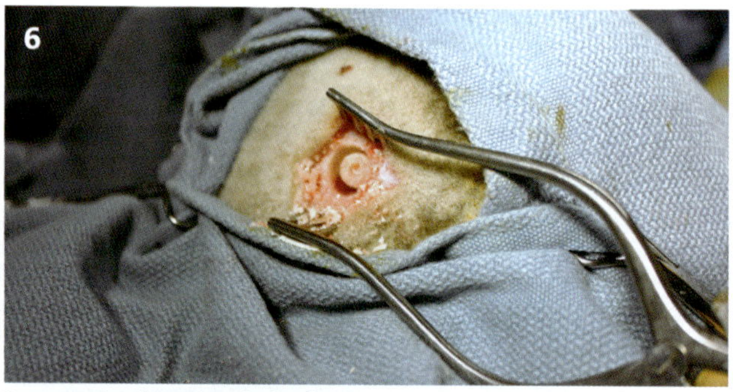

Stop sawing into the skull when you feel a slight give, which indicates that you have penetrated the full thickness of the skull. Remove the trephine.

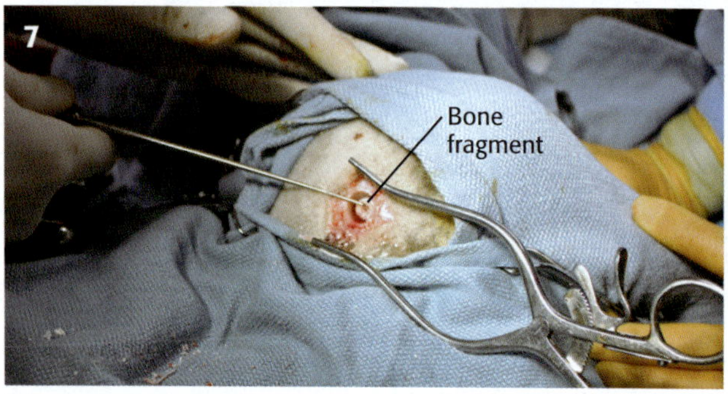

If the bone fragment does not come out in the trephine, use toothed forceps or a hooked instrument to remove it. Preserve the bone fragment in sterile saline.

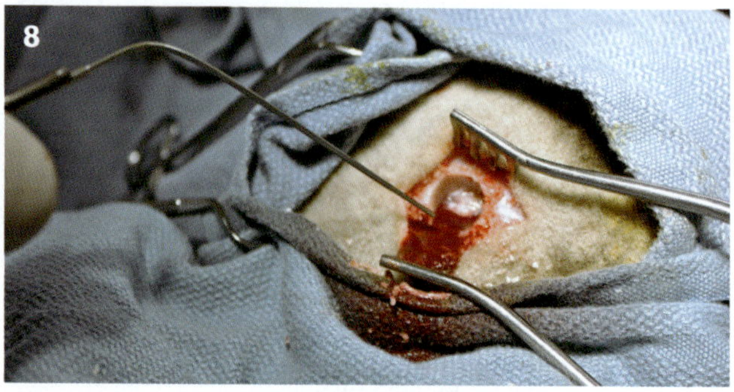

Allow the clot and blood to extrude from the burr hole. Apply gentle suction as needed to assist evacuation of the clot. A small suction catheter can be left in place during transport if needed.

Fig. 60.11 Emergency skull trephination. This technique is for patients with epidural hematomas in the temporal region. It should not be used for parietal or occipital hematomas. If a subdural hematoma is present, the dura must be opened. If no blood is encountered on a blind procedure done on the same side as a blown pupil, repeat it on the opposite side. *CT*, Computed tomography.

Emergency Skull Trephination

Indications

Acute epidural hematoma and both of the following:

1. Deteriorating findings on neurologic examination (e.g., decreasing level of consciousness, anisocoria, hemiparesis)
2. Delay in obtaining definitive neurosurgical care (e.g., remote-practice environments)

Contraindications

Parietal or occipital epidural hematomas (high risk for hemorrhage and air embolism because of dural venous sinuses)

Subdural hematomas (requires an incision through the dura mater and is less realistic for the non-neurosurgeon)

Complications

Bleeding

Infection

Brain parenchymal injury

Equipment

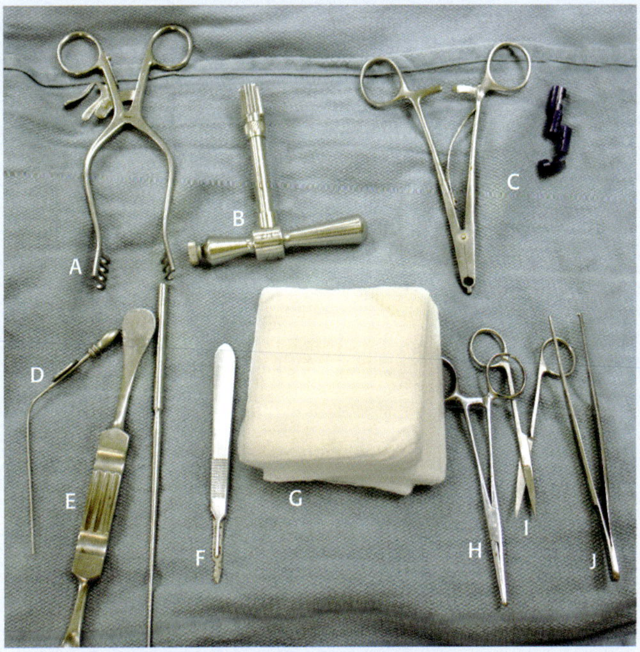

A. Self-retaining scalp retractor
B. ½-inch Galt trepine
C. Raney clips and applier
D. Suction
E. Periosteal elevator
F. Scalpel
G. Gauze 4- × 4-in pads
H. Kelly clamp
I. Scissors
J. Adson (toothed) forceps

Review Box 60.1 Emergency skull trephination: indications, contraindications, complications, and equipment.

for signs of improvement. In a significant minority of patients, false localizing signs may lead the clinician to suspect a hematoma on the wrong side. Thus if no improvement is noted with trephination on the side of the suspected hematoma, the procedure may be repeated on the opposite side. However, in all cases, the delay in definitive neurosurgical care caused by attempts at trephination must be weighed against the possible benefits of the procedure. Moreover, trephination should ideally be performed after consultation with the accepting neurosurgeon.[44]

Case reports of using more commonly available tools such as intraosseous intravenous drills have been published.[45] Complications of the procedure include bleeding, infection, and injury to the brain parenchyma.

Operative Management

Operative management is the definitive treatment of increased ICP secondary to a space-occupying lesion. This entails either craniotomy or ventriculostomy with drainage of blood and CSF.

INTRACRANIAL SHUNTS

Intracranial shunts are used for the long-term management of increased ICP. The basic principle behind an intracranial shunt is to divert excess CSF into a body cavity from which it can be absorbed.

The essential elements of the shunt system include a proximal and a distal catheter, valves, and a reservoir. The valves allow unidirectional flow away from the ventricles, incorporate a pumping chamber, and regulate the pressure at which flow will occur across it. The reservoir is usually located between two valves. The proximal valve allows flow from the ventricles to the reservoir, whereas the distal valve allows flow from the reservoir to the distal catheter (Fig. 60.12). In most cases, the reservoir allows for measurement of pressure, testing for patency, fluid sampling, and injection of medication or contrast material. In rare cases, other equipment is incorporated into the shunt system for specific purposes, including an on-off switch, a telemetric pressure sensor, and an anti-siphon device. Many different types of shunt systems, incorporating a variety of designs, are available (Fig. 60.13).

Most intracranial shunts drain CSF from the lateral ventricles into the peritoneum (ventriculoperitoneal or VP) shunts. They are the mainstay for treatment of hydrocephalus in infants and children because of the ease of insertion of the catheter and the capacity of the peritoneal cavity to absorb CSF. Other types of shunts include ventriculovenous, ventriculoatrial, ventriculopleural, and lumboperitoneal. These types of shunts tend to have a higher rate of complications and are usually reserved for circumstances in which VP shunting has failed or when the patient has a history of multiple abdominal surgeries or peritoneal infections.

In the VP shunt system, a ventricular catheter is placed in the right frontal horn of the lateral ventricle (nondominant

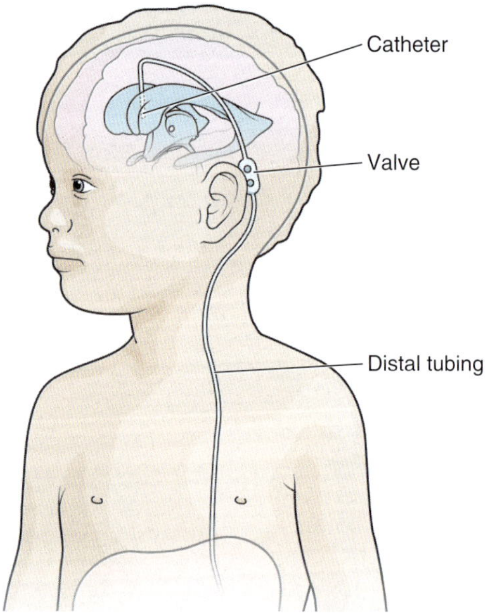

Fig. 60.12 The basic tripartite ventricular shunt system is composed of a ventricular catheter, valve mechanism, and distal tubing. A slit valve may be used in the far end of the distal tubing instead of a more proximally placed valve, as shown.

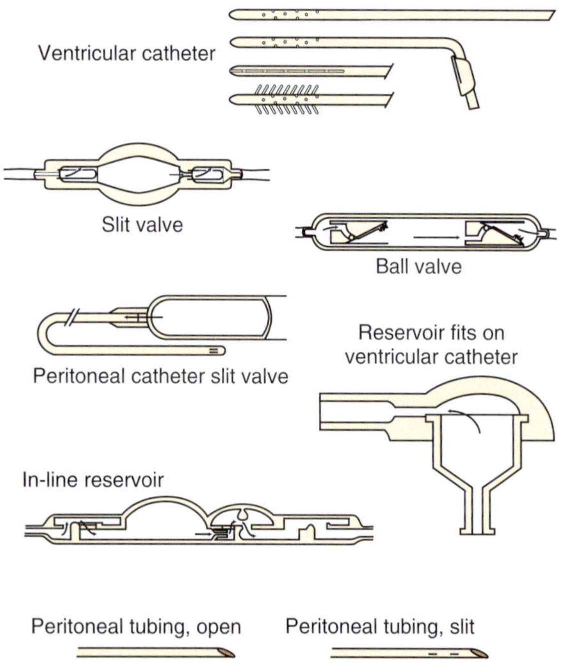

Fig. 60.13 Shunt components. (From Rengachary SS, Wilkins RH, eds. *Principles of Neurosurgery*. Mosby; 1994.)

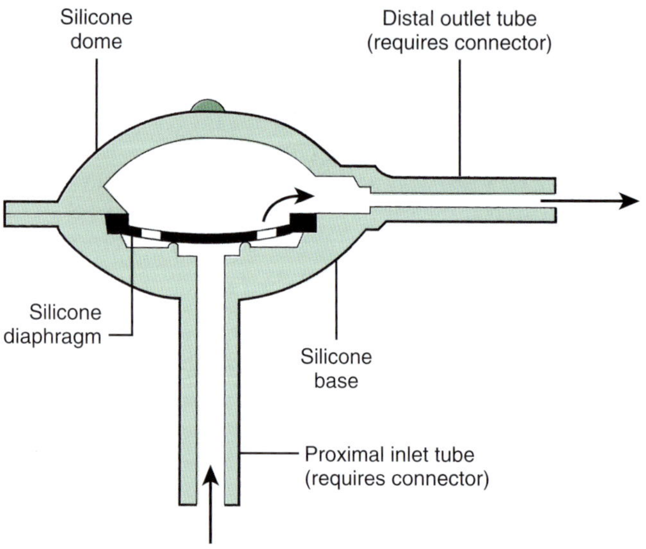

Fig. 60.14 Cross section of a Pudenz flushing valve illustrating the diaphragm valve. The proximal inlet tube and silicone base are placed in the bur hole so that only the reservoir (silicon dome) protrudes above the skull. (Courtesy PS Medical, Goleta, CA.)

hemisphere) and connected to a subcutaneous valve traversing the temporal aspect (Fig. 60.14). This valve is then connected to a distal catheter threaded subcutaneously into the neck and finally into the peritoneum (Fig. 60.15). Ventricular catheters can be either straight or angled, with the latter having the option of a reservoir component attachment. Valves come in four different types (ball, diaphragm, miter, slit), each with unique flow characteristics. The distal catheter has either an open or closed end. Identifying the type of shunt in place is often difficult unless the patient or caretaker has the information available. Moreover, the skin overlying the subcutaneous component of the shunt in the temporal regions can scar, thus rendering palpation of the shunt type impossible.

Programmable VP shunts have recently become more popular and several different brands are now available. Unlike a traditional shunt, which has a fixed pressure threshold for CSF drainage, the opening pressure of the valve in a programmable shunt can be adjusted transcutaneously using a magnetic coding device.

Shunt Failure

VP shunts represent the mainstay of treatment for chronic IIH in both children and adults, with an estimated 30,000 intracranial shunts placed every year in the United States.[46] The rate of complications and shunt failure is high. In one retrospective series, 84.5% of pediatric patients required one or more shunt revisions and nearly 5% of patients required 10 or more.[47] A shunt failure rate of 30% to 40% within the first year is consistently reported in the literature and approximately 80% of patients will require at least one revision in the span of 20 years; more than half of these occur within the first 2 years after shunt placement.[48] Indications for intracranial shunt placement may occur at any age: 8% of patients are neonates, 26% children and 66.2% are adults.[49] Neonatal and pediatric patients tend to be at higher risk of complications.[47,49] Shunt failure can occur because of mechanical obstruction, fracture or migration of the shunt, excessive CSF drainage or infection.[50]

Mechanical Obstruction

The most common cause of shunt malfunction is catheter obstruction. This usually occurs at the ventricular catheter tip or at the valve and the peritoneal catheter.[51] The proximal blockage may be due to choroid plexus within the ventricular catheter or tissue debris within the valve itself. Some evidence suggests that delayed hypersensitivity to the shunt material is also an occasional cause of obstruction. Identifying the location of the obstruction is important for the neurosurgeon as the individual malfunctioning components of the shunt may

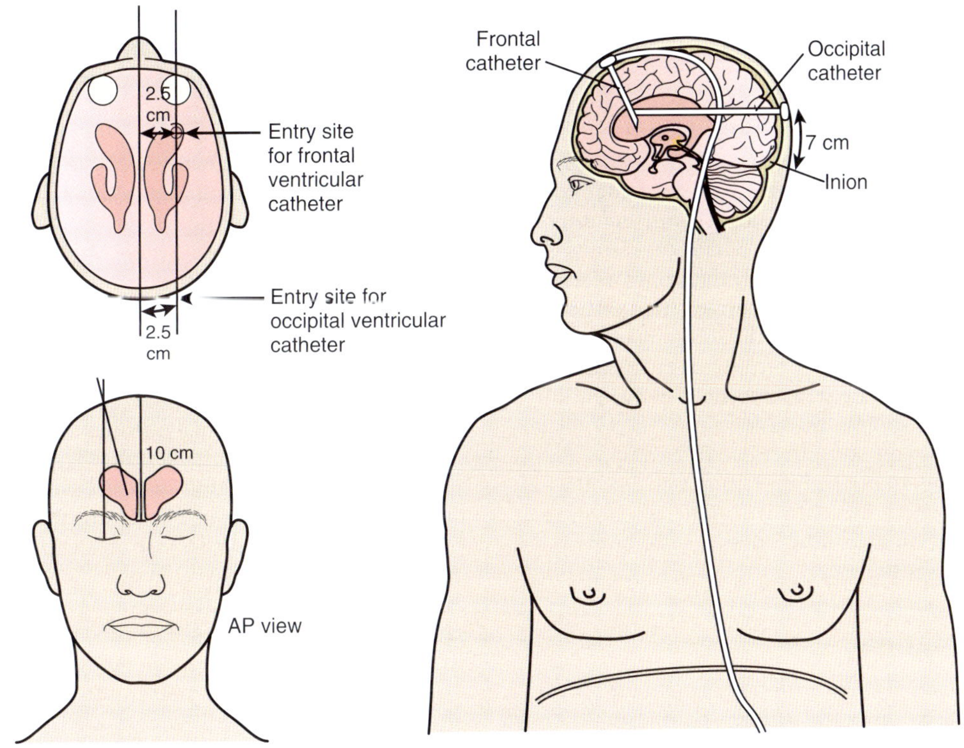

Fig. 60.15 Ventriculoperitoneal shunt and alternative occipital placement. *AP,* Anteroposterior. (From Rengachary SS, Wilkins RH, eds. *Principles of Neurosurgery.* Mosby; 1994.)

be replaced while preserving the rest of the device but is beyond the scope of the emergency physician.

Shunt Fracture

Often a late complication of shunt placement, fracture of the shunt may be due to a combination of aging of the components of the shunt itself and undue stress caused by tethering of the shunt by surrounding scar tissue. It generally occurs in the distal portion of the catheter in proximity of the clavicle or lower ribs. Catheter disconnection, migration, and misplacement are other less common forms of mechanical VP shunt failure.[51] Fracture and migration of the catheter usually present with subtle signs of elevated ICP and are clinically similar to shunt obstruction.[51]

Excessive CSF Drainage

Extra-axial fluid collection may occur in response to rapid decompression of enlarged ventricles. This is a relatively rare cause of shunt failure and is estimated to occur in approximately 3.4% of cases. Although most commonly due to a benign collection of CSF, at times a subdural hematoma may form in response to the sudden decompression of the ventricles, which leads to tearing of the bridging veins as the brain pulls away from the dura. Slit ventricle syndrome (SVS) can also occur in response to chronic over-drainage in children and is characterized by small ventricles demonstrated on CT scan with symptoms suggestive of shunt malfunction. In contrast to shunt obstruction, symptoms of SVS are typically influenced by postural changes and improve after resting supine.[52]

Abdominal Complications

Abdominal complications including the presence of ascites as well as the development of a pseudocyst surrounding the distal portion may affect the function of the VP shunt. A potentially lethal complication of the immediate postoperative period is perforation of intraabdominal viscera due to instrumentation of the peritoneum during the catheter placement.

Shunt Infection: Treatment and Prevention

Of all the potential complications associated with shunting procedures, infection is the most notorious and occurs in 2% to 10% of VP shunts.[51] This is the second most common cause of shunt failure. Both the diagnosis and the treatment may be elusive, and no clear evidence-based guidelines exist for the management of CSF infections in the presence of VP shunts. Rarely, infection can be due to skin organisms overlying the valve that may ulcerate the skin and colonize the shunt. The most common cause of shunt infection is thought to be colonization at the time of shunt placement.[53] Typical organisms include *Staphylococcus epidermidis* and *Staphylococcus aureus*, as well as gram-negative bacilli, which are thought to be introduced into the system during manipulation of the site.[52] Approximately 70% of these infections are seen within 2 months of shunt placement. Other risk factors associated with shunt infection include perioperative infection and dental or urologic instrumentation. Premature infants, who have an immature immune system, are substantially more vulnerable to shunt infections.[54] Most shunt infections are caused by otherwise nonvirulent bacteria such as *S. epidermidis*. In the presence of the shunt, these organisms exhibit unusual virulence. This reflects a variety of factors, including the ability to adhere to shunt surfaces, as well as production of mucoid substances that protect the bacteria from host defenses. The silicone elastomer shunt material itself has an adverse effect on the immune system. Specifically, leukocytes cannot adhere to such surfaces as well as bacteria can.

The diagnosis may be obvious in patients with variable systematic signs, wound infection, meningitis, peritonitis, or septicemia. However, the shunt may harbor an indolent infection without symptoms or signs. Culture of CSF obtained from a shunt tap may be negative even when the shunt is ultimately shown to be infected.

A 2014 systematic review and evidence-based guidelines for the treatment of pediatric hydrocephalus recommend removal of the shunt "with a moderate degree of clinical certainty" in the presence of shunt infection. However, controversy still exists over the need for complete or partial shunt removal.[55] Nevertheless, many neurosurgeons still recommend replacement of the entire shunt after the infection is eradicated.

If a shunt infection is suspected, empiric systemic antibiotics should be given as soon as possible in the ED. Consultation with a neurosurgeon and infectious disease specialist is recommended before administering antibiotics directly into the CSF, as the available evidence is insufficient to support intrathecal administration of antibiotics in addition to those administered systemically.[55]

Clinical Presentation

Patients with intracranial shunt malfunctions frequently present to the ED. In many cases, the patient's significant other or caretaker provides the subtle clues that lead to the diagnosis. Depending on the age of the patient, symptoms of increased ICP may include changes in behavior and level of consciousness. Headache, nausea, vomiting, and visual disturbances are also common. In children, lethargy, poor feeding, vomiting, ataxia, decreased or increased activity level, fussiness, fever and diaphoresis, as well as bulging fontanelles can all be indications of shunt malfunction. Bradycardia not associated with hypertension is also suggestive of increased ICP and shunt malfunction. Fever, particularly within the first 6 months after surgery, is strongly associated with shunt infection.[50] In children, lethargy and shunt site swelling are the most predictive signs of shunt malfunction.[56] Failure of upward gaze is another sign ("sunset eyes" or Parinaud syndrome). Cranial nerve, visual field, and fundoscopic examination and evidence of ataxia should be routine in the assessment of older, cooperative patients with intracranial shunts.[51]

Symptoms of shunt malfunction may be difficult to interpret, particularly if the symptoms are atypical or nonspecific or if they occur in young children. Likewise, asymptomatic shunt obstruction can occur in children in whom shunt independence has developed. Clinical evaluation of a child may not always be diagnostic of a shunt malfunction.

Shunt Assessment

Inspection and palpation of the accessible portions of the VP shunt can at times reveal the cause of dysfunction (fluid collection, scarring, fracture of the distal catheter).[51] The characteristics of the valve reservoir on compression or "pumping" the shunt may be useful in diagnosing shunt malfunction in some cases, although the utility of this technique has been challenged by some experts.[50] Partial shunt valve compression should be done because full depression and release may lead to suction and entrapment of the choroid plexus within the ventricular catheter. If the CT scan shows narrow (slit) ventricles, indicative of over-drainage, further valve compression should be avoided and may similarly cause blockage of the shunt. When compressing the shunt, a normal refill time of 15 to 30 seconds should be observed. If the valve fills more slowly than this but can be compressed easily, the obstruction is proximal to the valve. If the valve is not compressible, the blockage is either at the valve or distal to it. Proximal obstruction is more common than distal obstruction. The entire shunt tract and all surgical incisions should be examined for signs of wound infection, disruption of the tubing, or CSF leakage around the tract. Definitive treatment usually requires shunt revision.

Radiographic imaging is the cornerstone of shunt evaluation when dysfunction is suspected in the ED. A non–contrast-enhanced head CT is the initial imaging modality of choice. Radiographic findings indicative of hydrocephalus include enlarged ventricles and evidence of flow of CSF from the ventricle into the brain parenchyma. It should be noted, however, that the finding of enlarged ventricles on CT reveals little about shunt function unless comparison with previous images or serial scans shows progressive ventricular expansion. Head CT has a sensitivity of 83% in detecting shunt obstruction and a negative predictive value of 93%.

Although shunt series radiographs have long been a mainstay in the evaluation of VP shunts, evidence challenges the role of these radiographs as a routine part of the diagnostic workup for shunt malfunction in the setting of a normal CT or radionuclide imaging. Findings of an abnormal shunt series alone changed management only in 0.3% of cases in a retrospective review.[57]

Patients with intracranial shunts are subjected to repeat radiological evaluation over the course of their lifetime and excessive exposure to ionizing radiation is a very real concern. Therefore sparing additional unnecessary exposure to radiation has been advocated by certain experts.[57] Other techniques, such as low-dose CT scan obtained with decreased tube current and a lower number of CT slices (as low as three), have significantly decreased radiation exposure (up to 87%) while still accurately diagnosing shunt malfunction.[58] Modified magnetic resonance imaging (MRI) protocols have also decreased the use of ionizing radiation in the evaluation of shunt function. One note of caution: MRI studies may interfere with the settings of programmable VP shunts; consultation with the patient's neurosurgeon is advised before proceeding with MRI in these patients.[59]

Shunt series radiographs consist of anteroposterior (AP) and lateral skull, AP chest, and AP abdominal radiographs (Figs. 60.16 and 60.17). They still have an essential role in the setting of an abnormal CT as these films may reveal kinking, breakage, or disconnection of the catheter (Fig. 60.18) and help localize the site of shunt malfunction. Shunt series radiographs have a sensitivity of 20% and a negative predictive value of 22%.

If the distal catheter is in the peritoneum and a distal obstruction is suspected or if the patient complains of abdominal pain, abdominal ultrasound should be obtained. Ultrasound may reveal a pseudocyst at the distal portion of the catheter or an abnormal fluid collection. Ultrasound has also been used to rapidly identify the cause of catheter discontinuity malfunction at the bedside, particularly if radiographic studies are not readily available.[60]

Tapping the reservoir proximal to the distal valve allows percutaneous testing of proximal shunt patency. Although this is useful in most instances, it can be difficult to assess the rate of inflow or runoff adequately with a small-bore needle, particularly if the patient is a child or is unable to cooperate.

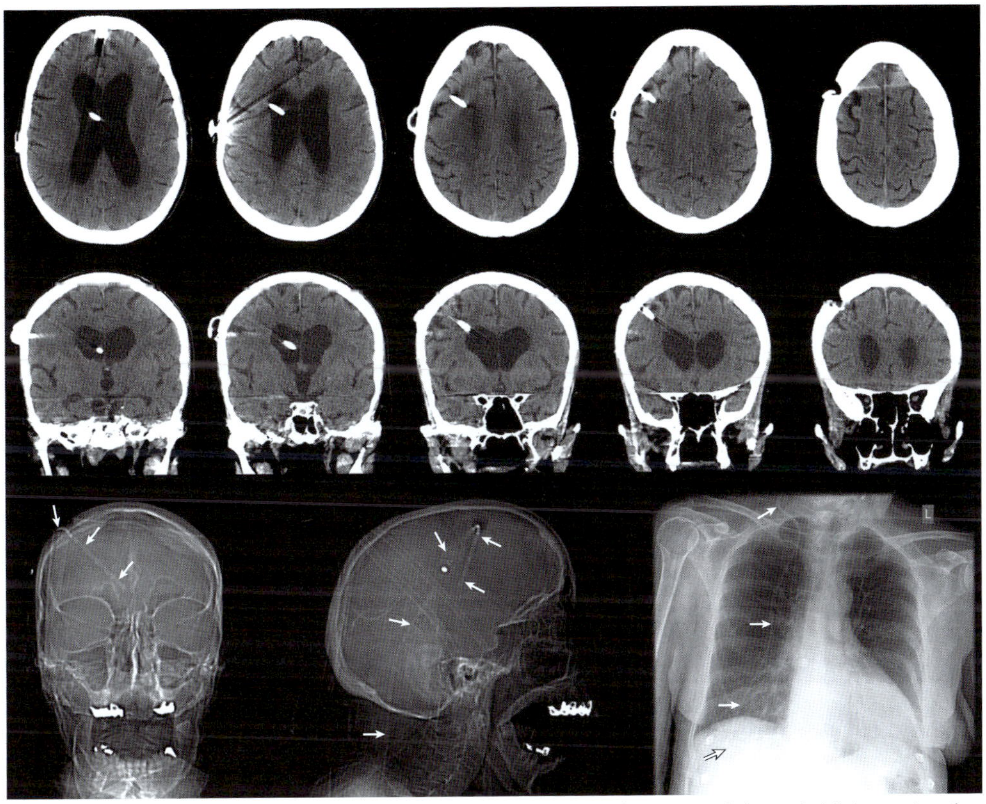

Fig. 60.16 Computed tomography (CT) evaluation of a ventriculoperitoneal shunt. Axial *(top row)* and coronal *(middle row)* CT images reveal the intracranial portion of the shunt. Mild ventriculomegaly is noted; however, this reveals little about shunt function without comparison to previous scans. The shunt *(arrows)* can also be visualized on the CT scout images *(bottom row, left and middle)*. A companion chest radiograph *(bottom row, right)* demonstrates continuity of the shunt *(arrows)* through to the peritoneal cavity.

CSF should be sent for analysis, including cell count, glucose, protein, Gram stain, and culture, when infection is suspected. The potential for introducing infection is a concern when accessing the VP shunt and strict sterile technique should be maintained throughout the procedure.

Other invasive techniques include injection of either radionuclide or contrast material into the shunt as a marker of flow; however, these techniques are rarely of use in the ED. If ventricular fluid pressure is low, there may be little evidence of flow, thus giving a false indication of shunt malfunction.

Various noninvasive techniques have been devised for assessing shunt function. Changes in visual evoked potentials associated with elevated ICP have been suggested as a means of determining function. Thermographic and doppler detection of shunt flow is also possible. MRI techniques can likewise assess CSF flow and shunt patency.

Shunt Tapping

See Videos 60.1 and 60.2. Percutaneous access of the VP shunt is generally performed by a neurosurgeon; however, if neurosurgical consultation is not available, the emergency physician may need to perform the procedure as described.

Clip the scalp hair over and around the reservoir, prepare the skin with a surgical scrub brush for 10 minutes, followed by the application of a povidone-iodine solution, and then allow it to fully dry. After appropriate draping, infiltrate the skin with 1% plain lidocaine to a level of adequate local anesthesia. Use a 25-gauge butterfly needle with tubing and enter the reservoir percutaneously at a 20- to 30-degree angle (Fig. 60.19). Lack of CSF flow from the reservoir indicates a proximal obstruction unless the ventricles are completely deflated (SVS). Even so, a small amount of CSF should be obtained within the tubing, thus ensuring that entry into the lumen of the reservoir has been accomplished. If the ventricles are deflated and only a small amount of CSF is aspirated, hold the end of the tubing 5 cm to 10 cm below the level of the reservoir to see whether CSF will fill the tubing and eventually begin to drip at the rate of 2 to 3 drops/min. If CSF is readily aspirated from the reservoir, hold the tubing vertically to obtain an indication of intraventricular pressure. This pressure reading, as well as the ease with which CSF is aspirated, will give some indication of proximal obstruction. To assess runoff or patency of the distal end, apply pressure to the tubing proximal to the reservoir and then deflate the reservoir without any resistance. If any resistance is encountered when deflating the reservoir, suspect a distal obstruction.

It is essential to send any aspirated CSF for laboratory analysis, including a cell count, protein, glucose, and most importantly, Gram stain, and culture to evaluate the system for infection.

Endoscopic Third Ventriculostomy

The diagnosis of shunt malfunction remains challenging and delays in diagnosis can cause permanent neurologic sequelae and death. An alternative CSF diversion technique not reliant on intracranial shunt devices is an endoscopic third ventriculostomy (EVT). This procedure creates an opening in the third

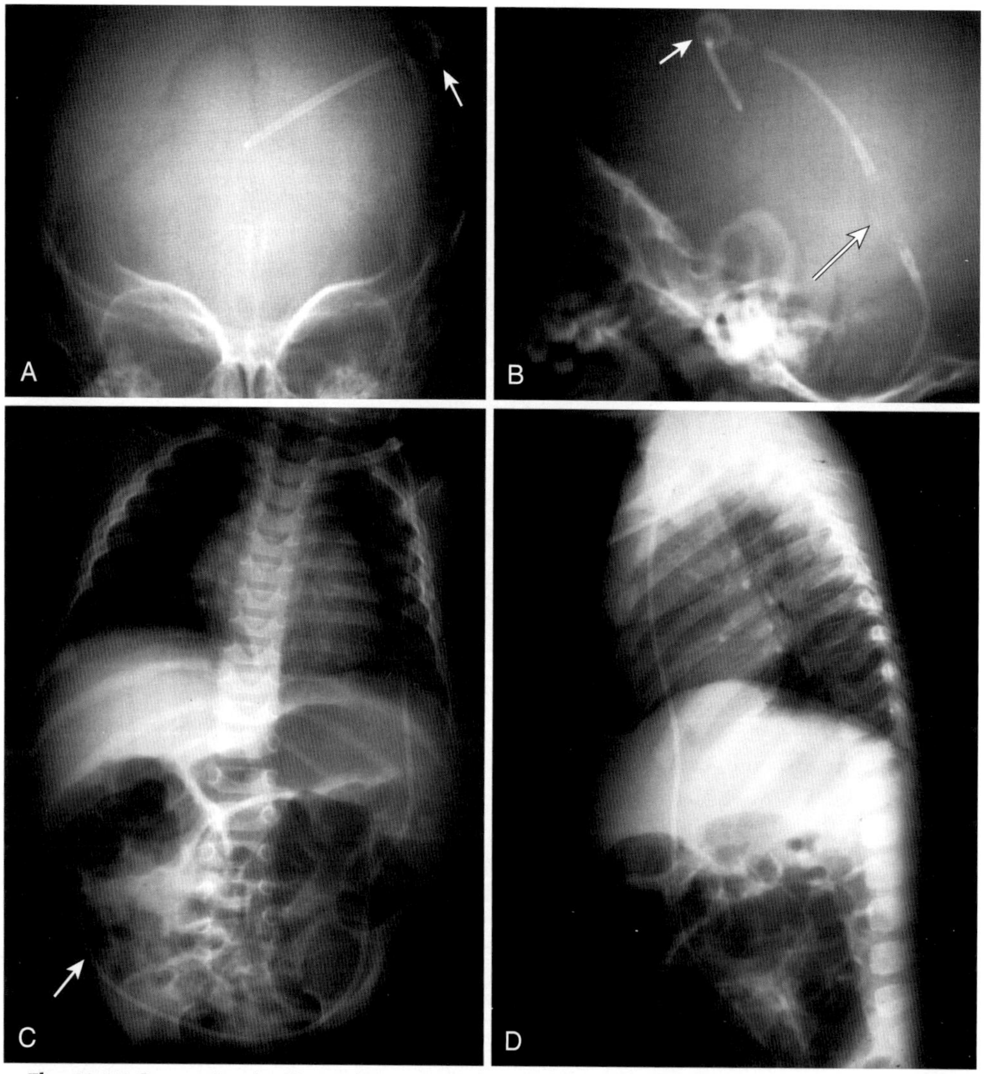

Fig. 60.17 Conventional radiography standard shunt series. A standard shunt series includes skull, chest, and abdominal radiographs. (A) This anteroposterior (AP) skull radiograph reveals the proximal intracranial portion of the shunt and a Rickham reservoir *(arrow)* over the burr hole. A companion non–contrast-enhanced head CT scan (see Fig. 60.16) is usually performed to further evaluate shunt function. (B) The lateral skull radiograph better reveals a cylindrical Holter valve *(long arrow)* several centimeters distal to the Rickham reservoir *(short arrow)*. (C) This AP chest and abdominal radiograph reveals the distal portion of the shunt *(arrow)*. Note the length of the catheter to allow patient growth. (D) The lateral chest and abdominal view demonstrate the course of the shunt.

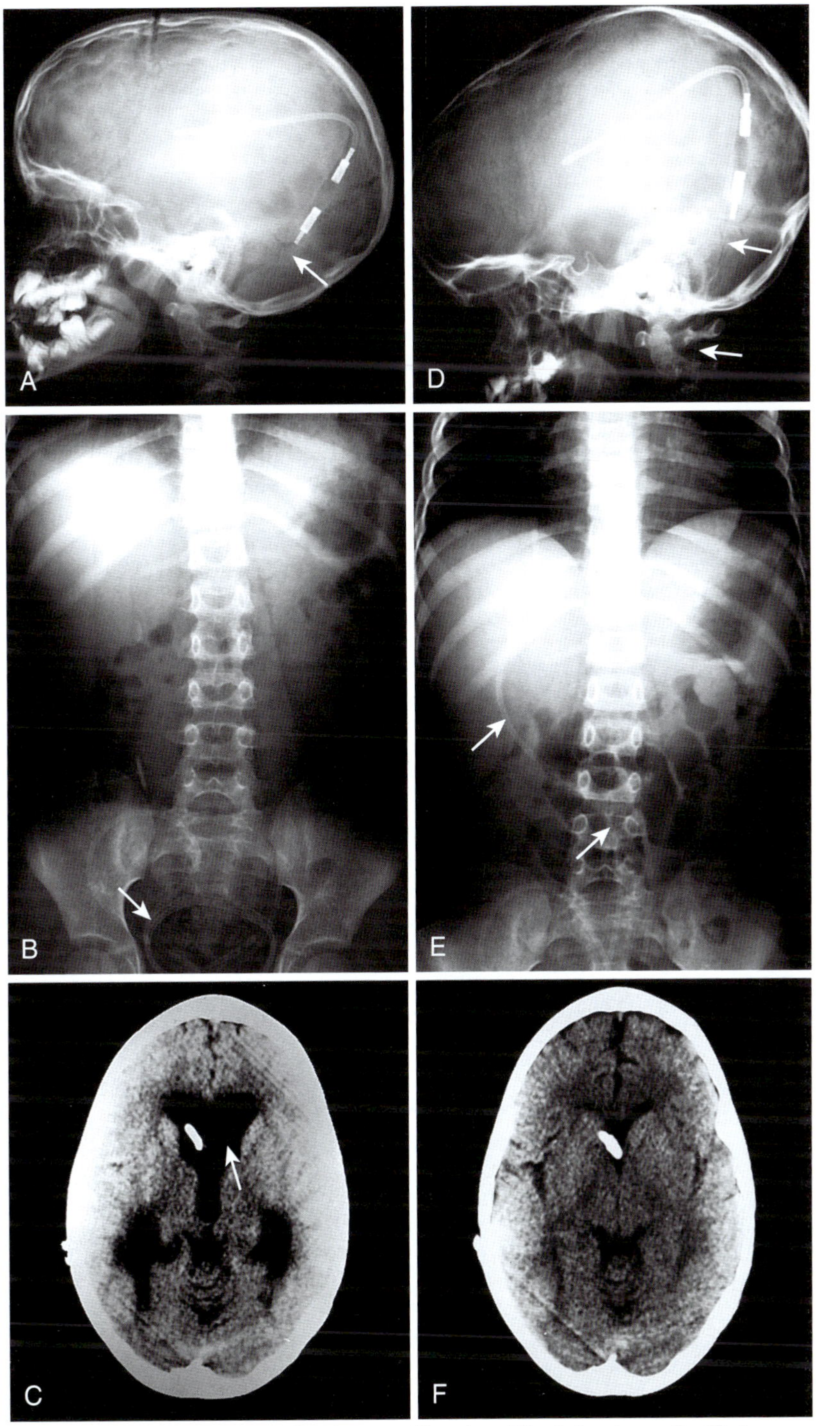

Fig. 60.18 Before and after series of a shunt malfunction. The left column (A–C) demonstrates a malfunctioning shunt. The right column (D–F) is the same patient after shunt revision. (A) The shunt has become disconnected at the valve; no efferent catheter tubing is seen coming from the inferior portion of the valve *(arrow)*. (B) The catheter has migrated inferiorly and has coiled in the pelvis *(arrow)*. (C) Head computed tomography (CT) scan showing ventriculomegaly *(arrow)*, a direct result of the shunt malfunction. (D) After shunt revision, the lateral skull radiograph shows that a catheter is now connected to the valve *(arrows*, difficult to appreciate on this film). (E) The catheter is seen coursing through the abdomen *(arrows)*. (F) Repeated head CT shows resolution of the ventriculomegaly.

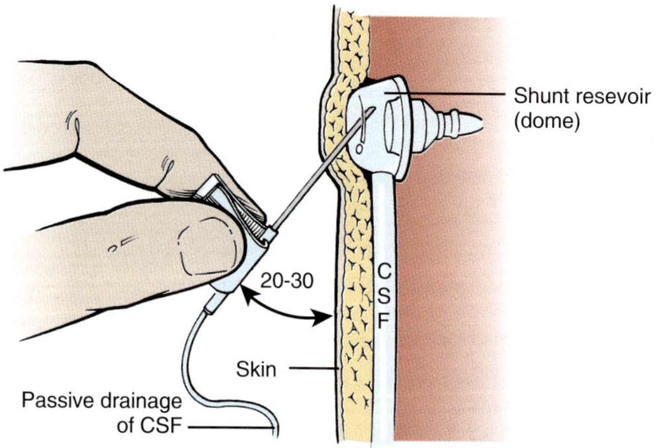

Fig. 60.19 Tapping a ventriculoperitoneal shunt. Use a 25-gauge butterfly needle to puncture the reservoir. To avoid damage to the reservoir, the angle should be approximately 20 to 30 degrees. Note that the dome reservoir is under the skin. Before passing the butterfly needle, the skin is anesthetized, sterilized with povidone-iodine, and nicked with a No. 11 scalpel blade or a larger needle. Fluid is not aspirated but is allowed to drain passively. *CSF,* Cerebrospinal fluid.

ventricle using an endoscope placed through a burr hole. This allows drainage of CSF into the basal cisterns bypassing the obstruction. EVT has several advantages over traditional shunts including lower cost, lack of implanted foreign body leading to less long-term complications (malfunction, infection, need for revision). However, patient selection is key as the procedure is dependent on the age of the patient, etiology of hydrocephalus, and prior shunt complications. Some patients will ultimately require traditional CSF shunting due to failure of the procedure. A systematic review of the evidence has found that ETV is a viable treatment option for pediatric hydrocephalus, with equivalent outcomes in determined clinical scenarios.[61]

ACKNOWLEDGMENTS

We thank Jessica L. Osterman, MD, and Megan L. Rischall, MD, as well as Frederick K. Korley, MD, Khosrow Tabassi, MD, and Cecile G. Silvestre, MD, for their contributions to this chapter in previous editions, as well as special thanks to Stuart P. Swadron, MD.

REFERENCES ARE AVAILABLE AT Elsevier eBooks+

CHAPTER 61

Spinal Puncture and Cerebrospinal Fluid Examination

Brian D. Euerle and Alexis Salerno

Cerebrospinal fluid (CSF) examination is performed in the emergency department (ED) to obtain information relevant to the diagnosis and treatment of specific disease entities. Many urgent and life-threatening conditions require immediate and accurate knowledge of the nature of the CSF. However, on rare occasions, certain harmful consequences may result from a spinal puncture. Perform a careful neurologic examination before the procedure and give special thought to the risks and merits of the procedure in each situation.

HISTORICAL PERSPECTIVE

In 1885 Corning punctured the subarachnoid space of a living patient to induce cocaine anesthesia.[1] In 1891 Quincke first removed CSF in a diagnostic study and introduced the use of a stylet.[2] He studied the cellular contents and measured protein and glucose levels. Quincke was also the first to record CSF pressure with a manometer. Subsequently, increasingly sophisticated bacteriologic, biochemical, cytologic, and serologic techniques were introduced. In 1919 Dandy reported on replacing CSF with air to determine normal brain anatomy and to identify pathologic changes.[3] Water-soluble contrast media have since been used to delineate the spinal subarachnoid space and cerebral cisterns. Other uses of spinal dural puncture include drainage of fluids and injection of anesthetic agents, chemotherapeutic agents, and antibiotics.

ANATOMY AND PHYSIOLOGY

In adults, CSF occupies approximately 140 mL of the spinal and cranial cavities, with approximately 30 mL in the spinal canal. This volume is the result of a balance between continuous secretion (primarily by the ventricular choroid plexus) and absorption into the venous system (mainly by way of the arachnoid villi). After formation, the fluid passes out of the ventricles via the midline dorsal foramen of Luschka and the lateral ventral foramina of Magendie. The fluid then flows into the spinal subarachnoid space, the basilar cisterns, and the cerebral subarachnoid space. The rate of production is approximately 0.35 mL/min, and ventricular production of CSF is such that there is a net flow out of the ventricles of 50 to 100 mL/day. The usual volume of CSF (4 mL to 10 mL) removed at lumbar puncture is commonly regenerated in approximately 1 hour.

CSF may have an embryologic nutritive function; at maturity, CSF most likely acts as a mechanical barrier between the soft brain and the rigid fibro-osseous dura, skull, and vertebral column. It also appears to support the weight of the brain.[4] When buoyed by CSF, the functional weight of the brain is reduced from 1400 g to 50 g. Contraction and expansion of CSF accommodate changes in brain volume.

Spinal Puncture

Indications

Suspected central nervous system infection (meningitis)
Suspected spontaneous subarachnoid hemorrhage
Suspected central nervous system syphilis
Suspected idiopathic intracranial hypertension

Contraindications

Absolute:

- Presence of infection near the puncture site

Relative:

- Coagulopathy
- Presence of increased intracranial pressure caused by a space-occupying lesion
- Severe thrombocytopenia

Complications

Brain herniation
Cauda equina syndrome
Cranial nerve VI palsy
Epidermoid tumor
Epidural cerebrospinal fluid collection
Epidural hematoma
Intrathecal pump catheter
Meningitis
Minor backache
Postdural puncture headache
Retroperitoneal abscess
Subarachnoid hemorrhage
Subdural hematoma

Equipment

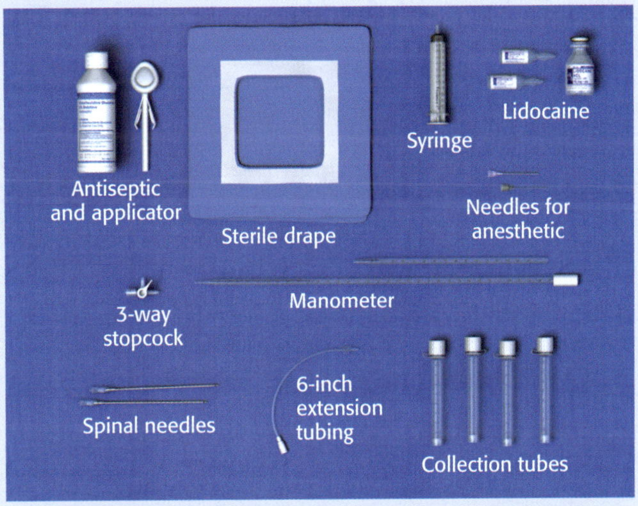

The equipment for spinal puncture is most commonly found in a prepackaged kit.

Review Box 61.1 Spinal puncture: indications, contraindications, complications, and equipment.

INDICATIONS FOR SPINAL PUNCTURE

General Indications

The indications for spinal puncture have been reduced with the introduction of noninvasive diagnostic procedures, that is, magnetic resonance imaging (MRI) and computed tomography (CT). A few clinical situations require early or even emergency spinal puncture. The primary indication for an emergency spinal tap is the possibility of central nervous system (CNS) infection (meningitis), with the exception of a suspected brain abscess or a parameningeal process. The need for early detection of meningitis results in the performance of many more lumbar punctures than ultimate diagnoses of infection.[5] No other method can be used to completely exclude meningitis.

The mere presence of a fever does not mandate lumbar puncture. However, CSF examination should be considered in patients with a fever of unknown origin, especially if consciousness is altered or the immune system is impaired, even in the absence of meningeal irritation. Meningeal signs may not be present in patients who are old, debilitated, or immunosuppressed; are receiving antiinflammatory drugs; or have had partial treatment with antibiotics.[6,7] In a newborn, even a fever is not a dependable sign because temperatures may be normal or even subnormal. For infants younger than 1 year, a high index of suspicion is required to make the diagnosis of meningitis.

Approximately 25% of infants with meningitis will not have nuchal rigidity, but many appear toxic or moribund. A tense and bulging fontanelle is somewhat more reliable, although this sign may be absent in a dehydrated child. Neonatal meningitis occurs in 25% of sepsis cases. In addition, 15% to 20% of infants with meningitis have negative blood cultures.[8,9] In a child between the ages of 1 month and 3 years, fever, irritability, and vomiting are the most common signs of meningitis. Typically, handling is painful for the child, and the child cannot be comforted. In addition, an older child may complain of a headache. At all ages, patients generally appear ill and drowsy with a dulled sensorium. Physical signs become more useful in diagnosing meningitis in children older than 3 years[10] and include nuchal rigidity, Kernig's sign (effort to extend the knee is resisted), and Brudzinski's sign (passive flexion of one hip causes the other leg to rise, and effort to flex the neck makes the knees come up), although both of these last two signs are rarely found on examination. The jolt accentuation test is a more sensitive sign of meningeal irritation.[11] This test is considered positive when the patient's pain is exacerbated by lateral rotation of the head to either side. A petechial rash in a febrile patient should also raise suspicion for *Neisseria* meningitis[12] or *Streptococcus pneumoniae*. Previous use of antimicrobial agents may modify the clinical and CSF findings; partially treated children are less likely to be febrile or exhibit an altered mental status. In addition, patients in the early stages of meningitis may lack the classic features associated with advanced disease.

The second indication for emergency spinal puncture is suspected spontaneous subarachnoid hemorrhage (SAH). The diagnosis is usually made by imaging (head CT) or by the direct finding of blood in CSF obtained by spinal puncture.[13,14] Before a major hemorrhage, 20% to 60% of patients with aneurysmal SAH have had a "sentinel thunderclap" or "warning leak" headache (i.e., an unusual sudden headache caused by a "minor" leak of blood from the aneurysm). The headache may precede a major rupture by hours to months. The goal of early clinical recognition is surgical or other interventional therapy before a recurrent major hemorrhage. After a warning leak, head CT is more likely to be falsely negative (especially if the patient is anemic or the CT scan is delayed by more than 6 hours), thus giving added importance to the performance of a lumbar puncture.

The usual clinical picture of SAH is a rapid-onset headache. Patients generally recall the exact moment that the headache occurred. The location of the headache is variable and does not necessarily indicate the site of hemorrhage. Nausea, vomiting, and a decreased level of consciousness are common (although not universal) symptoms, with approximately one-third of patients becoming unconscious at the onset. Examination usually reveals an acutely ill patient with irritability or overtly altered mental status. Meningeal signs may be present at the time of initial examination, but may take 2 to 3 days to develop, if they develop at all. The meningeal signs may become more severe during the first week after hemorrhage and correspond to the breakdown of blood in CSF. During the first week, patients may be febrile, a reflection of chemical hemic (blood-related) meningitis.[15] Failure to detect blood on CT imaging in an awake patient may indicate a small hemorrhage or a predominant basal accumulation of blood. If a patient is initially seen several days after the hemorrhage, the blood may have become isodense with brain tissue and may no longer be visible on CT. The proper diagnosis would then require additional testing with either spinal puncture or CT angiography.

Modern CT scanners detect recent SAH quite accurately.[16] However, because acute SAH is not detected by the initial CT scan in all patients, lumbar puncture has been used to rule out the diagnosis with certainty.[17–19] A 2011 study conducted at academic medical centers found that a noncontrast head CT done with a third-generation scanner within 6 hours after onset of the headache and read by a qualified radiologist was 100% sensitive for the detection of SAH.[20] Another study performed at nonacademic hospitals determined the negative predictive value for the detection of SAH of a head CT done within 6 hours after the onset of headache to be 99.9%.[21] An American College of Emergency Physicians clinical policy from 2019 gave a level B recommendation to the use of a normal head CT scan (minimum third-generation scanner) performed within 6 hours of headache onset to rule out nontraumatic SAH.[22] If the neurologic picture demonstrates localizing findings, the presence of a large intracranial hematoma should be suspected, and spinal puncture is contraindicated until imaging studies delineate the nature of the lesion.

Other nonemergent reasons for examination of CSF include evaluation for CNS syphilis, unexplained seizures, instillation of chemotherapy and contrast agents, assessment for a suspected demyelinating or inflammatory CNS process, and treatment of headache from SAH. Carcinomatous meningitis and suspected spinal cord compression from metastatic disease may require spinal puncture for myelography and cytologic examination. MRI is a suitable alternative for identifying compressive myelopathy and has largely replaced contrast-enhanced myelography in developed countries.

Idiopathic Intracranial Hypertension (Pseudotumor Cerebri)

Idiopathic intracranial hypertension (IIH) is a rare condition of unclear etiology. Patients with IIH have a marked elevation in opening pressure (usually >25 cm H_2O) without hydrocephalus or mass lesions in the setting of normal CSF composition. Findings on neuroimaging studies are typically normal, and most cases are idiopathic. Because of the nonspecific signs and symptoms, many cases initially escape detection by clinicians. IIH has been associated with hypervitaminosis A, tetracycline, estrogen therapy, and a plethora of other conditions such as sarcoidosis, tuberculosis, and carcinomatosis. IIH is most common in adolescent girls with an elevated body mass index and young females, but it can also occur in children and males. Patients suffer from chronic headaches, typically worse with maneuvers that increase intracranial pressure (ICP) (e.g., Valsalva maneuver, squatting, bending, coughing). Papilledema is frequently present. Cranial nerve palsies, particularly of the sixth cranial nerve, are caused by increased ICP alone and may be falsely localizing.[23]

IIH may regress spontaneously after a few months. The major concern is visual loss, which may be permanent. The diagnosis can be made only by lumbar puncture performed after neuroimaging. This condition underscores the need to measure opening pressure during lumbar puncture whenever possible. Many cases can be controlled with medication, but occasionally, lumbar puncture is required to lower ICP. In cases of rapid visual decline, one way to lower ICP in the ED is to drain CSF via lumbar puncture by removing 5- to 10-mL aliquots of CSF and checking ICP after each removal until a pressure lower than 20 cm H_2O is achieved. Herniation does not occur despite the elevated pressure in IIH, probably because ICP is uniform in all CNS compartments. As spinal fluid is regenerated rapidly, the procedure may need to be repeated every few days to keep CSF pressure at this level. Analysis of CSF should demonstrate all parameters to be normal. Drug therapy, in the form of acetazolamide, glycerol, diuretics, or corticosteroids, has been advocated and may negate the need for repeated lumbar puncture. Resistant cases may require shunting procedures.

CONTRAINDICATIONS TO SPINAL PUNCTURE

Spinal puncture is absolutely contraindicated in patients with infection in the tissues near the puncture site.[4,24] Spinal puncture is relatively contraindicated in the presence of increased ICP caused by a space-occupying lesion. Caution is particularly advised when lateralizing signs (hemiparesis) or signs of uncal herniation (unilateral third-nerve palsy with an altered level of consciousness) are present. In such cases, a tentorial or cerebellar pressure cone may be precipitated or aggravated by the spinal puncture. Cardiorespiratory collapse, stupor, seizures, and sudden death may occur when pressure is reduced in the spinal canal.[25]

The risk for herniation seems to be particularly pronounced in patients with brain abscesses.[26,27] Brain abscesses are frequently manifested as expanding intracranial lesions that induce headache, mental disturbances, and focal neurologic signs rather than as an infectious process with signs of meningeal irritation. Fever is often absent. In 75% of cases, a primary source of chronic suppuration is present. Common predisposing factors for brain abscess include craniofacial trauma, craniocerebral trauma, penetrating injuries that push bone fragments into the brain, large animal bites of infants' skulls, neurosurgical procedures, cardiovascular disorders with right-to-left shunts, bacterial endocarditis, gram-negative sepsis in neonates, dental infections, chronic sinusitis, otitis, mastoiditis, chronic abdominal, pulmonary, or pelvic infection, bacterial meningitis, and immunosuppression. Abscesses may also develop in infarcted brain tissue in septic patients if the blood-brain barrier is compromised.[28] Although the CSF is usually abnormal (elevated pressure, elevated white blood cell [WBC] count, and elevated protein concentration), spinal puncture in patients with a known or suspected abscess is contraindicated. Brain herniation markedly reduces the patient's likelihood of survival. If the history suggests abscess, CT can rapidly diagnose and localize the lesion (Fig. 61.1).[29] Because the appearance of brain abscesses on CT is similar to that of neoplastic and vascular lesions, false-positive reports of brain abscess are possible.[29]

Spinal epidural hematomas are very rare but may occur in certain subpopulations of patients undergoing lumbar puncture. Those most at risk are individuals with a bleeding diathesis, including those treated with anticoagulants either before or immediately after lumbar puncture and those with abnormal clotting mechanisms, especially thrombocytopenia. The condition can rarely occur in the setting of an atraumatic tap and in the absence of a coagulation defect.[30] Spinal subdural hematomas after lumbar puncture are more rare.[31,32] Lumbar puncture can injure the dural or arachnoid vessels, which may result in minor hemorrhage into the CSF.

In a coagulopathic patient, attempt to correct the clotting deficiency if clinically feasible and time permits. The procedure should be performed by experienced clinicians, who are less likely to traumatize the dura. After the procedure, monitor the patient carefully for progressive back pain, lower extremity motor and sensory deficits, and sphincter impairment. Thoroughly investigate any complaints of motor weakness, sensory loss, or incontinence after lumbar puncture. Lumbar puncture may be performed in patients with a coagulation defect if the procedure is expected to

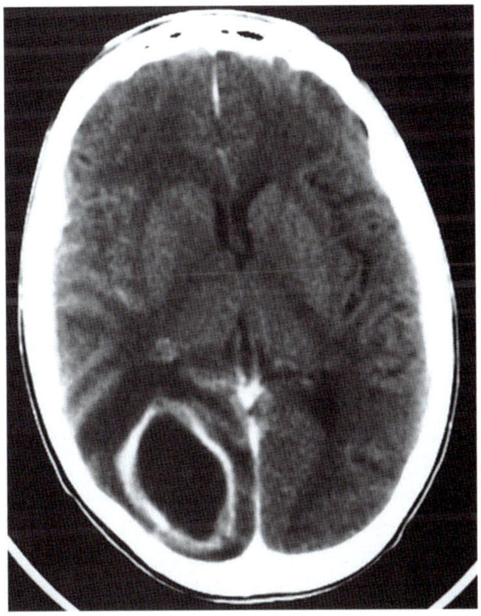

Fig. 61.1 This computed tomography scan demonstrates a low-density mass lesion with an enhancing rim and surrounding edema in an immunosuppressed patient with an *Aspergillus* abscess. Lumbar puncture in such a patient would be contraindicated. (From Zitelli BJ and Davis HW. *Atlas of Pediatric Physical Diagnosis.* 5th ed. Elsevier; 2007.)

provide essential information, such as in the diagnosis of meningitis and the pathogen. Correct warfarin-induced coagulopathy with prothrombin complex concentrate or fresh frozen plasma (FFP) together with vitamin K. Using prothrombin complex concentrates is preferred over FFP because the vitamin K–FFP protocol might need 12 to 24 hours to reverse the effect of warfarin. Correct the coagulopathy before a puncture if the clinical situation permits such delay. Butler has described the off-label use of low-dose prothrombin complex concentrate for the correction of warfarin-induced coagulopathy prior to lumbar puncture in one patient.[33] Lumbar puncture can be performed safely in patients with hemophilia A or B whose deficient clotting factor is replenished before the procedure.[34] Additional replacement of the clotting factor after the procedure is of unknown value.

Direct oral anticoagulants (DOACs) are increasingly being used for long-term anticoagulation in lieu of warfarin. There is no significant difference in the periprocedural bleeding risk in patients on DOACs as compared to warfarin.[35] Therefore the same considerations apply when planning a lumbar puncture on a patient on a DOAC. The American Society of Regional Anesthesia Pain Medicine (ASRA) offers guidance on managing periprocedural anticoagulation for neuraxial procedures. In general, patients on therapeutic doses should hold DOACs 3 to 5 days prior to a lumbar puncture. The duration of holding is agent-specific and assumes normal renal and hepatic functions. Patients with poor metabolism or delayed clearance of DOACs may need to hold DOACs for longer period.[36] When the lumbar puncture must be performed more urgently, the reversal agents idarucizumab (for dabigatran) and andexanet alfa (for apixaban and rivaroxaban) may be used. If these specific agents are not available, prothrombin complex concentrate or FFP may be used.[37] The risk of thrombosis precipitated by rapid reversal of anticoagulation should always be considered prior to administration of anticoagulation reversal agents.

In general, patients on aspirin and other nonsteroidal anti-inflammatory agents may continue their usual doses in relation to the procedure. Prophylactic subcutaneous heparin administration (i.e., 5000 units twice to three times daily) should be held for 4 to 6 hours or a normal activated partial thromboplastin time (aPTT) confirmed prior to the procedure. Normal aPTT should be used to guide optimal timing for the procedure in patients on higher doses of heparin. Hold times are even longer in patients taking P2Y12 receptor blockers (e.g., clopidogrel – 5 to 7 days, prasugrel – 7 to 10 days) and the use of these agents should cause the clinician to proceed with caution. One scenario is the need to diagnose meningitis because of an unusual or difficult-to-treat pathogen in a patient taking clopidogrel. It is necessary to withhold clopidogrel up to 1 week before the antiplatelet effect has fully dissipated, making the decision for emergency lumbar puncture in such a patient a risk-benefit scenario with no firm guidelines. Pharmacologic data suggest that cessation of the GP IIb/IIIa receptor antagonist tirofiban may allow lumbar puncture after 8 hours and cessation of abciximab after 24 to 48 hours. A recent study reported that among 100 patients on dual antiplatelet therapy who underwent lumbar puncture, there were no serious complications and no cases of epidural hematoma.[38] Because of the small number of patients the authors caution that their study was not powered to detect an increased risk of spinal hematoma. Spinal hematoma may develop in 1% to 2% of patients who receive full anticoagulant therapy *after* undergoing lumbar puncture. A 2023 study looked at 159 patients that were taking an adenosine-diphosphate receptor antagonist (ADPra) and had a lumbar puncture while taking the medication or after a brief period (median 2 days) of withholding the medication.[39] Approximately half the patients were taking the ADPra alone, the other half in combination with aspirin. No patients developed spinal hematoma or any neurological deficit.

Proceed with caution in a patient with prior lumbar fusion or laminectomy. It is technically difficult to enter the subarachnoid space in the presence of significant postoperative changes. It would be acceptable to perform the puncture in an applicable space above or below the surgical scar; otherwise, opting for fluoroscopic guidance is prudent.

Performance of lumbar puncture in patients with leukemia and low platelet counts has also been studied. Howard and coworkers reported on 5223 lumbar punctures performed on 958 children with newly diagnosed acute lymphoblastic leukemia.[40] The platelet count was $10 \times 10^9/L$ or lower in 29 children, 11 to $20 \times 10^9/L$ in 170 children, and 21 to $50 \times 10^9/L$ in 742 children. No serious complications were reported in any group. The overall rate of traumatic taps was 10.5%, but such taps were not associated with adverse sequelae. The authors concluded that in children with acute lymphoblastic leukemia, prophylactic platelet transfusion for lumbar puncture is not required if the platelet count is higher than $10 \times 10^9/L$. The number of patients with platelet counts lower than $10 \times 10^9/L$ was too small to allow any conclusion about this group. A 2010 review concluded that in the absence of additional risk factors, a platelet count of $40 \times 10^9/L$ is "safe" for lumbar puncture. Lower counts are probably safe as well, but there was insufficient evidence to make recommendations.[41] The 2015 clinical guidelines from the AABB (formerly the American Association of Blood Banks) include a weak recommendation for prophylactic platelet transfusion for patients having elective diagnostic lumbar puncture with a platelet count less than $50 \times 10^9/L$, acknowledging that the position was based on very-low-quality evidence.[42]

Attempts have been made to link bacterial meningitis to a lumbar puncture procedure in a bacteremic patient. Presumably, the procedure introduces bacteria into the CSF. This phenomenon is rare, difficult to substantiate, and not supported by clinical data. Bacteremia should not be used as a criterion to forego lumbar puncture if meningitis is suspected.

If the history and physical examination suggest a treatable illness such as meningitis or SAH, the clinician may perform a spinal puncture after careful consideration of the entire clinical picture. In all cases, undertake the study after careful thought regarding how the results will contribute to the evaluation and treatment of the patient. It is unlikely that spinal puncture will beneficially alter management in patients with neoplastic disease, intracranial hematoma, abscess, a completed nonembolic infarction, or cranial trauma. Moreover, even when acute life-threatening emergencies such as SAH or meningitis are suspected, delaying CSF examination temporarily while empirical treatment proceeds is an important management option when there are concerns about the safety of the procedure.

EQUIPMENT

Assemble the standard equipment for a spinal puncture before starting the procedure. Place it where the operator can easily access it. A standard-point Quincke cutting needle is most often used and supplied with the kit. Some operators prefer to use a Sprotte needle (Havel's, Inc.) or a Whitacre needle (Becton Dickinson and Company) to minimize any dural injury associated with passage of the needle (Fig. 61.2). These styletted needles have a side port for withdrawal of fluid and, theoretically, are more likely to separate than cut the dural tissue. Although commercial kits provide most of the items needed for lumbar puncture, the operator should bring additional supplies, including supplemental spinal needles, specimen tubes, gauze, antiseptic solution, additional local anesthetic, needles and syringes, and extra sterile gloves of the appropriate size (Review Box 61.1).

PROCEDURE

See Videos 61.1–61.4. Lumbar puncture is commonly carried out with the patient in the lateral recumbent position (Fig. 61.3). A line connecting the posterior superior iliac crests intersects the midline at approximately the L4 spinous process (Fig. 61.4). Spinal needles entering the subarachnoid space at this point are well below the termination of the spinal cord, and the only important neurologic structure is the cauda equina. Generally, the needle pushes isolated nerves to the side during advancement. The adjacent interspace above or below may be used, depending on which area appears to be most accessible to palpation. The space between the lumbar posterior spinous processes is relatively accommodating with proper patient positioning. In the thoracic region, the spinous processes overlap and are directed caudally. Therefore there is no midline area free of overlying bone. In adults, the spinal cord extends to the lower level of L1 or the body of L2 in 31% of persons, thus eliminating higher levels as sites for puncture. Puncture in adults and older children may be performed from the L2-L3 interspace to the L5-S1 interspace.

Developmentally the spinal canal and the spinal cord are of equal length in the fetus. Growth of the cord does not keep pace with the longitudinal growth of the spinal canal. At birth, the cord ends at the level of the L3 vertebra. Consequently, in infants the needle should be placed at the L4-L5 or L5-S1 interspace. The subarachnoid space extends to the S2 vertebral level; however, the overlying bony mass prevents entry into this lowermost portion of the subarachnoid space.

When performed with appropriate sedation and proper local anesthesia, a spinal tap is neither overly distressing nor very painful to most patients. Almost all patients are likely to have some anxiety about a spinal puncture for several reasons, including the stories commonly told of severe complications. Explain the procedure in advance and announce each step while performing it to reduce the patient's anxiety. Inquire about any history of allergies to local anesthetic agents and topical antiseptics. Obtain written informed consent whenever possible. In all cases, include a detailed procedural note that documents the process of patient or guardian education regarding the indications, procedural techniques, risks and benefits, alternatives to the procedure, and the patient's or guardian's consent for the procedure. Abridge this step when the patient is critically ill or eliminate it when the patient is mentally incapacitated, and no guardian is present. Many patients greatly fear lumbar puncture, and hence some clinicians provide routine preprocedural sedation or analgesia if not clinically contraindicated. Midazolam and fentanyl are useful adjuncts, but practices vary and there is no consensus on standard medications.

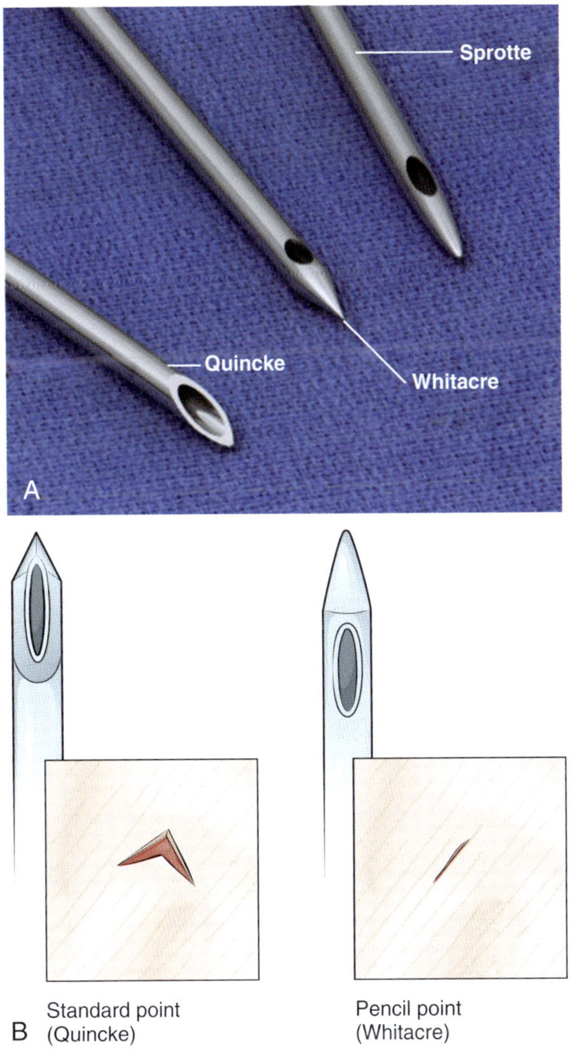

Fig. 61.2 (A) Various spinal needles. (B) Penetration of the dura by Whitacre (pencil-point) and Quincke (cutting) needles. The Whitacre needle separates the fibers of the dura without cutting them, whereas the Quincke needle cuts the fibers. The Quincke needle leaves a hole in the dura through which cerebrospinal fluid can leak until the hole heals several days or weeks later. Use of the Whitacre needle has been associated with a lower incidence of post–lumbar puncture headache. (A, From Thomsen T, Setnik G, eds. *Procedures Consult—Emergency Medicine Module*. Elsevier; 2008. All rights reserved.)

The next important step is positioning the patient. Generally, place older children and adults in the lateral decubitus position for the procedure. Give the patient a pillow to keep the head in line with the vertebral axis. Position the shoulders and hips perpendicular to the stretcher or table. Use a firm table or bed when available. Because flexion of the neck does not facilitate the procedure to any great extent and severe flexion may add to the patient's discomfort, this step may be omitted. Severe flexion of the neck in an infant may cause airway compromise. Arch the lower part of the patient's

Spinal Puncture

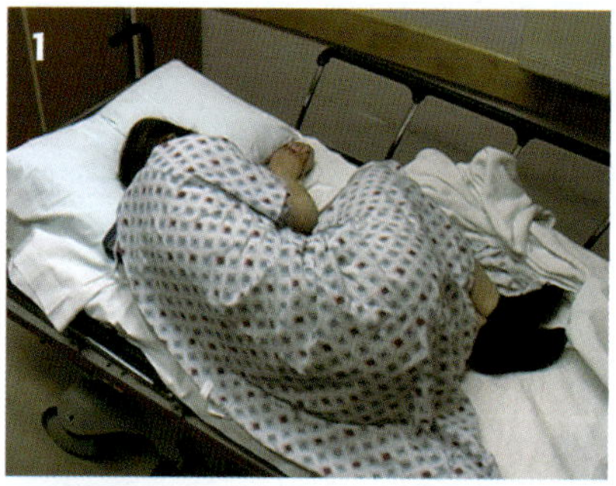

Position the patient in the bed. Generally, the lateral decubitus position is preferred. Arch the patient's back towards you.

Consider mild sedation or analgesia when clinically appropriate.

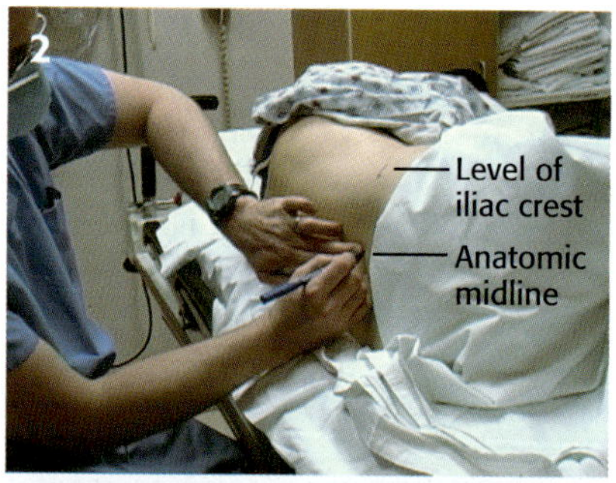

Identify and mark anatomic landmarks. The L4 spinous process is at the level of the posterior-superior iliac crests.

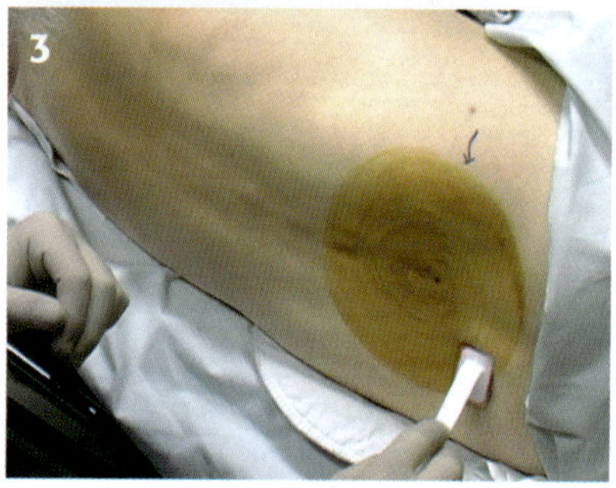

Prepare the skin with antiseptic solution. Apply in a circular motion with a gradually increasing circumference.

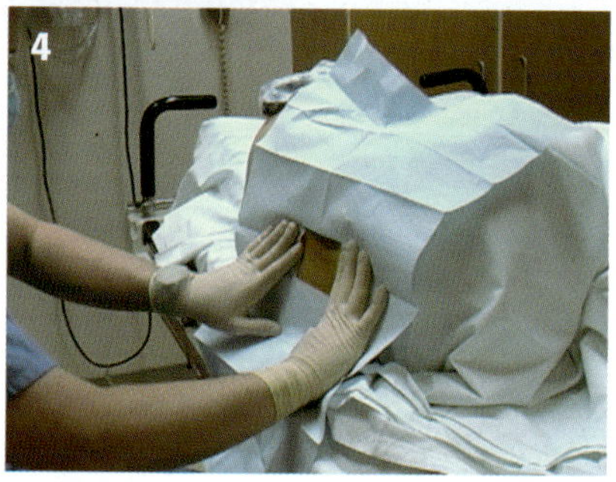

Apply a sterile drape.

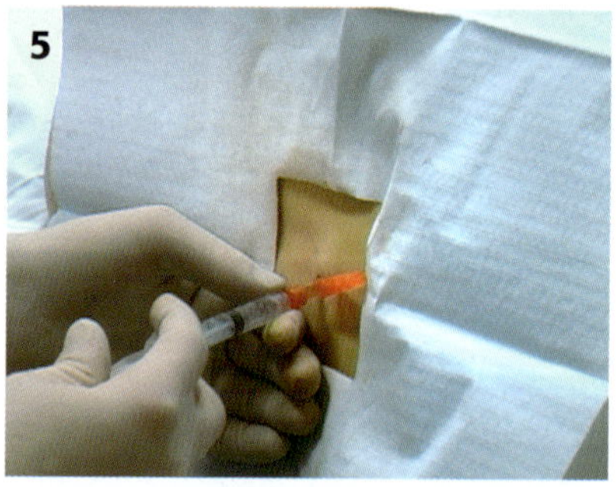

Create a wheal with anesthetic in the skin overlying the entry site. Then, infiltrate and anesthetize the deeper tissues.

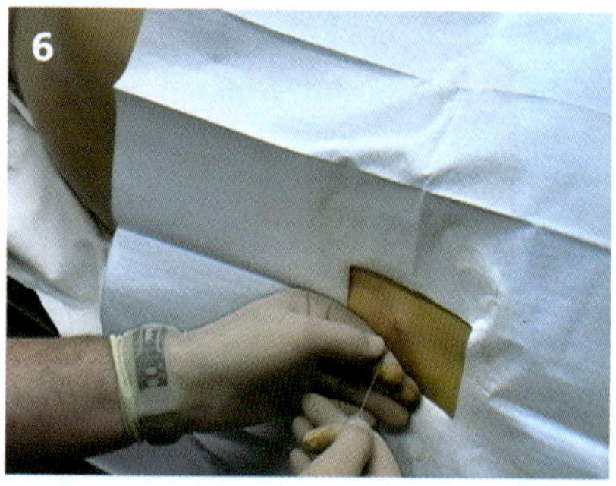

Insert the needle in the midline. Hold the needle parallel to the bed, and advance it toward the umbilicus. Remove the stylet periodically to check for CSF.

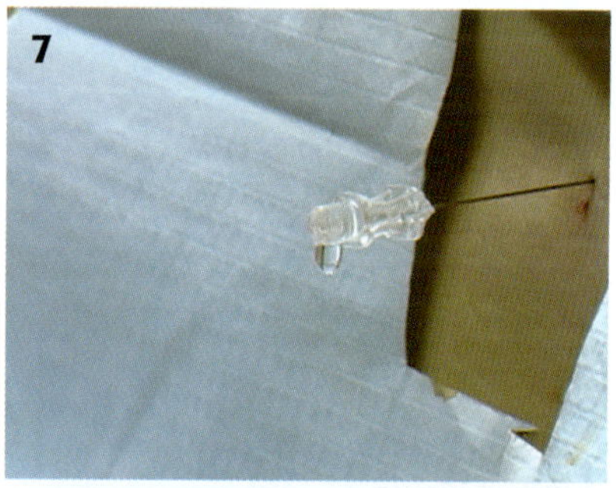

CSF will flow from the needle hub when the subarachnoid space has been penetrated.

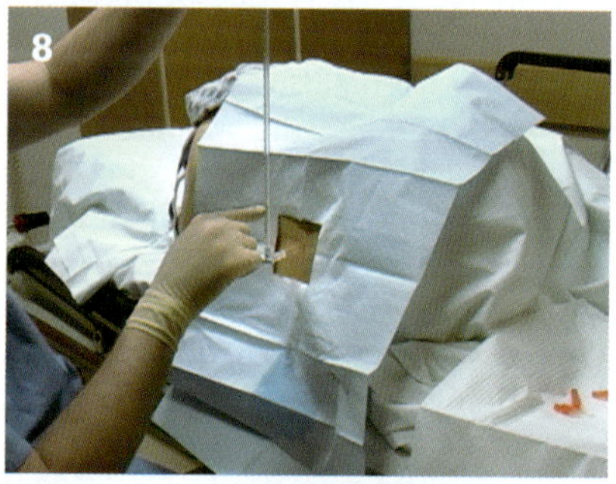

Attach the manometer and measure the opening pressure.

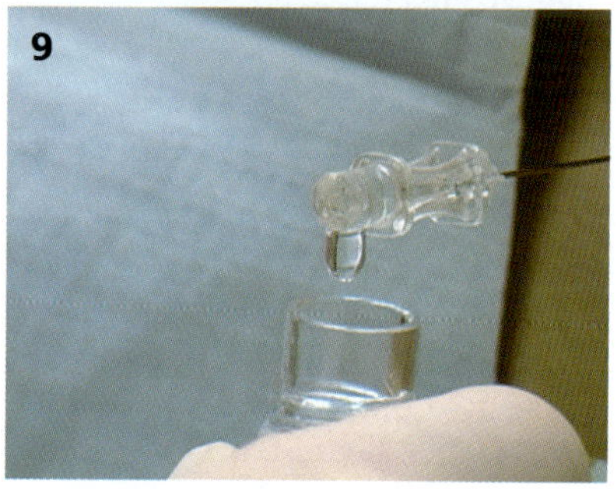

Collect the CSF sample in sequential, numbered vials.

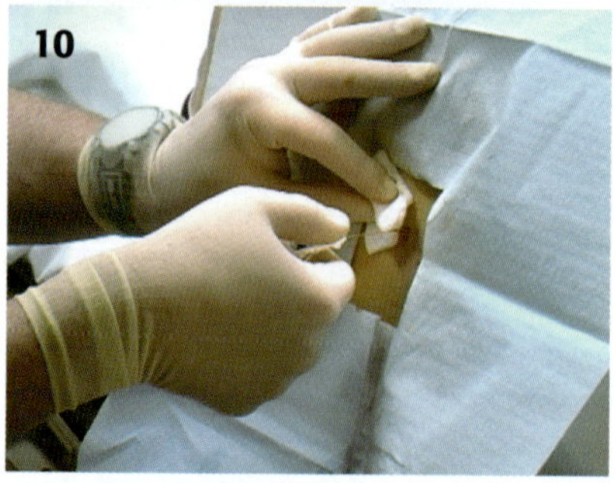

Replace the stylet before removing the needle.

Fig. 61.3 Spinal puncture. *CSF,* Cerebrospinal fluid.

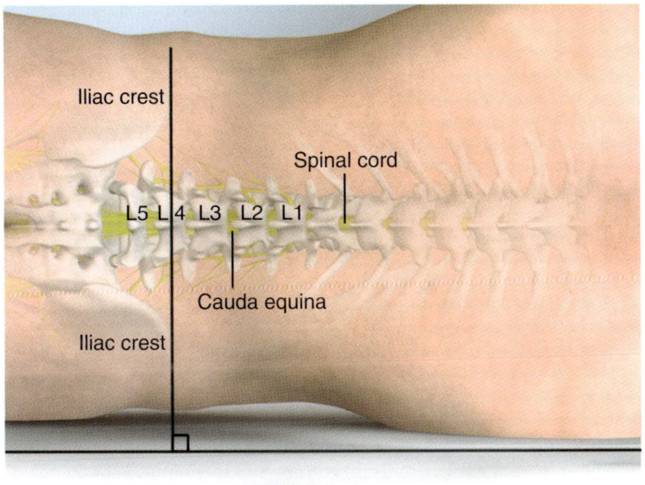

Fig. 61.4 The L4 spinous process is at the level of the posterior superior iliac crest. The spinal cord ends approximately at the level of L1 or L2 in adults; fibers of the cauda equina extend inferiorly from there. When the patient is positioned correctly for lumbar puncture, an *imaginary line* connecting the iliac crests will be exactly perpendicular to the bed, and the spine will be parallel to the bed.

back toward the clinician by having the patient's knees drawn toward the chest.

Some clinicians place the patient in an upright sitting position because the midline is more easily identified. This position can be used in both adults and infants (Fig. 61.5). The higher CSF hydrostatic pressure while sitting may aid flow of CSF in a dehydrated patient. Observe caution regarding orthostatic changes in blood pressure and airway maintenance. Generally, allow a sitting patient to lean onto a bedside stand and use a pillow to rest the head and arms. Have an assistant support the patient during the procedure. Radiographic studies by Fisher and colleagues have demonstrated the advantages of hip flexion when the sitting position is used.[43] To accomplish hip flexion, use a stool to support the patient's feet, which pulls the knees up toward the chest. This increases lumbar interspinous width, which may increase the success and ease of needle passage. Recent studies in both children and adults have shown that lumbar puncture is equally successful whether it is performed in the lateral decubitus or upright position.[44,45]

After the patient is positioned, but before antiseptic skin preparation, the intended entry site of the spinal needle should be marked. This has traditionally been done with an ink pen or specialized marker. An alternative technique involves applying pressure to the skin, causing an indentation that will remain visible during the procedure. One recent report described the use of a 10-mL syringe held against the skin and aspirated to 5 mL, and held in place for 1 minute, resulting in a mark that remained visible for 30 minutes and was not affected by antiseptic agents or ultrasound gel.[46] Alternatively a needle cap can be used to indent the skin for a few seconds and accomplish the same visible mark.

Iatrogenic infection after lumbar puncture is extremely rare. Use sterile gloves during the procedure; the need for face masks is debatable.[47–49] Some authors have suggested applying the same guidelines for control of central line infection (caps, gowns, gloves, and masks) to lumbar puncture.[50] Sterilize the patient's skin with an antiseptic solution applied

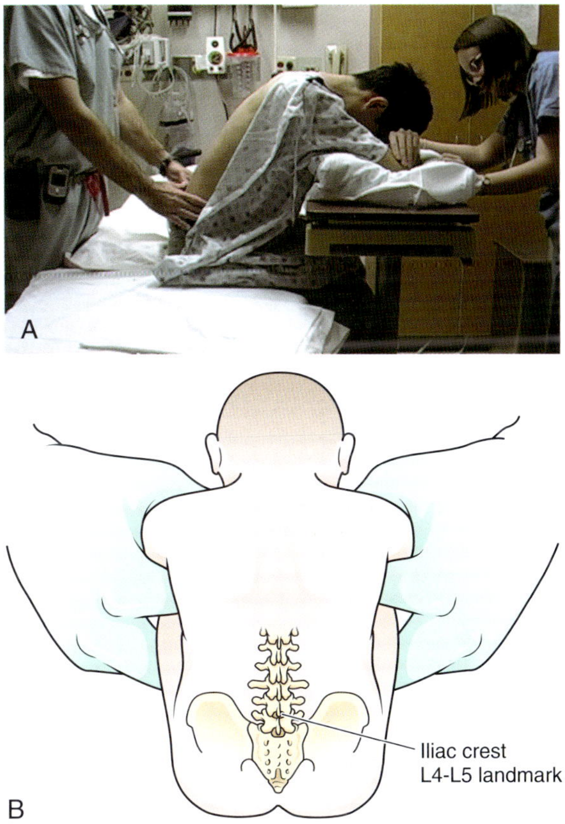

Fig. 61.5 (A) Many clinicians prefer the sitting position for lumbar puncture because of the ease of entering the dural space. However, the opening pressure obtained in this position is not accurate. If possible, place the patient in the lateral decubitus position for measurement of pressure, usually after fluid has been collected. (B) Upright positioning in an infant. (A, From Thomsen T, Setnik G, eds. *Procedures Consult—Emergency Medicine Module.* Elsevier; 2008. B, From Dieckmann R, Selbst S, eds. *Pediatric Emergency and Critical Care Procedures.* Mosby; 1997.)

in a circular motion and increase the circumference of the cleansed area with each motion. Place a sterile towel or drape between the patient's hip and the bed. Commercial trays have a second sterile drape with a hole that may be centered over the site selected for the procedure.

Infiltrate the skin and deeper subcutaneous tissue generously with local anesthetic. Warn the patient about transient discomfort from the anesthetic. Anesthetizing the deeper subcutaneous tissue significantly reduces procedural discomfort. Merely raising a skin wheal is insufficient anesthesia. Some operators not only anesthetize the interspinous ligament but also apply local anesthetic in a vertically fanning distribution on both sides of the spinous processes near the lamina. Such a field block on each side of the spinous processes anesthetizes the recurrent spinal nerves that innervate the interspinous ligaments and muscles.

While waiting for the anesthetic to take effect, connect the stopcock and manometer and ensure that the valve is working. Commonly, a 3.5-inch, 22-gauge needle is used in adults, and a 2.5-inch, 22-gauge needle is used in children (a 1.5-inch, 22-gauge needle is available for infants). A longer length needle may be required for patients with significantly high body mass indices. Needles of these sizes have enough rigidity to allow

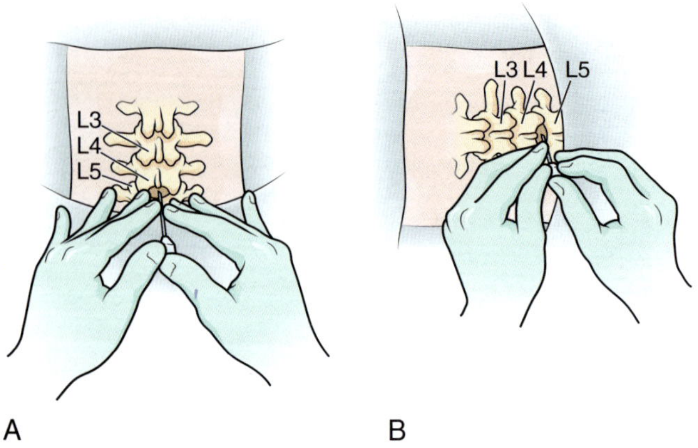

Fig. 61.6 Ways to hold the spinal needle. (A) Fingers extended. (B) FIngers flexed.

the procedure to be accomplished easily but make less of a dural tear than larger needles do. Patients should be told to report any pain and should be informed that they will feel some pressure.

With the patient in the lateral decubitus position, place the needle into the skin in the midline, parallel to the bed. Hold the needle between both thumbs and index fingers (Fig. 61.6). After the subcutaneous tissue has been penetrated, angle the needle toward the umbilicus. The bevel of the needle should be facing straight up toward the ceiling (bevel facing flank). The supraspinal ligament connects the spinous processes, and the interspinal ligaments join the inferior and superior borders of adjacent spinous processes. The ligamentum flavum is a strong, elastic membrane that may reach a thickness of 1 cm in the lumbar region. The ligamentum flavum covers the interlaminar space between the vertebrae and assists the paraspinous muscles in maintaining an upright posture (Fig. 61.7). The ligaments are stretched in a flexed position and are more easily crossed by the needle. The ligaments resist the needle, and a "pop" is often felt as they are penetrated. This "pop" may be subtle and not necessarily felt in all patients. Some clinicians choose to advance the needle in small increments, removing the stylet to check for CSF flow. If no fluid flows, the stylet is replaced and the needle is advanced. Hold the stylet in place during advancement, until the subarachnoid space has been reached. An important infection prevention point is not to keep your finger on the needle while replacing the stylet.

If bone is encountered, partially withdraw the needle to subcutaneous tissue. Palpate the back and ascertain that the needle is in the midline. Directing the tip of the needle toward the navel often enhances navigation of the interspinal space. If bone is encountered again, slightly withdraw and reangle the needle so that the point is placed at a more cephalad angle (Fig. 61.8). This approach should avoid the inferior spinous process.

Normal CSF is a clear fluid and will flow from the needle when the subarachnoid space has been penetrated and the stylet is removed. If opening pressure measurement is desired, immediately replace the stylet to prevent the flow of CSF. In normal patients, the dura will be penetrated when the needle is advanced approximately one-half to three-fourths of its length. In patients with an increased body mass index, inserting the entire length of the needle may be required to reach the subdural space (Fig. 61.9).

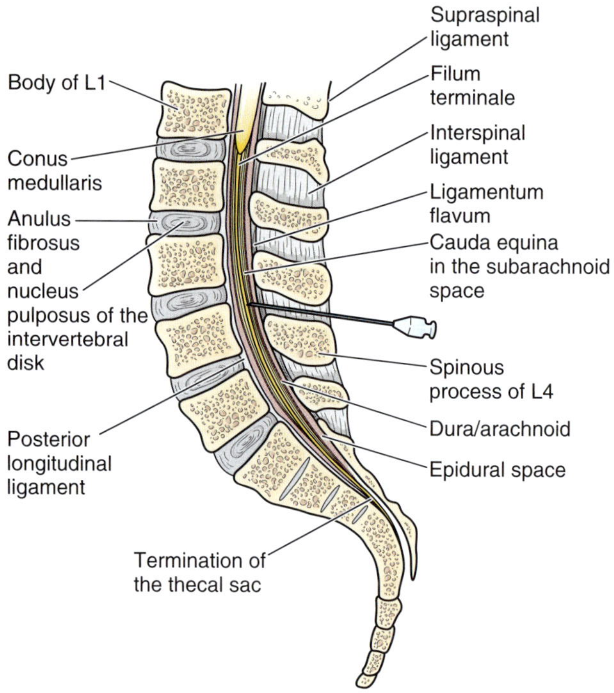

Fig. 61.7 Midsagittal section through the lumbar spinal column with a spinal puncture needle in place between the spinous processes of L3 and L4. Note the slightly ascending direction of the needle. The needle has pierced three ligaments and the dura/arachnoid and is in the subarachnoid space. (From Lachman E. Anatomy as applied to clinical medicine. *New Physician*. 1968;17:145.)

If feasible, attach the manometer and record the opening pressure (Fig. 61.10). Pressure readings from a struggling patient may be inaccurate. Readings are valid only if taken with the patient relaxed and in the lateral decubitus position (not the sitting position). A three-way stopcock, supplied in disposable kits, allows both collection of CSF and measurement of opening pressure with a single needle. Positioning of the manometer is often more convenient if an extension tube connects the needle hub to the stopcock, which in turn is attached to the manometer. Position the manometer so that the "zero" mark is at the level of the spinal needle. Then ask the patient to relax. Changing position from a straight to a fully extended position increases CSF pressure minimally, by 2 cm to 8 cm H_2O Extending the legs after needle placement does not meaningfully decrease opening CSF pressure.[51] CSF flow is enhanced if the patient straightens or extends the legs following confirmation of proper needle position. The observation of phasic changes in the fluid column with respirations and arterial pulsations confirms needle placement in the subarachnoid space. If the needle is against a nerve root or is only partially within the dura, the pressure may be falsely low, and respiratory excursions will not be reflected in the manometer. Minor rotation of the needle may solve these problems. Hyperventilation will reduce the pressure readings because of hypocapnia and the resultant cerebral vasoconstriction.

After measuring the pressure, turn the stopcock toward the patient (off to patient) and collect the fluid in the manometer tube. Then, the stopcock can be turned toward the manometer or alternatively taken off to collect enough CSF to perform all the studies desired. It is generally advised that CSF should be collected by a free flow from the needle, and not by aspiration.

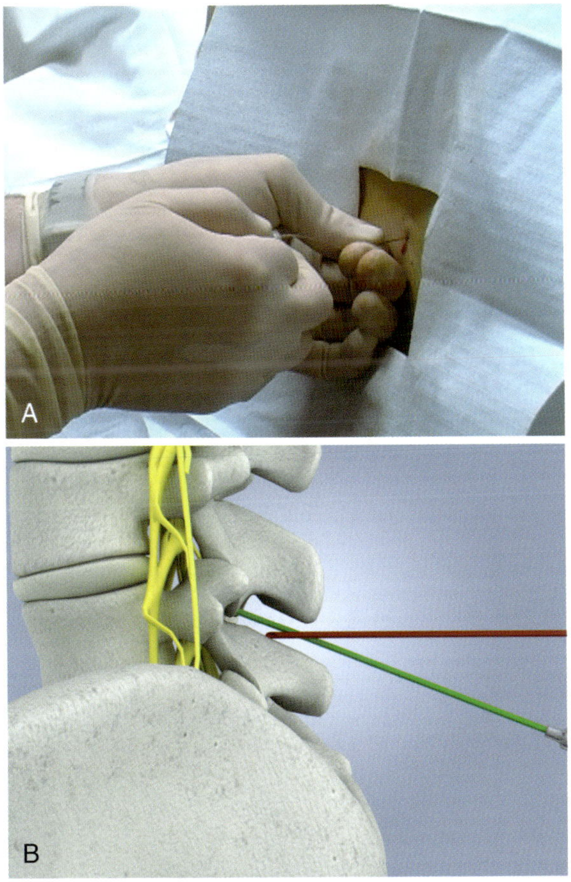

Fig. 61.8 (A) This 22-gauge spinal needle has struck bone during advancement (notice the bend in the needle) and needs to be repositioned. (B) If bone is encountered, it is usually the inferior spinous process *(red spinal needle)*. The needle must be partially withdrawn into subcutaneous tissue and then readvanced in a more cephalad direction *(green needle)*.

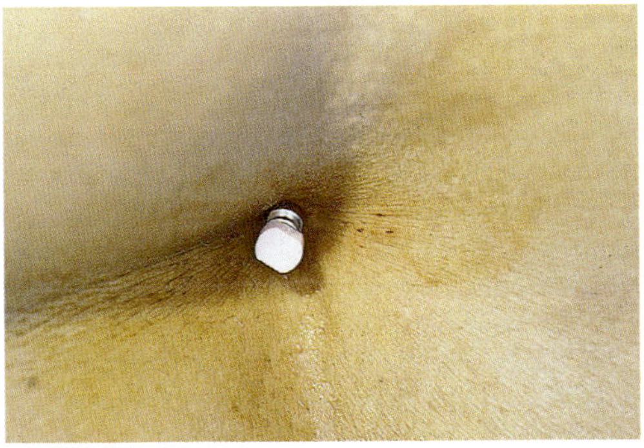

Fig. 61.9 The spinal needle is usually advanced one-half to three-fourths of its length before the spinal canal is reached. In this patient with an increased body mass index, the needle was advanced all the way to the hub of the needle before spinal fluid was returned. (Image shows needle inserted to the hub in the patient's lower lumbar area, indenting the tissues.)

The first sample of fluid exits from the manometer if pressure has been measured, and then additional fluid flows from the spinal canal. Replacing the stylet into the needle before withdrawing it may decrease the risk of post–dural lumbar puncture headache.

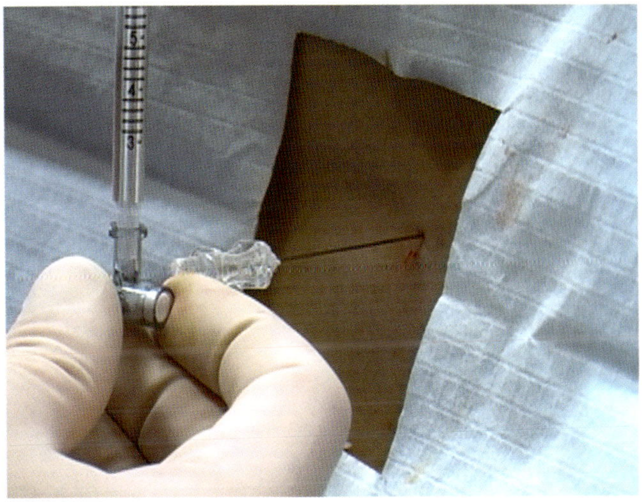

Fig. 61.10 To measure the opening pressure, attach the manometer to the needle hub with a three-way stopcock. The "zero" mark of the manometer should be level with the site of needle entry.

Commercial kits generally supply four specimen tubes. One tube is commonly used for determining protein and glucose levels and for electrophoretic studies, another is used for microbiologic and cytologic studies, and a third is used for serologic tests. Cell counts should be performed in the first and fourth tubes to help differentiate traumatic taps from true SAH. Depending on the clinical scenario, additional tests may be indicated. Use special stains, such as India ink for suspected *Cryptococcus* infection in patients with acquired immunodeficiency syndrome (AIDS), acid-fast stain in patients with possible tuberculous meningitis, viral studies in patients with suspected encephalitis, and various polymerase chain reaction studies. The remaining tube can be stored under refrigeration in the laboratory for any additional studies that may be required after the initial assessment.

Traumatic taps are common and usually clinically inconsequential. Nevertheless, they can be minimized by proper patient and needle positioning. A traumatic tap most commonly occurs when the subarachnoid space is transfixed at the entrance of the ventral epidural space, where the venous plexus is heavier. A plexus of veins forms a ring around the cord, and these veins may be entered if the needle is advanced too far ventrally or is directed laterally (Fig. 61.11). If blood is encountered and the fluid does not clear, repeat the procedure at a higher interspace with a fresh needle. A traumatic tap, per se, is not a particularly dangerous problem in a patient with normal coagulation, and no specific precautions are needed if blood-tinged fluid is obtained. However, observe for signs of cord or spinal nerve compression from a hematoma developing within the first several hours in patients with a coagulopathy.

Lateral Approach for Lumbar Puncture

The supraspinal ligament might be calcified in older persons, making a midline perforation difficult. A calcified ligament may deflect the needle. In this case, use a slightly lateral approach. Because the lower lamina rises upward from the midline, direct the needle slightly cephalad to miss the lamina and slightly medially to compensate for the lateral approach.

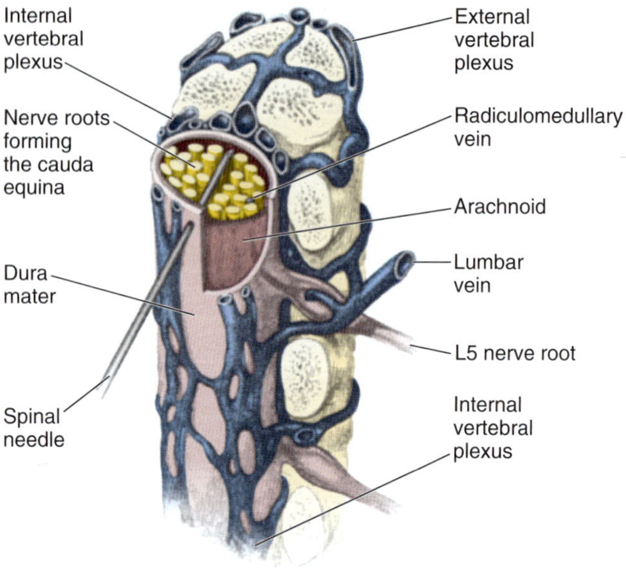

Fig. 61.11 The spinal contents at L4 and L5 show the relationship of a lumbar puncture needle to the major vessels at this level. The major radiculomedullary vein, shown accompanying the L5 nerve root, is situated far lateral to a needle correctly positioned in the midline of the dural sac. Note the avascular subdural space. (From Edelson RN, Chernik IVL, Rosner JB. Spinal subdural hematomas. *Arch Neurol.* 1974;31:134. Illustration by Lynn McDowell.)

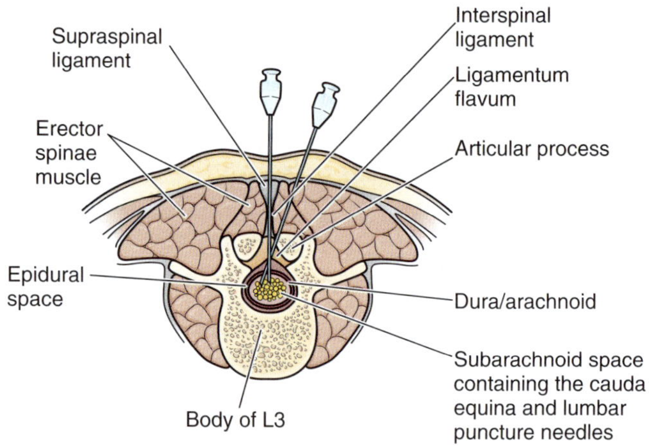

Fig. 61.12 Horizontal section through the body of L3. Note the two puncture needles in the subarachnoid space. The medial needle is in the midline. The lateral needle exemplifies the lateral approach, which avoids the occasionally calcified supraspinal ligament. Note the lateral needle piercing the intrinsic musculature of the back and only one ligament, the ligamentum flavum. (From Lachman E. Anatomy as applied to clinical medicine. *New Physician.* 1968;17:745.)

The needle passes through the skin, superficial fascia, fat, the dense posterior layer of the thoracolumbar fascia, and the erector spinae muscles. The needle then penetrates the ligamentum flavum (bypassing the supraspinal and interspinal ligaments), the epidural space, and the dura before CSF is obtained (Fig. 61.12). Lateral cervical puncture is an alternative approach that can be performed utilizing an insertion site 1 cm inferior and 1 cm dorsal to the mastoid process.[52] Ideally this approach is performed by experienced specialists using fluoroscopy.

Lumbar Puncture in Infants

See Videos 61.5–61.8. Lumbar puncture in infants is usually performed to exclude meningitis or encephalitis. The sitting position may allow the midline to be identified more easily. Use of a needle without a stylet has been suggested for small infants because this device allows the pressure to be estimated as the needle punctures the dura.[53] However, failure to use a stylet may cause the subsequent development of an intraspinal epidermoid tumor.[54] Use of a butterfly infusion set needle simplifies the procedure, which is helpful when managing a squirming or hyperactive patient.[53] In general, a stylet is recommended primarily at the time of skin penetration and on needle withdrawal, although many operators use the stylet during any advancement of the needle.

If the child's neck is very tightly flexed, CSF might not be obtained, and this position risks respiratory compromise in infants and small children and is discouraged. However, if the head is held in midflexion, CSF usually flows briskly. If CSF fails to flow, gently suction with a 1.0-mL syringe to exclude a low-pressure syndrome. Because pressure readings are inaccurate in a struggling child, measurement of pressure is not commonly attempted in infants and young children.[55]

Avoid prolonged severe flexion of the neck in an infant because it may produce dangerous airway obstruction. If the infant suddenly stops crying, check the airway immediately.[56] Proper positioning is best accomplished by an assistant, who maintains the spine maximally flexed by partially overlying the child and using the chest and body weight to immobilize the thorax and hips while holding the child behind the shoulders and knees.[57] Infants have poor neck control; therefore the assistant must also ensure that the child maintains an open airway. Pay particular attention to avoiding marked neck and trunk flexion. Incorrect positioning usually results in multiple punctures and a bloody tap.

Newborn and preterm infants may experience significant hypoxia and clinical deterioration during lumbar puncture; a sitting position appears to be preferable.[58] Lumbar puncture in infants with respiratory distress syndrome may pose greater risk than benefit.[59] This is a problem primarily in neonates but may also apply to younger infants with sepsis. Closely monitor all infants with serious cardiopulmonary disease during the procedure. Preoxygenation with or without monitoring oxygen saturation and end-tidal capnometry may be used as a precaution.

Although local anesthesia or sedation is not a routine practice during lumbar puncture in an infant or child, it should be considered.[60,61] Neonates perceive pain, and local anesthesia neither produces physiologic instability nor makes the procedure more difficult.[62,63] The use of topically applied eutectic mixture of local anesthetics (EMLA) (AstraZeneca) reduces the pain associated with needle insertion in newborns.[64] Sedation of an anxious child may be considered, but sedatives are relatively contraindicated in an obtunded patient without a protected airway and in the setting of hemodynamic instability.

The Difficult Lumbar Puncture

The traditional approach to lumbar puncture depends on palpation of bony landmarks to determine the correct location for insertion of the needle. However, landmarks are difficult to palpate in overweight and obese patients.[65] When lumbar puncture fails, the usual alternative has been fluoroscopic guidance, which necessitates movement of the patient out of the ED, as well as the availability of an appropriately trained radiologist.[65] Brook found CT guidance to be comparable to fluoroscopy in the facilitation of lumbar puncture in obese patients with a previously unsuccessful attempt.[66] Bedside ultrasound is being used increasingly in emergency and critical care medicine, and its scope of practice has expanded to include guidance for a number of procedures, including lumbar puncture (see Ultrasound Box).[66–70] Ultrasound can be used in adults as well as neonates and infants.[71]

ULTRASOUND: Lumbar Puncture

by Christine Butts, MD

See Video 61.9. When ultrasound is used to guide lumbar puncture, it is generally done in a static manner: the ultrasound probe is used to determine the site of skin entry, the skin is marked, and the probe is then set aside.

Equipment

A linear probe is preferred, although for patients with an extremely high body mass index, a curvilinear probe may be required because of the distance between the skin and the spine.

Image Interpretation

The bony spinous process will appear as a hyperechoic crescent-shaped structure with posterior acoustic shadowing. In the transverse view, acquisition of a perfectly symmetric image will provide assurance that the probe is in the anatomic midline (Fig. 61.US1). In the longitudinal view, multiple spinous processes can be visualized, along with the interspaces between them (Fig. 61.US2).

Procedure and Technique

To perform ultrasound-guided lumbar puncture, position the patient in the usual manner. Place the ultrasound probe over the spine in a transverse orientation at the level of the iliac crests such that the shadow caused by the spinous process is centered on the screen. Use a pen to mark the skin on each side of the transducer, exactly at the midpoints (Fig. 61.US3). These two marks can then be connected to mark the midline of the spine. Next, rotate the transducer 90 degrees to obtain a midline longitudinal view and position it until the gap between two spinal processes is in the center of the screen. Mark the skin at the midpoint of each side of the transducer and then connect the marks to form a single line (Fig. 61.US4). The intersection of the two lines is the site for entry of the needle which can be marked with a needle cap indented into the skin (Fig. 61.US5). Cleanse the skin with antiseptic solution and perform the remainder of the procedure in the usual fashion.

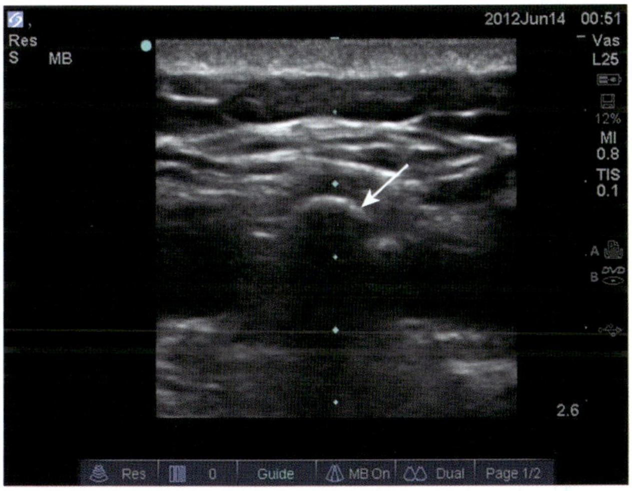

Fig. 61.US1 Transverse image of the lumbar spine. The crescent-shaped hyperechoic structure *(arrow)* is a spinous process. Note the presence of posterior acoustic shadowing. Align the probe so that the spinous process is directly centered in the image. The general symmetry of the image provides additional assurance that the probe is centered correctly.

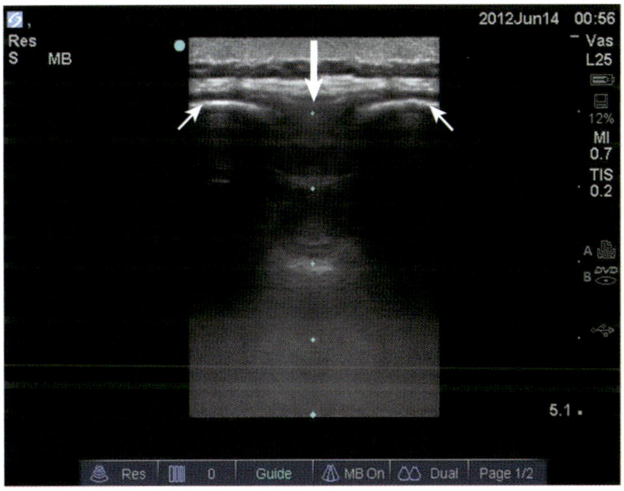

Fig. 61.US2 Longitudinal image of the lumbar spine. The spinous processes *(small arrows)* are visible again, and appear as crescent-shaped hyperechoic structures with acoustic shadowing. In between each spinous process is the interspinous space *(large arrow)*. Note how this space is bordered on either side by the acoustic shadow of the spinous process. Note also how the probe is centered directly over the interspace.

Continued

ULTRASOUND: Lumbar Puncture—cont'd

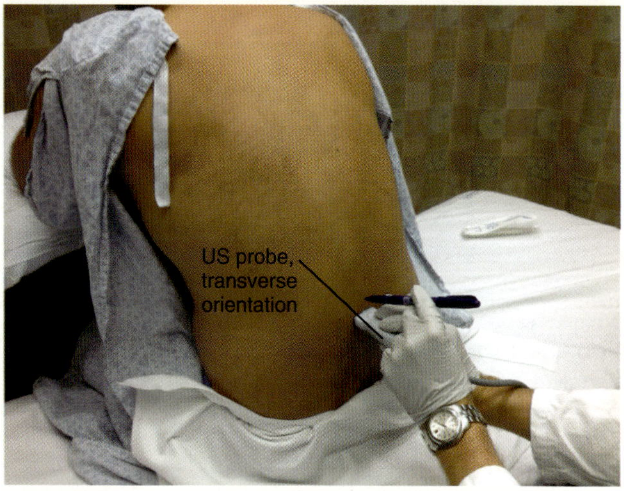

Fig. 61.US3 First use the ultrasound *(US)* probe in the transverse orientation at the level of the iliac crest and obtain an image with the shadow of the spinous process centered on the screen (as in Fig. 61.US1). Mark the skin at the exact midpoint of the transducer. This represents the anatomic midline.

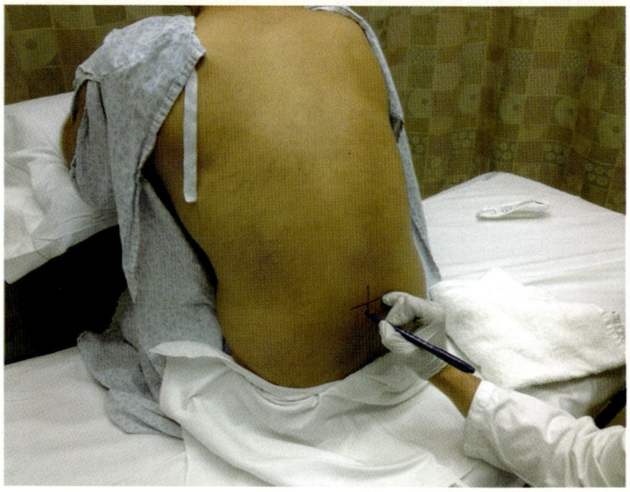

Fig. 61.US5 The intersection of the anatomic midline and the level of the interspinous space is the site of needle entry.

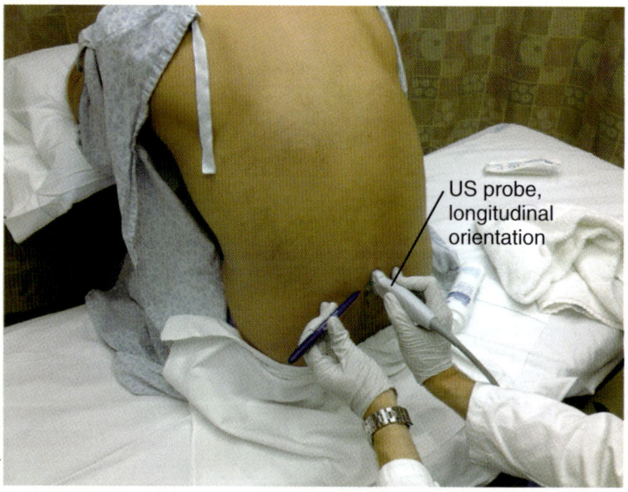

Fig. 61.US4 Rotate the ultrasound *(US)* probe 90 degrees and obtain a midline longitudinal view. Position the probe so that the interspace is centered on the screen (as in Fig. 61.US2). Mark the skin at the midpoint of the transducer. This represents the level of needle entry.

COMPLICATIONS

Headache after Lumbar Puncture

There are several complications from lumbar puncture.[72] One of the most common is headache, which occurs after 1% to 70% of spinal taps.[73–83] The syndrome most commonly starts within 48 hours after the procedure (although a case occurring 12 days after the procedure has been reported[84]) and usually lasts for 1 to 2 days (occasionally as long as 14 days). Cases lasting months have been described. The headache usually begins within seconds after the patient arises and characteristically ceases as soon as the patient lies down. The pain is mild to incapacitating and is generally cervical and suboccipital in location but might involve the shoulders and the entire cranium. Exceptional cases include nausea, vomiting, vertigo, blurred vision, ear pressure, tinnitus, and stiff neck. The headache may change to a positional backache or neck ache.

The technique of spinal puncture probably has little to do with the development of a post–dural procedure headache, but the type of needle used may affect the likelihood of this complication. The syndrome is widely thought to be caused by leakage of fluid through the dural puncture site. This results in a reduction in CSF volume below the cisterna magna and downward movement of brain tissue, along with displacement and stretching of pain-sensitive structures such as the meninges and vessels and causes a traction headache. The recumbent position brings relief because the weight of the brain is shifted cephalad. Another proposed mechanism is cerebral vasodilation. Another hypothesis suggests that the headache is caused by an altered distribution of craniospinal elasticity and acute intracranial venous dilation.[85] Some authors have commented on the incidence and severity of post–dural puncture headache in relation to the orientation of the spinal needle bevel and its type and size.[86–96] The incidence of post–dural puncture headache is lower when the bevel of the needle is oriented parallel to the longitudinal axis of the spine. The traditional explanation for this was that the parallel bevel would separate rather than cut the longitudinal dural fibers and thus produce a smaller dural hole and less CSF leakage. However, the dural fibers are oriented randomly, not longitudinally.[97] Even with random fiber orientation, back flexion is more likely to close a dural hole in the longitudinal plane than a hole in the horizontal plane.

The two basic types of spinal needles are cutting (Quincke; Becton, Dickinson and Company) and noncutting or pencil-point (Sprotte; PAJUNK Medical System L.P. and Whitacre; Becton, Dickinson and Company) (see Fig. 61.2). A recent systematic review and meta-analysis concluded that atraumatic (noncutting) needles were associated with significant reductions in the risk of post–dural puncture headache, and had similar efficacy to conventional needles.[98] It has traditionally been thought that the dural hole resulting from puncture with a noncutting needle is smaller than that created by puncture with a cutting needle; however, this may not be true. The important difference may be that the cutting needle causes a clean-cut opening in the dura, whereas the noncutting needle produces a jagged opening with rough edges.[99] The jagged opening may produce a more intense inflammatory response that results in edema and more complete closure of the hole. The use of noncutting spinal needles is not routine.[100] As more spinal kit manufacturers include them in kits, their use might increase.[101] A single-institution study suggested that routine use of noncutting needles yields a potential cost saving.[102] However, in thick-skinned individuals, passage of a thin, noncutting needle may be technically difficult. The solution is to make the initial pass with a thicker cutting needle to the level of the interspinal ligament or alternatively using a No. 11 blade to make a small stab incision beyond the dermis, followed by removal and advancement of a noncutting needle in the same soft tissue tract, can be helpful.

Use of a smaller-diameter needle is one intervention that will probably cause a lower incidence of post–dural puncture headache because it creates a smaller dural hole. If diameter were the only consideration, as small a needle as possible would be used. However, a needle must provide adequate CSF flow rates to allow timely CSF collection and pressure measurement. With a very small needle, a syringe may be needed to withdraw fluid, and pressure cannot be recorded easily. In addition, technically, a small needle such as a 25-gauge is difficult to place and manipulate as it is too malleable. A 2014 randomized crossover trial compared the use of 22-gauge and 25-gauge needles in children and found no difference in the incidence of post–dural puncture headache, but the 25-gauge needles were found to be flimsy and difficult to use, with fluid collection taking much longer.[103] When these characteristics are considered, a 20- to 22-gauge atraumatic needle seems to be the best overall choice for diagnostic lumbar puncture.[89]

Despite common beliefs about techniques and postprocedure interventions, lumbar puncture headaches may not be completely preventable. Studies of the influence of directives such as strict bed rest on postpuncture headache have yielded contradictory results, with no consensus on any specific preventive intervention forthcoming concerning the worsening of, improvement in, or effect on the incidence. Brocker reported a reduction in the incidence of headache from 36.5% to 0.5% when patients lie prone instead of supine for 3 hours after puncture with an 18-gauge needle.[104] He postulated that the prone position caused hyperextension of the spine and disrupted alignment of the holes in the dura and the arachnoid, making leakage less likely. Theonnissen and coworkers concluded that there was no evidence that longer bed rest after lumbar puncture was better than immediate mobilization or short bed rest in reducing the incidence of headache.[105] There appears to be no reason to enforce bed rest following lumbar puncture.[106]

Other factors that might influence the incidence of a post–dural spinal puncture headache were reviewed by Fishman and by Lin and Giederman.[24,107] The incidence is higher in young patients than in older patients and is also increased in females and individuals with a history of headache.

Many medications have been advocated for the treatment of headache after lumbar puncture: barbiturates, codeine, neostigmine, ergots, diphenhydramine, dimenhydrinate, caffeine, amphetamine sulfate, ephedrine, intravenous fluids (normal saline, lactated Ringer's solution), magnesium sulfate, vitamins, and aminophylline.[24,108–111] Niraj and colleagues tested the use of greater occipital nerve block in patients with post-procedural headache, a less invasive alternative to epidural blood patch, and achieved modest success in a small trial.[112]

Traditionally, caffeine has often been used as the initial intervention for post–dural puncture headache, and it appears to be of benefit.[110] Although caffeine may decrease headache, there is a high recurrence rate. Caffeine can be administered in the ED, bringing pain relief within a few hours. It is thought to result from caffeine's vasoconstrictive effect on the cerebral vasculature. One suggested regimen is 500 mg of caffeine (sodium benzoate) diluted in 1000 mL of normal saline infused over a 1- to 2-hour period. A second dose can be given if the headache is not relieved. If successful, consumption of caffeinated beverages may be continued as an outpatient. A cup of coffee contains 50 mg to 100 mg of caffeine.

Most post–dural puncture headaches can be managed by bed rest with the head in the horizontal position. Avoid dehydration because it lowers CSF pressure and might aggravate the headache. Although dehydration should be avoided, the role of fluid supplementation in the prevention of post–dural puncture headache remains uncertain.

Simple analgesics are commonly prescribed, but they have no apparent advantage over bed rest and fluid intake. A patient with a prolonged headache after spinal puncture should be reassessed to rule out structural causes. Because a spinal headache has classic signs and symptoms, if the headache is not postural, consider other causes.

Most post–dural puncture headaches are mild and self-limited, so conservative therapy for the first 24 to 48 hours is recommended. Bed rest and oral analgesics, including opioids, are usually effective, as well as, perhaps, oral caffeine drinks, usually suffice. In cases refractory to conservative measures, an epidural blood patch is recommended. For patients with a prolonged low-pressure headache, placement of an epidural blood patch by experienced operators (typically an anesthesiologist) is highly successful and often provides dramatic relief.[113–117] Consider a blood patch for all patients with seriously symptomatic spinal headaches.

To perform a blood patch, do an epidural tap at the level of the previous lumbar puncture. Use the loss-of-resistance technique with sterile saline to locate the epidural space.[118] Draw 10 mL to 20 mL of autologous blood into a syringe aseptically and slowly inject it (1 mL to 2 mL every 10 seconds) into the epidural space at the site of the dural puncture.[119] Slow or discontinue the injection if back pain or paresthesia develops. Keep the patient supine for 1 hour while hydration is administered intravenously. Relief usually occurs within 20 to 30 minutes after the procedure. Epidural patches are less likely to be effective if symptoms have been present for more than 2 weeks. Pain is relieved when the blood patch forms a gelatinous tamponade that stops the CSF leak and immediately elevates CSF pressure. Patch failures (15% to 20%) are believed to be caused by improper needle placement, injection of an inadequate quantity of blood (after which a second patch is usually successful), or an incorrect diagnosis.

Complications reported after placement of an epidural patch include back stiffness, paresthesia, radicular pain, subdural hematoma, adhesive arachnoiditis, and bacterial meningitis.[120] The procedure should be used in patients with refractory headaches that do not respond to conservative therapy, and it should be performed by clinicians trained in its use.

Infection

Spinal puncture is contraindicated in the presence of local infection at the puncture site (cellulitis, suspected epidural abscess, or furunculosis) because of the danger of inducing meningitis. A large concentration of bacteria in the bloodstream at the time of CSF examination is associated with meningitis. The meningitis could be coincidental ("spontaneous") or could result from leakage of blood containing bacteria into the subarachnoid space after lumbar puncture ("induced"). It is likely that many cases of puncture-induced meningitis emerge after a cautious clinician performs a lumbar puncture early in the course of meningitis, before the infection has had time to be reflected in CSF. A 2006 review concluded that the majority of cases of postpuncture meningitis are probably caused by contamination of the site with aerosolized bacteria from medical personnel, contamination from skin flora, or least commonly, direct or hematogenous spread from an endogenous infectious site.[50] Suspected bacteremia is not a contraindication to lumbar puncture. Delay in diagnosis because of concern regarding the risks associated with lumbar puncture is probably more serious than the risk of causing meningitis with the procedure.[121,122]

Herniation Syndromes after Lumbar Puncture

Generally, when the patient has symptoms consistent with bacterial meningitis but not increased ICP, it is safe to perform lumbar puncture without a preceding head CT scan. Lumbar puncture may also be the best initial procedure to diagnose SAH, thus reducing the need for routine CT scanning in certain low-risk patients with acute sudden headache.[123] However, in patients with severely altered mentation, focal neurologic findings, papilledema, immunosuppression, or a suspected intracranial mass lesion, one should perform a CT scan before lumbar puncture to rule out increased ICP or mass effect. Others have considered a recent seizure an indication for CT scan prior to lumbar puncture. When meningitis remains in the differential diagnosis, antibiotics are best administered after blood is obtained for culture and before the CT scan. In patients with suspected elevated ICP based on clinical features, head elevation, hyperventilation, and intravenous mannitol have been recommended.

In patients with supratentorial masses, there may be a large pressure gradient between the cranial and lumbar compartments. When brain volume is increased because of a mass or edema, rostrocaudal displacement may occur after lumbar puncture if the skull is intact.

The question of whether lumbar puncture precipitates brain herniation in cases in which herniation would not have occurred spontaneously cannot be answered with certainty. Controversy still exists regarding the risk for brain herniation from lumbar puncture in patients with acute bacterial meningitis, and data continue to be sparse.[124] Herniation may occur in the absence of lumbar puncture in the setting of acute bacterial meningitis and has been temporally related to the procedure. Brain herniation is usually fatal and occurs in approximately 5% of patients with acute bacterial meningitis and accounts for approximately 30% of the deaths associated with the disease.[124] Although CT imaging may reveal contraindications to lumbar puncture, normal findings on CT do not eliminate the risk for herniation and do not necessarily mean that a lumbar puncture is safe.

Lowering pressure in the lumbar spinal canal by removing CSF can increase the gradient between the cranial and lumbar compartments and thereby theoretically promote both transtentorial and foramen magnum (cerebellar) herniation. The frequency with which lumbar puncture causes or accelerates transtentorial herniation is unknown because herniation might have developed spontaneously in a seriously ill patient without the procedure. With the current use of small-caliber spinal needles, herniation appears to be extremely rare; nonetheless, it is not fully predictable by CT or the opening CSF pressure readings.

A careful neurologic examination should precede all spinal punctures. When the patient has a history of headache and fever with progressive deterioration in mental status and localizing neurologic signs, spinal puncture should not be performed as the initial diagnostic procedure. Gopal and colleagues identified three statistically significant predictors of new intracranial masses: papilledema, focal abnormalities on neurologic examination, and altered mental status.[125] Greig and Goroszeniuk made similar recommendations.[126] Hasbun and associates demonstrated that in adults with suspected meningitis, the presence of any of 13 clinical features is predictive of abnormal findings on CT (Box 61.1).[127] Theoretically, the presence of abnormal findings on CT portends potential herniation, with or without lumbar puncture. The absence of abnormal findings suggests the patient is a good candidate for immediate lumbar puncture because the risk for brain herniation as a result of the procedure is low (see Box 61.1). Joffe argues that clinical signs of impending herniation are the most appropriate criteria on which to base decisions regarding the timing of lumbar puncture in patients with acute bacterial meningitis.[124] Such signs include a significantly decreased level of consciousness (Glasgow Coma Scale score ≤11), brain stem findings (pupillary changes, posturing, irregular respirations), and a very recent seizure.[124] It is recommended that these patients undergo neuroimaging (CT or MRI) and receive antibiotics empirically while awaiting

BOX 61.1 Clinical Characteristics Associated With Abnormal Findings on Head CT in Adults With Suspected Meningitis

Age 60 years or older
Immunocompromised state[a]
History of central nervous system disease[b]
Seizure within 1 week before initial evaluation
Abnormal level of consciousness
Inability to answer two questions correctly
Inability to follow two commands correctly
Gaze palsy
Abnormal visual fields
Facial palsy
Arm drift
Leg drift
Abnormal language[c]

CT, *Computed tomography.*
[a]*Includes patients with human immunodeficiency virus infection or acquired immunodeficiency syndrome, patients receiving immunosuppressive therapy, and patients who have undergone transplantation.*
[b]*Mass, stroke, or focal infection.*
[c]*Aphasia, dysarthria, or extinction.*
From Hasbun R, Abrahams J, Jekel J et al. Computed tomography of the head before lumbar puncture in adults with suspected meningitis. N Engl J Med. *2001;345:1727.*

the results of imaging, which will help in assessment of the safety of a subsequent lumbar puncture. Measures to lower ICP before spinal puncture may also be considered. Appropriate cultures of blood and more easily accessible body fluids should be obtained before the administration of antibiotics. Blood cultures are positive in 80% of infants with meningitis.

Critically ill patients with acute bacterial meningitis often deteriorate rapidly and experience fatal brain herniation, both shortly after lumbar puncture and in the absence of the procedure. A direct cause-and-effect relationship between lumbar puncture and brain herniation in the setting of suspected meningitis is obscure and probably cannot be defined prospectively in the ED when clinical decisions must be made. A 2007 review identified 22 case reports of rapid deterioration and herniation after lumbar puncture in adults and children with acute bacterial meningitis.[124] The consensus is that less ill patients (clearly a subjective clinical judgment) with a clinical scenario that includes meningitis as a possibility can be evaluated safely with lumbar puncture. In critically ill patients, especially those with localizing neurologic signs, severely depressed level of consciousness, or papilledema, diagnostic lumbar puncture may be delayed until the risk for herniation is lower, and aggressive and empirical treatment with meningitis doses of antibiotics should proceed.

Head CT can identify hemorrhagic lesions and most neoplasms. Its results should contribute to the decision regarding the need for and the risk involved with spinal puncture. Head CT can identify patients with unequal pressure between intracranial compartments, who are at greater risk for cerebral herniation. Findings that suggest unequal pressure include (1) lateral shift of midline structures, (2) loss of the suprachiasmatic and perimesencephalic cisterns, (3) shift or obliteration of the fourth ventricle, and (4) failure to visualize the superior cerebellar and quadrigeminal plate cisterns with sparing of the ambient cisterns.[128] The presence of a mass in the posterior fossa is a strong contraindication to lumbar puncture. Unfortunately, because of bone and motion artifact, the posterior fossa may be a difficult area to visualize on CT.

Although there is no clear standard with respect to the use of CT before lumbar puncture, a reasonable and logical approach is to avoid initial lumbar puncture and first perform head CT when a mass lesion is suspected or if the patient has signs and symptoms of increased ICP (see Box 61.1). The 2016 European Society of Clinical Microbiology and Infectious Diseases guidelines similarly recommend neuroimaging before lumbar puncture in patients with prior CNS disease, recent seizure, abnormal immunity, abnormal neurologic examination, or papilledema.[129]

Epidermoid Tumor

An epidermoid tumor or cyst is a mass of desquamated cells containing keratin within a capsule of well-differentiated stratified squamous epithelium. Congenital lesions arise from epithelial tissue that becomes sequestered at the time of closure of the neural groove between the third and fifth weeks of embryonic life, but such lesions are rare. Acquired intraspinal epidermoid tumors result from the implantation of epidermoid tissue into the spinal canal at the time of lumbar puncture performed with needles without stylets or with ill-fitting stylets. The clinical syndrome consists of pain in the back and lower extremities developing years after spinal puncture. Failure to use a stylet on needle withdrawal might also result in aspiration of a nerve root into the epidural space.

Backache and Radicular Symptoms

Minor backache from the trauma of the spinal needle occurs in 90% of patients. Frank disk herniation has been reported from passage of the needle beyond the subarachnoid space into the anulus fibrosus. Transient sensory symptoms from irritation of the cauda equina are also common.

Other reported complications include transient unilateral or bilateral sixth-nerve palsies caused by stretching or displacement of the abducens nerve as it crosses the petrous ridge of the temporal bone, SAH, subdural and epidural hematoma, epidural CSF collection, cauda equina syndrome, anaphylactoid reactions to local anesthetics, settling of cord tumors, and retroperitoneal abscess produced by laceration of the dura in patients with meningitis.[130–136] Most of these complications are rare and seldom encountered; however, they should be considered if a patient returns after a lumbar puncture with worsening back pain or abnormal findings on neurologic examination.

The complications associated with lateral cervical and cisternal puncture are similar to those encountered with lumbar puncture. Perforation of a large vessel with resultant cisterna magna hematoma or obstruction of vertebral artery flow has been described. Puncture of the medulla oblongata may cause vomiting or apnea, and puncture of the cord may be associated with pain. Long-lasting side effects of cord puncture seem to be rare.

Spinal Epidural Hemorrhage

Rarely, serious bleeding leading to spinal hematoma after lumbar puncture can produce spinal cord compromise and permanent significant neurologic deficits, such as cauda equina syndrome.[30] This may occur more frequently in coagulopathic patients but can also arise in those with a normal coagulation profile and a seemingly atraumatic tap. Aspirin and nonsteroidal medications are not associated with an increased bleeding risk after lumbar puncture. The bleeding is concealed and might be suspected only because of persistent severe backache or neurologic findings. Weakness, numbness, and incontinence after spinal puncture must be investigated, usually with MRI, for a possible spinal hematoma. Surgical intervention, including laminectomy and evacuation of blood, may be required and must occur in a timely manner to avoid permanent loss of neurologic function. Those with mild symptoms and progressive recovery may be managed conservatively with close monitoring.

INTERPRETATION

Pressure

CSF pressure is clinically important.[137] Measure it accurately whenever feasible. Unfortunately, in some cases it will be logistically impossible to obtain. If the lumbar puncture is being performed with the patient in a seated position, place the patient in the lateral decubitus position before a measurement is obtained. This can be accomplished by replacing the stylet and ensuring that the sterile field is maintained while an assistant guides the patient to lay on their side from the sitting position. Accurate measurement depends on the cooperation of the patient. Measurements from struggling or agitated patients will probably be inaccurate; in such cases, sedation may allow more accurate readings to be obtained.

Normal CSF pressure is between 7 and 20 cm H_2O. Patients with increased body mass index may have a CSF pressure of up to 25 cm H_2O. Elevated pressure is abnormal. Opening pressure is taken promptly, thereby avoiding falsely low values caused by leakage through and around the needle. Herniating cerebellar tonsils may occlude the foramen magnum and prevent increased ICP from being reflected in the lumbar pressure reading. Increased ICP can result from expansion of the brain (edema, hemorrhage, or neoplasm), overproduction of CSF (choroid plexus papilloma), a defect in absorption, or obstruction of flow of CSF through the ventricles. Cerebral edema may be associated with meningitis, CO_2 retention, SAH, anoxia, congestive heart failure, or superior vena cava obstruction. Pressure may be falsely elevated in a tense patient when the head is elevated above the plane of the needle and, possibly, in markedly obese patients and those experiencing muscle contraction.[24] Pressure is not usually measured in neonates because a struggling or crying child will have a falsely elevated pressure. Avery and colleagues concluded that for most children (1 to 18 years of age), an opening pressure above 28 cm H_2O should be considered elevated.[138]

Low pressure suggests obstruction of the needle by the meninges. Low pressure can also be seen with a spinal block. Rarely, a primary low-pressure syndrome occurs in a setting of trauma, after neurosurgical procedures, secondary to subdural hematoma in older patients, with barbiturate intoxication, and in cases of CSF leakage through holes in the arachnoid.[139,140]

Appearance

If the CSF is not crystal clear and colorless, a pathologic condition of the CNS should be suspected. The examiner should compare the fluid with water and view down the long axis of the tube or by holding both tubes against a white background. A glass tube is preferred because plastic tubes are frequently not clear. CSF will appear grossly bloody if more than 6000 red blood cells (RBCs)/μL are present. Note that the fluid may appear clear with as many as 400 RBCs/μL and 200 WBCs/μL.[24] Xanthochromia, a yellow-orange discoloration of the supernate of centrifuged CSF, is generally considered to be the result of SAH of at least a few hours' duration and has been used to differentiate prior bleeding from a traumatic tap. A traumatic tap does not usually exhibit xanthochromia (see the later section on "The Traumatic Tap"). Xanthochromia is produced by red cell lysis and is caused by one or more of the following pigments: oxyhemoglobin, bilirubin, or methemoglobin.

Traditionally, CSF samples have been assessed for xanthochromia by visual inspection by a laboratory technician after centrifugation of a sample of CSF. Most hospitals still use this method.[141] Recently, spectrophotometry, designed to demonstrate both oxyhemoglobin and bilirubin, has been advocated as a more precise way of determining xanthochromia, but most hospitals do not have spectrophotometry available for this purpose. Oxyhemoglobin alone without bilirubin in a CSF sample is thought to be artifactual (traumatic). Visually, bilirubin and oxyhemoglobin cannot be differentiated. Therefore detection of bilirubin by spectrophotometry should define xanthochromia and prompt additional investigation for SAH. Relying on spectrophotometry to identify xanthochromia without pigment differentiation will cause a high false-positive interpretation. The absence of both oxyhemoglobin and bilirubin by spectrophotometry does not support the diagnosis of SAH. Oxyhemoglobin causes red coloration; bilirubin, yellow; and methemoglobin, brown. Oxyhemoglobin is seen within 2 hours after subarachnoid bleeding and red cell lysis, but it may be detected immediately if the bleeding is profuse. Formation of oxyhemoglobin peaks 24 to 48 hours after hemorrhage, and the discoloration disappears in 3 to 30 days.[4]

Blood must be present in CSF (in vivo) for several hours for bilirubin to appear; it will not appear spontaneously once CSF is in the collection tube. The appearance of bilirubin in CSF involves the conversion of oxyhemoglobin by the enzyme heme oxygenase. The enzyme is found in the choroid plexus, the arachnoid, and the meninges. Enzyme activity appears approximately 12 hours after the hemorrhage.[4] Bilirubin may persist in CSF for 2 to 4 weeks. Moreover, bilirubin in CSF caused by hepatic or hemolytic disease does not appear until a serum level of 10 mg to 15 mg of total bilirubin per 100 mL is reached, unless underlying disease associated with high CSF protein levels is present. Xanthochromia may also be seen with CSF protein values above 150 mg/dL. CSF may clot in patients with a complete spinal block and very high CSF protein.

Graves and Sidman noted that an RBC concentration of 5000/μL, created by adding RBCs to acellular CSF, will produce xanthochromia evident on spectrophotometry by 2 hours.[142] The addition of RBCs to achieve RBC concentrations of 20,000/μL and 30,000/μL will produce xanthochromia by 1 hour or immediately, respectively. Therefore xanthochromia may occur with a traumatic tap and does not always indicate SAH.

Methemoglobin is a reduction product of oxyhemoglobin that is characteristically found in encapsulated subdural hematomas and in old intracerebral hematomas.

Cells

In adults, WBC counts higher than 5 cells/μL indicate the presence of a pathologic condition. A large multicenter study by Thomson and colleagues in 2018 determined upper bound WBC reference values in infants: 15 cells/μL for infants 28 days of age or younger and 9 cells/μL for those between the ages of 29 and 60 days.[143] A median CSF WBC count of 271 WBCs/μL has been reported in infants with group B *Streptococcus* in the era of intrapartum antibiotic prophylaxis. The CSF WBC count in infants is higher with gram-negative meningitis than with gram-positive CNS infections. In general, polymorphonuclear leukocytes are never seen in normal adults. However, with use of the cytocentrifuge, an occasional specimen from an otherwise normal individual may show one to two neutrophils.[144] More than three neutrophils is always abnormal in an adult. Moreover, as many as 30% of patients exhibit CSF pleocytosis after a generalized or focal seizure. Nonetheless, such a finding should prompt culture of CSF because the presence of neutrophilic pleocytosis is commonly associated with bacterial meningitis or the early stages of viral or tuberculous meningitis. Small lymphocytes may be seen in normal individuals. Small and large immunocompetent cells are found with a variety of bacterial, fungal, viral, granulomatous, and spirochetal diseases.

Eosinophils always indicate an abnormal condition, most commonly a parasitic infestation of the CNS. They may also be seen after myelography and pneumoencephalography and, to a minor degree, with other inflammatory diseases, including tuberculous meningitis and neurosyphilis. Normal CSF RBC counts are lower than 10 cells/μL. Herpes simplex virus (HSV) encephalitis may elevate the RBC count. Finally, myeloid and RBC precursors may contaminate CSF with bone marrow cells from an adjacent vertebral body.[145]

Glucose

Glucose enters CSF by way of the choroid plexus, as well as by transcapillary movement into the extracellular space of the brain and the cord via carrier-mediated transport. It then equilibrates freely within the CSF subarachnoid space. Once in the CSF, glucose undergoes glycolysis and there is an invariable rise in CSF lactate levels. Glucose levels remain subnormal for 1 to 2 weeks after effective treatment of bacterial meningitis.

The normal range of CSF glucose is 50 to 80 mg/dL, which is 60% to 70% of the glucose concentration in blood. Ventricular fluid glucose levels are 6 to 8 mg/dL higher than in lumbar fluid. A ratio of CSF glucose to blood glucose of less than 0.5 or a CSF glucose level below 40 mg/dL is invariably abnormal. The ratio is higher in infants, in whom a ratio of less than 0.6 is considered abnormal. Hyperglycemia may mask a depressed CSF glucose level; when present, the ratio of CSF glucose to blood glucose should be measured routinely. With extreme hyperglycemia, a ratio of less than 0.3 is abnormal.[146] Between 90 and 120 minutes is required before CSF glucose reaches a steady state with changes in blood glucose (e.g., after an intravenous injection of glucose). When CSF glucose is of diagnostic importance, obtain CSF and blood samples, ideally after a 4-hour fast.

Low CSF glucose levels may be associated with several diseases of the nervous system (Box 61.2). Only low concentrations of glucose are of diagnostic value; elevated CSF glucose levels generally have little significance and usually reflect hyperglycemia. A rapid estimate of the CSF glucose level can be obtained by using bedside reagent strip testing with a commercial autoanalyzer. Formal laboratory testing is recommended for confirmation of the bedside levels.

BOX 61.2 Low CSF Glucose Syndromes

Bacterial meningitis
Tuberculous meningitis
Fungal meningitis
Sarcoidosis
Meningeal carcinomatosis
Amebic meningitis
Cysticercosis
Trichinosis
Syphilis
Chemical meningitis
Subarachnoid hemorrhage
Mumps meningitis
Herpes simplex encephalitis
Hypoglycemia

CSF, *Cerebrospinal fluid.*

Protein

The normal range of lumbar CSF protein is 15 to 45 mg/dL. Infants normally have a lower level than adults, and protein levels may drop after lumbar puncture. The concentration is lower in the ventricles (5 to 15 mg/dL) and the basilar cisterns (10 to 25 mg/dL) as a result of a gradient in the permeability of capillary endothelial cells to proteins in blood. Levels of CSF protein in premature infants and full-term neonates are higher than in adults, with a mean of 90 mg/dL; protein levels decline by the age of 8 weeks because of maturation of the blood-brain barrier.

Most of the proteins in CSF come from blood, which normally has a protein concentration of up to 8000 mg/dL. Protein entry is determined by its molecular size and the relative impermeability of the blood-CSF barrier. A full range of serum proteins is found in CSF at a several hundred-fold dilution.

An increase in the total CSF protein level is a nonspecific abnormality associated with many disease states. Levels higher than 500 mg/dL are uncommon and seen mainly with meningitis, SAH, and spinal tumors. The high levels that occur with cord tumors result from an increase in local capillary permeability. At high levels (generally 1000 mg/dL), CSF may clot (Froin syndrome).

Hemorrhage into CSF or the introduction of blood by a traumatic tap increases CSF protein levels. If the serum protein concentration is normal, the CSF protein level should theoretically rise by 1 mg/dL for every 1000 RBCs, but this relationship varies. The inflammatory effect of hemolyzed RBCs may also significantly increase CSF protein.

Selective measurement of immunoglobulin fractions in CSF has proved to be of diagnostic value in suspected cases of multiple sclerosis. Elevated CSF immunoglobulin levels may reflect disruption of the blood-brain barrier or a local antibody response to a CNS immune response.[147] Stimuli may be infectious or antigenic and produce an inflammatory response. Elevated immunoglobulin levels have been found in many conditions, including syphilis, viral encephalitis, subacute sclerosing panencephalitis, progressive rubella encephalitis, tuberculous meningitis, sarcoidosis, cysticercosis, and acute inflammatory demyelinating polyneuropathy (Guillain-Barré syndrome).

The Traumatic Tap

The incidence of a traumatic tap is 10% to 30%, depending on the criteria used to define the condition.[148–150] Currently, there is no consensus on what constitutes a traumatic tap. Traditionally, the number of RBCs in CSF, the rate of clearance of RBCs from tube 1 to tube 4, and the presence or absence of xanthochromia have guided clinicians in attempts to define the need for further investigation of possible SAH when blood is detected during lumbar puncture.

Absolute Number of RBCs

The current literature makes no firm recommendations regarding the absolute CSF RBC count that can be used as a cutoff to differentiate SAH from a traumatic tap. However, SAH consistently produces more RBCs in CSF than a traumatic tap does. In tube 3 or 4, an absolute RBC value of 400 to 500 RBCs/μL or less is very suggestive of a traumatic tap, and this value has been traditionally used by clinicians.[13] In a retrospective study of 300 patients, Gorchynski and coworkers reported a 100% negative predictive value for SAH with an RBC count in tube 4 of 500 RBCs/μL or less, with a sensitivity of 100% for SAH.[151] No radiographically normal subject had an RBC count higher than 10,000 RBCs/μL, suggesting that results above this number are suspicious for radiographically detectable SAH. When the RBC count in tube 4 ranged between 500 and 10,000 RBCs/μL, SAH could not be ruled out without further study. Perry and colleagues concluded that the combination an RBC count of fewer than 2000×10^6 in the final tube and no xanthochromia reasonably excluded the diagnosis of aneurysmal SAH with a sensitivity of 100% and 95% confidence interval of 74.7% to 100%.[152] They added that patients with a high pretest probability of SAH might need further investigation.

Any attempt to define precisely how low an RBC count must be to eliminate the possibility of SAH would result in an arbitrary threshold. As the foregoing discussion suggests, SAH is exceedingly unlikely with RBC counts lower than 500 RBCs/μL and becomes progressively less likely as this number decreases.

RBC Clearance from First to Last Tubes

In traumatic punctures, the fluid generally clears of RBCs between tubes 1 and tubes 4 as the needle is washed by CSF. In fact, a decrease in the RBC count between the first and last tubes of at least 25% to 30% has traditionally been considered strong evidence of a traumatic tap.[2,153] However, it must be remembered that a traumatic tap may also occur in a patient with true SAH. Thus regardless of the change in RBC count from the first to last tubes, SAH cannot be excluded unless the RBC count approaches zero in either tube. If this is not the case and xanthochromia is not present (see next section), it may be most prudent to repeat the puncture at a different interspace or site. To help avoid this situation, when a clinician encounters what is suspected to be a traumatic tap (e.g., a streak of blood flowing into an otherwise clear-appearing stream of CSF), wasting the first 2 or 3 mL of CSF while positioning the needle to obtain the clearest possible sample will increase the odds of an RBC count approaching zero.

Xanthochromia

RBCs undergo hemolysis in CSF after a few hours and xanthochromia is produced. Xanthochromia persists for up to 4 weeks, depending on the number of RBCs originally present. Xanthochromia is suggestive of but not pathognomonic for SAH.[154] An early CSF examination may show clear fluid before the development of hemolysis, even after spontaneous subarachnoid bleeding. However, xanthochromia may be detected immediately after a traumatic tap if the RBC count exceeds 30,000/μL.[151] The presence of a clot in one of the tubes strongly favors a traumatic tap. With SAH, clotting does not occur because blood is defibrinated at the site of the hemorrhage. Lumbar puncture performed several days after a traumatic tap may also yield stained fluid. Collection of clear CSF from an immediately repeated puncture at a higher interspace also indicates a traumatic tap. The fluid from a traumatic tap should contain approximately 1 WBC per 1000 RBCs if the complete blood cell count is normal, but this ratio is highly variable.[155] All blood-contaminated CSF should be cultured, especially samples from uncooperative infants and children being evaluated for sepsis.

A D-dimer test on CSF can be used to determine SAH by identifying local fibrinolysis.[156] Other conditions such as disseminated intravascular coagulation, a previous traumatic tap, or prior thrombolytic therapy may produce false-positive results.

Fluoroscopically guided lumbar puncture in patients with suspected SAH and negative findings on CT is another option that may reduce the frequency of traumatic punctures, but it requires specific expertise and is frequently performed in the radiology suite.[157]

CSF Analysis with Infections

Bacterial Infections

The CSF findings are essential to establish a provisional diagnosis of acute bacterial meningitis.[158] CSF analysis establishes not only the diagnosis but also the causative organism and therefore the choice of antibiotics (Table 61.1). CSF must be transported to the laboratory immediately and examined at once. CSF cells begin to lyse within 1 hour after collection; this process can be slowed by refrigeration. In cases of meningococcal infection, a delay in processing may cause the diagnosis to be missed because the organism tends to autolyze rapidly. For other organisms, speed is less important but still warranted.

Gram stain results may help direct antibiotic therapy. Gram-negative intracellular or extracellular diplococci are indicative of *Neisseria meningitidis*. Small gram-negative bacilli may indicate *Haemophilus influenzae*, especially in children. The presence of gram-positive cocci indicates *S. pneumoniae*, other *Streptococcus* species, or *Staphylococcus*. Twenty percent of Gram stains are falsely negative because too few organisms are present. The Gram stain smear is more likely to be positive in patients who have not received prior antibiotic therapy. Acridine orange stain may improve the yield with gram-negative organisms.[159]

TABLE 61.1 CSF Analysis in Bacterial and Viral Meningitis[a]

	BACTERIAL MENINGITIS	VIRAL MENINGITIS
Opening pressure	Usually elevated	Usually normal
White blood cell count (per mm^3)	Elevated, 500–10,000+	Elevated, 6–1000
Differential count	Polymorphonuclear predominance	Lymphocytic predominance
Glucose level	Decreased, 0–40 mg/dL	Usually normal
Protein level	Elevated, >50 mg/dL	Normal or slightly elevated

[a]This is only a guide. Care must be taken when interpreting these parameters, especially early in the clinical course.
CSF, Cerebrospinal fluid.
Adapted from Fong B, Van Bendegem J. Lumbar puncture. In: Reichman E, Simon R, eds. *Emergency Medical Procedures.* McGraw-Hill; 2004:875.

For culture, blood and chocolate agar are required. *N. meningitidis* and *H. influenzae* grow best on chocolate agar. The plates are incubated under 10% CO_2. Thioglycolate medium is used for possible anaerobic organisms. Cultures are examined at 24 and 48 hours, but the plates should be kept for at least 7 days. Large volumes of CSF may improve yields.

While the culture results are pending, bacterial infection should be suspected in patients with an elevated opening pressure and marked pleocytosis, often ranging between 500 and 20,000 WBCs/μL. The differential count with bacterial infections is usually neutrophil-predominant. Viral infections have a lower cell count, usually 1000 cells/μL or less. Occasionally, acellular fluid may be collected from a severely immunosuppressed patient. Moreover, repeated lumbar puncture may be required in febrile patients whose clinical features remain compatible with meningitis.[146,160,161] In such scenarios, broad-spectrum empirical antibiotics should be continued until the results of repeated testing or bacterial culture are available.

CSF glucose levels of 40 mg/dL or lower, or less than 50% of a simultaneous blood glucose level, should raise the question of bacterial meningitis, even in the presence of a negative Gram stain and a low cell count. Glucose levels with bacterial meningitis are occasionally below 10 mg/dL but are normal in a small percentage of patients.[146] The CSF protein content with bacterial meningitis usually ranges from 500 to 1500 mg/dL and typically returns to normal by the end of therapy. Of note, previous antibiotic therapy may adversely affect the sensitivity of cultures and Gram stain for bacterial meningitis but does not significantly affect WBC counts, the ratio of CSF glucose to blood glucose, or CSF protein values.[162] Spanos and colleagues developed a useful nomogram to help distinguish bacterial from viral infections.[163] However, no technique or tool is perfect in this regard. In general, the clinician should err on the side of diagnosing bacterial meningitis until the results of culture are available.

Microbial Antigens and PCR

In 50% to 80% of cases of bacterial meningitis, blood cultures are positive for the etiologic agent.[164] In addition to Gram stain and cultures, several tests are available to establish a bacterial cause of meningitis, including CSF counterimmunoelectrophoresis (CIE), CSF latex agglutination, and coagglutination CIE.[6] In general, these ancillary tests have low sensitivity for bacterial meningitis, limiting their use.

CIE uses wells in two rows of agarose gel. A different antiserum is placed in each well. A current is passed through the gel, which causes the reactants to move toward each other by electrophoretic mobilization of the antigen. The appearance of a line of precipitation in 1 to 4 hours represents a positive reaction between antiserum and antigen.[165] Commercial kits are available to detect *S. pneumoniae*; *Listeria monocytogenes*; *H. influenzae*; *N. meningitidis* A, B, C, and W135; group B streptococci; K1 strains of *Escherichia coli*; *Klebsiella;* and *Pseudomonas* species.[166]

Particle agglutination involves staphylococcal coagglutination and latex agglutination. Antibodies on the surface of a colloid combine with antigen-binding sites to cross-link the colloid-forming antigen bridges. A matrix forms and appears as a macroscopic agglutination. Agglutination tests can detect levels of antigen that are approximately 10 times lower than CIE is capable of detecting. False-positive results can occur in the presence of rheumatoid factor, serum complement components, and possibly other serum proteins. The technique may be used for infections with *H. influenzae*, *S. pneumoniae*, *N. meningitidis*, and group B streptococci.

Another technique that has some potential use for identification of bacterial meningitis is the enzyme-linked immunosorbent assay. This technique may detect levels of antigen 100 to 1000 times lower than agglutination tests can but is technically more difficult and requires 4 hours to perform.

A positive CSF antigen test may be expected in 70% to 90% of patients with *Neisseria* meningitis. This compares with a positive Gram stain in approximately 70% of patients. Positive latex antigen tests have been reported in approximately 60% of *S. pneumoniae* meningitis cases, with a positive Gram stain in 80%. A positive latex test and Gram stain are reported in approximately 85% of *H. influenzae* meningitis cases.[164,165] Group B streptococci can be detected with 60% to 90% sensitivity.

Bacterial antigens may persist in CSF for several days after antibiotic therapy. With appropriate antimicrobial therapy, 25% to 33% of positive tests convert to negative per day. A negative test, however, does not rule out bacterial meningitis.[166] In addition, blood and urine can be examined for antigen. Frequently, antigen is found only in urine. Urine needs to be concentrated and may have the disadvantage of reflecting urinary tract infections. Moreover, the particle agglutination test for *H. influenzae* type B may be positive up to 10 days after children have received *H. influenzae* polysaccharide vaccine. Antigen tests are not useful in diagnosing gram-negative bacillary, staphylococcal, and *Listeria* meningitis. In addition, although antigen tests may identify the bacterial pathogen, they do not provide information about the antibiotic susceptibility of the organism.

Polymerase chain reaction (PCR) is the latest technology leading to rapid diagnosis of CNS infections. PCR amplifies target nucleic acid in CSF using repeated cycles of DNA synthesis. PCR requires the use of flanking DNA sequences at the opposite ends of the target DNA. Synthetic primers anneal to their respective recognition sequences at the opposite end of the target sequence; they serve as primers for new DNA synthesis. PCR allows detection and quantification of organisms whose genetic material is DNA or messenger RNA. PCR permits the diagnosis of infectious disease with a high degree of sensitivity and specificity and allows rapid reliable detection of microbes present in small numbers. Some laboratories now routinely apply PCR technology to test CSF for the presence of common pathogen (bacterial, viral, and fungal) DNA and can yield a result within hours.

Empirical Antibiotic Use before Lumbar Puncture

Many patients are transported within a facility or to a referral center for a CT to rule out an intracranial mass after clinical concern for meningitis is raised. In such instances, CSF examination might not be performed before transport because of technical problems (an uncooperative or a large patient) or concerns regarding the safety of lumbar puncture in an obtunded patient with possible increased ICP.[146,167] The initial clinician may have to decide whether to initiate empirical antibiotic therapy. Antibiotic administration could obscure the bacterial source, whereas a delay in initiating therapy increases morbidity and mortality. It may be difficult to identify individuals at risk for a fulminant course, and bacterial meningitis cannot always be diagnosed with confidence; some cases might be misdiagnosed as SAH or metabolic encephalopathy.

After administration of parenteral antibiotics, CSF cultures are not adversely affected for 2 to 3 hours. Twenty-four hours after treatment, as many as 38% of patients with meningitis could still have positive CSF cultures. Kanegaye and associates demonstrated that CSF sterilization may depend on the infecting organism.[168] They reported CSF sterilization after antibiotic administration within the following time frames: meningococcal, less than 2 hours; pneumococcal, less than 4.3 hours; and group B streptococcal, longer than 8 hours.

Whenever possible, blood should be obtained for culture immediately before the administration of antibiotics. When CSF is cultured more than a few hours after parenteral antibiotics are administered, antigen and PCR tests may be helpful. Occasionally, lymphocytic pleocytosis may develop in response to antibiotic therapy, but in most cases, the cell count, differential, glucose, and protein concentrations are unchanged in the first 2 to 3 days of antibiotic therapy.[146] It is thus reasonable to initiate therapy on the premise that a delay might be harmful. If a lumbar puncture cannot be performed, consultation with clinicians at a referral center seems appropriate. If a lumbar puncture is performed before transfer, a portion of the CSF (chilled on ice) should be sent with the patient or held in the referring hospital laboratory.

Bacterial meningitis may be caused by *H. influenzae*. Fortunately, this organism is easy to grow in early post antibiotic cultures and is likely to be associated with positive blood cultures and antigen tests. In the pediatric population, a single dose of an antibiotic before transport is unlikely to prevent identification of bacteria. In neonates, adults, and immunosuppressed patients, the sensitivity of blood cultures and immunologic tests is less reliable. CSF examination as early as possible in the course of treatment is preferred.

For suspected or confirmed cases of acute bacterial meningitis, antimicrobial therapy can be started and based on the most likely causative organism with respect to the age of the subject, associated diseases, and renal function. Tables 61.2–61.4 offer guidelines for emergency antibiotic therapy. For immunocompromised patients and after neurosurgery, a third-generation cephalosporin (cefotaxime, ceftizoxime, or ceftriaxone) plus ampicillin and vancomycin should be used for coverage against staphylococci, *L. monocytogenes*, and gram-negative organisms.[6] The third-generation cephalosporins are efficacious in many empirical regimens or situations in which the organism is known, but reliance on third-generation cephalosporins alone for all cases of bacterial meningitis would result in treatment failure for all *Listeria* species and increasing numbers of *Enterobacter*, *Serratia*, and *Pseudomonas* groups.

Dexamethasone Therapy for Bacterial Meningitis

In acute bacterial meningitis, bacterial cell wall components, including lipopolysaccharides and teichoic acid, initiate and exacerbate the host response. These substances stimulate the production of cytokines, including interleukin-1 and tumor necrosis factor, from macrophages and monocytes. Cytokines may injure vessels, diminish cerebral perfusion, and stimulate cerebral swelling.[167] The outcome of acute bacterial meningitis has been related to the severity of the inflammatory process in the subarachnoid space.

TABLE 61.2 Empirical Therapy for Purulent Meningitis[a]

PREDISPOSING FACTOR	ANTIMICROBIAL THERAPY[b]
Age	
0–4 weeks	Ampicillin plus cefotaxime or ampicillin plus an aminoglycoside
4–12 weeks	Ampicillin plus a third-generation cephalosporin[c]
3 months–50 years	Vancomycin plus a third-generation cephalosporin[c,d]
>50 years	Vancomycin plus ampicillin plus a third-generation cephalosporin[c]
Immunocompromised state	Vancomycin plus ampicillin plus ceftazidime
Basilar skull fracture	Vancomycin plus a third-generation cephalosporin[c]
Head trauma; post neurosurgery	Vancomycin plus ceftazidime
Cerebrospinal fluid shunt	Vancomycin plus ceftazidime

[a]Consider corticosteroids before administration of antibiotics (see text). Also, consult local antibiogram to determine local bacterial resistance rates and susceptibilities.
[b]Vancomycin should be added to all empirical therapeutic regimens when strains of *Streptococcus pneumoniae* that are highly resistant to penicillin or cephalosporin are suspected.
[c]Cefotaxime or ceftriaxone. (Of note, cefotaxime is not available in the United States.)
[d]Add ampicillin if meningitis caused by *Listeria monocytogenes* is suspected.

Studies have suggested benefit from adjunctive dexamethasone therapy in reducing neurologic sequelae, especially hearing loss, in children with *H. influenzae* meningitis and in lowering the mortality rate and providing a better overall outcome in adults with community-acquired acute bacterial meningitis caused by *S. pneumoniae*.[169] There appear to be few adverse sequelae from steroid therapy. The adjunctive benefit of corticosteroids during treatment of meningitis caused by other viral, fungal, or parasitic organisms is unknown. A Cochrane review concluded that "the corticosteroid dexamethasone leads to a major reduction in hearing loss and death in both children and adults with bacterial meningitis, without major adverse effects."[170] Interestingly, in children in low-income countries, the use of corticosteroids was associated with neither benefit nor harmful effects.

The dosage of dexamethasone is 0.15 mg/kg (maximum of 10 mg intravenously in adults) every 6 hours for 4 days. It is recommended that the corticosteroid be given before or simultaneously with antibiotic use, but the exact timing and specific benefits are unclear. It has been suggested that caution be exercised when administering corticosteroids to immunocompromised and leukopenic patients with bacterial meningitis, but no specific recommendations have been published.

A moderate inflammatory response in the meninges is required for penetration of the CNS by many antibiotics. Reducing meningeal inflammation decreases the concentration of antibiotics in CSF. Corticosteroids should be discontinued after approximately 4 days of treatment, at which time the meningeal inflammation should be reduced.[171,172]

TABLE 61.3 Recommended Total Daily Dose (With Divided Dosing Intervals in Hours) of Antimicrobial Agents for Meningitis in Adults With Normal Renal and Hepatic Function[a]

ANTIMICROBIAL AGENT	TOTAL DAILY DOSE (IV)	DOSING INTERVAL (h)
Ampicillin	12 g/day	4
Cefotaxime	8–12 g/day	4–6
Ceftazidime	6 g/day	8
Ceftriaxone	4 g/day	12
Chloramphenicol[b]	50–100 mg/kg/day	6
Gentamicin[c]	5 mg/kg per day	8
Tobramycin[c]	5 mg/kg per day	8
Vancomycin[d]	30–60 mg/kg per day	8–12

[a]Consider corticosteroids before the administration of antibiotics (see text).
[b]High dose recommended for pneumococcal meningitis.
[c]Peak and trough serum concentrations must be monitored.
[d]Trough concentrations must be monitored.

TABLE 61.4 Recommended Total Daily Doses with Divided Dosing Intervals in Hours of Antimicrobial Agents for Meningitis in Neonates, Infants, and Children With Normal Renal and Hepatic Function

ANTIMICROBIAL AGENT[a]	NEONATES (0–7 DAYS)[b]	NEONATES (8–28 DAYS)[b]	INFANTS AND CHILDREN
Amikacin[c]	15–20 mg/kg per day IV divided q12h	30 mg/kg per day IV divided q8h	20–30 mg/kg per day IV divided q8h
Ampicillin	300 mg/kg per day IV divided q8h	300 mg/kg per day IV divided q6h	300–400 mg/kg per day IV divided q4–6h (max dose 10–12 g/day)
Cefotaxime	100–150 mg/kg per day IV divided q8–12h	150–200 mg/kg per day IV divided q6–8h	225–300 mg/kg per day IV divided q6–8h (max 12 g/day)
Ceftazidime	100 mg/kg per day IV divided q12h	150 mg/kg per day IV divided q8h	150 mg/kg per day IV divided q8h (max 6 g/day)
Ceftriaxone	—	—	100 mg/kg per day IV divided q12h
Chloramphenicol	25 mg/kg per day IV q24h	50 mg/kg per day IV divided q12–24h	75–100 mg/kg per day IV divided q6h (max 4 g/day)
Gentamicin[c]	4–5 mg/kg per dose IV q24–48h	5 mg/kg per dose IV divided q24–36h	7.5 mg/kg per day IV divided q8h
Tobramycin[c]	4–5 mg/kg per day q24–48h	5 mg/kg per day IV divided q24–36h	7.5 mg/kg per day IV divided q8h
Vancomycin[c]	30–45 mg/kg per day IV divided q8–12h	30–45 mg/kg per day IV divided q8–12h	60 mg/kg per day IV divided q6h

[a]Consider corticosteroids before the administration of antibiotics (see text).
[b]Doses and intervals may need adjustment based on weight, gestational and postnatal ages.
[c]Peak and trough serum concentrations must be monitored.

Viral Meningitis

The organisms most isolated in viral meningitis are the enteroviruses (coxsackieviruses, echoviruses) and mumps virus. Enteroviruses are most commonly seen in the summer and fall, and mumps appears most frequently in the winter and spring. Viral cultures in most hospitals are not available and play little role in acute decisions regarding diagnosis and treatment. A serial rise in CSF antibody titers may be helpful but are difficult to obtain in patients who have recovered clinically. Intrathecal production of organ-specific antibodies (IgM, IgG, and IgA isotopes) may be diagnostic of neurologic infection if there is no history of infection. Serum and CSF antibody titers must be measured in a specialized laboratory. Viral meningitis is diagnosed when bacterial culture and Gram stain are negative. A tentative diagnosis may be based on analysis of CSF.

The WBC count in viral meningitis and encephalitis is characteristically 10 to 1000 cells/μL. The differential cell count is predominantly lymphocytic and mononuclear in type. In the early stages of meningoencephalitis, however, polymorphonuclear cells may predominate, making the distinction between viral and bacterial infection difficult. In such cases, a tap repeated in 12 to 24 hours will assist in clarifying the diagnosis. Protein levels are usually mildly elevated, but normal levels may be seen. Antibiotic coverage pending the results of culture may be reasonably initiated if the diagnosis of viral meningitis is in doubt.[146] The CSF glucose concentration is characteristically normal; notable exceptions include some cases of mumps meningoencephalitis and HSV encephalitis. CSF pleocytosis and elevated protein levels have also been found in asymptomatic HIV-seropositive individuals.[173]

If CSF cannot be delivered to the viral laboratory in 24 to 48 hours, it should be refrigerated at 4°C. Members of the enterovirus group are occasionally isolated from CSF. Herpesviruses and arboviruses are also found in CSF. PCR is the diagnostic test of choice for HSV meningoencephalitis and will be used increasingly for the diagnosis of other CNS viral infections. Although most cases of viral meningitis are self-limited and have a good outcome, HSV encephalitis is a rapidly progressive and life-threatening emergency that responds to treatment with intravenous acyclovir. Thus in an acutely ill patient in whom the diagnosis of acute meningoencephalitis is being considered, a negative Gram stain and pleocytosis are sufficient grounds to initiate empirical acyclovir therapy until the results of more definitive diagnostic data from PCR are available.[174]

CSF Analysis in Immunocompromised Patients

The number of immunocompromised individuals has increased because of the HIV epidemic and the increased survival of patients with cancer, organ transplants, and autoimmune disorders. The nervous system is a major target of the HIV virus: neurologic disease develops in 40% to 60% of infected individuals during their lifetime. One-third of HIV-infected patients have neurologic complaints as the initial manifestations of AIDS, and an even higher incidence of nervous system involvement is found at autopsy.[175] The risk for CNS infection depends on the underlying disease, treatment, duration, and type of immune abnormality. Abnormalities include defects in T-lymphocyte and macrophage cellular immune function, defects in humoral immunity, defects in the number and function of neutrophils, and loss of splenic function with an inability to remove encapsulated bacteria.[176]

Patients with defective cell-mediated immunity include those with lymphoma or organ transplants, those taking corticosteroids daily, and patients with AIDS. These individuals are vulnerable to infections with microorganisms that are intracellular parasites. A common source of acute bacterial meningitis in such patients is *L. monocytogenes*. Clinical findings include fever, headache, seizures, focal neurologic deficits, and brain stem encephalitis.

Patients with defective humoral immunity include those with chronic lymphocytic leukemia, multiple myeloma, and Hodgkin disease after radiotherapy or chemotherapy. These patients have difficulty controlling infection by encapsulated bacteria. A fulminant meningitis caused by *S. pneumoniae*, *H. influenzae* type B, or *N. meningitidis* may develop. After splenectomy, patients are at risk for the development of meningitis for the same reason. Neutropenic patients are at risk for meningitis caused by *Pseudomonas aeruginosa* and the *Enterobacteriaceae*.

Establishing a specific diagnosis in HIV and organ transplant patients may be difficult or impossible because of overlapping clinical and radiographic findings, the presence of simultaneous infections with more than one organism, and changes in CSF that may be nonspecific. The immune response can be altered, with absence of the usual signs of meningeal irritation. Patients might have diffuse encephalopathy or focal neurologic deficits. CSF is abnormal in 60% of asymptomatic HIV-infected individuals, complicating correlation of the CSF and clinical findings.[175]

Neurosyphilis in Patients Infected With HIV

Syphilis and HIV infection can both be transmitted sexually, and patients with syphilis are at increased risk for HIV infection. CNS invasion is probably no more common in patients with HIV than in those not infected with the virus.[177] Both diseases may cause an elevation in CSF WBC counts, protein levels, and γ-globulin levels. The incidence of syphilitic meningitis, meningovascular syphilis, and ocular syphilis seems to be increasing. HIV-infected patients treated for syphilis may have viable organisms in CSF after therapy or have persistent CSF VDRL titers. Treatment failures are more likely to occur with single-dose benzathine penicillin therapy.

Neurosyphilis may be more difficult to diagnose in HIV-infected patients. A small number of patients with secondary or ocular syphilis have negative serum reagin tests. Positive treponemal tests may revert to nonreactivity after treatment, particularly in individuals with advanced symptomatic HIV disease and a low VDRL titer at the time of diagnosis. CSF pleocytosis and increased γ-globulin levels may not help to distinguish between HIV infection and CNS syphilis.

HIV-infected patients should undergo serum treponemal and nontreponemal tests early in their illness to minimize the likelihood of false-negative results.[177] Infected patients should undergo a CSF examination. Previously treated patients who did not have a CSF examination at the time of initial syphilis treatment should undergo lumbar puncture because of a probable increased risk for neurosyphilis, even with a decline in serum nontreponemal titers.

Cryptococcal Meningitis

The most common cause of CNS fungal infection is *Cryptococcus neoformans*. Infection with this fungus develops in approximately 5% of AIDS patients. Clinical findings in AIDS and non-AIDS patients include nonspecific symptoms of headache and altered mental status with or without meningeal signs. Most patients have increased ICP. Immunocompetent patients show a lymphocytic pleocytosis with CSF WBC counts lower than 500/μL. Glucose levels are depressed, with elevation of CSF protein. India ink preparations are positive in 50% of cases. CSF is less likely to have abnormal cell counts and chemistries in patients infected with HIV. However, CSF cultures and cryptococcal polysaccharide capsular antigens are almost always positive. False-positive antigen tests are rare but may be seen in the presence of rheumatoid factor. Blood cultures are frequently positive in AIDS patients. Cisternal puncture for fluid analysis may be helpful in undiagnosed cases of lymphocytic meningitis in which multiple lumbar punctures have not established a diagnosis.[175]

Toxoplasmosis

Toxoplasma gondii, an intracellular protozoan, is associated with CNS infection in up to 30% of AIDS patients who have antibodies to this organism. Most adults have antibodies against this organism; infection is believed to represent reactivation of latent primary infection. *Toxoplasma* encephalitis usually develops within the first 2 years after the diagnosis of AIDS. Cerebral toxoplasmosis is usually accompanied by the acute or subacute development of focal disease, including seizures. MRI or CT scanning often reveals multiple abscesses that might represent multiple pathogens. Toxoplasmosis and lymphoma can be difficult to distinguish clinically. Less commonly, the manifestation is one of chronic meningitis with confusion, memory loss, and lethargy similar to the AIDS-dementia complex. CSF in these patients is nonspecific with increased protein, mononuclear pleocytosis (<100 cells/μL), and, rarely, a reduced glucose concentration. Serum and CSF serology may be either positive or negative and does not help make a diagnosis, although most patients with encephalitis have detectable IgG antibodies. The diagnosis is usually based on clinical and imaging responses to antibiotics (pyrimethamine or sulfadiazine) or on brain biopsy. Treatment failures with relapse occur in 50% of patients with AIDS and in 15% to 25% of patients without AIDS and necessitate lifelong treatment.

Mycobacterial Tuberculosis

CNS mycobacterial infection is almost always the result of infection with *Mycobacterium tuberculosis*. Infection typically occurs in the setting of disseminated tuberculosis. Atypical *Mycobacterium* infection in HIV-infected individuals uncommonly affects the CNS.

The clinical manifestation is meningitis (particularly meningitis involving the basal cisterns), encephalitis, or abscess formation. If tuberculosis is suspected, a large volume of CSF (10 mL) is required for adequate culture. The cell count varies from 100 to 400 cells/μL, with a lymphocytic predominance; 30% may show predominantly neutrophils early in the course of infection. Protein levels are elevated (100 to 500 mg/dL), and the CSF glucose level may be depressed. Acid-fast stains should be examined by experienced technicians. Fluid is inoculated onto Löwenstein-Jensen medium, and the absence of visible growth on the medium should not be considered negative until 8 weeks has elapsed. CSF cultures are more sensitive than stains.

Primary CNS Lymphoma

CNS lymphoma develops in 2% of AIDS patients. The signs and symptoms resemble those of diffuse encephalopathy, although focal neurologic deficits occur occasionally. Leptomeningeal spread of malignancy is reflected in a modest lymphocytic pleocytosis with slightly elevated protein and decreased glucose levels. Cytologic yield is improved by repeated lumbar punctures and submitting large quantities of CSF or fluid obtained by cisternal puncture.[175]

Progressive Multifocal Leukoencephalopathy

Progressive multifocal leukoencephalopathy, an uncommon disorder in individuals with impaired cell-mediated immunity, is caused by reactivation of JC papovavirus in the kidney. Progressive demyelination is manifested as dementia, blindness, aphasia, hemiparesis, and seizures, which progress until death. MRI and CT demonstrate nonenhancing white matter lesions without a mass effect. Definitive diagnosis is made by brain biopsy, but CSF may show the presence of myelin basic protein, increased IgG, and an acellular or a mild CSF pleocytosis (<50 WBCs/μL). Average survival is 4 months.[176]

Cytomegalovirus Infection

Cytomegalovirus is detected in the brains of 30% of HIV-infected persons at autopsy. A distinct CNS disorder has not been defined. CSF pleocytosis may be minimal. Retinitis and painful polyradiculopathies are recognized, with a prominent CSF pleocytosis found in the latter condition.[175]

ACKNOWLEDGMENTS

The editors and authors acknowledge the contributions of Jon Kooiker to this chapter in previous editions. The authors would like to thank Eileen O'Brien for copyediting the manuscript and incorporating revisions into the final document.

References are available at Elsevier eBooks+

CHAPTER 62

Special Neurologic Tests and Procedures

Danya Khoujah and Wan-Tsu W. Chang

PROCEDURES TO EVALUATE AND TREAT DIZZINESS

Dizziness is a common complaint in the emergency department (ED), and encompasses a wide variety of descriptions, such as spinning, lightheadedness, giddiness, vertigo, and so forth. Vertigo is the illusory sensation of movement, sometimes experienced by patients as self-motion, other times as motion of the environment. Despite historical dogmatic teaching, the specific description of "dizziness" does not reliably predict the underlying etiology, whether cardiovascular or neurological.[1] Among neurological disorders, there are a wide variety of diseases that can cause vertigo, including dysfunction of the labyrinth, vestibular nerve, or central vestibular structures in the brain stem. Disease processes of relevance in the ED include benign paroxysmal positional vertigo (BPPV), cerebellar ischemia, and vestibular neuritis.

BPPV is a common mechanical disorder of the inner ear in which certain head movements precipitate vertigo; nystagmus, nausea, and vomiting commonly accompany the vertigo. Although patients may have quite dramatic symptoms, the actual episodes of vertigo are brief and typically last less than 1 minute.[2] Patients may describe a residual sensation of dizziness, nausea, or anxiety in between episodes (akin to the sensation that one would feel after stepping out of an amusement park spinning attraction), but will not have the nystagmus at rest or severe symptoms.[3]

In contrast, cerebellar ischemia and vestibular neuritis (along with other disorders) present with acute vestibular syndrome (AVS), which is characterized by an onset of vertigo, nausea, vomiting, and gait instability that lasts for days to weeks.

Dix-Hallpike Test and Supine Head Roll

Background

In BPPV, it is thought that small crystals of calcium carbonate, or canaliths (or otoliths), are displaced from the utricle, where they normally reside, into the endolymph of one of the three semicircular canals. Head movement shifts the canaliths, which induce movement in the endolymph fluid that persists after the head movement has stopped. The desynchrony of the signals from the affected and unaffected semicircular canals create the sensation of persistent movement and spinning, thus triggering the vertigo, and nystagmus of BPPV.[3,4] The posterior semicircular canal is most commonly affected,[4–6] followed by the lateral (or horizontal) canal.[5–8] The anterior (superior) semicircular is rarely involved and therefore not discussed in this chapter.

Indications and Contraindications

The diagnosis of BPPV is confirmed by moving the head through a series of positions that shift the canaliths within the suspected canal and provoke the nystagmus typical of this diagnosis. The Dix-Hallpike test is used to confirm the diagnosis of posterior BPPV, whereas the supine head roll is used to confirm the diagnosis of lateral BPPV. The Dix-Hallpike maneuver is recommended by major otolaryngology, neurology, and emergency medicine societies for the initial evaluation of BPPV.[2,3,9] Some experts recommend avoiding this maneuver in patients with severe cervical spine disease, unstable spinal injury, vascular problems like vertebrobasilar insufficiency and carotid sinus syncope, despite the limited evidence for such recommendations.[9] Premedicating patients with an antiemetic (such as ondansetron) may facilitate this procedure in patients with intense nausea and vomiting, as it is not expected to alter the findings and would enhance patients' comfort. If nystagmus is present at rest without any provocation, the diagnosis of BPPV is unlikely and the maneuver should not be performed.

Dix-Hallpike Test

Procedure

The Dix-Hallpike maneuver is illustrated in Fig. 62.1 and Video 62.1. Place the patient initially in the upright-seated position on the stretcher with the head turned 45 degrees to one side. Instruct the patient to keep the eyes open and focused on the examiner, then quickly lay the patient down flat so the head hangs over the edge of the bed by 30 degrees and observe the eyes for nystagmus. Start with the side that the patient believes may be involved—ask the patient if they recall which head direction triggers their symptoms. If one side does not illicit a nystagmus and vertigo within 30 seconds, repeat the entire maneuver with the head turned 45 degrees toward the opposite side.[6] An important step is to inform the patient that you are trying to induce the vertigo they experienced in order to make the diagnosis. Assure them that if vertigo is triggered it will not last more than 30 to 60 seconds.

Common pitfalls include not waiting long enough after the final position for the nystagmus, not coaching the patient sufficiently before and during the procedure, and performing in patients with nystagmus at rest.

Interpretation

The typical positive response in patients with posterior canal BPPV is dizziness that develops after a brief delay which is called the latency period. Usually this dizziness lasts for 3 to 5 seconds but occasionally can be up to 30 seconds. The examiner will note a rotatory (torsional) nystagmus, where the upper pole of the eye beats toward the dependent ear. The nystagmus may have a vertical upward component as well, with the rapid phase of the nystagmus beating toward the forehead. This will also reproduce their symptoms of dizziness, nausea, and/or vomiting.[2,3,6,9] The side with the ear in the downward position during the Dix-Hallpike test that shows vertical upward, torsional nystagmus toward the downward ear is the affected ear. The Dix-Hallpike maneuver on the other side should no produce nystagmus or vertigo. If the positional nystagmus produced is atypical (i.e., horizontal), or if the maneuver fails to elicit nystagmus in a patient with typical symptoms of BPPV, the supine head roll test should be performed to assess for possible lateral canal BPPV.

Dix-Hallpike Maneuver

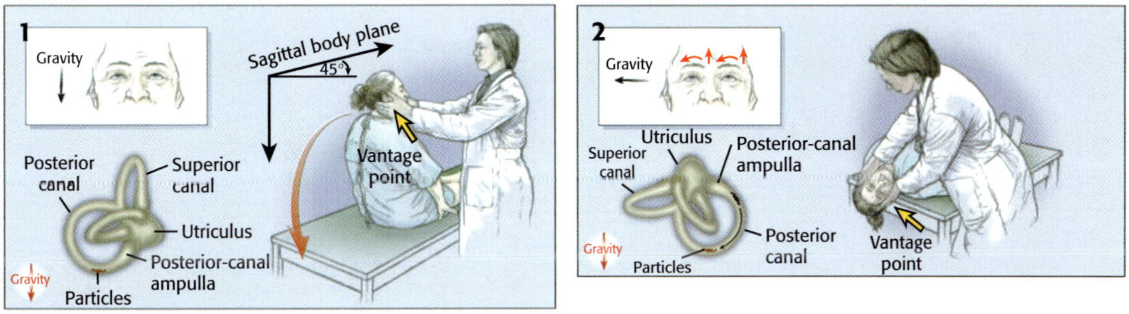

The examiner stands at the patient's head, 45 degrees to the right, to align the right posterior semicircular canal with the sagittal plane of the body.

The examiner moves the patient, whose eyes are open, from the seated to the supine, right-ear-down position and then extends the patient's neck slightly so that the chin is pointed slightly upward. The latency, duration, and direction of nystagmus, if present, and the latency and duration of vertigo, if present, should be noted. *Inset:* The *arrows* over the eyes depict the direction of nystagmus in patients with typical BPPV. The presumed location in the labyrinth of the free-floating debris thought to cause the disorder is also shown.

Fig. 62.1 Dix-Hallpike test for evaluating a patient complaining of dizziness from benign paroxysmal positional vertigo *(BPPV)* affecting the right ear. (Adapted from Furman C. Benign paroxysmal positional vertigo. *N Engl J Med.* 1999;341:1590.)

Some patients may have very subtle nystagmus rendering it difficult to see, necessitating the use of Frenzel glasses and/or video-oculography. A more feasible alternative would be capturing the eye response on a phone camera and reviewing the video in slow motion. It is important for clinicians to only diagnose posterior canal BPPV when the typical vertical upwards, torsional nystagmus is seen during the Dix-Hallpike maneuver. Rarely, atypical nystagmus during the Dix-Hallpike test can be seen in central mimics, leading to potential misdiagnosis.[3]

Supine Head Roll

Procedure

The supine head roll (Pagnini-Lempert or Pagnini-McClure roll test) is illustrated in Fig. 62.2. Have the patient lie supine and position the head in a neutral position. Quickly rotate the head 90 degrees to one side (warn the patient and ask them to move their head to avoid neck injury) and observe the patient's eyes for the typical nystagmus. After the nystagmus subsides (or if there's no nystagmus), return the head to the midline and repeat the maneuver on the other side.[9]

Interpretation

The typical positive response in patients with lateral BPPV is dizziness that develops after a brief delay (usually a few seconds but up to 30 seconds), generally lasting less than a minute and with horizontal nystagmus. Most commonly, the direction of the nystagmus will be toward the undermost ear, therefore termed "geotropic nystagmus" (beating toward the earth). Less commonly, the nystagmus will be toward the upper most ear, therefore termed "apogeotropic nystagmus" (beating away from the earth). Sometimes apogeotropic nystagmus will persist for as long as the patient is in the provoking position. Symptoms and nystagmus will be most intense when the patient's head is turned toward the affected ear in geotropic horizontal nystagmus. For apogeotropic horizontal nystagmus, the symptoms and nystagmus will be more intense when the head is turned away from the affected ear. This results in a direction-changing positional nystagmus, and determining the affected side depends on the intensity of the nystagmus, rather than its direction.[9]

If the provoked nystagmus is atypical, or if the maneuver fails to elicit nystagmus, consider the diagnosis of posterior canal BPPV, or another mimic, as noted previously.

Complications

The maneuver, by definition, will precipitate brief intense vertigo and nausea in patients with BPPV.

Summary

The Dix-Hallpike and supine head roll tests are useful in confirming the diagnosis of posterior and lateral BPPV, respectively, and in localizing the affected ear. Accurate identification of BPPV is important because canalith-repositioning therapeutic maneuvers may be used.

Canalith-Repositioning Maneuvers

Background

If the clinical evaluation of a patient with vertigo is consistent with the diagnosis of BPPV, the patient may be a candidate for canalith-repositioning maneuvers. Based on the theory that stray material in the semicircular canal causes the symptoms of BPPV, these maneuvers involve sequential head movements to reposition the debris.[4,6,10,11] Manipulation of head position allows the canaliths to sequentially move from the problematic location in the semicircular canal into the utricle from which they originated. The most commonly recommended maneuvers are the Epley maneuver for posterior BPPV,[3,4,9,12] and Lempert maneuver (or barbeque roll) for

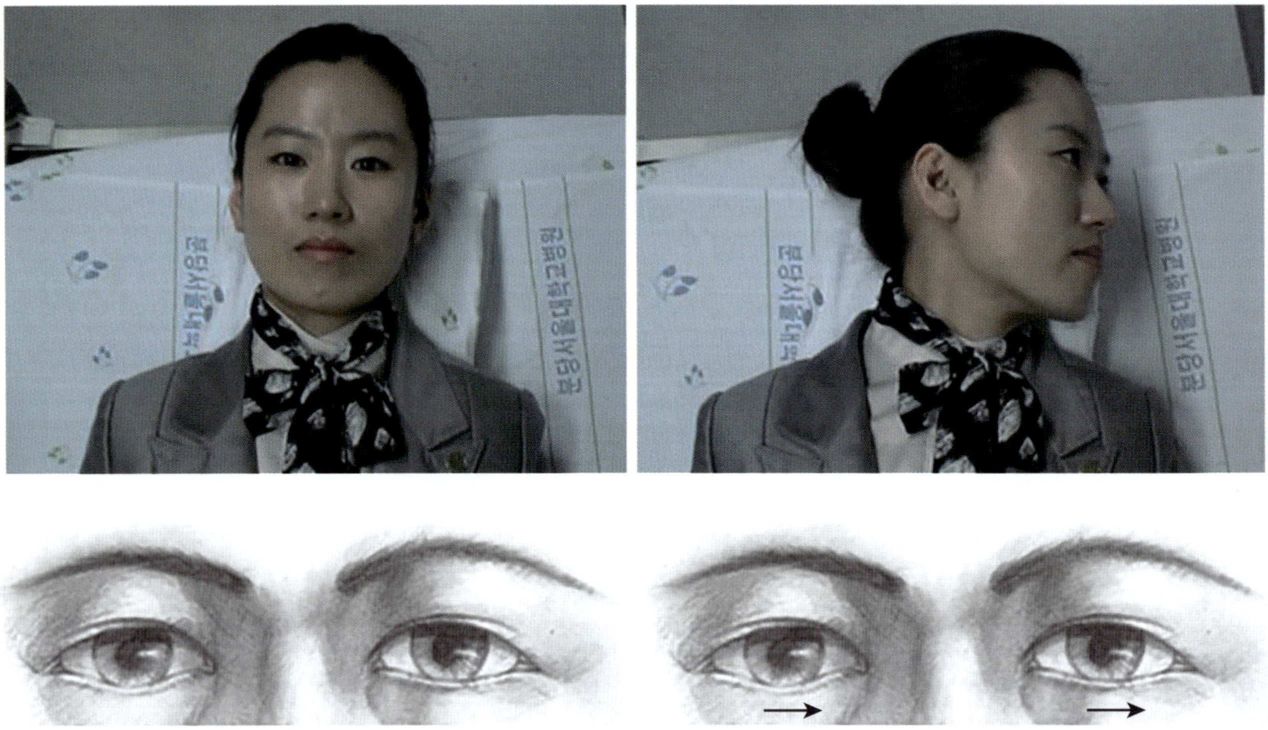

Fig. 62.2 The supine head roll test (Pagnini-McClure maneuver) for the diagnosis of benign paroxysmal positional vertigo involving the lateral semicircular canal (left). The head is turned 90 degrees to the affected side while supine. The corresponding illustrations demonstrate the direction of the induced nystagmus *(arrows)*. (Adapted from Lee SH, Kim JS. Benign paroxysmal positional vertigo. *J Clin Neurol.* 2010;6(2):51-63.)

lateral BPPV.[9] Patients undergoing the Epley maneuver are seven times more likely to have resolution of their symptoms at 1 week than those who received a sham maneuver or other treatment, with a number needed to treat of 3.[12] Canalith-repositioning maneuvers are recommended by major otolaryngology, neurology, and emergency medicine societies for the treatment of BPPV,[2,3,9] yet are underutilized in the ED.[13] The Semont (liberatory) maneuver has also been described for the treatment of posterior BPPV.[10] It may have a similar efficacy to the Epley maneuver, although the Semont is less well studied.[14]

Indications and Contraindications

The indication for canalith-repositioning maneuvers is the clinical diagnosis of BPPV as confirmed by the history and physical examination, including the Dix-Hallpike or supine head roll maneuvers. Careful patient selection is key to the success of these maneuvers, as well as correct identification of the impaired ear, which will dictate the initial position and movement of the patient. Contraindications are the same as for the Dix-Hallpike maneuver, including severe cervical spine disease, unstable spinal injury, and high-grade carotid stenosis.

Premedicating patients with antiemetics and/or vestibular suppressants (such as antihistamines or benzodiazepines) improve patients' comfort and therefore tolerance of the procedure, although most tolerate the maneuvers without medication.

Procedure

Epley Maneuver (for Posterior Canal BPPV)

The Epley procedure is illustrated in Fig. 62.3 and Video 62.2. The first step is the same as the Dix-Hallpike maneuver; lay the patient down flat with the head hanging over the edge of the bed by 30 degrees and the head turned 45 degrees toward the affected side. Wait an additional 30 seconds after the provoked nystagmus and vertigo subside (total of at least one minute), rotate the patient's head 90 degrees so that it faces the opposite shoulder while maintaining the head-hanging orientation. This position is the same as the position that was negative during the Dix-Hallpike maneuver. Wait another 60 seconds and then roll the patient further onto their side and rotate the head further into a facedown position. Again, after the provoked symptoms subside (60 seconds), return the patient to a seated position for a full minute, while keeping the patients head facing downward.[4]

The original description of the Epley maneuver included applying vibration to the mastoid region,[4] but a Cochrane review has shown it to be unnecessary.[15]

The success of the procedure can be confirmed by repeating the Dix-Hallpike maneuver on the affected side after the patient has been sitting still for 15 minutes. If the patient no longer develops vertigo symptoms, then the Epley maneuver was successful. The most significant pitfall is rushing the procedure and not allowing sufficient time for the canalith to travel in the viscous fluid of the semicircular canal. The maneuver may be repeated a few times (ensuring adequate time between each step) until it is successful.[16] Postprocedure restrictions, such as sleeping upright and wearing a neck brace, have been described with limited evidence of their efficacy, and therefore are not necessary.[15] Patients who are unable to undergo the maneuvers due to neck and body mobility limitations may require referral to specialists with specific procedure equipment (tilt tables).

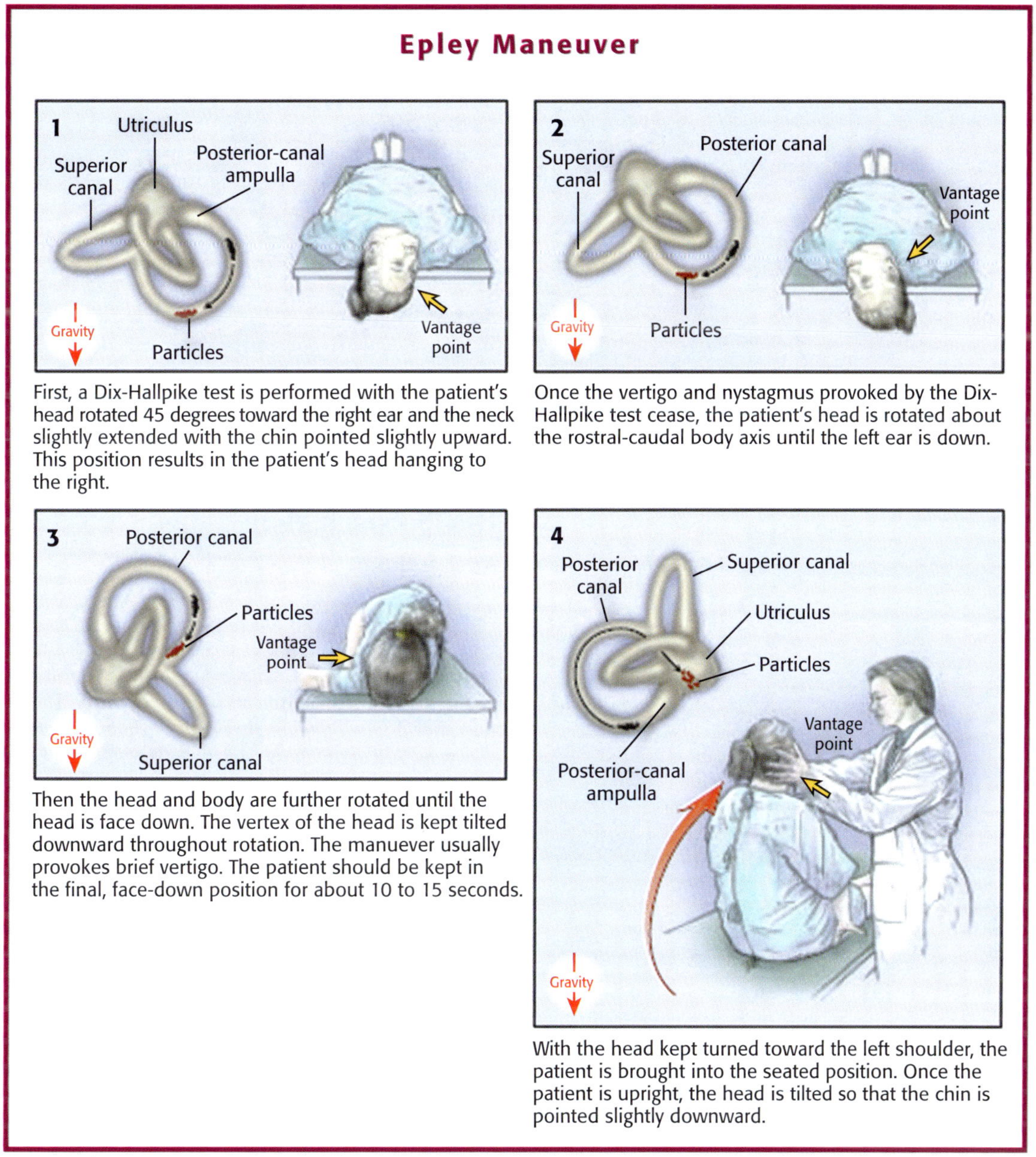

Fig. 62.3 The Epley procedure, a bedside maneuver for the treatment of a patient with benign paroxysmal positional vertigo affecting the right ear. The presumed position of debris within the labyrinth during the maneuver is shown in each panel. (Adapted from Furman C. Benign paroxysmal positional vertigo. *N Engl J Med.* 1999;341:1590.)

Semont Maneuver (for Posterior Canal BPPV)

The Semont maneuver involves larger and more abrupt body movements (Fig. 62.4). It is often referred to as a "liberatory maneuver." With the patient seated on the side of an examination table or bed, turn the patient's head 45 degrees toward the unaffected side; the head will maintain this position throughout the entire maneuver. Quickly lay the patient down into a side-lying position onto the affected side, keeping the head turned 45 degrees so the patient's head is directed partially toward the ceiling. This should reproduce the symptoms as well as the nystagmus. After the symptoms subside by at least 20 seconds, move the patient abruptly through the sitting position to the opposite side-lying position, maintaining the head position so that now the head faces down partially toward the floor. Keep the patient there until at least 30 seconds after the symptoms subside. Slowly, return the patient to the upright position.[9,10]

Lempert Maneuver (for Lateral Canal BPPV)

See Video 62.3. The Lempert maneuver, also known as the barbeque roll, is the treatment for geotropic lateral canal BPPV. The first step is the same as the supine head roll test. Have the patient lie supine and position the head in a neutral position. Quickly rotate the head 90 degrees to the affected side. Wait an additional 30 seconds after the provoked nystagmus and vertigo subside (total of at least 1 minute), then rotate the patient's head back to the supine position and wait for 60 seconds. Continue to rotate the head in this direction by 90 degrees (patient is now facing opposite their initial supine head roll) and wait 60 seconds. Next, the patient will roll on

Semont Maneuver

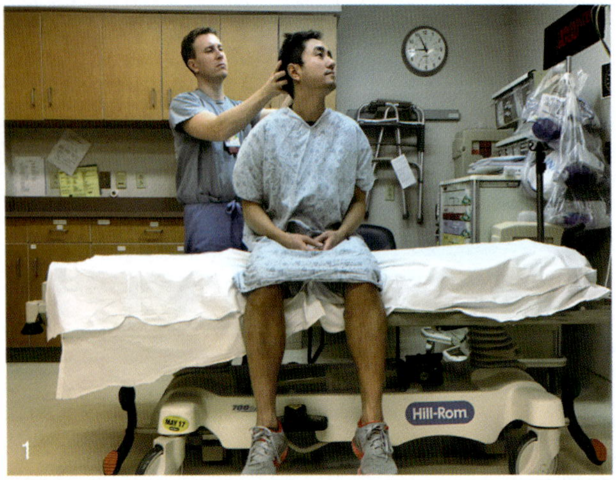

1

Sit the patient on the side of the bed, with his head turned 45 degrees toward the unaffected side.

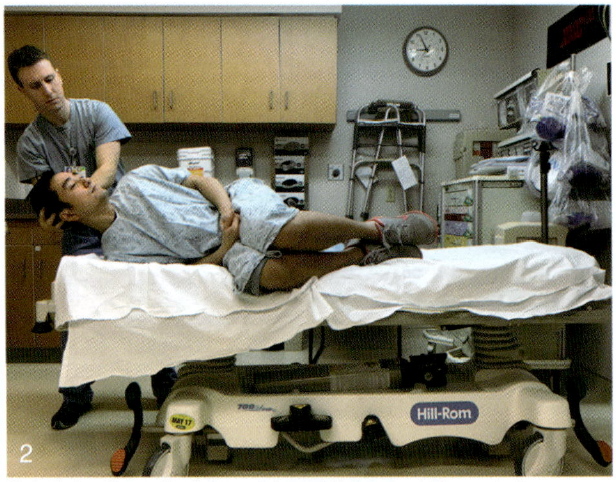

2

Quickly lay the patient down into a side-lying position onto the affected side; keep the head rotated 45 degrees, so he is looking at the ceiling.

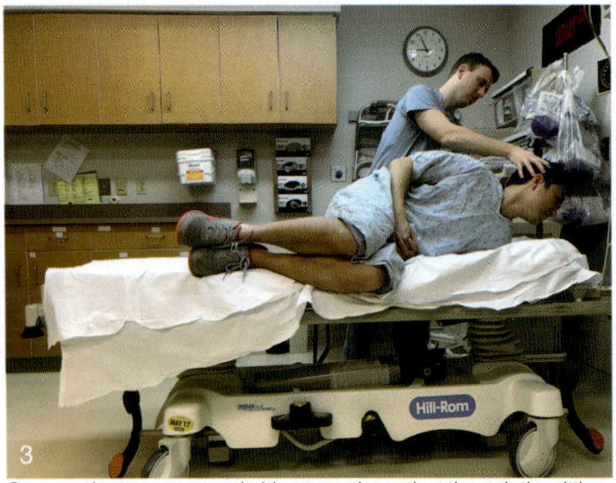

3

Once vertigo symptoms subside, move the patient through the sitting position to the opposite side-lying position, head pointed towards the floor. After symptoms subside, return to the upright sitting position.

Fig. 62.4 Semont maneuver. See text for details.

their chest and turn their head another 90 degrees such that they are looking down at the ground (wait 60 seconds). The roll is completed once the patient turns a final 90 degrees and ends in the original supine head roll position. After 60 seconds the patient can be helped into a seated position. Successful maneuver will result in a supine head roll test no longer triggering lateral canal BPPV.

Complications

Nausea and vomiting can occur in up to one-third of patients during canalith-repositioning maneuvers.[17] Conversion from posterior to lateral BPPV may occur.[18] Symptoms of vertigo may recur in up to one-third of patients;[14] early treatment significantly decreases the risk of recurrence.[19]

Summary

In patients with correctly identified BPPV, canalith repositioning improves outcomes with minimal side effects and resource utilization and results in marked patient satisfaction.[3] Patients can also be taught to do these maneuvers at home if they develop a recurrence.

HINTS Examination

Background

See Video 62.4. Whereas the majority of AVS conditions are the result of a peripheral neuropathy (such as vestibular neuritis), approximately 20% of AVS presentations are due to a central pathology, most of which are ischemic strokes of the brainstem or cerebellum.[20] It can be difficult to distinguish a peripheral from a central process in patients with AVS using the standard neurologic examination. The "HINTS" examination was created for this very purpose and is intended to assist clinicians in distinguishing central from peripheral causes of AVS. The HINTS examination is composed of three separate tests: the head impulse test, a test of nystagmus, and a test of skew (HINTS).[21]

Indications and Contraindications

The HINTS examination is only indicated in patients with AVS without new neurological deficits. Consideration of the following is important; the patient should not have new significant headache or neck pain, focal weakness or paresthesia, diplopia, dysarthria, dysmetria, dysphagia, dysphonia, vertical nystagmus at rest, and they should be able to walk unaided. By definition, patients must have constant vertigo and nystagmus observable at rest at the time of assessment. *Performing the head impulse test on a patient without nystagmus and or vertigo at the time of evaluation will result in misleading conclusions.* The head impulse test should not be performed in patients with severe cervical spine disease, unstable spinal injury, high-grade carotid stenosis, or unstable heart disease due to theoretical concerns of exacerbating these conditions.

Procedure

Although named and described as "head impulse, nystagmus, and test of skew," the optimal sequence is testing for nystagmus first, followed by test of skew, and finally the head impulse test. If any one component of the HINTS is consistent with a central lesion, then the test is considered abnormal, independent of the results of the other components. For example, if nystagmus is absent or indicative of a central cause of AVS, you should stop; there is no need to continue with the rest of the HINTS examination.

Test of Nystagmus

See Video 62.5. This is the first step of the HINTS examination. If the patient does not have a unidirectional horizontal nystagmus, the HINTS examination should not be performed. Ask the patient to gaze at a blank space on the wall about 30 degrees to the left and right. Note that fixation on a close object may diminish the amplitude of noted nystagmus. Having the patient look through a blank piece of paper placed close to the side of their head may bring out nystagmus. Avoid extreme lateral gaze as end-gaze nystagmus is a normal occurrence and may be confused for direction-changing nystagmus. Peripheral nystagmus from vestibular neuritis increases when the patient looks away from the affected ear. When gaze is directed toward the affected ear, it may decrease or cease, but it will always beat in the same direction, which is away from the affected ear. Unilateral horizontal nystagmus is illustrated in Video 62.5.

Test of Skew

See Video 62.6. Ask the patient to fixate on an object directly ahead. Alternately cover each eye in rapid succession. Look closely for subtle vertical or diagonal refixation of the eyes (i.e., the eye moves up or down as it is uncovered to compensate for misalignment). Test of skew is shown in Video 62.6.

Head Impulse Test

See Video 62.7. Have the patient seated in a comfortable position and stand in front of the patient. Ask the patient to always gaze directly on the examiner's nose and relax their neck as much as possible. Place hands on either side of the patient's head and slowly rotate the head by approximately 30 degrees to one side and then rapidly back to midline. Observe the eyes for loss of fixation on the examiner's nose. If the eyes move off target when the head is rotated rapidly toward the affected side, a corrective saccade to resume visual fixation on the central target occurs; this represents an abnormal head impulse test and is suggestive of a peripheral etiology. The abnormal saccade should be seen when the head is turned in the opposite direction of the fast component of the nystagmus. A patient with a central etiology will be able to fix their eyes on target when the head is rotated laterally (they will not have a corrective saccade).

Randomly alter the speed and direction of rotation to generate an unpredictable sequence so the patient cannot anticipate the direction of rotation. Normal and abnormal head impulse test maneuver are simulated in Fig. 62.5. Head impulse test with corrective saccade (consistent with peripheral etiology) is shown in Video 62.7.

Interpretation

Head Impulse Test

The terminology used to describe the results of the head impulse test can be confusing, as the test was initially designed to detect peripheral vestibular disease.[22] Therefore a "positive" (abnormal) test is suggestive of a peripheral lesion,

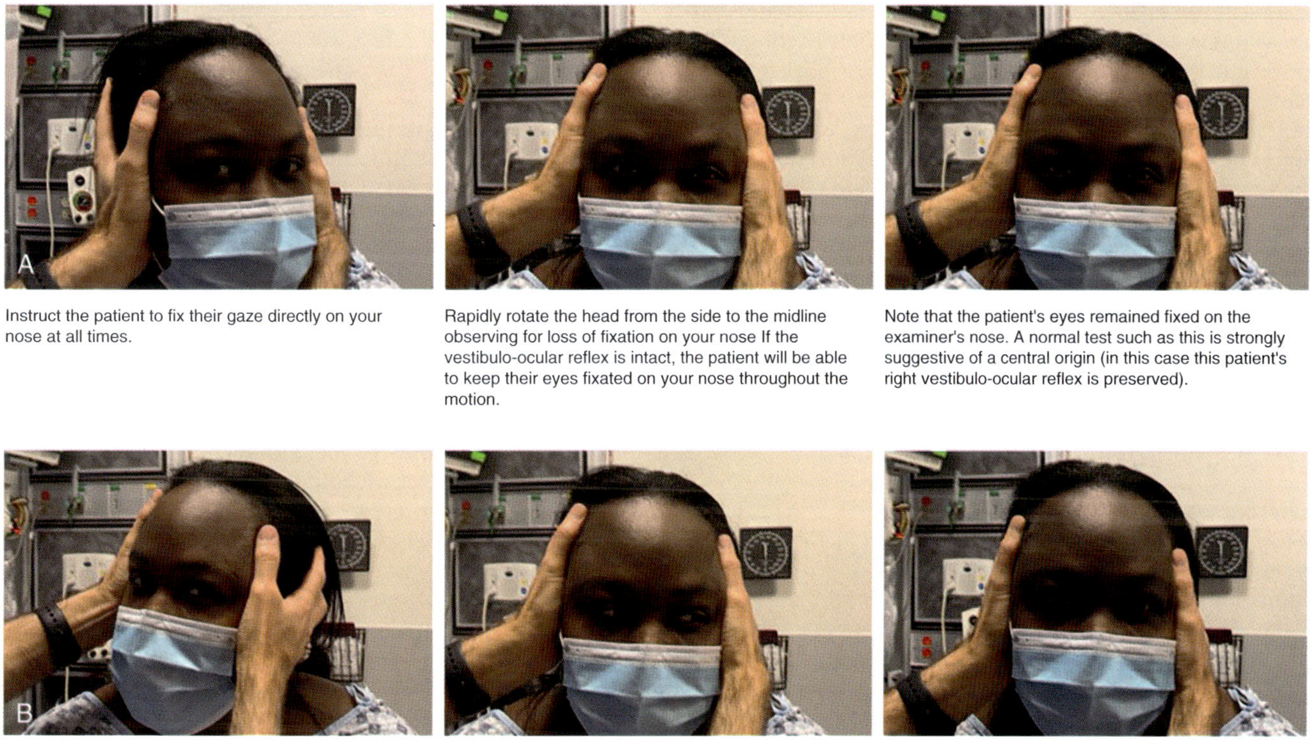

A Instruct the patient to fix their gaze directly on your nose at all times.

Rapidly rotate the head from the side to the midline observing for loss of fixation on your nose If the vestibulo-ocular reflex is intact, the patient will be able to keep their eyes fixated on your nose throughout the motion.

Note that the patient's eyes remained fixed on the examiner's nose. A normal test such as this is strongly suggestive of a central origin (in this case this patient's right vestibulo-ocular reflex is preserved).

B Rapidly rotate the head from the side to the midline observing loss of fixation on your nose. Patients with a peripheral vestibular lesion will not be able to keep their eyes fixated on your nose during the maneuver.

As the head is rapidly turned to the midline in the direction of the affected side, the patient cannot maintain fixation and their eyes briefly go in the direction of head movement.

A corrective saccade (fast jerking eye movement) will be noted at the end of the maneuver as the patient tries to regain fixation on the examiner's nose.

Fig. 62.5 The horizontal head impulse test (h-HIT). In the setting of acute vestibular syndrome, a normal horizontal head impulse test result strongly suggests a central origin (e.g., brain stem or cerebellar stroke). (A) A normal h-HIT result is suggestive of a central lesion (e.g., cerebellar stroke). The intact vestibular-ocular reflex causes the patient's eyes to smoothly track the examiner as the head is quickly turned to one side. (B) An abnormal h-HIT result is suggestive of a peripheral lesion (e.g., vestibular neuritis). A patient with a peripheral vestibular lesion does not track the examiner when the head is turned to the affected side, resulting in a quick, corrective saccade back to the examiner.

whereas a "negative" (normal) test is concerning central a lesion. Therefore using the terminology of positive/negative, or abnormal/normal, may be confusing, and may be better replaced by "consistent with peripheral/central etiology."

In the setting of AVS symptoms, the inability to maintain fixation during the head impulse test suggests a peripheral vestibular lesion. This is presumed to occur because there is decreased afferent input from the affected eighth cranial nerve when the head is rotated to the affected side. If a patient with AVS symptoms maintains fixation during the head impulse test, it suggests a central pathology. Please note that asymptomatic patients will also not have a corrective saccade emphasizing the importance of only performing the HINTS examination on patients with AVS and nystagmus at rest. In rare instances, patients with lateral pontine and cerebellar stroke syndromes can have a positive horizontal head impulse test that erroneously suggests a peripheral lesion (this is why all components of the HINTS examination must be met to rule out a central cause of AVS).[21,23]

Test of Nystagmus

If the patient does not have nystagmus at rest, the HINTS examination cannot be performed. The nystagmus that results from a peripheral lesion is horizontal and unidirectional. There is sometimes a torsional component seen as well. The direction of the nystagmus is determined by the fast phase. With gaze toward the affected side, the nystagmus may decrease in intensity or disappear, but the direction of the fast beats will not change. If the direction of the nystagmus differs with horizontal gaze to either side (e.g., left-beating when looking left and right-beating when looking right), a central cause should be suspected.[24] Nystagmus that is purely vertical or rotatory is consistent with a central cause as well. This is not to be confused with the provoked nystagmus seen during the Dix-Hallpike maneuver, where vertical and torsional nystagmus is an expected finding.

Test of Skew

Skew deviation refers to a vertical misalignment of the eyes (e.g., one eye is looking straight ahead, while the other eye is deviated downward or upward); it is usually associated with a central lesion. Although skew deviation can be subtle, it can be unmasked by alternately covering each eye in rapid succession while the patient fixes their gaze on the examiner.[25]

HINTS Examination

If any one of the components of the HINTS examination suggests a central cause, the overall HINTS examination is suggestive of a central lesion. Several studies have examined the diagnostic accuracy of the HINTS examination for identifying central causes of AVS. The original study describing the use of HINTS by neuro-otologists in 101 patients with new onset AVS showed a sensitivity of 100% (95% confidence interval [CI] 95% to 100%) and specificity of 96% (95% CI 80% to 99%) for a central cause.[21] Subsequent studies of the HINTS examination performed by various clinicians showed variable sensitivities and specificities. A meta-analysis of nonneurologists (including family practitioners and emergency physicians) showed a sensitivity of 83.4% and specificity of 88.9%.[26]

HINTS+ Examination

See Video 62.8. The addition of a bedside test of hearing utilizing the finger rub to the HINTS examination is termed HINTS+.[27] The purpose is to assess for the rare possibility of an anterior inferior cerebellar artery stroke, which can lead to ischemia of the eighth cranial nerve causing both hearing loss and a corrective saccade. The HINTS+ examination is 99.4% sensitive for stroke (95% CI 95.7% to 99.9%).[26] Confounders to consider include cerumen impaction and preexisting hearing loss. The hearing test is illustrated in Video 62.8.

Complications

The head impulse test may exacerbate injury in improperly selected patients with unstable cervical spinal injury or, theoretically, with severe carotid and vertebral artery atherosclerotic disease, although no reports of such complications have been reported.

Summary

The HINTS+ examination may be useful in identifying patients with a central cause of vertigo among those presenting with AVS. Proper patient selection and correct test interpretation are necessary, including recognizing those with equivocal HINTS examination who require further testing.

EVALUATION OF WEAKNESS

Background

Myasthenia gravis (MG) is the most common disease of neuromuscular transmission, with an annual incidence of 2 to 21 new cases per million.[28] Patients with MG most commonly have extraocular muscle weakness. Diplopia and/or ptosis, present in 80% to 85% of patients, may be the only symptoms, and termed ocular MG. Many patients have limb weakness, involving the proximal muscles more than the distal, with the upper limbs affected more than the lower limbs. Fifteen percent of patients with MG will also have bulbar weakness, such as dysphagia, hoarseness, or difficulty chewing. Fatigue is the hallmark of the disease; the symptoms typically wax and wane, worsening toward the end of the day.

Under normal circumstances, when the nerve terminal is stimulated, acetylcholine (ACh) is released and diffuses across the synaptic cleft in the neuromuscular junction to transiently interact with the ACh receptor (Fig. 62.6). This leads to an action potential that is propagated along the muscle membrane, followed by muscle fiber contraction. The ACh is rapidly hydrolyzed by acetylcholinesterase in the synaptic cleft. Of the millions of receptors at each neuromuscular junction, only a fraction must depolarize to stimulate muscle fiber contraction.

Any factor that decreases the interaction of ACh with ACh receptors decreases the probability of an action potential being generated and may lead to failure of neuromuscular transmission with resulting weakness. MG results from immune-mediated destruction of postsynaptic ACh receptors, with variable failure of neuromuscular transmission.[29] Weakness due to inhibition of ACh is termed *myasthenic crisis*. Whereas immunotherapy and thymectomy are significant advances in the treatment of MG, acetylcholinesterase inhibitors remain the first-line therapy for symptomatic MG. Of note, excessive inhibition of acetylcholinesterase from these agents can also cause weakness, termed *cholinergic crisis;* persistence of ACh in the synaptic cleft leads to continuous depolarization of the receptor, which also manifests as weakness. Other cholinergic findings (excess salivation, cramps, diarrhea, and blurred

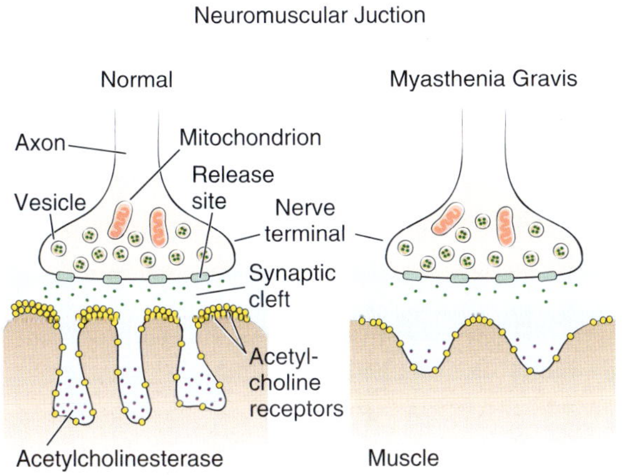

Fig. 62.6 Neuromuscular junctions. Acetylcholine is released from presynaptic vesicles and diffuses across the synaptic cleft to the postsynaptic receptors. Acetylcholinesterase, located deep within the synaptic folds, hydrolyzes acetylcholine. In myasthenia gravis there are a reduced number of postsynaptic acetylcholine receptors, which can lead to failed neuromuscular transmission and weakness.

vision) will help differentiate the two causes of weakness in these patients.

Several tests can be used for the assessment of a patient with suspected MG, but many are not available to the emergency clinician. Serologic testing for ACh receptor antibodies has a sensitivity of 90% to 96%, but has a turnaround time of several days and is more likely to be negative in patients with isolated ocular MG.[30] Repetitive nerve stimulation and single-fiber electromyography tests are available in the electrophysiology laboratory.[31] Multiple bedside tests have been used to aid in the diagnosis of suspected MG, including parenteral administration of neostigmine or curare, as well as the ice-pack test. The test that appears to have the most ED relevance is the ice-pack test, because it is safe and noninvasive.[32]

Ice-Pack Test

Background

Patients with MG have exacerbations of weakness with environmental heat and improvement in strength with cold temperatures, possibly because lower temperatures inhibit acetylcholinesterase function.[33] Utilizing this simple concept at the bedside to evaluate improvement of ptosis with cold exposure, specifically a pack of ice, is called the ice-pack test.[32–34] An ice pack is placed lightly over the closed eyelid for 2 minutes. Ptosis has been noted to improve in 80% or more of patients with ocular MG.[33,35,36] In addition, its safety, speed, and ease of administration make it an attractive ED application (Fig. 62.7).

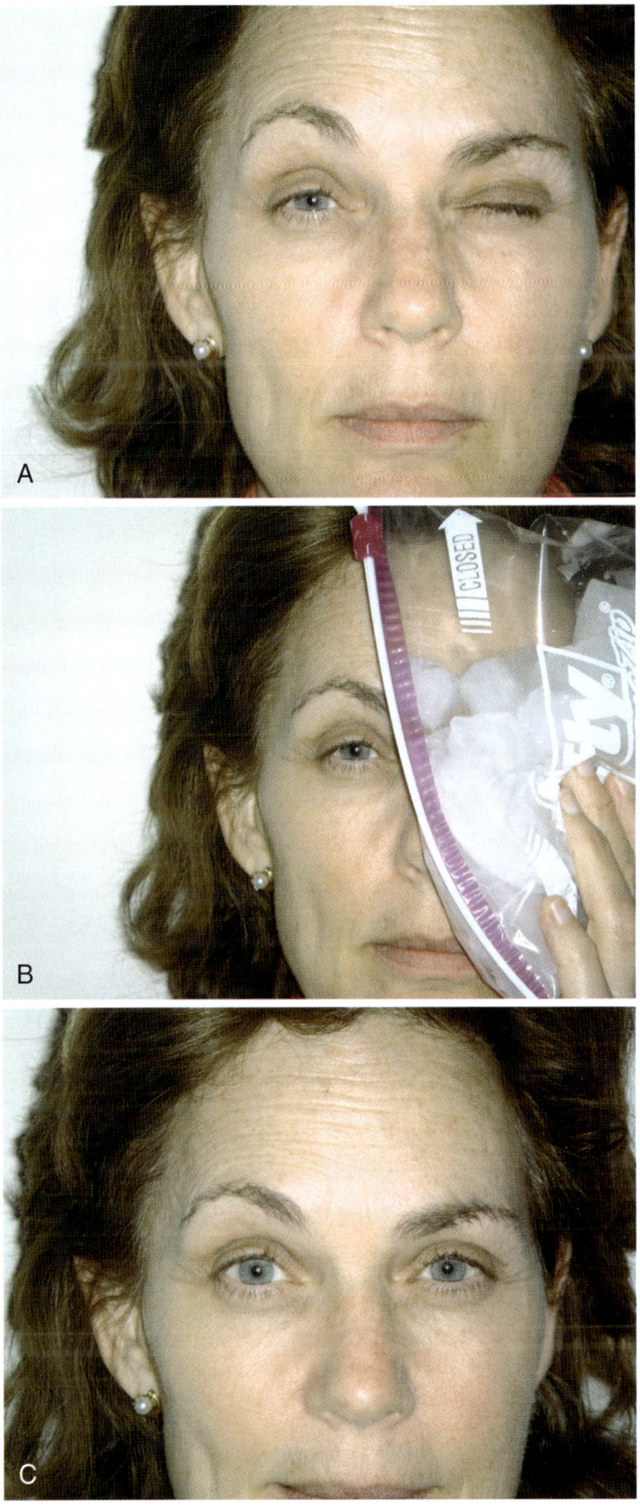

Fig. 62.7 The ice-pack test for myasthenia gravis. (A) Before placement of an ice pack. (B) Ice pack placed over the eyelid for approximately 2 minutes. (C) After placement of an ice pack, improvement is noted in ptosis of the right eye. (For details, see Sethi et al.[33])

Indications

Unilateral or bilateral ptosis of uncertain etiology in patients being evaluated for ocular MG.

Procedure

Ice and a bag (or a surgical glove) are the only equipment required. A digital camera to record a response is optional. Measure or photograph the degree of the patient's ptosis prior to the test. Studies have used the vertical distance between the upper and lower lid, or palpebral fissure, as an objective measure of the degree of ptosis.[36] If bilateral ptosis is present, test the more affected eye. Fill a bag (or surgical glove) with ice and place gently on the patient's closed eyelid for 2 minutes or until patient discomfort limits its application. After removing the ice, immediately assess the width of the palpebral fissure and compare with the pretest width.

Complications
Patient discomfort from ice pack application may limit cold exposure time to less than 2 minutes but may still allow a test to be successfully performed.

Interpretation
A clear improvement in ptosis in the cooled eye constitutes a positive test, commonly defined as 2 mm or more of improvement in the width of the palpebral fissure.[36,37] The effect should be reproducible. The ice-pack test is 80% to 92% sensitive and 79% to 100% specific for ocular MG,[30,37–39] and has similar diagnostic accuracy to electromyography.[35] False-negative results do occur, more commonly in patients with complete ptosis, and probably at approximately the same frequency as with Tensilon testing. Normal individuals show no change in width of the palpebral fissure after cold exposure. False-positive results are uncommon.[33,34,36]

Summary
MG is typically diagnosed by serologic testing for autoantibodies and electrodiagnostic studies in the ambulatory setting.[31,40,41] However, when diagnosis in the ED is desired, the ice-pack test may provide valuable information at the bedside. False-negative results do occur, and additional testing should be performed if clinical suspicion for MG persists.

EVALUATION OF SEIZURES

Electroencephalography

Background
Electroencephalography (EEG) measures electrical activity arising from the brain between pairs of electrodes. This real time, continuous, dynamic electrophysiological measurement is commonly used for the evaluation and characterization of seizures, though it can also be used in the detection of cerebral ischemia and to monitor depth of anesthesia.

There has been an increase in the rapid or limited EEG technology that has become commercially available in the recent years. Most of the current devices attempt to address two major gaps in the evaluation and management of patients with possible nonconvulsive seizures—the limited availability of electroencephalographic monitoring at most hospitals and the limited availability of specialty-trained epileptologists to interpret EEG recordings.

Indications and Contraindications
EEG is commonly used for the evaluation of clinical seizure–like activity to determine whether they correspond with electrographic epileptiform activity. This may occur in the inpatient or ambulatory setting. It may also occur in specialized epilepsy monitoring units. In the ED, EEG is often used for the evaluation of nonconvulsive seizures in patients with alterations in mental status.

Scalp wounds may limit the placement of EEG electrodes in the standardized array. Skull defects affect the proximity of the electrodes to the cortical cerebral activity, thereby affecting the morphology of the electrophysiological rhythm.

Equipment
Conventional EEG utilizes 21 scalp electrodes in a standardized array called the International 10-20 System.[42] Rapid EEG technology generally incorporates a reduced number of electrodes embedded in a headset or cap to simplify placement of the device on the patient's head. This allows application by clinicians other than trained EEG technicians. While these devices are easy to apply on patients, they may not accommodate different head sizes and shapes, skull deformities, or hair thickness and texture. Some of the currently available rapid EEG technology also includes an automated processing and analysis algorithm for seizure detection.

Complications
Prolonged EEG monitoring can result in scalp injuries as application of the electrodes may require abrasive cleaning of the scalp and adhesive conductive paste depending on the type of electrodes used.

Interpretation
Interpretation of EEGs are typically provided by neurologists subspecialized in neurophysiology and epilepsy. An advantage of automated analysis algorithms is their ability to answer straightforward clinical questions such as the presence of seizures.[43,44] However, it is important to note that determination of epileptiform activity on EEG needs to take into context the patient's background electrographic activity; thus patients with underlying brain injuries often require nuanced interpretation of their EEG patterns.

One of the biggest limitations of rapid EEG systems as a diagnostic tool is the reduced number of electrodes; therefore they do not provide the same level of detail on the electrophysiological activity of the brain. An analogy would be the difference between a 6-lead versus 12-lead electrocardiogram.

Summary
EEG is a useful dynamic assessment of cerebral activity and has applications beyond the evaluation of seizures. Current rapid EEG technology may serve as a valuable tool in the triage and risk stratification of appropriately selected patients and clinical questions.

EVALUATION OF THE COMATOSE PATIENT

Coma is defined as a state of deeply reduced consciousness from which a patient cannot be aroused by verbal, tactile, or noxious external stimuli.[45] This subsection will review procedures that have important diagnostic and prognostic significance in the comatose patient: caloric testing and the evaluation of brain death.

Caloric Testing

Background
In a comatose individual with normal brain stem and cranial nerve function, stimulation of the vestibular labyrinth results in well-described and reproducible extraocular movements through the vestibulo-ocular reflex (VOR). Pathologic conditions involving the labyrinth, vestibulocochlear nerve, or the oculomotor reflex pathways in the brain stem will alter or abolish the VOR.

Physiology and Functional Anatomy

The anatomic pathways underlying the VOR begin in the lateral semicircular canal of the inner ear. Movement of endolymphatic fluid within the canal results in changes in polarization in the underlying hair cells, which in turn are relayed via cranial nerve VIII (vestibular) to the brain stem (Fig. 62.8).

There are two main pathways between the vestibular and oculomotor nuclei in the brain stem. The direct pathway travels from the vestibular complex to the nuclei of the ipsilateral third cranial nerve (oculomotor) and contralateral sixth cranial nerve (abducens), and ultimately to the ipsilateral medial rectus and contralateral lateral rectus muscles. The indirect pathway occurs over multisynaptic circuits in the tegmental reticular formation.[46]

Rotation of the head generates flow of endolymphatic fluid within the semicircular canals; the direction of flow increases or decreases stimulation of the vestibular neuron, which results in conjugate deviation of the eyes away from or toward the affected side, respectively. This principle forms the physiologic basis of caloric testing. When the lateral canal is in the vertical position (head elevated 30 degrees above horizontal) and ice water is infused into the ear, the endolymph nearest the canal cools and sinks, which results in decreased stimulation of the vestibular neuron, and the eyes deviate conjugately toward the side of irrigation. When warm water is used in the same position or when the canal is inverted 180 degrees, the opposite occurs.

Indications and Contraindications

Caloric testing is infrequently used in ED settings in the United States where advanced neuroimaging is readily available. However, in resource-limited settings, caloric testing at the bedside may assist in the evaluation of comatose patients by differentiating structural, metabolic, and psychogenic causes of unresponsiveness.

Few contraindications exist to caloric testing of an unresponsive patient. An absolute contraindication is the presence of a basilar skull fracture, either documented radiologically or suspected by clinical signs, because of the risk of introducing infection into the central nervous system (CNS) through an associated dural tear. If active bleeding or cerebrospinal fluid otorrhea or rhinorrhea is present in a trauma patient, defer caloric testing and evaluate the patient for a potential basilar skull fracture. Tympanic rupture, hemotympanum, or step-off deformities of the auditory canal may indicate fracture of the temporal bone, which is a contraindication to caloric testing. Signs of active ear infection and perforation of the tympanic membrane are relative contraindications to caloric testing.

Equipment

A 30- or 50-mL plastic syringe is ideal for irrigation. The syringe may be used as is, or a short length of soft plastic tubing (e.g., a butterfly catheter with the needle cut off) may be attached. At least 100 mL of ice water should be available, although larger quantities of cool tap water (<25°C) can be used with similar results if ice is unavailable. Saline or tap water may be used. A small, curved plastic emesis basin is useful to collect water as it drains from the ear canal. Other equipment required includes an otoscope, ear specula, and equipment for removal of cerumen. Towels and a thermometer may be helpful.

Procedure

Inspect the ears before inserting the otoscope. Remove excess cerumen and foreign material. Clearly visualize the tympanic membrane. Leave the ear speculum in the canal as a guide for irrigation. Perform the test with the patient supine and the head and upper part of the body raised to 30 degrees, if possible. Drape the patient with a towel and position a small emesis basin below the ear to collect the outflow of water from the ear. Fill a container with ice water and place it near the bedside.

Fill a syringe and catheter system (without the needle) with 10 mL of ice water and direct the irrigation stream toward the tympanic membrane. Because the goal of qualitative caloric testing is to induce a maximum response, the amount and rate of infusion are not critical. As a general guide, infuse 5 mL to 10 mL of ice water initially over a period of 5 to 10 seconds. Amounts less than 5 mL may be advisable in suspected cases of light coma or psychogenic unresponsiveness. If no response is noted at first, infuse at least 100 mL before declaring that there is no response. Ask an assistant to hold the patient's eyelids open, which makes it easier to observe for eye deviation. Movement usually occurs after a latency of 10 to 40 seconds, with the response persisting for as long as 4 to 5 minutes. Focusing on a scleral vessel makes small deviations easier to detect. Wait at least 5 to 10 minutes after the eyes have returned to their original position before testing the contralateral ear.

Complications

Carefully selecting equipment can avoid the few complications that are possible with caloric testing. Using plastic syringes and soft catheter tubing instead of needles to irrigate the ear will reduce the risk of perforation of the tympanic membrane or canal wall injury if the patient moves unexpectedly.

As mentioned in the contraindications section, caloric testing should not be performed in patients with possible basilar skull fractures, due to the theoretical risk of meningitis. Other potential complications include otitis media and induction of vomiting with subsequent aspiration. Although ice water irrigation might produce nausea and emesis in awake patients, vomiting with aspiration has not been reported as a complication of caloric testing in comatose patients. Nevertheless, some may prefer to delay testing until the patient's airway is protected.

Interpretation

After irrigation, ocular movements should be observed for any response to the stimulus. Typically, there is a latency of response of 10 to 40 seconds. Reactions to ice water irrigation may be divided into four categories: (1) caloric nystagmus, (2) conjugate deviation, (3) dysconjugate deviation, and (4) absent responses (Fig. 62.8).

The first reaction, caloric nystagmus, is seen in normal, alert individuals. Ice water infusion induces a rhythmic jerking of the eyes that includes a slow deviation toward the irrigated side followed by a quick compensatory saccade toward the midline. In an apparently comatose individual, caloric nystagmus usually signifies psychogenic unresponsiveness due to catatonia, conversion reactions, schizophrenia, or feigned coma, but can also be present in patients with very mild organic disturbances in consciousness. The response is present in more than 90% of children by 6 months of age and declines in magnitude only after the seventh decade of life.[47]

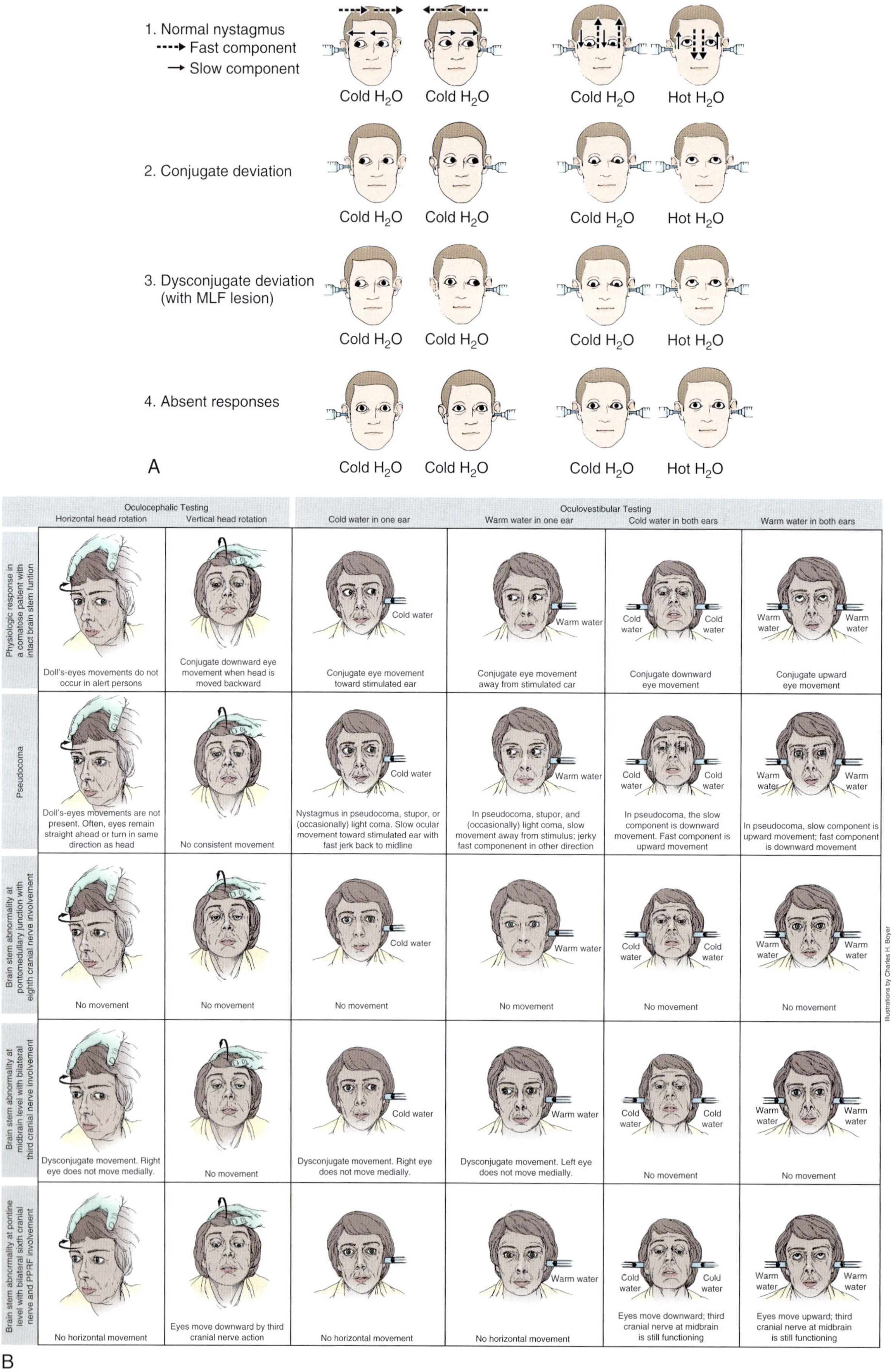

Fig. 62.8 (A) The four types of caloric responses seen with unilateral and bilateral irrigation. *1*, Normal nystagmus. *2*, Conjugate deviation. *3*, Dysconjugate deviation. *4*, Absent caloric responses. (B) Oculocephalic and oculovestibular testing in patients with selected clinical conditions. *MLF,* Medial longitudinal fasciculus; *PPRF,* pontine paramedian reticular formation. (A, Modified from Plum F, Posner JB, eds. *The Diagnosis of Stupor and Coma.* 3rd ed. Davis; 1980:55. B, From Smith M, Bleck T. Techniques for evaluating the cause of coma. *J Crit Illness.* 1987;2:51.)

In the second type of response to cold caloric stimulation, conjugate deviation, the eyes deviate conjugately toward the side of ice water stimulation (they "look" toward the source of irritation). When present, this reaction indicates intact brain stem function, as well as intact afferent and efferent limbs of the VOR. This is seen during general anesthesia, in supratentorial lesions without brain stem compression, and with many metabolic and drug-induced comas.

Dysconjugate reactions constitute the third type of caloric response to ice water stimuli. The most common dysconjugate reaction is internuclear ophthalmoplegia, in which a lesion of the medial longitudinal fasciculus causes weakness or paralysis of the adducting eye after caloric irrigation. Internuclear ophthalmoplegia can be due to acute damage to the rostral pons or as a manifestation of multiple sclerosis or stroke. With acute supratentorial lesions, the development of dysconjugate caloric responses is a significant sign that may indicate compression of the brain stem and impending herniation. Caloric responses of this type are less common with metabolic and drug-induced coma. Reversible internuclear ophthalmoplegia has been reported in patients with hepatic coma and may occur during toxic responses to phenytoin, barbiturates, or amitriptyline.

Absent caloric response is the fourth category of reactions to ice water stimuli. Loss of caloric responses in comatose patients with structural lesions is usually a sign of brain stem damage. The VOR may also be transiently absent or decreased on the side opposite massive supratentorial damage during the first hours after injury.[48] Whereas the initial absence of the VOR is generally a poor prognostic indicator, it does not uniformly predict a poor outcome when performed in the first 24 hours after presentation.[49] This has particular relevance in cases of traumatic coma, where testing in the first 24 hours after injury may generate variable responses and is of less prognostic value.[50] Absent caloric responses may occur with any infratentorial lesion that affects the vestibular reflex pathways, including pontine hemorrhage, basilar artery occlusion, cerebellar hemorrhage, or infarction with encroachment on the brain stem, and with any expanding mass lesion within the posterior fossa. Caloric responses may disappear in patients with deep coma resulting from subarachnoid hemorrhage, perhaps because of pressure on the brain stem.

The VOR is usually retained until the late stages of metabolic coma. Nevertheless, caloric responses may be transiently absent in certain types of drug-induced coma, with eventual complete recovery of the patient. The VOR seems to be particularly sensitive to the effects of sedative-hypnotic drugs, antidepressants (e.g., amitriptyline, doxepin), and anticonvulsants (e.g., phenytoin, carbamazepine).[51,52] As one would expect, neuromuscular blocking agents (e.g., succinylcholine) will abolish caloric-induced ocular movements.

Finally, the caloric response may be absent for reasons other than the neurologic causes responsible for the coma. Inadequate irrigation because of excessive cerumen or poor technique and unilateral or bilateral dysfunction of the peripheral vestibular apparatus must be considered. Bilateral loss of the caloric response *(areflexia vestibularis)* is uncommon in conscious patients, constituting 1.7% and 0.2% in two large series of patients.[53,54]

Summary

Caloric testing is a simple, easily performed bedside procedure that may enhance the neurologic assessment of comatose patients. In the ED this test should be reserved for stable patients undergoing secondary assessment. The examination requires minimal equipment and can be particularly useful in settings where access to advanced neuroimaging is limited or delayed. Complications are few if patients are properly selected and correct technique is used.

Brain Death Testing

Background

Brain death is defined as irreversible and complete loss of cerebral and brain stem function with preserved cardiac function.[55] It is only in the very rare occasion that an emergency physician may be asked to perform a brain death examination. Even in those cases, a second physician, usually a neurologist, intensivist or neurosurgeon, should be consulted to also perform the evaluation and both parties should concur before the patient is declared brain-dead. Although it occurs rarely, emergency clinicians may be asked to perform a brain death examination to identify potential organ and tissue donors.

It should be noted that a determination of brain death is not necessary for withdrawal of life-supporting measures. If a cause of coma or severe neurologic injury is identified and a poor prognosis is shared with the family, withholding or withdrawing life-sustaining treatment may be appropriate and formal determination of brain death need not be performed.

Indications and Contraindications

Evaluation for brain death implies that severe CNS dysfunction has been identified, that the cause of the CNS dysfunction is known, and that reversible causes of coma have been confidently excluded.[56] Prior to declaring brain death, the cause of the brain injury should be definitively identified, as some toxicologic syndromes may mimic brain death. Complex medical issues that may confound the assessment should be considered and ruled out, including severe electrolyte disturbances, hypothermia (defined as a core temperature <32°C), hypotension, drug intoxication or poisoning, and pharmacologic neuromuscular blockade.[56] Neuroimaging studies should be carefully reviewed. Hospital policy regarding determining brain death should be sought out and followed.

Procedure

The clinical neurologic examination remains the standard for determination of brain death.[56] Most hospitals have a specific policy regarding determined brain death and often outline the exact findings necessary to declare a patient brain-dead, so these policies should be sought out and followed. Determining brain death typically involves assessment for cerebral function, brain stem reflexes, and respiratory drive. The emergency clinician should be familiar with local practices and policies, which may also require ancillary testing such as electroencephalogram, documentation of absent cerebral blood flow by angiography or radioisotope brain scan, or other techniques. The following components of the clinical examination are generally utilized to establish brain death.

Coma Assessment

While holding the patient's eyes open, give loud verbal commands such as "Look up!" and assess for voluntary eye movements; this assessment is particularly important to identify patients with locked-in syndrome. Additionally, deliver a strong painful stimulus by forcefully pressing on the brow, sternum, or nail bed. Any purposeful response to stimuli in any extremity indicates the patient is not brain-dead. The absence of responses documents the presence of coma. It is important to apply noxious stimuli above and below the neck if there is concern for concomitant spinal cord injury.

Brain Stem Reflex Testing (Fig. 62.9)

Pupillary Reflex. The pupils in brain-dead patients are unreactive and mid-position to dilated. Shine a bright light into the pupil and observe for a reaction; none will be seen in a brain-dead patient.

Corneal Reflex. Stimulate the cornea with a cotton wisp or applicator. Any eye closure indicates an intact cranial nerve V to VII reflex and excludes the diagnosis of brain death.

Oculocephalic Reflex. Hold eyelids open and rotate the head abruptly from side to side in the horizontal plane. If the eyes do not turn with the head and appear to maintain visual fixation on a point in space, the oculocephalic reflex is present and brain death is excluded.

Acoustic Reflex. Deliver a loud handclap into each ear. Observe for eye blink or other reaction. Any reaction establishes that some brain stem function remains and excludes brain death.

Vestibulo-ocular Reflex (Caloric Testing). Perform cold-water irrigation of the external auditory canals with large volumes (≥100 mL) to elicit any eye movements through the VOR. In a brain-dead patient, there will be no movement of the eyes in response to irrigation.

Cough Reflex. Stimulate the trachea or main stem bronchi by deep tracheal suctioning and observe for coughing. A cough excludes brain death.

Gag Reflex. Stimulate the posterior oropharynx by deep oral suctioning and observe for contractions of the pharyngeal muscles. This should be tested bilaterally. A gag response excludes brain death.

Apneic Oxygenation Test. If brain stem reflexes are absent, apnea is formally tested to evaluate the function of the medulla, where respiratory drive originates. As hypercapnia (and not hypoxia) triggers respiratory effort, simply disconnecting the ventilator to allow hypercapnia to develop may lead to hypoxia and should therefore be avoided.[57] The most commonly described technique to avoid hypoxia while generating hypercapnia is to (1) disconnect the patient from the ventilator, (2) deliver oxygen at 10 to 15 L/min through a catheter inserted into the trachea, and (3) observe for respiratory effort for 8 to 10 minutes. An alternative technique is to set the ventilator rate to zero while allowing continuous

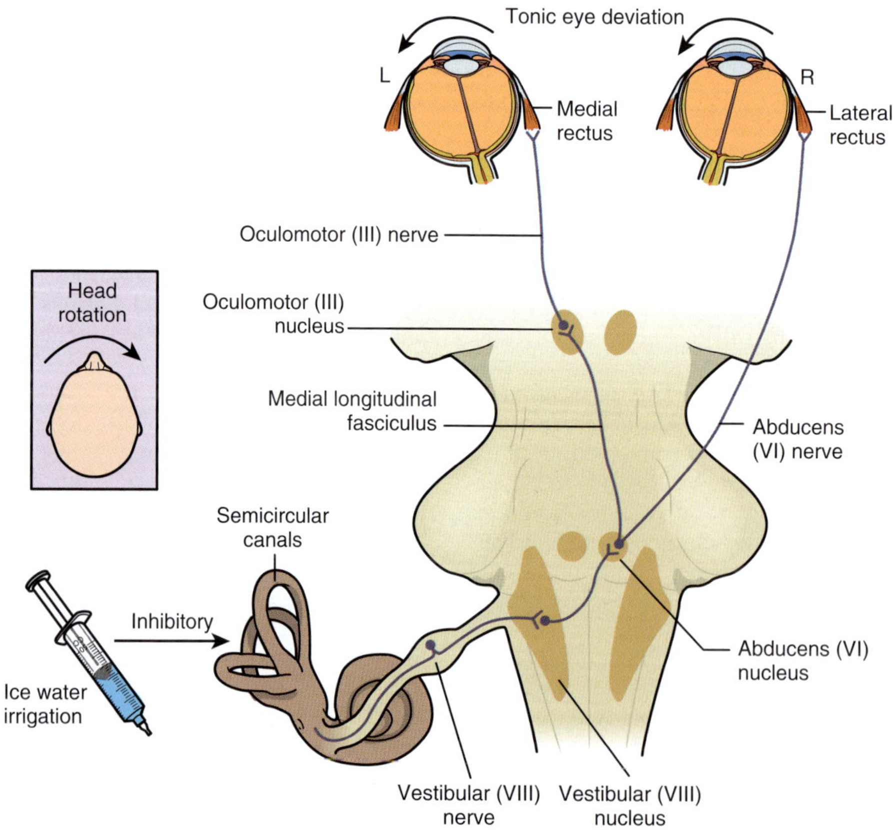

Fig. 62.9 Brainstem pathways mediating the vestibulo-ocular reflex. Rotational acceleration of the head to the right results in excitatory projections that travel to the contralateral sixth cranial nerve and lateral rectus, as well as the ipsilateral third cranial nerve and medial rectus, resulting in eye deviation to the left. In a similar manner, inhibitory projections are sent to the antagonist ipsilateral lateral rectus and contralateral medial rectus. (From Simon RP, Aminoff MJ, Greenberg DA, eds. *Clinical Neurology.* 4th ed. Appleton & Lange; 1999:313.)

oxygen flow to continue and maintaining any necessary continuous positive pressure through the ventilator.[58] Any observed excursion of the abdomen or chest sufficient to produce a tidal volume suggests that brain death is not present. If no respiratory excursions are observed, an arterial blood gas analysis should be obtained, and artificial ventilation resumed pending results. An arterial partial carbon dioxide pressure (Pco_2) of 60 mm Hg or higher and the absence of respiratory excursions are the criteria for a positive apnea test (i.e., that the patient lacks spontaneous respirations).[59] In patients with chronic CO_2 retention, a rise in PCO_2 of at least 20 mm Hg and the absence of respiratory effort are needed to meet the criteria for apnea testing.

Declaration of Death

If the criteria for brain death are satisfied, the family and all clinicians involved in patient care should be informed to allow further management decisions. At some institutions, the patient is declared dead at the time that the criteria are met, and further care is assumed by the transplant services if that is the anticipated course. Some institutions require evaluation by two independent clinicians with specific specialty training, or repeated examinations several hours apart; however, the need for a second brain death determination has been questioned.[60,61] Families are generally given the option of being present at the bedside when mechanical ventilation is discontinued, although some advise against this practice because spontaneous reflex movements may occur and disturb the family.[62]

Brain death in the pediatric population is more complex, with varying recommendations for repeated examinations and ancillary tests; such discussion is outside the scope of this chapter but is summarized in other resources.[36,56,63,64] A model for direct family conversation in this sensitive interaction has been described and includes a sample script and procedure.[65]

Complications

A substantial proportion of brain-dead patients (33% to 75%) may exhibit movements originating in the spinal cord or peripheral nerves.[66,67] These movements can be spontaneous or provoked by tactile stimuli and may falsely be interpreted as evidence of cerebral or brain stem function. Among the most frequently observed movements are finger jerks, the undulating toe flexion response (slow and repetitive flexion/extension of the toes), and the triple flexion reflex (flexion of thigh, leg, and foot); however, many other movements have been described.[66,68–72]

Summary

The emergency clinician may become involved in the assessment of patients for brain death. The cause of irreversible coma should be identified prior to initiating a systematic brain death examination, which includes an assessment of cerebral function, brain stem reflexes, and apnea. The clinician should be familiar with local practices and policies in this complex medicolegal process, and should strongly consider consulting another physician (usually a neurologist, intensivist or neurosurgeon) before declaring a patient brain-dead.

ACKNOWLEDGMENTS

We thank J. Stephen Huff, MD, Paul B. Baker, MD, and Mikaela L. Chilstrom, MD, for their significant contributions to this chapter in prior editions. The editor would like to recognize the expert contributions to the BPPV and HINTS+ sections by Peter Johns, MD, Associate Professor, University of Ottawa.

REFERENCES ARE AVAILABLE AT Elsevier eBooks+

SECTION XI

Ophthalmologic, Otolaryngologic, and Dental Procedures

CHAPTER 63

Ophthalmologic Procedures

Kevin J. Knoop, Timothy S. Forsythe, and Michael J. Shallcross

The following discussion focuses on procedures performed by emergency clinicians during the evaluation and treatment of injuries and diseases of the eye. Emphasis is placed on practical application of the techniques; cautions to be heeded by the emergency clinician are included. Not all procedures are mandated to be performed by the emergency clinician, and if beyond the expertise available in the emergency department (ED), they may be referred to a specialist.

ASSESSMENT OF VISUAL ACUITY

See Video 63.1. Evaluation of visual acuity may initially be deferred with simple, obvious, or straightforward cases, such as a stye, periorbital laceration, or minor eye irritation; however, assessment of visual acuity should be the first procedure performed in the majority of patients seen in the ED with an eye complaint). Even though it may initially be deferred in the triage or trauma room setting or under other relevant scenarios, the emergency clinician must ensure that visual acuity or function is assessed adequately as part of the initial evaluation.

Indications

Visual acuity should be assessed as soon as practicable and before the patient is examined with bright lights. In the event of blepharospasm from an injury (e.g., abrasion, chemical exposure), a topical anesthetic may facilitate the examination. Patients with eye complaints often say that they "can't see." In these instances, emergency visual acuity assessment should be performed first, beginning with evaluation of light perception, then hand motion, and finally counting fingers at 3 ft (Fig. 63.1). When asking patient to count fingers, place fingers no closer than about 14 inches as presbyopic patients may miscount fingers due to inability to accommodate. Also, use one, two, or four fingers. Three fingers may be confused as two or four due to proximity, whereas two and four fingers have distinct differences. Thumbs should not be used. If the patient succeeds in performing these assessments, measure visual acuity at the bedside with a near card as described later. In emergency circumstances, detailed formal vision testing is not essential; however, some form of visual acuity assessment is needed. In this situation, the ability to count fingers or read newsprint gives some indication of gross visual function. The patient's visual acuity and pupillary examination are the "vital signs" of the eye and when accurately obtained aid in differentiating a true eye emergency. Formal visual acuity testing should never delay critical therapeutic interventions such as eye irrigation in the case of eye exposures.[1,2]

Near Visual Acuity Procedure

Perform near visual acuity assessment in the ED at the bedside or at triage. Hold a pocket-sized near vision card (see Fig. 63.2C) or any printed material in good light at a distance of approximately 14 inches in front of the patient and occlude each eye alternately as described earlier. Alternately, an "app" may be used from a smartphone device, but directions vary and not all apps measure near distance.[3] When using available printed material in lieu of a near vision card, measure the size of the letters that are discerned by the patient. At a later time compare these letters with the size of the letters on the near vision card to deduce the patient's actual visual acuity. When near vision is decreased, it is usually caused by either loss of visual function or poor accommodation as a result of advancing age (presbyopia). Less commonly, it is caused by traumatic mydriasis. Thus examine patients with presbyopia with their reading correction in place to obtain the best corrected near visual acuity.

For patients who cannot communicate or in whom factitious blindness or malingering is suspected, check for optokinetic nystagmus (OKN) to determine whether the visual pathway is intact. To test for OKN, pass a regularly sequenced pattern in front of the eyes. If an optokinetic drum is available, rotate the drum in front of the patient (Fig. 63.3). This is not available in many EDs; however, multiple apps are available for use with smartphones which show a moving stripe that elicits nystagmus. In place of the drum, substitute a printed piece of paper such as newsprint (without photographs or large areas with no print) or a standard tape measure. Pass it in front of the patient's eyes at reading distance while instructing the patient to look at it as it moves rapidly by. Evaluate for tracking as demonstrated by involuntary nystagmus-like eye movements seen when the test object is moved from side to side in front of the patient. Such movement indicates an intact visual pathway. Finally, another effective method is to hold a mirror in front of the patient and slowly rotate the mirror to either side of the patient. Patients with an intact visual pathway will maintain eye contact with themselves as demonstrated by eye movement as the mirror is moved. A large mirror that reflects the patient's entire face is most effective for this purpose.

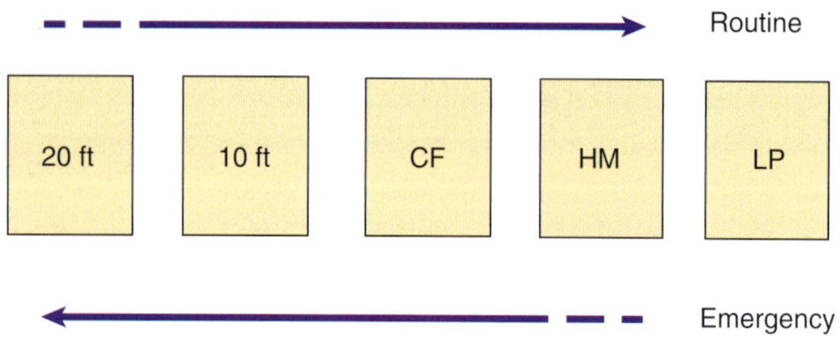

Fig. 63.1 The "routine" progression for assessing visual acuity is reversed in an emergency situation. Assessment of an intact visual pathway begins with quickly discerning whether the patient has light perception *(LP)*, can see hand motion *(HM)*, and can count fingers at 3 ft *(CF)*. Subsequent progression to assess vision at 10 and then 20 ft from a standard eye chart ensues.

Distant Visual Acuity Procedure

For formal vision testing, ask the patient to face a well-lit standard Snellen or similar eye chart from a premeasured distance of 20 ft. Use a card, tissues and a patch, or the palm of the hand to occlude one eye at a time. If possible, examine all patients while wearing their current lens correction to obtain the best corrected distant visual acuity. If not available, measure visual acuity first without correction and then with a pinhole device, and note any improvement in visual acuity. The pinhole device functions as a corrective lens by eliminating divergent light rays and allowing light only through the center of the lens, thus reducing corneal refractive error. In general, visual acuity is improved with the pinhole device. Decreased visual acuity that is not improved with this device suggests that corneal refractive error is not the cause. Construct a pinhole device by punching one to several holes in the center of a card (3 × 5 inch index card) with an 18-gauge needle. Devices with one or more pinholes drilled into an eye cover are available commercially (Fig. 63.2A–B) or can be constructed from readily available material in the ED, such as the index card with holes just mentioned (Fig. 63.4). Fig. 63.2C presents a chart for testing visual acuity while the patient is on a stretcher or in a chair. The chart can be used directly from this text if held 14 inches from the eye. Begin by testing the affected eye or the one presumed to have the worst visual acuity. First, instruct the patient to read the smallest letters on the chart that can easily be seen. Then ask the patient to read letters that can just barely be made out (i.e., they do not have to be clear). If the patient is unable to read the largest letter on the chart, move the patient to half the distance from the chart (10 ft), or if using the figure in this text, move it 7 inches closer to the eye and repeat the procedure. Record the results reflecting the change in distance (e.g., 10/200). The numerator in the vision ratio is the distance of the patient from the chart and the denominator is the distance at which a patient with normal vision can read the line of letters. For patients who still cannot read the letters on the chart, test vision progressively as follows: the ability to count fingers, detection of hand motion, and perception of light (with or without projection; i.e., the ability to perceive the direction of light), and finally, the inability to perceive light (no light perception [NLP]).

All patients with decreased visual acuity from baseline require routine referral for further ophthalmologic follow-up; however, patients with moderately or severely decreased visual acuity not explained by refractive error require ophthalmologic consultation in the ED.

USE OF OPHTHALMIC ANESTHETIC AND ANALGESIC AGENTS

Topical anesthetic agents are widely used in the ED setting. Their use is essential in achieving adequate pain control and to evaluate and treat painful eye conditions. Two agents most commonly used are tetracaine and proparacaine. Comparative studies suggest that proparacaine is less painful on instillation, whereas tetracaine is longer lasting, and thus possibly more effective. Additional clinical data are available in Moshirfar et al., Tables 63.1 and 63.2, discusses duration of onset and action.[4,5] Topical anesthetic agents have been used in the outpatient setting following ophthalmic surgery and are considered safe and effective for this condition. Although still controversial, there is a growing body of evidence that supports their use for brief outpatient pain management (24 to 72 hours) of corneal abrasions. A recent observational study supports prescribing tetracaine for 24 hours of analgesic control, administered as frequently as every 30 minutes while awake. Use is strictly for simple corneal abrasions and appropriately limiting the supply of the prescription on ED discharge is recommended. Complications reported are not due to short-term use of anesthetic agents such as tetracaine or proparacaine but from application to nonsimple corneal abrasions or misdiagnosis. Underlying conditions such as herpes keratitis, iritis, retained rust rings, recurrent corneal erosions, large corneal abrasions (greater than 4 mm), chemical abrasions, or episcleritis are examples of diagnoses that have resulted in complications with prolonged anesthetic use. With appropriate short-term use of dilute topical anesthetics, potent pain control is achieved and no adverse effects have been reported on limited studies available; however, high-quality studies are still lacking.[6–9]

Nonsteroidal antiinflammatory drugs (NSAIDs) ophthalmic drops have been evaluated for their effectiveness and in the treatment of traumatic corneal abrasions. Commonly used examples include ketorolac, diclofenac, indomethacin, and flurbiprofen, with diclofenac and ketorolac most commonly prescribed. These agents are thought to be safe to use and effective for the relief of pain associated with corneal abrasions.[10–13] Topical ophthalmic NSAIDs have also previously been shown to be safe and effective when used for the treatment of corneal abrasions in conjunction with bandage contact lenses.[14] However, recent systematic reviews have reported lack of strong evidence in supporting the use of topical ophthalmic NSAIDs for the relief of pain. Pain reduction with topical application is not as potent as breakthrough oral analgesics. In addition, high cost and patient-reported pain with application limit adherence and efficacy of the prescribed treatment regimen. Long-term use is associated with complications such as surface keratopathy and corneal melting. Despite similar potential complications (delayed corneal healing), topical NSAIDs have gained widespread acceptance compared with topical anesthetic agents in their use for treatment of corneal abrasions as they are thought to provide some pain relief. However, studies available do not always report clinically relevant pain reduction as a trial measure. Thus evidence for support of use is seen as weak through meta-analysis.[15]

Indications and Contraindications

Application of topical anesthetic agents can be both diagnostic and therapeutic. Relief of discomfort with a topical anesthetic strongly suggests, but does not ensure, a conjunctival or

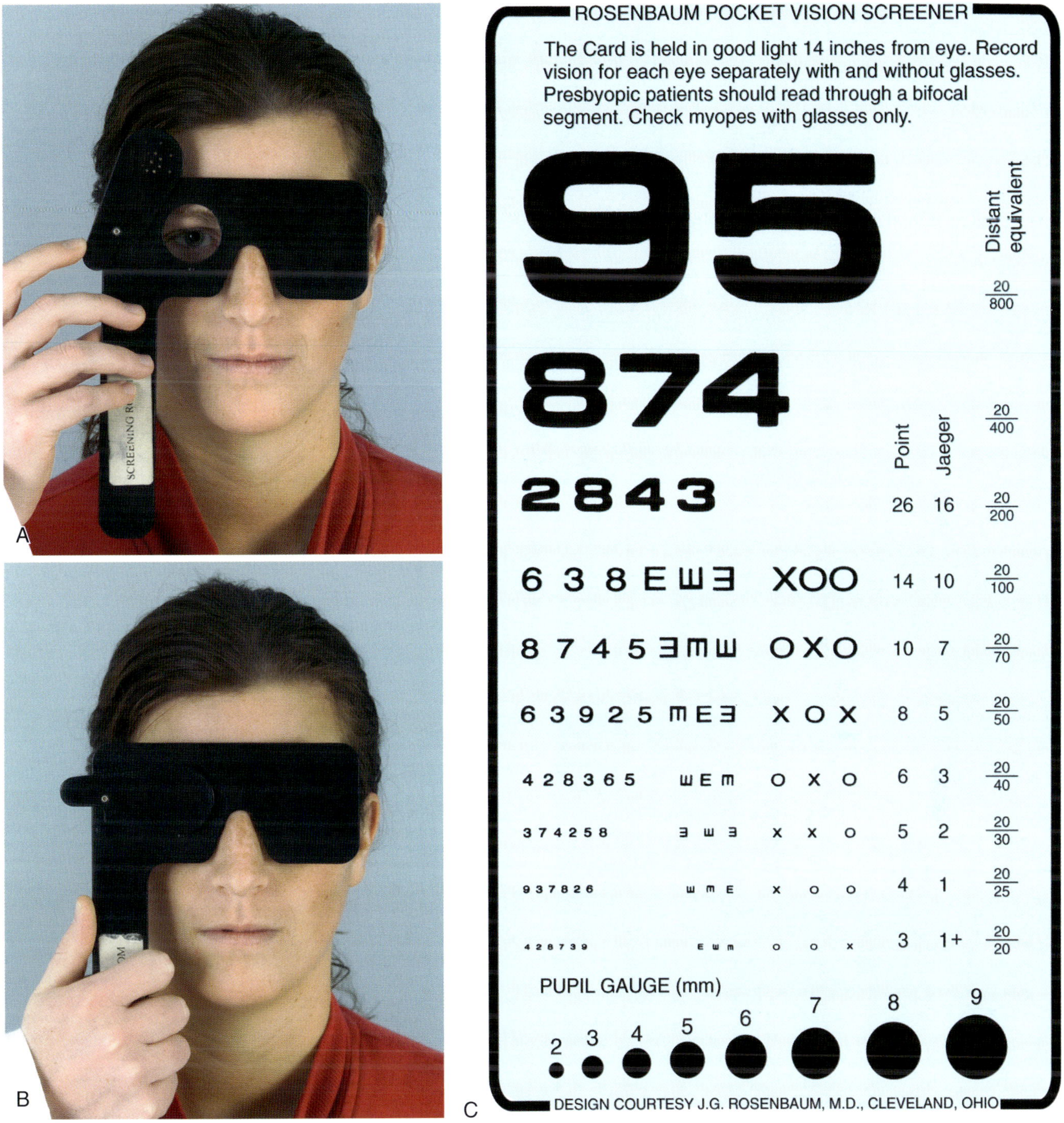

Fig. 63.2 A commercial pinhole device reveals refractive error caused by corneal aberration (excessive tearing or nearsightedness). The pinhole device functions as a corrective lens by eliminating divergent light rays and allowing light only through the center of the lens, thus reducing corneal refractive error. In general, visual acuity is improved with the pinhole device. Decreased visual acuity that is not improved with this device suggests that corneal refractive error is not the cause. (A) First measure visual acuity without the device. (B) Measure again with the patient looking through the pinhole. Document the acuity with and without the pinhole device. (C) If the patient cannot stand or a formal eye chart is not available, ask the patient to read this "distance equivalent" chart by holding the card 14 inches away from the patient.

corneal injury. An ocular irritant may also be masked by the use of these agents. Classic teaching is that patients should not self-administer anesthetic preparations. It is thought that they delay wound healing by disrupting surface microvilli and result in a decrease in the tear film layer and tear break-up time.[16] Self-administered topical anesthetic agents are now routinely used after photorefractive keratectomy for the first 3 or 4 postoperative days. This likely safe technique is becoming more common in ED practice.[17]

As evident from Table 63.1, the anesthetic solutions commonly used have a duration of action of less than 20 minutes, though tetracaine may have a slightly longer clinical effect.[4] Patients with a large corneal lesion may need a more extended period of pain relief and may require bed rest, opioid analgesics, and/or appropriate sedatives.

A final word of caution should be added regarding the use of ophthalmic solutions. Guaiac solutions are commonly supplied in dropper bottles similar in size and appearance to those containing ophthalmic solutions. Well-intentioned ED personnel may store the guaiac reagent bottles with the ophthalmic bottles. One should encourage both color coding of the bottles and examination of them and their labels before each use to avoid corneal injury from inadvertently instilling guaiac reagent into the eye. A typical guaiac reagent contains 5% hydrogen peroxide and 75% denatured ethyl alcohol. Inadvertent eye exposure to guaiac solution requires prompt treatment. Immediately and thoroughly irrigate the affected eye with water or 0.9% normal saline for at least 10 to 15 minutes.[18]

Procedure

Instillation of anesthetic or analgesic agents is similar to the administration of other eye solutions as described later. Forewarn the patient that the medication will sting transiently on instillation but will quickly offer relief. Repeat instillation in 1 minute to ensure maximum effect. Instruct the patient not to rub the insensate eyes to avoid causing or worsening an abrasion. Provide the patient with material to blot the eyes gently, if needed, as tearing occurs.

Complications

Open bottles can harbor bacteria and introduce infection. Out-of-date medication may not be effective and result in inadequate anesthesia. The absence of protective reflexes while the patient is under the effect of the medication may

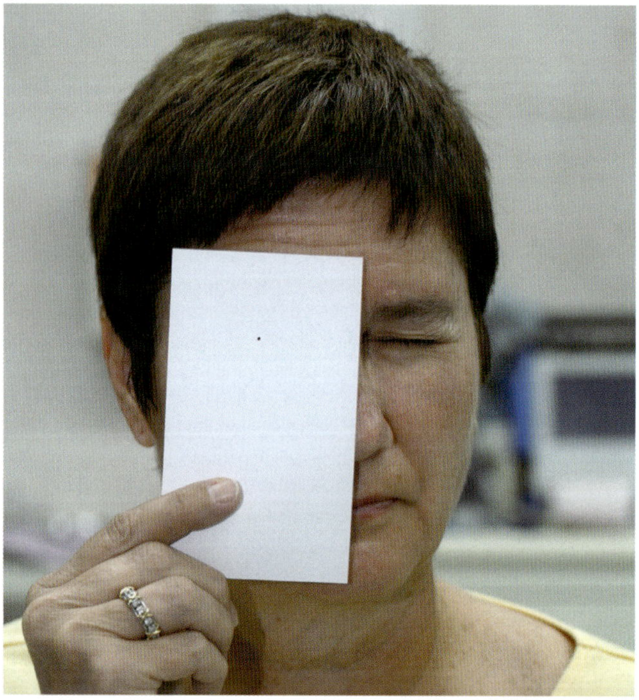

Fig. 63.3 Optokinetic nystagmus (OKN) testing will determine whether the visual pathway is intact. It will be normal in a patient with factitious blindness or malingering. Induce OKN by passing a regularly sequenced pattern in front of the eye such as this commercially available drum. Hold the drum in front of the patient. Direct the patient to look at the drum as you rotate it slowly. Alternatively, draw a tape measure across the line of sight while asking the patient to look directly at it as it passes.

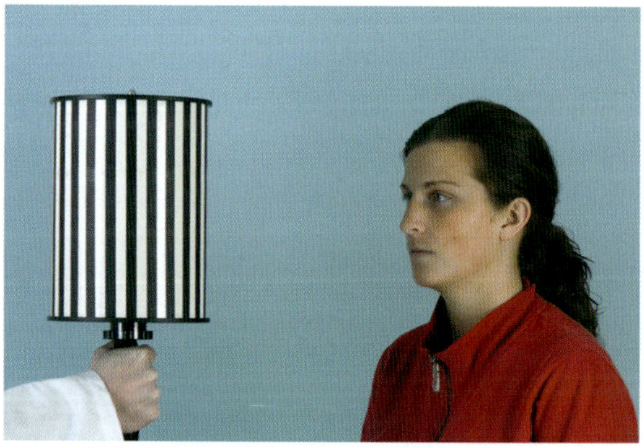

Fig. 63.4 A bedside pinhole device can be easily fashioned if commercial devices are not available. In this image, a single hole was crafted from a needle and an index card. Multiple holes work effectively as well. When assessing visual acuity with a handmade pinhole device, have the patient hold the device in front of the eye tested, while covering the other eye. (Courtesy Mary Jo Chandler, PA-C.)

TABLE 63.1 Ophthalmic Anesthetic Agents

GENERIC NAME	TRADE NAME	CONCENTRATION (%)	ONSET OF ANESTHESIA	DURATION OF ANESTHESIA (min)	COMMENTS
Tetracaine	Pontocaine	0.5–1.0	<1 min	15–20	Marked stinging; ointment and preservative-free unit dose available
Proparacaine	Ophthaine, Ophthetic	0.5	<20 s	10–15	Least irritating; no cross-sensitization with other agents
Benoxinate	Dorsacaine	0.4	1–2 min	10–15	Contains fluorescein in solution

TABLE 63.2 Mydriatic Agents[a]

AGENT	MAXIMUM MYDRIASIS	DURATION OF MYDRIASIS[b]	COMMON TRADE NAME
Sympathomimetics			
Phenylephrine,[c] 2.5%[d]	20 min	3 h	Neo-Synephrine
Cocaine, 5% or 4%	20 min	2 h	—
Parasympatholytics (Cycloplegics)			
Atropine, 1%	40 min	12 days	—
Scopolamine, 0.25%	30 min	7 days	—
Homatropine, 5%[e]	30 min	1–3 days	—
Cyclopentolate, 1%	30 min	6–24 h	Cyclogyl
Tropicamide, 1%	30 min	4 h	Mydriacyl

[a]Bottle caps of all these agents except cocaine are usually red.
[b]The duration of effect shows considerable individual variation. These are general estimates.
[c]Preferred for funduscopic examination.
[d]A 10% solution may produce cardiovascular reaction and hence should not be used.
[e]Preferred for iritis or corneal abrasion therapy.

encourage use of the eye and result in further corneal injury from the foreign body (FB) or corneal infection.

A systemic review of the safety of topical anesthetics in the treatment of corneal abrasions found corneal erosions, edema, or iritis reported when agents were used for prolonged periods of time (up to 10 weeks), too often (up to every 15 minutes), and with higher concentrations.[19] Delayed corneal healing has been long taught as a significant complication of topical anesthetic and analgesic agents, but several well-designed randomized clinical trials in the ED-based and ophthalmology (PRK surgery) literature report no adverse events from topical anesthetic use and corneal reepithelialization occurring by 72 hours, indicating that any delay in healing does not appear to be clinically significant.[20–22] Thus though not currently used for routine outpatient treatment, topical anesthetic drops can be considered for use safely for 2 to 3 days without documented adverse effects in selected patients.

DILATING THE EYE

Dilating the eye is useful for both diagnostic and therapeutic purposes. Be advised, however, that an attack of narrow-angle (angle-closure) glaucoma may be precipitated by dilating the pupil. The most common form of glaucoma, however, is open-angle glaucoma, and this type is not precipitated by dilating the pupil. Some patients may have a "mixed mechanism" glaucoma with both open-angle and narrow-angle components. Systemic reactions, such as bradycardia or even heart block from β-blocker eye drops, can be induced by mucosal absorption of dilating medications.

There are two types of dilators: sympathomimetic agents, which stimulate the dilator muscle of the iris, and cycloplegic agents, which block the parasympathetic stimulus that constricts the iris sphincter. Cycloplegic agents also block contraction of the ciliary muscles, which control focusing of the lens of the eye. This effect of cycloplegic agents blocking contraction (and painful spasm) of the ciliary muscle is beneficial as a therapeutic agent in iritis.

Indications and Contraindications

There are several diagnostic and therapeutic indications for dilating the pupil. Dilation is indicated for diagnosis when the fundus cannot be examined adequately through an undilated pupil. An older patient with miotic pupils and cataracts is an example of a patient in whom dilation may facilitate funduscopic examination. Dilation is therapeutically useful for many ophthalmic conditions, including inflammation of the eye. In the emergency setting, corneal injury with secondary traumatic iritis is a common example. Dilation helps the inflamed eye in two ways. First, it may help to prevent adhesions (synechiae) from forming between the iris and other ocular structures. Such adhesions eventually limit movement of the pupil and may precipitate glaucoma. Second, cycloplegic dilating agents relax the ciliary muscle spasm that often accompanies an inflamed eye and thus may reduce the pain associated with inflammation. Though traditionally used for these purposes, both benefits are largely theoretical with little formal evidence to support or refute their use in the ED.

Dilation is discouraged in patients with head injury who are at risk for herniation when it is necessary to monitor pupil findings. Dilation is contraindicated in the presence of narrow anterior chamber angles. Patients predisposed to having narrow angles may be unaware of this condition. Evaluate the depth of the anterior chamber before this procedure and do not dilate the eye if there is any question of a narrow angle.

To estimate the depth of the anterior chamber, shine a penlight tangentially from the lateral side of the eye. When the depth of the anterior chamber is normal, uniform illumination of the iris is seen. However, when the iris has a forward convexity as in the case of a narrow anterior chamber, only a sector of iris is illuminated and there will be a shadow on the medial (nasal) side of the iris (Fig. 63.5). With a slit lamp, the depth of the anterior chamber angle can be assessed directly. The definitive test for assessing the anterior chamber angle is gonioscopy, in which the anterior chamber angle structures are viewed directly by means of a special mirrored contact lens

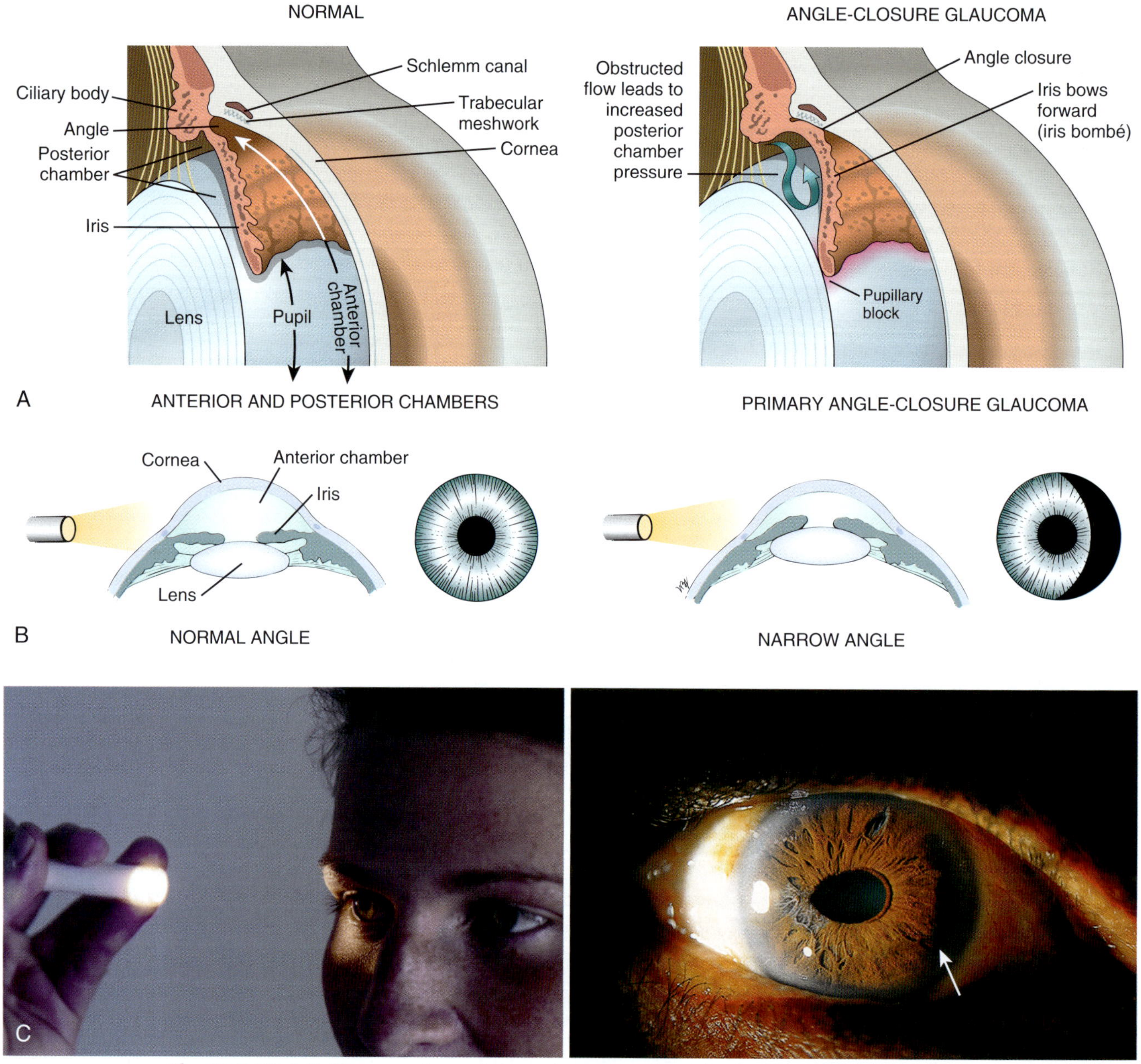

Fig. 63.5 (A) *Left,* The normal eye. Aqueous humor, produced in the posterior chamber, flows through the pupil into the anterior chamber. The major pathway for the egress of aqueous humor is through the trabecular meshwork into Schlemm's canal. *Right,* Primary angle-closure glaucoma. In anatomically predisposed eyes, transient apposition of the iris at the pupillary margin to the lens during pupil dilation blocks the passage of aqueous humor from the posterior chamber to the anterior chamber. Buildup of pressure in the posterior chamber bows the iris forward and occludes the trabecular meshwork. (B) *Left,* Normal anterior chamber with a negative transillumination test. Note that the entire iris is illuminated. *Right,* Shallow anterior chamber with a positive transillumination test. Note the shadow on the outer half of the iris. (C) *Left,* Clinical use of the penlight examination to assess the depth of the anterior chamber of the right eye. The examiner sits face to face with the patient to ensure that the light source is perfectly perpendicular to the line of vision. *Right,* The axial anterior chamber depth of the right eye is less than normal. This can be demonstrated by shining a light across the eye from the temporal side. Because of the convexity of the iris–lens diaphragm, the nasal iris manifests a crescentic shadow (eclipse sign). (A, From Kumar V, Abbas AK, Fausto N et al., eds. *Robbins & Cotran Pathologic Basis of Disease.* 8th ed. Saunders; 2009. B, From Swartz MH. *Textbook of Physical Diagnosis.* 6th ed. Saunders; 2009. C, From Kanski JJ. *Clinical Diagnosis in Ophthalmology.* Mosby; 2006.)

and a slit lamp. Gonioscopy is not a technique normally performed by emergency clinicians.

Systemic effects can develop after the application of eye drops.[23–26] Review the following sections on agents and complications before using these drugs in patients with compromised cardiovascular function.

Agents

Only two dilating agents are really needed in the ED. Phenylephrine (Neo-Synephrine) 2.5%, a potent sympathomimetic, is used for diagnostic dilation of the pupil and visualization of the fundus. The drug is short acting, and because accommodation is not affected, the patient's vision is not altered. Phenylephrine 10% should *not* be used because it can be systemically absorbed and, in rare cases, has caused hypertensive crisis, myocardial infarction, and death.[27,28]

For therapeutic cycloplegia in patients with iritis, 5% homatropine works well. Even though Table 63.2 indicates a maximum duration of 3 days, 24 hours is more common. Therefore 5% homatropine is a useful therapeutic agent for traumatic iritis. Avoid using atropine for traumatic iritis because the undesirable effects of pupillary dilation and blurred vision persist for a week or longer after the associated corneal abrasions have healed. Atropine drops may be prescribed as part of the therapy for nontraumatic iritis after appropriate ophthalmologic consultation. Individuals with lightly pigmented irises tend to have greater sensitivity to cycloplegic agents than do individuals with greater pigmentation; the cycloplegic effect might therefore be more prolonged in people with light eyes. It might be difficult to dilate some patients with deeply pigmented irises, however, and numerous applications of drops might be required.

Malingerers may use mydriatic agents to dilate a pupil unilaterally for the purpose of feigning neurologic disease. Normally, the pupillary dilation caused by intracranial compression of the third cranial nerve will constrict with 2% pilocarpine eye drops. A mydriatic-treated eye can be identified by full motor function of the third cranial nerve and absence of miosis after the instillation of pilocarpine. A fixed and dilated pupil in an awake and alert patient cannot be secondary to brain herniation. Although other neurologic problems may be present, in a normal-appearing patient with a fixed and dilated pupil, a pharmacologic cause is highly likely. It should be noted that legitimate patients may not recall the name of an eye medicine that they used but will usually recall whether the bottle had a red cap, as is found on all cycloplegic solutions marketed in the United States, though these agents are marketed in some countries (e.g., Greece, Türkiye, India) with different colored caps. An unexpected mydriasis in a trusted patient may be the result of such an agent. Medications that constrict the pupil, such as pilocarpine, generally have a green cap. Pressure-lowering drops for glaucoma may be yellow or blue topped (β-blockers), purple topped (adrenergic agents), or orange topped (topical carbonic anhydrase inhibitors).

A fixed and dilated pupil from a pharmacologic cause may be encountered after both nasotracheal and orotracheal intubation (Fig. 63.6). In such ill or injured patients, cerebral herniation must be considered. When phenylephrine is used to constrict the nasal mucosa before nasal intubation (endotracheal tube, nasogastric tube), inadvertent spread to the eye can result in a fixed and dilated pupil. The same scenario may occur during resuscitation when endotracheal epinephrine has been instilled into the lungs and cardiopulmonary resuscitation has expelled epinephrine into the eye. In such scenarios, the affected pupil will not constrict after intraocular pilocarpine administration. Finally, a fixed and dilated pupil might occur as a result of inadvertent contamination of the eye with scopolamine after the application of a scopolamine patch behind the ear.

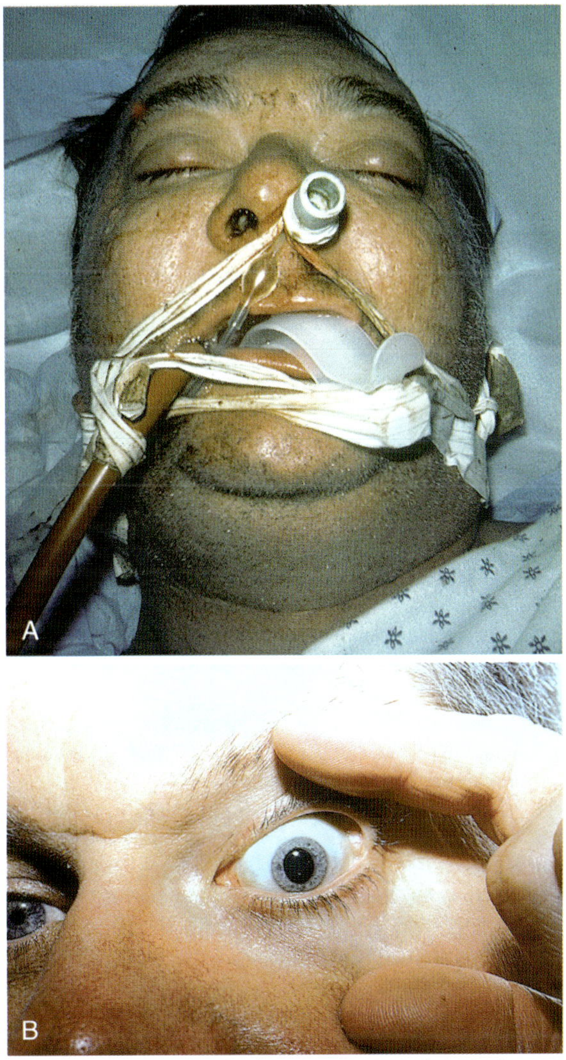

Fig. 63.6 (A) After phenylephrine (Neo-Synephrine) drops were instilled in the nose to facilitate passage of a tube, this comatose patient was nasotracheally intubated for his drug overdose. (B) On a subsequent examination, a unilateral fixed and dilated pupil was noted. Cerebral herniation was suspected. The pupil dilation resulted from Neo-Synephrine nose drops that were snorted from the nose into the eye during intubation and simulated cerebral herniation. Other unusual causes of a fixed and dilated pupil are endotracheal epinephrine expelled from the lungs and splashed onto the eye during cardiopulmonary resuscitation and inadvertent contamination of the eye after the application of a scopolamine patch behind the ear.

Procedure

Instillation of mydriatic agents is similar to the administration of other eye solutions. For medicolegal purposes, note the patient's visual acuity before instillation of the medicine. This documents that any decreased vision noted prior to the procedure is not the result of the mydriatic agent. Whenever

BOX 63.1 Treatment Options for Acute Angle-Closure Glaucoma[a]

Place patient supine; administer analgesics (such as IV morphine titrated to effect) and antiemetics (such as ondansetron 8 mv IV):

1. β-Blocker[b]: Timolol 0.5% (Timoptic), 1 drop to the affected eye, wait 1 minute, and then
2. α-Agonist: Apraclonidine 1% (Iopidine), 1 drop to the affected eye, wait 1 minute, and then
3. Miotic agent: Pilocarpine 2% (Isopto Carpine), 1 drop to the affected eye every 15 minutes for 2 total doses, wait 1 minute after first dose, and then
4. Prednisolone acetate 1%, 1 drop to the affected eye every 15 minutes for 4 total doses
5. Acetazolamide 500 mg IV (may give by mouth, two 250-mg tablets, if IV medication not available)

[a]*Empiric therapy, no controlled trials, based on clinical experience.*
[b]*Relative contraindications: severe bronchospasm, second- to third-degree heart block, uncompensated congestive heart failure.*
Modified from Shields SR. Managing eye disease in primary care. Part 3. When to refer for ophthalmologic care. Postgrad Med. *2000;108(5):99-106.*

dilation is performed, note on the patient's chart the dose and time that agents have been given to avoid confusion during subsequent neurologic evaluation.

Place the patient in a supine or a comfortable semirecumbent position. Instruct the patient to gaze at an object in the upper visual field, such as a fixture on the ceiling. Gently depress the lower lid with a finger on the epidermis. Instill a single drop of the solution into the lower lid fornix and ask the patient to blink to spread the medication. Do not use more than a single drop because it produces reflex tearing and reduces the concentration in contact with the conjunctiva. Forewarn the patient that the medication is uncomfortable when it goes into the eyes. After the medication has been instilled, the patient may blot the eye when it is closed but should not rub it with a tissue. If the desired effect is not noted in 15 to 20 minutes, repeat the dose, but this is seldom required.

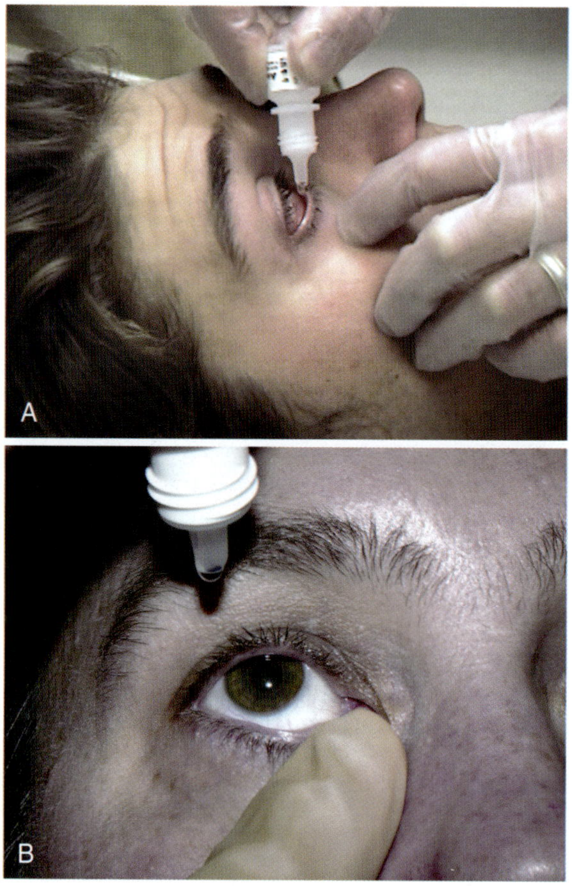

Fig. 63.7 (A) Administration of eye drops. Position the patient with the head tilted back. Direct the patient's gaze upward. Pull the lower lid downward and instill a single drop of medicine in the lower conjunctival fornix. Ensure that the tip of the dropper does not touch the lid or lashes. Instruct the patient to close the eyelids for 1 minute to increase contact of the medicine with the globe and to decrease outflow of medication down the tear duct and over the lid margin. (B) If administering large amounts of eye drops that have systemic effects, such as β-blocker drops, place the operator's index finger under the inferior eyelid along the nasal borders of the eye and firmly compress the nasolacrimal duct against the globe for a few minutes, thereby preventing migration of the drops into the nose and reducing systemic absorption.

Complications

Any dilator can precipitate an attack of angle-closure glaucoma in susceptible patients.[29] In the case of angle-closure glaucoma, it may take several hours before symptoms become evident. The patient often complains of smoky vision with "halos" around lights, as well as an aching pain that at times can be quite severe. Nausea and vomiting may occur. If the affected eye becomes injected in association with a hazy cornea, exhibits elevated pressure on tonometry, or develops an oval shape or fixed pupil on reassessment, consult an ophthalmologist immediately. Place the patient supine and administer analgesics and antiemetics. Treatment usually includes the agents suggested in Box 63.1, and later, definitive laser or surgical procedures.

Be aware that if contaminated, an eye medication can introduce infection. Most solutions contain bactericidal ingredients, but contamination of the tips of droppers can still occur (Fig. 63.7A).[30] Use only newly opened bottles of eye medication or single-use vials, particularly if the patient has a deep corneal injury or has recently undergone eye surgery. Promptly discard out-of-date drops and those in which crust or other material is found around the nozzle.

Forewarn the patient that any cycloplegic (in contrast to a sympathomimetic) will blur a patient's near vision. Vision will be less blurred in adults older than 45 years, who generally have a reduced ability to focus for near vision. Although most adults will be able to drive safely, even with both eyes affected, it is advisable to have someone else drive whenever feasible. Light sensitivity caused by pupillary dilation may also be bothersome; sunglasses are sufficient for this problem.

Systemic reactions are rare if using appropriate dilutions of sympathomimetic and cycloplegic eye drops.[23–29] In one report of 33 cases of adverse reactions associated with 10% phenylephrine, there were 15 myocardial infarctions (11 deaths), 7 cases of precipitation of angle-closure glaucoma, and a variety of systemic cardiovascular or neurologic reactions.[28]

After instillation of eye drops into the conjunctival sac, systemic absorption can occur through the conjunctival capillaries. Systemic absorption may also occur via nasal mucosa, the oral pharynx, and the gastrointestinal tract after passage through the lacrimal drainage system. Mucosal hyperemia enhances absorption. Symptoms can often be avoided by maintaining digital pressure on the nasal canthus to occlude the puncta for several minutes after administration (see Fig. 63.7B).[23]

FLUORESCEIN EXAMINATION

See Video 63.2. Perform fluorescein staining of the eye as part of the evaluation of patients with eye trauma and concern for infection. It is a quick and easy technique that is crucial for the proper diagnosis and management of common eye emergencies. View the fluorescein-stained cornea and conjunctiva under a "blue" light and ideally in conjunction with slit lamp magnification (see later section on "Slit Lamp Examination").

Sodium fluorescein is a water-soluble chemical that fluoresces. It absorbs light in the blue wavelengths and emits the energy in the longer green wavelengths. It fluoresces in an alkaline environment (such as in Bowman's membrane, which is located below the corneal epithelium) but not in an acidic environment (such as in the tear film over intact corneal epithelium). Thus it is useful in revealing even minute abrasions on the cornea.

Fluorescein solutions should be avoided in the ED due to possible contamination with *Pseudomonas*.[31] Use fluorescein-impregnated paper strips.

Indications and Contraindications

Fluorescein staining is indicated for the evaluation of suspected abrasions, FBs, and infections of the eye, including "simple" cases of conjunctivitis, which may actually be herpetic keratitis. Exposure of the face to pepper spray has been associated with corneal abrasions. These patients should undergo fluorescein staining and be subsequently evaluated under magnification, ideally with a slit lamp.[32] Corneal defects may be seen after even a few seconds of unprotected viewing of a welder's arc flame.

Fluorescein permanently stains soft contact lenses. Therefore when fluorescein is used soft contact lenses should be removed before instilling the fluorescein. Caution patients to avoid replacing contact lenses for several hours after the procedure to avoid accidental contamination and possible visual disturbance. Topically administered fluorescein is considered nontoxic, although reactions to a fluorescein-containing solution (not impregnated strips) have been described. These reports, which consist of vagal reactions[33] and generalized convulsions,[34] are rare, not rigorously supported, and believed to be caused by agents other than fluorescein in the solution.

In addition, be aware that fluorescein dye may enter the anterior chamber of the eye in patients with deep corneal defects. This form of intraocular fluorescein accumulation is nontoxic. When the anterior chamber is viewed under the blue filter of the slit lamp, a fluorescein "flare" is visible and should not be confused with the flare reaction noted with iritis.

Procedure

Theoretically, one should avoid use of topical anesthetics before fluorescein staining because superficial punctate keratitis may develop in some patients from the anesthetic, which can confuse the diagnosis. However, in patients who are tearing profusely and squeezing their eyes shut from an abrasion or an FB, the examination is often impossible if a topical anesthetic is not first used. Thus it is practical to apply a local anesthetic before instilling fluorescein.

Grasp the fluorescein strip by the nonorange end and wet the orange end with 1 drop of saline. Several convenient forms are available, including a small bottle of artificial tears or a 5-mL "bullet" or "fish" of normal saline commonly used for nebulizer treatments. Alternatively, wet the strip with tap water or the recently used local anesthetic drops. Once the strip is moistened, place it gently on the inside of the patient's lower lid (Fig. 63.8, *step 1*). The patient should be instructed not to blink with the strip in place. Withdraw the strip and ask the patient to blink, which spreads the fluorescein over the surface of the eye. The key to a good examination is to have a thin layer of fluorescein over the corneal and conjunctival surfaces. If the strip is too heavily moistened before placing it in the lower fornix, the eye may become flooded with the solution, which makes evaluation difficult. If too much dye accumulates, the patient can remove the excess dye by blotting the closed eye with a tissue. Conversely, placing a dry strip in an unanesthetized eye may be irritating. Next, use a Wood's lamp (magnification ×4), the blue filter of a slit lamp, or simply a penlight with a blue filter to examine the eye in a darkened room (see Fig. 63.8, *step 2*). Check for areas of bright green fluorescence on the corneal and conjunctival surfaces. The naked eye may not be able to see small defects. Ideally, use a slit lamp with magnification ×10 or ×25 to examine the stained cornea before ruling out a pathologic process. A handheld magnification device, the Eidolon Bluminator ophthalmic illuminator (Eidolon Optical, LLC), produces an intense blue light from a light-emitting diode with 7.5× magnification (see Fig. 63.8, *step 3*). After completion of the fluorescein examination, irrigate excess dye from the eye to minimize damage to the patient's clothing from dye-stained tears.

The Seidel test uses fluorescein to detect perforation of the eye.[35] To perform this test, instill a large amount of fluorescein onto the eye by profusely wetting the strip. Examine the eye for a small stream of fluid leaking from the globe (see Fig. 63.8, *plate 4*). This stream will fluoresce blue or green, in contrast to the orange appearance of the rest of the globe flooded with fluorescein.

Interpretation

Fluorescein is used primarily for evaluation of corneal injuries. Although conjunctival abrasions pick up the stain, most of the staining on the conjunctiva represents patches of mucus rather than a real pathologic condition. Corneal staining is more specific for injury, and the pattern of injury often reflects the original insult.

Corneal staining patterns are illustrated in Figs. 63.8 and 63.9. Abrasions usually occur in the central part of the cornea because of the limited protection of closure of the patient's eyelids. The margins of the abrasions are usually sharp and linear if seen in the first 24 hours (see Fig. 63.8, *plate 6*). Circular defects are seen about embedded FBs and may persist for up to 48 hours after removal of a superficial foreign object. Deeply embedded objects may be associated with defects persisting for longer than 48 hours. Objects under the upper lid (including some chalazia) often produce vertical linear lesions on the upper surface of the cornea (see Fig. 63.8, *plate 7*). When

Fluorescein Examination

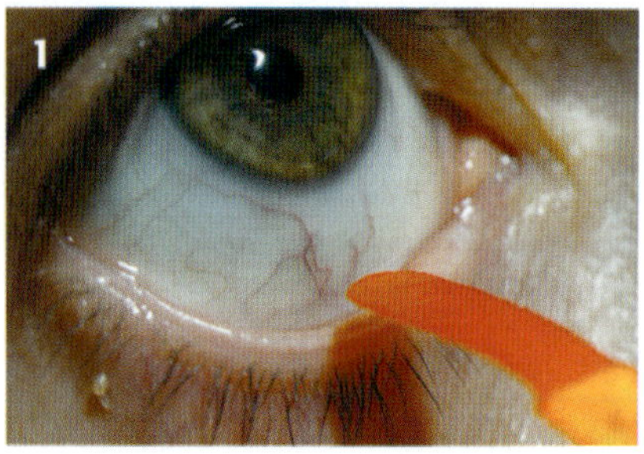

Moisten the fluorescein strip with 1 drop of saline or topical anesthetic. Depress the lower lid and gently place a wetted strip onto the inside of the patient's lower lid so that only the smallest amount is instilled.

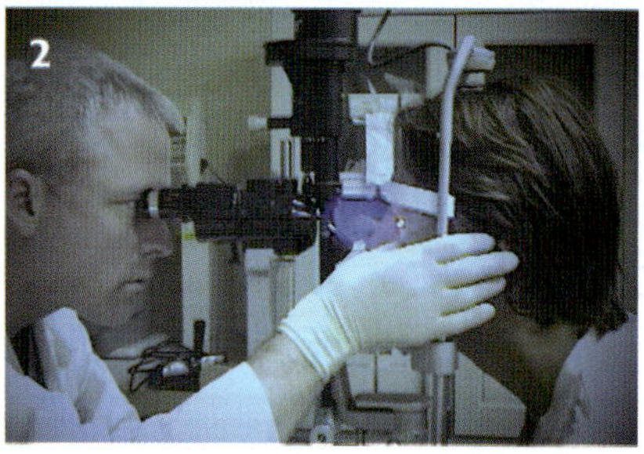

Examine the eye with a Wood's lamp or a slit lamp with a cobalt blue filter (shown). Check for areas of bright green fluorescence on the corneal and conjunctival surfaces. Because the naked eyes may not be able to appreciate small defects, magnification should be used.

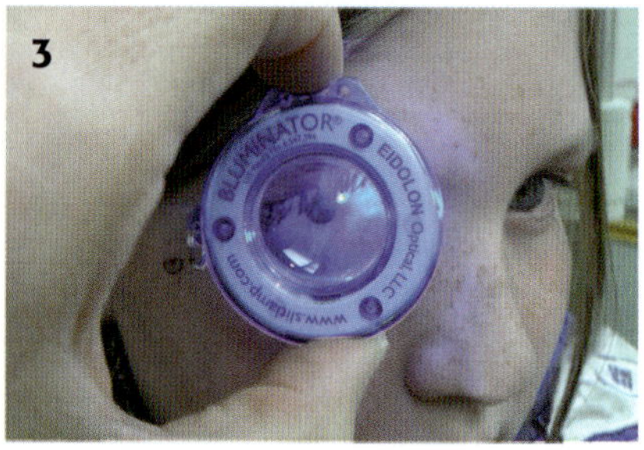

The Eidolon Bluminator ophthalmic illuminator provides an intense blue LED light with 7· magnification.

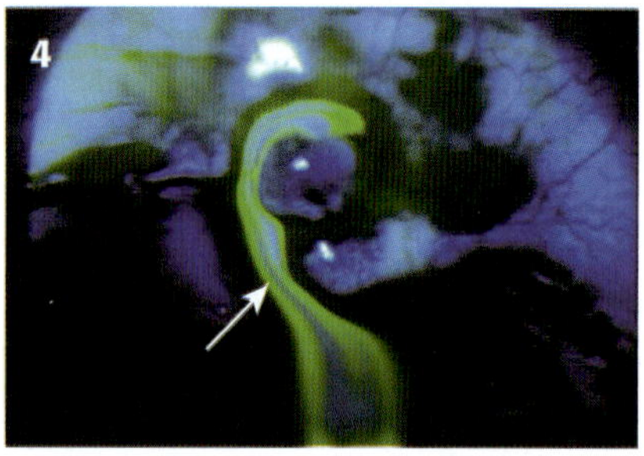

Positive Seidel test. Fluorescein seen streaming down the cornea indicates an open-globe injury.

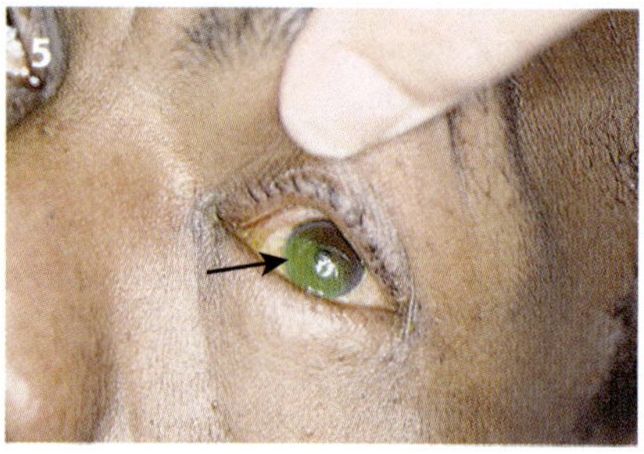

Large corneal abrasion seen with the naked eye. Smaller abrasions or corneal injuries produced by keratitis or a welder's arc flash require slit lamp evaluation to identify minor corneal defects.

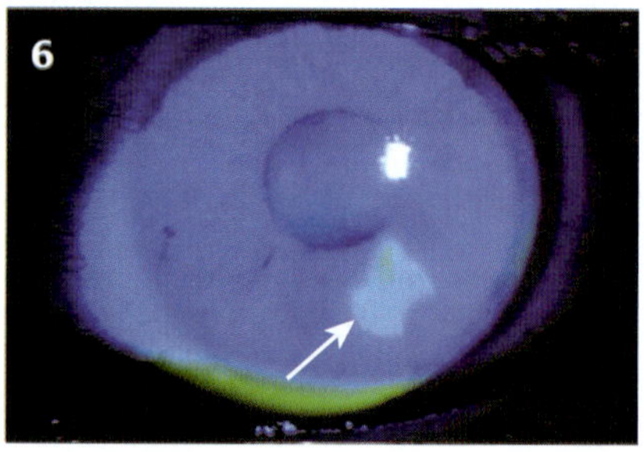

Corneal abrasion as seen via a slit lamp. A moderate-sized abrasion *(arrow)* is revealed by fluorescein staining and blue light.

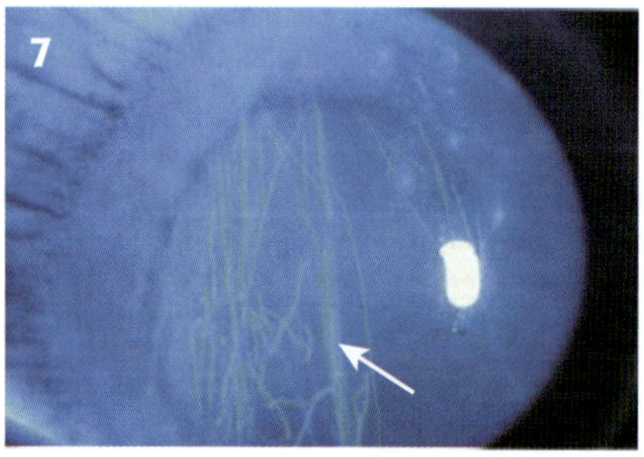

Vertical linear abrasions. These types of abrasions are typically caused by a foreign body trapped under the upper eyelid.

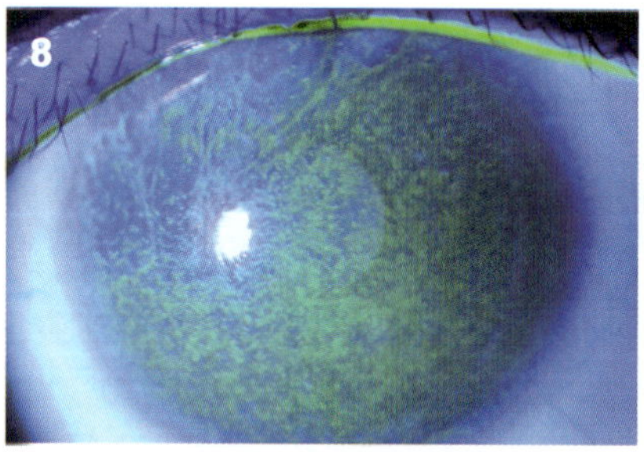

Superficial punctate keratitis. These diffuse, shallow corneal irregularities are caused by chemical irritation, viral illnesses, exposure to bright light, and many other conditions.

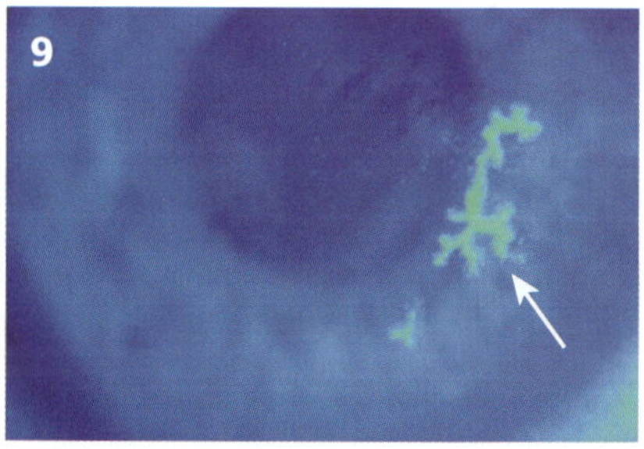

Herpes simplex keratitis. A classic herpetic epithelial dendritic lesion is seen on this fluorescein examination.

Fig. 63.8 The fluorescein examination. Excessive fluorescein may obscure subtle findings and thus should be avoided. Fluorescein will permanently stain contact lenses if they are not removed. *LED*, Light-emitting diode. (Panel 4, From Krachmer JH, Mannis M, Holland E, eds. *Cornea*. 3rd ed. Mosby; 2010. Panel 6, From Friedman NJ, Raiser PK, Pineda R. *Massachusetts Ear & Eye Infirmary Illustrated Manual of Ophthalmology*. 3rd ed. Saunders; 2009. Panel 7, From Kliegman R, Stanton B, Behman R et al., eds. *Nelson Textbook of Pediatrics*. 19th ed. Saunders; 2011. Panel 9, From Palay DA, Krachmer JH, eds. *Primary Care Ophthalmology: Concepts and Clinical Practice*. 2nd ed. Mosby; 2005.)

vertical lesions are noted, search diligently for a retained FB under the upper lid. Overuse of hard contact lenses diminishes the nutrient supply to the cornea. The central part of the cornea sustains the most injury and thus fluoresces brightly when stained. Excessive exposure to ultraviolet light as a result of sunlamp abuse, snow blindness, or welding flashes produces a superficial punctate keratitis, which in its mildest form may not be visible without a slit lamp (see Fig. 63.8, *plate 8*). The central part of the cornea is the least protected by the lids, and a central, horizontal band–like keratitis can result. Herpetic

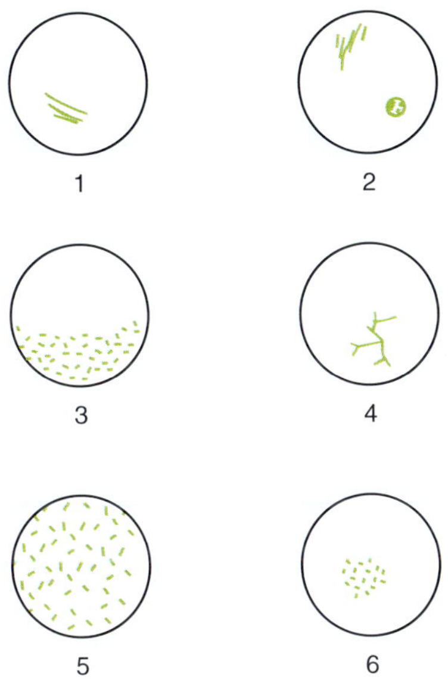

Fig. 63.9 Patterns of acute corneal injury. *1*, Traumatic abrasion, usually with linear features and sharp borders when seen early (<24 hours), occurs more in the central part of the cornea. *2*, Abrasion from a foreign body (FB). Vertical abrasions on the upper part of the cornea are seen when an FB is embedded in the upper lid. Also shown is a rust ring with a metallic FB. *3*, Exposure pattern seen with prolonged exposure to ultraviolet light (e.g., welding flash, sunlamp exposure). A bandlike keratitis is produced over the lower half of the cornea. Squinting in the setting of the bright light protected the upper corneal surface. *4*, Herpes simplex keratitis, classic dendritic pattern. *5*, Adenovirus keratitis. Diffuse minute corneal staining is seen in patients with epidemic keratoconjunctivitis approximately 7 days after the onset of symptoms. *6*, Contact lens overuse, central punctate staining. (From Knoop K, Trott A. Ophthalmologic procedures in the emergency department—part III: slit lamp use and foreign bodies, *Acad Emerg Med.* 1995;2:227.)

lesions may develop anywhere on the cornea. Classically, these lesions are dendritic, although ulcers may also be punctate or stellate (see Fig. 63.8, *plate 9*).

Any area of corneal staining with an infiltrate or opacification beneath or around the lesion should alert the practitioner to the possibility of a viral, bacterial, or fungal keratitis (see Fig 63.9). Obtain urgent ophthalmologic consultation so that cultures of the possible etiologic agents can be procured, and appropriate treatment initiated.

Many *Pseudomonas* organisms fluoresce when exposed to ultraviolet light[36]; therefore the presence of fluorescence before the instillation of fluorescein in a red eye should suggest the possibility of infection with this organism.

Summary

Fluorescein staining is a quick and easy diagnostic procedure that should be considered for every eye evaluation. The extra time that the examination takes provides a wealth of diagnostic information on patients with eye trauma or infection. No complications are associated with the procedure with the exceptions being reactions noted with the fluorescein solution, possible discoloration of soft contact lenses, and the potential for infection when premixed solutions rather than fluorescein-impregnated paper strips are used.

EYE IRRIGATION

See Videos 63.3 and 63.4. The crucial first step in the treatment of chemical injuries to the eye is irrigation. Irrigate as clinically appropriate for the severity, length of exposure, and causative agent. Serious chemical injury to the eye requires irrigation as soon as possible. Irrigation at the site where the exposure occurred should be performed before the patient is brought to the ED. Corneal injury can occur within seconds of contact, especially with an alkaline substance. Continue eye irrigation in the ED.

This section discusses methods of irrigation. Although it is best to irrigate liberally, copious irrigation is not needed when the patient's eye has been exposed to a small amount of a noncaustic, nonalkaline compound in the eye.

Indications and Contraindications

Irrigation is indicated for all acute chemical injuries involving the eyes. Irrigation may also be therapeutic in patients with an FB sensation but no visible FB. Small, unseen foreign material in the conjunctival tissues may be flushed out with irrigation. There is no contraindication to eye irrigation, but in patients with a possible perforating injury, perform the irrigation especially gently and carefully.

Equipment

The following equipment is necessary for eye irrigation:

- Topical anesthetic, such as 0.5% proparacaine
- Sterile irrigating solution (warmed intravenous saline or lactated Ringer's [LR] solution* or Balance Saline Solution Plus [Alcon Laboratories] in a bag with tubing)
- A basin to catch the fluid
- Cotton-tipped applicators
- Gauze pads to help hold the patient's lids open
- Lid retractors
- Irrigating device (e.g., nasal cannula tubing [Morgan Therapeutic Lens], modified central venous catheter [Eye Irrigator]) for prolonged irrigation
- Optimal: 10 mL of 1% lidocaine added to a liter of irrigating fluid

Procedure

Basic Technique

First, instill a topical anesthetic into the eye (Fig. 63.10, *step 1*). Evert the eyelid and sweep out any particulate matter in the conjunctival fornices with a moistened, cotton-tipped applicator (see later section on "Ocular FB Removal" and Fig. 63.10, *step 2*). Hold the eyelids open during irrigation (see Fig. 63.10, *step 3*). The easiest method is to use gauze pads to grasp the wet, slippery lids and hold them open. If the patient has severe blepharospasm, consider using lid retractors (Desmarres [Sklar Surgical Instruments]) or paper clip retractors (Fig. 63.11). When lid retractors are used, be certain that the eye is well anesthetized, that the retractors do not injure the globe or the lids, and that chemicals are not harbored under

*A balanced salt solution designed for eye irrigation is preferred by some (when available) and may produce less corneal edema with chemical injuries. Readily available normal saline and lactated Ringer's solution are equally well tolerated.

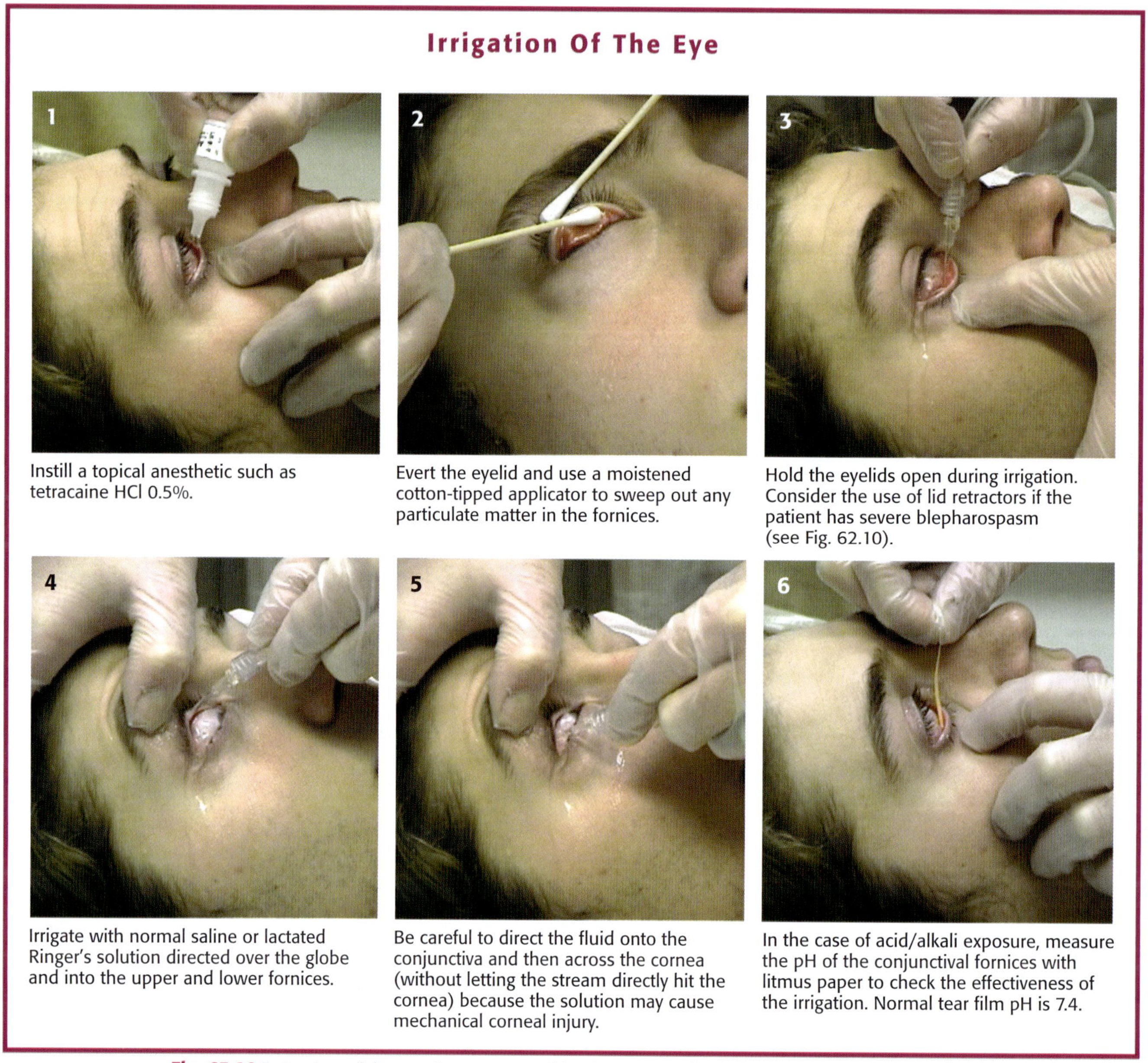

Fig. 63.10 Irrigation of the eye. Intravenous tubing is connected to a liter bag of saline or Ringer's solution, and irrigation occurs at a wide-open rate.

the retractors. Be aware that simple retractors fashioned from metal paper clips (especially those that are nickel plated and shiny) may have surface chipping, which can create an ocular FB.[37] Exercise caution to avoid ocular injury when utilizing a makeshift retractor.

An ipsilateral facial nerve block may be used for severe blepharospasm (Fig. 63.12). To avoid swelling of periorbital tissue, block the facial nerve just anterior to the condyloid process of the ipsilateral mandible. Place a subcutaneous line of anesthetic (2% lidocaine without epinephrine) to temporarily paralyze the orbicularis muscle.

Irrigate with normal saline or LR solution directed over the globe and into the upper and lower fornices (see Fig. 63.10, *step 4*). The choice of fluid initially is less important than initiating irrigation as rapidly as possible. If tap water is available at the scene of the injury, begin irrigation immediately with copious amounts of fluid before transporting the patient to the hospital. Teach out-of-hospital care providers to irrigate all acid injuries of the eye for at least 5 minutes at the scene and to irrigate all alkali injuries for at least 15 minutes.[38] LR or normal saline solution is preferred over tap water or 5% dextrose in free water for eye irrigation because these solutions are isotonic and do not contain dextrose. Dextrose can be quite sticky if spilled and might serve as a nutrient for an opportunistic bacterial infection. Although one clinical trial found a balanced salt solution less painful in patients with a chemical eye injury,[39] another volunteer study on uninjured eyes found that LR solution is better tolerated than normal saline and balanced saline solution when used with a Morgan lens.[40] Warmed fluids are also better tolerated than fluids at room temperature.[41] Warmed LR solution should be considered as first line when readily available for emergent eye irrigation.

Be careful to direct the irrigating stream onto the conjunctiva and then across the cornea without letting the stream splash directly onto the cornea because striking the eye with

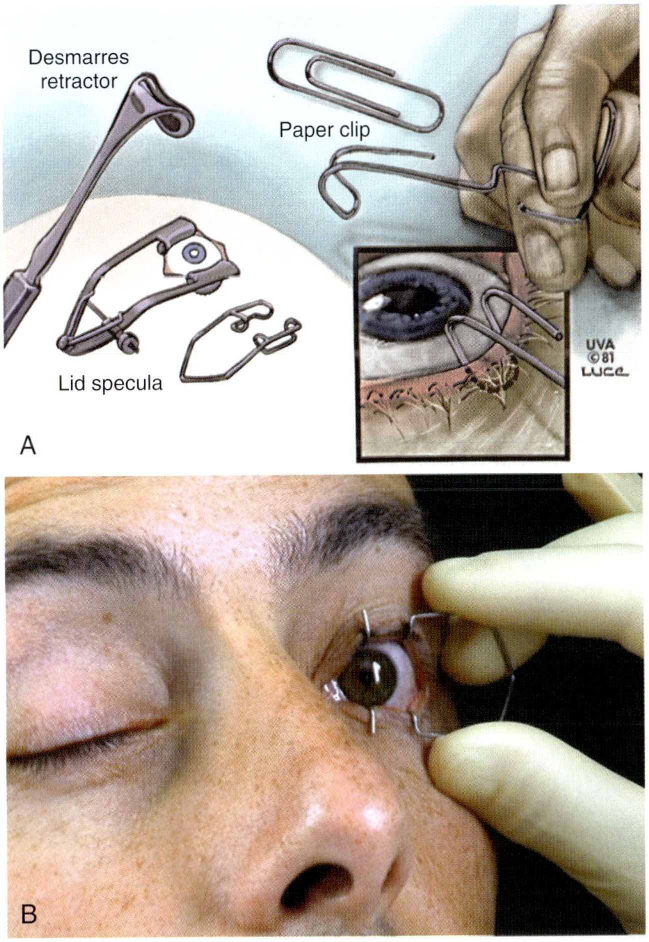

Fig. 63.11 Devices for separating eyelids. (A) A Desmarres retractor, lid specula, or retractor improvised from a paper clip allows active manipulation of the lids. Free-standing specula may require a seventh nerve block to reduce the blepharospasm. (B) Lid retractor in place. (A, From Fogle JA, Spyker DA. Management of chemical and drug injury to the eye. In: Haddad LM, Winchester JF, eds. *Clinical Management of Poisoning and Drug Overdose*. 2nd ed. Saunders; 1990.)

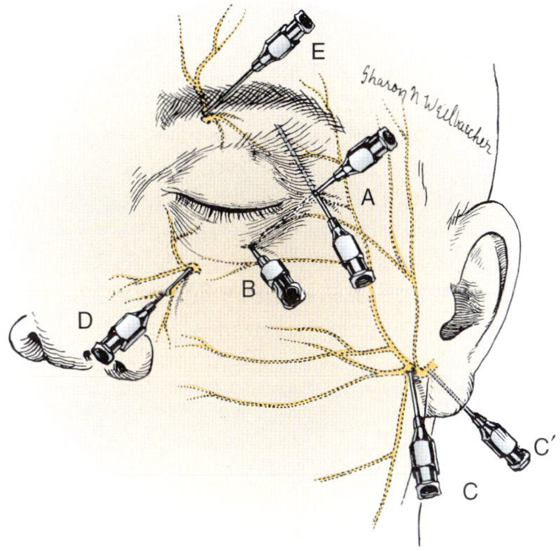

Fig. 63.12 Injection points for facial and orbital anesthesia and akinesia. *A*, Van Lint technique for infiltration of the orbicularis. *B*, Retrobulbar injection site. *C*, O'Brien facial nerve block. *C′*, Alternative facial nerve block by injection into the tympanomastoid fissure. *D*, Infraorbital sensory block. *E*, Supraorbital sensory block. Injection of the orbicularis (*A*) or facial nerve (*C* or *C′*) permits examination and treatment of the eye in the setting of severe blepharospasm. Anesthetic is placed within several millimeters of the nerves. (From Deutsch TA, Feller DB, eds. *Paton and Goldberg's Management of Ocular Injuries*. 2nd ed. Saunders; 1985:17.)

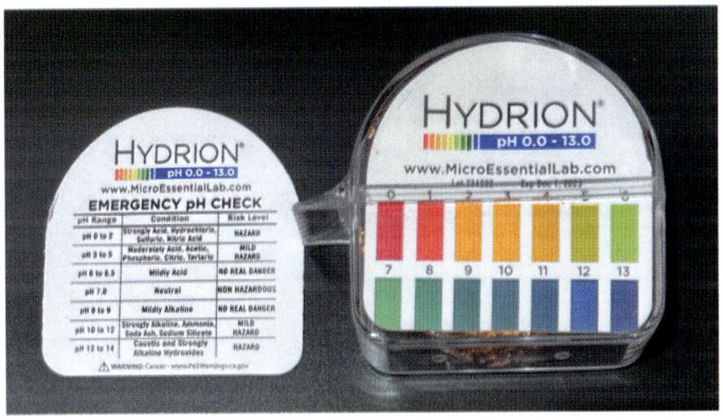

Fig. 63.13 Full-spectrum pH paper for use in chemical eye exposure.

the solution can in itself be harmful and cause mechanical injury (see Fig. 63.10, *step 5*). Direct irrigation of the cornea can result in the development of a superficial punctate epithelial keratopathy.

Before irrigation, instill anesthetic eye drops, such as 0.5% tetracaine. Adding 10 mL of 1% lidocaine to a liter of irrigating fluid can decrease the patient's discomfort during prolonged irrigation.

Duration of Irrigation

The duration of irrigation is best determined by the extent of the exposure and the causative agent. Acids are quickly neutralized by proteins in the surface tissues of the eye and, once irrigated out, cause no further damage. The only exceptions are hydrofluoric and heavy metal acids, which can penetrate through the cornea. Alkalis can penetrate rapidly and, if not removed, will continue to produce damage for days because of slow dissociation of the cation from combination with proteins. Therefore prolonged irrigation is indicated and at least 2 L of solution should be used. Although rapid flushing with the first 500 mL is prudent, slow continuous irrigation, as discussed later, at a rate sufficient to generate a continuous trickle is often more effective and better tolerated than continued high-volume flushing. If the nature of the offending agent is unknown or in question, use prolonged irrigation.

Consult ophthalmology for all alkaline, hydrofluoric acid, and heavy metal acid injuries. Irrigation on an inpatient basis may be required for a period of 24 hours or longer, especially when the cornea is hazy or obviously thickened. Note that the magnesium contained in sparklers combines with water from tears to produce magnesium hydroxide.[42] Treat such fireworks injuries as alkaline injuries rather than as thermal injuries. Treat eye damage from hair straighteners,[43] phosphate-free detergents,[44] and automobile air bags[45] as alkaline injuries as well.

Measure the pH of the conjunctival fornices with a pH paper strip to check the effectiveness of irrigation (see Fig. 63.10, *step 6*). Use full-spectrum pH paper (nitrazine paper present in many EDs to assess rupture of membranes in pregnant patients has a narrow range of 4.5 to 7.5) (Fig. 63.13). Also, the pH indicator on urine multi-indicator sticks can be used after cutting off distal indicator squares with scissors, leaving the pH indicator at the end of the stick. Normal tear film is slightly alkalotic with a pH of 7.4. Use the noninjured eye as a control if the results are equivocal. If the pH measured in the conjunctival fornices is still abnormal after the initial irrigation, continue to irrigate. If the pH is normal after irrigation, wait 20 minutes and check it again to make sure that it remains normal, especially if alkaline contamination has occurred. Delayed changes in pH are usually the result of incomplete irrigation and inadequate swabbing of the fornices. In anticipation of this deficiency, measure the pH deep in the fornices. Consider double-lid eversion with a lid elevator to expose the upper fornix for swabbing, irrigation, and pH testing.

Prolonged Irrigation

Alkaline burns may require prolonged irrigation, and it is essential to consult ophthalmology in such cases. The Morgan Therapeutic Lens is a contact lens–type irrigation device that can provide slow, continuous irrigation once the more vigorous initial irrigation has been completed (Fig. 63.14). First, anesthetize the eye with topical anesthetic drops. Then place the device carefully on the surface of the eye with the lids closed around the intravenous tubing adapter. Attach the intravenous tubing to the adapter and provide continuous flow through the device onto the cornea and into the fornices. As the local anesthetic agents wash out during the irrigation process, the device can become uncomfortable, so reapply the anesthetic drops frequently during irrigation for patient comfort. Such short-term use of local anesthetics will not inhibit healing of the cornea.

Another option for prolonged irrigation if a Morgan Therapeutic Lens is not available, or not tolerated by the patient, is nasal cannula prongs with IV tubing. Connect standard nasal cannula oxygen tubing to IV fluid tubing. The oxygen

Morgan Lens Irrigation

1

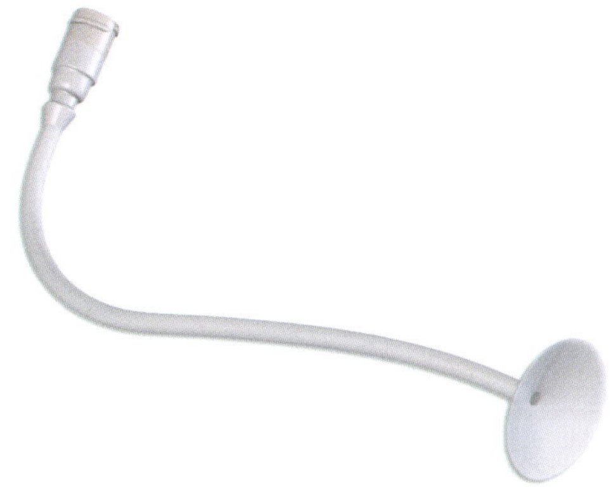

The Morgan therapeutic lens is a contact lens–type irrigation device that can provide slow, continuous irrigation once the more vigorous initial irrigation has been done.

2

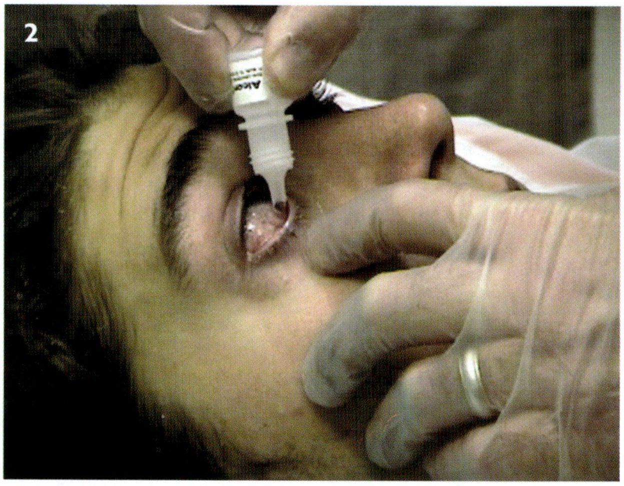

Prior to insertion, anesthetize the eyes with topical anesthetic drops such as tetracaine HCl 0.5%. The anesthetic will wash out during the irrigation process, so reapply frequently for patient comfort.

3

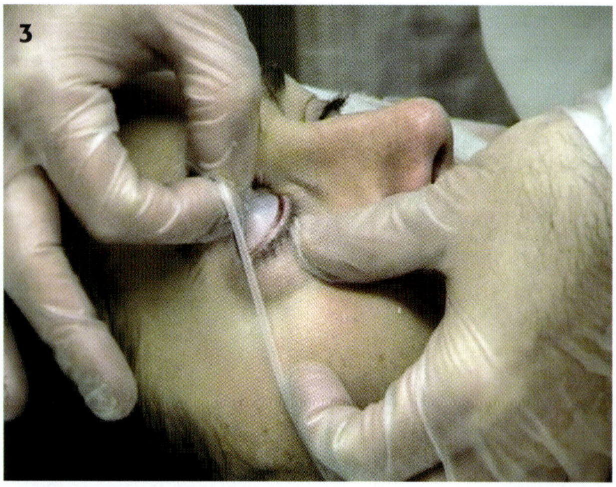

Carefully place the device on the surface of the eye with the lids closed around the intravenous tubing adaptor.

4

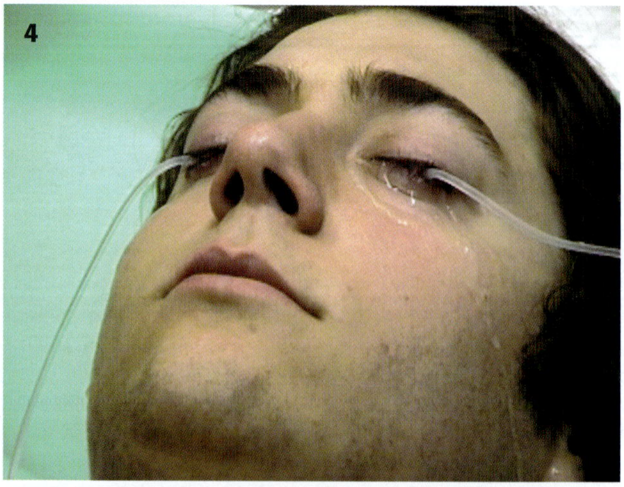

Attach the adaptor to intravenous tubing and provide continuous flow through the device onto the cornea and into the fornices. Bilateral irrigation is easily achieved with this technique.

Fig. 63.14 Morgan lens irrigation. A liter bag of saline or Ringer's solution is connected to the Morgan lens with intravenous tubing and irrigated at a wide-open rate.

connection site of the nasal cannula should fit snuggly into the IV fluid tubing extension. Connect the opposite end of the IV fluid tubing to a sterile irrigation solution of your choosing, as you would for IV fluid infusion. Rest the nasal cannula prongs over the bridge of the patient's nose with the prongs pointing toward the epicanthal folds. Allow the irrigation solution to hang on an IV pole and flow to gravity. Placing the patient in a supine position with towels and a basin behind the head can avoid excess pooling of fluid on the patient or surrounding area.

Complications

The only significant complication from irrigation is abrasion of the cornea or the conjunctiva. This can be a mechanical injury from trying to keep the lids open in an uncooperative patient, a small corneal epithelial defect from a Morgan irrigating lens, or fine punctate keratitis from the irrigation itself.[46] For this reason, do not direct the stream directly onto the cornea. If a superficial corneal defect occurs, treat it in the usual manner. Deep or penetrating corneal injuries are likely to be a result of the caustic chemical and require emergency ophthalmologic consultation. Continue to provide slow continuous irrigation pending arrival of the ophthalmologist. Some experimental evidence suggests that massive parenteral or oral ascorbic acid supplementation may prevent the development of deep corneal injury,[47] but such treatment has not gained universal acceptance.

Summary

Eye irrigation is easy, and complications associated with the technique are usually minimal. At times the clinician may be unsure whether a chemical injury is toxic enough to warrant irrigation. If any doubt exists, err on the side of irrigating the eye rather than omitting this vital procedure and risking progression of the eye injury.

GLOBE PROTECTION AND EVALUATION

In the evaluation of a patient in whom a penetrating injury to the globe is suspected, perform a careful expeditious examination of the eye, preferably with a slit lamp. Avoid any pressure on the eye or rapid eye movements. If perforation is obvious (e.g., teardrop pupil, flaccid globe, flat anterior chamber, prolapsed iris) or confirmed by slit lamp (positive Seidel test; see Fig. 63.8, *plate 4*), do not perform any procedures (except perhaps irrigation or ultrasound; see later) and consult ophthalmology early for definitive diagnosis and care (Fig. 63.15). Until the ophthalmologist arrives, protect the eye from further harm by keeping the patient quiet, elevating the head of the bed, and placing a protective shield over the eye. Commercial shields are available for this purpose. When a metal shield is not available, construct a makeshift protective shield with the material available (e.g., paper, plastic, or Styrofoam cups; Fig. 63.16). The protective shield helps avoid pressure on the globe and overlying tissue and assists in preventing extrusion

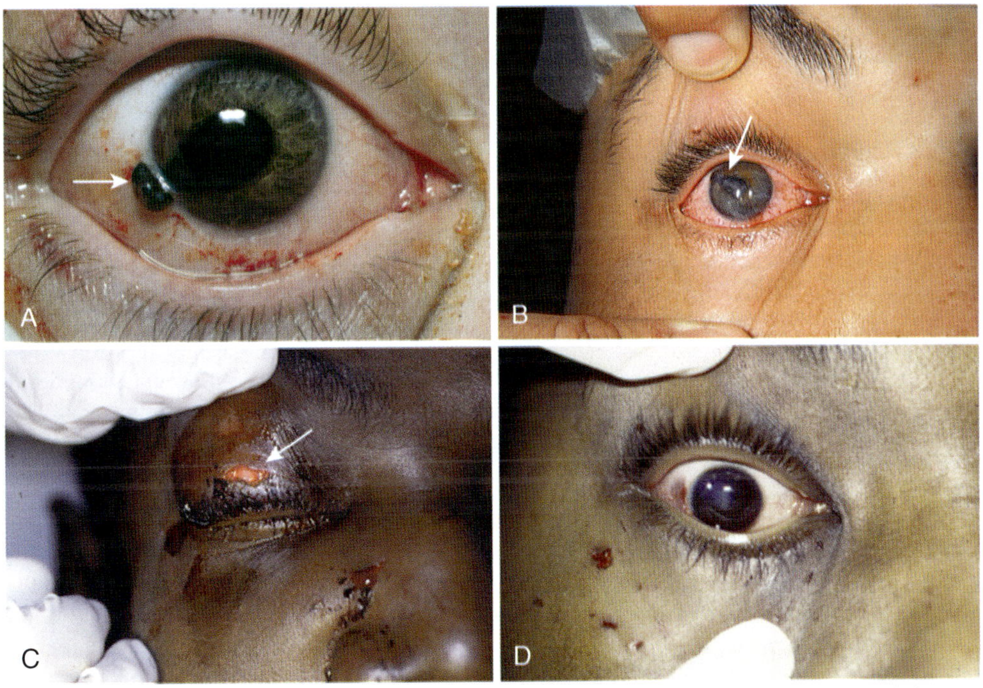

Fig. 63.15 Serious eye injuries. (A) Corneal laceration with prolapse of the iris. The extruded iris is dark and mimics a corneal foreign body *(arrow)*. Frequently, the only clue is an abnormal pupil, and the extruded iris may not be appreciated as intraocular tissue. The pupil is irregular (often pear or teardrop shaped) and points toward the laceration. (B) A pear-shaped pupil without protrusion of the lens is a more subtle, yet characteristic indication of a perforated globe *(arrow)*. (C) Another indication of a penetrating globe injury is periorbital fat protruding from an upper eyelid laceration *(arrow)*. This patient was stabbed with a knife. (D) This patient has an obviously cloudy lens soon after trauma. A projectile entered the temporal portion of the globe and produced a seemingly minor scleral hemorrhage. Patients with penetrating injuries to the globe should be treated with systemic antibiotics (such as a combination of cefazolin and gentamicin), tetanus toxoid if indicated, and antiemetics to control vomiting (which raises intraocular pressure). (A, Courtesy Lawrence B. Stack, MD.)

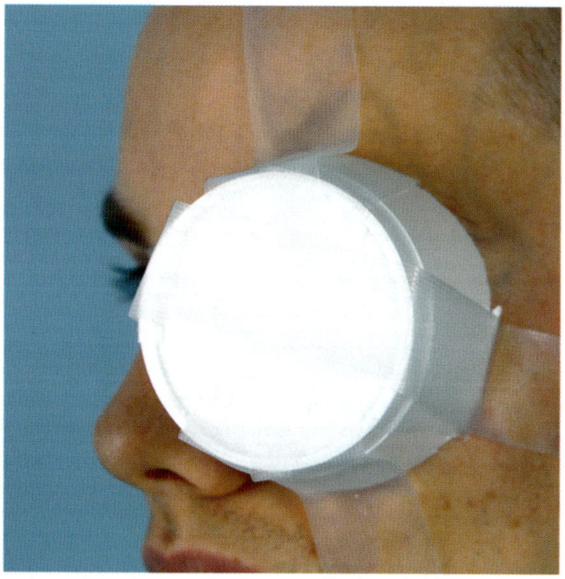

Fig. 63.16 When a penetrating globe injury is suspected and a metal shield is not available in the emergency department or prehospital setting, a makeshift shield can be fashioned with available material. A paper cup was used to fashion this shield.

of vitreous and other ocular contents. Extend the edges of the shield up to or beyond the bony orbital rim for this purpose. Apply adhesive tape over the shield from the forehead to the cheek to secure the shield in position.

If a patient has a globe perforation, treat with systemic antibiotics (a combination of cefazolin and gentamicin is a good initial choice), tetanus toxoid, and antiemetics in doses aggressive enough to halt vomiting.

OCULAR ULTRASOUND

See Videos 63.5 and 63.6. ED ocular ultrasonography has markedly advanced the emergency physician's (EP's) ability to quickly address important ocular conditions. Many studies have demonstrated that with proper training and equipment, EPs are competent, and care is improved by using this noninvasive technology at the bedside.[48–51]

Indications and Contraindications

Bedside ED ocular ultrasonography may be appropriately used as an adjunct in the evaluation of altered vision, suspected FB, ocular pain, headache, eye trauma, head injury, or altered mental status. Conditions that are reliably diagnosed include globe rupture, intraocular FB, vitreous hemorrhage, lens dislocation, retinal detachment, vitreous detachment, and elevated intraocular pressure (IOP).

The only absolute contraindications for bedside ED ocular ultrasound is an obvious open globe. Given proper equipment, an experienced sonographer, and a cooperative patient, an ED ocular ultrasound can be performed. The evaluation of a potential open globe deserves special mention. Whereas it is generally true that the eye should be protected from further manipulation after suspecting an open globe, evaluation with bedside ED ocular ultrasound is the exception. It is imperative that the EP performing the bedside ultrasound be mindful of the possibility of an open globe and utilizes the *no-pressure technique* described later. An immediate benefit is gained when the EP carefully uses this technique to avoid a delay in diagnosis and treatment. Any delay incurs an increased risk of adverse outcome. In general, the benefit obtained from the use of bedside ED ocular ultrasound outweighs the risk of further examination of the eye in this setting. However, if the physical examination obviously suggests open globe pathology, the clinician is discouraged from performing this procedure, as it carries the risk of vitreous extrusion (even with minimal globe compression) with little benefit to the diagnostic evaluation.

Equipment

Appropriate ultrasound machine with linear array transducer, 7.5 to 10 MHz or higher.

Procedure

Ensure ultrasound equipment is clean and disinfected. Adjust the setting on the machine for ocular ultrasound. Place the patient in a recumbent or semireclined position to minimize runoff of gel. Instruct the patient to keep eyes closed, but not clenched, to look straight ahead, and not to move the eyes. It has been suggested that the closed eye be covered with a large piece of clear Tegaderm dressing (3M) to facilitate the ultrasound examination without contaminating it with gel or the probe. However, a randomized study by Marks et al found that Tegaderm was associated with reduced image quality and there was no significant difference in patient discomfort, suggesting that ocular ultrasound is best performed without the use of Tegaderm.[52] Place a copious amount of gel over the closed eyelid to be examined, enough to completely fill the sulcus formed by the eye so that the transducer can touch the gel in a transverse plane without touching the eyelid and without breaking contact of the transducer with the gel (Fig. 63.17). Hold the transducer in such a way so that the examiner's hand can stabilize the probe against movement by resting the hand on the patient's forehead, bridge of the nose, or maxilla (Fig. 63.18). Barely touch the probe to the gel without applying pressure to the eyelid (no-pressure technique) (Fig. 63.19 and Video 63.7). Maintain this contact throughout the examination. As soon as the probe touches the gel, the ocular structures should immediately come into view. Adjust probe position to obtain a clear cross section of the eye showing anatomic structures (anterior chamber, iris, lens, vitreous, retina, nerve sheath). Adjust gain for a clear image, starting with maximal settings and reducing it until structures come into view again. Position the optic nerve in the middle of the screen and adjust the depth to view approximately 1 cm of the optic nerve. Identify the optic structures (Fig. 63.20A). Identify abnormal findings (see Fig. 63.20B–C) and describe abnormal findings in the caption. Use multiple planes to clarify normal and abnormal findings. A direct and consensual pupillary light reflex can be observed by viewing the pupillary response to light via ultrasound.

To measure optic nerve sheath diameter, ask the patient to adjust the gaze of the examined eye, approximately 10 degrees laterally. When viewed at this angle, the optic nerve is aligned with the ultrasound beam and decreases the possibility of obtaining a falsely widened measurement. This can occur if the optic nerve is imaged at an angle. Measure the width of the optic nerve sheath 3-mm deep to the retina (Fig. 63.21). Obtain at least two measurements and average for a final measurement. A diameter of greater than 5 mm is considered to be widened and suggests increased intracranial or IOP.

Complications

Inadvertent pressure applied to an eye with a ruptured globe could result in further damage to the globe. Excessive scan times could exceed exposure limit guidelines.

Findings

Globe rupture, intraocular FB, vitreous hemorrhage, retinal detachment, dislocated lens, and elevated IOP may be seen. These findings will be obscured if periorbital or orbital emphysema is present or if there is excessive air in the gel pocket placed over the eye.

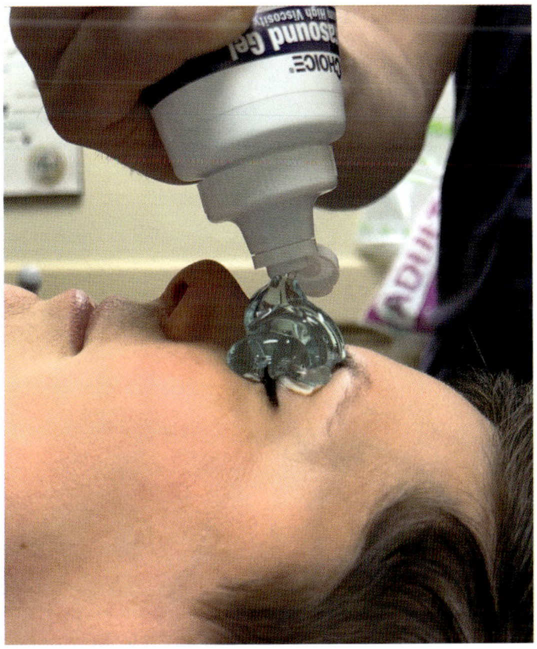

Fig. 63.17 The large amount of gel placed over the closed eyelid forms an acoustic window for the ultrasound probe. This allows an image to be obtained without additional pressure applied to the eye.

Summary

ED bedside ocular ultrasound is a valuable technique that can be used by the EP to discover important findings in the ED setting. It offers significant advantages for evaluation of ocular and central nervous system complaints, and it is particularly applicable to a possible open globe injury. It can be performed reliably at the bedside by EPs trained in its use.

OCULAR FOREIGN BODY REMOVAL

See Videos 63.8 and 63.9. Patients with an external FB in the eye are frequently seen in EDs. They are often in pain and desperate for help. Maintain a high degree of suspicion for FB injuries and perforation of the eye because such injuries may be occult and not readily detected. Not all FB injuries are associated with pain. Glass embedded in the cornea may be particularly difficult to detect. This section reviews procedures for locating and removing extraocular FBs and for appropriate postprocedural care. Finally, a brief discussion covering evaluation of the eye for potential perforation of the globe and detection of the presence of an intraocular FB is provided.

Indications and Contraindications

Extraocular FBs must always be removed. The timing of removal and the technique required vary according to the patient's clinical status and the type of injury. For the most part, the emergency clinician can proceed directly to removal of the object via the techniques described in this section. When the patient is extremely uncooperative (e.g., an intoxicated patient, a mentally deficient patient, or a young child)

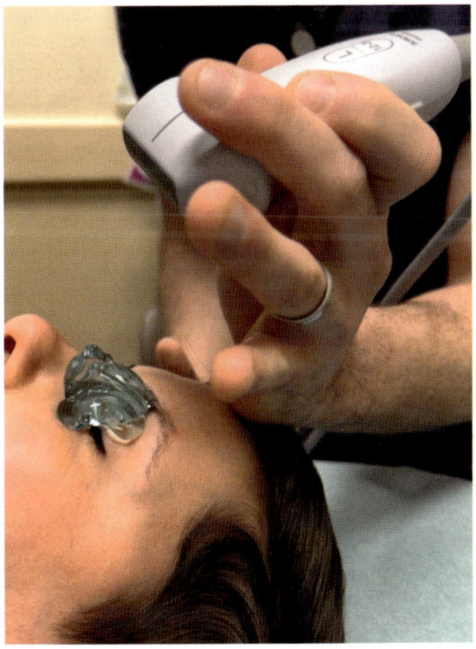

Fig. 63.18 It is essential that the sonographer maintain situational awareness about the position and weight of the probe at all times. This is accomplished by always maintaining stabilization of the probe against the patient's forehead or face.

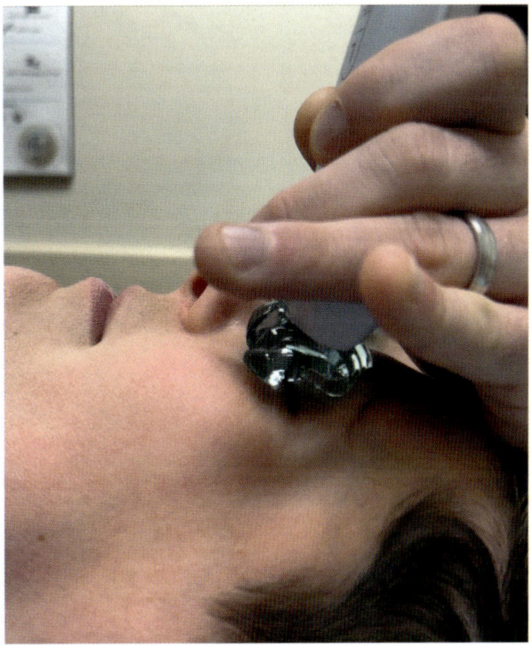

Fig. 63.19 Probe stabilization is accomplished by resting the sonographer's hand on the patient's nose and face while the probe is gently touched to the surface of the gel. The acoustic window can be seen underneath the probe.

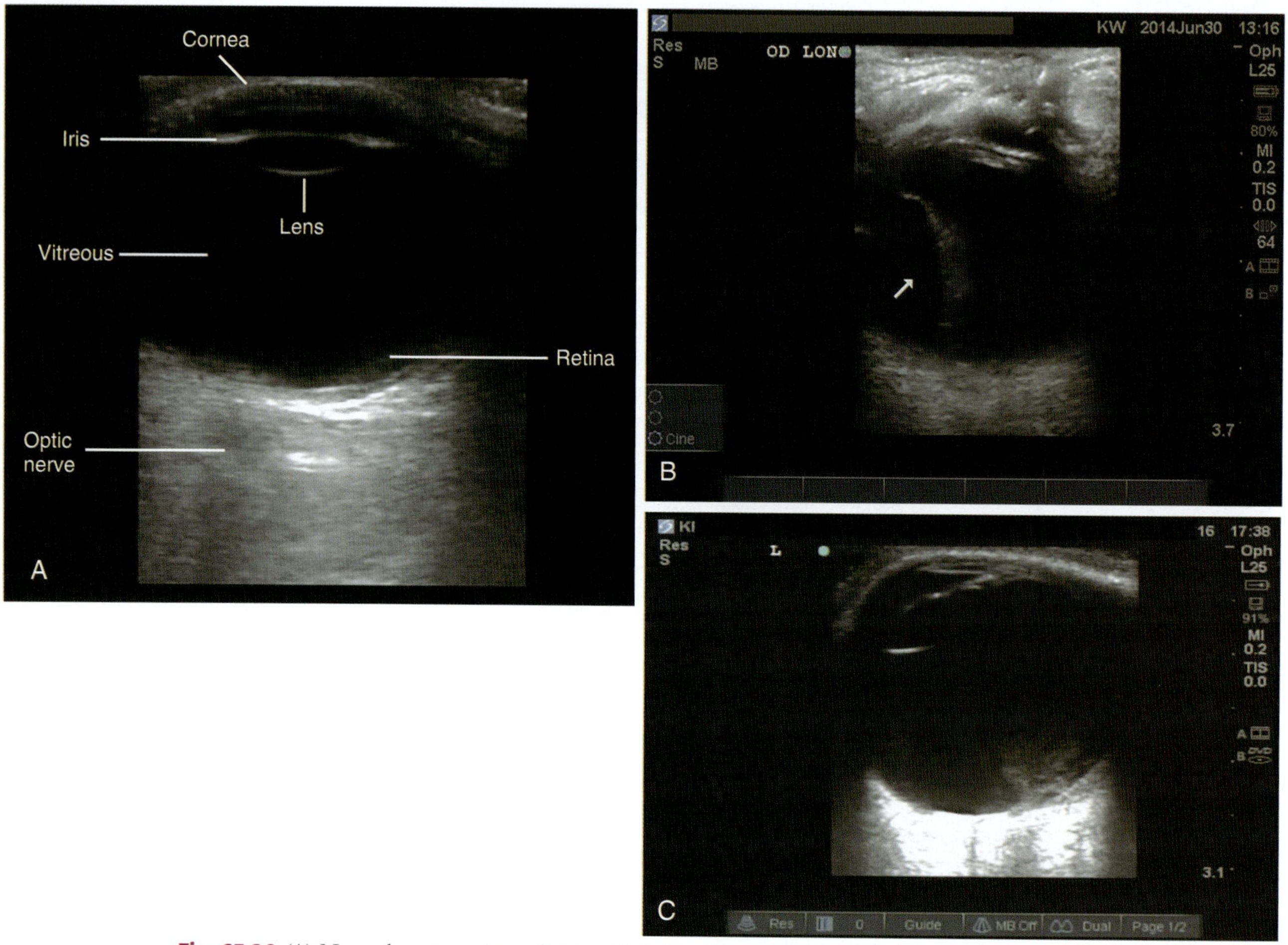

Fig. 63.20 (A) Normal anatomy is easily identified. Findings shown include (B) retinal detachment and (C) vitreous hemorrhage. (Courtesy Lauren Oliveira, MD.)

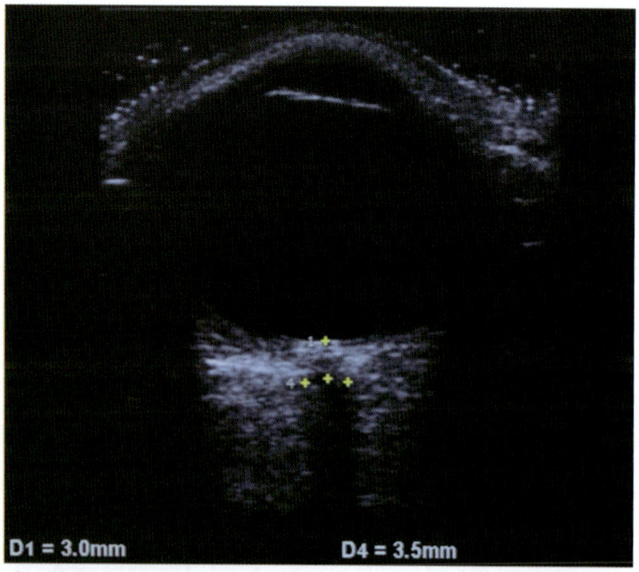

Fig. 63.21 Optic nerve sheath diameter measurements are shown for a normal eye. (Courtesy Lauren Oliveira, MD.)

or when the injury is complicated (e.g., deeply embedded object, multiple foreign objects from a blast injury, or possible globe penetration), consult ophthalmology immediately. A patient with a suspected FB or abrasion after exposure to a projectile (e.g., grinding wheel, hammering, metal objects colliding) should be rigorously evaluated for the presence of a deep intraocular FB. See further discussion later in this chapter. A penetrating injury of the cornea is of particular concern because the iris tissue may prolapse and have an appearance similar to a corneal FB (see Fig. 63.15). Hence, in addition to the history of projectile exposure, an irregular pupil, especially a pear-shaped pupil, should alert the clinician that a penetrating injury might have occurred.

Equipment

The following equipment is necessary for removal of an extraocular FB:

- Topical anesthetic, such as 0.5% proparacaine
- Sterile cotton-tipped applicators
- Fluorescein strips
- Magnification: loupes plus a Wood's lamp (×4), Eidolon Bluminator ophthalmic illuminator (×7.5), or slit lamp (×10 to ×16)
- Eye spud, 18- to 27-gauge needle attached to a 1- or 3-mL syringe or to the tip of a cotton-tipped applicator
- Dilator drops, such as 5% homatropine
- Antibiotic ointment, such as erythromycin

Consideration of an Intraocular Foreign Body

When examining a patient with an ocular FB sensation, always remain cognizant of the potential for an intraorbital or

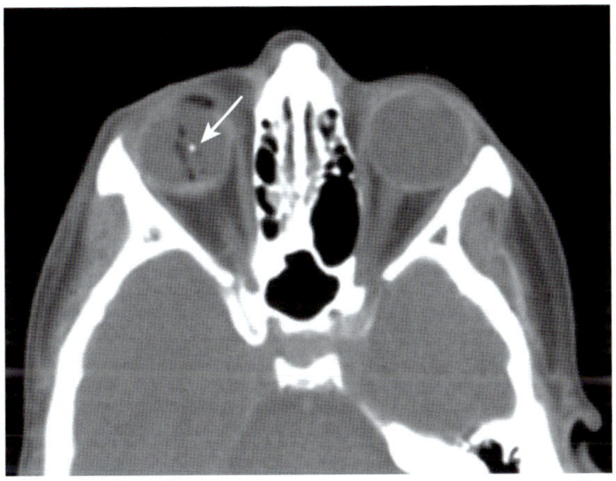

Fig. 63.22 Computed tomography scan showing a right intraocular foreign body (a BB pellet, *arrow*). (From Marx JA, Hockberger RS, Walls RM, eds. *Rosen's Emergency Medicine: Concepts and Clinical Practice*. 7th ed. Mosby; 2009.)

intraocular FB. Penetrating injuries represent a greater threat to visual loss than an extraocular FB does and can be disastrous if overlooked. Note that an intraocular FB can be deceptively subtle on initial evaluation and magnification with a Wood's lamp is only ×4. Bedside ED ultrasound is a useful adjunct for identification of intraocular FBs (see "Ocular Ultrasound" section).

The clinical findings are most helpful in determining which patients are at risk for a penetrating injury to the globe. An individual who complains of an FB sensation in the absence of trauma or one whose history is simply that something "fell" or "blew" into the eye is at low risk for perforation of the globe. Conversely, there is a greater probability of globe penetration in an individual who has sustained a high-velocity wound to the eye (e.g., drilling, hammering, grinding metal, blasting rock). The presence of any of the following findings on physical examination should alert the clinician to a probable intraocular FB: irregular pupil, shallow anterior chamber on slit lamp examination, prolapsed iris, positive Seidel test (see earlier section on "The Fluorescein Examination"), focal conjunctival swelling, hemorrhage, hyphema, lens opacification, and reduced IOP. Do not perform tonometry if penetrating injury to the globe is suspected. Be aware that a penetrating injury may not be associated with eye pain. If there is strong historical evidence and physical findings to support a diagnosis of globe penetration, obtain emergency ophthalmologic consultation.

An intraocular FB is often not visible on direct ophthalmoscopy. Although orbital radiography for radiopaque objects and ultrasonography of the globe have been used for indirect FB localization, computed tomography of the orbit is considered the most useful technique (Fig. 63.22).[53,54] When plain orbital radiography is performed to look for an intraocular FB, be aware that an eyelid FB may mimic an intraocular FB.[55] Patients with a suspected metallic FB should not undergo magnetic resonance imaging if the FB may be intraocular. Therapy for intraocular and intraorbital FBs must be individualized. Frequently, an ophthalmologist can localize an intraocular FB (if the vitreous is clear) with indirect ophthalmoscopy. The role of the emergency clinician is to suspect the diagnosis, protect the eye from further harm, and obtain ophthalmologic consultation. The remainder of this section addresses the problem of extraocular FBs.

Procedure

Foreign Body Location

The first step is to locate the FB. Apply a drop of topical anesthetic to the inside of the lower lid as described previously (see Fig. 63.7A). The presence of vertical corneal abrasions from FBs under the lids is helpful in localizing these hidden foreign objects (see Fig. 63.8, *plate* 7). Use a penlight and loupes or a slit lamp to examine the bulbar conjunctiva by having the patient look in all directions. Examine the inside of the lower lid by pulling it down with the thumb while asking the patient to look up. Evert the upper lid by asking the patient to look down as the end of an applicator stick is pressed against the superior edge of the tarsal plate of the upper lid. Meanwhile, grasp the lashes and pull down, out, and then up to flip the eyelid over (Fig. 63.23 and Video 63.10).

Minute FBs under the lid may be missed with simple visual inspection. Ideally, examine the everted lid under magnification with loupes or a slit lamp. With simple lid eversion, it is still not possible to see the far recesses of the upper conjunctival fornix. Although double eversion of the upper lid is helpful, the best way to rule out an FB in the upper fornix is to sweep the anesthetized fornix with a moistened applicator as the upper lid is held everted. Examine the tip of the applicator for removed foreign material. Small conjunctival FBs not hidden by the lids are often best removed with a moistened nasopharyngeal swab (e.g., nasopharyngeal Calgiswab [Puritan]).

Reexamine the cornea. Most corneal FBs have an area of fluorescein staining around them. Use a slit lamp or other magnification device such as the Eidolon Bluminator to make the examination easier. If the clinician is limited to loupes and a penlight, shine the light diagonally on the cornea to locate the FB. With a history of a high-speed projectile hitting the eye, rule out an intraocular FB. In the case of a blast injury, multiple FBs may penetrate the eye. If an FB cannot be found on the surface despite a suggestive history, examine the eye for physical evidence of penetration, as discussed earlier. Dilate the pupil and examine the fundus. Though not foolproof, bedside ultrasonography may identify the presence of a metallic FB (sensitivity of 87.5%, specificity of 95.8%, and positive and negative predictive values of 96.5% and 85.2%, respectively).[56] If in doubt regarding an intraocular FB, consider computed tomography and ophthalmologic consultation.

Foreign Body Removal

Once an extraocular FB is located, the technique for removal depends on whether it is embedded. If the FB is lying on the surface, eject a stream of water from a syringe through a plastic catheter, which will usually wash the object onto the bulbar conjunctiva. Once the FB is on the inner lid or bulbar conjunctiva, gently touch a wetted cotton-tipped applicator to the conjunctiva and the object will adhere to the tip of the applicator. Be aware that overzealous use of an applicator for removing corneal FBs can lead to extensive corneal epithelial injury. A spud device is required for removal of objects that cannot be irrigated off the cornea.

To remove embedded corneal FBs (Fig. 63.24), use a commercial spud device, a bur drill, a short 18- to 27-gauge needle on a small-diameter syringe (e.g., insulin or tuberculin syringe), or a cotton-tipped applicator. Use the applicator or syringe as a handle for the attached needle. Contrary to what one might expect, it is difficult to penetrate the sclera or the cornea with a needle, especially when it is applied tangentially

Lid Eversion and Foreign Body Removal.

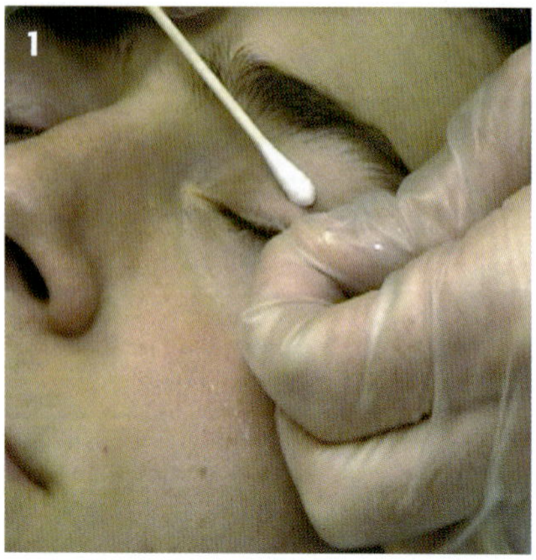

To evert the upper eyelid, place a cotton-tipped applicator against the superior edge of the tarsal plate.

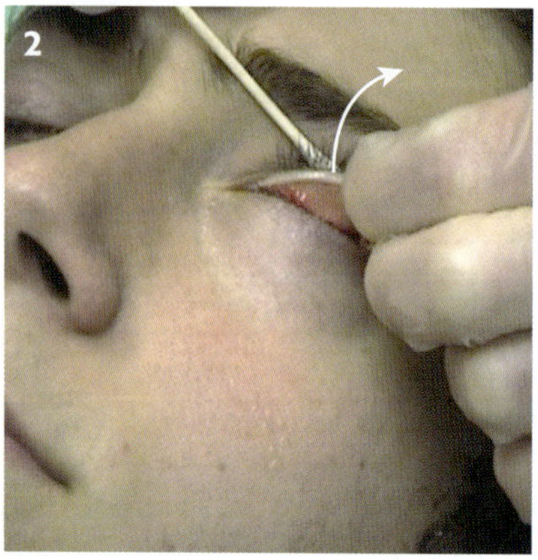

Grasp the eyelashes and pull them down, then out, and then up and over the applicator.

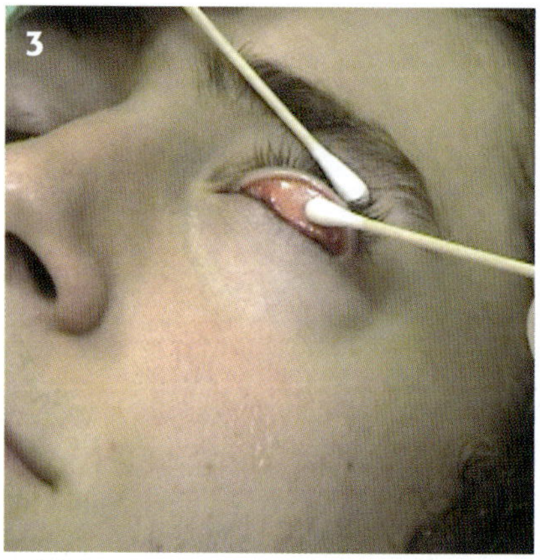

Hold the everted lid in place with the applicator. Use a second applicator to sweep the interior surface of the lid.

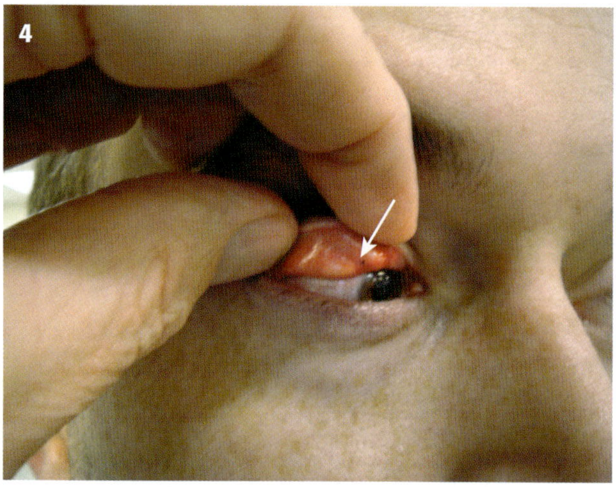

This patient complained of an FB in the eye despite irrigation. Lid eversion revealed a small speck *(arrow)* under the upper lid. This could cause a cornea abrasion characterized by vertical striations (see Fig. 63.8, *plate 7*).

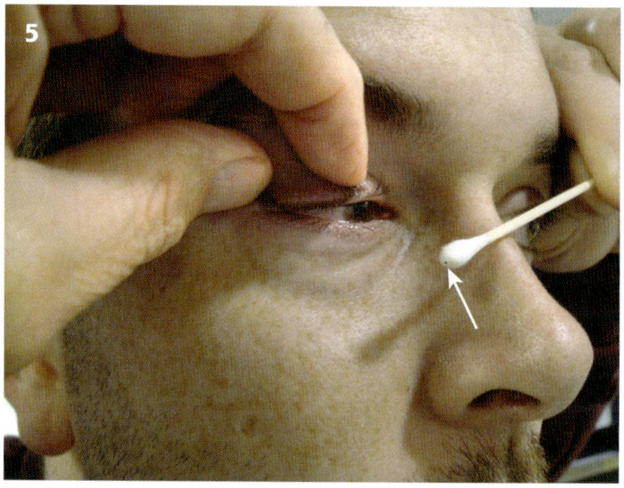

The foreign body was easily removed (*arrow*) by touching it with a moistened cotton-tipped applicator.

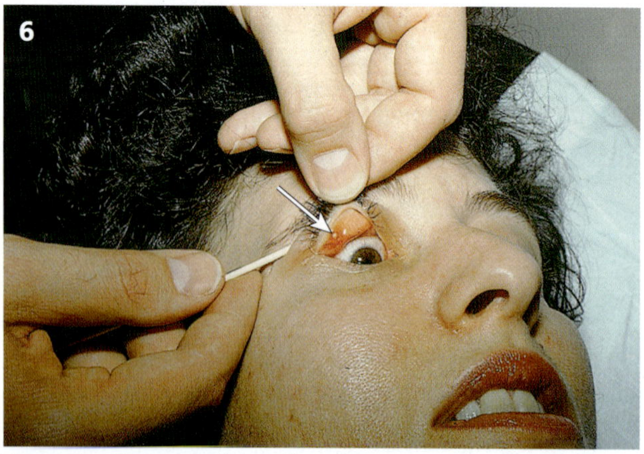

This patient had a swollen and tender upper eyelid thought to be secondary to a stye. With lid eversion, a small pustule *(arrow)* was found under the upper eyelid.

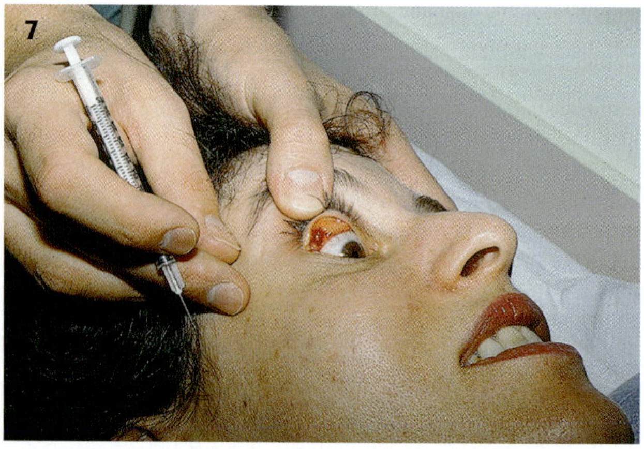

With a 27-gauge needle, the pustule was incised and a drop of pus was expressed; she made a rapid and uneventful recovery.

Fig. 63.23 Lid eversion and foreign body *(FB)* removal.

Corneal Foreign Body Removal

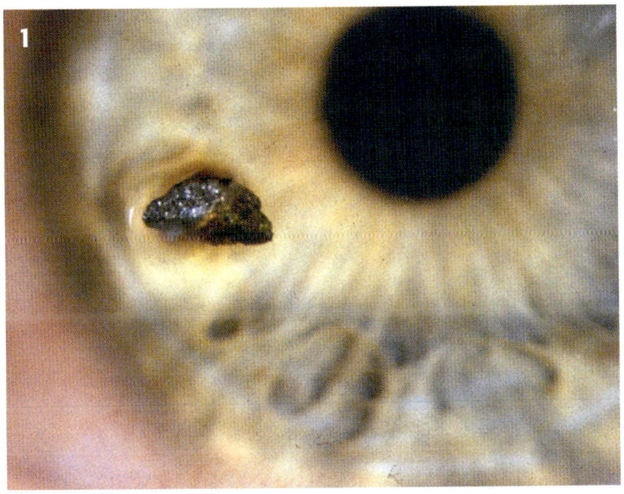

This embedded corneal FB is readily seen under slit lamp examination. A removal device (needle, spud, or bur drill) should be used for careful removal. A rust ring will remain if the FB has been there for only a few hours.

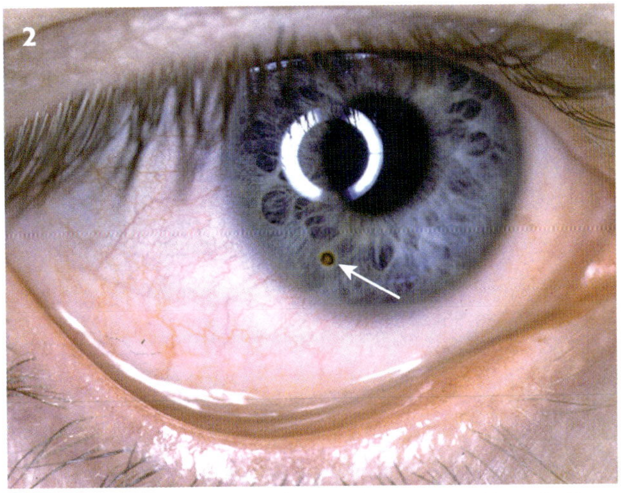

Rust rings *(arrow)* are retained FBs and are removed in a similar manner. Most rust rings should be removed, but there is no urgency. Small ones out of the line of sight may remain. A bur drill can be used for attempted removal, which if unsuccessful, can be reattempted in 24 hours. Alternatively, a small needle can be used to loosen the edges and then the ring scooped out. Both procedures will leave a corneal abrasion.

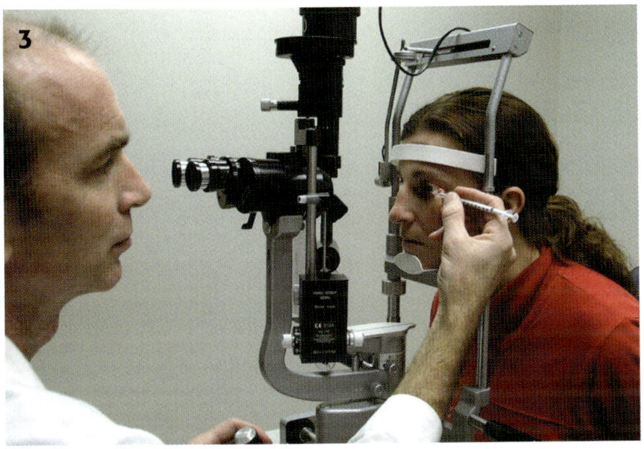

Under direct vision (not looking through the slit lamp), bring the syringe close to the eye while resting the hand on the patient's cheek. Be sure that the patient's forehead maintains continual contact with the crossbar on the slit lamp.

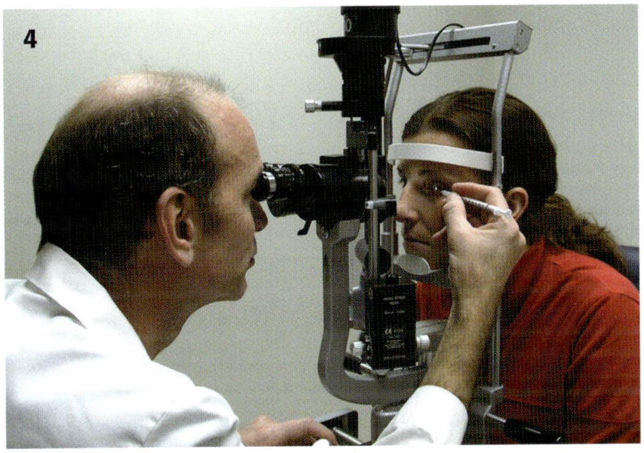

While looking through the slit lamp, bring the needle to the cornea and remove the FB.

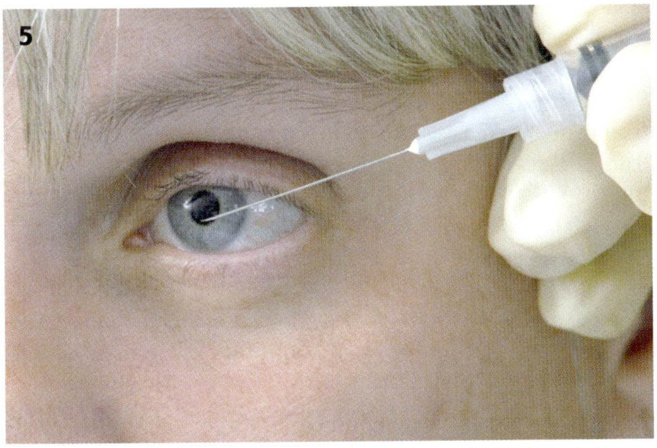

Hold the side of the instrument (drill bit or beveled edge of the needle) tangential to the cornea.

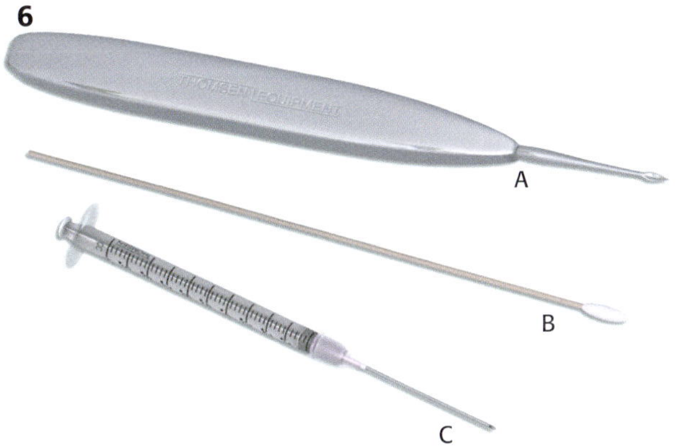

A variety of instruments may be used for FB removal, including an eye spud *(A)*, a cotton-tipped applicator *(B)*, and a 25- or 27-gauge needle on a tuberculin syringe *(C)*.

Fig. 63.24 Corneal foreign body *(FB)* removal.

to the cornea.[41] As with removal of conjunctival FBs, anesthetize the eye. Position the patient so that the head is well secured (preferably in a slit lamp frame). At this point, provide a simple explanation of the procedure, which usually ensures excellent compliance on the part of the patient. Rest your hand on the patient's cheek so that unexpected movements by the patient will not result in large movements of the removal device. Instruct the patient to gaze at an object in the distance (e.g., the practitioner's ear when a slit lamp is used) to further stabilize the eye. Bring the removal device close to the eye under direct vision; then while it is in focus, manipulate it under the magnification device (e.g., Wood's lamp, Eidolon Bluminator ophthalmic illuminator [see Fig. 63.8], or slit lamp) to remove the FB. Hold the device tangential to the globe, and pick up or scoop out the foreign object. If a bur drill is used, press the side of the drill against the FB until removal is accomplished.

During removal, rest your hand against the patient's face. It may also be helpful to brace the elbow with a pad or half-full tissue box to provide further support for the arm while removing the FB. If right-handed, place the lower part of your hand against the left maxillary bone when removing a foreign object from the patient's left eye and against the bridge of the patient's nose or infranasal area when removing an object from the right eye. If left-handed, reverse these positions. Using loupes or a slit lamp for magnification is highly recommended to minimize further injury during removal. In particular, corneal contact with the spud device is more readily discerned when magnification is used. Only topical anesthesia is required to remove FBs from the cornea. Although patients may feel pressure during removal of FBs, pain should not be felt after the eye is anesthetized.

Rust Rings

A common problem with metallic FBs is that rust rings can develop (see Fig. 63.24, *plate 2*). They can develop within hours because of oxidation of the iron in the FB. There are two preferred techniques for removal of a rust ring. The most direct technique is to remove the ring at the same time as the FB, either with repeated picking away with a needle, spud device, or with a rotating bur. The second approach is to let the iron of the rust ring oxidize and kill the surrounding epithelial cells during a 24- to 48-hour period. After that, the rust ring will be soft and often comes out in one solid plug. Generally, a small rust ring produces little visual difficulty unless it is directly in the line of sight. If large, a rust ring may delay corneal healing. Close follow-up is important to ensure healing of the cornea and total removal of the rust ring and FB.

Multiple Foreign Bodies

If multiple FBs are present in the eye, such as from an explosion, refer the patient to an ophthalmologist. One technique that may be chosen by the ophthalmologist is to denude the entire epithelium with alcohol and remove the superficial FBs. The deeper FBs gradually work their way to the surface, sometimes years later.

Aftercare

After removing the FB, an antibiotic ointment is frequently instilled. Though commonly used, the value of the ointment for superficial corneal defects after removal of an FB is unproved, and no specific standard of care is supported by scientific evidence. Contrary to previous techniques, conjunctival and corneal abrasions do not need patching. Data suggest that eye patching offers no benefit in healing corneal abrasions secondary to FBs.[57] If a superficial injury is sustained from the FB, instruct the patient to return only if the eye does not feel completely normal or if there is any blurred vision. The majority of superficial injuries heal without difficulty. The patient should be warned that the FB sensation might return temporarily when the anesthetic agent wears off. One animal study involving direct ocular exposure to *Clostridium tetani* organisms suggested that nonpenetrating ocular injuries are unlikely to lead to tetanus.[58] Tetanus prophylaxis after corneal FB removal is not standard, but it should be considered. However, tetanus prophylaxis appears to be essential for injuries that penetrate through the cornea or sclera.

Complications

Complications associated with ocular FB removal are rare. The most frequent problem is incomplete removal of the FB. In such cases, the epithelium has difficulty healing over the affected area, and thus the eye stays inflamed. Eventually, the diseased epithelium either sloughs off and heals or heals over the FB remnants, which are gradually absorbed. In either case, adverse effects on the eye are minimal; a minute scar on the cornea, even directly in the center, will rarely affect vision. Nonetheless, incomplete removal of a corneal foreign object warrants ophthalmologic follow-up.

Conjunctivitis may develop after removal of an extraocular FB. In most cases, the bacteria producing the infection are introduced by the patient rubbing the irritated eye.

Although perforation of the globe by the clinician's spud device is theoretically possible, this complication is exceedingly rare. Treatment of this type of corneal puncture wound consists of antibiotics, placement of an eye shield, and ophthalmologic consultation. In the absence of resultant endophthalmitis, permanent sequelae are unlikely to develop.

Epithelial injury can occur when cotton-tipped applicators are used to vigorously remove corneal FBs. Indeed, the use of cotton-tipped applicators for embedded corneal FB removal is condemned.

Summary

Ocular FBs are one of the most common eye emergencies. Searching for and removing the FB is usually straightforward. The only real trap is missing an intraocular FB. This must be ruled out if there is a history of a high-speed projectile hitting the eye or if the findings on physical examination suggest globe penetration.

EYE PATCHING

The use of eye patches has traditionally been the last step in the treatment of a number of common eye emergencies; however, multiple studies have shown that eye patching offers no benefit in pain relief or healing rates in patients with conjunctival or corneal abrasions.[59–61]

A meta-analysis of studies on eye patching and corneal abrasions or ulcers showed that patching might actually slow healing rates and patients might actually have worsening of their pain. This was found to be true in children as well.[1,14,62–64] Patching is also contraindicated in contact lens wearers and in situations in which the abrasion or ulcer may be infected.[60] In summary, eye patching is no longer indicated and might actually worsen the ophthalmologic process that it once was thought to help. Application of a therapeutic bandage contact lens directly to the cornea has been recommended as a possible treatment of corneal epithelial defects. Evidence from several small studies suggests that a bandage contact lens is safe, effective, and well tolerated and allows a significant number of patients to immediately resume their regular activities while maintaining baseline visual acuity. Further study on the application of this modality in the ED setting is needed.[14,65–67]

CONTACT LENS PROCEDURES

Removal of contact lenses in the ED may be required to permit further evaluation of the eye or to prevent injury from prolonged wear. Emergency clinicians also evaluate patients for "lost" contact lenses, which may be trapped under the upper lid. At times, patients may request that the clinician remove a lens that they have failed to extract from the cornea. Corneal ulcers can occur in patients who wear contact lenses and may require prompt treatment. This section on contact lens procedures addresses these concerns and discusses injuries associated with attempts at removal, the mechanism of injury from prolonged wear, and instructions to be given to patients at discharge. Furthermore, this section introduces the use of bandage contact lenses for the treatment of acute corneal abrasions.

Corneal Injury From Contact Lens Wear

Hard Contact Lenses

Oxygenation of the cornea is dependent on the movement of oxygen-rich tears under hard contact lenses during blinking. During the "adaptation" phase of early wear, a wearer of hard contact lenses produces hypotonic tears as a result of mechanical irritation from the lens. This results in corneal edema, which reduces subsequent tear flow under the lens during blinking. Overwearing a lens at this time leads to corneal ischemia, with superficial epithelial defects found predominantly in the central corneal area (see Fig. 63.9), where the least tear flow occurs. With adaptation, the tears become isotonic and the blinking rate normalizes, thus permitting increased wearing time. During early adaptation, blinking is more rapid than normal and then slows to a subnormal rate during late adaptation. Mucous delivery to the cornea in the tear film may also play an important role in maintaining corneal lubrication. Tight-fitting contact lenses may never permit good tear flow despite an adaptation phase; individuals with tightly fitted lenses may never be able to wear their original contact lenses for longer than 6 to 8 hours. Lenses that are excessively loose can also cause irritation by moving during blinking. Rough or cracked edges can cause corneal abrasions.

In the ED, a patient with eye irritation caused by prolonged contact lens wear may be either a new or an adapted wearer. An adapted wearer may have been exposed to chemical irritants (e.g., smoke), which reduces the tonicity of tears and leads to corneal edema and decreased tear flow. Alternatively, an adapted wearer with irritation may have ingested sedatives (e.g., alcohol) or may have fallen asleep wearing the contact lenses, thus decreasing blinking and tear flow. Another possibility is that the patient may actually be wearing tight-fitting contact lenses that have never allowed true adaptation despite many months of wear.

A patient with overwear syndrome usually awakens a few hours after removing the lenses. The patient experiences intense pain and tearing similar to that caused by a FB. The delay in onset of the symptoms until after removal of the lenses is caused by a temporary corneal anesthesia produced by the anoxic metabolic by-products that build up during extended lens wear. A second factor is the slow passage of microcysts of edema, which are pushed up to the corneal surface by mitosis of the underlying cells. When the cysts break open on the surface, the corneal nerve endings are exposed.

Most patients with overwear syndrome can be managed with reassurance, frequent administration of artificial tears, oral analgesics, and advice to "wait it out" in a darkened room. In the past, some patients required patching for comfort. A patient who has experienced no problems with contact lenses before an overwear episode can return to using the lenses after 2 or 3 days of wearing glasses but should be advised to build up wearing time gradually. A patient who was having chronic problems with lens comfort before the episode should check with an ophthalmologist before using the contact lenses again.

Soft Contact Lenses

The majority of contact lenses in use today are disposable soft contact lenses which come in a variety of types, including extended and daily wear. Although the cornea is also oxygenated by way of the tear film with soft contact lenses, only approximately one-tenth of the flow behind the lens that occurs with a hard lens is present during soft contact wear. The high degree of lens gas permeability permits the majority of oxygenation to occur directly through the lens. A hydrogel lens is more comfortable than a hard contact lens because lid motion over the lens is smooth. The minimization of lid and corneal irritation allows a more rapid adaptation phase because the initial reflex-induced changes in tearing and blinking are reduced. Nonetheless, the lenses may still lead to corneal edema and secondary hypoxic epithelial changes if worn for an excessive period when blinking is inhibited. Some individuals can tolerate the lenses for extended periods and may on occasion sleep with the contact lenses in place, although this practice is not encouraged. Newer extended-wear hydrogel lenses permit wear for up to 1 week without injury. These lenses are not discernible from standard soft lenses on examination.

Although the acute overwear syndrome that occurs with hard contact lenses can also occur with soft lenses, it is infrequent. More commonly, ocular damage from soft contact lenses falls into one of three categories:

1. Corneal neovascularization (Fig. 63.25A). Frequently, the patient is asymptomatic, but on slit lamp examination, fine vessels are seen invading the periphery of the cornea. Refer the patient to an ophthalmologist for refitting with looser or thinner lenses or with contact lenses that are more gas permeable.
2. Giant papillary conjunctivitis (see Fig. 63.25B).[68] The patient notes decreased lens tolerance and increased mucous production. On examination of the tarsal conjunctiva (best seen with eversion of the upper lid), large papillae are seen. These papillae appear grossly as a cobblestoned surface. Instruct the patient to discontinue wearing the lenses until the process reverses and to see an ophthalmologist to have the lenses refitted.
3. Sensitivity reaction to contact lens solutions (usually thimerosal or chlorhexidine).[69,70] Diffuse conjunctival infection and sometimes superficial keratitis develop. Advise the

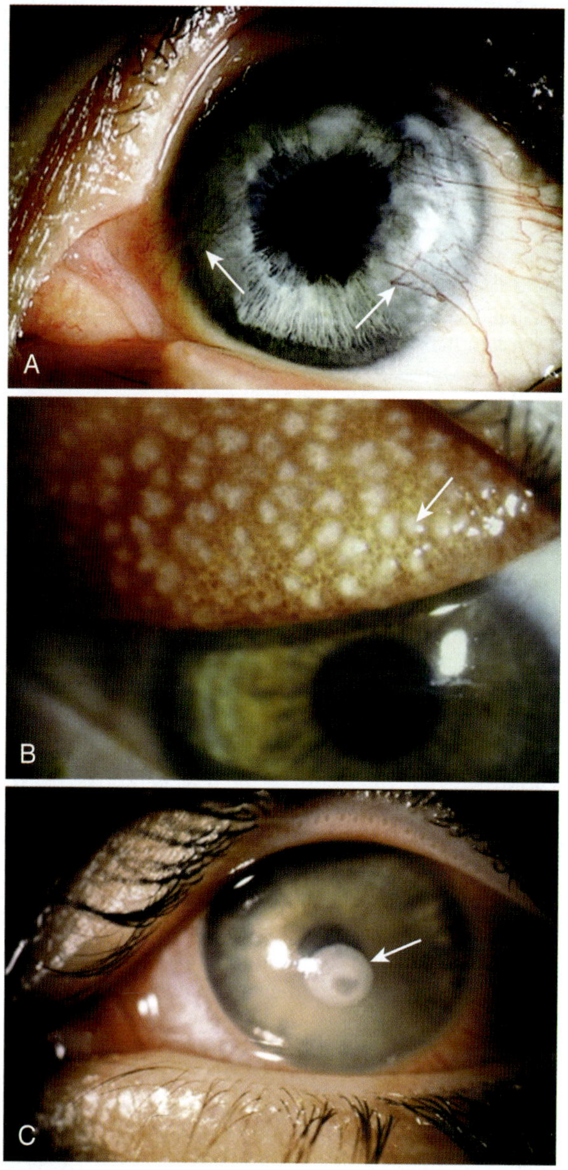

Fig. 63.25 Complications from contact lenses. (A) Corneal neovascularization. (B) Giant papillary conjunctivitis. (C) Corneal ulcer. See text for details. (A, From Friedman NJ, Kaiser PK, Pineda A. *Massachusetts Ear & Eye Infirmary Illustrated Manual of Ophthalmology*. 3rd ed. Saunders; 2009. B, From Krachmer JH, Mannis M, Holland E, eds. *Cornea*. 3rd ed. Mosby; 2010. C, From Yanoff M, Duker JS, eds. *Ophthalmology*. 3rd ed. Mosby; 2008.)

patient to switch to preservative-free saline with the use of heat sterilization. Frequently, the contact lenses will need to be replaced before lens wear can be resumed.

All these problems with soft lenses have a bilateral, subacute onset and do not require emergency treatment. The only form of ocular damage associated with soft contact lenses that is a true emergency is a bacterial or fungal corneal ulcer (often *Pseudomonas* or *Acanthamoeba* with soft contact lenses) (see Fig. 63.25C).[71–73] Because the nature of soft contact lenses is to absorb water, they can also absorb pathogens, which then can invade the cornea, especially if the soft lens is worn continuously for extended periods. The patient has a painful, red eye with associated discharge and a white infiltrate on the cornea. Immediately consult an ophthalmologist for appropriate culturing and antimicrobial treatment. These infections can permanently affect the patient's visual acuity.

Indications for Removal

Remove a contact lens in the following situations:

- *Contact lens wearer with an altered state of consciousness.* The emergency clinician should always be aware that a patient with a depressed or acutely agitated sensorium might be unable to express the need to have the contact lenses removed. Furthermore, it is likely that patients with a depressed sensorium will have decreased lid motion. During the secondary survey of these patients, identify the presence of the lenses and arrange for their removal and storage to prevent harm from excessive wear or possible accidental dislodgment at a later time. Without magnification, soft contact lenses may be difficult to see. Examine the eye with an obliquely directed penlight to reveal the edge of the soft lens 1 to 2 mm from the limbus on the bulbar conjunctiva.
- *Eye trauma with lenses in place.* After measurement of visual acuity with the patient's lenses in place, remove them and perform a more detailed examination of the cornea. Fluorescein may discolor hydrogel lenses; when possible, remove extended-wear lenses before using this chemical. After the dye is instilled, flush the eyes with normal saline. Advise the patient to wait at least 1 hour before reinserting the lenses.[14] The availability of single-use droppers of 0.35% fluorexon (Fluoresoft, Alden Optical) has permitted safe staining of eyes when soft lenses are to be worn immediately after the examination. Limited eye irrigation after the use of fluorexon drops is still recommended before the reinsertion of soft contact lenses.
- *Inability of the patient to remove the contact lens.* A patient may have a hard contact lens that cannot be removed because of corneal edema from prolonged wear. Alternatively, the patient may have a "lost" contact lens believed to be located behind the upper lid. Because there is no urgency for removal of the contact lens in the out-of-hospital setting, it can wait until the patient has been evaluated by a clinician.

Contraindication to Removal

The only major problem with contact lens removal occurs when the cornea may be perforated. In this case, the suction cup technique of removal, described later, is preferred.

Procedure

Hard Contact Lens Removal

A number of maneuvers have been devised for removal of a corneal lens. One technique is to first lean the patient's face over a table or a collecting cloth. Pull the lids temporally from the lateral palpebral margin to lock the lids against the edges of the contact lens. Ask the patient to look toward the nose and then downward toward the chin. This movement works the lower eyelid under the lower edge of the lens and flips the lens off the eye. The technique requires a cooperative patient because the clinician must pull the patient's lids tightly against the edge of the contact lens. The movement of the patient's eye then flips the contact free.

In an unresponsive patient in the supine position, modify the technique. Take a more active role in lid movement by using the following procedure (Fig. 63.26A). Place one thumb on the upper eyelid and the other on the lower eyelid near the margin of each lid. With the lens centered over the cornea,

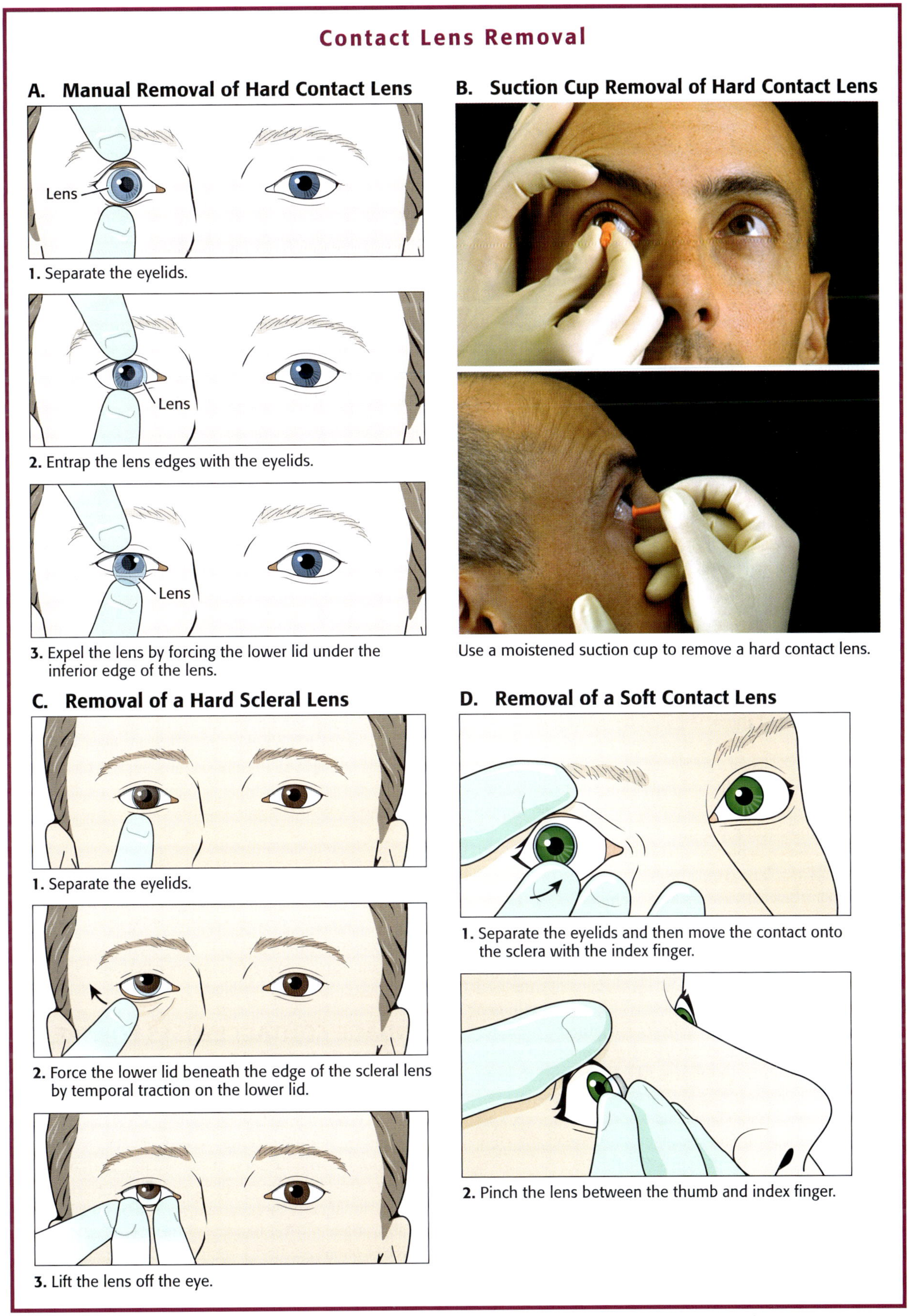

Fig. 63.26 Contact lens removal. (A, C, and D, From Grant HD, Murray RH, Bergeron JF, eds. *Brady Emergency Care*. 5th ed. Prentice Hall; 1990:338.)

open the eyelids until the margins of the lid are beyond the edges of the lens. Then press both eyelids gently but firmly on the globe of the eye and move the lids so that they are barely touching the edges of the lens. Press slightly harder on the lower lid to move it under the bottom edge of the lens. As the lower edge of the lens begins to tip away from the eye, move the lids together, which allows the lens to slide out sufficiently so that it can be grasped. Remember to use clean hands (and preferably wear examination gloves that have been rinsed in tap water or saline) when removing the lens.

Alternatively, move the lens gently off the cornea with a cotton-tipped applicator to guide the lens onto the sclera. Force the tip of the applicator under an edge of the lens and flip the contact loose. Apply topical anesthetic when using an applicator if the patient is awake. Take care with this technique to avoid contact of the applicator with the cornea when the lens is moved off the eye. Perhaps the easiest technique is to use a moistened suction-tipped device and simply lift the lens off the cornea (see Fig. 63.26B).

Scleral lenses (hard contact lenses that cover both the cornea and an amount of the sclera) can be removed by an exaggeration of the manual technique described earlier (see Fig. 63.26C). Elevation of the lens with a cotton-tipped applicator or a suction-tipped device is also an effective technique. Soft contact lenses should not be removed with a suction-tipped device because tearing or splitting of the lens might occur.

Soft Contact Lens Removal

With clean hands (preferably using gloves rinsed in saline or tap water), pull down the lower eyelid with the middle finger. Place the tip of the index finger on the lower edge of the lens. Slide the lens down onto the sclera and compress it slightly between the thumb and index finger. This pinching motion folds the lens so it can be removed from the eye (see Fig. 63.26D). Alternatively, use a cotton-tipped applicator instead of a gloved hand. Occasionally, a tight-fitting lens will be difficult to remove. One potential method is the use of topical anesthetic drops, lubricating eye drops (e.g., Refresh Celluvisc [Allergan] lubricant eye drops), and a cotton-tipped applicator to lift the edge of the lens from the limbus. This breaks the seal of the lens on the cornea and allows removal.

Lens Storage

Always attempt to use the patient's own storage container and lens solution if available. If it is not easily accessible, you can improvise by using a sterile urinalysis specimen container filled with sterile normal saline. A variety of alternative sterile containers are available for use in the ED. Be certain to keep the right and left lenses separate and in appropriately labeled containers. The containers should be kept with the patient until a friend or family member can procure them, or they should be locked up with the patient's valuables.

Evaluation of a "Lost" Contact Lens

A patient may request examination for a "lost" contact lens. The patient may be unsure whether the lens is hidden under a lid, remains on the cornea, or is truly outside the eye. Evaluation of a patient with a lost contact should begin, as should all eye examinations, with measurement of visual acuity. Measure visual acuity preferably with a 20-ft eye chart. Diminished visual acuity in the eye with the lost contact is convincing evidence that the lens is missing. Though transparent, soft contact lenses in proper position are usually seen when viewed closely with loupes or a slit lamp. The lens forms a fine line at the point where it ends on the sclera several millimeters peripheral to the limbus. Hard contact lenses are even more evident as they change in position on the cornea.

If the contact lens is not evident on initial inspection, evert the lids as discussed in the earlier section on "Ocular FB Removal" (double eversion of the upper lid). If the lens is still not visible, place a drop of topical anesthetic in the eye. Gently sweep the upper fornix with a moistened cotton-tipped applicator while the patient looks toward the chin. If the lens is still not evident even though the patient remains insistent that it is in the eye, perform a fluorescein examination after explaining that the dye will color the lens (permanently). Evert the upper lid again and examine with an ultraviolet light source.

If the lens remains elusive, reassure the patient that a thorough examination was performed and that no object was located under the eyelids or on the cornea. Next, examine the cornea for defects that warrant antibiotic ointment for treatment of corneal abrasion. Follow-up with the patient's eye specialist for a replacement lens and provision of further reassurance is advised. Ask the patient to retrace their movements at the time the contact began to cause trouble or was missed. Check the clothing being worn at that time and look for the lens there. A final possibility is that the patient may have accidentally placed the two lenses together in the same side of the carrying case, thereby causing them to stick together. Take a methodical approach, as outlined earlier, to ensure that no lens remains hidden in the eye.

Complications of Lens Removal

A corneal abrasion can occur during lens removal. It is difficult at times to determine whether the injury was produced by the patient or was a result of removal by the clinician. Fortunately, the corneal injury is generally of a superficial nature and responds well to symptomatic care.

Summary

Contact lens removal is usually simple. Challenging situations include identifying patients at risk for corneal injury from overuse, helping patients who have lost a contact lens in the eye, and providing aftercare instructions for patients with contact lens–related problems.

BANDAGE CONTACT LENSES FOR TREATMENT OF CORNEAL ABRASIONS

Acute corneal abrasions can cause significant pain, limit function, and result in lost days of work. Several studies have shown that bandage contact lenses are very effective in reducing pain without a requirement for narcotic analgesia. Their use decreases time away from work, and aids in returning to baseline functional status when used for uncomplicated acute corneal abrasions.[74–76] Yet bandage contact lenses are seldom used in the ED. An immediate benefit can be gained when the emergency practitioner selectively uses this treatment modality.

Indications and Contraindications

Bandage contact lenses may be used appropriately as an adjunct for the treatment of acute corneal abrasions resulting from minor trauma when symptomatic relief or rapid return of functionality is desired. Obtain a clear history of an acute traumatic abrasion and a fluorescein stain pattern consistent with this diagnosis.

Bandage contact lenses are contraindicated when the cause of the corneal epithelial defect is suspected to be due to infection. Ensure that a corneal ulcer is not present. The hallmark fluorescein stain pattern consistent with a corneal ulcer is a round stain with blurred margins, commonly in the central visual axis (midpupil region) (see Fig. 63.25C). Pain is disproportionate to the findings. An intense ciliary flush and anterior chamber reaction (cells and flare) may also be present. Avoid the use of bandage contact lenses in patients with a history of soft contact lens use and a nontraumatic abrasion in the central part of the cornea. Follow-up for removal of the bandage contact lenses and reevaluation of the eye are required to confirm improvement and identify complications. Unreliable patients who are not likely to be compliant with follow-up are at increased risk for infection and thus not good candidates for this modality.

Equipment

Hydrophilic bandage contact lenses are available and include, but are not limited to, Biomedics 55 (Ocular Sciences, Inc.), −0.50 dioptric power, 8.6 posterior curvature, and 14.2 diameter of the lens, and Acuvue Oasys BC (Johnson & Johnson Vision Care, Inc.), zero power (plano) or −0.50 diopter, 8.4 posterior curvature, and 14.0 diameter. Acuvue Oasys has been approved by the US Food and Drug Administration (FDA) for up to 1 week of continuous wear.

Procedure

Assess and document pain score. Instill 1 drop of a fluoroquinolone ophthalmic solution in the affected eye as prophylaxis against infection at the time of lens placement. Use of topical anesthetics is not required, but they have often been used in the evaluation of abrasions. Use a gloved hand that has been rinsed with water to remove the talc. Orient the contact lens on the tip of the examiner's index finger. Ensure that the lens is not inverted. The normal configuration of the lens resembles a cup, whereas an inverted lens resembles a saucer with its edges flaring outward. Another method to determine orientation of the lens is to try to close the edges or have them meet together with your fingers. If the edges curve away from each other, the lens is inverted. Direct the patient's gaze upward and then pull the lower lid slightly downward while inserting the lens over the cornea. Ask the patient to gently blink and then assess for placement. After a few minutes, reassess and again document whether pain is present. Instruct the patient to return for follow-up in 1 day. On return, remove the soft lens as described earlier, assess vision, document pain, and reevaluate the eye.

Complications

Because of the hypoxic microenvironment of the cornea, covering the cornea with a bandage contact lens could increase the opportunity for an infection to occur. Patients who do not disclose the use of soft contact lenses are at increased risk for corneal ulcers. Some patients may experience "tight lens syndrome" because of a lens that does not fit well or from drying out as the lens is exposed to the elements. Bandage contact lenses are usually of a generic size and thus do not offer a precise fit, but they are in place only for a short duration. Signs and symptoms of a tight lens may include redness, eye irritation, burning, a dry sensation, blurry vision, halos around objects, and lack of mobility of the contact lens over the cornea. Lack of mobility can reduce oxygen tension and thereby cause corneal edema and an even tighter lens. Rewetting solutions can improve hydration. Removal of a tight-fitting lens was described earlier.

Summary

Bandage contact lenses have been shown to be safe, effective, and comfortable in the treatment of corneal abrasions. Careful patient selection and proper technique will optimize this treatment modality when appropriately indicated for routine ED use. Patients will experience significantly decreased pain without the use of narcotic analgesics, significantly increased functionality, and decreased time away from work.

INFECTIOUS KERATITIS

Infectious keratitis with corneal ulceration can have a variety of causes and commonly includes overwear of contact lenses. Diagnosis of a corneal ulcer requires the use of a slit lamp and accurate determination of the patient's history. Infectious keratitis is a frequent problem in ophthalmic practice. Herpes simplex is a common corneal pathogen. *Acanthamoeba* is another pathogen particularly associated with contact lens use and exposure to organism-tainted environments. When a patient is seen in the ED with a corneal ulcer, promptly refer the patient to an ophthalmologist. When immediate referral is not possible, obtain telephone guidance from an ophthalmologist for initiation of therapy and arrange for ophthalmology follow-up within 24 hours.

Patients with herpes simplex keratitis often give a history of previous episodes of the disease. Patients who undergo almost any form of corneal stress may sustain an activation of preexisting corneal disease. Herpes simplex keratitis is classically recognized by its dendritic pattern on fluorescein staining (see Fig. 63.8, *plate 9*).

Acanthamoeba keratitis is a disease with potentially devastating consequences. Its frequency seems to be increasing, particularly in contact lens wearers, and its pathophysiology is not completely understood. Patients often have a red eye in which the initial bacterial culture results are negative.

Bacterial keratitis occurs in a variety of settings. Organisms range from the relatively common *Staphylococcus* (including methicillin-resistant *Staphylococcus aureus*) or *Streptococcus* to *Mycobacterium*, which can be difficult to identify. A variety of antibiotics are used against bacterial agents. Ciprofloxacin is a quinolone that has demonstrated efficacy against most of the common causative agents. Bacterial organisms in the cornea can develop resistance to any antibiotic, and resistance to fluoroquinolones has also been observed.[77] Ideally, treatment follows acquisition of material from the ulcer for culture.

Fungal keratitis is a rare, but life-threatening infection with significant ocular morbidity. Its incidence is increasing globally and should be considered in immunocompromised individuals as well as geographic populations in Africa and Asia. Filamentous fungi are the most common pathogens identified, and natamycin of the polyene drug class is considered first-line therapy. Severe keratomycosis cases have shown drug resistance, and non-*Fusarium* cases have shown response to voriconazole. Imidazole derivatives such as echinocandin may also be considered. Targeted therapy in the form of intrastromal injections and intranasal administrations has proven effective. The role of systemic treatment is controversial. Ultimately, treatment should be tailored on a case-by-case basis with consideration of geographic location, local antibiograms, culture sensitivities, drug availability, and specialist consultation.[78,79]

In instances in which a cellular infiltrate is seen on slit lamp examination, and there will be a delay of hours before an ophthalmologic consultant can perform the culture, it is prudent to initiate therapy with topical fluoroquinolones such as ciprofloxacin. In such circumstances, obtain corneal samples for culture under the telephone guidance of the consultant before starting the antibiotic. One approach is to lightly touch a culture medium–moistened cotton-tipped swab against the ulcer and then streak standard culture media. If the ulcer is chronic or the patient is immunocompromised, a fungal organism may be the causative agent. Finally, a saline-moistened cotton-tipped swab may be used to obtain a Gram stain of the ulcer. Initiation of therapy before obtaining specimens for culture makes subsequent identification of an organism difficult. For this reason, consider the circumstances of the individual case before initiating treatment.

TONOMETRY

See Video 63.11. Tonometry is the estimation of IOP. It is obtained by measuring the resistance of the eyeball to indentation by an applied force. Prolonged elevated IOP is associated with visual field loss and blindness. A sudden elevation in IOP can result from trauma or primary angle-closure glaucoma. Patients with primary angle-closure glaucoma are often seen in the ED with systemic complaints, including nausea, vomiting, and headache. Occasionally, these patients are surprisingly free of pain in or about the eye. The emergency clinician must determine the IOP and its relationship to the systemic symptoms.

Ophthalmologists depended on tactile estimation of eye pressure until the 1860s, when von Graefe developed the first mechanical tonometer. Applanation tonometry was introduced in 1885 by Maklakoff[80] but was not popularized until Goldmann[81] improved the instrument. Schiøtz[82] developed an impression tonometer in 1905 and modified it in the 1920s; this form is still in use today. Aside from modifications in configuration, current tonometers closely resemble the devices popularized by Schiøtz[82] and Goldmann.[81] Pocket-sized tonometers using the principle of the MacKay-Marg tonometer are available. One such device is the Tono-Pen XL (Reichert Inc).[83] These devices are portable, lightweight, and relatively accurate, with built-in provisions for calibration. They have the advantage of a one-time-use replaceable cover that eliminates concern about the possible transmission of an infectious agent. The Icare (Tiolat Oy) is a rebound tonometer that has recently appeared for use in clinical practice. This device uses a newer technology that calculates IOP from the rebound of a lightweight disposable plastic-covered magnetized metal rod that is bounced off the cornea. Its advantages include portability and lack of need for corneal anesthesia and correlate closely with the Tono-PenXL.[84,85] Whereas the Schiøtz and Tono-Pen XL tonometers are the most commonly used devices for measuring IOP in the ED, the Icare shows promise to be useful in the ED and primary care settings.

Tonometric Techniques

Four tonometric techniques are reliable and clinically useful for estimating IOP:

1. The impression method uses a plunger (3 mm in diameter) to deform the cornea, and the "indentation" is then measured. This technique was popularized by Schiøtz[82] and commonly bears his name.
2. The MacKay-Marg method[86] is a refined version of the impression technique in which smaller amounts of cornea are indented.
3. In the applanation method, a planar surface is pressed against the cornea.
4. Rebound tonometry is an induction-based impact method in which a very lightweight magnetized probe is bounced off the cornea.[87]

The Schiøtz tonometer actually measures total IOP (initial pressure plus the pressure added by the weight of the tonometer and the plunger). Friedenwald[88] empirically found that a "rigidity coefficient" could be introduced to allow an estimation of the true IOP. One must be aware, however, that calculated conversion tables for Schiøtz tonometers use an average estimate of the rigidity coefficient and hence are not accurate when eye rigidity is altered (e.g., after scleral buckle procedures for retinal detachment or with extreme myopia).

Measurement of IOP in the ED by tonometry is a technique available to most emergency clinicians. Tonometry is not a standard procedure for many eye-related complaints, but in the following special situations, tonometry may be particularly helpful:

- Confirmation of a clinical diagnosis of acute angle-closure glaucoma. For example, a middle-aged or older patient with acute aching pain in one eye, blurred vision (including halos around lights), and a red eye with a smoky cornea and a fixed midposition pupil needs a pressure reading (Fig. 63.27A). Sometimes the findings are less dramatic, and sometimes the patient complains mostly of nausea and vomiting, which suggests "flu" rather than an eye disorder.
- Determination of a baseline ocular pressure after blunt ocular injury. Patients with hyphema often have acute rises in IOP because of blood obstructing the trabecular meshwork (see Fig. 63.27B).[89] Later, angle recession can cause a permanent form of open-angle glaucoma. Arts and colleagues[90] suggested that an IOP greater than 22 mm Hg or a difference of 3 mm Hg or greater between the eyes is a good marker of "ocular injury" in the setting of an orbital fracture.

Tonometry may also be considered in the following scenarios:

- Determination of a baseline ocular pressure in a patient with iritis. Both open- and closed-angle glaucoma, as well as corticosteroid-induced glaucoma, can develop in patients with iritis. Because most cases of iritis are referred, tonometry may also be deferred unless signs of increased IOP are present.
- Documentation of ocular pressure in a patient at risk for open-angle glaucoma. All patients older than 40 years with a family history of open-angle glaucoma, optic disc changes, visual field defects, and pressure of 21 mm Hg or higher should be referred to an ophthalmologist for further workup. Referral should also be made for patients with suspiciously cupped discs who have normal pressure; some of these patients may have "low-pressure" glaucoma associated with visual field defects. This is usually part of an ophthalmologist's examination.

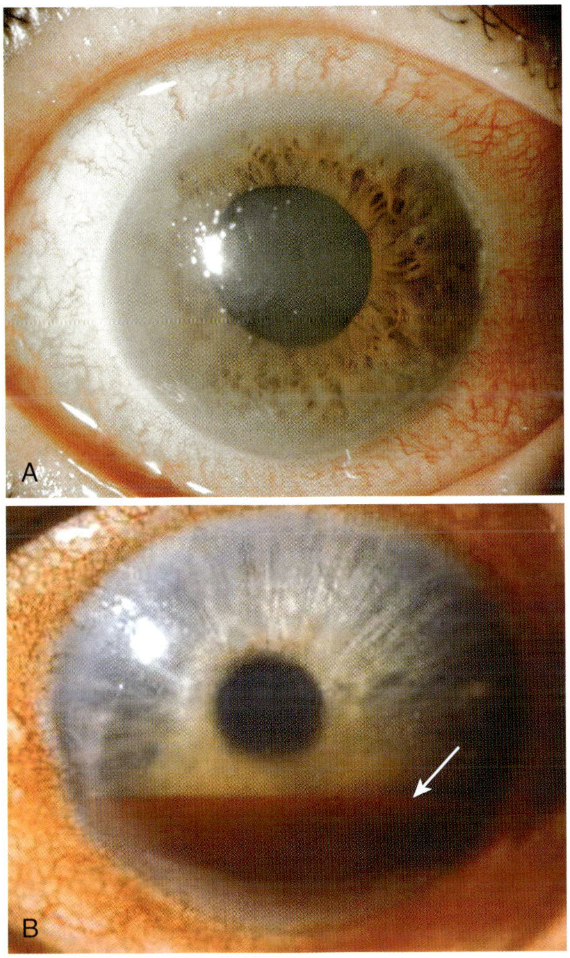

Fig. 63.27 Indications for tonometry. (A) This patient complained of severe headache, nausea, and blurry vision. The eye was obviously inflamed, with corneal edema (note the fragmented light reflex) and a mid-dilated pupil. This is acute angle-closure glaucoma. (B) Hyphema (layering of red blood cells in the anterior chamber) *(arrow)* in a patient who was struck in the eye with a racquetball. (From Palay DA, Krachmer JH, eds. *Primary Care Ophthalmology*. 2nd ed. Mosby; 2005.)

Contraindications to Tonometry

Tonometry is relatively contraindicated in eyes that are infected unless one is using a device such as the Tono-Pen XL or Tono-Pen Avia which use a sterilized cover'. Sterilize a tonometer before and after applying it to a potentially infected eye. Measure infected eyes with either a noncontact tonometer or a device with a covered tip (e.g., Tono-Pen). Swab the contact portions of any device with alcohol and allow it to dry before use on another eye. Not all viruses are destroyed by cleansing with alcohol. Hydrogen peroxide is effective in deactivating the human immunodeficiency virus (HIV) responsible for acquired immunodeficiency syndrome (AIDS). Ultraviolet sterilization, cold sterilizer bathing of the footplate and plunger, and ethylene oxide sterilization have all been advocated as alternatives to sterilizing the tip of the Schiøtz tonometer. The Schiøtz tonometer may also be used with sterile disposable coverings (marketed as Tonofilm). Nonetheless, defer measurement of IOP in an obviously infected eye until a subsequent visit to the ED, or private clinician, unless the red eye demands an immediate determination of IOP.

Examples of indications for immediate tonometry in the setting of a red eye are suspected angle-closure glaucoma (acute onset of redness and pain in the eye with smoky vision, a cloudy cornea, and a fixed pupil in mid-dilation, often with headache and nausea) and iritis (ciliary injection with photophobia), in which secondary angle-closure glaucoma or corticosteroid-induced changes in pressure may occur. Reported cases of conjunctivitis spread by tonometry predominantly tend to be viral infections. Particular effort should be made to avoid use of the instrument on patients with active facial or ocular herpetic lesions or those who may have AIDS.

The presence of corneal defects also represents a relative contraindication to tonometry. Use of a tonometer on an abraded cornea may lead to further injury and is commonly deferred until a subsequent visit. Patients who cannot maintain a relaxed position (e.g., because of significant apprehension, blepharospasm, uncontrolled coughing, nystagmus, or uncontrolled hiccups) are unlikely to permit an adequate examination and can sustain a corneal injury when sudden movements occur during an examination. Furthermore, tonometric examination, with the exception of the palpation technique (through the lids) and the noncontact method, should not be performed on a cornea without complete anesthesia.

Tonometry should not be performed on a patient with a suspected penetrating ocular injury. Globe perforation may be exacerbated by pressure on the globe with resultant extrusion of intraocular contents. Slit lamp examination can be used for detection of a possible perforation.

Procedure

Palpation Technique

All forms of tonometry are essentially ways of determining the IOP; an eye that is easily depressed or deformed has lower pressure. The most direct way to do this is simply to press on the sclera through the lids and grossly compare one eye with the other. One can easily distinguish the rock-hard eye of acute glaucoma from the normal opposite eye by this method. Direct the patient to look down without closing the lids. Rest both hands on the patient's forehead and apply just enough digital pressure on the involved eye to indent it slightly with one index finger. With the other index finger, alternately feel and compare the compliance of the other eye (Fig. 63.28, *plate 1*). An experienced examiner is able to estimate IOP within 3 to 5 mm Hg of the actual IOP with the palpation technique, but most emergency clinicians do not have enough experience to trust this method.[41]

Another method is to anesthetize the eyes topically and press a wetted applicator on the sclera of each eye. Again, eye deformation is inversely related to ocular pressure. Rigidity of the globe is also a factor in this crude method of tonometry.

Impression (Schiøtz) Technique

Use of the Schiøtz tonometer requires relaxation on the part of the patient and steadiness on the part of the clinician. After placing the patient in either a supine or a semi-recumbent position, instruct the patient to gaze at a spot directly above the eyes. A spot on the ceiling should suffice; alternatively, patients can stretch their arm up over their head and gaze at their thumb. Place a drop of topical anesthetic in each eye. After the irritation of the drop passes, allow the patient to blink while blotting the tears away with a tissue. Rubbing the

Tonometry: Palpation And Schiøtz Techniques

1

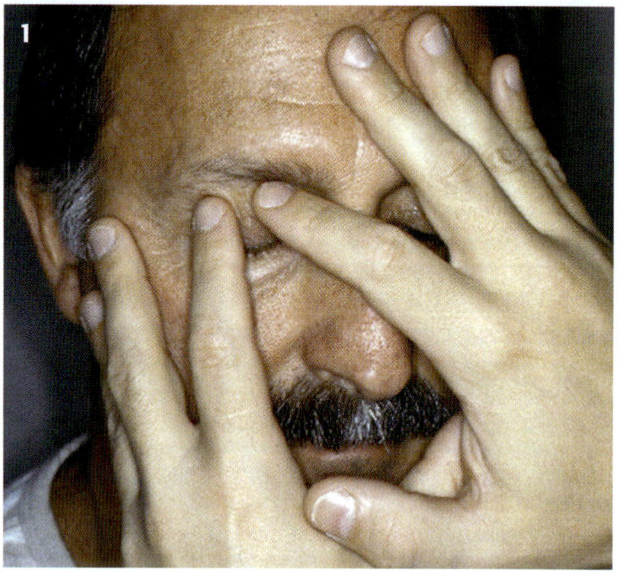

A relatively unskilled examiner can detect the very high intraocular pressure of acute angle-closure glaucoma with tactile tonometry. The examiner rests both hands on the patient's forehead and alternately applies just enough digital pressure on the globe to indent it slightly with one index finger while feeling the compliance of the globe with the other.

2

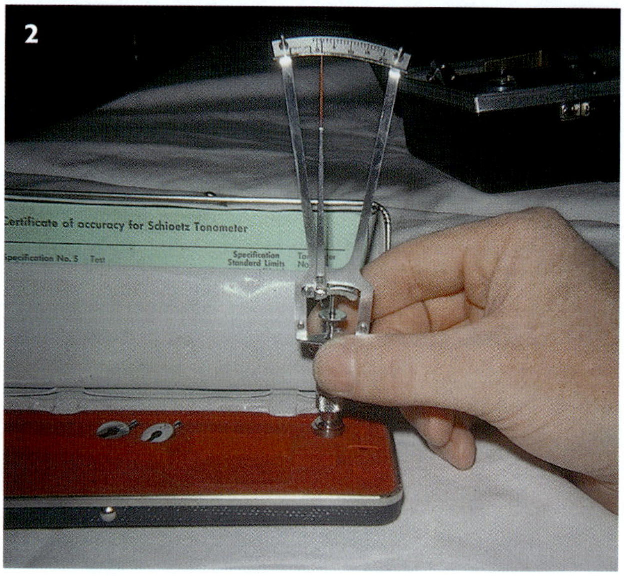

Before using the Schiøtz tonometer, test it on a flat surface to ensure smooth motion of the device and that the zero line is achieved.

3

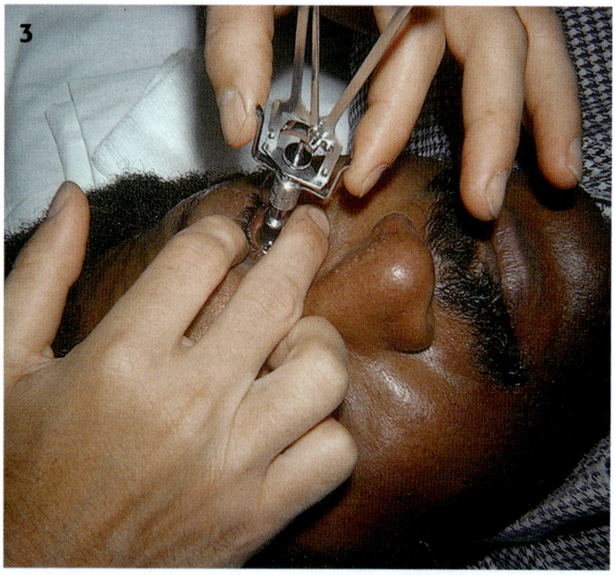

Apply lid separation pressure to the bony orbital rims. An assistant may separate the lids while you concentrate on proper placement of the tonometer. Hold the tonometer vertically during use, and rest your hand against the patient's facial bones. After anesthetic drops are instilled, the patient will not experience any pain from this procedure. It is important to have a relaxed patient because squinting and blepharospasm may interfere with the reading. Note: Gloves should be worn.

4 Schiøtz Tonometry*

Tonometer Scale	Tonometer Weights (g)		
Reading (Units)	5.5 (mm Hg)	7.5 (mm Hg)	10 (mm Hg)
2.50	27	39	55
3.00	24	36	51
3.50	22	33	47
4.00	21	30	43
4.50	19	28	40
5.00	17	26	37
5.50	16	24	34
6.00	15	22	32
6.50	13	20	29
7.00	12	18	27
7.50	11	17	25
8.00	10	16	23
8.50	9	14	21
9.00	8	13	20
9.50	8	12	18
10.00	7	11	16

* The table porvides estimates of intraocular pressure to the nearest mm Hg for the different weight of the Schiøtz tonometer. Accuracy is most dependable with scale readings greater than 5. If the scale reading is less than 5, use the next highest weight that will give a reading of 5 or more.

Use the above chart to determine the converted reading based on the reading and the amount of weight on the scale.

Fig. 63.28 Tonometry: palpation and Schiøtz techniques.

eyes lowers IOP. Reassure the patient that further discomfort will not occur during the procedure.

Ask the patient to keep both eyes wide open and fixed on an object. Separate the eyelids on the side where you are standing. Test the tonometer on a flat surface to confirm smooth movement of the device (see Fig. 63.28, *plate 2*). Take care to direct pressure onto the orbital rims rather than the orbit because pressure directed into the orbit falsely raises the reading. Hold the tonometer momentarily over the open eye, and inform the patient that the instrument will block vision in that eye. Instruct the patient to continue to gaze at the fixation point as though the instrument were not there. After the patient relaxes the involuntary muscle contraction that occurs when the instrument is first placed in the line of sight, gently lower the instrument onto the middle portion of the cornea (see Fig. 63.28, *plate 3*). This is a painless experience for patients with an anesthetized cornea. Vertically align the instrument with the footplate resting on the cornea; the reading should be in midscale. Should the reading be on the low end of the scale (<5 units), place additional weight on the plunger after the instrument has been removed. Repeat the process as before with the additional weight.

Measure the opposite eye in the same fashion. Use the chart provided to determine the converted reading based on the reading and amount of weight on the scale. Refer to ophthalmology if the converted scale reading is higher than 21 mm Hg (see Fig. 63.28, *plate 4*). Patients with elevations in IOP of 30 mm Hg or greater require more urgent consultation and initiation of therapy. Associated symptoms or signs of angle-closure glaucoma (primary or secondary) represent an ophthalmologic emergency.[91]

Errors With Impression Tonometry

Inaccurate readings can occur with the Schiøtz tonometer for a variety of reasons. Falsely low readings may occur if the plunger is sticky. Check plunger motion and the zero point of the tonometer on a firm test button before use. If the plunger is sticky, clean it with isopropyl alcohol and dry it with a tissue. Inadvertently directing pressure onto the orbit when the lids are held open may elevate IOP and provide a falsely elevated reading. The following eye movements have been found to elevate IOP: closing the lids (increases by 5 mm Hg), blinking (increases by 5 to 10 mm Hg), accommodation (increases by 2 mm Hg), and looking toward the nose (increases by 5 to 10 mm Hg).[92] Repeated or prolonged measurements have been found to lower IOP approximately 2 mm Hg and may also lower pressure in the opposite eye.[93] As mentioned in the introduction to this section, calibration of the Schiøtz tonometer is based on a mean rigidity coefficient. Factors that produce a reduction in ocular rigidity falsely lower the measured pressure. Such factors include high myopia, anticholinesterase drugs, overhydration (e.g., large cup of coffee or several cans of beer), and scleral buckle operations.[94,95] Ocular pressure measurements can vary with ocular perfusion. When measured after a premature ventricular contraction, IOP may be reduced as much as 8 mm Hg.[92] Similarly, decreased venous return as produced by breath holding, the Valsalva maneuver, or a tight collar can increase IOP.[92]

Impression (Tono-Pen XL, Tono-Pen AVIA) Technique (Fig. 63.29)

When using these devices, the preparations for testing are similar to those for the Schiøtz device. Encourage the patient to relax, and apply a topical anesthetic to numb the cornea. Ask the patient to stare with both eyes at a distant object during testing. As noted previously, help separate the eyelids but do not apply direct pressure on the globe. One major advantage of using the Tono-Pen is that the patient may be evaluated in any position as long as the device is applied perpendicular to the corneal surface. Another advantage is that the devices can be used in patients with irregular or high corneal astigmatism.

Ideally, the complete instructions provided with the device should be consulted before each use; however, the following synopsis is provided to help in circumstances in which instructions are unavailable.

First, spray the tip of the probe with compressed gas to clean the mechanism and ensure free movement. Place an Ocu-Film (latex; Reichert) cover snugly (but without tension) over the probe tip.

Calibration

To perform calibration of the Tono-Pen XL (required before use at least once each day), depress and release the activation switch momentarily. The liquid crystal display (LCD) should show a single dashed line "—". If the device beeps and double dashed lines "= =" appear on the LCD, push the activation switch again so that the single line reappears. If the previous calibration shows "bAd" on the LCD, a long beep sounds, followed by "CAL" on the LCD. A short beep follows and then the desired single line is displayed. Once a single line is displayed, hold the probe vertically with the tip pointing straight down. Press and release the activation switch twice in rapid succession. Two beeps will then sound, and "CAL" will appear on the LCD. Hold the probe in this position (up to 20 seconds) until a beep sounds and "-UP-" appears on the LCD. Immediately turn the probe 180 degrees so that the tip points straight up. In a few seconds, another beep occurs and the LCD changes. If the LCD reads "Good," the calibration was successful. If the LCD reads "bAd," the calibration was unsuccessful.

With an unsuccessful calibration, repeat the calibration steps described earlier until two consecutive "Good" readings are obtained. If further attempts are unsuccessful, loosen the Ocu-Film tip cover and repeat the calibration process. If attempts are still unsuccessful, press the reset button and repeat the process. If still unsuccessful, use compressed air to clean the uncovered tip of the probe and repeat the process. If still unsuccessful, the battery should be replaced, and the process repeated. Continued failure warrants contacting Reichert Technical Support.

The Tono-Pen AVIA (Fig. 63.30) does not require daily calibration but can be "verified" if spurious readings are suspected in a manner similar to the calibration described previously. The procedure is abbreviated and begins with pressing and holding the activation button for 5 seconds. A beep occurs with each passing second followed by the display showing "dn." At this point, continue as in the previous instructions for calibration. A properly functioning device will read "Pass" and will go into the applanation mode with one press of the activation button. Verification should be repeated if a reading of "Fail" is shown.

Measurement

To proceed to measurement, prepare the patient as outlined earlier. Depress and release the activation switch to obtain double dashed lines on the LCD. A beep will occur when ready. If the switch is not depressed long enough, the LCD will be blank. If a blank screen is seen, press and release the activation switch again to obtain double dashed lines on the LCD. Hold the probe like a pen and touch it to the cornea briefly and lightly. Touch the cornea four times. A click will sound and a reading will appear on the LCD each time that a valid reading is obtained. In the Tono-Pen XL, after four valid readings, a final beep will sound and the averaged measurement will appear on the LCD. The number represents IOP in millimeters of mercury. The associated bar reflects statistical reliability (a reading >20% reflects an unreliable measurement and should be repeated). In the Tono-Pen AVIA, after depressing the activation button, a green light and beep signal that the unit is ready for measurement. The dual-sided LCD display shows double dashed lines and the unit can be operated as described earlier. When 10 readings are obtained within 15 seconds, the LCD displays an IOP with a statistical confidence indicator (Fig. 63.31).

If single dashes appear on the LCD after the final beep, too few valid readings were obtained. In such a case, reactivate the probe (without recalibration) and repeat the measurement procedure. If the probe is not reactivated within 20 seconds, the LCD will clear, but the device can be activated as noted previously without recalibration.

The values are interpreted as outlined earlier for the Schiøtz device. Readings may be affected by the same features noted as causes of error with impression tonometry via the Schiøtz device. Store the device with an unused Ocu-Film cover protecting the tip of the probe. As with any device, be familiar with the manufacturer's instructions for use.

Impression/Rebound (Icare) Technique

When using the Icare tonometer, the preparations for testing are similar to the Tono-Pen described earlier, except that this device can be used without topical anesthetic drops. Review the user's manual to become familiar with the instructions before use. The following brief synopsis is provided if instructions are not available. Various parts of the tonometer are shown in Fig. 63.32 and referred to in these instructions.

Use of the wrist strap is recommended. Press the measuring button to turn on the device. When the display shows "LoAd," load the single-use probe into the probe base, being careful not to drop the probe out of the tonometer. Again, press the measuring button which will magnetize the probe, preventing it from falling out. The display should then indicate "OO" when the tonometer is ready to use. Align the tonometer with the patient's eye, ensuring that the central groove is in a horizontal position (Fig. 63.33). Keep the tip of the probe at a distance from the cornea of 4 to 8 mm, or ⅙ to ⅓ inch (Fig. 63.34). Adjust the forehead support wheel if necessary. To initiate measuring, lightly press the measuring button repeatedly for six measurements. The probe will be activated and bounce off the cornea for each measurement. A video demonstration can be viewed at https://www.youtube.com/watch?v=fqmFRpYXrxY. It is not necessary to look at the LCD display during measurements. A short beep will sound with each measurement and a longer beep will sound and the letter "P" with

Tonometry: Tono-Pen Technique

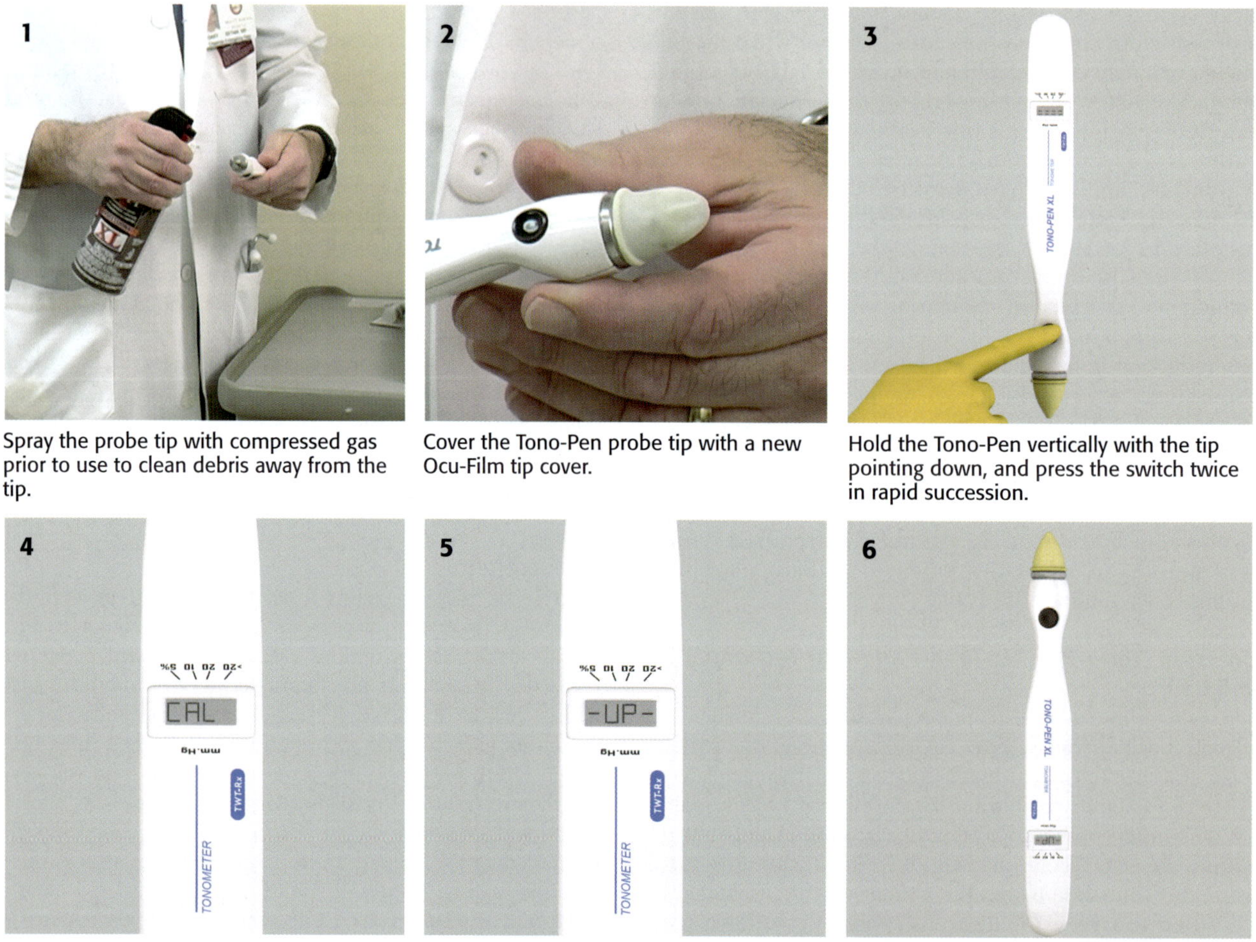

1. Spray the probe tip with compressed gas prior to use to clean debris away from the tip.
2. Cover the Tono-Pen probe tip with a new Ocu-Film tip cover.
3. Hold the Tono-Pen vertically with the tip pointing down, and press the switch twice in rapid succession.
4. After pressing the switch, 2 beeps will sound and "CAL" will appear on the screen.
5. Wait (up to 20 seconds) until a beep sounds and "-UP-" appears on the screen.
6. Quickly turn the probe so that the tip is pointing straight up.

Fig. 63.29 Tonometry: Tono-Pen technique. *IOP,* Intraocular pressure; *LCD,* liquid crystal display.

Tonometry: Tono-Pen Technique

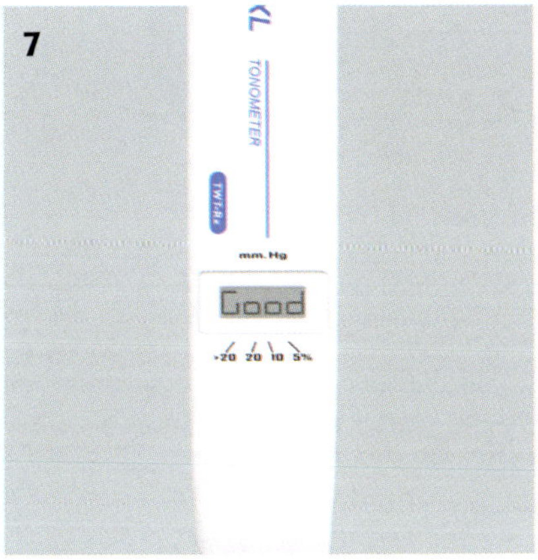

Wait a few seconds. If the calibration was successful, a beep will sound and "Good" will appear on the LCD screen.

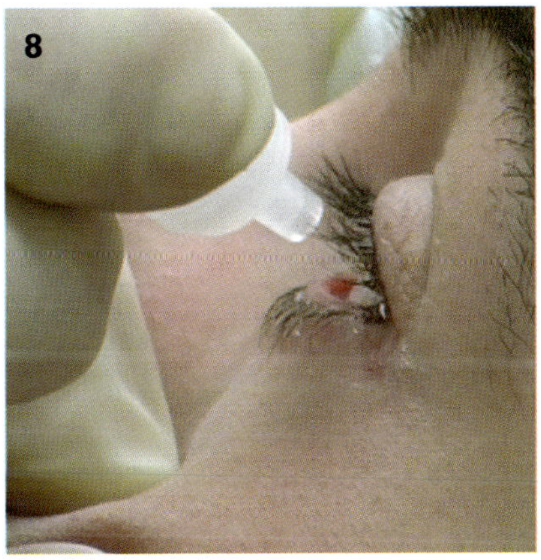

Instill a drop of topical anesthetic (e.g., tetracaine 0.5%) into both eyes.

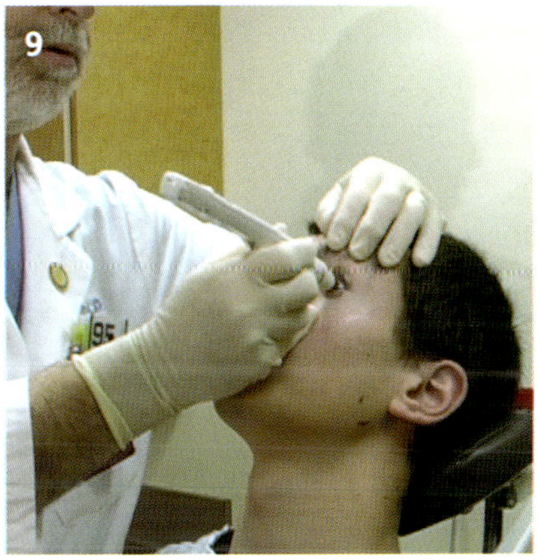

Hold the Tono-Pen as you would hold a pencil, and brace your hand against the patient's cheek for stability.

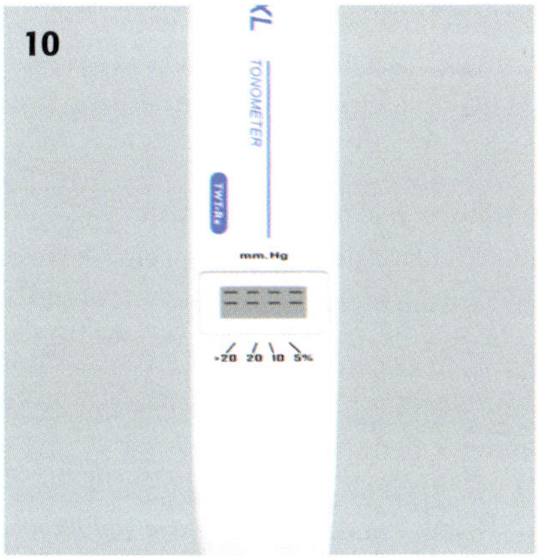

Activate the Tono-Pen by pressing the switch. A beep will sound and "= = =" will appear on the LCD screen.

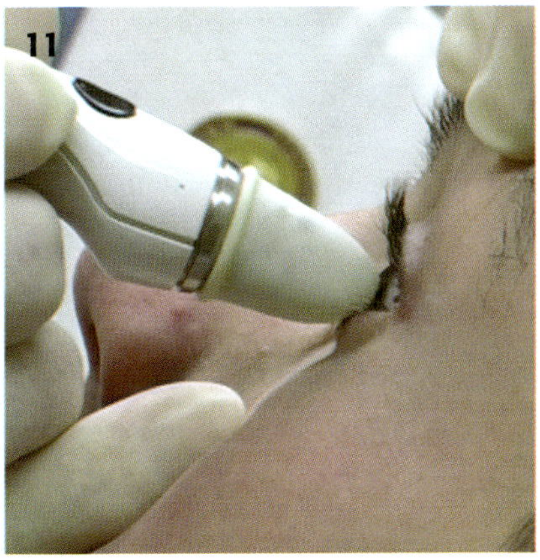

Touch the Tono-Pen against the cornea lightly and briefly. Repeat several times; a click will sound every time that a pressure is measured. After four valid readings, a final beep will sound, and the averaged measurement will appear on the LCD.

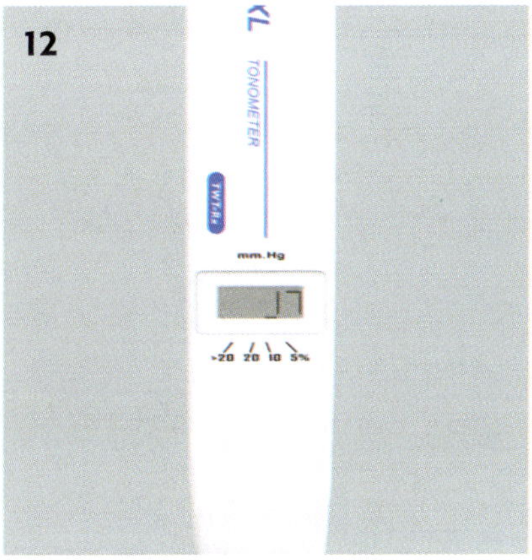

Check the reading on the screen. The number represents IOP in mm Hg. The bar below the number represents the statistical reliability. (A reading > 20% reflects an unreliable reading and should be repeated.)

Fig. 63.29, cont'd

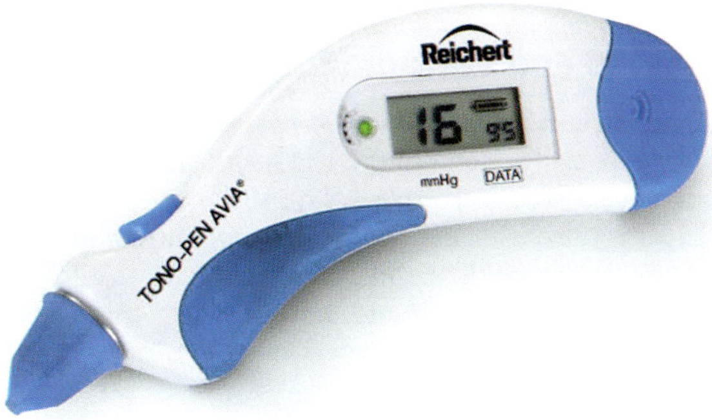

Fig. 63.30 The Tono-Pen AVIA is designed to fit comfortably in the hand and has a large dual-sided liquid crystal display.

APPLANATION MODE - USER INTERFACE SEQUENCE OF EVENTS		
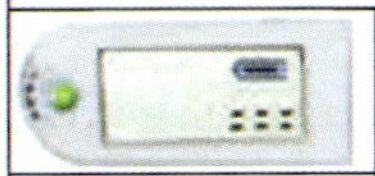	User Interface Ready to Measure	LED On, 1 Beep Ready to Begin IOP Testing (15 seconds for testing before Time Out)
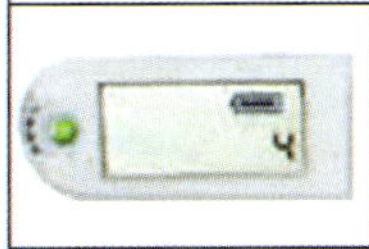	User Interface Testing Display	LED On During Test, screen shows number of applanations achieved (in this case 4 of 10) Each applanation taken equals 1 Chirp
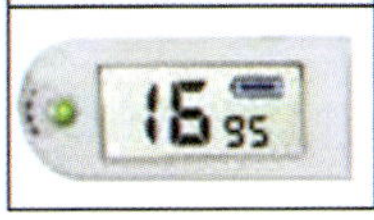	User Interface Test Complete	LED Off, 1 Beep Test Complete Patient has an IOP of 16 with a statistical confidence indicator of 95

Fig. 63.31 The Tono-Pen AVIA liquid crystal display indicates that the device is ready to measure with double dashed lines *(top)*. During the measuring mode, the display indicates the number of successful measurements *(middle)*. Once 10 measurements are completed successfully, the display will show the intraocular pressure *(IOP)* (large number) and a statistical confidence indicator *(bottom)*. *LED*, Light-emitting diode.

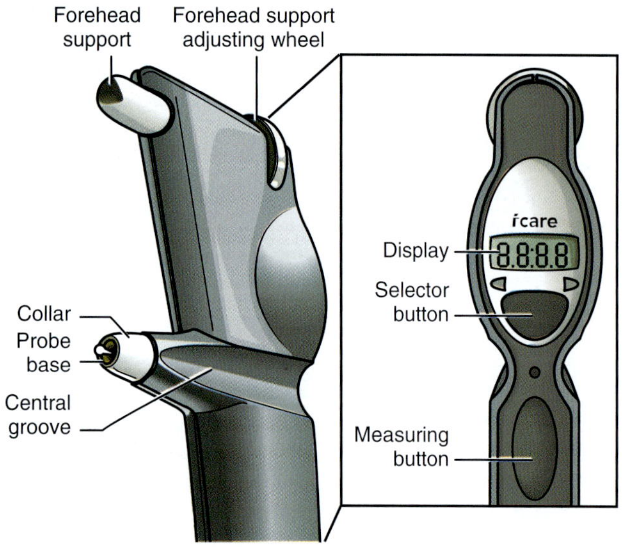

Fig. 63.32 Various parts of the Icare. (Courtesy Icare USA, Inc. http://www.icare-usa.com.)

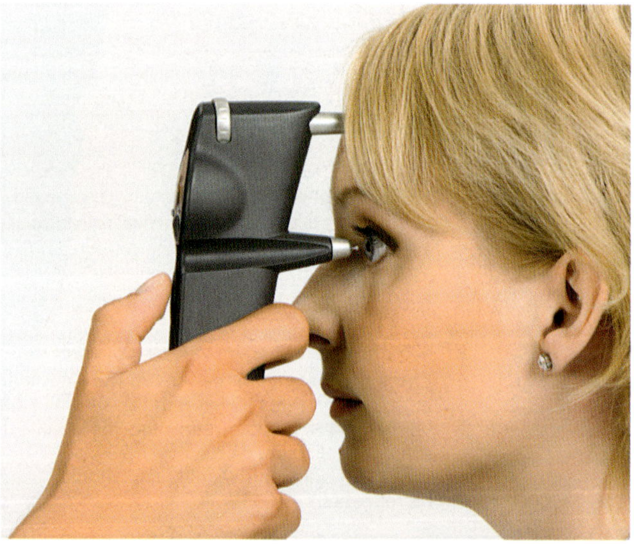

Fig. 63.33 Note the proper alignment of the device in relation to the patient. The central groove should be in a horizontal position for an upright patient. (Courtesy Icare USA, Inc. http://www.icare-usa.com.)

the IOP shown on the display when the required six measurements are made. If the "P" is blinking, or if there is a dash next to the middle or top of the "P" then a repeat measurement is indicated. A line near the bottom of the "P" indicates a slightly different, but insignificant standard deviation of the combined measurements. A double beep will sound if an incorrect measurement is made. Common reasons for an error code are holding the probe too far away from the cornea and aligning the tonometer incorrectly. Clear the error code by pressing the selector button once, then proceed with further measurements. See instruction manual for additional error codes. Abnormal findings should prompt a repeat measurement. The device will power off if not used after 2 minutes of inactivity but can be manually turned off by pressing either selector or measuring button once. After the LCD shows "byE," pressing either button again will turn off the device.

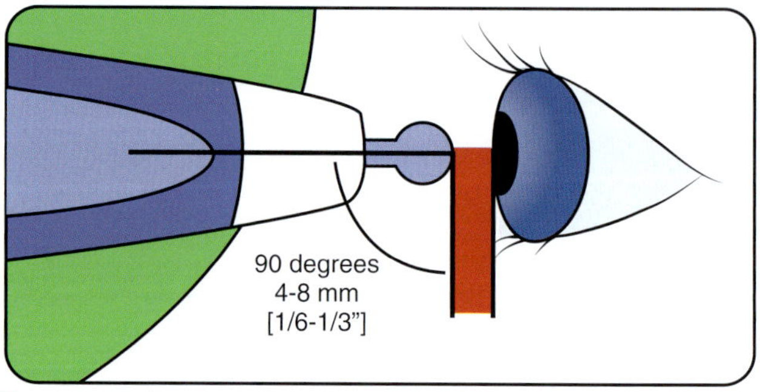

Fig. 63.34 The probe position should be 90 degrees to the frontal plane of the eye so that the probe will contact the central cornea. The distance of the probe to the cornea must be between 4 and 8 mm or ⅙ to ⅓ inch for a successful measurement to occur. (Courtesy Icare USA, Inc. http://www.icare-usa.com.)

Complications

When tonometric instruments are used properly and reasonable precautions are taken, complications are unusual. An eye with preexisting corneal injury should be spared the additional trauma of tonometer placement. Corneal abrasions can be produced or worsened by ocular movement during testing. In particular, patients with uncontrollable nystagmus, hiccups, coughing, or those who are extremely apprehensive should not be subjected to tonometry. Infection can be transmitted by use of the instrument. Careful cleansing of the device and avoidance of tonometry in patients with obvious conjunctivitis, corneal ulcers, or active herpetic lesions should minimize the risk of spreading the infection to the unaffected eye or to subsequent patients. Although protective coverings can be placed over the tonometer contact, tonometry can usually be postponed in the aforementioned individuals until the risk for infection is minimal. Extrusion of ocular contents with penetrating injuries is a potential, but rare complication.

SLIT LAMP EXAMINATION

See Videos 63.12–63.14. The slit lamp is an extremely useful instrument for examination of the anterior segment of the eye. The instrument can reveal pathologic conditions that would otherwise be invisible, such as minor corneal defects, anterior chamber hemorrhage, and inflammation.

Indications and Contraindications

The slit lamp can be used in the majority of eye examinations. It is especially useful in the ED for the diagnosis of corneal abrasions, FBs, and iritis.[41] The slit lamp facilitates FB removal and is also used in conjunction with most applanation tonometers. Portable slit lamp instruments are readily available, relatively inexpensive, and easily used in the ED (Fig. 63.35), but emergency practitioners may have access only to a stationary, upright device. Therefore in the absence of a portable device, a slit lamp examination is contraindicated in patients who cannot tolerate an upright sitting position (e.g., those with orthostatic syncope).

Equipment

The slit lamp has three essential components: a binocular microscope mounted horizontally, a light source that can

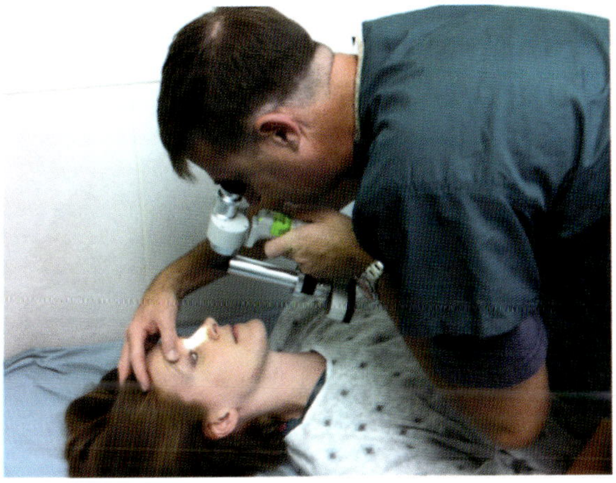

Fig. 63.35 A portable slit lamp can be used to evaluate patients who cannot tolerate an upright sitting position or cannot be easily moved to the examination chair.

create a beam of variable width, and a mechanical assembly to immobilize the patient's head and manipulate the microscope and light source. The location and arrangement of the knobs that control these components vary in devices made by different manufacturers. Usually, by simply turning each knob and watching the results, one can quickly master a new machine. Fig. 63.36 illustrates the location of the functional controls on one particular instrument.

First, locate the on/off switch for the instrument. Frequently, this switch incorporates or is adjacent to a rheostat that provides two or three different power settings. The lowest setting is adequate for routine examination and will preserve bulb life. One can use a high-intensity setting when examining the anterior chamber with a narrow-slit beam. Often, these controls are located on a transformer placed beneath the table to which the slit lamp has been attached. The second knob that one should find is the locking nut for the mechanical assembly. Loosen the nut so that the assembly can be moved relative to the stand.

Make adjustments so that the patient is comfortable while sitting with the head in the device. Ask the patient to press the forehead firmly against the headrest with the chin in the chin rest. By varying the height of the table and height of the chin rest, one should be able to maximize comfort of the patient's neck and back. Adjust the chin rest to align the patient's eye level with the mark on the headrest support rods.

The binocular microscope has a control for varying the magnification. Usually, low powers such as 10× or 16× are the most useful. Use a higher power to examine the anterior chamber for cells and flare and when the cornea is examined in minute detail. Adjust the binocular interpupillary distance to match that of the examiner. Focus the eyepieces by moving the instrument forward and backward until the narrowed vertical beam is sharpest on the patient's cornea when viewed with the unaided eye. Then, while viewing through each eyepiece individually, adjust the focus of each to produce a sharp image of the anterior surface of the cornea.

Notice that the light source is mounted on a swinging arm. Find the knobs that adjust the width and the height of the light beam. Click various filters in as needed, usually white and blue filters for standard examination. Alter the angle of the slit lamp beam to vertical from horizontal. The vertical alignment is preferred for routine examinations in the ED.

Both the microscope and the light source are mounted on swivel arms linked at their base to the movable table. Change the position of this table by pushing on any part of it. Use the joystick on the table for finer movements. Vary the height of the microscope and the light source by twisting either the joystick or a separate knob at the base, depending on the design of the instrument.

Procedure

There are three parts to every slit lamp examination that every operator must consider performing. The *first part* is for an overall screening of the anterior segment of the eye. For examination of the patient's right eye, swing the light source to your left at a 45-degree angle while the microscope is directly in front of the patient's eye. Set the slit beam to the maximum height and the minimum width using the white light. To scan across the patient's cornea, first focus the beam on the cornea by moving the entire base of the slit lamp forward and backward. Then move the whole base of the mechanical apparatus left and right to scan across the cornea while keeping the cornea in focus. The 45-degree angle between the microscope and the light source is the default position. The most common mistake is to try to scan by swinging the arm of the light source in an arc; this does not work because the light beam will remain centered on the same point of the patient's eye. Scan across at the level of the conjunctiva and the cornea and then push slightly forward on the base or joystick to focus and scan at the level of the iris. The depth of the anterior chamber is easily appreciated with this low-magnification setup (Fig. 63.37). When the depth of the anterior chamber is reduced, suspect a corneal perforation or a predisposition to angle-closure glaucoma.

Use this basic examination to examine the conjunctiva for traumatic lesions, inflammation, and FBs. Examine the eyelids for hordeolum, blepharitis, or trichiasis. Completely evert the lids (as described in the earlier section on "Ocular FB Removal") in conjunction with the slit lamp examination to permit evaluation of the undersurface of the upper lid for FB retention.

Corneal FB removal can be enhanced by use of the slit lamp. In particular, the instrument allows stabilization of the patient's head. Magnification also minimizes corneal injury during FB or rust ring removal. The upper eyelid may be immobilized with a cotton-tipped applicator, as discussed previously. The clinician's hand can be steadied against the patient's nose, cheek, or forehead or against the support rods of the headrest. The patient should be instructed to stare straight ahead at a fixed light or at the clinician's ear during removal of the FB.

The *second part* is essentially the same as the first but uses the blue filter to identify any areas of fluorescein staining. After fluorescein is applied, "click" the blue filter into position and widen the beam to 3 or 4 mm. A patient can tolerate a wider beam without photophobia if it is blue. Search for corneal defects (as discussed in the earlier section "The Fluorescein Examination") with this setup. The blue filter may also be used with applanation tonometry, as discussed in the earlier section on "Tonometry."

The purpose of the *third part* is to search for cells in the anterior chamber, either the white cells of iritis or the red cells of a microscopic hyphema. Shorten the height of the beam to 3 or 4 mm and make it as narrow as possible. Switch the

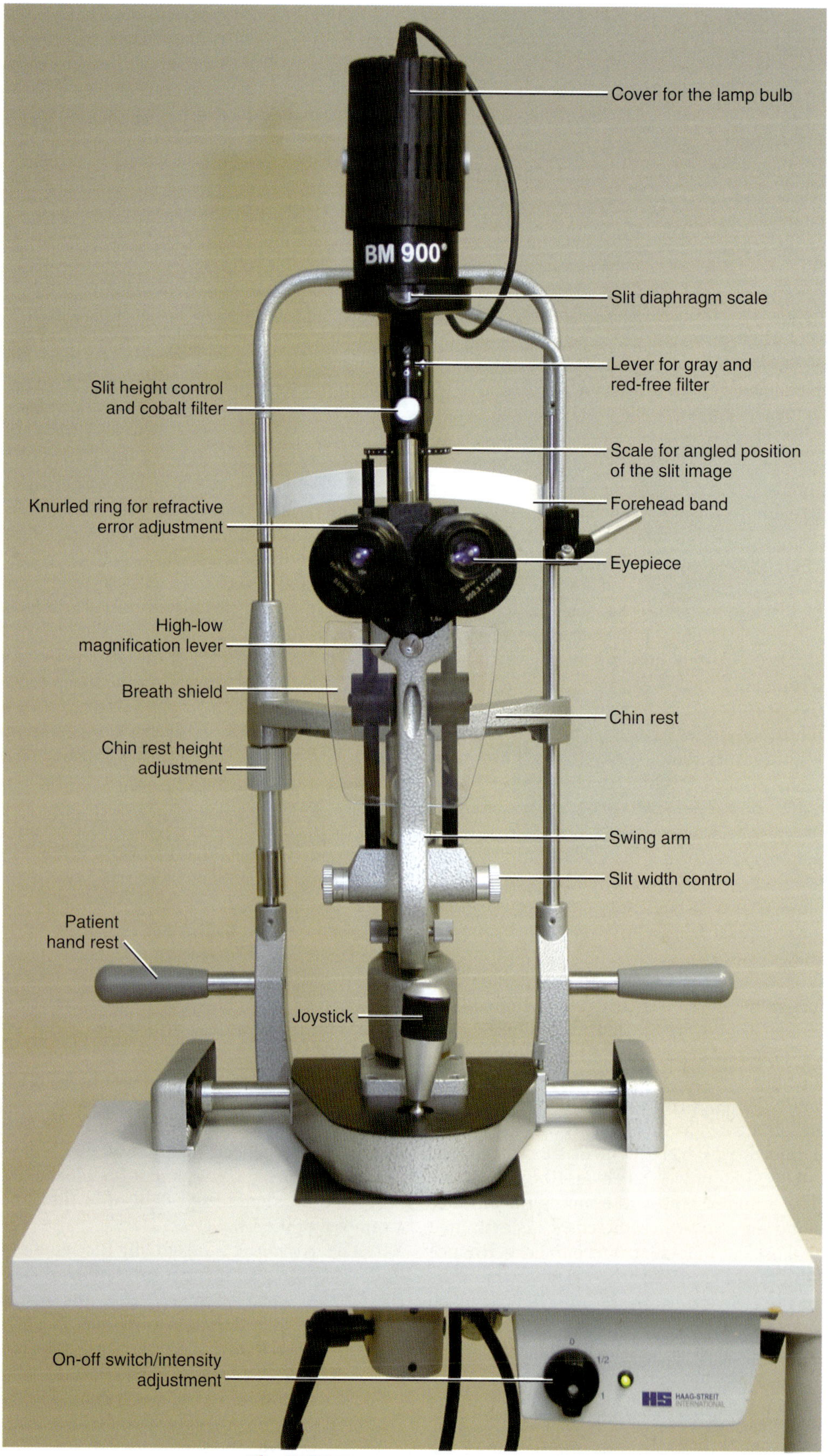

Fig. 63.36 Haag-Streit BM 900 slit lamp.

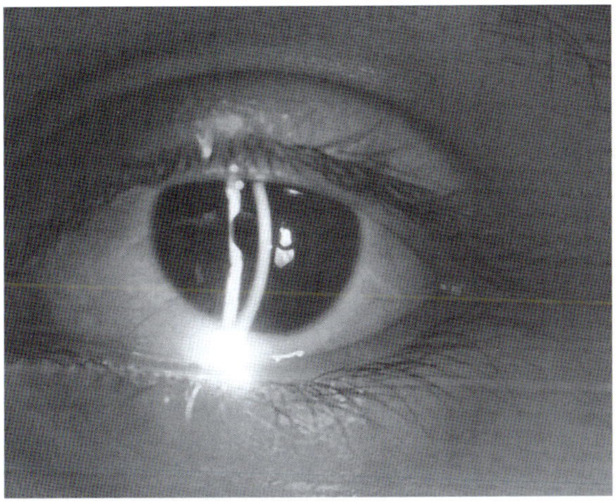

Fig. 63.37 Slit lamp photograph of a normal left eye under low power. The curved slit of light on the right is reflected off the cornea and the slit on the left is reflected off the iris. The depth of the anterior chamber can easily be appreciated under this low-magnification setup. Note that the light source is on the patient's left side to examine the left eye, with the path of the light going in a temporal-to-nasal direction. (Courtesy D. Price.)

microscope to high power. Focus the beam on the center of the cornea and then push forward slightly so that it is focused on the anterior surface of the lens. Pull the joystick back again to a focus point midway between the cornea and the lens, where it will be focused on the anterior chamber (Fig. 63.38). Keep the beam centered over the pupil so that there is a black background. Normally, the aqueous humor of the anterior chamber is totally clear. Small particles seen floating up or down through the beam are usually circulating cells. If the beam lights up the aqueous like a searchlight in the fog, the examiner has found the protein flare that accompanies iritis. Note that fluorescein can penetrate an abraded cornea and produce a fluorescein flare on slit lamp evaluation. To avoid confusion, some clinicians prefer to examine for anterior chamber flare before the stain is used. A variety of conditions evaluated by the slit lamp are pictured in Fig. 63.39.

Portable Slit Lamp

The indications and steps for using a portable slit lamp are the same as for a conventional slit lamp, thus follow the procedures already stated. The following differences, however, need to be taken into account. Ensure that the battery is charged. Familiarize yourself with the controls that adjust aperture width and height, intensity, and filters, especially the white and fluorescein filters. Check the device for a stabilizing bar, which has the same function as the forehead strap on the conventional slip lamp to hold the patient's head still. Without the stabilizing bar, it becomes very difficult to see any magnified object (Fig. 63.40). Start with low-power lenses (magnification ×10), which should allow for most of the examination needed in a portable setting. Portable units may have a separate set of lenses that can be exchanged readily if examination using high power is needed.

UNILATERAL LOSS OF VISION

There are a variety of reasons why an individual may sustain complete loss of vision in one eye, but most commonly, such loss is caused by occlusion of the central retinal vein, occlusion of the central retinal artery, or optic nerve damage. Less commonly, pressure on the orbit from a retroorbital hemorrhage may compromise the ophthalmic artery.

Although discussion of all the potential causes of unilateral loss of vision is beyond the scope of this text, amaurosis fugax deserves special mention. Amaurosis fugax is a transient loss of vision that is most commonly due to cholesterol or platelet emboli from atherosclerotic carotid occlusive disease. When plaques are visualized in the retinal vasculature, auscultate the neck for carotid bruits and consider referring the patient for a more thorough evaluation including ultrasound examination of the carotid artery.[96,97]

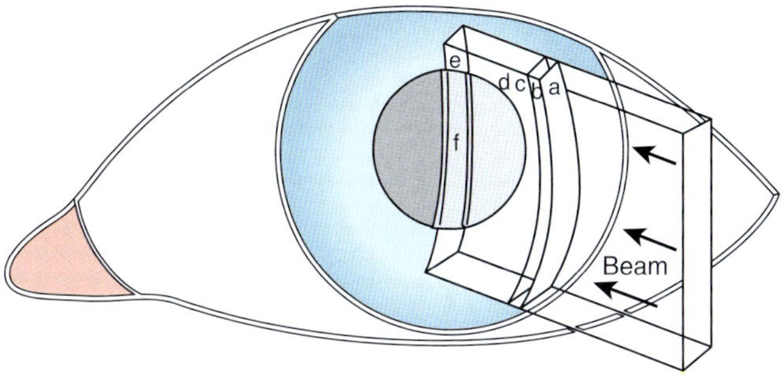

Fig. 63.38 Appearance of the left eye during examination of the anterior chamber under low power: *a*, corneal epithelium; *b*, corneal stroma; *c*, corneal endothelium; *d*, anterior chamber (potential location of cells or flare); *e*, iris; *f*, lens reflection. The slit of light shines in the temporal-to-nasal direction at a 45-degree angle to the anterior surface of the cornea. The depth of the cornea and anterior chamber examinations are best done under high power in a dark room.

Central Renal Artery Occlusion

A patient with central retinal artery occlusion (CRAO) has generally experienced a recent sudden painless (complete or nearly complete) unilateral loss of vision. On examination, there is an afferent pupillary defect (APD) (i.e., sluggish or nonreactive pupil in the affected eye with direct illumination and a normal consensual response) and reduced visual acuity. Immediately after the event the fundus may appear nearly normal; however, it soon becomes pale and a classic "cherry-red spot" in the macula may be evident as a result of patent choroidal vessels showing through the transparent fovea (Fig. 63.41).

Therapy

Visual recovery has been noted to occur up to 3 days after CRAO. Start treatment if the patient is seen within 24 hours after the onset of symptoms.[98] Consult ophthalmology while initiating therapy. In many centers, CRAO is considered an ischemic event and neurology as well as ophthalmology are often involved in acute management. In some stroke centers, patients with CRAO are admitted to neurology on confirmation of the diagnosis.

Most of the emergency techniques suggested for treating vascular insults to the eye in the ED are theoretically sound but are not supported or refuted by rigorous scientific data. No specific standard of care has been promulgated for these interventions by emergency clinicians. Techniques discussed later are probably safe and possibly useful and may be

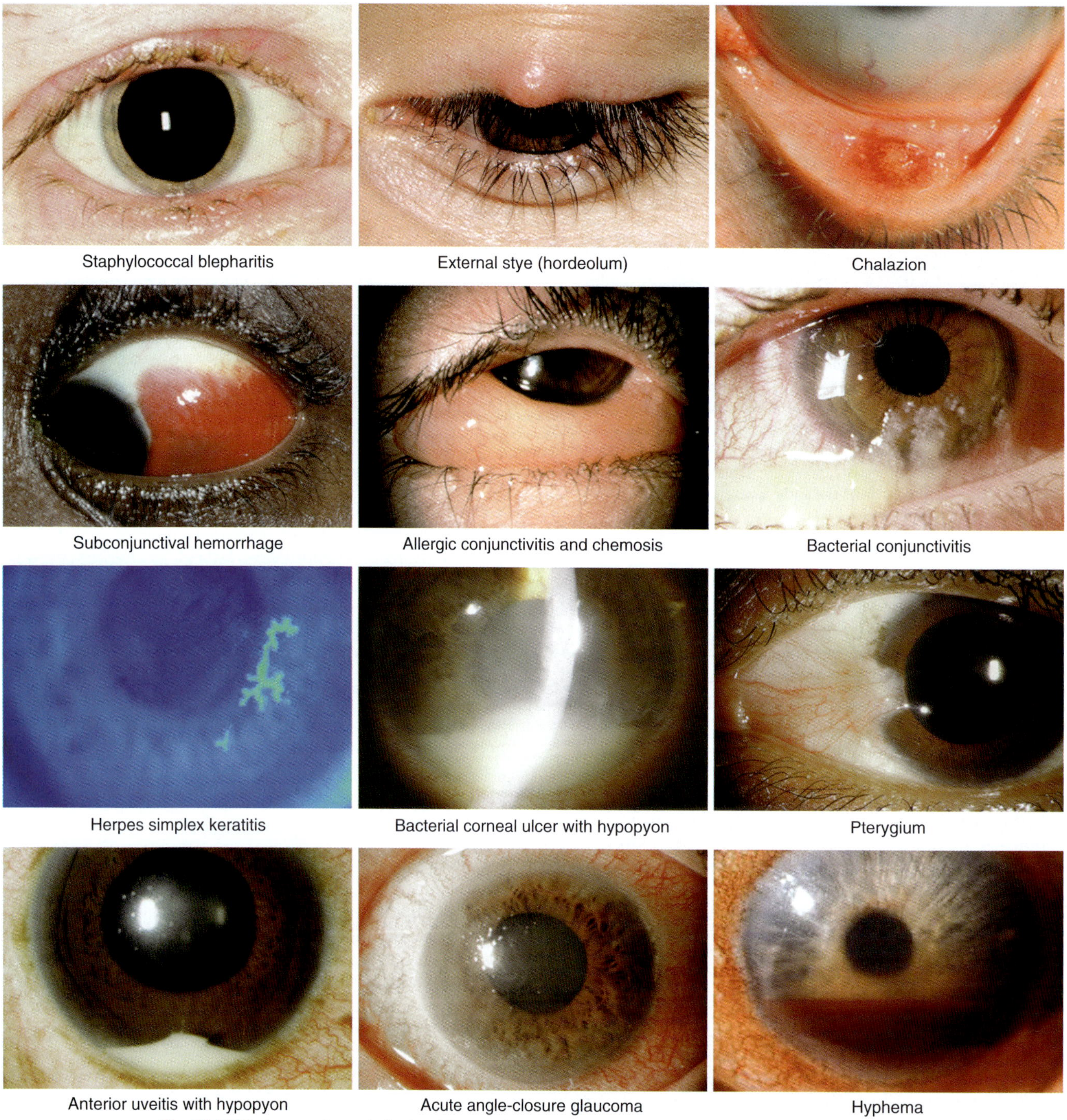

Fig. 63.39 Various ocular pathologies. (From Palay DA, Krachmer JH, eds. *Primary Care Ophthalmology*. 2nd ed. Mosby; 2005.)

attempted in an emergency situation. It is unknown whether these interventions will be vision saving.

Slow rebreathing into a paper bag is believed to increase the arterial carbon dioxide level, thus aiding vasodilation, permitting the occlusion to move more peripherally, and possibly reducing the ischemic area, although its effectiveness and safety in the presence of additional comorbidities has not been well elucidated. In the past, this was often accompanied by digital globe massage, and can certainly be applied without the paper bag rebreathing. *Digital massage* can be accomplished with the patient lying supine and applying firm steady pressure with the thumbs to the affected globe over the patient's closed lids. Apply pressure for 5 seconds and then abruptly release it (Fig. 63.42). Immediately repeat this maneuver several more times for up to 20 minutes. The objective of this technique is to help break up the occlusion and encourage movement of it more peripherally.

A more aggressive therapy, generally performed only by ophthalmologists, is *anterior chamber paracentesis*. In the absence of available consultation, consider this technique when CRAO is recent and unresponsive to the previously described therapeutic approaches. For this procedure, keep the patient supine with the head and eyelids secured. Anesthetize the cornea with topical anesthetic drops (e.g., 0.5%

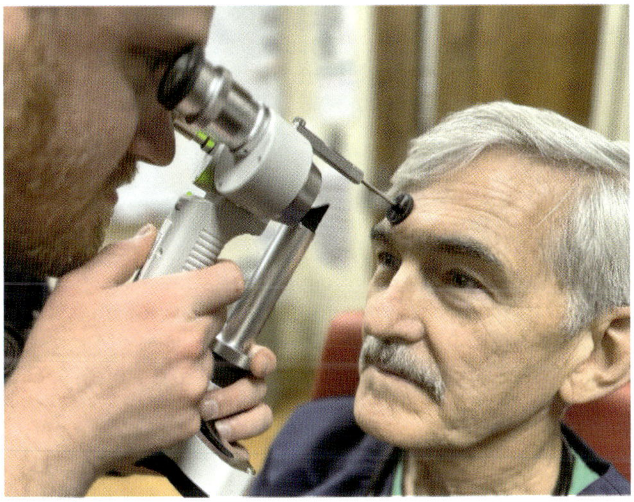

Fig. 63.40 Portable slit lamp with stabilizing bar in use.

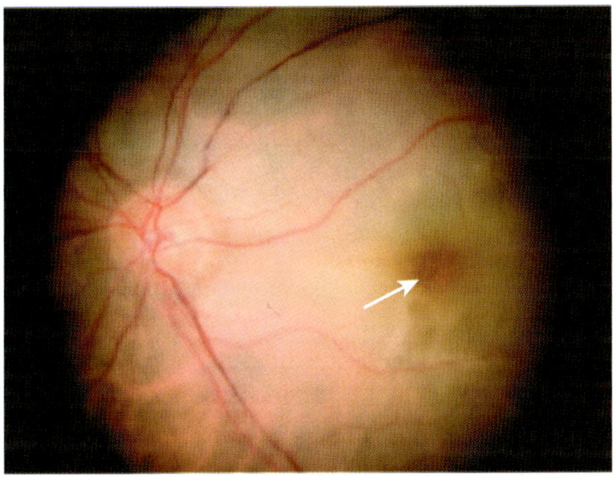

Fig. 63.41 Central retinal artery occlusion with a cherry-red spot in the fovea *(arrow)*. (From Friedman NJ, Kaiser PK, Pineda A. *Massachusetts Ear & Eye Infirmary Illustrated Manual of Ophthalmology*. 3rd ed. Saunders; 2009.)

proparacaine drops). Inject the conjunctiva adjacent to the limbus with a 27- or 30-gauge needle until the entire perilimbal area is infiltrated and has the appearance of chemosis in all quadrants. During the remainder of the procedure, ask an assistant to firmly grasp the conjunctiva with toothless forceps at the 3 and 9 o'clock positions to stabilize the eye. Insert a 30-gauge needle on a tuberculin syringe obliquely just adjacent to the limbus at either the 4:30 or the 7:30 position, and direct it toward the 6 o'clock position to avoid the lens (Fig. 63.43). Apply gentle pressure on the globe and, after 1 to 2 drops of aqueous are expressed, withdraw the needle.[99] As stated earlier, this procedure is best performed by the consultant ophthalmologist rather than the EP.

A recent retrospective study analysis reviewed data from patients treated for CRAO receiving standard inpatient therapy with and without paracentesis at the Dr. Horst Schmidt Clinics in Wiesbaden, Germany. Due to the retina's low tolerance to ischemia, irreversible damage occurs shortly after arterial occlusion, severely affecting visual acuity. The primary endpoint was visual acuity improvement 72 hours after intervention. This study revealed no significant improvement in mean visual acuity comparing patients receiving paracentesis

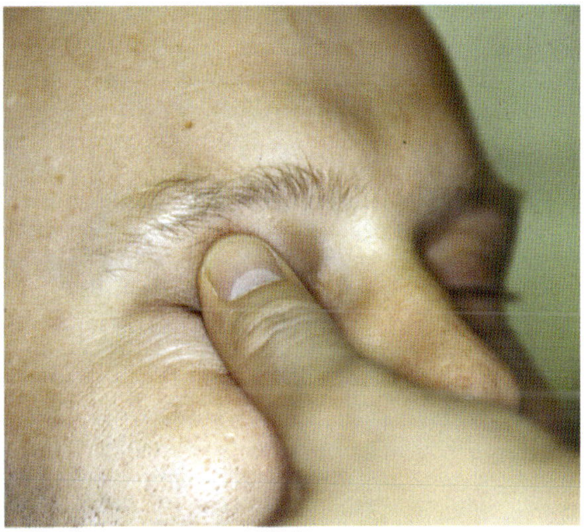

Fig. 63.42 To perform digital globe massage, apply firm steady pressure with the thumb on the globe for approximately 5 seconds and then abruptly release the pressure for 5 to 10 seconds. Repeat the process for up to 20 minutes or until improvement in vision is observed.

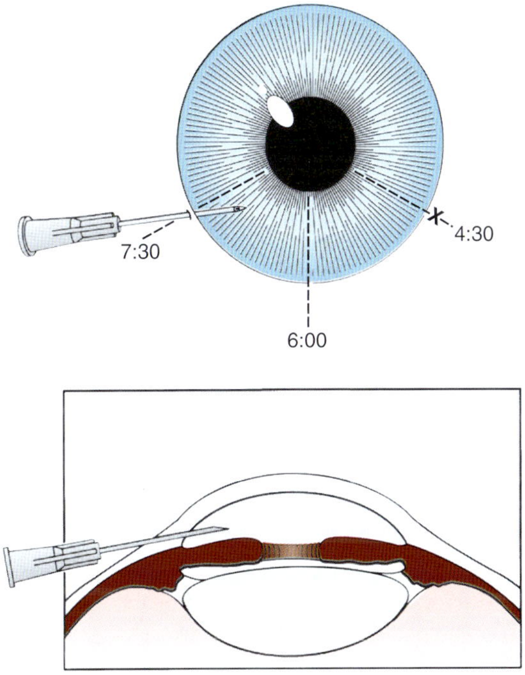

Fig. 63.43 Anterior chamber paracentesis. After topical and subconjunctival anesthesia (see text), a 30-gauge needle is directed obliquely from the 4:30 or 7:30 position toward the 6 o'clock position to avoid the lens. An assistant stabilizes the globe with forceps and grasps the conjunctiva (see text). *Top*, Anteroposterior projection; *bottom*, tangential projection. (From Knoop K, Trott A. Ophthalmologic procedures in the emergency department: I. Immediate sight-saving procedures. *Acad Emerg Med*. 1994;1:408.)

within 6 hours, 6–24 hours, or greater than 24 hours from initial symptom onset in comparison to conservative management. As a result, anterior chamber paracentesis was not recommended therapeutically at any time point following diagnosis of arterial occlusion. One argument in favor of performing anterior chamber paracentesis is reducing IOP, which theoretically increases retinal artery perfusion and oxygenation.

Ultimately, decision to treat with this procedure should be in consultation with an ophthalmologist on a case-by-case basis involving a team multidisciplinary approach.[100,101]

It should also be noted that CRAO can be considered as an acute vascular event near enough to the central nervous system that neurology should be involved as soon as the diagnosis is entered. In published literature, CRAO is considered the ocular equivalent of a cerebral stroke. Some hospital centers will include CRAO as part of a stroke syndrome involving both neurology and ophthalmology emergent consultations. If first symptom onset is within the time window for thrombolytic administration, systemic use of tissue plasminogen activator (t-PA) can be considered with consultation involvement. Due to the small caliber of the central retinal artery, academic centers have studied the use of targeted thrombolytic therapy as the risks of systemic therapy potentially outweigh its benefits. One multicenter randomized controlled trial compared targeted intraarterial fibrinolysis with t-PA to conservative management in 84 patients. Similar outcomes were reported in both treatment arms; however, the trial was concluded prematurely due to adverse reactions in the intraarterial fibrinolysis group (37%) compared with the control (4%).[102,103] In addition, antiplatelet agents are utilized for protection against intracranial embolism in conjunction with Stroke Neurology consultation. Secondary to the relative infrequency of CRAO compared with other ischemic events, large-scale randomized controlled trials are limited and well-designed prospective trials are needed.

A novel approach to treatment of CRAO within the first 24 hours of symptom onset is hyperbaric oxygen (HBO) therapy. Because the retina has a dual blood supply, it is thought initiation of HBO therapy increases choroidal oxygen levels. This leads to a downstream effect of oxygen perfusion to the inner retinal layers to maintain viability and boost oxygen supply to ischemic retinal regions. Initially supported by animal models, many patient case series report a significant mean increase in visual acuity after initiation of HBO therapy ranging from 2 to 3 lines on a Snellen eye chart. Protocols vary among institutions and standardization regarding duration and treatment frequency varies. The side effect profile is minimal and notable for barotrauma, but if treatments are limited to 120-minute duration and oxygen pressure is less than 3 atmospheres, HBO therapy is generally viewed as safe and benign. Absolute contraindications include an untreated pneumothorax and certain chemotherapeutic regimens. Relative contraindications include an existing pregnancy, epilepsy, severe claustrophobia, and acute upper respiratory tract infections. Studies available show promise of early HBO therapy improving visual acuity outcomes; however, prospective randomized trials are necessary.[102,104]

One study described a systematic approach in which ocular massage, sublingual isosorbide dinitrate, 10 mg; acetazolamide, 500 mg intravenously; 20% mannitol (1 mg/kg); or oral 50% glycerol (1 mg/kg); anterior chamber paracentesis; methylprednisolone, 500 mg intravenously; streptokinase, 750 kIU; and retrobulbar tolazoline, 50 mg, were given until the visual symptoms improved or all steps were complete.[105] Of the 11 patients in this arm of the study, eight had improved visual acuity. In those who improved, all had their symptoms improved in 12 hours or less. The presumed cause was either a platelet-derived or cholesterol embolus from atheroma or glaucoma.[95] Although this study is small, it supports emergency ophthalmology consultation and aggressive treatment of patients seen within 12 to 24 hours of the onset of symptoms. With no effective or definitive treatment available for CRAO, it is imperative to identify risk factors and causes, with a focus on preventive measures and risk factor modifications.

Complications

Overzealous globe massage has the potential to produce intraocular trauma, including retinal detachment and intraocular hemorrhage. Anterior chamber paracentesis may produce hemorrhage, infection (endophthalmitis), or mechanical injury to the cornea, iris, or lens.[106] Administration of systemic or targeted thrombolytic therapy carries the risk of intracranial hemorrhage or intravascular injury. Although these complications are rare, ophthalmologic consultation for assistance with the underlying CRAO and surveillance for these potential complications should be initiated on an emergency basis.

Orbital Compartment Syndrome

Acute facial trauma or recent retrobulbar anesthesia may produce retrobulbar hemorrhage with sufficient pressure to compromise the ophthalmic artery and result in an orbital compartment syndrome (Fig. 63.44). A form of posttraumatic glaucoma may also occur when the retrobulbar hematoma forces the globe against the eyelids. In this case, IOP rises precipitously because the globe is in a relatively closed space as a result of the firm attachment of the eyelids to the orbital rim by the medial and lateral canthal ligaments. The optic nerve, its vascular supply, and the central retinal artery are compressed, which can result in ischemia and subsequent visual loss. In this situation, emergency lateral canthotomy may be considered for relief of the pressure on the eye. Although not a commonly performed procedure for many EPs, in the proper scenario, it may be a prudent sight-saving intervention.

In this situation, ophthalmoscopic evaluation reveals a blanched ophthalmic artery in the presence of obvious retrobulbar pressure and ecchymosis around the eye. The patient exhibits decreased visual acuity, and an afferent pupil defect is often seen. IOP is markedly elevated but may be relieved by emergency lateral canthotomy and cantholysis. Such a procedure needs to be performed quickly because the ischemic retina will not retain function if it is deprived of blood for a long period.

Technique: Lateral Canthotomy and Cantholysis

See Fig. 63.45 and Videos 63.15 and 63.16. The goals of the procedure are to release pressure on the globe and decrease IOP sufficiently to reinstitute retinal artery blood flow. Because retinal recovery is unlikely to occur if rapid relief of ischemia is not accomplished, taking extra time to clean the eye beyond simple saline cleansing of the lids and lateral canthus must be carefully considered. Stabilize the patient's head and lids and anesthetize the lateral canthus by injecting 1% to 2% lidocaine with epinephrine. Before incising, crush the lateral canthus with a small hemostat for 1 to 2 minutes to minimize bleeding. Incise the canthus with iris or Steven's scissors. Take precautions to avoid injury to the protruding globe. Begin the incision at the lateral canthus and extend it toward the orbital rim. Find the superior and inferior crura of the lateral canthal tendon and release them from the orbital rim. Some operators prefer to release the inferior crus and reassess IOP before considering release of the superior crus.

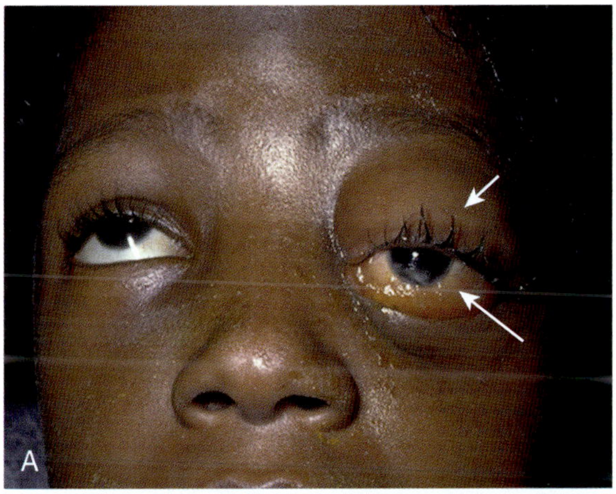

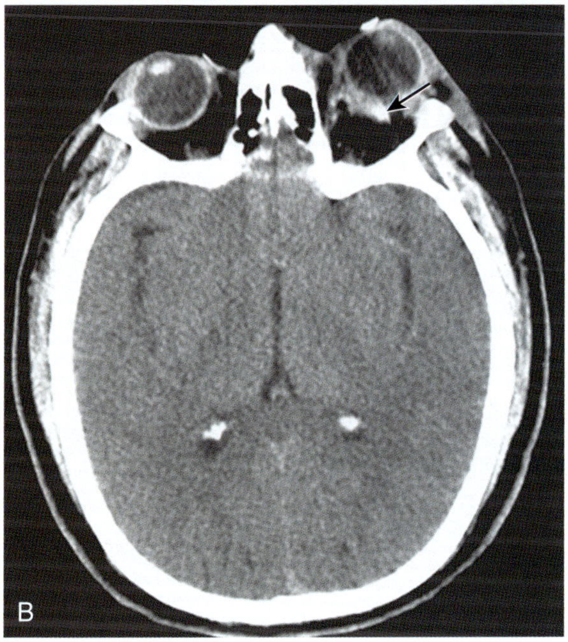

Fig.63.44 (A) Retrobulbar hemorrhage of the left eye demonstrating proptosis, lid swelling *(short arrow)*, chemosis *(long arrow)*, and restricted extraocular motility on upgaze. (B) Computed tomography scan demonstrating significant proptosis and radiodensity posterior to the left eye (retrobulbar hemorrhage indicated by the *arrow*). The intraocular pressure was measured to be 40 mm Hg and was rapidly lowered to 20 with a lateral canthotomy and cantholysis. Indications for lateral canthotomy and cantholysis include decreased visual acuity, ocular pressure greater than 40 mm Hg, proptosis, afferent papillary defect (Marcus Gunn pupil), cherry-red macula, ophthalmoplegia, optic nerve pallor, and severe eye pain. A ruptured globe is a contraindication.

An instructional video of the procedure on an actual ED patient can be found at https://www.youtube.com/watch?v=bUAagMd_Q8A.

Complications

Although hemorrhage, infection, and mechanical injury might result from the procedure, these complications generally respond to therapy better than retinal injury from prolonged ischemia. Emergency ophthalmologic consultation should be obtained, although when the procedure is indicated, it may be considered by the emergency clinician. Lateral canthotomy incisions generally heal without suturing or significant scarring.

REDUCTION OF GLOBE LUXATION

Although luxation of the globe is uncommon, the emergency clinician should be aware of the condition and its mechanisms, know how to reduce the globe, and know when to prioritize ophthalmologic consultation. With luxation of the globe there is extreme proptosis, which permits the lids to slip behind the globe equator (Fig. 63.46). Subsequent spasm of the orbicularis oculi muscles sustains the luxation and limits extraocular movement. Traction on the optic nerve and retinal vessels may produce direct or indirect injury to the optic nerve and retina.

Luxation may be spontaneous, voluntary, or traumatic. A variety of conditions (e.g., orbital neoplasms, Graves disease, histiocytosis X, cerebral gumma, and craniofacial dysostoses) may predispose the patient to luxation. Triggering events include maneuvers that increase IOP (e.g., Valsalva maneuver), trauma to the orbit or forehead, or eyelid manipulation.

Indications and Contraindications

Early globe reduction is indicated to relieve symptoms and minimize visual impairment. Attempts at reduction in the ED are relatively contraindicated when there is obvious rupture of the globe.

Technique

Before globe reduction, perform a rapid eye examination to document visual acuity, range of eye motion, pupillary reactivity, and any evidence of globe rupture (see earlier discussion).[107] Place the patient in a recumbent position and administer a topical ocular anesthetic agent. When the lashes are visible, ask an assistant to apply steady outward and upward traction while the globe is gently pushed behind the lids. Use gloved fingers to apply steady scleral pressure and to manipulate the globe back into the orbit. When the lashes cannot be grasped, introduce a lid retractor behind the lid to provide countertraction. Others recommend placing a suture through the anesthetized skin of each lid to provide countertraction.

After the procedure, repeat the eye examination to document visual acuity and extraocular movement. It is not uncommon for return of full visual function to be delayed for several days or occasionally longer.

Complications

It is common with this procedure for lashes to be retained in the conjunctival fornices. Evaluate for and remove any free lashes to prevent corneal injury. Edema, retrobulbar hemorrhage, or orbital deformity may prevent outpatient reduction. When reduction is not possible in the ED, saline drops should be applied to the globe and a noncontact eye shield used.

Aftercare

Patients with spontaneous luxation and no visual impairment in whom the globe is easily reduced warrant follow-up within 24 to 48 hours. Instructions to avoid potential triggering maneuvers should be given. Recurrent luxation may warrant lateral tarsorrhaphy. Further evaluation of potential precipitating factors can be pursued on an outpatient basis.

Patients with traumatic luxation are at greater risk for underlying ophthalmic injury and warrant emergency

Lateral Canthotomy And Cantholysis

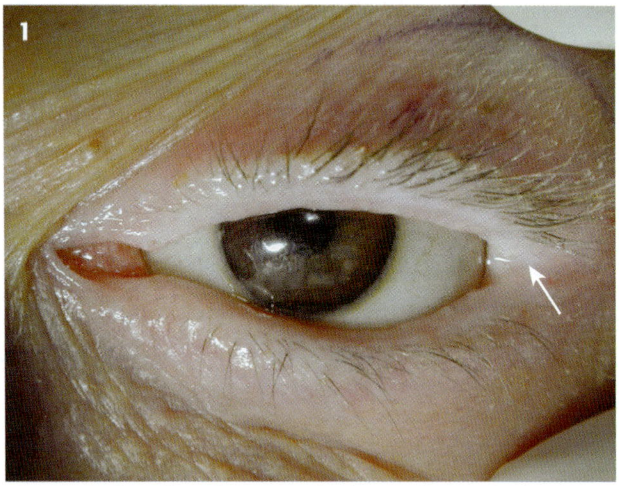

Identify the lateral canthus *(arrow)*. Cleanse the area with antiseptic and anesthetize with 1% lidocaine with epinephrine. (The left eye is depicted in this image sequence.)

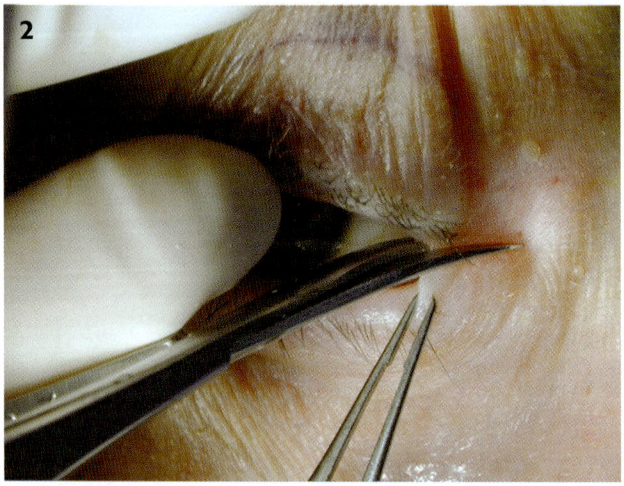

Crush the lateral canthus with a hemostat for 1 to 2 minutes to reduce incisional bleeding (not shown). Then, cut through the crushed tissue with iris scissors (as depicted above) to perform the canthotomy.

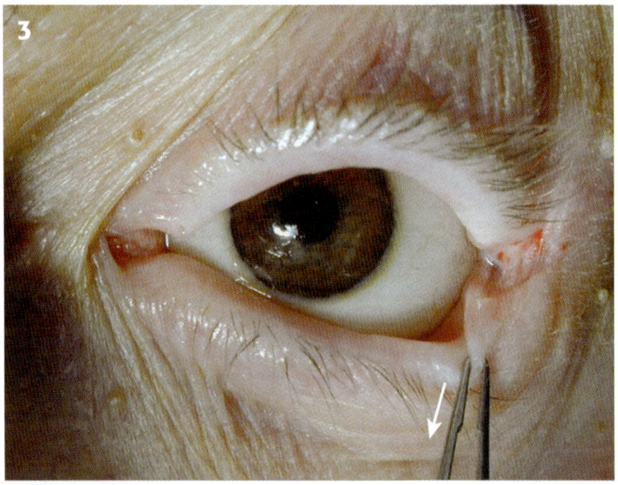

Pull the lower eyelid away from the globe with toothed forceps *(arrow)*.

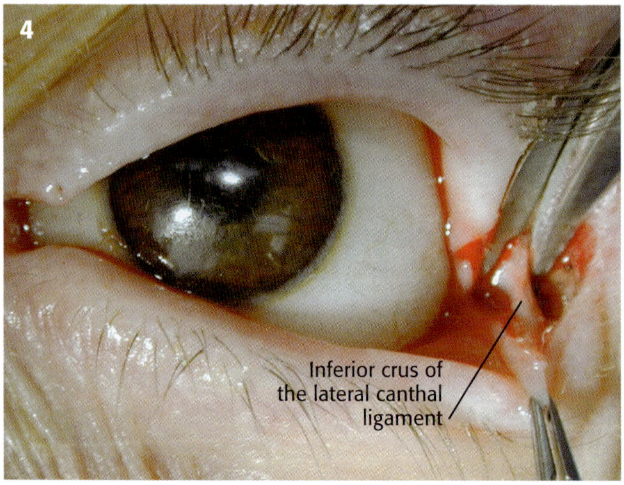

"Strum" the tissue under the canthotomy with the scissors to identify the inferior crus of the lateral canthal ligament. Cut through this ligament with scissors to perform the inferior cantholysis. Note that the scissors are directed inferiorly during this step, perpendicular to the canthotomy incision.

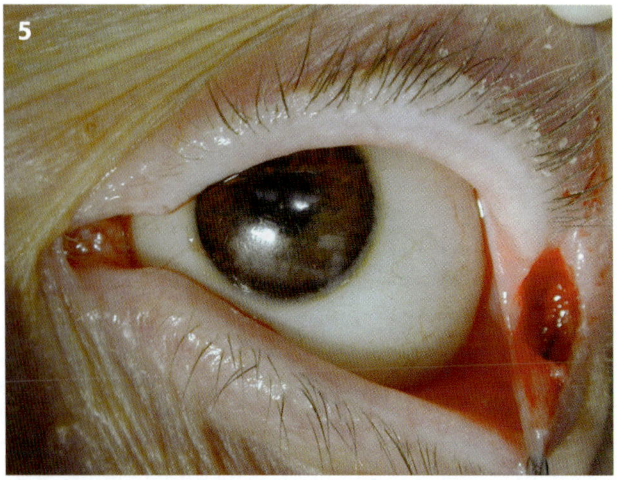

The eye after canthotomy and cantholysis. This procedure relieves increased intraocular pressure by allowing the globe and orbital contents to move forward.

NOTE:
If intraocular pressure remains elevated after inferior cantholysis, the superior crus of the lateral canthal ligament may be released in a similar fashion.

Fig. 63.45 Lateral canthotomy and cantholysis. (From Eisele OW, Smith RV, eds. *Complications in Head and Neck Surgery*. 2nd ed. Mosby; 2008.)

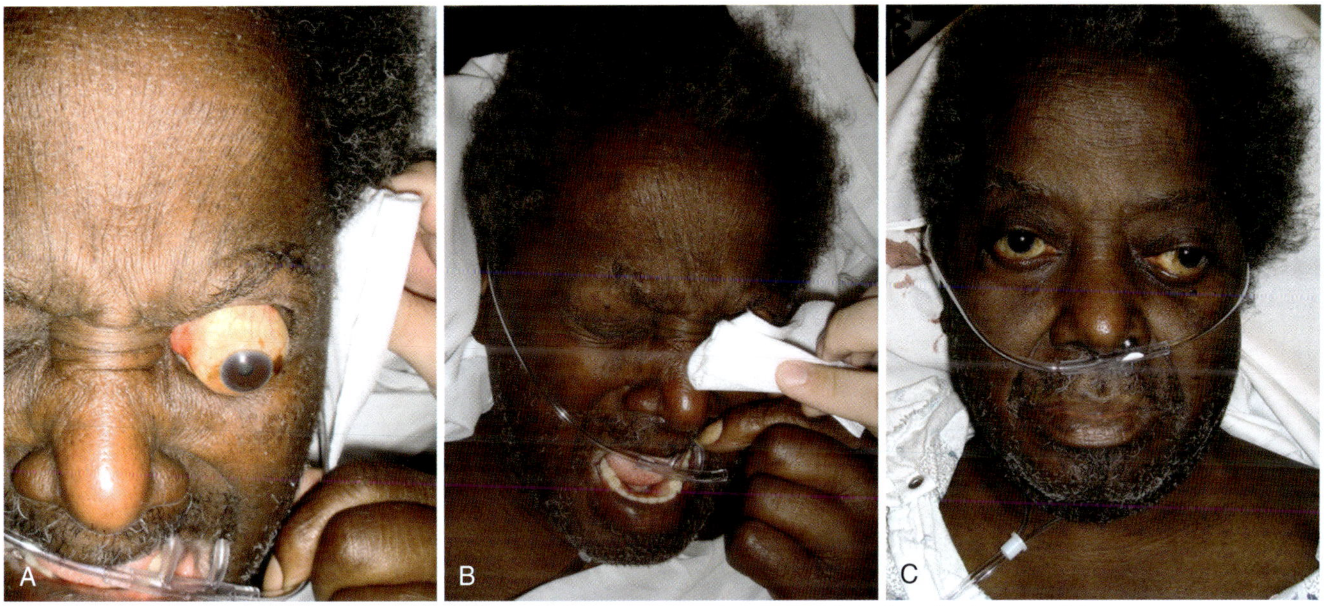

Fig. 63.46 Appearance of a luxated globe. (A) This globe protruded when the lower eyelid was retracted downward to examine the conjunctiva for anemia. (B) It was easily reduced with slight manual pressure on the closed upper lid. (C) Afterward, the patient had no eye or vision complaints. This is a normal variant in some people.

consultation. A computed tomography scan of the orbit is helpful for evaluating both the soft tissue and the bony structures about the globe.

STYE

See Video 63.17. A stye, or hordeolum, is an acute purulent inflammation (bacterial infection) of the eyelid characterized by pain, swelling, and redness. It can be quite annoying and painful to the touch. A small nodule or abscess first develops in an eyelid hair follicle or a modified sebaceous gland at the margin of the eyelid. This may be external (pointing at the lid margin) or internal (pointing under the conjunctival lid; Fig. 63.47). An obvious pustule may be seen, and if so, incising it with a small needle and expressing pus produces a faster cure. The lid may be inverted to find a small pustule on the inner surface of the lid that can be nicked with a 25-gauge needle (see Fig. 63.23, *plates* 6 and 7). *S. aureus* is the organism most frequently isolated from the infection.[1] Treat with warm compresses on the eyelid as frequently as possible. One method is to fill a sink with very hot water and alternate wet washcloths for 15 to 20 minutes. Topical ophthalmic antibiotics (drops every 2 hours or ointment five to six times a day) are usually prescribed. Erythromycin ointment is often suggested. Topical treatment is generally sufficient, but antistaphylococcal oral antibiotics (dicloxacillin, cephalosporins) might occasionally be needed, especially in patients with significant surrounding lid cellulitis. More formal incision and drainage may be necessary if the infection is unresponsive to conservative therapy. Spread of the infection can lead to preseptal cellulitis.

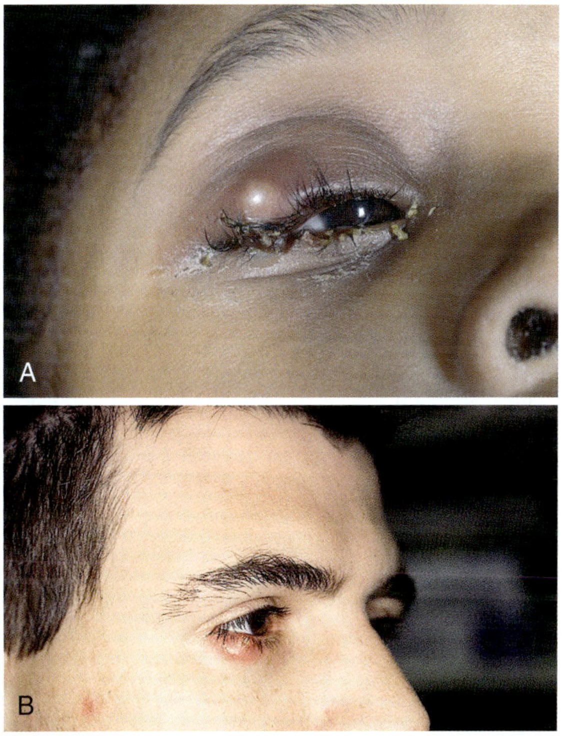

Fig. 63.47 Stye (hordeolum). (A) External hordeolum. An erythematous, tender swelling at the lid margin points externally. (B) Internal stye. This may form a pustule on the inner surface of the lid that may be incised and pus expressed (see also Fig. 63.39).

APD OR MARCUS GUNN PUPIL

An APD, or Marcus Gunn pupil, is caused by a variety of diseases of the afferent, or "in-going," pathways of the eye. It is produced by a *unilateral* lesion of the retina or optic nerve. Causes include optic neuritis (as seen with multiple sclerosis), ischemic optic neuropathy, optic tumor, and retrobulbar hematoma (an indication for lateral canthotomy). To evaluate for an APD, the swinging flashlight test may be used (Fig. 63.48).[108] Normally, shining a light in either eye causes bilateral pupil constriction. To evaluate for an APD (no light

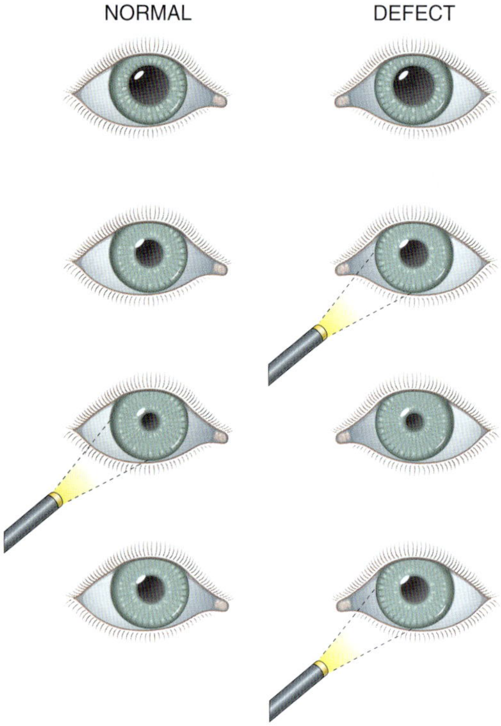

Fig. 63.48 Relative afferent pupillary defect (Marcus Gunn pupil). This patient has an abnormal left optic nerve. In ambient light *(top row)*, the pupils are equal. As the abnormal eye is illuminated *(second row)*, only modest constriction is noted. As the light is swung to the normal eye *(third row)*, the pupils constrict briskly. When the light is swung back to the abnormal eye *(bottom row)*, paradoxical dilation is noted. (From Friedman NJ, Kaiser PK, Pineda A. *Massachusetts Ear & Eye Infirmary Illustrated Manual of Ophthalmology*. 3rd ed. Saunders; 2009.)

reaching the brain via the optic nerve on the affected side), record the pupil size at baseline. Shine a light into the affected eye. Record the direct response (constriction of the illuminated pupil in response to light) and the indirect or consensual response (constriction of the opposite pupil in response to light). Next, shine the light into the other eye and record the direct and indirect responses. Repeat this procedure back and forth until the pattern of response to light is identified. With an APD, there is a decreased direct response to light along the afferent or in-going pathways, whereas the efferent or "outgoing" pathways to the opposite eye are preserved. Thus light shined into the affected eye will cause neither a direct nor a consensual response, but light shined into the unaffected eye will cause bilateral pupillary constriction.

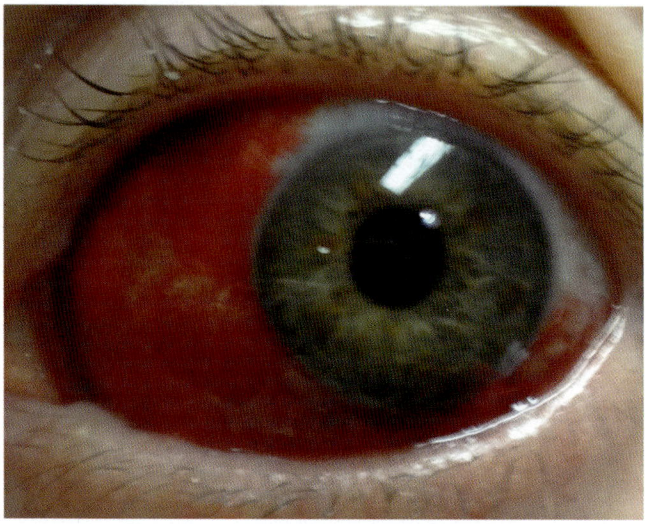

Fig. 63.49 Subconjunctival hemorrhage. Although very alarming to most patients, a spontaneous subconjunctival hemorrhage or the development after vomiting or coughing is a benign condition; no treatment is indicated. A painless bright red hemorrhage of the sclera is noted. The cornea and anterior chamber are unaffected, and there are no visual symptoms.

SUBCONJUNCTIVAL HEMORRHAGE

Subconjunctival hemorrhage may occur spontaneously (often noticed on awakening) or after straining, vomiting, or severe coughing. The patient notices a painless bright red hemorrhage in the eye (sclera). It may be bilateral (Fig. 63.49). Vision is not affected. Although this is concerning to the patient, it is benign. No laboratory evaluation is required unless the patient has taken anticoagulants, in which case clotting studies should be considered. The hemorrhage will disappear spontaneously over a few weeks and turn various colors as it recedes. No treatment will hasten resolution.

ACKNOWLEDGMENT

We recognize the many contributions by Jerris R. Hedges, MD, to this chapter through the first five editions of the textbook, and by William Dennis, MD, for the last two editions.

REFERENCES ARE AVAILABLE AT Elsevier eBooks+

CHAPTER 64

Otolaryngologic Procedures

Mark T. Foster and Ralph J. Riviello

The procedures presented in this chapter are most effectively performed with special equipment and techniques. Some are within the realm of general emergency medicine clinical expertise; others are not. They are reviewed from the perspective of the emergency clinician who must decide whether the patient needs treatment acutely in the emergency department (ED), can be managed with timely referral, or requires urgent consultant expertise.

PHARYNX AND LARYNX

Examination of the Larynx

Visualization of the larynx and pharynx is a critical part of the complete evaluation of patients with complaints of sore throat, hoarseness, foreign body (FB), or changes in phonation including stridor.

Anatomy

The pharynx is the part of the throat located posterior to the mouth and the nasal cavity and superior to the esophagus and larynx. It is commonly divided into three sections, the nasopharynx, the oropharynx, and the laryngopharynx (hypopharynx). The nasopharynx is the most cephalad portion and extends from the base of the skull to the upper surface of the soft palate. The oropharynx is behind the oral cavity and extends from the uvula to the level of the hyoid bone. Its anterior wall consists of the base of the tongue and the vallecula; its lateral wall consists of the tonsils, tonsillar fossa, and pillars; and its superior wall is formed by the inferior surface of the soft palate and the uvula. Pharyngeal branches of the ascending pharyngeal artery, ascending and descending palatine arteries, and pharyngeal branches of the inferior thyroid artery supply blood to the pharynx. The pharyngeal plexus and the maxillary and mandibular nerves innervate the pharynx.

The larynx in adults is located in the anterior part of the neck at the level of the C3–C6 vertebrae. It connects the inferior portion of the pharynx (hypopharynx) with the trachea. The larynx extends vertically from the tip of the epiglottis to the inferior border of the cricoid cartilage. It consists of nine cartilages. Branches of the vagus nerve, the superior laryngeal nerve, and the recurrent laryngeal nerve innervate the larynx. The relevant anatomy is depicted in Fig. 64.1.

Laryngoscopy Indications and Contraindications

Laryngoscopy is indicated for the evaluation of patients with complaints of dysphagia or odynophagia. More specifically, it should be performed in patients complaining of dysphagia, hoarseness, FB ingestion or sensation in the throat, angioedema, and in patients who require assessment of their airway status. In general, laryngoscopy can be used to evaluate a problem, to exclude airway compromise, and to diagnose several other diseases such as gastroesophageal reflux, cancer, and allergy.[1]

Laryngoscopy has traditionally been discouraged in patients with impending airway compromise; however, it may be performed carefully in stridulous patients as long as a predesignated team (usually consisting of an anesthesiologist, otolaryngologist, or another physician skilled in the management of a difficult airway) is readily available and able to intervene if necessary. Care should be taken to avoid accidental trauma to the laryngopharynx, which may exacerbate swelling and further compromise the airway.

Equipment

The equipment required depends on the type of laryngoscopy procedure performed. For flexible laryngoscopy a standard flexible nasopharyngolaryngoscope (NPL), a light source (alternatively, a digital display for more modern devices) (Fig. 64.2A–B), gloves, a nasal speculum, surgical lubricant, antifogging solution, decongestant spray, anesthetic spray, and a wall suction setup with a Frazier suction-tip catheter are needed (see Fig. 64.2, *plate 1*). Many choices of decongestant are available; however, 0.05% oxymetazoline (Afrin) or 0.1% to 1% phenylephrine is commonly used. Lidocaine (4%) is typically used as the anesthetic. If nasal spray formulations are not available, medication-soaked cotton pledgets, an atomizer bottle, or a syringe atomizer may be used.

Mirror laryngoscopy requires a curved dental mirror, an external light source (preferably a headlamp), 4 × 4-inch gauze, and an antifogging solution. If antifogging solution is not available, hot water can be used to prevent fogging of the mirror. Anesthetic solution may be required if the patient cannot tolerate the procedure.

Procedure

Flexible Laryngoscopy

See Videos 64.1 and 64.2. Attach the NPL to its light source (or digital display) and the suction tubing to its port (if available). Ensure that both are functioning properly before beginning. Before inserting the scope, adjust the eyepiece to your visual acuity; it is helpful to check the focus on newsprint or a small object. If using a modern digital display this step is not required. Review the scope's directional controls. Examine both nares and choose the more patent one to enter. Anesthetize and vasoconstrict the naris (see Fig. 64.2, *plate 2*). Because this procedure is irritating, allow enough time for these medications to become effective. You may also anesthetize the pharynx to minimize gagging (see Fig. 64.2, *plate 3*). Warm the end of the scope in warm water to help prevent fogging (alternatively you can use the patient's tongue). Place the patient in the seated position with the head placed against a headrest in the "sniffing position." Insert the tip of the lubricated scope just inside the naris. (Some authors recommend a series of soft nasal trumpets to gradually dilate the nasal cavity and allow easier passage of the scope.) Movement of the scope against the inside of the nasal passage may be irritating to the patient. Minimize this sensation by resting your fourth and fifth fingers on the bridge of the patient's nose while stabilizing and guiding the scope between your thumb and index finger (see Fig. 64.2, *plate 4*).

While visualizing, slowly advance the endoscope past the middle turbinate into the nasopharynx or through the lumen of a nasal trumpet. To clear fogging or mucus off the lens, ask the patient to swallow, wipe the lens against the pharyngeal mucosa, or use the suction. Once the scope is in the nasopharynx, direct the tip inferiorly by using the thumb control. Use the thumb control to accomplish up and down movements of the scope. Rotate the scope about its axis and then apply thumb control to provide lateral movement and visualization. At this point the base of the tongue and the tonsils will come into view. Slide the scope farther caudad to bring the larynx into focus. Once again, systematically view the patient's anatomy and function during both respiration and phonation (see Fig. 64.2, *plate 6*).

If the NPL will not pass through either naris, pass it through the oropharynx. Properly anesthetize the oropharynx and avoid contacting the posterior portion of the tongue to prevent gagging. A plastic bite block can be used. Alternatively, cut a 10-mL syringe (without the plunger) in half and ask the patient to hold it in the mouth between the incisors (see Fig. 64.2, *plate 5*). Pass the fragile endoscope through this tube into the oropharynx to prevent accidental biting of the scope.

Mirror Laryngoscopy

Otolaryngologists most commonly use mirror laryngoscopy, but it can be used in the ED setting if the necessary equipment is readily available. Clinicians unfamiliar with this method should practice frequently because significant eye-to-hand coordination is required to reflect the light beam off the angulated mirror onto the larynx. When this procedure is properly performed, most patients can tolerate it without anesthesia of the oropharynx. Fiberoptic nasopharyngoscopy has largely replaced mirror laryngoscopy in the ED when the equipment is available.

Establish rapport with the patient by explaining how the examination will be performed. Have the patient sit erect in the sniffing position, with the feet flat on the floor and leaning slightly forward. Attach your headlamp and adjust the beam of light. Warm the mirror with warm water to prevent fogging, but check the temperature of the mirror with your hand before placing it into the oropharynx so that the patient is not burned. Alternatively, apply an antifogging solution to the mirrored side. Wrap the patient's tongue with gauze to prevent it from slipping or being injured by the lower incisors and then grasp it with the nondominant hand (Fig. 64.3). Apply gentle traction on the tongue with your thumb and index finger and

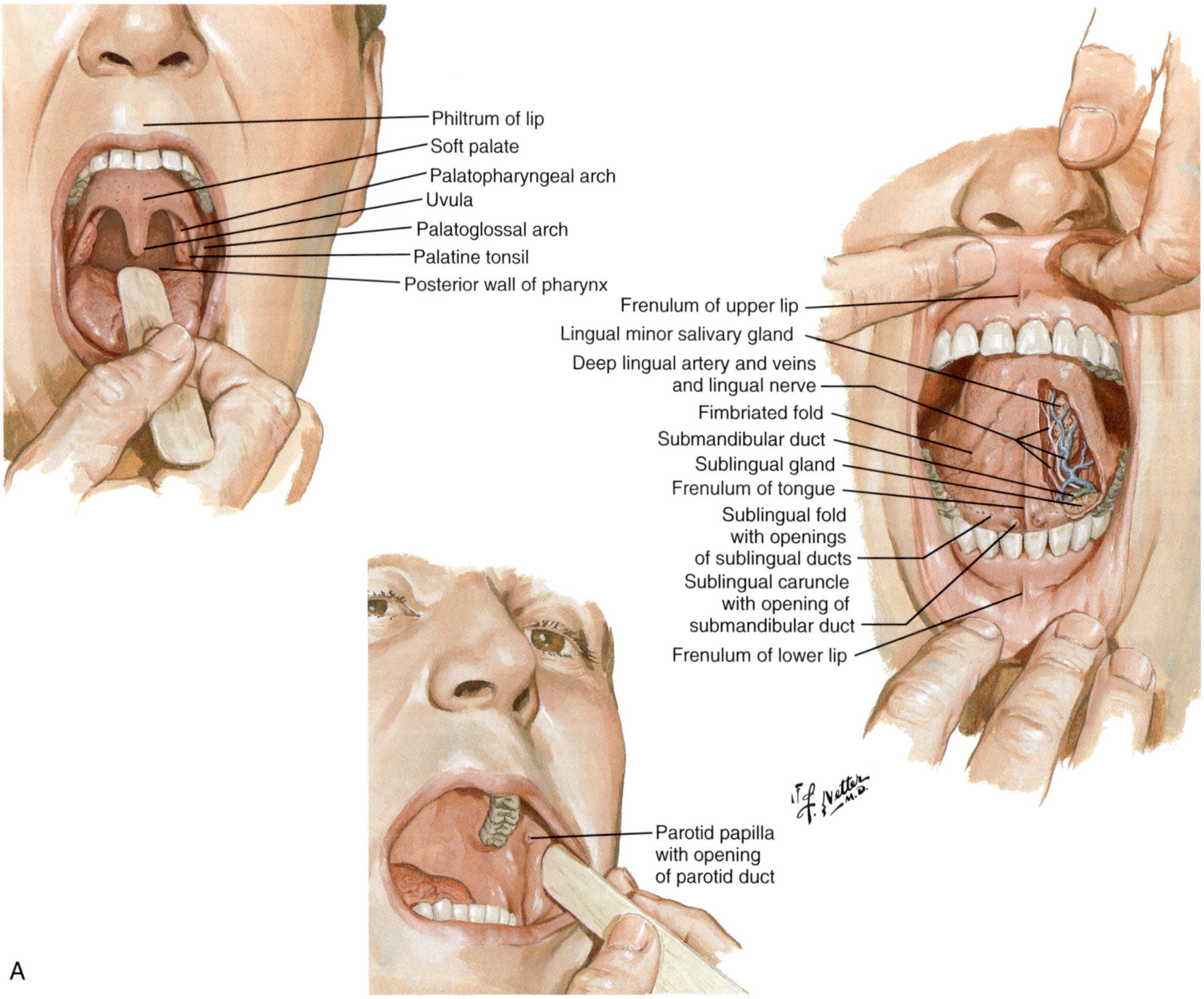

Fig. 64.1 (A) Anatomy of the oropharynx.

Continued

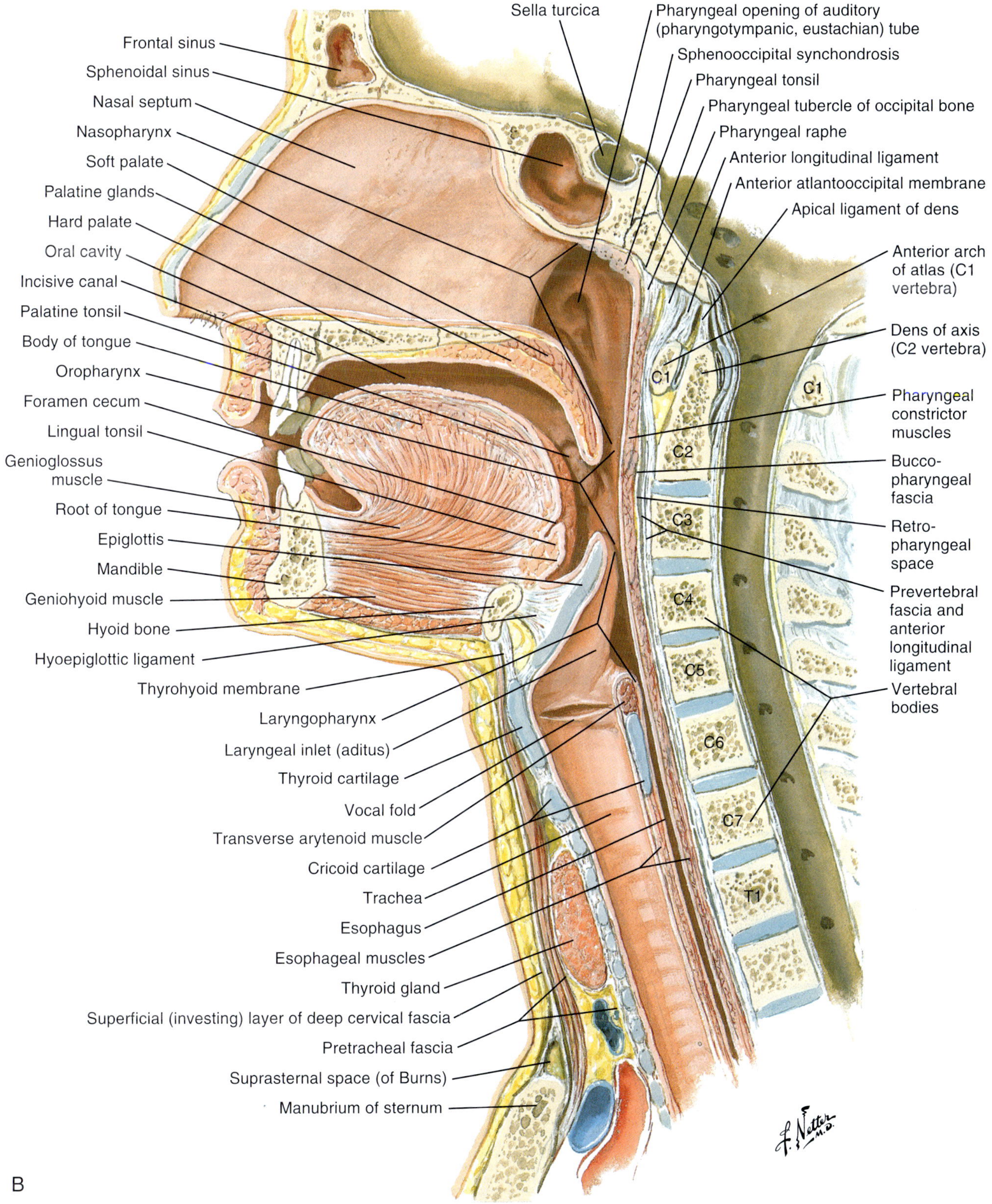

B

Fig. 64.1 cont'd (B) Sagittal section of the neck. (Netter illustration from www.netterimages.com. Elsevier, Inc. All rights reserved.)

lift the patient's upper lip with your middle finger. Slide the mirror into the oropharynx with the glass surface parallel to the tongue but not touching it. Place the back of the mirror against the uvula and soft palate and smoothly lift until the larynx is visualized. Although this should not induce gagging, try to make only slight changes in the mirror's position to inspect the appropriate structures.

In patients who cannot tolerate this procedure without gagging, apply topical anesthetic to aid in the examination. Reassure the patient beforehand that although this may make

Flexible Laryngoscopy

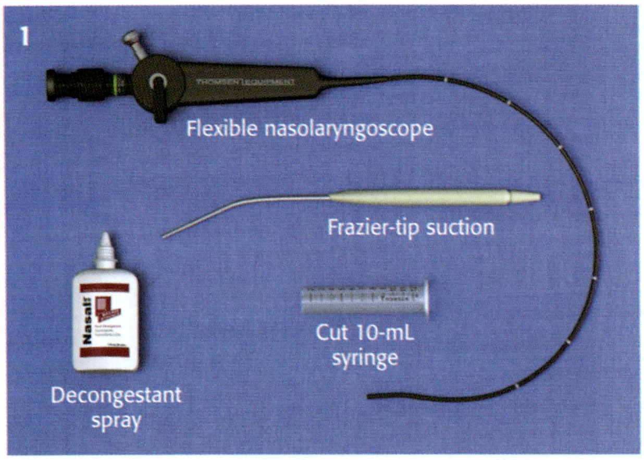

Basic equipment required for flexible laryngoscopy. Additional items include anesthetic spray, a nasal speculum, surgical lubricant, and antifogging solution.

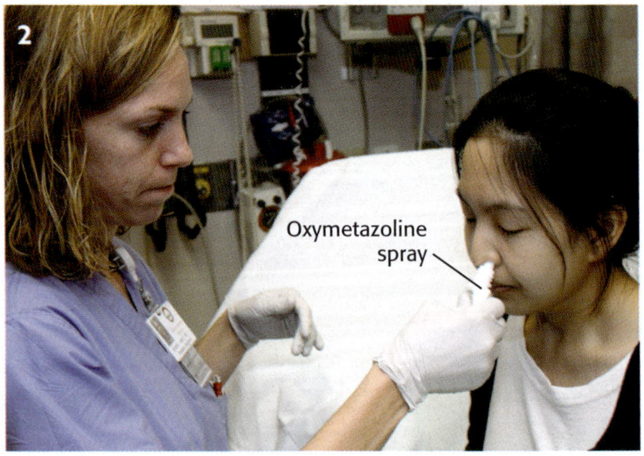

Anesthetize and vasoconstrict the naris before inserting the scope. Oxymetazoline (e.g., Afrin) spray is an ideal vasoconstrictor. Atomized 4% lidocaine can be use as an anesthetic.

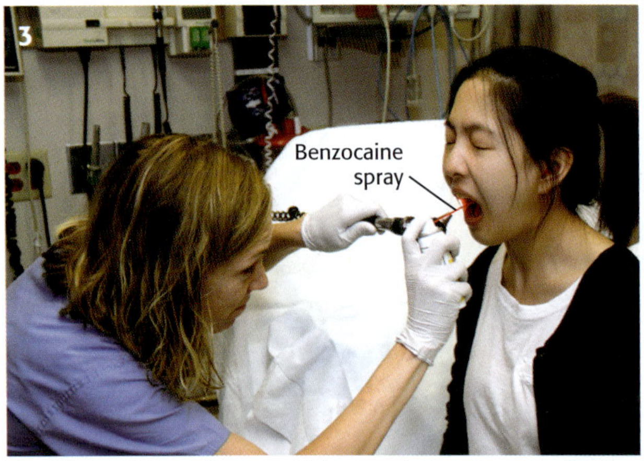

Anesthetize the oropharynx with benzocaine spray or atomized 4% lidocaine to prevent gagging.

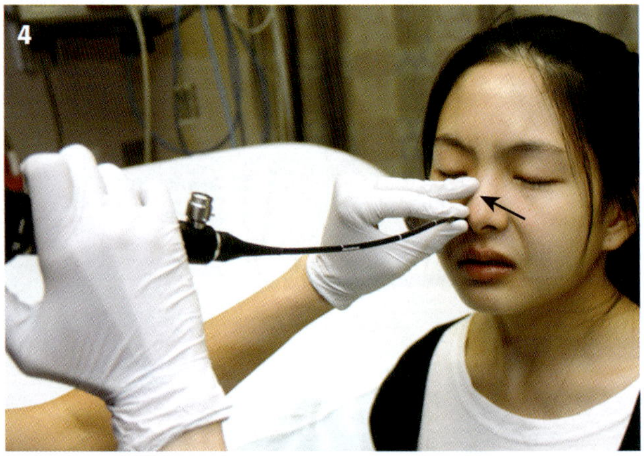

Rest your fingers on the bridge of the patient's nose while stabilizing and guiding the scope between the thumb and middle finger.

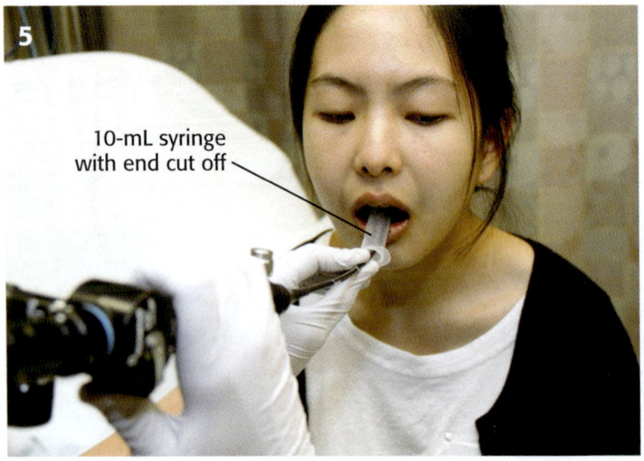

To pass the scope orally, first anesthetize the oropharynx (with atomized 4% lidocaine or benzocaine spray). Use a plungerless 10-mL syringe with the end cut off as a bite block to prevent accidental biting of the scope.

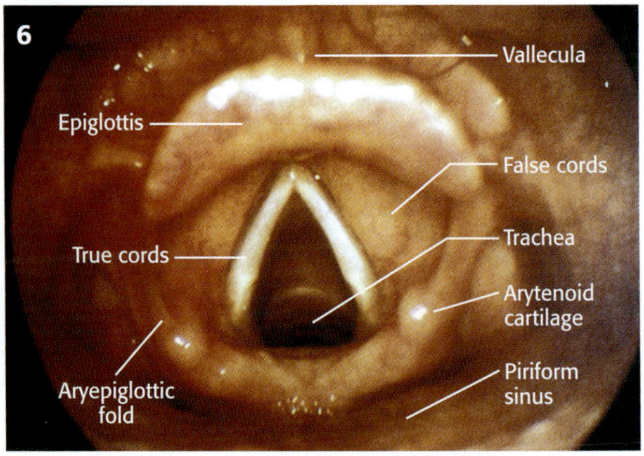

Laryngeal anatomy as seen through the nasopharyngoscope.

Fig. 64.2 Flexible laryngoscopy. (A) Disposable intubating nasopharyngolaryngoscope (NPL) with digital video display.

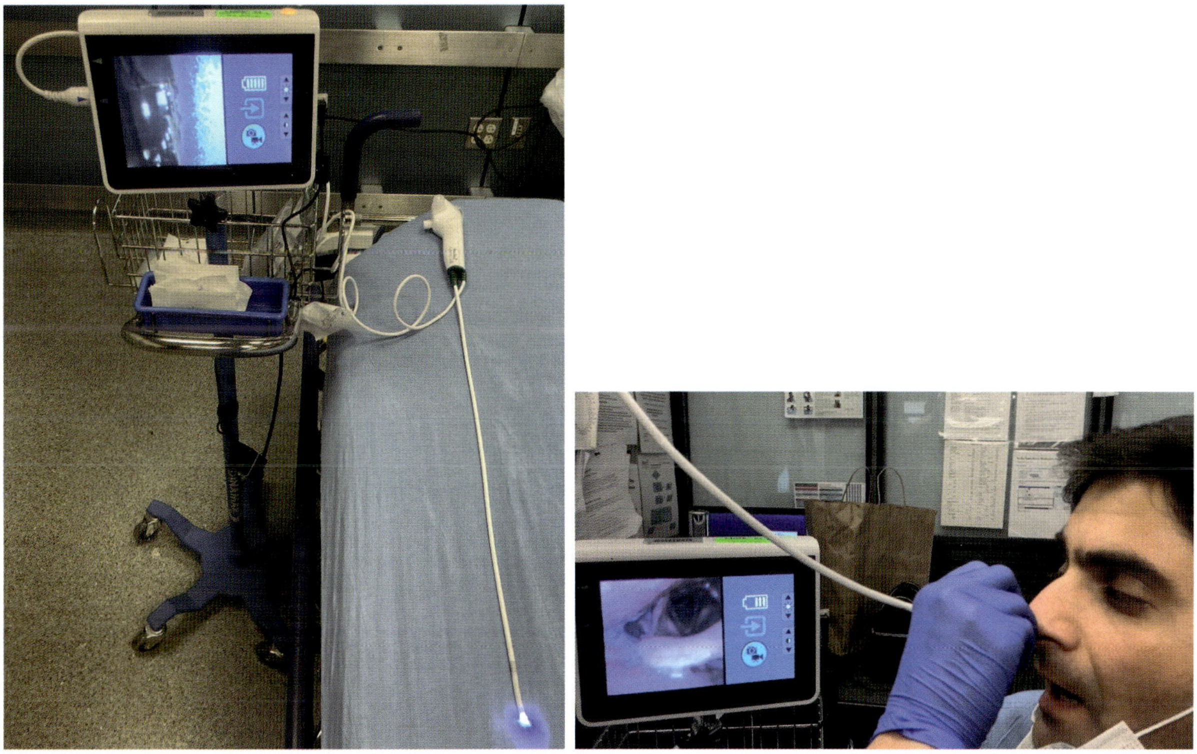

Fig. 64.2 cont'd Flexible laryngoscopy. (A) Disposable intubating nasopharyngolaryngoscope (NPL) with digital video display. (B) Glottic view on digital display during an NPL.

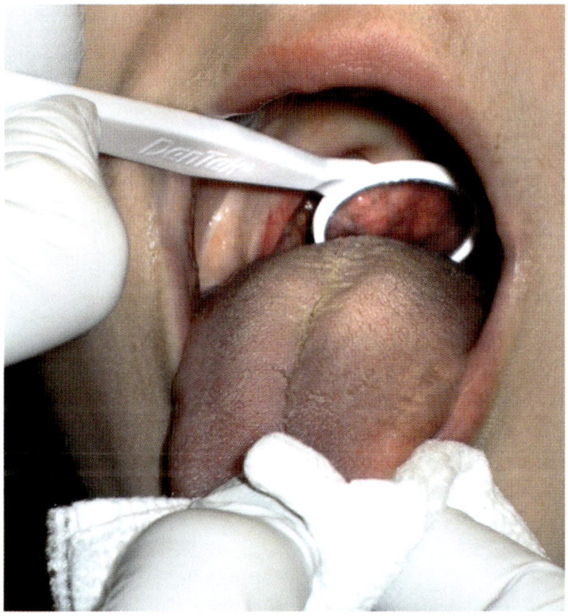

Fig. 64.3 Indirect mirror evaluation of the oropharynx. Grasp the patient's tongue between the thumb and first finger while using a gauze pad to provide traction. Elevate the upper lip with the middle finger. Advance the warmed (prevents fogging) laryngeal mirror into the posterior of the oropharynx while taking care to not stimulate the posterior part of the tongue or pharynx. Remember that the structures in the mirror will be reversed. Always follow universal precautions.

the throat feel as though it is swelling or paralyzed it is just the numbness that accounts for the sensation. The tendency to gag can also be minimized by having the patient concentrate on breathing efforts and keep the eyes open and fixed on an object in the distance.

Once the patient is anesthetized, repeat the steps described earlier and position the mirror against the soft palate. Rotate the angle of the mirror and systematically inspect the base of the tongue, valleculae, epiglottis, piriform recess, arytenoids, false and true vocal cords, and if possible, the superior aspect of the trachea (see Fig. 64.2, *plate 6*). Observe for masses, evidence of infection, asymmetry, or FBs. Further evaluate the anterior structure of the larynx and function of the vocal cords by having the patient say "eeee" in a high-pitched voice. This should move the epiglottis away from blocking the view of the larynx and bring the true cords together at the midline (Fig. 64.4). See Video 64.2.

Complications

There are very few complications with laryngoscopy. Occasionally, it may not be possible to complete the procedure because of a prominent gag reflex or patient apprehension and discomfort. Complications include traumatic abrasions and bleeding anywhere along the path of the laryngoscope or on the soft palate or pharynx if a mirror is used. Epistaxis and hemoptysis are uncommon. In patients with head injury, there is always a slight risk of passing the scope intracranially if a basilar skull fracture has occurred; use of a soft nasal trumpet significantly reduces this risk. Laryngospasm and acute airway compromise can be induced in patients with paraglottic infections; ensure backup airway equipment is readily available.

PERITONSILLAR ABSCESS

Introduction

Peritonsillar abscess (PTA), also known as quinsy, is a collection of pus between the palatine tonsil capsule and the pharyngeal muscle.[2,3] It has an annual incidence of approximately 30 per 100,000 in patients aged 5 to 49 years. The highest incidence is in 15- to 19-year-olds (167 per 100,000).[4,5] This makes PTA the most common head and neck abscess in patients over the age of 5 years.[2,4,5]

If untreated, patients are at risk for significant morbidity and mortality.[6] Complications of untreated infection include descending mediastinitis, parapharyngeal and retropharyngeal abscess, necrotizing fasciitis, internal jugular vein suppurative thrombophlebitis, and airway obstruction. In patients with a complication, mortality rates can approach 10%.[6]

Early diagnosis and treatment are critical to improving patient outcomes. Drainage of the abscess is usually required and should be performed in conjunction with the administration of antibiotics and pain control medication. Three options for surgical drainage include needle aspiration (most common), incision and drainage, and immediate (quinsy) tonsillectomy.

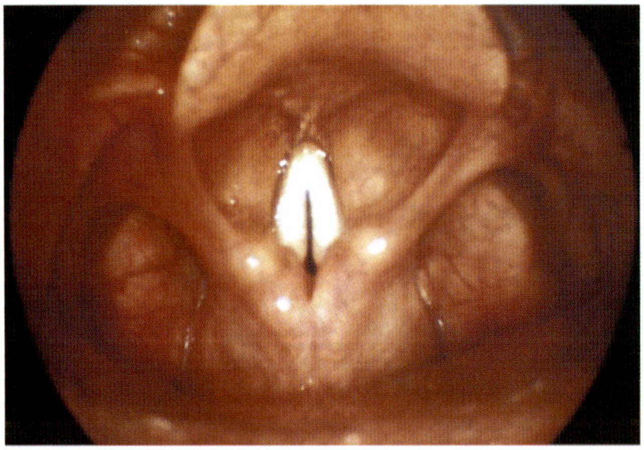

Fig. 64.4 Instruct the patient to say "eeeeee" in a high-pitched voice during the examination. This lifts the epiglottis out of your field of view and allows excellent visualization of the glottis. In this picture the vocal cords close with phonation. A paralyzed cord is easily discerned from one that is normal (see Video 64.2).

Anatomy

Understanding the relative anatomy before attempting to treat PTA is important (Fig. 64.5). The palatine tonsils are located between the anterior and posterior pillars of the throat, bound in a capsule, and covered by mucosa. The superior pharyngeal constrictor muscle defines the lateral wall of the tonsil. Of great importance is the internal carotid artery, which lies approximately 2.5 cm posterolateral to the tonsil.

The abscess usually forms between the tonsillar capsule, the superior constrictor muscle, and the palatopharyngeus muscle (Fig. 64.6). The abscess is not within the tonsil itself. It most commonly affects the superior pole of the tonsil, followed by the middle, then inferior poles.

Pathophysiology and Clinical Findings

PTA may be preceded by pharyngitis or tonsillitis but may occur without a preceding infection as a result of obstruction of the Weber glands.[7] Abscesses are often polymicrobial, including streptococcal species, staphylococcal species, and respiratory anaerobes (e.g., *Fusobacterium necrophorum*).[2,4,6–8] There are no data proving that antibiotics, even the correct ones in proper doses, invariably prevent the progression of tonsillitis to abscess formation. The abscess is generally unilateral, and bilateral involvement is rare.[9,10]

Patients with PTA have a sore throat, odynophagia, low-grade fever, and a variable degree of trismus. The trismus develops secondary to irritation of the pterygoid muscle. The patient may also complain of ipsilateral otalgia. As the abscess expands, the patient may experience dysphagia with drooling. Patients may be dehydrated secondary to poor oral intake. Changes in voice are common ("hot-potato voice") and caused by transient velopharyngeal insufficiency and muffled oral resonance. Rancid breath is also common. Tender ipsilateral anterior cervical lymphadenopathy is usually present.

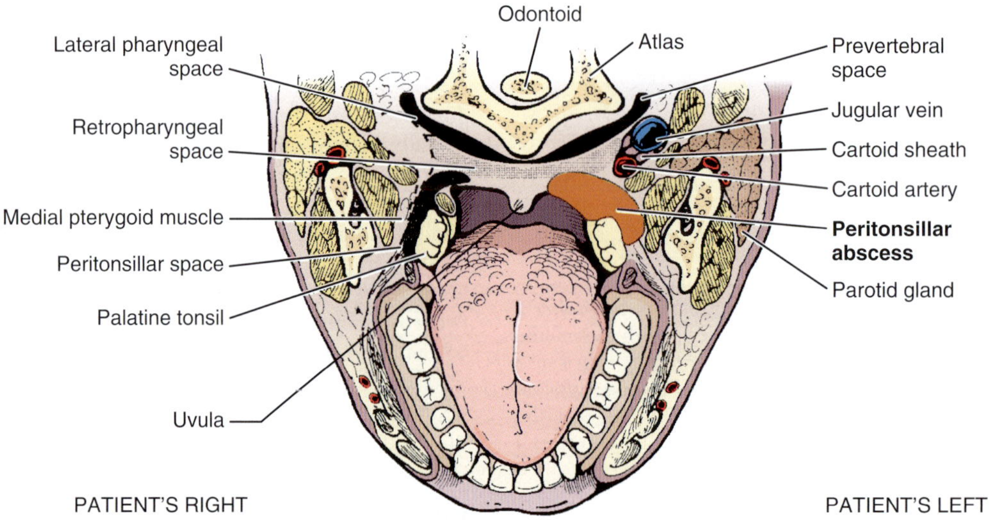

Fig. 64.5 Anatomy of a peritonsillar abscess. The palatine tonsil and peritonsillar space are identified on the patient's right. A peritonsillar abscess is shown on the patient's left. Note that the abscess can extend medially and displace the uvula. The carotid artery and jugular vein are posterior and lateral to the abscess. Avoid lateral angulation of the aspirating needle and use a needle guard to limit depth of penetration.

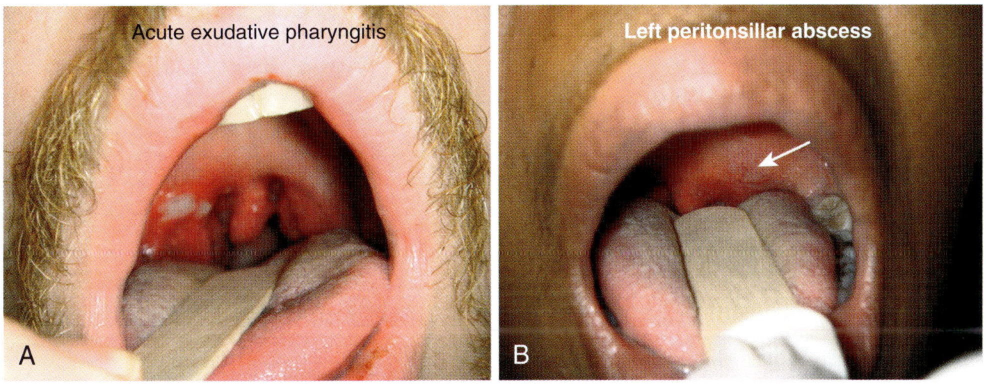

Fig. 64.6 Exudative pharyngitis versus peritonsillar abscess. (A) Acute exudative pharyngitis is characterized by bilateral tonsillar edema, erythema, and exudate. Note that the edema is for the most part symmetric and that the uvula lies in the midline. (B) A peritonsillar abscess *(arrow)* is characterized by asymmetric tonsillar bulging, with the uvula deviated away from the side of the abscess.

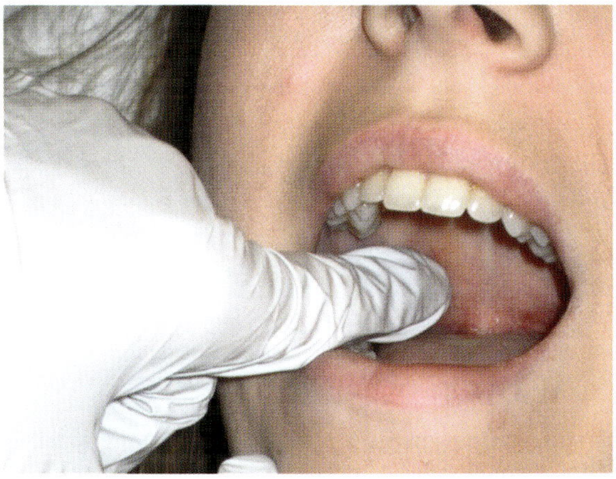

Fig. 64.7 Clinical symptoms and visual inspection may not be sufficient to differentiate a peritonsillar abscess from cellulitis. The clinician's gloved index finger is used to palpate the peritonsillar area to search for fluctuance and localized swelling. Computed tomography or ultrasound will further elucidate the diagnosis, but they are not needed in straightforward cases.

Although leukocytosis is often present, a complete blood count and other laboratory tests are nonspecific.

The differential diagnosis for this acute process includes unilateral tonsillitis, peritonsillar cellulitis, retropharyngeal abscess, infectious mononucleosis, epiglottitis, herpes simplex tonsillitis, retromolar abscess, neoplasm, FB, and internal carotid artery aneurysm. Chronic conditions include leukemia, carcinoma, and tumor in the parapharyngeal space. Differentiation of PTA from peritonsillar cellulitis may be difficult, especially in the early stages of an abscess. The history and time course of these two disease processes are quite similar. Trismus and uvular deviation are uncommon with peritonsillar cellulitis.[2] It may be difficult to differentiate cellulitis from abscess. To diagnose PTA prior to imaging, palpation of the peritonsillar region with a gloved index finger for evaluation of fluctuance may be helpful (Fig. 64.7).

Diagnostic Imaging

When PTA is clinically apparent, imaging is not necessary. It may be used if the diagnosis is unclear to differentiate PTA from other conditions (e.g., tonsillitis, retropharyngeal abscess) and to evaluate for complications. Point-of-care ultrasound (POCUS) should be used as the first-line imaging modality (Fig. 64.8).[11–16] POCUS can be used to confirm the presence of a PTA, identify the proximity of the carotid artery to the abscess, guide real-time drainage, and confirm abscess resolution. Gibbons and Costantino have published evidence demonstrating POCUS has transformed evaluation and treatment of PTAs with improved accuracy in diagnosis and successful aspiration while reducing CT usage as well as reduced consultation of specialists.[14] They demonstrated successful aspiration in 89% of patients using POCUS versus 24% without ultrasound (US). CT usage was 26.9% for US, versus 64% without POCUS. Only 4.5% of patients treated using US had a return visit compared to 12% of those without US in their study. Of note, blind PTA drainage with landmark guidance alone has a false negative (failure) rate of 10% to 24%.[13]

There are two approaches for POCUS imaging: intraoral with an intracavitary transducer (Fig. 64.8B) and extraoral (transcutaneous) using a linear or curvilinear transducer in the transcervical/submandibular location (see Fig. 64.8C).[16] The sensitivity of the intraoral approach ranges from 90% to 100%, whereas the sensitivity of the transcutaneous approach ranges between 80% and 91%. Specificity for both approaches range between 79% and 100%.[11–16]

When POCUS imaging is nondiagnostic, or another deep-space infection is suspected, CT with intravenous (IV) contrast of the neck should be obtained (Fig. 64.9). The sensitivity of CT with IV contrast approaches 100%, with a specificity of approximately 75%.[17–19] However, CT is associated with radiation exposure, longer time to diagnosis, and higher cost; therefore, POCUS remains preferable in most instances.

Indications and Contraindications

The indication for PTA drainage is usually straightforward, but some advocate that initial medical options exist, especially in children. If obviously present in an adult, the PTA should be drained. An alternative to immediate drainage in nontoxic-appearing patients with early and small PTA, is admission to the hospital for 24 hours of hydration, empirical IV antibiotics (clindamycin or penicillin with beta-lactamase inhibitor is often used), corticosteroids (dexamethasone 10 mg IV/IM/PO or methylprednisolone 125 mg IV), and analgesia (nonsteroidal antiinflammatory and/or opioids). Corticosteroids

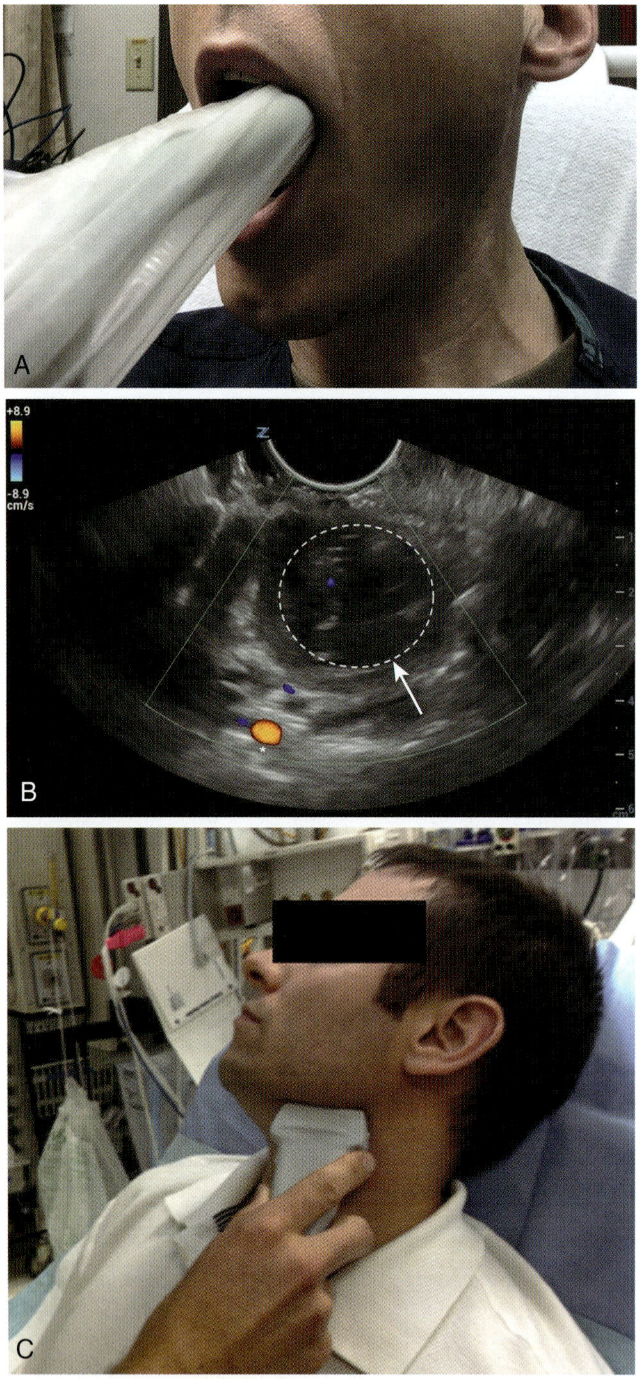

Fig. 64.8 Ultrasound (US) use in peritonsillar abscess (PTA). (A) Use of the intracavitary probe to diagnose and localize peritonsillar abscess. (B) Intraoral US, transverse view, of a peritonsillar abscess showing a hypoechoic, heterogeneous abscess *(dashed line with arrow)* using an intracavitary probe. Color Doppler can be used to delineate the vascular structures (*asterisk*, carotid artery). (C) Transcutaneous (submandibular) US approach. (From, Secko M, Sivitz A. Think ultrasound first for peritonsillar abscess. *Am J Emerg Med*. 2015;33(4):569-572)

have been shown to reduce pain and shorten recovery times compared with placebo.[20] If a rapid response to medical therapy is not seen, drainage should be performed.

Medical management alone may suffice. A few retrospective observational studies comparing medical therapy versus surgical drainage found no significant differences in treatment

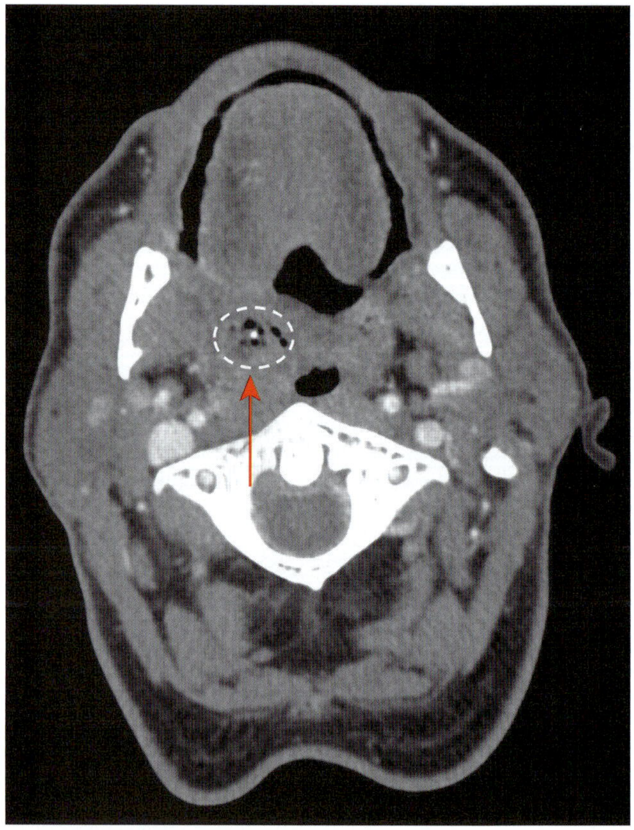

Fig. 64.9 Computed tomography scan with IV contrast demonstrating peritonsillar abscess *(dashed line with arrow)*.

success or complications.[21–23] One study reported that medical therapy patients had fewer sore days (4.5 vs. 5.7 days), received fewer opioid prescriptions (31 vs. 78), and required fewer days off work (3.4 vs. 4.9 days).[21] Of note, while one retrospective study found that those with a PTA size ≥2 cm were more likely to experience treatment failure in the medical therapy group, a separate study found no correlation with PTA size.[22–24] Although data suggest there may be a role for medical management among small abscesses, clinicians should engage in shared decision-making with patients and discuss the risks and benefits of medical management alone (particularly for larger abscesses).

There are very few, if any, contraindications to draining a PTA. One contraindication is the absence of a PTA; however, needle aspiration may be performed to confirm the presence of an abscess. Other contraindications can include severe trismus, coagulopathy, and inability of the patient to cooperate with the procedure. Fig. 64.10 demonstrates a potential management algorithm for PTA.[2]

Equipment

The equipment required depends on the technique that is going to be used to drain the PTA. For needle aspiration, you will need a light source, a tongue blade (alternatively a direct laryngoscope can serve as both a tongue depressor and light source), injectable (1% lidocaine with 1:100,000 epinephrine), topical (Cetacaine spray or 4% lidocaine) anesthetic, a 3-mL syringe with a long 25-gauge needle for injection of anesthetic, and a standard or long 18-gauge needle on a 10-mL syringe for aspiration (see Review Box 64.1). Long needles

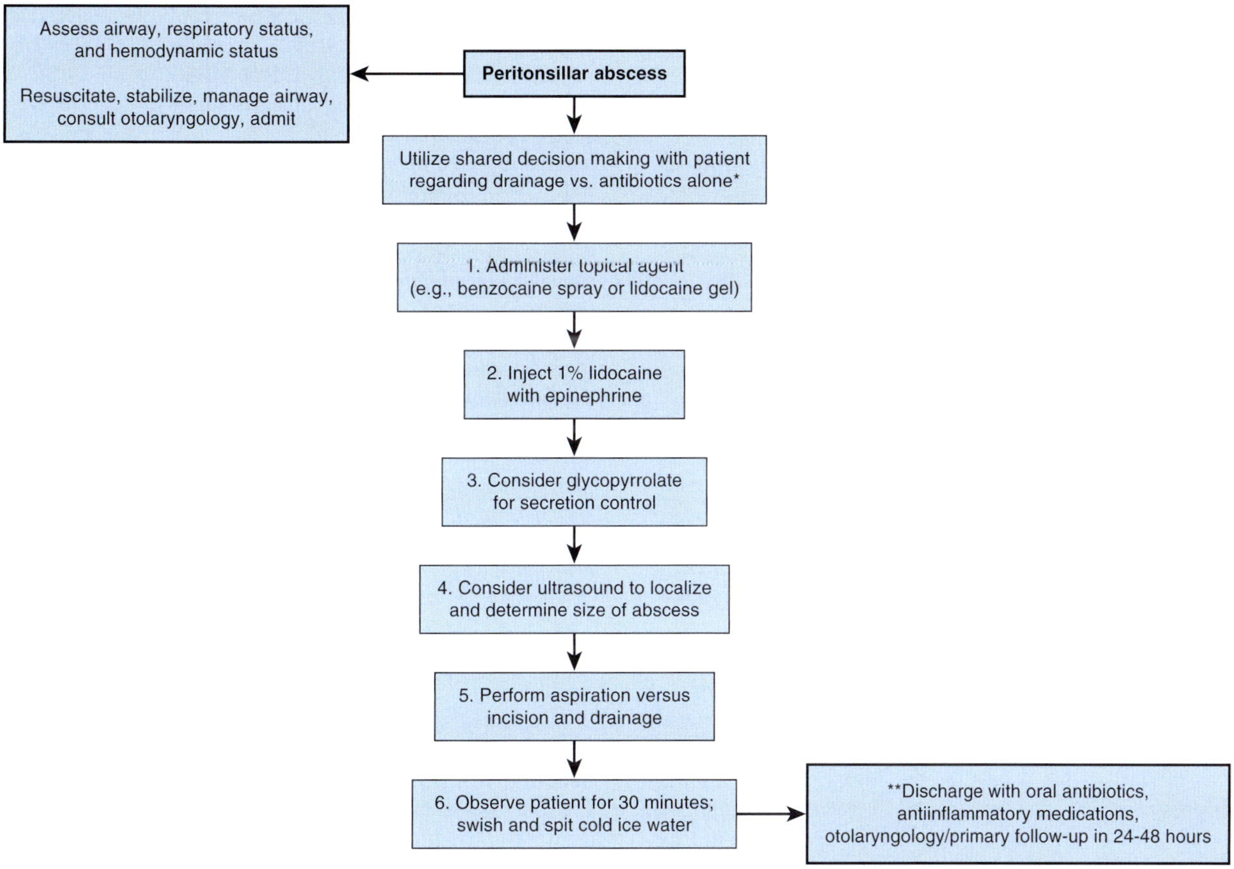

Fig. 64.10 Proposed algorithm for the management of peritonsillar abscess. *Medical management alone may be effective for an abscess <2 cm. **Patient must be able to tolerate oral intake, and symptoms must be controlled. If these criteria are not met, admission is recommended. (From Long B, Gottlieb M. Managing peritonsillar abscess. *Ann Emerg Med.* 2023;82:101-107.)

Peritonsillar Abscess Drainage

Indications

Clinical suspicion of peritonsillar abscess (PTA)
Signs and symptoms of PTA include
- Asymmetric tonsillar bulging
- Uvular deviation (away from the bulging)
- "Hot potato" voice

Contraindications

Severe trismus
Coagulopathy
Uncooperative patient

Complications

Failure to completely drain the abscess
Aspiration of pus and/or blood
Hemorrhage
Carotid artery puncture

Equipment

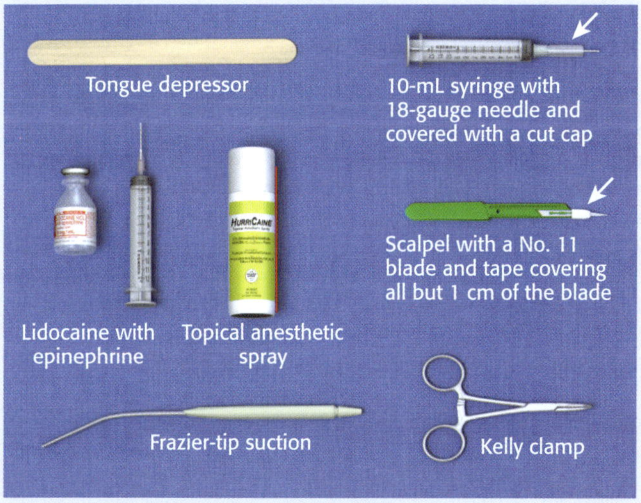

Review Box 64.1 Peritonsillar abscess drainage: indications, contraindications, complications, and equipment. Use a long 25- to 27-gauge needle and a 3- to 5-mL syringe for local anesthesia and a 10-mL syringe for aspiration. Larger syringes obscure the operator's view of the anatomy.

and small syringes will not obscure the operator's view of the anatomy. It is also helpful to have wall suction with a Frazier or Yankauer suction-tip device available.

For incision and drainage, the same examination, suction, and anesthetizing equipment are required. In addition, a No. 11 or 15 scalpel blade and Kelly forceps will be required.

Some patients may require mild or procedural sedation. Glycopyrrolate can be used to decrease secretions. The combination of midazolam, ketamine, and glycopyrrolate is reported to be safe and effective for outpatient peritonsillar drainage in children.[25]

Procedure

See Video 64.3. The emergency medicine drainage options include needle aspiration (most common) and incision and drainage. They should be performed only in a cooperative patient without severe trismus. As the carotid artery is located 2.5 cm behind and lateral to the tonsil, there is minimal room for error, patient movement, or poor anesthesia. Such complex cases should be drained in the operating room by a qualified surgeon.

Needle aspiration is relatively simple, can be performed by emergency clinicians, does not require special equipment, and is relatively time efficient. Other benefits of needle aspiration over incision and drainage include decreased pain and trauma. Many believe that this should be the initial surgical drainage procedure for adults and children. The recurrence rate after aspiration is 10%,[2] and its cure rate is 93% to 95%.[25] Approximately 4% to 10% of patients require repeated aspiration.[2,25,26] One drawback is that needle aspiration may miss the PTA and therefore lead to a misdiagnosis of peritonsillar cellulitis. This is less likely to occur with POCUS and CT imaging utilization.

The incision and drainage procedure is commonly done on an outpatient basis under local anesthesia. It is usually performed after pus is obtained by needle aspiration, but occasionally it is the primary procedure. It seems most logical to first attempt needle aspiration and follow with incision and drainage only if additional pus is suspected or other extenuating circumstances are present. The success rate for incision and drainage is high, with a recurrence rate similar to or lower than that with aspiration alone.[25]

Treatment guidelines based on a review of the literature[2,3,25–27] suggest that patients with PTA should initially be treated by needle aspiration. Incision and drainage and immediate tonsillectomy should be reserved for treatment failures or recurrences. These procedures can be performed in conjunction with hospital admission and administration of IV antibiotics or as outpatient treatment with oral antibiotics. One evidence-based review analyzed 42 articles, 5 of which were clinical studies on surgical technique.[25] Needle aspiration, incision and drainage, and tonsillectomy approaches were found to be effective in treating PTA, and the recurrence rate was low (grade C recommendation). The approach depends on the patient's clinical status, medical history, and clinician experience/comfort level. The emergency clinician makes decisions about the treatment of PTA in the ED, but as local protocols dictate, consultation with an otolaryngologist may be appropriate.

Needle Aspiration

See Fig. 64.11. Have the patient sit upright with a support behind the head. This is best done as a two-person procedure. Ask an assistant to retract the cheek laterally to maximize visibility. A headlamp provides optimal lighting; a double–tongue blade setup aids in visualization of the operative area. Other lighting options include using a laryngoscope with curved blade, a disposable vaginal speculum with light source, and video laryngoscope (Fig. 64.12A–B).[28,29] The laryngoscope blade is inserted into the patient's mouth as far posteriorly as the patient can tolerate. The blade shines light from inside the mouth onto the posterior aspect of the pharynx. In addition, it provides better exposure of the area because the handle is below the patient's mouth and the holding hand does not obscure the view. Moreover, the curved blade sweeps the tongue out of the way and the weight of the handle will help overcome trismus. A video laryngoscope can be used as well and has the advantage of procedural visualization by learners. Braude and Shalit described a similar process involving the use of a disassembled disposable vaginal speculum with a fiberoptic light (see Fig. 64.12C).[29] One advantage of both techniques is that the patient or an assistant can hold the light source without getting in the way of the operator.

Use digital palpation to locate the fluctuant area of the abscess. Anesthetize the area topically or with local infiltration. Infiltrate with 1 to 2 mL of 1% lidocaine with epinephrine via a 25- to 27-gauge needle. Use a 3-mL syringe (a larger syringe can block the operator's view) with a long needle so it is possible to visualize the area to be injected (see Fig. 64.11, *step 1*). Displacing the tongue with a finger rather than a tongue blade may provide a better view. Infiltrate the lidocaine intramucosally for the best results but be careful not to increase the size of the abscess by direct injection into the abscess cavity. The area should blanch. With proper local infiltration, the patient will not feel the penetration of the aspirating needle. If the trismus is so pronounced that it prevents adequate anesthesia, it will probably be too difficult to aspirate or incise the abscess properly. Chang and Hamilton reported that performing the procedure with the patient in the Trendelenburg position and the operator seated behind the patient's head provides comparable success rates and increased patient comfort.[30]

For abscess aspiration, attach a long 18- to 20-gauge needle to a 10-mL syringe. Fashion a needle guard by cutting off the distal 1 cm of the plastic needle cover, replace the cover on the needle, and securely attach this guard to the needle and syringe with tape to prevent inadvertent displacement (see Fig. 64.11, *step 2*).

Ensure that the needle protrudes only 1 cm beyond the cover to limit the depth of needle penetration and lessen the risk of entering any major vascular structures. If pus is not obtained at a 1-cm depth, deeper penetration is discouraged. Insert the needle into the most fluctuant (or prominent) area as previously determined, which is most commonly the superior pole of the tonsil (see Fig. 64.11, *step 3*).

Importantly, advance the syringe and needle in the sagittal plane only; do not angle to the side toward the carotid artery. Do not aspirate the tonsil itself because the abscess develops in the peritonsillar space surrounding the tonsil. Continually aspirate while advancing the needle in the sagittal plane and do not direct it laterally, where it could injure the carotid artery. If the aspirate yields pus, remove as much purulent material as possible. If the aspirate is negative, attempt aspiration again in the middle pole of the peritonsillar space, approximately 1 cm caudal to the first aspiration. If still negative, perform a third

Peritonsillar Abscess: Needle Aspiration

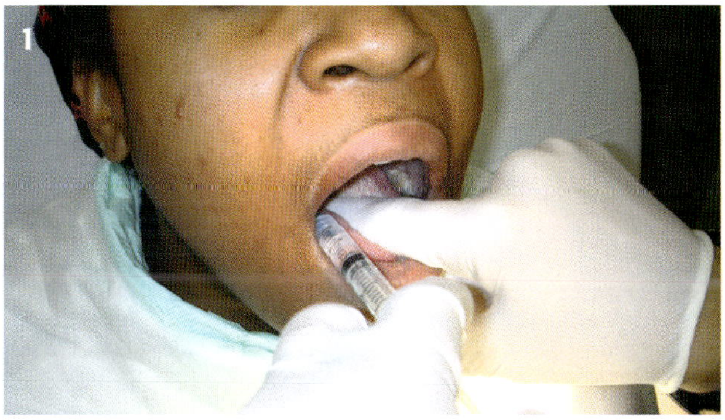

Use a 25- to 27-gauge needle to inject the mucosa with 1–2 mL of lidocaine with epinephrine; observe for blanching. Often, the tongue is best displaced with the finger rather than a tongue blade. Topical anesthetic spray (e.g., Hurricaine) may be used prior to injection.

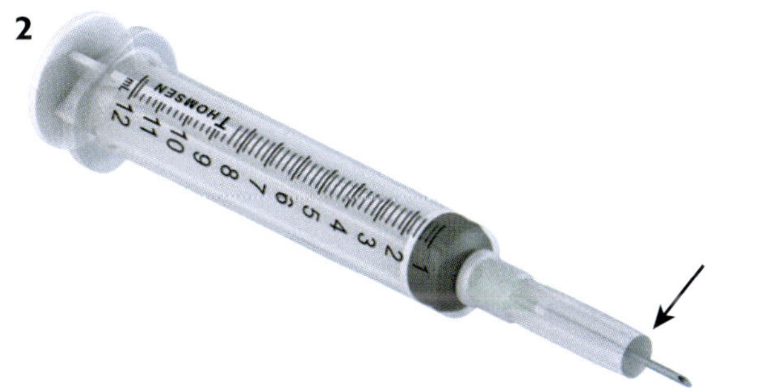

Use a long 18- to 20-gauge needle for aspiration. As a safeguard to prevent overpenetration of the needle, remove the plastic needle guard and cut off the distal 1 cm. Then, replace the cut-off guard on the needle *(arrow)* and secure it to the hub.

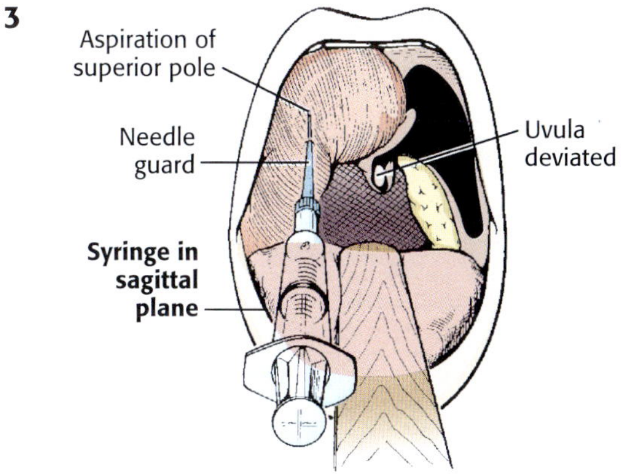

While applying continuous suction, direct the needle in the sagittal plane only (directly anterior to posterior), not to the side toward the carotid artery. Aspirate the superior pole initially.

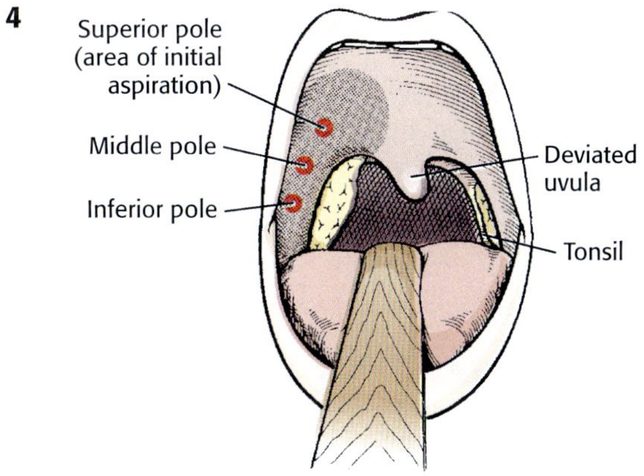

If pus is not obtained from the superior pole, next try the middle pole. The inferior pole may be aspirated last if needed. Note that the tonsil itself is not aspirated.

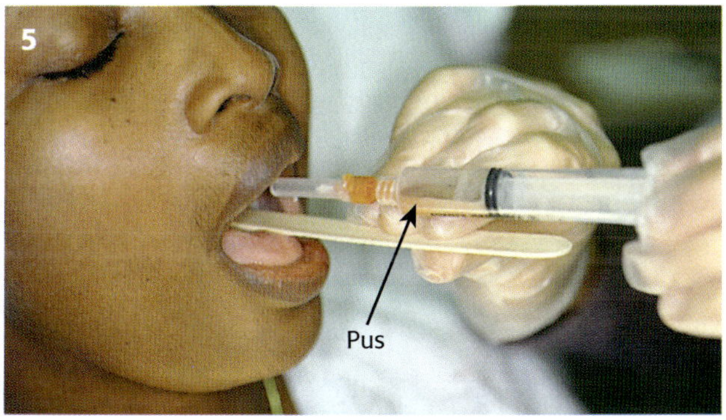

Usually, 2–6 mL of pus is obtained. It is unusual to recover more than 8–10 mL. If substantial amounts of pus are obtained, the patient usually notices immediate improvement in symptoms.

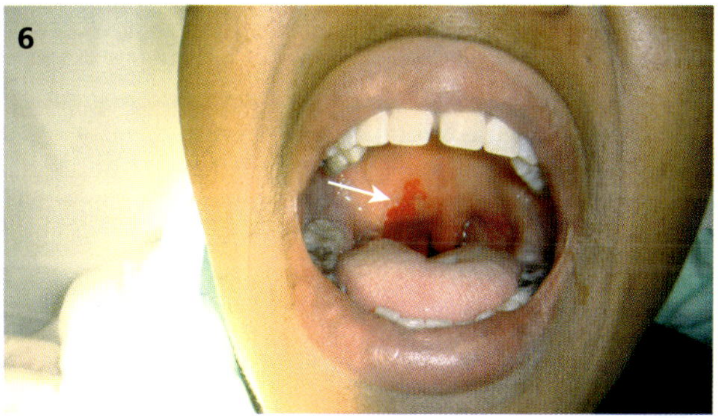

After needle removal, some bleeding will be noted *(arrow)*. Slight oozing of blood and pus may continue for several hours. Significant additional drainage may be an indication for repeated aspiration, incision and drainage, or hospital admission.

Fig. 64.11 Drainage of a peritonsillar abscess: needle aspiration technique.

and final attempt at the inferior pole (see Figs. 64.11, *step 4* and 64.13). It must be stressed that a negative aspiration does not rule out a PTA.

Usually, 2 mL to 6 mL of pus is obtained. It is unusual to recover more than 8 to 10 mL (see Fig. 64.11, *step 5*). Although culture is recommended, the results rarely alter subsequent therapy. When significant amounts of pus are aspirated, the patient usually feels immediate improvement in pain and dysphagia. After the needle is removed, some bleeding will be noted (see Fig. 64.11, *step 6*). Slight oozing may occur for a few hours. Drainage of pus may continue and is often sensed as a foul taste by the patient. Significant additional drainage of

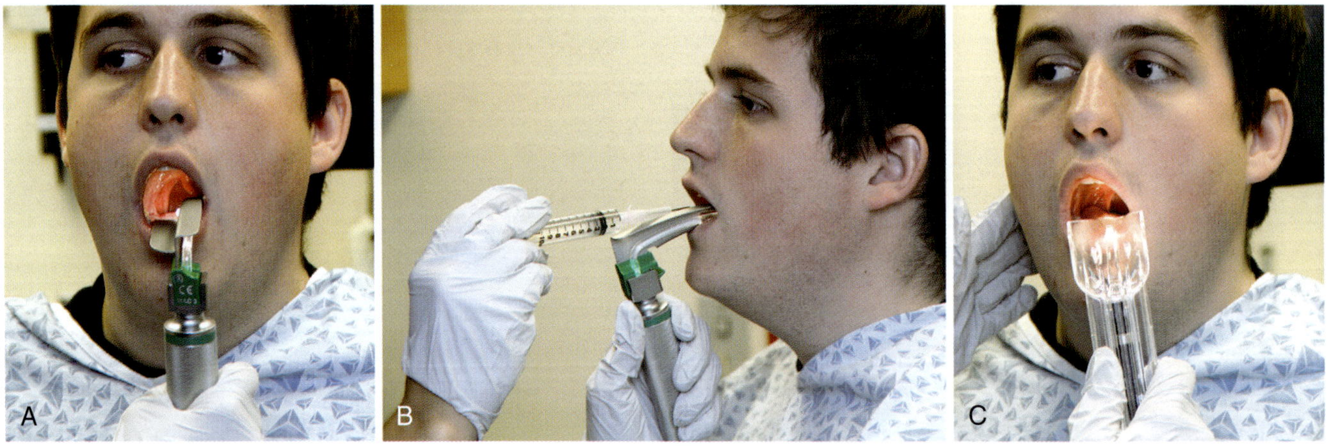

Fig. 64.12 (A–B) Laryngoscope and blade used to illuminate the posterior aspect of the pharynx. (C) Disassembled disposable plastic speculum with a fiberoptic light source used to illuminate the posterior aspect of the pharynx.

pus may be an indication for repeated aspiration, incision and drainage, or hospital admission.

Some clinicians advise a formal incision and drainage procedure if frank pus is obtained, whereas others now accept needle aspiration (with close follow-up) as the definitive initial treatment. Combined aspiration and formal drainage in the same visit may be indicated if large amounts of pus are obtained (>5 to 6 mL) or if pus continues to drain from the aspiration site.

There are no agreed standards regarding the best practice for this issue.

Incision and Drainage

To incise a PTA, anesthetize the area as described earlier. Prepare a No. 11 or 15 scalpel blade by taping over all but the distal 0.5 cm of the blade to prevent deeper penetration (Fig. 64.14, *step 1*). Incise the area of maximal fluctuance or the area where a preceding aspiration (if one was performed) located pus. Do not incise the tonsil itself; instead, incise the peritonsillar area where pus accumulates. Incise the mucosa in an area 0.5 cm long in a vertical direction (see Fig. 64.14, *step 2*). Warn the patient that the pus will flow posteriorly and must be expectorated. Expect bleeding because this is a vascular area. Suction the incised area with a No. 9 or 10 Frazier suction tip or a tonsil suction tip to aid in removal of the purulent material. Place a closed Kelly clamp into the opening and gently open it to break up the loculations (see Fig. 64.14, *step 3*). Allow the patient to rinse and gargle with water. Packing is not used in the drainage of this abscess.

Aftercare

Following successful drainage, the patient should be observed for 30 minutes to an hour. The patient should be encouraged to swish and spit ice water to reduce pain, bleeding, swelling, and to enhance further drainage. If the patient can tolerate oral intake and symptoms are controlled (pain, bleeding). ED discharge is appropriate. The patient can be discharged with primary care or otorhinolaryngology follow-up in 24 to 48 hours. A 10-day course of antibiotics is recommended. Clindamycin or amoxicillin/clavulanic acid are typical.[2,8] If not contraindicated, acetaminophen and antiinflammatory medications should be prescribed. At home, patients should keep hydrated, follow a soft diet, and swish and spit several times a day. Return precautions for fever, neck stiffness, bleeding, enlarging neck mass, worsening neck or throat pain, or worsening trismus should be provided.[4,6]

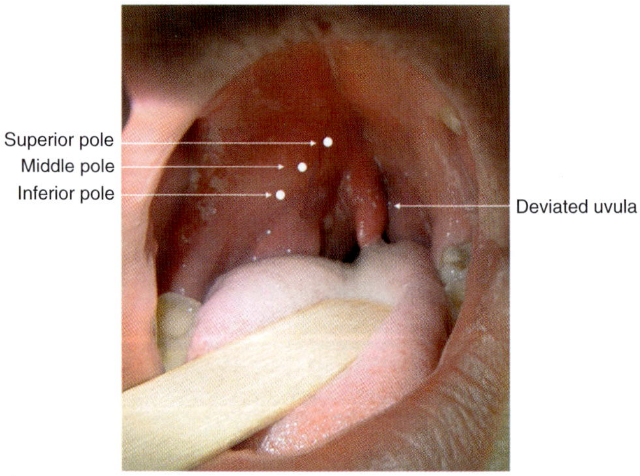

Fig. 64.13 Superior, middle, and inferior poles for drainage of peritonsillar abscess by needle aspiration.

Toxic patients, those with excessive volumes of aspirate, those with persistent bleeding, and those unable to take oral antibiotics are candidates for admission or more prolonged observation.

Complications

Needle aspiration is an accepted, safe, and effective technique for treatment of PTA in the ED. There is an approximate 10% failure rate and need for subsequent drainage.[2,25,26] Complications can include aspiration of pus or blood and hemorrhage. If the patient has cellulitis, the aspiration will be of no help, but it will not worsen morbidity. Failure to obtain pus in a setting where diagnostic imaging (CT, US) is unavailable should prompt consideration of transfer of care. If transfer is not feasible, empiric antibiotics and reevaluation (and possible aspiration reattempt) in 24 hours is warranted. Though often feared, injury to the carotid artery has not been reported as a complication of needle aspiration of PTA. Catastrophic hemorrhage may result from the extremely rare and largely theoretical aspiration of a pseudoaneurysm mimicking a PTA or similarly rare necrosis of the carotid artery. In addition, incisions

Peritonsillar Abscess: Incision and Drainage

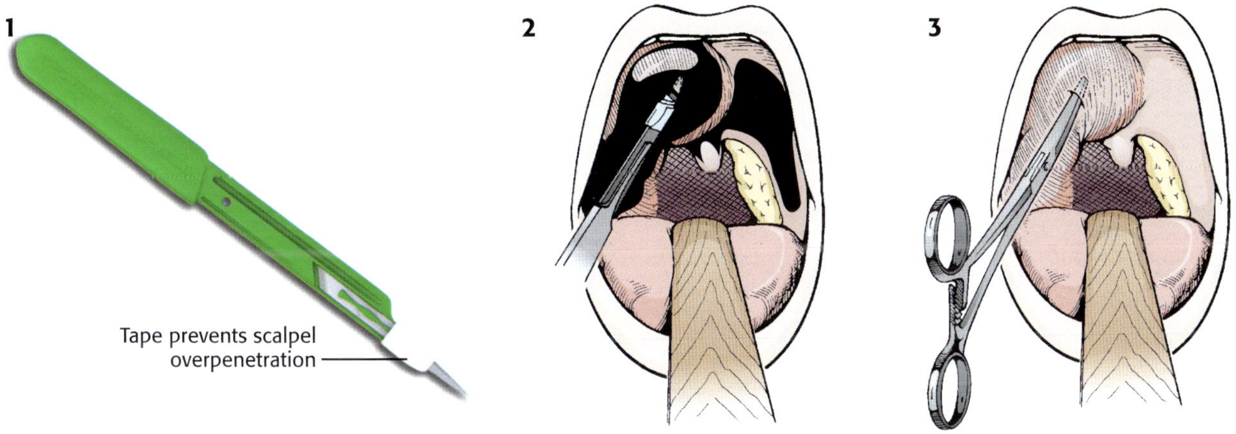

1. Place adhesive tape around a No. 11 or 15 scalpel blade so that only the distal 0.5–1 cm is exposed. This prevents overpenetration.

2. Incise the area of maximal fluctuance (or the area where previous aspiration located pus). Expect pus and blood to flow from the incision; have suction ready to remove the purulent material.

3. Use a Kelly clamp to gently break up loculations. Packing is not used. Observe the patient for about an hour to watch for complications such as bleeding.

Fig. 64.14 Drainage of a peritonsillar abscess: incision and drainage technique. Aspiration is often the only procedure required to successfully treat a peritonsillar abscess, but it has a 10% failure rate. In some instances the clinician will opt for incision and drainage of a peritonsillar abscess. This procedure may be used initially or after aspiration if copious pus is aspirated or pus continues to drain or reaccumulate.

that are too large or too small may lead to poor healing or an inability to completely evacuate the abscess, respectively.

Antibiotic Therapy

After drainage, empirical oral antibiotics are used in outpatients and IV antibiotics are administered to inpatients. PTAs are often polymicrobial, and hence culture of aspirated pus is prudent, although the results rarely affect subsequent treatment. The predominant bacterial species are *Streptococcus pyogenes* (group A streptococcus), *Staphylococcus aureus* (including in rare cases methicillin-resistant *S. aureus* [MRSA]), and various respiratory anaerobes (including *Bacteroides*, *Fusobacterium*, *Prevotella*, and *Veillonella* species). *Haemophilus* species are found occasionally. Aerobes and anaerobes may be recovered simultaneously if appropriate culture techniques are used. Appropriate oral antibiotics for outpatient therapy in areas where *S. aureus* remains susceptible to methicillin include amoxicillin-clavulanate or clindamycin. For inpatients, administer ampicillin-sulbactam or clindamycin. Penicillin plus metronidazole is also a recommended antibiotic regimen. In septic patients, it is prudent to also cover for MRSA. Although clindamycin may be adequate for MRSA, some clinicians add vancomycin or linezolid to the aforementioned initial antibiotic regimens if MRSA is suspected or predominant in the population.

Glucocorticoid Therapy

It is common practice for clinicians to administer short-term corticosteroids, such as IV dexamethasone or methylprednisolone, as an adjunct to other therapies to provide relief from the symptoms of PTA. Evidence of the benefits of glucocorticoids in the management of PTA is inconsistent, but such intervention may hasten improvement of symptoms in adolescent and adult patients treated with needle aspiration and antimicrobial therapy. The benefits may be marginal, but as there are no significant complications, it is reasonable to empirically treat adults with short-term corticosteroids. A single intramuscular or IV dose of dexamethasone (10 mg) is a common protocol.

EAR

Anatomy

The ear consists of three sections, the outer, middle, and inner ear. The outer ear includes the pinna (auricle), the external auditory canal (EAC), and the tympanic membrane (TM) (Fig. 64.15A). In this chapter, only the parts of the external ear will be discussed. The pinna (visible portion of the outer ear) is flesh-covered cartilage and serves both hearing and cosmetic functions. The EAC extends from the head to the external auditory meatus in the skull and measures approximately 2.5 cm in adults. It is relatively short and straight in early infancy but begins to take on its adult S-shape and overall anterocaudal orientation at 2 years of age. Initially, the EAC is almost entirely cartilaginous, but by adulthood its medial two-thirds are composed of bony support with an overlying thin, stratified squamous epithelium. The lateral third has a less sensitive, thicker hairy epithelium that produces cerumen and retains its cartilage as support. The arterial supply to the EAC originates from the external carotid artery via the posterior auricular, maxillary, and superficial temporal branches. The mandibular branch of the fifth cranial nerve (V3) and the vagus nerve innervate the ear.

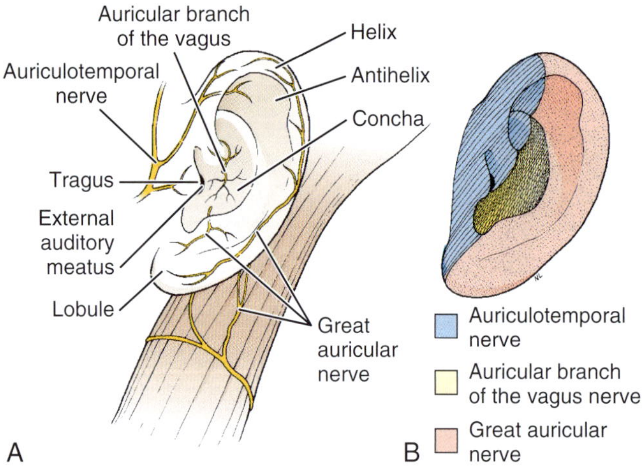

Fig. 64.15 (A) Anatomy of the ear and innervation of the auricle. (B) Sensory distribution of nerves of the ear.

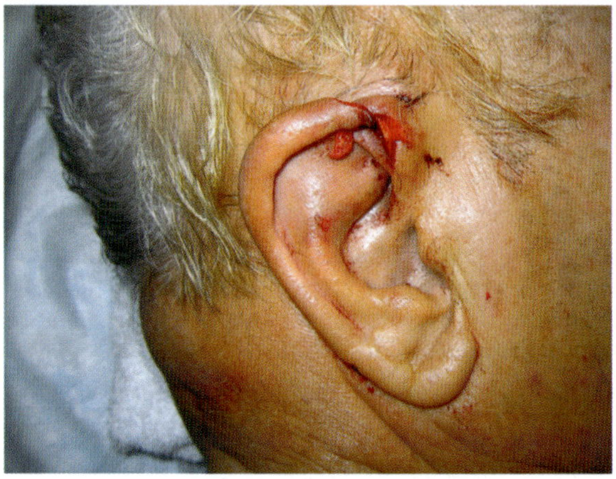

Fig. 64.16 Closure of extensive lacerations of the ear require a nerve block of the auricle.

Other important anatomic considerations include two natural narrowings in the EAC, which are important when considering FBs. One is located at the junction of bone and cartilage and the other lies just lateral to the TM. A blind spot may occur in the tympanic sulcus (inferior and anterior to the TM) because of the oblique orientation of the TM. An examiner using a simple otoscope may not visualize an FB in this sulcus.

Anesthesia of the External Ear

Auricle

See Video 64.4. Indications for local anesthesia of the auricle include closure of extensive lacerations or performance of other painful procedures such as incision and drainage of hematomas (Fig. 64.16). Four nerve branches supply the external ear; knowledge of their anatomy is required to understand the location for injection of anesthetic (see Fig. 64.15B). The great auricular nerve (branch of the cervical plexus) innervates most of the posteromedial, posterolateral, and inferior aspects of the auricle. A few branches of the lesser occipital nerve may contribute to this area. The auricular branch of the vagus supplies the concha and most of the area around the auditory meatus. The auriculotemporal nerve (from the mandibular branch of the trigeminal nerve) supplies the anterosuperior and anteromedial aspects of the auricle.

Procedure

Fill a 10-mL syringe with either 1% lidocaine or 0.25% bupivacaine. Mix with epinephrine if a regional block is planned in an area without evidence of traumatized vascularity. Attach the syringe to a 25- or 27-gauge needle (5 cm to 7 cm in length). One of several methods may be used to induce partial or complete anesthesia, depending on the area of concern. To anesthetize the great auricular and lesser occipital nerve branches, inject between 3 and 4 mL of anesthetic into the posterior sulcus (Fig. 64.17, *plate 1*). Insert the needle behind the inferior pole of the auricle and gradually aspirate and inject toward the superior pole along the crescent-shaped contour of the posterior aspect of the auricle. Anesthetize the auriculotemporal nerve anteriorly by placing 3 mL to 4 mL of anesthetic just superior and anterior to the cartilaginous tragus. Provide anesthesia to the auricular branch of the vagus nerve and the more central areas of the auricle by using the technique shown in Fig. 64.17, *plates 3 and 4*.

Another and possibly more effective option is the regional block shown in Fig. 64.17, *plate 2*. Insert the needle subcutaneously approximately 1 cm above the superior pole of the auricle and direct it to a point just anterior to the tragus. Be sure to inject the skin of the scalp while avoiding the auricular cartilage. Aspirate and then slowly withdraw the needle while injecting anesthetic until the needle is almost to the puncture site. Redirect the needle posteriorly and repeat the process while aiming at the skin just behind the mid-auricular area. Remove the needle and perform the same procedure but insert the needle just inferior to the insertion of the ear lobule and anesthetize it in a superior direction. Again, block the auricular branch of the vagus as described in Fig. 64.17, *plates 3 and 4*, if additional anesthesia of the concha is required.

Use caution if adding epinephrine to the anesthetic solution when performing regional nerve blocks of the ear, especially if the blood supply has already been traumatically reduced. Do not include epinephrine when directly infiltrating wounds of the auricle because restriction of blood flow through the end-arteries may result in tissue necrosis. Other complications related to local anesthesia and regional blocks of the head and neck are reviewed elsewhere in this text.

EAC and TM

The EAC is innervated by the auricular branch of the vagus nerve (inferiorly and posteriorly) and by the auriculotemporal nerve (superiorly, anteriorly, and inferiorly). The primary indication for local anesthesia of the auditory canal is for removal of FBs, including debridement of otitis externa or removal of significantly impacted cerumen. It is nearly impossible for even the most cooperative patient to be able to tolerate even minimal manipulation of the auditory canal or TM. It is very difficult to achieve adequate anesthesia of the inner ear and TM for painful procedures. Simply stated, no easy and completely effective procedure consistently works well. If total anesthesia is required, general anesthesia, especially in children, is often the only alternative. Ketamine is an ideal agent for short procedures, especially for children with foreign objects in the ear. Topical anesthetics are inadequate because of their poor absorption through the rather impermeable and keratinized epithelial surface of the EAC. Though effective for some procedures, injection of local anesthetics into and around the auditory meatus is quite

Anesthesia of the Ear

Auricular Field Blocks

1

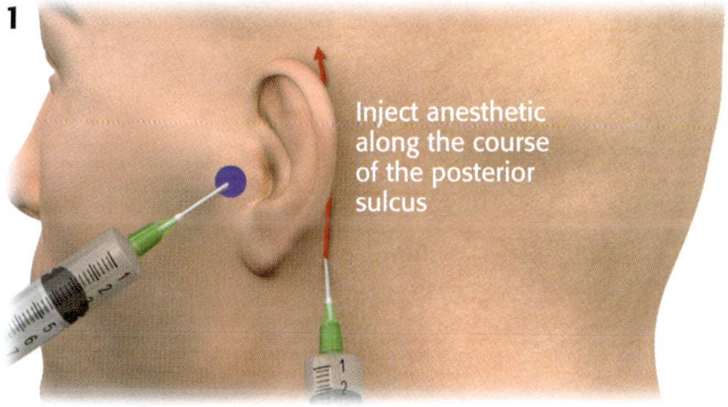

One method of auricular block uses approximately 3–4 mL of anesthetic injected both at the posterior sulcus *(red arrow)* and at a point just anterior to the tragus *(blue circle)*.

2

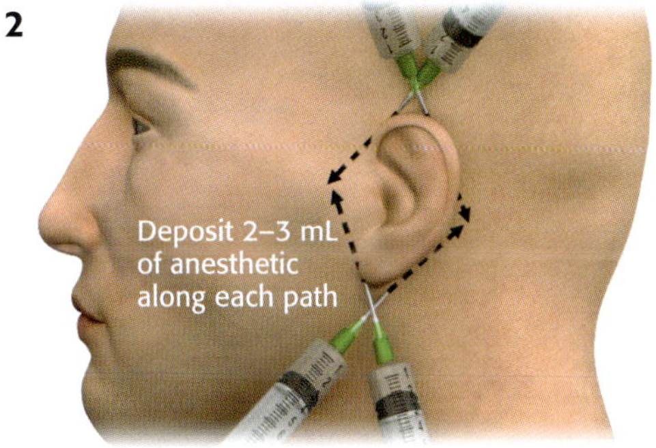

An alternative auricular block deposits 2–3 mL of anesthetic in four separate injections that encircle the ear. Begin each new injection in a region that is already anesthetized.

External Auditory Canal Blocks

3

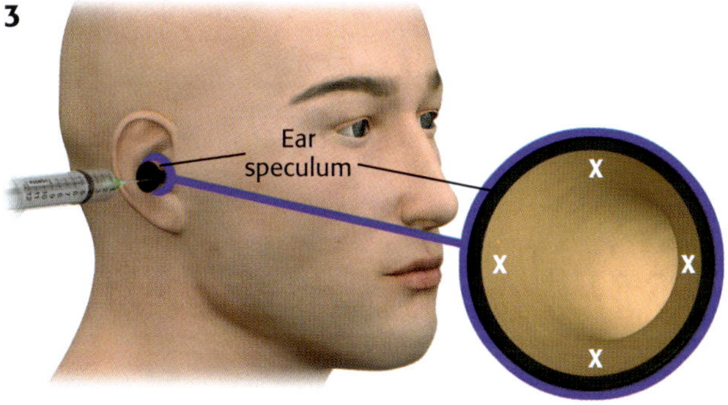

Four-quadrant field block. Inject anesthetic subcutaneously in the four quadrants of the lateral portion of the ear canal. Use the largest speculum that will fit to guide the injections. Withdraw the speculum, tilt it toward each of the four quadrants, and insert the needle subcutaneously *(x)*. Inject 0.25–0.50 mL of anesthetic to produce a slight bulge in the soft tissue. A total of 1.5–2.0 mL of anesthetic is usually sufficient to anesthetize the ear canal and permit painless removal of a foreign body. Ketamine procedural sedation may facilitate the procedure.

4

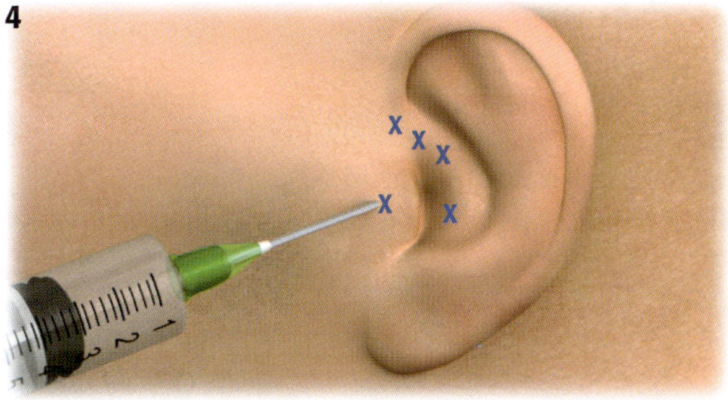

Diagram of injection sites for an alternative technique to anesthetize the ear canal and central concha. Inject each site with approximately 0.5 mL of 1% lidocaine. Do not inject if external signs of infection are present.

Fig. 64.17 Anesthesia of the ear.

painful and often difficult to perform in a struggling and uncooperative patient. Certain instances warrant adjunctive use of procedural sedation.

Procedure

For local anesthesia use a 25- or 27-gauge needle (3 to 5 cm in length) attached to a syringe containing 1% lidocaine with epinephrine. A 1:10 mixture of 8.4% sodium bicarbonate to lidocaine helps reduce pain during injection in this sensitive area. Place a speculum just inside the auditory meatus, inject 0.3 to 0.5 mL of the anesthetic into subcutaneous tissue, and stop after a small bulge is raised in the skin. Inject all four quadrants in this manner by moving the speculum after each injection (see Fig. 64.17 *plate 3*).

If additional anesthesia is necessary, give two more small injections. Inject the same amount slightly farther into the canal, once along the anterior wall and again at the posterior wall at the bone-cartilage junction.

Another similar technique involves depositing the anesthetic just lateral, or exterior, to the external auditory meatus. Using the same size of needle and type of anesthetic solution as just described, inject approximately 0.5 to 1.0 mL into each of five points around the auditory meatus and tragus (see Fig. 64.17, *plate 4*).

Examination

Several methods can be used to examine the EAC and TM. In all methods, grasp the superior aspect of the pinna and pull cephalad and posterior to straighten the slightly tortuous EAC. Examination is most commonly done with a fiberoptic otoscope (Fig. 64.18). Place a plastic or metal speculum into the auditory meatus for examination and use a headlamp or head mirror/lightbulb as a light source. After inspection, the operating hand can be used to pass instruments into the EAC and to maneuver them more easily. Although this technique

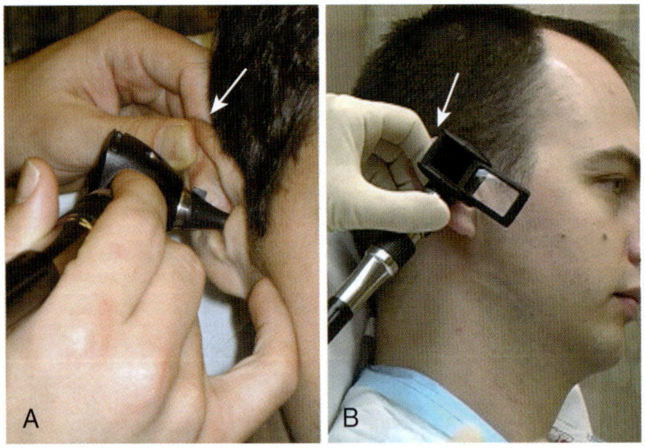

Fig. 64.18 Examination of the ear canal. (A) Retract the pinna in a superior and posterior direction to straighten out the ear canal *(arrow)*. Hold the scope in the other hand and stabilize it against the patient's head. This prevents inadvertent injury if the patient moves unexpectedly. (B) The pinna can be retracted and the scope held with a single hand that is also resting against the patient's head *(arrow)*. This technique is useful if instruments are to be passed through the otoscope.

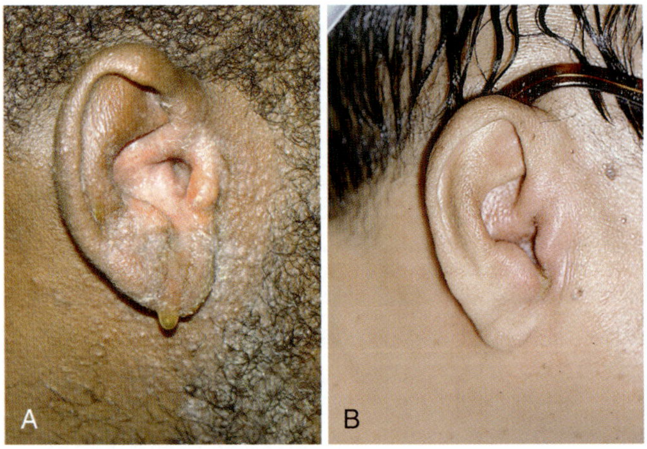

Fig. 64.19 (A) Extensive contact dermatitis from the use of neomycin-containing ear drops. (B) Malignant otitis externa in a diabetic patient developed after the patient manually removed cerumen with a cotton swab and a pencil, but it may develop without manipulation of the canal.

provides excellent illumination, the use of magnifying loupes can improve visualization during procedures. The ideal setup for removal of cerumen or an FB consists of an operating microscope and a speculum. This provides binocular vision and frees the examiner's hands for instrumentation. Unfortunately, this equipment is seldom found outside the otolaryngology clinic setting. If using a standard otoscope, stabilize the hand holding the otoscope against the temporal part of the patient's skull to prevent inadvertent injury to the canal if the patient moves unexpectedly.

Removal of Impacted Cerumen

Excretions from the ceruminous or apocrine and sebaceous glands, together with cells exfoliated from the EAC, combine to form cerumen. One study found that cerumen is composed of lipids, complex proteins, and simple sugars.[31] Cerumen repels water, has documented antimicrobial activity, and forms a protective barrier against infection. Cerumen often becomes impacted, which results in complaints of a "blocked" ear, sudden-onset impaired hearing, or dizziness.

Indications and Contraindications

Symptomatic impaction is an indication for removal, although symptoms are rare until complete obstruction is present. Sudden loss of hearing is a common complaint in patients with totally occluding, impacted cerumen. Cerumen obstructs visualization of the TM and can be evacuated as a part of the evaluation of a febrile child or a patient complaining of ear pain. However, removal of cerumen in a child is rarely indicated in the ED simply to visualize the TM. There are few, if any, true contraindications to removal of impacted cerumen. Cerumen is usually impacted for prolonged periods, and vigorous attempts to remove it may precipitate otitis externa. It is reasonable to instill antiseptics (acetic acid otic solution) (VoSol [ECR Pharmaceuticals Co., Inc.] and others), dilute hydrogen peroxide solution or antibiotic ear drops for a few days after removal of the cerumen to prevent otitis externa. Neomycin-containing ear drops are best avoided because of precipitation of a contact dermatitis (Fig. 64.19A). Caution should be used in removing impacted cerumen in patients with diabetes who commonly experience otitis externa after seemingly minor manipulation of the ear canal (see Fig. 64.19B).

Contraindications to irrigation include the following[32]:

- Patient aversion to or a history of injury from previous syringe irrigation
- History of middle ear disease
- History of ear surgery
- Known or suspected perforated TM
- Severe otitis externa
- Narrow ear canals
- FBs, especially sharp objects and vegetable matter
- Uncooperative patient
- Occluding aural exostoses
- Known inner ear disturbance, especially if the patient has severe vertigo
- History of radiation therapy encompassing the external or middle ear, base of the skull, or mastoid

Procedure

See Videos 64.5 and 64.6. Removal of cerumen can be accomplished by irrigation, manual extraction, or a combination of both. Generally, the procedures used to remove cerumen are safe; however, otologic injury has occurred after this "minor" procedure and has even resulted in litigation.[33]

Irrigation is an effective approach for removal of cerumen and has the advantage of being painless and simple to perform. It is usually most successful after the instillation of a cerumenolytic (see later). Because the patient does not have to remain completely still, it is ideal for the pediatric population. It is estimated that 150,000 ears are irrigated in the United States each week.[33] Though usually more time-consuming and messier than manual extraction, irrigation is an appropriate initial method to attempt and can be performed by technicians with guidance from the clinician.

Whichever of the following techniques are used, some tips for successful removal of cerumen include proper lighting, attention to patient comfort, and abrupt cessation when the patient's comfort level is breached.

Cerumenolytics

These products may break down the hardened or impacted cerumen and lessen the need for irrigation or manual removal. They are used as adjuncts to other procedures; simply instilling cerumenolytics into the canal will not remove enough cerumen to aid the emergency clinician. Data have shown that no cerumenolytic agent has been more effective than water or saline and either is recommended to be used initially. As a second-line option, mineral oil or docusate sodium may be trialed where water or saline has been ineffective.[34,35] Hydrogen peroxide is another commonly used cerumenolytic, but its use has not been systematically studied. An evidence-based review of agents found that docusate sodium administered 15 minutes before irrigation was most effective in facilitating removal of cerumen.[20]

If irrigation fails, continued outpatient use of cerumenolytics is often prescribed, usually combined with home irrigation via a bulb syringe or a repeated visit in a few days. Place the patient in the supine position with the affected ear up, instill the solution, and wait at least 15 to 30 minutes before attempts at removal (Fig. 64.20, *step 1*). Repeat the instillation between attempts at manual extraction or irrigation.

Irrigation (Ear Syringing)

After a cerumenolytic has been instilled and left in the canal for 15 to 30 minutes, irrigation of the canal is often effective in flushing out impacted cerumen. Ask the patient to sit upright and hold an emesis basin flush tightly against the skin just below the earlobe. Attach a 30- to 60-mL syringe to an 18-gauge IV catheter (with the needle removed). Insert the irrigation tip into the EAC only as far as the cartilage-bone junction and direct the stream of warm water superiorly to wash the impacted cerumen away from the TM (see Fig. 63.20, *step 2*). It is important to warm the water to body temperature to prevent caloric stimulation. Multiple attempts may be necessary, and intermittent attempts at manual removal of loosened cerumen may help hasten the process. During the irrigation, ask an assistant to apply traction to the pinna to straighten the canal for more efficient irrigation. Patients usually feel some discomfort with forceful irrigation, but not severe pain.

After irrigating the EAC, apply several drops of isopropanol to the EAC to facilitate evaporation of residual moisture. Do not use isopropanol if the TM is ruptured. Furthermore, topical steroid-containing suspension drops (ciprofloxacin/hydrocortisone) may be soothing after prolonged irrigation. Because severe otitis externa can develop in patients with diabetes after irrigation, some clinicians routinely prescribe antibiotic ear drops (e.g., fluoroquinolones) for a few days after irrigation in high-risk patients.

Manual Instrumentation

Manual instrumentation is more advantageous because it is usually quicker, and the examiner may more easily remove hardened or larger concretions of cerumen under direct visualization. However, it is difficult to manually remove cerumen without causing significant pain, so irrigation is preferred. Manual removal may be the initial procedure in some cases, followed by irrigation when the cerumen is partially disrupted. Place the diagnostic or operating head of the fiberoptic otoscope or a speculum as a protective port through which instruments are passed and manipulated (see Fig. 64.20, *step 3*). An operating microscope works best in this situation but, again, is not usually available. To prevent startling or agitating an already anxious patient, allow the patient to experience the sensation of an instrument in the canal by first placing it softly against the wall of the ear canal.

Instruments used for removal of cerumen include flexible plastic or wire loops, right-angle hooks, suction-tipped catheters, or plastic scoops (see Review Box 64.2 and Fig. 64.20, *steps 4–6*). The spoonlike instruments and irrigation are both more effective in removing softer cerumen. Firm cerumen is ordinarily more easily withdrawn with loops or right-angle hooks. Gently tease the cerumen off the canal wall with loops and then pass hooks or loops around the cerumen and withdraw it slowly. Take care to keep both hands in contact with the patient's head because any sudden movement may cause trauma to the canal or the TM.

Complications

Complications from removal of cerumen are rare but can have serious consequences. Although complications from ear syringing are more common with jet irrigators, they may occur with any method of ear irrigation and include otitis externa, TM perforation, or middle ear injury from a preexisting defect in the TM. If the patient is experiencing sudden pain, tinnitus, hearing loss, nausea, or vertigo, stop the irrigation and examine the TM. If the membrane is ruptured, give prophylactic oral antibiotics for otitis media, keep the ear canal perfectly dry with cotton, and refer the patient to an otolaryngologist. This complication is usually benign.

Complications from manual extraction most commonly occur when inadvertent contact is made with the thin, friable skin of the bony canal. Trauma may cause EAC laceration, otitis externa, or perforation of the TM.

Ear Canal Debridement and Wick Placement

Debridement of the ear canal and wick placement are essential components in the management and treatment of otitis externa or "swimmer's ear," an acute inflammation of the skin of the EAC. This is essentially cellulitis of the ear canal. Precipitants of otitis externa include water exposure and trauma. Excessive moisture in the canal raises the pH and removes the cerumen. Keratin cannot absorb water, thereby creating a medium for bacterial growth. Trauma, especially self-manipulation with FBs (e.g., cotton swabs, fingernails), causes abrasions in the ear canal and introduces infection. Removal of cerumen by water irrigation is a well-recognized risk factor for the development of otitis externa.[18]

Patients with diabetes and other immunocompromised patients, are susceptible to malignant (necrotizing) otitis externa, a life-threatening form of otitis externa caused by *Pseudomonas* (see Fig. 64.19B). Deep tissue necrosis, osteomyelitis, intracranial extension, and systemic toxicity are hallmark features. Malignant otitis externa is difficult to treat and the mortality rate can be as high as 53%.[36] The diagnosis of malignant otitis externa should be considered in a diabetic or immunocompromised patient with significant symptoms who does not respond to initial outpatient treatment.

Indications and Contraindications

In patients with suspected otitis externa, attempts should be made to clean debris from the canal to aid in healing. In addition, wick placement will be helpful in delivering antibiotic medications to the swollen canal. It has been touted that the key to successful treatment is adequate removal of canal debris. However, vigorous attempts to remove debris

Cerumen Impaction Removal

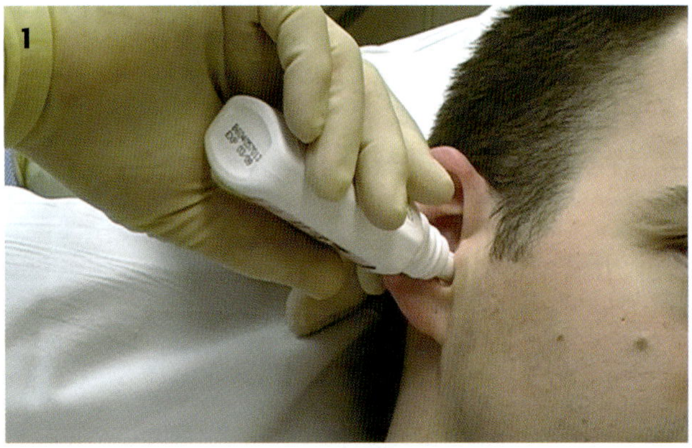

Instill a ceruminolytic solution into the ear at least 15 minutes before attempts at removal (see text for discussion of various agents). Repeat the instillation between attempts.

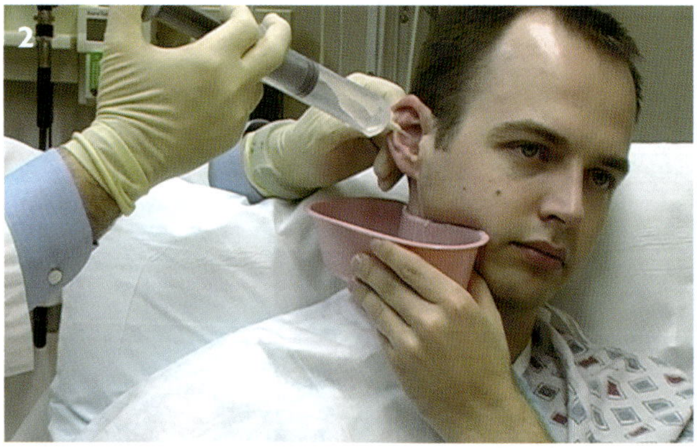

Irrigate with body-temperature water via a syringe with a plastic IV catheter (with the needle removed). Apply traction to the pinna during irrigation to straighten the ear canal. Periodic attempts at manual removal of loosened cerumen may be beneficial.

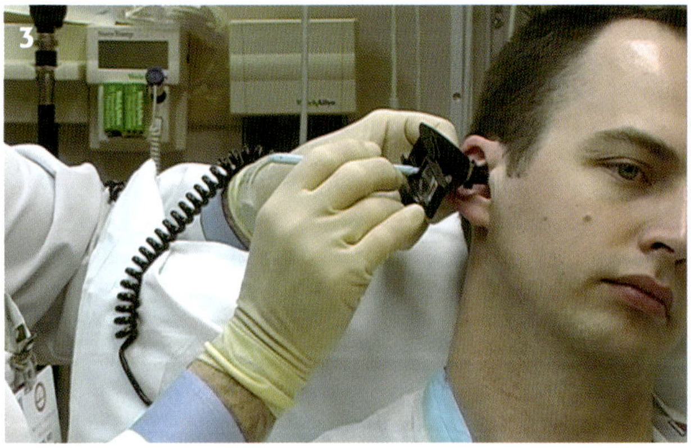

For manual removal, use the otoscope (with the view piece retracted) as a port for passage of the instrument.

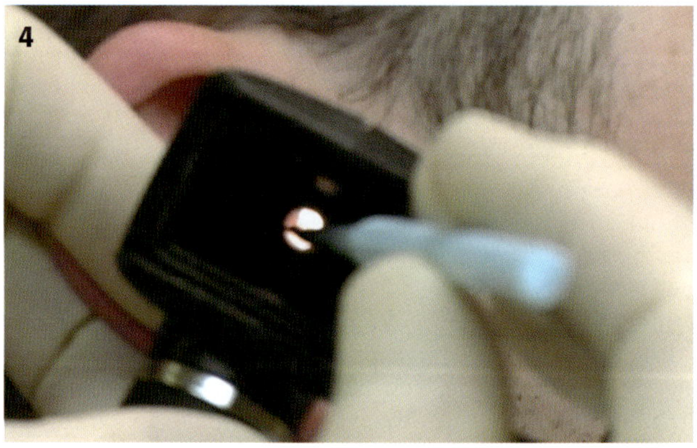

Gently tease the cerumen off the canal wall with a loop or plastic ear scoop. This should be performed only under direct visualization.

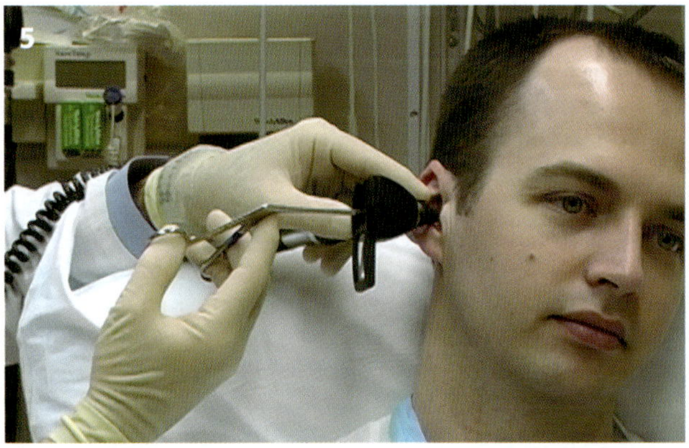

Remove dislodged pieces of cerumen from the canal with an instrument such as alligator forceps.

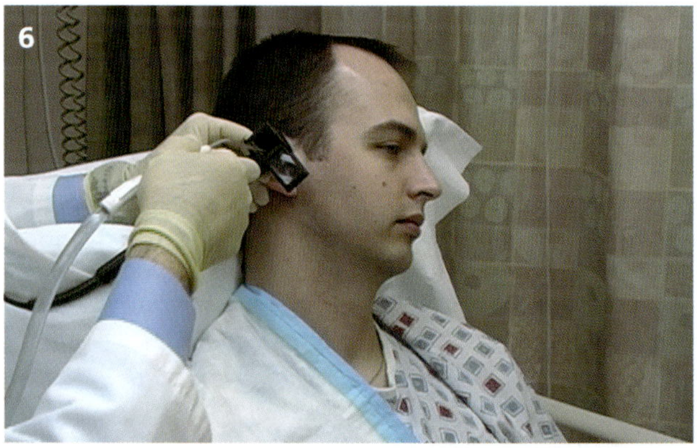

A suction-tip catheter may also be used. However, this should be done under direct visualization only to prevent iatrogenic injury to the fragile ear canal.

Fig. 64.20 Cerumen impaction removal. Place liquid Dulcolax or other cerumenolytic into the canal for 20 to 30 minutes prior to wax removal. Most wax is removed with irrigation alone, but multiple irrigations may be required. When removal of cerumen is unsuccessful in the emergency department, discharge the patient with a cerumenolytic and attempt irrigation again in 24 to 48 hours.

Cerumen Impaction Removal

Indications

Symptomatic cerumen impaction
Sudden hearing loss in the setting of cerumen impaction
Evaluation of otitis media in the setting of cerumen impaction

Contraindications

Few if any absolute contraindications
Contraindications to irrigation:

Patient aversion to irrigation	Foreign bodies
History of middle ear disease	Uncooperative patient
History of ear surgery	Occluding aural exostoses
Perforated tympanic membrane	Inner ear disturbance
Severe otitis externa	Radiation therapy in the area
Narrow ear canals	

Complications

Otitis externa
Tympanic membrane perforation
Middle ear injury
External auditory canal trauma

Equipment

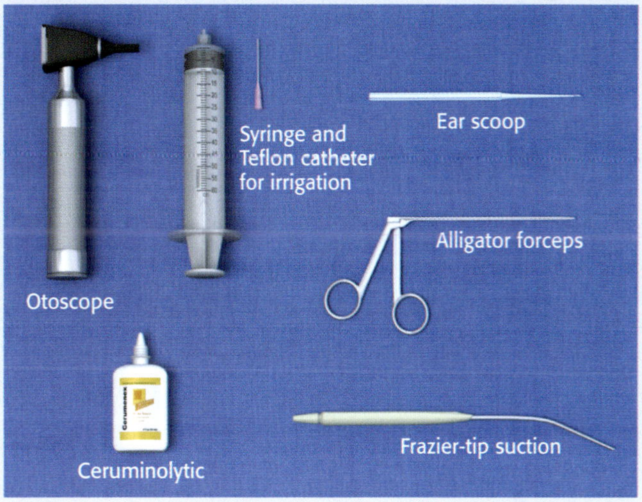

Review Box 64.2 Cerumen impaction removal: indications, contraindications, complications, and equipment.

on the first visit are frequently painful, of unproven value, and often eschewed.

Removal of debris is contraindicated in cases of suspected malignant otitis externa and otolaryngology consultation is required.

Procedure

See Video 64.7. Because of patient discomfort and canal swelling, use small swabs (e.g., urethral swabs) to gently remove debris. Irrigate the canal gently recognizing that many patients can be treated without extensive débridement. Perform irrigation only in the absence of TM perforation.[32,37]

Because the inflamed canal is susceptible to trauma, removal of debris by suctioning under direct visualization with the open or operating otoscope head and a 5- or 7-Fr Frazier suction tip may be a better option (see Fig. 64.20, *step 6*).

For more advanced cases with significant exudate and edema, removal of debris is necessary but intensely painful. Filling the ear canal with lidocaine and waiting 20 minutes for effect will often anesthetize the canal enough for gentle manipulation. Another approach is to use a local block of the EAC (see Fig. 64.17) as long as the cellulitis has not extended to the tragus or concha. Administer parenteral analgesics if additional control of pain is required.

When edema, debris, and exudate are marked enough to impede antibiotic drops from contacting the skin of the canal, use an ear wick. The wick works as a conduit to deliver antibiotic solutions to the ear canal. The true benefit of wick implantation is unknown, and it is often not performed because it is painful. One approach is to place a 0.25-inch strip of Nu-Gauze dressing (Johnson & Johnson) covered with an antibiotic and steroid cream (Cortisporin Otic cream, Monarch Pharmaceuticals, Inc.) into the external acoustic canal in a fashion similar to the technique used for anterior nasal packing. Using an otoscope and alligator forceps, place the leading edge of the gauze deeply in the canal until it is fully packed. Withdraw the otoscope and finish by also packing the lateral aspect of the canal. Cotton may be used as well (Fig. 64.21A).

An easier alternative is to use commercially available ear wicks, such as the Pope Merocel ear wick (Medtronic). Place this dehydrated and trimmed wick into an edematous canal and apply antibiotic/hydrocortisone drops onto it (see Fig. 64.21B). The wick swells and helps reduce edema by the antimicrobial and antiinflammatory effects of the solution and through pressure exerted against the walls as it expands. Keep the wick moist with drops and leave it in place until the patient is seen again in 24 to 48 hours for removal and further evaluation. Though relatively safe to use, the ear wick is designed for short-term use. Generally, these wicks will fall out of the canal as the edema subsides. However, wicks can harbor bacteria with prolonged retention and cause tissue ingrowth, which results in long-term problems for the patient.[38]

Complications

There are very few complications with canal debridement and ear wick placement. Usually, the wick will fall out as edema in the canal subsides; if not, it may become a FB of the EAC. Care should be taken to not injure the already friable skin of the EAC, which can lead to bleeding and possible infection or cellulitis of the EAC when placing or removing a wick.

Ear Canal Foreign Body

Despite its small size, the EAC may play host to numerous types of FBs.[39,40] Living insects account for most FBs found in adults. Children frequently place food (e.g., peas, beans), organic matter (e.g., grass, leaves, flowers), and inorganic objects (e.g., beads, rocks, dirt) into their ear canals during

Ear Wick Placement

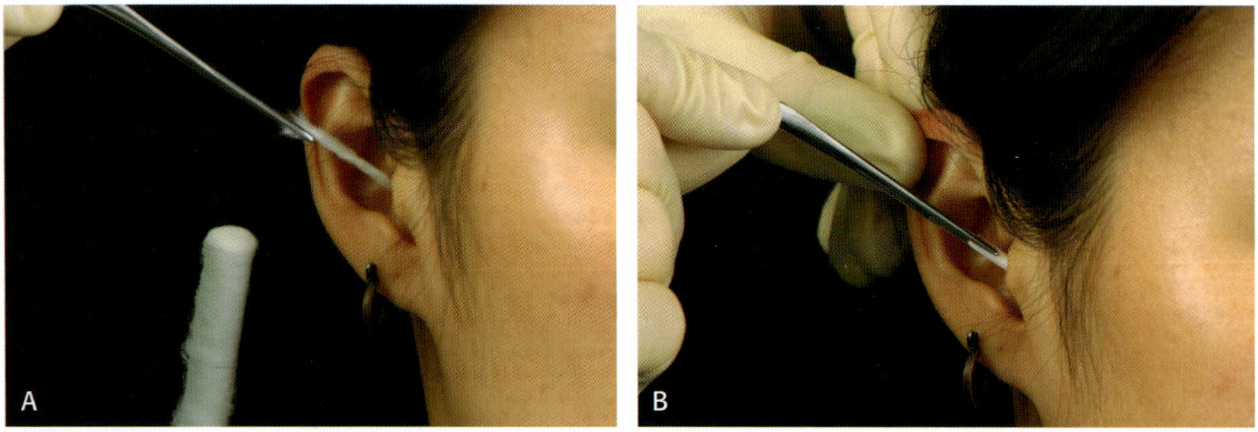

A: Cotton or 0.25-inch Nu-Gauze packing strip can be coated with Cortisporin Otic cream and placed into the external auditory canal with alligator forceps.

B: An easier solution is to use a Merocel ear wick. Place the dehydrated wick into the canal and apply Cortisporin Otic drops to it. Instruct the patient to place the drops directly on the wick until the follow-up visit.

Fig. 64.21 Placement of an ear wick. Ear wicks are used for the treatment of otitis externa and function to deliver antibiotic medications to the swollen external auditory canal.

play, and they often fail to admit this to parents. Button batteries may cause significant tissue destruction in a matter of hours, and it is vital to immediately obtain otolaryngology consultation for removal if the button battery is not easily extracted. Symptoms of FB retention usually consist of ear pain, fullness, or impaired hearing in adults; pediatric patients may not be encountered until an associated otitis externa with a purulent discharge has developed.

As described previously, the anatomy of the EAC predisposes to entrapment of FBs in either a lateral or a deeper position. Removal of more medial objects can be much more painful, and anesthesia is usually required. Even the most cooperative patient may become difficult after feeling pain during manipulation of the ear canal. It is probably impossible to adequately immobilize the head of an uncooperative awake child and to delicately extract an FB.

Anesthesia of the EAC may be difficult to achieve. Topical anesthetics have a partial effect, and a four-quadrant injection technique may not produce complete anesthesia, especially of the TM (see Fig. 64.17, *step 3*).[39,40] The simplest approach is to fill the ear canal with 1%, 2%, or 4% lidocaine and wait 20 minutes for some degree of topical anesthesia to occur (a caveat is that organic matter may absorb the fluid at increase in size and become more lodged). Procedural sedation (preferably an analgesic-sedative combination or dissociative anesthetic) can aid in the removal of FBs in a distraught child by preventing further struggling and potential canal trauma. Ketamine is an excellent option for simple FB removal in the outpatient setting. The care provider must weigh the inherent risks related to procedural sedation against those of general anesthesia and the cost of operating room intervention.

Adequate visualization of the object is needed for successful removal. One study showed that canal lacerations occurred in 48% of patients in whom removal was attempted without a microscope and in 4% when it was used.[40] The otoscope is the traditional ED instrument for viewing FBs in the ear canal. It is less likely to be useful for retrieval because it is difficult to insert the instrument through or around the end of the speculum. A specialized speculum allows more space for instrumentation. A headlamp provides a good light source and leaves both hands free. Magnifying loupes also provide hands-free magnification.

Indications and Contraindications

In most cases, removal of an FB should be attempted in the ED. Before initiating removal, the clinician should set realistic limits on the number of attempts to be made. Even the best clinician can become too aggressive as frustration builds with failed attempts to extract the object. Early consultation with an otolaryngologist should not be considered a failure with difficult FBs. Indeed, with the proper equipment and experience, most objects can be removed atraumatically.

Severely impacted objects and concomitant EAC infection are relative contraindications to removal, and ear, nose, and throat (ENT) consultation should be obtained. In addition, patient cooperation is essential for successful removal. The only other contraindication to removal of FBs from the EAC involves certain circumstances when irrigation will be the technique used. Irrigation should not be performed in cases of known or suspected TM rupture (tinnitus, vertigo, significant hearing loss, or bleeding from behind the object). In addition, irrigation should not be performed if the object is soft or if it is a seed or other vegetable or organic matter because the water may cause the object to swell.

Procedures

See Videos 64.8–64.16. Make a judicious effort to remove an ear FB in the ED setting. Avoid prolonged traumatic attempts because this often terrifies the patient, complicates subsequent attempts, and can cause bleeding and swelling, thus making subsequent efforts more difficult. Most approaches to removal of FBs are anecdotal and found in the literature as case reports or case series rather than as prospective clinical trials. Familiarize yourself with several techniques because the most appropriate choice depends on the size, shape, consistency, and depth of impaction of the object.

Irrigation

Irrigation is the least invasive method; the techniques were explained in detail earlier in this chapter (see section on "Removal of Impacted Cerumen" and Fig. 64.20). Irrigation works particularly well with small rocks, dirt, or sand that lie deep in the canal next to the TM. It is not recommended for organic material like popcorn or beans.

Suction-Tipped Catheters

This technique works well with objects that are round and difficult to grasp. Suction is readily available in the ED but should provide 100 to 140 mm Hg of negative pressure to be useful. To avoid iatrogenic injury, inform the patient of the impending noise to prevent sudden movements caused by a startle reflex. Place either the blunt or the soft plastic tip against the object and withdraw it slowly. If using a suction instrument with a thumb-controlled release valve (as with the Frazier suction tip), remember to cover the port to activate the suction.

The Schuknecht Foreign Body Suction Tip Remover (Olympus America) (Fig. 64.22A) is a commercially available device that is essentially a Frazier suction device with a soft flared tip. This device is especially useful for smooth and spherical FBs; and less for hard, irregularly shaped objects. The VacuTIP Foreign Body Suction Tip (Innovia Medical) (Fig. 64.22B is a disposable, nonsterile device that fits on most 7-Fr Baron or Frazier suction devices). The device is actually a suction cup that can conform to almost any shape and can be used for nasal or EAC FBs.

Manual Instrumentation

This approach can be attempted with various instruments (Fig. 64.23, *plate 1*). Use the diagnostic or operating head of a fiberoptic otoscope for illumination and magnification. Ask an assistant to hold the pinna back and out so that you can hold the otoscope with one hand and manipulate the instrument with the other. A speculum and either a headlamp or a head mirror/light source can also provide illumination; magnifying loupes are usually required for adequate visualization. Use small alligator forceps to remove objects with edges that can be grasped but avoid trying to encircle an impacted round FB because this may cause trauma to the canal wall. A small right-angle hook is another choice. Place the tip past the object, rotate it 90 degrees, and then pull the object from the canal. Fine tissue or Adson forceps, curets, and skin hooks are other instruments used occasionally. Use of these instruments is commonly associated with abrasions and bleeding of the ear canal.[39,40] Instruments should be used only on compliant, cooperative patients. Direct visualization of the object is essential.

Fogarty Catheters

Small Fogarty catheters (biliary or vascular) are balloon tipped and may be used in a manner like that described later in this chapter, in the section on nasal FB removal. Attach the tip of the catheter to a 3-mL syringe. Pass the catheter beyond the FB. Once the tip is past the object, gradually inflate the balloon and drag the FB out along with the balloon. Immediately deflate the balloon if pain suddenly occurs because rupture of the TM is a potential complication.

Cyanoacrylate (Superglue)

The use of glue to remove FBs was first reported in India in 1977.[40,41] Glue is most effective in removing smooth, round objects that are difficult to grasp (see Fig. 64.23, *plate 2*). The FB should be dry and easily visualized. Apply a small amount of glue to the tip of a thin paintbrush, a straightened paper clip, or the blunt end of a wooden cotton-tipped applicator. Allow the glue to become tacky. Place the tip against the object, allow it to dry, and then carefully withdraw the FB. Minor complications are possible if the tip dries against the canal wall (abrasion, excoriation) or if the glue spills or drips onto the wall (thereby creating a new FB). These can be prevented by placing an ear speculum in the canal first and inserting the applicator through it. This technique may be more useful in adults because cooperation is required.[41]

If glue does get into the canal, instill acetone into the ear canal (provided TM is intact) and allow it to stay for 5 minutes, and attempt to remove the glue. Repeat applications of acetone may be needed.

Removal of Insects

Small roaches are the most commonly found insects in the ear (see Fig. 64.23, *plate 3*). For patient comfort and to lessen distress from insect movement, the insect should be immobilized.

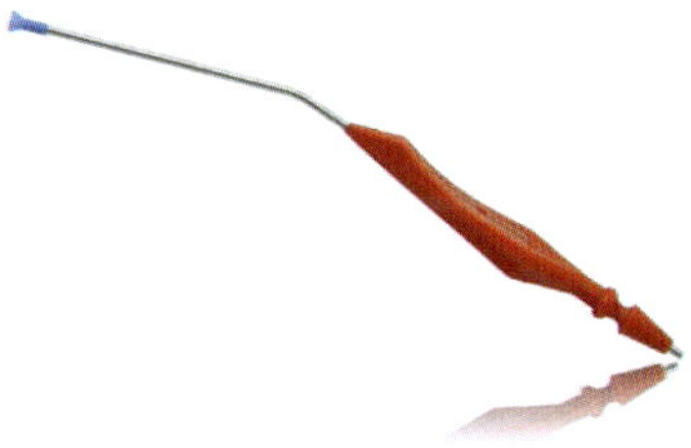

A

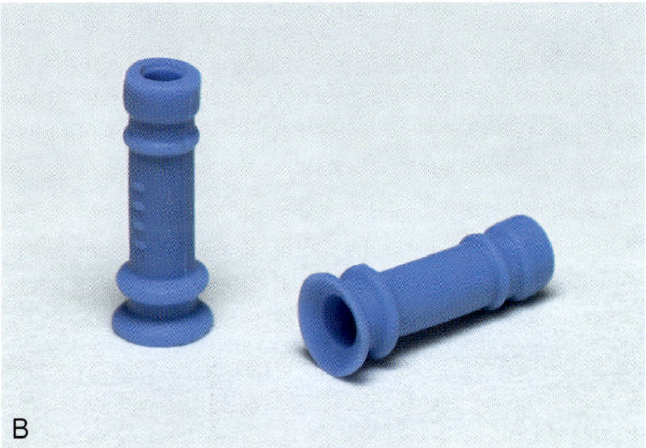

B

Fig. 64.22 Suction devices for foreign body removal. (A) Schuknecht Foreign Body Remover. (B) VacuTIP Foreign Body Suction Tip which can be attached to suction device.

Ear Canal Foreign Body Removal

1

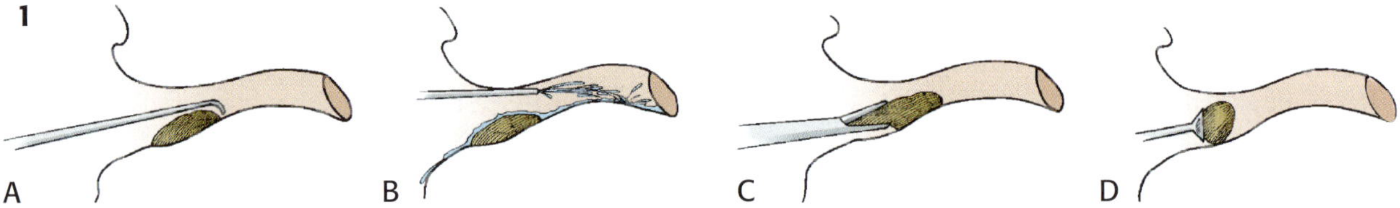

Various devices for FB removal from the ear canal. ***A,*** Right-angle hook. ***B,*** Irrigation. ***C,*** Alligator forceps. ***D,*** Soft-tipped suction. Direct visualization of the canal is mandatory, as is patient cooperation. Abrasions of the ear canal and subsequent bleeding are common.

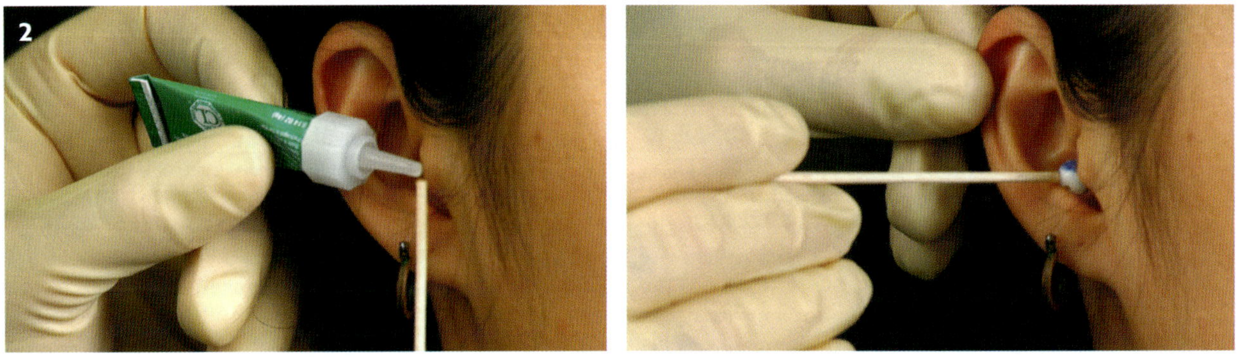

Putting superglue on a stick and allowing it to attach to an FB may be successful. This technique is most effective in removing smooth, round objects that are difficult to grasp. The FB should be dry and easily visualized. A high degree of patient cooperation is required.

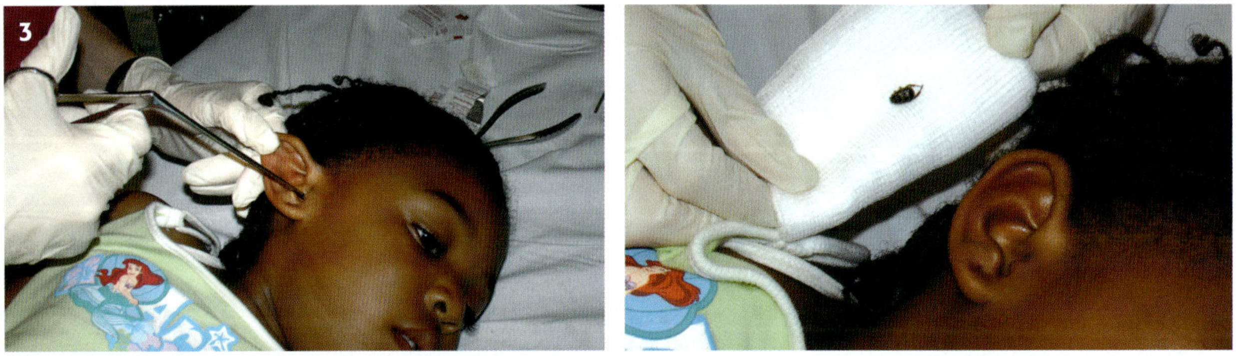

Removal of an insect can be a disaster or relatively easy. An easy way is to use ketamine anesthesia with careful direct extraction. No patient can cooperate with more than minimal manipulation of the inner ear canal. Instilling mineral oil or lidocaine into the canal to kill the insect before extraction is recommended.

Fig. 64.23 Removal of a foreign body from the ear canal. Avoid excessive and prolonged attempts in the emergency department to remove difficult FBs. For difficult-to-extract insects, it is appropriate to prescribe outpatient antibiotic drops for 24 to 48 hours and again try to irrigate the insect or refer to a specialist. Adequate anesthesia is essential because no patient can fully cooperate with painful deep ear canal manipulation. *FB,* Foreign body.

This can be easily accomplished by instilling lidocaine into the canal. Other substances (isopropanol, water, succinylcholine, hydrogen peroxide) were shown to be ineffective in killing the roaches in a reasonable amount of time.[42] Once disabled, insects are removed by mechanical extraction as described previously; pieces can be suctioned out if fragmentation occurs.

If an insect cannot easily be removed or if parts remain, it is quite acceptable to prescribe outpatient antibiotic drops for 24 to 48 hours and try irrigation again or refer to a specialist. As with any FB in the ear canal, prolonged attempts at removal in the ED are counterproductive.

Complications

Hearing should be evaluated before and after removal of an FB, especially in patients with suspected TM or middle ear injuries. Also examine the opposite ear and the nose of children to search for the rare but possible second FB. Minor lacerations or excoriations of the canal usually heal quickly with or without antibiotic ear drops, as long as the canal is kept clean and dry. Document preexisting canal trauma or suspected TM rupture before attempts at removal; otherwise, this may be falsely attributed to iatrogenic causes later.

Indications for otolaryngology referral include failed removal of the object in the ED, injury to the EAC or TM, TM rupture, EAC infection, object wedged in the medial part of the EAC or up against the TM, glass or other sharp-edged FBs, and special circumstances (disk batteries and putty). Generally, no routine follow-up is necessary except in cases of infection, severe trauma, or perforation of the TM. Parents should be educated to reduce the exposure of children to potential FBs.

Drainage of Auricular Hematomas

Auricular hematoma occurs from trauma and is an accumulation of blood under the perichondrium of the ear separating it from the cartilage. Occasionally the hematoma may arise from the cartilage itself. They are most commonly seen in wrestlers, boxers, and rugby players. Recurrent or untreated injuries allow the development of new cartilage, which subsequently deforms the auricle (cauliflower ear).

Indications and Contraindications

Diagnosis of an auricular hematoma is based on the history and physical examination (Fig. 64.24). The presence of tender, anterior auricular swelling following trauma that deforms the anatomy of the pinna should prompt drainage of the hematoma. The goal is to prevent cartilage damage and deformation of the pinna.

If the patient is initially seen more than 7 days after injury, drainage may be difficult because of the formation of granulation tissue, and these patients should be referred to an otolaryngologist. In addition, patients with concomitant cellulitis, perichondritis, or recurrent and chronic hematomas should be referred to a specialist.

Equipment

- Sterile gloves
- Local and topic anesthetic
- Antiseptic skin solution
- 11- or 15- blade scalpel and/or 18-gauge needle with 10-cc syringe
- Suction cannister
- Suction instrument (Frasier)
- Hemostat
- Toothed forceps
- Suture supplies
- Bolster material and dressings
- Light source

Procedure

See Videos 64.17–64.19. Treatment of an auricular hematoma is complete evacuation of the subperichondrial hematoma and approximation of the perichondrium to the cartilage.

Needle Aspiration

Though used widely, this technique is no longer recommended by most authorities because of the high risk for reaccumulation of the hematoma. Aspiration is often inadequate and other management is required. Other sources recommend needle aspiration followed by incision and drainage if reaccumulation occurs.[27]

Aspiration of an auricular hematoma is performed by perforating the hematoma with a 20-gauge needle. "Milk" the hematoma between the thumb and forefinger until the entire hematoma is evacuated. Apply a pressure dressing. Reexamine the ear frequently for reaccumulation of the hematoma. Reaccumulation of blood requires repeat aspiration. For small hematomas that are acute, needle aspiration alone with a bolster dressing is adequate therapy.[27]

A newer variation of needle aspiration has been described by Brickman and coworkers.[28] In their method, after preparation and local anesthesia, needle aspiration was performed using an 18-gauge angiocath and 10-mL syringe. After the collection was aspirated, the syringe and needle were removed, leaving the plastic catheter in place. A compressive dressing was then applied and patients were closely followed up. The catheter was removed in 5 days. Of the 53 patients enrolled, 94.3% initially had adequate hematoma drainage with excellent long-term results. In the initial 72 hours, six patients had catheter dislodgement, with hematoma reaccumulation in three patients (5.6%). These were successfully drained by reaspiration and there were no further recurrences.

Incision

An auricular hematoma may be incised along the natural skin folds (see Fig. 64.24). Anesthetize the pinna by local infiltration of 1% lidocaine or with an auricular block (described earlier). Incise the skin with a No. 15 blade at the edge of the hematoma and follow the curvature of the pinna. Gently peel the skin and perichondrium off the hematoma and underlying cartilage. Completely evacuate the hematoma and irrigate the remaining pocket with normal saline.

After removing the hematoma, apply antibiotic ointment and reapproximate the perichondrium to the cartilage with a pressure dressing. A compression dressing, noninvasive or surgical, must be applied because a simple dressing will allow the hematoma to reaccumulate. First, dry cotton should be placed into the EAC. Next, fill all external auricular crevices with mineral oil, saline-soaked gauze, or Vaseline gauze. Then place three to four layers of gauze behind the ear as a posterior pack. Cut a V-shape out of the gauze first to allow a snug fit. Cover the packed external ear with multiple layers of fluffed gauze. Bandage the fluffed gauze in place with Kerlix or an elastic wrap.

A surgical compressive dressing involves suturing dental rolls over the area. To accomplish this, pass a 4-0 nylon suture through the entire thickness of the ear and over the hematoma. Wrap the suture around a dental roll on the posterior aspect of the ear and then pass the needle back through the pinna. Wrap and tie the suture around a second dental roll on the anterior aspect of the pinna. The dressing should firmly reapproximate the perichondrium to the cartilage without compromising the vasculature. Remove the dressing in 1 week.

Prescribe antistaphylococcal antibiotics and instruct the patient to inspect the wound frequently for evidence of vascular compromise and infection. The wound should be reevaluated in 24 hours by the ED or otolaryngology for recurrence or infection. Reaccumulation is treated by repeat aspiration or incision-drainage. Treat infection by removal of the bandage, surgical drainage, and IV antibiotics. Patients should be advised to return to the ED at any time for recurrence, fever, or signs of infection.

Complications

There are a few complications associated with management of auricular hematomas. The first is incomplete evacuation of the hematoma, which can lead to destruction of cartilage (cauliflower ear). Reaccumulation is another complication. Local site infection can develop resulting in chondritis. Finally, scar formation leading to deformity is possible.

Auricular Hematoma Evacuation

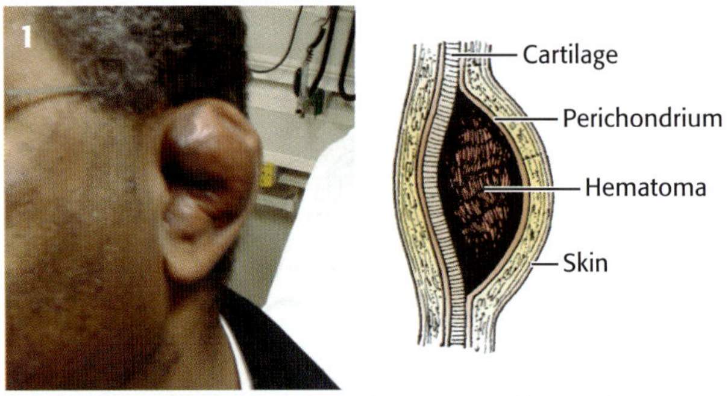

Auricular hematomas manifest after trauma with anterior auricular swelling. The hematoma forms between the cartilage and perichondrium and will lead to permanent deformity if not treated.

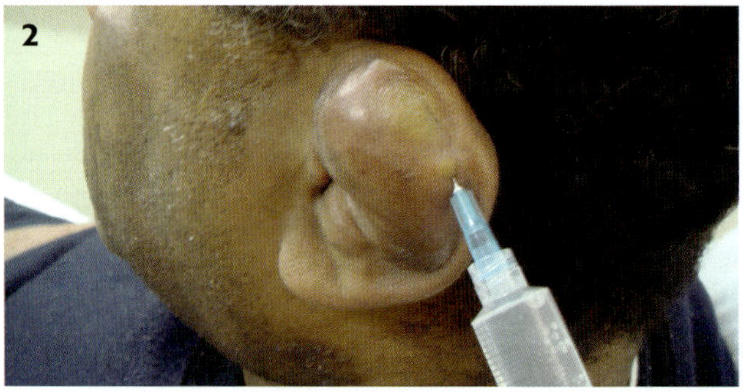

Anesthetize the pinna via local infiltration of 1% lidocaine without epinephrine or via an auricular block.

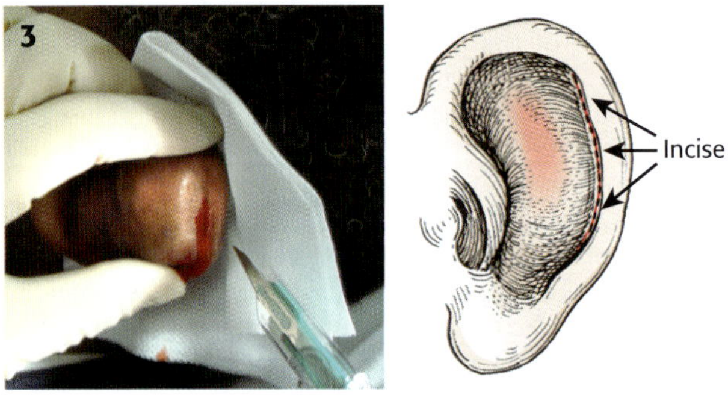

Use a scalpel to incise the skin along the natural skin folds at the edge of the hematoma. Follow the natural curve of the pinna.

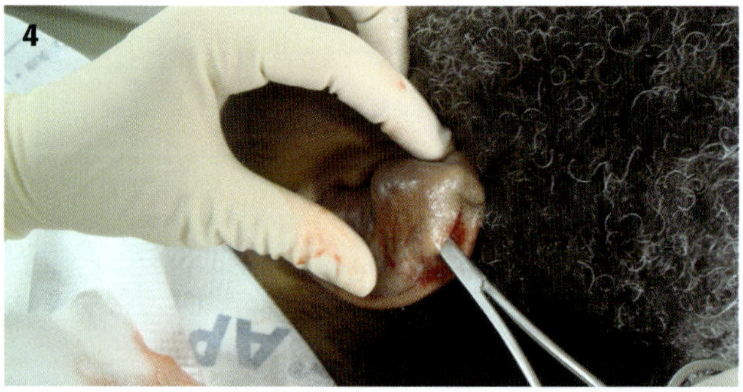

Gently peel the skin and perichondrium off the hematoma and underlying cartilage. Completely evacuate the hematoma and irrigate the pocket with normal saline.

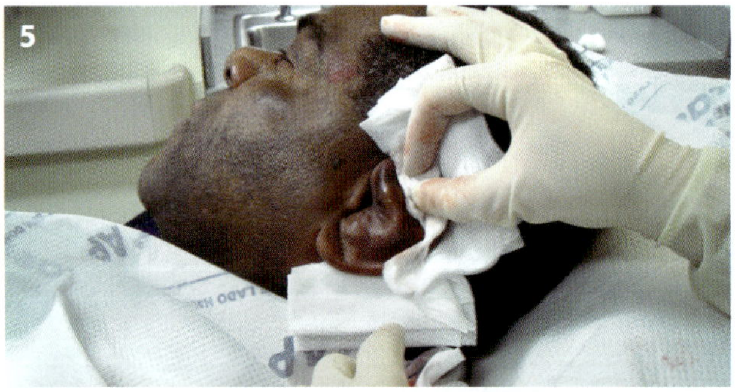

A compression dressing must be placed to prevent reaccumulation of the hematoma. Place dry cotton into the EAC and fill all external auricular crevices with saline-soaked or Vaseline gauze.

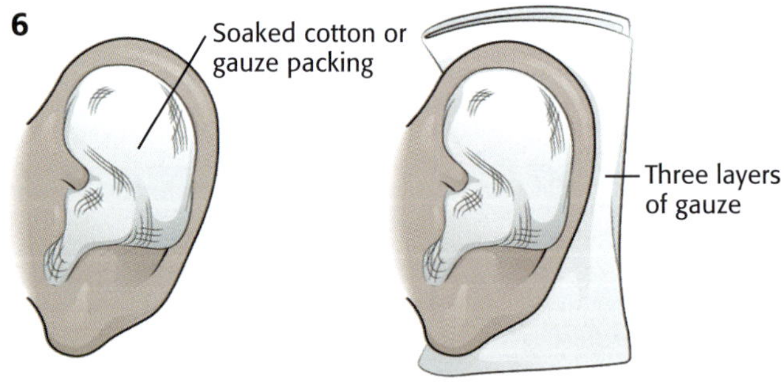

Carefully conform the material into all the convolutions of the auricle. Vaseline gauze, saline-soaked 1/4-inch packing gauze, or saline-soaked cotton may be used. Place gauze behind the ear.

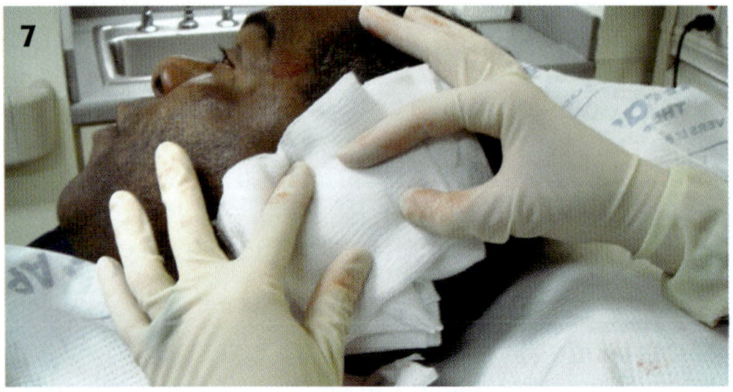

Place three to four layers of gauze behind the ear as a posterior pack, and then cover the entire ear with multiple layers of fluffed gauze.

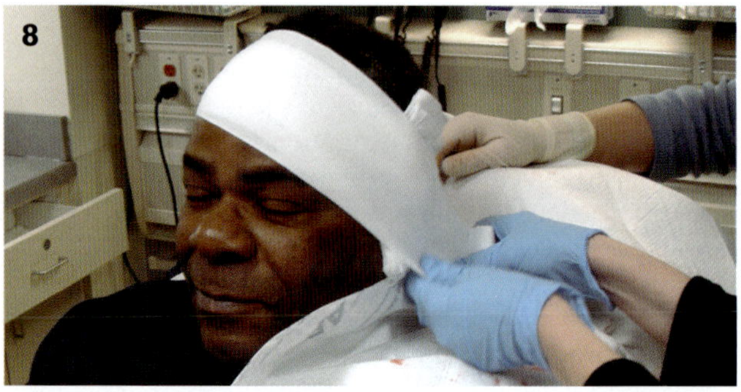

Secure the dressing to the head with Kerlix or an elastic wrap.

Fig. 64.24 Evacuation of an auricular hematoma. *EAC*, External auditory canal.

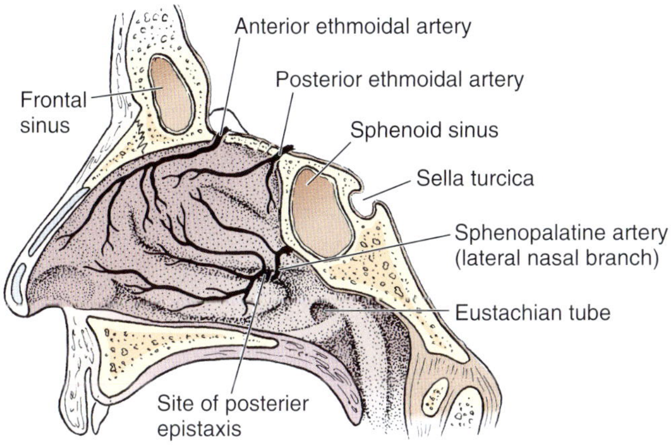

Fig. 64.25 Vascular supply to the lateral wall of the nose. The most common site of posterior epistaxis is the sphenopalatine artery as it emerges posterior to the middle turbinate. (From Maceri DR. Epistaxis and nasal trauma. In: Cummings CW, ed. *Otolaryngology—Head and Neck Surgery.* 2nd ed. Mosby–Year Book; 1993:728.)

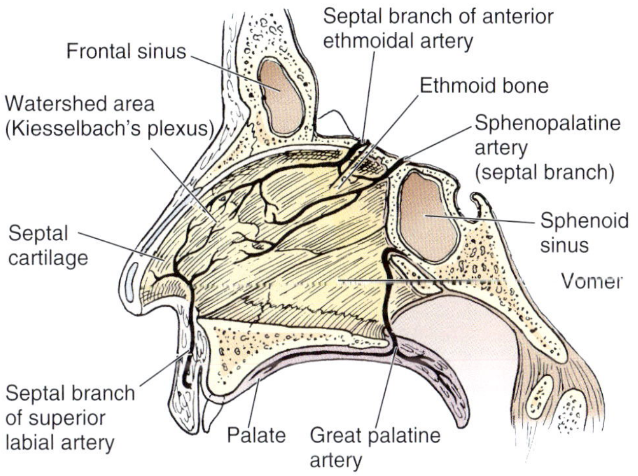

Fig. 64.26 Vascular supply to the nasal septum. The most common site of anterior epistaxis is within the area labeled *Kiesselbach's plexus.* (From Maceri DR. Epistaxis and nasal trauma. In: Cummings CW, ed. *Otolaryngology—Head and Neck Surgery.* 2nd ed. Mosby–Year Book; 1993:728.)

NOSE

Anatomy

The nose consists of the vestibule, nasal septum, lateral wall, and nasopharynx. The vestibule is the anterior-most portion of the nares and is composed of skin and hair follicles. The nasal septum is the midline structure and is composed of cartilage anteriorly and bone posteriorly. The lateral wall of the nose contains the superior, middle, and inferior turbinates, as well as the auditory tube opening.

Three major arteries supply the nose and conjoin via anastomoses. The sphenopalatine artery emerges from the sphenopalatine foramen, which is located at the posterior aspect of the middle turbinate (Fig. 64.25). This is the most common source of posterior epistaxis. This artery supplies the lateral turbinates and the posterior septum. The anterior and posterior ethmoidal arteries branch off the ophthalmic artery and penetrate the cribriform plate to supply the superior nasal mucosa. The superior labial branch of the facial artery completes the triad and supplies the nasal septum and vestibule. The watershed area on the anterior septum, also known as Kiesselbach's plexus, is the most common source of anterior epistaxis (Fig. 64.26).

Anesthesia of the Nose

Most nasal anesthesia can be accomplished topically. Numerous preparations are available and are often combined with a vasoconstrictor, especially when epistaxis is present. Cocaine (4% solution), the once preferred agent for both vasoconstriction and anesthesia, is often not routinely available. Topical lidocaine 4% is quite effective for anesthesia of the nose and commonly available. Alternatively, 2% lidocaine with epinephrine (local anesthetic solution) may be used but is less effective. Be aware of the total amount of lidocaine being administered and stay within recommendations for the maximum safe dosage. This is an issue primarily with older patients who have cardiovascular disease. LET solution (lidocaine 4%, Epinephrine 0.1%, Tetracaine 0.4%) or Benzocaine spray may also be used.

Apply the local anesthetic and vasoconstrictor to cotton swabs (Fig. 64.27). If a larger area of anesthesia is needed, use cotton pledgets. Fig. 64.28 describes the procedure of making pledgets. Soak each pledget in an anesthetic or vasoconstrictor and then squeeze the excess fluid out of the pledget. Place each pledget horizontally on the floor of the nasal cavity and stack the next pledget on top. Three pledgets are usually required to pack the nasal cavity. They can be replaced with new pledgets in 5 minutes if the desired anesthetic effect is not achieved. Remind the patient that excess anesthetic may numb the throat but will not inhibit swallowing.

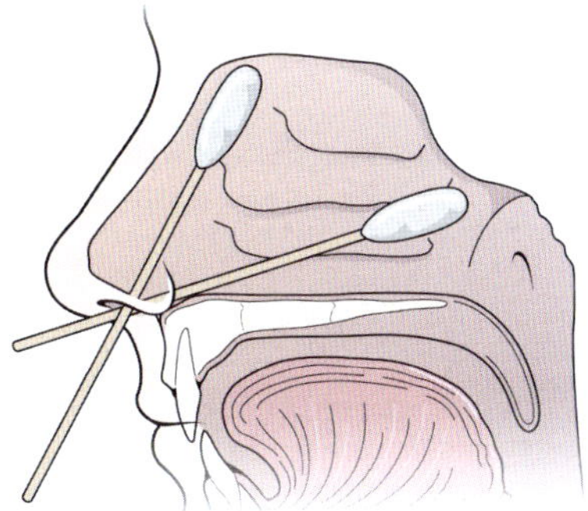

Fig. 64.27 Placement of local anesthetic in the nose to block the anterior ethmoidal nerve superiorly and the sphenopalatine ganglion at the posterior end of the middle turbinate before reducing a nasal fracture. (From Schuller DE, Schleuning AJ, DeMaria TF et al., eds. *DeWeese and Saunders Otolaryngology: Head and Neck Surgery.* 8th ed. Mosby; 1994:152.)

A local nasal block can be performed for more painful and prolonged procedures. The sensory innervation of the nose is illustrated in Fig. 64.29. It begins with topical anesthetic as just described. Next, using a thin 25- or 27-gauge needle, inject 1% lidocaine with 1:100,000 epinephrine along the septum, lateral walls, and nasopalatine nerves. Depending on the procedure, it may be necessary to anesthetize both sides. First, inject along and beneath the soft tissue of the nasal dorsum (infratrochlear nerve). Next, inject around the infraorbital foramen to anesthetize the infraorbital nerve. Finally, inject at the base of the columella (base of the nose between the nasal septa) and along the floor of the nasal cavity. Interestingly, studies have shown

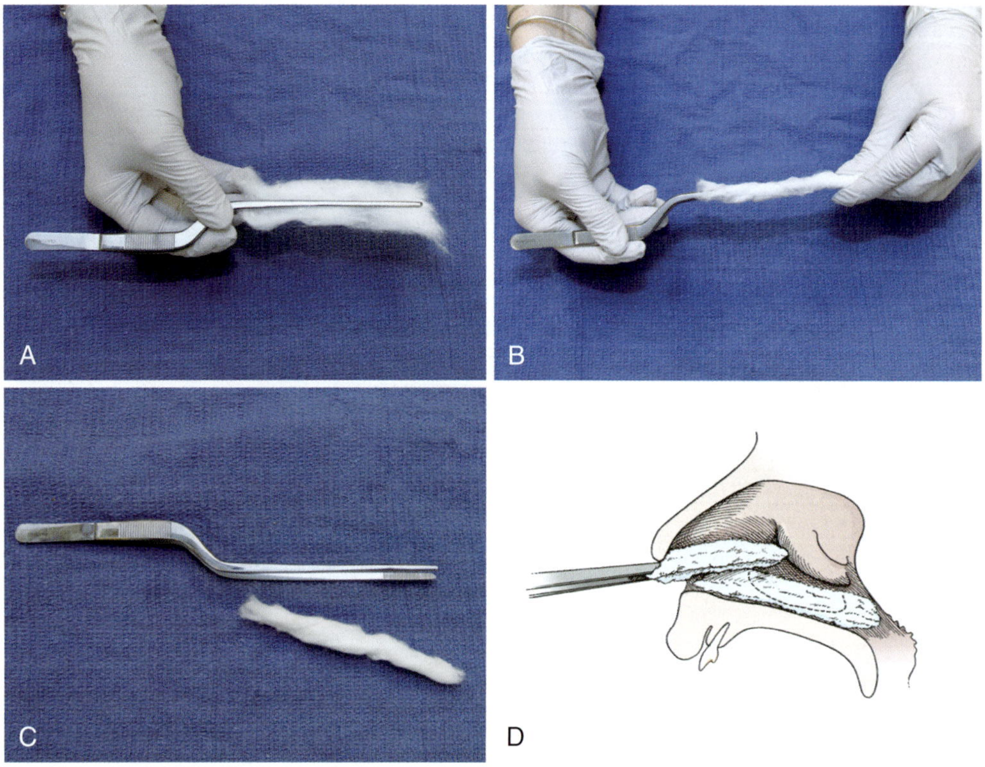

Fig. 64.28 Topical anesthetic and vasoconstrictors are applied on individually made cotton pledgets. The size of the pledget may be changed according to the extent of the nasal cavity to be anesthetized and the size of the patient. (A) Grasp an appropriately sized cotton pledget with bayonet forceps. (B) Then grasp the cotton with the opposite hand and rotate the forceps. (C) The pledget is removed and is ready for insertion. (D) To completely anesthetize the nasal cavity, three pledgets are necessary. The first is placed on the floor of the nose, the second in the middle meatus between the inferior and the middle turbinates, and the third in the roof of the nasal cavity and the anterior nasal vestibule. Note: This pledget technique can be used to make a cotton wick for the treatment of otitis externa.

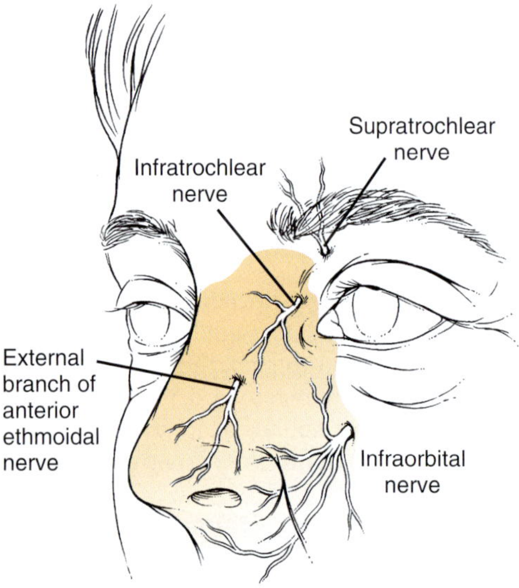

Fig. 64.29 Sensory innervation of the nose. (From Flint PW, Haughey BH, Lund VJ et al., eds. *Cummings Otolaryngology: Head and Neck Surgery*. 5th ed. Elsevier; 2010.)

that the use of EMLA (eutectic mixture of local anesthetics) cream applied over the nose 1 hour before reduction, in combination with topical intranasal anesthetic, provides similar nasal anesthesia for reduction of nasal fractures with less discomfort than occurs with needle infiltration.[43]

Examination

Examination of the nares is relatively straightforward, albeit often quite stressful to the patient. When using a nasal speculum, insert it into the naris with the handle parallel to the floor and slowly open the blades in a superior-to-inferior direction. It is a common error to attempt to spread the nares horizontally. Stabilize your hand on the patient's nose to prevent damage to the mucosa from unexpected movement (Fig. 64.30). When attempting to visualize the nasal passageway, remember to have the patient keep the floor of the nose parallel to the ground. Tilting the head allows a view of only the anterosuperior area. A nasopharyngoscope may be used to view the nasal passageways as well, and its use is described in the previous section on examination of the pharynx.

Management of Epistaxis

Patients with nasal hemorrhage are commonly seen in the ED and account for approximately 1 in 200 visits.[44] Epistaxis occurs more frequently in the young (<10 years) and old (70 to 79 years).[44,45] Most cases are atraumatic and occur in the winter months.[44,45] Approximately 6% require hospitalization.[46] The etiology of nosebleeds is divided into local (e.g., dryness, trauma, use of intranasal medications, infection, inflammation, tumors) and systemic (blood dyscrasias, leukemia, atherosclerosis, medications).[47]

Epistaxis is further divided into anterior and posterior bleeding. Anterior bleeds are much more common and originate in

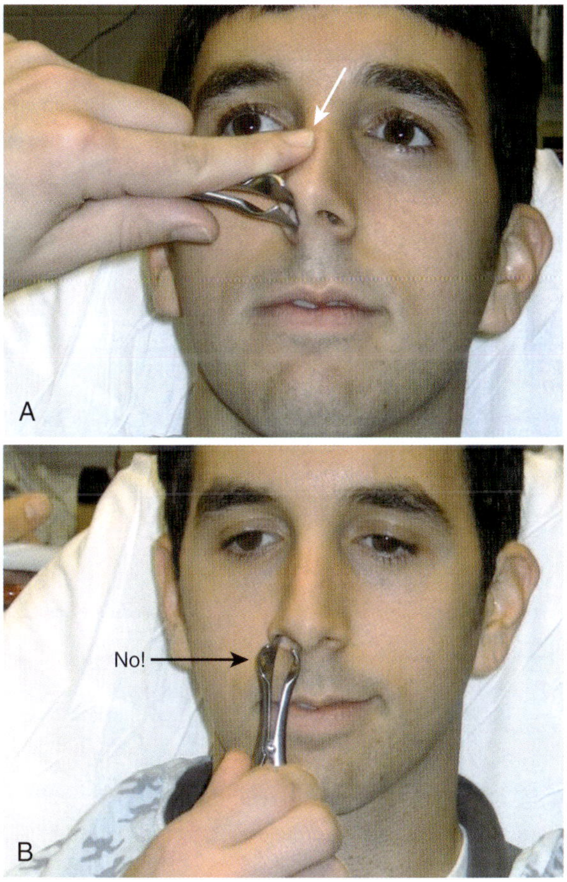

Fig. 64.30 To properly examine a nose, use a nasal speculum. (A) The clinician rests the index finger on the bridge of the nose *(arrow)* and spreads the speculum in an inferior-to-superior direction. (B) It is incorrect to spread the speculum laterally or to use the instrument in an unsupported manner.

the anteroinferior septum, where the Kiesselbach's plexus is located.[3] This location is easily visualized on nasal speculum examination. Posterior epistaxis occurs in 5% to 10% of cases and may be difficult to diagnose and control.[48,49]

Identification of the source of bleeding and subsequent control are paramount to the treatment of epistaxis. Although this can be frightening to both the clinician and patient, a systematic approach with the proper equipment will lessen the anxiety associated with the situation (Fig. 64.31). The goal of the procedure is to tamponade or cauterize the bleeding site. If the source is anterior, this may be the final treatment. For posterior bleeding, temporizing maneuvers are generally used until the process stops or a consultant can complete a definitive hemostatic procedure. The procedures can be performed in the ED with proper lighting and the equipment listed later in this section. Controlling epistaxis may be a time-consuming process without proper equipment or patient cooperation. In preparation for any procedure to treat epistaxis, evaluate the patient's hemodynamic status by assessing vital signs and orthostatic symptoms and by quantifying the amount of blood lost. If the patient is symptomatic in any of these areas or if the blood loss is deemed significant, consider starting a large-bore IV line for administration of fluid boluses. Hematologic testing is rarely useful and not required for most patients, but in extenuating circumstances, obtain a complete blood count and consider a type and screen. Coagulation studies are not routinely indicated but should be undertaken in patients taking

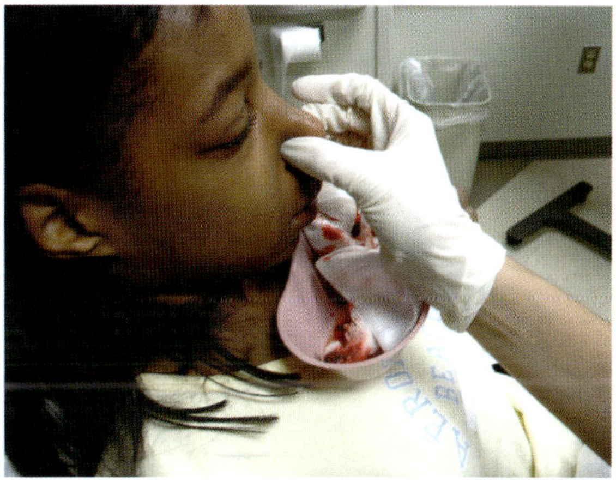

Fig. 64.31 A nosebleed is frightening and interventions are most unpleasant. Judicious use of parenteral sedation and analgesia, with attention to aesthetics, results in a more rewarding encounter. If required, intravenous morphine is a good choice.

anticoagulants, those with underlying hematologic abnormalities, or individuals with recurrent or prolonged epistaxis.

Indications and Contraindications to Treatment of Epistaxis

The vast majority of nosebleeds can be controlled with any of the methods listed. Uncontrollable bleeding would be an indication for ENT consultation. Massive facial trauma with the possibility of a basilar skull fracture is a contraindication to the use of an intranasal balloon or packing because it may travel into the skull cavity.

Equipment

Preparation is the key to successful management of a patient with epistaxis. The following list of equipment should be readily available to the emergency clinician (see Review Box 64.3):

- Chair with a headrest or gurney with an inclinable back
- Headlight with a light source and head mirror
- Wall suction with multiple suction catheters
- Gloves, mask, and gown for the clinician
- Gown or drapes for the patient
- Topical anesthetic
- Topical vasoconstrictor
- Nasal speculum
- Tongue depressors
- Small red rubber catheters
- Bayonet forceps
- Scissors
- Kidney basin
- Gauze (4 × 4 inch, 2 × 2 inch), dental rolls or cotton, No. 2 surgical silk ties
- 1.2-cm-wide Vaseline gauze or 0.5-inch-wide Nu-Gauze (Johnson & Johnson) packing
- Antibiotic ointment
- Silver nitrate sticks or electrocautery
- Foley catheters (10, 12, 14 Fr)
- Nasal compression devices
- Dual-balloon pack

Procedure

See Videos 64.20 and 64.21. Because most patients are frightened by continued epistaxis and because nasal instrumentation

Epistaxis Management

Indications
Persistent epistaxis

Contraindications
Massive facial trauma with the possibility of a basilar skull fracture

Complications
Cautery
- Nasal septal injury/perforation
- Rebleeding

Anterior packing
- Sinusitis
- Nasolacrimal bleeding
- Nasal mucosa pressure necrosis

Posterior packing
- Infection
- Dysphagia
- Eustachian tube dysfunction
- Tissue necrosis
- Dislodgment
- Hypoxia
- Hypercapnia
- Aspiration
- Hypertension
- Arrhythmias
- Myocardial infarction
- Death

Equipment

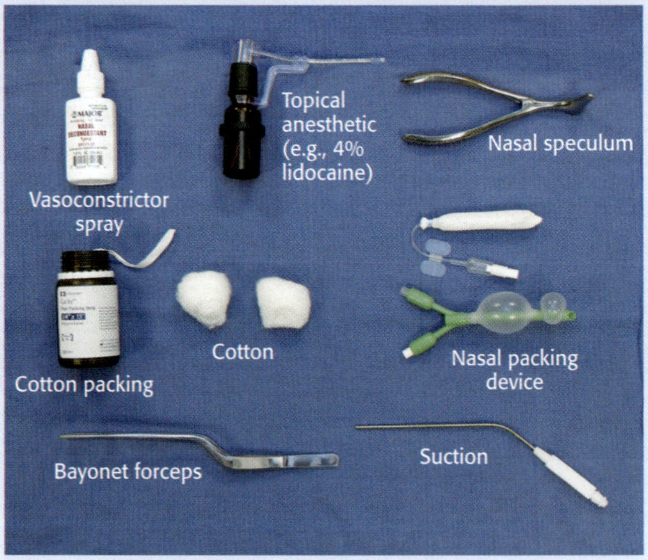

Other equipment not depicted: light source/headlight, protective equipment, tongue depressors, kidney basin, gauze, silver nitrate sticks, 12-Fr Foley catheters. See text for details.

Review Box 64.3 Epistaxis management: indications, contraindications, complications, and equipment.

can be annoying or painful, provide reassurance to the patient that the bleeding can be controlled with minimal discomfort. Judicious use of parenteral sedation or narcotic analgesia is well supported to make the entire interaction more palatable to the patient and ultimately more successful. Drape the patient with a gown to protect clothing from the bleeding. Have the patient hold an emesis basin to collect any continued bleeding and as a precaution to emesis of swallowed blood. Minor anterior bleeding is usually easily controlled with minimal techniques. There are several options to control epistaxis and can be used in a stepwise progression. A proposed algorithm is presented in Fig. 64.32.[47–49]

Ask the patient to sit upright in the sniffing position with the neck flexed and the head extended (see Fig. 63.30). The base of the nose should remain parallel to the floor. After putting on a face shield, gown, and protective gloves, position yourself in front of the patient, level with the patient's nose. Have the patient blow the nose to remove clots or suction the nasal passageway carefully. This may temporarily increase bleeding but can aid in identifying the bleeding site. Suction from front to back along the nasal septum and then laterally. If the bleeding is minimal, attempt to locate the specific bleeding source. If the bleeding is too profuse for visualization of the source, administer a topical anesthetic and vasoconstrictor.

Pressure Technique
This technique can be initiated at triage with the nurse instructing the patient on how to perform it or applying a device.

- Sit the patient upright and leaning forward to prevent aspiration of blood (Fig. 64.33). The base of the nose should remain parallel to the floor.
- Apply direct pressure to the cartilaginous portion of the nasal bridge just distal to the nasal bone(Fig. 64.34A).[50]
- Alternatively, nasal clips or two tongue blades taped together can be used to apply pressure (may be more effective than fingers) (see Fig. 64.34B).[50]
- Apply pressure for at least 15 minutes.

Topical Vasoconstrictor
If bleeding continues after manual compression, topical vasoconstriction can be used (see Fig. 64.33). Commonly used vasoconstrictors include: oxymetazoline 0.05%, phenylephrine 0.5%, and epinephrine 1:1000). Have patient blow their nose to remove clots to allow more surface area to contact vasoconstrictor. Apply vasoconstrictor by spraying or atomizing, or by soaking cotton pledgets and placing in nasal cavity. After vasoconstrictor is applied, continue manual compression for 15 minutes.

Cautery
Cauterization should be performed if there is a bleeding site visualized and there is no excessive bleeding (see Fig. 64.35).[51,52] Cauterization has been shown to be more effective and less painful than nasal packing.[53,54] Chemical cautery with silver nitrate is most commonly available in the ED.[47,51] However, electrocautery may be used.

Because most cases of anterior epistaxis occur in Kiesselbach's plexus, inspect this area closely for areas of bleeding, ulceration, or erosion. Dry the area with suction or a cotton pledget. The silver nitrate stick tip should be applied to a small area surrounding the bleeding site, starting on the periphery and moving centrally. The tip is left on for 4 to 5 seconds at a time until a gray eschar forms. Once hemostasis is obtained, apply petroleum jelly or antibiotic ointment to

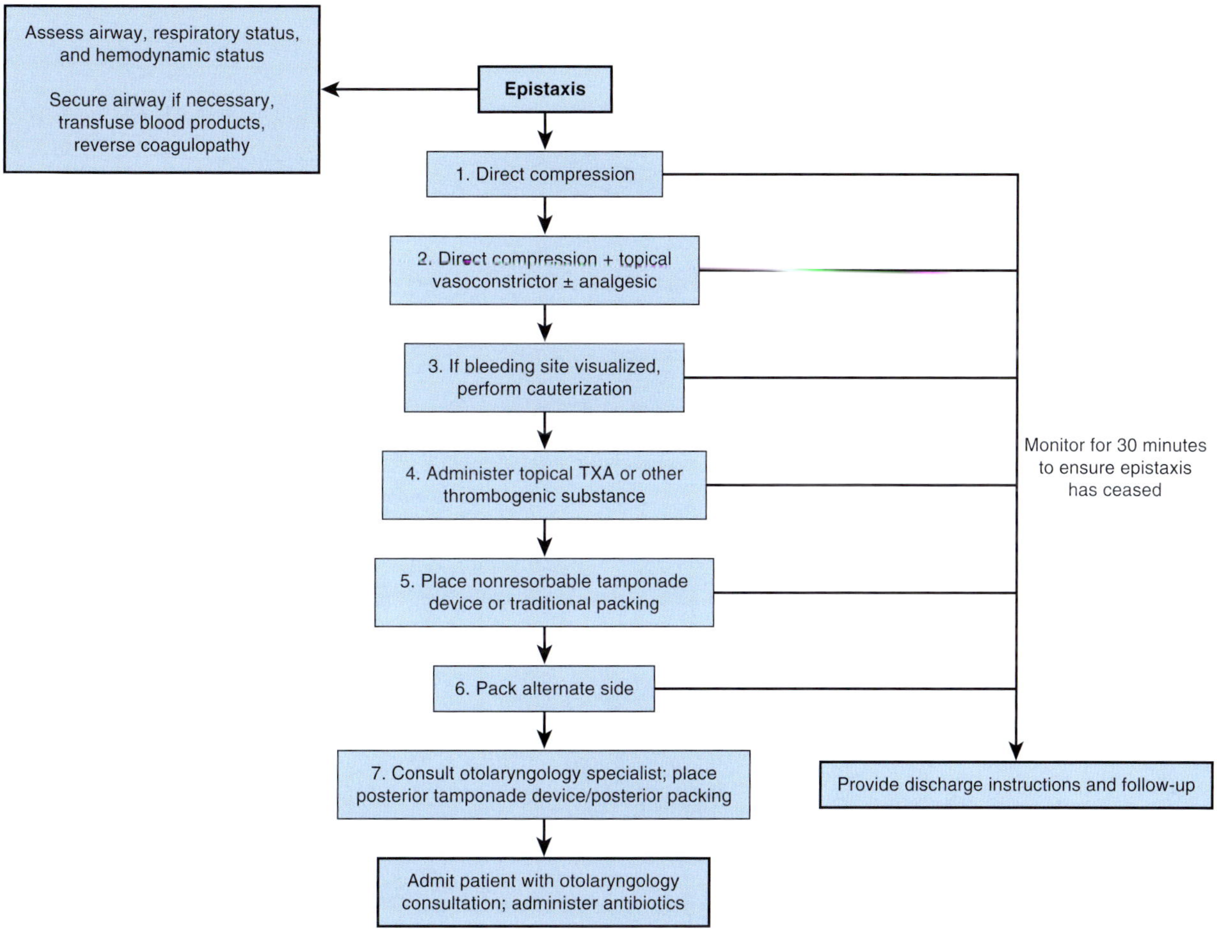

Fig. 64.32 Proposed algorithm on the management of epistaxis. *TXA*, Tranexamic acid. (From Gottleib M, Long B. Managing epistaxis. *Ann Emerg Med*. 2023;81(2):234-240.)

the area to prevent desiccation. If unsuccessful after two to three attempts, another method is required. Avoid cauterizing large areas or both sides of the septum due to the risk of perforation.[55,56]

Tranexamic Acid

See Video 64.22. If cautery is unsuccessful or the bleeding is not amenable to cautery, tranexamic acid (TXA) can be used next. TXA reversibly binds to plasminogen and inhibits binding to fibrin. In turn, this prevents plasminogen activation and transformation to plasmin. Initial studies on the use of TXA for epistaxis were controversial[57–59]; however, a recent study found TXA reduced the need for packing with a number needed to treat of 8.[60] Topical use is recommended. Soak cotton pledget in 500 mg of TXA. Insert pledget into the nasal cavity for 10 minutes.[59] Remove pledget and reassess for bleeding. TXA can be used with other devices such as Merocel packing.[61]

Resorbable Packing

There are several available thrombogenic resorbable foams and gels that promote thrombogenesis and tamponade at the bleeding site.[3,62] These materials are more comfortable and do not require removal.[3] Floseal (Baxter) is a thrombin-based, high-viscosity gel that does not require the activation of platelets. The material is left in the nose and degrades within 3 to 5 days. This product is as effective as traditional packing.[63,64] Fibrin sealants contain purified human cryoprecipitate and thrombin.[55] Fibrin sealants provide rapid hemostasis with greater reduction in mucosal atrophy, edema, and nasal discharge.[65] Other agents such as Surgicel, Gelfoam, Avitene are hemostatic materials that are cut to fit the naris and directly applied to the area followed by 1 minute of direct pressure.[62,66,67]

Tamponade Devices

Tamponade devices are useful in refractory cases of epistaxis and are effective in 90% to 95% of cases.[68–70] Commonly available devices are the Rapid Rhino, Rhino Rocket, and Merocel. These easier-to-use commercial devices have largely supplanted traditional petrolatum gauze.

The Rapid Rhino (ArthroCare ENT; see Fig. 64.37) is a high-volume, low-pressure balloon device with an open lumen air passage, a pilot cuff to check pressure, and a specialized Gel-Knit (carboxymethyl cellulose) covering designed to promote platelet aggregation.[71] Numerous variations for anterior, posterior, and combination packs are available. The Rapid Rhino causes less discomfort, is easier to insert, but has no difference in epistaxis control.[72–74] Submerge device in sterile water (not saline) for 30 seconds. Insert device parallel to the hard palate along the septal floor. Once fabric ring is fully within naris, inject up to 20 mL of air until the pilot cuff is firm. Inject the air slowly to reduce discomfort. Wait 10 to 15 minutes to reassess the pilot cuff. If no longer firm, add additional air. Tape the plastic butterfly to the patient's cheek.

Epistaxis Management: Initial Steps

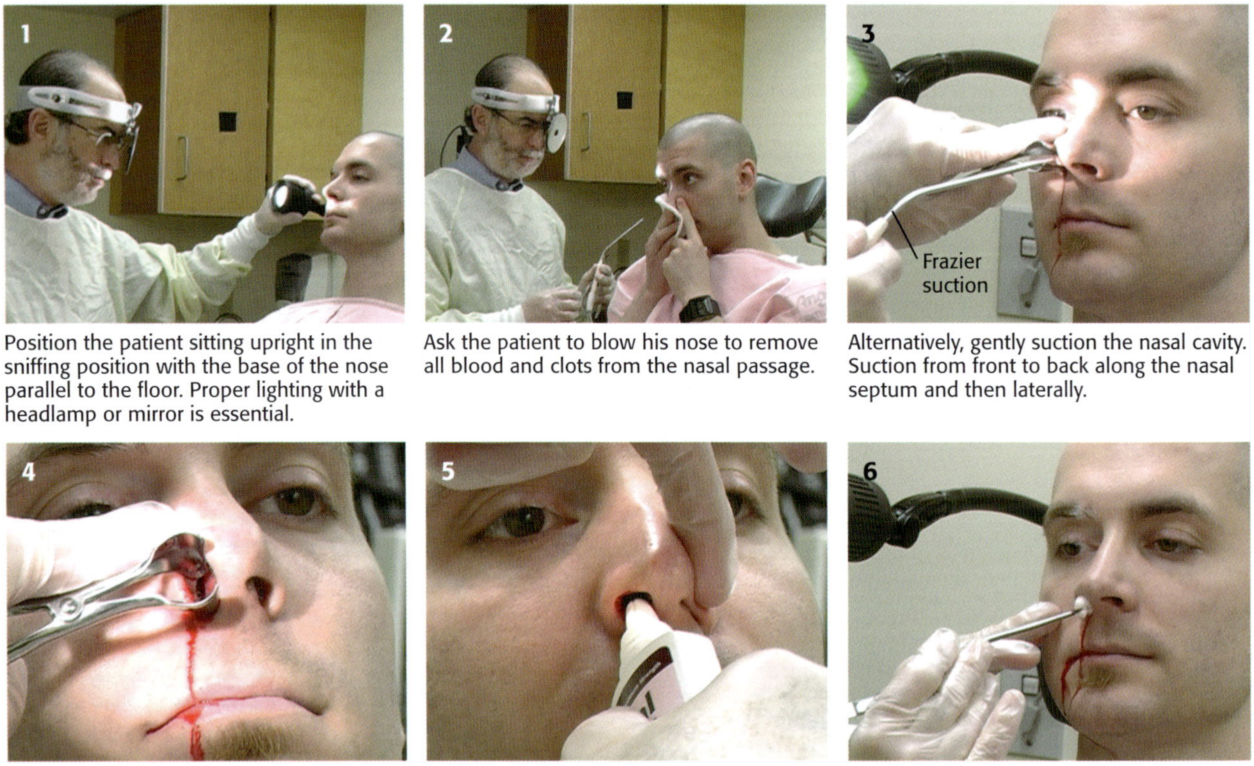

1. Position the patient sitting upright in the sniffing position with the base of the nose parallel to the floor. Proper lighting with a headlamp or mirror is essential.
2. Ask the patient to blow his nose to remove all blood and clots from the nasal passage.
3. Alternatively, gently suction the nasal cavity. Suction from front to back along the nasal septum and then laterally.
4. If bleeding is minimal, attempt to locate the specific bleeding source. Use a nasal speculum to maximize visibility.
5. If bleeding is too profuse for visualization, apply a topical vasoconstrictor such as oxymetazoline.
6. Alternatively, cotton pledgets soaked with tranexamic acid may be inserted into the nasal cavity with bayonet forceps.

Fig. 64.33 Management of epistaxis: initial steps.

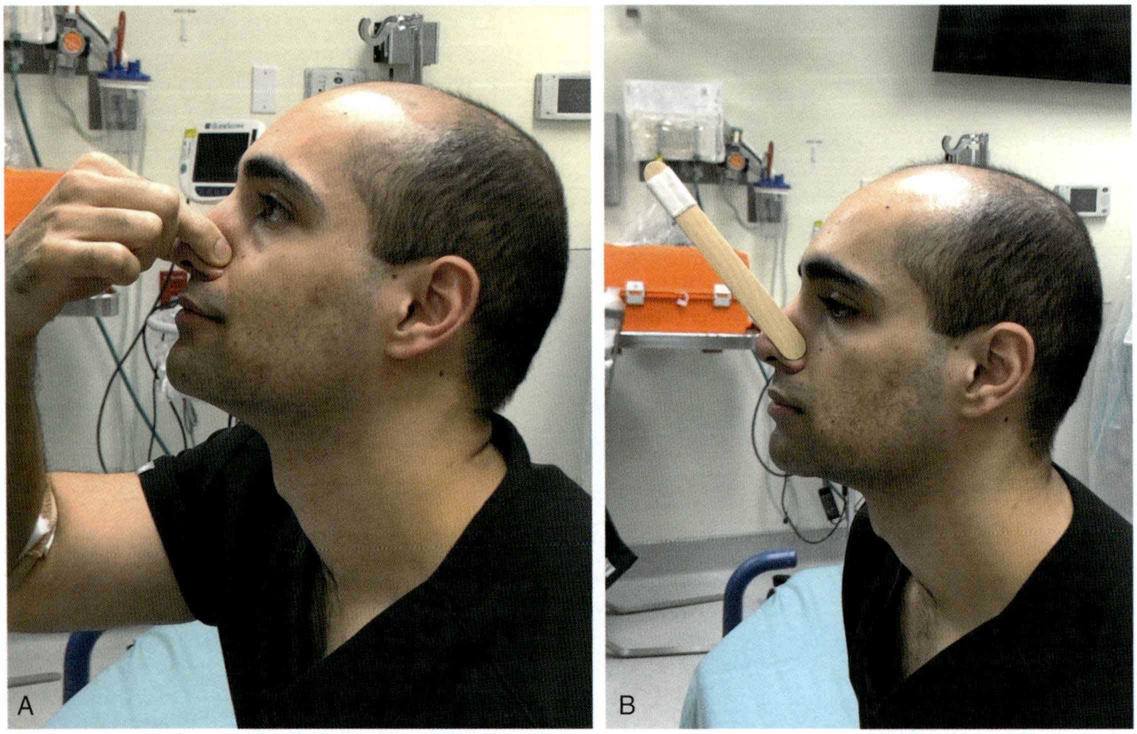

Fig. 64.34 Compression techniques for epistaxis management. (A) Patient squeezes nose. (B) Use of two tongue blades.

Epistaxis Management: Cautery

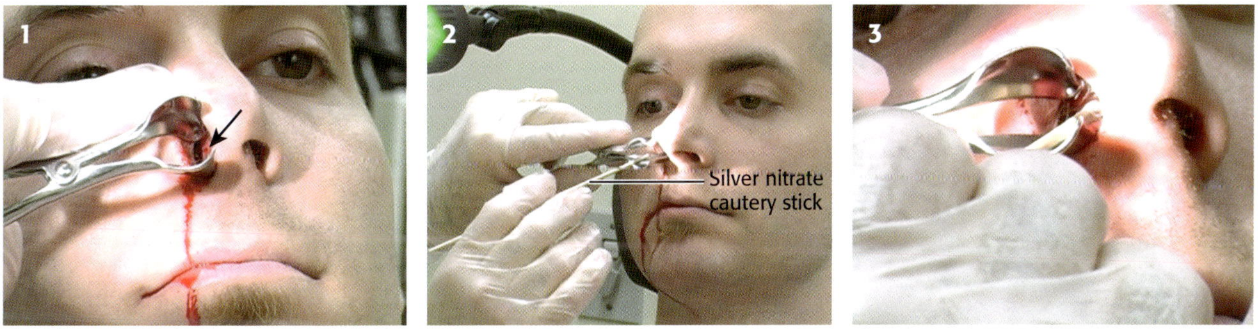

1. Cautery is used if an anterior bleeding source is identified. If no bleeding source is seen, brush the septum with a cotton swab under direct vision to stimulate the bleeding site. If there is active bleeding, cautery will not work and should not be attempted.

2. Cautery should be attempted only under direct vision; do not blindly cauterize. To apply, hold the tip of the silver nitrate stick against the site for 4 to 5 seconds. Most patients will sneeze after the application of silver nitrate.

3. The cauterized area will turn whitish gray. If bleeding restarts, the initial cautery was insufficient and should be reapplied. Avoid multiple cautery attempts and bilateral cauterization because these practices may lead to septal injury or perforation.

Fig. 64.35 Management of epistaxis: cautery.

The Rhino Rocket is a polyvinyl acetate Expanacell foam contained in a patented, syringe-like applicator that aids in its placement.[31] Insert gently into the naris along the floor of the nose. Push on plunger to advance and expel the foam from the applicator while withdrawing the syringe from the nasal cavity. Moisture from the naris should expand the foam. If not, moisten with sterile water.

Merocel is an absorbent nasal tampon made of compressed polyvinyl acetate with or without a drawstring that markedly expands on contact with fluid and thereby exerts pressure on the bleeding site.[75,76] The pack can be trimmed with scissors or a scalpel before insertion. The Merocel Doyle nasal pack (Medtronic) has an airway tube in the center of the compressed material and a more anatomic shape. Each is available in various sizes. Coat the device with a water-soluble antibiotic (e.g., bacitracin). Insert the device along the floor of the nasal cavity similar to the Rapid Rhino. Two tampons should be used for large nares; smaller nares may require a pediatric-sized tampon or an adult one trimmed. Wait 30 seconds for tampon to expand. If not expanded, 10 mL of normal saline should be infused using a 22-gauge angiocath. Once inserted, the device should be moistened with saline or water three times a day.[61] Device is usually left in place for a minimum of 24 hours.[61,68]

Traditional Nasal Packing

Commercially available products have mostly replaced the need for traditional anterior nasal packing. When not available a traditional packing technique may be done. Essentially, antibiotic-soaked gauze or lubricated-ribbon gauze is placed into the naris in an accordion-like fashion so that each layer extends the entire length of the nasal cavity.[47,61,68] This method is more time-consuming, difficult, and requires additional equipment. The gauze is placed as far back as possible without touching the nasopharynx (8 to 10 cm deep).

Properly insert nasal speculum into the affected naris to allow visualization of the nasal cavity floor. Grasp the packing material with the bayonet forceps and lay a strip of it across the nasal floor with the starting end of the gauze at the naris. Gently pack the gauze strip into the floor of the nose. Measure the gauze so that it is twice the length of the nasal cavity. Grasp the gauze at the midpoint and insert this point all the way to the posterior aspect of the nasal cavity. Attempt to place the layer without displacing the underlying layer. Continue this pattern until the cavity is filled. Reposition the nasal speculum after each layer to keep underlying layers in place. Packing is applied in an "accordion" fashion so that each layer extends the entire length of the nasal cavity (Fig. 64.36A).

When compared with gauze packing, compression devices are easier to place, better tolerated, and very successful. These are preferred over gauze packing by the editors. Preformed nasal packing products are convenient alternatives to anterior nasal packing (Figs. 64.37 and 64.38).

Corbridge and colleagues[31] found no significant difference in efficacy, patient tolerance, or complications between commercial products and gauze packing. Singer and associates[33] found that the Rapid Rhino nasal tampon is less painful to insert and easier to remove than the Rhino Rocket (Shippert Medical Technologies) and that both were similarly effective in stopping nosebleeds.

Anterior packs are usually left in place for 3 to 5 days. Premature removal may result in rebleeding. Decongestants are also prescribed to decrease secretions. Practices vary and no common standards exist.

During use and before removal, keep the nasal tampon hydrated with saline. If it contains an airway tube, first remove the tube, irrigate the space once occupied by the tube, and then remove it. To remove the Rapid Rhino, first remove the air and then slide the device out.

Posterior Nasal Packing

If no bleeding source is found anteriorly and the patient continues to hemorrhage down the posterior aspect of the pharynx, or experiences high-volume bleeding, the patient most likely has a posterior epistaxis (Fig. 64.39) requiring posterior packing. A posterior pack directly compresses the sphenopalatine artery and prevents the passage of blood or anterior packing into the nasopharynx. Posterior packing is painful and the patient may require IV pain control or procedural sedation (Fig. 64.40).

Epistaxis Management: Anterior Packing

A Accordion Petroleum Gauze Pack

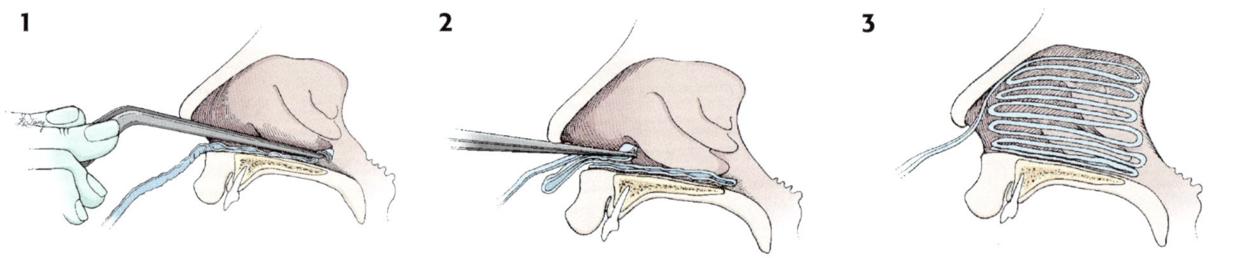

1. Place the packing in accordion fashion so that part of each layer lies anteriorly, which prevents it from falling posteriorly. Place the first layer on the floor of the nose and then remove the bayonet forceps.
2. Place a second layer on top of the first in an identical manner. After several layers have been placed, use the forceps to push the previous layers down onto the floor of the nose and pack them tighter.
3. A complete anterior nasal pack can tamponade a bleeding point anywhere in the anterior nasal cavity and will stay in place until the clinician or patient removes it.

B Nasal Tampon (Merocel)

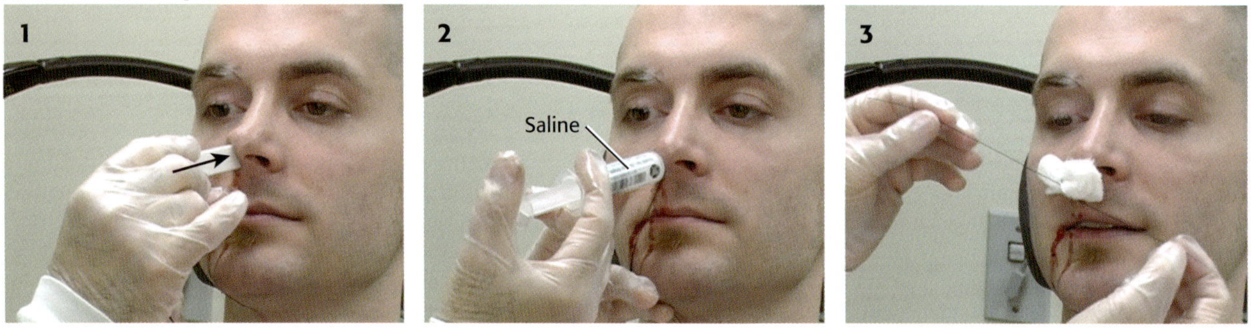

1. Trim the length and width of the tampon to fit the nose, lubricate with antibiotic ointment, and advance posteriorly, parallel to the nasal floor.
2. Once inserted, expand the tampon with 5–10 mL of saline.
3. If the tampon comes with a drawstring, it can be tied around a piece of gauze to prevent posterior displacement.

C Rapid Rhino Device

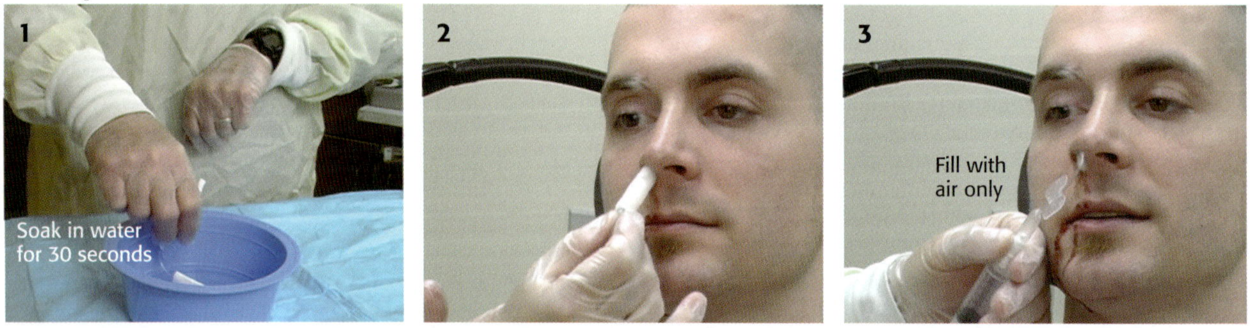

1. Soak the device in sterile water for 30 seconds. Do not soak in saline because this can inhibit its gelling characteristics.
2. Insert the Rapid Rhino along the floor of the nasal cavity parallel to the hard palate until the plastic ring is well within the nasal cavity.
3. Inflate the device with air (do not use water or saline) until the pilot cuff becomes rounded and feels firm to the touch.

Fig. 64.36 Management of epistaxis: anterior packing.

Posterior Gauze Pack

A posterior nasal gauze pack is the classic method of treating posterior epistaxis (Fig. 64.41). However, because balloon devices are easier to use and less distressing to the patient, formal posterior nasal packing is less commonly used. To place a formal traditional posterior nasal gauze pack: Anesthetize the patient's nares and posterior pharynx with topical anesthetic. Prepare a roll of gauze with two silk ties (2-0) secured around the middle and extending in opposite directions. One set of ends will be used to place the posterior pack and the second will remain extruding from the oral cavity to remove the pack. Place a No. 10 red rubber catheter through the bleeding nostril. When it is seen in the posterior of the pharynx, grasp it with forceps and guide it out of the mouth. Attach it to one set of the ends of silk ties secured to the gauze pack. Retract the red rubber catheter, thus carrying the No. 2 silk tie through the nasopharynx and out of the nose. Grasp the suture and pull the pack into the nasopharynx. Guide the pack swiftly into the oral cavity and nasopharynx with the other hand. Attach the silk tie that remains in the oropharynx to the patient's cheek

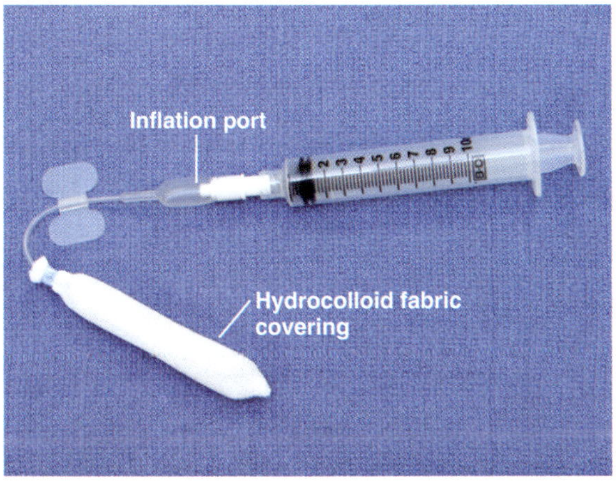

Fig. 64.37 Preformed nasal packing devices. Preformed devices are easier to place and better tolerated than traditional gauze packing. The Rapid Rhino epistaxis device shown here has an air-inflatable balloon covered by a hydrocolloid fabric covering that allows easy insertion and removal. Various lengths and configurations are available. A wide variety of similar products are offered by other vendors. Although insertion techniques for preformed devices follow the same basic steps, review the package inserts of the equipment available at your institution before use.

to aid in removal or rescue of the posterior pack. Use the silk ties exiting the nostril to maintain the position of the posterior pack. Pack the anterior passage as described for anterior epistaxis. Secure the silk ties over a gauze pad or dental roll.

Inflatable Balloon Packs

Either a Foley catheter or commercial device can be used. A Foley catheter is often used as a posterior pack because of its availability, ease of use, and successful tamponading effect (Fig. 64.42A). Insert a lubricated Foley catheter (10, 12, or 14 Fr) through the bleeding naris along the floor of the nasal cavity into the posterior aspect of the pharynx. Before insertion, trim the tip of the catheter to minimize irritation. Inflate the balloon halfway with approximately 10 mL of normal saline or water. Slowly retract the Foley catheter into the posterior part of the nasopharynx (choana) and secure it against the posterior aspect of the middle turbinate. If pain or inferior displacement of the soft palate occurs, deflate the balloon until the pain resolves. Ensure proper placement before completely inflating the balloon because the balloon will remain too posterior in the nasopharynx and fail to achieve hemostasis. While maintaining constant gentle anterior tension on the Foley catheter, pack the anterior cavity with a tamponade device or layered ribbon gauze. Pack the opposite nasal cavity to counteract septal deviation. A padded umbilical clamp or small c-clamp should be applied across the catheter to maintain gentle traction to prevent displacement and alar necrosis. Be careful to not exert undue pressure on the nasal alae to avoid causing necrosis.

Commercial Balloon Device. The second type of inflatable balloon pack is the premade dual-balloon tamponading system (see Fig. 64.42B). These devices have been a significant advance in the treatment of posterior epistaxis. Several balloon devices are available (e.g., Epistat [Medtronic], Epi-Stax [Summit Medical]). These devices typically have an anterior and posterior balloon. Each device may vary slightly. The following steps outline their use:

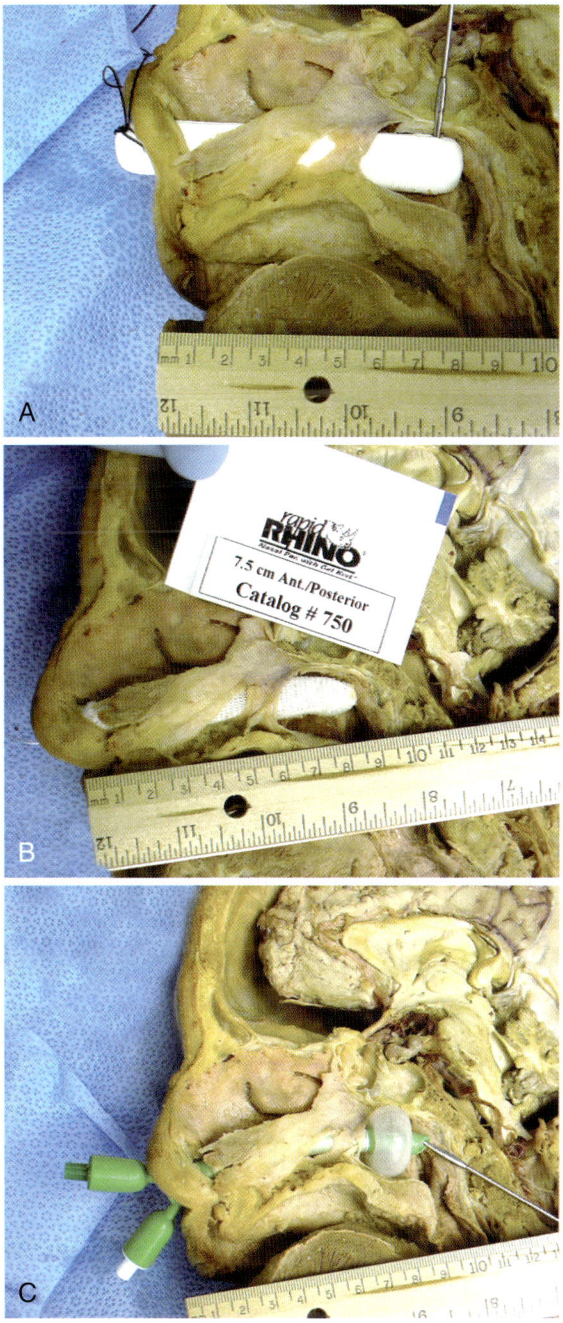

Fig. 64.38 Various packs for epistaxis in a cadaver model. (A) A posterior Merocel sponge, not inflated, will stop most nosebleeds and is more comfortable than some balloon devices. (B) Anterior/posterior Rapid Rhino in place. (C) Double-balloon posterior pack with the balloon inflated.

- Appropriately anesthetize the naris.
- Place the lubricated pack along the floor of the affected naris as far back as possible.
- Inflate the posterior balloon with 7 to 10 mL of sterile water and then retract the device to lodge the posterior balloon against the posterior choana.
- Slowly inflate the anterior balloon with 15 mL to 30 mL of sterile water to tamponade the anterior nasal cavity. Halt inflation if the patient experiences increasing pain or deviation of the nasal septum.
- Some authors suggest packing the opposite naris to prevent such septal deviation.

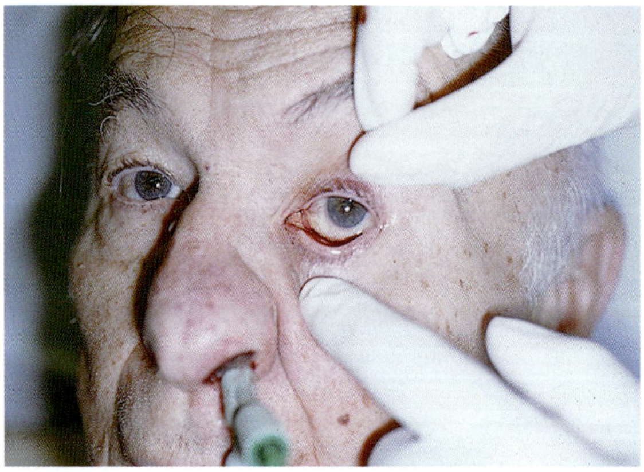

Fig. 64.39 After packing, blood coming from a nosebleed exiting via the nasolacrimal duct gives the appearance that the eye is bleeding. Though benign, it can be alarming to the patient.

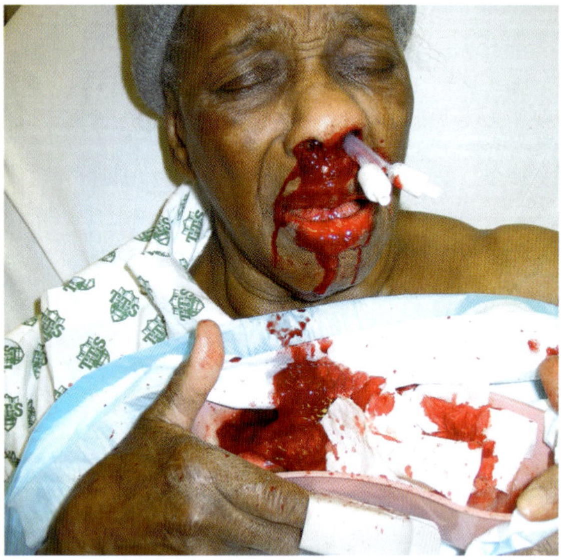

Fig. 64.40 Posterior bleeding is usually readily controlled, but blood loss can be significant. Epistaxis is rarely a feature of nasopharyngeal neoplasm, unknown blood dyscrasias, nasal foreign body, cocaine use, or aneurysm of the carotid artery. This older adult patient was very anxious and quite hypertensive, and judicious use of intravenous morphine made the procedure tolerable and reduced blood pressure. Hypertension alone is not a cause of epistaxis.

- Place a small piece of gauze between the nose and the external catheter hub to decrease skin irritation.

Most patients with a posterior pack, especially older adults and those with pulmonary and cardiovascular diseases, should be admitted to the hospital for sedation and monitoring. This recommendation was common for formal posterior packs, but the ease and safety of balloon devices now allow selected patients to be treated as outpatients despite the presence of posterior packing.

Other Techniques

ENT consultation may be required for posterior nosebleeds that do not respond to the posterior packing techniques. Other treatment options that consultants may consider include posterior endoscopic cautery, surgical ligation, or angiographic embolization of the sphenopalatine, anterior ethmoid, or internal maxillary artery.[48]

Special Considerations

Hypertension. No direct causal correlation between hypertension and overt epistaxis has been proved.[77,78] Many patients with epistaxis are hypertensive. This is most likely a response to the stress and anxiety of bleeding, and not an inciting event.[78–80] Treating the epistaxis may be enough to lower the blood pressure (BP). The Academy of Otolaryngology-Head and Neck Surgery Foundation recommends directing acute treatment at bleeding control and not emergent BP reduction.[51] However, any patient exhibiting other signs of a true hypertensive emergency needs immediate antihypertensive treatment in addition to control of the epistaxis.

Anticoagulated Patients With Epistaxis. Anticoagulated patients are at high risk for nosebleeds. However, the need for cessation and reversal of oral anticoagulants is not recommended unless there is severe, refractory bleeding. In patients with a mildly to moderately elevated international normalized ratio (INR), dose cessation may be sufficient. For those on warfarin who need reversal, 4-factor prothrombin complex concentrate with vitamin K should be used.[81] For patients on newer anticoagulants, the specific reversal agent should be used. In patients taking factor Xa inhibitors, 4-factor prothrombin complex concentrate (4-factor PCC) or andexanet alfa can be used.[81,82] Patients with hemophilia will require specific factor replacement and consultation with hematology is recommended.

Antibiotics. It was once thought a nasal pack or device may stimulate mucous production and act as an impetus for infection. There was also a concern about the packing/device leading to toxic shock syndrome (TSS). Data do not suggest a benefit to prophylactic antibiotics for patients who receive an anterior nasal pack or device due to the very low rate of infection with a number needed to treat of 571.[82,83] If the decision is made to provide antibiotics, oral antibiotic choices include cephalexin, amoxicillin, or trimethoprim-sulfamethoxazole.

Posterior packing is associated with a risk for infection, including nasopharyngitis, sinusitis, and rarely, TSS.[84,85] Packing blocks the sinus ostia, which prevents proper drainage of the sinuses. TSS is rare with nasal packing and is estimated to occur in approximately 16 per 100,000 posterior packings.[84] A systematic review did not find any methodologically rigorous studies evaluating the incidence of TSS following posterior nasal packing.[85] None of the studies reported TSS as a complication of nasal packing. There is no strong evidence to support or refute the practice of prescribing antibiotics. The choice is left up to the provider. It may be reasonable to provide prophylaxis to patients at greater risk for infection, such as those with diabetes, advanced age, or an immunosuppressed state. If used, an antibiotic with staphylococcal coverage should be selected, such as amoxicillin-clavulanate.

Aftercare

Once the bleeding is controlled, the patient should be observed for at least 30 minutes to monitor for any recurrence.[68,86] If no packing was required, patients can follow up with their primary care provider or ENT. Patients with anterior packing should follow up with ENT in 3 to 5 days for removal.[47] Patients with posterior packing require ENT consultation for further management and possibly hospitalization. Persistent posterior bleeding may require surgical or interventional

Epistaxis Management: Traditional Posterior Packing

1

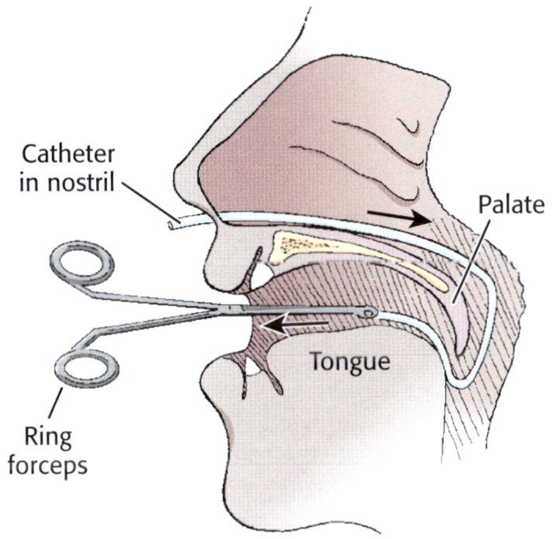

After applying topical anesthetic, pass a red rubber catheter through the nose, carefully grasp it in the oropharynx with ringed forceps, and bring it out through the mouth.

2

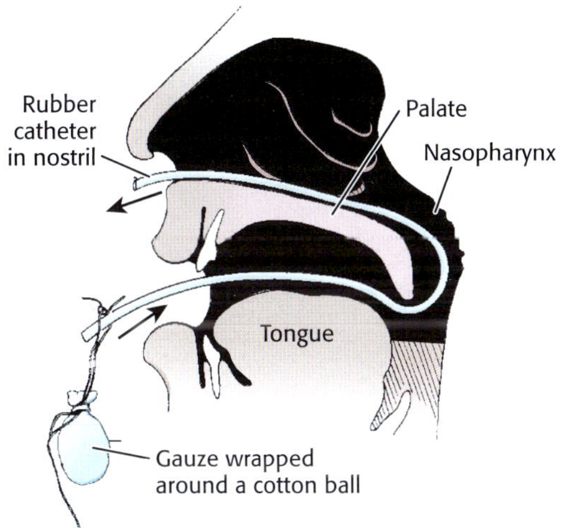

Make a posterior nasal pack by wrapping a cotton ball in a 4 x 4-inch gauze pad and tying two long silk sutures or umbilical tape around the neck of the pack. Leave one tie long so that it can be taped to the cheek until needed for removal of the pack.

3

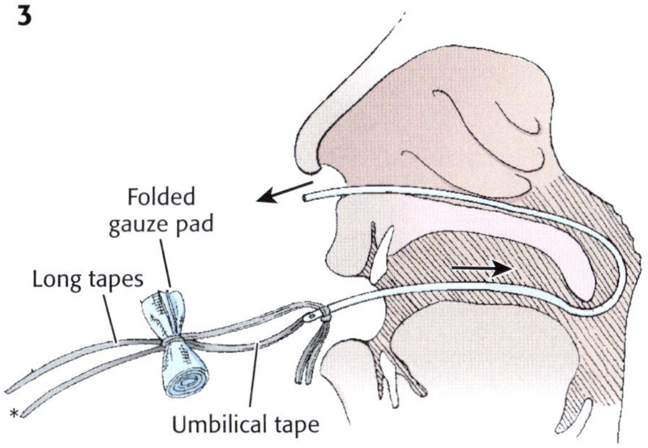

Alternatively, fold a gauze pad, roll it into a cylinder, and tie it with two strings. Use two of the long strings to tie the pack to the tip of the catheter, and use the other two to remove the pack.

4

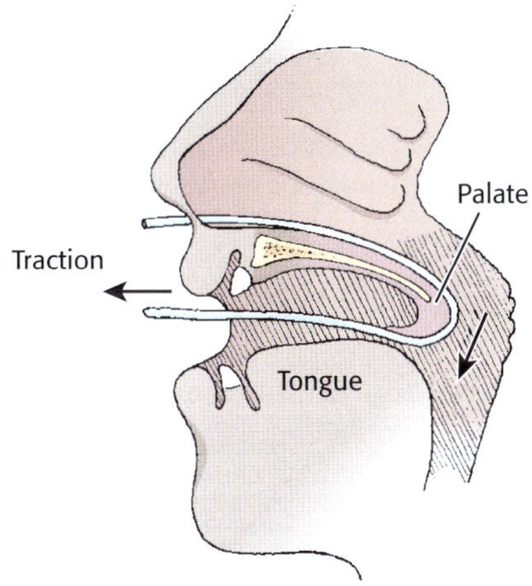

As an option, use a second catheter that has been passed through the nonbleeding side and brought out the mouth to retract the palate forward to aid in placement of the pack.

5

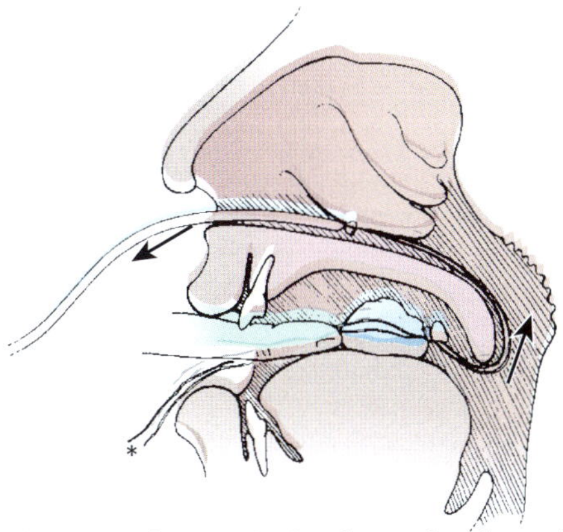

Remove the optional "retraction" catheter after the pack is in the proper position. Digitally guide the pack into the nasopharynx.

6

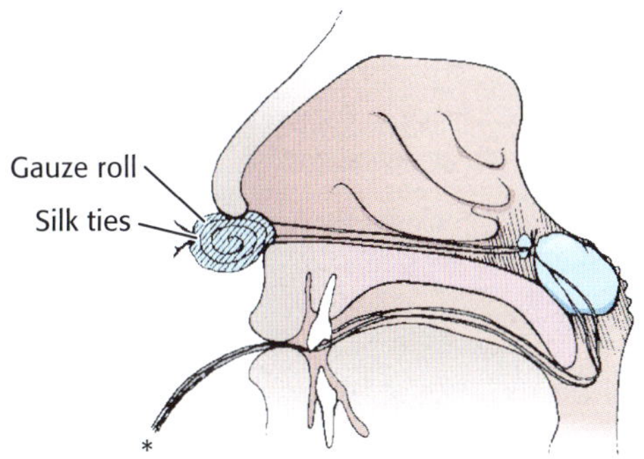

Use a gauze roll to secure the pack to the nose, and tape the rescue ties to the cheek.

Fig. 64.41 Management of epistaxis: traditional posterior packing.

Epistaxis Management: Posterior Packing With Inflatable Devices

A Foley Catheter Technique

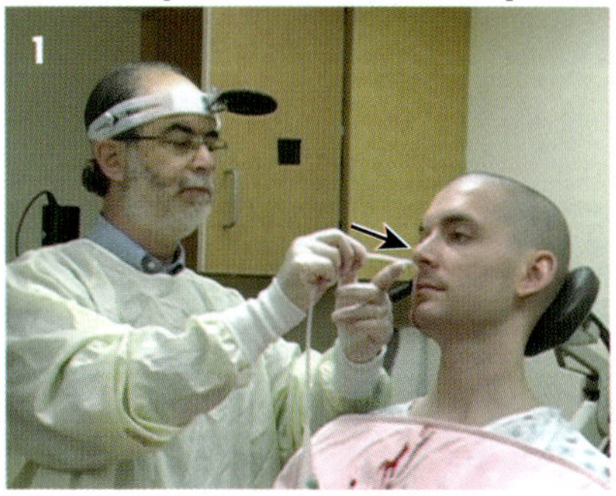

Insert a 12-Fr Foley catheter through the naris and into the posterior pharynx.

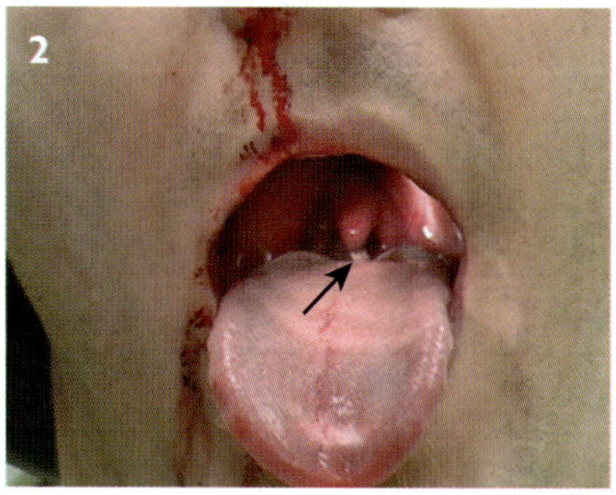

Look into the mouth to confirm that the catheter is properly positioned.

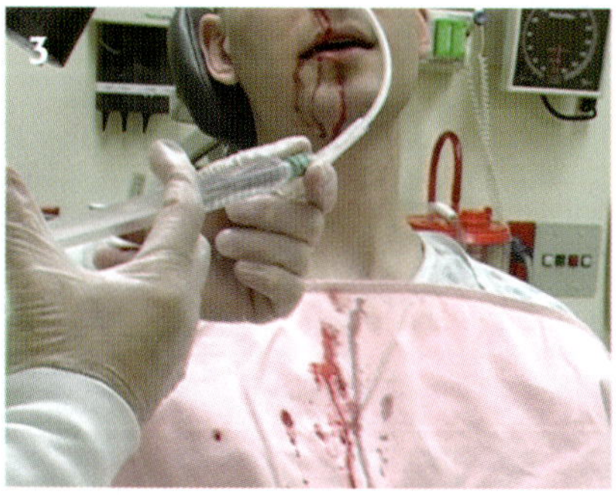

Inflate the balloon halfway with about 5–7 mL of water.

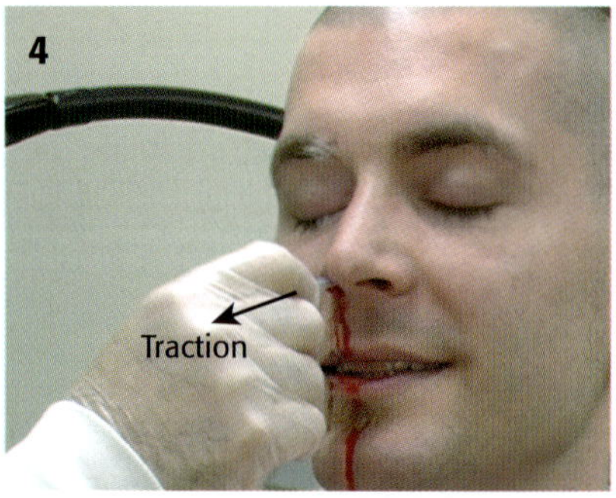

Slowly pull the catheter into the posterior nasopharynx up against the posterior aspect of the middle turbinate.

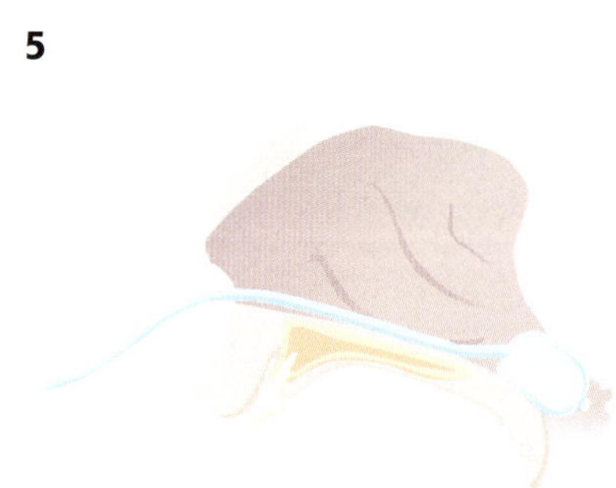

Foley catheter in proper position in the posterior nasopharynx. Inflate the balloon with another 5–7 mL of water.

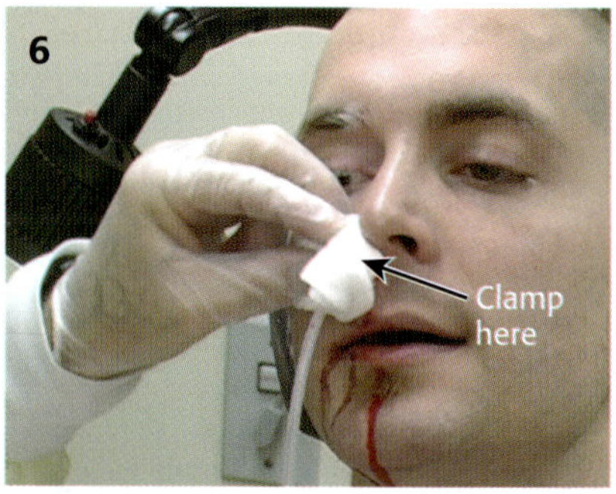

While maintaining traction, place anterior packing with layered gauze. Packing of the opposite side may be required to prevent septal deviation. Place a piece of gauze on the exposed catheter and secure with an umbilical clamp.

B Dual-Balloon Tamponade Catheter

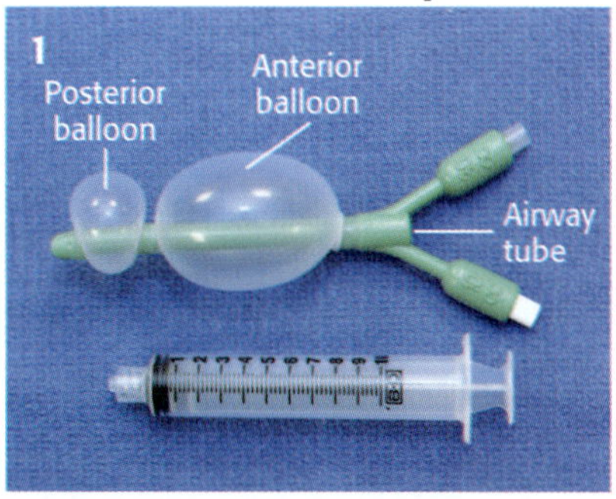

Double-balloon epistaxis catheters have both an anterior and posterior balloon, and some have an integral airway tube. These devices serve as both an anterior and a posterior pack. They are easily inserted and are often successful in temporary control of posterior epistaxis in the ED.

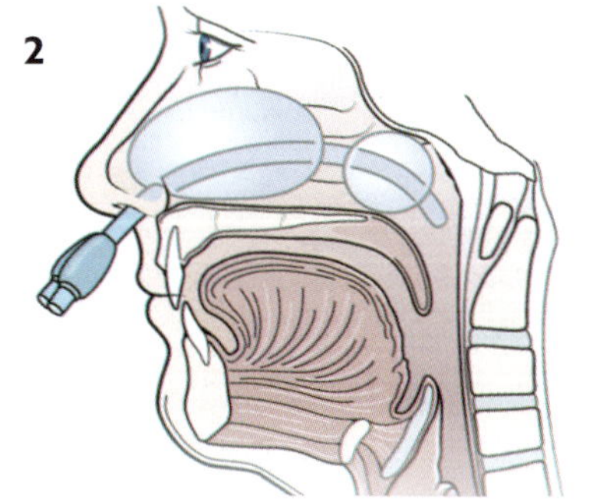

Insert the lubricated device along the nasal floor as far back as possible. Inflate the posterior balloon halfway with air, apply traction to pull the balloon up against the middle turbinate, and then complete the inflation. Maintain the position of the balloon and then inflate the anterior balloon with 30 mL of air.

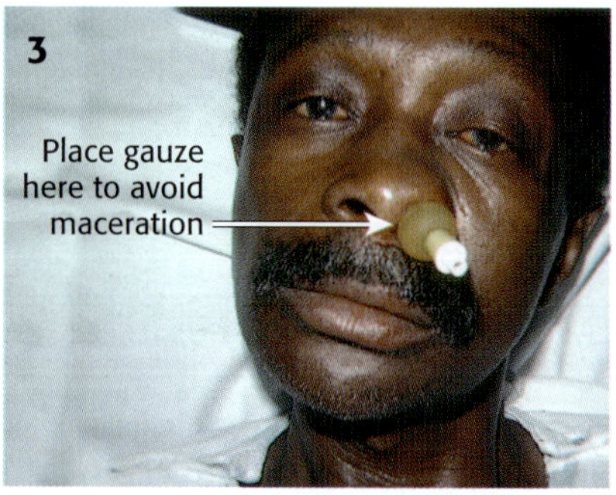

This patient with posterior epistaxis was successfully treated in the ED and discharged. Historically, most patients with posterior packs were admitted to the hospital; however, the ease and safety of balloon devices allow selected patients to be treated as outpatients. Consider admission for the elderly, and those with pulmonary or cardiovascular disease.

Fig. 64.42 Management of epistaxis: posterior packing with inflatable devices. *ED*, Emergency department.

radiology treatment.[87,88] In general, patients should avoid aspirin and nonsteroidal agents for 3 to 4 days. They should be advised to avoid nose blowing, strenuous activity, heavy lifting, and picking within the nose for at least 1 week.[47] They should also be advised to sneeze with an open mouth. Return to the ED precautions should be provided as well. Patients can be counseled on how to prevent nosebleeds with humidified air, saline nasal spray, and lubricating ointments.

TABLE 64.1 Complications in the Management of Epistaxis[55,56,97,102,103]

TECHNIQUE	COMPLICATIONS
Vasoconstrictors	Allergic reaction Transient BP increase
Tranexamic acid	Allergic reaction Venous thromboembolism, myocardial infarction, stroke[a]
Anterior nasal packing/ device	Pain Oozing Sinusitis Blood from nasolacrimal duct (Fig. 64.36) Nasal mucosal pressure necrosis Aspiration of packing Pneumocephalus Ethmoid fracture
Posterior nasal packing/ device	Pain and discomfort Infection Dysphagia Eustachian tube dysfunction Tissue necrosis (nasal ala, mucosa, and soft palate) Hypoxia Hypercapnia Aspiration Elevated BP Dysrhythmia/bradycardia

[a]Complications are more commonly seen with intravenous use. No reported cases with topical use.

BP, Blood pressure.

Data from Kucik CJ, Clenney T. Management of epistaxis. *Am Fam Physician*. 2005;71:305-311; Middleton PM. Epistaxis. *Emerg Med Australas*. 2004;16:428-440; Bledsoe RD. Case report: magnetically adherent nasal foreign bodies: a novel method of removal and case series. *Am J Emerg Med*. 2008;26:839.e1-839.e2; Navitsky RC, Beamsley A, McLaughlin S. Nasal positive-pressure technique for nasal foreign body removal in children. *Am J Emerg Med*. 2002;20:103-104; McNamee J, Jeong J. How to perform positive pressure technique for nasal foreign body removal. *ACEP Now*. 2014. Available at: http://www.acepnow.com/article/perform-positive-pressure-technique-nasal-foreign-body-removal/2/.

Complications

Complications are rare in the management of epistaxis and are based on the method used to control the bleeding. Rebleeding can occur with any method. Table 64.1 describes complications of the various management techniques for epistaxis control.[47,48,85,89,90]

Septal Hematoma

Trauma to the anterior portion of the nasal septum may cause a hematoma to form. A buckling stress tears the submucosal blood vessels. If the mucosa remains intact, the blood will accumulate between the mucoperichondrium and the septal cartilage. Stagnant blood is an excellent medium for bacterial growth and the formation of an abscess. Common bacteria include *S. aureus*, *Streptococcus pneumoniae*, and group A β-hemolytic streptococci. Other complications of an untreated hematoma include septal perforation and cartilage destruction with a resultant saddle nose deformity. Septal hematomas may occur immediately after the trauma or, more commonly, in the first 24 to 72 hours after the injury.[91] The hematoma can cause significant destruction of the nasal cartilage and result in a cosmetic deformity.

Indications and Contraindications

The presence of a nasal septal hematoma requires drainage to prevent cosmetic defects, septal necrosis, and other complications. The most common symptoms of septal hematoma are nasal obstruction, pain, rhinorrhea, and fever. Most patients will complain of an inability to breathe through the affected side, but the absence of nasal obstruction does not rule out a septal hematoma. It is usually possible to diagnose a septal hematoma by inspecting the nasal septum with a speculum for swelling, pain, and a fluctuant area (Fig. 64.43). The presence of septal asymmetry with a bluish or reddish hue of the mucosa is suggestive of septal hematoma. To some it looks like a grape. Inspect both sides because bilateral hematomas are possible. Direct palpation with the littlest finger may be necessary because newly formed hematomas may not yet be ecchymotic. Palpation can further differentiate septal hematoma from septal deviation, which may appear to be similar because of asymmetry. The best way to palpate for a septal hematoma is to insert the gloved small fingers in each side of the nose and palpate the entire septum to feel swelling, fluctuance, or widening of the septal space.

There are no absolute contraindications to drainage of nasal septal hematoma. Caution should be used in those with known bleeding diathesis or those who are taking anticoagulants.

Equipment

A topical or injectable anesthetic should be used. For the procedure itself, a light source, a nasal speculum, a No. 11 scalpel blade, suction apparatus, scissors, nasal saline, small Penrose drain, and some form of nasal packing material are all that are needed.

Procedure

Treatment of a septal hematoma consists of evacuation of the clot with subsequent reapproximation of the perichondrium to the cartilage (Fig. 64.44). To drain the hematoma, incise the mucosa over the hematoma horizontally after adequate anesthesia is achieved. Suction out all the clot and then irrigate with normal saline. Excise a small amount of mucosa to prevent premature closure of the incision and place a section of a sterile rubber band to act as a drain. Pack the nostril, as for anterior epistaxis, to reapproximate the perichondrium to the cartilage. Prescribe broad-spectrum antibiotic therapy. Inspect the septum daily for signs of infection, recurrent hematoma, or necrosis. Evacuate recurrent hematomas. When there is no further hematoma formation over a 24-hour period, remove the drain. Pack the affected naris for one more day to complete the apposition of perichondrium to cartilage where the drain had been. If any evidence of infection is present, admit for IV antibiotics and surgical debridement.

Complications

Though rare, nasal septal abscess formation is the most common complication of septal hematomas. The infection can

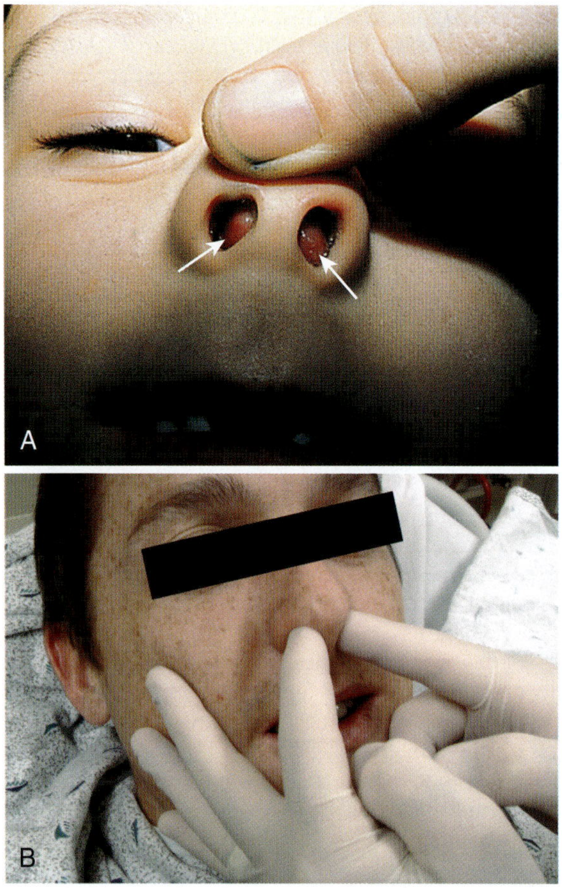

Fig. 64.43 Septal hematoma. (A) Bilateral septal hematoma in a 6-year-old child. Obstruction is present on both sides of the nose *(arrows)*. There was no response to vasoconstriction. (B) If visual inspection of the nose with a speculum does not rule out a septal hematoma, the clinician's gloved fingers, passed posteriorly along both sides of the septum, may feel bulging or fluctuance. A normal septum is thin and smooth. (A, Courtesy Robert Hickey, MD, Children's Hospital of Pittsburgh. B, From Flint PW, Haughey BH, Lund VJ et al., eds. *Cummings Otolaryngology: Head and Neck Surgery*. 5th ed. Elsevier; 2010.)

spread to the sinus cavities and lead to meningitis, cavernous sinus thrombosis, intracranial abscess, and orbital cellulitis.

A large or rapidly expanding hematoma may cause pressure on the septum and lead to avascular necrosis of the septal cartilage. The nasal septum can collapse and lose its shape, which causes a noticeable cosmetic defect.

After drainage, the hematoma may recur and should be treated by repeated drainage to prevent cartilage damage. Reaccumulation can be prevented by incising a piece of mucosa before packing the nasal cavity.

Nasal FB Removal

Nasal FBs most frequently occur in pediatric patients, but it is not uncommon to find them in psychiatric or cognitively impaired patients as well. Usually, a family member has witnessed the event or the patient complains of discomfort from the FB. Patients may also have unilateral purulent or bloody nasal discharge, unilateral sinusitis, or recurrent unilateral epistaxis. Retained FBs, especially plastic ones, often initially fail to cause pain or other symptoms.[92] The lack of a history of FB insertion is of little value in children because many will not admit it. Therefore emergency clinicians need to maintain a high level of suspicion for nasal FBs.

Types of nasal FBs vary widely and include food (e.g., meat, nuts, beans), rubber erasers, paper wads, pebbles, marbles, sponges, beads, jewelry, hardware (e.g., nuts, screws), and even certain living larvae or worms.[92,93]

Alkaline button batteries pose a unique problem because they may cause significant nasal injury within hours to days.[94,95] They are composed of heavy metals such as mercury, zinc, silver, nickel, cadmium, and lithium. Injuries can occur and include mucosal burns, ulcerations, liquefaction necrosis, septal perforation, synechiae, and stenosis of the nasal cavity.[94,95] It is imperative that these batteries be removed promptly before tissue damage occurs because of leakage of the battery contents, electrical currents, or direct pressure.

An increasingly common nasal FB is the magnetic nose ring. These small, commercially available earth magnets are

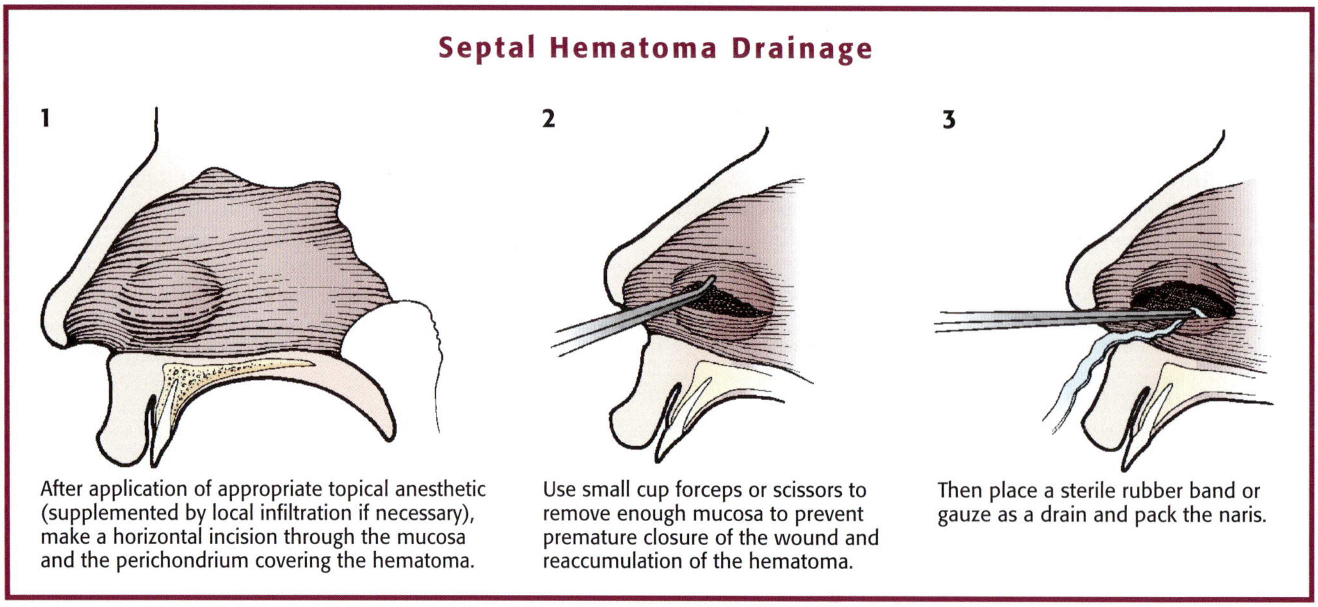

Fig. 64.44 Drainage of a septal hematoma.

usually worn on either side of the alar cartilage and give the appearance of a pierced nasal stud. The magnets can be displaced and become polarized across the nasal septum. The magnetic attraction can be quite strong and may lead to pressure necrosis of the nasal mucosa and possibly septal perforation. This attraction can also make removal difficult, as well as painful for the patient.[95,96] Suggested techniques include using polarized or nonferromagnetic tools.[97]

Many nasal FBs come to rest on the floor of the anterior or middle third of the nose. Metallic or calcified objects may show up on radiographs, but physical examination remains the most reliable means for diagnosis. Maxillary, ethmoid, or sphenoid sinusitis may also accompany FB retention. Plain radiographs or facial CT scanning may be of value in detecting sinusitis, although these studies are not usually necessary with an acutely retained object.

Inability to remove a nasal FB should necessitate ENT consultation and may result in admission for removal under anesthesia; therefore, it behooves emergency clinicians to be skilled in this procedure. Although admission incurs increased cost, has inherent procedural risks, and causes psychological stress in parents and patients, providers should be prepared to call a consultant after several attempts. As with the removal of auricular FBs, removal of nasal FBs can be both frustrating and time-consuming.

Indications and Contraindications

Attempt removal of a nasal FB only if it is likely to be retrieved. ENT consultation is needed if there is any doubt about the ability to successfully retrieve the object. Repeated attempts may result in trauma and displacement of the object into a less favorable location.

Do not attempt mechanical removal if the object appears to be out of range of the instruments. In addition, do not attempt removal in an uncooperative patient unless sedation is provided. Use sedation cautiously because it may increase the risk for aspiration, especially when using agents that blunt the protective airway reflexes.

Equipment

Most of the equipment used for removing FBs in the ear canal can also be used for nasal FB removal. Topical nasal anesthetic and vasoconstrictor solutions, such as oxymetazoline, can greatly aid in the removal of nasal FBs.

Procedure

See Videos 64.23 and 64.24. A cooperative patient is essential. Weigh the risks and benefits of using simple or procedural sedation. Ketamine anesthesia works well for children. Before attempting removal, anesthetize and vasoconstrict the mucosa of the affected naris topically. Ask an assistant to stabilize the patient's head and immobilize a younger patient if necessary. Place more cooperative patients in the sniffing position and use a headlamp for proper illumination. Several of the techniques previously mentioned for removing an FB from the EAC can also be used in the management of a nasal FB, including the use of cyanoacrylate glue.

Manual Instrumentation

Use alligator forceps or bayonet forceps to retrieve anteriorly lodged FBs that have edges amenable to grasping (Fig. 64.45, *plate 1*). For harder or larger objects, carefully pass a wire loop (one can be made using 24-gauge wire loop grasped by a hemostat),[98] a right-angle hook (if unavailable, one can be made out of an 18-gauge needle), or even a properly bent paper clip. Carefully insert it beyond the object and rotate it to allow the FB to be pulled from the naris. Direct mucosal trauma and epistaxis may occur with any of these methods. For a nasal FB with smooth, round edges that are difficult to grasp or get behind, attempt to extract it with a suction-tipped catheter in a manner similar to that described earlier for FBs in the EAC (see Figs. 64.22 and 64.23).

Balloon Catheter

For an object that cannot be removed with anterior instrumentation, one consideration is to attempt removal with a balloon catheter. A Fogarty catheter can be highly effective in removing a nasal FB (see Fig. 64.45, *plates 2 and 3*). A No. 4 or 5 vascular Fogarty catheter, a 12-Fr Foley catheter, and a No. 6 biliary Fogarty catheter have all been described in the literature for this use.

Place the patient in the supine position and apply a vasoconstrictor and anesthetic to the nasal mucosa. With a 5-mL syringe attached and the catheter lubricated with lidocaine gel, pass the tip above the object and into the nasopharynx. Inflate the balloon with air or water (≈2 mL in small children and 3 mL in older children) and control the syringe plunger and balloon size with your thumb. Withdraw the catheter until resistance is felt, and then slowly pull the object out. The Katz Extractor otorhinologic FB remover (InHealth Technologies; see Fig. 64.45, *plate 4*) is a disposable, single unit composed of a flexible catheter with a balloon tip attached to a syringe. The procedure is like that for the Fogarty catheter.

Complications mentioned in the literature include mild posttraumatic bleeding, as well as the theoretical risk for airway obstruction by the balloon or aspiration from further displacement of the object.

Positive Pressure

Another approach to a posteriorly placed nasal FB is to blow the object out with positive air pressure. The simplest way is to ask patients to blow their nose while occluding the unaffected nostril. Alternatively, a bag-valve-mask (BVM)[93] device can be used. Place the BVM over the child's mouth (without covering the nares) to provide positive pressure (see Fig. 64.45, *plate 5*). Occlude the opposite nostril and apply the Sellick maneuver (manual displacement of the cricoid ring posteriorly) to prevent passage of air into the esophagus. This technique often requires restraint and can also be threatening to a young child.

The "parent's kiss" technique may be used in children.[93,99,100] First gain the child's cooperation by saying that parent is going to "give them a big kiss." The technique is performed by having the child lie supine. Ask the parent to occlude the child's unaffected nostril with the thumb (see Fig. 64.45, *plate 6*). Next, as in mouth-to-mouth resuscitation, ask the parent to make a firm seal with their mouth over the child's open mouth and then give a short, sharp puff of air briskly into the mouth to produce outward pressure behind the object. Keep the opposite nostril occluded throughout the procedure. If successful, the object will move within grasping reach of an instrument or pop completely out of the naris. If it fails, the technique can be repeated. Studies of the parent's kiss technique have found it to be highly effective, nontraumatic, and preferable to restraint or instrumentation.[99,100] A modification of the technique, that may be easier for some parents to master, uses a drinking straw placed between the

NASAL FOREIGN BODY REMOVAL

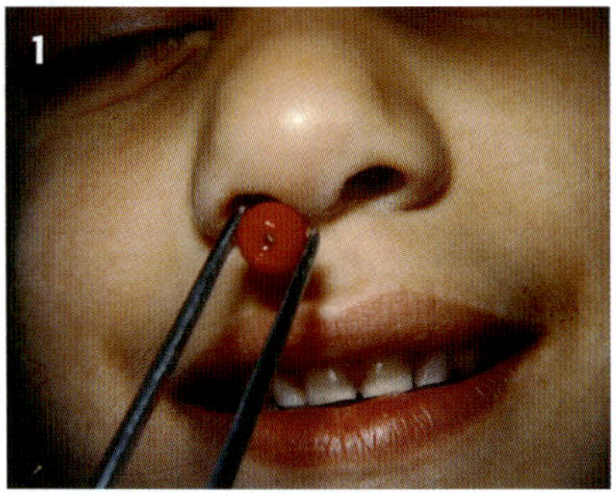

Following vasoconstriction and anesthesia (2% lidocaine with epinephrine was dripped into the nose), some FBs may be easily extracted with forceps.

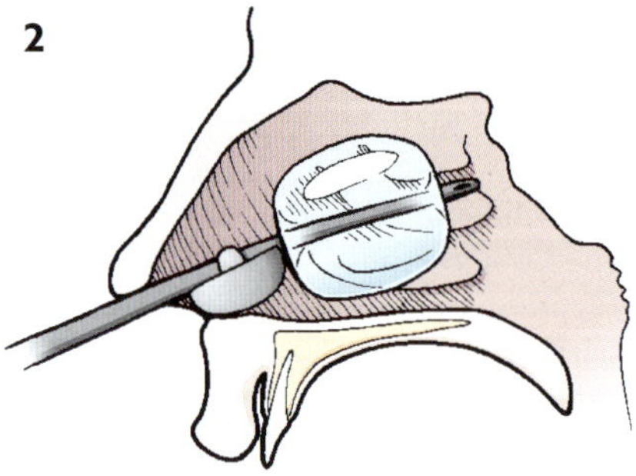

A Fogarty catheter may be used to extract a nasal FB. Insert the lubricated catheter tip above the FB and then gradually inflate the balloon.

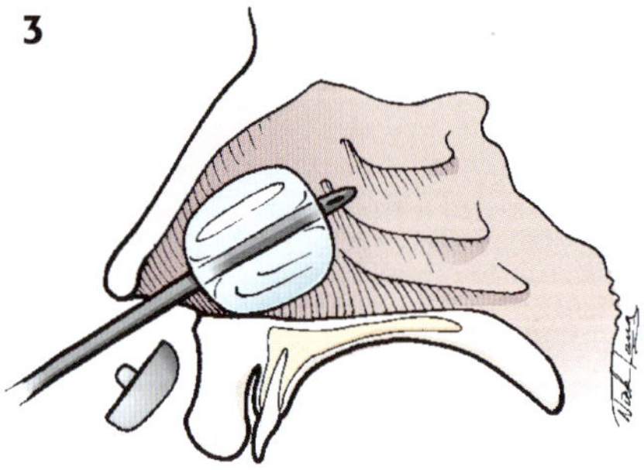

Slowly withdraw until resistance is met and then pull the object out of the naris.

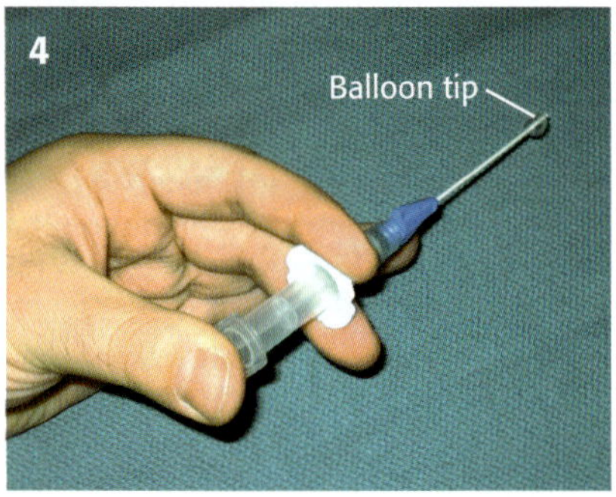

The Katz Extractor. This device is used in an analogous fashion to the Fogarty catheter.

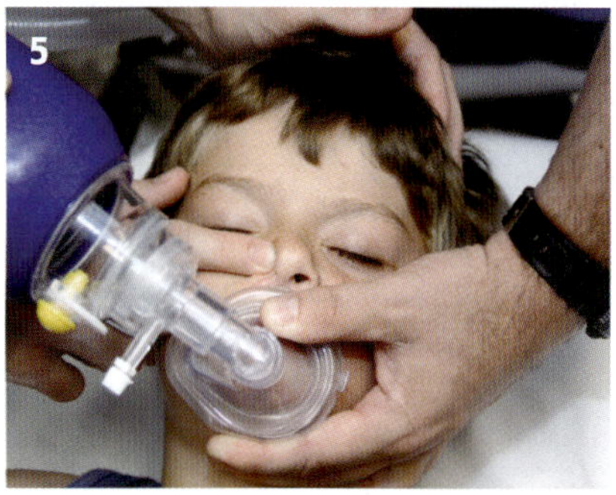

Bag-valve-mask technique to blow an FB out of the naris. Ensure that the face mask forms a tight seal around the patient's mouth and that the unaffected nostril is completely occluded. Attempt to firmly compress the bag as the patient exhales (an assistant is helpful to hold the mask snugly and to occlude the other nostril). This technique works best with objects that completely occlude the nostril.

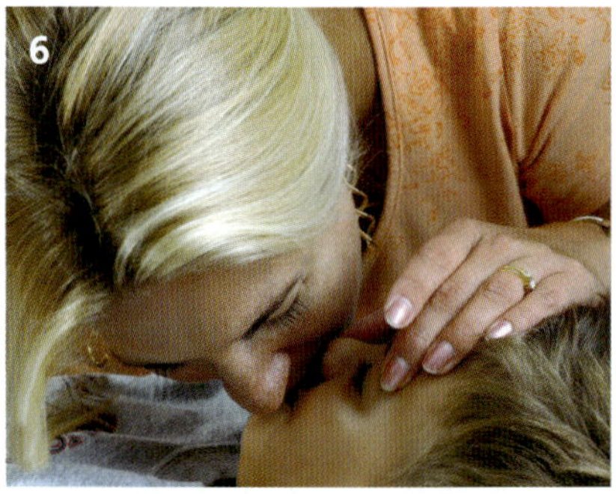

To blow an FB out of the nose, have the parent blow into the mouth while occluding the unaffected side with the thumb.

Fig. 64.45 Removal of a nasal foreign body *(FB)*.

parent's mouth and the child's mouth. Instruct the child to make a tight seal, as though drinking, and ask the parent to deliver a quick puff.

Another similar technique may be successful.[101]After a nasal decongestant is instilled into the affected side, place a 6- to 10-inch section of ¼- or ⅛-inch-wide rubber or soft vinyl tubing into or at the contralateral nostril and hold the tubing in place with the fingers of one hand. Place the free hand gently over the child's mouth, take a good-sized breath, and blow forcefully through the tubing. This step may be repeated up to four times. In one study, success was reported in 40 of 41 cases.[101] Navitsky and colleagues modified this technique to reduce the risk of disease transmission.[102]

Turn a wall oxygen source to a flow of 10 to 15 L/min. Use a male-to-male adapter at the end of oxygen tubing to direct the flow of oxygen into the contralateral (nonobstructed) nostril.

Two other techniques using positive pressure have been described and use simple equipment and oxygen or medical air. In the first technique,[103] wall oxygen or medical air, suction tubing, and a suction-tubing adapter are needed (Fig. 64.46A). Have the patient sit upright and lean forward with the head tilted down. Attach one end of standard suction tubing to the wall oxygen or compressed air unit. The plastic suction-tubing adapter should be firmly placed into the opposite end of the suction tubing. Insert the tubing with the adapter into the contralateral nostril. Titrate the oxygen to high flow (usually 10 to 15 L/min) until the foreign object is expelled.

The other technique uses a disposable stethoscope earpiece, 8-Fr suction catheter or feeding tube, oxygen, and oxygen tubing (see Fig. 64.46B–C).[104] Attach the earpiece to the 8-Fr suction catheter. Connect the set to a standard oxygen wall setup. At 15 L/min of oxygen, a pressure of 100 to 160 mm Hg is achieved. Patient positioning is determined by patient age. If the patient is older than 3 years, place the patient in a lateral position with the nostril containing the FB face down. If the patient is less than or equal to 3 years old, have the child sit in the parent's lap. Connect the device to the oxygen source with tubing and set the oxygen to 15 L/min. Bend the hose to occlude passage of pressure. Next, place the device in the unaffected nostril, release the pressure, and

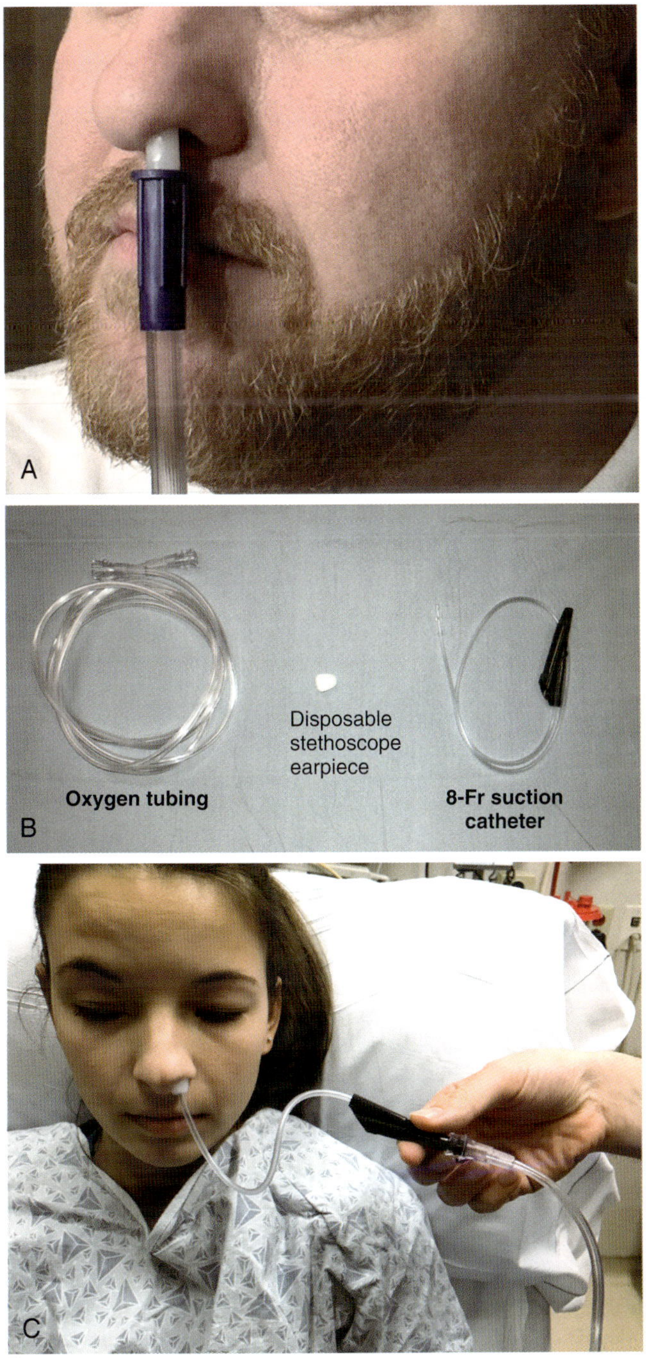

Fig. 64.46 Additional techniques for positive pressure removal of nasal foreign bodies. (A) Attach suction tubing to wall oxygen or medical air and use a suction adapter inserted in the contralateral naris. (B) An alternative technique uses oxygen tubing, an earpiece from a disposable stethoscope, and an 8-Fr suction catheter. (C) Equipment assembled and positioned for use.

immediately remove the device. If the object is not removed, make another attempt. In a study of 18 patients, the device was successful in 94.4% of patients on the first attempt. If an 8-Fr feeding tube is not available, an 8-Fr suction catheter may be used as an alternative.

Complications

Most complications are due to the FB itself and include pain, obstruction, rhinorrhea, ulceration of the nasal mucosa, septal perforation, infection, and nasal or choanal stenosis. Bleeding and mucosal laceration are the most reported complications of removal. The bleeding is usually minor and generally resolves with simple pressure. It may occur as a result of the object itself or from trauma during removal. Inadvertent posterior dislodgement of the object may occur and result in ingestion or aspiration of the object. Theoretically, barotrauma to the lungs and TMs may occur with positive-pressure techniques.

Temporomandibular Joint Dislocation

The temporomandibular joint (TMJ) joint is a hinge and sliding joint with a dense fibrocartilaginous disc lying between the joint and the glenoid fossa. Dislocation occurs when the mandibular condyle(s) is displaced from its normal position in the mandibular fossa of the temporal bone and becomes locked in an abnormal position resulting in muscle spasm and preventing mouth closure.[105,106] Although dislocation may result from trauma, it more commonly follows extreme opening of the mouth such as may occur while eating, signing, chewing, vomiting, laughing, or yawning (Fig. 64.47). Patients with a previous history of TMJ dislocation are more prone to repeated dislocations. Bilateral dislocation and anterior dislocation are the most common forms.[105–108] Lateral, posterior, and superior joint dislocations are rare and more often associated with high-energy trauma resulting facial fractures.[105–108] This section will focus on the management of anterior TMJ dislocations.

Risk factors for TMJ dislocation include conditions resulting in increased ligament laxity (Ehlers-Danlos, Marfan Syndrome), prior TMJ dislocation, medications with dystonic reactions, post-procedures (endoscopy, intubation), and neurodegenerative conditions (multiple sclerosis, Huntington disease).[105–121] Predisposing factors include anatomic disharmony between the mandibular fossa and the articular eminence and weakness of the capsule and the temporomandibular ligaments.

Indications and Contraindications

The presence of TMJ dislocation is the indication for reduction. The diagnosis is usually straightforward, but the condition can be misinterpreted as an acute dystonic reaction (see Fig. 64.47C). With dislocation, patients cannot close their mouth, and speech is affected. Pain varies, and patients are often very anxious. With unilateral dislocation, the jaw will deviate to the opposite side. More commonly, bilateral dislocation occurs. With traumatic dislocation, radiographic evaluation should be performed to exclude a fracture.[109,110] Maxillofacial CT is the preferred imaging. Plain radiographs (mandible series or panoramic jaw view) can be used if CT is not available, but are less desirable because of improved fracture visualization and anatomic localization with CT.

Contraindications to reduction include non-anterior TMJ dislocation, open dislocation, or those with associated facial fractures. In such cases, facial specialty (ENT or [oral and maxillofacial] OMF) consultation should be obtained.

Equipment

Gloves, gauze, and a bite block should be available. Items to protect the operator's fingers such as tongue blades or plastic finger splints can be used. Depending on the technique chosen, common ED supplies may be needed (syringe, tongue blades).

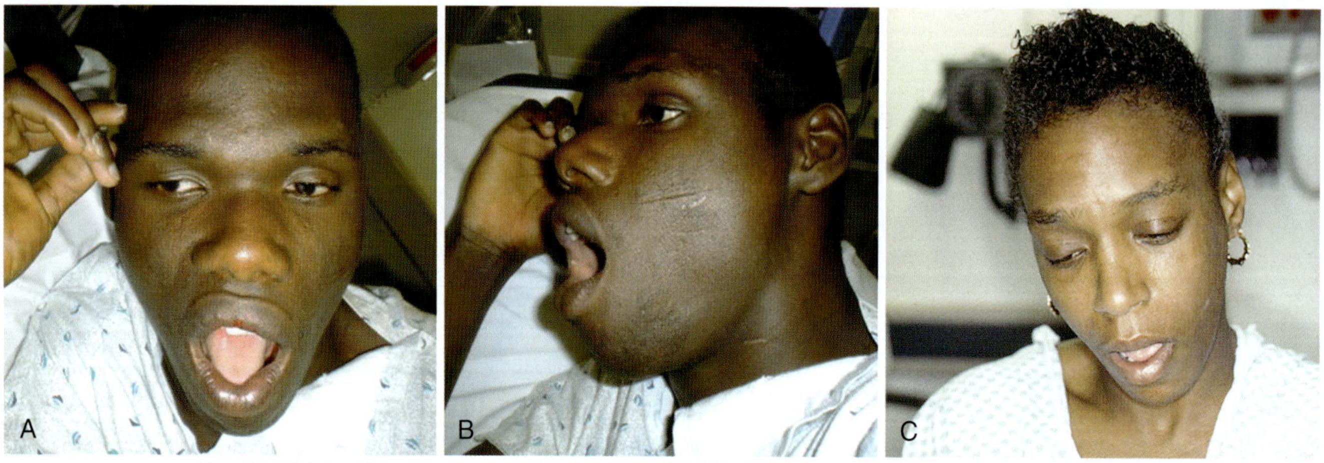

Fig. 64.47 Mandible (temporomandibular joint [TMJ]) dislocations. (A–B) This patient yawned and then could not close his mouth. This was a recurrent bilateral mandible dislocation. (C) This patient was suspected of having a dystonic reaction because she could not speak and her mandible was misaligned. It was a unilateral mandibular dislocation.

Procedure

See Videos 64.25–64.27. Reduction of a TMJ dislocation is straightforward. Because anterior dislocations are far more common, these techniques will be discussed here. The key to reduction is to direct the mandibular condyle out of its displaced location anterior to the articular eminence (Fig. 64.48A).[105] Because dislocation is painful, and there is a high degree of muscle spasm, pain control and muscle spasm reduction are key to successful reduction. This can include IV medications ranging from analgesia and/or anxiolysis to procedural sedation. Procedural sedation, however, is not required for all patients. One study reported only 39% required procedural sedation.[111] In addition, intraarticular injection of a local anesthetic, nerve block (masseteric, deep temporal nerve block), or pterygoid muscle injection can be performed. For TMJ injection, prepare the skin anterior to the ear, and introduce the needle into the TMJ space at the palpable depression caused by the dislocated condyle. Direct the needle anteriorly and superiorly onto the inferior surface of the glenoid fossa and inject 2 mL of local anesthetic. For the pterygoid muscle, inject 2 to 3 mL of anesthetic into the muscle posterior to the maxillary tuberosity.

There are several techniques that can be used for reduction. Clinicians should use the technique they are most familiar and have had success with. A potential algorithm is provided in Fig. 64.49.[106]

Classic/Traditional Bimanual Technique

This is also known as the Hippocratic technique and is one of the oldest, most common techniques and has a reported 86.2% to 86.7% success rate (see Figs. 64.48B and 64.50).[112,113] The patient is seated with their head stabilized against a headrest. Ask the patient to open their mouth as wide as possible to help relax the mandibular elevator muscles. Stand and face the patient and place your thumbs in the patient's mouth along the lower molar teeth. The level of the mandible should not be higher than the operator's elbow. Once the thumbs are positioned on the molars as far posteriorly as possible, curve the fingers and hand around the angle and body of the mandible along the jaw and chin. Then exert steady, constant downward pressure on the lower molar region, and direct the mandible inferiorly and posteriorly back into the temporal fossa. Be careful because once reduced, reflex spasm of the jaw muscles can suddenly snap the mandible shut and injure your thumbs. Additional upward force can be applied to the mentum with the third and fourth fingers to help rotate the inferior mandible anteriorly and facilitate the reduction.[1,112] A variation of this procedure is to have the patient sit on the ground with their head against the wall and stand over them for added leverage. It is also beneficial to have an assistant apply steady massage of the masseter muscles while simultaneously reducing the dislocation. (See Video 64.27.)

Posterior Approach

With the patient seated, stand behind the patient. Place your thumbs posterior to the last molar on the retromolar gum and along the ramus of the mandible.[114] Exert downward force in this position.

This procedure carries less risk of the fingers being bitten, but proper positioning of the thumbs may be difficult to accomplish.

Lever Technique

See Fig. 64.51.[115]A 3-cm diameter roll of gauze is placed in the posterior aspect of the patient's mouth near the third molar. Next, push upward on the mentum, using the gauze as a lever to disengage the mandible and rock it posteriorly. The original authors reported a 100% success rate.[115]

Syringe Technique

See Figs. 64.52C and 64.53.[5,116–118] The syringe technique is relatively novel, hands-free method for reduction of nontraumatic mandible dislocations that is fast, safe, effective, and does not require procedural sedation. In one study, 97% of patients were successfully reduced, with the majority occurring in less than 1 minute.[7,119] The syringe acts as a rolling fulcrum while the mandible and maxilla apply pressure on the syringe. With the patient seated, place a 5- or 10-mL syringe between the posterior upper and lower molars or the gums on the affected side. Instruct the patient to bite down and grasp the syringe between the teeth or gums. Next, ask the patient to roll the syringe back and forth, resulting in reduction of the dislocated TMJ joint. Syringe size varies with each patient and is determined by the distance between the upper and lower

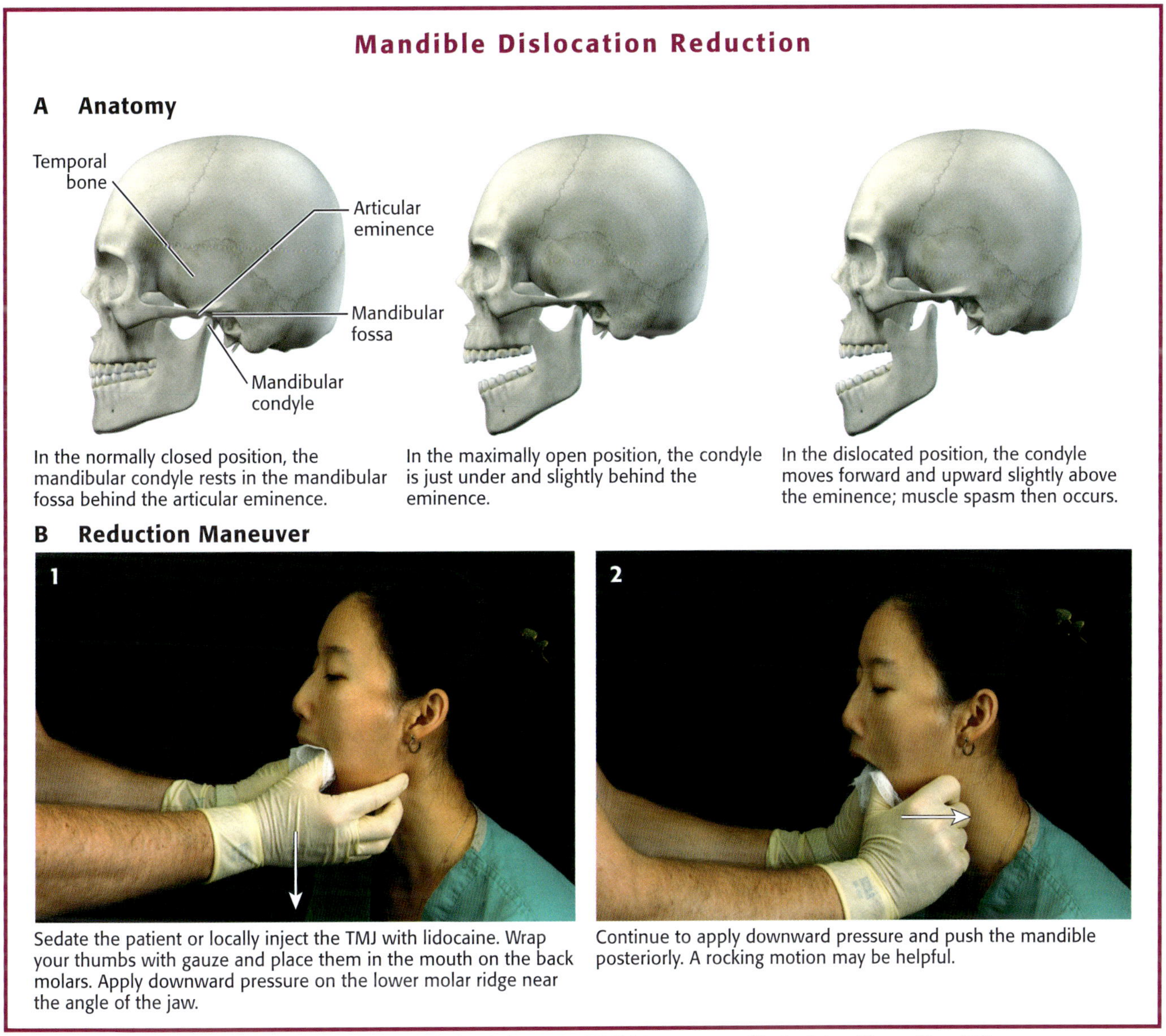

Fig. 64.48 Reduction of mandibular dislocation. *TMJ*, Temporomandibular joint. (From Chan TC, Harrigan RA, Ufberg J et al. Mandibular reduction. *J Emerg Med.* 2008;34:435-440.)

molars or gums and the ability to open the mouth on the affected side to allow syringe placement. The syringe acts as a rolling fulcrum. The mandible and maxilla apply pressure on the syringe. As the molars or gums move over the syringe, the gliding action moves the mandible posteriorly. The displaced condyle moves posteriorly to allow the condyle to slide back into its normal position. In bilateral dislocations, reducing one side will spontaneously reduce the other.

Stacked Tongue Blade

See Fig. 64.54.[119] This technique uses a large stack of tongue blades secured together and inserted into the open mouth to slightly over exaggerate the dislocation and to overcome the muscle spasm. Sedation is typically not required.

First, estimate the number of tongue blades that can fit in the mouth. Next, tape the tongue blades together and place in the mouth between the teeth. As the spasm is overcome and the mouth opens wider, additional tongue blades are inserted. When no more can be added, quickly remove the stack. There is a brief window where the muscles are relaxed and the dislocation may reduce spontaneously or by using one of the other described techniques.

Aftercare

In uncomplicated cases, postreduction imaging is not required as the patient will feel back to baseline and will be able to close their mouth. However, in cases of pain or when unsure, imaging (plain film, Panorex, or CT) is recommended to confirm reduction and to assess for fractures.[120,121] A bandage may be placed around the patient's head and mandible (Barton bandage, Fig. 64.55).[105,106,120] Alternatively, a rigid cervical collar can be used to provide support along the mandible. Upon discharge, the patient should be advised to avoid extreme mouth opening and to eat soft food for 1 week. Warm compresses, nonsteroidal antiinflammatory agents, and muscle relaxants may be helpful. The patient may be referred to an ENT or OMF surgeon for further care. Patients with chronic dislocation may require surgical fixation.

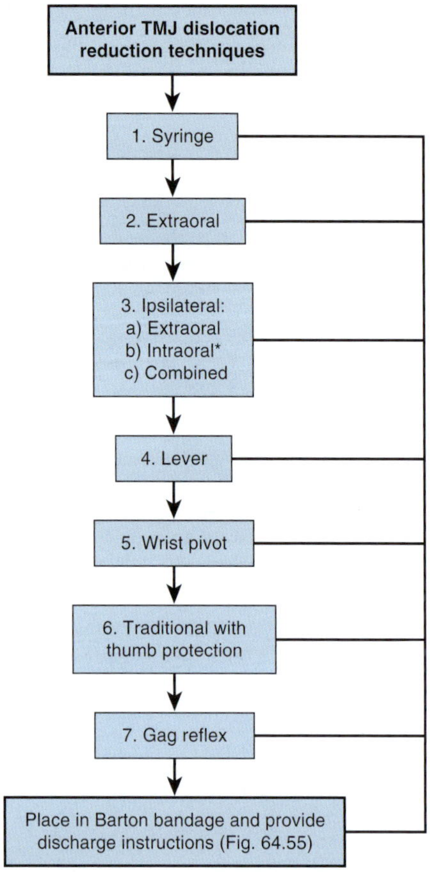

Fig. 64.49 Proposed algorithm for the management of temporomandibular joint dislocation *(TMJ)*. *Single hand or unified hand. (From Gottlieb M, Long B. Managing temporomandibular joint dislocations. *Ann Emerg Med*. 2022;80:539-547.)

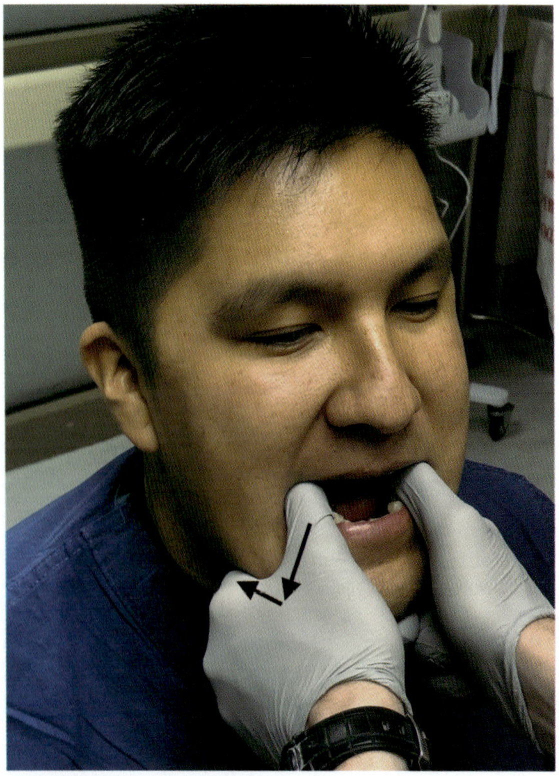

Fig. 64.50 Classic/traditional/bimanual reduction technique.

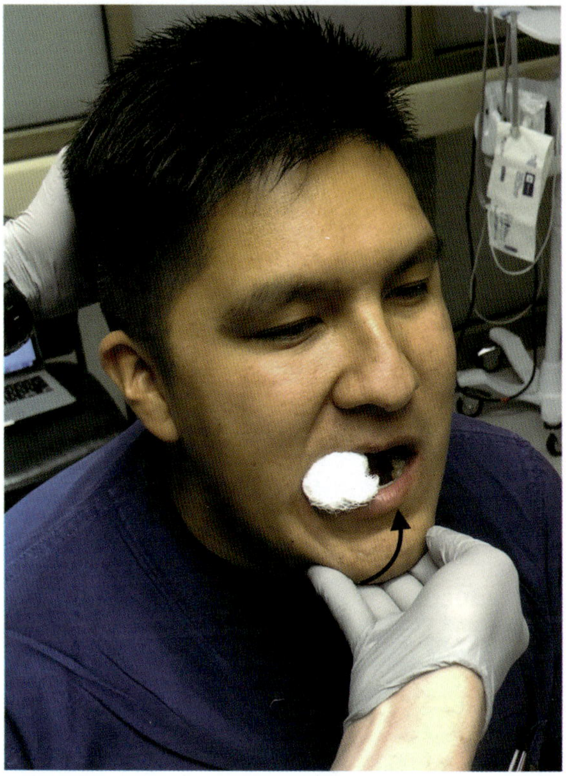

Fig. 64.51 Lever technique.

Complications

The most common complication is recurrent dislocations. Other complications include injuries to both the patient and operator. Patient injuries include repeat dislocation, mandibular fracture (rare), joint cartilage injuries, torn ligaments or muscles, and dental or gum injuries as a result of trauma from the attempt at reduction. There may be complications associated with procedural sedation as well.

Operator injuries are prominent in techniques that require placement of the operator's fingers in the mouth or on the teeth. These are usually caused by sudden masseter spasm after reduction. This results in the patient involuntarily biting down on the operator's thumbs. Take measures such as gauze and plastic finger splints to prevent such injuries to the thumbs.

Posttonsillectomy Bleeding

Hemorrhage is the most serious complication of adenotonsillectomy, with reported rates of 0.5% to 10%, depending on the technique (Fig.64.56).[59,121] Bleeding is categorized as intraoperative, primary (within 24 hours), and secondary (between 24 hours and 10 days). Bleeding is always serious and must be evaluated and controlled quickly. The most common time for patients to be seen in the ED with delayed bleeding is between the fifth and seventh postoperative days. Although some bleeding is minor, sudden severe hemorrhage can be fatal if not managed appropriately. If active bleeding is confirmed by physical examination, consult otolaryngology. Minor bleeding 5 to 10 days postoperatively secondary to eschar separation may be evaluated and treated in the ED. However, multiple bleeding episodes are common in those who bleed, and minor bleeding may herald more significant subsequent hemorrhage. A severely bleeding patient should

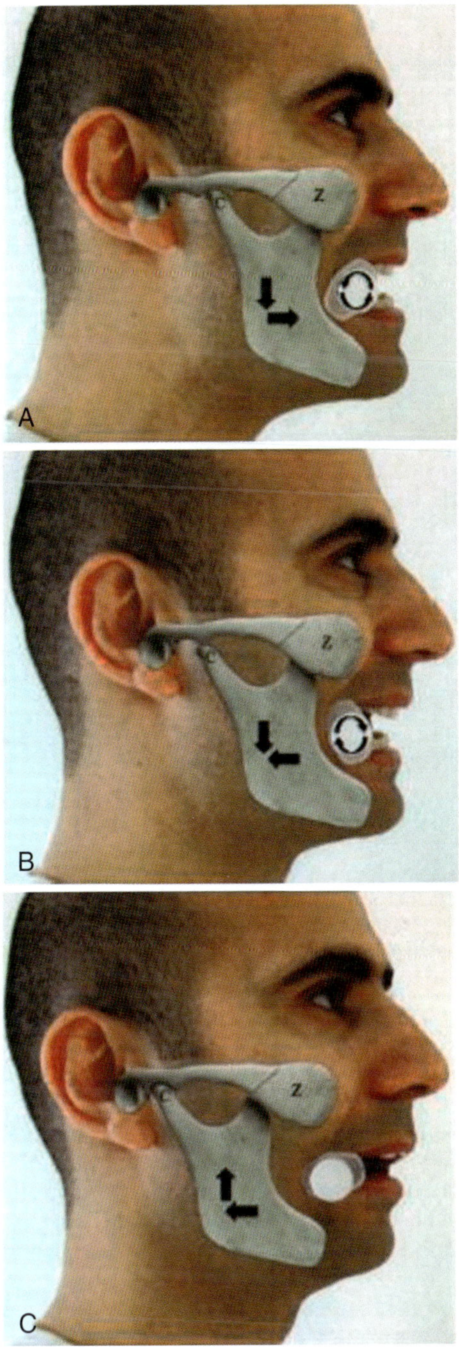

Fig. 64.52 (A) Dislocated temporomandibular joint (TMJ) where the condyle is displaced anterior to the articular eminence with syringe placement between the posterior molars. (B) Gliding of the mandible posteriorly as the molars roll over the syringe. (C) Normal TMJ with syringe placement. *C*, Condyle; *Z*, zygomatic bone. (From Gorchynski J, Karabidian E, Sanchez M. The "syringe" technique: a hands-free approach for the reduction of acute nontraumatic temporomandibular dislocations in the emergency department, *J Emerg Med.* 2014;47(6):676-681,.)

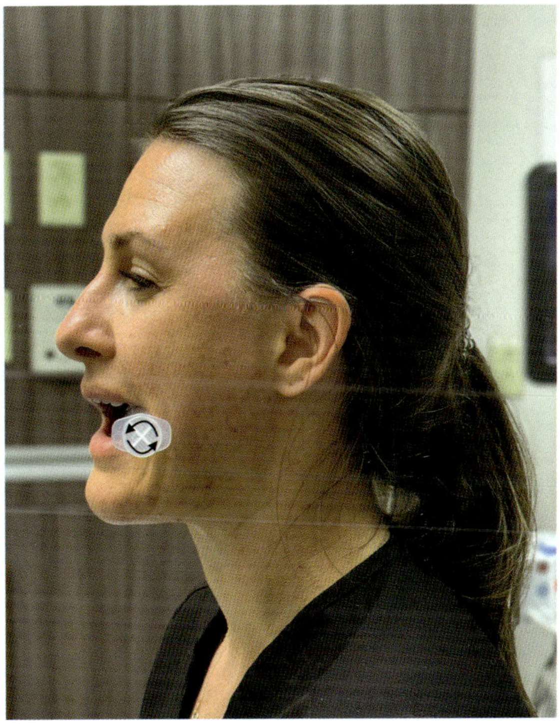

Fig. 64.53 Syringe technique.

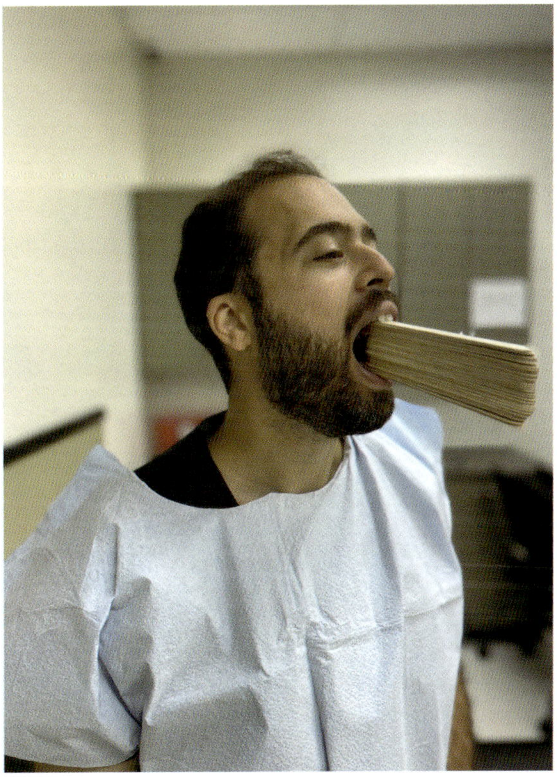

Fig. 64.54 Stacked tongue blade technique. Stacked tongue blades are inserted into the open mouth and as patient will allow, more are inserted until masseter muscle spasm is overcome and the dislocation can be reduced.

be taken to the operating room immediately for hemostasis. Up to 50% of patients who have major postoperative bleeding require control in the operating room.[121] It is difficult and occasionally impossible to even initially control severe hemorrhage in the ED. ED management includes airway control, medications, and direct pressure/local hemostatic maneuvers. Do not hesitate to intubate a massively bleeding patient to protect the airway and more easily perform local maneuvers. First administer TXA intravenously, 1 g in adults and 15 mg/kg in children. Until the surgeon arrives, apply pressure directly on the bleeding area with a sponge on a long

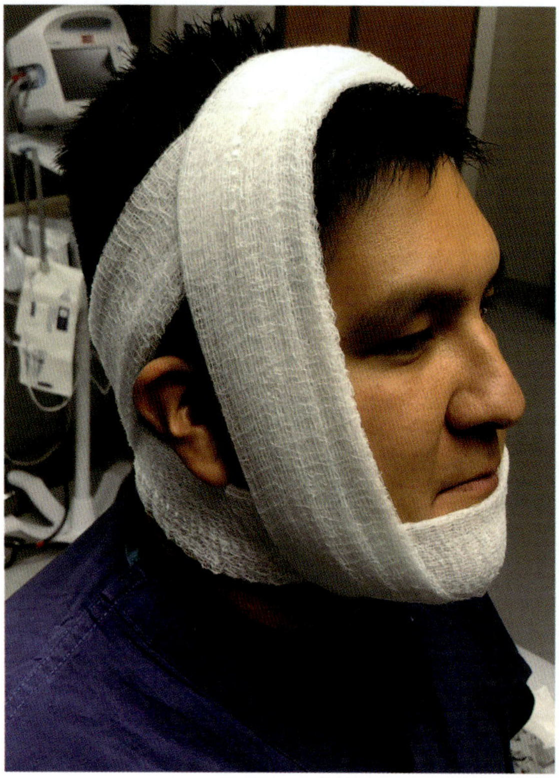

Fig. 64.55 Barton dressing/bandage placement after successful reduction.

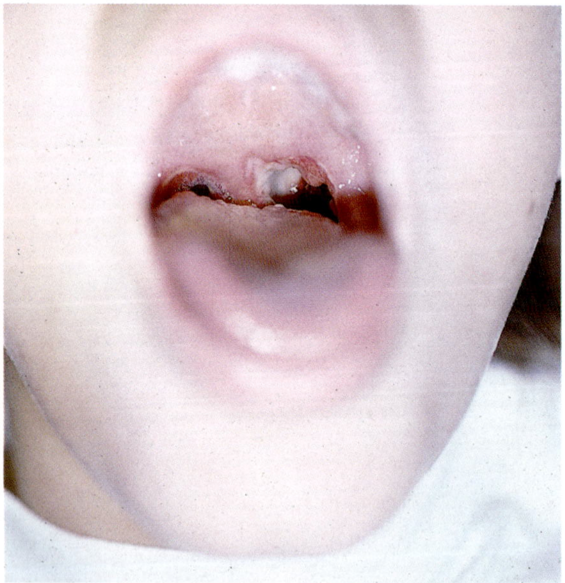

Fig. 64.56 Typical appearance of the oral cavity 5 to 7 days after bilateral tonsillectomy. This is a common time for bleeding.

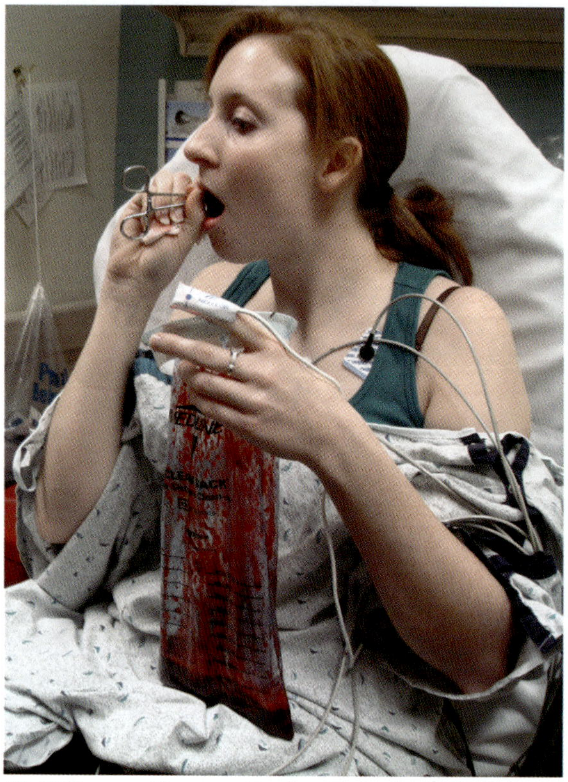

Fig. 64.57 Posttonsillectomy bleeding is a serious complication that is difficult to control in the emergency department; an ear, nose, and throat surgeon and the resources of the operating room are often required. Massive bleeding can be fatal. This cooperative patient tried to tamponade her bleeding with direct pressure with a 4 × 4-inch pad on a hemostat, without success. She eventually became hypotensive and required urgent tracheal intubation and control of the bleeding in the operating room.

clamp (Fig. 64.57). The sponge may be dipped in epinephrine or thrombin powder if available. This is often not tolerated by patients. The bleeding area can also be infiltrated with lidocaine with epinephrine.

If a patient is seen in the ED with a complaint of posttonsillectomy bleeding but no active bleeding is found on examination and a blood clot is present, do not remove the clot. It may be tempting to discharge stable patients, but definitive treatment and disposition are best made by the surgeon. If bleeding is present, or has temporarily stopped, it is prudent to admit the patient for observation. Obtain a sample of blood for a coagulation profile and a complete blood count. Blood transfusions may be required. Specific factor replacement or component therapy can be used for patients with hematological disorders.

REFERENCES ARE AVAILABLE AT ELSEVIER EBOOKS+

CHAPTER 65

Emergency Dental Procedures

Merle Carter

INTRODUCTION

The emergency department (ED) commonly evaluates and treats complaints pertaining to the teeth and supporting maxillofacial structures. Patient complaints may range in scope from a simple chipped tooth to an odontogenic deep space infection or a maxillofacial injury. Many emergency clinicians and other acute care providers do not receive instruction dedicated to dental emergencies during their training, yet it is important for them to be able to recognize and treat a wide range of dental and related maxillofacial problems. It is critically important for emergency providers to be able to recognize and treat a wide range of dental and maxillofacial problems, and know when referral or urgent consultation is warranted. Some dental emergencies can lead to significant morbidity such as loss of teeth, chronic pain, infection, and craniofacial abnormalities, while others can lead to life-threatening airway compromise.

Management of specific dental emergencies requires a thorough understanding of adult and pediatric dentition. This chapter reviews the relevant anatomy of adult and pediatric dentition, as well as techniques for the management of common conditions, often to temporize until definitive dental consultation or maxillofacial surgery referral can be obtained. Conditions that require emergency consultation are discussed. Topical, local, and regional anesthesia are discussed, as well as the initial stabilization of fractured, subluxed, luxated, and avulsed teeth; bleeding; dry sockets; abscesses; and infections. Topical, local, and regional anesthesia are of particular importance in the management of odontogenic emergencies, so the clinician should be very familiar with these techniques (Videos 65.1–65.3).

Although this chapter describes the diagnosis and treatment of dental injuries that may confront emergency clinicians, it is important to note that standard of care does not mandate that complex dental problems (e.g., replacement of avulsed teeth, drainage of deep space infections, etc.) be definitively treated in the ED. However, most simple oral or dental infections or injuries can be initially managed in the emergency setting. Advances in ED equipment and clinician training, as well as the introduction of dental skills laboratories into resident education, are gradually raising the existing standard of care for emergency providers. The initial stabilization of fractured, subluxed, luxated, and avulsed teeth, as well as bleeding and dry sockets, is now within the treatment realm of the emergency clinician. Likewise, abscesses and infections should be properly identified and drained where indicated. It is appropriate to consult or refer all significant or complicated dental pathology to an appropriate specialist.

TEETH

The adult dentition normally consists of 32 teeth: 8 incisors, 4 canines, 8 premolars, and 12 molars. From the midline to the back of the mouth on each side, there is a central incisor, a lateral incisor, a canine (cuspid), two premolars (bicuspids), and three molars, the last of which is called the wisdom tooth (Fig. 65.1). The 20 primary or deciduous (baby) teeth include 8 incisors, 4 canines, and 8 molars. From the midline to the back of the mouth, there is a central incisor, a lateral incisor, a canine, and two molars (Fig. 65.2). There are no premolars in the primary dentition. *Agenesis*, or lack of proper formation of a tooth or teeth, is not uncommon, especially in the maxilla. Likewise, *supernumerary*, or extra, teeth may also occur. The adult teeth are numbered from 1 to 32. Numerous classification and numbering systems of the teeth exist. However, given the possibility of missing or extra teeth, many consultants simply prefer the description of the involved tooth (or teeth) rather than the numbering convention (e.g., right lower lateral incisor, left upper second molar, etc.). For our purposes, the first tooth is the right upper third molar and the 16th tooth being the left upper third molar. The left lower third molar is the 17th, and the 32nd tooth is the right lower third molar.

A tooth consists of the central pulp, the dentin, and the enamel (Fig. 65.3). The pulp contains the neurovascular supply of the tooth, which is responsible for carrying nutrients to the dentin, a microporous substance that consists of a system of microtubules. The dentin makes up the majority of the tooth, is a primary determinant of tooth color, and cushions the tooth during biting or chewing. The enamel is the relatively translucent, outermost portion of the tooth and the hardest part of the body. The tooth may also be described in terms of the crown (coronal portion) and the root (apex portion). The crown is the portion covered in enamel; the root is the part that serves to anchor the tooth in the alveolar bone.

The following descriptive terminology is used for the different anatomic surfaces of the tooth and helpful when describing injury or other pathology in the medical record or to a consultant or colleague:

- *Facial*: the part of the tooth that faces the opening of the mouth. This is the part that you see when somebody smiles. It is a general term applicable to all teeth.
- *Labial*: the facial surface of the incisors and canines.
- *Buccal*: the facial surface of the premolars and molars.
- *Oral*: the part of the tooth that faces the tongue or the palate. This is a general term applicable to all teeth.
- *Lingual*: toward the tongue; the oral surface of the mandibular teeth.
- *Palatal*: toward the palate; the oral surface of the maxillary teeth.
- *Approximal/interproximal*: the contacting surfaces between two adjacent teeth.
- *Mesial*: the interproximal surface facing anteriorly or closest to the midline.
- *Distal*: the interproximal surface facing posteriorly or away from the midline.
- *Occlusal*: biting or chewing surface of the premolars and molars.
- *Incisal*: biting or chewing surface of the incisors and canines.
- *Apical*: toward the tip of the root of the tooth.
- *Coronal*: toward the crown or the biting surface of the tooth.

PERIDONTIUM

The *periodontium*, also known as the attachment apparatus, consists of two major subunits and is necessary for maintaining the integrity of the normal dentoalveolar unit.

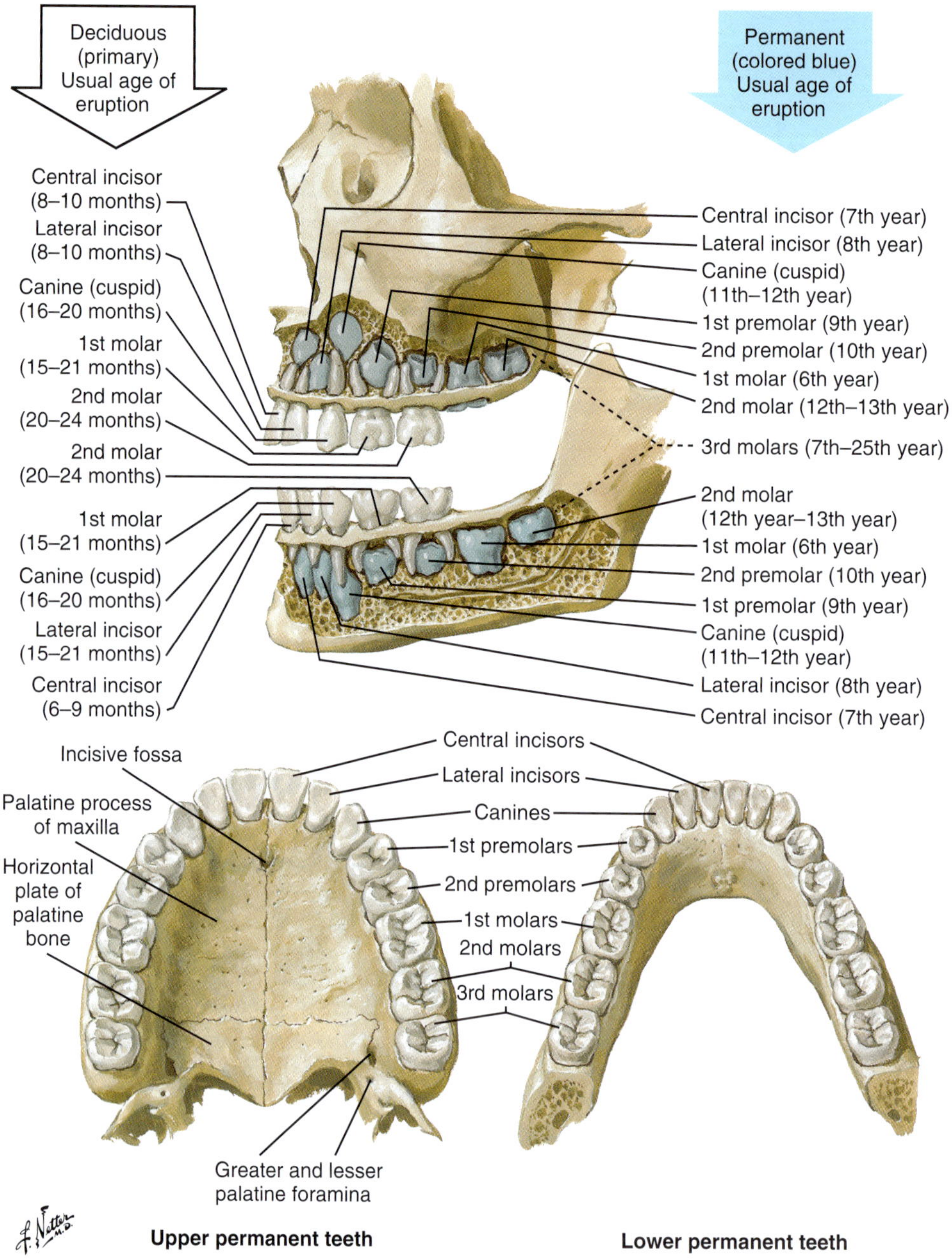

Fig. 65.1 Anatomy of the teeth, primary and permanent. *Note*: an avulsed primary tooth need not be reimplanted if it is lost traumatically. (Netter illustrations from www.netterimages.com. Elsevier, Inc. All rights reserved.)

The *gingival subunit* consists of the junctional epithelium and gingival tissue. Gingival tissue is composed of keratinized, stratified squamous epithelium; it can be divided into the free gingival margin and the attached gingiva. The free gingiva is the cuff of tissue formed around the neck of the tooth. The gingival sulcus is the space between the free gingiva and the tooth. It is rarely greater than 2 mm to 3 mm in depth in normal healthy dentition. The attached gingiva is the portion of gingiva attached to alveolar bone and extends apically (away from the tooth) to the mucogingival junction (or the mucobuccal fold). At this point the tissue, loose and nonkeratinized, is called the alveolar mucosa (or buccal mucosa).

The *periodontal subunit* includes the periodontal ligament, alveolar bone, and the cementum of the root of the tooth. The periodontal ligament consists of collagen that extends from the alveolar bone to the root of the tooth. One end of the periodontal ligament inserts into the alveolar bone and the other end into the cementum.

The gingival subunit is primarily responsible for maintaining the integrity of the periodontal subunit. Certain disease states such as gingivitis weaken the attachment apparatus and can result in loss of a tooth.

ACUTE TOOTHACHE IN THE ED

Patients with facial pain or swelling often seek evaluation and relief of symptoms. These symptoms are often odontogenic. In addition to direct trauma, several causes for dental pain exist. Postsurgical pain is a common dental complaint in the emergency setting and typically follows an expected course to

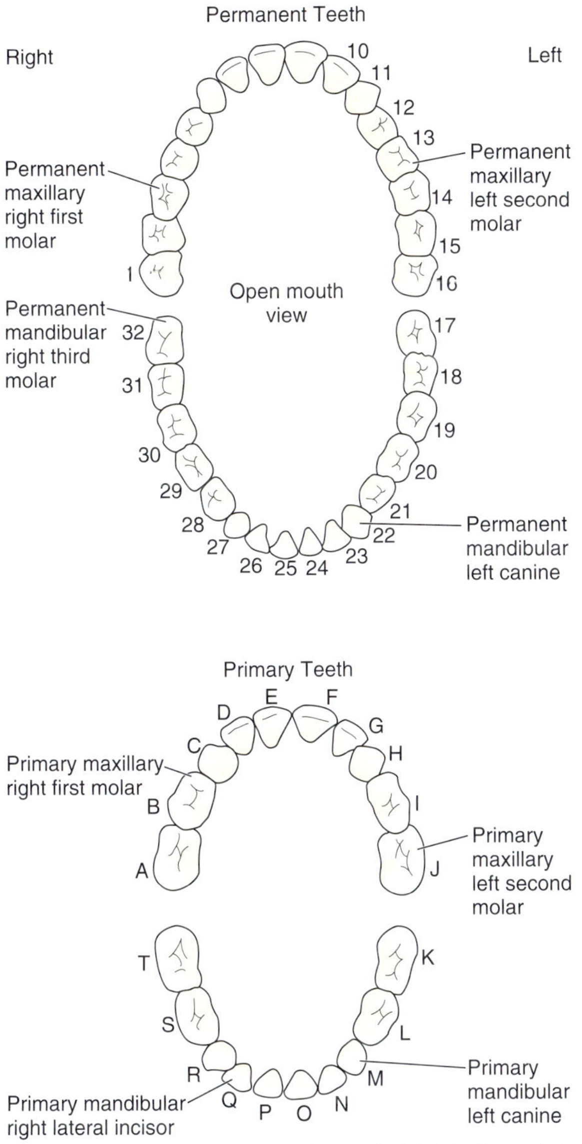

Fig. 65.2 Identification of teeth, adult and child. Each tooth has a number assigned to it. By 14 years of age, all primary teeth should normally be lost. Do not reimplant an avulsed primary tooth; instead, refer to a dentist to prevent future misalignment of the permanent teeth.

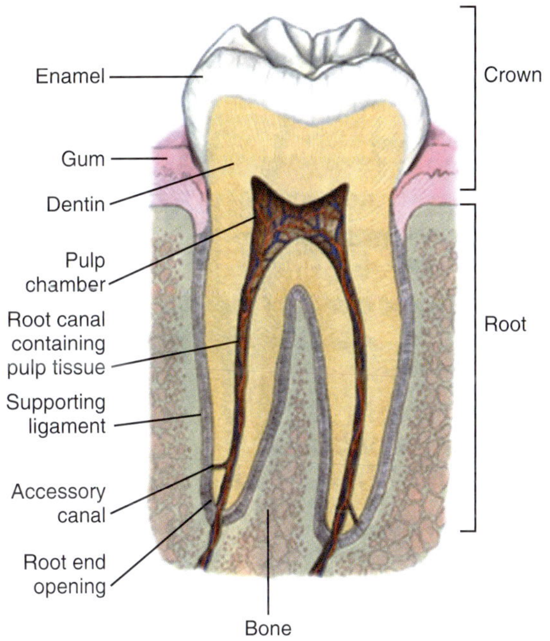

Fig. 65.3 The dental anatomic unit.

resolution depending on the procedure. Pain in a tooth when exposed to hot liquids usually indicates pulpal inflammation. Sensitivity to cold can signify simple sensitivity, gum recession, or indicate decay. Pain while biting down or to percussion can indicate a fractured tooth or supporting structure, abscess, or decay. Dental fillings can leak over time and cause significant pain. Microcracks can also occur and may not be apparent to a practitioner who is not a dentist or oral surgeon. Another cause of microcracks or a fractured tooth is the constant trauma from intraoral piercings. Although multiple problems can initially cause pain in the teeth or gums, the cause is usually pulpitis, infection, abscess, or dental trauma. Pulpitis can be either acute or chronic and the cause, treatment, aftercare, and prognosis are different for each patient. Unfortunately, by the time many patients seek emergency care they have irreversible pulpitis composed of a complex microbial environment.[1] For cases beyond the scope of the emergency clinician, immediate consultation or referral to a dentist or other appropriate oral care specialist (e.g., oral-maxillofacial surgeon, ear, nose, and throat [ENT] surgeon) is the definitive course of action. However, pain relief and antibiotics (where appropriate) should be initiated in the ED.

Oral analgesics and local anesthetic injections are common strategies for pain relief. Nonopioid and nonsteroidal antiinflammatory agents are the most commonly prescribed agents. More recently, the early use of oral steroids like dexamethasone as an adjunct to these conventional analgesics has been shown to reduce time to pain resolution in dental abscesses.[2]

For many years, those seeking more natural alternatives have turned to topical olive oil[3] or eugenol-containing clove oil[4] as reasonably effective short-term home remedies for acute toothache, inflamed gingiva, or postextraction pain. For a cavity or gingival pain without obvious infection, gauze saturated in clove or olive oil and placed directly into the cavity or along the gumline can provide relief for a few hours until definitive management is undertaken by a specialist. Clove oil should not be used more than two to three times because of irritation and possible nerve damage. Viscous lidocaine is another simple method of pain control when applied directly onto the tooth or by saturating a small cotton ball with the gel and placing it into a cavity. This treatment is temporary, and caution should be exercised if reapplication is considered. Do not exceed the total recommended dosage of lidocaine. A case report by Hile and Linklater[5] reported significant pain relief in a fractured tooth by applying 2-octylcyanoacrylate tissue adhesive (Super Glue) directly to the tooth. This specific intervention in fractured teeth has not been prospectively studied. However, case reports identify cyanoacrylate adhesive as an effective desensitizing agent[6] and may also provide temporary relief for patients with open decay when air and temperature exacerbate the pain. To apply, dry the tooth thoroughly with gauze, and generously apply two to three layers of the product to the affected area. This intervention lasts less than 24 hours before enzymatic breakdown occurs in the oral cavity and its effectiveness declines. It is important to note

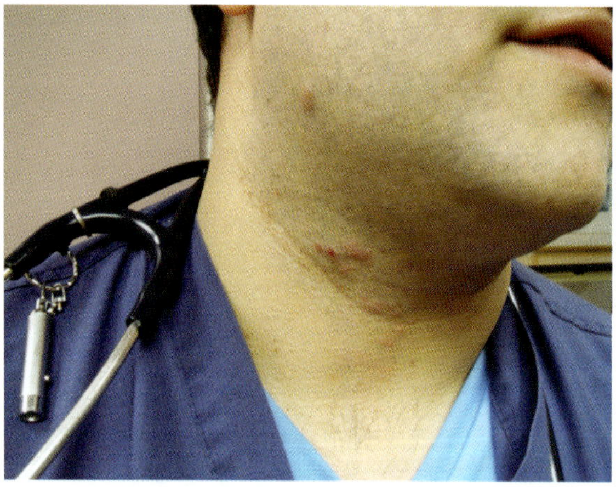

Fig. 65.4 This patient had severe pain in his jaw thought to be related to a dental problem. Two days after onset of the pain, the rash of herpes zoster appeared, which was the cause of the pain.

that while the use of skin adhesives for this purpose has been increasing, it is not currently approved for intraoral use.

Acute dental pain may also be referred pain, so a complete evaluation should be conducted if the intraoral or facial anatomy in question appears to be normal (Fig. 65.4). For example, acute sinusitis can cause dental pain and vice versa. Patients complaining of ear pain may have dental infection, and someone complaining of a posterior toothache may have otologic pathology. Antibiotics should be initiated when an obvious intraoral or dental infection exists until the patient receives definitive care from the appropriate specialist. Antibiotics provide no benefit for pain from a simple toothache, dental cavity, or pulpitis, although some clinicians prescribe them because follow-up dental care may be delayed or difficult to obtain.[7] The emergency clinician may not be able to confirm whether a periapical abscess exists or if definitive care is likely to be delayed. In these cases, prescribing an antibiotic may be a reasonable choice. Penicillin, clindamycin, and amoxicillin-clavulanate (or ampicillin-sulbactam) are still considered the mainstays for these polymicrobial infections.

It is important to inquire about duration of symptoms and the amount of analgesics used by patients prior to presenting to the ED. Chronic acetaminophen overdose is a known complication of overaggressive use of analgesics by patients unable to obtain dental care for an acute toothache.[8] Individual teeth (except the posterior molars) can be temporarily anesthetized with total pain relief by a supraperiosteal injection of a local anesthetic (see Chapter 30). Molars are more difficult to anesthetize with supraperiosteal injections. However, they can be anesthetized via different nerve block techniques, such as the inferior alveolar nerve block. Of the local anesthetics, bupivacaine has a long duration of action (4 to 12 hours) and has been shown to decrease the narcotic requirement of postoperative oral surgery patients even after the anesthetic properties of the medication have worn off.[9]

DENTOALVEOLAR TRAUMA

Dental Fractures

See Video 65.4. Maxillofacial and dentoalveolar trauma are common reasons for ED visits and can result in fractures, displacement of a tooth from its position in the alveolus (luxation), total avulsion, or injury of the supporting structures. Missing the diagnosis can lead to delayed treatment and poor outcomes. Frequent causes include sports-related injuries, motor vehicle or bicycle accidents, falls, and interpersonal violence. Studies have shown that 48% of facial injuries involve the oral cavity.[10] The incidence of dentoalveolar trauma has been linked to socioeconomic and insurance status, race, and age[11] which can impact aftercare and anticipated outcomes. Traumatic dental injuries involving primary teeth has a worldwide prevalence of 22.7%, occurring in young children as they learn to crawl, walk, and run.[12] More than 75% of tooth fractures are in the upper jaw, and more than half of these involve central incisors, followed by lateral incisors and canines. The maxillary central and lateral incisors are the most frequently fractured teeth because of their anatomic position in the oral cavity.[13–15] For these reasons, a high index of suspicion is required when evaluating patients with maxillofacial injury, particularly in children where management depends on whether the injury involves primary or permanent teeth.

Some general principles apply to the evaluation and management of dental trauma. Dentoalveolar fractures are often classified into four groups: (1) crown/root fractures, (2) luxation/displacement of teeth, (3) avulsion, and (4) alveolar fractures.[10] First, identify all fracture fragments and mobile teeth. Percuss each tooth surface for mobility and sensitivity. If an empty socket is present, do not assume that the tooth has been avulsed and missing. Teeth can be aspirated into the respiratory tract, swallowed into the gastrointestinal tract, or fully intruded into the maxillary sinus, alveolar bone, or nasal cavity. Appropriate radiographs may be required if there is a suspicion of aspiration or ingestion of tooth fragments, or intrusion of fragments into the gingiva or alveolar bone. Second, the oral cavity is more easily evaluated and managed if the patient is not in significant discomfort. Analgesia and common dental or regional anesthesia used early should be part of the emergency clinician's armamentarium. Third, long-term use of topical tooth remedies and analgesics, both over-the-counter and prescribed, should be discouraged as this can lead to the development of sterile abscesses and soft tissue irritation. Fourth, administer tetanus vaccine and/or antibiotics as indicated.

Acute trauma to the teeth is not usually life-threatening; however, outcomes are largely based on time from injury to immediate management, then to definitive treatment. The morbidity associated with poorly managed dental fractures can be significant and includes failure to complete eruption, change in color of the tooth, abscess, pulp necrosis, loss of space in the dental arch, ankylosis, abnormal exfoliation, tooth loss, and root resorption. Dental injuries are often associated with intraoral lacerations. When a tooth is chipped or missing, there is often a concomitant intraoral laceration and risk that the missing portion of the tooth is embedded in the laceration (Fig. 65.5).

Management of fractured teeth depends on the extent of fracture with regard to the pulp, the degree of development of the apex of the tooth, and the age of the patient. Early consultation or referral is essential and can significantly improve outcomes. Dentoalveolar injuries and, in particular, tooth fractures have been classified in several ways.[16] The Ellis classification is one system commonly cited in the emergency medicine literature; however, some dentists and maxillofacial surgeons do not use this nomenclature making the terminology less than ideal when discussing these injuries with specialists (Fig. 65.6).[16] The most easily understood method

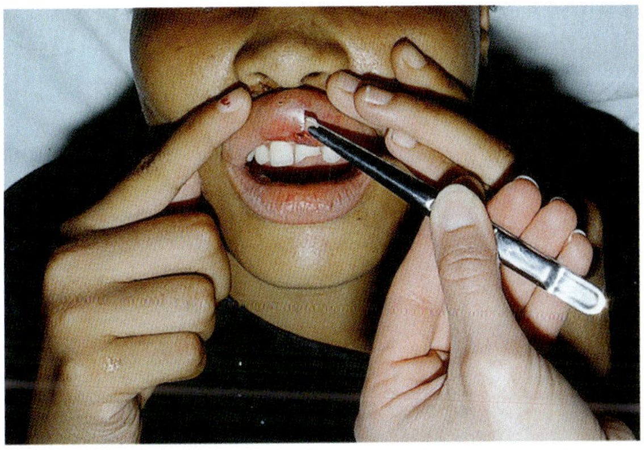

Fig. 65.5 A chipped front tooth after a punch to the mouth can result in a piece of tooth being aspirated or embedded in the surrounding tissue. When this lip laceration was explored, a piece of tooth was found within the laceration. If this foreign body is not removed, an infection is certain to occur within a few days. Note the obvious chipped upper tooth, the source of the piece found in the upper lip laceration.

of classification is one based on description of the injury and parts of the tooth exposed or injured.

The most common traumatic dental injury to permanent teeth are crown fractures.[17,18] Crown fractures may be divided into uncomplicated and complicated categories. Uncomplicated crown fractures result from injuries to the enamel alone or to a combination of the enamel and dentin. Complicated crown fractures extend into the pulp. Common complications of traumatic dental injuries are pulp necrosis, pulp infections, pulp space obliteration, root resorption, and breakdown of the gingiva and underlying bone.[17]

Ellis Class I Fractures

Uncomplicated crown fractures through only the enamel are known as *Ellis class I fractures* (see Fig. 65.6B) and are not sensitive to either temperature or forced air. These fractures generally pose minimal threat to the health of the dental pulp; however, follow-up with a dentist should be undertaken following ED evaluation. Ellis I fractures may feel sharp to the patient's tongue, lips, or buccal mucosa. Immediate treatment is not often necessary but may consist of smoothing the sharp edge of the tooth with an emery board or rotary disk sander. Nonurgent follow-up is important to ensure the integrity of the tooth and surrounding tissue is maintained. These patients can be reassured that a dentist can restore the tooth to its normal appearance with composite resins and bonding material and to watch for any progression that might occur.

Ellis Class II Fractures

Uncomplicated fractures through the enamel and dentin are called *Ellis class II fractures*. Fractures that extend into the dentin are at higher risk for pulp necrosis and therefore require more aggressive treatment by the emergency clinician (see Fig. 65.6C). The risk for pulp necrosis in these patients is less than 10%; however, it increases as treatment time extends beyond 24 hours.[16] These patients often complain of sensitivity to heat, cold, or forced air. Physical examination reveals the yellow tint of the dentin in contrast to the white hue of the enamel. With fractures closer to the pulp cavity, the dentin will have a pink tinge. The tooth is usually sensitive to percussion with a tongue depressor. The porous nature of dentin allows passage of bacteria from the oral cavity to the pulp, which may result in inflammation and infection of the pulp chamber. This is more likely to occur after 24 hours of dentin exposure but occurs sooner if the fracture site is closer to the pulp. Likewise, patients younger than 12 years have a pulp-to-dentin ratio larger than that in mature adults and are at increased risk for pulp contamination and infection. For this reason, younger patients should be treated aggressively and be seen by a dentist within 24 to 48 hours.[19,20]

The goal of treating dentin fractures is twofold: (1) to cover the exposed dentin and thus prevent secondary contamination or infection, and (2) to provide pain relief. After the tooth is covered, the patient can follow up with a dentist who can use modern composites to rebuild the tooth directly over the cap that was placed in the emergency setting. The most commonly used compound to cap these fractures is a paste composed of calcium hydroxide (CaOH) (Dycal [Dentsply Sirona], Preline [Henry Schein], or other similar products) (Fig. 65.7). Prior to any manipulation of the tooth, anesthetize the area using a supraperiosteal injection or a regional nerve block. This will make application of the paste less painful and therefore easier to apply. Other pastes/dressings that may be applied to the surface of the tooth include zinc oxide and liquid skin adhesives.[5] Many dental dressings come as a base and a catalyst which require mixing, but are often available in premixed formulations as well. Resin-based composites and glass ionomer cements have been proposed in the dental literature as additional options for treating dentin fractures.[21] However, the cost and availability make them less optimal for use in the emergency setting particularly when other options are readily accessible. While bone wax and skin adhesives are not recommended as long-term solutions, they may be required in the emergency setting when CaOH paste or other compounds are not available.

To use CaOH, combine the catalyst and the base in equal portions to create the paste. The surface of the tooth must be dry to ensure adherence of any applied paste or dressing. To dry the surface of the tooth, have the patient bite into gauze pads or mouth breathe for a few minutes. Likewise, connecting a nasal cannula to high-pressure wall O_2 and aiming it at the tooth will facilitate drying, but maintain it at a pressure that does not cause discomfort. Once the tooth is dry, place a small amount of paste on the exposed area using a cotton-tipped applicator or another appropriate instrument (see Fig. 65.7). CaOH will dry within minutes even after being exposed to the moist environment of the mouth. Although placing dental foil over the CaOH dressing is recommended in some texts, it is not necessary if the patient plans to follow up with a dentist within 24 to 36 hours. It is also not technically easy to perform. To prevent dislodgment of the CaOH dressing, instruct the patient to eat only soft foods until seen by a dentist. Although there is no evidence to support antibiotic therapy for fractured teeth in the ED, some recommend antibiotics until definitive dental care is obtained.[22]

Many patients who sustain a fracture through the dentin will require a root canal or other definitive endodontic treatment. Timely application of an appropriate dressing in the ED, however, may prevent contamination and infection of the pulp and therefore make a painful root canal therapy unnecessary. As with any significant trauma to the teeth, explain to the patient that disruption of the neurovascular supply is possible and that long-term complications such as pulp necrosis, color change, and resorption of the root may occur, and that timely dental follow-up is paramount.

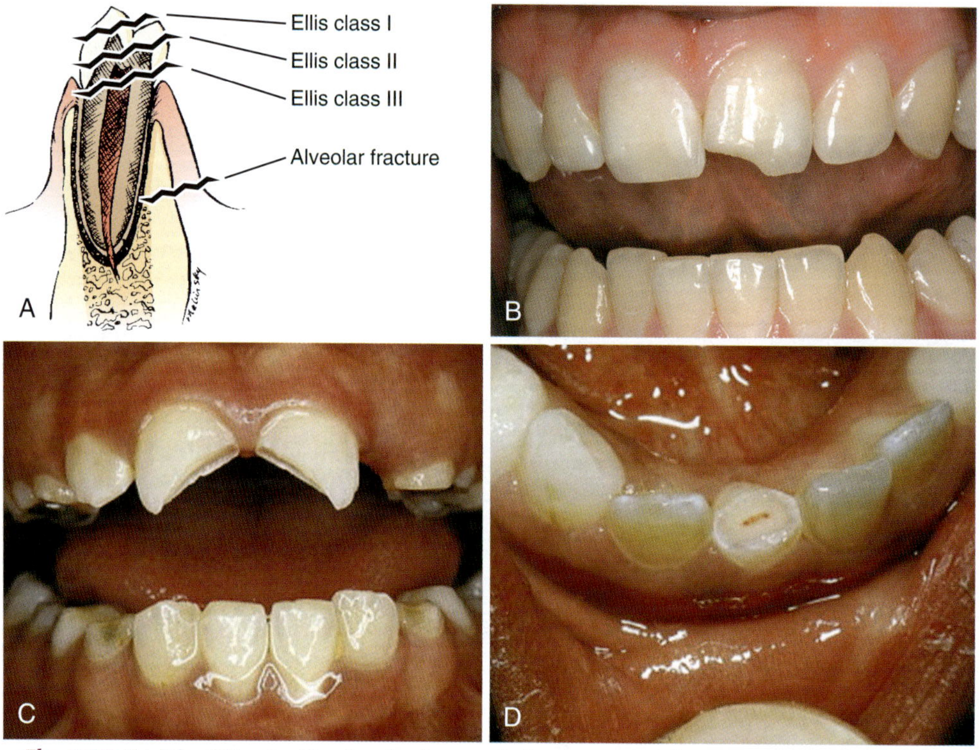

Fig. 65.6 (A) The Ellis classification for fractured alveolar teeth. The easiest method to classify fractured teeth is by description (e.g., fracture through the dentin of the first upper right molar). (B) Ellis class I: only the enamel is fractured. These fractures pose no threat to the dental pulp and are not sensitive to temperature or forced air. (C) Ellis class II: the crown fracture demonstrates involvement of the enamel and dentin, without exposure of the pulp. Immediate dental referral is necessary to prevent contamination of the pulp through the dentinal tubules. (D) This crown fracture involves enamel, dentin, and the soft tissue of the pulp as well. Immediate dental referral is mandatory to save the tooth. (C–D, from Zitelli BJ McIntire SC, Nowalk AJ, eds. *Zitelli and Davis' Atlas of Pediatric Physical Diagnosis.* 6th ed. Saunders; 2012.)

Calcium Hydroxide Application

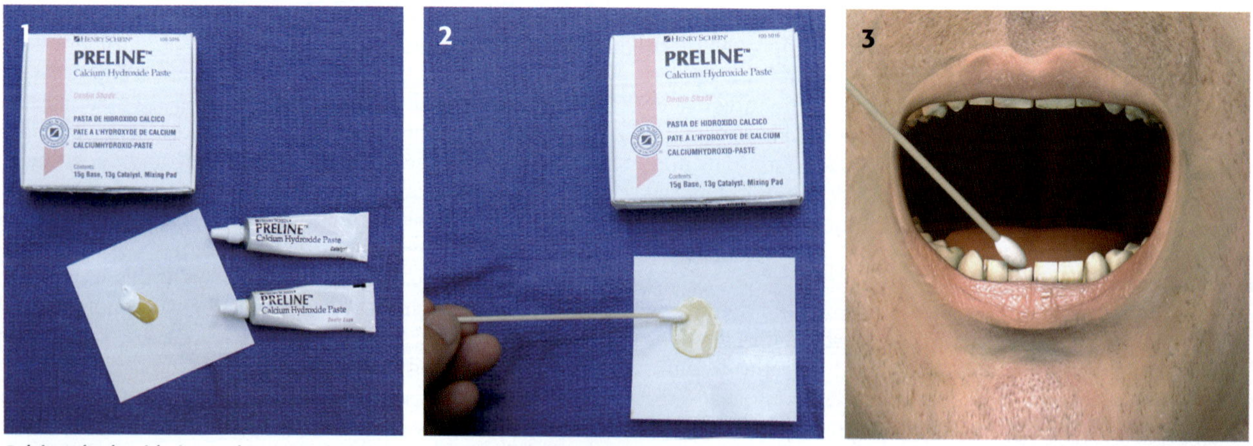

1. Calcium hydroxide is used to treat dentin fractures and aids in prevention of infection and pain relief. It is supplied in separate tubes of catalyst and base.

2. Mix equal portions of catalyst and base on the mixing pad that is supplied with the product. A dental spatula is an ideal tool; however, a simple cotton applicator will suffice.

3. Dry the tooth surface prior to application by having the patient bite down on a gauze pad. Then place a small amount of the paste onto the exposed surface. It will dry within minutes.

Fig. 65.7 Calcium hydroxide (CaOH) application for the treatment of dentin fractures.

Ellis Class III Fractures

Complicated fractures involving the pulp are also known as *Ellis class III fractures* (see Fig. 65.6D). Complicated fractures of the crown that extend into the pulp of the tooth are true dental emergencies. Pulp necrosis is a known potential complication of Ellis III fractures even with appropriate treatment. Therefore many of these injuries will end up with root canal therapy.[23] Ellis III fractures can be distinguished from fractures of the dentin by the pink color of the pulp. Wipe the fractured surface of the tooth with a clean gauze and observe for frank bleeding or a pink blush which indicates exposure of the pulp. Fractures through the pulp are often excruciatingly painful, but occasionally there is lack of sensitivity secondary to disruption or concussion of the neurovascular supply of the tooth.

Immediate management for these fractures includes consultation or referral to a dentist, oral surgeon, or endodontist. The patient usually requires pulpectomy (complete removal of the pulp) or, in the case of primary teeth, pulpotomy (partial removal of the pulp) as definitive treatment.[17] The longer the pulp is exposed, the greater the likelihood of contamination, infection, and abscess formation. If a dentist cannot see the patient immediately, provide pain relief and cover the exposed pulp as shown in Fig. 65.8 and ensure the patient can follow-up with a dentist within 24 to 48 hours. If significant pain is present, a supraperiosteal injection can provide sufficient relief to apply dressing until oral pain relievers take effect. Apply paste or composite as described earlier. These injuries are prone to bleeding which can be brisk at times. Control bleeding by having the patient bite onto a gauze pad that has been soaked with a topical anesthetic containing a vasoconstrictor such as epinephrine. Alternatively, instill a small amount of anesthetic/vasoconstrictor onto the pulp to control bleeding. After the bleeding has stopped and a covering is applied, instruct the patient to follow up as soon as possible with a dentist. Antibiotics with coverage directed at oral flora (including anaerobes) should be considered, with recommendations to eat only soft food and avoid chewing or biting on the affected side. Removal of the exposed pulp by emergency clinicians is not recommended as it can result in significant complications. It is best left to the expertise of a dentist or oral surgeon.

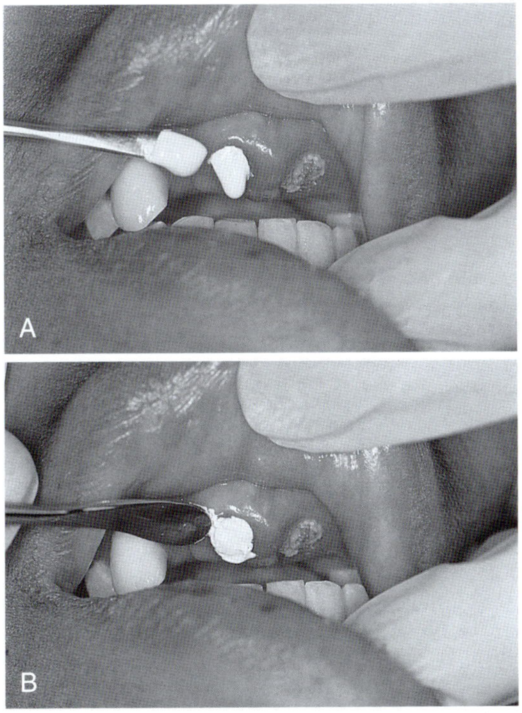

Fig. 65.8 (A) Application of periodontal calcium hydroxide (CaOH) paste to the fractured surface of the tooth. (B) The paste hardens quickly even in the moist intraoral environment.

Luxation, Subluxation, Intrusion, and Avulsion

Luxation and Subluxation

See Videos 65.5–65.7. *Subluxation* refers to teeth that are mobile but not displaced. *Luxation* refers to teeth that are displaced, either partially or completely, from their sockets. Luxation injuries are divided into four types (Fig. 65.9):

1. *Extrusive luxation* is an injury in which the tooth is forced partially out of the socket in an axial direction (see Fig. 65.9A).
2. *Intrusive luxation*, or intrusion, occurs when the tooth is forced apically. It may be accompanied by crushing or fracture of the tooth apex (see Fig. 65.9B).
3. *Lateral luxation* occurs when the tooth is displaced either facially, lingually, medially, or distally (see Fig. 65.9C). This injury is often associated with injuries to the alveolar wall.
4. *Complete luxation*, also known as complete avulsion, results in loss of the entire tooth from the socket.

Even minor trauma to the oral cavity requires meticulous examination for loose or missing teeth, intraoral lacerations, as well as jaw or facial instability. Examine each tooth for mobility by applying a back-and-forth motion on each side of the tooth surface with either the fingertips or two tongue depressors. Any blood in the gingival crevice (area where the gingiva touches the tooth) suggests a traumatized tooth.

Teeth that are minimally mobile and are not displaced do very well with just conservative treatment. The tooth will restabilize in the socket if not reinjured in any way. Instruct patients to eat only a soft diet for 1 to 2 weeks and see their dentist as soon as possible. A thorough examination is necessary as a seemingly lost or avulsed tooth may have been aspirated, swallowed, or intruded into neighboring tissue or sinuses creating potential for deformity or infection (Fig. 65.10).

Grossly mobile teeth require some form of stabilization as soon as possible. Stabilization is best performed by a dental specialist with enamel bonding material or wire ligation. Several different "home remedies" exist for splinting loosened teeth in the ED. The clinician must be aware of the possibility of splint failure, and avoid using unapproved devices or compounds in the mouth due to aspiration risk or further injury. For some patients with poor gingival health, luxated teeth may not be salvageable because of preexisting disease of the attachment apparatus. Splinting techniques are suitable for the emergency clinician to perform as temporizing measures until definitive care can be arranged. Teeth that are luxated in either the horizontal or the axial plane, or are slightly extruded, can also be splinted after repositioning to original position with the splinting techniques described in the following paragraph.

One simple technique for emergency use is to apply periodontal paste, commercially available as Coe-Pak (GC America Inc.) or other similar commercial products (Fig. 65.11).

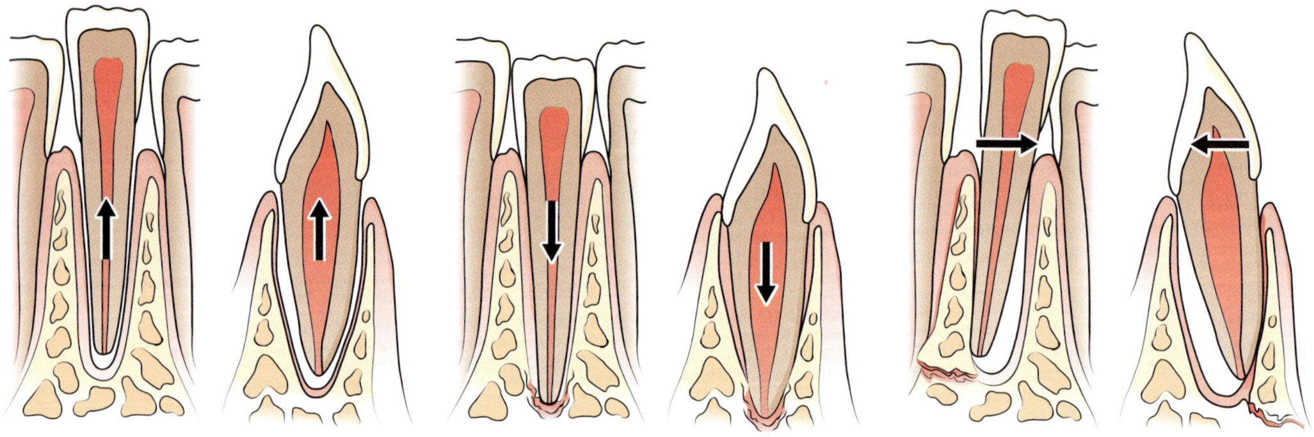

Fig. 65.9 Classification of tooth trauma. (A) Extrusive luxation occurs when the tooth is forced partially out of the socket in an axial direction. (B) Intrusive luxation of a tooth compresses the periodontal ligament and vascular supply of the pulp. It may even crush the apical bone. (C) Lateral luxation occurs when the tooth is displaced in a lingual, mesial, distal, or facial direction. Fractures of the alveolus frequently accompany lateral luxation injuries. (A–C, Adapted from King R. Orofacial infections. In: Montomery MT, Redding SW, eds. *Oral-Facial Emergencies—Diagnosis and Management*. JBK Publishing; 1994.)

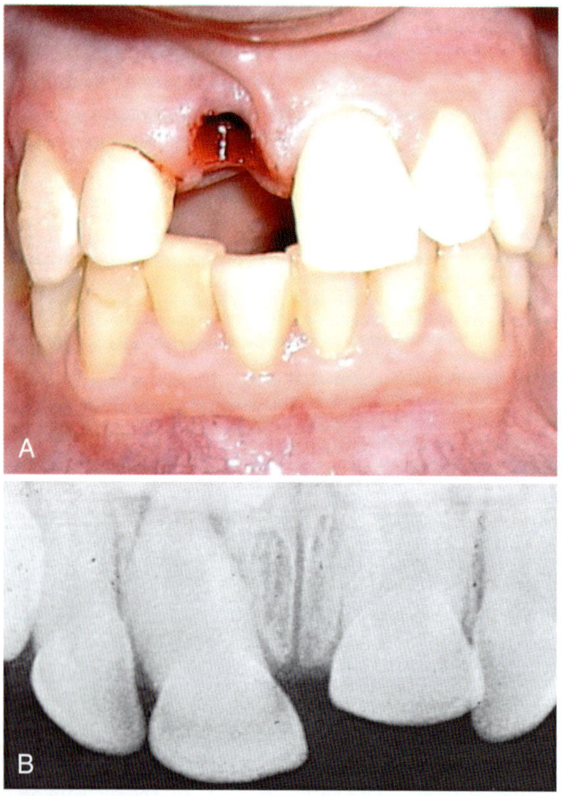

Fig. 65.10 Intruded tooth secondary to trauma. (A) On superficial examination it appears that the tooth was simply knocked out. This missing tooth could be lost, fully intruded, aspirated, or swallowed. (B) In some cases a dental radiograph or computed tomography scan is necessary to determine intrusion or avulsion. Intruded teeth create the potential for infection or cosmetic deformities. Intrusion of an upper tooth into the maxillary sinus can cause recurrent sinusitis. Teeth can also intrude into the nasal cavity and cause infection or bleeding, or they can be aspirated into the airway. The incisors are the teeth most commonly intruded.

These products usually consist of a base and a catalyst that when mixed, form a moderately sticky claylike dressing that becomes firm after application. It is typically applied over the enamel and gingiva, as well as the adjacent teeth, to splint the subluxed tooth into place. However, some have recommended keeping composites and bonding agents away from the gingiva where possible to avoid plaque retention and secondary infection.[17] Although the splint performs best if placed on the facial and buccal surfaces of the teeth, it is usually sufficient to apply the paste only to the front (facial) surface of the teeth. Make sure that the enamel and gingiva are completely dry prior to application. Lubricate gloves with water or lubricating jelly before applying the dressing to promote transfer of the paste to the injured area. Apply the paste into the grooves between the teeth, as well as on the adjacent teeth. Remind the patient to eat a soft diet until seen in follow-up within 24 to 48 hours. Periodontal pastes are usually fairly simple for the dentist to remove during formal evaluation and restoration. They are also useful in treating difficult-to-repair gingival lacerations that are not associated with alveolar ridge fractures. These lacerations may be covered with periodontal paste and removed in 5 to 7 days by the dentist at follow-up.

Intrusion and Avulsion

Intruded teeth are those that have been forced apically into the alveolar bone. This often results in disruption of the attachment apparatus or fracture of the supporting alveolar bone, especially in permanent teeth with mature roots.[10,17,20] Intruded teeth are usually immobile and do not require stabilization in the ED although frequently require endodontic treatment because of risk of pulp necrosis. It is important to consider the possibility of an intruded tooth anytime there is a space in the dentition (see Fig. 65.10). Undiagnosed intrusion of the teeth can lead to infection and craniofacial abnormalities. Obtain imaging when it is uncertain whether a tooth is intruded or simply avulsed. Intruded teeth are best managed

Dental Splint (Coe-Pak) Application

1

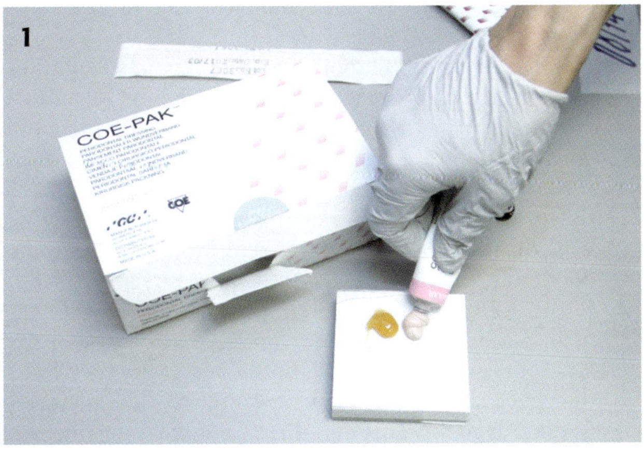

Coe-Pak is a periodontal paste used to splint loosened or avulsed teeth. Like calcium hydroxide, it is supplied as a catalyst and a base.

2

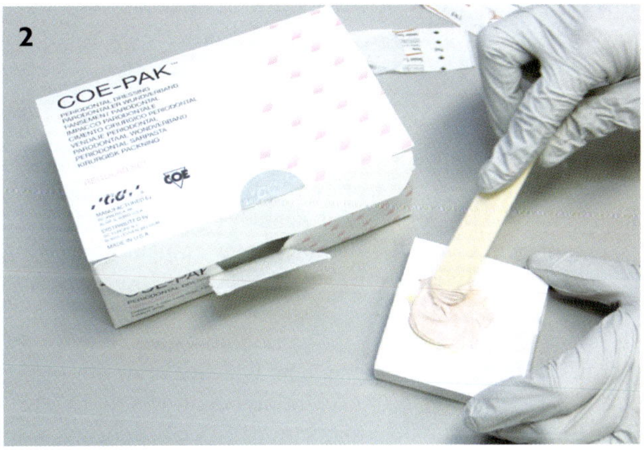

Mix equal parts of the catalyst and base on the mixing pad supplied with the product.

3

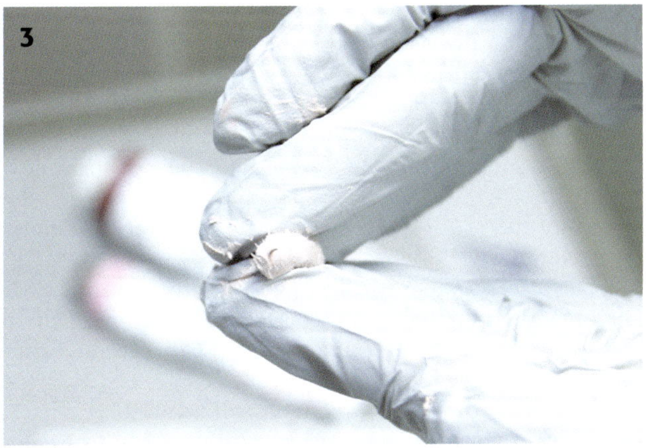

Roll the claylike mixture between your fingers into an elongated roll. Apply lubricating jelly to your gloves prior to handling the product to prevent it from sticking.

4

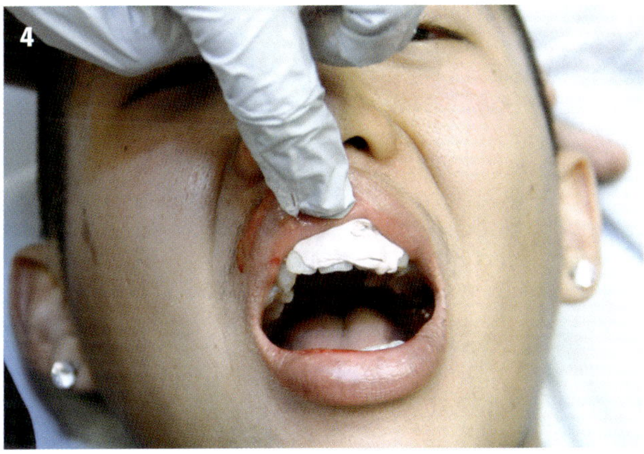

Dry the teeth and gingiva with gauze prior to application. Press the Coe-Pak into the grooves between the teeth, as well as across the adjacent teeth and gingiva. This type of splint works best when applied to both the front and back surfaces of the teeth, although it is usually sufficient to apply it only to the front.

Fig. 65.11 Dental splint application.

by a dentist or oral surgeon; referral should take place within 24 hours. Permanent teeth often require repositioning and immobilization (splinting), but primary teeth are usually given a trial period to erupt on their own before any intervention is taken.

Primary teeth are not replaced after avulsion because they can fuse to the alveolar bone and potentially cause craniofacial abnormalities or infection. Reimplanted primary teeth may also interfere with eruption of the secondary teeth. Reassure parents of these patients that, if desired, a prosthetic replacement for the avulsed teeth can easily be made and worn until the permanent teeth erupt. See Figs. 65.1 and 65.2 as a guide to identifying permanent versus primary teeth.

Avulsed permanent teeth are those that have been completely removed from their ligamentous attachments. These are true dental emergencies. The majority of patients seen in the ED with an avulsed tooth will lose that tooth, so patient and physician expectations should not be overly optimistic. Under ideal circumstances, such as arrival at a dentist's office with a properly stored tooth avulsed less than 60 minutes previously, this situation may result in successful reimplantation 80% to 90% of the time but often requires specialized procedures and endodontics (root canal). Emergency clinicians are not expected to save an avulsed tooth, but prompt action may give the replanted tooth some chance for survival.

The first consideration in treating dental avulsions is to ask, "Where is the tooth?" Missing teeth may have been intruded, fractured, aspirated, swallowed, or embedded into the soft tissues of the surrounding mucosa. Therefore imaging should be considered whenever an avulsed tooth cannot be located. Management of an avulsed tooth in the ED depends on a number of factors, including the age of the patient, the amount of time that has elapsed since the tooth was avulsed, associated trauma to the oral cavity such as alveolar ridge fractures, and the overall health of the periodontium.[17]

Time is the other important consideration when deciding whether to replace an avulsed tooth. In general, the longer the tooth is out of the socket, the higher the incidence of necrosis of the periodontal ligament and subsequent failure of reimplantation. Periodontal ligament cells generally die within 60 minutes outside the oral cavity if they are not placed in an appropriate transport medium.[24] A significant amount of research has been conducted on different media used to keep cells of the periodontal ligament alive.[25] Various transport media have been studied, including milk, Hank's Balanced Salt Solution (Thermo Fisher Scientific), Save-A-Tooth (Phoenix Lazarus), saliva, cell culture media, saline, and water. Although certain cell culture media have been developed to stimulate cells of the periodontal ligament to proliferate and remain viable, milk and the commercially available Save-A-Tooth and EMT ToothSaver (Smart Practice, Inc.) are the best and easiest for both prehospital care and ED storage (Fig. 65.12)[24,25] Milk will preserve the periodontal ligament for 4 to 8 hours; the commercial products will preserve the ligament for 12 to 24 hours. However, reimplantation should take place at the earliest possible opportunity after the socket has been adequately prepared. The key is to get the tooth into the transport medium immediately because even 10 minutes outside some type of storage medium can cause desiccation and death of the periodontal ligament cells. Use saliva if milk or any of the commercially available products are not immediately accessible.

In the prehospital setting, the patient should reimplant the tooth if milk or other appropriate medium is not available. The patient should NOT place the tooth in the cheek or lip during transport as this risks aspiration. The principles cited here should be followed when providing instructions to prehospital providers or to a patient who calls for advice prior to seeking treatment. It is always preferable to refer such patients directly to a dentist rather than the ED if this is feasible. Patients should be counseled to do the following:

- Determine whether this is a permanent tooth. By 14 years of age, all primary teeth should have been replaced by permanent teeth.
- Handle the tooth by the crown only because handling the tooth by the root can damage the periodontal ligament.
- Do not replace the tooth if it is fractured or if significant maxillofacial trauma has occurred.
- If the tooth can be replaced in the prehospital setting, gently rinse off the root first to remove any debris. Do not wipe off the root because this removes or injures the periodontal ligament.
- If the tooth cannot be reimplanted successfully in the field, place it in a transport medium as described earlier. Do not transport the tooth in the oral cavity such as inside the cheek or lip due to risk of aspiration. The buccal space is not ideal for keeping the periodontal ligament alive because of the bacterial flora and low osmolality of saliva.

Once the patient arrives in the ED, confirm proper placement and alignment. It is not important that the tooth be in perfect position because the dentist can make final adjustments. Splinting the repositioned tooth with periodontal paste or composite as outlined earlier may be necessary if mobility is present.

Should reimplantation be unsuccessful in the prehospital setting, it must be done in the ED according to the following guidelines:

- Store the tooth in an appropriate medium if reimplantation is delayed for any reason.
- Perform supraperiosteal injection with a local anesthetic before manipulating or replacing teeth to make the procedure more comfortable for the patient and easier to perform.
- Check the oral cavity for trauma. If an alveolar ridge fracture is present or the socket is significantly damaged, do not reimplant the tooth.
- Gently suction the socket first with a Frasier suction tip to remove any accumulated clot. Be careful not to damage the walls of the socket because this can further damage periodontal ligament fibers. Irrigate gently with normal saline after suctioning. If the clot is not removed, reimplantation and realignment will be difficult. Rinse off any debris on the tooth with saline but do not scrub it. Implant the tooth into the socket with firm, but gentle pressure. Remember to handle the tooth only by the crown.
- Ask the patient to bite down gently on gauze to help positioning and alignment of the tooth. The tooth may require splinting after replacement. This can be performed in the ED with periodontal paste as described earlier.
- Update the patient's tetanus status as necessary.
- Prescribe a liquid diet until the patient is seen in follow-up.

Antibiotics are controversial in the treatment of fractured and avulsed teeth. Although the American Association of Endodontics does not recommend the routine use of antibiotics for fractures or avulsion, others recommend the use of antibiotics effective against oral flora to decrease inflammatory resorption of the root particularly in those patients with poor oral health.[17] It is reasonable to use antibiotics if the root or socket is heavily soiled; otherwise, treatment should be tailored to the individual patient and discussed with an experienced consultant. Ideally, the patient is immediately referred to a dentist or oral surgeon, and the reimplanted tooth is held

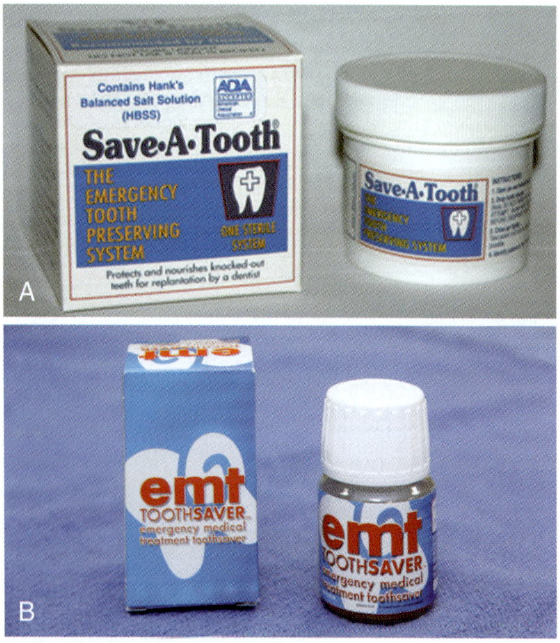

Fig. 65.12 With the (A) Save-A-Tooth or (B) EMT Toothsaver systems, an avulsed permanent tooth is placed into the container and closed. Avulsed primary teeth are not replanted. The preservative will increase the lifespan of traumatized periodontal ligament cells. Unpreserved teeth replanted after 60 minutes rarely survive; those that do survive require root canal procedures and close follow-up. This system prolongs the time to successful reimplantation but does not ensure success.

in place by biting on gauze, by periodontal paste (see Fig. 65.11), or by the suture technique described in Fig. 65.13.

Prognosis

The prognosis of a reimplanted tooth depends on several factors. As discussed earlier, the time to reimplantation is critical. Likewise, the age of the patient, the stage of development of the root (younger is better), and the overall health of the gingiva are also very important. An individual with gingival disease is more likely to have an unsuccessful reimplantation.

Management goals in any tooth avulsion or fracture is to salvage and reimplant the native tooth if possible. It is not uncommon for an avulsed and reimplanted tooth to lose the majority of its neurovascular supply. This causes pulp necrosis of the tooth, necessitating root canal therapy. However, if the periodontal ligament remains intact, there is a greater chance of a functional tooth. It is important that the patient be aware that some root resorption is likely to occur after reimplantation and the possibility of tooth loss exists. It is therefore important to set appropriate expectations in the ED regarding aftercare and prognosis.

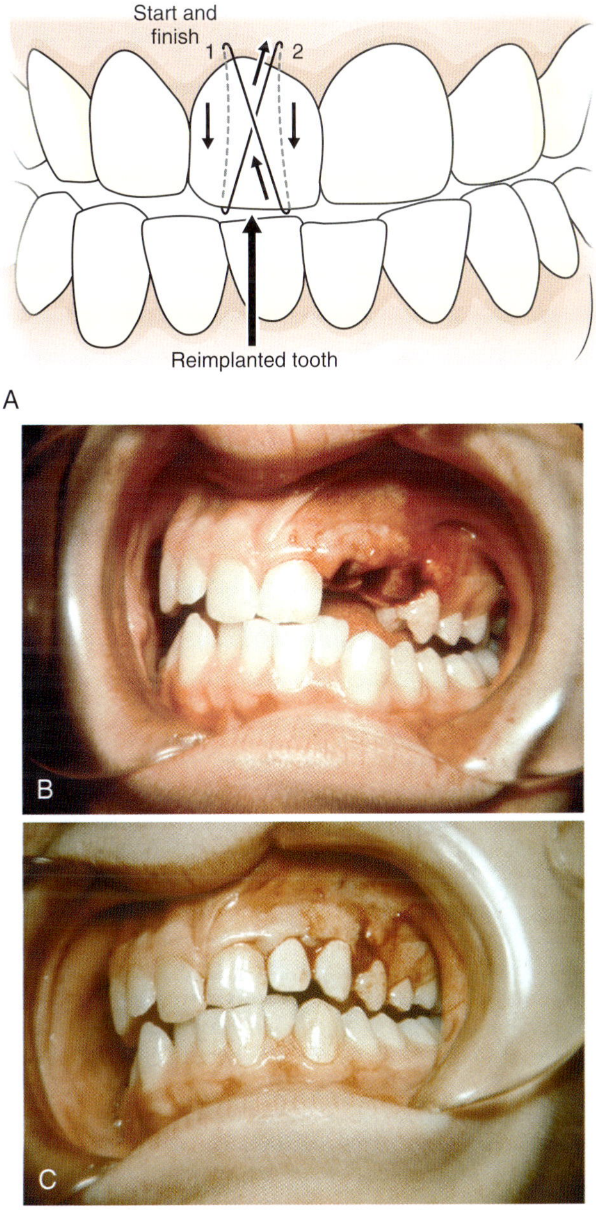

Fig. 65.13 Temporary suturing to hold a replanted tooth in place. (A) Use a nonabsorbable monofilament suture. Start by puncturing the gingiva at the border of the replaced tooth *(1)*. Bring the suture behind the tooth and then cross over the front of the tooth to the other side. Penetrate the gingiva *(2)*, go behind the tooth, cross over the front again, and tie the suture with at least 4 to 5 square knots to ensure the suture does not untie. (B–C) Multiple teeth can be reimplanted.

Alveolar Bone Fractures

Trauma involving the anterior teeth may be associated with fracture of the alveolus, which is the tooth-bearing portion of the maxilla or mandible. Alveolus or alveolar ridge fractures often occur in multi-tooth segments and will vary in the number of teeth involved, the amount of displacement, and the mobility of the affected segment. The patient generally complains of pain, as well as malocclusion. The diagnosis is usually clinically apparent and is notable for a section of teeth that are misaligned and variable in mobility (Fig. 65.14). Avulsed teeth, fractured teeth, or displaced teeth may be present within the alveolar segment itself. In the ED, facial or Panorex x-rays may show the fracture line just apical to the root of the involved teeth; however, these films are often inconclusive or may have normal findings. Maxillofacial computed tomography (CT) may provide more detailed information (Fig. 65.15) to assist in management decisions, as well as type and urgency of consultation or referral required. At follow-up, the dentist or oral surgeon also has several radiographic options to confirm the diagnosis.

Definitive treatment of alveolar ridge fractures involves rigid splinting after repositioning the involved segment. The displaced alveolar ridge should not be repositioned by the emergency clinician as this often converts a nonmobile displaced segment into a mobile displaced segment. Repositioning of alveolar ridge fractures is beyond the scope of the emergency clinician, and urgent consultation with an oral surgeon or dentist is necessary. The role of the emergency clinician is to identify the injury, as well as any avulsed or fractured teeth, and preserve as much of the alveolar bone and surrounding mucosa as possible. Alveolar bone that is debrided or missing is difficult to restore properly.[26] Alveolar ridge fractures, if not mobile or bleeding, may be discharged if urgent follow-up is arranged for within 24 hours. If there is ongoing or significant bleeding, or if movement of the segment is a risk, specialty consultation will need to take place within the hospital or urgent transfer to a facility with specialists available to manage this injury.

Lacerations and Dentoalveolar Soft Tissue Trauma

Trauma to the face and perioral region is often associated with soft tissue injuries such as abrasions or lacerations. Before any repair can take place, all wounds must be thoroughly inspected to determine the extent and depth of the wound and whether foreign bodies are present. Through-and-through lacerations are easily overlooked, as are small foreign bodies and debris such as tooth fragments. Obtain radiographs if there is any question of tooth fragments or other foreign bodies. Evaluate the patient for potential airway obstruction or compromise.

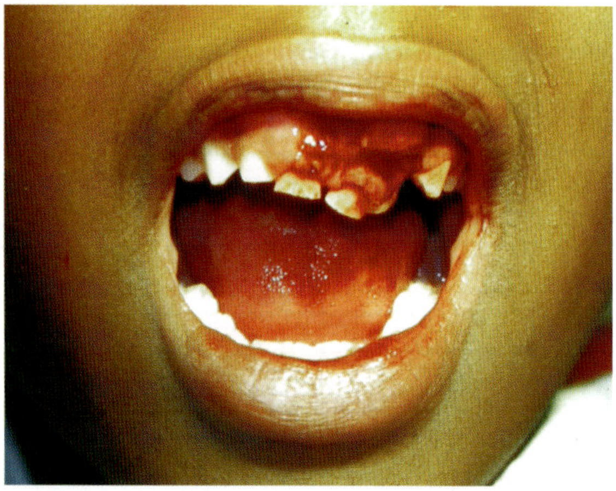

Fig. 65.14 Alveolar ridge fracture. Note that a section of teeth is misaligned. Clinically, the section is mobile and malocclusion will be present. (From Baren JM, Rothrock SG. Brennan J et al., eds. *Pediatric Emergency Medicine*. Saunders; 2007.)

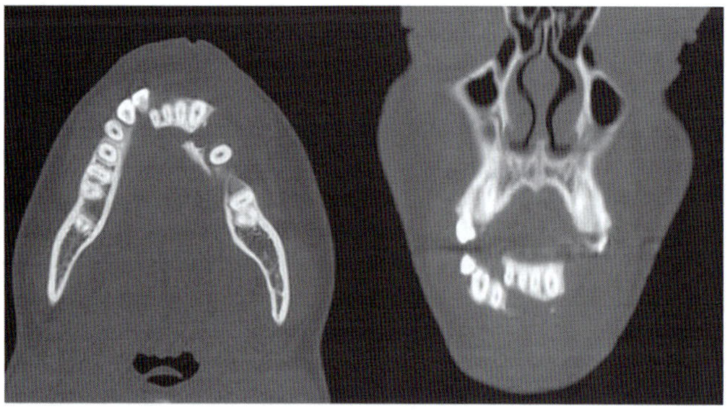

Fig. 65.15 Facial computed tomography provides a definitive diagnosis of alveolar fracture. Here, axial and reformatted coronal images show a comminuted displaced fracture of the mandible with involvement of the alveolar ridge. (From Soto JA, Lucey B. *Emergency Radiology: The Requisites*. Mosby; 2009.)

As a general rule, manage any injured teeth before undertaking soft tissue repair because manipulating the soft tissue while splinting, dressing, or repositioning teeth may damage sutures already in place in the soft tissues. Begin repair in the perioral region with standard wound care. After appropriate local or regional anesthesia, debride devitalized, crushed, or macerated tissue. Irrigate profusely with normal saline. The role of antibiotic prophylaxis in mucosal trauma has not been conclusively established, and there is no definitive standard of care in this regard.[27] A reasonable guideline to follow is to use antibiotics if a significant amount of devitalized or crushed tissue is present, if there is significant wound contamination, if the wound is a through-and-through laceration, if the injury is the result of an animal bite,[28] or if timely access to follow-up cannot be assured. Coverage of oral flora is appropriate for intraoral lacerations, and additional coverage should be considered for through-and-through lacerations or if caused by an animal bite. Dentoalveolar trauma may present the emergency clinician with several different injuries at once, and each should generally be managed as follows.

Buccal Mucosa

Most small lacerations and abrasions of the buccal mucosa heal quickly without repair, but large lacerations (>1 to 2 cm) should be repaired. In the mouth, use absorbable sutures such as gut, chromic gut, or Vicryl, and it is recommended to place the sutures so that the knots are buried wherever possible. While the optimal choice of suture material remains under debate, these suture materials have been used effectively for decades for intraoral repair and have excellent absorbability, tensile strength, and less tissue reactivity.[29,30] Practitioners often have their preferred material when working in such a tight space. Silk is an alternative; however, it has higher tissue reactivity, is not absorbable, and is not recommended for these repairs. Nylon sutures are generally not preferred for buccal mucosal repair because their ends are sharp, more apt to untie, and irritating to tissues.

Through-and-through lacerations of the oral cavity present a special challenge. Clinicians must evaluate for damage to the salivary ducts (Wharton's and Stensen's ducts) and to the facial nerve. If they are intact, it is generally safe to proceed with the repair. Guidelines for closure are controversial, but larger lacerations (>1 to 2 cm) should generally be closed. Close the mucosa surface first with absorbable sutures as noted earlier, then close the skin with an appropriate suture material (e.g., 5-0 or 6-0 Ethilon, Prolene, or a rapidly absorbable suture). Closing the mucosa first results in approximation of the skin layer, thus facilitating skin closure and an improved cosmetic outcome. If the mucosal wound is small or only a puncture wound, it is reasonable to close only the skin layer. Large, gaping, or complicated mucosal lacerations should be referred to an oral surgeon.

Large, complicated, or through-and-through lacerations repaired in the ED should be rechecked in 2 to 3 days either by the patient's dentist or in the ED. Remove nonabsorbable sutures in 7 to 10 days. Advise the patient to rinse four to six times a day with saline solution or a prescribed chlorhexidine gluconate (0.12%) oral rinse (e.g., Peridex). Instruct the patient to eat only a soft diet until sutures are removed. Apply thin layer of topical antibiotic ointment for the first 24 to 48 hours, unless parenteral antibiotics are indicated as described earlier in this section.

Gingiva

Small lacerations of the hard gingiva overlying the maxillary or mandibular alveolus usually heal uneventfully without repair. If the laceration is large, if a flap is present, or if bone is exposed, approximate the gingiva with 5-0 or 6-0 absorbable suture as discussed in the previous section. As mentioned earlier, silk and nylon are not recommended for intraoral repairs. It can be difficult to suture gingiva because there is little supporting soft tissue underneath. A helpful technique is to wrap the suture around the teeth circumferentially and use the teeth as anchors (Fig. 65.16). Large lacerations should be repaired to approximate the gingiva and cover the base of the teeth (Figs. 65.17 and 65.18). Nongaping, nonbleeding gingival lacerations may be covered with periodontal paste as described earlier in this chapter in lieu of suturing, as long as dental or maxillofacial follow-up is assured.

Frenulum

The maxillary frenulum rarely requires sutures for simple lacerations. The lingual frenulum is very vascular in nature and will often need a suture or two to control hemostasis. If the laceration is extensive or extends significantly into the surrounding mucosa or gingiva, approximate it with chromic, Vicryl, or Dexon suture. These wounds are often significantly

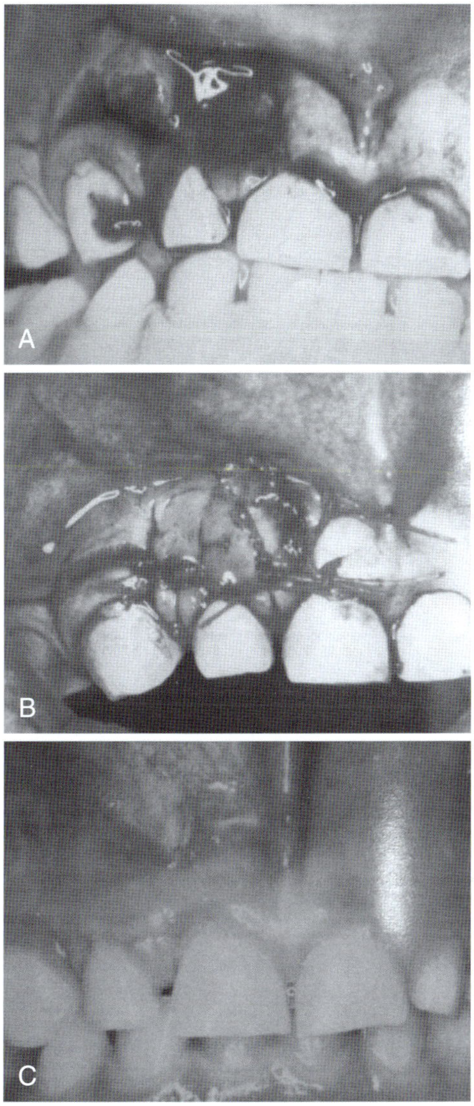

Fig. 65.16 (A) Gingival lacerations sometimes leave little tissue for approximation. (B) The teeth can be used as anchors for sutures and to help approximate the lacerated tissue. (C) Gingival lacerations usually heal rapidly.

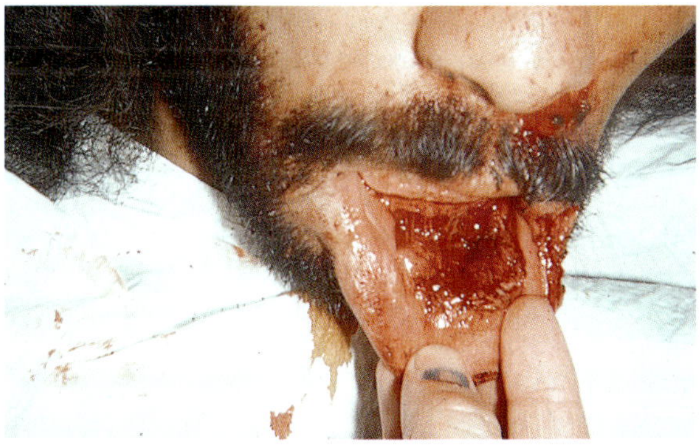

Fig. 65.17 Large gingival avulsions should be approximated to an anatomic position with interrupted absorbable sutures.

painful and may require topical or local anesthesia with a vasoconstrictor to facilitate repair and hemostasis. In rare circumstances, a lingual nerve block might be required. Analgesic medications are recommended after discharge even if the injured frenulum does not require repair.

The Tongue

See Video 65.8. Tongue lacerations are challenging. Although they may be tempting to suture, most large lacerations of the body of the tongue, such as those that occur from a seizure, will heal well without suturing (Fig. 65.19). Tongue lacerations with approximated wound edges do not require repair. Larger lacerations, or those that gape, require repair because the cleft left by the open wound will epithelialize leaving a grooved, bifid, or lateral flap appearance. Approximate wounds that are bleeding profusely, are flap shaped, involve muscle, or are on the edge of the tongue. Small avulsions (divots) or those in the center of the tongue usually heal without intervention.

Explain the procedure in detail to the patient before repairing these wounds. Ask an assistant to secure the tongue by holding it with gauze. An assistant can also hold a tongue depressor vertically between the upper and lower molars to keep the mouth open. Children with tongue lacerations that need repair generally require sedation or repair by a specialist in the surgical suite, but many of these lacerations are small and heal uneventfully on their own.

Begin the repair with either local injection of an anesthetic or a lingual nerve block (see Chapter 30). To promote hemostasis, infiltrate locally with lidocaine with epinephrine. Use absorbable sutures such as 5-0 or 6-0 chromic, Vicryl, or Dexon. Silk and nylon sutures are not recommended as they are irritating and can result in significant inflammatory response of the tongue and surrounding tissues. For lacerations extending through muscle, close with one deep absorbable stitch penetrating both the mucosa and the muscle. Whenever possible, bury the knots of absorbable suture because they will often work their way loose.

Full-thickness lacerations of the tongue can be closed in a number of ways. Place a suture through all three layers or close the top mucosa and muscle together and do the same thing on the underside of the tongue. Bleeding from large lacerations is almost always controlled with the primary repair. In many instances, hemostasis can be achieved without the use of sutures by using topical hemostatic sponge (e.g., Gelfoam), cellulose-based products (e.g., Surgicel) or gauze impregnated with topical thrombin (Fig. 65.20)[31]

ORAL HEMORRHAGE

Bleeding from the oral cavity is not uncommon and is often associated with oral trauma or dental procedures, such as tooth extractions. It is important to determine whether any recent dental work has been performed and what was done. Spontaneous bleeding of the gingiva or oral cavity not associated with dental manipulation or trauma is suggestive of advanced periodontal disease or an underlying systemic process. Ask the patient about other medical conditions that predispose to bleeding (e.g., liver disease, platelet abnormalities), as well as historical factors that may suggest a bleeding abnormality or clotting factor deficiency. Find out whether the patient is taking aspirin or other anticoagulants. Consider laboratory testing if pathologic coagulopathy is a significant concern, but not routinely indicated in a patient seen after dental manipulation.

Control gingival bleeding after dental procedures with direct pressure and saline or hydrogen peroxide rinses. Persistent bleeding from the gingival areas despite pressure and rinses raises suspicion of a bleeding abnormality. A much more common cause of oral hemorrhage seen in the ED is postextraction bleeding. Minor oozing after dental extractions, such

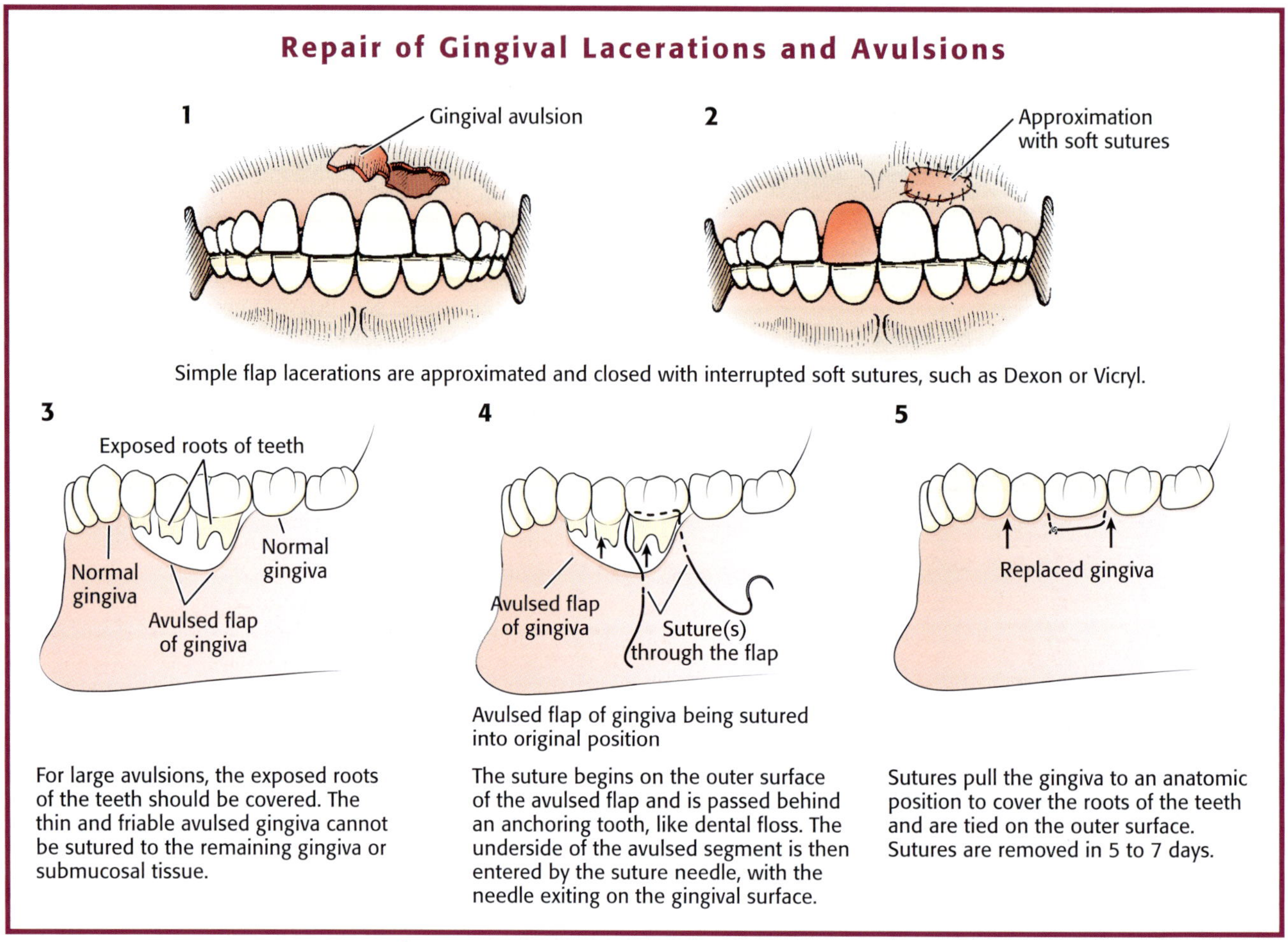

Fig. 65.18 Repair of gingival lacerations and avulsions.

as wisdom tooth extraction, is normal for 2 to 4 days after surgery, but many patients become concerned when bleeding persists despite warnings from the oral surgeon. Patients often go to the ED when their dentist is not available and after futile attempts to stop the bleeding at home. The emergency clinician has a number of options to achieve hemostasis from postextraction bleeding.

Direct Pressure

Although the patient may have been using this technique at home, a few simple procedures may make it more effective in the emergency setting. If a clot is present inside a recently removed tooth socket, leave it intact. If excessive clot has built up around the oozing site, remove the excess clot with a Frasier suction catheter and then gently irrigate the area. Once the clot is removed, place gauze as firmly as possible directly onto the bleeding site. Insert the gauze directly over the bleeding site and then cover it with 2× 2-inch gauze. Commercially available dental gauze fits more precisely between the teeth and therefore affords more pressure; however, 2× 2-inch gauze can be easily substituted. Moisten the gauze with a topical vasoconstrictor before placing it over the bleeding site. Instruct the patient to bite down and hold pressure for 15 minutes or so.

If active bleeding persists after 15 minutes, infiltrate the bleeding area and the gingiva surrounding the socket with lidocaine and epinephrine (1:100,000) until blanching occurs. Reapply the gauze over the site and instruct the patient to bite down for 15 more minutes. The injection serves two purposes: it causes vasoconstriction and it anesthetizes the area so that adequate pressure can be generated during biting.

If bleeding still persists, insert topical hemostatic sponge (e.g., Gelfoam), cellulose-based product (e.g., Surgicel) or gauze impregnated with topical thrombin into the socket. Then loosely close the gingiva surrounding the socket with a 3-0 or 4-0 absorbable figure-of-eight suture. Instruct the patient to bite down on gauze placed over the sutures (see Fig. 65.20). Topical tranexamic acid (TXA) used as a soaked pledget (500 mg/5 mL) is also a useful strategy for control of oral and nasal bleeding. TXA is an antifibrinolytic agent that blocks conversion of plasminogen to plasmin, and is an effective adjunct in the control of intraoral bleeding.[32] If these measures fail to control the bleeding, consult a specialist and consider checking blood counts and coagulation profiles.

Patients whose bleeding is controlled can be safely discharged and instructed not to take anything by mouth for 4 hours, and then only liquids and soft foods until followed up by their dentist or oral surgeon.

ALVEOLAR OSTEITIS (DRY SOCKET)

See Videos 65.9, 65.10. The pain associated with a tooth extraction can be significant, but usually manageable with over-the-counter or prescribed medication and typically

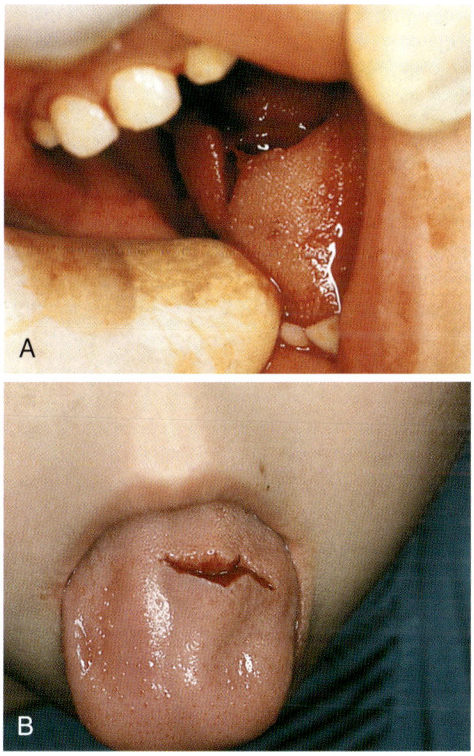

Fig. 65.19 Tongue lacerations. (A) A large gaping tongue laceration in a toddler produced by the upper front teeth being forced through the tissue by a fall with the tongue protruded. This type of injury requires suturing. (B) This small laceration, though gaping slightly, does not require surgical closure. (From Zitelli BJ, McIntire SC, Nowalk AJ, eds. *Zitelli and Davis' Atlas of Pediatric Physical Diagnosis.* 6th ed. Saunders; 2012.)

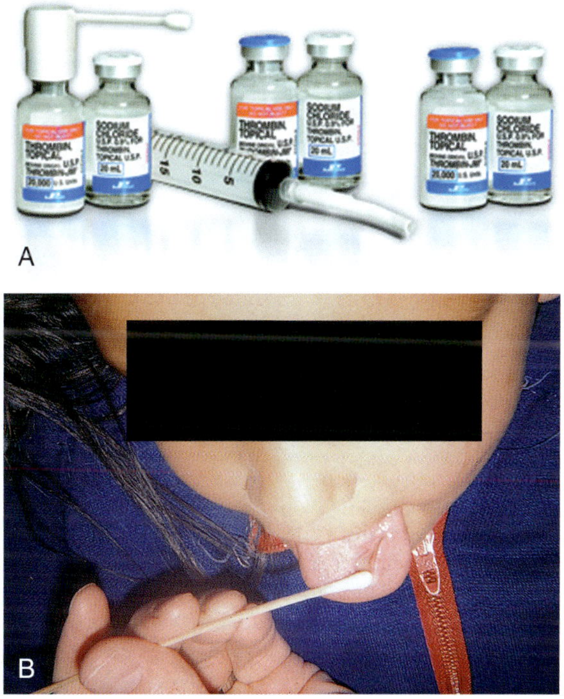

Fig. 65.20 (A) For persistent bleeding of a tongue, mucosa, or dental extraction site, topical thrombin (e.g., Thrombin-JMI) or the antifibrinolytic agent tranexamic acid (TXA) can be used. These products are available as a reconstituted powder or liquid to saturate absorbable Gelfoam to place at bleeding site. (B) A tongue laceration such as this one will heal well without sutures once the bleeding is controlled. Topical thrombin may be an option if hemostasis is problematic.

follows a predictable pattern. The pain associated with a dry socket, however, can be very severe and often requires more aggressive intervention. Alveolar osteitis (AO), or dry socket, is a localized inflammation that occurs when exposed alveolar bone becomes inflamed. It occurs when the fibrin clot fails to develop after the extraction, or becomes dislodged or dissolves before the socket has a chance to heal. AO usually begins within 2 to 4 days of the extraction and can last up to 4 to 6 weeks. The incidence been reported between 0.5% and 5%, however some studies have noted it as high as 68% in patients with risk factors.[33,34] Examination of the patient's oral cavity is essentially unremarkable with the exception of a missing clot where the tooth was extracted. Signs and symptoms of dry socket include the following:

- Moderate to severe pain localized to the area or radiating to the ear
- A foul odor or taste in the absence of purulence or suppuration
- Symptoms most commonly occurring 3 to 5 days following the extraction
- Absence of swelling, purulence, or lymphadenitis
- Duration of 5 to 40 days

Anything that increases negative intraoral pressure in the mouth (e.g., smoking, excessive rinsing, spitting, drinking from a straw), as well as oral contraceptives, hormone replacement, and periodontal disease, predispose patients to developing a dry socket. The risk increases with traumatic extractions or impacted third molars.[33,34]

As mentioned previously, only a small percentage of patients will develop a dry socket. However, the following increase the risk of developing a dry socket:

- Excessive trauma during extraction
- Inadequate blood supply to the extraction site
- Preexisting localized infection
- Loss of clot from sucking, straw use, rinsing, or smoking
- Foreign bodies remaining in the socket
- Use of oral contraceptives
- Use of corticosteroids
- Pericoronitis

The pain associated with a dry socket can be extremely severe. If a patient is seen several days after an extraction in severe pain with relatively normal findings on examination, it is likely a dry socket. However, this must be distinguished from osteomyelitis, which is characterized by fever, leukocytosis, malaise, and nausea. The pain related to a dry socket is typically not relieved with traditional pain medications. Dental nerve blocks are usually necessary to provide relief. Once the nerve block is performed, the AO can be treated. Irrigate the socket with normal saline and gently suction out any accumulated debris. Normal saline is preferred over chlorhexidine solutions as the intraalveolar irrigation solution of choice in the setting of AO.[34,35]

Following irrigation, fill the socket to prevent the recurrence of pain and allow healing to begin. Gauze (¼ inch) impregnated with eugenol (oil of cloves) or a local anesthetic may be used. The gauze should be packed into the socket to the level of the gingival cusps. Follow-up with the patient's dentist or oral surgeon should take place within 24 to 36 hours

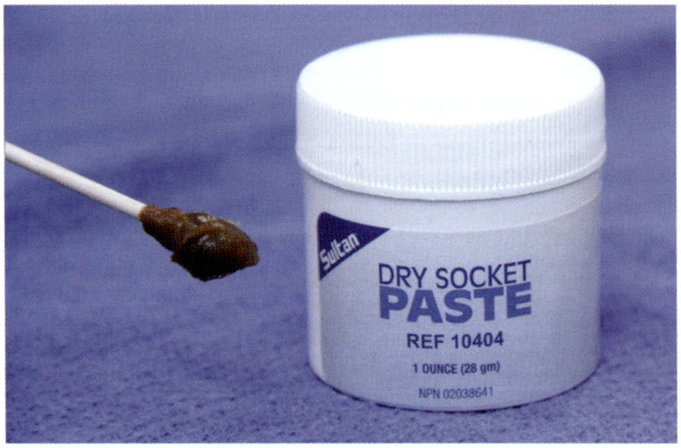

Fig. 65.21 Dry socket paste.

as the gauze tends to dry out and loosen. The socket may also be packed with a slurry of Gelfoam and eugenol. The Gelfoam acts as a matrix to hold the eugenol in the socket. Commercial products, such as Dry Socket Paste (Sultan Healthcare) or Dressol-X (Rainbow Specialty and Health Products Inc.) (Fig. 65.21), can be applied into the socket alone or in conjunction with Gelfoam. Dry Socket Paste is a very sticky thick paste containing eugenol. It may stay in place longer than gauze and does not dry out. Whichever packing material is used for a dry socket, one or more packings might be necessary before healing is complete. Therefore the patient must be referred back to the dentist or oral surgeon who performed the extraction within 1 to 2 days.

Although antibiotics may be given to prevent AO, they are not usually necessary once the socket has been packed and should be prescribed at the discretion of the patient's oral surgeon or dentist.[20,26] Over-the-counter or prescribed analgesia should be provided at discharge.

DENTOALVEOLAR INFECTIONS

Infections of the oral cavity run the spectrum from minor, easily managed abscesses to severe, life-threatening, deep space infections that require airway management and operative drainage. Although dental infections of all severities are encountered in the ED, the most common are those related to pulp disease. Others are associated with the attachment structures of the teeth such as the gingiva, periodontal ligament, and alveolar bone. These infections are often chronic conditions, but can progress to periodontal abscesses and emergency treatment is required.

Emergency clinicians will be called on to drain abscesses of dental origin that do not extend into the deep spaces and that have well-defined boundaries easily accessible by intraoral or external drainage. Remember that not all infections in and around the oral cavity are the result of a simple dental infection. Osteomyelitis of the mandible, various tumors, sinus infection, salivary gland disorders, and other diseases can simulate a dental infection.

Disease of the Pulp

Disease of the pulp can occur as a result of trauma, intraoral procedures, or other unknown causes. The most frequent cause is invasion of microorganisms after carious destruction of the enamel. As the enamel is destroyed, caries progress more rapidly through the dentin and into the pulp chamber causing an inflammatory response referred to as *pulpitis*. If the path of carious destruction through the tooth is adequate for drainage of the developing inflammation, the patient may be only mildly symptomatic or even asymptomatic for a long period of time. If drainage is blocked, however, the process may progress and rapidly involve the entire pulp cavity and the periapical space. The involved tooth is often exquisitely tender at this point. Abscesses in the periapical region are typically identified on specialized imaging in the dentist's or oral surgeon's office. Panoramic ("Panorex") and periapical x-rays are the most commonly used for evaluation and identification of oral trauma as well as dental infections and abscesses because they provide detailed imaging of pathology inside each tooth, under the gum line, and between each tooth.

However, these imaging options are often unavailable to the emergency clinician and CT imaging is often the preferred modality when deep space infections are suspected.

Point-of-care ultrasound (POCUS) has been extensively used in the evaluation of soft tissue swelling, fluid collections, and abscesses, including those of the head and neck.[36] However, its utility (and comparison to panoramic and CT imaging) in dental infections has not been extensively studied or widely adopted. Recent literature reports specific POCUS techniques to increase visibility of tissue planes in suspected dental abscesses (as well as deep space infections) having the added advantage of decreased radiation exposure, cost, decreased time to diagnosis, and ED length of stay.[37–39]

Unless extension through the cortex exists, it is not important for the emergency clinician to make the distinction between pulpitis and a periapical abscess. Examination may reveal gross decay of one or several teeth and tenderness of the abscessed tooth to percussion. A periapical abscess will follow the path of least tissue resistance if not treated. Infections may travel through alveolar bone and the gingiva and into the mouth or into the deep structures of the neck or face. If the infection has progressed apically through alveolar bone and localized swelling and tenderness are present, incision and drainage should be performed (discussed later in this chapter).

In the emergency setting it can be unclear whether a periapical abscess or simple pulpitis exists, and often dental x-rays are not available. In the absence of trauma or recent instrumentation, it is prudent to begin antibiotic coverage for typical oral flora when abscess or pulpitis is suspected. Dentoalveolar infections and abscesses are polymicrobial (e.g., streptococci, fusobacteria, *Prevotella*, *Staphylococcus*, *viridans* group). Penicillins, clindamycin, and metronidazole remain good choices to cover these infections; however, it is important to check for emerging resistance in your region. Analgesia should be provided as well. In most cases, a supraperiosteal block at the involved tooth with a long-acting anesthetic (e.g., bupivacaine) provides immediate and long-lasting relief, and decreases the requirement for narcotic analgesics once the anesthetic effect has dissipated. Avoid performing a supraperiosteal injection if the abscess has extended through gingival tissue and is present near the injection site. In this case a regional block away from the infected tissue may be more appropriate and lessens the risk of iatrogenic spread of the infection.

Disease of the Periodontium

See Videos 65.11 and 65.12. *Periodontal disease* is very common and refers to infection of the attachment apparatus of the teeth: the gingiva, periodontal ligament, and alveolar bone. Unlike pulpal disease, periodontal disease is typically asymptomatic and therefore rarely a primary reason to seek emergency treatment. *Gingivitis* is an inflammation of the gingiva caused by bacterial plaque. In advanced disease, the gingiva becomes red and inflamed and tends to bleed easily. With chronic periodontal disease, an abscess can form when organisms become trapped in the periodontal pocket. The purulent material can escape through the gingival sulcus; however, it occasionally invades the supporting tissues, the alveolar bone, and the periodontal ligament (periodontitis). Periodontal abscesses that are not draining spontaneously through the sulcus can be drained in the ED. Saline rinses are encouraged to promote drainage. Antibiotics should be reserved for severe cases or when abscesses cannot be drained. If it is uncertain whether the abscess originates from the pulp or the periodontium, prescribe antibiotics even if the abscess has been drained.[20,26]

Pericoronitis is a localized inflammation that occurs when the gingiva overlying erupting teeth becomes traumatized and inflamed. Third molars are especially susceptible; however, any tooth can be affected. The gingiva overlying the crown may entrap bacteria and debris, and infection may develop. Typical signs of inflammation and infection in this area include erythema, edema, pus, and foul breath. Examination of the overlying gingiva with a tongue depressor or finger will elicit tenderness and may produce drainage from the underlying the tissue. The pain may be moderate to severe, and commonly referred to the ear, neck, or jaw on the effected side. The localized infection occasionally spreads to deeper areas such as the pterygomandibular or submasseteric spaces. Clinically, patients with significant spread of a pericoronal infection will have trismus secondary to irritation of the masseter and pterygoid muscles.

ED treatment of pericoronitis is directed at ruling out regional spread to the deeper spaces. Trismus or other systemic signs of advanced infection require intravenous antibiotics and urgent consultation for drainage procedures. These usually require extraction of the offending tooth or other surgical intervention outside the scope of the emergency clinician. If pericoronal infection is localized, local or regional anesthesia is followed by removal and irrigation of the submucosal debris. Saltwater, saline, and/or prescribed chlorhexidine gluconate (0.12%) oral rinses and oral antibiotics are prescribed along with dental follow-up in 24 to 48 hours.

Drainage of Dentoalveolar Infections

Dental infections are not always obvious and can be mistaken for sinusitis, or vice versa (Figs. 65.22 and 65.23). The important determination for the emergency clinician to make is whether the odontogenic infection is localized, confined, and easily accessible, or whether it is complex and involves several deep potential spaces. Likewise, determine whether the patient appears to be in a toxic state, has trismus, or exhibits any signs or symptoms of potential airway compromise. These patients require IV antibiotics and admission or transfer to a facility with appropriate dental or oral-maxillofacial specialists for definitive treatment. Patients not meeting these criteria can be managed as an outpatient with specialist referral within 24 to 48 hours or return to an ED if symptoms do not improve or worsen.

Several anesthetic techniques can make the drainage process more comfortable. Regional nerve blocks and local injections work best. Benzocaine 20% gel, 5% lidocaine gel, or a combination of lidocaine, prilocaine, and tetracaine generally provide good topical anesthesia before injection (Fig. 65.24). Application of these medications to the dry mucosa before injection of the local anesthetic decreases the pain associated with injection. After applying the topical anesthetic, slowly infiltrate local anesthetic with a vasoconstrictor until the tissue blanches. Either a short-acting anesthetic (2% lidocaine) or a longer-acting anesthetic (0.5% bupivacaine) may be used, depending on the clinical circumstances. Regional or dental blocks may be performed instead of local infiltration if needle placement would transfer infection from infected tissues into

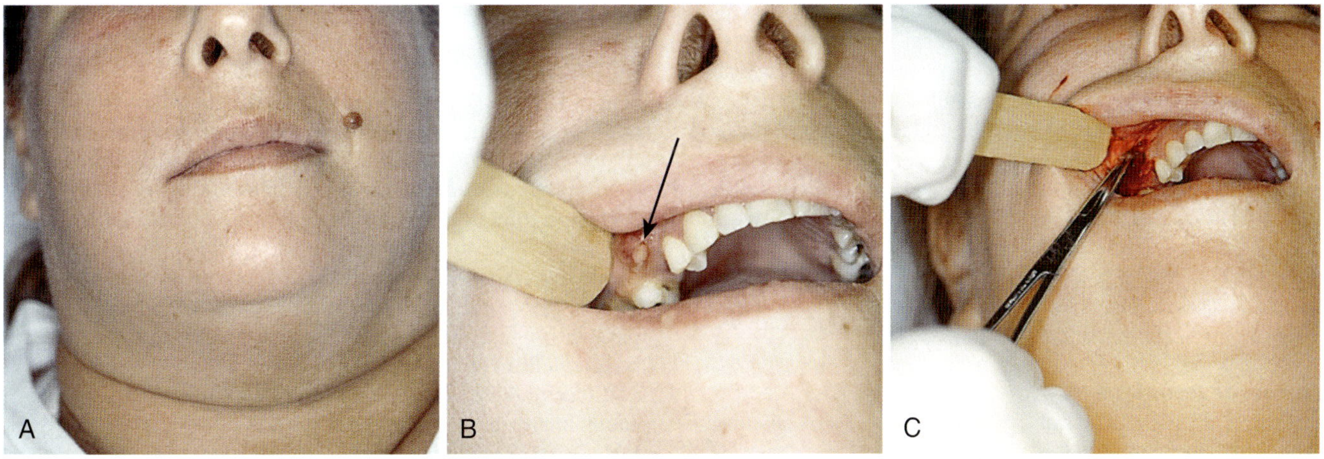

Fig. 65.22 (A) This patient had facial swelling up to the right eye and stated that her sinusitis had returned. She had minor tooth pain but mostly complained of an ache in her face. Radiographs revealed maxillary sinusitis with an air-fluid level. (B) Intraoral examination revealed a pea-sized pointing abscess *(arrow)* at the base of an upper tooth, the cause of the sinusitis. After a local anesthetic was applied, a No. 11 scalpel was used to puncture the abscess, and copious pus was drained. (C) A hemostat was inserted into the abscess cavity and spread open to drain more pus. Intravenous antibiotics (clindamycin) were administered followed by oral antibiotics, and the patient saw her dentist the next day. She recovered fully.

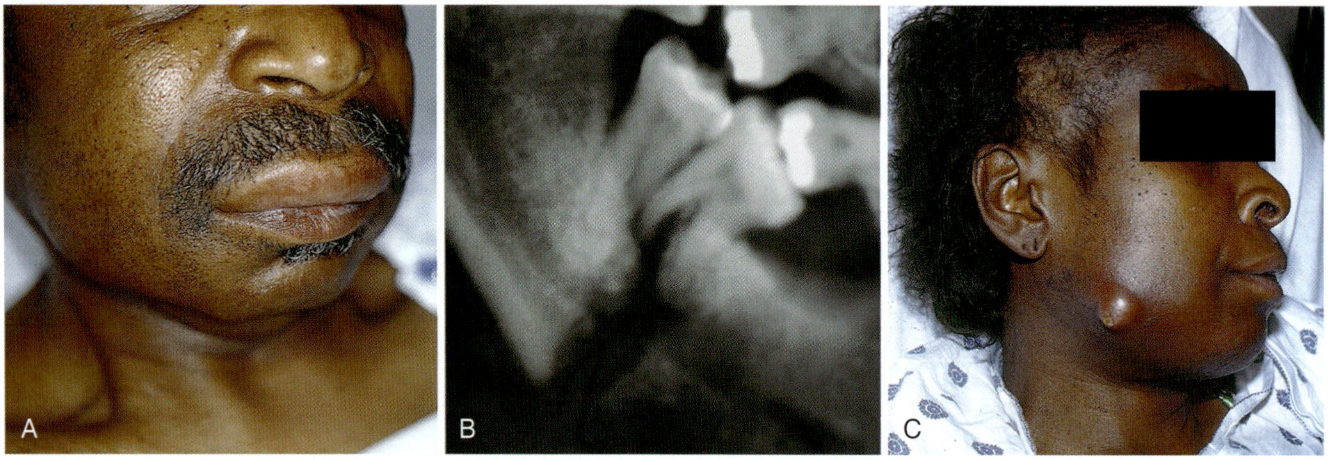

Fig. 65.23 Osteomyelitis manifested as a dental infection. (A) This patient had a chronic toothache for months and got minimally better with antibiotics from numerous emergency departments. No history of trauma. There was diffuse soft tissue swelling with malocclusion. (B) A panoramic (Panorex) x-ray revealed nonunion of a fractured mandible with osteomyelitis. (C) In this case a fractured mandible with osteomyelitis produced an obvious abscess. She had been treated for a presumed dental abscess many times in the past but only had temporary relief.

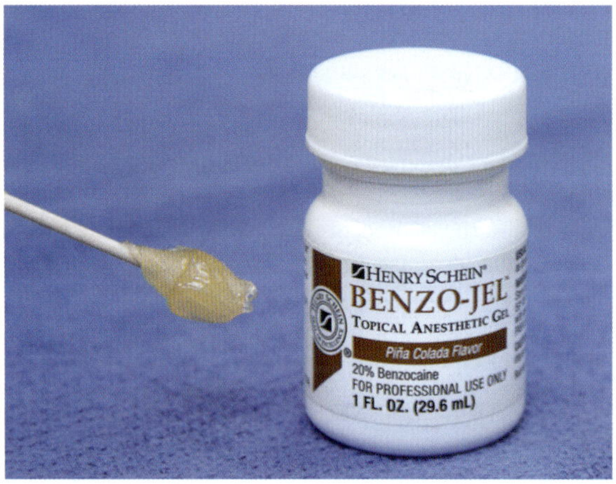

Fig. 65.24 Apply a dollop of 20% benzocaine gel to dry mucosa before injection of local anesthetic to decrease the pain of infiltration.

healthy areas. Otherwise, consider local infiltration over the site of the abscess being careful not to spread infection to surrounding tissues. Supplies necessary for drainage of dentoalveolar abscesses are those usually found in a standard incision and drainage kit and include hemostats, scalpel (No. 15 or 11), saline flushes, procedure drape, and packing material (¼ inch gauze). Packing of small abscesses like those in the oral cavity has not been shown to provide any significant benefit after incision and drainage and likely unnecessary in these infections. However, large gaping abscess pockets may require packing.

Intraoral Technique

Intraoral abscesses do not routinely require any antiseptic preparation of the mucosa before drainage. After anesthetizing the region, make a small incision (0.5 to 1.0 cm) over the area of fluctuance while keeping the point of the blade directed toward the alveolar bone. Use a hemostat to gently dissect the abscess and break up any loculations. Cultures are not necessary unless the patient is immunocompromised. Irrigate the wound profusely with normal saline. If the wound is gaping or large and requires gauze packing, to avoid aspiration tack one end to the mucosa with an absorbable or nylon suture. Advise the patient to perform saltwater rinses hourly and arrange follow-up in 24 to 48 hours with a dentist or oral surgeon provide ongoing management and remove any packing and sutures that were placed. Because the origin of the abscess is not always known to the emergency clinician, it is prudent to prescribe antibiotics after incision and drainage.

Extraoral Technique

Most simple dental infections can be drained intraorally, but occasionally, an abscess spreads to the face and requires drainage through the skin. It is important to realize that most dental infections should be drained from the inside of the mouth, if possible, because any extraoral drainage can cause significant scarring of the face. Never make any incisions on the face in direct proximity to important structures such as the facial nerve or the parotid gland and duct. Refer to Chapter 37 for more details on the incision and drainage technique.

Deep Space Infections of the Head and Neck

It is not unusual for odontogenic infections to spread into the fascial planes and potential spaces of the face and neck (Fig. 65.25). Common signs and symptoms include fever, chills, pain, difficulty with speech or swallowing, and trismus. Although infections of certain teeth usually spread to contiguous spaces, the rapid spread of these infections often makes localizing the exact origin difficult. Any space, including the buccal, temporal, submasseteric, sublingual, submandibular, parapharyngeal, and others, may be involved and present with facial swelling (Fig. 65.26).

Odontogenic infections of the head and neck region can cause life-threatening conditions, including airway compromise, diffuse inflammatory processes, necrotizing infections, meningitis, cerebrospinal abscesses, mediastinitis, sepsis, and septic shock.[40] Maxillary extension of periapical abscesses can spread into the infraorbital space and, subsequently, to the cavernous sinus through the ophthalmic veins and result in cavernous sinus thrombosis. Cavernous sinus involvement is associated with orbital cellulitis, as well as meningeal signs or a decreased level of consciousness. Periapical infections of

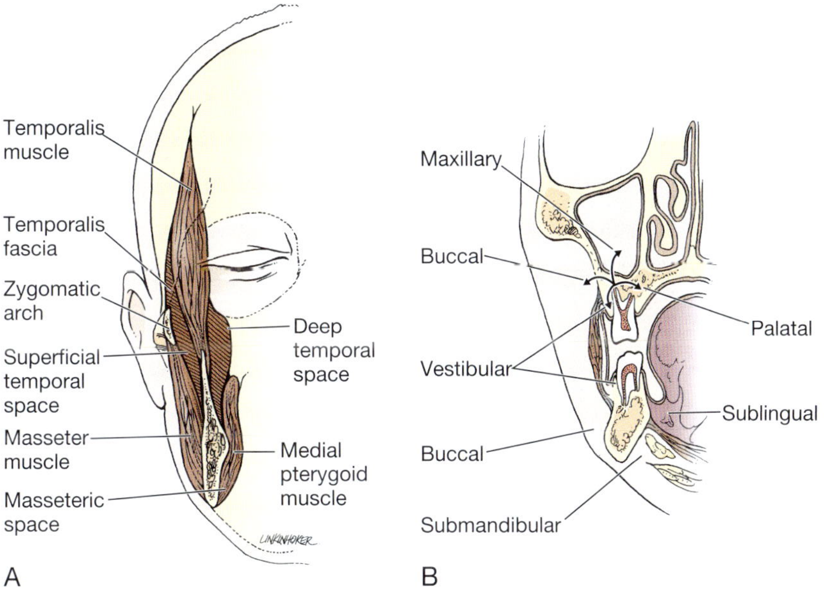

Fig. 65.25 (A) Location of temporal space abscesses. (B) Route of infection into the buccal space, vestibular spaces, submandibular space, sublingual space, and palatal space. (From Eisele D, McQuone S, eds. *Emergencies of the Head and Neck*. Mosby; 2000.)

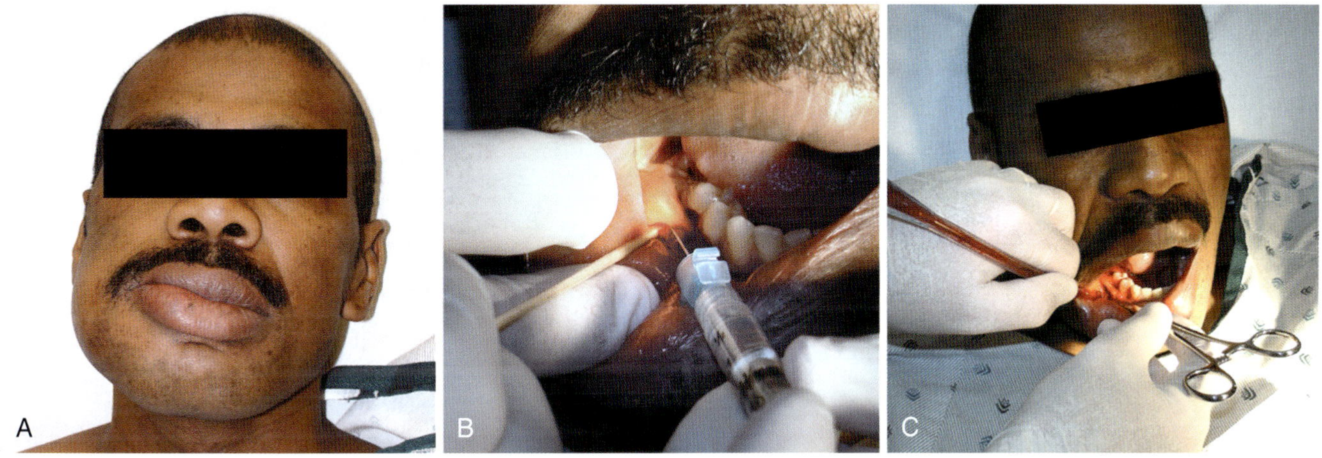

Fig. 65.26 (A) Advanced dental infection with characteristic facial swelling, likely involving the masseter space. (B) Local anesthetic (lidocaine with epinephrine) is injected with a 27-gauge needle into an area of obvious fluctuance (shown by the probe). A mandibular nerve block is an alternative to local injection. (C) After the site is punctured with a No. 11 blade, a hemostat is inserted into the cavity and spread. Copious pus is drained with a suction catheter. Initial intravenous antibiotics (clindamycin), followed by oral antibiotics, and outpatient follow-up yielded good results. The offending tooth was extracted once the infection was controlled.

the anterior mandibular teeth often spread to the buccinator space or the sublingual space, whereas those of the mandibular molars tend to spread into the submandibular space.

The submandibular space connects with the sublingual space. Infection involving both of these spaces is known as *Ludwig angina*, which can be life-threatening. The source is usually a decayed lower tooth, with the tooth itself being relatively asymptomatic (Fig. 65.27). Initially, this infection may be subtle, but it can progress rapidly. As the infection progresses, the submandibular, submental, and sublingual spaces all become edematous and painful, and there may be elevation of the tongue and the soft tissues of the mouth (Fig. 65.28). Ludwig's angina is not a simple abscess that can be drained in the emergency setting, and is considered a true oral emergency. Interventions include definitive airway management, intravenous antibiotics, and emergency ENT or oral surgery consultation for emergency operative intervention. Patients with established cases of Ludwig's angina are admitted to the hospital and undergo operative intervention often involving multiple drains. Minor early cases can be treated and observed for 6 to 8 hours in the ED with close follow-up if the infection is deemed benign, but care must be taken as Ludwig's angina sometimes presents rather unimpressively and can progress quickly. The soft tissues of the posterior aspect of the pharynx can also become involved. Securing the airway becomes of paramount importance in this setting. The suprahyoid region of the neck appears tense and indurated, and landmarks may be obscured. A CT scan is usually used to clarify deep space involvement, but emergency oral and maxillofacial (OMF) or ENT consultation, initiation of antibiotic therapy, and

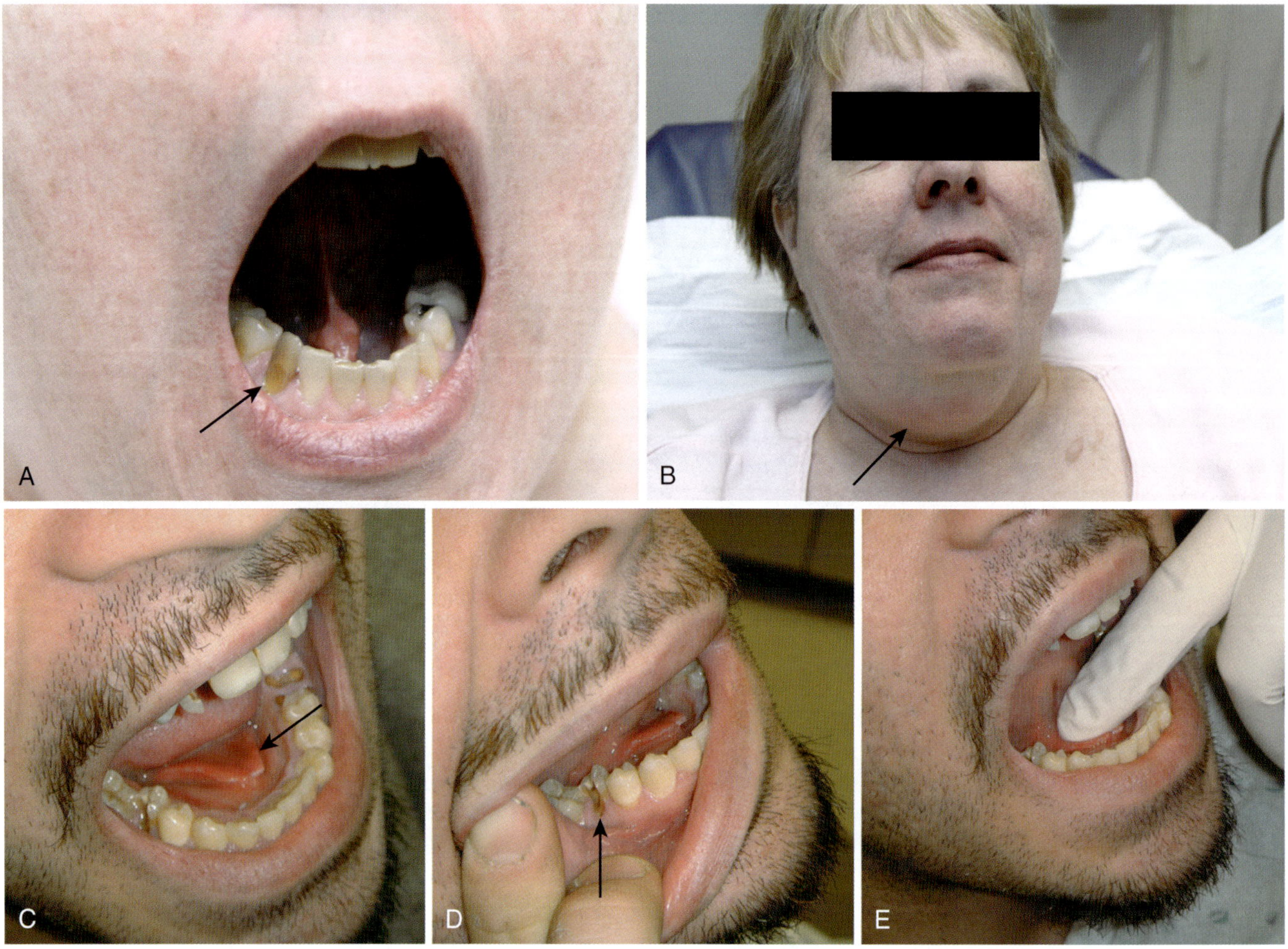

Fig. 65.27 Ludwig angina may initially appear to be benign. (A) This patient's main complaint was dental pain. Tooth No. 27 *(arrow)* was noted to be decayed and a probable source of the infection. (B) Physical examination revealed erythema and edema of the submandibular space, consistent with early Ludwig's angina. She was admitted to the hospital for intravenous antibiotics (clindamycin). A high index of suspicion and early treatment are mandated in such patients because this infection can progress rapidly. (C) This patient had the beginnings of an infection as manifested by elevation of the tongue and swelling of the floor of the mouth, which characteristically raises the openings of the submandibular (Wharton's) ducts *(arrow)*. (D) The cause was a badly decayed lower tooth *(arrow)*. (E) Tenderness and induration can be palpated in the floor of the mouth.

definitive airway management should be instituted immediately. This rapidly progressive disease can cause unexpected or rapid-onset of airway compromise and clinical deterioration. Surgical intervention of this infection is warranted, as is consultation with the team that handles difficult or surgical airways.

Treatment of complicated odontogenic head and neck infections, including Ludwig's angina, centers on airway management, surgical drainage, and antibiotics. If it is uncertain whether the deep spaces are involved, obtain a CT scan to delineate any extension of the infectious process. Involve the appropriate consulting services as soon as possible. Perform airway interventions early if there is any question of compromise and be prepared to perform a surgical airway if conventional methods of airway management are unsuccessful. Consult an OMF or ENT surgeon early because drainage and removal of necrotic tissue might be necessary. Administer IV antibiotics to slow spread of the infection and decrease risk of hematogenous dissemination. The bacteria involved are typically polymicrobial, involving both aerobic and anaerobic bacteria from the primary source. Antimicrobials of choice for complicated odontogenic infections usually include the broad-spectrum penicillins (ampicillin-sulbactam, ticarcillin–clavulanic acid, piperacillin-tazobactam) effective against β-lactamase–producing bacteria and also cover the anaerobe *Bacteroides fragilis*. Penicillins plus metronidazole is another option. Clindamycin is an effective choice in patients who are allergic to penicillin. It should be used in combination with a cephalosporin, such as cefotetan or cefoxitin, to cover recently emerging resistant organisms. It is important to realize that for many of these infections, antibiotics are an adjunctive therapy and not a substitute for surgical intervention and airway management. Likewise, if the source of the infection is likely otogenic or rhinogenic, the antibiotic regimen should be adjusted.

DENTAL SUPPLIES AND EQUIPMENT

As a general rule, EDs should have a well-stocked supply of basic dental material. Commercially available products can

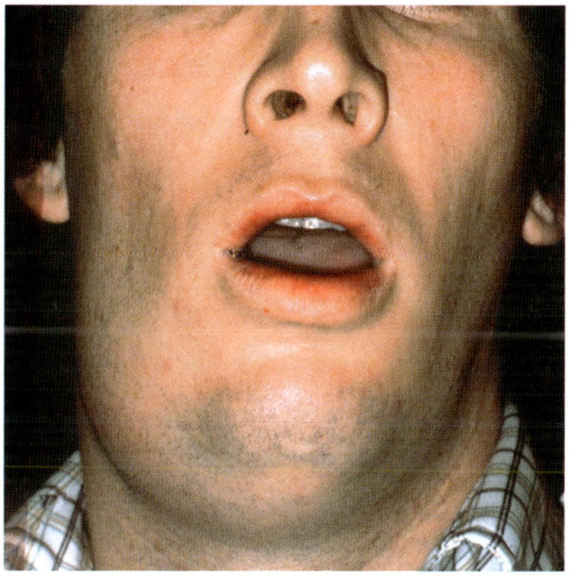

Fig. 65.28 Ludwig angina may progress rapidly and compromise the airway in a few hours. Notice how the massive submandibular edema elevates the tongue in the oral cavity.

be used interchangeably with many of the items listed here. These products can often be kept in a dedicated cart or in another appropriate easily accessible location.

The following is a basic list to have available:

- Gauze: medical (2 × 2, 4 × 4) and packing (1/4 inch, noniodinated). Dental gauze is also commercially available.
- Tongue depressors and cotton-tipped applicators
- CaOH paste (e.g., Pulpdent)
- Zinc oxide/eugenol temporary cement (e.g., Temrex), or glass ionomer cement
- Dry socket paste or eugenol paste
- Topical anesthetic gel (20% benzocaine or 5% lidocaine)
- Periodontal paste (e.g. Coe-Pak) or self-cure composite
- Save-A-Tooth Tooth Preservation System (Phoenix Lazarus), EMT Toothsaver (Smart Practice, Inc.), or fresh milk
- Topical thrombin and/or TXA
- Injection syringes
- Stainless steel spatula and mixing pads
- Incision and drainage tray or kit
- No. 11 or 15 scalpels
- Gelfoam, Surgicel, or HemCon (Tricol Biomedical)

Regional dental supply companies are good sources for these items. The Dental Box Emergency Kit (SmartPractice) is a commercially available kit that contains many of these items and is designed for ED use (Fig. 65.29). It is available at https://www.thedentalbox.smartpractice.com. Dentrauma Emergency Dental Kit is another kit available to emergency clinicians and available at https://www.dentrauma.com.

INTRAORAL PIERCING

Dating back to antiquity, body piercing has been practiced in many countries and cultures as part of ceremonial and religious rites. In recent years, body and intraoral piercing has gained popularity throughout the world as a means of self-expression. In the ED, clinicians may see patients with intraoral piercings of the lips, gums, tongue, frenulum, and even uvula. Repeated trauma from metal or stainless steel intraoral, tongue, or cheek piercings can be quite detrimental to oral

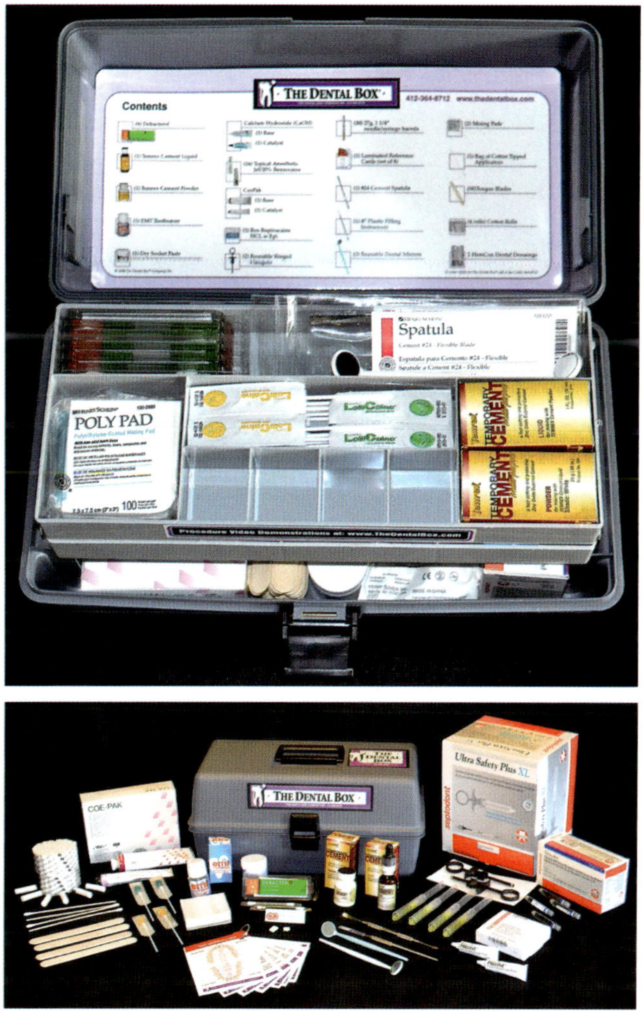

Fig. 65.29 The Dental Box. This commercially available kit contains most of the items required for dental care in the emergency department. It is available at https://www.thedentalbox.smartpractice.com.

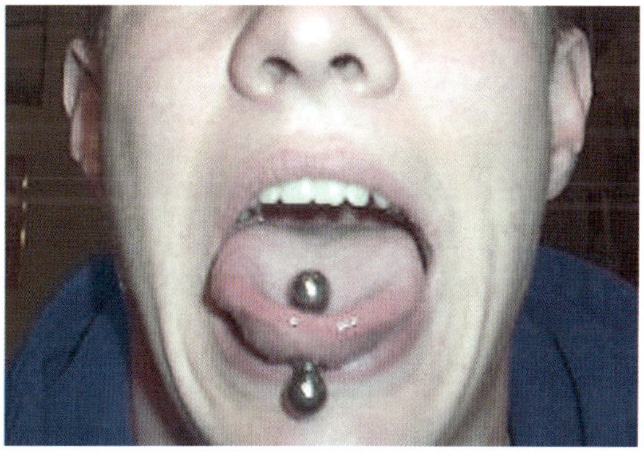

Fig. 65.30 Tongue and lip piercing can cause dental and gingival problems. A metal tongue ball and other intraoral piercings can have significant detrimental effects on the teeth and gums. Piercings can cause microfractures leading to a suddenly shattered tooth and gingival recession. The longer the post, the greater the potential damage.

health and teeth, and cause microfractures, enamel cracks, or a sudden shattered tooth (Fig. 65.30). Complications of oral piercing on the gums and teeth include pain, infection, bleeding, ulceration, increased salivary flow, difficulty swallowing, gingival recession, gingival trauma, and chipped or fractured teeth.[41]

ACKNOWLEDGMENTS

The contributions of Kip R. Benko, MD, and Robert H. Benko, DDS, to this material are greatly appreciated. The editors and author also wish to acknowledge the contributions of Drs. Benko and Dr. James T. Amsterdam to this chapter in previous editions and thank Michael B. Pavel, DMD, for his review of this manuscript.

REFERENCES ARE AVAILABLE AT Elsevier eBooks+

SECTION XII

Special Procedures

CHAPTER 66

Procedures Pertaining to Hypothermia and Hyperthermia

Pavitra Kotini-Shah, Sean McCann, and Heather Marie Prendergast

PROCEDURES PERTAINING TO HYPOTHERMIA

This chapter critically reviews approaches and procedures appropriate to the management of several categories of hypothermic patients. The recommendations combine treatment efficacy with safety. Before describing procedures and making recommendations, essential terms are defined, and the pathophysiology of hypothermia is briefly reviewed.

Definitions

Accidental hypothermia (AH) has been defined as an unintentional decrease in core (vital organ) temperature to below 35°C (<95°F).[1] Victims of hypothermia can be separated into the following categories: *mild hypothermia*, 35°C to 32°C (95°F to 90°F); *moderate hypothermia*, lower than 32°C to 28°C (<90°F to 82°F); and *severe hypothermia*, colder than 28°C (<82°F).[1] Other factors that may be useful in separating groups of patients with AH include the presence of underlying illness, altered neurologic state on arrival at the emergency department (ED), hypotension, and the need for prehospital cardiopulmonary resuscitation (CPR). A hypothermia outcome score has been developed that incorporates some of these factors and may permit comparison of outcomes in patient groups treated with different modalities.

With an increase in outdoor activities, changing weather patterns, and the growing epidemic of homelessness in our country, issues pertaining to hypothermia remain in the forefront. Hypothermia is not only a common diagnosis in rural areas but has also become more commonplace in urban centers across the nation secondary to inadequate housing or lack of preparation for cold weather changes.[2] It is also important to note that numerous cases of AH are reported each year in areas typically considered warm weather locales such as Florida, Texas, California, Alabama,[3–5] and even the Sahara desert.[6] Every year, many recreational and elite athletes participate in outdoor sporting events. The higher the environmental stress, the greater the potential for failure in performance and the development of hypothermia.[7]

Neonates are at particular risk of hypothermia due to large surface area-to-mass ratio, deficient subcutaneous tissue, and inefficient shivering.[8] Acute neonatal hypothermia after emergency delivery or resuscitation can alter thermoregulation causing bradycardia, and other clinical parameters that needed to be interpreted in the context of the core body temperature of 25.7°C.[9]

Despite some advances in AH management resulting in less mortality, optimal treatment of hypothermia remains controversial. A deeply hypothermic person may appear dead, but if treated properly, there is still a chance of being resuscitated.[1] It is a well-accepted practice to carry out resuscitation of these individuals for extended periods.[10] The medical literature contains numerous anecdotal reports of profoundly hypothermic individuals who are successfully resuscitated and discharged neurologically intact,[11,12] the longest being in cardiac arrest for 8 hours and 40 minutes.[13] Despite these spectacular reports of survival, both morbidity and mortality from hypothermia are common.[14] Hypothermia continues to be a significant contributor to weather-related deaths, with death rates doubling from 689 deaths per year between 1972 and 2002, to an average of 1300 deaths per year by 2011.[15] The US Centers for Disease Control and Prevention (CDC) reported that in the United States during the years of 2018–2020, death rates attributed to hypothermia were higher in rural areas and males had higher death rates than females in each category of urbanization. [16] The actual number of patients seen in EDs with hypothermia is unknown. In a recent 2019 National Hospital Ambulatory Medical Care Survey of Emergency Department visits, frostbite was presented as having less than 30 cases for the sample data. [17]

Risk factors for the development of AH include burn injuries, extremes of age, ethanol intoxication, dehydration, major psychiatric illness, trauma, use of intoxicants, significant blood loss, sleep deprivation, malnutrition, and concomitant medical illnesses.[18,19] Risk factors for the development of hypothermia indoors include these as well as advanced age, low body mass index (BMI), coexisting medical conditions, being alone at the time of illness, being found on the floor, and abnormal perception or regulation of temperature.[20]

Core body temperature is tightly regulated by central and peripheral thermoregulation processes. Ethanol intoxication in particular is a critical risk factor in thermoregulation, where moderate ethanol use results in activation of brown and white adipose tissue thermal dysregulation.[21] Shivering, an involuntary muscle contraction and relaxation in rapid succession is the body's natural response to restore the core body temperature. Shivering has been observed down to 31°C and may not cease until 30°C. Additionally, albeit rare, there are case reports of patients being verbally responsive at 25°C and having signs of life at temperatures less than 24°C.[22] Despite these extreme cases, Pasquier et al. have shown a positive linear correlation between core temperature and relationship to vital signs.[23]

Because signs and symptoms may be vague and nonspecific, mild to moderate hypothermia may easily be overlooked in the ED. It is particularly important to maintain a high degree of suspicion for AH when caring for older patients or those with unexplained illness. A common error is failure to routinely obtain an accurate core temperature in all patients at risk. The diagnosis is frequently delayed because of false reliance on standard oral temperatures. Symptoms such as confusion in older individuals and combativeness in intoxicated patients might not initially be recognized as symptoms of hypothermia. Hypothermic patients frequently will not feel cold or shiver, particularly the older population, who have impaired thermoregulatory responses because of their advanced age.[24,25] Paradoxical undressing, a cold-induced psychiatric dysfunction, has been described in confused patients in whom a sensation of heat develops at lowered body temperatures. It occurs as a result of constricted blood vessels near the surface of the body that suddenly dilate. In many cases, these patients are mislabeled as psychotic, thereby leading to further delays in appropriate treatment. Cases have been reported with paradoxical undressing mistaken for sexual promiscuity and assault.[26]

Measurement of Core Temperature

Because of the nonspecific nature of the symptoms of hypothermia, accurate assessment of core body temperature is a necessity when considering this diagnosis. Core body temperature is a critical vital sign and indicator of health. It is of paramount importance not only for confirmation of the diagnosis but also for guidance in further diagnostic and therapeutic decisions. Any thermometer that does not record temperatures in the hypothermic range is *inappropriate* for evaluating significant hypothermia. Standard glass/mercury thermometers generally cannot record temperatures lower than 34°C (<93.2°F), although some models are available that record temperatures as low as 24°C (75.2°F) (Dynamed, Inc.). An electronic probe with accompanying calibrated thermometer is recommended when monitoring this vital sign. Examples of thermometers with accompanying accuracy at various temperature ranges are shown in Fig. 66.1.

Core temperature is traditionally estimated with a rectal probe, but due to large gradients within the body, rectal temperature often lags behind core temperature by up to 1 hour, reading higher than esophageal temperature during cooling and lower than esophageal temperature during rewarming.[27,28] Esophageal probes may be used, although they may be affected by warm humidified air therapy. Other possible sites for measurement of temperature include the tympanic membrane, nasopharyngeal tract, and urinary bladder.[29,30] Bladder temperature measurements lagged behind the esophageal temperatures during targeted temperature management (TTM) in patients after cardiac arrest.[28] Recording both esophageal and bladder dynamic temperature measurements is a reliable and easily accessible way of tracking dynamic changes, but the esophageal method of temperature measurement most rapidly reflects the core temperature changes.[28] Forehead skin temperature measurement as is not a reliable method of core body temperature as it is susceptible to ambient temperature fluctuations.[31] Noncontact infrared tympanic temperatures have not demonstrated consistent accuracy clinically either.[32] In comparison of forehead and tympanic temperature measurements via infrared technology, the forehead method of measurement showed poor precision and low accuracy.[33] Caution should be used in relying on these tools, especially for monitoring extreme temperatures. For continuous core body temperature monitoring purposes, esophageal temperature probes are preferred given its proximity to the left side of the heart, followed by bladder, and least preferred are rectal probes given the significant delays in core temperature as well as poor correlation.[30] One should remember that temperature gradients exist in the human body and therefore consistently monitoring more than one site to reflect the physiological changes would best guide clinical decision-making. Insertion of a rectal probe should be at least 15 cm beyond the anal sphincter, a nasopharyngeal probe should have an insertion depth of 10 to 20 cm; bladder probe should not be used in patients with reduced urine output, and the esophageal probe should be inserted to the level of T8–T9.[30] A chart and formula that converts centigrade to Fahrenheit temperatures will assist the clinician in assessing the severity of hypothermia (see Fig. 66.1C).

Pathophysiology

AH results from failure of the body's thermoregulatory responses to generate enough heat to compensate for heat losses. These thermoregulatory responses include shivering, tachycardia, tachypnea, increased gluconeogenesis, peripheral vasoconstriction, and shunting of blood to central organs (Fig. 66.2).[34] As core temperature drops despite these compensatory mechanisms, the patient becomes poikilothermic and cools to ambient temperature.[8]

Four methods of heat loss affect the body: radiation, conduction, convection, and evaporation. Radiation involves transfer of heat from a warmer body to a cooler environment and accounts for approximately 60% of heat loss in a normothermic individual. Conduction refers to loss of heat from direct contact with a cooler surface. These losses are most profound with immersion hypothermia. Convection occurs when cool air currents pass by the body and this accounts for 15% of heat loss, especially with a wind chill factor. Evaporation refers to significant loss of heat through sweating and insensible water loss.[34] With hypothermia, the enzymatic rate of metabolism decreases twofold to threefold with each 10°C (18°F) drop, and cerebral blood flow decreases 6% to 7% per 1°C (1.8°F) drop. The overall functioning of all organ systems is impaired by the cold, but the greatest effects are seen in the cardiovascular, neurologic, and respiratory systems and vary according to the degree of hypothermia (Table 66.1). As core body temperature drops below 33°C (<91.4°F), the patient becomes confused and ataxic.[25] The initiation of involuntary motor activity (shivering) prevents the reduction in core temperature.[34] Shivering thermogenesis in skeletal muscle operates on acute cold stress. In a malnourished patient, the mechanism may be rendered ineffective secondary to reduced muscle mass.[35] Shivering stops at approximately

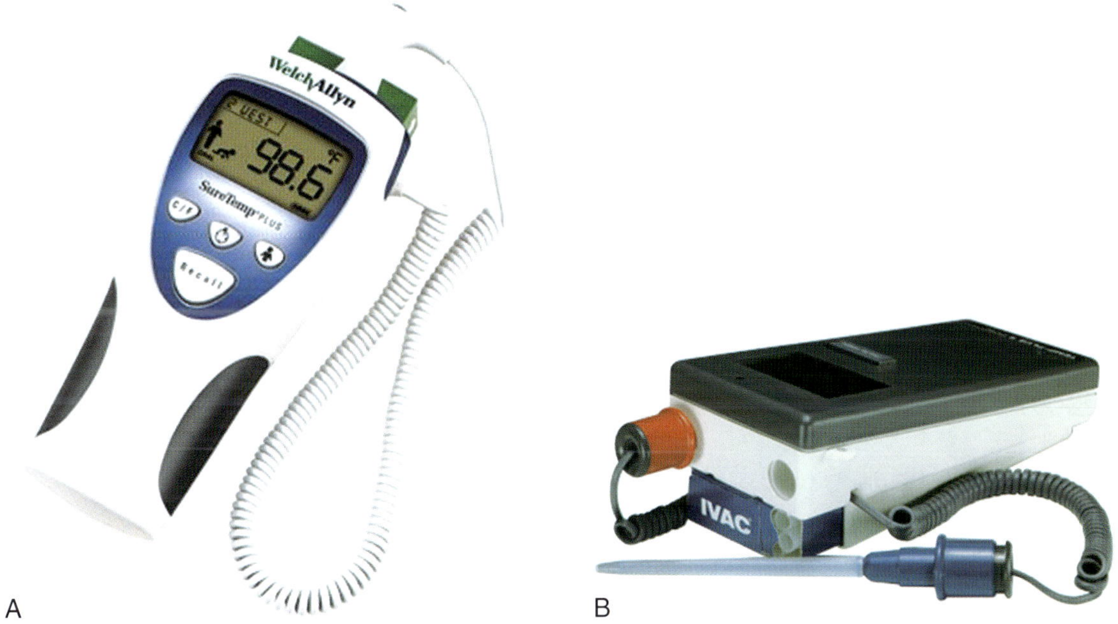

NORMAL BODY TEMPERATURE RANGES

°F	0–2 years	3–10 years	11–65 years	>65 years
Oral	—	95.9 99.5	97.6 99.6	96.4 98.5
Rectal	97.9 100.4	97.9 100.4	98.6 100.6	97.1 99.2
Axillary	94.5 99.1	96.6 98.0	95.3 98.4	96.0 97.4
Ear	97.5 100.4	97.0 100.0	96.6 99.7	96.4 99.5
Core	97.5 100.0	97.5 100.0	98.2 100.2	96.6 98.8

C

Fig. 66.1 Electronic thermometers provide accurate temperatures over various ranges. (A) The Welch Allyn Model 692/690 SureTemp Plus (oral, axillary, rectal) is accurate from 80°F to 110°F. Note the various ranges for normal temperatures from various sites by age. *It is generally accepted that a rectal temperature higher than 100.3°F represents a fever and that oral readings can be misleading.* (B) The IVAC electronic thermometer is also commonly used in the emergency department (accurate from 88°F to 108°F). For severe hypothermia or hyperthermia, it is important to know the accuracy of the thermometer being used. (C) The graph demonstrates variations in normal body temperature by site and age. (A–B, Courtesy Welch Allyn, Inc.)

32°C (89.6°F), and shivering artifact on an electrocardiogram has been associated with increased survival of individuals with severe hypothermia.[36] Atrial fibrillation occurs frequently as the temperature continues to drop and the patient loses consciousness. A J wave on the electrocardiogram often appears before ventricular fibrillation (VF) (Fig. 66.3).[37,38] Though classically considered pathognomonic for hypothermia, the J or "Osborne" wave has no prognostic or predictive value in cases of hypothermia and is not specific to hypothermia. Studies have found that Osborne waves are present in 36% of AH survivors and in 38% of nonsurvivors.[36,37] VF may occur below 29°C (<84.2°F) and becomes common as the core temperature drops to 25°C (77°F).[39] The electroencephalogram flattens at 19°C to 20°C (65.2°F to 68°F).[36] Asystole commonly develops at 18°C (64.4°F) but has been seen at higher temperatures. Initial core temperature does not necessarily correlate with patient outcome. The lowest recorded temperature in a survivor of AH is 4.2°C (39.6°F).[40]

Initial Evaluation and Stabilization of Hypothermic Patients

Several guidelines for the treatment of AH exist. The State of Alaska Cold Injuries Guidelines were last updated in 2014 and include a section on AH.[41] Additionally, in 2014, the Wilderness Medical Society developed practice guidelines for out-of-hospital care of AH.[42] Treatment of hypothermia can be divided into prehospital care and ED management.

Prehospital Care

In the prehospital setting, focus primarily on removing the patient from the current environment to prevent further decreases in core temperature. Handle these patients with special care and anticipate the presence of an irritable myocardium because aggressive measures can inadvertently trigger cardiac dysrhythmias. Studies have shown that oral temperatures are sufficiently accurate for field use; however, infrared tympanic thermometers may not be reliable in the prehospital

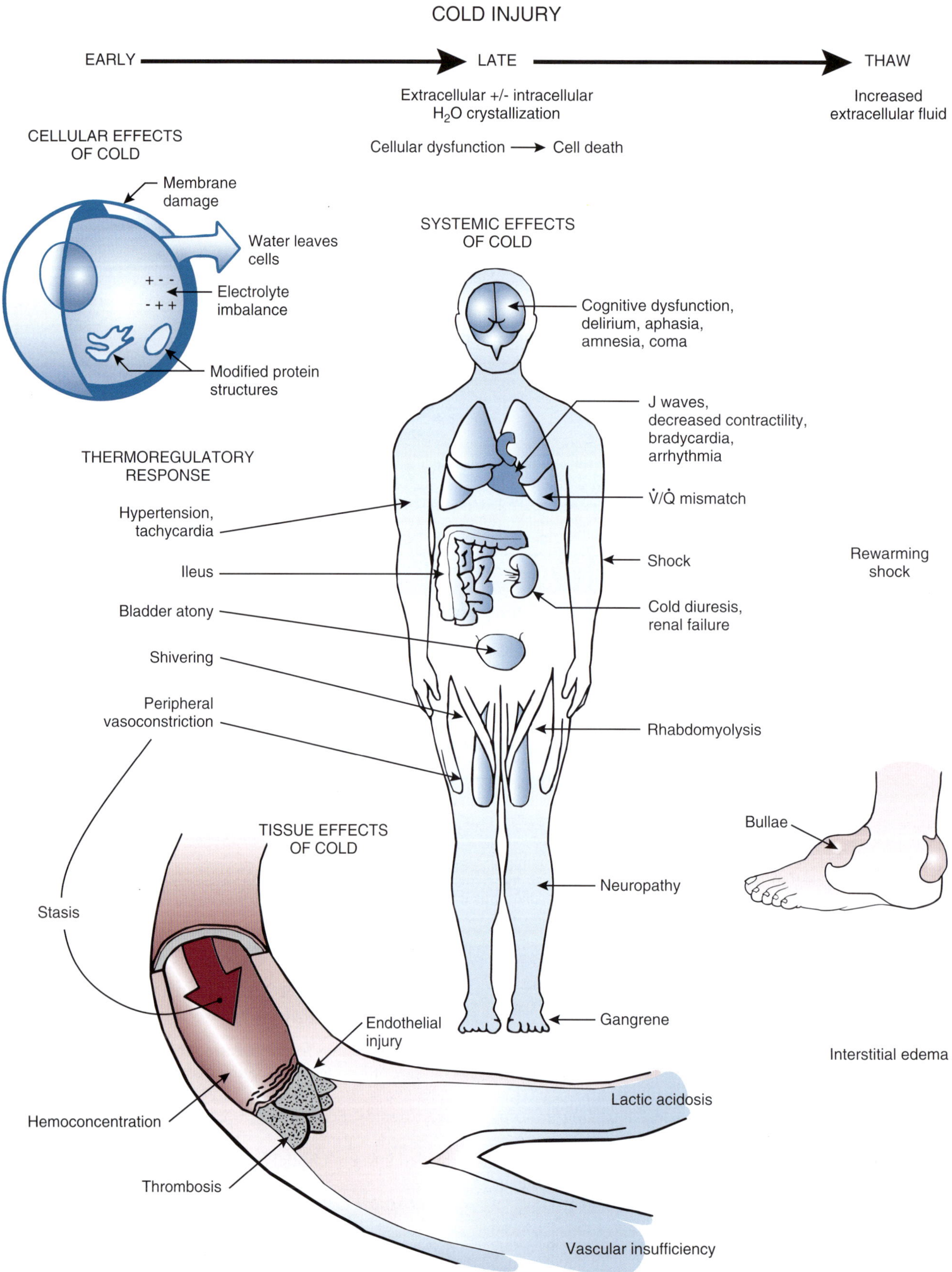

Fig. 66.2 Cold-induced injuries such as hypothermia and frostbite lead to a thermoregulatory response (e.g., shivering and increased sympathetic activity), cellular and tissue effects (e.g., membrane damage, electrolyte imbalance, endothelial injury, and thrombosis), and systemic effects (e.g., shock, arrhythmia, and neuromuscular dysfunction). (From Coughlin MJ, Zumwalt R, Fallico F, eds. *Surgery of the Foot and Ankle*. 8th ed. Mosby; 2006.)

TABLE 66.1 Signs and Symptoms of Hypothermia

CORE TEMPERATURE (°C)	CARDIOVASCULAR SYSTEM	RESPIRATORY SYSTEM	CENTRAL NERVOUS SYSTEM
35–32 (mild)	Tachycardia Increased afterload Increased systemic blood pressure	Tachypnea Increased minute ventilation	Conscious Lethargy Mild confusion Loss of fine motor coordination
32–28 (moderate)	Progressive bradycardia Decreased cardiac output Hypotension Lengthening of cardiac conduction Atrial/ventricular dysrhythmias (atrial fibrillation is common when <32°C)	Increased bronchial secretions Diminished gag reflex Depressed cough response	Impaired consciousness Delirium Slowed reflexes Muscle rigidity Abnormal EEG findings
<28 (severe)	Spontaneous ventricular fibrillation susceptibility greatest at <22°C[a] Osborne waves at 25°C Loss of vital signs typically <24°C	Respiratory rate decreased to 5 breaths/min	Unconscious/coma Areflexia Fixed pupils Rigidity EEG silent at 19°C

[a]Defibrillation may be ineffective at core temperatures less than 30°C. Limit shocks to a maximum of three defibrillations and wait for rewarming to 30°C as active rewarming may correct the dysrhythmia.
EEG, Electroencephalogram.
From Paal P, Gordon L, Strapazzon G, et al. Accidental hypothermia—an update: the content of this review is endorsed by the International Commission for Mountain Emergency Medicine (ICAR MEDCOM). *Scand J Trauma Resusc Med*. 2016;24(1):111.

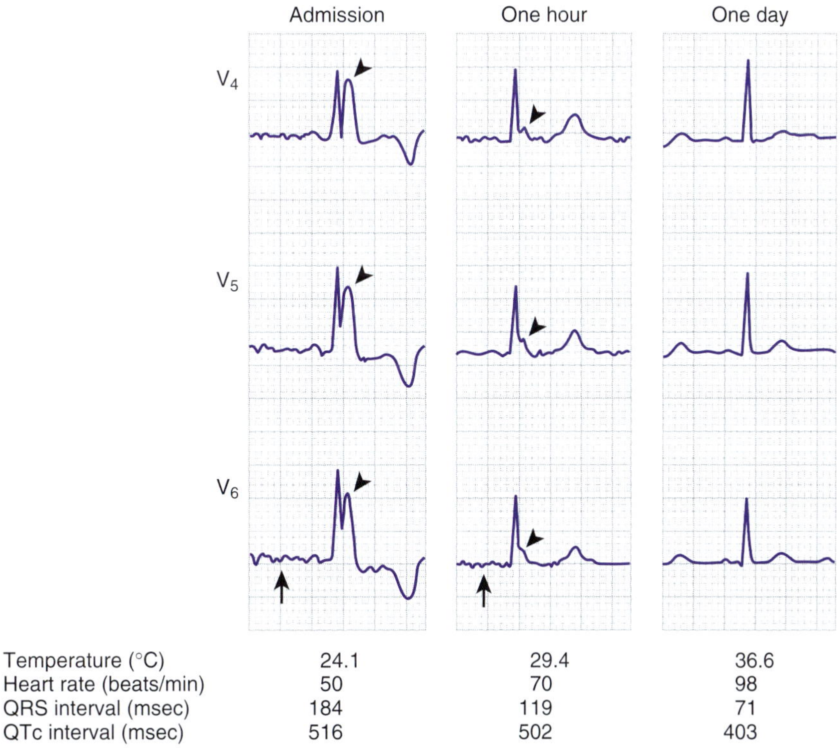

Fig. 66.3 In severe hypothermia, the ECG exhibits marked elevation of the J deflection, so-called Osborne waves *(arrowheads)*. The height of the J wave is proportional to the degree of hypothermia, and this finding is usually most marked in the midprecordial leads. This ECG is from a patient with sinus bradycardia, but in approximately half the patients with a temperature below 32°C (89.6°F), slow atrial *(arrows)* fibrillation develops, a rhythm that usually converts spontaneously with rewarming. (Adapted from Krantz MJ, Lowery CM. Giant Osborne waves in hypothermia. *N Engl J Med*. 2005;352:184.)

setting.[32,33] Avoid aggressive field management and prolonged transport times.[43,44] After removing the patient's wet clothing, wrap the patient in dry blankets or sleeping bags. Field rewarming is a misnomer because adding significant heat to a hypothermic patient in the field is extremely difficult.[45] Studies have shown that for mild hypothermia, resistive heating (e.g., warming blankets) can be used safely in the prehospital setting. Resistive heating augments thermal comfort, increases core temperature by approximately 0.8°C/h (33.4°F/h), and reduces patient pain and anxiety during transport.[46] However, there were no differences in rewarming rates, postcooling afterdrop, or metabolic heat production when electric resistive heating was compared with forced-air rewarming.[46] With longer transport times, use active rewarming methods limited to heated inhalation and truncal heat application. In more remote settings, another option is to use a modified forced-air warming system in the field, which can cover the patient's trunk and thighs and can adapt to various transport vehicle power sources. The Portable Rigid Forced-Air Cover is heated with a Bair Hugger heater/blower (Augustine Medical, Inc.). In addition, place insulated hot water bottles near the patient's axilla or groin. The Res-Q-Air device (CF Electronics, Inc.) is lightweight, portable, and delivers heated humidified air or oxygen at temperatures ranging from 42°C to 44°C (107.6°F to 111.2°F) and down to ambient conditions of −20°C (−4°F). Note that in patients with chest wounds or ongoing chest compressions, it is difficult to do rewarming of the torso, but head rewarming has been shown to be just as effective in rewarming rates in the setting of shivering inhibition medications.[47]

Immobilize patients with potential traumatic injuries to the spine or extremities before transport. Pay continuous attention to airway maintenance. Initiate fluid resuscitation with intravenous (IV) crystalloid, preferably 5% dextrose in normal saline (D_5NS). Alternatively, give warmed oral glucose-containing drinks to a patient who is awake and alert. Most hypothermic patients are dehydrated because fluid intake is reduced and cold causes diuresis. Avoid using lactated Ringer's solution because it can theoretically decrease the metabolism of lactate by cold-induced hepatic dysfunction. If possible, use of warmed IV fluids to physiological temperature of 40°C to 42°C is recommended.[48] If available, use a flameless heater, which is currently being used by military medical units and provides an easy and expedient means of warming fluids in the prehospital setting.[48] There is notable significant variation in battery-operated fluid warmers.[49]

Intubate unresponsive patients but recognize that there is no universal agreement on when to intubate a hypothermic patient who has detectable vital signs. Pulse oximetry is not usually helpful because vasoconstriction limits blood flow to the periphery and readings may be inaccurate or not possible. Prehospital providers should assess for pulses and initiate CPR at a standard rate of 100 compressions per minute if no pulses are palpable after 1 minute. Delayed or intermittent CPR can be associated with good outcomes with neurologically intact survivors after prolonged chest compressions[50] but should be used only if evacuation efforts necessitate the need for intermittent CPR.[50] Some authors suggest that pulseless patients with core temperatures below 32°C (<89.6°F) should be transported with continuous CPR and use of mechanical chest-compression can be used if available.[51] There are no universally accepted standards for intubation or CPR in hypothermic patients with detectable vital signs.[52]

Definitive prehospital determination of cardiac activity requires a cardiac monitor. Cardiac arrest is a common misdiagnosis because peripheral pulses are difficult to palpate when extreme bradycardia is present along with peripheral vasoconstriction. Some authors report that asystole is a more common rhythm than VF. In the field, differentiating between VF and asystole may be impractical. Successful defibrillation has been reported at 20°C but attempted defibrillation is often unsuccessful until the core temperature is above 30°C. If the defibrillation attempt is unsuccessful, initiate active rewarming while continuing CPR and defibrillation. These attempts can be given occasionally during the rewarming process.[52,53]

Transport cold, stiff, cyanotic patients with fixed and dilated pupils because the treatment dictum for prehospital personnel remains, "No one is dead until warm and dead." Some patients are actually cold and dead. It is useful and humane if they can be safely identified. Because human physiologic responses are variable, it is difficult to predict outcome.[10] A succinct summary of the prehospital care of a hypothermic patient is rescue, examine, insulate, and transport.[54] In the majority of cases, evacuation, resuscitation, and transport should be initiated, provided that doing so does not endanger prehospital responders.[52,55]

ED Management

See Videos 66.1 and 66.2. There are no universally established standards of care regarding the use of specific techniques for rewarming a hypothermic patient or cooling a hyperthermic patient. This chapter describes all potentially useful modalities. Many are not applicable for general use in the ED, whereas others are safe, beneficial, and easily accomplished in the general ED setting. Some invasive procedures, however, such as cardiopulmonary bypass and irrigation of the peritoneal or thoracic cavity, may be overly aggressive or of anecdotal or theoretical benefit only. When to institute any given intervention is best determined by the resources available, the initial scenario, and clinical judgment individualized for each patient.

Treatment priorities in the ED setting are to prevent further decreases in core body temperature; establish a steady, safe rewarming rate; maintain stability of the cardiopulmonary system; and provide sufficient physiologic support.[44] Adjust the rate of rewarming and the techniques used according to the degree of hypothermia and the severity of the patient's clinical condition (Table 66.2). Anticipate and prevent complications.

In a pulseless, apneic patient, initiate CPR and continue until the core temperature is above 34°C (>93.2°F).[54,55] Profound hypothermia results in coma, hyporeflexia, fixed and dilated pupils, severe bradycardia, and often an unobtainable blood pressure. With severe hypothermia, a pulse might not be palpable, and measurement of blood pressure might require the use of a Doppler device. If available, use ultrasound to detect the presence of cardiac wall motion. Follow the heart rate and rhythm with electrocardiographic monitoring. In patients who have anything more than minimal impairment, perform arterial blood gas analysis frequently to determine oxygenation, ventilation, and acid-base status. If feasible, establish large-bore IV lines. Avoid central lines if possible because insertion of such lines may exacerbate the myocardial irritation. Give maintenance IV fluids. Warm all IV fluids to 40°C to 42°C (104°F to 107.6°F), but be aware that the usual volumes administered will not contribute significant heat

TABLE 66.2 Rewarming Techniques

CORE TEMPERATURE (°C)	METHOD AND TECHNIQUES
>32	Passive external rewarming Dry blankets, clothing Heated intravenous solutions (43°C), D_5NS Warm fluids if fully alert
≤32	Active external rewarming Heated blankets, heating pads, warm air convection Radiant heat sources Alcohol-circulating blankets Active core rewarming Peritoneal dialysis Bladder, gastric, or colonic lavage with warm fluids (43°C) Heated intravenous fluids Heated humidified oxygen Thoracic cavity lavage (43°C) Extracorporeal blood rewarming Hemodialysis Ultrasonic and low-frequency microwave diathermy Arteriovenous anastomoses rewarming

calories.[56] With long standard IV tubing, the heated IV fluids may actually cool to room temperature before entering the patient's IV site.

With a mild to moderate reduction in core temperature, the level of mentation correlates with the severity of the AH, associated illnesses, or both. Noteworthy exceptions are patients with alcohol use disorder or diabetes, who can be in a coma at higher core temperatures because of concomitant hypoglycemia. Perform bedside glucose measurements on patients when they arrive in the ED. A high correlation exists between alcohol consumption and the development of hypothermia, especially in colder climates.[20] In other urban cases of AH reviewed, the majority were alcoholics. This study noted glycosuria in patients, even when low serum glucose values were evident, and described renal tubular glycosuria in patients with AH. Glycosuria in AH is no guarantee of an adequate serum glucose concentration. This supports the routine use of supplemental IV glucose unless a normal serum glucose value can be quickly ensured. Consider administering IV thiamine (100 mg) and a trial dose of 0.4 to 2 mg of IV naloxone (Narcan) in a comatose patient. Although failure to rewarm spontaneously has been noted in patients with hypothyroidism and other endocrine deficiencies, reserve the use of thyroid hormones and corticosteroids for patients with suspected thyroid and adrenal insufficiency, respectively.

Although antibiotics are not routinely indicated for patients with uncomplicated mild hypothermia, some authors advocate the routine empirical initiation of broad-spectrum antibiotic therapy on admission of severely hypothermic patients. In animal models, hypothermia appears to decrease leukocyte sequestration within the brain parenchyma, thus offering some resistance to meningitis.[57] However, in the setting of hypothermia, detection and treatment of the underlying cause, such as infection, may be more critical than treatment of the hypothermia.

Management Guidelines

Hypothermia affects virtually every organ system because of generalized slowing of the body (see Fig. 66.2). Management goals depend on the severity of the hypothermia, but in all cases the primary goal is to increase core temperature and prevent further loss. In a patient with mild hypothermia, a conservative approach to rewarming is generally advocated. Overly aggressive methods may be more harmful to the patient by causing worsening hypotension, a paradoxical decrease in core temperature, and cardiac dysrhythmias. Other complications may include bleeding and infection of surgical incisions.[56] The optimal rewarming rate remains unclear and varies with each case. Standard rewarming rates are a 0.5 to 2.0°C/h (0.9 to 3.6°F/h) rise in temperature in an otherwise stable patient (Table 66.3). Carefully consider and individualize invasive therapy to the severity of the hypothermia and the condition of the patient. Avoid overtreating and overusing invasive techniques in an otherwise stable hypothermic patient.[56] In patients with severe underlying problems such as hypoglycemia, hyperglycemia, sepsis, adrenal crisis, drug overdose, or hypothyroidism, treat these conditions appropriately in addition to treating the hypothermia. Long-term outcome may depend more on treatment of the underlying illness than on treating the hypothermia.[54]

Passive External Rewarming

The cornerstone of the effectiveness of passive external rewarming relies on the body's ability to restore normal body temperature through its own mechanisms for heat production. Stop further heat loss with insulation and manipulation of the environment. Give warm fluids containing glucose to patients who are fully alert. For patients with mild AH, remove wet clothing and then provide passive external rewarming with blankets. The technique is simple, but the patient must be capable of generating enough body heat for this method to be successful. Give warmed IV fluids to counteract the cold-induced diuresis. Internal heat generation is required for rewarming, and this effect will be relatively slow. In an otherwise stable patient, aggressive intervention with drugs and invasive monitoring might be more harmful than beneficial. Patients who cannot shiver, those who are hypotensive, or those who are intoxicated or malnourished may not have this capability. Survival rates with passive external rewarming have ranged from 55% to 100%.[43,54]

For patients in the moderate or severe category of hypothermia, a more aggressive approach may be warranted. The options available are active external rewarming and active core rewarming. Active core rewarming techniques can be further divided into less invasive and more invasive techniques. The aggressiveness of therapy depends more on the patient's underlying health, hemodynamic status, and response to initial therapy than on the initial temperature.[52,54,55,58]

Active External Rewarming

The application of heat to the skin of a hypothermic patient has been termed active external rewarming.

TABLE 66.3 Warming Rates (°C/h)

HOUR	PASSIVE EXTERNAL	ACTIVE EXTERNAL	INHALATION OF WARM AIR	PERITONEAL LAVAGE	BLADDER LAVAGE
1	1.4	1.5	1.5	1.5	1.3
2	1.4	2.4	2.0	2.5	1.7
3	1.8	2.0	1.9	3.2	1.8

Thoracic lavage had a median rewarming rate of 2.95°C/h (see Plaisier[54]).
From Danzl D, Pozos RS. Multicenter hypothermia study. *Ann Emerg Med*. 1987;16:1042.

Indications

Although there is some suggestion that active external rewarming of profoundly hypothermic patients by immersion may be associated with an increase in mortality over other treatments, other studies suggest that this technique is highly effective for mild hypothermia.[59] Use it selectively and limit it to the trunk. Other forms of active external rewarming are increasingly being used in the ED as adjunctive care of moderately hypothermic, otherwise healthy individuals.

Active external rewarming is most beneficial when the heat supplied by the external source is greater than the loss of rewarming heat incurred by the cessation of shivering. In more remote wilderness settings where more aggressive warming techniques are precluded because of the lack of equipment or personnel, active external rewarming with body-to-body contact may be the only option. The rewarming contribution of body-to-body contact appears to be limited, however.[60]

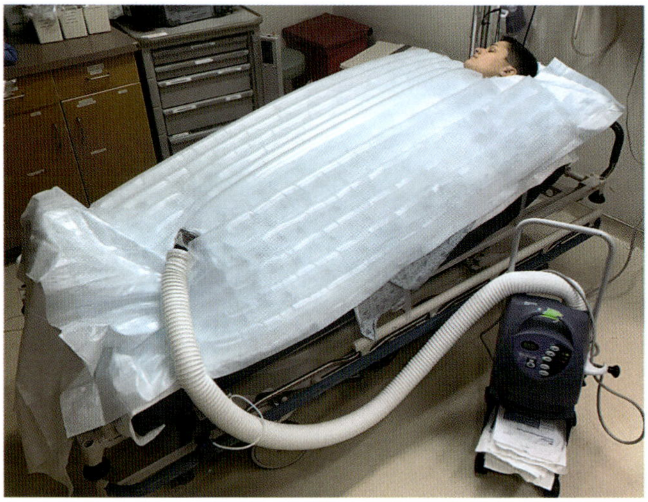

Fig. 66.4 Forced warm air convection systems, such as the Bair Hugger may be used for active external warming of patients with accidental hypothermia.

Equipment

Traditionally, immersion therapy has used a heated (40°C to 42°C [104.0°F to 107.6°F]) water tank of the types present in most burn units. Generally, immerse a hypothermic patient entirely except for the extremities and head, but immersion of the extremities may hasten rewarming. A major drawback is the inability to closely monitor patients undergoing immersion. Alternatively, use a warm water-filled heat exchange blanket (e.g., Blanketrol, Cincinnati Sub-Zero Products) for conduction warming. Intraoperative studies have demonstrated excellent results using a forced warm air convection system (Bair Hugger, Augustine Medical; Snuggle Warm Convective Warming System, Sims Level 1, Inc.).[61,62] This approach has also been used successfully for ED-based AH therapy (Fig. 66.4). Rewarming by warm air convection permits continued monitoring in the ED and is better tolerated than immersion because of the less rapid development of vasodilation in peripheral tissues. As an alternative for noninvasive active external rewarming, there are case reports describing rewarming hypothermic patients with a device called Arctic Sun (Medivance, Inc., Arctic Sun, Temperature Management System), a system also used to induce therapeutic hypothermia (TH). The system circulates warm water through gel pads placed on areas of the body with large surface areas (e.g., the trunk and thighs) and is an easy to use, feasible system for prolonged resuscitations for severe hypothermia.[63]

Technique

Because profound fluid shifts can occur with conduction warming, give the patient supplemental IV fluid warmed to 40°C (104.0°F; Hotline Fluid Warmer, Sims Level 1, Inc.) at a rate sufficient to generate a urinary output of 0.5 to 1.0 mL/kg per hour. Give an initial fluid bolus of 500 mL of D_5NS. Note that blood pressure is not an accurate means of gauging fluid resuscitation because serious hypothermia is always accompanied by "physiologic" hypotension. Because patients requiring mechanical ventilation have rarely been subjected to tank immersion, it cannot be recommended for hypothermic patients who require intubation. Rewarming rates ranging from 0.9°C to 8.8°C (1.6°F to 15.8°F) per hour have been reported with immersion therapy.

A heat exchange blanket allows the patient to receive other treatments that may be difficult or impossible to carry out in a tub, such as defibrillation, CPR, or more invasive warming techniques. Place the heating blanket and overlying cloth sheet underneath the patient. Set the blanket temperature to 40°C to 42°C (104.0°F to 107.6°F), and initiate the measures described in the section on Passive Rewarming Techniques. Forced-air rewarming (convection) uses a blanket cradle to create an environment through which heated air is blown. Access to the patient is quite good with this system because the overlying blankets can be raised temporarily to evaluate the patient or perform procedures. Perioperative use of force air rewarming systems has been helpful in preventing hypothermia.[64] Experience with mild immersion-induced hypothermia in volunteers suggests that the forced-air technique warms at a rate comparable to that of vigorous shivering, but with less metabolic stress and less afterdrop.[44,59]

Arteriovenous Anastomoses Rewarming

Arteriovenous anastomoses rewarming (AVR) involves immersion of the distal end of the extremities (hands, forearms, feet, and lower part of the legs). Advantages include rapid rewarming rates. A study of AVR immersion at temperatures of 45°C and 42°C (113.0°F and 107.6°F) in healthy volunteers demonstrated rewarming rates of 9.9°C/h (±3.2°C/h) for the former and 6.1°C/h (±1.2°C/h) (43.0°F ± 34.2°F/h) for the latter.[65] AVR is well tolerated by patients because of the rapid rise in core temperature, a decrease in postcooling afterdrop, and the shortened period of shivering.[65] There is also a case report of severe hypothermia management using venovenous hemofiltration.[66]

Complications

There is concern that surface warming with accompanying vasodilation may produce relative hypovolemia in a hypothermic patient. Other complications described with the active external rewarming method include core temperature afterdrop and rewarming acidosis. In core temperature afterdrop, colder peripheral blood is transported to the warmer core organs, thereby further reducing core temperature. In rewarming acidosis, colder blood and lactic acid return to the core organs and worsen the acidosis. To limit these complications in patients with moderate hypothermia, some authors advocate using active external warming only after active internal techniques have been initiated.[42] Others suggest that core afterdrop is inevitable regardless of the rewarming method, as temperature will temporarily decrease in any object with a warm core and cool periphery, due to conductive properties.[67]

CPR and other advanced cardiac therapy and monitoring are impossible with immersion rewarming. Until studied further, active external rewarming should be considered only in a clinically monitored setting for mildly hypothermic patients who can protect their airways. When using a heating device, also monitor the potential for burns in areas that have the greatest contact with the heating source.

Active Core Rewarming

There is evidence that active core rewarming may decrease mortality from severe hypothermic exposure when compared with other techniques. In the face of circulatory failure, often the best chance of survival is treatment with extracorporeal circulation (ECC) and warming of the blood.[55] Several methods have been described, including the use of warm humidified air through an endotracheal (ET) tube or mask, peritoneal lavage, gastric or bladder lavage with warm fluid, thoracic tube lavage, cardiopulmonary bypass, AVR, peripheral vascular extracorporeal warming, hemodialysis, and thoracotomy with mediastinal lavage.[54] These techniques transfer heat actively to the body core and achieve varying rewarming rates. The specific techniques and some of the advantages and disadvantages for each procedure follow.

Emergency Warming of Saline in a Microwave

Under ideal circumstances, keep saline in a standard warming device. Warm IV fluids especially perioperatively has been shown to maintain normothermia or prevent inadvertent hypothermia.[68] When large amounts of saline are required for such procedures as peritoneal lavage, warm 1 liter saline bags rapidly in a standard microwave oven (Fig. 66.5). Although devices vary, a 650 W microwave oven has been demonstrated to warm 1 L of room temperature non–dextrose-containing saline from 21.1°C to 38.3°C (70°F to 101°F) in 120 seconds on the high setting. At midcycle (i.e., after 60 seconds), interrupt the heating with agitation, and repeat the agitation at the end of the cycle before infusion. Fluids containing dextrose should not be warmed in this manner, as glucose caramelizes at 60°C. Fluids in glass bottles and blood products are also not safe to be warmed with this method.[69]

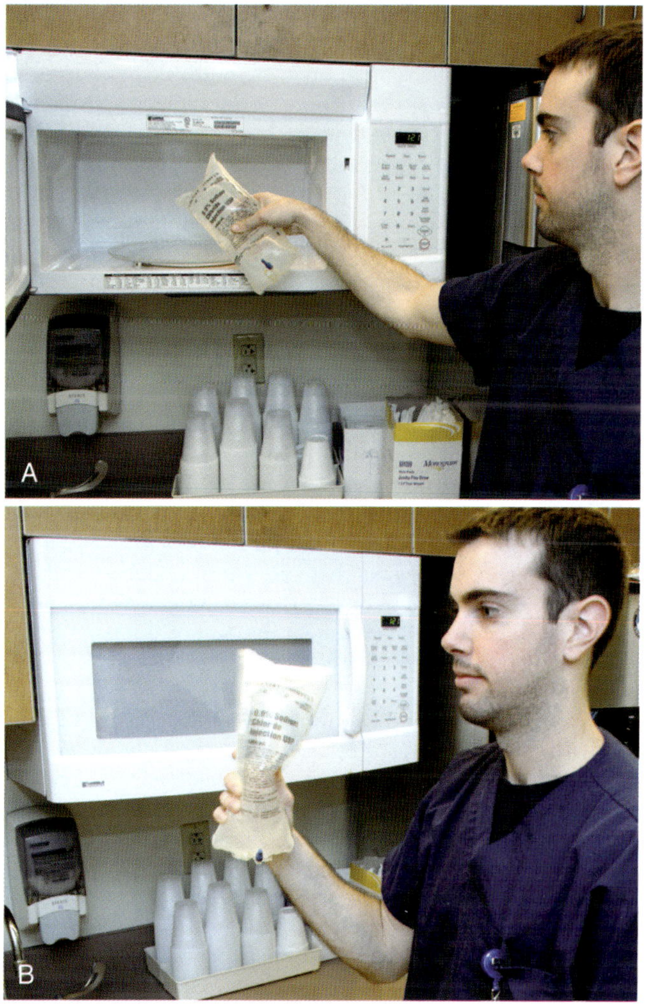

Fig. 66.5 (A) To rewarm hypothermic patients with intravenous heated saline, a standard 650 W microwave oven, on high for 120 seconds, will raise the temperature of a non–dextrose-containing liter of saline (in a plastic bag) to approximately 100°F. (B) Agitate the bag halfway through the warming and again before infusion.

Inhalation of Heated Humidified Oxygen or Air

The use of warm humidified oxygen to treat hypothermia has been well established. Average rates of rewarming of 1°C/h (33.8°F/h) via mask and 1.5 to 2.0°C/h (34.7 to 35.6°F/h) via ET tube with heated aerosol at 40°C (104.0°F) can be obtained.[70] Faster rewarming rates may be accomplished with a maximum safe aerosol temperature of 45°C (113°F). Core rewarming with this technique occurs through the following mechanisms. The warmed alveolar blood returns to the heart and warms the myocardium. The heated, humidified air delivered to the alveoli also warms contiguous structures in the mediastinum by conduction. Warming the inhaled air or oxygen eliminates a major source of heat loss.

Indications and Contraindications. Optimally, the use of heated humidified air or oxygen is a simple technique that should be used routinely in all patients with hypothermia, regardless of severity.[71] If the correct equipment is available, it can be used in the field and in the hospital. One must address the risk for burns during the inhalation of warm air in the field environment. Mouth-to-tube ventilation in an intubated hypothermic prehospital patient has the theoretical advantage of providing warm humidified air without special equipment. A ventilating rescuer can inhale oxygen and then expire it into the patient's ET tube to provide air with increased oxygen content. There are no contraindications to or reported complications from the use of warm humidified air for hypothermia, and there is no afterdrop.

Technique. Use a heated cascade nebulizer with a mask for patients with spontaneous respirations. Use a volume ventilator for intubated patients. Monitor the inspired air to maintain a temperature of approximately 45°C (≈113.0°F). Temperatures higher than 50°C (122°F) may burn the mucosa, and temperatures lower than 45°C (<113°F) do not deliver the maximum heat. Humidify the air or oxygen and note that the heater module may need modification because many units have feedback mechanisms that shut off at a given temperature. It may be difficult to deliver oxygen at the recommended temperature because of equipment limitations. In many cases, the air temperature is only 30°C (86°F).

Summary. Inhalation of warm humidified air or oxygen results in gradual rewarming of the core and should be the mainstay of all rewarming therapy. Studies have suggested that the rewarming rate of inhalation therapy is inferior to that of peritoneal lavage, thoracic lavage, and bath rewarming.[71] Inhalation therapy can be combined with any and all other methods of rewarming and is relatively noninvasive and inexpensive. This therapy should be considered as the initial treatment of choice for hypothermic patients.

Peritoneal Dialysis (Lavage)

Peritoneal dialysis (lavage) is an attractive treatment for severe hypothermia because it is available in most hospitals and does not require any unusual equipment or training. Rewarming rates of 2 to 3°C/h (3.6 to 5.4°F/h), depending on the dialysis rate, can be achieved without sophisticated equipment that may delay therapy or require transfer of the patient to a tertiary care facility. This technique can also be used to help correct electrolyte imbalances. Peritoneal lavage is useful primarily in severe cases in combination with other rewarming techniques for patients without spontaneous perfusion but has also been used alone in patients undergoing CPR in whom ECC was felt to be contraindicated or not available.[72,73]

Peritoneal lavage works via transfer of heat from lavage fluid to the peritoneal cavity. The peritoneal great vessels and abdominal organs provide a large surface area for exchange of heat. The use of warmed peritoneal lavage fluid is an effective approach to rewarming. There have been reports in the literature of success with rapid high-volume peritoneal lavage in pediatric patients.[74] The technique involves the use of an infraumbilical "mini-laparotomy" incision followed by placement of a large silicone peritoneal dialysis catheter. The catheter is connected to a rapid infusion device with delivery of 1 L of warmed normal saline every 90 seconds.

Indications and Contraindications. Peritoneal dialysis is appropriate therapy in a severely hypothermic patient. Peritoneal lavage rewarms the liver and restores its synthetic and metabolic properties. Rewarming by indwelling peritoneal dialysis has been successful in severely hypothermic patients with end-stage kidney disease as well.[75] It is theoretically useful in hypothermic patients who have overdosed with a dialyzable toxin. In practice, it is often omitted if other measures appear to be successful. There are no universally established criteria for performing peritoneal lavage in hypothermic patients who have detectable vital signs. Though theoretically less effective than other techniques that directly warm the thorax in the setting of cardiac arrest, it has been used successfully in that situation. Other less invasive methods, such as gastric or bladder lavage or warm nebulized air or oxygen inhalation, may be preferred in stable patients with temperatures higher than 26°C to 28°C (>78.7°F to 82.4°F).[76] Peritoneal dialysis should not be performed on patients with previous abdominal surgery. It should be used with extreme caution in patients with coagulopathy.

Equipment. Use the Seldinger technique with a commercially available disposable kit (e.g., Arrow Peritoneal Lavage Kit) because of the ease of performance and minimal morbidity associated with this procedure.

Technique. In a noncritical patient, obtain a coagulation profile before the procedure, but in life-threatening situations, initiate the procedure immediately before laboratory studies. Place the patient in the supine position with a Foley catheter and nasogastric tube in place. After infiltrating with lidocaine, make an infraumbilical stab incision with a No. 11 scalpel blade, and place an 18-gauge needle into the peritoneal cavity directed toward the pelvis at a 45-degree angle. Insert a standard flexible J wire through the needle, then remove the needle. Pass the 8-Fr dialysis catheter over the wire with a twisting motion, then remove the wire.

Lavage rates of 4 to 12 L/h can be achieved with two catheters. Warm the fluid with a standard blood warmer to 40°C to 45°C (104.0°F to 113.0°F). Use a standard 1.5% dextrose dialysate solution. Add potassium (4 mmol/L) if the patient becomes hypokalemic. Saline has also been used successfully. The rate should be at least 6 L/h and preferably 10 L/h.

Complications. The Seldinger method has a complication rate of less than 1%. A "mini-lap" performed via direct dissection may also be used but might have a higher complication rate. Further discussion of potential complications is provided in Chapter 43.

Summary. Peritoneal dialysis is a useful method because it entails readily available fluid and can be done with a self-contained disposable kit.[72] If a hospital also treats trauma patients, the lavage kit can be the same as that used for evaluation of abdominal trauma. If this technique is combined with warm nebulized inhalation, warming rates of 4°C/h (7.2°F/h) can be achieved.

Hemodialysis

Hemodialysis was first described for the management of AH in 1965.[77] It is a rapid and efficient modality for rapid internal rewarming of patients with moderate to severe AH, but it is uncommonly used in clinical practice.[77,78] Temporary dialysis catheters are readily available and relatively easy to place. Core rewarming by hemodialysis has been achieved after placement of a dialysis catheter or with the use of an existing shunt. Some of the potential advantages and drawbacks of cardiac bypass also apply to this procedure, although slower warming rates have been reported.[77,78] A range from 0.6°C/h (33.1°F/h) to rates as high as 4.5°C/h (40.1°F/h) have been achieved with fluid warmed to 40°C (104.0°F). For patients who have ingested a dialyzable toxin (such as barbiturates and toxic alcohols), hemodialysis can be used to both remove the toxin and rewarm the blood.

Gastrointestinal and Bladder Rewarming

Gastric or bladder irrigation offers some of the same advantages as peritoneal dialysis without invading the peritoneal cavity.[54] Heat is delivered to structures in close proximity to the core. In the Multicenter Hypothermia Study, gastric/bladder/colon lavage had a first-hour rewarming rate of 1.0 to 1.5°C/h (33.8 to 34.7°F/h) and a second-hour rewarming rate of 1.5 to 2.0°C/h (34.7 to 35.6°F/h) for severe hypothermia.[79] Although the amount of heat delivered with gastric lavage appears to be less than that delivered with peritoneal dialysis, it is somewhat easier to use and less invasive. When combined with other methods, gastric or bladder lavage provides significant warming. Serum electrolyte levels should be monitored if large volumes of tap water are used because dilutional electrolyte disturbances may occur. Children and geriatric patients might be more susceptible to electrolyte changes with tap water irrigation.

Indications and Contraindications. Warmed gastric or bladder lavage may be used as adjunctive therapy for moderate or severe hypothermia. It can be combined with other warming techniques when rapid rewarming is needed.[54] Patients who are obtunded and lack protective airway reflexes should undergo ET intubation before gastric lavage to prevent aspiration of gastric contents. Refer to the appropriate chapters concerning nasogastric tube placement (see Chapter 41), gastric lavage (see Chapter 41), and urethral catheterization for specific contraindications to these procedures.

Equipment. Use a large-diameter 32- to 40-Fr lavage tube with normal saline solution warmed to 40°C to 45°C (104.0°F to 113.0°F) in a microwave or blood warmer with verification of temperature before use. Although smaller tubes are easily passed nasally, use oral placement of the large lavage tubes. A modified Sengstaken tube with gastric and esophageal balloons may also be used.

Technique. Instill 200- to 300-mL aliquots of fluid into the stomach before removal by gravity drainage. For bladder irrigation, the optimal volume is not known but avoid distention of the bladder (100- to 200-mL aliquots should be sufficient). The amount of time that the irrigant should be left in place before removal is not known, but use of rapid exchanges with a dwell time of 1 to 2 minutes is suggested.

Complications. Complications of lavage include trauma to the nasal turbinates, gastric and esophageal perforation, dilutional hyponatremia, inadvertent placement of the tube in the lungs, and pulmonary aspiration, all of which can be minimized by careful, proper technique. Fluid overload and electrolyte disturbances when using tap water are potential complications in pediatric and geriatric patients.

Summary. Gastrointestinal and bladder lavage with heated fluids is easily performed with equipment and solutions available in any hospital. Although these methods are not as effective given the small surface area of heat exchange, because of its ease and availability, it can be started early in the resuscitation and be combined with any other rewarming method to significantly rewarm. Specific effect on morbidity and mortality is not known.

Thoracic Cavity Lavage

Thoracic cavity lavage can be performed either by closed means, through chest tubes placed in one hemithorax, or in open fashion, after resuscitative thoracotomy.[80] The former approach offers the advantages of being less invasive and is an effective form of treatment in hospitals not equipped for cardiopulmonary bypass. Furthermore, closed-chest CPR can be continued while this technique is used. The open thorax approach offers the theoretical advantage of direct warming of the heart and the option of open-chest cardiac massage. Rapid warming rates of 6°C to 7°C (42.8°F to 44.6°F) in 20 minutes have been described. Pleural irrigation results in cardiac rewarming and might be the method of choice, particularly in patients with an arrhythmia.[81]

Indications and Contraindications. Thoracic cavity lavage should be considered for patients requiring rapid core rewarming in the setting of cardiac arrest or inadequate perfusion (e.g., shock, during CPR) when cardiac bypass is not available.[81] Open thoracic lavage should be considered in patients who will receive open-chest massage or thoracotomy for other reasons (e.g., hypothermic arrest with penetrating trauma). Thoracic lavage is not necessary for patients with mild or moderate hypothermia who can be rewarmed by other less invasive methods. Avoid the technique in patients with a coagulopathy unless required as a lifesaving measure.

Closed Thoracic Lavage. An alternative that is more practical in the ED is pleural rewarming by repeatedly using warmed saline placed intermittently and then withdrawn through a chest tube. Place two large-bore thoracostomy tubes (e.g., 36- to 38-Fr in 70-kg adults) in one hemithorax. Infuse one chest tube with 3-L bags of heated normal saline (40°C to 41°C [104°F to 105.8°F]) via a high-flow fluid infuser (e.g., Level 1 Fluid Warmer). Collect the effluent with an autotransfusion thoracostomy drainage set (e.g., Pleur-evac, Deknatel A-5000-ATS). Empty the removable reservoir as needed. Alternatively, use a single-chest tube system with a Y-connector arrangement similar to that used for gastric lavage. Place aliquots of 200 mL to 300 mL with a 2-minute dwell time followed by suction drainage (at 20 cm H_2O).

Provide closed-chest massage until adequate spontaneous perfusion occurs. Perform closed-chest defibrillation if the patient is warmed to 30°C (86°F) and has persistent VF. Continue thoracic lavage until the patient's temperature approaches 35°C (95°F).

Open Thoracic Lavage. Perform a left thoracotomy and pour saline warmed to 40°C to 41°C (104.0°F to 105.8°F) continuously into the thoracic cavity to bathe the heart while an assistant suctions the excess fluid from the lateral edge of the thoracotomy. Alternatively, add fluid to the thorax and mediastinum intermittently and suction after several minutes. Follow this with more warmed saline and repeat. This technique also allows direct monitoring of myocardial temperature. Perform direct cardiac massage until adequate spontaneous perfusion occurs. Perform direct cardiac defibrillation in a patient warmed to 30°C (86°F) with persistent VF. When defibrillation is successful, continue direct myocardial warming until the patient's temperature approaches 35°C (95°F). If defibrillation is unsuccessful at a core temperature of 30°C (86°F), continue warming while oxygenation, perfusion, and other physiologic parameters are optimized before further attempts at defibrillation.

Summary. Thoracic lavage is an effective form of active core rewarming that is usually reserved for hypothermic arrest patients.[80–82] Thoracic lavage may be considered when vital signs are inadequate or unstable enough to severely limit perfusion. Precise indications have not been clarified beyond patients in cardiac arrest.

Cardiac Bypass

The use of cardiac bypass or an extracorporeal shunt through either the femoral artery-femoral vein or the aortocaval procedure can result in rapid rewarming but requires surgical expertise, the availability of appropriate equipment, and technical support.[54,55] Cardiopulmonary bypass or extracorporeal membrane oxygenation (ECMO) appears to reduce the risk of intractable cardiorespiratory failure or severe pulmonary edema after rewarming.[83] This procedure has not been compared with other rewarming methods in a controlled fashion, and few centers have this modality available in a time frame that would affect survival rates. Its main advantages appear to be the rapid rate of warming that it produces and optimal patient oxygenation and perfusion. Femoral flow rates of 2 to 3 L/min with the warmer set at 38°C to 40°C (100.4°F to 104°F) will raise the core temperature 1°C to 2°C (33.8°F to 35.6°F) every 3 to 5 minutes. Drawbacks include potential delays in assembling the appropriate team and equipment, delays because of the time necessary to complete the operation, complications from the operation, the expense of the procedure and bypass equipment, and the potential for infection. Its use in extreme situations that may include cardiac arrest should be based on individual characteristics of the patient, clinician team, and hospital resources. If readily available, it should be strongly considered in hypothermic patients with asystole or VF.[84]

Veno-arterial ECMO provides an efficient warming technique for severe hypothermia. Multiple studies showing positive benefit have led to expert consensus recommending the use of veno-arterial ECMO as a gold standard therapy in severe hypothermia.[85]

This equipment needs to be assembled before patients with hypothermia arrive. When compared with adults, children, especially smaller ones, require special consideration with regard to IV cannulation because drainage can be inadequate with femoral-femoral cannulation.[86] In smaller hypothermic children, some sources recommend a more aggressive emergency median sternotomy for cardiopulmonary bypass.

Cardiopulmonary bypass is indicated in the following situations: (1) cardiac arrest or hemodynamic instability with a temperature lower than 32°C (<89.6°F), (2) no response to less invasive techniques, (3) completely frozen extremities, or (4) rhabdomyolysis with severe hyperkalemia.[55,87] A 47% long-term survival rate was obtained in a Swiss study of 32 young, otherwise healthy individuals, including mountain climbers, hikers, and survivors of suicide attempts. Cardiopulmonary bypass is unlikely to confer similar benefit in older, poorly conditioned populations with underlying chronic diseases. Favorable and adverse prognostic factors need to be ascertained and taken into account to predict survival. The HOPE and ICE score are two scoring systems available to the clinician, and only recently has the HOPE score been externally validated.[83,88,89]

Experimental Techniques

Ultrasonic, radio wave, and low-frequency microwave diathermy rewarming appears to be a rapid, safe, noninvasive technique that has shown promise in animal studies. Frequencies of 13.6 MHz to 40.7 MHz are typically used. In a volunteer study, the technique seemed to be less effective than immersion therapy and equivalent to passive rewarming techniques.[90] Total liquid ventilation with warmed oxygenated perfluorocarbon is currently being studied in animals as a method of rapidly rewarming the core. Benefits include shorter rewarming times than with warm humidified oxygen (1.98 ± 0.5 hours vs. 8.61 ± 1.6 hours; $P < .0001$), no afterdrop phenomenon, and no increase in lactate dehydrogenase and aspartate transaminase.[78]

Very hot IV fluids (65°C [149°F]) have been used in animals with little vascular damage or hemolysis. Trials in humans undergoing burn debridement have been successful in preventing hypothermia during operative procedures. Saline heated to 60°C (140°F) with modified fluid warmers was infused through central venous access. There was no evidence of intravascular hemolysis or coagulopathy after the infusions. The role of hot IV fluids in the management of AH is currently undefined and other methods are preferred.

Special Situations

Cardiac Arrest

Cardiac arrest secondary to AH requires immediate treatment for the best chance of a successful outcome. Rapid rewarming and restoration of cardiac rhythm are essential for patients in cardiopulmonary arrest and can best be achieved with a combination of passive and multiple active core rewarming techniques. Because of numerous cases of survival from hypothermic cardiac arrest with prolonged external cardiac compression, thoracotomy is not mandatory.[53,83,91] The optimal rate of cardiac compressions in hypothermic patients is not known. Because of decreased oxygen consumption by vital organs, the rate required in hypothermic cardiac arrest is less than that recommended for normothermic cardiac arrest. Cardiac compressions should be initiated at half the normal rate in profoundly hypothermic patients. Guidelines developed by the American Heart Association and the Wilderness Medical Society recommend that CPR be initiated in patients with AH unless any of the following conditions exist: a "do-not-resuscitate" status is documented and verified, obvious lethal injuries are present, chest wall depression is impossible, no signs of life are present, or rescuers are endangered by delays in evacuation and altered triage conditions.[52,92]

The duration of CPR depends on the time required to raise the core temperature to a level at which defibrillation should be successful (i.e., >30°C [>86°F]). Previously, it was recommended that patients not receive a set of three countershocks until a core temperature above 30°C (>86°F) could be attained. There have been reports of successful defibrillation in patients with profound hypothermia with core temperatures of 25.6°C (78.1°F).[90,93,94] The decision to terminate resuscitative efforts remains a clinical one, but there are certain poor prognostic factors. Certainly, survival is unlikely in patients who persist in asystole or go from VF to asystole as they are warmed past 32°C (>89.6°F). Some prognostic markers include potassium levels elevated to above 10 mmol/L (mEq/L) and pH levels below 6.5. Presenting rhythm of asystole, advanced age, underlying illness (including infection) and elevated serum lactate may also be poor prognostic indicators. Multiple reviews have shown that asphyxia prior to hypothermia arrest (as seen in avalanche and drowning accidents) is a poor prognostic factor.[95] Ultimately, the decision to continue resuscitative efforts should not be based solely on specific laboratory values or the initial core temperature.

Isolated reports of survival of hypothermic patients with prolonged CPR make extended efforts to resuscitate such patients reasonable. Children may be the best candidates for heroic measures. Under ideal conditions, hypothermic cardiac arrest patients may reasonably be admitted to an intensive care unit for a 4- to 5-hour trial of rewarming with CPR in progress. Manual CPR should be replaced by mechanical methods if the equipment is available. The oxygen-powered "thumper" has been successful during prolonged hypothermic resuscitation. Absence of responsiveness to treatment, in conjunction with a highly elevated potassium level, is an indication for termination of resuscitative efforts.

Airway Management

Maintain a secure functioning airway for hypothermic patients, just as in any critically ill patient. With mild hypothermia, deliver heated, humidified oxygen by face mask. Recognize that a hypothermic patient can be combative and uncooperative and may require arm restraints if a mask is used. Intubate patients with decreased sensorium who cannot reliably maintain their airway or hypothermic patients who may be hypoxic. ET intubation may be performed safely without the added risk of ventricular dysrhythmias. The technique for ET intubation depends on the specific circumstances and the expertise of the operator. Once an ET tube has been placed and secured, use it to provide warm humidified oxygen. There is no evidence that tracheal intubation is detrimental in severely hypothermic patients, and it should be considered if indicated for ventilation, oxygenation, or airway protection.

Acid-Base Disturbances

Acid-base disturbances are variable and can lead to metabolic acidosis from carbon dioxide retention and to lactic acidosis or metabolic alkalosis from decreased carbon dioxide production or hyperventilation.[52] Interpretation of arterial blood gases in a hypothermic patient has been the cause of some confusion. Previously, it was suggested that all blood gases be corrected for temperature with correlation factors (with a decrease in temperature, pH rises 0.015, carbon dioxide pressure (Pco_2) drops by 4.4%, and oxygen pressure (Po_2) drops 7.2% relative to values that would be obtained with blood analyzed under normal conditions[8]). Despite the conversion guide, optimal or normal values in hypothermia have not been well documented. Gradual correction of acid-base imbalance will allow increased efficiency of the bicarbonate buffering system as the body warms. Arterial pH should not be used as a prognostic guide to resuscitation.

Coagulopathies

Abnormal clotting occurs frequently in hypothermic patients, probably because cold inhibits the enzymatic coagulation cascade.[96] Hypothermia-induced coagulopathy does not result from excessive clot lysis, but rather from impaired clot formation.[97] Platelet function is also impaired during hypothermia because production of thromboxane B_2 is inhibited. Such patients often have bleeding that is difficult to control. Replace appropriate clotting factors and use warm blood to limit further blood loss and worsening of the hypothermia.

Trauma and Hypothermia

Mortality is increased in trauma patients with temperatures below 32°C (<89.6°F). It is not clear whether this increased mortality is actually a result of the hypothermia or whether the hypothermia is merely an indicator of severe injury and response to a massive transfusion of cold fluid.[98] Patients with severe trauma are prone to hypothermia because their injuries often expose them to environmental heat loss. Patients with hemorrhagic shock are often acidotic and coagulopathic, leading to the "lethal triad" of acidosis, coagulopathy, and hypothermia.[98] These patients are at extremely high risk for multisystem organ failure and death. Patients with severe injury also lose heat because of inadvertent exposure during resuscitation and rapid administration of cold fluids. Concurrent alcohol misuse may add to the heat loss as a result of its vasodilatory effects on cutaneous vasculature and the prolonged cold exposure secondary to altered mental status from the intoxication.[99] There is a documented predisposition to acute pancreatitis in AH that has been reported.[100] There is a correlation between initial body core temperature, especially if it is below 28.5°C, and serum amylase level, indicating increased risk for acute pancreatitis in AH.[101]

It is unknown to what degree correcting hypothermia improves outcome. Nevertheless, devices to rapidly infuse warm fluids such as the Level 1 fluid warmer and the Thermostat 900 (Arrow International) are frequently used to warm large-volume fluid transfusions. Use of these devices seems reasonable to prevent the hypothermia associated with massive transfusions (see Chapter 28). Their use for hypothermia not associated with severe trauma is limited by the relatively low fluid requirements of patients with environmental exposure. Another Thermostat device (Aquarius Medical Corp.) is used to accelerate recovery from hypothermia by mechanically distending blood vessels in the hand, thereby increasing transfer of exogenous heat to the body core.

Pharmacotherapy and Monitoring

Hypothermia alters the pharmacodynamics of various drugs. It markedly alters drug kinetics, but not enough is known about this phenomenon to define specific therapeutic guidelines. Administer drugs with caution to hypothermic patients (Table 66.4). The negative effects of hypothermia on both hepatic and renal metabolism by reducing metabolism and clearance can lead to toxic levels of medications. Therefore medications can accumulate rapidly after repeated use, so loading dose and frequency of administration should be adjusted.[102] Vasopressors should be used with care, perhaps in much smaller doses than usual, because of the arrhythmogenic potential and the delayed metabolism of these agents. Avoid certain drugs, such as digitalis. Sinus bradycardia and most atrial arrhythmias do not require pharmacologic treatment because the cardiovascular response is physiologic, and the majority will resolve with rewarming. Transient ventricular dysrhythmias also do not require treatment. Amiodarone is the preferred agent for

TABLE 66.4 Commonly Used Medications for Hypothermia

CLINICAL SITUATION	MEDICATION	DOSAGE
Hypoglycemia	$D_{50}W$	1 mg/kg IV
Alcoholic/ malnourished	Thiamine	100 mg IV
Altered mental status	Naloxone	0.4–2 mg IV
Ventricular fibrillation	Bretylium[a] Magnesium sulfate	5 mg/kg IV 100 mg/kg IV

[a]The role of more available antidysrhythmics such as amiodarone in patients with hypothermia remains to be determined; available data is limited and consists primarily of animal studies.
$D_{50}W$, 50% dextrose in water; *IV*, intravenously.

patients requiring medication for ventricular dysrhythmias, but lidocaine, magnesium, and isoproterenol have also been used.[103] Studies have shown that the use of epinephrine was ineffective in cases of moderate hypothermia, and there was no advantage to repeated doses of epinephrine or high-dose epinephrine in hypothermic cardiac arrest.[103,104]

Administer IV fluids slowly to prevent fluid overload potentiated by the decreased cardiac output. Fluids should be started early because intravascular volume is depleted in most hypothermic patients. D_5NS has been advocated as the ideal initial resuscitation fluid.[68,71] Avoid potassium until electrolytes are measured and normal renal function is confirmed. Check serum levels of creatine phosphokinase in hypothermic patients, which may indicate rhabdomyolysis. If elevated, carefully monitor renal function. Replace fluids aggressively because this may help prevent the development of renal failure.

It should be emphasized that hypothermic patients exhibit a "classic physiologic response" that may be somewhat protective. This response depends on the severity of the decrease in core temperature and classically consists of hypotension, hypoventilation, depressed mental status, and bradycardia. This prohibits a precise recommendation of the indications and use of medications, intubation, CPR, and other resuscitative interventions, which are better defined in normothermic patients. Hypothermic patients with a blood pressure, respiratory rate, or mental status that would prognosticate certain morbidity in normothermic patients may recover with minimal intervention on their normal prehypothermic state. Avoid aggressive therapies or medications aimed at providing hypothermic patients with vital signs that would be desirable in normothermic patients but may be supraphysiologic in hypothermic patients.

Frostbite

Hypothermic patients frequently have other forms of cold-related injuries in addition to their systemic hypothermia. The mildest form of frostbite is termed *frostnip*, a condition that involves only the skin and spares subcutaneous tissue. The skin is blanched and numb, but the injury is immediately reversible with no permanent sequelae if the area is quickly rewarmed. Rewarm rapidly in a water bath at 37°C to 39°C (98.6°F to 102.2°F). Frostnip occurs most frequently on the distal ends of the extremities, the nose, and the ears. Nonfreezing temperatures also produce *trench foot*, an intermediate step in the progression to true frostbite. Trench foot (immersion foot) is the result of prolonged immersion in cold water. Rewarm patients and apply dry dressings.[105,106]

In frostbite, the body parts most susceptible are those farthest away from the body's core: the hands, feet, earlobes, and nose. Exposure of the fingers to severe cold leads to cold-induced vasodilation.[107] Apical structures rich in arteriovenous anastomoses can shunt blood flow away from tissues. Freezing of the corneas has been reported to occur in individuals who keep their eyes open in high wind chill situations without protective goggles (e.g., snowmobilers and skiers).[108]

The pathophysiology of frostbite includes three pathways of tissue freezing: (1) through the extracellular formation of ice crystals, (2) hypoxia as a result of cold-induced local vasoconstriction, and (3) release of inflammatory mediators. These pathways often occur simultaneously and intensify the tissue damage. At the early stages of frostbite, the "hunting reaction" is observed whereby the body alternates between periods of vasoconstriction and periods of vasodilation. As the temperature continues to decrease, the reaction stops, and vasoconstriction persists. Cold also increases blood viscosity, promotes vasospasm, and precipitates the formation of microthrombi. Release of the inflammatory mediators, prostaglandin F_2 and thromboxane A_2, causes further vasoconstriction leading to cell death. Release of these mediators peaks during rewarming, and cycles of recurrent freezing and rewarming only increase their tissue levels.[109]

The clinical signs and symptoms of frostbite vary according to the degree of injury. Though useful clinically, the degree classification does not predict the extent of further tissue damage.[110] The appearance of the affected extremity depends on the extent of the frostbite. With superficial frostbite, the affected extremity appears pale, waxy, and numb. The limb has poor capillary refill and is very painful on rewarming. With deeper frostbite, the affected extremity is hard, solid, and blanched. Hemorrhagic blisters may be present (Fig. 66.6). Initially, there is no pain or feeling in the frostbitten extremity. After rewarming, severe edema and blistering develop in the affected areas, and patients eventually exhibit dry gangrene, mummification, and ultimately tissue sloughing.[109]

Favorable prognostic signs for frostbite include intact sensation, normal color, warm tissues, early appearance of clear blisters, and edema. Early intervention is critical in terms of the ultimate outcome. Delay in seeking medical care for more than 24 hours is associated with an 85% likelihood that surgical intervention will be required. Patients seen within the first 24 hours require surgery less than 30% of the time. The predictive value of the initial physical examination is limited, but the presence of nonblanching cyanosis, hemorrhagic blisters, and impaired sensation appears to indicate a poor prognosis.[111]

Based on scoping review of studies, researchers from a NATO task force proposed a classification for consistent description of cold injuries.[110] Four degrees of severity are defined. With *first degree*, there is complete recovery. *Second degree* often leads to soft tissue amputation. With *third degree*, bone amputation is needed, and with *fourth degree*, systemic effects occur.[110] It is critical to stabilize hypothermia and other life-threatening conditions before warming frostbitten extremities.[112–114]

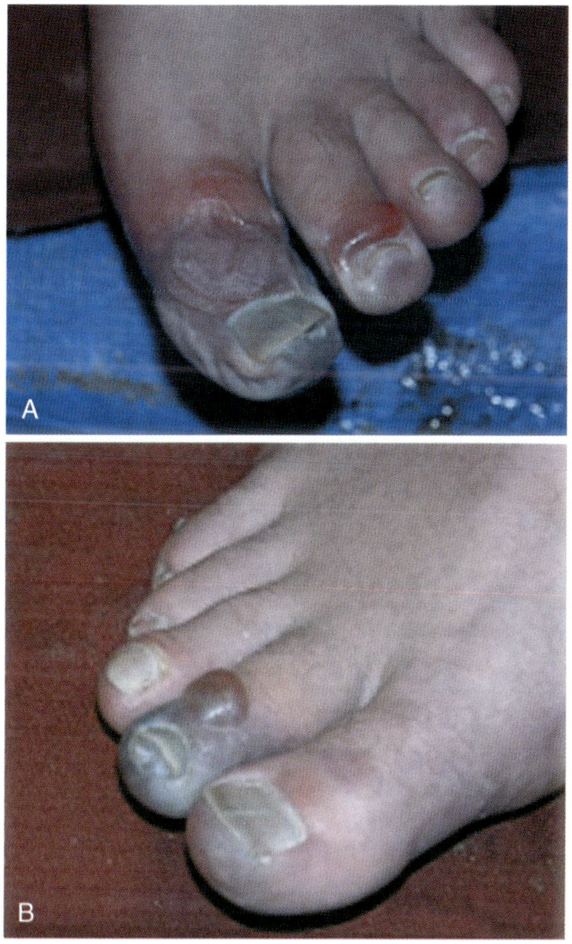

Fig. 66.6 Frostbite. Rapid rewarming is the treatment of choice; immersion in warm water (40°C to 42°C) for 15 to 30 minutes is a practical method. A conservative approach to frostbite debridement is suggested, with many alternatives acceptable. One approach is to debride white or clear blisters and leave hemorrhagic or dark blisters intact.

Rapid rewarming is the treatment of choice for frostbite. The aim is to limit the length of time that the tissue remains in the frozen state. The most practical way to rewarm an extremity is to totally immerse the area in warm water at 37°C to 39°C (98.6°F to 102.2°F) for 15 to 30 minutes. Carefully protect the affected area to ensure that the tissue is not additionally injured by contact with the sides or rim of the container. After thawing, meticulously protect the area from injury. Elevate the extremity and place cotton or gauze between the toes or fingers to limit maceration. At some point, necrotic tissue should be debrided, most often after the ED encounter has allowed identification of viable tissue; however, the ideal timing and best method or intervention have not been elucidated. A conservative approach is advocated. One method is to debride white or clear blisters. Leave hemorrhagic or dark blisters intact because disruption may theoretically cause damage to the vascular supply and viable tissue.[106,111]

Use topical aloe vera, a thromboxane inhibitor, and administer systemic antiprostaglandins such as ibuprofen. Aspirin and ibuprofen inhibit the arachidonic acid cascade, although there is no evidence of efficacy for either agent. Some prefer ibuprofen because it also produces fibrinolysis.[113] The use of semiocclusive dressings has shown promising results in the management of deep frostbite injuries of the fingertips. Provide tetanus prophylaxis. Adjuvant therapies involving the use of heparin or low-molecular-weight heparin, warfarin, vasodilators, and corticosteroids have failed to improve outcomes.

There has been good success in salvaging fingers with the use of thrombolytics but mixed success with the use of hyperbaric oxygen.[115,116] Administration of tissue plasminogen activator (tPA) within 24 hours of frostbite injury improved tissue perfusion and reduced amputations.[115,117] The protocol included intraarterial (IA) tPA included a bolus dose followed by infusion to the affected limb, administered at an initial rate of 0.15 mg/kg to 4 mg to 5 mg via a femoral or brachial arterial catheter sheath, followed by maintenance dose of tPA per infusion catheter ranged from 0.25 to 2 mg/h.[118] Heparin is also administered at 500 Units/h into the IA catheter. IV tPA has also been used and was administered with a bolus of 0.15 mg/kg and maintenance dose of 0.15 mg/kg per hour up to a total dose of 100 mg, followed by systemic anticoagulation or antiplatelet therapy.[119] Thrombolytic therapy for frostbite is encouraging and is the first significant therapeutic intervention in preventing amputations.

In a small study of patients with frostbite, Twomey and coworkers suggested the following treatment algorithm for severe frostbite[119a]: (1) rapid rewarming; (2) assessment of the patient's clinical appearance; (3) early-phase ^{99m}Tc scintiscan to assess the distal circulation; (4) administration of tPA, 0.15 mg/kg by IV bolus, followed by 0.15 mg/kg per hour to a maximum dose of 100 mg over a 4- to 6-hour period, for patients with digits or limbs showing no flow and an absence of contraindications; (5) therapeutic heparin for 3 to 5 days; (6) administration of warfarin to an international normalized ratio two times control for 4 weeks; (7) pain management as needed; (8) ibuprofen, 400 mg to 600 mg orally four times daily; (9) light dressings with topical antimicrobials; and (10) no ambulation on frostbitten feet.[116]

Iloprost, a prostacyclin analog, has vasodilatory properties that mimic a chemical sympathectomy. The risk of amputation was found to be significantly lower in patients with severe frostbite who received IV iloprost or iloprost with tPA after thawing.[120] Iloprost is advantageous over tPA as it can administered without the need for interventional radiology to administer it.[106,121]

Another aspect to consider is the level of oxygen supplementation. AH physiologically reduces global reduction in oxygen demand, and so oxygen delivery should be tempered. Close monitoring of Pao_2 levels via blood gases is judicious to prevent hyperoxia. Hyperoxia especially in older individuals, those with cardiovascular diseases, or severe hypothermia to below 28°C was shown to be most harmful, and Pao_2 levels greater than 300 mm Hg or higher, before rewarming was initiated, was associated with worse mortality at 28 days.[122]

The use of antibiotics continues to remain controversial, although some authors advocate agents effective against gram-positive bacteria such as *Staphylococcus* and *Streptococcus* (e.g., cephalosporins, penicillins). Empiric broad-spectrum antibiotics may be considered in cases of severe trauma or unexplained hypothermia where sepsis may be an underlying etiology. It is also appropriate to administer tetanus prophylaxis, especially with severe frostbite injuries.[113,120]

Cold Water Immersion and Submersion

One of the leading causes of hypothermia remains cold water immersion or submersion.[123] Cold water immersion results in a convective heat loss, making cold water immersion the most common mechanism for AH.[124] Unlike cases of AH caused by cold exposure, risk factors are harder to identify because of the high mortality from drowning.[97] Studies have shown that at cold water temperatures (8°C [46.4°F]), core cooling occurs at slower rates in persons with increased body mass and subcutaneous fat and at faster rates with increased voluntary activity (e.g., treading water). Risk factors for submersion hypothermia include impaired performance and the initial cardiorespiratory response to immersion. Studies have demonstrated that, in healthy volunteers, swimming efficiency and length of stroke decreased whereas the rate of stroke and swim angle increased as the water temperature dropped.

The body's response to cold water immersion (head out) has previously been described as occurring in three phases. The initial phase involves the "cold-shock response," which typically occurs within the first 4 to 6 minutes. Signs include peripheral vasoconstriction, gasp reflex, hyperventilation, and tachycardia. At this stage, there is a higher incidence of sudden death resulting from hypocapnia, inability to hold one's breath, and increased cardiac output. After the initial cold-shock response, the body undergoes profound cooling of the peripheral tissues. The peripheral cooling tends to be the greatest in the hands, which leads to incoordination and difficulty grasping. With prolonged immersion in cold water, heat is lost from the body quicker than it is produced, with the individual quickly progressing to hypothermia.[8,34]

In cases of cold water submersion, researchers have found that rapid cooling is protective against neurologic impairment and increases the chance of survival.[125] There are numerous reports in the literature of survival in children after cold water submersion but very few reports in adults. There are also reports of survival after up to 75 hours of cold water submersion.[126] Reports of hypothermia and drowning in fishing boat accidents and airplane crashes in water noted a strong protective association with the use of personal flotation devices, particularly immersion suits, in surviving cold water–related events in adults.[126]

Various mechanisms of brain and body cooling during submersion hypothermia have been described, including the mammalian dive reflex, cold-induced changes in release of neurotransmitters, and water ventilation. The mammalian dive reflex prevents or delays aspiration or ventilation until the body has cooled to a point at which protection against hypothermia occurs. Much attention has focused on the theory of water ventilation as a key component of accelerated brain cooling. The body also undergoes relative bradycardia as another protective measure. Bradycardia is inversely proportional to the water temperature, with heart rates reaching 18 beats/min in water at 10°C (50°F). Many authors advocate therapies aimed at symptoms resulting from water immersion rather than severe hypothermia because in fatal cases of submersion, death occurs too rapidly for hypothermia to be a significant contributor. Complications of water immersion include pneumonia, lung edema, hemorrhagic pancreatitis, and skin edema.[125]

Environmental Hypothermia Conclusion

Mortality rates from AH are decreasing, and this is linked to increased recognition, better classification of AH and associated injuries, and advanced therapy options. With the exception of severe hypothermia, the prognosis correlates mostly with the presence or absence of underlying disease states. Studies have shown that the prognosis is excellent in patients in whom no hypoxic event precedes hypothermia and no serious underlying disease states exist. Previously healthy individuals usually have full recovery, but patients with coexisting medical illnesses reportedly have mortality rates approaching 50%.[92]

As a general guideline, take a conservative approach to rewarming stable hypothermic patients, with avoidance of overtreatment and selective and careful use of invasive monitoring. Evaluate a hypothermic patient's "physiologic" hypotension, hypoventilation, and bradycardia with regard to that expected for the given core temperature.

With moderate hypothermia, underlying problems should be sought, passive rewarming and basic support started, and less invasive core rewarming begun. This approach should include mask ventilation with warm humidified air or oxygen in conscious patients and intubation and ventilation in unconscious patients. In selected patients, gastric or peritoneal lavage with warm fluid may be considered. For severely hypothermic, *unstable* patients, cardiac bypass and thoracic lavage may offer additional benefits. The benefits should be weighed against the institutional capabilities, time, expense, and the danger for complications that these procedures entail. Although these patients often require tremendous time and resources, the literature is clear on one point: incredible recoveries are possible.

Targeted Temperature Management for Cardiac Arrest

In contrast to environmental hypothermia or AH, TH (cooling to 32°C to 34°C) or TTM (cooling to 32°C to 36°C) refers to the intentional lowering of temperature in patients for clinical benefit. Whereas lowered temperature may be protective for several diseases, particularly following an ischemic injury, the greatest benefit of active cooling has been demonstrated in the clinical context of out-of-hospital cardiac arrest (OHCA). Application of hypothermia as a therapeutic agent dates back to over 5000 years ago.[127] In 1700 the first systematic experimental studies were done on humans to determine the effects of cooling on the body.[127] However, it was not until 1958 that the first clinical trial of hypothermia on four comatose cardiac arrest patients (two adult and two pediatric) was conducted.[128] Since then TTM (a term that now encompasses TH) has proven to be one of the few treatment options for cardiac arrest patients that significantly improves neurologically intact survival.[129]

Two landmark trials set the stage for TTM. In 2002 the Hypothermia After Cardiac Arrest (HACA) trial[130] and the Bernard and colleagues trial[131] became the largest randomized trials at that time to report the effect of cooling to 32°C to 34°C within 6 hours for up to 18 to 24 hours following OHCA in patients with initial rhythms of VF/tachycardia (VF/VT) on survival to discharge. Both trials showed that hypothermia improved neurological outcome. The HACA trial demonstrated significantly improved neurologically intact survival at 6 months after OHCA, with a number needed to treat of only six, suggesting a profound clinical benefit. Based on the evidence from these two prospective randomized trials, the International Liaison Committee on Resuscitation (ILCOR) incorporated TH into the post–cardiac arrest recommendations in 2003.[132] In 2013 Neilsen and colleagues conducted a prospective randomized trial comparing active cooling to 33°C versus 36°C for 24 hours following OHCA, with further temperature control to prevent fever of less than 37.5°C for an additional 72 hours.[133] Both groups demonstrated a similar mortality and neurological benefit at 180 days comparable with that seen in the HACA trial. However, the Nielsen study enrolled patients who survived to the ICU (vs. ED in the HACA trial), and who had the benefit of higher rates of bystander CPR and higher rates of ST-elevation myocardial infarction that could be treated by percutaneous intervention. Nielsen patients overall appeared less injured than HACA patients as demonstrated by lower rates of hypotension. Thus the use of TTM (32°C to 36°C) for OHCA patients in the most recent ILCOR treatment guidelines[134] allows for a wider range of target temperatures that can be based upon level of injury and whether patient characteristics are more comparable to those seen in the HACA or Nielsen studies.[135] Although the Nielsen study has been cited to suggest that cooling after OHCA is no longer necessary because it was a null study, it is important to emphasize that active cooling was still utilized to attain a target temperature of 36°C.[133] In 2019 Lascarrou et al. indicated that patients in coma following *nonshockable* cardiac arrest (in-hospital or out-of-hospital) who received hypothermia to 33°C for 24 hours had significantly improved favorable neurological outcome compared with the control group who received normothermia at 36.5°C to 37.5°C for 48 hours.[136] Most recently, in 2021, Dankiewicz et al. published an international, multicenter, parallel-group randomized control trial (RCT) for OHCA patients comparing the intervention of target temperature of 33°C to control group of device-controlled temperature of 37.5°C.[137] There was no difference between the groups in all-cause mortality at 6 months nor any difference in the secondary outcome measures of functional outcomes.[137] In light of this additional new data from the largest RCT pointing toward no benefit from TTM, the European Resuscitation Council have amended their recommendations to suggest active monitoring of post-cardiac resuscitation temperature to prevent a fever (less than 37.7°C), while also acknowledging that lower temperature ranges may be of benefit to certain patients.[138] Emerging observational studies have alluded to the possibility of refining the application of TTM based on severity of postcardiac injury.[139] When comatose patients after OHCA were stratified by severity, the moderate severity group was found to have better neurological recovery with TTM to 33°C versus 36°C , but the mild and severity groups did not show any difference between the two temperature groups.[140]

A similar study was conducted for pediatric patients through the Therapeutic Hypothermia After Pediatric Cardiac Arrests Out of Hospital (THAPCA-OH) to evaluate for the efficacy of TH (TTM to 33) versus therapeutic normothermia (TTM to 36.8).[141] Primary outcome of good neurological outcome at 12 months resulted in no significant difference between the groups. It must be noted that there are grave differences in the pediatric patients; the leading cause of arrest in pediatric patients was respiratory (72%) and the proportion of patients with shockable rhythms was only 8% versus 80% in the Neilsen study. Therefore a potentially important clinical benefit cannot be ruled out. Many unanswered questions remain about the depth (higher temperature vs. lower temperature), duration (longer vs. shorter) and timing of TTM in pediatric patients. However, as of 2020, the American Heart Association national recommendations conclude that for comatose children who achieve return of spontaneous circulation (ROSC), temperature should be monitored closely and fever treated aggressively (see Table 66.5 for specific recommendations for OHCA).[142]

The clinical implementation of TTM for OHCA occurs within hours after a patient has had ROSC and is generally maintained for 24 hours. There are multiple modalities available, from surface cooling to intravascular cooling devices, each with its own advantages and disadvantages.[143]

In summary, the role of environmental hypothermia and hyperthermia in causing human injury is well known and treatment strategies have advanced. In parallel, interest in intentional cooling and fever control for preventing the human injury of disease has a long history in medicine, with tremendous advances made in its application to OHCA patients. The time-sensitive care of patients that involves achieving optimal temperature for protection from injury remains a unique aspect of emergency medicine, with great potential to save the lives of some of our sickest patients.

A concise overview of all the recent TTM recommendations for adult,[144] pediatric,[142] and neonatal[145] guidelines for OHCA are listed in Table 66.5.

PROCEDURES PERTAINING TO HYPERTHERMIA

As a result of global climate change, it is projected that average global temperature will rise more than 3°C above pre-industrial levels, resulting in a significant increase in the number and intensity of heat waves worldwide with resultant deaths from hyperthermia and heat-related illness.[146,147] Temperature extremes and variability will remain important determinants of overall health, especially in the vulnerable populations of older adults, children, and those with chronic illness. The mortality associated with heat-related illness accounts for more than 700 deaths per year in the United States.[148] In the United States from 2004 to 2018, a total of 6220 deaths were attributed to extreme heat exposure.[148] Excess deaths have been reported during heat wave events around the globe including in the United States,[149] Turkey,[150] India,[151] China,[152] France, and Korea.[153] Morbidity associated with heat-related illness is on the rise. Nationally, heat-related illness accounted for over one million ED visits from 2008 to 2020, with an average increase in annual incidence rate of 2.85% per year.[146] Social determinants of health affect populations' vulnerability to heat-related illness with factors such as age >65, lower income, lack of access to air conditioning, participation in high-risk outdoor occupations such as agriculture and construction work increasing susceptibility to heat-related mortality.[148]

Other important causes of hyperthermia include malignant hyperthermia (MH), neuroleptic malignant syndrome (NMS), serotonin toxicity, and sympathomimetic toxicity. Both MH and NMS are largely iatrogenic and are mostly triggered by modern pharmacologic therapy.[154,155] Serotonin toxicity can be iatrogenic, occur due to substance abuse or misuse, or from a combination thereof.[156,157] Sympathomimetic toxicity generally occurs from abuse of psychostimulant drugs. Hyperthermia can also be seen in toxicity of anticholinergic agents but is a relatively uncommon feature of the anticholinergic toxidrome and tends not to be severe.[158] However, antimuscarinic medication use could predispose susceptible individuals to heat-related illness.

TABLE 66.5 AHA TTM Guidelines and 2020 Updates

AHA TTM Guidelines	2020 Updates
Initial TTM	All comatose (i.e., lacking meaningful response to verbal commands) adult patients with ROSC after cardiac arrest should have TTM, with a target temperature between 32°C and 36°C for at least 24 hours using a cooling device with feedback loop.
Beyond 24 hours	Actively preventing fever in comatose patients after TTM is reasonable.
Neuroprognostication	The earliest time to prognosticate a poor neurologic outcome using clinical examination in patients not treated with TTM is 72 hours after cardiac arrest, but this time can be even longer after cardiac arrest if the residual effect of sedation or paralysis is suspected to confound the clinical examination.
Prehospital cooling	The routine prehospital cooling of patients with rapid infusion of cold IV fluids after ROSC is not recommended.
Pediatric TTM	For comatose infants and children (24 hours to 18 years of age) resuscitated from OHCA, it is reasonable to use either TTM of 32°C to 34°C, followed by TTM maintenance of 36°C to 37.5°C or only use TTM of 36°C to 37.5°C.
Neonatal TTM (resource-limited setting)	Evidence suggests that use of therapeutic hypothermia in resource-limited settings (lack of qualified staff, inadequate equipment, etc.) may be considered and offered under clearly defined protocols similar to those used in published clinical trials and in facilities with the capabilities for multidisciplinary care and longitudinal follow-up.
Neonatal TTM (resource-abundant setting)	It is recommended that infants born at more than 36 weeks of gestation with evolving moderate-to-severe hypoxic-ischemic encephalopathy should be offered therapeutic hypothermia under clearly defined protocols similar to those used in published clinical trials and in facilities with the capabilities for multidisciplinary care and longitudinal follow-up.

AHA, American Heart Association; *IV*, intravenous; *OHCA*, out-of-hospital cardiac arrest; *ROSC*, return of spontaneous circulation; *TTM*, targeted temperature management.
Data from the 2020 American Heart Association (AHA) Guidelines Update for Cardiopulmonary Resuscitation (CPR) and Emergency Cardiovascular Care (ECC).

As with hypothermia, it is important to use the proper thermometer capable of detecting a wide range of body temperatures. Heatstroke remains a common clinical problem with significant morbidity and mortality. A variety of cooling techniques have been advocated since World War II. Although some cooling techniques have been compared in controlled human and animal models of heatstroke, our practice decisions are not based solely on the theoretical rate of cooling. Other important factors include ease of use, rapidity of initiation, and safety.

Before considering the various cooling techniques, a clear understanding of the underlying disorders of hyperthermia is essential. Heat illness represents a broad spectrum of disease ranging from mild heat exhaustion to severe heatstroke and other severe hyperthermic illnesses such as MH and NMS. Treatment of this spectrum of disease requires a discriminating approach, but in most cases where patients present with severely elevated body temperatures, aggressive and rapid cooling should be started while determining the cause of the patient's hyperthermia. Some causes may require specific treatment in addition to cooling measures (e.g., treating MH with dantrolene). A brief discussion of hyperthermic disorders is necessary before describing cooling techniques.

Normal Thermoregulation

Body temperature is typically tightly regulated with typical core temperature ranging from approximately 36°C to 38°C.[159] Fluctuations in temperature can occur with daily circadian rhythm, monthly menstrual cycles and over a lifetime with aging.[34] Exertion can cause elevations in core temperature in the range of approximately 38°C to 40°C generally without adverse effect.[160] Heat is produced as a by-product of metabolic processes and when ambient temperature exceeds body temperature. Body temperature increases when the rate of heat production exceeds the rate of heat dissipation. The brain's thermal center is located in the preoptic nucleus of the anterior hypothalamus. In response to rising core temperature, this thermal center activates efferent fibers of the autonomic nervous system to produce vasodilation and increase the rate of sweating. Vasodilation dissipates heat by convection and sweat dissipates heat by evaporation.

Hyperthermia occurs when the thermoregulatory mechanisms are overwhelmed by excessive metabolic production of heat, excessive environmental heat, or impaired heat dissipation. Different age-related thermoregulation strategies are used when dealing with heat stress. Children have a greater surface area-to-mass ratio and a lower sweating rate and rely more on "dry" heat exchange to dissipate heat. On the contrary, adults use evaporative heat loss as the primary heat dissipation technique. With primary aging, the reflex cutaneous vasoconstriction and vasodilation capabilities are impaired, thereby allowing increased susceptibility to complications from heat-related exposure.[160] Fever occurs when the hypothalamic set-point is increased by the action of circulating pyrogenic cytokines, which cause peripheral mechanisms to conserve and generate heat until the body temperature rises to the elevated set-point. Hyperthermia and fever cannot be differentiated clinically on the basis of the magnitude of temperature or on the pattern of its changes.[161]

Types of Hyperthermia

Mild to Moderate Heat Illness

Heat cramps and heat exhaustion are induced by a hot environment.[162] The body's heat dissipation mechanisms are generally able to keep up with heat production and absorption in these disorders. Symptoms are largely due to the mechanisms used by the body to dissipate heat, and body temperatures remain at or near normal. Rapid cooling techniques are *not* required, and supportive care and hydration in a cool environment are usually adequate therapy.

Heat cramps are intensely painful but generally benign involuntary skeletal muscle spasms. The pain most often occurs in the calf, hamstring, or quadriceps muscles but may also involve the arms and back. The cramps may be severe and prolonged but only rarely lead to rhabdomyolysis. Heat cramps occur after strenuous exercise or heavy labor in a hot environment. Heat cramps were previously thought to be the result of dehydration associated with significant loss of sodium chloride, but some clinical observations have proved that heat cramps can occur at rest or during exercise under any environmental conditions, possibly due to neuromuscular fatigue and abnormal spinal control of motor neurons.[163] Resting in a cool environment plus vigorous oral fluid replacement with isotonic solutions is usually adequate therapy.[162] The benefits of oral rehydration over IV hydration directly relate to oropharyngeal stimulation, which influences the release of antidiuretic hormone (arginine vasopressin), cutaneous vasodilation, thirst sensation, and mean arterial pressure.[164] A common mistake is to rely on thirst to indicate dehydration. The pain of severe cramping may be resistant to narcotics in the absence of adequate fluid replacement.

Heat exhaustion is a poorly defined syndrome with nonspecific symptoms that occur after heat exposure.[165] Some have suggested replacing the current terminology of heat exhaustion with the term exercise-associated collapse.[166] Malaise, flu-like symptoms, orthostasis, dehydration, nausea, headache, and collapse may all occur. Previously it was believed that heat exhaustion is the result of dehydration-induced heat retention that is not severe enough to cause heatstroke.[167] There is modern evidence that postural hypotension developing after exercise is the result of exercise-induced changes in blood pressure regulation. These changes involve recalibration of the arterial baroreflex to lower pressures after exercise, impaired sympathetic vascular regulation, and H_1 and H_2 receptor–mediated vasodilation.[25,167] When compared with the more severe heat disorder of heatstroke, mental status is normal and body temperature is normal or mildly elevated with heat exhaustion. There does not appear to be any thermoregulatory failure in persons with heat exhaustion. Rehydration, rest, and supportive care in a cool environment are adequate therapy for heat exhaustion.[162,165] Some authors advocate cooling and placing the patient either in the supine position with the legs elevated or seated with the head between the knees to decrease skin blood flow and increase venous blood flow to the heart.[162] Recovery is usually evident within a few minutes to hours. Occasionally, heat exhaustion is accompanied by heat cramps, thus presenting a confusing scenario if the diagnosis is not suspected. Rapid cooling techniques, IV hydration, and advanced therapies are not usually required, but patients should be observed for progression to heatstroke because heat exhaustion and heatstroke are a continuum of one disease process.[162,165]

Heatstroke

When the body's normal heat dissipation mechanisms are overwhelmed, core temperature elevation and heatstroke develop rapidly. Heatstroke is a state of thermoregulatory failure.[168] Previously, the morbidity and mortality associated with heatstroke were attributed to the magnitude of the hyperthermic response.[167] Recent literature has described a more complex interaction between cytokines, coagulation, and the systemic inflammatory response syndrome (SIRS), with endotoxin and cytokines being implicated as key mediators of heat-induced SIRS.[169] Two forms of heatstroke are described in the literature. *Classic* (*nonexertional*) *heatstroke* usually occurs during summer heat waves. The poor, urban older adults, infants, homeless, and persons with impaired mobility are at greatest risk.[162,168] Dehydration, lack of air conditioning, obesity, neurologic disorders, hyperthyroidism, cardiovascular disease, impaired mentation, and medications that interfere with heat dissipation (e.g., phenothiazines, diuretics, and anticholinergics) predispose this population to heatstroke. *Exertional heatstroke*, a consequence of strenuous physical activity, usually afflicts a younger segment of the population. Highly motivated, poorly acclimatized, or unconditioned athletes and overweight military recruits are commonly affected, as are individuals who perform heavy physical labor in hot, humid conditions (Fig. 66.7).[169,170] With exertional heatstroke, no single risk factor predisposes an individual to exertional heat illness, rather it appears that greater risk is associated with a combination of risk factors.[171]

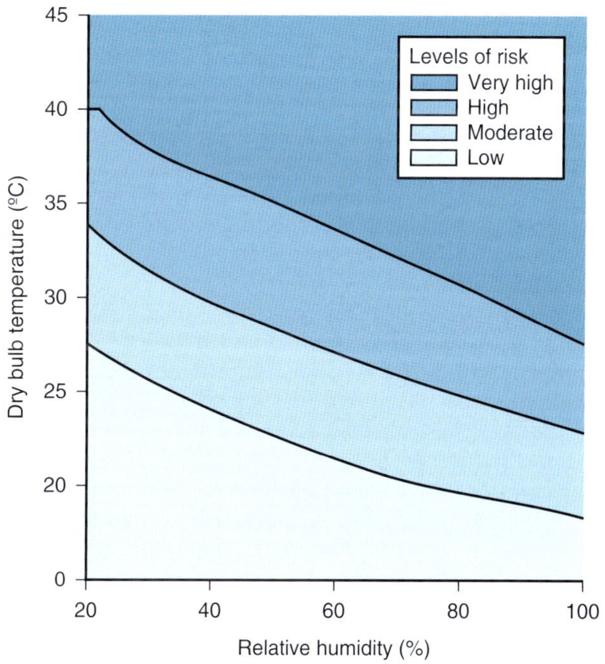

Fig. 66.7 Risk for heat exhaustion or heatstroke during intense work in the heat (adjusted to the American College of Sports Medicine position statement on the prevention of thermal injuries during distance running[227]). (Adapted from Epstein Y, Moran D. Environmental aspects of travel medicine. In: Keystone JS, Kozarsky P, Freedman DO, et al., eds. *Travel Medicine*. 3rd ed. Saunders; 2013.)

The degree of hyperthermia necessary to produce heatstroke in humans is unknown. In tissue culture cells, thermal injury is observed with temperatures in the range of 40°C to 45°C (104°F to 113°F). Studies of hyperthermia in patients undergoing cancer therapy have revealed that tissue sensitivity to heat is increased by relative hypoxia, ischemia, and acidosis.[172]

The key clinical findings in the diagnosis of heatstroke are (1) a history of heat stress or exposure, (2) a rectal temperature higher than 40°C (>104°F), and (3) central nervous system (CNS) dysfunction (altered mental status, disorientation, stupor, seizures, or coma). The cerebellum is very sensitive to heat, and ataxia may be an early clue. Although anhidrosis is described as a classic sign of heatstroke, investigations have demonstrated that cessation of sweating may be a late finding. Failure to consider the diagnosis of heatstroke in a diaphoretic patient with changes in mental status could prove disastrous.[162]

The sequelae of heatstroke are caused by thermal damage to multiple-organ systems.[169] Whole-body hyperthermia decreases pulmonary capillary wedge pressure and cerebral blood flow; however, the autonomic and cardiovascular response will depend on the duration, magnitude, and context (exertional or passive) of exposure to hyperthermia.[173] After a hyperthermic event, a systemic inflammatory response with associated tissue injury continues.[168] Delirium, seizures, and coma can result from the direct effects of heat on the CNS. The cerebellum is particularly sensitive to heat and ataxia or dysmetria may be an early sign of CNS injury in hyperthermia.[174] Miosis is a common finding, and combined with reduced level of consciousness or coma might be mistaken for opioid intoxication. Severe hyperthermia can lead to disruption of the blood-brain barrier leading to cerebral edema, hemorrhage, and herniation.[174] Cardiovascular collapse results from dehydration, maximal cutaneous vasodilation, and direct heat-induced myocardial depression.[175] Coagulopathies and liver dysfunction (elevated levels of bilirubin and transaminases) occur as a consequence of thermal breakdown, consumption of serum proteins, and direct heat damage to hepatic cells. Children often demonstrate diarrhea. Reduced intestinal blood flow causes barrier dysfunction and endotoxemia.[168,175,176] Development of an acute abdomen, bloody diarrhea, dilated loops of bowel on radiographic studies, and unexplained shock should raise suspicion for colonic ischemia and pending colonic perforation.[177] Renal failure can result from myoglobinuria (related to rhabdomyolysis) and acute tubular necrosis.[175] Hyperventilation can lead to respiratory alkalosis and the hypermetabolic state causes metabolic acidosis leading to a mixed acid-base disturbance, particularly in classic heat stroke. Metabolic acidosis tends to predominate in exertional heat stroke.[175]

In cases of suspected heat stroke, it is critical to initiate cooling measures as soon as possible to prevent further damage and reverse the heat stress. The more rapidly that rectal temperature is reduced to 38°C (100.4°F), the better the prognosis.[168] The human body tolerates hyperthermia poorly. Unlike patients with hypothermia, in whom slow, gentle rewarming and supportive care often result in a favorable outcome, patients with severe heatstroke must be treated aggressively with measures designed to rapidly lower core temperature. Studies investigating precooling techniques have demonstrated increased exercise tolerance but inconsistent results with small sample sizes with regard to prevention of heatstroke.[178–181] All other sequelae should be treated in the usual fashion.

Malignant Hyperthermia

MH is a pharmacogenetic disease attributable to a medication that triggers a life-threatening, hypermetabolic syndrome. It results from a rare inherited autosomal dominant abnormality in the skeletal muscle membrane and has an incidence ranging from 1 in 10,000 to 1 in 250,000.[155,182] Mutations in the *RYR1* gene, encoding for the ryanodine receptor, as well as the *CACNA1S* gene, encoding the main subunit of the dihydropyridine receptor have been linked to MH.[155] Development of MH requires genetic susceptibility and exposure to a triggering agent: a volatile anesthetic, depolarizing neuromuscular blocker, or in rare cases vigorous exercise or heat exposure.[155] Patients with this disorder sustain a potentially lethal hypermetabolic reaction with massive efflux of calcium from the skeletal muscle sarcoplasmic reticulum. This results in contraction of the sarcomeres, skeletal muscle rigidity, increased skeletal muscle metabolism, elevated serum creatine kinase levels, heat production, and finally, systemic hyperthermia.[155,182,183] Hyperthermia is a late development and occurs after rigidity has been present for some time and the body's normal heat dissipation mechanisms are overwhelmed. The earliest signs of MH are increased carbon dioxide production, muscle rigidity, and tachycardia.[155] Cardiac output and cutaneous blood flow also increase to maximize the heat loss. Diagnosis of MH is based on the clinical triad of (1) exposure to an agent or stress known to trigger the condition, (2) skeletal muscle rigidity, and (3) hyperthermia.

MH is usually encountered in the operating room while patients are undergoing general anesthesia, particularly with halogenated inhalational agents and depolarizing muscle relaxants. Cases of MH may be encountered anywhere general anesthetics or neuromuscular blocking agents are used. A massive increase in creatine kinase may indicate a MH reaction but is not sufficient alone to make the diagnosis, and treatment should not be delayed while awaiting laboratory results.[155]

As with heatstroke, treatment of MH requires rapid cooling and supportive care for the sequelae described previously. Unlike heatstroke, MH requires specific pharmacologic therapy to stop excessive heat production by skeletal muscle. Dantrolene sodium induces muscle relaxation in patients with MH by blocking release of calcium from the muscle cell sarcoplasmic reticulum.[155,182] In all cases of MH, the inciting stimulus should be discontinued immediately and dantrolene therapy administered. A dantrolene bolus of 2.5 mg/kg should be started and repeated at 5-minute intervals until normalization of the hypermetabolic state is achieved and all MH symptoms disappear. If a dose of 10 mg/kg is reached without improvement of symptoms, the diagnosis of MH should be reconsidered.[155]

It has been suggested that dantrolene administration speeds cooling of heatstroke patients by reducing skeletal muscle heat production.[184] An RCT of dantrolene use for heatstroke found no difference between the treatment and placebo groups in terms of cooling time, complications, or length of stay.[185] In 2005 a meta-analysis concluded that there was no role for the use of dantrolene in the management of heatstroke.[186] Currently, dantrolene administration is best reserved for patients with clinical muscle rigidity and suspected MH. Routine use of this drug in heatstroke patients is not recommended.[175]

Neuroleptic Malignant Syndrome

First described in the late 1960s,[187] neuroleptic malignant syndrome (NMS) is characterized by hyperthermia, muscle rigidity, altered level of consciousness, and autonomic instability. Mortality from NMS has been estimated at 10%[188]; however, a more recent study estimated a slightly lower mortality rate of 5.6% from a nationwide sample of US inpatients from 2002 to 2011, with the mortality rate appearing to decrease over that period.[189] This idiosyncratic disorder generally follows the therapeutic use of dopamine antagonists, both typical antipsychotics (including phenothiazines, butyrophenones, and thioxanthenes) and newer atypical antipsychotics. Although previously thought to be more common with older antipsychotics, it now appears that atypical antipsychotics confer similar risk of developing NMS and their widespread use translates to a majority of reported cases occurring in the context of atypical antipsychotic therapy.[190] A 2008 review identified a potential increased risk of NMS with concurrent use of selective serotonin reuptake inhibitors (SSRI) and atypical antipsychotics.[191] The syndrome can also be seen with sudden discontinuation of pro-dopaminergic medications used in the treatment of Parkinson's disease.[154] Lithium has been implicated in development of NMS, possibly through modulation of dopaminergic neurotransmission,[192] as have carbamazepine, metoclopramide, paroxetine, sertraline, and tricyclic antidepressants (Box 66.1).[190]

Hyperthermia develops in NMS likely through a combination of effects resulting in impaired thermoregulation including interference with hypothalamic dopaminergic neurotransmission, increased heat generation from muscle contraction, sympathetic nervous system activation, and increased acute phase reactants.[154,193] Muscle rigidity, described as "lead pipe" rigidity in its most severe form,[190] can be manifested as oculogyric crisis, dyskinesia, akinesia, dysphagia, dysarthria, or opisthotonos. Recent studies estimate NMS occurs in 0.02% to 0.9% of patients who take neuroleptic agents either chronically or acutely.[190] Temperatures can exceed 42°C (107.6°F). Mental status changes are almost always present, initially manifesting as agitation, psychosis, or catatonia and can progress to stupor and coma. Autonomic instability occurs as tachycardia, labile blood pressure, sweating, and incontinence. Ventilations are impaired by the chest wall rigidity.

This syndrome can occur at any point after the drug is initiated, but it is more likely to occur at the initiation of or after an increase in neuroleptic dosage. Researchers suggest that NMS typically occurs over a period of several days. NMS resembles MH but usually lasts longer (3 to 14 days) after use of the inciting drug is discontinued.[190] The syndrome may be misinterpreted as worsening of an underlying psychiatric disorder, drug intoxication (e.g., cocaine and amphetamines), a severe dystonic reaction, tetanus, or a variety of CNS infections. In addition to agents with increased dopaminergic blocking activity, other risk factors for NMS include dehydration, elevated ambient temperature, patient restraint, increasing age, number of medical comorbidities, and personal or family history of dystonia or NMS.[154,190] The mortality rate is high, and respiratory failure, renal failure, cardiovascular collapse, or disseminated intravascular coagulation (DIC) usually causes death.[194]

Treatment of NMS involves discontinuation of the triggering agent, rapid correction of hyperthermia, decreasing sympathetic excess, decreasing skeletal muscle hyperactivity, and supportive treatment of the ensuing organ failure.[154,190,193] Treatment of severe NMS must often be maintained for several days. Many cases of NMS can be managed with discontinuation of the triggering agent, supportive care, and benzodiazepines to limit sympathetic tone and skeletal muscle hyperactivity.[193] Benzodiazepines have the added benefit of being safe and effective when the diagnosis is unclear and conditions such as malignant catatonia[195] or serotonin toxicity are on the differential. Dopaminergic agonists, such as bromocriptine, cause indirect serotonin release and could theoretically worsen serotonin toxicity. Resumption of dopaminergic agonists is clearly beneficial in treatment of NMS precipitated by withdrawal of antiparkinsonian medication. Pharmaceutical therapy directed at overriding the dopaminergic blockade caused by neuroleptic agents is often recommended but more controversial. Bromocriptine and amantadine have been reported as effective in case series and case reports.[154] Dantrolene therapy, aimed at reducing skeletal muscle hyperactivity, has also been described as efficacious in case reports and case series.[154] These therapies have alternatively been associated with worse outcomes when compared with supportive care alone.[196] An approach utilizing stepwise inclusion of benzodiazepines, dopamine agonists, and dantrolene based on case severity has been proposed.[197] There are reports of successful treatment of NMS with high-dose benzodiazepines without dopamine agonists or dantrolene.[198] The use of dexmedetomidine and electroconvulsive therapy in the treatment of NMS has also been described,[199] and further study may demonstrate these as useful adjunctive treatments.

BOX 66.1 Triggers of Malignant Hyperthermia

DRUGS

Halothane
Methoxyflurane
Enflurane
Diethyl ether
Cyclopropane
Succinylcholine
Tubocurarine
Lidocaine
Mepivacaine
Isoflurane
Ketamine
Trichloroethylene
Chloroform
Gallamine
Nitrous oxide

CONDITIONS

Heat stress
Vigorous exercise
Emotional stress

Serotonin Toxicity (Serotonin Syndrome)

A disorder often confused with NMS is commonly referred to as serotonin syndrome, but more accurately described as serotonin toxicity, since toxicity presents on a spectrum rather than with a consistent collection of symptoms as occurs in a true syndrome.[200] Serotonin toxicity can result from therapeutic use, abuse, or misuse of prescription medications or street drugs with serotonergic agonist properties, which induce a clinical picture somewhat similar to NMS. Serotonin toxicity most often occurs when two or more drugs that interfere with serotonin signaling act synergistically on various serotonin receptors and lead to overstimulation.[156] A selection of medications implicated in inducing serotonin toxicity are listed in (Box 66.2). The range of symptoms varies from mild gastrointestinal upset, insomnia, tremor, and agitation to more severe symptoms that include muscle spasms, seizures, ataxia, rhabdomyolysis, and autonomic instability including hyperthermia. Impaired thermoregulation in serotonin toxicity occurs via direct nonshivering thermogenesis in brown fat, psychomotor hyperactivity, and constriction of cutaneous vasculature.[193,201] Hyperreflexia and clonus are the hallmark findings on examination that help distinguish serotonin toxicity from similar entities like NMS, anticholinergic toxicity, and sepsis. Hyperreflexia was present in 100% of patients in a recent case series.[202] Clonus can be inducible in mild disease, and with increasing severity, inextinguishable, spontaneous, and ocular clonus can be seen. In severe cases, profound muscle rigidity can mask hyperreflexia and clonus, confounding clinical differentiation from other entities like NMS. Clinical diagnostic criteria have been proposed by Sternbach[203] and Dunkley et al. (the Hunter Criteria)[204]; however, these criteria may be insensitive in both mild and severe toxicity and rely on patient history which may be limited by altered mentation. Therefore clinical criteria should not be used to definitively exclude the diagnosis and the gold standard for diagnosis is the clinical judgment of a toxicologist.[204]

BOX 66.2 Selected Agents Associated With Serotonin Toxicity

SEROTONIN PRECURSORS

L-Tryptophan

SEROTONIN AGONISTS

LSD
Triptans
Metoclopramide

AGENTS THAT AUGMENT SEROTONIN RELEASE

MDMA and other phenylethylamines
Cathinones
Buspirone
Cocaine
Lithium
Mirtazapine
L-Dopa

SEROTONIN REUPTAKE INHIBITORS

SSRIs
SNRIs
TCAs
Bupropion
Tramadol
Cocaine
Dextromethorphan
Fentanyl
Meperidine
Pentazocine
Milnacipran
Trazodone
Nefazodone

INHIBITORS OF SEROTONIN METABOLISM

MAOIs
St. John's Wort
Linezolid
Methylene blue
Harmine and harmaline (from Ayahuasca or Syrian Rue)

OTHER

Ginseng
Ritonavir
Valproic acid
Yohimbine

LSD, *Lysergic acid diethylamide*; MDMA, *3,4-methylenedioxymethamphetamine*; SSRI, *selective serotonin reuptake inhibitor*; SNRI, *serotonin and norepinephrine reuptake inhibitor*; TCA, *tricyclic antidepressant*; MAOI, *monoamine oxidase inhibitor*.

Treatment is primarily supportive and consists of prompt recognition and withdrawal of the offending agent. Adequate sedation, usually with benzodiazepines, is essential in controlling serotonin toxicity. Onset and resolution are generally faster than in NMS and many cases resolve within 24 hours; however, severe toxicity can persist for days.[193] For the most severe cases, aggressive intensive management, including rapid cooling of hyperthermia, is warranted to prevent organ failure and death. Benzodiazepines titrated to control of agitation and tachycardia are first-line pharmacotherapy. Given the contribution of psychomotor activity to development of hyperthermia, the use of neuromuscular blocking agents in refractory severe toxicity has been advocated.[156,193]

Pharmacotherapy with serotonin receptor antagonists has been investigated and recommended; however, data supporting efficacy in humans is limited. The most commonly recommended drug is cyproheptadine, which is an antihistamine with antagonist effects at all serotonin receptor subtypes. Theoretically, antagonism at serotonin receptor subtypes 1, 3, and 7 could be detrimental in treatment of serotonin-induced hyperthermia,[205] but case series of treatment with cyproheptadine have shown improvement after cyproheptadine administration with few adverse events.[206–208] These case series are limited by lack of control groups, and improvement after initiation of cyproheptadine may reflect the natural course of serotonin toxicity rather than therapeutic benefit. A recent retrospective review of cyproheptadine use in serotonin toxicity cases reported to the California Poison Control System over 11 years found no significant difference in severe outcomes between patients treated with and without cyproheptadine, but also found no major adverse effects attributable to cyproheptadine administration.[209] Cyproheptadine use may not be practical in some cases since it is only available in an oral form, though it may be crushed and given through a nasogastric or orogastric tube. In cases in which serotonin syndrome and NMS cannot be differentiated, benzodiazepines represent the safest therapeutic option.[193]

Hyperthermia and Psychostimulant Overdose

Psychostimulants reflect a broad class of pharmacologic agents including prescription drugs, illicit substances, and nonprescription medications and supplements. These agents produce stimulant effects through a variety of mechanisms promoting wakefulness, alertness, and energy.[210] Toxicity typically manifests in a sympathomimetic toxidrome with psychomotor agitation, tachycardia, hypertension, mydriasis, diaphoresis, and hyperthermia. Many psychostimulant medications have serotonergic agonist properties with potential to precipitate serotonin toxicity as well as sympathomimetic toxicity. Hyperthermia is a concerning finding and often portends impending arrhythmia, seizure, or death. Common agents include cocaine, amphetamines (including methamphetamine and 3,4-methylenedioxymethamphetamine [MDMA]), cathinones, ephedrine, and many novel psychoactive substances (NPS).[211] An estimated 9.2 million people in the United States and 75 million people worldwide abused or misused CNS stimulants in the prior year.[212,213]

Hyperthermia is a common feature of these potentially severe to lethal poisonings with sympathomimetic psychostimulant drugs and may be the primary cause of fatality or MDMA toxicity.[214] Methamphetamine use is of particular concern in the United States given rising levels of use, increasing severity of exposure, and increasing number of associated deaths.[215,216] Cocaine exposures have shown similar trends in the United States[217] and cocaine use is rapidly expanding worldwide.[213] In addition to profound hyperthermia (>42°C [>107.6°F]), acute rhabdomyolysis, DIC, psychiatric and cognitive dysfunction, renal failure, coma, seizures, and death have been described in these patients.[210,215,217] As demonstrated by Roberts and associates,[218] even a patient with a core temperature of 45.5°C (114°F) because of acute cocaine intoxication may survive with aggressive cooling methods.

Thermoregulation is impaired in sympathomimetic toxicity through a variety of mechanisms including disruption of central hypothalamic thermoregulatory function, increased metabolic rate, psychomotor agitation, dehydration, and vascular constriction.[210,219] Treatment requires prompt recognition, maintenance of adequate hydration, rapid cooling, and the aggressive use of sedatives or paralyzing agents (or both) to control agitation. Importantly, the longer that psychostimulant-overdosed patients remain hyperthermic, the higher their morbidity and mortality rates.[214] Agitation and seizures must be chemically controlled because they lead to continued generation of heat and muscle injury. Therefore liberal doses of benzodiazepines are recommended.[210] Dantrolene use has been advocated in sympathomimetic toxicity, but human and animal studies have shown no evidence of benefit and so cannot be recommended.[220,221] Bromocriptine should be avoided due to its indirect serotonergic agonism, which could worsen toxicity.

Hemorrhagic Shock and Encephalopathy Syndrome

The condition of hemorrhagic shock and encephalopathy syndrome in children (mainly infants, but some older children also) resembles heatstroke in adults. The full-blown syndrome includes hyperthermia, coagulopathy, encephalopathy, and renal and hepatic dysfunction.[222,223] Although there may be an association with concurrent viral illness, the condition generally follows an elevation in temperature, which may be triggered by "bundling" of a child with a low-grade fever. Pathogenesis is thought to occur from hypercytokinemia and acute necrotizing encephalopathy.[222]. Therapy is largely supportive and includes volume replacement with rapid cooling of the hyperthermic child while sources of bacterial infection are sought and treated.

Cooling Techniques

General Considerations

Heatstroke morbidity and mortality are proportional to the magnitude and duration of thermal stress measured in degree-minutes.[224,225] Delay in cooling may be the single most important factor leading to death or residual disability in those who survive.[175] In addition, advanced age and underlying disease states are significant contributing factors, though a recent review reported that the majority of patients who died or experienced long-term neurologic morbidity had no premorbid health conditions.[226]

Many patients with exertional heatstroke are volume depleted and may exhibit hypotension. Initial stabilization with cooled (room temperature) IV fluids and correction of electrolyte abnormalities are valuable in hypotensive patients. Traditional sources recommend a rate of 1200 mL over the first 4 hours.[227] Others advise a 2-L bolus over the first hour, with an additional 1 L/h for the following 3 hours.[228] Seraj and colleagues challenged this more aggressive recommendation.[229] In their study of pilgrims who had heatstroke, 65% had normal or above-normal central venous pressure (CVP) on arrival. These authors found that an average of 1 L of saline was sufficient to normalize CVP during the cooling period in their patients, who had a mean age of 55 years (range, 31 to 80 years). In older patients, fluid resuscitation should be monitored carefully to avoid pulmonary edema. Regarding antipyretics, there is no indication for salicylates, nonsteroidal antiinflammatory drugs (NSAIDs), or acetaminophen in the setting of heatstroke because their efficacy depends on a normally functioning hypothalamus. Overzealous use of acetaminophen could potentiate hepatic damage, and salicylates may promote bleeding tendencies.[230] A study comparing acetaminophen and physical cooling methods found that in patients treated with antipyretics only, mean body temperature increased by 0.2°C (32.4°F) on average.[231]

Given that rapid cooling is accepted as the cornerstone of effective heatstroke therapy, the clinician must choose which cooling technique to use. Studies in animal models are based on the assumption that the fastest cooling technique is the best. In clinical patient care, other factors also influence the choice of technique. Patient access, monitoring, safety, ease of use, availability, and speed are all considerations.[232] A technique that may not be the most rapid but allows easy patient access and is readily available may be preferable to more cumbersome (albeit more rapid once established) cooling techniques in some clinical settings.

The cooling rates achieved in selected human and animal studies of heatstroke are summarized in Table 66.6.[233–268] The advantages and disadvantages of various cooling techniques are outlined in Table 66.7.

In addition to the cooling procedures outlined, it is imperative that the clinician institute the judicious use of sedation, muscle paralysis, or both to control agitation, suppress shivering, reduce energy expenditure, and make the patient receptive to sometimes unpleasant therapies.[269] In general, IV benzodiazepines are the easiest and safest first-line drugs used for sedation.

Indications for Rapid Cooling

Rapid cooling should be instituted as soon as the diagnosis of heatstroke (rectal temperature >40°C [104°F], altered mental

TABLE 66.6 Cooling Rates Achieved With Various Cooling Techniques

TECHNIQUE	REFERENCE	MODEL	RATE (°C/min)
Evaporative	Daily and Harrison,[240] 1948	Rat	0.93
	Wyndham et al.,[267] 1959	Human	0.07
	Weiner and Khogali,[264] 1980	Human	0.31
	Kielblock et al.,[249] 1986	Human	0.09
	Al-Aska et al.,[281] 1987	Human	0.087
	Poulton and Walker,[257] 1987	Human	0.10
	Sinclair et al.,[259] 2009	Human	0.06
	Hee-Nee et al.,[247] 2010	Human	0.14
Immersion	Daily and Harrison,[240] 1948	Rat	1.86
	Wyndham et al.,[267] 1959	Human	0.14
	Magazanik et al.,[253] 1980	Dog	0.27
	Weiner and Khogali,[264] 1980	Human	0.11
	Armstrong et al.,[233] 1996	Human	0.20
	Proulx et al.,[258] 2003	Human	0.35
	Taylor et al.,[263] 2008	Human	0.18
	Lemire et al.,[250] 2009	Human	0.17
	Gagnon et al.,[244] 2010	Human	0.16
	Flouris et al.,[243] 2014	Human	0.26
	Demartini et al.,[241] 2015	Human	0.22
	Miller et al.,[255] 2015	Human	0.23
	Luhring et al.,[252] 2016	Human	0.14
	Nye et al.,[256] 2017	Human	0.07
	Caldwell et al.,[237] 2018	Human	0.62
	Divine et al.,[242] 2018	Human	0.22
Selective immersion	Clapp et al.,[238] 2001	Human	
	Torso immersion		0.25
	Hand/foot immersion		0.16
	Clements et al.,[239] 2002	Human	
	Torso immersion		0.16
	Barwood et al.,[234] 2009	Human	
	Hand immersion		0.04
Ice packing (whole body)	Kielblock et al.,[249] 1986	Human	0.034
Strategic ice packs (or towels)	Kielblock et al.,[249] 1986	Human	0.028
	Armstrong et al.,[233] 1996	Human	0.11
	Sinclair et al.,[259] 2009	Human	0.06
	Lissoway et al.,[251] 2015	Human	
	Neck, groin, axilla		0.17
	Glabrous skin surfaces		0.30
	Yang et al.,[268] 2017	Human	0.02
Evaporative with strategic ice packs	Kielblock et al.,[249] 1986	Human	0.036
	Pease et al.,[276] 2009	Human	0.005
	Singh et al.,[260] 2017	Human	0.06
Cold gastric lavage	Syverud et al.,[261] 1985	Dog	0.15
	White et al.,[266] 1987	Dog	0.06
	Szold et al.,[262] 2002	Human	0.07
Cold peritoneal lavage	Bynum et al.,[236] 1978[1]	Dog	0.56
	Horowitz,[248] 1989	Human	0.11
	White,[265] 1993	Dog	0.14
Cyclic lung lavage	Harris et al.,[246] 2001	Dog	0.5
Intravascular cooling devices	Mégarbane et al.,[254] 2004	Human	0.01
	Broessner et al.,[235] 2005	Human	0.01
	Hamaya et al.,[245] 2015	Human	0.1

TABLE 66.7 Advantages and Disadvantages of Various Cooling Techniques

TECHNIQUE	ADVANTAGES	DISADVANTAGES
Immersion	Noninvasive Relatively fast Low mortality rates	Cumbersome Patient access and monitoring difficult Shivering Poorly tolerated by conscious patients
Evaporative	Simple Readily available Noninvasive Easy monitoring and patient access	Constant moistening of skin required Relatively slow without specialty equipment
Ice packing	Noninvasive Readily available	Shivering Poorly tolerated by conscious patients
Strategic ice packs	Noninvasive Readily available Can be combined with other techniques	Relatively slower cooling Shivering Poorly tolerated by conscious patients
Cold gastric lavage	Can be combined with other techniques	Relatively slower cooling Invasive Requires airway control Human experience limited
Cold peritoneal lavage	Rapid cooling	Invasive Human experience limited

status, history of heat stress or exposure) is made. Rapid cooling is also indicated for the treatment of MH and NMS but should be instituted concurrently with discontinuation of the triggering agent or drug and administration of dantrolene in MH. There are no high-quality data to guide the optimal rate or endpoint of cooling, but because studies show that the degree of organ damage correlates with the degree and duration of temperature elevation above 40°C (>104°F), a reasonable clinical goal is to reduce the temperature to below 39°C (<102.2°F) within 30 minutes to an hour after the start of therapy.[175,225,232]

Contraindications to Rapid Cooling

Rapid cooling is never contraindicated in patients with heatstroke. Immersion cooling may be relatively contraindicated when cardiac monitoring of an unstable patient is required or when limited personnel make constant patient supervision impossible. Iced gastric lavage is contraindicated in patients with depressed airway reflexes unless the airway is protected by ET intubation. Gastric lavage is also contraindicated by conditions that preclude placement of an orogastric or nasogastric tube. Cold peritoneal lavage is relatively contraindicated when multiple previous abdominal surgeries make placement of a lavage catheter risky.

Immersion Cooling

It would seem obvious that the fastest way to cool a heatstroke patient would be immersion in ice water. In a recent meta-analysis of cooling methods for heatstroke, iced water immersion cooled patients at an average rate of 0.2°C/min, faster than any other method analyzed.[270] A 2010 study found that cold water immersion for 9 minutes in a 2.0°C circulated water bath until a rectal temperature of 38.6°C was achieved avoided any risk associated with overcooling.[244] Costrini reported no fatalities in 252 consecutive young marine recruits with exertional heatstroke who were treated by ice water immersion within 20 minutes of diagnosis.[271] Most contemporary sources recommend ice water immersion as the cooling technique of choice for heatstroke.[225,270,272] Plattner and associates demonstrated cooling rates with ice water immersion that were six times faster than rates seen with forced air or circulating water.[273]

In clinical trials, cold water immersion remains one of the fastest noninvasive cooling techniques available (see Table 66.6). Cold water immersion takes advantage of the high-conductance property of water, which is 25 times that of air.[274] Several factors are important in maximizing the rate of immersion cooling. Conductive heat loss depends on cutaneous blood flow to maintain a heat gradient from skin to water. Theoretically, contact with ice water causes skin and subcutaneous vasoconstriction, which blocks heat exchange and turns these structures into insulators.[258] Experimental and observational evidence suggests that this theoretical effect is not clinically significant, as ice water (1°C to 5°C) appears to result in faster cooling than temperate (20°C to 26°C), cold (14°C to 17°C), or colder (8°C to 12°C) water.[270] Mekjavic and coworkers reported that motion sickness potentiates core cooling during immersion by attenuating the vasoconstrictor response to skin and core cooling, thereby augmenting heat loss and the magnitude of the decrease in deep body temperature.[275] Careful monitoring is required because this may predispose patients to hypothermia.

Increasing surface area exposed to a conductive temperature gradient increases conductive heat loss. Maximizing the body's surface area in contact with water will increase cooling rates with immersion cooling. In clinical practice, this means that complete immersion of the trunk and extremities will cool the patient faster than partial immersion of the trunk (i.e., back only) with the extremities extended out of the bath.

Some investigators suggest the inclusion of skin massage as a crucial component of immersion cooling techniques.[276]

Procedure

For immersion cooling, undress the patient completely and transfer the patient to a tub of water with a depth sufficient to cover the torso and extremities. Support the patient's head out of the tub at all times.

Various water containers may be used. A regular bathtub can be used. Most clinical reports describe tubs that can be moved to the emergency treatment area when needed. A child's plastic wading pool and a decontamination tub or stretcher with waterproof sides and drainage capability are examples of the latter approach. When tubs are unavailable, place patients on water-impermeable sheets and in a sling apparatus while ice and water are poured into the sling. Securely attach temperature and electrocardiogram leads to the patient if monitoring is to be continued during immersion. Remove the patient from the bath when rectal temperature reaches 39°C (102.2°F) because core temperature will continue to drop for a short period even after the patient is removed. If available, use an electronic temperature monitor with a long flexible rectal probe for continuous monitoring of temperature during immersion. Studies show cooling rates with ice water immersion (1°C to 5°C [33.8°F to 41.0°F]) in heatstroke patients of 0.14 to 0.26°C/min.[243,252,270] Caldwell and colleagues reported the fastest rate of immersion cooling with cold water (14°C) immersion at 0.62°C/min[237]; however, this is far beyond anything reported in clinical settings and likely is not a realistic expectation for speed of cooling with immersion, or any other external cooling technique.[270] These findings invite future research investigating the ideal water temperature for immersion cooling.

Complications

The common complications of immersion cooling are shivering, cutaneous vasoconstriction, discomfort, and loss of monitoring capability. Shivering generates considerable heat through muscle metabolism. Cutaneous vasoconstriction theoretically impedes conductive heat loss. If significant shivering does occur, it can be reduced with benzodiazepines. A 2009 study found that high-dose IV diazepam facilitates core cooling during cold saline infusion in healthy volunteers. Subjects were randomized to receive high-dose (20-mg) or low-dose (10-mg) diazepam or placebo during cold saline infusion. Administration of high-dose diazepam decreased the shivering threshold without compromising respiratory or cardiovascular status.[277] Benzodiazepines are also valuable if the patient is hyperthermic secondary to sympathomimetic agents such as cocaine. Magnesium sulfate and dexmedetomidine have been used to control shivering in the context of TTM[278] and may be reasonable options, but safety and efficacy are unclear in the setting of hyperthermia. Other pharmacologic agents used for seizure control in TTM should be avoided in the context of hyperthermia. Meperidine could precipitate seizures, worsening hyperthermia via increased heat generation. Serotonin agonists such as buspirone would be absolutely contraindicated in cases of possible serotonin syndrome. The use of phenothiazines such as chlorpromazine has been advocated for shivering in the past. They are currently discouraged because administration of these agents may impair heat loss through anticholinergic effects on sweat glands, contribute to hypotension via α-adrenergic blockade, lower the seizure threshold, and cause dystonic reactions. In addition, phenothiazines possess central dopamine-blocking effects, which may exacerbate symptoms of NMS. In intubated and mechanically ventilated patients, neuromuscular blockade could be considered, but the benefit must be weighed against the risks including loss of ability to monitor the neurologic exam.[278]

Patient monitoring can be difficult during immersion. Electrodes can be used on the non-immersed upper part of the shoulders, but electrocardiographic artifact often becomes a problem during vigorous shivering. Immersion cooling is not recommended for patients with unstable cardiac rhythms or those at risk for the development of these rhythms. A significant change in cardiac rhythm might go undetected during the labor-intensive process of immersion cooling.

Patient access for resuscitative procedures is also a major problem when using this technique. Should VF develop, the patient must be removed from the bath and dried before defibrillation. Invasive and diagnostic procedures (e.g., IV access and radiography) cannot be performed during the cooling period. Diagnostic imaging should not delay management of severe hyperthermia, which is immediately life threatening. Care must be taken to avoid displacement of IV lines during placement into and removal from the bath.

As body temperature drops, mental status will improve in many patients with heatstroke. When awake, most people find ice water immersion difficult to tolerate. IV sedation may be required, but a core temperature should be checked as the patient may have become cool enough to be removed from the bath, eliminating the need for sedation. Finally, this technique is labor-intensive. Several caregivers must be present throughout the process. The patient's head must be maintained out of the bath. If massage is used, one or more individuals will need to immerse their own hands in water to continuously massage the patient. Medications should be given IV, and constant attention to temperature and electrocardiogram monitors is also necessary. This cooling technique should be used only if adequate personnel are available.

Evaporative Cooling

Evaporating water is thermodynamically a much more effective cooling medium than melting ice, given an appropriate water-vapor gradient. Evaporating 1 g of water requires 540 kcal. Melting 1 g of ice requires only 80 kcal. In theory, evaporative cooling should be approximately seven times more efficient than ice packing. In practice, data on the efficacy of evaporative cooling are mixed. In separate human studies, Weiner and Khogali, and Wyndham and colleagues found that evaporative cooling rates were substantially greater than cooling rates with water immersion at 14.4°C (57.9°F).[264,267] Studies in primate models demonstrated faster cooling rates with evaporative cooling as an adjunct to ice bag placement.[279] Methods using convection and evaporation were more effective than those involving conduction for the treatment of hyperthermia. In clinical practice, ice water immersion or ice packing causes heat loss by conduction and heat consumption by the phase change of melting ice. In healthy volunteers, evaporative cooling techniques (e.g., facial fanning) were associated with decreased thermal sensation and improved thermal comfort.[279] Two controlled studies, however, failed to demonstrate rapid cooling via evaporative techniques.[249,280]

To maximize evaporative cooling rates, several factors must be optimized. Airflow rates must be high and therefore large fans are required. The air must be warm but *not* humid because evaporation is decreased at lower temperatures. The entire body surface must be exposed to airflow and continuously moistened with water. Ideally, the patient is suspended in a mesh sling to expose the back to airflow and moisture. Finally, the temperature of the water used to moisten the skin must be tepid (15°C [59°F]). Warm forced air is essential for effective evaporation. It maintains good peripheral perfusion and prevents shivering by warming the skin.[186] If the water is ice cold, evaporation will be slowed. Conversely, if it is hot, conductive heat gain may occur.

Weiner and Khogali constructed a sophisticated "body cooling unit" (BCU) to maximize evaporative cooling.[264] Patients in the BCU are suspended in a mesh net. High airflow rates (30 m/min) at a temperature of 45°C (113°F) are maintained both anterior and posterior to the mesh net. Atomized water at 15°C (59°F) is continuously sprayed on all body surfaces. For EDs without access to a BCU,[247] temporary units can be set up with shower sprays and fans, provided that the ambient temperature in the ED is relatively cool. An alternative less expensive, portable device developed at King Saud University involves covering the patient with a gauze sheet soaked in water at 20°C (68°F) while two fans direct room air over the patient.[281] Cooling rates obtained with this device (0.087°C/min [32.2°F/min]) were nearly four times slower than rates achieved with the BCU developed by Weiner and Khogali.[264]

The realities of clinical practice make these conditions hard to reproduce. Half the body surface, the back, will usually be unavailable for evaporative cooling. Airflow rates and temperatures are usually limited by the ambient temperature in the treatment facility and by the size and power of the fan available. These realities are reflected by the slower cooling rates achieved with evaporative cooling in a clinical setting. Another report of rapid cooling with evaporative technique utilized a helicopter downdraft for air movement,[257] which may be feasible in military and certain prehospital environments but is likely impractical or impossible in most ED settings.

Procedure

For evaporative cooling, undress the patient completely. Position a fan at the foot of the bed or stretcher as close to the patient as possible. Then sponge or mist the patient's skin with tepid water (15°C [59°F]). Spray water continuously over the skin to create a warm microclimate around the skin and to promote water evaporation. A single care provider can continue the technique and monitor the patient once cooling has been initiated. It is important to keep as much of the body surface area as moist as possible and exposed to airflow. Do not cover with sheets or clothing because this will impede skin evaporation and cooling. Studies of evaporative cooling in heatstroke patients show cooling rates of 0.06 to 0.31°C/min.[259,264]

Complications

Complications of evaporative cooling are rare and more often a result of the underlying disorder than the cooling technique. Wet skin may interfere with electrocardiographic monitoring, but this can usually be avoided by placing electrodes on the patient's back. Shivering occurs infrequently with this technique when compared with other cooling methods because the water is relatively lukewarm. Because rectal temperature lags core (esophageal) temperature, evaporative cooling should be discontinued when rectal temperature reaches 39°C (102.2°F). Continued cooling beyond this temperature may lead to subsequent "overshoot hypothermia" as a result of a continued drop in core temperature after active evaporative cooling is discontinued.

Whole-Body Ice Packing

Packing a heatstroke victim in ice may enhance conductive heat loss without the attendant logistic problems caused by water immersion (Figs. 66.8 and 66.9). Constant attendance, as required for skin moistening with evaporative cooling and as described for immersion cooling, may not be necessary with ice packing. Kielblock and associates demonstrated in a human study of mild, exercise-induced hyperthermia that whole-body ice packing cooled just as fast as evaporative cooling did (see Table 66.6).[249]

Procedure

For whole-body ice packing, undress the patient completely and then cover the extremities and torso with crushed ice. A

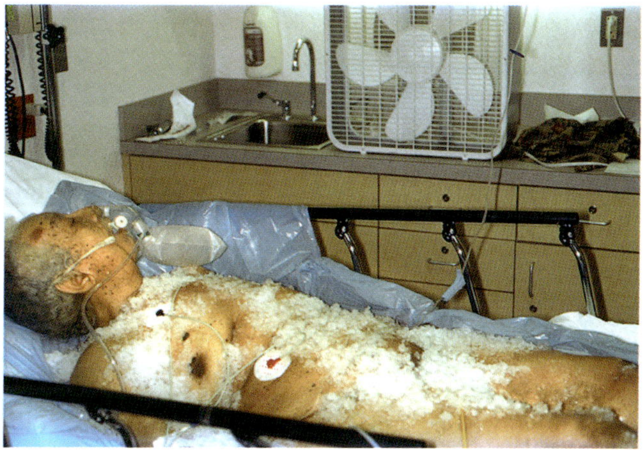

Fig. 66.8 It is essential to rapidly lower the core temperature of a severely hyperthermic patient by instituting cooling techniques as soon as possible. Evaporative cooling (see text) is usually quite effective and technically easy. Note the fan for additional cooling. Many such patients require sedation, paralysis, and mechanical ventilation. An alternative aggressive method shown here, in a patient with a rectal temperature of 110°F, is to literally pack the patient in ice. As is often the case, this older patient did not survive.

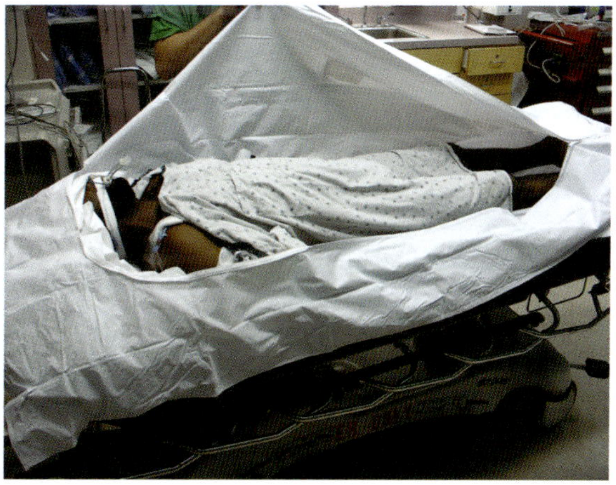

Fig. 66.9 A body bag or plastic sheets may keep water from flooding the floor when packing the patient in ice.

fan blown over the patient may increase cooling. As with any cooling technique, monitor the patient's temperature constantly with an electric thermometer and a long, flexible rectal probe. A large supply of crushed ice will be needed whenever this technique is used. Logistically, ice packing may be problematic. Whole-body ice packing can usually be performed on an ED stretcher without additional equipment. Ideally, the patient is placed in a container that facilitates contact of ice with the skin and prevents water from dripping onto the floor. A body bag makes an ideal device. Iced cooling may also be accomplished by placing the patient in a child's lightweight plastic pool, available in toy stores. Lacking this equipment, plastic cloths or trash bags may be placed under the patient with the edges curled up to form a sling-like apparatus. As with immersion cooling, electrocardiographic monitoring can potentially be difficult because of shivering artifact and displacement of electrodes. If the patient is alert and cannot tolerate the ice packing, use IV sedation or restraint. Treat excessive shivering with benzodiazepines if needed. Once rectal temperature reaches 39°C (102.2°F), remove the ice and dry the patient off. Studies show cooling rates of 0.34°C/min in heatstroke patients with whole-body ice packing.[249]

Strategic Ice Packs

Several reports have investigated strategic placement of ice packs over areas of the body where large blood vessels run close to the skin.[233,249,251,259,268] Cooling in these areas occurs despite cutaneous vasoconstriction because of direct conductive heat loss from blood within the vessel and across the vessel wall, subcutaneous tissue, and skin to ice. The most common areas used for strategic ice packing are the anterior aspect of the neck (carotid and jugular vessels), the axilla (axillary artery and vein), and the groin (femoral vessels). There have been numerous reports of successful cooling using ice packs as primary or adjunctive therapy, though other reports have demonstrated no more rapid cooling than occurs with passive cooling (see Table 66.6). Interestingly, Lissoway et al.[251] demonstrated relatively rapid cooling with application of ice packs to glabrous skin surfaces, which was more effective than typical strategic ice pack placement to the neck, axilla, and groin. Glabrous skin, located on the palms, soles, and ears, plays a role in normal thermoregulation and contains retia venosa, densely packed arteriovenous anastomoses with capacity for high blood flow to facilitate heat loss. Other studies utilizing hands and feet for cooling have shown this as a relatively ineffective approach, however.[270] Application of ice packs, though easier to perform than immersion or total-body ice packing, limits the conductive cooling offered by the latter two procedures.

A study in pigtail monkeys demonstrated that a combination of strategic ice packs with evaporative cooling results in faster cooling than either technique alone, although the relative increase achieved by adding ice packs to evaporative cooling was small.[279] In unconscious patients or in awake patients who can tolerate ice packs without excessive shivering, this technique could be added to evaporative cooling. Kielblock and associates found that the combination of strategic ice packs and evaporative cooling yielded higher cooling rates than did either method individually (0.036°C/min vs. 0.027°C/min and 0.034°C/min).[249] The clinical value of strategic ice packs alone or in combination with other techniques remains to be determined. Anecdotally, during the Chicago heat wave of 1995, the majority of heatstroke patients who went to EDs survived after being effectively cooled with the evaporation method accompanied by strategic placement of ice packs.[282]

Procedure

Place large plastic bags filled with crushed ice or an ice and water mixture in both axillae and over both femoral triangles. If the neck is used, place the packs laterally so that they do not compress the trachea or apply excessive weight over the carotid arteries. Do not pack the neck if the patient has carotid bruits or a history of cerebrovascular disease. Some sources advocate rubbing the body surface briskly with plastic bags containing ice after the body has been wet down with water. Studies show ranges of cooling rates of 0.028 to 0.3°C/min in heatstroke patients with strategic ice packs.[233,249,251,259,260,268,276]

Complications

Complications of strategic ice packing are limited to shivering and patient discomfort, as described previously for whole-body ice packing. As discussed, complications theoretically could develop from compression of anterior neck structures if ice bags are applied incorrectly. The ice packs are removed when rectal temperature reaches 39°C (102.2°F) to avoid an excessive drop in core temperature.

External Versus Core Cooling

All the external cooling techniques described previously are noninvasive and involve heat loss by evaporation or conduction across the skin as the primary cooling mechanism. With each of these techniques, central temperature will continue to drop even after the technique is discontinued and the skin is dried. This is due to a delay in establishment of an equilibrium between the cold skin and the core. The amount of "core afterdrop" can exceed 2°C (>35.6°F).[186,247] For this reason, cooling is discontinued when the core temperature reaches 39°C (102.2°F).

Because the sites of significant cell damage with heatstroke are centrally located (e.g., liver, kidney, heart), central cooling techniques are theoretically preferable to external techniques. Core cooling techniques studied in both animal and human models include iced gastric lavage, intravascular cooling, bladder lavage, and peritoneal lavage.[236,248,261,262,265,266] Central venous cooling is effective in rapidly decreasing core temperatures.[283] Studies conducted in healthy volunteers have demonstrated that reductions in core temperature vary according to the temperature of the infused fluid. Subjects receiving 30-minute infusions of fluid at 4°C (39.2°F) experienced decreases in core temperature of 2.5°C ± 0.4°C (36.5°F ± 32.7°F). Subjects receiving 30-minute infusions of fluid at 20°C (68°F) experienced decreases of 1.4°C (±0.2°C [34.5°F ± 32.4°F]).[283] Clinical trials investigating this method showed that cooling via the respiratory tract had no significant impact on temperature changes when used exclusively but did demonstrate effectiveness as an adjunctive measure to other external cooling techniques.[274] Cool air (10°C [50°F]) was administered via a hood or mask. Cooling via the respiratory tract has been studied in animals but not investigated clinically.[284,285] The use of cold hemodialysis and hemodiafiltration has been described,[286] but challenges in rapid initiation of such procedures likely limit their general usefulness. Central cooling techniques are necessarily more invasive than external techniques and have the potential for more significant complications.

Cold Gastric Lavage

The stomach lies in close proximity to the liver, great vessels, kidneys, and heart. The gastric mucosa is not subject to the intense vasoconstriction observed on exposure of the skin to ice water.[261] For these reasons, lavage of the stomach might be expected to be an effective central cooling method. Studies of cold gastric lavage in a canine model produced cooling rates five times greater than in controls exposed to ambient air at room temperature (0.15 vs. 0.03°C/min).[266] Humans with heatstroke have been cooled successfully with gastric lavage, but only in combination with external techniques.[248] Cold gastric lavage seems to be best suited for use in patients with severe hyperthermia who are cooling at a slow rate with external techniques alone. The presence of an ET tube and passage of a large-bore gastric tube make rapid lavage without aspiration possible. This technique should be reserved for patients whose airway is already protected by ET intubation and who do not have contraindication to gastric tube placement. Given the associated risks, it cannot be recommended to perform ET intubation for the sole purpose of performing cold gastric lavage.

Procedure

For cold gastric lavage, instill 10 mL/kg of iced tap water into the stomach as rapidly as possible (usually over a 30- to 60-second period). After a 30- to 60-second dwell time, remove the water by suction or gravity. Cooling will theoretically be faster if a high-temperature gradient is maintained in the stomach. A faster lavage rate can be maintained if suction is used to withdraw the instilled fluid. A large container of ice-temperature water maintained 1 m to 1.5 m above the patient's body will facilitate the instillation of fluid. Connect this container directly to the lavage tubing and ideally allow passage of water, but not ice, which may occlude the tube. Because large volumes of water are needed, it is helpful if additional ice can be added to the container without interrupting the lavage. A large syringe can be used as an alternative to gravity instillation, but this is usually slower.

A simple system that accomplishes this procedure can be devised from equipment readily available in most EDs. Use a standard lavage setup (for use in drug overdoses) and a large-bore gastric tube. Cut the lavage bag open at the top to allow water and ice to be added. Suspend this bag above the patient's body and connect it to the orogastric tube by Y tubing with clamps. Connect the other arm of the Y tubing to suction. Using the clamps, intermittently instill ice water by gravity and withdraw it by suction.

Complications

A major potential complication of cold gastric lavage is pulmonary aspiration. Use of a cuffed ET tube minimizes the incidence of this complication. Because of the large volume of water used and the frequent depression of airway reflexes seen with severe heatstroke, this technique should rarely be used in a patient who is not endotracheally intubated.

If tap water is used, water intoxication, hyponatremia, and other electrolyte disturbances are *potential* complications, particularly in pediatric or geriatric patients. Water is absorbed from the stomach and, with large-volume lavage, may pass the pylorus into the small intestine. In canine studies, large-volume gastric lavage with tap water did not cause electrolyte abnormalities.[261] The actual incidence of these potential complications in human heatstroke has not been determined.

Theoretically, passage of cold water through the esophagus, located directly behind the heart, has the potential to induce cardiac dysrhythmias. Dysrhythmias have not been observed in canine studies or in case reports of humans with heatstroke cooled with this technique.[248,261,262,266] Passage of a large-bore gastric tube has the potential to cause traumatic esophageal injury, and therefore may be contraindicated in patients with known esophageal pathology and should be performed by clinicians with experience in the procedure.

Cold Peritoneal Lavage

The surface area and blood flow of the peritoneum greatly exceed those of the stomach. Peritoneal lavage is expected to exchange heat much faster than possible with gastric lavage. Peritoneal lavage achieves some of the fastest cooling rates ever reported in large animal or human studies (see Table 66.6). As with gastric lavage, this central cooling technique offers the advantage of directly cooling the core organs that are most susceptible to thermal damage. Unlike gastric lavage, ET intubation is not required. Horowitz describes using peritoneal lavage (along with other techniques including gastric lavage and external cooling) and achieving a cooling rate of 0.11°C/min.[248] Canine models have achieved significantly higher rates of cooling up to 0.56°C/min,[236] but the applicability of this to humans with heatstroke is unclear.

Peritoneal lavage is a more invasive cooling technique. Because heat exchange is more efficient across the peritoneum, smaller volumes of fluid can be used. Surgical placement of the lavage catheter is necessary. This cooling technique is relatively contraindicated by conditions that preclude placement of a lavage catheter (e.g., multiple abdominal surgical scars).

Peritoneal lavage is the most rapid central cooling technique. It can theoretically be combined with other techniques to speed cooling of heatstroke patients with refractory hyperthermia. As the most invasive cooling technique, it requires time, proper equipment, and surgical expertise to institute. Its use is probably best suited to situations in which heatstroke patients are not responding to external cooling and adequate equipment and personnel are readily available.

Procedure

To institute cooling by peritoneal lavage, immerse 2 to 8 L of sterile saline in an ice water bath to cool while the catheter is being placed. Place a standard peritoneal lavage catheter (as for diagnostic use in trauma patients) via any of the techniques described in Chapter 43. Standard contraindications apply. Use of a larger peritoneal dialysis catheter may speed instillation and withdrawal of fluid. Actual lavage volumes and rates have not been established, however. One approach is to instill and withdraw 500 mL to 1000 mL every 10 minutes until adequate cooling is achieved. Rectal temperature may be falsely low during lavage because of the presence of cold water around the rectum at the level of the rectal temperature probe. It may be preferable to also monitor temperature in the tympanic membrane or esophagus when using this technique. Stop the lavage when core temperature reaches 39°C (102.2°F) to avoid excessive core temperature "afterdrop."

Complications

The potential complications of peritoneal lavage cooling are primarily related to placement of the catheter and include bowel or bladder perforation and placement into the rectus sheath rather than the peritoneum.

Other Cooling Techniques

"Forced-air warming" techniques are used to minimize ongoing heat loss via the respiratory tract in patients undergoing general anesthesia,[287] demonstrating the role of the respiratory tract in heat exchange with the environment. Although high-frequency jet ventilation (HFJV) achieves core cooling in critically ill patients,[284] efforts to use the respiratory tract to cool patients with heatstroke have been unsuccessful. In a canine model of heatstroke, HFJV was shown to be a relatively ineffective cooling technique.[285] Heat loss by convection (air transfer) is relatively inefficient when compared with the conductive heat loss mechanism used by other cooling techniques.

In human trials, ice water lavage of the bladder (300 mL of iced Ringer's solution every 10 minutes) provided only minimal cooling at rates of approximately 0.01°C/min.[249] Iced water lavage of the rectum would theoretically provide faster cooling rates secondary to the increased surface area and better perfusion, but it has not been investigated in human trials.

Hemodialysis or partial cardiopulmonary bypass could theoretically be used to cool heatstroke patients. Before the availability of dantrolene in 1979, partial cardiopulmonary bypass was one of the treatments of MH.[288] Drawbacks include the need for technical expertise and preparation time for the procedure. A 2005 case report described successful treatment of a heatstroke patient with multiple-organ failure refractory to conventional cooling techniques with cold hemodialysis initially at 30°C (86°F) and later at 35°C (95°F), followed by continuous hemodiafiltration with cold dialysate (35°C [95°F]) at a high flow rate of 18,000 mL/h. Within 3 hours of starting this particular technique, the patient's body temperature was below 38°C (<100.4°F).[286]

Cyclic lung lavage with cold perfluorochemicals has been investigated in animal models. Benefits include rapid cooling rates of 0.5°C/min (32.9°F/min) and minimally invasive nature in already mechanically ventilated subjects.[246,289]

Intravascular cooling catheters have demonstrated efficiency as cooling devices. They circulate temperature-controlled sterile saline placed in the bladder or inferior vena cava. Several case reports describe successful treatment of hyperthermia with intravascular devices,[235,245,254] though only the report by Hamaya et al. describes rates of cooling comparable with immersion and other methods above. Another promising cooling technique involves the use of a hypothermic retrograde jugular vein flush (HRJVF) for heatstroke. HRJVF has been studied only in animal models thus far. This technique involves the infusion of 4°C (39.2°F) isotonic sodium chloride solution through the external jugular vein (1.7 mL/100 g of body weight over a 5-minute period). Use of HRJVF was found to increase survival in rats during heatstroke by attenuating cerebral oxidative stress, tissue ischemia or injury, systemic inflammation, and activated coagulation.[290–292]

Conclusion

Rapid cooling is the key step in the emergency management of heatstroke patients. Survival rates approach 90% to 97% when elevated temperatures are lowered in a timely fashion.[175,276] Immersion cooling appears to be the most effective method of rapidly cooling hyperthermic patients and should be the method of choice when possible since both degree and duration of hyperthermia appear to be the primary determinates of morbidity and mortality.[270] Recent international consensus guidelines[272] recommend whole-body water immersion techniques as first-line treatment for hyperthermia.

Evaporative cooling has previously been advocated as the treatment of choice[293] due to simplicity, noninvasiveness, and published cooling rates. Studies demonstrating the highest rates of evaporative cooling, however, often use equipment not accessible in most ED settings, such as helicopter rotors or specialty BCUs.[247,257,264]. Evaporative cooling or other external cooling techniques are reasonable alternatives when immersion cooling is contraindicated or impractical due to lack of available supplies or personnel.

If a patient is not cooling rapidly with immersion cooling, other techniques can be added. If the patient is endotracheally intubated, gastric lavage can be instituted. If facilities and personnel are available, peritoneal lavage cooling can be used as a rapid central cooling technique. If MH is suspected, dantrolene sodium should be administered. In addition, the clinician should have a heightened index of suspicion for NMS, serotonin toxicity, and toxicity from sympathomimetic drugs. Regardless of the cause, a reasonable clinical goal is to reduce rectal temperature to 39°C (102.2°F) or below within 30 minutes of instituting therapy.[272,276]

Central venous cooling with iced saline is a promising technique for rapid cooling of patients with severe hyperthermia. Other cooling techniques require further study before a clear recommendation regarding their efficacy can be made.

ACKNOWLEDGMENTS

The authors thank Heather Prendergast for her contribution and guidance. We also thank Timothy Erickson, Dwight E. Helmrich, Scott A. Syverud, David Doezema, and David P. Sklar for their contributions and authorship in previous editions.

REFERENCES ARE AVAILABLE AT Elsevier eBooks+

CHAPTER 67

Ultrasound

Emily Neill and Christine Butts

Bedside ultrasound has become an indispensable tool in the emergency department (ED). It enables physicians to make a rapid diagnosis at the bedside and formulate a plan of care. Perhaps most importantly, ultrasound has revolutionized procedures performed in the ED. Use of ultrasound gives the physician the advantage of viewing the anatomy and directly imaging the procedure while it is being performed. Procedures that had previously been performed "blindly" can now be performed with the added assurance of monitoring the procedure while it is in progress. This has resulted in greater safety in both common and uncommon procedures.[1,2]

Ultrasound is now routinely applied to procedures in the ED ranging from the common, such as incision and drainage of an abscess, to the rare, such as drainage of a pericardial effusion. This chapter covers the basic principles of ultrasound that can be applied to any procedure. Ultrasound applications for specific procedures can be found in the appropriate procedure chapter. Videos on various aspects and applications of ultrasound are available online (Videos 67.1–67.8).

PHYSICS

Ultrasound operates on the *pulse echo principle*. Electrical energy created by the ultrasound machine causes crystals in the tip of the transducer to vibrate, also known as the *piezoelectric (sound-electricity) effect*. This vibration emits high-frequency sound waves that travel through a conduction medium (usually ultrasound gel, although other liquids or gel-like substances can suffice) into the body. The sound waves are reflected back to the transducer at varying intensities and speeds, depending on the nature of the object that they encounter. The ultrasound machine is able to interpret this information and plot an image on the screen.

Objects in the body that are liquid or water-like, such as a full bladder, reflect very few sound waves and allow most of the energy to pass through them. These objects are presented on-screen as black by ultrasound and are described as *anechoic* (i.e., without echoes) (Fig. 67.1). Conversely, objects that are dense and have very little water content, such as bones, reflect almost all the sound waves back. These objects are presented on-screen as white by ultrasound and are described as *hyperechoic* (i.e., producing a lot of echoes) (Fig. 67.2). Objects that lie between these two extremes present as varying shades of gray, depending on the water content of the object, and are described as *hypoechoic*. For example, the liver contains a large amount of blood, a water-like substance, and is not completely liquid, appearing on-screen as dark gray (Fig. 67.3). An object that contains less water and is not completely solid would appear as a lighter shade of gray.

These properties of objects also account for two important artifacts. *Acoustic shadowing* is an artifact that is encountered when dealing with hyperechoic objects. These objects reflect almost all the sound waves back to the transducer. As a result, the ultrasound machine "senses" an absence of information deep to the hyperechoic object. The absence of information is represented by a strong, dark vertical line emanating deep to the object (Fig. 67.4). This type of shadowing is referred to as a *clean shadow*. This shadow can be frustrating to the sonographer when attempting to obtain the best image possible, classically, when imaging over the ribs. Alternatively, it can also be helpful in identifying hyperechoic objects, such as gallstones or foreign bodies.

Air is a poor conductor of sound, resulting in a characteristic appearance on ultrasound. Air causes the ultrasound beam to scatter and creates a hazy, gray appearance on the image. In contrast to a clean shadow, the presence of smaller pockets of air may create a phenomenon known as *dirty shadowing* (Fig. 67.5). This can be an anticipated finding, such as when viewing bowel gas within the abdomen, or an indication of an abnormality, such as when viewing gas within subcutaneous tissue.

Acoustic enhancement, or an *acoustic window*, is the artifact created by an anechoic object. As noted earlier, sound waves pass through anechoic objects well and therefore lose less of their energy. This enables more ultrasonic energy to be available when the sound reaches the object on the other side of the fluid. This results in a brighter, clearer image immediately behind the fluid-filled object. As an example, a full bladder enables a clearer image of the pelvic organs (Fig. 67.6).

INDICATIONS AND CONTRAINDICATIONS

Although vascular access was one of the first uses of ultrasound for ED procedures, the list of procedures that can be facilitated by ultrasound is growing rapidly and continuously (Box 67.1). Even when a procedure cannot be directly observed with ultrasound, bedside ultrasound can frequently be used to diagnose the abnormality and to plan the approach for the procedure.

Ultrasound is a very safe modality for imaging at the bedside. It can be used in a variety of populations (pediatrics, pregnancy), without concern for radiation exposure. The only absolute contraindication to using bedside ultrasound for procedural guidance is lack of training or experience in its use. Lack of adequate training or experience may result in an incorrect diagnosis and erroneous evaluation of the anatomy. This may result in harm and unnecessary complications in patients.

EQUIPMENT

The nature of the image obtained depends on the type of transducer used. In general, transducers fall into two categories: high frequency and low frequency, referring to the type of ultrasound waves generated by the transducer.

High-frequency sound waves do not penetrate very far into the tissue and thus are limited to use in evaluation of superficial structures, but they provide excellent resolution. A linear or vascular transducer and an intracavitary transducer are examples of specific types of high-frequency transducers (Figs. 67.7 and 67.8). Examples of examinations that are best evaluated with a high-frequency transducer are central or peripheral vascular access, evaluation of the pleura for pneumothorax, and evaluation of soft tissue for an abscess or foreign body. These examinations rely on a high degree of resolution (Fig. 67.9).

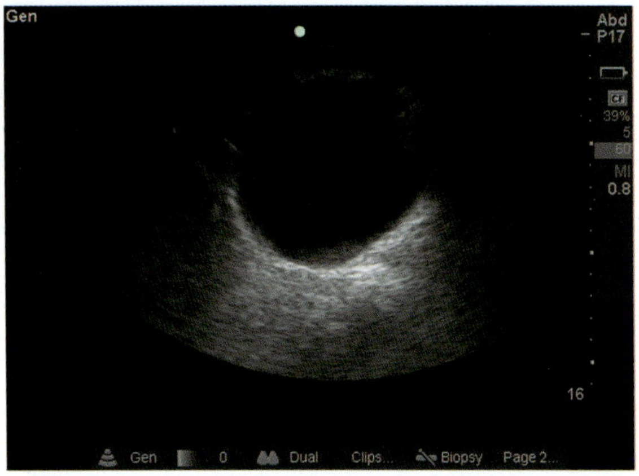

Fig. 67.1 A fluid-filled bladder appears black, or anechoic, when viewed with ultrasound.

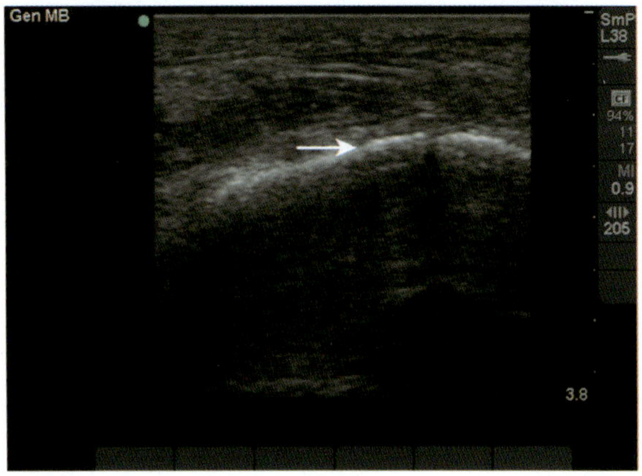

Fig. 67.2 The cortex of a bone *(arrow)* appears white, or hyperechoic, when viewed with ultrasound.

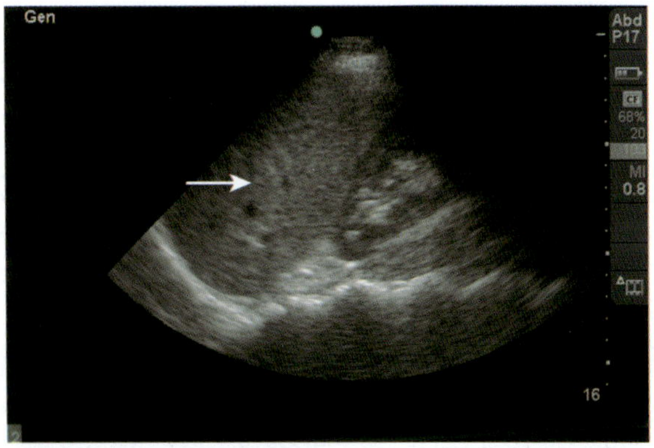

Fig. 67.3 The liver *(arrow)* contains a large amount of blood (a water-like substance) but is not completely liquid and appears on-screen as dark gray. Note the kidney adjacent to the liver. Fluid in the abdomen (blood, ascites) will often collect in the space between the liver and kidney and appear as a black collection (see Fig. 67.24).

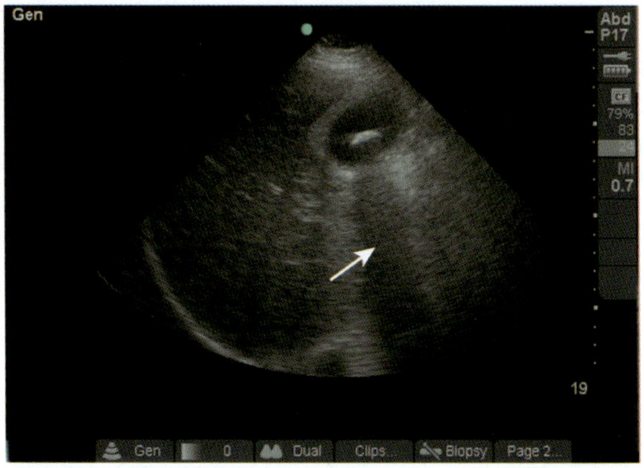

Fig. 67.4 Acoustic shadowing *(arrow)* occurs when ultrasound encounters a hyperechoic, or hard, object. All the sound waves are returned to the transducer, which results in absence of information behind the hyperechoic object.

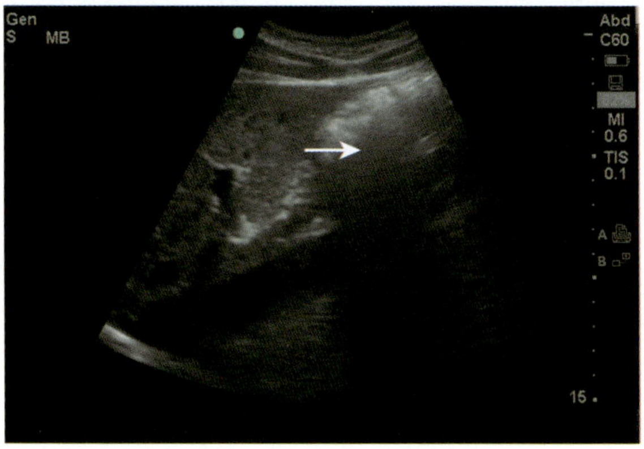

Fig. 67.5 In contrast to clean shadowing, the presence of air causes a dirty shadow *(arrow)*.

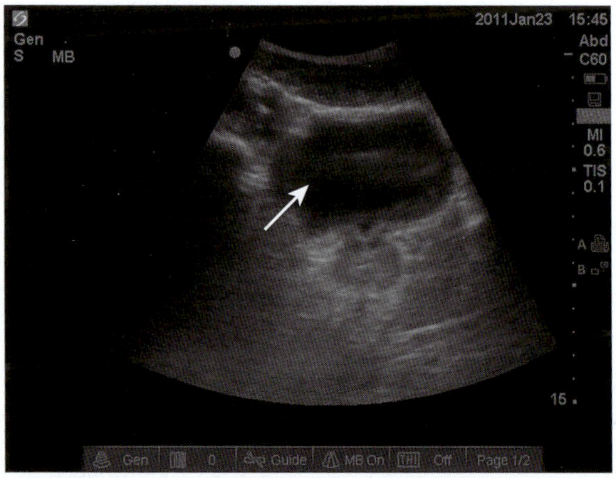

Fig. 67.6 The presence of a fluid-filled object (in this case a full bladder) creates an acoustic window effect *(arrow)*. This effect causes objects behind, or deep, to the window to appear brighter (posterior acoustic enhancement) and allows them to be seen more clearly.

Low-frequency sound waves penetrate farther into tissues, providing greater image depth, but do not provide as much resolution as high-frequency waves. Curvilinear, phased-array, and microconvex transducers are examples of specific types of low-frequency transducers (Figs. 67.10 and 67.11). They are distinguished from each other by the shape of the footprint of the transducer, the part that directly touches the patient, and by the layout of crystals in the tip of the transducer. Examples of the types of examinations that are best evaluated with a low-frequency transducer are evaluation of the pleural or peritoneal cavities for fluid drainage, evaluation of the bladder for aspiration or suprapubic catheter placement, and evaluation of the pericardium for pericardiocentesis. These examinations are not as dependent on resolution and typically require greater penetration (Fig. 67.12).

The growing use of ultrasound for procedures has prompted the development of echogenic needles and needle guidance

BOX 67.1 Examples of Procedures Performed With Ultrasound Guidance

Abscess incision and drainage
Arterial line placement
Arterial puncture
Arthrocentesis
Central venous catheter placement
Foreign body localization and removal
Nerve block
Paracentesis
Pericardiocentesis
Suprapubic catheter placement
Thoracentesis
Transvenous pacemaker insertion

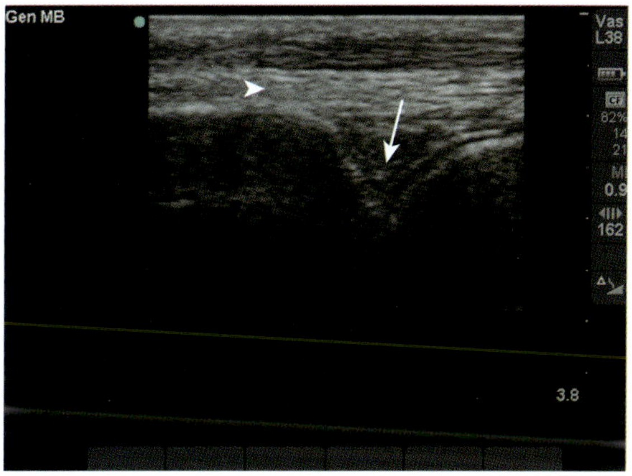

Fig. 67.9 An image as seen with a high-frequency transducer. In this case soft tissue and tendon *(arrowhead)* can be seen overlying the ankle joint *(arrow)*.

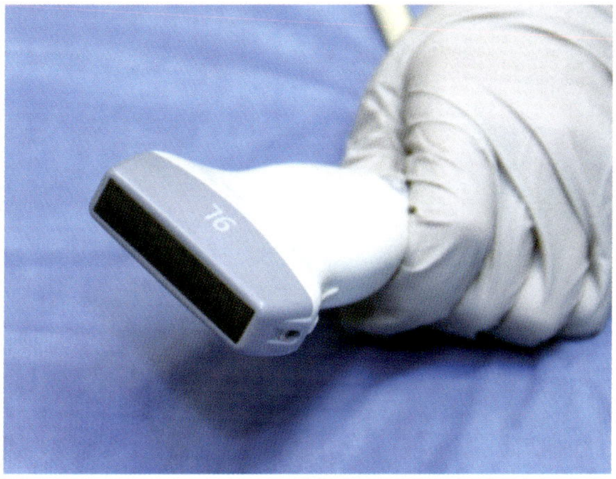

Fig. 67.7 Linear, or vascular, transducer.

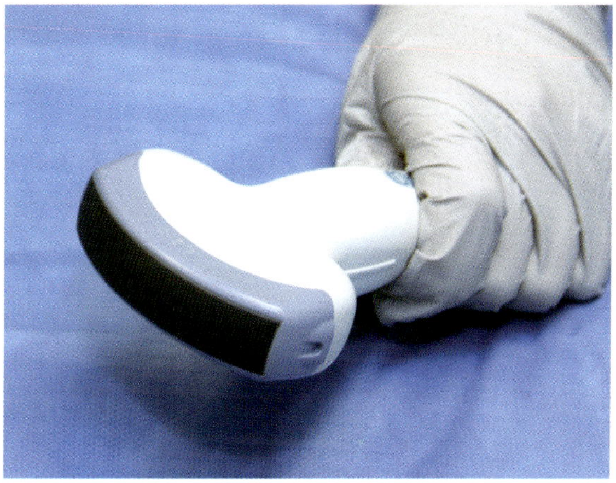

Fig. 67.10 Curvilinear transducer.

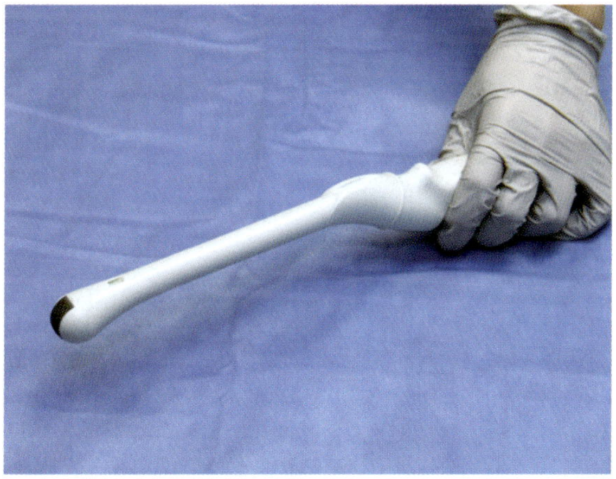

Fig. 67.8 Intracavitary transducer.

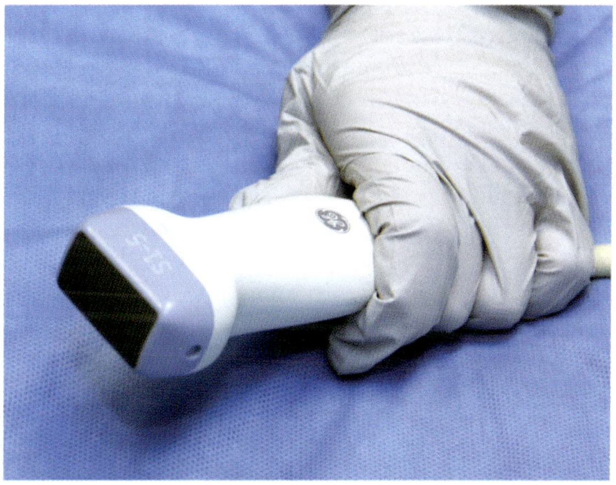

Fig. 67.11 Phased-array transducer.

systems. Both these advances are designed to improve the ease and accuracy of ultrasound-guided procedures, but this depends on the operator's familiarity with their properties and the correct use.

Additionally, many procedures require sterile conditions. Commercially designed sterile transducer covers are available and allow the operator to completely cover both the transducer and cord and are preferred for sterile technique. In the absence of these covers, the transducer can be placed inside a sterile glove, with a sterile drape wrapped around the cord.

GENERAL APPROACH

Although each procedure has unique techniques, there are several general principles that apply when using ultrasound. Selection of the correct transducer is of the utmost importance for adequate visualization of the anatomy and pathology. This process is described in the preceding section, and in general the degree of resolution and required depth of penetration should guide selection of the transducer.

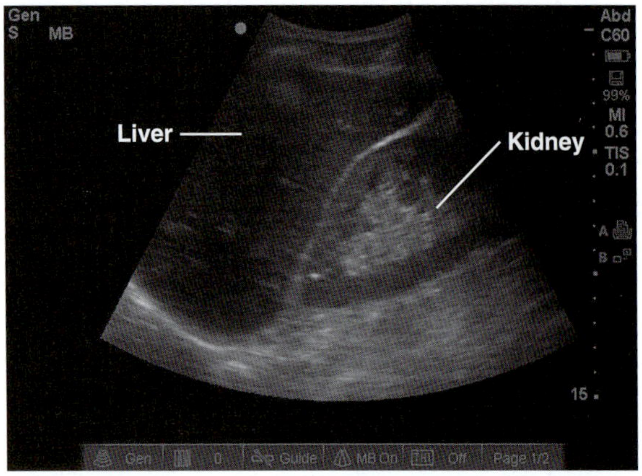

Fig. 67.12 An image as seen with a low-frequency transducer. In this case the liver and kidney can be seen in the right upper quadrant.

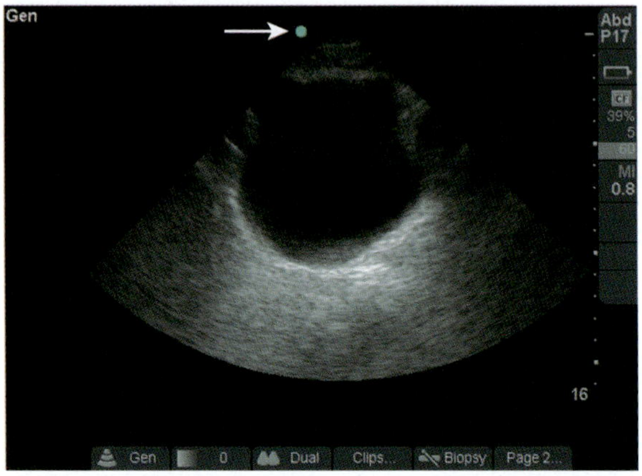

Fig. 67.14 Indicator on screen *(arrow)*, which corresponds to the indicator on the side of the transducer.

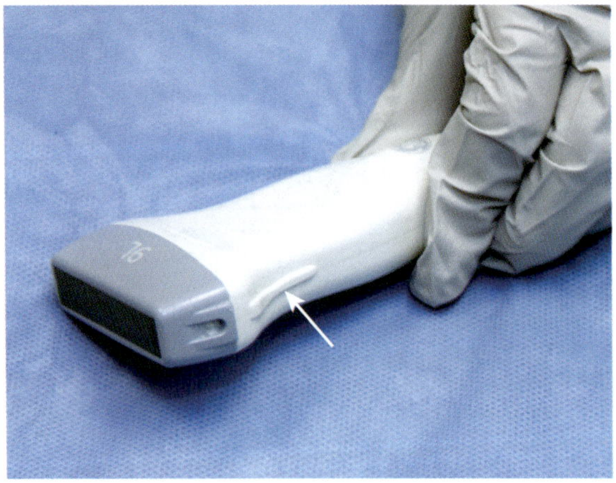

Fig. 67.13 Indicator on the transducer *(arrow)*.

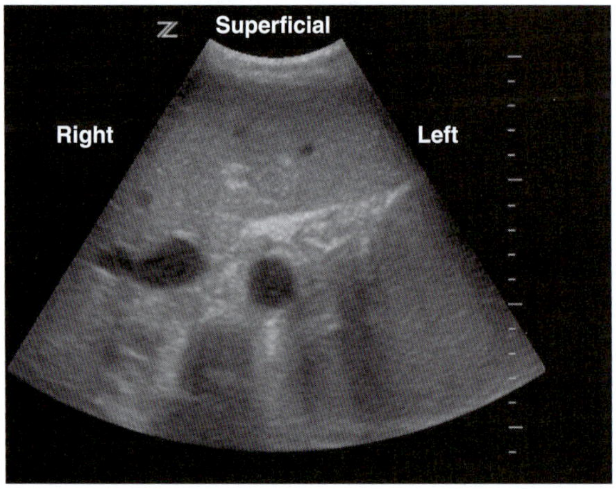

Fig. 67.15 Relationships in the transverse orientation. As the indicator points toward the patient's right, objects on the left side of the screen are toward the patient's right (toward the indicator). Objects on the right side of the screen are toward the patient's left (away from the indicator). As in all images, objects closer to the top of the image are closer to the surface, whereas objects at the bottom of the image are deeper in the body.

Once the correct transducer has been selected, evaluate the area of interest. This step is key when evaluating the nature of the pathology. For example, understanding the size and position of a subcutaneous abscess and the surrounding anatomy is essential. Determining the correct orientation of objects on the screen can be challenging, and it is crucial for success with ultrasound-guided procedures. All transducers have a dot or mark on one side (Fig. 67.13). This mark corresponds to an indicator on the left-hand side of the screen (Fig. 67.14). By convention, with standard ultrasound, the indicator is pointed toward either the patient's head or toward their right side. When the indicator on the transducer is pointing toward the patient's right, a transverse image will be generated (Fig. 67.15). Objects on the right of the screen are closer to the patient's left side and objects on the left side, near the on-screen indicator, are closer to the patient's right side. Objects near the top of the screen (near field) are closer to the skin and objects near the bottom of the screen (far field) are deeper in the body. When the indicator is turned toward the patient's head, a longitudinal image (either sagittal or coronal plane) is generated (Fig. 67.16). Objects on the right side of the screen are closer to the patient's feet and objects on the left side of the screen (near the on-screen indicator) are closer to the patient's head. As with the transverse image, objects near the top of the screen are closer to the skin surface and objects at the bottom of the screen are deeper in the body.

It can be helpful to think of the ultrasound like a flashlight, with the sonographic beam as the rays of light extending from the transducer. The operator can envision "shining" the beam toward the area of interest to capture its image on screen. While performing an ultrasound examination is highly individualized to both the operator and the specific study, there are four cardinal movements of ultrasonography that form the foundation of all scans: (1) *sliding* the transducer across the patient's body to cover a larger anatomic area. (2) *Rotating* the transducer clockwise or counterclockwise to change the angle (particularly useful when trying to avoid acoustic shadowing, such as when trying to maneuver between ribs for cardiac ultrasonography). (3) *Fanning* the transducer by moving left to right along the long axis of the transducer, so as to change the angle of the sonographic beam. (4) *Rocking* the transducer to put more pressure on one end or the other, again to change the angle of the beam (mostly used with the curvilinear transducer, which is shaped like the curved rockers of a rocking chair).

Once the initial evaluation has been completed, make a decision whether to use ultrasound to directly guide the procedure ("ultrasound-guided") or to simply "mark the spot" beforehand ("ultrasound-assisted"). Some procedures, such as paracentesis of large fluid collections, may not require direct guidance. In this case, ultrasound can be used to locate the most optimal puncture site, away from important structures.

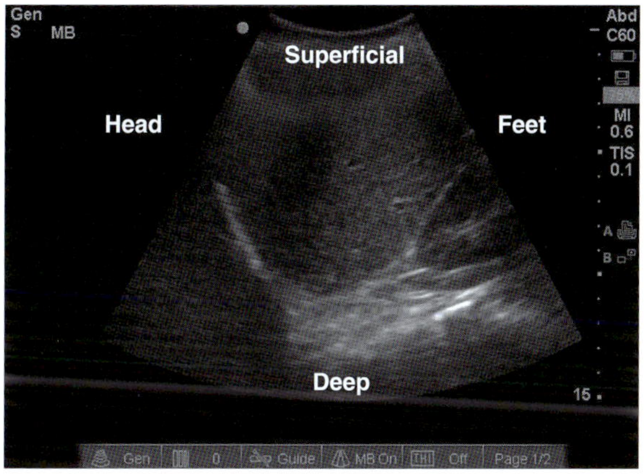

Fig. 67.16 Relationships in the longitudinal, or sagittal, orientation. As the indicator on the transducer points toward the patient's head, objects on the left side of the screen are toward the patient's head. Objects on the right side of the screen are toward the patient's feet. As in all images, objects closer to the top of the image are closer to the surface, whereas objects at the bottom of the image are deeper in the body.

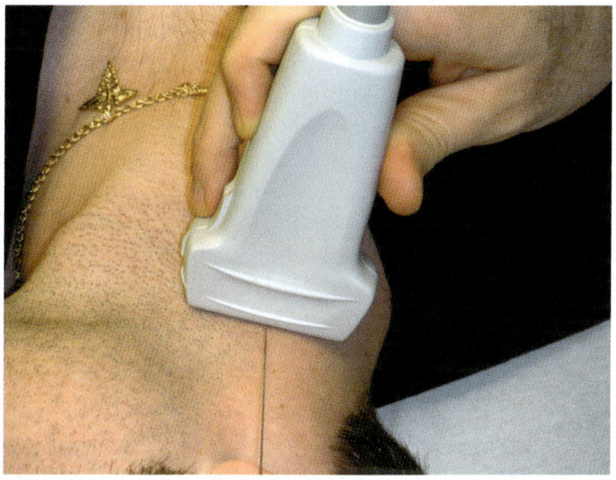

Fig. 67.17 Inserting a needle in the transverse or out-of-plane approach. In this technique the needle is inserted at the midpoint of the transducer. This image is for demonstration purposes only and does not demonstrate sterile technique.

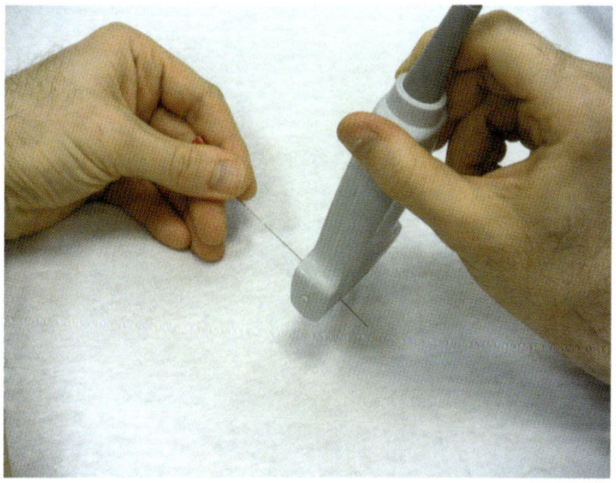

Fig. 67.18 As the needle is advanced in the out-of-plane approach, the transducer can be seen to transect only a small portion of the needle. The tip of the needle is now away from the transducer and will not appear on-screen.

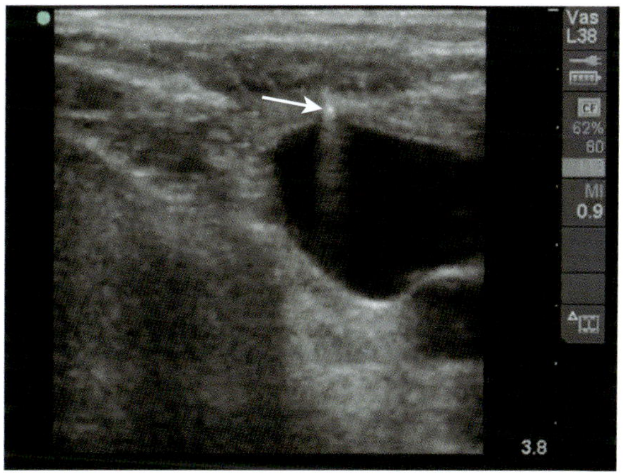

Fig. 67.19 Real-time image of the needle as it approaches the vein. The needle *(arrow)* is seen as a hyperechoic object with strong shadowing extending behind it. The portion of the needle seen will correspond to the portion of the needle that is underlying the transducer, as shown in Fig. 67.18.

Once that site has been marked, proceed with the procedure in the usual fashion. For other procedures, such as central line placement, direct visualization throughout the entire procedure may be more important.

When direct visualization is desired, the orientation of the needle to the transducer must be considered. The two main techniques are the out-of-plane and in-plane approaches. In the out-of-plane approach, the needle is introduced at the midpoint of the transducer at a right angle to the transducer beam. This approach is easier to learn, but the tip of the needle may be difficult to visualize (Fig. 67.17). The operator may have difficulty following the tip of the needle because only a small portion of the needle intersects the ultrasound beam at any given time (Figs. 67.18 and 67.19). Conversely, in the in-plane approach, the needle is introduced from either end of the transducer, and the needle can be visualized in its entirety (Figs. 67.20 and 67.21). However, this approach is technically more difficult, as slight movements of the transducer may result in losing the view of the needle. Consider each potential approach in the context of the particular procedure.

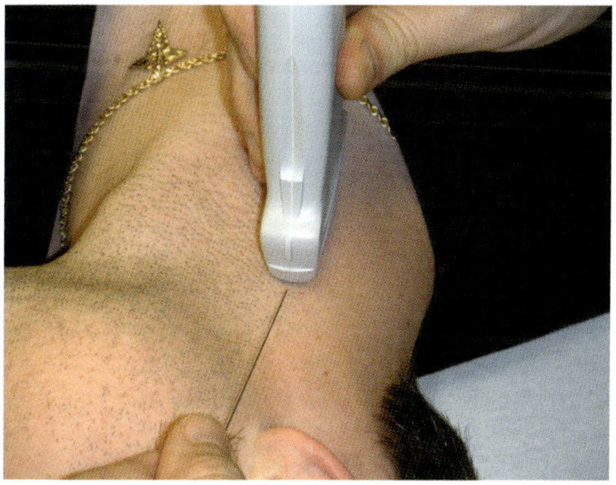

Fig. 67.20 Inserting a needle in the longitudinal or in-plane approach. In this technique the needle is inserted at the end of the transducer. This image is for demonstration purposes only and does not demonstrate sterile technique.

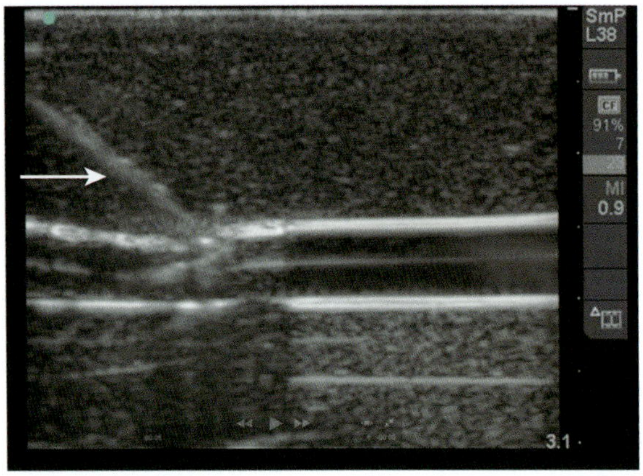

Fig. 67.21 Real-time image of the in-plane needle as it approaches the vein. The needle *(arrow)* can be identified as a hyperechoic object with reverberation artifact. In this orientation it can be seen in its entirety as it progresses toward the vein.

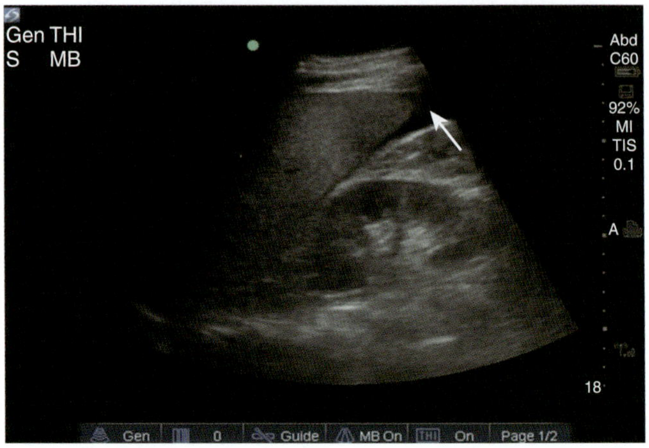

Fig. 67.22 Free fluid *(black)* seen surrounding the inferior tip of the liver *(arrow)*.

COMPLICATIONS

In general, the incidence of complications should be reduced with the use of ultrasound, but complications may occur even when performed by an experienced sonographer. Complications may be related to one of several factors. To maximize success, obtain an optimal image of the structure in question. Evaluate the anatomic relationships to ensure that the target object (e.g., the femoral vein versus the femoral artery) is correctly identified and pursued. Once the procedure begins, pay constant attention to the orientation and location of the needle. Errors, including inadvertent arterial puncture, can occur when the position of the tip of the needle is not closely followed.[3,4] Techniques to minimize these errors are addressed in the individual chapters.

FAST, E-FAST, AND RUSH EXAMINATIONS

No discussion about bedside ultrasound would be complete without a reference to the FAST (Focused Assessment with Sonography for Trauma), E-FAST (Extended Focused Assessment with Sonography for Trauma), and RUSH (Rapid Ultrasound in Shock) examinations.

The FAST examination was one of the first applications of ultrasound at the bedside, performed by nonradiology physicians. The FAST examination was first developed in the 1970s outside of the United States and spread to the United States in the 1980s, with rapid growth thereafter.[5,6] The FAST examination was first developed as an alternative to diagnostic peritoneal lavage (DPL) in patients with blunt trauma. In contrast to DPL, FAST is noninvasive, repeatable, and can be performed on any patient, from infants to pregnant females. Due to these advantages, FAST has not only largely replaced DPL for evaluation of hemorrhage following blunt trauma, but has been adapted for use in other scenarios, such as penetrating trauma and critical medical cases (such as in the case of a ruptured ectopic pregnancy). The E-FAST examination builds upon the traditional thoracoabdominal views of the FAST to include evaluation of the pleura and lung.

The effectiveness of the FAST and E-FAST examinations as diagnostic tools varies depending on the scenario in which they are used. The expertise and experience of the examiner plays a significant role and although the basic examination appears to be easily mastered, examiners with more experience are more capable of diagnosing small free-fluid collections.[7] FAST appears to be most sensitive when evaluating hypotensive blunt trauma patients.[8,9] Multiple studies have determined that the sensitivity for detecting free fluid in these patients approaches 100%.[10–12] In patients who are normotensive following blunt trauma, the sensitivity and specificity for FAST is more questionable, with most studies finding between 42% to 86% and 98% to 99%, respectively.[13–15] There is a role for the FAST examination in penetrating trauma, although the sensitivity is not as high as in blunt trauma patients.[16] In an unstable patient with penetrating trauma, a quick E-FAST examination to evaluate the pericardium and lungs can yield important information to help aid the operating room course.[17] Ultrasound for pneumothorax is extremely sensitive, particularly in comparison to traditional supine chest radiography.[18] Supine radiographs demonstrate sensitivities ranging from 47% to 75%, even with moderately sized pneumothoraces.[19,20] Ultrasound is also reliable for identifying pleural fluid.[21] Identifying a hemothorax can be difficult in the supine patient, as fluid can layer on chest radiographs, making rapid diagnosis challenging. Ultrasound at the costophrenic angles can quickly identify as little as 10 mL of fluid.[22]

The basis of the FAST examination relies on the principle that intraperitoneal free fluid will settle into dependent areas within the peritoneum when the patient is supine. These dependent areas form the four views that are the foundation of a basic FAST examination. The right and left upper quadrants, as well as the pelvis, are evaluated for free fluid. The pericardium is easily viewed from either the subxiphoid region or the anterior chest wall, identifying pericardial effusions. This view is helpful in determining if cardiac motion is present, particularly when deciding whether to continue resuscitation. Additional views of the bilateral pleura from the anterior chest can be added to perform the E-FAST to evaluate for pneumothorax and hemothorax

A full description of the FAST and E-FAST examinations is outside of the scope of this text, but the dependent areas of the abdomen should be evaluated for the presence of free fluid, which will typically appear anechoic or black (Figs. 67.22 and 67.23). A low-frequency transducer (2 mHz to 5 mHz) is usually optimal for evaluation of the abdomen. A curvilinear or phased-array transducer can be used, depending on availability and examiner preference. For evaluation of the pleura, a high-frequency transducer (6 mHz to 13 mHz) is optimal for maximum resolution, although a low-frequency transducer will suffice if no high-frequency transducer is available. The pericardium can be assessed for effusion from either the subxiphoid region of the chest or from the left anterior chest wall (Fig. 67.24), using either a low-frequency curvilinear transducer or a high-frequency phased-array transducer. In the supine patient, a pneumothorax will rise and be best seen on the anterior-medial aspect of the chest wall. A more detailed description of components of this examination can be found within this text:

- Evaluating the dependent portions of the abdomen in trauma is similar to evaluating dependent portions of the abdomen for ascites and paracentesis; see Chapter 44.
- Evaluating the pericardium for effusion following trauma is similar to evaluating effusions in anticipation of pericardiocentesis; see Chapter 16.
- Evaluating the pleura for evidence of a pneumothorax is covered in Chapter 10.

The RUSH examination was developed as a means to quickly assess a hypotensive patient at the bedside, utilizing ultrasound. The goals of the RUSH examination are to attempt to identify treatable causes of shock, such as pericardial tamponade, and also to attempt to classify the type of shock present.[23] Distinguishing between cardiogenic, obstructive, distributive, and hypovolemic shock is important, as the treatment strategies can vary widely. For example, determining that cardiogenic shock is present early in the evaluation of a hypotensive patient can assist the physician in narrowing the differential diagnosis and in avoiding unnecessary (and potentially harmful) initial treatments such as large fluid boluses. The RUSH examination is divided into components: the "pump", the "tank", and the "pipes" and should be evaluated in a step-wise fashion (Box 67.2). Each component of the RUSH examination should be evaluated for specific findings to guide management (Box 67.3). A

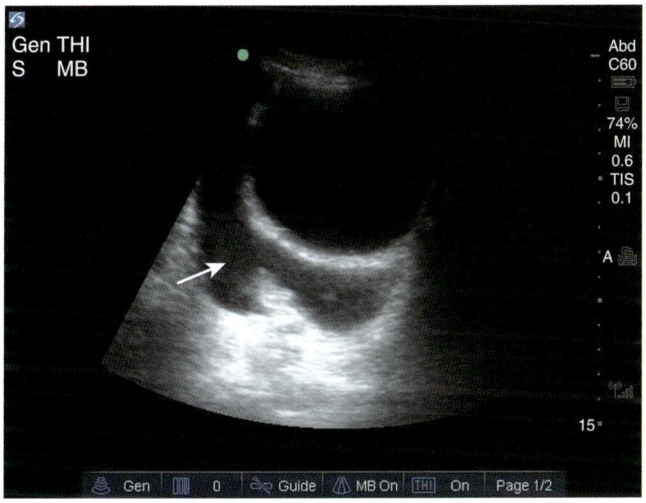

Fig. 67.23 Large amount of free fluid seen deep to the bladder *(arrow)*.

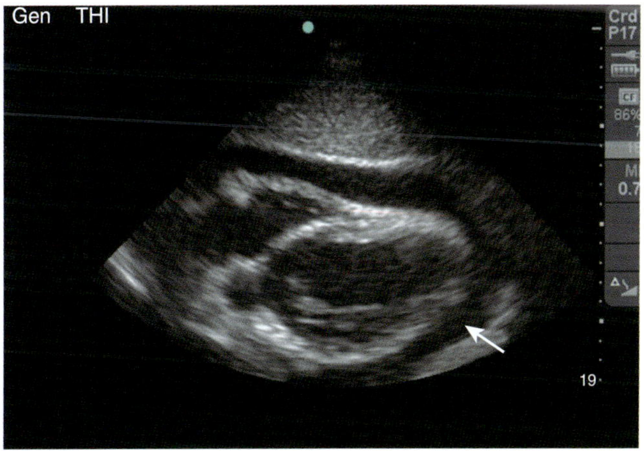

Fig. 67.24 Pericardial effusion seen surrounding the heart in the subxiphoid view *(arrow)*.

BOX 67.2 Components of the RUSH Examination

Pump	**Tank**	**Pipes**
Heart	Inferior vena cava	Aorta
	FAST examination	Lower extremity veins
	Pleura/lungs	—

FAST, Focused Assessment with Sonography for Trauma; *RUSH*, Rapid Ultrasound in Shock.

BOX 67.3 Findings Sought in Each Component of the RUSH Examination

Pump	**Tank**	**Pipes**
Estimate contractility of the heart to evaluate for cardiogenic shock and to determine ability to tolerate volume resuscitation	Determine the size and collapsibility of the inferior vena cava as a marker of volume status	Evaluate the thoracic and abdominal aorta for the presence of either an aneurysm (AAA) or dissection
Identify the presence of pericardial effusion and tamponade	Assess for the presence of free fluid in the peritoneum to indicate hypovolemic shock	Study the deep veins of the lower extremities to identify thrombus (DVT) when PE is a consideration
Evaluate for signs of right heart strain to indicate possible PE	Identify the presence of pneumothorax/tension pneumothorax	—
	Evaluate the lung parenchyma for evidence of pulmonary edema associated with cardiogenic shock	—
	Assess the costophrenic angles for evidence of pleural effusion/hemothorax	—

AAA, Abdominal aortic aneurysm; *DVT*, deep vein thrombosis; *PE*, pulmonary embolus; *RUSH*, Rapid Ultrasound in Shock.

BOX 67.4 Sonographic Views Used to Evaluate the Components of the RUSH Examination

Pump	Tank	Pipes
Parasternal long axis	IVC near entry into the right atrium	Thoracic aorta: parasternal long axis
Parasternal short axis	FAST: RUQ	Thoracic aorta: apical
Apical	FAST: LUQ	Abdominal aorta: proximal through bifurcation at umbilicus
Subxiphoid	FAST: pelvis	DVT: common femoral vein, superficial femoral vein, and popliteal veins
	Anterior pleura for sliding	—
	Anterior and lateral chest wall for signs of pulmonary edema	—

DVT, Deep vein thrombosis; *FAST,* Focused Assessment with Sonography for Trauma; *IVC,* inferior vena cava; *LUQ,* left upper quadrant; *RUQ,* right upper quadrant; *RUSH,* Rapid Ultrasound in Shock.

detailed overview of the technique is outside of the scope of this text. Box 67.4 lists the specific views that can be used to evaluate each component.

REFERENCES ARE AVAILABLE AT Elsevier eBooks+

CHAPTER 68

Bedside Laboratory and Microbiologic Procedures

Jason Chu and Samantha Selesny Klein

ASSESSMENT OF URINE

Obtaining a Urine Specimen

Several methods are available for obtaining a urine specimen. They can be found in Table 68.1 and are listed in order of increasingly precise collection techniques. They come at the cost of increasing difficulty, patient discomfort, or both.

General Considerations Regarding Urine Collection

The advantages and disadvantages of each of the techniques listed in Table 68.1 can be determined only by the purpose of the urine test and the clinical context. The clinical context influences interpretation of the results. For the majority of clinical scenarios, the basic dichotomy is between specimens obtained for infectious versus noninfectious reasons. Apart from testing for red blood cells (RBCs) and white blood cells (WBCs), most of the noninfectious tests (e.g., ketones, glucose, bilirubin, protein) are not affected by the collection method. Urine specimens collected to diagnose infection can be contaminated in several ways, and the clinical scenario intricately influences the choice and interpretation of tests.

Urinary tract infections (UTIs) can be asymptomatic or symptomatic, and the symptoms determine which collection method is required (Fig. 68.1). The standard for diagnosing UTIs is growth of greater than 10^5 colony-forming units (CFUs)/mL in urine culture and holds for asymptomatic patients.[1] However 30% to 50% of symptomatic patients can have UTIs at lower levels of bacteriuria (10^2 CFUs/mL), with up to 50% having polymicrobial infections.[2] Symptomatic female patients without potential complications who present for the first time require no further urine testing and should be treated empirically based on local patterns of susceptibility for urinary pathogens. Risk factors for acute UTI in females include recent sexual intercourse, use of spermicide, history of recent UTI.[3] The presence of dysuria, hematuria, frequency, or back pain increase the probability of UTI while the absence dysuria or back pain or history of vaginal discharge or vaginal irritation decrease the probability of UTI.[1] It is important to note that history and physical examination findings cannot rule in or out UTI. The presence of nitrite and leukocyte esterase on urine dipstick and the presence of moderate pyuria on microscopic examination (WBC >5) increase the probability of UTI.[4]

Symptomatic patients constitute a clinically distinct group who require a urine test that is much more sensitive and thus will render a false-positive result with much lower levels of contaminants. Although many studies do not show a statistically significant increase in contamination rates with less stringent urine collection techniques, most show increased accuracy with more meticulous or invasive collection methods.[5–8]

Patients with classic symptoms need the most careful urine collection method because they have the most riding on the outcome of the test. This group of patients should include those with systemic signs of infection (e.g., fever and chills) who are unable to accurately report their symptoms and patients in whom failure to diagnose asymptomatic bacteriuria would be potentially dangerous (e.g., the immunocompromised, neonates and infants, pregnant patients, patients with diabetes) or for whom urine cultures are going to be necessary because of a history of relapsing, recurrent, complicated, or childhood UTI.[9,10]

In cooperative, motivated males and females with symptoms of uncomplicated lower UTI or pyelonephritis who are capable of diligently performing the necessary maneuvers, a midstream clean catch (MSCC) specimen is as accurate as a catheterized specimen, especially when the possibility of urethral or prostatic trauma and patient discomfort are considered.[5] Lower resource utilization and avoidance of urethral or prostatic trauma and patient discomfort are additional advantages to an MSCC specimen. In patients who are unable to provide an MSCC specimen, or in children in whom thorough cleansing is more difficult, the increased accuracy afforded by a catheterized specimen is usually warranted.[11]

If no symptoms of UTI are present, the urine examination can be considered a screening test. In asymptomatic patients, routine screening for bacteriuria is unwarranted in all but two clinical situations: pregnant females and all patients scheduled for urologic surgery.[12,13] If only a urine culture is to be performed, some would argue that any spontaneously voided specimen would suffice because the diagnosis of asymptomatic bacteriuria depends on 10^5 or more CFUs of a single pathogen per milliliter of urine. With such criteria, contaminants are usually easily identified.[8] Because performing cultures on all such patients is prohibitively costly, dipstick testing, urinalysis (UA), or both are commonly used for screening.[14,15] With these tests, contamination by bacteria, leukocytes, or erythrocytes results in diagnostic confusion. The advantages of a less-contaminated specimen are worth the minimal, extra effort of asking the patient to provide an MSCC sample. The approach in Fig. 68.1 covers most situations. A few circumstances and techniques deserve special mention.

Bladder Percussion and the Midstream Specimen in Infants

Suprapubic bladder aspiration (SPA) has been the gold standard for urinary collection but is invasive. MSCC urine samples are a reasonable alternative to SPA samples but are challenging to obtain in infants. Several techniques can facilitate MSCC collection. For circumcised male infants, cleaning the penis with an antiseptic solution produced a MSCC sample within 10 to 20 minutes.[16] Another technique uses the Perez spinal reflex to induce urination.[17] After cleansing the genitalia, hold the infant in one hand while stroking the paraspinal muscles in a cephalad to caudad direction. This causes extension of the back and flexion of the hips and induces micturition in less than 5 minutes in most cases.[17] The bladder is stimulated with suprapubic finger tapping at a frequency of 60 to 100 taps/min for 1 minute and 1 minute of rest with a mean time to a MSCC urine sample of 5 minutes.[18] A combined method using finger tapping for 30 seconds alternating

TABLE 68.1 Urine Collection Methods Listed in Order of Increasing Precision

METHOD	DESCRIPTION AND COMMENTS
Random voided	Any specimen provided by the patient.
Midstream voided	No skin preparation, container placed in the urinary stream 2–3 s after initiation of micturition.
Clean catch	Same as above, plus antiseptic cleansing of the urethral area. This is performed by retraction of the prepuce in males and the labia in females and then cleansing the meatus in an anterior-to-posterior direction. Use three swabs soaked in povidone-iodine (or some other antiseptic solution). For female patients who are physically capable, the ideal position is sitting astride a toilet, facing backward. This helps separate the labia and position the cup for collection of the specimen.
Midstream clean catch	Cleansing as for clean catch, with midstream collection as for midstream voided.
Catheterized	Obtained from a newly placed catheter after cleansing of the meatus.
Suprapubic aspiration	See Chapter 56.

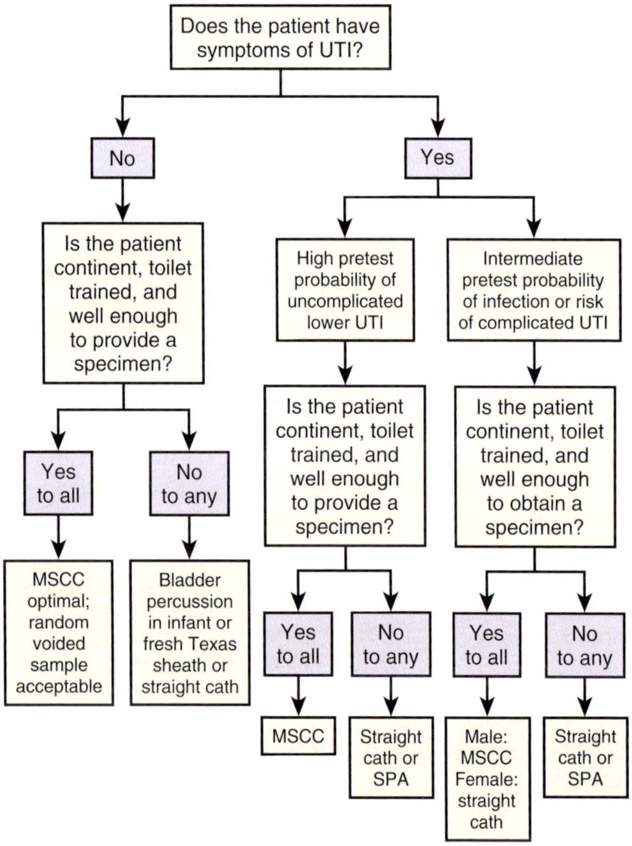

Fig. 68.1 Algorithm for deciding method of obtaining urine specimen for evaluation of possible urinary tract infection. For initial presentation with symptoms in otherwise healthy females: no urine testing indicated; see text. *MSCC*, Midstream clean catch; *SPA*, suprapubic aspiration; *UTI*, urinary tract infection.

with lumbar stimulation with a light circular motion for 30 seconds after oral hydration provided urine collection within 2 minutes.[19,20]

Bag Collection in Non–Toilet-Trained Children

The incidence of unsuspected UTI in a febrile neonate or infant is approximately 5%.[21] Similar rates are found in asymptomatic children less than 5 years of age who present to the emergency department (ED) with nonspecific symptoms of acute illness.[22] A true UTI in an infant or child requires subsequent evaluation with renal bladder ultrasound and/or voiding cystourethrography for urinary tract pathology, and the disease may produce significant morbidity (e.g., hypertension, renal disease). The costs of overdiagnosis with a false-positive UA are significant and include bacterial resistance that leads to the use of increasingly expensive/broad antibiotic medications.[23] Numerous studies have demonstrated false-positive rates of urine specimens obtained for culture from a collection bag stuck to an infant's perineum, and this method should not be used for ill-appearing children.[17,18,24–26]

In febrile children with a low likelihood of UTI, a bag urine specimen for UA is acceptable.[27] A positive result (presence of leukocyte esterase, nitrite, or bacteriuria) should be confirmed with UA from a catheterized or SPA specimen. Treatment should only be initiated if the UA is positive and urine culture has more than 50,000 CFU/mL.[27,28]

If a urine specimen is needed solely for chemical analysis (e.g., glucose, ketones, specific gravity), a bag specimen will suffice.

Urine Specimens from Patients with Chronic Urinary Drainage Systems

Urine obtained from any part of a chronic urinary drainage system is highly inaccurate for bacteriologic purposes. If UTI is suspected, insert a new catheter and obtain a fresh bladder urine specimen. In most cases, a Foley catheter should be used to obtain urine from patients with sheath catheters who have signs or symptoms of acute UTI and are unable to provide an MSCC specimen.[29]

Catheterization and Suprapubic Aspiration

The low levels of bacteriuria found in 2% to 8% of patients after straight catheterization are generally below the threshold that defines the presence of UTI.[30] Catheterization can cause minor local injury, as reflected by low-level hematuria in 15% of patients.[30,31] SPA continues to be advocated by some for neonates in cases in which accurate diagnosis is essential and the risk for infection must be minimized. Both SPA (see Chapter 56) and catheterization have an approximately 25% failure rate as a result of an empty bladder.[32] This problem and associated complications can be avoided by performing bedside ultrasound before the procedure.[33,34] SPA may spuriously lower leukocyte or bacterial colony counts because of the necessity of filling the bladder before performing the procedure.[35] A study in infants demonstrated that the discomfort associated with SPA is greater than that with catheterization.[36] Surprisingly, however, older males who underwent both catheterization and SPA strongly preferred SPA.[5]

Urine Dipstick

Urine dipstick tests are available to test 10 separate parameters. The unassuming appearance and commonplace use of the urine dipstick might lead one to mistakenly underestimate its technical sophistication. Each colored square on a urine dipstick involves a biochemically complex assay, and therefore it is essential to meticulously follow the manufacturer's instructions for storage and use.[37] Even with optimal storage and testing conditions, the false-negative and false-positive rates of these tests are problematic. In addition, most of the tests are susceptible to interference from a variety of substances (Table 68.2).

Method

Test urine specimens as soon as possible after they are collected. If the urine has been standing, stir or shake the specimen well because cells sink rapidly in a container. Immerse the test strip completely for 1 second. Draw the edge of the strip along the rim of the specimen container and lightly tap it to remove excess urine, thus avoiding mixing the reagents between different test patches. Next, hold the strip horizontally or place it on a clean pad until the recommended time has elapsed. Most strips are designed so that all the test results can be read together after 1 to 2 minutes (Fig. 68.2).

Interpretation

Glucose

The urine glucose test is normally negative. Urine glucose testing has limited usefulness in quantitative testing because the serum glucose level at which spillage occurs varies (although in most patients it starts at between 180 and 200 mg/dL).[38,39] Changes in urine glucose lag behind changes in blood glucose by approximately half the interval between voids.[40] Glycosuria in the absence of hyperglycemia suggests renal tubular dysfunction. Glycosuria may occur in hypothermic patients in the absence of hyperglycemia and indeed may actually occur with hypoglycemia in such patients.[41]

Ketones

Ketones are found in the urine of patients with starvation, inadequate carbohydrate intake, diabetic and alcoholic ketoacidosis, isopropyl alcohol poisoning, or glycogen storage disease. Tests for urine ketones are 5 to 10 times more sensitive to acetoacetate than to acetone, similar to the serum tests. Dipsticks do not detect beta-hydroxybutyrate, which accounts for 80% to 95% of the three ketone bodies and is the predominant form in the setting of ketoacidosis.[42] Urine ketone testing is significantly more sensitive than serum ketone testing.[43] There is generally no need to obtain serum acetones to diagnose or manage diabetic ketoacidosis when urine ketone monitoring is coupled with blood gas and anion gap analysis.

Leukocyte Esterase

This portion of the dipstick test is designed to detect indoxyl esterase activity from the azurophilic granules in neutrophils.[42] Studies report a wide and clinically important range of thresholds for the sensitivity of dipstick testing, from 10 to 100 WBCs/μL urine.[14,15] Studies suggest that the test is between 50% and 96% sensitive in detecting infection.[44–46] Its specificity for the presence of WBCs is between 91% and 99%. The most common cause of a false-positive leukocyte test is vaginal contamination.

Nitrites

Normally, urine does not contain nitrites. Nitrites are specific (≈ 95%), but not sensitive (≈ 45%) indicators of UTI.[12,47,48] Urinary nitrates are converted to nitrites most strongly by enteric coliform bacteria, thus explaining the nitrite test's 90% sensitivity in detecting UTI caused by *Escherichia coli*. *Enterococcus*, a moderately frequent urinary pathogen, *Pseudomonas* species, and *Acinetobacter* lack the reductase enzyme and are not detected by nitrite testing. False-negative results also occur because of the lack of dietary nitrate, frequent voiding, and diuresis. Early morning–voided specimens are ideal because they allow time for conversion of nitrate to nitrite, but they are rarely available in the ED. If possible, a specimen obtained more than 4 hours after the last voiding is preferred.

Protein

Proteins with a molecular weight below 50,000 to 60,000 Daltons can pass through the glomerulus to be reabsorbed in the proximal tubule. Normal passage of protein in urine is less than 150 mg/24 hours, or approximately 10 mg/dL of urine. Approximately 10% to 33% of urinary protein is albumin, 33% is Tamm-Horsfall glycoprotein (secreted by renal tubular cells), and the balance is made up of a variety of immunoglobulins and other proteins. The dipstick is most sensitive to albumin and not very sensitive for tubular or light chain proteins (Bence-Jones proteins).[49] The urine dipstick test is falsely positive for protein with pyuria of greater than 6 WBCs/high-power field (HPF).[50] Hematuria only slightly elevates urine protein levels. Less than 1.5% of patients with asymptomatic proteinuria have significant renal disease.[51] Proteinuria may be benign secondary to postural proteinuria (proteinuria when standing but not when recumbent).[49]

A study of ED patients with severe acute hypertension identified renal dysfunction, defined as elevated serum creatinine, with 100% sensitivity when using urine dipstick detection of 1+ proteinuria or hematuria.[52] Along similar lines, in patients being considered for radiographic contrast-enhanced studies who do not have a serum creatinine measurement, a negative dipstick test for protein or blood combined with the absence of prior renal disease, hypertension, diabetes, congestive heart failure, and age younger than 60 years effectively excludes renal insufficiency.[53]

In assessing a patient with proteinuria, it is helpful to divide the list of causes into those that are and those that are not associated with hematuria. These are listed in Box 68.1. Elevated urinary protein is more commonly due to renal than systemic causes. The source is either glomerular, with passage of normally unfiltered proteins, or tubular, with failure to reabsorb physiologically filtered, low-molecular-weight globulins. The former condition causes albuminuria. Renal tubular proteinuria is characterized by low levels of urinary albumin and is therefore more likely to be missed.

TABLE 68.2 Overview of Urine Dipstick Tests

	FALSE POSITIVE	FALSE NEGATIVE	COMMENTS
Glucose	Peroxide, hypochlorite, ketonuria, levodopa, and the dipstick exposed to air	Ascorbate, ketones, uric acid, alkaline pH, tetracycline, and high specific gravity	Hypothermia may cause glycosuria despite hypoglycemia Glycosuria without hyperglycemia suggests renal tubular dysfunction
Ketones	Ascorbate, low pH urine, high specific gravity, levodopa, valproate, phenazopyridine, *N*-acetylcysteine, high-protein diet, phenylketonuria, phthalein compounds, sulfhydryl groups	Delay in examination	Very susceptible to deterioration with humidity and delay in analysis, which can cause false-negative results Does not detect hydroxybutyric acid
Nitrites	Phenazopyridine	High specific gravity, frequent urination, ascorbate, high urine pH, and urine standing in the specimen cup >2 h	75% false-negative rate when exposed to air for 15 days Does not detect reductase-negative bacteria
Protein	Alkaline urine, chlorhexidine, phenazopyridine, quaternary ammonium compounds	Low pH, very dilute urine	Only reliable for albumin (glomerular proteinuria) Does not detect Bence-Jones protein Positive with pyuria, rarely with hematuria
Blood/heme	Povidone-iodine, certain peroxidase-producing bacteria, hypochlorite	High specific gravity, high concentrations of urinary nitrites, ascorbate, or captopril	Positive test with speckles or dots implies nonhemolyzed blood Positive test with a diffuse pattern implies hemolyzed red blood cells or high levels of myoglobin
Bilirubin	Iodine, stool contamination, chlorpromazine, etodolac, mefenamic acid, phenazopyridine	Prolonged standing—UV light exposure, elevated nitrite, ascorbate, rifampin	Hard to read with agents causing marked urine discoloration
Urobilinogen	Phenazopyridine, sulfisoxazole, sulfonamides, porphyrin, methyldopa, procaine, aminosalicylic acid, 5-hydroxyindolacetic acid	Sulfisoxazole, phenazopyridine, formalin, nitrate	Use a fresh specimen: rapidly broken down by light and in acidic urine
Leukocyte esterase	Vaginal contamination, alkaline pH, oxidizing agents, eosinophils in urine, *Trichomonas*	High glucose, ketones, protein (especially albumin), pH, and specific gravity, cephalexin, nitrofurantoin, tetracycline, tobramycin, oxalates, ascorbic acid, neutropenia	Sterile pyuria seen with tuberculosis, nephrolithiasis, interstitial nephritis
pH	High pH—urea-splitting bacteria, type I renal tubular acidosis (RTA) Low pH—dietary protein, acidic fruits, type II RTA Runoff from the protein strip can falsely lower pH		Use a fresh specimen: standing raises pH by loss of CO_2
Specific gravity	Overestimates specific gravity with low pH, ketoacidosis, and protein Underestimates specific gravity with glucose, urea, or pH >7		Not reliable at specific gravity >1.025 Elevated with use of dextran, intravenous contrast material, proteinuria

Blood

The pseudo-peroxidase activity of heme in erythrocytes, myoglobin and free hemoglobin catalyzes a reaction of peroxide with chromogens on the dipstick causing a color change.[42]

Studies have shown that the urine dipstick is very sensitive to 10 RBCs/mL. False-negative results are confined to clinically insignificant hematuria.[54] Moderate intravascular hemolysis does not cause hemoglobinuria because hemoglobin is tightly bound to haptoglobin and is therefore not filtered. Massive intravascular hemolysis gives rise to free plasma hemoglobin with a molecular weight of 32,000 Daltons, which easily passes through the glomerulus. Myoglobin has a molecular weight of 17,000 Daltons, which also allows easy glomerular passage, but the dipstick has been shown

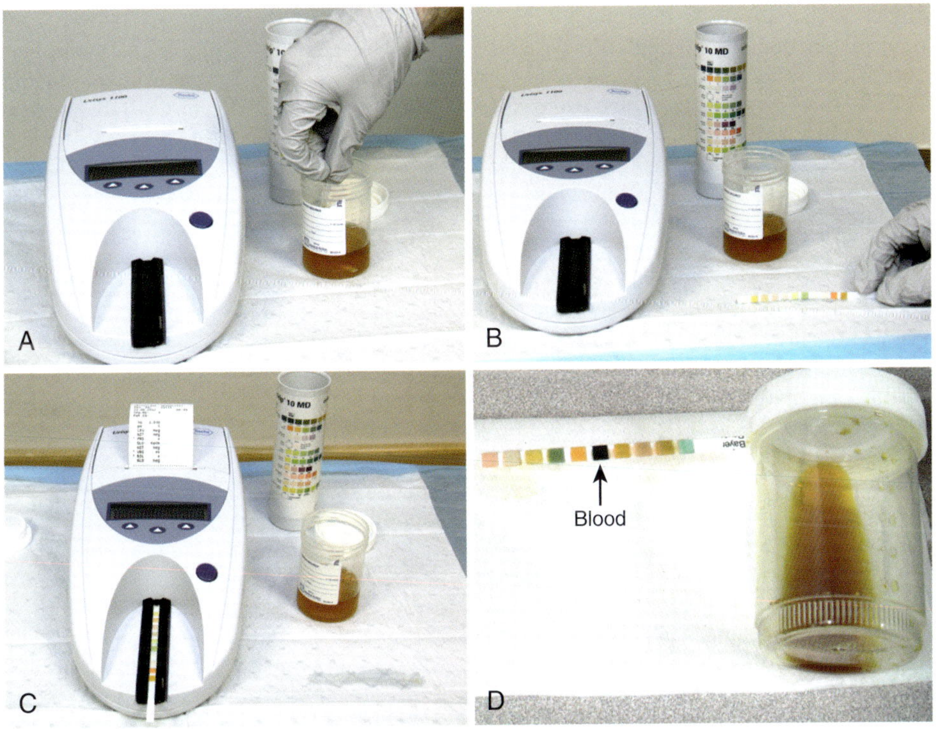

Fig. 68.2 Urine dipstick testing. (A) Completely immerse the dipstick in urine for a few seconds. (B) Place it on its side on a paper towel to allow drainage of urine and limit cross-contamination of the individual testing squares. Note that the bottle of test strips should be closed immediately because prolonged exposure to air can produce false results. (C) Formal reading of the test strip is accomplished electronically rather than only by the naked eye for quality assurance and a permanent record. (D) Myoglobinuria: strongly positive for blood on the dipstick with no red blood cells on microscopy.

BOX 68.1 Proteinuria

PROTEINURIA USUALLY WITH HEMATURIA

Usually indicates glomerular disease

Most etiologies in early stages can present without hematuria

Infectious Diseases

Poststreptococcal glomerulonephritis, pneumococcal pneumonia, bacterial endocarditis, meningococcemia, secondary syphilis, HIV, hepatitis B, severe viral infections, malaria, toxoplasmosis, Guillain-Barré syndrome

Multisystem Diseases

Vasculitides: Henoch-Schönlein purpura, polyarteritis nodosa, granulomatosis with polyangiitis, Kawasaki disease, etc.

Connective tissue diseases (lupus, rheumatoid arthritis, scleroderma)

Neoplasia

Rhabdomyolysis (artifactual hematuria)

Goodpasture syndrome

Cryoglobulinemias

Toxemia of pregnancy

Serum sickness

Primary Glomerular Diseases

PROTEINURIA USUALLY WITHOUT HEMATURIA

Generally indicates tubular/interstitial disease, or high serum levels causing "overflow"

In advanced disease, can develop hematuria

Systemic Conditions

Physiological: postexercise, postural (with standing)

Pathological: fever, shock states, severe hypovolemia, dehydration, congestive heart failure

Diabetes

Amyloidosis

Sarcoidosis

"Overflow states": multiple myeloma, lymphoma, leukemia, rhabdomyolysis

Renovascular hypertension

Medications, Drugs, and Toxins

Nonsteroidal anti-inflammatory drugs, gold, penicillamine, probenecid, captopril, lithium, cyclosporin

Heroin

Heavy metal nephropathy: lead, mercury, or cadmium

Renal Diseases

Chronic pyelonephritis

Interstitial nephritis

Fanconi syndrome

to have a low sensitivity in diagnosing rhabdomyolysis.[55,56] Guidelines for distinguishing hematuria, hemoglobinuria, and myoglobinuria are outlined in Table 68.3.

Dipsticks are vitiated by humidity and air, which can cause false-negative results after improper storage.[57] Because RBCs may lyse rapidly, delays in performing UA may misleadingly suggest myoglobinuria or hemoglobinuria. Microscopy or dipstick testing of a freshly obtained specimen can clarify this issue. Conversely, high specific gravity or low pH can inhibit lysis of erythrocytes, which is necessary for the dipstick chemical reaction to occur, thus causing false-negative results.[58] A study reproducing clinical conditions has demonstrated that povidone-iodine does not cause false-positive results on the dipstick.[59] Iatrogenically caused trace positive results may occur after catheterization in 15% of cases.[31]

Urine Bilirubin

Urine bilirubin represents the filtered, soluble, conjugated form of bilirubin. Unconjugated bilirubin is bound to protein and does not pass through the glomerulus. Bilirubinuria is therefore due to intrahepatic or extrahepatic cholestasis. Bilirubinuria will be detected significantly earlier than clinical jaundice. Urinary bilirubin excretion is enhanced by alkalosis. A fresh sample of urine should be tested because bilirubin glucuronide is hydrolyzed when exposed to light. Ascorbic acid and high levels of urinary nitrites decrease the sensitivity of the test to bilirubin.

Urobilinogen

In a healthy person, conjugated bilirubin is excreted in bile. In the colon it is broken down into a few compounds, including urobilinogen. Most of these compounds are excreted in stool, which is the source of its characteristic color. A small amount of urobilinogen is absorbed from the colon, and if it is not taken up on the first pass through the liver, it enters the circulation. Ultimately, some of this urobilinogen may enter the urine, so it is normal to have zero to moderate levels of urinary urobilinogen on dipstick testing. Hepatocellular disease (hepatitis, cirrhosis, passive liver congestion, etc.) or hemolysis increase urinary urobilinogen excretion by impairing hepatic uptake of urobilinogen.[42] As a qualitative test with a wide range of normal values it is rarely helpful, but in evaluating a patient with jaundice it can have diagnostic significance (Table 68.4).

pH

The average daily excretion of 50 mmol to 100 mmol of H^+ in urine gives rise to a typical urine pH of approximately 6 with a range from 4.5 to 8. Dietary citrate lowers urinary pH, whereas proteins, acidic fruit and vegetables tend to raise it.[49] In most states of alkalosis and acidosis, healthy kidneys maintain homeostasis by conserving or excreting H^+. Failure to do so suggests renal disease, especially renal tubular acidosis. An exception is the *paradoxical aciduria* of hypokalemic alkalosis secondary to volume contraction, hypercortisolism, or diuretics, where the highest priority of the renal tubule is to conserve sodium. pH is elevated by the action of urea-splitting bacteria, especially *Proteus* species. This can occur with stasis of urine, either in the bladder or in specimen cups. A persistently alkaline urine is seen in patients with struvite (triple phosphate) urolithiasis.

Specific Gravity

The dipstick test for urine specific gravity assays for the primary urinary cations, sodium, and potassium. True specific gravity, which is also dependent on anions, albumin, proteins, urea, and glucose, is therefore not measured. Artifactually low specific gravity readings are obtained with alkaline urine, whereas acidic urine and albumin falsely elevate the specific gravity reading. Consequently, some investigators believe that these strips on the dipstick test are of marginal clinical utility.[60] Other clinical indicators of a patient's hydration status are probably more reliable. If necessary, a refractive specific gravitometer or a hygrometer should be used.

Microscopic Urinary Analyses

Microscopic UA is performed to identify cells, bacteria, and other microbes, as well as formed elements such as casts and crystals (Fig. 68.3). Various cutoffs have been used to diagnose UTI ranging from more than 3 to 10 WBCs/HPF, more than 5 RBCs/HPF, or more than 15 bacteria/HPF.[61,62]

The presence of WBCs with bacteria distinguishes infection from colonization (bacteriuria without pyuria). Some authorities state that significant infection without pyuria occurs in less than 5% of cases, thus making pyuria alone a sensitive marker of infection.[57,63] Other studies do not support reliance on pyuria by itself as an indicator of infection.[5,44,64,65] The presence of WBC casts distinguishes pyelonephritis ("upper UTI") from cystitis ("lower UTI").

TABLE 68.3 Aids in Distinguishing Hematuria, Intravascular Hemolysis, and Myoglobinuria

	HEMATURIA	MYOGLOBINURIA	INTRAVASCULAR HEMOLYSIS
Serum findings	Color: clear	Color: clear Haptoglobin: normal	Color: pink Haptoglobin: low
Urine appearance	Color: clear to brown; clears with centrifugation	Color: clear to red/brown; no clearing with centrifugation	Color: clear to brown; no clearing with centrifugation
Urine microscopy	RBCs, RBC casts, and protein: glomerular source RBCs, no RBC casts, tubular cells, small protein: nephron source RBCs alone: source distal to the nephron (e.g., ureterolithiasis)	Possible occasional RBCs and tubular cells secondary to rhabdomyolysis-induced renal damage	Usually unremarkable

RBC, Red blood cell.

TABLE 68.4 Relationship Between Urinary Bilirubin, Urobilinogen, and Stool Color in Jaundiced Patients

	HEALTHY NORMAL	COMPLETE BILIARY OBSTRUCTION	INTRAVASCULAR HEMOLYSIS	HEPATOCELLULAR DISEASE
Urinary bilirubin	None	Elevated	None	Elevated
Urinary urobilinogen	None or present	None	Present, sometimes large	Normal early, increased late
Stool color	Normal	Acholic	Normal	Normal

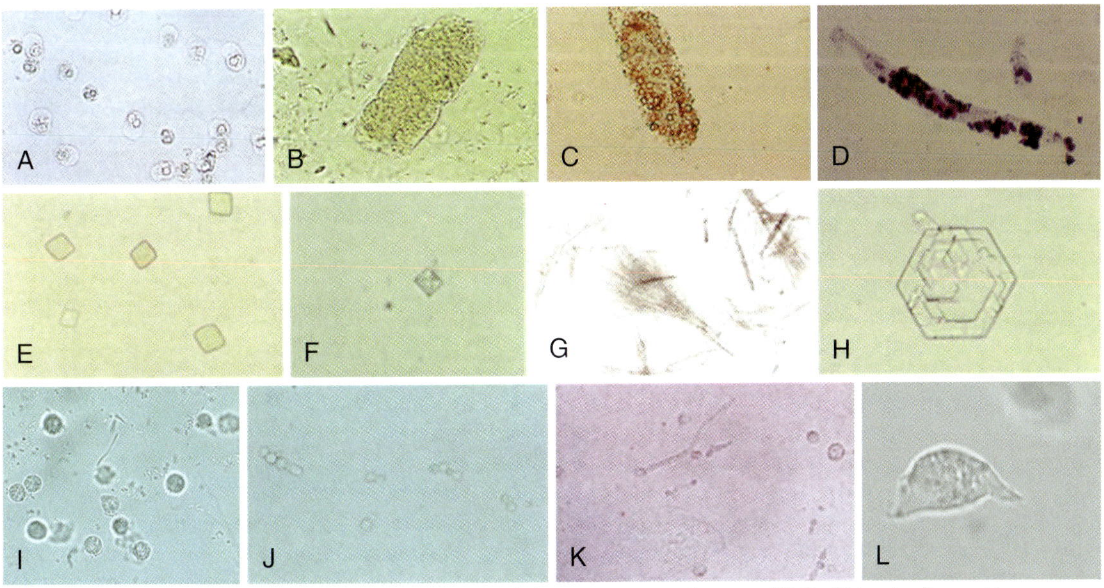

Fig. 68.3 Microscopic urinalysis. (A) Neutrophils. (B) Fine granular cast. (C) Red blood cell cast (the distinct and uniformly spherical shape of the erythrocyte is visible). (D) White blood cell cast (seen with intrinsic renal diseases such as pyelonephritis and glomerulonephritis; note the discernible nuclei and cell boundaries). (E) Uric acid crystals. (F) Calcium oxalate crystals. (G) Calcium phosphate crystals. (H) Cysteine crystal (indicative of cystinuria). (I) Bacteria and leukocytes. (J) *Candida*, budding yeast. (K) *Candida*, pseudohyphae. (L) *Trichomonas vaginalis*. (A–K, From McPherson RA, Pincus MR, eds. *Henry's Clinical Diagnosis and Management by Laboratory Methods*. 22nd ed. Saunders; 2011. L, From Bieber EJ, Sanfilippo JS, Horowitz IR, eds. *Clinical Gynecology*. Churchill Livingstone; 2006.)

Summary of Tests Used in the Diagnosis of UTI

The three tests commonly used to evaluate a patient for the presence or absence of UTI are urine dipstick, microscopic UA, and urine culture. Each represents an increasing degree of expense, delay, and resources.[66] A brief discussion of their relative strengths and weaknesses ensues.

Urine Dipstick

Dipstick testing of urine is faster than microscopic UA, is less labor-intensive, cheaper, and circumvents multiple sources of potential and proven error. It is sufficiently accurate to replace microscopic UA; however, if either leukocyte esterase or nitrites are used to indicate infection, the dipstick is only 50% to 90% sensitive for culture-proven infection.[14,46,47,67,68] This is not adequate to rule out infection in symptomatic patients, in whom the prevalence of disease is high, but may be acceptable in asymptomatic patients, in whom the test has a high negative predictive value of 95% to 99%. A large retrospective series demonstrated laboratory-performed UA (with microscopy) in children to be 8% more sensitive than dipstick testing in the ED, with similar specificity of approximately 80% for both tests.[23] In symptomatic males, sensitivity is enhanced by taking a positive result in any one (or more) of either leukocyte esterase, nitrites, protein, or blood as an indication of UTI.[14,69–71] This process can be augmented by allowing extra time before reading the strip. For females with classic symptoms of UTI, empirical treatment is recommended because no test can rule out infection.[66] A negative dipstick test in a patient with a high pretest probability of UTI should prompt a search for an alternative source of the patient's symptoms.

Microscopic UA

In various studies a range between 3 and 15 organisms/HPF or 5 WBCs/HPF has been considered a "positive" test (as the threshold number rises, so does specificity, at the price of sensitivity). In aggregate, the accuracy of microscopy in the diagnosis of UTI is similar to that of the dipstick alone, with 22% false-positive and 23% false-negative rates when compared with culture.[57,66,72] Microscopic UA, like the dipstick, cannot rule out infection in symptomatic patients. The specificity of pyuria is improved when viewed as a marker of all genitourinary infections, including urethritis, prostatitis, epididymitis, vaginitis, and cervicitis. These diagnoses should always be entertained in patients with urinary symptoms, especially those with sterile pyuria.

Urine Culture

Cultures are indicated for any potentially complicated UTI, including infections in children; males; females with recurrences or relapses; immunocompromised individuals; patients with urinary tract pathology, including stones and possible pyelonephritis; and pregnant patients. Cultures are usually recommended at approximately the 16th week of gestation. Every effort should be made to obtain a high-quality specimen because of the difficulty in distinguishing contamination from significant low-count bacteriuria in symptomatic patients and in view of the expense of cultures and treatment if the culture is positive.

The Bottom Line

It is well established that female patients with symptoms of uncomplicated lower UTI can be treated without culture because the prevalence of disease is 50% or greater in females with classic urinary symptoms.[13,48,73,74] Treatment is generally benign, and 95% of urine cultures that are positive will yield a limited number of organisms with predictable antibiotic susceptibilities. Some authors recommend dipstick, microscopic UA, or both because a negative test might prompt more careful consideration of alternative diagnoses in this group, with a high incidence of sexually transmitted disease.[13,48] If none is found, such patients can be treated empirically.

The Infectious Diseases Society of America recommends 5 days of nitrofurantoin, single dose of fosfomycin, or 3 days of trimethoprim-sulfamethoxazole 160/800 mg (if the prevalence of resistance is less than 20%) in females with uncomplicated UTI.[75] If these agents are not options, oral cephalosporins or fluoroquinolones (limited by rising resistance rates) can be substituted.[75,76]

Urine testing is more likely to influence clinical management in patients with an intermediate pretest probability of infection.[9] Urine microscopy may also help in distinguishing pyelonephritis (WBC casts), vaginitis (absence of pyuria or hematuria in a meticulous MSCC or catheterized specimen), and urethritis (pyuria, rarely hematuria) from cystitis (pyuria and often hematuria).[13,48] In the ED, the ease of performing a dipstick test argues for its use without UA because it is equally sensitive unless formed elements such as casts, crystals, *Trichomonas*, or other parasites are suspected. In patients with pyelonephritis, urine cultures are warranted because they alter therapy in approximately 5% of cases.[77] In most asymptomatic patients, a negative dipstick or UA result has sufficient negative predictive value to rule out disease unless the patient is pregnant or undergoing urologic surgery. Special clinical considerations in some patients (e.g., the immunocompromised, diabetic females at high risk for UTI) may mandate adjustments to this approach.[14] Recommendations vary regarding infants. Cultures are recommended for all febrile infants younger than 2 months and for children who appear sick or have a high pretest probability of infection.[24,26] In a 2009 study, combined microscopic and dipstick UA was only 64% sensitive (and 91% specific) for culture-proven UTI in febrile infants younger than 24 months, thus suggesting the use of culture unless an alternative source of infection is clear.[78]

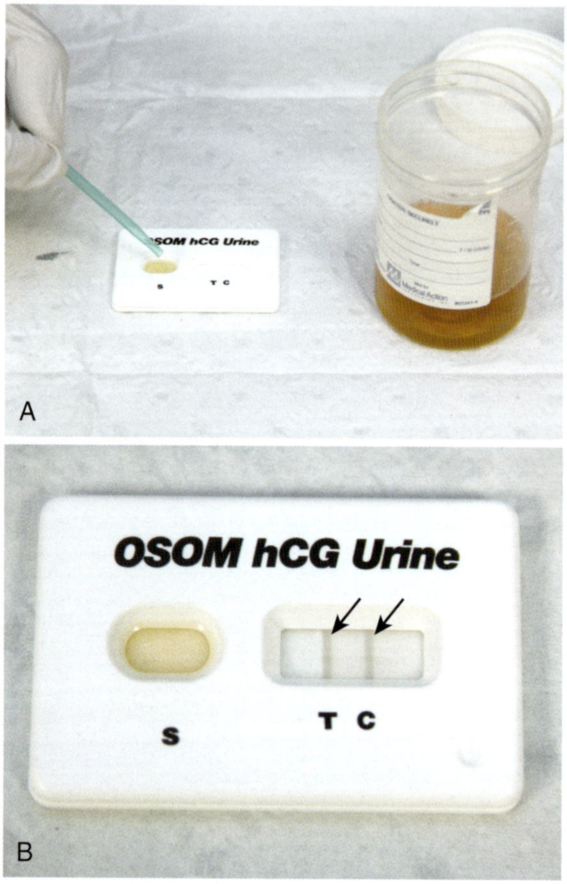

Fig. 68.4 Urine β-human chorionic gonadotropin (β-hCG) testing. (A) The concentration of β-hCG is usually lower in urine than in serum, thus making the urine test slightly less sensitive for the detection of early pregnancy. Whole blood specimens can also be used in these kits (see text). (B) This test is positive, as indicated by the dark stripe in both the test *(T)* and control *(C)* positions *(arrows)*.

TESTING FOR PREGNANCY

Pregnancy tests are based on the detection of β-human chorionic gonadotropin (β-hCG) in serum or urine. β-hCG is secreted by trophoblastic cells of the placenta starting from the time of implantation of the blastocyst. Qualitative serum and urine tests can detect β-hCG levels of between 15 and 25 mIU/mL (Fig. 68.4)[79] The concentration of β-hCG is usually lower in urine than in serum, which accounts for the slight advantage of serum tests in detecting early pregnancy. Optimal results on urine pregnancy tests are obtained with first-voided, concentrated morning specimens. β-hCG in urine binds both antibodies to form an antibody-antigen-antibody sandwich and gives a positive test. False negatives can occur with low levels of β-hCG (between 20 and 300 IU/L) or excessively high levels of β-hCG, which prevents the antibody-antigen-antibody sandwich from forming (Hook effect).[80,81]

Although not US Food and Drug Administration (FDA) approved, whole blood can be used in place of urine with urinary point-of-care immunoassay bedside tests with 99.6% concordance between whole blood and urine samples and similar sensitivities (95.8% whole blood, 95.3% urine) and negative predictive values (97.9% whole blood, 97.6% urine).[82,83]

The same volume of blood is placed in the testing well(s) as when performed with urine. This alternative may be lifesaving in timely recognition of an ectopic pregnancy in a hypotensive female with pelvic complaints and unknown pregnancy status when a urine specimen is unavailable or results in significant delay. Currently there are US FDA–approved whole blood quantitative bedside tests such as the Abbott i-STAT system (Total β-hCG cartridge) with a range of detection of 8 to 2000 IU/L without dilution.[84]

If fertilization has occurred, β-hCG levels of 5 to 8 mIU/mL (the threshold of the quantitative serum test) correspond to the 9th to 11th day after ovulation (23 to 25 days after the first day of the last normal menstrual period). In a viable intrauterine pregnancy (IUP), the β-hCG level doubles approximately every 2.5 days during the first 4 weeks of gestation and reaches a serum level of greater than 25 mIU/mL, which is detectable by virtually all pregnancy tests on the first day of the missed menstrual period. The doubling rate declines to every third day thereafter.[85,86] β-hCG reaches a peak of between 100,000 and 200,000 mIU/mL between the 10th and 14th gestational weeks and declines to 10,000 to 20,000 mIU/mL for the rest of the pregnancy (Table 68.5).[87,88] There is a wide range of β-hCG levels in different females at the same stage of gestation, thus making definite clinical determination on the basis of a single quantitative test impossible.[89,90] False-positive test results have been described in association with molar pregnancy, choriocarcinoma, teratoma, occasional malignancies outside the genitourinary tract, and very high levels of proteinuria.

Although a previous quantitative β-hCG level is rarely available to the emergency clinician, doubling rates are an important part of the assessment of a healthy first-trimester pregnancy. Fetal nonviability, ectopic pregnancy, and intrauterine demise are signaled by abnormalities in the predicted rise in quantitative β-hCG.[91,92] A 2-day increase of the β-hCG of less than 35% or a 2-day decrease of 36% to 47% (depending on the initial level) had a sensitivity of 83.2% and a specificity of 70.8% in predicting ectopic pregnancy.[93] β-hCG levels in a healthy IUP and associated sonographic findings are listed in Table 68.5.

The rate of decline in quantitative β-hCG after gestation depends on the reason for the conclusion of the pregnancy. After a term delivery, β-hCG falls to zero in 2 weeks; after surgery for an ectopic pregnancy, the range is 1 to 31 days, with a median of 8.5 days; after a first-trimester spontaneous miscarriage, the range is 9 to 35 days (median, 19 days); and after a first-trimester elective abortion, the range is 16 to 60 days (median, 30 days).[38]

The association between β-hCG levels and gestational dates has led to the concept of the "discriminatory zone." In a normal pregnancy, a quantitative β-hCG level of 1000 to 2000 mIU/mL should be reflected by the presence of a double decidual sac (at the least) on transvaginal ultrasound (and on transabdominal ultrasound with levels higher than 6500 mIU/mL).[94] The clinician should beware of several potential pitfalls in applying this concept. First, it applies only to the double decidual sign, itself subject to interobserver variation among sonographers. The discriminatory zone cannot be extrapolated to the expected levels at which any of the more definitive sonographic signs of IUP such as yolk sac, fetal pole, or cardiac motion should be seen. Second, although it is true that if the double decidual sign is absent at these thresholds, the pregnancy is almost certainly abnormal with a significant possibility of being ectopic, the converse—that it is pointless to perform ultrasonography if the quantitative β-hCG level is lower than 1000 mIU/mL—is not correct. This is because the discriminatory zone does not preclude the possibility of identifying an ectopic pregnancy (or an IUP) before the quantitative β-hCG level reaches 1500 mIU/mL. Ectopic gestational sacs are pathological and therefore do not display β-hCG levels according to nomograms established for normal IUPs, and advanced ectopic pregnancies may have low β-hCG levels. One percent of ectopic pregnancies have a quantitative β-hCG level of less than 10 mIU/mL, and approximately a third of ectopic pregnancies are diagnosed in patients with a quantitative β-hCG level lower than 1000 mIU/mL.[95–98] Even if no definitive diagnosis can be made, the clinician should be aware that pregnant ED patients with pelvic complaints and a β-hCG level of 1000 mIU/mL or lower have a fourfold increased risk for ectopic pregnancy in comparison to those with the same symptoms and a β-hCG level higher than 1000 mIU/mL.[99]

TABLE 68.5 Relationship Between Gestational Age, Qβ-hCG Levels, and Ultrasound Findings

TIME ELAPSED FROM THE FIRST DAY OF THE LAST NORMAL MENSTRUAL PERIOD	Qβ-hCG LEVEL (mIU/mL) USING THE IRP	ULTRASOUND FINDINGS
<28 days	5–50	
4–5 w	50–500	From approx. 4.5 w and Qβ-hCG level of 1000–1500 EVU can show a nonspecific intrauterine sac
5–6 w	100–10,000	Definitely abnormal if no DDS seen on TVU with a Qβ-hCG level >2000 or by TAU with a Qβ-hCG level >6500 Abnormal if no YS with an MSD >10 mm
6–7 w	1000–30,000	FP, cardiac activity 5.5–7 w, Qβ-hCG level >10,000 Abnormal if no FP with an MSD >18 mm
7–8 w	3500–115,000	—
8–14 w	12,000–270,000	—
>10 w	270,000–15,000	—

DDS, Double decidual sac; *EVU*, endovaginal ultrasound; *FP*, fetal pole; *IRP*, international reference preparation; *MSD*, mean sac diameter; *Qβ-hCG*, quantitative β-human chorionic gonadotropin; *TAU*, transabdominal ultrasound; *TVU*, transvaginal ultrasound; *YS*, yolk sac.

In summary, the discriminatory zone provides a basis for interpreting the ultrasound image, but not a basis for deciding whether to perform it.[94,96,100]

Although the percentage of patients below the discriminatory zone who will receive a definitive diagnosis by ultrasound is much lower than the percentage in those above the discriminatory zone (25% vs. 90%), even a 25% diagnosis rate would seem to merit pursuit for a life threatening condition, especially as follow-up for patients whose evaluation is indeterminate on their ED visit is time-consuming and resource-intensive.[96,101]

BLOOD CULTURES IN THE ED

Indications

Blood cultures are indicated when the clinical findings suggest an otherwise unidentifiable bacteremic state (Box 68.2). Twenty-five percent of patients with documented bacteremia have periods without fever.[102] In older patients the proportion is even higher, with 50% of bacteremic patients older than 65 having a temperature between 97.1°F (36.2°C) and 100.9° F (38.3°C) and at least 13% with no documented temperature higher than 99.1°F (37.3°C) at any time.[103–107] In older patients, increasing age, vomiting, altered mental status, urinary incontinence, presence of a Foley catheter, or greater than 6% leukocyte band forms is predictive of a positive blood culture.[104,107] The presence of chills in a febrile patient has a higher likelihood ratio for bacteremia while a subjective report of fever is not predictive of bacteremia.[108] Prediction models to optimize the use of this costly and resource-intensive test have been explored but are cumbersome, add little to educated clinical judgment, and lack widespread validation or acceptance.[109–112] Many studies have shown that blood cultures in patients with uncomplicated pneumonia or pyelonephritis are of very limited clinical value,[113–124] although a prospective investigation of patients with upper UTI found that malignancy, an indwelling urinary catheter, and ongoing antimicrobial treatment were clinical conditions that made it significantly more likely that blood cultures would be discordant with urine cultures and that they would reveal clinically important additional information.[125] Blood cultures are obtained during 2.8% of all ED visits in the United States, and in a single 3-year period this rate increased by 33%.[126] As disease prevalence is unlikely to have changed so rapidly, this increase is probably due to changes in practice. These changes have been coincident with regulatory agency–mandated blood cultures in patients being evaluated for pneumonia and have led to calls for more stringent criteria for obtaining blood cultures. Similarly, the implementation of the Severe Sepsis and Early Septic Shock Management Bundle (SEP-1) by the Centers for Medicare and Medicaid Services in 2015 led to a 76.2% increase in blood cultures ordered for discharged ED patients.[127]

In children, the traditional teaching that blood cultures are indicated for all patients younger than 2 years with fever higher than 38.6°C (>101.5°F) and without an obvious source has been modified by the widespread use of pneumococcal conjugate (PC) and *Haemophilus influenzae* type b (HIB) vaccines.[128,129] In the post-PC and post-HIB vaccine era, the incidence of occult bacteremia in otherwise well-appearing febrile children is probably lower than 1%, thus making the false-positive rate at least four times as high.[128–130] It seems reasonable to withhold blood cultures and empirical antibiotic coverage in otherwise well-appearing febrile children with reliable parents. The risk for bacteremia in a child is positively correlated with the degree of fever, WBC count, and rapidity of onset of the illness. It is inversely proportional to the patient's age.[131–134] In infants younger than 2 months with temperatures higher than 38°C (>100.5°F), some authorities would recommend blood cultures regardless of the presence or absence of a source, although this approach is subject to modification by experienced clinicians based on the patient's age and clinical setting. A child with a normal temperature in the ED and a history from the parents of a tactile fever needs to be approached in the same way as a patient with fever documented on physical examination. Parents' tactile impression of fever is reliable, and bacteremic children, like adults, have intermittent fever, with up to 50% afebrile rates in children with demonstrated bacteremia.[135,136]

BOX 68.2 Summary of Indications for Obtaining Blood Cultures

PATIENTS WITH FEVER AND ANY OF THE FOLLOWING:

- Unexplained alterations in mental status, functional status, or autonomic status in a previously healthy patient between the ages of 5 and 65
- No source found and younger than 2 years, older than 65, or immunocompromised
- Age younger than 2 months

PATIENTS WITH OR WITHOUT FEVER AND ANY OF THE FOLLOWING:

- Rigors
- Toxic or "septic" appearance (e.g., unexplained hypotension, altered mental status, shock)
- Suspicion of infectious endocarditis
- Serious focal infections (e.g., meningitis, septic arthritis, osteomyelitis)

Controversy Regarding Outpatient Blood Cultures

There is a long-standing debate regarding the utility of outpatient blood cultures (i.e., blood cultures on patients who are discharged from the ED pending results). Arguments for and against outpatient blood cultures are summarized in Box 68.3. Opponents cite medicolegal issues, problems with follow-up, high contamination rates, low rates of positive cultures, and even lower rates of frequency in patients in whom therapy is changed because of culture results.[137–140] Proponents also cite medicolegal concerns, positive rates similar to those seen with inpatient blood cultures, cost savings, and the benefit of diagnosing significant, yet subtle bacteremic states (such as endocarditis).[141–143] Patients discharged with occult bacteremia generally have a benign clinical course.[143,144] It should be noted that "occult" may be something of a misnomer in this setting, because some aspect of the patient's clinical state prompted the decision to obtain blood cultures. Proponents of outpatient blood cultures also point out that the high false-positive rates seen in many ED series should be an indictment of poor technique, not of the test itself.

BOX 68.3 Summary of Arguments for and Against the Performance of Outpatient Blood Cultures

ARGUMENTS AGAINST OUTPATIENT BLOOD CULTURES

Low true-positive rates
True positives are rarely clinically significant.
False positives are expensive and time-consuming for both the patient and the health care system.
Unreliability of emergency department follow-up makes positive results a medicolegal liability.

ARGUMENTS FOR OUTPATIENT BLOOD CULTURES

Permits outpatient evaluation and management of patients with a low probability of disease (especially infectious endocarditis).
Patients: financial, psychological, and nosocomial cost savings from spared admissions
Society: financial and nosocomial cost savings from spared admissions
Allows initiation of antibiotics for possible alternative infectious diagnoses without irrevocable loss of the opportunity for blood cultures

Based on current data, it may be costly to admit all patients in whom bacteremia is suspected and injudicious to withhold blood cultures solely on the basis of a patient not appearing "toxic enough" to warrant admission. Societal and economic pressures to avoid hospital admission buttress these clinical considerations. Outpatient blood cultures, with due attention to collection technique, patient selection, and arrangements for follow-up, have a place in emergency practice. This approach is reflected by the fact that fully half of ED blood cultures are obtained from patients who are not admitted to the hospital.[126]

Technique for Obtaining Blood for Culture

False-positive blood cultures obtained in the ED can result in significant costs, with an average increase in hospital length of stay of 1 day per patient.[145] Studies have demonstrated sources of contamination at every stage of the process of performing and processing blood cultures. In addition to obvious sources of contamination from the patient's and phlebotomist's skin, antiseptic agents and gloves have been implicated.[146,147] Some authorities have argued that the primary source of contamination is in the laboratory processing of specimens.[148] The consensus is that the most common source of contamination is the process of phlebotomy and inoculation of blood culture bottles.[145,149] Obviously, this is the single step over which emergency clinicians have control, either directly or via protocols of technique for blood culture phlebotomy. Contamination rates are typically between 1.5% and 3%,[128,150,151] although many ED series show much higher rates.[139,145,152] Conversely, settings in which there are rigorous protocols for obtaining blood cultures have contamination rates as low as 1%.[153]

A high degree of sensitivity is required for blood cultures. Many significant bacteremic illnesses have been documented with as little as 1 CFU/10 mL of blood.[39,154] In a cadaver study, human skin has been shown to have a bacterial concentration of between 10^3 and 10^6 CFUs/mL on the forearm and groin, respectively.[155] Designed to detect vanishingly low concentrations of bacteria, the test is clearly susceptible to false-positive results (impaired specificity) when blood must necessarily be obtained by passing a needle through the skin. Eighty percent of the skin flora is transient, superficial, and removable with cleansing; 20% inhabit the sebaceous ducts and hair follicles and cannot be removed without destroying the skin.[155,156] The former group consists of predominantly gram-positive and gram-negative aerobes and is the target of skin disinfectants.

The primary agents for skin disinfection are iodine compounds, alcohols, chlorhexidine, and hexachlorophene. Iodine solution remains a gold standard and kills bacteria, fungi, protozoa, and viruses but has been replaced in many institutions because of concern about skin burns and allergic reactions. Reports of the former were probably due to the use of 7% solution. The risk for a burn or an allergic reaction is thought to be negligible with the currently available 2% preparation.[149] The most effective cleansing agent is tincture of iodine, which is a mixture of 2% iodine solution and 70% alcohol.[157,158] Povidone-iodine 10% solution has a much lower free-iodine concentration than iodine solution and is therefore less potent. Iodine is superior to hexachlorophene and chlorhexidine in killing gram-negative bacteria. Iodine, like other antiseptic agents, is inhibited by the presence of organic matter and thus requires thorough skin cleansing before the application of any skin disinfectant.

Ethyl or isopropyl alcohol should be used in a 60% to 80% solution. Alcohol prep pads, which generally contain 70% isopropanol, have solved traditional concerns regarding evaporation of alcohol from cotton balls stored in jars. Alcohol is a less powerful germicide than iodine in vitro and kills only 90% of surface bacteria after a full 2 minutes with reapplication to prevent drying.[159] Alcohol foam applicators can avoid premature drying. Alcohol is inactive against fungi, spores, and viruses, but in vivo studies of blood culture contamination rates have shown it to compare favorably with iodine.[157,160] Because iodine solution is often not available and iodophor solutions are less potent, alcohol still has an important place in skin antisepsis. In addition, alcohol is an excellent solvent, so alcohol pads may assist in skin preparation by removing dirt- and microbe-laden skin oils before the application of iodine compounds.

Chlorhexidine and hexachlorophene are antiseptics that are more effective against gram-positive than gram-negative bacteria. Both agents are absorbed intradermally, thereby offering prolonged antimicrobial activity, which is the basis of their popularity as surgical scrub and operative site preparations. This also makes them preferable agents when indwelling lines, especially central lines, are being placed.[161] For routine blood culture phlebotomy, they are not as effective as alcohol and iodine combinations, although they are superior to povidone-iodine solution.[151] Most studies show chlorhexidine to be more potent than hexachlorophene, and it has not been associated with induction of seizures in infants.

The current acceptable blood culture contamination rate is less than 3%. Meta-analyses of skin antiseptics reported contamination rates less than 2% with alcoholic iodine tincture, 2% with alcoholic chlorhexidine, and greater than 3% with aqueous povidone-iodine.[162] Alcohol alone was not inferior to iodinated products, and alcoholic chlorhexidine was superior to skin antiseptics without alcohol.[161,162,165]

Box 68.4 presents a skin preparation protocol. Optimal results seem to be obtained with alcohol-iodine mixtures.[155,158,163,164] The most important concept in skin disinfection is that bacteria are not destroyed at the instant of contact with disinfectant agents. Iodine (2%), which is twice as potent as 10% povidone-iodine, requires at least 90 seconds in contact with the skin to kill 90% of surface bacteria.[159] Alcoholic chlorhexidine needs 15 to 30 seconds to dry; iodine tincture dries in 30 seconds, whereas povidone-iodine needs about 2 minutes.[162,165] In many ED patients it will be necessary to use alcohol prep pads to remove gross dirt and debris from phlebotomy sites before initiating the steps of formal skin preparation.

Dedicated phlebotomy teams and direct venipuncture as opposed to obtaining blood cultures from indwelling IV catheters decreased blood culture contamination rates.[166] Prepackaged blood culture kits and cleaning of blood culture tops had mixed effectiveness on blood culture contamination rates, but cleaning of blood culture tops is common practice.[166,167]

Special Considerations in Obtaining Blood for Culture

Changing the Needle after Phlebotomy

In considering this issue it is important to emphasize the distinction between needle changing and needle recapping.[168] The latter is a well-established risk to health care workers. It contravenes standard recommendations for universal precautions and should not be performed. Needle replacement using the standard needle removal device on sharps containers is an unquantified risk, but clearly much less dangerous than recapping.

BOX 68.4 Skin Preparation and Technique for Drawing Blood for Culture

Cleanse the skin with alcohol swabs three times or until the swabs appear entirely free of surface dirt.

Allow to dry.

Apply 10% povidone-iodine or (preferably) 2% iodine solution or (ideally) 2% tincture of iodine in 70% alcohol three times in centrifugal circles from the anticipated site of venipuncture.

After the third swab, allow to dry for at least 60 seconds. During this period:

- Remove the covers and sterilize the rubber stoppers of blood culture bottles with iodine, alcohol, or both.
- Lay out sterile gloves.
- Use a paper glove wrapper as a sterile field for the needle and syringe (not necessary if using a Vacutainer system).

Wipe off dry iodine at the venipuncture site with alcohol. Substitute chlorhexidine if placing an indwelling catheter.

Obtain at least 20 mL of blood to place in two bottles.

- If short, use at least 10 mL for an aerobic bottle.
- If more than 20 mL, use additional aerobic bottles. Place no more than 10 mL of blood per bottle.

Inoculate bottles without changing needles between bottles.

However many bottles are filled, this is one set of blood cultures. Another set cannot be obtained from this site, regardless of how many bottles are filled.

Based on little scientific data it was long considered essential to change the phlebotomy needle before inoculating blood culture bottles. With increasing awareness of the risks associated with needlestick injuries, this practice has come under scrutiny. A meta-analysis reported contamination rates of 2% with changing needles prior to inoculation of the blood culture bottle compared with 3.7% using the same needle.[169] However other studies generally show trends toward lower contamination rates with needle change without reaching statistical significance.[169–172] In one study, the type of antiseptic, the application of antiseptic solution to the top of collection bottles before inoculation, and the use of a double-needle collection method did not affect contamination rates.[173] Thus not changing needles before inoculation of blood culture bottles is acceptable practice for routinely obtaining blood for culture. In situations in which the results of blood cultures are of paramount importance (e.g., suspected infectious endocarditis, where empirical antibiotics are to be started immediately), needles can be changed before inoculation of culture bottles (without recapping). Alternatively, blood can be drawn directly into the culture vial using modern closed collection systems (a set of culture vials will be the first blood drawn, followed by traditional phlebotomy of various needed tubes via a Vacutainer system).

Special Access Sites

Most studies show that newly placed intravenous (IV) catheters are an acceptable source of blood specimens for culture, provided that the usual measures are taken in skin preparation.[150,172] Chronically placed lines either trend toward or show statistically significant increases in contamination rates.[166,174–176] An exception can be made for carefully tended central venous access ports in cancer patients. These cultures may have increased sensitivity in identifying bacteremia, possibly because the catheters themselves are often a source of bacteremia in these patients.[177]

Heel Stick in Neonates

This technique resulted in recovery rates of bacteria equivalent to those with phlebotomy in two studies.[178,179] As approximately 25% of bacteremic infants have fewer than 5 CFUs/mL of blood, this proportion (25%) will be missed if less than 0.2 mL is obtained for culture. For this reason, heel stick should be considered a source of last resort for blood culture.

Intraosseous Specimens

This technique may also be considered when traditional phlebotomy is not possible (see Chapter 25).[180]

Timing of Blood Cultures

In most circumstances the timing of blood cultures is moot in the ED. Patients are sick enough to warrant the initiation of empirical antibiotics or are well enough for discharge, so two or more sets of blood need to be drawn immediately. The timing of blood cultures might become a consideration in a patient requiring admission but in whom the diagnosis of bacteremia is in doubt such that empirical antibiotic therapy is withheld. Contrary to medical lore, true-positive blood cultures are more likely if blood is drawn in the 12 hours before a fever spike.[149,181] Furthermore, except for infectious endocarditis, most clinically significant bacteremia is thought to be intermittent, so multiple sets of specimens obtained at one time for culture would heighten the risk for missing the period of bacteremia.[182] For patients admitted to the hospital with the tentative diagnosis of sepsis, it is theoretically advantageous to draw the three sets of blood for culture over the first 12 to 24 hours of admission.[183] If immediate administration of antibiotics is indicated, the two or three sets of blood for culture should be obtained before initiation of antibiotic therapy.

Blood Culture Volumes

Volumes in Adults

A large number of studies almost uniformly demonstrate that the sensitivity of blood cultures is directly related to the volume of blood cultured.[184–189] In a representative study, Ilstrup and Washington showed that 20 mL and 30 mL of blood yielded, respectively, 38% and 62% more true-positive results than 10 mL did.[186] Mermel and Maki showed that each additional milliliter of blood yields an average of 3% more true-positive results.[189] This finding is also consistent with the fact that 40% of adults with bacteremia have less than 1 CFU/mL of blood and that 20% have less than 1 CFU/10 mL.[154]Alternatively expressed, if 10 mL of blood is obtained for culture, 20% of patients with continuous bacteremia will be missed. As most bacteremia is intermittent and endogenous factors in blood will cause some inhibition of bacterial growth even with modern lysis and filtration centrifugation techniques, the false-negative rate in clinical practice will always be significantly higher. On purely mathematical grounds, 10 mL per set of blood cultures is a bare minimum for culture. In adults, most authorities recommend at least 30 mL of blood per culture site or set.[190–192] To ensure dilution of the blood's antibacterial properties (e.g., immunoglobulins, complement, WBCs), culture bottles should contain a concentration of blood of less than 1 part blood to 10 parts medium.[192] In addition to improving sensitivity of blood cultures, larger volumes collected decrease blood culture contamination rates in adults and children.[173,193]

Volumes in Children

A blood volume of 30 mL from a 70-kg adult is equivalent to 0.5 mL of blood from a 3.5-kg neonate. Fortunately (for the utility of blood cultures), levels of bacteremia are typically 10-fold higher in neonates than in adults.[194] The sicker the child, the greater the likelihood of a high level of bacteremia.[178,194] As the immune system matures during infancy, levels of bacteremia might be expected to fall toward those seen in adults, so small culture volumes are at increased risk for false-negative results.[195–197] As a rule of thumb, a similar volume of blood with respect to body mass should be drawn from children as is drawn from adults: approximately 1 mL/2.5 kg, or 4 mL blood per 10-kg body mass.[114,198]

How Many Sets of Blood Cultures Are Needed?

A set of blood cultures is the sample obtained from a single site. A 1-mL specimen from a neonate placed in an aerobic bottle and a 30-mL specimen from an adult divided between fungal, aerobic, and anaerobic bottles are both a single set of blood cultures (Fig. 68.5). Two or more sets of blood cultures make up a series.[188] The information derived from the blood culture sets is pooled in such a way to make both the

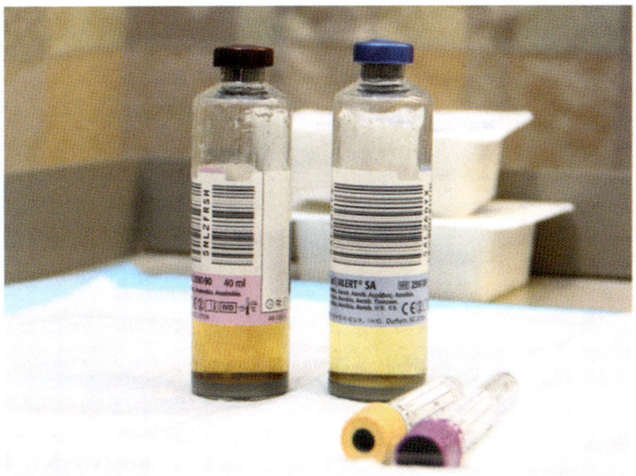

Fig. 68.5 These two blood culture bottles (anaerobic and aerobic) represent a single set of blood cultures, provided that they are filled with a sample from a single site. Two or more sets of blood culture bottles (each obtained from a different site) represent a series of cultures.

sensitivity and specificity of the series greater than that of the component sets. Sensitivity is enhanced because, as discussed earlier, an individual set is typically not more than 80% sensitive.[199] Specificity is improved for microbes that can act as both pathogens and contaminants by determining whether they appear in all sets (pathogen) or in only some (more likely a contaminant).

Although this conceptual process is applied to all blood culture series, the focus of inquiry depends on the infectious process being ruled in or out. For example, in an older patient with sepsis and a chronic indwelling Foley catheter, it is extremely unlikely that the causative organism is a typical skin contaminant. The usual causes of false-positive blood cultures will therefore be easily recognized, thus lowering the false-positive rate for the series and yielding a test with intrinsically higher specificity. At the same time, with the typical pathogens in this clinical context being nonfastidious organisms, sensitivity is typically at approximately 99% with two sets consisting of 20 mL of blood per set.[191] Conversely, in a patient with a prosthetic heart valve, fever, and signs of septic emboli, many probable pathogens are also skin contaminants, thereby lowering the specificity of each individual blood culture set. Thus at least two sets of cultures must be positive with such organisms before the overall test (i.e., the series) is considered positive. At the same time, this clinical picture makes the pretest probability of disease very high (diminishing the negative predictive value of a negative set), so an extremely sensitive overall test (i.e., series) will be needed to adequately rule out disease. In this setting, most authorities would recommend four sets of blood culture bottles, with good volumes in each. [182,199] Except in infants, single sets of blood for culture are of insufficient sensitivity or specificity to be of any utility and should not be drawn.[149,182,199–202] The recommended numbers of sets of blood cultures as they relate to the pretest probability of disease and causative organism are summarized in Table 68.6.

Aerobic Versus Anaerobic Versus Other Bottles

Anaerobic infections tend to occur in poorly perfused tissues or locations and frequently evolve into abscesses. Both

TABLE 68.6 Numbers of Blood Culture Sets to Be Obtained in Various Clinical Situations in Adults

NUMBER OF SETS (MINIMUM)	CLINICAL CONTEXT
Two sets	A true positive is likely to be easily distinguished from contaminants and pretest probability of bacteremia is low to moderate.
Three sets	Skin contaminants are possible causes of the infectious process, the pretest probability of bacteremia is high, or infectious endocarditis is a consideration, but with a low to moderate pretest probability.
Four sets	Infectious endocarditis AND either a moderate to a high pretest probability or the patient has recently been taking antibiotics.

TABLE 68.7 Blood Culture Types to Be Used in Various Clinical Settings

CLINICAL SITUATION	BOTTLES TO BE OBTAINED
Children <12 y	Aerobic bottles only unless the patient has peritonitis or fasciitis (in which case draw blood for standard aerobic and anaerobic culture).
Adults and children >12 y	Anaerobic infection unlikely, immunocompetent patient: aerobic bottles only. Anaerobic infection unlikely, immunocompromised patient: aerobic bottle, one bottle for fungal culture (usually effective in aerobic bottles; consult the laboratory for guidance). Possibility of anaerobic infection: one aerobic and one anaerobic bottle per set.

characteristics mean that these infections tend to be isolated or separated from the bloodstream, thereby decreasing the likelihood of bacteremia and detection by blood culture. For these reasons it is not surprising that anaerobic isolates account for 0.5% to 12% of positive blood cultures.[182,203–205] Blood cultures in general have a typical true-positive rate of approximately 5%; with 5% or less of positive blood cultures being anaerobic, more than 400 patients need to have a complete series of blood drawn for culture to detect one case of anaerobic bacteremia.[206–210] If more than 50% of anaerobic infections are clinically evident before culture, at least 800 blood culture series are needed to generate a single anaerobic result that would alter clinical management. Anaerobic cultures may also have the unintended consequence of compromising the sensitivity of aerobic cultures in situations in which less than the ideal 20 mL of blood is drawn for a blood culture set.[189,205] Allocation of blood to anaerobic bottles will also diminish the likelihood of detecting fungal infections, which are increasingly common in the rising population of immunocompromised patients.[211] In addition to these pathophysiologic considerations, there was a widely reported decrease in the positive anaerobic blood culture rate in the 1980s and 1990s, although some authors have recently suggested a resurgence of anaerobic bacteremia rates.[203–205,207,209,212] A review from the Mayo Clinic showed a 74% increase of anaerobic blood cultures from 1993 to 2004.[210] Based on a review of this topic, Table 68.7 suggests a possible approach to the allocation of blood specimens to various blood culture media after phlebotomy.[211–213] Clinical features that place a patient at high risk for anaerobic bacteremia are listed in Box 68.5.

BOX 68.5 Clinical Settings at Higher Risk for Anaerobic Bacteremia

INFECTIOUS FOCI

Abdominal or pelvic infections
Soft tissue or wound infections (e.g., myofasciitis)
Sepsis with decubitus ulcers or necrotic tissue
Aspiration pneumonia
Odontogenic head and neck infections

PREDISPOSING CLINICAL FEATURES

Malignancy
Immunosuppressive medications
Recent abdominal or pelvic surgery
Diabetes

Identifying Contaminants

The emergency clinician may receive calls from the laboratory about the results of positive blood cultures obtained on previous shifts. These may be true positives, a result of contamination or may be caused by the intermittent bacteremia that occurs in normal, healthy people. This situation has been complicated by the increasingly common identification of *Staphylococcus epidermidis*, *Streptococcus viridans*, and fungi as real pathogens in blood culture series.[177,214–216] The expense associated with false-positive blood cultures has been noted earlier. These costs emphasize the importance of good technique in obtaining blood for culture.[217,218] Distinguishing contaminants from clinically significant bacteremia is based on both microbiologic information and the patient's clinical condition. Features of false-positive blood culture results are listed in Box 68.6.[191,199,219] It is prudent to contact discharged patients with positive blood cultures, even when contamination is suspected on a microbiologic basis, to ensure that their condition is improving.

Fungal Cultures

Generally, fungi are difficult to isolate in blood cultures, and it may take 4 to 6 weeks to obtain a positive yield. If fungemia is suspected, it is best to discuss culture media and technique with the laboratory before blood is taken for culture. Cultures of bone marrow are occasionally positive for mycoses when blood cultures are negative.

BOX 68.6 Features Suggestive of Contaminant (False-Positive) Blood Culture Results

Coagulase-negative staphylococci (*Staphylococcus epidermidis*) and *Staphylococcus viridans* in a single bottle in patients not suspected of having infectious endocarditis and without chronic indwelling intravenous access catheters are usually contaminants.

Corynebacteria (previously known as *diphtheroids*), *Bacillus* species (except *Bacillus anthracis*), *Micrococcus* species, and as *Propionibacterium acnes*, *Cutibacterium acnes* and related species are usually contaminants but can be pathogenic in the immunocompromised.

Multiple organisms in a series suggest contamination.

Species that grow after prolonged culture have a higher likelihood of being contaminants. Conversely, early growing bacteria have a much higher likelihood of being pathogens.

The patient's symptoms have resolved or are inconsistent with sepsis (beware with infectious endocarditis, which can have an indolent course).

A primary source (e.g., sputum or urine) has a different pathogen isolated.

TABLE 68.8 Artifactual Causes of False Values of the CBC[a]

	ARTIFACTUAL INCREASE	ARTIFACTUAL DECREASE
White blood cell count	Nucleated red blood cells	Multiple myeloma and other monoclonal gammopathies
Hemoglobin and hematocrit	Severe leukocytosis (>30,000), hyperlipemic serum, giant platelets, cryoproteins	In vitro hemolysis Microcytic anemia will demonstrate true low values despite normal RBC count

[a]Improper collection techniques are the most common cause of errors in all categories.

CBC, Complete blood count; *RBC*, red blood cell.

Polymerase Chain Reaction

Polymerase chain reaction (PCR) is the latest technology leading to rapid diagnosis of bloodborne pathogens. PCR amplifies target nucleic acid in blood using repeated cycles of DNA synthesis. PCR allows detection and quantification of organisms whose genetic material is DNA or messenger RNA. PCR permits the diagnosis of infectious disease with a high degree of sensitivity and specificity and allows rapid reliable detection of microbes present in small numbers. Some laboratories now routinely apply PCR technology to test blood for the presence of common pathogen (bacterial, viral, and fungal) DNA and can yield results (including specific species) within hours.

PRINCIPLES AND PITFALLS IN PHLEBOTOMY FOR BLOOD TESTING

Several blood tests are ordered as a part of emergency practice, but by far the most common are the complete blood count (CBC) and serum chemistries. Many medications, substances, and diseases have been identified as causes of hematologic abnormalities besides the familiar categories of infectious, inflammatory, stress-related, neoplastic, and hematopoietic processes. These include antibiotics (especially sulfonamides), antineoplastic and therapeutic drugs, immunosuppressives, and toxins (mercury and black widow spider envenomation causing leukocytosis and arsenicals causing leukopenia). There are also substances and disease processes that cause purely artifactual errors by interfering with the equipment or procedures used to perform the tests. Examples include in vivo and in vitro hemolysis, cellular clumping, and markedly elevated platelet, leukocyte, or triglyceride levels, all of which can perturb proper functioning of the machinery used to perform blood assays. The less common causes of laboratory abnormalities (both pathophysiologic and artifactual) are numerous. It is necessary for most clinicians, when encountering a confirmed laboratory abnormality, to resort to standard reference texts or online sources to review potential causes or sources of error. Some of the analytical causes of false laboratory values on the CBC are listed in Table 68.8.

Blood samples are collected or filled (if using a syringe) into various colored-top tubes with different additives depending on the test required. The color schemes vary across manufacturers and sites despite calls for uniformity.[220] To decrease cross-contamination from tube additives, some have advocated an order in tube collection: blood culture, sodium citrate (light blue or blue), nonadditive (red), serum separation tube (SST—red/gray or gold), lithium/sodium heparin (light green or green), K_2EDTA (lavender), acid-citrate-dextrose (ACD) (yellow), K oxalate or Na fluoride (gray) (Fig. 68.6).[221] Recent studies found that using closed collection systems (Vacutainer system) decreased cross-contamination rather than the order of tube collection or open collection systems (needle and syringe).[222]

Before checking for obscure or uncommon causes of laboratory abnormalities, one should bear in mind that the most common source of error in laboratory blood tests is in the preanalytical phase.[223–226] This is the part of the laboratory process that actively involves the practicing clinician. Preanalytical errors have been broken down into problems with specimen loss and handling, clotting, hemolysis, inadequate volume, and patient identity.[225] In one series, more than 90% of these errors related to specimen collection.[80,227] These key components and their most common pitfalls are as follows:

1. Preparation of the site. The importance of aseptic technique in the preparation of a site to draw blood for culture has been discussed. For hematologic and serum analysis, enough time should be allowed for drying of the alcohol because trace amounts can cause hemolysis. Povidone-iodine can cause errors in several chemistry assays. When used, it should be cleaned off with alcohol, as described in the section "Technique for Obtaining Blood for Culture".
2. Venous occlusion. Both intracellular and chemical changes start occurring in blood as soon as a tourniquet is applied, not, as is often thought, only after it has passed through a needle into a specimen container. Serum potassium levels may increase by 6% in a vessel that has been occluded for only 3 minutes.[226] Venous access sites, if visually

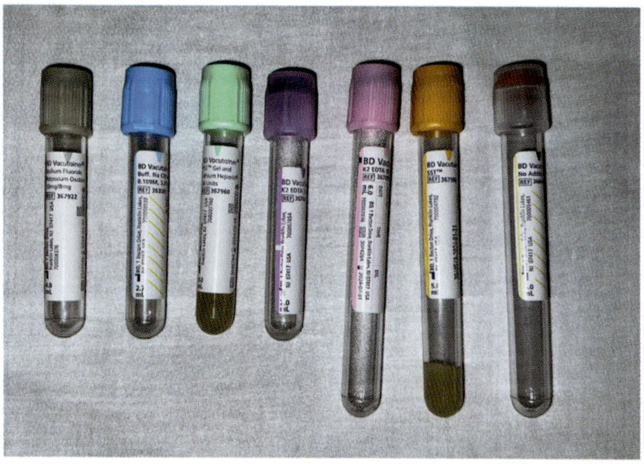

Fig. 68.6 Blood collection tubes and additives. Gray (K oxalate or Na fluoride); light blue or blue (sodium citrate); light green or green (lithium/sodium heparin); lavender (K_2EDTA); pink (K_2EDTA); gold or red/gray (serum separation tube [SST]); red (nonadditive).

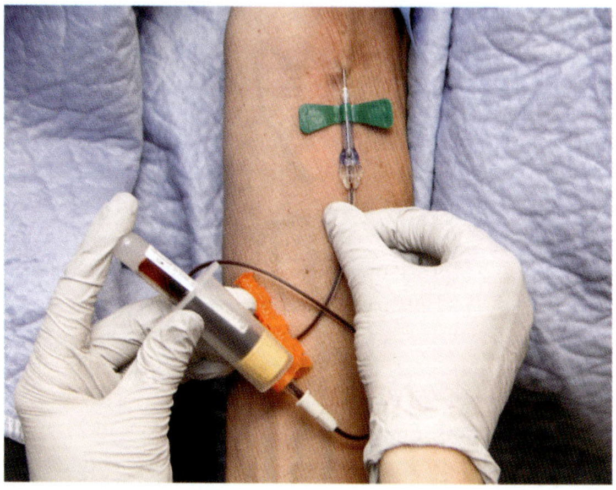

Fig. 68.7 Phlebotomy using a butterfly needle and Vacutainer system.

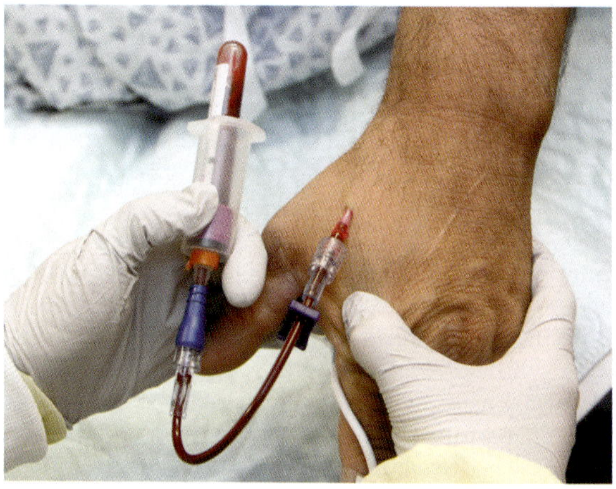

Fig. 68.8 Phlebotomy via a freshly placed intravenous catheter and Vacutainer system.

identifiable, should be prepared before placement of a tourniquet. After tourniquet application, phlebotomy and sample acquisition should proceed as rapidly as possible, ideally within 30 seconds.[228] Clenching the fist should be avoided if possible because it increases serum concentrations of calcium, chloride, creatinine kinase, lactate, magnesium, phosphate, potassium, and sodium.[226,229]

3. Routine phlebotomy. Smaller-gauge needles and higher suction pressure are associated with hemolysis.[225] Overexuberant application of suction on a syringe is doubly counterproductive because in addition to causing hemolysis, the needle is likely to be occluded by the wall of the vein. This increases the likelihood of unsuccessful phlebotomy and iatrogenic injury to the patient. When applying negative or positive pressure to a syringe, a given amount of force on the plunger causes higher pressure within the chamber of a smaller-diameter syringe (pressure is proportional to 1/radius^2). Blood drawn into either a standard Vacutainer or a syringe via a butterfly needle and tubing causes similar hemolysis rates (Fig. 68.7).[228] Consistent with experience, the perception of difficult access or phlebotomy is associated with higher hemolysis rates.[230,231]
4. Phlebotomy through a freshly placed IV catheter. The American Society of Clinical Pathology best practice benchmark for hemolysis is 2% or less.[232] Routine phlebotomy typically causes a hemolysis rate of less than 2%.[225] Reported hemolysis rates in ED patients range from 7% to 15%.[231,233–235] This may be due to any or all of the reasons considered here, but one contributing factor is the number of blood specimens drawn in the ED through a catheter being placed for therapeutic use (Fig. 68.8). Several studies have shown that this arrangement significantly increases rates of hemolysis.[231,234,236] The popularity of this technique in emergency care is most probably due to limitations of personnel and temporal resources, ease of access, and enhancement of patient comfort by avoiding an extra needlestick. As tourniquet times are probably longer with catheter placement than with simple phlebotomy, it is likely that this contributes to hemolysis, although it has never been experimentally verified. Perceived ease of blood aspiration, larger-bore catheters, and small aliquots drawn through the catheter are associated with lower rates of hemolysis.[234,236] Laboratory results of specimens obtained in this manner are accurate within clinically acceptable margins of error except for lower mean values for platelets and bicarbonate and higher mean values for chloride for IV compared to venipuncture specimens.[232]
5. Phlebotomy through an established IV catheter. An established IV line appears to be a reliable source of blood for analysis, although success rates are lower and hemolysis rates are higher than for phlebotomy from a fresh site.[237,238] Box 68.7 lists common blood tests that are accurate when drawn through an established IV line.[238,239] As with the use of a freshly placed catheter, results are accurate within clinical tolerances except for platelets, bicarbonate, and chloride.[232,237,240] If fluids are being administered through the catheter, it should be turned off for at least 3 minutes before the application of a tourniquet for phlebotomy. Several methods are described each with advantages and disadvantages. Discard method: (the IV catheter can be initially flushed or not) withdraw a discard sample that is at least three times the volume of the IV catheter volume. If using a syringe, change to a fresh syringe to obtain the sample(s) for lab analysis. If using a Vacutainer system, the initial tube of blood withdrawn is the discard sample, and subsequent tubes will be used for laboratory analysis. This method is more commonly described in the literature but runs the risk of anemia with repeated use. The following

BOX 68.7 Accurate Values Using Venous Blood Obtained From an Indwelling Intravenous Catheter or Saline Lock

CBC	Serum Chemistry	Other
Hemoglobin	Sodium	Creatine phosphokinase
Hematocrit	Potassium	Troponin I
	Bicarbonate	
	Chloride	
	Glucose	

CBC, Complete blood count.

methods decrease the risk of anemia but have other disadvantages. Reinfusion method: similar to the discard method but reinfuses the discard sample back into the catheter which can introduce clots into the patient. Push pull or mixing method: Withdraw up to 6 mL of blood with a syringe, then push the blood back into the catheter, and this cycle is repeated several times. A fresh syringe is then used to obtain the sample for laboratory analysis. There is an increased risk of hemolysis with this method.[241,242] Use of the standard distal port of the IV tubing (usually 25 cm from the end) is not recommended. The IV tubing has a volume (combined with the heparin well and catheter) of approximately 1.6 mL, thus making it necessary to discard large volumes of blood, in addition to the risk of contamination from IV fluids entrained in the specimen from the main IV line during aspiration through the port.

6. Disposition of the specimen after phlebotomy. If blood has been drawn into a syringe, it should be promptly decanted into the appropriate tubes for the laboratory although this step is not necessary when using a Vacutainer system. If it has already started to clot, it should not be forced because this can cause hemolysis of the specimen. As cells and platelets are fragile, specimens requiring agitation (all except red and speckled, red-topped tubes) should be rocked gently, not shaken. If specimens are sent to the laboratory in pneumatic tubes, they should be surrounded by shock-absorbing material. Progressive hemolysis of blood occurs with prolonged standing, and it is likely that specimens are of little utility after more than 2 to 3 hours of typical ED storage conditions.

BEDSIDE TESTS FOR GASTROINTESTINAL HEMORRHAGE

Detection of Blood in Stool (Fecal Occult Blood Testing)

Bedside guaiac-based fecal blood tests make use of the peroxidase-like activity of heme in hemoglobin or free heme. The test card is impregnated with guaiac that exhibits a blue color reaction when oxidized. The developer contains 5% hydrogen peroxide and 75% alcohol to act as an oxygen donor. Oxidants such as the peroxidases of heme will turn the guaiac card blue.[243] A positive test should be considered evidence of the presence of blood until proven otherwise.

Testing for occult blood in stool is associated with false-positive and false-negative results, but in its primary role in emergency medical practice, the test is usually reliable in detecting significant acute gastrointestinal (GI) hemorrhage (Fig. 68.9).[40] Low pH, heat, dry stools, reducing substances (including antioxidants such as vitamin C), and antacids can cause false-negative findings.[244–246]

Slow bleeding in the upper GI tract with prolonged transit through the gut results in heme being converted (denatured) to porphyrin may not be identified by fecal occult blood guaiac testing because porphyrin lacks peroxidases. False-positive results have been attributed to the ingestion of large quantities of meat (dietary sources of myoglobin and hemoglobin) and peroxidase-rich food.[246,247] However a systematic review of case series of challenge diets only showed false positives with large meat consumption while diets with peroxidase-rich fruits and vegetables did not have any increase of false positives.[248] Most vegetables and some fruits contain peroxidase, including (in decreasing order) broccoli, turnips, cantaloupe, red radishes, horseradish, cauliflower, parsnips, Jerusalem artichokes, bean sprouts, beans, lemon rind, mushrooms, parsley, and zucchini.[217,247] A simple in vivo study convincingly called into question the possibility of peroxidase passing through the stomach without being denatured.[218,249] False-positive tests resulting from exposure to povidone-iodine were reported in the 1970s and 1980s, but this substance is not usually a potential contaminant in a rectal examination.[219] If in doubt, the practitioner should determine the effects of povidone-iodine on the product used in their institution prior to performing the test on the patient's stool. Oral iron medications and bismuth in some antacids and antidiarrheal medications can cause dark or black stools but do not turn fecal occult blood guaiac tests blue.[243,250–252]

Normal GI blood loss is limited to less than 2.5 mL/day, which translates to less than 2 mg of hemoglobin per gram of stool (0.2% by weight).[253] The sensitivity of the Hemoccult test varies both with the concentration of hemoglobin present in stool and with the extent of hemoglobin exposure to the proteolytic effects of the digestive tract. A meta-analysis of guaiac fecal occult blood tests showed a sensitivity of 58% and specificity of 83% for diagnosing iron deficiency anemia.[254] The test is much more likely to detect lower GI hemorrhage than an identical rate of upper GI bleeding because of the 100-fold diminution in the peroxidase activity of blood during transition through the GI tract.[243] Impaired detection of hemoglobin may also occur as a result of dilution because of diarrheal illness.[38,40,255] Regulatory attempts in the United States to improve quality control in bedside occult blood testing seem to have had the unintended consequence of discouraging digital rectal examination in patients for whom they are indicated.[256,257] In the event of a trace positive Hemoccult test that is not the source of an emergency illness, notification to the patient and advice regarding further outpatient evaluation should not be overlooked.[245]

Method

Smear the stool specimen onto the reagent area on the card and add a drop of developer. Because the reaction must occur in an aqueous medium, add a drop of water to very dry specimens and allow it to moisten the specimen before adding the developer. Adding water increases the false-positive rate.[245,246] Formation of a blue color on the paper anywhere around or under the specimen within 60 seconds should be considered a positive result.

Testing for Gastric Blood

Heme tests designed for use on stool specimens can be unreliable when applied to gastric juices, with increasing inaccuracies

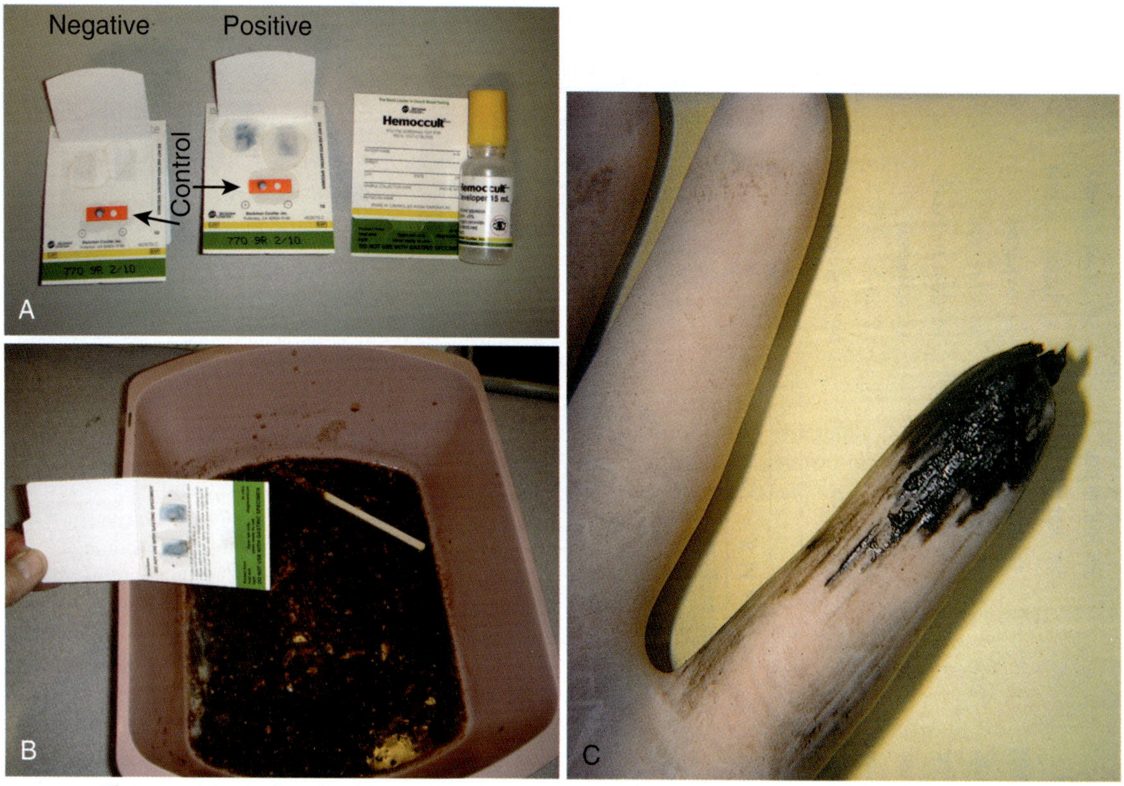

Fig. 68.9 (A) Hemoccult testing (see text). Two areas of stool can be tested. Add a drop of water to dry specimens. The positive and negative control areas *(arrows)* demonstrate that the test is working properly. Color change should occur on the paper under the stool sample. Brand instructions should be followed regarding time allowed before calling a negative test (positive results usually occur rapidly). Any blue color is a positive test. (B) Although Hemoccult may also detect gastric blood, the Gastroccult card/developer performs better on gastric specimens (see text). (C) Iron- and bismuth-containing products (such as Pepto-Bismol or Kaopectate) cause a black stool but not a reaction on the Hemoccult test. Do not attribute a positive test for blood in stool to iron therapy.

being reported as the pH decreases.[258,259] Although a positive test of gastric contents with a fecal Hemoccult card is likely to be accurate, a negative result with the fecal Hemoccult card does not rule out the presence of blood. The Gastroccult card uses a modified guaiac developer containing buffers to neutralize gastric acid, thereby facilitating accurate detection of hemoglobin. The test works on the same basis as the fecal guaiac test in that it uses the properties of hemoglobin as a peroxidase. In product testing, the Gastroccult card was 100% sensitive in detecting specimens with greater than 500 ppm of blood by volume, equivalent to 0.05% or 0.25 mL of blood in 500 mL of gastric contents.

Method

Apply a drop of gastric aspirate onto the test area and two drops of developer onto the sample. Look for the formation of a blue color within 1 minute. Do not use fecal blood test developer. In a specimen that is already a bilious green, the test is considered positive only if new blue color is formed. The Gastroccult card also contains a pH testing strip located close to the occult blood testing area, which might be useful in testing emesis after an acidic or alkaline ingestion. Inaccurate results might be anticipated in the presence of the same substances that can confound the Hemoccult test: meats, peroxidase-rich foods, and reducing substances such as ascorbic acid. The accuracy of Gastroccult should not be affected by the presence of cimetidine or sucralfate.[259]

BLOOD GLUCOSE METERS

Bedside testing of capillary blood for glucose levels is a common procedure performed in the ED and is generally an excellent substitute for venous blood testing. The US FDA recommends glucometer result accuracy in terms of accurate, more accurate, and most accurate as ±15% of laboratory result, ±10% of laboratory result, ±5% of laboratory result respectively.[260] A variety of meters are available and they are reasonably accurate (±10%) when a small drop of blood is electronically analyzed. Glucometers utilize glucose oxidase or glucose dehydrogenase enzymatic reactions to produce an electrochemical reaction in test strips when a small drop of blood is electronically analyzed (Fig. 68.10).[260,261] Factors affecting glucometer accuracy include temperature, humidity, oxygen, very low hematocrit, and interfering substances. Test strips exposed to high temperatures can give higher glucose levels. If exposed to humidity, test strips produce higher or lower readings depending on the brand.[262] Glucose oxidase meters are more affected by oxygen, with high oxygen (arterial blood sample, oxygen therapy) giving lower readings and low oxygen (severe chronic obstructive pulmonary disease [COPD], venous blood sample) giving higher readings.[262] Both glucose oxidase and glucose dehydrogenase meters can have inaccurate readings in critically ill patients with hypotension and poor perfusion due to increased glucose tissue extraction leading to lower glucose readings (Table 68.9).[263,264]

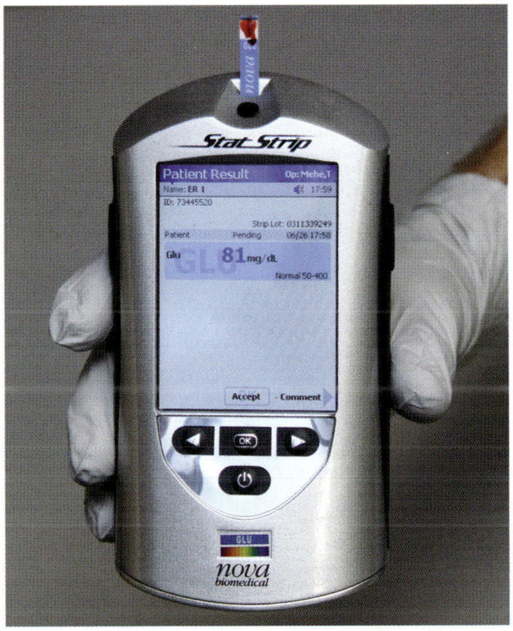

Fig. 68.10 Bedside glucose meters analyze capillary blood samples and are generally an excellent substitute for venous blood testing. Errors may occur in patients with poor tissue perfusion or in cases of extreme hypoglycemia or hyperglycemia. Additional errors may be due to the operator, including improper calibration, dirty meters, and improper storage of test strips.

Very low hematocrit can give falsely higher glucose levels.[262] Bedside testing is also less accurate in patients with extreme hypoglycemia or hyperglycemia, but readings are sufficiently accurate to alert the clinician to very high or very low glucose levels.[265]

In patients with poor tissue perfusion, the accuracy of determining hypoglycemia is less precise and may vary up to approximately 5% from venous blood. In the setting of hypoperfusion, bedside measurement of whole blood is preferable.

Most errors in bedside glucose testing are, however, due to operator error, including improper calibration, dirty meters, and improperly stored test strips. Meters should be calibrated frequently to ensure quality readings. Glucose strips have batch-to-batch variation. A common error in testing is due to leaving the lid off glucose strips for prolonged periods because inaccuracies on test strips can result from exposure to heat, moisture, and humidity.

Continuous glucose monitors are increasingly used in the outpatient and inpatient settings. Currently, inpatient use is primarily in the intensive care unit (ICU) but may extend to the ED in the future.[266]

OTHER POINT-OF-CARE TESTS

With new technology, there are now whole blood point-of-care tests (POCTs) systems which can provide rapid results on traditional laboratories and infectious disease POCTs available in the ED. Two such systems, i-STAT (Abbott Point of Care) and GEM Premier ChemSTAT, provide quantitative results on blood gas values (pH, pCO_2, pO_2, HCO_3, TCO_2, base excess, oxygen saturation), metabolic panel (sodium, potassium, chloride, glucose, BUN, creatinine, ionized calcium), lactate, hemoglobin, hematocrit, troponin I, brain natriuretic peptide (BNP), prothrombin time (PT), international normalized ratio (INR), and quantitative β-hCG

TABLE 68.9 Factors Affecting Blood Glucose Meters

	EFFECT ON GLUCOSE METER READINGS
High temperature	Increase
Humidity	Variable change depending on brand of test strip
High oxygen (arterial blood, oxygen therapy)	Decrease
Low oxygen (venous blood, severe COPD)	Increase
Low hematocrit	Increase
Hypotension	Decrease
Bilirubin	Decrease
Monoclonal gammopathies	Decrease
Triglycerides	Decrease glucose readings
Uric acid	Decrease glucose readings
Medications	
Acetaminophen	Variable change
Ascorbic acid	Variable change
Dopamine	Increase
Icodextrin (peritoneal dialysate)	Increase
L-dopa	Variable change
Mannitol	Increase

COPD, Chronic obstructive pulmonary disease.

(Fig. 68.11).[267–269] Rapid availability of these results can decrease the time to interventions for patients.[269,270]

Infectious disease POCTs include rapid streptococcal, influenza, respiratory syncytial virus (RSV), respiratory, and COVID-19 tests. In children, rapid antigen strep tests had pooled sensitivity of 85.6% and specificity of 95.4%.[271] In adults, sensitivities were 86% and 91% and specificities were 97% and 91% for enzyme immunoassay and immunochromatographic methods, respectively.[272] Newer POCTs are molecular assays using a variety of nucleic acid amplification tests with greater sensitivity and specificity compared to traditional rapid antigen tests.[273,274]

Rapid viral testing has expanded from influenza to RSV and respiratory multi-pathogen panel tests. Rapid antigen tests for influenza and RSV have poor sensitivities ranging from 50% to 70%.[273] Second generation antigen and molecular based tests have much improved sensitivities and specificities.[274] A meta-analysis found decreased chest radiography rates, a non-significant trend to lower antibiotic usage, but no change in ED length of stay, blood or urine testing.[275]

The gold standard for diagnosis of COVID-19 are nucleic acid amplification tests (NAATs) such as real-time reverse transcription polymerase chain reaction (real-time RT-PCR) but are time-consuming, and rapid antigen tests, while faster,

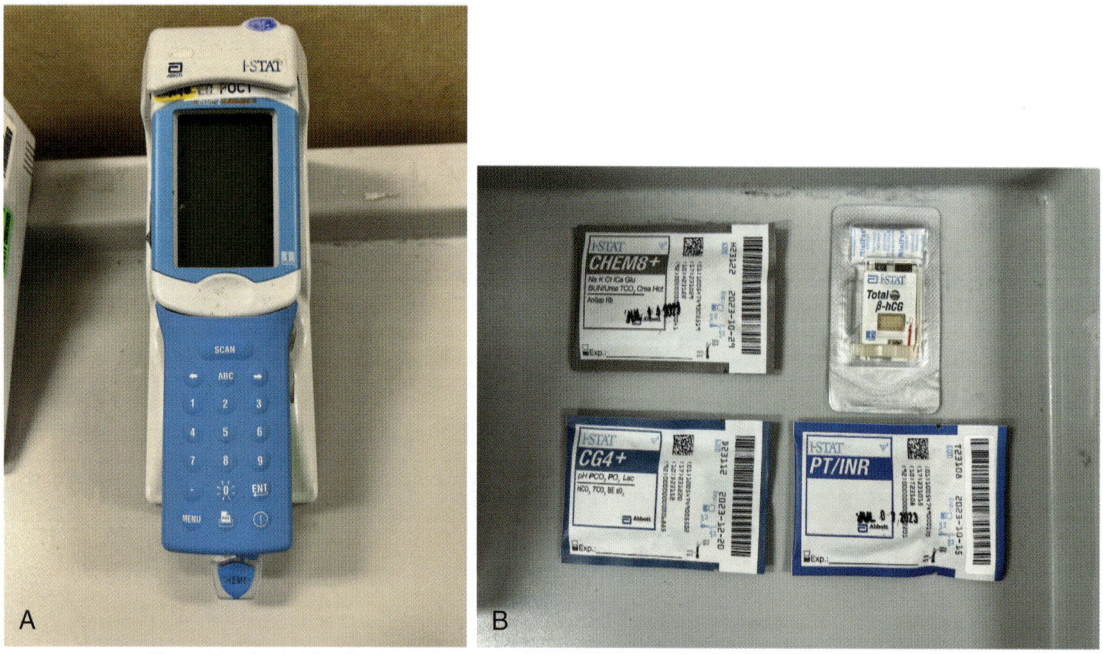

Fig. 68.11 (A) i-STAT point-of-care machine. (B) Various cartridges for i-STAT device.

have lower sensitivities. Several POCTs such as the Cobas Liat and Cepheid GeneXpert systems utilizing rapid RT-PCR were developed and have excellent test concordance with laboratory RT-PCR tests but other systems like the Abbott ID Now COVID-19 had poorer concordance.[276–278]

DIAGNOSTIC AND THERAPEUTIC TOXICOLOGIC BEDSIDE PROCEDURES

Diagnosis and management of the potentially poisoned patient can pose unique challenges. Often nominal history is available, and the information provided, such as the dose of toxin ingested or timeline of exposure, can be inaccurate. Clinicians must rely heavily on physical examination and other sources of information to diagnose or confirm their clinical suspicion of poisoning or overdose. The hospital-based toxicology laboratory can be valuable in select cases. Determining concentrations of specific xenobiotics (e.g., acetaminophen, lithium, digoxin, phenytoin) is useful in guiding management when a particular substance is suspected to be the source of toxicity. However, hospital-based laboratories are not equipped to perform timely analytical procedures for the thousands of possible toxins available. Furthermore, screening panels for drugs of abuse have a significant false positive and false negative rate, making the results of limited value in managing adult patients in the ED. Use of these toxicology screens in selected pediatric patients may have more of an impact on medical management in the correct clinical context. For example, a positive urine cannabinoid screen in a child who presents with altered mental status after exposure to a cannabis containing product, may help avoid subsequent invasive diagnostic procedures.

Certain diagnostic bedside tests (POCTs) for specific toxins have the advantage of being cost-effective and timely. When applied appropriately, certain bedside tests provide immediate information to the clinician and can influence medical management in a timely manner. Of note, bedside laboratory testing underwent stricter oversight after the establishment of the Clinical Laboratory Improvement Amendments of 1988 (CLIA). This federal regulation has jurisdiction on any laboratory tests performed on humans, or specimens obtained from humans, and has added a layer of complexity to bedside testing. Tests that are not performed on humans, such as the Meixner test or mothball testing, are not covered by the CLIA act. This section discusses bedside diagnostic and therapeutic toxicologic procedures.

Noninvasive Diagnostic Procedures

Amatoxin: Meixner Test

Cyclopeptide containing mushrooms are responsible for the most mushroom-related fatalities worldwide.[279] *Amanita phalloides* contains 15 to 20 cyclopeptides, the most toxic of which are amatoxins. Patients exhibiting toxicity from amatoxin containing mushrooms typically present with delayed gastrointestinal symptoms consisting of nausea, vomiting, diarrhea, and abdominal cramping beginning 6 to 8 hours after ingestion. They may bring in specimens of the mushrooms chopped, crushed, cooked, or mixed with stool or gastric contents. Furthermore, identification of poisonous mushrooms is challenging even for experienced mycologists.[279] Mushroom identification software on smart-phone applications have been found to be unreliable in properly identifying poisonous mushroom species.[280] Standard hospital laboratories cannot confirm or exclude the diagnosis of amatoxin poisoning. Thus treatment decisions are usually based on clinical grounds.

A colorimetric test for detecting amatoxins called the Meixner test can be used on gastric contents, stool, or actual mushroom samples. The basis of this test is the acid-catalyzed color reaction of amatoxins with lignin, a complex organic compound found in wood pulp (Fig. 68.12). Cheaper, old grades of paper (e.g., old newsprint or the whiter pages of a telephone book) contain high amounts of lignin. Although there have been no extensive reports of in vivo studies, in vitro tests have shown this method to be somewhat sensitive but

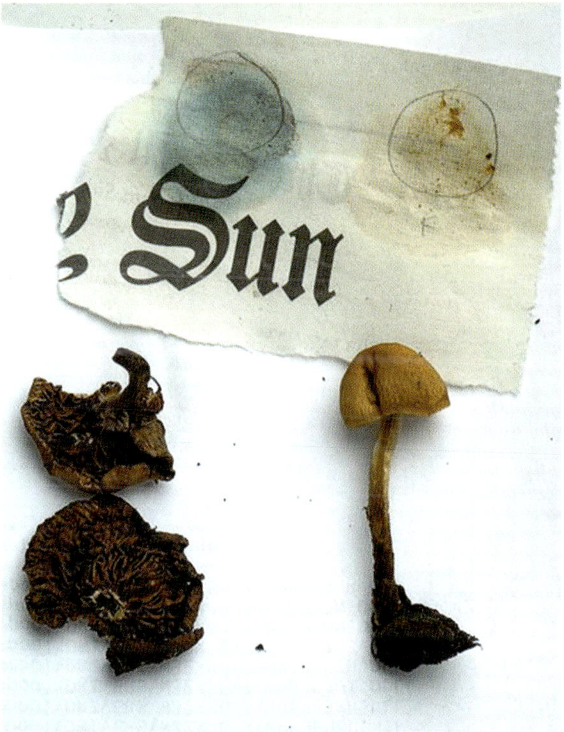

Fig. 68.12 The Meixner test is a crude assay for amatoxins. Place portions of the unknown dried mushroom on low-grade newsprint and add 10-N hydrochloric acid. The dried-up mushroom (*left*) is *Galerina marginata*, which yields a blue reaction (positive, probably deadly poisonous); the little brown mushroom (*right*) does not (negative, toxicity uncertain). This test is the only one readily available but has varying accuracy and depends on the paper being used (regular newsprint is shown here). (Courtesy Kathie T. Hodge and Kent Loeffler [photographer], Cornell University. Available at ht tp://blog.mycology.cornell.edu.)

not relatively specific for amatoxins. Thus it should be considered an adjunctive test only. Psilocybin-containing mushrooms can cause false-positive results for amatoxin given their similar structures.[281] A positive test result always requires further verification of mushroom identity. Furthermore, the test must be performed with older types of paper, which may not be readily available in modern clinical settings thus limiting the utility of this test.

The procedure for the qualitative detection of amatoxin consists of squeezing a drop of liquid from a fresh mushroom sample or squashing a piece of fresh mushroom onto a piece of newspaper. If stool or gastric samples are the only specimens available, mix the sample with reagent-grade methanol (99.8%) to extract the amatoxin. If the samples are mixed with methanol, centrifuge and filter them. Then place a drop of the liquid extract on newspaper. Gently air-dry all specimens at room temperature and avoid direct sunlight. Add two to three drops of concentrated hydrochloric acid (37%) to the dried specimen. Use an adjacent area for control. High amounts of amatoxin in the dried samples produce a blue color in 1 to 2 minutes. Small amounts of amatoxin yield a blue color in the sampled area in 10 to 20 minutes. This procedure has not been proven to be effective with other bodily secretions, such as blood or urine.[281] A lateral flow immunoassay POCT for amatoxin is now commercially available and inexpensive. It can be performed with the patient's urine, or a small fragment of the mushroom suspended in saline.[279,282]

Mothball Identification

At present, commercial mothballs are composed of either relatively nontoxic paradichlorobenzene or potentially toxic naphthalene. Paradichlorobenzene is familiar to many as a cake of disinfectant used in urinals and diaper pails. Naphthalene can cause a hemolytic anemia and methemoglobinemia in neonates and patients with glucose-6-phosphate dehydrogenase (G6PD) deficiency.[284] In the past, mothballs were produced from camphor, which can cause central nervous system (CNS) depression and seizures. Fortunately, camphor mothballs are no longer commercially available in the United States, although they may still exist in older households and may be obtained in other countries. Camphor is also easily obtainable in other formulations such as in blocks or tablets. Rapid differentiation between these groups of mothballs can expedite patient management and disposition. For example, identifying a moth repellent as paradichlorobenzene may allow for outpatient management and prevent unnecessary use of hospital resources. Several bedside tests have been reported to facilitate differentiation between mothballs.

1. Float tests: Paradichlorobenzene is heavier than naphthalene. In turn, naphthalene is heavier than camphor. In lukewarm tap water, camphor will float and naphthalene and paradichlorobenzene will sink. In a solution of 3 tbsp of table salt thoroughly dissolved in 4 oz of lukewarm water, camphor and naphthalene will float and paradichlorobenzene will sink. In a solution of 50% dextrose, camphor and naphthalene will float and paradichlorobenzene will sink.[283]
2. Melting point test: Paradichlorobenzene has a lower melting point than naphthalene. Paradichlorobenzene mothballs will melt in a water bath at 53°C, whereas naphthalene requires a water bath hotter than 80°C. Even in the absence of a thermometer, boiling water will cool rapidly below 80°C after 2 minutes at room temperature. When transferred to a glass container, it can drop a total of 20°C after 15 minutes, thus facilitating differentiation between melting points.[284]
3. Radiograph test: On a plain radiograph, paradichlorobenzene will be densely radiopaque, whereas naphthalene is faintly radiopaque and camphor is radiolucent.[285]

Based on these tests, a simple algorithm with materials readily available in most EDs can help differentiate between moth repellants: Place the unknown mothball in a solution of 50% dextrose. If it sinks, the mothball can be identified as paradichlorobenzene. If it floats, place the mothball in lukewarm tap water. If it floats, it can be identified as camphor and if it sinks, it can be identified as naphthalene.[283]

Body Secretion Analysis

Careful analysis of bodily secretions, the odor emanating from poisoned patients, and the color of their urine can help identify certain toxins. Some characteristic odors and urine colors are listed in Table 68.10 and Box 68.8.

Bedside Toxicologic Tests on Urine

Ethylene Glycol

Confirming ingestion of a toxic alcohol such as ethylene glycol can pose a diagnostic challenge as many hospital laboratories do not have the equipment required to measure serum

TABLE 68.10 Diagnostic Odors

CHARACTERISTIC ODOR	RESPONSIBLE DRUG OR TOXIN
Automobile exhaust	Carbon monoxide (odorless, but associated with exhaust)
Bitter almond	Cyanide
Carrots	Cicutoxin (water hemlock)
Coal gas (stove gas)	Carbon monoxide (odorless, but associated with coal gas)
Disinfectants	Phenol, creosote
Eggs (rotten)	Hydrogen sulfide, carbon disulfide, mercaptans, disulfiram, *N*-acetylcysteine
Fish or raw liver (musty)	Aluminum phosphide, zinc phosphide
Fruitlike	Acetone, chloral hydrate, chloroform, ethanol, isopropyl alcohol, methylbromide, paraldehyde, nitrites (e.g., amyl, butyl), trichloroethane
Garlic	Organic phosphorus compounds (parathion, malathion), tellurium, arsenic, selenium, dimethyl sulfoxide, thallium
Hay	Phosgene
Mothballs	Naphthalene, *p*-dichlorobenzene, camphor
Peanuts	*N*-3-pyridyl-methyl-*N*-*p*-nitrophenyl urea (Vacor)
Pepper-like	2-chlorobenzylidene malononitrile (tear gas)
Rope (burned)	Marijuana, opium
Shoe polish	Nitrobenzene
Tobacco	Nicotine
Vinegar	Acetic acid
Violets	Turpentine (metabolites excreted in urine)
Wintergreen	Methyl salicylate

Adapted from Takematsu M, Chiang WK. Otolaryngologic principles. In: Nelson LS, Howland M, Lewin NA, Smith SW, Goldfrank LR, Hoffman RS, eds. *Goldfrank's Toxicologic Emergencies*. 11th ed. McGraw Hill; 2019.

concentrations of these compounds. Thus surrogate markers including serum osmolar gap and anion gap, along with clinical suspicion are used to establish a diagnosis in a suspected toxic alcohol poisoning. Evaluating the urine of a patient with a suspected ethylene glycol ingestion can be helpful.

Oxalic acid, a metabolic byproduct of ethylene glycol metabolism, can precipitate as either envelope-shaped calcium dihydrate or needle-shaped calcium monohydrate crystals in urine (Fig. 68.13; see also Fig. 68.3F). While detection of calcium oxalate crystals in the urine supports diagnosis of ethylene glycol poisoning, it is neither sensitive nor specific. False positives may occur in patients with high dietary intake of foods containing oxalates or vitamin C.[286] Furthermore, calcium monohydrate crystals can easily be confused with sodium urate crystals.[287] Lack of these crystals does not rule out significant ethylene glycol ingestion because excretion of these crystals can occur late in the ingestion (>6 hours) and may not occur at all.

Visual inspection of urine under a Woods lamp or ultraviolet light to ascertain fluorescence may also be helpful in the diagnosis of ethylene glycol poisoning if performed within the first 6 hours of ingestion.[288]. Fluorescein is often placed in commercially available antifreeze (the most common source of ingested ethylene glycol) to enable mechanics to detect radiator leaks with a Woods lamp or other ultraviolet light source. Fluorescein is a nontoxic, inert vegetable dye that is eliminated unchanged in urine. Therefore high concentrations of fluorescein in urine suggest significant ethylene glycol ingestion. To perform this procedure, place the test urine sample and control samples onto white gauze or paper. Inspect for fluorescence under a Woods lamp in a dark room. It is preferable to perform this test with controls that include urine that does not contain fluorescein and urine that does contain fluorescein.[289] Fluorescein is readily available because fluorescein-containing strips are commonly used in ophthalmologic procedures.

This test has several limitations. Lack of fluorescein does not exclude a significant exposure because not all antifreezes contain fluorescein or high concentrations of fluorescein relative to ethylene glycol. Because fluorescence is time dependent, with sensitivity dropping markedly 4 to 6 hours post ingestion, this technique is unreliable for late presentations or those with unknown time of ingestion.[288] Fluorescence is also pH dependent and will be absent in urine that has a pH of less than 4.5.[286] False-positive findings can occur if certain plastic or glass urine containers are used because of the

BOX 68.8 Selected Toxins That Color Urine

RED
Anthraquinone (in alkaline urine)
Hydroxocobalamin
Deferoxamine

RED-BROWN
Chloroquine
Intravenous lipid emulsion
Levodopa
Methyldopa
Nitrofurantoin
Phenazopyridine
Phenothiazines
Phenytoin

ORANGE-RED
Aminopyrine
Aniline dyes
Antipyrine
Chlorzoxazone
Doxorubicin
Ibuprofen
Idarubicin
Phenacetin
Phenazopyridine
Phenothiazines
Phenytoin
Rifampin
Sulfasalazine

YELLOW
Fluorescein
Phenacetin
Quinacrine (in acidic urine)
Riboflavin (large doses)
Santonin

YELLOW-ORANGE
Aminopyrine
Anisindione
Sulfasalazine
Vitamin A
Warfarin

YELLOW-BROWN
Aloe
Cascara (in acidic urine)
Chloroquine
Nitrofurantoin
Primaquine
Sulfamethoxazole

BLUE-GREEN
Amitriptyline
Cimetidine
Indomethacin
Methocarbamol
Methylene blue
Metoclopramide
Mitoxantrone
Phenol
Promethazine
Propofol
Thymol
Triamterene
Zaleplon

BROWN-BLACK
Carbidopa/levodopa
Cascara (in alkaline urine)
Iron
Metronidazole
Senna (in alkaline urine)

WHITE
Propofol

Adapted from Chu J: Genitourinary principles. In: Nelson LS, Howland M, Lewin NA, Smith SW, Goldfrank LR, Hoffman RS. eds. *Goldfrank's Toxicologic Emergencies*, ed 11e. McGraw Hill; 2019.

inherent fluorescence of these materials. In a controlled study of healthy, human volunteers whose urine was tested after ingesting sodium fluorescein, the sensitivity and specificity of urine fluorescence were only 49% and 75%, respectively.[289]

Salicylates

Several bedside tests have been developed to qualitatively detect salicylates in urine, including 10% ferric chloride solution, Trinder's solution, and Phenistix reagent strips. All are rapid, inexpensive, sensitive tests that give a qualitative rather than a quantitative result. Although historically a mainstay of toxicologic testing, these bedside spot tests have mostly been replaced by quantitative serum salicylate measurements. They rely heavily on visual interpretation by the examiner; thus they are subject to interindividual variability. Furthermore, some of these tests are performed with hazardous chemicals (i.e., mercuric chloride and ferric chloride) and are not permitted in the United States under the CLIA, thus limiting their utility in modern facilities.

To perform the ferric chloride test, add several drops of 10% ferric chloride to 1 mL or 2 mL of urine that has been collected in a test tube. The immediate appearance of a bluish-purple color signifies that salicylates are present in the urine (Fig. 68.14). This test is very sensitive, and just one aspirin tablet taken within 12 to 24 hours will give a positive result. The reaction may take 60 to 120 minutes from the time of ingestion to become positive in patients with normal renal function, so early test results may be misleading. A negative urine ferric chloride test effectively excludes the diagnosis of salicylism.[290]

The Trinder test uses a mixture of mercuric chloride and ferric nitrate in deionized water. To perform this test, mix 1 mL of urine with 1 mL of Trinder's solution. A violet or purple color signifies the presence of salicylates.

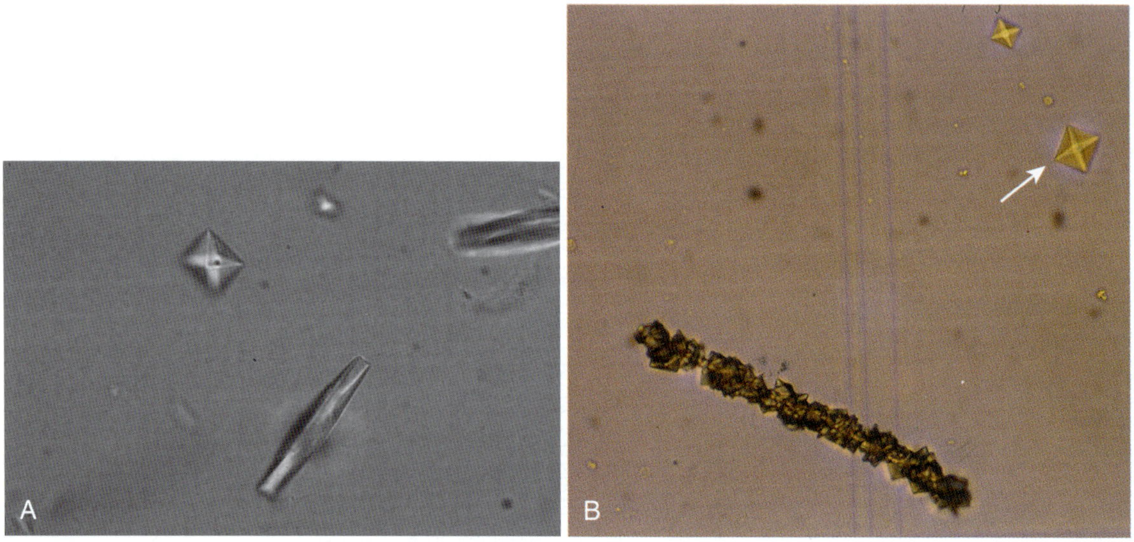

Fig. 68.13 (A) Monohydrate (needle- or prism-shaped) and dihydrate (envelope- or tent-shaped) calcium oxalate crystals from a patient poisoned with ethylene glycol. The dihydrate form is more specific for ethylene glycol toxicity because the monohydrate form can easily be confused with urate crystals. (B) Calcium dihydrate crystal *(arrow)* and a pseudocast of a crystal.

Ferric chloride and the Trinder reaction both have sensitivities of 100% with serum salicylate concentrations of 5 mg/dL. False positives can occur with both tests. Acetoacetic acid, acetone, and phenylpyruvic acid seen in diabetic, alcoholic or starvation ketoacidosis will cause false-positive results.[291,292] Phenol-containing drugs such as diflunisal, sulfasalazine, and salicylamide as well as phenothiazines (i.e., chlorpromazine and thioridazine) can also produce false positives. Any positive result requires a confirmatory quantitative serum salicylate assay.[291]

Phenistix reagent strips were originally developed to detect phenylketonuria. However, Phenistix strips also turn brown in the presence of salicylates. False-positive findings for salicylates can occur if phenothiazines are present.[293]

Paraquat and Diquat

Paraquat, a nonselective bipyridyl herbicide, is one of the most toxic herbicides available worldwide, and ingestion of only 10 to 20 mL of the 20% wt/vol solution is sufficient to cause death. It carries a mortality rate between 50% to 90% and in cases of intentional self-poisoning with concentrated formulations, mortality approaches 100%.[290] An increasing number of countries are banning the sale of paraquat, thus it is primarily only available in resource-poor areas. Diquat is structurally related to paraquat and can cause significant toxicity, though it is less widely used in agriculture.[294]

Diagnosis is typically based on history of exposure, as availability of serum testing is limited. A urinary dithionite test is a simple bedside method for confirming paraquat or diquat poisoning.

In the presence of the reducing agent dithionite, paraquat will turn blue and diquat will turn green.

In this colorimetric test, a combination of alkaline media (sodium bicarbonate or sodium hydroxide) and sodium dithionite are added to the patient's urine and a color change confirms presence of paraquat or diquat.[295]

Place 10 mL of the patient's urine in a clear container. Add 1 g to 2 g of sodium bicarbonate and shake gently. Then add 1 g of sodium dithionite and shake the solution again. Hold up the sample to a white background. The color of the solution will turn blue in the presence of paraquat or green in the presence of diquat. A darker color corresponds to a higher serum concentration of either herbicide.

Some hospitals are equipped with prepackaged paraquat test kits containing the necessary materials.[295] Since outcomes of paraquat poisoning are primarily determined by dose ingested, identifying those with high paraquat concentrations can be useful in assessing whether aggressive interventions will be futile.

Bedside Toxicologic Tests on Oral Secretions and Breath: Ethyl Alcohol

Several bedside devices have been developed to measure alcohol concentrations via noninvasive methods. Measurements of the alcohol concentration in expired air or saliva have been shown to correlate well with blood alcohol concentrations in the appropriate settings.

Breath alcohol analyzers were originally developed in the 1950s and are currently used in law enforcement.[296] There are several types of devices that are used to determine the concentration of alcohol in expired air. The most common methods use infrared spectral analysis (Intoxilyzer), colorimetric measurement of a catalytic reaction with alcohol (breathalyzer), or detection via chemical reaction of alcohol in a fuel cell (Alcosensor III or IV).[297,298] Almost all the alcohol found in expired air at the level of the mouth is secondary to alcohol diffused from the bronchial system rather than the alveolar system.[296] Minor alterations in breathing patterns can cause large variations in readings. Thus uncooperative patients who do not exhale properly can cause an inaccurate reading. Other causes of inaccurate readings include the recent ingestion of alcohol-containing products, belching or vomiting, poor technique, or restrictive pulmonary pathology.

Alcohol concentrations in saliva have been shown to correlate with serum concentrations.[298–300] They are a rapid, noninvasive alternative to breath alcohol analyzers that do not require regular calibration and can be used with patients who

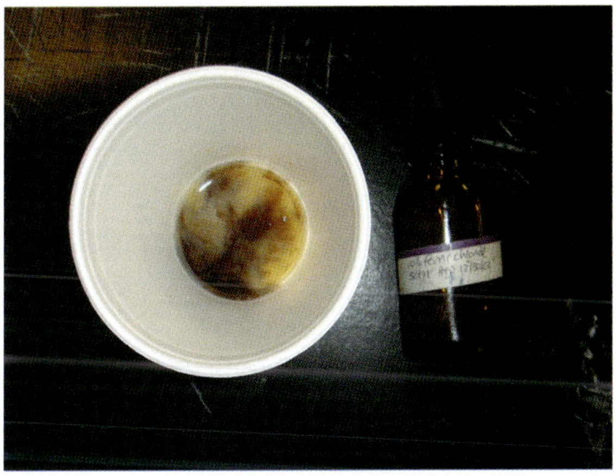

Fig. 68.14 Adding ferric chloride (10%) to a few milliliters of urine immediately turns it a deep purple color in the presence of very small quantities of aspirin. Beware of other changes in color, such as gray or brown, which are not positive tests. This test is also positive in ketoacidotic states such as diabetic ketoacidosis.

BOX 68.9 Drugs That Have Increased Elimination With Urinary Alkalinization

Chlorpropamide
2,4-Dichlorophenoxyacetic acid
Formate
Methotrexate
Phenobarbital
Salicylates

are unable to cooperate with examination such as those with significant CNS depression.[299] Bedside measurement of salivary alcohol concentrations can be obtained with a dipstick-like device. These devices use an enzymatic reaction involving alcohol dehydrogenase to measure alcohol concentrations.[301] Patients who are volume depleted (a common occurrence in alcohol-intoxicated patients) are often unable to provide adequate saliva samples, thus leading to inaccurate readings.[301,302]

Breath and saliva alcohol analyzers may provide a relatively cost-effective alternative in resource-poor areas or public health settings where intoxicated patients are frequently encountered.[300] Additionally, these approaches mitigate the possibility of needle stick injury compared with the traditional serum alcohol evaluation. All bedside quantitative tests should be evaluated in conjunction with the patient's clinical examination.

Metal Phosphides

Metal phosphides (including aluminum and zinc phosphide) are potent fumigants that act by releasing phosphine gas (PH_3) when exposed to ambient moisture. These pesticides are used throughout the world because they are highly effective, inexpensive, and do not leave toxic residue.[303] Unfortunately, intentional self-poisonings from metal phosphides have become increasingly common in agricultural and resource-poor areas. Metal phosphides produce PH_3 upon contact with hydrochloric acid in the stomach. These chemicals are highly potent carrying a mortality between 76% and 100% in intentional ingestions. Most deaths occur within 12 to 24 hours.[303]

Though diagnosis is typically made by history and clinical suspicion alone (including the smell of rotten fish on examination), the presence of PH_3 is suggested by a positive silver nitrate test. This test can be performed on exhaled breath to aid in confirming diagnosis.

To perform this test, place a surgical mask over the patient's face. Place a piece of filter paper impregnated with silver nitrate inside the mask for 10 to 15 minutes. The paper will turn black in the presence of phosphine gas as it forms silver phosphide.[304]

This test is specific, but less sensitive for the presence of PH_3 when small doses are ingested. In one study, the silver nitrate paper only turned black in patients who reported taking at least 2.5 tablets of aluminum phosphide. The test will also likely lead to a negative result if not performed within 8 to 12 hours of the ingestion. Hydrogen sulfide can cause a false-positive result. False negatives can occur in the presence of administered oxygen as PH_3 will form phosphorus pentaoxide.[304,305]

The silver nitrate test can also be performed with gastric contents and is significantly more sensitive (up to 100%); however, it requires more materials that may not be readily available in a typical ED. Place 5 mL of gastric contents in a flask and mix with 15 mL water. Place a filter paper impregnated with silver nitrate over the mouth of the flask. Heat the flask to 50°C (122°F) for 10 to 15 minutes. Remove the filter paper and let it dry. Once completely dry it will turn black if it has been exposed to PH_3.

Bedside Toxicologic Tests on Blood: Methemoglobinemia

Methemoglobin is formed when the iron molecules in hemoglobin are converted from a reduced ferrous form (Fe2+) to an oxidized ferric state (Fe3+). A small amount of methemoglobin (<1%) is physiologic. In the presence of oxidative stressors, particularly in patients with impaired ability to compensate for oxidative stress (such as those with G6PD deficiency), the amount of methemoglobin can rise to a level that significantly impairs overall oxygen transport to the point that it becomes clinically apparent.

Patients with methemoglobinemia will classically present with cyanosis, a low pulse oximeter reading, failure to respond to supplemental oxygen administration, and a normal partial pressure of oxygen (PO_2) on arterial blood gas analysis. Although modern co-oximetry analysis of venous or arterial blood can reliably measure methemoglobin levels, bedside visual inspection of venous or arterial blood in the correct clinical context may help diagnose methemoglobinemia. Rapid diagnosis of methemoglobinemia is essential, as the antidote, methylene blue, is effective and can help stave off unnecessary invasive measures like intubation in patients with significant respiratory symptoms.

To evaluate for methemoglobinemia, place a drop of sample blood on a white background (i.e., a piece of gauze) in a well-lit environment. Next to this, place a drop of normal blood as a comparison control sample. Blood with methemoglobinemia appears darker or chocolate brown. This method relies on the ability of the examiner to distinguish changes in color and may therefore have a degree of interobserver variance. Methemoglobin levels of less than 10% may alter the color of blood only slightly and thereby cause a false-negative finding. Methemoglobin levels of between 12% and 14% may cause a false-negative reading 50% of the time. Methemoglobin levels greater than 15% are reported to cause a cyanotic appearance in patients. With levels of 35% or greater, identification of methemoglobinemia by visual inspection of the color of blood is quite accurate.[306] At this level, almost all patients are obviously cyanotic and symptomatic.

Snake Venom–Induced Coagulopathy

A significant complication of certain snakebites is venom-induced consumption coagulopathy (VICC). The most common snakes capable of inducing this pathology are true vipers and pit vipers (Viperidae family) as well as Australasian elapids (Elapidae family).[307] VICC has historically been likened to disseminated intravascular coagulation (DIC) because both present with prolonged PT, elevated D-dimer, and low fibrinogen. However, VICC has distinct pathophysiology from DIC, including its rapid onset and resolution, lower mortality, lack of end organ failure or systemic microthrombi.

Laboratory hematologic and coagulation tests can aid in accurately diagnosing VICC and can determine when treatment with antivenom is necessary. However, in resource-poor areas, or in hospitals where these coagulation tests may take a prolonged period of time, a simple bedside clotting test can aid in diagnosing significant coagulopathy.[307] There are several methods used around the world including the 20-minute whole blood clotting test (WBCT20).

To perform this test place a few milliliters of the patient's freshly drawn venous blood into a new, clean, dry glass vessel (tube or bottle). Leave the container undisturbed for 20 minutes at room temperature. If the container is unable to stand on its own, it may be taped to the wall at the patient's bedside. Besure to label the specimen before leaving it alone. Tip the vessel once at 20 minutes and if the blood is not clotted, this is a positive test and suggests a diagnosis of VICC.

The WBCT20 performs well and had a sensitivity and specificity of 100%, in one cohort study, however only a small number of cases with VICC were included.[308] In another clinical study, the sensitivity and specificity were 82% and 98%, respectively when compared with an INR of 1.4 as the gold standard.[309]

The WBCT20 test is recommended by the World Health Organization to help diagnose VICC and determine whether a patient should receive antivenom in low resource health settings that lack readily available laboratory studies.[310]

Invasive Therapeutic Procedures

Orogastric Lavage

Orogastric lavage is a GI decontamination technique that is used to prevent toxicity of an ingested substance by blocking or decreasing absorption. The procedure involves passing a large bore orogastric tube and the sequential administration and aspiration of aliquots of liquid with the intent of removing a toxic substance from the stomach.[290,311] The decision to perform a gastric lavage requires a risk-benefit assessment in each individual case. Generally, a lavage should be performed when there is a high risk of mortality from the specific toxin ingested if there is no antidote available or if other removal techniques such as hemodialysis will not be effective. The substance must also be likely to fit through the lumen of the lavage tube and there must be reason to believe that the toxin is still located in the stomach. Thus patients who present many hours after ingestion may not benefit from this procedure. However, in overdose, GI motility is decreased, particularly when the drugs ingested include opioids or antimuscarinics, and thus can be present in the stomach several hours after ingestion.[312–315]

Clinicians must also evaluate for potential contraindications to this procedure which primarily include risk of perforation (history of gastric surgery) or hemorrhage (history of esophageal varices). The other potential risk of this procedure includes aspiration, thus in general, intubation for airway protection prior to the procedure is suggested. Though there are several different approaches available, the following is a general recommendation for the technique of a gastric lavage.[290]

1. Select the correct tube size. In adults the recommended size would be 36 to 40 Fr and in pediatric patients 22 to 28 Fr.
2. Measure the tube prior to insertion so that the distal end will pass beyond the lower esophageal sphincter.
3. Place the patient in the left lateral decubitus position as this will point the pylorus upward and help prevent the toxin from advancing through the pylorus during the procedure.
4. After inserting the tube, confirm that the distal end is in the stomach by aspirating gastric contents, injecting air into the stomach, or by using radiographic confirmation.
5. Withdraw any material present in the stomach.
6. Administer aliquots of 250 mL 0.9% saline lavage solution via funnel or lavage syringe. In pediatric patients, aliquots should be 10 to 15 mL/kg to a maximum of 250 mL.
7. Continue to lavage for at least several liters, (pediatric patients 0.5 to 1 L) or until the lavage effluent solution is clear.
8. After completing the lavage, administer activated charcoal through the same tube, if indicated.
9. Withdraw the tube and discard.

Ethanol Infusion for Toxic Alcohol Poisoning

Before fomepizole (4-methylpyrazole) was approved by the US FDA, ethanol was used for the treatment of toxic alcohol poisoning.[316] Both fomepizole and ethanol act by inhibiting alcohol dehydrogenase (ADH) and preventing the formation of toxic metabolites by ethylene glycol and methanol.[317] Fomepizole has several advantages including ease of use, fewer side effects than ethanol, and ability to maintain therapeutic concentrations without monitoring serum antidote concentrations or the need for continuous infusion. While fomepizole is now considered to be the antidote of choice, ethanol is recommended when fomepizole is not available or in limited supply such as in resource-poor areas or mass casualty situations. Therapeutic blockade with fomepizole or ethanol infusions are not indicated in the treatment of isopropyl alcohol poisoning because it does not form toxic metabolites.

Ethanol can be used as a therapeutic intervention in patients with methanol or ethylene glycol poisoning because ethanol has much greater affinity for alcohol dehydrogenases compared with methanol or ethylene glycol. With serum ethanol concentrations of 100 mg/dL, minimal amounts of ethylene glycol or methanol are metabolized by alcohol dehydrogenases.[318]

Ethanol can be administered orally or intravenously (Table 68.11). All dosing regimens begin with a loading dose, followed by a maintenance dose. IV ethanol has the advantages of achieving therapeutic concentrations rapidly, ensuring complete absorption, limiting the chance of

TABLE 68.11 Use of Ethanol for Methanol or Ethylene Glycol Poisoning

Intravenous Ethanol: Loading Dose (Using a 10% Ethanol Solution)[a] (A 10% Volume/Volume Concentration Yields Approximately 100 mg/mL)						
	Volume of Loading Dose (Given Over 1–2 h as Tolerated)					
	10 kg	15 kg	30 kg	50 kg	70 kg	100 kg
Loading dose of 1000 mg/kg of 10% ethanol (infused over 1–2 h as tolerated); assumes a zero-ethanol concentration to start. Aim is to produce a serum ethanol concentration of 100–150 mg/dL	100 mL	150 mL	300 mL	500 mL	700 mL	1000 mL
Oral Ethanol: Loading Dose (A 20% Volume/Volume Concentration Yields Approximately 200 mg/mL)						
	Volume of Loading Dose					
	10 kg	15 kg	30 kg	50 kg	70 kg	100 kg
Loading dose of 1000 mg/kg of 20% ethanol[b] diluted in juice; may be administered orally or via nasogastric tube; assumes a zero-ethanol concentration to start. Aim is to produce a serum ethanol concentration of 100–150 mg/dL	50 mL	75 mL	150 mL	250 mL	350 mL	500 mL
Intravenous Ethanol: Maintenance Dose (Using a 10% Ethanol Solution)[c] (A 10% Volume/Volume Concentration Yields Approximately 100 mg/mL; Infusion to be Started Immediately Following the Loading Dose; Aim Is to Maintain a Serum Ethanol Concentration of 100–150 mg/dL[d])						
	Infusion Rate (mL/h for Various Weights)[a]					
	10 kg	15 kg	30 kg	50 kg	70 kg	100 kg
Normal Maintenance Range (mg/kg per hour)						
80	8	12	24	40	56	80
110	11	16	33	55	77	110
130	13	19	39	65	91	130
Approximate Maintenance Dose for Patients With Alcohol Use Disorder						
150[e]	15	22	45	75	105	150
Range Required During Hemodialysis						
250[e]	25	38	75	125	175	250
300[e]	30	45	90	150	210	300
350[e]	35	53	105	175	245	350
Oral Ethanol: Maintenance Dose (A 20% Volume/Volume Concentration Yields Approximately 200 mg/mL; Infusion to be Given Each Hour Immediately Following a Loading Dose; Aim Is to Maintain a Serum Ethanol Concentration of 100–150 mg/dL[d]; Each Dose may be Diluted in Juice and Given Orally or via Nasogastric Tube)						
	Infusion Rate (mL/h[f] for Various Weights[g])					
	10 kg	15 kg	30 kg	50 kg	70 kg	100 kg
Normal Maintenance Range (mg/kg per hour)						
80	4	6	12	20	28	40
110	6	8	17	27	39	55
130	7	10	20	33	46	66

TABLE 68.11 Use of Ethanol for Methanol or Ethylene Glycol Poisoning—cont'd

Approximate Range for Chronic Alcoholics or for Patients Receiving Continuous Oral Activated Charcoal						
150	8	11	22	38	53	75
Range Required During Hemodialysis						
250	13	19	38	63	88	125
300	15	23	46	75	105	150
350	18	26	52	88	123	175

[a]If a 5% ethanol solution is used, double the volume of the loading dose.
[b]Equivalent to a 40-proof solution.
[c]If a 5% ethanol solution is used, double the volume rate; monitor closely for potential volume overload.
[d]Serum ethanol concentrations should be monitored closely.
[e]At higher infusion rates it may be necessary to administer by volume rather than by milliliters per hour.
[f]For a 30% concentration, divide the amount by 1.5.
[g]Rounded off to the nearest milliliter.
Ethanol concentrations higher than 10% are not recommended for intravenous administration. Ethanol concentrations higher than 30% are not recommended for oral administration. The dose schedule is based on the premise that the patient initially has zero-ethanol concentrations. The aim of therapy is to maintain serum ethanol concentrations of 100 to 150 mg/dL, but constant monitoring of the ethanol concentrations is required because of wide variations in endogenous metabolic capacity. Ethanol is removed by dialysis, and the infusion rate of ethanol must be increased during dialysis. Prolonged ethanol administration may lead to hypoglycemia. Note that 10% ethanol for infusion may be difficult to find in the hospital pharmacy. To formulate 10% ethanol for infusion, (1) remove 50 mL from a 1-L bottle of 5% ethanol/5% dextrose in water (D_5W) and replace it with 50 mL of 100% ethanol, or (2) remove 100 mL from a 1-L bottle of D_5W and replace it with 100 mL of 100% ethanol.

aspiration, and avoiding gastritis. However, IV ethanol has several downsides including increasing the risk of phlebitis at the infusion site and hyponatremia. Furthermore, a 5% concentration of ethanol, which can be given in a peripheral vein, requires the use of larger fluid volumes than 10% ethanol. For example, in a 70-kg patient, a loading dose requires 1.4 L of a 5% solution, with a maintenance dose of 700 mL/h. If IV ethanol is given, careful attention must be paid to the cardiopulmonary status. From a practical standpoint, commercial preparations of both 5% and 10% ethanol in 5% dextrose have been discontinued, thus infusions must be compounded by the pharmacy upon request.[316] This process increases the risk of preparation-related medication errors and further delays administration of this time sensitive antidote.

In contrast, oral loading of ethanol can be achieved with much lower volumes. However, administration can be difficult in an uncooperative or unconscious patient or if vomiting or GI hemorrhage is present. Additionally, a therapeutic ethanol concentration is reached more slowly with an oral loading dose.

Ethanol metabolism can vary widely, and ethanol is dialyzable. Therefore it may be difficult to maintain appropriate ethanol concentrations during hemodialysis for ethylene glycol or methanol poisoning. Frequent serum ethanol concentrations should be obtained along with close blood glucose and electrolyte monitoring. An increase in anion gap or decrease in bicarbonate concentration indicates that the ethanol concentration is inadequate, and the ethanol dose should be adjusted accordingly. Ethanol administration is associated with several adverse effects, including worsening CNS depression, hypothermia, hypotension, hypoglycemia, pancreatitis, hepatitis, gastritis, and phlebitis.[319,320] Furthermore, unlike fomepizole monotherapy, ethanol monotherapy has been associated with treatment failure in cases with high ethylene glycol concentrations. This may be due to fomepizole's greater affinity for ADH and better efficacy compared with ethanol.[321]

REFERENCES ARE AVAILABLE AT Elsevier eBooks+

CHAPTER 69

Standard Precautions and Infectious Exposure Management

Nida F. Degesys and Peter E. Sokolove

Contamination of health care workers (HCWs) with body fluids is a constant risk in the emergency department (ED). A survey of ED and trauma staff found that almost half reported a needlestick injury within the preceding year.[1] Body fluids may contain various transmissible infectious diseases, and the prevalence of human immunodeficiency virus (HIV) infection, hepatitis B virus (HBV), hepatitis C virus (HCV), and other communicable diseases has been shown to be significant in ED patient populations.[2,3]

Routine opt-out HIV screening of ED patients identifies approximately 1% of patients with previously undiagnosed HIV infections.[2,4] Of such patients, many (20%) have no identifiable HIV risk factors, making it more difficult to identify patients who pose a risk to HCWs.[5] This makes widespread use of standard precautions in the ED essential. However, compliance with standard precautions, formerly known as universal precautions, is far from universal.[6–8] Less than 20% of ED nursing staff comply with all standard precautions procedures.[9] In a video-taped review of pediatric trauma resuscitations, compliance with barrier precautions was 81.3%.[8] Similarly, ED staff have low observed compliance rates with standard precautions during cardiopulmonary resuscitation, with the lowest rates for wearing gowns (20%) and highest for wearing masks (90%).[10] Even during the early phase of the coronavirus disease (COVID) pandemic personal protective equipment (PPE) compliance rates were far below 100%.[11,12]

In 1985 the combination of high-risk illness with low-compliance barrier use prompted the Centers for Disease Control and Prevention (CDC) to recommend guidelines for the protection of HCWs.[13] In 1991 these recommendations were enacted into law by mandate of the Occupational Safety and Health Administration (OSHA).[14] The primary focus of the CDC guidelines is to reduce mucocutaneous exposure to body fluids by encouraging hand washing and barrier protection. These measures do little to protect from percutaneous exposure, which is the most efficient method of transmission of hepatitis and HIV.[15,16] The current strategy for risk reduction in the ED includes immunization against HBV, use of standard precautions (including reengineered safety products such as blunt tip suture needles), and prompt initiation of postexposure prophylaxis (PEP) when appropriate.

GUIDELINES FOR STANDARD PRECAUTIONS

Appropriate precautions for all patient contact must be viewed as a consistent practice or "way of life" in the ED. The following guidelines, based on 2022 World Health Organization (WHO) and CDC recommendations, should be used when there is any possibility of contact with body fluids.[17]

Hand Hygiene

Hand hygiene adherence is frequently low in emergency settings.[18–21] If performed properly, both soap and water and alcohol-based products are generally efficacious in removing bacteria and preventing the spread of communicable diseases.[21,22] Alcohol-based formulations have shown both bactericidal and virucidal activity.[23,24] However, soap and water perform better in removing *Clostridium difficile* spores.[25] See Box 69.1.

Barrier Precautions

1. Use gloves for any patient contact with a risk for exposure to body fluids (Fig. 69.1). Both cutaneous and percutaneous exposure can be reduced using gloves. Gloves have been shown to reduce disease transmission in needlestick injuries, with greater reduction seen with double-gloving in animal models and in a case crossover study of HCWs.[16] A systematic review looking at the practice of wearing multiple layers of gloves found moderate-quality evidence that double-gloving reduces perforations and blood stains on the skin, indicating a decrease in percutaneous exposure incidents.[26] Never wear the same pair of gloves for the care of more than one patient.
2. Wear a mask and protective eyewear when exposure to body fluid aerosols is possible (e.g., wound irrigation, traumatic chest wound) (Fig. 69.2). According to current CDC recommendations, an N95 respirator is indicated for HCW during aerosol-generating procedures, and for infectious diseases when airborne precautions should be followed (e.g., measles, tuberculosis [TB]).[27]
3. Wear a gown and shoe covers when there is a risk for large volumes of splashed body fluids (e.g., chest tube, thoracotomy) (Fig. 69.3).

BOX 69.1 Hand Hygiene Recommendations

USE AN ALCOHOL-BASED HAND SANITIZER

- Immediately before touching a patient
- Before performing an aseptic task (e.g., placing an indwelling device) or handling invasive medical devices
- Before moving from work on a soiled body site to a clean body site on the same patient
- After touching a patient or the patient's immediate environment
- After contact with blood, body fluids, or contaminated surfaces
- Immediately after glove removal

WASH WITH SOAP AND WATER

- When hands are visibly soiled
- After caring for a person with known or suspected infectious diarrhea
- After known or suspected exposure to spores (e.g., *B. anthracis*, *C. difficile* outbreaks)

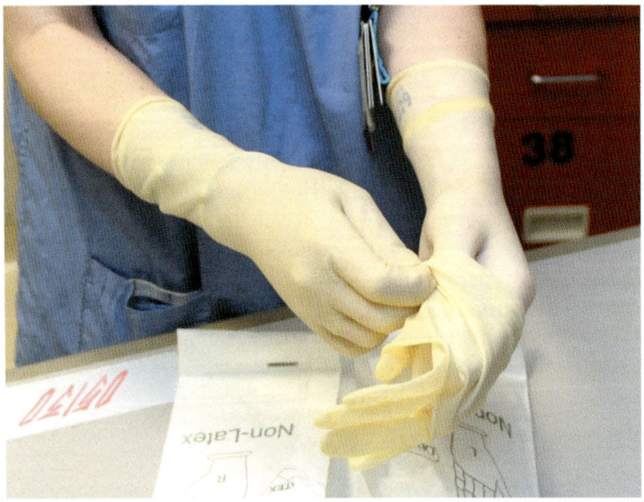

Fig. 69.1 Gloves are mandatory for any patient contact with a risk for exposure to body fluids. Double-gloving may confer additional protection and should be considered in high-risk situations.

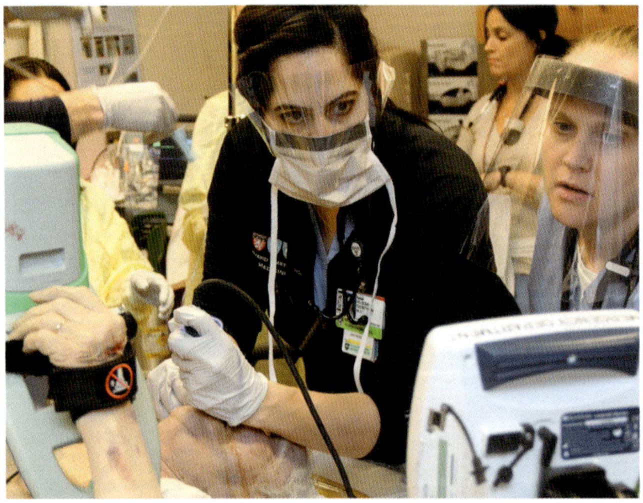

Fig. 69.2 A mask and protective eyewear are mandatory when exposure to body fluid aerosols is possible. A gown is also suggested. This patient vomited profusely during intubation, which may have led to an exposure if proper protective gear had not been worn.

Respiratory Hygiene/Cough Etiquette

In 2022 the CDC updated new elements to its standard precautions in response to outbreak investigations. The elements of "Respiratory Hygiene/Cough Etiquette" include (1) education of health care facility staff, patients, and visitors; (2) posted signs, in language(s) appropriate to the population served, with instructions to patients and accompanying family members or friends; (3) source control measures (e.g., covering the mouth/nose with a tissue when coughing and prompt disposal of used tissues, using surgical masks on the coughing person when tolerated and appropriate [respirators such as N95 or above are not necessary for this purpose]); (4) hand hygiene after contact with respiratory secretions; and (5) spatial separation, ideally >3 feet, of persons with respiratory infections in common waiting areas when possible.[28]

Safe Injection Practices

Most importantly, sharps precautions mean no recapping, bending, or breaking of needles. Most needlestick injuries occur during needle disposal.[29] If needle recapping is deemed necessary, use a single-handed technique (Fig. 69.4). A safer alternative is to immediately dispose of the needle in an approved sharps container without recapping. In an observational study of ED employees, the rate of needle recapping was 34%, with most practitioners incorrectly using a two-handed technique.[30] Various reengineered products are available for use in the ED, including retracting scalpels, auto-capping needles, and needleless intravenous systems (Fig. 69.5). Reviews of studies looking at these safety devices have found they are associated with a reduction in needlestick injuries.[31,32] US federal law now requires the use of safety-engineered sharps devices to protect HCWs. The Needlestick Safety and Prevention Act of 2000 required the use of safety-engineered sharps devices to protect HCWs from needlestick injuries.[33] A review of data from the Exposure Prevention Information Network (EPINet) sharps injury surveillance program estimated that needlestick injuries have decreased by 34% overall, with a 51% decline in nurses since the implementation of federal legislation.[34] In addition to the federal legislation, some states have enacted additional, more stringent laws,[35] in an effort to improve HCW safety. As each state law differs, HCWs should consult their own local regulatory agencies. To further prevent transmission of blood-borne infections, whenever possible use single-dose vials with a single-use disposable needle and syringe for each injection.[28]

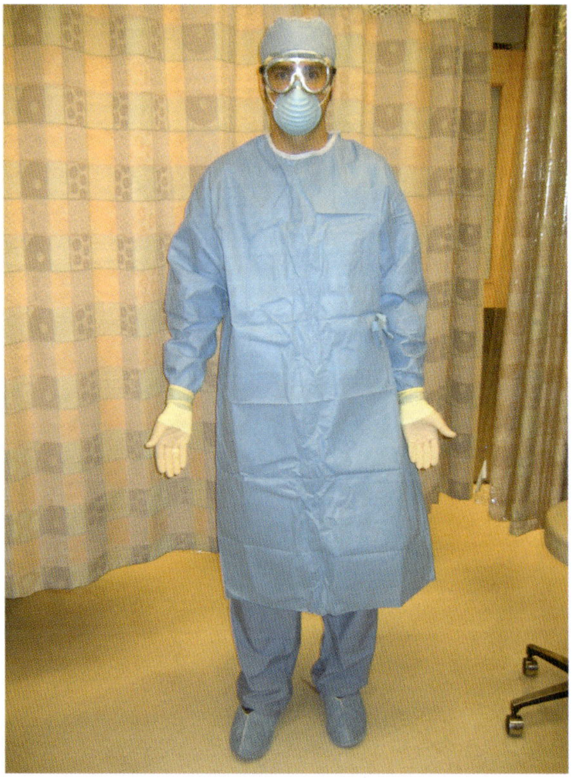

Fig. 69.3 Full protective gear (eye protection, face mask, impervious gown, gloves, and shoe covers) should be worn when there is a risk for large volumes of splashed bodily fluids (e.g., emergency thoracotomy).

Respiratory Precautions

ED patients commonly present with respiratory syndromes that require respiratory precautions in addition to standard precautions (Table 69.1).[28] For example, patients

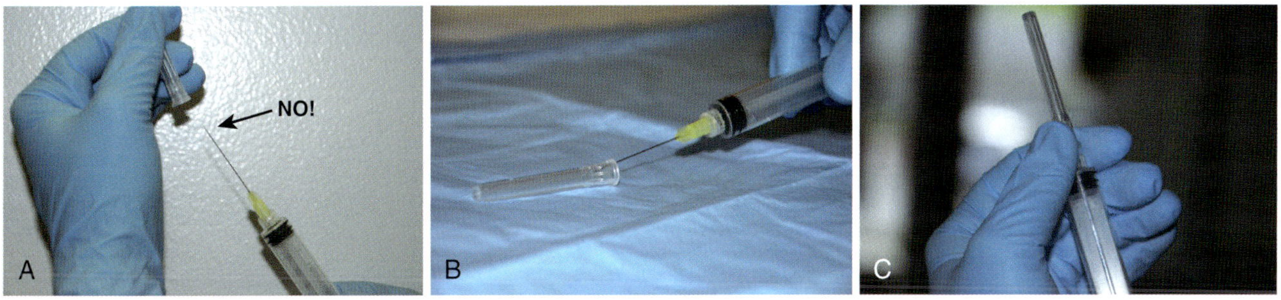

Fig. 69.4 (A) Recapping a needle by holding the cap in the hand is the most common way to sustain a needle puncture and should never be done. (B) It is best to discard the needle/syringe without recapping, but if deemed absolutely necessary, use a single-handed technique to partially recap without holding the needle cap. (C) Make sure that at least 80% of the needle is covered before completing the recapping with the second hand (by holding the base of the needle cap).

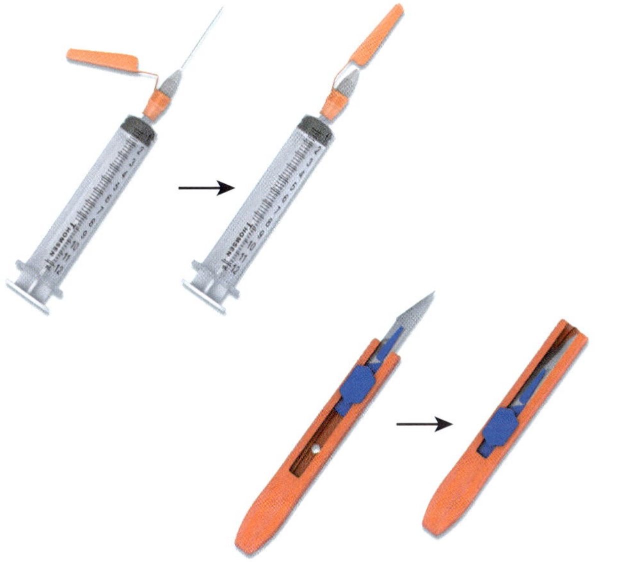

Fig. 69.5 Using safety systems such as auto-recapping needles and retracting scalpels dramatically reduces percutaneous injuries to health care workers, and US federal law now mandates their use.

with suspected or confirmed pulmonary TB, rubeola virus (measles), severe acute respiratory syndrome virus (SARS), COVID, or avian influenza should be isolated with airborne precautions, plus contact precautions with eye/face protections during any aerosol-generating procedures or if any contact with respiratory secretions is anticipated.[28] During contact with patients who require airborne precautions, wear a National Institute for Occupational Safety and Health (NIOSH)–approved N95 particulate respirator (Fig. 69.6). These masks are designed to efficiently filter 1- to 5-μm particles and are less costly and more comfortable than high-efficiency particulate air (HEPA)–filtered masks. In addition, place such patients in a respiratory isolation room with negative pressure, high circulation (optimally at least 12 air changes per hour), and external exhaust. If possible, source control of the patient, including the patient wearing a surgical mask is advised. When performing aerosol-generating procedures (such as intubation or sputum induction) that result in increased release of infectious droplets, add extra face/eye protection.[28] However, even during outbreaks, adherence to isolation precautions is variable. A survey of medical students and residents at a Washington, DC, hospital (November–December 2009) showed that only 13% of medical students and 21% of residents would wear an N95 respirator when caring for a patient with influenza symptoms.[36,37] During the COVID-19 pandemic, some studies have shown that strict adherence to N95 use was limited,[38] although extenuating circumstances such as supply chain shortages as well as controversy about whether or not the virus required airborne precautions were also factors that influenced HCW behaviors.

For patients with respiratory infections such as suspected or confirmed respiratory syncytial virus (RSV), parainfluenza virus, adenovirus, or human metapneumovirus, the CDC recommends droplet precautions (Table 69.1). Droplet precautions consist of placing the patient in a private room or a special separation of >3 feet. HCWs should don a surgical mask on entering the patient's room.[28] If transport or movement is necessary, such as to radiology, instruct the patient to wear a mask and follow Respiratory Hygiene/Cough Etiquette.[28]

Reuse and Extended Use of N95 Respirators

The Centers for Disease Control and Prevention recommends that HCWs dispose of N95s after a single patient encounter. However, during critical shortages, it recommends N95 extended use (wearing the same N95 for multiple patient encounters) and limited reuse (storing an N95 between encounters for use over multiple encounters).[39,40] Among HCWs, the safety of N95 extended use and reuse in clinical settings is not well understood, and some studies suggest that fit failure is unacceptably high with reuse.[41]

Personal Protective Equipment

Isolation gowns are worn in combination with gloves only if contact with blood or body fluid is anticipated. The need for and the type of isolation gown selected is based on the nature of the patient interaction, including the anticipated degree of contact with infectious material and the potential for blood and body fluid penetration of the barrier.[28] The CDC updated its PPE guidelines when contacting pox viruses (such as monkeypox)[42] as well as hemorrhagic fever viruses (such as the Ebola virus) in response to new data gained during outbreaks. CDC guidance emphasizes the importance of training, practice, competence, and observation of HCWs in correct donning and doffing of PPE.[43] Procedures recommended by the CDC for donning and doffing PPE are aimed at preventing skin or clothing contamination and are shown in Figs. 69.7 and 69.8.[43]

TABLE 69.1 Respiratory Syndromes That Require Respiratory Precautions in Addition to Standard Precautions[a]

CLINICAL SYNDROME OR CONDITION[b]	POTENTIAL PATHOGENS[c]	EMPIRIC PRECAUTIONS (ALWAYS INCLUDES STANDARD PRECAUTIONS)
Respiratory Infections		
Cough/fever/upper lobe pulmonary infiltrate in an HIV-negative patient or a patient at low risk for HIV infection	*Mycobacterium tuberculosis*, respiratory viruses, *Streptococcus pneumoniae*, *Staphylococcus aureus* (MSSA or MRSA)	Airborne precautions plus contact precautions
Cough/fever/pulmonary infiltrate in any lung location in an HIV-infected patient or a patient at high risk for HIV infection.	*M. tuberculosis*, respiratory viruses, *S. pneumoniae*, *S. aureus* (MSSA or MRSA).	Airborne precautions plus contact precautions. Use eye/face protection if aerosol-generating procedure performed or contact with respiratory secretions anticipated. If tuberculosis is unlikely and there are no AIIRs and/or respirators available, use droplet precautions instead of airborne precautions. Tuberculosis more likely in HIV-infected individual than in HIV-negative individual.
Cough/fever/pulmonary infiltrate in any lung location in a patient with a history of recent travel (10–21 days) to countries with active outbreaks of SARS, COVID, avian influenza.	*M. tuberculosis*, SARS-CoV1 and CoV2, avian influenza	Airborne plus contact precautions plus eye protection. If SARS, COVID, and tuberculosis unlikely, use droplet precautions instead of airborne precautions.
Respiratory infections, particularly bronchiolitis and pneumonia, in infants and young children.	Respiratory syncytial virus, parainfluenza virus, adenovirus, influenza virus, human metapneumovirus	Contact plus droplet precautions; droplet precautions may be discontinued when adenovirus and influenza have been ruled out.

[a]Infection control professionals should modify or adapt this table according to local conditions. To ensure that appropriate empiric precautions are always implemented, hospitals must have systems in place to evaluate patients routinely according to these criteria as part of their preadmission and admission care.
[b]Patients with the syndromes or conditions listed below may present with atypical signs or symptoms (e.g., neonates and adults with pertussis may not have paroxysmal or severe cough). The clinician's index of suspicion should be guided by the prevalence of specific conditions in the community, as well as clinical judgment.
[c]The organisms listed under the column "Potential Pathogens" are not intended to represent the complete, or even most likely diagnosis, but rather possible etiologic agents that require additional precautions beyond the standard precautions until they can be ruled out.
AIIR, Airborne infection isolation room; *CoV*, coronavirus; *COVID* coronavirus disease from SARS-CoV-2; *HIV*, human immunodeficiency virus; *MRSA*, methicillin-resistant *S. aureus*; *MSSA*, methicillin-sensitive *S. aureus*; *SARS*, severe acute respiratory syndrome.
Adapted from Siegel JD, Rhinehart E, Jackson M, Chiarello L, and the Healthcare Infection Control Practices Advisory Committee. *2007 Guideline for Isolation Precautions: Preventing Transmission of Infectious Agents in Healthcare Settings*. https://www.cdc.gov/infectioncontrol/guidelines/isolation/index.html

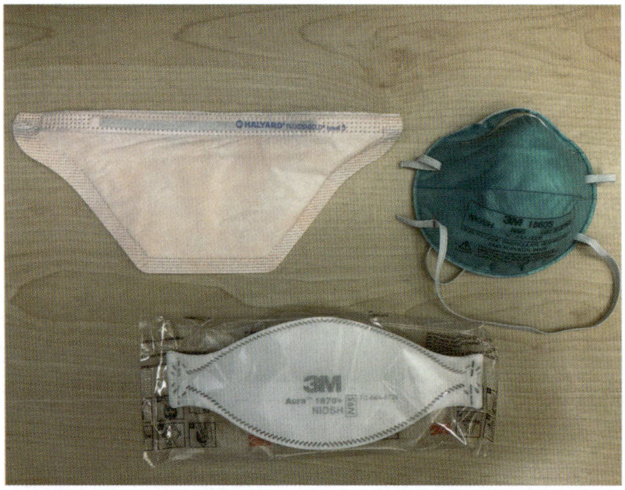

Fig. 69.6 Respiratory precautions. Surgical masks are appropriate to protect against pathogens that are larger than 5 μm, such as influenza and *Neisseria meningitidis.* N95 respirators are required for pathogens smaller than 5 μm, such as tuberculosis.

Contamination during removal of PPE occurs frequently, thus training and practice are important to reduce the risk of contamination during PPE removal.[44] The CDC recommends the following sequence for donning and doffing PPE when evaluating persons under investigation for Ebola specifically.[43,45]

Donning PPE

See Fig. 69.7. This donning procedure applies to PPE recommended for evaluating and managing persons under investigation, who are clinically stable and do not have bleeding, vomiting, or diarrhea. There is a lower risk of splashes and contamination in these situations. An established protocol, combined with proper training of the HCW, helps to facilitate compliance with PPE guidance.

1. Remove personal clothing and items. The HCW should wear surgical scrubs. No personal items (e.g., jewelry [including rings], watches, cell phones, pagers, pens) should be worn under PPE or brought into the patient room. Long hair should be tied back. Eyeglasses should be secured with a tie.

Donning Personnel Protective Equipment

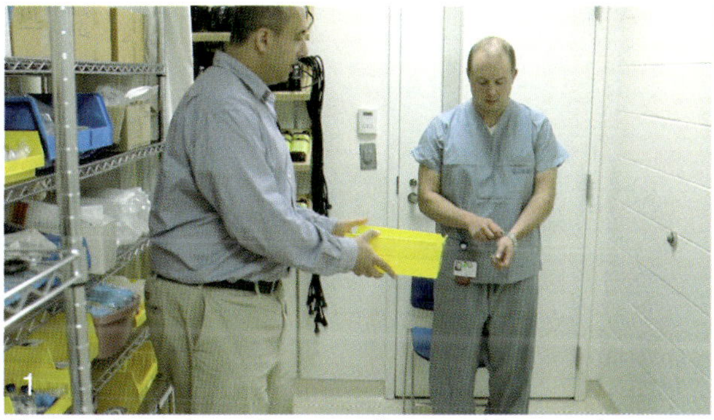

Change into scrubs, and remove all personal items such as jewelry and watches.

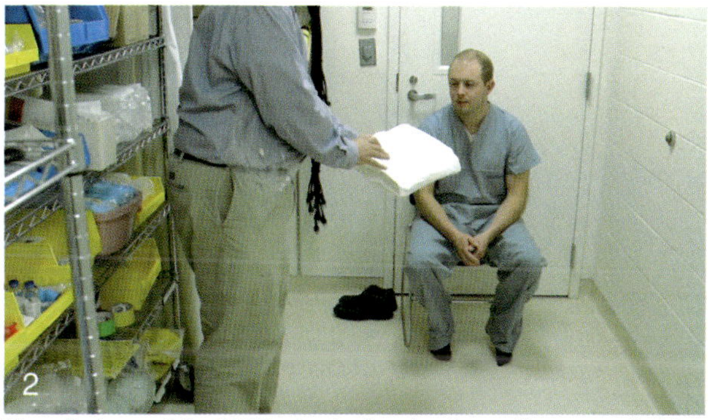

Visually inspect the PPE prior to donning to confirm correct sizing and ensure its structural integrity.

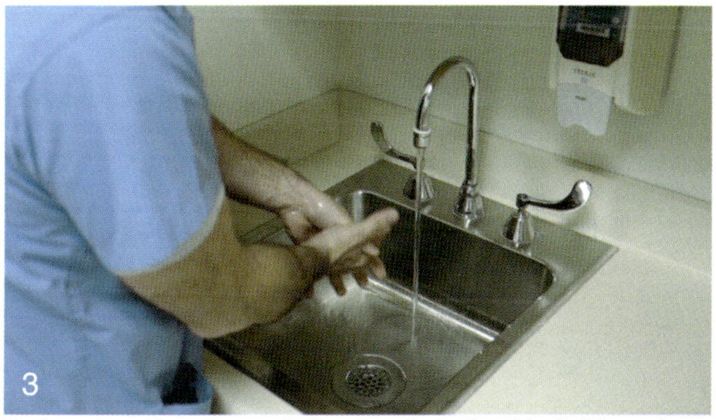

Perform hand hygeine and allow hands to dry. Alcohol-based hand rub is preferred if available.

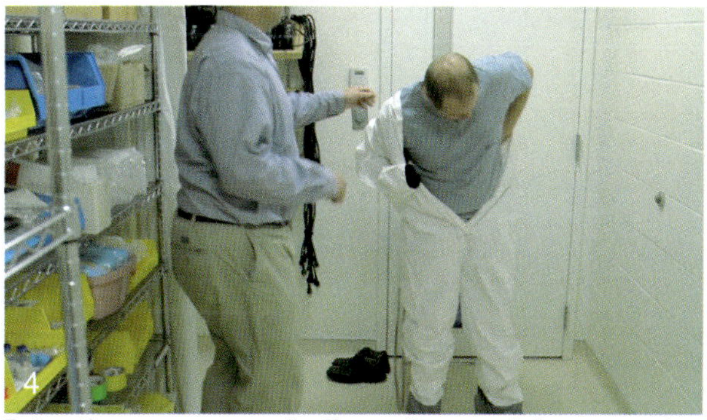

Put on the gown or coveralls. Ensure the gown is large enough to allow unrestricted movement.

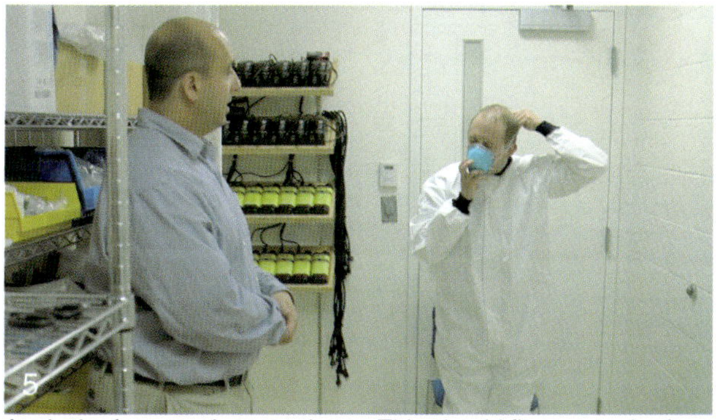

Apply the face mask or respirator. This should fit snug to the face and below the chin.

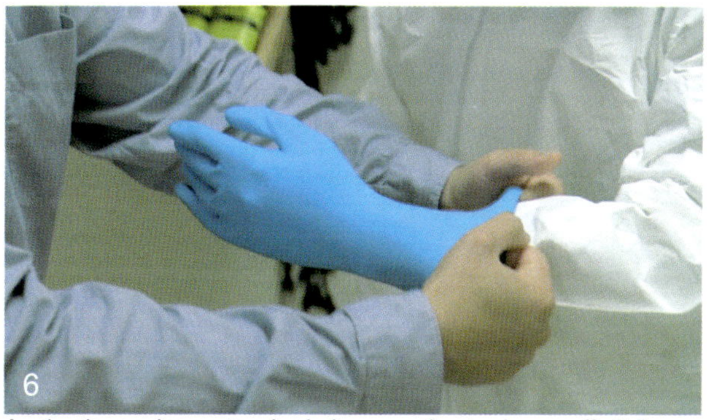

Apply gloves. Inner standard gloves and outer long-cuff nitrile gloves should be worn.

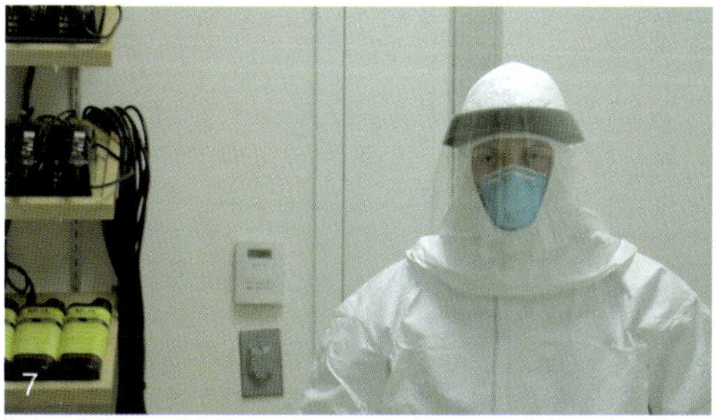

Put on full face shield over the surgical face mask to protect the eyes and front and sides of the face.

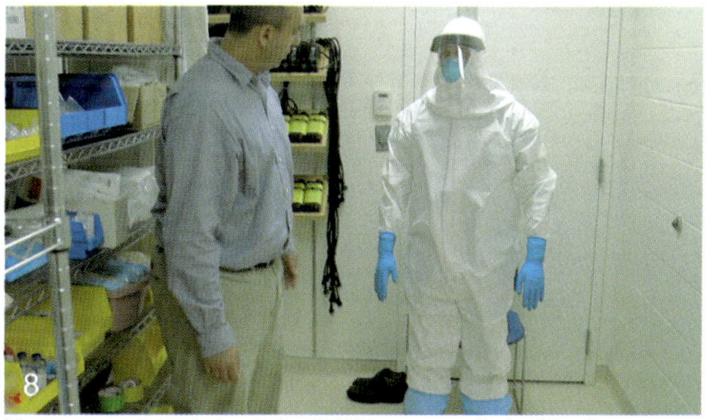

Have an assistant check the PPE to assure that all body areas are properly protected.

Fig. 69.7 Donning personal protective equipment. A trained safety observer should be present to help apply and inspect the equipment. *PPE*, Personal protective equipment.

Doffing Personal Protective Equipment

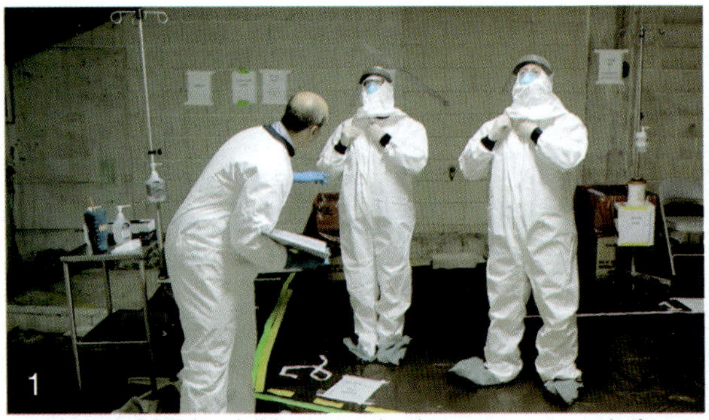

Inspect the PPE for visible contamination, cuts, or tears before starting to remove.

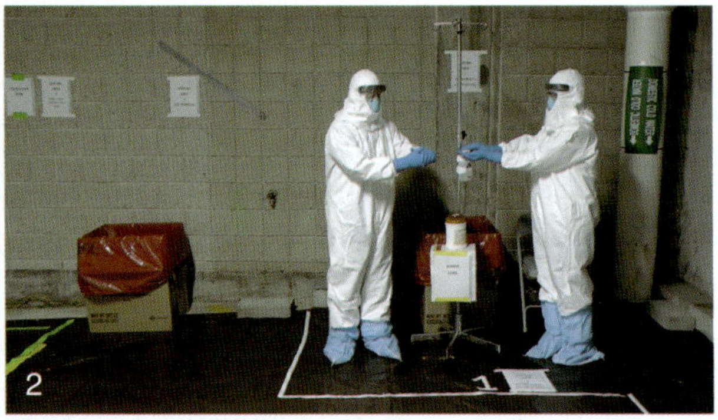

Disinfect outer-gloved hands with either a disinfectant wipe or ABHR, and then remove.

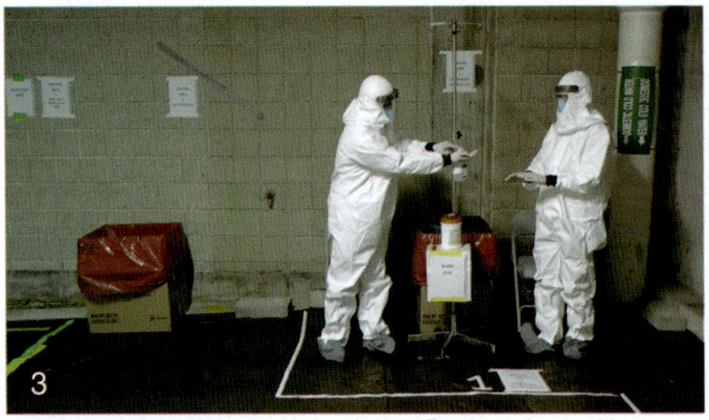

Inspect and disinfect the inner gloves. Replace them with a new pair if visibly soiled.

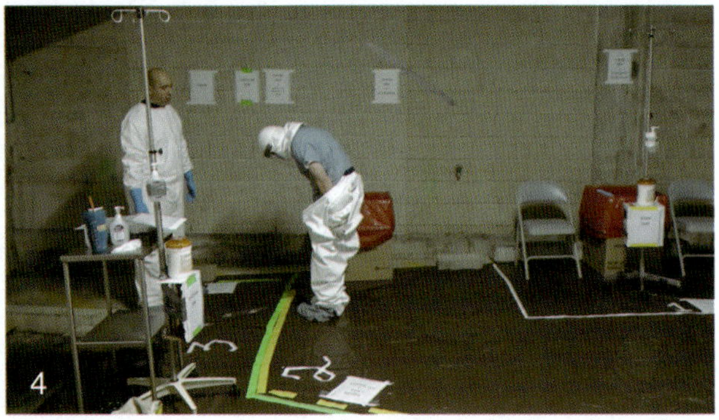

Remove the outer gown, avoiding contact with the outer surface. Disinfect and replace gloves.

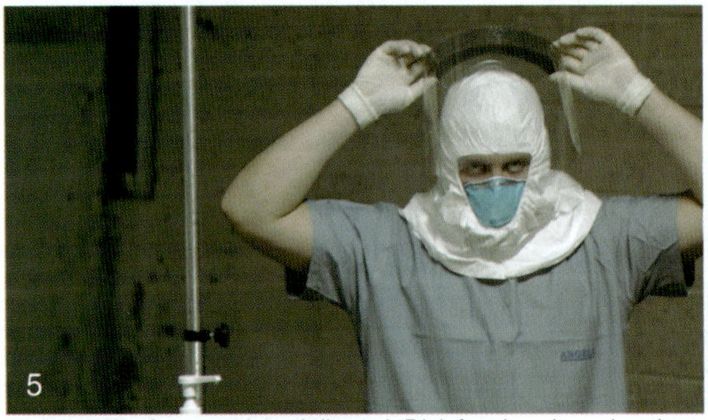

Remove the face mask and discard. Disinfect hands and replace gloves after face mask removal.

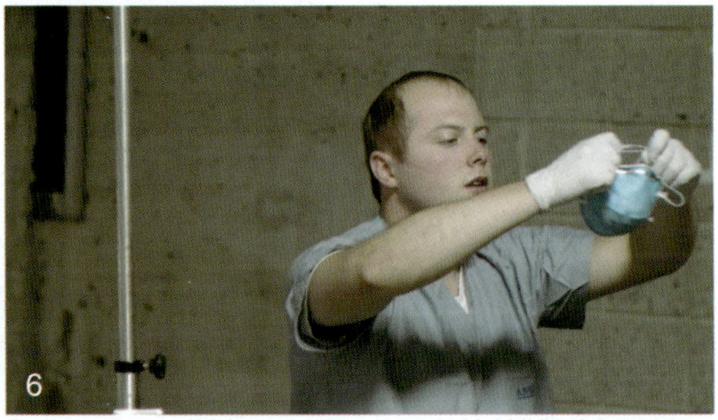

Remove the surgical or respiratory mask. Hold it by the straps and avoid touching the front of the mask.

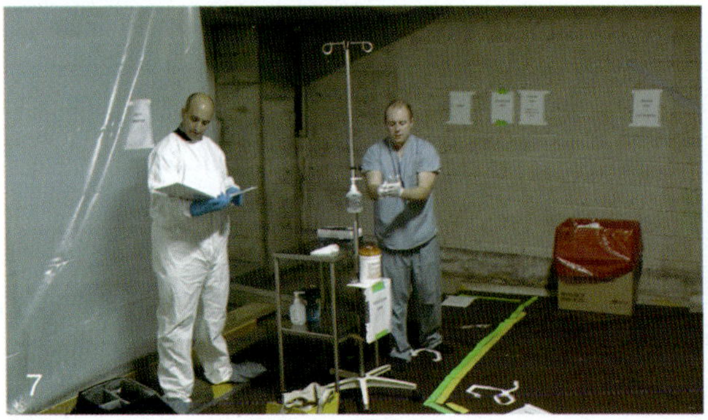

Disinfect and remove the inner gloves.

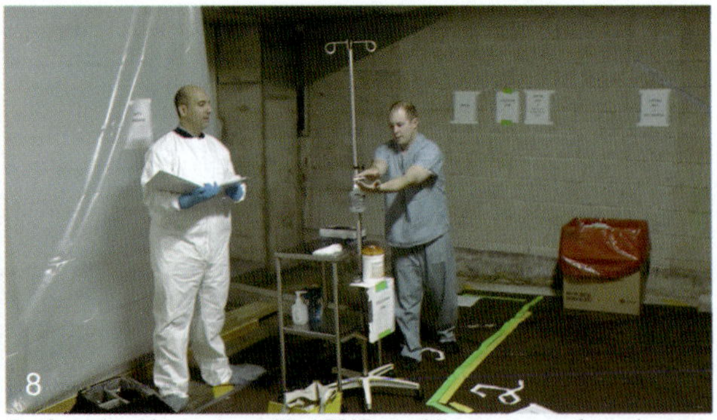

Perform hand hygeine with ABHR, and have your safety observer inspect your scrubs for contamination.

Fig. 69.8 Doffing personal protective equipment. *ABHR*, Alcohol-based hand rub; *PPE*, personal protective equipment.

2. Inspect PPE prior to donning. Visually inspect the PPE ensemble to ensure that it is in serviceable condition (e.g., not torn or ripped), that all required PPE and supplies are available, and that the sizes selected are correct for the HCW.
3. Perform hand hygiene. Perform hand hygiene with alcohol-based hand rub (ABHR). When using ABHR, allow hands to dry before moving to the next step.
4. Put on inner gloves. Put on the first pair of gloves.
5. Put on gown or coverall. Ensure the gown or coverall is large enough to allow unrestricted movement. Ensure cuffs of inner gloves are tucked under the sleeve of the gown or coverall.
6. Put on the face mask.
7. Put on outer gloves. Put on a second pair of gloves (with extended cuffs). Ensure the cuffs are pulled over the sleeves of the gown or coverall.
8. Put on a face shield. Put on a full face shield over the surgical face mask to protect the eyes, as well as the front and sides of the face.
9. Verify. After completing the donning process, the integrity of the ensemble should be verified by the HCW (e.g., there should be no cuts or tears in the PPE). The HCW should be comfortable and able to extend the arms, bend at the waist, and go through a range of motions to ensure there is sufficient range of movement while all areas of the body remain covered. A mirror in the room can be useful for the HCW while donning PPE.

Doffing PPE (See Fig. 69.8)

1. PPE is doffed in the designated PPE removal area in the health care facility. As with all PPE doffing, meticulous care should be taken to avoid self-contamination. Place all PPE waste in a leak-proof infectious waste container.
2. Inspect. Inspect the PPE for visible contamination, cuts, or tears before starting to remove. If any PPE is visibly contaminated, disinfect by using an Environmental Protection Agency (EPA)–registered disinfectant wipe. If the facility conditions permit and appropriate regulations are followed, an EPA-registered disinfectant spray can be used, particularly on contaminated areas.
3. Disinfect and remove outer gloves. Disinfect outer-gloved hands with either an EPA-registered disinfectant wipe or ABHR. Remove and discard outer gloves, taking care not to contaminate inner gloves when removing the outer gloves. Dispose of outer gloves into the designated leak-proof infectious waste container.
4. Inspect and disinfect inner gloves. Inspect the inner gloves' outer surfaces for visible contamination, cuts, or tears. If an inner glove is visibly soiled, disinfect the glove with either an EPA-registered disinfectant wipe or ABHR, remove the inner gloves, perform hand hygiene with ABHR on bare hands, and don a new pair of gloves. If a cut or tear is seen on an inner glove, immediately review occupational exposure risk per hospital protocol. If there is no visible contamination and no cuts or tears on the inner gloves, then disinfect the inner-gloved hands with either an EPA-registered disinfectant wipe or ABHR.
5. Remove face shield. Remove the full face shield by tilting the head slightly forward, grabbing the rear strap and pulling it over the head, gently allowing the face shield to fall forward. Avoid touching the front surface of the face shield. Discard the face shield into the designated leak-proof infectious waste container.
6. Disinfect inner gloves. Disinfect inner gloves with either an EPA-registered disinfectant wipe or ABHR.
7. Remove gown or coverall. Remove and discard.
   a. Depending on the gown design and location of fasteners, the HCW can either untie or gently break fasteners. Avoid contact of scrubs or disposable garments with the outer surface of the gown during removal. Pull the gown away from the body, rolling it inside out and touching only the inside of the gown.
   b. To remove the coverall, tilt the head back to reach zipper or fasteners. Unzip or unfasten the coverall completely before rolling down while turning inside out. Avoid contact of scrubs with outer surface of coverall during removal, touching only the inside of the coverall. Dispose of gown or coverall into the designated leak-proof infectious waste container.
8. Disinfect and change inner gloves. Disinfect inner gloves with either an EPA-registered disinfectant wipe or ABHR.
   a. Remove and discard gloves, taking care not to contaminate bare hands during the removal process.
   b. Perform hand hygiene with ABHR.
   c. Don a new pair of inner gloves.
9. Remove surgical face mask. Remove the surgical face mask by tilting the head slightly forward, grasping first the bottom tie or elastic strap, then the top tie or elastic strap, and remove the front of the surgical face mask without touching it. Discard the surgical face mask into the designated leak-proof infectious waste container.
10. Disinfect and remove inner gloves. Disinfect inner-gloved hands with either an EPA-registered disinfectant wipe or ABHR. Remove and discard gloves, taking care not to contaminate bare hands during the removal process. Dispose of inner gloves into the designated leak-proof infectious waste container.
11. Perform hand hygiene. Perform hand hygiene with ABHR.
12. Inspect. The HCW should inspect for any contamination of the surgical scrubs or disposable garments. If there is contamination, shower immediately, and then immediately inform the infection preventionist, occupational safety and health coordinator, or their designee.

OCCUPATIONAL DISEASE EXPOSURE

Occupationally acquired infections cause considerable morbidity and mortality among HCWs, despite OSHA requirements for precautions. Given the often occult manifestation of disease in the ED patient population, emergency HCWs are at high risk for exposure to infectious diseases. There is a high prevalence of HIV, HBV, HCV, pulmonary TB, and respiratory viruses in ED patients, as well as associated high morbidity and mortality. This section focuses on these particular diseases and provider risks.

HBV

Transmission

HBV is a well-recognized occupational risk for health care providers, and multiple studies have documented the high prevalence of hepatitis in ED patients.[46–48] Despite the attention focused on transmission of HIV, the infectivity of HBV is significantly higher. HBV is a more virulent organism and requires a relatively small inoculum for transmission.[49] Percutaneous injuries are the most efficient mode of HBV transmission and the risk of transmission is 6% to 30% depending on source serology and HCW vaccination/immunity status.[50,51] Many body fluids other than blood contain hepatitis B surface antigen (HBsAg), and levels of infectious HBV particles in blood-free body fluids are 100 to 1000 times lower than in blood itself. Implementation of the CDC's standard precautions, along with the OSHA regulations for barrier protection and preexposure vaccination, has led to a decrease in the incidence of HBV transmission.[52]

To understand the risk of HBV transmission resulting from occupational exposure, an understanding of a few key serologic markers for HBV is essential. HBsAg is a marker of active infection in the source patient. From a practical standpoint, HBV can be transmitted when HBsAg is present, and it is not generally transmissible when this marker is absent. Hepatitis B surface antibody is a protective antibody against HBV. In vaccinating HCWs, the goal is to stimulate the immune system prior to accidental exposure, to produce a sufficient quantity of this antibody to protect the individual if exposed to the virus. Hepatitis B e antigen (HBeAg) can be found in the bloodstream of HBV-infected individuals during times of peak virus replication. The risk for clinical hepatitis is approximately 2% (range, 1% to 6%) if HBeAg is absent, as opposed to a risk of 22% to 31% if HBeAg is present.[53] Yet testing occupational exposure–source patients for HBeAg is not recommended.[53]

Postexposure Management

Wounds and skin sites that have been in contact with blood or body fluids should be washed with soap and water; mucous membranes should be flushed with water. Using antiseptics (e.g., 2% to 4% chlorhexidine) for wound care or expressing fluid by squeezing the wound further have not been shown to reduce the risk for HBV transmission; however, the use of antiseptics is not contraindicated.[54] PEP following exposure to an HBsAg-positive source may require hepatitis B vaccine, hepatitis B immunoglobulin (HBIG), both, or neither (Table 69.2). This depends on the vaccination and antibody response status of the exposed HCW. HBIG is derived from pooled human plasma and provides passive immunization for nonimmune-exposed individuals. When HBIG is used for PEP, give it ideally within 24 hours after exposure, and note that it is of questionable value beyond 7 days.[53,54] PEP for HBV is remarkably effective, and infection is unlikely to develop in individuals who receive PEP.[53] Hepatitis B vaccine may also be given with PEP. Individuals who have not previously been vaccinated or who have not demonstrated an adequate response should receive the hepatitis B vaccine.[54] Adverse reactions to the hepatitis B vaccine are generally mild,

TABLE 69.2 Postexposure Management of Health Care Personnel After Occupational Percutaneous and Mucosal Exposure to Blood and Body Fluids, by Health Care Personnel: HepB Vaccination and Response Status

	Postexposure Testing		Postexposure Prophylaxis		
HCP STATUS	SOURCE PATIENT (HBsAg)	HCP TESTING (ANTI-HBS)	HBIG[a]	VACCINATION	POSTVACCINATION SEROLOGIC TESTING[b]
Documented responder[c] after complete series (≥3 doses)	No action needed				
Documented nonresponder[d] after six doses	Positive/unknown	—[e]	HBIG × 2 separated by 1 month	—	No
	Negative	No action needed			
Response unknown after three doses	Positive/unknown	<10 mIU/mL[e]	HBIG × 1	Initiate revaccination	Yes
	Negative	<10 mIU/mL	None		
	Any result	≥10 mIU/mL	No action needed		
Unvaccinated, incompletely vaccinated, or vaccine refusers	Positive/unknown	—[e]	HBIG × 1	Complete vaccination	Yes
	Negative	—	None	Complete vaccination	Yes

[a]HBIG should be administered intramuscularly as soon as possible after exposure when indicated. The effectiveness of HBIG when administered >7 days after percutaneous, mucosal, or nonintact skin exposures is unknown. HBIG dosage is 0.06 mL/kg.
[b]Should be performed 1–2 months after the last dose of the HepB vaccine series (and 4–6 months after administration of HBIG to avoid detection of passively administered anti-HBs) using a quantitative method that allows detection of the protective concentration of anti-HBs (≥10 mIU/mL).
[c]A responder is defined as a person with anti-HBs ≥10 mIU/mL after ≥3 doses of HepB vaccine.
[d]A nonresponder is defined as a person with anti-HBs <10 mIU/mL after ≥6 doses of HepB vaccine.
[e]HCP who have anti-HBs <10 mIU/mL, or who are unvaccinated or incompletely vaccinated, and sustain an exposure to a source patient who is HBsAg-positive or has unknown HBsAg status, should undergo baseline testing for HBV infection as soon as possible after exposure, and follow-up testing approximately 6 months later. Initial baseline tests consist of total anti-HBc; testing at approximately 6 months consists of HBsAg and total anti-HBc.
Anti-HBc, Hepatitis B core antibodies; *anti-HBs*, antibody to hepatitis B surface antigen; *HBIG*, hepatitis B immune globulin; *HBsAg*, hepatitis B surface antigen; *HCP*, health care personnel.
From Schillie S, Vellozzi C, Reingold A et al. Prevention of hepatitis B virus infection in the United States: recommendations of the Advisory Committee on Immunization Practices. *MMWR Recomm Rep*. 2018;67(No. RR-1):1-31.

and it is safe to give during pregnancy. For primary immunization, give an initial intramuscular injection, followed by subsequent intramuscular vaccinations at 1 and 6 months. There is no need to provide vaccination or to check titers in individuals who have previously had an adequate titer.[52,54] PEP with these agents is not contraindicated during pregnancy or lactation. HCWs who have previously been infected with HBV are immune to reinfection, so PEP is not indicated.

HCV

Transmission

The estimate of the number of US residents with active HCV from 2013 to 2016 was at least 2.4 million,[55] and many individuals are unaware of their infection.[56] ED patients have a high prevalence of HCV.[3] HCV is acquired through exposure to infected blood: injection drug use, birth, uncommonly sexually, unregulated tattoos/piercings, and rarely through blood transfusions. Mucous membrane transmission of HCV is possible but much less common.[57] Percutaneous transmission is the most efficient route. The incidence of seroconversion after an HCV-positive needlestick is approximately 0.2% based on recent analysis of several studies[57] (estimates previously ranged from 0% to 7%).[58,59] When seroconversion does occur, 80% of patients will demonstrate antibodies at 15 weeks and 97% at 6 months after exposure. Although the clinical course of HCV is often asymptomatic or mild, cirrhosis develops in 10% to 20%, and in those patients, the annual risk of hepatocellular carcinoma is 1% to 5%.[60]

Postexposure Management

Currently, PEP for HCV exposure is not approved or available. Instead, both the source patient and the HCW should be tested for HCV RNA or hepatitis C antibodies within 48 hours.[61] HCWs who become infected with HCV should be referred for care consistent with current AASLD/IDSA guidelines for evaluation and treatment of all persons with acute or chronic HCV infection.[62] The HCV exhibits a high degree of genetic heterogeneity and a very rapid mutation rate, making the development of a vaccine challenging but work is ongoing.[63,64] There is now an effective treatment for HCV, direct-acting antivirals (DAAs). While costly, these treatments have shown high rates of safety, tolerability, and efficacy against HCV,[65] are curative in 95% of cases, and have been shown to decrease mortality.[66]

HIV

Transmission

The number of occupational exposures to HIV reported to the CDC has steadily decreased. As of December 2013, 58 confirmed occupational transmissions of HIV had been reported since 1985 and only 1 since 1999.[67] In 2010 one additional case of occupational HIV transmission was reported to the CDC.[68] The risk for contracting HIV from working in the ED depends on the prevalence of HIV in the local patient population. The overall risk for HIV seroconversion is approximately 0.23% after a needlestick injury and 0.03% for mucocutaneous transmission. Unless visibly bloody, saliva, vomitus, urine, feces, sweat, tears, and respiratory secretions do not transmit HIV. The risk of HIV infection through intact skin is negligible.[69] Cardo and colleagues[70] demonstrated that the risk for HIV seroconversion after needlestick injuries is not uniform. Seroconversion was found to be more likely for deep injuries (odds ratio [OR] = 15), if blood was visible on the device (OR = 6.2), if the needle had been used in a source patient's artery or vein (OR = 4.3), or if the source patient had terminal acquired immunodeficiency syndrome (OR = 5.6). It is essential to gather information regarding the nature of the injury to risk-stratify the exposure.

When seroconversion occurs, HIV antibodies can be detected as early as 3 weeks after exposure and are almost always present by 6 months. Acute retroviral syndrome is a clinical manifestation of HIV seroconversion that occurs in approximately 80% of newly infected individuals at a median of 25 days after exposure. The signs and symptoms of acute retroviral syndrome are similar to those of mononucleosis and consist of fever, lymphadenopathy, and rash.

Postexposure Management

Evidence Supporting PEP

In 1998 the US Public Health Service first recommended using PEP for selected HIV exposures.[71,72] These recommendations were based on a single case-control study.[70] Currently, a large placebo-controlled trial would be considered unethical. The CDC-sponsored case-control study, undertaken in the United States, France, the United Kingdom, and Italy, compared 33 HCWs who seroconverted after exposure to HIV with 665 control HCWs who did not seroconvert after exposure to HIV. Approximately 90% of the patients in this study were exposed via hollow-bore needles.[70] When postexposure zidovudine (azidothymidine) was used, the risk for HIV infection was reduced by 81% (95% confidence interval, 48% to 94%).

Selecting Patients for PEP

In 2018 the US Public Health Service published updated recommendations regarding the use of HIV PEP.[71] In general, the decision to use PEP depends on the type of exposure and the source's HIV status. The first step in determining whether PEP is indicated is to assess the severity of exposure. Percutaneous exposure can be categorized as "less severe" or "more severe." A less severe exposure involves a solid needle, a superficial injury, and no blood visible on the device. All other percutaneous injuries are categorized as more severe. Exposure to mucous membranes and nonintact skin is categorized as either "small volume" (a few drops of blood) or "large volume" (a major blood splash). There are no reported cases of HIV seroconversion after exposure of intact skin to blood.[70,71] After assessing the severity of exposure, determine the potential infectivity of the source. The US Public Health Service emphasizes the importance of determining the HIV status of the exposure source.[71] Consider PEP only for exposure to blood and body fluids from a source known or likely to be HIV positive. Exposure from an HIV-negative source does not require PEP. Do not test sharp instruments for HIV because this is not reliable or recommended. Note that drug development is ongoing and recommendations change rapidly. The clinician is urged to periodically check for updates. The most reliable source is the CDC website or the *Morbidity and Mortality Weekly Report* journals, most easily found via an Internet search under various topics.

A number of special circumstances may arise when determining the need for HIV PEP. Rapid HIV testing of the source can be used to help determine the need for PEP, but the patient's risk for having the infection or possibly recently

TABLE 69.3 HIV PEP Regimens

Preferred HIV PEP regimen	Truvada 1 tablet by mouth once daily (co-formulated Tenofovir DF [Viread; TDF] 300 mg + emtricitabine [Emtriva; FTC] 200 mg) *plus* Raltegravir (Isentress; RAL) 400 mg by mouth twice daily *or* Dolutegravir (Tivicay; DTG) 50 mg by mouth once daily *Note: Dolutegravir should not be given to females in their first trimester of pregnancy or females of childbearing potential.*
Preferred in renal dysfunction (CrCl < 60 mL/min)	Zidovudine plus lamivudine (co-formulated as Combivir) Plus Raltegravir or dolutegravir
Alternative regimens[a] *May combine one drug or drug pair from the left column with one pair of nucleoside/nucleotide reverse transcriptase inhibitors from the right column.* Raltegravir (Isentress; RAL) Dolutegravir (Tivicay; DTG) Darunavir (Prezista; DRV) + ritonavir (Norvir; RTV) Etravirine (Intelence; ETR) Rilpivirine (Edurant; RPV) Atazanavir (Reyataz; ATV) + ritonavir (Norvir; RTV) Lopinavir/ritonavir (Kaletra; LPV/RTV)	Tenofovir DF (Viread; TDF) + emtricitabine (Emtriva; FTC); available co-formulated as Truvada Tenofovir DF (Viread; TDF) + lamivudine (Epivir; 3TC); available co-formulated as Cimduo Zidovudine (Retrovir; ZDV; AZT) + lamivudine (Epivir; 3TC); available co-formulated as Combivir Zidovudine (Retrovir; ZDV; AZT) + emtrictabine (Emtriva; FTC)

[a]The alternative regimens are listed in order of USPHS preference. Newer antiretroviral medications have become available since the USPHS occupational PEP guidelines were updated in 2018, and other alternatives using these newer medications may be reasonable based upon patient and clinician preference. http://nccc.ucsf.edu/clinician-consultation/pep-post-exposure-prophylaxis/.

For consultation or assistance with HIV PEP contact the National Clinicians' Post-Exposure Prophylaxis Hotline at telephone number 888-448-4911 or visit its website at http://nccc.ucsf.edu/clinician-consultation/pep-post-exposure-prophylaxis/.

HIV, Human immunodeficiency virus; *PEP,* postexposure prophylaxis.

Data from Kuhar DT, Henderson DK, Struble KA et al. Updated US Public Health Service guidelines for the management of occupational exposures to human immunodeficiency virus and recommendations for postexposure prophylaxis, *Infect Control Hosp Epidemiol.* 2018;34(9):875-892.

being infected must be taken into account. When a source is known but an individual's HIV status is pending, decide about the use of PEP on a case-by-case basis. When the source is high risk, initiate PEP and then stop or modify it later once the HIV status of the source is determined. When a source can be identified but the HIV status of the source is unknown and will not become available, PEP is not generally recommended. However, if it is unknown whether the source constitutes a significant risk and consultation is not available within a few hours, it is recommended to begin PEP and obtain consultation later.[71]

Choice of PEP Medications

The US Public Health Service recommends that PEP medication regimens begin as soon as possible, and within 72 hours, after the exposure and should be continued for 4 weeks. When HIV PEP is administered, a minimum of three drugs is recommended.[71] The current preferred three-drug HIV PEP regimen includes raltegravir, tenofovir, and emtricitabine (Table 69.3).

A number of second-line and alternative agents may be chosen for HIV PEP including for patients with renal dysfunction. Expert consultation is recommended, especially if antiretroviral (ARV) resistance is suspected. Pregnancy and breastfeeding are not contraindications to taking ARV agents and PEP is recommended.[71–73] Consult an infectious diseases or occupational health specialist when treating pregnant and lactating patients, as alternative regimens may be considered. Enter all pregnant females starting ARVs in the Antiretroviral Pregnancy Registry, a database designed to collect information on the outcomes of ARV-exposed pregnancies regardless of HIV status: http://www.apregistry.com. ARV agents can be used in pediatric patients for occupational and nonoccupational exposure; however, consultation is recommended.[74,75] For consultation or assistance with HIV PEP, contact the National Clinicians' Post-Exposure Prophylaxis Hotline, telephone number 888-448-4911 or visit its website at http://nccc.ucsf.edu/clinician-consultation/pep-post-exposure-prophylaxis/.

Timing, Duration, and Side Effects of PEP

HIV exposure should be considered a true emergency. Administer PEP as soon as possible after exposure, ideally within hours of exposure. Animal studies indicate that the efficacy of PEP diminishes with a delay in initiation.[76,77] HIV PEP regimens consist of a 28-day course of therapy. In the ED, patients can be prescribed the first 3 days of medications, and outpatient follow-up should be arranged within 72 hours.[71] Side effects from the medications used for HIV PEP are not insignificant. However, the current recommended three-drug regimen is better tolerated than earlier zidovudine-containing regimens.[78] Depending on the choice of PEP medications, patients should also be prescribed antiemetics and antidiarrheal agents when PEP is initiated.

Tuberculosis

Transmission

During the mid-1980s the United States experienced a resurgence in TB, especially among HIV-positive patients. The incidence of TB cases has declined gradually in the United States since 1993, with a slight rise in reported cases in 2022 of 8300,[79] and the risk of acquiring TB from occupational exposure is now very low.[80] TB is transmitted by infectious droplets 1 µm to 5 µm in size. Primary infection occurs when one to three organisms are inhaled into the alveoli, where they begin to replicate. Host defenses usually stop infection within 2 to 10 weeks, and the patient enters the latent period. During this time, patients are asymptomatic and not contagious. Reactivation occurs when cell-mediated immunity wanes, and patients are again contagious. This can be due to advancing age, HIV infection, steroid use, malignancy, malnutrition, or other causes of suppression of the immune system. The lifetime risk for reactivation is 5% to 10%, with approximately half this risk occurring in the first few years after primary infection. Patients with increased infectivity include those with pulmonary or laryngeal TB, an active cough, positive sputum smears for acid-fast bacilli, cavitary lesions on chest radiographs, and inadequate therapy. Overall, children are less contagious than adults, but can still transmit the disease. Extrapulmonary TB is contagious only in cases of an open skin lesion or involvement of the oral cavity.[81]

Depending on the patient population and geographic location, ED personnel may be at higher risk for occupational TB infection than other HCWs. In a 1993 study at a county hospital in Los Angeles, it was reported that 31% of ED workers became positive for purified protein derivative (PPD) during their employment.[82] EDs typically care for higher-risk patients: those who are experiencing homelessness, foreign born, recently incarcerated, or chronically debilitated. Overcrowding can lead to extended waiting periods and delays in admission. The clinical manifestation of TB in ED patients is often atypical, which can lead to a delay in diagnosis.[83,84] Delayed ED diagnosis of pulmonary TB is associated with factors such as the COVID pandemic, recent antibiotics, older age, renal insufficiency, preexisting chronic lung disease, HIV, homelessness, or substance abuse.[85–89] While overall rates in the United States may be declining, a 14-year review of the US National Tuberculosis Surveillance System showed that rates of advanced pulmonary TB may be on the rise in populations without traditional risk factors.[90] These data suggest that substantial delays in diagnosis and misdiagnosis of pulmonary TB may be increasing.

Preventing exposure to TB requires a multifaceted approach.[81] Proper ED ventilation plays a key role; inadequate ventilation has been a contributing factor in many nosocomial outbreaks. Ideally, install single-pass airflow from waiting rooms to the outside. Within the ED, make sure that air flows from clean areas to less clean areas, not vice versa. If patients with TB are seen frequently, provide at least one true respiratory isolation room in the ED. Make sure that such rooms have at least 12 air changes per hour and that they are "negative pressure" rooms in which air flows into the room from other ED areas. Other engineering approaches for control of TB infection include using HEPA filters and upper-room ultraviolet light irradiation.

Familiarize all ED personnel with the appropriate use of respiratory protection against TB. Provide surgical masks for source control. Place these masks on potentially contagious patients to decrease the passage of infectious droplets into the air. Because air can leak around such masks, they are not optimal for protection of HCWs. N95 respirators[91] filter particles 1 µm in size with at least 95% efficiency and are the preferred mask for HCWs (Fig. 69.9) especially when source patients are undergoing cough-inducing or aerosol-generating procedures. HCWs should undergo occupational health N95 fit testing to ensure appropriate N95 selection.

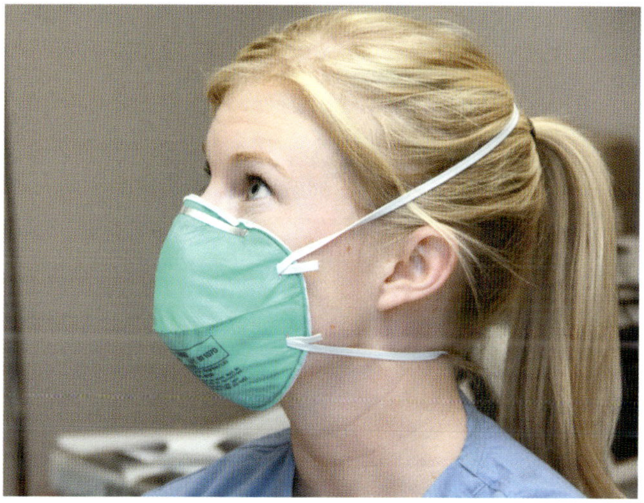

Fig. 69.9 N95 particulate respirators are the preferred mask for health care workers caring for patients who potentially have tuberculosis.

Initiate early respiratory isolation of patients with suspected pulmonary TB as soon as possible in the ED, ideally at triage. Screening protocols at triage can detect patients with more classic signs and symptoms of TB, but reported protocols are only moderately sensitive and somewhat cumbersome.[83,84] Consider immediate respiratory isolation for patients with high-risk chief complaints and those with hemoptysis, weight loss, or a prolonged cough. Also be aware of patients with HIV, with a history of TB, or from high-risk populations who have a cough or fever.[81] The best guideline is to initiate respiratory isolation as soon as TB is a possible diagnosis. Place masks on such patients before obtaining chest radiographs. Consider isolating patients with chest radiograph findings of an apical infiltrate, cavitary lesions, extensive hilar or mediastinal lymphadenopathy, pleural disease, or a miliary pattern.[92–95]

Postexposure Management

All HCW personnel should have baseline TB screening and individual risk assessment.

If HCWs without proper PPE are exposed to patients with active pulmonary TB, refer them to either employee health care or their primary care clinician for follow-up testing and treatment.

For HCWs with a baseline negative TB test and no prior TB disease/latent TB, either an interferon-gamma release assay or a tuberculin skin test (TST) should be performed within days after exposure. If that test is negative, perform another test (of the same type) 8 to 10 weeks after the last exposure. A positive TST (≥10-mm induration) indicates previous exposure or infection. A positive TST consists of 5-mm induration after a negative baseline test or an increase to at least 10-mm induration after a baseline test of 1- to 9-mm induration.

HCWs in whom a TB test converts to positive after an exposure should undergo symptom evaluation and chest radiography to screen for active pulmonary TB.[96] HCWs with a prior positive TB test and a documented normal chest radiograph do not require a repeat radiograph unless they are symptomatic or are starting treatment.[97] If active disease is present, initiate treatment with at least four antituberculous medications. In TB test converters who do not have active disease on radiography, chemoprophylaxis is strongly recommended unless contraindicated.[98,99] Both the CDC and the National Tuberculosis Controllers Association (NTCA) recommend short-course, 3- or 4-month rifamycin-based treatment regimens over the 6- to 9-month isoniazid treatment due to higher adherence rates and less hepatotoxicity.[100] The options for short-course regimens include:

- Three months of once-weekly isoniazid plus rifapentine (3HP)
- Four months of daily rifampin (4R)
- Three months of daily isoniazid plus rifampin (3HR)

Some HCWs may become exposed to strains of TB that are resistant to these treatment options because of the continued emergence of multidrug-resistant and extensively drug-resistant strains of TB.[101] For exposure to multidrug-resistant TB, consult an expert when selecting an individualized chemoprophylaxis regimen. Baseline and serial liver function testing is not necessary for administration of chemoprophylaxis in most cases, but the HCW must be monitored closely for clinical symptoms suggestive of hepatotoxicity.

In the absence of TB exposure, updated CDC guidelines no longer recommend routine annual HCW screenings.[96] Health care facilities may consider using serial TB screening of certain groups that may be at increased occupational risk for TB exposure (e.g., pulmonologists or respiratory therapists) or in certain settings if transmission has occurred in the past (e.g., EDs).

Novel Respiratory Pathogens

Transmission

There have been multiple worldwide outbreaks from novel respiratory pathogens including the 2002–2004 outbreak of SARS caused by a coronavirus (SARS-CoV-1) as well as the more recent worldwide COVID-19 pandemic from another coronavirus, SARS-CoV-2. While transmission of most respiratory pathogens is via droplets, there has been concern about the potential for airborne transmission, especially for novel viruses.

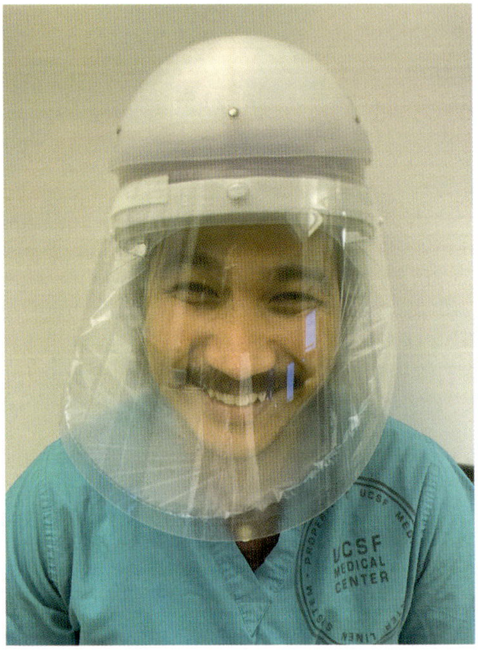

Fig. 69.10 Powered air purifying respirator.

Prevention

Due to the concern that novel respiratory viruses may be spread via airborne route, when there are an absence of data at the start of an outbreak, it is recommended that HCW utilize full airborne PPE with powered air purifying respirator (PAPR) (see Fig. 69.10) or N95 mask plus eye protection especially when performing aerosol-generating procedures, plus droplet precautions, plus contact precautions with all patient encounters.[102] Prevention guidelines often change as more information is learned about novel viruses, how they are transmitted and the development and administration of vaccinations. It is essential for HCWs to closely follow the recommendations provided by local and national guidelines, as they are regularly updated to reflect the most current knowledge and understanding of novel respiratory viruses.

REFERENCES ARE AVAILABLE AT Elsevier eBooks+

CHAPTER 70

Physical and Chemical Restraint

J. Michael Kowalski

INTRODUCTION

Emergency clinicians often face the challenge of caring for agitated, uncooperative, and violent patients who are unable to participate in their care, make rational health care decisions, and/or are a danger to themselves and others.[1,2] Psychiatric illness, acute chemical intoxication or withdrawal, delirium, medical illness, uncontrolled rage, hypoxia, and, rarely, central nervous system infection are causes of agitated or violent behavior in the emergency department (ED).[1]

BACKGROUND

Patients more likely to exhibit severe uncontrolled agitation are those who are experiencing intoxication or who have ingested sympathomimetic agents such as cocaine or methamphetamines, designer drugs such as ecstasy (3,4-methyle nedioxy-*N*-methamphetamine [MDMA]), mephedrone, or methylone (bath salts). or hallucinogenic drugs such as phencyclidine (PCP). Patients can also experience toxicity after accidental and intentional ingestion of medications. Drug-associated delirium may be related to anticholinergic toxicity, serotonin syndrome, or intoxication with sympathomimetics. Alcohol withdrawal may progress to delirium tremens, a condition typified by excessive agitation and confusion.

Patients who are agitated, confused, and combative are often the most difficult to manage and at high risk for significant morbidity and mortality. Causes of undifferentiated agitated delirium may include manic-depressive disorder, psychosis, decompensated schizophrenia, intoxication with sympathomimetics or anticholinergics, cocaine intoxication, alcohol or benzodiazepine withdrawal, hypoglycemia, the postictal state, or head trauma. Some causes are idiopathic, but many are due to a combination of underlying psychiatric illness and stimulant drugs or alcohol (or both). Because of the variety of causes, management of agitated and combative patients requires a systematic approach (Fig. 70.1).

Schizophrenia, schizoaffective disorder, and the manic phase of bipolar disorder can all lead to an impaired perception of reality. Paranoid delusions, hallucinations, and hostile moods that can easily lead to severe agitation often develop in patients with these disorders.

Any medical condition that leads to brain dysfunction may also result in agitated, combative, or violent behavior (Box 70.1). Well-documented examples include hypoglycemia, hypoxia, medication intoxication, encephalitis, meningitis, intracranial hemorrhage, thyrotoxicosis, traumatic brain injury, febrile illnesses in older adults, and dementia.[3]

It is essential to achieve control of an agitated patient as quickly as possible. Goals of management include preventing patients from harming themselves and others, identifying the underlying cause, and initiating medical treatment. Early intervention allows caregivers to implement appropriate monitoring, perform a physical examination, initiate diagnostic testing, and institute timely treatment. When more conservative measures fail (e.g., reasoning, de-escalation techniques), achieving these goals often necessitates physical and chemical restraint.

During the late 1980s and early 1990s, reports of restraint-associated deaths in psychiatric and extended care facilities[4] led lawmakers to pass legislation establishing regulations for the use of restraint.[5] Since then, the Joint Commission for Accreditation of Healthcare Organizations (TJC) and the Center for Medicare and Medicaid Services (CMS) have created standards governing the use of restraint in a variety of health care settings, including EDs and tertiary care facilities (Box 70.2).[6,7] The aforementioned standards allow the use of physical restraint for a limited period. A licensed practitioner must evaluate the patient and determine that less restrictive interventions have been ineffective and physical restraint is required to ensure the patient's well-being. The standards also include requirements for written policies and procedures governing the use of restraint that must address indications, staff training and education, patient assessment and reevaluation, appropriate documentation, and patient-focused issues such as maintaining dignity and respect. Hospitals and extended care facilities are required by law to report any death or adverse event related to the use of restraint.[6]

Some authors have advocated "restraint-free" environments in nursing homes, extended care facilities, and acute care hospitals.[8] Although this concept is laudable, mandating a restraint-free ED is impractical and potentially dangerous. Clinicians should recognize the risks associated with restraining a patient; however, they should not be deterred from using either physical or chemical restraint when patients demonstrate dangerous behavior toward themselves or others. Indeed, the American College of Emergency Physicians (ACEP) recently revised and approved their policy statement in 2020 by supporting the careful and appropriate use of chemical and physical restraint.[9]

Hyperactive Delirium with Severe Agitation

The term excited delirium syndrome (ExDS) has become increasingly controversial since the last publication of this text. Concerns have been raised by communities and national medical organizations that the use of this term contributes to bias and further endangers vulnerable patients.[10] The American Psychiatric Association (APA) highlighted their concern in a 2020 position statement in which they state that ExDS, "has been invoked to explain or justify injury or death to individuals in police custody".[11]

The term ExDS was first used in the 1980s to explain deaths in police custody. In 2009 an ACEP task force published a multiauthored White Paper Report on ExDS.[12] The task force sought to legitimize a heretofore poorly defined serious medical scenario that was familiar to law enforcement, emergency medical services, and emergency physicians. It was the consensus of the task force that ExDS was a unique syndrome that may be identified by the presence of a distinctive group of clinical and behavioral characteristics that can be recognized in the premortem state. The report supported the aggressive and potentially lifesaving use of chemical sedation.

Recent controversy surrounding ExDS prompted a reevaluation of the terminology used to describe patients in this state of confusion.[13] Many in the medical and legal

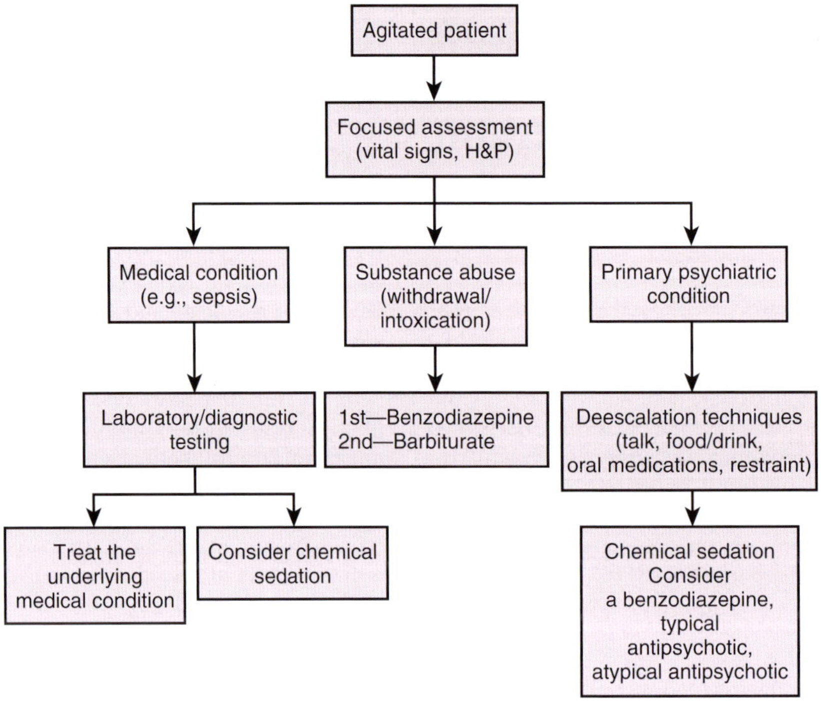

Fig. 70.1 Approach to undifferentiated delirium in the emergency department. Intramuscular benzodiazepines and antipsychotic agents (alone or in combination), and intramuscular/intravenous ketamine may be used for the treatment of acute agitation or violence in the emergency department. *H&P,* History and physical examination. (Adapted from Rund DA, Ewing JD, Mitzel K, et al. The use of intramuscular benzodiazepines and antipsychotic agents in the treatment of acute agitation or violence in the emergency department. *J Emerg Med.* 2006;31:317-324.)

communities are seeking to ban use of the term ExDS. The American Medical Association adopted a policy in 2021 opposing use of "excited delirium" as a medical diagnosis.[10] The ACEP recruited a Hyperactive Delirium Task Force that issued a new report in 2021.[14] In this paper, *Hyperactive Delirium with Severe Agitation* was proposed as a descriptive term to alert the medical team that a potentially fatal constellation of symptoms exists and requires immediate intervention. The ACEP Board of Directors approved this term in 2021, and for uniformity, the remainder of this chapter will replace ExDS with hyperactive delirium with severe agitation.

Features of hyperactive delirium with severe agitation may include aggression and agitation, pain tolerance, tachypnea, tachycardia, sweating, tactile hyperthermia, inability to follow directions, endurance, being inappropriately clothed, and an attraction to reflective surfaces.[14] Individuals are unable to engage in rational discussion or understand or deescalate their abnormal aggressive, violent, and threatening behavior. Potential laboratory findings may include acute kidney injury, hyperkalemia, acidosis, rhabdomyolysis, or disseminated intravascular coagulation.[14] A scenario characterized by a period of extreme delirium, increasing agitation, and inability to reason or comply with efforts to control their agitated state may be followed by a struggle with law enforcement that involves vigorous physical restraint (choke holds, hog-tying, prone positioning, knee to the throat), and noxious chemicals and can lead to death. The exact role that restraint plays in these cases has yet to be elucidated.[13,15–17] The use of the TASER device to control violent and markedly agitated individuals has been temporally related to death, but the role of this device in causing death is also unproven. Intervention may be followed by a sudden cessation of struggling that may herald death by cardiopulmonary arrest.

Fatalities in patients with hyperactive delirium with severe agitation may be related to underlying but unknown pathology (such as cardiomyopathy, conduction abnormalities, and metabolic disturbances). Lack of complete prior medical information, especially underlying cardiac abnormalities, hampers determination of a true cause of death.

Stimulant drug use, including cocaine, methamphetamine, and PCP, has a well-established association with hyperactive delirium with severe agitation and is usually implicated as being closely linked to, if not causative of, fatalities. Persons with psychiatric illnesses represent the second largest, but distinctly smaller cohort of hyperactive delirium with severe agitation cases. The combination of drugs, alcohol, and psychiatric illness is well recognized.

Currently, this disease state is identified by clinical features, has different inciting factors, and is sometimes handled exclusively prehospital. These factors render it difficult to ascertain the true incidence. Though not universally fatal, a proportion of individuals exhibiting hyperactive delirium with severe agitation can progress to cardiac arrest and death regardless of medical intervention.

The specific precipitants of fatal hyperactive delirium with severe agitation remain unclear, though epidemiologic and clinical reports provide some understanding of the underlying pathophysiology. The clinical picture is one of an agitated and delirious state with severe autonomic dysregulation. When available, cardiac rhythm analysis demonstrates bradycardic asystole; ventricular dysrhythmias are rare. Severe acidosis and hyperthermia appear to play a prominent role in lethal hyperactive delirium with severe agitation–associated

BOX 70.1 Conditions That May Cause Agitated and Violent Behavior

ENDOCRINE
Hypoglycemia
Hyperglycemia
Thyrotoxicosis, thyroid storm
Myxedema

INFECTIOUS
Meningitis
Encephalitis
Sepsis
Urinary tract infection

TOXICOLOGIC
Acute alcohol intoxication
Sympathomimetic intoxication
Anticholinergic intoxication
Delirium tremens
Alcohol withdrawal
Benzodiazepine withdrawal
Narcotic withdrawal

TRAUMATIC
Intracranial hemorrhage
Diffuse axonal injury
Hypoxia
Low-flow states secondary to systemic hemorrhage

METABOLIC
Hypoxia
Hypercapnia
Hyponatremia
Hypernatremia

NEUROLOGIC
Status epilepticus
Postictal states
Acute delirium
Subarachnoid hemorrhage
Cerebral vascular accident

cardiovascular collapse. Another potential cause is thought to be excessive central dopamine stimulation.

Use of the term "hyperactive delirium with severe agitation" should alert the care team of the existence of a disease process that, if left untreated, could progress to a fatal condition. This is analogous to a toxidrome or syndrome, a predictable constellation of symptoms, which serves to conjure a mental picture that facilitates the medical team to intervene, stabilize, and seek out reversible causes before the patient deteriorates. This condition should be considered undifferentiated and an inciting etiology should be sought and treated. The care team should promote a stepwise, respectful approach to the patient who is confused, agitated, and potentially unstable. If safe to do so, use verbal or nonverbal de-escalation techniques first. If unsuccessful, proceed to physical and/or chemical restraint. All this should occur while concurrently seeking a reversible etiology that can be treated.

BOX 70.2 The Joint Commission Requirements for Patient Restraint Protocols and Documentation

RESTRAINT PROTOCOLS SHOULD INCLUDE
Guidelines for assessing the patient
Criteria for applying restraint
Criteria for monitoring the patient and reassessing the need for restraint
Monitoring at least every 2 hours or sooner based on patient needs
Criteria for terminating restraint

DOCUMENTATION SHOULD INCLUDE
Relevant orders for use
Results of patient monitoring
Reassessment
Significant changes in the patient's condition

MEDICOLEGAL CONCERNS

Emergency clinicians need to be cognizant of the potential legal ramifications stemming from physically restraining patients. The risk for litigation may be mitigated by strict adherence to written institutional and departmental policies regarding the use of restraint and medications. Unfortunately, no one-size-fits-all protocol is realistic, and each case must be individualized by a clinician at the bedside, often with little data or background on which to base a specific intervention. Emphasis should be placed on timely and comprehensive assessment before restraint, regular patient reevaluation, limitations on the time spent in restraint, and detailed documentation in the ED record. Furthermore, clinicians need to recognize that *patients with decision-making capacity* have the legal right to refuse medical treatment even if the result of their refusal is death or serious bodily harm. Capacity, however, may be difficult to evaluate or ascertain in the time frame required to make important clinical decisions. There are many gray areas that cannot simply be solved by attempting to obtain a formal psychiatric consultation. In fact, there are no data proving that a psychiatrist is any better than an emergency physician in determining capacity in an ED patient within the time frame of the ED evaluation, when important decisions must be made. Individuals with true hyperactive delirium with severe agitation are clearly mentally incompetent, but coercive measures, including physical restraint or the threat of physical restraint, should not be used simply because a patient with capacity refuses treatment or as retaliation for perceived disruptive behavior.[18] Restraining patients can leave them feeling dehumanized and emotionally traumatized, whereas chemical sedation has helped to maintain a sense of dignity and respect.[19] Implicit bias may also influence who is placed in restraints. In an effort to minimize subjectivity and ensure patients are treated equally, a "restraint checklist" has been proposed for the emergency setting (Box 70.3).[20]

PATIENT ASSESSMENT

Emergency clinicians must avoid ascribing agitated or abusive behavior to drug or alcohol intoxication or underlying

BOX 70.3 Restraint Checklist Designed to Minimize Bias and Ensure Equal Treatment

- Have I tried to listen to the patient's desires, employ verbal de-escalation, and other alternatives to chemical/physical restraints (e.g., food/drink)?
- Is a different staff member, outside of myself or the patient's primary care team, better at de-escalating this patient based on demographic similarities?
- Is my fear of this patient exaggerated by their appearance?
- Are there cultural differences in the patient's expression of frustration and control?
- Am I using racial, gender/sex, socioeconomic, or other potentially harmful bias in determining my agitation care plan for this patient?

From Five restraint checklist questions. FOCUS. *American Psychiatric Association; 2023;21(1):100-105.* *All rights reserved.*

BOX 70.4 Recommended Areas to Assess During Reevaluation of Restrained Patients

NEUROLOGIC STATUS

Level of alertness
Degree of agitation
Pupillary examination
Motor examination
Sensory examination

VASCULAR STATUS

Capillary refill
Distal pulses

VITAL SIGNS

Blood pressure
Heart rate
Respiratory rate
Oxygen saturation
Temperature

PATIENT COMFORT

Skin under and around the restraints
Hydration
Personal hygiene
Toileting needs

ASSESSMENT FOR RESTRAINT REMOVAL

psychiatric disease before considering severe, life-threatening diagnoses (see Box 70.1). Every attempt should be made to obtain a detailed history of issues related to the patient's condition, as well as the patient's past medical and psychiatric history, including medications, drug and alcohol use, and previous similar events. Such information is rarely available or accurate, thus leaving only the clinician's clinical judgment to guide therapy.

Five groups of patients have been identified as being at increased risk for an underlying medical problem: older adults, those with a history of substance abuse, patients without a previous psychiatric disorder, those with preexisting or new medical complaints, and individuals from lower socioeconomic groups.[21,22] Of these, patients with new psychiatric symptoms are especially worrisome and require careful evaluation for underlying medical illness.[23]

Physical examination should be aimed at identifying organic causes of the patient's behavior such as trauma, infection, and metabolic derangements. Rapid bedside serum glucose determination should be performed on any patient with agitated or combative behavior. Temperature measurements, preferably rectal, should be obtained as soon as possible because hyperthermia may be indicative of an underlying central nervous system infection or drug-induced toxidrome. Suspected head trauma in a patient who appears intoxicated warrants further evaluation to exclude traumatic brain injury.

Once a patient has been restrained, frequent periodic reevaluation is paramount to the patient's safety and is required by TJC (see Box 70.2).[24,25] Reevaluation of restrained patients should include a reassessment of vital signs, neurologic status, respiratory status, skin condition, and perfusion of the extremities (Box 70.4). Physical restraints should be removed as soon as the clinician has determined that patients are no longer a risk to themselves or others.

DE-ESCALATION TECHNIQUES

Coburn and Mycyk described three phases of escalating violence: anxiety, defensiveness, and, finally, physical aggression.[26] Recognition of this somewhat predictable pattern may help in defusing a difficult situation before physical or chemical restraint is necessary. Indeed, several de-escalation techniques have been shown to assist in quelling agitated and violent patients.[2]

One simple, yet effective technique is verbally engaging the patient by asking, "how can we help you?" This display of compassion on the part of the treating clinician and staff may calm the patient. Similarly, offering food and drink will often soothe an agitated patient. Along with these displays of caring and empathy, it is important to impress on the patient that violent behavior will not be tolerated and will be dealt with quickly and firmly.[2] If the patient continues to demonstrate agitated or violent behavior, enlist the aid of a family member or a specially trained individual, such as a social worker, psychiatric counselor, or member of the clergy.

If these conservative measures fail, summon hospital security to ensure the safety of the patient and staff. In these situations, security staff should not rush to the patient's bedside but instead should gather outside the door or close by, within eye contact of the patient's room. A strong show of force may calm a potentially violent patient without the need for restraint.

TYPES OF PATIENT RESTRAINT

Seclusion

The ACEP supports the appropriate use of seclusion as well as restraint when applied in a thoughtful, respectful manner and only when de-escalation measures have failed.[9] The utility of seclusion in psychiatric evaluation units and inpatient hospital wards is well documented in both adult and pediatric populations.[27–30] In the mid-1980s, seclusion was commonly used to calm combative and violent ED patients, but its popularity has declined since then.[1,31] Reasons for this decline are unclear but probably include lack of adequate space and concerns regarding provision of medical care and compliance with regulatory agencies.[31] Nevertheless, at institutions with adequate physical space and well-designed policies and procedures, seclusion may be effective for selected patients. However, it should only be utilized when other measures to ensure patient and staff safety have been unsuccessful.[32]

Seclusion involves placing agitated and violent patients in an isolated space and confining them to dedicated hospital stretchers or beds that are secured in place to prevent injury. Seclusion is often used in conjunction with chemical sedation, physical restraint, or both.[32] The seclusion room should be located near ED staff to allow continuous patient observation. Regularly reassess patients who are placed in seclusion, similar to physically restrained patients (see Box 70.4).

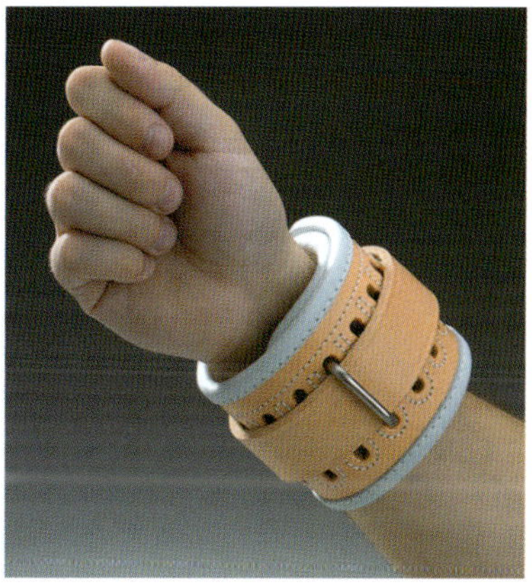

Fig. 70.2 Leather extremity restraint. (Courtesy Posey Company, Inc.)

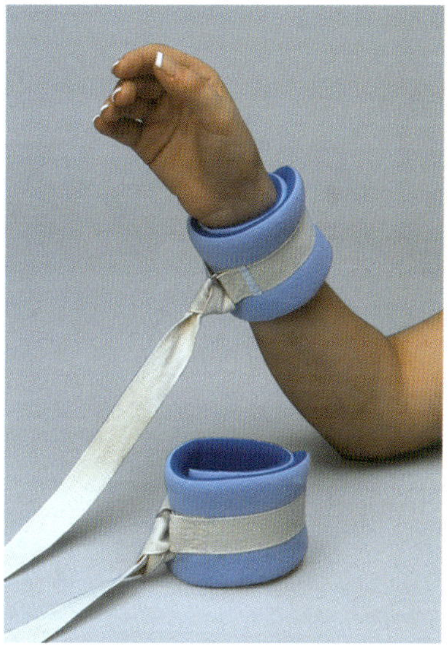

Fig. 70.3 Cotton extremity restraint. (Courtesy Posey Company, Inc.)

Physical Restraint

Research regarding the application of physical restraint in the ED is limited. In one prospective study of restraint-associated complications in 298 ED patients, minor complications occurred in only 7% of patients, and there were no serious complications or deaths.[33] The author of this study concluded that the dangers of ED patient restraint promulgated by professional organizations and health care regulators may be overstated.[33] Moreover, this study supports the safe use of restraint by emergency clinicians, who by virtue of their training and experience are experts in recognizing signs of deterioration and skilled in airway management and resuscitation. It should also be noted that TJC sentinel event tracking has demonstrated a decreased rate of complications when patients are restrained on their sides.[26]

Although the actual prevalence of patient restraint in EDs is unknown, it has been estimated that 25% of teaching hospitals physically restrain at least one person per day.[1]

Restraint Devices

Limb Holders (Restraints)

Restraining a patient's extremities is the primary method of physical restraint used in the ED. Limb restraints are constructed from a variety of materials, including leather, synthetic leather, cotton, and single-use foam material. These materials provide restraint that differs in strength, ease of removal, and cleaning.

Hard leather and synthetic leather limb holders are virtually impossible to break or tear but are difficult to sterilize if they become soiled with blood or body fluids (Fig. 70.2). They are more rigid than soft restraints, which also makes them somewhat more difficult and time-consuming to apply. More importantly, most leather limb holders require a key to unlock and, as a result, might take longer to remove after an adverse event such as vomiting or respiratory arrest. Leather limb holders are generally used to restrain combative and violent patients in whom the need for indestructible secure restraints outweighs the more time-consuming application and removal process.

Soft limb restraints are usually made from cotton or foam material, or both (Fig. 70.3). They are single-use devices, which obviates the need for cleaning and sterilization. Soft limb restraints are less rigid than leather limb restraints, which makes them easier to apply. In addition, because they are fastened without the use of a key, soft limb restraints are more easily removed. Soft restraints are typically used for agitated but less combative patients because they are not as secure as leather limb holders.

Belts/Fifth-Point Restraint

A fifth-point restraint is a belt apparatus used to supplement the use of four limb restraints by holding down the thighs, chest, or pelvis (Fig. 70.4). A fifth-point restraint is used on patients who continue to be at risk for harming themselves despite adequate limb restraint and whose continued combative behavior interferes with diagnostic or therapeutic interventions. When patients are restrained across the thighs, chest, or pelvis, they may not be able to sit up or turn onto their sides, thus placing them at higher risk for aspiration should vomiting occur. Always keep the side rails of the stretcher in the upright position and place the belt snugly enough to prevent the patient from slipping under the device and thereby increasing the risk for accidental suffocation. Fifth-point restraints are usually made of synthetic material and are available with both quick-release and key-release locks.

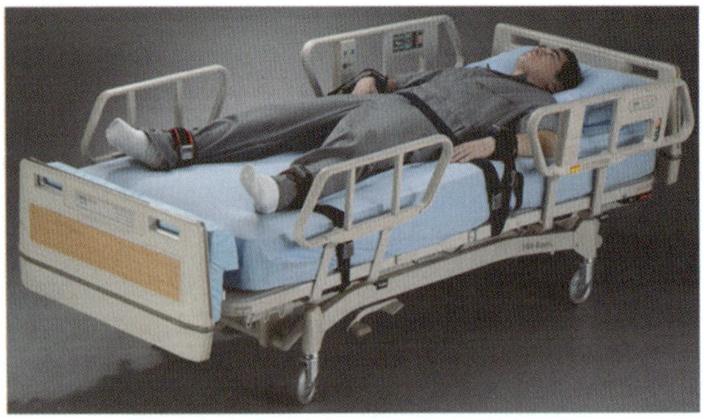

Fig. 70.4 Fifth-point restraint. (Courtesy Posey Company, Inc.)

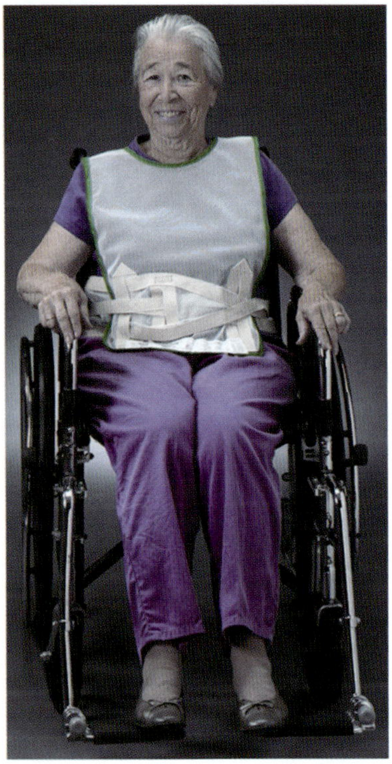

Fig. 70.5 Restraint vest. (Courtesy Posey Company, Inc.)

Jackets and Vests

Jackets and vests are generally used on inpatient wards and extended care facilities for the prevention of falls; they have little utility in the ED (Fig. 70.5). Moreover, these products have been implicated in several restraint-associated deaths secondary to choking and suffocation. The use of restraint jackets and vests in the ED is not recommended.

Hobble Leg Restraints

Hobble leg restraints limit movement by securing the patient's ankles with connecting locking cuffs (Fig. 70.6). Hobble leg restraints are commonly used by law enforcement agencies because they impede running and kicking, which makes them an effective method of transporting potentially violent patients and those who pose a risk for flight. Hobble leg restraints are seldom used in the ED, but their use by law enforcement agencies and prison authorities means that most emergency clinicians will encounter patients placed in these devices. The combination of prone positioning, hobble leg restraints, and binding a patient's hands behind the back, commonly referred to as *hog-tying*, was a common method of restraining prisoners and violent psychiatric patients (Fig. 70.7). However, this practice is no longer widely used because of the risk for suffocation (see later section on "Positional Asphyxia").

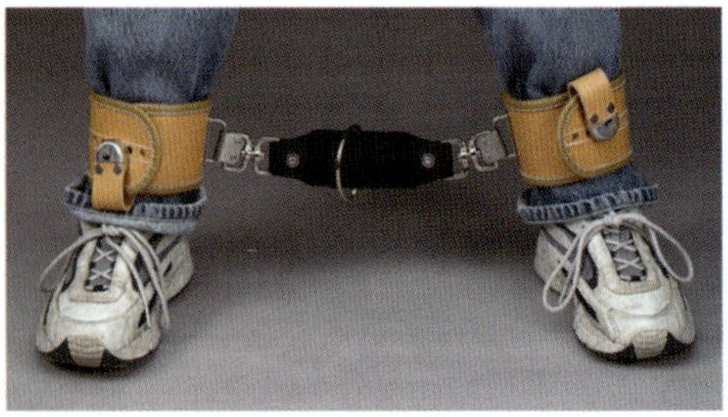

Fig. 70.6 Hobble leg restraint. (Courtesy Posey Company, Inc.)

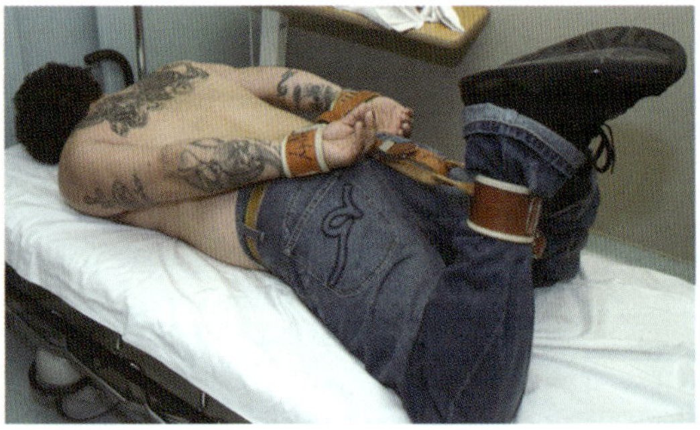

Fig. 70.7 *NOT TO BE USED:* The "hog-tie" method of restraint. The combination of prone positioning, hobble leg restraints, and binding a patient's hands behind the back is commonly referred to as a hog tie. Although this was a common method of restraining prisoners and violent psychiatric patients in the past, the hog tie is no longer recommended. The exact physiologic and metabolic derangements from this position by itself are probably minimal, but the practice is strongly discouraged.

Indications

Use limb restraints to prevent agitated, combative, or violent patients from harming themselves or others. Frequently, the use of restraints can be delayed while verbal de-escalation techniques are attempted (see earlier section on "De-escalation Techniques"). However, if a patient is deemed an immediate threat to themselves or others, restrain them without delay. Patients with altered mental status may require limb restraints so that diagnostic testing can be completed or appropriate treatment rendered, or both. Limb restraints also prevent patients from interfering with devices, such as endotracheal tubes, cardiac monitors, and indwelling intravenous (IV) lines and catheters.

Contraindications

When appropriate, delay physical restraint in favor of trying verbal de-escalation techniques. Do not place limb restraints on extremities with fractures, open wounds, or acute skin and soft tissue infections. Use caution to avoid ischemia in patients who exhibit tenuous perfusion of extremities, such as those with peripheral vascular disease or previous arterial injury or surgery.

Avoid fifth-point restraint of the abdomen and pelvic region in patients with pelvic fractures, suprapubic tubes, ostomies, and percutaneous feeding tubes. In addition, it is

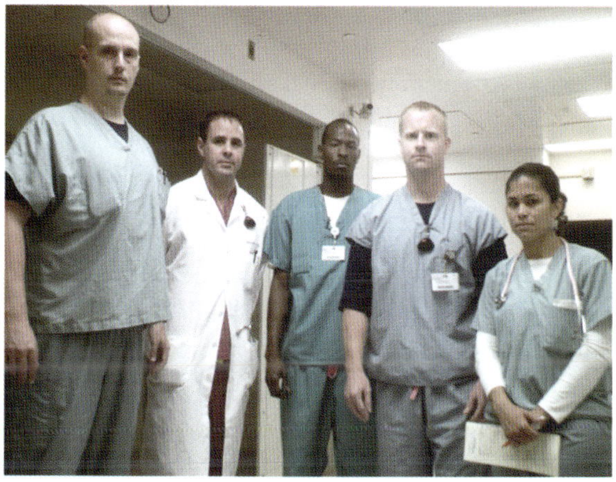

Fig. 70.8 Show of force. A minimum of five well-trained individuals should be available to restrain a patient. This show of force may help discourage the patient from resisting and is an important part of the restraint process.

important to note that patients with underlying pulmonary or cardiac disease may not tolerate restraint of their thorax.

Procedure

Use a minimum of five people, all trained in restraint techniques and patient safety, to restrain the patient if possible (Fig. 70.8). This show of force may help discourage the patient from resisting and is an important part of the restraint process. The individuals making up the restraint team may include clinicians, nurses, technicians, and police or hospital security. When possible, undress and place the patient in a hospital gown before attempting to apply physical restraint. When this is not practical, restrain the patient, but promptly search for weapons and potentially harmful belongings. Confiscate these items and account for them in accordance with institutional policies.

Always restrain patients in the supine rather than the prone position because the prone position increases the risk for suffocation. Assign one person to hold each limb firmly against the stretcher by applying direct pressure proximal to the elbows and knees. The fifth member of the team places restraints around the wrists and ankles (Fig. 70.9). Control above the elbows and knees reduces the risk for injury to these joints and concentrates force closer to the patient's center of gravity for better control.

Apply the limb holders snugly enough to control movement and prevent escape, but not so tight that they cause pain or impair circulation. If necessary, place a fifth-point restraint across the patient's thighs, pelvis, or chest to further limit motion. Place a surgical mask temporarily over the patient's mouth to prevent the patient from spitting at members of the restraint team or ED staff. If leather restraints are used, keep a restraint key readily available in the event that the restraints need to be removed urgently.

If four-point (Video 70.1) rather than five-point restraints are applied (i.e., use of extremity restraints only), consider placing one arm up alongside the head and the opposite arm down along the side of the body. In this position, it is less likely the patient will be able to overturn the stretcher.[26]

Once the patient has been safely restrained, frequently assess pulses, capillary refill, skin color and temperature, and motor and sensory function. Reevaluate frequently in accordance with your institution's policies and procedures because this is key to preventing complications. In general, restraints should have well-defined time limits and should be removed as soon as the patient's condition has changed sufficiently that the patient is no longer a threat to self or others. For further details regarding rules, regulations, and recommendations for restraint procedures and patient assessment, the reader is referred to the TJC website at https://www.jointcommission.org.

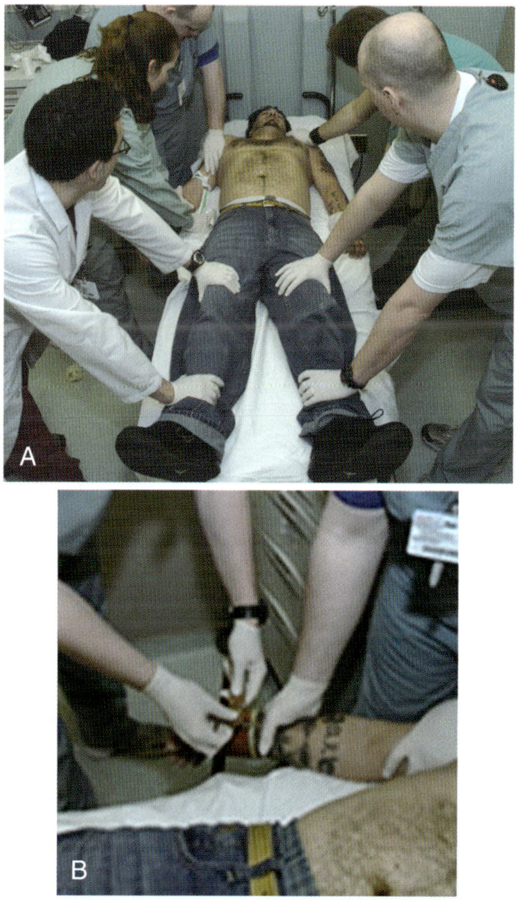

Fig. 70.9 Technique to physically restrain a violent patient. Adequate chemical restraint should be used early in the emergency department course, either before or after physical restraints, to limit acidosis, rhabdomyolysis, and hyperthermia. (A) Patients should always be restrained in the supine position. One person is assigned to each limb, which is held firmly against the stretcher by applying direct pressure proximal to the elbows and knees. (B) The fifth member of the team places restraints around the wrists and ankles. The limb holders should be applied snugly enough to control movement and prevent escape, but not so tight that they cause pain or impair circulation. If necessary, a fifth-point restraint may be placed across the patient's thighs, pelvis, or chest to further limit motion.

Complications

Increased Agitation

For some patients, placement in physical restraints is so emotionally disturbing that it paradoxically increases agitation and combative behavior. Patients who continue to struggle despite restraints are at risk for several potentially serious adverse events, including skin damage, ischemia, metabolic acidosis, rhabdomyolysis, hyperthermia, and even death (see later section on "Other Complications"). In these patients, the addition of chemical sedation is highly recommended (see later section on "Chemical Restraint"). In contrast, the use of extremity restraints alone is often effective in an alcohol-intoxicated patient because the natural progression of alcohol intoxication is sedation and sleep. Intoxicated patients may benefit from a brief period of observation before a decision is made to administer chemical sedation. Most of these patients will fall asleep, thereby obviating the need for sedation and the accompanying risks.

Local Skin

Restraints may cause skin irritation or breakdown. Risk factors include restraints that are too tight and those that have been left on for prolonged periods. Leather restraints are more likely than soft restraints to cause skin damage, particularly in patients who continue to struggle despite being placed in restraints. To help prevent skin complications, use soft restraints whenever possible, avoid overly tight restraints, limit restraint time, and reevaluate the patient frequently. In addition, use chemical restraint judiciously to help avoid skin damage in patients who continue to struggle. It is important to not ignore a patient's complaints of restraint pain without first evaluating the possibility of an adverse event.

Vascular Compromise

Restraints have the rare potential to impede blood flow to the hands and feet. In extreme cases, this could result in ischemia of the distal end of the extremity. Ischemia is more likely to occur in patients whose restraints are placed too tightly and in those in whom swelling develops as a result of a known or occult injury. Struggling against the restraints may further increase this risk. A thorough search for occult injuries, attention to proper fit, and limited restraint time will help avoid ischemia. Frequent assessment of pulses, capillary refill, skin color and temperature, and motor and sensory function is also extremely important. As mentioned previously, it is also important to not ignore a restrained patient's complaints regarding extremity pain without first evaluating for the possibility of ischemia.

Respiratory Compromise

Restraints may impair respiratory mechanics in some patients. This is more likely to occur in patients restrained in the prone or hog-tied positions and in those with underlying pulmonary disease.[34–38] Patients with chronic obstructive pulmonary disease (COPD) may not tolerate a fifth-point restraint across the chest. Avoid respiratory complications by not restraining patients in the prone or hog-tied position. In addition, use adequate chemical sedation to help negate the need for a supplemental restraint belt in patients with underlying COPD.

Positional Asphyxia

Positional asphyxia is a poorly elucidated respiratory complication often attributed to the use of restraints that results in asphyxia and eventually death. The specifics of respiratory dysfunction secondary to physical restraint are vague and unproven and have not been reproduced in volunteers, who do not experience severe pulmonary compromise from restraint. Thus, though often implicated, the exact contribution of restraint to sudden death is unclear. Obesity, underlying cardiac and pulmonary disease, prone positioning, and concurrent stimulant use are thought to be contributing factors.[34,36,38–41] The hog-tied position (see Fig. 70.7), in which a patient's hands and feet are bound behind the back, places a patient at theoretical risk for positional asphyxia and should therefore not be used in the ED.[34–36,41–44] Placing restrained patients in the supine position and frequently reevaluating them will help prevent positional asphyxia. Continuous monitoring of respiratory status, including oxygenation, ventilation, and tidal volume, is indicated in all physically restrained and chemically sedated patients, especially those with obesity, COPD, or intoxication from stimulant drugs.

Cocaine-Associated Agitated Delirium

Cocaine-associated agitated delirium is a syndrome consisting of hyperthermia with delirium and severe agitation that can progress to multisystem failure, coagulopathy, respiratory arrest, and death.[36,38,40,42,45] Much of the pathology may be due to cocaine alone, but restrained patients appear to be at particularly high risk for this syndrome. The syndrome was first described in 1985, but its incidence increased significantly in the 1990s because of the popularity of crack cocaine.[42,43]

The pathophysiology of cocaine-associated agitated delirium is a complex process involving downregulation of dopamine receptors with subsequent dopamine excess during times of cocaine binges.[42,46–48] When patients with cocaine-associated agitated delirium are restrained, especially in the prone position, interference with normal respiratory mechanics increases the likelihood of hypoventilation, hypercapnia, and hypoxemia and ultimately leads to asphyxia and death. It has also been suggested that the stress caused by the restraining process increases the risk for fatal cardiac arrhythmias secondary to catecholamine surge in an already cocaine-sensitized myocardium.[42] Chronic stimulant use leads to adrenergic-induced cardiomyopathy, which is often clinically silent until the individual is severely stressed. The potential for malignant arrhythmias is unknown, but they have been implicated in some cases of sudden death in restrained patients.

Metabolic Acidosis

In patients who have been restrained, continued agitation and struggling can lead to severe metabolic acidosis.[45] Their pH is often lower than 7.0. The etiology of this acidosis is unclear but probably involves the production of lactic acid from physical exertion compounded by sympathetic-induced vasoconstriction. Such vasoconstriction may result from agitation or cocaine (and other stimulant) use and is believed to enhance exercise-induced lactic acidosis by impeding clearance of lactate by the liver.[49,50] In some patients the buildup of lactate is further increased by the presence of psychosis and delirium, which may alter pain sensation and allow exertion far beyond normal physiologic limits.[45] In addition, some restraint positions (e.g., prone, hog-tied) may not allow adequate respiratory compensation, thereby resulting in further enhancement of the acidosis. Recently, animal models have demonstrated a correlation between prone positioning and cardiac arrest, referred to as prone restraint cardiac arrest (PRCA). PRCA is thought to be due to reduced ventilation in the prone position[51,52] However, it is worth noting that sudden cardiac death has occurred in a variety of positions and situations. Moreover, human studies examining ventilation and circulatory parameters in restrictive positions have been equivocal; thus PRCA remains unproven.[53] A common scenario is an out-of-hospital cardiac arrest in which a severely agitated individual suddenly stops struggling and experiences a bradycardic, asystolic death that is not immediately recognized. Such patients may have been subdued by force, by TASER, by mace or by pepper spray, which has led to unproven speculation that these interventions may have caused the change in patient status.

Regardless of the etiology, profound metabolic acidosis has been associated with cardiovascular collapse and sudden and unexpected death in restrained patients.[45] Individuals demonstrate bradycardia, pulseless electrical activity and experience asystolic cardiac arrest; resuscitation is unlikely once cardiac arrest ensues. Patients who remain combative despite restraints, especially those who have used cocaine or other sympathomimetic agents, are at particularly high risk for death.[45] Clues to the presence of metabolic acidosis include severe agitation, abnormal vital signs (e.g., persistent tachycardia, tachypnea, and hyperpyrexia), and decreased or concentrated urine output despite adequate IV fluid administration. Laboratory testing, including arterial or venous blood gas analysis, serum electrolytes, and serum creatine phosphokinase, is recommended in patients with signs and symptoms suggestive of metabolic acidosis and in those with potentially lethal co-ingestion (e.g., salicylates and toxic alcohols).

Restrained patients with severe metabolic acidosis should receive aggressive hydration and chemical sedation to counteract the sympathetic hyperactivity.[45] The utility of sodium bicarbonate is unknown and it is probably best reserved for patients with a pH below 7.0.

Chemical Restraint

Agitation leading to delirium and culminating in hyperactive delirium with severe agitation is a continuum with no rigidly defined parameters. This chapter discusses the treatment of mild agitation, as well as life-threatening hyperactive delirium with severe agitation, but it is important to realize that the recommendations are subject to alteration or modification depending on the degree of impairment and the necessity of the clinician to intervene differently in individuals with varying degrees of impairment. The exact role of chemical restraint will always be a clinical judgment made at the bedside and based on the scenario at hand. It is, however, axiomatic that chemical restraint is mandated when physical restraint and other modalities have failed. Medically compromised patients who appear mentally incompetent, are unable to comprehend or participate in the evaluation or treatment of a serious medical condition, or are otherwise unable to cooperate with required diagnostic or therapeutic medical interventions should be chemically restrained.

Chemical restraint, more aptly termed chemical sedation, describes the act of quelling an agitated patient by the administration of sedative-hypnotic, antipsychotic, or dissociative medications. Early, liberal use of appropriate anxiolytic and sedating medications permits thorough evaluation of a patient's medical condition. In some cases, administration of anxiolytic drugs (e.g., benzodiazepines [BZDs]) may be the optimal treatment of a person with an undifferentiated delirious state such as delirium tremens.[54] This is supported by Khan and associates, who identified an association between the use of physical restraint and death in patients with delirium tremens.[55] Although a clear causal relationship between restraint and death is lacking, early use of sedation may be safer than physical restraint for treatment of an undifferentiated delirium.

The CMS states that chemical restraint is "a medication used to control behavior or to restrict the patient's freedom of movement and is not a standard treatment for the patient's medical or psychiatric condition."[6] Curiously, TJC defines chemical restraint as "the inappropriate use of a sedating psychotropic drug to manage or control behavior."[24] These definitions lack perspective on the use of chemical sedation in the ED, where these medications are typically used after all other measures fail and the health and safety of the patient or staff are threatened. Such statements do not reflect standard care in the ED and should not be interpreted as prohibition of the appropriate short-term use of chemical sedation.

The pathogenesis of agitation is poorly understood; however, the advent of anxiolytic and antipsychotic medications has revolutionized the treatment of acute agitation. Not only has sedation become safer, but many of these new agents also have the added benefit of treating underlying psychotic states.[3] BZDs, with rare exception, have replaced barbiturates for the treatment of acute agitation. Recently, intramuscular (IM) preparations of "atypical antipsychotic" medications such as olanzapine, ziprasidone, and aripiprazole have provided additional treatment options for rapid control of acute psychosis.[56,57]

Oral administration is a reasonable first-line option in the cooperative patient and is the preferred route as consent is implied when the patient willingly ingests it.[58,59] Previous reports have shown that patients prefer oral formulations during the treatment of psychotic episodes because they are participating in their own care plan.[60,61] Oral lorazepam and oral risperidone have demonstrated increased efficacy when compared with the IM administration of haloperidol.[62] However, in the uncooperative agitated patient, where rapid tranquilization is usually the goal, medications are typically administered IV or IM. Obtaining early IV access allows titration of rapidly acting medications but may not be possible in some patients. When IV access is not possible, IM administration is recommended and, in some cases, has been shown to be as efficacious and safe as IV administration.[63] Other routes (oral, transmucosal) may be used when parenteral administration is not practical or feasible.

An ideal drug for chemical sedation in the ED should have multiple routes of administration (e.g., IV, IM, transmucosal), a rapid onset of action, negligible hemodynamic effects, and a good safety record with minimal adverse effects. Although no medication fits this profile perfectly, with proper patient assessment and careful drug selection, most ED patients can be rapidly and safely sedated. The remainder of this chapter discusses the safety, efficacy, side effect profile, and recommended dosages of the medications most used for chemical sedation. Recommendations for drug selection are also discussed (Table 70.1).

Other Methods of Drug Delivery

Under ideal circumstances, sedative medications are best administered IV. A peripheral vein is adequate but may be difficult to access or maintain in a struggling patient. Although an indwelling catheter is preferable to titrate escalating doses, the first dose may be directly administered into a peripheral vein via a syringe/needle, so-called "mainlining" (Fig. 70.10). A large extremity vein in the arm or leg is usually available if the extremity can be adequately immobilized. The external jugular vein presents another route. The head can often be more easily stabilized than a muscular extremity, and the external jugular vein is usually quite prominent in a struggling patient. Note that some antipsychotics, such as olanzapine and ziprasidone, have indications only for use IM. Droperidol is

TABLE 70.1 Drugs Used for Chemical Restraint in the ED

AGENT	DOSAGE	ONSET/DURATION OF ACTION	CONTRAINDICATIONS/ CAUTIONS	ADVERSE EVENTS	COMMENTS[a]
Haloperidol	Adults: 5–10 mg IM/IV/ PO q1–4h Children/adolescents: 0.05–0.15 mg/kg IM/IV q1h (max 5 mg)	Onset: IM/IV: 30–45 min Duration: IM/IV: 4–24 h	Patients with a history of QT prolongation, thyrotoxicosis, Parkinson's disease, and severe hepatic disease	EPSs, QTc prolongation, NMS, hypotension, cholinergic blockade	Can be given alone or in combination with a benzodiazepine; may lower the seizure threshold
Droperidol	Adults: 5–10 mg IM/IV	Onset: IM/IV: 3–10 min Duration: IM/IV: 2–12 h	Patients with a history of QT prolongation, thyrotoxicosis, Parkinson's disease, severe hepatic disease, and intoxication with LSD	EPSs, QTc prolongation, NMS, hypotension, cholinergic blockade	Black box warning regarding QT prolongation and serious arrhythmias; rapid-onset IM; use with caution in children
Lorazepam	Adults: 1–4 mg IM/IV/ PO q30–60 min Children: 0.05–0.1 mg/kg (max 4 mg/dose) Geriatric: <2 mg/dose	Onset: IM: 15–20 min IV: 2–3 min Duration: IM/IV: 8–10 h	Patients with respiratory depression and pregnant women	Respiratory depression, ataxia, hypotension	First-line therapy for children; use with caution in patients with alcohol intoxication because of the risk for respiratory depression
Diazepam	Adults: 2–10 mg IV/ IM/PO Children: 0.04–0.3 mg/ kg per dose IM/IV (max 0.6 mg/kg in 8 h) Geriatric: 2 mg PO	Onset: IV: 1–5 min Duration: IM/IV 15–60 min	Patients with respiratory depression and pregnant women	Respiratory depression, ataxia, hypotension	Use with caution in patients with alcohol intoxication because of the risk for respiratory depression
Midazolam	Adults: 1–5 mg IM/IV Children: 0.1–0.2 mg/kg IV/IM (max 0.5 mg/kg or 10 mg) Geriatric: 1–3 mg IM/IV	Onset: IV: 3 min IM: 5 min Duration: IM/IV: 30–120 min	Patients with respiratory depression and pregnant women	Respiratory depression, ataxia, hypotension	First-line therapy for children; rapid onset IM; use with caution in patients with alcohol intoxication because of the risk for respiratory depression
Ziprasidone	Adults: 10 mg IM q2 h, 20 mg IM q4h (max 40 mg/day) Children ≥5 years: 0.2 mg/kg/dose IM (not to exceed 20 mg)	Onset: 15–30 min Duration: 4 h	Patients with dementia	QT prolongation, somnolence, EPSs	Lower incidence of EPS than with haloperidol and droperidol; black box warning regarding use in older adults with dementia

Continued

TABLE 70.1 Drugs Used for Chemical Restraint in the ED—cont'd

AGENT	DOSAGE	ONSET/DURATION OF ACTION	CONTRAINDICATIONS/ CAUTIONS	ADVERSE EVENTS	COMMENTS[a]
Olanzapine	Adults: 5–10 mg IM Children <10 years: 1.25–5 mg IM; ≥10 years: 5–10 mg IM Geriatric: 2.5–10 mg IM	Onset: 15–30 min Duration: 2–24 h	Patients with dementia	Somnolence, EPSs	Lower incidence of EPS than with haloperidol and droperidol; black box warning regarding use in older adults with dementia
Ketamine	Adults/children: 1–2 mg/kg IV, 4–5 mg/kg IM	Onset: IV: <1 min IM: 3–5 min Duration IV:15 min (recovery 1–2 h) IM: 30 min (recovery 3–4 h)	Acute upper respiratory infection, children <3 months of age	Emergence phenomenon, potential increased intracranial and intraocular pressure, hypertension, tachycardia, salivation, vomiting, laryngospasm	Doses provided are for achieving a dissociative state; use ketamine when rapid sedation is required for lifesaving interventions

[a]Many of the caveats concerning the safety and efficacy of long-term use cannot be equated to short-term ED use. These medications are currently often used in doses far exceeding those recommended by the manufacturer or under other clinical circumstances; safety and efficacy for short-term sedation have been demonstrated in clinical ED practice.

ED, Emergency department; *EPSs*, extrapyramidal symptoms; *IM*, intramuscularly; *IV*, intravenously; *LSD*, lysergic acid diethylamide; *NMS*, neuroleptic malignant syndrome; *PO*, per os (oral).

experiencing a resurgence and can be given IM or IV. Haloperidol is commonly administered IV, although it has no formal indication for this route. Intranasal midazolam is another alternative route of administration that may also have prehospital utility but may be impractical in a noncooperative patient.

Indications

Chemical sedation is used to prevent patients from injuring themselves or others, attenuate psychosis, decrease the time spent in physical restraint, and calm patients enough to permit a medical history, physical examination, diagnostic testing, and procedures.

Contraindications and Adverse Effects

Absolute and relative contraindications, as well as adverse effects, vary by medication and are discussed separately for each drug.

First-generation Antipsychotics (Neuroleptic Agents)

First-generation or "typical antipsychotics," also known as neuroleptic agents, have been used safely and effectively for years to manage patients with undifferentiated agitated delirium in the ED. Agents such as droperidol or haloperidol are preferred because they lack tolerance after repeated uses, have a low addiction potential, and possess a high therapeutic index.[64] Droperidol, once again gaining in popularity, has been shown to be equal to or more effective than haloperidol in several studies.[65,66] Low-potency antipsychotics (e.g., chlorpromazine) are less desirable because of a higher incidence of hypotension, seizures, and anticholinergic effects.[64]

Contraindications

Haloperidol and droperidol should be avoided in patients with thyrotoxicosis (neurotoxicity may develop), Parkinson's disease, or severe hepatic disease. These drugs can lower the seizure threshold, so they should be used with caution or be avoided altogether in patients with a history of seizures or those who may be at known risk for the development of seizures (e.g., meningitis, sympathomimetic intoxication). Nevertheless, droperidol has been used safely to manage patients with known seizure disorders.[67] Haloperidol and droperidol can cause QT prolongation and should be used with caution in patients at risk for QT prolongation and torsades de pointes (Box 70.5). Droperidol has also been associated with serotonin syndrome in patients taking lysergic acid diethylamide (LSD) and should be avoided in these patients.[64,68]

Adverse Effects

Adverse effects related to droperidol and haloperidol include extrapyramidal symptoms (EPSs), QTc prolongation, neuroleptic malignant syndrome (NMS), hypotension, and cholinergic receptor antagonism.

EPSs include akathisia (restlessness), dystonia (muscular spasms of the neck, eyes [oculogyric crisis], tongue, or jaw), drug-induced parkinsonism (muscle stiffness, shuffling gait, drooling, tremor), and tardive dyskinesia. These effects are due to the drugs' antidopaminergic action and, though distressing to the patient, are seldom life-threatening. In the acute setting, anticholinergic agents such as diphenhydramine (25 to 50 mg orally [PO], IM, or IV) or benztropine (1 mg to 2 mg PO, IM, or IV) are effective in preventing or minimizing dystonia while BZDs may be used for treatment of akathisia.

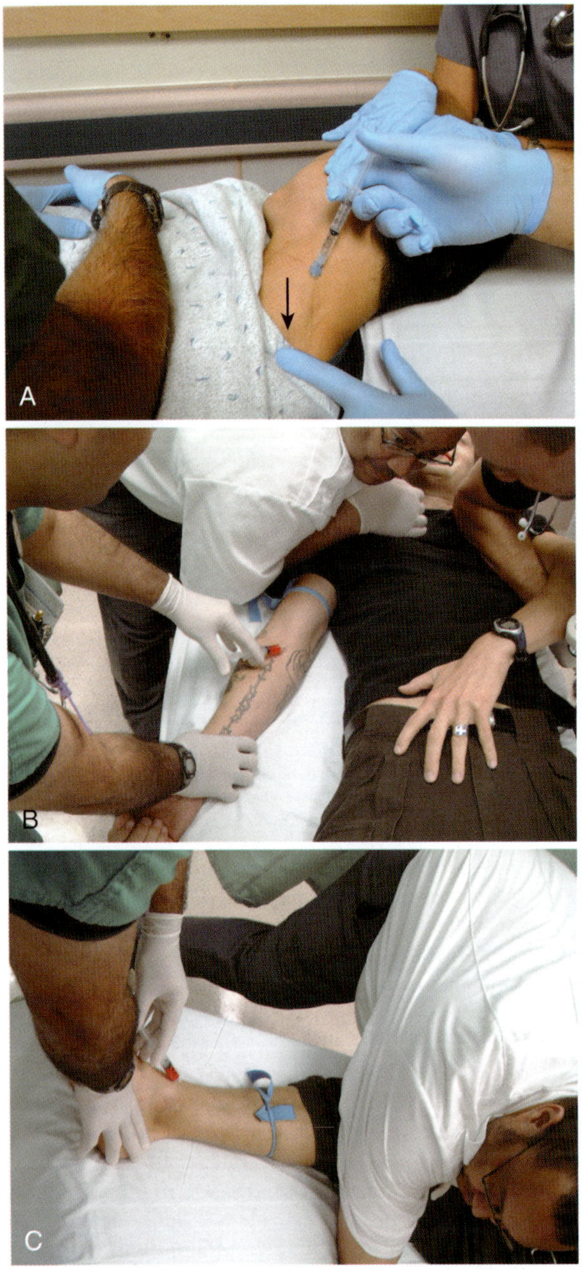

Fig. 70.10 When intravenous (IV) access is problematic in a patient in urgent need of IV sedation, an alternative is to mainline medication into a large vein directly from a syringe. (A) The external jugular vein is usually prominent in a struggling patient, and the head and upper part of the torso are easier to control than an extremity. A finger occluding the distal end of the vein *(arrow)* allows better access. (B) Other options include the antecubital fossa and (C) the greater saphenous ankle vein, if the respective extremity can be temporarily immobilized. Use a 23- to 25-gauge needle. When blood is aspirated, push the medication. Ketamine is effective within 1 to 2 minutes by the intramuscular route (anterior thigh or deltoid area) and is an option to IV benzodiazepines and antipsychotic medications.

A potentially deadly, but exceedingly rare effect of neuroleptic drug use is prolongation of the QTc interval, which can lead to torsades de pointes, a polymorphic ventricular arrhythmia that can progress to ventricular fibrillation and sudden death.[3] Droperidol has been the most publicized agent associated with QTc prolongation. It is currently the only neuroleptic agent that has received a "black box warning" for its alleged propensity to cause QTc prolongation and sudden death.[69] Despite the black box warning, the risk of clinically significant QT prolongation from therapeutic droperidol administration is now believed to be low.[14] In addition, a number of case reports and small case series have documented QTc prolongation and torsades de pointes after the administration of haloperidol as well.[70] Risk factors for QTc prolongation and torsades de pointes are listed in Box 70.5.

BOX 70.5 Risk Factors for QTc Prolongation and Torsades de Pointes

NONPHARMACOLOGIC

Congenital long QT syndromes
Cardiac disorders (ventricular hypertrophy, heart failure, bradycardia)
Electrolyte imbalance (especially hypokalemia)
Overdose of an antipsychotic drug
Female sex
Use of restraints and psychological stress
Substance abuse
Miscellaneous factors (obesity, hypothyroidism)
Adults 65 years of age or older
Renal and hepatic impairment

PHARMACOLOGIC

Pharmacokinetic Factors

Inhibition of specific cytochrome P-450 enzymes
Competition for specific cytochrome P-450 enzymes

Pharmacodynamic Factors

Independent QTc prolongation

Patients in whom symptoms of NMS develop exhibit autonomic instability, including rigidity of the extremities, hyperthermia, and delirium. Treatment includes cooling measures, sedation with BZDs, and in severe cases, bromocriptine, dantrolene, neuromuscular paralysis, and endotracheal intubation.[64]

Hypotension is usually orthostatic in nature and tends to be more pronounced when the drugs are administered IV. In general, haloperidol and droperidol have a lower incidence of hypotension and anticholinergic effects (e.g., confusion, dry mouth, blurred vision, urinary retention).

Haloperidol

Haloperidol is a commonly used first-generation antipsychotic. It is categorized as a high-potency neuroleptic because of its strong antidopaminergic activity. The antidopaminergic activity is responsible for both its intended effects against delusions, hallucinations, and psychomotor agitation and its unintended parkinsonian symptoms. Administration of haloperidol both alone and in combination with BZDs has been evaluated in a large number of clinical trials.[71–76] These studies have demonstrated the use of haloperidol IM to be both safe and effective for the management of acute agitation.

Dosage and Administration. Haloperidol can be administered PO, IV, and IM and has a low incidence of oversedation regardless of which route is chosen.[3] Despite a lack of US Food and Drug Administration (FDA) approval for IV use, haloperidol is often administered IV. The recommended starting dosage to achieve sedation is 5 mg IM or IV, titrated to effect. There is no absolute maximum dose, and in cases of severe hyperactive delirium and severe agitation, doses of 10 mg to 30 mg are common. Occasionally, extrapyramidal reactions occur but are easily treated. The dose should be halved or reduced further when administered to older adults. In children 6 to 12 years of age, the dosage is 0.5 mg to 2 mg IM every 4 to 8 hours with a maximum of 0.15 mg/kg per day. Children older than 12 years can receive the adult dosage. Haloperidol administered IM has a peak clinical effect within 30 to 45 minutes and may last up to 24 hours when given for acute agitation.

Droperidol

Droperidol, an analog of haloperidol, is a high-potency butyrophenone with rapid sedating effects. It also possesses significant antidopaminergic activity. Droperidol acquired FDA approval in 1970 first as an antiemetic and antipsychotic agent. Soon thereafter, psychiatric EDs found it useful for chemical sedation.[77] Many physicians prefer droperidol to haloperidol because of its more rapid onset and shorter duration of action.

Use of droperidol as a chemical sedative continued until 2001, at which time the FDA issued a black box warning regarding the potential for fatal dysrhythmias.[78] Many hospitals subsequently sought to restrict or prohibit its use. However, two large retrospective studies encompassing more than 15,000 patients did not demonstrate increased morbidity or mortality associated with the use of droperidol for the management of acute agitation.[67,77] This controversy prompted an independent review of the data submitted to the FDA that led to the black box warning. The authors of this review found several anomalies and duplicate reports. They, and others, concluded that droperidol is a safe drug when used at the recommended dosage (i.e., 5 mg to 10 mg).[79,80,81] As a result, the use of droperidol is again gaining popularity, particularly in the ED where rapid sedation is often needed.[82]

Studies comparing a variety of agents for rapid sedation have found that droperidol provides more rapid and effective control than do lorazepam,[83] haloperidol,[72] midazolam,[84,85] and ziprasidone.[84] In addition, in a retrospective study of patients with head injuries, alcohol and cocaine intoxication, and seizure disorders, those given droperidol had few serious reported adverse events with questionable causality.[67]

Dosage and Administration. The initial dosage used for sedation is 5 mg IV or IM. Its onset of action is 3 to 10 minutes with a peak clinical effect achieved in 30 minutes. The elimination half-life is 2 to 4 hours, but the sedative effects of droperidol may last up to 12 hours.

Benzodiazepines

All BZDs enhance the neurotransmission of γ-aminobutyric acid and thereby result in anxiolysis, sedation, hypnosis, and muscle relaxation. This combination makes them an excellent choice for calming of agitated patients. Because of a desirable safety profile, BZDs are a reliable choice for sedating medically undifferentiated patients. The differences in clinical effects (e.g., onset, duration, adverse effects) are primarily related to dosage, route of administration, and pharmacokinetics. BZDs are used as single agents or in combination with an antipsychotic drug, though combination therapy does not offer a clear benefit over monotherapy.[14] Midazolam and lorazepam are the BZDs most commonly used for chemical sedation. This is probably due to their rapid and predictable absorption when given IV or IM, as well as a long history of safety and efficacy. Unlike antipsychotics, BZDs do not treat underlying psychiatric disorders. Some clinicians prefer to administer diazepam IV for the treatment of delirium related to sedative-hypnotic withdrawal.[54] Phenobarbital is a suitable alternative to BZDs in cases of delirium from alcohol withdrawal, especially in the setting of drug shortages.[86,87]

Contraindications

There are few contraindications to the use of BZDs as a chemical sedating agent. Because of the possibility of respiratory depression, use BZDs with caution in patients in respiratory distress or identified pulmonary pathology like obstructive sleep apnea.

Adverse Effects

BZDs may cause respiratory depression. Additionally, hypotension, deep sedation, and paradoxical agitation have been reported. However, when administered in the doses recommended for agitation, adverse events are rare, thus making BZDs the drugs of choice in most circumstances.

Respiratory compromise is dose dependent and typically occurs only in the presence of other respiratory depressants.[88,89] Because of an increased risk for respiratory depression, administer BZDs cautiously to older adults and those with underlying pulmonary diseases such as apnea and COPD. In healthy patients, particularly those experiencing agitated delirium, respiratory depression is very unlikely to occur, even when large doses of BZDs are used. End-tidal carbon dioxide monitoring (e.g., capnography) may assist the practitioner in detecting the onset of respiratory depression before it becomes clinically significant.[90,91]

The most appropriate BZD is the one that the clinician is most comfortable administering and that has a duration of action most appropriate for the clinical situation. Titrate IV-administered BZDs until the desired level of sedation is reached. In the setting of severe delirium, there is no maximum dose described for any BZD, and doses more than the manufacturer's recommendation, and even those considered toxic under other circumstances, are commonly used. Of note, propylene glycol is a solvent found in non–water-soluble BZD (e.g., lorazepam, diazepam). In large doses, propylene glycol can cause an increased osmolar gap and metabolic acidosis and may precipitate or contribute to hypotension in some patients.[92]

Lorazepam

Lorazepam is the BZD most frequently studied for the management of acute agitation. It enjoys popularity as part of the well-known "five and two" treatment regimen, which consists of haloperidol, 5 mg IM, and lorazepam, 2 mg IM.[93] In a number of clinical trials, lorazepam was shown to be an effective drug for rapid chemical sedation.[73,76,77,83] In these studies, lorazepam had no extrapyramidal effects and was better tolerated than the antipsychotics. However, when compared with haloperidol, droperidol, midazolam, and a combination of haloperidol and lorazepam, the onset of sedation after administering lorazepam IM was more delayed.[73,76,83]

Dosage and Administration. When used alone, lorazepam is usually given in 2- to 4-mg doses and can be administered PO, sublingually, IM, IV, or rectally. No maximum dose has been established. Following an injection of lorazepam IM, adequate sedation is usually achieved in 30 to 45 minutes.[83] When given IV, sedation occurs in 15 to 20 minutes.[76] The elimination half-life is 12 to 15 hours, which produces a duration of effect of 8 to 10 hours. This makes lorazepam a better choice when long-term sedation is the goal. Lorazepam is rapidly conjugated to an inactive glucuronide. This does not require involvement of the cytochrome P-450 system, so lorazepam has few drug-drug interactions. Preparations of lorazepam intended for use IV or IM must be refrigerated, thus potentially limiting its use in the prehospital or low-resource settings.[3]

Midazolam

Midazolam has been shown to be effective for rapid sedation.[75,76,84,85] It has a more rapid onset and shorter duration of action than other BZDs, which makes it a good choice when rapid short-term sedation is desired. Midazolam also compares favorably with haloperidol, droperidol, olanzapine, and ziprasidone for the treatment of acute agitation in the ED.[75,76,85] With the exception of droperidol, which has a similar time until onset (5 to 10 minutes), midazolam has a more rapid onset of sedation than the other drugs in these studies. The studies also noted that midazolam, as expected, has a shorter duration of sedation.

Dosage and Administration. The initial dosage of midazolam for an agitated adult is 5 mg IV or IM, and it may be repeated at 5- to 10-minute intervals. No maximum dose has been established. Nasal administration is also an option, but oftentimes impractical. The onset of sedation occurs approximately 3 minutes after IV administration, 5 minutes after an IM injection, and 15 minutes after nasal administration. Midazolam is hydroxylated by the cytochrome P-450 system to its primary metabolite, α-hydroxymidazolam, which undergoes glucuronide conjugation before being excreted in urine. Its duration of action is between 30 and 120 minutes and does not vary significantly by route of administration.[76,94]

Diazepam

Diazepam has a long history of safe use in the management of agitated delirium, especially delirium tremens and alcohol withdrawal.[54,95] For patients experiencing delirium tremens the usual dose is 5 to 10 mg IV every 5 to 10 minutes until the desired level of sedation is achieved (lower doses are appropriate for less severe agitation or agitation from other causes). No maximum dose has been established, and doses of up to 2000 mg have been used over a 24-hour period in patients experiencing delirium tremens.[54,96] Because of erratic absorption, IM administration of diazepam is not recommended. Following the administration of diazepam, peak sedation is reached in approximately 5 to 6 minutes, which allows additional titrated doses if the desired clinical effect is not achieved initially.

Second-Generation Antipsychotic Agents

Second-generation or atypical antipsychotic agents generally have high affinity for 5-HT (serotonin) receptors and less affinity for D_1 and D_2 receptors. As a result, they have a lower incidence of EPSs than haloperidol and droperidol. Most common second-generation agents include ziprasidone, olanzapine, and aripiprazole. When administered IM, all three drugs are effective for the treatment of acute agitation.[97] However, the delay in sedation onset following IM administration may be a disadvantage in circumstances that require rapid sedation. Often sedation is markedly prolonged from the relatively high doses required. However, the combination of IM administration and the low incidence of EPSs makes these newer agents an attractive option for sedation of ED patients with undifferentiated agitation. This is particularly true for patients with a history of psychiatric disorders, for whom this class of medications is now considered appropriate first-line management.[98]

Contraindications

In 2005 a meta-analysis of placebo-controlled trials demonstrated an increased risk for death associated with the atypical antipsychotic agents used to treat older adults with dementia-related psychosis.[99] This report led the FDA to issue a black box warning regarding the use of atypical antipsychotics for "behavioral disorders" in older adults with dementia. Such warnings have not resulted in the prohibition of such agents for short-term use in the ED. The FDA has also advised caution with ziprasidone because of its tendency to prolong the QTc interval, especially when used in patients taking other drugs or with medical conditions that increase the risk for prolongation of the QTc interval (see Box70.5).[99] Ziprasidone prolongs the QTc interval more frequently than haloperidol, droperidol, and olanzapine do,[3] but the degree of prolongation is considered minor and is rarely greater than 500 ms.[100] To date, there have been no clinical reports of adverse events as a result of QTc prolongation with the short-term ED use of atypical antipsychotic agents. Experience with these agents in undifferentiated acutely agitated patients in the ED is increasing, and as a result, they are now considered reasonable options for treating agitation in the setting of hyperactive delirium with severe agitation.[14]

Adverse Effects

Atypical antipsychotic agents may cause somnolence, EPSs (though less often than with haloperidol and droperidol), QTc prolongation, and rarely, anticholinergic symptoms and NMS.

Ziprasidone

Ziprasidone is a benzylisothiazolylpiperazine antipsychotic agent whose effects are the result of dopamine and serotonin 5-HT_{2A} receptor antagonism.[3,97,101] This was the first atypical antipsychotic agent available in a fast-acting preparation administered IM. In a double-blind, randomized study, Martel and associates noted that ziprasidone was as effective as midazolam and droperidol in controlling acute agitation. Patients receiving ziprasidone and droperidol took longer to be sedated (30 minutes as compared with 15 minutes for midazolam) but were more deeply sedated at 60 and 120 minutes.[84] In a prospective, open-label study, ED patients receiving ziprasidone exhibited progressive improvement in anxiety, hostility, and cooperativeness starting at 15 minutes and continuing through the 90-minute study period.[57] In an observational study of agitated psychiatric ED patients with nonspecific psychosis, alcohol intoxication, or substance-induced psychosis, ziprasidone 20 mg IM was effective in sedating patients as quickly as 15 minutes.[102] Ziprasidone has not been approved by the FDA for the treatment of dementia-related psychosis.[101]

Dosage and Administration. The recommended dosage of ziprasidone is 10 mg IM, which can be repeated at 2 hours, or 20 mg IM, which may be repeated at 4 hours. The recommended maximum IM daily dose is 40 mg. The drug reaches peak plasma concentrations in 30 to 45 minutes and has an elimination half-life of 2 to 4 hours. Following an IM injection, sedation usually begins within 15 to 30 minutes and peaks at approximately 2 hours. The clinical effects usually last at least 4 hours.[103]

Olanzapine

Olanzapine is a second-generation thienobenzodiazepine antipsychotic agent that is thought to exert its effects through antagonism of both dopamine and serotonin type 2 receptors. Olanzapine in an IM formulation has been approved by the FDA for the treatment of agitation in acutely psychotic patients. Olanzapine has a more rapid onset than ziprasidone and is less likely to require rescue sedation than haloperidol.[66,104] Olanzapine is comparable to haloperidol or lorazepam monotherapy for acute agitation associated with schizophrenia and dementia[74,105,106] and superior to lorazepam monotherapy in the management of agitation associated with bipolar disorder.[107] Recent evidence supports olanzapine as a first-line antipsychotic for severe agitation in the ED.[14,108,109]

Dosage and Administration. The recommended dosage for olanzapine is 5 to 10 mg IM. Additional doses may be considered 2 to 4 hours after the preceding dose with a maximum recommended IM daily dose of 30 mg. Olanzapine reaches peak plasma concentrations in 15 to 45 minutes and has an elimination half-life of 21 to 54 hours. The onset of sedation usually begins 15 to 30 minutes after IM administration and typically lasts at least 2 hours. In some patients, the clinical effects have lasted as long as 24 hours. The drug is metabolized via direct glucuronidation and cytochrome P-450–mediated oxidation.[110] Post-marketing reports show an increased risk of respiratory depression associated with the concomitant parenteral administration of BZDs and IM olanzapine. Some providers avoid administration of IV/IM BZDs within 1 to 2 hours from IM olanzapine.

Dissociative Agents

Ketamine

Ketamine is a dissociative agent that has been used safely throughout the world for major surgery and with minimal monitoring.[111] Many clinicians are familiar with ketamine as a safe and rapidly effective dissociative agent for tracheal intubation and for both adults and children undergoing painful procedures in the ED. It inhibits the reuptake of catecholamines, promoting bronchodilation and increases in both heart rate and blood pressure. Commonly raised as a caution, there is no proven issue with ketamine causing harmful increased intracranial pressure.[112,113] Possible side effects of ketamine include salivation, vomiting, laryngospasm, and emergence phenomena consisting of nightmares, short-lived bizarre thoughts, and hallucinations. Fortunately, serious emergence phenomena have not been described as significant issues following ED use.

Literature supporting ketamine for the control of agitated and delirious patients has grown over the past decade. Ketamine is a desirable option as it can be given via IM administration, has a rapid onset of sedation, and generally maintains airway reflexes.[114] The drug's pharmacologic profile lends itself for use in acute, potentially violent situations. For example, ketamine has been used successfully in aeromedical transport as a sedative agent for patients with agitation.[115] It has also been reported as effective in the prehospital management and transport of patients with severe agitation and in combative trauma patients (including those with head injury),[116,117] acutely agitated cocaine-intoxicated patients,[118] and agitated suicidal patients.[119]

Dosage and Administration. The dose of ketamine to produce dissociation is 1.5 to 2.0 mg/kg IV or 4 to 5 mg/kg IM. IM administration is ideal in the ED when access for IV administration is not readily available. The anterior aspect of the thigh is a preferred site of injection for rapid tranquilization. Time of onset may vary slightly, but both routes have a rapid onset of action (30 seconds IV, 3 to 5 minutes IM).

Choosing the Best Agent

Undifferentiated Agitation

The most utilized agent for undifferentiated agitation in the ED has traditionally been a parenteral benzodiazepine, often combined with judicious doses of haloperidol. Chan and associates demonstrated the combination of an antipsychotic and midazolam had a shorter time to sedation than midazolam alone.[120] Administering escalating doses of BZDs is a prudent choice in such circumstances when the clinician is comfortable prescribing a drug from this class. There is little concern for respiratory or cardiovascular depression with the prudent use of carefully titrated IV BZDs in the monitored setting. Fig. 70.1 suggests a possible management approach to an acutely agitated patient in the emergency setting. It must be emphasized that benzodiazepine doses considered exceedingly high or even toxic by other standards are routinely and safely administered in the ED when aggressive sedation and chemical control are mandated as clinical priorities. In severe cases, BZDs alone may not be fully effective.

Agitation Caused by Alcohol and Drugs of Abuse

For patients who are suspected of intoxication from alcohol or other sedative agents, droperidol, haloperidol, olanzapine, or ziprasidone will provide rapid, safe, and effective tranquilization.[67,78,85] BZDs should be administered with caution to patients with alcohol intoxication and those taking sedative agents due to an increased risk of respiratory depression.[88,89] In contrast, BZDs and phenobarbital, are the drugs of choice in patients who are agitated as a result *of alcohol or benzodiazepine withdrawal.* Large doses may be required, and the safety profile is wide. Patients who are agitated because of sympathomimetic agents such as cocaine, methamphetamines, or hallucinogens, such as PCP or LSD, may be treated safely with escalating doses of BZDs, butyrophenones, or a combination of the two.[67,73,83] Droperidol has been associated with serotonin syndrome in patients taking LSD and should be avoided in these patients.[64,69]

Agitation Caused by Medical Illness

In patients whose agitation is due to medical illness, treatment should be aimed at correcting the underlying pathology. If rapid sedation is required, typical antipsychotics or BZDs should be used as first-line therapy. If the patient is frail, an older adult, or is known to have renal impairment, consider using smaller doses of a single agent.

Agitation Caused by an Underlying Psychiatric Disorder

Patients with an established psychiatric history and agitation attributed to schizophrenia, schizoaffective disorder, or the manic phase of bipolar disorder may be treated with typical antipsychotic agents, atypical antipsychotic agents, or BZDs. However, a growing body of evidence seems to support the use of atypical antipsychotic agents in this circumstance.[57,74,84,102,105,106,118,121,122] Ketamine administration in patients with schizophrenia has been criticized for a theoretical risk of exacerbating psychosis. Ketamine may be a viable alternative in patients with schizophrenia where the benefit of immediate calming outweighs this risk.[123]

Agitation in Children

Because of years of experience and a proven safety record, BZDs are considered first-line therapy for the management of agitation in children. The IM dose of lorazepam is 0.05 to 0.1 mg/kg and the IM dose of midazolam is 0.1 to 0.2 mg/kg. Antipsychotics have also been used to manage agitation in children. The IM dose of haloperidol is 0.025 to 0.075 mg/kg, with a maximum dose of 2.5 mg. Children older than 12 years can receive the adult dose, usually 2.5 to 5 mg IM (see Table 70.1). Although droperidol is a highly effective drug for rapid sedation of adults, there is a paucity of literature supporting its use in children. The pediatric dose of droperidol is 0.03 to 0.07 mg/kg with a maximum initial dose of 2.5 mg.[64] Combination therapy is not generally recommended for children.[93] Ketamine has been used for sedation in pediatric cases refractory to BZDs.[124]

Agitation in Pregnancy

Psychotropic and anxiolytic medications should be used during pregnancy only when the potential risk to the fetus from exposure is outweighed by the risk of not treating the disorder in the mother.[125] Based on years of accumulated clinical experience but very little scientific data, conventional antipsychotic agents such as haloperidol and droperidol are recommended to control agitation in pregnant females.[126] In pregnancy, BZDs may be associated with teratogenicity (especially craniofacial abnormalities) when used for an extended period.[127] Although clear causation has not been proved, BZDs are generally avoided during the first trimester to minimize the risk for fetal malformation.[128] Nevertheless, judicious benzodiazepine administration should be considered a viable option for controlling agitation at all stages of pregnancy if needed.

Agitation in Older Patients

Patients 65 years or older are particularly susceptible to adverse drug reactions because of coexisting medical illness, use of multiple prescription medications (which increase the risk for drug-drug interactions), and age-associated changes in pharmacokinetics and pharmacodynamics. Research suggests that conventional antipsychotic medications such as haloperidol and droperidol are safe and effective for both psychotic symptoms and nonpsychotic agitated behavior.[129] Low doses (e.g., half the usual dose) of BZDs may also be used but require close observation for respiratory depression. BZDs may also exacerbate delirium in older adults. Continued use (>8 to 10 weeks) of atypical antipsychotic agents has been associated with increased rates of death in cases of dementia-related psychosis.[99]

Conducted Electrical Weapons

Conducted electrical weapons (CEWs), including TASERs and stun guns, are used by law enforcement agencies throughout the world. These nonlethal weapons use a temporary high-voltage low-current electrical discharge to overcome a body's voluntary muscle-triggering mechanisms, which results in widespread involuntary muscle contractions that incapacitate the individual. The current is delivered by direct contact with a handheld device (i.e., electric shock prods) or via a small dart-like electrode fired from a gun using small gas charges (e.g., TASER) similar to some air rifle propellants. There are also electrical weapons that cause intense pain without incapacitating the target, so-called drive stun devices. Law enforcement and correctional personnel typically use drive stun devices as a pain compliance technique. A TASER may deliver approximately 1200 V with direct skin contact.[130]

The exact street scenario of hyperactive delirium with severe agitation, physical restraint, and a TASER-linked death will probably never be studied with unchallenged scientific accuracy, and hence one is left with animal and human volunteer data to intuit the cause and effect of untoward events. Despite claims of lethality in the press, emotional testimony and unscientific reports from human rights organizations, and poorly documented claims in case reports, there have been no documented deaths directly and indisputably attributable to a TASER discharge in humans.[131] Volunteer studies and animal models failed to provoke cardiac arrest, significant cardiopulmonary, or metabolic derangements after standard electrical discharges, even when animal models included stimulant toxicity and human volunteers were exercised to exhaustion.[130] Nevertheless, CEWs have been temporally linked to a number of fatalities.[130–132] The majority of these cases involved sympathomimetic drug intoxication (e.g., cocaine, methamphetamines), prolonged physical exertion, or both.[132] The role of severely altered metabolic and autonomic parameters, drug intoxication, or underlying comorbid conditions, including cardiomyopathy, obscures the exact contribution of CEW use in unexpected deaths. A complete discussion of this topic is beyond the scope of this chapter, but it has been well reviewed elsewhere.[133,134] Darts from a CEW often penetrate the skin and must be removed, so the remainder of this section focuses on the procedure for removing embedded TASER electrodes.

Electronic Control Devices

TASER is an acronym for "Thomas A. Swift's Electric Rifle" and has been in existence since the early 1990s (Fig. 70.11). More than 15,000 law enforcement, correctional, and military agencies in 44 countries deploy TASER devices, and many municipalities in the United States allow civilians to purchase and carry these weapons for personal protection. A TASER uses compressed nitrogen to propel two electrode-tipped barbs at 180 ft/s at the target. The electrode-tipped barbs are

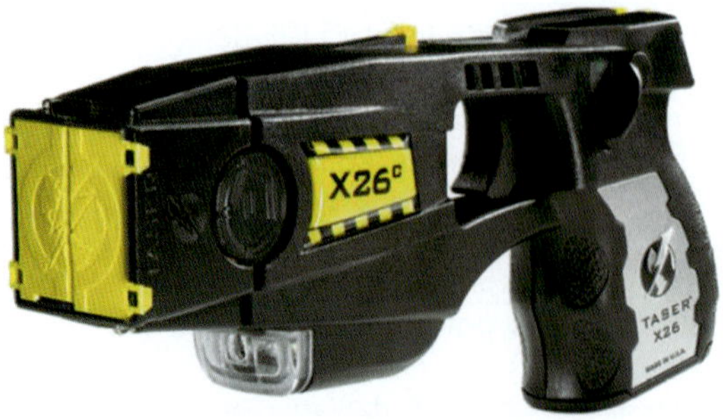

Fig. 70.11 TASER electrical control device.

attached to the electric device via two thin 21-foot wires and are similar in size to a No. 8 fishhook measuring 4 mm in length (Fig. 70.12). The barbs may attach to clothing and fail to penetrate the skin, or they may become embedded in skin and must be removed.

Removal Techniques

Barbs embedded in soft tissue can easily be removed with direct pressure. Place one hand on the skin surrounding the barb to hold the skin taut and use the other hand to apply direct pressure to the barb (Fig. 70.13).[129,130] If the patient cannot tolerate the procedure, inject a small amount of local anesthetic near the barb and use a No. 11 scalpel blade to cut down through the soft tissue to the tip of the barb. Because of the small size and linear shape of the barb, there is no need to advance the barb through the skin to remove the tip as is commonly performed during the removal of fishhooks.[135] A fulcrum technique can be used to remove barbs that have penetrated osseous structures. Grasp the base of the barb with pliers and use a 10-cc syringe placed below the pliers as a fulcrum to remove the barb (Fig. 70.14).[136] After removal, clean and dress the wound (see Chapter 34), but do not suture it. Analgesics (e.g., nonsteroidal anti-inflammatory drugs, acetaminophen) may be administered.

At discharge, provide standard wound care instructions (see Chapter 34). Advise the patient to watch for signs of infection; a 48-hour wound check may be prudent with contaminated wounds, when the barb was difficult to remove, or if there is concern for a retained foreign body. Tetanus status should be reviewed and updated if necessary. Significant infection after barb removal is rare, and prophylactic antibiotics are unnecessary. Following removal of a TASER dart, the disposition of the patient is based on the individual social scenario, and long-term ED observation is not required.

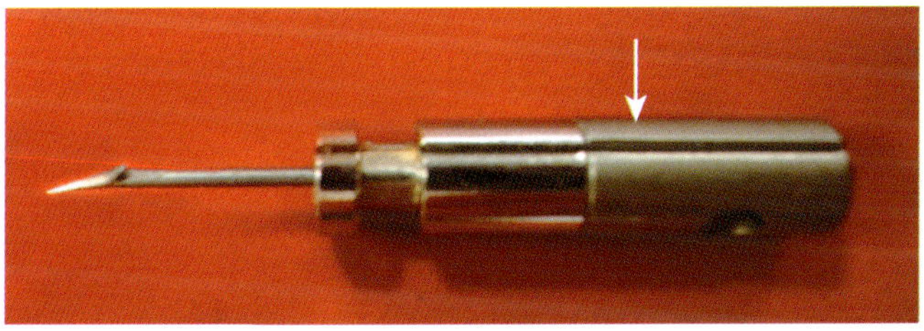

Fig. 70.12 TASER dart/electrode-tipped barb. The groove in the shaft *(arrow)* lines up with the barb tip to aid in removal.

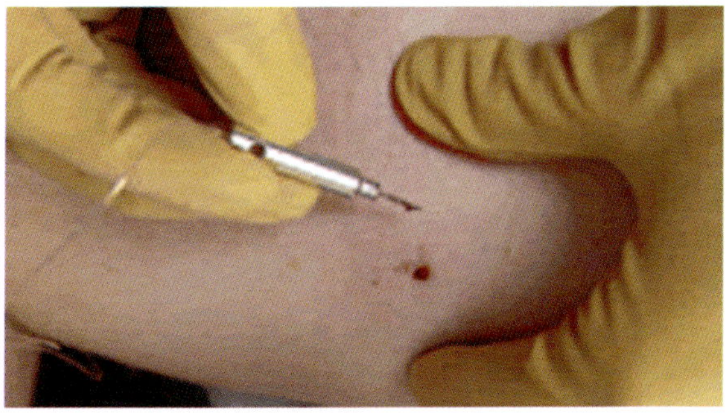

Fig. 70.13 Removal of an electrode-tipped barb. Barbs embedded in soft tissue can easily be removed with direct pressure. Place one hand on the skin surrounding the barb to hold the skin taut and use the other hand to apply direct pressure to the barb.

Complications

The risk for penetrating injury to the heart, lungs, or bowel from a TASER device is minimal, because of the small size of the barb. There are, however, increasing case reports of scrotal trauma, frontal sinus penetration, intraocular, osseous, and intracranial injuries resulting from TASER barbs.[136–145] Management will depend on the specific structure affected and can carry significant morbidity if not recognized. A barb embedded in a vascular structure can probably be removed with in-line manual traction followed by direct pressure on the wound because the size of the barb is similar to the size of devices used to obtain central venous access.[135] Consultation with an appropriate consultant can help manage these rare but potentially serious penetrating injuries.

Severe involuntary muscle contractions from the electrical discharge have been implicated as a cause of acute thoracic compression fractures.[146,147] Based on a literature review in 2019 by Vilke and colleagues, there is currently no indication for routine diagnostic or laboratory testing, monitoring, or hospitalization in awake, asymptomatic patients following short-duration exposure (<15 seconds) to a CEW.[148] However, there should be careful consideration for secondary injuries that may result from being incapacitated and falling.

TASER Use in the ED

Although data are difficult to confirm, it has been estimated that approximately 150 hospitals allow hospital security guards to carry TASERs. Those equipped with TASERs should have specific training, and policies on the use of the TASER in the hospital setting should be in place and training periodically updated. CMS regulations do not disallow TASERs in the hospital, but CMS and most states do not sanction the use of such devices to restrain a patient or to make them comply with medical treatment. Whenever possible, the least restrictive methods should be used to de-escalate aggressive behavior, or to calm agitated or disruptive individuals, such as a quiet and low-stimulation environment, reasonable bargaining, redirection of the patient, involvement of family, reality orientation, talk down, or a show of force. It is a gray area, indeed, as to when, or to what extent, any intervention is considered necessary to restrain a patient, or to protect a patient or medical personnel from harm. Every situation is somewhat unique so dogmatic approaches cannot be used. When a mentally incompetent or potentially suicidal patient wants to leave the ED against medical advice and does not have insight into the adverse effects of such an egress, involuntary commitment is initiated. Effective measures are usually initiated by the emergency physician because psychiatric evaluation on such short notice is impractical or unavailable and important decisions must be made immediately with limited data. Such patients may assault those attempting to keep them from leaving the ED in their incompetent mental state, when medical consequences, suicide, or harm to others could be the ultimate outcome.

Per CMS guidelines, the use of weapons by security staff is considered a law enforcement action, not a health care intervention. CMS does not support the use of weapons by any hospital staff as a means of subduing a patient to place that patient in restraint or seclusion. CMS interpretive guidelines to section 482.13(e) of the State Operations Manual say:

> *If a weapon is used by security or law enforcement personnel on a person in a hospital (patient, staff, or visitor) to protect*

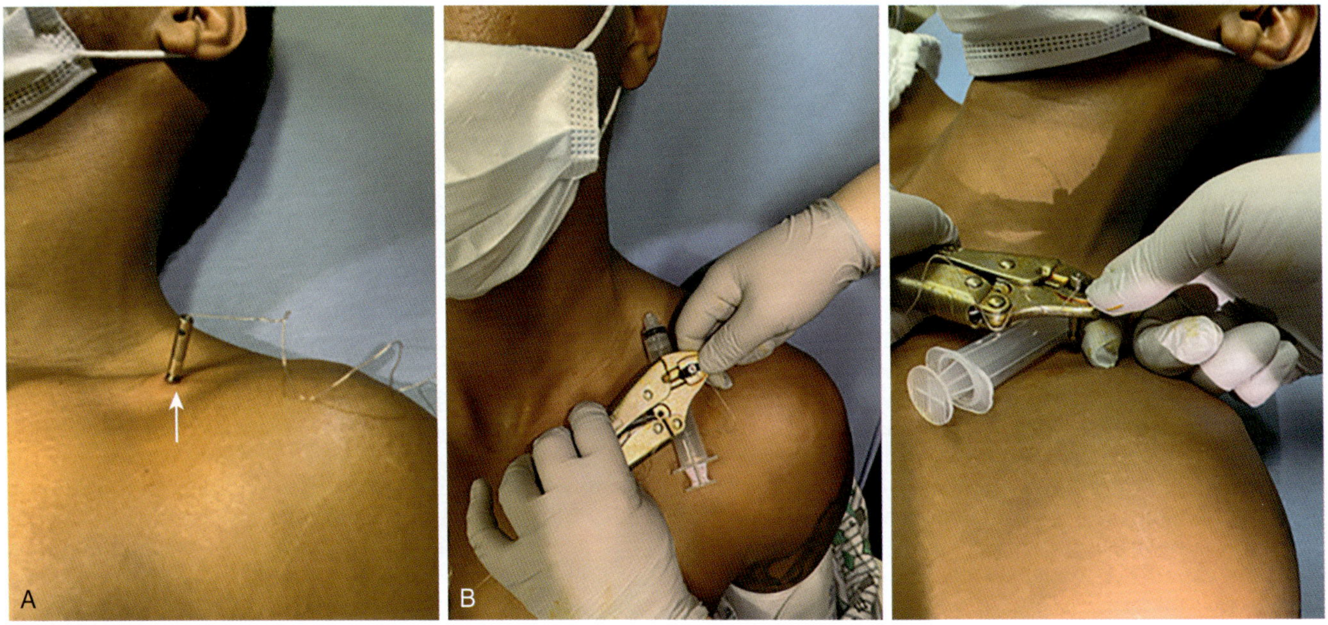

Fig. 70.14 Fulcrum technique to remove an electrode-tipped barb embedded in the clavicle. (A) Barb embedded in the left, anterior, mid-clavicle *(white arrow)*. (B) Pliers are used to grasp the base of the barb and a 10-mL syringe placed below the pliers is used as a fulcrum for easy removal (From Willoughby L, Peyton K, Gorgas D, Li-Sauerwine S. Leveraging resources to remove a Taser barb embedded in bone: Case report. *Clin Pract Cases Emerg Med.* 2022;6(1):29-31.)

people or hospital property from harm, we would expect the situation to be handled as a criminal activity and the perpetrator placed in the custody of local law enforcement.

In one small nonvalidated study, Ho and colleagues[149] concluded that the introduction of the TASER into the health care setting (a large urban tertiary care teaching hospital) demonstrated the ability to avert and control situations that could result in injury to medical personnel and patients, by simple TASER presentation or rarely actual use. In that study, there was a reduction in personnel injury rates and the contention that one suicide was averted. Further study is required before definitive statements can be made. In summary, the use of the TASER in the ED has not yet been clarified, and there are advocates as well as critics. Any weapon, including the TASER, should not be used to force a patient to comply or to induce restraint in the absence of reasonable suspicion of impending harm or actual assault of medical personnel.

REFERENCES ARE AVAILABLE AT ELSEVIER EBOOKS+

CHAPTER 71

Noncardiac Implantable Devices

Paul Jhun and Christopher R. Peabody

In addition to cardiac pacemakers and defibrillators, a number of noncardiac devices have been developed for electronic neuromodulation and drug delivery.[1] Although these devices are placed by a variety of subspecialists for the treatment of chronic illnesses, if the devices malfunction, patients may arrive at the emergency department in an acute state, thereby necessitating intervention by the emergency provider.

INSULIN INFUSION DEVICES

Background

External insulin infusion devices have become increasingly popular since their introduction in 1974. By 2007, there were more than 375,000 external insulin infusion pumps in use in the United States.[2]

Anatomy

An external insulin infusion pump device consists of a portable, programmable infusion pump connected to a subcutaneously implanted catheter that is maintained in place with adhesive tape (Fig. 71.1). The implanted catheter site varies, but it is commonly placed in the subcutaneous tissue of the abdomen in adults and the buttocks in young children. The thighs, hips, and upper part of the arms are other common sites. It is recommended that the infusion site be changed every 2 to 3 days.[3]

Device Complications

A 2023 study of 2429 insulin pump-associated adverse events reported that the highest percentage of these events resulted from problems with device components (27.3%), followed by alarms or alerts (16.7%), pump tasks (9.1%), and user error (3.4%). Box 71.1 lists the most frequently reported root causes in descending frequency. Box 71.2 lists the most frequently reported patient-oriented clinical consequences, which include hyperglycemia, hypoglycemia, and hospitalization.[4]

Procedure

If the device appears to be functioning normally, the American Association of Clinic Endocrinologists recommends that, should the patient be unable to manage their own pump while in the emergency department (ED), "the specialist(s) responsible for the patient's ambulatory pump management should be contacted promptly to make decisions about infusion adjustments."[2] Moreover, device malfunction should be considered in patients with insulin infusion devices who present to the ED with symptoms that may be related to blood glucose. In addition to medical management, troubleshoot the device and remove it in cases of uncertainty or emergency.

To remove the catheter, simply peel off the adhesive and embedded catheter together to discontinue the flow of injected medication into the patient. There are a variety of proprietary pump manufacturers, each with their own device programming. Call the appropriate manufacturer to troubleshoot the device, visit the manufacturer's website for an online troubleshooting manual, or simply instruct the patient to discontinue use of the device and return to a standard calculated insulin schedule by manual injection until the device-related complication is investigated and resolved.

INTRATHECAL DRUG DELIVERY SYSTEMS

Background

Intrathecal (spinal canal/subarachnoid space) drug delivery systems (IDDSs) have been in clinical use since the 1980s. The Food and Drug Administration (FDA) approved the use of intrathecal baclofen in 1992 for severe spasticity secondary to spinal cord injury, multiple sclerosis, cerebral palsy, or stroke. Subsequently, the FDA approved the use of intrathecal morphine in 1995 and intrathecal ziconotide in 2004 for chronic pain refractory to traditional medical therapies. Ziconotide is a nonopioid calcium channel blocker, but its use may be complicated by confusion, somnolence, and other neurologic side effects. Although data demonstrate efficacy of intrathecal morphine and ziconotide in relieving refractory pain[5–7] and efficacy of intrathecal baclofen in reducing spinal cord injury-induced spasticity,[8] more quality clinical evidence is needed.[9] IDDS devices are also used for the delivery of chemotherapeutic medications for specific oncologic conditions. Moreover, there are several off-label uses of various intrathecal medications.[9] Pumps are often used to deliver analgesics to patients with intolerable side effects from oral or parenteral analgesics, such as nausea, pruritus, and cognitive dysfunction. Other medications used include bupivacaine, hydromorphone, fentanyl, sufentanil, clonidine, midazolam, and ketamine. Some patients will receive a combination of medications. There are minimal data comparing various medications and current regimens have been empirically derived.

The advantage of IDDSs for chronic pain is the ability to get medication directly to receptors in the spinal cord by placing the medication into the subarachnoid space. For intrathecal morphine infusions, the recommended starting dose is 0.1 to 0.5 mg per day.[9] Such small intrathecal doses reduce systemic concentrations and minimize side effects. Patients in chronic pain may also use oral analgesics on a rescue basis.

Anatomy

There are two types of IDDS: continuous infusion devices and programmable devices. In the United States, the Codman 3000 (Codman & Shurtleff, Inc.) was an FDA-approved continuous infusion device, whereas the Medtronic SynchroMed III" and the Flowonix Prometra II are FDA-approved programmable devices. IDDS devices consist of an infusion pump connected to an intrathecal catheter (Fig. 71.2A). Codman's infusion pump was available with a refillable reservoir of either 16, 30, or 50 mL.[10] Both Medtronic's and Flowonix's refillable reservoirs are available in either 20 or 40 mL,[11] whereas Flowonix's refillable reservoir has

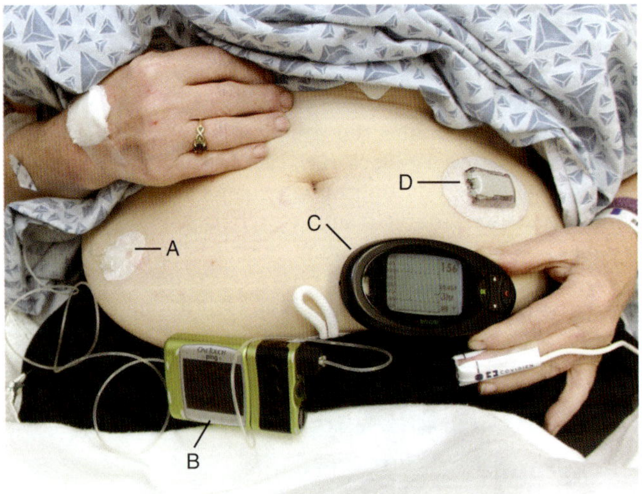

Fig. 71.1 External insulin infusion pump. Components include a subcutaneously implanted catheter *(A)* and a programmable infusion pump *(B)*. To discontinue the flow of insulin into the patient, simply peel off the adhesive and embedded catheter together. Also shown is a wireless continuous glucose monitoring receiver *(C)*, along with its sensor and transmitter *(D)*.

BOX 71.1 Most Frequent Adverse Event Narratives Citing the Root Causes With Insulin Infusion Pump Devices

1. Unknown (49.7%)
2. Device component: pump or pod reservoir/cartridge (8.9%)
3. Alarms, alerts, and notifications: obstruction of flow alarm (8.3%)
4. Device component: infusion set or site (8.2%)
5. Device component: continuous glucose monitor (4.3%)
6. Pump task: programming the pump (4.1%)
7. Device component: battery or power (4.0%)
8. Pump task: changing the pod/infusion set, including reservoir/cartridge (3.1%)

BOX 71.2 Most Frequent Adverse Event Narratives Citing the Clinical Consequence With Insulin Infusion Pump Devices

1. Blood glucose >400 mg/dL (47.3%)
2. Blood glucose <54 mg/dL (23.9%)
3. Hospital/ICU admission (15.2%)
4. Diabetic ketoacidosis (8.8%)

a 20-mL capacity.[12] The Codman 3000 does not utilize a battery and does not need to be replaced. SynchroMed III's battery life lasts up to 7 years, whereas Flowonix's battery life is 10 years. Normal refill intervals vary based on usage, typically on the order of every few months.

Intrathecal catheters are placed surgically and under general anesthesia by either neurosurgeons, interventional pain management physicians, or orthopedic spine specialists.[13]

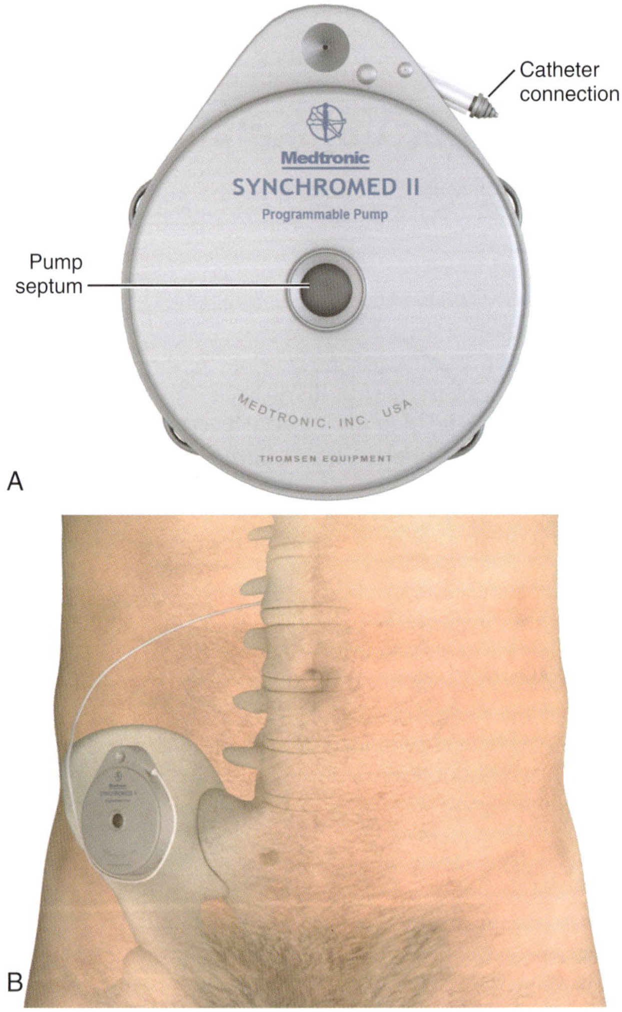

Fig. 71.2 (A) The Medtronic SynchroMed III programmable infusion pump is used primarily for intrathecal (cerebrospinal fluid) administration of opioids, baclofen, calcium channel blockers, or other medications used alone or in combinations. (B) The pump is usually implanted in a subcutaneous pocket in a lower abdominal quadrant, with the catheter tunneled subcutaneously to an appropriate lumbar interspace. Severe and difficult to treat withdrawal may occur if opioids or baclofen infusions are interrupted by a drained drug reservoir or pump malfunction.

A small incision is made in the back and the catheter tip is placed into the cerebrospinal fluid (CSF). The catheter is advanced to the desired level of medication delivery, based on symptoms. The catheter is then tunneled around the abdomen, placed in the lower abdominal wall, and attached to the subcutaneous pump. The pump has a port in the center that can be accessed by a needle placed through the skin. Medications are placed into the pump and refilled as needed (see Fig. 71.2B).

Continuous infusion devices, such as those made by Codman, are regularly refilled via manual bolus injections. Programmable devices are interrogated and programmed via an external manufacturer-specific device.

Device Complications

IDDS device complications requiring surgical intervention were found to occur with a frequency of 10.5% per year, with 35% pump related and 65% catheter related.[14,15]

In the perioperative period, complications can be serious and include a pump pocket hematoma, as well as epidural or intrathecal bleeds. A developing hematoma can present with sudden increase in back pain and neurologic symptoms consistent with cord injury including numbness and weakness in the lower extremities and loss of control of the bladder and bowels. If this condition is suspected, MRI or CT myelogram must be obtained and treatment is emergent surgical decompression.[13]

The most frequent and serious adverse events related to the device and implant procedures are catheter dislodgement from the intrathecal space, catheter fracture, implant site infection, and meningitis. Internal device programming errors that cause underdosing or overdosing are less common. If the drug supply is depleted, systemic symptoms related to acute drug withdrawal will occur. This is characteristic for the specific drug being delivered and should be anticipated.

A unique complication related to IDDSs that is the subject of a warning by the FDA is the formation of a granuloma at the tip of the intrathecal catheter. This space-occupying lesion can lead to temporary or permanent neurologic deficit or dysfunction, ranging from paresthesia to paralysis.[16] Interestingly, catheter-tip granuloma formation appears to be primarily associated with intrathecal opioids, and discontinuation of the offending agent is recommended in asymptomatic patients, with the expectation of granuloma resolution in 2 to 5 months.[16]

Common adverse effects related to intrathecal opioids include centrally mediated respiratory depression, nausea, vomiting, sedation, pruritis, constipation, and urinary retention.[17–19] One 2009 study using post-marketing data estimated a mortality rate of 3.9% at 1 year in IDDS patients being treated with an intrathecal opioid. The deaths were associated with respiratory arrest, although not causally proven.[19] A 2022 device manufacturer post-marketing analysis of 10,053 total targeted drug delivery system patients determined no deaths were a direct result of a product performance event.[20]

Intrathecal ziconotide may result in dizziness, nausea, vomiting, urinary retention, gait imbalance, nystagmus, and confusion. Although respiratory depression is uncommon, ziconotide may be associated with rare cases of rhabdomyolysis and psychosis.[7,17]

Common adverse effects related to intrathecal baclofen include hypotonia, somnolence, headache, dizziness, urinary retention, nausea, and paresthesias. It is more common to have an underdose of medication due to pump malfunction or a break or dislodgement of the catheter than to have an overdose. In the ED, it is usually impossible to accurately determine the exact cause of reduced medication delivery. In such cases, withdrawal syndromes will occur. In patients experiencing opioid, baclofen, or other medication withdrawal, treatment may be quite difficult because large doses of systemic medications are required to equal the effects of intrathecal medications. Hospital admission with specialty consultation and careful monitoring is often the most prudent tactic. Acute intrathecal baclofen withdrawal, which may resemble serotonin syndrome can be serious and difficult to manage.[21]

Baclofen withdrawal can lead to hemodynamic instability or seizures. As withdrawal is due to loss of medication at the spinal level, it may not be possible to safely deliver enough medication systemically to quell baclofen withdrawal symptoms. A propofol infusion has been suggested to treat baclofen withdrawal, but the patient may need to be intubated to facilitate a sufficient amount of propofol.[22] Specialty consultation, preferably by the specialty service who placed the pump, is required to address most complications of intrathecal pumps.

BOX 71.3 Drainage of the Infusion Pump Reservoir

EQUIPMENT

Antiseptic agent
22-gauge noncoring needle
20-mL Luer-Lok syringe or syringes

PROCEDURE

1. Palpate and locate the pump on the patient (typically in the lower abdominal subcutaneous layer). The reservoir fill port is located in the center of the pump.
2. Cleanse the injection site with the antiseptic agent.
3. Attach the 20-mL syringe to the 22-gauge needle and insert the needle through the skin into the center of the reservoir fill port until the needle touches the metal needle stop (see Fig. 71.3).
4. Use negative pressure to withdraw fluid from the reservoir. Empty the reservoir until backflow has stopped. Depending on pump volume, more than one syringe may be needed. Intrathecal drug delivery systems vary in their reservoir capacity from 15 to 50 mL.[11,12]
5. Remove the needle from the reservoir fill port.
6. Record the amount of medication fluid removed from the reservoir.

Procedure for Treating Medication Overdose

When there is concern for medication overdose secondary to the rare malfunction of the device, in addition to emergency medical management, the emergency physician can empty the pump reservoir by using the steps outlined in Box 71.3 if the relevant specialty service is not available.

One may also access the manufacturer-specific online manuals to review the steps necessary to remove the contents of the pump reservoir and thus prevent further infusion of intrathecal medication (Fig. 71.3).[11] Published guidelines suggest, in the absence of contraindications, withdrawal of an additional 30 mL to 40 mL of CSF by lumbar puncture to reduce the drug's concentration in CSF.[23]

VAGAL NERVE STIMULATORS

Background

Since the 1930s, several studies have shown the effects of vagal nerve stimulation on cerebral activity. In 1985, Zabara demonstrated the anticonvulsant effect of vagal nerve stimulation through animal studies.[24] In 1997 the FDA approved use of the vagal nerve stimulator (VNS) as an adjunctive treatment of medically refractory partial-onset epilepsy.[25] Subsequently, in 2005 the FDA approved use of the VNS as an adjunctive therapy for treatment-resistant depression.[26,27]

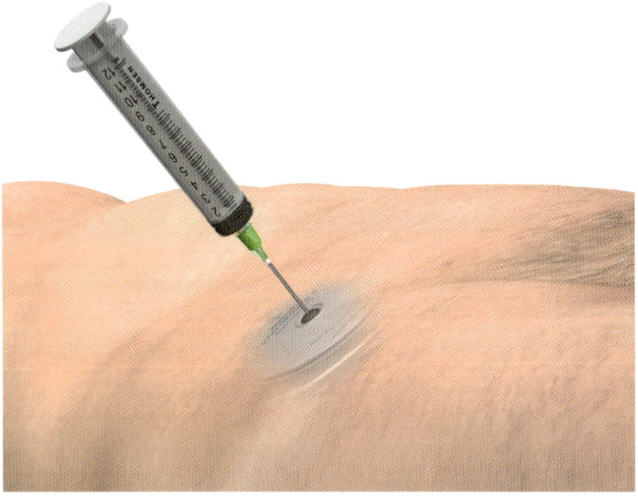

Fig. 71.3 The contents of the intrathecal pump reservoir can be removed with a syringe and 22-gauge needle (see Box 71.3). Cerebrospinal fluid may be withdrawn directly from a side port on the pump if a lumbar puncture is required.

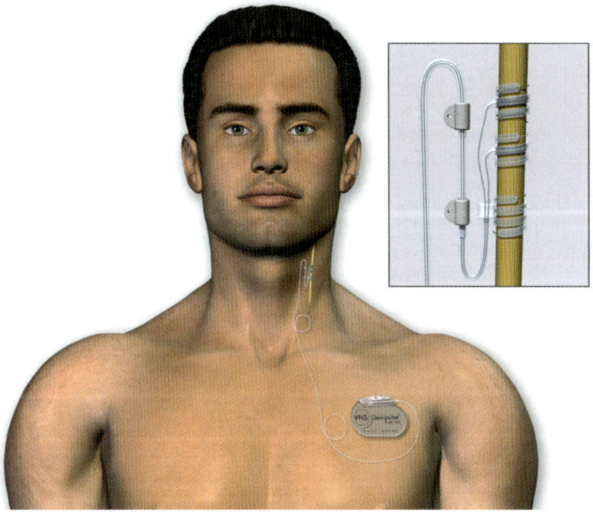

Fig. 71.4 Vagal nerve stimulator.

Anatomy

Currently in the United States, FDA-approved VNSs include Vivistim by MicroTransponder Inc. and VNS Therapy by LivaNova.

The device is composed of a generator attached to a bipolar VNS lead. Fig. 71.4 shows how the generator is surgically implanted into subcutaneous tissue in the left upper part of the chest, with the electrode lead being attached to the left cervical vagus nerve trunk. Interrogation and programming of the device are conducted with an external programming wand connected to a handheld computer. The variable settings that can be adjusted include current output, signal frequency, pulse width, and on/off stimulation times.[28]

Assuming normal parameters and output, the VNS generator has a projected battery life ranging from 5 to over 10 years. Of note, VNS devices are implanted only on the left vagus nerve because the right vagus nerve directly innervates cardiac tissue and may have undesired cardiac effects if stimulated.

BOX 71.4 Vagal Nerve Magnet Applications

TO DELIVER ON-DEMAND STIMULATION

Place the magnet over the generator for at least 1 second and then quickly remove it. The generator turns off and then immediately on again, thereby delivering a burst of vagal nerve stimulation based on the preprogrammed settings.

This maneuver can be repeated as needed.

TO TURN OFF THE STIMULATION

Hold and maintain the magnet over the pulse generator. If the device is properly turned off, the patient should notice loss of episodic adverse effects, such as stimulation-induced voice alteration or pain.[27,31]

Device Complications

The device is typically turned on 14 days after implantation to allow adequate wound healing. Be aware that patients seen postoperatively during the first 2 weeks after implantation may not have had their device activated yet.

In addition to surgery-related risks and complications, if the patient complains of severe neck pain, worsening hoarseness, choking, or difficulty breathing, consider device-specific complications. Voice alteration or hoarseness is the most common device-specific adverse effect, with more than 50% of patients being affected.[29–31] Other common side effects include increased coughing, shortness of breath, and pharyngitis. Less common device-specific adverse effects reported during clinical studies include ataxia, dyspepsia, dysphagia, hypoesthesia, infection, insomnia, laryngismus, nausea, pain, paresthesia, and vomiting.[28]

Procedure

In cases of emergency, diagnostic uncertainty, or significant adverse effects, turn off the pulse generator temporarily by holding a magnet over the generator (Box 71.4). Holding a magnet over the pulse generator (for at least 30 seconds for Vivistim and between 5 to 65 seconds for different VNS Therapy models) will turn *off* any ongoing stimulation while the magnet is held in place. Once the magnet is removed, the normal operation will resume. Alternatively, manual on-demand stimulation may be triggered by passing the external VNS magnet over the generator for at least 1 second and then immediately removing it. This on-demand stimulation, if initiated at the onset of an aura or seizure, may abort the attack or, if initiated during a seizure, may halt its progression.[28]

Unlike the typical donut-shaped magnet of a cardiac pacemaker, the VNS magnet is bar shaped, as shown in Fig. 71.5. Be aware that patients with VNSs may be provided with two magnets: one fitted with a wristband and the other fitted with a belt clip.

OTHER IMPLANTABLE DEVICES

There are several additional noncardiac implantable devices that the emergency provider may encounter, which are

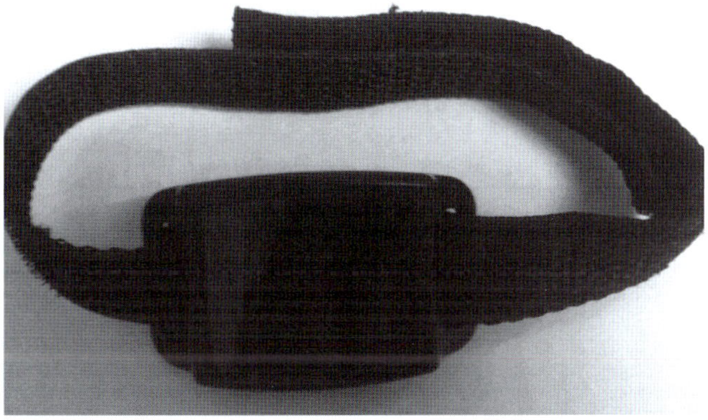

Fig. 71.5 Vagal nerve stimulator magnet.

TABLE 71.1 Additional Noncardiac Implantable Devices

DEVICE	DESCRIPTION	MALFUNCTION
Bladder stimulator or sacral nerve stimulator	Stimulator wire is inserted into the S3 sacral foramen adjacent to the sacral nerve for the treatment of urinary incontinence in the setting of severe neurologic disease[32]	Hardware complications include infection, pain, and lead migration.[33]
Deep brain stimulator	Stimulator implanted into the thalamus for treatment of Parkinson's disease, tremor, and dystonia[1]	Hardware complications include infection and lead migration.[33]
Gastric pacemaker	Neurostimulator with implanted leads into the gastric musculature to improve gastroparesis[34]	Gastric wall perforation, infection, and lead migration.[34]
Peritoneovenous (Denver) shunt	A shunt that drains peritoneal fluids directly into the venous system to treat refractory ascities[35]	Shunt occlusion, pulmonary edema, pulmonary embolism, disseminated intravascular coagulopathy, superior vena cava thrombosis, infection, tumor emboli.[36,37]
Phrenic nerve stimulator or diaphragmatic pacemaker	Electrodes implanted into each phrenic nerve with a receiver implanted into subcutaneous tissue. An external transmitter controls the receiver. Used to treat respiratory insufficiency secondary to upper motor neuron paralysis or respiratory drive dysfunction.[38,39]	Pneumothoraces have been described immediately after implantation. Infection and wire migration have been described.[38,39] Failure of the pacemaker is treated by ventilatory support.

outlined in Table 71.1. However, should these devices malfunction, there may not be specific procedures to be aware of in the emergency setting beyond supportive treatment.

MRI AND IMPLANTABLE DEVICES

The issue of MRI compatibility with implantable devices is very complex. In the event that MRI appears to be necessary, a case-by-case risk-benefit analysis involving the relevant subspecialist and radiologist is recommended.

For patients with implanted medical devices, the FDA requires labeling to include MRI safety information.[40] Given the existence of several generations of models and evolving technology, manufacturer device manuals and support websites should be reviewed. Of note, there are a number of clinical series and case reports indicating the compatibility of certain devices with MRI. For VNSs, both Vivistim and VNS Therapy are MR conditional devices under specific conditions,[27,27a] as it may cause heat injury and damage the device. Both SynchroMed III and Prometra II pumps are MRI conditional. However, the Prometra device is only MRI compatible after complete removal of medication from the reservoir, whereas there is no need to remove medication from the SynchroMed II device under certain conditions.[11,12] As detailed earlier in the chapter, insulin pumps may easily be removed in the event that MRI is required. Preferably, insulin pump removal occurs with knowledge of the provider who manages the patient's diabetes, as a manual insulin regimen may be needed temporarily until the device can be reimplanted.

REFERENCES ARE AVAILABLE AT Elsevier eBooks+

CHAPTER 72

Radiation in Pregnancy and Clinical Issues of Radiocontrast Agents

Kathlene Babalola and Ayo Igun

INTRODUCTION

In recent years, the increase in diagnostic radiation exposure has led to a concerted effort by several organizations including the Food and Drug Administration (FDA)[1] and American College of Radiology (ACR) to reduce radiation exposure and therefore risks to patients. Ionizing radiation is a known carcinogen; an estimated 1:270 females who undergo CT coronary angiography will develop cancer.[2]

Between 1980 and 2009, there was a 750% increase in population-wide radiation exposure due to diagnostic studies[3]; however, subsequent years have seen a substantial decrease in exposure.[4] Between 2006 and 2016, exposure from nontherapeutic studies decreased 15% to 20% due to reduced dose/study and a decline in the overall number of studies performed. Concepts such as "as low as reasonably achievable" or ALARA,[5,6] as well as the Imaging Wisely and Image Gently initiatives,[7,8] have led to greater awareness of the impact of radiation exposure on patients and the need for greater stewardship when contemplating the necessity of diagnostic studies. The Joint Commission sentinel event alert summarizes the recommendations for reducing ionizing radiation exposure to patients and medical staff "by providing the right test and the right dose through effective processes, safe technology and a culture of safety."[9]

Despite these efforts, the effects of radiation exposure remain a concern among pregnant females, including those in the medical field. Nearly 33% of females under 40 reported radiation exposure as a deterrent to choosing fields of practice such as interventional cardiology and interventional radiology.[10] Patients are often provided with inaccurate information from clinicians regarding the risks of radiation exposure to the unborn fetus[11] which can lead to unwarranted fears of harm that are not supported by scientific evidence.[12] According to the American College of Obstetricians and Gynecologists, "With few exceptions, radiation exposure through radiography, CT scan, or nuclear medicine imaging techniques is at a dose much lower than the exposure associated with fetal harm. If these techniques are necessary in addition to ultrasonography or MRI or are more readily available for the diagnosis in question, they should not be withheld from a pregnant patient."[13] This is of obvious importance in the emergency department (ED) where the decision to obtain testing must be quickly weighed against the risks, and where the consequences of not obtaining an appropriate study can be deleterious.

To determine the risk to both the mother and the fetus when evaluating the pregnant patient, several factors must be considered. This includes gestational age, type of radiation, dose of radiation, and the anatomical focus of evaluation. This chapter provides a review of ionizing and nonionizing radiation, its uses in diagnostic radiological examinations, the risks of its use, and strategies for minimizing risk to assist the clinician in counseling the patient to arrive at the most appropriate shared decision.

TYPES OF RADIATION

According to the Nuclear Regulatory Commission, radiation is "the transfer of energy through a medium."[14] The medium can be anything, such as air, water, or tissue and the radiation can take many forms as well. This includes electromagnetic waves in the spectrum of visible light, x-ray, gamma ray, or infrared; particle radiation such as alpha, beta, and neutrons; and acoustic radiation such as with ultrasonography or the radiofrequency (RF) energy used in MRI. As radiation propagates through space, it can impart or give-up some or all of its energy to surrounding material or tissues, and detection of this energy or its absence forms the basis of diagnostic medical imaging.

Radiation is further classified as ionizing or nonionizing based on the effect that the absorbed energy has on the absorbing medium. Both ionizing and nonionizing radiation deliver energy to the surrounding medium. However, nonionizing radiation lacks sufficient energy to liberate electrons, and its deposited energy subsequently manifests as heat, whereas ionizing radiation is of sufficient energy to liberate electrons, thereby breaking chemical bonds, forming highly reactive free radicals, and damaging DNA and cellular machinery.

RADIOBIOLOGY AND RADIOPHYSICS

Measurement of the effect of radiation exposure begins with measurement of radiation dose. The amount of energy that is imparted by radiation on a material per unit of mass is called the absorbed dose (D); this dose is quantifiable and measurable. The average dose over a material (e.g., an organ or tissue) is called the mean absorbed dose (D_T). Both are defined using the System Internationale (SI) unit of gray (Gy), which is measured in joule/kilogram (J/kg).

Prior to the adoption of the joule and the newton, the centimeter-gram-second (CGS) units of energy and force—the erg and the dyne respectively—were typically used in physics derived equations. The CGS unit of rad is derived from those antiquated units with the measure of erg/gram (erg/g) and is related to the Gy as such:

$$1\,\text{erg} = 10^{-7}\,\text{joules}$$

$$1\,\text{rad} = 100\,\text{erg/g} = 10^{-5}\,\text{J}/10^{-3}\,\text{kg} = 10^{-2}\,\text{J/kg} = 10^{-2}\,\text{Gy} = 0.01\,\text{Gy} = 10\,\text{mGy}$$

The rad is still used in the United States and in some other countries. However, for the sake of uniformity, the measure of Gy, which is more ubiquitous, will be used throughout this chapter.

Various forms of radiation can transfer energy to tissue and cause ionizing events. Heavy particles (those particles which are heavier than an electron), such as alpha particles, protons, neutrons, and carbon ions, move more slowly, have higher rates of energy loss in matter, produce less radiation scatter, and therefore produce more densely packed ionizing events. Conversely, light-charged particles such as beta particles and electromagnetic radiation move quickly through matter with less energy transfer, and more radiation scatter, producing ionizing events that are less densely packed.

The many forms of radiation differ in their abilities to impart energy to the absorbing material and cause ionizing events. Neutrons, alpha particles, and other heavy charged particles (e.g., carbon ions) impart their energy more readily, thereby producing more densely spaced ionizing events, whereas the converse is true for electromagnetic radiation and light-charged particles (e.g., beta particles). Another quantity, the *equivalent dose* (H_T), is therefore necessary and derived from the mean absorbed dose by scaling with a *radiation weighting factor* (w_R), $H_T = w_R D_T$, and the *effective dose* for an organism is the tissue-weighted sum of the equivalent doses for all tissues, radiation sources, and energies. The radiation weighting factor, previously called the quality factor, is dependent only on the type of radiation (and for neutrons, its energy) and is dimensionless. Per the International Committee on Radiological Protection, $w_R = 1$ for all photons and electrons; $w_R = 2$ for protons and charged pions; $w_R = 20$ for alpha particles, heavy ions, and fission fragments; and w_R is a continuous function of energy for neutrons. Equivalent dose and effect dose therefore have SI units of J/kg with the special name sievert (Sv). In CGS, they have units of *roentgen equivalent in man* (rem), and 1 rem = 100 erg/g = 0.01 J/kg = 0.01 Sv = 10 mSv. As diagnostic radiology examinations involve essentially only photons, the equivalent and effective doses have essentially the same magnitude as the absorbed dose. As an example, a mean absorbed dose of 100 mGy results in an effective dose of 100 mSv if the source is electromagnetic radiation or 2 Sv if the source is alpha radiation. Different tissues in the body have different tissue weighting factors, as noted in Table 72.1.

TABLE 72.1 Tissue Weighting Factors of Various Human Organs/Tissues

TISSUE	TISSUE WEIGHTING FACTOR w_T
Brain	0.01
Skin	0.01
Tissue[a]	0.01
Bladder	0.04
Thyroid	0.04
Tissue[b]	0.04
Gonads	0.08
Heart	0.12
Uterus/cervix	0.12
Lung	0.12
Breasts	0.12
Tissue[c]	0.12

[a]Bone surface, salivary glands.
[b]Esophagus, liver.
[c]Adrenals, gallbladder, kidneys, lymph nodes, muscle, oral mucosa, pancreas, prostate, small bowel, colon, spleen, thymus.
Adapted from International Commission on Radiological Protection. The 2007 Recommendations of the International Commission on Radiological Protection (Users Edition). *ICRP Publication 103* (Users Edition). *Ann ICRP*. 2007;37:2-4.

Radioactive decay or radioactivity is the process by which the nucleus of an unstable atom emits energy in the form of radiation. This rate is defined by the decay of the unstable atom by emission of alpha particles, protons, or neutrons, which results in a more stable ion and the emission of ionizable radiation. The SI unit of radioactivity is the becquerel (Bq) and is defined as one nuclear decay event per second. The unit of measure is therefore in inverse seconds, s^{-1}. This measure is independent of the type of radioactive material or the type of radiation that is emitted. The non-SI unit of radioactivity is the curie (Ci) which is equivalent to 3.7×10^{10} Bq. Doses of radioactive substances used in nuclear medicine are usually of the order of MBq or mCi.

EFFECTS OF RADIATION

The harmful effects of radiation can be divided broadly into two categories: stochastic effects and non-stochastic or tissue reactions (Table 72.2). Tissue reactions occur as a result of ionizing radiation exposure with an identifiable threshold below which effects are not observed and above which they are reliably observed. The severity of the effect rises with dose.[15] The effects of tissue reactions result *directly* from radiation exposure causing cell death that can lead to lethality, CNS abnormalities, organ dysfunction/malformation, growth retardation, and behavioral disorders.[16] Stochastic effects include heritable effects and cancer. These effects are indirect, and the probability of occurrence increases with dose; however, there is no identifiable threshold dose and severity is independent of dose. In addition to dose, the duration of exposure also impacts the effect. A single, high-intensity exposure is more likely to have an effect than a protracted exposure of low intensity. Fractionation of the dose (e.g., multiple radiographs over a period of hours or days) increases the threshold for tissue reactions and decreases the severity of the effect.[17]

STAGES OF FETAL DEVELOPMENT

Fetal development is divided into three major stages: (1) preimplantation and implantation phase, which comprises conception until the first 2 weeks of pregnancy; (2) organogenesis, which occurs primarily during weeks 2 to 8 of pregnancy; and (3) the fetal phase, which occurs from week 8 until term. The risks of harm from radiation exposure are most significant during organogenesis and the early portion of the fetal phase, when CNS development is most prominent. The risks decrease steadily after the 25th week of pregnancy and are decidedly low in the third trimester. The relationship between gestational age and radiation effects is illustrated in Fig. 72.1 and summarized in Table 72.3.[18]

Preimplantation and Implantation

The preimplantation and implantation phase has been designated an "all-or-none" period, as embryonic cells are few in number and totipotent, and can replace damaged neighboring cells.[17] It is in this stage of development that the embryo is least likely to be malformed, and the predominant effect of radiation exposure is failure to implant, resulting in abortion.[17–19] The threshold for mortality in this stage of development is quite high, estimated at 100 to 200 mGy and rises with fetal age such that at term the threshold for mortality is 1 Gy to 1.5 Gy[5] (see Table 72.3).[17–19] Embryos that survive exposure

TABLE 72.2 Stochastic and Tissue Reaction (Threshold) Comparison

PHENOMENON	PATHOLOGY	DISEASES	RISK	DEFINITION
Stochastic	Damage to a single cell may result in disease	Cancer, germ-cell mutation	Some risk exists at all dosages; at low doses the risk may be less than the spontaneous risk	The incidence of the disease increases with dose, but the severity and nature of the disease remain the same
Tissue reactions	Multicellular injury	Intrauterine death, organ malformations, mental impairment, growth retardation	No increased risk below the threshold dose	Both the severity and the incidence of the disease increase with the dose

Modified from Brent RL. Utilization of developmental basic science principles: the evaluation of reproductive risks from pre- and postconception environmental radiation exposures. *Teratology*. 1999;54:182.

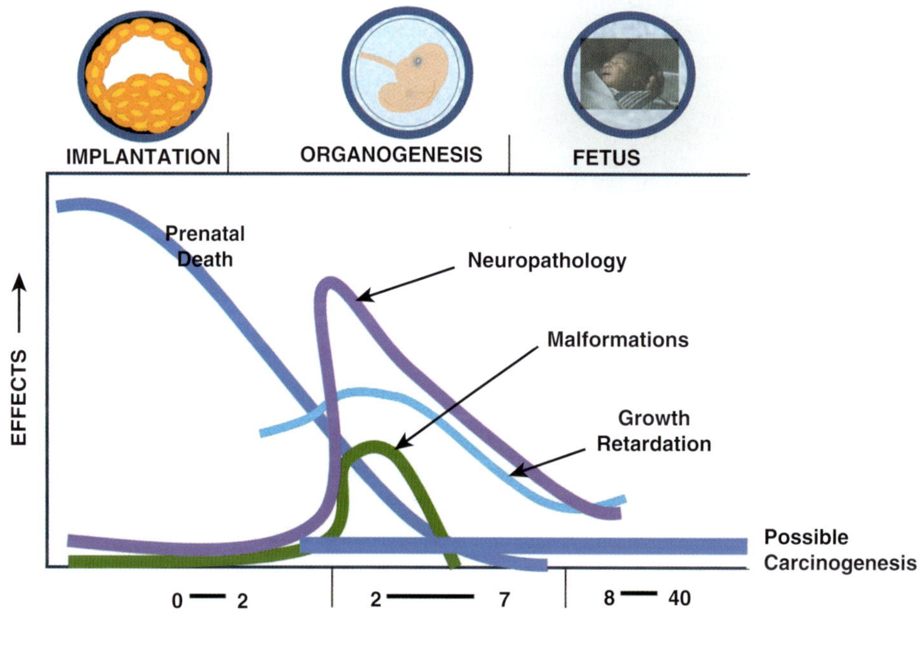

Fig. 72.1 Schematic presentation of the various adverse effects associated with high-dose radiation and their relative incidence at different stages of gestation. (Modified from Mettler FA, Upton A. *Medical Effects of Ionizing Radiation.* 3rd ed. Elsevier; 2008.)

in this period of development demonstrate no increased risk for malformations or growth retardation.[17]

Organogenesis

The potential for radiation induced abnormality is highest during the phase of organogenesis (between week 2 and week 8) and results from reduced ability to replace those cells damaged or killed by the exposure. Studies done on data collected during the Hiroshima and Nagasaki incidents[20] measured dose-response relationship with any intellectual disability; though previously a linear relationship with no threshold was assumed, this study showed a minimum threshold between 61 and 310 mGy with a linear-exponential relationship and unknown dose rate. However, no notable incidence of severe intellectual disability was observed with an acute exposure less than 610 mGy. Though any organ system can be affected during this stage, the most observed effects were microcephaly and growth retardation.[17–19,21]

The minimum dose threshold for observation for any of these effects was between 50 and 200 mGy.[18,19] Between 100 and 250 mGy, growth retardation effects tend to be temporary and infants experience normal growth through adulthood.[21] Permanent growth retardation is observed at gestational age 4

TABLE 72.3 Risks and Threshold Doses of the Main Effects of Prenatal Irradiation

GESTATIONAL AGE (WK)	POSTCONCEPTION AGE (WK)	MINIMUM LETHAL DOSE TO EMBRYO OR FETUS (Gy)	APPROXIMATE LD50	MINIMUM DOSE FOR PERMANENT GROWTH RETARDATION IN THE ADULT (Gy)	MINIMUM DOSE FOR GROSS ANATOMIC MALFORMATIONS (Gy)	INCREASED INCIDENCE OF MENTAL IMPAIRMENT(Gy)
3–4	1–2	0.15–0.2	>1	No increased incidence of GR in survivors	No increased incidence of congenital malformation in survivors	
5–7	3–5	0.25–0.5	1.4–2	0.2–0.5	>0.2 but most malformations require >0.5	
8–15	6–13	>1	>2	0.25–0.5		
16–Term	14–Term	>1.5	Same as mother	>0.5		
10–27	8–25					Severe at doses >0.5; (lower 95% CI value of ~0.3)

CI, Confidence interval; *GR*, growth retardation; *LD50*, lethal dose for 50% of the population.
Modified from National Council on Radiation Protection and Measurements. *Preconception and prenatal radiation exposure: health effects and protective guidance*. NCRP;2013:174.

to 6 weeks with a dose threshold of 200 to 500 mGy; at 7 to 15 weeks with a dose threshold of 250 to 500 mGy and at a dose threshold >500 mGy at 16 weeks and above (see Table 72.3).[17] No effects were seen below 50 mGy, which is higher than the fetal radiation dose of commonly ordered diagnostic studies.

Fetal Phase

At the end of organogenesis is the commencement of the fetal phase, which starts at around 8 weeks postconception. The CNS begins developing in the 8th week and continues through the 25th week, during which the fetus can be seriously affected by high doses of ionizing radiation, resulting in developmental delay, intellectual disability, neurobehavioral effects, and convulsive disorder.[17] CNS sensitivity to ionizing radiation is not uniform throughout its development, with highest sensitivity from the 8th through 15th week[18] during which there is a rapid increase in the number of neurons that migrate and differentiate, losing their ability to divide.[18] This process is largely concluded by the 15th week, at which point and lasting until the 25th week, further differentiation and architectural definition occur,[11] and the CNS becomes slightly less susceptible to damage.[22]

Growth Restriction

Fetal exposure to 100 mGy or less of radiation is not associated with grown retardation or congenital malformation.[16] Though intrauterine growth restriction was most commonly observed in animal studies when radiation exposure occurred during organogenesis, growth was largely recoverable, with permanent effects on postnatal growth requiring early fetal phase exposure upwards of 1 Gy.[23] The most commonly seen abnormality is microcephaly with the threshold dose for observation between 100 and 200 mGy.[24]

Intellectual Disability

At baseline, a child has a background risk of 3% of being born with an IQ <70. Fetal exposure to 100 mGy or less of radiation is not associated with a reduction in IQ.[18] Clinically observed IQ reductions require fetal-absorbed doses in excess of 500 mGy.[18,21] The most susceptible period occurs during weeks 8 to 15 and with a dose threshold of 1 Gy. Much of what we know about this effect of fetal exposure was from epidemiological studies done on survivors of the Hiroshima and Nagasaki atomic bomb attacks. In studying survivors, it was found that a 3-point drop in IQ for every 100 mGy of exposure was observed with a minimum threshold of 500 mGy.[20,21] No clinically observed incidence of exposure associated intellectual disability was seen at doses below 500 mGy except during organogenesis.

Convulsive Disorders

Convulsive disorders are a broad category encompassing various diagnoses, etiologies, and manifestations. The risk for convulsive disorder following in utero radiation exposure was evaluated in several studies on Japanese survivors of the atomic bombing.[20,25] Among these survivors, no convulsive disorders were identified in those receiving a dose less than 100 mGy. Those at highest risk for seizure disorder were those exposed in the 8th through 15th weeks postconception and who also had intellectual disability. The association of convulsive disorders with radiation exposure between the 8th and 15th weeks postconception without intellectual disability was borderline significant. There is no increase in convulsive disorders from exposure before the 8th week or after the 25th week.[17]

STOCHASTIC EFFECTS

The remaining effects (cancer and hereditary effects) are stochastic, notably in that risk exists at all levels of exposure (see

Table 72.2). The risk of childhood cancer is overall low, with the cumulative (all cause) risk being 1 to 2.5 per 1000 to age 15.[17] Childhood cancers make up less than 1% of all cancer diagnoses and the most common malignancies are CNS tumors, leukemia, and lymphoma.

Cancer

In 1956 Alice Stewart et al. published a study after working on the Oxford Child Health Surveys, which was initially set up by Professor John Ryle. At the time, she observed that child cancer rates were increasing and commenced the Oxford Survey of Childhood Cancers.[26] Abdominal pelvimetry was, at the time, used to assess the position of the fetus. The study showed that there was a nearly 1.5- to 2.0-fold increase in childhood cancers over the background occurrence in the children who had been exposed to antenatal x-ray. These results were met initially with skepticism and criticized on the basis of recall bias, but the effect persisted in later studies in which a 1.3- to 1.5-fold risk was reported.[17,27] As a result, prenatal pelvimetry was abandoned in favor of ultrasound (US) diagnostic imaging.[28,29] These findings are consistent with an analysis of later epidemiologic studies that found a relative risk of 1.4 for childhood cancer after exposure to 10 mGy.[18] Efforts were undertaken to estimate the risk per Gy from exposure and to determine the excess absolute risk coefficient of ~6% per Gy (2.5% per Gy for leukemia).[18,19,30] These results must be interpreted in the context of the background incidence; for a fetus exposed to 1 mGy, the risk for carcinogenesis is 0.006%, or 3 additional diagnoses for every 50,000 exposures, as compared with the background incidence of 0.2% to 0.3%, or 100 to 150 per 50,000. Exposure to 50 mGy, the generally accepted upper limit for exposure in utero, may double the risk for childhood malignancy in the offspring, but this absolute risk remains low (0.5% to 0.6%).[18,19,30]

Heritable Effects

Early research with flies and animals demonstrated ionizing radiation can induce germ-cell mutations, but these findings have failed to be demonstrated in humans[30] and were so small in the irradiated Japanese survivors as to be statistically insignificant.[24] Others report an excess absolute risk for hereditary disease of 1% per Gy.[21,31] In the context of a background incidence of 3%, an exposure of 50 mGy might then be expected to raise this risk to 3.05%.[32]

Computed Tomography and Radiography

The largest source of exposure to ionizing radiation in diagnostic imaging in the ED is from radiography, followed closely by CT.[33] Multisite imaging trends saw an overall decrease from 2010 to 2016 in a multisite comparative study of pregnant patients, but with similar trends of usage: 58/1000 patients radiography versus 10.6/1000 CT.[34] The overwhelming majority of these diagnostic imaging studies do not result in a significant risk of exposure to the fetus (Table 72.4), though CT scans of the pelvis have the potential to approach or even exceed the safe threshold of 50 mGy.[18] In addition to the relationship between the fetus and the imaged anatomy, other factors affect the amount of ionized radiation the fetus is ultimately exposed to. Variables such as slice thickness, helical movement pattern, etc. all impact the total level of exposure. Protocol-specific scanning parameters, such as wider beam collimation, pitch, and lower mAs, kV, and scan volume are selected to further reduce the fetal and maternal effective dose.[35,36] Multidetector CT offers diagnostic image quality faster than conventional spiral CT (0.37 s/rotations vs. 1 s/rotation), in addition to advances in image reconstruction that can result in reduction of effective dose.[37] Lead shielding is no longer recommended because (1) radiation dose reduction is modest at best and (2) increased radiation internal scatter after shielding can actually increase the effective dose absorption in the gravid uterus (Fig. 72.2).[36,38]

CT Contrast Agents

Contrast agents, IV and oral, are often required for optimal image clarity and improved detection rates. Iodinated contrast solutions are used for CT imaging and are typically classified as ionic versus nonionic with the former having five to seven times the osmolality of normal serum versus the latter, which is two to three times the osmolality.[39] Ionic contrast agents have a higher incidence of contrast-related reactions and are generally not used for typical CT studies done in EDs. Instead, EDs normally employ low molecular weight, low osmolality nonionic agents such as iohexol (Omnipaque) and iodixanol (Visipaque).[40]

Most studies of fetal exposure to iodinated contrast material have focused on fetal thyroid function. By the early portion of the second trimester, the fetal pituitary-thyroid axis is functioning independently of the mother and fetal thyroxine is produced by stimulation of fetal thyroid-stimulating hormone (TSH).[41] To date, no study has shown an adverse effect on neonatal thyroid function after the administration of maternal IV nonionic contrast; oral contrast is minimally absorbed in the gut and poses no risk to the fetus.[39,42] A minimal amount of contrast is present in breast milk of nursing mothers and a minimal fraction of it is absorbed in the gut of neonates.[41] Nursing mothers are advised that they do not need to interrupt nursing after receiving IV contrast.[13]

Contrast-induced nephropathy (CIN) is defined as an increase in creatinine by 0.3 mg/dL within 48 hours after IV contrast, a relative increase in creatinine of 1.5 to 1.9 within 7 days, or decreased urine output of <0.5 mg/kg for at least 6 hours post contrast administration.[39] Patients with chronic kidney disease (CKD) are at increased risk of developing nephropathy and no studies have found an increased susceptibility in pregnant patients compared with the general population.[39] Protocols for prevention of CIN are listed in Table 72.5. There are no studies showing an adverse effect on fetal kidney function after antenatal maternal IV contrast administration.

Nuclear Medicine Studies

Nuclear medicine studies use "radioactive tracers (radiopharmaceuticals) to assess bodily functions and to diagnose and treat disease."[43] Unstable isotopes are introduced into the body and emit alpha, beta, or gamma radiation which can then be detected by gamma detectors. Overall, the most common

TABLE 72.4 Estimated Fetal and Gonadal Exposure From Various Diagnostic Imaging Methods and Radiopharmaceuticals

TYPE OF PROCEDURE	DESCRIPTION	TYPICAL DOSE TO EMBRYO OR FETUS (mGy)[a]	DOSE TO GONADS (OVARIES, TESTES) (mGy)
Radiography and fluoroscopy	Skull	<0.01	<0.01, <0.01
	Chest	<0.01	<0.01, <0.01
	Thoracic spine	<0.01	<0.01, <0.01
	Mammography	<0.1	<0.01, NA
	Pelvis	0.1–1.1	2, 4
	Lumbar spine	1–2	4, 0.6
	Abdomen	1–3	2.5, 0.7
	Upper GI series	7	1, 0.1
	Barium enema	7–8	10, 4
CT	Brain	<0.1	<0.1
	Chest, angiography of coronary arteries	0.1–1	<0.1, <0.1
	Abdomen	4–16 (avg: 8; max: 49)[b]	1, 1
	Pelvis[a]	Avg: 25; max: 79	
	Lumbar spine[a]	Avg: 2.4; max: 8.6	
Nuclear medicine	Lung-ventilation study; ^{133}Xe (740 MBq)	0.02–0.3	0.5, 0.5
	Lung-perfusion study; ^{99m}Tc-MAA (148 MBq)	0.4–0.7	0.27, 0.16
	White cell scan; ^{111}In (18.5 MBq)	1.7–2.4	2.2, 0.8
	Renal scan; ^{99m}Tc-MAG3 (370 MBq)	1.9–6.7	2, 1.4
	Bone scan; ^{99m}Tc-MDP (740 MBq)	1.5–4.4	2.7, 1.8
	Cerebral blood flow; ^{99m}Tc-HMPAO (740 MBq)	3–6.7	4.9, 1.9
	Positron emission tomography; ^{18}F-FDG (740 MBq)	13–16	10, 8.1
	Myocardial perfusion; ^{99m}Tc-sestamibi (1110 MBq)	5–6	9.0, 4.1
	Cancer therapy—5% uptake; ^{131}I (3,700 MBq)	66–1000	163, 107
	Benign therapy—50% uptake; ^{131}I (555 MBq)	40–150	23, 14

[a]Modified from National Council on Radiation Protection and Measurements. *Preconception and prenatal radiation exposure: health effects and protective guidance.* NCRP;2013:174.

[b]Modified from International Commission on Radiological Protection. Pregnancy and medical radiation. *Ann ICRP*. 2000;30(iii):1-43.

CT, Computed tomography; *FDG,* fludeoxyglucose; *GI,* gastrointestinal; *HMPAO,* hexamethylpropyleneamine oxime; *MAA,* macroaggregated human albumin; *MAG3,* mercaptoacetyltriglycine; *MDP,* methylene diphosphonate; *NA,* not applicable.

imaging modalities most used for detection are positron emission tomography (PET) scans and single photon emission CT (SPECT) scans. In the ED, the most frequent modality is 2D scintigraphy used for $\dot{V}/\dot{Q}$ scans.

While most imaging studies are designed to provide an anatomical view of the body for the purpose of diagnoses, nuclear medicine studies rely on the physiological variations associated with certain disease processes to provide diagnostic information. Substrates with radioactive isotopes are inhaled, ingested, or injected into the body and the spatial/temporal distribution of the radiopharmaceuticals relative to normal tissue provides the basis of nuclear medicine studies. The different types of isotopes used in nuclear medicine studies are listed in Table 72.4.

Each isotope is absorbed/metabolized differently, and the selection of the appropriate radiopharmaceutical/isotope is dependent on the disease process being monitored. As expected, the absorbed dose and the effect on the fetus varies, but in general, the use of therapeutic radiopharmaceuticals is contraindicated in pregnancy and breast feeding.[44]

Some radiopharmaceuticals contain ^{131}I or ^{32}P which cross the placenta, emit beta radiation, and are generally not used in pregnant patients.[18,44] ^{131}I is a radioisotope of iodine that is often used for the detection and treatment in hyperthyroidism and thyroid cancer. Use is contraindicated in pregnancy and breastfeeding because of the potential for destroying fetal/neonatal thyroid tissue.[44] For the remainder, the dose to the fetus is derived from the activity in maternal tissues, the proximity of these tissues to the fetus, and the excretion of the radiopharmaceutical. For example, the ventilation portion of a ventilation-perfusion ($\dot{V}/\dot{Q}$) study for pulmonary embolism (PE) can be done with either ^{133}Xe or ^{99m}Tc-DTPA. Use of ^{133}Xe results in little fetal exposure, as its activity is confined to the maternal lungs, remote from the fetus or embryo, but ^{99m}Tc-DTPA is excreted by the kidneys and can collect in the urinary bladder, where it, and other renally excreted radiopharmaceuticals, can expose the fetus or embryo.[12] Strategies for reducing fetal exposure therefore include maternal hydration and frequent voiding, considering the use of smaller administered doses and longer

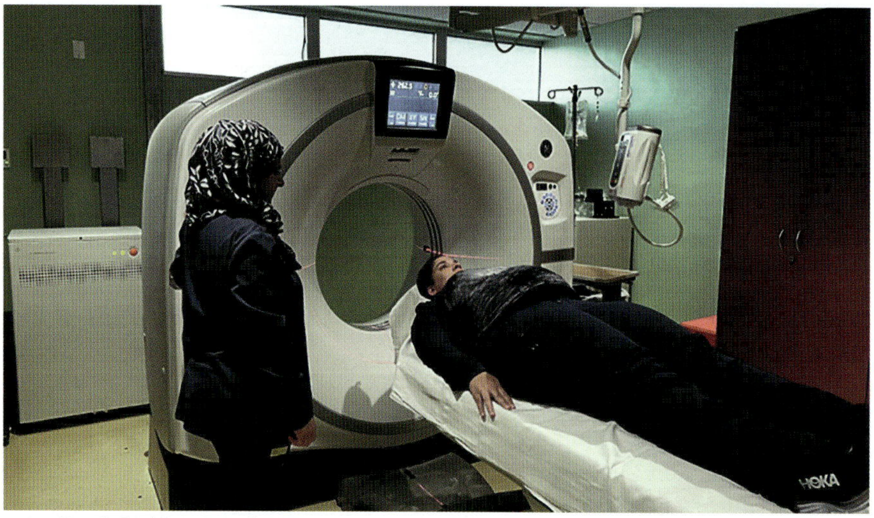

Fig. 72.2 Lead shielding is no longer recommended because (1) radiation dose reduction is modest at best and (2) increased radiation internal scatter after shielding can actually increase the effective dose absorption in the gravid uterus. (From American College of Radiology. *ACR-SPR practice parameter for imaging pregnant or potentially pregnant patients with ionizing radiation. Resolution 39.* American College of Radiology; 2023. https://www.acr.org/-/media/acr/files/practice-parameters/pregnant-pts.pdf.)

imaging times, selecting alternative radiopharmaceuticals (e.g., ^{133}Xe vs. ^{99m}Tc-DTPA), and adjusting the examination protocol (e.g., obtaining the perfusion portion of a $\dot{V}/\dot{Q}$ study first which, if normal, precludes obtaining the ventilation portion).[46,47]

Nonpregnant females may inquire about delaying pregnancy after undergoing a nuclear medicine examination. It is advised that pregnancy be delayed until the dose from the remaining radiopharmaceutical is less than 1 mGy, which is generally not a consideration except for ^{59}Fe (metabolism studies) and ^{75}Se (adrenal studies), for which delays of 6 and 12 months, respectively, are advised.[18] Lactating females must also be counseled to cease breastfeeding for at least 12 hours for ^{99m}Tc, except for labeled red blood cells, phosphates, and diethylenetriamine pentaacetic acid (DTPA), for which a period of at least 4 hours is advised.[18] Breastfeeding should be delayed in those undergoing nuclear medicine studies for 3 weeks for most isotopes but can be resumed after 12 hours for iodine-labeled hippurates and ^{99}TC-containing medicines.[18]

The clinician may also encounter a patient undergoing a nuclear medicine examination who is also the household contact of a pregnant female. These individuals pose no risk to the pregnant female, the fetus, or any other household contact, as the total decay dose measure at 0.5 m and 1 m is 0.02 to 0.25 mGy and 0.05 to 0.1 mGy, respectively.[12]

NONIONIZING RADIATION

MRI and ultrasonography are the preferred modalities of imaging in pregnant females, assuming that adequate diagnostic utility is uncompromised, because they do not utilize ionizing radiation.[17] Neither is completely without risks; however, there have been no studies that have shown increased harm to the embryo or fetus with exposure to MRI or with diagnostic ultrasonography.[48–50]

MRI

Nuclear magnetic resonance (NMR) has been in use since the early 1950s, when 1D spectra were generated by exploiting an anatomical property called spin and its response to externally applied magnetic field.[51] Over the next few decades, several advances led to the development of the diagnostic imaging modality we know today as MRI; nuclear was dropped from the name because of the layperson association of the term with dangerous radiation.

Nuclear spin refers to the intrinsic angular momentum of elemental particles, such as protons, electrons, or neutrons. Spin exists in two states, +1/2 or −1/2, and elements that have even protons or neutrons have a net spin of zero. MRI exploits both intrinsic net spin of the hydrogen ion (thus called a proton because it has lost its only electron) and the abundance of hydrogen ions in nature, particularly in water.

The proton has its own intrinsic magnetic properties which is called its nuclear magnetic moment. This can be thought of as a small magnet whose axis is randomly aligned in space. When placed in a large magnetic field, all the small magnets, the protons, align with that magnetic field and produce a net magnetic vector. Once aligned, these protons are then exposed to a nonionizing radiofrequency (RF) pulse which causes the proton to switch alignment within the field. Magnetic field gradients can also be employed to alter the field around a specific anatomic site. Once the pulse is turned off, protons relax back to their original spin alignment, releasing the electromagnetic energy that it absorbed from the RF pulse. The amount of energy absorbed is dependent on the environment of each proton and this difference can then be used by computers to generate anatomic images. The amount of time that it takes for the sum magnetic vector to relax to its original alignment is T1; the amount of time for each proton to return to its original spin orientation is T2.[52]

TABLE 72.5 Prevention of Contrast-Induced Nephropathy

Renal Failure: Radiocontrast Agents
Radiocontrast-induced acute renal failure is more likely to occur in the presence of advanced age, renal insufficiency, diabetes mellitus, severe congestive heart failure, multiple myeloma, volume depletion, low—cardiac output states, and high-dose contrast-enhanced studies (>125 mL). The incidence of nephrotoxicity depends on the underlying risk factors and the sensitivity of the measure used to determine nephrotoxicity. When a rather sensitive index of renal dysfunction (an increase in the level of serum creatinine to >0.3 mg/dL and >20% on day 1, 2, or 3 and day 5, 6, or 7) is used, the incidence of nephrotoxicity is approximately 2% in nondiabetic, nonazotemic patients and 16% patients with azotemia and diabetes. Patients with azotemia and diabetes had approximately a 38% incidence of nephrotoxicity. In a study of 59 patients with diabetes and advanced azotemia (mean serum creatinine level, 5.9 mg/dL) undergoing coronary angiography, contrast-related nephrotoxicity developed in 30 (51%), as defined by a serum creatinine level that was 25% above baseline 48 h after angiography. Nine patients (15%) required hemodialysis.
Risk Factors for Radiocontrast Nephrotoxicity
Advanced age
Renal insufficiency
Decreased absolute and effective circulatory volume
Diabetes mellitus
Multiple myeloma
Coadministration of other nephrotoxic agents
From Brenner BM, ed. *Brenner and Rector's The Kidneys.* 7th ed. Saunders; 2004, Table 34.3; from MD Consult. Note: Renal failure may be oliguric or nonoliguric, with nonoliguric renal failure being more common in patients with previously nearly normal renal function. Most episodes of contrast-induced nephrotoxicity are mild and characterized by a reversible 1- to 3-mg/dL rise in serum creatinine; dialysis therapy is rarely needed and usually only in patients whose baseline serum creatinine level is high, for example, >3 mg/dL.
Prevention of Radiocontrast Nephropathy
The development of acute renal failure significantly complicates the use of intravascular contrast medium (CM) and is linked with high morbidity and mortality. The increasing use of CM, an aging population, and an increase in chronic kidney disease (CKD) will result in an increased incidence of contrast-induced nephropathy (CIN), unless preventive measures are used. At the current time there is no universally accepted, agreed, or proven intervention to totally prevent CIN. However, the Canadian Association of Radiologists has developed guidelines as a practical approach to risk stratification and potential prevention of CIN. The major risk factor predicting CIN is preexisting CKD, which can be predicted from the glomerular filtration rate (GFR). In terms of being an absolute measure, serum creatinine is an unreliable measure of renal function. Patients with a GFR >60 mL/min have a very low risk for CIN, and preventive measures are generally unnecessary. With a GFR <60 mL/min, preventive measures should be instituted. The risk for CIN is greatest in patients with a GFR <30 mL/min. As preventive measures, alternative imaging that does not require CM should be considered. Fluid volume loading is the single most important protective measure. Nephrotoxic medications should be discontinued 48 h before the study. CM volume and the frequency of administration should be minimized, but satisfactory image quality should still be maintained. High-osmolar CM should be avoided in patients with renal impairment. There is some evidence to suggest that isosmolar CM reduces the risk for CIN in patients with renal impairment, but further study is necessary to determine whether isosmolar CM is superior to low-osmolar CM. N-acetylcysteine (NAC) has been advocated to reduce the incidence of CIN; however, not all studies have shown a benefit, and it is difficult to formulate evidence-based recommendations at this time. Use of NAC may be considered in high-risk patients but is not thought to be mandatory.
Additional Caveats
1. Metformin use is not a contraindication to the use of CM, but metformin should be withheld for 48 h after CM and after evaluation of renal function.
2. Although the GFR is the best way to predict renal dysfunction after CM, patients with normal creatinine are at minimal risk.
From Benko A. Canadian Association of Radiologists: consensus guidelines for the prevention of contrast-induced nephropathy. *Can Assoc Radiol J.* 2007;58:79.
Potential Prevention of Contrast-Induced Nephropathy[a] *NAC*
Suggested regimen for oral NAC: 600 mg (3 mL of a 20% solution in liquid) twice a day for 24 h before and 24 h after procedure.
Suggested IV (intravenous) NAC: 150-mg/kg IV bolus over 30 min, followed by a 50-mg/kg infusion over 4 h.[b]
Example in an 80-kg patient: 12,000 mg NAC in 500 mL normal saline over 30 min, followed by 4000 mg NAC in 500 mL normal saline over 4 h.

TABLE 72.5 Prevention of Contrast-Induced Nephropathy—cont'd

Hydration
Suggested regimen for fluid therapy in elective cases: normal saline, at least 1 mL/kg per hour 12 h before and 12 h after the procedure.
Alternative if an emergency procedure is required: 5-mL/kg bolus of normal saline 1 h before and 1 mL/kg per hour for 12 h after the procedure.
Alternative fluid regimen with bicarbonate: add 154 mL of 1000 mEq/L sodium bicarbonate to 850 mL of 5% dextrose in water (D_5W) (or add 3 ampules of standard bicarbonate to 1 L D_5W). Initial bolus of 3 mL/kg for 1 h before injection of contrast material, followed by 1 mL/kg per hour for 6 h after the procedure.

[a]Suggested but unproven, minimal downside.
[b]From Baker CS, Wragg A, Kumar S, et al. A rapid protocol for the prevention of contrast-induced renal dysfunction: the RAPPID study. *J Am Coll Cardiol.* 2003;41:2114.
From Merten GJ, Burgess P, Gray LV, et al. Prevention of contrast-induced nephropathology with sodium bicarbonate: a randomized controlled trial. *JAMA.* 2004;291:2328.

Dispensing and Administration Guidelines for CIN

NAC + Hydration

ORAL NAC DOSING	*ORAL NAC DOSING*
Give NAC, 600 mg liquid (3 mL of a 20% solution) in 9 mL ginger ale or cola	0.9% sodium chloride IV fluid at 1 mL/kg per hour 12 h before and after catheterization (normal saline preferred, but 0.45% has also been used with success)

IV Sodium Bicarbonate (154 mEq/L) Mixed in 1 L of D_5W

	3-mL/kg IV BOLUS OVER 1 h	*1 mL/kg per hour × 6 h IV INFUSION*	*TOTAL mL INFUSED*
60 kg	180 mL	360 mL (60 mL/h)	540
70 kg	210 mL	420 mL (70 mL/h)	630
80 kg	240 mL	480 mL (80 mL/h)	720
90 kg	270 mL	540 mL (90 mL/h)	810
100 kg	300 mL	600 mL (100 mL/h)	900
≥110 kg	330 mL	660 mL (110 mL/h)	990

From Merten GJ, Burgess WP, Gray LV, et al. Prevention of contrast-induced nephropathy with sodium bicarbonate: a randomized controlled trial. *JAMA.* 2004;291:2328.

IV NAC

	150-mg/kg IV BOLUS OVER 30 min	*50-mg/kg IV INFUSION OVER 4 h*
60 kg	9000 mg/500 mL NS	3000 mg/500 mL NS
70 kg	10,500 mg/500 mL NS	3500 mg/500 mL NS
80 kg	12,000 mg/500 mL NS	4000 mg/500 mL NS
90 kg	13,500 mg/500 mL NS	4500 mg/500 mL NS
≥100 kg	15,000 mg/500 mL NS	5000 mg/500 mL NS

NS, Normal saline.
From Baker CS, Wragg A, Kumar S, et al. A rapid protocol for the prevention of contrast-induced renal dysfunction: the RAPPID study. *J Am Coll Cardiol.* 2003;41:2114.

Continued

TABLE 72.5 Prevention of Contrast-Induced Nephropathy—cont'd

UMMC Pharmacy Cost Comparisons With Treatment Regimens for CIN

REGIMENS	*REGIMENS*
600 mg NAC × 8 doses (oral)	$17.84/day
2 L NS	$4/day
Sodium bicarbonate, 154 mEq/L D_5W	$24/day
70-kg patient: 10,500 mg NAC/500 mL NS by IV bolus	$67/day
70-kg patient: 3500 mg NAC/500 mL NS by IV infusion	$67/day

UMMC, University of Maryland Medical Center.

Most diagnostic studies employ use of MRIs with a static field strength of 1.5 Tesla (T), though field strengths up to 3 T are also common for clinical diagnostic studies, and magnets up to 11.7 T are generally reserved for special studies and animal research. The RF field produces frequencies in the 10s to 100s MHz range; the time-dependent magnetic field gradient produces changes on the orders of 10 T/s. Thus, the fetus is exposed to energy from these three separate sources.

The concern for harm arises from the effect of the dissipated energy from the absorbed RF pulse which manifests as heat within the tissue. The greater the amount of energy dissipated in a shortened interval of time the greater the potential for injury. The energy deposited by the RF pulse is called the average specific absorption rate (SAR), and it is dependent on the MRI protocol being used. It is measured as a function of energy per unit time per unit mass:

$$\text{SAR} = \text{J/s/kg} = \text{W/kg}$$

This value is calculated using the whole-body mass; the FDA imposes a limit of SAR ≤4 W/kg averaged over 15 or more minutes and 3.2 W/kg for the head averaged over 10 minutes or more.[53] MRI scanners have three modes of operations with limits defined by the International Electrotechnical Commission (IEC): (1) normal—whole-body SAR ≤2 W/kg Δ temperature up to 0.5°C; (2) first level controlled—whole-body SAR ≤4 W/kg, Δ temperature up to 1°C, requires radiologist approval and supervision; and (3) second level controlled—SAR can exceed 4 W/kg, Δ temperature >1°C, requires IRB-approved protocol.

Several other factors, such as medication use, BMI, underlying disease, and basal body temperature also affect the patient's thermoregulatory ability. Also, RF energy absorption is heterogeneous and local SARs often differ from whole-body SAR. As such, the FDA limits local SAR to 8 W/kg for any 5-minute period in 1 g of tissue, and the IEC limits local SAR to 10 W/kg for any contiguous 10 g of tissue. To reduce risk of harm, it is advised that MRI operation only be used in normal mode to scan pregnant patients. Further, patients should be screened and scanning should be avoided in patients with altered thermoregulatory function.[54]

Magnetic gradient fields can cause painful nerve and muscle stimulation. The IEC/FDA previously limited magnetic field gradients to a max of 20dB/s; however, presently the guidance recommends "any time rate of change of gradient fields (dB/dt) sufficient to produce severe discomfort or painful nerve stimulation." Using normal operation modes and maximum scan times of 30 minutes, no difference in SAR has been detected between 1.5 and 3 T scanners.[55] The FDA therefore limits the field strength of the static magnetic field to 4 T for neonates and infants aged 1 month or less, and to 8 T for patients aged more than 1 month.[53] The risk of harm to the fetus when using scanners with magnetic fields >3 T is unclear.

MRI Contrast Agents

Like CT studies, MRI studies are often done with contrast agents. These agents are used to highlight vasculature or interstitium (note: contrast is not always needed for MR angiography), enhance or decrease the signal of bowel, or for enhancement in hepatobiliary studies. Both paramagnetic agents—gadolinium (Gd)-based contrast agents (GBCA), ferric chloride, ferric ammonium citrate—and diamagnetic agents (e.g., barium) are administered orally and, owing to their different properties, allow for varied uses for anatomical evaluation. Barium contrast works by using displacement of water protons with barium in the gut, causing signal loss in the gut that improves visualization of the pancreas.[56] Paramagnetic agents work by decreasing T1 relaxation time, resulting in enhanced, brighter T1 signal and decreased T2 relaxation time which results in hypointense T2 signal. These are more suitable for bowel evaluation.[57]

GBCAs are the most commonly intravascularly administered agents for hepatobiliary studies and general intravascular or interstitial enhancement. Gd is a rare earth metal which, in its ionic form, has a high magnetic moment that makes it suitable for MRI. However, this ion is also potentially toxic as a free ion and is thus administered with a chelating agent. This chelator helps to make contrast water-soluble and aids in excretion of the contrast, which occurs primarily renally. Some Gd, however, remains unbound and can be found deposited in tissue months to years after administration. The overall level of harm of this is still unknown (Box 72.1).[58] GBCAs are categorized by the type of chelating agent it is paired with: linear versus macrocyclic, ionic versus nonionic (Table 72.6).[59]

Adverse reactions are rare with GBCAs; however, the most concerning reaction associated with GBCA is nephrogenic systemic fibrosis, which is potentially fatal. This is generally observed in patients with chronic renal disease. Though still overall rare, the ACR has developed a classification system of GBCAs based on risk of development of nephrogenic systemic fibrosis: Group I has the greatest number of reported cases; Group II has few if any cases; Group III has few if any cases but there are limited data on these agents (See Table 72.6).[60]

BOX 72.1 Guidelines for ED Diagnostic Imaging During Pregnancy

- Fetal risk of anomalies, growth restriction, or abortion have not been reported with radiation exposure of less than 50 mGy, a level above the range of exposure for diagnostic procedures.
- Use of CT and associated contrast material should not be withheld if clinically indicated, but a thorough discussion of risks and benefits should take place.
- Ultrasonography and magnetic resonance imaging (MRI) are not associated with risk and are the imaging techniques of choice for the pregnant patient, but they should be used prudently and only when use is expected to answer a relevant clinical question or otherwise provide medical benefit to the patient.
- Whether for diagnostic or therapeutic treatment purposes, iodine 131 should not be used during pregnancy. If a diagnostic scan of the thyroid is essential, technetium 99m is the isotope of choice.
- If a pregnant female undergoes multiple imaging studies using ionizing radiation, it is prudent to consult with a radiation physicist to calculate the total dose received by the fetus.
- It generally is recommended that contrast only be used if absolutely required to obtain additional diagnostic information that will affect the care of the fetus or female during the pregnancy.

Committee on Obstetric Practice. Guidelines for diagnostic imaging during pregnancy. *ACOG Committee Opinion No. 723. 2021.*
CT, *Computed tomography;* ED, *emergency department.*

TABLE 72.6 Gadolinium-Based Contrast Agents/Classifications

COMPOUND	BRAND NAME	ACR GROUP CATEGORY
Linear-Ionic		
Gd-DTPA (gadopentetate dimeglumine)	Magnevist[a]	I
Gd-BOPTA (gadobenate dimeglumine)	MultiHance[a]	II
Gd-EOB-DTPA, gadoxetate disodium	Eovist[a], Primovist[a]	III
Linear-Nonionic		
Gd-DTPA-BMA (gadodiamide)	Omniscan[a]	I
Gd-DTPA-BMEA (gadoversetamide)	OptiMARK[a]	I
Macrocyclic-Ionic		
Gd-DOTA (gadoterate meglumine)	Dotarem[a], Artirem[a]	II
Macrocyclic-Nonionic		
Gd-HP-DO3A, (gadoteridol)	ProHance[a]	II
Gd-BT-DO3A (gadobutrol)	Gadovist, Gadavist[a]	II
Gadopiclenol[b]	Elucirem, Vueway	

[a]FDA-Approved brand name.
[b]Gadopiclenol demonstrates kinetic stability and a long dissociation half-life that are comparable to other Group II macrocyclic agents. Based on the most recent scientific and clinical evidence the ACR Committee on Drugs and Contrast Media considers the risk of NSF among patients exposed to standard or lower than standard doses of gadopiclenol is sufficiently low or possibly nonexistent such that it has been classified as a Group II agent.
ACR has developed a classification system of GBCAs based on risk of development of nephrogenic systemic fibrosis: Group I has the greatest number of reported cases; Group II has few if any cases; Group III has few if any cases but there is limited data on these agents.
BT-DO3A, 2-[4,10-bis(carboxylatomethyl)-7-(1,3,4-trihydroxybutan-2-yl)-1,4,7,10-tetrazacyclododec-1-yl]acetate; *DTPA*, diethylenetriaminepentaacetic acid; *DTPA-BMA*, 2-[bis[2-[carboxymethyl-[2-(methylamino)-2-oxoethyl]amino]ethyl]amino]acetic acid; *DTPA-BMEA*, 2-[bis[2-[carboxylatomethyl-[2-(2-methoxyethylamino)-2-oxoethyl]amino]ethyl]amino]acetate; *DOTA*, 1,4,7,10-Tetraazacyclododecane-1,4,7,10-tetraacetic acid; *EOB-DTPA*, 2-[[(2S)-2-[bis(carboxymethyl)amino]-3-(4-ethoxyphenyl)propyl]-[2-[bis(carboxymethyl)amino]ethyl]amino]acetic acid; *HP-DO3A*, 2,2',2"-[10-(2-hydroxypropyl)-1,4,7,10-tetraazacyclododecane-1,4,7-triyl]triacetate; *BOPTA*, (2R)-2-[2-[2-[bis(carboxymethyl)amino]ethyl-(carboxymethyl)amino]ethyl-(carboxymethyl)amino]-3-phenylmethoxypropanoic acid.
From American College of Radiology. *ACR Manual on Contrast Media*. https://www.acr.org/-/media/ACR/Files/Clinical-Resources/Contrast_Media.pdf. 2023.

The potential impact on the unborn embryo or fetus after maternal administration of GBCA has also been studied. One such study showed that while first-trimester MRI was not associated with adverse fetal outcomes, prenatal GBCA exposure was associated with increased risk of rheumatologic or inflammatory conditions and possibly stillbirth or neonatal death.[49] A subsequent study, however, found no significant increase in fetal or neonatal death or neonatal intensive care unit (NICU) admission after prenatal GBCA exposure compared with unexposed fetuses.[61] Questions still remain on the long-term effects of fetal tissue deposition of Gd, and as such, the ACR "recommends avoidance of routine administration of GBCAs to pregnant patients. A decision to administer GBCAs to a pregnant female should only be made when there is the potential for significant clinical benefit that outweighs the unknown risk of fetal exposure and should be the product of discussion that involves the referring provider and patient."[60,62]

Ultrasonography

Ultrasonography remains the screening modality of choice for evaluation of the maternal pelvis and the fetus because of its real-time capability, relative low cost, and safety profile. Though US studies have not been shown to convey significant risks to the mother or fetus, most of the safety data collected on US were conducted prior to 1992, when the US acoustic intensity output power limits were increased by the FDA from 94 mW/cm^2 to 720 mW/cm^2.[63,34] Increased power leads to concern for biological effects via mechanical or thermal changes in the tissue. Indirectly, the risk of thermal temperature increase can be decreased by on-screen monitoring of the thermal index and mechanical index while scanning, maintaining a value less than 1.0.[65] Typically, B-mode scans, which produce the 2D images, produce output powers <50 mW/cm², [66] with M-mode studies (e.g., used for observing fetal heart tones) producing slightly higher output[67] and Doppler studies producing output approaching and sometimes exceeding the limit of safety. Animal studies suggest that temperature increases related to increased power can lead to liver cell apoptosis and functional neuronal cell changes, though this affect has not yet been observed in humans.[68] Along with increased use of point-of-care US (POCUS) in the ED, which portends lower risk and the gaining popularity of 3D and 4D images which require higher power output, more studies are needed to assure the ongoing safety of US for prenatal diagnostic studies. POCUS studies should be limited to first-trimester studies using B-mode and M-mode scanning; Doppler imaging at this stage is discouraged.[69] The principle of ALARA[5,6] is generally supported and promotes a balance between obtaining the necessary medical information while using minimal settings and examination time. Generally, US is considered a safe procedure in pregnancy.

The American College of Obstetricians and Gynecologists has reviewed the effects of radiography, ultrasonography, and MRI during pregnancy and suggested guidelines for radiographic examination during pregnancy (Box 72.2).[13]

DIAGNOSIS OF PE

The possibility of PE during pregnancy poses a challenge for both the clinician and the patient. Pregnancy increases susceptibility to developing thromboembolism due to increased clotting in pregnancy (to prevent blood loss during labor and delivery), as well as decreased blood return from the legs in latter stages of pregnancy because of compression of pelvic veins by the gravid uterus.[70] During pregnancy there is continuous coagulation and fibrinolysis during the development of the placenta that causes D-dimer levels to rise.[71] During pregnancy and until 2 days postpartum, D-dimer levels have been found to increase by 20 percentile points in 50% of females. The established D-dimer threshold of 0.50 mg/L would be exceeded by 4.8% of pregnant females in the second trimester and 23.8% of pregnant females in the third trimester.[72] This has led to established D-dimer first, second, and third trimester reference intervals of 0.11 to 0.40 mg/L, 0.14 to 0.75 mg/L, and 0.16 to 1.3 mg/L, respectively. These factors cause pregnant females to be five times more likely to develop deep vein thrombosis (DVT). In the immediate postpartum period, the risk of venous thromboembolism (VTE) is up to 20-fold higher. Eighty percent of VTE events during pregnancy are DVT, compared with 20% being PE.[73]

Diagnosis of PE during pregnancy poses several challenges. Many of the presenting symptoms of PE such as shortness of breath and lower limb edema are also reported in almost 50% of females during physiological pregnancy.[74] Clinical suspicion of PE is therefore increased by the onset of symptoms, prior history of VTE, and other common risk factors such as recent travel and decreased mobility. In the general nonpregnant population diagnostic pathways are based on clinical scoring systems, D-dimer levels, US imaging, $\dot{V}/\dot{Q}$, or CT scans.[75] There have been two studies, the CTPE Pregnancy study and the ARTEMIS study, that have prospectively assessed diagnostic strategies in pregnant females with suspected PE. These two studies utilized two different pretest probability models: the Geneva score and a pregnancy-adapted YEARS model.[76,77]

BOX 72.2 Technique of $\dot{V}/\dot{Q}$ Scanning

This test uses both intravenous (perfusion) and aerosolized (ventilation) agents.

PERFUSION

1. Before injection, prepare the intravenous technetium. Mix sodium pertechnetate 99mTc with macroaggregated human albumin (MAA) to form 99mTc-MAA, the substance that is injected intravenously to investigate blood flow in the lungs. If the preparation is not used within 8 hours, discard it.
2. The usual dose is 37–111 MBq (1–3 mCi). Doses as low as 37 MBq are used in pregnancy.
3. Within 5 minutes of injection, more than 90% of the Tc-albumin aggregate is trapped in the arterioles and capillaries of the lung. The particle size determines where the 99mTc will be localized in the body.
4. Accumulation in the lung is temporary, and the fragile albumin aggregate quickly breaks down, thereby allowing Tc to enter the general circulation.
5. Once in the body, the half-life of 99mTc is 6 hours.
6. The majority of 99mTc is excreted in urine. If it remains in the urinary bladder, it is in close proximity to the fetus.
7. Technetium in the bladder exposes the fetus to small amounts of radiation.
8. Frequent voiding or bladder catheterization after the study will lessen exposure of the fetus to radiation.
9. Technetium is relatively contraindicated in patients with severe pulmonary hypertension (because 99mTc-MAA temporarily blocks blood flow in the lungs).
10. Allergic reactions to technetium and human serum albumin are extremely rare.
11. The radiation exposure to the total body from 92.5 MBq (2.5 mCi) is extremely low: less than 1 mGy.

VENTILATION

1. Some radiologists forgo the ventilation portion of the $\dot{V}/\dot{Q}$ scan in pregnancy to limit the total radiation exposure.
2. Most hospitals use 133Xe for the ventilation portion of the $\dot{V}/\dot{Q}$ scan.
3. Fetal radiation exposure from xenon is extremely low, and the 50 mGy threshold is not reached until more than 125 scans have been performed.
4. The estimated dose to the fetus of the standard 370 MBq (10 mCi) of xenon used in a $\dot{V}/\dot{Q}$ scan is 0.4 mGy.
5. If Tc-based aerosol is the marker used for the ventilation portion, fetal exposure is higher than with xenon aerosol.

$\dot{V}/\dot{Q}$, *Ventilation-perfusion.*

The CTPE study used the Geneva score to risk stratify pregnant females who were being evaluated for PE. However, the original Geneva score includes criteria such as age >65 years and cancer that are not generally relevant to the pregnant population. In addition, physiologic changes of pregnancy may change the acceptable limits of some variables included in the Geneva score, such as heart rate.[77] The pregnancy-adapted Geneva score utilizes only objective items that are relevant to all pregnant females in an effort to stratify pregnant females into low, intermediate, and high-risk categories (Table 72.7). Low and intermediate risk patients would then proceed with

TABLE 72.7 Geneva Score and Pregnancy-Adapted Geneva Score

Geneva Score		Pregnancy-Adapted Geneva Score	
COMPONENT	**POINTS**	**COMPONENT**	**POINTS**
Age >65	+1	Age 40 years and older	+1
Active malignant condition	+2		
Surgery (under general anesthesia) or lower limb fracture in past month	+2	Surgery (under general anesthesia) or lower limb fracture in past month	+2
Unilateral lower limb pain	+3	Unilateral lower limb pain	+3
Hemoptysis	+2	Hemoptysis	+2
Heart rate 75–94	+3	Heart rate >110 bpm	+5
Heart rate >95	+5		
Pain on lower limb palpation and unilateral edema	+4	Pain on lower limb palpation and unilateral edema	+4
Previous DVT or PE	+3	Previous DVT or PE	+3
Maximal point number	22	Maximal point number	20
Pregnancy-Adapted Geneva Score Categories			
POINTS	**PTP CATEGORY**	**PE PREVALENCE**	**95% CI**
0–1	Low	2.3%	1.0–4.9%
2–6	Intermediate	11.6%	6.9–18.9%
≥7	High	61.5%	35.5–82.2%

CI, Confidence interval; *PTP*, pretest probability; *PE*, pulmonary embolism.
Adapted from Robert-Ebadi H, Moumneh T, Le Gal G, Righini M. Diagnosis of pulmonary embolism during pregnancy. *Diagnostics (Basel)*. 2022;12(8):1875.

D-dimer testing. If elevated, imaging would start with bilateral lower extremity Doppler and then to CTPE if Doppler studies were negative or treatment if positive. Patients with negative dimers were effectively ruled out for PE.

High-risk patients would skip dimer testing and proceed directly to Doppler studies. This study has not yet been validated for clinical use as of the published date of this text.

The YEARS criteria are used in hemodynamically stable patients ≥18 years of age who are suspected of acute PE.[78] The algorithm includes three criteria: clinical sign of DVT, hemoptysis, and PE as the most likely diagnosis. In the ARTEMIS study, the pregnancy adaptation to this algorithm includes *first* ruling out DVT in patients with clinical signs of DVT.[74] If the DVT study was positive, patients were treated with anticoagulation. If the study was negative, or a patient had either of the other two YEARS criteria, a D-dimer level was obtained. If the level was <500 ng/mL, PE could be reasonably excluded without further imaging. If the patient did not meet any of the initial YEARS criteria, then PE could be excluded with a dimer level <1000 ng/mL. If PE could not be excluded as a diagnosis based on those guidelines, then CTPE study was recommended. See Fig. 72.3 for the pregnancy-adapted YEARS criteria algorithm from the ARTEMIS study.

Imaging modality decisions in diagnosing PE are complicated in pregnancy due to clinician and patient concern of radiation exposure to fetus. Fetal exposure of doses above 100 mGy are viewed as the minimum dose in which there are negative consequences.[36,79] Increased fetal gestational age confers more resistance to radiation, as the embryo/fetus is most susceptible to radiation during organogenesis and in the first trimester.[36] $\dot{V}/\dot{Q}$ scintigraphy leads to higher absorbed radiation doses than CT of the pulmonary arteries (CTPA, sometimes referred to as CTPE) and an isolated perfusion scintigraphy.[71] CTPA and perfusion-only scintigraphy have estimated breast-absorbed doses of 44 mGy and 0.28 mGy, respectively; both have an estimated fetal-absorbed dose of 0.25 mGy. $\dot{V}/Q$ scintigraphy has an estimated breast-absorbed dose of 0.37 mGy, and a fetal-absorbed dose of 0.40 mGy. Although the CTPA has a higher breast-absorbed dose, its lower fetal dose often makes it the preferred imaging modality (Boxes 72.3 and 72.4).[71]

DIAGNOSIS OF APPENDICITIS

The leading cause of nongynecological or obstetric-related emergency surgeries in pregnant females is acute appendicitis.[79] There is an occurrence rate of 0.05% to 0.07% of pregnancies with the highest frequency of cases during the second trimester.[79] Pregnancy complicates the diagnosis of appendicitis. The gravid uterus as well as the classical symptoms of nausea and vomiting that occur in pregnancy make the diagnosis of appendicitis more difficult. This lack of diagnostic certainty

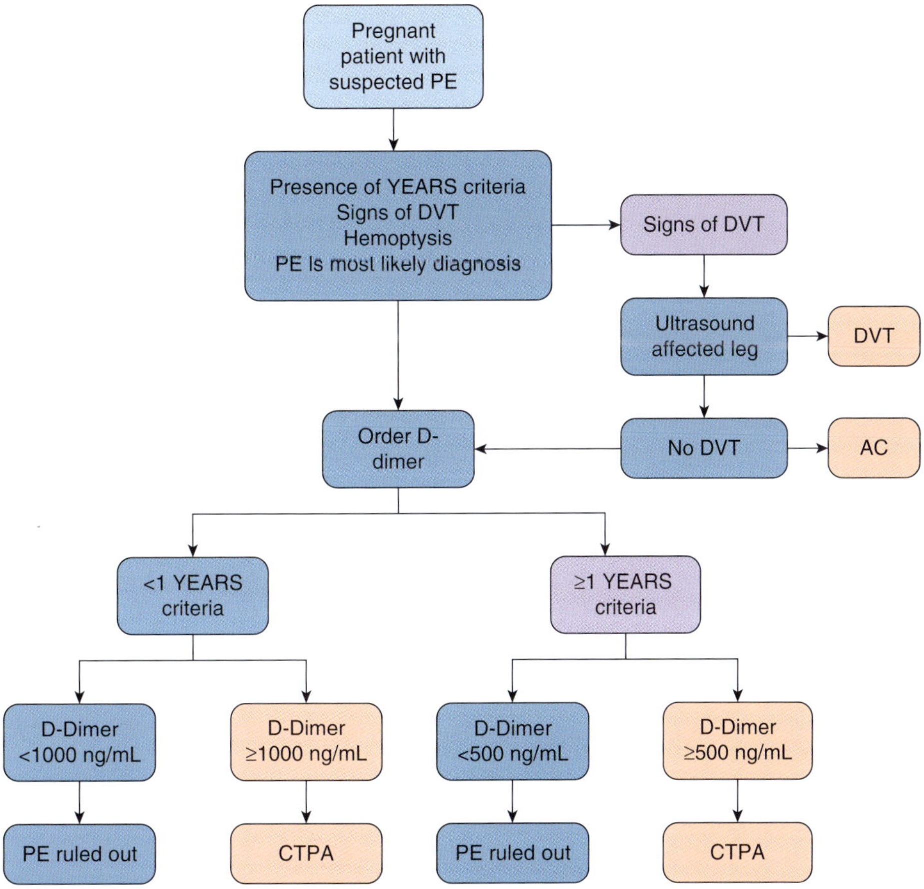

Fig. 72.3 Pregnancy-adapted YEARS algorithm for the management of suspected acute pulmonary embolism in pregnant patients. *AC*, Anticoagulation; *CTPA*, computed tomography of the pulmonary arteries; *DVT*, deep venous thrombosis; *PE*, pulmonary embolism. (Adapted from van der Pol LM, Tromeur C, Bistervels IM, et al. Pregnancy-adapted YEARS algorithm for diagnosis of suspected pulmonary embolism. *N Engl J Med*. 2019;380(12):1139-1149.)

BOX 72.3 Dose Reduction Methods When Using CT Pulmonary Angiography to Image Suspected Pulmonary Embolic Disease in Pregnancy

- Reduce tube current (mA)[a,b]
- Reduce peak tube kilovoltage (kVp)[a,b]
- Increase pitch[a,b]
- Reduce the field of view[a,b]
- Increase detector and beam collimation[a]
- Reduce z-axis scan volume (caudal extent limited to the top of the diaphragm)[a]
- Eliminate frontal and lateral scout views[a]
- Iterative reconstruction postprocessing[b]
- *Do not use circumferential shielding of the abdomen and pelvis*[b]

[a]*From Scarsbrook AF, Evans AL, Owen AR, Gleeson FV. Diagnosis of suspected venous thromboembolic disease in pregnancy.* Clin Radiol. *2006;61:1.*
[b]*From Nguyen ET, Hague C, Manos D, et al. Canadian Society of Thoracic Radiology/Canadian Association of Radiologists best practice guidance for investigation of acute pulmonary embolism, part 1: Acquisition and safety considerations.* Can Assoc Radiol J.*2022;73(1):203-213.*

is heightened given the severity of appendicitis, especially in pregnancy. Appendicitis is associated with premature labor, fetal morbidity and mortality, and an increased rate of perforation. Pregnant females are more likely to experience perforation of the appendix, with rates as high 55%, compared with 4% to 19% in the general population[80] Concern for appendicitis in a pregnant patient warrants early surgical consultation and discussion of the need and type of imaging. Several practical scores have been identified to facilitate the prompt diagnosis of acute appendicitis, including the Alvarado criteria (Fig. 72.4). One retrospective study found that an Alvarado score >7 presented specificity and sensitivity of 80% and 79% respectively. Use of the Alvarado score in pregnant patients with suspected appendicitis is still under investigation.[81]

Patel et al. published an algorithm that uses US and MRI techniques before exposing patients to ionizing radiation.[82] They recommended the use of graded-compression US followed by abdominal/pelvic US to search for other pathology if needed. If the US studies are negative, the authors recommend MRI of the abdomen and pelvis (Fig. 72.5). Notably, some authors have found that using a nonionic oral contrast agent (a mixture of ferumoxsil and barium sulfate) improved sensitivity and specificity of MRI in detecting appendicitis

BOX 72.4 Key Statements on Diagnostic Imaging Modalities During Pregnancy

RADIOGRAPHS AND COMPUTED TOMOGRAPHY

- "The vast majority of routine diagnostic studies (including nuclear medicine studies) typically deliver far less than 20 mGy to the uterus." American College of Radiology and the Society for Pediatric Radiology."
- ACR–SPR practice parameter for imaging pregnant or potentially pregnant patients with ionizing radiation. Resolution 39. American College of Radiology; 2023.
- "Almost all diagnostic radiological procedures involve doses that are below the no adverse-effect level for these developmental effects, especially when pregnant women have diagnostic x-ray studies of the head, neck, chest or extremities However, most diagnostic radiological studies that expose the abdomen do not result in a dose to the embryo or fetus of >0.1 Gy."
- National Council on Radiation Protection and Measurements. Report No. 174. *Preconception and prenatal radiation exposure: Health effects and protective guidance.* NCRP; 2013.
- "Prenatal doses from most properly done diagnostic procedures present no measurable increased risk of prenatal death, malformation, or impairment of mental development over the background incidence of these entities."
- International Commission on Radiological Protection. *Pregnancy and medical radiation. Ann ICRP.* 2000; 30(iii):1.
- "With few exceptions, radiation exposure through radiography, computed tomography (CT) scan, or nuclear medicine imaging techniques is at a dose much lower than the exposure associated with fetal harm. If these techniques are necessary in addition to ultrasonography or MRI or are more readily available for the diagnosis in question, they should not be withheld from a pregnant patient."
- Committee on Obstetric Practice. *Guidelines for diagnostic imaging during pregnancy.* ACOG Committee Opinion No. 723. ACOG; 2021.

MAGNETIC RESONANCE IMAGING

- "Ultrasonography and magnetic resonance imaging (MRI) are not associated with risk and are the imaging techniques of choice for the pregnant patient, but they should be used prudently and only when use is expected to answer a relevant clinical question or otherwise provide medical benefit to the patient."
- Committee on Obstetric Practice. *Guidelines for diagnostic imaging during pregnancy.* ACOG Committee Opinion No. 723. ACOG; 2021.

ULTRASONOGRAPHY

- "There have been no reports of documented adverse fetal effects for diagnostic ultrasonography procedures, including duplex Doppler imaging."
- Committee on Obstetric Practice. *Guidelines for diagnostic imaging during pregnancy.* ACOG Committee Opinion No. 723. ACOG; 2021.

in pregnancy.[83] The authors noted that US imaging of the appendix was more easily done during the first and early second trimester and that the left lateral decubitus position assisted in visualization of the appendix in third-trimester patients. Finally, if US and MRI are still inconclusive, CT of the abdomen and pelvis may be considered. Definitive surgical exploration should be discussed with a general surgeon before proceeding to ionizing radiation. These guidelines are consistent with the ACR's appropriateness criteria that suggest US should be performed first, followed by MRI if inconclusive, and reserves CT as a last resort that should not be withheld if needed for diagnostic certainty.[13]

DIAGNOSIS OF PREGNANCY AND CONSENT

If exposure to less than 50 mGy does not measurably affect the exposed embryo, why should the clinician determine the pregnancy status of the patient? Brent reported sound reasoning for diagnosing pregnancy before a radiographic study.[16] The principle of informed consent must remain paramount. It is beneficial and more sound ethically to have the patient informed of her pregnancy status before imaging. An informative discussion about the risk-benefit aspects of the test before the study conveys concern for the patient and fetus. Discussing the risk-benefit aspects of imaging after the study may be misconstrued as "backpedaling" and has the potential to upset the patient. Many lawsuits are stimulated by the factor of surprise. Frank discussion before imaging may prevent misguided litigation. More importantly, having patients both understand the problem (imaging in pregnancy) and take part in the management discussion can help them become more empowered and potentially reduce the anxiety associated with their condition and with their pregnancy.

Determination of pregnancy by the history and physical examination alone can be problematic. The menstrual history by itself may not be totally reliable in determining pregnancy. Amenorrhea and physical changes in the size and shape of the uterus may be consistent with pregnancy. While a history of recent menstruation, use of an intrauterine device, tubal ligation, absence of coitus, or proper use of birth control pills can result in a suggestion of nonpregnant status, these factors are not accurate enough to exclude pregnancy. If the diagnosis of pregnancy is in the differential or imaging is ordered, or both, definitive determination of the patient's pregnancy status should be strongly considered if the clinical scenario is reasonable. A menstrual history and other information should be obtained whenever possible, and a confirmatory urine pregnancy test should be considered. Urine pregnancy tests to detect early pregnancy are quite sensitive and reliable, and it is not necessary to routinely order a quantitative serum test. Theoretically, there will be a few days' window between fertilization and implantation, a period when no method will confirm the presence or absence of early pregnancy.

A pregnant patient has the right to know the magnitude and type of risks that might result from in utero exposure to radiation. The Annals of the International Commission on Radiological Protection Publication[18] summarized the need for informed consent as follows:

The need and degree of disclosure is usually measured by what a reasonable person believes is material to the mother's decision to be exposed to radiation. The level and degree of disclosure should be related to the level of risk. For low-dose

ALVARADO SCORE FOR ACUTE APPENDICITIS	
SIGNS	
Right lower quadrant tenderness	2
Elevated temperature (>37.3°C or 99.1°F)	1
Rebound tenderness	1
SYMPTOMS	
Anorexia	1
Nausea or vomiting	1
Migration of pain to right lower quadrant	1
LABORATORY VALUES	
Leukocytosis (>10k WBC)	2
Left shift (>75% neutrophils)	1
Total	10

1-4
30% Appendicitis
Consider other diagnosis

5-7
66% Appendicitis
Monitoring/admission

8-10
93% Appendicitis
Consider surgery

Fig. 72.4 The Alvarado score is a clinical scoring system based on the eight signs and symptoms of acute appendicitis. Risk stratification and subsequent clinical management. *WBC,* White blood cells. (From Ohle R, O'Reilly F, O'Brien KK, Fahey T, Dimitrov BD. The Alvarado score for predicting acute appendicitis: a systematic review. *BMC Med.* 2011;9,139.)

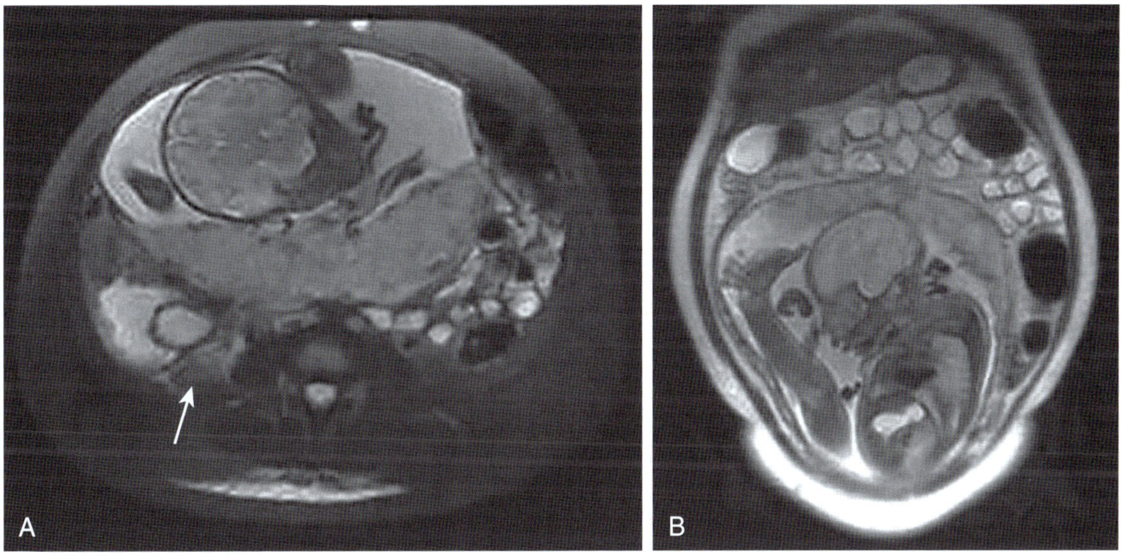

Fig. 72.5 Magnetic resonance imaging (MRI) for appendicitis in pregnancy. Right lower quadrant pain presents a diagnostic dilemma in pregnant patients, and abdominal computed tomography is generally eschewed in favor of modalities that do not use ionizing radiation. Ultrasound may be utilized but the appendix is often difficult to visualize, especially in the third trimester. (A) MRI (fast spin echo, fat saturated) of a patient who is 33 weeks pregnant. A dilated appendix (12 mm) and periappendiceal edema are noted adjacent to the right psoas muscle *(arrow)*, indicative of acute appendicitis. (B) A coronal section from the same study reveals the fetus in a frank breech presentation. MRI is thought to present no risk to the fetus at any stage of pregnancy.

procedures, such as chest x-rays, <100 mrad, the only information that may be needed is a verbal assurance that the risk is judged to be extremely low. When fetal doses are >100 mrad, usually a more detailed explanation is given. The information should include potential radiation risks and potential alternative modalities, as well as the risk of harm from not having the medical procedure. The degree of documentation of such explanations and consent is variable, but many clinicians will include a note of any such counseling or consent in the record of the patient.

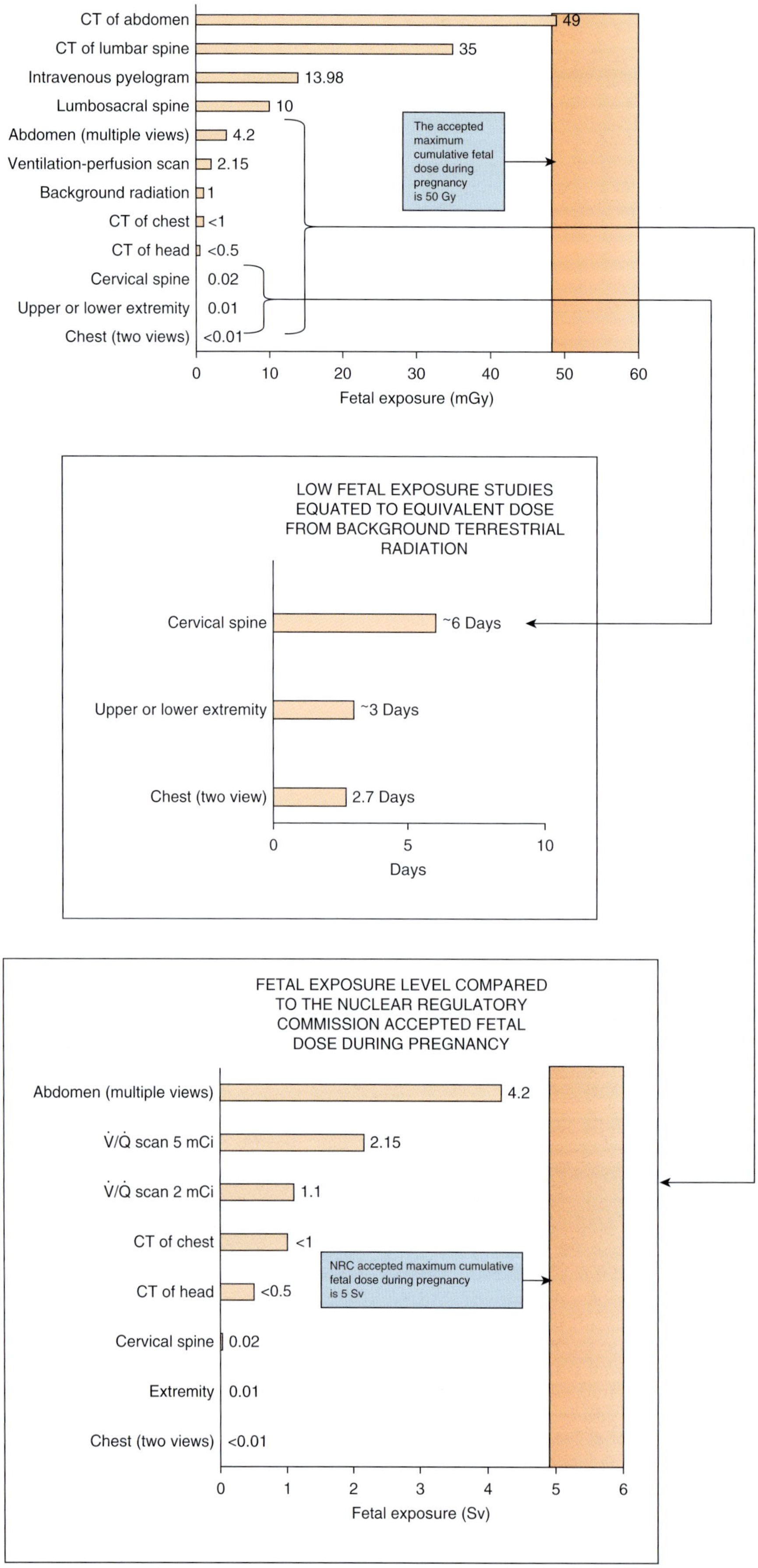

Fig. 72.6 *Top*, Comparison of common radiographic studies with the accepted 50 mGy (5 rad) cumulative fetal exposure limit. *Middle*, Low fetal exposure studies equated to the equivalent dose from background terrestrial radiation. *Bottom*, Fetal exposure level compared with the fetal dose during pregnancy accepted by the Nuclear Regulatory Commission (NRC). *CT*, Computed tomography; *$\dot{V}/\dot{Q}$*, ventilation-perfusion.

TABLE 72.8 Probability of Bearing Healthy Children as a Function of Radiation Dose

RADIOGRAPHIC STUDY	FETAL EXPOSURE (mGy)	INCREASED RISK FOR ABORTION, GROWTH RETARDATION, MENTAL IMPAIRMENT, AND MALFORMATION	PROBABILITY THAT A CHILD WILL HAVE NO MALFORMATION (%)	PROBABILITY THAT A CHILD WILL HAVE NO GENETIC DISEASE PRESENT AT BIRTH[a] (%)	PROBABILITY THAT CANCER WILL NOT DEVELOP IN A CHILD (AGE 0–19 y)[b] (%)
No study	0	None	97	97	99.7
Chest x-ray	0.007	None	97	97	99.7
Extremity x-ray	0.01	None	97	97	99.7
C-spine x-ray	0.02	None	97	97	99.7
Head CT	<0.5	None	97	97	99.7
Chest CT	<1	None	97	97	99.7
$\dot{V}/\dot{Q}$ scan 3 mCi	1.45	None	97	97	99.7
$\dot{V}/\dot{Q}$ scan 5 mCi	2.15	None	97	97	99.7
Multi studies	10	None	97	97	99.6
Multi studies	50	None	97	97	99.4

[a]Rounded values. The radiation risk for genetic mutation is assumed to be 0.01%/rad fetal dose with a linear dose-response relationship. The background rate for genetic mutation is estimated to be 3%. From Osie IK. Fetal doses from radiological examinations. *Br J Radiol*. 1999;72:773.

[b]Rounded values. The radiation risk for fatal cancer is assumed to be 0.06%/rad fetal dose with a linear dose-response relationship. Many epidemiologic studies suggest that the risk may be lower than that assumed here. The background risk for childhood cancer is calculated from National Cancer Institute. *Surveillance, epidemiology and end results cancer statistics review 1973–1991: tables and graphs*. National Cancer Institute; 1994.

CT, Computed tomography; $\dot{V}/\dot{Q}$, ventilation-perfusion.

Modified from International Commission on Radiological Protection. *Publication 84: Pregnancy and medical radiation*. *Ann ICRP*. 2000;30(iii):1-43.

BOX 72.5 MRI Contrast Agent Concerns and Contraindications

INFORMATION FOR HEALTHCARE PROFESSIONALS:

FDA warns that gadolinium-based contrast agents (GBCAs) are retained in the body; this requires new class warnings.

FDA ALERT (12-19-2017, updated 5/16/2018): The U.S. Food and Drug Administration (FDA) is requiring a new class warning and other safety measures for all gadolinium-based contrast agents (GBCAs) for magnetic resonance imaging (MRI) concerning gadolinium remaining in patients' bodies, including the brain, for months to years after receiving these drugs. Gadolinium retention has not been directly linked to adverse health effects in patients with normal kidney function, and we have concluded that the benefit of all approved GBCAs continues to outweigh any potential risks.

However, after additional review, we are requiring several actions to alert health care professionals and patients about gadolinium retention after an MRI using a GBCA, and actions that can help minimize problems. These include:

- Requiring a new patient *Medication Guide*, providing educational information that every patient will be asked to read before receiving a GBCA.
- We are also requiring manufacturers of GBCAs to conduct human and animal studies to further assess the safety of these contrast agents.

To date, the only known adverse health effect related to gadolinium retention is a rare condition called nephrogenic systemic fibrosis (NSF) that occurs in a small subgroup of patients with preexisting kidney failure. We have also received reports of adverse events involving multiple organ systems in patients with normal kidney function. A causal association between these adverse events and gadolinium retention could not be established.

We are continuing to assess the health effects of gadolinium retention in the body and will update the public when new information becomes available. We are requiring the following specific changes to the labeling of all GBCAs:

- A *Warning* and *Precaution*
- Changes related to gadolinium retention in the Adverse Reactions, Pregnancy, Clinical Pharmacology, and Patient Instructions sections

We urge patients and health care professionals to report side effects involving GBCAs or other medicines to the FDA MedWatch program, using the information in the "Contact FDA" box at www.fda.gov/medwatch/index.html or by calling 800-332-1088 (800-FDA-1088).

CONTRAINDICATIONS TO MRI

Because this is an area of continuing change and there are rapid advancements in the technology to produce MRI-safe materials, consultation with the radiology department is suggested if any questions arise concerning the safety of MRI.

Overview

There are few contraindications to MRI. Overall, no biologic adverse effects are associated with conventional MRI. Most contraindications to MRI are relative and essentially precautions

BOX 72.5 MRI Contrast Agent Concerns and Contraindications—cont'd

related to the effect of MRI on devices and material within the body that may be affected by the magnetic field of MRI.

Implanted Devices and Foreign Bodies

Electronic devices and magnetizable material represent potential hazards to the patient. Titanium objects are safe for MRI.

- *Intracoronary stents:* It is considered safe to perform MRI at any time after placement of coronary artery stents of any type.
- *Sternal wires after sternotomy:* Sternal wire sutures are considered safe for MRI.
- *Mechanical cardiac valves:* It is safe to scan most prosthetic cardiac valves because at most, they experience only a mild torque. An exception involves the pre-6000 series Starr-Edwards caged ball valves; devices rarely used now.
- *Pacemakers, implantable defibrillators, and implanted electronic devices:* The risks of scanning patients with cardiac pacemakers are related to possible movement of the device, magnetically induced changes in programming, electromagnetic interference, and induced currents in lead wires leading to heating and/or cardiac stimulation. It is currently considered inadvisable for patients with pacemakers or other intracardiac wires to undergo MRI. Nerve stimulators, insulin pumps, cochlear implants, and other implanted electronic devices may also be affected by MRI and are considered unsafe.
- *Implanted vagal nerve stimulator:* Brain MRI performed at less than 2 T, with a send and receive head coil and the stimulator turned off, appears to be safe under guidelines published by the manufacturer. Other MRI studies are not known to be safe.
- *Aneurysm clips and magnetizable material:* Any ferromagnetic object within the body represents a potential hazard when exposed to the large magnetic field of an MRI system. The hazard primarily reflects the possibility of deflecting the foreign body sufficiently to injure vital structures. For example, certain older-model vascular clips used for cerebral aneurysms are ferromagnetic and could be moved by the magnetic field, with obviously dire consequences.
- *Intraorbital or intraocular metallic fragments,* such as might be acquired from machining, are a potential risk and generally a contraindication to MRI.
- *Cutaneous metal objects:* Although most metallic biomaterial is now nonferrous and nonmagnetizable, any metallic device within or connected to the patient needs to be evaluated for safety. Dental alloys, wires, splints, dental braces, and prostheses do not appear to pose a risk to the patient, although such material may result in artifactual changes. Cutaneous burns can result from contact of the skin with metal objects, including neurosurgical halo pins, pulse oximetry probes, and drug-eluting medical patches that contain metal foil (e.g., nicotine patch), although the mechanism of this injury is unclear.
- *Orthopedic/neurosurgical hardware:* It is safe to perform MRI in patients with titanium implants, screws, rods, and artificial joints.
- *Bullets/shrapnel:* These foreign objects within the body are relative contraindications to MRI. Many bullets are safe, but those with metal (specialized bullets, such as metal jackets) may pose a risk.
- *Tattoos:* The majority of professionally obtained tattoos are safe for MRI; however, tattoos containing lead, such as those obtained in prison, can burn the skin if exposed to MRI.
- *Oxygen cylinders:* Standard metal oxygen cylinders should not be used in the MRI suite. Safe oxygen cylinders are available.
- *Credit cards:* Credit card and other information-containing strips may be destroyed in the MRI scanner.

PATIENT COUNSELING

When a pregnant patient requires an imaging study, be prepared to discuss the risk associated with the test. Counseling can be done after attempting to estimate the dose received by the conceptus from the procedure and comparing the radiation risk with other risks of pregnancy. It is important to use terminology that is easily understood by the patient. Fig. 72.6 depicts three different strategies to inform the patient about the level of exposure from her study and established limits. Table 72.8 compares the level of exposure with established background risks.

The top bar graph in Fig. 72.6 compares the fetal exposure level for various radiographic studies with the maximum accepted fetal dose during pregnancy (50 mGy). A patient's particular study may be plotted on this graph to show the clear margin of safety that exists for all single hippurates diagnostic tests.

The middle graph equates the exposure from low-level diagnostic studies to the number of hours needed to accumulate a similar exposure dose from background terrestrial radiation. One of the most commonly ordered studies in pregnancy is a chest radiograph. The potential risk to the fetus can be put into perspective for the patient by comparing the absorbed dose for the chest radiograph with the natural background radiation exposure. The environmental background radiation over a 9-month period results in a cumulative dose of 1 mGy.[84] The fetal dose exposure for a chest radiograph (two views) is estimated to be less than 0.1 mGy. Therefore, the exposure dose to the fetus from a chest radiograph is equivalent to the same amount of naturally occurring background radiation to which the patient was exposed in the previous 2.7 days.

The lower graph depicts the upper limit of the Nuclear Regulatory Commission (NRC) for cumulative gestational dose versus various diagnostic studies. The NRC has established occupational radiation dose limits for pregnancy. Its recommendation is that the dose to the fetus not be allowed to exceed 5 mSv during gestation. Brent noted that this factor-of-10 lowering of the widely accepted threshold is "extremely conservative."[16] One can explain to the patient that the level of exposure from her radiograph is below the conservative cumulative acceptable dose for a pregnant employee at a nuclear facility in the United States.

Another useful approach is to indicate to the patient the probability of not having a child with either a malformation or cancer and how that probability is affected by radiation. Table 72.8 depicts the probability of bearing healthy children as a function of radiation dose. This discussion should be coupled with the fact that a nonexposed fetus has a baseline incidence of spontaneous abortion, multiple developmental abnormalities, and subsequent childhood cancer.

Numerous organizations have declared fetal exposure to less than 50 mGy as being safe. Box 72.5 presents various conclusions from key organizations on the use of radiation and pregnancy. The International Commission on Radiological Protection concluded that fetal doses below 100 mGy should not be considered a reason for terminating a pregnancy.[18] If a patient still has considerable concern or has possibly received greater than 50 mGy, referral to a radiation physicist or genetic specialist for further counseling is reasonable.

SUMMARY

In summary, the threshold dose for the tissue reactions from ionizing radiation throughout the gestational period is greater than 50 mGy. Prenatal doses of less than 50 mGy present no measurable increased risk for prenatal death, malformation, growth retardation, or impairment of mental development over the background incidence of these entities. The risk for stochastic effects, carcinogenesis, or mutagenesis, is related to the fetal-absorbed dose and is very low in comparison to the natural background incidence of childhood cancer and genetic disease for most diagnostic procedures. The vast majority of radiographic imaging obtained in the ED exposes the fetus to 100 times less than the threshold for adverse effects. The 50 mGy threshold for onset of concern for adverse fetal effects is quite conservative, and any statistically significant change in fetal outcome probably requires at least several times this dose. One of the methods put forth in this chapter can be used to counsel pregnant patients in need of diagnostic imaging. For females inadvertently exposed to radiation before pregnancy is recognized, open and frank discussion can help educate patients and alleviate their fears.

CLINICAL USE OF RADIOCONTRAST MATERIAL

Emergency clinicians must frequently initiate studies with the use of radiocontrast material. A full discussion of these procedures is not within the scope of this chapter, but basic issues of contrast material–induced nephropathy, the possible prevention thereof, and recent concern over the use of gadolinium for MRI studies have been included for completeness and ready reference (See Table 721.5 and Box 721.1).

REFERENCES ARE AVAILABLE AT Elsevier eBooks+

CHAPTER 73

Procedures in the Setting of Anticoagulation

Caroline Kaigh and Rita McKeever

INTRODUCTION

Performing an invasive procedure on an anticoagulated emergency department (ED) patient can be challenging for the emergency provider (EP). Depending on the procedure, some anticoagulated patients may be at risk of hemorrhage from the procedure. However, emergency reversal of anticoagulation to perform the procedure may also place the patient at risk for serious thrombotic complications. When deciding to perform a procedure on an anticoagulated ED patient, the EP must weigh the urgency of the procedure and the risks of bleeding from the procedure with the risk of disrupting or reversing anticoagulation. If the procedure is not needed for life-saving therapy, postponing the procedure or providing empiric treatment may be a reasonable choice. In contrast, emergency procedures to reverse an imminent life-threatening condition need to be performed and emergency reversal of anticoagulation may be required. This chapter reviews current literature and recommendations for select ED procedures including lumbar puncture (LP), central venous catheterization, arthrocentesis, paracentesis, thoracentesis, and tube thoracostomy in the anticoagulated patient.

ASSESSING RISK OF BLEEDING AND THROMBOSIS

All anticoagulants inhibit stable clot formation and increase the risk of bleeding. Routine coagulation testing (prothrombin time [PT], partial thromboplastin time [PTT], international normalized ratio [INR], and platelet count) may be recommended prior to performing an invasive procedure. Despite this recommendation, depending on the anticoagulant the patient is taking, these tests may not reflect the patient's degree of anticoagulation. PT and INR conveniently assay the extrinsic pathway to monitor the quantitative effect of warfarin therapy. PTT or activated PTT (aPTT) accurately monitors the anticoagulant effect of heparin. Direct oral anticoagulants (DOACs) were developed to have predictable pharmacokinetics with minimal interactions to avoid the need for routine laboratory testing. Coagulation assays to quantify the effect or presence of a DOAC would be useful in many clinical circumstances such as in active bleeding, suspected overdose, and the perioperative period, but do not exist for many. The direct measurement of drug concentration is not suitable in clinical practice because of the time required to perform the laboratory analysis. Standard coagulation assays can be useful in extreme scenarios but are generally insufficient in determining drug concentration or degree of anticoagulant effect of DOACs (Table 73.1).

Normal thrombin time is suitable for excluding significant dabigatran levels but is too sensitive for determining the degree of anticoagulant effect.[1–4] Dilute thrombin time, ecarin chromogenic assay, and ecarin clotting time may be useful to determine the degree of anticoagulant effect but are not standardized across laboratories. Although using standard coagulation assays to quantify dabigatran effect is not recommended, an elevated PT/INR suggests a supratherapeutic dabigatran effect. However, a normal PTT may not exclude below or on-therapy drug levels that are clinically relevant.[5,6] Unfortunately, none of these tests are accurate predictors of bleeding risk with dabigatran and patients may have bleeding when these tests are within the normal range.[5,6]

Antifactor Xa activity is valuable to determine the effect of factor Xa inhibitors such as rivaroxaban and apixaban, but this test is not widely available. Although it is not recommended to use standard coagulation assays to quantify drug effect, a normal PT and INR level virtually excludes supratherapeutic rivaroxaban effect.[4]

For patients on vitamin K antagonists (VKAs) such as warfarin, understanding how INR correlates to the risk of bleeding is important. Spontaneous bleeding events are uncommon when the INR is normal or within a therapeutic range (i.e., 2 to 3).[7,8] The relative risk for bleeding with an INR between 3 and 5 is 2.7 (95% confidence interval [CI] 1.8 to 3.9). However, when the INR is above 5, the relative risk of a spontaneous hemorrhagic event increases dramatically to 21.8 (95% CI 12.1 to 39.4). These findings are similar to a previous retrospective review in 1995 that also showed adverse events occurred in 75 per 100 patient-years for an INR greater than or equal to 6.5.[9] Patients with severe coagulopathy (INR greater than 9) have a higher risk of bleeding and mortality, with 67% experiencing spontaneous hemorrhagic events and a 74% mortality rate.[10]

Patients without a history of bleeding or anticoagulant use do not require routine coagulation studies prior to performing a procedure unless history or physical examination suggests a bleeding disorder or use of anticoagulation.[11] A 2005 systematic review failed to demonstrate the utility of routine coagulation studies on nonanticoagulated patients prior to the performance of a procedure.[12] Abnormal laboratory findings such as thrombocytopenia, an elevated INR, or other coagulation abnormalities are not necessarily absolute contraindications to performing an invasive procedure. Numerous studies have demonstrated that select procedures can safely be performed even in the setting of anticoagulation with a VKA.[13–15]

Determining a patient's risk for bleeding involves the bleeding risks of the procedure to be performed, the anticoagulant medication, the last dose of the medication, and the level of anticoagulation. Unfortunately, there are no validated systems available to quantify risk of bleeding.

The risk of thrombosis after anticoagulant reversal is significant for a subset of ED patients. These patients include those with a recent diagnosis of pulmonary embolism, significant clot burden, or those with mechanical hardware such as a prosthetic cardiac valve. When clinically feasible, it is best to allow the anticoagulant effect of a medication to wane rather than emergently reversing the medication in these patients. This approach may not be possible in the ED, so timing of the procedure should be coordinated with the inpatient provider if the patient requires admission.

Many procedures report contraindications with severe coagulopathy (INR greater than 9) and disseminated intravascular coagulation (DIC). Effective coagulation is significantly disrupted in these clinical settings and invasive procedures

TABLE 73.1 Summary of Anticoagulant Testing and Management

ANTICOAGULANT	LABORATORY TESTING TO CONSIDER	PHARMACOLOGY	AGENTS TO REVERSAL OF REMOVAL
Heparins			
Low-molecular-weight heparin (LMWH)	Antifactor Xa	3–6 h	Consider protamine sulfate or rVIIa in life-threatening bleeding
Unfractionated heparin	PTT, aPTT	60–90 min	Protamine sulfate
Vitamin K Antagonist			
Warfarin	PT/INR	20–60 h (duration of action 2–5 days)	Prothrombin complex concentrate (PCC), vitamin K, fresh-frozen plasma (FFP), recombinant factor VIIa
Direct Thrombin Inhibitors			
Argatroban	Activated clotting time (ACT), aPTT	39–51 min	Consider hemodialysis, rFVIIa or FFP but generally not indicated due to short half-life
Dabigatran	Thrombin time (TT), dilute TT, ecarin chromogenic assay (ECA), and ecarin clotting time (ECT), PT/INR, PTT	12–17 h	Idarucizumab, PCC, hemodialysis
Commonly Used Factor Xa Inhibitors			
Apixaban Rivaroxaban	Antifactor Xa, PT/INR	12 h 5–9 h	PCC, andexanet alfa infusion
Antiplatelet Agents			
Aspirin Clopidogrel Prasugrel Ticagrelor	Platelet function testing	Duration of action 7–10 days, irreversibly inhibits platelet 7–10 h	Platelet transfusion

aPTT, Activated partial thromboplastin time; *INR*, international normalized ratio; *PT*, prothrombin time; *PTT*, partial thromboplastin time.

may lead to severe bleeding. However, life-saving measures such as thoracostomy, central venous catheterization, and endotracheal intubation are sometimes required even in these severe conditions. An additional life-saving procedure that may carry a high risk of bleeding in the setting of anticoagulation, but should not be withheld, is pericardiocentesis. The gravity of the clinical scenario is important to keep in mind when weighing the risk of performing a procedure in the setting of anticoagulation.

DOACs have now become the most widely prescribed oral anticoagulants in the United States.[16,17] In comparison to VKAs, DOACs have been shown to have less incidence of major bleeding and have simplified perioperative management in the non-emergent setting.[16,17] Idarucizumab (Praxbind), used for reversal of dabigatran, and andexanet alfa (Andexxa), used to reverse factor Xa inhibitors, are two specific Food and Drug Administration (FDA)–approved DOAC reversal agents. Other reversal agents include off-label activated prothrombin complex concentrate (aPCC) and prothrombin complex concentrate (PCC), which are approved for reversal of VKAs but not for DOAC reversal.[16,17] Limited data are available on the safety of performing procedures on patients taking newer DOACs. Patients may not require reversal agents and may be treated with supportive measures, such as antifibrinolytic treatments, activated charcoal, transfusion and resuscitation measures, and discontinuation of the DOAC. The Anticoagulation Forum guidelines recommend to reserve reversal agents for situations such as life-threatening bleeding, critical site bleeding, or major bleeding that does not respond to the aforementioned supportive measures.[16]

MANAGEMENT OF ANTICOAGULANT-ASSOCIATED BLEEDING

Although periprocedural bleeding is typically not life threatening and can often be controlled with direct pressure, predicting which anticoagulated patients will bleed from a procedure is difficult. Furthermore, the simple act of controlling periprocedural bleeding may not entirely end the risk of serious harm. For instance, periprocedural bleeding with percutaneous coronary intervention is associated with an increased short- and long-term morbidity and mortality, including major adverse cardiovascular events and readmission rates well after the bleeding is controlled.[18,19]

When managing spontaneous, periprocedural, or postprocedural bleeding associated with anticoagulation, there are a few principles to consider. Most importantly, emergency life-saving procedures such as endotracheal intubation, tube thoracostomy, cardiac defibrillation, pericardiocentesis, or vascular access should be performed when necessary, regardless of the patient's anticoagulation status.

Stabilization with supportive treatments such as oxygenation, intravascular volume resuscitation, and repletion of blood products via transfusion are the initial steps of assessment and management of bleeding in the anticoagulated patient. Patients with prolonged or severe bleeding may have presenting symptoms in various stages of circulatory shock. Poor blood supply and intravascular volume leads to poor tissue perfusion. Cellular hypoxia, damage, and resulting inflammatory response from hypoperfusion can exacerbate the patient's clinical status. Adequate resuscitation and stabilization are key to the initial phase of management.

Hemostatic measures such as direct compression of a bleeding or oozing vessel, wound, or region should be performed concurrently with stabilization to prevent further blood loss. Additional measures may be needed to control bleeding when compression fails or when the bleeding originates from a noncompressible site. These measures include the use of topical hemostatic agents, systemic hemostatic agents (i.e., tranexamic acid), procedural intervention, operative management, or intra-arterial embolization.

The clinician can assess the severity of coagulopathy with laboratory analysis. Patients may experience bleeding at subtherapeutic, therapeutic, or supratherapeutic levels of anticoagulation. Determining a qualitative level of anticoagulation may help guide therapy. However, as mentioned above, many anticoagulants do not have an associated diagnostic test that is accurate, timely, and clinically relevant to determine severity of coagulopathy like warfarin or heparin. Obtain routine coagulation assays (i.e., PT, PTT, and INR) when no relevant study exists. Routine coagulation assays may sometimes be helpful in determining the lack of a supratherapeutic anticoagulant effect but are often difficult to interpret.

When bleeding is severe, life-threatening, refractory to hemostatic efforts, or the coagulopathy is determined to be severe, restoring the ability to generate an effective clot by administration of an antidote, coagulation factor, blood product, or removal of the offending anticoagulant (i.e., hemodialysis) may be necessary. Consideration for the anticoagulant's duration of action is also important when deciding whether to reverse anticoagulation.

Withholding further doses of anticoagulation may be necessary after stabilization and disposition. When the clinical decision to withhold anticoagulant is not clear, consultation with the prescribing physician (e.g., cardiologist prescribing aspirin and clopidogrel for cardiac stent) or hematologist may be warranted.

Reversal of Anticoagulation

The decision to discontinue or reverse anticoagulation prior to a procedure is difficult. Although there are no validated data that can accurately stratify risk for peri- or postoperative thromboembolism, the American College of Chest Physicians (ACCP) has published guidelines that stratify patients into low-, moderate-, and high-risk groups.[20] These guidelines are listed in Table 73.2.

Risk factors that increase the likelihood of a thromboembolic event with anticoagulant disruption include a prosthetic heart valve, atrial fibrillation, recent cerebrovascular accident (CVA) or transient ischemic attack, recent venous thromboembolism (VTE), the presence of a VTE risk factor (i.e., protein C/S deficiency, antiphospholipid antibody), and a high $CHAD_2$ score (congestive heart failure, hypertension, age, diabetes mellitus, CVA).[20–22] Patients with mechanical valves are at higher risk for thromboembolic events when anticoagulation is disrupted than patients with bioprosthetic valves. Mitral valves present a higher risk of thromboembolic events

TABLE 73.2 Suggested Patient Risk Stratification for Perioperative Arterial or Venous Thromboembolism: Indication for VKA Therapy

RISK STRATUM	MECHANICAL HEART VALVE	ATRIAL FIBRILLATION	VTE
High	Any mitral valve prosthesis Older (caged-ball or tilting disc) aortic valve prosthesis Recent (within 6 months) stroke or transient ischemic attack	CHADS2 score of 5 or 6 Recent (within 3 months) stroke or transient ischemic attack Rheumatic valvular heart disease	Recent (within 3 months) VTE Severe thrombophilia (e.g., deficiency of protein C, protein S or antithrombin, antiphospholipid antibodies, or multiple abnormalities)
Moderate	Bileaflet aortic valve prosthesis and one of the following: atrial fibrillation, prior stroke or transient ischemic attack, hypertension, diabetes, congestive heart failure, age >75 years	CHADS2 score of 3 or 4	VTE within the past 3 to 12 months; nonsevere thrombophilic conditions (e.g., heterozygous factor V Leiden mutation, heterozygous factor II mutation); Recurrent VTE; active cancer (treated within 6 months or palliative)
Low	Bileaflet aortic valve prosthesis without atrial fibrillation and no other risk factors for stroke	CHADS2 score of 0–2 (and no prior stroke or transient ischemic attack)	Single VTE occurred 12 months ago and no other risk factors

CHADS2, Congestive heart failure-hypertension-age-diabetes-stroke; *VTE*, venous thromboembolism.
From Douketis JD, Spyropoulos AC, Murad MH, et al. Perioperative management of antithrombotic therapy: an American College of Chest Physicians Clinical Practice Guideline. *Chest*. 2022;164(1):267.

than aortic prosthetic valves. The postoperative period just after (less than 3 months) mechanical valve placement is also a high-risk time for thromboembolic events.[22]

Procedures on patients with prosthetic valves typically require a delayed approach to operative management, except when there is an emergency. In general, discontinuing anticoagulation in a patient with a prosthetic valve is safer than reversal of anticoagulation to perform a procedure. Reversal of anticoagulation puts patients at higher risk for thromboembolic events than does simply discontinuing the anticoagulant. When possible, discontinue anticoagulation and delay invasive procedures on patients with prosthetic valves until coagulation status returns to near normal. For patients with low-risk bioprosthetic valves that require discontinuation of anticoagulation, warfarin should be discontinued 48 to 72 hours prior to the procedure or until the INR drops below 1.5.[22] Anticoagulation may then be restarted 24 hours following the procedure. High-risk patients with prosthetic valves (e.g., mitral valve) require bridging therapy to reduce the time off anticoagulation.[22]

For patients taking VKAs that require reversal of anticoagulation for an urgent procedure, administration of oral vitamin K is recommended.[20] If more immediate reversal is required for a procedure, administration of PCC (preferred) or fresh-frozen plasma (FFP) in addition to oral vitamin K is recommended.[20] For patients taking antiplatelet agents such as aspirin or clopidogrel, platelet transfusion is recommended for reversal of the effect (Fig. 73.1).[20]

DOACs generally have shorter half-lives compared to VKAs, and in most bleeding events that are non–life threatening, they may be controlled with supportive measures, such as withholding DOAC temporarily or blood product transfusion.[16,17,23] However, in cases where life-threatening bleeding occurs, reversal of a DOAC with a specific reversal agent may be necessary in addition to surgical control of bleeding if direct pressure is not possible, as well as other stabilizing measures such as 3 or 4 F-PCC, aPCCs, FFP, hemodialysis in the case of dabigatran, and activated charcoal.[16,17,23]

PROCEDURES

Lumbar Puncture (See Chapter 61)

The decision to perform a LP in an anticoagulated patient should be individualized and based on an assessment of the risks and benefits of the procedure. When the risks of an LP are high, the procedure can be delayed and treatment initiated, such as empiric antibiotic therapy for cases of suspected meningitis. When the condition is difficult to diagnose or treat, LP may be necessary. In these cases, hold doses of the anticoagulant before the procedure as long as it is safe to do so. In addition, reversal using specific anticoagulant-appropriate agents (PCCs, idarucizumab, or andexanet alfa) consultation with interventional radiology, anesthesiology or appropriate specialists may be warranted to reduce the risk of hemorrhage.

When an LP is performed in an anticoagulated ED patient, it is critical to monitor for complications. The most important complication associated with LP in the setting of anticoagulation is a spinal epidural hematoma (SEH). This rare, but catastrophic, complication is more likely to occur with a difficult or traumatic LP in anticoagulated patients or those with a platelet disorder.[24–27] An emergency magnetic resonance image should be performed if there is suspicion for an SEH. If an SEH is diagnosed, immediate decompression with a laminectomy should be performed to avoid irreversible spinal cord ischemia.[26]

Many clinicians feel that spinal procedures such as an LP may be safely performed on patients taking aspirin or a nonsteroidal antiinflammatory drug (NSAID) without discontinuing the medication or transfusing platelets.[27–32] It is important to consider the specific medication. Aspirin irreversibly inactivates cyclooxygenase-1 (COX-1) and blocks thromboxane production for the life of a platelet (7 to 10 days) within an hour of ingestion. Therefore platelet function does not return to normal until the permanently inhibited platelets are replaced by enough newly synthesized active platelets. The ability for platelets to aggregate can be seen after 4 days following aspirin cessation, as it requires only a few uninhibited platelets (newly synthesized or transfused) to recruit aspirin-treated platelets to action.[33,34] Horlocker and colleagues studied 391 patients undergoing spinal anesthesia and also on antiplatelet therapy including aspirin, naproxen, piroxicam, ibuprofen, indomethacin, dipyridamole, and sulindac.[29] There were 113 patients on multiple antiplatelet agents preoperatively. No SEHs were reported in this study. The authors concluded that preoperative antiplatelet medication was not a contraindication to spinal anesthesia. Importantly, it is not recommended to perform an LP on patients who are using aspirin or an NSAID concurrently with another anticoagulant such as heparin, low-molecular-weight heparin (LMWH), a DOAC, or other antiplatelet agents.[32]

The safety of performing an LP in patients receiving newer antiplatelet agents, including clopidogrel, ticlopidine, abciximab, eptifibatide, or tirofiban is not well studied. The American Society of Regional Anesthesia and Pain Medicine (ASRA) recommends discontinuation of these medications prior to LP.[32] Reversing the effect of these medications and the period of discontinuation prior to the performance of the procedure depends on the medication. Pharmacologically, normal platelet activity is expected 8 hours after discontinuing tirofiban and eptifibatide, 24 to 48 hours after discontinuing abciximab, and 1 to 2 weeks after discontinuing clopidogrel and ticlopidine.[32] The ASRA, ACCP, and the American Heart Association (AHA) recommend discontinuing clopidogrel for 7 days in medium- to high-risk procedures. For those with a high risk of developing thromboembolic events, a 5-day discontinuation period in conjunction with platelet function testing that shows adequate platelet function, if available, has been recommended. Other organizations recommend a 5-day washout period prior to giving spinal injections in patients receiving these medications.[20,27,32–35]

Heparin increases the risk of SEH. In a study from 1981, 2% (7 of 342) of patients receiving heparin for anticoagulation developed SEH after LP. Risk for SEH increased with a traumatic procedure, starting anticoagulation within an hour of the LP, and concomitant aspirin therapy.[36] Patients with preexisting coagulopathy were excluded from this study. This study suggests that the risk of SEH in patients on heparin prior to the LP is at least 2%. In a study by Tryba and colleagues, the risk of SEH increased tenfold in patients receiving heparin or aspirin who experienced a traumatic LP.[37] As intravenous (IV) heparin has a short duration of action, it should be discontinued for at least 4 hours prior to the LP and the aPTT has normalized.[27] Heparin infusion should not be resumed for at least an hour after an LP is performed.[36] The risk for SEH from LP in patients on twice daily subcutaneous

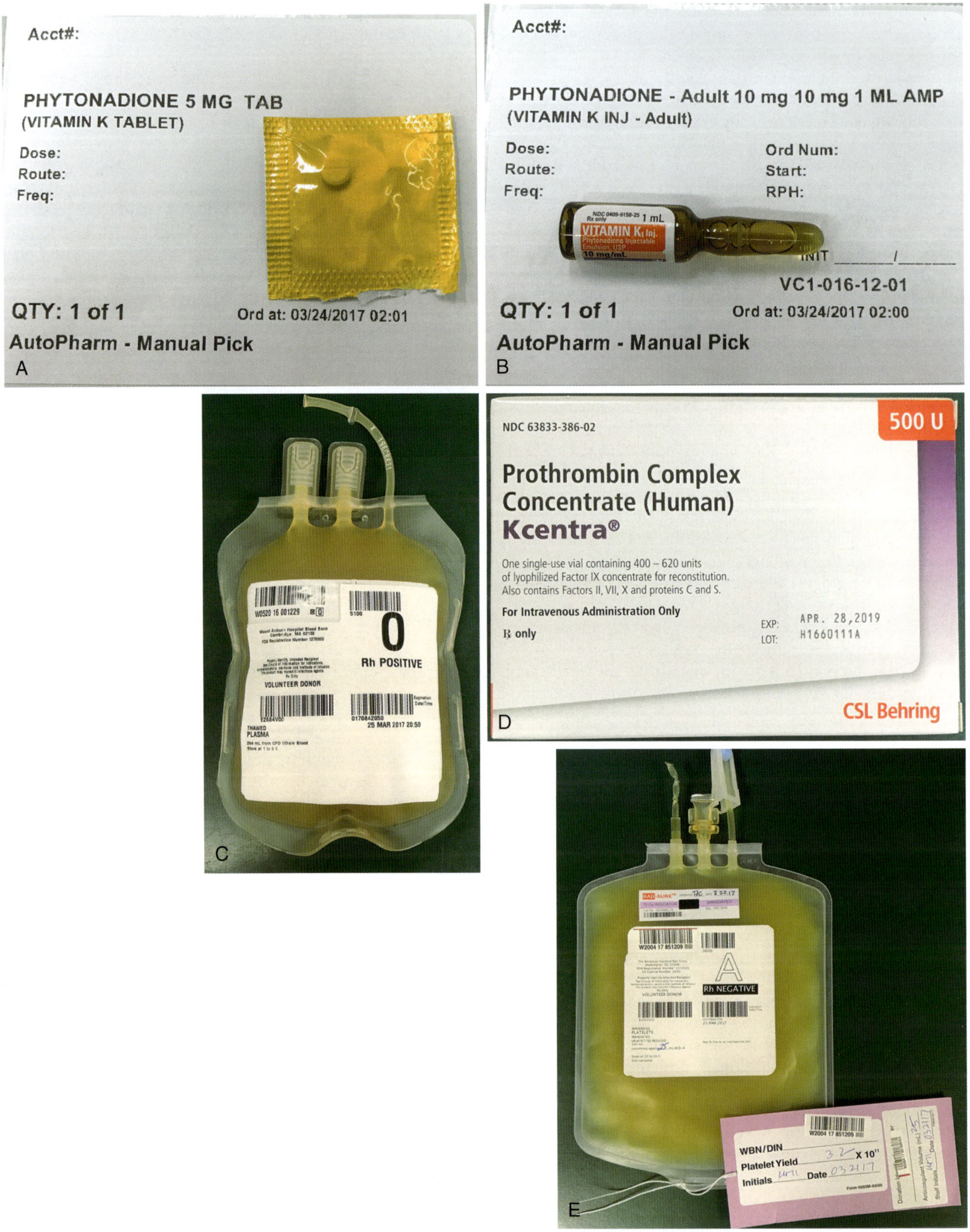

Fig. 73.1 Anticoagulant and coagulopathy reversal agents. (A) Oral vitamin K reverses the effect of vitamin K antagonists, such as warfarin. Onset of action ranges from hours to days. (B) Intravenous vitamin K can be used in patients who require emergency procedures; however, onset of action is measured in hours, as the liver must regenerate coagulation factors. There is a risk of anaphylaxis with intravenous vitamin K, and it should be administered via slow infusion (over 20 to 60 minutes). (C) Fresh-frozen plasma (FFP) can be used to reverse the effect of vitamin K antagonists in emergency situations. (D) Prothrombin complex concentrates (such as the four-factor PCC Kcentra) provide rapid international normalized ratio correction and may be safer than FFP. PCCs can also be used to reverse the effects of direct thrombin inhibitors (e.g., dabigatran) and factor Xa inhibitors (e.g., apixaban). (E) Platelet transfusions can be used to reverse the effects of antiplatelet medications such as aspirin or clopidogrel, and also to correct thrombocytopenias.

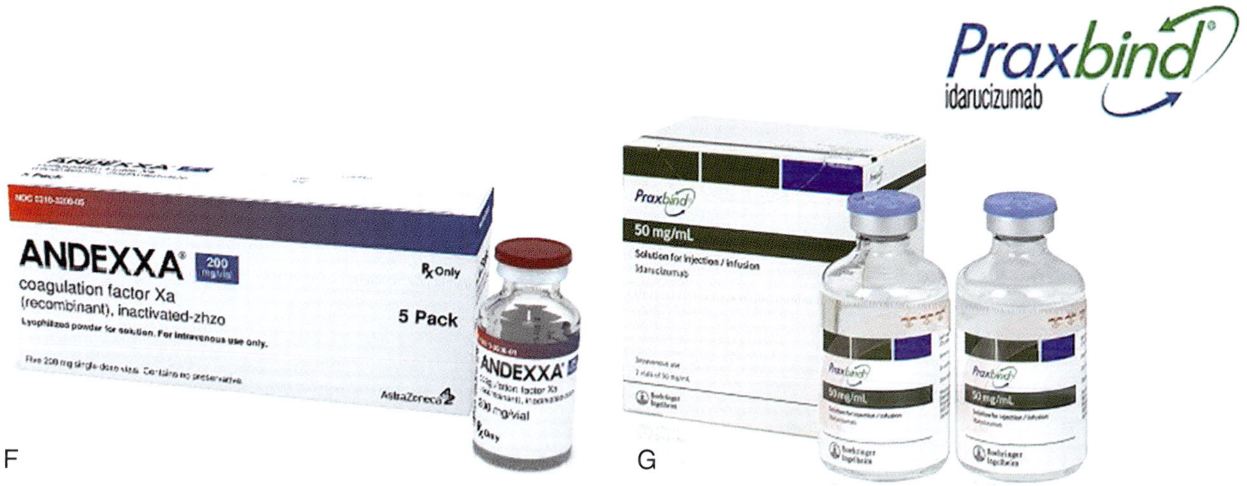

Fig. 73.1 cont'd (F) Andexanet alfa (Andexxa), used to reverse factor Xa inhibitors. (G) Idarucizumab (Praxbind), used to reverse the direct thrombin inhibitor dabigatran.

heparin for the prophylaxis of deep venous thrombosis is low.[38] Nonetheless, it is recommended to discontinue for at least 8 hours prior to neuraxial procedures.[27]

LMWH has a half-life that can range between 2 and 6 hours depending on the dose, route of administration, and renal function. The ASRA guidelines recommend discontinuing LMWH 12 hours prior to neuraxial procedures when used at doses intended for deep vein thrombosis prophylaxis and 24 hours when used at doses intended for anticoagulation.[27] Anticoagulation with LMWH should be withheld for 18 to 24 hours after the LP to prevent SEH.[31]

Warfarin is associated with a high risk of SEH following an LP. Warfarin should be stopped for 5 days and the INR normalized prior to performing an LP.[27] Administration of PCCs or vitamin K with FFP is recommended for complete warfarin reversal.

There are no evidence-based guidelines regarding patients on DOACs in need of an LP, although the available data suggest a lower risk of major bleeding complications in patients on DOACs as compared to warfarin. It has been suggested that, if possible, a diagnostic LP should be postponed by 24 hours for patients who are on DOACs; however, if it is truly emergent a consideration can be made to proceed with the LP without delay.[39]

Performing an LP in patients with hemophilia is safe following 100% factor replacement. In a study by Silverman and colleagues, 30 of 33 patients (91%) with severe factor deficiency had no serious complications with LP after adequate factor replacement.[24] In a review of six articles that evaluated neuraxial procedures in patients with hemophilia, there were no SEHs in 107 procedures on 85 patients, of which 53 of the procedures were diagnostic LPs in the ED. In 105 of the 107 procedures (98%), factor levels were replaced to normal. One case of an SEH with neurologic impairment occurred in a patient with undiagnosed hemophilia.[40]

There is scant literature on the performance of an LP in patients with select platelet disorders, including von Willebrand disease (vWD) and idiopathic thrombocytopenic purpura (ITP). Choi and colleagues conducted a literature review of studies from 1975 to 2008 that performed neuroaxial procedures (lumbar epidural anesthesia, other spinal anesthesia, and LPs) for patients with hemophilia, vWD, and ITP. The most relevant study for ED practice in the review evaluated LPs conducted in the ED in patients with hemophilia A and B. It found no bleeding complications when factor was replaced to normal levels in advance of the procedure. The other included studies were not ED-based and evaluated spinal epidural and other forms of spinal anesthesia for obstetric or other surgical procedures, and are thus less relevant.

Performing an LP in the setting of thrombocytopenia has been well studied in the pediatric oncology population. In 2000 Howard and colleagues reported on the safety of performing LPs in children with platelet counts greater than 10 × 10^9/L without transfusing platelets. Procedures were performed on 941 patients with platelet counts below 50 × 10^9/L without the development of an SEH. Procedures were performed on 29 patients with platelet counts less than or equal to 10 × 10^9/L. No complications were reported, although the study was not powered to determine patient safety. Nonetheless, the authors recommended platelet transfusion for an LP when the platelet count is less than or equal to 10 × 10^9/L.[41]

A 2010 systematic review by van Veen states that with a platelet count greater than or equal to 40 × 10^9/L, it is safe to perform an LP provided that the platelet count is stable, the patient does not have an acquired or congenital coagulopathy, the platelet function is normal, and the patient is not receiving an antiplatelet or anticoagulant medication. The authors also stated that it may be safe to perform an LP at lower platelet counts (20 to 40 × 10^9/L); however, there were insufficient data to recommend safety at this platelet level without transfusion.[42] The American Association of Blood Banks recommends a slightly higher threshold for prophylactic platelet transfusion for patients having an elective diagnostic LP (platelet count less than 50 × 10^9/L).[43] However, this is a weak recommendation based on very low-quality evidence.

Vascular Access (See Chapter 22)

Patients frequently require central venous access for resuscitation, medication administration, or hemodynamic monitoring. Critically ill patients are sometimes anticoagulated or develop a coagulopathy secondary to their illness. Providers are oftentimes hesitant to perform central venous cannulation in anticoagulated patients or those with a coagulopathy because of the risk of bleeding.

Bleeding complications during central venous catheterization in patients with abnormal hemostasis are relatively low.[44,45] Arterial puncture is the most common complication associated with central venous catheter insertion and occurs in 3% of catheters placed in the internal jugular vein and 0.5% of catheters placed in the subclavian vein.[46] Numerous studies have demonstrated that central venous cannulation is safe in patients with a coagulopathy or disorder of hemostasis.[12,43,44,46–48] Emergency reversal of anticoagulation prior to the insertion of a central venous catheter is common practice but does not appear to be evidence-based.[12,44,45,49,50] In one study, central venous access procedures were performed on 76 consecutive patients with various disorders of hemostasis (i.e., thrombocytopenia, anticoagulation with heparin, anticoagulation with warfarin, and abnormalities in coagulation assays). Of the 104 procedures, only one patient required an intervention beyond 20 minutes of site compression to control bleeding.[44] The authors noted that bleeding problems are uncommon and serious bleeding is rare. Providers should make a case-based clinical decision weighing the risk of hemorrhage versus the risk of thrombosis and fluid overload associated with reversal.

In a 2000 study evaluating the complications of central venous catheter placement in patients with various hemostasis disorders, thrombocytopenia (platelet count less than 50×10^9/L) was the only significant predictor for bleeding complications.[45] However, the authors call into question the utility of platelet transfusion because the complications were easily addressed with compression and suturing. Other studies have also found that a platelet count less than 50×10^9/L is an independent risk factor for bleeding.[44,45,51] Further studies are required to assess the benefit of preprocedural platelet transfusion for central venous catheter insertion.[52] Platelet transfusion to maintain counts greater than 50×10^9/L is recommended in patients with evidence of postprocedural bleeding at catheter insertion site until hemostasis is achieved.[53]

In 1999 Fisher and colleagues demonstrated a low incidence of major vascular complications in patients with cirrhosis and an elevated INR. Of 658 cannulations, there was one major event (hemothorax) caused by accidental subclavian artery puncture. The mean INR was 2.4 (range 1 to 16) and no attempt was made to reverse coagulopathy prior to the procedure.[51] Similar results were found in two additional studies on coagulopathic patients including patients with liver disease receiving central venous access.[44,49]

Patients with DIC should have vigorous correction of coagulation abnormalities in conjunction with hematology consultation prior to central venous catheterization when patient stability allows for it.[53] Targets for correction include PT less than 1.5 times normal and fibrinogen greater than 1.0 g/L.

Factor replacement is recommended for patients with hemophilia prior to central venous cannulation.[54,55] The goal of management is to achieve a circulating factor level of 100% prior to the procedure followed by a continuous factor infusion for 2 to 3 days afterward to prevent serious bleeding complications.

In nonurgent situations, IV heparin infusion should be discontinued for 3 hours prior to central venous cannulation.[53] In patients receiving therapeutic anticoagulation with subcutaneous LMWH, the recommendation is to wait 18 hours after the last injection before performing nonurgent central venous cannulations.[53] Similarly, nonurgent central venous cannulation in patients on warfarin should be withheld until the INR is less than 1.5.[53]

The use of ultrasound for the placement of central venous catheters is well established and has been shown to increase success rates and decrease complication rates.[56–60] The use of ultrasound in patients with disorders of hemostasis is safe and preferred when available.[56,60] There are no data comparing ultrasound-guided versus traditional approach in the setting of anticoagulation.[59]

In emergency situations, site selection for central venous cannulation may improve outcomes. The safest technique in an anticoagulated patient appears to be an ultrasound-guided internal jugular approach. The lower risk of malposition, ease of ultrasound-guided technique, and the ability to manually compress a bleeding vessel in the event of a bleeding complication make the internal jugular access the favored approach over the subclavian approach.[46] Though the subclavian approach is associated with fewer arterial punctures, the provider is unable to manually compress bleeding vessels effectively. The femoral approach is also suitable for emergency central venous access because it is amenable to ultrasound-guided technique, and the provider is able to manually compress a bleeding vessel. Importantly, femoral venous catheters are less favorable long-term because of an increased risk of infection.

The use of intraosseous access is not contraindicated in anticoagulated patients. The manufacturer of the EZ-IO (Arrow) device notes that applying pressure to the site for 1 to 2 minutes controls bleeding after needle removal, but more time may be required for patients on anticoagulant therapy.[61]

Patients requiring temporary placement of a hemodialysis catheter for emergency hemodialysis may have an increased risk of complications with central venous access because of comorbid conditions leading to anticoagulation or impaired hemostasis, particularly uremia-induced platelet dysfunction. Dialysis catheters generally have larger diameters than standard triple lumen catheters and require more dilation. These catheters are also firmer and have less flexibility. If a patient requires emergency access for hemodialysis and is coagulopathic, the preferred approach site is the femoral vein due to compressibility, although placement in this location will limit patient mobility and requires the longest available catheter (19 to 24 cm). Whereas complication rates are similar to typical central venous catheter placement, inadvertent dilation of the artery or unrecognized arterial puncture with a hemodialysis catheter can lead to massive bleeding. Although there are no data or guideline specifically targeted for the placement of hemodialysis catheters in the setting of anticoagulation, mechanical errors may be complicated by anticoagulation.

ARTHROCENTESIS (SEE CHAPTER 54)

Although prior conventional wisdom indicated the need to reverse anticoagulation prior to arthrocentesis for patients receiving anticoagulation with warfarin, more recent data suggest that this is not necessary. In a large 2023 systematic review, there were only 5 reported cases of bleeding out of 871 joint injection/aspiration procedures on patients receiving warfarin. The authors' meta-analysis suggested that it is safe to perform arthrocentesis in patients receiving warfarin, even without first obtaining INR.[62]

There is no available literature evaluating the safety of arthrocentesis in patients receiving an antiplatelet agent or a non-VKA.

Similarly, while data are somewhat limited on the safety of performing arthrocentesis in patients receiving DOAC medications, the studies available suggest that the procedure is likely safe. A 2021 systematic review found only one bleeding complication among 688 patients who underwent joint injection/aspiration procedures and who were receiving rivaroxaban, apixaban, or dabigatran. The affected patient was receiving dabigatran. The authors suggest that DOACs can safely be continued during arthrocentesis.[63]

Hemarthrosis is a common presentation for patients with bleeding disorders such as hemophilia. It is typically recommended that patients or parents replace factors to achieve circulating factor activity of 40% to 50% at the first sign of acute bleeding episodes. Arthrocentesis is not always required to make the diagnosis of hemarthrosis in this clinical setting. However, if performing an arthrocentesis in the setting of hemophilia is required, the recommendation is to perform the procedure after appropriate factor replacement.

Spontaneous nontraumatic hemarthrosis is an infrequent complication with supratherapeutic anticoagulation and may even occur within the target therapeutic range.[64] Routine coagulation studies are recommended if hemarthrosis is suspected in an anticoagulated patient. Temporary discontinuation of anticoagulants is typically recommended as part of treatment of hemarthrosis. If arthrocentesis is required, reversal of anticoagulation is not recommended if the INR is less than 4.5.[15] Although arthrocentesis can safely be performed in the setting of supratherapeutic anticoagulation as previously mentioned, there are no safety data for the setting of hemarthrosis.[14] Clinical judgment should be used to determine the necessity of this procedure.

PARACENTESIS (SEE CHAPTER 44)

Paracentesis is a relatively safe procedure. The frequency of complications such as minor bleeding or major complications such as abdominal hematoma that require a transfusion is low. In the era of ultrasound guidance for procedures, hemorrhagic complication rates for paracentesis are vanishingly low, even among patients with coagulopathies commonly seen in cirrhosis such as thrombocytopenia and elevated INR.[65–67] Generally it is not recommended to correct mild to moderate coagulopathy (PT or PTT up to twice normal) or thrombocytopenia (platelet count 50 to 99 × 10^9/L) prior to low-risk procedures such as paracentesis, and blood products such as FFP or platelets should be used sparingly given their associated risks such as increased portal pressure and transfusion complications.[68,69]

In a 2009 prospective study evaluating the complication rate of paracentesis in cirrhotic patients, local bleeding occurred in 2.3% of cases and major bleeding requiring a medical or surgical intervention occurred in 1% of cases. Two of the five patients with major bleeding included a major hematoma, whereas three cases involved bleeding into the peritoneal cavity. A nonsignificant trend toward increased risk of complications was seen in patients with a platelet count less than 50 × 10^9/L. Therefore the authors advised caution when performing paracentesis on patients with a platelet count less than 50 × 10^9/L.[70]

While paracentesis has been well studied in the setting of coagulopathy due to cirrhosis, there are minimal data available for the safety of paracentesis in the setting of anticoagulation with DOAC drugs. A small 2019 retrospective study of hemorrhagic complications among patients who underwent ultrasound-guided paracentesis while being treated with DOAC drugs or clopidogrel concluded that the risk of significant hemorrhage in this population was low.[71]

THORACENTESIS AND TUBE THORACOSTOMY (SEE CHAPTERS 9 AND 10)

The major procedural complication associated with thoracentesis is pneumothorax, not bleeding.[72] Numerous studies have failed to demonstrate an increased risk of bleeding with thoracentesis in the setting of anticoagulation.[73,74] When performed under ultrasound guidance, the risk of bleeding is low even when coagulation studies or the platelet count are abnormal.[73–75]

Additionally, the correction of abnormal coagulation laboratory values prior to the procedure is unlikely to have benefit.

In a 2013 retrospective study of 1009 ultrasound-guided thoracenteses, Hibbert and colleagues evaluated patients treated with and without preprocedural transfusion of FFP or platelets for abnormal coagulation profiles.[74] The authors found no statistical difference in the bleeding complication rate (overall 0.4%) between those treated with transfusion prior to the procedure and patients not treated with blood products. In this study, the patients who did not receive FFP or platelet transfusions had a mean INR of 1.9 prior to the procedure. Of the 74 patients (14%) who were not treated with a transfusion had a platelet level of less than 50 × 10^9/L. There were no bleeding complications seen in the group that did not receive FFP or platelets compared with four bleeding complications that occurred in the group that received transfusions.

Recent studies have raised concerns about the risk of bleeding when thoracentesis is performed on patients taking clopidogrel. One prospective study of 25 consecutive patients noted a low rate of clinically significant hemorrhage in patients receiving thoracentesis while on clopidogrel, but further studies are required to determine safety. In that study, one patient developed a significant hemothorax requiring blood transfusion and tube thoracostomy.[76] A 2013 case report also raised similar concerns as a patient on clopidogrel and aspirin developed a hemothorax after chest tube insertion.[77] However, there are no data to support this recommendation. In fact, two studies failed to demonstrate a high risk for bleeding in patients taking clopidogrel especially when using small bore chest tubes.[78,79]

In patients with a tension pneumothorax, there are no absolute contraindications to tube thoracostomy. In stable patients undergoing chest tube placement, the need for anticoagulation reversal should be considered. Several clinicians have recommended that coagulopathies and platelet defects be corrected prior to tube thoracostomy.[80,81]

DENTAL PROCEDURES (SEE CHAPTER 65)

Managing postoperative bleeding after a dental procedure can be a challenging task for EPs especially in the setting of anticoagulation. Dental procedures such as extractions are commonly performed without the cessation of anticoagulants. Multiple studies and authors have concluded that the risk of cessation of anticoagulation including antiplatelet therapy is much greater than the risk of significant bleeding with continued anticoagulation for dental procedures.[82–86] Multiple organizations including the AHA, ACCP, American College of Surgeons, American Dental Association, and The American College of Cardiology all agree that single or dual antiplatelet therapy should not be interrupted for dental procedures. It also appears to be safe to continue DOAC medications such as dabigatran or rivaroxaban for dental procedures.[87–89]

Bleeding and oozing from a dental procedural site is common after extractions such as wisdom tooth extractions even in the setting of normal coagulation. Patients commonly come to the ED after futile attempts to control the bleeding at home. Simple local therapy such as compression, packing, and vasoconstrictor infiltration is typically sufficient to control bleeding, even in the anticoagulated patient. Although none are specific for anticoagulated patients, there are multiple commercially available products that can be utilized to achieve hemostasis. Thrombin-soaked gelatin sponges, oxidized cellulose material, chitosan coated gauze dressing, and topical tranexamic acid have all been described for this purpose.

Patients with hemophilia and vWD have an increased risk of bleeding during and after dental procedures. In addition to utilizing standard therapies, IV or local tranexamic acid and epsilon-aminocaproic acid in patients with hemophilia may also aid in achieving hemostasis, as has been described in a limited number of trials.[90–92] However, a 2019 Cochrane review was unable to definitively conclude its efficacy.[93]

Although no studies exist looking specifically at the safety of performing simple oral and dental procedures in the ED such as incision and drainage of a dental abscess, they are likely benign, considering the safety data for more invasive dental procedures such as extraction.

EPISTAXIS (SEE CHAPTER 64)

Epistaxis is a common presenting symptom in the ED and may be complicated by anticoagulant use. When the bleeding occurs in the setting of excessive anticoagulation, achieving hemostasis may be more difficult than normal clinical scenarios. Evaluation of coagulation parameters (PT, INR, PTT, platelet count, or other anticoagulant-specific laboratory assays) should be routinely ordered for anticoagulated patients presenting with epistaxis. A complete blood count or point-of-care hemoglobin is also suggested for patients with prolonged or severe bleeding with epistaxis.

Anticoagulant reversal is rarely necessary unless the patient has severe, symptomatic, or life-threatening bleeding. Specific factor replacement is necessary for patients with hemophilia and severe bleeding.

A variety of topical hemostatic agents are available and can be applied to the nasal cavity for the management of epistaxis in the anticoagulated patient when standard therapy is not adequate. Cellulose, gelatin, and thrombin compounds can be placed directly on the bleeding site to promote clot formation even in fully anticoagulated patients. Both topical and IV use of tranexamic acid has also been described in the management of epistaxis, but there is a lack of evidence-based data supporting its efficacy.[94–96] A case report described the successful use of topical tranexamic acid in the management of rivaroxaban associated epistaxis after failure with a thrombin-soaked inflated nasal tampon.[97]

NASOGASTRIC TUBE INSERTION (SEE CHAPTER 41)

There is a lack of information available about the safety of placing a nasogastric tube (NGT) in the setting of anticoagulation. Severe coagulopathy is a commonly stated relative contraindication of NGT passage for risk of epistaxis without reference to evidence-based data.

Similarly, the often-stated NGT placement contraindication of esophageal varices is unproven. Although mechanical or chemical irritation is thought to cause esophageal varices rupture and bleeding, there are limited data that stratify the risk of NGT placement in this clinical circumstance. In a study of patients with esophageal varices requiring NGT placement, less than 15% of patients had subsequent gastrointestinal bleeding. Bleeding was associated with higher model of end-stage liver disease (MELD-Na) scores and varices in the distal third of the esophagus.[98] Additional research is required to prove or disprove the link between bleeding and NGT placement.

Thrombocytopenia is a common finding in cirrhosis and may be associated with risk of future gastrointestinal hemorrhage.[99] Unfortunately, routine coagulation assays are not reliable indicators of coagulation status in patients with cirrhosis. Whereas platelet transfusion is commonly recommended prior to endoscopy for a platelet count of less than 30×10^9/L, there is no analogous recommendation for NGT insertion.[100]

LABOR AND DELIVERY (SEE CHAPTER 57)

Delivery of a newborn in the ED is a relatively rare event. Postpartum bleeding and hemorrhage are complications exacerbated by maternal factors such as anticoagulation and bleeding disorders. Tranexamic acid administration has been shown to reduce mortality due to postpartum hemorrhage in a large cohort of females independent of anticoagulation or inherited bleeding disorder status.[101]

Pregnant patients diagnosed with VTE are typically treated with LMWH. In the final weeks of pregnancy, obstetricians occasionally switch patients to unfractionated heparin to reduce time to normalization of coagulation studies when labor begins. However, fully anticoagulated patients may present with precipitous labor and develop postpartum hemorrhage. Reversal of anticoagulation may be necessary in the event of refractory bleeding. There is no recommendation for prophylactic reversal of anticoagulation for delivery.[102]

Patients with vWD are at increased risk for postpartum hemorrhage. These patients have a higher risk of delayed postpartum hemorrhage reported up to 2 to 3 weeks after delivery. According to case reports, postpartum hemorrhage may still occur despite prophylaxis with factor VIII, cryoprecipitate, FFP, and desmopressin acetate (DDAVP). Expert opinion recommends that a von Willebrand factor activity of greater than or equal to 50 IU/dL should be achieved before delivery and maintained for at least 3 to 5 days afterward. There are no randomized trials that have studied DDAVP's efficacy to prevent or treat postpartum hemorrhage.[103,104]

Although hemophilia rarely affects females because of its X-linked nature, replacement of factors is recommended for pregnant females with severe hemophilia A or B in labor. Although high-quality clinical trials are lacking, the available evidence suggests that history of bleeding may be more strongly correlated with risk for peripartum hemorrhage than specific factor levels.[105]

WOUND MANAGEMENT

Control of Hemorrhage

Hemostasis is an essential step in wound management. Inadequate hemostasis can lead to the formation of a hematoma within a closed wound, which may cause dehiscence of wound edges, impaired healing, and increased risk for wound infection. Anticoagulated patients may come to the ED for prolonged or severe episodes of bleeding from an acute traumatic wound. Most bleeding wounds are effectively managed with routine application of direct pressure and elevation. However, anticoagulants may impair the integral mechanisms of hemostasis and prevent adequate spontaneous hemostasis.

There are multiple techniques that can be utilized to control a bleeding wound including compression, vessel crushing, ligation, electrocautery, or application of a vasoconstrictor or hemostatic agent. These traditional techniques are not specific to anticoagulated patients, but they may be useful in achieving hemostasis. There are a few topical hemostatic agents that have been shown to be effective in the setting of anticoagulation.

Chitosan is a complex carbohydrate derived from chitin that interacts with platelets and red blood cells to form a gel-like clot independent from coagulation factors. In a heparinized swine model, Millner showed chitosan granules (Omni-Stat, Medtrade Products Ltd.) and dressings (Celox Gauze, Medtrade) were both efficacious in providing hemostasis over plain gauze compression.[106] The long-term stability of the clot is not well established and therefore these products are used as temporary management if definitive therapy such as surgical intervention is required. Chitosan-based dressings (Hemcon, Tricol Biomedical) have also been used externally for hemostasis in pediatric patients with bleeding tendencies from congenital or acquired bleeding disorders.[107]

Topical thrombin has also shown efficacy as a topical hemostatic agent in anticoagulated patients, in particular heparin and clopidogrel therapy.[108,109] These commercially available topical thrombin products aid in the production of fibrin in one of the final steps of the coagulation pathway to create a stable clot.

IV tranexamic acid has been shown in one study to be efficacious in trauma patients, especially when given early after injury.[110] However, the study did not include anticoagulated patients. The use of topical tranexamic acid for the control of bleeding has been promising in many clinical scenarios but remains unproven especially in the setting of anticoagulation.

INCISION AND DRAINAGE (SEE CHAPTER 37)

There is no literature reporting complications in anticoagulated patients who undergo incision and drainage. Although bleeding is a risk with incision and drainage, local therapy alone is typically sufficient to provide hemostasis. EPs should make a case-based clinical decision weighing the risk of hemorrhage for patients requiring incision and drainage.

SUMMARY

Procedures in the setting of anticoagulation present a unique complexity in the ED. The EP should be mindful of potential bleeding complications and should be prepared to identify and treat these events. Reversal of anticoagulation is not always necessary prior to performing a procedure and the EP should be attentive to the risk of thrombosis. In some instances, the risk-benefit ratio may favor delaying a procedure until the patient's coagulation status returns to normal range with time, or the use of medications or blood products. Lastly, emergency procedures to correct an imminent life-threatening life-saving condition should never be withheld in the setting of anticoagulation.

ACKNOWLEDGMENT

The authors thank Dr. Joseph D'Orazio for his work on previous editions of this chapter.

REFERENCES ARE AVAILABLE AT Elsevier eBooks+

CHAPTER 74

The Impact of Health Inequities on Medical Procedures

Kaitlen Howell

INTRODUCTION: SOCIAL DETERMINANTS OF HEALTH

This chapter reviews what is known about the impact of health inequities on medical procedures by presenting information about a selection of the emergent and urgent medical procedures covered in this book. Health inequities affect medical procedures in many ways including by increasing a patient's risk of requiring a procedure, influencing clinician decision-making about medical procedures, and increasing risks of procedural complications and poorer outcomes. While covering each of these aspects, when possible, this chapter will highlight the interplay between health inequities and procedural management, to identify practices that individual clinicians as well as the field of emergency medicine can change.

Social determinants of health, the historical and present-day external factors that impact a person's health, contribute heavily to health inequities and are estimated by the World Health Organization to determine 30% to 55% of an individual's health.[1] The health inequities and related procedures that are the focus of this chapter were selected based on having a thorough evidence base in the medical literature, including their documented direct impacts on medical procedures.[2–10] Race and ethnicity,[11] gender and biological sex,[12] and income and socioeconomic status[13] have been especially well studied to date and are key contributors to health inequities. However, it should be noted that there are many additional causes and effects of these health inequities that could be covered in this chapter, as well as additional characteristics that can lead to inequities including spoken language, gender identity, sexual orientation, age, disability, education level, housing status, health care access, food availability, geographic residence, among others.

Presumed genetic and biological determinants are often used to explain worse outcomes for racial and ethnic minority patients after various medical procedures, but the reality is more complex. Races are groupings that are socially assigned based on physical or cultural characteristics, and have no genetic basis.[14,15] Patients of the same "race" are not more genetically similar to one another than patients of different races, and patient "race" also does not correlate to nation of origin.[16–18] As race is a social grouping and not an intrinsic quality, medical research on "racial" disparities reflects differences in exposures (including racism) experienced by people who have been grouped in different ways by society. Exposures also include social determinants of health, as well as differences in health care availability, access, triage, and resource allotment, and differences in provider treatment and clinical decision-making that can be due to implicit biases.[19]

Disparities across patients who have been socially grouped as belonging to different races are evidenced in many procedures discussed in this chapter. Most differences in procedural outcomes attributed to race and ethnicity would be most accurately reported as being due to structural and societal racism, rather than to race. With this awareness, the term "race" is referred to throughout this chapter due to the limitations of existing medical research groupings. Please note that the use of the word race is intended to highlight important health disparities, not to indicate biologic difference between people groups. Where possible, the term *ethnic minorities* is preferentially used in this chapter in recognition of there being no biologic basis for different races among human beings.

The United States is featured prominently as it has some of the world's greatest health inequities according to international standards.[20] Race and ethnicity correlate with many social determinants of health and thus begin to impact health inequities before a patient ever presents to care. They are also associated with worse health care metrics in the emergency department. Racial and ethnic minority patients receive lower triage scores for the same complaint and vital signs,[21] wait longer to see a provider for a given triage score,[22] are less likely to queue jump,[23] are disproportionately transported by emergency medical services (EMS) to under-resourced hospitals,[24] and face a longer wait before getting their first electrocardiogram (ECG) in the setting of ST-elevation myocardial infarction (STEMI).[25] Before the emergency clinician sees a patient and considers whether a procedure is indicated, they must consider that emergency care for these populations may have already been deprioritized and delayed on a systemic level.

PROCEDURAL MONITORING

Health care inequities have been shown to influence medical procedures in many ways, including the ways patients are monitored to determine need for procedures[26–28] and during procedures.[29,30] Emergency providers rely on vital signs as objective measures of a patient's status; however, one of the health care disparities illuminated by the global COVID-19 pandemic was the fact that pulse oximetry monitors overrepresent arterial oxygen concentration in patients with increased dermal melanin content;[31] as a result, many of these patients did not meet hypoxemic criteria for COVID-19. Therapies were delayed,[26,32] opportunities for antiviral treatment were missed,[33] supplemental oxygen was not administered,[34] and there was delayed escalation to providing critical care.[35] Consequently, patients with occult hypoxemia were found to have increased organ dysfunction and increased mortality.[36,37] The pandemic revealed that the problem was not malfunctioning equipment, but the fact that ethnic minority individuals are routinely undersampled in validation trials for medical equipment.[38] US census data reported 39.9% of the population was made up of ethnic minority individuals at the time that the Food and Drug Administration (FDA) approved that only 15% of patients included in studies of medical grade pulse oximeters' performance needed to have non-White skin tones.[37] While subsequent investigations have shown that pulse oximetry readings can, depending on patient skin tone, overestimate arterial oxygen concentrations to the degree that they fall outside of FDA clearance requirements,[39] at the time of publication of this edition there has been no resolution of this health care inequity.

RESPIRATORY PROCEDURES

The COVID-19 Pandemic Impact on Health Inequities

Throughout the world, the COVID-19 pandemic accentuated existing health inequities. Ethnic minorities and those with fewer economic resources were disproportionately affected by more severe disease,[40] and many required intubation and mechanical ventilation.[41] Yet even before the pandemic, certain populations already faced higher risks of needing these invasive respiratory procedures. For example, in the United States, Black and Hispanic patients experience more frequent severe asthma exacerbations and increased risk of requiring intubation and invasive ventilation procedures.[3] Socioeconomic status has also been shown to have a similar impact, with lower socioeconomic status associated with increasing rates of intubation and ventilation.[4]

Inequities Upon Inequities: Racial Disparities in Procedures for Asthma

The procedural disparities related to asthma provide an example of social determinants of health determining health inequities. Asthma severity correlates closely with air quality levels,[42] and air pollution exposure in the United States disproportionately impacts ethnic minorities and those of low socioeconomic status,[43,44] even after accounting for city versus rural residence.[45] In addition, historical "redlining" has created health inequities related to asthma over decades. "Redlining" was the practice from the 1930s to 1960s by the US government–sponsored Home Owners' Loan Corporation of marking predominantly Black neighborhoods as regions where they would not offer loans.[46] This kept Black people from purchasing homes and acquiring assets that might improve their own and their descendants financial prospects. While this practice ended in the late 1960s, today the risk of Black adults in the United States having severe or uncontrolled asthma matches closely to whether they live in a region that was historically redlined, as does the degree of air pollution to which they are exposed.[47,48]

Racial and Ethnic Disparities in Airway and Ventilation Mechanics

Provider mechanics of intubation and ventilation also vary for ethnic minority patients. For example, EMS providers are more successful when attempting to intubate White adults in cardiac arrest compared with adults of all other ethnicities[49] and with the intubation of White infants compared with Black or Hispanic infants.[50] For patients mechanically ventilated in the emergency department, female and Hispanic patients are less likely to receive low tidal volume ventilation,[51] which is associated with better outcomes and lesser barotrauma.[52] This finding is mediated by height: patients with shorter heights are less likely to receive lung-protective tidal volumes. In addition to lower success levels of intubation by EMS, research has also shown that Hispanic and Asian patients have higher death rates associated with failed intubation.[53] Furthermore, despite that prehospital intubation success rates are consistently significantly higher for female patients, females in cardiac arrest receive fewer attempts,[49,54–56] indicating deprioritization of an indicated medical procedure for certain populations. These examples demonstrate some of the harmful effects of medical standards having been created studying White male patients, which may lead to missed recognition of clinically indicated procedures and higher risk for certain procedures when performed for non-White or nonmale patients.

CARDIAC PROCEDURES

Cardiopulmonary Resuscitation

Cardiopulmonary resuscitation (CPR) and resuscitation procedures for cardiac arrest are affected by similar health inequities as other medical procedures. Overall, members of racial and ethnic minority groups and poor patients are at higher risk for needing these procedures and, along with female patients, have worse outcomes. For patients requiring CPR, survival after cardiac arrest is lowest in the United States for Black,[57] Hispanic,[58] and Native American people;[59] in the United Kingdom, for Black and Asian people;[60,61] in Singapore, for the ethnic minority group of Malay people;[62] and in New Zealand, for the ethnic minority groups of the Māori and Pacific peoples.[63] Social determinants of health impact each link in the American Heart Association's (AHA's) "chain of survival" for out-of-hospital cardiac arrest care.[64]

Rapid Recognition of Cardiac Arrest and Activation of EMS

Emergency dispatchers play a crucial role in decreasing the interval from arrest to start of chest compressions.[65] Despite uniform dispatcher training to help callers initiate CPR in suspected cardiac arrest,[65–67] large registry-based studies of witnessed out-of-hospital cardiac arrest show this varies with social determinants of health. In South Korea, dispatchers were far less likely to instruct callers to initiate CPR in calls from communities with lower levels of education.[66] In a study in Taiwan, for calls from poorer neighborhoods, dispatchers were slower to recognize cardiac arrest and guide callers to initiate CPR.[67] This time delay was associated with less frequent return of spontaneous circulation (ROSC) in the field as well as worse neurologic function at hospital discharge.[67]

Bystander CPR

Bystander CPR increases survival rates in out-of-hospital cardiac arrest.[68] Patients who receive bystander CPR are more likely to be in a shockable rhythm at first opportunity for defibrillation.[68] A patient's likelihood of receiving bystander CPR is closely related to social determinants of health. Many studies in the United States report that Black adult[57] and pediatric[69] patients receive less bystander CPR and conclude that worse outcomes for Black cardiac arrest patients simply reflect that communities with higher percentages of racial and ethnic minority populations perform less bystander CPR.[70–73] However these outcome disparities are not quite so simple. When an adult Black patient has a witnessed cardiac arrest in a public location in a wealthy or predominantly White neighborhood, they are significantly less likely to receive bystander CPR than a White person arrested in that location.[5,74] This exemplifies the importance of evaluating the scientific literature critically.

Early Defibrillation

Earlier defibrillation leads to improved survival, but access to an automated external defibrillator before EMS arrival is dependent on social determinants of health as these resources are unevenly distributed and favor neighborhoods with higher income levels. Patients who have a cardiac arrest in predominantly Black neighborhoods are less likely to have an automated external defibrillator available and less likely to receive potentially life-saving defibrillation prior to ambulance arrival.[70] Survival depends on EMS arriving quickly,[75] and shorter ambulance arrival time increases likelihood of a good neurologic outcome.[76] In the United States, the longest delays until ambulance arrival in cardiac arrest tend to occur in areas with the lowest mean income and are often inconsistent with AHA recommendations.[77] In addition, lower income neighborhoods have been shown to have fewer ambulances after accounting for population density,[78] illustrating how inequalities in resource distribution often disproportionally harm patients of lower socioeconomic resources and patients who are ethnic minorities.[77]

ROSC and Post-ROSC Care

The social determinants of health associated with race continue to play a role in the final link in the chain of survival and reveal persistent race-based disparities in American health care. Black patients have worse outcomes after out-of-hospital cardiac arrest. One reason is that Black individuals are more likely to be treated at lower quality hospitals, and research has shown that White patients cared for in these hospitals after out-of-hospital cardiac arrest also have worse outcomes.[79] Black and Hispanic patients are disproportionately transported to safety-net hospitals, in comparison to White patients living in the same zip code, regardless of the acuity of their complaint, where they previously have received care, or distance to nearest facility.[24] When treated at extracorporeal membrane oxygenation (ECMO)-capable facilities, racial and ethnic minorities, as well as female patients, are significantly less likely to have ECMO initiated during cardiac arrest.[80] When evaluating intrahospital variations in procedures for cardiac arrest care, Black and Brown patients often receive less frequent mechanical circulatory support procedures, which is associated with worse neurologic outcomes and decreased survival.[60]

Electrocardioversion: Procedural and Periprocedural Disparities

Wealth or poverty has a powerful impact on access to health care and medical procedures; however, even when patients of lower socioeconomic status access care, they often are treated differently. In Finland, a country with universal health care for all inhabitants, patients with lower income were far less likely to receive electrocardioversion or other forms of rhythm control for new atrial fibrillation,[81] which is associated with better symptom control and has increasing evidence for better safety outcomes than rate control.[82] In the United States, when ethnic minority or female patients do receive electrocardioversion for acute atrial fibrillation, they are less likely to be treated with postprocedural anticoagulation according to current professional guidelines,[83,84] and more likely to experience a stroke, arterial embolism, or death within 90 days.[85]

ECGs and Acute Care Syndrome: an Example of Protocolization to Reduce Disparities

Health care inequities are present in even the most fundamental everyday emergency department procedures, such as obtaining an ECG. Examination of over 178,000 STEMI patients in the United States over a 6-year period showed multiple disparities in health care provision and timing.[25] Black and Hispanic patients with STEMI were less likely to have any ECG performed by EMS and less likely to meet AHA guidelines for ECG performed in <10 minutes from emergency department arrival.[25] Similar delays in care occur in patients who do not speak English[86] or are female.[6] STEMI mortality correlates with time to ECG,[25] as well as to time to coronary reperfusion. STEMIs are an important example of geography-related health disparities, as outcomes are worse in rural regions due to longer EMS transit time and fewer percutaneous coronary intervention (PCI-) capable facilities.[87] A randomized controlled trial in Australia demonstrated that a quality improvement intervention successfully reduced missed or delayed STEMI diagnoses in rural hospitals with no emergency medicine or cardiology physicians on-site by a creative protocol targeting the source of the disparity—the need for clinicians who could evaluate for STEMI. The intervention involved an automated consultation from triage to a more resourced regional facility including immediate transmission of ECG for any patient presenting to triage with symptoms that could be consistent with ACS.[87] This intervention improved the hospitalized randomized to the intervention from high missed STEMI rates to zero misses. This example demonstrates that thoughtful consideration of intervenable targets and dedication of resources are necessary to meaningfully reduce disparities from social determinants of health for vulnerable populations.[88]

TRANSFUSION PROCEDURES

Blood transfusion is a critical part of managing traumatic injuries and other causes of acute hemorrhage. Indications for transfusion procedures include objective measures of very low hemoglobin values or clinical signs of hemodynamic instability. Despite clear guidelines,[89] there is still tremendous room for bias to skew management; and, in fact, sometimes it is the guidelines themselves that provide bias.

Bias in Trauma Indications for Transfusion

Recent studies indicating whole blood transfusions may have better outcomes than separated blood products for trauma patients show promise, but are preliminary.[90] Whole blood, however, is less available than other blood products, increasing the pressure to make appropriate clinical decisions to prevent waste of a precious resource. A prospective observational study of 14 trauma centers evaluated how race interacted with these pressures in all trauma patients receiving blood products. Controlling for severity of injury and shock, Black patients were significantly less likely to receive whole blood transfusions. This study found that mortality was twice as high among Black patients who did not receive whole blood compared with their non-Black counterparts.[91]

Bias in Medical Indications for Transfusion

Despite blood hemoglobin criteria for transfusion for hemodynamically-stable anemia,[89] a large registry of almost 5000 patients in the United States with significant anemia revealed disparities in transfusion guideline adherence for Black and White patients.[7] Black patients were transfused at a lower average hemoglobin threshold than their White counterparts and furthermore received less blood products than White patients did for the same hemoglobin level.[7]

Bias in Obstetric Indications for Transfusion

Postpartum hemorrhage is one of the most common causes of maternal death worldwide.[92] This is also true in the United States, where Black females are five times more likely than White females to die from postpartum hemorrhage.[93] For many years, well-intended clinicians did not realize they were contributing to that risk. Until 2021,[94] the American College of Obstetricians and Gynecologists (ACOG) recommended a race-based correction to lower the hemoglobin level required to diagnose anemia in the third trimester for Black pregnant females to <10.2g/dL, rather than <11.0 as in non-Black females, based on observational data sets showing lower mean hemoglobin levels in Black females during pregnancy. The standard of care was that Black females with hemoglobin levels from 10.2 to 10.9g/dL were not treated for anemia, while non-Black females with this hemoglobin level were. In 2021, a study showed that pregnant Black females with untreated hemoglobin levels of 10.2 to 10.9g/dL in the third trimester were more likely to have hemoglobin <11.0g/dL at delivery, which was associated with three times increased odds of requiring blood transfusion.[8]

Until 2021, postpartum hemorrhage risk was also increased for racial and ethnic minority patients by a clinical risk score that predicted lower success of trialed vaginal birth after cesarean delivery for Black and Hispanic females.[95] Similar to the prior ACOG guidelines for diagnosis of anemia, this tool was built based on observational data where different rates of vaginal birth after cesarean were interpreted to represent natural or biological differences between racial groups, rather than considering disparities due to underlying health inequities.[94,95] As a result, use of this tool diverted more Black and Hispanic females to cesarean delivery and its associated higher risks of postpartum hemorrhage.[96]

PROCEDURAL SYMPTOM MANAGEMENT

While most clinicians do not identify themselves as racist or biased against certain patient populations, they may not realize how their unconscious beliefs impact their view of patients, communication with patients, and medical decision-making. For instance, even though false beliefs that Black patients have thicker skin are often referred to as historical, there is strong evidence that many clinicians still believe in variable pain sensitivity based on race or ethnicity.[97] Unconscious biases such as these can contribute to poor outcomes for minority patients.[11]

Pain Perception

There is a preponderance of evidence that racial or ethnic minority patients receive lesser pain control from EMS[98] and during an emergency department visit[99] in the United States. Clinicians are not exempt from unconscious false beliefs about race-based "biological" differences in patients—including regarding pain perception[97] as well as prejudice about opioid misuse risk.[100] Understanding unconscious biases can allow the clinician to reflect on their clinical interactions and decisions regarding pain management when caring for patients at higher risk of receiving inadequate pain control. For all procedures and with all patients, it is essential that clinicians attend to procedural pain assessment and management using the same standards.

Procedural Excellence Entails Excellence in Periprocedural Pain Management

Procedural pain management is inseparable from procedural performance quality. A study evaluating procedural management of joint dislocations at 53 emergency departments in the United States showed that despite no difference in reduction success, Black patients were significantly less likely than White patients to receive both opioid and nonopioid analgesic medication. Furthermore, White patients who received pain medication received it faster than Black patients who received pain medication.[9]

Advancements in Emergency Medicine Procedures

As emergency medicine continues to expand its repertoire of procedures and pain relief modalities, they will be subject to the same biases and disparities as the rest of medicine until underlying health inequities are recognized and addressed. Disparities in ultrasound-guided nerve blocks have not yet been studied in emergency medicine; however, within anesthesia practice, racial and ethnic minority patients and those of lower socioeconomic status receive less frequent perioperative regional anesthesia.[101] Language barriers likely exacerbate the effects of race and ethnicity, as Hispanic patients were least likely to receive regional anesthesia, and perceived extra effort and time for interpreter services is postulated to contribute to this disparity.[102]

Procedural Sedation

Disparities associated with skin color cause similar health inequities for pediatric patients as for adults. In both pediatric and general emergency departments, procedural sedation is utilized less frequently for painful skin and soft tissue infection–related procedures in Hispanic,[10] Black, nonprivately insured, and male children.[103] Similar disparities in use of procedural sedation were seen for ethnic minority children as well as children of lower socioeconomic status needing laceration repairs.[104] Similar to anesthesiologist-performed nerve blocks described earlier, language barriers likely contribute to these differences, with one study showing non-Hispanic children to be 1.6 times more likely to receive procedural sedation than Hispanic children for the same procedure.[10]

SKIN AND SOFT TISSUE PROCEDURES

Disproportionate use of photos of people with light-toned skin in medical education is increasingly recognized as a problem in the United Kingdom,[105,106] Canada,[107] and the United States.[108] Preferentially featuring images of White patients' skin extends past medical school lecture halls into United States Medical Licensing Exam preparation materials,[109,110] general medical education textbooks,[111] dermatologic specialty textbooks,[112] and online resources.[113] Misrepresentation of the range of patient skin phenotypes is not without consequence. In the United States, a survey of 46 dermatology residency programs revealed that residents felt significantly less confident in their ability to accurately care for Black and Brown patients' skin.[114]

Emergency medicine clinicians must be able to identify abnormalities such as cutaneous signs of inflammation in patients of all skin tones, and the materials used during their education and training may underrepresent different skin colors. For example, the classic focus on erythema as "redness" is less helpful in highly pigmented skin, and many clinicians are unaware that erythema in darker skin tones may have a more violaceous or hyperpigmented appearance.[115] Not recognizing dermatologic inflammatory changes may cause providers to miss skin and soft tissue infections, including abscesses that would benefit from incision and drainage procedures. While this disparity can be ameliorated by using ultrasound to assess for findings associated with abscesses such as a discrete fluid collection, it is essential that clinicians be educated to distinguish normal and abnormal skin findings across the full range of possible skin pigmentation.

Skin tone representation in medical education has never been representative of the US population, and the demographic changes in the last 30 years in the United States[116] or England[117] (the producers of most of the medical textbooks evaluated in the studies cited in this section) are not reflected in the images in the majority of medical textbooks today. Even new modern-day examples continue to show White skin bias. An evaluation of primary literature about COVID-19 dermatologic manifestations performed in 2020 identified 36 articles with 130 published images, none of which depicted darkly pigmented skin, and few depicted anything but light-toned skin.[116a]

Urologic and gynecologic specialty textbooks also predominantly feature genital, perineal, and perianal findings in people with White skin,[112] limiting clinicians' ability to recognize abnormalities versus normal findings on skin and mucosal inspection, genital examinations, and during associated procedures. The one notable exception where Brown and Black skin are grossly overrepresented relates to skin lesions associated with sexually transmitted infections,[112] which have been historically stigmatized illnesses.[118] In order to better care for all patients, there are increasing calls for diverse representation of skin tones in medical education images and for making this a mandatory requirement for medical school accreditation.[119]

CONCLUSION

Health and health care inequities clearly influence the landscape of emergency medicine procedures. From the initial decision-making process regarding what procedure to perform to the final procedural outcomes, disparities rooted in perceived "race," ethnicity, gender, socioeconomic status, spoken language, and other social determinants of health are pervasive and global. Health inequities not only heighten the risk of requiring emergency procedures but also skew the quality of care and outcomes for marginalized groups. Emergency clinicians should be aware of how these inequities impact the health of their patients, the medical interventions they receive, and the care delivered in the emergency department.

REFERENCES ARE AVAILABLE AT Elsevier eBooks+

CHAPTER 75

The Mass Casualty Incident

Jeanne Noble and Mary Mercer

INTRODUCTION

Simply stated, a mass casualty incident (MCI) is an incident where the number of patients exceeds the healthcare resources available.[1] The Centers for Disease Control and Prevention (CDC) has suggested that, in the hospital setting, this may generally correlate to a hospital operating at 20% above licensed bed capacity.[2]

An MCI may be declared by a hospital's incident command center or more broadly by county or state officials. MCIs may be due to natural disasters (e.g., earthquakes, fires, floods, hurricanes, tornadoes); human-caused accidents (e.g., airline, train, or bus crash; building collapse); or from intentional attacks using conventional, chemical, or biological weapons, or other means such as vehicles or improvised explosives (e.g., active shooter, vehicle driven into crowd, bombings, warfare). Although it is impossible to prepare for every conceivable type of MCI, having realistic, easy-to-follow, easy to find protocols in place, and having those practiced by core staff at regular intervals, will increase the probability of an effective response to an MCI. This coordination will help to save as many lives as resources allow, while minimizing missed opportunities for providing life-sustaining care due to chaos and communication breakdowns.

The scope of this chapter will include the essentials of what every emergency physician needs to know about the provision of emergency medical care during an MCI, from "re-triage" to create capacity for incoming patients, to sorting and treating MCI victims with an effective distribution of human and material resources across your department, to communication protocols with your hospital's incident command structure and other clinical services that should be working to support the emergency department (ED).

CONSIDERATIONS WHEN PREPARING FOR A MASS CASUALTY INCIDENT

Many hospitals operate at or near capacity on a regular basis, making rapid deployment of resources to care for a surge of ill or injured patients a daunting task. Even with an established framework and a detailed plan, meeting the demands of an MCI is challenging. Without a plan, an MCI is likely unmanageable.

All hospitals should have an Emergency Operations Plan that encompasses how the entire facility will respond to a disaster, including the location and staffing of the Hospital Incident Command Center (HCC), and the person who will activate (and announce) "Code Triage" or a similar designation that an MCI is underway. All pertinent emergency personnel should be familiar with the specific criteria required to declare an MCI and whether they have the right and responsibility to declare one. This varies by type and size of institution. At smaller hospitals, the attending emergency physician onsite may serve as the Disaster Medical Officer in charge of all hospital resources until a command center is established. At larger institutions, activation of MCI protocols may be determined by the Director of Emergency Management or the senior "Administrator on Call" (AOC).

If the ED has an MCI plan, it should be reviewed at least once per year to ensure that the plan, supplies, and key personnel information remain up-to-date.

When revising an existing plan, or creating a plan de novo, be sure that the following questions are addressed:

- Are MCI equipment and supplies stored near the ED and readily accessible to ED staff?
- Where can treatment supplies and equipment be deployed and who will deploy them?
- Where can victims be treated safely?
- Who is best suited to staff external treatment areas?
- What is your emergency communication system for mobilizing offsite staff and is it regularly tested?
- For onsite communication, are an adequate number of walkie-talkies available and maintained, with staff trained in their use?
- Where and how can staff surge to an alternate location when the ED is full?
- What specific logistical challenges need to be overcome to implement your MCI plan?

Emergency Physicians as MCI Leaders

Emergency medicine (EM) physicians play a crucial role in disaster planning and response and are commonly called upon to lead both clinical and organizational response to MCIs.[3–6] Their active engagement in disaster preparedness leadership offers numerous benefits to hospitals, patients, and communities. The first and most practical reason EM physicians participate in preparedness efforts is their proximity to and likelihood of being present during an MCI: the ED is the most common front line of the hospital's response to an MCI. Moreover, EM physicians regularly collaborate with various hospital departments and disciplines, and possess comprehensive knowledge of throughput and clinical operations across the hospital.[7–9] This familiarity makes EM physicians natural MCI leaders, facilitating the triage, treatment, and flow of all affected patients. Additionally, EM physicians have experience leading diverse teams with varying clinical skills and abilities during routine resuscitations, such as nurses, ED techs or medical assistants, pharmacists, and other physicians, and they can effectively apply these skills to real-time response and preparedness efforts.

EMS and Special Operations Physicians

Some EM physicians have specialized training and expertise in supporting management of MCIs. These include physicians trained or working in emergency medical services (EMS), disaster medicine, or urban search and rescue (USAR) teams.[10–12] Collaborating with these specialists can greatly enhance the preparedness and real-time response efforts of a hospital or first response system. Engaging with EMS professionals is crucial for seamless implementation of protocols regarding triage, distribution, and treatment of multiple casualties. Emergency physicians should familiarize themselves with local EMS policies and protocols for MCIs, as patient transport procedures may differ from usual protocols. For example, during an MCI, hemodynamically stable patients with anatomical injuries, who would normally be transported efficiently to a trauma center, might instead receive delayed transport or be directed to non-trauma centers for initial evaluation. EMS and special operations physicians may also oversee specialized field response teams, such as USAR or tactical units, and provide pre-event trainings on commonly encountered conditions or specialized protocols.

MCI PLANNING TOOLS

Individuals charged with writing or reviewing an ED's MCI plan can incorporate one of the following existing frameworks.

The "Dual Wave Phenomenon" Framework

The dual wave phenomenon anticipates patients' arrival timing and injury severity. The first wave includes the early arrival of a larger number of victims, often within 15 to 30 minutes of the disaster's onset, who are less severely injured, sometimes known as the "walking wounded." The second wave includes more severely injured victims, those requiring EMS transport, arriving 1 to 2 hours after the onset of the disaster. According to the CDC Mass Casualty Predictor (Box 75.1), the number of patients arriving in the first hour multiplied by two estimates the total number of patients in the surge. In other words, approximately half of all patients will arrive in the first hour, with the severity of illness and trauma spiking significantly in the second hour. Triage tags (sort-assess-lifesaving treatment/transport [SALT] and simple triage and rapid treatment [START], Fig. 75.1) are used to designate injury severity and are discussed in more detail later in the chapter. The distribution of victims is likely to be 10% to 20% with immediate life-threatening conditions (red-tagged patients), 30% with serious conditions requiring treatment that can be delayed by hours (yellow-tagged patients), and 50% to 60% with minor conditions (green-tagged patients), who may be discharged after minimal care, seeking more definitive care outside of the disaster zone as needed.[2] If the receiving hospital is close to the disaster, these time intervals will be compressed. This means less time to clear green-tagged patients out of triage and treatment areas, in order to prioritize the second wave of more critically injured patients. Staff ratios based on the size of the MCI should be anticipated as part of planning (Fig. 75.2), as well as the likely need for increased staffing during the second wave, when more higher acuity patients arrive.

The "15 Minutes Until 50 Patients" Framework

The MCI Framework "15 Minutes Until 50 Patients," or "15 'til 50," is another way to frame patient arrivals and was developed by emergency planners at Providence Little Company of Mary Medical Center Torrance and Henry Mayo Newhall Hospital in southern California. It is a useful tool for organizing your hospital's MCI preparedness plan (Fig. 75.3). It can be downloaded and populated with any given hospital's information.[2] The 15 'til 50 framework includes a detailed planning process that includes prepositioning of equipment and supplies, coverage of operational details during an MCI activation, and the transition back to routine care. It focuses on the critical preparatory steps needed before the arrival of the first patient (within the first 15 minutes of notification of an MCI) and continues through the first 2 hours of response, during which the Hospital Incident Command System (HICS) should be activated and establish its Incident Action Plan. While the ED will initiate logistical and communication responsibilities, it is expected that the HICS should assume the majority of these responsibilities within 2 hours of the MCI notification.

By following the 15 'til 50 framework, an ED's MCI planning will include:

- Identification of a secure location that allows for pedestrian and ambulance traffic.
- Setting aside specific equipment and supplies for MCI deployment.
- Securing a rapidly accessible storage location for MCI supplies.
- Designating key personnel who will respond to an MCI.
- Designating specific personnel from departments outside of the ED who need to be part of the immediate response (e.g., surgery, anesthesia, medicine).
- Identifying and incorporating ancillary services that regularly support the ED (e.g., patient transport, material services) into MCI planning.

Either the START (Fig. 75.4) or the SALT triage algorithms can be utilized within the 15 'til 50 framework. Each is appropriate for both adult and pediatric patients.[13] The template is intended to supplement, not replace, your institution's Emergency Operations Plan.

BOX 75.1 CDC Mass Casualty Predictor

Total expected casualties = total number of casualties arriving in a 1-hour window multiplied by 2.

Approximately 50% of acute casualties may arrive at closest medical facilities within 60 minutes.

50% to 80% may arrive within 90 minutes.

Most arrive within 1–4 hours.

CDC, *Centers for Disease Control and Prevention.*

MCI TRAINING FOR EMERGENCY PHYSICIANS AND HOSPITAL LEADERSHIP

In addition to drafting or refining the department's MCI plan, all emergency physicians should consider participating in in-person MCI training. For hospital and departmental leaders, FEMA (Federal Emergency Management Agency) offers the Healthcare Leadership for Mass Casualty Incidents (HCL) course.[14] The 4-day HCL course defines management roles and responsibilities within HICS for all-hazards disasters, including supply distribution, decontamination requirements, mass fatality management, and public information and risk communications messaging. The course concludes with a 2-day functional exercise.

For emergency physicians and other healthcare providers likely to respond to an MCI, FEMA offers the Hospital Emergency Response Training for Mass Casualty Incidents (HERT) course.[15] The 3-day HERT course includes training on differentiating between different illnesses and injuries that may result from an MCI, appropriate decontamination strategies, deployment of emergency treatment areas, MCI triage practice using SALT procedures, providing treatment in appropriate personal protective equipment (PPE), and the formation and utilization of a Hospital Emergency Response Team. Both courses are free and offered multiple times per

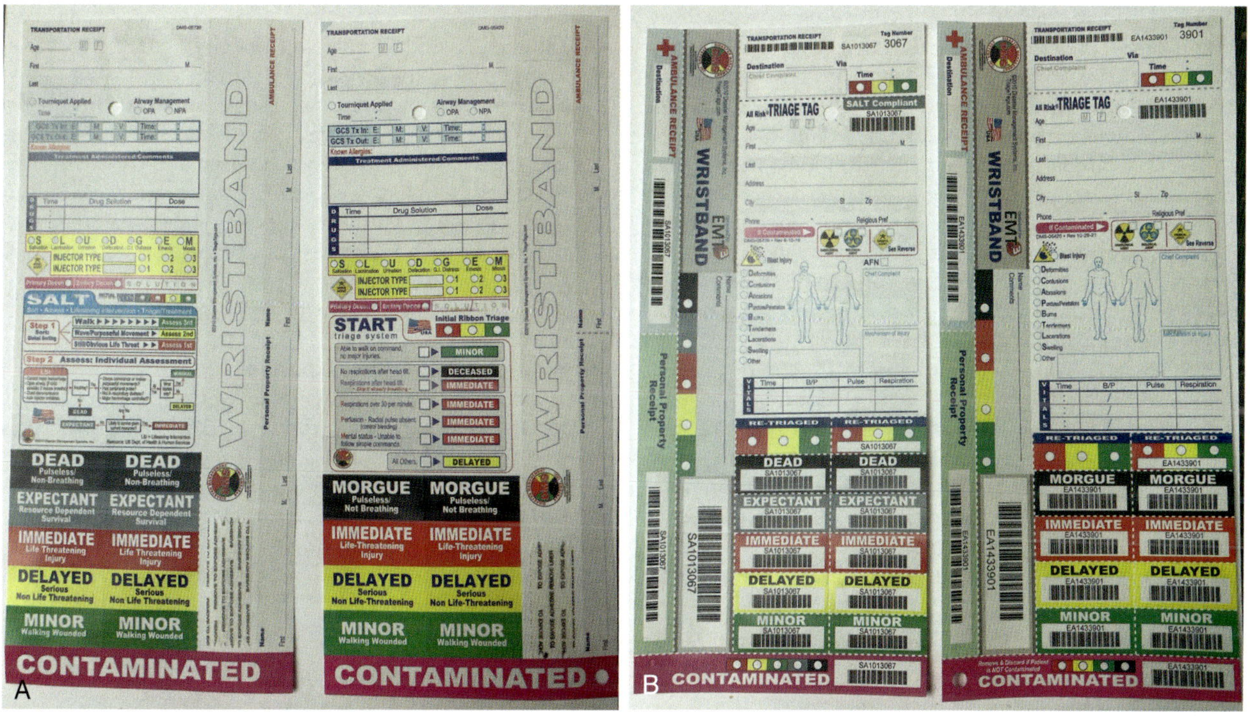

Fig. 75.1 SALT and START triage tags.

Staffing	Minimum activation	Level I (10-30 patients)	Level II (30-50 patients)	Level III (50+ patients)
Clinical/Licensed	5	10	15	20
Support	15	20	25	30

Fig. 75.2 Ideal staffing based on mass casualty incident (MCI) level.

year, taking place at FEMA's Center for Domestic Preparedness in Anniston, Alabama. Costs of travel and lodging on the FEMA campus are also covered by the program, making this an accessible option for organizations of all resource levels. There are several other on-line and in-person training options, including ICS-100 through ICS-800, which can be found either on-line or regionally through state disaster offices.

MCI CHECKLIST: 10 ESSENTIAL STEPS TO INCLUDE IN AN MCI PROTOCOL

Upon receiving emergency communication of an impending MCI, the EM attending physician, together with the charge nurse, will need to quickly alert all ED staff; work to rapidly increase the capacity of the ED to treat new patients (by implementing rapid discharge or admission protocols); assign roles for sorting, triaging, and treating incoming patients; and deploy immediately available supplies to meet the needs of the incoming patients, while calling for additional human and material resources as quickly as possible.

Whether using a template, such as 15 'til 50, or revising a protocol already in place, the essentials of the MCI protocol should be represented in an easily usable MCI Checklist. The items on the checklist may be carried out chronologically during an MCI drill; however, several steps should occur simultaneously during an actual MCI. The 10 steps should occur immediately after the ED receives notice of an MCI via ReddiNet or a similar emergency communications system.

- **Step 1**: **Locate MCI protocol.** The charge nurse and attending physician briefly review "disaster binder" or equivalent documents, determining MCI role assignments based on current staffing.
- **Step 2**: **ED huddle.** An immediate department-wide huddle is held. The charge nurse gives a brief description of the impending MCI with the estimated number of potential victims. Job action sheets, vests, and walkie-talkies are distributed. Paper triage tags (e.g., SALT tags) are given to the triage team.
- **Step 3**: **Reverse triage.** Providers and bedside nurses perform "reverse triage," rapidly reviewing all ED patients, designating each patient as "pending admission," or "pending discharge" if the patient is able to safely leave the ED and seek medical care outside the MCI zone, creating capacity to triage and treat an influx of new patients. If appropriate, high-acuity patients (e.g., ESI level 2s) currently in the waiting room should be included in the reverse triage process. Otherwise, waiting room patients may be seen by the external MCI triage team.
- **Step 4**: **Clear ED.** Noncritical patients pending admission are moved out of ED rooms to a predesignated area, preferably adjacent to the ED, pending transfer to inpatient

floors. An ED registered nurse (RN) remains with these patients until inpatient hospital staff (MDs/RNs) arrive and assume care. Patient transporters physically move all patients pending discharge to a predesignated safe location outside of the ED. An ED case manager should be assigned to the MCI discharge zone to help facilitate transportation and safe discharge for these patients. If needed, ED MCI leadership should engage with hospital leadership to designate locations outside of the ED that can be used for patients who are stabilized and awaiting admission or other MCI assessment and treatment activities that may not be possible within the physical space of the ED.

- **Step 5: Waiting room announcement.** Triage RN makes waiting room announcement that no additional patients will be triaged indoors and advises waiting patients to seek care outside the disaster area if they feel they can safely postpone medical care for 24 hours. If they cannot postpone care, they will be triaged by the MCI triage team, typically in an external location outside of the ED. Patients and visitors should be alerted to move their cars out of the ED parking lot immediately to make way for incoming ambulances and pedestrians, and that unmoved cars will be inaccessible until the disaster is over.
- **Step 6: Deploy external triage and treatment zones.** The MCI triage team and zone leaders deploy equipment and supplies to predesignated triage and treatment areas.
- **Step 7: ED lock down.** Security personnel secure all access points to the ED and set up cones and/or barriers to guide the safe ingress and egress of ambulances and pedestrians. Ideally, the ED should have a single ingress and egress point for enhanced security and to facilitate accurate tracking of patient flow.
- **Step 8: Deploy MCI patient tracking system.** Clerical workers deploy downtime quick registration systems for tracking patients without detailed electronic registration. A large dry-erase board should be deployed at the ED entrance, allowing rapid real-time accounting of MCI patients by SALT color treatment zones, until the electronic track board can be updated by a predesignated staff member (Fig. 75.5).

---

15 'til 50

Mass Casualty Incident Plan Template

TEMPLATE INSTRUCTIONS

The Plan Template provides an easy-to-populate document that can be used to create a Mass Casualty Incident (MCI) Plan for your facility.

This Plan Template should be used in conjunction with the companion 15 'til 50 MCI Guide. The Guide offers step-by-step instruction on how to develop your plan. For each section and subsection within this Plan Template, corresponding page numbers are provided to the Guide with tips and an explanation of the information that should be provided in that area. Bracketed text is provided where healthcare facility specific information should be inserted.

Insert healthcare entity name
Insert plan version number
Insert date of last revision
Insert healthcare entity logo

Fig. 75.3 15 'til 50 template contents.

15 'til 50 Mass Casualty Incident Plan
[INSERT NAME OF HOSPITAL]

Table Of Contents

See Guide, p. 20

Fig. 75.3, cont'd

- **Step 9**: **Emergency call for backup staff.** Emergency communication is sent to offsite ED staff (clinical and non-clinical) requesting backup support. Predefined numbers of backup staff requested are based on the anticipated size of MCI (see Fig. 75.2).
- **Step 10**: **Emergency call for logistics support.** Facilities management or other predetermined personnel are activated to bring MCI emergency equipment and supplies to the ED including pop-up tents, gurneys, emergency cots, wheelchairs, folding chairs, wound care carts, pharmacy carts, and decontamination supplies (if indicated).

MASS CASUALTY INCIDENT PLANNING

Prepare Staff Job Action Sheets

ED staff, both clinical and non-clinical, need specific job assignments during an MCI. The number of roles and division of responsibilities will vary by the size of your institution. Job action sheets should be prepared to cover all major roles in the ED. A sample configuration of nursing and physician roles is found in Table 75.1.

Prepare MCI Equipment and Supplies

Finding a suitable location for MCI equipment and supplies can be challenging. Items should be stored onsite: items stored offsite may not be accessible, particularly in the event of a natural disaster. Creating administrative buy-in to purchase essential equipment and allocate storage for a low-frequency event such as an MCI can be challenging. The 15 'til 50 toolkit includes an executive briefing PowerPoint presentation underscoring the importance of this investment.[16]

Essential equipment includes 20 to 40 cots, 10 to 20 wheelchairs, 20 folding chairs, an external shower for decontamination, and canopies to cover outdoor treatment areas. Signage or colored tarps to clearly indicate each treatment zone are also needed.

Essential supplies should include: a large supply (~100) tourniquets and hemostatic dressings, wound care carts and

IV carts for each treatment zone, 20 oxygen tanks, and 10 or more hand-held radios (walkie-talkies) regularly checked to ensure they are in working order. In addition, SALT or START triage supplies will be needed (see the section on "MCI Triage System").

Medication carts, either pre-stocked, or with an agreed-upon list for rapid stocking, should be deployed in both the internal and external treatment areas. Medication carts should include RSI packs, narcotic and nonnarcotic analgesics, naloxone, injectable anesthetics, bronchodilators, antibiotics, benzodiazepines, anticonvulsants, and anti-emetics.[17] Coordination with the hospital pharmacy is vital to ensure regular monitoring of supplies and expiration dates for medications that need to be rotated.

Prepare MCI Documentation Forms

Electronic systems may become nonoperable during a natural disaster, and paper or other forms of nonelectronic documentation during an MCI should be the default. The ED needs a way to track the flow of patients into and out of the ED in real time without using the electronic medical record (EMR)

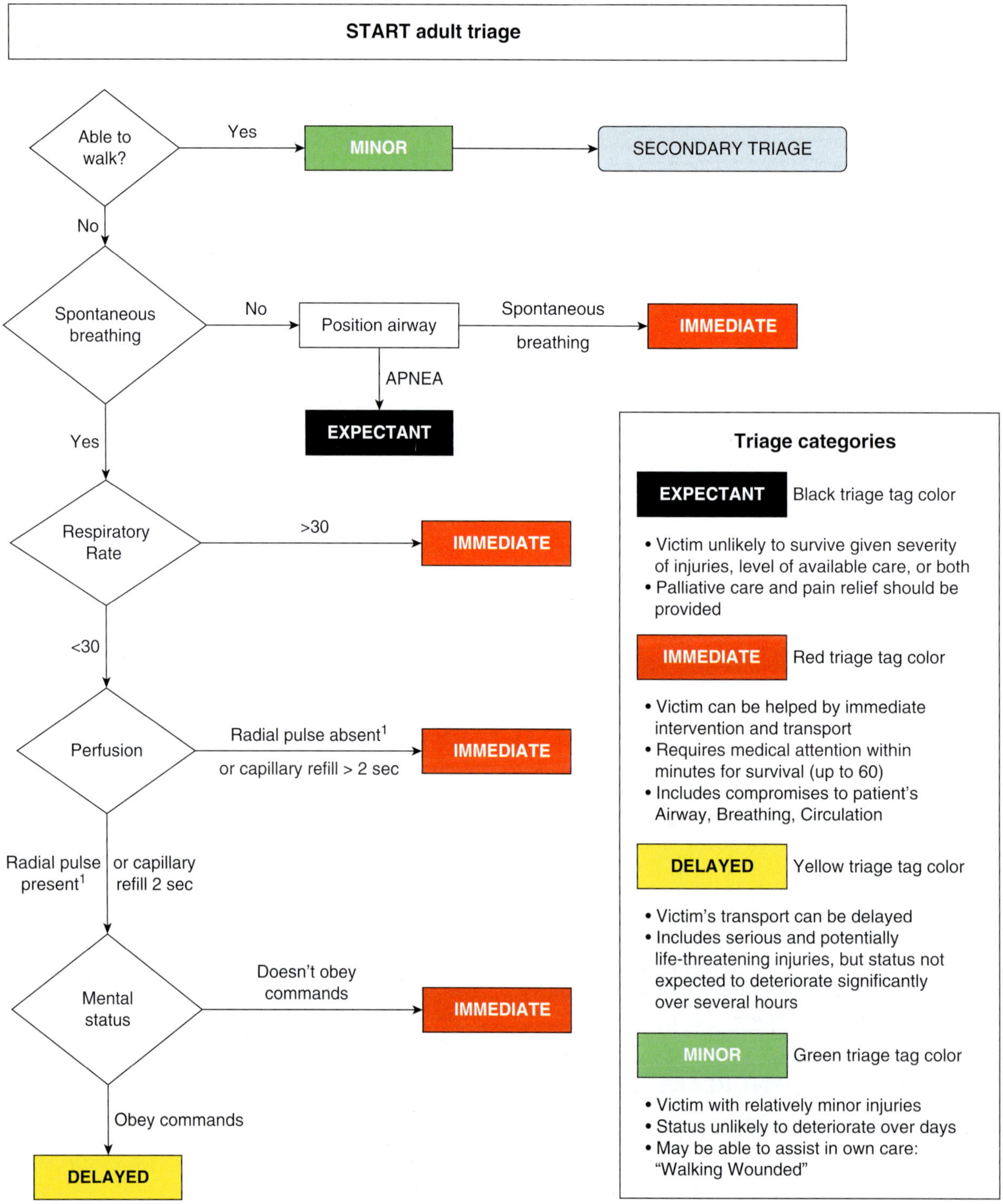

Fig. 75.4 (A) START triage algorithm.

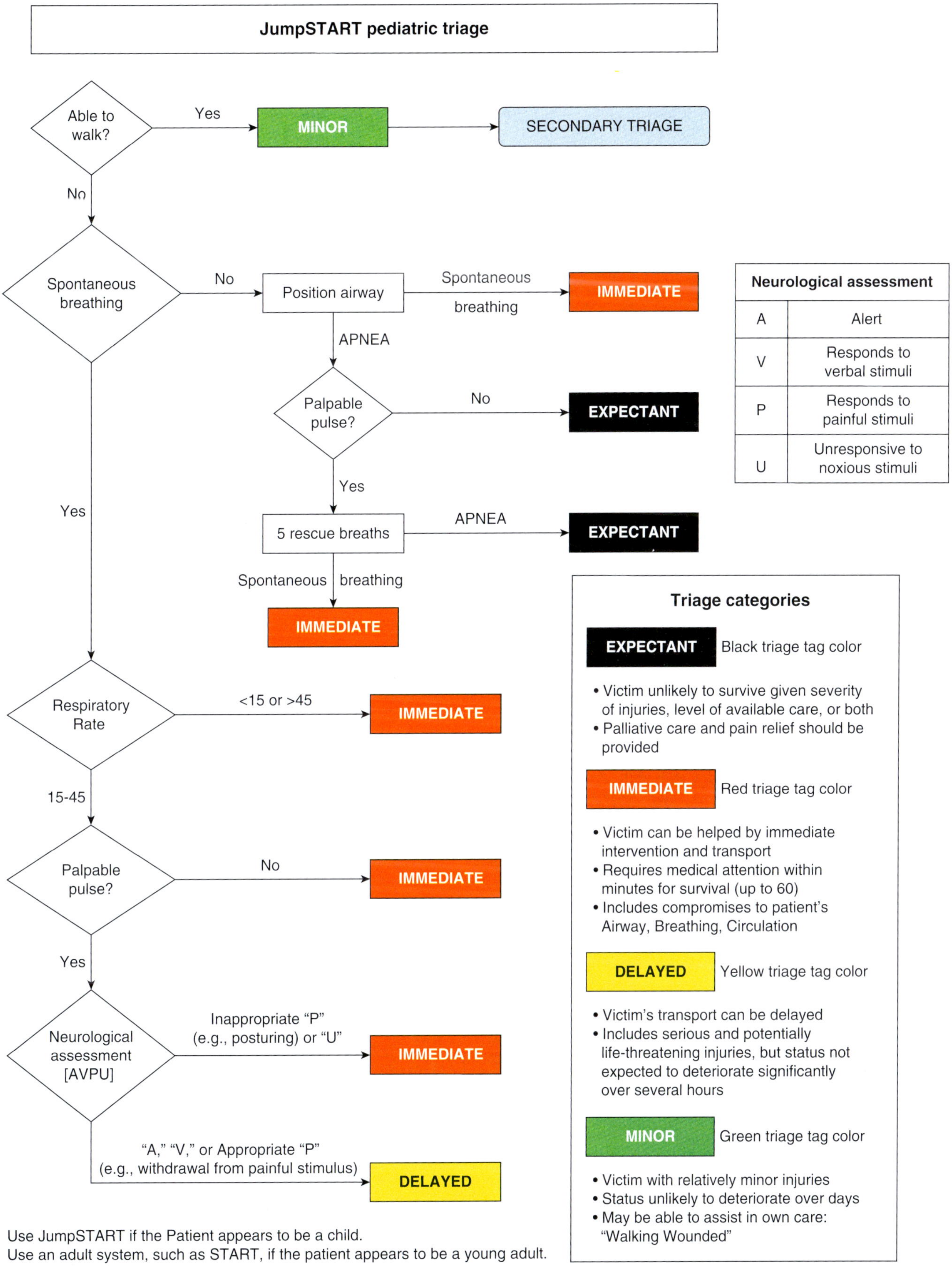

Fig. 75.4, cont'd (B) JumpSTART triage algorithm.

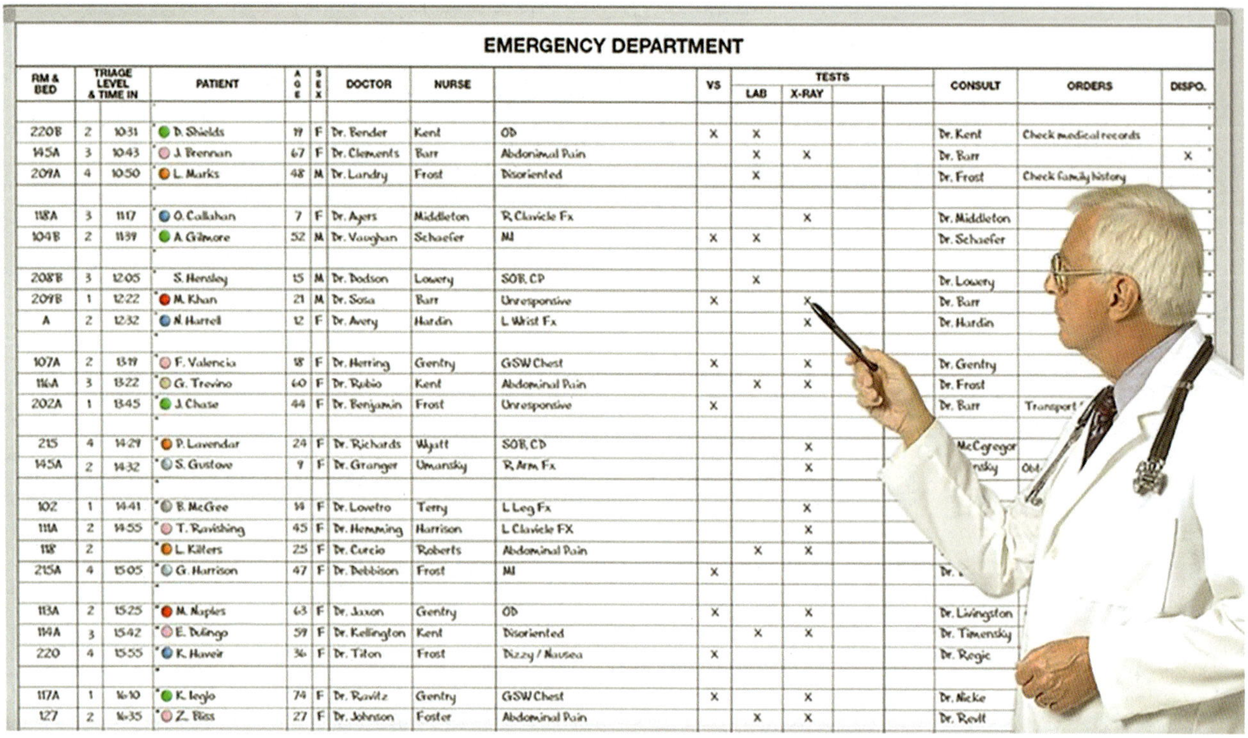

Fig. 75.5 Dry-erase board for downtime tracking.

TABLE 75.1 Sample Configuration of Physician and Nursing Roles During a Mass Casualty Incident (MCI)

Charge RN	1. Call Nursing Supervisor to activate Code triage: MCI. 2. Call bed control to inform them of MCI. Request that all available beds be allocated to ED patients. 3. Call huddle with all ED staff: • Give brief description of situation, including MCI level denoted on ReddiNet, and anticipated number of incoming patients. Remind staff not to talk to the media. • Designate initial ED treatment zones (Red/Yellow/Green/Gray/Black). • Distribute job action sheets. 4. Perform reverse triage with MD/provider team. • Identify patients with imminent risk of deterioration within 24 hours if not hospitalized. All others should be discharged according to Crisis Standards of Care receiving generic MCI discharge instructions. 5. Update ReddiNet polling. 6. Continue communication/coordination with ED Attending and Medical Branch Director (once HICS established) to ensure ED staff have adequate resources. 7. Initiate Incident Log in Disaster Binder.
MCI disposition RN	1. Consult with ED charge RN and ED provider team at tracking board to determine which patients can be discharged during reverse triage. 2. Discharge patients meeting reverse triage criteria, using generic MCI discharge instructions. (Do not wait for patient-specific instructions.) Move patients to external discharge area staffed by Case Manager. 3. Move stable admitted patients to external hallway (admission launch pad) while awaiting transfer to inpatient beds, using wheelchairs (not gurneys) whenever possible. Patients who can safely sit upright may be transferred to chairs placed in launch pad hallway while awaiting transport upstairs. 4. Group launch pad patients by admitting service (e.g., medicine, surgery), and indicating "Admitted with orders" vs. "Pending orders" vs. "Pending presentation" visible on patient's wearable pouch (see Fig. 75.7). 5. Monitor patients in launch pad area until relieved by a nurse from the inpatient labor pool.

TABLE 75.1 Sample Configuration of Physician and Nursing Roles During a Mass Casualty Incident (MCI)—cont'd

MCI triage RN	1. Deploy colored triage tarps, surge response kits, and treatment supplies from the MCI storage area. 2. Sort and tag patients using SALT triage together with MCI triage MD. 3. Perform basic lifesaving interventions (e.g., tourniquet application) as part of SALT triage. 4. Communicate with MCI Flow RN for placement of red-tagged patients in internal ED.
MCI flow RN	1. Direct external triage team where to send red-tagged patients via radio. 2. Coordinate patient flow between all other treatment zones. 3. Coordinate patient flow to ICU, OR, inpatient floors, and outside facilities.
Red zone treatment RN	1. Discharge current ED patients who meet reverse triage criteria, utilizing generic MCI discharge instructions. 2. Assist Disposition RN in moving stable admitted/pending admission patients to admission launch pad and discharged patients to discharge zone. 3. Ensure treatment rooms have ambu bag, suction, and IV supplies. 4. Be prepared to place airway adjuncts and perform BVM for airway management, and control hemorrhage with tourniquet application. 5. Complete Zone Report Form every 30 to 60 minutes.
Yellow/green zone treatment RN	1. Deploy supplies to treatment zone. 2. Assess, provide, and document care to patients in treatment zone. 3. Monitor for change in patient condition, requiring a higher level of care. 4. Notify Disposition RN of patients needing admission. 5. Discharge patients as appropriate, transporting patients to discharge area. 6. Complete Zone Report form every 30 to 60 minutes.
MCI triage MD	1. Deploy MCI triage station external to ED at single point of ED ingress, limiting entrance to internal ED by acuity. 2. Ensure tourniquets, QuikClot, and airway adjuncts are available at MCI triage station. 3. Triage nonambulatory patients first. • If a crowd has amassed outdoors, you will need to perform global sorting by asking patients to walk toward a specified area. Patients who cannot walk and appear unresponsive are triaged first. Nonambulatory patients with purposeful movement are triaged second. Ambulatory patients are triaged last. • Provide lifesaving interventions at MCI triage station, limited to: insertion of oral airway/nasal trumpet, 2 rescue breaths for pediatric patients, needle compression with 14- to 16-G catheter for suspected tension pneumothorax, tourniquet application, and use of autoinjector antidotes (atropine and 2PAM) in case of nerve agent/organophosphate exposure. 4. Tag each patient for entry in the ED by acuity: red, yellow, green, gray, or black. Add additional details to triage tag when time allows. 5. Patients arriving in extremis may proceed directly into ED (red zone) without external triage if space/resources allow. In this case, triage MD must radio RN dedicated to patient flow (Flow RN) and red zone leader in real time of patient coming straight into ED. Flow RN will ensure that patient will be registered inside ED. 6. When no further patients are awaiting triage, enter main ED to help treat red zone patients. Anticipate radio call back to external triage by triage RN if more patients arrive.
MCI treatment MDs and NPs/PAs (assign to zones)	1. All attend ED huddle and participate in reverse triage. 2. All ED residents stay in red zone if possible—choose zone leader. 3. NPs/PAs assigned to yellow zone—choose zone leader. 4. Off-service residents assigned to yellow and green zones choose zone leader. 5. Following reverse triage, all providers move to treatment zones and prepare supplies. (Wound care cart, IV cart, tourniquets, and QuikClot should be staged in external yellow and green zones.) 6. Stabilize/treat/disposition patients according to acuity within each zone. 7. Communicate directly with other treatment zone leaders when patients' status changes require movement to different treatment zone. 8. Be prepared to redistribute job assignments based on acuity and number of patients arriving in each triage category.

ambu bag, Artificial manual breathing unit; *BVM*, bag-valve mask; *ED*, emergency department; *HICS*, Hospital Incident Command System; *I&D*, incision and drainage; *ICU*, intensive care unit; *MCI*, mass casualty incident; *MD*, medical doctor; *NP*, nurse practitioner; *OR*, operating room; *PA*, physician assistant; *RN*, registered nurse; *SALT*, sort, assess, lifesaving interventions, treatment/transport; *2PAM*, pralidoxime.

system. SALT-colored magnetic disks added to a standard dry-erase board used for downtime patient tracking can suffice (see Fig. 75.5). In addition, four essential forms should be prepared as a part of the department's MCI protocol. These forms will facilitate rapid discharge during reverse triage, rapid admission during reverse triage and during the MCI, and communication with the central command structure for hospital capacity decisions and ED resupply. While disaster protocols and forms should be uploaded to the department's communication platform, ample hard copies of these four documents should be stored within your disaster binder in case of electronic system failure.

- *MCI after visit summary*: this form should be given to all patients discharged during the reverse triage process. This discharge paperwork should reiterate the incomplete nature of the patient's evaluation and treatment, with encouragement to seek further medical care outside of the disaster area.
- *MCI Rapid Admit Form*: this should include:
    1. Patient's name, date of birth, and medical record number (MRN) or SALT triage tag number
    2. Clinical impression
    3. Designation as stable versus unstable
    4. Vital signs, blood glucose, and GCS
    5. Dispo: OR/SICU/medical ICU/TCU/telemetry/floor/comfort care
    6. Special considerations: C-spine precautions/full spine precautions/5150/other
    7. Diet: NPO/regular
    8. Allergies
    9. Meds/drips
    10. Pertinent physical/lab/imaging findings
    11. Interventions performed
    12. Plan/pending interventions
    13. Physician name/time/pager or phone number
- *Patient log of disaster-related injuries and illnesses* should be completed by the ED charge nurse and provided to HICS at regular intervals. This will help the central command make real-time decisions regarding resource allocation, including the need to transfer patients to other facilities. Data on the patient log should include time of arrival, patient identifiers (name, DOB, age, gender, MRN, or SALT triage tag number), type of injury or illness (polytrauma, burn, fracture, chest trauma, abdominal trauma, head injury, vascular injury, other, unknown), stable versus unstable, and disposition (OR, ICU, TCU, floor, transfer, home).
- *ED status report form:* To optimize ED resources, each ED treatment zone should be equipped with a form for quickly reporting staff and supply needs at 30- to 60-minute intervals and should designate a staff member to communicate these needs to the ED charge nurse and, if needed, to HICS. This form should include: number of open beds (noting any limitation in function/safety), critical staff needs, critical equipment and supply needs, and environmental/engineering needs. When there is no change in zone needs between reporting intervals, the form should include a check box for "No change" to prevent wasting time on unnecessary documentation.

Decide on an MCI Triage System

During an MCI, patients may be triaged multiple times, beginning at the scene of the disaster, during transit, and upon arrival to the hospital or other treatment facility. Accurate and efficient triage is needed to achieve the greatest good for the greatest number when demand for care outstrips supply. Ideally, triage determinations should take less than 1 minute per patient without sacrificing accuracy for speed. (Both under- and over-triage can result in increased morbidity and mortality by delaying critical care to those who need it most.) Multiple triage systems exist for rapid assessment of MCI victims and there are no randomized controlled trials to suggest the superiority of one system over another.

To address the lack of uniformity in MCI response across the United States, the National Association of EMS Physicians (NAEMSP) convened a workgroup in 2006 to examine the evidence supporting existing mass casualty triage systems and to make a recommendation for the adoption of a single system as a national standard.[18] This became known as the SALT workgroup, which found deficiencies in all existing systems and instead designed a new system to be promoted as the new national standard, since known as SALT (Fig. 75.6). In 2009, to encourage greater uniformity in MCI triage regardless of the system used, the CDC supported the development of the Model Uniform Core Criteria (MUCC) for Mass Casualty Triage, consisting of 24 criteria forming the essential elements of an MCI triage system. Only SALT meets all 24 criteria and is designed for both adult and pediatric patients. If an alternative triage system is used, it is recommended that it be revised to be MUCC-compliant.

While SALT is endorsed as a national standard, START, developed in 1983, is potentially the most widely used protocol in the United States (see Fig. 75.4). It uses the same basic assessments as SALT: ability to walk, respirations, circulation, and mental status to assess individuals >8 years of age. The JumpSTART Pediatric Triage Algorithm, developed in 1995, uses the same assessments as START with the addition of the AVPU neurologic assessment (A = alert, V = verbal, P = pain, U = unresponsive) for patients less than 8 years of age (see Fig. 75.4).

There is simulation-based evidence that SALT has significantly lower under-triage rates compared with START (9% vs. 20%), and both systems have similar rates of over-triage (17% vs. 21%).[13] In addition, SALT has been endorsed by several leadership bodies including the American College of Emergency Physicians, the American College of Surgeons Committee on Trauma, the National Association of EMS Physicians, and the National Disaster Life Support Education Consortium.[19]

SALT and JumpSTART performed similarly in at least one MCI simulation of pediatric patients,[20] although JumpSTART was performed 8 seconds faster than SALT. A systematic literature review of JumpSTART compared with other triage systems concluded that all protocols suffer from limited accuracy without clear superiority of one system over another.[20,21]

SALT versus START and JumpSTART: Similarities

In the United States today EM providers are most likely to be trained in either SALT or START (coupled with JumpSTART for pediatric patients). In both SALT and START/JumpSTART, lowest priority is given to patients who can walk, are deemed non-salvageable, or are deceased. These groups are rapidly identified during initial sorting and do not receive immediate care. The remaining patients are assessed for immediate versus delayed treatment (or transport to a

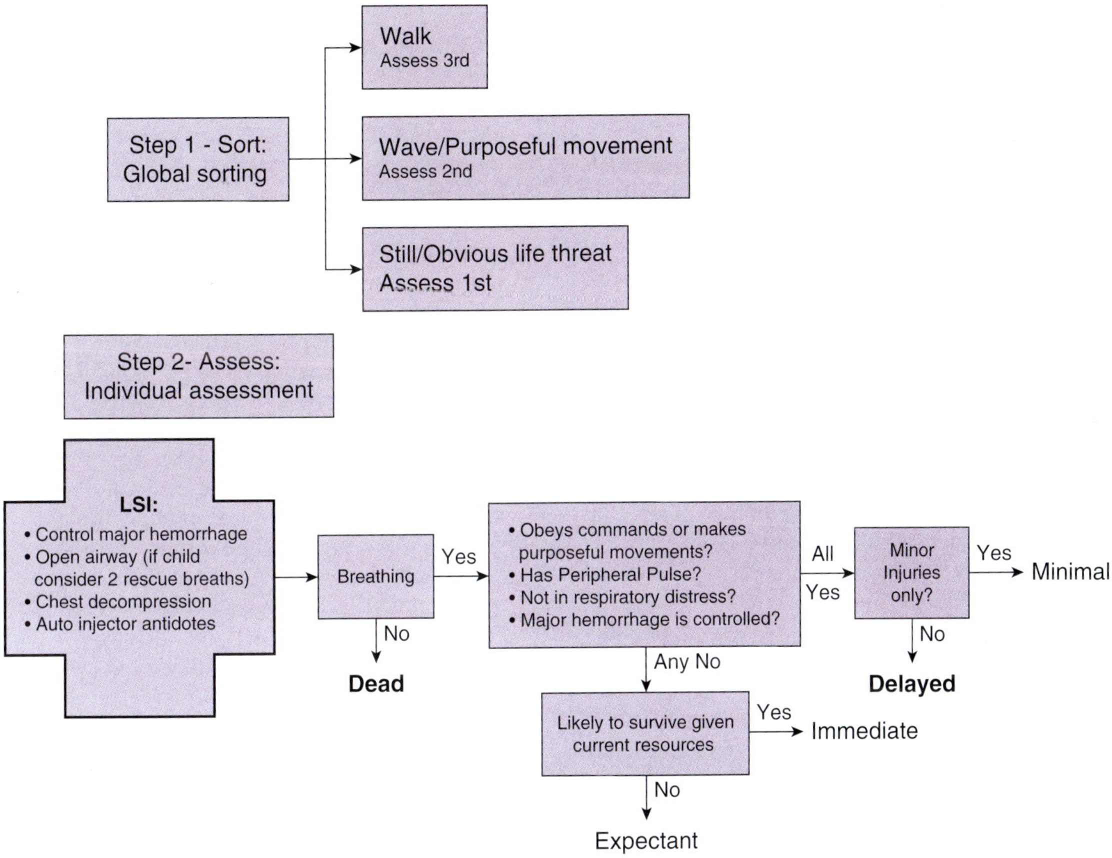

Fig. 75.6 SALT triage algorithm. *LSI*, Life-saving intervention.

medical treatment facility if performed in the field). Both SALT and START use the same color codes for triage destinations: black, red, yellow, and green signifying deceased, immediate care, delayed care, and minor conditions, respectively. Under the SALT system, the additional color gray is used to signify patients who are not salvageable (referred to as "expectant," meaning expected to die). Expectant patients are coded as black in the START/JumpSTART protocols.

Both protocols are divided into two steps: global sorting and individual assessment. Global sorting is based on ambulatory status. Those who can walk are assigned last priority for the individual assessment. In SALT, individual assessment begins with immediate lifesaving interventions for those with obvious life-threatening conditions. The four immediate interventions are: tourniquet application or direct pressure for hemorrhage control; airway repositioning and placement of basic airway adjuncts, including two rescue breaths for pediatric patients; needle decompression of pneumothorax; and autoinjector antidote administration (e.g., atropine, pralidoxime) in case of nerve agent or organophosphate poisoning. Thereafter, both protocols converge, designating patients as black if spontaneous breathing does not begin after airway repositioning (and 2 to 5 rescue breaths for pediatric patients). Patients with spontaneous respirations are triaged for immediate care (red) if: they are in respiratory distress, have delayed cap refill or an absent radial pulse, or do not follow commands or show purposeful movement. If they do not meet these criteria, they are triaged as yellow (delayed care) or green (minor ailments), who may safely seek care outside of the disaster zone if appropriate.

SALT Versus START and JumpSTART: Key Differences

There are several key differences between the two triage algorithms:

- **Global sort is more refined in SALT:** SALT and START both begin with a global sort, asking patients to walk and assessing ambulatory individuals last. SALT includes an extra step in the global sort, asking individuals who cannot walk to wave. Under SALT, individuals who fail to show any purposeful movement are assessed first, followed by nonambulatory patients showing purposeful movement, with ambulatory patients being assessed third. START begins individual assessments of all nonambulatory persons as a single, undifferentiated group.
- **Lifesaving interventions earlier in SALT:** In SALT, the individual assessment begins with immediate application of four lifesaving interventions when appropriate (hemorrhage control, basic airway maneuvers, needle decompression of pneumothorax and antidote autoinjector use in the case of a chemical MCI). In START, the provider completes the individual assessment before providing any emergent treatment.
- **Number of rescue breaths consistent with standard CPR in SALT:** In both SALT and START, the individual assessment begins by checking for spontaneous breathing. If absent, airway repositioning is performed for adults and, if apnea persists, the patient is coded as black. Under SALT, apneic pediatric patients are given two rescue breaths. If apnea persists, the patient is coded black. In JumpSTART, children who remain apneic after airway repositioning are checked for a pulse and if pulseless, they are coded black. If

a palpable pulse is present, five rescue breaths are given. If apnea persists, they are coded black. The use of five rescue breaths (vs. two) stems from the hypothesis that providers might need five attempts in order to deliver two effective ventilations in infants.

- **Hemorrhage control emphasized in SALT:** In SALT, spontaneously breathing patients must meet four criteria to qualify for delayed care (yellow): no respiratory distress, palpable pulse, hemorrhage controlled, and following commands. Any patient with respiratory distress, absent pulse, ongoing hemorrhage, or inability to follow commands is coded red. In START and JumpSTART, hemorrhage control is not used as a criterion for red versus yellow designation.
- **Determination of respiratory distress by gestalt in SALT:** Using SALT, the providers simply decide whether the patient is in respiratory distress. In contrast, respirations need to be counted in START (a respiratory rate >30 for adults is considered distress) and JumpSTART (a respiratory rate less than 15 or greater than 45 is considered respiratory distress in children).
- **Use of capillary refill time is *not* a proxy for a peripheral pulse in SALT:** The presence of a peripheral pulse, without reference to capillary refill time, is used in SALT. In START, capillary refill greater than 2 seconds can be used instead of the presence or absence of radial pulse for adults (but not for children in JumpSTART).
- **Neurologic status can be based on observation, rather than testing, in SALT:** In SALT, neurologic status is more broadly defined as the ability to follow commands **or** observation of purposeful movement. In START, neurologic status is determined by an adult's ability to follow commands, while in JumpSTART the neurologic assessment for children is based on whether the child reacts to noxious stimuli, where lack of reaction (or posturing) designates the child as red.

BEYOND MCI TRIAGE: MCI TREATMENT, PATIENT TRACKING, AND REASSESSMENT

Post-assessment move: After patients have been sorted and assessed during an MCI, they move to their designated treatment areas. SALT and START triage tags (see Fig. 75.1B) contain spaces for recording vital signs, examination findings, and key interventions as well as bar codes for tracking patients. It is essential that there is a system in place to track patients in and out of treatment areas, as their medical needs evolve, interventions are performed, and their ultimate dispositions are determined.

Reassessment and continued treatment: When a patient arrives to their treatment zone, whether being placed on a cot or in a chair, vital signs should be taken and recorded on their triage tag. For persistent respiratory distress, additional airway adjuncts should be considered while placing the patient on oxygen. Any ongoing bleeding should be controlled with tourniquet application or a pressure dressing, with leg elevation for patients in shock. Fluid and blood transfusions may be initiated. Other identified treatment or medication needs should be reported to the zone leader, and specialty care providers (e.g., surgery, ENT) should be consulted.

Testing: It may be necessary to order available testing, such as x-rays and bloodwork, by paper. If so, a physical drop box system should be created to consolidate paper orders and reporting of results, with regular runners to the laboratory and radiology suites, reporting back critical results as rapidly as possible.

Physical indication of post-ED destination: Following initial treatment, patients should be identified for transport to other areas of the hospital (e.g., operating room, inpatient bed) or for transfer to outside facilities. Ideally, patients should have a wearable medical pouch where a Rapid History and Physical Form, Rapid Admit form (see earlier), and MCI triage tag can be safely kept, and not easily separated from the patient. Consider writing the patient's diagnosis and disposition in large block letters on the outside of the pouch (Fig. 75.7), allowing consultants and rotating staff to quickly identify patients' needs in a rapidly changing and potentially chaotic care environment.

Registration: Only after initial stabilization, quick registration should be completed for each patient, and may be limited to name, age, date of birth, and address/cellphone. A patient identification number should be assigned, and for those who arrived by ambulance, the EMS triage tag number should be included to facilitate family reunification

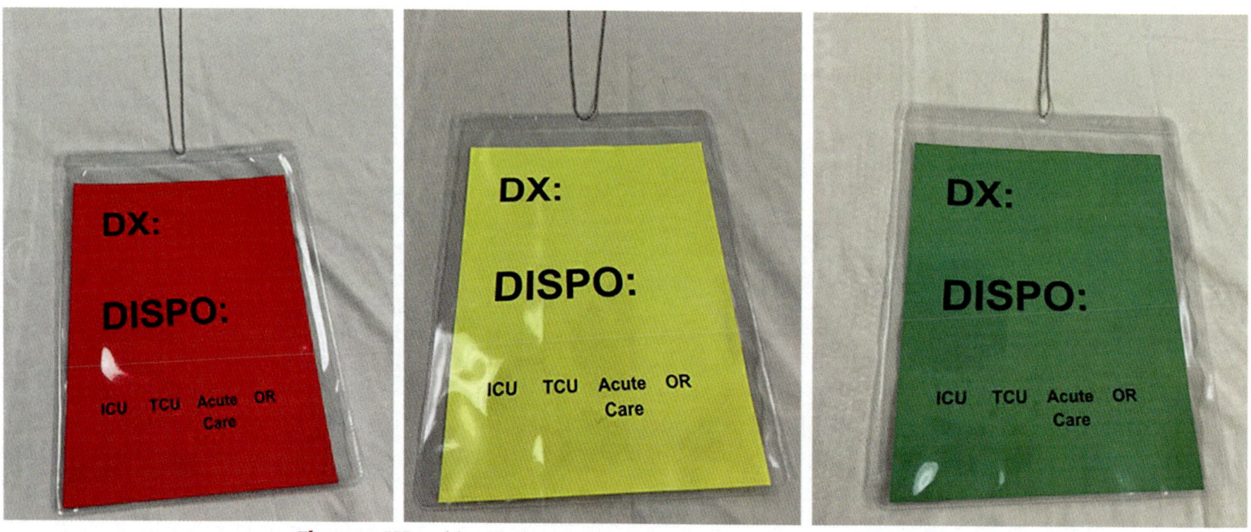

Fig. 75.7 Wearable pouch containing triage tags and other MCI forms.

(see below). The patient's belongings should be placed in a fluid-resistant bag which includes the tear-off personal property receipt from the triage tag.

Patient Tracking and Family Reunification

For patients who arrived via EMS, every effort should be made to link their registration to the EMS triage tag number. During particularly large or complex MCIs, family members may become separated across multiple hospitals and direct communication (mobile devices) or hospital-based patient information phone lines may become incapacitated or overwhelmed. Many jurisdictions will have family unification processes and can assist with patient identification and family reunification by linking patient identifiers from field to hospital and sharing with a central coordinating center (such as a contracted organization like the American Red Cross) in a HIPPA-compliant manner.

Monitoring and Reassessment of Patients and Treatment Areas

Expect patients' conditions to change rapidly, necessitating frequent reevaluation and movement of patients between treatment zones. Zone leaders must remain in close communication, typically using walkie talkies, alerting one another of the need for patient transfers.

The leader of each treatment zone should report the status of their zone to the charge nurse at 30- to 60-minute intervals. This report should include the number of patients in the treatment zone, number of patients awaiting transport to inpatient or outside facilities, existing bed capacity, equipment and supply needs, staffing needs, security needs, and any other support needs. The charge nurse will collect reports from all zones and in turn communicate status reports to HICS so that human and material needs can be met as quickly as possible.

Verify Outside Departments (e.g., Medicine and Surgery) are Ready to Support the ED

Collaborate with departmental leaders from medicine and surgery to ensure that they are ready to send specific personnel to the ED in the event of an MCI. Medicine colleagues will be needed to rapidly and proactively absorb medical admissions during reverse triage and after the arrival of MCI victims with nonsurgical needs. ED and Medicine disaster leads should collaborate with hospital leadership during MCI planning to designate spaces for stabilized patients pending admission to move outside the ED if needed in order to allow for influx of new critically ill patients. Surgical colleagues will be needed to assist with triage and initial treatment of traumatized patients once the MCI is underway. In collaboration with surgical colleagues, the MCI protocol might include surgery and anesthesia attendings, or senior residents, immediately reporting to the ED to assist in red zone assessment and triage to the OR.

During protocol planning and practice, ensure that outside departments are familiar with the rapid admit forms and designated treatment areas.

MASS CASUALTY INCIDENTS: A SYSTEM-WIDE APPROACH

Coordination With EMS

Effective preparation in the ED, both internally and in collaboration with external partners, is a vital but challenging component of timely response to MCIs.[22–24] Coordinating with EMS partners is an important aspect of pre-event preparation. During an MCI, EMS systems often employ triage protocols and communication methods that may differ from routine practices. For instance, during an MCI, EMS may follow an Incident Command System (ICS) organizational structure at the scene, with designated roles for triage, transportation prioritization, and patient reassessment and stabilization. Communication patterns between the field and hospitals may be modified to minimize radio traffic and streamline transportation logistics. Instead of individual prearrival notifications from the prehospital team directly caring for a patient, an EMS supervisor or MCI-transportation lead may provide a brief report to the hospital, indicating the number of patients expected from the incident scene and their general triage severity without extensive injury-specific details, or rely solely on triage tag/paper communication to convey basic injuries assessed in the field.[23,24]

Due to resource scarcity in the prehospital setting during MCIs, EMS providers, like hospitals, often implement mitigation strategies to stretch resource utilization. These strategies include transporting multiple patients in a single ambulance, utilizing non-ambulance transport vehicles for lower acuity patients (e.g., buses or law enforcement vehicles), and requesting mutual aid from neighboring jurisdictions.[6,25] These mitigation measures result in changes in the speed and level of detail during the prehospital-to-hospital hand-off process, requiring emergency clinicians to adapt accordingly. Moreover, hospital flow issues such as security, traffic, and potential decontamination procedures implemented during an MCI can impact EMS patient off-loading procedures and environmental safety for personnel and patients. Integrating EMS personnel into hospital-based disaster planning and drills is a valuable strategy for identifying workflow changes, educating staff about expectations, and improving processes.

Coordination With HICS

Clear communication and organizational interoperability are vital for efficient and effective responses to MCIs involving multiple organizations or jurisdictions. Understanding the ICS and its hospital-based counterpart, the HICS, is crucial for emergency physicians involved in either the direct clinical care or administrative oversight of MCI response. The ICS is a management system adopted by the US federal government as well as regional and local jurisdictions. It operates on a broader scale than the individual hospital, and provides a function-based organizational structure for managing teams during complex emergencies. Its purpose is to facilitate efficient communication, decision-making support, and resource mobilization. The ICS is designed to ensure streamlined communication from field responders to the incident commander or unified command leadership team.[26,27]

The ICS and HICS have similar structures, and consist of four functional groups—Operations, Logistics, Planning, and Finance—that report to the incident commander and command team. The command team includes the incident commander (or unified command for multi-organization responses) and various cross-functional leaders and advisers, such as the Public Information Officer, Liaison Officer, Safety Officer, and technical specialists.[26–28] Increasingly, incident command teams may also include an equity officer who is responsible for ensuring that principles of diversity, equity, and inclusion are incorporated into response planning, enactment, and outcome assessment.[29]

Within the HICS (hospital-based) structure, the ED functions as the "Casualty Care Unit" within the medical branch of the operations section.[26–28] The unit manager, who may be the charge nurse, nursing manager, medical director, or an on-duty physician, oversees the ED's operations and resources and communicates needs and updates to higher HICS leadership. Establishing predetermined roles and responsibilities aligned with the HICS organizational structure is a best practice for effective performance. Typically, the ED charge nurse assumes the operational role of casualty care unit leader to report up the chain of command on operational needs, while on-duty emergency physicians provide clinical expertise and guidance. However, emergency physicians may be called on to serve in any role within the HICS structure during a response. In addition, over the course of a prolonged response they may serve in multiple roles. Given this reality, additional training in ICS/HICS principles and terminology may benefit emergency clinicians.[26,27] Conducting in-person simulations of MCIs and disasters facilitates interdisciplinary teams' familiarity with HICS terminology and enhances teamwork and collaboration through simulated problem-solving activities, leading to improved performance during actual events.[26,27,30]

Coordination With Inpatient and Outpatient Services

In addition to collaboration between hospital and ED leadership on crisis management best practices such as HICS, triage processes, or simulated MCIs, it is critical for ED leadership to coordinate regularly with inpatient and outpatient services in planning and practicing protocols and critical actions needed during and immediately following an MCI. Efficient patient flow through the ED during an MCI is a critical need that impacts the availability of bed, staff, and supplies to triage and treat critically ill and injured patients. Patient flow can mean the difference between whether an ED and hospital adapts within a state of "contingency care" or whether the state of resource scarcity progresses to "crisis care" and severe rationing.

Advance planning: Best practices for coordinating with inpatient services include engaging stakeholders in the planning and exercise processes and identifying triggers and protocols for rapid admission, patient management (e.g., holding orders), and rapid discharge procedures. Some hospitals have reported on the safety and efficacy of frequent simulated and "tabletop" exercises in which inpatient services simulate "reverse triage" of current inpatients. Reverse triage is defined as active "down-grading of care due to strained resources in order to create additional triage spaces."

Census sharing: Additionally, census sharing agreements between services during disasters may be helpful for balancing workloads during events that may require one specialty significantly more than others. For example, during an event with significant traumatic injuries such as an earthquake or mass shooting, a census sharing arrangement in which nonsurgical specialists manage patients with non-emergent conditions that traditionally would be cared for by a surgical specialty (e.g., non-ruptured appendicitis) allows surgical specialists to focus on emergency triage and management of those acutely involved in an MCI, while maintaining quality and safety for patients with less urgent surgical conditions (e.g., ensuring antibiotics administration and monitoring for a change in symptoms).[6,31]

Access to follow-up care: Similarly, follow-up access to care after an initial, but possibly abbreviated, evaluation and treatment period in the ED may impact quality of outcomes for patients with minor or intermediate injury or illness following an event with multiple casualties. For example, ensuring adequate return precautions and access to timely, outpatient services can provide the means for receiving definitive procedures, catching missed diagnoses, and identifying other health and wellness needs for individuals who have experienced a traumatic event.

TRAINING AND MAINTENANCE OF MCI MANAGEMENT SKILLS

As with all critical skills and procedures, practicing MCI management skills is critical for maintenance of proficiency. As discussed earlier, emergency physicians should involve key internal and external stakeholders in planning and practice of MCI-related processes. Both tabletop and functional exercises can play an important role in testing processes. The Joint Commission, the national accrediting body for acute care hospitals, requires an annual disaster exercise at each facility.[32] A mix of both types of exercises (tabletop and functional) is helpful for probing different parts of disaster preparedness efforts. Tabletop exercises are helpful for examining multisystem processes and agreements over a short time period. For example, tabletop exercises can bring together leaders from multiple organizations including hospitals, EMS, and city government officials to discuss high-level policy, decision-making, or governance practices that would take effect during an MCI. Tabletop exercises can also be used to test one component of a specific skill-set or technical component of a response such as triage categorization or scarce resource contingency or rationing plans. Functional exercises are very useful for training front-line staff in specific processes and testing the operational details and sticking points in a real-life scenario. A functional exercise can be limited to one or two specific processes (e.g., patient registration or reverse triage hand offs). Or they can be full-scale functional exercises with moulaged patients and full staff enacting a simulated response with observer documentation of critical actions and assessment of areas for improvement. It is helpful to schedule exercises (tabletop and functional) at different times of day so that different teams can participate.[3,6,30] Allocating sufficient time to debrief and document lessons learned as well as next steps is essential for improving future performance around MCIs. If an education or training gap is identified or an electronic process is revealed to have a glitch, identify a champion and timeline to correct and re-test the issue. Key findings and takeaways from the exercise should be disseminated to the rest of the ED.

SPECIAL CONSIDERATIONS: DECONTAMINATION, LAW ENFORCEMENT, AND FORENSICS

There are several types of special circumstances that may need to be considered during an MCI, requiring specialized components or teams for response. The following section reviews additional considerations for EDs when managing specific types of MCIs.

Chemical, Biological, Radiological or Nuclear and Explosives Emergencies and Decontamination Procedures

Chemical, biological, radiological or nuclear and explosive (CBRNE) emergencies encompass a range of scenarios in which an agent that is harmful to the general public has been released intentionally or accidentally and is circulating in a community. In many cases, the agent may go undetected until patients become symptomatic, and similarly, it frequently has the potential to contaminate others including first responders or healthcare workers. Examples of such CBRNE include everything from an infectious disease outbreak such as Ebola, COVID, or anthrax to a nerve-agent attack, such as Sarin gas, a dirty bomb, a nuclear waste disruption, or a chemical spill. EDs should include these scenarios and specific needs in their all-hazards approach to preparedness.[30,33–35] The ED and hospital may have little to no warning of the event, nor an early indication of what the agent is. Therefore in cases where a CBRNE event is suspected, it may be best to proceed with a conservative approach including high-level PPE and precautions until further information about the agent can be ascertained and safety guidance tailored to the specific agent. More information about specific agents as well as levels of PPE can be found from sources such as the CDC and the U.S. Department of Health and Human Services (HHS).[36]

Managing high-level PPE is a complex psychomotor skill with physiologic implications for the wearer. Regular training in the appropriate methods for donning and doffing PPE is essential for ED staff to be prepared to respond to CBRNE events safely. Doffing PPE represents one of the times of greatest risk for a first responder to contaminate themselves or others. High-level PPE may include chemical resistant suits and powered air purifying respirators (PAPRs) or self-contained breathing apparatus (SCBAs) that limit the motion, visual fields, and hearing capabilities of the provider. Additionally, the extra, impermeable clothing worn during decontamination procedures and treatment can limit the number of patient interventions that can be performed, while placing additional strain on medical staff, raising body temperatures, heart rate, and causing insensible water losses. For these reasons, it is important to have a time limit for those serving in full PPE and an assigned safety monitor to observe the high-risk periods of donning and doffing PPE to minimize risk of contamination.[34,36]

When an ED is alerted that it will be receiving patients from an MCI with a CBRNE component, appropriate decontamination and containment protocols must be put into effect with close safety monitoring of PPE. The ED's external and internal treatment areas should be partitioned to clearly indicate where decontamination is occurring, where equipment is being doffed, and where usual care treatment is occurring.[34,37] In technical terms, the exposure zone is known as the "exclusion zone" or "hot zone" where everything is contaminated, and rescue personnel are limited. Near the contamination site and in the ED, there are two other zones. The first area reached by a patient is called the "Contamination reduction or decontamination zone" (also called a "warm zone"), where contaminated or potentially contaminated individuals are coming to be decontaminated. The core ED treatment area is the "support zone" (or "cold zone"), where no contamination should occur, and usual treatment practices and standard PPE is worn. (Fig. 75.8) Security barriers (e.g., doors, partitions, staff) should be in place to ensure both one-way patient flow through these areas and to ensure appropriate PPE are worn in each zone. This will minimize the risk of bringing contaminated materials or patients into a cold zone, while allowing maximum flexibility for staff and patients and the usual level of care in the cold zone.[37,38]

All ED staff should be trained in standard decontamination processes in which patients enter through one entryway. A bifurcation between ambulatory and nonambulatory patients is required, with similar processes in each category.

The first stage of decontamination is "dry decontamination" in which clothing is removed and any large dry substances are removed or brushed off. Ambulatory patients can be directed to remove their own clothing. Nonambulatory patients should have clothing cut off. Clothing should be placed into hazardous materials containers. Avoid attempting to wring out materials.

The second phase of decontamination is referred to as "wet decontamination," in which patients are showered with warm water. Several decontamination procedures

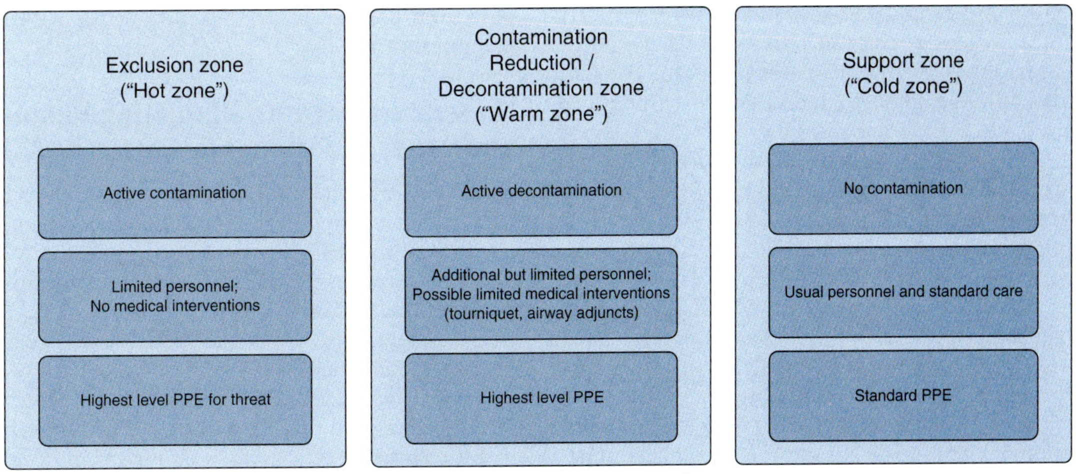

Fig. 75.8 Decontamination zones of care.

involve multiple showering steps. After the final shower step, a patient is provided with toweling and clean clothes or a hospital gown prior to evaluation. Front-line workers involved in active decontamination procedures should follow the same decontamination procedure prior to doffing their PPE. During the decontamination process, hospitals and EDs should maximize privacy for patients and staff and minimize exposure to the elements to avoid hypothermia.

Depending on the size of the MCI and the number of persons requiring decontamination, minimal lifesaving maneuvers should be performed in the decontamination zone. The contamination areas may have basic life support devices such as tourniquets or clotting interventions but airway and other circulation management, including placement of IVs and definitive airways, is extremely limited due to mobility in PPE. Most of these procedures should be deferred to the support zone.

Crime Scenes, Law Enforcement Engagement, and Forensics

Certain types of MCIs are due to criminal activity (i.e., mass shooting, bomb, or chemical event). Depending on the perpetrator's motivations and scale of the event, multiple law enforcement or government agencies, from local police to the FBI or Homeland Security, may need to be involved in the response to the MCI, in some cases working alongside medical personnel in the prehospital or hospital setting. Multiple considerations may impact the medical response.

Tactical Teams, Hot Zones, Warm Zones, and Law Enforcement–Physician Collaboration

In some scenarios where there is an active threat to the general public, law enforcement is involved in the immediate response to contain the threat and restore scene safety. Most tactical (SWAT) teams are trained and have supplies present to initiate basic measures for hemorrhage control (tourniquets, pressure dressings, or QuikClot). Some teams include an EMT, paramedic, or physician in their group to help address medical needs encountered by tactical team members as well as by victims or perpetrators of an attack.[4,24,25] As with CBRNE events, similar terminology is used in active threat scenarios regarding treatment areas.[38] For example, during an incident in which a threat is still considered to be present, such as an active shooter scenario, the unsecured area in which the threat is present is considered the "hot zone." In general, medical first responders are not allowed into the hot zone unless part of a tactical unit. The "cold zone" or area of safety is outside of the police line. This is usually where medical personnel including ambulances will stage for initial triage, treatment, and transport of patients from the scene. The area immediately outside of the active area but inside of the police line is often referred to as a "warm zone." These "zones" are depicted in Fig. 75.9. Over the last few decades, as mass shootings have become increasingly common, EMS and law enforcement have worked more closely to stage treatment areas behind the police line in the so-called warm zone where treatments such as tourniquets, and initial triage can take place more efficiently.[38]

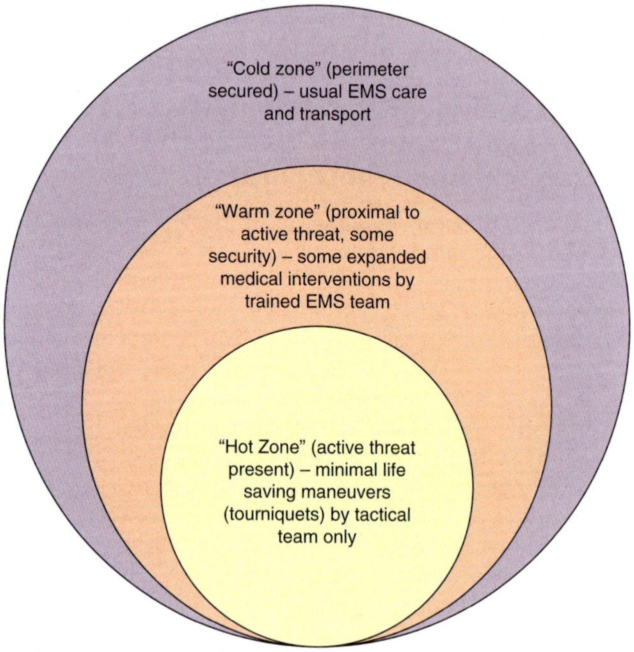

Fig. 75.9 Tactical emergency medical services (EMS) response.

ED and Hospital Considerations for Law Enforcement-Associated Events

In rare cases, such as a mass shooting, an ED or hospital may become the primary scene of a crime and MCI. It is important for hospitals and EDs to include preparedness plans and exercises to prepare staff on how to respond in those unique instances, not only for the treatment of the injured but also to ensure the safety of as many staff and patients as possible. Most of the time, the ED and hospital are a destination for EMS and patients following an MCI with a criminal component. In those instances, the ED and hospital must be prepared to work alongside a continuing investigation. Several issues may intersect with ED care including the potential for a perpetrator to be among the injured being triaged or treated, and evidence collection from the event. Assuming a secured hospital environment, medical stabilization is the priority and should be the focus of ED staff. While it is not the duty of the medical staff to participate in any aspect of investigation, EM providers and administrators should be aware of the potential concurrent missions and how to activate administrative support from hospital leadership to interface with law enforcement personnel.

Understanding and Mitigating Resource Shortages, Contingency Care, and Crisis Care

During mass casualty events or prolonged disasters, available resources (including staff, supplies, and therapeutics) are often insufficient to meet all patient needs. In the acute phase, limited staff for assessments, stabilization, and transport usually becomes the first critical resource, necessitating the usage of triage systems that prioritize patient access based on acuity. However, as an incident unfolds or becomes more prolonged, additional resources may become more limited. Emergency physicians require real-time strategies and preparedness plans to address resource shortages equitably and prevent the full progression to a state of "crisis care."

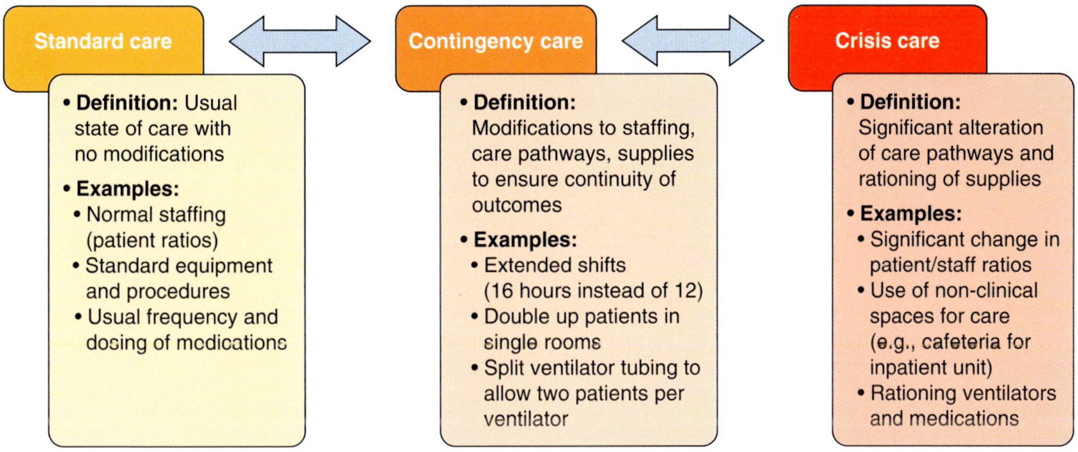

Fig. 75.10 Framework for progression between standard, contingency, and crisis care.

Understanding how ethical frameworks apply to scarce resource management intentionally and during the planning and preparedness phases of crisis response is essential for ensuring equitable application of resources. As Rawlings et al. wrote: "Beneficence, justice, autonomy, and non-maleficence are generally accepted as the four fundamental ethical principles that guide health care delivery."[39] Beneficence is defined as acting in the best interest of others and with intent to do good. Justice is defined as treating people fairly and equitably. Autonomy means self-determination, and ability to make one's own choices. Non-maleficence is defined as doing no harm or acting to avoid harm. Persad, Emanuel, Fauci, and their collaborators have elaborated on additional ethical frameworks that can be applied during disasters to ethically allocate scarce resources and maintain the core principles of health care.[40,42]

While much has been said about the concept of "Crisis Standards of Care," it is important for emergency clinicians to work and train within frameworks that seek to prevent and mitigate full progression to crisis conditions. As laid out by Hanfling et al. in a report on "Framework for Evaluating Crisis Care" for the National Academies of Medicine and in other texts, it is most helpful to consider scarce resource utilization along a spectrum that runs from "standard care," through "contingency care," and ends in "crisis care."[43,44] This framework is described in Fig. 75.10. "standard care" refers to the provision of usual complexity of care, using adequate resources, ensuring timely patient access, preventing staff overload, and maintaining equipment functionality. "Contingency care" denotes the utilization of limited resources through extended, reused, or multipurpose applications to sustain the usual level of interventions. Examples of contingency care include extending staff shifts from 8 to 12 hours per day, expanding patient-to-clinician ratios, doubling patients in hospital rooms or hallways but with access to usual equipment, and bifurcating ventilation tubing in order to utilize one ventilator for multiple patients. "Crisis care" signifies the depletion of resources and contingency options, necessitating resource rationing and limited application of definitive care. Instances of crisis care involve deferred or significantly delayed care based on triage status or prioritizing certain patients for ventilator assignments or medications based on age or comorbidity criteria.

To prevent the progression to full or prolonged crisis care, various stages of resource mitigation can be implemented within the realm of contingency care. Disaster preparedness entails the anticipation of factors that may lead to resource scarcity, enabling EM clinicians and other clinical leaders to plan and practice resource mitigation strategies until resources are replenished or patient care demands return to normal. As part of a robust MCI preparedness plan, EM physicians and their hospital counterparts should consider developing a formalized framework and plan for scarce resource allocation and enhancing peer education on the issue. Cao and Huang demonstrated that a simulation approach to scarce resource allocation education may be effective in demonstrating these core principles.[45]

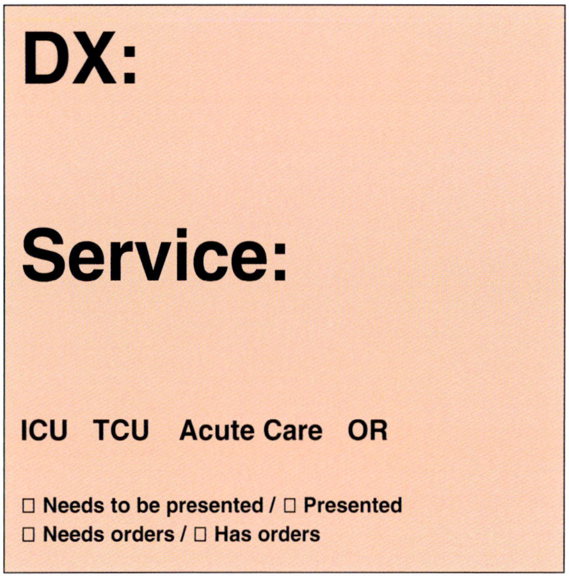

Fig. 75.11 Sample face sheet for patients requiring admission during reverse triage.

ENSURING AN EQUITABLE DISASTER RESPONSE

Ensuring equitable outcomes for patients and implementing contingency mitigation strategies are essential in preventing the progression along the continuum of contingency or crisis care. Vulnerable patient populations, including extremes of age, those with limited English proficiency, and historically marginalized groups based on race, gender, sexual identity, or socioeconomic status, are at a higher risk of experiencing disparities in standard and contingency care. These disparities can be exacerbated during crisis care and resource rationing. Emergency clinicians involved in disaster preparedness and response should familiarize themselves with existing hospital policies on resource management and actively engage in the ethical review and revision of these policies as part of ongoing preparedness efforts to ensure equitable response.

Several best practices have been identified for developing a scarce resource management policy. First, proactive planning and framework development prior to an event facilitate the inclusion of diverse internal and external stakeholders, allowing sufficient time for ethical review. Second, establishing a multidisciplinary team with representatives from various specialties (e.g., EM, critical care, inpatient, surgical services) and professions (physicians, nurses, respiratory therapists), as well as engagement of internal and external stakeholders such as community and patient advocates, and union representatives, can help to provide broad and diverse input. Third, grounding the challenge of scarce resource management in clear ethical principles that are consistent with other aspects of clinical practice is crucial for equitable patient access.

As outlined earlier, MCI preparation is a complex and multifaceted process involving numerous stakeholders. Ensuring that adequate protocols are in place and familiarity with the roles of key ED staff during an MCI will help ensure that your department maximizes opportunities to provide the best care possible for the greatest number of patients.

REFERENCES ARE AVAILABLE AT Elsevier eBooks+

CHAPTER 76

Recognition and Response to Human Trafficking

Wendy L. Macias-Konstantopoulos

BACKGROUND

Human trafficking, also known as trafficking in persons, constitutes a pervasive criminal, human rights, and public health problem of global concern that is associated with a broad range of significant adverse health outcomes. Recognizing human trafficking as a form of interpersonal abuse and exploitation with negative health implications for affected adults and children is an essential foundation from which emergency practitioners can understand their role in identifying and caring for patients who are trafficked.

Definition

There are many misconceptions about the term *human trafficking*, including its synonymous use with *sex trafficking*, excluding other labor forms, and its conflation with *human smuggling*.

The US Trafficking Victims Protection Act of 2000 and its subsequent reauthorization acts, as amended (22 USC § 7102) defines "severe forms of trafficking in persons" as labor trafficking and sex trafficking (Box 76.1).[1,2] In both cases, human trafficking involves the use of *force, fraud, or coercion* for the purpose of exploiting an individual for labor. Furthermore, the US Justice for Victims of Trafficking Act of 2015 amended the legal definition of "child abuse and neglect" under the Child Abuse Prevention and Treatment Act of 1988 to include "sex trafficking" and other "severe forms of trafficking in persons" of a minor.[3] While emergency practitioners need not establish whether a situation satisfies the legal definition of human trafficking, the definition is helpful in anchoring the physical and psychological health impact.

EPIDEMIOLOGY

Prevalence

The true prevalence of human trafficking is difficult to determine, and prevalence figures are based on fragmented and incomplete data. The reliability of prevalence figures is challenged by multiple factors including the lack of common databases and reliance on local data sources focused on specific types of trafficking or using varying definitions of trafficking to collect data, as well as the clandestine nature of human trafficking and difficulty in identifying marginalized trafficking victims.[4]

Using a methodology that combined multiple data sources and system dynamics modeling to develop global estimates of human trafficking, the United Nations International Labour Organization, Walk Free, and the International Organization for Migration estimated that 49.6 million people were trapped in situations of modern slavery on any given day in 2021.[5] Of these, approximately 21 million were trapped in forced labor, 6 million in forced commercial sexual exploitation, and 22 million in forced marriage.[4] The study further determined that females and girls accounted for 52% of persons in modern slavery and one in every four victims was a child.[4] While most prevalence estimates are inadequate, the National Human Trafficking Hotline, supported by the US Department of Health and Human Services, tracks reports of human trafficking across the 50 states, the District of Columbia, and US territories and can serve as a proxy for understanding the scope and severity of the problem in the United States.[6]

Typologies

An analysis of over 32,000 human trafficking cases reported to the National Human Trafficking Hotline identified 25 different types of labor and sex trafficking in the United States.[7] Manifestations of human trafficking in the United States include forced labor in both formal and informal industries such as agriculture, construction, and landscaping, as well as hospitality services like restaurants and hotels.[7] Persons trafficked for domestic work and in-home health care services are harbored in the privacy of residential homes, although there is increasing recognition of labor trafficking occurring in nursing homes.[7] The commercial sex industry impacts minors and adults and includes establishment-based, street-based, and technology-based venues of adult sexual entertainment.[7–9] Bodywork businesses such as health spas and massage parlors have been associated with individuals who are trafficked both for labor and commercial sex.[7]

Risk Factors

Although any person may be trafficked, numerous factors increase an individual's vulnerability and risk for trafficking. Factors that impact risk exist at the societal, community, interpersonal, and individual levels of the socioecological model.[4,10–17] Societal or structural risk factors can include systemic poverty, sex-based discrimination, early sexualization of children, and migration due to mass displacements in settings of political unrest, armed conflict, and natural disasters. Community factors are those that place an entire community at risk, such as the lack of resources (e.g., afterschool programming), the presence of street gangs, and a tolerance for sexual violence and exploitation. Interpersonal risk factors may be associated with family dysfunction, violence, and criminality; caregiver mental health disorders; cultural expectations that children financially assist the family; and migration of adolescents and young adults for kinship placements with distant family and acquaintances. Push and pull factors at the individual level of the socioecological model include a personal history of child abuse and neglect, sexual violence, early substance use, child protective services involvement, difficulty in school (e.g., bullying, learning/developmental disabilities), identification with the LGBTQ+ community, housing instability due to running away or being thrown out, and poor self-esteem. An awareness of the risk factors associated with human trafficking can improve the emergency practitioner's competence in recognizing patients who may be trafficked or at elevated risk for trafficking.

Indicators

As may be the case in intimate partner violence, trafficked persons presenting for care in the emergency department (ED)

BOX 76.1 Legal Definition of Human Trafficking[1,2]

The US Trafficking Victims Protection Act (TVPA) of 2000, and its subsequent reauthorizations, define:

1. *Labor trafficking* as "the recruitment, harboring, transportation, provision, or obtaining of a person for labor or services, through the use of *force, fraud, or coercion* for the purposes of subjection to involuntary servitude, peonage, debt bondage, or slavery," and
2. *Sex trafficking* as "the recruitment, harboring, transportation, provision, obtaining, patronizing, or soliciting of a person for the purposes of a commercial sex act,[a] in which the commercial sex act is induced by *force, fraud, or coercion*, or in which the person induced to perform such an act has not attained 18 years of age."

[a]*Pursuant to the TVPA of 2000, a* commercial sex act *is defined as "any sex act on account of which anything of value is given to or received by any person."*

may not feel safe or ready to attempt an exit due to the threats and violent tactics typically employed by traffickers to maintain control. Thus whether presenting alone or accompanied by a perpetrator, trafficked persons infrequently disclose their situation. As a result, the identification of patients who may be experiencing trafficking requires the proactive efforts of emergency practitioners and other health professionals. While no single sign, symptom, or indicator is unequivocally pathognomonic of human trafficking, emergency practitioners can develop a high index of suspicion for trafficking when able to recognize the convergence of multiple red flags.

Box 76.2 provides a list of potential indicators of human trafficking and, while not meant to be exhaustive, it highlights the wide array of signs and symptoms that can be seen across the spectrum of human trafficking experiences.[16–18] The long-standing recommendation that emergency practitioners engage in trafficking assessments selectively, rather than universally, requires an understanding of human trafficking and the potential indicators in the health care setting in order to recognize patients at high risk.[17]

Health Problems

Human trafficking is associated with a broad range of physical, reproductive, and mental health problems.[16–25] Due to the tactics employed by traffickers to gain and maintain control over an individual, physical health problems associated with trafficking may be the direct result of sexual and physical violence including injuries related to strangulation, burns, and blunt force and penetrating trauma, as well as industry-specific occupational injuries. Physical health problems may also be related to chronically untreated common health conditions, such as asthma, diabetes, and hypertension, in the absence of regular primary and preventive care. From a reproductive perspective, health problems may be associated with unintended pregnancies, maternal and fetal complications of pregnancy, unsafe abortions, and recurrent sexually transmitted infections (STIs) as well as the advanced disease states of untreated STIs (e.g., hepatitis C virus–associated hepatocellular carcinoma, human papillomavirus–associated cervical cancer). Finally, the mental health burden of trafficking is extensive and may result in anxiety, depression, posttraumatic stress disorder, night terrors, dissociative disorders, and high-risk health behaviors including substance use and self-harm.

Due to the myriad health problems that may arise while trafficked, 28% to 88% of survivors within cohorts surveyed report having sought medical attention during the course of their exploitation.[26–29] Emergency/urgent care practitioners (56%)[28] and EDs (63%)[29] were the most frequently reported health professionals and health care access points visited. Because trafficking victims infrequently self-identify and their chief complaints are not necessarily distinct from those of any other patient, emergency practitioners need to rely on their knowledge of human trafficking—risk factors, violent tactics, and indicators—to recognize patients who may be potentially trafficked.

ASSESSMENT FOR HUMAN TRAFFICKING

Setting the Stage

Familiarity with the potential indicators of human trafficking (Box 76.2) establishes a foundation of knowledge from which the emergency practitioner can recognize suspicious presentations and patterns of behavior. Using a trauma-informed approach, the emergency practitioner can care for the health needs of their patients and pursue a more focused trafficking assessment when indicated. Consistent with a trauma-informed approach, however, disclosure of human trafficking is not the goal of the assessment. Disclosures may be hampered by guilt, shame, fear of stigma or judgment, threats of retaliation, threats of harm to loved ones, and fear of being reported to the authorities, including reports to child protective services, law enforcement (LE), and immigration and customs enforcement.[4,17,18,30] In the face of such barriers, aggressive attempts to obtain a disclosure can be harmful to the patient and detrimental to a therapeutic relationship and should not be pursued without a compelling reason. Instead, practitioners should regard the patient encounter as an opportunity to build rapport, establish trust, validate experiences of trauma, and create a safe space where disclosures might follow.[17]

Trauma-Informed Approach to Care

Experiences of trauma—which can include neglect, abuse, and violence—are ubiquitous and occur throughout the lifespan from early childhood to late adulthood. Previous and current experiences of physical and psychological trauma may impair an individual's ability to (1) regulate sympathetically driven posttraumatic stress reactions to perceived threats (e.g., irritability, hostility, anger), (2) cope with emotional stressors and triggers, (3) trust authority figures, and (4) experience health care as positive and beneficial.[13,16] Using a trauma-informed approach throughout the care encounter can help practitioners to promote physical and psychological safety, establish trust, and forge a therapeutic relationship with an individual experiencing the impacts of trauma.

A trauma-informed framework understands the wide-ranging impact of trauma on individuals, acknowledges that there are triggers of psychological and emotional distress in the regular course of care, resists retraumatization through deliberate efforts to avoid or minimize triggers, and promotes safety, well-being, and recovery by fully integrating knowledge about trauma into all aspects of care including policies, procedures, and practices.[31] In emergency care, understanding

BOX 76.2 Potential Indicators of Human Trafficking[16–18]

INDICATORS OF CONTROL

- Accompanied by a person who is dominating the conversation, answering questions, correcting the child, and overall controlling the encounter
- Accompanied by a person who obstructs provider attempts to meet with the child alone
- Accompanied by a person who resists the use of a professional interpreter
- Scripted or restricted communications
- Frequent glances at the accompanying person for signs of approval or disapproval after speaking
- Avoidance of eye contact with the accompanying person or providers
- Appears fearful, subordinate, or hypervigilant
- Preoccupied with responding promptly to frequent texts

INDICATORS OF ABUSE OR NEGLECT

- Delayed presentation for medical care
- Signs of medical/dental neglect
- Signs of malnourishment
- Signs of physical/sexual trauma
- HIV and recurrent sexually transmitted infections
- Multiple pregnancies
- Complications of unsafe abortions
- Intravaginal/rectal foreign bodies
- Atypical material to stop menses flow
- Discrepancy between the history provided and clinical presentation
- Discrepancy between reported and apparent age (i.e., lying about age)
- Tattoos or branding indicating ownership
- Hypervigilance
- Hyper-startle reflex

INDICATORS OF TRAUMA

- Sudden personality changes
- Somatic complaints
- Sleeping difficulties
- Changes in appetite
- Sexualized talk and behaviors
- New onset substance use
- Self-aggrandizing and brazen attitude to demonstrate strength and control
- Interprets neutral words and facial expressions as irritation or judgment
- Signs of traumatic stress
    - Anxiety
    - Panic attacks
    - Social withdrawal
    - Anhedonia
    - Chronic disobedience
    - Chronic running away
    - Irritability
    - Defensiveness
    - Distrusting
    - Aggression/hostility
    - Self-injurious behaviors
    - Suicidal ideation

the psychological and behavioral manifestations of trauma can equip practitioners with the knowledge necessary to engage compassionately and effectively with patients who exhibit pronounced trauma-related symptoms and outcomes (e.g., poor coping skills, feelings of being judged, substance use disorder, and mental illness).[32]

Finally, practitioners will rarely have confirmation that patients are exhibiting the short- or long-term harmful impacts of trauma. Given traumatic experiences are commonplace, emergency practitioners are advised to care for all patients using a trauma-informed approach as a universal precaution, similar to using hand sanitizer before every patient encounter.[33,34]

Professional Language Interpreters

In the case of language barriers, emergency practitioners should secure the services of a professional interpreter rather than relying on accompanying persons for interpretation. When the resources are available, patient requests for interpreters of a specific gender should be considered. Practitioners are discouraged from engaging a potential victim of human trafficking in a language other than English unless they possess advanced or native fluency in the language (*Note:* institutions may require certification as a qualified bilingual practitioner). Asking patients to repeat themselves due to gaps in language comprehension, particularly when discussing sensitive matters, can not only be retraumatizing to patients but can strain the patient—provider relationship and lead to distrust and loss of confidence in the health sector's ability to assist.

Privacy and Confidentiality

Ensuring privacy and confidentiality is of paramount importance in patient—provider encounters and this is especially true when broaching sensitive matters as is the case with assessments for human trafficking. To protect the physical and psychological safety of trafficking victims and survivors, emergency practitioners should refrain from exploring the possibility of trafficking or any other form of abuse until the patient is in a private space, out of earshot, and separated from any accompanying persons who may be complicit in the trafficking.[16,17]

The question of wanting or needing privacy should not be left to the patient as they may not be at liberty to request that the person(s) accompanying them leave the examination room. Instead, emergency practitioners must address privacy and take responsibility for creating opportunities to speak to the patient alone without alerting the other person(s) of their concerns. In some cases, this can be achieved by simply encouraging the other person(s) to step out momentarily for the physical examination as a matter of privacy practices. In other cases, where the practitioner meets initial resistance, more creative means become necessary such as walking the patient to the bathroom, asking the accompanying person to assist with paperwork at the registration desk, and meeting with the patient while in the radiology suite where visitors are prohibited by safety hazard protocols.[17]

Additionally, patients should be reassured of their right to have the information they share kept confidential. Likewise, it is important to inform patients of the limits of confidentiality, as is the case when mandatory reporting laws apply.[35] A brief, carefully worded statement that other professionals may need to be engaged for assistance under certain circumstances can generate trust and instill confidence in the practitioner's ability to assist, while also encouraging the patient to make an informed decision about the information they choose to share. This simple yet powerful communication demonstrates transparency, conveys respect for patient autonomy, and, theoretically, guards against significant relationship rifts when patients are informed of the legal requirement to disclose certain information they shared.

Screening Versus Assessment

Although a number of human trafficking screening tools exist, these are either lengthy and resource-intensive or have yet to be validated for use in the health care setting. As a result, experts have conventionally recommended that emergency practitioners conduct selective, rather than universal, assessments for human trafficking in patients who exhibit signs, symptoms, and indicators suggestive of trafficking. Recent research, however, suggests that two screening tools are emerging as promising for use in emergency departments—the *Short Screen for Child Sex Trafficking* (SSCST) tool for adolescents with specific high-risk chief complaints (Box 76.3)[36,37] and the *Rapid Appraisal for Trafficking* (RAFT) for clinically stable adult patients (Box 76.4).[38,39]

The SSCST tool is a six-item screening tool that has been validated on English-speaking adolescents 11 to 17 years of age seeking care in a teen clinic with any chief complaint, a child advocacy center with a chief complaint related to abuse or neglect, and a pediatric ED with a chief complaint related to sexual violence or high-risk sexual or social behaviors. A positive screen, defined as positive answers to two or more questions, indicates a high risk for trafficking and, according to the developers, does not necessarily mean the child is actually being trafficked. Consequently, a positive screen should prompt an additional formal assessment to determine whether a child is being trafficked (keeping in mind that disclosure is not the goal) or whether the level of risk is high enough that mandatory reporting laws apply based on a reasonable degree of suspicion for sex trafficking.

The RAFT tool is a four-item screening tool that has been validated on clinically stable adults 18 years of age or older speaking any language and seeking care in an ED. An affirmative response to any one of the four questions constitutes a positive screen, however, like the SSCST, a positive RAFT screen is not necessarily indicative of human trafficking and, when unclear, should prompt a more comprehensive assessment to determine the need for antitrafficking resources or interventions. Similarly, a negative screen does not exclude human trafficking and may occur in a trafficked patient actively withholding information to conceal their situation or when the circumstances of the patient's trafficking situation are not captured by any of the screener questions.

While there is increasing interest in broadened screening, decisions to implement universal screening protocols must take into consideration the limited utility of the currently validated tools, which are designed to detect a narrow scope of trafficking and may require additional assessments. Experience with universal screening for trafficking in all-comers is scarce. The effectiveness of rote screening in identifying and assisting victims of trafficking is unknown, and active screening for traumatic experiences is not without the risk of retraumatization and harm. Thus the evidence to support, or lack thereof, and the potential unintended impacts of implementing universal screening for human trafficking should be carefully considered before recommending and adopting such an approach.

BOX 76.3 SSCST Tool

The *Short Screen for Child Sex Trafficking*[36] (SSCST) is a six-item screening tool validated for use among 11- to 17-year-old pediatric emergency department patients presenting with chief complaints related to sexual violence or high-risk sexual or social behaviors. SSCST items include the following six questions:

1. Have you ever broken any bones, had any cuts that required stitches, or been knocked unconscious?
2. Some kids have a hard time living at home and feel that they need to run away. Have you ever run away from home?
3. Kids often use drugs or drink alcohol, and different kids use different drugs. Have you used drugs or alcohol in the last 12 months?
4. Sometimes kids have been involved with the police. Maybe for running away, for breaking curfew, for shoplifting. There can be lots of different reasons. Have you ever had any problems with the police?
5. If you have had sex before, how many sexual partners have you had? (Choices: 0, 1–5, 6–10, and >10 partners)[a]
6. Have you ever had a sexually transmitted infection, like herpes or gonorrhea or chlamydia or trichomonas?

An affirmative answer to any two of the six SSCST questions constitutes a positive screen. A positive screen does not necessarily indicate a trafficking situation and a negative screen does not exclude it.

[a]*Question 5 is considered "positive" when the child reports ≥6 sexual partners.*

BOX 76.4 Rapid Appraisal for Trafficking (RAFT) for Clinically Stable Adult Patients RAFT Tool

The *Rapid Appraisal for Trafficking*[38] (RAFT) is a four-item screening tool validated for use among clinically stable emergency department adult patients (≥18 years old). RAFT items include the following four questions:

1. It is not uncommon for people to stay in work situations that are risky or even dangerous, simply because they have no other options. Have you ever worked, or done other things, in a place that made you feel scared or unsafe?
2. In thinking back over your past experience, have you ever been tricked or forced into doing any kind of work that you did not want to do?
3. Sometimes people are prevented from leaving an unfair or unsafe work situation by their employers. Have you ever been afraid to leave or quit a work situation due to fears of violence or threats of harm to yourself or your family?
4. Have you ever received anything in exchange for sex (e.g., a place to stay, gifts, or food)?

An affirmative answer to any one of the four RAFT questions constitutes a positive screen. A positive screen does not necessarily indicate a trafficking situation and a negative screen does not exclude it.

Additionally, emergency practitioners and trafficked patients are better served when response protocols are developed prior to instituting any screening protocols. Adequate and carefully planned policies, procedures, and partnerships with community-based service organizations are critical to ensuring a safe and effective response to the identification or disclosure of trafficking in the ED. Ideally, response protocols facilitate a multipronged, interdisciplinary, and intersectional approach to addressing the vast needs of identified adult and child trafficking victims and survivors.[18]

Conducting the Assessment

Once privacy has been established, the emergency practitioner may proceed with building rapport, establishing trust, performing a focused physical examination as indicated, and conducting an assessment for human trafficking.

Nonverbal Communication

Emergency practitioners must be vigilant of their nonverbal communication, including posture, gestures, gaze, facial expressions, and tone of voice. According to Mehrabian's Communication Model, facial expressions carry the most weight among the elements of human communication, followed by tone of voice, especially in situations dealing with emotions.[40] The words spoken carry the least weight as evidenced by the finding that nonverbal elements of communication can change how verbal communications are interpreted in situations where incongruence exists between the two messages.[40] Thus nonverbal cues are constantly being communicated and interpreted by the receiver. Body language is a continuous source of nonverbal communication that is subconscious and can either convey respect and put others at ease or offend and contradict verbal communication.

Spatial Empathy

As with all patients, but especially with persons who have experienced abuse and violence, respect for personal space is crucial to the promotion of physical and psychological safety. Standing too close, too soon, may invoke memories of a traumatic experience, causing the patient to feel intimidated, physically threatened, or frightened. This type of retraumatization in the health care setting can trigger an emotionally dysregulated response and may be especially harmful to the development of a therapeutic patient-provider relationship.

To avoid the inadvertent invasion of personal space and other physical or psychological triggers, emergency practitioners may choose to engage respectfully with the patient from a reasonable distance while building rapport. When a physical evaluation is necessary, there are specific procedures that could be followed to help minimize retraumatization. Before physically entering a patient's personal space and touching them, practitioners may want to: (1) provide an overview of the steps entailed and the reason for the exam; (2) invite and respond to clarifying questions until all the patient's concerns have been addressed; (3) ask the patient for consent to perform the exam; and (4) encourage the patient to request a break or stop the examination if at any point it begins to feel unsafe. In situations where a medical chaperone is advisable, the practitioner should inform the patient, ask if the patient has a gender preference, and introduce the chaperone to the patient in advance of the examination. The medical chaperone could be coached to introduce themself to the patient, confirm how the patient wants to be addressed, and ask the patient to share ways in which their comfort could be maximized during the examination.

Empathic Listening

To engage effectively in a formal assessment for human trafficking, the emergency practitioner will need to be attentive and engaged. Sitting at eye level with the patient and maintaining appropriate eye contact can communicate a genuine interest in what the patient may share, and a commitment of the time and effort needed to build rapport and establish trust.

Empathy has been identified by both patients and practitioners as fundamental to humane patient-centered health care.[41] Patients who perceive their physicians as having empathy and positive attitudes toward psychosocial issues have been found to have lower levels of anxiety, decreased reports of physical pain, increased levels of patient satisfaction, improved treatment plan adherence and health outcomes, and greater confidence in their own ability to cope and change.[41,42]

Empathic listening is a structured technique of active listening and supportive questioning that promotes the development of relationships based on empathy and a stronger understanding of what is being communicated both verbally and nonverbally.[43] Empathic listening strategies include, but are not limited to, developing an awareness of body language, resisting distractions, waiting patiently for the speaker to complete their thoughts, interjecting brief phrases that validate the speaker's feelings and experiences, and offering summary responses when needed to ensure a proper understanding.[43] When offering summary responses, empathic listeners should mirror the words and reflect the statements of the speaker accurately while mindful of not passing judgment inadvertently, make premature assumptions, jump to conclusions, or criticize. Once proper understanding is confirmed, the empathic listener uses the information shared to formulate appropriately bounded, open-ended prompts that facilitate reflection or advance the conversation to deeper levels. Interrupting, filling the silence, competing for attention, disputing the facts, and attempting to complete the other person's thoughts to move the conversation along can convey impatience, disinterest, and lack of understanding.

Trafficking Inquiry

Once rapport has been developed and the limits of confidentiality discussed, if the practitioner has concerns about human trafficking, inquiries can begin with a broader conversation about safety that is framed as the standard of care, explaining the rationale and normalizing the process of addressing safety with all patients. To the extent possible, the assessment should be conducted in a conversational manner to minimize the patient's experience of the interaction as an interrogation. Sitting at or below the patient's level may help diminish the patient—provider power differential and create a sense of a more equal alliance. As the details surrounding any given situation of human trafficking are unique, the actual prompts or questions used to elicit information about a patient's personal circumstances and experiences will vary from one case scenario to another. The conversation should advance from more generic questions about the patient's life and work circumstances to less invasive inquiries about their general safety. Finally, as the conversation progresses, more sensitive queries related to abuse, violence, exploitation, and trafficking can be broached and should be done gently and nonjudgmentally.

Allowing the patient to set the pace can go a long way to building rapport and establishing trust. Individuals who are trafficked are constantly evaluating what and how much information to share with any given person at any given time. In the health care setting, trafficked patients are balancing the potential risks and benefits of disclosure through a wider lens view than is available to the practitioner. Their decisions take into account their understanding of the severity and legitimacy of threats made by the trafficker, their readiness logistically to undertake an attempt to leave the situation, and their degree of confidence in the health care system's ability to assist them. Thus patients' decisions to avoid certain threads of conversation, withhold information, and decline printed material should be respected. For the emergency practitioner, creating a safe space for victims and survivors of interpersonal violence entails validating not only their traumatic experiences and the impact of trauma, but also honoring their decision-making and autonomy even when their course of action may be difficult to understand and accept.

RESPONSE TO HUMAN TRAFFICKING

How emergency practitioners respond to an unconfirmed or confirmed suspicion of human trafficking assessment can be a defining moment for the patient and may have long-term implications for future engagement with health care.

Responding to a Nondisclosure

The notion that all trafficked patients want and will accept assistance is predicated on the myopic assumption that all trafficked persons (1) view themselves as "victims" in need of help and (2) believe that disclosing the circumstances of their situation will automatically lead to guaranteed safety and exit. There are many reasons why a victim of human trafficking may choose to withhold information and forego assistance, and these may include fear of deportation, fear of retaliation by the trafficker, credible threats made against loved ones, concerns over an implanted hearing device, and concerns that the emergency practitioner would not be able to keep them safe or assist them.

The spur-of-the-moment calculation that trafficked persons must make when asked if someone is hurting them or compelling them to work under the threat of harm is further complicated by guilt, fear, shame, and in some cases, trauma bonds toward their traffickers. Even with patients in whom there is a high suspicion of being trafficked, emergency practitioners must respect the patient's decision not to disclose their situation and refrain from aggressive attempts to obtain a disclosure. Emergency practitioners can instead focus on addressing any immediate safety concerns and offering information about local social service resources to address their needs. Emergency practitioners should convey an open door by assuring the patient that they can return for assistance if ever their situation takes a turn for the worse or they experience any form of abuse or violence.

Responding to a Disclosure

First and foremost, the emergency practitioner should recognize the sheer magnitude of such an outcome. Eliciting a disclosure of human trafficking is no easy feat—remember that the patient has just entrusted a stranger with consequential information. By the same token, the patient has placed their trust and hopes for change in an emergency practitioner who will need to respond confidently and decisively.

Reassurance

Following disclosure, the patient may experience a moment of panic when they realize there is no way to put the information revealed back in the box. Although they certainly retain control over the next steps, notwithstanding cases in which mandatory reporting laws apply, they may fear having set into motion a cascade of events from which there is no going back and over which they will have no control. It is critical for the practitioner at this point to thank the patient for trusting them with such personal information, followed by reassurance that they are still in control of their trajectory and that nothing will happen without their consent.

Clinical Reassessment

If the suspicion of human trafficking is confirmed, the emergency practitioner must consider the possibility of missed diagnoses. In the case of physical trauma, a patient may have initially provided an alternative explanation about the mechanism of the injury, and it would be important for practitioners to revisit the trauma and develop a full understanding of the range of possible injuries, including strangulation and sexual assault. In addition, screening and treatment for STIs such as chlamydia, gonorrhea, syphilis, viral hepatitis, and human immunodeficiency virus may be indicated and should be pursued with the patient's consent. Emergency contraception to prevent pregnancy may also be indicated.

Mandatory Reporting

Although human trafficking may not be a reportable event, special circumstances or components of the trafficking situation may be reportable to authorities depending on state statutes. For example, trafficking that involves the physical or sexual abuse of a minor (≤18 years of age) would be a reportable event under child maltreatment statutes. Burns, firearm injuries, sexual assault, and strangulation are examples of events that may be reportable in certain states. Some cases of human trafficking can resemble domestic violence on the surface and may end up being reported as such in states where domestic violence is a reportable event.

When mandated reporting laws apply, and especially if outside authorities need to become involved, emergency practitioners will need to communicate this information to patients with the utmost sensitivity and provide patients with an overview of what to expect. An open and honest discussion that, to the extent possible, offers options, is critical to preserving the patient's sense of autonomy and control. Emergency practitioners can approach decisions about the sequence and timing of the next steps in concert with the patient as a means of strengthening rapport, preserving trust, and conveying genuine concern. Consulting a hospital-based child protection team or social worker can help ensure that a health professional with the skills and training to guide the process is intimately involved at each step of the intervention from start to finish.

Law Enforcement

In some states, mandated reporting laws may require the involvement of LE. Practitioners should be aware that trafficked persons may be fearful of LE officers due to fear of arrest or deportation, previous arrests, and perceptions of LE as complicit in their trafficking. Emergency practitioners can help minimize retraumatization by ensuring a transparent and predictable process, and requesting that LE officers do the same, for the sake of the patient's sense of control and safety. Outside of mandated reporting protocols, the involvement of LE should be limited to explicit patient requests and situations of imminent life-threatening danger to the patient or staff.

Social Assessment

Survivors of human trafficking can access the National Human Trafficking Hotline 24/7 by texting "INFO" or "HELP" to BeFree (233733) or calling 1-888-373-7888 to request immediate assistance or information about local antitrafficking resources. Emergency practitioners can offer the patient access to a phone in a private space to place the call or help the patient memorize the phone number for future reference. Pointing out that the hotline number spells 1-888-ER-ER-888 may help individuals recall the number. Emergency practitioners and social workers in the ED are encouraged to familiarize themselves with any available resources for human trafficking survivors in their communities or contact the National Human Trafficking Hotline for a current list of resources in their region.

In addition to assisting in cases of mandatory reporting, social workers have the knowledge and expertise to perform a danger assessment, engage the patient in safety planning, and secure the resources needed for a safe ED discharge (e.g., emergency shelter). A danger assessment may help to identify situations of imminent life-threatening danger by exploring the frequency and severity of physical assaults, the use or possession of certain weapons, and any new or escalating threats or erratic behavior. By mentally practicing a step-by-step plan for executing a run for safety and creating a list of essentials (e.g., identification documents, prepaid phone, cash), safety planning can be of great benefit to the patient in a moment of escalating violence. Finally, social workers can place warm referrals by directly contacting a resource service on behalf of a patient to advocate for urgent or special attention to specific needs.

Disposition

In some cases, unresolved security concerns may preclude a safe ED discharge and require admission until they are properly addressed, especially in the case of minors or persons with disabilities. Safe discharges are critical to the physical safety of patients experiencing trafficking who have requested assistance leaving their situation.

Resources

- National Human Trafficking Hotline: 888-373-7888 toll-free hotline operated by Polaris with support from the US Department of Health and Human Services. https://humantraffickinghotline.org/en.
- SOAR Training: Health professional training administered by the Office of Trafficking in Persons at the US Department of Health and Human Services, through the National Human Trafficking Training and Technical Assistance Center. https://www.acf.hhs.gov/otip/training/soar-health-and-wellness-training.
- HEAL Trafficking: Network of multidisciplinary professionals dedicated to ending human trafficking and supporting survivors from a health perspective. https://healtrafficking.org/.
- National Center for Missing and Exploited Children (NCMEC): Provides services, resources, training, and technical assistance focused on assisting child victims of abduction and sexual exploitation and serving families and professionals. Hotline: 800-843-5678. https://missingkids.com/home.

REFERENCES ARE AVAILABLE AT Elsevier eBooks+

APPENDIX 1

Commonly Used Formulas and Calculations

Zlatan Coralic and Diane Birnbaumer

INTRODUCTION

This Appendix presents a list of calculations commonly used by emergency physicians and clinicians. It is not all-inclusive and purposely does not include decision tools or scales that do not require algebraic calculations. Many of these equations can be found in online calculators on websites such as https://www.mdcalc.com or http://reference.medscape.com/guide/medical-calculators.

GENERAL CALCULATIONS

English-to-Metric Conversions, Fahrenheit-to-Celsius Conversions

It is vital to pay careful attention to whether numbers are reported in English or metric measures to assure appropriate interpretation of this information and to deliver care such as medication doses. Please see Table A1.1 for conversion factors and simple examples.

Ideal Body Weight

Ideal body weight (IBW) is used in many applications including mechanical ventilator settings, drug dosing, and renal function measurement. Many equations have been described but the Devine formula is the most widely used. This formula, however, cannot be used for patients less than 5 feet (60 in) tall.

$$\text{IBW (male)} = 50 \text{ kg} + [2.3 \times (\text{height (in)} - 60)]$$
$$\text{IBW (female)} = 45.5 \text{ kg} + [2.3 \times (\text{height (in)} - 60)]$$

TABLE A1.1 Standard-to-Metric Calculations

Fahrenheit to Celsius °C = (°F – 32)/1.8	A patient's temperature is 100.4°F" (100.4°F – 32)/1.8 = 38°C
Pounds to kilograms kg = lb/2.2	A patient reports his weight to be 154 lb" 154 lb/2.2 = 70 kg
Inches to centimeters cm = inches × 2.54	The patient's height is 72 inches" 72 inches × 2.54 = 182.9 cm
Fluid ounces to milliliters mL = oz × 30	The child drinks 4 oz of formula at a sitting" 4 oz × 30 = 120 mL

CARDIOPULMONARY

Mean Arterial Pressure

Calculation of mean arterial pressure (MAP) provides a weighted average of systolic blood pressure (SBP) and diastolic blood pressure (DBP). It is a determination of tissue perfusion pressure and is normally 70 to 100 mm Hg in adults. To determine MAP:

$$\text{MAP} = \left[\text{SBP} + (2 \times \text{DBP})\right]/3$$

Example: A hypertensive emergency is diagnosed in an older, hypertensive patient. Current recommendations are to reduce MAP by 10% to 20% in the first hour. The patient's blood pressure is 240/120. To calculate the current MAP:

$$\text{MAP} = \left[240 + (2 \times 120)\right]/3 = 160 \text{ mm Hg}$$

QT AND QTC INTERVALS

The QT interval on the electrocardiogram (ECG) represents the period of ventricular electrical activity from activation to repolarization. The most important determinant of the QT interval is the heart rate. As the heart rate increases, the QT interval shortens. Many ECG machines calculate this; however, the presence of U waves or other ECG abnormalities can result in inappropriate readings. To calculate the rate-corrected QT interval (QTc) using Bazett's formula, divide the QT interval by the square root of the R-R interval (the interval between the R wave on two consecutive QRS complexes). The R-R interval may be measured from the ECG or calculated as 60 divided by the heart rate (in beats/min). The interval is represented in seconds or milliseconds:

$$\text{QTc} = \text{QT} / \sqrt{(\text{R} - \text{R})}$$

The QTc is normally less than 0.46 second in males and 0.44 second in females. This may be calculated online at: http://www.medical-calculator.nl/calculator/QTc/. The QTc is also reported on most ECGs.

Table A1.2 shows the normal range of the QT interval in adults.

Example: A 21-year-old male ingested a large quantity of amitriptyline (tricyclic antidepressant) tablets. His ECG revealed a QT interval of 0.37 second and a heart rate of 120 beats/min. The QTc is calculated as:

$$\text{R} - \text{R interval} = 60/120 = 0.50$$
$$\text{QTc} = 0.37/\sqrt{0.5} = 0.523 = 523 \text{ ms}$$

The patient's QTc is significantly prolonged for his heart rate and indicates significant cardiac effects from overdose of a tricyclic antidepressant.

TABLE A1.2 Normal Range of the QT Interval in Adults

HEART RATE (beats/min)	NORMAL QT RANGE (s)
40	0.42–0.53
50	0.37–0.48
60	0.34–0.44
70	0.31–0.41
80	0.29–0.38
90	0.28–0.36
100	0.27–0.34
110	0.25–0.32
120	0.24–0.31
130	0.23–0.30
140	0.22–0.29
150	0.21–0.28

PREDICTED PEAK EXPIRATORY FLOW RATE

The peak expiratory flow rate (PEFR), measured in liters per minute, is a useful means of assessing airway obstruction. It is measured by having a patient exhale maximally through a peak-flow meter. Normal values range from 350 to 600 L/min. Comparison between the initial and post-treatment PEFR in patients with exacerbations of asthma helps determine the degree of severity. Patients with an initial PEFR of less than 20% of predicted or with a subsequent value of less than 60% of predicted after initial therapy may require further evaluation, treatment, or both.

Many patients monitor PEFR on themselves and are able to state a personal best, which is the preferred standard for that individual. Other patients may be monitored with an estimated PEFR. Estimations are based primarily on a patient's sex, age, and height. Although graphs and tables are available to provide values across a range of ages and heights, the PEFR can also be approximated by using the following formulas:

$$\text{Adults}: \text{PEFR} = 13 \times (\text{height (in)} - 40) + 110$$

$$\text{Female children / adolescents}$$
$$\text{PEFR} = \text{height (m)} \times 5.5 - \text{age} \times 0.03 - 1.11$$

$$\text{Male children / adolescents}:$$
$$\text{PEFR} = \text{height (m)} \times 6.14 - \text{age} \times 10.043 + 0.15$$

These may also be found online in many places including: http://www.mdcalc.com/estimatedexpected-peak-expiratory-flow-peak-flow/.

NEUROLOGY

Glasgow Coma Scale

For head-injured patients, the Glasgow Coma Scale (GCS) is a frequently referenced assessment of neurologic function. It is calculated by using the best result of neurologic testing of eye opening, motor function, and verbal function. Each of the three subscores is determined by using verbal and painful stimuli. Point assessments are listed in Table A1.3, with adjustments noted for pediatric patients. Points are given for the best response observed for each category. For example, a person with right-sided motor deficits but otherwise normal function would have a normal GCS score because left-sided function is normal. Scores of 13 to 15 correlate with mild brain injury, 9 to 12 with moderate brain injury, and 3 to 8 with severe brain injury.

TABLE A1.3 Glasgow Coma Scale Score (Adults/Children <5 years When Different)

POINTS	BEST EYE RESPONSE	BEST VERBAL RESPONSE	BEST MOTOR RESPONSE
1	No eye opening	No verbal response	No motor response
2	Opens eyes to pain	Incomprehensible/moans to pain	Extension to pain
3	Opens eyes to command/opens eyes to verbal cues	Inappropriate words/cries to pain	Flexion to pain
4	Spontaneous eye opening	Confused/decreased verbal ability, irritable crying	Withdrawal from pain
5	—	Orientated/age-appropriate speech or cooing	Localizes pain/localizes pain or withdraws from touch
6	—	—	Obeys commands/normal spontaneous movements

Example: An intoxicated male is involved in a motor vehicle crash and is brought to the emergency department (ED). He opens his eyes only to painful stimuli, is muttering incomprehensibly, and localizes pain on the left and withdraws from pain on the right. What is his GCS score, and what severity of injury does this score represent?

$$\text{GCS} = \text{eye opening} + \text{verbal response} + \text{motor response}$$

$$\text{Eye opening to pain} = 2 \text{ points}$$

$$\text{Incomprehensible sounds} = 2 \text{ points}$$

Localizing pain is 5 points and withdrawal from pain is 4 points. The better score is used.

$$2 + 2 + 5 = 9 \text{ points}$$

National Institutes of Health Stroke Score

The full National Institutes of Health (NIH) stroke scale is shown in Table A1.4.

The scale includes directions for patient assessment, as well as recommended adjustments for special situations that might impair the ability of the patient to respond to the assessor. Training scenarios and the NIH Stroke Scale can be found at http://www.nihstrokescale.org/.

The scale itself, in unedited format, is presented in Table A1.4.

Scores range from 0 (normal neurologic function) to 34 (maximal injury). Use of thrombolytics has been suggested for patients with scores between 8 and 26 who have no contraindications and can receive the intervention within a specified time of onset; for many sites the time of onset should be within 3 hours.

Example: A 74-year-old, left-handed female arrives at the ED 90 minutes after the onset of left-sided arm and leg weakness. She has no headache. By 2 hours from symptom onset, she has confirmed normal findings on head CT and does not have contraindications to thrombolytics. Her symptoms have not changed in any way since onset. Using the NIH Stroke Scale, she is determined to have the following findings. On cognitive

TABLE A1.4 National Institutes of Health Stroke Scale

Administer stroke scale items in the order listed. Record performance in each category after each subscale examination. Do not go back and change scores. Follow the directions provided for each examination technique. Scores should reflect what the patient does, not what the clinician thinks that the patient can do. The clinician should record answers while administering the examination and work quickly. Except when indicated, the patient should not be coached (i.e., repeated requests to patient to make a special effort). If any item is left untested, a detailed explanation must be clearly written on the form. All untested items will be reviewed by the medical monitor and discussed with the examiner by telephone.

Instructions	Scale Definition
1a. *Level of Consciousness (LOC):* The investigator must choose a response, even if a full evaluation is prevented by obstacles such as an endotracheal tube, language barrier, or orotracheal trauma or bandages. A 3 is scored only if the patient makes no movement (other than reflexive posturing) in response to noxious stimulation.	0 = Alert; keenly responsive 1 = Not alert but arousable by minor stimulation to obey, answer, or respond 2 = Not alert, requires repeated stimulation to attend, or is obtunded and requires strong or painful stimulation to make movements (not stereotyped) 3 = Responds only with reflex motor or autonomic effects or is totally unresponsive, flaccid, areflexic
1b. *LOC Questions:* The patient is asked the month and his or her age. The answer must be correct—there is no partial credit for being close. Aphasic and stuporous patients who do not comprehend the questions will score 2. Patients unable to speak because of endotracheal intubation, orotracheal trauma, severe dysarthria from any cause, language barrier, or any other problem not secondary to aphasia are given a 1. It is important that only the initial answer be graded and that the examiner not "help" the patient with verbal or nonverbal cues.	0 = Answers both questions correctly 1 = Answers one question correctly 2 = Answers neither question correctly
1c. *LOC Commands:* The patient is asked to open and close the eyes and then to grip and release the nonparetic hand. Substitute another one-step command if the hands cannot be used. Credit is given if an unequivocal attempt is made but not completed because of weakness. If the patient does not respond to command, the task should be demonstrated (pantomime) and the result scored (i.e., follows none, one, or two commands). Patients with trauma, amputation, or other physical impediments should be given suitable one-step commands. Only the first attempt is scored.	0 = Performs both tasks correctly 1 = Performs one task correctly 2 = Performs neither task correctly

Continued

TABLE A1.4 National Institutes of Health Stroke Scale—cont'd

2. *Best Gaze:* Only horizontal eye movements will be tested. Voluntary or reflexive (oculocephalic) eye movements will be scored, but caloric testing is not done. If the patient has a conjugate deviation of the eyes that can be overcome by voluntary or reflexive activity, the score will be 1. If a patient has an isolated peripheral nerve paresis (cranial nerve III, IV, or VI), score a 1. Gaze is testable in all aphasic patients. Patients with ocular trauma, bandages, preexisting blindness, or other disorders of visual acuity or fields should be tested with reflexive movements and a choice made by the investigator. Establishing eye contact and then moving about the patient from side to side will occasionally clarify the presence of a partial gaze palsy.	0 = Normal 1 = Partial gaze palsy. This score is given when gaze is abnormal in one or both eyes but forced deviation or total gaze paresis is not present 2 = Forced deviation or total gaze paresis not overcome by the oculocephalic maneuver
3. *Visual:* Visual fields (upper and lower quadrants) are tested by confrontation, with finger counting or by visual threat used as appropriate. Patient must be encouraged, but if they look at the side of the moving fingers appropriately, this can be scored as normal. If there is unilateral blindness or enucleation, visual fields in the remaining eye are scored. Score 1 only if a clear-cut asymmetry, including quadrantanopia, is found. If the patient is blind from any cause, score 3. Double simultaneous stimulation is performed at this point. If there is extinction present, the patient receives a 1 and the results are used to answer question 11.	0 = No visual loss 1 = Partial hemianopia 2 = Complete hemianopia 3 = Bilateral hemianopia (blind, including cortical blindness)
4. *Facial Palsy:* Ask or use pantomime to encourage the patient to show his or her teeth or raise the eyebrows and close the eyes. Score the symmetry of grimace in response to noxious stimuli in a poorly responsive or noncomprehending patient. If facial trauma, bandages, an orotracheal tube, tape, or other physical barrier obscures the face, these impediments should be removed to the extent possible.	0 = Normal symmetric movement 1 = Minor paralysis (flattened nasolabial fold, asymmetry on smiling) 2 = Partial paralysis (total or nearly total paralysis of the lower part of the face) 3 = Complete paralysis of one or both sides (absence of facial movement in the upper and lower parts of the face)
5 and 6. *Motor Arm and Leg:* The limb is placed in the appropriate position: extend the arms (palms down) 90 degrees (if sitting) or 45 degrees (if supine) and the leg 30 degrees (always tested supine). Drift is scored if the arm falls before 10 seconds or the leg before 5 seconds. An aphasic patient is encouraged by using urgency in the voice and pantomime, but not noxious stimulation. Each limb is tested in turn, beginning with the nonparetic arm. Only in the case of amputation or joint fusion at the shoulder or hip may the score be "9," and the examiner must clearly write the explanation for scoring as a "9."	0 = No drift; the limb holds 90 (or 45) degrees for a full 10 seconds 1 = Drift; the limb holds 90 (or 45) degrees but drifts down before a full 10 seconds; does not hit the bed or other support 2 = Some effort against gravity; the limb cannot get to or maintain (if cued) 90 (or 45) degrees, drifts down to the bed, but has some effort against gravity 3 = No effort against gravity; the limb falls 4 = No movement 9 = Amputation, joint fusion; explain 5a. Left Arm 5b. Right Arm 0 = No drift; the leg holds a 30-degree position for a full 5 seconds 1 = Drift; the leg falls by the end of the 5-second period but does not hit the bed 2 = Some effort against gravity; the leg falls to the bed by 5 seconds but has some effort against gravity 3 = No effort against gravity; the leg falls to the bed immediately 4 = No movement 9 = Amputation, joint fusion; explain 6a. Left Leg 6b. Right Leg

TABLE A1.4 National Institutes of Health Stroke Scale—cont'd

7. *Limb Ataxia:* This item is aimed at finding evidence of a unilateral cerebellar lesion. Test with the eyes open. In case of a visual defect, ensure that testing is done in the intact visual field. The finger-nose-finger and heel-shin tests are performed on both sides, and ataxia is scored only if present out of proportion to weakness. Ataxia is absent in a patient who cannot understand or is paralyzed. Only in the case of amputation or joint fusion may the item be scored "9," and the examiner must clearly write the explanation for not scoring. In the case of blindness, test by touching the nose from an extended arm position.	0 = Absent 1 = Present in one limb 2 = Present in two limbs. If present, is ataxia in the
	Right arm: 1 = Yes, 2 = No 9 = Amputation or joint fusion; explain
	Left arm: 1 = Yes, 2 = No 9 = Amputation or joint fusion; explain
	Right leg: 1 = Yes, 2 = No 9 = Amputation or joint fusion; explain
	Left leg: 1 = Yes, 2 = No 9 = Amputation or joint fusion; explain
8. *Sensory:* Sensation or grimace in response to a pinprick when tested or withdrawal from a noxious stimulus in an obtunded or aphasic patient. Only sensory loss attributed to stroke is scored as abnormal, and the examiner should test as many body areas (arms [not hands], legs, trunk, face) as needed to accurately check for hemisensory loss. A score of 2, "severe or total," should be given only when severe or total loss of sensation can be clearly demonstrated. Stuporous and aphasic patients will therefore probably score 1 or 0. A patient with a brain stem stroke who has bilateral loss of sensation is scored 2. If the patient does not respond and is quadriplegic, score 2. Patients in coma (item 1a = 3) are arbitrarily given a 2 on this item.	d = Normal; no sensory loss 1 = Mild to moderate sensory loss; the patient feels that a pinprick is less sharp or dull on the affected side or there is a loss of superficial pain with pinprick but the patient is aware of being touched 2 = Severe to total sensory loss; the patient is not aware of being touched on the face, arm, and leg
9. *Best Language:* A great deal of information about comprehension will be obtained during the preceding sections of the examination. The patient is asked to describe what is happening in the attached picture, to name the items on the attached naming sheet, and to read from the attached list of sentences. Comprehension is judged from responses here, as well as to all the commands in the preceding general neurologic examination. If visual loss interferes with the tests, ask the patient to identify objects placed in the hand, repeat, and produce speech. An intubated patient should be asked to write. A patient in coma (question 1a = 3) will arbitrarily score 3 on this item. The examiner must choose a score in a patient with stupor or limited cooperation, but a score of 3 should be used only if the patient is mute and follows no one-step commands.	0 = No aphasia; normal 1 = Mild to moderate aphasia; some obvious loss of fluency or facility of comprehension, without significant limitation in ideas expressed or form of expression. Reduction in speech and/or comprehension, however, makes conversation about the material provided difficult or impossible. For example, in conversation about the materials provided, the examiner can identify a picture or naming card from the patient's response. 2 = Severe aphasia; all communication is through fragmentary expression; great need for inference, questioning, and guessing by the listener. The range of information that can be exchanged is limited; the listener carries the burden of communication. The examiner cannot identify materials provided from the patient's response. 3 = Mute, global aphasia; no usable speech or auditory comprehension
10. *Dysarthria:* If the patient is thought to be normal, an adequate sample of speech must be obtained by asking the patient to read or repeat words from the attached list. If the patient has severe aphasia, the clarity of articulation of spontaneous speech can be rated. Only if the patient is intubated or has another physical barrier to producing speech may the item be scored "9," and the examiner must clearly write an explanation for not scoring. Do not tell the patient why he or she is being tested.	0 = Normal 1 = Mild to moderate; the patient slurs at least some words and, at worst, can be understood with some difficulty 2 = Severe; the patient's speech is so slurred that it is unintelligible in the absence of or out of proportion to any dysphasia or is mute or anarthric 9 = Intubated or other physical barrier; explain

Continued

TABLE A1.4 National Institutes of Health Stroke Scale—cont'd

11. *Extinction and Inattention (Formerly Neglect):* Sufficient information to identify neglect may be obtained during the prior testing. If the patient has a severe visual loss preventing visual double simultaneous stimulation and the cutaneous stimuli are normal, the score is normal. If the patient has aphasia but does appear to attend to both sides, the score is normal. The presence of visual spatial neglect or anosognosia may also be taken as evidence of abnormality. As the abnormality is scored only if present, the item is never untestable. This is an additional item, not a part of the NIH Stroke Scale score.	0 = No abnormality 1 = Visual, tactile, auditory, spatial, or personal inattention or extinction to bilateral simultaneous stimulation in one of the sensory modalities 2 = Profound hemi-inattention or hemi-inattention to more than one modality. Does not recognize own hand or orients to only one side of space
A. *Distal Motor Function:* The patient's hand is held up at the forearm by the examiner and the patient is asked to extend the fingers as much as possible. If the patient cannot or does not extend the fingers, the examiner places the fingers in full extension and observes for any flexion movement for 5 seconds. The patient's first attempts only are graded. Repetition of the instructions or of the testing is prohibited.	0 = Normal (no flexion after 5 seconds) 1 = At least some extension after 5 seconds, but not fully extended. Any movement of the fingers that is not command is not scored 2 = No voluntary extension after 5 seconds. Movements of the fingers at another time are not scored a. Left Arm b. Right Arm

NIH, National Institutes of Health.

testing she is keenly responsive (0 points), knows her age and the current month (0 points), and can follow two-step commands with the unaffected side (0 points). She has a partial gaze palsy without forced deviation (1 point); partial hemianopia (1 point); unilateral, complete paralysis of her face (3 points); no drift on her right arm (0 points); no movement of her left arm (4 points); no drift on her right leg (0 points); and some effort of her left leg against gravity, although it falls to the bed within 2 seconds of elevation (2 points). She has no ataxia (0 points). Her sensation to pinprick is decreased, although she is aware of the testing (1 point). She has a mild expressive aphasia but is easily comprehensible (1 point), has some slurring of words but is still comprehensible (1 point), and exhibits no evidence of neglect (0 points). Her total NIH score is 14, and as a result she may be a candidate for thrombolytic therapy.

LABORATORY

Absolute Neutrophil Count

The absolute neutrophil count (ANC) is the total number of neutrophils in the blood, both mature and immature. The value represents the actual number of neutrophils as compared to a percentage of white blood cells (WBCs). It can be an important measure in an immunocompromised patient as it can help to assess a patient's risk for developing opportunistic infections and guide treatment. Immunocompromised patients who are neutropenic and present with fever are at high risk of developing sepsis. It is calculated as:

$$\text{ANC} = [(\%\ \text{neutrophils} + \%\ \text{bands})\ /\ 100] \times \text{WBC count}$$

Normal: >1500 cells/μL
Mild neutropenia: 1000 to 1500 cells/μL
Moderate neutropenia: 500 to 1000 cells/μL
Severe neutropenia: <500 cells/μL

WHITE BLOOD CELL CORRECTION IN CEREBROSPINAL FLUID

When performing a lumbar puncture (LP) on a patient to evaluate for meningitis, the number of WBCs in the cerebrospinal fluid (CSF) is an important value for diagnosis. However, a traumatic LP can falsely elevate this value. A formula using the WBCs and red blood cells (RBCs) in CSF and in blood can correct the WBCs in CSF. The normal value for WBCs and RBCs in CSF is <5 cells/μL. All values are in cells/μL except RBCs in blood, which is cells $\times 10^6$/μL.

$$\text{Adjusted WBC}_{\text{CSF}} = \text{WBC}_{\text{CSF}} - [(\text{WBC}_{\text{blood}} \times \text{RBC}_{\text{CSF}} / (\text{RBC}_{\text{blood}} \times 10^6)]$$

Example: A 25-year-old male presents with fever, sore throat, and headache. Meningitis is suspected. His blood shows elevated WBC at 15,000 cells/μL. An LP is completed and results show elevated WBCs of 25 cells/μL. The rest of his CSF values are unremarkable. His RBC in blood is 5 × 10^6/μL.

$$\text{Adjusted WBC in CSF} = 25 - \left[(15,000 \times 7000)\ /\ 5 \times 10^6\right]$$

$$\text{Adjusted WBC in CSF} = 4\ \text{cells}\ /\ \mu\text{L}$$

His WBCs in CSF are actually within normal range and the elevation is likely due to a traumatic LP.

RENAL FUNCTION

Creatinine clearance (Cr_{Cl}) occasionally needs to be calculated by emergency physicians to risk-stratify patients undergoing imaging studies requiring intravenous (IV) contrast material, as well as to determine the severity of renal failure in patients without a known baseline. Cr_{Cl} is best calculated from a collection of urine over a 24-hour period. However, if the patient's Cr_{Cl} is in steady state (i.e., without recent change), it is possible to estimate Cr_{Cl} by using a formula that incorporates serum creatinine (S_{Cr}) in mg/dL, lean body weight (LBW) in kg, age in years, and gender:

$$Cr_{Cl}\ (\text{males}) = [(140 - \text{age}) \times (\text{LBW})] / [72 \times S_{Cr}]$$
$$Cr_{Cl}\ (\text{females}) = 0.85 \times [(140 - \text{age}) \times \text{LBW}] / [72 \times S_{Cr}]$$

Normal values: 74 to 160 mL/min.
Mild renal impairment: 40 to 60 mL/min.
Moderate renal impairment: 15 to 40 mL/min.
Severe renal impairment: <15 mL/min (indication for renal dialysis).

The following examples illustrate the importance of calculating Cr_{Cl}:
Example 1: A 71-year-old female needs a medication whose dose is adjusted based on renal function, so the clinician needs to know her Cr_{Cl} to determine the correct dose. The patient's S_{Cr} is 1.4 mg/dL and she weighs 55 kg. To calculate her Cr_{Cl}:

$$Cr_{Cl}\,(\text{females}) = 0.85 \times \left[(140 - 71) \times (55\,\text{kg}) / (72 \times 1.4)\right]$$
$$= 32.0\ \text{mL/min}$$

The patient has moderate renal impairment.
Example 2: A 21-year-old male needs a medication whose dose is adjusted based on renal function, so the clinician needs to know his Cr_{Cl} to determine the correct dose. The patient's S_{Cr} is 1.4 mg/dL, and he has an LBW of 100 kg. To calculate his Cr_{Cl}:

$$Cr_{Cl}\ (\text{males}) = (140 - 21) \times (100\ \text{kg}) / (72 \times 1.4)$$
$$= 118\,\text{mL/min}$$

The patient has adequate Cr_{Cl}. Note that despite an identical serum creatinine level, the second patient has normal renal function, whereas the first has renal insufficiency.

FRACTIONAL EXCRETION OF SODIUM

Acute kidney injury (AKI) can have many etiologies. Calculating the fractional excretion of sodium (FE_{Na}) can help to differentiate prerenal disease, intrinsic renal disease, and postrenal disease. The calculation measures the percent of filtered sodium that is excreted in the urine. Low values of FE_{Na}, less than 1%, in the setting of AKI suggests a prerenal etiology as the kidneys are appropriately retaining sodium in response to decreased perfusion. Higher values of FE_{Na}, greater than 2%, suggests an intrinsic etiology of AKI. The higher values can be caused by either salt wasting by damaged nephrons or an appropriate response by remaining nephrons to volume expansion. FE_{Na} greater than 4% can be suggestive of a postrenal cause of AKI. To calculate FE_{Na} a serum creatinine (S_{Cr}), serum sodium (S_{Na}), urine creatinine (U_{Cr}), and urine sodium (U_{Na}) need to be measured.

$$FE_{Na} = (S_{Cr} \times U_{Na}) / (S_{Na} \times U_{Cr}) \times 100$$

Example: A 65-year-old previously healthy male had a syncopal episode while working outside on a hot day. He was found to have AKI with an S_{Cr} of 2.0 mg/dL. His S_{Na} is 150 mEq/L, U_{Na} is 18 mEq/L, and U_{Cr} is 30 mg/dL.

$$FE_{Na} = (2.0 \times 18) / (150 \times 30) \times 100$$
$$FE_{Na} = 0.8\,\%$$

The patient's FE_{Na} is less than 1%, which suggests a prerenal cause, likely hypovolemia.

SODIUM DEFICIT

The following formula may be used to calculate the Na^+ deficit in hyponatremia:

$$Na^+\ \text{deficit}\ (\text{males}) = 60\% \times \text{weight}\ (\text{kg}) \times \left(\text{desired}\ Na^+ - \text{measured}\ Na^+\right)$$

$$Na^+\ \text{deficit}\ (\text{females}) = 50\% \times \text{weight}\ (\text{kg}) \times \left(\text{desired}\ Na^+ - \text{measured}\ Na^+\right)$$

Symptoms related to hyponatremia are variable, and the severity of symptoms should guide therapy. Sodium replacement is most commonly given as isotonic saline, which contains 154 mmol of Na^+/L. Patients who are severely symptomatic may require 3% saline solution, which contains 513 mmol of Na^+/L. The volume of solution needed to replace the Na^+ deficit (in mmol) can be calculated by using the concentrations in the saline solutions listed earlier.
Example: A young male is seizing on arrival at the ED. He is known to have schizophrenia and compulsive water drinking. His Na^+ is 116 mmol/L. He weighs 65 kg. To determine his sodium deficit:

$$Na^+\ \text{deficit} = 0.6 \times 65\ \text{kg} \times (140 - 116) = 936\ \text{mmol of}\ Na^+$$

This amount of Na^+ deficit can be corrected by administering approximately 6 L of isotonic saline or 1.8 L of hypertonic saline. Na^+ should be replaced very slowly to avoid the possibility of inducing central pontine myelinolysis, which results from overaggressive correction of sodium. Most recommendations state a rise in serum sodium of 4 to 6 mmol/L in a 24-hour period is ideal.

Calculate sodium deficit and replacement rate online: http://www.mdcalc.com/sodium-correction-rate-in-hyponatremia/.

CORRECTED SERUM SODIUM

Factitious hyponatremia may be due to hyperglycemia. In this hyperosmolal state, glucose tends to stay in extracellular fluid and draws water out of cells into extracellular fluid. Serum sodium is decreased by approximately 1.6 mmol/L for each 100 mg/dL of excess glucose. To calculate the corrected sodium:

$$\text{Corrected}\ Na^+\,(\text{mmol/L}) = \text{measured}\ Na^+\,(\text{mmol/L}) + \left[0.016 \times \left(\text{glucose}\,(\text{mg/dL}) - 100\right)\right]$$

Many laboratories automatically make this adjustment, so it is important to check with your laboratory to determine the necessity for this correction.
Example: An obtunded older male appears dehydrated. His sodium level is 126 mmol/L and his glucose is 1000 mg/dL.

$$\text{Corrected}\ Na^+ = 126\ \text{mmol/L}\left[0.016 \times (1000 - 100)\right]$$
$$= 126 + 14.4 = 140.4\ \text{mmol/L}$$

His corrected Na^+ suggests that he has factitious hyponatremia because of hyperglycemia.

TOTAL BODY WATER DEFICIT

Elevation of the serum sodium concentration is proportionate to the free water deficit when volume is depleted. Because

60% of the adult body is water, the total-body free water deficit is calculated by using measured Na^+, desired Na^+, and body weight in kilograms. To calculate the free water deficit:

$$\text{Ideal total body water (TBW)} = 60\% \times \text{weight (kg)}$$

$$\text{TBW deficit} = \left[(\text{measured Na}^+ - \text{normal Na}^+)/\text{normal Na}^+\right] \times \text{TBW}$$

(assume normal Na^+ to be 140 mmol/L)

Example. An older male is brought to the ED in a coma. He has severe dehydration, his IBW is 70 kg, and his serum Na^+ level is 165 mmol/L. To determine his free water deficit:

$$\text{Ideal TBW} = 0.6 \times 70 \text{ kg} = 42 \text{ L}$$

$$\text{Free water deficit} = [(165 - 140)/140] \times 42 = 7.5 \text{ L}$$

In general, fluid correction for hypernatremia should take place over a 48- to 72-hour period to avoid the potential for cerebral edema.

Calculate free water deficit and fluid rate online: http://www.medcalc.com/sodium.html.

POTASSIUM LEVELS WHEN THE PH IS ABNORMAL

Serum potassium (K^+) levels change with acid-base status. In acidotic states, K^+ moves out of cells as H^+ moves in, thus raising serum K^+ levels. In alkalotic states, K^+ moves into cells as H^+ moves out, thus lowering serum K^+ levels. The change in K^+ varies inversely with pH at the following rates:

The serum K^+ concentration increases 0.6 mmol/L for each 0.1-unit decrease in pH.

The serum K^+ concentration decreases 0.6 mmol/L for each 0.1-unit increase in pH.

CORRECTED SERUM CALCIUM

Approximately 50% of serum calcium is bound to serum proteins (primarily albumin), 40% is in the free ionized state (the physiologically active form), and 10% is mixed with serum anions (phosphate, bicarbonate, citrate, and lactate). For this reason, serum calcium is lowered approximately 0.8 mg/dL for every decrease in albumin of 1 g/dL. To correct for decreased albumin (at levels <4 g/dL), the following formula can be used:

$$\text{Corrected Ca}^{2+}\ (\text{mg/dL}) = \text{serum Ca}^{2+}\ (\text{mg/dL}) + \left(0.8 \times \left[4.0 - \text{serum albumin}\ \{\text{g/dL}\}\right]\right)$$

Example: A malnourished male has a serum calcium level of 7.5 mg/dL and a serum albumin level of 2 g/dL. To calculate his corrected calcium level:

$$\text{Corrected Ca}^{2+}\ (\text{mg/dL}) = 7.5\ \text{mg/dL} + \left[0.8 \times (4.0 - 2.0\ \text{g/dL})\right] = 9.1$$

ANION GAP

The anion gap (AG) is an estimate of the amount of unmeasured negatively charged ions in serum that are not bicarbonate (HCO_3^-) and chloride (Cl^-). The AG is calculated by subtracting the sum of HCO_3^- and Cl^- values from sodium (Na^+), which is the major positive charge in serum. An elevated AG usually means that there is some unmeasured anion, toxin, or organic acid in the blood. Box A1.1 lists many substances that can cause an AG acidosis. The AG is normally 8 to 12 mmol/L:

BOX A1.1 Substances Associated with a High Anion Gap[a]

Aspirin
Methanol, metformin
Uremia
Diabetic ketoacidosis
Paraldehyde, phenformin
Isoniazid, iron
Lactate (multiple causes)
Ethylene glycol/propylene glycol (diluent)
Carbon monoxide, cyanide
Alcoholic ketoacidosis
Toluene

[a] *Follows the mnemonic A MUDPILE CAT.*

$$AG = Na^+ - (Cl^- + HCO_3^-) = 8 - 12\ \text{mmol/L}$$

Example: A suicidal young male drank an unknown amount of antifreeze. His electrolyte levels are Na^+, 144; K^+, 3.1; Cl^-, 108; and HCO_3^-, 14. The AG is calculated as follows:

$AG = [144 - (108 + 14)] = 22$ mmol/L. His AG is abnormally elevated presumably because of ingestion of ethylene glycol.

OSMOLAL GAP

Serum osmolality can be measured in the laboratory by freezing point depression. The measured serum osmolality is usually higher than the calculated osmolality, and the difference is termed the *osmolal gap* (OG). The OG is normally 5 to 10 mOsm/kg. If there is a higher gap, the osmols unaccounted for may represent methanol, ethylene glycol, isopropyl alcohol, or other solutes (Table A1.5). Large doses of medications such as lorazepam contain propylene glycol diluent that can raise the OG. To calculate serum osmolality (Osm_{calc}) and the OG:

$$Osm_{calc} = 2 \times Na^+ + [\text{BUN (mg/dL)}/2.8] + [\text{glucose (mg/dL)}/18]$$

$$OG = Osm_{meas} - Osm_{calc}$$

where BUN is the blood urea nitrogen.

Calculate online: https://www.healthcare.uiowa.edu/path_handbook/Appendix/Calculators/OsmoGap.html.

Table A1.5 shows the effect of some solutes on serum osmolality. The increase in osmolality caused by a solute can be calculated by dividing its serum concentration by the tabulated value.

Example: An intoxicated patient has serum chemistry results as follows: Na^+, 142; K^+, 4.5; Cl^-, 100; HCO_3^-, 22; glucose, 90; BUN, 14. His ethanol level is 240 mg/dL and his measured serum osmolality is 354. You want to know whether he has

TABLE A1.5 Effect of Some Solutes on Serum Osmolality

EACH mg/dL OF	INCREASES SERUM mOsm/kg BY	FOR EACH SERUM mOsm/kg INCREASE DUE TO	THE CORRESPONDING mg/dL CHANGE IS (≈ Mol Wt/10)
Methanol	0.31	Methanol	3.2
Ethanol	0.22	Ethanol	4.6
Acetone	0.17	Acetone	5.8
Isopropyl alcohol	0.17	Isopropyl alcohol	6.0
Ethylene glycol	0.16	Ethylene glycol	6.2
Glycerol	0.11	Glycerol	9.2
Mannitol	0.05	Mannitol	18.2

Modified from Kullig K, Duffy JP, Linden CH, etal. Toxic effects of methanol, ethylene glycol and isopropyl alcohol. *Top Emerg Med*. 1984;6(2):16.

ingested other osmotically active substances. His calculated serum osmolality is:

$$Osm_{calc} = 2 \times 142 + (14/2.8) + (90/18) = 294$$

To evaluate for the effect of ethanol on osmolality, refer to Table A1.5 and add the alcohol level divided by 4.6:

$$240/4.6 = 52$$

$$Osm_{calc} = 294 + 52 = 346$$

Finally, calculate the OG:

$$OG = Osm_{meas} - Osm_{calc} = 354 - 346 = 8$$

His elevated osmolality is explained by the ethanol.

ACID-BASE DISORDERS

A thorough understanding of blood gas interpretations is crucial for critically ill patients but is beyond the reach of this section. Unfortunately, most online calculators either struggle with mixed acid-base disorders or cannot handle different units (kPa vs. mm Hg).

By using the combination of an arterial blood gas (ABG) sample and serum electrolyte levels, a patient's acid-base status can be evaluated. A single acid-base disorder may be present as a primary disorder (respiratory acidosis, respiratory alkalosis, metabolic acidosis, or metabolic alkalosis), or several disorders may be present at the same time. When an acid-base disorder is present, the body will try to compensate to preserve the pH as close to normal as possible. The compensatory responses in relation to the primary disorder are as follows:

Primary Disorder	Compensatory Response
Metabolic acidosis	Increased ventilation
Metabolic alkalosis	Decreased ventilation
Respiratory acidosis	Increased renal reabsorption of HCO_3^- in the proximal tubule Increased renal excretion of H^+ in the distal tubule
Respiratory alkalosis	Decreased renal reabsorption of HCO_3^- in the proximal tubule Decreased renal excretion of H^+ in the distal tubule

TABLE A1.6 Acidosis and Compensatory Response

PRIMARY DISTURBANCE	PREDICTED COMPENSATORY RESPONSE
Metabolic acidosis	↓ in Pco_2 = 1.3 × ↓ in HCO_3^-
Metabolic alkalosis	↑ in Pco_2 = 0.6 × ↑ in HCO_3^-
Respiratory acidosis	*Acute:* For every Pco_2 ↑ of 10 mm Hg, HCO_3^- ↑ by 1 mmol/L *Chronic:* For every Pco_2 ↑ of 10 mm Hg, HCO_3^- ↑ by 4 mmol/L *Acute:* For every Pco_2 ↓ of 10 mm Hg, HCO_3^- ↓ by 2 mmol/L *Chronic:* For every Pco_2 ↓ of 10 mm Hg, HCO_3^- ↓ by 5 mmol/L

Modified from Rutecki GW, Whittier FC. Acid-base interpretation. *Consultant*. 1991;31:44–59.

When interpreting acid-base disorders, the following basic steps are suggested:

Knowledge of normal values:

Normal serum pH = 7.40
Normal partial pressure of carbon dioxide (Pco_2) = 40 mm Hg

First, determine the patient's pH status. Acid-base changes are either metabolic or respiratory. Simple disturbances are categorized by examining pH, Pco_2, and HCO_3^- (Table A1.6). If pH is less than normal (<7.35), the patient is acidemic. If pH is above normal (>7.45), the patient is alkalemic. If the patient is acidemic and Pco_2 is elevated (>45 mm Hg) as a primary disorder, respiratory acidosis is present. If the patient is alkalemic and Pco_2 is decreased (<35 mm Hg) as a primary disorder, respiratory alkalosis is present. If the patient is acidemic and the arterial HCO_3^- level is less than normal (<22 mEq/L) as a primary disorder, metabolic acidosis is present. If the patient is alkalotic and the HCO_3^- level is greater than normal (>26 mEq/L) as a primary disorder, metabolic alkalosis is present.

Acid-base homeostasis is normally maintained because a change in pH will usually trigger a compensatory change to minimize the change in pH, although the compensation is never complete. The degree and timing of compensation are determined by the primary disturbance itself and by

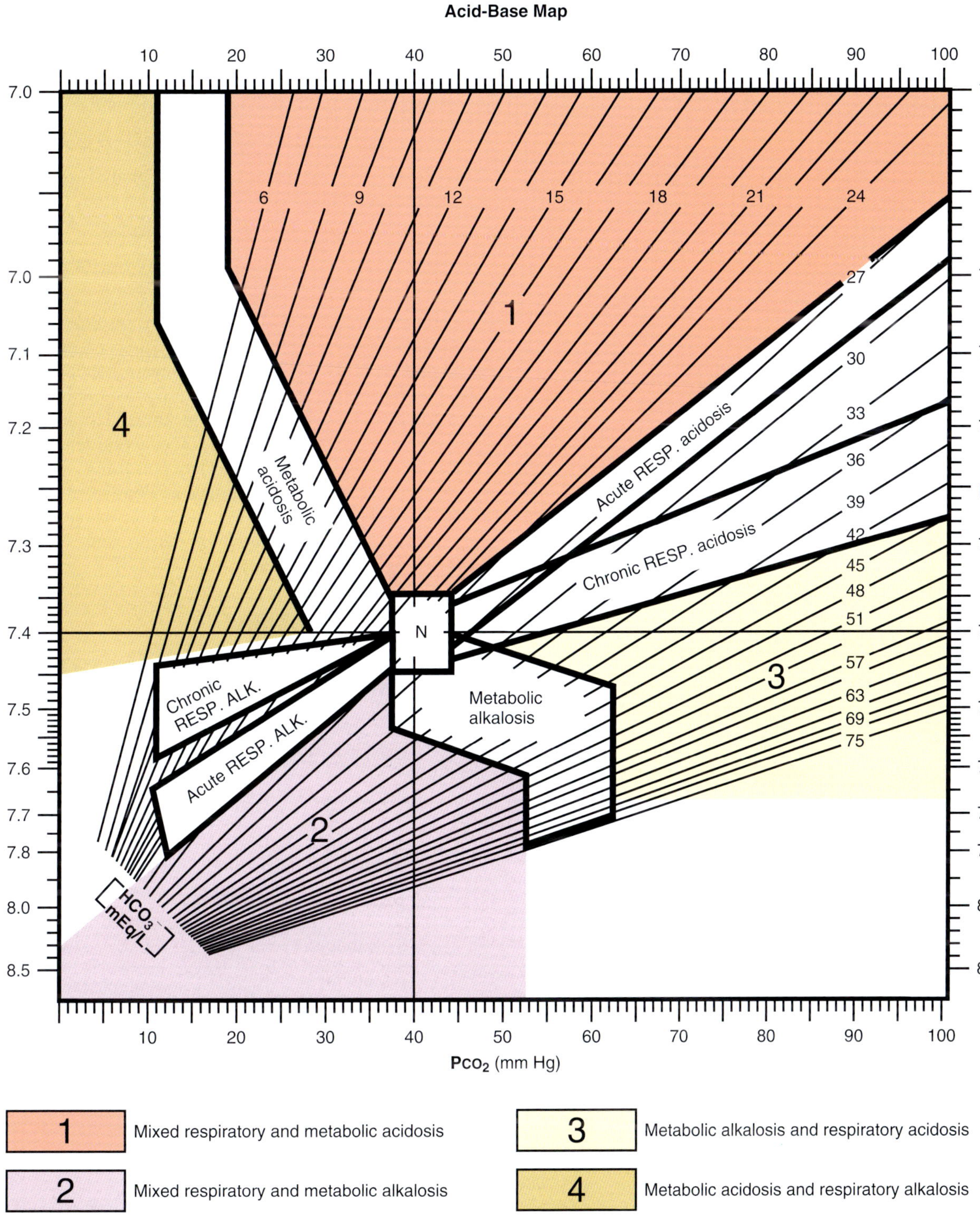

Fig. A1-1 Acid-base map.

individual physiology. Respiratory compensation for metabolic disorders is more rapid and occurs through a change in the respiratory rate, which in turn adjusts the Pco_2. Metabolic compensation for a respiratory disturbance requires renal adjustment of HCO_3^- and can take 3 to 5 days. The predicted compensatory responses for the primary disturbances are shown in Table A1.6. It is important to remember that physiologic compensatory mechanisms may themselves be compromised or overwhelmed by the acid-base disorder (Fig. A1.1).

Example 1: A 58-year-old female has had profuse diarrhea for 1 week. Initial laboratory data include the following: Na^+, 133; K^+, 2.8; pH 7.26; Cl^-, 118; Pco_2, 13; HCO_3^-, 5.

1. Acidosis is present (pH < 7.40).
2. The primary process is metabolic (HCO_3^- < 22 mmoL, and Pco_2 is not increased).

3. Compensation. In primary metabolic acidosis, the formula that checks for compensation is:
The actual P_{CO_2} is 13 mm Hg.

The respiratory compensation is predicted by the equation and suggests that no other acid-base disorder is present.

Example 2: A 74-year-old nursing home resident is admitted to the hospital with hypotension (96/70) and fever (39°C). He has had a positive urine culture for *Escherichia coli* and two positive blood cultures with the same organism. His laboratory values are as follows:

Sodium, 138 mmol/L.
Potassium, 3.2 mmol/L.
Chloride, 105 mmol/L.
pH, 7.49.
P_{CO_2}, 25 mm Hg.
HCO_3^-, 22 mmol/L.

1. Alkalosis is present (pH > 7.44).
2. The primary process is respiratory (P_{CO_2} < 40 mm Hg and HCO_3^- was not increased).
3. Compensation. The decrease in P_{CO_2} is 40 to 25, or 15 mm Hg. The formula for an expected decrease in HCO_3^- is 2 mmol for every 10-mm Hg decrease in P_{CO_2}. In this instance, the expected decrease in HCO_3^- for the 15-mm Hg decrease in P_{CO_2} is 3 mmol/L, which is nearly identical to the actual decrease (i.e., 25 to 22). Therefore only acute respiratory alkalosis is present with normal compensation.

WINTER'S FORMULA

In a pure primary metabolic acidosis, the body's normal response is a change (decrease) in P_{CO_2}. The expected compensation can be predicted by Winter's formula:

$$\text{Expected } P_{CO_2} = 1.5 \times HCO_3^- + 8 \pm 2$$

Example: HCO_3^- calculated from ABG analysis is 10 mEq/L. With pure metabolic acidosis the expected P_{CO_2} is:

$$\text{Expected } P_{CO_2} = 1.5 \times 10 + 8$$

$$\text{Expected } P_{CO_2} = 23 \text{ mm Hg (range 21 to 25 mm Hg)}$$

If the measured P_{CO_2} is higher than the expected P_{CO_2}, a concomitant respiratory acidosis is also present. Normocapnia or hypercapnia in the presence of severe metabolic acidosis may be a harbinger of impending respiratory failure and suggests the possible need for mechanical ventilation.

A lower P_{CO_2} would suggest a concomitant respiratory alkalosis, such as seen with salicylate poisoning.

Another useful tool in estimating P_{CO_2} in metabolic acidosis is the recognition that P_{CO_2} is approximately equal to the last two digits of the pH. In the previous example, the expected pH should be 7.23.

Diagnostic Probability

Table A1.7 shows the definitions and ways to calculate various epidemiologic terms.

TABLE A1.7 Definitions of Commonly Used Epidemiologic Terms

Prevalence	= (a + c)/(a + b + c + d)	= Incidence of disease in the population tested
Sensitivity	= a/(a + c)	= Probability of a positive test result, disease present
Specificity	= d/(b + d)	= Probability of a negative test result, disease absent
False-negative rate	= c/(a + c)	= Probability of a negative test result, disease present
False-positive rate	= b/(b + d)	= Probability of a positive test result, disease absent
Positive predictive value	= a/(a + b)	= Probability of a disease present, test positive
Negative predictive value	= d/(c + d)	= Probability of a disease absent, test negative
Overall accuracy	= (a + d)/(a + b + c + d)	= Probability of a "true" test result

	Disease State		
Test Result	*Present*	*Absent*	
Positive	a (true positive)	b (false positive)	a + b = All positive tests
Negative	c (false negative)	d (true negative)	c + d = All negative tests
	a + c = All patients with disease	b + d = All patients without disease	a + b + c + d = All patients tested

Modified from Goldman L. Quantitative aspects of clinical reasoning. In: Isselbacher KJ, Braunwald E, Wilson JD, eds. *Harrison's Principles of Internal Medicine*. 13th ed. McGraw-Hill; 1994: 44.

No medical test is totally accurate. The parameters listed in Table A1.7, when available, can help guide a clinician's test selection. When this information is not available, it may be difficult to identify random laboratory errors or detect failures. Knowledge of disease prevalence, combined with the sensitivity and specificity of the test, yields the positive (or negative) predictive value of that test. For a given sensitivity and specificity, predictive value is directly proportional to prevalence. Hence, even a test with high sensitivity and specificity may not detect a rare disease. This underscores the importance of pretest clinical evaluation.

ACKNOWLEDGMENT

The editors and authors acknowledge the contributions of Matthew Veltkamp, Eric D. Katz, Brent E. Ruoff, and M. John Mendelsohn to this Appendix in previous editions.

APPENDIX 2

Toxicology and Precautions

Michael Hayoun and Diane Birnbaumer

INTRODUCTION

This appendix is meant as a reference and while it is comprehensive it is not all inclusive. This appendix does not replace the guidance and recommendations of a well-trained and experienced expert clinician. Included are many commonly used formulas, but this is not an exhaustive list. Please follow local protocols and guidelines.

TOXIDROMES

There are five classically taught toxidromes that can be used to guide management in the event of an unknown exposure or to gauge toxicity in a known agent exposure (Table A.1). There are other toxidromes described in specialty literature but may not be applicable to the general audience.

Ingestions/Exposures and Antidotes

Ingestions and exposures are commonly seen in the emergency department. Clinicians need to be aware of antidotes available to treat them, as some must be given early to maximally manage the patient (Table A.2).

TABLE A.1 Toxidromes

TOXIDROME	HR AND BP	RESP	TEMP	PUPILS	BOWEL SOUNDS	SKIN
Anticholinergic	Increased	Increased or normal	Increased	Dilated	Decreased	Dry
Cholinergic	Increased HR + BP (nicotinic), decreased HR (muscarinic)	Normal; may see wheezing and/or bronchorrhea	Normal	Pinpoint	Increased	Wet
Sympathomimetic	Increased	Increased	Increased	Dilated	Increased	Wet
Opioid	Decreased	Decreased	Decreased	Pinpoint	Decreased	Dry
Sedative-hypnotic	Decreased	Decreased	Decreased	Normal	Decreased	Dry

BP, Blood pressure; *HR*, heart rate; *resp*, respiration.

TABLE A.2 Antidotes for Ingestions and Exposures

ANTIDOTE	INGESTION OR EXPOSURE
Acetylcysteine	Acetaminophen toxicity
Antivenom (*Latrodectus mactans*)	Black widow spider envenomation
Atropine	Bradydysrhythmias, cholinesterase inhibitor toxicity
Benztropine	Acute dystonia
Botulinum antitoxin/trivalent ABE	Botulism
Bromocriptine	Neuroleptic malignant syndrome
Calcium disodium EDTA	Lead, copper, zinc, cobalt, cadmium toxicity
Calcium gluconate 10%	Hydrofluoric acid exposure, calcium channel blocker toxicity
Crotalinae polyvalent immune fab	Crotalinae (rattlesnake) envenomation
Cyproheptadine	Serotonin syndrome
Dantrolene	Malignant hyperthermia, neuroleptic malignant syndrome

Continued

TABLE A.2 Antidotes for Ingestions and Exposures—cont'd

ANTIDOTE	INGESTION OR EXPOSURE
Deferoxamine mesylate	Iron toxicity
Diazepam/lorazepam	Seizures, severe agitation; stimulant toxicity
Digoxin-specific antibody fragments	Digoxin and other cardiac glycoside toxicity
Dimercaprol(BAL)	Arsenic, lead, mercury toxicity
Diphenhydramine	Acute dystonia; histamine receptor blockade
Flumazenil	Benzodiazepine toxicity
Folic acid	Methanol toxicity
Fomepizole	Ethylene glycol, methanol toxicity, adjunct for acetaminophen
Glucagon	Beta-blocker toxicity
Hydroxocobalamin	Cyanide exposure/smoke inhalation
Insulin (high dose)	Calcium channel and beta-blocker toxicity
Idarucizumab	Dabigatran reversal
Leucovorin calcium	Methotrexate toxicity
Levocarnitine	Valproic acid toxicity
Methylene blue 1%	Methemoglobinemia
Naloxone	Opioid toxicity
Octreotide	Sulfonylurea toxicity
Physostigmine	Anticholinergic toxicity
Phytonadione/vitamin K1	Oral anticoagulant/rodenticide toxicity
Pralidoxime(2-PAM)	Cholinesterase inhibitor (organophosphate/carbamate) toxicity
Protamine	Heparin reversal
Protein complex concentrate	Direct oral anticoagulant reversal, warfarin
Pyridoxine/vitamin B6	Ethylene glycol/isoniazid/gyromitra mushroom toxicity
Sodium bicarbonate	Cyclic antidepressant/salicylate toxicity, metabolic acidosis
Silibinin	Amanita phalloides
Succimer/DMSA	Arsenic, lead, mercury
Thiamine/vitamin B1	Wernicke-Korsakoff syndrome, ethylene glycol toxicity

EDTA, Ethylenediaminetetraacetic acid.

Precautions

Protecting healthcare workers and other patients is critical when assessing and treating patients with various infectious diseases. The specific precautions needed depend on the infectious agent involved, as summarized in Table A.3.

It is prudent to review the possible causes when caring for a patient in cardiac arrest. A common way to assure evaluating for these causes is to use the "Five H's" and "Five T's."

TABLE A.3 Precautions

PRECAUTION	EQUIPMENT
Airborne	Negative pressure room N95 or higher respirator Mask on the patient Door must remain closed
Droplet	Mask Eye protection Gloves Gown Mask on the patient
Contact	Gloves Gown Dedicated or disposable equipment
Enhanced Contact	Reserved for *C. diff* and other high-risk infections Gloves Gown Dedicated/disposable equipment Soap and water hand washing

TABLE A.4 Cardiac Arrest: The H's and T's

Hypovolemia	Toxins
Hypoxia	Tamponade (cardiac)
Hyper/hypokalemia	Tension pneumothorax
Hypothermia	Thrombosis
Hydrogen cation excess (acidosis)	Trauma

Roberts and Hedges'
Clinical Procedures in Emergency Medicine and Acute Care

Index

A

Note: Page numbers followed by "f" refer to illustrations; page numbers followed by "t" refer to tables; page numbers followed by "b" refer to boxes.

B

C

D

E

F

I

J

K

L

M

N

Q

R

S

T

U

V

W

X

Y

Z